FOUNDATIONS OF NURSING

*To Joy Fleming, RN, colleague and friend,
who has consistently worked for and
assisted others in improving the education
of vocational nursing students in Texas.*
L.W.

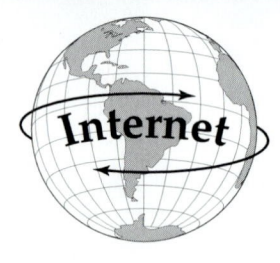

FOUNDATIONS OF NURSING

Caring for the Whole Person

Lois White, RN, PhD

Former Chairperson, Professor
Department of Vocational Nurse Education
Del Mar College
Corpus Christi, Texas

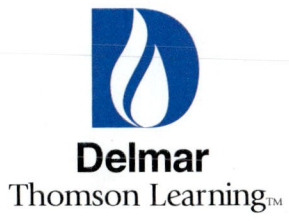

Delmar
Thomson Learning™

Notice to the Reader

Delmar Staff:

Business Unit Director: William Brottmiller

Executive Editor: Cathy L. Esperti

Acquisitions Editor: Matthew Filimonov

Developmental Editor: Elisabeth F. Williams

Editorial Assistants: Darcy M. Scelsi and Brian R. Haines

Executive Marketing Manager: Dawn F. Gerrain

Channel Manager: Tara Carter

Executive Production Manager: Karen Leet

Project Editors: Patricia Gillivan, Elizabeth B. Keller, and Stacey Prus

Production Coordinator: James Zayicek

Art/Design Coordinator: Timothy J. Conners

Cover Design: Cummings Advertising

Copyright © 2001

Delmar is a division of Thomson Learning. The Thomson Learning logo is a registered trademark used herein under license.

Printed in the United States

1 2 3 4 5 6 7 8 9 10 XXX 05 04 03 02 01 00

For more information, contact Delmar, 3 Columbia Circle, PO Box 15015, Albany, NY 12212-0515; or find us on the World Wide Web at http://www.delmar.com

International Division List

Asia:

Thomson Learning

60 Albert Street, #15-01

Albert Complex

Singapore 189969

Tel: 65 336 6411

Fax: 65 336 7411

Japan:

Thomson Learning

Palaceside Building 5F

1-1-1 Hitotsubashi, Chiyoda-ku

Tokyo 100 0003 Japan

Tel: 813 5218 6544

Fax: 813 5218 6551

Australia/New Zealand:

Nelson/Thomson Learning

102 Dodds Street

South Melbourne,

  Victoria 3205

Australia

Tel: 61 39 685 4111

Fax: 61 39 685 4199

UK/Europe/Middle East:

Thomson Learning

Berkshire House

168-173 High Holborn

London

WC1V 7AA United Kingdom

Tel: 44 171 497 1422

Fax: 44 171 497 1426

Thomas Nelson & Sons LTD

Nelson House

Mayfield Road

Walton-on-Thames

KT 12 5PL United Kingdom

Tel: 44 1932 2522111

Fax: 44 1932 246574

Latin America:

Thomson Learning

Seneca, 53

Colonia Palanco

11560 Mexico D.F. Mexico

Tel: 525-281-2906

Fax: 525-281-2656

South Africa:

Thomson Learning

Zonnebloem Building

Constantia Square

526 Sixteenth Road

P.O. Box 2459

Halfway House, 1685

South Africa

Tel: 27 11 805 4819

Fax: 27 11 805 3648

Canada:

Nelson/Thomson Learning

1120 Birchmount Road

Scarborough, Ontario

Canada M1K 5G4

Tel: 416-752-9100

Fax: 416-752-8102

Spain:

Thomson Learning

Calle Magallanes, 25

28015-MADRID

ESPANA

Tel: 34 91 446 33 50

Fax: 34 91 445 62 18

International Headquarters:

Thomson Learning

International Division

290 Harbor Drive, 2nd Floor

Stamford, CT 06902-7477

Tel: 203-969-8700

Fax: 203-969-8751

Library of Congress Cataloging-in-Publication Data

Contents

SECTION 1 PERSPECTIVES IN NURSING

UNIT 1 Nurse Skills for Success

UNIT 2 History and Nursing Organizations

UNIT 3 Legal and Ethical Issues

UNIT 4 Communication

SECTION 3 AREAS OF NURSING PRACTICE

UNIT 10 Medical–Surgical Nursing

Chapter 44 Nursing Care of the Client: Responding to Emergencies 1151

UNIT 11 Mental Health and Substance Abuse

Chapter 45 Nursing Care of the Client: Mental Illness .1174

Chapter 46 Nursing Care of the Client: Substance Abuse 1212

Contributors

Joy E. Ache-Reed, RN, MS
Assistant Professor of Nursing
Indiana Wesleyan University
Marion, Indiana
Chapter 12, Cultural Diversity and Nursing

Carol A. Fetters Andersen, RN, MSN
Director of Mental Health Services
St. Anthony Regional Hospital and Nursing Home
Carroll, Iowa
Chapter 55, Nursing Care of the Older Client

Carma Andrus, RN, MN, CNS
Dauterive Primary Care Clinic
St. Martinville, Louisiana
Chapter 43, Nursing Care of the Client: Sensory System

Diane R. Behrens, RNCS, MA, MSEd
Instructor
University of Saint Francis
Fort Wayne, Indiana
Chapter 39, Nursing Care of the Client: Immune System

Lenore Boris, RN, BSN, MS, JD
New York State Public Employees Federation Organizer (nurse)
Albany, New York
Chapter 57, Leadership/Work Transition

Susan L. Bredemeyer, RN, MS
Assistant Professor
Lutheran College of Health Professions
Fort Wayne, Indiana
Chapter 25, Assessment

Ali Brown, RN, MSN
Assistant Professor
College of Nursing
University of Tennessee
Knoxville, Tennessee
Chapter 9, Nursing Process

Gyl A. Burkhard, RN, BSN, MS
Instructor
OCM BOCES
Syracuse, New York
Chapter 42, Nursing Care of the Client: Urinary System

Donna J. Burleson, RN, MS
Chair of Health Occupations
Cisco Junior College
Abilene, Texas
Chapter 2, Critical Thinking

Ann H. Cary, RN, PhD, MPH, A-CCC
Professor and Coordinator, PhD in Nursing Program
College of Nursing and Health Sciences
George Mason University
Fairfax, Virginia
Chapter 4, Nursing History, Education, and Organizations

Diana L. Case, RN, MA, FNP
Neighborhood Health Clinic
Fort Wayne, Indiana
Chapter 29, Nursing Care of the Surgical Client

Judy Conlin
Chapter 20, Safety/Hygiene

Jan Corder, RN, DNS
School of Nursing
Northeast Louisiana University
Monroe, Louisana
Chapter 9, Nursing Process

Julie Coy, RNC, MS
Pain Consultation Service
The Children's Hospital
Denver, Colorado
Chapter 19, Rest and Sleep
Chapter 26, Pain Management

Sue C. DeLaune, RN, C, MN
Adjunct Faculty
Loyola University
New Orleans, Louisiana *and*
President, SDeLaune Consulting
Mandeville, Louisiana *and*
Health Education Coordinator
Southeast Louisiana Hospital
Mandeville, Louisana
Chapter 4, Nursing History, Education, and Organizations
Chapter 5, The Health Care Delivery System
Chapter 7, Ethical Responsibilities
Chapter 9, Nursing Process
Chapter 11, Client Teaching
Chapter 14, The Life Cycle

Chapter 16, Stress, Adaptation, and Anxiety
Chapter 17, Loss, Grief, and Death

Gena Duncan, RN, MS, MSEd
Director of Associate Degree Program
University of Saint Francis
Fort Wayne, Indiana
Chapter 32, Nursing Care of the Client: Cardiovascular System
Chapter 33, Nursing Care of the Client: Blood and Lymph Systems

Mary Elias, RNC, BSN, CCE
Instructor
Practical Nursing Program
Ivy Tech State College
Fort Wayne, Indiana
Chapter 35, Nursing Care of the Client: Reproductive System

Cheryl Erickson, RN, BSN, MA
Associate Professor
Lutheran College of Health Professions
Fort Wayne, Indiana
Chapter 25, Assessment

Mary Ellen Zator Estes, RN, MSN, CCRN
Former Assistant Professor
School of Nursing
Marymount University
Arlington, VA *and*
Former Critical Care Nursing Education Coordinator
The George Washington University Medical Center
Washington, D.C.
Chapter 25, Assessment

Michael A. Fiedler, CRNA, MS
Assistant Professor
Applied Health Sciences
University of Alabama at Birmingham
Birmingham, Alabama
Chapter 28, Anesthesia

Mary Frost, RN, BSN
Covington, Louisiana
Chapter 13, Alternative/Complementary Therapies

Norma Fujise, RN, C, MS
School of Nursing
University of Hawaii
Honolulu, Hawaii
Chapter 40, Nursing Care of the Client: Integumentary System

Cathy Greer, RN, MS
Instructor
Lutheran College of Health Professions
Fort Wayne, Indiana
Chapter 29, Nursing Care of the Surgical Client

Margaret L. Griffin, RN, BSN, MS
Instructor
Lutheran College of Health Professions
Fort Wayne, Indiana
Chapter 40, Nursing Care of the Client: Integumentary System

Susan Halley, RN, MS, FNP
Instructor of Nursing
Ball State University
Muncie, Indiana
Chapter 7, Ethical Responsibilities

Mary Jane Hamilton, RN, C, PhD
Professor of Nursing
Texas A&M University-Corpus Christi
Corpus Christi, Texas
Chapter 52, Basics of Pediatric Care

Beverly F. Hildebrand, RN, BSN, MS
Former Health Occupations Coordinator
Washington, Saratoga, Warren, Hamilton, & Essex Counties BOCES
Saratoga, New York
Chapter 42, Nursing Care of the Client: Urinary System

Lucille Joel, RN, EdD, FAAN
Professor
College of Nursing
Rutgers, The State University of New Jersey
Newark, New Jersey
Chapter 5, The Health Care Delivery System

Janet Leah Joost, RN, BSN
Instructor
Front Range Community College
Boulder, Colorado
Chapter 31, Nursing Care of the Client: Respiratory System

Denise M. Jordan, RN, BSN, MA
Instructor
Practical Nursing Program
Ivy Tech State College
Fort Wayne, Indiana
Chapter 6, Legal Responsibilities

Janet E. Keith, RN, MSEd
Instructor
Practical Nursing Program
Ivy Tech State College
Fort Wayne, Indiana
Chapter 38, Nursing Care of the Client: Musculoskeletal System

Vicki L. Khouli, RN, BSN, MA, IBCLC
Instructor
Practical Nursing Program
Ivy Tech State College
Fort Wayne, Indiana
Chapter 36, Nursing Care of the Client: Sexually Transmitted Diseases

Patricia K. Ladner, RN, MS, MN
Consultant for Nursing Practice
Louisiana State Board of Nursing
New Orleans, Louisiana
Chapter 4, Nursing History, Education, and Organizations
Chapter 6, Legal Responsibilities
Chapter 10, Documentation
Chapter 18, Basic Nutrition
Chapter 23, Fluid, Electrolyte, and Acid–Base Balance
Chapter 24, Medication Administration
Chapter 25, Assessment
Chapter 27, Diagnostic Tests

Mary E. A. Laskin, RN, CS, MN
Clinical Nurse Specialist
Surgical/Orhopedic Services
Kaiser Permanente
San Diego, California
Chapter 26, Pain Management

Celinda Kay Leach, RN, BS, MPH
Program Chair, Practical Nursing
Practical Nursing Program
Ivy Tech State College
Bloomington, Indiana
Chapter 30, Nursing Care of the Oncology Client

Sandra Liming, RN, MN
Nursing Instructor
North Seattle Community College
North Seattle, Washington
Chapter 35, Nursing Care of the Client: Reproductive System

Judy Martin, RN, MS, JD
Nurse Attorney
Louisiana Department of Health and Hospitals
Health Standards Section
Baton Rouge, Louisiana
Chapter 6, Legal Responsibilities

Linda McCuistion, RN, PhD
Assistant Professor
School of Nursing
Our Lady of Holy Cross College
New Orleans, Louisiana
Chapter 9, Nursing Process

Cheryl McGaffic, RN, PhD
Clinical Instructor
College of Nursing
The University of Arizona
Tucson, Arizona
Chapter 39, Nursing Care of the Client: Immune System

Robin Theresa McKenzie, RN, MSN, CCRN
Assistant Chairman
Navy Medical Center
San Diego, California
Chapter 43, Nursing Care of the Client: Sensory System

Betty Miller
Staff Development Coordinator
Meadowcrest Hospital
Gretna, Louisiana
Chapter 17, Loss, Grief, and Death

David K. Miller, RNC, BSN, MSEd
ICU/Medical–Surgical Manager
W.S. Major Hospital
Shelbyville, Indiana
Chapter 39, Nursing Care of the Client: Immune System

Barbara S. Moffett, RN, PhD
Associate Professor of Nursing
School of Nursing
Southeastern Louisiana University
Hammond, Louisiana
Chapter 9, Nursing Process

Mary Anne Mordcin-McCarthy, RN, PhD
Associate Professor and Director of the Undergraduate Program
College of Nursing
University of Tennessee–Knoxville
Knoxville, Tennessee
Chapter 9, Nursing Process

Barbara Morvant, RN, MN
Louisiana State Board of Nursing
Metairie, Louisiana
Chapter 4, Nursing History, Education, and Organizations

Joan Fritsch Needham, RNC, MS
Director of Education
DeKalb County Nursing Home
DeKalb, Illinois
Chapter 17, Loss, Grief, and Death
Chapter 55, Nursing Care of the Older Client
Chapter 56, Rehabilitation, Home Health, Long-Term Care, and Hospice

Rebecca Osterhaut
Chapter 1, Holistic Care

Brenda Owens, RN, PhD
Associate Professor
School of Nursing
Louisiana State University Medical Center
New Orleans, Louisiana
Chapter 24, Medication Administration

Raymond Phillips, RN, MS, CCRN
Clinical Nurse Specialist
Staff Development Coordinator
U.S. Naval Hospital
Rota, Spain
Chapter 43, Nursing Care of the Client: Sensory System

Demetrius Porche, RN, CCRN, DNS
Associate Professor and Director
Bachelor of Science in Nursing Program
Nicholas State University *and*
Adjunct Assistant Professor
Tulane University
School of Public Health and Topical Medicine
New Orleans, Louisiana

Chapter 20, Safety/Hygiene
Chapter 21, Infection Control/ Asepsis
Chapter 22, Standard Precautions and Isolation

Susan Reinhart, RN, MS
Assistant Professor
Department of Registered Nurse Education
Del Mar College
Corpus Christi, Texas
Chapter 45, Nursing Care of the Client: Mental Illness

Suzanne Riche, RN
Charity School of Nursing
Delgado Community College
New Orleans, Louisiana
Chapter 9, Nursing Process

Kathy Rockwell, RN, BSN, MA, MSN, PNP
Professor
Department of RN Education
Del Mar College
Corpus Christi, Texas *and*
Supervisor, Surgical Services
94th General Hospital
Seagoville, Texas
Chapter 44, Nursing Care of the Client: Responding to Emergencies

Martha Ann Rust, RN, BSN, MSN
Instructor
Lutheran College of Health Professions
Fort Wayne, Indiana
Chapter 41, Nursing Care of the Client: Nervous System

Mary Kay Schultz, RN, MSN, ANP
Instructor
Department of Nursing
Regis University
Denver, Colorado
Chapter 37, Nursing Care of the Client: Endocrine System

Leslee R. Sinn, RN, BSN
Instructor
Front Range Community College
Boulder, Colorado
Chapter 34, Nursing Care of the Client: Gastrointestinal System

Russlyn A. St. John, RN, MSN
Associate Professor & Coordinator, Practical Nursing
St. Charles Community College
St. Peters, Missouri
Chapter 37, Nursing Care of the Client: Endocrine System

Maureen Straight, RN, BSN, MSEd
Regents College
Albany, New York
Chapter 3, Student Nurse Skills for Success

Susan Stranahan, RN, PhD
Chair, Nursing Department
Indiana Wesleyan University
Marion, Indiana
Chapter 12, Cultural Diversity and Nursing

John M. White, PhD
Former Chairperson, Professor
Biology Department
Del Mar College
Corpus Christi, Texas
Chapter 23, Fluid, Electrolyte, and Acid–Base Balance

Donna Wofford RN, PhD
Professor
Department of RN Education
Del Mar College
Corpus Christi, Texas
Chapter 53, Infants with Special Needs: Birth to 12 months
Chapter 54, Common Problems: 1–18 years

Lorrie Wong, RN, MS
School of Nursing
University of Hawaii
Honolulu, Hawaii
Chapter 40, Nursing Care of the Client: Integumentary System

Rothlyn Zahourek, RN, CS, MS
Certified Clinical Nurse Specialist
Amherst, Massachusetts
Chapter 13, Alternative/ Complementary Therapies

Procedure Contributors

Gaylene Bouska Altman, RN, PhD
Director of the Learning Lab *and* Faculty
School of Nursing
University of Washington
Seattle, Washington
Procedures B24, B25, I8

Barbara Brillhart, RN, PhD, CRRN, FNP-C
College of Nursing
Arizona State University
Tempe, Arizona
Procedures B8, B9, B10, B11, B12, B13, B14, B15, I27

Bethany Campbell, RN, MN, OCN
University of Washington Medical Center
Seattle, Washington
Procedure B7

Pat Carroll, RN, C, CEN, RRT, MS
Owner and Consultant
Educational Medical Consultants
Meriden, Connecticut *and*
Per Diem Staff Nurse, Emergency Department
Manchester Memorial Hospital
Manchester, Connecticut
Procedures B2, B33, B38, B39, B40, I8

Beth Christensen, RN, MN, CCRN
Touro Infirmary
New Orleans, Louisiana
Procedures B36, B37, I21, I22, I23, I24

Cheryl L. Cooke, RN, MN
Student Services Coordinator
University of Washington
School of Nursing
Seattle, Washington
Procedure B34

Valerie Coxon, RN, PhD
Affiliate Assistant Professor
University of Washington
Seattle, Washington *and*
CEO

NRSPACE Software, Inc
Bellevue, Washington
Procedure B34

Mary Ellen Zator Estes, RN, MSN, CCRN
Assistant Professor
School of Nursing
Marymount University
Arlington, Virginia *and*
Former Critical Care Nursing Education Coordinator
The George Washington University Medical Center
Washington, D.C.
Procedures B3, B4, B5, B6

Tom Ewing, RN, BSN
Hematology-Oncology
University of Washington Medical Center
Seattle, Washington
Procedure B23

Norma Fujise, RN-C, MS
School of Nursing
University of Hawaii
Honolulu, Hawaii
Procedures I17, I18, I19, I20

Mikel Gray, PhD, CURN, CCCN
Nurse Practitioner/Clinical Investigator
Associate Professor
Department of Urology
University of Virginia Health Sciences Center
Charlottesville, Virginia *and*
Adjunct Professor
Lancing School of Nursing
Bellarmine College
Louisville, Kentucky
Procedures B26, B27, B28, I3, I4, I5, I6, I7

Patricia K. Ladner, RN, MS, MN
Consultant for Nursing Practice
Louisiana State Board of Nursing
New Orleans, Louisiana
Procedures B3, B4, B5, B6, B29, B30, B31, I9, I10, I11, I12, I13, I14, I15, I16, I25, I26, I28, A2, A3, A4, A5, A6, A7

Kathryn Lilleby, RN
Clinical Research Nurse
Fred Hutchinson Cancer Research Center
Seattle, Washington
Procedures B32, B33

Joan M. Mack, RN, MSN, CS
Nebraska Medical Center
Omaha, Nebraska
Procedure B20

Brenda Owens, RN, PhD
Associate Professor
School of Nursing
Louisiana State University Medical Center
New Orleans, Louisiana
Procedures I9, I10, I11, I12, I13, I14, I15, I16, A6

Demetrius Porche, RN, DNS, CCRN
Associate Professor and Director
Bachelor of Science in Nursing Program
Nicholas State University *and*
Adjunct Assistant Professor
Tulane University
School of Public Health and Topical Medicine
New Orleans, Louisiana
Procedures B1, B16, B17, B18, B19, B21, B22, B35, I1, I2, A1

Lorrie Wong, RN, MS
School of Nursing
University of Hawaii
Honolulu, Hawaii
Procedures I17, I18, I19, I20

Martha Yager, RN
Assistant Director of Nurses
Bennington Health and Rehabilitation Center
Bennington, Vermont
Procedures B26, B27, B28, I3, I4, I5, I6, I7

Reviewers

Terri Ardoin, RN, CCM
Louisiana Technical College
Charles B. Coreil Campus
Ville Platte, Louisiana

Kay Baker, RN, MS
Instructional Faculty (Nursing)
Pima Community College
Tuscon, Arizona

Lou Ann Boose, RN, BSN, MSN
Harrisburg Area Community College
Harrisburg, Pennsylvania

Susan Brooks, RN, BSN, MS, MN
Community College of Southern
 Nevada
Las Vegas, Nevada

Gyl A. Burkhard, RN, BSN, MS
Instructor
OCM BOCES
Syracuse, New York

Kay Rice Francis, RN, BSN, MSN
Woman's Health Nurse Practitioner
Nursing Instructor
Lake Michigan College
Benton Harbor, Michigan

Judith L. Gisondi, RN, BSN, MPS
Career Education Center Hamilton
 Fulton Montgomery BOCES
Johnstown, New York

Ester Gonzales, RN, MSN, MSEd
Del Mar College
Corpus Christi, Texas

Lisa Greenwall
PN Coordinator
Frackville, Pennsylvania

Sheila Guidry, RN, LPN, BSN, DSN, PhD
Wallace Community College
Dothan, Alabama

Ruth Hall, BA, MA
Augusta Technical Institute
Augusta, Georgia

Renee Harrison, RN, BSN, MS
Tulsa Community College
Tulsa, Oklahoma

Suellen Klein, RN, BSN, MSN
Nursing Instructor
Lake Michigan College
Benton Harbor, Michigan

Hope Laughlin, RN, BSN, MS, MSN, EdD
Pensacola Junior College
Pensacola, Florida

Netta Moncur-Bowen, RN, BSN, MS
ADN Program
Seminole Community College
Sanford, Florida

Carol J. Nelson, RN, BSN, MSN
Spokane Community College
Spokane, Washington

Dr. Carol Rafferty
Northeast Wisconsin Technical
 College
Green Bay, Wisconsin

Gail J. Smith, RN, BSN, MSN
Miami-Dade Community College
School of Nursing
Miami, Florida

Preface

Foundations of Nursing: Caring for the Whole Person is a textbook developed to cover the entire curriculum of a practical/vocational nursing program (fundamentals, growth and development, nutrition, microbiology, medical–surgical nursing, mental health/mental illness, maternal/child health, gerontological nursing, and personal/vocational adjustments). Since the complete curriculum is covered, the reader can see how the subject matter from the different areas is interrelated. Readers will also find this text helpful by having all information in one book.

An anatomy and physiology review opens each of the medical–surgical system chapters. Pharmacology basics and medication administration are presented. A chapter on critical thinking lays a foundation for the nursing process, which is woven throughout all of the care chapters. The concept of holistic care is a unifying thread underlying the entire text.

Organization

Foundations of Nursing consists of 57 chapters grouped into 15 units, and an Atlas of Nursing Procedures:

- **Unit 1, Nurse Skills for Success,** discusses holistic care, critical thinking, time management, study skills, and organizational skills.
- **Unit 2, History and Nursing Organizations,** presents an overview of the history of nursing and the development of educational programs and nursing organizations. A synopsis of various nursing organizations is provided.
- **Unit 3, Legal and Ethical Issues,** addresses the legal aspects of nursing and the responsibilities of the LP/VN. Ethical responsibilities are presented and explored.
- **Unit 4, Communication,** addresses the process of communication, how communication is used in the nurse–client relationship, and the technical and legal aspects of documentation. Each component of the nursing process is explained in a clear, concise manner. The client teaching process is presented as a major nursing intervention for clients throughout the life cycle.
- **Unit 5, Cultural Aspects of Nursing,** focuses on the cultural diversity of clients and coworkers. Alternative and complementary treatment modalities are described.
- **Unit 6, Human Development Over the Life Span,** describes the growth and developmental changes throughout the life cycle.
- **Unit 7, Health Promotion,** addresses wellness concepts and coping behaviors as well as grief, loss, and death. Basic nutrition, rest and sleep, and safety and hygiene are presented as methods of promoting health.

- **Unit 8, Infection Control,** presents the chain of infection, describes various types of pathogenic microorganisms, explains the concept of asepsis and aseptic technique, and outlines Standard Precautions and isolation measures.
- **Unit 9, Homeostasis,** thoroughly discusses fluid, electrolyte, and acid–base balance. Medication administration is presented in a nursing process format. Also included are legal considerations of medication administration, dose equivalents, and dosage calculations.
- **Unit 10, Medical–Surgical Nursing,** includes chapters on assessment, pain management, diagnostic tests, anesthesia, care of the surgical client, care of the oncology client, as well as chapters devoted to care of the client with disorders of the various body systems, including a separate chapter on clients with sexually transmitted diseases. In the body system chapters, there is an anatomy and physiology review and a presentation of each disorder, with medical–surgical management, pharmacological, dietary, and activity aspects of treatment. The nursing process identifies subjective and objective data, possible nursing diagnoses, goals, interventions, and evaluation. A chapter on responding to emergencies completes this unit.
- **Unit 11, Mental Health and Substance Abuse,** centers on the care of clients with common psychiatric illnesses. Chapter 46, "Nursing Care of the Client: Substance Abuse," describes substances that are commonly abused, the signs and symptoms of abuse, and treatments available.
- **Unit 12, Maternal/Child Health Nursing,** covers preconception education, prenatal care and fetal development, complications of pregnancy, the birth process, postpartum care, and care of the newborn. The basics of pediatric care, including procedure adaptations, are presented in a very concise manner. Chapter 53, "Infants with Special Needs: Birth to 12 Months" and Chapter 54, "Common Problems: 1–18 Years" address the major situations of pediatric care.
- **Unit 13, Gerontological Nursing,** presents myths and realities of aging, physiologic changes of aging, common health problems of an aging population, and methods of meeting the needs of the elderly client.
- **Unit 14, Health Care in the Community,** discusses the scope of care provided in rehabilitation, home health, long-term care, and hospice settings.
- **Unit 15, Leadership/Work Transition,** focuses on the skills related to actual working situations and the changes encountered when shifting from the role of student to that of employee. Job skills such as preparing a resume and applying for a position are explained in detail.

- **Atlas of Nursing Procedures** addresses nursing skills in three levels: basic, intermediate, and advanced care. Procedures are presented in a step-by-step format, with a rationale for each step. Numerous figures and illustrations add to the clarity of the presentation.

Features

Each chapter opens with a **Making the Connection** box which guides the reader to other key chapters related to the current chapter. This highlights the integration of the text material. Procedures used for the care of clients with the disorders discussed in the chapter are identified as appropriate. **Learning Objectives** are provided to guide the reader's learning.

The content of each chapter is presented in a nursing process format. Where appropriate, a **Sample Nursing Care Plan** is provided in the chapter. **Case Studies** are presented at the conclusion of the body system and specialty chapters.

A bulleted list **Summary**, multiple choice **Review Questions**, and **Critical Thinking Questions** at the end of each chapter assist the student in remembering and using the material presented.

Special boxed features are used throughout the text to emphasize key points and to provide specific types of information. Boxed features include:

 Life Cycle Considerations provide information related to the care of specific age groups during the life span.

 Client Teaching identifies specific items that the client should know related to the various disorders.

 Professional Tip offers tips and technical hints for the nurse to ensure quality care.

 Home Health Care describes factors to consider when providing care in a client's home and adaptations in care that may be necessary.

 Infection Control outlines methods to prevent the spread of infection.

 Cultural Considerations share beliefs, manners, ways of providing care, communication, and relationships of various cultural and ethnic groups as a way to provide sensitive and holistic care.

 Safety emphasizes the importance of safety and describes ways to maintain safe care.

 Web Flash! guides the student to the Internet for the latest information related to the chapter content.

Back matter in the text includes References/Suggested Readings organized by chapter, which allows the student to find the source of the material presented in each chapter and also to find additional information concerning the topics covered. Resources are also listed by chapter and provide names, addresses, and/or telephone numbers of organizations specializing in a specific area of health care. Internet addresses are included as available. A master listing of all Abbreviations, Acronyms, and Symbols used in the text is also provided.

Complete Teaching/Learning Package

The supplements package for *Foundations of Nursing* will assist students in learning the essential skills and information needed to secure a position as an LP/VN, and will assist instructors in planning and developing their programs and classes for the most efficient use of time and resources.

Classroom Manager (order # 0-7668-0828-9) components:

- *Instructor's Guide* includes Instructional Approaches, Student Learning Activities, Resources, and Additional Web Activities.
- *Computerized Test Bank and Electronic Gradebook* contains approximately 1,000 multiple choice questions with answers in NCLEX-style format. The online testing feature allows exams to be administered on-line via a school network or stand-alone PC. The *Electronic Gradebook* automatically calculates grades, tracks student performance, and provides other aids to simplify administrative tasks.
- *Image Library* is a software tool that contains hundreds of images from the text. A Windows™98 application, it can be used with the most common graphics file formats (BMP, TIFF, GIF) to add new images, create additional libraries, sort art by categories, and pull images into Microsoft® Power-Point™ presentations.
- *Procedures Checklists* correspond to the Atlas of Nursing Procedures from the text. These contain key steps for every procedure to help evaluate students' comprehension and execution of the procedures.
- *Answers* are included for the Case Studies and Review Questions from the text.

Student Study Guide (order # 0-7668-0827-0) components:

- *Learning Objectives* are drawn from the text.
- *Key Terms Review* is a matching exercise designed to encourage understanding of new terms presented in text.
- *Abbreviations Review* tests the reader's knowledge of abbreviations, acronyms, and symbols used in the text.

- *Exercises and Activities* provide short scenarios with related questions.
- *Self-Assessment* includes multiple choice questions in NCLEX format and draws on the key ideas in the chapter.

Acknowledgments

Many people must work together to produce any textbook; a comprehensive book such as this requires an even greater effort and coordination of more people with various areas of expertise. I would like to thank all of the contributors for their time and effort to share their knowledge gained through years of experience in both the clinical and academic settings.

The reviewers, I thank for their time spent critically reading the manuscript and providing the valuable suggestions that have added to this text. A special thank you to Pat Carroll for reviewing all the procedures. Thank you to the consultants Captain Alston Kirk, CHC, USN (retired) and John White, PhD for providing their expertise in religions and anatomy and physiology respectively.

To my husband John, a huge thank you for graciously reading the manuscript and delaying travel plans until the completion of this book.

I would like to acknowledge and sincerely thank the entire team at Delmar Publishers who have worked to make this textbook a reality. Beth Williams, developmental editor, is a gem who worked tirelessly and whose knowledge, guidance, humor, and attention to detail kept me motivated and on track throughout this project. Cathy Esperti provided one-on-one instruction relating to art manuscript preparation. Darcy Scelsi and Brian Haines compiled the master glossary and abbreviations appendix. The rest of the team—Tim Conners, Pat Gillivan, Jim Zayicek, Liz Keller, Stacey Prus, Danya Plotsky, Linda Ireland, Anne Matera, Harriet Hart, and Peter Toop all worked diligently to bring this textbook to the faculty and students in practical/vocational nursing. My heartfelt thanks goes to each person.

About the Author

Lois Elain Wacker White earned a diploma in nursing from Memorial Hospital School of Nursing, Springfield, Illinois; an Associate degree in Science from Del Mar College, Corpus Christi, Texas; a Bachelor of Science in Nursing from Texas A & I University-Corpus Christi, Corpus Christi, Texas; a Master of Science in Education from Corpus Christi State University, Corpus Christi, Texas; and a Doctor of Philosophy degree in educational administration-community college from the University of Texas, Austin, Texas.

She has taught at Del Mar College, Corpus Christi, Texas in both the Associate Degree Nursing program and the Vocational Nursing program. For 14 years she was also chairperson of the Department of Vocational Nurse Education. Dr. White has taught fundamentals of nursing, nutrition, mental health/mental illness, medical–surgical nursing, and maternal/newborn nursing. Her professional career has also included 15 years of clinical practice.

Dr. White has served on the Nursing Education Advisory Committee of the Board of Nurse Examiners for the State of Texas and the Board of Vocational Nurse Examiners, which developed competencies expected of graduates from each level of nursing. She maintains membership in the Texas Association of Vocational Nurse Educators, Sigma Theta Tau, American Nurses Association, and the National League for Nursing.

Dr. White has been listed in *Who's Who in American Nursing*. She currently serves on the Vocational Nursing Financial Aid Advisory Committee for the Texas Higher Education Coordinating Board.

How to Use this Text

This text is designed with you, the reader, in mind. Special elements and feature boxes appear throughout the text to guide you in reading and to assist you in learning the material. Following are suggestions for how you can use these features to increase your understanding and mastery of the content.

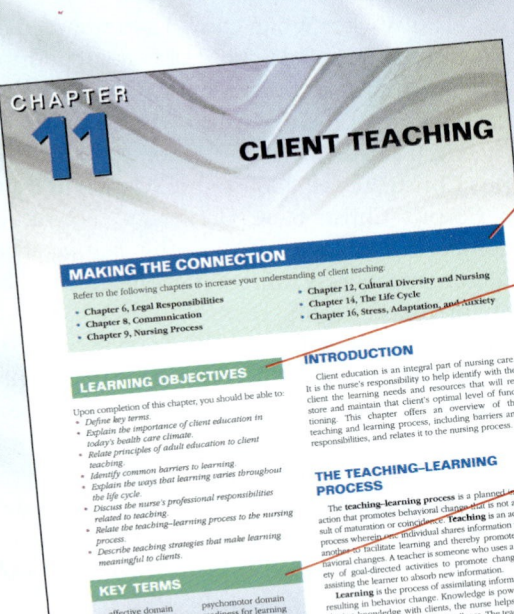

Making the Connection

Read these boxes before beginning a chapter to link material across the holistic care continuum and to tie new content to material you have already encountered.

Objectives

Read the chapter objectives before reading the chapter content to set the stage for learning. Revisit the objectives when preparing for an exam to see which entries you can respond to with "yes, I can do that."

Key Terms

Review this list before reading the chapter to familiarize yourself with new terms and to revisit those terms you already know to link them to the content of the new chapter.

Home Health Care

Read these boxes before making a home visit to a client with a given disorder. You can also use these boxes to prepare for client discharge to ensure that all necessary self-care topics have been covered with a client.

Professional Tip

Use these boxes to increase your professional competence and confidence, and also to expand your knowledge base.

Client Teaching

Read these boxes to gain insight into client learning needs related to the specific disorder or condition. You may want to make up your own index cards listing these teaching guidelines to use when you are working with clients.

Infection Control

When reading a chapter, stop and pay attention to these features and ask yourself, "Had I thought of that? Do I practice these precautions?"

Cultural Considerations

Test your sensitivity to cultural and ethnic variations by scanning these boxes and incorporating their guidelines and suggestions into your practice. You may also want to ask yourself what biases or preconceptions you have about different cultural practices before reading a chapter and then read these boxes for information that may help you be more sensitive in your nursing care and approach to clients.

Safety

Pause while reading to consider these elements and do a self-quiz: "Do I take steps such as these to ensure my own and the client's safety? Do I follow these guidelines in every practice encounter?"

Life Cycle Considerations

Use these boxes to increase your awareness of variations in care based on client age; this will help you deliver more effective and appropriate care.

Nursing Care Plan

Use these features to test your understanding of application of the content presented. Ask yourself, "Would I have come up with the same nursing diagnoses? Are these the interventions that I would have proposed? What other interventions would be appropriate?"

Case Study

Read over these boxes within text. Draw on the knowledge you have gained and synthesize information to develop your own educated responses to the case study challenges.

Review Questions

When you finish reading a chapter, use these questions to critically test your understanding of concepts covered. You might also read these questions before beginning a new chapter to gauge how much you already know or need to learn about the topic.

Critical Thinking

Visit these boxes after reading the entire chapter to check your acquisition and understanding of the concepts presented.

Web Flash!

Use these boxes to tap into the power of the Internet and enhance your research and technology skills.

Procedures

Reference the procedures as you read the chapters. Study the techniques, review the figures, and be prepared for your clinical days with questions of clarification for your instructor.

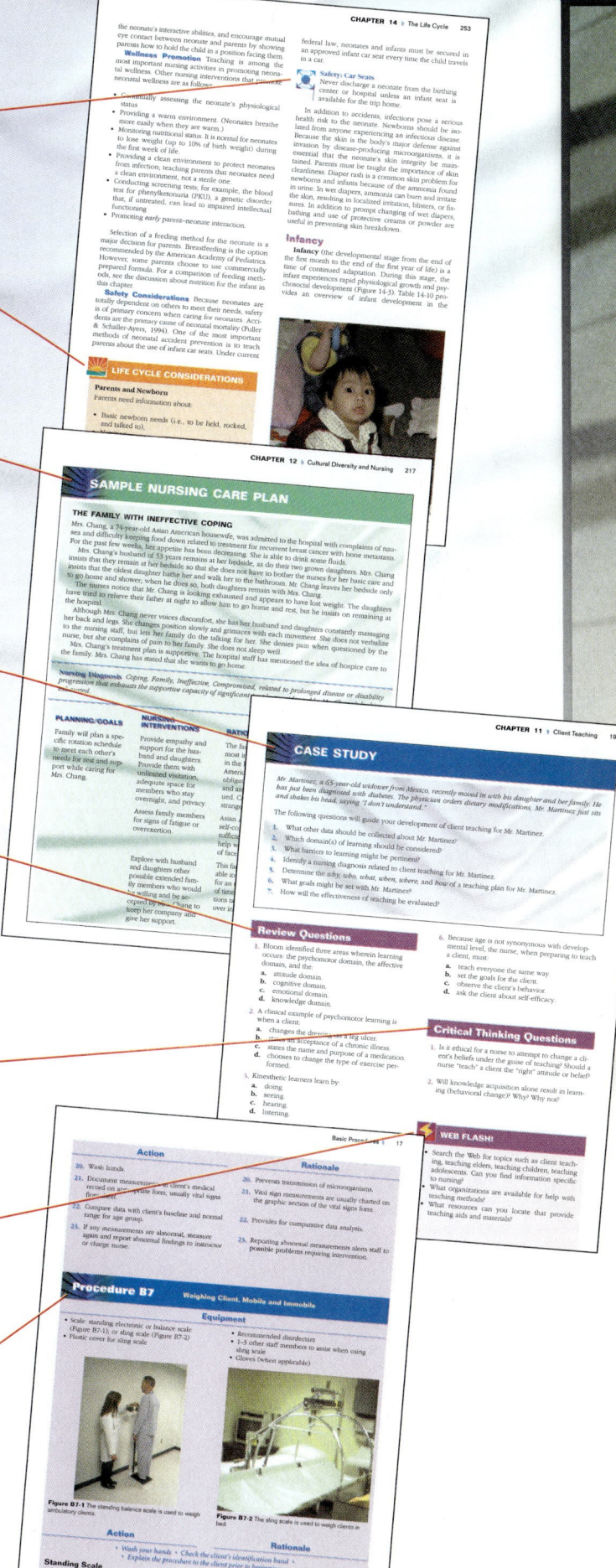

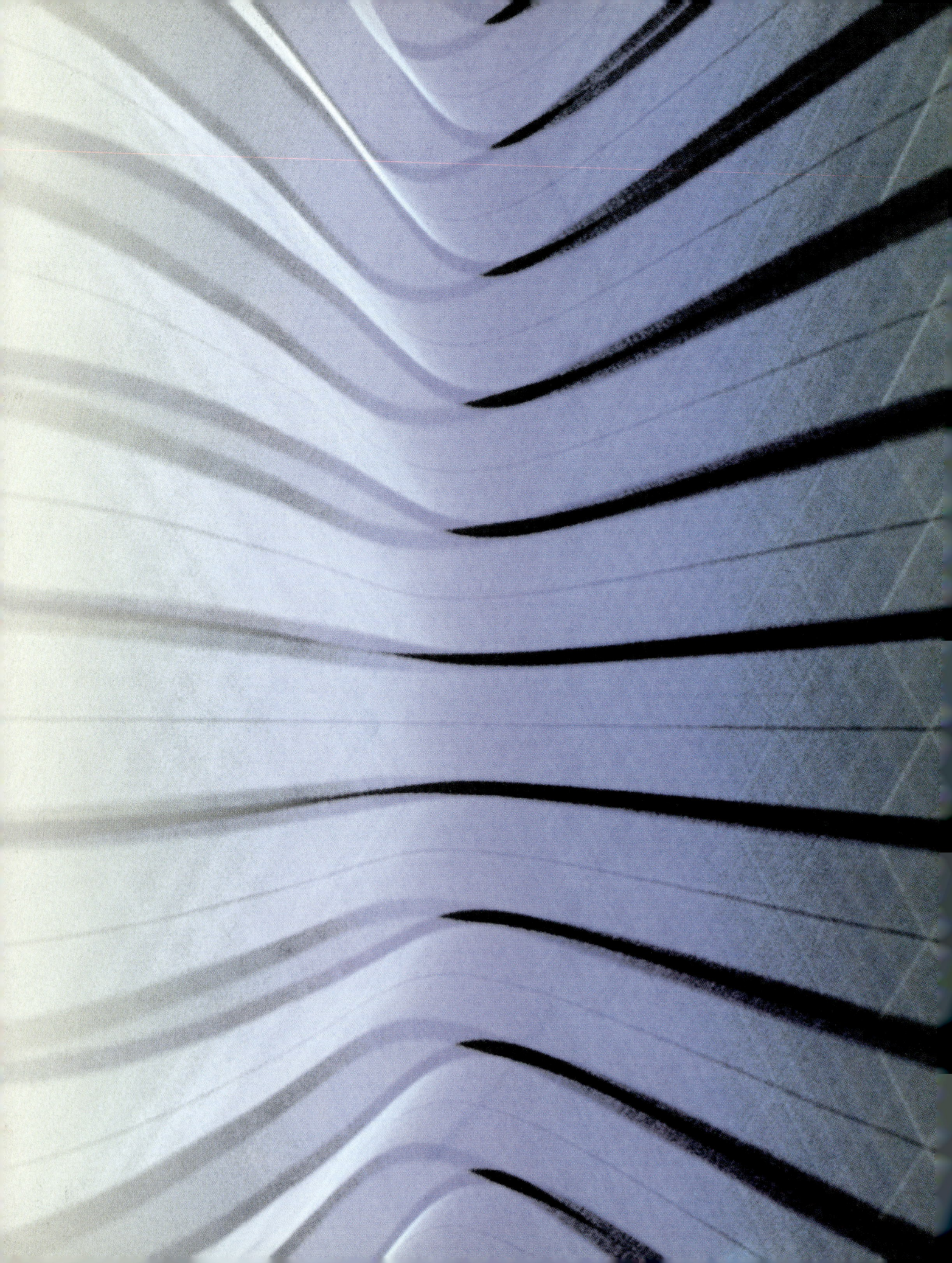

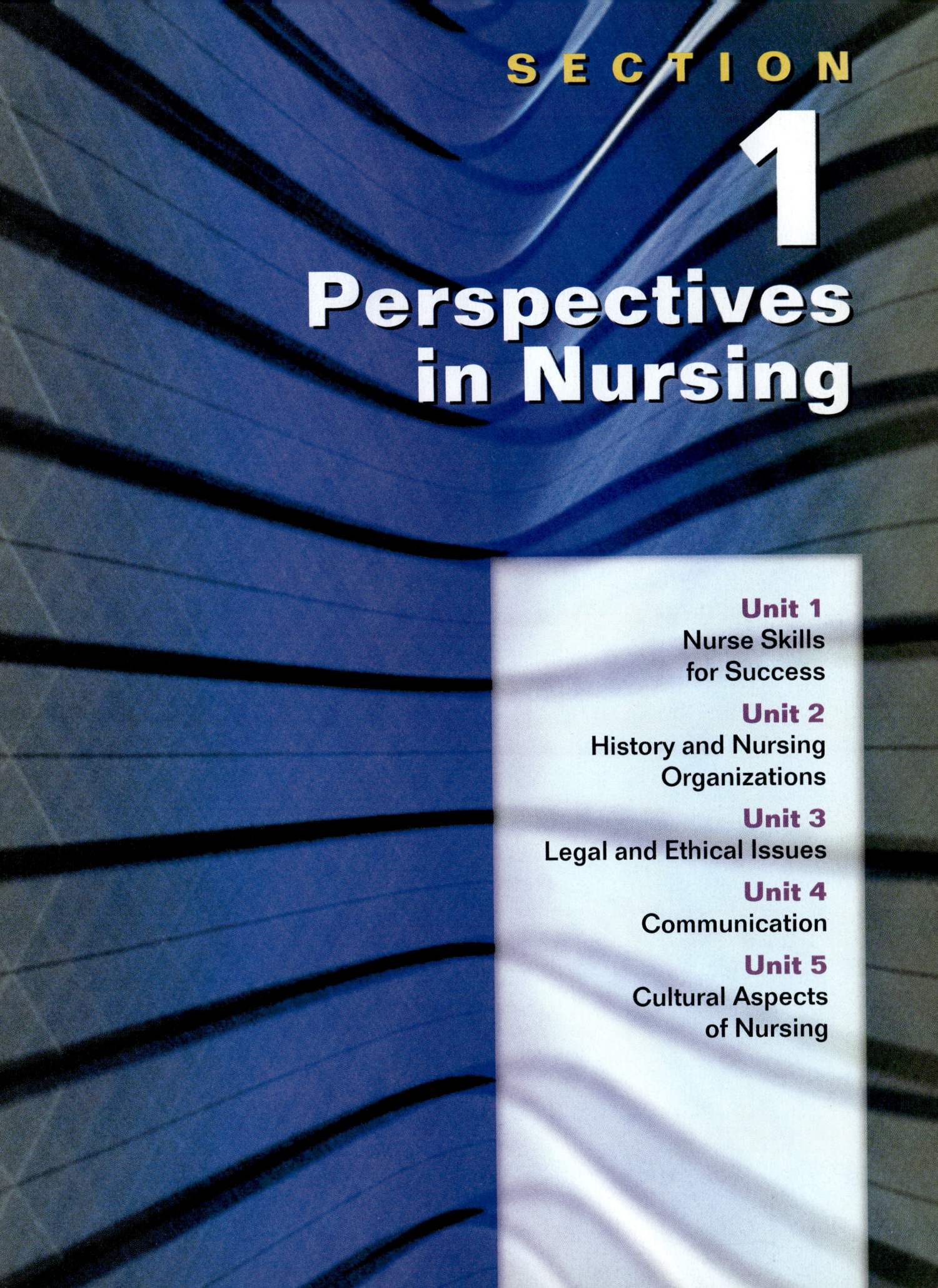

Nurse Skills
for Success

HOLISTIC CARE

MAKING THE CONNECTION

Refer to the following chapters to increase your understanding of holistic care:

- **Chapter 6, Legal Responsibilities**
- **Chapter 12, Cultural Diversity and Nursing**
- **Chapter 13, Alternative/Complementary Therapies**
- **Chapter 16, Stress, Adaptation, and Anxiety**
- **Chapter 18, Basic Nutrition**
- **Chapter 20, Safety Hygiene**

- **Chapter 22, Standard Precautions and Isolation**
- **Chapter 23, Fluid, Electrolyte, and Acid-Base Balance**
- **Chapter 46, Nursing Care of the Client: Substance Abuse**
- **Procedures:** B1, Handwashing; B8, Practicing Proper Body Mechanics

LEARNING OBJECTIVES

Upon completion of this chapter you should be able to:
- *Define key terms.*
- *Define health as it relates to the whole person.*
- *List and discuss the five aspects of total wellness.*
- *List and discuss Maslow's Hierarchy of Needs.*
- *Describe self-awareness and why it is important to nurses.*
- *Describe self-concept.*
- *Discuss the concept of personal responsibility for one's own illness.*
- *Discover personal attitudes about health and illness and take responsibility for personal well-being.*
- *Identify the components of a healthy lifestyle.*

KEY TERMS

attitude
body mechanics
culture
health
health continuum
holistic
homeostasis
intellectual wellness
Maslow's Hierarchy of Needs
physical wellness
psychological wellness
self-awareness
self-concept
sociocultural wellness
spiritual wellness
wellness

INTRODUCTION

Welcome to practical/vocational nursing. You have chosen one of life's rewarding careers. The next few months of your life will be challenging, exhilarating, frustrating, and full of new experiences. When you consider the difficulty of the nursing program's admission process, being a member of this nursing class is no small achievement. The fact that you have survived admissions demonstrates that you are capable of overcoming the challenges that lie ahead. Balancing family, community, and school responsibilities may prove the most difficult task you have yet to face.

As a nurse, you are a professional caregiver. Your intimate contact with clients allows you the opportunity not only to provide physical and emotional support, but also to teach ways to take an active role in maintaining health.

You may have contact with hundreds of clients, each needing specialized treatment and care. The care you provide will vary from routine, to critical, to emergency. You will be part of a multidisciplinary team

3

of caregivers including registered nurses, physicians, nursing assistants, physical therapists, respiratory therapists, laboratory technicians, dietitians, and social workers. All caregivers work together to promote and maintain client health.

Because the caregiver's goal is promoting and maintaining health, understanding the concept of health is paramount. Most simply, **health** means that an organism is performing its vital functions normally and properly (*Webster's*, 1997).

INTERRELATED CONCEPTS OF HEALTH

In 1948 the World Health Organization (WHO) was founded. The WHO, which functions as an arm of the United Nations, places particular emphasis on combating communicable diseases, educating health care workers, and improving the health of all people of the world. The WHO defines health as follows: "Health is a state of complete physical, mental, and social well-being and not merely the absence of disease or infirmity" (WHO, 1974).

Many people believe that health or wellness is the absence of disease. In its truest form, however, health refers to the total well-being of the whole person.

Holistic Health

Holistic is a term derived from the Greek word *holos,* meaning "whole." Holistic health views the physical, intellectual, sociocultural, psychological, and spiritual aspects of a person's life as an integrated whole. These five aspects cannot be separated or isolated; anything that affects one aspect of a person's life also affects the other aspects. The environment within which a person lives and the manner whereby the person interacts with that environment are also considerations.

The American Holistic Nurses' Association (AHNA) (1994) describes health as the maintenance of harmony and balance among body, mind, and spirit. **Homeostasis** is the balance or stability that the body strives to achieve among these aspects of a person's life by continuous adaptation. Internal physiologic homeostasis is balance of the body's fluids.

Nurses must understand the integration of these aspects of a person's life in order to help clients through healing processes. Figure 1-1 illustrates the holistic perspective.

Holistic Care

Dossey (1998) reports that the use of holistic modalities is gradually becoming integrated into mainstream client care. The National Institutes of Health (NIH) has established an Office of Alternative Medicine (OAM) to investigate holistic modalities. The NIH defines holistic care as care that "considers the whole person,

including physical, mental, emotional, and spiritual aspects." The final goal of investigating holistic modalities is to allow the validated therapies to be further integrated into general client care.

Success in using holistic modalities in client care requires an awareness of a fundamental principle of holism: The nurse *facilitates* the client in attaining the best state for healing to occur. Among the holistic modalities most frequently used in nursing are the following:

- Biofeedback
- Exercise and movement
- Goal-setting
- Humor and laughter
- Imagery
- Journaling
- Massage
- Play therapy
- Prayer

Nurses must be open to new ideas and must not allow holistic modalities to become just another technology. They must work on developing personal healing qualities and become more aware of healing in their own lives. Among other qualities, a healer:

- Demonstrates awareness that self-healing is a continual process.
- Is familiar with self-development.
- Recognizes personal strengths and weaknesses.
- Models self-care.
- Demonstrates awareness that personal presence is as important as technical skills.
- Respects and loves clients.

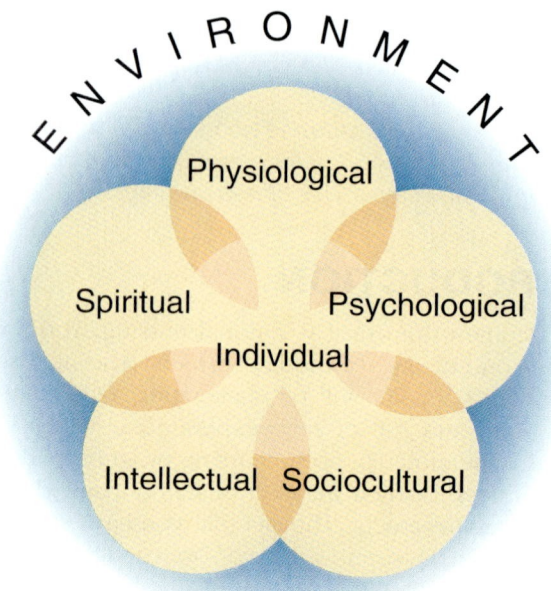

Figure 1-1 Holistic Perspective of Individuals

- Presumes that clients know the best life choices.
- Guides clients in discovering creative options.
- Listens actively.
- Shares insights without imposing personal values and beliefs.
- Accepts client input without judgment.
- Views time spent with clients as an opportunity to serve and share (adapted from Dossey, 1998).

Nursing the Whole Person

Nursing the whole person, or holistic health care, is a comprehensive approach to health care. It considers physical, intellectual, sociocultural, psychological, and spiritual aspects, the response to illness, and the effect of illness on a person's ability to meet self-care needs. Also taken into account is the individual's responsibility for personal well-being. Teaching preventive care is always a focus (Figure 1-2).

Nurses work with people throughout life to promote wellness and prevent illness. The highest level of wellness should be the goal of each nurse and every client.

Wellness

Wellness is a responsibility, a choice, a lifestyle design that helps maintain the highest potential for personal health (Hill & Howlett, 1997). The **health continuum** is a way to visualize the range of an individual's health, from highest health potential to death (Figure 1-3).

An individual's place on the continuum may change daily or even hourly depending on what is happening to that individual. Constant effort is required to balance all aspects of life and to maintain the highest level of health. A person at the highest level of wellness is one who demonstrates good physical self-care, emotional well-being, creative expression, and positive relationships with others.

Wellness incorporates physical, intellectual, sociocultural, psychological, and spiritual wellness. To provide holistic care, all aspects of the individual's wellness must be addressed.

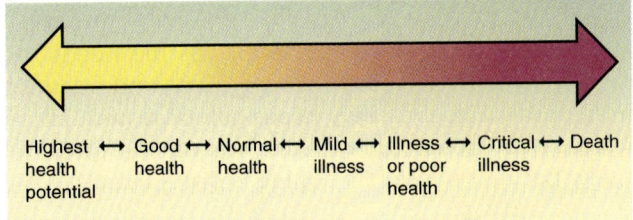

Highest ↔ Good ↔ Normal ↔ Mild ↔ Illness ↔ Critical ↔ Death
health   health   health   illness or poor illness
potential   health

Figure 1-3 Health Continuum

Maslow's Hierarchy of Needs

Abraham Maslow developed a theory of behavioral motivation based on needs. This theory is often referred to as **Maslow's Hierarchy of Needs**. There are five levels in this hierarchy. The basic physiological needs must be met to maintain life. The rest of the needs are related to quality of life. They are safety and security, love and belonging, self-esteem, and self-actualization. The needs of the lower levels must be met before a person is motivated to meet the needs of the next higher level (Figure 1-4).

Many nursing programs use Maslow's Hierarchy of Needs as a basis for planning the care of clients. This ensures that basic physiological needs as well as the other needs are assessed and addressed in individualized care plans.

Physiological Needs

Although Maslow (1954) did not specifically identify the physiological needs, they are generally accepted to be the needs of oxygen, food, water, elimination, rest (sleep)/activity (exercise), and sex. With the exception of sex, all of these needs must be met for the life of the individual to be maintained. Satisfying the sexual need, while not necessary for individual survival, is necessary for survival of the human race. The basic physiological needs must be met before higher-level needs become motivators of behavior. For example, a person who is truly hungry is motivated by that need, and behavior is focused on getting food.

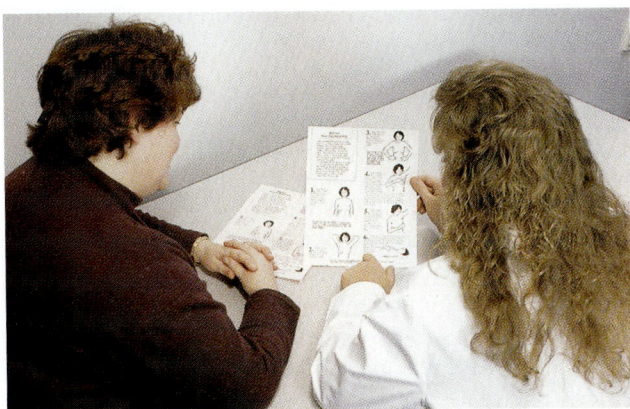

Figure 1-2 Teaching Preventive Care

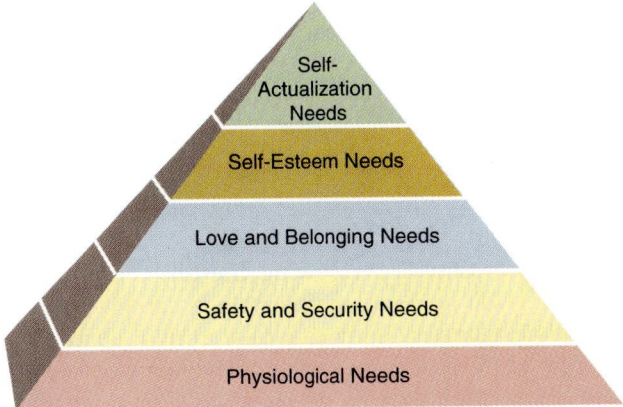

Figure 1-4 Maslow's Hierarchy of Needs

Safety and Security Needs

The next level, safety, encompasses the needs for shelter, stability, security, physical safety, and freedom from undue anxiety. Safety needs comprise both physical and emotional aspects. Illness is often a threat to safety because the stability of life is disrupted.

Love and Belonging Needs

The third level of the hierarchy, love and belonging, incorporates not only the giving of affection but also the receiving of affection. Having friends and participating with others in groups and organizations are two ways to meet these needs. Meeting these needs is extremely important for mental health.

Self-Esteem Needs

The needs of the self-esteem level are met by achieving success in work and other activities. Recognition from others increases self-esteem and feelings of pride in one's accomplishments.

Self-Actualization Needs

Self-actualization is the highest level of the Maslow hierarchy. A person who has met these needs is confident, self-fulfilled, and creative; looks for challenges; and sees beauty and order in the world.

Maslow contends that because most people are so busy meeting the physiological and the safety and security needs, little time or energy is left to meet the love and belonging, self-esteem, and self-actualization needs; thus, most people are less than satisfied at higher levels of the hierarchy. Even when the lower two levels are met without much trouble, many people have personalities and attitudes that make meeting the needs of the three higher levels difficult if not impossible.

An individual does not move steadily up the hierarchy. As life situations change, a person's unmet needs change, and behavior is motivated by different levels of the hierarchy. For example, if a person who is working to meet the self-esteem need is suddenly laid off at work, the safety and security need of providing financially for self and family suddenly becomes the unmet need that motivates that person's behavior.

PROVIDING QUALITY CARE

The first step in providing quality client care is to be aware of yourself. What kind of personality do you have? Is your self-concept positive, or do you have self-doubts and lack self-confidence? What are your beliefs and attitudes? Knowing the answers to such questions will help you in your role as caregiver.

The next step is taking care of your own needs (see the preceding section on Maslow's Hierarchy of Needs). When you attend to the needs in your own life, you can then be free to concentrate on caring for others. Your example of self-care inspires your clients to have confidence that you will provide quality care. Thus, self-care is a factor in your effectiveness as a caregiver.

Self-Awareness

Self-awareness is consciously knowing how the self thinks, feels, believes, and behaves at any specific time. Being self-aware is a constant process that is focused on the present. A person's thoughts, feelings, and beliefs are interrelated and greatly influence behavior. Being self-aware influences a person in several ways.

Self-awareness may make a person uncomfortable. Awareness allows the person to either accept or alter feelings, beliefs, and behavior. One can learn to be self-aware. Begin now to concentrate on becoming aware of your thoughts and actions. Take note of your reactions to any given situation. What makes you anxious? What makes you happy? Listen to yourself when you respond to questions and when you visit with friends. Realize that everyone has strengths and weaknesses. Focus on your strengths. Spend your energies on today. Do not dwell on past mistakes; rather try to learn from them, and then forget them. Stop periodically and pay attention to what you feel and believe. Listening not only to those words one speaks but also to the way those words are spoken assists in self-awareness. Use the word *I*, and take ownership of feelings and beliefs. Say, "I am so happy," instead of "That makes me happy."

Self-awareness is extremely important for nurses. Nurses must understand themselves so that their personal feelings, attitudes, and needs do not interfere with providing quality client care. The nurse who is self-aware is more likely to make decisions in response to the client's needs rather than the nurse's own needs. For example, student nurses—and even experienced nurses—are often anxious about caring for a client. By taking some time to practice self-awareness, the nurse might discover that the anxiety stems from never having performed the procedure in question. The nurse can then deal directly with the situation by reviewing the procedure and requesting assistance from an instructor or supervisor. All decisions about client care must be made in response to the client's needs, not the nurse's needs.

Development of Self-Concept

Self-concept is how a person thinks or feels about himself. These thoughts and feelings come from the experiences the person has with others and reflect how the person thinks others view him.

Self-concept begins forming in infancy. An infant whose needs are met feels satisfied and "good." Experiences, both positive and negative, influence a person's self-concept (Figure 1-5). Interactions with significant others, such as parents, extended family, and friends, have a great impact on self-concept. This is true not only during the developing years, but also throughout

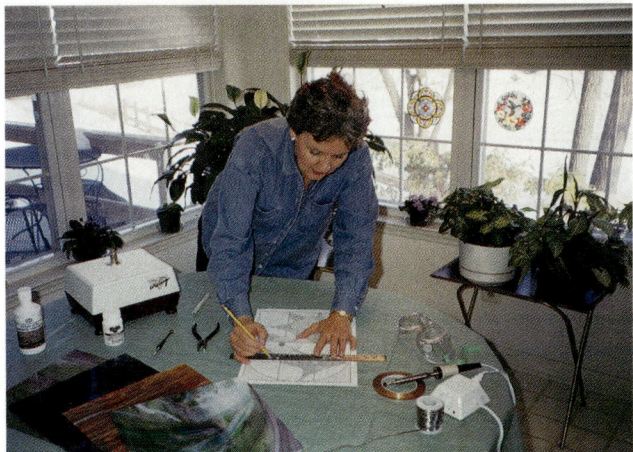

Figure 1-5 Self-concept and self-esteem can be enhanced by learning new skills.

life. Because of its influence on client care, it is important for the nurse to be aware of how her own self-concept has developed. Self-concept develops through feedback from others. The nurse is responsible for providing feedback that will not negatively affect the client's self-concept. A client who is constantly ignored or who receives messages such as "Don't bother me," "Can't you do anything right?", or "You don't have any sense" may very well begin to view himself in these terms, with the likely result being a negative self-concept. On the other hand, a person who is shown caring and who hears messages such as "Let me help you in a minute," "Let's try it this way," or "Have you thought about . . . ?" will move toward a positive self-concept.

SELF-CARE AS A PREREQUISITE TO CLIENT CARE

The most effective means to teach wellness is by positive example. By first practicing good health habits as a nursing student, you will become, by example, an important factor in your clients' overall well-being and good health. Remind yourself and your clients that health is a personal choice and that each person has control over his or her own wellness.

You will be helping clients recognize how their own actions can prevent many of the conditions that cause illness. Choosing to exercise regularly, to eat a balanced diet, to eat breakfast each day, to control fat content, and to select from the basic food groups are good rules for wellness (Figure 1-6). Choosing to not smoke, to practice moderation in the use of alcohol, to avoid all nontherapeutic drugs, and to practice safe sex can help prevent many of the conditions that cause disease and death.

While emphasizing health promotion and client education, the nurse must also encourage and respect the client's responsibility for wellness. This respect allows

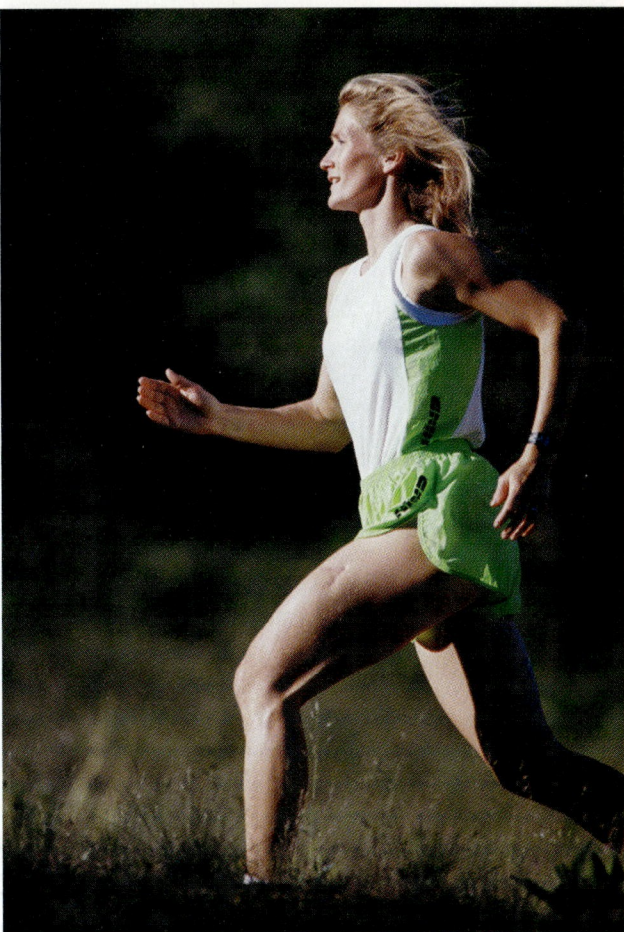

Figure 1-6 Through exercise, this woman is demonstrating a lifestyle choice that will enhance her health status.

the client to become an active partner in, rather than a passive recipient of, health care. It is not enough to tell a client *what* can be done to improve health; the nurse must also be prepared to explain *why*. If a client understands the reason behind an action, the likelihood of compliance increases.

Just as you are aware of yourself as a whole person with many components, help your clients see themselves and their health care as more than physical health. Help clients understand how physical, intellectual, sociocultural, psychological, and spiritual health are all related and can lead to an overall sense of well-being. This is the full meaning of holistic care.

Physical Wellness

Physical wellness refers to a healthy body that functions at an optimal level. To achieve physical wellness a person must practice good grooming; use proper body mechanics; have good posture; refrain from smoking and the use of drugs and alcohol; and have adequate nutrition, sleep, rest, relaxation, and exercise.

Grooming

The nurse should communicate a message of health and well-being. To do so, the nurse must be clean and

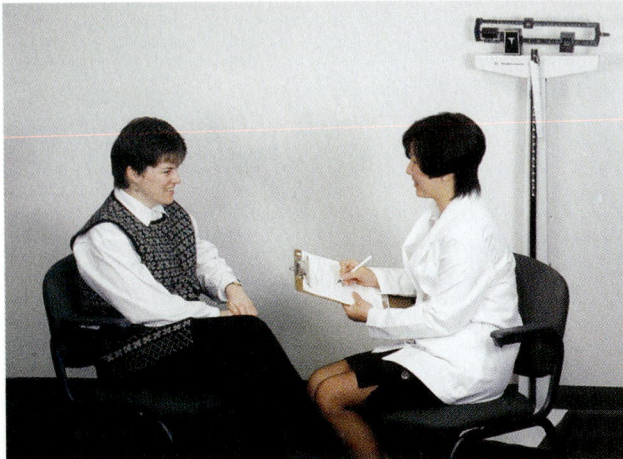

Figure 1-7 The well-groomed nurse sends a message of health and well-being.

neatly dressed (Figure 1-7). A daily bath or shower and the use of a deodorant form the basis of good grooming. Hair should be clean, combed, and neatly styled. Perfume should not be worn, as it may be offensive to clients. Frequent brushing and regular dental checkups also contribute to good grooming and overall wellness.

While important for client safety, good handwashing is also crucial to the nurse's wellness. Antiseptic hand lotion can be used to prevent cracked, dry skin. Fingernails should be kept short, as long nails not only harbor dirt and microorganisms, but also can scratch clients.

Standard Precautions have been established by the Centers for Disease Control and Prevention (CDC) in Atlanta, Georgia. These precautions are designed to protect all health care workers and their clients from the transmission of communicable disease. Good handwashing is an integral part of the Standard Precautions. As soon as you have been taught the skill of handwashing, practice it. Make it a part of your daily life. Encourage your clients to establish good handwashing habits.

Jewelry, which can harbor bacteria, and excessive makeup are both inappropriate for the nurse in uniform. Clothing should be clean and free of stains and wrinkles. Clients will have confidence in the nurse who maintains a professional appearance and who practices good hygiene.

Body Mechanics

Wellness involves more than just good grooming practices. It also requires proper **body mechanics**, that is, using the body in the safest and most efficient way to move or lift objects. The use of proper body mechanics is very important because many of the skills and tasks you will perform as a nurse involve lifting or moving clients or objects (Figure 1-8). Bending, lifting, or stooping can cause injury if done incorrectly. One of the first skills you will study involves the practice of proper body mechanics to prevent physical disability, including safe methods for bending, lifting, and moving.

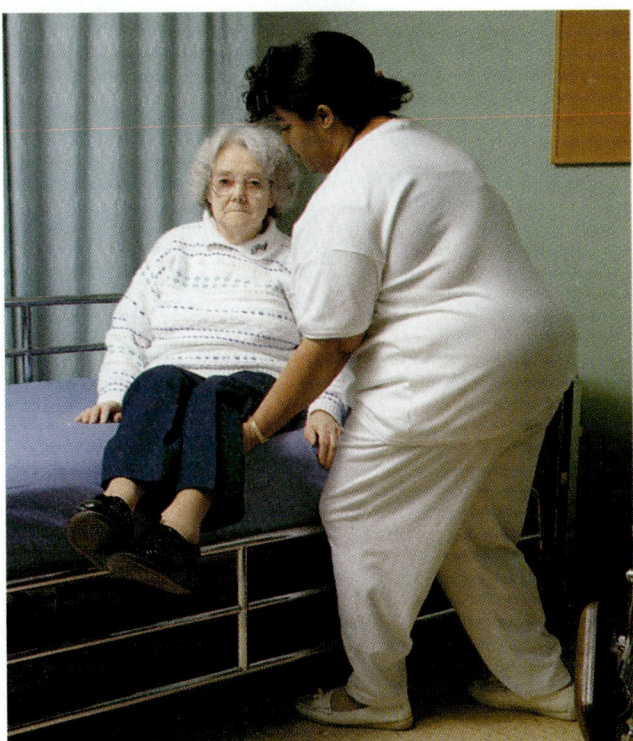

Figure 1-8 Use of Proper Body Mechanics

Posture

Good posture is the basis for proper body mechanics. Good posture means the ability to carry oneself well and in correct body alignment. Posture also can send messages about a person. A person who stands with feet spread apart and with hands on hips, for example, may be perceived as aggressive or authoritative, whereas one who holds the arms tightly folded over the chest may be viewed as closed minded.

Observe those around you as they communicate with others. Notice the differences in posture. Does the person who stands in good alignment, with shoulders back and head up, convey self-confidence and capability? Does the individual whose shoulders are drooped and head bowed convey depression, sadness, or lack of self-confidence?

As you continue your studies and begin client care, you will realize that clients appreciate having nurses who appear confident in their own abilities and decision making. When you are with clients, you must be particularly careful of the way you stand. Remember that your posture sends messages about your attitude and feelings. The client should feel that you are confident, caring, relaxed, and willing to listen.

Smoking

Smoking contributes to many health hazards and illnesses. It also may be personally offensive to clients. The odor of cigarette, pipe, or cigar smoke on clothing or the breath may precipitate allergic reactions or lead to a feeling of nausea in some clients. Most health care facilities have strict rules about smoking by clients and staff. Many facilities are "smoke free." The nurse should never smoke in a client's room. Further, great care should be taken to ensure that no offensive tobacco odors remain should the nurse use or be in close proximity to tobacco products. In each situation, every effort should be made to enforce all safety rules for clients and visitors. "No smoking" signs should be posted and strictly enforced when oxygen is in use.

Drugs and Alcohol

A frightening trend in the United States is the increasing rate of alcohol and drug abuse. Drug abuse has become so widespread within the health professions themselves that impaired caregiver programs have been implemented. Many states now provide access to treatment for the impaired nurse through state boards of nursing. A nurse should never give or make available to another person any drug without the written order of a physician or other person who can legally prescribe medications, such as a nurse practitioner. If you believe that a colleague is abusing drugs, you have an obligation to let your supervisor know so that the colleague can receive help through the impaired nurse program in your state. Should you yourself become addicted, you have a duty to your clients, your peers, and yourself to accept help through a recovery program.

Nutrition

Nursing is emotionally, mentally, and physically demanding. Nurses must be able to think clearly and work efficiently. A balanced diet including fruits and vegetables, whole grains and cereals, milk and milk products, and meats or other protein foods is required for optimal body function.

Nursing students may be tempted to skip meals, omit breakfast, eat snacks, and follow fad diets. This is never a wise practice. While you are in school, your success depends upon your functioning at your best. Skipping meals, especially breakfast, leaves a person tired, weak, and hungry. It is impossible to think efficiently when hungry. Remember Maslow's Hierarchy of

Needs: The need for food must be satisfied before you will be motivated to meet the need to learn or to study.

Always eat a balanced breakfast. Pastries and coffee, although satisfying in the moment, elevate the blood sugar level only for a short while before the level plummets. This reaction leaves a person drained, irritable, and hungrier than before. Try to avoid snacking on "junk foods," which contain "empty" calories, or those having very little nutritional value. Instead, plan to eat fruit or high-protein snacks.

Plan a routine for mealtimes, and stick to it. Doing so helps prevent the urge to binge on unhealthy snacks. Also, drink plenty of water. Water is the body's most important nutrient (Figure 1-9). A human being can survive for weeks without food, but only for a few days without water. By weight, approximately 60% of the adult body is water. In order to maintain proper fluid balance and to facilitate the elimination of body wastes, it is necessary to drink plenty of fluids. Most authorities agree that the average adult needs six to eight (8-ounce) glasses of water each day. It is important to maintain a balance in the diet for optimal wellness. See the accompanying display for suggestions on maintaining proper nutrition.

Sleep, Rest, Relaxation, and Exercise

Wellness implies more than eating balanced meals, avoiding harmful substances, and practicing good grooming. Wellness also means taking time to enjoy yourself. It means making time for sleep, rest, relaxation, and exercise.

Sleep is the time for the body to replenish its energy reserves and to heal itself. The amount of time needed

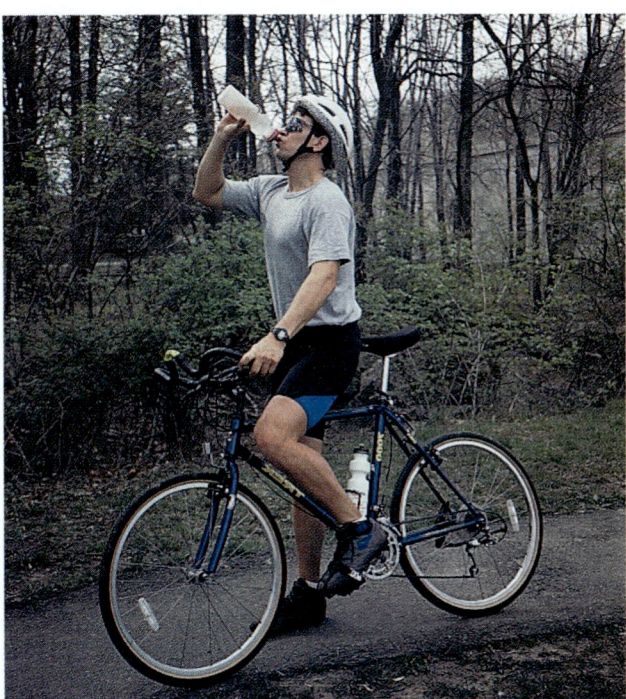

Figure 1-9 Drinking plenty of water is an important element of proper nutrition.

LIFE CYCLE CONSIDERATIONS

Nutrition

- Children's appetites vary with their growth spurts and growth plateaus.
- Healthy eating habits should be established during childhood.
- The amount of food eaten generally declines in the elderly person.
- Proper food choices are more important than quantity for the elderly person.

CLIENT TEACHING

Tips on Maintaining Proper Nutrition
- Read product labels.
- Avoid foods high in fat, sugar, and salt.
- Work to maintain or attain your ideal weight.
- If you drink alcohol, do so in moderation.
- Always eat breakfast.
- Make between-meal snacks healthy, such as raw fruits and vegetables.

may vary with the individual or even with the day. One person may need 8 hours of sleep after a heavy work day but need only 6 after a less strenuous day. An infant, of course, needs more sleep than does a young adult. Sleep is necessary to allow the body's organs to function at their most minimal levels. This period of rejuvenation for the body is necessary for total wellness.

Rest, meaning conscious freedom from activity and worry, is just as important as sleep. Rest is a time of inner quiet and physical inactivity. Only when a person is relaxed and at inner peace can that person rest.

Relaxation means doing something for the fun of it. That which is relaxing to one person may not be relaxing to another. Examples of relaxation activities include reading a novel, reading to children, playing cards or other games, fishing, painting, or sewing or other handwork.

Many experts agree that the best rest follows planned exercise. During exercise, heart rate and breathing increase, circulation improves, and muscles stretch. Exercise is also a time to free the mind of anxiety-producing thoughts. Sometimes after a day's work, a brisk walk frees the mind and allows the body to relax in preparation for rest.

Whichever form of exercise, rest, and relaxation is best for you, make time for it in each day. Rest and relaxation as well as regular sleep and exercise are essential ingredients for wellness and result in reduced fatigue and irritability and possibly increased resistance to colds, flu, and serious infections. Furthermore, the capacity to concentrate increases, which should make a significant difference in your studies.

Intellectual Wellness

Intellectual wellness is the ability to function as an independent person capable of making sound decisions. Such decisions are based on the individual's needs but at the same time take into account the needs of others. Clear thinking, problem-solving skills, good judgment, and the desire to continually learn are all qualities found in the person who is intellectually well.

Nursing requires making many decisions, some of which may mean life or death to the client. The nurse must have intellectual wellness to be able to make the best decisions possible with regard to client care.

Sociocultural Wellness

Sociocultural wellness is the ability to appreciate the needs of others and to care about one's environment and the inhabitants of it. As a nurse, you will care for clients of all ages and races who speak different languages and come from various cultural groups. Each client's **culture** (behavior, customs, and beliefs of the family, extended family, tribe, nation, and society) influences the way that person views wellness and responds to illness.

It is important that the nurse understand that while everyone's basic needs are the same, the ways that those needs are met may vary based on the client's culture. Today's population is working, playing, and contributing to society for more years than ever before. People are more health conscious, better educated, and more involved in making health choices than perhaps any previous generation. Nurses should encourage such involvement and work to dispel discrimination by accepting each person as an individual.

Psychological Wellness

Psychological wellness encompasses the enjoyment of creativity, the satisfaction of the basic need to love and be loved, the understanding of emotions, and the ability to maintain control over emotions. Emotions are an integral part of the balance sought in life and are important factors in the way a person relates to others. They are measures of inner thoughts and feelings and are apparent in actions or behaviors.

CULTURAL CONSIDERATIONS

Sociocultural Wellness
Nurses and nursing students come from various cultural backgrounds and are thus excellent resources for you to learn about cultural variations.

Wellness requires that individuals recognize emotions and control their reactions in various situations. By controlling their emotions, nurses help create a therapeutic environment within which to help clients.

Another aspect of emotional wellness is a positive attitude. An **attitude** is a feeling about people, places, or things that is evident in the way one behaves. It can be positive or negative. Many books have been written and hundreds of studies have described the role that a positive attitude plays in helping to conquer illness. Many authorities believe having a positive attitude is at least as important as having the best treatment for an illness.

Nursing requires that you see the best in people

during the worst of times. In order to survive and function well, the nurse needs to see life as a challenge and as a gift to cherish and enjoy.

Because a positive attitude is so important when caring for your clients, it is vital that you share yours with them. An attitude can become a habit. If you repeatedly think positively, soon you will unconsciously find yourself seeing the positive aspects in any given situation. For example, you may find yourself at work when the usual number of staff does not show up. You can say to yourself at the beginning of your shift; "There is no way I will ever finish my work on time," or you can tell yourself, "This is the perfect opportunity to get organized early and work together as a team." Either way you will have the same number of staff members. But whereas having a negative attitude will increase your chances of being miserable and unsuccessful, having a positive attitude will help the day go smoother and increase the likelihood of your coworkers being cheerful and willing to help.

Having a positive attitude will also help you in your studies. It will help to open your mind and will spill into your daily life, making that life more enjoyable.

Spiritual Wellness

Spiritual wellness manifests as inner strength and peace. Spirituality is a broader concept than religion and involves one's relationship with self, others, the natural order, and a higher power. It manifests as meaningful work, creative expression, familiar rituals, and religious practices (Wright, 1998). Spirituality involves finding meaning in everything including life, illness, and death. Spiritual needs include love, meaning in life, forgiveness, and hope. The human spiritual dimension is a major healing force. It can mean the difference between life and death, wellness and illness (Dossey, Keegan, Guzzetta, & Kolkmeier, 1995).

Florence Nightingale spoke boldly about the importance of the spiritual aspect of client care. Dossey and Dossey (1998) state that the richness of a person's interactions with others correlates with positive health outcomes, and that practice of any religion correlates with greater health and increased longevity.

Nurses are not asked to take over the role of spiritual counselors. Rather, nurses are encouraged to integrate a holistic approach by extending love, compassion, and empathy; motivating clients to address the spiritual issues; and suggesting how they might do so (Dossey & Dossey, 1998).

Cerrato (1998b) has two suggestions regarding nursing and spiritual wellness: (1) Nurses who have strong religious convictions should not impose those convictions on their clients and (2) nurses should never assume that clients who have no religious interests have no interest in spiritual values. Clients not interested in religion can be encouraged to become involved in some humanitarian endeavor or to look at life's everyday wonders in a different way.

Because they play a key role in helping clients find hope and meaning in life, it is important that nurses understand spirituality. For many, religious practices are an expression of their spirituality. An important function for the nurse is to respect the religious beliefs of clients, provide clients with privacy to practice those beliefs, and make spiritual guidance available through the client's minister, priest, rabbi, or other representative, when requested.

NURTURE YOURSELF

The worthy and demanding profession of nursing requires unselfish caring for others. Those who select nursing as a career generally want to make a difference in people's lives. The demands of clients, employers, and coworkers can cause stress for the nurse. The nurse's personal life may also be a source of stress. Many caregivers do not know how to care for themselves. Those who do not nurture themselves will suffer stress symptoms and illnesses.

Persons who are well physically, intellectually, socioculturally, psychologically, and spiritually lead productive creative lives. They are better able to meet life's challenges and to control their stressors. For nurses, wellness means practicing wellness habits daily. As role models for clients, nurses should be examples of the holistically healthy individual.

SUMMARY

- Wellness includes physical, intellectual, sociocultural, psychological, and spiritual health.
- The keys to wellness are prevention and education.
- Each individual must learn to accept responsibility for his own wellness.
- Nurses are teachers. The most effective means to teach wellness is by positive example.
- There are five levels in Maslow's Hierarchy of Needs: physiological, safety and security, love and belonging, self-esteem, and self-actualization.
- Self-awareness is important for nurses so that their own needs do not interfere with providing quality client care.

PROFESSIONAL TIP

Self-Nurturing
- Develop activities that recharge the body, mind, and spirit.
- Make time for fun. Any activity that brings happiness or joy is beneficial.
- Schedule a few minutes each day to do at least one fun thing.

CLIENT TEACHING

Tips for Wellness

Encourage clients to adopt the following tips for wellness:

- Eat healthy meals and healthy snacks.
- Eat breakfast.
- Do not use tobacco products.
- Exercise regularly.
- Do not use drugs.
- Do not drink alcoholic beverages or drink only in moderation.
- Focus on one problem at a time.
- Get enough sleep every night.
- Practice having a positive attitude.
- Think before speaking.
- Make a list of goals for each day.

- Nurses should get to know themselves by becoming aware of their thoughts, actions, and reactions to situations.
- Good posture is necessary for personal and client safety.
- Dental health is necessary for overall wellness and professionalism.
- Wellness tips include exercising regularly, getting enough sleep, and finding a quiet time each day for relaxing.
- A positive attitude is helpful in looking for the best in everyone.
- All nurses should learn to laugh at themselves and enjoy life's little pleasures.

Review Questions

1. Rest is defined as:
    a. sleeping.
    b. physical inactivity.
    c. playing games with family or friends.
    d. conscious freedom from activity and worry.

2. According to many experts, the best rest follows:
    a. eating.
    b. reading.
    c. exercise.
    d. studying.

3. Regular mouth care and avoiding refined sugars will help control:
    a. acne.
    b. malocclusion.
    c. dental caries.
    d. mononucleosis.

4. What responsibility does the nurse have who believes a colleague is abusing drugs?
    a. Report it to the supervisor.
    b. Ignore it; it is not the nurse's concern.
    c. Tell the colleague to stop or the nurse will call the police.
    d. Assist the nurse to receive help through the local drug treatment program.

5. What can be the result when breakfast is omitted?
    a. The person loses weight faster.
    b. The person is left tired, weak, and hungry.
    c. The person eats more at the noon and evening meals.
    d. The person's mind is sharper, and study time is more productive.

6. Positive or negative feelings about people, places, or things are called:
    a. culture.
    b. empathy.
    c. symptoms.
    d. attitudes.

7. The nurse who smokes may have:
    a. mitosis.
    b. meiosis.
    c. halitosis.
    d. arthrosis.

8. The aspects of total wellness are:
    a. rest, exercise, and good grooming.
    b. physical, psychological, spiritual, intellectual, and sociocultural.
    c. self-awareness; rest; balanced, nutritious diet; good grooming; dental care.
    d. physiological; safety and security; love and belonging; self-esteem; self-actualization.

Critical Thinking Questions

1. What are your own attitudes about health and wellness?

2. What are you doing or what can you do to take responsibility for your own well-being?

WEB FLASH!

- How many references do you find on the Web for "holistic care"?
- Visit the American Holistic Nurses' Association on the Internet.
- Visit the Web site of NIH's Office of Alternative Medicine. What is the latest information on holistic modalities?

CRITICAL THINKING

MAKING THE CONNECTION

Refer to the following chapters to increase your understanding of critical thinking:

- **Chapter 8, Communication**
- **Chapter 9, Nursing Process**

LEARNING OBJECTIVES

Upon completion of this chapter you should be able to:
- *Define key terms.*
- *State five characteristics of the person who uses critical thinking.*
- *Identify behaviors that illustrate the traits of a nurse who is a critical thinker.*
- *Assess personal strengths and weaknesses in relation to critical thinking skills.*
- *Develop a personal plan for the enhancement of personal critical thinking and reasoning skills.*

KEY TERMS

concept	logic
critical thinking	opinion
discipline	reasoning
disciplined	reflective
judgment	standard
justify	

INTRODUCTION

Thinking as a nurse involves much more than gathering an assortment of facts and skills. Critical thinking in nursing education is not a separate component of the curriculum. It is "an approach to inquiry where both students and faculty examine clinical and professional issues and search for more effective answers" (Miller & Malcolm, 1990).

Nursing is part of a rapidly changing and increasingly complex society. Anyone who expects to have a successful career in nursing, at any level, must be able to compete effectively. This means that practical/vocational nurses must have good problem-solving skills and make quality decisions related to the client care they deliver. Over the past 15 years, increasing attention has been paid to the need for graduates of educational programs at every level and in every **discipline** (branch of learning, field of study, or occupation requiring specialized knowledge) to develop better thinking skills. Nurse educators have been among the leaders in the current movement to find ways to improve the thinking ability of their students. Nurses in clinical practice have also been challenged to improve their ability to reason clearly and logically. Because of these movements, you, as a beginning nursing student, will need to develop your critical thinking skills.

CRITICAL THINKING

The first step in improving your ability to think well is to develop an understanding of **critical thinking**. This involves much more than memorizing a simple definition of this process. The ability to think critically requires a great deal of effort and time. There are many definitions, all of which may be valuable, as you begin the process of learning to assess your own thinking and the quality of the thinking of others (see Figure 2-1). In fact, memorizing an exact definition of critical thinking would be detrimental to the full development of an understanding of this **disciplined** (trained by instruction and exercise) type of thinking. The **concept** of critical thinking includes the basic idea that one becomes a better thinker by developing specific attitudes, traits, and skills. A concept is a mental picture of abstract phenomena that serves to organize observations related to that phenomena. Each

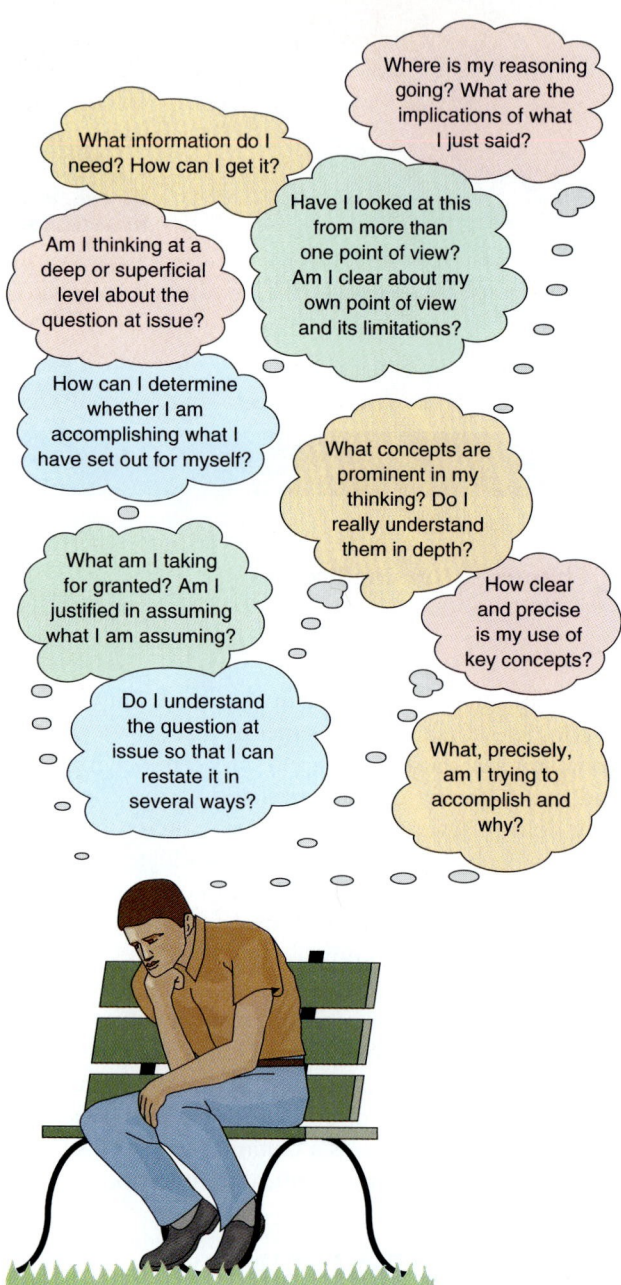

Figure 2-1 Assessing Our Own Thinking (*Courtesy of The Foundation for Critical Thinking, Santa Rosa, CA*)

person must learn to be **reflective**, or introspective, about his or her own thinking. Critical thinking was briefly described in this way in a workshop presented by Richard Paul (Paul & Willsen, 1993): "Critical thinking is that mode of thinking—about any subject, content, or problem—in which the thinker improves the quality of his or her thinking by skillfully taking charge of the structures inherent in thinking and imposing intellectual **standards** (or a level or degree of quality) upon them." To ensure integrity and consistency of the presentation in this chapter, the criteria, standards, and

materials developed by the Center for Critical Thinking have been used as the organizing framework.

Penny Heaslip (1994), in a newsletter designed for nurse educators interested in the use of critical thinking within the nursing curriculum, presents a definition of critical thinking. This definition serves as a basis for your development of strategies and tactics as you begin the exciting experience of learning to think more clearly, and in a disciplined manner, about nursing. A comprehensive definition of critical thinking is the disciplined, intellectual process of applying skillful clinical **reasoning** (use of the elements of thought to solve a problem or settle a question) and self-reflective thinking as a guide to belief or action in nursing practice (Heaslip, 1994; Norris & Ennis, 1989; Paul, 1990).

Table 2-1 presents some definitions of critical thinking. Review them and compare the elements that are common to all of them and the elements that are different.

Most of the authors who have written about critical thinking have addressed instructors. This chapter is written for you, the student. It is designed to guide your process of reflecting on and evaluating your own thinking. While your instructors want to help you with the process, you are ultimately responsible for your own thinking.

Many students enter nursing programs unprepared to think critically. Many educators believe this inability may be the result of a lack of instruction in thinking. The result is similar to what would happen to you if you tried to play soccer without knowing the rules or having had a chance to learn the basic skills of the game. Quality thinking is like any skill; it takes practice and discipline to learn. This is a good time to do a self-evaluation related to your current ability to perform the four basic critical thinking processes: reading for meaning, listening critically, writing clearly, and speaking in a logical, coherent manner. These four skills are discussed in the next section. If your basic education program did not emphasize all of these skills, decide now to develop these abilities.

Table 2-1 DEFINITIONS OF CRITICAL THINKING

- "Reflective and reasonable thinking that is focused on deciding what to believe or do" (Ennis, 1985).
- "An investigation whose purpose is to explore a situation, phenomenon, question, or problem to arrive at a hypothesis or conclusion about it that integrates all available information and that can therefore be convincingly justified" (Kurfiss, 1988).
- "The attentive commitment to a self-reflective process of examining one's thoughts, ensuring that the thinking occurring meets intellectual standards" (Heaslip, 1993).

New Information

The quantity of new information that you must be prepared to master may be a barrier to the development of critical thinking skills. Many students (and instructors) focus so intently on the content of a course that they allow little time to think about the material. The ability to think critically about the knowledge base of nursing is essential for learning the content of your nursing courses. The discipline of nursing has an organizing **logic**, or formal principles of a branch of knowledge, that serves to define the appropriate facts and methods required to produce effective nursing practice. This logic serves as a framework within which the student can construct a unique, meaningful system for the practice of nursing. Your nursing program probably has a philosophy and a statement of the main concepts that the nursing faculty uses to present the course material in a logical framework.

Activity

If you have not yet reviewed your program's philosophy and main concepts for the purpose of helping you understand your program of study, this would be a good time to do so. Most programs of nursing include a philosophy statement, organizing concepts, and program outcomes in the student handbook or other document provided to students. To use these resources to help you use your own logic to discover the logic of nursing as presented in your program, try the following activities:

1. Identify the major concepts (such as nursing, learning, caring) that provide structure for your program's philosophy and organization.
2. Discuss the components, or parts, of each major theme with your classmates and instructors.
3. Use your own words to see how your mental pictures of these ideas may be the same or different from those in your program materials.
4. Review the material you have already covered in your nursing program to identify how the major parts of each course relate to these concepts.
5. Look at the objectives for this course and the topics in this textbook to see how they will relate to the main ideas you have discovered in this activity.

Student Responsibility

Finally, many students find the process of becoming responsible for their own thinking painful. For many students the education processes that were part of their basic school preparation were based on a very structured approach to acquiring selected facts and skills; the students' recall was then tested by "objective" tests. If this was your experience, you may view learning as being the result of the teacher's presenting what must be learned and devising "fair" tests. You may thus believe your own input to the learning process to be of less importance than that of the teacher. You, along with many other students, may find that you are uncomfortable when asked to decide what is important or to be able to defend your **opinions** (subjective beliefs) and **judgments** (conclusions based on sound reasoning and supported by evidence). You may prefer to be told, with no ambiguity, what you need to know.

Nursing, however, does not take place in predictable, highly structured situations. Practical/vocational nurses are required to make decisions at many levels. Knowing how to make good decisions begins with developing the essential skills, traits, and attitudes associated with critical thinking.

SKILLS OF CRITICAL THINKING

Four basic skills are necessary for the development of higher-level thinking skills. These skills are part of the process of developing and using thinking for problem-solving and reasoning. Your abilities in these four areas can be measured by the extent to which you are achieving the universal intellectual standards (UIS). These standards are discussed in the following section and are illustrated in Table 2-2. The four basic skills are critical reading, critical listening, critical writing, and critical speaking.

Critical Reading

Reading for meaning is basic to the acquisition of knowledge from textbooks and journals. The student who can read critically will also do better on tests. Study time will be reduced and retention of material

Table 2-2 THE SPECTRUM OF UNIVERSAL INTELLECTUAL STANDARDS

Clear	Unclear
Precise	Imprecise
Specific	Vague
Accurate	Inaccurate
Relevant	Irrelevant
Consistent	Inconsistent
Logical	Illogical
Deep	Superficial
Complete	Incomplete
Significant	Insignificant
Adequate	Inadequate
Fair	Unfair

Adapted from The Foundation for Critical Thinking, Santa Rosa, CA.

will be enhanced. An exercise that can help build reading skills is to use a highlighter pen to mark the main idea of a sentence. Students who have not learned to read critically will find that they have marked most of the text. Joining a study group may help you identify main ideas by comparing with others the various main ideas each of you have derived from the same material. During test reviews, you can make sure to note when misreading or misinterpretation caused you to make an error on the test. By making a conscious effort to identify your individual weaknesses, you will improve your critical reading skills.

Another tactic you can try is to practice restating the main idea to yourself or to another student. As you read the text, have a dialogue with yourself, which could go something like this: "What is the reason for studying this material? How does this relate to what I already know? This does not seem to fit. Did I misunderstand? Can I say this in my own words?" Worrell (1990) has developed a useful tool for guiding your dialogue. It is illustrated in Table 2-3.

Critical Listening

Communication skills, especially listening skills, receive a great deal of emphasis in the nursing curriculum. Even so, many persons do not have effective listening skills. One reason is that many persons have developed the habit of tuning in only occasionally to orally presented material. The result is that the meaning of the oral communication is lost. A way to improve your listening skills is to try to restate the points made in a discussion with another student and have that student give feedback about how accurately you have restated her position. Critical listening also requires that you carry on a mental dialogue with the speaker. For instance, as you listen, focus on what the speaker is saying, listen for key points, notice anything that seems confusing to you as well as those points you already understand (Figure 2-2).

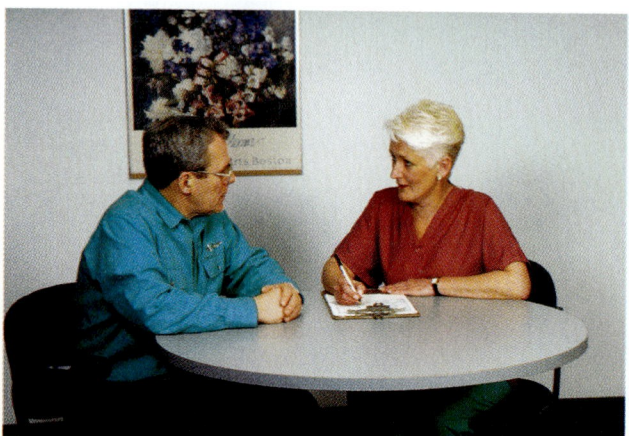

Figure 2-2 Effective listening skills are essential to all client interactions.

Table 2-3 STRATEGIC READING LIST

The following questions serve as a guide for self-talk when reading texts or journal articles. An effective reader is an active, strategic reader! Soon you will find yourself automatically using these and other questions that you have developed, no longer needing the checklist.

PREREADING QUESTIONS

___ 1. Have I previewed (skimmed) the title, headings, subheadings, objectives, and overview?

___ 2. Do the headings/subheadings identify main ideas?

___ 3. What is the chapter about?

___ 4. How is the content related to what I already know?

___ 5. How has the author organized the material? How will this organization help me?

___ 6. Will I need other resources as I read?

___ 7. Based on previewing, what questions should I formulate to guide my reading?

QUESTIONS DURING READING

___ 1. Does this make sense to me?

___ 2. Do I need to look up any unfamiliar words?

___ 3. Do I need to reread difficult material? Or will this be explained further if I read on?

___ 4. Is the author using signal words (*first, next, therefore, as a result,* etc.)?

___ 5. How is this information related to what I know?

___ 6. How is this section linked to the previous section?

___ 7. Can I summarize this section before going any further?

___ 8. Can I answer my prereading questions? Can I formulate new questions?

QUESTIONS AFTER READING

___ 1. Do I understand the main points?

___ 2. Can I outline the content?

___ 3. How is this related to previous learning?

___ 4. How would I use or apply this information?

___ 5. Are there points that I need to clarify? How will I do this?

___ 6. What questions would likely be on an exam from this material?

___ 7. Can I answer my questions, paraphrase the content, and link main points without looking at my notes or text?

From Metacognition: Implications for Instruction in Nursing Education, *by P. J. Worrell, 1990,* Journal of Nursing Education, *29(4), pp. 170–175. Reprinted with permission of Journal of Nursing Education, SLACK Incorporated, Thorofare, NJ.*

Critical listening requires that you make a conscious commitment to focus on the topic of discussion. This means that you should actively attend to the words and meanings of the speaker. Your ability to recognize things that distract your attention is valuable in increasing your listening skills. Some typical distractions for students include attempting to take word-for-word notes, focusing on the mannerisms or appearance of the speaker, and daydreaming. As in all areas, a good thinker is not afraid to identify weaknesses and strengths in order to improve.

Critical Writing

The ability to state one's thoughts coherently, clearly, and concisely is basic to good thinking skills. Many students arrive at college unable to write well. The quality of thinking is improved by the discipline required to state facts and judgments well. Many students are afraid to write down their thoughts, because they feel that writing is too revealing. Writing is important for the improvement of thinking because it can be reviewed using the UIS to evaluate the quality of the thinking reflected in the writing (Figure 2-3). These standards are discussed in greater detail later in the chapter. You may also refer back to Table 2-2.

One technique for improving the quality of your thinking through writing is to summarize, in your own words, the main idea in a reading assignment. Next, use that main idea in relation to a client care problem from the material you are studying. Then, put the writing away until the next day and reread it. Can you understand it? Submit it to a friend for critique. Can your friend understand what you meant to say? How could you improve what you have written? Improving your writing skills may not seem like fun, but it is an effective and vital process for improving the quality of your own thinking.

Critical Speaking

Perhaps the most neglected skill is disciplined speaking. We do not hear many examples of clear, logical, accurate spoken communication. Oral communication is different from written communication. It is usually more spontaneous and must be carefully presented because, unless recorded, it is present only for the moment. Ambiguous statements are misleading. Personal biases influence what the other person hears. Practicing in a small group and soliciting feedback from the listeners can help a student assess and improve this skill.

STANDARDS FOR CRITICAL THINKING

The simple definition of critical thinking used in the preceding section includes the provision that the assessment of your own thinking relies on the use of universal standards for quality thinking. As you begin to develop and apply critical thinking to nursing, the first requirement is to become familiar with these standards. The Spectrum of Universal Intellectual Standards developed by The Center for Critical Thinking is used in this discussion because it provides a valid and

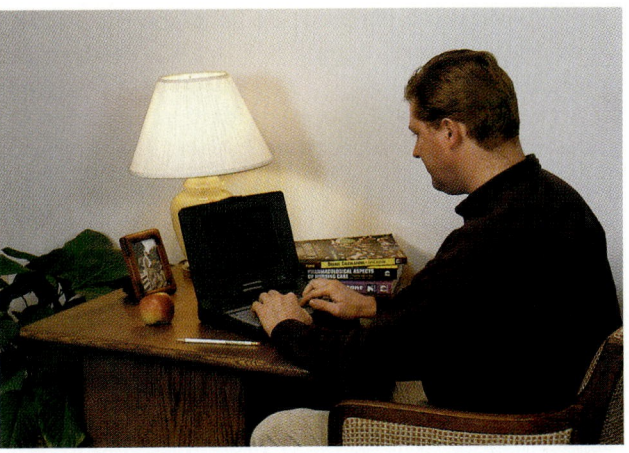

Figure 2-3 Effective writing skills are integral to critical thinking.

reliable measure for the quality of thinking. Whether you are reading the assigned material from a textbook, listening to an oral presentation, writing a paper, answering test questions, or presenting ideas in oral form, the following standards should be applied.

Clarity vs. Lack of Clarity

Fundamental to quality thinking is the ability to think clearly. Thinking clearly means that you can place the facts and ideas of course content into a logical and coherent framework. The measure for the degree to which this is true is the degree to which you can state these relationships orally or in writing so that others can understand your position. One tactic for increasing your clarity of thought is to pay particular attention to the exact meaning of the words encountered. The year that you spend in the practical/vocational nursing program is filled with many new terms and concepts. Time spent in practicing the proper use of these terms and in applying concepts appropriately will result in improved clarity of thought and increased retention of content. You can use small study groups to challenge one another to write and speak clearly as you review content together.

A review of the words used in the preceding paragraph may illustrate how the meaning of words can be misunderstood. For example, think about the word *clarity*. When you look up this word in a dictionary, you find that there are several shades of meaning. Look up the word for yourself and decide which of the definitions applies to the use of clarity in describing a standard for critical thinking.

Think about some expressions you use every day. Would someone who is from another part of the country understand them? An example is the use of the term *this evening*, which is common in some parts of the country. If someone told you that she would visit you "this evening," when would you expect her? In some places, the person might arrive in the early afternoon; in other places, at night. When speaking to clients, families, and other health team members, the nurse must be sure that the words used clearly express the intended message. When reading or listening, do not assume that you understand a term. Take the time to verify the meaning.

Precision vs. Imprecision

Sometimes, we have a "ballpark" mentality. That is, we learn enough about a subject to be "in the ballpark," but not enough to hit a home run. The result is a general idea of the meaning of a fact or idea, but not enough understanding to apply it or to use the information for problem-solving or promoting communication of an idea to someone else. You may be making this mistake if you find yourself saying something like this: "I knew that, but on the test, it was stated differently." Precision of thought means that the meaning of a concept is clearly understood in terms of its relationship to other concepts and to its practical implications, so that the thought is exact, accurate, and definite (Paul & Willsen, 1993).

Specificity vs. Vagueness

Specificity means that the student can be concrete or exact in stating or applying a fact. An example of vagueness, which can be commonly ascribed to nursing students, occurs during the use of the planning phase of the nursing process when students do not write concrete nursing interventions. For example, a student may state that the nursing action will "provide support to the client and his family." It is difficult to explain exactly what this statement means, either in general or in relation to this client and this nurse. Appropriate planning involves deciding on definite, well-stated nursing diagnoses, goals, and nursing actions. The use of the nursing process requires that the student learn the degree of specificity required for each nursing situation. State or itemize the nursing actions to be performed.

Accuracy vs. Inaccuracy

Accuracy means being correct and within the proper parameters. Nursing students can readily understand the need for accurate calculation of a drug dose or accurate measurement of blood pressure. In the same way, the collection and interpretation of data must be accurate. Accuracy usually implies the use of some measuring instrument. In the case of blood pressure, this is easy to see. In the case of accuracy in thinking, it may be harder to conceptualize. An example would be when the nurse uses the term *hypertension* to mean someone who is anxious and hyperactive instead of the actual meaning, an elevation of blood pressure above the accepted normal maximum. When dealing with more abstract concepts, accuracy of interpretation and understanding are equally important. Students can

improve the accuracy of their thinking by trying to write new information in their own words and having another student interpret the meaning. Inaccurate information will become evident.

Accurate recording of findings during client care is essential to quality care. Accurate understanding of the concepts underlying each part of your nursing courses, plus understanding of the ways whereby each part of your nursing course relates to any given client, will enable you to be more accurate in your thinking.

There are degrees of accuracy. For example, you might measure a client's temperature using a thermometer that can measure to the 0.01 degree, but this degree of accuracy may be unnecessary. On the other hand, when figuring a pediatric dosage, a difference of 0.01 can be important. One of your challenges is to increase your awareness of the degree of accuracy required in given nursing situations.

Relevance vs. Irrelevance

Relevance refers to needed information as opposed to information that is not needed at the moment. Students must be able to separate the two; otherwise, they may spend time arguing for a position that does not matter. For instance, students may get sidetracked from the purpose of an exercise by failing to limit their responses to the central issue or heart of the question or problem to be solved. It is also important to be able to recognize when sufficient relevant information is not available. An example of failing to recognize relevant information might be ignoring a client's comment that his rash began the day after starting a new medication. On the other hand, the nurse may assume that a client is depressed about being in the hospital and so may fail to ask him why he seems sad.

During the study process, you can ask yourself how a particular concept is relevant to the application of the nursing process to client care. **Justify** (prove or show to be valid) your ideas to yourself and to another student.

Consistency vs. Inconsistency

Consistency means using principles and concepts appropriately for related applications. For instance, if you are using a particular nursing diagnosis based on accepted indicators, it should be applied when those indicators are present and should not be used when the indicators are not present. Failure to follow this standard results in inconsistent use of the nursing diagnosis.

Consistency can also refer to recognizing and using basic concepts appropriately whenever they apply. For example, knowing the basic actions of epinephrine will enable you to predict client responses to the administration of the drug. It will also help you understand that the client has the same response when an increased secretion of epinephrine is released by the client's kidneys.

Logical vs. Illogical

To be logical means to build one idea upon another so that the conclusion is based on a sequence of steps. Each step should be reasonable and related to the step before it and the step after it. Many symptoms that clients exhibit can be understood logically based on your knowledge of normal physiology and the changes produced by the client's given disease or malady. The successful student will make more efficient use of study time by identifying the logical basis of the material being presented.

The author of a nursing textbook uses nursing logic to organize the content of the book. You must use your own logic to grasp the meaning of the material. Do this by discovering the logic of the author. In this way you will begin to think within the logic of nursing.

Depth vs. Superficiality

Busy students may be tempted to rely on the specific learning objectives and the teacher's pre-test review as indicators of the amount of material they must master. This, however, may result in only a superficial understanding of basic processes and principles. Students can improve their ability to recognize the depth to which they must explore concepts and ideas. There is no easy way to do this, but knowing that different material requires different depth of study can assist the student. With time, these decisions will be easier to make. Your instructor and the learning aids within your textbook are useful guides. The more you use them, the better you will become at identifying relevant information and the appropriate depth of knowledge required to make good clinical decisions.

Completeness vs. Incompleteness

During the assessment phase of client care it is important that the nurse know when the client database is sufficient. Proper nursing care is based on identification of priority needs. The nurse will provide care only for those problems that have been identified. Although the physician orders treatments related to the medical diagnosis, these orders are not meant to direct all required care. Nursing care is essential to client well-being. Incomplete information or analysis of client needs will result in inappropriate or inadequate nursing care. Of course, your ability to identify and prioritize client care problems depends on the completeness of your knowledge base. This standard is related to accuracy. An incomplete database leads to inaccurate conclusions.

Significance vs. Triviality

When making decisions or sorting out information it is important for the nurse to identify information that is necessary for good decision making. Being able to recognize irrelevant facts or data that are not helpful for the problem at hand is an important skill. It is easy for a student to view all the material in a textbook as equally significant. Learning to identify significant (important) concepts will minimize the chances of your being distracted by trivial materials.

Adequacy vs. Inadequacy

In solving problems or exploring a subject, adequacy refers to the degree to which the available information is sufficient for the purpose and the amount of time and effort spent on the matter. When making clinical decisions, the nurse must be able to recognize when there is sufficient information upon which to base a decision. Premature closure of the process or the inability to decide because of fear that there is not enough information are equally detrimental to quality thinking.

As you study each chapter you will be given information that will help you identify the basic information required to care for each client. Knowing that good client care decisions are based on good preparation by the nurse can help you fit information into the logic of nursing.

Fairness vs. Bias

You, along with other students, come to the educational setting with a set of beliefs, opinions, and points of view. People are predisposed to believe that what they think is true must be true. The improvement of the quality of your thinking depends on your ability to identify the biases present in your thinking and the biases present in the thinking of others. Commitment to fairness will lead a person to challenge conclusions in the light of the presence or absence of personal bias. A nursing example would be the assessment of a person in pain. Each individual has learned a way to respond to pain: Some become quiet, some complain loudly, some are stoic, and some are emotional. When a nurse who has a stoic response to pain assesses a person who has an emotional response to pain, it is possible that the nurse will allow personal values to influence the assessment. This can lead to stereotyping of a client as a "cry baby," with the result being that the nurse provides inadequate pain control for the client.

REASONING AND PROBLEM-SOLVING

Reasoning has been defined as the process of figuring things out by using critical thinking skills. Although reasoning involves thinking, all thinking is not reasoning. A human being is thinking when daydreaming, jumping to conclusions, stereotyping, or deciding to listen to music. None of these activities can be called reasoning. In order to use reasoning, to figure things out, or to problem-solve, the student must become

Table 2-4 THE ELEMENTS OF THOUGHT IN REASONING

1. All reasoning has a PURPOSE.
   - Take time to state your purpose clearly
   - Distinguish your purpose from related purposes
   - Check periodically to be sure you are still on target
   - Choose significant and realistic purposes
2. All reasoning is an attempt TO FIGURE SOMETHING OUT, TO SETTLE SOME QUESTION, TO SOLVE SOME PROBLEM.
   - Take time to clearly and simply state the question at issue
   - Express the question in several ways to clarify its meaning and scope
   - Break the question into subquestions
   - Identify whether it is a factual question, a preference question, or a question that requires reasoning
3. All reasoning is based on ASSUMPTIONS.
   - Clearly identify your assumptions and check for their probable validity
   - Check the consistency of your assumptions
   - Reexamine the question at issue when assumptions prove insupportable
4. All reasoning is done from some POINT OF VIEW.
   - Identify your own point of view and its limitations
   - Seek other points of view and identify their strengths as well as their weaknesses
   - Strive to be fairminded in evaluating all points of view
5. All reasoning is based on DATA AND INFORMATION.
   - Restrict your claims to those supported by sufficient data
   - Lay out the evidence clearly
   - Search for information against your position and explain its relevance
6. All reasoning is expressed through, and shaped by, CONCEPTS.
   - Identify each concept that is needed to explore the problem, and precisely define it
   - Explain the choice of important concepts and the implications of each
   - Define when concepts are used vaguely or inappropriately
7. All reasoning contains INFERENCES by which we draw CONCLUSIONS and give meaning to data.
   - Tie inferences tightly and directly from evidence to conclusions
   - Seek inferences that are deep, consistent, and logical
   - Identify the relative strength of each of your inferences
8. All reasoning leads somewhere and has IMPLICATIONS AND CONSEQUENCES.
   - Trace out a variety of implications and consequences that stem from your reasoning
   - Search for negative as well as positive consequences
   - Anticipate unusual or unexpected consequences from various points of view

Courtesy of The Foundation for Critical Thinking, Santa Rosa, CA.

familiar with the components of reasoning. These elements are purpose, the question at issue, assumptions, point of view, data and information, concepts, inferences and conclusions, and implications and consequences (Paul & Willsen, 1993). Table 2-4 illustrates the elements of thought in reasoning.

Purpose

All reasoning is directed toward some specific purpose. This is one way whereby reasoning is different from daydreaming. In the case of the nursing student, the purpose of reasoning is to effectively solve client care problems. During your formal education process, you will use reasoning to discover the logic of the practice of nursing.

The Question at Issue

The reasoning process has as its purpose the solution to some problem. This problem must be clearly defined. At the beginning of each study period, you must be able to state clearly the particular problems presented by this particular material. In the clinical setting, good clinical judgment begins with the clear statement of the problems presented by each client. One purpose of the nursing process is to identify client problems in a sufficiently clear and simple manner to enable appropriate responses by the nurse.

Assumptions

Assumptions are those ideas or things that are taken for granted. In the process of reasoning, you must be aware of the assumptions that are made in contrast to the facts that are known. Assumptions are accepted as being true without examination. Assuming certain things may be helpful in problem-solving, but an attempt should be made to recognize the assumptions. An example of an assumption is that nursing makes a difference in the outcome of a client's illness. It is evident that this is a necessary assumption for the nurse to make in order to engage in problem-solving related to client care needs; but it is also important for the nurse to examine this assumption from time to time. One of the issues in nursing today is the question of what nurses do and what preparation is necessary.

It is important to remember that assumptions that have proven reliable can help in decision making. It is just as true that faulty assumptions may cause you to draw faulty conclusions and may lead to poor problem-solving. Learn to recognize your own assumptions and those of others. Never be afraid to challenge your own assumptions or to ask others to clarify the assumptions they are using.

Point of View

Each person reasons using his own logic. Logic consists of previous experience, the quality of thinking already acquired, available information, and many other factors. These factors work together to give each person a unique way of thinking and a unique perspective. This unique perspective determines the individual's point of view. This can be conceptualized by thinking about what a person can see from a small window as compared to a view of the same landscape from an airplane. Each person will see things differently. They may both see a house but each person's view of the house may differ. In the same way, the individual's point of view determines what facts and information will be noticed, the relative importance assigned to each bit of information, and even the acceptable solutions to the problem. You must take the time to recognize your own point of view and to affirm the right of others to have their own points of view (Figure 2-4).

Data and Information

Data and information are the basic materials of reasoning. These are needed in order to define the problem under consideration and to find the solution. During the nursing education program, you may often feel overwhelmed by the quantity of data and information that is presented to you. The result may be that you attempt to practice rote memorization. If data and information are seen as the evidence for reasoning and for problem-solving, however, the process will be more than an exercise in memory. There is a logical relationship between the ideas and facts that compose the content of the nursing course. This logic can be discovered by reasoning. Once the logic is found, the

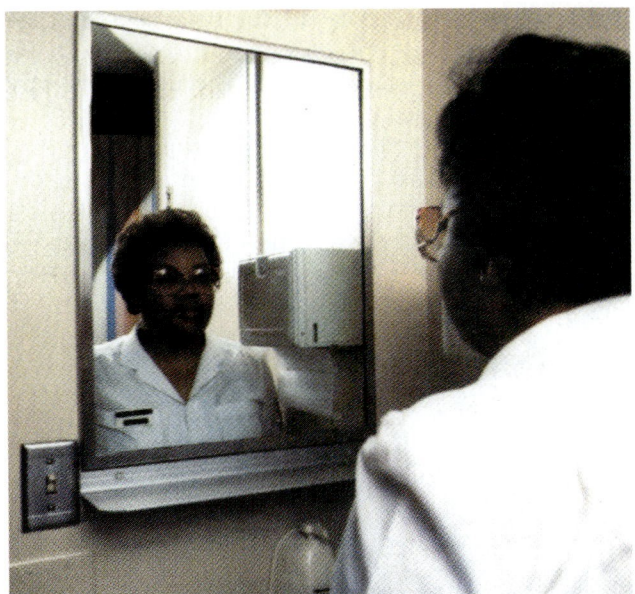

Figure 2-4 To be effective problem-solvers and critical thinkers, nurses must first take a good look at their own ideas and beliefs.

information can be used for problem-solving. Be sure to also look for evidence against your position.

Concepts

The evidence given in support of a conclusion consists of one or more statements relating the conclusion to the problem and to the supporting facts. Reasons must be logically related to the information; in other words, the conclusion cannot be based on something apart from the reasoning process. The concepts (such as pain, adaptation, and so on) that support the nursing process must be part of the evidence supporting a nursing judgment.

Inferences and Conclusions

Reasoning requires interpretation of facts and information. The interpretation must be justifiable in light of the relevant facts. It must be supported by logical connections to the problem and to appropriate data and information. Such interpretation can be called a judgment or inference. Too many times, students state opinions as judgments or inferences. This occurs when interpretations are based on personal preferences rather than on the information that is pertinent to the solution of the problem and on accepted authoritative information.

Properly drawing judgments or inferences is basic to thinking well. An inference results from the following kind of thinking: "Because that is true, then this must be true." For example, you have learned that when the body's temperature goes above normal, the body's metabolic rate increases. You also know that increased metabolism requires more oxygen for the tissues. One way more oxygen can be delivered to the tissues is to increase the heart rate. From these facts, you can infer that an elevated body temperature may result in an increased heart rate.

The product of reasoning is a conclusion in regard to the problem. The conclusion is the answer to the question that began the process. The conclusion must be logical and must answer the question. It must be based on the proper information and be logically related to the question.

Implications and Consequences

As an outcome of the reasoning process, more than one solution will usually be apparent. At this point, it will be necessary to examine the implications of each solution. This may require thinking about the ease with which a solution can be applied, the ability of a person to carry out the required actions, or the risks involved.

The outcomes of a particular approach to a problem under consideration are important. Consequences can result from action or inaction. Responsible problem-solving requires that all known consequences be acknowledged. Of course, it is not possible to predict all consequences; but the possible outcomes should be examined as completely as possible.

TRAITS OF A DISCIPLINED THINKER

The presentation in this chapter of some of the requirements of critical thinking will not make anyone think critically. By incorporating the idea that thinking about the quality of your own thinking in relation to

PROFESSIONAL TIP

Critical Thinking

Critical thinking is far more than an academic exercise. As a nurse, you are responsible for helping clients achieve and maintain their optimal level of health. To help sharpen your critical thinking skills, get in the habit of asking yourself several times throughout the day while caring for clients questions such as "Why is this procedure being done?", "What are its benefits?", and "Do I see alternatives that might result in better client outcomes?" Training yourself to think critically about all client care and interactions will help you to become a more skilled and compassionate professional.

UIS is a desirable goal, you can improve your own thinking. Improved thinking is not something that can be acquired in a day or two. It is like any high-level skill; it takes time, effort, and disciplined practice. The result is well worth it, however. Consistent efforts to improve your thinking can result in the acquisition of the traits of an educated person (Paul & Willsen, 1993). These traits or habitual characteristic ways of thinking can be recognized by others and can enable a person to compete successfully in the high-tech world.

Reason

The educated person will be reasonable. This simply means that the person values reasoning in himself and in others. This person will not be interested in placing blame or dodging responsibility. There will be a commitment to problem-solving and to cooperative efforts aimed at logically solving the problems encountered in the workplace.

Humility

Another quality that results from consistent efforts to practice disciplined thinking is intellectual humility. To be intellectually humble means that an individual is aware of how much he does not know. There will be a willingness to examine conclusions and beliefs based on new evidence. There will be respect for the thoughts and ideas of others and a sense of continually learning and improving one's own thinking.

Courage

The thinking person will be intellectually courageous. One of the characteristics of this trait is a willingness to take unpopular positions based on reasoning. Conclusions and beliefs that direct activities will thus be the result of disciplined thinking, rather than the opinions of the group.

Integrity

Integrity refers to the constancy of one's actions, meaning that based on reasoning, the same standards are applied consistently and are not changed to suit circumstances or personal prejudices. The result is a person whose behavior is in harmony with his thinking.

Perseverance

Finally, the thinking person will be capable of intellectual perseverance; meaning a willingness to undertake the challenge of completing hard intellectual tasks. Not giving up, pursuing a solution until its conclusion, and maintaining the quality of thinking are the qualities related to this trait.

CASE STUDY

At this point in subsequent chapters, you will be given a client scenario or case study. This activity is designed to give you an opportunity to apply the knowledge and skills you have gained. This means that you will be expected to use critical thinking skills as you explore selected nursing situations. For this chapter, the scenario is to be written by you and about you.

1. Review the four basic skills of critical thinking: reading, writing, listening, and speaking.

2. Identify specifically the precise skills you want to improve. Write in your own words what you want to accomplish in terms of positive skills you will possess when you have implemented your plan and accomplished your goal. This means that you will identify both specific performance measures for your reading, writing, speaking, and listening skills, and time frames for points at which you will evaluate your performance. For example, if you set a goal of being able to identify the main points of an assigned reading, how would you measure that? In comparison with others in your study group? By your test performance? Write down your evaluation criteria and the time frames for evaluation.

3. When you have clearly stated in writing which basic skills you will work on, review the material in this chapter or from other resources to identify possible ways to work on those skills. Choose the most appropriate methods for you. Write down your plan. Be precise and specific.

4. Your next step is to actually put your plan into action by doing what you have planned to do.

5. Evaluate your actions to see whether they have resulted in the desired outcome. In order to perform a valid evaluation, you must evaluate your performance based on the evaluation criteria and goals you outlined in number 2.

6. Realize that you must know yourself well. If the processes of critical thinking and reasoning are new to you, select only one or two things on which to work. If you feel more adventurous, use the suggested process to explore your thinking in relation to the universal standards of thought and to the traits of a thoughtful person. Assess your problem-solving style in relation to the elements of thought in reasoning.

SUMMARY

- Critical thinking is a disciplined way of thinking that the nursing student can begin to develop. The effective use of the nursing process depends on the ability to think well.

- There are many ways to define critical thinking. Essential components of any definition should emphasize self-assessment of the quality of one's own thinking according to standards of excellence and careful use of the elements of reasoning.

- Four basic intellectual skills are essential to quality thinking: critical reading, critical listening, critical writing, and critical speaking.

- The spectrum of Universal Intellectual Standards (UIS) can be the measure of competence in each of the basic skills.

- Reasoning is the process of applying critical thinking to some problem so as to find an answer or to figure something out. Therefore, reasoning has a purpose. The process of reasoning requires that attention be paid to the elements of thought in reasoning and to the UIS.

- When students begin to be aware of their own thinking and begin to assume responsibility for it, they will begin to use their own logic to discover the logic of nursing. The result will be better learning and the ability to make high-quality decisions related to client care.

- Consistent attention to improving the quality of thinking will produce the traits of an educated nurse. The student will become intellectually reasonable, humble, and courageous and will possess intellectual integrity and perseverance.

Review Questions

1. A branch of learning or field of study is called a:
   a. career.
   b. movement.
   c. principle.
   d. discipline.

2. Fundamental to quality thinking is the ability to think:
   a. clearly.
   b. effectively.
   c. quantitatively.
   d. with ambiguity.

3. The person who is concrete or exact when stating or applying a fact is practicing the standard for critical thinking called:
   a. accuracy.
   b. precision.
   c. consistency.
   d. specificity.

4. The person who has the ability to separate needed information from information not needed at the present time is practicing the standard for critical thinking called:
   a. logic.
   b. relevance.
   c. adequacy.
   d. significance.

5. Ideas or things that are taken for granted are called:
   a. evidences.
   b. inferences.
   c. assumptions.
   d. implications.

6. The person who is willing to take an unpopular position based on reasoning is said to have:
   a. courage.
   b. humility.
   c. integrity.
   d. perseverance.

WEB FLASH!

- Search the Web for sites dealing with critical thinking. What date is the oldest entry? What date is the newest entry?
- Search the web using the names of the major nursing organizations such as National Federation of Licensed Practical Nurses (NFLPN), National Association of Practical Nurse Education and Service, Inc. (NAPNES), and the National League for Nursing (NLN). Do they have web sites that include pages that might offer information on critical thinking?

Critical Thinking Questions

1. Of the four basic skills of critical thinking, which one are you able to do best? Why? How do you know?

2. How do you take responsibility for your own thinking?

STUDENT NURSE SKILLS FOR SUCCESS

MAKING THE CONNECTION

Refer to the following chapters to increase your understanding of student nurse skills for success:

- **Chapter 2: Critical Thinking**
- **Chapter 11: Client Teaching**
- **Chapter 16: Stress, Adaptation, and Anxiety**

LEARNING OBJECTIVES:

Upon completion of this chapter, you should be able to:
- *Define key terms.*
- *Outline strategies for developing a positive attitude toward the learner role.*
- *Identify strategies for developing proficiency in basic skills.*
- *Identify learning-style methods that can be incorporated for effective study.*
- *Design a time-management plan.*
- *Design a personal study plan.*
- *Identify strategies for improving test-taking outcomes.*
- *Complete a stress-reduction exercise using guided imagery.*

KEY TERMS

ability	learning style
anxiety	metacognition
attitude	mnemonic
attribute	perfectionism
encoding	procrastination
learning	time management
learning disability	

INTRODUCTION

Learning is defined as the act or process of acquiring knowledge and/or skill in a particular subject. An individual never stops learning. This is especially true in the field of nursing and health care. The amount of information within the health care domain has expanded exponentially in just the past several years. Consider, for example, the advances in drug therapies, alternative therapies, and genetics. By the time you graduate, some of the information you learned in the beginning of your program will have been displaced by new information and discoveries. We are living in the information age and have constant access to thousands of pieces of information through various media, including television and the Internet. Knowledge is never static. Learning is defined as the act of acquiring knowledge, thus, learning is also not static, but, rather, is a lifelong process.

Individuals seek knowledge to effect some type of change. As a student, you are seeking knowledge to learn skills and to prepare yourself for a career in nursing. Referring to yourself as a learner implies that you are an active participant in the learning process, as opposed to a passive recipient of information. You bring to this new adventure yourself, your past experiences, your abilities, and your motivation to master the knowledge necessary to reach your goals. You have already learned much in your lifetime and are ready to continue the process. It is important that you take some time to think about the competencies needed for the role of learner. It is equally important that you realize that *you* are in charge of developing those competencies that will enable you to learn.

The learning you are seeking will afford you the knowledge and skills necessary to become a nurse and, thus, to demonstrate your ability to competently provide care to clients who seek your professional talents. Nursing education is different from many other college majors in the turnaround time allowed for learning. Few other disciplines require the student to apply on Thursday that which was acquired on Monday. Nursing

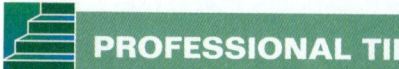

students must acquire a greater depth of understanding in a short amount of time; to achieve this, basic learning processes will need to be well developed.

This chapter addresses *how* you learn rather than *what* you learn. It focuses on competencies necessary to master the learning process: attitude, basic skills, learning style, time management, study strategies, critical thinking, and test-taking strategies. Assessing which habits you already practice and which ones you have yet to incorporate, internalize, and utilize will assist you in improving your process of learning. As you do so, your potential for attaining your goals will increase.

DEVELOP A POSITIVE ATTITUDE

Attitude is defined as a manner, feeling, or position toward a person or thing. In order to effect change in your behavior, you must first develop a positive attitude about this experience you are about to begin. You are in charge of setting yourself up for success. This is your opportunity to acquire the knowledge and skills that will make it possible for you to reach the goal of becoming a licensed practical/vocational nurse. You must develop a positive attitude toward yourself as a person and a learner, as well as a genuine desire to learn. To maintain this attitude late at night when you are struggling over the names of the latest drugs and writing client assessments, you must be convinced that you have the capability of completing your task, that some intrinsic factor will be able to support you in your pursuit of your goal. This positive self-attitude sustains the question "Why am I doing this?" Among the strategies you can practice to help you build a positive attitude are the following:

• Create positive self-images, and visualize yourself attaining your goals
• Recognize your abilities
• Identify realistic expectations

Create Positive Self-Images

To begin to create a positive self-image, you must know those attributes that are unique to you. An **attribute** is a characteristic, either positive or negative, that belongs to you. For instance, some positive attributes that are typical to nurses including caring and compassion. Attributes are sometimes also referred to

My attribute chart	
Positive Attributes	Negative Attributes

Figure 3-1 Attribute Chart

as strengths and weaknesses. Whatever you call them, you must actively engage in listing and recalling these qualities about yourself. Using a chart like the one presented in Figure 3-1, list as many words describing your attributes as you can. List both positive and negative qualities.

Which side has more entries? Did you start with the negative list? It is unfortunate that sometimes we can recall the negatives faster than the positives. We often speak about ourselves in negative terms, which creates negative self-images. For example, you may recall thinking some of the following: "I wish I were thinner . . . ," "I hope I can do this, I'm not very good at math." Neither of these statements draws a positive image of the speaker. You may need to lose 10 pounds, or improve your math skills, but these are not the total measure of your attributes. If they are the only qualities you recall, they might become the overall image you see of yourself. Regardless of where you started, you must concentrate on the positive side of the chart. You must actively recall your positive side at least as often as you recount the things that could be improved.

Begin to speak of yourself in positive terms and accept compliments from yourself! You will be building the sustenance to get through the rough parts of the new role you have taken on. When an assignment is particularly difficult you can refocus from "I hope I can do this. I have never been good at math" to "I can read and follow the chapter instructions on how to complete the problems." This simple restatement can sometimes make the difference in whether we succeed or fail at our attempts to acquire new knowledge.

The list does not have to stop at just the words you write today. Continue to practice and do periodic self-assessments. You will add more and more words to the positive side and begin to complement yourself more often. When things go awry you will be able to draw on these positive attributes and know that you have these strengths.

Recognize Your Abilities

Recognizing your abilities is also an attitude builder. **Ability** can be defined as competence in an activity. An ability is something you can learn; competency is proficiency in a task. Your degree of competence as a nurse will depend on such factors as prior exposure, motivation, how often and with whom you practice, expectations of those things that you should be doing, and a willingness to laugh at attempts and learn from mistakes.

You have abilities and skills that you perform well. To acquire these things took courage, discipline, and hard work. Recalling these abilities and the ways you developed competency in them not only adds to your positive self-image, but showcases your strengths. Begin to practice recalling your abilities by completing the exercise described in Figure 3-2. Under each of the columns (A and B), write an ending to each statement and place it in the big box. Next, list all of the skills you need to be able to be "really good" at that task. Write these skills in the smaller boxes. Do not worry if you cannot fill all the small boxes or if you run out of boxes.

As an example for column A, maybe you wrote, "I am really good at cooking." Following are some skills you could have included in the smaller boxes:

- *Arithmetic:* You must have an understanding of fractions and the relationships of parts to the whole.
- *Reading:* You must comprehend the words in the recipe in order to follow all the steps.
- *Prioritizing:* You must know with what to start in order to have all of the food ready at the same time.

- *Risk taker:* You may worry about whether your guests will like your dish, but you persist, confident in your ability to turn the raw ingredients into a delicious meal.

Now look at column B, using math as an example. Mathematics is an ability you must develop in order to safely administer medications to your clients. If you view this skill only as something to avoid, you start out with a negative attitude toward an ability you will need. You are creating a negative image of yourself completing this task. Instead, look to your past experiences for your strengths; you may realize that you already possess much of the mathematical knowledge you need to correctly compute medication dosages. Realizing this puts a positive slant on this ability.

Now you must develop mathematical competency. Begin by asking yourself which skills are needed to perform mathematical operations. You must pay attention to details, understand the way parts relate to the whole, and have solid skills in arithmetic (addition, subtraction, division, and multiplication). Mathematics requires you to choose appropriate formulas to solve a variety of real-world problems. For example, to give the correct dose of medication to your client, you must know the correct formula to use for the calculation. This is a real-world problem for which you must both choose the correct formula and understand it. You must then accurately perform the arithmetic operations.

Identify Realistic Expectations

As mentioned earlier, developing a positive self-image is of primary importance to learning. Your expectations regarding how you will perform in the role as a learner will affect your attitude toward both yourself and learning. You have an expectation about the way you will progress through this program. Ideally, you

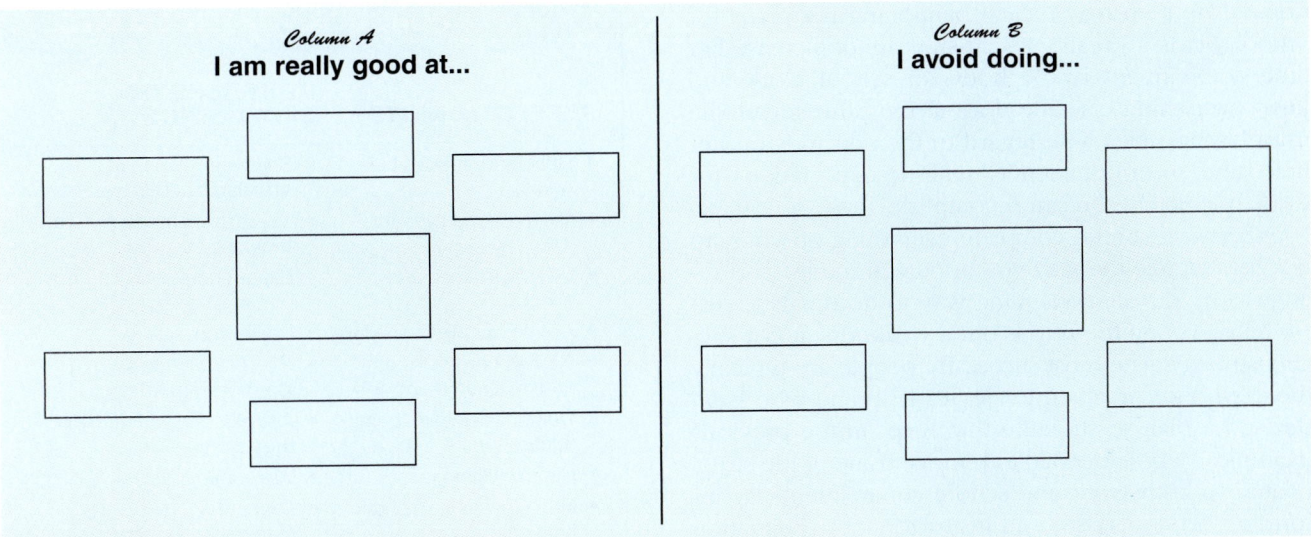

Figure 3-2 Recognizing Your Abilities

will attend all classes, pass all exams, and graduate. Further, your current life responsibilities will cooperate with and support this plan. You will likely, however, encounter at least some obstacles. When you hit that first "speed bump" to your plan, your ability to look at the reality of your expectations will be important in regaining a positive focus. Consider the following example:

Marissa is a 25-year-old enrolled full time in a nursing program for the fall. She did well in high school and has already attended a college part time prior to this program. Marissa expects that she will get grades in the B and A range, as she did in prior course work. She works full time and has a 4-year-old daughter. When the class schedule is published, the times conflict with one of the days that she works. This will cause her to be 20 minutes late to work on that day. She has not shared with her employer that she is attending school. She has child care for her daughter, but the need to arrive at the clinical site at 7 A.M. means that she must rearrange her child care and that she will be 30 minutes late for clinical on Fridays. She does not tell her instructors of her time constraints for child care. She has always needed quiet time for study and is a morning person. Marissa finds her reading assignments take twice as long as she had planned. With all her other responsibilities, her only time for study is after her daughter goes to bed. She has a family that lives close by, but she does not like to burden them with baby-sitting. She has always found a way to do things on her own in the past.

Marissa is a capable person, but her expectation of being able to control all the various facets of her life in perfect harmony is unrealistic. Maintaining a positive attitude while in the midst of the stress of completing all the tasks at hand is difficult if not impossible, and the plan is often abandoned. In Marissa's case, abandoning the plan may mean abandoning her plans for school. Marissa's reality is that she cannot increase her time commitment by 30 hours of school work and keep everything else she does at the same level. She must set priorities with regard to the demands on her time, and she must identify realistic expectations for those things that she can accomplish.

When you cannot complete everything on your "to do" list, change the way you approach the list and realign your expectations. One way to do this is to ask for help. Asking for help is not a weakness, it is a success strategy. The most successful people are typically those who know when to ask for help and who have devised a plan to structure that help. In the previous example, Marissa needed to remove some of the stress related to both work and school commitments by informing her supervisor and instructors of her situation and asking for their help in guiding her to manage her

many demands. Help may mean something as simple as talking to your instructors so that they know you must leave on Thursdays at 3 P.M., due to work commitments. Present a proactive plan of how you will get the notes and make up the time and then ask them to accommodate you.

If you do not set realistic expectations for yourself, you may fall victim to a positive attitude's biggest enemy, perfectionism. **Perfectionism** is not synonymous with excellence, but rather is an overwhelming expectation of being able to get everything done. This is setting yourself up for failure, as it is a standard no one can live up to. Table 3-1 suggests some behaviors of perfectionists versus those of pursuers of excellence. Which list describes you most accurately? Remember to strive to be as realistic with your expectations as possible; be patient with yourself and ask for help when needed.

DEVELOP YOUR BASIC SKILLS

Dirkx and Prenger (1997) list the following skills as basic for success in academics and life: reading, arithmetic and mathematics, writing, listening, and speaking. They further describe each of the skills in terms of characteristics that provide a sense of what is expected from the learner in each area (Table 3-2).

When you consider these characteristics, the basic skills do not seem so basic but, rather, take on a new importance. Look at the list and make a quick note of your strengths and weaknesses. You must have a strong foundation in these basic skills to advance your knowledge beyond the level of memorization. You

Table 3-1 BEHAVIORS OF PERFECTIONISTS AND PURSUERS OF EXCELLENCE	
PERFECTIONISTS	**PURSUERS OF EXCELLENCE**
• Reach for impossible goals	• Enjoy meeting high standards within reach
• Value themselves for what they do	• Value themselves for who they are
• Get depressed and give up	• Experience disappointment but keep going
• Are devastated by failure	• Learn from failure
• Remember mistakes and dwell on them	• Correct mistakes, then learn from them
• Can only live with being number one	• Are pleased with knowing they did their best
• Hate criticism	• Welcome criticism
• Have to win to maintain high self-esteem	• Do not have to win to maintain high self-esteem

Table 3-2 BASIC SKILL COMPETENCY LIST

SKILL	BASIC COMPETENCY
Reading	Locate, understand, and interpret written information in prose and documents, including manuals, graphs, and schedules, to perform tasks; learn from a text by determining the main idea or essential message; identify relevant details, facts, and specifications; infer or locate the meaning of unknown or technical vocabulary; judge the accuracy, appropriateness, style, and plausibility of reports, proposals, or theories from other writers
Arithmetic and mathematics	Perform basic computations; use basic numerical concepts such as whole numbers and percentages (fractions, decimals) in practical situations; approach practical problems by choosing appropriately from a variety of mathematical techniques
Writing	Communicate thoughts, ideas, information, and messages; record information completely and accurately; compose and create documents and use language, style, organization, and format appropriate to the subject matter, purpose, and audience; include supporting documentation; attend to detail and check, edit, and revise for correct information, appropriate emphasis, form, grammar, spelling, and punctuation
Listening	Receive, attend to, interpret, and respond to verbal messages and other cues, such as body language, in ways that are appropriate to the purpose in order to comprehend, learn, evaluate critically, appreciate, or support the speaker
Speaking	Organize ideas and communicate oral messages appropriate to listeners and situations; use verbal language and other cues such as body language appropriate in style, tone, and level of complexity to the audience and occasion; speak clearly and communicate a message; understand and respond to listener feedback and ask questions when needed

Adapted from Planning and implementing instruction for adults *(pp. 133–134), by J. Dirkx and S. Prenger, 1997, San Francisco: Jossey-Bass. Copyright 1997 by Jossey-Bass.*

reading encompasses vocabulary building, which includes the skill of identification and understanding of both English and medical terminology. Investing in quality medical and English dictionaries is a good step to understanding both these languages. Another strategy is simply to take the time when reading to look up the words you do not know (Figure 3-3).

The primary reason for building a strong medical vocabulary is that words are the tools for thinking about and understanding your world, and you are entering the new world of nursing: You must therefore take the time to learn its language. Developing the habit of vocabulary building takes time initially, but as you persist in practicing this skill, your comprehension of the material will increase.

Comprehension goes beyond rote memorization. One sign of true comprehension is the ability to summarize the writer's message. When you summarize, you must recite the material in your own words (Phillips & Sotiriou, 1996). Unless you understand the words you have read, you will not be able to advance your level of knowledge from rote memorization to comprehension. When you are actively reading your nursing textbook and you realize that you are not understanding what you are reading, you may find it helpful to use one, some, or all of the five strategies outlined in Table 3-3.

Reading level is another element of your reading skills. Reading level is not related to what you can understand, but, rather, refers to the length of the words and the sentences used in a text to explain, describe, and convey information. It does not have anything to do with your intelligence, but it has a great deal to do with the length of time it takes you to read.

Arithmetic and Mathematics

The next skill you must develop competency in is that of arithemtic and mathematics. You will be responsible for correctly calculating dosages and safely

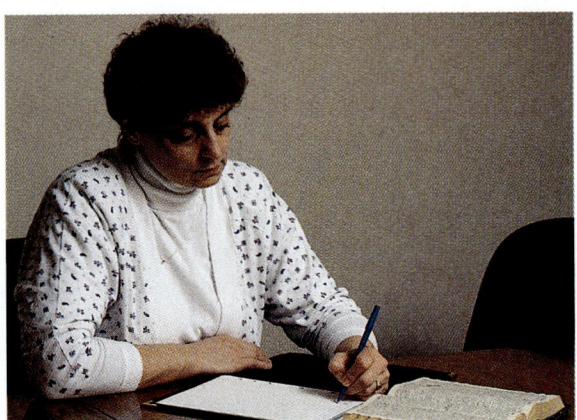

Figure 3-3 Keep a notebook of new terms to expand your vocabulary. Review your notebook and try to use the words in practice daily.

must advance your knowledge level from memorization to comprehension and application. If you are struggling with these basic skills, you will have difficulty advancing. Developing these skills is basic to the habits of successful learners.

Reading

Ninety percent of your program is in written format. To study effectively, you must be highly adept in the basic skill of reading. Among the several strategies you can effectively implement in your reading and study plan to improve this skill are vocabulary building, comprehension, and reading level. Your basic skill of

Table 3-3 STRATEGIES TO IMPROVE COMPREHENSION

STRATEGY	EXPLANATION
Reread	Do this after reading one section of the text, or even after one paragraph.
Define new words	Write the definitions of each new word in the margin of your text and then reread the paragraph. Use a small notebook to build your own glossary. Make your own flashcards for further study.
Visualize	Create mental pictures of the material you are reading. You may even want to draw a simple stick figure, and as you continue to read, adjust the picture.
Research	Many times the reason you are unable to comprehend the material presented is that you have insufficient background in the subject. A solution may be to consult another text that is specific to that knowledge base. Use a dictionary, anatomy and physiology text, general subject text (like a psychology text) or a nursing journal to increase your background knowledge in a subject area (Meltzer & Marcus-Palau, 1993)
Summarize	Use your own words to "tell" yourself what you just read and how this connects to what you are going to be doing. Ask yourself, "Why might I need to know this material?"

administering medications to your clients. You must therefore be able to recognize whether your calculations are correct and, upon looking at the amount on a medication order, estimate whether your answer is logical and correct. In nursing, your mastery of mathematical basic skills cannot be overemphasized. Consider the following excerpt from a study of medication errors done in 1998 at a tertiary care teaching hospital; this excerpt underscores the importance of mathematical competency among nurses.

> Forty-two percent of dosage errors were considered to put the patient at risk for a serious or severe preventable adverse outcome. Errors in decimal point placement, mathematical calculation, or expression of dosage regime accounted for 59.5% of the dosage errors. The dosage equation was wrong in 29.5% (Lesar, 1998).

Give yourself a reality check on your competency in mathematics and commit to improving those areas where you are weakest. You may want to investigate a resource such as the learning services center at your school, enlist the assistance of a tutor, or use a programmed-learning text to refresh your skills. There are also numerous texts written to assist nursing students in developing these essential skills. Consider also using computer-assisted instruction (CAI) programs or self-paced study modules to hone these skills. Whatever means you use, an honest assessment of your compe-

tency in mathematics and a commitment to improvement is essential to your practice in the profession.

Writing

In your role as a student and as a professional, you will need writing skills. Contrary to popular opinion, the influx of the computer into health care has not removed the need for this skill (Figure 3-4). You will be writing client assessments, transfer summaries, discharge summaries, and client-teaching plans, as well as contributing to development of policies and, possibly, even publishing your experiences in a journal. The skill of writing can be practiced and improved. Follow the steps outlined in Table 3-4 as a checklist for your writing assignments.

Listening

The old saying " I know you can hear me, but are you listening?" can be applied to all of us. You must be listening, understanding, and processing information, as opposed to just hearing, when you are in class, as well as when you begin working with clients. When listening during any lecture or demonstration, you receive, interpret, and respond to verbal messages and other cues such as body language. You are attempting to both comprehend the information and evaluate the

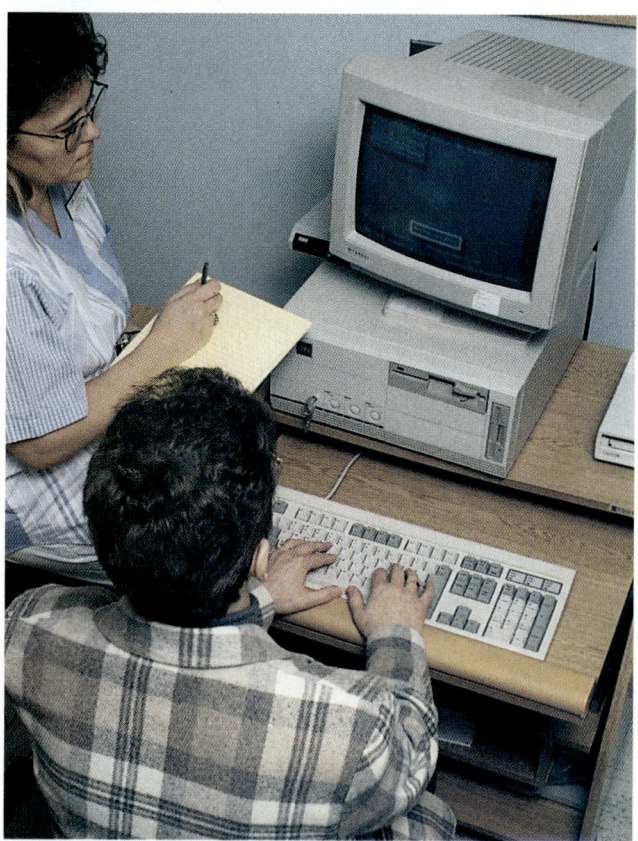

Figure 3-4 Although computers are being used more and more in health care, this does not replace the need for competent writing skills.

Table 3-4 STEPS TO CLEAR WRITING

STEP	EXPLANATION
Prewrite	Select a subject, collect details about that subject, and develop your writing plan
Establish a writing plan	Answer the following questions in outline form: • *What* are you writing (essay, test, questionnaire, dialogue)? • *Why* are you writing (to persuade, describe, explain, and narrate)? • *For whom* are you writing (peers, instructors, colleagues)? • *How* are you writing (alone, with a classmate, in a group, on computer)? • *Where* are you writing (on the bus, in the library, at the computer lab)? • *When* will you be writing (consider the time frame for this writing project)?
Write first draft	Organize your writing plan ideas into phrases, sentences, and paragraphs as appropriate to the task, content, and audience. Obtain feedback from your intended audience as to the accuracy, relevance, and understandability of your materials
Revise	Make changes to improve your writing so it conveys your main idea and purpose
Edit	Examine critically for errors in spelling, punctuation, grammar, or style

Adapted from Learning Strategies for Allied Health Students, *by M. Meltzer and S. Palau, 1996b, Philadelphia: W. B. Saunders. Copyright 1996 by W. B. Saunders.*

speaker. You may need to polish up on ways that you can improve listening and evaluation skills to make the most of your class time. Class time is a time for learning. Listening effectively can make efficient use of this time to increase your comprehension of the content.

Among the many strategies that can be used to improve listening skills are the following:

• *Being interested in the subject.* Make a connection with the reason you are going to this lecture. What is the connection between the information and your need for the information? Have you prescanned the information and come with questions about the subject that tie in to how you will use the information presented?

• *Being open to the information.* When you hear a topic and immediately react with your instinct, you often miss the point and some aspect of the presentation you did not consider before. Listening does not automatically mean you will change your mind on topics, but it will allow you to evaluate and incorporate those aspects that are beneficial to you.

• *Not being critical of the speaker.* Focus on the message, not the messenger. The speaker is not there as a member of a theatrical company to entertain you. The speaker's role is to impart information. It is up

to you to concentrate on the information that you need to know and apply it properly.

• *Concentrating on the information.* Be present to the lecture. If you find yourself falling asleep, do muscle flexes or breathe deeply to try to stay alert and aware. Imagine test questions that might be asked on the information.

• *Evaluating the information.* Not every word is critical. Relate the information to what you know, where you may use it, and whether you agree with what is said. If you have difficulty with what is being said, use the next strategy to maintain your concentration.

• *Writing down questions as you listen.* This allows you to follow the speaker to the end of her thoughts. Many of your questions may be answered. If not, you have them written down and can refer later to the list. This promotes concentration on the information presented. You will not be distracted trying to remember questions you wanted to ask.

Speaking

Learning to speak or present in front of a group is one of the most-feared activities of many students. Yet as a nurse, you have entered one of the most "speaking"-oriented professions. You will communicate daily with your clients, their families, instructors, peers, ancillary staff members, and the multiple members of the health care team. Learning to do this well will free you from worry about doing it and allow you to use this skill to your advantage in your classes as well as in the professional environment.

Most of the fear of speaking in public arises from our fear of appearing the fool. Many students will not ask questions during a lecture specifically because they believe themselves incapable of speaking clearly and identifying exactly the information they need. We have all heard the saying, "There is no stupid question"; we must believe it. You must develop the confidence to speak up when you have a question; consider the potential consequences to your clients should you fail to clarify a medical order or question a procedure that is unclear.

The following strategies may help when you want to ask a question:

• *Understand why you are asking the question.* Instead of saying, "I don't understand," say, "I was with you on the physiology of the kidney until you traveled into the Bowman's capsule. Can you connect this particular part of the kidney with osmosis for me?" This puts you and the speaker in a positive light; you have not attacked the speaker's explanation, and you acknowledge your skill in listening. You are communicating what you need and asking the speaker to help by connecting the two concepts for you.

• *Know when to ask the question.* Writing down those topics on which you need further information may

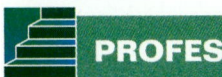

help you decide the correct time to ask a question. If the instructor begins by saying, "Today we will be speaking about pharmacokinetics," and you do not understand the word, stopping her before she has a chance to define the word may not be the most effective strategy. If instead you write down, "What does pharmacokinetics mean?" and listen for the meaning of that word in the context of the lecture, you will most likely hear clues as to the word's meaning. The instructor will use other words, such as *absorption, distribution, metabolism,* and *excretion* to describe what happens to a drug as it goes through the body. When an appropriate time in the presentation comes, review those things that have been said and clarify: "So, Prof. Z., am I correct when I say that pharmacokinetics has to do with the movement of drugs through all the systems of the body?" You will get your answer because your instructor will know from your question that you have been listening.

You must speak clearly and articulate those things you need daily as you attend classes; listen to your instructors; listen to your clients; and transmit information to instructors, colleagues, support staff, doctors, and allied health care team members. Practice both the skills of listening and speaking equally and keep asking questions.

DEVELOP YOUR LEARNING STYLE

The term **learning style** refers to the ways you best receive, process, and assimilate information (knowledge) about a particular subject. In your life as a stu-

dent, you have probably had both of the following experiences.

You attend class with Professor A for Course 100. The professor arranges the room casually in small groupings and breaks up class time to alternate short lectures with small group work. There is time for a hands-on demonstration of the principle along with actual work-related items used as examples. Professor A allows for student–teacher interchange of ideas and gives credence to experiences of the students during the class discussions. You leave the class exhilarated and with ideas, aware that this content connects with your desired outcome. You plan a review of the notes with a fellow student you met in your class group. You continue to prepare throughout the course and prior to the final, on which you get a B.

The next day you attend Course 200 with Professor B. The room is arranged in rows. Professor B puts up the class outline on the overhead, lectures for 40 minutes, then allows 10 minutes at the end for questions. If you hand him a written question, he will answer it during the next class. You dread his boring presentation and wish that Professor B was more like Professor A. You really do not know anyone in the class with whom to study, you cannot understand the text, and your grades are in the low C to D range. You know you need this class for your major. You try to do your part, but you just can't "get into it."

Think about Professor A, who presents information in a variety of methods—short lecture, small group, hands-on demonstration. As a student, you can grasp the information from whichever method appeals to you. You come away feeling connected to the subject and your classmates and want to continue learning about the subject. You are rewarded for your efforts through the academic grade system.

Now consider Professor B, who knows just as much about the subject as does Professor A, but who presents it using only one method—lecture. Lecture is not your preferred learning style, and your ability to clarify your understanding through questions is limited by the class format. Your outcomes on tests are less rewarding, and you begin to avoid putting time into studying the subject all together. You end up thinking that you really do not do well in that subject and consider changing your major.

The difference in the outcomes of the two examples lies in the perceived role of the learner. In these examples, the student relied heavily on the *teacher's* ability to present material in the student's preferred learning style. Remember that *you* are in charge of your learning. Teacher presentations vary in ways that may not appeal to your primary learning style, but you can still learn the information. You must take charge of

PROFESSIONAL TIP

Learning Disabilities

According to the National Center for Learning Disabilities, Inc. (NCLD 1999), 15% to 20% of the population have some form of learning disability. **Learning disability** is a generic term that refers to a heterogeneous group of disorders manifested as significant difficulties in the acquisition and use of listening, speaking, reading, writing, reasoning, or mathematical abilities.

If you think that having a learning disability will prohibit your success, you are incorrect; you must, however, understand your different abilities. You must know those types of accommodations that will enhance your learning capabilities, and you must be comfortable asking for those things that you need. Accommodations in postsecondary programs are mandated by the federal government, however the onus to disclose, provide documentation, and request accommodations is on the student. Accommodations are determined on a case-by-case basis. Reasonable accommodations in the classroom may be as simple as having the instructor wear a microphone, being able to use a tape recorder or note taker, or requesting textbook tapes. In the clinical area, all reasonable accommodations are made within the confines of client safety and essential skills needed to participate in a program of study for nursing. A quiet work area and ear protectors may provide quiet for students who are hypersensitive to background noise. Using a computer for writing assignments, note taking in class, and studying may assist students who have difficulty handwriting reliably. Getting a tutor skilled at working with students with learning disabilities may be another intervention to consider.

Whatever you suspect your needs to be, getting professional testing to ascertain both whether you in fact have a disability and those specific accommodations you will need is crucial. Seek the assistance of your instructors, student service personnel, learning center personnel, or call the special education coordinator at the nearest high school. These resources will help you locate an accredited testing agency to provide you with further resources and documentation.

Classification of Learning Styles

Learning styles are cognitive (mental) functions. They refer to the ways whereby you perceive, remember, think, and solve problems: Their focus is *how* you learn as opposed to *what* you learn. Your preference for one style over another can be argued to be both genetic and developmental. Regardless, your awareness of the ways you best learn will affect your learning outcomes.

Learning styles are classified in many different ways. One classification method focuses on the route by which students best perceive and remember information: visual, auditory, or kinesthetic. These divisions are not mutually exclusive; we possess all three, and we use all of them to garner our information. Visual learners make up approximately 65% of the population, auditory learners approximately 30%, and kinesthetic learners approximately 5% (Mind Tools, 1998). To do a quick self-assessment, read the descriptions of the different styles in Figure 3-5 and note the one(s) that come closest to describing the way you prefer to receive information.

You may have selected two or three styles from Figure 3-5, because we sometimes use one style over another in certain learning situations. If all of the noted styles were "close," you may want to rank them to gain

☐ **Visual** learners think in pictures. It does not matter whether they are hearing the information, reading the information, or feeling the information. They take in the information through the senses and store it as visual images. When visual learners want to recall information, they "play the movie" in their brain. Visual learners also relate best to information they have seen written down in texts, in their own notes, in diagrams, and in pictures. A statement such as "I see," or "I get the picture" reflects the style of the visual learner.

☐ **Auditory** learners learn best by hearing and listening. They do not make mental pictures but filter information through listening and repeating skills. They relate best to the spoken word. They may not take notes in class, but rather may ask to tape the lecture. These learners prefer classroom discussion and oral presentations over writing assignments. Speech patterns represent exactly how the auditory learner thinks, "I hear you," "That clicks," "That sounds right," "That rings a bell".

☐ **Kinesthetic** learners learn by touch, movement, imitation, and practice. These learners will process and remember information well if they can touch or feel that which they are learning about. These students are easily distracted during lectures, do not think in pictures, and can appear slow in understanding didactic material as it is being presented. They may have to go away and process (manipulate) material by rewriting the notes in a condensed format. These learners like to speak about learning in terms of their feelings, saying things like, "I feel" or "I'd like to get a better handle on this information."

Figure 3-5 Division of Learning Styles *(Adapted from Center for New Discoveries in Learning Personal Learning Style Inventory, 1998)*

developing your abilities, increasing your awareness of your preferred learning styles, and implementing some simple strategies to enhance those styles. As you increase your skills in your preferred methods and strengthen those in your weaker ones, you will change your outcomes.

a better understanding of your overall learning style. All of us have the capacity to learn in all three modes. You naturally gravitate to one over the others based on which style has lead to your greatest learning successes.

Another way to classify learning styles is according to brain-hemisphere dominance. The left hemisphere of the brain is associated with analytical activities, such as logic, structure, speech, reasoning, numbers, verbal expression, verification of data, and analysis of parts of the whole. The right side is associated with creativity and synthesizing parts to form a whole idea. The right side is also considered the more emotional side and links to insight, intuition, daydreams, visualization, music, rhythm, and color visualization.

We need both sides of the brain to function and learn. Numerous studies demonstrated that individuals with left-brain dominance are primarily auditory learners and those with right brain dominance are primarily visual. Additional studies show that right-brain–dominant learners process, recall, and retain more from information presented in computer-assisted instructional programs, whereas left-brain–dominant learners derive more success from a lecture format. To overlook or use one style to the exclusion of the other is using only part of your overall potential learning ability.

Strategies for Learning

By determining your preferred learning style you will be able to adopt strategies to enhance that style when you study. You want to effectively move the required information into long-term memory and increase your knowledge level from memorization to comprehension and, finally, to application. To accomplish this you must know which strategies work with which learning styles. Refer to Table 3-5 and note all of the listed strategies that you consistently use in your study routine. Start with the style you previously ascertained to be your preferred learning style.

Are strategies listed under your preferred style that you currently do not use? To enhance your acquisition of material, begin to incorporate these into your study plan. Are these strategies listed under any of the other styles that you could use in addition to your usual strategies when the material you are learning is especially difficult for you?

One way to incorporate more than one learning style into your study program is to employ a CAI program. Many texts now come with an accompanying disk designed to enhance learning style. Such disks may contain the total text along with testing materials, exercises that accompany the text, and/or resource material for the text. For example, several medical terminology packages come as program-instruction texts with disks and provide audio pronunciation in the computer programs. The student can read the text, manipulate the information on the computer, and hear the correct pronunciation.

To begin to incorporate new learning styles related to the way you receive and recall information, review the list in Table 3-6 and think about ways to add the study strategies to your study plan. You will notice that the three basic learning styles (visual, auditory, and kinesthetic) are expanded on in this list.

When faced with a particularly difficult passage or concept, incorporate more that one style and one strategy to process the information. The more action you put into your learning methods, the more effective your time and outcomes will be.

DEVELOP A TIME-MANAGEMENT PLAN

Somewhere in your decision-making process to go to school, you decided you would have the time to do so. You now must make that a reality by actively engaging in a time-management plan. **Time management** is a system to help meet goals through problem solving. Practicing time-management strategies will not eliminate the need to perform tasks you do not like, but it will make doing so more manageable. Active application of time-management strategies will make a difference in what you can accomplish in the time you have.

Table 3-5 SAMPLE LEARNING STRATEGIES

VISUAL LEARNER	AUDITORY LEARNER	KINESTHETIC LEARNER
Takes notes in class	Reads aloud	Takes notes and rewrites them to condense
Writes notes in margin of book	Reads into a tape recorder and plays it back to self	Expresses self with hands, even while reading
Looks for reference books with pictures, graphs, and charts	Discusses ideas about class content with others	Handles visual aids during class
Draws own illustrations	Requests explanations of illustrations	Requests to do a demonstration

Table 3-6 ADDITIONAL LEARNING STYLES AND STRATEGIES

STYLE	STUDY TECHNIQUES
Linguistic (word smart: uses words as cues, likes poems)	Speaks out loud, uses audiotapes of text information, uses workbooks, makes up **mnemonics** (words or phrases used to aid memory)
Logical/math (number smart: looks for patterns, enjoys science)	Needs to have a connection for information; uses charts, diagrams, note taking; may use mapping rather than straight words to see connections
Spatial (picture smart: visualizes, good at puzzles)	Draws diagrams; uses flash cards; chooses books with pictures, charts, and diagrams rather than total text, workbooks with pictures; uses highlighters in multiple colors to indicate special things and help information take hold in mind
Body/kinesthetic (body smart: rides a bike, walks, moves, loves the outdoors)	Tapes lectures, walks and listens, watches a video while on the treadmill, goes to a unit to "see" the information, goes to the library to get information, drives and listens to taped lectures or notes (allotted time takes on importance)
Music (music smart: listens to/ loves music, plays an instrument)	Makes up songs and rhymes, uses audio tapes of information or makes up own, listens to music while studying
Interpersonal (people smart: talks things though, likes to chat over coffee)	"Teaches" the material to somebody, studies in a group, runs material by mentor or coworkers
Intrapersonal (self smart: uses quiet time to process, a hobby person)	Uses examples from own experience to apply information, may process material from audio tape while doing a hobby

Adapted from Learning Out of the Box, "Tuning in to Your Unique Cluster of Intelligences," *by K. H. Matthews, 1997, Fall, 22–27* The Next Step Magazine.

Strategies for time management include the following:

- Analyzing your time commitments
- Knowing yourself
- Clarifying your goals
- Setting priorities and identifying one or two valued goals to achieve
- Disciplining yourself to adhere to the plan through changes and until the goal is reached

Analyze Time Commitments

To analyze your time commitments, start by listing them. You should provide yourself with both a big-picture plan and a daily plan. Creating a year-at-a-glance calendar that lists all of your important time commitments can provide a quick illustration of the way the months ahead will be used. Start by putting in your graduation date in red capital letters. This will give you an instant visual reminder of your current goal. Next, using a pencil, insert all important dates including holidays, birthdays, work, and organizational obligations. Remember to also include activities for those in your household that will require your participation, such as carpooling, special school programs, after-school activities, and child care. Use your academic program calendar as the source for the dates classes, as well as vacations, begin and end, financial aid forms and tuition payments are due, and the like. Use your individual class schedules as the sources for dates of exams, special review or clinical days, field trips, or any other time commitments that you must meet in order to complete the courses. This exercise will give you a big-picture view of your time commitments and will also point out any conflicts.

Conflicts are not impossible obstacles. Knowing about them in advance will allow you to take steps now to prioritize and reschedule. When prioritizing, think about delegating some tasks to other people. Do not always solve a conflict by removing those tasks you enjoy or that will renew you. Taking care of yourself during this time will be very important. Never give up the time you need to refresh and renew, even if it is just a hot bath, a brisk 15-minute walk, or a dinner out with family and friends. Place yourself near the top of the priority list to complete your goal.

Each learner's big-picture map will differ. The struggle is to mesh your map with your other relationships and keep yourself toward the top of the list. One strategy is to prominently display your big-picture calendar in an area where all of the members of your household can see it—including and especially you. Everyone will then have the opportunity to see that they are on the list and that they contribute to helping you reach your goal.

The next step is daily planning. Using a week-at-a-glance planner helps illustrate more concrete expectations of those things you plan to do and the amount of time you actually have (Figure 3-6). You should include time to sleep, eat, drive, work, attend class, and study.

You may find that you must rearrange your schedule. This does not mean continuing to do all of the things you have listed but just on different days; rather, it means choosing two valued goals on which to work.

	Monday	Tuesday	Wednesday	Thursday	Friday	Saturday	Sunday
7 AM	Work	Carpool	Carpool	Carpool	Clinical	House Chores	
9 AM	Work	Class	Class	Class		House	Sunday school
11 AM	Work	Class	Class	Class		Chores	Church
1 PM	Work	Class	Class	Class			
3 PM	Work				Work	Work	
5 PM	Carpool Dinner				Work	Work	
7 PM					Work	Work	

Figure 3-6 Week-at-a-Glance Calendar

One must be to be a learner. The other will be unique to you. This does not mean that you replace all other goals with these two valued goals. Rather, it means that these goals must take precedence when choosing ways to use your time. If you choose child care and learner as your most valued goals, you could refine them even further to complement each other. For example, you may opt to keep driving the carpool, but negotiate to drive every morning, because doing so will afford you 2 hours to study prior to class. You may then have to make child care arrangements for after school, which might mean asking your neighbor or

PROFESSIONAL TIP

Time Wasters

Are you a time waster? We all sometimes behave in ways that sabotage the best of plans. Following are some examples of time wasters along with some strategies for helping you reclaim those wasted hours.

1. *Clutter:* Wisdom holds that you can save 1 hour each day by just clearing your work area of clutter and keeping it clean. This time can be put to good use in the form of study. Organize your study area so that when you arrive it is ready for work, and take a few minutes at the end of your session to prepare your area for the next session.

2. *Interruptions:* Intrusions into your study or work hours (from either people or things) can be real time wasters. Try the following:

   • Learn to say, "no." You do not have to agree to every request. Learn to pick your involvements carefully and according to those which are most important to you reaching your goals.

   • Put your answering machine on, and turn the phone's ringer off. Delegate a time to listen and respond to messages after studying.

   • Open your mail over the garbage can. Respond, delegate, or throw it out.

   • Organize your papers. For instance, have a folder for each child's paper/notes. Keep your class notebooks, your calendar, and phone lists in one three-ring binder, so you have all your essentials together.

3. *Procrastination:* This refers to intentionally putting off or delaying something that should be done. **Procrastination** is a time waster because it does not afford effective use of time. Time management is not necessarily finishing everything at one sitting, but, rather, scheduling time to return to the task until you complete it; whereas procrastination is intentionally delaying the task without good cause or a plan to complete it in a time-efficient manner. Breaking the task down into manageable segments and rewards will encourage you to return to it again and again until it is complete.

4. *Perfectionism:* Very often we do not stick to a plan because it does not give us results immediately or does not give the results we expected. Perfectionism affects your time-management plan by prohibiting you from accepting anything less than perfection; it also damages your positive attitude of yourself by setting unrealistic expectations. Focus on your positive accomplishments, look for ways to improve, accept your failures, and build on your experiences.

contracting with an after-school program. You may also have to set aside 1 hour each evening to get everything laid out for the next day, a task you might ask someone else in the household to do each night so that you can gain an extra hour of study time. That extra hour, in turn, might mean that you dedicate Saturdays for nothing but family commitments. Regardless of the way you choose to solve such problems, the solutions must be designed to help you reach your goals.

Know Yourself

To develop your system you must know yourself. You must be honest with yourself about your work habits and preferences. Consider the time of day when you are at your intellectual best. Is it early in the morning, or do you come alive at 10 P.M.? You must be able to focus and concentrate when you are studying. Deciding you are going to carpool in the morning to get to school early to study will not be effective if you cannot concentrate until after noon. If this is the case, it would be better to do the more mechanical and less intellectually demanding tasks, such as the shopping or laundry, in the 2 hours before class. Are you a person who is more left-brain oriented (logical, orderly, structured, and plays by the rules)? Then writing out lists of tasks and crossing them off may be your time-management strategy to stay on track. Perhaps you are a more right-brain personality (creative, resists rules, has own sense of time)? Scheduling your task within a specific time frame that has a time-sensitive goal/reward at the end may assist you to use your available time more effectively.

Clarify the Goal

Without setting goals, we cannot know whether we are making any progress. Goals are like grocery lists. Think about when you go to the store without a list. You may purchase many items, but when you get home you often discover that, you did not get all the things you needed. If the next time you go to the store, you make a list, however, you will likely get all the items you want.

Just like the grocery list, goals must be written down. They must be based on reality and broken down into manageable parts. Say your goal is to provide study time each week that will allow you to be successful in each unit exam of your program. This time will comprise the time you need to prepare and review material, prepare for clinical assignments, view information in the library, and practice new skills in the lab. As a rule, you will need 1 to 2 hours of study time for each hour you spend in class. If you are in class 12 hours per week, you will thus need to find 24 more hours to study; and if you are in clinical 6 hours 3 days per week for a total of 18 hours, you will need to fit in 36 hours of study. As a rough estimate, this would mean 12 class hours plus 24 study hours plus 18

clinical hours plus 36 preparation hours for a total of 90 hours per week (30 class hours plus 60 study hours) for the ideal study week and 30 hours (class attendance only) for a week without any study. So now you know what amount of time you are aiming for. You can now take this goal of 60 study hours per week and compare it to your written schedule and calendar to determine how to best arrange the demands on your time in order to meet your goals.

Set Priorities

Another part of setting goals is prioritizing tasks into general categories. Look at your daily calendar and list the general categories. Some examples might be as follows:

- Work
- Study
- Personal (eating, sleeping)
- Household chores (shopping, budget)
- Transportation (self, others)
- Supervising children
- Decision making (planning, outside organizational responsibility, time for self, time for spouse, friends, and children)

Next, rank these general categories in order of priority, keeping in mind that not everything is a primary priority. If you uncover conflicts, try to further clarify which items take top priority.

Another way to prioritize is to group tasks according to the time frame in which you wish them to be accomplished. To do this, divide a sheet of paper into three parts. Label the first part column A, the second, column B, and the third, column C. Under column A, write "I must work on these tasks now." This list includes your priority tasks that need immediate attention. Under column B write "I can do these after A is done." Under column C write "I can delay, eliminate, or delegate these until after B is done" (Figure 3-7).

If you placed your entire list under column A, go back to your original two goals—one of which includes your new role as learner—and rethink your list. You must prioritize your activities in order to reach your goal. *You cannot be all things at all times to all people.* You also must know how to work smarter, not longer or harder, to remain focused on the priority task.

Discipline Yourself

The hardest strategy to commit to may be the last one. The idea that you must actively engage in using the plan sounds simple. In practice, the plan will not always work. When this happens, you may be tempted to abandon the plan instead of changing it. If the plan is not working, you must ascertain the reasons. Maybe you lack resources, have not scheduled enough time, or need to revisit and re-evaluate your goal. Build time

A	B	C
I must work on these tasks now	I can do these after A is done	I can delay, eliminate, or delegate until after B is done
school/study	*supervise children*	*organization*
child care		*shopping*
self-care		
work		

Figure 3-7 Prioritizing Tasks

to plan into your weekly schedule. If you really want to use a time-management system, your ability to go back to the plan and revise it will be very important.

DEVELOP A STUDY STRATEGY

Developing a study plan involves more than just buying a textbook and reading it. Several strategies that will assist you to study more efficiently and effectively are discussed following.

Set Up the Environment

Where and when you study are as important as how. The fact that you assign a specific behavior to your study space will set you up for success. The space should fit your style. Do you like everything organized in neat spaces, or do you just need it near you? What type of lighting, seating, or noise level will assist or detract from your concentration? Consider your preferred learning style when setting up your study space (Figure 3-8). If you are a kinesethic learner, you may want to put motion into your space by, for instance, using a treadmill in your study plan. You may want to spend a percentage of your study time sitting to read and take notes and then switch to walking or running on the treadmill to recite and reflect on the material. You will be increasing comprehension and making connections, all while walking 2 miles! Regardless of the way you arrange your space, take into consideration the type of learner you are and your biological and personality preferences.

Gather Your Resources

Your resources should all be easily accessible from your study space. In some homes, the kitchen table serves as the study space. If your study space serves more than one function, as would the kitchen table, consider keeping your study resources in a milk crate or box so they are portable yet readily at hand when needed.

Gathering your resources is your start to building a library of textbooks, which will serve you throughout your program. These resources become a reference library for you when you study. Some general resources to keep on hand include the following:

- A recent edition of an unabridged dictionary
- A medical dictionary
- An anatomy and physiology text

Additional resources you will need as you progress through your program may include texts on pharmacology, nutrition, and the nursing process. Depending on your personal knowledge base, you may need further resources in the foundation sciences—biology, psychology, and sociology. These areas serve as the knowledge base for your future profession.

Keeping your learning style in mind, consider also purchasing accompanying workbooks or other study aids that come with the text and research CAI or videotapes available in your nursing program library. Using varied and multiple resources enhances your knowledge base and will increase your comprehension of

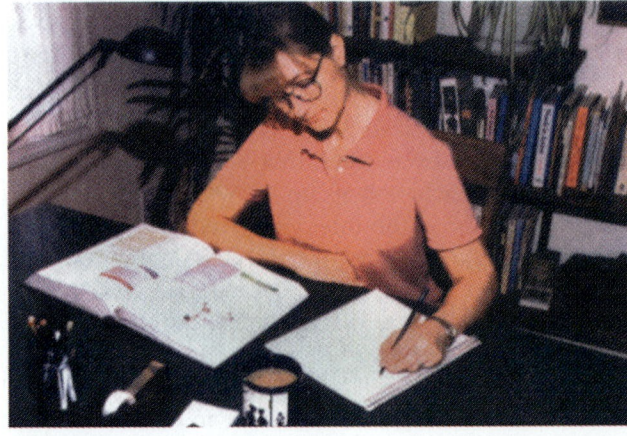

Figure 3-8 Create a study space that reflects your learning style. Ensure that all the resources you need to study are close at hand.

the content. You must go beyond memorization, beyond amassing facts, to comprehension of this knowledge base in order to answer the questions on the exams. Keep in mind that you are studying for the program examination, the National Council Licensure Examination (NCLEX-PN), and, ultimately, to apply your knowledge base to provide safe, effective care to your clients.

Remember to use journals as resources. The articles and related client situations can assist you in understanding the application of content to the clinical area. Your ultimate goal is to apply your content information to client care. Consider getting a subscription to your nursing journal, *The Journal of Practical Nursing*. Nursing organizations such as the National Federation of Licensed Practical Nursing are also valuable resources, and many have Web sites, which you can visit.

Whatever resources you ultimately choose, gathering them and having your resources readily at hand are simple strategies that will make the time you have allotted for study more efficient and effective.

Minimize Interruptions

Interruptions to your study time decrease the actual time you can focus on the material and affect your concentration. Interruptions may also become your procrastination "triggers." If you allow your study time to be constantly interrupted, you will soon be doing something other than studying. At the very least, these interruptions minimize your efficient use of time. When you plan your time to study, do not set yourself up for interruptions. Look realistically at your time schedule and do not schedule your study time around the household's "naturally" busy times of the day—typically mornings, mealtimes, early evenings, and bedtimes.

This is where you put the strategies listed in the section on time management to work. If you have set aside a time and a space for study, make it known that you are not to be interrupted unless there is an emergency. Hang a sign on the door that reads, "Think, before you knock." Planning on studying in 1 or 1½ hour blocks is also a way to cut down on interruptions. This is a reasonable time period for you to put the world on hold in order to accomplish your task.

Get to Know the Textbook

Your textbook is not intended to be read like the latest mystery novel, from beginning to end in one sitting. It has both directions on the way to use it (introduction, preface) and built-in references (glossary, appendix, summary questions). It is arranged in sections, each dealing with a major topic, and then subdivided into the parts (chapters) that make up the sum of that topic. Getting to know your textbook and its resources and the author's approach to writing may constitute the first part of your study plan. Having this information gives you some insight into the way the material has been grouped and connected.

Another author may have written the book in totally stand-alone chapters and may encourage students to review the table of contents and start anywhere they feel they need to. Self-instruction modules or texts in math often give students instructions to first take all of the post-tests in the chapters and as long as a certain score is reached, to go on. This is a means of giving students credit for knowledge already learned and facilitating recall of knowledge in preparation for new learning.

Take a look at various parts of this text. How is the information organized? What built-in references can assist you? Consider the cues the author gives you about the way to use this text to help you organize the big picture.

Set Up the Study Plan

Each time you enter your study "space," your study plan should be with you. You should have a plan or a specific goal for that time. Each time you enter the space, bring a positive attitude toward reaching that goal. Your nursing course outline will drive your study plan. You will have a certain amount of material to cover in a specific time span. You first must know those things that are expected of you. Your course outline, curriculum, and instructors will give you this information.

As an example, consider a unit on vital signs, which is assigned to be completed in 1 week. The components of the unit include understanding the theory base about vital signs as well as learning the psychomotor skills involved in actually measuring these indicators. You are expected to acquire the knowledge by reading the chapter in the text, attending the lecture and demonstration, and practicing in the lab. You will be tested on your ability to apply your knowledge through a pencil-and-paper test and a redemonstration of your psychomotor skills. Now that you know the information you must cover, the sources of the information, and the way you will be tested, you can map out a study plan. Consider the following steps:

1. *Preview the material to be studied.* Your assigned reading from the text on the content of the unit may be contained in one chapter or may span several chapters. Always preview the assigned chapter(s). Often, the student reads only the pages assigned, thinking that this is the most efficient way to study. By not spending the 5 or 10 minutes to preview the entire chapter, the connections between the content may be lost. Previewing can be done very quickly by scanning the chapter headings, art, and tables.

2. *Consider the chapter heading.* The material about vital signs may be contained in a chapter labeled "Baseline Assessment" or "Measurement of Baseline Values" or "Physiologic Functions of the Body." All of these give you a cue as to what you are about to study.

3. *Read the objectives for the chapter.* The objectives list those things you should be able to do when you are finished learning the content of the chapter.

4. *Scan the vocabulary section and the end-of-chapter summary and questions.* Read the key terms and the summary and questions at the chapter's end. Doing so gives you an overview of the scope of the reading you will need to do and should take no more than 5 to 10 minutes

5. *Set up your questions.* Beginning at the chapter objectives, write down those things you already know, questions about those things you must learn for each objective, and some additional resources that you think you should check. For example, in a chapter about vital signs, the initial page may look like the one in Figure 3-9. Jot down your current knowledge, your questions. The resources note relates to the reasons you are trying to learn this material. Connecting the material to your role in the profession is most important. You are now ready to read the chapter critically for the answers to your questions. You may uncover more and have more questions at the end; but you have a plan and can move on to the next step.

6. *Read and take notes.* Answer your questions and check your vocabulary knowledge as you read.

7. *Reread when necessary.* Remember your basic skills and concentration.

8. *Reflect on the connections you can make between the material and client care.* Identify the reasons the information is important and the way you will use it.

9. *Recite or create your individual style cues.* This is where you will put your individual unique learning styles to work. Make up songs. Create mnemonics. Design flash cards for items that must be memorized. Try to create a logical connection when recalling information.

10. *Review or summarize the information.* Answer the objectives. Use your own words to answer your initial questions. Do you have more questions? Must you consult a second resource to answer them?

11. *End the session with a critical thinking question.* What would the client look like if his temperature were 103°F? What other body systems would be affected? What nursing measures might I use to support the client with this level temperature (e.g., monitor the client's fluid intake and output because the body would be losing fluid as a result of the thermoregulation [sweating and evaporation that would reduce the temperature]), and why? Write these down in your notes. You will soon have a collection of "client scenarios" that you will be able to build on as you increase your knowledge base.

The Measurement of Vital Signs

At the completion of this chapter, you should be able to:

1. Describe the physiologic mechanisms controlling temperature, pulse, respiration, and blood pressure.

   Temp = ?, Pulse = heart, Respiration = lungs, Blood pressure = arteries need to find out about temp.

2. Identify the normal range for vital sign measurements.

   For adults? Children?

3. Select the appropriate equipment used to take vital signs.

   Thermometer, stethoscope, blood pressure cuff

4. Demonstrate the correct psychomotor technique used in measuring vital signs.

   I do this in the lab/get procedure from book or instructor? Ask in class.

5. Document the normal findings of the measurement of blood pressure.

   Temp = 98.6, p = 60-80, bp = 120/80
   I need to know this to be able to tell if the client is normal or having trouble.

Figure 3-9 Start with the chapter objectives and devise questions and answers to determine those things that you know and those things that you will need to give more attention.

The preceding steps require skill in five areas: reading, rereading, reflecting, reciting, and review. With each step, you are engaging in the process of encoding the material. **Encoding** is thought of as actually laying down tracks in the areas of your brain. Each time you read, reread, reflect, recite, and review, you increase the depth of the tract, and your ability to recall and utilize the information increases. You move the information from short-term to long-term memory, and you increase your level of knowledge. The more senses and action you put into your study plan, the more you are able to utilize the information.

You move your level of knowledge from the memorization of a group of facts to the comprehension of the facts in a logical, organized fashion that allows you to relate the information to clients to whom you will provide care. Each time you sit down to study, this should be your goal. You can preview, question, and quickly outline the major points in the chapters prior to class. Listen to the lecture and take notes. Approach

PROFESSIONAL TIP

Mnemonics

Create your own mnemonics to group the steps of a procedure. A mnemonic is simply a method for helping your association and recall; it consists of a memorable word or phrase created from the letters of the list of items you are trying to recall. For example, to remember all of the areas to include when assessing a client to whom a cast has been applied (pulse, circulation, sensation, movement, and temperature), you might make up a silly sentence to help you remember, such as *"Paul Can Shine My Tuba."* This type of statement will help you group these facts together (pulse, circulation, sensation, movement, temperature) and assist you in recalling them. You could sing this also. Do whatever you can to be active in moving material from short-term to long-term memory.

new material with the read, reread, reflect, recite, and review steps before moving on to the next topic.

Note Taking

Note taking is an action that connects you to the content of written material or a lecture presentation and will assist you in identifying the main ideas and their connection to the overall topic.

Keep materials for each of your classes or topics in a separate three-ring binder. Take notes on loose-leaf paper and write on one side only, as this allows you to arrange your preview notes and lecture notes chronologically. You can also insert handouts from the class in the appropriate order as you receive them. Using this method, you can also review notes against additional information you have from other resources to assist you when it is time to review for the examinations.

When you are taking notes from the text, read with a pencil in your hand to put yourself in the action mode. You will thus be ready to receive and process information. You may also take notes from text readings on your computer, which facilitates editing and re-arranging material.

Prior to class, preview your chapter material and divide your paper, leaving a 3-inch border on the left side. From the assigned reading, identify the main topic to be covered, list the main section and the sub headings, and summarize the information in the left column. Then write your questions in this column. This prepares you for more active participation in the lecture; in the right column, you will take the actual notes from the lecture.

Regardless of the way you choose to take notes, note taking while you study sets you up for connecting with the content. It positions you as an active participant in the learning process, and any time you increase your active participation in the learning process, you increase your learning.

When taking notes in class, listen attentively, lean forward, and concentrate on the information the speaker is imparting (Figure 3-10). Take notes on the following:

- The topic, as stated by the speaker; write it on the top of the page
- The main ideas and the details that support the topic
- The most important points, based on the speaker's organization and emphasis

PROFESSIONAL TIP

Memory and Activity

Remember the following as a guide for a study plan when you want to learn new material:

People Remember	Learner Activity
10% of what they READ	Reading
20% of what they HEAR	Hearing the words
30% of what they SEE	Watching still pictures (charts, diagrams)
50% of what they SEE and HEAR	Watching moving pictures (video or a demonstration)
70% of what they SAY and WRITE	Giving a presentation making up a story (case studies)
90% of what they SAY AS THEY PERFORM THE EXPERIENCE	Talking your way through a demonstration Teaching someone else.

Adapted from Audiovisual Methods in Teaching, *(p. 43), by E. Dale, 1954, New York: Dryden Press.*

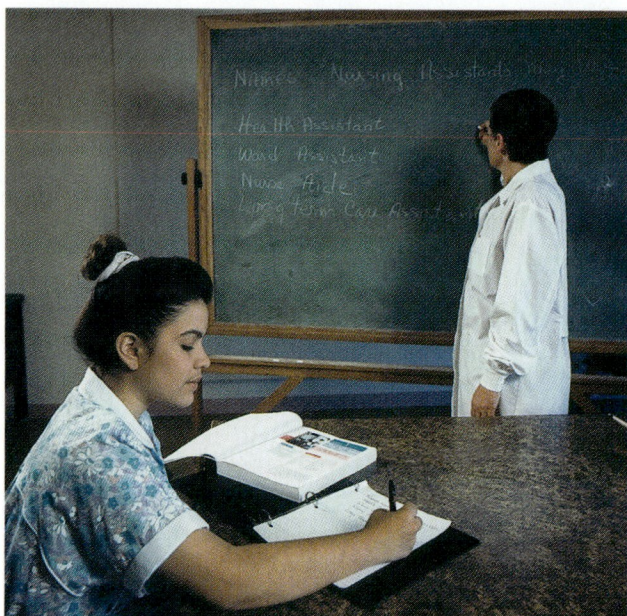

Figure 3-10 Note taking is an important component of increasing your comprehension of the material.

- Other students' questions and the responses from the speaker, which often will be the very questions you had

Look for visual and auditory cues from the speaker, for example, if the speaker says, "This is important" or writes steps on the board. Do not form an opinion of what is being said until you have heard the entire lecture. As stated earlier, a good strategy is to write your questions as you think of them. They may be answered by the time the lecture is over.

The purpose of note taking during a lecture is not to create a transcript of the information imparted, but, rather, to record what you understand. The combination of attending lecture, listening, and note taking can provide you with much knowledge that you will then not have to learn elsewhere. Previewing the material to be covered further contributes to this dynamic. When taking notes, consider the following guidelines to make your note taking efficient and effective:

PROFESSIONAL TIP

Attending Lectures

In general, the best strategies for getting the most from lectures are to:

- Get to class on time.
- Get a front row seat, and
- Listen attentively with a pencil in your hand and take notes.

- Do not take notes with the intent of writing them over. This is a waste of time and, contrary to what you may expect, it does not improve recall. Using the Cornell system of note taking or making a note map of your notes is a more effective recall tool. Examples of both follow.
- If your handwriting is sloppy, print or use a laptop computer.
- Condense the amount of actual writing you do by using symbols and abbreviations and leaving out everything but necessary words. For instance, instead of writing "If the client's blood pressure reading is greater than 140 systolic and 90 diastolic, . . ." write "If BP > 140/90 . . ."
- Write definitions and mathematical formulas exactly as you heard them in lecture.
- In mathematics and science lab courses, write the process step by step exactly as explained. Indicate which formulas are used with which problems, for example

    "Use ratio/proportion for word problems"

- Pick an abbreviation system and stick to it.
- Review the notes as soon as possible after class. Many studies have demonstrated that even a brief review of notes after class increases retention of the material by 50%.

Prepare for Exams

The final plus of having a study plan is the ability to review for exams. Reviewing for exams is not studying all of the material over from the beginning. The subject matter you are going to cover on the exam you have already studied; now, you are reviewing and recalling it through a series of exercises designed to increase your comprehension and facilitate application. Most nursing examinations are written at the comprehension or recall level. The NCLEX-PN is written at the application level. On this exam you will not see many questions about naming where the pulse points are (comprehension, recall), for instance. You will instead find questions about which of the pulse points of the body are most appropriate for assessing an infant (application). Making decisions about which fact or groups of principles you have learned will be the basis for most nursing examination questions.

Depending on the curriculum, you may have examinations every week or every month, a weekly quiz, a midterm, and a final. Regardless, you will know the schedule, and you must set aside review time for preparation. If you are to have weekly quizzes, you must build a time for review into your daily study plan. One way to do so is to set aside the last 30 minutes of each study session for review. Take each objective of your course outline and without looking at your notes or text, turn them into questions and then answer them. If you are weak in one area, refer to your notes and devise a technique for recall, such as the use of flash cards, rhythms, mnemonics, pictures, or graphic drawings. Work through each of the objectives for the content that will be covered.

If your examinations are by unit, you must divide the material up over the time you will need to cover it, leaving at least 2 days for review and recall prior to the examination. Each of these review sessions will also serve as preparation for both your final examination and the NCLEX-PN. As you are successful in each of your examinations and continue to see further connections in your clinical application, your depth as well as breadth of content mastery will increase.

PRACTICE THINKING CRITICALLY

Most of this chapter thus far has been devoted to presenting strategies for the effective and efficient acquisition of knowledge. Your ultimate goal is to be able to use this knowledge to provide safe client care. To do so, you must go beyond the initial stage of simply acquiring information. In delivering nursing care, facts alone do not constitute a sufficient knowledge base for making sound decisions about client care. You must internalize these facts and be able to manipulate them when presented with new situations. In the early 1950s, Bloom and other psychologists identified six learning-achievement levels involved in cognitively processing information. These six levels are listed in Table 3-7.

Your progress in this cognitive arena will be evaluated by testing. Practicing thinking critically will enhance your ability to increase your level of knowledge

You must think about *how* you think. Thinking is a process: It is the way you move information from one point to another to get something accomplished. Have you ever been asked, "How did you arrive at that conclusion?" Your explanation was an example of your thinking process. This process of examining how we think is called **metacognition** (from m*eta,* meaning "among" plus *cognition,* meaning "the process of knowing").

Consider all of the problem solving you have done in your life. How did you arrive at your decisions? Why did you make the choices you did? Given more information, would you have made different decisions? Have you made decisions you regretted?

To make sound decisions, you must consider the knowledge you have and choose that which is relevant given the unique parameters of the given situation. Each client situation is unique. Your text and instructors present information about nursing practice within what is called *predictable parameters,* but clients are anything but predictable.

In considering which actions you may need to take in a new situation, you must consider past experience

Table 3-7 LEARNING ACHIEVEMENT LEVELS

COGNITIVE LEVEL	LEARNER ACTIONS
Knowledge	Memorize specifics; ways of dealing with specifics; trends and sequences; classifications and categories.
	Return exact definitions or statements as taught.
	"Blood pressure is always written as systolic over diastolic" or *"One principle of teaching is to assess readiness to learn."*
Comprehension	Understand concepts or principles, and use them.
	Able to see the relationship of the parts.
	Draw inferences from data as to what might happen within a limited range.
	"What does 'maintain fluid and electrolyte balance' mean?"
Application	Able to use concepts, rules, methods, laws, principles, and theories to arrive at the solution of the problem, when neither the solution nor the method is given.
	"John has serum potassium of 5.6. If this is not reduced to normal, what physiological effects can be expected and why?"
Analysis	Able to divide something into its basic parts and examine them, sort important information from less important, assemble information into meaningful order, and draw a conclusion using the entire problem solving process.
	"Your client has a third degree burn of 24-hour duration. What effect would this have on his laboratory values?"
Synthesis	Able to create new solutions that are unique, as in devising a new teaching tool (a new procedure or a new theory).
	Use pieces of prior knowledge that are re-formed into a new approach.
	Able to develop a research hypothesis (educated guess) about relationships among abstract concepts.
Evaluation	Able to use standards and principles to compare the results of an action in order to make a judgment of its validity.
	Use internal and external criteria as evidence of whether an action/statement or theory is of merit.

From How To Categorize Questions According to the "New" NCLEX-RN Test Plan, *by P. Arnett, 1988, SC: Arnett Development Corporation.*

and principles of care, postulate possible outcomes from a variety of interventions, and seek additional information from colleagues, clients, and resource materials. This process is called *thinking critically,* and it is what you will be expected to do with the knowledge you are acquiring.

How do you foster this type of thinking and knowledge advancement as you are studying? The following strategies used during your study process will help develop your critical thinking skills.

1. *Recall the facts.* Remind yourself of those things you already know about the targeted topic. (***Example:*** The cardiovascular system is made up of the heart, the arteries, and the veins; it carries the blood to the cells.)

2. *Group facts into a pattern and organize the data.* (***Example:*** The heart is the center of this system. The arteries carry blood from the heart to the cells, the veins carry blood from the cells to the heart. The blood's function is to transport nutrients and oxygen to the cells and to take waste and carbon dioxide from the cells.)

3. *Associate this information with an experience or an action.* (***Example:*** The cardiovascular system is like a plumbing system, with the heart as the main pumping station, the arteries as the carriers of the hot water, and the veins as the carriers of the cold water.)

4. *Practice "what if" scenarios.* Imagine a person in your life and analyze the facts that you have learned in light of this person. Confirm whether the facts are applicable. If not, what was significant in this situation to alter your conclusion? What action might you take? (***Example:*** What happens when the pump doesn't work [as in Uncle Joe's pacemaker]? What causes this? What runs the heart's electrical system? What else can cause the main pump to stop working—no food [nutrients] or no oxygen? Where does the heart get its oxygen? How does this affect Joe's lifestyle? How could I tell whether a person has a pacemaker? What would I do if the pacemaker stopped?)

5. *Discuss these questions with peers and your instructor.* Conferring with others increases your experience and the variety of ways you look at a problem and promotes increased comprehension of the subject.

6. *Postulate new solutions.* Allow yourself to consider all possible solutions without assigning merit. There is no need to label an idea as "good" or "bad" before the idea has even been discussed. Often, such flashes of insight come when we are daydreaming, on the verge of sleep, or as we awaken. Our mind is free to roam and process during these times.

The last strategy will involve taking some risk, but students who take that risk quickly develop a thick skin and are the most likely to contribute innovatively to the clinical practice as a result of their thinking process. Chapter 2 on critical thinking provides much more information on this particular process, but the subject bears inclusion here. Practice this habit as you study, and never stop asking, "Why?" and "What about this?"

DEVELOP TEST-TAKING SKILLS

Testing is not studying; however, the skills you need for testing are similar to those needed for studying. The task involved in taking a test is not to pass it; to pass the test is the *outcome.* You cannot achieve the outcome if you do not know the task. The task is to read the question, understand what the question is asking, and make a decision about a correct response.

To hone your test-taking behaviors, you must first perform a personal analysis with regard to your attitudes, preparation methods, and behaviors related to a testing situation. Only after you have identified these variables can you initiate strategies to improve your outcomes.

Attitude and Expectations

If you are like most students, you may feel quite anxious about taking a test. You may think of each test as the final chance to show your worth. Or you may consider receiving less than an A grade on an examination as being the same as failing. Neither of these is a reasonable expectation for testing. Testing is a useful tool for both measuring your level of knowledge and showing what you still need to learn. Have you ever considered that receiving a grade of C on an examination usually indicates that you know 75% of all of the knowledge that was tested? And the knowledge on any given test does not represent all the knowledge you possess. Your attitude toward testing is very important if you are to improve your outcome. Maintaining a reasonable expectation regarding both the purpose of the test as well as the meaning of your grade is often a key factor in improving your test performance.

Preparation

In analyzing your preparation for test taking, you must critically examine your study habits. Review the section in this chapter on a study strategies and consider whether you are on task when it comes to your study habits. There may be some areas where you can improve. If you know of an area of weakness, make a conscious effort to develop this part of your preparation. Be reasonable in your expectations and do not expect to see results overnight. Building your study habits takes time and persistence. Persevere and your outcome on tests will improve.

Next, consider the way you review for an examination. Do you cram the night before, or are you consistently planning for questions in your study plan and adding time for review of material prior to the examination? One strategy is to use the technique of note mapping to help you organize the material into manageable parts. Taking each part and developing a more detailed one-page outline that you can take with you to review for 15 to 20 minutes at a time is another method to try. Another suggestion is to change your study place and times. Instead of 1-hour sessions, break your review sessions into 30-minute recall sessions. You must draw an imaginary line between studying and reviewing. Studying is the learning of new knowledge; reviewing comprises recall, organization, and summary of information.

Do not study only just prior to the test. This represents poor technique. What are the odds that prior to the examination you would hit upon just the right information that would be on the test in just the exact form that you would see it on the test? Approaching preparation in this manner serves only to put a few facts into short-term memory. Better to spend the time before the examination relaxing with a good book or good friends or at the spa or gym. You must be confident and rested and come to the testing area with that "good" feeling that results from doing something you like.

Consider the rest you get the night prior to the examination. Physical stamina is needed for concentration. If you cram for a test by "pulling an all-nighter," you are setting yourself up for possible errors on the examination. Be reasonable, revisit your study plan, and keep this behavior to a minimum.

Next, consider whether you have enough energy to take the test. You can eat what you want, but eat. The cells of the brain require glucose to function; this glucose is supplied in the calories you consume. Try not to increase caffeine intake immediately prior to a test, as doing so may make you jittery.

Finally, ask yourself whether surrounding yourself with positive people helps keep you focused, or whether talking to students prior to a test only makes you more anxious. If the latter is the case, you should arrive with just enough time to walk into the testing room and you should not speak to anyone.

Minimize Anxiety

Anxiety is the physiologic response of the autonomic nervous system to a perceived stressful situation. As the situation becomes more stressful, the body's response increases. This affects the ability to process information and make rational choices. People are often not good at identifying what they are feeling and are often unaware of the degree to which stress affects the ability to take tests.

You must develop a plan to deal with anxiety. Anxiety about our performance is always with us. Past experience with testing often contributes to the development of test anxiety. If our expectation regarding our performance on a test is not mirrored in the grade we receive, our confidence in our ability is shaken, and we approach the whole experience with more and more anxiety.

To deal with anxiety, consciously develop an activity to counter the feeling that anxiety evokes. Some people listen to music, pace, or do deep breathing to combat feelings of stress and anxiety. All of these are good strategies, even if all of them cannot be done *while you are actually taking the test.*

PROFESSIONAL TIP

The 30-Second Vacation

For those of you who need an "anxiety buster," consider a "30-second vacation." The 30-second vacation is based on a guided imagery technique that is used often in the client care arena. This technique takes practice. Start by doing the following:

Sit in a comfortable spot where you will not be disturbed, close your eyes, and think of an event or a place that evokes in you a feeling of calmness (not necessarily happiness). This is an event or place that when it happened or when you were there, you felt like everything was right with the world and you. It can be from any time in your life.

It may take some time to settle on the right event or place. Relax and take a few minutes now and think.

Once you have it, don't tell anyone! This is your secret place, your place of peace, and when you go there, no one can find you.

Once you have selected this event or place, start to give it "life." To do this, you must begin to recall this event or place regularly. Practice doing so at the beginning of your study sessions, when you are stuck in traffic, when you are at the dentist, when you have something difficult to do, at the beginning of your test-taking exercises, or at the beginning of your real tests.

Each time you recall your event or place, give it more "life." Recall the time of day, the setting, the colors of that day. Was it raining, was it sunny, was it snowing? If it was raining, was it a summer rain or an autumn rain? Recall what you were wearing and what colors you had on. Were you alone or with others? Were you eating something? What did the food smell like?

Improve Test-Taking Skills

How do you improve your test-taking skills? You practice, practice, practice and analyze, analyze, analyze. Consider the following:

> *Treat every wrong answer as a treasure. Examine it and discover the secret of why you got it wrong*

This is the only way to know which errors you are making. From this point forward, always request to review your examinations, and track your incorrect responses using the analysis worksheet presented in Figure 3-11. Initially when you review your tests, do not concern yourself with the content of the questions. Simply write the number of the question in the row that indicates the reason you got that question incorrect. You will also notice that there is a heavy black line before the last row of the worksheet. The first four rows represent what are known as *mechanical errors;* these can be eliminated by developing positive habits and revising current practices. You will notice after 3 or 4 quizzes that a pattern starts to emerge. Imagine that you just took a 100-question test and received a score of 60/100. You then use the worksheet to categorize your incorrect responses.

Of the 40 incorrect answers you provided, you see that 10 of them fell in "did not read carefully," 2 in "did not know the vocabulary," 7 in "inferred additional data," 4 in "identified priorities incorrectly," and 7 in "did not know the material." If you could eliminate the bad habits that resulted in the first 23 errors, this would improve your test score immediately. Your grade would be 83/100. More importantly, tests would truly represent only what you did not know, not areas where bad habits resulted in poor test scores.

After you have identified your error patterns, you can work on developing the counter habits that will eliminate them. Work first on the one that is the most glaring.

Read Carefully

Reading carefully is a test-taking behavior that must be practiced. The section on study strategies noted the value of scanning in looking for important words when you read. When you are reading a test question, however, you must *never* scan. Many students choose incorrect responses for test questions, because they miss key words, scan the question for familiar terms, infer what the question is, or misinterpret words they read too quickly. Incorrect responses resulting from any of these actions represent poor reading habits rather than a substandard knowledge base. The following exercise will help improve your reading habits.

Exercise for Improving Your Literal Reading Skills

You will need

- A timer (stove/egg).
- An NCLEX-PN review text or any comparable question and answer book. It is important that you have the answers and the rationales for each answer in a review text.
- Two sheets of paper: one to take the test on and one to make your analysis worksheet.

Test Question Analysis Worksheet

Reason for Incorrect Response	Test 1 Date	Test 2 Date	Test 3 Date	Test 4 Date	Test 5 Date	Test 6 Date	Test 7 Date	Test 8 Date
Did not read carefully (missed details, missed key words)								
Did not know the vocabulary (medical terminology, English vocabulary)								
Inferred additional data (made assumptions, "read into the question")								
Identified priorities incorrectly (placed events in wrong order)								
Did not know the material								

Figure 3-11 Test Question Analysis Worksheet

• Pencil or pen.
• Dictionary.

1. Pick a time and a place where there will be no interruptions for 20 minutes. You may neither speak to anyone nor get up to use any other resources. You are taking a test.
2. Randomly pick a page of the review book and choose five questions from that page. It does not matter whether you have not yet studied the content in your program.
3. Set the timer for 5 minutes.
4. Start the test. Read each question out loud.
   a. If you read "over" a word, stop reading, make a mark next to that word, and begin again from the beginning.
   b. If you mispronounce a word, stop reading, make a mark next to that word, and begin again from the beginning.
   c. If you do not know the meaning of a word (English or medical), stop and look it up.
5. At the end of the question, restate what is being asked of you.
6. Read the choices, connect each to the question, and choose the most correct answer.
7. When the timer goes off, score your questions.
8. Analyze why you got questions correct or incorrect.
9. Repeat this exercise with five different questions three or four times a week.

The object of this exercise is not to finish all the questions, nor is it even to get all the answers right. Rather, the object is to consciously practice reading every word literally. Each time you do this exercise, you must treat it as a test—no food, no talking, no music, no interruptions. You must associate this type of reading with taking a test, so that each time you take a test, this literal reading habit is instinctual.

Know the Vocabulary

If vocabulary is your weak area, there is only one thing to do—learn the vocabulary. Look up the word (English and medical) in the appropriate dictionary, write the definition on the back of your analysis sheet, and review the definition during your next study session. Add additional time in your study plan for vocabulary building. Use additional modes of learning such as audio or flashcards to master your vocabulary skills.

Do Not Infer Additional Data

The more experiences you have in life, the easier it is to infer additional data in any given situation. You must realize, however, that for the moment, the only relevant information is the information on the test paper—no more, no less. Based on that information alone and the given choices, you must decide on the correct responses. You base your decision on those things you have learned about the topic of the question, on standards of care, on the nursing process, and on your base of knowledge. If you read into the question, you have in essence rewritten it and may not choose the correct answer. One strategy for overcoming this habit is to recognize whenever you begin to interject information upon getting to the last word in a question. In any such instance, you must stop, take some physical action to call your attention to the fact that you are adding information, and clear your mind—take a breath, clear your throat, wear a rubber band and snap it! Then start over again, concentrating on reading the question literally.

Identify Priorities Correctly

When questions concern priorities, ask yourself which of the given choices would result in serious consequences if not done first. When you are being questioned about procedural tasks, ask which of the given choices must be done before the others.

Know the Material

Not knowing the material represents a lack of knowledge base. Write down the content area of each of the questions you miss, then go back and review the concept or facts in question. If the same content areas are problematic over several tests, seek additional assistance from your instructor. You need clarification regarding your understanding of both the information and the questions.

Behaviors in the Testing Room

Setting yourself up in the testing room for a positive experience can make a difference in your outcome. Be sure to practice the following behaviors:

1. **Get a good seat.** Unless your seat is assigned, sit in an area that is quiet, has good light, and where you can "zone in" on the test and "zone out" the rest of the room. If you are a student who gets anxious when you are the last one left in the room, pick a seat in the front row and farthest from the door and turn your seat slightly toward the wall. You will be less apt to notice as people leave.
2. **Set the mood.** As you wait for the test to be passed out, take your 30-second vacation. Adopt the most positive attitude possible. Identify the task ahead of you. Take a breath and repeat the following:

   "I have prepared. I am able to read the questions, process the information, and, from the choices given, make the best choice and move on."

3. ***Read—do not scan.*** You must read literally every word in the question. Every word counts!

4. ***Read the question to determine the following:***
   - *Who is the question about?* This will affect your chosen answer. If you automatically assume that all of the questions relate to the nurse, you may miss a question that asks you to decide those things the father might say to demonstrate his understanding of the discharge instructions, for example.
   - *What is the question about?* You must determine to which part of the knowledge base the question refers. Is the question about the way to teach a 9-year-old juvenile diabetic to check his blood glucose? To answer this question, you must consider the learning style of the 9-year-old, his cognitive development and manual dexterity, and any significant others who should be involved in the session. The correct choice must support all of these principles.
   - *When is the question about?* The time frame of the question is also significant in terms of the client's continuum of care. Is this the acute session? Is this a client who has had diabetes for 20 years and is now developing pulmonary vascular disease? Is this a new mother with her first child or a new mother with her fifth? Are you in the assessment phase of the nursing process, are you in the planning stage, or are you evaluating the effects of a treatment or a drug?
   - *Where is the question about?* The focus of the nurse in the acute care institution is different from that of the nurse in the community clinic. This will affect your choice.

5. ***Do not argue with the question.*** Whether you agree with the question is irrelevant. The task is to read the question, put your mind to the question, and, given the choices offered, make your choice based on principles and the application of your knowledge base.

6. ***Plan your time.*** Do not spend an inordinate amount of time on one question. There are some things you will not know, and if you spend so much time on one question, you can sabotage your success on others. You can come back to any question, but you must be able to clear your mind of this question before moving on to tackle another. This is a good place for a 30-second vacation to put you back on task! If you cannot let a question "go," you will be unable to concentrate on the next few questions and, very likely, will get several questions in a row incorrect. It is best to read, choose, and move on.

7. ***Do not panic.*** When you come to a question to which you do not immediately know the answer, do not panic. Use your 30-second vacation to counter your anxiety and facilitate your ability to process. Recite again, "I have prepared, I am able to read, process, choose, and move on." Remember, the answer is on the paper.

SUMMARY

- Developing a positive attitude will enhance your learning experience.
- Strategies for developing a positive attitude include creating a positive self-image, recognizing your abilities, and identifying realistic expectations for meeting those goals.
- Nurses must develop competency in the basic skills of reading, arithmetic and mathematics, writing, listening, and speaking.
- It is important to build your vocabulary and comprehension of medical terminology to better enable you to meet your clients' learning needs.
- Should you suspect that you have a learning disability, it is important to identify the disability so that you can seek the right tools to help compensate for the disability.
- The most common learning styles are visual, auditory, and kinesthetic.
- Identifying your preference for a particular learning style will help you identify the strategies you need to be a successful student.
- Organizing your study space and decreasing interruptions will increase your efficiency and facilitate your sticking to your study plan.
- Several methods can be used to take notes. Note taking in lectures and from your text is a strategy to help you retain the information presented.
- Critical thinking is the ability to apply your knowledge base.
- Developing a strategy to minimize anxiety when taking tests will improve your performance.
- To successfully complete a test, read each question thoroughly, do not infer additional information, and identify priorities.

⚡ WEB FLASH!

- Visit your professional association's Web site and gather information on your profession.
- Visit one of the learning sites to take a learning-style assessment.

Review Questions

1. Ninety percent of your program is based on which basic skill?
   a. Listening
   b. Writing
   c. Reading
   d. Mathematics

2. What is a sign of true comprehension of material?
   a. The ability to repeat a paragraph word for word
   b. Memorization of the material
   c. The ability to recite the material
   d. The ability to summarize the material using your own words

3. If you suspect you have a learning disability, it is important that you:
   a. ignore it; you will be able to work around it on your own.
   b. be tested to determine the assistance you will need to compensate for the disability.
   c. keep it to yourself; you will not be able to pass the program if you tell anyone about it.
   d. use it as an excuse to put less work into the program.

4. A kinesthetic learner:
   a. learns by using the senses and visual images.
   b. learns by movement and imitation.
   c. learns by hearing and listening.
   d. learns by example.

5. The best way to study is to:
   a. read only the assigned material.
   b. take notes in the lecture only.
   c. read, reread, reflect, recite, and review.
   d. read and attend lectures.

6. What is the best way to deal with any anxiety you may experience during a test?
   a. Jogging
   b. Listening to music
   c. Practicing deep breathing and imagery
   d. Asking for more time to take the test

Critical Thinking Questions

In the section on Practicing Thinking Critically, you were asked, "How did you arrive at that conclusion?" Recall the last fairly crucial decision you made and outline your thinking process.

NURSING HISTORY, EDUCATION, AND ORGANIZATIONS

MAKING THE CONNECTION

Refer to the following chapters to increase your understanding of nursing history, education, and organizations:

- **Chapter 7, Ethical Responsibilities**
- **Chapter 57, Leadership/Work Transition**

LEARNING OBJECTIVES

Upon completion of this chapter you should be able to:
- *Define key terms.*
- *Define nursing as an art and a science.*
- *Identify major historical and social events that have shaped current nursing practice.*
- *Describe Florence Nightingale's impact on current nursing practice.*
- *Discuss the contributions of early nursing leaders in the United States.*
- *Discuss the impact of selected landmark reports on nursing education and practice.*
- *Define the role of the RN.*
- *Define the role of the LP/VN.*
- *Describe select nursing organizations and their purposes and functions.*
- *Differentiate between program approval and program accreditation.*

KEY TERMS

accreditation	history
autonomy	morbidity
clinical	mortality
didactic	nursing
empowerment	primary care provider
health maintenance	primary health care
organization	staff development

INTRODUCTION

Nursing is an art and a science by which people are assisted in learning to care for themselves whenever possible and are cared for by others when they are unable to meet their own needs.

Nursing has evolved from an unstructured method of caring for the ill to a scientific profession. The result has been movement from the mystical beliefs of primitive times to a "high-tech, high-touch" era. Nursing combines art and science. By using scientific knowledge in a humane manner, nursing combines critical thinking skills with caring behaviors.

Nursing focuses not on illness but, rather, on the client's *response* to illness. Nursing promotes health and helps the client move to a higher level of wellness. This aspect of nursing also includes providing assistance to the client with a terminal illness with the goal of maintaining comfort and dignity in the final stage of life.

This chapter traces the evolution of nursing by exploring its rich heritage and the social forces that have affected its development. Nursing education and nursing organizations are also discussed.

HISTORICAL OVERVIEW

To understand the present status of nursing, it is necessary to have basic historical knowledge about nursing. By studying nursing history, the nurse is better able to understand such issues as **autonomy** (being self-directed), unity within the profession, supply and demand, salary, education, and current practice. **History** is a study of the past, including events, situations, and individuals. By learning from historical role models, nurses can enhance their abilities to create positive change in the present and set a course for the future.

Learning from the past is the major reason for studying history. Ignoring nursing's history can be detrimental to the future of the profession (Ogren, 1994). By applying the lessons gained from a historical review, nurses will continue to be a vital force in the next millennium.

The study of nursing history offers another advantage: learning how the profession has advanced from its beginnings. **Empowerment** is the process of enabling others to do for themselves. Only when nurses are empowered are they truly autonomous. Autonomy has historically been difficult for nurses to achieve. Empowerment and autonomy go together and are necessary if nursing is to bring about positive changes in health care today. Personal power comes to individuals who are clear about what they want from life and who see their work as essential to the contributions they wish to make.

Evolution of Nursing

Nursing has evolved alongside human civilization. While it is not possible to present a complete history of nursing and health care within the scope of this text, it is necessary for all nurses to have some understanding of their profession's heritage and of those pioneers who led the way on the path to modern nursing. Table 4-1 is a chronological listing of events in the evolution of nursing.

Primitive Times

Primitive humans may very well have derived early nursing care practices from observing the animal world. Many animals care for their sick and injured. For example, wild turkeys feed their young wild berries to ward off the chill of inclement weather, much as we use vitamin C (found in wild berries) today; the snipe (a small bird) has been observed splinting an injured leg with sticks and straw; and many animals eat grass

Table 4-1 HISTORICAL EVENTS INFLUENCING THE EVOLUTION OF NURSING

DATE	EVENT	DATE	EVENT
4000 B.C.	Primitive societies	1871	Founded: New York State Training School for Nurses, Brooklyn Maternity, Brooklyn, New York
2000 B.C.	Babylonia and Assyria		
800–600 B.C.	Health religions of India		
700 B.C.	Greece: source of modern medical science	1872	New England Hospital for Women's one-year program for nurses yields America's first trained nurse, Linda Richards
460 B.C.	Hippocrates		
3 B.C.	Ireland: pre-Christian nursing	1873	Founded: first three Nightingale schools in United States: Bellevue (New York City), Connecticut, and Massachusetts General
A.D. 390	Fabiola: first hospital founded		
390–407	Early Christianity, deaconesses		
711	Field hospital with nursing, Spain	1881	Founded: American Red Cross, by Clara Barton
1096–1291	Military Nursing Orders (Knights Hospitalers of St. John in Jerusalem)	1892	Founded: Ballard School at YWCA Brooklyn, NY; first practical nursing school
1100	Ambulatory clinics, Spain (Moslems)	1893	Founded: American Society of Superintendents of Training Schools for Nurses
1440	First Chairs of Medicine, Oxford and Cambridge	1899	Founded: International Council of Nurses (ICN)
1500–1752	Deterioration of hospitals and nursing, "dark ages of nursing"	1900	*American Journal of Nursing* (AJN) established
1633	Founded: Daughters of Charity	1903	New York: efforts fail to pass a nurse licensing law
1820	Florence Nightingale born		North Carolina: first state nurse registration law passes
1836	Kaiserswerth, Order of Deaconesses reestablished		Founded: Army Nurse Corps
1841	Founded: Nursing Sisters of the Holy Cross	1907	Thompson Practical Nursing School in Brattleboro, VT established
1848	Women's Rights Convention, Seneca Falls, New York	1910	Flexner report
1854–1856	Crimean War	1911	Founded: American Nurses Association (ANA), formerly the Associated Alumnae
1859	Nightingale's *Notes on Nursing* published in England		
1860	Founded: first Nightingale School of Nursing, St. Thomas Hospital, London	1912	Founded: National League of Nursing Education, formerly the Superintendents' Society
1861–1865	Civil War, United States		
1861	Dorothea Dix appointed Superintendent of the Female Nurses of the Army	1914	Mississippi becomes first state to license practical nurses

continued

Table 4-1 HISTORICAL EVENTS INFLUENCING THE EVOLUTION OF NURSING *continued*

DATE	EVENT	DATE	EVENT
1917	Smith-Hughes Act passes (provided federal funds for practical nursing programs in vocational schools)	1955	Practical nursing established under (Title III) Health Amendment Act
1918	Household Nursing Association School of Attendant Nursing in Boston, MA, established		All states pass licensure laws affecting practical/vocational nursing
1920s	First prepaid medical plan established, Pacific Northwest	1959	National Association of Practical Nurse Education (NAPNE) changes name to National Association for Practical Nurse Education and Service (NAPNES)
	Hospitals offer a prepaid plan	1960s	Established: Medicare and Medicaid
	Baylor Plan (prototype of Blue Cross) established	1961	National League for Nursing establishes a Council for Practical Nursing Programs
1921	Women get the right to vote		Surgeon General's Consultant Group
1923	Goldmark Report: Nursing and Nursing Education in the United States	1965	First nurse practitioner program, pediatric
1935	Social Security Act passes		ANA position paper on entry into practice
1941	Founded: Association of Practical Nursing Schools	1966	Educational opportunity grants for nurses
1942	Association of Practical Nursing Schools becomes National Association of Practical Nurse Education (NAPNE)	1970	Secretary's commission to study extended roles for nurses
	Practical nursing curriculum planned and advocated across United States	1973	Health Maintenance Organization Act
1944	U.S. Department of Vocational Education commissions intensive study to differentiate tasks of the practical nurse	1977	Rural Health Clinic Service Act
		1980	Omnibus Budget Reconciliation Act (OBRA)
1945	New York only state to have mandatory licensure law for practical nurses	1982	Budget cut to Health Maintenance Organization Act
1948	Brown Report: Future of Nursing		Tax Equity Fiscal Responsibility Act (TEFRA)
1949	Founded: National Federation of Licensed Practical Nurses (NFLPN)	1983	Institute of Medicine Committee on Nursing and Nursing Education study
		1987	Secretary's Commission on Nursing
1952	National League of Nursing Education changes name to National League for Nursing (NLN)	1990s	Health care reform
		1996	Certification Examination for Practical and Vocational Nurses in Long-term Care

Adapted from Fundamentals of Nursing: Standards and Practice, *by S. DeLaune and P. Ladner, 1998, Albany, NY: Delmar Publishers. Copyright 1998 by Delmar Publishers. Adapted with permission.*

as an emetic when they have stomach problems. Early humans were closely associated with the animals.

Early Civilizations

The evolution of nursing dates back to 4000 B.C., to primitive societies wherein mother–nurses worked with priests. In 2000 B.C., the use of wet nurses is recorded in Babylonia and Assyria.

Ancient Greece

The ancient Greeks built temples to honor Hygiea, the goddess of health. These temples were more like health spas than hospitals in that they were religious institutions governed by priests. Priestesses (who were not nurses) attended to those housed in the temples. The nursing that was done by women was performed in the home.

Hippocrates, a Greek physician born in 460 B.C., is considered the father of medicine. He used a system of physical assessment, observation, and record keeping in his care of the sick. Hippocrates wrote about many aspects of medicine, including pathology, anatomy, physiology, diagnosis, prognosis, mental illness, gynecology, obstetrics, surgery, client-centered care, bedside observation, hygiene, and professional ethics. Case histories that he wrote are still used as examples today. He emphasized the importance of caring for the client and thus laid a foundation for nursing. The Hippocratic Oath, based on his principles, is still taken by physicians today.

Roman Empire

Hospitals were first established in the Eastern Roman Empire (Byzantine Empire). St. Jerome was responsible, through one of his disciples, Fabiola, for introducing hospitals in the West. Western hospitals were primarily religious and charitable institutions housed in monasteries and convents. The caregivers had no formal training in therapeutic modalities and volunteered their time to nurse the sick (Bullough & Bullough, 1993).

Middle Ages

During the medieval era, hospitals in large Byzantine cities were staffed primarily by paid male assistants and male nurses. These hospitals were established as almshouses, and care of the sick was only secondary (Bullough & Bullough, 1993).

Medical practices in Western Europe remained basically unchanged until the 11th and 12th centuries, when formal medical education for physicians was required in a university setting. Although there were not enough physicians to care for all the sick, other caregivers were not required to receive any formal education or training. The dominant caregivers in the Byzantine setting were men; however, this was not true in the rural parts of the Eastern Roman Empire and in the West. In these societies, nursing was viewed as a natural nurturing job for women.

Renaissance

During the Renaissance (A.D. 1400–1550), interest in the arts and sciences emerged. This was also the time of many geographic explorations by Europeans. As a result, the world literally expanded.

Because of renewed interest in science, universities were established, but no formal nursing schools were founded. Because of social status and customs, women were not encouraged to leave their homes; they instead continued to fulfill the traditional role of nurturer/caregiver in the home.

Enlightenment and the Industrial Revolution

With the beginning of the Industrial Revolution came technology that led to a proliferation of factories. Conditions for the factory workers were deplorable. Long hours, grueling work, and unsafe conditions prevailed in the workplace. The health of laborers received little, if any, attention.

Medical schools were founded, including the Royal College of Surgeons in London in 1800. In France, men who were barbers also functioned as surgeons by performing procedures such as leeching, giving enemas, and extracting teeth.

At the end of the 18th century, there were no standards for nurses who worked in hospitals. In the early to mid-1800s, nursing was considered unseemly for women, even though some hospitals (almshouses) relied on women to make beds, scrub floors, and bathe the poor. Most nursing care was still performed in the home by female relatives of the ill.

Religious Influences

The strong influence of religions on the development of nursing started in India in 800–600 B.C. and flourished in Greece and Ireland in 3 B.C. via male nurse–priests.

In 1836, Theodor Fleidner, a pastor in Kaiserswerth, Germany, revived the Lutheran Order of Deaconesses to care for those in a hospital he had founded. He established the first real school of nursing to educate the deaconesses in the care of the sick. These deaconesses of Kaiserswerth became famous because they were the only ones formally trained in nursing. Pastor Fleidner had a profound influence on nursing through Florence Nightingale, who received her nurse's training at the Kaiserswerth Institute.

The Catholic Church established religious orders that were devoted to caring for the sick and poor. Secular nursing was not an acceptable option for women. Only nurses who functioned within a religious order received social approval. Social conditions and the need for nurses in the mid-19th century, however, set the stage for the reforms instituted by Florence Nightingale (discussed following).

The order of the Nursing Sisters of the Holy Cross was founded in LeMans, France by Father Bassil Moreau in 1841. Also in 1841, a Father Sorin brought four sisters to Notre Dame in South Bend, Indiana. In 1844, these sisters established St. Mary's Academy in Bertrand, Michigan. In 1855, the school was moved to Notre Dame and became known as Saint Mary's College, which later had a strong influence on the emerging role of women (Wall, 1993).

Florence Nightingale

Florence Nightingale (1820–1910) is considered the founder of modern nursing. She grew up in a wealthy, upper-class family in England during the mid-1800s. Unlike other young women of her era, Nightingale received a thorough education, including studies in Greek, Latin, history, mathematics, and philosophy. She had always been interested in relieving suffering and caring for the sick. Social mores of the time made it impossible for her to consider caring for others because she was not a member of a religious order. After receiving encouragement from a family visitor, Dr. Samuel Gridley Howe, however, she became a nurse over the objections of society and her family.

After completing the 3-month course of study at Kaiserswerth Institute, Nightingale became active in reforming health care. Britain's war in the Crimea presented her with the opportunity to volunteer with 38 other nurses to serve in the battle-site hospital (Figure 4-1). The physicians in charge relegated the nurses to nonclient care duties. Florence Nightingale persisted in advocating cleanliness, good nutrition, and fresh air. When battle casualties mounted, the nurses were presented with the chance to prove their worth. They worked around the clock, caring for the wounded, carrying oil lamps to light their way in the darkness. The symbol of the oil lamp is still used today in nursing and is responsible for Florence Nightingale being called the "Lady With The Lamp." The implementation

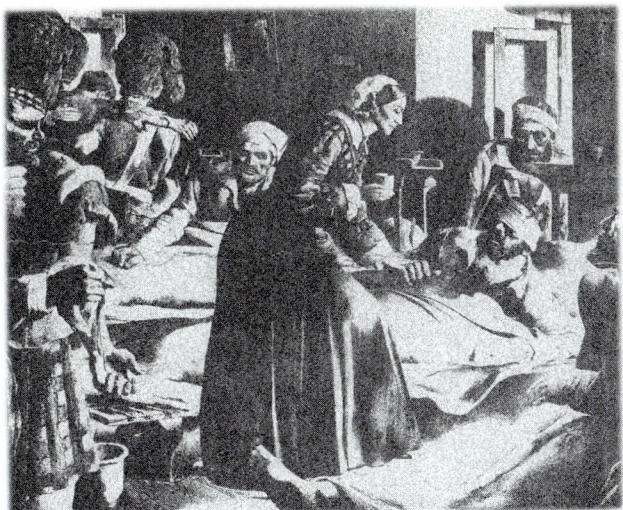

Figure 4-1 Florence Nightingale in the Crimea *(Photo courtesy of Parke, Davis & Company, a division of Warner-Lambert Company)*

of her principles in the areas of nursing practice and environmental modifications resulted in reduced **morbidity** (illness) and **mortality** (death) rates during the war.

Nightingale worked to further develop the public's awareness of the need for educated nurses and forged the future of nursing education as a result of her experiences in training nurses to care for British soldiers. She established the Nightingale Training School of Nurses at St. Thomas' Hospital in London. This was the first school for nurses that provided both theory-based knowledge and clinical skill building. She revolutionalized not only the public's perception of nursing but also the method for educating nurses. Some of Nightingale's novel beliefs about nursing and nursing education were the need for:

- A holistic framework inclusive of illness and health;
- A theoretical basis for nursing practice;
- A liberal education as a foundation of nursing practice;
- An environment that promotes healing; and
- A body of nursing knowledge distinct from medical knowledge (Macrae, 1995).

Nightingale introduced many other concepts that, although unique in her time, are still used today. Specifically, she advocated (1) a systematic method of assessing clients; (2) individualizing care on the basis of the client's needs and preferences; and (3) maintaining confidentiality.

Nightingale also recognized the influence of environmental factors on health. She advocated that nurses provide clean surroundings and fresh air and light to improve the quality of care (Nightingale, 1969). Nightingale believed that nurses should be formally educated and should function as client advocates (Se-

landers, 1993). She is credited with being the originator of modern nursing because many of these beliefs and concepts are still advocated in nursing schools today.

Nursing and the Civil War

America's need for nurses increased dramatically during the Civil War (1861–1865). The Sisters of the Holy Cross were the first to respond to the need for nurses during this war. Answering a request from Indiana's governor, 12 sisters started caring for wounded soldiers. By the end of the war, 80 sisters had cared for soldiers in Illinois, Missouri, Kentucky, and Tennessee (Wall, 1993).

During the Civil War, nursing care was provided by the Sisters of Mercy, Daughters of Charity, Dominican Sisters, and the Franciscan Sisters of the Poor. These sisters were influenced by the roles assigned to women during the 19th century. Although they were submissive to authority, they were willing to take risks when human rights were threatened (Wall, 1993). Other women also volunteered to care for the soldiers of both the Union and Confederate armies (Figure 4-2). These women performed various duties, including the implementation of sanitary conditions in field hospitals.

Dorothea Dix (1802–1887), a New England schoolteacher, was appointed Superintendent of the Female Nurses of the Army in 1861; no woman had ever before been appointed to an administrative position by the federal government. As a result of her recruitment efforts, more than 2,000 women cared for the sick in the Union Army. After the Civil War, Dix concentrated her energies on reforming treatment of the mentally ill (Johnson, 1997).

Clara Barton (1821–1912) volunteered her nursing services during the Civil War and, in 1881, organized the Red Cross in the United States.

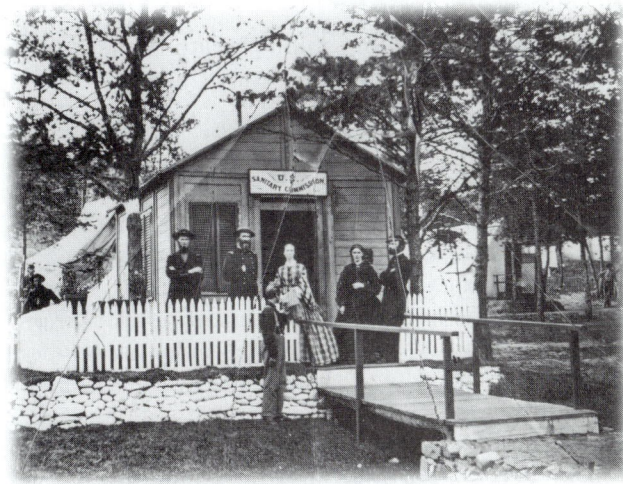

Figure 4-2 During the Civil War, women were instrumental in the effort to minimize the risk of spreading contagious diseases among wounded soldiers. *(Photo courtesy of Corbis-Bettmann)*

The Women's Movement

In 1848, the Women's Rights Convention in Seneca Falls, New York, signaled the beginnings of social unrest. Women were not considered equal to men, society did not value education for women, and women did not have the right to vote. With suffrage, not only were the rights of women advocated, but the nursing profession itself advanced. By the mid-1900s, more women were being accepted into colleges and universities, even though only limited numbers of university-based nursing programs were available.

Nursing Pioneers and Leaders

Modern nursing was forged by the contributions of many outstanding nurses through the years. The establishment of public health nursing, the provision of rural health care services, and the advancement of nursing education occurred as a result of the work of nurse pioneers and leaders, some of whom are discussed following. Note that the term *trained nurse* was used historically as the predecessor of *registered nurse*.

Lillian Wald

Lillian Wald (1867–1940) spent her life providing nursing care to the indigent population. In 1893, as the first community health nurse, she founded public health nursing with the establishment of the Henry Street Settlement Service (Figure 4-3) in New York City (Silverstein, 1994). Wald was a tireless reformer who:

- Improved housing conditions in tenement districts;
- Supported education for the mentally challenged;
- Advocated passage of more lenient immigration regulations; and
- Initiated change of child labor laws and founded the Children's Bureau of the U.S. Department of Labor.

In addition to initiating public health nursing, Wald also established a school of nursing.

Isabel Hampton Robb

Isabel Hampton Robb (1860–1910) founded several nursing organizations, including the Superintendents' Society in 1893 and the Nurses' Associated Alumnae of the United States and Canada in 1896 (Figure 4-4). She recognized the necessity of nurse participation in professional organizations to establish unity on positions and issues across the profession. She was instrumental in establishing both the American Nurses Association (ANA) and the National League of Nursing Education, the predecessor of the National League for Nursing (NLN). Robb was also an early supporter of the rights of nursing students. She called for shorter working hours and emphasized the role of the nursing student as learner instead of employee.

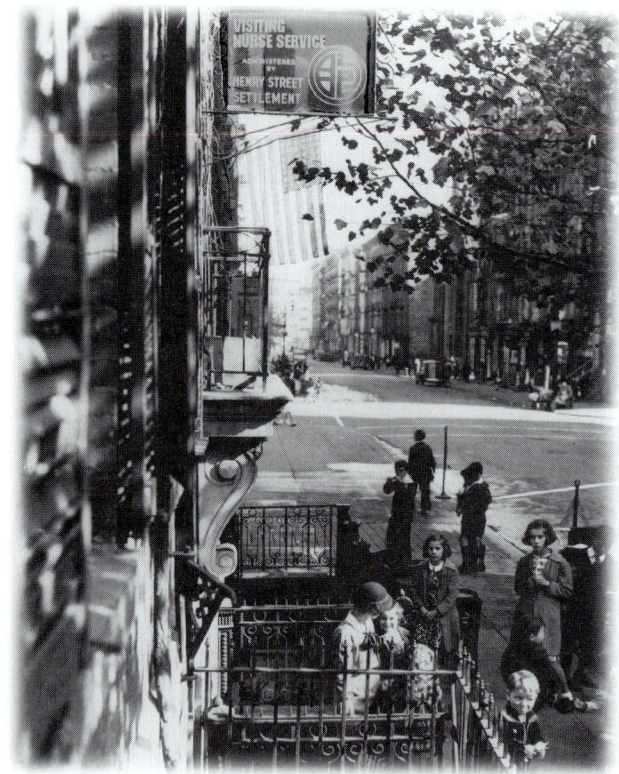

Figure 4-3 Nurses at the Henry Street Settlement in New York City *(Photo courtesy of Visiting Nurses Service of New York)*

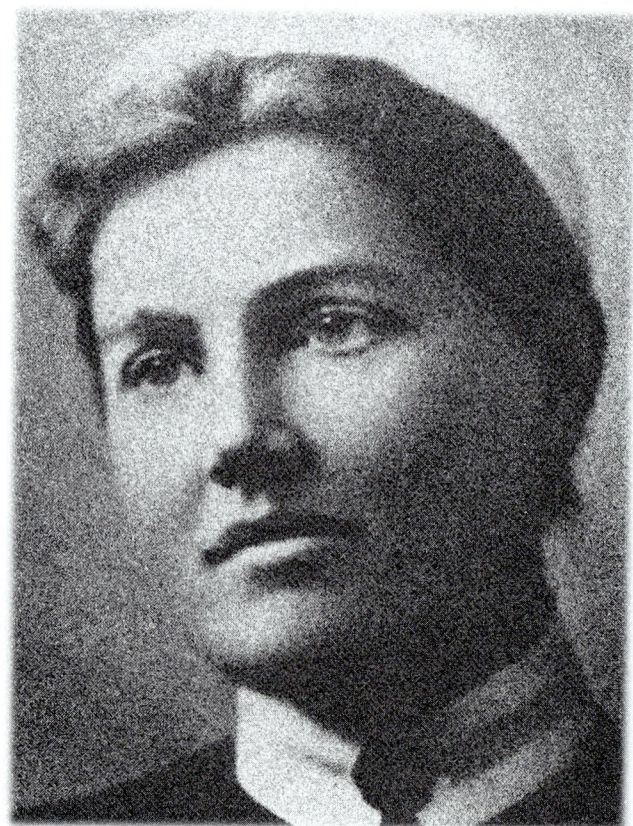

Figure 4-4 Isabel Hampton Robb *(Photo courtesy of the American Nurses Association)*

Adelaide Nutting

Adelaide Nutting (1858–1947) was a nursing educator, historian, and scholar. She actively campaigned for the education of nurses in university settings and was the first nurse to be appointed to a university professorship.

Lavinia Dock

An influential leader in nursing education was Lavinia Dock (1858–1956), who graduated from Bellevue Training School for Nurses in 1886. Early in her nursing practice, she worked at the Henry Street Settlement House in New York City, providing visiting nursing services to the indigent. She wrote one of the first nursing textbooks, *Materia Medica for Nurses*. Dock wrote many other books and was the first editor of the *American Journal of Nursing* (*AJN*).

Mary Breckenridge

In 1925, Mary Breckenridge (1881–1965) introduced a system of delivering health care to rural America. This decentralized system for primary nursing care services in the Kentucky Appalachian Mountains, called the Frontier Nursing Service, lowered the childbirth mortality rate in Leslie County, Kentucky, from the highest in the nation to below the national average.

Mamie Hale

In 1942, Mamie Hale was hired by the Arkansas Health Department to upgrade the educational programs for midwives (Figure 4-5). Hale, a graduate of Tuskegee School of Nurse–Midwifery, gained the support of granny midwives, public health nurses, and obstetricians. Through education, Hale decreased superstition and illiteracy among those functioning as midwives. Hale's efforts resulted in improved mortality rates for both mothers and infants (Bell, 1993).

Mary Mahoney

America's first African American professional nurse, Mary Mahoney (1845–1926), was a noted nursing leader who encouraged a respect for cultural diversity. Today, the ANA bestows the Mary Mahoney Award in recognition of individuals who make significant contributions toward improving relationships among multicultural groups.

Linda Richards

In 1873, the first diploma from an American training school for nurses was awarded to Linda Richards (1841–1930). Richards established numerous hospital-based training schools for nurses. She also introduced the practice of keeping nurses' notes and physicians' orders as part of medical records, and began the practice of nurses' wearing uniforms. As the first Superintendent of Nurses at Massachusetts General Hospital, she demonstrated that trained nurses gave better care than those without formal nursing education.

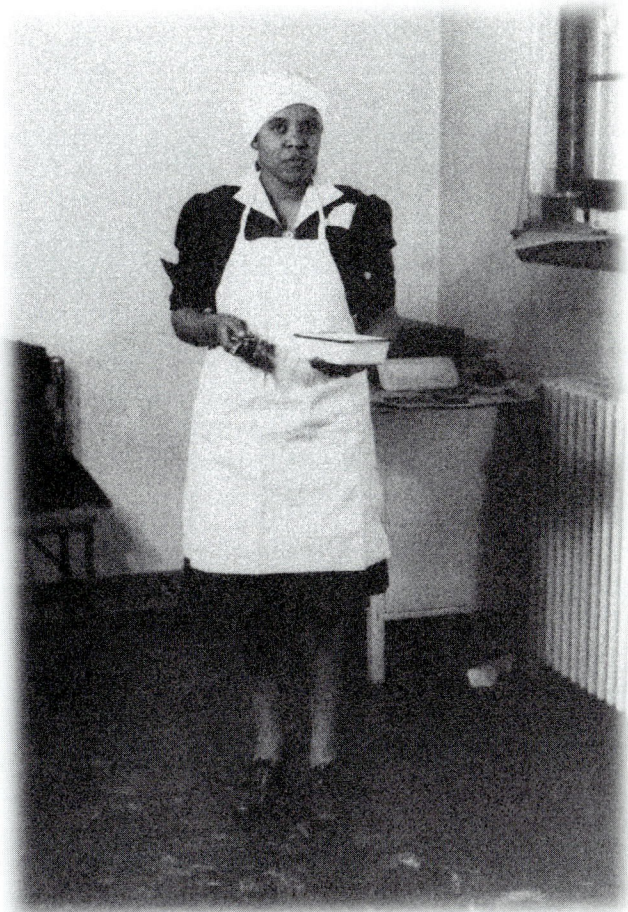

Figure 4-5 Mamie Hale *(Photo courtesy of Historical Research Center, University of Arkansas for Medical Sciences Library, Little Rock, RG 515, Box 47)*

PRACTICAL NURSING PIONEER SCHOOLS

Women who cared for others, but who had no formal education, often called themselves "practical nurses." Formal education for practical nursing began in the 1890s. The first schools were Ballard School, Thompson Practical Nursing School, and Household Nursing Association School of Attendant Nursing.

Ballard School

In 1892, the Ballard School, funded by Lucinda Ballard, was opened in New York City by the YWCA. It offered several courses for women, one of which was practical nursing. The 3-month course in simple nursing care focused on the care of infants, children, elders, and disabled persons in their own homes. The course included cooking, nutrition, basic science, and basic nursing procedures. When the YWCA was reorganized in 1949, the school closed.

Thompson Practical Nursing School

Thomas Thompson of Brattleboro, Vermont, left money in his will to help women who were making shirts for the army and were receiving only one dollar per dozen. His executor, Richard Bradley, saw the need for nursing service and, in 1907, established a practical nursing school in Brattleboro. It is still operating today and is accredited by the NLN.

Household Nursing School

In 1918, a group of women in Boston were concerned about providing nursing care for people who were sick at home. After talking with Richard Bradley, they opened the Household Nursing Association School of Attendant Nursing. The name was later changed to Shepard-Gill School of Practical Nursing. It closed in 1984.

NURSING IN THE 20TH CENTURY

The beginning of the 20th century brought about changes that have influenced contemporary nursing. Several landmark reports about medical and nursing education, as well as some contemporary reports, are discussed following. The establishment of visiting nurse associations and their use of protocols are also discussed.

Flexner Report

In 1910, Abraham Flexner, supported by a Carnegie grant, visited the 155 medical schools in the United States and Canada. The goal of the resulting Flexner report, which was based on his findings, was to impose accountability for medical education. Flexner's study resulted in the following changes: closure of inadequate medical schools, consolidation of schools with limited resources, creation of nonprofit status for remaining schools, and establishment of medical education in university settings and based on standards and strong economic resources.

Seeing the value and impact of the Flexner report on medical education, Adelaide Nutting, together with colleagues from the Superintendents' Society, presented a proposal to the Carnegie Foundation in 1911 to study nursing education. Although the foundation never allocated monies to study nursing education, it did support educational studies in other disciplines such as law, dentistry, and teaching.

Although the efforts of Nutting and other nursing leaders went unheeded, in 1906 Richard Olding Beard successfully established a 3-year diploma school of nursing at the University of Minnesota under the College of Medicine.

Early Insurance Plans

At the turn of the 20th century, there were more than 4,000 hospitals and 1,000 schools of nursing. It was at this time that the concepts of third-party payments and prepaid health insurance were instituted. Third-party payment refers to payment made by someone other than the recipient of health care (usually an insurance company) for the health care services provided. Prepaid medical plans were started in lumber and mining camps of the Pacific Northwest, where employers contracted for medical services, for which they paid a monthly fee. This led to the establishment of the Bureau of Medical Services, where the employer contracted for medical services and the subscriber selected one of the physicians in the bureau.

Lillian Wald suggested the establishment of a national health insurance plan when she was the first president of the National Organization for Public Health Nursing.

Blue Cross and Blue Shield

The Depression provided the main impetus for the growth of insurance plans. The philosophy in the United States of health care for all further contributed to the growth of insurance plans. In 1920, American hospitals offered a prepaid hospital plan; this, in turn, led to the Baylor Plan, which eventually became the prototype of Blue Cross.

The American Hospital Association pioneered the development of an insurance company to provide benefits to subscribers who were hospitalized. Blue Shield was developed by the American Medical Association to provide reimbursement for medical services provided to subscribers. In 1933 the American Hospital Association endorsed Blue Cross, and in 1938 the American Medical Association endorsed Blue Shield.

The federal government became more involved in health care delivery in 1935 with the passage of the Social Security Act, which provided for (among other things) benefits for elderly persons, child welfare, and federal funding for training of health care personnel. During World War II, the U.S. government extended the benefits for military personnel to include health care for veterans and their dependents.

Visiting Nurses Associations

In 1901, at the suggestion of Lillian Wald, the Metropolitan Life Insurance Company, which provided visiting nursing services to its policyholders, entered into an agreement with the Henry Street Settlement. Wald worked with Metropolitan to expand the services of the Henry Street Settlement to other cities; thus, one form of managed care began.

Nurses providing care in the home environment experienced greater autonomy of practice than did hospital-based nurses (Figure 4-6). This led to conflicts with some physicians regarding the scope of medical

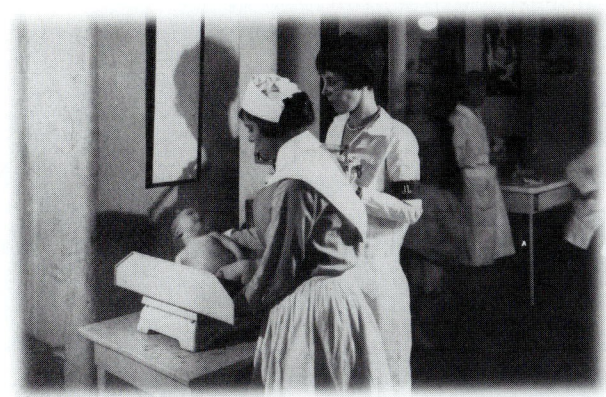

Figure 4-6 A Baby Being Weighed by a Student Nurse and a Junior League Volunteer in 1929 *(Photo courtesy of Touro Infirmary Archives, New Orleans, LA)*

practice versus that of nursing practice. Some physicians thought nurses were taking over their practice, whereas other physicians encouraged nurses to do whatever was necessary to care for the sick at home.

In 1912, in an effort to provide direction to home health staff nurses, the Chicago Visiting Nurse Association developed a list of standing orders for nurses to follow in providing home care. These orders were to direct the nursing care of clients when the nurse did not have specific orders from a physician. Thus, the groundwork for nursing protocols was established.

Landmark Reports in Nursing Education

During the first half of the 20th century, a number of reports were issued concerning nursing education and practice. Three of these reports, the Goldmark, the Brown, and the Institute of Research and Service in Nursing Education, are discussed following.

Goldmark Report

In 1918, Adelaide Nutting (relentless in her efforts to document the need for nursing education reform) approached the Rockefeller Foundation for support. Funding was provided, and, in 1919, the Committee for the Study of Nursing Education was established to investigate the training of public health nurses. Josephine Goldmark, a social worker, served as the secretary to the committee.

As secretary, Goldmark developed the methodology of data collection and analysis for a small sampling of the 1,800 schools of nursing in existence. The study of 23 of the best nursing schools across the nation represented a cross sample of schools—small and large, public and private.

The Goldmark report, entitled Nursing and Nursing Education in the United States, was published in 1923. Goldmark identified the major weakness of the hospital-based training programs as that of putting the needs of the institution (service delivery) before the needs of the student (education). Nursing tradition and the apprenticeship form of education reinforced putting the needs of the client before the learning needs of the student.

Some major inadequacies in nursing education as identified by the study were limited resources, low admission standards, lack of supervision, poorly trained instructors, and failure to correlate clinical practice with theory. The report concluded that for nursing to be on equal footing with other disciplines, nursing education should occur in the university setting.

Brown Report

In 1948, Esther Lucille Brown, a social anthropologist, published *Nursing for the Future and Nursing Reconsidered: A Study for Change*. Several recommendations were put forth in this study, including the need for nurses to demonstrate greater professional competence by moving nursing education from the hospital to the university setting.

Although published 20 years after the Goldmark report, the Brown report identified many of the same problems in diploma education; for instance, nursing students were still being used for service by the hospitals, and inadequate resources and authoritarianism in hospitals still prevailed in nursing education.

Brown recognized that the university setting would provide the proper intellectual climate for educating the professional nurse. Visionary nurse educators were securing libraries, laboratories, and clinical facilities as necessary learning resources. Professional endeavors such as research and publication were being implemented by nurse leaders.

Institute of Research and Service in Nursing Education Report

The 1950s addressed different aspects of nursing. Post World War II, a deficit in the supply of nurses coincided with an increased demand for nursing services. Hospital closures were one result of the nursing shortage. Some contributing factors to the scarce supply of nurses were the low esteem of nursing as a profession, long hours combined with a heavy workload, and low salaries.

The Institute of Research and Service in Nursing Education Report resulted in the establishment of practical nursing under Title III of the Health Amendment Act of 1955. This led to a proliferation of practical nursing schools in the United States.

Other Health Care Initiatives

In the 1960s, health care services were provided to the elderly and the indigent populations with the federal programs of Medicare and Medicaid.

This era also saw passage of the Nurse Training Act (1964), which provided federal funds to expand enrollments in schools of nursing. Federal funds were used to construct nursing schools, and student loans and scholarships were made available to nursing students.

The Health Maintenance Organization Act of 1973 provided an alternative to the private health insurance industry. **Health maintenance organizations** (HMOs) are prepaid health plans that provide primary health care services for a predetermined fee. Because fees are set in advance of services being rendered, HMOs provide cost-effective services. **Primary health care** refers to the client's point of entry into the health care system and includes assessment, diagnosis, treatment, coordination of care, education, preventive services, and surveillance.

The National Commission for Manpower Study, released in 1977, resulted in amendments to the House of Representatives 2504 of Title XVIII of the Social Security Act, which provided payment for rural health clinic services. Through the efforts of Anne Zimmerman, former President of the ANA, the bill was amended to substitute the term **primary care providers** (health care providers whom a client sees first for health care) for *physician extenders,* thereby, allowing nurse practitioners to be paid directly for their services. This represented the first time that nurses could be directly reimbursed for care they rendered.

Costs and Quality Controls

During the 1970s, the cost-control systems of various federal health programs were inadequate because of the rapid escalation of health care expenditures. Consequently, the Tax Equity Fiscal Responsibility Act (TEFRA) of 1982 was created in response to the $287 billion spent on health care in 1981. At the same time that the federal government was trying to control costs with TEFRA and prospective payment legislation, concern was also growing regarding the quality of health care.

Although business and industry embraced quality control systems in the 1940s and 1950s, the health care industry failed to see the need for such controls until the 1980s. The Joint Commission on Accreditation of Healthcare Organizations' (JCAHO) agenda for change in the late 1980s emphasized monitoring quality for outcomes rather than process, thus advocating change from a static quality assurance system to dynamic quality improvement. The JCAHO (1996) views quality of care as an ongoing process of continuously looking for ways to improve the care provided.

Health Care Reform

With an ever-increasing number (over 60 million) of Americans being uninsured or underinsured, health care access and costs have become a major focus of attention in the 1990s (Edleman & Mandle, 1998). Children are especially at risk for having their health care neglected, with one in five children in the United States being uninsured (Baker, 1994).

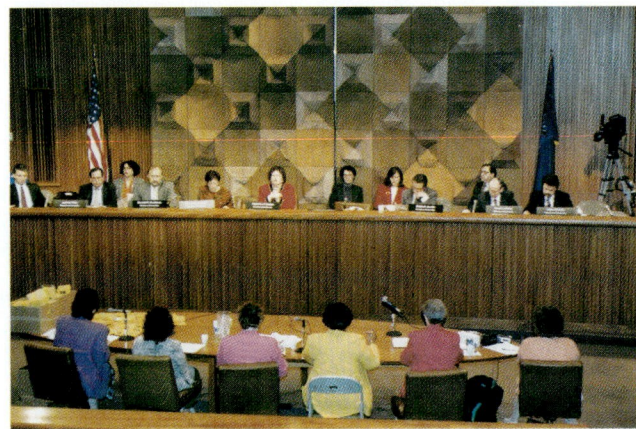

Figure 4-7 Nurses Making a Presentation Before a State Legislature *(Photo courtesy of the New York State Nurses Association)*

Nursing as a profession has made great strides in effecting federal and state health care legislation (Figure 4-7). Hospitals are moving away from the controlling, bureaucratic entities they once were and instead are more often being characterized by an environment of shared governance, where nurses have a voice in both administrative and clinical decision making. Nurses are serving as case managers and are working in collaboration with physicians and other health care providers.

Nurses are working to obtain prescriptive privileges for all advanced practitioners. Differentiated practice models are being developed and should settle the issue of educational preparation for entry into practice. The foundation has been laid for nursing to move forward with alternate client care delivery models that will allow access to care at a reasonable cost.

Health care providers are managing their organizations as does industry, focusing on quality management systems and competitive measures to market their services, and on information systems to facilitate data collection and cost efficiency.

NURSING EDUCATION

Educational programs that prepare graduates to take a licensing examination must be approved by a state board of nursing. Boards approve entry level programs to ensure the safe practice of nursing by setting minimum educational requirements and guaranteeing that the graduate of the program is an eligible candidate to take a licensing examination. In the United States, candidates must pass the National Council Licensure Examination (NCLEX) to obtain a license to practice nursing.

Types of Programs

Two types of entry level nursing programs are available in the United States: licensed practical or vocational nurse (LPN or LVN) and registered nurse (RN).

An entry level educational program is one that prepares graduates to take a licensing examination. Graduates of the licensed practical/vocational programs take the NCLEX for practical nurses (NCLEX-PN), and graduates of registered nurse programs take the NCLEX for registered nurses (NCLEX-RN).

Postgraduate programs prepare nurses to practice in various roles as advanced practice registered nurses (APRNs). Individual states have varying statutory provisions for APRNs.

Licensed Practical/Vocational Nursing

Licensed practical nurses (LPNs) or licensed vocational nurses (LVNs, as they are called in Texas and California), work under the supervision of an RN or other licensed provider such as a physician or dentist. The LP/VN, like the RN, was first trained in hospitals. The Smith Hughes Act passed by Congress in 1917 gave impetus to the formation of vocational-school–based practical nursing programs. Today, there are more than 1,000 hospital, vocational school, and community college licensed practical/vocational programs in the United States. Programs are state approved and in some cases also have accreditation by the NLN. **Accreditation** is a process by which a voluntary, nongovernmental agency or organization appraises and grants accredited status to institutions and/or programs or services that meet predetermined structure, process, and outcome criteria. These educational programs are generally 1 year in length and provide both **didactic** (systematic presentation of information) and **clinical** (observing and caring for living clients) experience. The education is focused on basic nursing skills and direct client care. Although the majority of clinical experience is in hospitals, long-term care facilities, physician's offices, home health agencies, and ambulatory care facilities are also used.

Admission generally requires a high school diploma or General Education Development (GED) certificate. Schools may require a preentrance examination that assesses such skills as math, reading, and writing.

Once licensed, the LP/VN is prepared to work in structured settings such as hospital, long-term care, home health, medical office, and ambulatory care facilities. Just as the RN has been delegated duties previously considered the domain of the physician, the LP/VN has been assigned duties once considered the domain of the RN. Many hospitals offer programs that provide levels of advancement for the LP/VN.

The National Federation of Licensed Practical Nurses, Inc. has written standards of nursing practice for LP/VN. They are listed in Table 4-2.

Registered Nursing

Registered nurses are graduates of state-approved and, in many cases, NLN-accredited programs. They are typically prepared for entry into practice in one of three ways: associate degree nursing programs, hospital diploma programs, or baccalaureate degree nursing programs.

Associate Degree Programs Associate degree programs are typically 2 years in length and are offered through community colleges but may also be offered as options at 4-year–degree-granting universities. The graduate receives an Associate Degree in Nursing (ADN). In 1997, 876 associate degree programs produced 60% of nurse graduates, as compared to 3% of graduates in 1960 (NLN, 1998). Traditionally, program content reflected basic skill preparation and emphasized clinical practice in the hospital setting. Because of the decreasing demand for hospital beds, however, students are now likely to spend a higher number of clinical hours in community-based institutions (e.g., ambulatory settings, schools, and clinics).

Diploma Programs Diploma nursing programs are typically 3 years in length and are offered by hospitals. Most diploma programs are now affiliated with colleges or universities that grant college credit for select courses. Graduates of these programs receive a diploma as opposed to a college degree.

Program content prepares the graduate in basic nursing skills particularly suitable for hospitalized clients. In 1994, however, the majority of diploma schools reported using community-based settings such as physicians' offices, clinics, visiting nurse services, and health departments as training sites (NLN, 1998).

Although prominent in the early history of nursing education, diploma nursing programs today produce only 6% of graduates (NLN, 1998). However, 24% of RNs working in 1996 were initially educated in diploma programs (U.S. Department of Health and Human Services [USDHHS], 1996).

Baccalaureate Degree Programs Baccalaureate degree programs, typically 4 years in length, are offered through colleges and universities. The graduate receives a Bachelor of Science in Nursing (BSN). These programs emphasize more preparation for practice in nonhospital settings, broader scientific content, and systematic problem-solving tools for autonomous and collaborative practice. In 1997, 523 baccalaureate programs produced 34% of all nursing graduates (NLN, 1998).

Staff Development and Continuing Education

Once a nurse is in practice, both staff development and continuing education are used to maintain the needed knowledge and skills for contemporary practice. **Staff development** typically occurs in the setting of employment and is described as the delivery of instruction to assist the nurse to achieve the goals of the employer. It is guided by the accreditation standards of the JCAHO and ANA's *Standards for Nursing Staff Development* (ANA, 1990).

Orientation is an important organizational tool for

Table 4-2 NURSING PRACTICE STANDARDS FOR THE LICENSED PRACTICAL/ VOCATIONAL NURSE

Education

The licensed practical/vocational nurse:

1. Shall complete a formal education program in practical nursing approved by the appropriate nursing authority in a state.

2. Shall successfully pass the National Council Licensure Examination for Practical Nurses.

3. Shall participate in initial orientation within the employing institution.

Legal/Ethical Status

The licensed practical/vocational nurse:

1. Shall hold a current license to practice nursing as an LP/VN in accordance with the law of the state wherein employed.

2. Shall know the scope of nursing practice authorized by the Nursing Practice Act in the state wherein employed.

3. Shall have a personal commitment to fulfill the legal responsibilities inherent in good nursing practice.

4. Shall take responsible actions in situations wherein there is unprofessional conduct by a peer or other health care provider.

5. Shall recognize and commit to meet the ethical and moral obligations of the practice of nursing.

6. Shall not accept or perform professional responsibilities that the individual knows (s)he is not competent to perform.

Practice

The licensed practical/vocational nurse:

1. Shall accept assigned responsibilities as an accountable member of the health care team.

2. Shall function within the limits of educational preparation and experience, as related to the assigned duties.

3. Shall function with other members of the health care team in promoting and maintaining health, preventing disease and disability, caring for and rehabilitating individuals who are experiencing an altered health state, and contributing to the ultimate quality of life until death.

4. Shall know and utilize the nursing process in planning, implementing, and evaluating health services and nursing care for the individual patient or group.

   a. Planning: The planning of nursing includes:

      1) Assessment of health status of the individual patient, the family, and community groups

      2) Analysis of the information gained from assessment

      3) Identification of health goals

   b. Implementation: The plan for nursing care is put into practice to achieve the stated goals and includes:

      1) Observing, recording, and reporting significant changes that require intervention or different goals

      2) Applying nursing knowledge and skills to promote and maintain health, to prevent disease and disability, and to optimize functional capabilities of an individual patient

      3) Assisting the patient and family with activities of daily living and encouraging self-care as appropriate

      4) Carrying out therapeutic regimens and protocols prescribed by an RN, physician, or other persons authorized by state law.

   c. Evaluation: The plan for nursing care and its implementations are evaluated to measure the progress toward the stated goals and will include appropriate persons and/or groups to determine:

      1) The relevancy of current goals in relation to the progress of the individual patient

      2) The involvement of the recipients of care in the evaluation process

      3) The quality of the nursing action in the implementation of the plan

      4) A reordering of priorities or new goal setting in the care plan

5. Shall participate in peer review and other evaluation processes.

6. Shall participate in the development of policies concerning the health and nursing needs of society and in the roles and functions of the LP/VN.

Continuing Education

The licensed practical/vocational nurse:

1. Shall be responsible for maintaining the highest possible level of professional competence at all times.

2. Shall periodically reassess career goals and select continuing education activities that will help to achieve these goals.

3. Shall take advantage of continuing education opportunities that will lead to personal growth and professional development.

4. Shall seek and participate in continuing education activities that are approved for credit by appropriate organizations, such as the NFLPN.

Specialized Nursing Practice

The licensed practical/vocational nurse:

1. Shall have had at least one year's experience in nursing at the staff level.

2. Shall present personal qualifications that are indicative of potential abilities for practice in the chosen specialized nursing area.

3. Shall present evidence of completion of a program or course that is approved by an appropriate agency to provide the knowledge and skills necessary for effective nurisng services in the specialized field.

4. Shall meet all of the standards of practice as set forth in this document.

Reprinted with permission of the National Federation of Licensed Practical Nurses, Inc.

recruitment and retention. Orientation sessions typically occur at the initiation of employment and whenever positions and roles change. The sessions include information unique to the institution of employment, such as philosophy, goals, policies and procedures, role expectations, facilities, resources and special services, and assessment and development of competency with equipment and supplies used in the work setting (ANA, 1990).

In-service education occurs after orientation and supports the nurse in acquiring, maintaining, and increasing skills to fulfill assigned responsibilities.

Nurses are responsible for their own continuing education. Continuing education offers both personal and professional growth to the nurse and constitutes an essential dimension of lifelong learning. In some states, license renewal depends on acquiring continuing education units (CEUs) according to the board of nursing's rules. Lifelong learning is essential to career development and competency achievement in nursing practice.

Trends in Nursing Education

Trends in nursing education reflect issues in nursing, nursing education, delivery of care, and the public's health. At the heart of many of these trends are two fundamental issues: competency development and delivery of care.

Competency Development

Debate concerning multiple education levels for entry level nursing practice will continue. The focus on basic competency demonstration by all entry level graduates regardless of educational level is likely to gain much greater support from nursing because it allows for both consensus about the outcome (competency) and diversity (innovation) about the process of achieving the competency (Figure 4-8). Competency development in nursing education is stimulating many changes in nursing education.

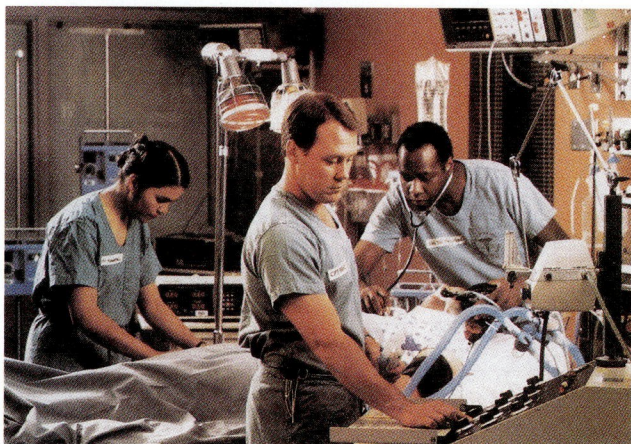

Figure 4-8 Competent nurses deliver highly advanced care to clients. *("Be All You Can Be" courtesy of the U.S. Government, as represented by the Secretary of the Army)*

Delivery of Care

The demand for nursing care will continue to be driven by a larger aging population that makes use of long-term care and home health services. Other changes will include: expansion of primary and preventive care which focuses on health promotion and wellness; an increased use of ambulatory care services because they are less expensive; increased complexity of health care delivery which requires well-educated nurses; and increased demand to provide health services such as prenatal care, well child clinics, adolescent clinics, and neighbor care clinics, to underserved populations (such as inner city residents).

Managed care arrangements are the delivery systems of the future. They emphasize wellness, disease prevention, and health promotion. What a natural fit for nursing practice! Nursing has long been aware that health behaviors, genetics, the environment, and biological factors all contribute to health. As additional contributing factors of disease point to health behaviors and preventive interventions, nursing education must provide a strong scientific base in health-seeking and health behavior frameworks that can prevent premature morbidity and mortality. The Healthy People 2000 objectives (Table 4-3) will be accomplished only through the intervention of nursing in collaboration with other disciplines.

NURSING ORGANIZATIONS

Nursing organizations exist for LP/VNs and RNs. Some organizations also welcome as members those who are interested in nursing but who are not nurses. There are also many specialty nursing organizations. Table 4-4 provides pertinent information about the various general nursing organizations.

American Nurses Association

The ANA represents registered nurses through its constituent state organizations. The ANA fosters high standards of nursing practice, promotes the economic and general welfare of nurses in the workplace, projects a positive and realistic view of nursing, and lobbies Congress and regulatory agencies on health care issues affecting nurses and the public (ANA, 1998).

National Association of Practical Nurse Education and Service, Inc.

Originally called the Association of Practical Nurse Schools, this organization was dedicated exclusively to practical nursing. The multidisciplinary membership planned the first standard curriculum for practical nursing. The name was changed to National Association of Practical Nurse Education (NAPNE) in 1942. In 1945, they established an accrediting service for

Table 4-3 HEALTHY PEOPLE 2000 OBJECTIVES

Goals

- Increase the span of healthy life
- Reduce health disparities
- Achieve access to preventive services

Objectives

Health Promotion

1. Physical activity and fitness
2. Nutrition
3. Tobacco
4. Alcohol and other drugs
5. Family planning
6. Mental health and mental disorders
7. Violent and abusive behavior
8. Educational and community-based programs

Health Protection

9. Unintentional injuries
10. Occupational safety and health
11. Environmental health

12. Food and drug safety
13. Oral health

Prevention Services

14. Maternal and infant health
15. Heart disease and stroke
16. Cancer
17. Diabetes and chronic disabling conditions
18. Human immunodeficiency virus infection
19. Sexually transmitted diseases
20. Immunization and infectious diseases
21. Clinical preventive services

Surveillance and Data Systems

22. Surveillance and data systems

Age-Related Objectives

- Children
- Adolescents and young adults
- Adults
- Older adults

From Healthy People 2000: National Health Promotion and Disease Prevention Objectives *(DHHS Publication No. PHS 91-50212),* by U.S. Department of Health and Human Services, 1990, Washington, DC: Author. Copyright 1990 by the U.S. Department of Health and Human Services.

Table 4-4 SELECTED NURSING ORGANIZATIONS

ORGANIZATION	DESCRIPTION
American Nurses Association (ANA)	Established: 1911 Purpose: To improve the quality of nursing care Activities: • Establish standards for nursing practice • Establish a professional code of ethics • Develop educational standards • Promote nursing research • Oversee a credentialing system • Influence legislation affecting health care • Protect the economic and general welfare of registered nurses • Assist with the professional development of nurses (i.e., by providing continuing education programs) Membership: • Registered nurses only • Federation of state nurses' associations • Individual, by joining respective state nurses' association Publications: • *American Journal of Nursing* • *American Nurse*

continued

Table 4-4 SELECTED NURSING ORGANIZATIONS *continued*

ORGANIZATION	DESCRIPTION
National Association for Practical Nurse Education and Service, Inc. (NAPNES)	Established: 1941 Purpose: To improve the quality, education, and recognition of nursing schools and LP/VNs in the United States Activities: • Provide workshops, seminars, and continuing-education programs • Evaluate and certify continuing-education programs of others • Provide individual student professional liability insurance program • Inform legislatures and public on LP/VN issues • Authorize those who pass the CEPN-LTC to use the initials *CLTC* Membership: • LP/VNs • RNs, physicians, and caregivers in all fields • Practical/vocational nursing students Publications: • *Journal of Practical Nursing* • *NAPNES Forum*
National Federation of Licensed Practical Nurses, Inc. (NFLPN)	Established: 1949 Purpose: • Provide leadership for LP/VNs • Foster high standards of practical/vocational nursing education and practice • Encourage continuing education • Achieve recognition for LP/VNs • Advocate effective utilization of LP/VNs • Interpret role and function of LP/VNs • Represent practical/vocational nursing • Serve as central source of information on practical/vocational nursing education and practice Activities: • Promote continuing education of LP/VNs • Establish principles of ethics • Offer members an opportunity to participate in activities of the organization • Keep members informed on matters of interest and concern • Offer members best type of low-cost insurance • Represent and speak for LP/VNs in Congress • Encourage fellowship among LP/VNs • Develop mutual understanding and good will among members, other allied health groups, and the general public Membership: • Three-tier concept of local, state, and national enrollment • LP/VNs • Practical/vocational nursing students • Affiliate (person who has an interest in the work of NFLPN but is neither an LP/VN nor an LP/VN student) Publication: • *AJPN* (quarterly newsletter)
National League for Nursing (NLN)	Established: 1952 Purpose: To identify the nursing needs of society and to foster programs designed to meet these needs Activities: • Accredit (through voluntary participation from schools) nursing education programs • Conduct surveys to collect data on education programs

continued

Table 4-4 SELECTED NURSING ORGANIZATIONS *continued*

ORGANIZATION	DESCRIPTION

National League for Nursing (NLN) (*continued*)	• Provide continuing-education programs
	• Offer testing services, including:
	   Achievement tests for use in nursing schools
	   Preadmission testing for potential nursing students
	Membership:
	• Open to any individual or agency interested in improving nursing services or nursing education
	• Composed of both nurses and non-nurses
	Publication:
	• *Nursing & Health Care*

National Council of State Boards of Nursing, Inc. (NCSBN)	Established: 1978 Purpose: Provide an organization through which boards of nursing act and counsel together on matters that are of common interest and concern and that affect public health, safety, and welfare, including the development of licensing examinations in nursing Activities: • Develop and administer licensure examinations for registered nurse and licensed practical/vocational nurse candidates • Conduct job analyses that provide data required to support the NCLEX examinations and the test development process • Maintain a national disciplinary data bank • Monitor and analyze issues and trends in public policy, nursing practice, and nursing education that impact nursing regulation • Serve as the national clearinghouse of information on nursing regulation • Offer educational conferences and regional meetings Membership: • Boards of nursing in the 50 states, the District of Columbia, and five United States territories Publications: • *Issues* • *NCLEX-RN Program Reports* • *NCLEX-PN Program Reports*

Data from American Nurses Association Bylaws, by American Nurses Association, 1991, Washington, DC: Author; History of NAPNES, by National Association for Practical Nurse Education and Service, Inc., 1998, Silver Spring, MD: Author; All About NFLPN (On-line), by National Federation of Licensed Practical Nurses, 1998, Available: http://www.nflpn.org/allaboutnflpn.htm; Bylaws, by National League for Nursing, 1995, New York: Author; National Council Mission and Purpose (On-line), by National Council of State Boards of Nursing, Inc., 1998a, Available: http://www.ncsbn.org/files/aboutnc/mission.asp; Overview: Programs and Services of the National Council (On-line), by National Council of State Boards of Nursing, Inc., 1998b, Available: http://www.ncsbn.org/files/aboutnc/overview.asp

practical/vocational nursing schools. This service has been discontinued for some years. In 1959, the name was changed to National Association of Practical Nurse Education and Service (NAPNES, 1998).

National Federation of Licensed Practical Nurses, Inc.

The National Federation of Licensed Practical Nurses (NFLPN) was founded in 1949 by a group of LPNs who recognized that to gain status and recognition in the health field and to have a channel through which they could officially speak and act for themselves, they needed an organization of their own.

Since 1991, affiliate membership (lacking the rights to vote and hold office) has been available to anyone who is interested in the work of NFLPN but who is neither a practicing LP/VN nor an LP/VN student. The NFLPN is the official organization for LP/VNs (NFLPN, 1998a; NFLPN, 1998b).

National League for Nursing

The National League of Nursing Education changed its bylaws in 1952 to become the NLN. Because of the growth of practical/vocational nursing programs, the NLN established a Department of Practical Nursing Programs (now called Council of Practical Nursing

Programs, [CPNP]) in 1961. The NLN offers accreditation services to all nursing programs through an independent subsidiary called the National League for Nursing Accrediting Commission (NLNAC) (National League for Nursing History, 1997).

National Council of State Boards of Nursing

The National Council of State Boards of Nursing (NCSBN) was established in 1978 to assist member boards, collectively and individually, to promote safe and effective nursing practice in the interest of protecting public health and welfare. They have developed the NCLEX-PN and NCLEX-RN to test the entry level nursing competence of candidates for licensure as LP/VNs and RNs (National Council of State Boards of Nursing, 1997).

In 1996, they began the administration of the first large-scale, national certification examination available to LP/VNs. It is named the Certification Examination for Practical and Vocational Nurses in Long-Term Care (CEPN-LTC™). Those who pass the examination are certified in long-term care and are authorized by NAPNES to use the initials *CLTC* to signify their new status (National Council of State Boards of Nursing, 1996).

THE FUTURE OF NURSING

History is being made daily for nurses and other health care providers as the citizens of this country decide which way to move with health care reform initiatives. Pressing issues for nursing (e.g., third-party reimbursement and prescriptive privileges for advanced practitioners) will be determined by legislative outcomes. Nurses can make the most of this time of transformation, a time driven by societal needs (Mason & Leavitt, 1995).

PROFESSIONAL TIP

Professional Memberships

Every nurse should become involved in a nursing organization. Membership means more political clout for passing legislation to improve health care for all citizens and to improve the profession of nursing.

Nursing students must stay abreast of current issues and meet with local nursing leaders to discuss health care reform, alternative health care delivery models, and other issues. Then as graduates, they will be able to share this information with both the public and legislators.

SUMMARY

- Nursing is an art and a science whereby people are assisted in learning to care for themselves whenever possible and are cared for when they are unable to meet their own needs.
- By studying nursing history, the nurse is better able to understand such issues as autonomy, unity within the profession, supply and demand, salary, education, and current practice, and can thus promote the empowerment of nurses.
- Nursing's early history was heavily influenced by religious organizations and the need for nurses to care for soldiers during wartime.
- Florence Nightingale forged the future of nursing practice and education as a result of her experiences in training nurses to care for soldiers.
- Early American leaders, the professional organizations, and the landmark reports of nursing determined the infrastructure of current nursing practice.
- Influential nursing leaders such as Lillian Wald, Isabel Hampton Robb, Adelaide Nutting, and Lavinia Dock were instrumental in the advancement of nursing education and practice.
- Other nursing leaders such as Mary Breckenridge, Mary Mahoney, and Linda Richards made important contributions to both nursing education and practice.
- In 1923, the Goldmark Report concluded that for nursing to be on equal footing with other disciplines, nursing education should occur in the university setting.
- The Brown Report (1948) addressed the need for nurses to demonstrate greater professional competence by moving nursing education to the university setting.
- The Health Maintenance Organization Act of 1973 provided an alternative to the private health insurance industry.
- Title III of the Health Amendment Act of 1955 resulted in the establishment of practical nursing.
- Types of programs that currently prepare nurses for entry level practice are practical/vocational, diploma, associate degree, and baccalaureate degree.

Review Questions

1. The founder of modern nursing is considered to be:
   a. Lillian Wald.
   b. Dorothea Dix.
   c. Florence Nightingale.
   d. The Nursing Sisters of the Holy Cross.

2. The founder of the American Red Cross is:
   a. Lavinia Dock.
   b. Clara Barton.
   c. Linda Richards.
   d. Adelaide Nutting.

3. The first practical nursing school was:
   a. Ballard School.
   b. Thompson Practical Nursing School.
   c. Bellevue Training School for Nurses.
   d. Household Nursing Association School of Attendant Nursing.

4. Practical nursing was established under:
   a. Bureau of Medical Services, 1908.
   b. Health Maintenance Organization Act of 1973.
   c. Title III of the Health Amendment Act of 1955.
   d. Nursing and Nursing Education in the United States, 1923.

5. Staff development includes:
   a. recruitment.
   b. license renewal.
   c. continuing education.
   d. orientation and in-service.

6. The nursing organization that accredits schools of nursing is:
   a. ANA.
   b. NLN.
   c. NFLPN.
   d. NAPNES.

7. The National Council of State Boards of Nursing began administering a national certification examination available to the LP/VN. It is for:
   a. licensure.
   b. acute care.
   c. accreditation.
   d. long-term care.

8. The major recommendation of both the Goldmark and Brown reports was to:
   a. recruit more people into the nursing profession.
   b. compensate nurses with higher salaries and more comprehensive benefits.
   c. place nursing education within institutions of higher learning.
   d. increase the amount of clinical practice in nursing education programs.

Critical Thinking Questions

1. Think of some lessons you have learned from the past. Can you identify some life experiences that have been excellent teachers? List two lessons gained from these experiences or situations.

2. Florence Nightingale has been described as being strong minded and assertive. In what ways would it be helpful for you to develop such characteristics?

 WEB FLASH!

- Search for nursing history, nursing education, and nursing organizations on the Web. How many resources do you find for each topic?
- What type of information is provided about the nursing organizations? Is it enough to make a decision about becoming a member of an organization?

THE HEALTH CARE DELIVERY SYSTEM

MAKING THE CONNECTION

Refer to the following chapters to increase your understanding of the health care delivery system:

- **Chapter 4, Nursing History, Education, and Organizations**
- **Chapter 7, Ethical Responsibilities**
- **Chapter 15, Wellness Concepts**

LEARNING OBJECTIVES

Upon completion of this chapter you should be able to:
- *Define key terms.*
- *Describe the types of services in the U.S. health care delivery system.*
- *Discuss the various health care settings through which health care services are delivered.*
- *Identify the members of the health care team and their respective roles.*
- *Describe the differences among financial programs for health care services and reimbursement.*
- *Explain the factors that influence health care delivery.*
- *Identify the challenges to providing care.*
- *Discuss nursing's role in meeting the challenges within the health care system.*
- *Describe the emerging trends and issues for the health care delivery system.*

KEY TERMS

capitated rates
comorbidity
exclusive provider
 organization
fee-for-service
health care delivery
 system
health maintenance
 organization
managed care
medical model
preferred provider
 organization

prescriptive authority
primary care
primary care provider
primary health care
prospective payment
secondary care
single-payer system
single point of entry
subacute care
tertiary care

INTRODUCTION

A **health care delivery system** is a mechanism for providing services that meet the health-related needs of individuals. The U.S. health care delivery system is currently experiencing dramatic change. Health care institutions that once flourished economically are now searching for ways to survive. Health care providers are seeking cost-effective ways to deliver an ever-increasing range of services to consumers. Consumers are demanding greater accessibility to quality health care services that are also affordable.

Nursing is a major component of the U.S. health care delivery system. Consequently, nurses must understand the changes occurring within this system, as well as nursing's role in shaping those changes. This chapter explores the types of health care services available, the various settings where those services are offered, and the members of the health care team. The economics of health care and the challenges within the health care delivery system are also addressed, as is nursing's role in meeting those challenges.

TYPES OF HEALTH CARE SERVICES

Health care services can be classified into three levels: primary, secondary, and tertiary. The complexity of care varies according to the individual's need, the provider's expertise, and the delivery setting. Table 5-1 provides an overview of the types of care. The trend is toward holistic care, that is, care of the entire person including physiological, psychological, social, intellectual, and spiritual aspects.

Table 5-1 TYPES OF HEALTH CARE SERVICES

TYPE OF CARE	DESCRIPTION	EXAMPLES
Primary	*Goal:* To decrease the risk to a client (individual or community) for disease or dysfunction *Explanation:* General health promotion Protection against specific illnesses	Teaching Lifestyle modification for health (e.g., smoking cessation, nutrition counseling) Referrals Immunization Promotion of a safe environment (e.g., sanitation, protection from toxic agents)
Secondary	*Goal:* To alleviate disease and prevent further disability *Explanation:* Early detection and intervention	Screenings Acute care Various therapies Surgery
Tertiary	*Goal:* To minimize effects and permanent disability associated with chronic or irreversible conditions *Explanation:* Restorative and rehabilitative activities to attain optimal level of functioning	Education and retraining Provision of direct care Environmental intervention (e.g., advising on necessity of wheelchair accessibility for a person who has experienced a cardiovascular accident [stroke])

Primary Care

The major purposes of **primary care** are to promote wellness and prevent illness or disability. Care is coordinated by the office of the primary care provider, usually a family practice physician, pediatrician, internal medicine physician, or family nurse practitioner. Traditionally, the U.S. health care system focused on illness treatment rather than wellness promotion. Within the past two decades, however, focus has shifted to health-promoting behaviors such as regular exercise, reducing fat in the diet, reducing air pollution, and monitoring cholesterol level. Illness prevention activities may be directed toward the individual, the family, or the community.

Under the traditional **medical model**, our health care delivery system was not a *health* care system at all, but, rather, an *illness* care system. Services have traditionally been directed toward caring for an individual after disease or disability has developed rather than emphasizing preventive aspects of care (Pruitt & Campbell, 1994). Today, however, there is more of an emphasis on the holistic promotion of wellness and on the preventive aspects of care.

Secondary Care

Services within the realm of **secondary care**—diagnosis and treatment—occur after the client exhibits symptoms of illness. Acute treatment centers (hospitals) still constitute the predominant site for the delivery of these health care services. However, there is a growing movement to provide diagnostic and thera-peutic services in locations that are more easily accessed by the population. These are often satellite care centers of a major hospital, where holistic care is promoted.

Tertiary Care

Restoring an individual to the state of health that existed before the development of an illness is the purpose of **tertiary** (rehabilitative) **care**. In situations where the person is unable to regain previous functional abilities, the goal of rehabilitation is to attain the optimal level of health possible, for example, a client regaining partial use of an arm after experiencing a stroke. Restorative care is holistic in that the physiological, psychological, social, and spiritual aspects of the person are all addressed in the provision of care.

HEALTH CARE DELIVERY SYSTEM

The U.S. health care delivery system is complex, involving myriad providers, consumers, settings, personnel, and services.

Providers/Consumers

Health care services in the United States are delivered by public (including official and voluntary), public/private, and private sectors. Consumers are the individuals who receive the health care services.

Public Sector

Public agencies are financed with tax monies; thus, these agencies are accountable to the public. The public sector includes official (or governmental) agencies and voluntary agencies. Figure 5-1 shows the hierarchy of the official agencies in the public sector of health care delivery.

At the national level, the U.S. Department of Health and Human Services (USDHHS) is administratively responsible for health care services delivered to the public. The U.S. Public Health Service (USPHS) is the major agency that oversees the actual delivery of care services. Table 5-2 lists the USPHS agencies and their purposes. The Veterans Administration (VA) has hospitals and clinics that provide services to veterans of the armed services. These services are also financed with tax monies.

Each state varies in the provision of public health services. Generally, a state department of health coordinates the activities of local health units.

At the local level, services provided include immunizations, maternal–child care, and activities directed toward control of chronic diseases.

Voluntary agencies also constitute an important part of the public sector of the health care delivery system. These not-for-profit agencies (e.g., the National Federation of Licensed Practical Nurses [NFLPN], the American Nurses Association [ANA], the National League for

Table 5-2 AGENCIES OF THE U.S. PUBLIC HEALTH SERVICE	
AGENCY	**PURPOSE**
Health Resources and Services Administration (HRSA)	Provide health-related information Administer programs concerned with health care for the homeless; people with human immunodeficiency virus (HIV) and acquired immunodeficiency syndrome (AIDS); organ transplants; rural health care; and employee occupational health
Food and Drug Administration (FDA)	Protect the public from unsafe drugs, food, and cosmetics
Centers for Disease Control and Prevention (CDC)	Study and prevent the transmission of communicable diseases
National Institutes of Health (NIH)	Conduct research and education related to specific illnesses
Alcohol, Drug Abuse, and Mental Health Administration (ADAMHA)	Serve as clearinghouse for information on substance abuse and mental health issues
Agency for Toxic Substances and Disease Registry (ATSDR)	Maintain registry of certain diseases Provide information on toxic agents Conduct mortality and morbidity studies on defined population groups
Indian Health Service (IHS)	Provide health care services to Native Americans, including health promotion, disease prevention, alcoholism prevention, substance abuse prevention, suicide prevention, nutrition, maternal–child health
Agency for Health Care Policy and Research (AHCPR)	Serve as primary source of federal support for research related to quality of health care delivery

Nursing [NLN], and the American Medical Association [AMA]) can exert significant legislative influence. Other voluntary agencies, such as the American Cancer Society and the American Heart Association, provide educational resources to the general public and to health care providers, such as dietary suggestions along with corresponding recipes. Voluntary agencies are funded in a variety of ways including individual contributions, corporate philanthropy, and membership dues.

Public/Private Sector

A blending of the public and private sectors in many areas of health care has gradually occurred following the inception of Medicare and the diagnosis-related groups (DRGs), discussed in an upcoming section. Federal regulations guide both the care provided to clients in private non-profit and for-profit agencies by private physicians and the reimbursement to both the agencies and the physicians.

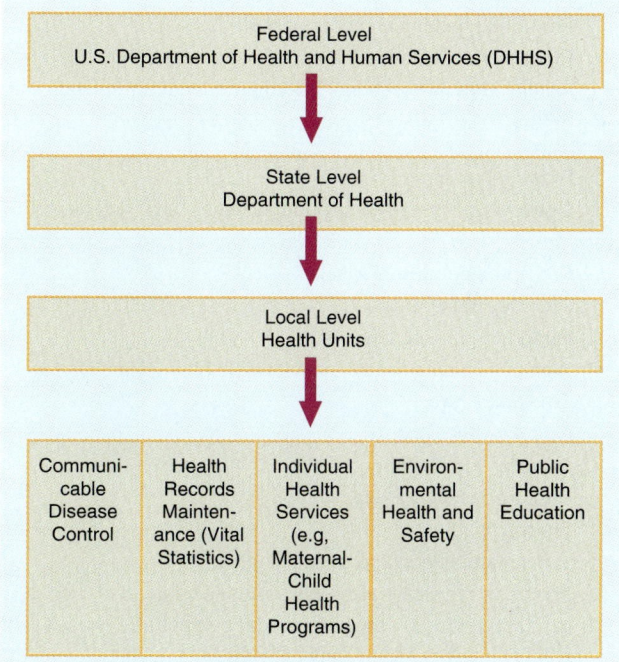

Figure 5-1 The Public Sector of Health Care Delivery (*From Fundamentals of Nursing: Standards & Practice, by S. DeLaune & P. Ladner, 1998, Albany, NY: Delmar Publishers. Copyright 1998 by Delmar Publishers. Reprinted with permission.*)

Private Sector

The private sector of the health care delivery system is composed primarily of independent health care agencies and providers who are reimbursed on a **fee-for-service** basis (whereby the recipient directly pays the provider for services as they are provided). Fee-for-service clients may have private insurance or use their own financial resources to pay the provider for services rendered.

Settings

The variety of settings where health care is delivered and the roles of nurses in these settings are presented in Table 5-3.

Table 5-3 HEALTH CARE SETTINGS

SETTING	SERVICES PROVIDED	NURSE'S ROLE
Hospital	Diagnosis and treatment of illnesses (acute and chronic) Acute inpatient services Ambulatory care services Critical (intensive) care Rehabilitative care Surgical interventions Diagnostic procedures	Serves as caregiver Educates clients Provides ongoing assessment Coordinates care and collaborates with other health care providers Maintains client safety Initiates discharge planning Can specialize in a variety of areas: • Cardiology • Oncology • Critical care • Orthopedics • Dialysis • Pediatrics • Emergency • Psychiatry • Geriatrics • Rehabilitation • Infection control • Surgery • Neurology
Extended-care (long-term care) facilities (e.g., nursing homes, skilled nursing facilities)	Intermediate and long-term care for people who have chronic illnesses and are unable to care for themselves Restorative care until client is ready for discharge home	Provides care directed toward meeting basic needs (e.g., nutrition, hydration, comfort, elimination) Provides teaching and counseling Plans and coordinates care Administers medications, treatments, and other therapeutic modalities
Home health care agencies	Wide range of services, including curative and rehabilitive	Provides skilled nursing care Coordinates health-promotion activities (e.g., education)
Hospices	Care of individuals who have terminal illnesses Improving the quality of life until death	Promotes comfort measures Provides pain control Supports grieving families
Out-patient settings (clinics, physician's offices, ambulatory treatment centers)	Treatment of illness (acute and chronic) Diagnostic testing Simple surgical procedures	*Traditional role:* Checks vital signs Assists with diagnostic tests Prepares client for examination *Expanded role:* Provides teaching and counseling Performs physical (or mental status) examination In some settings, advanced practice registered nurses (APRNs) act as primary care providers
Schools (school-based clinics [SBCs])	Federally funded to provide physical and mental health services in middle and high schools	Coordinates health-promotion and disease prevention activities Treats minor illnesses Provides health education

continued

Table 5-3 HEALTH CARE SETTINGS *continued*

SETTING	SERVICES PROVIDED	NURSE'S ROLE
Industrial clinics	Maintain health and safety of workers	Coordinates health-promotion activities Provides education for safety Provides urgent care as needed Maintains health records Conducts ongoing screenings Provides preventive services (e.g., tuberculosis testing)
Managed care organizations	Reimbursement for health care services	Serves as case manager Uses triage to determine the most appropriate intervention for various clients
Community nursing centers	Direct access to professional services	Treats client's responses to health problems Promotes health and wellness
Rural primary care hospitals (RPCHs)	Stabilize clients until they are physiologically able to be transferred to more-skilled facilities	Performs assessments and provides emergency care

Personnel and Services

Many personnel and services exist within the various health care settings. Large hospitals provide the greatest number of services. Other health care settings may provide some but not all of these same services. The service departments most commonly found in the various settings include nursing units, specialized client care units, diagnostic departments, therapy departments, and support services.

Nursing Units

Nursing units are composed of client rooms, where most nursing care is provided. Units often serve one particular type of client such as cardiac, orthopedic, diabetic, surgical, pediatric, or obstetric. The nurse responsible for the unit may be called by several different titles, such as unit coordinator, nurse manager, or head nurse. Registered nurses (RNs), licensed practical/vocational nurses (LP/VNs), and nursing assistants provide the nursing care.

Specialized Client Care Units

Specialized units provide nursing care for specific needs of the clients. The LP/VN may work in these areas depending on experience, further education, the size and location of the hospital, and the number of RNs available. Examples of specialized units include the following:

- Emergency department (ED): provides care to clients involved in all types of accidents and those confronted with medical emergencies such as heart attack or stroke
- Intensive care unit (ICU): provides care to critically ill clients until they are stabilized and can be managed with routine nursing interventions on a regular nursing unit
- Coronary care unit (CCU): provides care to clients who have had a heart attack or who have had heart surgery such as coronary artery bypass or valve replacement
- Mental health unit: provides care to clients who are having difficulty with relationships, coping with everyday demands, or dealing with a crisis
- Psychiatric unit: provides care to clients diagnosed as having mental illness
- Rehabilitation unit: provides care to clients who must learn to regain the highest level of self-care possible following injury, accident, or illness such as heart attack or stroke
- Dialysis unit: provides care to clients who need dialysis because of renal failure
- Hospice unit: provides both care to clients who are dying and support to their families; may be a unit in a hospital or a free standing unit
- Outpatient unit: provides care to clients when admission to the hospital is unnecessary
- Home care: provides care to clients in their homes when professional supervision and/or minimal care is required; has been added to many hospitals to provide continuity of care
- Client education unit: provides teaching to clients, either individually or in groups, about specific client conditions or other health-related issues

Surgical Units

Care of the client just before, during, and after surgery is performed by the operating room (OR) and recovery room (RR) personnel. In addition to the main surgical unit, many hospitals also have a day surgery/ambulatory surgery unit. Clients come in a couple of hours before their scheduled surgeries and leave when recovered from the anesthesia. Total length of stay is shorter than 24 hours.

Diagnostic Departments

Diagnostic departments provide specialized tests that assist the physician in making a diagnosis for the client.

Clinical Laboratory Clinical laboratory personnel examine specimens of tissues, feces, and body fluids such as blood, sputum, urine, amniotic fluid, and spinal fluid. Testing assesses values of normal components as well as abnormal components of these specimens.

Radiology Department X-ray studies are performed in the radiology department, sometimes called nuclear medicine. This department also performs computed tomography (CT) scans, mammography, ultrasound, arteriograms, venograms, echocardiograms, and magnetic resonance imaging (MRI).

Other Diagnostic Services Other diagnostic services may include the following:

- Sleep center: provides observation, testing, and monitoring of clients as they sleep, to identify sleep-related problems
- Electroencephalography (EEG): records brain waves and ascertains electrical activity in the brain
- Electrocardiogram (ECG): records electrical activity in the heart
- Electromyogram (EMG): records electrical activity in body muscles

Therapy Departments

The function of the various therapy departments is to provide specialized treatments and/or rehabilitation services to clients to improve functional level in a specific area. Most hospitals have respiratory therapy and physical therapy departments. Some large teaching hospitals also have occupational therapy and speech therapy departments.

Support Services

Support services meet various other needs in providing care to clients.

Pharmacists mix and dispense medications to the various client care units. Nurses then administer the medications to the clients.

Dietitians supervise food preparation for all clients. They specifically choose the foods and calculate the amounts for special diets and provide client teaching for those clients on special diets.

Social workers help clients deal with psychosocial problems, providing assistance in areas such as housing, finances, and referrals to support groups.

Chaplains provide individual counseling to clients and support to families and assist clients in meeting spiritual needs.

The admission department handles the admission process by preparing necessary paperwork and ensuring that the ordered preadmission laboratory testing and x-rays are performed.

The business office oversees insurance and financial affairs upon client discharge from the health care agency.

Medical records, also called health information systems, maintains and stores all medical records for every client ever cared for by the health care agency.

Housekeeping and maintenance keep the physical facilities and equipment clean, in good repair, and in proper working order.

HEALTH CARE TEAM

Health care services are delivered by a multidisciplinary team (Figure 5-2). Table 5-4 lists the various health care team members, their educational requirements, and their roles. Because nurses work with the other team members on an ongoing basis, it is necessary to understand the role of each team member.

The nurse fulfills a variety of roles in assisting clients to meet their needs. Table 5-5 defines the most common roles of nurses. Nurses function in independent, interdependent, and dependent roles. In the independent role, the nurse requires no direction or order from another health care professional, for example, in deciding that a client's edematous arm should be elevated. In the interdependent role, the nurse works in collaboration with other health care professionals,

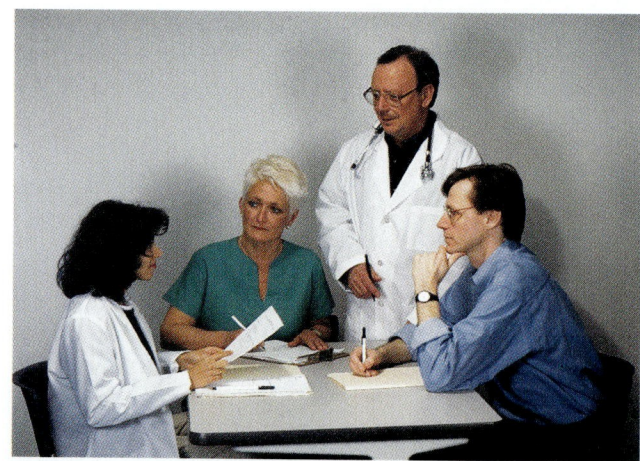

Figure 5-2 Members of the health care team work together for the benefit of the client.

Table 5-4 HEALTH CARE TEAM MEMBERS

TEAM MEMBER	EDUCATION	FUNCTION/ROLE
Nurse (both LP/VN and RN)	LP/VN: 1 year RN: 2 to 4 years	Emphasizes health (wellness) promotion With a holistic approach, assists clients in coping with illness or disability by providing nursing care, health and health care education, and discharge planning Formulates nursing diagnoses to guide plan of care Addresses the needs of the client (individual, family, or community) Assists physician
Physician (medical doctor [MD])	8+ years	Formulates medical diagnoses and prescribes therapeutic modalities Performs medical procedures (e.g., surgery) May specialize in a variety of areas (e.g., gynecology/obstetrics, oncology, surgery)
Physician assistant (PA)	2 years (plus a master's degree for PA licensure, required in many states)	Provides medical services under the supervision of a physician
Registered pharmacist (RPh)	5 to 6 years	Prepares and dispenses drugs for therapeutic use May be involved in client education
Dentist (both doctor of dental surgery [DDS] and doctor of dental medicine [DMD])	8+ years	Diagnoses and treats conditions affecting the mouth, teeth, and gums Performs preventive measures to promote dental health
Registered dietitian (RD)	4+ years	Plans diets to meet special needs of clients Promotes health and prevents disease through education and counseling May supervise preparation of meals
Social worker (SW)	4 years	Assists clients with psychosocial problems (e.g., financial, housing, marital) May assist with discharge planning Makes referrals to support groups
Respiratory therapist (RT)	2 years	Administers pulmonary function tests Performs therapeutic measures to assist with respiration (e.g., oxygen administration, ventilation) Provides various treatments for respiratory illnesses and conditions
Physical therapist (PT)	4 years	Works with clients experiencing musculoskeletal problems Assesses client's strength and mobility Performs therapeutic measures (e.g., range of motion, massage, application of heat and cold) Teaches new skills (e.g., crutch walking)
Occupational therapist (OT)	4 years	Works with clients who have functional impairment to teach skills for activities of daily living
Speech therapist	4 years	Assists clients who have speech impairments to speak understandably or to learn another method of communication
Chaplain	8 years	Assists clients in meeting spiritual needs Provides individual counseling Provides support to families Conducts religious services

Table 5-5 NURSING ROLES

ROLE	DESCRIPTION
Caregiver: **LP/VN and RN**	Traditional and most essential role
	Functions as nurturer
	Provides direct care
	Is supportive
	Demonstrates clinical proficiency
	Promotes comfort of client
Teacher: **LP/VN and RN**	Provides information
	Serves as counselor
	Seeks to empower clients in self-care
	Encourages compliance with prescribed therapy
	Promotes healthy lifestyles
	Interprets information
Advocate: **LP/VN and RN**	Protects the client
	Provides explanations in client's language
	Acts as change agent
	Supports client's decisions
Manager: **LP/VN and RN**	Makes decisions
	Coordinates activities of others
	Allocates resources
	Evaluates care and personnel
	Serves as a leader
	Takes initiative
Expert: **RN**	Advanced practice clinician
	Conducts research
	Teaches in schools of nursing
	Develops theory
	Contributes to professional literature
	Provides testimony at governmental hearings and in court
Case manager: **RN**	Tracks client's progress through the health care system
	Coordinates care to ensure continuity
Team member: **LP/VN and RN**	Collaborates with others
	Possesses excellent communication skills

ECONOMICS OF HEALTH CARE

The reform movement in health care has been motivated primarily by costs. Control of costs has shifted from the health care providers to the insurers, with the result being increasing constraints on reimbursement. For years, the predominant method of covering health care costs was fee for service, and there was little, if any, incentive for cost-effective delivery of care (Chamberlain, Chen, Osuna, & Yamamoto, 1995). All that is changing.

The U.S. health care system has a diverse financial base, composed of both private and public funding. As a result, administrative costs for health care reimbursement are higher in this country than in countries with a **single-payer system** (a model wherein the government is the only entity to reimburse health care costs, such as in Canada). The level of U.S. health care expenditures is higher than that of any other nation, and previous cost-containment measures have been ineffective in slowing the growth in expenditures (Schieber, Poullier, & Greenwald, 1997). Despite the enormous expenditure of public funds, the United States has not found a way to provide health care coverage for all citizens.

Private Insurance

The system for financing health care services in the United States is based on the private insurance model. Private insurance companies constitute one of the largest sectors of the health care system. Currently, more than 1,000 private insurance companies exist (Feldstein, 1999). Payment rates to health care providers vary among insurance companies. Figure 5-3 shows

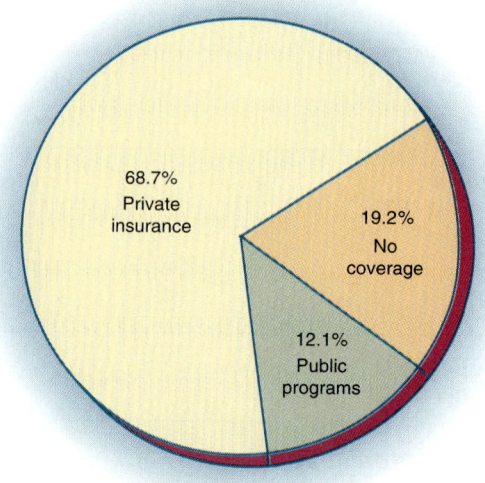

Figure 5-3 Health Insurance Coverage: U.S. Civilian, Non-institutionalized Population under Age 65 (*Courtesy of the Center for Cost and Financing Studies, Agency for Health Care Policy on Research,* Medical Expenditure Panel Survey Household Component, *1996 [Round 1]*)

for example, in a client care conference where several members of the health care team together plan ways to meet the client's needs. In the dependent role, the nurse requires direction from a physician or dentist, for example, medications must be ordered by a physician or dentist before a nurse may administer them to the client. The degree of autonomy nurses experience is related to client needs, nurse expertise, and practice setting.

the percentage of the U.S. population under age 65 that is covered by either private or public health insurance programs.

In the United States, insured individuals pay substantial monthly premiums for insurance coverage having high deductibles for health care services. For many, these costs may prove barriers to procuring necessary insurance coverage and health services. In addition, insurers will no longer pay for services that *they* deem unnecessary, effectively taking client care decisions out of the hands of physicians. The quality of care provided is now being monitored not only by providers (physicians), but by third-party payers (insurance companies) and, ever increasingly, by consumers.

Managed Care

Managed care is a system of providing and monitoring care wherein access, cost, and quality are controlled before or during delivery of services. The goal of managed care is the delivery of services in the most cost-efficient manner possible. Managed care organizations combine the financing and delivery of health care services. Managed care seeks to control costs by monitoring delivery of services and restricting access to expensive procedures and providers.

Managed care was designed to provide coordinated services with an emphasis on prevention and primary care (ANA, 1995). The rationale behind managed care is to give consumers preventive services delivered by a **primary care provider** (a health care provider whom a client sees first for health care; typically, a family practitioner, internist, or pediatrician). The primary care provider is responsible for managing or coordinating all care of a client when illness makes referrals necessary. This is supposed to result in less expensive interventions.

Managed care has been in existence for years; however, it is only within the past 20 years that it has enjoyed national prominence (Society for Ambulatory Care Professionals, 1994). The Health Maintenance Organization Act (passed in 1973) implemented two mandates. First, federal grants and loans were made available to **health maintenance organizations** (HMOs) (prepaid health plans that provide primary health care services for a preset fee and that focus on cost-effective treatment measures) that complied with strict federal regulations as opposed to the less-restrictive state requirements. Second, large employers were required to provide to employees an HMO as an option for health care coverage (Society for Ambulatory Care Professionals, 1994). From their inception, HMOs have constituted a viable alternative to the traditional fee-for-service system.

Managed care is not a place but, rather, an organizational structure with several variations. One such variation is the HMO, which is both provider and insurer.

Table 5-6 COMPARISON OF INDEPENDENT PRACTICE AND MANAGED CARE

TYPE	DESCRIPTION
Independent Practice	Fee for service or salary
	Functions within socially prescribed boundaries (professional ethics)
	Free choice of provider
	Disease-oriented philosophy
Managed Care	
Health maintenance organizations (HMOs)	Provide services to a group of enrolled persons
	Preset and prepaid fees
	Limited to certain providers
Preferred provider organizations (PPOs)	Networks of providers that give discounts to sponsoring organization
	Members' choice of physician not mandated, but lesser reimbursement if physician is outside of the network
Exclusive provider organizations (EPOs)	No benefit if member is treated outside of the network
	Usually regulated by state insurance laws

Other variations are **preferred provider organizations** (PPOs), wherein members must use providers within the system in order to obtain full reimbursement but may use other providers for lesser reimbursement, and **exclusive provider organizations** (EPOs) wherein care must be delivered by the providers in the plan in order for clients to receive any reimbursement. In the past decade, there has been a great shift on the part of the population from private insurance to HMOs and PPOs (Feldstein, 1999). Table 5-6 compares independent practice and managed care organizational structures.

Health Maintenance Organizations

Health Maintenance Organizations often maintain primary health care sites (although not necessarily) and commonly employ provider professionals. They use **capitated rates** (preset flat fees based on membership in, not services provided by, the HMO), assume the risk of clients who are heavy users, and exert control over the use of services. Health maintenance organizations have been noted for using advanced practice registered nurses (APRNs) as primary care providers and using precertification programs to limit unnecessary hospitalization. Further, HMOs emphasize client education for health promotion and self-care.

Another common feature of HMOs is the practice of **single point of entry** (entry into the health care system through a point designated by the plan), through which primary care is delivered. **Primary health care** is the client's point of entry into the health care system and includes assessment, diagnosis, treatment, co-ordination of care, education, preventive services, and surveillance. It comprises the spectrum of services provided by a family practitioner (nurse or physician) in an ambulatory setting. Primary care providers (PCPs) serve as "gatekeepers" to the health care system, in that they determine which, if any, referrals to specialists are needed by the client. To reduce costs, HMOs purposely limit direct access to specialists. Managed care plans assume a significant portion of the risk of providing health care and, consequently, encourage prudent use by both consumers and providers. In 1976, there were 175 HMOs in the United States; by 1995 there were 591 (Feldstein, 1999).

Preferred Provider Organizations

The most common managed care systems are PPOs. A PPO represents a contractual relationship between hospitals, providers, insurers, employers, and third-party payers to form a network wherein providers negotiate with group purchasers to provide health services for a defined population at a predetermined price (Feldstein, 1999). Care received within the network is associated with the highest reimbursement; care received outside the network is associated with lower reimbursement, with the client paying the difference. Preferred provider organizations have been very popular in the United States. In fact, the number of PPOs has increased from fewer than 10 in 1981 to over 700 in 1994 (Feldstein, 1999).

Exclusive Provider Organizations

Exclusive provider organizations create a network of providers (such as physicians and hospitals) and offer the incentive of consumer services for little or no copayment if the network providers are used exclusively. If a member receives treatment outside of the network, no benefit is paid. For instance, a member who becomes ill and receives treatment while visiting relatives in another state would receive no benefits for the treatment.

Federal Government Insurance Plans

The federal government became a third-party payer for health care services with the advent of Medicare and Medicaid in 1965. The Health Care Financing Administration (HCFA) is a federal agency that regulates Medicare, Medicaid, and Children's Health Insurance Program (CHIP) expenditures. There are many public programs for the financing of health care, with Medicare and Medicaid being the predominant ones. Medicare is the federally funded program that provides health care coverage for elderly persons and disabled persons. Medicaid pro-

vides health care coverage for the poor. Children's Health Insurance Program is a partnership between the federal and state governments to cover previously uninsured children.

With the ultimate goal of curtailing spending for hospitalized Medicare recipients, the federal government created diagnosis-related groups (DRGs) to categorize the average cost of care for each diagnosis. A prospective payment system was then created based on the DRGs. **Prospective payment** is a predetermined rate paid for each episode of hospitalization based on the client's age and principal diagnosis and on the presence or absence of surgery and **comorbidity** (simultaneous existence of more than one disease process in an individual). Hospitals are reimbursed the predetermined amount regardless of the actual cost of providing services to the client. The prospective payment system, originally designed for Medicare, has been adopted by other agencies and insurance companies.

Medicare

When Medicare was established in 1965, it was intended to protect individuals over the age of 65 years from exorbitant health care costs. In 1972, Medicare was modified to also cover permanently disabled individuals and those with end-stage renal disease. Because many individuals over the age of 65 do not have employee-paid insurance, public funds cover the majority of health care services for elderly persons (USD-HHS, 1993).

Medicaid

Medicaid is the largest third-party payer of nursing home health care expenditures (Feldstein, 1999). Medicaid is a shared venture between the federal and state governments. Each state has latitude in determining who is "medically indigent" and, thus, qualifies for pub-

PROFESSIONAL TIP

Impact of Prospective Payment System and DRGs

- Decreased length of client stay in hospitals
- More emphasis on preventive care
- Increased concern about consumer's (client's) response to care
- An increased number of critically ill clients in hospitals
- Clients sicker upon discharge from hospital
- An increase in outpatient care
- Client and family more responsible for care
- Greater need for home health care
- Mergers or closures of hospitals because of inordinate competition

lic monies. Minimal services covered by Medicaid are defined by the federal government and include inpatient and outpatient hospital services, physician services, laboratory services (including x-ray), and rural health clinic services. States may elect to cover other services, such as dental, vision, and prescription drug.

Children's Health Insurance Program

Children's Health Insurance Program was created in 1997 as part of the Balanced Budget Act. The program is designed to provide health care to uninsured children, many of whom are members of working families that earn too little to afford private insurance on their own but earn too much to be eligible for Medicaid.

FACTORS INFLUENCING HEALTH CARE

Despite cost-containment efforts (such as DRGs, established by the federal government, and managed care, established by the insurers), the U.S. health care system still has problems with issues of cost, access, and quality. These issues are important for nurses to understand and are integral to any effort toward health reform.

Cost

Cost has been a driving force for change in the health care system as evidenced by the strength and numbers of managed care plans, increased use of outpatient treatment, and shortened hospital stays. These market forces (to maximize profits by minimizing costs) are dominating the current changes in the health care system.

The cost of providing health care has risen dramatically during the past 15 years. The U.S. government spends more on health care per person than does any other country (O'Neil, 1993). The increasing consumption of federal funds for health care means that resources are being moved from other areas of need, such as education, housing, and social services (Grace, 1997). Figure 5-4 illustrates health care expenditures.

The most cost-efficient programs in terms of administration are Medicare and Medicaid, with administration costs being less than one cent of each dollar (HCFA, 1998). It should be noted that the administration of these programs is subcontracted to private agencies and organizations. In contrast, some private plans, particularly small business plans, use over 40 cents of each dollar for administration. The cost of employee health care benefits is thus an expensive commitment for small businesses.

Three major factors increase the cost of health care: (1) an oversupply of specialized providers (fees are raised to maintain provider income in light of fewer clients); (2) a surplus of hospital beds (empty beds are

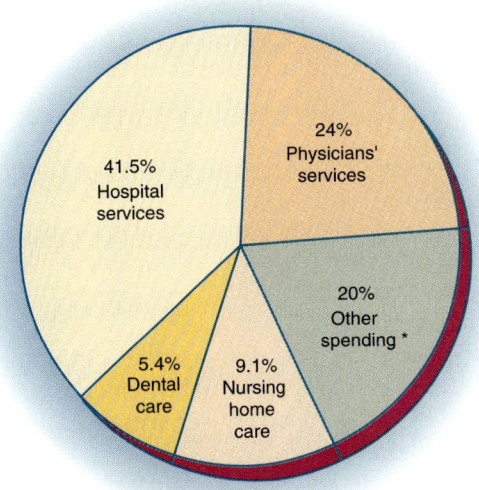

Figure 5-4 Health Care Expenditures. *Note:* Other spending = eye care services, services by other than physicians, lab tests, x-rays, repair of medical equipment, other medical care services. (*Adapted from* Health Care Economics, *by P. J. Feldstein, 1999, Albany NY: Delmar Publishers. Copyright 1999 by Delmar Publishers. Adapted with permission.*)

a cost liability); and (3) the passive role assumed by most consumers (when someone else pays the bill, consumers typically are less concerned about cost) (Feldstein, 1999). Other factors that contribute to the high cost of health care are the aging of the population, the increased number of people with chronic illnesses, the increase in health-related lawsuits and the associated unnecessary use of services (e.g., additional diagnostic testing), and advanced technology that has allowed more people to survive formerly fatal illnesses even though those people require extensive and lifelong care.

Access

Related to the issue of cost is that of access to health care services, which carries serious implications for the functioning of the health care system. As a result of high costs, health care for many people is crisis oriented and fragmented. Numerous people in the United States are unable to gain access to health care services because of inadequate or no insurance; thus, illness among these people may progress to an acute stage before intervention is sought. Services used by individuals during acute illnesses are typically provided by emergency departments. Emergency room and acute care services are expensive when compared to early intervention and preventive measures.

Only a small portion of the medically indigent are covered by Medicare. In addition, many individuals are underinsured. These people are neither poor nor old but, rather, are middle-class unemployed Americans or those who have jobs lacking adequate health care benefits. In addition to poverty and unemployment, other factors can hinder a person's ability to obtain insurance and/or health care services, including the following:

- Lack of insurance provision by employer because of prohibitive costs
- High costs of obtaining individual insurance
- Certain preexisting conditions making it difficult to obtain insurance
- Cultural barriers
- Shortages of health care providers in some geographic areas (especially rural or inner city areas)
- Limited access to ancillary services (e.g., child care and transportation)
- Status as single-parent or two-income family, making it difficult for parents to take time from work to transport children to health care providers

Quality

It is estimated that 30% to 40% of diagnostic and medical procedures performed in this country are unnecessary (Lee, Soffel, & Luft, 1997). This inappropriate use of resources can be traced to several factors, including:

- The litigious environment and resultant tendency toward defensive practice (e.g., ordering all possible tests instead of only those that the provider deems truly necessary).
- The widely held American belief that more is better.
- Lack of access to and continuity of services and the subsequent misuse of acute care services.

The greatest number of health care dollars are expended in the last days of life, with 40% of in-hospital days and 35% of prescription medications being used by elderly persons. Twelve percent of the U.S. population is aged 65 years or older and uses 33% of health care expenditures (Rowe, 1996).

In an attempt to provide universal access to services in a cost-effective manner, quality may be sacrificed. For example, hospitals that are reducing the numbers of nurses ("downsizing") risk endangering quality. Safety and quality are frequently compromised by the inappropriate substitution of unqualified personnel for LP/VNs and RNs in direct care of clients. Cross-training of staff, increased use of unlicensed personnel, and reductions in full-time positions for nurses are affecting the type of care delivered in hospitals. Any movement toward reform must focus on providing quality nursing care to all consumers.

CHALLENGES WITHIN THE HEALTH CARE SYSTEM

The major challenges facing the U.S. health care delivery system—which also happen to impact the control of costs—include the public's disillusionment with providers; providers' and consumers' loss of control over health care decisions; decreased use of hospitals and the accompanying negative impact on quality of care; changing practice settings; ethical issues; and vulnerable populations.

Disillusionment with Providers

Greed and waste have been identified as major problems of the U.S. health care system (Maraldo, 1997). Whether these problems are caused by defensive practice, consumer demand, or professional economics is irrelevant to the public. Success in reform depends on starting where the public expects reform should begin: eliminating the greed of providers and the waste in the health care system. Further, people in the United States have become suspicious of health care providers. The high level of esteem in which medicine has traditionally been held has eroded over the past few years. Consumers, increasingly tired of paying the high cost of care, are questioning medical practices and fees (Zerwekh & Claborn, 1997). However, the public is not disillusioned with nurses (Kellogg Foundation, 1994). This positive perception of nurses will be important as patterns of reform are established.

Positive Perception of Nurses

Several studies (ANA, 1993a; Kellogg Foundation, 1994) verify the public's trust in nurses. The public sees nurses as part of the solution, not the problem, and believes that if nurses were allowed to use their skills, they would significantly enhance quality and reduce costs. One survey (ANA, 1993a) inquired about consumer receptivity to nurses' taking on expanded

CULTURAL CONSIDERATIONS

Barriers to Health Care Services

Certain cultural beliefs and values may prevent individuals from seeking health care. These may include the following:

- Belief in Divine healing
- Refusal of care on holy days
- Belief that the individual taking the ill person to a health care facility is responsible for the ill person for the rest of that person's life after recovery
- Belief that illness is a result of sins committed in previous life
- View of prayer as a tool for deliverance from illness
- Belief that illness is God's punishment

responsibilities. Respondents supported **prescriptive authority** (legal recognition of the ability to prescribe medications) for RNs and endorsed the role of nurses in performing physical examinations and managing minor acute illnesses. Nurses should expand their focus on holistic care and spend as much time as possible on prevention of illness and wellness issues.

Loss of Control

Providers feel they have lost control over the care they provide to their clients. Increasingly, the insurance companies or the managed care organizations decide which care can and which care cannot be provided to the client.

Consumers express feeling terrorized by the health care delivery system. They feel they have lost personal control over their health care. Many stay in their current jobs because of their health care benefits or give up employment mobility out of fear of being denied a new policy because of preexisting conditions.

Decreased Hospital Use

In the early 20th century, hospitals focused on providing care to those who had no caregivers in the family or community. The focus of these early institutions was care as opposed to cure (Grace, 1997). The focus of hospitals changed in the mid-1940s as a result of technological changes and the passage by Congress in 1946 of the Hill–Burton Act, which provided funding for the renovation and construction of hospitals. One unanticipated outcome of this act was a substantial oversupply of hospital beds. Health care costs escalated because of the need to keep the hospital beds occupied: Everyone was put in the hospital, for everything from a complete physical examination, to specific diagnostic testing, to acute care or surgery.

From 1945 to 1982, the demand for hospital beds steadily increased. After 1982, however, a steady decline in the number of hospital admissions and the average length of stay occurred (Grace, 1997). In 1995, there were 23.7% fewer inpatient days than in 1985 (Feldstein, 1999). Many small hospitals have had to close their doors because they could no longer compete with the large hospitals.

Currently, hospitals continue to be the nucleus of the health care delivery system in the United States. Hospitals account for the largest proportion of expenditures and employ the majority of health care workers. Hospitals have fewer clients today because of the trend toward rapid discharge and a greater number of procedures being performed in outpatient settings. The clients who are hospitalized require more nursing care because of greater complexity of needs and severity of illness. Additional factors that have contributed to the decreased hospital population include:

- Shorter length of stays,
- Greater availability of outpatient facilities,
- Technological advances,
- An increased number of services available in outpatient settings, and
- Expectations/demands of third-party payers.

As a result of the changes in reimbursement practices, hospitals are restructuring (also referred to as redesigning and reengineering). Examples of restructuring activities include mergers with larger institutions; development of integrated systems that provide a full range of services focusing on continuity of care, such as preadmission, outpatient, acute inpatient, long-term inpatient, and home care; and the substitution of multiskilled workers for nurses.

Changing Practice Settings

Most nurses currently practice in hospitals and will continue to do so in the future (Aiken, 1995). The increasing presence of severely ill clients requires that nurses who work in hospitals possess technical expertise, critical thinking skills, and interpersonal competence. Outside the hospital setting, there is an ever-increasing need for nurses in different areas of practice. Home health services, in particular, will need to continue expanding in order to meet the growing needs of the steadily increasing elderly population (Hull, 1997). Social and political changes are affecting nurses by creating the need for expanded services and settings. Because of these changes, demand for nursing care fluctuates: For example, nursing employment outside the hospital continues to increase. More nurses will be needed in the future because:

- The growing elderly population will require more health care services.
- The number of people admitted to nursing homes is steadily growing.
- The number of homeless individuals, who are most often denied access to health care, is increasing rapidly.

As initial reform occurs, some nurses may be displaced from their current jobs. But overall, many more jobs will be created by the demand for greater access to health care services. Some examples of areas where larger numbers of nurses will be required are primary care, public health, extended care, and home care.

Ethical Issues

The United States is struggling with a major ethical conflict of cost containment versus compassionate care. According to Hicks and Boles (1997), no country, regardless of wealth, can provide all citizens with every health care service they desire or need. Today,

HOME HEALTH CARE

Cost of Home Health Care

- Since the advent of Medicare and Medicaid, home health care has grown rapidly. Because it is much less costly to provide home care, clients are sent home to recuperate.
- Expenditures for health care in the home are greatly increasing.

LIFE CYCLE CONSIDERATIONS

Health Care Needs

- One in five children lives in a family with income below the poverty level, and only one-half of these are covered by Medicaid (Uphold & Graham, 1993).
- More children will be declared ineligible for Medicaid as the government tries to curb health care expenditures.
- More then one-third of preschool children in the United States are not fully immunized (Kyle & Coulter, 1995).

the U.S. health care delivery system is faced with the dilemma of citizens' needs being greater than available resources. Thus, some difficult choices must be made to determine which needs will be met and which will remain unmet.

The national mentality reflected in the expectation that everything must be done to save a dying person has created an enormous drain on the health care resources of the United States and represents one example of ethical issues related to health care. As decisions are made regarding how scarce resources are to be allocated, there will be much debate about the ethics involved. The appropriateness of futile life-sustaining measures—those that only keep the client in a vegetative state—must be addressed (Rowe, 1996). Nurses must strongly advocate for just and ethical distribution of resources as health care reform progresses.

Vulnerable Populations

Meeting the health care needs of underserved populations is especially challenging. Groups that may be unable to gain access to health care services include children, rural residents, people with AIDS, and the homeless and others living in poverty. An increase in poverty further strains hospitals because Medicaid is no longer adequate to meet the needs of the medically indigent.

Our current health care system neglects the overall needs of children. Children are more likely than adults to be uninsured or underinsured. Children who are covered by health insurance have a greater degree of well-being.

Many parents have their children immunized only when the children are ready to start school, because immunization is a requirement for entry into the public school system. Preventive health care should be encouraged and made available to children of all ages, with an emphasis on early immunization. The ANA and a coalition of allied nursing associations are working together in an attempt to immunize all children in the United States.

Traditionally, rural areas have had fewer health care providers and facilities that are easily accessible than have their urban counterparts. Approximately 45% of

those over the age of 65 years live in rural areas (Vrabec, 1995). Because people in rural areas tend to work for small businesses or be self-employed, many of them have no health insurance.

As of December 1997, 641,086 people in the United States have been diagnosed with AIDS, and estimates suggest that 650,000 to 900,000 persons in the United States are now living with HIV (CDC, 1998). It is estimated that at least 40,000 new infections occur each year (CDC, 1998). The most rapid spread of the disease is occurring among women, children, and intravenous drug users and their sexual partners. Women who have AIDS have a higher mortality rate than do men, and decreased access to health care may be one contributing factor (Tlusty, 1994). Although the cost of this epidemic is unmeasurable in terms of human suffering, approximately $10.5 billion was spent on care of people with AIDS in 1994 alone (Hull, 1997). Not only will additional funding be necessary, but outpatient care settings (such as hospices, home care, and clinics) must be expanded to care for those affected by this epidemic.

The homeless and others living in poverty are often mobile, having no permanent address. They may not know which services are available to them or how to access the system except through inner city hospitals. This creates a significant financial burden on these health care agencies. Illegal aliens, because of fears of being arrested and deported, may enter emergency departments under false identities and in acute distress, receive treatment, and then disappear.

NURSING'S RESPONSE TO HEALTH CARE CHALLENGES

As the United States continues to look for ways to address the issue of health care reform, the implications for nursing will continue to increase. Some nurses feel threatened by impending changes, whereas

LIFE CYCLE CONSIDERATIONS

Rural Elders

Health care barriers experienced by elderly persons living in rural areas include the following:

- Inadequate financing of rural health care facilities. Medicare's lower reimbursement rates for rural hospitals than for urban hospitals has been a contributing factor to the closure of some hospitals in rural communities.
- Decreased availability of health care providers.
- Greater geographic distances that must be traveled in order to obtain services.

Table 5-7 NURSING'S AGENDA FOR HEALTH CARE REFORM

Nursing's agenda for health care reform includes several basic tenets, including the following:

- All citizens and residents of the United States must have equitable access to essential health care services.
- Primary health care services must play a very basic and prominent role in service delivery.
- Consumers must be the central focus of the health care system. Assessment of health care needs must be the determining factor in the ultimate structuring and delivery of programs and services.
- Consumers must be guaranteed direct access to a full range of qualified health care providers who offer their services in a variety of delivery arrangements at sites that are accessible, convenient, and familiar to the consumer.
- Consumers must assume more responsibility for their own care and become better informed about the range of providers and potential options for services.
- Health care services must be restructured to create a better balance between the prevailing orientation toward illness and cure and a new commitment to wellness and care.
- The health care system must ensure that appropriate, effective care is delivered through efficient use of resources.
- A standardized package of essential health care services must be provided and financed through an integration of public and private sources.
- Mechanisms must be implemented to protect against catastrophic costs and impoverishment.

From Nursing's Agenda for Health Care Reform, *by American Nurses Association, 1991, Kansas City, MO: Author.*

---

others are excited about the possibility of transforming the health care system into something better. The nursing profession has responded to the myriad challenges in health care delivery by proposing a plan for reform.

Nursing's Agenda for Health Care Reform

In 1991, in response to the problems of high cost, limited access, and eroding quality that were affecting the U.S. health care system, the nursing community created a public policy agenda that is currently endorsed by more than 70 organizations. *Nursing's Agenda for Health Care Reform* (ANA, 1991) provides a valid framework for change in health care policies and establishes nursing's legislative program, through which these changes can be implemented. Table 5-7 lists the major tenets of this agenda. A cornerstone of nursing's proposal is the delivery of health care services in environments that are easily accessible, familiar, and consumer friendly. Another essential part of nursing's agenda is the empowerment of consumers in the area of self-care. This goal has enormous implications for nurses as health educators and for the use of incentives for increasing personal accountability for one's own health status.

Standards of Care

Another approach to the challenges of the health care delivery system has been the move toward standardization of care. In December 1990, the Agency for Health Care Policy and Research (AHCPR) was established with the specific charge of achieving consensus within the medical/health care community regarding the usual treatment of high-volume and expensive disease conditions that differ in therapeutic management despite substantial research. More simply put, there is significant variation in the diagnosis and treatment of certain illnesses and diseases. The medical justification

for such variance has been that every client is an individual and that the choice of treatment is a private decision involving client and physician. Prostatic hypertrophy (enlarged prostate gland) and breast cancer are examples of high-volume diagnoses that have been studied by the AHCPR but for which appropriate diagnostic tests and treatments of choice have not yet been conclusively determined. The AHCPR aims to identify the standards of treatment to which the health care community can be held. Currently, 18 AHCPR-published guidelines are available to the public and should be integral to nursing practice.

Advanced Practice

The advanced practice of nursing has evolved as nursing has become more complex and specialized. Since the late 1960s, nurse practitioners (NPs), clinical nurse specialists (CNSs), certified nurse midwives (CNMs), and other advanced practice registered nurses (APRNs) have provided primary health care services to individuals, many of whom would have otherwise had inadequate or no access to services (Brown &

Grimes, 1993). The APRN possesses advanced skills and in-depth knowledge in specific areas of practice (Stafford & Appleyard, 1997). Although there are differences among various advanced practice roles, all APRNs are experts who work with clients to prevent disease and promote health.

There are currently more than 100,000 APRNs in the United States (ANA, 1995). Nurses in advanced practice are also moving toward independent practice. Data suggest that APRNs can independently diagnose and resolve over 80% of the primary health care problems of the American public (ANA, 1993a). The NP facilitates access to and continuity of care and provides high-quality care (Brown & Grimes, 1993). Advanced practice registered nurses prescribe less-expensive diagnostic tests, the length of their visits is comparable to that of physicians', and they charge less for services because of the comparatively lower cost of professional liability insurance (ANA, 1993b). Despite repeated proof of the cost efficiency and therapeutic effectiveness of APRNs, obstacles to this role for nurses persist. In a recent Division of Nursing report on APRNs, the single most formidable obstacle to practice is that most people are unaware of what APRNs offer (Washington Consulting Group, 1994).

Recent progress has been made on the access issues that constrain APRNs. Reimbursement is now available to some segments of the advanced practice community in every federal entitlement program (HCFA, 1998).

Currently, 44 states and the District of Columbia award APRNs some type of prescriptive authority (National Council of State Boards of Nursing [NCSBN], personal communication, 1998) (Figure 5-5). In 15 states, this authority is complete and unrestricted, is unassociated with physician oversight, and includes all classes of drugs (Pearson, 1996). The ANA (through the JCAHO and the HCFA) began the groundwork for

professional staff privileges for APRNs in its revision of the official definitions of professional staff that include a broad range of providers.

Public vs. Private Programs

The combination of public sector and private sector health care resources seems to be beneficial for U.S. residents. The competition between the two sectors has encouraged quality and progress. Each setting offers benefits as well as drawbacks to health care recipients.

The nursing profession supports an integration of public and private sector programs and resources. Public dollars are required to help the poor and those who do not receive health care benefits through the workplace. Actual services should be available through a variety of public and private sources. To safeguard the health care system from becoming a two-tiered process based on personal resources, both the poor and nonpoor and the privileged and nonprivileged must be enrolled in the same programs.

Finally, the basic required package of services must be defined in the same way in each state and required as the minimum for both public and private sector programs. Minimal national standards should be set, but local planning and implementation should be promoted.

The states' rights philosophy prevalent in the United States creates an obstacle to national standards, which are necessary for several areas of assurance. Some coast-to-coast consistency in the cost of services, with room for local adjustments, is needed.

Public Health

During the past several years, public health has perceptibly eroded. Public health includes services such as immunizations, prenatal care, environmental concerns (conditions that may affect health), and analysis of the prevailing disease patterns in a community. Current public health problems include:

- Appearance of new fatal diseases (e.g., AIDS and the Ebola virus),
- Emergence of drug-resistant strains of tuberculosis, and
- Presence of toxic environmental conditions.

Community Health

Parris and Hines (1995) recommend a commitment to a community-based approach to reforming the system of health care delivery. Community-based care focuses on prevention and primary care. Successful movement toward a healthy and empowered consumer requires access to community-based primary health care. Nursing has a rich heritage of providing such community services, as evidenced by the work of pioneers such as Lillian Wald and Mary Breckenridge.

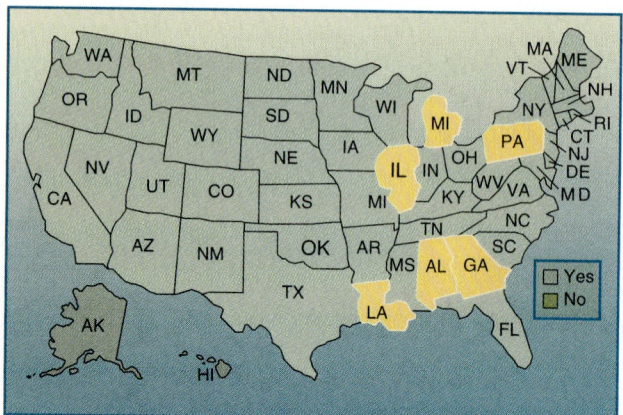

* States vary in degrees of independence in prescribing.

Figure 5-5 States with Some Form of Prescriptive Authority for Advanced Practice Nurses (*Data from National Council of State Boards of Nursing [NCSBN], 1996, Personal Communication, 1998.*)

Table 5-8 TRENDS AFFECTING DELIVERY OF HEALTH CARE SERVICES

- The aging of the U.S. population
- Increasing diversity in the U.S. population
- Increased number of single-parent families and of children living in poverty
- Continued growth in outpatient settings and a greater demand for primary care providers
- Advances in technology with resultant ability to perform more services in outpatient settings (including the home)
- More states using managed care models to deliver services to the medically indigent
- Incentives for individuals who participate in preventive activities
- Federal funding of health care provider education focusing on service to underserved populations and areas
- The system as a union of both public and private sector resources and services
- Managed care dominating as the context for service delivery
- Continued focus on quality improvement

TRENDS AND ISSUES

As current trends continue, the delivery of health care services will continue to change. Table 5-8 lists factors that will continue to shape reform of the health care delivery system.

As health care reform occurs, some professions will experience opportunities for growth whereas others will experience layoffs (O'Neil, 1993). The challenge is to improve the nation's delivery of health care services by positioning nursing to preserve its integrity and to guarantee its preferred future. Nurses must be at the forefront of change.

LIFE CYCLE CONSIDERATIONS

Meeting the Needs of Elderly Clients

In 1992, the HCFA funded community nursing organizations (CNOs) to help meet the needs of elderly persons in four communities. These four projects yielded the following results:

- A high degree of client satisfaction
- Decreased Medicare expenditures associated with home care
- Use of less-expensive equipment
- Decrease emergency department costs (ANA, 1995)

SUMMARY

- The three levels of health care services can be categorized as primary, secondary, and tertiary.
- Health care services are delivered and financed by the public (official, voluntary, and nonprofit agencies), public/private, and private (hospitals, extended-care facilities, home health care agencies, hospices, outpatient settings, schools, industrial clinics, managed care organizations, community nursing centers, and rural hospitals) sectors.
- The health care team is composed of nurses, physicians, physician's assistants, pharmacists, dentists, dietitians, social workers, therapists, and chaplains.
- Managed care organizations seek to control health care costs by monitoring the delivery of services and restricting access to costly procedures and providers.
- Managed care plans include health maintenance organizations, preferred provider organizations, and exclusive provider organizations.
- The primary federal government insurance plans are Medicare, the program that provides health care coverage for elderly persons and disabled persons, and Medicaid, the jointly administered program that provides health care services for the poor.
- To achieve equity for all Americans, health care reform must address the three critical issues of cost, access, and quality of health care services.
- The challenges that the health care delivery system must overcome are the public's disillusionment with providers; the public's loss of control over health care decisions; the decreased use of hospitals and the related impact on quality of care; the change in practice settings; ethical issues, and the health care needs of vulnerable populations.
- *Nursing's Agenda for Health Care Reform* outlines nursing's proposals for easing the current problems in health care delivery.
- The Agency of Health Care Policy and Research aims to identify therapeutic standards to which the health care community can be held.
- A primary goal of the nursing profession within the areas of public health, community health, and long-term care is to provide health care services that emphasize prevention and primary health care for clients in these settings and thus help reduce costs and increase quality of health care.

Review Questions

1. When the goal of a health care service is to decrease the risk to clients for a disease or dysfunction, the type of care is called:
   a. primary.
   b. tertiary.
   c. exclusive.
   d. secondary.

2. Identified members of the health care team include:

   a.   nurses, pharmacists, chaplains.
   b.   nurses, physicians, ward clerks.
   c.   therapists, housekeeping personnel, dietitians.
   d.   dentists, social workers, maintenance personnel.

3. The primary federal government insurance plan(s) is (are):

   a.   Medicaid and welfare.
   b.   Medicaid and Social Security.
   c.   Medicaid and diagnosis-related groups.
   d.   Medicare and Children's Health Insurance Program.

4. Cost, access, and quality of health care services are the three critical issues that must be addressed by:

   a.   schools.
   b.   hospitals.
   c.   health care reform.
   d.   managed care plans.

5. The nursing role that protects the client and supports the client's decisions is:

   a.   teacher.
   b.   advocate.
   c.   caregiver.
   d.   team member.

6. The major health care problem for children is:

   a.   living in poverty.
   b.   having no transportation.
   c.   receiving substandard health care.
   d.   not receiving immunizations as infants.

Critical Thinking Questions

1. The U.S. health care system is first in technological advances, biomedical research, and state-of-the-art clinical equipment and facilities. Yet, even given these advantages, many consider the system to be in crisis. From your perspective, is the health care system in a state of strength or weakness? Why or why not?

2. What factors do you think have contributed to a positive perception of nurses? A negative perception? What can you do specifically to promote positive images of nurses among the public?

3. Think about the ethical ramifications of determining medically necessary therapeutics. Is rationing of scarce resources the answer to our health care dilemma?

 ## WEB FLASH!

*   Search the Internet for information regarding Oregon's plan for allocating resources. What are the main points of the plan?
*   Research health care reform on the Web. What is its status? What are the future plans for health care reform?

UNIT
3

Legal and Ethical Issues

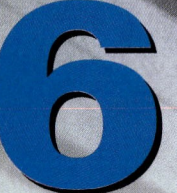

CHAPTER 6

LEGAL RESPONSIBILITIES

MAKING THE CONNECTION

Refer to the following chapters to increase your understanding of legal responsibilities:

- **Chapter 7, Ethical Responsibilities**
- **Chapter 10, Documentation**
- **Chapter 17, Loss, Grief, and Death**
- **Chapter 46, Nursing Care of the Client: Substance Abuse**

LEARNING OBJECTIVES

Upon completion of this chapter you should be able to:
- *Define key terms.*
- *Describe the difference between public law and civil law.*
- *State the purpose and identify various sources of standards of practice.*
- *Discuss the difference between intentional and unintentional torts.*
- *Discuss the importance of accurate documentation.*
- *Discuss ways that informed consent relates to nursing practice.*
- *Discuss the concept of advance directives.*
- *State the purpose and correct utilization of an incident report.*
- *Discuss ways the nurse can reduce personal liability.*
- *State the benefits of having one's own malpractice insurance policy.*
- *List steps to be taken when suspecting a colleague of being impaired by drugs or alcohol.*

KEY TERMS

administrative law	implied contract
advance directives	incident report
assault	informed consent
battery	law
civil law	liability
confidential	libel
constitutional law	living will
contract law	malpractice
criminal law	misdemeanor
defamation	negligence
durable power of	nursing practice act
attorney for health	peer assistance
care	programs
expressed contract	public law
false imprisonment	restraint
felony	slander
formal contract	standards of practice
fraud	statutory law
Good Samaritan Act	tort
impaired nurse	tort law

INTRODUCTION

Nursing, which embodies a concern for the client in every aspect of life, encompasses a great responsibility—one that requires knowledge, skill, care, and commitment. As society advances and technology changes, the issues that affect nursing practice also change. We continue to recognize the importance of informed consent, of the right to decide what is best for one's self, and of belief in the client's bill of rights. However, difficult issues, such as living wills, advance directives, do-not-resuscitate (DNR) orders, and impaired nurses, now confront the profession of nursing. Nurses in the past did not have to contend with these controversial topics. Today's nurse must be informed on these and other issues. This chapter provides a general overview of many legal concepts that affect nursing.

BASIC LEGAL CONCEPTS

Because it is useful to have working definitions of some basic legal concepts before applying them to a health care setting, a discussion of pertinent legal concepts follows.

Definition of Law

Laws are rules of conduct that guide interactions among people. Laws are binding, enforceable, and necessary so that people can live and work together. If laws are broken, a penalty is incurred.

The word **law** is derived from an Anglo-Saxon term meaning "that which is laid down or fixed." The two types of law are **public law**, which deals with the individual's relationship to the state, and **civil law**, which deals with relationships among individuals.

Sources of Law

The four sources of public law at the federal and state levels are constitutional, statutory, administrative, and criminal. The three sources of civil law at the federal and state levels are contracts, torts, and protective/reporting laws.

Public Law

Constitutional law, set forth in the U.S. and state constitutions, defines and limits the powers of government. **Statutory law** is enacted by legislative bodies. State boards and professional practice acts, such as nursing practice acts, are created and governed under statutory laws.

Administrative law (regulatory law) is developed by those persons appointed to governmental administrative agencies. These persons are entrusted with enforcing the statutory laws passed by the legislature. Administrative law gives state boards of nursing the power to make rules and regulations governing nursing as set forth in the nursing practice acts. In these administrative rules, nursing boards identify the specific processes for educational programs; licensure; grounds for disciplinary proceedings; and the establishment of fees for services and for penalties rendered by the board.

Criminal law, the most common example of public law, addresses acts or offenses against the safety or welfare of the public. Under criminal law, there are two types of crime: **felony** (crime of a serious nature that is usually punishable by imprisonment at a state penitentiary or by death or crime in violation of federal statute and involving punishment of more than 1 year incarceration) and **misdemeanor** (offense that is less serious than a felony and may be punishable by a fine or a sentence to a local prison for less than 1 year). Table 6-1 outlines the types of public law.

Civil Law

Civil law addresses crimes against a person or persons in such legal matters as contracts, torts, and protective/reporting law (Table 6-2). Most cases of malpractice fall under the civil law of torts (Flight, 1998).

Contract law is the enforcement of agreements among private individuals. There are three essential elements in a legal contract.

- Promise(s) between two or more legally competent individuals that state what each individual must do or not do
- Mutual understanding of the terms and obligations the contract imposes on each individual
- Compensation for lawful actions performed

The terms of a contract may be agreed on orally or in writing. However, a **formal** (written) **contract**

Table 6-1 TYPES OF PUBLIC LAW

TYPE	FEDERAL	STATE
Constitutional law	U.S. Constitution Civil Rights Act	State Constitutions Law
Statutory law	None	State boards and professional practice acts such as nursing practice acts
Administrative law	Food, Drug, and Cosmetic Act Social Security Act National Labor Relations Act	Rules and regulations governing nursing as set by state boards of nursing
Criminal law	Controlled Substance Act Kidnapping	Criminal codes (defining murder, manslaughter, criminal negligence, rape, fraud, illegal possession of drugs, theft, assault, and battery)

Adapted from Fundamentals of Nursing: Standards & Practice, *by S. DeLaune and P. Ladner, 1998, Albany, NY: Delmar Publishers. Copyright 1998 by Delmar Publishers. Adapted with permission.*

Table 6-2 TYPES OF CIVIL LAW

TYPE	FEDERAL	STATE
Contract law	None	Employment contracts
		Business contracts with clients
		Contracts with allied groups
		Uniform Commercial Code
Torts	Federal Torts Claims Act	State Torts Claims Act (allows claims against the state)
		Negligence (common law claim)
		Malpractice statutes (professional liability)
		Assault
		Battery
		False Imprisonment
		Invasion of privacy
		Defamation (libel and slander)
		Fraud
Protective/ reporting laws	Child Abuse Prevention and Treatment Act	Age of consent statutes (medical treatment, drugs, sexually transmitted disease)
	Privacy Act of 1974	Privileged Communication Statute
		Abortion statute
		Good Samaritan Act
		Abuse statutes (child, elderly, domestic violence)
		Involuntary Hospitalization Act
		Living will legislation

Adapted from Fundamentals of Nursing: Standards & Practice, *by S. DeLaune and P. Ladner, 1998, Albany, NY: Delmar Publishers. Copyright 1998 by Delmar Publishers. Adapted with permission.*

cannot be changed legally by an oral agreement. An **expressed contract** gives, in writing, the conditions and terms of the contract. An **implied contract** recognizes a relationship between parties for services.

In accord with U.S. Contract Law, the nurse is legally required to:

- Adhere to the employer's policies and standards unless they conflict with federal or state law,
- Fulfill the terms of contracted service with the employer, and
- Respect the rights and responsibilities of other health care providers, especially in areas that promote continuity of client care.

Along with these legal responsibilities, the nurse has a right to expect:

- Adequate and qualified assistance in providing care,
- Reasonable and prudent conduct from the client,
- Compensation from the employer for services rendered,
- A safe work environment with the necessary resources to render services, and
- Prudent, reasonable conduct from other health care providers.

A **tort** is a civil wrong committed by a person against another person or property (Zerwekh & Claborn, 1997). **Tort law** is the enforcement of duties and rights among individuals independent of contractual agreements.

The protective/reporting law may be considered criminal law, depending on the state classification. Two examples of protective law are The Americans with Disabilities Act (ADA) and the Good Samaritan Act.

The ADA was passed by the U.S. Congress in 1990. It prohibits discrimination in employment, public services, and public accommodations on the basis of disability. The ADA defines a disability as a physical or mental impairment that substantially limits one or more of the major life activities. Disabilities that may be covered by the ADA include the following:

- Mental impairments
  Learning disabilities
  Psychiatric disorders
  Organic brain syndrome
  Retardation
- Physical impairments
  Addiction
  Cancer

Cerebral palsy
Diabetes
Epilepsy
Heart disease
Human immunodeficiency virus (HIV, symptomatic or asymptomatic)
Multiple sclerosis
Muscular dystrophy
Orthopedic, visual, speech, and hearing impairments
Tuberculosis

The **Good Samaritan Act** provides protection to health care providers by ensuring immunity from civil **liability** (obligation one has incurred or might incur through any act or failure to act) when care is provided at the scene of an emergency and the caregiver does not intentionally or recklessly cause the client injury.

The Good Samaritan Act applies only in emergency situations, usually those outside the hospital setting. It stipulates that the health care worker must not be acting for an employer or receive compensation for care given.

In most states, health care professionals are not required to stop at the scene of accidents. If they do stop, however, they are held to higher standards than is a lay person. Health care professionals are expected to use their specialized body of knowledge when providing care. They are expected to act as would most other professionals with the same background and education.

PROFESSIONAL TIP

Good Samaritan Acts

Good Samaritan acts vary in coverage from state to state and may be amended periodically by legislation. It is the responsibility of caregivers to know the law for their respective jurisdictions (Zerwekh & Claborn, 1997).

NURSING PRACTICE AND THE LAW

Nursing practice falls under both public law and civil law. In most states, nurses are bound by rules and regulations stipulated by the **nursing practice act** as determined by the legislature. For licensed practical/vocational nurses (LP/VNs) four states, Texas, California, Tennessee, and South Dakota, have title acts as opposed to practice acts.

Public laws are designed to protect the public. If these laws are broken, the nurse can be punished by paying a fine, losing her license, or being incarcerated.

PROFESSIONAL TIP

Nursing Practice Act/Title Act
• Nursing practice acts state those things that the nurse can and cannot do.
• Title acts state who can be called an LP/VN.

An example would be a nurse guilty of diverting drugs, which is considered a crime against the state. The offending nurse could lose her license to practice and could be sent to jail.

Civil laws deal with problems that occur between a nurse and the client. For example, if a nurse catheterizes a client and perforates the bladder, the client may bring a civil suit against the nurse. No law affecting the population as a whole has been broken, but the client has sustained injury. This is a problem between individuals—the nurse and the client or the nurse, the client, and the nurse's employer. The client may receive compensation for injuries, but no jail time is incurred by the nurse.

Standards of Practice

The state boards of nursing have been assigned the responsibility of determining and regulating nursing practice. The boards indicate what nursing is and is not, defines registered nursing and practical nursing, and sets educational guidelines for each program.

The state boards of nursing also stipulate who may practice nursing in their respective states (licensure). The related criteria usually involve graduating from a state-approved or -accredited program, passing the National Council Licensure Exam (NCLEX), and meeting certain moral and legal standards. The boards have the authority to bring disciplinary action against a nurse for violation of its rules and regulations. Disciplinary action can include suspension or revocation of a nurse's license and/or a fine.

Under the auspices of the nursing practice acts, guidelines have been developed to direct nursing care. These guidelines are called **standards of practice** or standards of care.

Standards of practice are derived from a variety of sources. As stated, they are usually defined by the board of nursing and described in the nursing practice act. However, professional organizations like the American Nurses Association (ANA) for the registered nurse (RN) and the National Federation of Licensed Practical Nurses (NFLPN) for the LP/VN also develop standards of practice. Books on nursing care planning, especially for specialized areas, are additional resources for the development of practice standards.

Policy and procedure manuals also represent standards of practice. Each facility, based on a rigorous review process, has identified specific ways of performing procedures such as passing medications, inserting catheters, and collecting specimens. The nurse employed by the facility is expected to follow the guidelines as laid out by the policy and procedure manuals. For situations not covered in the policy and procedure manuals, the nurse is expected to exercise good judgment in the planning and providing of client care. In other words, the nurse is expected to act in a reasonable and prudent manner.

Liability

What is meant by reasonable and prudent? In the case of nursing, it means that the nurse is expected to act as would other nurses at the same professional level and with the same amount of education or experience. If most nurses would respond to a particular situation in a certain way, and the nurse in question does so also, the nurse would be acting in a reasonable and prudent manner. However, if most nurses would respond differently than the nurse in question, the nurse would not be behaving in a reasonable and prudent manner and can be held liable or responsible for damages. Liability is determined by whether the nurse adhered to the standards of practice.

Legal Issues in Practice

Many aspects relating to nursing practice and areas of nursing are subject to liability, including physician's orders, floating, inadequate staffing, critical care, and pediatric care.

Physician's Orders

The physician is in charge of directing the client's care, and nurses are to carry out the physician's orders for care, unless the nurse believes that the orders are in error or would be harmful to the client. In this case, the physician must be contacted to confirm and/or clarify the orders. If the nurse still believes the orders to be inappropriate, she should immediately contact the nursing supervisor and put in writing why the orders are not being carried out. A nurse who carries out an erroneous or inappropriate order may be held liable for harm experienced by the client. Nurses are responsible for their actions regardless of who told them to perform those actions.

Floating

Nurses sometimes are asked to "float" to an unfamiliar nursing unit. The supervisor should be informed about a float nurse's lack of experience in caring for the type of clients on the new nursing unit. The nurse should be given an orientation to the new unit and will be held to the same standards of care as are the nurses who regularly work on that unit.

Inadequate Staffing

The Joint Commission on Accreditation of Healthcare Organizations (JCAHO) has established guidelines for determining the number of staff needed for any given situation (staffing ratios) (JCAHO, 1993). When there are not enough nurses to meet the staffing ratio and provide competent care, substandard care may result, placing clients at physical risk and the nurse and institution at legal risk. The nurse in this situation should provide nursing administration with a written account of the situation. A nurse who leaves an inadequately staffed unit could be charged with client abandonment.

Critical Care

Because the monitors used in critical care units are not infallible, constant observation and assessment of the clients are required. This makes a one-to-one or a one-to-two nurse–client ratio imperative. Furthermore, equipment must be checked regularly, and on a schedule, by the biomedical department.

Pediatric Care

Legislation in each state requires that suspected child abuse or neglect be reported. Legal immunity is provided to the person who makes a report in good faith. When suspected child abuse or neglect is not reported by health care providers, legal action, civil or criminal, may be filed against them.

NURSE–CLIENT RELATIONSHIP

A variety of situations can develop between a nurse and a client that may require legal intervention. The following is a discussion of the types of torts that may arise.

Torts

When a case is brought against a nurse, it is usually a civil action that falls under tort law. Torts can be intentional or unintentional (Table 6-3). The person who commits an intentional tort violates the civil rights of another individual knowingly and willfully. Examples of intentional torts are assault and battery, defamation (libel and slander), fraud, false imprisonment, and invasion of privacy. Unintentional torts are those actions that cause harm to the client and that result from a carelessness or negligence on the part of the nurse. If found liable, the nurse generally must pay monetary damages. Prison terms are rare.

Intentional Torts

Assault and Battery Assault and battery, though frequently used together, are actually two separate terms. **Assault** is the threat to do something that may

Table 6-3 SELECTED TORTS: DEFINITIONS AND EXAMPLES

TYPE OF TORT	DEFINITION	EXAMPLE
Intentional		
Assault and battery	Threaten or attempt to touch another person. Unconsented touching.	Nurse who unjustifiably forces a treatment against the client's will and in the absence of consent
False imprisonment	Unwarranted restriction of the freedom of an individual.	Nurse who uses the restraints on a client who is of sound mind and is not in danger of inflicting injury on self or another
Quasi-intentional		
Invasion of privacy	All individuals have the right to privacy and may bring charges against any person who violates this right.	Nurse who either discloses information about a client that is considered private or photographs a client without consent
Defamation (libel and slander)	Verbal (slander) or written (libel) remarks that may cause the loss of an individual's reputation.	Nurse who makes a statement that could either ruin the client's reputation or cause the client to lose his or her job
Unintentional		
Negligence	Failure to use such care as a reasonably prudent person would use under similar circumstances, which leads to harm.	Nurse who loses client's property Nurse who makes a medication error Nurse who burns a client via the improper use of equipment Nurse who fails to observe and/or report a change in the client's condition. Nurse who inaccurately counts sponges in the operating room
Malpractice	Failure of a professional to use such care as a reasonably prudent member of the profession would use under similar circumstances, which leads to harm.	Nurse who makes an inaccurate nursing diagnosis and implements the wrong treatment Nurse who does not follow physician orders Nurse who does not question physician's clearly erroneous order

Adapted from Nursing Perspectives and Issues *(5th ed.), by P. R. Mitchell and G. M. Grippando, 1993, Albany, NY: Delmar Publishers. Copyright 1993 by Delmar Publishers. Adapted with permission.*

cause harm or be unpleasant to another person. **Battery** is the unauthorized or unwanted touching of one person by another.

Fear and intimidation are the key elements in assault. The person assaulted must believe that the threat made can and will be carried out, for example, a client who is confined to a wheelchair and told, "If you do not finish your meal, you are going to sit there all night." The client complies because he believes the health care worker will leave him to sit for an uncomfortable period of time. The worker is in a position to carry out this threat, and the client knows it.

The key factor regarding battery is consent. People have the right to be free of unwanted handling of their person. Striking a client is battery. Performing a procedure without the client's consent is battery. Forcing a person to take medication they do not want is battery. Any unwanted touching, regardless of outcome, can be construed as battery.

Defamation **Defamation** is the use of words to harm or injure the personal or professional reputation of another person. If the words are written down, they constitute **libel**. If the information is communicated verbally to a third party, it constitutes **slander**.

CULTURAL CONSIDERATIONS

Assault and Battery Charges

To prevent assault and battery charges:

- Respect the client's cultural values, beliefs, and practices with regard to "touching."
- To African Americans, touching another person's hair is sometimes viewed as offensive.
- Asian Americans usually do not touch others during conversations. Touching someone on the head is considered disrespectful because the head is considered sacred.
- European Americans employ handshakes for formal greetings.
- Hispanic Americans are very tactile and may embrace and shake hands when greeting one another.
- To Native Americans, touching dead body is prohibited and may leave the offender open to charges of assault.

Nurses must be discreet as to the ways that they characterize clients, peers, and other health care professionals. Negative or derogatory comments that are untrue leave the nurse no defense against charges of defamation. If comments are true, the relevance of the information is important. The most common examples of this tort are giving out inaccurate or inappropriate information from the medical record; discussing clients, families, or visitors in public areas; or speaking negatively about coworkers (Zerwekh & Claborn, 1997).

Fraud   **Fraud** is a wrong that results from a deliberate deception intended to produce unlawful gain. Common forms of fraud in health care include illegal billing and deceit in obtaining or attempting to obtain a nursing license (Flight, 1998).

False Imprisonment   **False imprisonment** refers to making the client wrongfully believe that she cannot leave a place. The most common example of this tort is telling a client not to leave the hospital until the bill is paid (Zerwekh & Claborn, 1997). Any mechanism used to confine a client or to restrict movement can be considered a restraint and a form of false imprisonment. This includes threats, locked doors, physical restraints such as wrist or vest restraints, side rails, geriatric chairs, and psychotropic drugs.

Nurses may find themselves in a quandary in situations where a client chooses to leave the health care facility, and no discharge order has been written. It is possible that the health care problem has not been resolved, and the nurse feels that it is not in the best interest of the client to leave. If the client is of sound mind, however, he has the right to make this decision, regardless of what others think is best. Detaining the individual could result in charges of false imprisonment.

Documentation is very important in these situations. The nurse should document the client's reasons for leaving the facility and include any teaching or interventions related to the situation. Facility policy usually requires that the client sign a form indicating that he is leaving against medical advice (AMA), which releases the facility of any liability. If the client is angry and refuses to sign the AMA form, the client's refusal should be documented, and the nursing supervisor and the client's physician should be notified.

As indicated, any device used to restrict movement is called a **restraint**. To safeguard against possible charges of false imprisonment, the nurse should carefully assess the situation and include the client or significant other in the care planning process. If it is determined that a restraint is needed, the purpose and use of the restraint should be explained, including the way the restraint fits into the plan of care, the length of time the restraint may be necessary, and the expected outcome. The planning session should be documented in the client's medical record.

The client in restraints must be assessed frequently. Documentation must show that:

- Restraints were checked hourly and released every 2 hours,
- The client was toileted,
- The client received food and water, and
- The client had position changes.

In acute care settings, restraints can usually be applied temporarily as a nursing measure for client safety; however, in most states, a physician's order must be immediately obtained. In long-term care settings, a physician's order is required prior to utilizing any restraints.

Invasion of Privacy   People are entitled to **confidential** (private) health care. All information gleaned from working with a client or his medical records must be kept confidential. Therefore, a client's health status may not be discussed with a third party, unless either the client is present and has given verbal permission or permission has been obtained in writing. This does not apply to nurses' discussing a client's health status with other health care workers involved in the care of the client.

Invasion of privacy occurs when a person's private affairs become public knowledge without the person's permission. Photographing a client without his consent is an invasion of privacy. Failing to pull curtains to shield the client when performing personal or intimate care also constitutes an invasion of privacy.

A common mistake made by health care personnel is discussing clients in public areas. It is difficult to gauge who may overhear when comments are made while sitting in the cafeteria or waiting for the elevator (Figure 6-1). The results can be detrimental if the client is embarrassed by this loss of privacy: The client's job

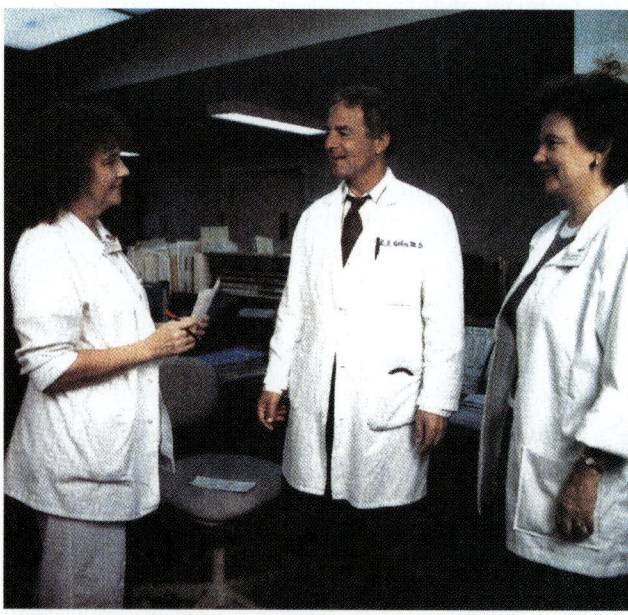

Figure 6-1 The nurse should not discuss clients, families, or coworkers in public areas

or family situation may be compromised, depending on the nature of the information. For example, news of an abortion, positive HIV status, or venereal disease may be socially damaging to some clients. Clients or their health care status should never be discussed in public areas or with those persons not directly involved in the care of the client.

All clients have the right to be free of unwanted public exposure. Permission should be obtained before going through a client's belongings. Doors should be kept closed and curtains pulled when providing personal care. People not involved in the performance of a procedure should not be invited to watch unless the client has given permission. Clients cannot be photographed or videotaped without their permission and a release form must be signed. Confidentiality should not be breached by using a client's full name on care plans, case studies, or other assignments that a student may have during clinical experience; only initials should be used. This helps protect the client's privacy should the papers be lost. The client's chart and other materials should not be left lying around, making a client's private information public knowledge.

Unintentional Torts

Negligence and malpractice are considered to be unintentional torts.

Negligence Negligence is a general term referring to negligent or careless acts on the part of an individual who is not exercising reasonable or prudent judgment. All nurses, including student nurses, are expected to use good judgment when providing client care. This means, for instance, that side rails should not be left down on confused clients' beds, and sedated clients should not be allowed to smoke unattended. To prevent falls, puddles and spills are cleaned up immediately, rather than waiting for housekeeping to take care of the matter. Any person, with or without the specialized knowledge required for nursing, could make these determinations. Should a nurse fail to protect a client in such a situation or in one requiring similar judgments, the nurse could be found negligent.

Malpractice Negligent acts on the part of a professional can be termed **malpractice**, or professional negligence. More specifically, malpractice relates to the conduct of a person while acting in a professional capacity.

Negligent or careless acts on the part of a nurse frequently come from not meeting the standards of care, in other words, from not doing what a reasonable and prudent nurse would do under similar circumstances. A nurse can be charged with malpractice for acts committed or acts omitted. Failure to properly assess a client or to act on assessment information are examples of omission. Giving a client the wrong medication because of improper identification procedures (not checking the armband) or improper setup (not using

the medication administration record) are acts of commission.

Malpractice can include attempting a procedure with which the nurse is unfamiliar or improperly performing a procedure that results in client injury. Malpractice differs from negligence in that anyone can be accused of negligence; only professionals can be accused of malpractice.

Several factors must hold true for a nurse to be found guilty of malpractice:

- The nurse owed a special duty to the client; in other words, a nurse–client relationship existed.
- The nurse failed to meet the standards of care. Policy, procedure, or standards of care were not followed.
- Injury occurred as a result of the nurse's action or inaction, a direct cause and effect.

The prudent nurse is protected by adhering to facility policy and procedure and attempting to meet the standards of care at all times. The case study discussed in Figure 6-2 illustrates some of the difficulties in distinguishing between malpractice and negligence.

Documentation

The source of information regarding the client's clinical history is the medical record, or the chart. The chart should accurately reflect diagnosis, treatment, testing, clinical course, nursing assessment, and intervention. According to the law, "If it was not charted, it was not done." If a chart ever winds up in court, this is the standard the jury applies when trying to determine what happened and who is at fault.

The nurse should not chart medications before they are given or treatments before they are completed. Either constitutes a direct violation of the standards of practice for documentation and medication administration. The standard of practice is that medications are documented *after* they are administered. All client care, including treatments, is documented after being provided.

Documentation must be accurate and objective. The nurse should describe what is seen and done. Nurses' notes should reflect facts, not inferences or opinions, about the client. Furthermore, it is not enough to chart nursing assessment or identified problems. The nurse must complete the task by documenting any actions taken, including nursing interventions and physician's orders implemented.

Entries must be neat, legible, spelled correctly, written clearly, and signed or initialed. It is illegal to go back and change a chart. If an error in charting is made, a line should be drawn through the incorrect entry and the nurse should initial it. Blacking out entries or using correction fluid is not acceptable, as this renders the original entry illegible. Sloppy, misspelled charting might discredit excellent nursing care.

Case Study: Standard of Care—Malpractice or Ordinary Negligence?

Facts: A 75-year-old client fell and fractured a hip while in the hospital. The client had been medicated with castor oil and a sleeping pill, and the nurse failed to raise the side rails on the bed. During the night, the client got out of bed to go to the bathroom and fell, fracturing the hip. The client sued, alleging that the nurse had been negligent in failing to raise the side rails and in failing to tell the client that a bedpan would be brought to the client when needed.

Holding: The nurse's conduct constituted negligence. Unlike a malpractice action, no expert testimony was necessary to establish the applicable standard of care. The duty to raise side rails on a bed and to instruct the client to use the call button beside the bed if assistance were needed did not involve the failure to render professional nursing or medical services requiring special skills. The jury, therefore, could evaluate the nurse's conduct under the standard of "the reasonably prudent person," rather than "the reasonably prudent nurse."

Norris v. Rowan Memorial Hospital, North Carolina Court of Appeals 1974

Comment: This case points out the difficulties even courts have in drawing the line between ordinary negligence and malpractice. Cases involving a nurse's failure to raise bed rails are decided under the standard of ordinary negligence as often as they are decided under the standard of professional malpractice.

Figure 6-2 Case Study: Standard of Care—Malpractice or Ordinary Negligence? *(Adapted from* Nursing Perspectives and Issues *[5th ed.], by P. Mitchell and G. Grippando, 1993, Albany, NY: Delmar Publishers. Copyright 1993 by Delmar Publishers. Adapted with permission.)*

Incomplete Documentation: Mrs. Drew

Mrs. Drew, 85 years old, was a resident on a transitional care unit. She lost 15 pounds over a 3 month period. When her chart was reviewed, the auditor targeted the weight loss as a problem. She examined the chart to discover what the nurses did to try to correct this situation.

The nurses had carefully documented the percentages Mrs. Drew had eaten at each meal, her lack of appetite, and the pattern of weight loss. They thought they had covered all bases. They were wrong.

The auditor referred to the standards of practice on weight loss in long-term care facilities. She questioned, "Did the nurses follow the guidelines?" No interventions were charted, so it was presumed that nothing was done.

In fact, the nurses had called the dietitian to see this client several times to discuss her food preferences and a calorie count was initiated. Student nurses assigned to Mrs. Drew sat with her at mealtimes to encourage her to eat. The nurses had spoken with the doctor and Mrs. Drew's family about their concern over her lack of appetite and loss of weight. However, none of this was charted. There was no proof, other than the dietitian's entries, that any attempt had been made to intervene in this client's nutritional deficit.

Figure 6-3 Incomplete Documentation: Mrs. Drew *(From* Medical–Surgical Nursing: An Integrated Approach, *by L. White and G. Duncan, 1998, Albany NY: Delmar Publishers. Copyright 1998 by Delmar Publishers. Reprinted with permission.)*

Figures 6-3 and 6-4 reflect situations where nurses identified client problems. In Figure 6-3, documentation was incomplete. In the situation presented in Figure 6-4, the nurses clearly identified the problem, the client's response, and the actions taken.

INFORMED CONSENT

Informed consent refers to a competent client's ability to make health care decisions based on full disclosure of the benefits, risks, potential consequences of a recommended treatment plan, and alternate treatments, including no treatment and the client's agreement to the treatment as indicated by the client's signing a consent form. This detailed explanation, provided by the physician, allows the client to make intelligent decisions about treatment options. The issue of informed consent deals with the right of the client to determine what happens to his or her person. Consent to treatment also helps protect the health care worker from unwarranted charges of battery.

Individuals who are declared incompetent have a guardian or someone who has **power of attorney** to make heath care decisions and give consent for treatment.

Nurses must obtain consent for nursing procedures. Each client, on admission, signs a general care consent form. The nurse is obligated to explain what is to be

Complete Documentation: Roberta Wilson

Roberta Wilson is a 44-year-old woman with a history of diabetes mellitus controlled by diet. She was admitted 2 days ago for abdominal pain. Ms. Wilson has been designated nothing by mouth (NPO) since midnight for an ultrasound scheduled at 9:30 A.M. The doctor instructed that she was to remain NPO until seen by a consultant. Her 11 A.M. accucheck revealed a blood sugar of 44. She was experiencing no symptoms of hypoglycemia.

What needed to be done and what needed to be documented to protect everyone involved? Hospital protocol stipulated giving 4 ounces of Coke for blood sugars less than 60, then repeating the accucheck in approximately 30 minutes. The nurses contacted the physician to cancel the NPO order, then administered the Coke. Roberta's blood sugar at 11:40 A.M. was 93. She was served an 1,800 calorie ADA (American Dietetic Association) diet for lunch.

What was charted?

2/08/XX	11:10 A.M.	Accucheck 44. Client's skin is warm and dry, denies nausea, tremors, or confusion. States she feels "fine." Physician notified of low blood sugar and client condition. Orders received to discontinue NPO status and resume previous orders.
2/08/XX	11:15 A.M.	4 ounces of Coke given.
2/08/XX	11:40 A.M.	Blood sugar 93. Served 1,800 calorie ADA diet for lunch. Blood sugar to be repeated at 4 P.M.

Figure 6-4 Complete Documentation: Roberta Wilson *(From Medical–Surgical Nursing: An Integrated Approach, by L. White and G. Duncan, 1998, Albany NY: Delmar Publishers. Copyright 1998 by Delmar Publishers. Reprinted with permission.)*

done to the client and to receive at least implied consent, as indicated by lack of objection on the part of the client. It is the physician's responsibility to obtain consent for medical or surgical treatment. The disclosure about the risks and benefits of treatment generally takes place at a time when the nurse is not present, often in the physician's office. It is usually on the basis of this discussion that the client decides whether to accept the treatment recommendation and sign the consent form. Confusion arises, however, because nurses are often delegated the duty of collecting the signature for invasive procedures such as surgery, cardiac catheterization, and other diagnostic procedures. Student nurses should neither ask the client to sign a consent form, nor witness a consent form.

When a nurse has a client sign a consent form, the nurse is verifying the following three things:

- The client's signature is authentic.
- The client has the mental capacity to understand the things discussed with the physician.
- The client was not coerced into signing the form.

If the nurse is unsure about the client's understanding or if the client still has questions, the client should not sign the form. The nurse should document the client's lack of understanding and contact the physician. Further clarification is needed, and it must come from the physician.

Clients over the age of 18 years may give consent for their own health care. Parents or guardians give consent for minor children. In most states, however, minors who are married, live on their own, become pregnant, or require treatment for sexually transmitted diseases, mental illness, or substance abuse may give consent for themselves.

Complex situations occur when minors refuse treatments to which parents have consented, or parents refuse consent or treatment that has been deemed medically necessary for their minor children. The court has had to intervene in such cases. In situations such as these, the child may be made a ward of the court and the decision-making capacity temporarily taken

CLIENT TEACHING

Informed Consent

Consent may be withdrawn, either verbally or in writing, at any time.

PROFESSIONAL TIP

Consent in Emergencies
- Consent is implied when immediate action is necessary to save a life or prevent permanent physical harm. Written consent is waived.
- After the emergency is over, consent must be obtained for further care.

CLIENT TEACHING

Advance Directives

- Advance directives should be discussed with the family and physician so that everyone understands the client's wishes, and conflicts are less likely to occur at a later time.
- An advance directive may be changed by the client as long as the client is competent.

away from the parents. An example would be the child of Jehovah's Witnesses who needs a blood transfusion but whose parents refuse treatment on the basis of religious beliefs.

Invasive procedures or those that may have serious consequences, such as surgery, cardiac catheterization, or HIV testing, require written consent. Figure 6-5 illustrates a typical consent form used to obtain client permission for the performance of invasive medical, surgical, or diagnostic procedures. Consent for procedures that are not invasive can be either given verbally or implied. The client implies consent when he cooperates with the procedure offered. For example, if the orderly says, "Mr. Jones, I am here to take you for your chest x-ray," and Mr. Jones gets into the wheelchair, consent is implied by Mr. Jones' cooperation.

ADVANCE DIRECTIVES

An **advance directive** is a written instruction for health care that is recognized under state law and is related to the provision of such care when the individual is incapacitated. Advance directives emphasize the right of the client to self-determination. They are instructions about health care preferences regarding life-

PROFESSIONAL TIP

Consent in Special Situations

- If a client is unable to consent and the family is too far away, consent may be received over the telephone, according to agency policy (usually, two persons must hear the consent being given).
- A client who has already received preoperative or preprocedure medication is not competent to sign a consent. When this situation arises, the surgery or procedure may have to be postponed.
- For blood transfusions, some facilities require that a denial form be signed if the client indicates *No* on the consent form.

sustaining measures. These instructions may indicate who may make health care decisions for the client should he become unable to do so for himself. In essence, they express the client's wishes about the kinds of medical treatment wanted and not wanted.

A client of sound mind retains the right to make all health care decisions and even reverse previous decisions. Should a situation arise when the person becomes incapable of making decisions, however, advance directives serve as a guide to family members concerning those kinds of treatment that should or should not be allowed. Advance directives permit those involved in the decision-making process to know what the client prefers. Although these instructions are best put in writing, this is not always done. Sometimes, health care preferences are shared verbally with family members or friends. Such verbal instructions can be interpreted differently by different people, creating difficulty for all involved—the physician, the health care facility, and the family. Thus, it is best to get this information in writing. When an advance directive indicates that the client does not wish to have cardiopulmonary resuscitation (CPR) performed in the event of cardiac arrest, the physician must write a DNR order, also referred to as a "No Code."

All health care facilities that receive Medicare or Medicaid monies are required to offer to all competent clients on admission the opportunity to execute advance directives. The client should also be told about the purpose and availability of a living will and durable power of attorney for health care (discussed following). If desired, assistance in completing these documents should be offered to the client. In addition, the medical record must show that the client was offered the opportunity to complete these documents. The documentation must indicate decisions made or not made at that time. Clients cannot be coerced into signing advance directives, nor can they be discriminated against should they choose not to sign an advance directive.

Facility policies vary as to who provides the information on advance directives. Many health care facilities assign this responsibility to the admissions office or social services; others have the nurses do it. Regardless of which department is assigned this task, the nurse is frequently called on to assist the client in understanding this information.

Before discussing advance directives with a client, the nurse must be familiar with the Patient Self-Determination Act of 1990. In the role of client advocate, the nurse explains the different types of advance directives to the client and family members. Terms such as *palliative care, supportive care, comfort measures,* or *nutrition and hydration* may not be understood by the client. The nurse can define those concepts more clearly and emphasize that the client has the right to choose what he believes is best for himself.

TO THE PATIENT: You have the right as a patient to be informed about your condition and the recommended surgical, medical, or diagnostic procedure to be used so that you may make the decision whether or not to undergo the procedure after knowing the risks and hazards involved. This disclosure is not meant to scare or alarm you, but is simply an effort to make you better informed so you may give or withhold your consent to the procedure. Any questions or concerns you may have with respect to the proposed procedure, its risks, complications, or benefits should be directed to your treating physician.

I (we) voluntarily request Dr. _____ as my physician, and such associates, technical assistants and other health care providers as they may deem necessary to treat my condition, which has been explained to me as: _____

_____

I (we) understand that the following surgical, medical, and/or diagnostic procedures are planned for me, and I (we) voluntarily consent and authorize these procedures: _____

_____

I (we) understand that my physician may discover other or different conditions which require additional or different procedures than those planned. I (we) authorize my physician, and such associates, technical assistants, and other health care providers, to perform such procedures which are advisable in their professional judgment.

I (we) [DO] [DO NOT] consent to the use of blood and blood products as deemed necessary.

I (we) understand that no warrant or guarantee has been made to me as a result or cure.

Just as there may be risks and hazards in continuing my present condition without treatment, there are also risks and hazards related to the performance of the surgical, medical, and/or diagnostic procedures planned for me. I (we) realize that common to surgical, medical, and/or diagnostic procedures is the potential for infection, blood clots in veins and lungs, hemorrhage, allergic reactions, and even death. I (we) realize that the following risks and hazards may occur in connection with this particular procedure:

_____

_____

_____

I (we) understand that anesthesia involves additional risks and hazards, but I (we) request the use of anesthetics for the relief and protection from pain during the planned and additional procedures. I (we) realize the anesthesia may have to be changed, possibly without explanation to me (us).

I(we) understand that certain complications may result from the use of any anesthetic, including respiratory problems, drug reaction, paralysis, brain damage, or even death. Other risks and hazards which may result from the use of general anesthetics range from minor discomfort to injury to vocal cords, teeth, or eyes. I (we) understand that other risks and hazards resulting from spinal or epidural anesthetics include headache, chronic pain, remote possibility of nerve injury, hematoma, infection, septic and aseptic meningitis, nausea, vomiting, itching, and urinary retention.

I (we) consent to the photographing of the operations or procedures to be performed, including appropriate portions of the body, for medical, scientific, or educational purposes, provided my identity is not revealed by descriptive texts accompanying the picture.

I (we) consent to the disposition by hospital authorities of any tissues or parts which may be removed.

I (we) have been given the opportunity to ask questions about my conditions, alternative forms of anesthesia and treatment, risks of non-treatment, the procedures to be used, and the risks and hazards involved, and I (we) believe that I (we) have sufficient information to give this informed consent.

I (we) certify that I (we) have discussed the proposed procedures and risks with my physician; that this form has been fully explained to me; that I (we) have read it or have had it read to me (us); that the blank spaces have been filled in; and that I (we) understand its contents.

DATE:_____   TIME:_____

                                                                                      A.M./P.M.

_____   _____
Patient/other legally responsible person   Witness Name
(Minor patient and parent/guardian signature)

SPOHN HEALTH SYSTEM CORPUS CHRISTI, TEXAS 78404 DISCLOSURE AND CONSENT- MEDICAL AND SURGICAL PROCEDURES PATIENT CARE SERVICES 2704980 NEW: 05/82 REVISED: 05/98	

Figure 6-5 Disclosure and Consent—Medical and Surgical Procedures *(Courtesy Spohn Health System, Corpus Christi, TX)*

The nurse may suggest that the client discuss personal preferences with the physician and family members. When the client does so, problems may be prevented later. If the wishes of the family are different from those of the client, the health care team is caught in the middle, the concern being that the family may bring a lawsuit against the facility and the physician. The advance directive serves as a guide from the client. The facility's ethics committee may also be involved. The nurse should emphasize that these advanced directives only go into effect should the individual become incompetent or have a terminal illness, or death is imminent.

Durable Power of Attorney

A **durable power of attorney for health care** (DPAHC) is a legal document designating who may make health care decisions for a client when that client is no longer capable of decision making. This health care representative is appointed by the client and is expected to act in the best interests of the client. This appointment can be revoked any time the competent client chooses.

For example, if a client lapses into a coma and the prognosis is poor, the health care representative or the person appointed DPAHC can either give consent for certain types of treatment or withhold consent for treatment, even if the lack of treatment results in the client's death. It is expected that the health care representative has discussed treatment preferences with the client and thus knows the client's wishes. The DPAHC is activated only when the client is no longer competent to make health care decisions.

The person who has power of attorney or the authority to make decisions for a client in some areas does not necessarily have the same authority regarding health care issues. The granting of the right to make health care decisions has to be specified in the power of attorney agreement, or a DPAHC must be signed (Figure 6-6). Because of a possible conflict of interest, the health care representative may be different from the individual assigned the power of attorney.

A person who stands to benefit from the client's estate cannot be appointed health care representative. If a decision to terminate life support would benefit the designee financially, for instance, a conflict of interest would exist. This person could have the right to make decisions about the client in matters not pertaining to health care, however.

Living Will

A **living will** is a legal document that allows a person to state preferences about the use of life-sustaining measures should she be unable to make her wishes known. These preferences can be expressed either with a living will or a Life-Prolonging Procedure Declaration. These documents allow the client to specify, in advance, those life-sustaining measures that are to be done or not done.

The living will states that certain life-prolonging treatments are not to be used and that the individual prefers to die naturally. Food, fluids, and comfort measures are continued, and the person is not abandoned. However, artificial means of sustaining life, such as ventilators or feeding tubes, are not to be used.

Although not all states currently recognize living wills, the client's requests should be given due weight when making health care decisions. The nurse must be knowledgeable about living will legislation in her state. A sample living will is shown in Figure 6-7.

The Life-Prolonging Procedure Declaration indicates that the person wants all possible procedures done to delay the dying process (Figure 6-8). This can include the use of ventilators and any other methods to keep the person alive by artificial means.

Where a form for a living will, durable power of attorney, and/or health care representative is provided by statute, it should be utilized, because health care providers are familiar with it. However, variations of the forms, if all the required elements are included, may also be legal.

INCIDENT REPORTS

An **incident report** is a risk management tool used to describe and report any unusual event that occurs to a client, visitor, or staff member. It is used to help the facility identify or track problem areas and alert the legal department to possible lawsuits. An incident report is not meant to be a punitive device, although it is often perceived in that manner.

Incident reports are completed to document such events as falls, medication errors, forgotten treatment, injuries—anything that happens out of the ordinary. Another name for an incident report is a variance report or an occurrence report. The following three examples illustrate the types of occurrences that should be documented in an incident report.

- Mrs. Duncan had blood drawn for various laboratory tests. It was later discovered that the laboratory work had been ordered on Mrs. Falson, not Mrs. Duncan. The requisition had been stamped with the wrong name.
- Mrs. Barnes was given Lasix 20 mg PO at 9 A.M. When reviewing the physician's orders, the evening nurse discovered that Losec 20 mg had been ordered. Mrs. Barnes received the wrong medication.
- Mrs. Gomez was visiting her daughter, who had just given birth to the family's first grandchild. While walking down the hall, Mrs. Gomez slipped and fell, injuring her right hip.

Part I. Durable Power of Attorney for Health Care

• If you do NOT wish to name an agent to make health care decisions for you, write your initials in the box

[Initials]

This form has been prepared to comply with the "Durable Power of Attorney for Health Care Act" of Missouri.

1. Selection of agent. I appoint:
Name:_____
Address:_____

| It is suggested that only one Agent be named. However, if more than one Agent is named, anyone may act individually unless you specify otherwise. |

Telephone:_____
as my Agent.

2. Alternate Agents. Only an Agent named by me may act under this Durable Power of Attorney. If my Agent resigns or is not able or available to make health care decisions for me, or if an Agent named by me is divorced from me or is my spouse and legally separated from me, I appoint the person(s) named below (in the order named if more than one):

First Alternate Agent   Second Alternate Agent

Name:_____   Name:_____

Address:_____   Address:_____

_____   _____

Telephone:_____   Telephone:_____

| This is a Durable Power of Attorney, and the authority of my Agent shall not terminate if I become disabled or incapacitated. |

Part I. Durable Power of Attorney for Health Care (Continued)

3. Effective date and durability. This Durable Power of Attorney is effective when two physicians decide and certify that I am incapacitated and unable to make and communicate a health care decision.

• If you want ONE physician, instead of TWO, to decide whether you are incapacitated, write your initials in the box to the right.

[Initials]

4. Agent's powers. I grant to my Agent full authority to:

A. Give consent to, prohibit, or withdraw any type of health care, medical care, treatment, or procedure, even if my death may result;

• If you wish to AUTHORIZE your Agent to direct a health care provider to withhold or withdraw artificially supplied nutrition and hydration (including tube feeding of food and water), write your initials in the box to the right.

[Initials]

• If you DO NOT WISH TO AUTHORIZE your Agent to direct a health care provider to withhold or withdraw artificially supplied nutrition and hydration (including tube feeding of food and water), write your initials in the box to the right.

[Initials]

B. Make all necessary arrangements for health care services on my behalf, and to hire and fire medical personnel responsible for my care;

C. Move me into or out of any health care facility (even if against medical advice) to obtain compliance with the decisions of my Agent; and

D. Take any other action necessary to do what I authorize here, including (but not limited to) granting any waiver or release from liability required by any health care provider, and taking any legal action at the expense of my estate to enforce this Durable Power of Attorney.

5. Agent's Financial Liability and Compensation. My Agent acting under this Durable Power of Attorney will incur no personal financial liability. My Agent shall not be entitled to compensation for services performed under this Durable Power of Attorney, but my Agent shall be entitled to reimbursement for all reasonable expenses incurred as a result of carrying out any provision hereof.

Part II. Health Care Directive

• If you DO NOT WISH to make a health care directive, write your initials in the box to the right, and go to Part III.

[Initials]

I make this HEALTH CARE DIRECTIVE ("Directive") to exercise my right to determine the course of my health care and to provide clear and convincing proof of my wishes and instructions about my treatment.

If I am persistently unconscious or there is no reasonable expectation of my recovery from a seriously incapacitating or terminal illness or condition, I direct that all of the life-prolonging procedures which I have initialed below be withheld or withdrawn.

I want the following life-prolonging procedures to be withheld or withdrawn:

| • artificially supplied nutrition and hydration (including tube feeding of food and water) . . . . | [Initials] |

• surgery or other invasive procedures. . . . . [Initials]

• heart-lung resuscitation (CPR) . . . . [Initials]

• antibiotic. . . . . [Initials]

• dialysis. . . . . [Initials]

• mechanical ventilator (respirator). . . . . [Initials]

• chemotherapy. . . . . [Initials]

• radiation therapy. . . . . [Initials]

• all other "life-prolonging" medical or surgical procedures that are merely intended to keep me alive without reasonable hope of improving my condition or curing my illness or injury. . . . . [Initials]

However, if my physician believes that any life-prolonging procedure may lead to significant recovery, I direct my physician to try the treatment for a reasonable period of time. If it does not improve my condition, I direct the treatment be withdrawn even if it shortens my life. I also direct that I be given medical treatment to relieve pain or to provide comfort, even if such treatment might shorten my life, suppress my appetite or my breathing, or be habit forming.

IF I HAVE NOT DESIGNATED AN AGENT IN THE DURABLE POWER OF ATTORNEY, THIS DOCUMENT IS MEANT TO BE IN FULL FORCE AND EFFECT AS MY HEALTH CARE DIRECTIVE.

Part III. General Provisions Included in the Directive and Durable Power of Attorney

YOU MUST SIGN THIS DOCUMENT IN THE PRESENCE OF TWO WITNESSES.
IN WITNESS WHEREOF, I have executed this document this_____day of _____, year____.

_____
Signature

Print name _____
Address _____

The person who signed this document is of sound mind and voluntarily signed this document in our presence. Each of the undersigned witnesses is at least eighteen years of age.

Signature_____   Signature_____

Print name _____   Print name _____

Address _____   Address _____

| ONLY REQUIRED FOR PART I — DURABLE POWER OF ATTORNEY |

STATE OF MISSOURI   )
) as
_____OF _____   )

On this _____day of _____, year_____, before me personally appeared to me known to be the person described in and who executed the foregoing instrument and acknowledged that he/she executed the same as his/her free act and deed.

IN WITNESS WHEREOF, I have hereunto set my hand and affixed my official seal in the County of _____, State of Missouri, the day and year first above written.

_____
Notary Public

My Commision Expires:

Figure 6-6 Durable Power of Attorney for Health Care and Health Care Directive *(Reprinted with permission of The Missouri Bar)*

Sample Living Will

Declaration made this ____ day of __________, year_____.

I, _______________________, willfully and voluntarily make known my desire that my dying not be artificially prolonged under the circumstances set forth below, and I do hereby declare:

If at any time I have a terminal condition and if my attending or treating physician and another consulting physician have determined that there is no medical probability of my recovery from such condition, I direct that life-prolonging procedures be withheld or withdrawn when the application of such procedures would serve only to prolong artificially the process of dying, and that I be permitted to die naturally with only the administration of medication or the performance of any medical procedure deemed necessary to provide me with comfort care or to alleviate pain.

It is my intention that this declaration be honored by my family and physician as the final expression of my legal right to refuse medical or surgical treatment and to accept the consequences for such refusal.

In the event that I have been determined to be unable to provide express and informed consent regarding the withholding, withdrawal, or continuation of life-prolonging procedures, I wish to designate, as my surrogate to carry out the provisions of this declaration:

Name: ______________________________
Address: ______________________________
______________________ Zip Code: __________
Phone: ______________________________

I wish to designate the following person as my alternate surrogate, to carry out the provisions of this declaration should my surrogate be unwilling or unable to act on my behalf:

Name: ______________________________
Address: ______________________________
______________________ Zip Code: __________
Phone: ______________________________

Additional instructions (optional):

I understand the full importance of this declaration, and I am emotionally and mentally competant to make this declaration.
Signed: ______________________________

Witness 1:
Signed: ______________________________
Address: ______________________________

Witness 2:
Signed: ______________________________
Address: ______________________________

Figure 6-7 Sample Living Will *(Courtesy Choice in Dying, 1034 30th Street NW, Washington, DC 20007)*

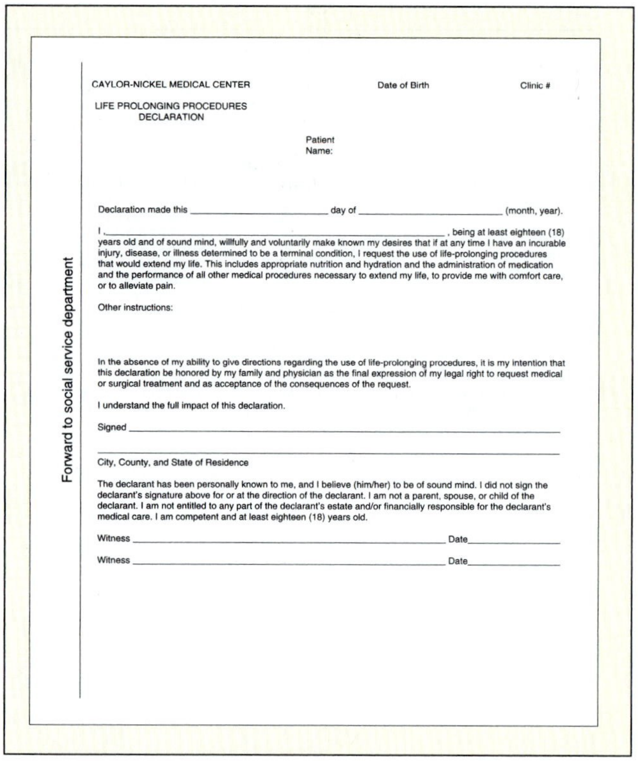

Forward to social service department

CAYLOR-NICKEL MEDICAL CENTER   Date of Birth   Clinic #

LIFE PROLONGING PROCEDURES DECLARATION

Patient Name:

Declaration made this ______________ day of ______________ (month, year).

I, ______________________, being at least eighteen (18) years old and of sound mind, willfully and voluntarily make known my desires that if at any time I have an incurable injury, disease, or illness determined to be a terminal condition, I request the use of life-prolonging procedures that would extend my life. This includes appropriate nutrition and hydration and the administration of medication and the performance of all other medical procedures necessary to extend my life, to provide me with comfort care, or to alleviate pain.

Other instructions:

In the absence of my ability to give directions regarding the use of life-prolonging procedures, it is my intention that this declaration be honored by my family and physician as the final expression of my legal right to request medical or surgical treatment and as acceptance of the consequences of the request.

I understand the full impact of this declaration.

Signed ______________________________

____
City, County, and State of Residence

The declarant has been personally known to me, and I believe (him/her) to be of sound mind. I did not sign the declarant's signature above for or at the direction of the declarant. I am not a parent, spouse, or child of the declarant. I am not entitled to any part of the declarant's estate and/or financially responsible for the declarant's medical care. I am competent and at least eighteen (18) years old.

Witness ______________________ Date__________

Witness ______________________ Date__________

Figure 6-8 Life-Prolonging Procedures Declaration *(Courtesy Caylor-Nickel Medical Center)*

All of the previous examples are incidents or variances that may typically occur in health care settings. For each situation, an incident report must be completed and channeled to the risk management department. Under the auspices of risk management, a subgroup comprising representatives from various departments, such as nursing administration, dietary services, environmental safety, and others, reviews the incident report. This group tries to identify those factors, if any, that contributed to the incident. Examples of questions asked include "Can the causal factors be eliminated or reduced?" "Does the possibility of a lawsuit exist as a result of the incident?" and "What can be done to prevent this incident from occurring again?"

Incident reports are filed by the person who was responsible for, who witnessed, or who discovered the incident. The report should state what was observed, as opposed to what is supposed. It should be factual and concise. In the third example given previously, if the nurse did not witness the actual fall, the correctly worded report would read: "Mrs. Gomez found lying on floor outside room 222. Several puddles of liquid found under and around her; paper cup lying nearby." An incorrect, presumptuous, and potentially damaging report might read: "Mrs. Gomez tripped and fell outside room 222. She slipped in a puddle of water." Mrs. Gomez may have spilled the cup of water she was carrying during the fall. However, this second note implies that Mrs. Gomez slipped in water that was already on the floor, thus implicating the facility.

Incident reports should include a description of the care given to the client or individual, and the name of the physician who was notified. The incident should be charted in the client's medical record, but the incident report should not be referred to in any way. Although the incident report is not a part of the medical record, the details described in the medical record and in the incident report should be the same.

When completing an incident report, the nurse should be sure to include the date and time of the incident; assessments; and interventions. The time that family members and physicians were notified should also be included. The nurse should refer to nursing administration policy and procedure regarding follow-up documentation.

PROFESSIONAL LIABILITY

Many nurses believe they do not need their own malpractice or liability insurance. They assume the coverage provided by their employer is adequate. This may be a misconception.

Nurses claim to be competent and knowledgeable health care providers. The health care consumer has heard this message and thus holds the nurse accountable for her actions. As a result, nurses are named as defendants in malpractice suits. Under the doctrine of *Respondeat Superior,* employers are responsible for the actions of their employees. However, this responsibility stops when the employee leaves work. Also, if the nurse violates policy and the employer is forced to pay damages, the employer has the right to sue the nurse to recover losses.

Having a professional liability policy provides the nurse with an attorney, someone who will represent that nurse in court. An attorney representing the facility or a group of employees will be most concerned about the employer; the needs of an individual nurse will be secondary. The decision to settle a case or pursue a particular course of action may be based on the needs of the employer. The individual nurse is better represented in court by private counsel.

Frequently, family members and friends ask a nurse for advice or assistance in health care matters. This advice is sought because of the nurse's knowledge, experience, and role. Should the family members or friends later take issue with the results of the advice or treatment given by a nurse, they might bring a suit against the nurse.

Despite the fact that no money was exchanged for information or services, the nurse is still accountable for the advice given. If the situation ends up in court, the nurse needs legal representation. Legal representation is costly as can be judgments against the nurse. A professional liability insurance policy protects the nurse by providing legal representation and paying the judgments.

There are two basic types of liability protection: the claims made policy and the occurrence policy. The claims made policy protects the nurse against claims made during the time the policy is in effect. If a claim is made after the policy has been terminated, the nurse is not covered. Occurrence policies protect the nurse against events that took place during the period of time the policy was active, even if a claim is filed after the policy is terminated. Occurrence policies seem to offer better protection for the nurse.

Opinions differ as to whether nurses should carry individual liability insurance. Some attorneys and health care professionals believe this practice encourages lawsuits. Nurses must compare the cost and the benefits of having professional liability insurance against the cost of potential legal fees and loss of personal assets. When securing liability insurance, the nurse should validate the company's reputation. Most nursing organizations offer group professional liability insurance.

IMPAIRED NURSE

One of the more sensitive issues in the nursing profession today is the subject of the impaired nurse. By definition, an **impaired nurse** is a nurse who is habitually intemperate or is addicted to the use of alcohol or habit-forming drugs. Although job performance may not be immediately compromised, substance abuse does eventually interfere with clinical judgment and performance. Because of the high level of job-related stress and the accessibility of drugs, the chemical dependency rate among nurses is greater than that among the general public.

In cases of impaired health care workers, the primary concern is client care. In the role of client advocate, a nurse cannot let loyalties to co-workers interfere with duty to the client. It is difficult reporting a coworker. No one wants to be a "squealer." In many states, however, the board of nursing requires nurses to report impaired coworkers. Nurses suspected of being under the influence of drugs or alcohol must be reported to the proper authority at the place of employment. The second consideration is getting help for the impaired nurse and taking action to correct the problem.

A nurse who suspects a coworker of diverting drugs or abusing alcohol should:

1. Document the dates, times, and observed behavior. Specific and descriptive accounts of what was observed are critical. For example:

   > January 3, 1996. P.P. working 3–11 shift. Client A and Client B verbalized unrelieved postoperative pain. Documentation by P.P. stated both clients were comfortable after administration of Demerol 75 mg IM. Narcotic count at shift change satisfactory.

January 4, 1996. Client C and Client D verbalized unrelieved pain. Documentation by P.P. indicated both clients stated pain was relieved after administration of Demerol 100 mg IM. Narcotic count at shift change okay.

January 5, 1996. Narcotic count showed 1 Demerol 100-mg syringe listed as broken and 1 Demerol 75-mg syringe listed as wasted, "client changed her mind." P.P. signed the narcotic sheet.

or

March 1–2, 1996. S.L. working the night shift. Strong odor of alcohol on his breath.

March 3, 1996. S.L. observed walking with unsteady gait, speech is slurred, strong odor of alcohol on breath.

2. Go to the supervisor and report concerns. Providing a copy of the documentation about the suspicious incidents is helpful. The supervisor will take responsibility for confronting the suspected employee. Intoxication requires immediate removal from the clinical area. In other situations, the supervisor will devise a plan before confronting the nurse.

3. Refrain from approaching or confronting the coworker. The impaired coworker may become defensive and deny the problem or make threats. Also, once aware that someone is suspicious, the nurse may become more secretive, making detection less likely. Frequently, the nurse will quit one facility and go to another, repeating the same pattern.

Some employers offer an employee assistance program to rehabilitate the impaired nurse. In addition, most states have **peer assistance programs** (rehabilitation programs designed to provide an impaired nurse with referrals, professional and peer counseling support groups, and assistance and monitoring for reentry into nursing). These peer assistance programs operate under the auspices of the state nurses association and in conjunction with the board of nursing. The goals of assistance programs are to protect the public from impaired nurses, provide the needed assistance to the impaired nurse, assist the nurse to reenter nursing, and monitor the nurse's compliance. With the help of the peer counselor, the impaired nurse develops a contract for treatment. Compliance is monitored, and confidentiality is ensured. Successful completion of the program allows the nurse to return to the practice setting.

Participation in employer and peer assistance programs is optional. If the nurse chooses not to cooperate, however, employment may be terminated, and sanctions by the board of nursing may follow, including revocation of the license to practice.

SUMMARY

- Laws are rules that guide personal interaction. They are derived from several sources and can be classified as public or civil.
- Within most states, the nursing practice act indicates the scope of practice for nurses. Standards have been developed to guide nursing practice.
- The nurse should be familiar with client rights. Care should be taken not to falsely imprison a client or violate the client's right to privacy.
- The client's chart is a legal document and should accurately reflect client status and care. Entries should be neat and timely.
- Informed consent is more than just signing a form. It requires an understanding of the risks, benefits, and alternatives to treatment.
- Whether to purchase malpractice insurance is a personal decision. However, having one's own policy provides both coverage off the job and individual legal counsel.
- Impaired nurses are everyone's concern. Dates and times of inappropriate behaviors should be documented and reported to the immediate supervisor.
- Incident reports are a risk management tool. They are not meant to be used for punitive purposes.
- Advance directives are instructions about health care preferences. They both protect the rights of the client and guide the family through difficult decisions.

Review Questions

1. Standards of practice are:
    a. different for each school of nursing.
    b. guidelines to direct nursing care.
    c. not legally binding.
    d. specific criteria on how to perform procedures.

2. Immunity for nurses giving care in emergency situations is provided under the:
    a. Care and Good Faith Act of 1937.
    b. Good Samaritan Act.
    c. state nursing practice act.
    d. Patient Self-Determination act.

3. Select the situation that violates client privacy.
    a. Copying information from the chart for a case study
    b. Discussing client status with clinical instructor
    c. Shutting the door and closing the curtain during a procedure
    d. Talking in the cafeteria about an interesting client

CASE STUDY

Mr. Jones is admitted for congestive heart failure. He is 66 years old, newly diagnosed, and acutely ill at this time. A student LP/VN is assisting the RN with the admission. The student notes that Mr. Jones has a living will. Later, she asks the RN, "Will you have to contact the doctor regarding a No Code status for Mr. Jones? He's got a living will, so he doesn't want anything done."

1. List factors that the nurse should explain to assist the student in understanding the concept of a living will.

2. Describe how a cardiac arrest might affect this situation.

Mr. Jones' wife speaks privately with the RN, stating, "I want everything possible done to save my husband. I don't care what it takes."

3. Describe how Mrs. Jones' statements may or may not affect the living will requests that Mr. Jones has made.

4. Delineate how the nurse might respond in this situation.

When Mr. Jones refuses a recommended treatment option, Mrs. Jones disagrees and tells the doctor to go ahead with the recommended treatment plan.

5. How does the Patient Self-Determination Act affect Mr. Jones' refusal of treatment?

6. List the parameters that allow Mrs. Jones to consent or refuse treatment for her husband.

Jamal Wilkins came to the hospital for outpatient diagnostic testing. Passing an open door, he saw his high school principal, Mr. Jones, lying in a bed. A respiratory therapist was giving Mr. Jones a treatment, and there seemed to be tubes and bags hanging everywhere. Alarmed, Jamal went to the nurse's station seeking information. He pointed to Mr. Jones' name and room number, which were listed on the board, and began asking questions.

7. Discuss ways to calm Jamal's fears without violating Mr. Jones' right to privacy.

8. Identify those ways that this client's privacy has already been violated.

---

4. To make the best use of time in the clinical area, the nurse should:
   a. chart events as they happen.
   b. chart in a block at the end of the shift.
   c. have a coworker who is not busy chart for her.
   d. sign off all meds at the beginning of the shift.

5. The responsibility for informed consent rests with the:
   a. nurse.
   b. client.
   c. physician.
   d. unit clerk.

6. Informed consent occurs when the:
   a. nurse discusses the surgical procedure with the client.
   b. client gives consent verbally.
   c. client understands the risks, benefits, and alternatives to treatment.
   d. client signs the consent form.

7. If a coworker is suspected of diverting drugs, the nurse should:
   a. approach the coworker and tell him what she thinks.
   b. document dates, times, and observed behavior and report same to the supervisor.
   c. say nothing; it is none of her business.
   d. tell coworkers what she thinks so that they can help watch for suspicious behavior.

8. Advance directives:

   a. are binding only if written.

   b. cannot be changed once they are notarized.

   c. guide family members through difficult decisions.

   d. prevent clients from determining the course of their health care.

9. The health care representative or durable power of attorney for health care:

   a. is appointed by hospital administrators to make medical decisions for the client.

   b. can give or withhold consent for treatment.

   c. is contacted to override the decisions the client makes for himself.

   d. is the client's physician or health care provider.

10. Which of the following situations reflects inappropriate use of an incident report?

   a. Mrs. Khamel falls in the hall while visiting her daughter.

   b. A student nurse gives Losec instead of Lasix.

   c. The safety committee reviews incident reports regarding falls on the 3–11 shift on A-wing.

   d. An instructor, frustrated with a disorganized student nurse, fills out an incident report because the student gave a 9 A.M. medication at 9:25.

Critical Thinking Questions

1. How would you explain advance directives to your family?

2. How would you know whether a client gave informed consent?

 WEB FLASH!

- What organizations or professional journals could you search to obtain information on nursing and legal issues?
- Search the Web sites of certain law schools, such as Harvard or the University of Texas, for information pertaining to nurses or health care.
- What resources are available on the Web for nurses needing legal advice?
- Search for information about the Good Samaritan Act, malpractice, and professional liability insurance.

ETHICAL RESPONSIBILITIES

MAKING THE CONNECTION

Refer to the following chapters to increase your understanding of ethical responsibilities:

- **Chapter 2: Critical Thinking**
- **Chapter 6: Legal Responsibilities**
- **Chapter 9: Nursing Process**
- **Chapter 12: Cultural Diversity and Nursing**

LEARNING OBJECTIVES

Upon completion of this chapter, you should be able to:
- *Define key terms.*
- *Explain the relationship among the concepts of ethics, morality, and law.*
- *Discuss the ethical theories of teleology and deontology.*
- *Describe the major ethical principles that have an impact on health care.*
- *Explain the link between ethics and values and the process involved in reconciling the potential conflicts between them.*
- *Relate the ethical codes developed by the National Federation of Licensed Practical Nurses and the International Council of Nurses to daily nursing practice.*
- *Identify the rights of the client as established by the American Hospital Association.*
- *Apply the steps identified in the framework for ethical decision making to issues such as euthanasia, refusal of treatment, and scarcity of resources.*
- *Discuss the roles of the nurse as client advocate and whistleblower in the delivery of ethical nursing care.*

KEY TERMS

active euthanasia	fidelity
assisted suicide	justice
autonomy	material principle of
beneficence	justice
bioethics	nonmaleficence
categorical imperative	passive euthanasia
client advocate	teleology
deontology	utility
ethical dilemma	value system
ethical principles	values
ethical reasoning	values clarification
ethics	veracity
euthanasia	whistleblowing

INTRODUCTION

Every day, nurses encounter situations wherein they must make decisions based on the determination of right and wrong. How do they make such decisions? Whose values determine the rightness of an action?

The delivery of ethical health care is becoming an increasingly difficult and confusing issue in contemporary society. Nurses are committed to respecting their clients' rights in terms of providing health care and treatment. This desire to maintain clients' rights, however, often conflicts with professional duties and institutional policies. Nurses must thus learn to balance these potentially conflicting perspectives so as to achieve the primary objective—the care of the client.

In considering the situations presented throughout this chapter, one must realize that there are no absolute right answers. Dealing with the gray areas (ambiguities) causes much discomfort for many nurses. Because clients and nurses are humans, no two situations, no matter how similar, can ever be exactly alike. This chapter explores the concept of ethics, including ethical principles and theories; ethics and values; ethical codes; the client's rights; ethical dilemmas; ethical decision making; and the application of ethical guidelines to nursing practice.

CONCEPT OF ETHICS

Ethics is the branch of philosophy concerned with determining right from wrong on the basis of a body of knowledge rather than on just the basis of opinions. Ethics deals with one's responsibilities (duties and obligations) as defined by logical argument. Ethics is *not* a religious dogma. Ethics looks at human behavior—which things people do under which types of circumstances. But ethics is not merely philosophical in nature; ethical persons put their beliefs into action.

Ethics in Health Care

The application of general ethical principles to health care is referred to as **bioethics**. Ethics affects every area of health care, including direct care of clients, allocation of finances, and utilization of staff. As Aroskar (1994) states:

> Ethics encompasses the whole of life: our conduct and behavior toward ourselves, toward others, and toward the environment. Ethics in nursing and health care is not just about terrible dilemmas at the beginning or end of life. Most human activity involves an ethical dimension even if it is not recognized or articulated.

Ethics does not provide easy answers, but it can help provide structure by raising questions that ultimately lead to answers.

Ethical practice is gaining ever-increasing importance in health care today. Several factors contribute to the increased need to provide health care in an ethical manner. Some of these factors are:

- An increasingly technological society. The nature of advanced technology creates situations involving complicated issues that never had to be considered before. As a result of technological advances:

    Many newborns are surviving at earlier gestational ages, and many of them have serious health problems.
    People are living much longer than ever before.
    Organ transplants and the use of bionic body parts are becoming more common.

- The changing fabric of our society. Family structure is moving from extended families to nuclear families, single-parent families, and nonrelated groups living together as families.

- Clients are becoming more knowledgeable about both their health and health-related interventions. As consumer demand for information increases, health care providers must adapt quickly. The result is a focus on the consumer-driven system.

Every day, nurses face situations wherein they must make decisions that transcend technical and professional concerns. These situations may or may not be life threatening. Such situations raise complex problems that cannot be answered completely with technical knowledge and professional expertise. The way that nurses relate to clients, families, and other health care providers is the true demonstration of ethical behavior.

ETHICAL PRINCIPLES

Ethical principles are codes that direct or govern actions. They are widely accepted and generally based on the humane aspects of society. Ethical decisions are principled, that is, they reflect what is best for the client and society. Table 7-1 summarizes the major ethical principles. Each principle is discussed in detail in the following paragraphs.

By applying ethical principles, the nurse can become more systematic in solving ethical conflicts. Ethical principles can be used as guidelines in analyzing dilemmas; they can also serve as justification (rationale) for the resolution of ethical problems. It should be emphasized that these principles are not absolute; there can be exceptions to each principle in any given situation.

Autonomy

The principle of **autonomy** refers to the individual's right to choose and the individual's ability to act on that choice. The individuality of each person is respected. This respect for personal liberty is a dominant value in U.S. society.

Nurses must respect the client's right to decide and must protect those clients who are unable to decide for themselves. Although the legal definition of competency varies among states, the ethical principle of autonomy reflects the belief that every competent person has the right to determine his own course of action. The right to free choice thus rests on the client's competency to decide.

Table 7-1 **OVERVIEW OF ETHICAL PRINCIPLES**	
PRINCIPLE	**EXPLANATION**
Autonomy	Respect for an individual's right to self-determination; respect for individual liberty
Nonmaleficence	The obligation to do or cause no harm to another
Beneficence	The duty to do good to others and to maintain a balance between benefits and harms
Justice	The equitable distribution of potential benefits and risks
Veracity	The obligation to tell the truth
Fidelity	The duty to do what one has promised

PROFESSIONAL TIP

Autonomy

- Competent clients have a right to self-determination, even if their decisions may result in self-harm.
- Probably one of the most difficult things for nurses to accept is that clients are ultimately responsible for themselves; they will do what they want to do.

Informed consent is based on the client's right to decide for herself. Upholding autonomy means that the nurse accepts the client's choices, even those choices that are not in the client's best interests or those choices that conflict with the nurse's values. Following are examples of autonomous behavior on the part of the client that can impair recovery or treatment:

- Smoking after a diagnosis of emphysema or lung cancer
- Refusing to take medication
- Continuing to drink alcohol after being diagnosed with cirrhosis of the liver
- Refusing to receive a blood transfusion because of religious beliefs

Nonmaleficence

Nonmaleficence is the obligation to cause no harm to others. Harm can take many forms: physiological, psychological, social, financial, and/or spiritual. Nonmaleficence refers to both intentional harm and the risk of harm. The principle of nonmaleficence helps guide decisions about treatment approaches; the relevant question is "Will this treatment modality cause more harm or more good to the client?" Determining whether technology is harmful to the client is not always a clear-cut process. Factors to consider when choosing a treatment include:

- A reasonable prospect of benefit, and
- Lack of excessive expense, pain, or other inconvenience.

Nonmaleficence requires that the nurse act thoughtfully and carefully, weighing the potential risks and benefits of research or treatment. It is sometimes easier to weigh the risk than to measure the benefit. Further, it is possible to violate this principle without acting maliciously and without ever being aware of the harm, making the principle of nonmaleficence closely related to the concept of negligence. When upholding the principle of nonmaleficence, the nurse practices according to professional and legal standards of care.

Table 7-2 VOCATIONAL NURSE'S PLEDGE

God being my Witness and Judge and the Light whereby my life is patterned, do solemnly pledge myself to keep the following vows:

I shall endeavor in all ways so to live and to conduct myself, at home and abroad, that my vocation shall be uplifted in the eyes of all people.

I shall help to elevate the standards of my vocation by doing my work, where ever I may be, at least a little better on each tomorrow than I was able to do it on each today.

I shall put the welfare of my patients above all else.

I shall not engage in idle talk about other vocational nurses, professional nurses, or doctors, for we are united in our care of the patient and gossip destroys unity.

So let me live that I may be of service to Him Who "so loved the world that He gave His only begotten Son that whosoever believeth in Him should not perish but have everlasting life."

Author unknown: Used over 30 years by the Department of Vocational Nurse Education, Del Mar College, Corpus Christi, TX

Nonmaleficence is considered a fundamental duty of health care providers. The Vocational Nurses's Pledge (Table 7-2), The Practical Nurse's Pledge (Table 7-3), and the Nightingale Pledge (Table 7-4) all profess the same basic philosophy of nursing care. Some clinical examples of nonmaleficence are:

- Preventing medication errors (including drug interactions),
- Being aware of potential risks of treatment modalities, and
- Removing hazards (e.g., obstructions that might cause a fall).

Table 7-3 PRACTICAL NURSE'S PLEDGE

Before God and those assembled here, I solemnly pledge:

To adhere to the code of ethics of the nursing profession.

To cooperate faithfully with the other members of the nursing team and to carry out faithfully and to the best of my ability the instructions of the physician or the nurse who may be assigned to supervise my work.

I will not do anything evil or malicious and I will not knowingly give any harmful drug or assist in malpractice.

I will not reveal any confidential information that may come to my knowledge in the course of my work.

And I pledge myself to do all in my power to raise the standards and the prestige of practical nursing.

May my life be devoted to service, and to the high ideals of the nursing profession.

Reprinted with permission of the National Association for Practical Nurse Education and Services Inc., Silver Spring, MD.

Table 7-4 NIGHTINGALE PLEDGE

I solemnly pledge myself before God and in the presence of this assembly: To pass my life in purity and to practice my profession faithfully.

I will abstain from whatever is deleterious and mischievous, and will not take or knowingly administer any harmful drug.

I will do all in my power to maintain and elevate the standards of my profession, and will hold in confidence all personal matters committed to my keeping, and all family affairs coming to my knowledge in the practice of my profession.

With loyalty will I endeavor to aid the physician in his work, and devote myself to the welfare of those committed to my care.

Beneficence

Beneficence is the duty to promote good and to prevent harm. Beneficence is often viewed as the core of nursing practice. The nurse serves as a client advocate and promotes the rights of the client. The nurse nurtures the client and incorporates the desires of the client into the plan of care. Sometimes, it is difficult to determine what is "good," especially when doing good causes the client discomfort. For example, a client who has been in a serious car accident may resist performing painful range of motion exercises and become angry at the nurse for insisting. The nurse understands the long-term value of performing the exercises, yet understands the client's physical and psychological pain.

Justice

The principle of **justice** is based on the concept of fairness extended to each individual. The major health-related issues of justice involve the way people are treated and the way resources are distributed. Justice considers action from the point of view of the least fortunate in society. As a result of equal and similar treatment of people, benefits and burdens are equally distributed. The distribution of scarce resources is commonly decided according to individual need (Davis & Aroskar, 1997).

The ethical principle of justice requires that all people be treated equally unless there is a justification for unequal treatment. The **material principle of justice** is the rationale for determining those times when there can be unequal allocation of scarce resources. This concept specifies that resources be allocated:

- Equally,
- According to need,
- According to individual effort,
- According to the individual's merit (ability), and
- According to the individual's contribution to society (DeLaune & Ladner, 1998)

An example of the application of the material principle of justice (according to the individual's contribution to society) is the Veterans Affairs (VA) Medical Centers. Only individuals who gave to their country by serving in the military are eligible to receive health care through the VA in ambulatory, acute care, and psychiatric facilities.

In health care institutions, the principle of justice is being strenuously tested on the issue of allocating one important resource: nursing personnel. Many institutions and agencies are downsizing their professional staff as a cost-containment measure. As a result, some health care facilities are so poorly staffed or have such a high ratio of underqualified personnel providing care, that quality of care is being severely compromised (Schildmeier, 1997).

Veracity

Veracity means truthfulness (neither lying nor deceiving others). Deception can take many forms: intentional lying, nondisclosure of information, or partial disclosure of information. Veracity often is difficult to achieve. It may not be hard to tell the truth, but it can be very hard to decide how much truth to tell. Exceptions to truth-telling are sometimes upheld by the principle of nonmaleficence, when the truth does greater harm than good. The act of giving placebo medications is an example of when telling the truth does greater harm than good.

Fidelity

The concept of **fidelity** (which is the ethical foundation of nurse–client relationships) means faithfulness and keeping promises.

Clients have an ethical right to expect nurses to act in their best interests. As nurses function in the role of **client advocate** (a person who speaks up for or acts on behalf of the client), they are upholding the principle of fidelity. Fidelity is demonstrated when nurses:

- Represent the client's viewpoint to other members of the health care team,
- Avoid letting their own personal values influence their advocacy for clients, and
- Support the client's decision, even when it conflicts with their own preferences or choices.

Within the nurse–client relationship, nurses should be loyal to their responsibilities, keep promises, maintain privacy, and meet resonable expectations of clients. Nurses also have a duty to be faithful to themselves. Conflict between commitments can complicate matters for the nurse, who may question who is owed fidelity. Although maintaining client centeredness may help clarify this question, it may not resolve the conflict. For example, if the mother of a frightened teenage girl tried to pressure the nurse into revealing the results of the daughter's pregnancy test after the daughter had already requested that her mother not be told, although the nurse may believe that the mother has the girl's best interests at heart, the nurse must protect the client's right to privacy.

ETHICAL THEORIES

Ethical theories were debated by ancient philosophers such as Plato and Aristotle, and the debate continues today. Whereas ethical theories can be used as a way to analyze ethical problems, no theory in and of itself can provide the "correct" answer to any single ethical conflict. Common ethical theories include teleology, deontology, situational theory, and caring-based theory.

Teleology

Teleology is an ethical theory that states that the value of a situation is determined by its consequences. Thus, the outcome of an action—not the action itself— is the criterion for determining the goodness of that action. An example would be immunizations—receiving an injection is not "good," but preventing the illnesses is.

This theory (also called the consequentialist theory) was advocated by the philosopher John Stuart Mill. The principle of **utility** is a basic concept of teleology; utility states that an act must result in the greatest degree of good for the greatest number of people involved in a given situation. "Good" refers to positive benefit. Thus, any act can be ethical if it delivers positive results. Concepts considered inherently good for all members of a society include health, strength, truth, freedom, security, and peace (Edge & Groves, 1999). Every alternative is assessed for its potential outcomes, both positive and negative. The selected action is the one that results in the most benefits and the least amount of harm for all those involved. A major disadvantage is that minority and individual rights may be ignored for the benefit of the masses.

Safety: Immunizations
- The outcome of immunizations is the prevention of given illnesses in the individual and, thus, the prevention of the spread of those illnesses to the community.
- The greatest good for the greatest number of persons is achieved with immunizations.

Deontology

Deontology is an ethical theory that considers the intrinsic significance of an act itself as the criterion for determination of good. That is, in determining the ethics of a situation, a person must consider not the consequences of the act, but the motives of the individual performing the act. This theory (also called formalism) was postulated by the philosopher Immanuel

Kant. Kant established the concept of the **categorical imperative**, which states that a person should act only if the action is based on a principle that is universal (that is, everyone would act in the same way in a similar situation). The categorical imperative also mandates that a person should never be treated as a means to an end. Adherence to this concept may pose an ethical problem for health care researchers, who sometimes might be willing to risk the well-being of a person participating in an experimental procedure for the sake of finding, for example, a drug that will save many victims from suffering.

Situational Theory

The situational theory holds that there are no set rules, norms, or majority-focused results. Each situation must be considered individually, with an emphasis on the uniqueness of the situation and a respect for the person involved. Decisions made in one situation cannot be generalized to another situation (Pappas, 1997).

Caring-Based Theory

Caring-based theory is founded on the premise that people do not make ethical decisions based on principles. Decisions are made with respect to relationships, caring, communication, a desire not to hurt others, and responsiveness. Caring-based theory focuses on emotions, feelings, and attitudes (Figure 7-1). This theory is sometimes referred to as the "voice of care" and is contrasted with the "voice of justice." Justice and caring are not considered mutually exclusive and can, in fact, be complementary (Beare & Myers, 1998).

ETHICS AND VALUES

The close relationship between ethics and values both illuminates and complicates the nurse's approach toward balancing the ethical principles of the health care profession with those of the client. Nurses must examine their own value systems to ascertain the best approach in managing the care of clients whose values may be different from their own. In order to practice ethically, nurses must understand their own values.

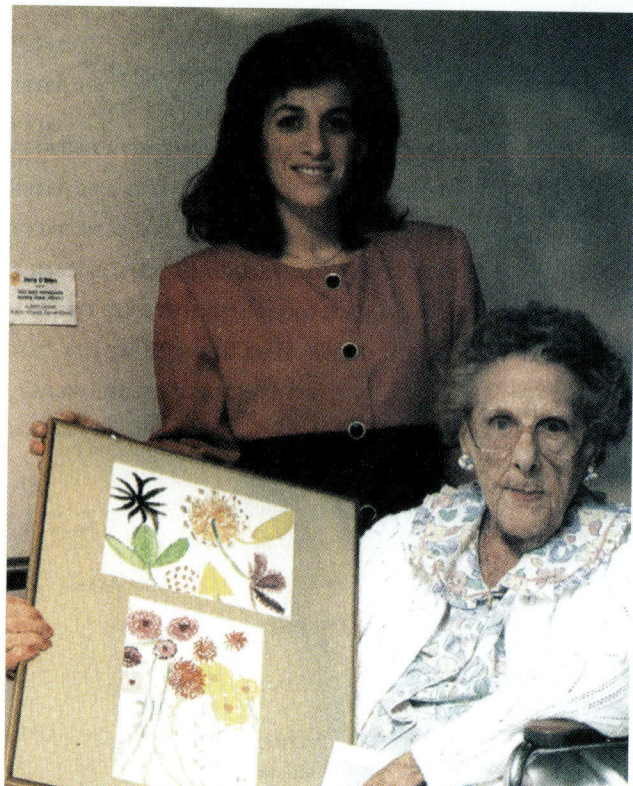

Figure 7-1 Caring-based theory is expressed by this nurse, who is supporting the client through caring.

Values are different from principles, in that they influence the development of beliefs and attitudes rather than behaviors, although they might, and usually do, indirectly influence behaviors. A **value system** is an individual's collection of inner beliefs that guides the way the person acts and helps determine the choices the person makes in life. Although nearly nothing in life is value free, the impact of values on decisions and resultant behaviors is often not considered. Values are similar to the act of breathing; one does not think about them until a problem arises.

Nurses often care for clients whose value systems conflict with their own. "Rarely do diagnostic and treatment decisions occur without reference to values" (Gordon, Murphy, Candee, & Hiltunen, 1994). For example, a client with a value system of "grin and bear it" may be insulted by a nurse's attempts to offer pain medications. In order to ascertain those things that are meaningful to the client, the nurse must have an understanding of the client's value system (Figure 7-2). Furthermore, nurses must be aware of their own values, especially when they conflict with the values of clients.

Values Clarification

Values clarification is the process of analyzing one's own values to better understand those things that are truly important. Through values clarification, nurses can increase self-awareness and become better

PROFESSIONAL TIP

Values Clarification

It is the nurse's responsibility to make known to the supervisor any personal values that may influence or interfere with client care. For instance, a nurse who believes abortions should not be performed would find a conflict in working on a unit where abortions are performed. The nurse with this belief should make her values known to the employer before employment so that an assignment to that unit would not be made.

able to care for clients whose values differ from their own. In their classic work *Values and Teaching*, Raths, Harmin, and Simon (1978) formulated a theory of values clarification and proposed a three-step process of valuing, as follows:

• Choosing: Beliefs are chosen freely (that is, without coercion) from among alternatives. The choosing step involves analysis of the consequences of the various alternatives.
• Prizing: The beliefs that are selected are cherished (that is, prized).
• Acting: The selected beliefs are demonstrated consistently through behavior.

Nurses must understand that values are individual rather than universal and that, therefore, the nurse should not try to impose personal values on clients. The provision of ethical nursing care is directly related to one's values. For example, the nurse who strongly

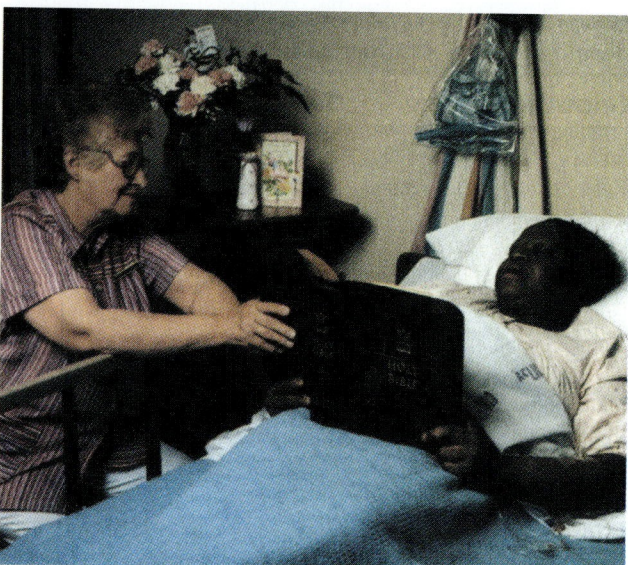

Figure 7-2 Clients' values determine those things that are meaningful to them.

values the sanctity of life may experience an ethical conflict when caring for a terminally ill client who refuses treatment that may extend life for a short time.

ETHICAL CODES

One hallmark of a profession is the determination of ethical behavior for its members. Several nursing organizations have developed codes as guidelines for ethical conduct. The Code for Licensed Practical/Vocational Nurses, developed by the National Federation of Licensed Practical Nurses (NFLPN), is presented in Table 7-5. This code, adopted by NFLPN in 1961 and revised in 1979 and in 1991, provides a motivation for establishing, maintaining, and elevating professional standards. Each LP/VN, upon entering the profession, inherits the responsibility to adhere to the standards of ethical practice and conduct as set forth in this code.

The Code for Nurses (Table 7-6) was developed by the International Council of Nurses (ICN). The American Nurses Association (ANA) has also established a code for ethical conduct of registered nurses. Although a code of ethics, which provides broad principles for determining and evaluating nursing care, is not legally binding, most state boards of nursing have authority to reprimand nurses for unprofessional conduct that results from violation of the ethical code.

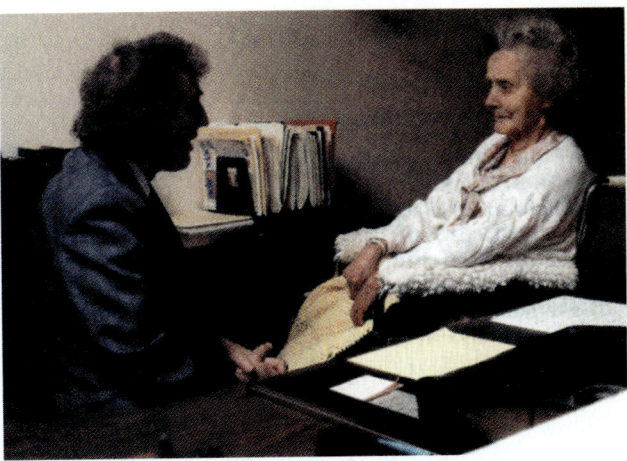

Figure 7-3 Clients have the right to information that will enable them to make decisions regarding their care.

THE CLIENT'S RIGHTS

The concept of rights is often misused, overused, and abused. Our society tends to take rights for granted. Rights and obligations are culturally defined. The dominant culture in the United States, however, holds the ethnocentric perspective that our rights and values are shared globally.

Clients have certain rights that apply regardless of the setting for delivery of care. These rights include, but are not limited to, the right to:

- Make decisions regarding their care (Figure 7-3),
- Be actively involved in the treatment process, and
- Be treated with dignity and respect (Figure 7-4).

When clients are admitted to short-term acute care agencies or extended care facilities, they are also entitled to certain rights. In 1972, the American Hospital Association (AHA) established *A Patient's Bill of Rights*, which outlines the rights and responsibilities of clients receiving care in hospitals (Table 7-7). This document, revised in 1992, increases health care providers' awareness of the need to treat clients in an ethical manner and encourages all health care providers to protect the rights of clients.

 HOME HEALTH CARE

The Client's Rights

The client's rights as outlined in Table 7-7 must be respected regardless of the setting for delivery of care. For care delivered in the home environment, for instance, the home health care nurse should discuss the client's rights with the client during the initial assessment (Figure 7-5).

Table 7-5	**THE CODE FOR LICENSED PRACTICAL/VOCATIONAL NURSES**

1. Know the scope of maximum utilization of the LP/VN as specified by the nursing practice act and function within this scope.
2. Safeguard the confidential information acquired from any source about the patient.
3. Provide health care to all patients regardless of race, creed, cultural background, disease, or lifestyle.
4. Refuse to give endorsement to the sale and promotion of commercial products or services.
5. Uphold the highest standards in personal appearance, language, dress, and demeanor.
6. Stay informed about issues affecting the practice of nursing and delivery of health care and, where appropriate, participate in government and policy decisions.
7. Accept the responsibility for safe nursing by keeping oneself mentally and physically fit and educationally prepared to practice.
8. Accept responsibility for membership in NFLPN and participate in its efforts to maintain the established standards of nursing practice and employment policies which lead to quality patient care.

From Nursing Practice Standards for the Licensed Practical/Vocational Nurse, by National Federation of Licensed Practical Nurses, Inc. (NFLPN), 1996, Garner, NC: Author. Copyright 1996 by Author. Reprinted with permission.

Table 7-6 INTERNATIONAL COUNCIL OF NURSES CODE FOR NURSES

The fundamental responsibility of the nurse is fourfold: to promote health, to prevent illness, to restore health, and to alleviate suffering.

The need for nursing is universal. Inherent in nursing is respect for life, dignity, and rights of man. It is unrestricted by considerations of nationality, race, creed, color, age, sex, politics, or social status.

Nurses render health services to the individual, the family, and the community and coordinate their services with those of related groups.

Nurses and People

The nurse's primary responsibility is to those people who require nursing care.

The nurse, in providing care, promotes an environment in which the values, customs, and spiritual beliefs of the individual are respected.

The nurse holds in confidence personal information and uses judgment in sharing this information.

Nurses and Practice

The nurse carries personal responsibility for nursing practice and for maintaining competence by continual learning. The nurse maintains the highest standards of nursing care possible within the reality of a specific situation.

The nurse uses judgment in relation to individual competence when accepting and delegating responsibilities.

The nurse, when acting in a professional capacity, should at all times maintain standards of personal conduct that reflect credit upon the profession.

Nurses and Society

The nurse shares with other citizens the responsibility for initiating and supporting action to meet the health and social needs of the public.

Nurses and Coworkers

The nurse sustains cooperative relationships with coworkers in nursing and other fields. The nurse takes appropriate action to safeguard the individual when his care is endangered by a coworker or any other person.

Nurses and the Profession

The nurse plays the major role in determining and implementing desirable standards of nursing practice and nursing education.

The nurse is active in developing a core of professional knowledge.

The nurse, acting through the professional organization, participates in establishing and maintaining equitable social and economic working conditions in nursing.

From ICN Code for Nurses: Ethical Concepts Applied to Nursing, by International Council of Nurses (ICN), 1973, Geneva, Switzerland: Imprimeries Populaires. Copyright 1973 by ICN. Reprinted with permission.

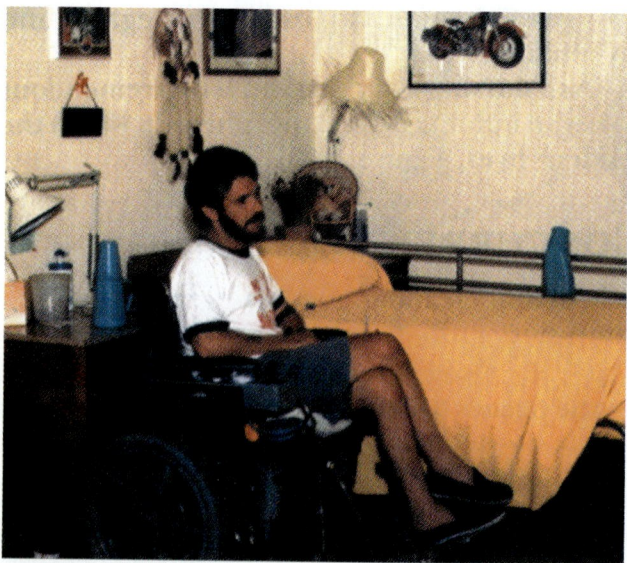

Figure 7-4 Clients have the right to dignity and respect and may keep personal articles in their rooms.

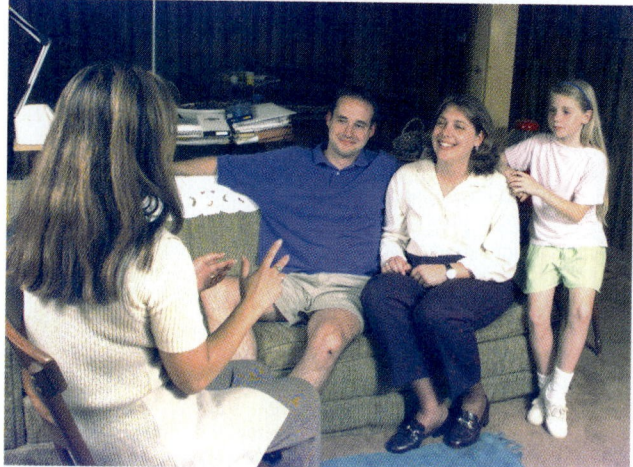

Figure 7-5 A home health nurse explains a client's rights.

Table 7-7 A PATIENT'S BILL OF RIGHTS

Introduction

Effective health care requires collaboration between patients and physicians and other health care professionals. Open and honest communication, respect for personal and professional values, and sensitivity to differences are integral to optimal patient care. As the setting for the provision of health services, hospitals must provide a foundation for understanding and respecting the rights and responsibilities of patients, their families, physicians, and other caregivers. Hospitals must ensure a health care ethic that respects the role of patients in decision making about treatment choices and other aspects of their care. Hospitals must be sensitive to cultural, racial, linguistic, religious, age, gender, and other differences as well as the needs of persons with disabilities.

The American Hospital Association presents *A Patient's Bill of Rights* with the expectation that it will contribute to more effective patient care and be supported by the hospital on behalf of the institution, its medical staff, employees, and patients. The American Hospital Association encourages health care institutions to tailor this bill of rights to their patient community by translating and/or simplifying the language of this bill of rights as may be necessary to ensure that patients and their families understand their rights and responsibilities.

Bill of Rights*

1. The patient has the right to considerate and respectful care.

2. The patient has the right to and is encouraged to obtain from physicians and other direct caregivers relevant, current, and understandable information concerning diagnosis, treatment, and prognosis. Except in emergencies when the patient lacks decision-making capacity and the need for treatment is urgent, the patient is entitled to the opportunity to discuss and request information related to the specific procedures and/or treatments, the risks involved, the possible length of recuperation, and the medically reasonable alternatives and their accompanying risks and benefits. Patients have the right to know the identity of physicians, nurses, and others involved in their care, as well as when those involved are students, residents, or other trainees. The patient also has the right to know the immediate and long-term financial implications of treatment choices, insofar as they are known.

3. The patient has the right to make decisions about the plan of care prior to and during the course of treatment and to refuse a recommended treatment or plan of care to the extent permitted by law and hospital policy and to be informed of the medical consequences of this action. In case of such refusal, the patient is entitled to other appropriate care and services that the hospital provides or transfer to another hospital. The hospital should notify patients of any policy that might affect patient choice within the institution.

4. The patient has the right to have an advance directive (such as a living will, health care proxy, or durable power of attorney for health care) concerning treatment or designating a surrogate decision maker with the expectation that the hospital will honor the intent of that directive to the extent permitted by law and hospital policy. Health care institutions must advise patients of their rights under state law and hospital policy to make informed medical choices, ask if the patient has an advance directive, and include that information in patient records. The patient has the right to timely information about hospital policy that may limit its ability to implement fully a legally valid advance directive.

5. The patient has the right to every consideration of privacy. Case discussion, consultation, examination, and treatment should be conducted so as to protect each patient's privacy.

6. The patient has the right to expect that all communications and records pertaining to his/her care will be treated as confidential by the hospital, except in cases such as suspected abuse and public health hazards when reporting is permitted or required by law. The patient has the right to expect that the hospital will emphasize the confidentiality of this information when it releases it to any other parties entitled to review information in these records.

7. The patient has the right to review the records pertaining to his/her medical care and to have the information explained or interpreted as necessary, except when restricted by law.

8. The patient has the right to expect that, within its capacity and policies, a hospital will make reasonable response to the request of a patient for appropriate and medically indicated care and services. The hospital must provide evaluation, service, and/or referral as indicated by the urgency of the case. When medically appropriate and legally permissible, or when a patient has so requested, a patient may be transferred to another facility. The institution to which the patient is to be transferred must first have accepted the patient for transfer. The patient must also have the benefit of complete information and explanation concerning the need for, risks, benefits, and alternatives to such a transfer.

9. The patient has the right to ask and be informed of the existence of business relationships among the hospital, educational institutions, other health care providers, or payers that may influence the patient's treatment and care. The patient has the right to obtain information as to the existence of any professional relationships among individuals, by name, who are treating him.

10. The patient has the right to consent to or decline to participate in proposed research studies or human experimentation affecting care and treatment or requiring direct patient involvement, and to have those studies fully explained prior to consent. A patient who declines to participate in research or experimentation is entitled to the most effective care that the hospital can otherwise provide.

11. The patient has the right to expect reasonable continuity of care when appropriate and to be informed by physicians and other caregivers of available and realistic patient care options when hospital care is no longer appropriate

12. The patient has the right to be informed of hospital policies and practices that relate to patient care, treatment, and responsibilities. The patient has the right to be informed of available resources for resolving disputes, grievances, and conflicts, such as ethics committees, patient representatives, or other mechanisms available in the institution. The patient has the right to be informed of the hospital's charges for services and available payment methods.

The collaborative nature of health care requires that patients, or their families/surrogates, participate in their care. The effectiveness of care and patient satisfaction with the course of treatment depend, in part, on the patient's fulfilling certain responsibilities. Patients are responsible for providing information about past illnesses, hospitalizations, medications, and other matters related to health status. To participate effectively in decision making, patients must be encouraged to take responsibility for requesting additional information or clarification about their health status or treatment when they do not fully understand information and instructions. Patients are also responsible for ensuring that the health care institution has a copy of their written advance directive if they have one. Patients are responsible for informing their physicians and other caregivers if they anticipate problems in following prescribed treatment.   *continued*

Table 7-7 A PATIENT'S BILL OF RIGHTS *continued*

Patients should also be aware of the hospital's obligation to be reasonably efficient and equitable in providing care to other patients and the community. The hospital's rules and regulations are designed to help the hospital meet this obligation. Patients and their families are responsible for making reasonable accommodations to the needs of the hospital, other patients, medical staff, and hospital employees. Patients are responsible for providing necessary information for insurance claims and for working with the hospital to make payment arrangements, when necessary.

A person's health depends on much more than health care services. Patients are responsible for recognizing the impact of their lifestyle on their personal health.

Conclusion

Hospitals have many functions to perform, including the enhancement of health status, health promotion, and the prevention and treatment of injury and disease; the immediate and ongoing care and rehabilitation of patients; the education of health professionals, patients, and the community; and research. All these activities must be conducted with an overriding concern for the values and dignity of patients.

*These rights can be exercised on the patient's behalf by a designated surrogate or proxy decision maker if the patient lacks decision-making capacity, is legally incompetent, or is a minor.

A Patient's Bill of Rights *was first adopted by the American Hospital Association (AHA) in 1973. This revision was approved by the AHA Board of Trustees on October 21, 1992. Copyright 1992 by the American Hospital Association, 840 North Lake Shore Drive, Chicago, Illinois 60611. Printed in the U.S.A. All rights reserved. Reprinted with permission of the American Hospital Association.*

ETHICAL DILEMMAS

An **ethical dilemma** occurs when there is a conflict between two or more ethical principles—when there is no "correct" decision. Ethical dilemmas are situations of conflicting requirements; something ought to be done and ought not to be done at the same time. When an ethical dilemma occurs, the nurse must make a choice between two alternatives that are equally unsatisfactory. Ethical analysis is not an exact science. In some cases, even after a dilemma seems to have been resolved, questions remain. This ambiguity makes it emotionally painful for the persons involved. Three areas where ethical dilemmas are possible are euthanasia, refusal of treatment, and scarcity of resources.

Euthanasia

Most people hope to experience a peaceful, gentle death when their "time comes." The word *euthanasia* comes from the Greek word *euthanatos*, which literally means "good, or gentle, death." In current times, **euthanasia** refers to intentional action or lack of action that causes the merciful death of someone suffering from a terminal illness or incurable condition.

Active euthanasia refers to taking deliberate action that will hasten the client's death, such as removing from a respirator a client who is in a vegetative state. In contrast, **passive euthanasia** means cooperating with the client's dying process. Passive euthanasia is "a decision made not to prolong life. . . . It is the omission of an action that would prolong the dying process" (Sumodi, 1995). An example is not putting in a feeding tube to provide nourishment when the client cannot or will no longer eat.

Assisted suicide is a form of active euthanasia whereby another person provides a client with the means to end his own life. Recently, physician-assisted suicide has been the topic of much controversy. Nurses have differing opinions regarding assisted suicide. Some look on it as a violation of the ethical principles on which the practice of nursing is based: autonomy, nonmaleficence, beneficence, justice, veracity, and fidelity. Regardless of a nurse's personal viewpoint, assisted suicide is still illegal. Other nurses may see assisted suicide as an ethical dilemma; they agree that it violates some ethical principles but question whether it violates others. For example, in answer to the question "Does assisted suicide violate the principle of autonomy?" one might argue that it is *refusal* to assist a suicide that violates a client's autonomy.

Refusal of Treatment

The client's right to refuse treatment is based on the principle of autonomy. In fairness, the client can refuse treatment only after the treatment methods and their consequences have been explained. A client's rights to refuse treatment and to die challenge the values of most health care providers.

> Honoring the refusal of treatments that a patient does not desire, that are disproportionately burdensome to the patient, or that will not benefit the patient is ethically and legally permissible (Curtin, 1995).

One possible ethical dilemma in this area relates to the use of ventilators for clients who would otherwise die. Medical technology makes it possible for these clients to continue breathing as long as they are connected to the machine. But one might ask "What are the emotional, physical, psychological, and fiscal costs?" and "What is the quality of a life prolonged by technology?"

Scarcity of Resources

With the current emphasis on containing health care costs, the use of expensive services is being closely examined. The use of specialists, organ transplants, and distribution of services are being influenced by social and political forces. For example, the length of stay in a hospital and the number of office visits allowable for individual clients are already predetermined by many third-party payers. In addition to economics, the availability of goods (such as organs) is contributing to a scarcity of resources.

In many situations, clients wait extended periods before receiving donated organs. The allocation of scarce resources is emerging as a major ethical dilemma: Who should receive the benefit of such a scarce and precious resource as a living organ? How should the determination be made? Currently, the selection of organ recipients is based on objective criteria such as organ availability, donor/recipient match, the degree of the recipient's need, and the recipient's willingness to commit to a lifetime of drug therapy and follow-up care. But should only objective criteria be used in determining who receives a donated organ, or should moral judgments also be made?

ETHICAL DECISION MAKING

Nurses must understand the basis on which they make their decisions. **Ethical reasoning** is the process of thinking through what one ought to do in an orderly, systematic manner based on principles. Ethical decisions cannot be made in a scattered, unorganized manner based entirely on intuition or emotions. Ethical decision making is a rational way of making decisions in nursing practice. It is used in situations where either the right decision is not clear or conflicts of rights and duties exist. A framework for resolving ethical dilemmas follows.

Framework for Ethical Decision Making

"After a moral conflict has been formulated, the nurse must differentiate the relevant parts of the conflict and resolve it" (Gordon et al., 1994). When making an ethical decision, the nurse must consider the following relevant questions:

- Which theories are involved?
- Which principles are involved?
- Who will be affected?
- What will be the consequences of the alternatives (ethical options)?

To resolve ethical dilemmas, the nurse must be able to make decisions in a systematic fashion. Figure 7-6 illustrates a method for making ethical judgments.

The first step of ethical analysis is to gather relevant

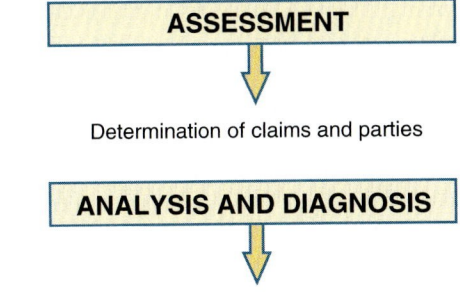

Determination of claims and parties

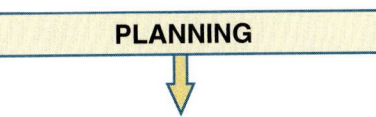

Identification of problem: Statement of the ethical dilemma

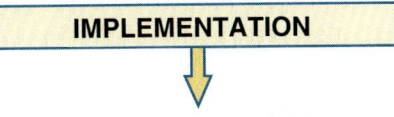

Consideration of priorities of claims;
Generation of alternatives for resolving the dilemma;
Consideration of the consequences of alternatives

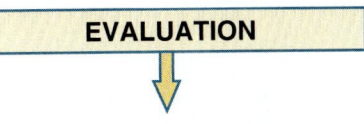

Carrying out selected moral actions

EVALUATION

Evaluation of the outcome of moral actions;
"Were the actions ethical?"
"What were the consequences?"

Figure 7-6 Ethical Decision-making Model *(Adapted from Fundamentals of Nursing: Standards & Practice, by S. DeLaune and P. Ladner, 1998, Albany, NY: Delmar Publishers. Copyright 1998 by Delmar Publishers. Adapted with permission.)*

data in order to identify the ethical problem and to determine which type of ethical problem exists: Do principles conflict with principles? Do actions conflict with actions? Do actions conflict with principles? What are the claims?

Next, all the people involved (the parties) must be considered. What are their rights, responsibilities, duties, and decision-making abilities? Who is the most appropriate person to make the decision? Whose problem is it? It is important to identify several possible alternatives and predict the outcome of each. Then, and only then, can a course of action be selected—one that, it is hoped, ends in resolution of the problem. The final step of ethical decision making is evaluation of the resolution process.

ETHICS AND NURSING

As professionals, nurses are accountable for protecting the rights and interests of the client. Consequently, sound nursing practice involves making ethical decisions. Ethics affects nurses in every health care setting, and each practice setting presents the nurse with its own set of ethical concerns. Whatever the setting, nurses must balance their ethical responsibilities to each client as an individual with their professional obligations. Often, there is an inherent conflict.

Ethics Committees

The provision of ethical health care requires both self-examination on the part of the care provider and dialogue among health care providers. Many health care agencies now recognize the need for a systematic manner whereby to discuss ethical concerns (Figure 7-7). Multidisciplinary committees (also referred to as institutional ethics committees) constitute one arena for dialogue regarding ethical dilemmas. In addition to serving as a forum where ethical issues are discussed, ethics committees can lead to the establishment of policies and procedures for prevention and resolution of dilemmas.

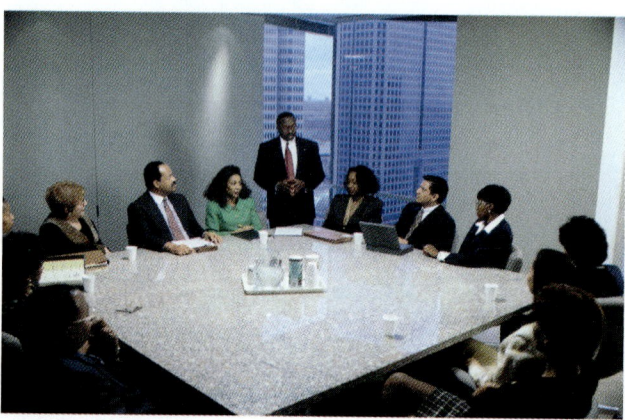

Figure 7-7 Ethics Committee Meeting *(Photo courtesy of Photodisc)*

HOME HEALTH CARE

Client Autonomy

With the increased acuity level of clients cared for in the home setting, home health nurses face ever-increasing ethical challenges.

Clients who are being cared for at home have more control over their decisions and actions than those who are institutionalized. . . . Client autonomy becomes a much stronger influence in the outcome of care than it does in institutional settings, because the provider has less control over what the client does on a day-to-day basis at home. . . . [Home health care] represents a power reversal in which the client's autonomy takes on greater significance. (Kristoff, Sellin, & Miller, 1994)

PROFESSIONAL TIP

Providing Ethical Care

- Initiate dialogue concerning the client's wishes. Do more listening than talking. (For example, the following is a question you might ask to help determine the client's wishes: "If your heart stopped, would you want us to try to start it again?")
- Assess the client's understanding of the illness and the available treatment options.
- Allow time for the client to explore values and to communicate.
- Facilitate communication of the client's desires to family and other health care providers.

Nurse as Client Advocate

When acting as a client advocate, the nurse's first step is to develop a meaningful relationship with the client. The nurse is then able to make decisions with the client based on the strength of the relationship. The nurse's primary ethical responsibility is to protect clients' rights to make their own decisions.

Nurses have an ethical obligation to do everything possible to prevent anyone from taking advantage of vulnerable patients—or clouding objectivity so that the patients' best interests fade from sight. (Haddad, 1995)

Nurse as Whistleblower

The term **whistleblowing** refers to calling attention to unethical, illegal, or incompetent actions of others. Whistleblowing is based on the ethical principles of veracity and nonmaleficence. As professionals, nurses are expected to monitor coworkers' abilities to perform their duties safely (Pinch, 1990). Although nurses are expected to "blow the whistle" on incompetent health care providers, many are reluctant to do so because there are inherent risks in whistleblowing. Curtin (1993) identifies some of the questions a person should consider before reporting unethical or incompetent behavior:

- Whose problem is this?
- Must I do anything about it?
- Is it my fault?
- Who am I to judge?
- Do I have the facts straight?
- Should I ignore the situation? Should I tolerate it?
- What do I get out of this?
- Is it worth the trouble?
- Is anything to be gained?
- What will it cost me?

CASE STUDY

Janice is a 45-year-old woman who is pregnant with her fourth child. The pregnancy was unplanned and distressed Janice and her husband at first, but now they have accepted it and look forward to the delivery of their child. Janice has been receiving prenatal care from her family practice physician since her second month of pregnancy. She is now in her seventh month.

During her sixth month of pregnancy, the physician ordered laboratory tests, and the results indicated a fetal abnormality. The physician requested to perform further diagnostic testing on the fetus during the seventh month. Janice and her husband refused further fetal testing. Although the physician explained the importance of the testing, the couple continued to refuse it.

After the couple left the office, the physician turned to the nurse and stated, "Since they will not follow my suggestions, write them a letter and tell them I am terminating our relationship. Tell her to see a specialist." No arrangements for a referral were made for Janice by the doctor, who feared that the high-risk delivery predisposed him to a lawsuit.

The following questions are related to the case study.

1. Based on the information presented, what are the primary ethical issues?
2. What are your personal values in relation to the situation?
3. What course of action would you recommend for the nurse and why? What ethical principles would guide you?
4. To what extent, in your opinion, is Janice noncompliant?
5. Was the medical intervention adequate? Is the nurse to judge medical care?
6. What is the nurse's responsibility to ensure follow-up care?

Federal law and state laws (to varying degrees) provide protection, such as privacy, to whistleblowers. Unfortunately, however, the inclination to protect one's coworkers and the fear of reprisal may deter a nurse from fulfilling the ethical obligation to report substandard behaviors.

SUMMARY

- Ethics is the branch of philosophy concerned with the distinction of right from wrong on the basis of a body of knowledge rather than on just opinions. It is the study of the rightness of conduct.
- Ethics examines human behavior—those things that people do under a given set of circumstances.
- There is a connection between acts that are legal and acts that are ethical. Professional nursing actions are both legal and ethical.
- Teleology is an ethical theory that states that the value of a situation is determined by its consequences.
- Deontology is an ethical theory that considers the intrinsic significance of an act itself as the criterion for determination of good.

- Ethical decisions are based on principles such as autonomy, nonmaleficence, beneficence, justice, veracity, and fidelity.
- Because ethics and values are so closely associated, nurses must explore their own values in order to acknowledge the value systems of their clients.
- Ethical codes that have been developed by nursing organizations such as the NFLPN, the ICN, and the ANA establish guidelines for the ethical conduct of nurses with clients, coworkers, society, and the nursing profession.
- The Patient's Bill of Rights is designed to guarantee ethical care of clients in terms of their decision making about treatment choices and other aspects of their care.
- Nurses must apply the process of ethical reasoning to resolve ethical dilemmas wherein conflict exists between principles and duties.
- The roles of client advocate and whistleblower enable nurses to protect their clients' rights and ensure the ethical and competent actions of their peers within the nursing profession.

Review Questions

1. Nurses would use the Code for Licensed Practical/Vocational Nurses to:

    a. solve an ethical dilemma.
    b. develop a nursing care plan.
    c. seek an answer to a client care problem.
    d. understand the professional expectations required of them.

2. Values influence the nurse–client relationship because:

    a. the client's values take precedence over the nurse's values.
    b. every individual has a personal value system that helps determine actions.
    c. the nurse must help the client clarify his values in order to ensure effective nursing care.
    d. the nurse cannot effectively care for a client who has values that differ from those of the nurse.

3. Values clarification is a useful exercise for the nurse to perform because it helps the nurse:

    a. make ethically sound decisions.
    b. stay informed of new developments.
    c. avoid conflicts with clients and coworkers.
    d. establish policies about proper and improper client care.

4. An ethical dilemma is a:

    a. choice to be made between right and wrong.
    b. problem with two equally unsatisfactory solutions.
    c. series of problems that the nurse encounters in each client care situation.
    d. problem the nurse cannot solve without the intervention of a physician.

5. Active euthanasia means a person:

    a. helps a client to die.
    b. has an advance directive.
    c. limits the amount of care.
    d. chooses to stop pain therapy.

Critical Thinking Questions

1. A client delivers a baby with multiple congenital defects. The prognosis is poor, with the infant not being expected to live longer than 12 months at most. The mother says, "We can't afford to pay for the baby's care." Who should determine the degree of intervention? Should the cost of care be the foremost basis for the decision?

2. An 80-year-old woman is in a persistent vegetative state as a result of a cardiovascular accident. She has always talked about "someday" signing a living will requesting that heroic measures not be taken, but her family wants "everything to be done that can be done." Whose wishes should prevail? What ethical principles would come into play in this decision process?

 WEB FLASH!

- What organizations or professional journals can you locate for information on nursing and ethical issues?
- What resources and references can you find when you search under healthcare ethics as related to organ donation, euthanasia, scarcity of resources, or refusal of treatment?

Communication

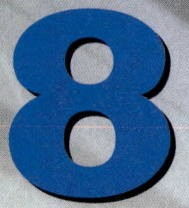

CHAPTER

8

COMMUNICATION

MAKING THE CONNECTION

Refer to the following chapters to increase your understanding of communication:

- **Chapter 2, Critical Thinking**
- **Chapter 6, Legal Responsibilities**
- **Chapter 12, Cultural Diversity and Nursing**
- **Chapter 17, Loss, Grief, and Death**
- **Chapter 25, Assessment**

LEARNING OBJECTIVES

Upon completion of this chapter you should be able to:
- *Define key terms.*
- *Describe the process of communication and factors that influence it.*
- *Differentiate between verbal and nonverbal communication.*
- *Utilize therapeutic communication.*
- *Understand the psychosocial aspects of communication.*
- *Demonstrate proper telephone communication.*
- *Communicate effectively with clients and families.*
- *Demonstrate communicating with special clients who are visually impaired, hearing impaired, speech impaired, unconscious, and non-English speaking.*
- *Communicate effectively with terminally ill clients and their families.*
- *Communicate effectively with other members of the health care team.*

KEY TERMS

active listening	hearing
aphasia	listening
communication	nonverbal communication
congruent	proxemics
dysarthria	rapport
dysphasia	telemedicine
empathy	therapeutic communication
feedback	verbal communication

INTRODUCTION

Why study communication? Students in a nursing program have generally had a minimum of 17 years of communicating. But have you ever told another person a story and then heard the story repeated by someone else? Or have you ever played the game of "telephone," where a message is whispered from one person to another and the last one states the message out loud? In both situations, when you hear the story or message again, it typically has changed from the original. When communicating with a client, family, or another member of the health care team, it is important that the message be sent and received accurately.

This chapter addresses the process of communication; methods of communicating, including verbal and nonverbal communication and factors that influence communication, such as age, culture, education, language, attention, emotions, and surroundings. Techniques that promote effective (therapeutic) communication are also described, as are barriers to communication, and examples of both are presented. Also explored are psychosocial aspects of communication, such as style, gestures, meaning of time, meaning of space, cultural values, and political correctness, and their importance to the health care system. Finally, communication with the client, family, and health care team as well as self-communication is discussed.

PROCESS OF COMMUNICATION

The simplest definition of **communication** is the sending and receiving of a message. The six aspects of communication are: sender, message, channel, receiver, feedback, and influences.

Sender

The sender of a message is the person who has a thought, idea, or emotion to convey to another person. Messages stem from a person's need to relate to others, to create meanings, and to understand various situations.

Message

The message is the thought, idea, or emotion one person sends to another person. It is a stimulus produced by the sender and responded to by the receiver.

Channel

The person sending the message must decide how to send the message. The channel, or medium, through which a message is transmitted may be auditory, visual, or kinesthetic.

The auditory channel involves the verbal (speaking) method for the sender and the **hearing** (act or power of perceiving sounds) and/or **listening** (interpreting sounds heard and attaching meaning to them) modes of transmission for the receiver.

The visual channel involves the verbal (writing) and/or nonverbal methods for the sender and the sight, reading, observation, and perception modes of transmission for the receiver.

The kinesthetic channel involves touch for the sender and experience of sensation for the receiver (Table 8-1).

Receiver

The physiological component involves the processes of hearing, seeing, and the reception of the touch stimulus. The psychological processes may enhance or impede the receiving of messages. For example, anxiety may cause an individual to experience alterations in hearing, sight, or feeling.

The cognitive aspect is the "thinking" part of receiving. It involves interpreting stimuli and converting them into meaning.

Feedback

Feedback is a response from the receiver that enables the sender to verify that the message sent was the message received. If this is not the case, additional messages are sent and received until an understanding of the primary message is reached between the sender and receiver.

Influences

Both the sender and receiver are influenced by their education, culture, emotions, and perceptions and by the situation within which they find themselves. These elements are collectively referred to as a person's frame of reference. Sometimes these influences help communication, and sometimes they hinder communication. Figure 8-1 shows the process of communication and the influences on the sender and receiver.

Table 8-1 COMMUNICATION CHANNELS

CHANNEL	MODE OF TRANSMISSION	OUTCOME	EXAMPLE
Auditory (verbal)	• Hearing	Receiving an auditory stimulus	Hearing the client say, "I feel fine"
	• Listening	Interpreting sounds heard and attaching meaning to them	Hearing loud moaning in a client's room, the nurse enters the room to check whether the client is in pain
Visual (nonverbal or verbal)	• Sight	Receiving a visual stimulus	Watching the rise and fall of a client's chest while counting respirations
	• Reading		Reading the client's record
	• Observation	Interpreting a visual stimulus by making note of accompanying sounds	Making note of sounds of labored breathing while counting respirations and concluding that breathing is abnormal
	• Perception	Assigning meaning to a visual event	Diagnosing an alteration in oxygenation related to respiratory distress
Kinesthetic (tactile or nonverbal)	• Procedural touch	Performing nursing procedures and techniques	Giving the client a bed bath
	• Caring touch	Conveying emotional support	Holding the client's hand

Adapted from Fundamentals of Nursing: Standards & Practice, *by S. DeLaune and P. Ladner, 1998, Albany, NY: Delmar Publishers. Copyright 1998 by Delmar Publishers.*

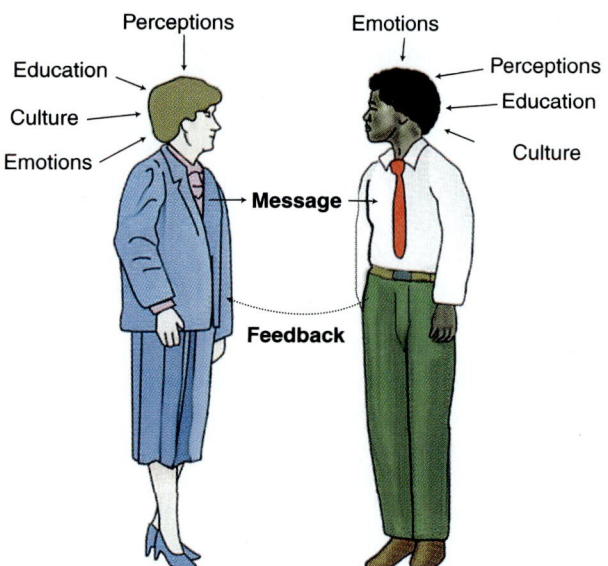

Figure 8-1 Process of Communication

METHODS OF COMMUNICATING

There are two methods of communicating: verbally and nonverbally. Which is better? The answer is neither, or more accurately, it depends on what the sender is trying to communicate. Seldom is a spoken message sent without some accompanying nonverbal aspects. Some experts believe that nonverbal communication is more honest than is verbal communication because it usually is conveyed unconsciously by the sender.

Verbal Communication

Verbal communication is the use of words, either spoken or written, to send a message. Methods of verbal communication include speaking, listening, writing, and reading.

Speaking/Listening

Most commonly, speaking is thought of as verbal communication. The receiver of a spoken message must listen. Speaking and listening must both occur in order for there to be communication. Have you ever sent a spoken message to someone in the same room with you and received nonmeaningful, senseless feedback from that person, or no feedback at all? More than likely, the other person was only hearing the message but not listening.

Communication experts say that people speak at a rate of 125 to 150 words per minute (WPM) but hear at a rate of 400 to 800 WPM. This extra time allows for distractions. Listeners are generally distracted because they are not concentrating on what is being said. Listening is one of the most difficult skills to learn and execute well.

Writing/Reading

The other mode of verbal communication is writing. The receiver of the written message must read the words. The reader must understand the words and attach meaning to them. With a written message, immediate feedback is generally not available. Therefore, great care should be taken to ensure clarity when composing a written message. Charting is a good example. The physician may read the chart after the caregivers who did the charting go off duty, allowing little chance for immediate feedback. In such an instance, if a chart read that a client was "uncooperative," for example, the physician would have little idea exactly what the caregiver meant. An entry of "refused to eat lunch, refused to get out of bed and sit in chair," however, is far more exact, illustrating the clarity in writing that is essential to good communication.

Nonverbal Communication

Nonverbal communication, sometimes called body language, is the sending of a message without using words. There are many ways we communicate without words, including gestures, facial expressions, posture and gait, tone of voice, touch, eye contact, body position, and physical appearance.

Nonverbal communication is generally unconscious—part learned behavior and part instinct. Because there is little conscious control involved in nonverbal communication, feelings are generally most honestly expressed nonverbally.

Clients seem to believe and are particularly sensitive to nonverbal messages. Nurses must thus make an effort to be aware of the nonverbal messages they may be sending to clients. For example, consider those aspects of nursing care that are not pleasant but must be done. Think how the client would feel if a nurse were to register an expression of disgust or revulsion on her face when changing a surgical dressing.

Nurses must also be sensitive to the client's nonverbal messages. Many clients do not want to bother "busy" nurses. Such clients may say they are fine or do not need anything when this is in fact not the case. An astute nurse, however, will observe nonverbal signs such as stiff posture, clenched fists, or a frowning facial expression and know that something is not right. Further assessment would then be undertaken to determine why the client is sending such nonverbal clues.

Gestures

Gestures are often referred to as "talking with hands." Gestures may be used to help clarify a verbal message, to emphasize an idea, to hold other's attention, or to relieve stress. Fingertapping, fidgeting, or ring twisting generally indicates tension, nervousness, or impatience. Shaking a fist indicates anger, whereas pointing may be used to clarify directions.

Facial Expressions

Although some people have very expressive faces, some do not. A big smile is easily interpreted as indicating happiness. Eyebrows can be very expressive, showing surprise, worry, thoughtfulness, or displeasure. The manner in which the forehead is wrinkled also sends a message.

Nurses must be very aware of their own facial expressions, especially when caring for a client under "unpleasant" conditions, such as when a client is vomiting or suffering from bowel incontinence. An expression of displeasure manifested as a "curled up" nose or disgust is easily identified by the client. The client, often already embarrassed at requiring such care, is likely to feel even worse should the nurse's facial expressions indicate anything but caring, concern, and empathy.

Posture and Gait

Good posture, with the head held up, and a purposeful gait are usually interpreted as meaning self-confidence, competence, and a positive self-image. Stooped shoulders, a downward-held head, and a shuffling gait generally convey low self-esteem, depression, and lack of confidence.

Tone of Voice

Tone of voice has been estimated to convey 23% of the context of a message. When the same words are said in different tones of voice, they can have very different meanings. Tone of voice might be pleasant, sincere, sorrowful, sarcastic, joyful, or angry.

Touch

Touch is a simple yet powerful form of nonverbal communication that even a newborn infant can understand. Touch can communicate caring, understanding, encouragement, warmth, reassurance, or affection. Of course, touch can also communicate anger, displeasure, or a lack or caring and understanding. Sometimes touch can hurt or be harmful to the person being touched.

While some people are natural "touchers," others are not. The use of touch can be learned, however. Many nursing tasks involve touching the client. If the nurse is uncomfortable touching a client, the touch along with other nonverbal communication such as facial expression, posture, eye contact, and tone of voice will all convey the nurse's discomfort. Most clients accept touch as an integral part of nursing care when it is done appropriately and professionally.

Eye Contact

Eyes, it is said, mirror the soul. Have you ever seen joy, sadness, pain, or laughter in someone's eyes? It is very difficult to control these messages of the eyes.

Eye contact is generally interpreted as indicating interest and attention, whereas lack of eye contact is thought to indicate avoidance, disinterest, or discomfort.

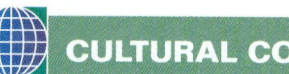

CULTURAL CONSIDERATIONS

Eye Contact
In some cultures it is considered rude or disrespectful to make direct eye contact.

Body Position

Body position is often a good indicator of a person's attitude. For example, crossed arms generally indicate withdrawal, although the person could just be cold. Open body positions, with the arms held freely at the sides, are usually taken to mean a receptive attitude.

Physical Appearance

A person's physical appearance says a great deal about that person. A clean, neat, appropriately dressed individual conveys a positive self-image, knowledge, and competence. A dirty, sloppy, or inappropriately dressed person conveys the message of "I don't care how I look," with the potential further implication of "maybe I am not too knowledgeable or competent," or "I am sloppy in what I do."

It is very important for every nurse to be clean, neat, and professionally dressed. Clients and families understand the nonverbal message that appearance conveys. Appearance does influence communication.

INFLUENCES ON COMMUNICATION

Communication involves more than just the sending and receiving of verbal and nonverbal messages. How a person sends or receives a message is influenced by such factors as age, education, emotions, culture, and language. Attention to the message and the surroundings are other influences. These factors must be taken into account for accurate communication to take place.

Age

Factors related to age affect communication. For instance, communicating with a child is different from communicating with an adult and is dependent on the age of the child. Nonverbal communication, particularly touch, and facial expression can be understood by infants. Before learning to understand words, a child can interpret tone of voice and gestures. Preschool children respond well to communication involving toys or play situations. They should be allowed some choices, but no more than two alternatives should be offered. As the child's vocabulary increases, more verbal communication can take place.

Elderly persons may have some degree of hearing loss or a slowed response time. The nurse should face the elderly client when speaking and allow time for a response. The client should be addressed as "Mr." or "Ms." unless he or she asks to be called by his or her first name. Elderly clients should be treated with respect and not talked to as if they were children; they are individuals with special needs (Figure 8-2).

Education

Education is another strong influence on communication. The more educated a person, the greater the vocabulary of that person. Highly educated persons are generally able to discuss and understand concepts and abstract ideas, whereas persons of lesser education generally communicate in a more literal and less abstract way.

Emotions

A person's emotional state greatly influences how messages are sent or received. Someone who is very anxious or upset, for example, may not hear what is said or may interpret the message differently than the sender intended. This same person typically speaks in an abrupt manner, loudly, and in harsh tones. The depressed person, on the other hand, typically says very little, speaking only one or two words or in very short sentences.

Culture

Each culture has its own standards of communication, especially with regard to nonverbal behavior. In the United States, for example, eye contact is considered a sign of openness and honesty. Those of Spanish heritage, however, believe eye contact to be disrespectful. Similarly, in many parts of Europe, a kiss on the cheek between two men is accepted. People from other parts of the world, however, may look suspiciously on this behavior.

Language

Language certainly influences communication. Speaking the same language assists people in understanding each other, although regional accents or dialects of a language can inhibit communication and understanding. When verbal communication comes to a standstill, nonverbal communication is often employed to assist. Any nurse who works in an area where there is a predominate second language should learn a few words or phrases in that language to help put clients at ease and to facilitate their understanding.

Attention

The amount of attention each individual focuses on a given communication greatly affects the outcome. In selective listening, the receiver hears only what he

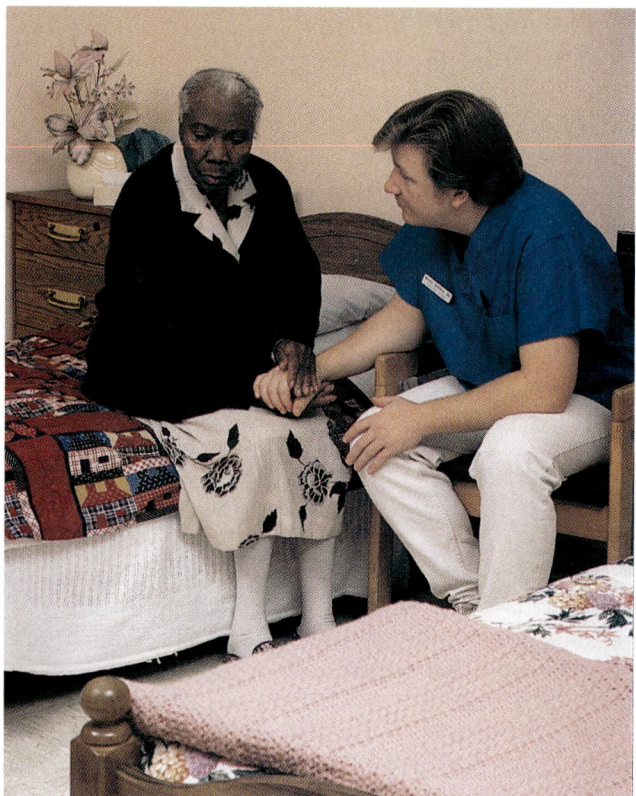

Figure 8-2 When addressing elderly clients, face them directly and allow adequate response time. A warm touch on the hand or arm will communicate caring and respect.

wants or expects to hear. Pain or discomfort, physical or mental, may result in preoccupation, limiting the attention given to the communication.

Surroundings

Most people do not want to talk about the intimate details of their health care concerns in public (Figure 8-3). Thus, privacy should be provided. If the client occupies a room alone, the nurse should close the room door; if the client shares a room, the nurse should take the client to a conference room or other private place, if possible, to discuss personal information.

The nurse should respect the client's current "home" (e.g., the hospital room) as she would any person's home, knocking on the door before entering the room, not sitting on the bed without permission, and asking before moving any personal articles that are in the way. These simple courtesies show respect for the client as a person. When the client feels respected, communication is enhanced.

CONGRUENCY OF MESSAGES

It is important that verbal and nonverbal communications be **congruent**, or in agreement. Saying, "I really appreciate what you just did," in a happy tone of voice while smiling is congruent and clear; saying the

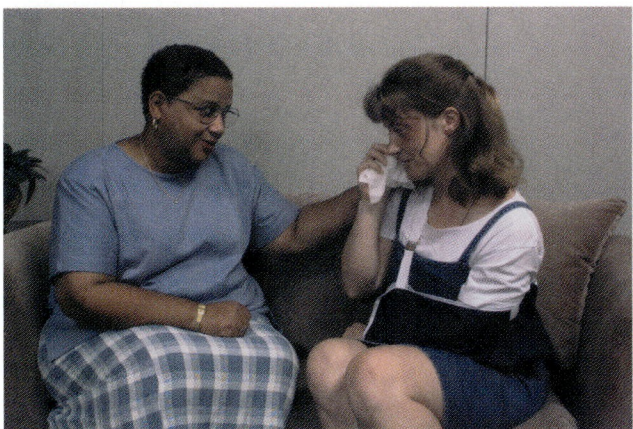

Figure 8-3 Provide privacy when discussing personal or intimate health concerns with clients.

same words in a disgusted tone of voice while frowning is incongruent and, thus, potentially unclear. The receiver may not know whether the sender is genuinely pleased with what was done or is displeased and being sarcastic. Messages such as these can confuse the receiver, who then may require feedback in order to correctly interpret the message.

It is important for the nurse to watch for congruency between verbal and nonverbal messages and to ask for clarification when incongruity exists.

LISTENING/OBSERVING

Listening and observing are two of the most valuable skills a nurse can have. These two skills are used to gather the subjective and objective data for the nursing assessment. Because the nursing diagnoses and nursing interventions are based on the assessment, it is imperative that the assessment be accurate.

The term **active listening** has been used to describe this behavior of listening and observing; it reflects the process of hearing spoken words and noting nonverbal behavior. It takes energy and concentration. The nurse who is at eye level with the client, who leans slightly forward toward the client, and who makes eye contact is showing undivided attention to the client and will be able to listen and observe more accurately. Responses from the nurse such as "go on," "tell me more," "yes," "what else?" or "mmhm" both encourage the client to continue and communicate that the nurse is really listening.

THERAPEUTIC COMMUNICATION

Therapeutic communication, sometimes called effective communication, is purposeful and goal directed, creating a beneficial outcome for the client.

One person is the helper (nurse) and the other is being helped (client). The focus of the conversation is the client, the client's needs, or the client's problems, not the needs or problems of the nurse.

Goals of Therapeutic Communication

There are several goals or purposes of therapeutic communication. One or more of these goals guide every therapeutic communication in the nurse–client relationship. The goals are: obtain or provide information, develop trust, show caring, and explore feelings.

Obtain or Provide Information

It is important for the nurse to obtain information from the client about general health and specific health problems. It is with this information that the nurse can make an accurate assessment and plan of care.

The nurse provides information to the client from admission to discharge, beginning with the orientation of a new client to the hospital policies and routines. Information provision continues throughout the hospital stay as the nurse explains procedures, treatments, and tests; teaches the client self-care; clarifies instruction from other health care workers; and answers client questions. The discharge instructions constitute the final stage of information provision.

Develop Trust

Client and nurse are generally strangers at the time of their first meeting. The nurse must work to establish trust with each client. Answering questions honestly, responding to call lights promptly, and following through are examples of ways to build trust. Trust develops faster when caring is shown.

Show Caring

Fluffing a pillow or offering a drink of water without being asked are two ways to show caring (Figure 8-4). Taking time to always greet the client by name and knocking on the room door before entering are other ways.

Mutual trust established between client and nurse is termed **rapport**.

Explore Feelings

Once rapport is established, the nurse can encourage the client to explore feelings. Generally, most clients are anxious about illness. Some fear the results of diagnostic tests, and some are anxious about the hospital environment. Many clients do not want to admit they are anxious or fearful. By using therapeutic communication techniques, the nurse is often able to help the client talk about feelings and reduce anxiety. Sometimes, a clarifying statement is all that is needed to alleviate fear or anxiety. Other times, allowing the client to talk about the fear or anxiety reduces that fear or anxiety.

Behaviors/Attitudes to Enhance Communication

Some behaviors and attitudes enhance therapeutic communication. Included are: self-disclosure, caring, genuineness, warmth, active listening, empathy, and acceptance and respect.

Self-Disclosure

Self-disclosure means sharing something about yourself such as thoughts, expectations, feelings, or ideas. It does not mean sharing your personal problems. When the nurse shares something, such as future goals in nursing, it shows that the client is trusted with that knowledge. The more the client feels trusted, the more the client will trust the nurse and therapeutic communication is enhanced.

Caring

Caring is not only a goal of therapeutic communication but also an attitude that enhances communication. Caring is the foundation of a nurse–client relationship (Figure 8-4). A caring attitude is easily identified by the client. The client is made to feel important. Table 8-2 gives some examples of ways to show caring.

Genuineness

Effective communication must be genuine. The nurse must be himself. It means being honest about one's feelings. Sometimes it is "ok" to cry with a client.

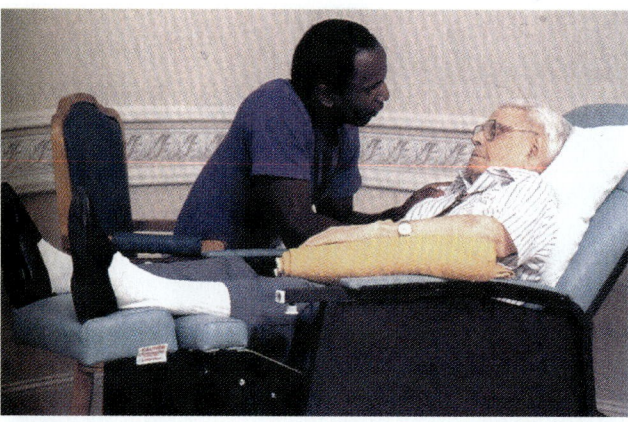

Figure 8-4 The nurse shows caring in everyday activities, such as ensuring client comfort.

It means being truthful and never attempting to answer a question when the answer is not known. The nurse should admit not knowing but offer to find the answer and then do so.

Being genuine builds trust. However, the nurse must use good judgment when expressing negative thoughts or confronting a client, family member, or another health care worker.

Warmth

Warmth makes the client feel welcomed, relaxed, and unjudged. It is expressed predominantly by nonverbal communication. A smile helps the client feel relaxed.

Touch is an important method to show warmth, but it must be used appropriately. Society dictates the type of touching that is appropriate in different situations. Holding a client's hand or putting a hand on the shoulder can greatly enhance communication by providing a connection between the nurse and the client. Touch may not always be welcomed by the client.

Active Listening

As the words imply, listening is an active process requiring energy and concentration. It involves listening to the words spoken as well as being aware of nonverbal messages. The nurse listens to both the words spoken and the nonverbal messages.

Active listening requires responses from the listener. This indicates that the nurse is really listening to the client. It is important for the nurse to concentrate on the interaction at hand and not let other thoughts become a distraction (Figure 8-5).

Empathy

Empathy is the capacity to understand another person's feelings or perception of a situation. It is an objective awareness of, or a sensitivity to, another person's feelings and thoughts. Although the nurse does not share the thoughts and feelings of the client, with empathy the nurse is able to understand and accept

Table 8-2 WAYS TO SHOW CARING

ACTIVITY	STATEMENTS TO USE WITH ACTIVITY
Cover the client with a blanket.	"It feels chilly in here. Perhaps this blanket will help."
Assist the client to dress.	"I noticed you're having a little trouble getting your robe on. Perhaps I can help."
Serve a tray to the client.	"It's time to eat. I hope you're hungry because it really looks good."
Offer assistance.	"Here, let me help you. Perhaps together we can arrange these flowers."
When leaving the room.	"Is there anything more I can do for you before I go?" or "I'm leaving now, but I'll be back in 20 minutes."
Move the client up in bed.	"You look so uncomfortable. Let me move you up in bed."
Make the client's bed.	"Now you have a nice fresh bed."
Regulate environmental temperature.	"It seems very warm in here. Perhaps if I turn the air conditioner up, it will help."
Turn the client in bed.	"Changing position really makes a difference, doesn't it?"
Straighten a pillow.	"Let me straighten your pillow for you."

Adapted from Mental Health Concepts (4th ed.), by C. Waughfield, 1998, Albany, NY: Delmar Publishers.

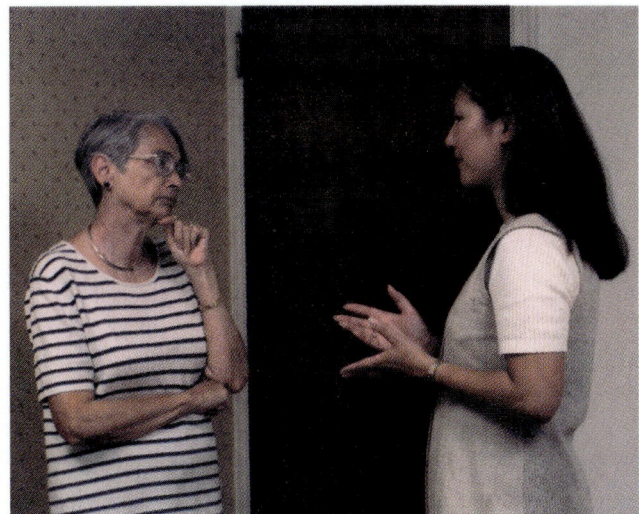

Figure 8-5 Active listening, concentrating on the interaction with the client, enhances communication.

the thoughts and feelings of the client. Sympathy and empathy are not the same. In sympathy, the nurse becomes involved in the feelings and thoughts of the client, which are generally related to a loss.

Acceptance and Respect

Accepting clients as individuals with beliefs and values of their own is an attitude that enhances communication. The nurse must be nonjudgmental, that is, accepting of the client at face value. It is acceptable to privately disagree with the client's values and beliefs, but the nurse must accept that the client has different values and beliefs.

The nurse shows acceptance by not expressing differing values or beliefs and by simply accepting the statements or complaints of clients. Clients may then feel free to communicate and cooperate in their care.

Respect follows acceptance. Accepting clients in a nonjudgmental way leads to understanding them as unique individuals. Acceptance and respect on the part of the nurse let clients know that they can be themselves; they can then feel that they will still receive the best quality care, even though they have different values and beliefs than the nurse. The nurse also shows respect by introducing himself and addressing the client by name (preceded by "Mr.," "Mrs.," or "Ms.").

Techniques of Therapeutic Communication

Certain techniques promote therapeutic communication. These techniques should be learned and incorporated into the nurse's manner of communicating.

Clarifying/validating

Clarifying or validating are used when the nurse is not sure of the meaning of a message. Clarifying is the technique used to understand verbal messages. For example:

"Do you mean . . . ?"

Validating is used to establish truth or accuracy. It is used for nonverbal as well as verbal messages. Examples are as follows:

"Are you saying that you did not get your medication today?"

"You are holding your side. Are you having pain there?"

Open Questions

Open questions encourage clients to express their own thoughts and feelings. *How, when, where,* and *what* are words with which to begin an open question. Open questions cannot typically be answered with "yes" or "no" or with just one or two words. For example:

"How has this medication affected your vision?"

"What did the doctor tell you about going home?"

Indirect Statements

An indirect statement calls for a response from the client. Because it is a statement and not a question, the client does not feel quizzed. Indirect statements allow the client to determine the direction of the conversation, thus helping the client maintain a feeling of independence. Examples of indirect statements are as follows:

"Tell me about your physical therapy today."

"You were telling me about. . . ."

Reflecting

Reflecting is repeating all or part of a message back to the sender. Often, reflecting focuses on feelings and helps the sender "hear" the message from the receiver. This allows the sender a chance to clarify the message and shows that the listener is trying to understand the message. Reflecting can be a very useful technique if not overused. Examples include the following:

Client: "I'm really nervous about my surgery tomorrow. My friend got an infection after her surgery. I'm very frightened."

Nurse: "You are anxious about your surgery and afraid of getting an infection?"

Paraphrasing

Paraphrasing is restating the message in the receiver's own words. This lets the sender know how the receiver interpreted the message. Clarification can then be done if necessary. The sender is aware that the receiver is listening and trying to understand the message. For example:

Nurse: "You are afraid that you might have complications from your surgery?"

Summarizing

Summarizing in a sentence or two the major points of a conversation lets the sender know what was heard. The sender can then add more information or clarify what was originally heard. An example might be as follows:

"Let me see, we have discussed. . . ."

Focusing

Keeping communication focused on the topic being discussed can sometimes be difficult. Clients may wander off to other topics, or the topic may shift to the nurse. It is important to keep the focus on the client and not the nurse. For example the nurse could say:

"We can discuss that in a minute, right now I'd like to discuss. . . ."

"A minute ago you mentioned that you'd had an upset stomach after taking your medication. Tell me more about that."

Silence

Silence is one of the most difficult techniques to use. In the dominant U.S. culture, most people are uncomfortable with silence and feel the urge to fill the gap by saying something. Silence can be a valuable therapeutic technique, however, allowing the client time to gather thoughts or check emotions. Silence also gives the nurse a chance to decide how best to continue the interaction. If the nurse employs behaviors to enhance communication during the silence, the client will often verbalize thoughts or feelings.

Barriers to Communication

Employing behaviors and attitudes to enhance communication will be of little use if the nurse also employs barriers to communication. Although the communication process is sensitive, it should not be threatening. The purpose in learning about those things that block communication is to enable the nurse to identify them and avoid using them. Many mistakes can be corrected when identified. A simple "I'm sorry, I shouldn't have said that" will often take care of the situation. Practice helps sharpen communication skills. The most common barriers are discussed following.

Closed Questions

Questions that can be answered with "yes" or "no" or with only one or two words are considered closed. After the one- or two-word answer, communication is usually ended; there is no other avenue for the communication to follow. This type of question is appropriate in certain circumstances, however, such as when taking a health history or in an emergency. Examples of closed questions are as follows:

PROFESSIONAL TIP

Therapeutic Communication

Practice the techniques of therapeutic communication with family, classmates, friends, and instructors. This may seem artificial and uncomfortable at first; but it will become easier with practice. If you begin using the techniques of therapeutic communication now, you will have incorporated them into your manner of communication by the time you begin clinical experience.

"Is the pain gone?"

"Did you sleep well?"

Clichés

Clichés are overused, trite phrases that are almost meaningless. They are impersonal and often used when individuals are at a loss for anything better to say. They are used without thinking of the impact on the other person, and often seem disrespectful of the client's individual circumstances. Examples include the following:

"Hang in there, tomorrow is another day."

"It could be worse."

False Reassurance

False reassurance is often used in an effort to cheer up the client regardless of the facts, giving false hope about the outcome of a situation. False reassurance can be especially traumatic to a terminally ill client who may be desperate to believe assurances even if they are not founded in reality. An example of false reassurance is as follows:

"Don't worry, I'm sure everything will be fine."

Judgmental Responses

Judgmental responses are based on the nurse's personal value system and imply right or wrong. Such responses allow no room for further discussion. For example:

"You shouldn't feel that way."

Agreeing/Disagreeing or Approving/Disapproving

Whether the nurse is agreeing/approving or disagreeing/disapproving, offering an opinion implies that one belief is right and the other wrong. Clients are thus prevented from sharing their feelings and may feel pressured to express the same values and opinions as the nurse. One example is as follows:

"I wouldn't do it that way."

Giving Advice

Giving advice involves offering personal rather than professional opinion. When the nurse does this, the client's responsibility for making decisions is diminished. Furthermore, some clients may end up feeling unable to make their own choices and may therefore become more dependent on the nurse. One example might be:

"I think you should. . . ."

Stereotyping

Stereotyping occurs when individual differences are ignored and a person is automatically put into a specific category. The stereotype may have either a positive or negative connotation. For example:

"Someone your age shouldn't worry about that."

"Boys aren't supposed to cry."

Belittling

Belittling conveys to a person that his thoughts or feelings really have no value, that it is silly to think or feel a certain way, or that he is no different from other individuals in similar circumstances. Examples include the following:

"Many people have it much worse."

"Yes, everyone feels like that."

Defending

Defending is a response to a feeling of being directly or indirectly threatened. The nurse may make statements in defense of self, another nurse, a doctor, or the health care facility. Defending implies that the client is not permitted to criticize or express feelings. This may be one of the most difficult communication barriers to overcome. No one likes to be criticized or to hear coworkers criticized. A natural first response is to defend why something was said, done, or not done. An example of defending is as follows:

"No one on this unit would say that."

Requesting an Explanation

It can be very intimidating for a client when a nurse asks for an explanation of behaviors, feelings, or thoughts. Often, the client does not know the "why." The usual results are increased anxiety and an end to communication. Examples are as follows:

"Why did you do that?"

"Why do you feel that way?"

PROFESSIONAL TIP

Understanding Communication Barriers
Take measures to become aware of communication barriers. For instance, join a classmate in pointing out the barriers that each of you use, then discuss how you each feel when confronted with these communication barriers.

Changing the Subject

An abrupt change of subject by the nurse generally indicates to the client that the nurse is uncomfortable or anxious about the topic under discussion. It often is used to avoid listening to a client's fear, distress, or problems and is interpreted by the client as a lack of interest.

Client: "I don't think I'll ever get well."

Nurse: "Isn't it a beautiful day?"

PSYCHOSOCIAL ASPECTS OF COMMUNICATION

The psychosocial aspects of communication include: style, gestures, meaning of time, meaning of space, cultural values, and political correctness. These aspects are based on individuality and culture and will influence the nurse–client relationship. It is important to understand these aspects and how they vary in different persons and cultures.

Style

Each person has a style of communication that reflects the personality and self-concept of that person. According to Jack (1997), style can be divided into three common types: passive, aggressive, and assertive. It is important to remember that a person's

PROFESSIONAL TIP

When Clients Block Communication
In instances when clients block communication, keep the following things in mind:

- The client may not wish to discuss the topic introduced by the nurse or may not wish to talk at all. Everyone needs time alone to think.
- Accept and respect the client's desires to not communicate at a particular time.
- Let the client know that you are ready to listen whenever she is ready to talk.

style of communication is learned and reinforced over the years. The fact that communication style is learned indicates it can change.

When a person becomes a client in the health care system, fear and anxiety may change the person's style of communication. Fear and anxiety may cause the client's communication style to become passive or aggressive.

Passive

The person who uses the passive style of communication does not stand up for himself, is not able to share feelings or needs with others, has difficulty asking for help, and feels hurt and angry at others for taking advantage of him. This person uses apologetic words; has a weak, soft voice; makes little eye contact; and is often fidgety. The person with a passive style of communication will often go along with others without expressing a personal desire for an alternate plan of action. The client who has a passive style of communication is generally very compliant, asks for nothing, and gets little attention.

Aggressive

The person who uses the aggressive style of communication puts his own feelings, rights, and needs first and communicates them in a haughty or angry way. The voice is often demanding, and the eyes expressionless. Such a person also has an attitude of superiority, works to control or manipulate others, and shows no concern for anyone else's feelings.

Assertive

The person who uses the assertive style of communication stands up for himself without violating the basic rights of others. He expresses true feelings in an honest, direct manner and does not allow others to take advantage of him. His voice is firm and confident, and he makes appropriate eye contact. Such a person also respects the rights, needs, and feelings of others; takes responsibility for the consequences of his actions; and behaves in a manner that enhances self-respect.

A person using the assertive style of communication effectively lets others know his thoughts, feelings, and needs. He also listens to and acknowledges the other person's thoughts, feelings, and needs. If the thoughts, feelings, or needs of the persons communicating are in conflict, a compromise acceptable to both can usually be worked out.

Gestures

Gestures are movements of the hands and arms. Some gestures are known globally, such as applause to indicate approval. Some gestures, however, have entirely different meanings in various countries. The nurse must be sensitive to cultural variances and exercise good judgment when caring for clients of different backgrounds and heritages.

CULTURAL CONSIDERATIONS

Gestures

The meaning of gestures is not universal. For instances, in many places, a small circle made with the thumb and forefinger means "okay." This is not true in Japan and France, however, where this gesture means "money" and "zero," respectively. And in Brazil and Turkey, this gesture is a symbol for female genitalia and is considered an insult.

Meaning of Time

In the United States, great emphasis is placed on time and schedules. Being on time is very important. Time is precious. The clock tells us what we are to do and where we are to be every hour of the day and night. A person is considered dependable when scheduled appointments are kept.

People of some cultures know a day has passed only because the sun has risen, set, and is rising again. In fact, some cultures do not even have an instrument for telling time. They have different ways of perceiving and dividing time. Scheduling in such cultures may mean "when they get around to doing it."

PROFESSIONAL TIP

Being Assertive

"I" messages—I think . . . , I expect . . . , I feel . . . , I need . . .—are excellent ways to begin practicing assertive communication. Such messages indicate ownership of the thought, feeling, or need—a fact with which no one can argue.

PROFESSIONAL TIP

Time Orientation

Be sensitive to the fact that clients of different cultural backgrounds may value time differently than you do. Do not jump to conclusions that the client who is always late is lazy or inconsiderate of schedules.

Meaning of Space

Edward T. Hall (1959) has for many years studied **proxemics**, the study of space between people and its effect on interpersonal behavior. Hall says that humans, like other animals, are territorial. Some examples of human territoriality include the following: On a beach, people mark territory with a towel or blanket; in waiting rooms, people mark space with a jacket, hat, luggage, or newspaper; in a classroom, students generally sit in the same place and expect others to respect that space.

How close do you like to be to another person? Generally, this distance varies with the person and the situation. Age, gender of those interacting, and cultural values all influence the distance at which one person is comfortable with another person. Hall (1959) categorizes these comfort zones as intimate, personal, social, and public space.

- Intimate—touch to 18 inches; usually limited to family and close friends; necessary when performing most nursing procedures.
- Personal—18 inches to 4 feet; used with friends and coworkers; effective for many nurse–client interactions involving interviewing or data gathering.
- Social—4 to 12 feet; preferred distance with casual acquaintances.
- Public—12 feet or more; generally used with strangers in public places.

The distances associated with the comfort zones vary from person to person. Some people are comfortable being quite close in space to the person with whom they are interacting. Others prefer a greater distance. Nurses must always be aware of the client's comfort level with regard to space (Figure 8-6).

Much of nursing care involves touching the client, yet on admission, the nurse and client generally do not know each other. Thus, in a very short span of time, the nurse moves from the client's public space to the client's intimate space when giving care. Care given competently and professionally will help the client feel comfortable when the nurse occupies the client's intimate space.

Cultural Values

It is important that the nurse be familiar with the cultural values of the people in the nurse's region of employment, especially when those values differ from the values of the dominant culture. For example, optimal health for all is the focus of the dominant U.S. culture. In some cultures, however, health is not a major concern, and little financial or political effort is dedicated to health. Likewise, individualism is stressed in our culture. In many other cultures, however, the social group, not the individual, is the primary focus.

As another example, consider that a number of cultural groups have learned to enjoy what they have and do not feel the need to keep working for some goal or material object. This contrasts with the dominant U.S. culture, where persons must work hard, achieve, and keep busy in order to be considered successful. Finally, in the dominant U.S. culture, cleanliness is closely related to optimal health and is a dominant value. Few cultural groups emphasize cleanliness in the way the U.S. culture does, however. In fact, many have no problem with being dirty, and some even see it as a positive value.

Political Correctness

To be politically correct in communication means to use language that shows sensitivity to those who are different from oneself. It is intended to help eliminate prejudice by avoiding the use of language that offends. Politically correct language is designed to replace terms that suggest inferior status for members of minority groups and terms that exclude women, older people, and those with handicaps. Racist and bigoted language perpetuates prejudice and false ideas and often leads to violence.

Importance to Health Care System

It is important for nurses to understand the psychosocial aspects of communication and be aware of them with regard to individual clients. Communication is more effective when these aspects are taken into consideration.

Effective communication has a positive influence on a client's well-being. Furthermore, clients often judge nurses' competence by their communication skills. Good communication skills also result in increased client satisfaction, and increased client satisfaction leads to increased compliance with the therapeutic regimen.

Communication, then, is a key factor in the client's perception and evaluation of the health care services provided.

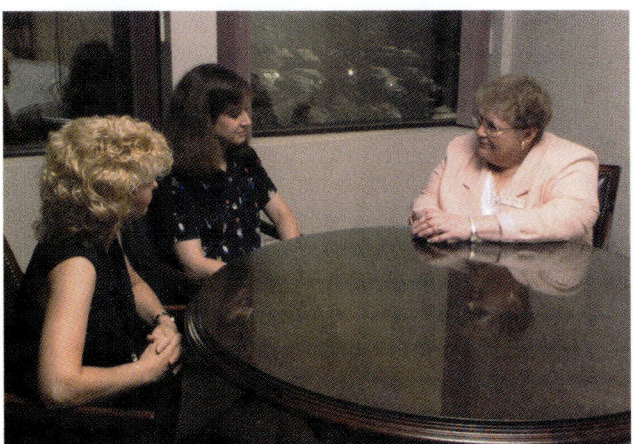

Figure 8-6 A distance of up to 4 feet is appropriate for interviewing and data gathering.

NURSE–CLIENT COMMUNICATION

One of the most important aspects of nursing care is communication. Whether the nurse is gathering admission information, taking a health history, teaching, or implementing care, good communication skills are essential.

Nurses have both an ethical and moral responsibility to use any information gathered from the client in the client's best interest. Information that affects the health status or care of the client should be shared with other members of the health care team. All information concerning a client is confidential and should never be discussed in elevators, the cafeteria, the hallways, or other public places outside the health care facility.

Formal/Informal Communication

Formal communication is purposeful and is employed in a structured situation such as information gathering on admission or scheduled teaching sessions (Figure 8-7). Specific items are covered in a planned sequence. In this way, more information can be given or received in the shortest amount of time.

Informal communication does not follow a structured approach, though it often reveals information that is pertinent to the client's care. For instance, a client may comment that the tape holding her bandage in place is irritating to her skin. This would lead the nurse to assess the wound area and take action to correct the problem. This interaction, although not planned or structured, was nonetheless helpful in ensuring quality nursing care.

Social Communication

Social communication is the everyday conversations held with family, friends, and acquaintances. Topics are generally those of interest to both parties and reflect the social relationship of those involved. Both parties share information, thoughts, and feelings. When getting acquainted with clients, social communication provides a way to learn about each other and to begin a nurse–client relationship.

Although social communication is not considered therapeutic communication, it is part of nurse–client communication. Because it is nonthreatening, social communication puts the client at ease; it also allows the nurse to get to know the client and what is important to the client. Clients often interpret social communication as expressions of caring on the part of the nurse—that is, the nurse cares enough about the client to spend some time communicating on a person-to-person level rather than on a nurse-to-client level.

Interactions

Nurse–client interactions and relationships progress through three phases. The amount of time spent on each phase depends on the purpose of the interaction.

Introduction Phase

The beginning of any interaction is usually fairly short. The client is greeted by name, and the nurse introduces himself and defines his role. Expectations of the interaction are clarified, and mutual goals are set. A good format might be:

"Good morning, Mrs. Jamal. My name is Paul Farrell. I am a student practical (vocational) nurse and I will be caring for you today and tomorrow. I would like to teach you some breathing and coughing exercises that you will be asked to do after your surgery tomorrow."

Working Phase

The working phase generally constitutes the major portion of any interaction. It is used to accomplish the goal or objective defined in the introduction. The nurse should always ask for feedback to ensure understanding on the part of the client. In the previously presented scenario, the client's demonstrating the breathing and coughing exercises and verbalizing why the exercises are necessary would indicate understanding.

Termination Phase

The final phase of any interaction is the termination phase. Seldom do nurses have unlimited time to spend with one client, and there are several ways for the nurse to indicate the end of an interaction. The nurse may ask whether the client has any questions about the topic discussed. Summarizing the topic is another good way for the nurse to indicate closure.

Factors Affecting Nurse–Client Communication

As mentioned previously, factors such as age, education, emotions, culture, language, attention, and surroundings, affect both parties in a communication. In

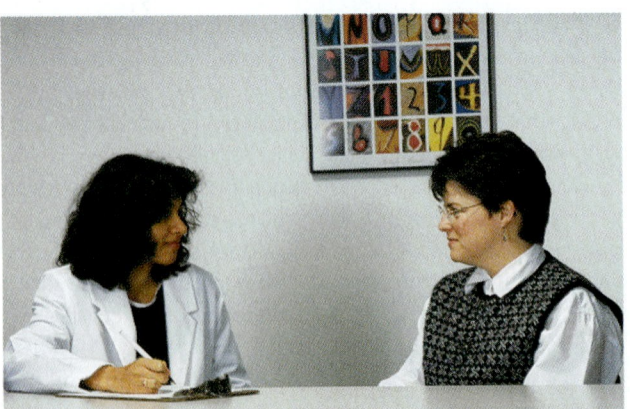

Figure 8-7 Formal Interaction, Admission Interview

nurse–client communications, additional factors relating to both the nurse and client also come into play. The nurse must be sensitive to these factors and to personal biases in order to provide appropriate nursing care.

Nurse

Many personal factors pertaining to the nurse can influence nurse–client communication. Past experiences as a nurse, state of health, home situation, workload, and staff relations can all impact the thinking, concentration, attitude, and emotions of the nurse. These in turn influence how the nurse sends and receives messages. Self-awareness is very important for the nurse when communicating.

Client

Factors related to the client that must be considered include: social factors, religion, family situation, visual ability, hearing ability, speech ability, level of consciousness, language proficiency, and state of illness.

Social Factors Some health concerns are easy to discuss because they are socially acceptable, such as having the gallbladder or appendix removed or having the flu. It may be more difficult, however, to communicate with a woman who is having a breast removed. The symbolic meaning of the breast may make its removal hard for the client to accept and may influence how she relates to others. A person with a sexually transmitted disease or one who is HIV positive may be very reluctant to discuss any aspect of the illness.

Religion Members of some religions seek healing through faith and not through conventional medical services. Others will not receive blood transfusions when an accident or disaster places these individuals in the health care system. When religious beliefs conflict with those of the health care team, communication can be difficult.

A client may have a priest, minister, or rabbi visit. Privacy for such visits should be provided if at all possible.

Family Situation Illness often unites family members around the client. If the family has not been close to or supportive of the client before the illness, communication between the family and client may be strained. Such stress may be noticed in the course of nurse–client interactions. If so, the nurse must be careful not to discuss aspects of the client's condition or treatment in front of family members. In fact, it is best to ask family members to step out of the room when any nursing care is being given. This applies whether assessing the client, providing physical care, or gathering information. The client's right to privacy and confidentiality is thus maintained.

Sometimes the client expresses a desire for a specific person to remain in the room. Unless contraindicated, this is usually allowed.

Visual Ability Communicating with clients who are visually impaired may not seem to be a challenge at first. However, because the nonverbal part of any message, such as facial expressions, gestures, and other body language, is missed, an important part of every message is lost to the client.

Persons who are visually impaired generally speak only when spoken to. Their speech may be loud if they are not sure where the other person is. Silence makes them uncomfortable if they are not sure of another person's presence in the room.

LIFE CYCLE CONSIDERATIONS

Nurse–Client Communication

Children

- Assess the child's level of language development.
- Talk directly to the child unless the child is an infant or very young, in which case communicate through the parents.
- Be especially aware of your nonverbal messages; children are very perceptive with regard to nonverbal communication.
- Communicate at eye level with the child.
- Use simple, direct language.
- Be honest and explain what is going to happen.

Elderly

- Assess for sensory disturbances.
- Face the client when speaking.
- Have patience, response may be slow.
- Show respect and be considerate of the older client's personal dignity.

PROFESSIONAL TIP

Caring for the Client Who Is Visually Impaired

- Look directly at the client when speaking.
- Use a normal tone and volume of voice.
- Advise the client when you are entering or leaving the room.
- Orient the person to the immediate environment; use clock hours to indicate positions of items in relation to the client.
- Ask for permission before touching the client.

Adapted from Health Assessment & Physical Examination, *by M. E. Z. Estes, 1998, Albany, NY: Delmar Publishers. Copyright 1998 by Delmar Publishers. Adapted with permission.*

The nurse must include an explanation of "hospital sounds" when orienting a new client who cannot see. The room must be described in detail and the client guided around the room if possible. It is important for nurses to always speak and identify themselves when entering the room. As with any client, all procedures should be explained. Each step of the procedure as well as any touching should be described before it is initiated. As with any client, the nurse should always inform the client who is visually impaired before touching so as not to startle him.

Hearing Ability Many persons who are hearing impaired can communicate by sign language, but few hearing persons can understand or use sign language. If the person who is hearing impaired is able to read, writing may be the easiest method of communication. Many persons who are hearing impaired have learned, at least to some degree, to speechread, formerly known as lipread. Communicating with a client who is hearing impaired requires time and patience.

The nurse should face the client and speak slowly and deliberately using slightly exaggerated word formation. Gesturing can also be very effective. Check to see whether the client has a hearing aid and, if so, encourage its use during the communication.

The frustration of trying to communicate can make the client who is hearing impaired stubborn or even hostile. Such frustration generally stems more from trying to understand others rather than from trying to be understood. Touching the client's arm when entering the room lets the client know that someone is there and helps prevent feelings of paranoia.

PROFESSIONAL TIP

Caring for the Client Who Is Hearing Impaired

- Check to see whether the client wears a hearing aid. Be sure it is in working order and turned on.
- Make every effort to move the client to a setting with minimal background noise.
- Always face the client.
- Speak in a normal tone and at a normal pace.
- Determine whether the client uses sign language. If signing is used, enlist the assistance of an interpreter.
- Pay particular attention to nonverbal cues of the client and to your own nonverbal behavior.
- Provide a pen and paper to facilitate communication, if necessary.

Adapted from Health Assessment & Physical Examination, *by M. E. Z. Estes, 1998, Albany, NY: Delmar Publishers. Copyright 1998 by Delmar Publishers. Adapted with permission.*

Speech Ability **Dysphasia**, the impairment of speech, and **aphasia**, the absence of speech, both can result from a brain lesion, although they are most commonly seen as the result of a stroke. Other neurological diseases such as Parkinson's disease may also cause dysphasia. A dysfunction of the muscles used for speech is termed **dysarthria**, which makes a person's speech difficult, slow, and hard to understand. Dysphasia, aphasia, and dysarthria create communication problems.

The person with dysphasia has difficulty both putting thoughts and feelings into words and sending messages. It should be noted, however, that seldom does the person with dysphasia have difficulty receiving and interpreting messages; thus, explanations should be given before doing anything. If the client can write, a magic slate or paper and pencil can be used for communication. A picture board, word board, or letter board may also be employed, as can a computer, assuming that one is available and that the client is able to use a computer. A person with any of these speech impairments may feel frustrated and helpless. Establishing some method of communication for the client provides hope and maintains self-esteem while at the same time minimizing or preventing feelings of depression, anger, and hostility.

Level of Consciousness True communication cannot be accomplished with unconscious or comatose clients. It should be remembered, however, that unconscious or comatose clients can hear even though they cannot respond. Caregivers should speak to these clients just as they would to alert clients. Always greet the client by name, identify yourself, and explain why you are in the room (i.e., what you are going to do). Then let the client know when you are leaving and, if possible, when you will return. Although one-sided, this interaction is important to the client.

Language Proficiency The client's ability to communicate effectively through the spoken language also influences the nurse–client interaction. Clients who do not speak English are generally from another culture. It is important to learn about the other culture, especially about the values and beliefs. Doing so will help prevent the nurse from violating those values and beliefs.

If a family member speaks English, that person could be used as an interpreter, as shown in Figure 8-8. Sometimes another health care worker on the nursing unit may speak the same language as does the client. As long as it does not interfere with his or her work, this person could also be used as an interpreter.

Pictures or a two-language dictionary are often helpful. If the other language is prevalent in the community, the nurse should learn some phrases in the language that are useful in client assessment and in care. Remember, gestures and other nonverbal communication send messages without the use of language.

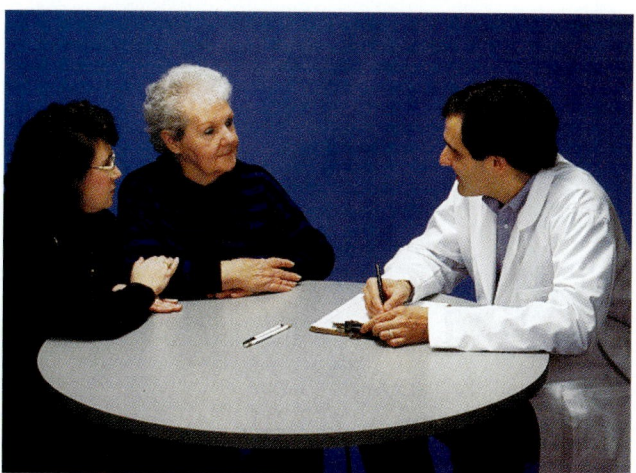

Figure 8-8 A family member interprets communications with non-English speaking client.

Stage of Illness The stage of a client's illness may influence the client's desire to communicate with the nurse. Clients in the early stages of illness may be eager to learn all they can about the illness or may express anger and resentment at their current state of health.

Terminally ill clients may pose special challenges for the nurse. Most terminally ill clients know they are dying and are concerned about those whom they love. It is thus important for the nurse to have the client identify those persons the client considers to be "family." Family and nurses often struggle with the proper way to speak with those who are dying; no one can escape death, but many people do not want to discuss it. Death is often considered a defeat by health care workers and therefore is not a prime subject for discussion. It is important to remember that listening and silence are both part of communication.

Anytime a client initiates a conversation regarding death the nurse must be willing to participate. Too often nurses hesitate to communicate with the terminally ill for fear of saying the wrong thing. When the client wants to talk, a good listener is needed. Let the client guide the conversation. Try not to give advice, just listen and accept what the client says. This may be very difficult to do.

CULTURAL CONSIDERATIONS

Family Interaction Patterns
- In some families the male members make all the decisions.
- In some families, decisions are made jointly, with all members (or all adults) participating.
- In some families, unrelated persons such as godparents or special friends are involved in decision making.

The nurse and the family must work together to understand the ways that the terminally ill client communicates. It can take persistence and insight to identify and decipher some messages. "Listening" to the client's gestures and facial expressions helps facilitate understanding of messages.

COMMUNICATING WITH THE HEALTH CARE TEAM

Providing care to clients is a team effort. For the team to work efficiently and effectively and to provide continuous quality care to clients, effective communication is necessary. This communication may be oral or written, individual or group, or even on computer.

PROFESSIONAL TIP

Objectivity
The nurse must remain objective and nonjudgmental when the client's idea of family is different from the nurse's idea of family.

Oral Communication

Oral communication among the health care team is necessary for the appropriate planned care of the client and for the efficient and effective functioning of the nursing unit. In order to provide continuity of care, all persons who provide direct care to clients must communicate orally with each other concerning that care.

Nurse–Nurse

Nurse–nurse communications can be either peer–peer or superior–subordinate communication. Peer–peer communication takes place many times every day. If each nurse uses effective communication with peers as well as clients, the unit will run more efficiently, and client care will be more effective. Superior–subordinate communication often directs the client care to be performed by the subordinate. The way whereby this communication is handled affects both the attitude of the subordinate and the client care given.

Nurse–Nursing Assistant

The nurse is responsible for informing the nursing assistants of their duties. Taking time to answer questions and providing reasons for specific activities requested helps establish a relationship of trust and mutual respect.

An experienced nursing assistant can be of considerable assistance to the new graduate (whether an RN or LP/VN). Nursing assistants are often much more comfortable and confident in providing bedside care.

Given that they also often have creative solutions to problems, they should be included in planning care.

Nurse–Student Nurse

Student nurses must communicate not only with the clinical instructor but also with the staff nurses. How well the staff nurses interact with student nurses depends on how the staff nurses were treated as students and on the experiences the staff nurses have had with other student nurses. Student nurses are involved in the clinical facility for specific learning experiences selected by the instructor and related to classroom topics. They must have time to review client records, observe others performing procedures, and communicate with and care for their clients. Students are limited in their nursing activities depending on how far they have progressed through the nursing curriculum. Because staff nurses retain responsibility for the care of clients even when clients are assigned to students, communication between student nurses and staff nurses is essential. Generally, a complementary relationship develops between nursing students and staff nurses.

Nurse–Physician

Nursing education and expertise have evolved over the years to a professional level. Nurses are responsible for their own actions even when under the direction of a physician.

When the term *nursing diagnosis* was introduced, many physicians had difficulty understanding how nurses could make a diagnosis. Whereas medical diagnoses focus on disease conditions, nursing diagnoses focus on human needs. Nurses must communicate openly and honestly with physicians, demonstrating their competence in assessments, nursing skills, and provision of quality care.

Nurse–Other Health Professionals

Communication with professionals in other departments should always be on a peer basis. Clarification of goals for each client and of ways to meet those goals should be the focus of communication. Listening to those in other departments and establishing mutual respect for each other's area of expertise provides the client with top quality care.

Group Communication

Client care conferences may be scheduled regularly or whenever the need arises. Some conferences may be solely for the staff of a particular nursing unit; others may include members of other departments. In either case, only those persons directly involved with the care of the client should be invited (Figure 8-9).

The conference leader should establish the objectives of the conference and make all necessary arrangements. A conference room or other private

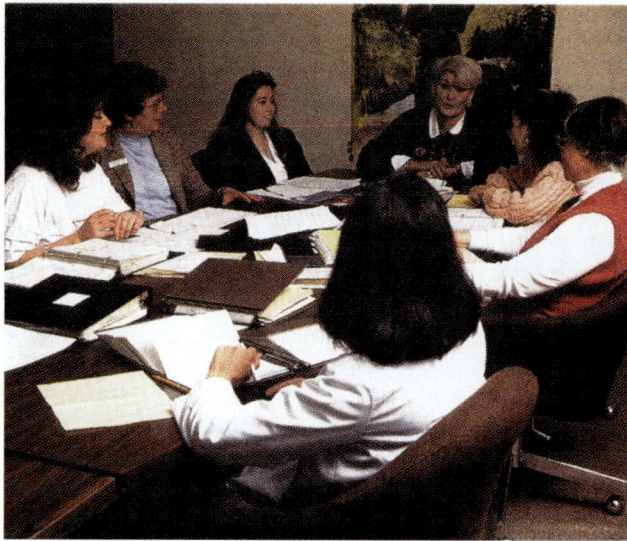

Figure 8-9 Nurses work together to plan client care.

place should be used as a meeting site. One person should be designated to record the discussion. If the conference is about a specific client, only facts should be documented on the client's chart. If the topic is general and not related to a specific client, only a record of the discussion is needed.

Telephone

When a student nurse is the only person available to answer a telephone call, the call should be answered with the name of the department or floor and the student's full name and position (i.e., student nurse). The caller should then be informed that an appropriate person will be found to take the call. If a message must be taken, the student nurse should write it down and read it back to the caller and ask for the caller's name and for the caller to spell out his or her name. The nurse must never give out any information about clients.

Written Communication

Most written communication relates to the client's chart. All aspects of a client's care are recorded on that client's chart.

Requisitions to x-ray or to physical or respiratory therapy and requests for laboratory services for a client are all forms of written communication. The reports resulting from these requests become a part of the client's chart.

One type of written communication not pertaining to a specific client is the interdepartmental memo requesting equipment, supplies, maintenance, or housekeeping. Such documents are necessary to keep the nursing unit functioning efficiently and effectively.

Electronic Communication

Computers are being used extensively in the business offices of health care agencies and have been so for years. The introduction of computers into the departments of direct client care has been slower, however. Nonetheless, in many places, computers are used by client care departments to send requisitions to other departments and to receive test results. Some hospital pharmacies use computer programs that show safe dosages and drug interactions. There are also programs to aid physicians in diagnosing and treating some conditions. With the expanding use of computers in health care and the corresponding potential for increased use, it is important for all health care workers to have some knowledge about computers.

Although the computerized patient record (CPR) as envisioned by the Institute of Medicine (IOM) is not yet available in the United States, parts of the CPR have been implemented. The IOM defines the CPR as an "electronic record that resides in a system specifically designed to support users through availability of complete and accurate data, practitioner reminders and alerts, clinical decision support systems, links to bodies of medical knowledge and other aids." This moves the client record from simply tracking client care to serving as a resource for health care delivery (Brandt, 1995).

Before there is widespread use of the CPR, many questions must be be answered, including: How can changes to the data entered be prevented? How will charting errors be corrected? What happens when the computers are down? How will security be maintained? What are the legal implications of electronic or digital signatures? According to Rhodes (1995), all client records must be confidential, accurate, secure, and protected from unauthorized access and disclosure, regardless of the form.

Telemedicine

The Telemedicine Research Center (1997) defines **telemedicine**, also called telehealth, as the use of communications technology to transmit health information from one location to another. Included is the transmission of radiographic (teleradiology) and pathologic (telepathology) images, telemetry, and telephone triage.

The use of two-way video allows the client and health care provider to see, hear, and talk to each other. A stethoscope or otoscope (called peripherals)

HOME HEALTH CARE

Use of Telemedicine

- From the office, a home health nurse can watch a client at home change a dressing or self-administer insulin.
- During a video consult, a home health nurse might assist by manipulating the peripherals or actually performing a physical assessment.

PROFESSIONAL TIP

Telemedicine Confidentiality

- Avoid sending or receiving client data by e-mail unless the computer has encryption capabilities.
- During a two-way video consultation, inform the client of any other people who are present in the room, but off camera. Try to ensure that only those persons who must know about the client's condition are present (Granade, 1997).

can be included in the hookup so that the sounds and visual images can be transmitted (Granade, 1997). This allows physician specialists in large medical centers to examine a client many miles away.

California and Arizona have both passed legislation requiring providers to obtain written and verbal informed consent before providing any nonemergency care via telemedicine. Oklahoma is also considering such legislation (Granade, 1997).

Nurses should document all activities, assessment findings, information provided by the client, and any instructions given to the client. All data transmissions (e.g., telemetry printouts or videotapes) should be stored in the client's record. Most telemedicine laws require that existing confidentiality rules be maintained.

COMMUNICATING WITH YOURSELF

Whether they admit it or not, people talk to themselves every day. Oftentimes, such communication takes the form of thoughts rather than spoken words. What people say to themselves influences their personalities and, therefore, how they interact with others. Sherman (1994) describes self-talk as positive or negative.

Positive Self-Talk

Practicing positive self-talk is the key to positive self-esteem. Send positive thoughts to yourself about yourself. Better yet, say the thoughts out loud. Thinking, saying, and hearing positive statements about oneself reinforces positive self-esteem. Remind yourself of your good attributes and accomplishments. When you have had a difficult day, whether in the classroom or clinical area, pat yourself on the back for what you did accomplish. Each day verbally tell yourself what you learned or what good care you gave to your client(s).

Positive self-talk reinforces the desire to succeed. Memories of successes can serve as positive influences, especially when things are not going well and frustration sets in.

CASE STUDY

Martha, a 25-year-old Mexican American female, is admitted for severe abdominal pain. Martha clings to her mother's arm when the nurse asks the mother to leave the room during the admission procedure. The mother asks to stay in the room. The nurse looks at Martha, who smiles but says nothing.

Consider the following:

1. What do you think may be causing Martha to cling to her mother?

2. What can the nurse do to communicate with Martha?

3. What subjective and objective data should the nurse gather?

Positive affirmation is a positive thought or idea on which a person consciously focuses to produce a desired result. Positive affirmation can be used to change negative inner messages to positive messages. Instead of saying, "I don't know if I can pass this test," for instance, say, "I know I can pass this test." Of course, positive affirmation is not a substitute for studying and preparing for the test. Positive affirmation merely serves to modify your attitude about the test—or about any other situation.

Negative Self-Talk

Whenever you say to yourself, "I can't do . . . ," you are decreasing your self-esteem with the negative self-talk. Negative self-talk may originate within you, or you may be replaying things that others have said about you. Negative self-talk is self-destructive. Your self-image is lowered by your own criticism, and you begin to see yourself as a failure.

SUMMARY

- Communication is influenced by age, education, emotions, culture, language, attention, and surroundings.
- Nonverbal messages are generally more accurate in communicating a person's feelings.
- Verbal and nonverbal messages must be congruent for clear communication to take place.
- Techniques of therapeutic communication should be practiced and incorporated into the nurse's communication.
- Barriers to communication should be identified and avoided when communicating.
- People have four comfort zones of closeness: intimate, personal, social, and public.
- Therapeutic communication is purposeful and goal directed.
- Psychosocial aspects of communication may aid or hinder communication.

- Almost every nurse–client interaction should involve therapeutic communication.
- Nurse–client communication is influenced by both the nurse and the client.
- The nurse is often a role model for the family in terms of communicating with the terminally ill client.
- Accurate communication among the health care team is necessary for continuity of care.

Review Questions

1. Mr. George is looking out the window, with his back to the door. A nurse opens the door and says, "You will not be able to eat or drink after supper because of tests tomorrow." Then the nurse leaves. Did communication take place?

a. No; there was no feedback.
b. No; there was no eye contact.
c. Yes; Mr. George had to hear the message.
d. Yes; there was a sender, receiver, and message.

2. What is the best way to communicate?

a. Verbally.
b. Nonverbally.
c. It depends on what the message is.
d. Verbally and nonverbally together.

3. Initial client assessment related to communication would include:

a. vital signs.
b. visual ability.
c. ambulatory ability.
d. complete health history.

4. When performing a nursing procedure on a client, the nurse should:

a. only listen to what the client says.
b. be aware of her own nonverbal messages.
c. always have someone witness the procedure.
d. tell the client how fortunate he is to be the nurse's client.

5. The nurse is aware that most nursing procedures are performed in which spatial comfort zone?

   a. Public
   b. Social
   c. Personal
   d. Intimate

6. Which of the following are all examples of verbal communication?

   a. Singing, dancing, smiling
   b. Reading, writing, listening
   c. Shaking hands, reading, grimacing
   d. Whispering, making eye contact, answering

7. When a client says, "I'm not sure how I'll handle all this;" which response of the nurse represents clarification?

   a. "Handle all this?"
   b. "Well, you can ask your sister to help."
   c. "Oh, you'll be able to handle things. You're an intelligent person."
   d. "I'm not sure I understand what it is you're concerned about being able to handle."

8. The statement "I'm sure you'll feel much, much better after your surgery" is an example of:

   a. advice.
   b. false reassurance.
   c. a judgment.
   d. excessive emotionalism.

9. That phase of an interview during which goals and objectives are identified is called the:

   a. working phase.
   b. interview phase.
   c. termination phase.
   d. introduction phase.

10. The most effective technique the nurse can use to facilitate communication is:

    a. giving.
    b. focusing.
    c. listening.
    d. questioning.

11. Which of the following represents the best way for a nurse to show caring?

    a. Constantly staying with the client
    b. Doing everything for the client
    c. Assisting the client in learning self-care
    d. Relaying to the physician everything the client says

12. A terminally ill client denies there is anything wrong and talks constantly about going back to work. The nurse should:

    a. listen but not comment.
    b. acknowledge the client's hopes and wishes.
    c. advise the client that it will be impossible to return to work.
    d. assist the client in planning when to return to work.

13. The nurse uses therapeutic communication with the client to:

    a. cure the client of fear.
    b. discuss personal problems.
    c. obtain or provide information.
    d. relieve the client of all concerns.

14. The nurse is aware that communication among members of the health care team is necessary because it:

    a. provides for continuity of care.
    b. identifies who provides better care.
    c. allows team members to become friends.
    d. promotes competition between departments.

15. Mrs. Banc tells the nurse that she would rather die than have radiation. To whom should the nurse report this communication?

    a. The physician only.
    b. Everyone on the nursing unit.
    c. The physician and charge nurse.
    d. No one; the communication is confidential.

Critical Thinking Questions

1. How can you communicate with an unconscious adult?

2. Which barriers to communication do you use? How can you change?

WEB FLASH!

- Search for information on the Web about the Telemedicine Research Center. What are the latest reports?
- How much information about telemedicine is available on the Internet?
- To what sites can a client go to find out about telemedicine?

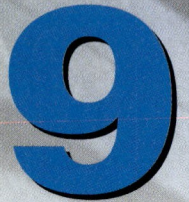

CHAPTER 9

NURSING PROCESS

MAKING THE CONNECTION

Refer to the following chapters to increase your understanding of the nursing process:

- **Chapter 1, Holistic Care**
- **Chapter 8, Communication**
- **Chapter 10, Documentation**
- **Chapter 25, Assessment**
- **Chapter 57, Leadership/Work Transition**

LEARNING OBJECTIVES

Upon completion of this chapter, you should be able to:
- *Define key terms.*
- *Describe the components of the assessment step of the nursing process.*
- *Describe the four types of nursing diagnoses.*
- *List the tasks involved in the planning and outcome identification step of the nursing process.*
- *Discuss the types of skills that nurses must possess in order to perform the nursing interventions during the implementation step of the nursing process.*
- *Identify factors that may influence evaluation.*
- *Explain the way that critical thinking is related to the nursing process.*
- *Relate the nursing process to the problem-solving method.*
- *Describe the nursing process as a tool for promoting multidisciplinary collaboration.*

KEY TERMS

actual nursing
  diagnosis
analysis
assessment
assessment model
assumptions
bias
comprehensive
  assessment
critical pathways
data clustering
defining characteristics
delegation
dependent nursing
  interventions
discharge planning
etiology
evaluation
expected outcome
focused assessment
goal
health history
implementation
independent nursing
  interventions
initial planning
interdependent
  nursing interventions
long-term goal
medical diagnosis
nursing audit
nursing care plan
nursing diagnosis
nursing intervention
nursing process
objective data
ongoing assessment
ongoing planning
planning
primary source
process
protocol
risk nursing diagnosis
secondary source
short-term goal
specific order
standing order
subjective data
synthesis
wellness nursing
  diagnosis

INTRODUCTION

The nursing process is a systematic method of providing care to clients. Use of the nursing process allows nurses to communicate their roles in planning and executing client-centered activities to clients, their families, and other health care professionals. It is a process that encourages orderly thought, analysis, and planning when working with clients to decide those things that need to be done. The nursing process consists of five steps: assessment, diagnosis, planning and outcome identification, implementation, and evaluation.

This chapter presents information about both the historical development of the nursing process and the elements that compose each step of the process. A discussion on the way the nurse uses critical thinking in each step of the nursing process is included. The relationship of the nursing process to problem solving, decision making, and collaboration is also discussed.

HISTORICAL PERSPECTIVE

Lydia Hall first referred to nursing as a "process" in a 1955 journal article, yet the term *nursing process* was not widely used until the late 1960s (Edelman & Mandle, 1998). Referring to the nursing process as a series of steps, Johnson (1959), Orlando (1961), and Wiedenbach (1963) further developed this description of nursing. At that time, the nursing process involved only three steps: assessment, planning, and evaluation. In their 1967 book *The Nursing Process,* Yura and Walsh identified four steps in the nursing process:

- Assessing
- Planning
- Implementing
- Evaluating

Fry (1953) first used the term *nursing diagnosis,* but it was not until 1974, after the first meeting of the group now called the North American Nursing Diagnosis Association (NANDA), that nursing diagnosis was added as a separate and distinct step in the nursing process. Prior to this, nursing diagnosis had been included as a natural conclusion to the first step, assessment. Currently, the steps in the nursing process are:

- Assessment
- Diagnosis
- Planning and outcome identification
- Implementation
- Evaluation

OVERVIEW OF THE NURSING PROCESS

A **process** is a series of steps or acts that lead to accomplishment of some goal or purpose. According to Bevis, "processes have three characteristics: (1) inherent purpose, (2) internal organization, and (3) infinite creativity" (1989). These characteristics can be applied to the nursing process. The **nursing process** is a systematic method of providing care to clients. The purpose is to provide client care that is individualized, holistic, effective, and efficient. Although the steps of the nursing process build on each other, they are not linear. Each step overlaps with the previous and subsequent steps (Figure 9–1).

The nursing process is dynamic and requires creativity in its application. Although the steps remain the same in each client situation, the application and results will differ. The nursing process is designed to be used with clients throughout the life span and in any care setting. It is also a basic organizing system for the National Council Licensure Examination for both practical/vocational nurses (NCLEX-PN) and registered nurses (NCLEX-RN).

Assessment

Assessment is the first step in the nursing process and includes systematic collection, verification, organization, interpretation, and documentation of data. It is a very important step because the completeness and correctness of the information obtained in this step are directly related to the accuracy of the steps that follow. Assessment involves several steps:

- Collecting data from a variety of sources
- Validating the data
- Organizing the data
- Interpreting the data
- Documenting the data

Purpose of Assessment

The purpose of assessment is to establish a database concerning a client's physical, psychosocial, and emotional health in order to identify health-promoting behaviors as well as actual and/or potential health problems. Through assessment, the nurse ascertains the client's functional abilities and the absence or presence of dysfunction. The client's normal activities of daily living and lifestyle patterns are also assessed. Identification of the client's strengths provides the nurse and other members of the treatment team information about the skills, abilities, and behaviors the client has available to promote the treatment and recovery process. The assessment phase also offers an opportunity for the nurse to form a therapeutic interpersonal relationship with the client. During assess-

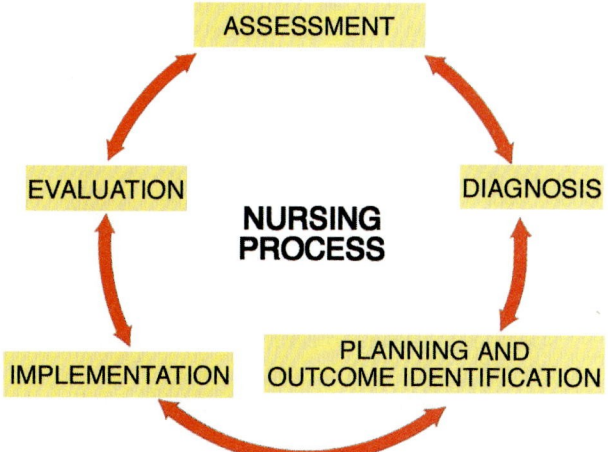

Figure 9–1 Components of the Nursing Process *(From Fundamentals of Nursing: Standards & Practice, by S. DeLaune and P. Ladner, 1998, Albany, NY: Delmar Publishers. Copyright 1998 by Delmar Publishers. Reprinted with permission.)*

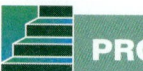

PROFESSIONAL TIP

The Nursing Process
- Rather than being linear, the nursing process involves overlapping steps.
- The steps are explained one after the other for ease of understanding, but in actual practice, there may not be a definite beginning or ending to each step.
- Work in one step may begin before work in the preceding step is completed.

ment, the client is provided an opportunity to discuss health care concerns and goals with the nurse.

Types of Assessment

The type and scope of information needed for assessment are usually determined by the health care setting and needs of the client. Three types of assessment are comprehensive, focused, and ongoing. Although a comprehensive assessment is most desirable in initially determining a client's need for nursing care, time limitations or special circumstances may dictate the need for abbreviated data collection, as represented by the focused assessment. The assessment database can then be expanded after the initial focused assessment, and data should be updated through ongoing assessment.

Comprehensive Assessment A **comprehensive assessment** provides baseline client data including a complete health history and current needs assessment. It is usually completed upon admission to a health care agency. This database provides a baseline against which changes in the client's health status can be measured and should include assessment of physical and psychosocial aspects of the client's health; the client's perception of health; the presence of health risk factors; and the client's coping patterns.

HOME HEALTH CARE

Ongoing Assessment
- In the home, ongoing assessment may involve specific questions to elicit specific information.
- Clients are more comfortable and feel in charge in their own homes as opposed to a health care facility.
- The client may have a tendency to spend a lot of time telling stories about past medical problems and treatment, as opposed to providing information relevant to the situation at hand (Humphrey, 1998).

Focused Assessment A **focused assessment** is an assessment that is limited in scope in order to focus on a particular need or health care concern or on potential health care risks. Focused assessments are not as detailed as comprehensive assessments and are often used in health care agencies where short stays are anticipated (e.g., outpatient surgery centers and emergency departments), in specialty areas such as labor and delivery, in mental health settings, or for the purpose of screening for specific problems or risk factors (e.g., well-child clinics).

Ongoing Assessment Systematic follow-up is required when problems are identified during a comprehensive or focused assessment. An **ongoing assessment** is an assessment that includes systematic monitoring and observation related to specific problems. This type of assessment allows the nurse to broaden the database or to confirm the validity of the data obtained during the initial assessment. Ongoing assessment is particularly important when problems have been identified and a plan of care has been implemented to address these problems. Systematic monitoring and observation allow the nurse to determine the response to nursing interventions and to identify any emerging problems.

Sources of Data

Although data are collected from a variety of sources, the client should be considered the **primary source** of data (the major provider of information about a client). As much information as possible should be gathered from the client, using both interview techniques and physical examination skills. Sources of data other than the client are considered **secondary sources** and include family members, other health care providers, and medical records.

Types of Data

Two types of information are collected through assessment: subjective and objective. **Subjective data** are data from the client's (sometimes family's) point of view and include feelings, perceptions, and concerns. The primary method of collecting subjective data (also called symptoms) is the interview. The **health history**, a review of the client's functional health patterns prior to the current contact with the health care agency, provides much of the subjective data.

PROFESSIONAL TIP

Clients Who Were Adopted
Keep in mind that clients who were adopted will have varying degrees of knowledge about their biological parents. Sensitivity to this issue is critical in gaining client trust during the interview process.

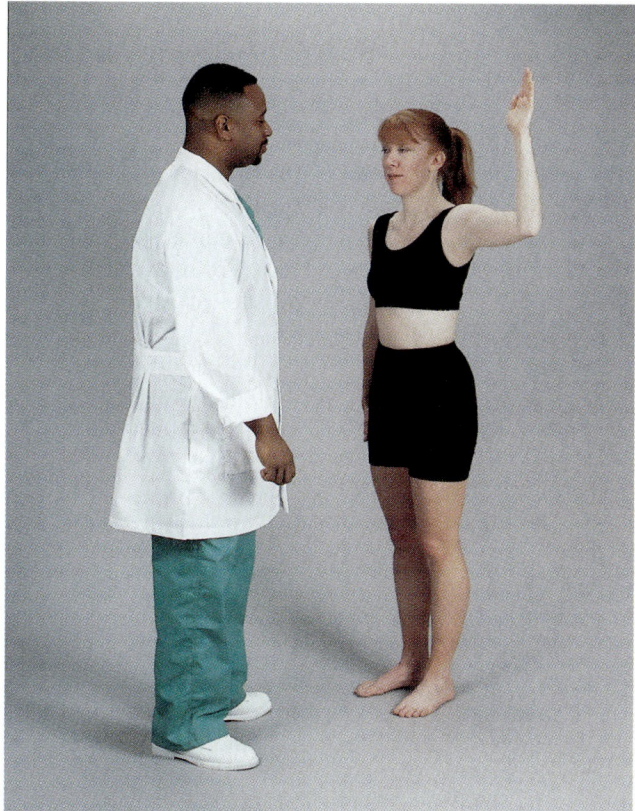

Figure 9–2 The nurse is gathering objective data through assessment of the client's ability to perform range-of-motion (ROM) activity.

Table 9–1 TYPES OF DATA

DATA

A client, age 47, has come to the clinic after "passing out" twice in the last 2 days. She tells the nurse that she becomes "lightheaded" after almost any type of activity. She has experienced some nausea since yesterday and vomited after eating breakfast this morning. She also tells the nurse that she is very nervous about these occurrences because she remembers her mother having similar symptoms when the mother suffered from a brain disorder. The nurse observes that the client's gait is unsteady and skin pale. The client also has large bruises on her right arm and on the right side of her face, which she states occurred when she fell.

TYPE OF DATA

Subjective	Objective
Report of fainting	Vomiting
Complaint of dizziness	Unsteady gait
Nausea	Pale skin
Verbalization of anxiety	Bruises on right side of face
Self-reported fall	and right arm

From Fundamentals of Nursing: Standards & Practice, *by S. DeLaune and P. Ladner, 1998, Albany, NY: Delmar Publishers. Copyright 1998 by Delmar Publishers. Reprinted with permission.*

Objective data (also called signs) are observable and measurable data that are obtained through both standard assessment techniques performed during the physical examination (Figure 9–2) and the results of laboratory and diagnostic testing. Table 9–1 provides examples of both types of data.

Validating the Data

Objective data may add to or validate subjective data. A critical step in data collection, validation prevents omissions, misunderstandings, and incorrect inferences and conclusions (Figure 9–3). This process is particularly important if data sources are considered unreliable. For example, if a client is confused or unable to communicate, or if two sources provide conflicting data, it is necessary to seek further information or clarification. Findings should also be compared with norms. Any grossly abnormal findings should be rechecked and confirmed.

Organizing the Data

Collected data must be organized so as to be useful to the health care professional collecting the data and to others involved in the client's care. After being organized into categories, the data are clustered into groups of related pieces. **Data clustering** is the process of putting data together in order to identify areas of the client's problems and strengths. Many health care agencies use an admission assessment format, which assists the nurse in collecting and organizing data.

An **assessment model** is a framework that provides a systematic method for organizing data. A few of the many assessment models available to nurses are described following.

Hierarchy of Needs Maslow's hierarchy of needs proposes that an individual's basic needs (physiological) must be met before higher-level needs can be met. Use of a hierarchy of needs model requires initial

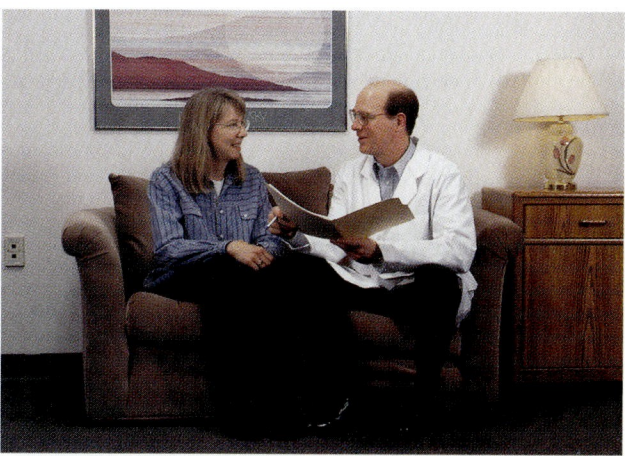

Figure 9–3 This nurse is validating information collected from the client during assessment.

assessment of all physiological needs followed by assessment of higher-level needs.

Body Systems Model The body systems model organizes data collection according to organ and tissue function in the various body systems (e.g., cardiovascular, respiratory, gastrointestinal). This method is sometimes referred to as the "medical model," because it is frequently used by physicians to investigate the presence or absence of disease.

Human Response Patterns In an effort to standardize terminology related to client problems, NANDA developed a taxonomy organized according to nine human response patterns. This framework suggests that a person's health status is evidenced by observable phenomena that can be classified into one of these response patterns, which can then be used as a model for organizing data collection. The nine response patterns are as follows:

- Exchanging: mutual giving and receiving
- Communicating: sending messages
- Relating: establishing bonds
- Valuing: assigning relative worth
- Choosing: selecting alternatives
- Moving: activity
- Perceiving: reception and information
- Knowing: meaning associated with information
- Feeling: subjective awareness of information (NANDA, 1999)

Functional Health Patterns Gordon's Functional Health Patterns (Gordon, 1997) provides a systematic framework for data collection that focuses on 11 functional health patterns. These functional health pattern areas allow the gathering and clustering of information about a client's usual patterns and any recent changes in order to ascertain whether the client's response is functional or dysfunctional. For example, the activity–exercise pattern is assessed for a client who recently experienced a stroke. Data collection would be focused on mobility and exercise patterns prior to the stroke, current muscle strength and joint mobility, and the effect of any changes on the client's lifestyle and functional ability. The eleven patterns are as follows:

- Health perception/health management pattern
- Nutritional/metabolic pattern
- Elimination pattern
- Activity/exercise pattern
- Cognitive/perceptual pattern
- Sleep/rest pattern
- Self-perception/self-concept pattern
- Role/relationship pattern
- Sexuality/reproductive pattern
- Coping/stress-tolerance pattern
- Value/belief pattern (Gordon, 1997)

Theory of Self-Care The theory of self-care, developed by Orem (1995), is based on a client's ability to perform self-care activities. Self-care is learned behavior and deliberate action in response to need. It includes activities that an individual performs to maintain health. A major focus of this theory is the appraisal of the client's ability to meet self-care needs and the identification of existing self-care deficits. Because this theory focuses on deficits in care, it primarily addresses illness states. The self-care requisites are as follows:

- Maintenance of a sufficient intake of air
- Maintenance of a sufficient intake of water
- Maintenance of a sufficient intake of food
- Provision of care associated with elimination processes and excrements
- Maintenance of a balance between activity and rest
- Maintenance of a balance between solitude and social interaction
- Prevention of hazards to human life, human functioning, and human well-being
- Promotion of human functioning and development within social groups in accord with human potential, known human limitations, and the human desire to be normal (Orem, 1995)

Interpreting the Data

After data have been collected, the nurse can begin to develop impressions or inferences about the meaning of the data. Organizing data in clusters helps the nurse to recognize patterns of response or behavior. When data are placed in clusters, the nurse can:

- Distinguish between relevant and irrelevant data,
- Determine whether and where there are gaps in the data, and
- Identify patterns of cause and effect.

Documenting the Data

Assessment data must be recorded and reported. The nurse must make a judgment about which data are to be immediately reported to the head nurse and/or physician and which data need only to be recorded at that time. Data that reflect a significant deviation from the normal (for example, rapid heart rate with irregular rhythm, severe difficulty in breathing, or a high level of anxiety) would need to be reported as well as recorded. Examples of data that need only to be recorded at the time include a report that prescribed medication has relieved a headache and a determination that an abdominal dressing is dry and intact.

Accurate and complete recording of assessment data is essential for communicating information to other health care team members. In addition, documentation is the basis for determining quality of care and should include appropriate data to support identified problems.

Diagnosis

The second step in the nursing process involves further **analysis** (breaking down the whole into parts that can be examined) and **synthesis** (putting data together in a new way) of the data that have been collected. Formulation of the list of nursing diagnoses is the outcome of this process. According to NANDA, a **nursing diagnosis**

> is a clinical judgment about individual, family, or community responses to actual or potential health problems/life processes. A nursing diagnosis provides the basis for selection of nursing interventions to achieve outcomes for which the nurse is accountable. (NANDA, 1999, p. 149)

The nursing diagnoses developed during this phase of the nursing process provide the basis for client care delivered through the remaining steps.

Clients receive both medical and nursing diagnoses. Table 9–2 compares the two categories of diagnoses. It is important to have a clear understanding of the nature of a nursing diagnosis as compared to a **medical diagnosis** (clinical judgment by the physician that identifies or determines a specific disease, condition, or pathological state). Table 9–3 compares selected nursing and medical diagnoses.

The nurse uses critical-thinking and decision-making skills in developing nursing diagnoses. This process is facilitated by asking questions such as:

- Are there problems here?
- If so, what are the specific problems?
- What are some possible causes of the problems?
- Is there a situation involving risk factors?
- What are the risk factors?
- Can a problem develop if preventive measures are not taken?
- If so, under what circumstances?
- Has the client indicated a desire for a higher level of wellness in a particular area of function?
- What are the client's strengths?
- What data are available to answer these questions?
- Are more data needed to answer the question?
- If so, what are some possible sources of the data that are needed?

Components of a Nursing Diagnosis

Several formats have been used to structure nursing diagnosis statements. Two formats that are frequently seen in the nursing literature are the two-part statement and the three-part statement. The two-part statement is NANDA approved and is used by most nurses mainly because of its brief and precise format. The three-part statement is usually required of nursing students and is preferred by those nurses desiring to strengthen the diagnostic statement by including specific manifestations. Table 9–4 lists the NANDA-approved nursing diagnoses.

Two-Part Statement The first component, the actual nursing diagnosis, is a problem statement or diagnostic label that describes the client's response to an actual or potential health problem or a wellness condition.

Table 9–2 COMPARISON OF MEDICAL AND NURSING DIAGNOSES

MEDICAL DIAGNOSIS	NURSING DIAGNOSIS
Identifies conditions the physician is licensed and qualified to treat	Identifies situations the nurse is licensed and qualified to treat
Focuses on the illness, injury, or disease process	Focuses on the client's responses to actual or potential health problems or life processes
Remains constant until a cure is effected	Changes as the client's response and/or the health problem changes
EXAMPLE: Breast cancer	EXAMPLE: *Knowledge Deficit; Powerlessness; Grieving, Anticipatory; Body Image Disturbance; Individual Coping, Ineffective.*

Adapted from Fundamentals of Nursing: Standards & Practice, *by S. DeLaune and P. Ladner, 1998, Albany, NY: Delmar Publishers. Copyright 1998 by Delmar Publishers. Adapted with permission.*

Table 9–3 COMPARISON OF SELECT NURSING AND MEDICAL DIAGNOSES

NURSING DIAGNOSIS	MEDICAL DIAGNOSIS
Breathing Pattern, Ineffective	Chronic obstructive pulmonary disease
Activity Intolerance	Cerebrovascular accident
Pain	Appendectomy
Body Image Disturbance	Amputation
Body Temperature, Risk for Altered	Strep throat

Adapted from Fundamentals of Nursing: Standards & Practice, *by S. DeLaune and P. Ladner, 1998, Albany, NY: Delmar Publishers. Copyright 1998 by Delmar Publishers. Adapted with permission.*

Table 9–4 NANDA-APPROVED NURSING DIAGNOSES

Activity intolerance

Activity intolerance, risk for

Adaptive capacity, intracranial, decreased

Adjustment, impaired

Airway clearance, ineffective

Anxiety

Anxiety, death

Aspiration, risk for

Body image disturbance

Body temperature, altered, risk for

Bowel incontinence

Breastfeeding
  effective
  ineffective
  interrupted

Breathing pattern, ineffective

Cardiac output, decreased

Caregiver role strain

Caregiver role strain, risk for

Communication, verbal, impaired

Confusion
  acute
  chronic

Constipation

Constipation, colonic

Constipation, perceived

Constipation, risk of

Coping, defensive

Coping: community
  ineffective
  potential for enhanced

Coping, family, ineffective
  compromised
  disabling
  potential for growth

Coping: individual, ineffective

Death anxiety

Decisional conflict

Decreased cardiac output

Denial, ineffective

Dentition, altered

Development, risk for altered

Diarrhea

Disuse syndrome, risk for

Diversional activity deficit

Dysreflexia

Dysreflexia, risk for autonomic

Elimination, urinary, altered

Energy field disturbance

Environmental interpretation syndrome, impaired

Failure to thrive, adult

Family processes, altered

Family processes, altered, alcoholism

Fatigue

Fear

Feeding pattern, ineffective infant

Fluid volume
  deficit
  excess
  imbalance, risk for
  risk for deficit

Gas exchange, impaired

Grieving

Grieving, anticipatory

Grieving, dysfunctional

Grieving, risk for altered

Growth and development, altered

Health maintenance, altered

Health-seeking behaviors

Home maintenance management, impaired

Hopelessness

Hyperthermia

Hypothermia

Incontinence, bowel

Incontinence, urinary
  functional
  reflex
  stress
  total
  urge
  risk for urge

Infant behavior, disorganized

Infant behavior, disorganized, risk for

Infant behavior, potential for enhanced organized

Infant feeding pattern, ineffective

Infection, risk for

Injury, risk for

Injury, risk for, perioperative positioning

Knowledge deficit

Latex allergy response

Latex allergy response, risk for

Loneliness, risk for

Management of therapeutic regimen
  community
  families, ineffective
  individuals, ineffective

Memory, impaired

Mobility, impaired
  bed
  physical
  wheelchair

Nausea

Noncompliance

Nutrition, altered
  less than body requirements
  more than body requirements
  risk for more than body requirements

Oral mucous membrane, altered

Pain

Pain, chronic

Parent/infant/child attachment, altered, risk for

Parental role conflict

Parenting, altered

Parenting, altered, risk for

Peripheral neurovascular dysfunction, risk for

Personal identity disturbance

Poisoning, risk for

Post-trauma syndrome

Post-trauma syndrome, risk for

Powerlessness

Protection, altered

Rape-trauma syndrome

Rape-trauma syndrome, compound reaction

Rape-trauma syndrome, silent reaction

Relocation stress syndrome

Retention, urinary

Role conflict, parental

Role performance, altered

Self-care deficit
  bathing/hygiene
  dressing/grooming
  feeding
  toileting

Self-esteem
  chronic low
  disturbance
  situational low

Self-mutilation, risk for

Sensory/perceptual alterations

Sexual dysfunction

Sexuality patterns, altered

Skin integrity, impaired

Skin integrity, impaired, risk for

Sleep deprivation

Sleep pattern disturbance

Social interaction, impaired

Social isolation

Sorrow, chronic

Spiritual distress

Spiritual distress, risk for

Spiritual well-being, potential for enhanced

Stress incontinence

Suffocation, risk for

Surgical recovery, delayed

Swallowing, impaired

Syndrome
  disuse, risk for
  environmental interpretation, impaired
  post-trauma
  rape-trauma
  relocation stress

Thermoregulation, ineffective

Thought processes, altered

Tissue integrity, impaired

Tissue perfusion, altered

Total incontinence

Transfer ability, impaired

Trauma, risk for

Unilateral neglect

Urge incontinence

Urinary elimination, altered

Urinary incontinence, reflex

Urinary retention

Ventilation, inability to sustain spontaneous

Ventilatory weaning response, dysfunctional

Violence, risk for
  directed at others
  self-directed

Walking, impaired

From Nursing Diagnoses: Definitions & Classification, 1999–2000, by North American Nursing Diagnosis Association, 1999, Philadelphia: Author. Copyright 1999 by North American Nursing Diagnosis Association. Reprinted with permission.

The second component of a two-part nursing diagnosis statement is the etiology. The **etiology** is the related cause or contributor to the problem and is identified in the complete NANDA diagnosis description. The diagnostic label and etiology are linked by the terminology *related to* (R/T). Because the NANDA list of nursing diagnoses is constantly evolving, there may be times when no etiology is provided. In such cases, the nurse should attempt to describe likely contributing factors to the client's condition. Examples of a two-part nursing diagnosis statement are *Body Image Disturbance R/T loss of left lower extremity* and *Activity Intolerance R/T decreased oxygen-carrying capacity of cells.*

Three-Part Statement The nursing diagnosis can also be expressed as a three-part statement. As in the two-part statement, the first two components are the diagnostic label and the etiology. The third component consists of **defining characteristics** (collected data, also known as signs and symptoms, subjective and objective data, or clinical manifestations). The third part is joined to the first two components with the connecting phrase *as evidenced by* (AEB). An example of a three-part nursing diagnosis statement is *Breathing Pattern, Ineffective R/T pain AEB respiratory rate less than 11 and use of accessory muscles.*

Writing The Nursing Diagnosis Statement

The nursing diagnosis selected from the NANDA list becomes the diagnostic label, the first part of the diagnosis statement. Etiologies are also chosen from the NANDA descriptions. The appropriate etiology is selected and joined to the first part of the statement with the "related to" phrase. Table 9–5 compares selected NANDA-approved diagnoses in two- and three-part formats.

Types of Nursing Diagnoses

Analysis of the collected data leads the nurse to make a diagnosis in one of three categories:

- An **actual nursing diagnosis** indicates that a problem exists; it is composed of the diagnostic label, related factors, and signs and symptoms. An example of an actual diagnosis is *Skin Integrity, Impaired, R/T prolonged pressure on bony prominence AEB Stage II pressure ulcer over coccyx, 3 cm in diameter.*
- A **risk nursing diagnosis** (potential problem) indicates that a problem does not yet exist, but that special risk factors are present. A risk diagnosis is composed of the diagnostic label followed by the phrase *Risk for* and a list of the specific risk factors. An example of a risk diagnosis is *Skin Integrity, Impaired, Risk for; risk factors include physical immobilization AEB inability to turn self from side to side in bed.*
- A **wellness nursing diagnosis** indicates the client's expression of a desire to attain a higher level of wellness in some area of function. It is composed of the diagnostic label followed by the phrase *Potential for Enhanced.* For example, a couple expecting their first child asks the nurse for suggestions on books to read and classes to attend so that they can be well prepared for their child. The nurse would

Table 9–5 EXAMPLES OF NURSING DIAGNOSES EXPRESSED IN TWO- AND THREE-PART STATEMENTS

TWO-PART STATEMENT	THREE-PART STATEMENT
Self-Care Deficit, Feeding R/T decreased strength and endurance	*Self-Care Deficit, Feeding R/T decreased strength and endurance AEB inability to maintain fork in hand from plate to mouth*
Anxiety R/T change in role functioning	*Anxiety R/T change in role functioning AEB insomnia, poor eye contact, and quivering voice*
Airway Clearance, Ineffective, R/T fatigue	*Airway Clearance, Ineffective, R/T fatigue AEB dyspnea at rest*
Knowledge Deficit (Insulin Injection Technique) R/T misinterpretation of information	*Knowledge Deficit (Insulin Injection Technique) R/T misinterpretation of information AEB inaccurate return demonstration of self-injection*
Spiritual Distress R/T separation from religious ties	*Spiritual Distress R/T separation from religious ties AEB crying and withdrawal*

Adapted from Fundamentals of Nursing: Standards & Practice, by S. DeLaune and P. Ladner, 1998, Albany, NY: Delmar Publishers. Copyright 1998 by Delmar Publishers. Adapted with permission.

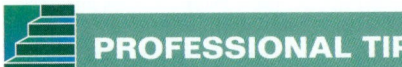

Nursing Diagnosis

- The nursing diagnosis must be developed from the data, never the other way around.
- Do not try to fit a client to a nursing diagnosis; rather, select the appropriate diagnosis from the data cues presented by the client. Failure to do so may result in errors in developing a nursing diagnosis.

make a wellness diagnosis of *Family Coping: Potential for Growth*.

Examples of the three types of diagnoses are shown in Table 9–6.

After formulation, the nursing diagnoses should be discussed with the client, if possible. If this is not possible, the diagnoses may be discussed with family members. Finally, the list of nursing diagnoses is recorded on the client's record. After this list has been developed and recorded, the remainder of the client's care plan can be completed. The list of nursing diagnoses is not static. It is dynamic, changing as more data are collected and as client goals and client responses to interventions are evaluated.

Planning and Outcome Identification

Planning combines with outcome identification to comprise the third step of the nursing process and includes both the formulation of guidelines that establish the proposed course of nursing action in the resolution of nursing diagnoses and the development of the client's plan of care. After the nursing diagnoses have been developed and the client's strengths have been identified, planning can begin.

The planning of nursing care occurs in three phases: initial, ongoing, and discharge. Each type of planning contributes to the coordination of the client's comprehensive plan of care. **Initial planning** involves development of a preliminary plan of care by the nurse who performs the admission assessment and gathers the comprehensive admission assessment data. Because of progressively shorter lengths of hospitalization, initial planning is important in addressing each problem and in correlating nursing care to hasten resolution of these problems. **Ongoing planning** entails continuous updating of the client's plan of care. As new information about the client is gathered and evaluated, revisions may be generated and the initial plan of care further individualized to the client. **Discharge planning** involves critical anticipation and planning for the client's needs after discharge.

Table 9–6 TYPES OF NURSING DIAGNOSES

NURSING DIAGNOSIS	EXAMPLE
Actual diagnosis	*Fluid Volume Deficit R/T nausea and vomiting AEB dry skin and mucous membranes and decreased oral intake of fluids*
Risk diagnosis	*Infection, Risk for, R/T presence of invasive lines (intravenous line and indwelling bladder catheter)*
Wellness diagnosis	*Spiritual Well-Being, Potential for Enhanced*

Adapted from Fundamentals of Nursing: Standards & Practice, *by S. DeLaune and P. Ladner, 1998, Albany, NY: Delmar Publishers. Copyright 1998 by Delmar Publishers. Adapted with permission.*

The planning phase involves several tasks:

- Prioritizing the list of nursing diagnoses
- Identifying and writing client-centered long- and short-term goals and outcomes (outcome identification)
- Developing specific nursing interventions
- Recording the entire nursing care plan in the client's record

Prioritizing the Nursing Diagnoses

Prioritizing the nursing diagnoses involves making decisions about which diagnoses are the most important and therefore require attention first. One of the most common methods of selecting priorities is to consider Maslow's hierarchy of needs, which leads the nurse to consider a life-threatening diagnosis more urgent than a non–life-threatening diagnosis. After basic physiological needs (e.g., respiration, nutrition, temperature, hydration, and elimination) are met to some degree, the nurse would then consider needs on the next level of the hierarchy (e.g., safe environment, stable living condition, affection, and self-worth) and so on up the hierarchy until all of the client's nursing diagnoses have been prioritized. Table 9–7 illustrates this process.

Identifying Outcomes

Outcome identification includes establishing goals and expected outcomes, which together provide guidelines for individualized nursing interventions and establish evaluation criteria to measure the effectiveness of the nursing care plan.

Goals A **goal** is an aim, intent, or end. Goals are broad statements that describe the intended or desired change in the client's condition or behavior. Client-centered goals are established in collaboration with

Table 9–7 PRIORITIZING NURSING DIAGNOSES

NURSING DIAGNOSIS	MASLOW'S HIERARCHY OF NEEDS	PRIORITY
Anxiety R/T hospitalization	Safety and security	Moderate
Coping, Individual, Ineffective, R/T situational crisis	Self-esteem	Low
Airway Clearance, Ineffective R/T excessive secretions	Physiological	High

Adapted from Fundamentals of Nursing: Standards & Practice, by S. DeLaune and P. Ladner, 1998, Albany, NY: Delmar Publishers. Copyright 1998 by Delmar Publishers. Adapted with permission.

Table 9–8 SHORT- AND LONG-TERM GOALS

Nursing Diagnosis: *Pain related to rheumatoid arthritis*

Short-term Goals (Focused on Etiology)	Long-term Goals (Focused on Problem)
Verbalizes the presence of pain	Verbalizes comfort
Identifies factors that influence the pain experience	
Client or significant other administers pain medication appropriately	

From Fundamentals of Nursing: Standards & Practice, *by S. DeLaune and P. Ladner, 1998, Albany, NY: Delmar Publishers. Copyright 1998 by Delmar Publishers. Reprinted with permission.*

the client whenever possible. Goal statements refer to the diagnostic label (or problem statement) of the nursing diagnosis. If the client or significant others are unable to participate in goal development, the nurse assumes that responsibility until the client is able to participate. Client-centered goals ensure that nursing care is individualized and focused on the client.

A **short-term goal** is an objective statement that outlines the desired resolution of the nursing diagnosis over a short period of time, usually a few hours or days (less than a week). Short-term goals focus on the etiology component of the nursing diagnosis. A **long-term goal** is an objective statement that outlines the desired resolution of the nursing diagnosis over a longer period of time, usually weeks or months. Long-term goals focus on the problem component of the nursing diagnosis. Table 9–8 provides examples of short-term and long-term goals.

Expected Outcomes After the goals have been established, the expected outcomes can be identified based on those goals. An **expected outcome** is a detailed, specific statement that describes the methods through which the goal will be achieved and includes aspects such as direct nursing care, client teaching, and continuity of care. Outcomes must be measurable, time limited, and realistic. Several expected outcomes may be required for each goal (Table 9–9). After goals and expected outcomes have been established, nursing interventions are formulated to enable the client to reach the goals.

Developing Specific Nursing Interventions

A **nursing intervention** is an action performed by the nurse that helps the client achieve the results specified by the goals and expected outcomes. Nursing inter-

ventions refer directly to the related factors in the actual or wellness nursing diagnoses and to the risk factors in risk nursing diagnoses. If the nursing interventions can remove or reduce the related factors and the risk factors, the problem can be resolved or prevented.

For each nursing diagnosis, there may be a number of nursing interventions. Nursing interventions are individualized and are stated in specific terms. Examples of nursing interventions are as follows:

- Assist client to turn, cough, and deep breathe q 2 h beginning at 0800, 2/10

Table 9–9 GOAL WITH EXPECTED OUTCOMES

Nursing Diagnosis: *Sleep Pattern Disturbance R/T sensory alterations: internal (illness) and external (social cues)*

Goal	Expected Outcomes
Client will sleep uninterrupted for 6 hours.	• When ready for bed, client will request back massage for relaxation. • By the next visit, client will have set limits for visits from family and significant others.

Nursing Diagnosis: *Tissue Perfusion, Altered (Peripheral) R/T interruption of flow, venous*

Goal	Expected Outcomes
Client will have palpable peripheral pulses in 1 week.	• Client will identify three factors to improve peripheral circulation within two days. • Client's feet will be warm to touch within two weeks.

From Fundamentals of Nursing: Standards & Practice, *by S. DeLaune and P. Ladner, 1998, Albany, NY: Delmar Publishers. Copyright 1998 by Delmar Publishers. Reprinted with permission.*

- Teach nipple care when breastfeeding at 1000, 2/11
- Weigh client at each visit

After interventions have been formulated for each diagnosis, they are recorded on the client's care plan. As is true with other steps in the nursing process, the list of interventions is not static. As the nurse interacts with the client, assesses responses to interventions, and evaluates those responses, interventions may change.

Categories of Nursing Interventions

Nursing interventions are classified into one of three categories: independent, interdependent, or dependent. **Independent nursing interventions** are nursing actions that are initiated by the nurse and do not require direction or an order from another health care professional. In many states, the nursing practice act allows independent nursing interventions with regard to activities such as daily living, health education, health promotion, and counseling. An example of an independent nursing intervention is the nurse's elevating a client's edematous extremity.

Interdependent nursing interventions are those actions that are implemented in a collaborative manner by the nurse in conjunction with other health care professionals. A client care conference with an interdisciplinary health care team results in interdependent nursing interventions. For example, the nurse may assist a client to perform an exercise taught by the physical therapist.

Dependent nursing interventions are those actions that require an order from a physician or another health care professional. An example of a dependent intervention is administration of a medication. Although this intervention requires specific nursing knowledge and responsibilities, it is not within the realm of legal practice for licensed practical/vocational nurses (LP/VNs) to prescribe medications. When administering medications, the nurse is responsible for knowing the classification, pharmacological action, normal dosage, adverse effects, contraindications, and nursing implications of the drug. Therefore, dependent nursing interventions, like all nursing actions, must be guided by appropriate knowledge and judgment.

Recording the Nursing Care Plan

The **nursing care plan** is a written guide that organizes data about a client's care into a formal statement of the strategies that will be implemented to help the client achieve optimal health. Nursing care plans usually include components such as assessment, nursing diagnoses, goals and expected outcomes, and nursing interventions. The nurse begins the nursing care plan on the day of admission and continually updates and individualizes the client's plan of care until discharge.

There are several types of care plans; including student-oriented, standardized, institutional, and computerized care plans. The student-oriented care plan promotes learning of problem-solving skills, the nursing process, verbal and written communication skills, and organizational skills. This comprehensive care plan offers great depth for teaching the process of planning care and usually includes a scientific rationale for each intervention. Although educational programs vary, the student-oriented care plan usually begins with assessment and proceeds in a sequential manner until it concludes with the evaluation of the care plan.

The standardized care plan is a preplanned, preprinted guide for the nursing care of client groups with common needs. This type of care plan generally follows the nursing process format. The nurse may use standardized care plans when a client has predictable, commonly occurring problems. Individualization may be accomplished by the inclusion of additional handwritten notes regarding unusual problems.

Institutional nursing care plans are concise documents that become a part of the client's medical record after discharge. The Kardex nursing care plan is an example of this type of care plan and is frequently used. The institutional nursing care plan may simply include the nursing diagnoses, nursing interventions, and evaluation. In addition, the Kardex nursing care plan may be expanded to include assessment, nursing diagnoses, goals, implementation, and evaluation. Figure 9–4 provides an example of an institutional care plan.

Computers are used for creating and storing nursing care plans and can generate both standardized and individualized nursing care plans. The nurse selects appropriate diagnoses from a menu suggested by the computer, which then lists possible goals and nursing interventions. The nurse has the option of reading the client's plan of care from the computer screen or printing an updated working copy. Figure 9–5 is an example of a computerized nursing care plan.

Implementation

The fourth step in the nursing process is implementation. **Implementation** involves the execution of the nursing care plan derived during the planning phase. It consists of performing nursing activities (interventions) that have been planned to meet the goals set with the client. It also involves the **delegation** (process of transferring a select nursing task to a licensed individual who is competent to perform that specific task) of some nursing interventions to staff members or to assistive personnel capable of competently performing the task. The nurse remains accountable for appropriate delegation and supervision of care provided by these individuals.

Requirements for Effective Implementation

Implementation involves many skills. The nurse must continue to assess the client's condition before, during,

NURSING DIAGNOSIS	NURSING INTERVENTIONS	EVALUATION
Ineffective breathing pattern R/T operative site/incisional pain.	1. Auscultate breath sounds q 4h. & PRN 2. Assist pt. to TCDB q 2h while awake.	1. Lungs clear on auscultation. 2. "It doesn't hurt as much to cough today."
Risk for infection R/T surgical incision & indwelling catheter	Assess for s/s of infection q 4h.	T-100.2°, incision site warm & pink, non-edematous. "It really hurts under the bandage."

Figure 9–4 Handwritten Institutional Care Plan *(From* Fundamentals of Nursing: Standards & Practice, *by S. DeLaune and P. Ladner, 1998, Albany, NY: Delmar Publishers. Copyright 1998 by Delmar Publishers. Reprinted with permission.)*

and after each nursing intervention. Assessment prior to intervention implementation provides the nurse with baseline data. Assessment during and after intervention implementation allows the nurse to detect positive or negative responses the client may have to the intervention. If negative responses occur during the intervention, the nurse must take appropriate action. If positive responses occur, the nurse adds this information to the database for use in evaluating the efficacy of the intervention.

The nurse must also possess psychomotor skills, interpersonal skills, and cognitive skills to perform the nursing interventions that have been planned. The nurse uses psychomotor skills to safely and effectively perform nursing activities. Nurses must be able to both handle medical equipment with a high degree of competency and perform such skills as giving injections, changing dressings, and helping the client perform range-of-motion (ROM) exercises.

Interpersonal skills are necessary as the nurse interacts with the client and the family to collect data, provide information in teaching sessions, and offer support in times of anxiety. The nurse–client relationship is established and maintained through the use of therapeutic communication. Interaction between and among members of the health care team promotes

---

Client Name: Margaret Jones
Age: 55   **Temp:** 98.8   **BP:** 150/90   **Pulse:** 90   **Sex:** F

Disease/Disorder/Condition: Diabetes

Client Health History

Mrs. Jones was diagnosed 2 years ago with type 2 (non-insulin-dependent) diabetes and takes metformin (Glucophage) 500 mg b.i.d (twice a day) with meals. She is being seen in the clinic for her 6-month visit. she says, "I hardly have the energy to get up and dress in the morning. I am thirsty all day and awaken several times during the night, having to go to the bathroom." She does not work outside the home and has not been involved in community activities for the past five years since her youngest child graduated from high school. Her daily routine involves cooking for her husband and brother, reading, and watching the TV for 6-8 hours. She says, "I eat because I have nothing else to do." She is concerned about her eating habits and her recent weight gain.

Assessment Findings

Weight, 177 lb.   Weight gain, 8 lb.
Height, 5'4"   Sedentary lifestyle
Triceps skinfold, 28mm   Eats in response to boredom
Elevated blood glucose

Nursing Diagnosis: Altered Nutrition: More than Body Requirements

Goals: Mrs. Jones will:
1. Come to clinic weekly for 4 weeks.
2. Modify eating habits to decrease amount of intake.
3. Lose 2 lb./month.
4. Participate in some exercise.
5. Begin involvement outside of home.

continued

Figure 9–5 Computer-Generated Nursing Care Plan

Intervention

1. Conduct a dietary history, using open-ended statements to assist the client in exploring psychological factors that may contribute to eating.

2. Encourage client to modify eating habits to decrease amount of intake (smaller servings, taking small bites and chewing each bite 12 times, putting the fork on the plate between bites, drinking water with meals, eating only at mealtime, chewing sugar-free gum when watching TV).

3. Assess client's motivation to lose weight.

4. Discuss risk factors and symptoms (thirst and urination) of diabetes.

5. Instruct client to maintain a daily dietary intake log; time of meals and snacks, type and amount of foods eaten.

6. Provide with dietary materials, review the Food Pyramid and Diabetic Exchange List; plan with client a 1600-kilocalorie per day diet for a week, taking into consideration food preferences.

7. Review with client age-appropriate exercises; emphasize need for daily walking.

8. Review with client community and church interests outside the home, unrelated to cooking and eating.

9. Schedule return visit with nurse in one week; Monitor progress and assess plan of care.

Rationale

1. Nonjudgmental approach to acquiring information will encourage client trust and honesty.

2. Healthy eating habits and tips on recognizing fullness during a meal will help the client eat to satisfy hunger, not boredom.

3. Having client's support for care plan will influence success.

4. Client understanding of her disease may increase motivation to manage it.

5. Helps client recognize her eating patterns and note healthy and unhealthy behaviors.

6. Ensures client has information necessary to plan healthy meals within recommended guidelines.

7. Changing sedentary lifestyle will increase self-esteem, burn calories, and increase energy level

8. Helps client focus on activities not involving food to decrease boredom and to increase self-esteem.

9. Close monitoring and follow-up will allow modification of plan of care as required to meet client needs.

Evaluation/Outcome

1. Client made return clinic appointment; noted phone number of nurse and dietitian to answer questions; agreed to 1800-kilocalorie meal plan for one week.

2. On return visit, the client reported drinking more water with meals, chewing her food slowly, and chewing gum while watching TV.

3. On return visit, the client was found to have lost 1.8 lbs.

4. On return visit, the client indicated that she now walks to the store 4-5 times a week (40 minutes round trip).

5. The client reported on return visit that she is now volunteering 2 hours 3 times a week at the church's child care center.

Format from Delmar's Electronic Care Plan Maker *by Susan Sheehy, 1998, Albany, NY: Delmar Publishers. Content from* Fundamentals of Nursing: Standards & Practice *by S. DeLaune and P. Ladner, 1998, Albany, NY: Delmar Publishers. Copyright 1998 by Delmar Publishers.*

Figure 9–5 *continued*

collaboration and enhances the holistic care of the client.

Cognitive skills enable the nurse to make appropriate observations, understand the rationale for the activities performed, ask the appropriate questions, and make decisions about those things that need to be done. Critical thinking is an important element within the cognitive domain because it helps the nurse analyze data, organize observations, and apply prior knowledge and experiences to current client situations.

Types of Nursing Interventions

Nursing interventions are written as orders in the care plan and may be nurse initiated, physician initi-

ated, or derived from collaboration with other health care professionals. Interventions can be implemented on the basis of specific orders, standing orders, or protocols.

A **specific order** is an order written in a client's medical record or nursing care plan by a physician or nurse especially for that individual client; it is not used for any other client.

A **standing order** is a standardized intervention written, approved, and signed by a physician that is kept on file within health care agencies to be used in predictable situations or in circumstances requiring immediate attention. Nurses can implement standing orders in these situations after assessing the client and

HOME HEALTH CARE

Standing Orders
Nurses in home health care agencies may have standing orders for administering certain medications or ordering laboratory tests when indicated.

---

identifying the primary or emerging problem. An example of a physician-initiated standing order on an inpatient unit would be specification of certain medications to be administered for a common headache.

A **protocol** is a series of standing orders or procedures that should be followed under certain specific conditions. The protocol defines those interventions that are permissible and those circumstances under which the nurse is allowed to implement the measures. Health care agencies or individual physicians frequently have standing orders or protocols for client preparation for diagnostic tests or for immediate interventions in life-threatening circumstances. These protocols prevent needless duplication of effort with regard to writing the same orders repeatedly for different clients, often saving valuable time in critical situations.

Documenting and Reporting Interventions

The implementation step also involves documentation and reporting. Data to be recorded include the client's condition prior to the intervention, the specific intervention performed, the client's response to the intervention, and client outcomes. This documentation not only constitutes a legal record, but also allows for valuable communication among other health care team members for purposes of ensuring continuity of care and evaluating progress toward expected outcomes. In addition, written documentation provides data necessary for reimbursement for services.

Verbal interaction among health care providers is also essential for communicating current information about clients. Communication between nurses generally occurs at the change of shift, when the responsibility for care changes from one nurse to another. Nursing students must communicate relevant information to the nurse responsible for their clients when they leave the unit. Information that should be shared in the verbal report includes:

- Those activities completed and those yet to be completed,
- Status of current relevant problems,
- Any abnormalities or changes in assessment,
- Results of treatments, and
- Diagnostic tests scheduled or completed (and results).

All communication—both written and verbal—must be objective, descriptive, and complete. All communication must include observations rather than opinions and be stated or written to convey an accurate picture of the client's condition. Thorough and detailed communication of implementation activities is fundamental to ensuring that client care and progress toward goals can be adequately evaluated.

Evaluation

Evaluation, the fifth step in the nursing process, involves determining whether the client goals have been met, partially met, or not met. If a goal has been met, the nurse must then decide whether nursing activities should cease or continue in order for status to be maintained. If a goal has been partially met or not met, the nurse must reassess the situation. Data are collected to determine both the reasons the goal has not been achieved and the necessary modifications to the plan of care. Among a number of possible reasons that goals are not met or are only partially met are the following:

- The initial assessment data were incomplete.
- The goals and expected outcomes were not realistic.
- The time frame was too optimistic.
- The goals and/or the nursing interventions planned were not appropriate for the client or situation.

Evaluation is a fluid process that is dependent on all the other components of the nursing process. As shown in Figure 9–6, evaluation affects, and is affected by, assessment, diagnosis, planning and outcome identification, and implementation of nursing care. Table 9–10 shows the way evaluation is woven into every phase of the nursing process. Ongoing evaluation is essential if the nursing process is to be implemented appropriately. As Alfaro-LeFevre (1995) states:

> When we evaluate early, checking whether our information is accurate, complete, and up-to-date, we're able to make corrections *early*. We avoid

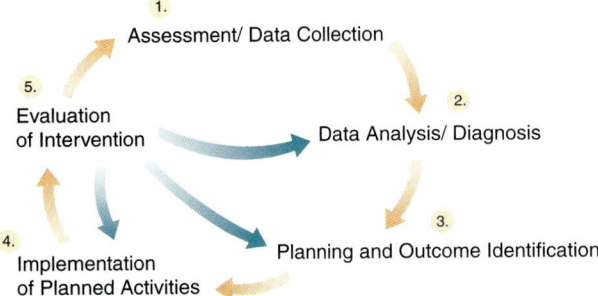

Figure 9–6 Relationship of Evaluation to the Nursing Process *(From Fundamentals of Nursing: Standards & Practice, by S. DeLaune and P. Ladner, 1998, Albany, NY: Delmar Publishers. Copyright 1998 by Delmar Publishers. Reprinted with permission.)*

HOME HEALTH CARE

Effectiveness of Care

When evaluating the effectiveness of care, the home health care nurse can use the following questions to examine client achievement of expected outcomes:

- Were the goals realistic in terms of client abilities and time frame?
- Were there external variables (for example, housing problems, impaired family dynamics) that prevented goal achievement?
- Did the family have the resources (for example, transportation) to assist in meeting the goals?
- Was the care coordinated with other providers to facilitate efficient delivery of care?

making decisions based on outdated, inaccurate, or incomplete information. Early evaluation enhances our ability to act safely and effectively. It improves our *efficiency* by helping us stay focused on priorities and avoid wasting time continuing useless actions.

Nursing Audit

A **nursing audit** is the process of collecting and analyzing data to evaluate the effectiveness of nursing interventions. A nursing audit can focus on implementation of the nursing process, on client outcomes, or on both in order to evaluate the quality of care provided. Health care facilities each have an ongoing nursing audit committee to evaluate the quality of care given. Nursing audits examine data related to:

- Safety measures,
- Treatment interventions and client responses to those interventions,
- Preestablished outcomes used as a basis for interventions,
- Discharge planning,
- Client teaching, and
- Adequacy of staffing patterns.

THE NURSING PROCESS AND CRITICAL THINKING

A number of skills are required of nurses in their use of the nursing process as a framework for providing client care. One important skill is critical thinking. Critical thinkers ask questions, evaluate evidence, identify assumptions, examine alternatives, and seek to understand various points of view.

Table 9–10 INTERACTION BETWEEN EVALUATION AND THE OTHER PHASES OF THE NURSING PROCESS

NURSING PROCESS PHASE	EVALUATION FOCUS
Assessment	Data collection was thorough and complete. Data were collected from multiple, varied sources. Data were relevant to client needs. Appropriate methods were used to obtain data. A systematic, organized method was used in collecting data.
Diagnosis	Nursing diagnoses were client centered, accurate, and relevant. Each nursing diagnosis was complete. Nursing diagnoses were comprehensive. Diagnoses were based on the collected data. Nursing diagnoses guided planning and implementation of care.
Planning and Outcome Identification	Outcomes were realistic and achievable. Nursing diagnoses were prioritized. Expected outcomes were relevant to nursing diagnoses. Resources (including team members) were used efficiently. Nursing plans were documented.
Implementation	Team members followed the plan of care. Necessary resources were available. Nursing actions assisted client in meeting expected outcomes. Client achieved expected outcomes. Care plan was revised according to the client's needs. Documentation reflected the client's status, including responses to nursing interventions.

Adapted from Fundamentals of Nursing: Standards & Practice, *by S. DeLaune and P. Ladner, 1998, Albany, NY: Delmar Publishers. Copyright 1998 by Delmar Publishers. Adapted with permission.*

Critical thinking is a skill that can be learned, just as other skills are learned. The skill of critical thinking is important and useful in all aspects of a person's life and is an especially vital tool for the nurse with regard to the nursing process. Critical thinkers develop a questioning attitude and delve into situations in order to seek possible explanations for what is happening. Examples of questions that the nurse as critical thinker might ask at each step in the nursing process are listed in Table 9–11.

Table 9–11 EXAMPLES OF CRITICAL THINKING QUESTIONS FOR USE WITH THE NURSING PROCESS	
NURSING PROCESS STEP	**CRITICAL-THINKING QUESTION**
Assessment	Are the data complete? What other data do I need? What are some possible sources of those data? What assumptions or biases do I have in this situation? What is the client's point of view? Are there other points of view?
Diagnosis	What do these data mean? What else could be happening? Are there any gaps in the data? How are these data similar, and how are they different? What assumptions or biases do I have in this situation? Have my assumptions affected my interpretation of the data? If so, in what way?
Planning and outcome identification	What are the goals for this client? How are my goals related to what the client wants to accomplish? What are the expected outcomes for this client? What interventions are to be used? Who is the best-qualified person to perform these interventions? How much involvement can the client and family or significant others have at this time? How much involvement does the client wish to have at this time?
Implementation	What is the client's current status? What are the most critical steps in this intervention? How must I alter the intervention to best meet this client's needs and maintain principles of safety? What is the client's response during and after the intervention? Is there a need to alter the intervention in any way? If so, why and how?
Evaluation	Were the interventions successful in assisting the client to achieve the desired goals? How could things have been done differently? What data do I need to make new decisions? Where will I get the data? Were there assumptions, biases, or points of view that I missed that affected the outcomes? What can be done about these assumptions, biases, or points of view?

From Fundamentals of Nursing: Standards & Practice, *by S. DeLaune and P. Ladner, 1998, Albany, NY: Delmar Publishers. Copyright 1998 by Delmar Publishers. Reprinted with permission.*

Assumptions are those beliefs or attitudes that one takes for granted in a situation that requires action or resolution; they are the things that one accepts as "givens." Assumptions are the implicit views one uses to filter and make sense of everyday experiences. Cause-and-effect relationships are understood within the context of these assumptions. Assumptions both are related to one's point of view and influence the way one looks at things.

Bias is a mental inclination or leaning. It can manifest in two ways. According to one interpretation of bias, a person's point of view causes that person to be more observant about certain things. According to another interpretation of bias, a person is blind to or unwilling to consider weaknesses in his own point of view. Critical thinkers attempt to be aware of both interpretations of bias and avoid the second.

THE NURSING PROCESS AND PROBLEM SOLVING

The steps in the nursing process and in problem solving are similar. People use problem solving in their daily lives. With the problem-solving method, problems are identified, information is gathered, a specific problem is named, a plan for solving the problem is developed, the plan is put into action, and results of the plan are evaluated. Problem solving, however, is frequently based on incomplete data, and plans are sometimes based on guesses. Conversely, the nursing process, which is used by nurses to identify and make decisions about client needs, is a systematic and scientifically based process that requires the use of many cognitive and psychomotor skills. Table 9–12 compares of the nursing process and the problem-solving method.

THE NURSING PROCESS AND DECISION MAKING

Nurses make decisions every day. It is important that those decisions be the best decisions possible, that

Table 9–12 COMPARISON OF THE PROBLEM-SOLVING METHOD AND THE NURSING PROCESS	
PROBLEM-SOLVING METHOD	**NURSING PROCESS**
Identify the problem	Assessment
Gather information	Assessment
Name the problem	Diagnosis
Develop a plan	Planning and outcome identification
Activate the plan	Implementation
Evaluate results	Evaluation

From Fundamentals of Nursing: Standards & Practice, *by S. DeLaune and P. Ladner, 1998, Albany, NY: Delmar Publishers. Copyright 1998 by Delmar Publishers. Reprinted with permission.*

they be based on reliable information, and that they be made with as much critical thought as possible. Nurses make decisions at each step of the nursing process. Through a process of problem solving, one arrives at the point at which decisions can be made. The nursing process is the specific problem-solving method used by nurses to arrive at the point at which decisions about client care can be made.

Because the nursing process is a dynamic, circular, and fluid process, decisions must be made at many points as the nurse implements the various steps. Each of these decisions, resulting from critical thought and problem-solving strategies, leads to the determination of appropriate nursing interventions for the client.

THE NURSING PROCESS AND HOLISTIC CARE

Nurses bring to each client situation a broad knowledge base. The theoretical base of nursing knowledge comes from many different fields, including the natural sciences, behavioral sciences, social sciences, arts and humanities, and nursing science. This broad knowledge base allows the nurse to interact with the client from a holistic viewpoint. Each nurse–client interaction adds to the client database and allows for individualized planning and care. The nursing process assists the nurse in determining client responses to situations, and critical-thinking and decision-making skills allow the nurse to prioritize client needs and decide which person can best meet certain client needs. Referral and collaboration among nurses and other health care professionals contribute to optimal achievement of client goals.

In some settings, the traditional nursing care plan formulated solely by nurses has been replaced by plans that are developed by a multidisciplinary team and referred to as critical pathways. **Critical pathways** are comprehensive, standard plans of care for specific case situations. Included in these plans are nursing interventions, medical interventions, interventions from other team members, specific client outcomes, and time lines for those outcomes. Because the nurse has a broad base of knowledge, the nurse is often the person who manages the care of the client through these critical pathways.

SUMMARY

- The nursing process is an organized method of planning and delivering nursing care. It is composed of five steps: assessment, diagnosis, planning and outcome identification, implementation, and evaluation.
- The nurse uses the process of assessment to establish a database about the client, to form an interpersonal relationship with the client, and to provide the client with an opportunity to discuss health care concerns.
- The second step in the nursing process involves further analysis and synthesis of the data and results in a list of nursing diagnoses.
- Nursing diagnoses contribute to a clearer conceptualization of knowledge unique to nursing, improved communication among nurses and other health care professionals, and promotion of individualized client care.
- The types of nursing diagnoses are actual, risk, and wellness.

CASE STUDY

Mr. Jona is a client on your unit. A 70-year-old widower, he was admitted 2 days ago with a broken left hip. While bowling with his church bowling league, Mr. Jona tripped, fell, fractured his hip, and sprained his right wrist. He recently retired from an administrative position with a large company and moved to Florida from his home in Iowa. He has two children: one son who lives in Shumak, Washington, and a daughter who lives in Ono, New York. Mr. Jona lives alone in a one-bedroom apartment approximately 10 blocks from the hospital. In 4 days, Mr. Jona will be discharged and referred to the home health division for follow-up care.

The following questions will guide your development of a nursing care plan for the case study.

1. What assessments must be done with regard to Mr. Jona's going home?
2. Which three nursing diagnoses may apply to Mr. Jona?
3. What goals and outcomes may be appropriate for Mr. Jona?
4. What nursing interventions may be appropriate to meet the goals?

- Planning and outcome identification, the third step in the nursing process, involves prioritizing nursing diagnoses, identifying and writing goals and client outcomes, developing nursing interventions, and recording the plan of care in the client's record.
- The nursing care plan documents health care needs, coordinates nursing care, promotes continuity of care, encourages communication among health care team members, and promotes quality nursing care.
- The implementation step of the nursing process is directed toward meeting client needs, resulting in health promotion, prevention of illness, illness management, or health restoration.
- Interventions can be nurse initiated, physician initiated, or collaborative in origin and, thus, are considered independent, dependent, or interdependent.
- Evaluation, the fifth step in the nursing process, measures the effectiveness of nursing interventions by the examination of the goals and expected outcomes, which provide direction for the plan of care and serve as standards against which the client's progress is measured.
- Critical-thinking, problem-solving, and decision-making skills are important in the use of the nursing process.

Review Questions

1. Mrs. Rose was admitted to your unit 2 hours ago. The following data are recorded on her chart. Which data are objective?

   a. Temperature 102°F
   b. Nausea
   c. Headache
   d. Pain in abdomen

2. Which of the following statements would describe the nursing process?

   a. It is a linear, static procedure.
   b. It is a circular, dynamic process.
   c. It is a hierarchy of steps to plan client care.
   d. It is a long, detailed form to be filled out for each client.

3. The nursing care plan includes:

   a. collected documentation of all team members providing care for the client.
   b. physician orders, demographic data, and medication administration and rationales.
   c. client's nursing diagnoses, goals, expected outcomes, and the nursing interventions.
   d. client assessment data, medical treatment regimen and rationales, and diagnostic test results and significance.

4. When establishing priorities of a client's plan of nursing care, the nurse should rank life-threatening diagnoses as the highest priorities and which as the lowest priorities?

   a. Safety-related needs
   b. Client needs regarding referral agencies
   c. The client's social, love, and belonging needs
   d. Needs of family members and friends who are involved in plan of care

5. What are the essential components of an expected outcome?

   a. Nursing diagnosis, interventions, and expected client behavior
   b. Target date, nursing action, measurement criteria, and desired client behavior
   c. Nursing client behavior, target date, and conditions under which the behavior occurs
   d. Client behavior, measurement criteria, conditions under which the behavior occurs, and target date

6. Which guideline is most appropriate when developing nursing interventions?

   a. Make intervention statements specific to ensure continuity of care
   b. Choose actions that a nurse can perform without leaving the unit or consulting with medical staff
   c. Make sure that nursing care activities receive priority over other aspects of the treatment regimen
   d. Write interventions in general terms to allow maximum flexibility and creativity in delivering nursing care

Critical Thinking Questions

1. How are goals and outcomes different?

2. Differentiate between the three categories of nursing interventions: independent, interdependent, and dependent.

⚡ WEB FLASH!

- Can you find specific sites or resources dealing with the nursing process?
- Do the resources listed for this chapter also have Web sites? What types of information do they provide?
- What resources on the Internet are available for nurses needing assistance with the nursing process or nursing diagnosis?

DOCUMENTATION

MAKING THE CONNECTION

Refer to the following chapters to increase your understanding of documentation:

- **Chapter 6, Legal Responsibilities**
- **Chapter 8, Communication**
- **Chapter 9, Nursing Process**

LEARNING OBJECTIVES

Upon completion of this chapter, you should be able to:
- *Define key terms.*
- *Explain the purposes of documentation in health care.*
- *Discuss the principles of effective documentation.*
- *Describe various methods of documentation.*
- *Recount various types of documentation records.*
- *Delineate the latest advances in computerized documentation.*

KEY TERMS

charting by exception (CBE)
critical pathway
documentation
focus charting
incident report
Kardex
narrative charting
Nursing Intervention Classification (NIC)
Nursing Outcome Classification (NOC)
Nursing Minimum Data Set (NMDS)
PIE charting
point-of-care charting
problem-oriented medical record
SOAP charting
source-oriented charting
variations
walking rounds

INTRODUCTION

Throughout the development of modern nursing, multiple documentation systems have emerged in response to changes in health care delivery. Systems of recording and reporting data pertinent to the care of clients have evolved primarily in response to the demand that health care practitioners be held to societal norms, professional standards of practice, legal and regulatory standards, and institutional policies and standards.

As with all facets of health care, advanced technology has affected the expectations for documentation. Activities in the areas of quality improvement and cost containment have also increased the demands on health care practitioners to create efficient documentation systems. Efficiency is measured in terms of time, thoroughness, and the quality of the observations being recorded. The documentation systems used today reflect the specific needs and preferences of the numerous health care agencies. Select systems and their ramifications are discussed in this chapter.

DOCUMENTATION AS COMMUNICATION

Communication is a dynamic, continuous, and multidimensional process for sharing information as determined by standards or policies. Reporting and recording are the major communication techniques used by health care providers in directing client-based decision making and continuity of care. The medical record serves as a legal document for recording all client activities initiated by all health care practitioners.

Documentation Defined

Documentation is defined as written evidence of:

- The interactions between and among health professionals, clients, their families, and health care organizations;
- The administration of tests, procedures, treatments, and client education; and
- The results of, or client's response to, diagnostic tests and interventions (Eggland & Heinemann, 1994).

Documentation provides written records that reflect client care provided on the basis of assessment data and the client's response to interventions.

In implementing the nursing process, nurses rely on the documentation tools of client charts and other documents that facilitate a logical sequencing of events. All the tools used by nurses to record their nursing care should form a system. Systematic documentation is critical because it presents the care administered by nurses in a logical fashion, as follows:

- Assessment data, obtained through interview, observation, and physical examination, identify the client's specific alteration and lay the foundation for the nursing care plan.
- The identified alteration in functional health pattern directs the formulation of a nursing diagnosis.
- The nursing diagnoses trigger the client's expected outcomes (both short- and long-term goals) and accompanying supportive nursing interventions—the planning and implementation phases.
- The effectiveness of the nursing interventions in achieving the client's expected outcomes becomes the criterion for evaluation, determining the need for subsequent reassessment and revision of the plan of care (Eggland & Heinemann, 1994; Iyer & Camp, 1995).

The system becomes a vehicle for expressing each phase of the nursing process. Nurses rely on systems that provide thorough, accurate charting reflective of the nurse's decision-making ability and the client's plan of care. The nurse's critical-thinking skills, judgments, and evaluations must be clearly communicated through proper documentation.

Purposes of Health Care Documentation

Professional responsibility and accountability are two primary reasons for documentation. Other reasons to document include communication; education; research; satisfaction of legal and practice standards; and reimbursement. The professional responsibility of all health care practitioners, documentation provides written evidence of the practitioner's accountability to the client, the institution, the profession, and society.

Communication

Documentation is a communication method that confirms the care provided to the client and clearly outlines all important information regarding the client. Thorough documentation provides:

- Accurate data needed to plan the client's care and to ensure continuity of care;
- A method of communication among the health care team members responsible for the client's care;
- Written evidence of those things done for the client, the client's response, and any revisions made in the plan of care;
- Evidence of compliance with professional practice standards (e.g., those of the American Nurses Association [ANA]);
- Evidence of compliance with accreditation criteria (e.g., those of the Joint Commission on Accreditation of Healthcare Organizations [JCAHO]);
- A resource for review, audit, reimbursement, education, and research; and
- A written legal record to protect the client, institution, and practitioner.

The client's medical record contains documents for record keeping. The type of document that constitutes the medical record in a given health care institution is determined by that institution. Throughout this chapter, various types of medical record documents are referenced. Table 10-1 outlines the content of these documents.

Education

The documentation contained in the client's medical record is used for the purpose of education. Health care students can use the medical record as a tool to learn about disease processes, complications, medical and nursing diagnoses, and interventions. The results from physical examinations and laboratory and diagnostic testing provide valuable information regarding specific diagnoses and interventions.

Nursing students can enhance their critical-thinking skills by examining the records in chronological order, analyzing the results, and following the health care team's plan of care, including the way it was developed, implemented, and evaluated. Students and all health care professionals must be aware of confidentiality issues before reading any client's chart; these issues are discussed later in the chapter.

Research

Researchers rely heavily on the client's medical record as a clinical data source to determine whether clients meet the research criteria for a study. Documentation also can direct the need for research. For example, if documentation demonstrates an increased infection rate in association with intravenous catheters,

Table 10-1 MEDICAL RECORD DOCUMENTS

DOCUMENT	INFORMATION
Face sheet	Lists biographical data (name, date of birth, address, phone number, Social Security number, marital status, employment, race, gender, religion, closest relative); insurance coverage, allergies, attending physician, admitting medical diagnosis, assigned diagnosis-related group (DRG), statement of whether the client has an advance directive
Consent form	Admit: gives the institution and physician the permission to treat. Surgery: explains the reason for the operation in lay terms; the risks for complications; and the client's level of understanding Blood transfusion: grants permission to administer blood or blood products Various others: grant permission to participate in research, have photograph taken, know HIV status
Medical history and physical examination	Details results of the client's initial history and physical assessment as performed by the physician
Physician's order sheet	Outlines medical orders to admit; the treatment plan
Physician's progress notes	Delineates physician's evaluation of the client's response to treatment; may also contain the progress recording of other practitioners, e.g., dietary or social services
Consultation sheet	Initiated by the physician to request the evaluation or services of other practitioners
Diagnostic results	Contains the results from laboratory and diagnostic tests, e.g., x-ray, hematology
Nursing admit assessment	Records data obtained from the interview and physical assessment conducted by the nurse
Nursing plan of care	Contains the treatment plan, e.g., nursing diagnosis or a problem list, initiation of standards of care, or protocols
Graphic sheet	Lists data related to vital signs and weight
Flow sheet	Contains all routine interventions that can be indicated via a check mark or other simple code; allows for a quick comparison of measurements
Nurse's progress notes	Details additional data that do not duplicate information on the flow sheet, e.g., client's achievement of expected outcome, revision of the plan of care
Medication administration record (MAR)	Contains all medication information for routine and prn (as needed) drugs: date, time, dose, route, site (for injections)
Client education record	Records both the nurses' educational efforts directed toward the client, family, or other caregiver and the learner's response
Health care team record	Serves as the treatment and progress record for nonmedical and nonnursing practitioners (e.g., respiratory, physical therapy, dietary) when the physician's progress notes are not used by those practitioners
Critical pathway	A multidisciplinary form for each day of anticipated hospitalization; identifies the interventions and achievement of client outcomes; in the progress notes, explains the practitioner's initial implementation and the variances from the norm
Discharge plan and summary	A multidisciplinary form used before discharge from a health care facility; contains a brief summary of care rendered and of discharge instructions (e.g., food–drug interactions, referrals or follow-up appointments)
Advance directive or living will	Federal law requires that health care providers discuss with the client the use of advance directives, a living will, or a durable power of attorney. Most states recognize the living will as a legal document. If the client has advance directives, they are reviewed at the time of admission and placed in the medical record.

Adapted from Fundamentals of Nursing: Standards & Practice, *by S. DeLaune and P. Ladner, 1998, Albany, NY: Delmar Publishers. Copyright 1998 by Delmar Publishers. Adapted with permission.*

researchers can identify and study the variables that may be associated with the increased infection rate.

Legal and Practice Standards

"Failure to document appropriately is a key factor in clinical mishaps and a pivotal issue in many malpractice cases" (Springhouse, 1995). The client's medical record is a legal document, and in the case of a lawsuit, it is the record that serves as the description of exactly what happened to a client. In 80% to 85% of malpractice lawsuits involving client care, the medical record is the determining factor in providing proof of significant events (Iyer & Camp, 1999). The legal issues of documentation require:

- Legible and neat writing,
- Proper use of spelling and grammar,
- Use of authorized abbreviations, and
- Factual and time-sequenced descriptive notations.

To focus attention on the importance of communicating and documenting all information, Fiesta (1991) cites *Ramsey v. Physician Memorial Hospital.* An emergency room nurse failed to communicate to the physician that the mother of two pediatric clients had found a tick on one of the two children. One of the children later died from Rocky Mountain spotted fever. The physician had questioned the health team about ticks because of the children's elevated temperature, but was told nothing. The court dismissed the hospital from liability, but the appeal court held the hospital liable because the nurse had failed to communicate to the physician the information obtained from the mother about the tick.

The nurse is responsible for documenting on the chart both that the physician was notified and the significant information that was orally communicated. If the physician does not respond in a way that indicates an understanding of the urgency of the information, the nurse must document the physician's response and notify the supervisor of the situation. Nurses are responsible for the care the client receives and can be held liable if appropriate interventions are not imple-

PROFESSIONAL TIP

The Importance of Communication
Important information obtained from an assessment and warranting immediate intervention should not only be documented in the medical record but also communicated orally to those other practitioners involved in the client's care. The element of time must direct decision making when critical information is obtained.

PROFESSIONAL TIP

Consent from Sedated Clients
Sedated clients should never be requested or allowed to sign an informed consent. Because the client may not be capable of understanding the nature of and risks associated with the procedure, the consent will be invalid, and the nurse and institution will be at legal risk. Instead, either wait for the client to be competent and free of sedation (usually, 4 hours after administration of the last medication that alters the level of consciousness) or have a legally acceptable family member brought into the decision.

mented in a timely manner when information is available that would dictate otherwise.

Informed Consent Informed consent is a competent client's ability to make health care decisions based on full disclosure of the benefits, risks, and potential consequences of a recommended treatment plan and of alternative treatments, including no treatment, and the client's agreement to the treatment as indicated by the client's signing a consent form. Although the physician who is to perform the procedure is responsible for obtaining the client's informed consent, the nurse is often the person who actually has the client sign the form.

Advance Directives An advance directive (i.e., living will and durable power of attorney for health care) is written instructions about an individual's health care preferences regarding life-sustaining measures that guides family members and health care professionals as to those treatment options that should or should not be considered in the event that the individual is unable to decide for herself. This effectively allows clients, while competent, to participate in end-of-life decisions and to choose the types of life-sustaining procedures they wish to be performed.

State Nursing Practice Acts In an attempt to recognize and control the practice of nursing, nursing practice acts, on a state-by-state basis, establish guidelines to ensure safe practice and to demonstrate accountability to society. The standards of care, as set forth in the practice acts, are based on the phases of the nursing process and require compliance as evidenced in documentation. Nurses should be familiar with the practice act of the state in which they work.

Joint Commission on Accreditation of Healthcare Organizations The JCAHO surveys health care facilities to measure compliance with its standards for safe health care provision. Although facilities voluntarily submit to this accreditation process, reimbursement eligibility for Medicare, Medicaid, and private funding is dependent on JCAHO accreditation.

The JCAHO no longer requires that health care organizations have traditional nursing care plans, but documentation of an individualized plan of care must be evident for each client (JCAHO, 1998). The JCAHO's standards require:

- The involvement of the client or family in the development of the plan, which must be documented in the medical record, and
- Interdisciplinary planning and implementation of all aspects of care.

The use of interdisciplinary tools has proved an effective approach to documenting client and family education for agencies not yet using critical pathways (discussed later in the chapter). By complying with JCAHO's client and family teaching standards, one medical center, through the use of an interdisciplinary record, increased its education documentation rate from 30% to 84% (Tucker, 1995).

During the accreditation survey (or process), the reviewer looks for evidence of an organized and systematic method of monitoring and evaluating client care as reflected through documentation in the medical record. Documenting the steps of the nursing process ensures compliance with JCAHO's plan of care requirements.

Reimbursement

Peer review organizations (PROs), consisting of physicians and nurses, are required by the federal government to monitor and evaluate the quality and appropriateness of care provided. Medical record documentation is the mechanism for the PRO review, which evaluates the intensity of services and the severity of illness on the basis of a comparison of sample medical records from different facilities against specific screening criteria.

The federal enactment of the diagnosis-related group (DRG) classification system changed the health care provider reimbursement process from a cost-per-case to a prospective payment system (PPS). With PPS, the medical record must provide documentation that supports the DRG and the appropriateness of care. Nursing documentation must also show evidence of client and family education and discharge planning.

From a hospital's perspective, when information in the medical record demonstrates compliance with Medicare and Medicaid standards, the reimbursement is maximized. If nurses fail to document the equipment or procedures used daily (e.g., feeding pump; daily weight, intake and output; intravenous therapy; drug additives), reimbursement to the facility can be denied.

Another federal law, the Comprehensive Omnibus Budget Reconciliation Act (COBRA), allows employees to temporarily carry their employer-provided health insurance benefits for 90 days after termination, reduc-

HOME HEALTH CARE

Documentation

Home health agencies also keep documents: physician orders, history and physical form, home care team records, and nursing records (initial assessment form, plan of care, problem list for daily progress notes, client teaching activities, and discharge summary). Home health care providers are required to comply with state and federal regulations that affect health care, documentation, and reimbursement.

tion in the work hours, or retirement. The law requires that for any COBRA client receiving care in an emergency room, the client's condition must be stabilized before the client can be transferred to another facility. If the client's condition is not stable, the institution cannot initiate a transfer.

Facilities in violation of COBRA laws are fined and stand to lose their eligibility for Medicare and Medicaid funding. Compliance with this law is evaluated through medical record review. The documentation concerning client transfers must include:

- Chronology of the event,
- Measures taken or treatment implemented,
- The client's response to treatment, and
- Results of measures taken to prevent the client's condition from deteriorating.

PRINCIPLES OF EFFECTIVE DOCUMENTATION

Documentation requirements differ depending on the health care facility (hospital, nursing home, home health agency), the setting within the facility (e.g., emergency room, perioperative unit, medical–surgical unit), and the specific client population (e.g., obstetric, pediatric, geriatric). Regardless of the client care administered, the documentation of that care must reflect the nursing process. General documentation guidelines are listed in Table 10-2.

PROFESSIONAL TIP

Chart Following the Nursing Process

Charting in accordance with the nursing process ensures thorough documentation in compliance with nursing practice acts and with reimbursement and accreditation criteria.

Table 10-2 GENERAL DOCUMENTATION GUIDELINES

- Ensure that you have the correct client record or chart and that the client's name and identifying information are on every page of the record.
- Document as soon as the client encounter is concluded to ensure accurate recall of data (follow institutional guidelines on frequency of charting).
- Date and time each entry.
- Sign each entry with your full legal name and with your professional credentials, or per your institutional policy.
- Do not leave space between entries.
- If an error is made while documenting, use a single line to cross out the error, then date, time, and sign the correction (follow institutional policy); avoid erasing, crossing out, or using correction fluid (Figure 10-1).
- Never change another person's entry, even if it is incorrect.
- The first entry of the shift should be made early (e.g., at 7:30 A.M. for the 7–3 shift, as opposed to 11:30 A.M. or 12 P.M.). Chart at least every 2 hours, or per institutional policy.
- Use quotation marks to indicate direct client responses (e.g., "I feel lousy").
- Document in chronological order; if chronological order is not used, state why.
- Write legibly.
- Use a permanent-ink pen (black is usually preferable because it photocopies well).
- Document in a complete but concise manner by using phrases and abbreviations as appropriate.
- Document all telephone calls that you make or receive that are related to a client's case.

Adapted from Health Assessment & Physical Examination *by M. E. Z. Estes, 1998, Albany, NY: Delmar Publishers. Copyright 1998 by Delmar Publishers. Adapted with permission.*

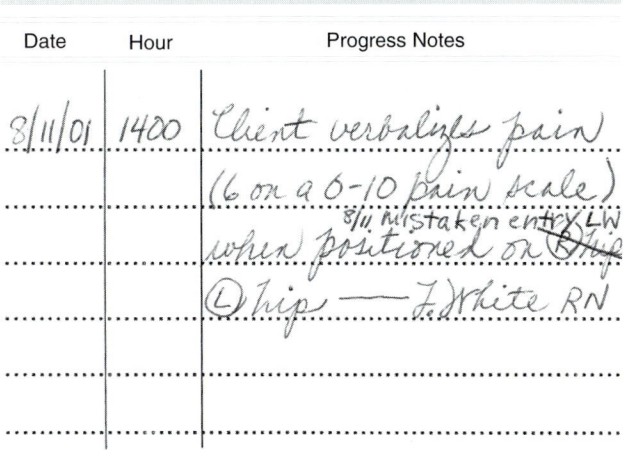

Figure 10-1 Correcting a Documentation Error

Nursing notes must be logical, focused, and relevant to care, and the outcomes must represent each phase in the nursing process (Simmons & Meadors, 1995; Thompson, 1995). Nursing documentation based on the nursing process facilitates effective care because client needs can be traced from assessment, through the identification of the problems, to the care plan, implementation, and evaluation. A brief outline of the elements of the nursing process as they relate to documentation follows:

- *Assessment:* Assessment data related to an actual or potential health care need are summarized without duplication. With reassessment, any new findings or any changes in the client's condition (e.g., increased pain) are highlighted.
- *Nursing diagnosis:* NANDA terminology to identify the client's problem or need.
- *Planning and outcome identification:* The expected outcomes and goals of client care as discussed with

the client and communicated to members of the multidisciplinary team should be documented on the care plan or critical pathway rather than in the progress notes.

- *Implementation:* After an intervention has been performed, observations, treatments, teaching, and related clinical judgments should be documented on the flow sheet and progress notes. Client teaching should include learning needs, teaching plan content, methods of teaching, who was taught, and the client's response.
- *Evaluation:* The effectiveness of the interventions in terms of the expected outcomes is evaluated and documented: progress toward goals; client response to tests, treatments, and nursing interventions; client and family response to teaching and significant events; questions, statements, or complaints voiced by the client or family.
- *Revisions of planned care:* The reasons for the revisions along with the supporting evidence and client agreement are documented.

Elements of Effective Documentation

Several factors are important in producing effective documentation. To ensure effective documentation, nurses should:

- Use a common vocabulary,
- Write legibly and neatly,
- Use only authorized abbreviations and symbols,
- Employ factual and time-sequenced organization, and
- Document accurately and completely, including any errors that occurred.

PROFESSIONAL TIP

Abbreviations

Avoid abbreviations that can be misunderstood (Figure 10-2). For example, what does the abbreviation *Pt* mean? Does it refer to the patient, prothrombin time, physical therapy, or part-time? Refer to your institution's approved abbreviations listing.

The following discussion of effective charting refers to all nursing documents, such as flow sheet, progress notes, and so on. An entry should be made in nursing documents when:

- The client's condition changes,
- The client's response to an intervention or expected outcome is measured, or
- The client or family voices a complaint.

Use of Common Vocabulary

During the past decade, nurse researchers have observed inadequacies in the clinical record that prevent data collection and comparison among large groups of clients. One such inadequacy relates to the vocabulary used. Documented clinical data cannot be correlated without a common vocabulary for addressing client outcomes related to specific nursing interventions (McCloskey & Bulechek, 1994). Nursing practice reflects the use of multiple terms for nursing interventions, thus preventing cross-institutional comparisons of nursing care. Current efforts to establish a taxonomy for nursing interventions determined by specific nursing diagnoses will both enhance the quality of documentation and support the efforts of researchers. Use of a common vocabulary will also improve intrateam communication and lessen the chance of misunderstandings.

Legibility

Whatever is charted must be easily readable, without any chance of error in interpretation due to poor penmanship.

Abbreviations and Symbols

Facilities usually have a list of abbreviations and symbols that is approved by the Medical Records Committee for use in documenting information in the client's record. The nurse should always refer to the facility's approved listing (see Appendix B).

Organization

Every entry should start with the date and time. Charting should be done in chronological order: assess-

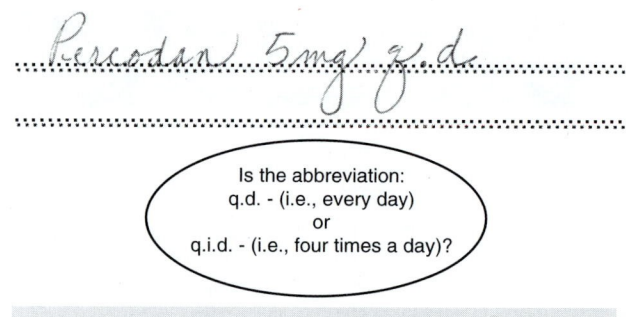

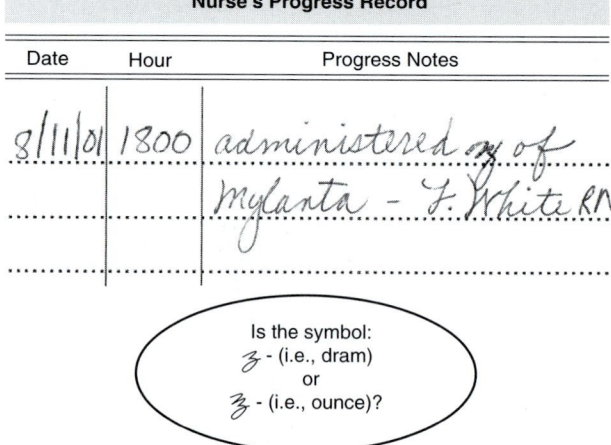

Figure 10-2 Misleading Abbreviation and Symbol

ment data, observation, intervention, and evaluation (Figure 10-3). The nurse should comply with the time frame indicated in the facility's guidelines for documentation, for example, the frequency of charting observations for a client with restraints or the time frame within which the admit assessment must be completed.

Charting should be done in a timely fashion to prevent omission of pertinent data. It is never good practice to wait until the end of the shift to chart on all clients. Should a client's condition suddenly deteriorate and documentation has not been performed during the shift, the nurse may forget to record a pertinent piece of information that may later become a legal issue. To prevent errors, the nurse should chart medications immediately after administration. The nurse should also sign her name after each entry.

When the nurse forgets to document significant data, it is appropriate and advisable to include these data at a later date (Fiesta, 1991). Examples of situations possibly necessitating late entries include the following:

- The chart was not available (e.g., the chart was with the client in special procedures lab).
- Entries had to be added after notes were completed.
- Information was documented on the wrong record.

As with other aspects of documentation, the nurse should follow the facility's policy for charting a late

Nurse's Progress Record

Date	Hour	Progress Notes
8/11/01	1730	Client reports a burning pain (5 on a 0-10 pain scale) in URQ, leaning forward; burning pain R/T gastric secretion reflux; admin. Mylanta 30 cc P.O. PRN as ordered; head of bed elevated 45°. —— F. White RN ——
8/11/01	1815	Client states burning pain 2 (on a 0-10 pain scale) — F. White RN

Figure 10-3 Charting a prn Medication

entry. Common practice is to enter the date and time and to notate "Late entry" to indicate that the entry is out of sequence. Then the date and time the entry should have been made is recorded in the body of the entry, as shown in Figure 10-4.

Nurse's Progress Record

Date	Hour	Progress Notes
8/11/01	2000	Late entry (8/11/01 - 1730) ⟵ *Time the entry should have been made* — Client stated "I received an upsetting phone call from my daughter 30" ago." —— F. White RN

Figure 10-4 Charting a Late Entry

Accuracy

"Accuracy is crucial if the documentation is to be useful either clinically or for research" (Hayes, Norris, Martin, & Androwich, 1994). Factual, descriptive terms must be used to chart exactly those things that were observed or done. For example, an entry reading "wound is 2.5 cm by 1.0 cm" is more accurate than is "wound appears the same." Likewise, "foul-smelling, yellowish drainage completely soaked two 4 × 4s in 20 minutes" is clearly more accurate than "large amount of drainage."

Correct spelling and grammar and complete sentences (following institutional policy) should be used. The nurse should differentiate who did what, for example, "Dr. Diaz inserted a triple-lumen, 20-gauge catheter into the right subclavian vein." To maintain continuity of care, the nurse should read the notes recorded by nurses on previous shifts and document the client's current status in the areas previously documented.

Documenting a Medication Error

Facilities require nurses to report medication errors on incident reports (discussed later in this chapter). The medication given in error should appear on the MAR and in the nurses' progress notes. It should be remembered that the purpose of the medical record is to report any care or treatment the client receives, including any errors made. However, no mention is made of an incident report being completed.

When a medication error occurs, the following should be done (Grane, 1995):

- The medication should be charted on the MAR to prevent other caregivers from giving the client additional doses of the same drug, doses of similar drugs, or doses of drugs that may be contraindicated.
- The error should be documented in the nurses' notes as follows: name and dosage of the medication; time it was given; client's response to the medication; name of the practitioner who was notified of the error; time of the notification; nursing interventions or medical treatment to counteract the error; and client's response to treatment.

METHODS OF DOCUMENTATION

Documentation must reflect the complexity of care and must embody accuracy, completeness, and evidence of professional practice. The clinical standards (structure, outcome, process, and evaluation) are used to develop a system that complies with legal, accreditation, and professional practice requirements of documentation.

Among the many methods used for documentation are the following:

- Narrative charting
- Source-oriented charting
- Problem-oriented charting
- PIE charting
- Focus charting
- Charting by exception
- Computerized documentation
- Critical pathways

Narrative Charting

Narrative charting, the traditional method of nursing documentation, takes the form of a story written in paragraphs and describing the client's status, interventions and treatments, and the client's response to treatments. Before the advent of flow sheets, this was the only method for documenting care.

Narrative documentation is easy to use in emergency situations, wherein a simple, chronological order is needed. With this type of documentation, however, subjectivity is a common problem, and analysis and critical decision making on the part of the nurse tend to be lacking. Narrative charting is now being replaced by other formats because:

- The flow of care is disorganized. It is difficult to show a relationship between data and critical-thinking skills. Each nurse writes in a unique style, making continuity of care difficult to identify.
- It fails to reflect the nursing process. The focus is on tasks rather than on assessment data or progress toward achievement of outcomes.
- It is time consuming. Because the paragraphs are free flowing, it takes more time both to accurately record information and to read information recorded by others.
- The information is difficult to retrieve, and because the same problems may not be addressed from shift to shift, it is difficult to track the client's progress.

Source-Oriented Charting

Source-oriented charting is described as a narrative recording by each member (source) of the health care team on separate records. Because each discipline uses a separate record, care is often fragmented, and communication between disciplines is time-consuming. Source-oriented charting has similar advantages and disadvantages to narrative charting, because both methods take an unstructured approach to documenting in the progress notes.

Problem-Oriented Charting

Problem-oriented medical record (POMR) focuses on the client's problem and employs a structured, logical format called **SOAP charting**:

- S: subjective data (what the client states)
- O: objective data (what is observed/inspected)
- A: assessment (conclusion reached on the basis of data)
- P: plan (actions to be taken)

SOAPIE and SOAPIER refer to formats that add the following:

- I: implementation
- E: evaluation
- R: revision

Figure 10–5 shows an example of SOAPIE charting. Some physicians use this format when writing progress notes.

There are four critical components of POMR/POR:

- Database (assessment data)
- Problem list (client's problems labeled as acute, chronic, active, or inactive)
- Initial plan (outline of goals, expected outcomes, and learning needs)
- Progress notes (charting based on the SOAP, SOAPIE, or SOAPIER format)

PIE Charting

After SOAP charting gained popularity, the problem, intervention, evaluation **(PIE) charting** system evolved to streamline documentation. The key components of this system are assessment flow sheets, nurses' progress notes, and an integrated plan of care. Figure 10-6 shows an example of PIE charting. This system eliminates the traditional care plan by incorporating an ongoing plan of care (problem, intervention, evaluation) into the daily documentation.

Focus Charting

Focus charting is a documentation method that uses a column format to chart data, action, and response (DAR). The column format of focus charting is used within the progress notes to distinguish the entry from other recordings in the narrative notes, as shown in Figure 10-7, page 173.

Charting by Exception

Charting by exception (CBE) is a documentation method that requires the nurse to document only deviations from preestablished norms. The CBE system has three key components:

- Flow sheets: highlight significant findings and define assessment parameters and findings
- Reference documentation: related to the standards of nursing practice
- Bedside accessibility: related to the documentation forms (Burke & Murphy, 1995)

Nurse's Progress Record		
Date	Hour	Progress Notes

Date	Hour	Progress Notes
10/14/01	0730	Problem #2 Ketoacidosis
		S: Client states "I feel sick all over." Client claims difficulty in breathing, abdominal pain + nausea.
		O: Lungs clear, R 38/min, labored. Abdomen distended, bowel sounds underactive all 4 quadrants. Abdominal pain 5 on a 0-10 pain scale.
		A: Alteration in nutrition + comfort R/T keto-acidosis. Blood glucose 458 mg/dl. Ketones strongly positive. pH < 7.3.
		P: Maintain IV infusion of 0.9% NS c̄ regular insulin as ordered. NPO. Oral hygiene hrly. Maintain accurate I+O. Assess for rales, hypotension, cardiac dysrhythmias. Monitor blood glucose electrolytes. — L. White RN

Date	Hour	Progress Notes
10/14/01	0730	**I:** Called Dr. Singh, blood glucose 458 mg/dl IV bolus regular insulin given as ordered. 1000 ml 0.9% N.S. infusing @ 17/H central line #1 via infusion pump. 50u regular insulin in 500 ml N.S. infusing @ 50ml/H central line #2 via infusion pump. EKG taken, placed on telemetry.
10/14/01	0835	**E:** Lungs clear, R 24/min, non-labored. NSR abdominal pain 3 on a 0-10 pain scale. Urinary output 750ml hr. Blood glucose 360 mg/dl. — L. White RN

Figure 10-5 Sample SOAPIE Charting

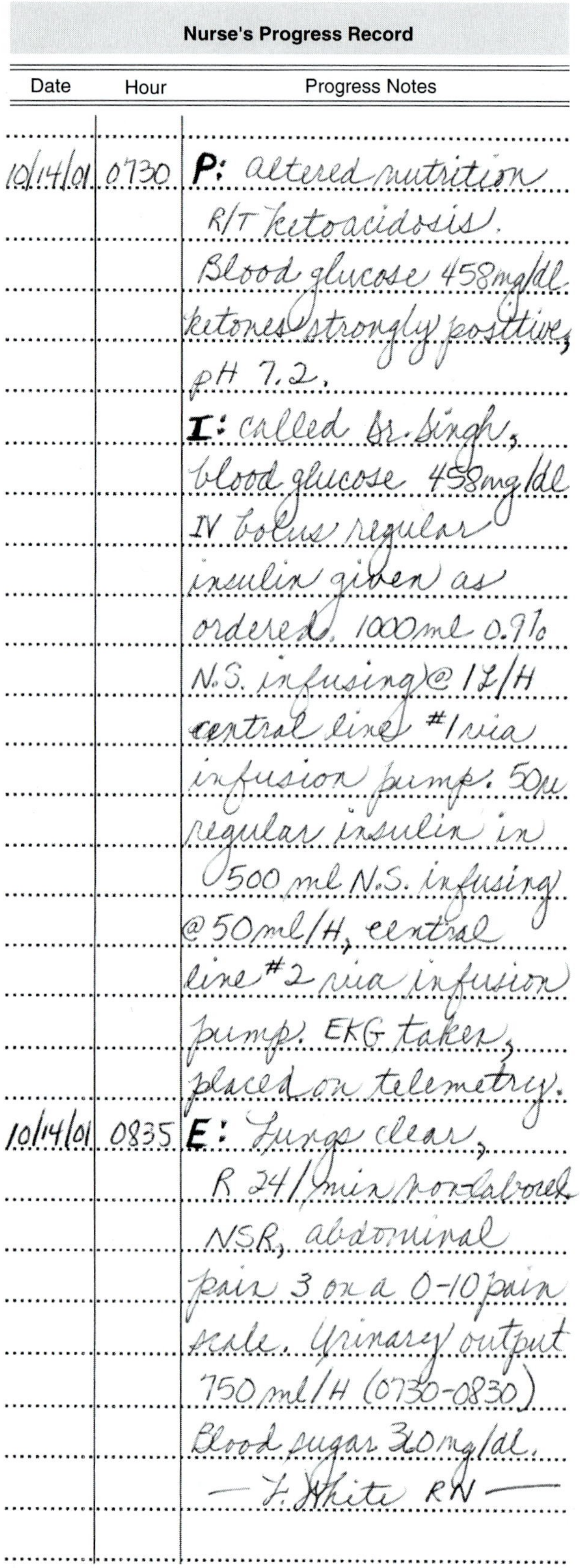

Nurse's Progress Record		
Date	Hour	Progress Notes
10/14/01	0730	**P:** altered nutrition R/T ketoacidosis. Blood glucose 458mg/dl. ketones strongly positive, pH 7.2. **I:** called Dr. Singh, blood glucose 458mg/dl IV bolus regular insulin given as ordered. 1000ml 0.9% N.S. infusing @ 1L/H central line #1 via infusion pump. 50u regular insulin in 500 ml N.S. infusing @50ml/H, central line #2 via infusion pump. EKG taken, placed on telemetry.
10/14/01	0835	**E:** Lungs clear, R 24/min nonlabored NSR, abdominal pain 3 on a 0-10 pain scale. Urinary output 750 ml/H (0730-0830) Blood sugar 320mg/dl. ─ T. White RN ─

Figure 10-6 Sample PIE Charting

Computerized Documentation

In response to the large demand for clinical, administrative, and regulatory information in today's health care system, nurse leaders are working to develop computerized records. The resultant nursing information systems (NIS) will complement existing hospital information systems (HIS). These NIS will collect, store, process, retrieve, display, and communicate timely information. Health care facilities work in collaboration with producers of computer software to design medical record documents that complement existing documentation systems.

Computerized documentation enhances the systematic approach to client care with standardized protocols, teaching documents, data management, and communication. The practical advantages to staff nurses are as follows:

- Decreased documentation time: Data entry needs to be done only once; the system eliminates duplication of effort. For example, a physician's medication order goes immediately to the pharmacy, eliminating the need to transcribe and transmit orders; the pharmacy receives the order and the client's MAR is immediately updated.
- Increased legibility and accuracy: A computer printout is easy to read and legible. Accuracy is achieved through standardized documents that prompt the nurse for information, making the charting more complete, thorough, concise, and organized. For example, the fall-prevention standard is automatically initiated for all high-risk clients. Bedside terminals allow for client care data to be entered in a timely fashion.
- Clear, decisive, and concise key words: Standardized nursing terminology provides for consistency in key words (e.g., "alert") and eliminates ambiguous phraseology (e.g., "appears to be").
- Statistical analysis of data.
- Enhanced implementation of the nursing process: Documentation tools provide an individualized plan of care (admission and nursing history data, diagnoses, goals, measurable outcomes, and interventions, inclusive of client teaching).
- Enhanced decision making: Quick electronic access to other data, such as laboratory results, facilitates correlation of that data with the nurses' assessment data. If a trend is developing (e.g., decreasing levels of oxygenation), the nurse will recognize it quickly.
- Multidisciplinary networking: Information is quickly coordinated and integrated by other departments; all departments have access to the data.

Disadvantages associated with computerized documentation include high installation cost, which limits the number of terminals at nursing stations; slow processing speed at peak usage times; and downtime

(time for routine servicing or sudden unexpected failure). Further, practitioners are often reluctant to change from the familiar "pen-and-paper" methods to high-tech electronic systems.

A series of legal issues has emerged in relation to computerized documentation: problems in protecting client confidentiality; sharing of access codes (passwords); determining who should have access to the clinical database and how it should be used. Computerized software can be designed to record all transactions, thus permitting the identification of all staff members who request sensitive information.

Point-of-Care Charting

Point-of-care charting is a computerized documentation system that allows health care providers to gain

Nurse's Progress Record			
Date	Hour	Focus	Progress Notes
10/14/01	0730	Altered nutrition R/T ketoacidosis	**D:** Client experiencing labored breathing, abdominal pain, 5 on a 0-10 pain scale, & nausea. Blood sugar 458 mg/dl; ketones strongly positive; pH 7.2. T 99.8, R 28, P 110, B/P 100/56. **A:** Auscultation reveals lungs clear + underactive bowel sounds in all 4 quadrants. Abdomen distended. Dr. Singh notified of blood glucose, ketones, & pH. IV bolus of regular insulin given as ordered. IVs infusing as ordered through central lines c̄ infusion pumps. STAT EKG done, telemetry, NPO, oral hygiene admin., measuring I & O. L. White RN —
10/14/01	0830		**R:** Within 1 H (0730-0830) blood glucose 360 mg/dl R 24 non-labored. Urinary output 750 ml/H. Client identifies abdominal pain as 3 on a 0-10 pain scale. — L. White RN —

Figure 10-7 Sample Focus Charting

immediate access to client information. The system allows for the input and retrieval of client data at the bedside through a handheld portable computer.

The advantages of point-of-care charting relate to the efficiency of the computer system. Because this documentation method allows health care providers to record client data at the point of care, it:

- Controls operating costs,
- Complements existing information systems,
- Eliminates redundant data entry,
- Allows the provider more one-on-one time for client care, and
- Provides crucial client information to all health care providers in a timely fashion.

Point-of-care computerized documentation also facilitates the transition to a managed-care system (an integrated health care team) by focusing on the continuum of care. Each health care practitioner is provided with all pertinent client data to ensure continuity of care without duplication. One final advantage of point-of-care charting is that it fosters compliance with accreditation and regulatory standards.

Disadvantages include all of the problems inherent in computerized storage of records, such as maintaining confidentiality, controlling who has access to which data, and correcting errors.

Critical Pathway

A **critical pathway** (or critical path) is a comprehensive, standard plan of care for specific case situations. The pathway is monitored to ensure that interventions are performed on time and that client outcomes are achieved on time.

Variations, sometimes referred to as variances, are goals not met or interventions not performed according to the established time frame. The nurse documents on the back of the critical pathway the unexpected event (e.g., medications not given because client in physical therapy), actions taken in response to the event, and appropriate discharge planning (Russell-Babin, 1994).

Critical pathways allow for the efficient use of time and increase the quality of care by having the expected outcomes identified on the plan. When clients have more than two diagnoses or variations, however, documentation becomes complicated because of limited space. This situation requires additional documentation forms to complement the pathway, such as intervention flow sheets and nurses' notes.

FORMS FOR RECORDING DATA

There are several types of forms used in record keeping: Kardex, flow sheets, nurses' progress notes, and discharge summaries. All of these forms are de-

signed to facilitate record keeping, minimize duplication of effort, and ensure quick and easy access to information.

Kardex

A **Kardex** is a summary worksheet reference of basic client care information that traditionally is not part of the medical record. A concise client data source, Kardex is used as a reference throughout the shift and during change-of-shift reports. Kardexes come in various sizes, shapes, and types, including computer-generated. The Kardex is designed to complement the care delivery setting and usually contains the following information:

- Client data: name, age, marital status, religious preference, physician, family contact with phone number
- Medical diagnoses: listed by priority
- Nursing diagnoses: listed by priority
- Allergies
- Medical orders: diet, medications, intravenous (IV) therapy, treatments, diagnostic tests and procedures (inclusive of dates and results), consultations, DNR (do-not-resusitate) order (when appropriate)
- Activities permitted: functional limitations, assistance needed in activities of daily living, and safety precautions

Flow Sheets

Flow sheets have vertical or horizontal columns for recording dates and times and related assessment and intervention information, making it easy to track changes in the client's condition. Client teaching, use of special equipment, and IV therapy are other aspects of the flow sheet. Because flow sheets have small spaces for recording, these forms usually contain legends that identify the approved abbreviations for charting data (Figure 10-8). It is important to fill out flow sheets completely because blank spaces imply that an intervention was not completed, attempted, or recognized.

Because they decrease the redundancy of charting in the nurses' progress notes, flow sheets are used as supplements to most documentation systems. They do

HOME HEALTH CARE

Home Health Kardex

In addition to the usual information, the home health Kardex contains information related to family contacts, practitioners (physician), other services, and emergency referrals.

Date:

Nutrition:	Hygiene:	7-3			3-11			11-7		
Diet □ NPO □ Hyperal □ Tube Fed □	Bath □ Sitz □ Shower□	self □ assist □ total refused □ □			self □ assist □ total refused □ □			self □ assist □ total refused □ □		
Breakfast: All >1/2 <1/2 0 □ □ □ □	Oral Care	self □	assist□	total □	self □	assist□	total □	self□	assist□	total □
	Shave	self □	assist□	total □	self □	assist□	total □	self□	assist□	total □
	Peri Care	self □	assist□	total □	self □	assist□	total □	self□	assist□	total □
Lunch: All >1/2 <1/2 0 □ □ □ □	Other:									
	Comments:									
Dinner: All >1/2 <1/2 0 □ □ □ □										
Snacks: All >1/2 <1/2 0 □ □ □ □										

Tube Feeding Residuals		Intake						Output			
Time	Amount	7-3	PO	IV	NG & Flush	Enteral	Other	Urine	Ng/Emesis	Stool	Drains
		7-3 Total									
Weight		3-11									
Today:											
Previous:											

Vital/Signs														
Time	T	P	R	B/P	3-11 Total									
					11-7									
					11-7 Total									
					24° Total									

4010

SPOHN HEALTH SYSTEM
SPOHN HOSPITAL
CORPUS CHRISTI, TEXAS 78404

FLOW SHEET - 24 HOUR RECORD
PATIENT CARE SERVICES

2705066

NEW: 07/94
REV: 06/26/98
.FM2

	Date:	7-3 Time:	3-11 Time:	11-7 Time:
Neuro	Normal: alert, oriented to time, place, person, follows command, speech clear	WNL: □ *	WNL: □ *	WNL: □ *
Respir-atory	Normal: Regular, unlabored symmetrical respirations, no abnormal lung sounds	WNL: □ *	WNL: □ *	WNL: □ *
Cardio-vascular	Normal: Heart rhythm regular, peripheral pulses easily palpable and strong bilaterally, no edema, capillary refill brisk	WNL: □ *	WNL: □ *	WNL: □ *
Musculo-Skeletal	Normal: Full ROM of All joints, no weakness, steady balance and gait, handgrips equal	WNL: □ *	WNL: □ *	WNL: □ *
G.I.	Normal: Abdomen soft, bowel sounds present all 4 quadrants, no nausea/vomiting, diarrhea/constipation Last BM:	WNL: □ *	WNL: □ *	WNL: □ *
G.U.	Normal: Voiding without difficulty, clear urine, no bladder distention	WNL: □ *	WNL: □ *	WNL: □ *
Skin	Normal: Skin warm, dry, intact, tugor elastic, oral cavity moist and intact Date of Last EZ Graph ______ Site: ______	WNL: □ *	WNL: □ *	WNL: □ *
Psycho-social	Normal: Thought processes logical, memory intact, behavior appropriate for situation	WNL: □ *	WNL: □ *	WNL: □ *
Incision	Normal: Incision clean, no redness, drainage Site:	WNL: □ *	WNL: □ *	WNL: □ *
Wound	Normal: Dry, no drainage, no odor Site:	WNL: □ *	WNL: □ *	WNL: □ *

SAFETY ASSESSMENT

STATUS: MENTAL/PHYSICAL	MEDICATIONS	HISTORY
D E N	D E N	D E N
□□□ (5) Confused/judgement impaired	□□□ (5) Diuretics	□□□ (5) Age greater than 60
□□□ (5) Sensory Impairment	□□□ (5) Laxatives/G.I. preps	□□□ (5) History of previous falls
□□□ (5) Combative/aggressive	□□□ (3) Antihypertensives	□□□ (3) from nursing home
□□□ (5) "Sundowners" syndrome	□□□ (3) Antiseizures	□□□ (3) Has had sitter/ companion at home
□□□ (5) Noncompliance/uncooperativeness	□□□ (5) Sedative/hypnotics	SAFETY LEVEL
□□□ (5) Paralysis/amputee	□□□ (3) Analgesics	D E N
□□□ (5) Urgent/frequent elimination needs	□□□ (3) Antipsychotics/ antidepressants	□□□ Level 1 (0-17)
□□□ (10) Restraints in use		□□□ Level 2 (18-24)
□□□ (5) Weakness/debilitation/mobility impaired		□□□ Level 3 (25 or greater)

TOTAL D ______ E ______ N ______

Figure 10-8 Assessment and Intervention Flow Sheet *(Courtesy of Spohn Health System, Corpus Christi, TX)*

PROGRESS NOTES

TIME	PROBLEM #	PROGRESS NOTES

PLAN OF CARE VERIFICATION

IV SITE ASSESSMENT

			RN _____ Time _____
Normal: IV Patent; No redness, drainage or edema	Site #1: Start Date:	WNL: ☐ *	WNL: ☐ *	WNL: ☐ *	WNL: ☐ *
# of IVAC's in use _____	Site #2: Start Date:	WNL: ☐ *	WNL: ☐ *	WNL: ☐ *	WNL: ☐ *

IV Site Care per hospital standard ☐   Time: _____ *
IV Tubing Change per hospital standard ☐   Time: _____ *

IV Start:	Time	Attempts	Site	Needle Size	S	U
					☐ ☐ ☐	☐ ☐ ☐

Site prep per Standard ☐

INITIALS	SIGNATURE	INITIALS	SIGNATURE

EDUCATION REASSESSMENT

Have the education needs of the patient changed in past 24 hours?	☐ Yes	☐ No
Is the patient scheduled for any new test or procedure today? Explanation given?	☐ Yes	☐ No
Patient/significant Other verbalizes understanding:	☐ Yes	☐ No
Patient desires/requires education on:	☐ Yes	☐ No

Have discharge Planning needs changed in past 24 hours?	☐ Yes	☐ No

If yes, send consult to Social Services and document changes below.
ALL EDUCATION MUST BE DOCUMENTED ON THE MULTIDISCIPLINARY EDUCATION FORM (#3177)

PROGRESS NOTES

TIME	PROBLEM #	PROGRESS NOTES

Figure 10-8 Assessment and Intervention Flow Sheet *continued*

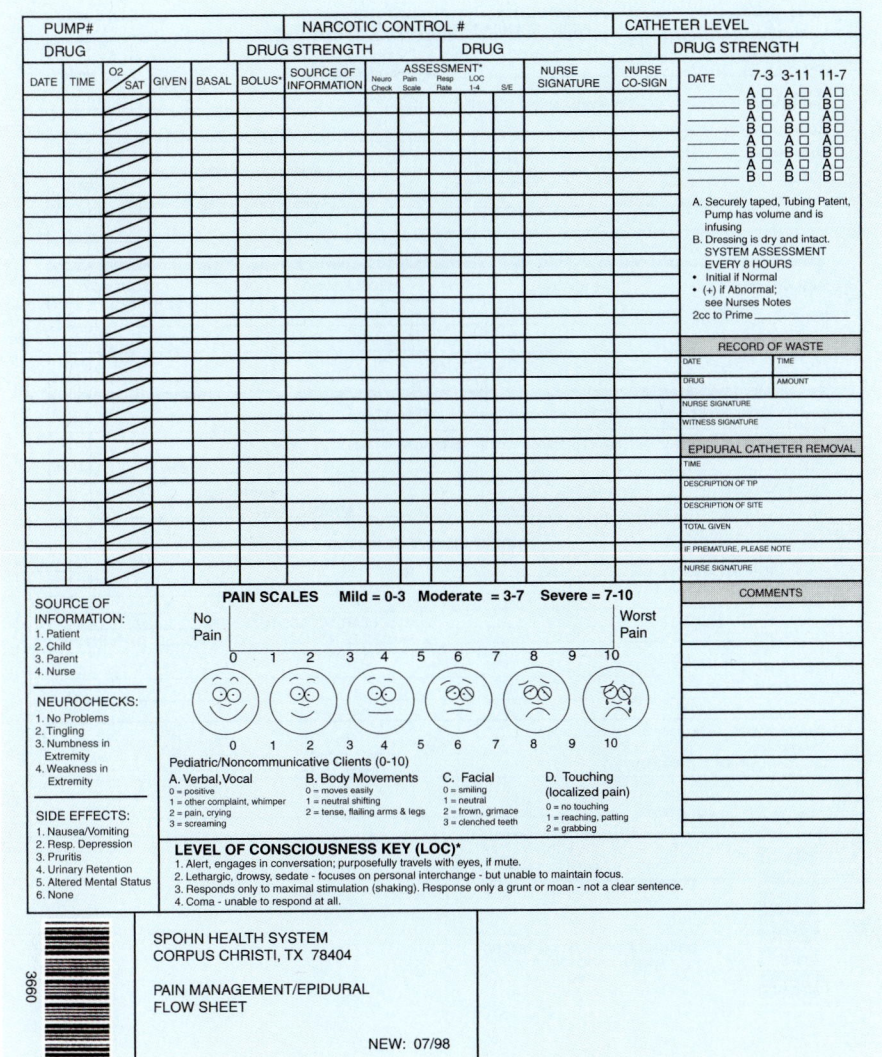

Figure 10-8 Assessment and Intervention Flow Sheet *continued*

not, however, replace the progress notes. Nurses still must document observations, client responses and teaching, detailed interventions, and other significant data in the progress notes.

Nurses' Progress Notes

Nurses' progress notes are used to document the client's condition, problems, and complaints; interventions; the client's response to interventions; and achievement of outcomes. Progress notes comprise the following elements: nurses' notes, MAR, personal care flow sheets, teaching records, intake and output forms, vital sign records, and specialty forms (e.g., diabetic flow sheet or neurologic assessment form) (Eggland & Heinemann, 1994). Progress notes can be either completely narrative or incorporated into a standardized flow sheet to complement SOAP(IE), PIE, focus charting, and other documentation systems.

Discharge Summary

The discharge summary highlights the client's illness and course of care. When a narrative discharge summary is entered into the progress notes, it includes:

- The client's status at admission and discharge;
- A brief summary of the client's care;
- Intervention and education outcomes;
- Resolved problems and continuing care needs for unresolved problems, inclusive of referrals; and
- Client instructions regarding medications, diet, food–drug interactions, activity, treatments, follow-up, and other special needs.

Many facilities have a documentation form that itemizes discharge and client instructions. The form has a duplicate copy for the client, with the original being placed in the medical record. Figure 10-9 shows the common elements of this tool.

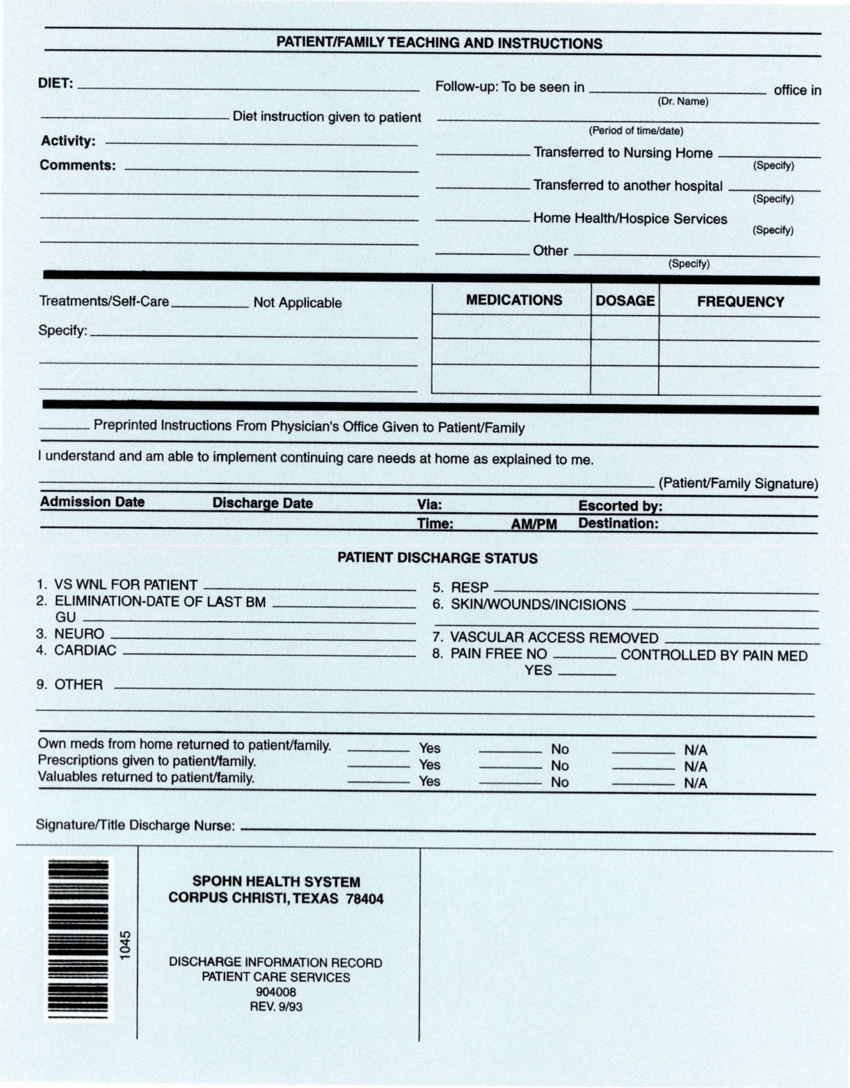

PATIENT/FAMILY TEACHING AND INSTRUCTIONS

DIET: ______ Follow-up: To be seen in ______ office in
(Dr. Name)
______ Diet instruction given to patient ______
(Period of time/date)
Activity: ______ ______ Transferred to Nursing Home ______ (Specify)
Comments: ______ ______ Transferred to another hospital ______ (Specify)
______ Home Health/Hospice Services (Specify)
______ Other ______ (Specify)

Treatments/Self-Care ______ Not Applicable
Specify: ______

MEDICATIONS	DOSAGE	FREQUENCY

______ Preprinted Instructions From Physician's Office Given to Patient/Family

I understand and am able to implement continuing care needs at home as explained to me.

______ (Patient/Family Signature)

Admission Date | Discharge Date | Via: | Escorted by:
Time: AM/PM | Destination:

PATIENT DISCHARGE STATUS

1. VS WNL FOR PATIENT ______
2. ELIMINATION-DATE OF LAST BM ______
   GU ______
3. NEURO ______
4. CARDIAC ______
5. RESP ______
6. SKIN/WOUNDS/INCISIONS ______
7. VASCULAR ACCESS REMOVED ______
8. PAIN FREE NO ______ CONTROLLED BY PAIN MED
   YES ______
9. OTHER ______

Own meds from home returned to patient/family. ______ Yes ______ No ______ N/A
Prescriptions given to patient/family. ______ Yes ______ No ______ N/A
Valuables returned to patient/family. ______ Yes ______ No ______ N/A

Signature/Title Discharge Nurse: ______

1045

SPOHN HEALTH SYSTEM
CORPUS CHRISTI, TEXAS 78404

DISCHARGE INFORMATION RECORD
PATIENT CARE SERVICES
904008
REV. 9/93

Figure 10-9 Discharge Summary *(Courtesy of Spohn Health System, Corpus Christi, TX)*

TRENDS IN DOCUMENTATION

Computerized charting has become one of the most widespread trends in nursing documentation. However, computerized nursing documentation can demonstrate the quality, effectiveness, and value of the services nurses provide only if standardized databases are developed that will ensure accuracy and precision in the information. At the 1991 conference of the National Center for Nursing Research of the National Institutes of Health, the need was identified for databases that would permit analysis of the effectiveness and costs of specific interventions in achieving desired outcomes for clients with a variety of nursing diagnoses (Ozbolt, Fruchtnight, & Hayden, 1994). The recommendations arising from this conference support the need to define and develop standard terminology for nursing data, nursing diagnoses, nursing interventions, and nursing outcomes.

Nursing Minimum Data Set

In 1985, Werley and Lang convened an invitational working conference at the University of Wisconsin—Milwaukee to identify the elements that should be included in a **nursing minimum data set** (NMDS). These are the elements that should be contained in clinical records and abstracted for studies on the effectiveness and costs of nursing care (Werley & Lang, 1988). The sixteen identified elements were grouped into the following three categories:

- Demographics: personal identification, date of birth, gender, race and ethnicity, and residence
- Service: unique facility or service agency number, episode admission or encounter date, discharge or termination date, disposition of client, expected payer, unique health record number of client, and unique number of principal registered nurse provider

- Nursing care: nursing diagnosis, nursing intervention, nursing outcome, and intensity of nursing care (Werley & Lang, 1988)

Several challenges are inherent in the development of the four nursing care categories: diagnoses, interventions, outcomes, and intensity (Hayes et al., 1994). For example, automated information systems must be capable of supporting cost-effective nursing practice through efficient, comprehensive documentation. Further, basic to standardizing databases is the consistent use of a taxonomy that promotes validity and reliability. The NMDS, however, does not specify for any of the four elements a taxonomy such as NANDA (1999) nursing diagnoses, Nursing Interventions Classification (NIC) (NIC, 1995), or acuity ratings. Nursing must achieve consensus of terminology in order for clinical data to be included in nursing care elements of a NMDS.

Nursing Diagnoses

A nursing diagnosis is a clinical judgment about individual, family, or community responses to actual or potential health problems or life processes (NANDA, 1999). The American Nurses Association (ANA) endorsed NANDA to develop a classification for nursing diagnoses, and in 1992, the NANDA terms were accepted into the Unified Medical Language System (UMLS). The UMLS was begun in 1986 by the National Library of Medicine as a way to help health professionals and researchers retrieve and integrate electronic biomedical information from a variety of sources (National Library of Medicine, 1998).

Nursing Intervention Classification

The **Nursing Intervention Classification (NIC)** is a comprehensive standardized language for nursing interventions organized in a three-level taxonomy (McCloskey & Bulechek, 1995). This taxonomy attempts to sort, label, and describe interventions used by nurses for various diagnostic categories. Initiated by a research team (Iowa Intervention Project) at the University of Iowa in 1987, the three-level taxonomy now comprises 6 domains, 26 classes, and 433 interventions. Each nursing intervention has a label, a definition, and a set of activities to carry out the interventions. *Activities are not interventions and should not be labeled as such in nursing information systems* (NIC, 1995).

Although continuing to evolve, this classification system already provides assistance in choosing interventions based on nursing diagnoses or problems. The NIC interventions have been incorporated into health care data sets and the computerized client medical record. The ANA has recognized NIC as one of the first nursing languages to be included in the National Li-

HOME HEALTH CARE

Taxonomy of Nursing Interventions
Grobe and colleagues at the University of Texas at Austin have been developing a lexicon and taxonomy of nursing interventions taken from home care records (Grobe, 1992).

brary of Medicine's Metathesaurus, one of four knowledge sources for the UMLS (McCloskey & Bulechek, 1995).

Nursing Outcomes Classification

A nursing outcome is defined as the resolution status of the nursing diagnosis according to the NMDS (Ozbolt et al., 1994). The Iowa Outcomes Project being conducted at the University of Iowa has developed a taxonomy of client outcomes for nursing care, called **Nursing Outcomes Classification (NOC)**. This classification system comprises 190 outcome labels and corresponding definitions, measures, indicators, and references (Johnson & Maas, 1997).

REPORTING

Reporting is the verbal communication of data regarding the client's health status, needs, treatments, outcomes, and responses (Eggland & Heinemann, 1994). A report must summarize the current critical information pertinent to clinical decision making and continuity of care. As with recording, reporting is based on the nursing process, standards of care, and legal and ethical principles. The nursing process provides structure for an organized report, a challenge inherent in verbal communications. In order to verbally communicate an efficient and well-organized report, the nurse must consider the following questions:

- What must be said?
- Why must it be said?
- How must it be said?
- What are the expected outcomes?

Considering these aspects of reporting before communicating the information provides for a concise, organized report.

Another critical element in reporting is listening. Reports require participation from everyone present. When receiving a report, the nurse must focus behaviors to enhance listening skills: The nurse eliminates distractions, puts thoughts and concerns aside, concentrates on those things being said, and does not anticipate the presenter's next statements. The reporting process is an integral component of developing effective interpersonal and intrapersonal relationships that promote continuity of client care. Regardless of the type of communication, planned presentation of client data is key to accurate, concise, effective reporting. Summary reports, walking rounds, telephone reports and orders, and incident reports are all types of reporting.

Summary Reports

Summary reports outline information pertinent to the client's needs as identified by the nursing process. Summary reports commonly occur either at the change of shift when a new caregiver is involved or when the client is transferred to another area. A summary, or end-of-shift, report should include the following information in the order indicated:

1. Background data obtained from client interactions and assessment of the client's functional health patterns
2. Primary medical and nursing diagnoses and priority problems
3. Identified client risks
4. Recent changes in condition or in treatments (e.g., new medications, elevated temperature)
5. Effective interventions or treatments of priority problems, inclusive of laboratory and diagnostic results (e.g., client's response to pain medication)
6. Progress toward expected outcomes (priority problems, teaching, or discharge planning)
7. Adjustments in the plan of care
8. Client or family complaints

This logical and time-sequenced format follows the nursing process and thus provides structure and organization to the data. In order to provide continuity of care, the new caregiver must receive an accurate, concise report about those things that have happened during the previous shift. Client and family complaints relative to each client should be addressed last, because these situations usually generate questions and discussion.

Walking Rounds

Walking rounds can take the form of nursing rounds, physician–nurse rounds, or multidisciplinary rounds. **Walking rounds** is a reporting method used when the members of the care team walk to each client's room and discuss care and progress with each other and with the client, as shown in Figure 10-10.

Nursing rounds are used most frequently by charge nurses as their method of report. During the rounds, the on-coming nurse is introduced to the client and the off-going nurse discusses with the client and the on-coming nurse changes in the plan of care. Although more time consuming than the end-of-shift report, walking rounds give the nurses and the client the opportunity to evaluate the effectiveness of care together.

Nursing rounds are also used as a teaching method. The instructor introduces the client to the student, and together they discuss the client's care. The instructor can also use this time to appraise the student's observation, communication, and decision-making skills.

Nurse–physician rounds involve the physician and either the staff nurse or the charge nurse. These rounds usually occur daily and provide the nurse, the physician, and the client the opportunity to evaluate the effectiveness of care.

Multidisciplinary rounds, which involve all disciplines, usually occur less frequently than the other types of rounds; primarily because it is difficult to schedule caregivers from all the disciplines for rounds. Multidisciplinary rounds are done most commonly in place of or to supplement case conferences and to discuss discharge planning. Multidisciplinary rounds support the concept of critical pathways and are seen most frequently in facilities that use pathways.

PROFESSIONAL TIP

Information for Shift Report
1. Client name, room and bed, age, and gender
2. Physician, admission date and diagnosis, and any surgery
3. Diagnostic tests or treatments performed in the past 24 hours; results, if available
4. General status, any significant change in condition
5. New or changed physician's orders
6. Nursing diagnoses and suggested nursing orders
7. Evaluation of nursing interventions
8. Intravenous fluid amounts, last prn medication
9. Concerns about the client

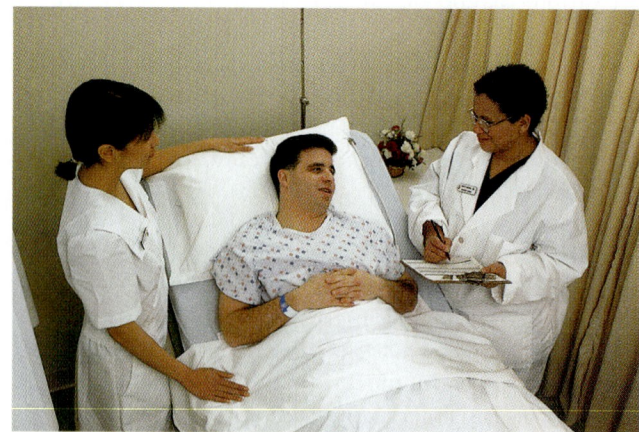

Figure 10-10 Nursing Rounds

Telephone Reports and Orders

Telephone communications are another way nurses report transfers, communicate referrals, obtain client data, solve problems, and inform a client's family members regarding a change in the client's condition. Nurses are expected to demonstrate phone courtesy and professionalism when initiating and receiving telephone reports.

When initiating a phone call, the nurse should organize the information to be reported or received. For example, the nurse should:

- Ensure all lab results are back; if they are not, the nurse should identify in advance those that are missing and should phone the lab or check the computer to ascertain whether other results are available. If phoning the lab, the nurse should spell the client's name and provide the client's medical record number to minimize the chances of receiving results for the wrong client. The nurse should write down those tests that have been performed and the results.
- Review her notes and have the client's assessment data readily available, especially any significant data related to abnormal results. If the nurse has not assessed the client, this should be done before telephoning the practitioner; otherwise, the practitioner might ask questions that the nurse is unable to answer.
- Inform the charge nurse or someone else at the nurses' station of plans to place the call, so as to minimize the chances of being interrupted while on the phone.

When placing the call, the nurse should state the reason for the call, for example, "I am calling Dr. Wojtal regarding the blood sugar results for Mrs. Beacon." The nurse should be brief, listen carefully, and repeat the test results and any orders the physician gives over the phone.

The date and time the phone call was placed, the client data reported by the nurse, the name of the person with whom the nurse spoke, and whether an order was obtained should be recorded accurately in the medical record. Rather than charting, "Physician notified, no orders obtained," The nurse should chart, "Dr. Wojtal notified by phone, blood sugar 260 mg (drawn by the lab at 1300), orders received and recorded on the physician order sheet." Telephone orders should be charted and the nurses' progress notes updated as soon as possible after the phone call to prevent another caregiver from posting an entry before the telephone orders have been posted.

Figure 10–11 demonstrates the way to write a telephone order on the physician order sheet: the entry is dated and timed; the order as given by the physician is recorded; and the order is signed beginning with t.o.

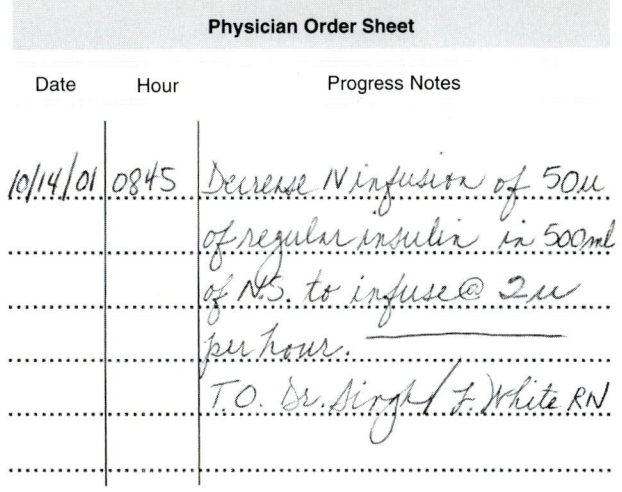

Figure 10-11 Documenting a Telephone Order

(telephone order), the physician's name is written, and the nurse's name is signed. If another nurse witnesses the phone order, that nurse's signature should follow the first nurse's signature.

The physician must countersign the order within a time frame specified by the facility's policy. Fax machines have decreased the need for lengthy or complicated telephone orders, both saving time and minimizing errors. The physician should be phoned to confirm the physician's identity as the initiator of the fax orders. The physician must countersign the fax orders according to agency policy.

Incident Reports

Incident reports, or occurrence reports, are used to document any unusual occurrence or accident in the delivery of client care, such as falls or medication errors. Incident reports are not a means of punishing the caregiver; rather, ethical practice requires that the nurse file an incident report to protect the client.

Incident reports are not merely an internal device for the facility; they are required by federal, national, and state accrediting agencies. For legal reasons, nurses are often advised not to document the filing of an incident report in the nurses' notes. As previously discussed, however, a medication error (Grane, 1995) necessitates both an incident report and documentation in the nurses' notes to ensure that the client receives safe care.

The incident report serves two functions:

- It informs the facility's administration of the incident, thereby allowing risk management personnel to consider changes that might prevent similar occurrences in the future.
- It alerts the facility's insurance company to a potential claim and the need for further investigation.

Each person with firsthand knowledge of the occurrence should fill out and sign a separate report. Although the incident report format varies from one facility to another, the following key elements must be addressed when filing a report:

- The date, exact time, and place the nurse discovered the occurrence should be recorded.
- The person(s) involved in the occurrence, including witnesses, should be identified.
- The exact occurrences witnessed by the nurse must be accurately and objectively documented; for example, "Found the client sitting on the floor, client stated that . . . ," rather than "Client fell."
- The exact details of what happened and the consequences for the persons involved must be recorded in time sequence.
- The nurse's actions to provide care and the results of the nurse's assessment for injuries and client complaints should be recorded.
- The supervisor on duty should be notified and the time and name of the physician notified recorded; if telephone orders were received from the physician, these should be documented as previously discussed and the orders implemented.
- The nurse should not record personal opinions, judgments, conclusions, or assumptions about what occurred; point blame; or suggest ways to prevent similar occurrences.
- The incident report should be forwarded to the designated person as defined by the facility's policy.

Iyer and Camp (1999) suggest an additional safeguard for the nurse: writing a brief, accurate description of the incident and keeping it at home. Included in the description should be the details of the incident and the names of the people who were involved, especially if these people can substantiate the nurse's description. Lawsuits may take several years from the time of the incident until the time that the case goes to court; thus, personal notes will help the nurse accurately recall the incident. Because they may be read by the plaintiff's attorney, the nurse's notes should reflect the same elements as are included in an incident report.

Special attention should be given to documenting falls, because current research shows that client falls

constitute 75% to 80% of all incident reports on clinical units (Springhouse, 1999). Client falls are the main reason nurses are sued (Iyer & Camp, 1999).

SUMMARY

- Documentation provides a system of written records that reflect client care provided on the basis of assessment data and the client's response to interventions.
- The medical record can be used by health care students as a teaching tool and is a main source of data for clinical research.
- Nurses are responsible for assessing and documenting that the client has an understanding of the treatment prior to the intervention.
- Accreditation and reimbursement agencies require accurate and thorough documentation of the nursing care rendered and the client's response to interventions.
- Effective documentation requires clear, concise, accurate recording of all client care and other significant events in an organized and chronological fashion representative of each phase of the nursing process.
- Client safety requires appropriate reporting and recording of medication errors and other occurrences, in compliance with the facility's policy.
- Narrative charting requires an organized, chronological presentation of the client's problems and responses to interventions.
- Problem-oriented charting provides structure when documenting the client's problems and responses in the nurses' progress notes.
- Computerized documentation saves time, increases legibility and accuracy, provides standardized nursing terminology, enhances the nursing process and decision-making skills, and supports continuity of care.
- Critical pathways are comprehensive, standard plans of care for specific cases. Variations are documented on the back.
- Incident reports are used to document any unusual occurrence in a health care facility.

PROFESSIONAL TIP

Documenting an Incident Report

The incident should be factually documented in the nurse's notes, but the notes should not say "incident report filed."

Review Questions

1. Systematic documentation is critical because it:
   a. is done every hour.
   b. shows the care given by all health care providers.
   c. identifies the planning and implementation phases.
   d. presents in a logical fashion the care provided by nurses.

2. The two primary reasons for health care documentation are:
   a. education and research.
   b. research and reimbursement.
   c. accountability and responsibility.
   d. fulfillment of legal and practice standards.

3. The legal issues of documentation require the use of:
   a. black ink pens.
   b. legible, neat writing.
   c. short, descriptive phrases.
   d. hourly recording of client status.

4. The person responsible for obtaining a client's informed consent is the:
   a. physician.
   b. staff nurse.
   c. admissions clerk.
   d. nurse supervisor.

5. The person responsible for ensuring that the client understands the procedure or intervention and has signed the informed consent is the:
   a. nurse.
   b. physician.
   c. social worker.
   d. admission officer.

6. Documentation of nursing care the client receives must:
   a. never have an error.
   b. be neatly spaced out.
   c. reflect the nursing process.
   d. be signed at the end of each shift.

7. A medication error is documented on the:
   a. graphic sheet.
   b. nursing plan of care.
   c. health care team record.
   d. medication administration record.

8. When a documentation error has been made, it should:
   a. be erased.
   b. be scratched out.
   c. have one line drawn through it.
   d. be whited out so as to keep the record neat.

Critical Thinking Questions

1. Of what value is a client's medical record in a court of law? How can it be used?

2. Why are there so many types of charting? Of what value is each?

WEB FLASH!

- Search the various methods of documentation; use search terms such as PIE, charting, and Kardex.
- Research what the Internet has to offer about computerized documentation.
- What can you find about NIC, NOC, and NMDS?

MAKING THE CONNECTION

Refer to the following chapters to increase your understanding of client teaching:

- **Chapter 6, Legal Responsibilities**
- **Chapter 8, Communication**
- **Chapter 9, Nursing Process**
- **Chapter 12, Cultural Diversity and Nursing**
- **Chapter 14, The Life Cycle**
- **Chapter 16, Stress, Adaptation, and Anxiety**

LEARNING OBJECTIVES

Upon completion of this chapter, you should be able to:
- *Define key terms.*
- *Explain the importance of client education in today's health care climate.*
- *Relate principles of adult education to client teaching.*
- *Identify common barriers to learning.*
- *Explain the ways that learning varies throughout the life cycle.*
- *Discuss the nurse's professional responsibilities related to teaching.*
- *Relate the teaching–learning process to the nursing process.*
- *Describe teaching strategies that make learning meaningful to clients.*

KEY TERMS

affective domain	psychomotor domain
auditory learner	readiness for learning
cognitive domain	self-efficacy
formal teaching	teaching
informal teaching	teaching–learning
kinesthetic learner	process
learning	teaching strategies
learning plateau	visual learner
learning style	

INTRODUCTION

Client education is an integral part of nursing care. It is the nurse's responsibility to help identify with the client the learning needs and resources that will restore and maintain that client's optimal level of functioning. This chapter offers an overview of the teaching and learning process, including barriers and responsibilities, and relates it to the nursing process.

THE TEACHING–LEARNING PROCESS

The **teaching–learning process** is a planned interaction that promotes behavioral change that is not a result of maturation or coincidence. **Teaching** is an active process wherein one individual shares information with another to facilitate learning and thereby promote behavioral changes. A teacher is someone who uses a variety of goal-directed activities to promote change by assisting the learner to absorb new information.

Learning is the process of assimilating information, resulting in behavior change. Knowledge is power. By sharing knowledge with clients, the nurse helps them achieve their maximum level of wellness. The teaching–learning process is familiar to nurses in that it mirrors the steps of the nursing process: assessment, identification of learning needs (nursing diagnosis), planning, implementation of teaching strategies, and evaluation of learner progress and teaching efficacy. These steps are discussed in greater detail later in this chapter.

According to Edelman and Mandle (1998), the goal of health education is to help individuals achieve optimal states of health through their own actions. Teaching, one of the most important nursing functions, addresses the client's need for information. Often, a knowledge deficit about the course of illness and/or self-care practices will hinder the client in recovering from illness or practicing health-promoting behaviors. The nurse's charge is to help bridge the gap between those things a client knows and those things a client needs to know to achieve optimal health.

Client teaching is done for a variety of reasons, including:

- Promotion of wellness
- Prevention of illness
- Restoration of health
- Facilitation of coping abilities

Client education focuses on the client's ability to practice healthy behaviors. The client's ability to care for self is enhanced by effective education. Client education has been credited with the following (Seley, 1994):

- Improved quality of care
- Shorter length of hospital stays
- Decreased chance of hospital readmission
- Greater compliance with prescribed treatment regimens

These benefits are enhanced through nurses' continued active participation as client educators.

Formal teaching is planned and goal directed, but informal teaching can occur in any setting at any time.

Formal Teaching

Formal teaching takes place at a specific time, in a specific place, and on a specific topic. It is planned and goal directed (Figure 11-1). The teacher prepares the information and/or activities related to the topic. Formal teaching may take place in a class setting with several learners, or it may be performed one-on-one. For example, many health care facilities provide formal classes related to diabetes. The same basic information is necessary for all clients with diabetes.

Informal Teaching

Informal teaching takes place any time, any place, and whenever a learning need is identified. In the course of providing nursing care, nurses have many opportunities for informal teaching, such as answering the clients' questions and explaining care being given to the client (Figure 11-2). Informal teaching may also occur in the midst of formal teaching. A comment or question from a learner in a formal setting may trigger some informal teaching in response. For example, during a class on diet for the diabetic client,

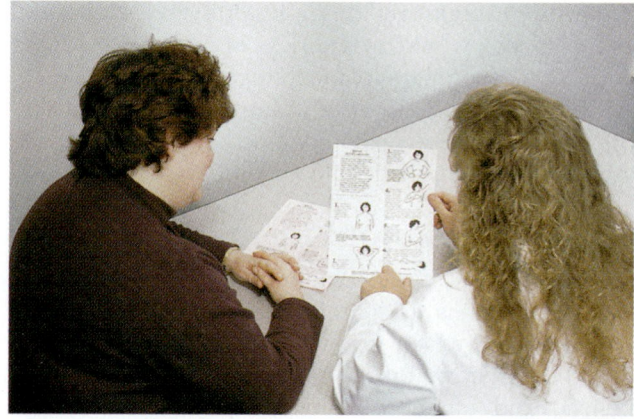
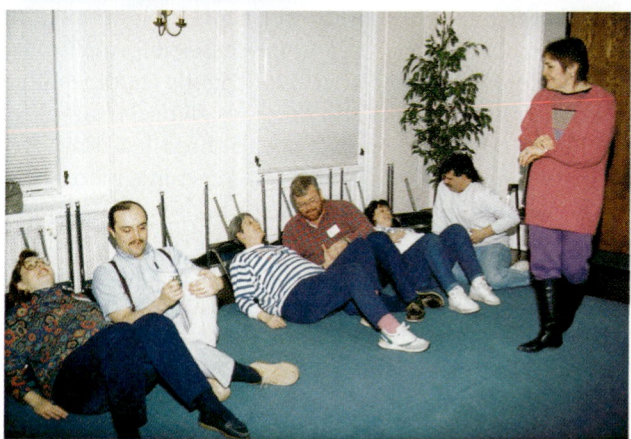

Figure 11-1 Nurses engage in formal teaching, with both individual and group clients. *(Second photo courtesy of Bellevue . . . The Woman's Hospital, Niskayuna, NY)*

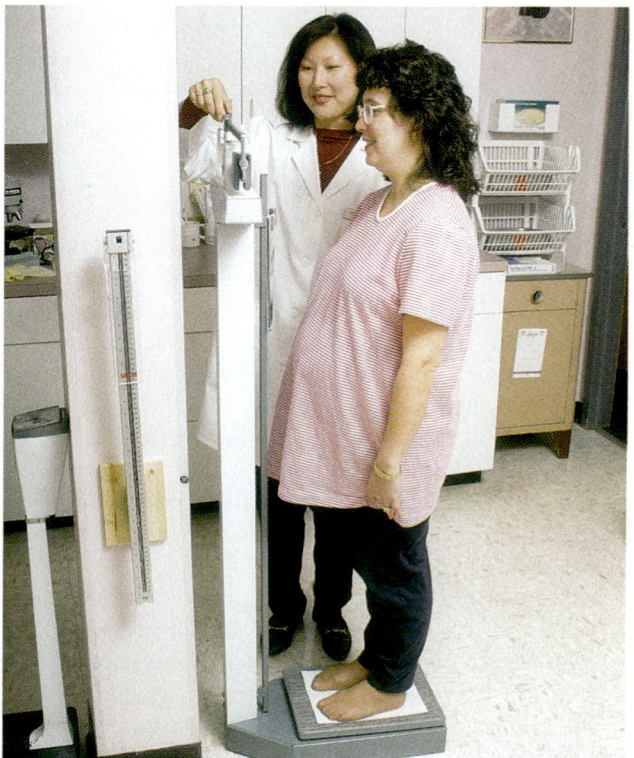

Figure 11-2 Informal teaching can occur during a routine procedure.

a question about dietary cholesterol may be asked. The response would be considered informal teaching because it was not the planned topic.

An understanding of learning domains, learning principles, learning styles, learning barriers, and teaching methods are also helpful and are discussed below.

Learning Domains

In his classic work, Bloom (1977) identifies three areas or domains wherein learning occurs: the **cognitive domain**, which involves intellectual understanding; the **affective domain**, which involves attitudes, beliefs, and emotions; and the **psychomotor domain**, which involves the performance of motor skills. Each domain responds to and processes information in very different ways. Table 11-1 briefly outlines the three learning domains and provides clinical examples.

Nurses must be sensitive to all three learning domains when developing effective teaching plans and must use **teaching strategies**, or techniques to promote learning, that will tap into each of the domains. For instance, teaching a diabetic client the reasons and way to measure the proper daily balance of insulin against the glucose level falls within the cognitive domain; helping the same client learn the way to self-administer insulin falls within the psychomotor domain; and encouraging the client to view diabetes as only one aspect of the individual falls within the affective domain.

Learning Principles

Certain fundamental learning principles can be used by nurses when teaching clients. Knowles, Holton, and Swenson (1998) cite four basic assumptions about adult learners, which are applicable to client education:

- *Assumption 1:* An individual's personality develops in an orderly fashion from dependence to independence. *Nursing application:* The nurse should plan teaching–learning activities that promote client participation, thus encouraging independence and increasing client control and self-care through empowerment.
- *Assumption 2:* Learning readiness is affected by developmental stage and sociocultural factors. *Nursing application:* The nurse should conduct a thorough psychosocial assessment before planning the teaching–learning activities.
- *Assumption 3:* An individual's previous learning experiences can be used as a foundation for further learning. *Nursing application:* The nurse should perform a complete assessment to ascertain what the client already knows and build on that knowledge base.
- *Assumption 4:* Immediacy reinforces learning. *Nursing application:* The nurse should provide opportu-

Table 11-1 LEARNING DOMAINS

DOMAIN	DEFINITION	EXAMPLE
Cognitive	Learning that involves the acquisition of facts and data; used in problem solving and decision making	Client states the name and purpose of prescribed medications.
Affective	Learning that involves changing attitudes, emotions, and beliefs; used in making judgments	Client starts to accept the nature of the chronic illness.
Psychomotor	Learning that involves gaining motor skills; used in physical application of knowledge	Client gives self an injection.

From Fundamentals of Nursing: Standards & Practice, *by S. DeLaune and P. Ladner, 1998, Albany, NY: Delmar Publishers. Copyright 1998 by Delmar Publishers. Reprinted with permission.*

nities for immediate application of knowledge and skills and should incorporate feedback as a continuous part of each nurse–client interaction.

Learning principles include relevance, motivation, readiness, maturation, reinforcement, participation, organization, and repetition.

Relevance

The material to be learned must be meaningful to the client, easily understood by the client, and related to previously learned information. Individuals must believe that they need to learn the information before learning can occur. Does the client perceive relevance (meaningfulness) in the current information to be taught? If an individual sees the information as being personally valuable, the information is more likely to be learned. If the client does not view the content as relevant, however, learning is not likely to occur. Because relevance is individually determined, the nurse must assess the personal meaning of learning for each client.

Motivation

The psychologist Bandura (1977) purports that **self-efficacy** (one's belief that one will succeed in attempts to change behavior) has a profound influence on motivation. Clients should perceive value in the information. If clients feel they will not achieve the goals, they will lack motivation to try. To maximize motivation, the nurse must keep the teaching–learning goals realistic by breaking the content down into small, achievable steps. For example, the cardiac client must see value in information about exercise, such as that the heart will be strengthened and the client will have more energy.

Readiness

The client should be able and willing to learn. Readiness is closely related to growth and development. For example, the client must have the requisite cognitive and psychomotor skills for learning a particular task, and the client must comprehend the information. One indicator of learning readiness is the client's asking questions; another is the client's becoming involved in learning activities, such as actively participating in return demonstration of a dressing change. Some indicators of lack of client readiness are anxiety, avoidance, denial, lack of participation in discussion or demonstration, and lack of participation in self-care activities.

Maturation

The client should be developmentally able to learn and have requisite cognitive and psychomotor abilities. The nurse assesses the client for characteristics that will hinder or facilitate learning. One such characteristic is the client's developmental stage. The nurse must asess the client's developmental stage and not automatically assume, for instance, that a client who is 34 years old has mastered the developmental tasks of earlier stages.

Maturity level greatly influences the client's ability to learn information. Each developmental stage is characterized by unique skills and abilities that affect the

response to various teaching tools. Developmental stage greatly determines the type of data to be taught, the method(s) to be used, the vocabulary to be used, and the location of teaching. In addition to developmental stage, the nurse should also evaluate the client's cognitive skills, problem-solving abilities, and attention span.

Reinforcement

Feedback provided to the learner should be positive and immediate in order to reinforce the client's motivation and readiness to learn. For example, the client who is learning to apply a sterile dressing to an open wound should be told during the application of the dressing that it is being done correctly (if it is) and should be praised upon completion for learning so quickly (or whatever is appropriate). If some aspect of the dressing application is lacking, the nurse must maintain a positive approach in guiding the client in correctly performing the application.

Participation

The client's active involvement in the learning process will promote and enhance learning. Client involvement is relatively easy to monitor when a psychomotor skill is to be learned, as the client is actively involved in practicing a physical skill. Learning that takes place in the cognitive or affective domain is also most effective when active involvement of the client is encouraged. For example, the client who is to be on a low-fat diet can be involved in learning to self-regulate with regard to diet by reading labels of foods and planning menus of low-fat meals.

Organization

The material to be learned should incorporate previously learned information and be presented in sequence from simple to complex and from familiar to unfamiliar. Again using the example of the client learning about a low-fat diet, the nurse should begin the teaching session by finding out what the client knows about the nutrient content of foods and should proceed to helping the client first learn to read food labels, then plan a meal, and then plan a menu for a day and a week, and so forth.

Repetition

Retention of material is reinforced with practice, repetition, and presentation of the same material in a variety of ways. The more often the learner hears or sees the material, the greater the chance that the material will be retained.

It is good to keep in mind that a **learning plateau**, or peak in the effectiveness of teaching and depth of learning, will occur in relation to the client's motivation, interest, and perception of relevance of the material. Frequent reinforcement of learning through immediate feedback and continual reassessment of effectiveness will enhance the value of the learning process for both the teacher and the learner. Making the information-acquisition process as user friendly as possible will also increase satisfaction and success. This can be done by organizing content from the simple to the complex and from the familiar to the new, making learning as creative and interesting as possible, and adopting a flexible approach to allow the learning process to be dynamic.

Learning Styles

Each individual has a unique way of processing information. The manner whereby an individual incorporates new data is called **learning style**. Some people learn by processing information visually (**visual learner**), others by listening to the words (**auditory learner**), and others by experiencing the information or by touching, feeling, or doing (**kinesthetic learner**). The nurse should use a variety of techniques, such as lecture, discussion, small-group work, role play, modeling, return demonstration, imitation, problem solving, games, and question-and-answer sessions, to match different learning styles of clients. A good way to discover learning style is for the nurse to ask the client, "What helps you to learn?" or "What kinds of things do you enjoy doing?" The nurse can then match teaching strategies with the client's learning style.

Barriers to the Teaching–Learning Process

The giving and receiving of information does not, in and of itself, guarantee that learning will occur. Several

PROFESSIONAL TIP

Common Beliefs about Learning
- Each individual has the capacity to learn, but learning ability varies among people and situations.
- The pace of learning varies from person to person.
- Learning is a continuous process, occurring throughout the life cycle.
- Learning can occur in formal and informal settings and interactions.
- Learning is an individualized process.
- Learning new information is based on previous knowledge and experiences.
- Motivation and readiness are necessary prerequisites for learning.
- Prompt feedback facilitates learning.

Table 11-2 LEARNING BARRIERS

EXTERNAL BARRIERS	INTERNAL BARRIERS
Environmental	**Psychological**
• Interruptions	• Anxiety
• Lack of privacy	• Fear
• Multiple stimuli	• Anger
	• Depression
	• Inability to comprehend
Sociocultural	**Physiological**
• Language	• Pain
• Value system	• Fatigue
• Educational background	• Sensory deprivation
	• Oxygen deprivation

From Fundamentals of Nursing: Standards & Practice, *by S. DeLaune and P. Ladner, 1998, Albany, NY: Delmar Publishers. Copyright 1998 by Delmar Publishers. Reprinted with permission.*

barriers can impede the teaching–learning process. In a nursing situation, the nurse, the client, or both may encounter one or more of these barriers. Learning barriers can be classified as either internal (psychological or physiological) or external (environmental or sociocultural). Examples of these barriers are listed in Table 11-2. To facilitate the learning process, the nurse must assess for the presence of learning barriers. Specific assessment information is presented later in this chapter.

Environmental Barriers

Both the nurse and client are subject to environmental barriers. As part of planning for a teaching session, the nurse should ensure necessary privacy and minimize interruptions and multiple stimuli.

Sociocultural Barriers

When language is a barrier to the teaching–learning process, several steps can be taken to ensure that learning does take place, such as using pictures, providing printed material in the appropriate language, or using an interpreter. Even when the nurse and client both speak the same language, a language barrier may exist when clichés, health care jargon, or value-laden terms are used. Furthermore, the meanings that the nurse and client attach to specific types of body language may differ depending on cultural influences. Nurses must be aware of their own value systems but focus client teaching within the client's value system. The educational background of the client must be kept in mind, and language should be tailored to the client's developmental level, without "talking down" to the client.

CULTURAL CONSIDERATIONS

Overcoming Sociocultural Barriers

* Use pictures whenever possible
* Provide written material in the appropriate language
* Use a culturally sensitive interpreter or a family member who understands health care terminology
* Avoid the use of clichés, jargon, or value-laden terms
* Learn about the cultural norms to which the client adheres
* Be aware of your own values
* Tailor teaching (information and questions) to the client's ability to read and write
* Have the client verbalize what has been understood from the teaching–learning session

Psychological Barriers

Nurses may be anxious about client teaching. Knowing the client's learning needs should help alleviate some of this anxiety, as should adequate preparation related to content, environmental and sociocultural aspects, and developmental ability of the client. What little anxiety is left will likely serve to make the nurse more alert and sensitive.

Clients and families are often upset about the health situation they are experiencing. They may be anxious, fearful, angry, or depressed. In addition to the client's words, the nurse should pay attention to body language and behavior. If clients or family members are obviously angry, the nurse should recognize and acknowledge the anger by saying something like "You appear to be very angry about something. Tell me what you are feeling." Allowing clients and family members to express their emotions clears the air and allows learning to take place.

PROFESSIONAL TIP

Overcoming Psychological Barriers

* Recognize your own emotions related to client teaching
* Prepare content of teaching and assess for environmental, sociocultural, psychological, and physiological barriers to learning
* Acknowledge the client's emotions but do not respond in kind

PROFESSIONAL TIP

Physiological Comfort and Learning

* Administer pain medication, as appropriate, before a teaching session to enable the client to concentrate on the information being presented
* Plan teaching sessions when the client is not fatigued, as might be the case after a physical therapy session, for example
* Ensure that the client is in a comfortable position and does not have to go to the bathroom

Physiological Barriers

Physiological situation affects the client's ability to learn. The client who is struggling to breathe, for example, is unable to pay attention to any teaching. A teaching session should be planned for a time when the client is rested and free from pain.

Teaching Methods

Many different teaching methods can be used depending on the client's learning need and the applicable learning domain.

Teaching Methods Applicable in the Cognitive Domain

Effective methods for promoting cognitive learning include discussion, formal lecture, question-and-answer sessions, role play, and games/computer activities.

Discussion Discussions may involve the nurse and one or several clients who need to learn the same information. Active participation is promoted in the topic of discussion. Group discussions allow peer support.

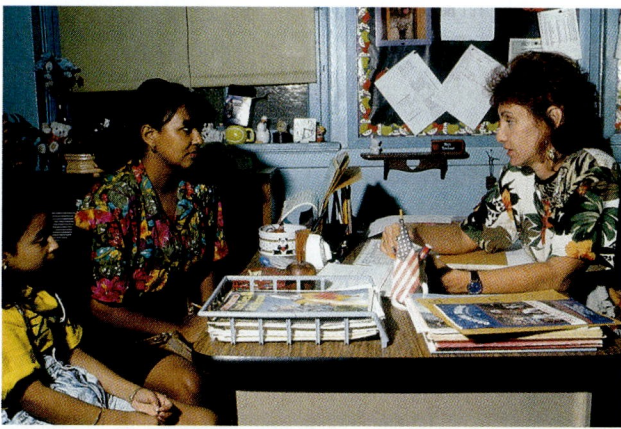

Figure 11-3 A Question-and-answer Session between School Nurse, Mother, and Child

Formal Lecture In formal lectures, the teacher presents the information to be learned, and learner participation is usually minimal.

Question-and-answer Sessions Question-and-answer sessions can take two forms. In one, the client's concerns are addressed by the client asking the questions and the nurse providing answers. In the other the nurse assists the client in applying the knowledge learned by asking the client questions that the client then answers (Figure 11-3).

Role Play Role play provides the client an opportunity to apply knowledge in a safe, controlled environment. In role play, the nurse and client each assume a certain role in order to play out different potential scenarios. For instance, the nurse teaching a client sex education information intended for an adolescent may have the client assume the role of parent, while the nurse assumes the role of the teenager. The two can then engage in practice discussion sessions to prepare the client for the actual parent–teen discussion.

Games/Computer Activities Via games and computer activities learning can be completed as the client is able. These methods allow the client to use the new information in various situations and to have fun while learning.

Teaching Methods Applicable in the Affective Domain

Role play and discussion are both effective methods for stimulating affective learning.

Role Play Role play allows expression of feelings, attitudes, and values in a safe, controlled environment. The client can "try out" different attitudes and values.

Discussion One-on-one discussion between nurse and client is effective for personal or sensitive topics related to values, feelings, attitudes, and emotions (Figure 11-4).

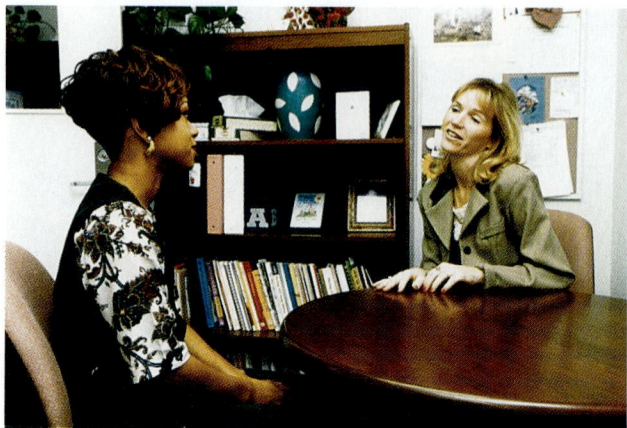

Figure 11-4 Sensitive topics are discussed in a one-on-one setting.

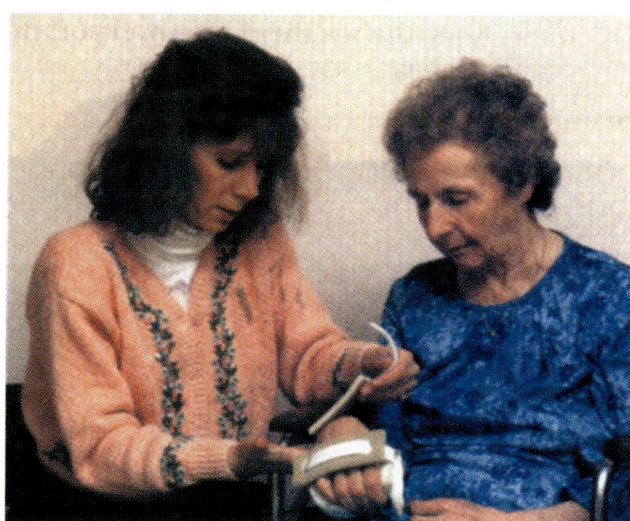

Figure 11-5 Demonstrating Application of a Splint

Teaching Methods Applicable in the Psychomotor Domain

Demonstration, supervised practice, and return demonstration assist the client to learn psychomotor skills.

Demonstration In demonstration, the nurse presents in a step-by-step manner the skill or procedure to be learned, explaining what is being done and why. In this way, the client sees not only the equipment and the way it is used, but also the nurse's attitude and behaviors (Figure 11-5).

Supervised Practice In supervised practice, the client uses the equipment and performs the skill or procedure while the nurse watches. The nurse gives suggestions and corrects the client as the practice proceeds. Repetition can continue until the client feels confident in performing the skill or procedure.

Return Demonstration In return demonstration, the client performs the skill or procedure without any coaching from the nurse. Upon completion of the task, the nurse provides feedback and reinforcement to the client.

LEARNING THROUGHOUT THE LIFE CYCLE

One basic assumption underlies teaching effectiveness: *All people are capable of learning.* However, the ability to learn does vary from person to person and from situation to situation. Further, learning needs and learning abilities change throughout life, and the client's chronological age and developmental stage greatly influence the ability to learn. The principles of learning discussed earlier in this chapter have relevance to learners of all ages. However, teaching approaches must be modified according to the client's developmental stage and level of understanding. Specific information for children, adolescents, and older adults is described in the following sections.

Children

Readiness for learning (evidence of willingness to learn) varies during childhood depending on maturation level. Responding to knowledge deficits of young children requires that the nurse work closely with the child's caretaker. Including the family or significant others in teaching is especially important when caring for young children.

Young children learn primarily through play. Incorporating play into teaching activities for children can therefore enhance learning (Figure 11-6). Puppets, toys, and coloring books can be effective teaching tools for the young child. Creativity is effective in encouraging the young child to be an active participant in the learning process.

Older children can also benefit from the use of art materials to express their emotions and their understanding of those things that are or will be happening to them. Using medical supplies (such as medicine cups or bandages), for example, the child may play at giving medicine to a doll or putting a bandage on the doll like the bandage that will be put on the child. While the child is involved in play, the nurse is both teaching the child what to expect regarding treatment procedures and alleviating anxiety.

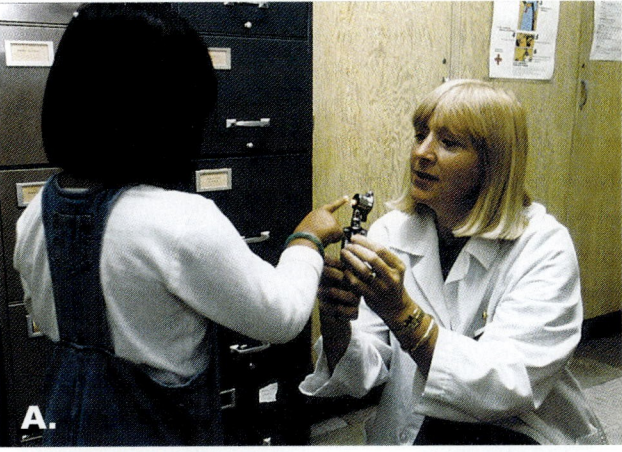

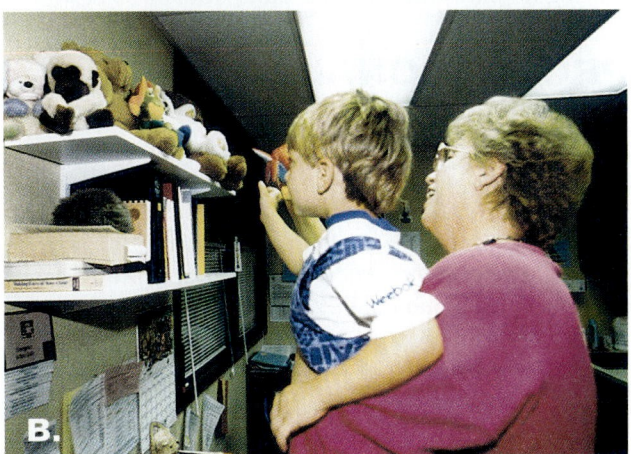

Figure 11-6 A. The nurse is at the child's level while the child learns about the instrument to be used in the examination; B. The nurse encourages a child to select a toy to help in teaching.

LIFE CYCLE CONSIDERATIONS

Teaching Children

- Ensure that the child is comfortable.
- Encourage caregiver participation.
- Assess the child's learning readiness, motivation, and developmental level. Do not equate age with developmental level.
- Assess the child's psychological status.
- Determine self-care abilities of the child and caregiver.
- Use play, imitation, and role play to make learning fun and meaningful.
- Use different visual stimuli, such as books, chalkboards, and videos, to convey information and assess understanding.
- Use terms that are easily understood by the client and caregiver.
- Provide frequent repetition and reinforcement.
- Develop realistic goals that are consistent with developmental abilities.
- In planning teaching approaches, remember that the goals of educating children are to "prevent excessive anxiety, improve cooperation, and hasten the recovery process" (Biddinger, 1993).

Adolescents

As individuals approach adolescence, they are better able to conceptualize relationships between things. Usually, reading and comprehension ability have advanced, and the adolescent can understand more complex information. Because one of the strongest influences on the adolescent is peer support, group meetings are often useful in teaching. The nurse can

CLIENT TEACHING

Do As I Do

- The adage "Do as I say, not as I do" goes against all wisdom. Individuals learn from examples set by role models.
- Adolescents are especially sensitive to discrepancies between an adult's words and actions.
- Encourage parents to model the behaviors they wish their children to develop.

often be a powerful teacher by acting as a role model. The accompanying display provides guidelines for teaching adolescents.

Older Adults

Aging is accompanied by many physiological changes. As a result of these changes, some older adults experience perceptual impairments such as vision and hearing impairments. The nurse must thus assess for perceptual changes and adjust teaching materials accordingly. For example, providing large-print written material and verifying that the client hears all instructions and directions are strategies helpful in teaching older clients. The accompanying display provides guidelines for teaching older adults.

PROFESSIONAL RESPONSIBILITIES RELATED TO TEACHING

Through teaching, the nurse empowers clients in their self-care abilities. Teaching is the tool for providing information to clients about specific disease processes, treatment methods, and health-promoting behaviors. Although each state has its own definition

LIFE CYCLE CONSIDERATIONS

Teaching Adolescents

- Show respect for adolescents by recognizing their struggle to gain the knowledge and experience of adulthood while breaking away from the grasp of childhood
- Boost adolescents' confidence by asking their input and opinions on health care matters
- Encourage adolescents to explore their own feelings about self-concept and independence
- Be sensitive to the peer pressure many adolescents face
- Help adolescents identify and build on their positive qualities
- Gear teaching to the adolescent's developmental level and use language that is clear yet appropriate to the health care setting
- To encourage independent and informed decision making, engage adolescents in problem-solving activities

LIFE CYCLE CONSIDERATIONS

Teaching Older Adults

- Ensure that the client is comfortable. Pain, fatigue, a full bladder, or hunger can impair learning.
- Assess the client's learning readiness, motivation, and developmental level. Do not equate age with developmental level.
- Assess the client's psychological status. Depression, severe anxiety, or denial can interfere with learning.
- Ascertain the client's self-care abilities.
- Use terms that are easily understood by the client. Avoid talking down to the client; a condescending, paternalistic manner impedes learning.
- Ascertain the time of day when the client is best able to concentrate.
- Present material slowly and use examples.
- Encourage client involvement and participation.
- Ask for feedback and employ active listening.
- Provide frequent feedback.
- Assess for perceptual impairments and individualize teaching strategies accordingly:

For memory-impaired clients:
- Use repetition
- Use a variety of cues (spoken words, written materials, pictures, and symbols)

For visually impaired clients:
- Provide large-print materials
- Provide magnifying glasses
- Be sure client is wearing prescription eyeglasses
- Provide adequate lighting and reduce glare

For hearing-impaired clients:
- Face the client directly when speaking
- Use short sentences and words that are easily understood
- Use signals to reinforce verbal information (point, gesture, and demonstrate)
- Eliminate distractions (noises or activities from the environment) as much as possible

Adapted from Principles and Practice of Adult Health Nursing, *by P. G. Beare & J. L. Myers 1998. St. Louis: Mosby; and from "Altered Patterns of Degenerative Origin," by S. C. Delaune, in* Mental Health and Psychiatric Nursing *[3rd ed.] by J. L. Davies [Ed.] 1991, Boston: Jones and Bartlett.*

of nursing practice, teaching is a required function of nurses in most states. Redman (1997) cites National League for Nursing documents dating back to 1918 as stating that "the nurse is essentially a teacher and an agent of health."

Providing client education is expected of all nurses. Freda (1997), is disturbed by reports that some nurses in the United States, however, are voluntarily giving up their client teaching responsibilities, mainly because of a perceived lack of time. She believes that if nurses give up their role as client educators in favor of spending that time performing additional tasks, nursing's worth to the health care system could greatly diminish. Client teaching requires the depth of information that only nurses possess; as such, it is one of the truly independent functions of nursing practice.

Client teaching is also mandated by several accrediting bodies including the Joint Commission for Accreditation of Healthcare Organizations (JCAHO, 1998). The American Hospital Association's *Patient's Bill of Rights* (1973) calls for the client's understanding of health status and treatment approaches. Informed consent for treatment procedures can be given only by clients who are well informed. The nurse assesses the client's level of understanding about treatment methods and corrects any knowledge deficits. The nurse often serves as an interpreter for the client—explaining in easily understood terms, clarifying, and referring.

Teaching supports behavioral changes that lead to positive adaptation by the client. Thus, teaching decreases the fear of change. Reducing anxiety and anticipatory stress is an important component of teaching.

Client teaching is an essential function of every nurse regardless of practice setting. All clients require information about disease prevention, growth and development, safety, first aid, nutrition, and hygiene. The client who is hospitalized needs information about his condition, the expected treatment, and the environment of the health care facility. By the time of discharge, clients must also have information about

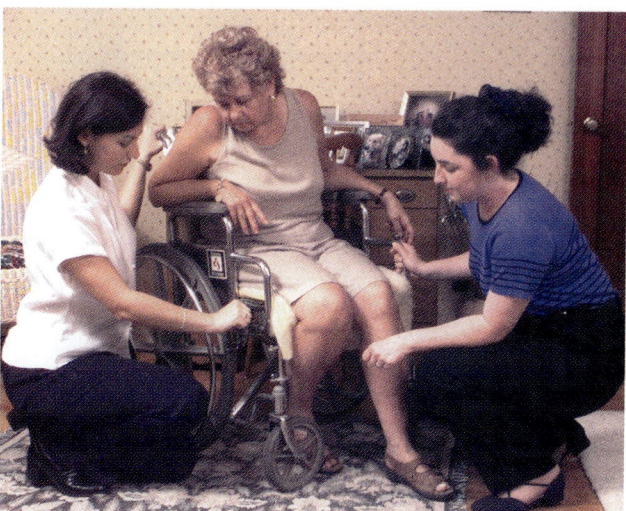

Figure 11-7 Nurse Teaching a Family Member To Provide Care

postdischarge care related to medications, dietary modifications, activity, complication prevention, and rehabilitation plans.

Clients who are recovering at home and their families also have significant learning needs. A primary role of the home health nurse is to teach the client about caring for himself at home. This often involves teaching family members ways to provide care (Figure 11-7). Home-based clients need information regarding their illness, accident, or injury. They also need to learn ways to achieve and maintain a maximum state of wellness. Accurate teaching plans for the home-based client and family are established by assessing multiple factors, some of which are listed in Table 11-3.

Self-Awareness

Several characteristics of nurses influence the outcome of the teaching–learning process. Nurse self-awareness with regard to the concepts discussed in the following sections is an all-important first step in teaching.

Knowledge Base

It is impossible for nurses to teach if they lack the knowledge or skills that are to be taught. Staying both current in knowledge and proficient in skills is the first step to maintaining efficacy and credibility as a teacher. Although it is impossible for one individual to be an expert in every area of nursing, knowing when to refer the client to others for teaching is an important critical-thinking skill.

Interpersonal Skills

Effective teaching is based on the nurse's ability to establish rapport with the client. The empathic nurse shows sensitivity to the client's needs and preferences. An atmosphere in which the client feels free to ask

HOME HEALTH CARE

Client Teaching Considerations

- Preparation of the client and family for home care begins at the time of hospital admission, not at the time of discharge.
- The nurse's effective teaching is the link to thorough follow-up care in the home.
- Discharge planning requires consideration of current learning needs of clients and caregivers as well as potential needs after discharge.
- Teaching involves consideration of community resources and possible referral.

Table 11-3	FACTORS AFFECTING LEARNING NEEDS OF HOME HEALTH CLIENTS
FACTOR	**EXAMPLE**
Environmental	• Accessibility of home to the client with a physical disability • Need for and availability of equipment and supplies • Space to accommodate special needs of the client • Need for information about environmental cleanliness as it relates to health • Need for assistance with self-care activities
Economic	• Ability to purchase medications, equipment, and supplies • Available financial assistance
Support system	• Persons available to assist with caregiving • Caregiver's knowledge deficits regarding necessary care
Community resources	• Resources in the immediate area • Awareness of and access to support services • Available respite for the family

From Fundamentals of Nursing: Standards & Practice, *by S. DeLaune and P. Ladner, 1998, Albany, NY: Delmar Publishers. Copyright 1998 by Delmar Publishers. Reprinted with permission.*

questions promotes learning. Activities that help establish an environment conducive to learning include:

• Showing genuine interest in the client,
• Including the client in *every* step of the teaching–learning process,

PROFESSIONAL TIP

Medical Jargon and Teaching

• Consider the language used by most nurses; think of the terms nurses take for granted. When a client is asked to "void," for example, does the client understand what is meant?
• Think of the following frequently used terms that can easily be misunderstood by clients and families: *ambulate, defecate, dangle, NPO, vital signs,* and *contraindicated.*
• Listen to the language nurses use when communicating with clients.
• How can you communicate without using professional jargon?

• Employing a nonjudgmental approach, and
• Communicating at the client's level of understanding.

Documentation

The reasonable and prudent standard calls for nurses to document client education. From a legal perspective, if the nurse teaches the client and fails to document it, the educational activities never occurred. Documentation of teaching promotes continuity of care and facilitates accurate communication to other health care colleagues involved in the client's care.

Many different approaches can be used to document client teaching. Figure 11-8 is an example of a documentation form related to client teaching in an inpatient setting; Figure 11-9 is a sample form for documenting teaching in the home setting.

Because client education is a standard and essential component of nursing practice, each nurse must document the teaching interventions used and the client's response. Elements to be documented in all practice settings include:

• Content
• Teaching methods
• Learner(s) (e.g., client, family member, other caretaker)
• Client/family response to teaching activities

TEACHING–LEARNING AND THE NURSING PROCESS

The teaching–learning process and the nursing process are interdependent. Both are dynamic and comprise the same phases: assessment, diagnosis, planning, implementation, and evaluation. Figure 11-10, page 197, compares the nursing process and the teaching–learning process.

Assessment

The nurse should assess each learning situation for each client. Primary (client) and secondary (family or significant other) sources are used by nurses to assess learning needs. Communication with the client and family or significant others is the foundation of assessment related to learning. Several factors must be considered during assessment:

• Actual learning needs
• Potential learning needs
• Client strengths and limitations
• Previous experiences

Actual Learning Needs

Everyone who receives health care services has some need for learning. Client teaching may be indicated when a client:

INITIAL EDUCATIONAL ASSESSMENT

EDUCATIONAL

Patient Family Learning Needs: (initial all that apply:)

___ Present Illness ___ Rehabilitation ___ Hypertension ___ Diabetes ___ Heart Disease ___ Cancer
___ Incontinence ___ Medications ___ Diet ___ Skin Care ___ Post-Op Care ___ Home Equipment
___ Community resources ___ Personal hygiene & grooming ___ * Other ___________

All "yes" answers require comment Patient/Family Ability to Learn:
*Physical Limitations: ___ No ___ Yes *Cognitive Limitations: ___ No ___ Yes *Emotional Barriers: ___ No ___ Yes
*Language Barrier: ___ No ___ Yes *Primary Language Spoken ___ English ___ Spanish ___ Other: ___________
Ability to read ___ English ___ Spanish ___ Other ___ None
Religious or cultural practices that may impact care of education ___ No ___ Yes
Financial implications of care choices. ___ No ___ Yes
COMMENTS: ___________
Patient/Family Preferences for Learning: (Initial all that apply:)
___ Video ___ Demonstration ___ 1 to 1 instruction ___ Handout material
___ Other (please comment) ___________
Patient/Family Readiness to Learn: ___ Express readiness ___ Express desire to delay learning (Comment) ___________
Date: ___________ Time: ___________ Signature: ___________

KEYS:

Learner		Teaching Methods	Limitations to Learning		Evaluation	
Patient [P] Spouse	[S]	Written Material [W] Video [V]	None [1] Pain [2] Anxiety	[3]	States Understanding	[S]
Family [F] Other	[O]	Demonstration [D] Explanation [E]	Physical Limitation	[4]	Reference (See CPG, Problem List Teaching Records)	[Ref]
Demonstration	[D]		Unable to Understand	[5]	No Indication Learning Has Occurred	[N]
Video	[V]		Disinterested	[6]	Return Demonstration	[R]
					Needs ongoing instruction	[O]

DATE	TIME	CONTENT	LEARNER	TEACHING METHODS	LIMITA TIONS	EVALU ATION	SIGNATURE/ DEPT.
		Explanation of disease process, diagnosis, or condition.(Specify)___________					
		Pre Op Teaching/Preparation for diagnostic tests/invasive procedure (Specify)___________					
		Food/Drug interactions (list drugs) ___________					
		Diet Education ___________					
		Medication Use (List drugs) ___________					
		Medical Equipment (List) ___________ ☐ No Need Identified					

Content continued on back if needed.

3189

SPOHN HEALTH SYSTEM
CORPUS CHRISTI, TEXAS 78404

MULTIDISCIPLINARY PATIENT/FAMILY
EDUCATION SUMMARY
PATIENT CARE SERVICES

NEW: 09/95
REV: 05/98 2705187.FM4

KEYS:

Learner		Teaching Methods	Limitations to Learning		Evaluation	
Patient [P] Spouse	[S]	Written Material [W] Video [V]	None [1] Pain [2] Anxiety	[3]	States Understanding	[S]
Family [F] Other	[O]	Demonstration [D] Explanation [E]	Physical Limitation	[4]	Reference (See CPG, Problem List Teaching Records)	[Ref]
Demonstration	[D]		Unable to Understand	[5]	No Indication Learning Has Occurred	[N]
Video	[V]		Disinterested	[6]	Return Demonstration	[R]
					Needs ongoing instruction	[O]

DATE	TIME	CONTENT	LEARNER	TEACHING METHODS	LIMITA TIONS	EVALUA TION	SIGNATURE/ DEPT.
		Rehabilitation (Describe) PT ______ TR ______ OT ______ Speech ______					
		Special Treatments (Describe)					
		Community Resources (Specify) ___________					
		Diabetes Teaching ☐ DM Medication ☐ Insulin Adm. Techniques ☐ Diet Guidelines ☐ Hypoglycemia – Sx., Tx, Prev. ☐ Foot Care ☐ Sick Day Guidelines ☐ Referred to OP Diabetes Class					
		Explanation of safety program, level precautions, and wristband					
		Tests and Procedures Education: (Specify) ___________					
		Topic ___________					
		Topic ___________					
		Topic ___________					
		Topic ___________					
		Topic ___________					

INITIALS	SIGNATURE	INITIALS	SIGNATURE	INITIALS	SIGNATURE

2705187.FM4 – 07/08/98

Figure 11-8 Documentation Form for Client Teaching: Inpatient Setting *(Courtesy of Spohn Health System, Corpus Christi, TX)*

RIVER REGION HOME HEALTH SERVICES, INC.
PSYCHIATRIC NURSE PROGRESS NOTE

PATIENT NAME _____ MR# _____ _____ IN_____ OUT_____

NURSE NAME _____ _____ DAY _____ DATE _____

VSBP _____ T _____ P_____ R _____ WT _____ DIET_____

Nutritional Status _____   Heart/Lung Status_____

Neuro Oriented X _____ PEERL_____   Homebound Status _____

Physical Status _____

_____

Assess Degree of Existing Problem: (1) Mild, (2) Moderate, (3) Severe

Somatic Concern	_____	Emotional Withdrawal	_____	Anxiety	_____
Depressive Mood	_____	Hostility	_____	Uncooperativeness	_____
Blunted Affect	_____	Lack of Insight	_____	Delusions	_____
Suicidal Ideation	_____	Motivational Disability	_____	Hallucinations	_____
Impaired Memory	_____	Rx Non–Compliance	_____	Socialization	_____
Communication	_____	Mannerisms & Posturing	_____		
ADL's	_____	Unusual Thought Concern	_____		
Conceptual Disorganization	_____				

SN Assessment/Intervention/Teaching: _____

_____

_____

Teaching: _____

_____

_____

Feedback to Teaching: _____

_____

Changes: Meds/Plan of Care:_____

Aide Supervision AS/PAS: _____

Reason HHA Needed: _____

Comments Regarding Care: _____

_____

HOME HEALTH ASSISTANT _____   PATIENT _____

Current Requisition in Home _____   Appearance _____   Dolpe _____

Completes Assignment _____   Bathed Completely _____

Rapport with Patient _____   Body Alignment _____

PT/FMY Satisfied _____

Room Tidy _____

Planning: Continue Same Plan_____   Personal Hygiene _____

Increase Visits _____

Decrease Visits _____

Discharge Planning _____

_____   _____
NURSE SIGNATURE   PATIENT OR CAREGIVER SIGNATURE

Figure 11-9 Documentation Form for Client Teaching: Home Health (*Courtesy of River Region Home Health Services, Inc., Louisiana*)

TEACHING-LEARNING PROCESS

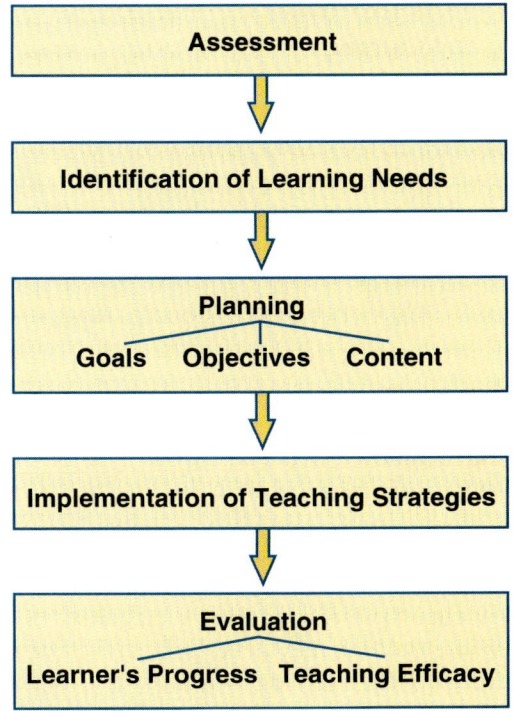

NURSING PROCESS

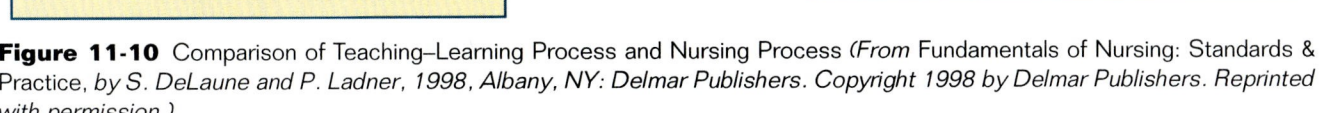

Figure 11-10 Comparison of Teaching–Learning Process and Nursing Process (*From* Fundamentals of Nursing: Standards & Practice, *by S. DeLaune and P. Ladner, 1998, Albany, NY: Delmar Publishers. Copyright 1998 by Delmar Publishers. Reprinted with permission.)*

- Expresses a need for information to make decisions,
- Needs new skills,
- Wants to make lifestyle modifications, or
- Is in an unfamiliar environment.

A crucial step in teaching is to determine the client's learning needs—those things the client needs to know and those things the client already knows. The nurse must evaluate the client's knowledge about the content to be taught. Previous knowledge can then be used as a foundation for new concepts. If the client is misinformed, the nurse must develop a remediation plan for learning. Determining the client's learning needs is accomplished in a variety of ways, including:

- Questioning the client directly,
- Observing client behaviors, and
- Interacting with the client's family or significant others.

It is imperative that the nurse first address the client's immediate need for knowledge by assessing the client's perception of learning needs and prioritizing those needs on the basis of client input and status. For example, preoperative clients must be taught deep breathing exercises and leg exercises before surgery so that they will be able to perform those exercises after

surgery and thereby prevent potential complications. After surgery, incision care to be performed at home can be taught. Comprehensive assessment is a mutual process between client and nurse. The client's opinion regarding the most pressing needs is a critical factor in prioritizing those needs.

Potential Learning Needs

The nurse also assesses for potential learning needs so that anticipatory planning can be done to avert a relapse in the recovery process and to maintain wellness. Following are two scenarios with related anticipatory learning needs noted:

- Mrs. Stone is pregnant for the first time. *Potential learning need:* Infant care.
- Mr. Carpenter has diabetes that is currently controlled by dietary modifications. He has just been told that he may have to take insulin daily in the future. *Potential learning need:* Self-administration of insulin.

Client Strengths and Limitations

Identification of the client's strengths and limitations provides a foundation for realistic expectations. An understanding of the client's strengths and weaknesses allows the nurse to plan successful teaching–learning

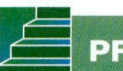

PROFESSIONAL TIP

Learning Needs Assessment

Questions to ask in assessing the client's learning needs include the following:

- Does the client express uncertainty over an up-coming procedure?
- Is the client able to tell you about medications, purposes, and side effects?
- Can the client describe necessary lifestyle modifications?
- Does the client correctly perform self-care activities?
- Is the client able to demonstrate necessary treatment procedures (e.g., colostomy irrigations, injections, blood glucose monitoring)?

CULTURAL CONSIDERATIONS

Learning and Culture

- Culture plays an important role in knowledge acquisition.
- Attitudes (which are derived from a cultural context) toward what is appropriate to learn and who should teach may require alterations in the nurse's approach.
- Sensitivity to cultural values affects every aspect of the teaching–learning process.

experiences. Determination of client strengths assists the nurse in selecting appropriate teaching methods. For example, a client who has limited vision should not be given pamphlets or other reading material in small print from which to learn the intended information.

Previous Experiences

The client has a knowledge base acquired through life experiences. Previous knowledge affects the client's attitudes about learning and the client's perception of the importance of the information to be learned. Previous knowledge is related to the client's type of educational experiences. A client who has had several experiences of hospitalization will have both a basis of knowledge and feelings (positive and negative) about those experiences. Current attitudes about this hospitalization will be influenced by prior hospital experiences.

Identification of Learning Needs (Nursing Diagnosis)

Several nursing diagnoses are pertinent to the learning process. When lack of knowledge is the primary learning need, the diagnosis of *Knowledge Deficit* is applicable. For example:

- A client who does not understand the way to use crutches for assisted ambulation may have the diagnosis of *Knowledge Deficit: Crutchwalking, related to inexperience as evidenced by multiple questions and hesitancy to walk.*
- A client who has had a colostomy and will be discharged soon may have a diagnosis of *Knowledge Deficit: Follow-up Care related to colostomy care and maintenance as evidenced by requests for information.*

Knowledge deficit may also be a component of many other nursing diagnoses that encompass risk or impaired behavior. For instance, *Risk for Infection* may relate to a client's compromised health status; this risk can be modified or reduced through certain physical and environmental changes and through proper client education. A client presenting with a diagnosis of a *Self-Care Deficit: Bathing* may need both assistance in acquiring the physical supplies to remedy the deficit and instruction in techniques related to present physical and mental abilities.

Planning

Learning does not just happen by chance—it is planned. An important part of planning in the teaching–learning process is goal setting. The client and family or significant others must be involved in the setting of goals. Mutually determined goals promote learning. Specific learning goals should include the following elements:

- Measurable behavioral change
- Time frame
- Methods and intervals for evaluation

Teaching–learning goals must be realistic, that is, based on the abilities of the learner and the teacher.

Establishing teaching–learning goals involves setting priorities. One way to set priorities with regard to goals is to teach "need-to-know" content (that which is necessary for survival) before moving on to "nice-to-know" content. For example, Mrs. Stone, who is in her first trimester of pregnancy, must be taught guidelines for diet and exercise ("need-to-know" content); information about infant care ("nice-to-know" content at this time) can be given later in the pregnancy.

Planning, an ongoing phase of the teaching process, involves consideration of the following:

- Why teach?
- What should be taught?
- How should teaching be done?
- Who should teach and who should be taught?

- When should teaching occur?
- Where should teaching occur?

Why Teach?

Client need is *why* teaching is done. The client may realize the need for knowledge about a given subject and ask for information or ask questions about the subject. The nurse should recognize the client's need for knowledge even when the client does not recognize that need. For example, the nurse should recognize that a preoperative client needs to know how to do deep breathing exercises and leg exercises after surgery. The nurse should then plan teaching for that purpose.

What Should Be Taught?

Determination of *what* to teach is accomplished through comprehensive assessment. The content to be taught depends greatly on the client's knowledge base, readiness to learn, and current health status.

How Should Teaching Be Done?

Deciding *how* to teach involves ascertaining which teaching strategies are best given the content and the client's learning style and abilities. The nurse who is an effective teacher uses methods that capture the client's interest. Selection of teaching methods is often influenced by the teaching location. For example, videos can often be used effectively in inpatient settings; however, the same information may need to be presented with flipcharts or brochures in the home setting.

Who Should Teach and Who Should Be Taught?

Planning also means deciding *who* will teach the client. Although effective client education is the result of a multidisciplinary effort, the nurse is the coordinator of the health care team's teaching activities. Responsibility for planning a comprehensive teaching approach, from admission to postdischarge, rests with the nurse. Continuity of care is greatly affected by the teaching plan. The "who" part of planning also relates to who should be taught. The nurse must determine who in addition to the client (e.g., family members, significant others) must be taught about the illness and recovery process.

When Should Teaching Occur?

When to teach should be carefully considered. The nurse should recognize that every interaction with the client is an opportunity for teaching. Whenever a client asks a question, there is an opportunity for teaching. These windows of teaching opportunity must be used. Nothing destroys a client's motivation to learn more quickly than hearing comments such as "Ask your doctor that" or "We'll talk about that later. Right now, take your medicine." The best time for teaching is when the client is comfortable—physically and psychologically.

Where Should Teaching Occur?

Where teaching occurs must also be well planned. The location of teaching affects the quality of learning. Some factors to be considered in determining the location of teaching include provision of privacy and availability of equipment.

Implementation

Katz (1997) suggests several strategies to achieve successful client teaching, as outlined in the following sections.

Get and Keep the Client's Attention

The nurse should begin a teaching session by letting the client know what is going to be taught and why it is important to the client. The nurse can retain the client's interest by varying the tone of voice and using assorted teaching methods to present the material. Making the abstract concrete by using realistic examples from the client's experience is also effective in keeping the client's attention.

Stick to the Basics

Because the average adult can remember only five to seven points at a time, the nurse must be specific about what the client is to learn. Simple, everyday language should be used, and the most critical information presented first.

Use Time Wisely

The nurse can incorporate teaching into client care by providing information during each nurse–client interaction. Involving the client's family and friends, allow-

PROFESSIONAL TIP

Guidelines for Effective Client Teaching

- Assess the client's knowledge and needs
- Focus on the client's perceived needs
- Relate material to the client's prior knowledge
- Encourage the client's active participation
- Provide opportunity for immediate application of knowledge or skill
- Expect learning plateaus
- Reinforce learning frequently
- Provide immediate feedback to facilitate learning
- Ensure a comfortable environment
- Organize content from the simple to the complex, building on what the client already knows
- Use a variety of teaching methods
- Emphasize oral instructions with the written word and pictures
- Maintain a flexible approach
- Be creative

ing them to discuss the material with the client, is also helpful. The nurse should consider supplementing teaching with written material for the client and/or family to read; doing so provides time for the learners to review the material and then ask questions to clarify understanding.

Reinforce Information

Repetition creates habits; the nurse can take advantage of this by reviewing the material with the client and serving as a role model. For example, when teaching a client a procedure, the nurse must be sure to do it correctly each time and to avoid taking shortcuts. The nurse can reward the client by giving positive reinforcement such as a smile, a nod, or a few words of praise.

Evaluation

Evaluation of teaching–learning is a twofold process:

1. Determining what the client has learned
2. Assessing the nurse's teaching effectiveness

Evaluation of Learning

In performing the continual process of evaluating what the client has learned, the nurse must determine whether a behavior change has occurred, whether the behavior change is related to learning activities, whether further change is necessary, and whether continued behavior change will promote health. The following strategies can be used to evaluate client learning:

- Oral questioning
- Observation
- Return demonstration
- Written follow-up (e.g., questionnaires)

Evaluation of Teaching

A major purpose of evaluation is to assess the effectiveness of the teaching activities and decide which modifications, if any, are necessary. When learning objectives are not met, reassessment is the basis for modifying teaching–learning activities. Evaluation is facilitated by the use of goals that are measurable and specific. Several activities can be used in evaluating teaching effectiveness:

- Feedback from the learner
- Feedback from colleagues
- Situational feedback
- Self-evaluation

SUMMARY

- Client education is designed to help individuals achieve optimal states of health.
- The teaching–learning process is a planned interaction that promotes behavioral change that is not a result of maturation or coincidence.

PROFESSIONAL TIP

Evaluation of Learning

- Did the client meet mutually established goals and objectives?
- Can the client demonstrate skills?
- Have the client's attitudes changed?
- Can the client cope better with illness-imposed limitations?
- Does the family understand the health problem and know ways to help?

PROFESSIONAL TIP

Evaluation of Teacher Effectiveness

- Was content presented clearly and at the client's level of comprehension?
- Was the presentation (session) interesting?
- Did the nurse use a variety of teaching aids?
- Were the teaching aids appropriate for the client and the content?
- Was client participation encouraged?
- Was the nurse supportive?
- Did the nurse communicate an interest in the client and in the material?
- Did the nurse give frequent feedback and allow for immediate return demonstration?
- Were learning objectives stated in behavioral terms (i.e., easy to evaluate)?

- Teaching supports behavior change leading to positive adaptation.
- Learning is the process of assimilating information, resulting in behavioral change.
- Learning occurs in three domains: the cognitive (intellectual), the affective (emotional), and the psychomotor (motor skills).
- Learning readiness is affected by developmental and sociocultural factors and is present throughout the life span and at every developmental stage.
- Elements of documenting client education include the content taught, the teaching methods used, the person(s) taught, and the response of the learners.
- The teaching–learning process and the nursing process are interdependent, dynamic processes.
- Evaluation of the teaching–learning process involves two aspects: determination of what the client has learned and assessment of teacher efficacy.

CASE STUDY

Mr. Martinez, a 65-year-old widower from Mexico, recently moved in with his daughter and her family. He has just been diagnosed with diabetes. The physician orders dietary modifications, Mr. Martinez just sits and shakes his head, saying "I don't understand."

The following questions will guide your development of client teaching for Mr. Martinez.

1. What other data should be collected about Mr. Martinez?
2. Which domain(s) of learning should be considered?
3. What barriers to learning might be pertinent?
4. Identify a nursing diagnosis related to client teaching for Mr. Martinez.
5. Determine the *why, who, what, when, where,* and *how* of a teaching plan for Mr. Martinez.
6. What goals might be set with Mr. Martinez?
7. How will the effectiveness of teaching be evaluated?

Review Questions

1. Bloom identified three areas wherein learning occurs: the psychomotor domain, the affective domain, and the:
   a. attitude domain.
   b. cognitive domain.
   c. emotional domain.
   d. knowledge domain.

2. A clinical example of psychomotor learning is when a client:
   a. changes the dressing on a leg ulcer.
   b. states an acceptance of a chronic illness.
   c. states the name and purpose of a medication.
   d. chooses to change the type of exercise performed.

3. Kinesthetic learners learn by:
   a. doing.
   b. seeing.
   c. hearing.
   d. listening.

4. It is important for the nurse to be aware that learning needs:
   a. change daily.
   b. are the same for everyone.
   c. change throughout the life cycle.
   d. change as teaching approaches are modified.

5. Nurses are required to provide teaching by:
   a. all state nursing practice acts.
   b. the National League for Nursing.
   c. the American Hospital Association.
   d. the Joint Commission for Accreditation of Healthcare Organizations.

6. Because age is not synonymous with developmental level, the nurse, when preparing to teach a client, must:
   a. teach everyone the same way.
   b. set the goals for the client.
   c. observe the client's behavior.
   d. ask the client about self-efficacy.

Critical Thinking Questions

1. Is it ethical for a nurse to attempt to change a client's beliefs under the guise of teaching? Should a nurse "teach" a client the "right" attitude or belief?

2. Will knowledge acquisition alone result in learning (behavioral change)? Why? Why not?

 WEB FLASH!

- Search the Web for topics such as client teaching, teaching elders, teaching children, teaching adolescents. Can you find information specific to nursing?
- What organizations are available for help with teaching methods?
- What resources can you locate that provide teaching aids and materials?

UNIT
5
Cultural Aspects of Nursing

CULTURAL DIVERSITY AND NURSING

MAKING THE CONNECTION

Refer to the following chapters to increase your understanding of cultural diversity and nursing:

- **Chapter 1, Holistic Care**
- **Chapter 7, Ethical Responsibilities**
- **Chapter 8, Communication**
- **Chapter 13, Alternative/Complementary Therapies**
- **Chapter 15, Wellness Concepts**
- **Chapter 18, Basic Nutrition**
- **Chapter 26, Pain Management**

LEARNING OBJECTIVES

Upon completion of this chapter, you should be able to:
- *Define key terms.*
- *Describe the components and characteristics of culture.*
- *Describe the impact of cultural beliefs on health and illness.*
- *Compare and contrast diverse health beliefs of major cultural groups in the United States.*
- *Describe specific differences of cultural groups in relation to time and space.*
- *Identify nutritional preferences held by various cultural groups.*
- *Identify the general beliefs that account for the differences among religions.*
- *Describe the way that the nurse's religious beliefs or lack thereof can influence nursing care.*
- *Discuss the nurse's role in meeting the spiritual needs of the client and family.*
- *Analyze personal cultural beliefs and values.*
- *Perform a cultural assessment.*

INTRODUCTION

Every aspect of one's life—including attitudes, beliefs, and values—is influenced by one's culture. Behavior, including behavior affecting health, is culturally determined. As the population of the United States continues to diversify, recognition of cultural differences and their impact on health care becomes more critical. Nurses provide health care to culturally diverse client populations in a variety of settings. Knowledge of culturally relevant information is thus essential for delivery of competent nursing care. This chapter discusses the various concepts related to culture, the influence of culture on health, the relationships between culture and health beliefs, cultural aspects and the nursing process, and illnesses associated with ethnic groups.

CULTURE

Each individual is culturally unique. Behavior, self-perception, and judgment of others all depend on one's cultural perspective. To provide holistic care, the nurse needs a thorough understanding of concepts relating to culture.

In society, **culture** refers to dynamic and integrated structures of knowledge, beliefs, behaviors, ideas, attitudes, values, habits, customs, languages, symbols,

KEY TERMS

acculturation	minority group
agnostic	oppression
atheist	race
culture	religious support system
cultural assimilation	spiritual care
cultural diversity	spiritual needs
dominant culture	stereotyping
ethnicity	yin and yang
ethnocentrism	

rituals, ceremonies, and practices that are unique to a particular group of people. This structure provides the group of people with a general design for living.

Individuals often acquire cultural beliefs unconsciously throughout the process of growth and maturation (Giger & Davidhizar, 1999). People are exposed to culture at an early age through the observance of traditions (established customary patterns of thought and behavior). Cultural beliefs, values, customs, and behaviors are transmitted from one generation to another through interaction, daily activities, and celebrations. For instance, the birth of a child is celebrated according to the family's cultural norms and customs, which may include prayers, blessings, special naming ceremonies, religious rites, and so forth. Grandparents, other elders, and parents all teach children cultural expectations and norms through role modeling, demonstration, and discussion (Figure 12-1).

Culture is not static nor is it uniform among all members within a given cultural group. Culture repre-

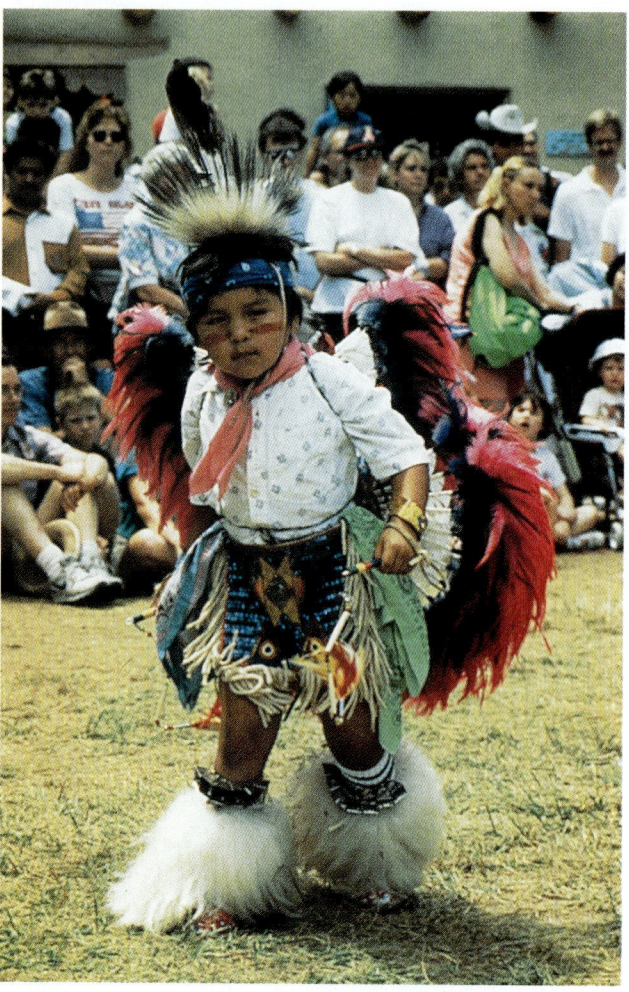

Figure 12-1 This child is celebrating his Native American heritage by participating in a traditional ceremony that has been passed down through the generations. *(Photo courtesy of Smithsonian Institution)*

 CULTURAL CONSIDERATIONS

Sharing Culture
Cultural messages are transmitted in a variety of settings such as homes, schools, religious organizations, and communities. The various media, such as radio and television, are also powerful transmitters and shapers of culture.

sents adaptive dynamic processes learned through life experiences. Diversity among and within cultural groups results from individual perspectives and practices. Consider, for example, the way that a family deals with a crisis. A crisis may cause a family that is part of a culture with a strong sense of responsibility to family and blood relatives to become closer; conversely, the same situation may cause a family that is from a culture that values independence and individuality to withdraw and create distance among its members. These reactions are rooted in the family's cultural background and heritage.

Ethnicity and Race

Ethnicity is a cultural group's perception of itself, or a group identity. Ethnicity is a sense of belongingness and a common social heritage that is passed from one generation to the next. Members of an ethnic group demonstrate their shared sense of identity through common customs and traits. Ethnic identity can be expressed in many ways, including dress; for instance, many African Americans display ethnic pride by choosing clothing that highlights their ethnic origin and shared heritage.

Race refers to a grouping of people based on biological similarities. Members of a racial group have similar physical characteristics such as blood group, facial features, and color of skin, hair, and eyes. There is often overlap between racial and ethnic groups because the cultural and biological commonalities support one another (Giger & Davidhizar, 1999). The similarities of people in racial and ethnic groups reinforce a sense of commonality and cohesiveness.

Cultural Diversity

Cultural diversity refers to the differences among people that result from racial, ethnic, and cultural variables. Within the United States exist a variety of rich cultural heritages. The vast potential of human resources with divergent viewpoints and behaviors enriches the sociopolitical climate. New and varied ideas, viewpoints, and problem-solving approaches and increased tolerance are all outcomes of a diverse population.

There are also some disadvantages associated with living and working in such a culturally diverse society.

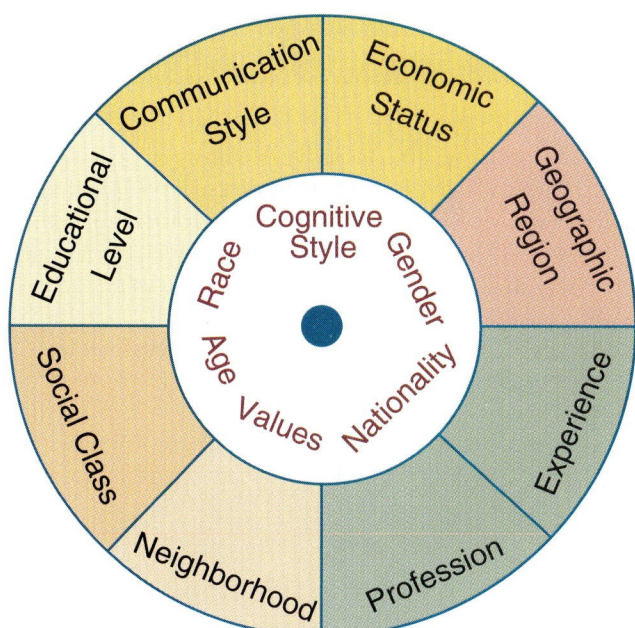

Figure 12-2 Areas of Cultural Diversity (*From* Fundamentals of Nursing: Standards & Practice, *by S. DeLaune and P. Ladner, 1998, Albany, NY: Delmar Publishers. Copyright 1998 by Delmar Publishers.*)

Problems arise when differences across and within cultural groups are misunderstood. Misperception, confusion, and ignorance often accompany people's expectations of others. Figure 12-2 illustrates the many areas in which individuals may differ.

Members of some cultural groups have historically and globally experienced bias or prejudice in the forms of racism (discrimination based on race and biological differences), sexism (discrimination based on gender), and classism (prejudice based on perceived social class). These biases are perpetuated (consciously and unconsciously) by society. The basic underlying premise of these biases is that one way is better or "right," and every other way is inferior. **Ethnocentrism**, an assumption of cultural superiority and an inability to accept other cultures' ways of organizing reality, results in oppression. **Oppression** occurs when the rules, modes, and ideals of one group are imposed on another group. Oppression is based on cultural biases, which stem from values, beliefs, traditions, and cultural expectations.

Stereotyping is the belief that all people within the same racial, ethnic, or cultural group will act alike and share the same beliefs and attitudes. Stereotyping results in labeling people according to cultural preconceptions, thereby ignoring individual identity.

A **dominant culture** is the group whose values prevail within a given society. The dominant culture of the United States is that composed of white, middle-class Protestants of European ancestry. The European value orientation has greatly influenced U. S. culture,

as illustrated by the following beliefs held by the dominant culture:

- Achievement and success
- Individualism, independence, and self-reliance
- Activity, work, and ownership
- Efficiency, practicality, and reliance on technology
- Material comfort
- Competition and achievement
- Youth and beauty

Frequently, these dominant values conflict with the values of minority groups. A **minority group** is a group of people that constitutes less than a numerical majority of the population. Because of their cultural, racial, ethnic, religious, or other characteristics, such groups are often labeled and treated differently from others in the society. Minority groups are usually considered to be less powerful than the dominant group (Giger & Davidhizar, 1999).

People assume the characteristics of the dominant culture through **acculturation**, which is the process of learning norms, beliefs, and behavioral expectations of a group. **Cultural assimilation** occurs when individuals from a minority group are absorbed by the dominant culture and take on the characteristics of the dominant culture.

Components of Culture

Stewart has identified five components of culture that organize the way people think about life (as cited in Lock, 1992).

- Activity: identifies how people organize and value work
- Social relations: explains the importance and structure of friendships, gender roles, and class
- Motivation: describes the value and methods of achievement
- Perception of the world: refers to the interpretation of life events and religious beliefs
- Perception of self and the individual: refers to personal identity, value, and respect for individuals

This model is particularly helpful to the nurse who is planning care for a client from another ethnic group.

 CULTURAL CONSIDERATIONS

Individuality
Remember that each person is first and foremost an individual, and secondly a member of a cultural group. While similarities may exist within an ethnic or culture group, individual differences must also be respected.

Work, social relationships, success, religion, and self-identity influence both the definition cultural groups attribute to health and illness and the cultural group's response to health events. For example, if a culture values relationships more than work, the culture may sanction an extended period of illness and a lengthy time away from the employment site. However, if a culture measures achievement by output at work, illness may be interpreted in a negative manner. Members of the latter culture may deny illness and delay seeking appropriate health care.

Characteristics of Culture

Spradley and Allender (1996) have identified five characteristics shared by all cultures.

- Culture is learned. Patterns of behavior are acquired as children imitate adults and develop actions and attitudes acceptable by others in society.
- Culture is not inherited or innate, but, rather, culture is integrated throughout all the interrelated components. Activities, relationships, motivations, world views, and individuality are permeated with consistent patterns of behavior to form a cohesive whole.
- Culture is shared by everyone who belongs to the cultural group. Behavioral patterns are not individually defined, but, rather, are accepted and practiced by all.
- Culture is tacit (unspoken), in that acceptable behavior is understood by everyone in the cultural group, regardless of whether beliefs are written down or spoken. Cultural beliefs are commonly known and adopted.
- Culture is dynamic; it is constantly changing. Each generation experiences new ideas that may generate different standards for behavior.

CULTURAL INFLUENCES ON HEALTH CARE BELIEFS AND PRACTICES

It is common for cultural groups to have a body of knowledge and beliefs about health and disease. Cultural practices can positively and negatively affect health and disease distribution. In cultures where raw foods are not consumed, for instance, the incidence of shigellosis may be lower than cultures where consumption of raw meat and fish is common. On the other hand, cultural taboos against eating protein during pregnancy have a harmful or destructive effect on fetal development. Human responses to illness are defined by cultural values. Whether an individual seeks professional care when ill and complies with prescribed treatment depends on cultural values.

Beliefs and patterns of behavior affect attitudes about various aspects of health. Beliefs about the defi-

PROFESSIONAL TIP

Cultural Sensitivity

Nurses must be able to provide culturally appropriate care to a diverse population of clients. Cultural diversity presents special challenges for nurses who must provide care that is incongruent with personal beliefs and values. Nurses caring for clients who differ from themselves must remember to ascertain the client's perception of the event (illness), including the significance (meaning) that the client assigns the event. The nurse must honor individual differences and understand that culture influences the way clients are viewed and treated within health care settings.

nition of health; etiology (cause and origin of disease); health promotion and protection practices; and health practitioners and remedies are all influenced by cultural background.

Definition of Health

The most widely accepted definition of health, developed by the World Health Organization (WHO), purports that health is not only the absence of disease, but also complete physical, mental, and social wellness. While this definition of health is broad enough to be global, that which is understood to be physical, mental, and social wellness is culturally defined. Any deviation from that which is culturally understood to be normal health is considered illness. For example, a biological disease of immediate etiology might not be interpreted as an illness by some cultures; intestinal parasites are so common in some areas in Africa that the presence of ascaris in stools is considered normal. When the cultural group does not recognize certain behaviors or symptoms as illness, individuals are not likely to seek medical intervention when these symptoms appear. In such cases, disease conditions may persist untreated to an irreversible state.

Etiology

Peter Morley, a noted medical anthropologist, presents four views of the origin of disease: supernatural, nonsupernatural, immediate, and ultimate (Morley & Wallis, 1978). The supernatural view of disease traces disease to metaphysical forces such as witchcraft, sorcery, and voodoo. In this view, an individual might ascribe illness to evil spirits or to a curse by a powerful spiritual person. The nonsupernatural view holds that diseases have an accepted cause-and-effect relationship, even though that relationship may lack scientific rationale. For example, people of many cultures believe that colic in an infant is caused by breast milk rendered impure when a nursing mother has sexual relations. In such cultures, sexual relations are prohibited for nursing mothers. The immediate view of disease traces diseases to known pathogenic agents, such as chickenpox is caused by *Herpes varicella;* and the ultimate view describes determinates for diseases, such as smoking resulting in lung cancer. Most cultural groups support a multietiologic origin, borrowing from three or all four explanations for how and why diseases occur.

Health Promotion and Protection

Strategies for achieving and maintaining good health vary by cultural group. For example, the dominant U.S. culture has come to endorse a low-fat, high-fiber diet; regular exercise; and appropriate immunizations as means to promote and protect health. Other cultures may place greater value on meditation, prayer, and restored relationships, particularly those cultures wherein health protection and disease prevention are closely linked to beliefs about disease etiology. For example, preventing disease may require paying homage to ancestral spirits in order to avoid offending them and provoking their revenge through illness.

Practitioners and Remedies

Variety in health/illness care providers is a natural extension of culturally diverse concepts of etiology and definitions of health and illness. Alternative remedies and practitioners are characteristic of culturally diverse groups. When a scientific rationale for the etiology of disease is not accepted by a cultural group, standard medicine may not be accepted as treatment. In order to enhance client compliance with treatment regimens health care providers must make efforts to base therapy and prescribe treatments that respect culturally traditional remedies. Clients who trace disease etiology to a supernatural cause are more likely to seek interventions from spiritual leaders or traditional healers.

The folk medicine system categorizes illnesses as either natural or unnatural (Giger & Davidhizar, 1999). The classification of an illness determines the type of treatment and healer used. Because the folk medicine system (also referred to as alternative medicine) can present challenges to nurses caring for clients from diverse cultures, knowledge of basic beliefs about illness, factors contributing to illness, and home remedies is necessary.

Folk healers are knowledgeable about cultural norms and customs (Edelman & Mandle, 1998). Table 12-1 lists both the various healers within the five dominant cultural groups in the United States (European American, African American, Hispanic American, Asian American, and Native American) and the common folk healing practices within these cultures. Nurses must be able to relate care and treatment to the client's cultural context and incorporate informal caregivers, healers, and other members of the client's support system as allies in treatment.

Beliefs of Select Cultural Groups

While the population of the United States encompasses innumerable ethnic groups—European Americans, African Americans, Hispanic Americans, Asian Americans, and Native Americans together represent a majority. These groups form the basis for the following brief discussion of specific health beliefs affected by culture.

European American

In 1990, Americans of European descent represented 75% of the U.S. population; this figure is expected to be only 53% by the year 2020, however (U.S. Department of Commerce, Bureau of the Census, 1992). The prevailing value system for many European Americans is based on what is referred to as the white, Anglo-Saxon, Protestant (WASP) ethic (Sue & Sue, 1990). This ethic traces its origins to the Caucasian Protestants who came to this country from Northern Europe over 200 years ago. Values that still dominate the Caucasian American middle-class ethic include independence, individuality, wealth, comfort, cleanliness, achievement, punctuality, hard work, aggression, assertiveness, rationality, orientation toward the future, and mastery of one's own fate (Andrews & Boyle, 1998; Edmission, 1997).

Traditionally, most Caucasian Americans have wanted to be recognized as individuals rather than as members of groups. Thus, Caucasian Americans, unlike members of many other cultures, tend to be competitive rather than cooperative with each other. Mainstream American culture also values the nuclear family and its traditions (Luckmann, 1999, p. 25).

African American

The African American population currently represents the largest minority group in the United States (U.S. Department of Commerce, Bureau of the Census, 1992). African American ancestors came to North America from various African countries and the Caribbean as either slaves or free immigrants. The different countries

CULTURAL CONSIDERATIONS

Subculture

Many Caucasian Americans do not belong to the mainstream culture, but, instead, belong to ethnic subcultures that hold strong values of their own (e.g., Irish, Jewish, German, Italian, Norwegian, Appalachian, and Amish subcultures).

Table 12-1 FOLK MEDICINE: HEALERS AND PRACTICES

CULTURAL GROUP	TRADITIONAL HEALERS	HEALING PRACTICES
European American	• Nurse • Physician	• Exercise • Medications • Modified diets • Amulets • Religious healing rituals
African American	• Elderly women healers • "Community Mother" or "Granny" • "Root doctor" • Voodoo healer ("Mambo" or "oungan") • Spiritualist	• Herbs, roots, oils • Poultices • Religious healing through rituals (e.g., laying on of hands) • Talismans worn around the wrist or neck or carried in a pouch to ward off disease
Hispanic American	• Curandero • Espiritualista • Yerbero (herbalist) • Brujo (healer who uses witchcraft) • Sobadora • Santiguadora	• Hot and cold foods to treat some conditions • Herbal teas, such as manzanilla, to treat gastrointestinal problems, insomnia, and menstrual cramps • Prayers and religious medals • Massage • Azabache, a black stone, worn as a necklace or bracelet to ward off the "evil eye" • Among some Haitian mothers, the "three baths" ritual (bathing for the first 3 postpartum days in water boiled with special leaves)
Asian American	• Herbalist • Physician	• Hot and cold foods • Herbs, soups • Cupping, pinching, and rubbing • Meditation • Acupuncture • Acupressure • Application of tiger balm (a salve) to relieve muscular pains • Energy to restore balance between yin and yang
Native American	• Shaman • Medicine man/woman	• Plants and herbs • Medicine bundle or bag filled with herbs that have been blessed by a medicine man/woman during a healing ceremony • Sweet grass (herbs) burned to purify the ill person • Estafiate (dried leaves) boiled to produce a tea for treating stomach disorders • The Blessingway ceremony (a healing ritual conducted by the medicine man/woman) • In some Navajo tribes, sand paintings made by the medicine man/woman for diagnostic purposes

Data compiled from Cultural Diversity and Community Health Nursing Practice, *by C. Degazon, in* Community Health Nursing: Promoting Health of Aggregates, Families, and Individuals *(4th ed.), by M. Stanhope and J. Lancaster (Eds.), 1996, St. Louis: Mosby-Yearbook;* Transcultural Nursing: Assessment and Interventions *(3rd ed.), by J. Giger and R. Davidhizar, 1999, St. Louis, MO: Mosby-Yearbook; and* Cultural Dimensions in Home Health Nursing, *by D. Grossman, 1996,* American Journal of Nursing, *96(7), 33–36.*

of origin as well as disparate educational levels, income, occupations, and religious beliefs explain the heterogeneous (different) cultural practices among African Americans today.

Some African American beliefs about health and illness are linked to either a supernatural or a nonsupernatural view of disease. In traditional African societies, disease may be viewed as caused by disharmony in relationships. Discord may occur between a client and ancestral spirits, evil spirits, or living relatives. For example, if, following a wedding, a man were to refuse to finish making bride-price payments to his in-laws and the man were subsequently to become ill, his illness may be attributed to the break in relations with his wife's family caused by his outstanding debt. Healing comes with restoration of harmony and may be achieved through prayer, meditation, or activities considered to be therapeutic, such as offering a gift, wearing a charm, or confessing a wrong.

Disease may also be viewed as sent by God or another higher power as a punishment for a serious infraction against Him or another person. Evil forces may be thought to account for illness in other cases. Treatments may be found in herbs and home remedies, consultation with a local healer, and prayer.

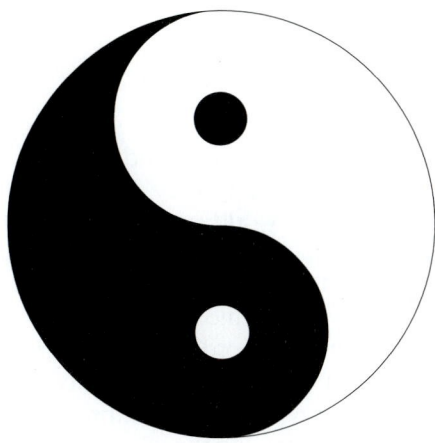

Figure 12-3 Yin and Yang

Hispanic American

Hispanic Americans constitute the second largest minority ethnic group in the United States. The majority of this group has origins in Mexico, Puerto Rico, and Cuba. Although the Spanish language is common to most Hispanics, cultural patterns vary due to the different countries of origin. In general, the Hispanic American belongs to a large extended-family system within which females are seen as subservient to males but as having a major role in family cohesiveness (Giger & Davidhizar, 1999).

The influence of religion on culture is particularly evident in Hispanic populations. Most Hispanic Americans have roots in Catholicism blended with traditional Indian beliefs. Illness may be viewed as having a natural cause, as "an act of God" as punishment for sin, or as the result of witchcraft or a curse by an enemy. Diseases may be traced to an imbalance between "wet" and "dry" or "hot" and "cold" forces. Treatment depends on the cause. Western medicine is appropriate for some diseases, whereas the native healer (curandera) may have to intervene for illnesses having supernatural causes. Treatment may consist of herbal potions, diets based on hot and cold foods, or religious ceremonies.

Asian American

Asian Americans have origins in the Pacific-rim countries: Korea, Vietnam, Laos, the Philippines, Cambodia, China, and Japan. Generalization of a specific Asian culture is not possible among peoples from such a diversity of countries; however, certain similarities exist. Asian cultures are typically patrilineal, that is, family relations are traced through males. Males are the heads of household, and elders are respected.

Asians hold to a yin (cold) and yang (hot) etiology of disease. **Yin and yang** are opposing forces that when in balance yield health (Figure 12-3). Illness occurs as a consequence of an imbalance in these forces. Foods are identified as either hot or cold and are used

in treatment. For example, if yang is overpowering yin, hot foods are avoided until balance is restored. Illness may also be viewed as being caused by supernatural powers such as God, evil spirits, or ancestral spirits. In this situation, healing might be attained through prayer or treatment by a traditional healer. Many Asian Americans rely on herbal remedies, acupuncture, and cupping and burning, a treatment that draws blood to the skin's surface when a warmed cup is placed on the skin. In cupping, the inside and rim of a cup are heated with a candle flame. The rim of the cup is then applied directly to the client's skin, and, as the cup cools, blood is drawn to the surface of the skin, causing a bruised appearance. Cupping is used to draw out evil or illness in order to restore yin and yang. The nurse must be aware of these cultural practices so they are not viewed as abuse but, rather, as important cultural customs.

Native American

The fourth major minority ethnic group in the United States is Native Americans (U.S. Department of Commerce, Bureau of the Census, 1992). These peoples form a very diverse group, stemming from over 200 different tribes across the United States. Although many Native Americans have assumed Euro-American practices with regard to health, some still use traditional practices. Health is believed to result from a harmonious relationship with nature and the universe. Illness is frequently traced to a supernatural origin and discord with the forces of nature. Use of witchcraft can cause illness, and treatment may require exorcism of evil spirits. Prevention may be attained through prayer, charms, and fetishes (objects having power to protect or aid the owner). Remedies often include herbal drinks. "Medicine men" are persons thought to have supernatural powers of healing. Through prayers, rituals, ceremonies, and herbal drinks, health may be restored.

CULTURAL AND RACIAL INFLUENCES ON CLIENT CARE

Clients' cultural backgrounds and preferences influence the manner whereby they interact with other people and with the world around them. In an unfamiliar situation, such as admission to a health care setting, cultural differences may seem even greater, because in times of stress, most people hold tightly to that which is familiar in order to protect themselves from the unknown. The nurse can show caring in such a situation by acknowledging the expression of these differences and encouraging the client to retain what is familiar.

The influences of culture and race can be viewed through the phenomena of communication, space and time orientation, social organization, and biological variations.

Communication

Although language is common to all human beings, not everyone shares the same language. This cultural difference can lead to misunderstanding and frustration. The nurse must realize that a client who speaks a different language or with an accent, simply has a different means of expressing needs. When communication is restricted because of language differences, alternative methods of communication such as gestures and flash cards can be used.

The client's family may be able to assist when there is a block in communication. Family members can interpret procedures and instructions for the client and communicate the client's thoughts and questions to the nurse (Figure 12-4). If no family members are

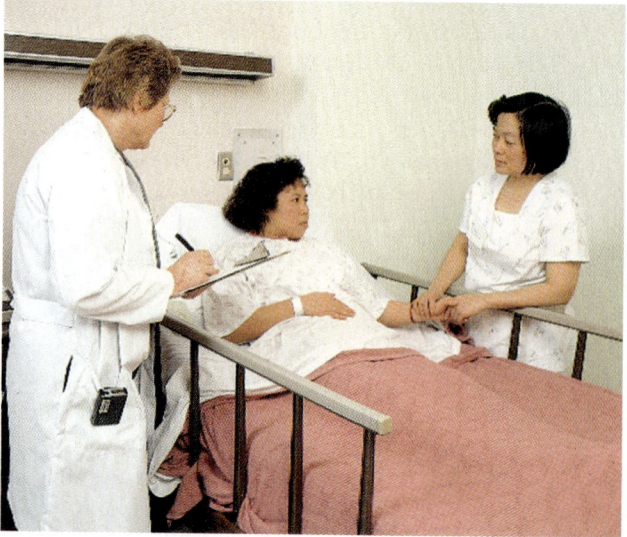

Figure 12-4 Family members can often serve as interpreters to help clients who do not speak English understand procedures and instructions and to communicate the client's thoughts and questions to the nurse.

PROFESSIONAL TIP

Non-native Speakers
When interacting with someone who does not understand English well, many people will try to compensate for the lack of understanding by speaking more loudly. Speaking slowly, distinctly, and in a normal volume are more effective measures to ensure communication.

available, the hospital social worker may be able to find an interpreter.

Orientation to Space and Time

Orientation with regard to space and to time represents two other culturally influenced variables that may affect a client's attitude toward care. Territoriality, or interpretation of personal space, is a pattern of behavior resulting from an individual's belief that certain spaces and objects belong to that person. The distance that a person prefers to maintain from another is determined by one's culture. In general, people of Arabic, Southern European, and African origin frequently sit or stand relatively close to each other (0 to 18 inches), whereas people from Asian, Northern European, and North American origin are more comfortable with a larger personal space (more than 18 inches).

Affection and caring behavior are not communicated by touch in some cultures. For instance, among Asians, adults seldom touch one another, and the head is believed to be sacred. The nurse should thus not touch an Asian client's head without permission to do so. When working with clients from cultures where personal touch is viewed negatively, the nurse should use the universal sign of caring: the smile.

People in U.S. society tend to be future oriented: They plan for the future, establish long-term goals, and, increasingly, are concerned with prevention of future illnesses. In daily life, they are oriented to time of day, constantly referring to clock time for everything from meal time to time of appointments with health care professionals as well as other obligations. The nurse must also be very attentive to time. Medications are given at scheduled times, and work begins and ends at specified times. Other groups that tend to be future oriented are Japanese, Jews, and Arabs. These groups tend to view time as a commodity for achieving future goals.

Not all cultural groups are future oriented, however. People of some cultures (e.g., Asians) may be oriented to the past. For Asians, this orientation is reflected in the roles that ancestor worship and Confucianism play in the present. Members of other cultural groups, such as Native Americans, tend to be present oriented.

Many Native Americans do not own clocks, and they live one day at a time, showing little concern for the future (Giger & Davidhizer, 1999). Mexican Americans and African Americans often value relationships with people in the present more than in the future. African Americans tend to be present oriented in health care behaviors as well. They often express the fatalistic belief that "it's going to happen anyway, so why bother" and fail to seek medical attention until a disabling condition occurs. The African American culture often teaches flexible attention to schedules; whatever is happening currently is most important. Explanations about the necessity of time scheduling, for instance, the need for strict schedules for medication requiring therapeutic blood level maintenance, must be given to the client.

How does time orientation affect health care? An individual's orientation to time may affect promptness or attendance at health care appointments, compliance with self-medication schedules, and reporting the onset of illness or other health concerns. Clients might not see the necessity for preventive health care measures if they experience no difference in their health today when they follow a special diet or exercise programs. The nurse must both teach clients when timing is critical in health care situations and practice patience when working with people whose background differs from that of the dominant culture.

Social Organization

Social organization refers to the ways whereby cultural groups determine rules of acceptable behavior and roles of individual members. Examples of social organization include family structure, gender roles, and religion.

Family Structure

The definition of family has changed dramatically through the years (Doherty, 1992). Until 1920 the norm was the "institutional family," which was organized around economic production and the kinship network. Marriage was a functional, not a romantic, relationship. Family tradition and loyalty were more

CULTURAL CONSIDERATIONS

Environmental Control

Environmental control refers to the relationships between people and nature and to a person's perceived ability to control activities of nature, such as factors causing illness. One's cultural background and heritage influence one's perception of environmental control.

PROFESSIONAL TIP

Families

Each individual defines family differently. These definitions are shaped by personal experience and observation of other families. You must remain objective and nonjudgmental when the client's family is different from your idea of family. Have the client identify family members, so you know exactly who the client considers to be family.

important than individual goals or romantic interests. The chief value was responsibility.

From 1920 to 1960, the norm was the "psychological family." Family affairs were more private and less tied to the extended kinship network. Family was based on personal satisfaction and fulfillment of the individual members in a nuclear, two-parent arrangement. The chief value was satisfaction.

The social changes of the 1960s, including gender equality and personal freedom, caused changes in the family. The increased divorce rate may have resulted from the sexual revolution and the attitude that the individual deserves more and owes less to the family.

Today, no single family arrangement has a monopoly. Many types of families have emerged and are accepted. The chief value is flexibility. Family no longer necessarily implies biological relation, but rather has come to mean members of a shared household who have similar values and participate in shared goals. Fawcett (1993) cites the following characteristics of family:

- Love and affection
- Caring and compassion
- A sense of belonging and connectedness
- A history and linkage to posterity
- Rituals of rejoicing
- A sense of place
- Acceptance of members, including shortcomings
- Honor of elders
- A system of earning and spending money
- A competent manner of parenting or caretaking
- Division of chores and labor

According to systems theory, families are considered to be interdependent, interacting individuals related by birth, marriage, or mutual consent (Sherman, 1994). Examples of families with varying lifestyles today are two-parent nuclear, single-parent, blended (through remarriage), extended (including grandparents), cohabitating (couple having never married), gay or lesbian, divorced, adoptive, multi-adult, and mixed or interracial families (Figure 12-5).

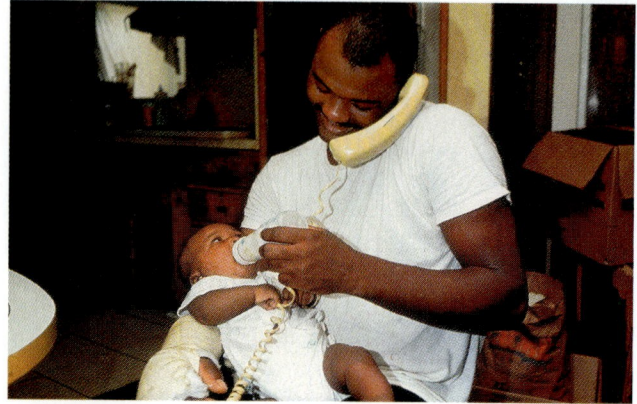

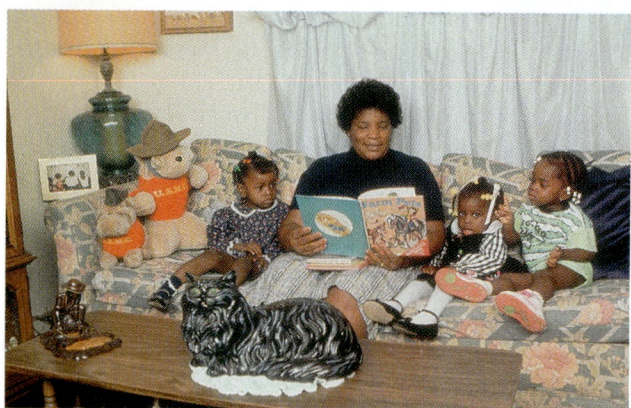

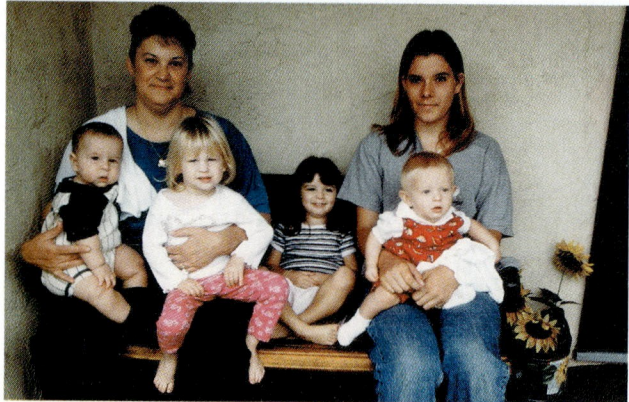

Figure 12-5 Families come in all shapes, sizes, and configurations.

Gender Roles

Gender roles vary according to cultural context (Figure 12-6). For example, in families organized around a patriarchal structure (with the man being the head of the household and chief authority figure), the husband/father is the dominant member. Such expectations are typically the cultural norm in Latino, Hispanic, and traditional Muslim families. The husband/father is the one who makes decisions regarding health care for all family members. Also, in such cultures, the wife is responsible for child care and household maintenance, whereas the father's role is to protect and support the family members (Grossman, 1996).

HOME HEALTH CARE

Culturally Sensitive Care

To provide culturally sensitive care in the home:

- Remember that the setting for care is controlled by the client and family, not by the health care provider.
- Be sensitive to the fact that the nurse is often viewed as a guest by the client and family. Social chatter may be necessary to facilitate rapport.
- Be nonjudgmental about the condition of the home (e.g., presence of clutter and disarray).
- Show respect and consideration for the client. For example:
  - Wipe your feet before entering the home.
  - Ask permission to use the sink or bathroom to wash your hands.
  - Ask permission before moving the client's belongings and replace items after you have finished the task.
- Take advantage of the home environment to assess cultural values and norms. Clues to cultural values may include:
  - Decor and possessions on display in the home.
  - Assignment of family roles and tasks.
  - Types of interactions among family members.
  - Value placed on privacy.
  - Value placed on possessions.

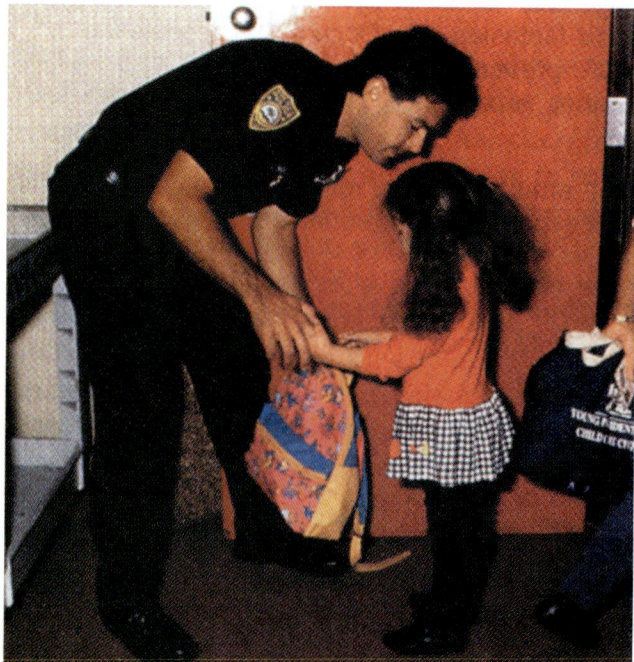

Figure 12-6 One example of changing gender roles is fathers assuming more responsibility in caring for children.

Religion

Anthropologists have identified the strength of the influence of religion on culture. In many cases, culture and tradition have been maintained and preserved through religious beliefs. Religion often includes the formal organizational structures for social behavior.

Spiritual and religious beliefs are important in many individuals' lives. These beliefs can influence lifestyle, attitudes, and feelings about life, pain, and death. Some organized religions specify practices about diet, birth control, and appropriate medical care. Spiritual beliefs often assume a greater significance at the time of illness than at any other time in a person's life. These beliefs help some people accept their own illnesses and help explain illness for others. Spiritual beliefs often help people plan for the future. Religion can both help people live fuller lives as well as strengthen or console people during suffering and in preparation for inevitable death. By providing meaning to life and death, religion can supply the client, the family, and the nurse with a sense of strength, security; and faith during a time of need.

Spiritual needs are identified as an individual's desire to find meaning and purpose in life, pain, and death. The spiritual realm is often considered a very private area. In order to provide holistic care, however, the nurse must pay attention to the spiritual dimension of each client, recognizing spiritual needs and assisting the client in meeting them (Figure 12-7).

Although spiritual needs are recognized by many nurses, **spiritual care** (recognition of spiritual needs and the assistance given toward meeting those needs) is often neglected. Spirituality is characterized as an individual's search to find meaning and purpose in life.

The goal of spiritual nursing care is to enable clients to identify and utilize their spiritual beliefs as coping mechanisms when faced with a health crisis. Among the reasons that nurses fail to provide spiritual care are the following:

- They feel that spirituality is a private matter.
- They are uninformed about the religious beliefs of others.
- They have not identified their own spiritual beliefs.
- They view meeting the spiritual needs of the client as a family or clergy responsibility, not a nursing responsibility.

Spiritual nursing care is appropriate when the nurse cares about the client's emotional, physical, and psychosocial health. The nursing diagnosis, *Spiritual Distress,* can be apparent in a client who is unable to practice religious or spiritual rituals due to illness or confinement in a health care institution.

The **religious support system** is a group of ministers, priests, rabbis, nuns, mullahs, shamans, or laypersons who are able to meet clients' spiritual needs in the health care setting. The nurse has the responsibility of working with these individuals, including them in the client care team (Figure 12-8).

Nurses must be aware of the general philosophies of their clients' spiritual beliefs, and also be aware that some individuals do not believe in a higher being or practice a specific religion. **Agnostics** believe that the existence of God cannot be proved or disproved, whereas **atheists** do not believe in God or any other deity.

It is important to identify particular beliefs from various religions that can influence client care activities.

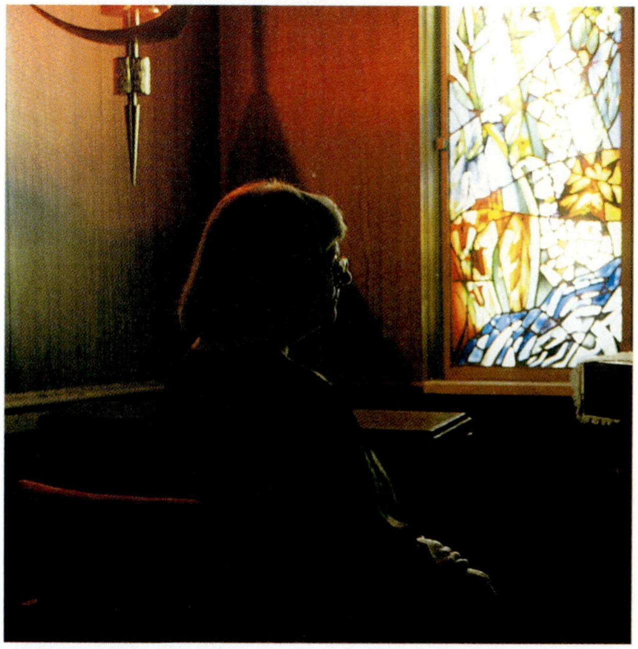

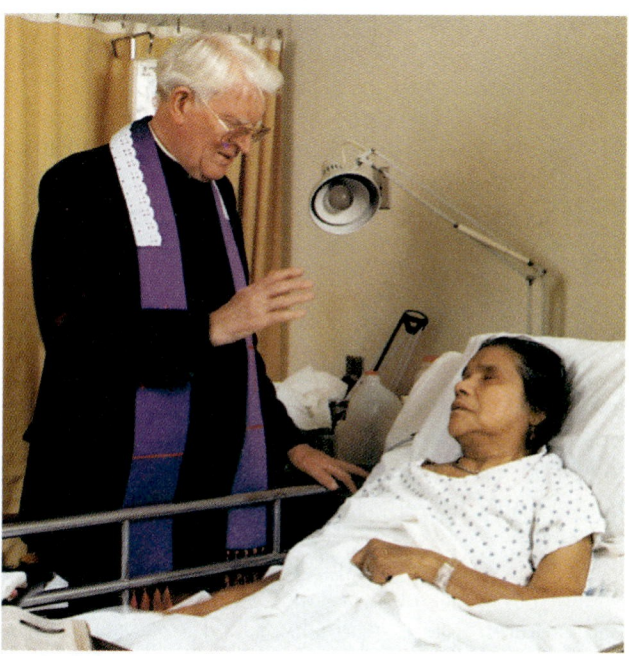

Figure 12-7 Spiritual needs often increase when individuals are sick.

Figure 12-8 A Catholic priest is a means of support and comfort to this dying client.

Some of these beliefs concern holy day practices, dietary restrictions, birth, death, and organ donation.

Protestant Many separate denominations (over 1,200) constitute the group known as Protestant. Protestant groups include such denominations as Baptist, Episcopal, Lutheran, Methodist, Presbyterian, and Seventh Day Adventist. The majority worship on Sunday, and their primary written reference is the Holy Bible.

Baptist Baptists do not practice infant baptism. For them, baptism is a rite to be performed only after a believer reaches an age of understanding and confesses his acceptance of the saving work of Jesus Christ. Communion is a spiritual act and symbolizes the suffering, death, and resurrection of the Lord.

Episcopal Episcopalians have a number of sacraments including confession, anointing of the sick (Holy Unction), communion, and baptism. Holy Unction is most often given as a healing sacrament. Episcopalians believe that a dying infant should be baptized, and the nurse may perform the rite. The usual administration of these sacraments is by an Episcopal priest.

Lutheran Traditionally, Lutherans practice baptism of infants and adults by sprinkling. Emergency baptisms may be performed by any baptized Christian. The Lutheran churches recognize two sacraments, baptism and Holy Communion. Holy Communion is understood as the body and the blood of the Lord and is often administered to those who are ill or awaiting surgery. Central to the Lutheran belief is the doctrine of "justification by faith." People are redeemed by God solely on the basis of God's grace, which they receive through faith or acceptance of what God has done for them.

Methodist Methodists practice both infant and adult baptism. They believe that religion is a matter of personal belief, and they use the conscience as a guide for living.

Presbyterian Presbyterians also practice communion, remembering the death of Jesus Christ for them and baptism. Salvation is believed to be a gift from God.

Seventh Day Adventist Seventh Day Adventists do not believe in infant baptism, but baptize individuals when they reach an age of accountability. They follow some dietary restrictions. Their Sabbath worship is observed from sunset on Friday to sunset on Saturday. They do not pursue their jobs or worldly pleasures during this time.

Roman Catholic Various rites known as Sacraments (sacred) are performed by the priest at appropriate times in the life of the Catholic. Sacraments that might be encountered in the health care setting are: baptism, the Eucharist (Communion), confession, and sacrament of the sick. Baptism, administered only once in the life of a Catholic, is believed to be absolutely necessary for salvation. A client preparing to take communion is normally asked to abstain from food or drink for an hour before the rite, although water and medications are allowed at any time. Con-

fession is a rite for the forgiveness of sins. It is a very private matter and should be respected. The Sacrament of the Sick, in which the client is anointed with holy oil, was formerly known as the "last rites" given to someone near death.

Orthodox The Orthodox churches express their love of God through worship liturgies. It is important to the church that they remain faithful to the teachings of the ancient church. Holy Unction is practiced using oil to anoint the body for healing of bodily and spiritual infirmities. Baptism is also important; in life-threatening situations involving an unbaptized child an emergency baptism is performed.

Jehovah's Witness Jehovah's Witnesses are prohibited from receiving any blood or blood products, including plasma. They also will not eat anything containing blood. Blood volume expanders are permissible if they are not derivatives of blood. In some cases, children have been made wards of the court so that they could receive blood when a medical condition requiring blood transfusion was life-threatening. They have a special observance of the Lord's Supper.

Mormon (Church of Jesus Christ of the Latter Day Saints) Mormons do not believe in baptizing infants, but will baptize at the age of eight years. If necessary, baptism of the dead will be performed for adults. Mormons wear a special undergarment that has special significance symbolizing dedication to God. This garment may be worn under the hospital gown.

Christian Science Christian Scientists generally believe that illness can be eliminated through prayer and spiritual understanding. Healing is considered an awakening to this belief. When a critically ill Christian Scientist client is admitted to a health care facility they may wish to have a Christian Science practitioner contacted to give treatment through prayer. Christian Scientists ordinarily do not use medicine, agree to surgical procedures, or accept blood transfusions.

American Indian Religions All life is sacred and all things are interconnected is the central belief of the various religions. Community importance is emphasized. The individual who is able to communicate with the spirits or the Great Spirit is the spiritual leader. There are no written religious books. Religious traditions are passed on orally and through participation in ceremonies and festivals. Illness may be the result of a sin or a spirit or god who is unhappy.

Judaism Judaism is both a religious faith and an ethnic identity. The religion is based on the five books of Moses called the Torah. Culture and religion are deeply interwoven in the Jewish faith. As a result, ritual, tradition, ceremony, religious and social laws, and the observance of holy days are major influences in the Jewish daily life.

There are three groups in Judaism: Orthodox, Conservative, and Reformed. All share the fundamental teachings of Judaism but vary in how strictly they follow the traditions. Orthodox Jews strictly observe all traditional practices. The Conservative group observes many of the traditional practices, and the Reformed group interprets traditions loosely.

The rabbi is the spiritual leader of the Jewish congregation and is the representative to be informed when a client of the Jewish faith requests it.

The Jewish Sabbath, the day of worship, begins at sunset on Friday and ends at sunset on Saturday.

Circumcision is a religious custom in Judaism that is performed on the male infant eight days after birth. It may be done by the pediatrician or by the Mohel who may be a rabbi.

Islam The religion of Muslims is Islam. They believe that Allah is the supreme deity and that Mohammed, the founder of Islam, is the chief prophet. The Muslim's holy day of worship extends from sunset on Thursday to sunset on Friday. Some Muslims may desire to pray to their god Allah five times a day (after dawn, at noon, at mid-afternoon, after sunset, and at night). If the client requests that he face Mecca, the holy city of Islam, a bed or chair may be positioned facing the southeast direction (if in the continental United States). The Muslim client may be wearing an article of writing from the Koran on a piece of string around his neck, arm, or waist. This should not be allowed to get wet or to be removed. Rules of cleanliness include eating with the right hand and cleansing self with the left hand after urinating or defecating. Medications or other materials should be handed to the Muslim client with the right hand so as not to offend them, as they consider the left hand dirty.

Some Islamic females prefer to be clothed from head to ankle. During the physical examination, they may prefer to undress one body part at a time. They may refuse to be cared for by male nurses or physicians.

Buddhism Buddhism is a general term that indicates a belief in Buddha, "the enlightened one." Nirvana, a state of greater inner freedom and spontaneity, is the goal of existence. When one achieves Nirvana, the mind has supreme peace, purity, and strength. Buddhism does not dictate any specific practices or sacraments. There are no religious restrictions for therapy or special holy days. Buddhists do not believe in healing through faith. The religious support system for the sick is the priest. The Buddhist believes in reincarnation.

Hindu Hinduism has no common creeds or doctrines that bind Hindus together. The major distinguishing characteristic is the social caste system. The religion of Hinduism is founded on the Scripture called the Vedas. Brahma is the principal source of the universe and the center from which all things proceed and to which all things return. Reincarnation is a central belief in Hindu thought. The goal of existence is freedom from the cycle of rebirth and death and entrance into what the Hindus, like the Buddhists, call Nirvana. Hindu temples are dwelling places for deities to which people bring offerings. Some Hindus believe

in faith healing; others believe that illness is God's way of punishing a person for sins.

Biological Variation

Biological variations distinguish one cultural or racial group from another. Common obvious biological variations include hair texture, skin color, thickness of lips, eye shape, and body structure (Degazon, 1996). Biological variations that are less obvious include enzymatic differences and susceptibility to disease (Andrews & Boyle, 1998; Giger & Davidhizar, 1999). Enzymatic differences account for diverse responses of some groups to dietary therapy and drugs (Table 12-2).

Table 12-2 EFFECTS OF BIOLOGICAL VARIATIONS ON SELECT DRUGS	
CULTURAL GROUP	**EFFECT OF BIOLOGICAL VARIATION ON DRUG ACTION**
European American	• Due to liver enzyme difference, caffeine is metabolized and excreted faster than by people of other cultural groups.
African American	• Isoniazid (drug used to treat tuberculosis) is rapidly metabolized, thus becoming inactive quickly: occurs in approximately 60% of population. • An enzyme deficiency interferes with metabolism of primaquine (used to treat malaria); occurs in approximately 35% of population. • Antihypertensive drugs (e.g., propranolol) must be administered in higher doses to produce same effects as in European Americans.
Hispanic American	None noted
Asian American	• Isoniazid is rapidly metabolized, thus becoming inactive quickly; occurs in approximately 85% to 90% of population. • Rapid metabolism of alcohol results in excessive facial flushing and other vasomotor symptoms. • Chinese men need only approximately half as much propranolol (antihypertensive drug) to produce same effects as in European American men.
Native American	• Isoniazid is rapidly metabolized, thus becoming inactive quickly; occurs in approximately 60% to 90% of population. • Rapid metabolism of alcohol results in excessive facial flushing and other vasomotor symptoms.

Data from Transcultural Nursing: Assessment and Intervention (3rd ed.), by J. Giger and R. Davidhizar, 2000, St. Louis: Mosby-Yearbook.

CULTURAL ASPECTS AND THE NURSING PROCESS

Each individual comes from a cultural background that, in some way, influences behavior and attitudes about health and illness. Personal attitudes and behaviors determine not only the ways that clients interpret health events and utilize health care, but also the ways that nurses interpret health events and provide health care. The central role that culture plays in determining perception compels health care providers to evaluate their personal views about health and illness before examining those of clients from other cultural groups. Nurses must be able to recognize the way that culture affects the health care needs of clients and respond appropriately.

Assessment

Culturally sensitive nursing care begins with an examination of one's own culture and beliefs. It is followed by an assessment of the client's cultural beliefs and background.

Personal Cultural Assessment

Spradley and Allender (1996) identify five areas to be examined in assessing one's own culture and the influence it may have on personal beliefs about health care.

- Influences from own ethnic/racial background
- Typical verbal and nonverbal communication patterns
- Cultural values and norms
- Religious beliefs and practices
- Health beliefs and practices

They suggest that the nurse should gather as much information as possible on each issue and then validate this information with one or two other persons from the same cultural group.

Client Cultural Assessment

Having examined one's own culture and the influences it may have had in developing personal beliefs about sickness and health, the next step to providing culturally appropriate care is to assess the client's cultural background (Figure 12-9). Data about various cultures may be collected from members of the culture to be studied, from others familiar with the culture, or from the local library.

Spradley and Allender (1996) identify six categories of information necessary for a comprehensive cultural assessment of the client. These categories may also be useful in organizing interviews with representatives from the culture.

- *Ethnic or racial background.* Where did the client group originate, and how does that influence the status and identity of group members?
- *Language and communication patterns.* What is the preferred language spoken, and what are the culturally based communication patterns?
- *Cultural values and norms.* What are the values, beliefs, and standards regarding such things as roles, education, family functions, child-rearing, work and leisure, aging, death and dying, and rites of passage?
- *Biocultural factors.* Are there physical or genetic traits unique to the ethnic or racial group that predispose group members to certain conditions or illnesses?
- *Religious beliefs and practices.* What are the group's religious beliefs, and how do they influence life events, roles, health, and illness?
- *Health beliefs and practices.* What are the group's beliefs and practices regarding prevention, causes, and treatment of illnesses?

PROFESSIONAL TIP

Culturally Diverse Coworkers

Many nursing units represent a mix of nationalities and cultures. While such a mix has the potential of improving nursing care, in practice it often leads to conflict and poor teamwork. The same cultural differences discussed in relation to clients may also be found among coworkers. Grensing-Pophal (1997) suggests five ways to successfully manage diversity in the workplace:

- Be aware of your own biases, and strive to avoid stereotyping others.
- Be aware of the way the things you do and say affect others.
- Help others to be more sensitive and help correct misconceptions.
- Learn to welcome different opinions and viewpoints.
- Be open to feedback.

Learn more about your coworkers and remember that respect for individual differences reflects acknowledgment of each person's uniqueness. Have a unit conference focusing on a cultural assessment of each other. Grossman and Taylor (1995) suggest having a potluck lunch, with everyone bringing a typical ethnic dish. Such strategies might also work well in a nursing program where various cultures are represented.

Cultural Assessment Interview Guide

Name: _____

Nickname or other names or special meaning attributed to your name: _____

Primary language:

    When speaking _____

    When writing _____

Date of birth: _____

Place of birth: _____

Educational level or specialized training: _____

To which ethnic group do you belong? _____

To what extent do you identify with your cultural group? _____

Who is the spokesperson for your family? _____

Describe some of the customs or beliefs that you have about the following:

    Health _____

    Life _____

    Illness _____

    Death _____

How do you best learn information?

    ☐ Reading

    ☐ Having someone explain verbally

    ☐ Having someone demonstrate

Describe some of your family's dietary habits and your personal food preferences: _____

_____

Are there any foods forbidden from your diet for religious or cultural reasons? _____

_____

Describe your religious affiliation: _____

What role do your religious beliefs and practices play in your life during times of good health and bad health? _____

_____

On whom do you rely on for health care services or healing, and to what type of cultural health practices have you been exposed? _____

_____

Are there any sanctions or restrictions in your culture about which the person taking care to you should know? _____

_____

Describe your current living arrangements: _____

How do members of your family communicate with each other? _____

Describe your strengths: _____

Who /what is your primary source of information about your health? _____

Is there anything else that is important about your cultural beliefs that you want to tell me? _____

Figure 12-9 Cultural Assessment Interview Guide (*From* Fundamentals of Nursing: Standards & Practice, *by S. DeLaune and P. Ladner, 1998, Albany, NY: Delmar Publishers. Copyright 1998 by Delmar Publishers.)*

Nursing Diagnosis

Any nursing diagnosis may be appropriate for a client of any cultural group. When cultural variables are identified during assessment, the nurse should be as specific as possible when asking questions and determining appropriate nursing diagnoses, so that interventions can be individualized with respect to the client's cultural beliefs. For instance, *Cardiac Output, Decreased* may be viewed by the nurse or physician as having a medical or physical cause, whereas the client may attribute the origin to an imbalance of yin and yang. Table 12-3 lists select nursing diagnoses that are most likely to have cultural implications.

Planning/Outcome Identification

Cultural variables must be taken into consideration when establishing goals and planning interventions. Care will be most effective when the client and family

Table 12-3 NURSING DIAGNOSES WITH CULTURAL IMPLICATIONS

Anxiety
Body Image Disturbance
Breastfeeding, Ineffective
Communication, Verbal, Impaired
Coping, Family, Ineffective, Compromised
Coping, Individual, Ineffective
Decisional Conflict
Fear
Grieving, Anticipatory
Health Maintenance, Altered
Health-Seeking Behaviors
Noncompliance
Nutrition, Altered, More Than Body Requirements
Pain
Role Performance, Altered
Sleep Pattern Disturbance
Social Interaction, Impaired
Spiritual Distress

CLIENT TEACHING

Culturally Sensitive Teaching Guidelines

When caring for clients from diverse cultures, consider the following guidelines for client teaching:

- Determine the client's cultural background.
- Evaluate the client's current knowledge base by asking the client to state what he knows about the specific topic.
- To identify the client's perception of need, ask the client and family what they need and want to learn.
- Observe the interaction between the client and family to determine family roles and authority figures. Ask the client whether the dominant family member should be included in teaching and care sessions.
- Use language easily understood by the client, avoiding jargon and complex medical terms.
- Clarify your verbal and nonverbal messages with the client.
- Have the client repeat the information. If feasible, have the client do a return demonstration of the material taught.

are active participants in planning care, and when cultural preferences are respected. Potter and Perry (1999) suggest the following goals to consider when cultural factors are involved:

- Client will express health care needs to family and caregiver.
- Client will maintain cultural health practices as appropriate.
- Client and family will understand the effect that health care beliefs have on health status.

Implementation

Cultural aspects are always a factor in a nursing care plan, and effective communication and client education are important nursing responsibilities that can enhance cultural understanding and appreciation. Interventions should be carried out in a manner that will respect, to the degree possible, the preferences and desires of the client. When a client does not speak or understand the native language well, the nurse should arrange to have an interpreter present to explain procedures and tests.

Evaluation

Evaluation should include feedback from the client and family to determine their reaction to the interventions. Revisions to the plan of care should be made with client and family input, and alternative sources and resources brought in when needed to enhance communication and exchange of information. Nurses should also perform self-evaluations to identify their attitudes toward caring for clients from diverse cultures.

PROFESSIONAL TIP

Culturally Appropriate Care

- Respect clients for their different beliefs.
- Be sensitive to behaviors and practices different from your own and respond accordingly.
- Accommodate differences if they are not detrimental to health. For example, a client might believe that eating onions will resolve his respiratory infection. While eating onions may not be therapeutic, it is also not likely to negatively impact health.
- Listen for cues in the client's conversation that relay a unique ethnic belief about etiology, transmission, prevention, or some other aspect of disease. For example, a client might say, "I knew I would be sick today. I heard an owl last night."
- Use the occasion to teach positive health habits if the client's practices are deleterious to good health. For example, when asked about her diet, a pregnant woman might reply that she never eats meat or eggs while pregnant because she believes that gaining too much weight will increase her risk of a difficult delivery. Such a situation offers the nurse an opportunity to provide nutritional instruction.

SAMPLE NURSING CARE PLAN

THE FAMILY WITH INEFFECTIVE COPING

Mrs. Chang, a 74-year-old Asian American housewife, was admitted to the hospital with complaints of nausea and difficulty keeping food down related to treatment for recurrent breast cancer with bone metastasis. For the past few weeks, her appetite has been decreasing. She is able to drink some fluids.

Mrs. Chang's husband of 53 years remains at her bedside, as do their two grown daughters. Mrs. Chang insists that they remain at her bedside so that she does not have to bother the nurses for her basic care and insists that the oldest daughter bathe her and walk her to the bathroom. Mr. Chang leaves her bedside only to go home and shower; when he does so, both daughters remain with Mrs. Chang.

The nurses notice that Mr. Chang is looking exhausted and appears to have lost weight. The daughters have tried to relieve their father at night to allow him to go home and rest, but he insists on remaining at the hospital.

Although Mrs. Chang never voices discomfort, she has her husband and daughters constantly massaging her back and legs. She changes position slowly and grimaces with each movement. She does not verbalize to the nursing staff, but lets her family do the talking for her. She denies pain when questioned by the nurse, but she complains of pain to her family. She does not sleep well.

Mrs. Chang's treatment plan is supportive. The hospital staff has mentioned the idea of hospice care to the family. Mrs. Chang has stated that she wants to go home.

Nursing Diagnosis *Coping, Family, Ineffective, Compromised, related to prolonged disease or disability progression that exhausts the supportive capacity of significant people as evidenced by Mr. Chang's looking exhausted.*

PLANNING/GOALS	NURSING INTERVENTIONS	RATIONALE	EVALUATION
Family will plan a specific rotation schedule to meet each other's needs for rest and support while caring for Mrs. Chang.	Provide empathy and support for the husband and daughters. Provide them with unlimited visitation, adequate space for members who stay overnight, and privacy.	The family is one of the most important factors in the life of the Asian American. A sense of obligation to intervene and assist is highly valued. Casual help from strangers is avoided.	Family is sharing bedside care responsibilities. Husband and eldest daughter remain at bedside during daytime hours. Youngest daughter rests at home during the day and exchanges places with the father and eldest sister at night. Mrs. Chang is agreeable.
	Assess family members for signs of fatigue or overexertion.	Asian Americans value self-control and self-sufficiency. To ask for help would mean loss of face and dignity.	
	Explore with husband and daughters other possible extended family members who would be willing and be accepted by Mrs. Chang to keep her company and give her support.	This family will not be able to keep up this vigil for an unknown period of time. Family obligations take precedence over individual desires.	

continued

PLANNING/GOALS	NURSING INTERVENTIONS	RATIONALE	EVALUATION
Client and family will maintain open communication.	Develop trusting and respectful relationships with Mrs. Chang and family members.	Asian Americans tend to be reserved with those whom they view as being in authority. The nurse should remember that this family needs to establish a caring, trusting relationship before they participate in self-disclosure.	Mr. Chang meets with both daughters to discuss their mother's plan of care. He includes the primary care nurse in the discussion.
	Encourage Mr. Chang to have family meetings as necessary to discuss realistic plans and expectations of other family members, using health care providers as needed.	Asians traditionally value authoritarian styles of leadership, where the father makes unilateral family decisions. Authority and communication come from the top down. Discouragement of verbal communication, avoidance of discussion of personal problems, and limited expression of emotion have been noted as common patterns in the traditional Asian family.	
	Encourage and assist family to explore outside resources to assist them in dealing with the crisis.	This family structure cannot maintain bedside attendance without help. The outside resource might take the form of extended family, sisters, brothers, nieces, or nephews of Mrs. Chang who live in the neighborhood.	
Family members will perform client care without compromising their own physical and emotional health.	Assess whether basic physical and emotional needs of Mrs. Chang and family members are being met.	The ideal pattern of communication in Asian society is silent communication. Stoic reactions to pain and other uncertain situations is common. Direct expression of negative feelings is unusual. The nurse will need to assess for nonverbal clues indicating the status of needs.	Mr. Chang and his daughters continue to provide the physical care for Mrs. Chang. Mr. Chang appears more rested and has gained back some weight. The daughters express gratefulness that their father is stronger and has taken on the leadership role.
	Monitor ability of family members to carry out treatment plan and provide safe care.	When care is provided by family members who are exhausted, safety is always an issue. The	

continued

PLANNING/GOALS	NURSING INTERVENTIONS	RATIONALE	EVALUATION
		nurse is ultimately responsible for the well-being of the client.	
	Teach coping strategies for managing tension and strain in the event of previous techniques losing their effectiveness.	Coping strategies to maintain healthy emotional and psychological health may be necessary. This is especially true for individuals from a culture that discourages placing individual needs or emotions ahead of those of the family.	

CASE STUDY

Maria Garcia brings her Catholic, 18-year-old sister, Rosa, to the hospital emergency room. Rosa has a high temperature and chills, is vomiting, and complains of right-lower-quadrant pain. Maria also brings her three children, ages 3, 2, and 1 year old, with her. Maria understands and speaks broken English, but Rosa is fluent in Spanish only. The nurse directs Maria to the waiting room with her children, then takes Rosa to the examination room. Rosa is examined by a male nurse, who promptly complains at the nurses' station about how uncooperative Rosa was during the physical examination. Rosa is admitted for inpatient care and is diagnosed with appendicitis requiring emergency surgery. Maria is left in the waiting room, unaware of the difficulty that the nursing staff has had in communicating with Rosa. Rosa is taken upstairs to her room to await her surgical preparation. Maria is notified that she can go upstairs for a few minutes but must then leave because her children do not meet the age requirement for visitor privileges. Maria finds Rosa weeping, nearly hysterical. The physician walks in and asks Maria why she waited so long to bring Rosa in for treatment. He informs her that Rosa's appendix was close to rupturing and that treatment should have been started 3 days ago, when her symptoms first began. Maria informs him that she had taken Rosa to the curandero, who had given her some herbal tea to drink. When that did not help, she had brought Rosa to the hospital.

The following questions will guide your development of a nursing care plan for the case study.

1. Why was communication among Maria, Rosa, and the health care professionals problematic?
2. What Mexican American cultural diversities were not addressed by the health care professionals?
3. What needs of Maria and Rosa are being ignored by the health care professionals?
4. What questions do you feel must be asked by the health care professionals to give them a better understanding of this situation?
5. Identify two individualized culturally sensitive nursing diagnoses and goals for Rosa.
6. Formulate pertinent nursing interventions for the diagnoses and goals identified in question 5.
7. List resources that the nurses could use to assist Rosa in her recovery.
8. List at least two successful client outcomes for Rosa.

SUMMARY

- Culture is composed of beliefs about activity, relations, motivation, perception of the world, and perception about self.
- Culture is learned, integrated, shared, unspoken, and dynamic.
- Beliefs about concepts of health, disease etiology, health promotion and protection, and practitioners and remedies are influenced by culture.
- Unlike opinions, preferences, and attitudes, which can change, cultural characteristics are deeply rooted and are thus difficult to change. Clients reflect their cultural and ethnic heritage every time they interact with the world around them.
- Culture is influenced by religion, which in turn affects beliefs and practices about health and illness.
- Spiritual and religious beliefs are important in many people's lives. They can influence lifestyle, attitudes, and feelings about illness and death.
- The nurse should not make assumptions about clients based on the client's religious and cultural affiliations. Individuality exists among all peoples.
- The focus of nursing care is to help the client maintain his own beliefs in the midst of a health care crisis and to use those personal beliefs to strengthen coping patterns.
- Understanding and encouraging client differences are important aspects of nursing.
- Response to health and illness varies depending on cultural origin.
- Culturally appropriate care begins with an understanding of one's own cultural beliefs.
- Client cultural assessment is a prerequisite to providing appropriate nursing care.

Review Questions

1. A mother is observed breastfeeding her 4-year-old son, who is a client in the pediatrics wing of the hospital. A nurse is overheard talking in the nursing station about the "weird" way the mother has continued to breastfeed a 4-year-old. She comments that the American way is the best. The nurse is guilty of:

   a. ethnocentrism.
   b. stereotyping.
   c. unusual break behavior.
   d. not insisting that the mother stop breastfeeding.

2. Which religious group teaches that physical healing comes exclusively through prayers and readings?

   a. Roman Catholic
   b. Jewish
   c. Christian Science
   d. Seventh Day Adventist

3. Which religious group observes the Sabbath from sunset Friday until sunset Saturday?

   a. Mormons
   b. Jews
   c. Presbyterian
   d. Muslims

4. A client of this religion would most likely refuse a blood transfusion, even if his life were in jeopardy.

   a. Hindu
   b. Jehovah's Witness
   c. Jew
   d. Mormon

5. The nursing diagnosis that might be used for a client who is hospitalized and has religious practices that conflict with hospital practice is:

   a. *Emotional Depression.*
   b. *Guilt and Misery.*
   c. *Spiritual Distress.*
   d. *Spiritual Manipulation.*

6. It is important for the nurse to know the client's religion in order to:

   a. chart it on his record.
   b. give holistic care.
   c. meet his physical needs.
   d. know how to pray for him.

7. Which of the following is a characteristic of culture?

   a. Culture is learned.
   b. Culture stays the same.
   c. Culture is biologically inherited.
   d. Culture is individually determined.

8. Which of the following is descriptive of Hispanic Americans?

   a. They are culturally homogeneous.
   b. Their culture is not based on religion.
   c. Illness may be viewed as a punishment from God.
   d. They always seek Western medical intervention.

9. When a client says to the nurse, "I need to pray with my pastor in order to get well," the most appropriate response from the nurse is:

   a. "The medicine you take will make you well."
   b. "When you are released from the hospital, you can go to church and pray."
   c. "May I call your pastor for you and ask him to visit you?"
   d. "Why do you think prayer will make you well?"

10. It is important to be aware of cultural aspects of health and disease because:

    a. some cultural groups are represented in greater numbers than others.
    b. cultural groups respond differently to illness.
    c. differences in care should not be based on culture.
    d. reimbursement is related to ethnicity.

Critical Thinking Questions

1. How does your culture influence your beliefs about health practices?

2. Suppose one of your clients practiced the custom of placing an amulet (religious icon and necklace) around a newborn's neck. You are concerned about the risk of strangulation this presents. How would you approach this client to discuss your concerns?

 WEB FLASH!

- Search "cultural diversity" on the Web. What related topics do you find?
- Can you locate health-related Web sites specific to European Americans, African Americans, Hispanic Americans, Asian Americans, and Native Americans?

CHAPTER 13

ALTERNATIVE/ COMPLEMENTARY THERAPIES

MAKING THE CONNECTION

Refer to the following chapters to increase your understanding of alternative/complementary therapy:

- **Chapter 1, Holistic Care**
- **Chapter 12, Cultural Diversity and Nursing**
- **Chapter 16, Stress, Adaptation, and Anxiety**
- **Chapter 18, Basic Nutrition**
- **Procedures:** B23, Giving a Backrub

LEARNING OBJECTIVES

Upon completion of this chapter, you should be able to:
- *Define key terms.*
- *Describe the historical influences on current alternative/complementary modalities.*
- *Discuss the connection between mind and body and the effect of this relationship on a person's health.*
- *Explain the concept of the nurse as an instrument of healing in holistic nursing practice.*
- *Identify the various mind-body, body-movement, energetic-touch healing, spiritual, nutritional, and other modalities that can be used as complementary therapies in client care.*
- *Discuss the use of alternative/complementary modalities throughout the life cycle.*

KEY TERMS

acupressure	healing touch
acupuncture	hypnosis
alternative therapies	imagery
antioxidants	instrument of healing
aromatherapy	meditation
biofeedback	neuropeptides
bodymind	neurotransmitters
centering	phytochemicals
complementary therapies	psychoneuro-immunology
curing	shaman
energetic-touch therapies	shamanism
free radicals	therapeutic massage
healing	therapeutic touch
	touch

INTRODUCTION

Western society tends to think of health and healing in terms of medical, surgical, and other technological interventions. However, in many other cultures—both past and present—healing has been promoted by faith, magic, ritual, and other nonmedical approaches.

The use of **alternative therapies** (therapies used *instead of* conventional or mainstream medical modalities) and **complementary therapies** (therapies used *in conjunction with* conventional medical therapies) is becoming more prevalent among the general public (Keegan, 1998).

This chapter addresses alternative/complementary treatment methods that are currently being used in ho-

listic nursing practice. Nurses are encouraged to think critically before recommending or implementing any of these approaches. Whether they simply discuss alternative/complementary therapies with clients or perform these therapies, nurses should understand the ramifications.

Because more and more states are regulating alternative/complementary therapies, nurses must know the laws that govern these therapies in the states in which they work. Some states have outlawed certain therapies or consider them experimental procedures, whereas other states require licensure or certain educational standards before allowing practitioners to perform alternative/complementary therapies. Nurses who perform alternative/complementary therapies not in accordance with the laws of their respective states could have legal charges filed against them (Brooke, 1998).

Employer policy and the nurse's job description must also be checked to confirm that performing alternative/complementary therapies is within the nurse's scope of practice at that agency. Employer malpractice insurance policies typically do not cover situations where a client is injured as a result of an alternative/complementary therapy. The financial risk of any nurse who engages in alternative/complementary therapies will be lowered by having insurance that specifically covers those therapies.

HISTORICAL INFLUENCES ON CONTEMPORARY PRACTICES

For as long as history has been recorded, people have tried to cure ills and relieve pain. Early cave drawings depict healers practicing their art. Primitive healers attributed the cause of mysterious diseases to magic and superstition; as a result, religious beliefs and health practices became intertwined. Remedies and practices that are based in ancient traditions are being rediscovered and used by contemporary holistic healers. A brief look at ancient Greek, Far Eastern, Chinese, Indian, and Shamanistic practices will highlight their influences on modern alternative/complementary modalities.

Ancient Greece

In the ancient Greek culture, health was perceived as the maintenance of balance in all dimensions of life. In Greek mythology, Asclepius was the god of healing. Temples (called Ascleipions) were beautiful places for people (regardless of ability to pay) to rest, restore themselves, and worship. The elaborate healing system consisted of myths, symbols, and rites administered by rigorously trained priest-healers. Illnesses were treated by restoring balance to a person's life through music, art, baths, massage, laughter, herbs, and simple surgery (Keegan, 1994). Many of our current therapies such as massage, art therapy, and herbal therapy have origins in ancient Greek traditions.

The Far East

Healing systems from the Far East have traditionally integrated mind, body, and spirit into a system of balanced energy between the individual and the universe. The concept of a life force or life energy "has been recognized in many cultural traditions. . . . What is universally agreed on is that the more [life energy] you have, the more vital your mental and bodily processes" (Chopra, 1993). The origins of some energetic-touch therapies can be traced to the Far East.

China

The traditional Chinese healing system is based on the belief in the oneness of all things in nature. Life energy (chi) flows through both the universe and the person, thus creating a wholeness among all things and people. Chi provides warmth, protection from illness, and vitality. Chi flows along an invisible system of meridians (pathways) that link the organs together and connect them to the external environment and, therefore, to the universe. Illness and injury can alter the flow of this energy. The energy flow can be influenced by stimulating points along the meridians.

Herbalism is an essential component of traditional Chinese healing practice. In seeking to promote balance, healers use herbs for dual purposes. For example, the herb dan qui relaxes the uterus when it is contracted (as in preterm labor) and tightens it if it is too relaxed (when normal labor needs to be enhanced). A complete discussion of the use of herbs in contemporary health practices appears later in this chapter.

Many contemporary Western health care providers are studying and now using traditional Chinese healing techniques. **Acupuncture**, one technique used in traditional Chinese medicine, is the application of heat and needles to various points on the body to alter the energy flow (Figure 13-1). Acupuncture is helpful in relieving headache and low back pain (Eisenberg, 1993) and is used to treat a variety of chronic and acute conditions.

India

Practiced for more than 4,000 years by the people of India, Ayurvedic medicine emphasizes prevention and a holistic approach to life (Keegan, 1994). The term *ayurveda* (meaning "the science of life") refers to India's traditional medicine and has an underlying spiritual basis. The life energy (prana) is transported through the body by a "wind" or vata. Vata regulates every type of movement.

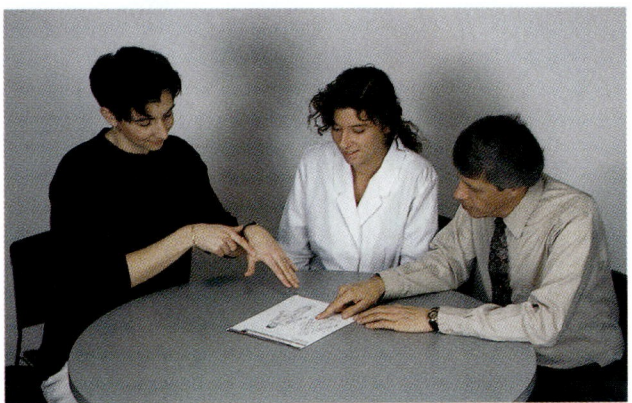

Figure 13-1 Acupuncturist, Nurse, and Client

Vata, Kapha, and Pitta are the three metabolic principles (doshas) that provide life to all living things (Chopra, 1993). Kapha is the energy responsible for body structure, and pitta is the transformative process between vata and kapha. Each person is born with a unique balance of the three doshas. One predominates, and that dosha determines body type, temperament, and susceptibility to certain illnesses.

In the Ayurvedic system, chakras are areas of energy concentration in the body. Like the Chinese pathways (or meridians), these areas can become stagnant and blocked, thus causing illness. Ayurvedic healers seek to activate chakra energy for self-healing.

Prevention of illness and restoration of health through inner search and spiritual growth are the primary goals in the Ayurvedic system. Union of the Divine and the Truth occurs through the physical and meditative practice of yoga. In contemporary practice, Ayurvedic intervention may consist of yoga, herbs, diet, and exercise; methods to cleanse the body, such as steam baths, cathartics, and detoxifying massage; and nasal purging.

Shamanistic Tradition

A need to understand and explain life processes (i.e., birth, health, illness, and death) is part of being human. In many cultures, both modern and ancient, ritualized practices have been used to keep peace with the great spirits, to harness their power, to promote power, and to prevent death.

Shamanism refers to the practice of entering altered states of consciousness with the intent of helping others. The **shaman** is a folk healer-priest who uses natural and supernatural forces to help others and who has an extensive knowledge of herbs, is skilled in many forms of healing, and serves as guardian of the spirits. Illness is considered to be the result of spirit loss; shamans have the power to heal by working with the spirits to encourage their full return to the individual. The shaman functions as both healer and priest and one who has access to the supernatural.

Seeking wisdom about the universe, establishing a relationship with the creator, and avoiding death are all feats accomplished through ritualized processes performed by the shaman (see Figure 13-2). The shaman's practice incorporates special objects such as power animals, totems, and fetishes as well as ritual songs, dances, food, and clothing. Sleep deprivation, ritual chants, isolation, imagery, drumming, and hallucinogenic drugs may be used to create a trance-like state that is the vehicle through which the shaman contacts the spirit world. The contemporary practices of hypnosis and guided imagery have roots in Shamanistic traditions.

MODERN TRENDS

The public perception of alternative/complementary treatment methods has been changing over the past few decades. In the late 1960s and early 1970s, the "natural," "new age," and "self-help" movements began to attract followers, first among consumers and later among health care practitioners. During that time period, there was a growing trend toward rejection of traditional medicine because of its perceived invasiveness, painfulness, cost, and ineffectiveness. A rekindled interest in Eastern religions, lifestyle, and medicine has fueled the development of contemporary holistic, alternative/complementary modalities. Clients are seeking out alternative/complementary therapies because most such therapies are noninvasive, holistic, and, in many instances, less expensive than going to a physician (Keegan, 1998).

In 1993, a landmark survey found that one-third of the U.S. population had used some nontraditional, alternative methods of treatment in addition to standard medical treatment (Eisenberg, Kessler, & Foster, 1993). In 1992, the U.S. government established the Office of Alternative Medicine (OAM) at the National Institutes of Health. "One of the reasons for the OAM's creation was the federal government's recognition that U.S. citizens are pursuing alternative methods of health care with unprecedented enthusiasm" (Dossey & Guzzetta, 1995).

In 1992, the OAM was allocated $2 million to investigate the use of nontraditional treatment methods. Congress increased the OAM's budget to $20 million for fiscal year 1998 (National Institutes of Health, 1998). A few of the therapies being investigated by the OAM (Swackhamer, 1995) include:

- Biofeedback to control pain,
- Acupuncture to relieve depression,
- Imagery to control asthma,
- Ayurvedic medicine to treat Parkinson's disease,
- Music therapy to treat brain-injured clients, and
- Shark cartilage to treat cancer.

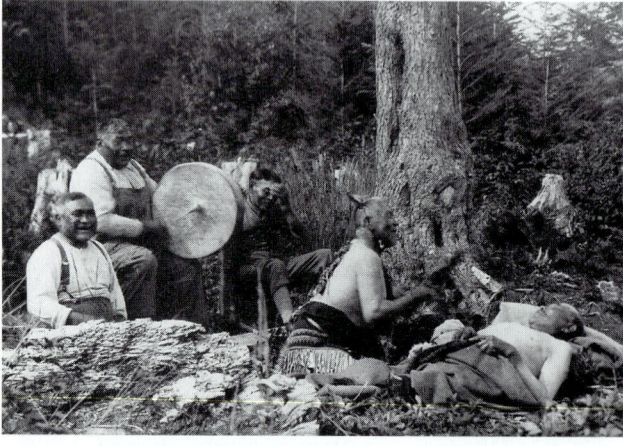

Figure 13-2 Shamanistic Healing Ritual (*Photo Courtesy of the Canadian Museum of Civilization, image number: 69617*)

Mind/Body Medicine and Research

The traditional medical model is founded on the belief that the mind, body, and spirit are separate entities. A relatively new field of science, however, called **psychoneuroimmunology** (PNI), is studying the complex relationship among the cognitive, affective, and physical aspects of humans. Psychoneuroimmunologists are investigating the way the brain transmits signals along the nerves to enhance the body's normal immune functioning. This research supports the idea that the human mind can alter physiology.

All body cells have receptor sites for **neuropeptides**, amino acids that are produced in the brain and other sites in the body and that act as chemical communicators. Neuropeptides are released when **neurotransmitters** (chemical substances produced by the body that facilitate nerve-impulse transmission) signal emotions in the brain. Pert, of the National Institutes of Health, wrote in 1986 that "the more we know about neuropeptides, the harder it is to think in the traditional terms of a mind and a body. It makes more sense to speak of a single integrated entity, a '*bodymind*'" (Pert, 1986).

Thus, it is possible for cells to be directly affected by emotions. In other words, people can affect their health by what they think and feel. There are many examples of terminally ill persons hanging on to life until the occurrence of a specific event such as a child coming to visit or a grandchild's graduation or marriage.

The intermeshed, complex system of psyche and body chemistry is now referred to as the **bodymind**, the inseparable connection and operation of thoughts, feelings, and physiological functions. According to psychologist Earnest Rossi (1993), because all body systems are interconnected, mental images can be converted into neurotransmitters in the autonomic nervous system, hormones in the endocrine system, and white blood cells in the immune system. These three systems (nervous, endocrine, and immune) are interactive, thus modulating the activity of each other (Rossi, 1993). This helps explain how some alternative/complementary therapies allow the calming influences of the parasympathetic system to take over during stress-inducing situations such as illness (Dossey, 1995c).

Holism and Nursing Practice

The expansion of the holistic health movement has been based on the growing acceptance of the concept that body, mind, and spirit are interconnected. Nursing in its broadest sense (theory, concept, and practice) is truly holistic in nature. Holism encompasses consideration of the physiological, psychological, sociocultural, intellectual, and spiritual aspects of each individual. Holistic nursing can be described as the art and science of caring for the whole person, knowing that each person is unique in all expressions of self. As holistic caregivers, nurses may employ alternative/complementary techniques to promote clients' well-being. The focus of care in these practices is healing, as opposed to curing.

The word **healing** is derived from the Anglo-Saxon word *hael,* meaning "to make whole, to move toward, or to become whole." It is important to establish that healing is not the same as **curing** (ridding one of disease), but is instead a process that activates the individual's forces from within. As a healing facilitator, the nurse enters into a relationship with the client and can assist the client by offering to be a guide, change agent, or **instrument of healing** (a means by which healing can be achieved, performed, or enhanced).

When the nurse serves as an instrument of healing, the objective is to help the client call forth inner resources for healing. In order to accomplish this goal, nurses must develop the following attributes:

- Knowledge base: initially established in nursing school and then continuously expanded through lifelong learning
- Intentionality: having a conscious direction of goals, essential in helping the healer to focus
- Respect for differences: demonstrated by honoring clients' culturally based health beliefs
- Ability to model wellness: tending to one's own needs and attempting to stay as healthy and balanced as possible

PROFESSIONAL TIP

Use of Alternative/Complementary Therapy

Practical ways for nurses to use alternative/complementary therapies include:

- Having a nonjudgmental attitude about these therapies;
- Asking clients whether they use any nontraditional therapies and, if so, asking which therapies, why, and how the therapies have worked;
- Getting adequate instruction in these therapies before trying to administer them;
- Trying one or two basic therapies such as massage or guided imagery; and
- Discussing a therapy with the client *before* using it (Keegan, 1998).

ALTERNATIVE/ COMPLEMENTARY INTERVENTIONS

Many alternative/complementary interventions are used in holistic nursing practice. These interventions are categorized as mind/body, body-movement, energetic-touch, spiritual, nutritional/medicinal, and other methodologies (Table 13-1). Although different in technique, many of the alternative/complementary therapies have common ideological threads, as follows:

- The *whole system* must be considered if the *parts* of the individual are to be helped to function.
- The person is integrated and related to the surroundings.
- There exists some life force or energy that can be used in the healing process.
- Ritual, prescribed practice and skilled practitioners are integral parts of holistic healing interventions.

Mind/Body (Self-Regulatory) Techniques

Self-regulatory techniques are methods by which an individual can, independently or with assistance, consciously control some functions of the sympathetic nervous system (for example, heart rate, respiratory rate, and blood pressure). When the client is learning the way to perform these techniques, an assistant is involved; later, however, the client can perform them independently. Self-regulatory techniques include meditation, relaxation, imagery, biofeedback, and hypnosis.

Meditation

The practice of **meditation**, quieting the mind by focusing the attention, can bring about remarkable physiological changes. People who meditate strive for a sense of oneness within themselves and a sense of relatedness to a greater power and the universe.

A person can be guided into a meditative or relaxed state with breath coaching (assisting the client to become aware of or focus on breathing and thus slow it). Meditation has proved particularly beneficial for clients in labor. Nurses can teach this modality to clients by using verbal cues, counting the client's inhalations and exhalations, and showing the client the way to take slow, deep breaths. According to Borysenko and Borysenko (1994), some therapeutic benefits of meditation are:

- Stress relief,
- Relaxation,
- Reduced level of lactic acid,
- Decreased oxygen consumption,
- Slowed heart rate,
- Decreased blood pressure, and
- Improved functioning of the immune system.

Relaxation

In 1975, cardiologist Herbert Benson studied the effects of meditation on individuals. He then incorporated the basic elements of meditation into the therapeutic process he called the *relaxation response* (Benson, 1975). Benson employed the relaxation response with individuals experiencing high blood pressure and heart disease. Benson discovered that the techniques were more effective if individuals focused on an inspirational prayer or phrase. The basic elements of the relaxation response are:

- A quiet environment,
- A comfortable position,
- Focused attention,
- A passive attitude, and
- Practice.

One method for achieving relaxation is progressive muscle relaxation (PMR), which is the alternate tensing and relaxing of muscles. Clients are instructed to concentrate on a certain body area (the jaw, for instance), tense the muscles for a count of five, then relax the muscles for a count of five. This process is repeated for

Table 13-1 CATEGORIES OF ALTERNATIVE/COMPLEMENTARY INTERVENTIONS

MIND/BODY	BODY MOVEMENT	ENERGETIC TOUCH	SPIRITUAL	NUTRITIONAL/ MEDICINAL	OTHER
Meditation	Movement and exercise	Touch	Faith Healing	Phytochemicals and antioxidants	Aromatherapy
Relaxation	Yoga	Therapeutic massage	Healing Prayer	Macrobiotic diet	Humor
Imagery	Tai chi	Therapeutic touch	Shamanism:	Herbal therapy	Pet Therapy
Biofeedback	Chiropractic therapy	Healing touch	• Sand painting		Music therapy
Hypnosis		Acupressure	• Sweat lodges		
		Reflexology	• Drumming		

From Fundamentals of Nursing: Standards & Practice, *by S. DeLaune and P. Ladner, 1998, Albany, NY: Delmar Publishers. Copyright 1998 by Delmar Publishers. Adapted with permission.*

CLIENT TEACHING

Progressive Muscle Relaxation

After explaining the purpose and process of progressive muscle relaxation, instruct the client to:

- Assume a comfortable position in a quiet environment.
- Close eyes and keep them closed until the exercise is completed.
- Breathe in deeply to a count of 4.
- Hold breath for a count of 4.
- Breathe out to a count of 4.
- Continue to breathe slowly and deeply.
- Tense both feet until muscle tension is felt.
- Hold a gentle state of tension in both feet for a count of 3.

Caution the client to tighten the muscles only until the muscles are tensed, not to the point of pain.

- Slowly release the tension from the feet.
- Fully experience the difference between tension and relaxation.
- Repeat the previous three steps.
- Gently tense the muscles of both lower legs.
- Continue this procedure with all the muscle groups in a toe-to-head direction.
- After tensing and releasing all muscle groups, take in a few more deep relaxing breaths and scan your body for any areas that remain tense. Concentrate on tensing and relaxing the muscles in those areas.
- Breathe in deeply to a count of 4.
- Hold breath for a count of 4.
- Breathe out to a count of 4.
- Resume your usual breathing pattern.
- Slowly stretch and open your eyes.

To be effective, this procedure requires approximately 20 to 30 minutes. Like all other relaxation exercises, progressive muscle relaxation is most effective with repetition.

muscle groups over the entire body until the client has achieved a state of overall relaxation.

Nurses can use relaxation techniques in their work with clients to reduce pain and stress. Relaxation techniques are also an essential aspect of cognitive behavioral therapy when treating people with phobias, fear, and depression.

Imagery

Imagery is a technique of using the imagination to visualize a pleasant, soothing image. The practitioner

encourages the client to use as many of the senses as possible in order to enhance the formation of vivid images. Table 13-2 presents examples of incorporating all five senses into imagery.

Nurses can create guided imagery for many clients who are capable of hearing and understanding the nurse's suggestions of meaningful and physiologically correct images. For example, a nurse can show a chart of the stages of bone healing to a client who has suffered a fracture and ask the client to imagine this sequential activity in his body.

"The nurse using guided imagery can promote a sense of well-being in clients and help them change their perceptions about their disease, treatment, and healing ability" (Dossey, 1995b). Studies have found that a combination of medication and guided imagery decreases physical tension, anxiety, and the adverse effects of chemotherapy (Keegan, 1998). In addition to being a tool for distraction when a person is confronting pain, discomfort, and fear, imagery is also a powerful mechanism for making decisions and for altering behaviors, as it allows the client to try out decisions and behaviors before actually implementing them. The power of the human imagination is limitless, and helping clients to use that power can be a rewarding role for the nurse.

Biofeedback

Biofeedback is a measurement of physiological responses that yields information about the relationship between the mind and the body and helps clients learn ways to manipulate those responses through mental activity. Biofeedback allows a person to see the effect of the mind on the body. While attached to sensitive devices that measure bodily responses such as skin temperature, blood pressure, galvanic skin resistance, and electrical activity in the muscles, the individual imagines stressful experiences. The individual's physiological responses are then measured and recorded, as are the individual's physiological responses to relaxation. The individual receives an interpretation

Table 13-2	**INCORPORATING ALL FIVE SENSES INTO IMAGERY**
SENSE	**IMAGERY**
Visual	See the dark blue sky
Auditory	Hear the babbling brook
Kinesthetic	Feel yourself floating on a cloud
Gustatory	Taste the tartness of a freshly cut lemon
Olfactory	Smell the salt air at the ocean

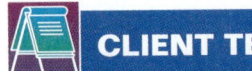

CLIENT TEACHING

Guided Imagery

After explaining the purpose and process of guided imagery, instruct the client to:

- Assume a comfortable position in a quiet environment.
- Close your eyes and keep them closed until the exercise is completed.
- Breathe in deeply to a count of 4.
- Hold breath for a count of 4.
- Breathe out to a count of 4.
- Continue to breathe slowly and deeply.
- Think of your favorite place and prepare to take an imaginary journey there. Select a place in which you are relaxed and at peace.
- Picture in your mind's eye your favorite place. Look around you and see all the colors, the light and shadows, and all the pleasant sights.
- Listen to all the sounds. Pay attention to what you hear.
- Feel all the physical sensations . . . the temperature . . . the textures . . . the movement of the air.
- As you take in a deep breath, smell the aromas of your favorite place.
- Taste the foods and drinks you usually consume in your favorite place. Savor each taste fully.
- Focus all your attention totally on your favorite place.
- Breathe in deeply to a count of 4.
- Hold breath for a count of 4.
- Breathe out to a count of 4.
- Resume your usual breathing pattern.
- Slowly open your eyes and stretch, if desired.

This procedure works best when all five senses are used. Like all other relaxation exercises, guided imagery becomes more effective with repetition.

of these responses and is taught methods for practicing relaxation to control reactions to stressful experiences.

Biofeedback is used as a restorative method in rehabilitation settings to help clients who have lost sensation and function as the result of illness or injury. Machines that can detect a person's internal bodily functions translate them into a form that the client can detect, such as a light or beep. After training with the machine, clients are able to alter their responses without the machine. Biofeedback also enhances relaxation in tense muscles, relieves tension headaches and backache, and reduces bruxism (grinding of the teeth) and the pain associated with temporomandibular joint

syndrome (Association of Psychophysiology and Biofeedback, 1998). Temperature biofeedback is useful in training clients to purposefully warm their hands to treat Raynaud's disease (a circulatory disorder), to lower blood pressure, and to prevent or relieve migraine headaches.

Hypnosis

The practice of hypnosis was once overshadowed by mystery and misconception. Today, with our expanding knowledge of the human mind, hypnosis is becoming a more common nursing intervention (Zahourek & Larkin, 1995). Therapeutic **hypnosis** induces an altered state of consciousness or awareness resembling sleep and during which the person is more receptive to suggestion. Hypnosis also enhances the client's ability to form images.

Nurses wishing to use hypnosis in their practices must be aware of the guidelines concerning this modality with regard to the scope of practice as defined by their respective state boards of nursing. They also should receive advanced training in the art of hypnosis (Kolkmeier, 1995).

Body-Movement (Manipulation) Strategies

As the name implies, body-movement therapies employ techniques of moving or manipulating various body parts to achieve therapeutic outcomes. Modalities such as movement and exercise, yoga, tai chi, and chiropractic treatment are discussed in the following sections.

Movement and Exercise

Movement, as a therapeutic intervention and health-promoting activity, is associated with athletic exercise, dance, celebration, and healing rituals. Although the primary goal of exercise is fitness (muscle strength, flexibility, endurance, and cardiovascular and respiratory health), there are many other positive outcomes of exercise, such as feeling more energetic and sleeping better.

Nurses can help clients use movement as therapy in a variety of ways such as range of motion exercises, water exercises, physical therapy, and stretching exercises.

LIFE CYCLE CONSIDERATIONS

Exercise and the Very Old

Those of very advanced ages (95 years and older) are achieving positive results from regular exercise and weight lifting, including increased physical strength and flexibility and improved mental status in areas such as memory and depression (Mills, 1994).

Movement is an effective method through which people of all ages can improve their level of functioning. Exercise has also been documented to improve functional ability in people with arthritis (Budesheim, Neuberger, Kasal, Vogel-Smith, Hassanein, & DeViney, 1994).

Yoga

Many cultures believe that particular forms of movement keep the body's life forces in correct balance and flow. Yoga and tai chi are examples of ancient ritual movements that enhance overall health including spiritual enlightenment and well-being. Both of these approaches require concentration and the use of symbolic movements.

A form of meditative exercise, yoga rejuvenates, promotes longevity and self-realization, and speeds the natural evolution of the person toward self-enlightenment. Traditional yoga has always been primarily concerned with healthy individuals and promoting health by maintaining the balance and flow of life forces.

Yoga therapy is an effort to integrate traditional yogic concepts and techniques with Western medical and psychological knowledge (Feuerstein, 1998). The focus of yoga therapy is to holistically treat various psychological or somatic dysfunctions ranging from back problems to emotional distress.

Both yoga and yoga therapy are based on the understanding that the human being is an integrated body/mind system that best functions in a state of dynamic balance (Feuerstein, 1998). Studies regarding benefits of yoga practice have found that mentally challenged individuals become more aware of their bodies and enjoy improved coordination, while clients with osteoarthritis of the hands experience less pain (Keegan, 1998). Claims made by yoga authorities range from a beneficial effect on physical flexibility, muscle tone, and stamina to a reduction in obesity, back pain, hypertension, various respiratory diseases, anxiety, and memory loss (Feuerstein, 1998).

Tai Chi

Tai chi is based on the philosophy of the quest for harmony with nature and the universe through the laws of complementary (yin and yang) balance. When perfect harmony exists, everything functions effortlessly, spontaneously, perfectly, and in accordance with the laws of nature. If one moves to the right, then one must also move to the left. Tai chi consists of a series of sequential, dance-like movements connected in a smooth-flowing process.

People who regularly perform tai chi believe that it enhances stamina, agility, and balance and that it boosts energy and confers a sense of well-being. Tai chi has been used as a complementary method to treat digestive disorders, stress, depression, and rheumatoid arthritis (Keegan, 1995a).

PROFESSIONAL TIP

Preparing for Chiropractic Therapy
As with any alternative/complementary intervention, nurses should encourage clients who are considering the use of chiropractic services to first undergo comprehensive health assessment to rule out any contraindications.

Chiropractic Therapy

The major principle underlying chiropractic therapy is that the brain sends vital energy to every organ in the body via the nerves originating in the spinal column. Dis-ease, body disharmony, or malfunction results from vertebral subluxation complex (spinal nerve stress). The body is rebalanced and realigned using chiropractic "spinal adjustment" techniques.

The goal of chiropractic care is to awaken the client's own natural healing ability by correcting any areas of vertebral subluxation complex. Vitality, strength, and health are thus promoted. Chiropractic Arts Center (1998) reports case histories of clients recovering from heart trouble, hyperactivity, fatigue, digestive problems, and many other conditions.

Stedman (1999) explains that chiropractic practitioners fall into one of two groups, the "straights" and the "mixers." The straights believe in the chiropractic therapy just described, despite the fact that no scientific evidence exists to support the claims. The mixers use spinal adjustments mainly to relieve back pain, neck stiffness, and headaches, conditions that have sometimes been shown to be alleviated by chiropractic therapy. Most mixers are willing to work closely with a client's medical doctor.

Chiropractic services have gained increasing acceptance in the United States. Chiropractors are licensed in all 50 states, and 41 states require insurance reimbursement for chiropractic services (Japsen, 1995).

Energetic-Touch Therapies

One category of alternative/complementary therapies that has been incorporated into nursing practice in the past 20 years is the **energetic-touch therapies**, techniques of using the hands to direct or redirect the flow of the body's energy fields and thus enhance balance within those fields. These modalities are effective interventions for many problems and can be used to restore harmony in all aspects of a person's health. Energetic-touch therapies can be used with persons of all ages and all stages of wellness and illness.

Energetic-touch therapies have their roots in traditional Chinese, ancient Eastern, and Native American philosophies. The fundamental concept is that individuals are composed of a life force, a source of energy

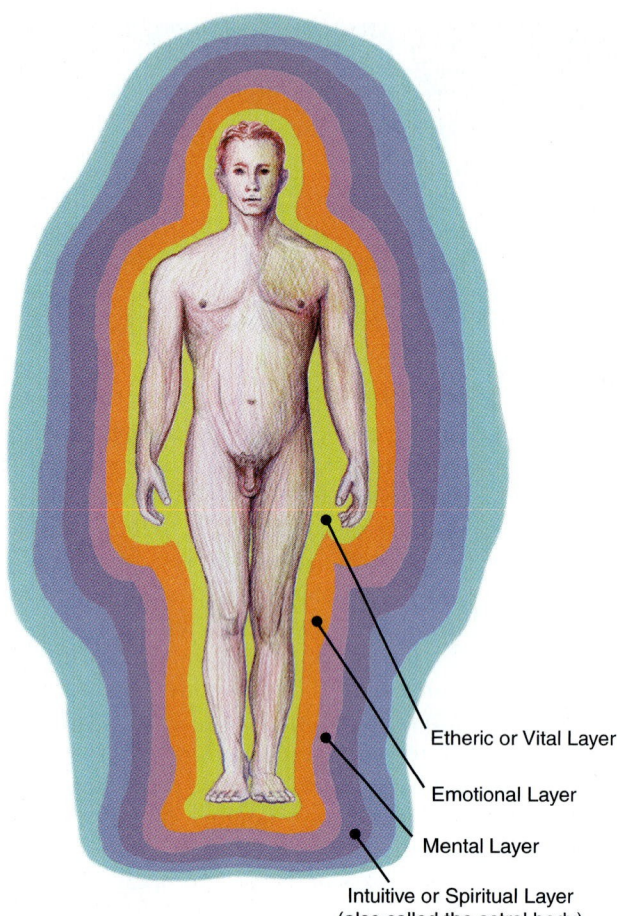

Etheric or Vital Layer

Emotional Layer

Mental Layer

Intuitive or Spiritual Layer
(also called the astral body)

Figure 13-3 Layers of the Human Energy Field Extending beyond the Physical Boundaries

that is not confined to physical skin boundaries. Figure 13-3 illustrates the energy field that extends beyond a person's physical body.

An individual's energy field consists of energy layers in constant flux. These energy layers can be diminished or otherwise adversely affected by any type of illness, trauma, or distress. The energy system can also be positively affected by the intentionally directed use of a practitioner's hands. The primary focus of the nurse using an energetic-touch therapy is "to restore the optimal flow of life energy through the field" (Cowens, 1996).

Many energetic-touch therapies are being used by nurses today. Touch, therapeutic massage, therapeutic

CULTURAL CONSIDERATIONS

Touch

- Ask permission before touching a client.
- Tell the client what is going to happen.
- The meaning of touch and the body areas acceptable to touch vary from culture to culture.

touch, and healing touch are some examples. Other modalities include acupressure and reflexology, techniques that involve deep-tissue body work and require advanced training on the part of practitioners.

Touch

One of the most universal alternative/complementary modalities is touch. **Touch**, simply defined, is the means of perceiving or experiencing through tactile sensation. Although it was used in all ancient cultures and shamanistic traditions for healing, the advent of scientific medicine and Puritanism led many healers away from the purposeful use of touch. It should be noted that touch carries with it taboos and prescriptions that are culturally dictated. Some cultures are very comfortable with physical touch; others specify that touch may be used only in certain situations and within specified parameters.

Because touch involves personal contact, the nurse must be sure to convey positive intentions. When in doubt, the nurse should withhold touch until effective communication with the client has been established. Touch has several important uses in nursing practice, in that it:

- Is an integral part of assessment;
- Promotes bonding between nurse and client (Figure 13-4);
- Is an important means of communication, especially when other senses are impaired;
- Assists in soothing, calming, and comforting; and
- Helps keep the client oriented.

Therapeutic Massage

Therapeutic massage is the application of pressure and motion by the hands with the intent of improving the recipient's well-being. It involves kneading, rubbing, and using friction.

Massage therapy is now recognized as a highly beneficial modality and is prescribed by a number of

PROFESSIONAL TIP

Contraindications for Touch

It is important to know when *not* to touch.

- It may be difficult for persons who have been neglected, abused, or injured to accept touch therapy.
- Touching those who are distrustful or angry may escalate negative behaviors.
- Persons with burns or overly sensitive skin may not benefit from touch.

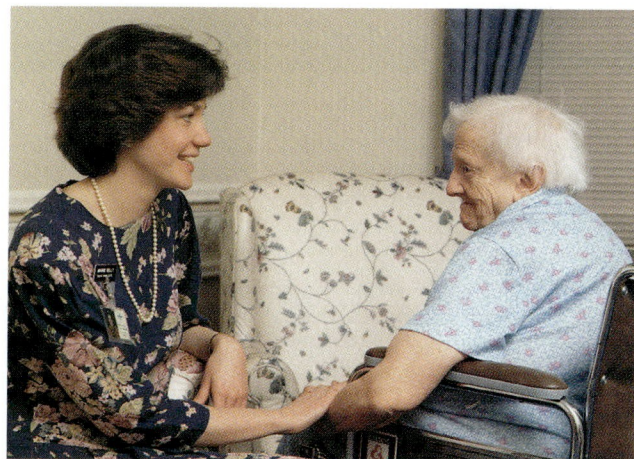

Figure 13-4 Touch promotes bonding between nurse and client.

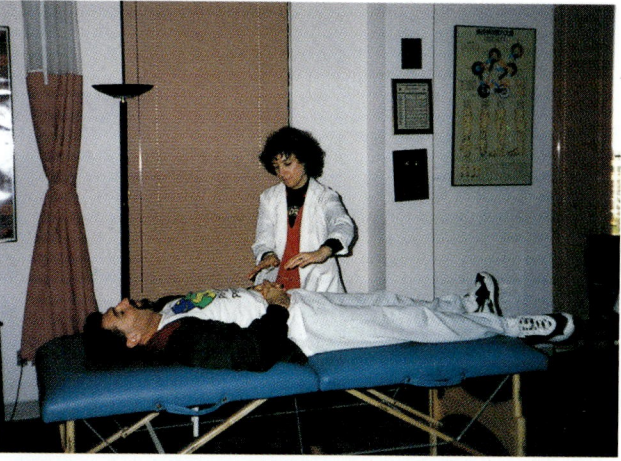

Figure 13-5 A Nurse Administering Therapeutic Touch to a Client

physicians. In addition, many states now have licensing requirements for massage practitioners.

Traditionally, back rubs have been administered by nurses to provide comfort to hospitalized clients. Massage techniques can be used with all age groups and are especially beneficial to those who are immobilized. A back rub or massage can achieve many results, including relaxation, increased circulation of the blood and lymph, and relief from musculoskeletal stiffness, pain, and spasm.

Safety: Precautions for Massage

- Massage should be used with caution on people with heart disease, diabetes, hypertension, or kidney disease, because increased circulation may be harmful in the presence of these conditions.
- Massage should never be attempted in areas of circulatory abnormality, such as aneurysm, varicose veins, necrosis, phlebitis, or thrombus, or in areas of soft-tissue injury, open wounds, inflammation, joint or bone injury, dermatitis, recent surgery, or sciatica.

Therapeutic Touch

Therapeutic touch, which is based on ancient healing practices such as the laying on of hands, consists of assessing alterations in a person's energy field and using the hands to direct energy to achieve a balanced state. Therapeutic touch is based on four assumptions:

- A human being is an open energy system.
- Anatomically, a human being is bilaterally symmetrical.
- Illness is an imbalance in an individual's energy field.
- Human beings have natural abilities to transform and transcend their conditions of living (Krieger, 1993).

The therapeutic touch process is readily learned in workshops, can be done with hands either on or off the body, complements medical treatments, and has demonstrated reasonably consistent and reliable results (Figure 13-5). Table 13-3 outlines the five-phase process of therapeutic touch.

The relaxation response may be apparent in the client as quickly as 2 to 5 minutes after a therapeutic touch treatment has begun, and some clients may fall asleep or require less pain medication after a treatment. When done correctly, the practice of therapeutic touch can be mutually beneficial, energizing and increasing feelings of wellness in the practitioner as well as in the client (Mackey, 1995).

Research has documented the effectiveness of therapeutic touch in numerous areas. Therapeutic touch has been shown to accelerate wound healing of infections after cesarean section delivery (Wetzel, 1993); promote relaxation, increase energy, enhance a sense of well-being, and improve immunological functioning (Quinn, 1993); decrease anxiety in hospitalized psychiatric clients (Gagne & Toye, 1994); reduce postoperative pain, thereby decreasing the need for medication (Meehan, 1993); enhance the relaxation response, pain management, and immune function (Wilson, 1995); and alleviate generalized anxiety (Olsen & Sneed, 1995).

Healing Touch

Healing touch is an energy-based therapeutic modality that alters the energy field through the use of touch, thereby affecting physical, mental, emotional, and spiritual health (Keegan, 1995b). Healing touch was developed in the 1980s by Janet Mentgen, a nurse. In 1990, healing touch was established as a certification program of the American Holistic Nurses' Association (AHNA). The curriculum includes varied techniques in general balancing of the body's energy field, relaxation, and specific problems such as headaches, spinal problems, and pain.

Table 13-3 PHASES OF THERAPEUTIC TOUCH

PHASE	DEFINITION	TECHNIQUES
Centering	• Bringing body, mind, and emotions to a quiet, focused state of consciousness • Being still • Being nonjudgmental	Become centered: • Controlled breathing, • Imagery, and • Meditation.
Assessment ("scanning")	• Using the hands to determine the nature of the client's energy field • Being attuned to sensory cues (e.g., warmth, coolness, static, pressure, tingling) to detect changes in the client's energy	• Hold the hands 2 to 6 inches from the client's energy field while moving the hands from the head to the feet in a rhythmic, symmetrical manner.
Unruffling ("clearing")	• Facilitating the symmetrical and rhythmic flow of energy through the field	• Use slightly more vigorous hand movements from midline while continuing to move in a rhythmic and symmetrical manner from the head to the feet.
Treatment ("balancing," "rebalancing," or "intervention")	• Projecting, directing, and modulating energy on the basis of the nature of the living energy field • Assisting to reestablish order in the system.	• Because each practitioner experiences the living energy field uniquely, the law of opposites serves as a guideline for intervening (e.g., if a pulling or drawing sensation is detected, energy is directed to the depleted area until it feels replenished). • Continue to assess, clear, and balance the field while remaining centered.
Evaluation	• Using professional, informed, and intuitive judgment to determine when to end the session	• Reassess the field. • Elicit feedback from the client. • Give the client an opportunity to rest and integrate the process.

The phases, although learned sequentially by beginners, are dynamic and often are performed concurrently and repetitively by experienced practitioners.

Adapted from Therapeutic Touch: Teaching Guidelines: Beginner's Level Krieger/Kunz Method, by Nurse Healers-Professional Associates, Inc., 1992. New York: Author.

Healing touch can be administered in a few minutes or, ideally, in a session lasting one full hour (Mentgen, 1995). Implicit in this therapy is the need for follow-up or sequential treatments as well as discharge planning and referral to assist the client in adequately meeting goals.

In both therapeutic touch and healing touch, the practitioner uses **centering** (a process of bringing oneself to an inward focus of serenity) before initiating treatment. Centering is a valuable tool to use before performing any treatment or before any situation that may be stressful or difficult (such as a major school examination).

Shiatsu and Acupressure

Shiatsu, from the word meaning "finger pressure," is a Japanese form of acupressure. Both shiatsu and acupressure are based on the Chinese meridian theory, which states that the body is divided into meridian channels through which energy (Qi, pronounced "chi") flows. Cold, damp, fire, bacteria, or viruses may block the flow of Qi, causing disease in the body. **Acu-**

pressure is a technique of releasing blocked energy within an individual when specific points (Tsubas) along the meridians are pressed or massaged by the practitioner's fingers, thumbs, and heel of the hands. When the blocked energy is freed, the disease subsides. The most commonly treated conditions include muscular pains, joint pains, depression, digestive disturbances, and respiratory disorders (Lanfranco, 1997).

Shiatsu primarily focuses on health maintenance rather than on treatment of illness (Keegan, 1995b); that is, it is used to make sure the Qi is able to flow freely so that the individual does not become ill. When practicing shiatsu, nurses must be self-aware and grounded (focused on their inner energy). This focus enables the practitioner to concentrate completely on promoting the client's comfort.

Reflexology

Reflexology is rooted in ancient healing arts. The fundamental concept of reflexology is that the body is divided into 10 equal, longitudinal zones that run the length of the body, from the top of the head to the tip of the toes. These 10 zones are correlated with the 10 fingers and toes. The foot is thus viewed as a microcosm of the entire body. Reflexology theory posits that illness manifests itself in calcium deposits and acids in the corresponding part of the person's foot. The pressing of specific points on the foot stimulates energy movement and produces relaxation, reduces stress, and promotes health by relieving pressures and accumulation of toxins in the corresponding body part (Figure 13-6).

Reflexology can be used as a complementary method for managing chronic conditions such as asthma, sinus infections, migraines, irritable bowel syndrome, kidney stones, and constipation. After the pressure points are learned, the nurse can massage the areas of the client's foot to relieve pain and produce relaxation.

Spiritual Therapies

A state of wholeness or health is dependent on one's relationship not only to the physical and interpersonal environments, but also to the spiritual aspects of self. The idea that there is a relationship between spirituality and health is not new. "From the earliest time of the shaman we have witnessed the mysterious spiritual element of healing . . . the connection of the healer with the divine" (Keegan, 1994).

The role of the spirit in healing is witnessed in all cultures. The inseparable link between the state of one's soul (life energy or spirit) and the state of one's health is accepted by many cultures. Scientists (especially psychoneuroimmunologists) are beginning to validate that individuals have inner mechanisms of healing. Many of the major religions have ideologies relating to health, illness, and healing.

Faith Healing

At the heart of spiritual or faith healing is the belief that practitioners must purify themselves and reach a state of unity with God or a Higher Power before faith healing can occur. This process, based on religious belief, is usually accomplished through prayer. During preparation for healing, the practitioner adapts a passive and receptive mood in order to be a channel for divine power. The ill person's belief enhances, but is not crucial to, the success of healing.

Healing Prayer

When individuals pray, they believe they are communicating directly with God or a Higher Power. Prayer is an integral part of a person's spiritual life and, as such, can affect well-being. Florence Nightingale recognized that prayer helps connect individuals to nature and the environment (Nightingale, 1969). Medical research is currently investigating the effects of prayer on physical health.

A study conducted by Byrd and Sherrill (1995) investigated the effects of prayer on clients in critical

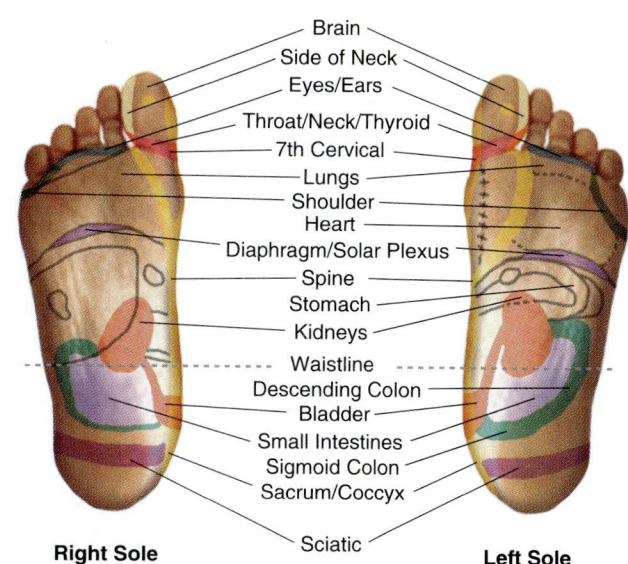

Figure 13-6 Foot Reflexology Charts *(Reproduced with permission from* Better Health with Foot Reflexology. *Copyright 1983 by Dwight C. Byers. Ingham Publishing, Inc., POB 12642, St. Petersburg, FL 33733-2642.)*

care units. The results showed that clients who received standard medical treatment with the addition of intercessory prayers had fewer complications, required less medication, and improved faster than did clients in the control group, who received standard medical care and no prayers. Findings reported by Marwick (1995) showed that religious involvement may lead to improved physical health status.

Shamanism

Shamanism was discussed earlier in this chapter.

Nutritional/Medicinal Therapies

In the past 20 to 30 years, nutritional interventions for prevention and treatment of disease have generated increasing interest among consumers and health care providers. This section addresses the alternative/complementary nutritional and medicinal approaches.

Phytochemicals

Currently, certain foods are being studied for their medicinal value. **Phytochemicals** are nonnutritive, physiologically active compounds present in plants in very small amounts (Simons, 1997). *Phyto* is the Greek word for "plant." Therefore, phytochemicals are plant chemicals. These chemicals have several functions including storage of nutrients and provision of structure, aroma, flavor, and color. Phytochemicals protect against cancer and prevent heart disease, stroke, and cataracts. Phytochemicals are found in fruits and vegetables.

No single fruit or vegetable contains all phytochemicals. The consumption of a wide variety of fruits and vegetables provides the best supply. The major sources of phytochemicals are onions, garlic, leeks, chives, carrots, sweet potatoes, squash, pumpkin, cantaloupe, mango, papaya, tomatoes, citrus fruits, grapes, strawberries, raspberries, cherries, legumes, soybeans, tofu, and the cruciferous vegetables (broccoli, cauliflower, brussels sprouts, and cabbage). Nurses can use this information to encourage clients to eat more fruits and vegetables.

Antioxidants and Free Radicals

Antioxidants are substances that prevent or inhibit oxidation, a chemical process whereby a substance is joined to oxygen. In the body, antioxidants prevent tissue damage related to **free radicals**, which are unstable molecules that alter genetic codes and trigger the development of cancer growth in cells. Vitamins C and E, beta-carotene (which is converted to vitamin A in the body), and selenium are antioxidants. Antioxidants may prevent heart disease, some forms of cancer, and cataracts. Free radicals contribute to cardiovascular disease by oxidizing low-density lipoproteins (LDLs) and allowing cholesterol to adhere to vessel walls. Antioxidants help repair eye tissue damaged from sunlight and thus prevent cataract formation (Simons, 1997). Other vitamins, minerals, trace elements, and enzymes are being investigated for their possible therapeutic value.

Macrobiotic Diet

In the 1960s, macrobiotic (from the Greek words *makro,* meaning "long," and *bios,* meaning "life") diets became popular because of a heightened interest in "natural" and more spiritual approaches to managing health and illness. The basis of macrobiotics is the Taoist concept of balance between opposites as achieved through food intake. Food has the qualities of *yin* (associated with death, cold, and darkness) and *yang* (associated with immortality, heat, and light). For example, tropical sweet foods are yin, and meat and eggs are yang. Overindulgence in either type causes difficulties; for example, too much yin food yields worry and resentment, whereas too much yang food leads to hostility and aggression. People need balance and, therefore, should consume foods that balance yin and yang.

Because brown rice and whole grains are categorized as balanced foods, they are major staples of a macrobiotic diet. The diet should be flexible and related to the season and should consist of foods indigenous to the area where the individual lives. Foods to be avoided include processed and treated foods, red meat, sugar, dairy products, eggs, and caffeine. The macrobiotic diet generally conforms to the recommendations of the American Dietary Association in terms of

the guidelines for low-fat, low-cholesterol, high-fiber diets (Guinness, 1993).

Herbal Therapy

Herbal medicine has been a powerful tool in folk healing for centuries. Medicinal herbs have been catalogued for thousands of years and have probably been used in every culture. Many drugs commonly used today were, in an earlier time, tribal remedies derived from plants. Herbal medicine, also known as botanical medicine or phytotherapy, uses plant extracts for therapeutic outcomes.

Learning about herbal treatment is similar to learning pharmacology. Many holistic practitioners incorporate the use of herbs into their practices. Herbs work because of their chemical composition. Different herbs contain different compounds that can strengthen the immune system, alter the blood chemistry, or protect specific organs against disease. Table 13-4 lists medicinal values of commonly used herbs.

Other Methodologies

The mind/body, body-movement, energetic-touch, spiritual, and nutritional/medicinal treatment modalities are not the only available alternative/complementary therapies. Others such as aromatherapy, humor, pet therapy, music therapy, and play therapy are also used by holistic practitioners.

Aromatherapy

Aromatherapy is defined as the therapeutic use of concentrated essences or essential oils that have been extracted from plants and flowers. When diluted in a carrier oil for massage or in warm water for inhalation, essences may be stimulating, uplifting, relaxing, or

Table 13-4 MEDICINAL VALUE OF HERBS

HERB	MEDICINAL VALUE
Aloe vera	• Promotes wound healing • Soothes minor cuts, abrasions, and burns
Calendula	• Promotes healing of cuts, abrasions, minor burns, sunburn, acne, and athlete's foot • Soothes oral thrush (as a mouthwash) and vaginal thrush (as a douche)
Celery	• Lowers cholesterol • Decreases dizziness • Relieves headache
Chamomile	• Produces a calming effect • Relieves nausea • Eases tension headache
Eucalpytus	• Acts as an antibacterial • Acts as a decongestant
Garlic	• Acts as an antimicrobial remedy for intestinal worms • Helps protect against and treat respiratory infections • Used as expectorant in cases of bronchitis or a cold
Ginger	• Eases nausea (especially effective for motion sickness and morning sickness associated with pregnancy) • Stimulates circulation in feet and hands • Acts as expectorant • Helps relieve indigestion and flatulence • Relieves diarrhea

HERB	MEDICINAL VALUE
Ginkgo	• Enhances cerebral blood flow • Helps lessen mild depression • Eases dementia • Combats impotence • Decreases peripheral vascular insufficiency • Relieves premenstrual syndrome symptoms • Decreases vascular fragility
Peppermint	• Relieves headache • Eases sinus congestion • Reduces muscle spasms
Sage	• Acts as an antibacterial
Saint John's Wort	• Relieves mild to moderate depression • Lessens severity of viral infections
Thyme	• Acts as an antimicrobial • Helps relieve symptoms of common cold • Acts as an antispasmodic on bronchioles • Relieves cystitis • Acts as an antifungal (especially when applied as a lotion for athlete's foot) • Used as a mouthwash for oral thrush

Note: This information is not intended to serve as a guide for self-medication or the treatment of others. Consult a health care practitioner trained in the use of herbs before consuming or giving any herb for medicinal purposes.

From "Herbs for Health," by S. Foster, 1995, The Herb Companion, 8(1), 63–86; "Down to Earth: An Ancient Herb for a Modern Garden," by J. Long, 1995. The Herb Companion, 8(1), 22; "Eight Healing Herbs, 1995–1996," by M. Polunin and C. Robbins, 1995, Holistic Health Directory, 30–34; The Backyard Medicine Chest: An Herbal Primer, by D. Schar, 1995, Washington, DC: Elliot & Clark; and Spontaneous Healing: How To Discover and Enhance Your Body's Natural Ability To Maintain and Heal Itself, by A. Weil, 1995b, New York: Alfred A. Knopf.

soothing. The following are some popular essential oils (Keville & Green, 1995):

- *Lavender* is said to have anti-inflammatory, antidepressant, and antibacterial effects.
- *Eucalyptus* is claimed to act as a decongestant, antimicrobial, and stimulant.
- *Chamomile* is believed to benefit the gastrointestinal tract, relieve allergies, and act as a sedative.
- *Marjoram* is purported to work as an antiseptic and anti-inflammatory agent and to relieve muscle spasms.
- *Peppermint* is believed to improve digestion and act as an antiseptic and decongestant.
- *Rosemary* is said to stimulate the circulation.
- *Geranium* is thought to balance the mind and body.

Aromatherapists use concentrated oils derived from the roots, bark, or flowers of herbs and other plants to treat specific ailments. The aromas cause physiological, psychological, and pharmacological reactions (Trevelyan, 1993). Some essential oils have antibacterial properties and are found in a wide variety of pharmaceutical preparations. Essential oils should be used intelligently and with caution.

A clinical study reported by Wilkinson (1995) concluded that massage oil that incorporated the essential oil Roman chamomile reduced anxiety and improved the quality of life of cancer clients to a greater extent than did unscented oil. Another study found that post-cardiac surgery clients receiving foot massages with neroli oil (from orange flowers) experienced greater and more lasting psychological benefits than did those

LIFE CYCLE CONSIDERATIONS

Essential Oils

Essential oils should be used with caution in children, pregnant women, and elderly persons. These clients are usually more sensitive to essential oils than are nonpregnant adults and teenagers and thus require smaller amounts and less-concentrated forms of the essence.

Table 13-5 AROMATHERAPY CONTRAINDICATIONS

ESSENTIAL OIL	CONTRAINDICATION
Sweet fennel	Epilepsy
Rosemary, sage, thyme	Hypertension
Peppermint, rose, rosemary	First trimester of pregnancy
	Use only in well-diluted form in later stages of pregnancy
Arnica, basil, celery, sage, cypress, jasmine, juniper, marjoram, myrrh, sage, thyme	Pregnancy
Camomile, lavender	Use with care in pregnancies carrying the risk of bleeding or miscarriage

From "Aromatherapy," by J. Trevelyan, 1993, Nursing Times, 89(25), 39.

receiving massages without neroli oil (Stevenson, 1994). Weiss and James (1997), however, report clients with allergic contact dermatitis to essential oils.

Some contraindications for aromatherapy are listed in Table 13-5.

Safety: Aromatherapy

- Essential oils are very potent and should never be used in an undiluted form, be used near the eyes, or be ingested orally.
- Because some people are allergic to certain oils, a small skin-patch test should be done before generalized application.

Humor

Of all the complementary interventions addressed in this chapter, humor is the one that can be used most often by nurses to benefit clients. "Humor is probably one of the least understood, easiest to do, and most beneficial of the nonpharmacologic interventions" (Mornhinweg & Voignier, 1995).

To avoid giving offense, it is important to determine the client's perception of what is humorous. Whether a given situation is considered humorous or offensive will vary greatly from culture to culture and person to person. Good taste and common sense should serve as guides.

Nurses can use humor with clients in a variety of ways. A humor cart (portable cart or carrier filled with cartoon and joke books, magic tricks, and silly noses) is easy to use and allows clients to select their own humor tools for health. A "humor room" may be made available, where clients can watch comedy videos or play fun games with visitors or other clients.

PROFESSIONAL TIP

Use of Humor

Never do or say anything that gives clients the idea that you are laughing *at* them as opposed to *with* them (McGhee, 1998).

Humor has many therapeutic outcomes. Norman Cousins, former chairman of the Task Force in Psychoneuroimmunology at the School of Medicine at UCLA, relates how he enhanced his recovery from an incurable connective tissue disorder, ankylosing spondylitis, by the daily watching of films and movies that made him laugh (Cousins, 1979). Humor can be used effectively to relieve anxiety and promote relaxation, improve respiratory function, enhance immunological function, and decrease pain by stimulating the production of endorphins.

Pet Therapy

The use of pets to enhance health status has a long history. In Britain in the 18th and 19th centuries, pets were used in institutions to give a sense of meaning and purpose to people institutionalized because of developmental delays (i.e., mental retardation). Pet therapy was also used during the Crimean War and World War II (Mornhinweg & Voignier, 1995). Pet therapy is currently used as adjunctive treatment for people in both acute and long-term care settings (Figure 13-7).

Pet therapy has many applications including overcoming physical limitations, improving mood, lowering blood pressure, and improving socialization skills and self-esteem.

Music Therapy

Music enters the bodymind through the auditory sense. Therapeutic use of music consists of playing music to elicit positive changes in behavior, emotions, or physiological response. Music complements other treatment modalities and encourages clients to become active participants in their health care and recovery.

Music is a good adjunct to use with imagery, as it can enhance the relaxation response and, therefore,

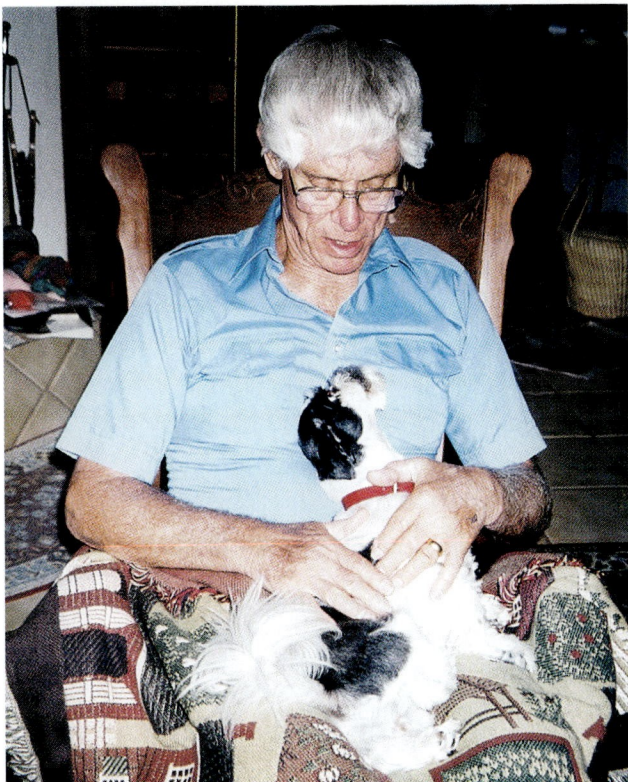

Figure 13-7 Pet therapy provides health benefits. *(Photo courtesy of John White)*

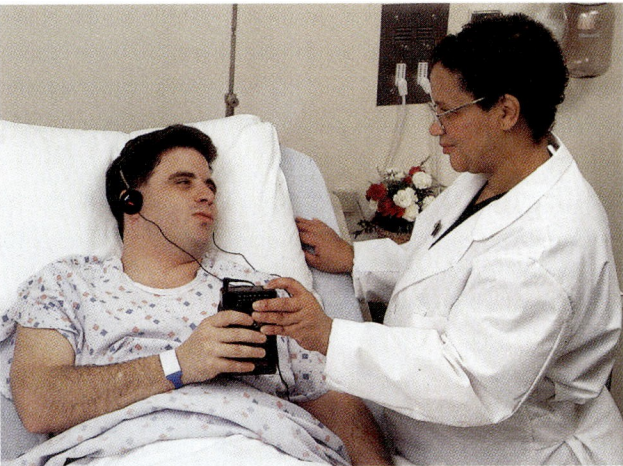

Figure 13-8 Music therapy helps client relax.

heighten images. Different types of music elicit different responses, but all music stimulates the neurotransmitters that evoke chemical changes in the bodymind (Achterberg, Dossey, & Kolkmeier, 1994). Music-thanatology is a holistic and palliative method of using music with dying clients (Schroeder-Shecker, 1994). It is used to help dissipate obstacles to the client's peaceful transition to death.

Music on audiocassette and heard via a tape player and headphones can be a very useful tool for clients who are immobilized, who must wait for diagnostic tests, or who are undergoing the perioperative experience (Figure 13-8). Some facilities allow clients to choose the type of music played while they undergo procedures such as cardiac catheterization. Clients

may request that their music and tape player accompany them during surgery. Pleasurable sound and music can reduce stress, perception of pain, anxiety, and feelings of isolation. Music can also be especially useful in helping adolescent clients relax.

Play Therapy

Play therapy is especially useful with children. Toys are used to allow children to learn about what will be happening to them and to express their emotions and their current situations. Drawing and art work also provide a way for children to share their experiences. When language ability is reduced or not yet well developed, play therapy and drawings constitute a method for children to communicate their needs and feelings to care providers.

NURSING AND ALTERNATIVE/ COMPLEMENTARY APPROACHES

Some methods labeled by Western society as "alternative" (e.g., acupuncture) have already been validated by having been used successfully for centuries. Other alternative/complementary methods such as biofeedback have been proven through research. Still other alternative/complementary modalities such as therapeutic touch need further investigation and validation. Nurses play an important role in educating consumers about nontraditional interventions appropriate throughout the life cycle (Table 13-6) by providing information about the safety and efficacy of such methods. The following are terms frequently used to describe various treatment modalities:

- *Proven:* have been scientifically tested in clinical trials
- *Experimental:* are undergoing Food and Drug Administration (FDA) investigations to ascertain safety and efficacy

CULTURAL CONSIDERATIONS

Music and Culture

- Each culture and each generation within each culture has its own preferred type of music.
- Music that is soothing to one client may be irritating to another.
- Either ask which type of music the client would prefer or allow the client to bring music.

- *Untested:* have not been investigated by the FDA with regard to safety and efficacy
- *Folklore:* have been passed from one generation to another as remedies, many of which have therapeutic value
- *Quackery:* have not proven effective, may result in harm to consumers, and are usually marketed with numerous unfounded promises (e.g., as "cure-all" products or therapies) (Brown, Cassileth, Lewis, & Renner, 1994)

According to Keegan (1998), research has documented the effectiveness of specific alternative/complementary therapies:

- Meditation combined with guided imagery decreases physical tension, anxiety, and the adverse effects of chemotherapy.
- Nutrition, exercise, and meditation—without the use of medication or surgery—can reverse coronary heart disease.

Table 13-6 CORRELATION OF STAGES OF LIFE CYCLE WITH RECOMMENDED COMPLEMENTARY THERAPIES

STAGE OF LIFE CYCLE	RECOMMENDED COMPLEMENTARY THERAPIES
Premature infants	• Massage (with modifications) • Energetic-touch therapies • Music (e.g., recorded human heartbeat) • Gentle movement • Touch (stroking, skin-to-skin contact)
Infants	• Massage (with modifications) • Energetic-touch therapies • Music (e.g., lullabies) • Movement (e.g., rocking)
Toddlers and preschoolers	• Massage • Energetic-touch therapies • Music (e.g., playing and listening to songs, singing) • Movement • Play (all activities should be age appropriate) • Humor • Imagery • Art/drawing • Aromatherapy (with precautions)
School-age children	• Massage • Energetic-touch therapies • Music (playing and listening) • Movement (e.g., dance) • Play (all activities should be age appropriate) • Humor (e.g., riddles, jokes) • Imagery • Art/drawing • Aromatherapy (with precautions) • Hypnosis • Yoga • Tai chi • Pet therapy
Adolescents	All modalities discussed in this chapter, as appropriate to the condition
Adults	All modalities discussed in this chapter, as appropriate to the condition
Women during childbirth	• Massage (emphasis on lower back) • Energetic-touch therapies • Breath coaching • Imagery • Hypnosis
Elders	• Massage (lighter pressure and other modifications for body's status) • Aromatherapy (with precautions) • Any other modalities discussed in this chapter, as appropriate to the condition and with precautions
Terminally ill	• Massage • Reflexology • Energetic-touch therapies • Music-thanatology • Prayer • Any other modalities discussed in this chapter, as appropriate to the condition and with precautions

From Fundamentals of Nursing: Standards & Practice, *by S. DeLaune and P. Ladner, 1998, Albany, NY: Delmar Publishers. Copyright 1998 by Delmar Publishers. Adapted with permission.*

- Yoga can help mentally challenged individuals become more aware of their bodies and improve coordination.
- Yoga can help reduce pain in clients with osteoarthritis of the hands.

Numerous alternative/complementary interventions can be incorporated into nursing practice. As Frisch (1997) states:

> While holistic nurses use many alternative and complementary approaches to care, it is not the alternative modality that makes us holistic; it is our presence, our caring, and our willingness to put the client first.

Putting the client first means individualizing every intervention on the basis of the client's unique needs. From the time before birth until the moment of death, people of all ages experience trauma, stress, and life challenges and have needs in all dimensions. Nurses are challenged to discover and meet those needs.

The power of the nurse's presence with any client should never be underestimated. Many of the alternative/complementary modalities require further study and advanced training. However, nursing students already have the ability to listen, to touch, and to care. Clients can benefit from intent, compassion, and something as simple as having another person present with them.

CASE STUDY

Mr. Vincent, who is receiving chemotherapy for colon cancer, tells the nurse that he is seeing both an aromatherapist to relieve his pain and nausea and a practitioner of healing touch to cure his cancer. He also says that he does not know whether he will come back for his next chemotherapy session because it makes him feel bad. The other therapies make him feel better.

Consider the following:

1. What should the nurse do with this information?
2. How should the nurse respond?
3. What assessments should the nurse make?
4. Identify a nursing diagnosis and goal for Mr. Vincent.
5. List three nursing interventions for this nursing diagnosis.
6. Identify sources for information about the therapies.

SUMMARY

- Ever-increasing numbers of health care consumers are using nontraditional treatment modalities.
- Psychoneuroimmunology is the study of the way that the body and mind are connected and the way that beliefs, thoughts, and emotions affect health.
- Holistic nursing practice encompasses consideration of each client as a unique and whole being with many aspects: physiological, psychological, sociocultural, intellectual, and spiritual.
- Healing is not curing but, rather, is regaining balance and finding harmony and wholeness as changes take place from within the individual.
- No one can heal another, but a nurse can act as a guide, support system, or instrument of healing for the client.
- Some of the mind/body modalities that nurses use are meditation, relaxation, imagery, biofeedback, and hypnosis.

- Body-movement modalities include movement and exercise and chiropractic therapy.
- Energetic-touch therapies can be used with persons of all ages and in various stages of illness and wellness.
- Energetic-touch therapies include therapeutic massage, therapeutic touch, healing touch, shiatsu, acupressure, and reflexology.
- Spiritual therapies such as faith healing, healing prayer, and laying on of the hands are helpful modalities to use in caring for clients.
- Nutritional/medicinal therapies include the use of antioxidants, macrobiotic diets, and herbal therapy.
- Other modalities such as aromatherapy, humor, pet therapy, music therapy, and play therapy are valuable adjuncts to conventional treatment.

Review Questions

1. Therapies that are used instead of mainstream medical practice are called:

   a. alternative therapies.
   b. contemporary therapies.
   c. complementary therapies.
   d. nontraditional therapies.

2. Therapies that are used in conjunction with conventional medical therapies are called:

   a. alternative therapies.
   b. contemporary therapies.
   c. complementary therapies.
   d. nontraditional therapies.

3. The Office of Alternative Medicine:

   a. investigates nontraditional treatment methods.
   b. refers persons to practitioners of nontraditional therapies.
   c. monitors the number of people using nontraditional therapies.
   d. grants a license to those who practice nontraditional therapies.

4. Healing is:

   a. curing a disease.
   b. treating a disease.
   c. making a client well.
   d. a process that activates internal forces.

5. Imagery is a:

   a. balancing of life forces.
   b. relaxation technique using the five senses.
   c. measurement of physiological responses when dreaming.
   d. blocking of the body's energy fields with unhappy thoughts.

6. One of the most universal alternative/complementary modalities is:

   a. touch.
   b. massage.
   c. nutrition.
   d. faith healing.

7. Learning about herbal treatments can be compared to learning about:

   a. hypnosis.
   b. nutrition.
   c. reflexology.
   d. pharmacology.

8. Clients using pet therapy:

   a. play with a cat.
   b. have no other companions.
   c. experience a decrease in blood pressure.
   d. show an increase in physical limitations.

9. The complementary therapy recommended for all ages in the life cycle is:

   a. massage.
   b. hypnosis.
   c. reflexology.
   d. aromatherapy.

Critical Thinking Questions

1. Your close friend has AIDS and is experiencing a great deal of pain and discouragement. She wants to find alternative methods to ease the pain. She confides in you that she believes there may be a cure available at the holistic health center. How do you best help your friend in this situation? What do you advise?

2. A client asks the nurse to rub his foot in a particular spot because that is where his reflexologist rubs to relieve his abdominal pain. How should the nurse handle this situation?

 WEB FLASH!

- Are there specific sites listed under alternative therapies or complementary therapies?
- Search the Web for the organizations listed as resources for this chapter at the end of the book. What information do they provide?
- What resources (books, videos, discussion forums) are available through the Internet for clients interested in a specific alternative/complementary therapy?

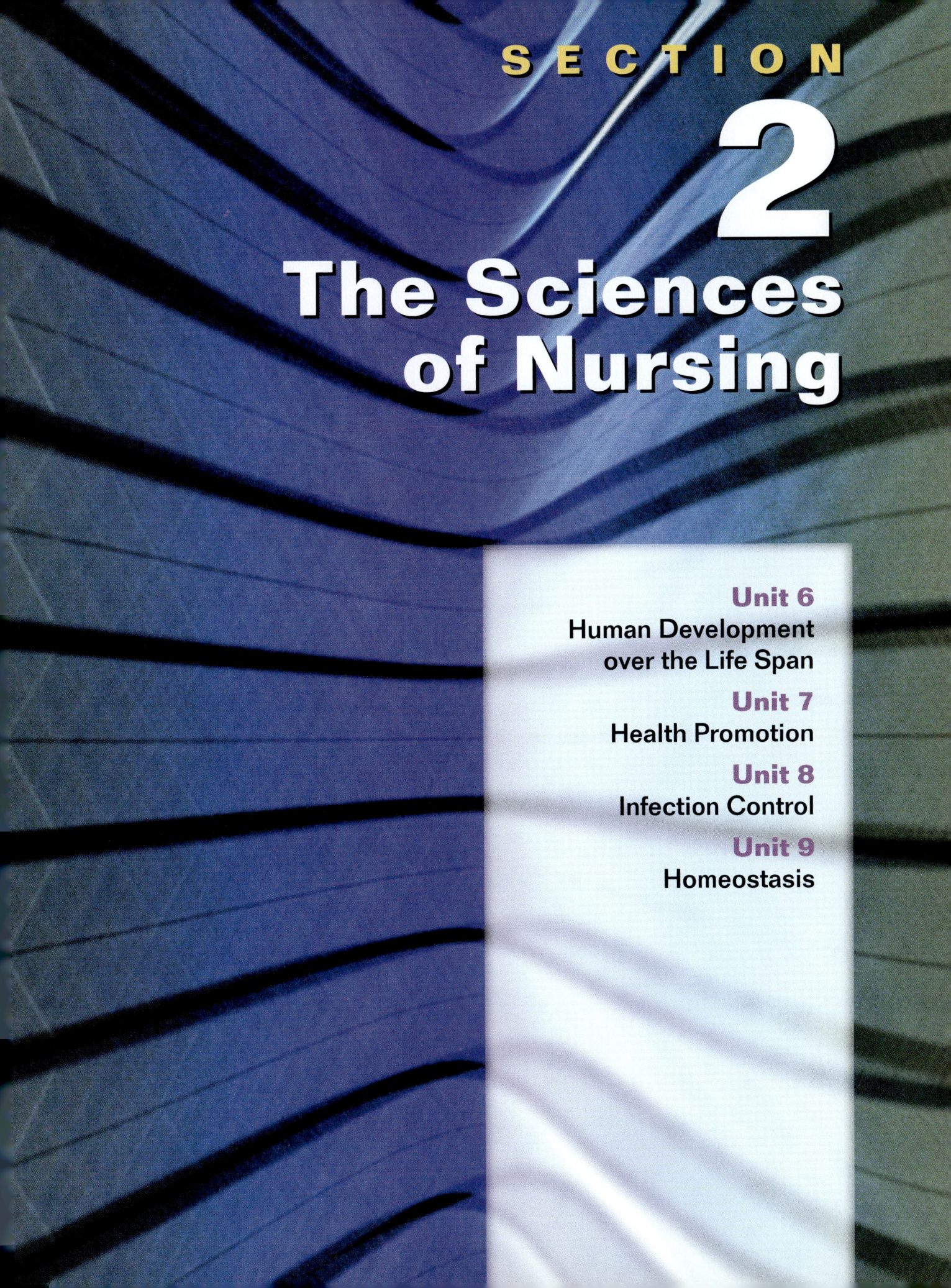

The Sciences of Nursing

UNIT
6
Human Development over the Life Span

Chapter 14
The Life Cycle

THE LIFE CYCLE

MAKING THE CONNECTION

Refer to the following chapters to increase your understanding of the life cycle:

- **Chapter 8, Communication**
- **Chapter 18, Basic Nutrition**
- **Chapter 20, Safety/Hygiene**
- **Chapter 35, Nursing Care of the Client: Reproductive System**
- **Chapter 36, Nursing Care of the Client: Sexually Transmitted Diseases**
- **Chapter 47, Prenatal Care**
- **Chapter 49, The Birth Process**
- **Chapter 51, Newborn Care**
- **Chapter 52, Basics of Pediatric Care**
- **Chapter 55, Nursing Care of the Older Client**

LEARNING OBJECTIVES

Upon completion of this chapter, you should be able to:
- *Define key terms.*
- *Discuss the basic principles of growth and development.*
- *Identify the factors that influence growth and development.*
- *Compare the major developmental theories.*
- *Discuss the importance of development as a holistic framework for assessing and promoting health.*
- *Identify the critical milestones of each developmental stage.*
- *Describe the specific nursing interventions that are relevant to each developmental stage.*

KEY TERMS

accommodation	maturation
adaptation	menarche
adolescence	middle adulthood
anorexia nervosa	moral maturity
assimilation	neonatal period
bonding	obesity
bulimia nervosa	older adulthood
critical period	preadolescence
development	prenatal period
developmental tasks	preschool period
embryonic stage	puberty
fetal alcohol syndrome	school-age period
fetal stage	self-concept
germinal stage	spirituality
growth	teratogenic substance
infancy	toddler period
intrapsychic theory	young adulthood
learning	

INTRODUCTION

From conception to death, individuals are constantly changing. Physical growth, psychological development, emotional maturation, cognitive development, moral development, and spiritual growth occur throughout life. Progression through each developmental stage influences health status. A thorough understanding of developmental concepts is essential for professional quality nursing practice. This chapter presents the types of changes that occur in each stage of the life cycle.

BASIC CONCEPTS OF GROWTH AND DEVELOPMENT

Development occurs continuously through the life span. Adults continue to have transition periods during which growth and development occur.

Growth is the quantitative (measurable) changes in the physical size of the body and its parts, such as increases in cells, tissues, structures, and systems. Examples of growth are physical changes in height, weight, bone density, and dental structure. Even though growth is not a steady process through the life cycle, growth patterns can be predicted. The growth rate varies from periods of rapid increase to periods of slower increase within each individual. Rapid growth is most common in the prenatal, infant, and adolescent stages.

Development refers to behavioral changes in functional abilities and skills. Thus, developmental changes are qualitative, that is, not easily measured. **Maturation** is the process of becoming fully grown and developed and applies to both physiological and behavioral aspects of an individual. Maturation depends on biological growth, functional changes, and **learning** (assimilation of information with a resultant change in behavior). During each developmental stage of the life cycle, certain goals (**developmental tasks**) must be achieved. These developmental tasks set the stage for future learning.

The **critical period** is the time of the most rapid growth or development in a particular stage of the life cycle. During these critical periods, an individual is most vulnerable to stressors of any type.

Growth, development, maturation, and learning are interdependent processes. For learning to occur, the individual must be mature enough to grasp the concepts and make required behavioral changes. Physical growth is also a prerequisite for many types of learning; for example, a child must have the physical ability to control the anal sphincter before toilet training skills are learned. Likewise, cognitive maturation precedes learning.

Principles of Growth and Development

All persons have individual talents and abilities that contribute to their development as unique entities. Thus, *there are no absolute rules in predicting the exact rate of development for any given individual*. There are, however, a few general principles regarding the growth and development of all humans (Table 14-1).

Although evidence of specific skills varies with each person, the sequence of development is predictable. For example, not all infants roll over at the same age, but most roll over before they crawl.

Table 14-1 PRINCIPLES OF GROWTH AND DEVELOPMENT

PRINCIPLE	EXAMPLE
Development occurs in a *cephalocaudal* (head-to-toe) direction.	An infant raises his head before sitting up.
Development occurs in a *proximodistal* manner. Functions closer to the midline (proximal) of the body develop before functions farther away from the body's midline (distal).	The infant is able to move his arms before picking up objects with hands and fingers.
Development occurs in an orderly manner from *simple to complex* and from the *general to the specific*. Gross motor control is achieved before fine motor coordination.	An infant crawls before walking. A child holds a crayon with the entire hand before being able to grasp it between thumb and finger.
The pattern of growth and development is continuous, orderly, and predictable. However, growth and development do not proceed at a consistent rate.	Periods of rapid growth (similar to the growth spurts of adolescence) alternate with periods of slower growth (as seen in middle adulthood).
All individuals go through the same developmental processes; individual differences occur but the process is consistent.	At a certain age in normal development, all individuals will learn how to smile.
Every person proceeds through stages of growth and development at an individual rate.	A child who grows more slowly may be shorter than other children of the same age.
Every stage of development has specific characteristics.	An infant is dependent on others for physical and emotional survival. Adolescence is characterized by a search for identity.
Each stage of development has certain tasks to be achieved or acquired during that specific time. Tasks of one developmental stage become the foundation for tasks in subsequent stages.	An infant must master the psychological task of developing trust to mature as an adolescent who can establish a separate identity.
Some stages of growth and development are more critical than others.	The first trimester of pregnancy is a critical time for embryonic development. During this critical phase, the developing human is most vulnerable to damage from toxins (e.g., drugs, chemicals, viruses).

From Fundamentals of Nursing: Standards & Practice, *by S. DeLaune and P. Ladner, 1998, Albany, NY: Delmar Publishers. Copyright 1998 by Delmar Publishers.*

Factors Influencing Growth and Development

Multiple factors such as heredity, life experiences, health status, and cultural expectations influence a person's growth and development. The interaction of these factors greatly influences how an individual responds to everyday situations; the choices a person makes regarding health behaviors are also greatly determined by these factors.

Heredity

A complex series of processes transmits genetic information from parents to children. The genetic composition of an individual determines physical characteristics such as skin color, hair texture, facial features, and body structure, as well as a predisposition to certain diseases (i.e., Tay-Sachs, sickle cell anemia). Heredity is a genetic blueprint from which an individual grows and develops; to a great extent, it determines the rate of physical and mental development.

Life Experiences

A person's experiences can also influence the rate of growth and development. For example, contrast the differences in physical growth rates between a child whose family can afford food, shelter, and health care and a child whose family has little, if any, resources. The child from an environment lacking in physical resources has a higher risk of experiencing physical and mental lags in growth and development.

Health Status

Individuals who experience wellness progress normally through the life cycle. Illness or disability can interfere with an individual's achievement of developmental milestones. Individuals with chronic conditions will often meet developmental milestones but will be delayed in doing so.

Cultural Expectations

Society expects people to master certain skills at each developmental period. The age at which an individual masters a particular task is determined in part by culture. For instance, cultures that discourage boys from showing tenderness and nurturance may well produce men who are reluctant or incapable of fully expressing these qualities.

CULTURAL CONSIDERATIONS

Growth and Development

The time for mastery of such developmental tasks as speaking and toilet training is as dependent on cultural norms as it is on physiological development.

THEORETICAL PERSPECTIVES OF HUMAN DEVELOPMENT

Nurses must have a thorough understanding of human growth and development in order to provide individualized care. Remember that chronological age and developmental age are not synonymous. An overview of the major developmental theories follows. These theories are discussed more fully in the specific sections about each developmental period.

Physiological Dimension

Physiological growth (physical size and functioning) of an individual is influenced primarily by interaction of genetic predisposition, the central nervous system (CNS), the endocrine system, and maturation. The role of heredity in human development is complex and not yet fully understood. Genetics is the foundation for achievement of specific tasks. Factors such as the psychosocial environment and health status help individuals live up to their genetic potentials.

Psychosocial Dimension

The psychosocial dimension of growth and development consists of subjective feelings and interpersonal relationships. A favorable **self-concept** (perception of one's self, including body image, self-esteem, and ideal self) is perhaps the most important key to a person's success and happiness. Following are characteristics of an individual with a positive self-concept:

- Self-confidence
- Willingness to take risks
- Ability to receive criticism without becoming defensive
- Ability to adapt effectively to stressors
- Innovative problem-solving skills

People with a healthy self-concept believe in themselves. As a result, they set goals that can be achieved. The achievement then reinforces the positive belief about one's self. Figure 14-1 illustrates this positive cycle of self-fulfilling beliefs and actions.

A person with a positive self-concept is likely to engage in health-promoting activities. For example, a person who values self is more likely to change unhealthy habits (such as smoking and sedentary lifestyle) to promote health. An individual with a negative or poor self-concept, on the other hand, is likely to have low self-esteem, a lack of confidence, and difficulty setting and achieving goals.

There are many and varied psychosocial theories that explain the development of self-concept. Following is a discussion of the intrapsychic and interpersonal theories of personality development.

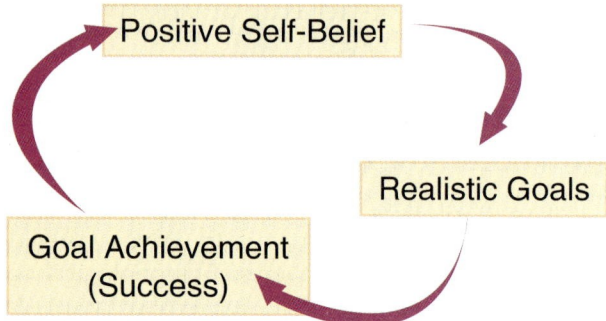

Figure 14-1 Self-Fulfilling Cycle in Positive Self-Concept

Intrapsychic Theory

Intrapsychic (also called psychodynamic) **theory** focuses on an individual's unconscious processes. Feelings, needs, conflicts, and drives are considered to be motivators of behavior, learning, and development. Sigmund Freud, Erik Erikson, and Robert Havighurst are three of the major intrapsychic theorists.

Freud's theories, developed in the early 1930s, continue to influence current concepts related to human development. A basic belief of the Freudian model is that all behavior has some meaning. According to Freud (1961), to mature, a person must successfully travel through five stages of development (Table 14-2). In each stage, there is a conflict to be mastered; if the conflict is not resolved, the individual is halted, developing a fixation at that stage. Fixation implies either inadequate mastery of or failure to achieve a developmental task. A fixation in earlier stages inhibits healthy progression through subsequent stages.

Erikson (1968) expanded Freud's concept of developmental stages by theorizing that psychosocial development is a lifelong process that does not end with the cessation of adolescence. Erikson also emphasized the importance of societal expectations on development. According to Erikson, certain psychosocial tasks must be mastered at each developmental stage. Erikson's model proposes that psychosocial development is a series of conflicts that can have favorable or unfavorable outcomes. These conflicts occur in eight developmental stages of life, described in Table 14-3.

Havighurst (1972) theorizes six developmental stages of life, each with essential tasks to be achieved. Mastery of a task at one developmental stage is essential for mastery of tasks in subsequent stages. When a task at one stage is mastered, it is learned for life, independent of subsequent neurological change (which may occur with disease or injury). Table 14-4 presents Havighurst's developmental stages and the associated tasks.

Interpersonal Theory

Interpersonal theory focuses on a person's relationships with those around him. Harry Stack Sullivan (1953) theorizes that relationships with others influ-

Table 14-2 FREUD'S STAGES OF PSYCHOSEXUAL DEVELOPMENT

STAGE	AGE	DESCRIPTION
Oral	Birth– 18 months	Management of anxiety by using mouth and tongue.
Anal	18 months– 3 years	Control of muscles, especially those controlling urination and defecation.
Phallic (Oedipal)	3 years– 6 years	Awareness of gender and genitalia.
Latency	6 years– 12 years	Exhibition of latent sexual development and energy.
Genital	12 years– adulthood	Emergence of sexual interests and development of relationships with potential sexual partners.

Data from Civilization and Its Discontents, *by S. Freud, 1961, New York: Norton. Copyright 1961 by Norton.*

ence how one's personality develops. Approval and disapproval from significant others shape the formation of one's personality. To form satisfying relationships with others, an individual must complete six stages of development, shown in Table 14-5.

Cognitive Dimension

The cognitive dimension is characterized by the intellectual process of knowing, which includes perception, memory, and judgment. It develops as an individual progresses through the life span. Intelligence is an adaptive process. Individuals use intelligence to adapt by changing the environment to meet their needs and by altering their responses to environmental stressors. The ability to change behavior in response to the demands of an ever-changing environment is characteristic of intelligent beings.

Jean Piaget (1963) studied the differences between children's thinking patterns at different ages and how intelligence is used to solve problems and answer questions. He theorized that children learn to think by playing. Four factors are catalysts to intellectual development:

- Maturation of the endocrine and nervous systems
- Action-centered experience that leads to discovery ("learning by doing")
- Social interaction with opportunities for receiving feedback
- A self-regulating mechanism that responds to environmental stimuli (Murray & Zentner, 1997)

Piaget and Inhelder (1969) enumerate four phases of intellectual development: sensorimotor, preoperational, concrete operations, and formal operations.

Table 14-3 ERIKSON'S STAGES OF PSYCHOSOCIAL DEVELOPMENT

STAGE	AGE	TASK TO BE ACHIEVED	IMPLICATIONS
Trust vs. mistrust	Birth–18 months	To develop a sense of trust in others.	To promote mastery, give consistent, affectionate care. Deficient, inconsistent care produces an unfavorable outcome at this stage.
Autonomy vs. shame and doubt	18 months–3 years	To learn self-control.	To facilitate the child's use of newly acquired skills of independence, provide support, praise, and encouragement. Shaming or insulting the child will lead to unnecessary dependence.
Initiative vs. guilt	3 years–6 years	To initiate spontaneous activities.	Give clear explanations for events and encourage creative activities. Threatening with punishment or labeling behavior as "bad" leads to development of guilt and fear of doing wrong.
Industry vs. inferiority	6 years–12 years	To develop necessary social skills.	To build confidence, recognize the child's accomplishments. Unrealistic expectations or excessively harsh criticism leads to a sense of inadequacy.
Identity vs. role confusion	12 years–20 years	To integrate childhood into a personal identity.	Help the adolescent make decisions. Encourage active participation in home events. Assist with planning for the future.
Intimacy vs. isolation	18 years–25 years	To develop commitments to others and to a life work (career).	Teach the young adult to establish realistic goals. Avoid ridiculing romances or job choices.
Generativity vs. stagnation	21 years–45 years	To establish a family and become productive.	Provide emotional support. Recognize individual accomplishments and provide appropriate praise.
Integrity vs. despair	45+ years	To view one's life as meaningful and fulfilling.	Explore positive aspects of one's life. Review contributions made by the individual.

Data from Childhood and Society, *by E. Erikson, 1968, New York: Norton. Copyright 1968 by Norton;* American Nursing Review of Psychiatric and Mental Health Nursing Certification, *by N. Randolph, 1998, Springhouse, PA: Springhouse. Copyright 1998 by Springhouse.*

Table 14-4 HAVIGHURST'S DEVELOPMENTAL STAGES AND TASKS

DEVELOPMENTAL STAGE	DEVELOPMENTAL TASK	
Infancy and early childhood	Eat solid foods Walk Talk Control elimination of wastes Relate emotionally to others	Distinguish right from wrong through development of a conscience Learn gender differences and sexual modesty Achieve psychological stability Form simple concepts of social and physical reality
Middle childhood	Learn physical skills required for games Build healthy attitudes toward oneself Learn to socialize with peers Learn appropriate masculine or feminine roles Gain basic reading, writing, and mathematical skills	Develop concepts necessary for everyday living Formulate a conscience based on a value system Achieve personal independence Develop attitudes toward social groups and institutions
Adolescence	Establish more mature relationships with individuals of the same age and of both genders Achieve a masculine or feminine social role Accept own body Establish emotional independence from parents	Achieve assurance of economic independence Prepare for an occupation Prepare for marriage and establishment of a family Acquire skills necessary to fulfill civic responsibilities Develop a set of values that guides behavior

continued

Table 14-4 HAVIGHURST'S DEVELOPMENTAL STAGES AND TASKS *continued*

DEVELOPMENTAL STAGE	DEVELOPMENTAL TASK	
Early adulthood	Select a partner Learn to live with a partner Start a family Manage a home	Establish self in a career/occupation Assume civic responsibility Become a part of a social group
Middle adulthood	Fulfill civic and social responsibilities Maintain standard of living appropriate to economic status Assist adolescent children to become responsible, happy adults	Relate to one's partner Adjust to physiological changes Adjust to aging parents
Later maturity	Adjust to physiological changes and alterations in health status Adjust to retirement and altered income Adjust to death of spouse	Develop affiliation with one's age group Meet civic and social responsibilities Establish satisfactory living arrangements

Data from Developmental Tasks and Education, *by R. J. Havighurst, 1972, New York: Longman. Copyright 1972 by Longman.*

Table 14-6 lists descriptions of these phases. Each phase is characterized by the ways that the child interprets and uses the environment. Approximate ages are indicated for each phase, although there is great variation among individuals.

The individual learns by interacting with the environment through three processes: assimilation, accommodation, and adaptation. **Assimilation** is the process of taking in new experiences or information. **Accommodation** allows for readjustment of the cognitive structure (mindset) to take in the new information thus increasing understanding. **Adaptation** refers to the changes that occur as a result of assimilation and accommodation (Murray & Zentner, 1997).

Moral Dimension

The moral dimension consists of a person's value system, which helps one differentiate right and wrong. **Moral maturity** (the ability to independently decide for oneself what is "right") is closely related to emotional and cognitive development. Lawrence Kohlberg (1977) established a framework for understanding how individuals determine a moral code to guide their behavior. Kohlberg's model states that a person's ability to make moral judgments and behave in a morally correct manner develops over a period of time.

According to Kohlberg, there are six stages of moral development, with each stage being built on the previous stage and becoming the foundation for successive stages. Moral development progresses in relationship to cognitive development. Individuals who are able to think at higher levels have the necessary reasoning skills on which to base moral decisions. Table 14-7 provides an overview of Kohlberg's stages of moral development. Kohlberg purports that although individuals move through the six stages in a sequential fashion; not everyone reaches the fifth and sixth stages in the development of personal morality (Kohlberg, 1977).

Table 14-5 SULLIVAN'S INTERPERSONAL MODEL OF PERSONALITY DEVELOPMENT

STAGE	AGE	DESCRIPTION
Infancy	Birth–18 months	Infant learns to rely on caregivers to meet needs and desires.
Childhood	18 months–6 years	Child begins learning to delay immediate need for gratification of needs and desires.
Juvenile	6 years–9 years	Child forms fulfilling peer relationships.
Preadolescence	9 years–12 years	Child relates successfully to peers of the same gender as the child.
Early adolescence	12 years–14 years	Adolescent learns to be independent and forms relationships with members of the opposite sex.
Late adolescence	14 years–21 years	Person establishes an intimate, long-lasting relationship with someone of the opposite sex.

Data from Interpersonal Theory of Psychiatry, *by H. S. Sullivan, 1953, New York: Norton. Copyright 1953 by Norton.*

Table 14-6 PIAGET'S PHASES OF COGNITIVE DEVELOPMENT

PHASE	AGE	DESCRIPTION
Sensorimotor	**Birth–2 years**	Sensory organs and muscles become more functional.
Stage 1: reflex use	Birth–1 month	Movements are primarily reflexive.
Stage 2: primary circular reaction	1 month–4 months	Perceptions center around one's body. Objects are perceived as extensions of the self.
Stage 3: secondary circular reaction	4 months–8 months	Becomes aware of external environment. Initiates acts to change the environment.
Stage 4: coordination of secondary schemata	8 months–12 months	Differentiates goals and goal-directed activities.
Stage 5: tertiary circular reaction	12 months–18 months	Experiments with methods to reach goals. Develops rituals that become significant.
Stage 6: invention of new means	18 months–24 months	Uses mental imagery to understand the environment. Uses fantasy ("make-believe").
Preoperational	**2 years–7 years**	Ability to think emerges.
Preconceptual stage	2 years–4 years	Thinking tends to be egocentric. Exhibits use of symbolism.
Intuitive stage	4 years–7 years	Unable to break down a whole into separate parts. Able to classify objects according to one trait.
Concrete Operations	**7 years–11 years**	Child learns to reason about events in here-and-now.
Formal Operations	**11+ years**	Child is able to see relationships and to reason in the abstract.

Data from The Origins of Intelligence in Children, *by J. Piaget, 1963, New York: Norton. Copyright 1963 by Norton.*

Table 14-7 KOHLBERG'S STAGES OF MORAL DEVELOPMENT

LEVEL AND STAGE	DESCRIPTION
Level I: Preconventional	Authority figures are obeyed.
(Birth–9 years)	Misbehavior is viewed in terms of damage done.
Stage 1: *punishment and obedience orientation*	A deed is perceived as "wrong" if one is punished; the activity is "right" if one is not punished.
Stage 2: *instrumental-relativist orientation*	"Right" is defined as that which is acceptable to and approved by the self. When actions satisfy one's needs, they are "right."
Level II: Conventional	Cordial interpersonal relationships are maintained.
(9 years–13 years)	Approval of others is sought through one's actions.
Stage 3: *interpersonal concordance*	Authority is respected.
Stage 4: *law and order orientation*	Individual feels "duty bound" to maintain social order. Behavior is "right" when it conforms to the rules.
Level III: Postconventional	Individual understands the morality of having democratically established laws.
(13+ years)	
Stage 5: *social contract orientation*	It is "wrong" to violate others' rights.
Stage 6: *universal ethics orientation*	The person understands the principles of human rights and personal conscience. Person believes that trust is basis for relationships.

Data from Recent Research in Moral Development, *by L. Kohlberg, 1977, New York: Holt, Rinehart, & Winston. Copyright 1977 by Holt, Rinehart, & Winston.*

Spiritual Dimension

The spiritual dimension is characterized by a sense of personal meaning. The term *spirit* is derived from the Latin word meaning breath, air, and wind. Thus, spirit refers to whatever gives life to a person. **Spirituality** refers to relationships with one's self, with others, and with a higher power or divine source. Spirituality does not refer to a specific religious affiliation; rather, it can be defined as the core of a person. Development of spirituality is an ongoing, lifelong process.

Fowler's theory of spiritual development was influenced by the works of Erikson, Piaget, and Kohlberg.

Fowler's theory is composed of a prestage and six distinct stages of faith development (Fowler, 1995). Although individuals vary in the age at which they experience each stage, the sequence of stages remains the same. Table 14-8 outlines Fowler's theory.

Although some clients seem to be unaware of their spiritual natures, each client has a personalized definition of spiritual self. Acknowledgment of a client's spirituality is essential to the practice of nursing. Caring for the whole being is the hallmark of a holistic nurse.

HOLISTIC FRAMEWORK FOR NURSING

Providing care to the whole person is a basic concept of nursing. Knowledge of growth and development concepts is essential for nurses because nursing interventions must be appropriate to each client's developmental stage. Nursing's holistic perspective recognizes the progression of individual development across the life span. Developmental progress, or lack thereof, in one dimension affects all other dimensions of life. Figure 14-2 shows the holistic nature of individuals.

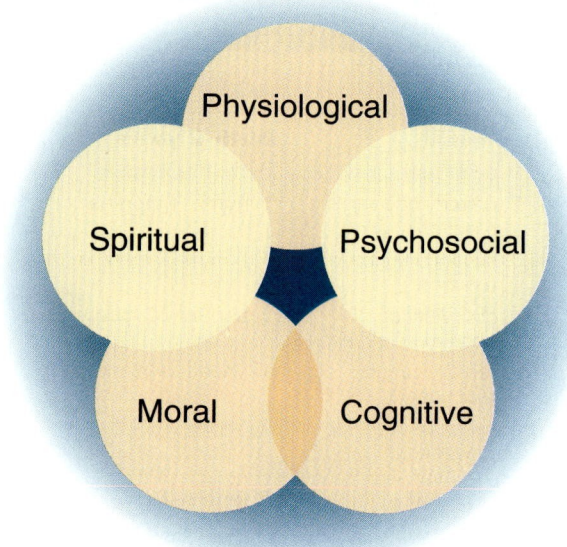

Figure 14-2 Holistic Nature of Human Beings

Growth and development theories are useful to nurses as assessment parameters. Alterations in expected patterns are indicators for early intervention. Examples of situations wherein knowledge of developmental milestones is essential for prompt identification of problems and comprehensive intervention include the following:

- The infant who does not sit, crawl, or walk at expected times
- The adolescent girl who has not experienced menarche by the expected time
- The adult who has failed to develop adequate problem-solving skills

STAGES OF THE LIFE CYCLE

For purposes of this discussion, eleven developmental stages are considered: prenatal, neonatal, infant, toddler, preschooler, school-age, preadolescent, adolescent, young adult, middle adult, and older adult. For each stage, the manifestations of growth and development in the physiological, psychosocial, cognitive, moral, and spiritual dimensions are discussed together with relevant nursing implications.

Prenatal Period

The **prenatal period** (the developmental stage beginning with conception and ending with birth) is a critical time in a human being's development and consists of three developmental phases: germinal, embryonic, and fetal. The **germinal stage** begins with conception and lasts approximately 10 to 14 days. This stage is characterized by rapid cell division and implantation of the fertilized egg in the uterine wall. In

Table 14-8 FOWLER'S STAGES OF FAITH		
STAGE	**AGE**	**CHARACTERISTICS**
Prestage: *undifferentiated faith*	Infant	Trust, hope, and love compete with environmental inconsistencies or threats of abandonment.
Stage 1: *intuitive-projective faith*	Toddler and preschooler	Imitates parental behaviors and attitudes about religion and spirituality. Has no real understanding of spiritual concepts.
Stage 2: *mythical-literal faith*	School-age child	Accepts existence of a deity. Religious and moral beliefs are symbolized by stories. Appreciates others' viewpoints. Accepts concept of reciprocal fairness.
Stage 3: *synthetic-conventional faith*	Adolescent	Questions values and religious beliefs in an attempt to form own identity.
Stage 4: *individuative-reflective faith*	Late adolescent and young adult	Assumes responsibility for own attitudes and beliefs.
Stage 5: *conjunctive faith*	Adult	Integrates other perspectives about faith into own definition of truth.
Stage 6: *universalizing faith*	Adult	Makes concepts of love and justice tangible.

Data from Stages of Faith: The Psychology of Human Development and the Quest for Meaning, *by J. W. Fowler, 1995, New York: Harper & Row. Copyright 1995 by Harper & Row;* Psychiatric-Mental Health Nursing: Adaptation and Growth *[4th ed.], by B. S. Johnson, 1997, Philadelphia: Lippincott. Copyright 1997 by Lippincott.*

this very early stage, the central nervous system (CNS) is already beginning to form.

The **embryonic stage** (weeks 2 to 8 after conception) is characterized by rapid cellular differentiation, growth, and development of the body systems. This critical period is when the embryo is most vulnerable to noxious stimuli, which may lead to a spontaneous abortion (i.e., miscarriage) (Murray & Zentner, 1997).

The **fetal stage** (the intrauterine developmental period from 8 weeks to birth) is characterized by rapid growth and differentiation of body systems and parts.

Nursing Implications

The pregnant woman needs physical examinations and screenings throughout pregnancy. Early prenatal care is essential for a positive pregnancy outcome.

Learning that one is pregnant can elicit many emotions including happiness, fear, sadness, excitement, and anxiety. Because emotions lead to alterations in biochemicals, the mother's emotional state can bring about biochemical changes in the fetus. By teaching pregnant women how to relax, the nurse can promote a supportive environment for the developing embryo and fetus.

Wellness Promotion The uterus is the primary environment affecting prenatal growth and development. Ideally, this environment nurtures positive growth of the embryo and fetus.

An ample supply of nutrients must be provided by the mother. For example, the rate of preterm and low birth weight infants among women who consume insufficient amounts of protein during pregnancy is high. Such infants are at risk for developmental alterations.

When teaching the pregnant woman about nutrition, the nurse must emphasize that vitamin supplements are not substitutes for adequate food intake. Other nursing interventions that promote prenatal health include:

- Screening (blood pressure, urine glucose, and albumin)
- Teaching (e.g., about nutritional guidelines)
- Counseling (e.g., providing guidance about bonding with the child and incorporating a child into the family unit)
- Promoting the use of alternative modalities to reduce stress
- Working with economically disadvantaged clients to obtain prenatal care

Safety Considerations The fetus is especially vulnerable to substances consumed by the mother. In addition to providing the fetus with wholesome nutrients, maternal blood can also transport deadly toxins.

Cigarettes contain several toxic substances, including nicotine, that cross the placental barrier and interfere with the transport of oxygen to the fetus. Such toxins often result in increased risk of premature birth, retarded growth, learning difficulties, and fetal death.

Use of alcohol during pregnancy can result in **fetal alcohol syndrome** (FAS), a condition wherein fetal development is impaired, as manifested by physical and intellectual problems. Typically, FAS infants are small, have facial abnormalities (such as thin upper lips and short, upturned noses), and may have some degree of brain damage (Levin, 1995). Alcohol consumption is most dangerous during the first 3 months of pregnancy, when the embryo's brain and other vital organs are developing. The effects of alcohol on the fetus are permanent. Fetal alcohol syndrome is considered to be the leading cause of mental retardation among infants, and the incidence continues to increase (Wong et al., 1999).

Safety: Tobacco and Alcohol Use During Pregnancy

Total abstinence from cigarette smoking is advised during pregnancy. Because a "safe" amount of alcohol consumption has not been determined, caution all pregnant women to abstain from drinking alcohol.

There are many other teratogenic substances in addition to nicotine and alcohol. A **teratogenic substance** is any substance that can cross the placental barrier and impair normal growth and development. The Food and Drug Administration requires that all manufactured drugs list their potential for causing birth defects. The use of illegal drugs by pregnant women presents a very serious threat to the unborn. Substance abuse prevention programs are effective in preventing or reducing this threat.

Neonatal Period

The **neonatal period** (the first 28 days of life following birth) is a time of major adjustment to extrauterine life. The energies of the neonate (newborn) are focused on achieving equilibrium through stabilization of major body systems. Table 14-9 outlines neonatal development.

The neonate's activities, which are reflexive in nature, consist primarily of sucking, crying, eliminating, and sleeping. The neonate blinks in response to bright light and demonstrates the startle reflex in response to

CLIENT TEACHING

Pregnancy and Medications

Teach pregnant women to check labels of *all* medicines for information about potential effects on the fetus. Encourage expectant mothers to call the practitioner with any questions about the safety of any drug taken during pregnancy.

Table 14-9 NEONATE: GROWTH AND DEVELOPMENT

DIMENSION	CHARACTERISTICS	NURSING IMPLICATIONS
Physiological	Circulatory function shifts from umbilical cord to heart.	Accurately assess neonate's cardiovascular status.
	Gas exchange (oxygen and carbon dioxide) is transferred from placenta to lungs.	Immediately after birth, hold the neonate with head lower than body to allow for drainage of fluids that may block respiratory passages.
	Seconds after birth, respiratory reflexes are activated.	If spontaneous respirations do not occur, resuscitate immediately.
	Neck and shoulder muscles are weak.	Carefully support the neonate's head.
	Temperature-regulating mechanism is immature.	To conserve heat: • Dry neonate immediately after birth and place in a warmed bassinet and • Place a stockinette cap on neonate's head.
	Ossification (process of cartilage changing to bone) is incomplete.	Protect the anterior fontanel on neonate's skull.
	Visual acuity is poor, and visual focus is generally rigid.	Instruct parents to be directly in front of the neonate (approximately 9 to 12 inches away from child's face) when communicating.
Motor	Reflexes direct the majority of movement.	Teach parents to recognize neonate's protective reflexes.
	The full-term neonate has some limited ability to hold the head erect and is able to lift the head slightly when lying prone.	Support neonate's neck and head when lifting.
Psychosocial	Crying is the neonate's method of communication. There is a reason for the cry.	Teach parents about the dynamics of crying so that they neither label the neonate as "fussy" nor develop the misconception that they are inadequate caregivers. Encourage parents to learn to discriminate crying patterns.
	The bonding process begins shortly after birth.	Teach parents the importance of interacting with the neonate during every contact (feeding, bathing, changing, cuddling).
Cognitive	Neonates learn through sensory experiences. Learning is enhanced by an environment that provides stimuli without bombarding the neonate. Learning occurs by repeated exposure to stimuli.	To promote learning, encourage parents to provide frequent sensory stimuli (touching, talking, looking the neonate in the eyes).

Data from Health Assessment: A Nursing Approach *(3rd ed.), by J. Fuller and J. Schaller-Ayers, 2000, Philadelphia: Lippincott. Copyright 2000 by Lippincott;* Health Assessment & Promotion Strategies through the Life Span *(6th ed.), by R. B. Murray and J. P. Zentner, 1997, East Norwalk, CT: Appleton & Lange. Copyright 1997 by Appleton & Lange;* Whaley & Wong's Nursing Care of Infants and Children *(6th ed.), by D. L. Wong, M. Hockenberry-Eaton, D. Wilson, M. L. Winkelstein, E. Ahmann, and P. DiVito-Thomas, 1999, St. Louis, MO: Mosby-Yearbook. Copyright 1999 by Mosby-Yearbook;* Fundamentals of Nursing: Standards & Practice, *by S. DeLaune and P. Ladner, 1998, Albany, NY: Delmar Publishers. Copyright 1998 by Delmar Publishers.*

loud noises. Neonatal reflexes play a major role in the ability to survive.

During the first month of life, the neonate progresses developmentally from a mass of reflexes to behavior that is more goal directed (purposeful). In addition to the major physiological adjustments necessitated by extrauterine life, the neonate also undergoes psychological adaptation.

The major psychological task of neonates is to adjust to the parental figure(s). **Bonding**, the formation of attachment between parent and child, begins at birth, when the neonate and parent make initial eye contact. The quality of parent–neonate bonding lays the foundation for the trust necessary for the development of future interpersonal relationships.

Nursing Implications

A complete and thorough assessment of the neonate is performed immediately after delivery. Evaluation of the neonate's reflexes should be performed at the same time or as soon as the neonate is physiologically stable.

In the first few hours after birth, the nurse should encourage the parents to cuddle the newborn, explain the neonate's interactive abilities, and encourage mutual eye contact between neonate and parents by showing parents how to hold the child in a position facing them.

Wellness Promotion Teaching is among the most important nursing activities in promoting neonatal wellness. Other nursing interventions that promote neonatal wellness are as follows:

- Continually assessing the neonate's physiological status
- Providing a warm environment. (Neonates breathe more easily when they are warm.)
- Monitoring nutritional status. It is normal for neonates to lose weight (up to 10% of birth weight) during the first week of life.
- Providing a clean environment to protect neonates from infection; teaching parents that neonates need a clean environment, not a sterile one.
- Conducting screening tests; for example, the blood test for phenylketonuria (PKU), a genetic disorder that, if untreated, can lead to impaired intellectual functioning
- Promoting *early* parent–neonate interaction.

Selection of a feeding method for the neonate is a major decision for parents. Breastfeeding is the option recommended by the American Academy of Pediatrics. However, some parents choose to use commercially prepared formula. For a comparison of feeding methods, see the discussion about nutrition for the infant in this chapter.

Safety Considerations Because neonates are totally dependent on others to meet their needs, safety is of primary concern when caring for neonates. Accidents are the primary cause of neonatal mortality (Fuller & Schaller-Ayers, 1994). One of the most important methods of neonatal accident prevention is to teach parents about the use of infant car seats. Under current

federal law, neonates and infants must be secured in an approved infant car seat every time the child travels in a car.

Safety: Car Seats
Never discharge a neonate from the birthing center or hospital unless an infant seat is available for the trip home.

In addition to accidents, infections pose a serious health risk to the neonate. Newborns should be isolated from anyone experiencing an infectious disease. Because the skin is the body's major defense against invasion by disease-producing microorganisms, it is essential that the neonate's skin integrity be maintained. Parents must be taught the importance of skin cleanliness. Diaper rash is a common skin problem for newborns and infants because of the ammonia found in urine. In wet diapers, ammonia can burn and irritate the skin, resulting in localized irritation, blisters, or fissures. In addition to prompt changing of wet diapers, bathing and use of protective creams or powder are useful in preventing skin breakdown.

Infancy

Infancy (the developmental stage from the end of the first month to the end of the first year of life) is a time of continued adaptation. During this stage, the infant experiences rapid physiological growth and psychosocial development (Figure 14-3). Table 14-10 provides an overview of infant development in the

CLIENT TEACHING

Parents and Newborn
Parents need information about:

- Basic newborn needs (i.e., to be held, rocked, and talked to),
- Nutrition,
- Infection control (especially handwashing and hygienic diaper changing practices),
- Care of the umbilicus,
- Incorporating the newborn into the family unit, and
- Growth and development milestones in order to provide appropriate stimulation and have realistic expectations for their newborn.

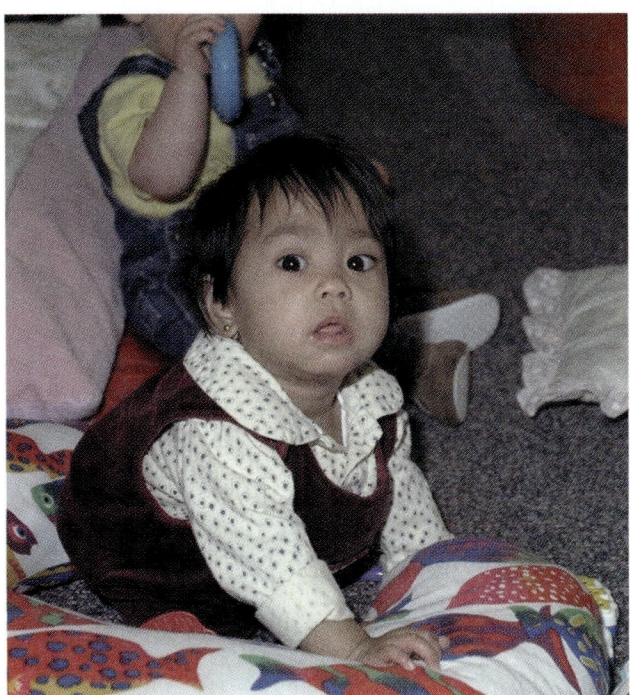

Figure 14-3 This child is exploring the world and is developing mastery of both the physiological and cognitive dimensions of development.

Table 14-10 INFANT: GROWTH AND DEVELOPMENT

DIMENSION	CHARACTERISTICS	NURSING IMPLICATIONS
Physiological	Physical growth is rapid. Birth weight usually triples by the end of the first year. Height increases by approximately 50%.	Inform parents of the developmental norms.
	Progressive maturation of all body systems occurs.	Encourage parents to have "well-baby" checkups as recommended.
	Body temperature stabilizes.	
	Heart rate slows (to approximately 80 to 130 beats per minute).	
	Blood pressure rises.	
	At approximately 4 to 6 months, eruption of teeth begins.	
	Brain grows rapidly (reaching approximately half the adult size).	
	Posterior fontanel closes at approximately 2 months.	Protect infant's skull.
	Eyes begin to focus.	
Motor	Physical maturation allows for development of motor skills.	Teach parents anticipated ages for motor skill development.
	Primitive reflexes are replaced by movement that is more voluntary and goal directed.	
	Motor skills develop rapidly:	
	• 6 months: rolls over voluntarily	
	• 6 to 7 months: crawls	
	• 8 months: sits alone	
	Grasping of objects, reflexive for the first 2 to 3 months, gradually becomes voluntary.	
Psychosocial	*Freud:* oral stage	Encourage parents to provide toys and objects for teething and sucking.
	Seeks immediate gratification of needs.	
	Receives pleasure and comfort through mouth, lips, and tongue.	
	Erikson: trust vs. mistrust stage	Encourage parents to feed in a prompt, consistent manner (feed on demand rather than a fixed schedule).
	A sense of self begins to develop.	
	Responds to caregiver's voice.	Other activities that promote trust are providing warmth, diapering, and comforting.
	Separation anxiety develops at approximately 6 months.	
	Havighurst: Developmental tasks include learning to eat solid food, crawl, walk, and talk.	Teach parents approximate ages that develop mental milestones are expected to occur.
Cognitive	*Piaget:* sensorimotor stage	Encourage parents to provide a variety of sensory stimuli: visual, sensory, auditory, and tactile (e.g., colorful mobiles; musical toys; soft, plush animals; rubbing, patting, and stroking of the infant's skin).
	Infant learns by interacting with the environment.	
	Language development includes babbling, repetition, and imitation.	Tell caregivers to talk to the infant often. Encourage caregivers to name objects that are the focus of the infant's attention.
Moral	*Kohlberg:* preconventional stage	Teach parents that now is the time to start teaching (by role modeling) the difference between "right" and "wrong."
Spiritual	*Fowler:* stage of undifferentiated faith	Encourage caregivers to model the values they want the infant to learn.

Data from Health Assessment & Promotion Strategies through the Life Span *(6th ed.), by R. B. Murray and J. P. Zentner, 1997, East Norwalk, CT: Appleton & Lange. Copyright 1997 by Appleton & Lange;* Whaley & Wong's Nursing Care of Infants and Children *(6th ed.) by D. L. Wong, M. Hockenberry-Eaton, D. Wilson, M. L. Winkelstein, E. Ahmann, and P. DiVito-Thomas, 1999, St. Louis, MO: Mosby-Yearbook. Copyright 1999 by Mosby-Yearbook;* Fundamentals of Nursing: Standards & Practice, *by S. DeLaune and P. Ladner, 1998, Albany, NY: Delmar Publishers. Copyright 1998 by Delmar Publishers.*

physiological, motor, psychosocial, cognitive, moral, and spiritual dimensions.

Nursing Implications

The nurse providing care to an infant must focus on safety, prevention of infection, and teaching parents about incorporating the child into the family. Teaching parents and other caregivers about developmental milestones is also essential. Nursing care involves the provision of support, reassurance, and information to the parents.

Wellness Promotion Nurses promote infant wellness by teaching growth and development concepts to parents and other caregivers. Knowledge of the type of behavior to expect at certain times during infancy serves to both guide and reassure parents. Three specific areas about which parents need guidance from the nurse in caring for their infants are nutrition, protection from infection, and promotion of sleep.

A major factor influencing health maintenance of the infant is the provision of adequate nutrients delivered in a loving, consistent manner. Caregivers should be taught that the nutrients must be germ free and must provide the recommended amounts of carbohydrates, protein, calcium, iron, and vitamins. The American Academy of Pediatrics recommends that infants be breastfed for the first 12 months (Murray & Zentner, 1997). Nurses can teach parents about the benefits of breastfeeding, including that it:

- Offers immunologic benefits (e.g., it contains immunoglobulins, lymphocytes, and other bacteria growth retardants),
- Is more easily digested because it contains smaller curds than those found in cow's milk and formula, and
- Enhances absorption of fat and calcium.

In addition, breastmilk is readily available and economical. Furthermore, the act of breastfeeding promotes maternal–infant bonding (Wong et al., 1999).

Special formulas are available for infants who are hypersensitive to protein, who have PKU, and who experience fat malabsorption. Soy-based formulas have been developed for the infant who is lactose intolerant or allergic to regular formula. Infants who are formula

CULTURAL CONSIDERATIONS

Choice of Infant Feeding Method

There are some cultural sanctions against breastfeeding, and some cultures view bottle-feeding as a status symbol. Be sensitive to the client's cultural background and norms when discussing choice of infant feeding method. Nurses can also teach parents about the benefits of bottle-feeding.

CLIENT TEACHING

Bottle Feeding

- Assume a comfortable position and place the baby in a semireclining position and cradled close to your body.
- Never prop a bottle in a baby's mouth because choking may result.
- Use care if heating bottles. Do not warm bottles in the microwave because the hot liquid can cause esophageal and oropharyngeal burns.
- Avoid using the bottle as a pacifier because this action may result in tooth decay and may set the stage for overeating in the future.

fed generally have greater deposits of subcutaneous fat (Murray & Zentner, 1997). Whole cow's milk is not recommended for infants under 1 year of age. Human milk and commercially prepared formula are more easily digested.

It is important for the nurse to provide accurate information about the types of feeding available and to support the parents' decision about the method chosen.

Solid foods are usually introduced at 3 to 4 months of age. Rice cereal is the first solid food of choice because it generates the fewest allergic responses (Murray & Zentner, 1997).

Infants are especially vulnerable to infections. Because the immune system is not fully matured, infections pose a great threat.

Infection Control: Handwashing and Infant Care

Handwashing is the most important action in preventing the transmission of microorganisms. This is especially true when caring for infants, whose immune systems are still immature.

Immunizations are of utmost importance in preventing infections. Nurses should advocate the administration of all necessary immunizations and should confirm those received by the infant. Refer to Appendix A for a recommended schedule for immunizations.

Parents often need information about normal sleep patterns of infants and how those patterns change with maturation. Activities that promote sleep include:

- Providing a quiet room for the infant,
- Scheduling feedings and other care activities during periods of wakefulness rather than drowsiness,
- Developing sensitivity to the unique sleep and rest periods established by the infant,
- Providing comfort and security measures (e.g., rocking, singing), and
- Establishing routine times for sleep.

Preventing Infant Accidents

- To prevent vehicular accidents: use infant seats and keep the infant out of the paths of automobiles and other vehicles.
- To prevent burns: keep the infant away from open heaters, furnaces, fireplaces, hot stoves, and matches.
- To protect from falls: keep crib rails up at all times, never leave the infant lying unattended on furniture, and use protective gates and barriers to block stairways.
- To prevent drowning: never leave the infant unattended near water (bathtubs, buckets, swimming pools).
- To prevent electrocution: when the infant begins to crawl, keep electrical cords out of the infant's reach and use plastic safety plugs to cover all electrical outlets.
- To prevent choking: closely monitor the infant who is exploring the environment. During this oral phase of development, the infant tends to test out the environment and seeks pleasure through the mouth. Aspiration accidents are common, with infants choking on objects such as buttons, coins, and food.

Safety Considerations Most infant injuries and deaths are related to motor vehicle accidents. The consistent and proper use of infant car seats is thus one of the most effective measures parents can take to ensure their infant's safety.

Safety: Aiding the Choking Infant
Never use the Heimlich maneuver on an infant who is choking. Instead, use alternating back blows and chest compressions to dislodge the object.

Toddler Period

The **toddler period** begins at 12 to 18 months of age, when a child begins to walk alone, and ends at approximately 3 years of age. The family is very important to the toddler in that the family promotes language development and teaches toileting skills. During this stage, the child becomes more independent and, when attempts to demonstrate autonomy are prevented, temper tantrums often result. This stage is thus often referred to as "the terrible twos." Parents must understand that the toddler's frequent use of the word *no* is an expression of developing autonomy.

Nurses can greatly influence the quality of parent–child interaction by teaching parents about developmental concepts. This information helps parents form realistic expectations of the toddler's behavior. The use of firm limits applied consistently both helps the toddler learn and provides parameters for safe and socially acceptable behavior. Table 14-11 outlines the toddler's growth and development in the physiological, motor, psychosocial, cognitive, moral, and spiritual dimensions.

Nursing Implications

Nurses who work with toddlers must be sensitive to the fact that children of this age are likely to be anxious and fearful when in the presence of strangers. The establishment of rapport with the child will help alleviate stranger anxiety. Play is an effective tool for building rapport with children of this age.

When toddlers are hospitalized, whether for an extended time or only a day, fear and anxiety can make the experience a negative one. The major stressor related to hospitalization is separation from the parents. An unfamiliar environment also results in stress for the toddler. Nurses can help reduce stress in the hospitalized toddler by teaching both the child and the parents about procedures. Preprocedural teaching lessens anxiety (Biddinger, 1993).

Toddlers need regular health examinations, and immunizations remain an essential part of health care. Parents should be involved during examinations and immunizations. Parents can alleviate the toddler's stress by holding the child and talking in a calm manner when in the presence of the health care provider.

Wellness Promotion Teaching involves both toddlers and their parents. Play can be used to establish an effective relationship with the child. Play is a valuable process for toddlers in that it is the primary mechanism for learning and socialization. To facilitate teaching, the nurse should approach toddlers at eye level and use terminology they can understand.

Respiratory infections are common health threats to the toddler. Parasitic diseases are also fairly common.

Health Care for Toddlers

- In a calm tone of voice, explain what is being done
- Use play to alleviate anxiety (e.g., demonstrate a procedure on a teddy bear or doll; allow the child to manipulate equipment, such as a stethoscope, prior to using it on the child)
- Give short, simple directions
- After a painful procedure, comfort the child (e.g., cuddle, rock)
- Encourage parents' active participation in the care

Table 14-11 TODDLER: GROWTH AND DEVELOPMENT

DIMENSION	CHARACTERISTICS	NURSING IMPLICATIONS
Physiological	Overall rate of growth slows. By 24 months of age, weight usually reaches four times that at birth. Brain grows rapidly. Bones in extremities grow in length. Physiological readiness for bowel and bladder control develops.	Instruct parents on need for vitamin D, calcium, and phosphorus. Recognize that "growing pains" are normal. Instruct parents of timing for toilet training and need for consistency and patience.
Motor	Child walks and runs. Child becomes more coordinated.	Tell parents to assess home environment for safety as toddler becomes more mobile.
Psychosocial	*Freud:* anal stage Receives pleasure from contraction and relaxation of sphincter muscles. *Erikson:* autonomy vs. shame and doubt stage *Havighurst:* Developmental tasks include: • Beginning to learn gender differences and • Learning to talk Toddler engages in parallel play (playing near other children but not necessarily interacting with them). A reemergence of separation anxiety often occurs. By age 3, most toddlers are able to tolerate being left with strangers.	Instruct parents to avoid overemphasis on toilet training. Teach parents to encourage toddler's attempts at independence (e.g., trying to feed and dress self). Explain that sexual curiosity is normal. Encourage parents to talk to child frequently. Provide opportunities for child to socialize with peers. Reassure child that parents will return.
Cognitive	*Piaget:* preoperational stage Child can follow simple directions. Child's thought processes are concrete. Child is able to anticipate future events. Child has short attention span. Child compreheneds self as a separate entity. *Language:* At approximately 1 year of age, the child can make two-syllable sounds (e.g., ma-ma, da-da) At approximately 2 years, the child can form short sentences and has a vocabulary of approximately 900 words.	Instruct parents to give only one direction at a time. Use a calendar to show today's date and the number of days until a significant event. Teach caregivers importance of calling child by name. Instruct caregivers to talk to child frequently and to avoid the use of "baby talk."
Moral	*Kohlberg:* preconventional stage Child learns to distinguish right from wrong.	Teach parents to be consistent in setting limits. Emphasize the significance of modeling desired behavior to the child.
Spiritual	*Fowler:* intuitive-projective stage of faith	Instruct parents to provide simple answers to questions related to religion, God, and church. Instruct on the importance of incorporating religious rituals and ceremonies into daily life.

Data from Health Assessment & Promotion Strategies through the Life Span *(6th ed.), by R. B. Murray and J. P. Zentner, 1997, East Norwalk, CT: Appleton & Lange. Copyright 1997 by Appleton & Lange;* Whaley & Wong's Nursing Care of Infants and Children *(6th ed.) by D. L. Wong, M. Hockenberry-Eaton, D. Wilson, M. L. Winkelstein, E. Ahmann, and P. DiVito-Thomas, 1999, St. Louis, MO: Mosby-Yearbook. Copyright 1999 by Mosby-Yearbook;* Fundamentals of Nursing: Standards & Practice, *by S. DeLaune and P. Ladner, 1998, Albany, NY: Delmar Publishers. Copyright 1998 by Delmar Publishers.*

Teaching parents about preventive measures such as frequent handwashing with antibacterial soaps is thus the focus of wellness promotion. The nurse should also verify which immunizations are needed.

As the rate of growth slows during the toddler period, nutritional needs change. Toddlers need fewer calories than do infants. The required amounts of pro-tein and fluids (Wong et al., 1999) also decrease; however, toddlers still need more protein than do older children. Because most toddlers become selective ("picky") about the foods they will eat, it is sometimes difficult to provide increased amounts of calcium and iron. The toddler should consume an average of 2 to 3 cups of milk per day to ensure adequate calcium

CLIENT TEACHING

Toddler Nutrition
- Avoid using food as a reward because doing so encourages overeating.
- Do not serve large helpings because doing so may overwhelm the child, possibly resulting in a refusal to eat.
- Expect sporadic eating patterns (e.g., the toddler eats a lot one day and very little the next, or the toddler enjoys one food for several days and then suddenly refuses to eat that food).
- Avoid power struggles related to meals. Trying to force a child to eat is counterproductive to establishing healthy eating habits.
- Establish a mealtime routine and follow it; rituals are comforting to toddlers.
- Provide nutritional snacks to meet dietary requirements.

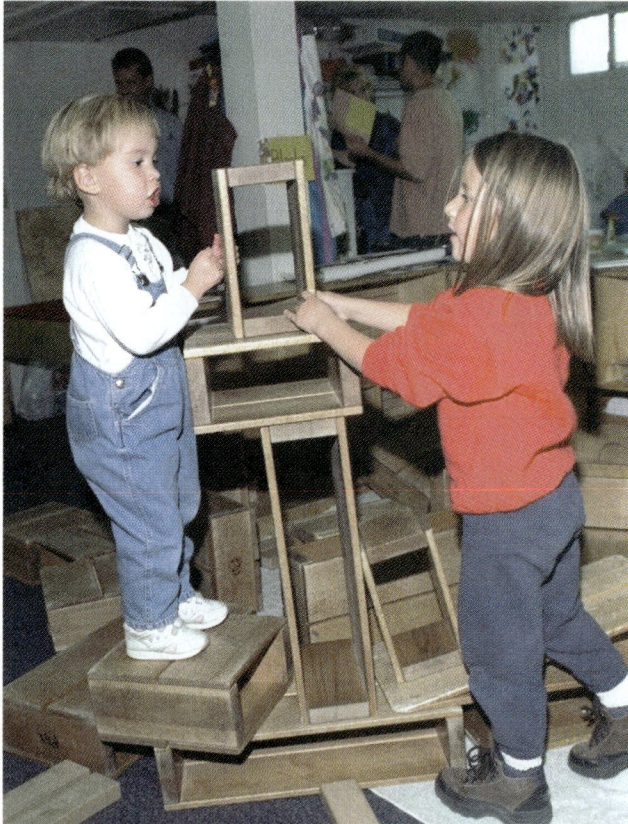
Figure 14-4 Toddlers enjoy playing with a variety of toys. Parents must be diligent in checking all toys for potential safety hazards—looking at not only the toy itself but the manner in which it is used—and must supervise toddler play at all times.

intake. The toddler who drinks more than a quart of milk per day, however, is at increased risk of developing anemia, because high milk consumption may limit the amount of other nutrients taken in (Wong et al., 1999). Nurses can play a key role in nutritional counseling for toddlers.

Safety Considerations Accidents (especially those involving automobiles) are the most frequent cause of disability and death among toddlers (Edelman & Mandle, 1998; Murray & Zentner, 1997). The information previously provided regarding use of car seats for neonates and infants also applies to toddlers.

Another common type of accident among toddlers involves toys. As children gain new skills, parents must reassess the safety of toys and of all environments where the toddler might play (Figure 14-4).

Safety: Toys for Toddlers
Teach parents to inspect toys for the following:

- Age appropriateness
- Sharp pieces or corners
- Small parts that can be swallowed
- Poisonous paint (e.g., lead-based paint)
- Flammable or toxic materials

With their increased mobility and curiosity, toddlers are especially prone to accidental poisoning (Figure 14-5). Parents should thus child-proof the home and carefully observe the toddler.

Preschool Period

The developmental stage from ages 3 years–6 years is called the **preschool period**. During this stage, physical growth slows, and psychosocial and cognitive

development accelerate. Table 14-12 outlines preschool development in detail.

During this period of childhood, curiosity becomes pronounced, and the child is better able to communicate. The nurse should teach parents that the child's

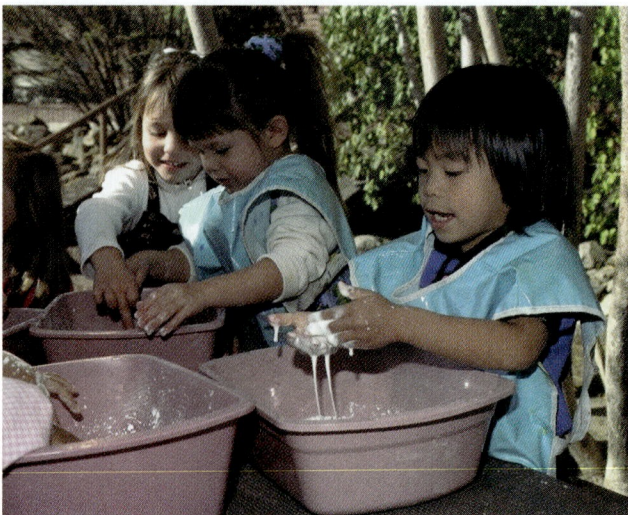
Figure 14-5 Parents must ensure that all materials with which a child plays are safe, nontoxic, and nonflammable.

Table 14-12 PRESCHOOLER: GROWTH AND DEVELOPMENT

DIMENSION	CHARACTERISTICS	NURSING IMPLICATIONS
Physiological	Physical growth slows; average weight at age 5 years is 45 pounds. Head size approximates that of an adult. Deciduous teeth come in fully; these "baby teeth" start to fall out about age 6 and will be replaced by permanent teeth.	Can eat larger meals and a variety of foods.
Motor	Fine motor skills develop, e.g., ability to skip, throw a ball over hand, use scissors, tie shoelaces.	Emphasize providing a safe environment for play and exploration. Tell parents to praise attempted independent activities.
Psychosocial	*Freud:* phallic stage Oedipal conflict leads to development of superego (conscience). *Erikson:* initiative vs. guilt stage *Havighurst:* Developmental tasks include: • Learning gender differences and modesty, • Language development and basic ability to formulate concepts, • Emerging reading readiness, and • Distinguishing right from wrong	Inform parents that preschoolers learn self-control through interacting with others. Encourage parents to provide sex education information at the child's comprehension level. Encourage parents to read to child.
Cognitive	*Piaget:* preoperational stage Increased curiosity coupled with improved ability to use reason and logic lead to frequent questioning. Play becomes more reality based. As a result of increased ability to communicate, socialization with peers increases.	Tell parents that children of this age learn through frequent use of the word *why.*
Moral	*Kohlberg:* preconventional stage A conscience begins to develop. Child fears wrongdoing. Child seeks parental approval.	Encourage parents to teach the child basic values, ideally by modeling. Encourage parents to provide consistent praise and acceptance of child.
Spiritual	*Fowler:* intuitive-projective stage of faith Child is not yet able to understand spiritual concepts and imitates parental behaviors.	Remind parents that teaching by example is the best approach for a child of this age.

frequent use of the word *why* is necessary for normal cognitive and psychosocial development.

The child's world continues to expand outside the immediate home environment. Play is the mechanism used by the preschooler to both learn about and develop relationships.

Nursing Implications

Play is a tool that can be used by nurses to help reduce fear and anxiety in the preschooler. Through the use of play, preschoolers learn about the environment, incorporate socially defined expectations for behavior, and reduce tension (Figure 14-6).

Wellness Promotion When working with a preschooler, it is important for the nurse to communicate at the child's level of comprehension while at the same time not talking down to the child. The nurse should include the child in activities and decisions as much as possible. The preschool years are the optimal time for the child to begin showing an interest in

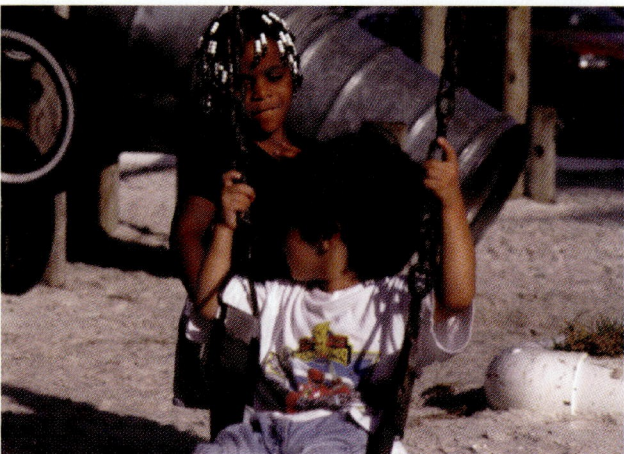

Figure 14-6 Play is an important vehicle for socialization among preschoolers.

health. In order to promote the development of lifelong health-promoting lifestyles, the astute nurse capitalizes on this opportunity by making health education fun. A major wellness intervention for preschoolers is immunization. The nurse should thus verify at each checkup that immunizations are up to date.

Safety Considerations Accidents are the leading cause of death among young children. Cognitive immaturity coupled with an eagerness to explore the environment lead to the preschooler's risk for accidents. Children in this stage often act impulsively and cannot be expected to remember and follow all safety rules. To prevent accidents, parents must understand the importance of teaching young children the meaning of the word *no*.

Common accidents among preschoolers include automobile accidents, burns, falls, drowning, animal bites, and ingestion of poisonous substances.

The nurse should place emphasis on educating parents about protecting preschoolers from potential hazards. The safety practices developed by the preschooler will tend to be lifelong. Adults can best teach preschoolers about accident prevention through modeling. For example, parents who buckle their seatbelts every time they get into a car are not only protecting themselves, but are also teaching their children an important accident prevention measure.

School-Age Period

During the **school-age period** (the developmental stage from the ages of 6 years–10 years), physical changes occur at a slow, even, continuous pace. Table 14-13 gives an overview of growth and development of the school-age child.

The school-age child's world expands greatly. Participation in school activities, team sports, and play contributes to an enlarging social network. As children continue to mature, their play time becomes more structured and less spontaneous. Communication levels

increase, and vocabulary expands greatly to accommodate the expression of needs, thoughts, and feelings.

As the school-age child's cognitive abilities expand, creativity is expressed in a variety of unique ways. Involvement in academic, sporting, and social activities stimulates the development of creativity and provides outlets for its expression.

Nursing Implications

The most common health problems among school-age children are accidents and minor illnesses such as upper respiratory infections. Health-promotion teaching is a major role of the nurse in caring for school-age children.

Wellness Promotion Lifestyles begin to be established during childhood; nurses can intervene to promote the development of healthy lifestyles among children in schools. Although school-age children and adolescents constitute 25% of America's population, only 10% of the national health care budget is allocated to their care (Baker, 1994). Schools are an area where health-promotion behaviors can be taught in a cost-effective manner.

Safety Considerations Many accidents experienced by school-age children occur during play. Injuries related to the use of skates, skateboards, in-line skates, and bicycles are common.

 Safety: Accidents and Abductions
- Children must know the safety rules for use of riding toys (e.g., use of protective equipment, see Figure 14-7).
- Parents must frequently remind children of the danger of playing near traffic.
- Children must also be taught to use caution with regard to strangers because of the possibility of abduction.

 CLIENT TEACHING

Promoting Wellness
- Encourage healthy lifestyles (nonsedentary activities, nutritious meals)
- Have children immunized
- Teach children appropriate hygienic measures
- Schedule regular checkups with the primary health care provider
- Keep immunizations up to date
- Schedule dental checkups and encourage daily brushing and flossing
- Teach safety precautions
- Establish sleep patterns alternating with periods of activity
- Report any symptoms of illness immediately to the health care provider

Table 14-13 SCHOOL-AGE CHILD: GROWTH AND DEVELOPMENT

DIMENSION	CHARACTERISTICS	NURSING IMPLICATIONS
Physiological	Physical growth is steady (approximately 3 to 6 pounds and 2 to 3 inches per year).	Emphasize to parents the need for a balanced diet to sustain growth requirements.
	Due to changes in amount and distribution of fat, body has an overall slimmer shape.	
	Maturation of the CNS is nearly complete. By age 12, all permanent teeth (except second and third molars) are present.	Teach parents about the need for dental hygiene (daily brushing and flossing) and regularly scheduled visits to the dentist.
		Instruct to change toothbrushes every 3 months.
Motor	Motor control continues to develop.	Encourage participation in physical activities.
	Child becomes less dependent on parents for activities of daily living.	Provide praise for independent activities.
Psychosocial	*Freud:* latency stage	To develop a sense of confidence, encourage child to:
	Same-gender companions are preferred.	• Participate in both group and individual activities and
		• Become involved in a variety of activities
	Erikson: industry vs. inferiority stage	
	Child develops initiative and high self-esteem as manifested in school and sports.	Encourage parents to praise child's efforts.
	Child exhibits less dependency on family.	
	Havighurst: Developmental tasks include the ability to perform more complex motor functions (e.g., ride a bicycle, catch a ball).	
Cognitive	*Piaget:* concrete operations stage	
	Ability to cooperate with others and to see others' points of view leads to more meaningful communication.	Encourage child to engage in group activities.
	Reasoning ability moves from intuitive to logical and rational.	
	Ability to think in the abstract is not fully developed.	Communicate at child's level of comprehension.
	Child develops the concept of time:	
	• Knows difference between past and present	
	• Begins to learn to tell time	
	• Better able to understand the process of aging	
	Child is able to order, categorize, and classify groups of objects as evidenced by increased interest in collections (e.g., coins, stamps, rocks).	
	Child sees relationships between objects.	
Moral	*Kohlberg:* conventional stage	Encourage parents to provide consistent limits.
	Child can understand what society deems as unacceptable behavior but cannot always choose between right and wrong without assistance.	Emphasize modeling appropriate behavior.
		Tell parents to praise appropriate behavior.
Spiritual	*Fowler:* mythical-literal stage	Encourage parents to discuss their beliefs.
	Child accepts existence of a diety.	Storytelling and use of parables can reinforce understanding of spiritual concepts.
	Beliefs are symbolized through stories.	

Data from Health Promotion throughout the Lifespan *(4th ed.), by C. L. Edelman and C. L. Mandle, 1998, St. Louis, MO: Mosby-Yearbook. Copyright 1998 by Mosby-Yearbook;* Health Assessment & Promotion Strategies through the Life Span *(6th ed.), by R. B. Murray and J. P. Zentner, 1997, East Norwalk, CT: Appleton & Lange. Copyright 1997 by Appleton & Lange;* Fundamentals of Nursing: Standards & Practice, *by S. DeLaune and P. Ladner, 1998, Albany, NY: Delmar Publishers. Copyright 1998 by Delmar Publishers.*

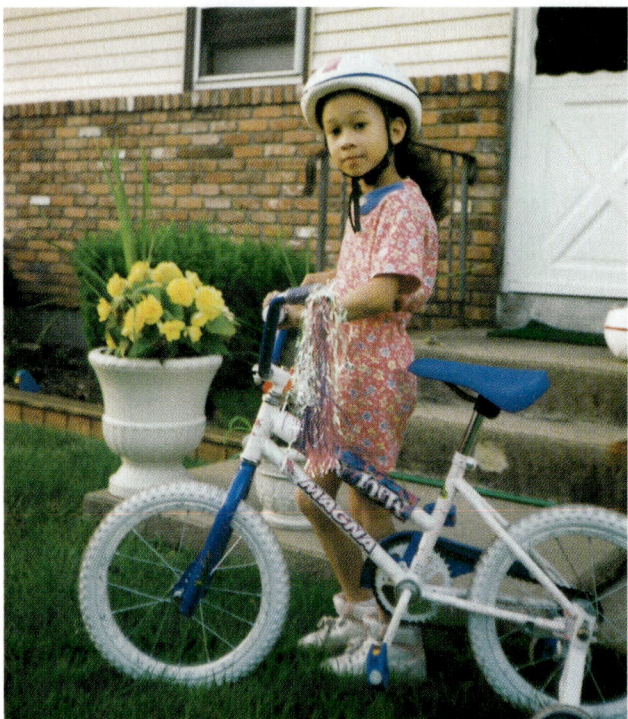

Figure 14-7 The use of equipment such as safety helmets helps protect school-age children from injury.

Preadolescence

Preadolescence (the developmental stage from the ages of 10 years–12 years) is marked by rapid physiological changes having psychological and social implications. The child begins to experience hormonal changes that will result in the onset of **puberty** (the emergence of secondary sex characteristics). Girls generally experience puberty at a younger age than do boys—approximately 9 to 10 years of age, as compared to 10 to 11 years of age for boys (Edelman & Mandle, 1998). Table 14-14 provides an overview of preadolescent development.

In girls, breast development begins between the ages of 10 and 11. Further breast development is stimulated by the release of estrogen, which occurs during puberty. Approximately 2 years after the appearance of breast buds, **menarche** (onset of the first menstrual period) occurs. The first menstrual periods are usually irregular, scant, and may or may not be accompanied by ovulation. The average age of menarche in the United States is 12.8 years. This number represents a gradual decline over the past century in average age of menarche; a decline probably due to improved general health status, particularly nutrition and sanitation (Wong et al., 1999).

The menstrual cycle is a complex blend of physiological and psychological changes that occur approximately every month. After approximately the first 6 to 12 months, a girl's cycle typically becomes established

in a regular pattern. Nurses must be aware that some girls may have received inadequate or incorrect information regarding the onset of menstruation. Client teaching should address the physiological changes, emotional changes, and hygienic practices and should emphasize that cyclical, hormone-induced changes are normal.

In preadolescent boys, the first signs of puberty are:

- Testicular enlargement,
- Penile enlargement,
- Thinning and reddening of the scrotum, and
- Pubic hair growth.

Nursing Implications

Sensitivity is essential in working with the preadolescent. To increase sensitivity, the nurse should use a nonjudgmental approach and attend to the preadolescent's body language.

Wellness Promotion The preadolescent needs information about nutrition, rest and activity, and the physiological changes being experienced. This client should be taught about the dramatic growth spurt, the sexual changes, and the psychosocial changes that characterize this life stage (Figure 14-8). By preparing the preadolescent for upcoming changes, the nurse promotes physical and emotional health. The nurse should also confirm that immunizations are current.

Safety Considerations The preadolescent is at risk for injury from sports and play activities. Another major health risk posed to many preadolescents is vio-

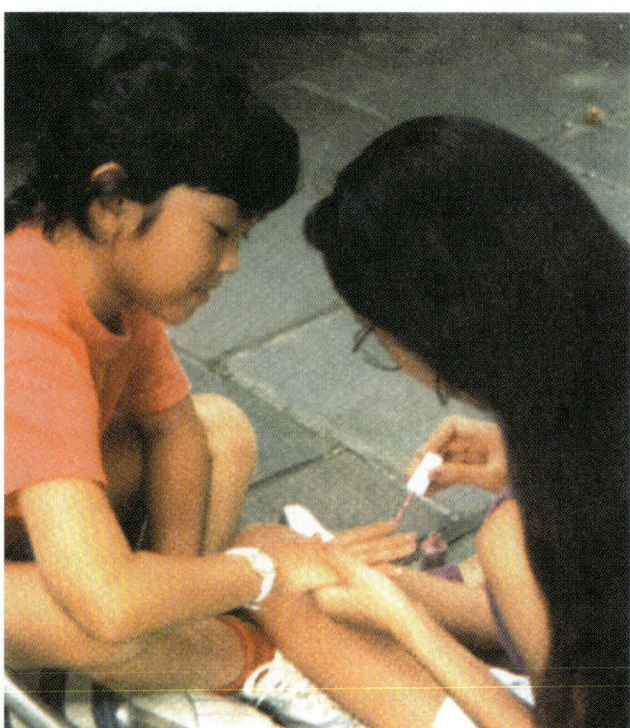

Figure 14-8 Preadolescence is a time of gender role discovery and of increasing independence.

Table 14-14 PREADOLESCENT AND ADOLESCENT: GROWTH AND DEVELOPMENT

DIMENSION	CHARACTERISTICS	NURSING IMPLICATIONS
Physiological	*Physiological changes:* Physical growth accelerates and is accompanied by changes in body proportion. Extremities grow first, then trunk and hips. Growth in skull and facial bones results in changes in physical appearance. *Endocrine changes:* Hypothalamus stimulates secretion of pituitary gonadotropins, leading to reproductive maturity. Both primary and secondary sex characteristics develop. Beginning of puberty is evidenced in girls by: • Breast development, • Pubic and axillary hair growth, • Menarche (onset of menses), and • Increases in height. Beginning of puberty is evidenced in boys by: • Genital development, • Growth of facial, pubic, and axillary hair, • Nocturnal ejaculations, • Height increases, and • Voice changes. *Musculoskeletal changes:* Bones ossify. Muscle mass and strength increase. *Cardiovascular changes:* Heart increases in size and strength. Heart rate decreases to adult norms. Blood volume and blood pressure increase. *Respiratory changes:* Rate decreases to an average of 15 to 20 respirations per minute. Respiratory volume and vital capacity increase. Larynx, laryngeal cartilage, and vocal cords grow; voice pitch deepens. *Gastrointestinal changes:* Spleen, liver, kidneys, and digestive tract enlarge but experience no functional changes. *Genitourinary changes:* Genitalia develop as described previously. *Dental changes:* Last four molars erupt. *Integumentary changes:* Skin becomes thicker and tougher. Activation of sebaceous glands possibly leads to acne. Pubic hair appears.	Teach the child and parents about expected growth spurts. Provide reassurance that it is not uncommon for facial appearance to change in only a few months. Provide support and information about sexual changes. Remember that the physiological changes are accompanied by psychological and social alterations. Encourage physical activities and intake of adequate amounts of calcium. Instruct about anticipated changes. Emphasize importance of continued dental hygiene. Teach proper skin care: • Wash two to three times per day with soap and water • Avoid vigorous facial scrubbing • Avoid cosmetics with a fat or grease base • Use sunscreen and avoid prolonged exposure to sunlight • Provide support to preadolescents experiencing acne
Motor	The adolescent displays complete independence with regard to performing self-care activities.	Encourage parents to allow some freedom of choice and expression.

continued

Table 14-14 PREADOLESCENT AND ADOLESCENT: GROWTH AND DEVELOPMENT *continued*

DIMENSION	CHARACTERISTICS	NURSING IMPLICATIONS
Psychosocial	*Freud:* genital stage	
	Erikson: identity vs. role diffusion stage	Offer support.
	The major task is to develop a sense of identity.	
	The adolescent develops a new body image.	
	Intimacy with members of opposite gender is established.	Provide sex education.
	Peer group is the primary mechanism of support.	
	The adolescent rebels against adult authority.	Inform parents that rebellion is a normal developmental experience.
	Havighurst: achievement of personal independence	Encourage attempts to achieve independence while providing assistance and support as needed.
	Relationships established with others are characterized by increased maturity.	
Cognitive	*Piaget:* formal operations stage	Teach parents expected developmental changes in thinking patterns.
	Approach to thinking is logical, organized, and consistent.	
	The adolescent thinks in terms of cause and effect.	
	Note: Not all adolescents achieve this level of cognitive development. Some are capable of flights from reality.	
	The adolescent tends to be extremely idealistic.	
	Egocentric (self-centered) thinking is common, as is a view of self as omnipotent.	
	The adolescent sees self as exceptional, special, and unique, and views self as being immune to problems.	Recognize that a false sense of immunity ("It can't happen to me" attitude) has an impact on health behaviors.
		Teach safety issues to preadolescents:
		• Safe sex practices
		• Safe driving practices (never mixing driving and use of alcohol)
Moral	*Kohlberg:* postconventional stage	
	The adolescent tends to support the morality of law and order in determining right from wrong.	Teach parents that questioning of values is normal.
	Adolescents begin to question and discard the status quo and to choose different values.	
	Moral maturity varies dependent on the context of the situation and the relationship.	
	Peer pressure may override the adolescent's own moral reasoning.	Teach preadolescent assertiveness skills to use in communicating with peers.
Spiritual	*Fowler:* synthetic-conventional stage	Inform parents that curiosity about other religious beliefs is normal.
	The adolescent questions values and beliefs.	

Data from Health Promotion throughout the Lifespan *(4th ed.), by C. L. Edelman and C. L. Mandle, 1998, St. Louis, MO: Mosby-Yearbook. Copyright 1998 by Mosby-Yearbook;* American Nursing Review of Psychiatric and Mental Health Nursing Certification, *by N. Randolph, 1998, Springhouse, PA: Springhouse. Copyright 1998 by Springhouse;* Fundamentals of Nursing: Standards & Practice, *by S. DeLaune and P. Ladner, 1998, Albany, NY: Delmar Publishers. Copyright 1998 by Delmar Publishers.*

lence both in and away from the home. Education is a major preventive approach to violence and is a tool for helping break the intergenerational pattern of child abuse (Johnson, 1995).

Other areas to be emphasized in promoting preadolescent safety are substance abuse prevention, sex education, and development of healthy lifestyles.

Adolescence

Adolescence (the developmental stage from the ages of 13 years–20 years) begins with the onset of puberty. During adolescence, the individual undergoes the major transition from child to adult. Numerous physiological changes and rapid physical growth occur during this stage. The rapid changes that occur

Preadolescent–Nurse Relationship

To encourage the preadolescent to ask questions about any health-related concerns it is imperative that the nurse establish a trusting relationship with the preadolescent.

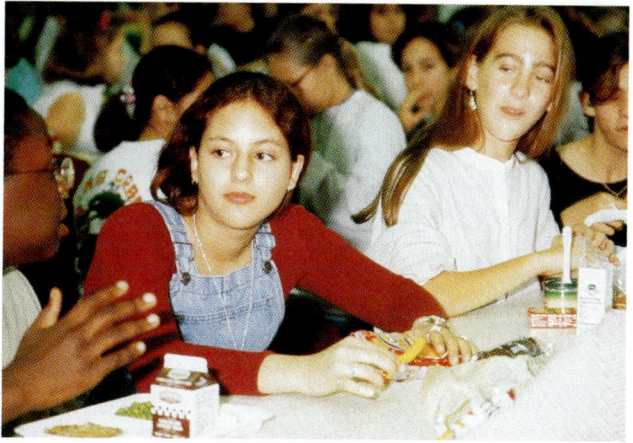

Figure 14-9 Peer group is very important during adolescence.

during adolescence are not only physical; many psychosocial adjustments must be made by the adolescent. Friendships become very important (Figure 14-9). Establishing a sense of personal identity takes up a great amount of the adolescent's psychic energy. Questions such as "Who am I?" and "What is *really* important?" are common ones among adolescents.

Most adolescents are greatly concerned about their appearance. This emphasis on physical attractiveness sometimes results in eating disorders, such as **anorexia nervosa** (self-imposed starvation that results in a 15% loss of body weight). It is projected that 1 out of every 200 girls in the United States will develop anorexia nervosa (Johnson, 1995). Male adolescents are also affected by eating disorders, but at a much lower percentage than are girls. Other types of eating disorders common in adolescents are **bulimia nervosa** (episodic binge-eating followed by purging) and **obesity** (weight that is 20% or more above ideal body weight).

Nursing Implications

The nurse can support the adolescent by providing information about the numerous bodily changes experienced during this developmental stage. The nurse should encourage adolescents to share their health concerns with parents, but must honor the adolescent's choice to withhold sensitive information from parents. The confidentiality of the client as well as of those in relationship with the adolescent (such as sexual partners) must be protected.

Wellness Promotion The nurse promotes the adolescent's wellness primarily through teaching. Areas to be emphasized in health education of adolescents include hygiene, nutrition, sex education, developmental changes, and substance abuse prevention.

The nurse should teach adolescents about the physical changes they are undergoing. Health teaching is often done by school nurses, and nurse-managed clinics in schools represent one avenue for promoting wellness among adolescents (Figure 14-10). School-based clinics are rapidly increasing, allowing the possibility of delivering care to 23 million children and their parents, the majority of whom are uninsured (Baker, 1994). *Nursing's Agenda for Health Care Reform* (American Nurses Association, 1990) calls for the delivery of primary health care services to individuals in convenient, familiar places. What better place to teach adolescents about health care than in the schools? Schools are ideal settings for nurses to institute cost-effective measures for improving the health of children (Baker, 1994).

Safety Considerations As a group, today's adolescents are less healthy than were their parents at the same age (Roye, 1995). Unhealthy behaviors contribute to the three major causes of adolescent death: accidents,

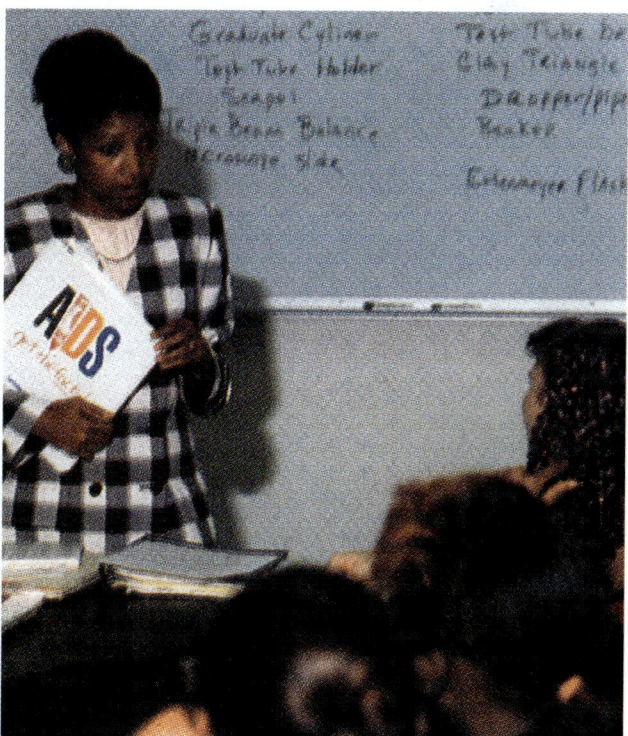

Figure 14-10 Wellness promotion for the adolescent may include in-school seminars by school nurses, such as this one on AIDS prevention.

PROFESSIONAL TIP

Working with Adolescents

- Use a nonjudgmental attitude to establish rapport when working with adolescents.
- Treat every adolescent in a respectful, dignified manner.
- Avoid using a condescending attitude when communicating with the adolescent.
- To form a collaborative partnership, treat the adolescent as an active participant in health care.
- Answer all questions honestly.
- Be especially sensitive to nonverbal clues. Adolescents are often too embarrassed to initiate discussion of their health-related concerns.
- Remember that the peer group is of major importance to the adolescent; thus, use group settings whenever possible to provide health education.
- Demonstrate acceptance of the adolescent even when limits must be established in the face of unhealthy or inappropriate behaviors.
- Questioning adult authority is a normal part of adolescent rebelliousness. Do *not* personalize such behavior. Nurses who do so become defensive and lose their interpersonal effectiveness and credibility with adolescents.

homicide, and suicide (Roye, 1995). The following factors increase the adolescent's risk for accidents:

- Impulsive behavior
- Sense of being invulnerable to accidents ("It can never happen to me!")
- Testing limits
- Rebelling against adult advice

As a result, many adolescents engage in unhealthy behaviors such as smoking, consuming alcohol and other drugs, reckless driving, violence, and unprotected sexual activity.

Many health problems in adolescents are related to sexual behaviors. For example, consider the following facts stated by Roye (1995):

- Acquired immunodeficiency syndrome (AIDS) is now the primary killer of individuals between the ages of 24 and 54 years; many of these people were infected during their adolescent years.
- Adolescents between the ages of 15 and 19 years have the highest rates of hospitalization for treatment of sexually transmitted diseases (STDs).
- Every year, more than 1 million adolescent girls become pregnant.

The effect of teen pregnancy on families and communities is great. Social programs that provide resources for meeting the special needs of pregnant adolescents are decreasing. A result for many pregnant teens is becoming trapped in a cycle of school failure (or dropout), limited employment opportunities, and poverty. Adolescents who become pregnant experience developmental difficulties in that they must make adult decisions. Infants born to adolescent mothers are likely to experience health-related problems such as preterm birth and low birth weight.

The pregnant adolescent needs expert prenatal care, a supportive environment, and information. Client teaching must emphasize the prevention of STDs because the pregnancy itself is evidence of high-risk (i.e., unprotected) sexual activity.

Sexually transmitted diseases present a serious health threat to adolescents. Diseases such as genital herpes, chlamydia, syphilis, and gonorrhea are spread through sexual contact. The human immunodeficiency virus (HIV), which causes AIDS, is also transmitted through unprotected sexual activity.

Nurses must educate adolescents about methods for preventing the spread of STDs. Nurses who teach adolescent clients about safe sex practices must be especially sensitive to cultural influences on sexual activity.

A major health problem during adolescence is the high risk of suicide. The rate of suicide is higher among adolescent males than females. Often, suicide is perceived by the adolescent as the only alternative to an overwhelming situation. Suicidal behavior can be traced to low self-esteem, lack of maturity, and resultant impulsive behaviors.

When assessing for suicide potential, the nurse should always directly question adolescents about any plans for harming or killing themselves. Nurses should be aware of the following signs of suicide risk in adolescents:

- Anorexia
- The writing of suicide notes
- Discussion of suicide
- Aggressive behavior
- Substance abuse
- Running away from home
- Preoccupation with death
- Neglect of personal hygiene
- The giving away of treasured objects
- Sudden changes in behavior
- Verbal cues (e.g., "You won't have to worry about me much longer.")
- Fatigue
- Social withdrawal

When teaching suicide prevention, the nurse should encourage *immediate* contact of a health care professional should someone exhibit any of the previously noted indicators of suicide risk. Most communities have a special telephone suicide-prevention line available.

Safety: Suicide Prevention
- Never leave the suicidal adolescent alone.
- Close observation is the best deterrent to suicide.

Another significant health problem for many adolescents is substance abuse. Use of alcohol or other drugs represents a common maladaptive attempt to cope with the stressors of adolescence. Indicators of substance abuse by adolescents include the following:

- Decline in academic performance
- Mood swings
- Changes in personality
- Fatigue
- Drowsiness
- Behaviors indicative of depression (e.g., appetite changes, insomnia, weight loss, apathy)

Nurses can play a key role in substance abuse prevention among adolescents. A comprehensive substance abuse prevention education program covers:

- Hazards of drug use
- Misuse of legal substances such as tobacco and alcohol
- Methods of boosting self-esteem
- Assertive communication skills (how to say "no" to peers)
- Adaptive coping mechanisms for dealing with stress

By providing such information, nurses can help adolescents make responsible, informed decisions before experimentation with drugs begins.

Young Adulthood

Physical growth stabilizes during **young adulthood** (the developmental stage from the ages of 21 years through approximately 40 years). The young adult continues to experience physical and emotional changes, but at a slower rate than does the adolescent. Table 14-15 outlines the development of young adults. Young adulthood is a time of transition from an adolescent to a person capable of assuming adult responsibilities and making adult decisions.

Table 14-15 YOUNG ADULT: GROWTH AND DEVELOPMENT

DIMENSION	CHARACTERISTICS	NURSING IMPLICATIONS
Physiological	*Physiological changes:* Physical growth stabilizes. Physical functioning is at an optimum and therefore less likely to be concerned with own health. Maturation of body systems is complete. *Cardiovascular changes:* Men are more likely to have an increased cholesterol level than are women. *Gastrointestinal changes:* After age 30, digestive juices decrease. *Dental changes:* By the mid-20s, dental maturity is achieved with the emergence of the last four molars ("wisdom teeth"). *Musculoskeletal changes:* At approximately age 25, skeletal growth is complete. *Reproductive changes:* System is completely matured. *Women:* Ages 20–30 are optimal years physically for reproduction. *Men:* Beginning at approximately age 24, male hormones slowly decrease (does not affect ability to reproduce).	Teach importance of health-promoting behaviors. Encourage development of healthy lifestyles.
Psychosocial	*Erikson:* intimacy vs. isolation stage Young adults engage in productive work. The young adult develops intimate relationships. *Havighurst:* The individual becomes part of a social group The young adult selects a partner. The person assumes civic responsibility.	Emphasize need for social support as the person assumes new roles. Teach time management skills. Provide sex education information, including information on prevention of STDs.

continued

Table 14-15 YOUNG ADULT: GROWTH AND DEVELOPMENT *continued*

DIMENSION	CHARACTERISTICS	NURSING IMPLICATIONS
Cognitive	*Piaget:* formal operations stage	Encourage the development and use of appropriate judgment.
	Problem-solving abilities are realistic.	
	The young adult demonstrates less egocentricism.	
	Many young adults engage in formal educational activities.	
Moral	*Kohlberg:* postconventional stage	Assess the person's value system and respect the person's beliefs.
	Right and wrong are defined in terms of personal beliefs and principles.	
Spiritual	*Fowler:* individuative-reflective faith stage	Encourage client to use spiritual support system.
	The young adult assumes responsibility for own beliefs.	

Data from Adult Health Nursing *(3rd ed.), by P. G. Beare and J. L. Myers, 1998, St. Louis, MO: Mosby-Yearbook. Copyright 1998 by Mosby-Yearbook;* Health Promotion throughout the Lifespan *(4th ed.), by C. L. Edelman, and C. L. Mandle, 1998, St. Louis, MO: Mosby-Yearbook. Copyright 1998 by Mosby-Yearbook;* Fundamentals of Nursing: Standards & Practice, *by S. DeLaune and P. Ladner, 1998, Albany, NY: Delmar Publishers. Copyright 1998 by Delmar Publishers.*

Pregnancy, a time of transition and lifestyle adjustment, is experienced by many young adults. Throughout pregnancy, women experience changes in self-concept and may need reassurance that such changes are normal.

Nursing Implications

Young adulthood is usually the healthiest time in a person's life. Consequently, concern for health is low among people in this age group, and wellness is taken for granted by many young adults. Preventive measures for young adults have two primary components:

- Avoidance of accident, injury, and violence
- Development of health-promoting behaviors (e.g., lifestyle modification, Figure 14-11).

By teaching and counseling, the nurse plays an important role in each of these areas of health promotion. Other developmentally appropriate topics for the nurse to address are vocational counseling and relationship establishment.

Wellness Promotion Decision making by young adults affects their health status. Because young adults tend to take excessive risks, they are at greater risk for violent death from accident, suicide, or homicide (Edelman & Mandle, 1998). Driving recklessly, driving while intoxicated, and engaging in unprotected sex are examples of activities that demonstrate the lack of fear demonstrated by many young adults.

Sexually transmitted disease is a leading cause of infection and resultant reproductive dysfunction among young adults. The information presented about STDs in the discussion of safety considerations for adolescents is also applicable to young adults. Nurses should teach women how to perform a monthly breast self-examination (BSE), and men must learn how to perform a testicular self-examination (TSE). The nurse should also confirm currency of tetanus/diphtheria (Td) immunization.

Safety Considerations Because vehicular accidents are a major cause of health problems among young adults, providing information about driving safety is a must. Another activity that poses a health risk to many young adults is sunbathing. Exposure to

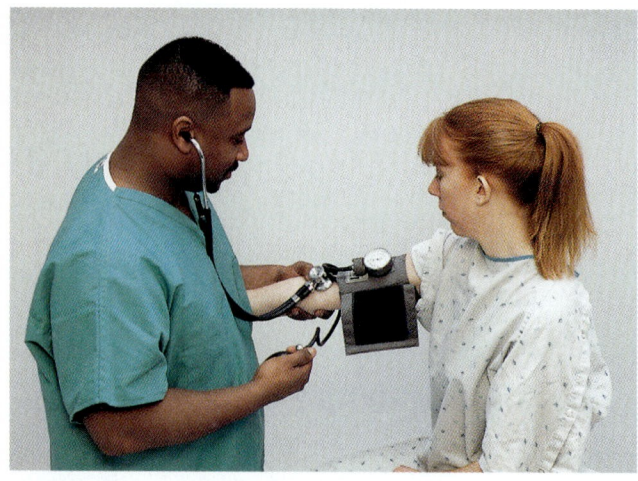

Figure 14-11 The assessment of this young adult's blood pressure is one part of a health-promotion program to help enhance this client's wellness.

the radiation resulting from direct sunlight or the lighting used in tanning salons is directly linked to skin cancer. According to the United States Public Health Service, approximately 400,000 cases of skin cancer occur every year (U.S. Department of Health & Human Services, 1990). Nurses can be influential in decreasing this rate through teaching and modeling safe behaviors.

Middle Adulthood

Middle adulthood (the developmental stage from the ages of 40 years–65 years) is characterized by productivity and responsibility. Many physiological changes occur during middle adulthood. Table 14-16 lists the major changes experienced by the middle-aged person. For most middle-aged adults, the majority of activity

Table 14-16 MIDDLE ADULT: GROWTH AND DEVELOPMENT		
DIMENSION	**CHARACTERISTICS**	**NURSING IMPLICATIONS**
Physiological	*Cardiovascular changes:* Decreased functional aerobic capacity results in decreased cardiac output and a decreased capacity for physical activity.	Instruct cardiac client about necessity of remaining physically active.
	Blood vessels become thicker and lose elasticity.	
	Hypertension (high blood pressure), coronary artery disease, and cerebral vascular accidents ("strokes") may appear.	Teach client about lifestyle modifications related to cardiovascular health: • Quitting smoking • Avoiding secondary tobacco smoke • Practicing good nutrition (low fat, low cholesterol) • Engaging in physical activity
	Neurological changes: Changes in cell regulation and repair occur gradually, as does cell atrophy.	Explain age-related changes. Provide support and reassurance.
	A gradual loss in efficiency of nerve conduction leads to impaired sensation of heat and cold.	Teach safety precautions regarding: • Exposure to sunlight, • Sensitivity to heat stroke, and • Sensitivity to frostbite.
	Gastrointestinal changes: Slower gastrointestinal motility results in constipation.	Teach client about: • Nutrition (increase high-fiber food intake; drink adequate amounts of fluid), and • Maintaining physical activity.
	Genitourinary changes: Nephron units diminish in number and size; diminishing blood supply to kidneys.	Teach normal age-related changes. Teach signs indicative of dehydration.
	Decreased glomerular filtration rate leads to decrease in urinary output and resultant dehydration.	Inform client of need to maintain adequate fluid intake.
	Integumentary changes: Decreased moisture and turgor of skin and loss of subcutaneous fat leads to development of wrinkles.	Instruct client about effects of sun and of cigarette smoking on the skin.
	Hair thins and turns gray.	Assess client for body image alterations. Employ nonjudgmental listening.
	Musculoskeletal changes: Bone mass and density decreases. Slight loss of height (from 1 to 4 inches) may occur. Intervertebral disks thin.	Instruct client about: • Need for calcium intake, • Importance of decreasing caffeine and alcohol consumption, and • Effects of sedentary versus active lifestyle on osteoporosis.
	There is a generalized decrease in muscle tone; appearance becomes "flabby," and agility lessens, leading to an increased risk of injury.	Instruct client of need for proper posture (especially when sitting), exercise, and adequate fluid intake. Instruct client on need for adequate physical activity.

continued

Table 14-16 MIDDLE ADULT: GROWTH AND DEVELOPMENT *continued*

DIMENSION	CHARACTERISTICS	NURSING IMPLICATIONS
Physiological (*continued*)	*Endocrine changes:* Decreased metabolism results in reduced production of enzymes and increased hydrochloric acid, leading to acid indigestion and belching.	Instruct client to: • Eat foods that are not spicy or fried, and • Avoid eating within 2 hours before bedtime.
	Reproductive changes: *Women:*	
	Estrogen and progesterone production cease during menopause.	Teach clients about age-related sexual/reproductive changes. Encourage responsible sexual behavior.
	Secondary sex characteristics regress (decreased breast size, loss of pubic hair).	Teach about prevention of sexually transmitted diseases.
	Vaginal secretions decrease.	
	Note: With no pregnancy risk, some postmenopausal women enjoy sexual activity more.	
	Men:	
	Testosterone level decreases. There is a reduction in the amount of viable sperm. Sexual energy declines, and it takes longer to achieve an erection; however, erection is sustained longer.	
	Adaptation to developing chronic diseases and sexual problems may diminish self-esteem.	
	Grown children leaving home may lead to happiness or depression ("empty nest syndrome").	
Psychosocial	*Erikson:* generativity vs. stagnation stage	
	Adults who have achieved generativity feel good about their lives and comfortable with themselves.	Provide support as the client deals with aging.
	Middle-aged adults become more involved in altruistic acts (e.g., community, volunteer work).	Encourage client to become involved in community activities. Teach leisure skills.
	Family roles usually change (become caregiver to aging parents, become grandparent).	Instruct in the need to care for self while caring for others.
	Havighurst:	
	The middle-aged adult fulfills social and civic responsibilities.	
	Middle-aged adults assist children in becoming independent.	
	The middle-aged adult maintains relationship with partner.	
Cognitive	*Piaget:* will use all stages, depending on the task (e.g., can move between formal operations, concrete operations, and problem-solving as needed).	Encourage middle-aged clients who are anticipating returning to school or engaging in other intellectually stimulating activities.
	The middle-aged adult is able to reflect on the past and anticipate the future.	
	Reaction time diminishes during late middle age.	
	Learning ability remains intact if person is motivated and material is meaningful.	
Moral	*Kohlberg:* postconventional stage	Use nonjudgmental approach when client discusses values.
Spiritual	*Fowler:* conjunctive faith stage	
	The middle-aged adult is able to appreciate others' belief systems.	Encourage use of spiritual support.
	Middle-aged adults are less dogmatic with regard to own beliefs.	Refer to clergy if desired by client.
	Religion is usually a source of comfort.	

Data from Adult Health Nursing. *(3rd ed.), by P. G. Beare and J. L. Myers, 1998, St. Louis, MO: Mosby-Yearbook. Copyright 1998 by Mosby-Yearbook;* Health Promotion throughout the Lifespan *(4th ed.), by C. L. Edelman and C. L. Mandle, 1998, St. Louis, MO: Mosby-Yearbook. Copyright 1998 by Mosby-Yearbook;* Health Assessment: A Nursing Approach *(3rd ed.), by J. Fuller and J. Schaller-Ayers, 2000. Philadelphia: Lippincott. Copyright 2000 by Lippincott;* Fundamentals of Nursing: Standards & Practice, *by S. DeLaune and P. Ladner, 1998, Albany, NY: Delmar Publishers. Copyright 1998 by Delmar Publishers.*

revolves around work and family, and success and achievement are measured in terms of career accomplishments and family life.

The primary developmental task of the middle-aged adult revolves around the conflict of generativity (a sense that one is making a contribution to society) versus stagnation (a sense of nonmeaning in one's life). When an individual successfully resolves this developmental conflict, acceptance of age-related changes results. Achievement of this developmental task is manifested by the following:

- Demonstrating creativity
- Guiding the next generation
- Establishing lasting relationships
- Evaluating goals in terms of achievement

Evaluation of goals often leads to a midlife crisis, especially if individuals feel they have accomplished little or have not lived up to earlier self-expectations.

Nursing Implications

Middle-aged adults constitute almost half the U.S. population (Edelman & Mandle, 1998). Individuals of the baby-boom generation have entered midlife and will thus require more nursing care to maintain wellness and cope with illness.

Nurses can help middle-aged clients improve their health status (and thus quality of life) by identifying risk factors and providing early intervention. The major risk factors for adults in the middle years can be changed because they are primarily environmental and behavioral. In assisting the middle-aged client to change unhealthy behaviors, the nurse can work on either a one-on-one or group basis.

Wellness Promotion As health educators, nurses can encourage middle-aged adults to assume more responsibility for their own health. The nurse should both encourage clients to obtain influenza and pneumococcal immunizations as recommended by their physicians and confirm currency of Td (tetanus/diphtheria) immunization.

Safety Considerations Automobile accidents, especially those involving the use of alcohol, are a serious health problem among middle-aged adults. Occupational health hazards such as exposure to environmental toxins constitute another significant problem.

Middle adulthood is also the time when a lifelong accumulation of unhealthy lifestyle practices, such as smoking, sedentary habits, and overuse of alcohol, begins to exert adverse effects.

Most middle-aged individuals have more leisure time than in the past, resulting in an increased risk of recreational accidents such as boating accidents, sports-related injuries, and jogging mishaps.

CLIENT TEACHING

Self-Care for Middle-Aged Adults

Self-care topics pertinent to the middle-aged adult include:

- Acceptance of aging,
- Nutrition,
- Exercise and weight control,
- Substance abuse prevention,
- Stress management, and
- Recommendations for health screening (cholesterol screening, prostate examination, mammogram, Pap test).

Older Adulthood

Older adulthood is the developmental stage starting at age 65 and extending to death. Table 14-17 provides an overview of growth and development in the older adult.

Older adults have several psychosocial tasks to accomplish, including:

- Developing a sense of satisfaction with the life that one has lived (finding meaning in one's life),
- Establishing meaningful roles,
- Adjusting to infirmities (if any exist),
- Coping with losses and changes, and
- Preparing for death.

Nursing Implications

Nursing care is important in assisting the aging person to develop a sense of well-being (Eliopoulos, 1997). Nurses who work with elderly clients must be especially sensitive to their own feelings, attitudes, and beliefs about aging and be aware of the potential effects of these responses on their care provided to older clients.

When assessing the older adult for health-related needs, the nurse must learn about the client's background, including family history, work history, hobbies, and achievements (Figure 14-12). Clients should be encouraged to talk about their life experiences. When planning care, it is important to build on the client's lifelong interests. By recognizing each client's unique experiences and assets, the nurse is more likely to individualize care.

When clients express dissatisfaction and regrets about the past, the nurse should listen in a nonjudgmental manner and not try to convince clients that things are really better than remembered or perceived. It is important, though, to help the elderly client put disappointments into perspective by balancing them

Table 14-17 OLDER ADULT: GROWTH AND DEVELOPMENT

DIMENSION	CHARACTERISTICS	NURSING IMPLICATIONS
Physiological	Refer to chapter 55 for a detailed discussion of physiological changes related to aging.	
Psychosocial	*Erikson:* integrity vs. despair stage	Ask the older person for advice.
	The older adult accepts own life as it is.	Identify and use the older adult's strengths.
	A sense of worth is garnered from helping others.	Encourage the use of reminiscence.
	Havighurst:	
	The older adult adjusts to a decline in physical strength.	
	The older adult fulfills civic responsibilities.	
	Older adults meet social obligations.	
	The older adult develops an affiliation with peers and age group (i.e., sees self as "old").	Encourage to express feelings concerning aging.
	Retirement from employment affects finances, activities, leisure time, and role identity (positively or negatively).	Promote socialization with peers.
	Potential for social isolation increases as significant others and peers die.	
Cognitive	*Piaget:* formal operations stage	Allow client time to respond to questions or instructions.
	There is no decline in IQ associated with aging.	Be alert for the possibility of medication-induced confusion and resultant impact on memory.
	Reaction time is usually slowed.	
	Memory:	
	Short-term: Capacity for recall decreases.	
	Long-term: Capacity remains unchanged.	
Moral	*Kohlberg:* postconventional stage	Support decision making.
	The older adult makes moral decisions according to own principals and beliefs.	Respect values even when different from own.
Spiritual	*Fowler:* universalizing stage	Listen carefully to determine spiritual needs.
	The older adult is generally satisfied with own spiritual beliefs.	Acknowledge losses and encourage appropriate grieving.
	Older adults tend to act on beliefs.	

Data from Women's Health: Instant Nursing Assessment, *by P. A. Firth and S. J. Watanabe, 1996, Albany, NY: Delmar Publishers. Copyright 1996 by Delmar Publishers;* Health Promotion throughout the Lifespan *(4th ed.), by C. L. Edelman and C. L. Mandle, 1998, St. Louis, MO: Mosby-Yearbook. Copyright 1998 by Mosby-Yearbook;* Health Assessment & Promotion Strategies through the Life Span *(6th ed.), by R. B. Murray and J. P. Zentner, 1997, East Norwalk, CT: Appleton & Lange. Copyright 1997 by Appleton & Lange.* Fundamentals of Nursing: Standards & Practice, *by S. DeLaune and P. Ladner, 1998, Albany, NY: Delmar Publishers. Copyright 1998 by Delmar Publishers.*

against accomplishments and achievements. The nurse should encourage family members to engage in a positive life review with the elderly client. Most nursing interventions for elders center around introspection and reflection on their lives. Life review (or reminiscence therapy) promotes a positive self-concept in older people (Heriot, 1995).

Wellness Promotion Health-promotion activities should be implemented with the elderly client to maintain functional independence. Elderly people who are independent are healthier (Campbell & Kreidler, 1994). Health-promotion activities are aimed at maximizing the elder's abilities and strengths. Specific topics that are developmentally appropriate for older clients are use of leisure time, increased socialization,

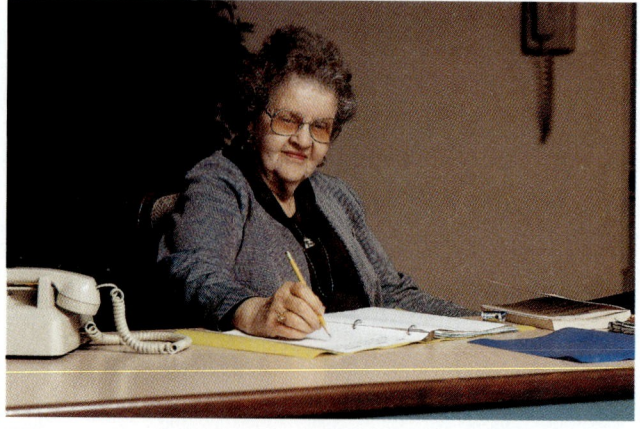

Figure 14-12 This older adult is able to maintain her independence and self-esteem through volunteer work.

regular physical activity, maintaining a positive mental attitude, and developing and maintaining healthy lifestyles. Many older people engage in more health-promoting behaviors than do younger people (Sapp & Bliesmer, 1995). The nurse should both encourage the client to obtain influenza and pneumococcal immunizations as recommended and confirm currency of Td immunization.

Safety Considerations Falls pose a major health threat to elderly persons.

HOME HEALTH CARE

Home Safety for Elders

The nurse can encourage the elderly client to create a safe home environment by:

- Ensuring adequate lighting,
- Removing all throw or loose rugs,
- Clearing all walking paths,
- Having a handrail on all stairs, and
- Installing hand-holds in tubs and showers.

CASE STUDY

Mary Jo, age 32, and her two daughters, Sara, age 14, and Katie, age 8, live with Mary Jo's grandmother, age 85. Mary Jo is having difficulty dealing with her daughters and her grandmother.

Consider the following:

1. At what stage of psychosocial development is each member of the household?
2. Compare the cognitive dimensions of these four people.
3. What is the focus of wellness-promotion for each person?
4. What are the safety considerations for each person?

SUMMARY

- Growth is the quantitative changes in physical size of the body and its parts. Development refers to behavioral changes in functional abilities and skills.
- Growth and development of an individual are influenced by a combination of factors including heredity, life experiences, health status, and cultural expectations.
- Maturation is the process of becoming fully grown and developed and involves both physiological and behavioral aspects of an individual.
- During each developmental stage, certain developmental tasks must be achieved for normal development to occur.
- According to Freud, certain developmental tasks must be achieved at each developmental stage; failure to achieve or a delay in achieving the developmental task is the result of a psychosexual fixation in a previous stage.
- Erikson purports that psychosocial development is a series of conflicts that occur during eight stages of life.
- Sullivan theorizes that personality development is strongly influenced by interpersonal relationships.
- Piaget's theory cites four stages of cognitive development: sensorimotor, preoperational, concrete op-

erations, and formal operations. Each stage is characterized by the ways whereby the child interprets and uses the environment.
- Kohlberg's theory describes six stages of moral development through which individuals determine a moral code to guide their behavior.
- Fowler's theory outlines six distinct stages of faith development, and though individuals vary in the age at which they experience each stage, the sequence of stages remains the same.
- Nurses have important roles in promoting the health and safety of individuals at each stage of the life cycle.

Review Questions

1. The fact that development occurs in a proximo-distal manner means that the infant is able to:

   a. crawl before he walks.
   b. raise his head before he is able to sit up.
   c. move his arms before picking up an object with his fingers.
   d. master psychological tasks before establishing a separate identity.

2. The task to be achieved in Erikson's stage of industry versus inferiority is to:

   a. learn self control.
   b. develop necessary social skills.
   c. develop commitments to others and to a career.
   d. view one's life as meaningful and fulfilling.

3. Piaget's theory relates to a child's:

   a. moral development.
   b. cognitive development.
   c. interpersonal development.
   d. spiritual development.

4. The nurse knows that at birth the neonate's activities are:

   a. reflexive.
   b. adjusting.
   c. purposeful.
   d. continuing.

5. The time for parents to begin teaching (by role modeling) the difference between "right" and "wrong" is during:

   a. infancy.
   b. childhood.
   c. toddler stage.
   d. preschool stage.

6. Immunizations are important during:

   a. infancy.
   b. childhood.
   c. adolescence.
   d. entire life.

7. The nurse working with preadolescent children should:

   a. offer opinions on the child's lifestyle choices.
   b. provide an opportunity for the child to ask questions about health-related concerns.
   c. finish the child's thoughts and sentences to avoid awkward silences.
   d. give a lecture on all the changes to be expected in the next few years; nutrition; and personal hygiene.

8. A great many health problems among adolescents are related to:

   a. nutrition.
   b. sexual behaviors.
   c. activity/exercise.
   d. sleep/rest behaviors.

9. The focus of wellness promotion during middle adulthood should be to:

   a. maintain functional independence.
   b. encourage use of fewer risk-taking behaviors.
   c. encourage client to assume responsibility for own health.
   d. teach about hygiene, nutrition, and substance abuse prevention.

10. The older adult has an increased risk of falls, burns, and other injuries because of:

    a. slower metabolism.
    b. diminished hearing.
    c. decreased ability to see colors.
    d. slower response to environmental changes.

Critical Thinking Questions

1. What is most important in determining a person's behavior: the person's genetic predisposition or the response of other people and socialization?

2. Our society labels certain characteristics as "masculine" or "feminine." How do you think these stereotypes influence the development of young boys and girls in our society?

3. Nurses often encounter clients whose value systems conflict with their own. How will you provide care to sexually active adolescents if you think their behavior is immoral or "wrong"? Is it ethical for you to try to change the adolescent's values so that they become congruent with yours? Should you change your values to be congruent with those of the client?

 WEB FLASH!

- Visit the American Academy of Pediatrics on the Web. What information do they offer on such topics as nutrition, safety, discipline, and growth and development?
- What Web sites are available for information on elders, adolescents, or middle-age adults?
- What information related to immunizations does the Centers for Disease Control and Prevention (CDC) offer on the Internet?

UNIT

7

Health Promotion

15

WELLNESS CONCEPTS

MAKING THE CONNECTION

Refer to the following chapters to increase your understanding of wellness concepts:

- Chapter 12, Cultural Diversity and Nursing
- Chapter 14, The Life Cycle
- Chapter 16, Stress, Adaptation, and Anxiety
- Chapter 17, Loss, Grief, and Death
- Chapter 18, Basic Nutrition
- Chapter 19, Rest and Sleep
- Chapter 20, Safety/Hygiene
- Chapter 35, Nursing Care of the Client: Reproductive System
- Chapter 46, Nursing Care of the Client: Substance Abuse
- Chapter 55, Nursing Care of the Older Client

LEARNING OBJECTIVES

Upon completion of this chapter, you should be able to:

- *Define key terms.*
- *Discuss guidelines for healthy living.*
- *Describe the scope of prevention.*
- *Explain the importance of Healthy People 2000.*
- *Make a teaching plan for ways to promote and maintain wellness.*

KEY TERMS

health
prevention
primary prevention
secondary prevention
tertiary prevention
wellness

INTRODUCTION

The responsibility for maintaining health rests squarely on the shoulders of each individual adult. Parents are responsible for maintaining their children's health and teaching them a healthy lifestyle. Health maintenance involves the whole person and the person's whole life. It includes the prevention of disease and the early detection and treatment of disease. Main-tenance of health requires constant effort and a focus on all aspects of a person's life.

Simon (1992) quotes Dr. Wood Hutchison, who wrote in the *Journal of the American Medical Association* that "our system's philosophy might be condensed in the motto 'millions for health care and not a penny for prevention'." This was written in 1896. Over 100 years have passed and we still spend less than 3 cents of each health dollar on prevention and education.

The United States is the world leader in medical science and education yet is only 16th among nations in life expectancy. We spend more for health care than any other country, yet we rank 24th in infant mortality. In 1991, there were 82,902 positions for residents in specialty areas and only 202 in preventive medicine. Many doctors have not incorporated preventive medicine into their practices (Simon, 1992).

There is no profit in prevention. Insurance premiums buy illness insurance, not health insurance, given that insurance companies often will not pay for preventive testing and treatment. Compensation for clinical care makes illness the priority, not wellness. Diagnosis and treatment of illnesses are what insurance pays for, not health maintenance.

HEALTH

A widely accepted definition of **health** comes from the World Health Organization (WHO), which defines health as a state of complete physical, mental, and social well-being, not merely the absence of disease or infirmity.

Other concepts of health focus on motivation. A eudaemonistic approach to health (from the Greek word *eudaimonia,* meaning "fortunate or happy") views the individual as being motivated by joy and self-fulfillment: Health is the full realization of potential, and illness is an impediment to that realization.

Those who hold the adaptive view of health are motivated by altering the risks in self or the environment through such means as dietary and exercise programs or reducing exposure to environmental hazards. Illness results when the individual is unable to cope with the risks and stresses of daily life.

Some individuals are motivated by being able to meet responsibilities at home, at work, at play, and in the community: Their health focus is role performance. Health is considered achieved when the individual fulfills the obligations and responsibilities to family, job, and community.

Other individuals are motivated by the absence of disease: Theirs is a clinical health focus. As long as no disease is present, the individual considers himself healthy. Personal definition of health influences life choices and personal health decisions.

WELLNESS

Wellness is defined as a state of optimal health wherein an individual moves toward integration of human functioning, maximizes human potential, takes responsibility for health, and has greater self-awareness and self-satisfaction. Floyd, Mimms, and Yelding-Howard (1995), Hafen and Hoeger (1994), and Seiger, Vanderpool, and Barnes (1995) describe the behaviors exhibited by individuals in a state of wellness. These researchers outline seven areas of wellness: emotional, mental, intellectual, vocational, social, spiritual, and physical wellness. Various areas of wellness overlap and none is mutually exclusive.

CLIENT TEACHING

Suppressed Anger in Women

Research has shown that middle-aged women who suppress anger and have hostile attitudes may be at greater risk for developing cardiovascular disease (Matthews, 1998). Nurses can help such women minimize this risk by encouraging them to learn to express negative feelings in a constructive manner, to talk calmly about their feelings, to find other women who may share some of the same concerns and stressors, and to engage in regular exercise routines to relieve stress and tension.

Emotional Wellness

Emotions bridge the gap between mind and body. The person who is emotionally well understands his own feelings and knows when to express them appropriately. This individual accepts his limitations, has the ability to adjust to change, copes with stress in healthy ways, enjoys life, is optimistic and happy, and shows respect and affection to others.

Mental Wellness

The individual who is mentally well is alert, creative, logical, curious, open-minded, clear thinking, and accepting of others. This person also exhibits common sense, a good memory, and a desire for continual learning.

Intellectual Wellness

Intellectual wellness manifests as the ability to think, to process information, and to solve problems. The intellectually well person questions and evaluates information and situations, learns from life experiences, and is flexible, creative, and open to new ideas.

Vocational Wellness

The individual who is satisfied in school and/or job and who works in harmony with others enjoys vocational wellness (Figure 15-1).

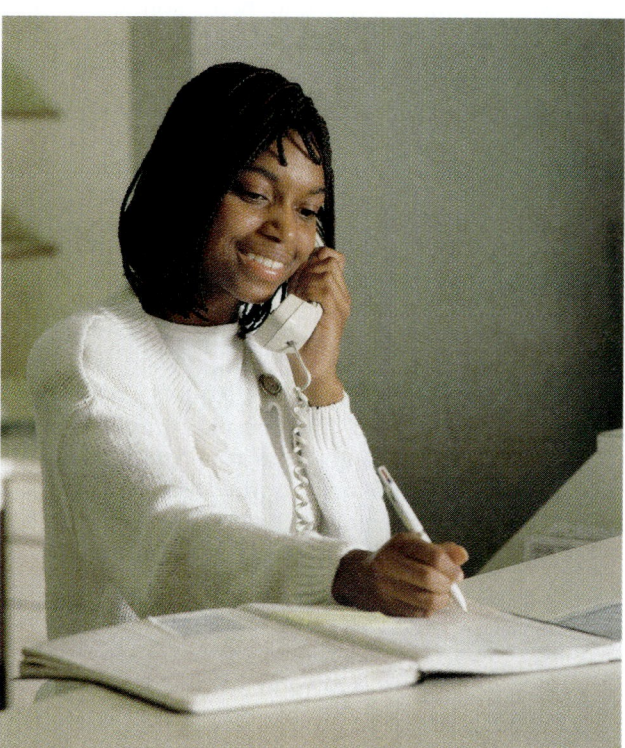

Figure 15-1 Vocational wellness means being content and satisfied with your occupation.

Social Wellness

Social wellness is evident when a person shows concern, fairness, affection, and respect for others; communicates effectively; has satisfying relationships; and interacts well with others. This person has a network of family and friends, is a member of various organizations, and works with a spirit of teamwork. Other behaviors exhibited are honesty, loyalty, confidence, and tolerance.

Spiritual Wellness

Spiritual wellness gives meaning, direction, and purpose to life by way of values, ethics, and morals. The spiritually healthy person has faith, optimism, and high self-esteem.

Physical Wellness

Physical wellness is noted in the person who avoids risky sexual behavior; tries to limit exposure to environmental contaminants; and restricts the intake of alcohol, tobacco, caffeine, and drugs. Regular exercise, a well-balanced diet, and regular physical examinations also enhance physical wellness (Figure 15-2).

HEALTH PROMOTION

Health promotion means more than preventing illness: It means assisting individuals to enhance their health, well-being, and functioning and to maximize their potential. Health promotion focuses on adopting healthy behaviors rather than on avoiding illness. The goal is for individuals to control and improve their health. Health promotion is appropriate for the individual and the population as a whole.

The concept of self-responsibility is important to health promotion, and it must be accepted and acted on in order for wellness to become a reality for an individual. No one else can make a person live a healthy life; self-responsibility is the only way to make changes. An individual can be given information relating to health and wellness, but only that person can change unhealthy or destructive habits. With the exception of small children, each individual must take responsibility

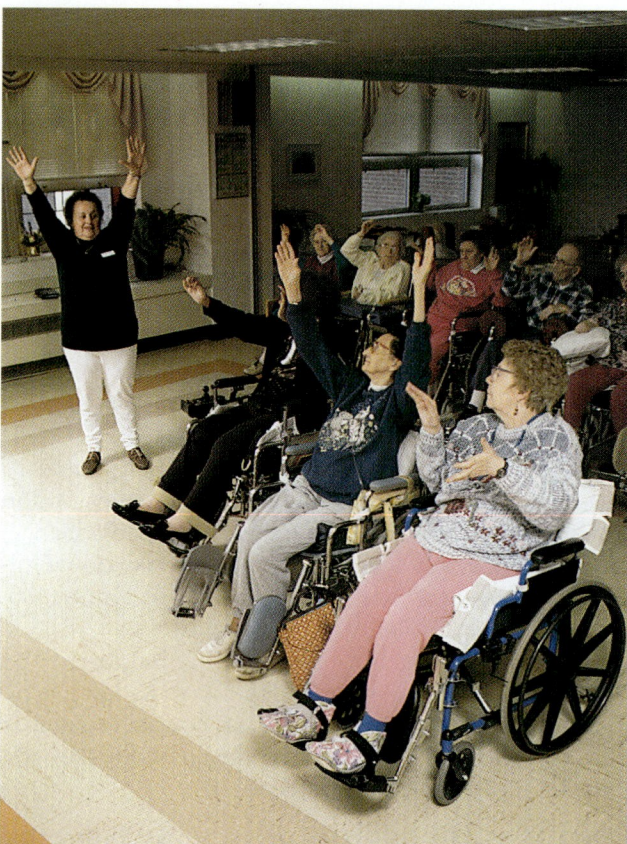

Figure 15-2 Individuals must learn to achieve physical wellness in a manner that accommodates their lifestyle and physical abilities.

for behaviors leading to health and wellness (Figure 15-3). Objectives for healthy living are outlined in the Healthy People 2000 and Healthy People 2010 documents issued by the federal government.

Healthy People 2000

In 1980 and again in 1990, the United States Department of Health and Human Services (USDHHS) released a list of objectives for disease prevention and health promotion in 22 priority areas (USDHHS, 1990). In 1990, more than 10,000 individuals representing 300

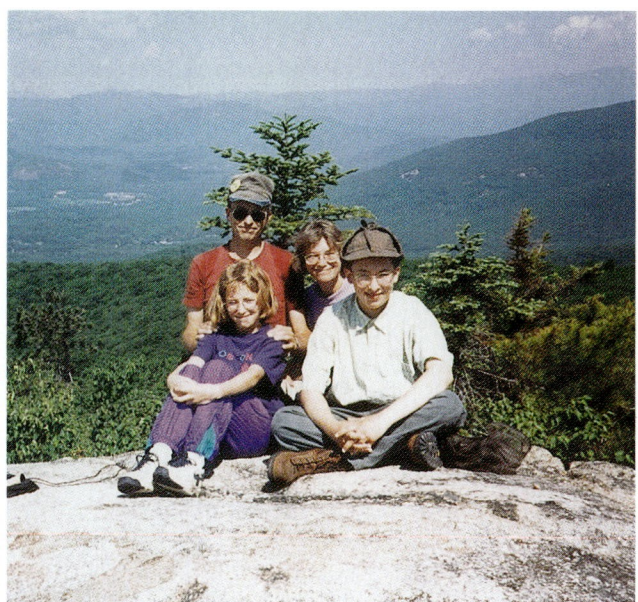

Figure 15-3 Families can work together to achieve wellness.

national organizations were involved in developing the health objectives for the year 2000. More than 300 health objectives for the nation to achieve by the year 2000 evolved. These objectives were published in a document titled *Healthy People 2000: National Health Promotion and Disease Prevention Objectives,* which addresses three important issues:

- Personal responsibility: Each individual must be health-conscious and must practice responsible, informed health behaviors.
- Health benefits for all people: Everyone must have health benefits in order for the nation to be healthy.
- Health promotion and disease prevention: Health care must change from a treatment focus to a prevention focus to cut costs and to increase the quality of life.

The overall goals include:

- Increasing the span of healthy life for Americans,
- Reducing health disparities among Americans, and
- Achieving access to preventive services for all Americans.

A sample of the objectives is found in Table 15-1. The entire document may be ordered from the United States Department of Health and Human Services, Washington, DC, DHHS Publication No. (PHS) 91–50212.

The USDHHS (1997–1998) reported on the progress made in meeting the 319 objectives of Healthy People 2000. In 1997, 13% of the goals had been reached or surpassed, and progress had been made in another 43%. Eighteen percent had fallen short of target, 7%

showed mixed results, and 2% showed no change. Fourteen percent now have baseline data but no data to evaluate progress, and baselines have not yet been established for 3% of these goals (USDHHS, Healthy People 2000).

Healthy People 2010

The Healthy People 2000 Consortium met in November of 1996 to discuss necessary improvements and modifications to be made for Healthy People 2010 objectives. Over the past 4 years, the consortium worked with a wide range of representatives of national membership organizations, state governments, managed care organizations, and private businesses through focus groups, public meetings, and the Healthy People 2010 website. Several themes that emerged from the meetings and focus groups were earmarked to be addressed in the revised objectives. These include the:

- need to address morbidity and mortality in setting objectives,
- value of packaging the 2010 document into different formats for multiple audiences,
- necessity of linking objectives to community-based health improvement initiatives, and
- importance of using language that is understandable to the general public.

Two goals for the 2010 objectives emerged as a result of these sessions: (1) "Increase Years of Healthy Life," which was retained from the Healthy People 2000 goal, and (2) "Eliminate Health Disparities," a stronger version of the Healthy People 2000 goal "Reduce Health Disparities." These two goals will be supported by four enabling goals concerned with promoting healthy behaviors, protecting health, achieving access to quality health care, and strengthening community prevention. A comparison of select 2000 objectives is presented in Table 15-1, along with baselines, targets, and 2010 objectives.

The 2010 objectives are grouped into 25 focus areas. New focus areas include disability; people with low income; race and ethnicity; chronic diseases; and public health infrastructure.

To expand the ability to track the objectives, new strategies are being developed to improve data collection, especially at the community level, and to improve the ability to measure access and quality of health services.

Healthy People 2010 was released in January 2000.

ILLNESS PREVENTION

Prevention (hindering, obstructing, or thwarting a disease or illness) incorporates both old and new ideas. The taboos, dietary laws, and traditions of various

Table 15-1 SELECTED OBJECTIVES FROM HEALTHY PEOPLE 2000 AND 2010

OBJECTIVE	BASELINE	YEAR 2000 TARGET	REPORT	YEAR 2010 TARGET
Physical Activity and Fitness				
• Increase the proportion of people who engage regularly in light to moderate physical activity for at least 30 minutes per day	22% (1985)	increase	23% (1995) (+)	30%
• Increase the proportion of young people in grades 9 to 12 who participate in daily school physical activity	42% (1991)	increase	25% (1995) (−)	50%
Nutrition				
• Increase the proportion of people aged 2 years and older who meet the Dietary Guidelines average daily goal of no more than 30% of calories from fat	34% (1989–91)	30%	33% (1994–96) (−)	75%
• Reduce the prevalence of BMI at or above 30.0 among people ages 20 years and older	24% males 27% females (1976–80)	20% both groups	34% males 37% females (1988–94) (−)	15%
Tobacco				
• Increase the proportion of cigarette smokers ages 18 years and older who stopped smoking cigarettes for a day	34% (1986)	50%	45.8% (1995) (+)	75%
• Increase the proportion of worksites with a formal smoking policy that prohibits smoking or limits it to separately ventilated areas at the workplace	NA	NA	59% of worksites with 50 or more employees (1992)	100%
Substance Abuse				
• Decrease alcohol-related motor vehicle crash deaths	9.8/100,000 (1987)	5.5/100,000	6.5/100,000 (1997)	3.5/100,000
• Reduce drug-related deaths	3.8/100,000 (1987)	3/100,000	4.7/100,000 (−)	1.3/100,000
Family Planning				
• Reduce the proportion of individuals ages 15 to 17 who have ever had sexual intercourse	33% of males 27% of females (1988)		43% of males 38% of females (1995) (−)	25%
• Increase the proportion of all females ages 15 to 44 at risk of unintended pregnancy who use contraception		95%	84% (1995)	95% (modified to "use effective contraception")
Mental Health and Mental Disorders				
• Reduce suicide rates	11.7/100,000 (1987)	10.5/100,000	11.2/100,000 (1995)	9.6/100,000
Injury/Violence Prevention				
• Reduce firearm-related deaths	14.6/100,000 (1990)	11.6/100,000	13.9/100,000 (1995)	Fewer than 11.6/100,000
• Increase use of bicycle helmets of 9th- to 12th-grade students who ride bicycles		50%	8% (1995)	50%
Maternal, Infant, Child Health				
• Increase the proportion of all pregnant women who begin prenatal care in the first trimester of pregnancy	78.9% (1993)	90%	81.3% (1995)	90%
• Reduce the cesarean delivery rate	24.4/100 (1987)	15/100	22/100 (1994)	15/100
Cancer				
• Reduce cancer deaths		130/100,000	130/100,000 (1995) (=)	103/100,000

continued

Table 15-1 SELECTED OBJECTIVES FROM HEALTHY PEOPLE 2000 AND 2010 *continued*

OBJECTIVES	BASELINE	YEAR 2000 TARGET	REPORT	YEAR 2010 TARGET
AIDS/HIV Infection				
• Confine annual incidence of diagnosed AIDS cases among adolescents and adults	29.8/100,000 (1994)		28/100,000 (1998) (+)	12/100,000
• Increase the proportion of those with positive HIV tests who return for counseling	72.5% (1989)	80%	83% (1995) (+)	none
Sexually Transmitted Diseases				
• Reduce prevalence of *Chlamydia trachomatis* infections among 14–24 year olds	12.5% (1996)	5%	11.2% (1997)	3%
• Eliminate sustained domestic transmission of primary and secondary syphillis	84% higher than 1997 (1990)	4/100,000	3.2/100,000 (1997) (+)	0.25/100,000
Immunizatons and Infectious Diseases				
• Reduce indigenous cases of vaccine preventable diseases				
– Diphtheria		0	4 (1997)	0
– Polio		0	0 (1997)	0
– Measles	3,058 (1988)	0	135 (1997)	0
– Rubella	225 (1988)	0	161 (1997)	0
– Mumps	4,866 (1988)	500	612 (1997)	0
– Pertussis	3,450 (1988)	1,000	6,568 (1997) (–)	2,000
• Increase proportion of contacts completing course of preventive therapy for tuberculosis	66.3% (1987)	85%	65.4% (1995) (–)	85%
Environmental Health				
• Reduce exposure of children age 6 and younger who are regularly exposed to tobacco smoke	39% (1986)	20%	27% (1994)	15%

(+) Exceeding target
(–) Receding from target
(=) Met target

Data from *Healthy People 2000: National Health Promotion and Disease Prevention Objectives, by U.S. Department of Health and Human Services, Public Health Service, 1991, Washington, D.C.: Author. Available on-line: http://web.health.gov/healthypeople*

cultural, ethnic, and religious groups were initiated for a reason. If scientific research has not proved these incorrect or harmful, there is no reason not to practice the old ways. New methods of illness prevention emerge as technology expands and health awareness increases.

All stages of life should embody the tenets of preventive health. It must begin before conception with healthy parents and prenatal care and continue through the life span. Scientific advice based on firmly established medical data and reasonable probability should be heeded. Interventions for disease prevention range from lifestyle changes that cost little or nothing to high-tech procedures that are very expensive.

Before the full impact of illness prevention can be discovered, major changes are needed in health care delivery, funding, and insurance coverage. The health care system must insist on more research relating to prevention and must then apply the results of the research to insurance practices. Prevention practices must be supported and funded by the health care system in order for a change from illness treatment to illness prevention to occur. The rewards of such a shift will be enhanced health, longer life expectancy, and a population that feels better, looks better, and functions better.

Illness prevention must be viewed according to the type of prevention and the health care team responsible for its implementation.

Types of Prevention

Prevention extends to all stages of health. There are three types of prevention: primary, secondary, and tertiary. Primary prevention has not historically been supported by our health care system, whereas secondary and tertiary prevention have been, and still are, the main focus. They are also the most expensive.

Primary Prevention

Primary prevention includes all practices designed to keep health problems from developing. Following recommended childhood immunization schedules, not smoking to prevent lung cancer, and eating calcium-rich foods to prevent osteoporosis are all examples of primary prevention. Primary prevention should be the focus for every individual and health care provider. It is usually the least expensive intervention and provides the greatest benefits.

Secondary Prevention

Secondary prevention refers to early detection, diagnosis, screening, and intervention to reduce the consequences of a health problem. That is, disease or illness is identified before the individual has any symptoms or functional impairment. Screening for tuberculosis and performing monthly breast self-examinations are both examples of secondary prevention. When no known methods of primary prevention exist for a specific disease or illness (such as breast cancer), the focus should be on performing self-examinations, and having a regular physical exam, and testing.

Tertiary Prevention

Tertiary prevention refers to caring for a person who already has a health problem; the illness or disease is treated after symptoms have appeared so as to prevent further progression. For example, taking antibiotics for an ear infection should eliminate the infection. Furthermore, potential complications and the disability of hearing impairment are prevented. Rehabilitation is an important aspect of tertiary prevention; this refers to preventing deterioration of a person's condition and minimizing the loss of function. One example is providing range of motion exercises to a client who has had a stroke, to encourage circulation and maintain function in the extremities.

Prevention Health Care Team

The prevention health care team consists of the individual assisted by nurses and the primary physician.

Individual

The individual is the center of the prevention health care team. It is the individual who must incorporate the knowledge related to preventive health care and make the behavioral changes necessary to live a more healthy life.

Individuals should decide those things that they want and expect from health care. Honesty with self, the nurses, and physician is necessary. Clients must be assertive and ask questions of the physicians and nurses and be active, informed health care consumers. The ultimate responsibility for health care belongs with the individual.

Nurses

Nurses, especially nurse practitioners, often do the initial health screening in clinics and physicians' offices. This provides a great opportunity to inquire about lifestyle and the preventive health habits of the client. Nurses can use their excellent listening skills to give clients time to discuss health care habits and ask questions. Nurses are also great teachers of preventive health habits and health promotion activities.

Primary Physicians

Primary physicians generally are family practitioners, pediatricians, or internists: These are the family doctors, the physicians seen on a regular basis. They have the opportunity and obligation to discuss and inquire about preventive health habits. When necessary, they refer clients to specialists for specific problems. After the problem has been resolved, the client returns to the primary physician for further care.

FACTORS AFFECTING HEALTH

A great many factors affect health. They can be categorized into four broad topics:

- Genetics and human biology
- Personal behavior
- Environmental influences
- Health care

Genetics and Human Biology

Inherited traits and the way the human body functions have an impact on an individual's state of health and wellness. An individual's genetic make up may include inherited disorders, such as sickle-cell anemia, or chromosomal anomalies, such as Down syndrome. Both of these may ultimately affect the individual's quality of life and level of health.

Human biology affects health because normal body functioning prevents some illnesses and makes us more susceptible to others. Production of the female and male hormones, estrogen and testosterone, respectively, are responsible for many of these effects (Hoffman, 1995) (Table 15-2).

Personal Behavior

Personal behavior is the area having the most factors affecting health and wellness, and they are controlled entirely by the individual. It is the individual's decision to use or not to use these factors to promote health and wellness. Factors typically deemed to be under the individual's control include diet, exercise, personal care, sexual relationships, level of stress, tobacco and drug use, alcohol use, and safety.

Table 15-2 EFFECTS OF ESTROGEN AND TESTOSTERONE ON SPECIFIC TISSUES

| Tissue | HORMONE | |
	Estrogen (Female)	Testosterone (Male)
Cardiovascular	• Increases arterial dilation • Causes vascular spasms • Improves cardiac function	• Increases size of heart
Liver	• Inhibits production of triglycerides, low-density lipoprotein (LDL) (bad) cholesterol, and free glucose • Decreases drug metabolism, prolonging action	• Produces triglycerides, LDL (bad) cholesterol, and free glucose • Increases drug metabolism, shortening action
Fat	• Encourates fat deposits in breasts, hips, and thighs and suppresses the movement of fat from these areas	• Encourages fat deposits in the abdomen
Gastrointestinal	• Slows motility and favors formation of gallstones	
Respiratory	• Increases respiratory rate and basal body temperature	
Musculoskeletal	• Enhances bone density	• Ensures bone density and strength
Immune	• Enhances antibody production and suppresses T cell-mediated processes (prevents rejection of sperm and fetus)	
Blood	• Suppresses red blood cell (RBC) development • Lowers hemoglobin (Hgb) level • Increases coagulation	• Increases RBC development • Increases Hgb level
Integumentary	• Enhances skin vitality • Increases collagen and water content	• Promotes body hair

Adapted from Our Health, Our Lives, *by E. Hoffman, 1995, New York: Pocket Books. Copyright 1995 by Pocket Books.*

Diet

Healthy eating habits and a proper diet greatly enhance an individual's overall state of health and well-being. Eating both fulfills the basic biological needs of sustenance, nutrition, and hydration and allows individuals to meet social and interpersonal needs (Figure 15-4). All of these factors contribute to overall wellness.

Exercise

Integrating physical activity into daily life is one of the best ways of promoting health. Exercise improves circulation, muscle strength, and emotional well-being; lowers blood pressure; increases endurance; and reduces the chances of heart attack, stroke, and osteoporosis. The individual who exercises regularly looks healthier and feels better.

Many people have joined health clubs in an effort to meet their need for exercise. Health clubs can be a wonderful source of regular exercise, but, also, a source

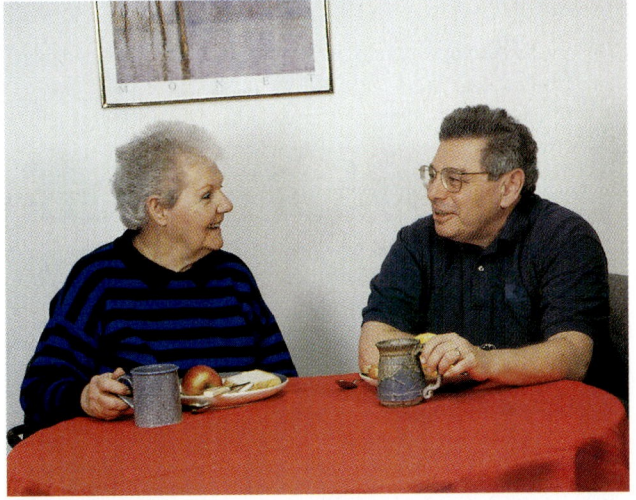

Figure 15-4 Sharing meals together is a wonderful means of meeting both physical and interpersonal needs.

CULTURAL CONSIDERATIONS

Parents' Beliefs about Feeding Children

Many parents:

- Begin feeding cereal and other solid foods earlier than recommended, believing that milk alone will not satisfy their babies' hunger,
- Use food to soothe or console children,
- Believe a heavier child is a healthier child, and
- View having a heavy infant or toddler as evidence of parental competence (Baughcum, 1998).

Nurses can work with these clients by respecting their cultural beliefs while enforcing the notion that a healthy child is a child who is satisfied following a meal and who shows a healthy, normal physical and emotional growth pattern. These factors, not plumpness, are indicators of wellness.

of disease, as reported in *Health-Club Hygiene* (Nov. 6, 1995). For example, perspiration on exercise machines is a prime source of impetigo. Clients should be made aware of such dangers so that they can practice safety precautions, such as wearing thigh-length shorts and always keeping a towel between the body and the exercise equipment.

Personal Care

The skin protects the body from outside elements. It works with the immune system to defend the body

CLIENT TEACHING

Dietary Guidelines for Americans

Teach clients to develop nutritional wellness by:

- Eating a variety of foods.
- Balancing the foods they eat with physical activity—maintaining or improving their weight;
- Choosing a diet with plenty of grain products, vegetables, and fruits;
- Choosing a diet low in fat, saturated fat, and cholesterol;
- Choosing a diet moderate in sugars;
- Choosing a diet moderate in salt and sodium; and
- Drinking alcoholic beverages only in moderation or not at all.

From Home and Garden Bulletin No. 232 *(4th ed.), by U.S. Department of Agriculture, U.S. Department of Health and Human Services, 1995.*

CLIENT TEACHING

Preventing Food-Borne Diseases

Share the following tips with clients to educate them in ways to prevent food-borne diseases:

- Allow cooked foods to sit at room temperature for no more than 2 hours
- Date leftovers, refrigerate, and eat within 5 days
- Wash dirty dishes in hot (120°F) water, as dirty dishes are an ideal place for bacteria to multiply
- Keep dishcloths and sponges clean and allow to dry between uses
- Use a bleach solution to clean cutting boards and countertops
- Wash all fruits and vegetables in a diluted bleach solution (a bleach to water ratio of 1:100)

against harmful bacteria, fungi, viruses, and allergens. Regular skin, hair, and nail care will enhance wellness and foster self-esteem. Personal care also includes such wellness habits as proper posture, proper body mechanics, adequate sleep, and dental hygiene.

Sexual Relationships

Establishing intimacy and a sexual relationship with another person is a natural step in growth and development. To maintain health and wellness, the individual will use values, ethics, and morals to guide the development of the relationship. A healthy sexual relationship is based on mutual satisfaction of the parties, a consensual approach to pleasurable activities, and mutual respect for preferences and personal choices.

Level of Stress

Not all stress is harmful. Limited stress makes one more alert and raises one's energy level. The way one responds to or copes with stressors dictates whether the situation is healthy or harmful. For instance, whereas one individual may enjoy the challenge of balancing work and family, another may feel torn by these seemingly conflicting demands and will therefore experience undue stress. Stress results not from an individual's life situation, but from that individual's reaction to and perception of the life situation.

Tobacco and Drug Use

Refraining from tobacco use is a strong step towards health promotion and maintenance. Even when a long-time smoker gives up the habit, the health risks begin to decrease at once; although it will take 10 to 15 years to eliminate all the effects of smoking from the lungs. The person who smokes exhales secondhand smoke, which presents a health risk to those who do not smoke.

PROFESSIONAL TIP

Moderate Exercise Reduces Stroke Risk

- Individuals who burn 1,000 to 1,999 calories per week by exercising moderately have a 24% lower risk of suffering a stroke than do those who burn less.
- Individuals who burn 2,000 to 2,999 calories per week by exercising moderately have a 46% lower risk.
- Burning over 2,999 calories a week through moderate exercise lowered the risk of having a stroke by only 20%.
- Moderate exercise includes activities such as brisk walking, dancing, and cycling (Lee & Paffenbarger, 1998).

Abuse of both illegal and prescription drugs is a serious medical and social problem in our society. Drugs prescribed by a physician are abused if they are not taken as directed, or if they are taken by anyone other than the client for whom they were prescribed. Many prescribed drugs can be addictive if not taken as directed. Health can be maintained when clients understand the effects, indications, side effects, and interactions of the prescription medications they are taking.

Alcohol Use

The decision to consume alcohol is a personal choice that can influence an individual's state of health. The amount of alcohol consumed will affect sobriety, decision-making ability, and, in many instances, safety. The use of alcohol can play a significant role in drownings, adult fire deaths, traffic fatalities, falling fatalities, and suicides.

Safety

Personal choices concerning safety affect many areas of an individual's life and can be viewed collectively more as a lifestyle choice than individually as separate acts to promote safety. For example, individuals who embrace safety as a fundamental element of health and well-being will ensure safety in their homes by having smoke detectors, fire extinguishers, carbon monoxide detectors, practiced escape plans, locked medicine cabinets, and gates blocking dangerous stairways. These individuals will also most likely buckle their car seat belts, secure their children in child car seats, and obey speed limits when driving. All these elements of safety add up to a healthy lifestyle.

Environmental Influences

Environmental factors that may influence health are numerous, can be natural or man-made, and vary de-

pending on geographic location and living conditions. Exposure to or ingestion of certain natural biological irritants can cause disease, such as results from exposure to poison ivy, and even death, such as results from ingestion of poison mushrooms. Exposure to chemicals such as asbestos in older buildings, lead in paint in older houses, and mercury in polluted water sources, can also pose health hazards. Radiation from the sun and certain types of machinery can be harmful in large doses; extreme, prolonged exposure to solar radiation can even result in death. Natural disasters such as hurricanes, floods, volcanic eruptions, droughts, heat waves, blizzards, and other extreme weather conditions pose health risks, as do man-made environmental crises including wars, bombings, pollution, and overpopulation.

Health Care

Most people use the health care system when they are ill, for the treatment of their disease or condition. A more effective use of the health care system, however, is health promotion and disease prevention. Routine physical examinations with minimal testing are invaluable for maintaining health and preventing disease (Figure 15-5). Healthy adults should consider health care services based on factors related to family health history, personal health history, personal habits, or the presence of symptoms that may alter the time frame for suggested health care services.

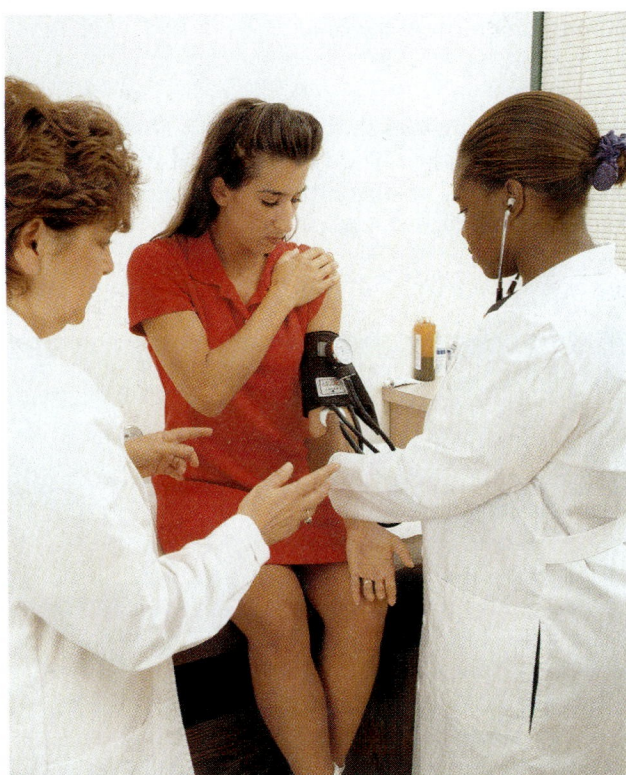

Figure 15-5 Routine physical examinations are essential to maintaining health and preventing disease.

Physical Exam

The physical examination should begin with a review of family health history, personal health history, personal habits (tobacco, alcohol, and drug use, sexual practices), and concerns or questions the client may have. Before visiting the physician, the client should write down questions and concerns so that none will be forgotten. Individuals between the ages of 20 and 39 years should have a complete physical exam every 1 to 3 years; those 40 to 49 years of age, every 1 to 2 years; and those over 50 years of age, every year. Women should have a breast exam with every physical exam obtained before age 40 and yearly thereafter. Men should have a testicular exam with every physical exam and should have a rectal exam to check the prostate at every physical exam obtained after age 40.

Immunizations

Adults who have not had the recommended immunizations as children should discuss this with their primary physicians. Depending on the client's risk factors, the physician may recommend having the immunizations as an adult.

Each adult should have a tetanus booster immunization every 10 years for life. Those at high risk of exposure, such as health care workers and college students; those who have chronic pulmonary, heart, or kidney disease; those who have diabetes; and those 65 years of age and older should have an influenza immunization every year and a pneumococcal pneumonia immunization every 6 years.

Tests

The following tests should be done with every physical exam: complete blood count, blood sugar, cholesterol, urinalysis, stool for blood, and, for women, a Papanicolau (Pap) smear. An electrocardiogram (EKG

PROFESSIONAL TIP

Hepatitis B Vaccine

Health care personnel who may be exposed to blood and body fluids are at risk for contracting the hepatitis B virus. Health care employers are required by law to offer the hepatitis B vaccination without cost to employees who are in direct care positions. Employees have the option of having or refusing this immunization. The vaccine is not contraindicated during pregnancy, and there are no apparent adverse effects to developing fetuses; however, the vaccine may cause shock in individuals who are allergic to baker's yeast.

PROFESSIONAL TIP

Mammograms

The Centers for Disease Control and Prevention (CDC) (1998) reports that 70.9% of insured women over 40 years of age had a mammogram in 1996–1997, but only 46.2% of uninsured women over age 40 had a mammogram in the same years.

or ECG) should be done at ages 20 years and 40 years and every 5 years thereafter (and yearly if the client is at high risk). Women should have a baseline mammogram (Figure 15-6) at age 40 and yearly thereafter. Men should have a testicular exam and rectal exam of the prostate at each physical exam. Each woman should perform a breast self-exam after every menstrual period. Each male should perform a testicular self-exam on a monthly basis.

Dental Exam

A dental exam, prophylaxis, and needed treatment should be performed every 6 to 12 months throughout life.

Eye Exam

An eye exam, including tonometry for glaucoma, should be performed every 2 to 3 years from ages 40 to 49 years and every 1 to 2 years after the age of 50.

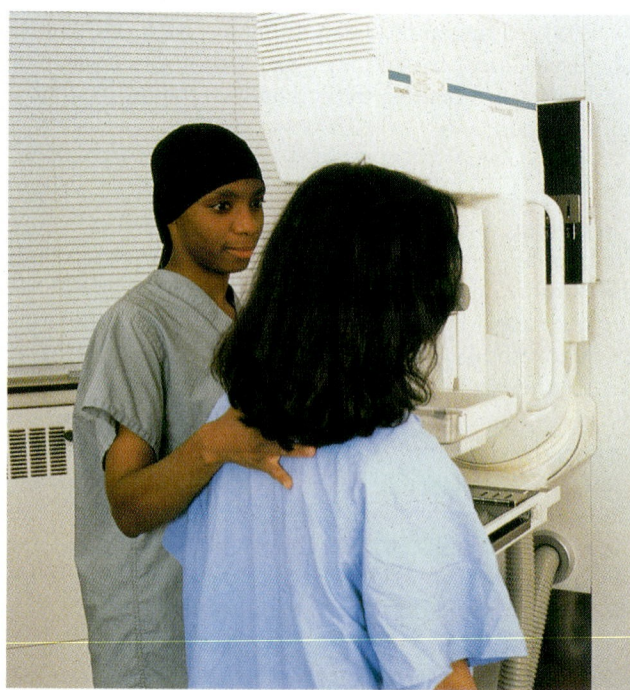

Figure 15-6 Mammograms are a key element to wellness promotion for all women over the age of 40 years.

CLIENT TEACHING

Crucial Health Practices

Simon (1992) states that all the medical progress in the United States from 1900–1990 increased the life span of an average adult by 4 years; but that simple lifestyle changes increased the life span of an average adult by 11 years. He describes 10 crucial health practices:

- Do not use tobacco and drugs.
- Do not consume more than 2 ounces of alcohol per day.
- Eat a diet low in fat, cholesterol, and salt but high in fiber, fruits, vegetables, and fish.
- Exercise regularly—1 hour each week is helpful, 3 is ideal.
- Stay lean.
- Drive cars with air bags and wear seatbelts; drive prudently, and never drink before driving.
- Avoid excessive stress.
- Minimize exposure to radiation, ultraviolet rays, chemical pollutants, and other environmental hazards.
- Protect self from sexually transmitted diseases.
- Obtain regular medical care including immunizations and screening tests.

GUIDELINES FOR HEALTHY LIVING

Because of their education and training, nurses are in a unique position to practice healthy living habits themselves and to promote such habits in their clients. Table 15-3 outlines select causes of death and the controllable lifestyle factors that most contribute to these types of deaths. While it is important to remember that certain health variables such as gender and race cannot be controlled or changed, others such as diet and tobacco use result from individual choice. These lifestyle choices are based on individual preference, and nurses can help clients make the best choices to promote wellness and optimal functioning. Following is a list of select guidelines, for nurses and their clients, to promote healthy living and wellness in daily life.

Heart Disease:
- Eat a diet low in fat and cholesterol and high in fiber
- Exercise regularly, 30 minutes three to five times a week (walking, swimming, cycling)
- Quit smoking or do not start to smoke
- Handle stress appropriately; use relaxation or meditation
- Do not use caffeine or alcohol excessively

Table 15-3 CONTROLLABLE FACTORS FOR LEADING CAUSES OF DEATH

CAUSE OF DEATH	CONTROLLABLE FACTORS
Heart disease	Tobacco use, high blood pressure, high cholesterol, lack of exercise, excessive stress, diabetes, obesity
Cancer	Tobacco use, radiation, alcohol abuse, improper diet, environmental exposure
Stroke	Tobacco use, high blood pressure, high cholesterol, lack of exercise
Accidents	Alcohol abuse, drug abuse, tobacco use, failure to use seat belts, fatigue, stress, recklessness
Chronic lung disease	Tobacco use, environmental exposures
Pneumonia and influenza	Chronic lung disease, environmental exposures, tobacco use, alcohol abuse, lack of immunization
Diabetes	Obesity, improper diet, lack of exercise, excessive stress
Suicide	Excessive stress, alcohol abuse, drug abuse
Liver disease	Alcohol abuse, exposure to toxins (ingested and environmental), lack of immunizations
Atherosclerosis	Tobacco use, high cholesterol, high blood pressure, lack of exercise

- Maintain appropriate weight for height
- Maintain normal blood pressure
- Have a regular physical exam

Osteoporosis:
- Throughout life, eat calcium-rich foods (milk and milk products) and a balanced diet
- Get plenty of exercise
- Discuss with the primary care physician the need for a calcium supplement and estrogen replacement therapy (females)
- Do not smoke

Cancer:
- Do not smoke
- Avoid exposure to unnecessary radiation
- Protect skin from ultraviolet rays; use sunscreen
- Avoid exposure to harmful chemicals
- Minimize exposure to pesticides, herbicides, and poisons

- Limit alcohol intake
- Eat a well-balanced diet with adequate fiber
- Exercise
- Practice safe sex
- Have cancer screening tests—mammogram, Pap smear, fecal occult blood test, and rectal exam—with each physical exam

Low-Back Pain:
- Exercise regularly
- Practice good posture
- Use proper body mechanics

Colds and Flu:
- Wash hands frequently
- Use paper tissues and dispose of properly
- Have flu shots yearly
- Follow the Dietary Guidelines for Americans for a balanced diet
- Drink plenty of fluids

Breast Cancer:
- Eat a diet low in fat
- Exercise regularly
- Limit alcohol and caffeine intake
- Perform monthly breast self-examinations
- Have mammograms as recommended by the American Cancer Society

Sexually Transmitted Diseases:
- Practice monogamous sex between noninfected individuals
- Use latex condoms

Tuberculosis (especially for health care workers):
- Mantoux test
- Isoniazid preventive therapy—any newly exposed and infected individual taking a full course of therapy (Reichman & Mangura, 1996)

Urinary Tract Infections:
- Drink plenty of water
- Empty bladder frequently, especially before and after sexual intercourse
- Wear underwear with a cotton crotch
- Wipe from front to back
- Drink cranberry juice
- Avoid bubble bath, douches, and scented or colored toilet paper

Sickle-Cell Anemia and Thalassemia:
- Request genetic screening and counseling if a high-risk group

Cataracts:
- Wear sunglasses and a hat with a brim
- Eat a well-balanced diet
- Do not smoke

Glaucoma:
- Have tonometry performed
- Have an optic nerve exam

Sunburn:
- Always wear suncreen (with a minimum SPF of 15) when out in the sun

Dental Caries and Periodontal Disease:
- Brush after each meal; floss daily
- Use fluoride toothpaste
- Have a professional cleaning twice a year
- Have a dental exam yearly

Home Safety:
- Lock cupboards containing medicines and cleaning materials
- Maintain working smoke alarms and fire extinguishers
- Use a carbon monoxide alarm in the presence of gas appliances and heaters
- Plan escape routes in case of fire and have fire drills
- Safety proof home against falls
- Know water safety rules

Work Safety:
- Follow workplace safety regulations
- Report unsafe equipment or practices

Travel Safety:
- Wear a seat belt
- Do not drink and drive
- Drive safely and defensively
- Use infant and child seats and restraints
- Wear a helmet when riding a bicycle or motorcycle
- Never swim alone

Weight:
- Follow the Dietary Guidelines for Americans for a balanced diet
- Exercise 30 minutes daily
- If overweight, eat the least number of servings recommended
- If needed, use raw fruits or vegetables as snacks between meals
- If underweight, eat the largest number of servings recommended
- Eat a nutritious snack between meals

Stress:
- Identify sources of stress
- Establish realistic goals and expectations
- Be flexible
- Express thoughts and feelings
- Do not depend on alcohol or drugs for relaxation
- Exercise
- Practice deep breathing and muscle relaxation
- Get enough sleep
- Have a sense of humor—laugh
- Obtain professional help when needed

SUMMARY

- Wellness includes prevention, early detection, and treatment of health problems.
- The best way to maintain health is to follow the Dietary Guidelines for Americans, exercise regularly, reduce stress, prevent accidents, and receive routine health exams.
- The leading causes of death can be significantly reduced by lifestyle changes.
- Physical, mental, emotional, social, and spiritual aspects play a key role in the ability to resist disease and maintain health and wellness.

Review Questions

1. The person responsible for health maintenance and disease prevention is the:
   a. nurse.
   b. physician.
   c. individual.
   d. nurse practitioner.

2. The Healthy People 2000 objectives:
   a. are related only to physical fitness.
   b. are related only to disease conditions.
   c. address the treatment of disease conditions.
   d. address the issue of personal responsibility for health behaviors.

3. Primary prevention:
   a. begins with the physician.
   b. is curing a disease in a week.
   c. takes place before disease begins.
   d. includes all diseases or conditions.

4. The prevention health care team is composed of the:
   a. dietitian, nurses, and pharmacist.
   b. individual, physician, and nurses.
   c. physician, pharmacist, and laboratory.
   d. radiology, laboratory, and individual.

5. Health is improved by:
   a. not smoking.
   b. drinking alcohol.
   c. eating more sweet foods.
   d. sleeping 3 to 4 hours each night.

6. How often should an individual have a physical exam?
   a. Every year.
   b. Every two years.
   c. Every three years.
   d. It depends on the person's age.

7. A genogram is used for:
   a. building a family tree.
   b. identifying potential health problems.
   c. preventing most diseases and illnesses.
   d. identifying the genes a person inherits.

8. Colds and flu can best be prevented by:
   a. smoking.
   b. staying warm and dry.
   c. washing hands frequently.
   d. having a flu shot every three years.

Critical Thinking Questions

1. How can you assist a client in identifying potential health problems?

2. What kind of preventive health care should be received by a person 20 years old, 42 years old, and 65 years old?

3. How does the nurse's state of health affect client care?

 WEB FLASH!

- What information does the Internet provide about Healthy People 2000 and Healthy People 2010?
- What information/resources can be found about wellness?

CHAPTER
16

STRESS, ADAPTATION, AND ANXIETY

MAKING THE CONNECTION

Refer to the following chapters to increase your understanding of stress, adaptation, and anxiety:

- Chapter 1, Holistic Care
- Chapter 2, Critical Thinking
- Chapter 8, Communication
- Chapter 13, Alternative/Complementary Therapies

- Chapter 21, Infection Control/Asepsis
- Chapter 26, Pain Management
- Chapter 40, Nursing Care of the Client: Integumentary System

LEARNING OBJECTIVES

Upon completion of this chapter, you should be able to:
- *Define key terms.*
- *Discuss stress, adaptation, and anxiety as they affect health.*
- *Identify factors contributing to the stress response.*
- *Describe the general adaptation syndrome.*
- *Detail the effects of stress on the whole individual.*
- *Explain stressors inherent in the change process.*
- *Discuss the role of the nurse as a change agent.*
- *Explain nursing interventions that promote positive adaptation to stress.*
- *Develop an individualized stress management plan for use as a nurse.*

KEY TERMS

adaptation	depersonalization
adaptive energy	distress
adaptive measures	endorphins
anxiety	eustress
burnout	fight-or-flight response
catharsis	general adaptation syndrome (GAS)
change	
change agent	homeostasis
cognitive reframing	local adaptation syndrome (LAS)
conditioning	
crisis	maladaptive measures
crisis intervention	stress
defense mechanisms	stressor

INTRODUCTION

Stress and anxiety are universal experiences that can be either catalysts for positive change or sources of discomfort and pain. Nurses are involved with stress management from a teaching perspective, helping clients learn to cope with the stress imposed by illness, injury, disability, or treatment approaches. Caring for clients who are experiencing high levels of anxiety can also be stress provoking for the nurse. Successful stress management is necessary for wellness of both clients and nurses. This chapter discusses the major concepts related to stress and anxiety, including strategies for coping with stress.

STRESS

According to Hans Selye (1974), **stress** is a nonspecific response to any demand made on the body. Selye termed such demands **stressors**. Any situation, event, or agent that produces stress is considered a stressor. A stressor is a stimulus that evokes the need to adapt. Stressors can be internal or external. For example, a headache is an internal stressor, whereas a difficult assignment is an external stressor.

Even pleasant events can be stressful in that they evoke the need to adapt. Stressors in themselves are neutral; in other words, a stressor is neither good nor bad. The individual's *perception* of the stressor greatly determines whether the effect on the individual is positive or negative. Any event can be stressful, depending on the person's interpretation of that event.

Response to Stress

Adaptive energy is the term Selye coined to describe the inner force an individual uses to respond or adapt to stress. All persons have adaptive energy; however, the amount of adaptive energy varies from person to person. After an individual has used all of his adaptive energy, the result may be illness, disease, or even death, as he is no longer able to change and adapt to the needs of his environment. Reactions to stress are typically categorized as either general (affecting the entire body) or local (affecting only the involved body part).

General Adaptation Syndrome

Stressors cause structural and chemical changes in the body as the body attempts to maintain **homeostasis,** which is the balance or equilibrium among the physiologic, psychological, sociocultural, intellectual, and spiritual needs of the body. Selye called these responses to stressors the **general adaptation syndrome** (GAS).

Selye divided the GAS into three stages, as illustrated in Figure 16-1. In the first stage, crisis or alarm, the body readies itself to handle the stressors. The physiologic changes may result in symptoms such as cool, pale skin;

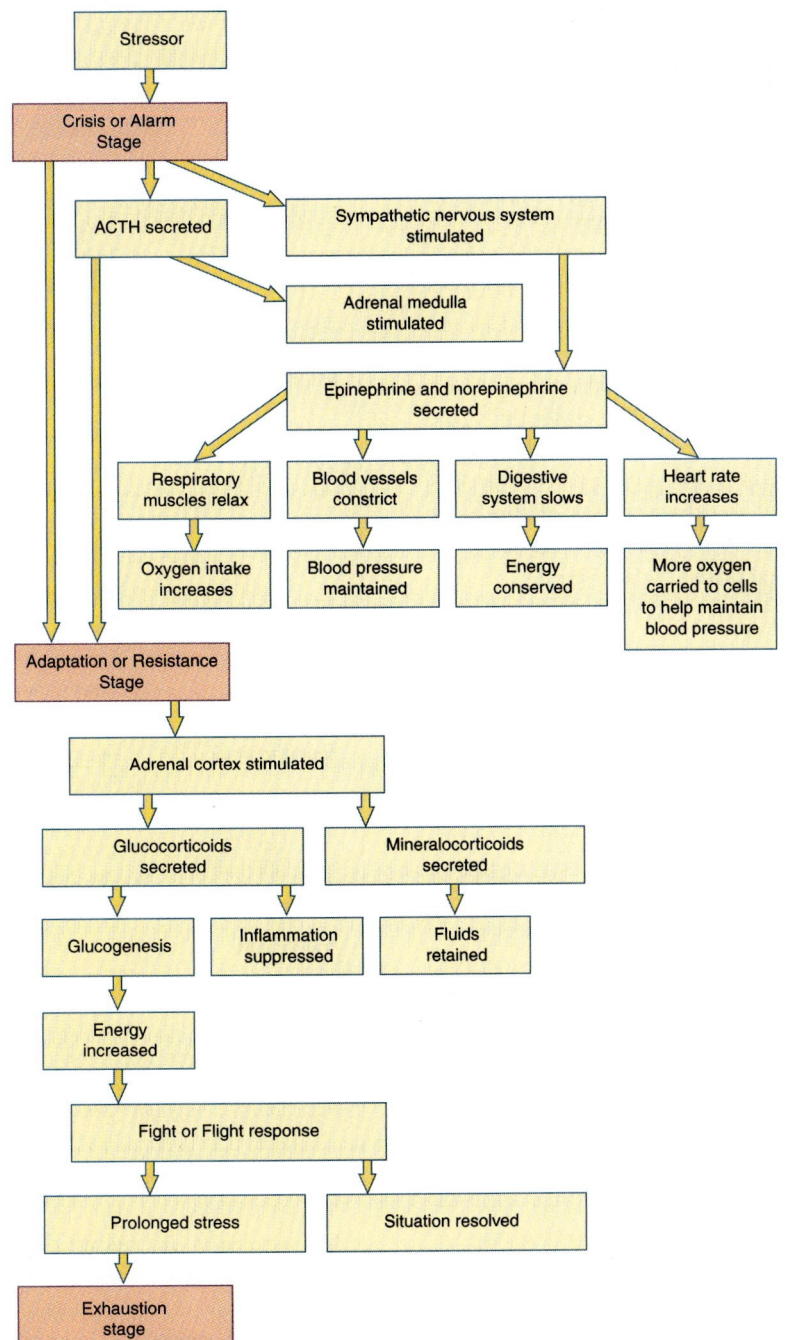

Figure 16-1 Physiological Effects of the General Adaptation Syndrome (GAS). *(Adapted from* Mental Health Concepts *by C. Waughfield, 1998, Albany, NY: Delmar Publishers. Copyright 1998 by Delmar Publishers.)*

PROFESSIONAL TIP

Anticipatory Stress

When a person worries about a situation, such as an upcoming exam, the thoughts are stressors that trigger the GAS. The body responds as if the person were *actually* experiencing the events in the present moment, and the individual may feel ill, nauseous, sweaty, or very jittery.

shivering; and sweating of the palms and of the soles of the feet. Severe stress may cause dilated pupils, dry mouth, pounding heart, nausea, and diarrhea.

During the second stage, adaptation or resistance, the body attempts to defend against the stressor through the **fight-or-flight response.** The body becomes physiologically ready to defend itself by either fighting or running away from the danger (stressor).

The third stage, exhaustion, occurs if adaptive energy is inadequate to deal with prolonged or overwhelming stress.

The GAS is the same whether the stressor is actual or imagined, present or potential. In other words, the physiologic reactions of the body are essentially the same regardless of the source of the stress. For example, the mind can imagine a stressor, and the physiologic response (GAS) will be the same as if the body had actually experienced the stressor. According to Selye (1976), all stress reactions involve similar physiologic reactions.

Local Adaptation Syndrome

Selye also described the **local adaptation syndrome** (LAS), which is the physiologic response to a stressor (e.g., trauma, illness) affecting a specific part of the body. For example, if a person experiences a puncture wound on the foot, the LAS is initiated, leading to localized inflammation: The classic symptoms of inflammation (redness, warmth, and swelling) occur at the injured site. The LAS is usually a temporary process that resolves when the traumatized area is restored to its pre-injury state. However, if the inflammation does not resolve with the LAS, the individual will then experience the GAS as the entire body becomes diseased.

Manifestations of Stress

The manifestations of stress are numerous and affect every dimension of a person. Common manifestations of stress are outlined in Table 16-1.

Outcomes of Stress

Stress is an experience that provides the individual with two possibilities: (1) an opportunity for personal growth or (2) the risk of disorganization and distress.

Table 16-1	MANIFESTATIONS OF STRESS
Physiologic	**Cardiovascular/ Respiratory Effects**
	• Increased pulse rate
	• Increased blood pressure
	• Rapid, shallow breathing
	Neurologic Effects
	• Dizziness
	• Headaches
	• Dilated pupils
	Gastrointestinal Effects
	• Nausea
	• Altered appetite
	• Diarrhea or constipation
	Genitourinary Effect
	• Polyuria
	Musculoskeletal Effects
	• Tension
	• Twitching
	Endocrine Effect
	• Increased levels of blood glucose and cortisol
Psychological	• Irritability
	• Increased sensitivity (feelings easily hurt)
	• Sadness, depression
	• Feeling "on edge"
Cognitive	• Impaired memory
	• Confusion
	• Impaired judgment
	• Poor decision making
	• Delayed response time
	• Altered perceptions
	• Inability to concentrate
Behavioral	• Pacing
	• Sweaty palms
	• Rapid speech
	• Insomnia
	• Withdrawal
	• Exaggerated startle reflex
Spiritual	• Alienation
	• Social isolation
	• Feeling of emptiness

From Fundamentals of Nursing: Standards & Practice, *by S. DeLaune and P. Ladner, 1998, Albany, NY: Delmar Publishers. Copyright 1998 by Delmar Publishers.*

When stressors are responded to appropriately, adaptation is successful, and the body returns to its normal steady state.

The term **eustress** is used to describe a type of stress that results in positive outcomes. Consider for example, students who have an examination scheduled the following week. The stress over the impending test motivates them to study early, and, as a result, they pass the examination. This stress was positive in that it produced motivation to change study habits (an example of growth) and resulted in positive or desired outcomes (high test scores).

When stressors evoke an ineffective response, **distress** is experienced. For example, consider students who have an examination scheduled for the next day. They had plenty of time to study, but because they put it off until the last minute, they take the examination unprepared. As a result of "cramming" all night, they are not alert, do not know the material, and fail the examination; they are experiencing distress.

ADAPTATION

Adaptation is an ongoing process whereby individuals use various responses to adjust to stressors and change. The nurse's goal is to identify and support the client's positive adaptive responses. Adaptation is a holistic response that involves all dimensions of an individual. Individuals, as holistic beings, seek to maintain a steady state in all dimensions of life: physiologic, psychological, cognitive, social, and spiritual. Wellness is an adaptive state; that is, the well person is one who is coping effectively with stressors and thus maintains a high level of well-being. Adaptation may be physiologic, psychological, cognitive, social, or spiritual.

Physiologic adaptation is the way the body responds to stressors affecting the functioning of the body. It may involve the entire body or only a specific area. An individual who lives in the mountains (high elevation) produces more red blood cells to carry enough oxygen to meet the body's needs. The chest also enlarges to allow the lungs to expand to accommodate the needed exchange of oxygen and carbon dioxide.

Psychological adaptation involves the use of defense mechanisms and learning to mentally accept new situations. A person's hardiness includes a sense of commitment, challenge, and control (Kobasa, 1979). A 55-year-old worker who suddenly finds himself unemployed will need to learn to adapt psychologically to the new situation and decide which steps to take next.

Cognitive adaptation involves education, communication, problem-solving ability, and perception of people and the world. A person gains these methods of adaptation as development occurs throughout life. For example, the high-school student will have a different perspective of the world and different problem-solving abilities than will this same individual as a college graduate, due to development and maturity.

Social adaptation involves social relationships with family, friends, and coworkers who may provide support in times of stress. A person unable to cope may withdraw socially. An example of social adaptation would be a couple moving to a new town and making new friends and modifying relationships with existing friends.

Spiritual adaptation involves beliefs about a supreme being and a positive sense of life's purpose and meaning. These beliefs are a personal resource for coping with stressors. Following the loss of a loved one, for instance, a family's spirituality and sense of faith may undergo changes.

Coping Measures

Coping measures include all the ways an individual may react to stress. Stress is an automatic response, but individuals can learn to conserve their adaptive energy through conditioning. **Conditioning** occurs when a person is taught a behavior until it becomes an automatic response. Some individuals who are conditioned to do so can handle a great deal of stress, whereas others cannot handle even a small amount of stress. Other factors that affect an individual's ability to cope with stress are the:

- Degree of danger perceived by the individual,
- Immediate needs of the individual,
- Amount of support from others,
- Individual's belief in his own ability to handle the stressful situation,
- Individual's previous successes and failures in coping, and
- Number of concurrent or cumulative stresses being handled by the individual (Waughfield, 1998).

Adaptive Measures

Measures for coping with stress that require a minimal amount of energy are called **adaptive measures** (Figure 16-2). They deal directly with the stressful

LIFE CYCLE CONSIDERATIONS

Coping Ability

An individual's ability to cope with stressors will depend in part upon age and developmental level.

CULTURAL CONSIDERATIONS

Adaptive Measures

Nurses must be sensitive to the fact that culture and ethnicity may influence an individual's choice of coping mechanisms. For instance, moaning and chanting may be an expected response to stress in some cultures; the nurse must be careful to view this behavior not as unhealthy, but as a culturally healthy response to a stressful stimulus.

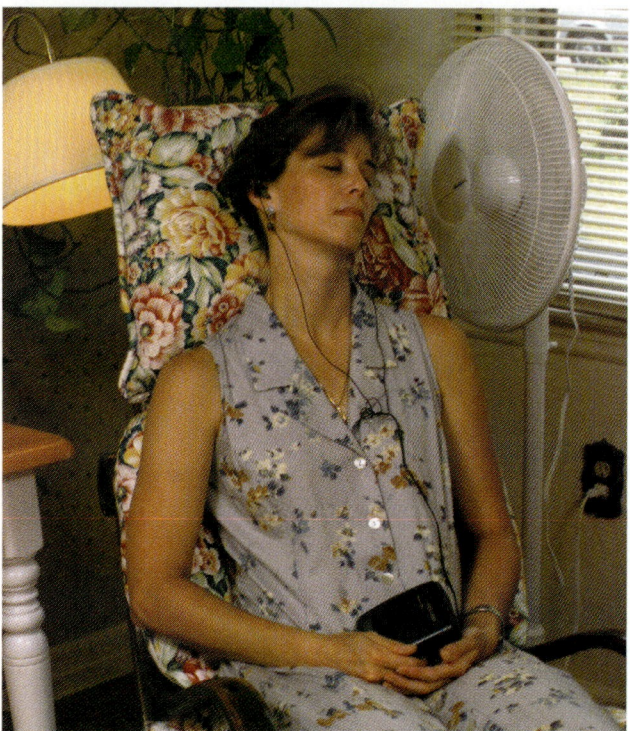

Figure 16-2 Listening to relaxation tapes is a way of coping with stress.

situation or the symptoms thereof. Adaptive measures useful in dealing with stressful situations include the following:

- Use of support people
- Relaxation to relieve tension
- Behavioral change
- Development of more realistic goals
- Problem solving

Defense Mechanisms

Just as the body has physiologic mechanisms (e.g., the immune system, the inflammatory response) to defend against infection and disease, the mind has psychological protective mechanisms. Most of these **defense mechanisms** are unconscious operations that protect the mind from anxiety. Defense mechanisms are employed to achieve and maintain psychological home-

PROFESSIONAL TIP

Defense Mechanisms

The nurse who is unfamiliar with defense mechanisms is likely to be judgmental about clients who do not respond according to the nurse's expectations. If, for example, the nurse tries to break through a client's denial (defense mechanism) too quickly by presenting reality, the client may be overwhelmed by anxiety and will panic.

ostasis, and in many cases, the individual does not consciously decide to use a defense mechanism, but, rather, it will automatically activate.

Defense mechanisms are universal. Their use does not indicate psychosocial imbalance or mental illness. Defense mechanisms are considered to be maladaptive when they become a stereotyped pattern, that is, the only way that an individual responds to a threat. Defense mechanisms are also considered to be maladaptive when they limit the individual's ability to function. Table 16-2 describes and gives examples of various defense mechanisms.

Maladaptive Measures

Measures used to avoid conflict and stress are considered **maladaptive measures**, because they prevent the individual from making progress towards resolving and accepting stress. They may include somatic disorders (transferring stress to an organ, as in an ulcer), rituals, excessive use of alcohol or drugs, excessive eating, or withdrawal from reality.

Crisis

When stressors exceed a person's ability to cope, a crisis occurs. A **crisis** (an acute state of disorganization) occurs when the individual's usual coping mechanisms are no longer effective. Crisis is characterized by extreme anxiety, inability to function, and disorganized behavior. A crisis is time limited; that is, no one can remain in acute disequilibrium for a long period of time because of the degree of discomfort that is experienced. Given the time-limited nature of crisis, a client experiencing a crisis needs immediate intervention to reach a successful resolution. Crisis intervention is discussed later in this chapter.

Crisis can be a negative experience, but it also can present an opportunity for growth and learning. The outcome is unique to each individual's perception and coping abilities. Nurses are challenged to help clients discover the opportunities in their crises, to adapt in positive, healthy manners.

Not every person will experience a crisis as a result of stressful events. Each crisis is unique to the individual; however, some characteristics are common to all crises (Table 16-3). A crisis is *not* a mental illness, even though it is not uncommon for persons experiencing the acute discomfort and anxiety of crisis to fear for their sanity.

ANXIETY

Anxiety is a subjective response that occurs when a person experiences a real or perceived threat to well-being; it is a diverse feeling of dread or apprehension. There is a close relationship between anxiety and stress. Anxiety is the psychological response to a threat, such as the worry that results when an individual oversleeps on a work day. This worry can translate

Table 16-2 DEFENSE MECHANISMS

DEFENSE MECHANISM	DESCRIPTION	EXAMPLE
Denial	Refusal to acknowledge the reality of threatening situations despite factual evidence	A person with heart disease continues to eat fatty foods and fried foods, despite medical advice to the contrary.
Displacement	Transfer of feelings or reactions from one object to another object, usually one that is "safer"	A husband who is angry with his wife yells at the dog instead of dealing with his anger at his wife.
Projection	Attribution of one's own thoughts, feelings, or impulses to others	An adolescent who does not want to go with the crowd states, "My parents won't let me go."
Rationalization	Intellectual explanation or justification of ideas, feelings, or behavior	A student responds after failing a test that "The test had many trick questions on it; I really know the material."
Reaction formation	Expression of a feeling that is the opposite of one's real feeling	A client brings a gift to the nurse at whom he is really angry.
Regression	A return to a previous developmental level	A child who has not sucked her thumb in 2 years starts to do so again when admitted to the hospital.
Repression	The unconscious blocking from awareness of material that is painful or threatening	Adult's claim, despite evidence, that "I never got angry with my parents; we lived in love and harmony."
Suppression	A conscious or unconscious attempt to keep threatening or unpleasant material out of consciousness	Failure to remember a house fire during childhood.
Sublimation	Channeling of socially unacceptable impulses into socially acceptable activities	A young man who deals with aggression by playing football.

Adapted from Psychiatric Mental Health Nursing, *by N. Frisch and L. Frisch, 1998, Albany, NY: Delmar Publishers. Copyright 1998 by Delmar Publishers.*

into stress, or the person's physiologic response to a stimulus, such as rushing, perspiring, and becoming careless. Anxiety can be both an activator of stress and a response to stress: It is usually activated by stress and may, in and of itself, lead to more stress. Anxiety is a major component of mental health disturbances.

Anxiety is the most common emotional (affective) response to stress. Individuals feel anxious whenever they are threatened, even if the threat is perceived rather than actual. Anxiety occurs on a continuum; some degree of anxiety is necessary, because it serves as a motivator for adaptation. High levels of anxiety, however, can overwhelm a person and impair the ability to think and function. As the severity of anxiety increases, the person is less and less able to function (Figure 16-3). Table 16-4 describes the levels of anxiety.

Table 16-3 CHARACTERISTICS OF CRISIS

- Loss is a component of every crisis. The loss can be actual or perceived and can be related to any significant aspect of the person's life.
- A crisis is experienced as a sudden event.
- A crisis has an identifiable precipitating event.
- The situation is perceived as overwhelming or life threatening.
- Communication becomes impaired.
- The situation cannot be resolved with usual coping skills.
- Intervention is required for equilibrium to be reestablished.

From Psychiatric Nursing *(5th ed.), by H. S. Wilson and C. R. Kneisel, 1996, Menlo Park, CA: Addison-Wesley. Copyright 1996 by Addison-Wesley.*

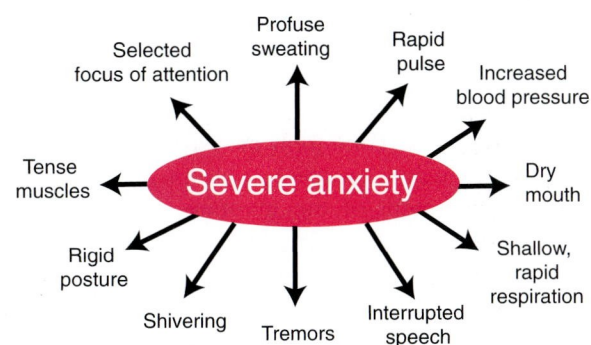

Figure 16-3 Physical and Mental Responses to Severe Anxiety. (*From* Mental Health Concepts *by C. Waughfield, 1998, Albany, NY: Delmar Publishers. Copyright 1998 by Delmar Publishers.*)

Table 16-4 LEVELS OF ANXIETY

ANXIETY LEVEL	CHARACTERISTICS OF THE ANXIOUS PERSON	NURSING IMPLICATIONS
Mild	• Increased degree of alertness • Increased vigilance • Increased motivation • Readiness for action • Slight increase in vital signs	• This is an optimal time for client teaching, because of heightened awareness and increased perceptual field.
Moderate	• Subjective distress (tension) • Decreased perception and attention • Alert only to specific information • Possible tendency to complain or argue • Possible headache, diarrhea, nausea, or vomiting	• Help the client to determine a cause-and-effect relationship between stressor and anxiety.
Severe	• Increased subjective distress • Feeling of impending danger • Selective attention • Distorted communication • Distorted perception • Feelings of fatigue	• Encourage verbalization. • Encourage motor activity. • Give specific directions.
Panic	• Major perceptual distortion • Immobilization; inability to function. • Feelings of terror • Possible harm to self and others	• Provide limits and structure. • Maintain client safety (both physical and psychological).

From Interpersonal Relations in Nursing *by H. E. Peplau, 1952, New York: Putnam and* The interpersonal theory of psychiatry *by H. S. Sullivan, 1953, New York: Norton.*

EFFECTS OF ILLNESS

Everyone experiences stress and accompanying anxiety. Anxiety increases during illness and the recovery process. Illness and stress are interwoven to such a degree that it is difficult to determine which precedes the other. When a person's adaptive attempts are unsuccessful, illness occurs. Also, a person who is ill has fewer adaptive resources available to cope with stressors. Even though some stressors may not directly cause illness, stress is a significant component in the onset and progression of many diseases. Table 16-5 lists some disorders commonly associated with stress.

One of the major outcomes of prolonged periods of stress is impairment of the immune system. As the body continues to fight off the actual or perceived threat, steroid production increases. Steroids impair the immune system's ability to function adequately. Thus, the body is less able to protect itself from disease. For example, consider the client recovering from the stress of surgery. Stress affects metabolism and protein synthesis and, thus, can result in inadequate wound healing (Poole, 1993).

All clients entering the health care system for hospitalization, surgery, or long-term care experience a change in their usual routine. Such changes may evoke anxiety, which can lead to stress.

Being in an unfamiliar environment, losing control over one's schedule, and being dependent on others for care are all issues with which hospitalized or institutionalized clients must cope. Each of these issues is a stressor that requires adaptation on the part of the client in order to maintain a steady state. Most clients

 HOME HEALTH CARE

Reducing Stressors

Remember, as a home health or visitng nurse, you are a guest in the client's home. If changes must be made in the home or the way it is kept, provide suggestions that are directly related to the client or the care of the client. Never criticize the home itself or the way it is kept.

Table 16-5 STRESS-RELATED DISORDERS

Respiratory disorders	• Emphysema • Chronic bronchitis • Asthma
Cardiovascular disorders	• Hypertension • Cardiac arrhythmias • Migraine headaches
Endocrine disorders	• Thyroid problems • Amenorrhea, anovulation • Diabetes • Excessive weight gain or weight loss
Musculoskeletal disorders	• Chronic back pain • Arthritis
Genitourinary disorders	• Enuresis • Urinary frequency
Sexual and reproductive disorders	• Low libido • Impotence • Menstrual irregularities
Gastrointestinal disorders	• Colitis • Chronic constipation • Ulcers • Gastritis
Integumentary disorders	• Eczema • Hives • Psoriasis

From Fundamentals of Nursing: Standards & Practice, *by S. DeLaune and P. Ladner, 1998, Albany, NY: Delmar Publishers. Copyright 1998 by Delmar Publishers.*

do not have the energy to cope with the numerous changes simultaneously with coping with their illnesses. Some cues that a person may be reacting adversely to hospitalization include the following:

• Increased stress response
• Increased level of anxiety
• Increased or impaired use of coping mechanisms
• Inability to function
• Disorganized behavior

Individuals do not have to be hospitalized to experience stressors associated with the client role. Consider for example the person having "minor" surgery at an outpatient center, the employee being treated at the industrial clinic for a work-related injury, or the adolescent being treated by the school nurse. Even clients who are treated through home health agencies experience stressors associated with having a health care provider enter their personal environment.

The greater the threat (or perceived threat), the greater the level of the client's anxiety. The nurse must be sensitive to stress and anxiety stemming from the multiple changes imposed by illness on the client, family, and/or significant others. The nurse's sensitivity to clients' stress reduces the risk of depersonalizing the client.

Depersonalization describes the process whereby an individual is treated as an object instead of a person. Literally, it involves taking away clients' unique aspects by treating them as nonhuman. Nursing interventions should focus on helping the client reduce feelings of unfamiliarity and loss of control.

EFFECTS OF CHANGE

Change, a dynamic process whereby an individual's response to a stressor leads to an alteration in behavior, is an inherent part of life; it is the process whereby individuals adapt. Whether it is planned or

PROFESSIONAL TIP

Promoting Client Control

• *Communicate clearly.* Use terms easily understood by clients and families. Avoid using medical jargon with clients.
• *Answer questions thoroughly.* Validate the client's and family's level of understanding.
• *Teach the use of relaxation techniques,* such as progressive muscle relaxation and guided imagery.
• *Instruct clients in the use of* **cognitive reframing** (a technique whereby the individual changes a negative perception of a situation or event to a more positive, less-threatening perception.)
• *Provide support and reassurance.* The nurse's presence ("being with" the client) can alleviate anxiety. The most therapeutic tool in alleviating client anxiety is the nurse's therapeutic use of self (Figure 16-4).
• *Break down the information shared with clients.* Providing too much information at one time can overwhelm the client, making him less likely to listen. When clients have adequate information, they can make informed decisions and maintain some degree of control over their lives.

From Fundamentals of Nursing: Standards & Practice, *by S. DeLaune and P. Ladner, 1998, Albany, NY: Delmar Publishers. Copyright 1998 by Delmar Publishers.*

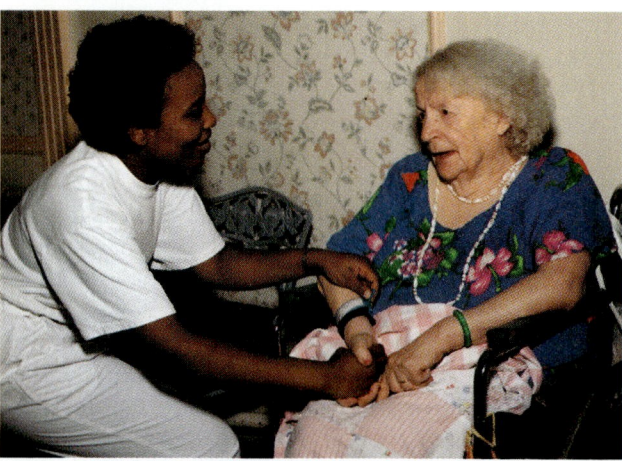

Figure 16-4 Through talking, listening, and touch, the nurse can help relieve the client's feelings of anxiety.

unplanned, change is both inevitable and constant. Change can be constructive or destructive and is stressful to individuals because it activates the GAS. Characteristics of change are that it:

- Is an inevitable part of life,
- May be eustressful or distressful,
- Can be self-initiated or externally imposed,
- Can occur abruptly or have a gradual onset and insidious progression, and
- Requires energy to effect, as well as to resist.

Nurses, and all health care providers, must be able to initiate and cope with change. Proficiency in critical-thinking and problem-solving skills is necessary for effectively initiating and coping with change.

The pace of change is rapidly increasing in health care agencies, which have been changing and continue to change in response to consumer demands. Gillies (1994) lists the following changes that have evolved from consumer demands and needs:

- Self-care units
- Abortion clinics
- Sports medicine clinics
- Substance-abuse treatment programs
- Day treatment programs for geriatric and psychiatric clients
- Weight control programs
- Exercise programs

Types of Change

Change is either planned or unplanned. Unplanned change is change that "just happens"; it is unpredictable and may be imposed by others or by uncontrollable natural events (e.g., losing one's home in a flood). Conversely, planned change results from a deliberate effort to alter a situation. A marriage is an example of a planned change. In addition to planned change and unplanned change, there are other types of change.

Developmental changes are physical and emotional alterations that occur at different stages of the life cycle. These are generally predictable and occur in a certain progression. For instance, a baby will first learn to roll over, then crawl, then walk. Whereas the exact age for each of these milestones will vary, the sequence generally does not: The majority of infants will crawl before they are able to walk.

Accidental or reactive changes are adaptive responses to external stimuli. These include an individual's efforts to cope with change imposed by others, such as a modification to one's working hours or reaction to a child's baseball game being rescheduled due to the weather.

Covert changes are often subtle and occur without a person's conscious awareness. These might include a gradual shifting of responsibilities as new skills are acquired or developed at work.

Overt changes are obvious and identifiable, and an individual is aware that they are occurring. Although overt changes are usually not under an individual's direct control, such as the restructuring of one's place of employment, the individual must adapt to and accept the new situation in order to continue functioning effectively.

Resistance to Change

Many people tend to resist change because of the energy required to adapt. Conversely, energy is also required to resist change, or to maintain the status quo. Individuals differ in their ability to tolerate (or even thrive on) change. As Gillies (1994) points out, "Most persons, even those who enjoy novelty, are discomfited by the change process, which generates anxiety by moving the person from the comfortable familiarity of the status quo to the painful uncertainty of an unknown future."

People tend to resist change for many reasons (Table 16-6). In particular, there are no absolute guarantees that the change activity will lead to positive outcomes. Uncertainty regarding outcomes is a major barrier to change.

It is risky to initiate change, to challenge one's own ideas and those of others. One of the first signs of the need for change is questioning. The nurse who wonders "Why?" "Why not?" or "What if?" is the nurse who will likely take the risk to initiate change activity. The risk taker who is effective is neither reckless nor overly cautious. Successful risk takers "weigh the costs and benefits of their actions. They consider possible outcomes in relationship to the expenditure of available resources" (Talbott, 1993).

Because change is inevitable, nurses must learn ways to deal with change. Resistance manifests as the individual rejecting proposed new ideas without criti-

Table 16-6 BARRIERS TO CHANGE

BARRIER	EXPLANATION
Conformity	Often referred to as "groupthink;" complying with the group's expectations; going along with others to avoid conflict.
Dissimilar beliefs and values	Differences in attitudes and expectations regarding health and illness behaviors; differences between client and nurse that can impede positive change.
Habits	Routine, "set" behaviors are often hard to change.
Satisfaction with status quo	Seeing only advantages to the present system can blind one to the possible need for change. Satisfaction with the way things are now reinforces resistance to change.
Threats to satisfying basic needs	Change may be perceived as a threat to self-esteem, security, or survival.
Fear	Fear of failure and fear of the unknown especially block change.
Unrealistic goals	Set up the individual for failure in change efforts.

From Fundamentals of Nursing: Standards & Practice, *by* S. DeLaune and P. Ladner, 1998, Albany, NY: Delmar Publishers. Copyright 1998 by Delmar Publishers.

cally thinking about the proposal. Nurses must be willing to take the time to research ideas and make informed decisions as to whether change is worthwhile. Coping with change of any type calls for flexibility, adaptability, and resilience.

The Nurse as Change Agent

Nurses are greatly affected by change. Nurses experience stress daily as a result of changes both within their immediate work environments and in the health care delivery system as a whole. The uncertainty over health care reform is very distressful to some nurses. Others, those with an eustressful outlook, see opportunity for positive change in the future.

In bringing about change to promote positive adaptation, the nurse serves as a **change agent** (a person who intentionally creates and implements change). True change agents constantly seek ways to make improvements. They use critical-thinking skills to develop creative, innovative solutions.

To be most effective, change should be planned and goal directed by people who are proactive. Proactive individuals initiate change rather than respond to change imposed by others. The proactive individual takes action rather than waiting for others to make decisions, solve problems, or become rescuers. On the other hand, a reactive person responds only to externally imposed change. Proactive nurses are change agents who affect the entire health care system as well as individual clients.

Change agents keep the change process moving toward a positive outcome. As an advocate for change, the nurse empowers the client to initiate change in order to adapt more successfully. Client education is a powerful tool for initiating change. Teaching a client about a disease process, a treatment modality, or a lifestyle alteration provides the client with an opportunity to change. Learning results in behavioral changes. Huebner and Nelson (1994) compare the change process to the nursing process, in that change involves assessment, planning, decision making, implementation, and evaluation.

NURSING PROCESS

Nurses can be very instrumental in helping clients both understand their anxiety and learn measures to cope with and control their feelings of stress.

Assessment

When caring for an anxious client, the nurse must first ascertain the client's perception of the situation. This is accomplished by directly asking for the client's input. The nurse must then carefully listen to the client's response. Because the nurse's nonverbal behavior can affect the client's anxiety level, nurses must be aware of their own body language. Because anxiety is a subjective experience, it cannot be directly observed. Therefore, the nurse must look for the signs indicative of anxiety (refer back to Table 16-4).

A thorough assessment of stress and anxiety levels includes eliciting client input to evaluate the following factors:

- Patterns of stressors
- Typical responses to stressful situations
- Cause-and-effect relationships among stressors and thoughts, feelings, and behaviors
- Past history of successful coping mechanisms

Assessing the client's coping abilities can be done in various ways. For example, open-ended questions can be used to determine previously used coping mechanisms. Some sample questions are as follows:

- What is the problem?
- What have you tried before?
- How well did it work?

Identification of the client's coping abilities assists in establishing appropriate nursing diagnoses and developing an effective plan of care. Assessment, which relies heavily on the nurse's observation and listening skills, provides the data necessary for formulating nursing diagnoses.

Nursing Diagnosis

Several nursing diagnoses may apply to clients experiencing anxiety; the most common of these are *anxiety; coping, ineffective individual; denial, ineffective;* and *powerlessness*. Additional North American Nursing Diagnosis Association (NANDA) (1999) diagnoses that may occur in response to stressors include:

- *Adjustment, Impaired*
- *Role Performance, Altered*
- *Thought Processes, Altered*
- *Coping, Defensive*
- *Fear*
- *Post-Trauma Syndrome*
- *Social Interaction, Impaired*
- *Spiritual Distress*
- *Hopelessness*
- *Fatigue*
- *Sleep Pattern Disturbance*

Planning/Outcome Identification

Client involvement in planning care is essential because helping clients learn to cope successfully is part of the empowerment process. Planning means exploring with the client self-responsibility issues. A major goal for intervening with an anxious client is to reduce anxiety to a level at which learning and problem solving can occur (Lehman, 1993).

Expected outcomes (goals) appropriate for clients experiencing stress or anxiety may be numerous. A good starting point is to assist the client to:

- Identify situations that increase stress and anxiety levels;
- Verbalize a plan to decrease the effects of common stressors;
- Differentiate positive and negative stressors in own life;
- Classify stressors into categories of those that can be eliminated, those that can be controlled, and those that cannot be controlled directly by self;
- Demonstrate the accurate use of select stress-management exercises (e.g., progressive muscle relaxation, guided imagery, thought stopping); and
- Verbalize a plan for stress management, including necessary lifestyle modifications.

 Safety: The Client Experiencing Panic
Never leave a panic-stricken client alone. When anxiety has reached the panic level, the client may inflict self harm. Stay with the highly anxious client or have someone else do so.

Nursing Interventions

Teaching, a major nursing intervention for managing stress, is inherent in holistic nursing practice. Stress management approaches can be taught to clients of every age and developmental stage in all health care settings: acute care (inpatient and outpatient), long-term care, and the home.

Teaching clients to reduce their own levels of stress is a major step in promoting self-care. Client education provides clients with options. Clients who have a thorough understanding of their options can make informed decisions about necessary lifestyle changes (Figure 16-5). Some of the many interventions that can be used with anxious clients follow.

Meeting Basic Needs

There is a close relationship between stress and basic physiologic needs. Anything that interferes with the satisfaction of basic needs evokes the stress response and attendant anxiety. Clients who are cold, hungry, or in pain have higher anxiety levels than do those who are comfortable. When anxiety levels increase, so does the perception of pain. Nurses who empower clients to meet basic needs are laying the foundation for a less stressful, more caring treatment process. By reducing anxiety, the nurse is actually improving the client's potential for recovery.

Minimizing Environmental Stimuli

An individual's immediate environment can influence stress levels. It is important for the nurse to decrease environmental stimuli that may contribute to anxiety. Some specific ways to limit environmental stimuli are to:

- Close the door to the client's room;
- Turn off the television;
- Lower the tone of the telephone ringer or take the phone off the hook, if feasible;
- Turn off the lights or close the blinds; and

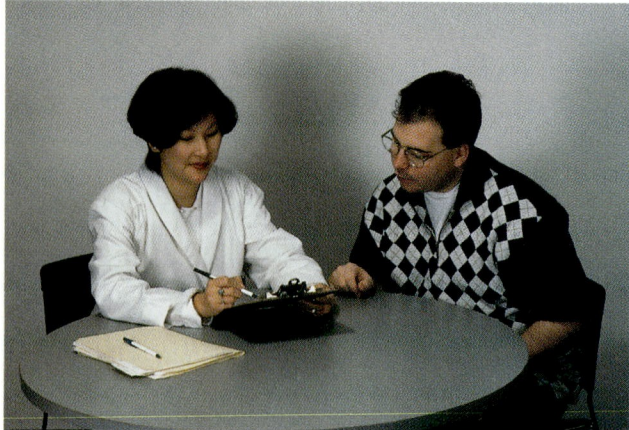

Figure 16-5 The nurse discusses the options for care and provides the client with the information needed to plan effective lifestyle changes.

• Limit the number of visitors (unless isolation increases the client's anxiety).

Verbalizing Feelings

Encouraging clients to express their feelings is especially valuable in stress reduction. Freud (1959) used the term **catharsis** to describe the process of talking out one's feelings. People instinctively know the value of "getting things off their chest" through verbalization. Verbalization promotes relaxation because: (1) when a feeling is described it becomes real, and after a problem is identified, the person can begin to deal effectively with it; and (2) the actual activity of talking uses energy and, therefore, reduces anxiety.

Involving Family and Significant Others

The client's developmental stage influences the type of intervention for stress management. Children and adolescents have varying coping skills; children of all ages need and rely on their parents or caretakers for security and support (Bru, Carmody, Donohue-Sword, & Bookbinder, 1993). It is important to include the entire family in the care of the client whenever possible (Figure 16-6). Such an approach is useful in decreasing the stress level of everyone involved, because families provide essential support for clients.

Family members who are extremely anxious often have a negative impact on the client's health status. Therefore, nurses often must help family members relax. One way to accomplish this is to provide explanations and information. Thus, it is often necessary for nurses to teach stress-management techniques to the client's family.

Using Stress-Management Techniques

A variety of stress-management techniques can easily be taught to clients, families, and significant others.

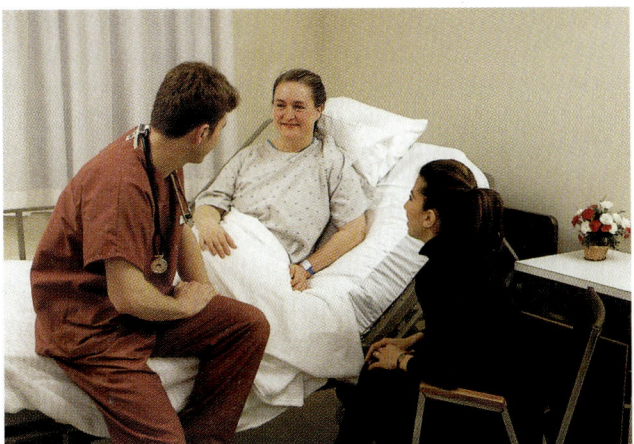

Figure 16-6 The nurse encourages the interaction of clients with family members and significant others. This involvement helps ease the client's anxiety about issues such as hospitalization and serves as a method whereby the family is kept informed about the client's care.

Some of the most common approaches for managing stress are discussed following.

Exercise   Physical exercise is a powerful way to reduce anxiety. Client teaching should emphasize the need for incorporating exercise into one's lifestyle. Guidelines for establishing an exercise program are:

• Explore the availability of different exercise programs,
• Consult with a health care provider about the safety of a specific exercise program,
• Set realistic goals,
• Plan a routine that allows for warm-up and cool-down periods using stretching exercises, and
• Engage in activity that increases heart rate for a period of time and is followed by a cool-down period.

In other words, if exercise is to reduce anxiety, it must be done on an ongoing and regular basis. The physiologic benefits of regular exercise are listed in Table 16-7. The psychological benefits of exercise include:

• Enhanced feelings of well-being,
• Improved concentration and memory,
• Reduced depression,
• Reduced insomnia,
• Reduced dependence on external stimulants or relaxants,
• Increased self-esteem, and
• Renewed sense of self-control over anxiety.

Relaxation Techniques   Several techniques can help individuals relax (Figure 16-7). Alternative and complementary interventions such as progressive muscle relaxation and guided imagery are useful in helping clients learn specific approaches to achieve relaxation. Meditation and hypnosis can also be very effective in inducing relaxation and relieving stress.

Cognitive Reframing or Thought Stopping   Cognitive reframing is a technique based on a theory

CLIENT TEACHING

Thought Stopping: A Cognitive Reframing Technique

• Listen to self-talk (thoughts).
• Recognize when the self-talk is negative.
• When a negative thought is detected, do something physical to stop the train of thought. For example, clap your hands or snap a rubber band on your wrist. Tell yourself, "Stop!"
• Replace the negative thought with one that is both positive and realistic.

Like all other relaxation exercises, thought stopping becomes more effective with repetition.

Table 16-7 PHYSIOLOGICAL BENEFITS OF EXERCISE

EFFECT OF EXERCISE	PHYSIOLOGICAL BENEFIT
Promotes metabolism of adrenalin and thyroxine	• Minimizes autonomic arousal and hypervigilance
Reduces musculoskeletal tension	• Reduces feelings of being tense and "uptight"
Improves circulation, resulting in better oxygenation of the bloodstream and the brain	• Increased alertness and concentration leading to enhanced problem-solving ability
Stimulates **endorphin** (a group of opiate-like substances produced naturally by the brain) production	• Raises the body's pain threshold, produces sedation and euphoria, and promotes a sense of well-being
Decreases cholesterol level	• Reduces the risk of atherosclerosis (a common form of arteriosclerosis characterized by the formation of plaques containing lipids, including cholesterol, on the inner walls of the arteries).
Decreases blood pressure	• Reduces risk of myocardial infarction (heart attack) and cerebral vascular accident (CVA) (stroke)
Increases acidity of blood (lowered pH)	• Improves digestion • Improves energy level • Improves utilization of food for energy (promotes metabolism)
Improves elimination (through lungs, skin, bowels)	• Reduces buildup of toxins in the body.

From "Nutrition, Exercise, and Movement," by L. Keegan, 1995, in B. Dossey, L. Keegan, C. Guzzetta, and L. Kolkmeier (Eds.), Holistic Nursing: A Handbook for Practice (2nd ed.), Gaithersburg, MD: Aspen and "Health Promotion and the Individual," by C. Mandle and R. Gruber-Wood, 1998, in C. Edelmen and C. Mandle (Eds.), Health Promotion Throughout the Lifespan (4th ed.). St. Louis, MO: Mosby.

proposed by Aaron Beck (1976), who purports that a person's emotional response is determined by the meaning attached to an event. For example, if an event is perceived to be threatening, the client is likely to feel anxious. If the interpretation of the event can be modified, the client will be less anxious. Reframing is a technique used to alter one's perceptions and interpretations by changing one's thoughts.

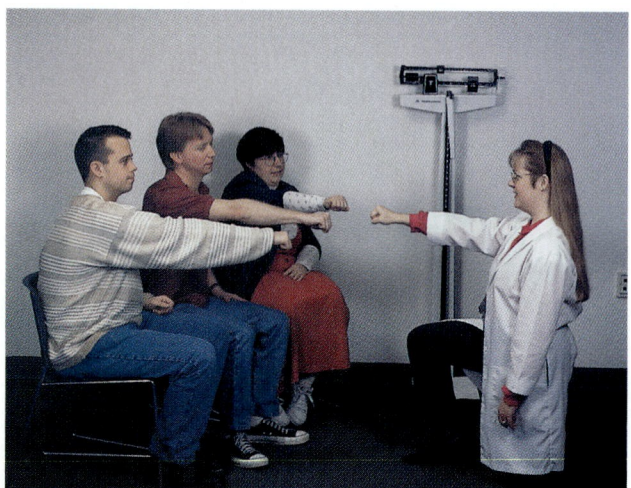

Figure 16-7 The nurse demonstrates the technique of progressive muscle relaxation in a client-education program.

Crisis Intervention

Some clients will be in an acute crisis state and require **crisis intervention**, a specific technique that helps clients regain equilibrium. Crisis intervention is a therapeutic strategy that views individuals as capable of personal growth and as having the ability to influence and control their own lives (Kneisl & Riley, 1996). The five steps of crisis intervention are illustrated in Figure 16-8).

Clients sometimes need more assistance than the nurse is able to provide. Recognition of such situations calls for prompt consultation with and, sometimes, referral to other health care providers, such as:

- Psychiatric clinical nurse specialists,
- Nurse psychotherapists,
- Psychologists,
- Social workers,
- Psychiatrists, or
- Clergy and other counselors.

Evaluation

Evaluating the effectiveness of the client's coping abilities is an ongoing, comprehensive process that must include client input. It is imperative that the nurse evaluate client outcomes as well as the process of delivering nursing care. The family can also be a

Identification of the Problem

It is necessary to be as specific as possible when naming the underlying issue(s). Being specific promotes clarity in planning.

Identification of Alternatives

Client and nurse need to list all the possible options for resolving the crisis. The greater the number of alternatives identified, the greater the likelihood of successful resolution.

Selection of an Alternative

The potential outcomes of each option are examined and one alternative is chosen.

Implementation

The selected alternative is carried out.

Evaluation

The overall effectiveness of the plan is evaluated in terms of process and outcome.

Figure 16-8 Steps of Crisis Intervention (*From* Fundamentals of Nursing: Standards & Practice, *by S. DeLaune and P. Ladner, 1998, Albany, NY: Delmar Publishers. Copyright 1998 by Delmar Publishers.*)

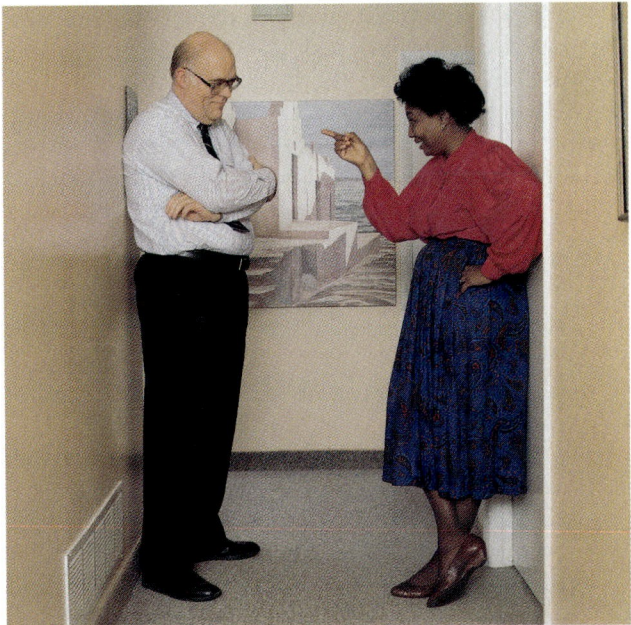

Figure 16-9 Sharing a light and humorous moment with a friend is a wonderful way to relieve stress and regain perspective.

valuable source of information when evaluating the effectiveness of different stress-reduction approaches.

PERSONAL STRESS-MANAGEMENT APPROACHES FOR THE NURSE

Many stressors are inherent in nursing. Learning to cope successfully with stressors is essential for nurses (Figure 16-9). Two major reasons nurses must cope successfully with stress are to maintain their own wellness and to model health-promoting behaviors to others. In order to help clients learn to manage stress, nurses must first be able to manage their own stress.

High stress levels among nurses are associated with **burnout**, a state of physical and emotional exhaustion that occurs when caregivers deplete their adaptive energy. Nurses who have experienced such an overwhelming degree of stress tend to treat clients in depersonalizing ways. Such nurses also lack feelings of personal accomplishment. Burnout exacts a high price not only on individual nurses themselves, but also on the profession: Highly qualified professionals leave nursing and, as a result, the quality of care declines.

Several work-related factors can contribute to the development of nursing burnout:

- Job-related stress (for example, the stress evoked by caring for dying people)
- Heavy workload
- Interpersonal conflict in the work environment
- Organizational barriers that "prohibit autonomous decision making and action" (Bowman, 1993).

Burnout prevention and recovery depend on stress management. A stress-management plan is a continuous process, not the occasional use of a technique or exercise. Development of such a plan begins with self-awareness. "A crucial first step to changing nonconstructive or self-defeating practices is the development of self-awareness" (Bowman, 1993). Nurses who care for clients extremely well often fail to take care of themselves. It is essential that nurses learn to care for themselves as well.

Other guidelines that are helpful in changing from a negative to a positive outlook (DeLaune, 1993) include the following:

- Expect to be successful
- Remember the power of self-fulfilling prophecies and deliberately focus on the positive
- Let go of the need to be perfect
- Listen to self-talk
- Encourage the use of appropriate humor in the workplace.

Nurses can use many strategies to help manage professional and personal stress, as outlined in Table 16-8

Nurses who cultivate the hardiness factor will likely be resilient to stress. Kobasa (1979) originated the concept of hardiness in the late 1970s. Hardiness consists of a set of attitudes, beliefs, and behaviors that result in individuals being more resilient (or hardy) to the negative effects of stress. There are three components to stress hardiness:

- *Commitment:* becoming involved in what one is doing
- *Challenge:* perceiving change as an opportunity for growth rather than as an obstacle or threat
- *Control:* believing that one is influential in directing what happens to oneself rather than feeling helpless and victimized

According to studies (Kobasa, 1979; Kobasa, Maddi, & Kahn, 1982), individuals who have higher degrees of hardiness are healthier than are individuals with low degrees of hardiness. Such people develop fewer illnesses when they experience multiple stressors.

PROFESSIONAL TIP

Managing Professional Stress

- Develop and maintain active support systems, both at work and away from work. Having friends who are not health care providers helps maintain a sense of balance and separateness between personal and professional domains.
- Develop time-management and decision-making skills. For example, break large tasks down into small, realistic, achievable objectives. This strategy prevents your becoming overwhelmed by the seemingly "impossible" task before you.
- Avoid consumption of noxious substances. Practice a substance-free lifestyle to effectively manage stress. Do not depend on unhealthy behaviors such as smoking, overeating, or consuming alcohol or caffeine as avenues to relaxation.
- Nourish your body with a healthy diet and adequate amounts of sleep and rest balanced with activity and exercise. Care for yourself as you would for clients.
- Maintain a sense of humor while you work. Humor helps a person maintain a positive outlook; therefore, it can be used to reframe situations so as to reduce distress.

(*From* Fundamentals of Nursing: Standards & Practice *by S. DeLaune and P. Ladner, 1998, Albany, NY: Delmar Publishers. Copyright 1998 by Delmar Publishers.*)

Many nurses must relearn the value of play and learn when to stop working. J. S. Borman (1993) refers to the 1990s as the "Age of Overwork" and states that many in the United States are adopting a 60-hour work week as normal. Nursing students, who spend many hours a week working and studying, may need to schedule some time for play. By doing so, the student nurse will make a start on managing stress and, thereby, become a more effective care provider.

Table 16-8 STRATEGIES FOR COPING WITH PROFESSIONAL STRESS

STRATEGY	RATIONALE
Using time management methods	When own needs are seen as priorities; you are more likely to schedule time to meet those needs. Time should especially be scheduled to meet highly valued needs.
Focusing on accomplishments instead of the uncompleted tasks	Focusing on unfinished business increases anxiety; paying attention to successes boosts self-esteem.
Practicing slow, focused breathing	Such breathing alleviates muscle tension by increasing the amount of oxygenated blood. Also, consciously thinking about own breathing serves as a diversionary tactic.
Avoiding assumption of responsibility where you have none	You will be less prone to play the role of rescuer who takes on the problems of others.
Knowing your limits	By clarifying your expectations, strengths, and limitations, you will learn to differentiate those things that are really important from the "small stuff" and know when a problem is beyond your control and find ways to accept the problem until you have the resources to deal with it.
Whenever possible, removing yourself from stressors that have a negative impact	Exposure to needless stress and subsequent draining of adaptive resources are minimized.
Identifying and changing the stressors that you can directly influence	Sense of personal power increases, and needless expenditure of energy decreases.
Varying tasks between physical and mental activities	You conserve energy, and the resultant reduction in fatigue helps restore a sense of balance.

From "Tips for Managing Stress on the Job," by J. Badger, 1995, American Journal of Nursing, *95(9), 31–33 and "Burnout: Why Do We Blame the Nurse?" by A. Cullen, 1995,* American Journal of Nursing, *95(11), 23–27.*

SAMPLE NURSING CARE PLAN

THE CLIENT EXPERIENCING ANXIETY

Kathryn is a 38-year-old female who is seeking treatment in the emergency department of a metropolitan hospital. She is tearful, pacing, and wringing her hands. She is complaining of severe chest pain, a pounding headache, and back pain. She is sweating profusely and exhibits fine hand tremors. Her blood pressure and pulse are elevated, and her respirations are rapid and shallow. She says that she hasn't slept well since her husband left her 3 months ago. She states, "I'm afraid I'm losing my mind! My heart is racing and I can't sit still. Help me! I feel like I'm going to die."

Assessment reveals autonomic hyperactivity (rapid pulse, elevated blood pressure), verbalized feelings of apprehension and uneasiness, and restlessness.

Nursing Diagnosis *Anxiety related to threat to self-concept and change in role functioning as evidenced by statement "I'm afraid I'm losing my mind" and the fact that husband left her 3 months ago*

PLANNING/GOALS	NURSING INTERVENTION	RATIONALE	EVALUATION
Kathryn will identify effective coping mechanisms.	Establish a trusting relationship.	Kathryn may perceive the nurse or emergency department as a threat, and, thus, anxiety will increase.	Kathryn is visibly relaxed. Vital signs are within normal limits. Kathryn verbalizes that she is calmer and no longer afraid that she is "losing her mind" or "going to die."
	Have Kathryn identify and describe physical and emotional feelings.	The first step in coping with anxiety is to recognize the anxiety and become aware of feelings in order to link emotions to maladaptive coping responses.	
	Help Kathryn relate cause-and-effect relationships between stressors and anxiety.	Increases Kathryn's sense of control and power over the situation.	
	Encourage Kathryn to use coping mechanisms that have been successful previously.	Increases confidence in own abilities to cope.	
Kathryn will report that anxiety is reduced to a manageable level.	Using therapeutic communication techniques, encourage Kathryn to talk about what has been happening in her life.	Talking about a situation often clarifies it.	

continued

Kathryn will demonstrate relaxation skills.	Teach Kathryn relaxation techniques (such as imagery and meditation).	The relaxation response is the opposite of the stress response and, therefore, counters the physiologic effects of the stress response. The relaxation response leads to lowered blood pressure, decreased heart rate, and deeper and slower respirations.

CASE STUDY

Miguel, a 35-year-old lawyer, comes to the emergency medical facility and describes vomiting small amounts of blood for the past several days. He also says that he has been having heartburn and epigastric pain for 3 weeks. The initial interview reveals that his wife asked for a divorce 6 weeks ago because of his long hours at work, which keep him away from the family. He also states that he is working on a very difficult lawsuit.

Vital signs are T 98.6, P 90, R 24, and BP 136/82. A complete blood count and upper GI exam are ordered. He is scheduled to see a clinical specialist to discuss the stressors in his life. At the initial screening, Miguel relates that he has been experiencing frequent headaches and is having difficulty concentrating on his court case, symptoms of moderate to severe anxiety.

(Adapted from Mental Health Concepts, *by C. Waughfield, 1998, Albany, NY: Delmar Publishers.)*

The following questions will guide your development of a nursing care plan for the case study.

1. What clinical manifestations indicate that Miguel is experiencing moderate to severe anxiety?
2. What two nursing diagnoses might be appropriate for Miguel?
3. What goal for each nursing diagnosis might be desirable?
4. What nursing interventions would be helpful to Miguel in meeting the goals?
5. How will the evaluation be determined?

SUMMARY

- Stress is an individual's physiologic response to stimuli.
- Individuals who experience prolonged periods of stress are at risk for developing stress-related diseases.
- Anxiety, the psychological response to a threat to the health and well-being of an individual, activates the stress response.
- An individual seeks equilibrium through the process of adaptation. When adaptation is effective, homeostasis (the body's self-regulation of physiologic processes) is maintained.
- Many factors, such as physiologic, psychological, cognitive, or environmental changes, contribute to stress.

- The general adaptation syndrome (GAS), the physiologic response to stress, consists of three stages: alarm, resistance, and exhaustion. The GAS is the same whether the stressor is actual or imagined, present or potential.
- Illness and hospitalization are major stressors for individuals and their families. To alleviate the stress of hospitalization, nursing interventions should reduce the client's feelings of unfamiliarity and loss of control.
- Change can be perceived as stressful because of a fear of failure, a threat to security, or a potential for loss of self-esteem.
- Nursing interventions that promote positive adaptation to stress are to empower clients to meet basic needs; minimize environmental stimuli; encourage verbalization of feelings; include family members

and significant others in client care; and use various stress-management techniques such as progressive muscle relaxation (PMR) and guided imagery.

- Burnout occurs when the nurse is overwhelmed by stress. As a result, the nurse experiences physical, emotional, and behavioral dysfunction, including decreased productivity.
- A stress-management plan for professional nurses involves maintaining support systems; developing time-management and decision-making skills; identifying and changing stressors that can be managed; and knowing personal limits.

Review Questions

1. Physiologic indicators of anxiety include:
   a. warm, dry skin.
   b. constricted pupils.
   c. increased pulse rate.
   d. decreased blood pressure.

2. The body's reaction to any demand made on it (stimulus) is called:
   a. stress.
   b. anxiety.
   c. stressor.
   d. stress response.

3. A major component of mental health disturbances is:
   a. worry.
   b. stress.
   c. anxiety.
   d. adaptation.

4. The general adaptation syndrome (GAS) is the:
   a. behavioral response to stress.
   b. sociocultural response to stress.
   c. psychological response to stress.
   d. physiologic response to stress.

5. The level of anxiety best for client learning is:
   a. no anxiety.
   b. mild anxiety.
   c. severe anxiety.
   d. moderate anxiety.

6. Most defense mechanisms are used unconsciously. The one that is consciously used is:
   a. projection.
   b. regression.
   c. repression.
   d. suppression.

7. The purpose of the first stage of the GAS is to:
   a. alert the individual to danger.
   b. determine the cause of the danger.
   c. mobilize energy needed for adaptation.
   d. prevent the individual from having an unpleasant experience.

8. Symptoms associated with the response to stress are the result of the body's attempt to:
   a. conserve energy.
   b. run from the impending threat.
   c. identify the impending danger.
   d. shield the person from an unpleasant experience.

9. Coping mechanisms to avoid dealing directly with stress are called:
   a. adaptive measures.
   b. maladaptive measures.
   c. nonadaptive measures.
   d. progressive measures.

Critical Thinking Questions

1. Describe the way that you would explain the relationship between stress and illness to a client.

2. A client is exhibiting panic-level anxiety, and you do not want him left alone. You are experiencing severe burnout because of very long work hours and stressful situations that have recently occurred with clients and with other nurses. Your stress level is so high that you feel you cannot even be in the same room with this upset client. If you leave the room to find another nurse to stay with him, he may injure himself; if you stay, you risk your own emotional well-being. How do you deal with this situation?

3. Society often labels people who take care of themselves as selfish. Do you agree? Why or why not? Consider how taking care of yourself can help you be a better care provider to others. What are some specific things you can do now to take better care of yourself?

WEB FLASH!

- Search the Web for information on stress and anxiety. What sites might you recommend to clients and families who are experiencing anxiety and looking for self-help and information sources?
- What resources are listed for caregivers and health care professionals?
- What organizations or professional journals might you search for information on anxiety or stress?

CHAPTER 17

LOSS, GRIEF, AND DEATH

MAKING THE CONNECTION

Refer to the following chapters to increase your understanding of loss, grief, and death:

- **Chapter 1, Holistic Care**
- **Chapter 6, Legal Responsibilities**
- **Chapter 7, Ethical Responsibilities**
- **Chapter 11, Client Teaching**
- **Chapter 12, Cultural Diversity and Nursing**

- **Chapter 13, Alternative/Complementary Therapies**
- **Chapter 16, Stress, Adaptation, and Anxiety**
- **Chapter 56, Rehabilitation, Home Health, Long-Term Care, and Hospice**

LEARNING OBJECTIVES

Upon completion of this chapter, you should be able to:
- *Define key terms.*
- *Describe various losses that affect individuals at different stages of the life cycle.*
- *Describe the characteristics of an individual experiencing grief.*
- *Differentiate adaptive grief and pathological grief.*
- *Discuss theoretical perspectives of loss, grief, and death.*
- *Discuss use of the nursing process with a grieving individual.*
- *Discuss the holistic needs of the dying person and his family.*
- *Define the purpose of hospice care.*
- *Develop a plan of care for a dying client.*
- *Discuss nursing responsibilities when a client dies.*
- *Describe ways that nurses can cope with their own grief.*

KEY TERMS

algor mortis	hospice
anticipatory grief	life review
autopsy	liver mortis
bereavement	loss
breakthrough pain	maturational loss
Cheyne-Stokes respirations	mortuary
complicated grief	mourning
death rattle	palliative care
disenfranchised grief	post-mortem care
dysfunctional grief	resuscitation
grief	rigor mortis
grief work	shroud
Health Care Surrogate Law	situational loss
	uncomplicated grief

INTRODUCTION

In contemporary society, individuals constantly experience loss. Frequent episodes of terrorism, natural disaster, and personal crises result in the universal experience of loss. It can be overwhelming to think about real and potential losses. Nurses must be aware of the potential for loss in today's world, as well as the processes whereby individuals react and adapt to losses.

Throughout the life cycle, people are faced with loss, without which growth would not continue. Many people consider loss only in terms of death and dying; however, loss of every type occurs daily.

Every day, nurses encounter clients who are responding to grief associated with losses. Nurses must have an understanding of the major concepts related to loss and grieving. Grief is a response to losses of all types. However, this chapter focuses on grief as a response to death. Nurses also care for dying clients. Thus, this chapter also provides information on meeting the special needs of terminally ill clients and their families.

LOSS

Loss is any situation, either actual, potential, or perceived, wherein a valued object or person is changed or is no longer accessible to the individual. Because change is a major constant in life, everyone experiences losses. Loss can be actual (e.g., a spouse is lost through divorce) or anticipated (a person is diagnosed with a terminal illness and has only a short time to live). A loss can be tangible or intangible. For example, when a person is fired from a job, the tangible loss is income, whereas the loss of self-esteem is intangible.

Losses also occur as a result of moving from one developmental stage to another. An example of such a **maturational loss** is the adolescent who loses the younger child's freedom from responsibility. Other examples of losses associated with growth and development are discussed later in this chapter. A **situational loss** occurs in response to external events usually beyond the individual's control (such as the death of a significant other).

Types of Loss

Not everyone responds to loss in the same way because the significance of the lost object or person is determined by individual perceptions. There are many types of loss, including:

- *Actual loss:* loss of someone or something, such as the death of a loved one or the theft of one's property.
- *Perceived loss:* sense of loss felt by an individual but not tangible to others, such as the perceived loss of self-esteem of a student who was not accepted into a nursing program.
- *Physical loss:* loss of a part or aspect of the body, such as the loss of an extremity in an accident, scarring from burns, or permanent injury.
- *Psychological loss:* emotional loss, such as a woman feeling inadequate after menopause and resultant infertility.

There are four major categories of loss: loss of external objects, loss of familiar environment, loss of aspects of self, and loss of significant other.

Loss of an External Object

When an object that a person highly values is damaged or changed or disappears, loss occurs. The significance of the lost object to the individual determines the type and amount of grieving that occurs. For instance, an individual who loses a family heirloom in a fire may react not only to the lost financial value of the piece, but also to the lost sense of history and heritage that the piece represented.

Loss of Familiar Environment

The loss of a familiar environment occurs when a person moves away from familiar surroundings, for instance to another home or a different community, to a new school, or to a new job. A client who is hospitalized or institutionalized may also experience loss when faced with new surroundings. This type of loss evokes anxiety related to fear of the unknown.

Loss of Aspect of Self

Loss of an aspect of self can be psychological or physiological. Examples of psychological aspects of self that may be lost include ambition, a sense of humor, or enjoyment of life. These feelings of loss may result from life events such as losing a job or failing at a task that the individual deems important. Physiological loss includes loss of physical function or loss resulting from disfigurement or disappearance of a body part, as is the case with amputation or mastectomy. Loss of a physiological aspect of self can result from illness, trauma, or treatment methodologies such as surgery.

Loss of Significant Other

The loss of a loved one is a significant loss. Such a loss can result from separation, divorce, running away, moving to a different area, or death. This chapter focuses on the loss of a significant other as a result of death.

GRIEF

Grief, a series of intense physical and psychological responses that occur following a loss, is a normal, natural, necessary, and adaptive response to a loss. Loss leads to the adaptive process of **mourning,** the period of time during which grief is expressed and resolution and integration of the loss occur. **Bereavement** is the period of grief following the death of a loved one (Figure 17-1).

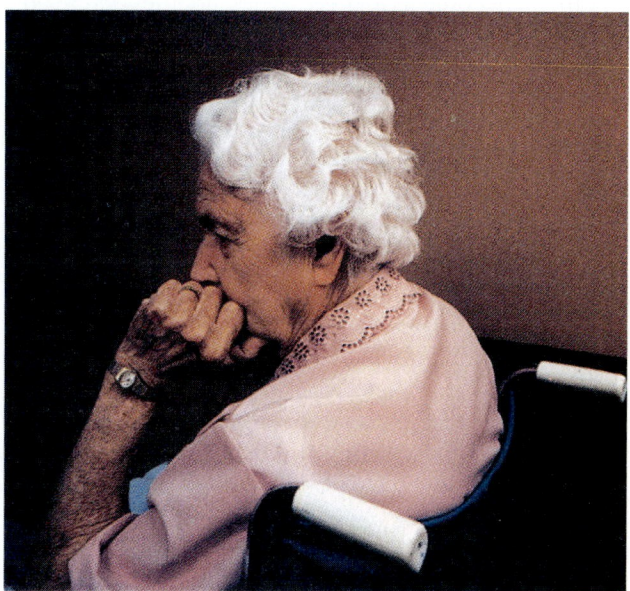

Figure 17-1 Older adults may grieve intensely over the loss of a person or situation that has been a part of their life for many years.

Theories of the Grieving Process

Several theoretical models describe grieving. The theories of Erich Lindemann, George L. Engle, John Bowlby, and J. William Worden are discussed in the following sections.

Lindemann

Following the Coconut Grove fire in Boston in 1944, Lindemann studied survivors and their families. Lindemann coined the phrase **grief work,** which is still used today to describe the process experienced by the bereaved. During grief work, the person experiences freedom from attachment to the deceased, becomes reoriented to the environment where the deceased is no longer present, and establishes new relationships (Lindemann, 1944). Lindemann's classic work is the basis of current crisis and grief resolution theories. Lindemann (1944) and Roach and Nieto (1997) describe Lindemann's theory of a person's reactions to normal grief as:

- *Somatic distress*: The bereaved experience episodic waves of discomfort in durations of 10 to 60 minutes; multiple somatic complaints; fatigue; and extreme physical or emotional pain.
- *Preoccupation with the image of the deceased:* The bereaved experience a sense of unreality, emotional detachment from others, and an overwhelming preoccupation with visualizing the deceased.
- *Guilt:* The bereaved consider the death to be a result of their own negligence or lack of attentiveness; they look for evidence of how they could have contributed to the death.
- *Hostile reactions:* The bereaved's relationships with others become impaired owing to the bereaved's desire to be left alone and the bereaved's feelings of irritability and anger.
- *Loss of patterns of conduct:* The bereaved exhibit generalized restlessness and an inability to sit still; they continually search for something to do.

Engle

Grief is a typical reaction to loss of a valued object. According to Engle, there are three stages of mourning, and progression through each stage is necessary for healing. The grieving process, which may take several years to complete, cannot be accelerated. The goal of the grieving process is for the mourner to accept the loss and let go of the deceased. Engle (1961, 1964) and Roach and Nieto (1997) outline Engle's theory of grief as follows:

- *Stage I: Shock and Disbelief* (can last from minutes to days)
    Disorientation
    Feeling of helplessness

Denial, which provides protection until the person is able to face reality

- *Stage II: Developing Awareness* (may last from 6 to 12 months)
    Guilt
    Sadness
    Isolation
    Loneliness
    Feelings of helplessness
    Possible anger and hostility toward others
    Increasing emotional pain in response to increasing reality of loss
    Recognition that one is powerless to change the situation

- *Stage III: Restitution and Resolution* (marks the beginning of the healing process; may take up to several years)
    Emergence of bodily symptoms
    Possible idealization of the deceased
    Beginnings of coming to terms with the loss
    Establishment of new social patterns and relationships

Bowlby

According to Bowlby, grief results when an individual experiences a disruption in attachment to a love object. His theory proposes that grief occurs when attachment bonds are severed. The four phases of grieving as cited by Bowlby are:

- Numbness,
- Yearning and searching,
- Disorganization and despair, and
- Reorganization (Bowlby, 1982)

Worden

Worden has identified four tasks that an individual must perform in order to successfully deal with a loss:

- Accept the fact that the loss is real
- Experience the emotional pain of grief
- Adjust to an environment without the deceased
- Reinvest the emotional energy once directed at the deceased into another relationship (Worden, 1991)

Types of Grief

Grief is a universal, normal response to loss. Grief drains people, both emotionally and physically. Because grief requires so much emotional energy, relationships may suffer (Wong, 1996). There are different types of grief, including uncomplicated ("normal"), dysfunctional, anticipatory, and disenfranchised grief.

Nurses play an important role in assisting mourners to develop and understand the normal grieving process and the complex feelings exhibited when grief becomes more complicated. Nurses with a sound knowledge base of both normal grief and dysfunctional grief are better prepared to assist survivors than are nurses who mistakenly believe that all grief is the same.

Uncomplicated Grief

Uncomplicated grief is what many individuals would refer to as *normal grief*. Engle (1961) states that the grief reaction is similar to other physical conditions and draws a parallel between a disease process and the grief process. Both include:

- A common etiologic factor (e.g., loss precipitates grief),
- A predictable symptomatology and course,
- Functional impairment for a period of time, and
- Distress and inability to function normally.

Engle (1961) proposed use of the term **uncomplicated grief** to describe a grief reaction that normally follows a significant loss. Uncomplicated grief runs a fairly predictable course that ends with the relinquishing of the lost object and the resumption of the duties of life. Some of the common reactions experienced by grieving individuals are cited in Table 17-1.

Many grieving people experience feelings of anger or blame; these feelings may be directed toward those perceived to have caused or contributed to the death. Often, the anger associated with grief is directed at one's self, that is, expressed as guilt or depression. Even though the bereaved have done nothing to cause the death, "they often believe that somehow they should have been able to prevent it" (MacGregor, 1994). Some survivors have a strong need to assign blame. If someone else can be blamed, the survivors can rid themselves of any responsibility (Figure 17-2).

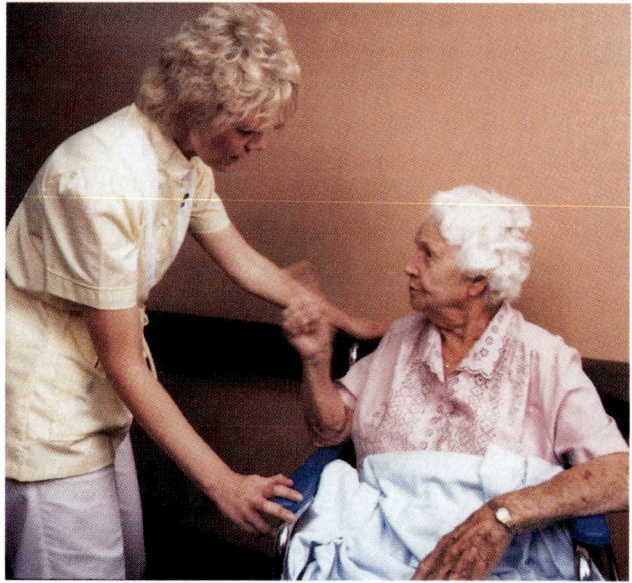

Figure 17-2 Anger is often a response to grief. This nurse is trying to help this client work through the anger she feels following a loss.

Dysfunctional Grief

Dysfunctional grief is a demonstration of a persistent pattern of intense grief that does not result in reconciliation of feelings. Persons experiencing dysfunctional (or pathological) grief do not progress through the stages of overwhelming emotions associated with grief and may fail to demonstrate any behaviors commonly associated with grief. The person experiencing pathological grief continues to have strong emotional reactions, does not return to a normal sleep pattern or work routine, usually remains isolated, and displays altered eating habits. The bereaved may have the need to endlessly tell and retell the story of loss but without subsequent healing. The pathologically

Table 17-1 REACTIONS COMMONLY EXPERIENCED DURING GRIEF (ENGLE)			
PHYSICAL REACTIONS	**PSYCHOSOCIAL REACTIONS**	**COGNITIVE REACTIONS**	**BEHAVIORAL REACTIONS**
• Loss of appetite • Insomnia • Fatigue • Decreased libido • Decreased immune functioning (increased susceptibility to illness) • Multiple somatic complaints (e.g., headache, backache) • Restlessness	• Profound sadness • Helplessness • Hopelessness • Denial • Anger • Hostility • Guilt • Nightmares • Ennui (overwhelming sense of emptiness) • Preoccupation with lost object • Loneliness	• Inability to concentrate • Forgetfulness • Impaired judgment • Decreased problem-solving ability	• Impulsivity • Indecisiveness • Social withdrawal • Distancing

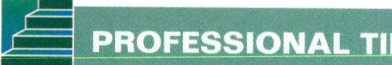

PROFESSIONAL TIP

Identifying Dysfunctional Grief

The difference between normal and dysfunctional grief is that the person experiencing dysfunctional grief is unable to adapt to life without the deceased person.

Dysfunctional grief can take several forms, specifically absent grief, distorted grief, or converted grief.

Absent grief is the inability of the person to incorporate the reality of the death into his life. This blocking of reality leads to an incapacity to feel.

Distorted grief blocks the progress of adaptive grieving. The person becomes "stuck" in feelings of guilt and anger, two emotions that are most likely to become distorted. This type of dysfunctional grief usually occurs when the relationship with the deceased was ambivalent or dependent and issues were left unresolved.

Converted grief occurs when the anxiety is expressed as distressing symptoms without the bereaved's being aware of the relationship between the symptom and the loss. The manifestations have no organic basis and can consist of:

- Somatic symptoms: fatigue, headache, tension, sleep changes, weight fluctuations, loss of libido;
- Psychological symptoms: anger, mood instability, diminished coping ability, depression, loss of sense of humor, inability to relax;
- Attitudinal changes: rigid thinking, cynicism, criticism, lack of concern, apathy; and
- Relational differences: irritability, decreased frustration tolerance, distancing.

grieving person is unable to reestablish a routine. Visits to the gravesite or mausoleum may be made often or not at all. A person experiencing dysfunctional grief continues to focus on the deceased, may overvalue objects that belonged to the deceased, and may engage in depressive brooding.

The professional caregiver must be aware of these behaviors and refer the pathologically grieving person to professional counseling.

Anticipatory Grief

Anticipatory grief is the occurrence of grief work before an expected loss actually occurs. Anticipatory grief may be experienced by the terminally ill person as well as the person's family. This phenomenon promotes adaptive grieving and, therefore, frees up the mourner's emotional energy necessary for problem solving. Although anticipatory grieving may be helpful in adjusting to the loss, it also has some potential disadvantages. For example, in the case of the dying client, anticipatory grieving may lead to family members' distancing themselves and not being available to provide support. Also, if the family members have separated themselves emotionally from the dying client, they may seem cold and distant, and, thus, not meet society's expectations of mourning behavior. This response can, in turn, prevent the mourners from receiving their own much needed support from others (Prichett & Lucas, 1997).

Disenfranchised Grief

Doka, Rushton, and Thorstenson (1994) describe **disenfranchised grief** as "grief that is not openly acknowledged, socially sanctioned, or publicly shared." Grief can become disenfranchised when an individual either is reluctant to recognize the sense of loss and develops guilt feelings or feels pressured by society to "get on with life." An example of disenfranchised grief is extreme sadness over the loss of a pet when this mourning might be viewed by others as excessive or inappropriate. A mother's sadness over a miscarriage might also be considered disenfranchised grief, as a lengthy period of mourning may not be publicly expected despite the mother's intense feelings of loss and despair.

Factors Affecting Loss and Grief

Studies (Corless, Germino, & Pittman, 1995) conducted to determine factors that influence grieving identify the following variables as possibly affecting the intensity and duration of grieving:

- Developmental stage
- Religious and cultural beliefs
- Relationship with the lost object
- Cause of death

Developmental Stage

Depending on the client's place on the age/development continuum, the grief response to a loss will be experienced differently. Nurses practice in many settings where children, adolescents, and adults, as a result of growth and development, experience changes that result in loss. For example, a pregnant woman will, to some degree, experience loss after delivery of a first child (loss of freedom, independence, and self-focused life), even when the child is normal and healthy. Certain kinds of loss at key developmental points may have a profound effect on a person's ability to both work through the resulting grief and achieve the tasks of the given developmental stage. For example, an adolescent who has lost a parent may have difficulty forming an intimate relationship with members of the opposite sex.

Childhood   Children vary in their reactions to loss and in the ability to comprehend the meaning of death. It is important to understand the way a child's concept of death evolves, because the concept varies with developmental level and may affect mastery of developmental tasks (Table 17-2).

Children who are grieving need explanations about death that are honest and in terms they can comprehend.

Adolescence   Most adolescents value physical attractiveness and athletic abilities. Grief may occur when the adolescent suffers the loss of a body part or function. Because of the strong influence of peer groups, adolescents seek approval of their friends, and they fear being rejected if a loss affects their acceptance by others (e.g., grief after a disfiguring accident is usually intense in adolescents). Even though they have an intellectual understanding of death, adolescents believe themselves to be invulnerable and, thus, immune to death; they reject the possibility of their own mortality.

Early Adulthood   In the young adult, grief is usually precipitated by loss of role or status. For example, unemployment or the breakup of a relationship

LIFE CYCLE CONSIDERATIONS

Talking with Children about Death

- *Avoid the use of euphemisms.* For example, telling a child that the deceased person has "gone away" may encourage the child to believe that the dead person will return. Also, telling a child that the deceased is "asleep" may lead to the development of sleep phobia in the child.
- *Do not overexplain.* Keep explanations factual and concise; do not offer lengthy explanations of medical conditions.
- *Use simple, concrete terms.* Young children are not able to conceptualize abstract ideas such as "grandma is in a better place now."
- *Show them.* Often, young children do not understand something until they see it. Take them to the funeral home and cemetery.

(*Data from* The 1996 National Directory of Bereavement Support Groups and Services, *by M. M. Wong, 1996, Forest Hills, NY: ADM Publishing.*)

Table 17-2 PERCEPTION OF DEATH BY CHILDREN AND ADOLESCENTS

DEVELOPMENTAL STAGE	PERCEPTION	POTENTIAL DEVELOPMENTAL DISRUPTIONS
Infancy, toddlerhood	• Is not aware of death • Is aware of disruptions in normal routine • Can react to family's expressions of grief	• Death of primary caregiver during the first 2 years of life may have significant long-lasting psychosocial implications.
Preschool	• Views death as temporary separation • Is able to react to the gravity of death in accordance with the reactions of parents or others	• Loss of either parent may have significant psychosocial implications, especially between ages 4 and 6 years (owing to *magical thinking,* wherein children may believe death is their fault). • Problems with development of sexual identity, depending on the gender of the parent lost, the child's identification with that parent, and the child's present state of sexual identity.
School-age	• Appreciates that death is final and inevitable • Fantasizes about and tends to personify death ("the boogie-man")	• Potential nightmares. • Potential death-avoidance behaviors (e.g., hiding under the covers, leaving the lights on, closing closet doors). • Possible intense guilt and a sense of responsibility for the death.
Preadolescence and adolescence	• Recognizes that death is final • Understands that death is inevitable • *Preadolescents:* tend to worry about dying; *adolescents:* tend to deny that death could happen to them	• Loss of a parent may interfere with mastery of the young-adulthood task of forming an intimate relationship with members of the opposite sex

From Fundamentals of Nursing: Standards & Practice, *by S. DeLaune and P. Ladner, 1998, Albany, NY: Delmar Publishers. Copyright 1998 by Delmar Publishers.*

may cause significant grief for the young adult. The concept of death in this age group is primarily a reflection of cultural values and spiritual beliefs.

Middle Adulthood   During middle adulthood, the potential for experiencing loss increases. The death of parents often occurs during this developmental phase. As an individual ages, it can be especially threatening when peers die, because these deaths force acknowledgment of one's own mortality.

Late Adulthood   During late adulthood, most individuals recognize the inevitability of death. It is challenging for elders to experience the death of age-old friends or to find themselves the last one of their peer group left living. Older adults often turn to their children and grandchildren as sources of comfort and companionship. Cultivating friendships in all age groups helps prevent loneliness and depression.

Religious and Cultural Beliefs

Religious and cultural beliefs can have a significant effect on an individual's grief experience. Every culture has certain religious beliefs about the significance of death, as well as rituals for care of the dying. Beliefs about an afterlife, a supreme being, redemption of the soul, and reincarnation are important aspects that can assist one in grief work.

Relationship with the Lost Object

In general, the more intimate the relationship with the deceased, the more intense the grief experienced by the bereaved. The death of a child poses a particular risk for dysfunctional grieving:

> One of life's saddest and deepest losses is the death of a child. . . . Without denying the seriousness of the loss in any death, there is an increased understanding that, at least in our culture, loss of a child represents a more severe and longer-lasting kind of injury and, because of this, is more difficult for the parents to process and resolve. (MacGregor, 1994)

The death of a child is generally thought to be exceptionally painful because it upsets the natural order of things; parents do not expect their children to die before them.

Individuals experiencing parental grief usually have intense reactions and responses (Figure 17-3). The uniqueness of parental grief for a deceased child may lie in the loss of the perceived potential of that child. It is the loss of the hopes of the parents for the child, for "the things that could have been." Table 17-3 lists characteristics of parents of infants and children who have died.

The death of a parent or a sibling can pose a major challenge for children. The child's feelings may often go unrecognized by adults who fail to understand the child's need to mourn. Normal reactions of a child

CULTURAL CONSIDERATIONS

Rituals following Death

- Judaism practices burial of the dead within 24 hours. A 7-day period of mourning, called *Shiva,* begins the day of the funeral.
- In the Muslim faith, men wash the body of a man and women wash the body of a woman after death.
- Buddhists believe that after death, the body should not be disturbed by movement, talking, or crying.
- Hindus pour holy water into the mouth of the dying person. The eldest son arranges for the funeral and cremation within 24 hours of death. Embalming is forbidden.
- Jehovah's Witnesses believe that the soul dies with the body, but 144,000 will be resurrected at the end-time and will be born again as spiritual sons of God.
- Native Americans believe that the spirit lives on after death. Ancestor worship is practiced.

(*From* Health Assessment & Physical Examination, *by M. E. Z. Estes, 1998, Albany, NY: Delmar Publishers. Copyright 1998 by Delmar Publishers.*)

whose sibling has died as an infant along with nursing responses to those reactions are delineated in Table 17-4.

Cause of Death

The intensity of the grief response also varies according to the cause of death, be it unexpected, traumatic, or a suicide.

Unexpected Death   The loss occurring as a result of an unexpected death poses particular difficulty for the bereaved in achieving closure. As Roach and

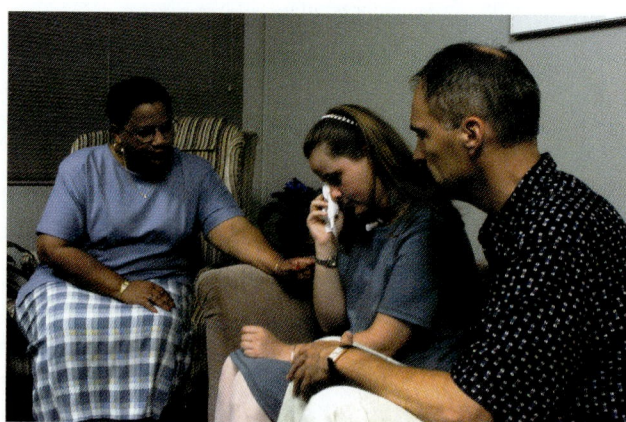

Figure 17-3 This couple discusses their grief over the loss of their child.

Table 17-3 CHARACTERISTICS OF PARENTS WHOSE CHILDREN DIE

TYPE OF DEATH	PARENTAL CHARACTERISTICS
Miscarriage and stillbirth	• Parents, especially the mother, may have feelings of intense sadness, anger, or guilt. The death is often inadequately recognized by others, especially if the loss occurs in early weeks of pregnancy. • The death may be considered a personal failure. • Parents may dwell on details, designating blame to themselves or others. • Grief from previous miscarriages may be relived. • Anticipatory grief may occur if the condition of the infant is known early in the pregnancy. • Ambivalence about being pregnant, experienced early in the pregnancy, may increase grief. • Hopes for the future must be modified or changed. • Despair may peak when the parents must leave the hospital or birthplace without the baby.
Neonatal death	• Feelings are similar to those associated with stillbirth. • Parents have had the time to form a bond with the infant, intensifying the grief. • Grief may be intense for both parents.
Sudden infant death syndrome (SIDS)	• Parents are in a state of shock. • Pain is increased by lack of knowledge and misinformation. • Because SIDS usually occurs during the first 6 months of life, parental bonding is complete. • Guilt may be present. • Police may investigate, adding to the guilt. • Grief is acute, because the death is sudden and the parents are not prepared for the loss. • Parents, especially the mother, may be preoccupied with the details of the death.
Abortion	• Shame, secrecy, and guilt may accompany grief. • Highly ambivalent feelings may be present. • Little support or comfort is offered by others. • Feelings of relief are expected, but despair and depression may surface. • No guilt may be felt, especially if the woman did not want a child.

From Healing and the Grief Process, *by S. S. Roach and B. C. Nieto, 1997, Albany, NY: Delmar Publishers. Copyright 1997 by Delmar Publishers.*

Table 17-4 REACTION OF SIBLINGS AFTER INFANT DEATH

NORMAL REACTION	NURSING RESPONSE
• Fear of separation from and loss of parents	• Provide reassurance that parents will not abandon them
• Guilt, secondary to feelings of jealousy and anger and to magical thinking in relation to a wish that the infant would go away	• Provide information (at the appropriate level of comprehension) to reassure them that they did not contribute to the cause of death
• Fear about personal needs (that the intensity of parental reactions will interfere with parents' ability to take care of them)	• Continue routine activities to provide assurance that life will go on
• Concern over own health and fear of dying soon	• Encourage parents to avoid overprotectiveness, which reinforces children's fears

Data adapted from "Supporting Families after Sudden Infant Death," by M. McClain and J. Shaefer, 1996, Journal of Psychosocial Nursing and Mental Health Services, *24(4), 30–34.*

Nieto (1997) state, any death, even an anticipated death, is a traumatic experience to the surviving loved ones. Unanticipated death, such as a death from a heart attack, aneurysm, or stroke, leaves survivors shocked and bereaved. Most often, the bereaved are capable of working through the grieving process without complications.

Traumatic Death   **Complicated grief** is associated with traumatic death such as death by homicide, violence, or accident. Although traumatic death does not necessarily predispose the survivor to complications in mourning, survivors often suffer emotions of greater intensity than those associated with normal grief.

When loved ones die violently, the bereaved may suffer from traumatic imagery, that is, reliving the terror of the incident or imagining the feelings of horror felt by the victim. Traumatic imagery is a common occurrence in cases of traumatic death. Such thoughts, coupled with intense grief, can lead to post-traumatic stress disorder (PTSD) in the survivors. Nurses must be aware of the possibility of PTSD and be alert for the presence of symptoms, which may include:

• Sleep disturbances, such as recurrent, terror-filled nightmares;
• Psychological distress; and
• Chronic anxiety.

Unless this problem is recognized and the survivors are encouraged to express their intense feelings, they will not be able to progress through the normal, adaptive grieving process.

Suicide The loss of a loved one to suicide is frequently compounded by feelings of guilt among the survivors. They feel guilty for failing to recognize clues that may have enabled the victim to receive help. These feelings of guilt and self-blame can transform into anger at the victim for inflicting such pain, at themselves, and at caregivers. Feelings of shame for having a suicide in the family may also be present. The negative stigma of suicide may prohibit survivors from successfully resolving their grief.

Nursing Care of the Grieving Client

Resolution of a loss is a painful process and must be done by clients in their own way. Nurses can assist by providing support as the client moves through the process of mourning. Grieving individuals have significant needs at the time of death of a loved one; these needs may continue for months or even years (Fauri & Grimes, 1994). Grief changes people by affecting self-esteem, triggering the development of new ways of coping, and precipitating a new lifestyle without the deceased.

Nurses can play an active role in assisting people to grieve by encouraging clients to do their grief work, that is, to experience their feelings to the fullest in order to work through them. Providing support and explaining to the bereaved that it will take time to grieve the loss and to gain some closure to the relationship are both important nursing responsibilities (Figure 17-4).

Assessment

A thorough assessment of the grieving client and family begins with a determination of the personal meaning of the loss. Another key assessment area is deciding the person's progress in terms of the grieving process. The nurse understands that the stages of grieving are not necessarily mastered sequentially, but, instead, that individuals may vacillate in progression through the stages of grief.

Nursing Diagnosis

The North American Nursing Diagnosis Association (NANDA) defines *Dysfunctional Grieving* as "extended, unsuccessful use of intellectual and emotional responses by which individuals, families, communities attempt to work through the process of modifying self-concept based upon the perception of potential loss" (NANDA, 1999). Another diagnosis that may be applicable is *Anticipatory Grieving,* defined as "intellectual and emotional responses and behaviors by which individuals, families, communities work through the process of modifying self-concept based on the perception of potential loss" (NANDA, 1999).

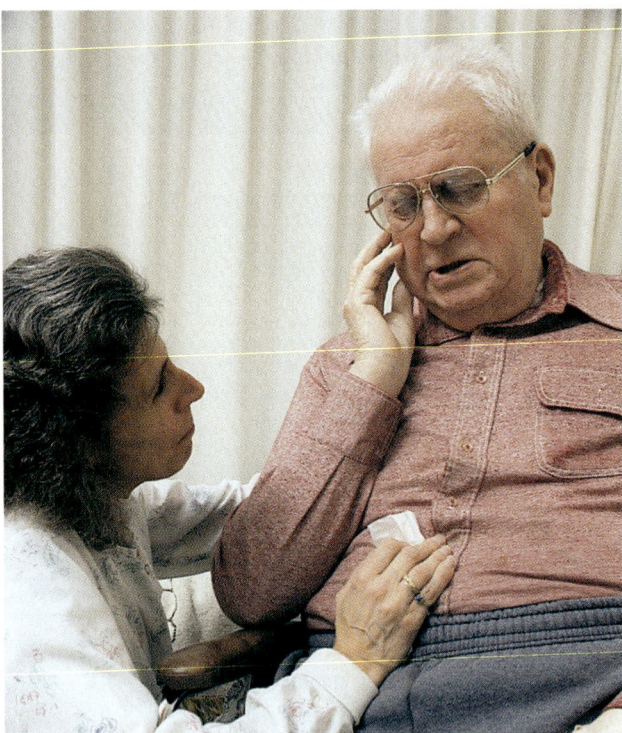

Figure 17-4 The nurse provides support to this client to help him through the grief process.

Planning/Outcome Identification

It is important to clarify the expected outcomes when planning care for the grieving client. Listed below are some expected goals for the person experiencing grief:

- Verbalize feelings of grief
- Share grief with significant others
- Accept the loss
- Renew activities and relationships

Some of these expected outcomes will take a long period of time to achieve, and some must be achieved before others are mastered. For example, to accept the loss, the person must begin to share grief with others by verbalizing those feelings. Two of the expected outcomes are discussed below.

Acceptance of the Loss Only by going through grief work are individuals able to reach some acceptance and, ultimately, resolution of feelings about the loss. Often, people try to find some meaning in their situations. This search involves introspection, for which spiritual support may be therapeutic.

Renewal of Activities and Relationships The very core of grief work revolves around acceptance of the fact that the needs met by key people in our lives can be met in other ways and by other people. The deceased cannot be replaced; however, enough healing must occur so that new relationships can be initiated.

Implementation

Therapeutic nursing care is based on an understanding of the significance of the loss to the client. To understand the client's perspective, the nurse must spend time listening. As the client expresses feelings, the nurse must demonstrate acceptance, even if the client is not responding according to the nurse's expectations or belief system. The nurse's nonjudgmental, accepting attitude is essential during the bereaved's expression of all feelings, including anger and despair. The nurse communicates an understanding of the client's anger and avoids personalizing and using defensive behaviors. "Caregivers must demonstrate, verbally and through nonjudgmental attitudes and behaviors, that the expression of grief is not only appropriate but essential for therapeutic resolution of the loss" (Mac-Gregor, 1994).

Grieving people need reassurance, counseling, and support. One mechanism of support on a long-term basis is support groups. The nurse must be informed about the availability of such groups within the community in order to make appropriate referrals. When bereaved people join support groups, they will be with others who have experienced similar losses. This sharing decreases the feelings of loneliness and social isolation so common in the grief experience.

Evaluation

People follow their own time schedule for grief work. In general, it takes months or years for grief resolution. Therefore, nurses usually do not have an opportunity to be with the bereaved family when grief work is completed. However, the nurse has a unique opportunity to lay the foundation for adaptive grieving by encouraging the bereaved to share their feelings and to continue to verbalize their experience with significant others. The goals mutually established with client and family are the foundation for evaluation. It is important for nurses to teach grieving individuals that resolution of the loss is generally a process of life-long adjustment.

DEATH

Historically, death has been considered as natural as birth, as simply the last stage of life. The last three decades have brought about significant changes in the cultural perception of death, however. In some cases, dying and death are no longer simple matters but are issues involving ethical concerns and, in some cases, legal intervention by the court system.

Just as each person lives a unique life, each person dies a unique death. Death may be sudden and unexpected, caused by heart attack or accident, for example, or death may be prolonged, coming after a distressing long-term illness. Death may come quietly for the older person who dies during sleep. And some deaths are planned by those who choose to die on their own terms by way of suicide.

Health care workers must understand the legal and ethical issues surrounding dying and death. Understanding the stages of death and dying and the signs of impending death will help prepare the nurse to render sensitive, effective care, both to the client and family and to the client's body after death. Nurses must also come to terms with their own mortality and feelings about death if they are to provide comfort to dying clients and their families. Health care workers can learn a great deal about life from the dying client.

Legal Considerations

The *Patient Self-Determination Act* (PSDA) was incorporated into the Omnibus Budget Reconciliation Act (OBRA) of 1990. The act was intended to provide a legal means for individuals to determine the circumstances under which life-sustaining treatment should or should not be provided to them. The individual's choices are validated by advance directives. An advance directive is any written instruction, including a living will or durable power of attorney for health care, that is recognized under state law (Taylor, 1995). The act applies to hospitals, long-term care facilities, home health agencies, hospice programs, and certain health maintenance organizations (HMOs). According to the PSDA, all clients entering the health care system through any of these organizations must be given information and the opportunity to complete advance directives if they have not already done so. Clients need to know that in many states, just signing these documents may not be adequate for carrying out their wishes. They may also need to indicate their wishes in regard to artificial feeding, intubation, chemotherapy, surgery, blood transfusions, and transfer to the hospital (for residents in skilled care facilities).

Although the living will and durable power of attorney for health care are legal documents, they do not preclude the need for **resuscitation** (support measures to restore consciousness and life). The medical record must have a written do-not-resuscitate (DNR)

CULTURAL CONSIDERATIONS

Cultural Influences and Advance Directive Decisions

African American Clients
- Are more likely to select aggressive interventions.
- Are less likely than European American or Hispanic American clients to have documented their end-of-life health care wishes

European American Clients
- Are much more likely to have written advance directives than are members of other cultures.
- Select "no code" more than do Hispanic American or African American clients but less than do Asian American clients

Asian American Clients
- Select "no code" more than do all other groups
- Are less likely to have advance directives

Hispanic American Clients
- Are less likely than are European American or Asian American clients to have written directives
- Are least likely of all groups to select "no code"

(*Data from "Meeting the Challenge of Advance Directives," by P. Haynor, 1998,* American Journal of Nursing, *98(3), 27–32.*)

PROFESSIONAL TIP

Care of the Dying Client

Dying was once considered to be a normal part of the life cycle. Today, it is often considered to be a medical problem that should be handled by health care providers. Technological advances in medicine have lead to depersonalized and mechanical care of those who are dying. Technological advances, the institutionalization of medical practice, legislative regulations, and societal changes have "in many ways depersonalized the process of dying, while engendering growing new fears of death" (Thompson, 1994).

Our highly technological world calls for application of high-touch interventions with the dying. In other words, appropriate care of the dying is administered by compassionate nurses who are both technically competent and able to demonstrate caring.

order from a physician if this is in agreement with the client's wishes and with the advance directives. In the absence of such an order, resuscitation will be initiated.

Many states also have a **Health Care Surrogate Law** which is implemented in the absence of advance directives. This law varies from state to state. Basically, it provides a legal means for specific individuals to make decisions for the client when the client can no longer do so. The law has developed a hierarchy of individuals who would act in the interests of the client. The spouse is the first person in the hierarchy, followed by children in the event that there is no spouse.

Ethical Considerations

Death is often fraught with ethical dilemmas that occur almost daily in health care settings. Many health care agencies have ethics committees to develop and implement policies to deal with end-of-life issues. Ethics committees are interdisciplinary and may have attorneys and clergy in addition to health care providers as members. Ethical decision making is a complex issue. One of the most difficult dilemmas is determining the difference between killing and allowing someone to die by withholding life-sustaining treatment methods.

The American Nurses Association (ANA) distinguishes relieving pain and mercy killing (euthanasia or assisted suicide). Pain relief is a central value in nursing, whereas euthanasia is viewed as unethical. The ANA's position is that increasing doses of medication to control pain in terminally ill clients is ethically justified, even at the expense of maintaining life (ANA, 1992).

Stages of Dying and Death

In her classic works, Elizabeth Kübler-Ross (1969, 1974) identified five possible stages of dying that are experienced by clients and their families (Table 17-5). Not every client moves sequentially through each stage. These stages are experienced in varying degrees and for varying lengths of time. The client may express anger, and then, a few minutes later, express acceptance of the inevitable, and then express anger again. The value in Kübler-Ross' work is that it helps increase sensitivity to the needs of the dying client.

Denial

In the first stage of dying, the initial shock can be overwhelming. Denial is a useful tool in coping. It is an essential and protective mechanism that may last for only a few minutes or may manifest for months.

In some clients, denial manifests as "doctor shopping" (not to imply that second opinions are not sometimes necessary) or insisting that there must have been a mix-up or mistake in the diagnostic tests. In other clients, denial manifests as simply avoiding the issue. They go about their daily routines as though nothing in their lives has changed. Most people, given the time, will eventually move past the stage of denial.

Clients may choose to be selective in the use of denial. For example, clients may use denial with certain

Table 17-5 KÜBLER-ROSS' STAGES OF DYING AND DEATH

STAGE	EXAMPLE
First Stage: **Denial**	*Verbal:* "This can't be happening to me!" *Behavioral:* Client is diagnosed with terminal lung cancer; client continues to smoke two packs of cigarettes daily.
Second Stage: **Anger**	*Verbal:* "Why me?" *Behavioral:* Client strikes out at caregivers.
Third Stage: **Bargaining**	*Verbal:* Client prays, "Please, God, just let me live long enough to see my grandchild graduate." *Behavioral:* Client tries to "make deals" with caregivers or god.
Fourth Stage: **Depression**	*Verbal:* "Go away. I just want to lie here in bed. What's the use?" *Behavioral:* Client withdraws and isolates self.
Fifth Stage: **Acceptance**	*Verbal:* "I feel ready. At least, I'm more at peace now." *Behavioral:* Client gets financial or legal affairs in order. Client says goodbye to significant others.

Data from On Death and Dying, *by E. Kübler-Ross, 1969, New York: Macmillan. Copyright 1969 by Macmillan.*

family members or friends because they are trying to protect those people from the truth. Clients may also use denial from time to time to set aside thoughts of illness and death in order to focus on living.

Anger

The initial stage of denial is often followed by anger. The client's security is being threatened by the unknown. All the normal daily routines have become disrupted. This stage is typically very difficult for family and caregivers because they may feel powerless or useless in terms of helping their loved one through the situation. The client has no control over the situation and, thus, becomes angry in response to this powerlessness. The anger may be directed at self, God, others, the environment, and the health care system. In the client's eyes, whatever is done is not the right thing. Family members may be greeted with silence or with outbursts of anger. Their response, in turn, may be anger, guilt, or despair.

Bargaining

The anticipation of the loss through death may bring about bargaining, through which the client attempts to postpone or reverse the inevitable. The client's bargaining represents an attempt to postpone death and usually has self-imposed limitations. For example, the client will ask to live just long enough to see her first grandchild born in exchange for a promise to perform some service for the church. Most clients bargain in silence or in confidence with their spiritual leader. Caregivers who have cared for terminally ill clients will agree that it is not uncommon for a client to live long enough for some special event (a wedding or birth), only to die shortly afterwards.

Depression

When the realization comes that the loss can no longer be delayed, the client moves to the stage of depression. This depression is different from dysfunctional depression in that it helps the client detach from life and, thus, be able to accept death. Depression in this sense is a therapeutic experience for the dying person. Clients sometimes feel abandoned, as persons who were once friends begin to visit less and less, sometimes severing ties with the client even before death; this may compound the client's feelings of depression and hopelessness.

Acceptance

The final stage, acceptance, may not be reached by every dying client. With acceptance comes growing peace and contentment. The feeling that all that could be done has been done is often expressed during this stage. Reinforcement of the client's feelings and sense of personal worth are important during this stage. Many clients will make an effort to get all of their personal and financial affairs in order.

The client may sleep more, not to avoid reality, but because sleep is needed to fill a physical and emotional

LIFE CYCLE CONSIDERATIONS

Reactions to Impending Death

- Persons of all ages generally experience the same feelings and emotions as they progress through a terminal illness.
- Persons of any age who have endured a long illness may view death as a release from their suffering.
- Persons of any age may find it difficult to reach acceptance if they have unfinished business.
- Many people receive satisfaction from **life review** (a form of reminiscence wherein a client attempts to come to terms with conflict or to gain meaning from life and die peacefully).
- Elderly clients may welcome death, especially if they have outlived everyone who was near and dear to them.

need. The client may limit visitors to a few people with whom he feels safe and comfortable. The most significant form of communication at this time is moments of silence.

Nursing Care of the Dying Client

Nursing care of clients who are terminally ill or who are facing and preparing for their own death can be both challenging and rewarding. The death process is typically a very emotional time for clients and their families; compassionate and sensitive nursing care that respects clients' wishes as well as meets their physical needs can help bring peace and dignity to this natural process.

Assessment

Nursing interventions are based on a thorough assessment of the client's holistic needs. Assessment of the dying client includes an ongoing collection of data regarding the strengths and limitations of the dying person and the family.

Nursing Diagnoses

The nurse's assessment of the dying client may lead to any number of diagnoses. One NANDA-approved nursing diagnosis that is applicable for many dying clients is *Powerlessness*, that is, "the perception that one's own action will not significantly affect an outcome; a perceived lack of control over a current situation or immediate happening" (NANDA, 1999). Another response that is often experienced by the dying is described by the diagnosis *Hopelessness*, "a subjective state in which an individual sees limited or no alternatives or personal choices available and is unable to mobilize energy on own behalf" (NANDA, 1999). The

PROFESSIONAL TIP

Information Needed in Assessment of the Dying Client

- Client and family goals and expectations
- Client's awareness of the terminal nature of illness
- Availability of support systems
- Current stage of dying
- History of previous positive coping skills
- Client perception of unfinished business to be completed

(*Adapted from Death and Dying, by K. Pritchett and P. Lucas, 1997. In* Psychiatric–Mental Health Nursing: Adaptation and Growth *(4th ed., pp. 206–207), by B. S. Johnson (Ed.), 1997, Philadelphia: Lippincott.)*

PROFESSIONAL TIP

Planning Care for the Dying Client

- Schedule time to be available to the client
- Identify areas that are of special concern to the client and make referrals if appropriate (e.g., social worker consult for information on financial assistance)
- Promote and protect individual self-esteem and self-worth
- Balance the client's needs for independence and assistance
- Meet the physiological needs of the client and family
- Respect the client's confidentiality
- Answer all questions and provide factual information to the client and family
- Offer to contact clergy or other spiritual leader

(*Adapted from Death and Dying, by K. Pritchett and P. Lucas. In* Psychiatric–Mental Health Nursing: Adaptation and Growth *(4th ed., p. 208), Philadelphia: Lippincott.)*

client may also exhibit *Death Anxiety*, or apprehension, worry, or fear related to death or dying (NANDA, 1999).

Planning/Outcome Identification

The major goals of nursing care are the physical, emotional, and mental comfort of the client. The goals of nursing care for the dying client are the same as those goals developed for all clients who are unable to meet their own needs. The dying client must be treated as a unique individual worthy of respect, rather than as a diagnosis to be cured. Many dying clients do not fear death but are anxious about a painful death or dying alone.

Promoting optimal quality of life means treating the client and family in a respectful manner and providing a safe environment for the expression of feelings. Planning focuses on meeting the holistic needs of the client and family. These needs are specified in the Dying Person's Bill of Rights (Figure 17-5), which is as relevant today as when it was written in 1975. In planning care, the nurse should make every effort to be sensitive to the dying client's rights.

Implementation

The nurse's first priority is to communicate a caring attitude to the client. A recent study (Czerwiec, 1996) quoted family members of recently deceased hospitalized clients as stating that "the factor that most strongly affects family satisfaction [is] perceiving the staff to have a caring attitude toward the patient and to be acting on his behalf."

The Dying Person's Bill of Rights

- I have the right to be treated as a living human being until I die.
- I have the right to maintain a sense of hopefulness, however changing its focus may be.
- I have the right to be cared for by those who can maintain a sense of hopefulness, however challenging this might be.
- I have the right to express my feelings and emotions about my approaching death in my own way.
- I have the right to participate in decisions concerning my care.
- I have the right to expect continuing medical and nursing attention even though "cure" goals must be changed to "comfort" goals.
- I have the right not to die alone.
- I have the right to be free from pain.
- I have the right to have my questions answered honestly.
- I have the right not to be deceived.
- I have the right to have help from and for my family in accepting death.
- I have the right to die in peace and dignity.
- I have the right to retain my individuality and not be judged for my decisions, which may be contrary to beliefs of others.
- I have the right to expect that the sanctity of the human body will be respected after death.
- I have the right to be cared for by caring, sensitive, knowledgeable people who will attempt to understand my needs and will be able to gain some satisfaction in helping me face my death.

Figure 17-5 The Dying Person's Bill of Rights *(From "The Dying Person's Bill of Rights," by A. J. Barbus, 1975,* American Journal of Nursing, *75(1), 99.)*

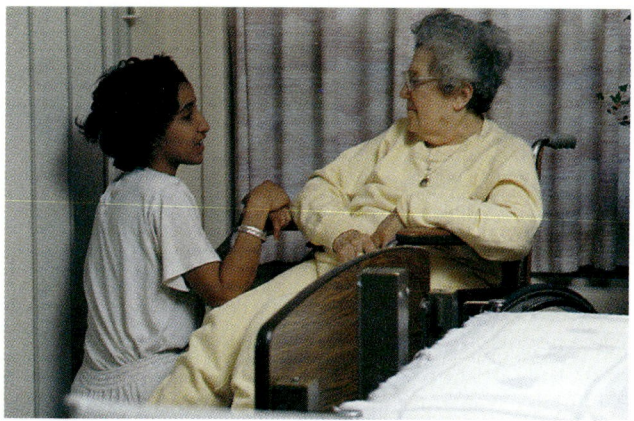

Figure 17-6 Establishing a caring and trusting relationship helps the client come to terms with a terminal illness.

When a client is in denial, it is important for the nurse to approach the client with understanding and the knowledge that moving between the stages of dying is enhanced by a trusting nurse–client relationship. Establishment of rapport facilitates the client's verbalization of feelings (Figure 17-6). The nurse establishes a safe environment wherein the client does not feel embarrassed or chastised for experiencing those feelings. Nurses must understand that clients are not angry with them, but, rather, with the situation they are experiencing.

Terminally ill clients are often given **palliative care,** or care that relieves symptoms, such as pain, but does not alter the course of disease. A primary aim of palliative care is to help the client feel safe and secure. The nurse can do much to increase the client's feelings of safety by being available when needed. Holding the client's hand and listening are therapeutic measures. Ufema (1995a) suggests asking the client three questions: What do you want? From whom do you want it? and When do you want it? The client needs to know that he has the nurse's support as an advocate for his care and well-being.

Physiological Needs   According to Maslow's hierarchy of needs, physiological needs must be met before others, because they are essential for existence. Areas that are often problematic for the terminally ill client are respirations; fluids and nutrition; mouth, eyes, and nose; mobility; skin care; and elimination.

Respirations   Oxygen is frequently ordered for the client experiencing labored breathing. Suctioning may be needed to remove secretions that the client is unable to swallow.

Fluids and Nutrition   The refusal of food and fluids is almost universal in dying clients. It is believed that the client is not feeling thirst and hunger. Although the issue of permitting dehydration in terminally ill clients is often met with great resistance, the literature supports the concept that forced nutrition has questionable value and may even exacerbate the client's condition (Taylor, 1995). Artificial nutrition often increases the client's agitation, leads to increased use of limb restraints, and increases the risk of aspiration pneumonia (Rhymes, 1993). Hospice nurses have indicated that withholding artificial nutrition is not painful. Regardless, in every situation, the client's own wishes must always take precedence. If the comatose client has not previously made his wishes known, family members must be given accurate and truthful information. For the person in irreversible coma, withholding of artificial nutrition does not cause death; rather, it allows life to take its natural course (Taylor, 1995). Several professional groups have issued statements regarding artificial nutrition and hydration. The

American Medical Association, the American Dietetic Association, and the ANA agree that it is legally, ethically, and professionally acceptable to discontinue nutritional support if the terminally ill client so requests (Taylor, 1995).

Mouth, Eyes, and Nose Oral discomfort is the only documented side effect of dehydration in the terminally ill client (Taylor, 1995). Both the administration of oxygen and mouth breathing increase the need for meticulous oral care. Caregivers can use saliva substitutes and moisturizers to alleviate discomfort. The regular use of toothpaste and a toothbrush may be adequate. The tongue must be given the same attention as is the rest of the mouth, with gentle brushing. Ice chips and sips of favorite beverages should be offered frequently, and petroleum jelly applied to the lips. Oral care must be given every 2 to 3 hours to maintain the client's comfort.

The eyes may become irritated due to dryness. Artificial tears can alleviate this discomfort. A cotton ball should be used to gently wipe the eye from inner to outer canthus (one wipe per cotton ball) to remove any discharge.

The nares may become dry and crusted. Oxygen given by cannula can further irritate the nares. A thin layer of water soluble jelly applied to the nares will help alleviate discomfort. The elastic strap of the oxygen cannula should not be applied too tightly, lest it cause discomfort.

Mobility As the client's condition deteriorates, mobility decreases. The client becomes less able to move about in bed or to get out of bed and requires more assistance. Physical dependence increases the risk of complications related to immobility, such as atrophy and pressure ulcers. Attentive nursing care can prevent the onset of these complications, which increase both client discomfort and the cost of care.

The client should be repositioned at least every 2 hours. It is important to keep in mind that the client may have other disorders that contribute to discomfort related to mobility, such as arthritis or lung disease. The nurse can help the client maintain body alignment with the use of pillows and other supportive equipment and can use positioning techniques to facilitate ease of breathing. Passive range of motion exercises should be performed at least twice a day to prevent stiffness and aching of the joints. The client may prefer to be assisted into a reclining type of chair at intervals throughout the day. Using a wheelchair can also increase the client's environmental space, giving the client more mobility, control, and independence.

Skin Care The prevention of pressure ulcers is a priority. Pressure ulcers are painful, can cause secondary complications such as sepsis, and are costly to treat. Regular repositioning and passive range of motion exercises are two preventive measures. In addition, keeping the skin clean and moisturized will promote healthy tissue. The skin should be inspected once or twice daily, with special attention paid to pressure points and areas where skin surfaces rub together. Gentle massages with soothing lotion are comforting. Bed baths are adequate if the client cannot get into the tub or sit in a shower chair.

Elimination Constipation may occur due to side effects of pain medications and to lack of physical activity. Fluids and foods with high-fiber content can be effective preventive measures for clients with adequate oral intake. Constipation can also be alleviated by maintaining a scheduled time for bowel elimination and administering suppositories, if necessary. A commode with padded arms can be more comfortable than a toilet.

The client may become incontinent of bladder and bowel, so the nurse must check the client frequently, clean the skin with peri-washes, and apply a moisture barrier after each incontinent episode. Incontinent undergarments may increase the client's comfort, especially when the client is out of bed.

Indwelling catheters are never a first choice for bladder management. However, for some clients, the need for frequent cleaning, the discomfort of using a bedpan, or getting out of bed to use the toilet or commode may cause agonizing pain. In these circumstances, the benefits of a catheter greatly outweigh the risks.

Comfort The primary activities directed at promoting physical comfort include pain relief, keeping the client clean and dry, and providing a safe, nonthreatening environment. The nurse who demonstrates a respectful, caring attitude promotes the client's psychological comfort by establishing rapport. The fear of a painful death is almost universal. Pain is a subjective, personal experience, and the client is the best judge of the severity of the pain. Many, though certainly not all, dying clients experience pain. In its position statement on pain relief for the terminally ill, the ANA states that promotion of comfort is the major goal of nursing care (ANA, 1992). Comfort should be maximized by management of pain and other discomforting factors.

The client needs to know that caregivers accept and believe complaints of pain and that they will intervene to prevent and alleviate the pain. The nurse should ask the client to rate the pain on a scale from 0 to 10, with 0 being no pain, and 10 being severe pain. Medication must be given around the clock and not "as needed." A nonnarcotic analgesic may be effective in early stages for mild, intermittent pain. As the pain increases, the client may need to be started on morphine, titrated at increments until adequate pain relief is achieved without severe side effects. Titrating the analgesic dose and interval means finding the lowest dose and the longest interval that will relieve pain. The dosage that should be used is the one that controls the pain to the satisfaction of the client and that causes minimal side effects. For some clients, this may be 10 mg of oral

PROFESSIONAL TIP

Adjuvant Therapy

Adjuvant therapy may be effective. Nonsteroidal anti-inflammatory agents are beneficial for bone metastases; tricyclic antidepressants and anti-seizure medications for neurogenic pain, and steroids for headaches related to cerebral edema (Rhymes, 1993). Nonpharmacological techniques can be used along with medication. Relaxation techniques, guided imagery, massages, and repositioning may enhance the action of the medications.

morphine sulfate (MS) every 4 hours. For other clients, it may be 480 mg MS intravenously per hour. The question for the nurse is, what dose can be safely given? No maximum number of milligrams applies to every individual.

The nurse must monitor the client's responses with regard to pain rating and respiratory rate. For example, 10 mg MS given IM may afford pain relief, but if the respiratory rate drops from 12 to 6 per minute, the next dose should be reduced. If the same dose given to another client provides minimal relief, and the client is alert and displays no change in respirations, the next dose should be increased (McCaffery & Pasero, 1999).

The client must be monitored for **breakthrough pain**, or sudden, acute, temporary pain that is usually precipitated by a treatment or procedure or by unusual activity of the client. A supplemental dose of medication is required. If the precipitating factor is known (dressing changes, for example), a dose should be given 30 to 60 minutes before the procedure.

Physical Environment A soothing physical environment can significantly increase the client's comfort. Soft lighting enhances vision without causing the discomfort associated with harsh, glaring light. Complying with the client's request for a night light is also helpful in creating a pleasant and non-threatening environment. If possible, the client should be offered the opportunity to have the bed or a chair near a window to increase the range of the environment. As the client's circulation becomes more sluggish, body temperature will fall. Lightweight comforters will increase warmth without adding uncomfortable weight. The nurse can help eliminate environmental odors by ensuring adequate ventilation, daily cleaning of the room, removal of leftover food, and frequent linen changes. Noise can be distracting and anxiety provoking, so the nurse and visitors should comply with the client's wishes with regard to the use of radio and television. The telephone can be removed from the room, if the client finds the ringing disturbing.

Psychosocial Needs Death presents a threat to not only one's physical existence, but to one's psychological integrity. As deBlois (1994) states:

We are all too familiar with the scene of the dying person tethered to tubes and electronic gadgetry in an intensive care unit. Held captive in a tangle of technology, the person is kept at a distance from the supportive presence and touch of family and friends by well-meaning but technologically oriented healthcare professionals.

Technology does not replace touch, concern, compassion, and human companionship. Nurses, through their presence, can humanize the dying person's environment. Families should be encouraged and invited to participate in the client's care, if they desire to do so and the client is willing.

For many clients, maintaining a well-groomed appearance is important. When the client can no longer make requests or give directions for care, caregivers should presume that the client would prefer to maintain the same grooming habits as were previously preferred. Shaving the male client's beard or cleaning and trimming the client's fingernails and toenails, for instance, will help the client maintain a well-groomed appearance and will also promote client dignity. Combing and brushing the hair not only improves appearance, but is also a comforting and relaxing activity for many clients.

HOME HEALTH CARE

Equipment To Increase Client Comfort

The following equipment can be rented and may qualify for payment by Medicare or private insurance.

- An electric hospital bed with overhead trapeze, to give the client more control of the environment
- A commode, to extend the client's independence in elimination
- A lifting device, to facilitate getting the dependent client out of bed
- Remote control, for the client who enjoys television
- Portable telephone
- Shower chair and hand-held shower for the bathtub
- Comfort devices such as special mattresses for the bed and cushions for chairs
- Overbed table, for eating or hand activities
- Comfortable chairs close to the bed, to facilitate visits of family and friends

Dressing and undressing may become a cumbersome, frustrating, and fatiguing activity. The client who spends time up and about may choose attractive pajamas, housecoats, dusters, or exercise suits. Nurses should advise individuals who may be purchasing clothing for the client to select items that are loose fitting, have few fasteners, and are washable.

Spiritual Needs   Nurses play a major role in promoting the dying client's spiritual comfort. "Dying persons are among the most vulnerable members of the human family. The moral health and integrity of the broader community can be measured in part by the way we respond to their needs" (deBlois, 1994). Dying persons may experience confusion, anger at their god, crises of faith, or other types of spiritual distress.

Dying is a personal and, frequently, lonely process. "People living impoverished spiritual, social, intellectual lives lack the resources for a meaningful experience with dying" (Thompson, 1994). Table 17-6 provides information on the views of various religions

Table 17-6 RELIGIONS AND DYING AND DEATH ISSUES

RELIGION	LIFE SUPPORT WITHDRAWAL	DEATH	ORGAN DONATION
Judaism	Allowed under the right circumstances (when life support is serving only to impede a natural death).	• Suicide is forbidden. • Burial should occur within 24 hours. • Cremation is forbidden.	• Permitted because the procedure saves life. • Rejected by Orthodox Jews. • Autopsy is permitted if it will save future lives.
Islam	Permitted if only serving to prolong death or if client's condition is medically hopeless.	• Suicide is forbidden. • Relatives and friends are present. • Autopsy is permitted to solve a crime or provide further medical knowledge.	• Permitted.
Catholicism/ Orthodoxy	Controversial; permitted if client's condition is hopeless.	• Prayers are offered at time of death. • Burial and cremation are permitted. • Autopsy is permitted.	• Permitted.
Protestantism	Permitted if client's condition is hopeless.	• Prayers are offered at time of death. • Burial and cremation are permitted. • Autopsy is permitted.	• Permitted, although may be rejected by some Baptists or Pentecostals.
Jehovah's Witnesses	Permitted if serving only to prolong death or if quality of life is nonexistent.	• Suicide is not approved. • Autopsy is permitted if legally necessary.	• Individual choice.
Buddhism	Acceptable for those on threshold of death.	• Suicide is criticized. • Cremation is common.	• Controversial.
Hinduism	Supported to allow a natural death.	• Prefer to die at home. • Embalming is forbidden. • Autopsy is discouraged. • Suicide is forbidden.	• Forbidden.
Mormons	A client or family decision.	• Cremation is discouraged. • Autopsy is a family decision.	• A family decision.
Native Americans	Life support is viewed as unnatural and, therefore, unnecessary.	• Complex beliefs about death and treatment of the body.	• Discouraged.

Data from Health Assessment & Physical Examination, *by M. E. Z. Estes, 1998, Albany, NY: Delmar Publishers. Copyright 1998 Delmar Publishers.*

with regard to withdrawal of life support; death; and organ donation. The nurse can serve as a sounding board for the client who expresses values and beliefs related to death. The following are therapeutic nursing interventions that address the spiritual needs of the dying client:

- Communicate empathy
- Play music
- Use touch
- Pray with the client
- Contact clergy, if requested by the client
- Read religious literature aloud, at the client's request.

Support for the Family   Family members need to be involved in the care of their dying loved one. Guilt may be increased by feelings of powerlessness. Involving family members in the treatment is a helpful intervention (MacGregor, 1994). Families facing the impending death of a loved one require much support from nurses and other caregivers. The nurse's presence, just being there with the family, is extremely important. A recent study showed that "family members indicated that when a loved one is dying, they'd like to know that a nurse will make a special effort to be . . . available" (Czerwiec, 1996).

Each family group has its unwritten rules, its leaders and followers, and its methods for coping with crises. The family's equilibrium is threatened by the impending death. If family members have limited coping skills and inadequate support systems, they need assistance and guidance from the caregivers. Nurses must remember that the rules and coping mechanisms used by the family may not always coincide with the values and beliefs of the staff and that the client's and family's wishes must be respected to the extent possible.

Each family member will grieve the approaching death in her own way. The nurse must be supportive and nonjudgmental. The family needs to know that the staff cares about them as well as the client.

The relationship with the family does not always end with the client's death. Staff members may attend visitations, funerals, or memorial services. If a hospice was involved, the family may participate in a bereavement support program. If the client was a resident in a long-term care facility, family members may return to visit other residents with whom they became acquainted.

Learning Needs   Bereaved families need much support and information. The nurse's role is to teach family members what they need to know. For instance, families must be assisted with acquiring the tools that will help them help their loved one. An example might be the need for the family to understand that the dying person needs to conserve energy. Some simple actions on the part of the family could be to schedule activities after a rest period or early in the morning, when the client is strongest. The nurse may need to

CLIENT TEACHING

Guidelines for Teaching a Family Caregiver

- Discuss the nature and extent of the disease process
- Use adult-education principles
- Reinforce material frequently
- Clearly explain the purpose of palliative care while maintaining a sense of realistic hope
- Inform client and family of available community resources; reassure them that they are not alone
- Teach steps for caregiver to follow if an emergency arises at home
- Provide written instructions for caregiver to follow, including important telephone numbers and persons to be contacted
- Inform about the purpose of hospice

point out to the family this type of common sense approach, as simple interventions such as these can be overlooked during this highly charged emotional time.

Client and family knowledge deficits can relate to:

- Insufficient information about physical condition,
- Information about the treatment regimen,
- Inability to anticipate medical crises,
- Inexperience with personal threat of death, and
- Unfamiliarity with protocol to follow in case of the need for emergency care outside of the hospital

Hospice Care   **Hospice,** a type of care for the terminally ill, is founded on the concept of allowing individuals to die with dignity and surrounded by those who love them. Clients enter hospice care when aggressive medical treatment is no longer an option or when the client refuses further medical intervention.

Home Care   A dying person is often not given the opportunity to be surrounded by family and friends. "More than 80% of all reported deaths in the United States occur in healthcare institutions where people die in unfamiliar, and sometimes intimidating, surroundings" (deBlois, 1994).

Impending Death

No one can predict how long a client will be in the terminal stages of illness. A client may exhibit signs of impending death and then rally to live for several more days. It is not uncommon for clients to endure until a member of the family arrives for a last goodbye. The client who has had a long and troublesome illness may be ready to die but needs "permission" to die from a loved one, who says, "It's okay, you can go now." A client may not wish to die when others are

HOME HEALTH CARE

An Alternative for the Dying Client

- Family members should be physically and emotionally able to provide care.
- Health care providers should share the responsibility of home care with the family. This sharing could include respite time and frequent visits.

HOME HEALTH CARE

When the Client Dies at Home (Expected Death)

The family must:

- Have a list of telephone numbers readily available,
- Have the name and telephone number of the funeral director,
- Know whom to call (physician or hospice nurse or funeral director),
- Know whom not to call (ambulance and emergency services),
- Record the time of death,
- Record the last medications given,
- Record the condition of the client during the last few hours, and
- Record the last time the client was seen by the nurse.

present and will wait to take the last breath until everyone has left the room.

Even when death is expected, it is never easy for the family. The family should be thoroughly informed, in simple terms, about what will happen before and after the client's death, including:

- Physical changes that will occur just before and following death
- Pronouncement of death
- Post-mortem care
- Removal of the body

Impending death is signaled by a series of irrevocable events (Durham & Weiss, 1997):

- The lungs become unable to provide adequate gas diffusion.
- The heart and blood vessels become unable to maintain adequate tissue perfusion.
- The brain ceases to regulate vital centers.

Cheyne-Stokes respirations (breathing characterized by periods of apnea alternating with periods of dyspnea) most often herald pulmonary system failure. Secretions accumulate in the larynx and trachea, causing noisy respirations, often called the "**death rattle**."

The heart fails in its pumping function, resulting in poor perfusion, ischemia, and cell death. The skin becomes cool and, possibly, very pale, cyanotic, jaundiced, or mottled. The pulse becomes rapid, irregular, weak, and thready. Death is several hours away if a peripheral pulse is strong and easily palpated. Cold, cyanotic extremities and irregular respirations indicate that death may be expected within an hour or two (Durham & Weiss, 1997).

Inadequate cerebral perfusion hinders the brain's ability to integrate vital functions. The client may be confused and lethargic and may respond only to direct visual, auditory, or tactile stimulation. Pupils no longer react to light and become fixed. The client may "talk" to dead loved ones. A frown or tight facial muscles may indicate pain or discomfort. A client in a coma will move only in response to deep pain. Analgesics should not be withdrawn from a client in a coma.

The care of the client does not cease during this final stage of life. The nursing actions previously de-

scribed should be continued. The nurse should tell the client in brief, simple terms what is happening as care is rendered. The family should be allowed and encouraged to continue their participation, if that is their wish. The nurse should caution family members that the dying client can hear even in the absence of verbal response, so all comments and conversation should continue to be respectful.

There may be other indications that death is near. The client may report seeing angels (Ufema, 1995b) or hearing beautiful music. These experiences should be accepted as a natural step in the process of dying. When the final breath is taken, the heart stops beating. Within a few minutes, cerebral death (the point at which brain cells die) occurs, and brain activity ceases.

Care after Death

Caring for the deceased body and meeting the needs of the grieving family are nursing responsibilities. The body of the deceased must be treated in a way that respects the sanctity of the human body (Barbus, 1975). Nursing care includes maintaining privacy and preventing damage to the body. **Post-mortem care** is given immediately after death but before the body is moved to the mortuary.

Several physiological changes occur after death. Body temperature decreases, resulting in a lack of skin elasticity (**algor mortis**). In order to avoid skin breakdown, the nurse must therefore use caution when removing tape from the body. Another physiological change, **liver mortis,** is a bluish-purple discoloration of the skin, usually at pressure points, that is a by-product of red-blood-cell destruction. This discoloration occurs in dependent areas of the body; the nurse should therefore elevate the head to prevent discoloration associated with pooling of blood. Approximately 2 to 4 hours after death, **rigor mortis** occurs: The body stiffens due to contraction of skeletal and smooth muscles. To prevent disfiguring effects of rigor mortis, as soon as possible after death, the nurse should close the client's eyelids, insert dentures (if applicable), close the mouth, and position the body in a natural position.

In preparing the body for family viewing, the nurse strives to make the body look comfortable and natural. This means removing all tubes (if allowed) and preparing and positioning the body as previously described. After the family has viewed the body, the nurse places identification tags on the body's toe and wrist. The body is then placed in a plastic or fabric **shroud** (a covering for the body after death), and the shroud is tagged. Next, the body is transported to the morgue according to the agency's policy, where it is kept until it can be transported to a **mortuary** (funeral home). In some institutions, the body is kept in the room until the funeral director arrives. The nurse is also responsible for returning the deceased's possessions, such as jewelry, eyeglasses, clothing, and all other personal items, to the family.

Legal Aspects

In most states, the physician is legally responsible for determining the cause of death and signing the death certificate. The nurse may, in certain situations, be the person responsible for certifying the death. It is important for nurses to know their legal responsibilities, which are defined by their respective state boards of nursing.

Autopsy

An **autopsy** (examination of the body after death, by a pathologist to ascertain the cause of death) is mandated in situations where an unusual death has occurred. For example, an unexpected death and a violent death are circumstances that would necessitate

an autopsy. Families must give consent for an autopsy to be performed in other situations. The funeral director must know whether an autopsy is to be performed.

Organ Donation

The donation of organs for transplantation is a matter that requires compassion and sensitivity from the caregivers. Health care institutions are required to have policies related to the referral of potential donors to organ procurement agencies. It is important that families of the deceased know the need for and process of organ donation. There is an inadequate supply of organs and tissues to meet the demand for transplants. The following organs and tissues are used for transplantation:

- Kidneys
- Heart
- Lungs
- Liver
- Pancreas
- Skin
- Corneas
- Bones (long bones and middle ear bones)

At the time that the family gives consent for donation, the nurse notifies the donor team that an organ is available for transplant. Time is of the essence, because the organ or tissue must be harvested and transplanted quickly to maintain viability.

Care of the Family

At the time of death, the nurse provides invaluable support to the family of the deceased. Informing the family of the circumstances surrounding the death is extremely important. The nurse provides information about viewing the body, asks the family about donating organs, and offers to contact support people (e.g., other relatives, clergy). Sometimes, the nurse must help the family with decision making regarding a funeral home, transportation, and removal of the deceased's belongings. Sensitive and compassionate interpersonal skills are essential in providing information and support to families.

Nurse's Self-Care

Working with dying clients can evoke both a personal and a professional threat in the nurse. Because many nurses are confronted with death and loss daily, grief is a common experience for nurses. Smith-Stoner and Frost (1998) describe a part of the psyche called the shadow self, where stresses are stored. Unresolved sadness is called shadow grief. Everyone has a shadow self and may have some shadow grief. Nurses often have a great deal of shadow grief, which, if not released, may cause illness and burnout. Frequent exposure to death can interfere with the nurse's effectiveness because of subsequent anxiety and denial.

Whether working in a hospice, a hospital, a long-term care facility, or the home, nurses are at particular risk for experiencing negative effects from caring for the dying. Often, nurses do not want to confront their grief and will use some of the common defenses against grieving: keeping busy, taking care of others, being strong, and suffering in silence. Nurses must avoid pretending that they do not experience grief and subsequent suffering and must instead talk about the intense emotions associated with caregiving. According to Smith-Stoner and Frost (1998), shadow grief may be starting to overwhelm a person if that person experiences the following:

- A loss of energy, spark, joy, and meaning in life
- Detachment from surroundings
- A feeling of being powerless to make a difference
- Increased smoking or drinking
- Unusual forgetfulness
- Constant criticism directed toward others
- Consistent inability to get work done
- Uncontrolled outbursts of anger
- Perception of clients and their families as objects
- Surrender of hobbies or interests

To cope with their own grief, nurses need support, education, and assistance in coping with the death of clients. Staff education should focus on decreasing staff anxiety about working with grieving clients and families; ways to seek support; and ways to provide support to coworkers. Smith-Stoner and Frost (1998) suggest the following ways to cope.

- Take time to cry with and for clients.
- Get physical: run, walk, bicycle, play tennis.

- Ask colleagues to help with tasks; do not try to be "Supernurse."
- Connect to place of worship; pray.
- Look for joy in work. Laughter is a great healer.
- Create a caring circle of friends.
- Listen to music.

Often, the nurse's fears and doubts about death and its meaning surface, causing anxiety related to feelings about mortality. Even though such feelings are normal, caring for the dying client and the client's family can be emotionally draining. Nurses must therefore remember to care for themselves.

PROFESSIONAL TIP

Care for Yourself during Grief

- Do what you do so well: care. By helping the family, you will counter your feelings of helplessness.
- Set aside some time for your own grieving.
- Allow for crying to help ease the pain.
- Know when to ask your coworkers for help.
- Call on someone you can trust, and express your feelings of grief to that person.
- Use support from within your agency—counselors, clergy, support groups.
- Find a way to say goodbye to the deceased client. Rituals bring closure, which is a necessary part of grieving.

(*Adapted from "Please Cry with Me: Six Ways to Grieve," by C. D. Reese, 1996, Nursing96, 26[8], 56.*)

SAMPLE NURSING CARE PLAN

THE CLIENT WITH A TERMINAL ILLNESS/CANCER OF THE LUNG

Mrs. O'Riley, a 78-year-old widow, was diagnosed with cancer of the lung 6 months ago. After a right lower lobectomy, she was discharged to a local skilled-care facility with plans to go home after completing her treatment. Mrs. O'Riley was transported to a cancer center for radiation therapy. After completing the treatments, she resisted the idea of going home, and discharge plans were discontinued. Mrs. O'Riley's condition is deteriorating. She now requires pain medication, is frequently short of breath, has dyspnea, and needs moderate assistance with activities of daily living because of fatigue. She frequently grimaces and says, "Oh, it hurts." Her nutritional intake is marginal because of difficulty swallowing. Mrs. O'Riley is in bed most of the day, getting up only to use the commode. She has two adult children and three grandchildren who live nearby and visit often. They are willing to help their mother get her affairs in order but she resists their efforts. The family very much wants to make their mother's remaining time as comfortable and serene as possible. However, Mrs. O'Riley sometimes defies their attempts to do so.

continued

Nursing Diagnosis 1 *Pain, Chronic, related to disease progression as evidenced by verbal statements, body language, and the need for pain medication*

PLANNING/GOALS	NURSING INTERVENTIONS	RATIONALE	EVALUATION
Mrs. O'Riley will verbalize relief from pain.	Give analgesics as ordered.	Administering regular doses of medication is more effective than waiting until the pain begins.	Mrs. O'Riley's body language and verbal statements indicate freedom from pain.
	Ask client to rate pain on a scale of 0 to 10, with 0 being no pain and 10 being severe pain, to assess the need for beginning morphine. Give morphine as ordered, titrated at increments until adequate pain relief is achieved.	Morphine is the drug of choice for severe pain associated with cancer. The client should begin morphine as soon as it is necessary.	
	Monitor for signs of sudden, acute, temporary pain (breakthrough pain). If the precipitating factor is known, give medication 30 to 60 minutes before the event. For unpredictable breakthrough pain, give the medication as soon as possible.	Breakthrough pain is often precipitated by activity or stress and requires supplemental medication.	
	Assure Mrs. O'Riley that the nurses will help her manage the pain and keep it under control. Give back massages and reposition as necessary for comfort. Assist with progressive relaxation techniques if client agrees.	Clients need reassurance that everything possible will be done to manage the pain.	
	Monitor bowel elimination.	Pain medication may cause constipation.	

continued

Nursing Diagnosis 2 *Breathing Pattern, Ineffective, related to diminished lung function as evidenced by dyspnea and shortness of breath*

PLANNING/GOALS	NURSING INTERVENTIONS	RATIONALE	EVALUATION
Mrs. O'Riley will be free from moderate or severe dyspnea.	Teach breathing exercises and effective coughing techniques.	Breathing exercises and coughing techniques enhance gas exchange in the alveoli.	Mrs. O'Riley breathes with ease. Dyspnea does not interfere with activities.
	Allow adequate time for physical activities. Postpone activity if dyspnea is present. Provide as much assistance as needed.	Physical exertion increases dyspnea.	
	Administer low-flow oxygen if blood gases indicate need.	Oxygen will ease the effort to breathe but will not be effective unless blood gases indicate the need.	
	Encourage client to drink 8 to 10 glasses of fluid each day.	Adequate fluid intake liquifies respiratory secretions and promotes hydration.	
	Humidify the air with a cold-water vaporizer.	Moisturized air enhances breathing.	
	Assess for signs of respiratory tract infection.	The client is at high risk for respiratory infection.	

Nursing Diagnosis 3 *Coping, Individual, Ineffective, related to terminal illness as evidenced by inability to communicate effectively with family members and to accept their help*

PLANNING/GOALS	NURSING INTERVENTIONS	RATIONALE	EVALUATION
Mrs. O'Riley will express her feelings openly.	Consult Mrs. O'Riley on all aspects of care, giving adequate information. Provide opportunities to express feelings. Acknowledge feelings and let Mrs. O'Riley know that crying and grieving are beneficial.	Mrs. O'Riley needs to be given as much control as she wishes to have. Letting Mrs. O'Riley express her feelings will validate those feelings—she needs to know her feelings are normal and expected.	Mrs. O'Riley is at ease with herself.

continued

| | Listen for clues indicating unfinished business that needs attention. Encourage the process of life review. | There may be something in Mrs. O'Riley's past that needs to be resolved before she can successfully cope with the business of dying. Life review is a process of reflection and pondering of one's past and accepting one's life as having had value and meaning. |
| Mrs. O'Riley will maintain a satisfying relationship with her family. | Encourage family visits. Provide privacy. | Families need privacy in order to feel free to express their emotions. |

CASE STUDY

Mrs. Jason, a 76-year-old with a history of heart failure, has been hospitalized twice within the last year and was critically ill both times. Both times, she was discharged to her home. A home health nurse and a nursing assistant make intermittent visits to monitor her condition and to help with her activities of daily living. Her husband manages the household chores. Mrs. Jason's condition is deteriorating, the shortness of breath becoming more severe. Her energy level is easily depleted, and she is having increasing difficulty getting out of bed. The family is concerned because Mrs. Jason does not have any advance directives. Any attempt to bring up the subject is met with avoidance and a change of subject.

The following questions will guide your development of a nursing care plan for the case study.

1. List the clinical manifestations you would expect Mrs. Jason to experience.
2. Identify four nursing diagnoses to utilize in planning her care.
3. Describe several nursing interventions for implementing palliative care.
4. Describe appropriate interactions with the family to ease their concerns.
5. Cite reasons that Mrs. Jason and her family might benefit from hospice services.

SUMMARY

- Loss is a universal response experienced when someone (or something) of value is no longer available.
- Grief is a psychological response to loss characterized by deep mental anguish and sorrow. Grieving people experience various stages of grief.
- The difference between normal and pathological grief is the inability of the individual to adapt to life without the loved one.
- There are five psychological stages involved in the dying process: denial, anger, bargaining, depression, and acceptance.

- Complicated grief is associated with traumatic death such as by accident, homicide, or suicide.
- Each person dies a unique death.
- Hospice care offers clients an alternative to hospitalization when aggressive medical treatment is no longer an option.
- After death, the nurse focuses on supporting the family and caring for the deceased body.
- Nurses must care for themselves in order to provide quality, compassionate care to the dying person and family.

Review Questions

1. Susan, age 11 years, was left with a distant relative 2 weeks ago. Her parents have not returned or called. Susan is experiencing a:

    a. physical loss.
    b. situational loss.
    c. maturational loss.
    d. anticipational loss.

2. Knowing that a loved one is terminally ill allows family members to begin the grieving process. This is called:

    a. complicated grief.
    b. anticipatory grief.
    c. dysfunctional grief.
    d. disenfranchised grief.

3. A defining characteristic of the NANDA nursing diagnosis *Anticipatory Grieving* is:

    a. prolonged denial or depression.
    b. unsuccessful adaptation to loss.
    c. social isolation or withdrawal from others.
    d. an expression of distress at potential loss.

4. Nursing interventions for a client who has experienced a loss are based on an understanding of:

    a. the degree of the client's depression.
    b. the anger expressed by the client.
    c. the significance of the loss to the client.
    d. the number of support groups available for the loss experienced by the client.

5. The purpose of the Patient Self-Determination Act is to:

    a. serve as an order for "do not resuscitate."
    b. designate a guardian for an incompetent client.
    c. provide a means, instead of a will, to designate what is to be done with a person's property, money, and personal possessions.
    d. provide a legal means for individuals to state those circumstances under which life-sustaining treatment should or should not be provided to them.

6. One of the major goals of hospice care is:

    a. freedom from pain and other symptoms.
    b. free care for all dying clients and their families.
    c. to cure the client using very aggressive medical treatment.
    d. to transfer all dying clients to the hospital when death is imminent.

7. Signs of impending death include:

    a. flushed skin.
    b. slower pulse rate.
    c. increased blood pressure.
    d. Cheyne-Stokes respirations.

8. The nurse must use caution when removing tape from a body because of:

    a. liver mortis.
    b. rigor mortis.
    c. algor mortis.
    d. rimas mortis.

Critical Thinking Questions

1. Find a classmate from a cultural background different from yours. How does your perception of death differ from that of your classmate?

2. Thompson (1994) asks, "Can we afford to leave death in the hands of science, or should we use the benefits of science to provide the dying with a nurturing spiritual environment that feeds the spirit while sustaining the body?" What is your response to this question? What are some ways nurses can promote a "nurturing spiritual environment"?

WEB FLASH!

- What key terms related to loss and death might you search for on the Internet (for instance grief, bereavement)?
- Is there a listing on the Internet of books, videos, or other media on self-care for caregivers to the terminally ill? Are these resources available in your local library?
- What sites can you find that offer information on hospice care?
- Search the Web for "Symptoms of terminal illness"; what can you find?

BASIC NUTRITION

MAKING THE CONNECTION

Refer to the following chapters to increase your understanding of nutrition:

- **Chapter 12, Cultural Diversity and Nursing**
- **Chapter 14, The Life Cycle**
- **Chapter 27, Diagnostic Tests**
- **Chapter 45, Nursing Care of the Client: Mental Illness**

Procedures: B1, Handwashing; B29, Measuring Intake and Output; I28, Administering Enteral Tube Feedings

LEARNING OBJECTIVES

Upon completion of this chapter, you should be able to:
- *Define key terms.*
- *Describe the role of the nurse in promoting proper nutrition.*
- *Explain the way the body uses nutrients.*
- *Discuss the six types of nutrients.*
- *Describe factors affecting kilocalorie needs.*
- *Explain the Food Guide Pyramid.*
- *Explain the purposes of the Dietary Guidelines for Americans and the Recommended Dietary Allowances (RDAs).*
- *Discuss factors influencing nutrition.*
- *Explain the dietary needs and nutritional assessments for infancy, childhood, adolescence, older adulthood, pregnancy, and lactation.*
- *Explain the relationship between health and nutrition.*
- *Discuss weight management.*
- *Explain the way to determine energy (kcal) needs.*
- *Describe three ways to promote food safety.*
- *Describe the standard hospital diets: regular, soft, liquid, mechanical, and pureed.*
- *Cite the proper procedure for serving a meal tray.*
- *List important points to follow when feeding a client.*

KEY TERMS

absorption	fortified
allergy	gluconeogenesis
anabolism	glycogenesis
anthropometric	glycogenolysis
measurements	hyperglycemia
atherosclerosis	hypoglycemia
basal metabolism	incomplete protein
body mass index	ingestion
calorie	insulin
catabolism	intracellular fluid
cholesterol	ketosis
chyme	kilocalorie
complete protein	lipid
deglutition	mastication
dehydration	metabolic rate
diet therapy	metabolism
dietary prescription/	nutrition
order	obesity
digestion	oxidation
empty calories	parenteral nutrition
enriched	peristalsis
enteral nutrition	phospholipid
euglycemia	satiety
excretion	triglycerides
extracellular fluid	villi
fat-soluble vitamin	water-soluble vitamin

INTRODUCTION

Nutrition encompasses all of the processes involved in consuming and utilizing food for energy, maintenance, and growth. These processes are ingestion, digestion, absorption, metabolism, and excretion. Much of the discussion throughout this chapter focuses on ingestion, because this is the process that the individual can control and with which the nurse can be of assistance to the client. This chapter presents basic information regarding proper nutrition and the role of the nurse in assisting clients to meet their nutritional needs. Topics covered include: specific nutrients and their functions in the body; phytochemicals; promoting proper nutrition; factors influencing nutrition; nutritional needs during the life cycle; nutrition and health; weight management; food labeling, quality, and safety; food allergies; and nutrition and the nursing process.

PHYSIOLOGY OF NUTRITION

Five processes are involved in the body's use of nutrients: ingestion, digestion, absorption, metabolism, and excretion.

Ingestion

Nutrition begins with **ingestion**, the taking of food into the digestive tract, generally through the mouth. In special circumstances, ingestion occurs directly into the stomach, through a feeding tube; this situation is discussed later in the chapter.

Digestion

Digestion refers to the mechanical and chemical processes that convert nutrients into a physically absorbable state. Mechanical digestion includes **mastication** (chewing), the breaking of food into fine particles and mixing it with enzymes in saliva; **deglutition** (swallowing of food), the peristaltic waves and mucous secretions that move the food down the esophagus. Chemical digestion is the process whereby enzymes, gastric and intestinal juices, bile, and pancreatic juices change food into the individual nutrients that can be used by the body.

Digestion begins in the stomach (except in the case of some starches, for which digestion begins in the mouth) and is completed in the intestines. **Peristalsis** (coordinated, rhythmic, serial contractions of the smooth muscles of the GI tract) forces **chyme** (an acidic, semi-fluid paste) through the small and large intestines. Only carbohydrates, proteins, and fats require chemical digestion to make the nutrients available for absorption. Figure 18-1 illustrates the basic elements and functions of the digestive system.

Absorption

Absorption is the process whereby the end products of digestion (i.e., individual nutrients) pass through the epithelial membranes in the small and large intestines and into the blood or lymph system. The nutrients are absorbed and taken to the parts of the body that need them. Most nutrients are water soluble and can be absorbed directly through the **villi** (finger-like projections that line the small intestine) and into the blood. Fats, which are not water soluble, are absorbed first into the lymph system and eventually enter the circulatory system.

Metabolism

The conversion of nutrients into energy by the body is called **metabolism**; this process is the sum total of all the biological and chemical processes in the body as they relate to the use of nutrients in every body cell. Metabolism involves two processes: anabolism and catabolism. **Anabolism** is the constructive process of metabolism, wherein new molecules are synthesized and new tissues are formed, as in growth and repair. This process requires energy. **Catabolism** is the destructive process of metabolism, wherein tissues or substances are broken into their component parts. This process releases energy. During metabolism, energy is also produced by the process of **oxidation**, which is the chemical process of combining nutrients with oxygen. The energy produced by the body is used in a number of ways: electrical energy for brain and nerve activities, chemical energy for metabolism, mechanical energy for muscle contractions, and thermal energy to keep the body warm.

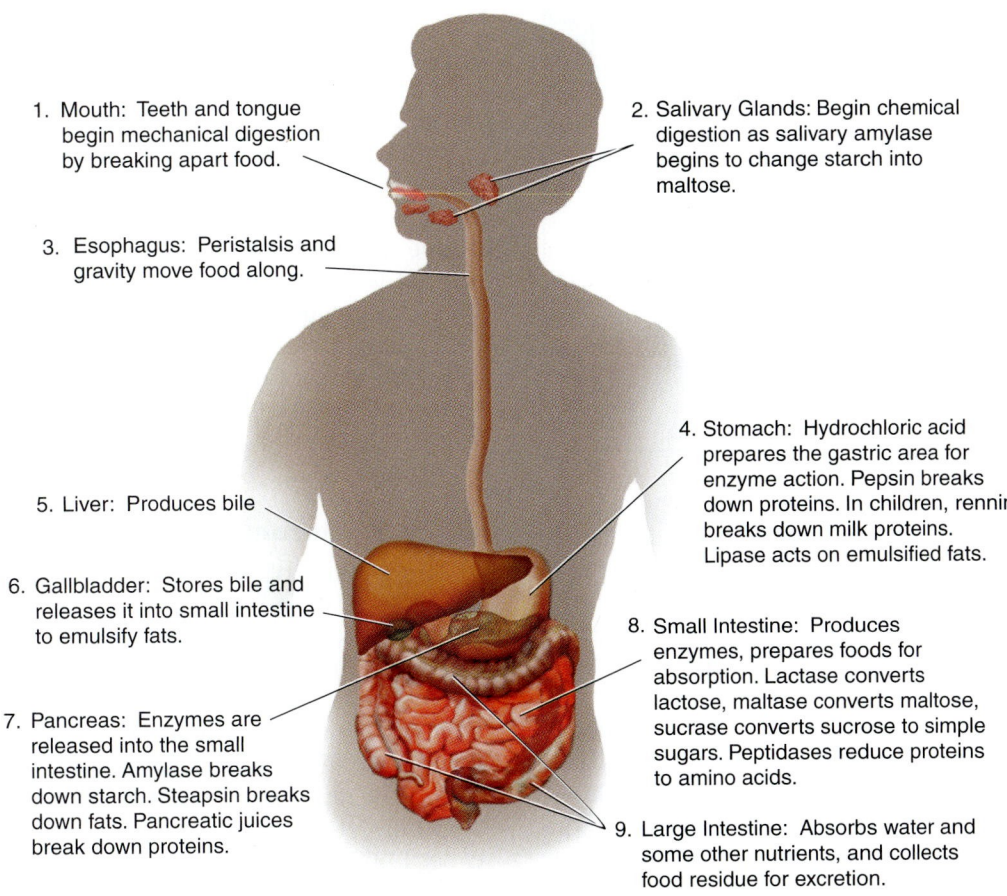

1. Mouth: Teeth and tongue begin mechanical digestion by breaking apart food.

2. Salivary Glands: Begin chemical digestion as salivary amylase begins to change starch into maltose.

3. Esophagus: Peristalsis and gravity move food along.

4. Stomach: Hydrochloric acid prepares the gastric area for enzyme action. Pepsin breaks down proteins. In children, rennin breaks down milk proteins. Lipase acts on emulsified fats.

5. Liver: Produces bile

6. Gallbladder: Stores bile and releases it into small intestine to emulsify fats.

7. Pancreas: Enzymes are released into the small intestine. Amylase breaks down starch. Steapsin breaks down fats. Pancreatic juices break down proteins.

8. Small Intestine: Produces enzymes, prepares foods for absorption. Lactase converts lactose, maltase converts maltose, sucrase converts sucrose to simple sugars. Peptidases reduce proteins to amino acids.

9. Large Intestine: Absorbs water and some other nutrients, and collects food residue for excretion.

Figure 18-1 Functions of the Digestive System

Metabolic rate is the rate of energy utilization in the body; it is expressed in units called calories. One **calorie** is the amount of heat required to raise the temperature of one gram of water by 1° Celsius. Because of the large quantity of energy released during metabolism, the energy is expressed in **kilocalories** (kcal), each of which is equal to 1,000 calories.

Basal metabolism is the amount of energy needed to maintain essential physiologic functions, such as respiration, circulation, and muscle tone, when a person is at *complete* rest, both physically and mentally.

The major factor affecting basal metabolism is body composition. Lean muscle tissue has a higher metabolic rate and thus produces more energy than does fatty tissue. Generally, women have a lower metabolism than men because they have a higher percentage of fat tissue. However, metabolism increases during menstruation, pregnancy, and lactation. Age is also an influence, because growth periods increase metabolism. Glandular activity, especially of the thyroid gland, affects metabolism. The rate of metabolism is governed primarily by the hormones triiodothyronine (T_3) and thyroxine (T_4). Hypothyroid activity, a decrease in the secretion of thyroid hormones, causes a lower rate of metabolism, whereas hyperthyroid activity, an increase in the secretion of thyroid hormones, causes a higher rate of metabolism.

Excretion

Excretion is the process of eliminating or removing waste products from the body. Dietary fiber and other indigestible materials, salts, and other products such as bile and water are formed into feces and excreted from the body as solid waste. Other excretory organs that aid the digestive system in the elimination of wastes includes the kidneys, bladder, sweat glands, skin, and lungs. Most liquid waste is sent through the kidneys and bladder to be excreted as urine. Some liquid waste is removed through the sweat glands of the skin as perspiration. Gaseous waste is eliminated through the lungs.

NUTRIENTS

The body must have six types of nutrients to function efficiently and effectively. These are water, carbohydrates, fats, proteins, vitamins, and minerals. If a person eats a well-balanced diet, all the nutrients the body requires are provided by the food. Table 18-1

Table 18-1 NUTRIENTS, FUEL VALUES, AND DAILY REQUIREMENTS

NUTRIENT	FUEL VALUE	DAILY REQUIREMENTS
Water	0	1,000 mL/1,000 kcal eaten
Carbohydrates	1g = 4 kcal	50% to 60% total kcal per day
Fats	1 g = 9 kcal	25% to 30% total kcal per day
Protein	1 g = 4 kcal	15% to 20% total kcal per day

offers an overview of the first four nutrients in relation to their fuel value (the amount of energy they supply) and their daily requirements.

Nutrients are classified as energy nutrients, organic nutrients, and inorganic nutrients, as shown in Table 18-2.

Energy nutrients release energy for use by the body. Organic nutrients build and maintain body tissues and regulate body processes. Inorganic nutrients provide a medium for the body's chemical reactions, transport materials, maintain body temperature, promote bone formation, and conduct nerve impulses.

The functions of the nutrients are interrelated. Intake changes in one nutrient may lead to functional changes in another. Some examples of interrelated functions are as follows: Iron is better absorbed when vitamin C is present, and calcium absorption depends on the presence of vitamin D.

Water

Water is the most important nutrient. It is more vital to life than is food. Virtually all body functions require water. An individual may live for weeks without food, but for only approximately 10 days without water.

Water is the major constituent in every cell of the body. Approximately 50% to 60% of an adult's weight is due to water, and approximately 70% to 75% of an infant's weight is water. The body's water content decreases with age.

Approximately two-thirds of the water in the body is **intracellular fluid** (ICF), fluid within the cells. The other one-third is **extracellular fluid** (ECF), fluid outside the cells, including plasma fluid, lymph, cerebrospinal fluid, interstitial fluid, and GI fluids.

Daily Requirements

The amount of water needed by the body varies based on environmental factors, such as temperature and humidity, and physical factors, such as activity level, metabolic need, functional losses (urine and feces), age, respiratory rate, and state of health. Higher environmental temperatures and vigorous physical activity cause more water loss as perspiration increases. Water lost must be replaced to maintain metabolism. Generally, 1,000 mL of water is needed to process every 1,000 kcal eaten.

A state of relative water balance exists when the body has adequate fluid distributed appropriately as ICF and ECF. A person's daily water intake and output should be equal (Figure 18-2). Excessive intake of fluids is not a problem in a healthy individual; more intake simply causes more output.

Table 18-2 CLASSIFICATION OF NUTRIENTS

CLASSES	NUTRIENTS
Energy nutrients	Carbohydrates
	Fats
	Proteins
Organic nutrients	Carbohydrates
	Fats
	Proteins
	Vitamins
Inorganic nutrients	Water
	Minerals

From Fundamentals of Nursing: Standards & Practice, *by S. DeLaune and P. Ladner, 1998, Albany, NY: Delmar Publishers. Copyright 1998 by Delmar Publishers.*

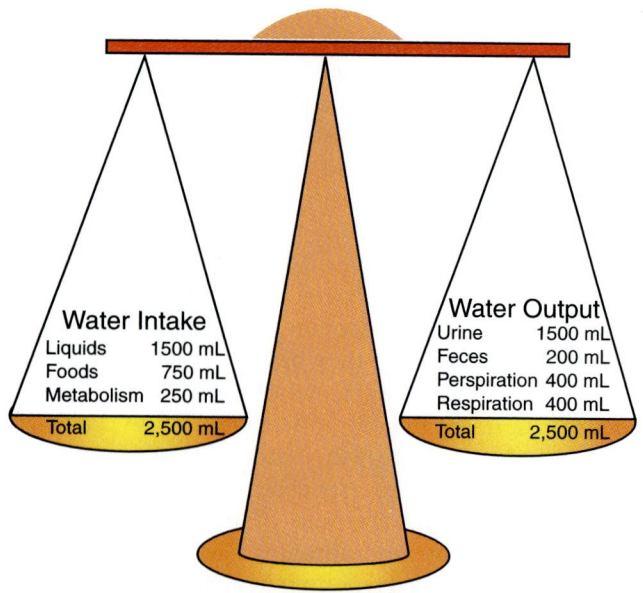

Figure 18-2 Body Water Balance (Approximate figures for a sedentary adult)

Functions

Water has many functions in the body:

- *Solvent:* Water is the liquid in which many substances are dissolved to form solutions.
- *Transportor:* Water carries nutrients, wastes, and other materials throughout the body and to and from each cell via blood, tissue fluids, and body secretions.
- *Regulator of body temperature:* Water is excreted as perspiration when the temperature goes up. Evaporation of perspiration cools the body.
- *Lubricant:* Water is a component of fluid within the joints, called synovial fluid, which provides for smooth movement of the many joints in the body.
- *Component of all cells:* Water gives structure and form to the body.
- *Hydrolysis:* Water breaks apart substances, especially in metabolism.

Classification and Sources

There are three sources of water for the body:

- Liquids consumed, including water, coffee, juice, tea, milk, and soft drinks.
- Foods consumed, especially vegetables and fruits.
- Metabolism, which produces water when oxidization occurs.

Digestion, Absorption, and Storage

Water is not digested but, rather, is absorbed and used by the body as we drink it. It cannot be stored by the body and is excreted daily. Water losses are classified as sensible, that is, the person is aware of the loss, or insensible, that is, the person is not generally aware of the loss. There are four ways the body normally loses water:

- *Urine:* accounts for the greatest amount of water lost from the body (sensible loss)
- *Feces:* contains a small amount of water (insensible loss, except in cases of diarrhea)
- *Perspiration:* varies with temperature, but some fluid is always lost (insensible or sensible loss)
- *Respiration:* releases moisture with every breath (insensible loss)

LIFE CYCLE CONSIDERATIONS

Dehydration

Infants, small children, and elders are more susceptible to dehydration. For them, dehydration occurs more rapidly and is more severe.

PROFESSIONAL TIP

Signs and Symptoms of Dehydration

- Health history reveals inadequate intake of fluids.
- Urine output is decreased.
- Urine specific gravity is > 1.035.
- Weight loss (% body weight) is 3% to 5% for mild, 6% to 9% for moderate, and 10% to 15% for severe dehydration.
- Eyes appear sunken; tongue displays increased furrows and fissures.
- Oral mucous membranes are dry.
- Skin turgor is decreased.
- Venous filling and emptying times are delayed (> 3 to 5 seconds).
- In infants, fontanels are sunken.
- Changes in neurological status may occur with moderate to severe dehydration.

(*From* Health Assessment & Physical Examination, *by M. E. Z. Estes, 1998, Albany, NY: Delmar Publishers. Copyright 1998 by Delmar Publishers.*)

Signs of Deficiency and Excess

Abnormal water losses from the body include profuse sweating, vomiting, diarrhea, hemorrhage, wound drainage (burns), fever, and edema. With edema, the water is still in the body, but is not useable.

A deficiency of water is called **dehydration**. Prolonged dehydration results in death.

Some conditions cause an excessive accumulation of fluid in the body. This condition is called *positive water balance.* It occurs when more water is taken in than is used and excreted, and edema results. Hypothyroidism, congestive heart failure, hypoproteinemia (low amounts of protein), some infections and cancers, and some renal conditions can cause such water retention because sodium is not being excreted normally.

Carbohydrates

Carbohydrates are made of the elements carbon, hydrogen, and oxygen. In nutrition, the first letters of these three elements are used as the abbreviation: CHO.

Carbohydrates constitute the chief source of energy for all body functions. They are also the major food source for all people, because they are the least expensive and the most abundant foods.

Daily Requirements

It is recommended that carbohydrates make up 50% to 60% of an individual's kcal intake per day. For example, if an individual's total energy requirement is 2,000 kcal, 50% of this number is 1,000; this number is then divided by 4 (the number of kcal in each gram of carbohydrate, refer to Table 18-1), for an estimated carbohydrate requirement of 250 g/day. It is estimated that current U.S. diets contain only 45% of their kcal from carbohydrates (Townsend & Roth, 2000).

Functions

Carbohydrates constitute the primary source of energy for the body. The body must maintain a constant supply of energy; therefore, it stores approximately one-half a day's supply of carbohydrates in the liver and muscles for use as needed. A sufficient supply of carbohydrates spares proteins from being used for energy, thus allowing proteins to perform their primary function of building and repairing body tissues. Carbohydrates are needed to oxidize fats completely and for the synthesis of fatty acids and amino acids. The central nervous system and erythrocytes rely solely on carbohydrates for energy.

Classification and Sources

Carbohydrates are classified as either simple or complex. Simple carbohydrates are single sugars (monosaccharides) such as glucose, fructose, and galactose found in fruits, honey, and corn syrup. Monosaccharides require no digestion and are quickly absorbed. They are either used immediately for energy or stored as glycogen.

Double sugars (disaccharides), such as sucrose, maltose, and lactose, are two single sugars joined together. They are found in milk, sweeteners, sugar, and molasses. Before they can be absorbed by the body, disaccharides must be separated into monosaccharides through digestion.

Complex carbohydrates (polysaccharides) are composed of many single sugars joined together. Those important in nutrition are starch, glycogen, and dietary fiber (cellulose). The most significant of these polysaccharides in the diet is starch, which is found in grains, grain products, legumes, potatoes, and other vegetables. Complex carbohydrates are digested much more slowly than the simple carbohydrates, and they thus supply the body with energy for a longer period of time.

Glycogen does not come from the foods we eat. Rather, it is a form of carbohydrate made by the liver and stored in the liver and muscles. The body keeps a 12- to 48-hour store of glycogen. This reserve is used between meals and during sleep to maintain **euglycemia** (normal blood glucose level) for body functions. **Glycogenesis** is the process of converting glucose to glycogen. **Glycogenolysis** is the process of changing the glycogen back to glucose when it is needed by the body for energy. **Insulin** is a pancreatic hormone necessary for cells to produce energy and the liver to produce and store glycogen. Glucose metabolism depends on the availability of insulin.

Dietary fiber has no nutritive value: The human body is unable to digest it. There are two types of di-

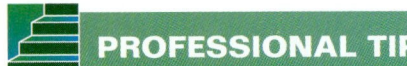

PROFESSIONAL TIP

Insulin Levels and the Client Who Is Diabetic

When the secretion of insulin is impaired or absent, the glucose level in the blood becomes excessively high. This condition is called **hyperglycemia** and is usually a symptom of diabetes mellitus. If control by diet is ineffective, insulin injections or an oral hypoglycemic must be used to control blood sugar. When insulin is given, the client's intake of carbohydrates must be carefully controlled to balance the prescribed dosage of insulin. When blood glucose levels are unusually low, **hypoglycemia** results. A mild form of hypoglycemia may occur if one waits too long between meals or if the pancreas secretes too much insulin. Symptoms include fatigue, shaking, sweating, and headache.

etary fiber: soluble and insoluble. Soluble dietary fiber slows gastric emptying and binds bile acids and cholesterol. This fiber provides **satiety** (a feeling of fulfillment from food) and lowers the cholesterol level in the blood. Insoluble dietary fiber holds water, which increases fecal bulk and stimulates peristalsis for better elimination. Good sources of both kinds of dietary fiber are whole grains, whole grain products, legumes, and fruits and vegetables with their skins.

Digestion, Absorption, and Storage

Digestion of cooked starches begins in the mouth, when the salivary enzyme ptyalin mixes with the starch in food during chewing. Little digestion takes place in the stomach. Carbohydrate digestion is completed in the small intestine by pancreatic and intestinal enzymes present there. Carbohydrates are used completely, leaving no waste for the kidneys to eliminate.

Glucose and other monosaccharides, the final products of carbohydrate digestion, are absorbed into the blood through the capillaries in the villi of the intestinal mucosa. Fructose and other monosaccharides are converted to glucose in the liver.

Glucose not needed for immediate energy is converted to glycogen by the liver and stored there and in the muscles. Any remaining glucose is then converted to fatty acids and stored as adipose tissue (fat). The body has no way to rid itself of excess carbohydrates; they are either used or stored.

Signs of Deficiency and Excess

A mild deficiency of carbohydrates can result in weight loss and fatigue. A diet seriously deficient in carbohydrates could cause **ketosis**, a condition wherein acids called *ketones* accumulate in the blood and urine, upsetting the acid–base balance. Ketones are produced

PROFESSIONAL TIP

Lactose Intolerance

Many adults are unable to digest lactose and suffer from bloating, abdominal cramps, and diarrhea after drinking milk or consuming milk-based food products such as processed cheese. This reaction is called lactose intolerance. It is caused by insufficient lactase, the enzyme required for digestion of lactose. Special low-lactose milk products can be used instead of regular milk. Lactase-containing products are also available.

CLIENT TEACHING

Fats

No more than 10% of total kcal should be provided by saturated fats in the diet.

Currently, it is estimated that most American diets obtain 40% to 45% of their kcal from fat.

---

when fat oxidation in cells is incomplete. This situation results from an inadequate intake of carbohydrates, which causes an emergency need for energy. Because there are insufficient carbohydrates to fulfill the body's energy needs, an abnormally large amount of fat is metabolized. Ketosis can result from uncontrolled insulin-dependent diabetes mellitus, starvation, or diets extremely low in carbohydrates. It can lead to coma and even death.

Excess carbohydrate consumption is one of the most common causes of obesity. Although some of the surplus carbohydrate is changed to glycogen, the major part of any surplus becomes adipose tissue. Too many carbohydrates may cause tooth decay, irritate the lining of the stomach, or cause flatulence.

Fats

Fats constitute the most concentrated source of energy in the diet. People in developed countries tend to eat diets relatively high in fat. Although fat is an essential nutrient, too much fat is a hazard to health. The descriptive word for fats of all kinds is *lipids*. **Lipids** are organic compounds that are insoluble in water but soluble in organic solvents, such as ether and alcohol, and include true fats and fat-like compounds such as lipoids and sterols. Fats provide slightly more than twice the calorie content of carbohydrates. Refer back to Table 18-1 for the fuel values and requirements of fats in the diet. Like carbohydrates, fats are composed of carbon, hydrogen, and oxygen, but they have a substantially lower proportion of oxygen.

Daily Requirements

It is recommended that fats make up no more than 25% to 30% of an individual's caloric intake per day. For example, assuming that one's total energy requirement is 2,000 kcal/day, one-quarter (25%) of this would be 500 kcal. Dividing 500 kcal by 9 (the number of kcal in each gram of fat; see Table 18-1) yields an estimated fat requirement of 55.5g/day.

Functions

Fat has many functions in the body. Fat:

- Provides a concentrated source of energy (more than twice the kcal of carbohydrates);
- Assists in the absorption of fat-soluble vitamins;
- Is a major component of cell membranes and myelin sheaths;
- Improves the flavor of food and delays the stomach's emptying time, providing a feeling of satiety;
- Protects and helps hold organs in place; and
- Insulates the body thus assisting in temperature maintenance.

Classifications and Sources

Fat is formed by one molecule of glycerol being joined to one, two, or three fatty-acid molecules. The most important lipids are as follows:

- **Triglycerides** (true fats), which are composed of one glycerol molecule attached to three fatty-acid molecules. Most dietary fat and body fat are triglycerides.
- **Phospholipids** (lipoids), which are composed of glycerol, fatty acids, and phosphorus. They are structural components of cells, for example myelin (insulating covering of many nerves) and lecithin (a part of cell membranes).
- **Cholesterol** (a sterol), which is not essential in the diet because the liver manufactures approximately 1,000 mg every day. Cholesterol is found in all cell membranes, in brain and nerve tissue, and in blood, and it is excreted in bile. Cholesterol is required for the production of several hormones including estrogen, testosterone, adrenalin, and cortisone. The intake of dietary cholesterol from such sources as animal food products may affect the serum (blood) cholesterol level.

Fats can also be classified by source, visibility, and saturation. The source of fats can be either animal or plant (vegetable). Examples of animal fat are lard, butter, milk, cream, egg yolks, and the fat in meat, poultry, and fish. Examples of plant fat are oils (corn, safflower, olive, cottonseed, peanut, palm, and coconut), nuts, and avocado.

Fats are either visible or invisible. Visible fats are easy to identify, such as butter, oils, margarine, lard, shortening, bacon, salt pork, and the fat around beef. Examples of hidden or invisible fats are those in egg yolks, whole-milk and whole milk products, cheeses, nuts, seeds, olives, avocados, many desserts, and baked goods.

The saturation of a fat refers to its chemical composition. When fatty acids, the main building blocks of fats, contain all of the hydrogen ions possible in the molecule, they are said to be saturated. Saturated fats tend to be solid at room temperature. Generally, animal fats are saturated. Plant fats that are saturated are coconut, palm kernel, and palm oils. Unsaturated fats are missing a hydrogen ion at one or more places in the molecule. They tend to be soft or liquid at room temperature. Plant fats are generally unsaturated, with the exceptions mentioned preceding. Unsaturated fats are subdivided into monounsaturated and polyunsaturated fats. **Monounsaturated fatty acids** are fatty acids that form glycerol esters with one double or triple bond; foods in this category are nuts, fowl, and olive oil. **Polyunsaturated fatty acids** form glycerol esters that have many carbons unbonded to hydrogen atoms. Foods such as fish, corn, sunflower seeds, soybeans, cottonseeds, and safflower oil contain polyunsaturated fat.

There are three essential fatty acids (linoleic, linolenic, and arachidonic) necessary for growth, cholesterol metabolism, and heart action. They are found primarily in vegetable oils, egg yolks, and poultry.

Digestion, Absorption, and Storage

No chemical breakdown of fats occurs in the mouth, and very little fat digestion takes place in the stomach. When fat reaches the small intestine, digestion begins. The digestive agents for fat are bile, from the gallbladder, and enzymes, from the pancreas and the small intestine. The final products of fat digestion are fatty acids and glycerol. Approximately 95% of dietary fat is absorbed in the small intestine.

Fats not immediately needed by the body are stored as adipose tissue. Approximately 5 g of fat are excreted daily in the feces.

CLIENT TEACHING

Blood Cholesterol

- Blood cholesterol level should not exceed 200 mg of cholesterol/dL of blood.
- To decrease the blood cholesterol level, the client must follow a diet low in saturated fat.
- Weight loss and exercise will also help lower blood cholesterol level.
- A diet high in saturated fat increases the blood cholesterol by 15% to 25%.

LIFE CYCLE CONSIDERATIONS

Children and Cholesterol

If children are not fed high-cholesterol foods on a regular basis, their chance of overusing these foods as adults lessens, as does their risk of heart attack and stroke.

Signs of Deficiency and Excess

Deficiency symptoms occur when fats provide less than 10% of the total daily kcal requirement. Gross deficiency may result in eczema (inflamed and scaly skin condition), retarded growth, and weight loss.

Excess fat in the diet can lead to overweight and heart disease. In addition, studies point to an association between high-fat diets and cancers of the colon, breast, uterus, and prostate.

An elevated level of cholesterol in the blood is thought to be a contributing factor in heart disease, because hypercholesterolemia (high serum cholesterol) is common in clients with atherosclerosis. **Atherosclerosis** is a cardiovascular disease wherein plaque (fatty deposits containing cholesterol and other substances) forms on the inside of artery walls, reducing the space for blood flow.

Protein

Proteins are made of the elements carbon, hydrogen, oxygen, and nitrogen. In nutrition, the first letters of these four elements are used as the abbreviation: CHON.

Protein is the only nutrient that can build, repair, and maintain body tissues. An adequate supply of proteins in the daily diet is essential. All tissues and fluids in the body with the exception of bile and urine, contain some protein. The basic building materials of protein are amino acids. Refer to Table 18-1 for the fuel value and requirements of protein.

Daily Requirements

Daily protein requirement is determined by size, age, gender, and physical and emotional condition. A large person has more body cells to maintain than does a small person. A growing child, a pregnant

LIFE CYCLE CONSIDERATIONS

Proteins

By the age of 4 years, body protein content reaches the adult level of approximately 18% of body weight.

woman, or a woman who is breastfeeding needs more protein for each pound of body weight than does the average adult. When digestion is inefficient, fewer amino acids are absorbed by the body; consequently the protein requirement is higher. This is sometimes thought to be the case with elderly clients. Extra proteins are usually required after surgery or severe burns or during infections in order to replace lost tissue and manufacture antibodies. In addition, emotional trauma can cause the body to excrete more nitrogen than it normally does, thus increasing the need for protein-rich foods.

The National Research Council of the National Academy of Sciences considers the average adult's daily requirement to be 0.8 g of protein for each kilogram of body weight. Daily protein requirement is determined by multiplying body weight in kilograms (weight in pounds divided by 2.2) by 0.8. For instance:

$$130 \text{ lb. woman} \div 2.2 \text{ lb/kg} = 59./\text{kg} \times 0.8 \text{ g/kg}$$
$$= 47.3 \text{g protein/day}$$

Appendix C lists recommended dietary allowances of protein.

Functions

The primary function of protein in the diet is to provide the amino acids necessary for the synthesis of body proteins, which are used to build, repair, and maintain the body tissues. Protein composes most of the muscles, skin, hair, nails, brain, nerves, and internal organs.

Another function of protein is to assist in regulating fluid balance. Proteins are a vital part of enzymes, hormones, and blood plasma. Many body processes are regulated by enzymes and hormones. Plasma proteins help control water balance between the circulatory system and surrounding tissues. Protein is also used to build antibodies, which help defend the body against disease and foreign substances.

In the event of insufficient stores of carbohydrate and fat (the body's primary and secondary sources of energy), protein, in the form of amino acids, can be converted into glucose and used for energy. This process is called **gluconeogenesis**. However, when protein is used for energy, it is not available for its primary function. Using protein for energy also results in waste products that are difficult for the kidneys to excrete.

Classification and Sources

Protein is classified by source and completeness. Animal sources include meat, fish, poultry, eggs, milk, and dairy products. Plant sources are grains, legumes, nuts, and seeds.

The completeness of a protein refers to its quality. Of the 22 amino acids, 9 are called essential amino acids, that is, they must be present in the diet because the body cannot synthesize them. **Complete proteins** contain all 9 essential amino acids. All animal proteins, with the exception of gelatin, are complete proteins; the only complete plant protein is soy beans.

Plant proteins (with the exception of soy beans) are **incomplete proteins**; that is one or more of the essential amino acids are missing. Because all plant proteins do not lack the same essential amino acids, they can be combined in various ways to provide all of the essential amino acids. When two plant protein foods are combined to provide the essential amino acids, they are said to be complementary. Some of the common complementary plant proteins are rice and beans (legumes); corn and beans; wheat bread and beans; toast and pea soup; and rice and lentils. Complementary proteins are a very important part of planning a healthy vegetarian diet.

Digestion, Absorption, and Storage

Chemical digestion of protein begins in the stomach, with hydrochloric acid activating the enzyme pepsin. However, most of the digestion takes place in the small intestine through the action of pancreatic and intestinal enzymes. The end products of protein digestion are amino acids. The body can then combine the amino acids to build, repair, and maintain body tissues.

The amino acids are absorbed into the blood by the capillaries in the villi of the intestinal mucosa. Amino acids not used to build proteins are converted to glucose, glycogen, or fat and are stored.

Signs of Deficiency and Excess

When people are unable to obtain an adequate supply of protein for an extended period, muscle wasting occurs, and arms and legs become very thin. At the same time, albumin (protein in blood plasma) deficiency causes edema, resulting in an extremely swollen appearance. The water is excreted when sufficient protein is eaten. People may lose appetite, strength, and weight, and wounds may heal very slowly. Clients suffering from edema become lethargic and depressed. These signs are seen in grossly neglected children or in the elderly poor or incapacitated.

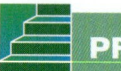

PROFESSIONAL TIP

Vegetarians and Protein

It is essential that clients following vegetarian diets carefully calculate the types and amount of protein in their diets so as to prevent protein deficiency.

People suffering from protein energy malnutrition lack both protein and energy-rich foods. Such a condition is not uncommon in developing countries where there are long-term shortages of both protein and energy foods. Children who lack sufficient protein do not grow to their potential size. Infants born to mothers eating insufficient protein during pregnancy can have permanently impaired mental capacities (Townsend & Roth, 2000).

Two deficiency diseases that affect children are caused by a grossly inadequate supply of protein, energy, or both. Marasmus, a condition resulting from severe malnutrition, afflicts very young children who lack both energy and protein foods as well as vitamins and minerals. The infant with marasmus appears emaciated but does not have edema; hair is dull and dry, and the skin is thin and wrinkled. Kwashiorkor results when there is a sudden or recent lack of protein-containing food (such as during a famine). This disease results in edema, painful skin lesions, and changes in the pigmentation of skin and hair (Townsend & Roth, 2000).

It is easy for people living in the developed parts of the world to ingest more protein than the body requires. There are a number of reasons this should be avoided. The saturated fats and cholesterol common to complete protein foods may contribute to heart disease and provide more kcal than are desirable. Some studies seem to indicate a connection between long-term high-protein diets and colon cancer and high calcium excretion, which depletes the bones of calcium and may contribute to osteoporosis. People who eat excessive amounts of protein-rich foods may ignore the also essential fruits and vegetables, and excess protein intake may put more demands on the kidneys than they can handle (Townsend & Roth, 2000).

Vitamins

Vitamins are organic compounds essential to life and health. They regulate body processes and are needed in very small amounts. They have no fuel value but are required for the metabolism of fats, carbohydrates, and proteins.

Daily Requirements

The Food and Nutrition Board of the National Academy of Sciences—National Research Council has pre-

LIFE CYCLE CONSIDERATIONS

Vitamins

Vitamin needs vary with the life cycle. Vitamin supplements are generally needed for pregnant or lactating women, infants, and elders.

pared a list of recommended dietary allowances for the 11 vitamins for which it considers current scientific research to be adequate for determining daily recommendations (Appendix C). Vitamin allowances are given by weight in milligrams (mg) or micrograms (μg or mcg).

Vitamins taken in addition to the vitamins received in the diet are called vitamin supplements. Lifestyle choices may affect the need for vitamin supplementation; refer to Table 18-3.

Functions

The functions of vitamins are unique to each individual vitamin. Table 18-4 and Table 18-5 list the functions of each type of vitamin.

Classification and Sources

Vitamins are commonly grouped according to solubility. Vitamins A, D, E, and K are fat soluble, and vitamin C and the B-complex vitamins are water soluble; refer to Tables 18-4 and 18-5.

Fat-Soluble Vitamins The **fat-soluble vitamins** (A, D, E, and K) require the presence of fats for their absorption from the GI tract into the lymphatic system and for cellular metabolism. They must attach to protein carriers to be transported through the blood. Excess intake is not excreted but, rather, is stored in the liver and adipose tissue. The body's stored reserve makes daily intake unnecessary. In fact, the reserve can result in toxic levels if large supplemental doses are taken, especially in the case of vitamin A. Deficiencies can occur in conditions that interfere with fat absorption.

Table 18-3 SUPPLEMENTS FOR LIFESTYLE CHOICES

LIFESTYLE CHOICE	SUGGESTED SUPPLEMENT
Restricted diets	B₁₂ (cobalamin)
Extensive exercise program	Riboflavin
Oral contraceptives	Pyridoxine, niacin, vitamin C
Smoking	Vitamin C
Alcohol	Thiamine, folate
Caffeine	B vitamins, vitamin C

Table 18-4 FAT-SOLUBLE VITAMINS

VITAMIN	FUNCTION	SOURCES	DEFICIENCY	TOXIC EFFECTS
A	• Aids in night vision • Promotes growth of bones and teeth • Maintains skin and mucous membranes	• Fish oils • Carrots • Sweet potatoes • Broccoli • Cantaloupe • Green leafy vegetables	• Night blindness • Dry, scaly skin • Diarrhea • Respiratory infections	• From supplementation: anorexia, diarrhea, hair loss, bone pain, liver damage
D	• Stimulates absorption of calcium and phosphorus for good bone mineralization	• Yeast • Fish liver oils • Fortified milk and cereals	• Rickets • Malformed teeth • Bone deformities	• Hypercalcemia • Kidney stones • Cardiovascular damage
E	• Acts as an antioxidant • Maintains cell membrane integrity • Protects red blood cells (RBCs) from hemolysis	• Vegetable oils • Leafy vegetables • Wheat germ	• Increased RBC hemolysis • Rare, except in cases of fat malabsorption	• Depression • Fatigue • Diarrhea • Cramps • Headaches
K	• Responsible for synthesis of prothrombin, needed for normal blood clotting	• Dark-green leafy vegetables • Made by intestinal bacteria	• Rare, except in newborns • Delayed blood clotting	• No toxic effects

Table 18-5 WATER-SOLUBLE VITAMINS

VITAMIN	FUNCTION	SOURCES	DEFICIENCY	TOXIC EFFECTS
C (asorbic acid)	• Builds and maintains strong tissues • Promotes wound healing • Aids in resisting infection • Enhances iron absorption	• Citrus fruits • Green and red peppers • Tomatoes • Melons • Cabbage • Broccoli • Strawberries	• Scurvy • Easy bruising • Delayed wound healing • Swollen, inflamed gums • Secondary infections	• Megadoses; excessive iron absorption • Nausea • Diarrhea
B_1 (thiamine)	• Promotes CHO metabolism • Ensures normal nervous system functioning	• Enriched grains and cereals • Pork • Legumes	• Beriberi • Mental confusion • Anorexia • Fatigue • Muscle weakness	• None known
B_2 (riboflavin)	• Promotes CHO, protein, and fat metabolism • Promotes deoxyribonucleic acid (DNA) synthesis • Aids in protein synthesis	• Milk and milk products • Meat, poultry, fish • Enriched grains and cereals	• Oral lesions • Dermatitis • Cheilosis • Red, swollen tongue • Reddening of cornea	• None known

continued

Table 18-5 WATER-SOLUBLE VITAMINS *continued*

VITAMIN	FUNCTION	SOURCES	DEFICIENCY	TOXIC EFFECTS
Niacin (nicotinic acid)	• Aids in oxidation • Promotes CHO, protein, and fat metabolism • Aids tissue protein building	• Meat, poultry, fish • Legumes • Enriched grains • Peanuts	• Pellegra • Anorexia • Apathy • Weakness • Dermatitis • Diarrhea • Dementia	• Large doses: flushing, itching, hypotension, tachycardia
B_6 (pyridoxine)	• Is necessary for amino acid metabolism • Promotes blood formation • Maintains nervous tissue	• Chicken, fish, pork • Eggs • Whole grains	• Depression • Dermatitis • Abnormal brain wave patterns • Convulsions • Anemia	• Clumsiness • Nerve degeneration
B_{12} (cobolomin)	• Promotes normal function of all cells, especially those of the nervous system • Promotes blood formation • Promotes CHO, protein, and fat metabolism • Aids in synthesis of ribonucleic acid (RNA) and DNA • Is necessary for folate metabolism	• Fresh shrimp, oysters, meats, milk, eggs, and cheese	• Pernicious anemia • Anorexia • Indigestion • Paresthesia of hands and feet • Poor coordination • Depression	• None known
Folate (folic acid)	• Is necessary for synthesis of ribonucleic acid (RNA) and DNA • Promotes amino acid metabolism, RBC and white blood cell (WBC) formation	• Green leafy vegetables • Milk • Eggs • Yeast	• Glossitis • Diarrhea • Macrocytic anemia	• None known
Pantothenic acid	• Promotes CHO, protein, and fat metabolism	• Animal tissues • Whole-grain cereals • Legumes • Milk	• Not observed in humans	• None known
Biotin	• Promotes CHO and fat metabolism • Is necessary for glycogen formation	• Egg yolk • Yeast • Milk • Soy flours • Cereals • Legumes • Made by intestinal bacteria	• Only induced with long-term total parenteral nutrition (TPN)	• None known

Water-Soluble Vitamins The **water-soluble vitamins** (C and the B-complex vitamins) require daily ingestion in normal quantities, because they are not stored in the body. They are absorbed by the capillaries in the intestinal villi directly into the circulatory system. When consumed in excess of the body's need, they are excreted in the urine. Deficiency symptoms develop quickly in response to inadequate intake. Foods should be cooked in the least amount of water possible, because the water-soluble vitamins are released

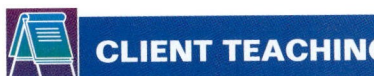

CLIENT TEACHING

Natural or Synthetic Vitamins

Some people believe that natural vitamins are superior in quality to synthetic vitamins. According to the U.S. Food and Drug Administration (FDA), however, the body cannot distinguish between a vitamin of plant or animal origin and one manufactured in a laboratory. The two types of the same vitamin are chemically identical.

PROFESSIONAL TIPS

Enriched or Fortified Foods

Foods that have synthetic vitamins added to them during processing are labeled as enriched, or fortified. An example is milk, which frequently has vitamins A and D added to it.

into the cooking water: When the water is discarded, the vitamins are lost.

Digestion, Absorption, and Storage

Vitamins do not require digestion. Fat-soluble vitamins are absorbed into the lymphatic system, whereas water-soluble vitamins are absorbed directly into the circulatory system. Excess amounts of fat-soluble vitamins cannot be excreted but are stored in the liver and adipose tissue. Water-soluble vitamins are excreted through urine, when excess amounts are taken into the body.

Signs of Deficiency or Excess

Vitamin deficiencies can occur and result in disease. Those persons inclined to vitamin deficiencies because they do not eat balanced diets include alcoholics; the poor; incapacitated elders; clients with serious diseases that affect appetite; mentally retarded persons; and young children who receive inadequate care. Deficiencies of fat-soluble vitamins occur in clients with chronic malabsorption diseases such as cystic fibrosis, celiac disease, and Crohn's disease.

Vitamins consumed in excess amounts can be toxic to the body; refer to Table 18-4 and Table 18-5.

Minerals

Minerals are inorganic elements that help regulate body processes and/or serve as structural components of the body. Like vitamins they have no fuel value (refer to Table 18-1).

Chemical analysis shows that the human body is made up of specific chemical elements. Four of these elements—oxygen, carbon, hydrogen, and nitrogen—make up 96% of body weight. All the remaining elements are minerals, which represent only 4% of body weight. Nevertheless, these minerals are essential for good health.

Daily Requirements

Major minerals are required in amounts greater than 100 mg/day. Trace minerals are those required in amounts less than 100 mg/day.

Functions

The functions of minerals are unique to each individual mineral. Table 18-6 outlines the functions of each mineral.

Classification and Sources

Minerals are generally classified as major minerals and trace elements (Table 18-7, p. 350). The major minerals occur in large amounts in the body and the required intake is greater than for the trace elements.

Table 18-6 MINERALS

MINERAL	FUNCTION	SOURCES	DEFICIENCY	TOXIC EFFECTS
Calcium (Ca)	• Aids in bone and teeth formation • Promotes muscle contraction and relaxation • Aids blood clotting • Aids in nerve transmission • Promotes normal heart rhythm • Needs vitamin D for absorption	• Milk • Cheese • Sardines • Salmon • Green leafy vegetables • Whole grains	• Rickets • Osteoporosis • Tetany • Poor tooth formation	• Kidney stones • Deposits in joints and soft tissue • May inhibit iron and zinc absorption

continued

Table 18-6 MINERALS *continued*

VITAMIN	FUNCTION	SOURCES	DEFICIENCY	TOXIC EFFECTS
Phosphorus (P)	• Aids in bone and teeth formation • Involved in energy metabolism • Regulates acid–base balance • Ensures structure of cell membranes • Is part of nucleic acids	• Fish, beef, pork, poultry • Cheese • Legumes • Milk • Carbonated beverages	• Rickets • Osteoporosis • Poor tooth formation • Disturbed acid base balance	• Low serum calcium • Kidney stones
Sodium (Na)	• Helps regulate fluid balance and acid–base balance • Regulates cell membrane irritability • Regulates nerve transmission	• Table salt • Milk • Meat • Processed foods • Carrots • Celery	• Hyponatremia • Nausea • Headache • Mental confusion • Hypotension • Anxiety • Muscle spasms	• Hypernatremia • Hypertension • Cardiovascular disturbance • Edema
Potassium (K)	• Maintains fluid balance • Maintains acid–base balance • Regulates muscle activity • Aids in protein synthesis • Aids in CHO metabolism	• Fruits, especially oranges, bananas, and prunes • Red meats • Vegetables • Milk and milk products • Coffee	• Hypokalemia • Fluid and electrolyte imbalances • Tissue breakdown • Cardiac weakness • Muscle cramps	• Hyperkalemia • Muscle weakness • Severe dehydration • Mental confusion • Hypotension • Cardiac arrest
Magnesium (Mg)	• Is necessary for muscle–nerve action • Regulates CHO, CHON, and fat metabolism • Activates enzymes • Aids in bone formation	• Green leafy vegetables • Whole grains • Legumes	• Hypomagnesemia • Tremors • Spasms • Convulsions	• Hypermagnesemia • Central nervous system (CNS) depression • Coma • Hypotension
Chlorine (Cl)	• Helps regulate fluid balance and acid–base balance • Aids digestion as part of hydrochloric acid in stomach	• Table salt • Milk • Meat • Processed foods	• Rare	• Rare
Sulfur (S)	• Serves as component of amino acids • Aids vitamin, enzyme, and hormonal activity • Is part of skin, hair, nails, and soft tissue	• Cheese • Eggs • Poultry • Fish	• None specific	• None specific
Iron (Fe)	• Aids in formation of hemoglobin • Aids in antibody formation	• Meat • Whole grains • Egg yolk • Legumes • Prunes • Raisins • Apricots	• Iron deficiency • Anemia	• Hemochromatosis • GI cramping • Vomiting • Nausea • Shock • Convulsions • Coma

continued

Table 18-6 MINERALS *continued*

VITAMIN	FUNCTION	SOURCES	DEFICIENCY	TOXIC EFFECTS
Iodine (I)	• Is a component of thyroid hormones	• Iodized salt • Seafood (salt water) • Milk	• Cretinism • Goiter	• Hyperthyroidism • Fatal in large amounts
Zinc (Zn)	• Is a component of DNA and RNA • Aids in physical and sexual development • Helps ensure normal taste and smell • Aids in wound healing	• Meats, oysters • Eggs • Milk • Whole grains	• Poor wound healing • Decreased taste and smell • Growth retardation	• Muscle incoordination • Vomiting • Diarrhea • Renal failure
Selenium (Se)	• Acts as an antioxidant • Works with vitamin E	• Seafoods • Meats	• Muscle weakness • Cardiomyopathy	• Selenosis • Nausea • Peripheral Neuropathy • Fatigue
Copper (Cu)	• Aids in bone and blood formation • Promotes iron absorption • Is part of myelin sheath	• Seafood • Nuts • Legumes	• Iron-deficiency anemia • Hypocholesterolemia	• None known
Manganese (Mn)	• Aids bone growth • Aids reproduction • Acts as enzyme activator	• Whole-grain cereals • Legumes • Tea	• Unknown	• Unlikely
Flourine (Fl)	• Protects against dental caries • Contributes to bone formation and integrity	• Flouridated water • Tea • Seafood	• Dental caries	• Mottled stains on teeth
Chromium (Cr)	• Associated with glucose metabolism	• Whole grains • Brewers yeast	• Insulin resistance • Impaired glucose tolerance	• Dietary: unlikely
Molybdenum (Mo)	• Helps ensure normal body metabolism	• Milk • Legumes • Whole grains	• Decrease production of uric acid	• Interferes with copper metabolism
Cobolt (Co)	• Is a component of vitamin B_{12} • Aids in RBC formation	• Meat, as B_{12}	• Associated with vitamin B_{12} deficiency	• Unknown

Minerals are found in water and in natural (unprocessed) foods, together with proteins, carbohydrates, fats, and vitamins. Minerals in the soil are absorbed by growing plants. Humans obtain minerals by eating plants grown in mineral-rich soil or by eating animals that have eaten such plants.

Highly processed or refined foods such as sugar and white flour contain almost no minerals. Iron, together with the vitamins thiamin, riboflavin, niacin, and folate is commonly added back to some flour and cereals, which are then labeled enriched.

Most minerals in food occur as salts, which are soluble in water. Therefore, the minerals leave the food and remain in the cooking water when foods are cooked in water. Foods should be cooked in as little water as possible or, preferably, steamed, and any cooking liquid should be saved to be used in soups, gravies, and white sauces. Using this liquid improves the flavor as well as the nutrient content of foods to which it is added.

Supplemental minerals may be required during growth periods and in some clinical situations. Individuals

LIFE CYCLE CONSIDERATIONS

Mineral Supplements
- During adolescence calcium may be needed, if the diet is insufficient.
- Pregnant and lactating women require added calcium, phosphorus, and iron.

with iron deficiency anemia require extra iron. Persons taking potassium-losing diuretics need a potassium supplement. Functions, sources, deficiencies, and toxic effects of minerals are listed in Table 18-7.

Digestion, Absorption, and Storage

Minerals are absorbed in their ionic forms (i.e., carrying a positive or negative electrical charge). The amount of a mineral absorbed by the body is influenced by three factors:

- *Type of food:* Minerals in foods that come from animals are more readily absorbed than those in foods that come from plants.
- *Need of body:* If there is a deficiency of a mineral in the body, more will be absorbed.
- *Health of absorbing tissue:* If absorbing tissue (intestine) is affected by disease, less will be absorbed.

Signs of Deficiency and Excess

Because it is known that minerals are essential to good health, some would-be nutritionists will make claims that "more is better." Ironically, more can be hazardous to one's health when it comes to minerals. In a healthy individual eating a balanced diet, there will be some normal mineral loss through perspiration

PROFESSIONAL TIP

Vitamins, Minerals, and Herbs
Since July 1994, the federal Food and Drug Administration has placed limitations on marketing claims for vitamins, minerals, and herbs. The rules are aimed at deterring false or unproven health claims and require that companies selling these products make only claims that are substantiated by broad scientific consensus. Labeling requirements of dietary supplements began in July 1995.

and saliva, and amounts in excess of body needs will be excreted in urine and feces. However, when concentrated forms of minerals are taken on a regular basis and over a period of time, they become more than the body can handle, and toxicity develops. An excessive amount of one mineral can sometimes cause a deficiency of another mineral. In addition, excessive amounts of minerals can cause hair loss and changes in the blood, hormones, bones, muscles, blood vessels, and nearly all tissues. Concentrated forms of minerals should be used only on the advice of a physician. Refer to Table 18-6 for specific signs of deficiency and toxicity of each mineral.

PROMOTING PROPER NUTRITION

Through the years, various ways to promote proper nutrition have been devised. The best known are the Four Food Groups, the Food Guide Pyramid, the Dietary Guidelines for Americans, the Recommended Daily Allowances, and the Dietary Reference Intakes.

Four Food Groups (Historical)

For many years, the four food group system constituted a plan to assist people in eating a well-balanced diet. Consuming foods from the four groups—milk, meat, fruit/vegetable, and bread/cereal—provided most nutrients required in a daily diet. The minimum servings given for the four food groups yielded approximately 1,200 kcal. Additional servings were to be added depending on the individual's age and activity level.

Food Guide Pyramid

In 1992, the United States Department of Agriculture introduced the food guide pyramid, which identifies the food groups from which additional servings should be obtained when calorie needs exceed the 1,200 kcal provided for by the minimum servings from the four food groups. The pyramid separates the fruit and vegetable groups and the suggested number of servings from each of these groups. The food guide

Table 18-7 MAJOR MINERALS AND TRACE ELEMENTS

MAJOR MINERALS	TRACE ELEMENTS	
	Essential	**Questionable**
Calcium (Ca)	Iron (Fe)	Arsenic (As)
Phosphorus (P)	Iodine (I)	Boron (B)
Sodium (Na)	Zinc (Zn)	Cadmium Cd)
Potassium (K)	Selenium (Se)	Nickel (Ni)
Magnesium (Mg)	Copper (Cu)	Silicon (Si)
Chlorine (Cl)	Manganese (Mn)	Tin (Sn)
Sulfur (S)	Fluorine (Fl)	Vanadium (V)
	Chromium (Cr)	
	Molybdenum (Mo)	
	Cobalt (Co)	

pyramid also focuses on fat, because most American diets are too high in fat. Figure 18-3 shows the Food Guide Pyramid.

Each food group of the food guide pyramid provides some, but not all, of the nutrients needed each day. Foods in one group cannot replace foods in another group. No one group is more important than another: All are needed.

Bread, Cereal, Rice, and Pasta Group

At the base of the pyramid is the bread, cereal, rice, and pasta group. The nutrients contributed by this group are complex carbohydrates, incomplete protein, the B vitamins, and iron, if the product is whole grain or **enriched** (nutrients that are removed during processing are added back) with iron. Six to eleven servings a day should come from this group. Examples of serving sizes from this group are one slice of bread, one tortilla, 1 ounce (1 cup) dry cereal, and ½ cup cooked cereal, rice, or pasta.

Fruit and Vegetable Groups

On the second level of the pyramid are the foods that come from plants: fruits and vegetables. Most people should eat more of these foods because of the vitamins, minerals, and fiber they supply.

The nutritional contributions of fruits and vegetables are carbohydrates, vitamins, minerals, water, and very small amounts of proteins and fats. Dietary fiber, important for elimination, is found in the skin or pulp of many foods in this group.

Fruits Each person should have two to four servings of fruit every day. Citrus fruits, melons, and berries should be eaten regularly as they are high in vitamin C. Examples of serving sizes from the fruit group are one medium size apple, pear, banana, or orange; ½ cup of cooked, chopped, or canned fruit, or ¾ cup of fruit juice.

Vegetables From the vegetable group three to five servings a day are suggested. Among the vegetables eaten daily, one should be a dark-green or deep-yellow vegetable to provide vitamin A. Sample serving sizes from the vegetable group include 1 cup of raw leafy vegetables; ½ cup of cooked or chopped raw vegetables; or ¾ cup of vegetable juice.

Milk and Meat Groups

On the third level are the foods that come mostly from animals. These foods have significantly greater amounts of saturated fat or added sugar than do the foods on the first and second levels. Fewer servings should be eaten from this level each day.

Milk The nutritional contributions of the milk group are calcium, protein, riboflavin, fat, carbohydrates, phosphorus, sodium, vitamin B$_{12}$, and vitamin A. If skim milk or skim milk products are used, there is no fat and significantly fewer kcal. All commercial milk

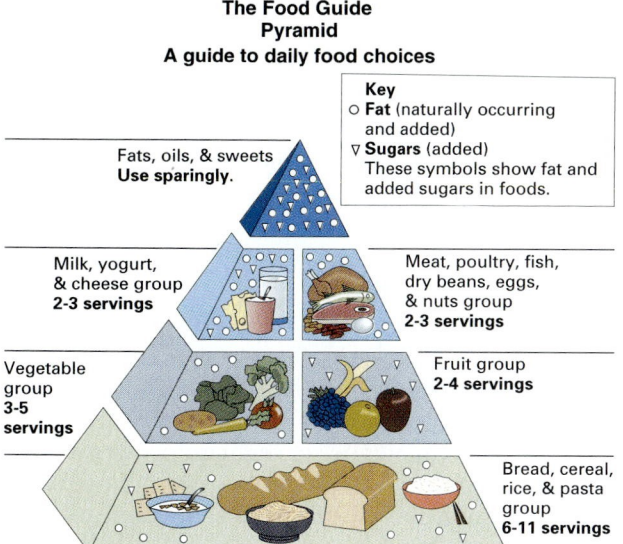

Figure 18-3 Food Guide Pyramid [*Courtesy of the U.S. Department of Agriculture, Human Nutrition Information Service, 1992. Food Guide Pyramid (Home and Garden Bulletin, No. 252). Washington, DC: USDA.*]

products are **fortified** (a nutrient not naturally occurring in a food is added to the food) with vitamin D. Vitamin D, not naturally found in milk, is added because the calcium provided by milk is better absorbed when vitamin D is present.

Two to three servings a day are suggested from the milk group. Eight ounces of milk is considered one serving. Other milk products and their serving sizes to provide the equivalent nutrients of 8 ounces of milk are 1½ ounces of cheese, 1 cup of yogurt, 1½ cups of cottage cheese, and 1½ cups of ice cream. The kcal content of these foods varies, with ice cream containing more kcal than do the other foods in the milk group.

Meat The meat group contributes protein (especially complete protein), fats, iron, most other minerals, and the B vitamins. Cheese and bacon are not considered part of this group because cheese has too little iron and bacon has too much fat.

The suggested number of servings from the meat group is two to three each day. A serving size is 2 to 3 ounces of meat, fish, or poultry. Other foods that can be substituted for one serving of meat are: two eggs, 4 tablespoons of peanut butter, or ½ cup cooked beans or peas (legumes). Legumes such as dried peas, beans, or lentils can be used instead of meat because of their high protein content. Peanuts as well as many other nuts are high in protein, but they are also typically high in fats and should thus be used sparingly.

Fats, Oils, and Sweets Group

Fats, oils, and sweets are placed at the very top of the pyramid because they do not fit into any of the other food groups. These other food items are considered to be **empty calories**, that is, they generally provide many calories but very few nutrients. Items included are potato chips, cookies, cakes, pies, soft drinks, alcohol, jelly, syrup, fats, oils, salad dressings, pickles, olives, catsup, and mustard. These foods are to be eaten in very small amounts and infrequently, as they have the most fat and added sugar and the least nutritional value of all the foods.

Number of Servings

The number of servings for an individual depends on the number of calories the individual needs. The number of calories needed by a person depends on age, gender, size, and activity. Almost everyone should have the minimum number of servings for each group. Three general calorie levels are suggested, the serving recommendations for which are listed in Table 18-8.

The Vegetarian Diet

There are several vegetarian diets. The common factor among them is that they do not include red meat. Some include eggs, some fish, some milk, and some even poultry. When carefully planned, these diets can be nutritious. They can even contribute to a reduction in obesity, high blood pressure, heart disease, some cancers, and, possibly, diabetes (Townsend & Roth, 2000). They must be carefully planned so that they include all the needed nutrients.

Lacto-ovo vegetarians use dairy products and eggs but no meat, poultry, or fish.

Lacto-vegetarians use dairy products but no meat, poultry, or eggs.

Vegans avoid all animal foods. They use soybeans, chickpeas, meat analogues, and tofu. It is important that their meals be carefully planned to include appropriate combinations of the essential amino acids. For example, beans served with corn or rice, or peanuts eaten with wheat, are complementary proteins. Vegans can show deficiencies of calcium; vitamins A, D, and B_{12}; and, of course, proteins.

Dietary Guidelines

The *Dietary Guidelines* developed by the U.S. Department of Agriculture and the U.S. Department of Health & Human Services were last revised in 1990. They are now stated in positive terms (i.e., "eat . . ."; "consume . . .") instead of negative terms ("avoid . . ."). These guidelines attempt to prevent overnutrition by incorporating some of the concepts of the food guide pyramid (Table 18-9).

Recommended Dietary Allowances

Recommended dietary allowances (RDAs) of essential nutrients are the recommended intake levels judged adequate to meet the known nutrient needs of practically all healthy people. Recommendations are grouped according to infants, children, males, females, and pregnant/lactating, and are subdivided within those groups according to age. Amounts are also recommended for pregnancy and lactation. The RDAs are compiled by the Food and Nutrition Board of the National Academy of Sciences and are periodically revised (refer to Appendix C).

Dietary Reference Intakes

The dietary reference intakes (DRIs), according to Barrett (1998), are nutrient-based reference values for use in planning and assessing diets. They are intended to replace the RDAs. The DRIs focus on decreasing the risk of chronic disease through nutrition, rather than on protecting against deficiency diseases, as do the RDAs.

The DRIs encompass four categories:

- Estimated average requirement (EAR) is the amount that meets the estimated nutrient need of 50% of the individuals in a specific group.
- Recommended dietary allowance (RDA) is the amount that meets the nutrient need of almost all (97% to 98%) of healthy individuals in a specific age and gender group. It is the EAR plus an increase, based on scientific evidence, to account for variation within the specific group. The RDA should be used to achieve adequate nutrient intake aimed at decreasing the risk of chronic disease.
- Adequate intake (AI) is set when there is insufficient scientific evidence to estimate an average re-

---

Table 18-8 SERVINGS FOR THREE CALORIE LEVELS

FOOD GROUP	TOTAL CALORIC INTAKE AND NUMBER OF SERVINGS PER GROUP		
	1,600 calories	**2,200 calories**	**2,800 calories**
Bread	6 servings	9 servings	11 servings
Vegetable	3 servings	4 servings	5 servings
Fruit	2 servings	3 servings	4 servings
Milk	2 to 3 servings	2 to 3 servings	2 to 3 servings
Meat	5 ounces	6 ounces	7 ounces

A 1,600-calorie diet is about right for sedentary women and older adults.

A 2,200 calorie diet is about right for most children, teenage girls, and active women and for many sedentary men. Pregnant and lactating women may need more calories.

A 2,800 calorie diet is about right for teenage boys, many active men, and some very active women.

Adapted from Food Guide Pyramid . . . Beyond the Basic 4, *by USDA Human Nutrition Information Service and Food Marketing Institute, 1992.*

Table 18-9 DIETARY GUIDELINES FOR AMERICANS

Eat a variety of foods. More than 40 different nutrients are needed for good health. These should come from a variety of foods, not from a few highly fortified foods or supplements. No single food can supply all nutrients in the amounts needed. Choose foods each day from the five major food groups as shown on the food guide pyramid.

Maintain healthy weight. Check to see whether you are at a healthy weight; if not, set reasonable weight goals and try for long-term success through better habits of eating and exercise. Have children's height and weight checked regularly by a physician.

Choose a diet low in fat, saturated fat, and cholesterol. Use fats and oils sparingly in cooking. Choose liquid vegetable oils most often because they are lower in saturated fat. Check labels on foods to see how much fat and saturated fat are in a serving. Trim fat from meat; take skin off poultry. Have cooked dry beans and peas instead of meat occasionally. Moderate the use of egg yolks and organ meats. Choose skim or low-fat milk and fat-free or low-fat yogurt and cheese most of the time.

Choose a diet with plenty of vegetables, fruits, and grain products. Choose three or more servings of vegetables, two or more servings of fruits, and six or more servings of grain products such as breads, cereals, pasta, and rice, with an emphasis on whole grains. These foods are generally low in fat. Increase fiber intake by eating more of a variety of foods that contain fiber naturally.

Use sugars only in moderation. Use sugars in moderate amounts—sparingly if your calorie needs are low. Avoid excessive snacking, and brush and floss your teeth regularly.

Use salt and sodium only in moderation. Use salt sparingly, if at all, in cooking and at the table. Use salted snacks, such as chips, crackers, pretzels, and nuts, sparingly. Check food labels for the amount of sodium in the product. Choose those lower in sodium most of the time.

If you drink alcoholic beverages, do so in moderation. If you drink, be moderate in your intake. Women should have no more than one drink per day, men should not have more than two drinks per day. Alcohol should not be consumed by women who are pregnant or trying to conceive, individuals who plan to drive or engage in other activities that require attention or skill, individuals using prescription or over-the-counter medicines, individuals who cannot keep their drinking moderate, and children and adolescents.

From Nutrition and Your Health: Dietary Guidelines for Americans *(3rd ed., Home and Garden Bulletin, No. 232), by the U. S. Department of Agriculture, and U. S. Department of Health and Human Services, 1990.*

quirement. It is derived through experimental or observational data that show a mean intake that appears to sustain a desired indicator of health, such as calcium retention in bone.

- Tolerable upper intake level (UL) is the maximum intake by an individual that is unlikely to pose risks of adverse health effects in almost all healthy individuals in a specified group. It is not intended to be a recommended level of intake. There is no established benefit for individuals to consume nutrients at levels above the RDA or AI.

FACTORS INFLUENCING NUTRITION

Many factors influence nutrition. Some of the major factors are culture, religion, socioeconomics, fads, and superstitions.

Culture

A person's culture encompasses a total way of life including values, attitudes, and practices. Food practices are a substantial part of a culture. These food habits are based on availability of foods, preparation techniques, methods of serving, and the personal meaning of food (Figure 18-4). American cuisine (cooking style) is a marvelous composite of countless national, regional, cultural, and religious food customs. Consequently, categorizing a client's food habits can be difficult. Nevertheless, it is sometimes helpful to be able to do so to a certain extent. People who are ill commonly have little interest in food, and sometimes foods that were familiar to them during their childhood and youth are more apt to tempt them than other types. The following section briefly discusses some food patterns typical of various cultures, regions, and countries. Of course, there can be and usually are enormous variations within any one classification.

Native American

It is thought that approximately one-half of the edible plants commonly eaten in the United States today originated with the Native Americans. Examples are corn, potatoes, squash, cranberries, pumpkins, peppers, beans, wild rice, and cocoa beans. In addition, wild fruits, game, and fish were used. Foods were commonly prepared as soups and stews or were dried. The original Native American diets were probably more nutritionally adequate than are current diets, which frequently consist of a too-high proportion of sweet and salty, snack-type, low-nutrient foods. Native American diets today may be deficient in calcium, vitamins A and C, and riboflavin (Townsend & Roth, 2000).

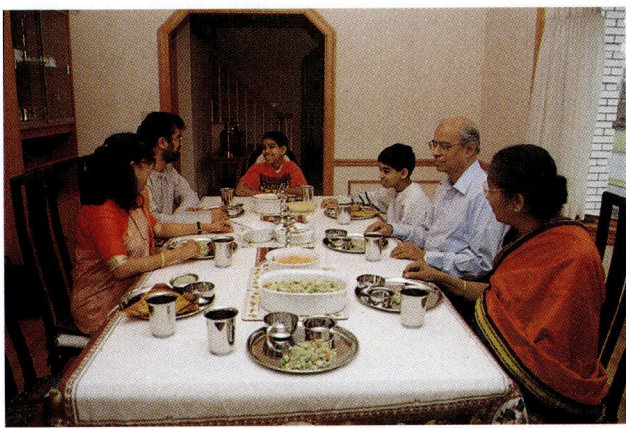

Figure 18-4 Family and cultural values often affect diet.

U.S. Southern

Hot breads such as corn bread and baking powder biscuits are common in the U.S. South because the wheat grown in the area does not make good-quality yeast breads. Grits and rice are also popular carbohydrate foods. Favorite vegetables include sweet potatoes, squash, green beans, and lima beans. Green beans cooked with pork are commonly served. Watermelon, oranges, and peaches are popular fruits. Fried fish is served often, as are barbecued and stewed meats and poultry. These diets have a great deal of carbohydrate and fat and limited amounts of protein in some cases. Iron, calcium, and vitamins A and C may be deficient (Townsend & Roth, 2000).

Mexican

Mexican food is a combination of Spanish and Native American foods. Beans, rice, chili peppers, tomatoes, and corn meal are favorites. Meat is often cooked with a vegetable, as in chili con carne. Corn meal or flour is used to make tortillas, which are served as bread. The combination of beans and corn makes a complete protein. Corn tortillas filled with cheese (called enchiladas) provide some calcium, but the use of milk should be encouraged. Additional green and yellow vegetables and vitamin C-rich foods would also make these diets more well-balanced.

Puerto Rican

Rice is the basic carbohydrate food in Puerto Rican diets. Vegetables commonly used include beans, plantains, tomatoes, and peppers. Bananas, pineapple, mangoes, and papayas are popular fruits. Favorite meats are chicken, beef, and pork. Milk is not used as much as would be desirable from the nutritional point of view (Townsend & Roth, 2000).

Italian

Pastas with various tomato or fish sauces and cheese are popular Italian foods. Fish and highly seasoned foods are common to southern Italian cuisine; whereas meat and root vegetables are common to northern cuisine. The eggs, cheese, tomatoes, green vegetables, and fruits common to Italian diets provide excellent sources of many nutrients, but additional fat-free milk and low-fat meat would make the diet more complete (Townsend & Roth, 2000).

Northern and Western European

Northern and Western European diets are similar to those of the U.S. Midwest, but with a greater use of dark breads, potatoes, and fish, and fewer green-vegetable salads. Beef and pork are popular, as are various cooked vegetables, breads, cakes, and dairy products. The addition of fresh vegetables and fruits would add vitamins, minerals, and fiber to these diets.

Central European

Citizens of Central Europe obtain the greatest portion of their calories from potatoes and grain, especially rye and buckwheat (Townsend & Roth, 2000). Pork is a popular meat. Cabbage cooked in many ways is a popular vegetable, as are carrots, onions, and turnips. Eggs and dairy products are used abundantly. Limiting the number of eggs consumed and using fat-free or low-fat dairy products would reduce the fat content in this diet. Adding fresh vegetables and fruits would increase vitamins, minerals, and fiber.

Middle Eastern

Grains, wheat, and rice provide energy in Middle Eastern diets. Chickpeas in the form of hummus are popular. Lamb and yogurt are commonly used as are cabbage, grape leaves, eggplant, tomatoes, dates, olives, and figs. Black, very sweet coffee is a popular beverage. There may be insufficient protein and calcium in this diet, depending on the amounts of meat and calcium-rich foods eaten. Fresh fruits and vegetables should be added to the diet to increase vitamins, minerals, and fiber.

Chinese

The Chinese diet is varied. Rice is the primary energy food and is used in place of bread. Vegetables are lightly cooked, and the cooking water is saved for future use. Soybeans are used in many ways, and eggs and pork are commonly served. Soy sauce is extensively used, but it is very salty and could present a problem for clients needing low-salt diets. Tea is a common beverage, but milk is not. This diet is typically low in fat (Townsend & Roth, 2000).

Japanese

Japanese diets include rice, soybean paste and curd, vegetables, fruits, and fish. Food is frequently served tempura style, which means fried. Soy sauce (shoyu) and tea are commonly used. Current Japanese diets have been greatly influenced by Western culture. Japanese diets may be deficient in calcium, given the near total lack of milk in the diet (Townsend & Roth, 2000). Although fish is eaten with bones, this may not supply sufficient calcium to meet needs. Japanese diets may contain excessive amounts of salt.

Indian

Many Indians are vegetarians who use eggs and dairy products. Rice, peas, and beans are frequently served. Spices, especially curry, are popular. Indian meals are not typically served in courses as Western meals are. They generally consist of one course with many dishes.

Thai, Vietnamese, Laotian, and Cambodian

Rice, curries, vegetables, and fruit are popular in Thailand, Vietnam, Laos, and Cambodia. Meats and fish are used in small amounts. The wok (a deep, round fry pan) is used for sautéing many foods. A salty sauce made from fermented fish is commonly used. Thai, Vietnamese, Laotian, and Cambodian diets may contain deficient amounts of protein and calcium (Townsend & Roth, 2000).

Religion

Religious beliefs often influence nutrition by placing restrictions on the foods eaten and their preparation. A few examples follow.

Jewish

Interpretations of the Jewish dietary laws vary. Persons who adhere to the Orthodox view consider tradition important and always observe the dietary laws. Foods prepared according to these laws are called *kosher*. Conservative Jews are inclined to observe the rules only at home. Reform Jews consider their dietary laws to be essentially ceremonial and thus minimize their significance. Essentially the laws require the following (Townsend & Roth, 2000):

- Slaughtering must be done by a qualified person and in a prescribed manner. The meat or poultry must be drained of blood, first by severing the jugular vein and carotid artery, then by soaking the meat in brine before cooking.
- Meat and meat products may not be prepared with milk or milk products.
- The dishes used in the preparation and serving of meat products must be kept separate from those used for dairy foods.
- Dairy products and meat may not be eaten together. Six hours must elapse after eating meat before eating dairy products, and at least 30 minutes to 1 hour must elapse after eating dairy products before eating meat.
- The mouth must be rinsed after eating fish and before eating meat.
- The following may not be eaten: animals without cloven (split) hooves or animals that do not chew their cud; hindquarters of any animal; shellfish or fish without scales or fins; birds of prey; creeping things and insects; and leavened (containing ingredients that cause it to rise) bread during Passover.

There are prescribed fast days: Passover Week, Yom Kippur, and Feast of Purim. Chicken and fresh smoked and salted fish are popular, as are noodles, eggs, and flour dishes. These diets can be deficient in fresh vegetables and milk.

Roman Catholic

Although the dietary restrictions of the Roman Catholic religion have been liberalized, meat is not allowed its adherents on Ash Wednesday and Fridays during Lent.

Eastern Orthodox

The Eastern Orthodox religion includes Christians from the Middle East, Russia, and Greece. Although interpretations of the dietary laws vary, meat, poultry, fish, and dairy products are restricted on Wednesdays and Fridays and during Lent and Advent.

Seventh Day Adventists

In general, Seventh Day Adventists are lacto-ovo vegetarians, meaning that they use milk products and eggs, but no meat, fish, or poultry. Nuts, legumes, meat analogues (substitutes), and tofu (made from soybeans) may be used. Coffee, tea, and alcohol are considered to be harmful.

Mormon (Latter Day Saints)

The only dietary restriction observed by the Mormons is the prohibition of coffee, tea, and alcoholic beverages.

Islamic

Adherents of Islam are called Muslims. Dietary laws prohibit the use of pork and alcohol, and other meats must be slaughtered according to specific laws. During the month of Ramadan, Muslims do not eat or drink during daylight hours.

Hindu

To the Hindus, all life is sacred, and animals contain the souls of ancestors. Consequently, most Hindus are vegetarians, and do not use eggs in food preparation because eggs represent life.

Socioeconomics

The amount of money available to purchase food certainly influences nutrition. More money, however, does not always mean better nutrition. Often, persons with less money plan their meals and buy food more carefully than do those with higher incomes. Expensive food does not mean better nutrition. Many times, persons with no monetary worries eat what they want, when they want, without paying attention to nutritional value, thereby shortchanging themselves nutritionally.

Fads

Food fads are beliefs that persist for a period of time about certain foods and that generally have no scientific basis. Often, these fads are translated into diets that can be harmful if basic nutrients are missing or are in excess. One of the most popular diets some years ago was the grapefruit and egg diet. One of the more recent fads was the liquid-protein diet. This diet overloaded the body with protein, yet other nutrients were lacking. The excessive amount of protein damaged the kidneys of many people. Indeed, some people died from this fad diet (American Heart Association, 1999).

Superstitions

Superstitions are irrational beliefs about a food that are generally passed down from generation to generation. The nurse should be aware of the beliefs and the facts that contradict them so as to be knowledgeable and respectful. Examples of such superstitions are as follows:

- **Superstition:** Toast is less fattening than bread.
  Fact: Only moisture is removed during toasting.
- **Superstition:** "Cravings" during pregnancy should be satisfied or the infant will be marked or deformed.
  Fact: Foods eaten or not eaten by the mother do not directly affect the infant, only the nutrients or lack thereof.

NUTRITIONAL NEEDS DURING THE LIFE CYCLE

As a person grows and develops from birth to old age, nutritional needs change. These changes generally are based on growth needs, energy needs, and utilization of nutrients. A nutritional assessment should be conducted to ascertain the nutritional status of the individual. The following basic assessment should be done for everyone over 1 year old.

- Nutritional status
- Height and weight
- Meal and snack pattern (food record or 24-hour recall)
- Adequacy of intake based on the food guide pyramid
- Food allergies
- Physical activity
- Cultural, ethnic, and family influences
- Use of vitamin/mineral supplements

Infancy

Food and its presentation are extremely important during the baby's first year. Physical and mental development are dependent on the food itself, and psychosocial development is affected by the time and manner whereby the food is offered.

Although babies have been fed according to prescribed time schedules in the past, it is preferable to feed infants on demand. Feeding on demand prevents the frustrations that hunger can bring and helps the child develop trust in people. The newborn may re-

PROFESSIONAL TIP

Nutritional Needs of Infants
It is important to remember that growth rates vary from child to child. Nutritional needs depend largely on a child's growth rate.

quire more frequent feedings, but, normally, the demand schedule averages approximately every 4 hours by the time the baby is 2 or 3 months old (Townsend & Roth, 2000).

Nutritional Requirements

The first year of life is a period of the most rapid growth in one's life. A baby doubles its birth weight by 6 months of age and triples it within the first year. This explains why the infant's energy, vitamin, mineral, and protein requirements are higher per unit of body weight than are those of older children or adults.

During the first year, the normal child needs approximately 100 kcal per kilogram of body weight each day. This is approximately two to three times the adult requirement. Infants who have suffered from low birth weight, malnutrition, or illness require more than the normal number of kcal per kilogram of body weight. The nutritional status of infants is reflected in many of the same characteristics as those of adults.

The American Academy of Pediatrics recommends breast milk for the first 12 months of life, although parents must decide on the method of feeding based on their lifestyle, values, and personal feelings.

Breast Milk Breastfeeding is nature's way of providing a good diet for the baby. It is, in fact, used as the guide by which nutritional requirements of infants are measured.

Mother's milk provides the infant with temporary immunity to many infectious diseases. It is sterile, easy to digest, and usually does not cause GI disturbances or allergic reactions. Breastfed infants grow more rapidly during the first few months of life than do formula-fed

CLIENT TEACHING

Breastfeeding
If the mother works and cannot be available for every feeding, breast milk can be expressed earlier, refrigerated or frozen, and used at the appropriate time, or a bottle of formula can be substituted. Never warm the breast milk in a microwave oven because the antibodies will be destroyed. Instead, warm a cup of water and place the bag of breast milk in the water to heat it.

CLIENT TEACHING

Cow's Milk

Infants under the age of 1 year should not be given regular cow's milk. Because its protein is more difficult and slower to digest than that of human milk, it can cause GI blood loss. The kidneys are challenged by its high protein and mineral content, and dehydration and even damage to the CNS can result. In addition, the fat is less bioavailable, meaning it is not absorbed as efficiently as that in human milk (Townsend & Roth, 2000).

CLIENT TEACHING

Nursing Bottle Syndrome

Infants should not be put to bed with a bottle. Saliva, which normally cleanses the teeth, diminishes as the infant falls asleep. The milk then bathes the upper front teeth, causing tooth decay. Also, the bottle can cause the upper jaw to protrude and the lower to recede. The result is known as the baby bottle mouth, or nursing bottle syndrome. It is preferable to feed the infant the bedtime bottle, cleanse the teeth and gums with some water from another bottle or cup, and then put the infant to bed.

babies, and they typically have fewer infections (especially ear infections). And, because breast milk contains less protein and minerals than does infant formula, it reduces the load on the infant's kidneys. Breastfeeding also promotes oral motor development in infants because sucking requires more and different muscles than does bottle feeding (Townsend & Roth, 2000).

One can be quite confident the infant is getting sufficient nutrients and kcal from breastfeeding if (1) there are six or more wet diapers per day; (2) there is normal growth; (3) there are one or two mustard-colored bowel movements per day; and (4) the breast becomes soft during nursing.

Formula If the baby is to be bottle-fed, the pediatrician will provide information on commercial formulas and feeding instructions. Formulas are usually based on cow's milk, because it is abundant and easily modified to resemble human milk. It must be modified because it has more protein and mineral salts and less milk sugar (lactose) than does human milk. Formulas are developed so that they are similar to human milk in nutrient and kcal values.

When an infant is extremely sensitive or allergic to infant formulas, a synthetic formula may be given. Synthetic milk is commonly made from soybeans. Formulas with predigested proteins are used for infants unable to tolerate all other types of formulas (Townsend & Roth, 2000).

Formulas can be purchased in ready-to-feed, concentrated, or powdered forms. Sterile water must be

mixed with the concentrated and powdered forms. The most convenient type is also the most expensive.

If the type purchased requires the addition of water, it is essential that the amount of water added be correctly measured. Too little water will create too heavy a protein and mineral load for the infant's kidneys; too much water will dilute the nutrient and kcal value such that the infant will not thrive.

Solid Foods The introduction of solid foods before the age of 4 to 6 months is not recommended. The child's GI tract and kidneys are not sufficiently developed to handle solid food before that age. Further, it is thought that the early introduction of solid foods may increase the likelihood of overfeeding and the possibility of the development of food allergies, particularly in children whose parents suffer from food allergies.

An infant's readiness for solid foods will be demonstrated by (1) the physical ability to pull food into the mouth rather than always pushing the tongue and food out of the mouth, (2) a willingness to participate in the process, (3) the ability to sit up with support, (4) having head and neck control, and (5) the need for additional nutrients. If the infant is drinking more than 32 ounces of formula or nursing 8 to 10 times in 24 hours, then solid food should be started.

Solid foods must be introduced gradually and individually. One food is introduced and then no other new food for 4 or 5 days. If there is no allergic reaction, another food can be introduced, a waiting period allowed, then another, and so on. The typical order of introduction begins with cereal, usually iron-fortified rice, then oat, wheat, and mixed cereals. Cooked and pureed vegetables follow, then cooked and pureed fruits, egg yolk, and, finally, finely ground meats. Between 6 and 12 months, toast, zwieback, teething biscuits, custards, puddings, and ice cream can be added.

When the infant learns to drink from a cup, juice can be introduced. Juice should never be given from a bottle because babies will fill up on it and not get

CLIENT TEACHING

Honey

Honey should never be given to an infant because it could be contaminated with *Clostridium botulinum* bacteria.

enough calories from other sources. Pasteurized apple juice is usually given first. It is recommended that only 100% juice products be given because they are nutrient dense (Townsend & Roth, 2000).

By the age of 1 year, most babies are eating foods from all the food guide pyramid's groups and may have most any food that is easily chewed and digested. However, precautions must be taken to avoid offering foods on which the child can choke. Examples include hot dogs, nuts, whole peas, grapes, popcorn, small candies, and small pieces of tough meat or raw vegetables. Foods should be selected according to the advice of the pediatrician.

Nutritional assessment for an infant should include the following:

- Height and weight
- Sleeping habits
- Type of feeding (breast- or bottle-fed)
- If breastfeeding, mother's nutritional status and use of alcohol, tobacco, caffeine, and drugs; infant's feeding schedule (how often fed and for how long)
- If formula feeding, type, frequency, and method of preparation and storage; feeding schedule; amount taken at each feeding
- Use of vitamin/mineral supplements
- If on solid foods, age at introduction, and any reactions or allergies
- Family attitudes about eating, food, and weight

Childhood

Although specific nutritional requirements change as children grow, nutrition always affects physical, mental, and emotional growth and development. Studies indicate that the mental ability and size of an individual are directly influenced by nutrition during the early years.

Eating habits develop during childhood. Once developed, poor eating habits are difficult to change. They can exacerbate emotional and physical problems such as irritability, depression, anxiety, fatigue, and illness. Good eating habits formed in early childhood will generally last a lifetime (Figure 18-5).

Parents should be aware that it is not uncommon for children's appetites to vary. The rate of growth is not constant. As the child ages, the rate of growth actually slows. The approximate weight gain of a child during the second year of life is only 5 pounds. Children between the ages of 1 and 3 years undergo vast changes: Their legs grow longer; they develop muscles; they lose their baby shape; they begin to walk and talk; and they learn to feed and generally assert themselves.

As children continue to grow and develop, their likes and dislikes may change. New foods should be introduced gradually, in small amounts, and as attractively as possible.

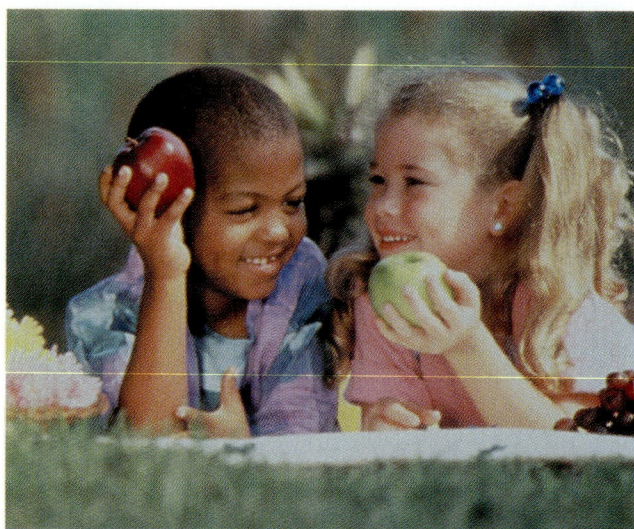

Figure 18-5 Good health radiates from these two children. (*Courtesy of USDA/ARS #K-48191*)

Children should be offered nutrient-dense foods because the amount eaten will be small. Fats should not be limited before the age of 2 years, but meals and snacks should not be fat-laden either. Whole milk is recommended until the age of 2, but low-fat or fat-free should be served from 2 years on. The guideline for fat intake after the age of 2 is 30% or less of total kcal per day, with no more than 10% coming from saturated fats. It is recommended that children not salt their food at the table or have foods prepared with a lot of salt (Townsend & Roth, 2000).

Children are especially sensitive to and reject hot (temperature) foods, but they like crisp textures, mild flavors, and familiar foods. They are wary of foods covered by sauce or gravy. Parents should set realistic goals and expectations as to the amount of food a child needs. A good rule of thumb for preschool children is one tablespoon of new food for each year of age. Table 18-10 details serving sizes according to age. Calorie needs depend on rate of growth, activity level, body size, metabolism, and health.

Nutritional Requirements

The rate of growth diminishes from the age of 1 year until about age 10, thus the kcal requirement per pound of body weight also diminishes during this period. For example, at 6 months, a girl needs approx-

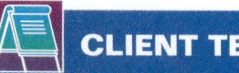

CLIENT TEACHING

Introducing New Foods

Allowing the child to assist in purchasing and preparing a new food is often a good way of arousing interest in the food and a desire to eat it.

Table 18-10 FOOD PLAN FOR PRESCHOOL AND SCHOOL-AGE CHILDREN BASED ON THE FOOD GUIDE PYRAMID

FOOD GROUP	NUMBER OF SERVINGS	APPROXIMATE SERVING SIZE*			
		AGE 1–2	AGE 3–4	AGE 5–6	AGE 7–12
Milk, yogurt, and cheese	3	½ to ¾ cup or 1 oz	¾ cup or 1½ oz	1 cup or 2 oz	1 cup or 2 oz
Meat, poultry, fish, dry beans, eggs, and nuts	2 or more	1 oz or 1 to 2 tbsp	1½ oz or 3 to 4 tbsp	1½ oz or ½ cup	2 oz or ½ cup
Vegetables	3 or more	1 to 2 tbsp	3 to 4 tbsp	½ cup	½ cup
Fruits	2 or more	1 to 2 tbsp or ½ cup juice	3 to 4 tbsp or ½ cup juice	½ cup or ½ cup juice	½ cup or ½ cup juice
Bread, cereal, rice, and pasta	6 or more	½ slice or ½ cup	1 slice or ½ cup	1 slice or ¾ cup	1 slice or ¾ cup

*Use as a starting point. Increase serving size as energy yields dictate, but maintain variety in the diet by making sure all food groups are still appropriately represented.

Adapted from Food and Nutrition Services, U. S. Department of Agriculture: Meal Plan Requirements and Offer versus Serve Manual, FNS-265, 1990.

imately 54 kcal per pound of body weight, but by the age of 10, she will require only 35 kcal per pound of body weight.

Nutrient needs, however, do not diminish. From the age of 6 months to 10 years, nutrient needs actually increase because of the increase in body size. Therefore, it is especially important that young children are given nutritious foods that they will eat.

In general, the young child will need 2 to 3 cups of milk each day, or the equivalent in terms of calcium. However, excessive use of milk should be avoided because it can crowd out other, iron-rich foods and possibly cause iron deficiency. The number of servings of the other food groups is the same as for adults, but the sizes will be smaller. The use of sweets should be minimized because the child is apt to prefer them to nutrient-rich foods. Sweetened fruit juices, especially, should be avoided. Children also need water and fiber in their diets. They need to drink 1 milliliter of water for each kcal. If food valued at 1,200 kcal is eaten, five

8-ounce glasses of water are needed. Fiber needs are calculated according to age. After age 3 years a child's fiber needs are "age + 5g" and no more than "age + 10g." A child who eats more fiber than that might be too full to eat enough other foods to provide all the kcal needed for growth and development. Fiber should be added slowly, if not already in the diet, and fluids must also be increased. Childhood is a good time to develop the lifelong good habit of getting enough dietary fiber to prevent constipation and diseases such as colon cancer and diverticulitis (Townsend & Roth, 2000). In addition to the basic nutritional assessments, dental health should also be assessed.

CLIENT TEACHING

Preventing Choking

Instruct parents to:

- Avoid the use of foods that may cause choking in infants and small children (up to 3 years old), such as corn, nuts, raw peas and carrots, celery, small candies, hot dogs, popcorn, and any other small, hard food
- Offer peanut butter only on bread or a cracker
- Stress the importance of sitting upright while eating
- Prohibit running with food or objects in the mouth

PROFESSIONAL TIP

Snacks

A child needs a snack every 3 to 4 hours for continued energy. Children often prefer finger foods for snacks. Snacks should be nutrient dense and as nutritious as food served at mealtimes. Cheese, saltines, fruit, milk, and unsweetened cereals make good snacks.

Adolescence

Adolescence is a period of rapid growth that causes major physiologic changes. The growth rate may be as much as 3 inches per year for girls and 4 inches for boys; nutrition plays a role in overall healthy adolescent development. Bones grow and gain density, muscle and fat tissue develop, and blood volume increases (Townsend & Roth, 2000).

Adolescents typically have enormous appetites. When good eating habits have been established during childhood and there is nutritious food available, the teenager's food habits should present no serious problem. However, peer pressure is great at this time, and good eating habits are often forgotten. Many adolescents skip breakfast and/or lunch and then eat at fast-food places (Figure 18-6). Adolescents are concerned with body image and often compare their bodies to those of their peers and of popular media figures. They often restrict food intake, leading to inadequate nutrient intake.

Nutritional Requirements

Because of adolescents' rapid growth, kcal requirements naturally increase. Boys' kcal requirements tend to be greater than do girls', because boys are generally bigger, tend to be more physically active, and have more lean muscle mass than do girls (Townsend & Roth, 2000).

Except for vitamin D, nutrient needs increase dramatically at the onset of adolescence. Because of menstruation, girls have a greater need for iron than do boys. The RDAs for vitamin D, vitamin C, vitamin B_{12}, calcium, phosphorus, and iodine are the same for both sexes. The RDAs for the remaining nutrients are higher for boys than they are for girls (Townsend & Roth, 2000).

In addition to the basic nutritional assessments, the following should be assessed for the adolescent client.

PROFESSIONAL TIP

Preventing Eating Disorders
- Encourage healthy dietary habits and adequate exercise
- Emphasize a healthy lifestyle over physical appearance and weight loss
- Encourage increased self-esteem and stress a positive self-worth
- Avoid pressuring children to achieve perfection or perform beyond their abilities
- Recognize signs and symptoms of eating disorders, and seek professional help when suspected

(From Health Assessment & Physical Examination, *by M. E. Z. Estes, 1998, Albany, NY: Delmar Publishers. Copyright 1998 by Delmar Publishers.)*

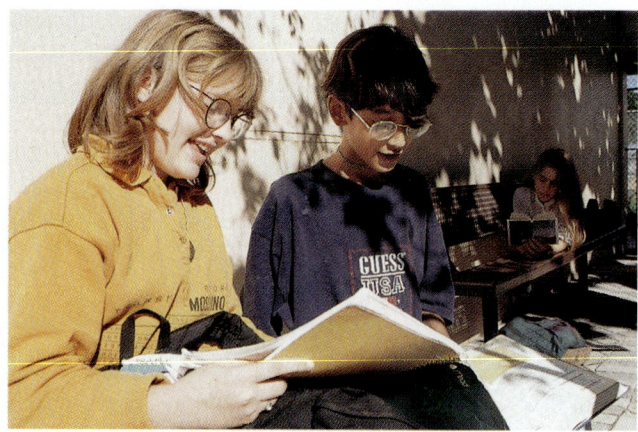

Figure 18-6 Adolescents are vulnerable to peer pressure.

- Use of alcohol, tobacco, caffeine, and drugs
- Use of fad diets
- Family attitude toward thinness and the adolescent's weight

Young and Middle Adulthood

The period of young adulthood ranges from approximately 18 years–40 years of age. Individuals are alive with plans, desires, and energy as they begin searching for and finding their places in the mainstream of adult life. They appear to have boundless energy for both social and professional activities. They are usually interested in exercise for its own sake and often participate in athletic events as well.

The middle adulthood period ranges from approximately 40 years–65 years of age. This is a time when the physical activities of young adulthood typically begin to decrease, resulting in lowered kcal requirement for most individuals. During these years, people seldom have young children to supervise, and the strenuous physical labor of some occupations may be delegated to younger people. Middle-age people may tire more easily than they did when they were younger. They may not get as much exercise as they did in earlier years. Because appetite and food intake may not decrease, there is a common tendency toward weight gain during this period (Townsend & Roth, 2000).

Nutritional Requirements

Physical growth is usually complete by the age of 25 years. Consequently, except during pregnancy and lactation, the essential nutrients are needed only to maintain and repair body tissue and to produce energy. During these years, the nutrient requirements of healthy adults change very little.

Despite men's generally larger size, only 11 of the given RDAs are greater for men than for women. Six of the RDAs are the same for both sexes. The iron requirement for women throughout the childbearing years remains higher than that for men. Extra iron is needed to replace blood loss during menstruation and to help build both the infant's and the extra maternal blood needed during pregnancy. After menopause, this requirement for women matches that of men (Townsend & Roth, 2000).

The kcal requirement begins to diminish after the age of 25 years, as basal metabolism is reduced by approximately 2% to 3% per decade. This is a small amount each year, but, after 25 years, a person will gain weight if the total kcal value of the food eaten is not reduced accordingly. An individual's actual need, of course, will be determined primarily by activity and amount of lean muscle mass. Those who are more active will require more kcal than those with a high proportion of fat tissue.

A normal healthy adult should eat a variety of foods as shown on the food guide pyramid. This, along with following the *Dietary Guidelines for Americans,* should provide a healthy diet for the adult. In addition to the basic nutritional assessment, the following should be assessed for the adult client:

- Use of alcohol, tobacco, caffeine, and drugs
- Use of fad diets
- Prescribed restricted diet

Older Adulthood

Physical changes of aging affect nutrition in several ways. The body's functions slow with age, and its ability to replace worn cells likewise diminishes. Metabolic rate slows; bones become less dense; lean muscle mass lessens; eyes do not focus on nearby objects as they once did and some grow cloudy from cataracts; poor dentition is common; the heart and kidneys become less efficient; and hearing, taste, and smell are less acute.

Digestion is affected because the secretion of hydrochloric acid and enzymes diminishes. This, in turn, decreases the intrinsic factor synthesis, which leads to a deficiency of vitamin B_{12}. The tone of the intestines is reduced, possibly resulting in constipation or, in some cases, diarrhea (Townsend & Roth, 2000).

Healthy eating habits throughout life, an exercise program suited to one's age, and social activities that please can prevent or delay physical deterioration and psychological depression during the senior years. The benefits of such pursuits can be said to be circular. The first two contribute largely to one's physical condition, and social activities can prevent or diminish depression, which, if unchecked, can also depress appetite. They give purpose to the day, joy to the heart, and zest to the appetite. Nutrition and lifestyle should be carefully reviewed in any elderly client suspected of having depression.

Food–drug interactions must be monitored closely in the elderly client. Frequently, specific foods will prevent, decrease, or enhance the absorption of a particular drug.

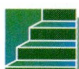

PROFESSIONAL TIP

Food–Drug Interactions

Dairy products should not be consumed within 2 hours of taking the antibiotic tetracycline or the drug will not be absorbed. A person taking a blood clot–reducing drug such as warfarin sodium (coumadin) must consume vitamin K–rich food in moderation, as this vitamin counteracts blood thinners. Even vitamin supplements can cause interactions. The antioxidant vitamins are not to be taken with blood clot–reducing medications, because they also have a tendency to thin the blood (Townsend & Roth, 2000).

Drug–drug interactions as well as food–drug interactions can contribute to decreased nutritional status. These interactions could affect both appetite and the absorption of nutrients from the food eaten. Careful monitoring is recommended.

Nutritional Requirements

In general, most elderly persons decrease their activity; thus their kcal needs also decrease.

The kcal requirement decreases approximately 2% to 3% per decade, because both metabolism and activity slow. If kcal intake is not reduced, weight will increase. This additional weight increases the work of the heart and puts increased stress on the skeletal system. It is important that the kcal requirement not be exceeded and just as important that the nutrient requirements be fulfilled to maintain good nutritional status. An exercise plan appropriate to one's age and health can be helpful in burning excess kcal and in toning and strengthening the muscles.

Protein needs remain the same or may increase during illness. A well balanced diet of a variety of foods should supply adequate amounts of vitamins and minerals. An increase in water and dietary fiber is often needed to maintain proper elimination.

In addition to the basic nutritional assessment, the following should be assessed for elderly clients.

- Undesirable change in weight
- Dentition and swallowing
- Appetite
- Vision
- Hand–eye coordination
- Adequacy of daily intake of food
- Ability to self-feed
- Prescribed restricted diet
- Use of alcohol, tobacco, caffeine, and drugs

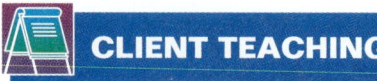

CLIENT TEACHING

Special Dietary Considerations for Elders

- Give special attention to water needs, regardless of physical activity, because the thirst mechanism is less responsive than in younger people.
- Decrease the kcal requirements in relation to activity: 10% for ages 51–75, and 20% to 25% for ages 75 and older. Bedridden and immobilized persons need a further reduction in kcal. Limit the quantities of empty-kcal foods (sugars, sweets, fats, oils, and alcohol).
- Maintain protein requirements, with 12% to 14% of kcal intake being derived from protein food (meat, eggs, poultry, milk, and cheese).
- Ensure adequate consumption of unsaturated fats, to provide a source of energy, provide the essential fatty acids, utilize the fat-soluble vitamins, and serve as a lubricating agent.
- Select carbohydrates as follows: limit concentrated sweets; use moderate amounts of simple sugars (candy, sugar, jams, jellies, preserves, and syrups); select most sources from complex carbohydrates (fruits, vegetables, cereals, and breads).
- Ensure adequate amounts of vitamin D, calcium, and phosphorus to maintain bone integrity (fortified milk is a good source).
- Consume high-fiber foods (dried fruits, whole-grain cereals, nuts, fresh fruit, and vegetables) to increase satiety and maintain intestinal motility and thereby prevent constipation.
- Maintain a safe, adequate intake of sodium, avoiding canned foods and salted or cured meats high in sodium content for those with cardiac problems and hypertension.
- Include foods from the food guide pyramid in the amounts that meet the RDAs for age 51 and older.

Pregnancy and Lactation

Good nutrition during the 38 weeks–40 weeks of a normal pregnancy is essential for both mother and child. In addition to her normal nutritional requirements, the pregnant woman must provide nutrients and kcals for the fetus, the amniotic fluid, the placenta, and the increased blood volume and breast, uterine, and fat tissue.

The pregnant woman who follows a nutritionally adequate diet is more apt to feel better, retain her health, and bear a healthy infant than does one who chooses her foods thoughtlessly (Townsend & Roth, 2000).

Studies have shown a relationship between the mother's diet and the health of the baby at birth. It is also thought that the woman who consumes a nutritious diet before pregnancy is more apt to bear a healthy infant than is one who does not. Malnutrition of the mother is believed to cause growth and mental retardation in the fetus. Infants with low birth weight (less than 5.5 pounds) have a higher mortality (death) rate than those of normal birthweight.

Nutritional Requirements

Despite the saying, the pregnant woman is not "eating for two." No increase in kcal is required during the first 12 weeks of pregnancy. After that time, an extra 300 kcal/day is recommended. This increase can almost be accomplished by drinking two *extra* 8-ounce glasses of 2% milk each day, which supplies 240 kcal. Those two extra glasses of milk also supply the extra calcium, protein, and vitamin D required during pregnancy. The other nutrients that should be increased during pregnancy are folic acid and iron. Folic acid is necessary to prevent neural tube deformities in the fetus. Folic acid has been approved as a supplement for pregnant women. Good sources of folic acid are beef, legumes, wheat germ, and eggs. Good sources of iron are red meat, dried fruit, egg yolk, and whole-grain products. Appendix C lists the RDAs during pregnancy and lactation.

To ensure that the nutritional requirements of pregnancy are met, vitamin supplements may be prescribed in addition to an iron supplement. However, it is *not* advisable for the mother to take any unprescribed nutrient supplement, as an excess of vitamins or minerals can be toxic to mother and infant. Excessive vitamin A, for example, can cause birth defects (Townsend & Roth, 2000).

The mother's kcal requirement increases during lactation. The kcal requirement depends on the amount of milk produced. Approximately 85 kcal are required to produce 100 mL (3⅓ oz) of milk. During the first 6 months, average daily milk production is 750 mL (25 oz), and for this, the mother requires approximately an extra 640 kcal a day. During the second 6 months, when the baby begins to eat food in addition to breast milk, average daily milk production slows to 600 mL (20 oz), and the kcal requirement reduces to approximately 510 extra kcal a day.

In addition to the basic nutritional assessment, the following should be assessed for the pregnant client:

- Weight and rate of weight gain
- Diet changes in response to pregnancy
- Cravings for foods or nonfoods (pica)
- Taking of supplemental vitamins/minerals
- Feeding plans (breast or formula)
- Use of alcohol, caffeine, tobacco, or drugs

NUTRITION AND HEALTH

An individual who embraces good nutrition is more likely to have good health than is someone who does not follow good nutritional practices. Of course, all situations of disease or ill health cannot be prevented by good nutrition.

The nutrients in the food we eat may be thought of as the building materials, fuel, and regulators necessary to keep the body functioning. When the body is supplied with nutrients in the proper amounts, it is most likely to function efficiently and effectively. The body is very adaptable and keeps functioning, though less effectively, even when it is not supplied with the proper amounts of nutrients. In this situation, however, the body can become more susceptible to some diseases.

Primary Nutritional Disease

A primary nutritional disease occurs when nutrition is the cause of the disease. Usually, there is an inadequate intake of one or more nutrients. Some examples of such diseases are scurvey, from inadequate intake of vitamin C; rickets, from insufficient intake of vitamin D; and anemia, from a deficiency of iron in the diet.

Excesses of nutrients can also cause illness. These, however, occur when nutrient supplements are taken in excess, rather than from food intake. For instance, excess vitamin D may cause nausea, diarrhea, weight loss, and calcification of the renal tubules, blood vessels, and bronchi. Excess niacin may cause flushing, itching, and hypotension.

Secondary Nutritional Disease

Most nutritional diseases are secondary diseases, that is, they are a complication of another disease or condition. The original disease or condition interferes with digestion or absorption, or there is an increased need for one or more nutrients. For instance, in pregnancy, the body's need for iron increases. Not receiving the increased amount may cause anemia in the mother. In malabsorption disorders, the body is unable to absorb sufficient amounts of certain nutrients. The amount ingested may be adequate, but the body is unable to use it. Rapid excretion from the body, as in diarrhea, does not allow the nutrients to be absorbed and utilized. Uncontrolled, diarrhea can lead to dehydration along with electrolyte and acid–base imbalance.

WEIGHT MANAGEMENT

Maintaining weight at a desired level can be very difficult for some people. Weight management is based on the relationship between the intake and the use of kcal. When these two elements are balanced, weight is maintained at a steady level. A range of 10% over or under the desired weight is considered appropriate.

Determining Caloric Needs

The number of kcal needed to achieve or maintain a desired weight is based on two factors: basal energy needs and total energy requirements.

Basal Energy Needs

Basal energy needs refers to the number of kcal required to keep an individual alive when at rest. There are two ways to determine basal energy (kcal) needs. One is based on the person's desired weight (Table 18-11), the other on the person's actual weight.

Calculation using desired weight is as follows:

$$\text{Basal energy needs} = \text{desired weight} \times 10$$
$$(\text{Table 18-11}).$$

Examples

Female: 5 ft 5 in tall
　　　　 5 ft　=　100 lb
　　　　 5 in　=　 25 lb
　　　　　　　　 125 lb desired weight

　　　　 $125 \times 10 = 1,250$
　　　　 Basal energy needs = 1,250 kcal

Male:　 5 ft 9 in tall
　　　　 5 ft　=　106 lb
　　　　 9 in　=　 54 lb
　　　　　　　　 160 lb desired weight

　　　　 $160 \times 10 = 1,600$
　　　　 Basal energy needs = 1,600 kcal

Calculation using actual weight is as follows.

Female weight in kg $\times 0.9 \times 24$ = basal kcal
Male weight in kg $\times 1 \times 24$ = basal kcal
(Weight in lb $\div 2.2$ = weight in kg)

Examples

Female weighs 130 lb
　 $130 \div 2.2 = 59.1$ kg.
　 59.1 kg. $\times 0.9 \times 24 = 1,276.6$
　 Basal energy needs = 1,276.6 kcal

Table 18-11	**DETERMINING DESIRED WEIGHT**	
BUILD	**WOMEN**	**MEN**
Medium	100 lb for 5 ft of height, plus 5 lb for each additional inch	106 lb for 5 ft of height, plus 6 lb for each additional inch
Small	Subtract 10%	Subtract 10%
Large	Add 10%	Add 10%

Male weighs 170 lb
   170 ÷ 2.2 = 77.3 kg.
   77.3 kg. × 1 × 24 = 1,855.2
   Basal energy needs = 1,855.2 kcal

Total Energy Requirements

People do not live their lives at rest. They are active! Kilocalories must be added to the basal metabolic requirements in order to meet the needs of activity. All activity is not equal in kcal needed, however. A person's overall activity level can be divided into sedentary (light, such as watching television), moderate (such as playing a tennis match), or strenuous (such as running a marathon). The following formulas can be used to determine the number of kcal to add given the activity level:

Sedentary: basal kcal × 1.3 = total kcal
Moderate: basal kcal × 1.5 = total kcal
Strenuous: basal kcal × 2.0 = total kcal

Example: The 125-lb woman in the preceding example who is planning on running a marathon would need the following:

1,250 kcal (basal kcal) × 2, or 2,500 kcal

Factors in addition to activity that have an effect on the total kcal need are state of health and climate. A person who is ill needs more kcal to repair tissue. A cold climate requires a person to take in more kcal to provide more thermal energy to maintain body temperature.

Overweight

A person is considered to be overweight when weight is 11% to 19% above the desired weight. **Obesity** is considered present in a person who is 20% or more above the desired weight. Overweight conditions can become serious health hazards by placing increased strain on the heart, lungs, muscles, bones, and joints. Overweight and obese people are more susceptible to diabetes and hypertension and tend to have a shortened life span.

According to the Centers for Disease Control and Prevention (1997), the Third National Health and Nutrition Examination Survey indicated that obesity is rising in the United States. Among children between the ages of 6 and 11 years, 13.7% are overweight; among adolescents ages 12 to 17, 11.5% are overweight. Among adults, 36.4% of men and 33.3% of women are overweight.

Causes

There is no single cause of obesity. Genetic, physiologic, biochemical, and psychological factors may all contribute to overweight conditions. Most often, the cause of being overweight or obese is an energy im-

balance. That is, more kcal are being taken in than are being used. When this occurs, the body stores the excess kcal as adipose tissue. Hypothyroidism is a possible, but rare, cause of obesity. In this condition, basal metabolism is low, thereby reducing the number of kcal needed for energy. Unless corrected, this condition can result in excess weight (Townsend & Roth, 2000).

Treatment

Treatment for an overweight person involves two parts: revised eating habits and exercise. Revised eating habits include reducing daily kcal intake at mealtime, limiting between-meal snacks to fresh fruits or vegetables, and restricting or eliminating empty calories.

One (1) pound of body weight equals 3,500 kcal. Therefore, to lose 1 pound per week, a person must reduce kcal intake by 500 kcal each day. Weight loss should be limited to 1 to 2 pounds per week, unless the client is under strict medical supervision. Diets should be planned according to the minimum servings of the food guide pyramid and should not be reduced to below 1,200 kcal/day in order for the dieter to receive adequate nutrients to sustain health.

Attention should also be given to the preparation of the food. Frying adds many kcal from fat to a food item. Broiling, grilling, baking, roasting, boiling, and poaching are healthy ways to prepare foods. Vegetables should be eaten raw or steamed; addition of butter, margarine, or sauces should be avoided. Eating habits may be adapted to decrease the amount eaten, and yet provide satisfaction: place food on a smaller plate; cut food into smaller bites; chew each bite at least 12 times; and place the fork on the plate between bites.

Exercise, particularly aerobic exercise, is an excellent adjunct to any weight-loss program. Aerobic exercise uses energy from the body's fat reserves, as it increases the amount of oxygen the body takes in. Examples of aerobic exercise are dancing, jogging, bicycling, skiing, rowing, and power walking. Such exercise helps tone the muscles, burns kcal, increases the basal metabolism so that food is burned faster, and is fun for the participant. Any exercise program must be begun slowly and increased over time so that no physical damage occurs.

Exercise alone can only rarely replace the need to be mindful of diet, however. The dieter should be made aware of the number of kcal burned by specific exercises so as to avoid overeating after the workout.

Underweight

Persons are considered to be underweight when their weight is 10% to 15% below the desired weight. An underweight person is more likely to have nutritional deficiencies because of the decreased intake of food. For women, this can cause complications during pregnancy, when there is an increased need for nutrients. Being underweight may lower a person's resistance to infection. Being severely underweight may even cause death.

Causes

There are several possible causes of being underweight, such as an inadequate intake of food, excessive exercise, poor absorption of nutrients, or severe infection. Occasionally, hyperthyroidism may be the cause. After the adequacy of food intake and the appropriate activity level are ascertained, specific diagnostic tests must be done to determine whether poor absorption, infection, or hyperthyroidism are present.

Treatment

Dietary treatment for an inadequate intake of food is to gradually increase the amount of food eaten. Also, higher-kcal foods can be eaten. Between-meal snacks and a bedtime snack can help increase the intake of food.

If the individual is to gain 1 pound per week, 3,500 kcal in addition to the individual's basic normal weekly kcal requirement are prescribed. This means an extra 500 kcal must be taken in each day. If a weight gain of 2 pounds per week is required, an additional 7,000 kcal each week, or an additional 1,000 kcal per day, are necessary. This diet cannot be immediately accepted at full kcal value. Time will be needed to gradually increase the daily kcal value. In this diet, there is an increased intake of foods rich in carbohydrates, some fats, and protein. Vitamins and minerals are supplied in adequate amounts. If there are deficiencies of some vitamins and minerals, supplements are prescribed (Townsend & Roth, 2000).

FOOD LABELING

In 1990, Congress passed the Nutrition, Labeling and Education Act (NLEA). This was the first legislation on labeling since the 1970s. Prior to this newest legislation, labeling was only required if a nutrient was added or a nutritional claim was made about the product. Now, labeling is required on virtually all retail food products, including bulk foods, fresh produce, and seafood. The nutrition information for fresh produce and seafood is to be displayed or made available at the point of purchase through counter cards, booklets, loose-leaf binders, signs, or tags.

The labels must follow the approved uniform format and use standard serving sizes and household measurements. Information on the label includes calories per serving; calories from fat; total fat, saturated fat, and cholesterol; total sodium; total carbohydrate, dietary fiber, and sugar; amount of protein; and percentages of vitamins A and C, calcium, and iron. A sample food label is shown in Figure 18-7.

Nutrition Facts

Serving Size ½ cup (114g)
Servings Per Container 4

Amount Per Serving

Calories 90	Calories from Fat 30

	% Daily Value
Total Fat 3g	5%
Saturated Fat 0g	0%
Cholesterol 0mg	0%
Sodium 300mg	13%
Total Carbohydrate 13g	4%
Dietary Fiber 3g	12%
Sugars 3g	
Protein 3g	

Vitamin A	80%	•	Vitamin C	60%
Calcium	4%	•	Iron	4%

• Percent Daily Values are based on a 2,000 calorie diet. Your daily values may be higher or lower depending on your calorie needs:

	Calories	2,000	2,500
Total Fat	Less than	65g	80g
Sat Fat	Less than	20g	25g
Cholesterol	Less than	300mg	300mg
Sodium	Less than	2,400mg	2,400mg
Total Carbohydrate		300g	375g
Fiber		25g	30g

Calories per gram:
Fat 9   •   Carbohydrate 4   •   Protein 4

Figure 18-7 Sample Food Label

Words used to describe nutrient content, such as *low, light, lean,* or *reduced,* now have specific, consistent definitions (Table 18-12).

The standardized label and word definitions make it easier for the consumer not only to know the amount of specific nutrients in a food or food product, but also to easily compare foods and food products.

FOOD QUALITY AND SAFETY

When planning an adequate diet, the quality and safety of the food must be considered in addition to the types of foods and serving sizes. To ensure the quality (nutrient content) and safety of food, proper storage, preparation, sanitation, and cooking are necessary; such measures will help prevent or reduce the risk of food-borne illnesses.

Quality of Food

Foods usually begin to lose nutrients when they are harvested, so they are best purchased when fresh in appearance and of bright color. Dates should be checked on all processed foods such as dairy products, lunch and other processed meats, crackers, and breads; all foods should be used prior to their expiration dates. All produce should be cooked until tender

Table 18-12 NUTRIENT CONTENT DESCRIPTORS

- **Free, without, no, zero:** The product contains only a tiny or insignificant amount of fat, cholesterol, sodium, sugar, and/or calories. For example, *fat-free* and *sugar-free* contain fewer than 0.5 g per serving. *Calorie-free* has fewer than 5 kcal per serving.
- **Low:** A food described as *low* in fat, saturated fat, cholesterol, sodium, and/or calories could be eaten fairly often without exceeding dietary guidelines. For instance, *low in fat* means no more than 3 g of fat per serving.
- **Lean:** *Lean* means that the product contains fewer than 10 g of fat, 4 g of saturated fat, and 95 mg of cholesterol per serving. *Lean* is not as lean as is *low*.
- **Extra Lean:** *Extra lean* means that the product has fewer than 5 g of fat, 2 g of saturated fat, and 95 mg of cholesterol per serving. *Extra lean* is still not as lean as is *low*.
- **Reduced, less, fewer:** Means a diet product contains 25% less of a nutrient or calories. For example, hotdogs might be labeled *25% less fat than our regular hotdogs.*
- **Light/lite:** Means a diet product with ⅓ fewer kcal or ½ the fat of the original. *Light in sodium* means a product with ½ the usual sodium.
- **More:** A food in which one serving has at least 10% more of the daily value of a vitamin, mineral, or fiber than usual.
- **Good source of:** One serving contains 10% to 19% of the daily value for a particular vitamin, mineral, or fiber.

Adapted from "Answering Your Questions on Nutrition and Nutrition Labeling," by M. Gravely, 1993, Spring/Summer, Food News for Consumers, USDA, Food Safety and Inspection Service, 8–9.

and thoroughly done, in the smallest amount of water possible to prevent loss of vitamins. Cooking meats via stewing increases mineral loss, so cooking methods that retain the most nutrients should be used instead; these include stir-frying, steaming, microwaving, or pressure cooking.

Safety of Food

There are three aspects to food safety: proper storage, proper sanitation, and proper cooking.

Proper Storage

Foods must be properly stored prior to and after purchase. Packages and jars should be tightly sealed, and cans should not leak or bulge. Any foods that look or smell unusual or show signs of mold or deterioration should be discarded. Hot foods should be kept hot—above 140°F—and cold foods should be kept below 40°F. Foods allowed to stand at temperatures between 40°F and 140°F provide an ideal breeding ground for pathogens. Leftovers must be refrigerated promptly and not allowed to cool before refrigerating.

Proper Sanitation

Proper sanitation means that all cooking utensils, pots, pans, and cutting boards, as well as the cook's hands, have been washed with soap and hot water before preparation begins. To prevent contamination of one food by another, cutting boards, utensils, and the cook's hands should be washed well with soap and hot water between preparation of different foods. A person who is ill should not prepare food. Good handwashing is a must prior to food preparation and following bathroom use.

Meat, fish, and poultry should be rinsed under cold running water and patted dry with several paper towels before preparing and cooking. A capful of chlorine bleach in a sink one-half full of water can be used to wash fruits and vegetables: leafy vegetables, cauliflower, broccoli, and other fruits and vegetables can be washed in the bleach water for a few minutes, rinsed, and then drained on paper towels.

Proper Cooking

Meats, fish, shellfish, and eggs should be cooked well done to ensure that harmful microorganisms are destroyed.

Food-Borne Illnesses

When proper storage, sanitation, or cooking are not maintained, food-borne illnesses often occur. These illnesses range in severity from fairly mild (such as staphylococcal food poisoning) to potentially fatal (such as botulism and E. coli). The important thing to remember is that food-borne illness is highly preventable with proper handling, preparation, and storage of food.

 HOME HEALTH CARE

Resources for Meal Preparation

Ensure that the family has:

- Hot and cold running water;
- A working refrigerator;
- A working oven and range;
- A clean, pest-free kitchen;
- Fresh perishables stored in the refrigerator;
- Adequate food supplies (including canned goods and staples, such as milk and bread), safely stored; and
- Appropriate adaptive equipment, if needed, such as low countertops that facilitate wheelchair access.

From "Home Health Nutrition" by M. Costello, 1996, MedSurg Nursing 5(4), 229–238.

It is important to emphasize that nutrition involves the appropriate kinds and amounts of a variety of available foods so that a properly functioning body can digest and use the nutrients in the foods. If the foods are unsafe, they cannot adequately nourish the body.

FOOD ALLERGIES

An **allergy** is an altered reaction of the tissues of some individuals to substances that, in similar amounts, are harmless to other people. The substances causing hypersensitivity are called allergens. A food allergy occurs when the immune system reacts to a food substance, usually a protein. When such a reaction occurs, antibodies form and cause allergic symptoms. An altered reaction to a specific food that does not involve the immune system is called (the specific *food*) *intolerance*.

Allergic Reactions

Allergic reactions are sometimes immediate, or sometimes several hours elapse before signs occur. Allergic individuals seem most prone to allergic reactions during periods of stress. Typical signs of food allergies include hay fever, hives, edema, headache, dermatitis, nausea, dizziness, and asthma (which causes breathing difficulties).

Allergic reactions are uncomfortable and can be detrimental to health. When breathing difficulties are severe, they are life threatening.

Allergic reactions to the same food can differ in two individuals. For example, the fact that someone gets hives from eating strawberries does not mean that an allergic reaction to strawberries will appear as hives in another member of the same family. Allergic reactions can even differ from time to time with the same individual.

Treatment of Allergies

The simplest treatment for allergies is to remove the item that causes the allergic reaction. However, because of the variety of allergic reactions, finding the allergen can be difficult.

When food allergies are suspected, it is wise for the client to keep a food diary for several days and to record all food and drink ingested as well as allergic reactions and the time of their onset. Such records can help pinpoint specific allergens. It is common for other foods in the same class as the allergens to cause allergic reactions as well. Cooking sometimes alters the foods and can eliminate allergic reactions in some people.

Laboratory tests may be used to find the allergen or allergens. The radio allergosorbent test (RAST), for example, may be used to determine which compounds are causing allergic reactions.

After completion of the allergy testing, the client is usually placed on an elimination diet. For 1 or 2 weeks, the client does not eat any of the tested compounds that gave a positive reaction. The client includes in the diet the foods that almost no one reacts to, such as rice, fresh meats and poultry, noncitrus fruits, and vegetables. Sometimes, these diets allow only a limited number of foods and can be nutritionally inadequate. If that is the case, vitamin and mineral supplements may be prescribed.

When relief is found from the allergic symptoms, the client is continued on the diet, and, gradually, other foods are added to the diet at a rate of only one every 4 to 7 days. Those foods most likely to produce allergic reactions are added last until an allergic reaction occurs. The allergy can then be pinpointed, and the offending foods eliminated from the diet. Knowing the cause of the allergy enables the client to lead a healthy, normal life, provided that eliminating these foods does not affect overall nutrition (Townsend & Roth, 2000).

If the elimination of the allergen results in a diet deficient in certain nutrients, suitable substitutes for those nutrients must be found. For example, if a client is allergic to citrus fruits, other foods rich in vitamin C to which the client is not allergic must be found. If the allergy is to milk, soybean milk may be substituted.

NURSING PROCESS

Collection of subjective and objective data regarding the client's nutrition serves as the basis for determining the type of nutritional care the client requires.

Assessment

Proper assessment allows the health care team to determine the degree to which the client's nutritional needs are being met. Assessment must be performed in a logical fashion and should include a nutritional history, physical examination, and the results of laboratory tests.

 CLIENT TEACHING

Allergies

The client must be taught the food sources of the nutrient or nutrients lacking so that other foods can be substituted that are nutritionally equal to those causing the allergy. It is essential that the client be taught to read the labels on commercially prepared foods and to check the ingredients of restaurant foods carefully. For instance, baked products, mixes, meatloaf, or pancakes may contain egg, milk, or wheat, which may be responsible for the allergic reaction.

Subjective Data

Subjective data can be obtained through a nutritional history by asking about food allergies; level of physical activity; cultural, socioeconomic, and religious influences; and the use of alcohol, caffeine, tobacco, drugs, and vitamin or mineral supplements. Several methods can be used in collecting these subjective data: 24-hour recall, food frequency questionnaire, food record, and diet history. Although the history data may indicate adequate nutrition, clients must be reassessed periodically to prevent nutritional problems.

24-Hour Recall The 24-hour recall requires client identification of everything consumed in the previous 24 hours. It is performed easily and quickly by asking pertinent questions. However, clients may be unable to accurately recall their intake or anything atypical in the diet. Family members can often assist with these data, if necessary.

Food-Frequency Questionnaire The food-frequency method gathers data relative to the number of times per day, week, or month that the client eats particular foods. The nurse can tailor the questions to particular nutrients, such as cholesterol and saturated fat. This method helps to validate the accuracy of the 24-hour recall and provides a more complete picture of foods consumed.

Food Record The food record provides quantitative information regarding all foods consumed, with portions weighed and measured for three consecutive days. This method requires full client or family member cooperation.

Diet History The diet history elicits detailed information regarding the client's nutritional status, general health pattern, socioeconomic status, and cultural factors. This method incorporates information similar to that collected by the 24-hour recall and food-frequency questionnaire. The history may require more than one interview because of the amount of data to be collected.

Objective Data

A physical examination may elicit findings that suggest nutritional imbalance. Table 18-13 lists physical indicators of nutritional status.

PROFESSIONAL TIP

Nutritional History

Food preferences are an expression of an individual's likes and dislikes. They may be related to the texture of food, how it is prepared, or what was served to the individual during childhood. However, preferences can also be an expression of the person's economic, ecological, ethical, or religious beliefs.

Peer pressures often dictate what teenagers eat. Stress, depression, and alcohol abuse alter the appetite. Medications can alter food absorption and excretion and affect the taste of food. Gastrointestinal disorders can cause anorexia, nausea, vomiting, diarrhea, constipation, discomfort, and pain, all of which may alter eating habits and food preferences.

The measurement of a client's intake and output and a daily weight are critical assessments, especially for hospitalized clients. **Anthropometric measurements** (measurement of the size, weight, and proportions of the body) are indicative of the client's calorie–energy expenditure balance, muscle mass, body fat, and protein reserves. The measurements used are body mass index (calculated using weight and height), skinfolds, and limb and girth circumferences.

Body Mass Index Body mass index (BMI) is a measurement used to determine whether a person's weight (in kilograms) is appropriate for height (in meters). It is calculated using a simple formula:

$$BMI = \frac{weight\ (kg)}{[height\ (m)]^2}$$

A BMI of 27 or greater indicates obesity. For example, a person who weighs 65 kilograms and is 1.6 meters tall would have a BMI of 65 kg/(1.6)², or 25.4. Using Table 18-14, find your height and follow the row across to find your weight; then follow the column up to determine your BMI.

Table 18-13 PHYSICAL INDICATORS OF NUTRITIONAL STATUS

BODY AREA	GOOD NUTRITION	INADEQUATE NUTRITION
General	Alert, responsive, sleeps well, energetic, seldom ill	Apathetic, easily fatigued, looks tired, often ill
Weight	Appropriate for age, height, body build	Overweight, underweight
Skeleton	Good posture, no malformations	Poor posture
Skin	Good color, no rashes or swelling, smooth, moist, good turgor	Rough, dry, pale, poor turgor
Muscles	Firm, good tone	Flaccid, poor tone
Nails	Pink, firm	Pale, brittle
Eyes	Clear, bright, moist	Dull, pale, dry
Hair	Shiny, smooth	Dull, dry, brittle
Elimination	Regular, soft	Diarrhea or constipation

Skinfold Measurement Skinfold measurement indicates the amount of body fat. The skinfold is measured by grasping the subcutaneous tissue and taking a reading using a special caliper. Measurements can be taken of the tricep, subscapular, bicep, and suprailiac skinfolds (Figure 18-8).

Other Measurements Mid–upper-arm circumference serves as an index of skeletal muscle mass and protein reserve. Abdominal-girth measurement serves as an index as to whether the abdomen is increasing, decreasing, or remaining the same. Both of these measurements should be made repeatedly over a span of time, for best assessment.

Laboratory Tests Several laboratory tests provide information about a client's nutritional status. These include the protein indices of serum albumin, pre-albumin, and serum transferrin; hemoglobin; total lymphocyte count; blood urea nitrogen (BUN); and urine creatinine. The serum albumin blood test is used to measure prolonged protein depletion that occurs in chronic malnutrition, liver disease, and nephrosis. The pre-albumin test indicates protein depletion in acute conditions such as trauma and inflammation. Serum transferrin also measures the protein level as indicated by iron stores. Hemoglobin is a measurement of the oxygen- and iron-carrying capacity of the blood. Total

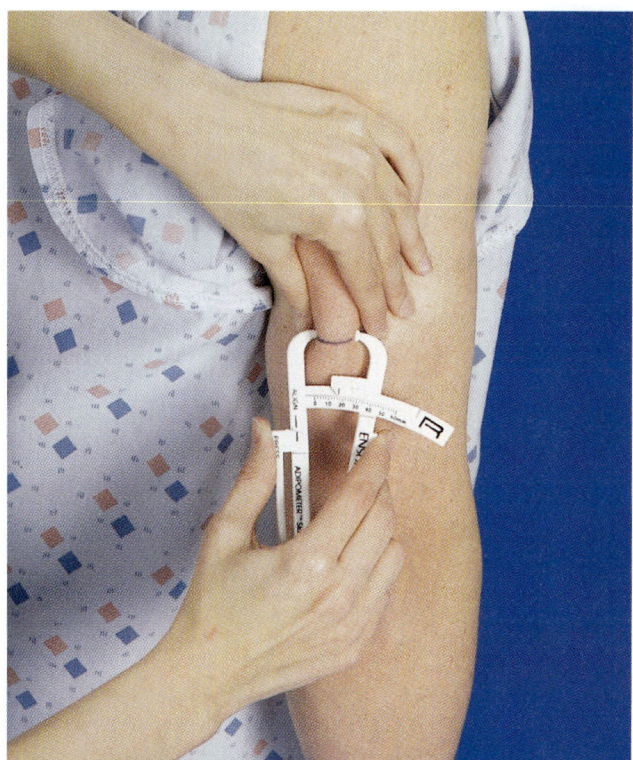

Figure 18-8 Measuring Triceps Skinfold at Midpoint of Upper Arm

Table 18-14 BODY MASS INDEX DETERMINATION

How to use this chart:

1. Look down the left column to find your height (*measured in feet and inches*).
2. Look across that row and find the weight nearest your own.
3. Look to the number at the top of the column to identify your BMI.
4. If your number is 27 or greater, you may be at risk.

BMI	25	26	27	28	29	30	31	32	33	34	35	36	37	38	39	40
4'10"	119	124	129	134	138	143	148	153	158	162	167	172	177	181	186	191
4'11"	124	128	133	138	143	148	153	158	163	168	173	178	183	188	193	198
5'	128	133	138	143	148	153	158	164	169	174	179	184	189	194	199	204
5'1"	132	137	143	148	153	158	164	169	174	180	185	190	195	201	206	211
5'2"	136	142	147	153	158	164	169	175	180	186	191	196	202	207	213	218
5'3"	141	146	152	158	163	169	175	180	186	192	197	203	208	214	220	225
5'4"	145	151	157	163	169	174	180	186	192	198	203	209	215	221	227	233
5'5"	150	156	162	168	174	180	186	192	198	204	210	216	222	228	234	240
5'6"	155	161	167	173	179	185	192	198	204	210	216	223	229	235	241	247
5'7"	159	166	172	178	185	191	198	204	210	217	223	229	236	242	248	255
5'8"	164	171	177	184	190	197	203	210	217	223	230	236	243	249	256	263
5'9"	169	176	182	189	196	203	209	216	223	230	237	243	250	257	264	270
5'10"	174	181	188	195	202	209	216	223	230	236	243	250	257	264	271	278
5'11"	179	186	193	200	207	215	222	229	236	243	250	258	265	272	279	286
6'	184	191	199	206	213	221	228	235	243	250	258	265	272	280	287	294
6'1"	189	197	204	212	219	227	234	242	250	257	265	272	280	287	295	303
6'2"	194	202	210	218	225	233	241	249	256	264	272	280	288	295	303	311
6'3"	200	208	216	224	232	240	247	255	263	271	279	287	295	303	311	319
6'4"	205	213	221	230	238	246	254	262	271	279	287	295	303	312	320	328

Used by permission of Knoll Pharmaceutical Company.

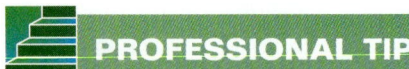

Creatinine Excretion
Record the client's height and gender on the laboratory request for a creatinine excretion test because the normal values are standardized on the basis of these variables.

lymphocyte count may reflect protein-calorie malnutrition, which inhibits lymphocyte synthesis. Blood urea nitrogen is a nitrogen balance study that indicates the degree to which protein is being depleted or replaced, and urine creatinine excretion indicates the amount of creatinine eliminated by the kidneys.

Nursing Diagnosis

Nursing diagnoses related specifically to nutrition include the following:

Nutrition, Altered, Less than Body Requirements
Nutrition, Altered, More than Body Requirements
Nutrition, Altered, Risk for More than Body Requirements

Other possible nursing diagnoses related to nutritional problems include the following:

Body Image Disturbance
Breastfeeding, Ineffective
Dentition, Altered
Knowledge Deficit
Oral Mucous Membrane, Altered
Pain
Self-Care Deficit, Feeding
Self-Esteem Disturbance
Skin Integrity, Impaired, Risk for

Planning/Outcome Identification

A plan should be formulated by the nurse and client to achieve mutually agreed-upon goals. The plan is individualized to meet the client's specific needs. These needs may include achieving desired weight, correcting nutritional deficiencies, maintaining a special diet, preventing nutritional disorders secondary to a particular therapy, or improving nutrition to promote health and prevent disease.

Goals for clients with nutritional alterations might be as follows:

Client will maintain intake and output balance.
Client will comply with diet therapy, avoiding high-sodium foods.
Client will gain 2 pounds in 4 weeks.

Implementation

The nurse and client actually carry out the plan through specific actions. Interventions to accomplish

the goals may include diet therapy, assistance with meals, weight and intake monitoring, and nutritional support.

Diet Therapy

Diet therapy is the treatment of a disease or disorder with a special diet. A **dietary prescription/order** is an order written by the physician for food, including liquids. This is similar to a medication prescription written for any medication a client receives. A client must not be given anything to eat or drink without an order. The dietary prescription is written for one or more of the following purposes:

- Provide the client with nutrients needed for maintenance or growth.
- Prepare a client for diagnostic tests.
- Treat the client with a disease or condition.

When the dietary prescription has been received, the dietary department must be notified so that the proper food will be sent to the client.

Many times a client needs some help in understanding changes in the diet and the reasons that the changes are necessary. A basic knowledge of nutrition and diet therapy contributes to the nurse's ability to competently answer the client's questions about nutrition and diet. It is important, however, for the nurse to recognize when to refer questions to the dietitian.

The dietary prescription may be for nothing by mouth, a standard diet, or a special diet.

Nothing By Mouth Nothing by mouth (NPO) status is a type of diet modification as well as a fluid restriction. This intervention is prescribed prior to surgery and certain diagnostic procedures, to rest the GI tract, or when the client's nutritional problem has not been identified.

Standard Diets Each health care agency has standard or house diets. The standard diets include general (sometimes called regular), soft, clear liquid, full liquid, mechanical soft, and pureed.

General, or Regular, Diet The general, or regular, diet is planned in accordance with the food guide pyramid. There are no restrictions of any kind. It is a very adequate diet providing approximately 2,000 kcal a day.

Soft Diet A soft diet provides foods that are easy to chew and swallow, thus promoting mechanical digestion of foods. Foods to be avoided include nuts, seeds (tomatoes and berries with seeds), raw fruits and vegetables, fried foods, and whole grains. The food guide pyramid is the basis for this diet, although fewer kcal, usually approximately 1,800, are provided.

Clear-Liquid Diet The clear-liquid diet, also called the surgical liquid diet, is ordered as preparation for diagnostic tests or as the first meal or two after surgery. It consists mostly of water and carbohydrates, providing approximately 500 kcal/day. This is a very nutritionally inadequate diet but does relieve thirst, aids in hydration, and mildly stimulates peristalsis. Liquids included are water; clear, fat-free broth; tea; coffee; clear and strained fruit juices; jello; popsicles; and carbonated drinks such as lemon-lime soda.

Full-Liquid Diet A full-liquid diet provides approximately 800 to 1,000 kcal per day. It includes all foods that are liquid at room temperature. In addition to the liquids on a clear-liquid diet; milk; milk drinks; cream soups; strained, cooked cereals; ice cream; puddings; all fruit and vegetable juices; and custard are included.

Mechanical Soft or Edentulous Diet A mechanical soft or edentulous diet consists of food fixed especially for a person who has no teeth or has difficulty chewing. The food is either ground or chopped into very small pieces and cooked very soft, to ease the work of chewing.

Pureed Diet A pureed diet provides food that has been blenderized to a smooth consistency. It is prescribed for clients who have difficulty swallowing.

Special Diets The purpose of a special diet is to restore or maintain a client's nutritional status. These diets are variations of the general diet; however, they still must provide all of the nutrients of the general diets. Special diets may provide specific amounts of nutrients or may increase or restrict certain foods. Low-residue, high-fiber, liberal bland, fat-controlled, and sodium-restricted are types of special diets.

Low-residue Diet The low-residue diet of 5 to 10 g of fiber a day is intended to reduce the normal work of the intestines by restricting the amount of dietary fiber and reducing food residue. In some facilities, this diet consists of foods that provide no more than 3 g of fiber a day and do not increase fecal residue. Some low-residue diets limit tough or coarse meats, milk, and milk products. The low-residue diet is prescribed to decrease GI mucosal irritation in clients with diverticulitis, ulcerative colitis, and Crohn's disease. Foods to be avoided include raw fruits (except bananas), vegetables, seeds, plant fiber, and whole grains. Dairy products are limited to two servings per day.

High-fiber Diet A high-fiber diet contains 25 to 35 g or more of dietary fiber. A high-fiber diet is an integral part of the treatment regimen for diverticulosis because it increases the forward motion of the indigestible wastes through the colon. This diet is believed to help prevent constipation, hemorrhoids, and colon cancer, along with helping in the treatment of diabetes mellitus and atherosclerosis.

The recommended foods for this diet include coarse and whole-grain breads and cereals, bran, all fruits, vegetables (especially raw), and legumes. The diet is nutritionally adequate. High-fiber diets must be introduced gradually to prevent the formation of gas and the discomfort that accompanies it. Eight 8-oz glasses of water also must be consumed along with the increased fiber.

PROFESSIONAL TIP

Opening a Food Tray
Remove the tray cover before moving the overbed table in front of the client, as the concentration of odors when the lid is first removed can be nauseating to the client.

Liberal Bland Diet A liberal bland diet eliminates chemical and mechanical food irritants such as fried foods, alcohol, and caffeine. This diet is prescribed for clients with gastritis and ulcers, because it reduces GI irritation.

Fat-Controlled Diet The fat-controlled diet reduces the total fat ingested by replacing saturated fats with monounsaturated and polyunsaturated fats and restricting cholesterol. This diet is prescribed for clients with atherosclerosis, heart disease, and obesity. Saturated-fat foods to be avoided include animal fats, gravies, sauces, chocolate, and whole-milk products.

Sodium-Restricted Diet Sodium-restricted diets tailor the level of sodium to mild (2 to 3 g); moderate (1,000 mg); strict (500 mg); or severe (250 mg). This diet is prescribed for clients with fluid volume excess, hypertension, heart failure, myocardial infarction, or renal failure.

Assistance with Meals

Assisting with meals consists of preparing the client, preparing the environment, serving the tray, and assisting with eating.

Preparing the Client Before taking a meal tray into a client's room, the nurse must ensure that the client is ready to eat. This means that the client has washed the face and hands, completed oral hygiene, and emptied the bladder, if necessary. The nurse may need to assist with these tasks. The nurse should also help the client into a comfortable eating position; this may be individualized to each client, as not everyone is allowed or able to sit up to eat a meal.

Preparing the Environment The nurse should make every effort to see that the physical environment is as conducive to a pleasant mealtime atmosphere as possible. This may necessitate cleaning and clearing the overbed table so that the tray can be placed on it, tidying the room to remove offensive sights and smells, and brightening the room.

Serving the Tray The nurse should check that the tray contains the diet ordered, that everything on the tray is appropriate for the diet, and that nothing has spilled. For example, if a low-sodium diet tray has a salt packet, the packet should be removed. The nurse should then check the client's ID band against the name on the tray; it is very important that the correct

PROFESSIONAL TIP

Feeding a Client

- Position yourself at the same level as the client (stand if the bed is high, sit if the bed is low)
- Allow time for prayer, if the client wishes
- Protect the client's clothing with a napkin
- Allow time for chewing (do not hurry the client)
- Give bite size portions
- Warn about hot foods (do not blow on food to cool)
- Use a separate straw for each liquid
- Allow the client to choose the order in which the food is eaten
- Offer pleasant conversation

PROFESSIONAL TIP

Feeding the Client Who Is Visually Impaired

Clients with impaired vision need established routines that facilitate feeding. For example, foods are usually placed on the plate in a clockwise order: bread at the 12 o'clock position, meat at 3 o'clock, starches at 6 o'clock, and vegetable at 9 o'clock. The plate should have a raised edge so that the food can be scooped to the outside of the plate. Serving liquids in either a glass or a cup with a plastic lid and straw may be helpful in preventing spills.

meal is served to each client. The nurse should prepare the food by opening cartons or cutting food, if necessary.

Assisting with Eating The client who needs assistance in eating should be served last. This way, the nurse will have ample time and not have to hurry the client through the meal (Figure 18-9).

Weight and Intake Monitoring

Measuring weight daily or weekly and measuring the amount of food and fluid intake monitors therapy effectiveness.

Recording and Reporting

After the client has finished eating, the tray should be promptly removed. The amount of food eaten should be recorded, usually as the percentage of the meal eaten. When a client with diabetes does not eat all the food on the tray, both the charge nurse and the dietitian must be notified so that a supplemental feeding can be sent later. If the client is on intake and output (I & O), the amount of fluids consumed during the meal must be recorded. Any problems or difficulty in eating as well as likes and dislikes should be reported and documented on the client's medical record.

Nutritional Support

There are two routes for delivery of nutritional support in adult clients: enteral nutrition and parenteral nutrition. **Enteral nutrition** includes both the ingestion of food orally and the delivery of nutrients through a GI tube, but is generally used to mean the latter. **Parenteral nutrition** refers to nutrients bypassing the GI system and entering the blood directly.

Enteral Nutrition When clients cannot or will not take food by mouth, but their GI tracts are working, they will be given tube feedings (TF). Sometimes, this may be necessary because of unconsciousness, surgery, stroke, severe malnutrition, or extensive burns. Tube feedings maintain the structural and functional integrity of the GI tract, enhance the utilization of nutrients, and provide a safe economical method of feeding.

Usually, for periods that do not exceed 6 weeks, tube feeding is administered through a nasogastric (NG) tube inserted through the nose and into the stomach or small intestine. When the tube cannot be placed in the nose or when tube feedings will be required for more than 6 weeks, an opening called an ostomy is surgically created into the esophagus (esophagostomy), the stomach (gastrostomy), or the intestine (jejunostomy) (Figure 18-10). The physician selects the route and type of feeding tube. The tubes used for these feedings are soft, flexible, and as small as they can be and still allow the feeding to pass through. Nu-

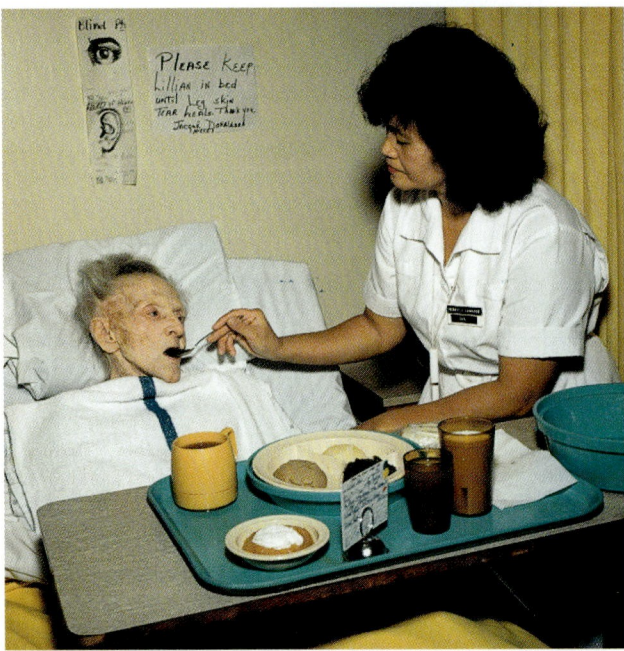

Figure 18-9 Older adults may have health problems that affect their ability to self-feed.

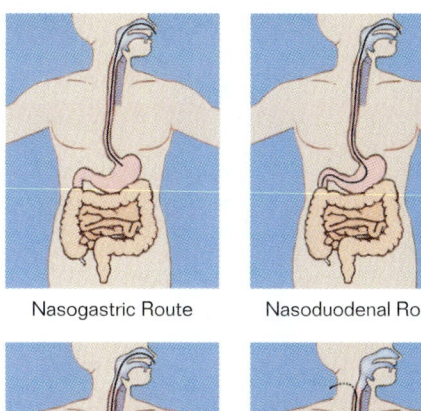

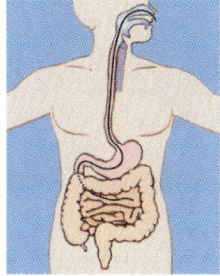
Nasogastric Route

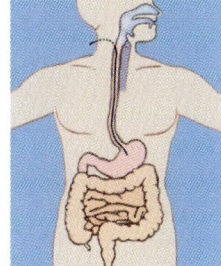
Nasoduodenal Route

Nasojejunal Route

Esophagostomy Route

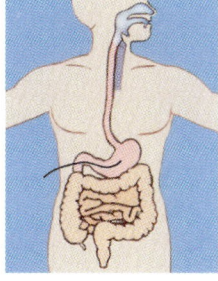
Gastrostomy Route

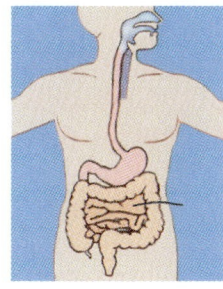
Jejunostomy Route

Figure 18-10 Enteral Feeding Routes

merous commercial formulas are available, with varying types and amounts of nutrients.

There are three methods for administering tube feedings: intermittent, bolus, and continuous. Usually tube feedings are administered by the continuous infusion method, preferably with a pump. This means the feeding is continuous over a 16- to 24-hour period. Sometimes, the formula is given at half strength at a rate of from 30 to 50 mL per hour. This rate may be increased by approximately 25 mL every 4 hours until tolerance has been established. As soon as the client tolerates the half-strength formula, a full-strength formula is initiated at the appropriate rate. When clients are ready to return to oral feedings, the transfer must be done gradually.

Parenteral Nutrition Parenteral nutrition is the infusion of a solution directly into a vein to meet the client's daily nutritional requirements. It is used if the GI tract is not functional or if normal feeding is not adequate for the client's needs. Formerly called hyperalimentation, it is now frequently referred to as total parenteral nutrition (TPN). The solution used in this intravenous infusion contains dextrose, amino acids, fats, essential fatty acids, vitamins, and minerals. Administration of TPN is generally a function of the registered nurse.

Evaluation

The effectiveness of the plan is evaluated in relation to attaining the desired goals. The nurse must assess whether the goals were met. The plan is continued or modified based on the evaluation.

SAMPLE NURSING CARE PLAN

THE CLIENT WITH ALTERED NUTRITION

Mrs. Vincent, age 58 years, is seen in the clinic for her yearly physical examination. She says, "I hardly have the energy to get up and dressed in the morning. Cleaning the house and doing the laundry makes me exhausted." She does not work and is not involved in community activities. Her daily routine involves cooking for her husband, reading, and watching TV for 6 to 8 hours. She loves to bake fresh breads and pastry. She has a history of being overweight and does not exercise. She says, "I eat because I have nothing else to do." Assessment reveals: height, 5′3″; weight, 166 pounds; weight gain, 14 pounds in the past year; sedentary lifestyle; eats in response to having nothing to do.

Nursing Diagnosis *Nutrition, Altered, More than Body Requirements, related to excess intake of high-calorie foods, eating in response to boredom, and sedentary lifestyle as evidenced by height–weight relationship and weight gain*

continued

PLANNING/GOALS	NURSING INTERVENTIONS	RATIONALE	EVALUATION
Mrs. Vincent will verbalize factors contributing to excess weight.	Conduct a dietary history, using open-ended statements to assist Mrs. Vincent in exploring factors that may contribute to excess eating.	A nonjudgmental approach to acquiring information will encourage client trust and honesty.	Mrs. Vincent verbalized boredom as the main reason for eating.
Mrs. Vincent will lose 1 to 2 pounds each week while eating well-balanced meals.	Assess Mrs. Vincent's motivation to lose weight.	Having the client's support for the plan will influence success.	Mrs. Vincent is drinking water with meals, chewing her food slowly, and chewing gum while watching TV. She has lost 1.5 pounds in 1 week.
	Suggest methods to adapt eating habits to decrease amount of intake (smaller servings, taking small bites and chewing each bite 12 times, placing the fork on the plate between bites, drinking water with meals, eating only at mealtime, chewing sugar-free gum when watching TV).	Healthy eating habits and tips on recognizing fullness during a meal will help the client eat to satisfy hunger, not boredom.	
	Instruct Mrs. Vincent to maintain a daily dietary intake log: time, food, and amount.	Helps the client recognize her eating patterns and note healthy and unhealthy behaviors.	
	Provide and review the food guide pyramid and *Dietary Guidelines;* plan with Mrs. Vincent a diet for 1 week, taking into consideration food preferences.	Ensures that the client has information necessary to plan healthy meals within recommended guidelines.	
Mrs. Vincent will engage in 20 to 30 minutes of exercise three times a week.	Review with Mrs. Vincent age-appropriate exercises; emphasize the need for walking.	Changing sedentary lifestyle will increase self-esteem, burn calories, increase energy level, and decrease boredom.	Mrs. Vincent now walks 30 minutes 4 days a week.
Mrs. Vincent will explore outside interests to decrease boredom and increase feelings of self-worth.	Review with Mrs. Vincent community interests outside the home, unrelated to cooking and eating.	Helps the client focus on activities not involving food, thereby decreasing boredom and increasing self-esteem.	Mrs. Vincent will begin volunteering 2 hours three times a week at the church's child care center.

CASE STUDY

Tom, age 27 years, has been HIV positive for 4 years. He is admitted to the hospital complaining of diarrhea and cramping for 3 weeks and a burn wound on his right forearm that will not heal. He states, "I do not have the energy to eat or get dressed. For the past month, I have eaten mainly bread, cereal, milk, and potatoes."

The following questions will guide your development of a nursing care plan for the case study.

1. What subjective and objective data should the nurse gather?
2. Which nursing diagnoses and goals would be appropriate for Tom?
3. List appropriate nursing interventions for helping Tom meet the goals.
4. List teaching Tom will need before leaving the hospital.

SUMMARY

- The LP/VN plays an important role in promoting proper nutrition.
- The six types of nutrients are water, fats, carbohydrates, protein, vitamins, and minerals.
- Water is the most vital nutrient.
- There must always be a balance between water intake and output to maintain health.
- Nutrients build, repair, and maintain body tissue; provide energy; and regulate body processes.
- The food guide pyramid identifies the five food groups for a well-balanced diet along with a range of servings to meet varying kcal needs.
- Nutritional needs vary as an individual moves through the life cycle.
- Nutrition is influenced by culture, religion, socioeconomics, fads, superstitions, age, and health.
- The kcal needs of an individual are based on basal energy needs and activity.
- Weight management is based on the relationship between the intake and the use of kcal.
- Food safety is based on proper storage, proper sanitation, and proper cooking.
- Food-borne illnesses can be fairly mild or fatal.

Review Questions

1. The role of the LP/VN in meeting the nutritional needs of the client includes:
   a. writing the diet order.
   b. preparing food for clients.
   c. preparing a complete diet plan.
   d. answering questions about nutrition.

2. Which of the following would most likely be on a clear liquid diet?
   a. Milk shake
   b. Tomato soup
   c. Orange juice
   d. Cranberry juice

3. What is the main function of carbohydrates?
   a. Build and repair tissue
   b. Provide the body with energy
   c. Provide a source of dietary fiber
   d. Insulate the body to prevent heat loss

4. What is the fuel value of protein?
   a. 3 kcal/g
   b. 4 kcal/g
   c. 8 kcal/g
   d. 9 kcal/g

5. Which of the following is a complete protein?
   a. Milk
   b. Gelatin
   c. Pinto beans
   d. Peanut butter

6. Which of the following is the best source of dietary fiber?
   a. Popcorn
   b. Chicken
   c. Tomato juice
   d. Macaroni and cheese

7. Which of the following is true of cholesterol?
   a. It is made in the body.
   b. It has no function in the body.
   c. It is not important in any disease.
   d. It should not be included in the diet.

8. A female client is 5 ft. 5 in. tall and weighs 180 lb. What would be her desired weight?

    a. 115 pounds
    b. 120 pounds
    c. 125 pounds
    d. 130 pounds

9. Why should the nurse advise a client to take an iron supplement with orange juice?

    a. To prevent heartburn
    b. To prevent constipation
    c. To improve absorption of the iron
    d. To improve digestion of the orange juice

10. Where is most of the water in the body found?

    a. Inside the cells
    b. In the intestines
    c. In the blood and lymph
    d. In the kidneys and bladder

Critical Thinking Questions

1. What recommendations should be made regarding vitamin supplements?

2. What should the nurse know about nutrition in order to properly care for an obese client?

 WEB FLASH!

- Search the Web for information about a vaccine for *E. Coli* O157:H7.
- What resources related to nutrition can be found on the Internet?

REST AND SLEEP

MAKING THE CONNECTION

Refer to the following chapters to increase your understanding of rest and sleep:

- **Chapter 8, Communication**
- **Chapter 9, Nursing Process**
- **Chapter 11, Client Teaching**
- **Chapter 13, Alternative/Complementary Therapies**
- **Chapter 16, Stress, Adaptation, and Anxiety**
- **Chapter 26, Pain Management**

LEARNING OBJECTIVES

Upon completion of this chapter, you should be able to:
- *Define key terms.*
- *Describe the stages of sleep.*
- *Discuss age-related sleep variations.*
- *State the outcomes of sleep deprivation.*
- *Delineate nursing interventions that promote rest and sleep.*

KEY TERMS

biological clock	REM movement
bruxism	disorder
cataplexy	rest
chronobiology	restless leg syndrome
circadian rhythm	sleep
hypersomnia	sleep apnea
insomnia	sleep cycle
jet lag	sleep deprivation
narcolepsy	snoring
parasomnia	somnambulism

INTRODUCTION

The quality of rest and sleep can have a significant impact on a client's health, including physical well-being, mental status, and effectiveness of coping mechanisms. This chapter explores both the importance of rest and sleep and the nursing care that will help clients maintain optimal health when disturbances in rest and sleep patterns threaten to compromise health status.

REST AND SLEEP

Rest and sleep are fundamental components of well-being. All individuals require certain periods of calm and lesser activity so that their bodies can regain energy and rebuild stamina. The need for rest and sleep varies with age, developmental level, health status, activity level, and cultural norms.

Rest refers to a state of relaxation and calmness, both mental and physical. Activity during rest periods can range from lying down to reading a book to taking a quiet walk. When discussing a client's rest patterns, the nurse should try to ascertain those activities and environments that the client defines as restful (Figure 19-1).

Sleep refers to a state of altered consciousness during which an individual experiences fluctuations in level of consciousness; minimal physical activity; and a general slowing of the body's physiologic processes. Sleep generally occurs in a periodic cycle and usually lasts for several hours at a time; disruptions in the usual sleep routine can be distressing to clients and will most likely impair further sleep. As a restorative function, sleep is necessary for physiologic and psychological healing to occur. It is important for clients, their significant others, and health care providers to understand both the normal sleep–wake cycle and the ways sleep affects mood and healing.

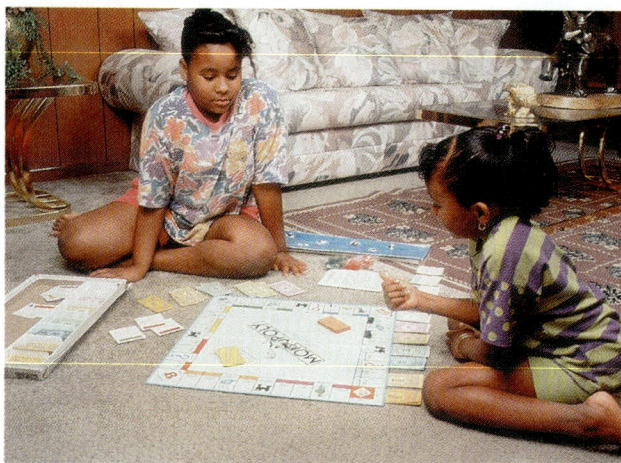

Figure 19-1 Playing a quiet board game can be a very relaxing activity for children.

Physiology of Rest and Sleep

The cycles of wakefulness and sleep are controlled by centers in the brain and are influenced by routines and environmental factors. An individual's biological clock also helps determine the specific cycles that will be followed for wakefulness and sleep.

Stages of Sleep

Electroencephalograph (EEG) patterns, eye movements, and muscle activity are used to identify stages of sleep. The stages of sleep are classified in two categories: non-rapid eye movement (NREM) and rapid eye movement (REM) sleep.

NREM Sleep With the onset of sleep, heart rate and respiratory rate slow slightly and remain regular. This first phase of sleep is referred to as non-rapid eye movement, or NREM, sleep. This sleep phase consists of four different stages. As the client enters *stage 1 sleep,* EEG frequency slows overall, but wave spikes occur; the eyes tend to roll slowly from side to side, and muscle tension remains absent except in the facial and neck muscles. In adult clients with normal sleep patterns, stage 1 sleep usually lasts only 10 minutes or so. Stage 1 NREM sleep is of a very light quality, meaning that during this stage, a sleeper can be easily awakened. If awakened, the sleeper often feels as if he has been daydreaming.

Stage 2 sleep is still fairly light sleep; EEG patterns slow further, slow-rolling eye movements stop, and relaxation heightens. Fifty percent of normal adult sleep may be spent in stage 2. After an initial 20 minutes or so of stage 2 sleep, a deep form of sleep, called stage 3 to 4, is entered.

Stage 3 and *stage 4 sleep* are frequently discussed together because of the difficulty in identifying and separating the two. Stage 3 refers to medium-depth sleep, and stage 4 signals the deepest sleep. Each stage lasts 15 to 30 minutes. During these stages, all cortical brain cells appear to be firing at the same time, resulting in large, slow waves on the EEG. Vital signs are significantly lower than during waking hours. When roused from stage 3 to 4 sleep, an adult can take 15 seconds or so to become fully awake. This difficulty in awakening is even more pronounced in children. Stage 3 to 4 sleep is when most sleepwalking, sleeptalking, enuresis, and night terrors occur.

Stage 3 to 4 sleep is felt to have restorative value, necessary for physical recovery. The majority of human growth hormone is secreted at night, peaking during stage 3 to 4 sleep, near the beginning of a sleep period. This growth hormone is required not only for growth but also for normal tissue repair in clients of all ages. Stage 3 to 4 sleep accounts for approximately 25% of sleep in children, declines slightly in young adulthood, gradually declines in middle age, and may be absent in elderly clients.

REM Sleep After the initial 90 minutes or so of NREM sleep in adults, the client enters rapid eye movement, or REM, sleep. The EEG pattern resembles that of the awake state; rapid, conjugate eye movements are present; heart rate and respiratory rate are irregular and often higher than when awake; and muscles, including those of the face and neck, are flaccid, leaving the body immobilized. Dreams occur 80% of the time clients are in REM sleep; these dreams serve as a vehicle for clients to consolidate memories,

PROFESSIONAL TIP

Sleep Deprivation

Sleep deprivation can be deadly, and the price tag is staggering. According to the National Sleep Foundation (NSF, 1998e), sleep-related accidents cost the U.S. government and businesses $46 billion each year. Drowsy drivers are blamed for 100,000 police-reported crashes each year in the United States, and 31% of commercial truck crashes that are fatal to the driver are caused by drowsiness.

Forty million people in the United States have serious sleep disorders that undermine the quality of their sleep and their health. Many of these sleep disorders are undiagnosed (NSF, 1998e). During the past century, the average time asleep for the typical American has been reduced by 20%. The person who is deprived of restful sleep is less alert, less attentive, less able to perform even simple tasks, more irritable, and has poorer concentration and judgment and mood problems that make relationships with family, friends, and coworkers difficult. No matter the cause of sleep deprivation, inadequate sleep reduces the quality of life and is harmful to health.

LIFE CYCLE CONSIDERATIONS

REM Sleep

- Rapid eye movement sleep accounts for 50% of sleep in the newborn. This percentage gradually declines to 20% to 25% of sleep by early childhood and remains fairly constant throughout the remainder of the life span.
- An adult typically has four to six REM-sleep periods during the night.

adapt behaviors, solve problems, and clarify thoughts and emotions. Unlike stage 3 to 4 sleep, which is most abundant during the early portion of a sleep period, REM-sleep periods become longer as the night progresses and the individual becomes more rested.

Sleep Cycle

A **sleep cycle** refers to the sequence of sleep that begins with the four stages of NREM sleep in order, with a return to stage 3 and then stage 2, followed by passage into the first REM stage (Figure 19-2). The duration of a sleep cycle is generally 70 to 90 minutes, and the typical sleeper will pass through four to six sleep cycles during an average sleep period of 7 to 8 hours.

The length of the NREM and REM periods of sleep will change as the overall sleep period progresses and

the sleeper becomes more relaxed and re-energized. There is less need for stage 3 to 4 sleep and more need for REM sleep as the sleep period progresses, and dreams during the REM phases of later sleep may become more vivid and intense. If the sleep cycle is broken at any point, a new sleep cycle will start, beginning again at stage 1 of NREM sleep and progressing through all the stages to REM sleep.

Biological Clock

The **biological clock** is an internal mechanism capable of measuring time in a living organism (Coleman, 1986). It controls the daily fluctuations in hundreds of physiologic processes, including body temperature, respiratory rate, performance, alertness, and a number of hormone levels. According to Coleman (1986), the major characteristics of biological clocks are:

- They are internal physiologic systems that can measure the passage of time;
- They have their own daily cycle length, which is close to, but not exactly, 24 hours;
- When exposed to normal environmental cues, such as the day–night cycle, they can adapt to a 24-hour day; and
- When free of environmental cues, such as the day–night cycle, the organism's internal cycle length determines its behavior.

When external time cues such as day–night, sleep–wake, and mealtimes are inconsistent, a desynchronization, or mismatching, of the circadian biological rhythms occurs. This internal desynchronization disrupts

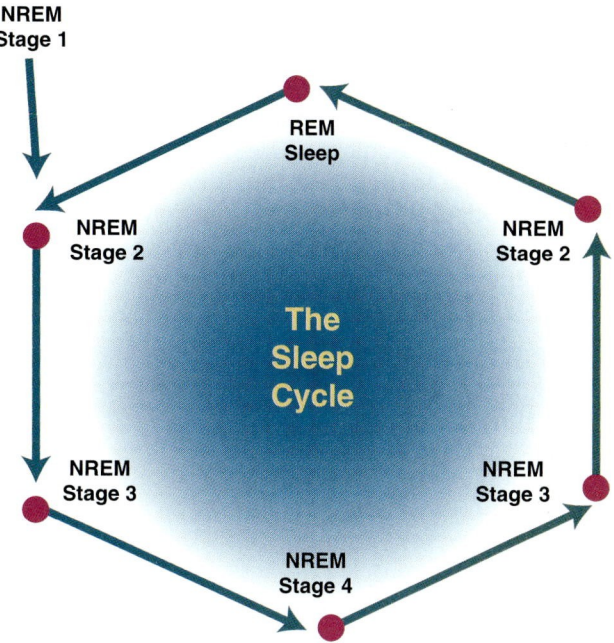

Figure 19-2 The Sleep Cycle (*From* Fundamentals of Nursing: Standards & Practice, *by S. DeLaune and P. Ladner, 1998, Albany, NY: Delmar Publishers. Copyright 1998 by Delmar Publishers. Reprinted with permission.*)

PROFESSIONAL TIP

Biorhythms

Chronobiology is a relatively new branch of science that studies biorhythms, or the rhythms that are controlled by our biological clocks. The most widely studied are the **circadian rhythms**, or those that cycle on a daily basis, such as the sleep–wake cycle. Other biological rhythms include the following:

- Ultradian: those lasting much shorter than a day, such as the milliseconds it takes for a neuron to fire
- Infradian: those lasting a month or more, such as the monthly menstrual cycle
- Circannual: those requiring approximately 1 year to complete, such as seasonal affective disorder, which causes depression in susceptible people during the short days of winter.

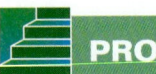

PROFESSIONAL TIP

Sleep in the United States

Statistics show that 90% of people in the United States require from 6 to 9 hours of sleep per day, with the average being 7 to 8 hours. Differing requirements in this biological circadian rhythm may be genetically programmed and may also be linked to longevity (Coleman, 1986).

the timing of physiologic and behavioral activity, which, in turn, causes chronic fatigue, disrupted sleep patterns, and decreased performance and coping abilities. An example of desynchronization is that of the newborn, whose biological rhythms are not established until 3 to 4 months of age. At this point, infants will start to develop longer sleep periods at night and become more predictable in their waking and sleeping patterns.

Factors Affecting Rest and Sleep

Several factors can influence the quality and quantity of both rest and sleep. Often, sleep problems result from a combination of many factors.

Degree of Comfort

Comfort is a highly subjective experience. The nurse must assess the degree to which the client's physical

 CLIENT TEACHING

Jet Lag

When traveling by plane through several time zones, a person must allow several days for his "biological clock" to adjust to the new time. This is known as **jet lag**. The body wants to go to sleep in daylight and wakes up during the night. Suggestions to minimize jet lag include the following:

- Getting up earlier and going to bed earlier for several days before a trip eastward and doing so later for a trip westward
- During the flight, changing your watch to the time at the destination
- Avoiding caffeine and alcohol for 4 hours before bedtime
- Avoiding strenuous exercise for 2 hours before bedtime
- Wearing ear plugs and a blindfold while sleeping
- Staying out in the sunlight as much as possible

(NSF, 1998d)

and psychological needs have been met. Whenever basic needs are not satisfied, the person experiences discomfort, which, in turn, leads to physiologic tension and resultant anxiety and, potentially, disturbed sleep and rest. For example, a client experiencing hunger or pain may become restless and irritable and will focus on getting these needs met as opposed to getting restful sleep.

Anxiety

A restless body and mind interfere with the ability to sleep. When trying to go to sleep, many individuals often have intrusive thoughts or muscular tension, which interferes with rest and sleep. Anxiety related to work pressures, family demands, and other stressors does not automatically cease when an individual attempts to go to sleep, and it often results in difficulty falling or staying asleep.

Environment

Environmental factors can either enhance or impair sleep. Lighting, temperature, odors, ventilation, and noise level can all interrupt the sleep process when they differ from the norms of the client's usual sleep environment. The comfort and size of the bed, firmness of the pillow, and habits (snoring or movements) of a sleep partner may all interfere with sleep.

Lifestyle

A fast-paced life filled with multiple stressors can result in a person's inability to relax easily or to fall asleep quickly. Relaxation precedes healthy sleep. Vigorously exercising within an hour of going to bed or performing mentally intense activities just before or after getting into bed often work against getting a good night's sleep.

Another lifestyle factor that interferes with sleep is having a work schedule that does not coincide with an individual's biological clock (e.g., working at times other than the day shift). Approximately 20% of employees in the United States are shift workers (NSF, 1998a). Individuals who frequently change work shifts

 CLIENT TEACHING

Methods To Reduce Anxiety

Teach clients the following methods to relieve anxiety:

- Progressive muscle relaxation
- Guided imagery
- Deep breathing
- Thought stopping
- Meditation
- Therapeutic massage

PROFESSIONAL TIP

Providing Environmental Comfort

A firm pillow is suggested for side-sleepers, a medium pillow for back-sleepers, and a soft pillow for stomach sleepers (*Pillow Firmness Key*, 1998).

CULTURAL CONSIDERATIONS

Cultural and Societal Expectations Affecting Sleep

Some people perceive sleep as a luxury to be indulged in when they are not too busy with "important" activities. Others view sleep as an absolute necessity. The amount of sleep that a person considers necessary is partially determined by the attitudes of family and culture.

or travel across several times zones face a real challenge in trying to stabilize their biological rhythms and rest comfortably.

Diet

The type of food consumed has an impact on the quality and quantity of sleep. Foods high in caffeine, such as coffee, colas, and chocolate, serve as stimulants and often disrupt the normal sleep cycle. Also, consuming a large, heavy, or spicy meal just before bedtime may cause indigestion, which will likely interfere with sleep. Conversely, going to bed when hungry can also result in sleep problems because the individual may be preoccupied with food and hunger pangs instead of concentrating on sleep.

Drugs and Other Substances

Alcohol and nicotine use can also impair sleep. Small amounts of alcohol may help some people fall asleep; in others, however, alcohol may interfere with REM sleep, causing very restless and nonrefreshing sleep. Nicotine, which is a stimulant, can also impair the sleep cycle by stimulating the body, resulting in difficulty falling and staying asleep. Many medications, both prescription and over the counter, list fatigue, sleepiness, restlessness, agitation, or insomnia as side effects, all of which will have an impact on the quality and quantity of rest and sleep.

Safety: Medications and Sleep

Some medications used to treat high blood pressure, asthma, or depression, may cause sleeping difficulties. For instance, captopril (Capoten) and theophylline (Theomar), used in the treatment of high blood pressure and asthma, respectively, may cause insomnia, whereas trazodone (Desyrel), an antidepressant, may induce drowsiness or insomnia.

Age/Aging

Although sleep and rest patterns are closely tied to lifestyle and other variables, some common variations are based on age.

The neonate (birth–1 month) sleeps in 3- to 4-hour intervals for a total of approximately 16 to 20 hours per day. The newborn usually is very passive, with little activity occurring during sleep ("sleeping like a baby"),

and typically sleeps very soundly. For the first few weeks or even months of life, a baby's biological clock is not attuned to regular day–night patterns, so there is often no difference in sleep patterns between day and night.

The infant averages approximately 12 to 16 hours of sleep per day. As the infant ages, the amount of sleep needed decreases. At approximately 2 months of age, infants can begin to sleep through the night and will typically nap two or three times during the day.

During toddlerhood, the daily average amount of sleep is 12 to 14 hours, which is usually broken down into 10 to 12 hours at night and one or two daytime naps (Figure 19-3). During this stage, bedtime rituals often develop and assume great importance in providing nighttime security. A repeated and predictable nighttime routine such as a bath, brushing teeth, and reading books is helpful in establishing expectations and comfort.

The preschool child sleeps approximately 10 to 12 hours per day. Daytime napping decreases or ceases, unless cultural norms dictate otherwise. Night sleep is often filled with vivid dreams and nightmares, which often awaken children several times during the night.

The school-age child also averages approximately 10 to 12 hours of sleep daily. Both resistance to bedtime

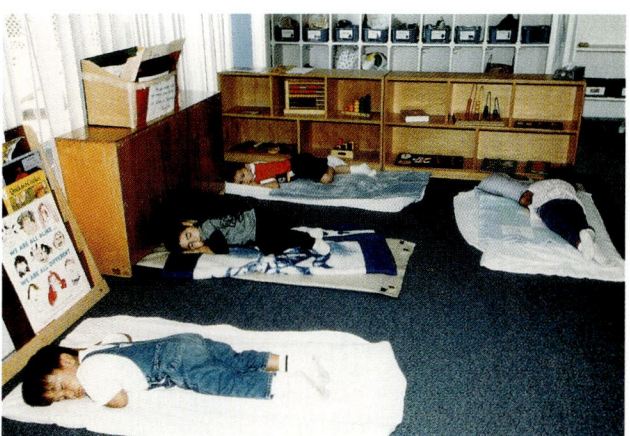

Figure 19-3 Young children require naps and rest periods throughout the day.

and struggles for independence are hallmarks of the school-age child. During this time, the child may develop fear of the dark and will need reassurance and methods to handle this fear.

Adolescents sleep approximately 8 to 10 hours per day and often decide their own bedtime routines and hours. A high activity level often interferes with regular sleep patterns, and irregular sleeping habits often become the norm at this stage.

The young adult averages approximately 8 hours of sleep per day. During this stage, sleep is often interrupted by young children in the home or by work responsibilities. Lifestyle patterns cause many young adults to experience difficulties falling or staying asleep.

The middle-age adult sleeps approximately 6 to 8 hours per day. Daily stressors may continue to result in insomnia, and use of sleep-inducing medications is common.

Most older adults sleep less at one time than do those who are younger, though overall sleep needs remain constant at 7 to 9 hours (NSF, 1998b). They may go to sleep earlier, wake up more often, get less "deep" sleep, and rise earlier (NSF, 1998a). Often, a daytime nap is taken. The quality of sleep may diminish due to frequent waking, physical pain, and less time spent in stage 3 to 4 sleep. The percentage of REM sleep remains fairly constant.

Physical Factors

The stress imposed by illness often disrupts sleep. Some physical problems can interfere with the ability to fall asleep or stay asleep. Conditions that cause discomfort or pain, such as arthritis, make it difficult to sleep well, as can breathing disorders such as sleep apnea and asthma. Hormonal changes that cause premenstrual syndrome (PMS) or menopause with its hot flashes can disrupt sleep. Even pregnancy, especially during the last few weeks, may make sleeping difficult.

Sleep is especially disrupted when a person is hospitalized. Some factors associated with hospitalization that lead to sleep impairment include:

- Physical or emotional pain,
- Loss of familiar surroundings,
- Loss of routine,
- Fear of the unknown,
- Timing of assessments, procedures, and treatments,
- Intrusive lighting or equipment,
- Noise level (especially unfamiliar noises), and
- Loss of privacy.

Alterations in Sleep Patterns

Sleep disturbances can take many forms and are quite common. Alterations in sleep patterns are generally viewed as either primary sleep disorders (those wherein the sleep alteration is the fundamental prob-

lem) or secondary sleep disorders (those wherein the alteration has a medical or clinical cause that results in or contributes to the sleep alteration). The most common sleep alterations include insomnia, hypersomnia, narcolepsy, sleep apnea/snoring, sleep deprivation, parasomnias, restless leg syndrome, and periodic limb movement disorder.

Insomnia

Insomnia refers to the inability to sleep or to inadequate quality of sleep resulting from sleep being prematurely ended or interrupted by periods of wakefulness. It affects one in three adults each year in the United States (Cooper, 1998). Insomnia is not a disease, but it may be a manifestation of many illnesses. Causes may include stress, depression, medical problems, caffeine, alcohol, pain, shortness of breath, poor sleep habits, or changes in sleep patterns related to travel or shift work. The person experiencing insomnia often gets caught up in a vicious cycle of not being able to sleep, trying harder to fall asleep, and experiencing increasing anxiety about not sleeping, which, in turn, increases the inability to fall asleep.

Symptoms of insomnia include difficulty falling to sleep, waking frequently during the night, waking very early and not being able to go back to sleep, feeling unrested in the morning and/or tired during the day, and becoming anxious and restless as bedtime arrives. Many who have insomnia actually sleep significantly more than they think they do; thus, there is a discrepancy between perception and reality.

Many times, insomnia may occur only for a night or two. If it continues for more than a few nights or is viewed as very disturbing or disruptive by the individual, a health care provider should be consulted for some relief. Treatment for insomnia is best directed at modifying those factors or behaviors that are causing it.

Hypersomnia

Hypersomnia is an alteration in sleep pattern characterized by excessive sleep, especially in the daytime. Persons suffering from hypersomnia often feel that they cannot get enough sleep at night, and, therefore, they sleep very late into the morning and nap several times throughout the day. Causes of hypersomnia can be physical (such as a disease or use of medications) or psychological (such as a self-imposed short sleep time); treatment depends on addressing the underlying cause.

Narcolepsy

Narcolepsy, another sleep alteration, manifests as sudden, uncontrollable urges to fall asleep during the daytime. Approximately 1 in 2,000 people have narcolepsy (NSP, 1998b). These "sleep attacks" can occur during a conversation or while driving, and they can last from a few seconds to more than 30 minutes. A common characteristic of narcolepsy is **cataplexy**, a sudden loss of muscle control, which may cause the person to fall. The person may also experience vivid dream-like images as they fall asleep or as they awaken (NSF, 1998b).

Individuals suffering from narcolepsy often achieve adequate sleep at night but are overwhelmed by sleepiness at unexpected and unpredictable periods during the day. There is no cure, but symptoms can be controlled by taking short daytime naps, taking prescribed stimulant medications, or avoiding substances or activities that cause sleepiness.

Sleep Apnea/Snoring

Sleep apnea is characterized by breathing pauses of 30 to 60 seconds during sleep, interspersed between loud **snoring** (noisy breathing during sleep) episodes. The trachea partially closes, and the individual grunts, snorts, and snores. Pulse rate slows and may become irregular. Receptors in the brain, sensing a loss of oxygen, struggle to awaken the sleeper. The unaware sleeper wakes up several hundred times a night for 5 to 10 seconds, takes a deep breath, rolls over, and goes back to sleep, only to start another cycle of apnea. More often than not, sleep apnea victims have no idea that they are not breathing or that they are continually waking up (Coleman, 1986).

The result of sleep apnea is REM-sleep deprivation, which may manifest as daytime sleepiness or chronic fatigue. Persons with sleep apnea have a three to seven times greater risk of falling asleep while driving (NSF, 1998c). Complications can include hypertension and an increased risk of heart attack or stroke. The first line of defense against apnea is treating its cause. Use of a nasal continuous positive airway pressure (CPAP) device, which maintains airflow with a small compressor, may give relief. Dental appliances that reposition the tongue may also help (NSF, 1998b). With some individuals, surgical intervention is required to correct the cause of the apnea.

Sleep Deprivation

Sleep deprivation is a term used to describe prolonged inadequate quality and quantity of sleep, either of the REM or the NREM type. Sleep deprivation can result from age, prolonged hospitalization, drug and substance use, illness, and frequent changes in lifestyle patterns. Sleep and dreaming have a restorative value necessary for mental and emotional recovery, and they appear to enhance the ability to cope with emotional problems. Therefore, sleep deprivation can cause symptoms ranging from irritability, hypersensitivity, and confusion to apathy, sleepiness, and diminished reflexes. Treating or minimizing the factors that cause the sleep deprivation is the most effective intervention.

Parasomnia

Parasomnia refers to a condition wherein a person suffers from profoundly disturbed sleep due to behavioral or physiological events. **Somnambulism** (sleepwalking), sleeptalking, night terrors, REM movement disorder, bed wetting, and **bruxism** (teeth grinding) are the most common parasomnias; the first four are discussed in more detail following. Treatment for parasomnias varies, and care should be focused on helping the client and family understand the given disorder and its potential safety risks.

Somnambulism Sleepwalking, mostly done by children, is typically not remembered by the individual the next morning. The sleepwalker usually moves around furniture very safely, though doors and windows must be kept locked at night to protect the sleepwalker from harm. Sleepwalkers are difficult to rouse during an episode and if awakened are often confused and without any specific recall of events that led to their behavior. Sleepwalking tends to run in families and usually stops at puberty (NSF, 1998b).

Sleeptalking Sleeptalking can occur at any age. It may be a word or two or a long speech, sometimes understandable and sometimes gibberish. The person has no memory of talking, but the sleep partner may have been awakened.

Night Terrors Night terrors, sometimes called sleep terrors, are more common in children and seldom continue into adulthood. Night terrors usually occur during NREM stage 3 to 4 sleep. The child suddenly appears to awaken, thrashes about, sweats, and may even cry. This can last anywhere from 1 minute to approximately 15 minutes. The child remembers nothing in the morning (Brown, 1997). Reassurance by the parents during the episode is the only treatment; the child will eventually outgrow the behavior.

REM Movement Disorder **REM movement disorder** results when the paralysis that normally occurs during REM sleep is absent or incomplete and the sleeper acts out the dream that is occurring. It is most common among older men. Violent behavior and injuries may result. The person *can* remember the dream in the morning. Medication usually is effective in controlling the physical movements.

PROFESSIONAL TIP

Sleep Apnea

Sleep apnea and snoring are more common in obese persons, although the obesity connection is much weaker among older people. Among middle-age people, 4% of men and 2% of women have sleep apnea. After the age of 65, the rate increases to 28% for men and 24% for women (NSF, 1998c).

Restless Leg Syndrome

Restless leg syndrome (RLS) is characterized by the uncomfortable sensations of tingling or crawling in the muscles and by twitching, burning, prickling, or deep aching in the foot, calf or upper leg when at rest (lying down or sitting) (Carter, 1997). Temporary relief is found by walking, standing, or moving or rubbing the legs (Figure 19-4). The sensations return in seconds or minutes. The legs frequently jump involuntarily if they are not moved. Symptoms worsen at night. If sleep does come, the leg movements awaken the person frequently.

Although the cause is unknown, some cases of RLS have been linked to iron deficiency, dialysis treatment, peripheral neuropathy, pregnancy, excessive caffeine intake, alcohol dependence, smoking, and rheumatoid arthritis (Carter, 1997; NSF, 1998c). The disorder is more common among women who have surpassed middle age. Avoiding or reducing both smoking and caffeine and alcohol intake may help. Symptoms may be relieved by the anti-Parkinson drug carbidopa/levodopa (Sinemet).

Periodic Limb Movement Disorder

Periodic limb movement disorder (PLMD) is a condition wherein the legs jerk every 20 to 40 seconds throughout the night (NSF, 1998c). It is typically not uncomfortable for the affected person, but may be distressing to the sleep partner. Multiple sleep interruptions occur, leading to daytime sleepiness and nighttime insomnia.

The disorder is quite common in persons over age 65 years. Approximately 45% of elders have at least a mild form of PLMD, which occurs only during sleep and is not as uncomfortable as RLS (NSF, 1998c). Most cases are successfully controlled with carbidopa/levodopa (Sinemet).

NURSING PROCESS

All standardized nursing history tools include questions related to a client's rest and sleep patterns. Care of the client who is diagnosed with a sleep disorder is collaborative, with the nurse participating in an interdisciplinary team providing treatment.

Assessment

Discussion of sleep habits is part of the regular health history. Any client acknowledging a sleep disturbance should be thoroughly assessed to determine sleep routines, sleep alterations, types of disturbance, and impact of sleep problems. Typically, the client is a reliable source for this information, but a spouse or partner who shares sleeping arrangements may be able to add valuable information to the client's report. Ques-

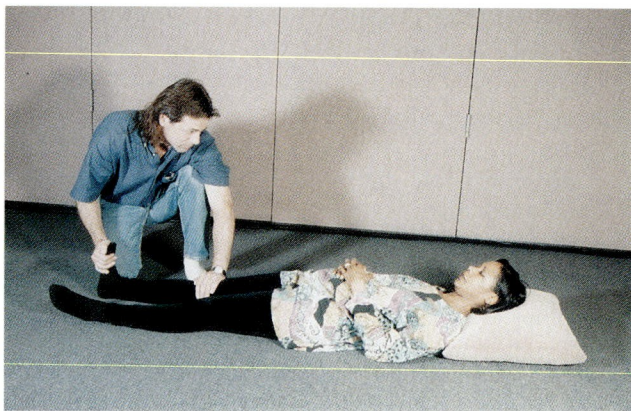

Figure 19-4 Massaging or rubbing the legs often helps relieve the sensations of restless leg syndrome.

tions regarding the client's usual sleep patterns should focus on the following:

- Nature of sleep (restful, uninterrupted)
- Quality of sleep (usual sleep pattern, schedules, hours of sleep, feeling on waking)
- Sleep environment (description of room, temperature, noise level)
- Associated factors (bedtime routines, use of sleep medications or any other sleep inducers)
- Opinion of sleep (adequate, adequate in terms of energy restoration, inadequate, problematic)

Questions regarding altered sleep patterns are intended to discover information such as the following:

- Nature of the problem (inability to fall asleep, difficulty remaining asleep, inability to fall asleep after awakening, restless sleep, daytime sleepiness)
- Quality of the problem (number of hours of sleep versus number of hours spent trying to sleep, number of hours of sleep per night, duration and frequency of naps or other compensatory measures, number of awakenings per sleep period)
- Environmental factors (lighting, bed, noise level, surrounding stimulation, sleep partner)
- Associated factors (relation to meals eaten, activity before retiring, life stressors, work stressors, anxiety level, pain, recent illness or surgery)

LIFE CYCLE CONSIDERATIONS

Sleep and Aging

- Sleep needs do not decline with age, but stay fairly constant at 7 to 9 hours per day.
- Middle-age and elderly clients are more likely to experience sleep apnea, restless leg syndrome, and periodic limb movement disorder (NSF, 1998c).

- Alleviating factors (mild diet, warm drink before retiring, reading, listening to quiet music, taking a hot bath)
- Effect of problem (fatigue, irritability, confusion)

A sleep questionnaire that can be used to assess a hospitalized client's sleep pattern is shown in Figure 19-5. The questionnaire focuses on sleep and common factors that may cause problems. In addition to the questionnaire, other factors such as age, medical diagnosis, occupation, allergies, and psychiatric disorders must also be considered when assessing sleep problems.

For clients whose sleep problems do not seem to be well defined, a daily journal of their sleep patterns may prove useful. This written account can mirror the preceding lists of information to obtain when asking a client about sleep.

The Sleep Questionnaire

At home, what do you do at bedtime to help you sleep? _____

_____

Some of the statements may *appear* to be the same, but each is different and should be rated as such.*

A. I think I have difficulty with sleep
   a. in the hospital
   b. at home
B. I sleep more at home than in the hospital.
C. When I awaken in the hospital, I feel fatigued and groggy.
D. It takes me longer than 30 minutes to fall asleep in the hospital.
E. Since I've been in the hospital, I awaken frequently at night.
F. In the hospital, if I wake up in the middle of the night it takes me longer then 30 minutes to fall back to sleep.
G. It bothers me that I now go to bed at a different time than I would like.
H. It bothers me that I get up at a different time each morning.
I. Hospital staff awaken me while I'm sleeping.
J. I am awakened at night for treatments.
K. During the day, there is little time for rest.
L. At night I am awakened by noises.
M. At night I am awakened by light.
N. The mattress in the hospital bothers my sleep.
O. The pillow in the hospital bothers my sleep.
P. Having a roommate in the hospital affects my sleep.
Q. I sleep in a very warm room.
R. I have pain at night.
S. The medicines I take keep me awake.
T. My illness keeps me awake at night.

1. I drink coffee, tea, cola, or cocoa during the day.
2. I drink coffee, tea, cola, or cocoa around sleeping time.
3. I exercise during the day.
4. I exercise around sleeping time.
5. I smoke during the day.
6. I smoke around sleeping time.
7. I have unpleasant conversation during the day.
8. I have unpleasant conversation around sleeping time.
9. I have negative thoughts during the day.
10. I have negative thoughts around sleeping time.
11. I think about what happened during the day and at sleeping time I plan for tomorrow.
12. I read during the day.
13. I read around sleeping time.
14. I eat around sleeping time.
15. I watch TV during the day.
16. I watch TV around sleeping time.
17. I have pleasant conversation during the day.
18. I have pleasant conversation around sleeping time.
19. I have positive thoughts during the day.
20. I have positive thoughts around sleeping time.
21. I drink alcohol around sleeping time.

* Response choices were: *Never, Rarely, Sometimes, Often, Very Often.*

Figure 19-5 Sleep questionnaire for hospitalized clients. Statements A through F elicit the client's perception of a sleep problem. Answers of "rarely" or "never" to statements A, B, and C indicate no sleep problem. Statements G through T identify the cause of the problem. Statements 1 through 21 identify both daytime and bedtime behaviors that induce or prevent sleep. *(From "I Didn't Sleep a Wink," by B. McNeil, K, Padrick, and J. Wellman, 1986,* American Journal of Nursing, 86*(1). Copyright 1986 by Lippincott-Raven Publishers. Reprinted with permission.)*

Nursing Diagnosis

After information about the sleep impairment has been collected, the data must be analyzed to formulate appropriate nursing diagnoses. Alterations in sleep can manifest as verbal complaints on the part of the client, physical signs such as yawning or dark circles under the eyes, or alterations in mood, such as apathy or irritability. The primary diagnosis for individuals experiencing sleep problems is *Sleep Pattern Disturbance*. According to the North American Nursing Diagnosis Association (NANDA) (1999), *Sleep Pattern Disturbance* is defined as "time-limited disruption of sleep (natural, periodic suspension of consciousness) amount and quality."

Another possible diagnosis related to rest and sleep is *Sleep Deprivation* (NANDA, 1999). This diagnosis is defined as "prolonged periods of time without sustained natural, periodic suspension of relative unconsciousness."

If the client presents with problems in addition to the sleep disturbance, the nurse must be alert to the possibility that the sleep disturbance is the *cause* (not the effect) of another problem. For example, a client may be experiencing *Activity Intolerance related to lack of sleep as evidenced by verbal complaint, extreme fatigue, disorientation, confusion, and lack of energy.*

Planning/Outcome Identification

The plan of care for the client experiencing a sleep-disorder must be individualized. For the nursing care to be effective, client input should be incorporated when developing the plan and goals. It is important to tailor the plan of care and the goals to the true cause related to the sleep disturbance or alteration. For example, if the client is experiencing *Sleep Pattern Disturbance* because of bedwetting, the bedwetting should be targeted for intervention.

Effective planning and goal identification will also take into account that many sleep disturbances require extended periods of time (weeks or months as opposed to days) to correct. Sleep patterns are by nature habitual and intertwined with lifestyle patterns, and these types of disturbances typically require interventions the results of which cannot be seen immediately. When planning care, the nurse should remember to time procedures and treatments in a manner that disturbs sleep time and routines as little as possible.

Nursing Interventions

Several interventions can promote rest and sleep in clients; these are discussed following.

Trusting Nurse–Client Relationship

The quality of the nurse–client relationship can enhance the client's ability to rest and sleep. Knowing that the nurse is a trustworthy individual who genuinely

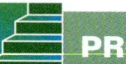

PROFESSIONAL TIP

Communicating with the Client Who Is Sleep-Impaired

- Thoroughly explain procedures before implementation
- Encourage the client and significant others to verbalize feelings and ask questions
- Answer questions honestly and completely
- Identify and support coping mechanisms of the client and family
- Spend adequate time with the client to facilitate communication
- Assess and incorporate the client's preferences as much as possible into the plan of care

cares about the client's condition allows the client to relax and feel secure. Anxiety can be minimized by the nurse's use of therapeutic communication skills. The therapeutic use of self helps allay client anxiety.

Relaxing Environment

Arranging the immediate surroundings to promote sleep is important for the sleep-impaired client. A place to sleep should be inviting. The nurse should ascertain the type of environment the client finds relaxing, then either provide this environment in the inpatient setting or help the client establish this type of environment in the home setting. For example, the nurse might suggest that the client in the hospital bring the preferred sleeping pillow from home, if doing so will aid in sleeping.

Relaxation Techniques

The client's mood before sleep is of utmost importance. The belief that one can and will sleep affects sleep quality and quantity to a significant extent. The client who is calm and relaxed is likely to fall asleep quickly and stay asleep all night. Relaxation techniques are useful sleep aids (Figure 19-6). Progressive muscle relaxation is especially therapeutic for the person who needs to lessen muscular tension and quiet the mind. A warm bath may be relaxing.

Appropriate Nutrition

Certain foods can actually enhance sleep. Tryptophan, a substance in milk, promotes sleep by stimulating the brain's production of the neurotransmitter serotonin. The old wives' tale that drinking warm milk promotes sleep is supported by scientific data. Other dietary considerations include avoiding large or heavy meals close to bedtime, refraining from eating spicy or other foods that cause gastrointestinal distress, and avoiding caffeine after noon.

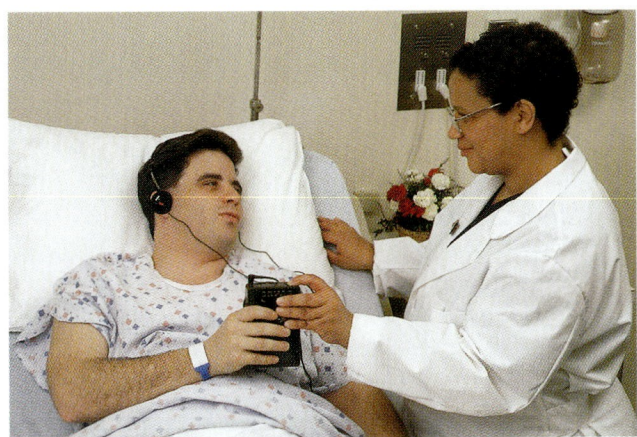

Figure 19-6 To help relieve this client's stress, the nurse is giving him a tape recorder and a relaxation tape.

Pharmacological Interventions

If unrelieved pain is a factor in the client's sleep disturbance, pain management should be the focus of initial interventions. Many of the nonpharmacological relaxation and imagery interventions can be effective in helping clients with sleep disturbances.

Pharmacological agents that may be therapeutic for clients with sleep disturbances include tricyclic antidepressants, antihistamines, and short-acting hypnotics

(McCaffery & Pasero, 1999). The tricyclic antidepressants of choice are amitriptyline (Elavil) or doxepin (Sinequan). Amitriptyline (Elavil) improves the client's ability to fall asleep and stay asleep by causing sedation when given 1 to 3 hours before bedtime. Doses of amitriptyline given for sleep disturbances are significantly lower than those given for treatment of depression.

Antihistamines such as hydroxyzine (Vistaril, Atarax) and diphenhydramine (Benadryl) have mild sedative effects that can promote sleep if given at bedtime. If anxiety throughout the day is of concern, low doses of these medications at regular intervals throughout the day may be effective.

The final group of pharmacological agents for sleep disturbances are the short-acting hypnotics. These are *not* recommended for routine or long-term use, as they have been associated with insomnia; however, they may be effective for short-term treatment. When they are used, it is recommended that a hypnotic with a short half-life be chosen.

Client Education

Educating the client about sleep-promoting activities is a good investment of the nurse's time. By providing clients with ways of promoting good sleep habits, the nurse helps them gain a sense of control over their sleep disturbances and boosts their confidence so that they can successfully meet their sleep and rest needs.

Evaluation

The plan of care must be individualized for and negotiated with the client and must be updated on a regular basis and additional interventions initiated as needed. One of the strongest supportive activities the nurse can perform is to ensure that clients understand that there is help for sleep problems and that they are not alone in having difficulty successfully managing their sleep patterns.

 CLIENT TEACHING

Managing Sleep Disturbance

To facilitate rest and sleep, the client should be encouraged to:

- Select regular times for going to bed and awakening and try to observe them.
- Avoid "sleeping in" on weekends, vacations, or holidays.
- Limit daytime naps to no more than 30 minutes.
- Take a warm bath before going to bed.
- Avoid stimulating activities, such as strenuous exercise or demanding intellectual activity, during the hour before bedtime and use the time instead to wind down with relaxing activities such as taking a warm bath, reading a book, or sitting by the fire.
- Use bedtime rituals on a consistent basis.
- Practice relaxation techniques, such as neck rolls and muscle relaxation, to release tensions before going to bed.
- Not watch television, study, or talk on the phone while lying in bed and instead accustom the body to using the bed only for sleeping.
- Follow dietary guidelines to avoid caffeine, spicy foods, and heavy meals in the several hours before bedtime

 PROFESSIONAL TIP

Noise Control in Hospitals

- Keep the door to the client's room closed
- Reduce the volume of paging and telephone systems, especially at night
- Ensure that unused equipment in the client's room is turned off
- Turn off or lower the volume on radios and televisions
- Workers should keep noises to a minimum, especially at night
- Hold discussions and conferences away from the client's room

PROFESSIONAL TIP

Variables To Consider in Evaluation

When evaluating the care of the client experiencing a sleep disorder, consider the following questions:
- Were the client's basic needs met?
- Did client education include the family or significant others?
- Was an environment conducive to rest maintained?

- Were therapeutic activities balanced with the client's need for rest and sleep?
- Were the client's bedtime rituals followed as closely as possible?
- Were anxiety-reduction techniques used appropriately?

SAMPLE NURSING CARE PLAN

THE CLIENT WITH TROUBLE SLEEPING

Six-year-old Jacques Porcheron is brought to your clinic by his father, who states that Jacques has trouble sleeping at night. In the evenings after a dinner of hot dogs, corn or baked beans, and chocolate milk, Jacques reads some books, then watches his favorite superhero video. Afterward, he runs and plays, mimics the actions he sees in the video, and refuses to take a bath or cooperate when getting ready for bed. After being put to bed at 9 P.M., he is up several times for any number of reasons and often is not asleep until midnight. When his father wakes him at 7 A.M. for school, Jacques is disagreeable, tired, and difficult to get moving.

Nursing Diagnosis *Sleep Pattern Disturbance (less than age-normal total sleep time) related to environmental factors (excessive stimulation) and parental lack of knowledge of sleep-promoting behaviors as evidenced by parental complaint, ineffective bedtime rituals, and insufficient hours of sleep for developmental age*

PLANNING/GOALS	NURSING INTERVENTIONS	RATIONALE	EVALUATION
Jacques and his family will determine those sleeping behaviors they would like to achieve.	Explain that the normal sleep requirement for a child of Jacques' age is 10 to 12 hours each day.	Helping the family understand Jacques' sleep requirements will help them be more effective in their management of his bedtime and sleeping habits.	Jacques and his family have decided they would like Jacques to cooperate in getting ready for bed and to be asleep in 30 minutes.
Jacques and his family will develop bedtime rituals to help Jacques wind down from the day.	Teach the family about the effect that certain foods can have on digestion and sleep habits, and identify with them those foods that are good choices for dinner.	Educating the family about the potential adverse effects of certain foods will help them plan meals more appropriately.	Together they have established a bedtime ritual that begins with playing quietly, followed by taking a warm bath, reading two books, brushing teeth, and then going to bed.
	Discuss those bedtime activities that can be detrimental to sleep induction.	Understanding those behaviors that can interfere with falling asleep will assist the family in modifying pre-bedtime behaviors	

continued

	Suggest appropriate bedtime rituals such as taking a bath, brushing the teeth, reading a book, or listening to calming music.	Focusing on quiet activities and having a routine helps the body and mind prepare for bedtime.	
Jacques and his family will identify behaviors that are helpful before bedtime.	Explain that overstimulation close to bedtime, such as watching superhero movies and engaging in rowdy play, prevents the body and mind from slowing down and preparing for sleep.	Understanding the psychological and physical implications of overstimulation before bedtime will help the family in choosing more appropriate bedtime activities.	The behaviors identified as helpful include no watching of stimulating videos after 7 P.M. and engaging in quiet play such as reading, arts and crafts, or writing. Some modification to Jacques' diet is planned for the next few weeks.
	Emphasize the importance of establishing a calming bedtime routine that is followed every night, especially for the school-age child.	Children Jacques' age are helped by ritual and knowing those things that are expected of them, and they need guidance in practicing routines that are appropriate for bedtime.	
	Describe an appropriate sleep environment for Jacques, such as a calm room kept at a comfortable temperature and lit only by a night light.	Such an environment promotes sleep and does not interfere with falling back asleep once awake.	

CASE STUDY

Mr. Leis, age 74, is hospitalized with deep vein thrombosis. His left thigh hurts when he moves. An intravenous line has been started in his right arm. Mr. Leis reports that it is difficult to fall asleep because of the pain in his leg. Hallway noises and nurses checking on him have awakened him the past 2 nights. He usually goes to bed at 9:30 P.M. but has not been able to fall asleep until 11:30 P.M. He states that he is tired and has been unable to take a nap.

The following questions will guide your development of a nursing care plan for the case study.

1. What other assessments should be done?
2. What nursing diagnosis is appropriate for Mr. Leis?
3. Identify three goals for Mr. Leis.
4. What nursing interventions would be appropriate to meet the goals?

SUMMARY

- Nonpharmacological interventions should be used in promoting rest and sleep.
- The amount of sleep required differs according to developmental stage.
- Pharmacological agents can be therapeutic for clients experiencing sleep pattern disturbances. However, the medications should not be the only interventions used.

Review Questions

1. The first phase of sleep is called:
   a. REM sleep.
   b. deep sleep.
   c. NREM sleep.
   d. light sleep.

2. A new sleep cycle for a client who is awakened during stage 4 NREM sleep will begin in:
   a. REM sleep.
   b. stage 1 sleep.
   c. stage 2 sleep.
   d. stage 3 sleep.

3. Individuals have several rhythms controlled by their biological clocks. The circadian rhythm cycle occurs:
   a. daily.
   b. every year.
   c. every month or so.
   d. several times a day.

4. Irregular sleeping habits often become the norm during:
   a. school-age.
   b. older adulthood.
   c. adolescence.
   d. young adulthood.

5. The older adult:
   a. needs less sleep.
   b. often takes a nap.
   c. experiences less REM sleep.
   d. experiences good-quality sleep.

6. Mitra is waking frequently at night and wakes very early in the morning. She may have:
   a. insomnia.
   b. parasomnia.
   c. narcolepsy.
   d. sleep apnea.

7. Jorge frequently falls asleep while sitting on the couch talking to his wife. He may have the sleep disturbance called:
   a. bruxism.
   b. narcolepsy.
   c. sleep apnea.
   d. hypersomnia.

8. Sleep apnea occurs mostly in:
   a. adolescents.
   b. young adults.
   c. middle-age adults.
   d. elders (those over age 65).

9. REM-sleep deprivation results from:
   a. sleep apnea.
   b. somnambulism.
   c. restless leg syndrome.
   d. periodic limb movement disorder.

Critical Thinking Questions

1. How are the stages of sleep related to the sleep cycle?

2. What age-related sleep variations should be considered when assessing the sleep habits of neonates, infants, toddlers, adolescents, and elders?

 WEB FLASH!

- Search the Internet for the topics of sleep and sleep disturbances. What information is available to clients and families?
- Search specific sleep disturbances on the Web. How much information can you find?

SAFETY/HYGIENE

MAKING THE CONNECTION

MAKING THE CONNECTION

Refer to the following chapters to increase your understanding of safety/hygiene:

- **Chapter 1, Holistic Care**
- **Chapter 6, Legal Responsibilities**
- **Chapter 8, Communication**
- **Chapter 9, Nursing Process**
- **Chapter 12, Cultural Diversity and Nursing**
- **Chapter 13, Alternative/Complementary Therapies**
- **Chapter 15, Wellness Concepts**
- **Chapter 16, Stress, Adaptation, and Anxiety**
- **Chapter 21, Infection Control/Asepsis**
- **Chapter 22, Standard Precautions and Isolation**
- **Chapter 25, Assessment**
- **Chapter 27, Diagnostic Tests**

- **Chapter 38, Nursing Care of the Client: Musculoskeletal System**
- **Chapter 41, Nursing Care of the Client: Nervous System**
- **Chapter 43, Nursing Care of the Client: Sensory System**
- **Chapter 45, Nursing Care of the Client: Mental Illness**
- **Chapter 55, Nursing Care of the Older Client**
- **Procedures:** B1, Handwashing; B16, Bedmaking: Unoccupied Bed; B17, Bedmaking: Occupied Bed; B18, Adult Bath; B19, Perineal Care; B21, Oral Hygiene; B22, Eye Care: Artificial Eye and Contact Lens Removal; B35, Application of Restraints; I27, Assisting a Client with Crutch Walking

LEARNING OBJECTIVES

Upon completion of this chapter, you should be able to:
- *Define key terms.*
- *Describe types of accidents that can occur in health care settings.*
- *Describe the importance of and procedure for correctly identifying clients.*
- *Identify safety factors to be considered before using equipment.*
- *Recount safety measures related to the use of protective restraints.*
- *Detail safety measures related to preventing fire when oxygen is in use.*
- *Discuss factors that influence a client's personal hygiene practices.*
- *Explain the role of assessment in maintaining a safe environment.*

KEY TERMS

body image
chemical restraints
client behavior accident
dental caries
equipment accident
gingivitis
halitosis
hygiene
perineal care

physical restraint
poison
pyorrhea
restraint
self-care deficit
sensory overload
stomatitis
therapeutic proce-
   dure accident

- *Describe the modifications that can be used to resolve environmental hazards in institutional and home settings.*
- *Cite nursing interventions that promote a client's personal hygiene.*

INTRODUCTION

Safe care is a basic need of all clients, regardless of setting. Nurses are responsible for providing the client with a safe environment through the delivery of professional, quality nursing care that incorporates safety precautions and hygiene assistance. This chapter describes the nurse's role in these areas.

SAFETY

Safety must be the number one priority in providing client care. The first step in maintaining safety is to raise nurses' awareness regarding risk factors. Prevention is the key to safety. Nurses must be aware of those factors that have the potential to endanger a client's safety. Constant attention to these factors enables the nurse to maintain a safe environment for the client.

A safety committee is required in all health care facilities, with the purpose of maintaining an overall safe facility for clients, employees, and visitors. The committee is composed of representatives from all departments of the facility. Responsibilities range from analyzing environmental safety in the facility to researching illness rates.

Safety is associated with health promotion and illness prevention. A safe environment reduces the risk of accidents and subsequent alterations in health and lifestyle; it also helps contain the cost of health care services (Figure 20-1). Many factors in the environment can threaten safety.

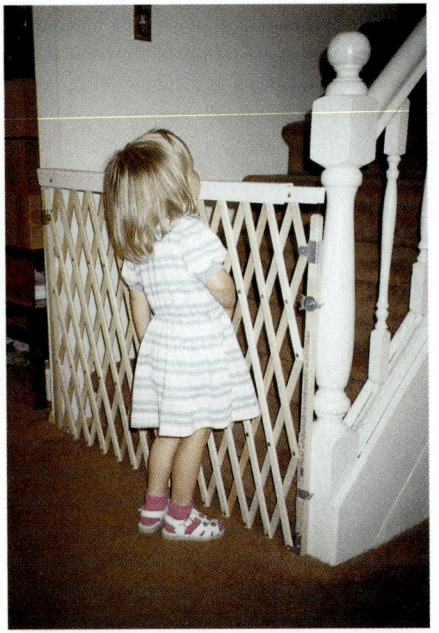
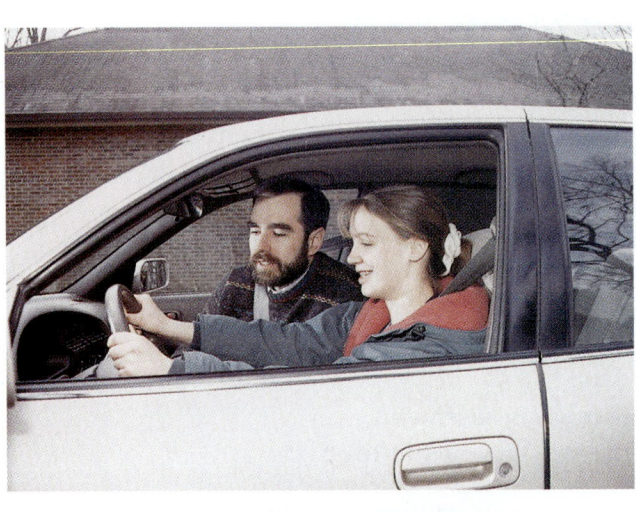
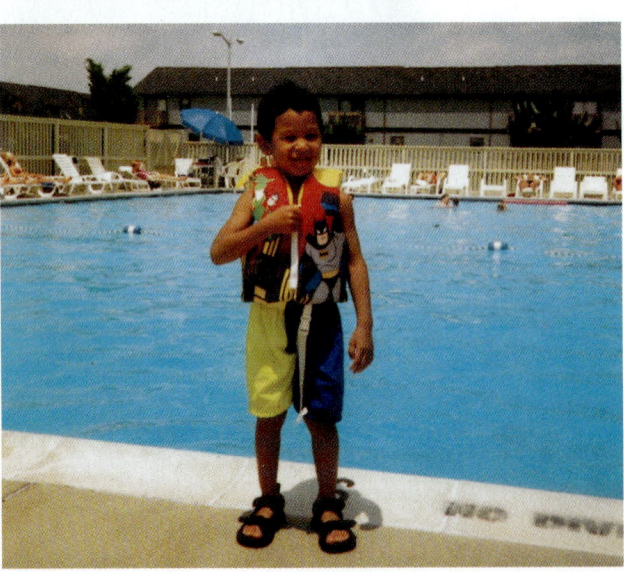
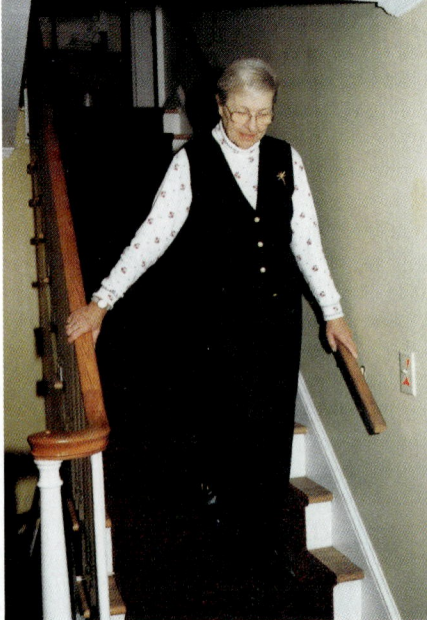

Figure 20-1 Use of stair gates, life vests, seat belts, and handrails minimizes safety risks.

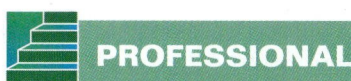

Workplace Safety

Employee Right-to-Know Laws

Under the authority of the Occupational Safety and Health Administration (OSHA) of the Department of Labor and Industry, several states have passed employee right-to-know laws, which state that employees are legally entitled to information regarding hazardous substances or harmful agents in the workplace. Such substances include skin and eye irritants, flammables, poisons, carcinogens, pathogens, and harmful rays (radiation).

Regulations Relating to Hazardous Materials

OSHA also outlines and enforces regulations that all health care facilities must follow with regard to employees' exposure to and handling of potentially infectious materials.

Material Safety Data Sheet

As part of conforming to OSHA regulations, all facilities must have a material safety data sheet (MSDS) for each hazardous substance. The MSDS describes the substance in question, including the associated dangers. Protective equipment, safe handling techniques, and first-aid information are also given. The MSDSs for toxic materials must be kept on site for no fewer than 30 years. All employees must know how to use the MSDS.

FACTORS AFFECTING SAFETY

Client safety and health are influenced by several factors including age, lifestyle, sensory and perceptual alterations, mobility, and emotional state.

Age

Risk for injury varies with chronological age and developmental stage. Health education about preventive measures can facilitate injury prevention among clients of various age groups.

As infants mature, their potential for injury increases. Infants, toddlers, and preschoolers are explorers of the environment. Most accidents involving those in these age groups can be prevented with careful adult supervision to reduce the risk of falls from bed; burns; electrical hazards; choking on small objects; suffocation; and drowning.

As school-age children explore the environment outside the home, their risk for injury increases. Preventive measures during this stage focus on stranger awareness; bicycle, skating, and swimming safety; traffic safety rules; protective equipment for sports; and avoidance of substance abuse.

Adolescents and young adults usually enjoy good physical health; however, their lifestyles put them at risk for injury. Because this age group spends much time away from home, collaborative educational efforts among parents, schools, and community health care providers must focus on environmental safety. High-risk factors for injury and death are automobile accidents, substance abuse, violence, unwanted pregnancies, and sexually transmitted diseases.

Adult risk for injury is generally related to lifestyle, work practices, and behaviors. Preventive measures for adults emphasize nutrition, exercise, and occupational safety. High-risk factors for those in this age group include fatigue, anxiety, sleep pattern disturbances, caregiver role strain, and altered health maintenance.

Because of poor vision and mobility; loss of muscle strength and flexibility; effects of medications and alcohol; chronic diseases such as osteoarthritis, Parkinson's disease, and Alzheimer's disease; and changes in the inner ear that upset the sense of balance, the older adult is prone to falls, especially in the bathroom, bedroom, and kitchen (Walker, 1998). Preventive measures for older adults emphasize slow position changes, good lighting, use of hand rails, application of skid-proof strips in the bathtub or shower, and removal of throw rugs and loose carpets.

Accidents in the Health Care Setting

In the health care setting, accidents are categorized by their causative agent: client behaviors, therapeutic procedures, or equipment:

- **Client behavior accidents** result from the client's behavior or actions. Examples include poisonings, burns, and self-inflicted cuts and bruises.
- **Therapeutic procedure accidents** result from the delivery of medical or nursing interventions. Examples include medication errors, client falls during transfers, contamination of sterile instruments or wounds, and improper performance of nursing activities.
- **Equipment accidents** result from the malfunction or improper use of medical equipment. Examples include electrocution and fire. National and institutional policies establish safety standards with regard to equipment. For example, a facility may attempt to maximize the risk of equipment accidents by requiring that the biomedical engineering department check the equipment inspection label prior to use.

All accidents and incident reports must be fully documented according to institutional protocol.

According to a study conducted by Alexander, Rivara, and Wolf (1992), approximately 30% of older adults fall each year, and 20% to 30% of those who fall suffer moderate to severe injuries that lead to loss of mobility and independence and to increased risk of death. Fall-related trauma among older adults in Washington State accounted for 5.3% of all hospitalizations, cost over $53 million, and required more nursing services after hospital discharge than did any other illness.

Lifestyle

Lifestyle practices, which reflect an individual's personal choices about those activities or habits to pursue, can increase a person's risk for injury and potential for disease. For instance, individuals who operate machinery; experience excessive stress, anxiety, and fatigue; use alcohol and drugs (prescription and nonprescription); and live in high-crime neighborhoods are at increased risk for injury and alterations to health. Risk-taking behaviors such as participating in daredevil activities, driving vehicles at high speeds, and not wearing seat belts are factors that pose a threat to an individual's safety and well-being. Unlike other factors such as age, however, lifestyle practices are modifiable.

Sensory and Perceptual Alterations

Sensory functions are essential for accurate perception of environmental safety. Clients who have visual, hearing, taste, smell, communication, or touch perception impairments are at increased risk for injury, as they are often not able to perceive a potential danger.

Mobility

The client whose mobility is impaired is at increased risk for injury, especially from falls. Mobility impairment may result from poor balance or coordination, muscle weakness, or paralysis. Immobility may also precipitate physiologic and emotional complications such as decubitus and depression.

Emotional State

Emotional states such as depression and anger affect a client's perception of environmental hazards and of the degree of risk associated with certain behaviors. These emotional states alter a client's thinking patterns and reaction time. Usual safety precautions may be forgotten during periods of emotional stress.

HYGIENE

Hygiene is the science of health. Care related to hygiene promotes cleanliness, provides for comfort and relaxation, improves self-image, and promotes healthy skin. Client hygiene is an extension of client safety in that proper hygiene protects the client's defense mechanisms against disease. The health of the body's first line of defense, the skin and mucous membranes, is promoted by proper hygiene. Nurses are responsible for ensuring that the client's needs with regard to hygiene are met. The type of care provided depends on the client's ability, needs, and practices.

Factors Influencing Hygiene Practice

Hygiene needs and practices are unique to each client; nurses should provide individualized care based on these needs and practices. Hygiene practices are influenced by several factors including body image, social and cultural practices, personal preferences, socioeconomic status, and knowledge.

Body Image

Body image is the individual's perception of physical self including appearance, function, and ability. Body image is associated with the client's emotions, mood, attitude, and values. A client's body image directly affects the type of personal hygiene practiced, which may change if the client's body image is altered because of illness or surgical procedures. At such times, the nurse should help the client maintain hygiene practices in accordance with the client's pre-illness level of hygiene and personal preferences.

Social and Cultural Practices

Social and cultural practices also directly influence hygiene practices. Clients are socialized to their hygiene practices by family practices in early childhood. As a person ages, hygiene practices are influenced by maturational development and socialization with people outside the family. For example, teenagers are usually concerned with peer acceptance and follow the latest trends in personal hygiene. In later adulthood, hygiene practices may be influenced by coworkers and social networks.

Cultural practices and beliefs are derived from family, religious, and personal values developed during maturation. Clients from diverse cultural backgrounds will have differing hygiene practices. Nurses should maintain a nonjudgmental attitude when assessing or providing hygiene care to clients from different social or cultural backgrounds.

Personal Preferences

Personal preferences influence the timing of bathing; those products that are used for bathing; and the type of bathing performed. For example, some male clients shave before bathing, whereas others prefer to do so after bathing. Some clients prefer to bathe in the morning to facilitate waking, whereas others prefer to bathe before bedtime to encourage relaxation and sleep. Un-

CULTURAL CONSIDERATIONS

Hygiene
- Some cultures do not permit women to submerge their bodies in water during the time of menstruation because of a fear that the woman may drown.
- In North America, people typically bathe daily and use numerous deodorant products.
- In Europe, many people do not bathe daily, nor do they use deodorant products. Europeans do not consider the smell of human perspiration as offensive as do North Americans.

less the client's health is adversely affected, the nurse should permit the client to practice usual routines and to use hygiene products preferred by the client. Individualized nursing care should incorporate the client's personal hygiene preferences.

Socioeconomic Status

A client's hygiene practices may also be influenced by socioeconomic status. Limited economic resources may affect the type, frequency, and extent of hygiene practiced. Assessment of socioeconomic status provides information about the availability of hygiene supplies. Some clients may not be able to afford deodorants, perfumes, soaps, shampoo, and toothpaste. The nurse can function as an advocate for the client by contacting social services, which can make referrals to community agencies that provide assistance to needy persons, for example, Catholic Charities or a local chapter of the American Association of Retired Persons (AARP).

Knowledge

Knowledge level influences the client's understanding of the relationship between hygiene and health. Thus, knowledge should influence a client's hygiene practices. In order for clients to perform basic hygiene, however, they must have more than such knowledge; they must also be motivated and believe that they are capable of self-care.

Frequently, an illness or surgical procedure results in a knowledge deficit about basic hygiene practices. In such situations, the client may not know the correct procedures or types of hygiene that can be performed. The nurse is responsible for providing the necessary education about hygiene during an illness. Sometimes, the nurse may have to perform all hygiene practices for a client during an illness until the client regains this ability and returns to the former level of independence.

NURSING PROCESS

The nursing process facilitates an understanding of the scope of challenges inherent in providing nursing care to clients at risk for injury or a self-care deficit.

Assessment

Assessment data direct the prioritization of the client's problems and accompanying nursing diagnoses. Clients at risk for injury require frequent reassessment of status, with appropriate changes being made in the plan of care and expected outcomes.

The health history and physical examination data are correlated with the laboratory indicators to identify those clients who are at risk for problems relating to safety, infection, or hygiene. Appropriate risk appraisals may be incorporated into the nursing health history interview.

Subjective Data

The nursing health history interview is the first step in assessment; wherein the client's subjective account of specific health data is elicited. It is important for the nurse to gather complete, pertinent, and relevant information at this point.

Health History Key elements of relevant data regarding the client at risk for injury and infection are obtained in the health history. The client is often asked to complete a health history questionnaire; depending on the client's status, however, the nurse may have to perform an interview to obtain these data. If the client is unable to provide the subjective data, the nurse must designate, either on the questionnaire or in the

PROFESSIONAL TIP

Key Interview Questions about Safety and Hygiene
- What things do you do to stay healthy?
- How do you typically spend a day (e.g., home or work)?
- Do you have any health care concerns?
- Do you need assistance with bathing and dressing?
- Do you regularly visit the dentist and eye doctor?
- Do you use dental floss on a regular basis?
- Do you wash your hands before preparing food?
- Do you keep meats and dairy products refrigerated until ready to use?
- Is there a smoke detector or fire extinguisher in your home?
- Are emergency phone numbers readily available?

nursing progress notes, the person who provided the information.

During the nursing health history interview, the client's general health perception and management status should be assessed to ascertain how the client manages self-care. This information will provide data regarding the client's routine self-care and health-promotion needs.

Objective Data

Objective data are gathered through the physical examination and the diagnostic and laboratory findings.

Physical Examination A complete health assessment includes a systematic physical examination, generally conducted from head to toes, in order to obtain objective data relative to the client's health status and presenting problems. When assessing the client to ascertain the level of risk for injury and hygiene deficits, the nurse should focus the physical examination on the following areas and signs:

- Level of consciousness: The Glasgow Coma Scale (GCS) is an objective measurement tool.
- Range of motion: Immobilization of an extremity and/or limited mobility are risk factors for development of joint contractures, skin breakdown, and muscle atrophy.
- Secretions or exudate of the skin or mucous membranes.
- Condition of the skin: Skin condition provides data concerning a client's nutritional and hydration status, continuity of intact skin, hygiene practices, and overall physical abilities.

Risk Factors A comprehensive nursing assessment involves using specifically developed risk assessment tools and appraising the client's environment to detect potential hazards. The client's self-care abilities, used for determining the level of assistance needed in providing hygiene care, are appraised during the health history. The analysis of relevant risk factors alerts the nurse to actual or possible risks. For instance, the risk of impaired skin integrity increases when a person is placed on bed rest. A skin integrity risk appraisal (Table 20-1) should be completed to assist with planning care.

Client in an Inpatient Setting Inpatient clients should be assessed for fall and infection risk factors. The hospitalized or institutionalized client's risk of falling is identified after compiling specific assessment data that are correlated with contributing factors as shown in Table 20-2. Each of these indicators carries a specific weight to determine the client's risk. For example, age over 65 years carries a weight of 3, and diuretic administration carries a weight of 7. The total risk factor for a 65-year-old client receiving a diuretic would thus be 10, placing the client at high risk for falls and requiring the implementation of special fall measures.

The inpatient client should be assessed for falls every shift or as designated by institutional policy. To minimize the chance of falls, the nurse must ensure that the client's environment is safe by keeping the bed in a low position, the side rails up, the nurse call light and personal belongings within easy reach, and

Table 20-1 SKIN INTEGRITY RISK APPRAISAL

AREA OF ASSESSMENT	SCORE
General Physical Condition (Health Problem)	
Good (minor)	0
Fair (major but stable)	1
Poor (chronic/serious, not stable)	2
Mental State/Level of Consciousness (to Commands)	
Alert (responds readily)	0
Lethargic (slow to respond)	1
Semicomatose (responds only to verbal or painful stimuli)	2
Comatose (no response to stimuli)	3
Activity	
Ambulates without assistance/infant	0
Ambulates with assistance	2
Chairfast/out of bed to chair	4
Bedfast/confined to bed	6
Mobility (Extremities)	
Full active range	0
Restricted movement (slightly limited)	2
Moves only with assistance	4
Immobile	6
Incontinence (Bowel and/or Bladder)	
None	0
Occasional (less than twice in 24 hours)	2
Usually (greater than twice in 24 hours)	4
Total (no control)	6
Nutrition (for Age and Size)	
Good (eats/drinks adequately)	0
Fair (eats/drinks inadequately)	1
Poor (unable/refuses to eat/drink)	2
Totally depleted	3

Assess the client's risk status for each indicator on the skin integrity risk appraisal form, then total the numbers from all six indicators. The risk rating is as follows:

   0 to 8: low risk

   9 to 16: moderate risk

   17 to 27: high risk

A rating greater than 8 usually requires implementation of special measures; for example, a protocol to prevent skin breakdown.

Patient Care Admission Sheet courtesy of Tulane University Hospital and Clinic, New Orleans, LA.

Table 20-2 FALL RISK APPRAISAL

AREA OF ASSESSMENT	SCORE
General Factors	1
Restraint (posey, arm, leg)	
Orthostatic changes	
History of falls/crawling out of bed/ syncope (brief loss of consciousness)	
Seizure disorder	
Elimination Function	2
Decreased bladder/bowel tone	
Urgency/frequency	
Incontinence	
Nocturia (excessive urination at night)	
Age	3
Over 65	
Level of Consciousness/Mental Status	4
Lethargy (slow to respond)	
Inability or refusal to follow directions	
Inability or refusal to call for help	
Impaired judgment, memory, awareness	
Confusion, disorientation	
Sensory Deficits	5
Diminished visual acuity, blind, blurred vision	
Slow reaction time	
Mobility/Physical Limitations	6
Decreased mobility in lower extremities	
Ability to rise with assistance	
Amputation/joint difficulties	
Weakness, dizziness, fatigability, vertigo (dizziness), syncope	
Cast, splint	
Use of crutches, cane, walker	
Hemiparesis (one-sided paralysis), paraparesis (loss of function), hemiplegia, paraplegia (loss of function in lower limbs)	
Ataxia (unsteady gait)	
Improperly fitting/smooth soled/no footwear	
Unsteady gait, decreased balance, imbalance	
Medications	7
Sedatives/hypnotics/tranquilizers	
Diuretics/antihypertensives/laxatives	
Narcotics/analgesics/anesthetics	
Antihistamines	
Antiseizures	
Barbiturates/phenothiazines	
Eye drops	
Antipsychotics/antidepressants	

Patient Care Admission Sheet courtesy of Tulane University Hospital and Clinic, New Orleans, LA

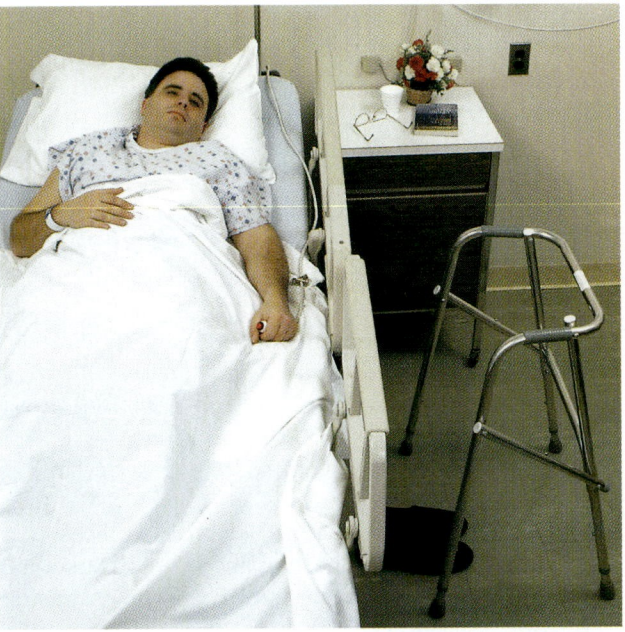

Figure 20-2 This client's risk of falls has been assessed and responded to through the measures shown here.

assistive devices (e.g., a walker) nearby, as shown in Figure 20-2.

Client in the Home An injury risk appraisal provides the nurse with assessment data to determine the client's level of safety knowledge. Injuries in the home primarily result from falls, fires, poisonings, suffocation, and malfunctioning household equipment (Stanhope & Knollnueller, 1996). Home health nurses may use a safety risk appraisal.

The safety risk data assessed in the home environment direct the nurse in planning for the client's and caregiver's education. The home health nurse must prioritize these data when planning the client's care. Assessment, teaching, and outcome evaluation of all safety hazards can take several home visits.

Diagnostic and Laboratory Data Appraising the client's risk for injury also involves evaluating laboratory findings related to an abnormal blood profile (e.g., altered clotting factors, anemic conditions, or leukocytosis). Malnourished clients are at risk for injury.

Nursing Diagnosis

After data collection and analysis, the nurse is able to formulate a nursing diagnosis. The main nursing diagnoses that relate to safety and hygiene deficits are *Injury, Risk for,* and *Self-Care Deficits.*

Injury, Risk for

The primary nursing diagnosis *Injury, Risk for* exists when the client is at risk for injury as a result of environmental conditions interacting with the individual's

HOME HEALTH CARE

Home Safety Risk Appraisal

Infants

- Crib side rails stay in the up position while the infant is in the crib.
- Infants are not left unattended, especially on elevated surfaces or in the bath.
- Bath water temperature is 37.8° to 40.6°C (100° to 105°F). Check temperature for comfort with wrist.
- Environment is kept warm and draft free at bath time.
- Bottles are washed with soap and hot water, and formula is refrigerated.
- Toys are soft and have no detachable pieces.
- Car seat has a restraint strap and is used consistently.
- Stroller and carry seat are sturdy and have a restraint strap.
- Fire, police, and poison control numbers are posted by telephones.
- Caregivers know infant cardiopulmonary resuscitation (CPR).

Toddlers/Preschoolers

- Sharp objects are placed out of reach and out of sight.
- Poisons are labeled and placed in a locked cabinet.
- Medications and other toxins have childproof lids and are stored in a locked cabinet.
- Small, hard food objects (peanuts, candy) are kept in locked cabinets.
- Stairs and floor furnaces have gates or barriers.
- Doors and windows have safety locks.
- Electrical outlets are covered.
- Burners on the stove are not left on and unattended.
- Pots with hot liquids are placed on back burners, handles facing toward the back wall.
- Home and yard are free of poisonous plants.
- Play equipment is kept in proper functioning condition; toys have no small parts; crayons are nontoxic.
- Outdoor play is supervised in a fenced area with locks on gates.
- Car seat or seat belt is used consistently.
- Children are supervised when crossing the street.
- Caregivers know child CPR and Heimlich maneuver.

School-Age Children

- Play and sports are supervised.
- Play equipment is kept in proper functioning condition and free of hazards.

- Outdoor play is limited to soft surfaces.
- Bicycle helmet is worn consistently.
- Children are taught not to open the door or speak to strangers while at play.
- Firearms are kept unloaded and in locked cabinets.
- Seat belt is worn at all times.
- Caregivers know child CPR and the Heimlich maneuver.

Adolescents

- Firearm safety is taught.
- Seat belt is worn at all times.
- Teenagers take drivers' education and are cautioned about drinking and driving.
- Caregivers know adult CPR and the Heimlich maneuver.

Adults

- Firearms have safety latches.
- Smoke detectors and fire extinguishers are installed in the home.
- A nondrinking designated driver is chosen.
- Emergency phone numbers are readily available.
- Caregiver knows adult CPR and Heimlich maneuver.

Older Adults

- Stairs have adequate lighting and nonskid surfaces, and rails are in good condition.
- Throw rugs are not present.
- Hallways are uncluttered.
- Carpets are free from frayed ends/pieces.
- Phone cords and other cords are behind furniture.
- Bathtub has rails and a nonslip surface.
- Shower stall has a seat.
- Bathroom is free of drafts.
- Shoes fit properly and have nonskid soles.
- Home is adequately ventilated and heated.
- Home is free of space heaters.
- Pilot lights on gas appliances are functional.
- Electrical appliances are in good working condition.
- Food is properly refrigerated.
- Medications are kept in properly labeled containers with readable print.
- Emergency phone numbers are readily available.
- Fire and police departments are aware that older adult is home alone.
- Caregiver knows adult CPR and Heimlich maneuver.

(From Fundamentals of Nursing: Standards & Practice, *by S. DeLaune and P. Ladner, 1998, Albany, N.Y.: Delmar Publishers.)*

adaptive and defensive resources (North American Nursing Diagnosis Association [NANDA], 1999). Although this diagnostic label does not have defining characteristics as set forth by NANDA, it is categorized as having either internal or external potential hazards. An internal biochemical risk factor for a client with impaired vision would be stated as *Injury, Risk for, related to the risk factor of sensory dysfunction (visual)*. In contrast, medications on a nightstand in a home with a toddler present should be identified by a home health nurse as creating an external chemical risk factor for the toddler; the related nursing diagnosis would be stated as *Injury, Risk for, related to the risk factor of medications in the environment*.

Seven subcategories of specific risk factors for this diagnostic labeling are defined by NANDA (1999):

Aspiration, Risk for: risk for entry of gastrointestinal secretions, oropharyngeal secretions, or solids or fluids into the tracheobronchial passages

Disuse Syndrome, Risk for: risk for deterioration of body or body systems as the result of prescribed or unavoidable musculoskeletal inactivity

Poisoning, Risk for: accentuated risk of accidental exposure to or ingestion of drugs or dangerous products in doses sufficient to cause poisoning

Suffocation, Risk for: accentuated risk of accidental suffocation

Trauma, Risk for: accentuated risk of accidental tissue injury (e.g., wound, burn, fracture)

Latex Allergy Response: allergic response to natural latex rubber products

Latex Allergy Response, Risk for: at risk for allergic response to natural latex rubber products

These seven subcategories of nursing diagnoses provide the nurse with the opportunity to relate specific nursing interventions to the diagnosed problem. For example, the specific nursing diagnosis for the situation of the toddler encountering medications on the nightstand in the home would be *Poisoning, Risk for, related to the risk factor of medications accessible to children*. The level of risk would be considered higher if the medications on the client's nightstand were in open containers or if the closed containers did not have childproof caps. This subcategory diagnosis provides for specific nursing interventions directed toward the level of risk for the toddler and toward the need for client teaching.

Self-Care Deficits

A **self-care deficit** exists when an individual is not able to perform one or more activities of daily living (ADL). Three self-care deficits related to hygiene practices are identified by NANDA (1999). These diagnostic labels, together with their defining characteristics and related factors, are presented in Table 20-3.

Table 20-3 SELF-CARE DEFICITS

NURSING DIAGNOSIS AND DEFINITION	DEFINING CHARACTERISTICS	RELATED FACTORS
Self-Care Deficit (Bathing/Hygiene): Impaired ability to perform or complete bathing/hygiene activities for oneself	Inability to get bath supplies; inability to wash body or body parts; inability to obtain or get to water source; inability to regulate the temperature or flow of bath water; inability to get in and out of bathroom; inability to dry body	Decreased or lack of motivation; weakness and tiredness; severe anxiety; inadequate to perceive body part or spatial relationship; perceptual or cognitive impairment; pain; neuromuscular impairment; musculoskeletal impairment; environmental barriers
Self-Care Deficit (Dressing/Grooming): Impaired ability to perform or complete dressing and grooming activities for oneself	Inability to choose clothing; inability to use assistive devices; inability to use zippers; inability to remove clothes; inability to put on socks; inability to put clothing on upper body; impaired ability to put on or take off necessary items of clothing; impaired ability to obtain or replace articles of clothing; impaired ability to fasten clothing; inability to maintain appearance at a satisfactory level; inability to put clothing on lower body; inability to pick up clothing; inability to put on shoes	Decreased or lack of motivation; intolerance to pain; severe anxiety; perceptual or cognitive impairment; neuromuscular impairment; musculoskeletal impairment; discomfort; environmental barriers; weakness or tiredness
Self-Care Deficit (Toileting): Impaired ability to perform or complete own toileting activities	Inability to manipulate clothing; unable to carry out proper toilet hygiene; unable to sit on or rise from toilet or commode; unable to get to toilet or commode; unable to flush toilet or commode	Environmental barriers; weakness or tiredness; decreased or lack of motivation; severe anxiety; impaired mobility status; impaired transfer ability; musculoskeletal impairment; neuromuscular impairment; pain; perceptual or cognitive impairment

From Nursing diagnoses: Definitions and classification 1999–2000, *by North American Nursing Diagnosis Association, 1999, Philadelphia: Author.*

Other Nursing Diagnoses

The client who is at risk for injury or has a self-care deficit may have other associated physiologic or psychological problems. The nursing diagnoses that often accompany diagnostic labels for risk for injury or self-care deficits are as follows:

Nutrition, Altered (specify less than body requirements or more than body requirements)

Protection, Altered

Tissue Integrity, Impaired

Skin Integrity, Impaired

Social Isolation

Loneliness, Risk for

Coping, Individual, Ineffective

Mobility, Impaired (specify bed, physical, or wheelchair)

Hopelessness

Powerlessness

Knowledge Deficit (specify)

Pain

Anxiety

Fear

Though not all-inclusive, this list gives an indication of the number of related problems that must be considered when planning care for clients identified as having safety or self-care deficits.

Planning/Outcome Identification

The primary nursing goal is to provide safe care through the identification of actual or potential hazards and the implementation of safety measures. The assessment data are reviewed with the client, and the nurse records the areas where the client indicates a need for change and health teaching, for example, age-related exercise or maintaining a safe environment. These findings are incorporated into the plan of care, reflecting the individualized needs of each client.

During the planning phase, the nurse collaborates with the client and other health care providers to determine the goals, outcomes, and interventions. Identified outcomes provide direction for the nursing care that is implemented to reduce the risk of injury.

Another critical element of the care plan is client/caregiver education related to the identification of potential hazards and health-promotion practices. The nursing care plan should include safety measures to educate the client about preventive actions and modification of an unsafe environment, for example, proper use of a call light or potential hazards related to the side effects of medications.

Table 20-4 outlines the basic components of care planning and outcome measurement for the client who is at risk for injury or has a self-care deficit. Nursing actions are discussed in detail in the following section.

Implementation

Implementation involves continual assessment of client health risks and prioritization of nursing interventions aimed at risk reduction, such as:

- Administration of prescribed medications,
- Provision of balanced nutritional intake,
- Promotion of adequate rest and exercise, and
- Teaching client about health hazards.

Implementation of safety measures may require an alteration in the physical environment as directed by the fall prevention protocol (Table 20-5).

Identify Client

In order to provide safe care, it is essential that nurses correctly match clients with the activity, medication, diet, or treatment ordered for them. The client's well-being can be placed in jeopardy by administration of incorrect care.

The identification (ID) band or bracelet is the primary means of correctly identifying a client. It lists the client's name, room number, bed number, hospital number, and doctor and may include other information such as age, sex, and religion.

This band is placed on the client's wrist upon admission to the hospital. Each time care is given, the band must be checked against the assignment sheet, order sheet, diet card, and medication and treatment sheet or card (Figure 20-3). The client's identity should always be further verified by one other method such as asking the client's name, asking the client to state his name, or obtaining a positive identification from another person. None of these methods is safe when used alone, but when used in conjunction with the ID band, any can help the nurse verify identity.

If a client is discovered without an ID band, care should be withheld until positive identification can be

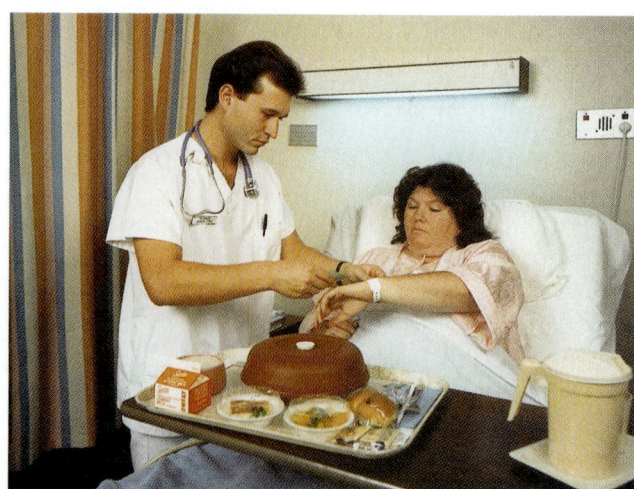

Figure 20-3 Checking the client's ID band ensures that the correct person receives care.

Table 20-4 PLANNING THE CARE OF THE CLIENT WHO IS AT RISK FOR INJURY AND/OR WHO HAS A SELF-CARE DEFICIT

NURSING DIAGNOSIS	GOALS	EXPECTED OUTCOMES	NURSING INTERVENTIONS
Injury, Risk for	The client will identify factors that increase the potential for injury.	The client will identify internal and external factors that increase the risk for injury.	Risk identification: analysis of potential risk factors, determination of of health risks, and prioritization of risk reduction strategies for an individual
	The client will remain free of bodily injury.	The client will identify and implement safety measures to decrease the risk for injury.	Fall prevention: instituting special precautions with the client at risk for injury
Self-Care Deficit Bathing/Hygiene and Dressing/ Grooming	The client will maintain an optimum functional level of hygiene practices in a safe and effective manner.	The client will participate physically and/or verbally in bathing, dressing, and toileting activities.	Bathing: cleaning of the body for the purpose of relaxation, cleanliness, and healing
			Perineal care: maintenance of perineal skin integrity and relief from perineal discomfort.
			Dressing: choosing, putting on, and removing clothes for a person who cannot do same for self.
	The client's skin will remain clean and intact.	The client's skin will remain free of drainage and secretions; intact; and free of redness.	Skin surveillance: collection and analysis of client data to maintain skin and mucous membrane integrity.
Knowledge Deficit related to health hazards	The client will not sustain injuries.	The client will verbalize both feedback of instructions and a willingness to comply.	Teaching, individual: Planning, implementation, and evaluation of a teaching program designed to address a client's particular needs.

Compiled from Nursing Interventions Classification (NIC) (2nd ed.), by J. C. McCloskey and G. M. Bulecheck (Eds.), 1996, St. Louis, MO: Mosby Yearbook and from Handbook of Nursing Diagnosis (7th ed.), by L. Carpenito, 1997, Philadelphia: Lippincott.

made. A new ID band should be placed on the client's wrist as soon as identity is verified.

Most nursing home residents also wear ID bands. Some, however, do not, and other methods of identification, such as photographs, are used. Nurses working in such long-term care facilities must learn to safely use the identification system. Whatever the system, client identification is essential before rendering any care.

Raise Safety Awareness and Knowledge

Nurses in all settings must demonstrate an awareness of safety hazards and must teach clients accordingly. Clients must be made aware of safety precautions in order to prevent injuries. Clients may also need specific safety information regarding the use of oxygen, intravenous equipment, heating devices, and automatic bed controls.

A 1995 Food and Drug Administration (FDA) safety alert addressed entrapment hazards with regard to side rails on hospital beds. The FDA received 102 reports of head and body entrapment incidents that resulted in 68 deaths, 22 injuries, and 12 entrapments without injury (FDA, 1995). These incidents occurred in hospitals, long-term care facilities, and private homes. All reported entrapments occurred in one of the four ways illustrated in Figure 20-4.

Prevent Falls

Most falls occur among clients who are weak, fatigued, uncoordinated, paralyzed, confused, or disoriented. The data obtained from the fall risk appraisal will identify those clients who require special nursing measures to prevent falls. The risk for falls can be reduced by the following:

- Proper supervision
- Orienting the client to the environment and the call system
- Providing ambulatory aids (e.g., a wheelchair or walker)
- Placing personal belongings and the call light within easy reach
- Keeping hospital beds in the lowest position and the side rails up
- Using nonslip mats and rugs
- Illuminating the environment

Specific nursing interventions aimed at preventing falls include wiping up spills; encouraging use of side rails; applying restraints; encouraging use of assistive devices for walking; using proper body mechanics; ensuring adequate lighting; and removing obstacles. These are discussed following.

Table 20-5 ADULT FALL PREVENTION PROTOCOL

Purpose

To direct the nursing management of the client at risk for falls

Supportive Data

Falls account for nearly 90% of injuries reported in hospitalized clients (Whedon & Shedol, 1989). Risk factors for falls include advanced age, dizziness, confusion, use of medications, and physical or mental alterations. Fall prevention is used to increase staff awareness of clients at risk for falls and to provide preventive safety measures.

Content

Assessment

1. Perform client injury risk appraisal and identify fall risks. Update (on nursing care plan) status of fall risks daily or as needed.
2. Assess effects of administered medications that increase the risk of falls.
3. Implement institution's fall prevention program.

Report to Physician

4. Notify physician of previous fall history and identify risk factors for falls.
5. Notify physician of adverse effects of medications that may increase the client's risk of falling.

Client Teaching

6. Orient client to surroundings on admission and as necessary.
7. Instruct client and significant others on safety measures.
8. Instruct client and significant others on correct use of hospital equipment.
9. Instruct client at risk for falls to call for assistance when ambulating or performing ADL.

Environmental Interventions

10. Keep bed in lowest position, brakes locked, and side rails up.
11. Keep call light and frequently used objects within easy reach at the bedside.
12. Keep environment clean and clutter free.
13. Provide adequate lighting at all times.
14. Lock wheels on wheelchair, bed, and stretcher at all times.
15. Provide nonslip footwear, mats, and rugs.
16. Keep hospital furniture in the same place throughout hospital stay.
17. Provide call cord in bathroom.
18. Encourage use of handrails in bathroom and hallways.
19. Provide nonslip mats in the tub or shower.
20. Place high-risk clients in a room near the nurse's station.

Direct Nursing Care

21. Respond promptly to call lights and verbal requests for assistance.
22. Provide assistance with ADL.
23. Maintain close supervision by performing hourly safety assessments.
24. Encourage significant others to stay with high-risk clients.
25. Provide proper equipment for ambulation and elimination needs.
26. Communicate client's injury risk status in shift report.
27. Provide protective devices, such as restraints, for client safety (physician's order necessary).

Evaluation

28. Evaluate client's knowledge of safety measures.
29. Evaluate effectiveness of environmental interventions.
30. Evaluate changes in client's injury risk status.
31. Evaluate effectiveness of direct nursing care.

Documentation

32. Document the following in the client's medical record:
a. Assessment of client's injury risk status
b. Nursing care plan
c. Safety measures implemented
d. Client education performed
e. Client outcomes

From "Prediction and Prevention of Patient Falls," by M. B. Whedon and P. Shedol, 1989, Image: Journal of Nursing Scholarship, *21(2), 108–114.*

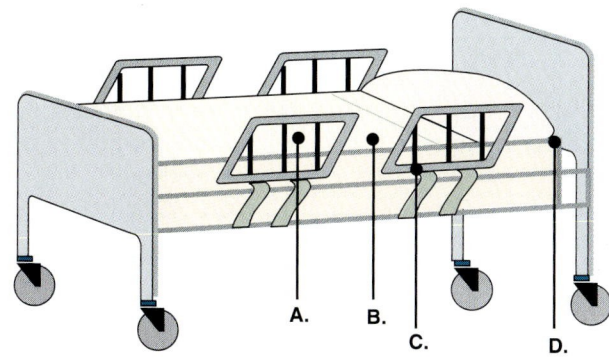

Figure 20-4 Entrapment Hazards Associated with Hospital Bed Side Rails: A. between the bars of a side rail; B. between two side rails; C. between the side rail and mattress; D. between the headboard or footboard, side rail, and mattress (*Source: Food and Drug Administration*, Safety Alert, *August 23, 1995*)

Wipe Up Spills Floors must be kept clean and free of spills. Although the housekeeping department usually does the actual washing of floors, it is the nurse's responsibility to either wipe up a spill at the time it occurs or to mark the area as a safety hazard and notify the appropriate person for immediate cleanup (Figure 20-5). Something wet or sticky on the floor can easily cause a weak, unsteady client to slip or trip.

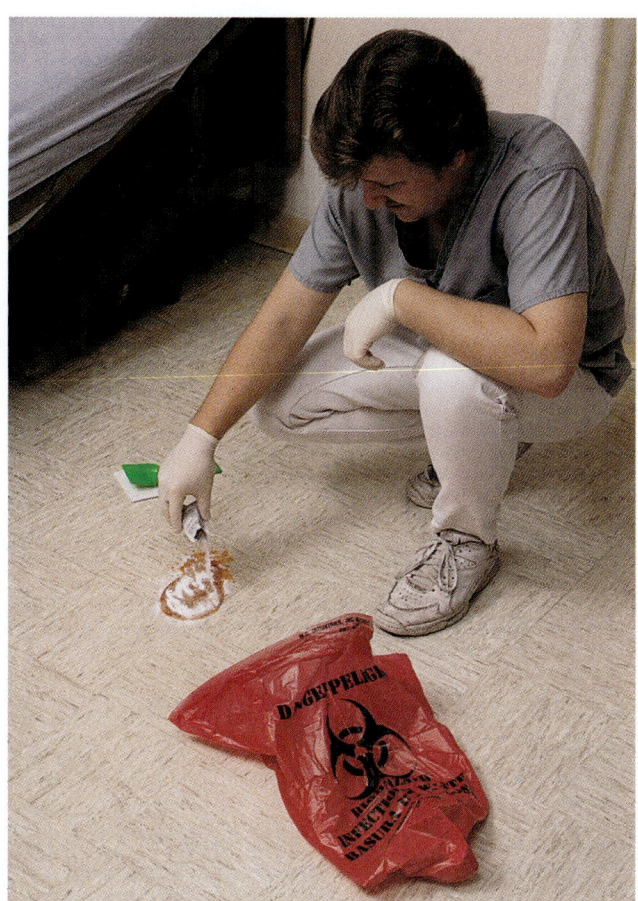

Figure 20-5 Wiping up spills is an important safety measure.

Even those unimpaired by illness, such as visitors and hospital personnel, are at risk.

Encourage the Use of Side Rails Falls from bed are the most common type of accident in hospitals (Easterling, 1990). The reasons are many and varied. Weakness due to illness is a major contributor to such accidents. Confusion and disorientation due to a strange environment, medication, anesthesia, or as a symptom of the client's condition increase the risk of falls.

Side rails are placed on the sides of hospital beds and stretchers to prevent falls. They can be raised and lowered and locked into place. Generally, side rails should be used most of the time (Figure 20-6). For those clients at risk for falls, the side rails should be used all the time.

Many clients resist the use of side rails because of an associated loss of self-esteem: They do not wish to be "treated like children" or to feel dependent. Thorough explanations from the nurse regarding the need for and purpose of side rails, coupled with a positive and respectful attitude will help neutralize resistance. Some facilities allow clients and/or families to sign a release form in the event that side rails are refused. Others may require that a family member or "sitter" provided by the family stay with the client at all times that side rails are not used.

The use of side rails should not give nurses a false sense of security. Beds must still be placed in the lowest position to reduce the height of a fall, should one occur, and clients at risk for falls should still be closely monitored.

Apply Restraints **Restraints** are protective devices used to limit the physical activity of a client or to immobilize a client or extremity. Restraints are used to protect the client from falls, protect a body part, keep the client from interfering with therapies (e.g., pulling out tubes, disconnecting intravenous setups, or removing wound coverings), and reduce the risk of injury to others. Restraints should *never* be used as a substitute

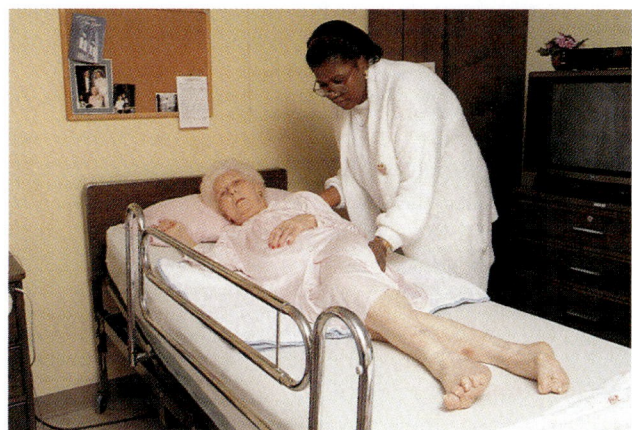

Figure 20-6 The use of side rails can contribute to a safe and secure environment.

PROFESSIONAL TIP

Key Elements of Restraint Documentation
- Reason for the restraint
- Method of restraint
- Explanation given to client and family
- Date and time of and client's response to application
- Duration
- Frequency of observation and client's response
- Safety (release from the restraint along with periodic, routine exercise and assessment for circulation and skin integrity)
- Assessment of the continued need for the restraint
- Client outcome

for close observation and supervision by nursing personnel.

The use of restraints has become very controversial because of client injuries related to these devices. In response, the Omnibus Budget Reconciliation Act (OBRA) of 1987 defines clients' rights and choices and states the following as acceptable reasons for the use of physical restraints:

- Restraints are part of the medical treatment.
- All other interventions have been tried first.
- Other disciplines have been consulted for assistance with the problem.
- Supporting documentation has been provided (Sullivan-Marx, 1994).

The Joint Commission on Accreditation of Healthcare Organizations (JCAHO) has also updated its guidelines on physical restraints. Citing studies, JCAHO stated that the use of restraints may violate clients' rights and cause "physical and psychological harm, loss of dignity . . . and even death" (JCAHO, 1998). Nurses must know the risks they face when physical restraints are or are not used (Richman, 1998).

Once restrained, clients are rendered less able to care for their own basic needs; thus, the nurse's responsibility in meeting these needs increases. Facility policy regarding the use of restraints, the care of the client in restraints, and the method of documentation must be followed precisely.

Restraints used either to limit physical activity or to immobilize a client can be physical or chemical. **Physical restraints** reduce the client's movement through the application of a device. Most states require a physician's order for the application of physical restraints. **Chemical restraints** are medications used to control the client's behavior. Commonly used chemical restraints are anxiolytics and sedatives. Discussion following is limited to the common types of physical restraints (Figure 20-7):

- Jacket (body restraint): a sleeveless vest with straps that cross in front of the client and are tied to the bed frame or around a chair or wheelchair.
- Belt: straps or belts applied across the client to secure to a wheelchair, stretcher, or bed.
- Mitten or hand: enclosed cloth material applied over the client's hand to prevent injury from scratching.
- Limb or extremity: cloth devices that immobilize one or all limbs by securely tying the restraint to the bed frame or chair.
- Elbow: a combination of fabric and plastic or wooden tongue blades that immobilize the elbow to prevent flexion.
- Mummy: a blanket or sheet that is folded around the child to limit movement and is used when performing procedures on children.

The nursing plan of care should include safety measures to reduce the potential for injury from restraints. Additional safety measures to observe when using restraint devices are as follows:

- Restraints should neither interfere with any treatment (e.g., intravenous therapy) nor aggravate the client's health problem.
- There should be enough slack in the straps to allow the client to move both arms and legs and perform range-of-motion exercises.
- At least once every 2 hours, the nurse must perform circulation and neurological examinations, assessing the color, sensation, temperature, motion, and capillary refill in the area distal to the restraint.
- The client and significant others should be provided psychological support, as needed (Easterling, 1990; Stillwell, 1991).

 Safety: Restraints
- Jacket or belt restraints should not restrict respiratory effort. Placing a restraint too tightly on the diaphragm will inhibit the expansion of the lungs.

- To avoid accidental injury to the extremity in the event that the side rail is released, the restraint strap should be secured to the bed frame, *not* to the side rail.

Encourage the Use of Assistive Devices for Walking
Devices used to assist walking include canes, crutches, walkers, and wheelchairs.

Canes Canes are curved walking devices that provide support to one side of the body that is weak. Three common types of canes are the single stick, the tripod (three footed), and the quad (four footed). All types should have a sturdy grip and rubber tips. The tips should be checked frequently for signs of wear.

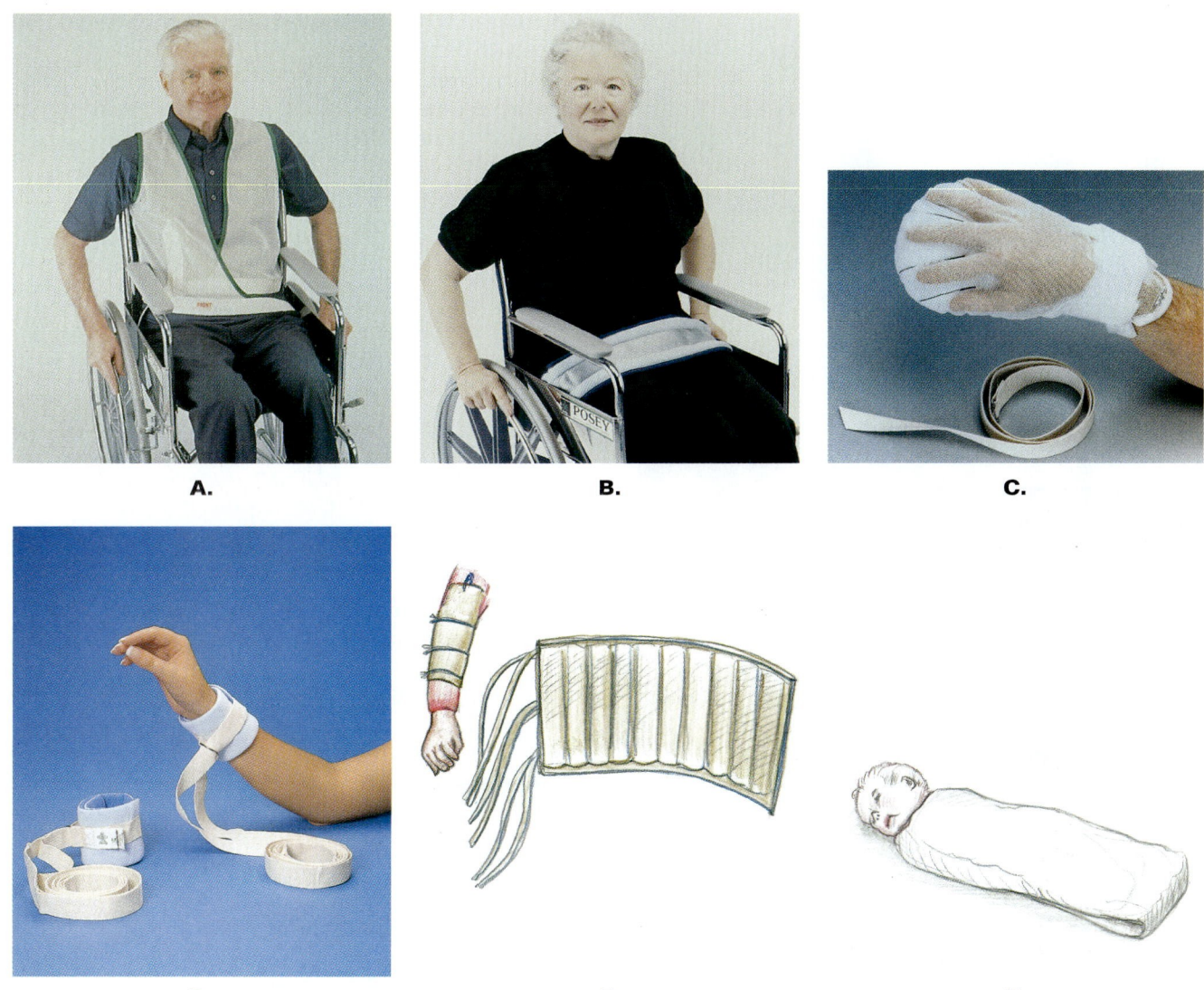

Figure 20-7 Types of Restraints: A. Jacket or vest restraint; B. Belt restraint for chair; C. Mitten, or hand, restraint; D. Limb, or extremity, restraint; E. Elbow restraint; F. Mummy restraint. (*Parts A and B courtesy of J.T. Posey Co., Inc.*)

Canes should be held on the strong side of the body (Figure 20-8). The affected side and the cane should move simultaneously while the weight is supported on the strong side. The strong side is moved while the weight is supported on the cane and the weaker side.

Crutches Crutches are wooden or metal staffs used either temporarily or permanently to increase mobility. There are two types of crutches: the axillary crutch and the Lofstrand, or forearm, crutch. The axillary crutch, the type most commonly used, fits under the axilla, with the weight being placed on the handgrips. The Lofstrand crutch has a handgrip and a metal cuff that fits around the arm. This type of crutch is more convenient but not as stable as the axillary crutch.

To prevent slipping, crutches have rubber tips, which must be kept dry. The tips should also be inspected regularly. If tips become loose or worn, they must be replaced immediately. The structure of the

crutch must also be inspected regularly. The person's weight will not be properly dispersed if there are cracks or bends in the crutch.

Walkers A walker is a waist-high metal tubular device with a handgrip and four legs. Some walkers have wheels on the front two legs, whereas other walkers have rubber tips on all four legs. Walkers give a sense of security and extra support, as well as independence, to clients. The client first moves the walker forward and then takes a step while balancing the weight on the walker.

Wheelchair A wheelchair is a means of ambulation for clients who are unable to support their weight while standing. The nurse should instruct the client in the safe use of a wheelchair by reminding the client to keep the wheelchair locked when not moving and to lift the footrests out of the way when getting in or out of the wheelchair. The wheelchair should be pushed

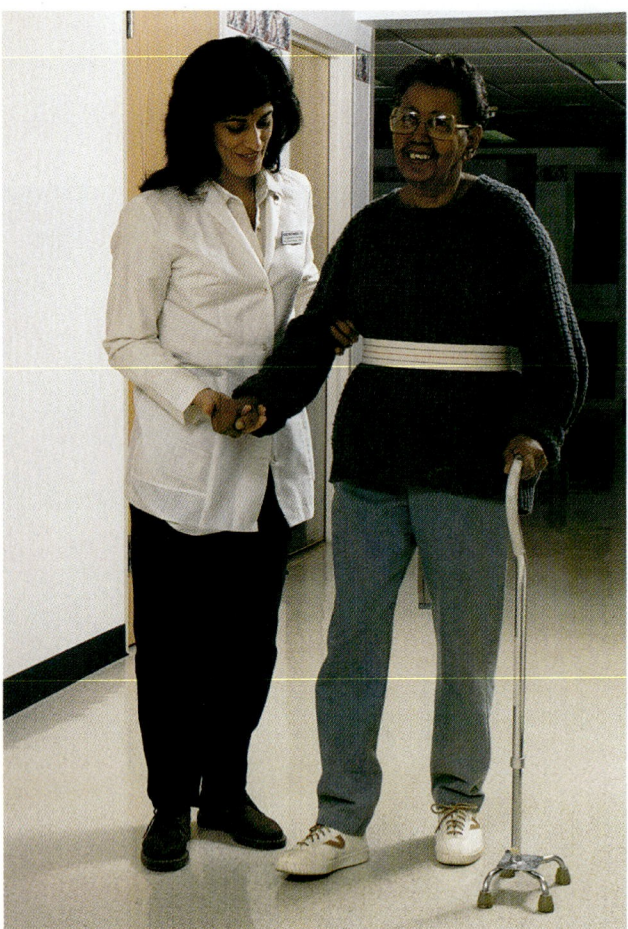

Figure 20-8 A nurse ensures the safety of a client using a quad cane.

slowly from behind and should be backed into doorways and into and out of elevators.

Use Proper Body Mechanics The human body is able to move in many different ways, some more efficient than others. The most effective, safest way of lifting and moving things is through using the principles of body mechanics; including center of gravity, base of support, and body alignment.

Center of Gravity The center of gravity is located in the center of the body, in the pelvic area. Body weight is approximately equal above and below this area. All movement should pivot around this central point. This keeps the weight over the base of support, making it easier to stay balanced. Keeping the back straight and bending at the knees and hips helps to maintain the center of gravity in the pelvic area. If the center of gravity shifts, the body tends to fall.

Base of Support Feet are the base of support. The feet should be kept wide apart when lifting heavy items, as it is easier to stay balanced with a wide base of support. Further, one foot should be kept a little forward of the other to give stability from front to back. Keeping the knees slightly bent allows for quick movement and for jolts to the body to be absorbed.

When turning, the feet rather than the body should be moved, in order to prevent injury to the back.

Body Alignment Proper body alignment requires that the various parts of the body be kept in proper anatomic relationship to each other.

Safety: Body Mechanics

- Stoop to lift objects from the floor: bend at the hips and the knees, keeping the back straight and base of support wide. The large muscles of the legs can then be used to straighten the body and lift the object.
- Avoid bending from the waist, as doing so strains the lower back muscles.
- To prevent undue stress and strain on the back when caring for clients, adjust the height of the bed to one of comfort and ease.
- Carry objects close to the midline of the body.
- Avoid stretching to reach objects.

Ensure Adequate Lighting Adequate lighting facilitates visualization of environmental hazards. Rooms should be adequately lit so that the client can safely perform ADL and the health care providers can perform procedures. Lighting can be supplemented by lamps and nightlights.

Remove Obstacles Obstacles in heavily traveled areas of health care facilities or homes represent a risk to the client's safety. Older adults or persons who are unfamiliar with the environment are at greatest risk of injury from obstacles. The risk that obstacles pose can be reduced by keeping hallways clear; removing excess furniture from heavily traveled areas; either removing all electrical cords or taping them securely to the floor; removing throw rugs; cleaning up spills immediately; and moving objects that could fall.

Reduce Bathroom Hazards

Bathrooms pose a threat to the client in the home because of the presence of water and the storage of medication. Accidents common to the bathroom are falls, scalds or burns, and poisonings. Such accidents can be reduced with the use of grab bars near the tub, shower, and toilet; nonslip mats in the tub and shower; and a secured bathroom rug near the tub or shower. Other safety measures include checking the temperature of the water before entering the tub or shower; checking the thermostat setting on the water heater; and storing medications in a locked cabinet, out of the reach of children and disoriented or confused adults.

Prevent Fire

Fire is a potential danger to all people in an institutional or home environment. Fire requires the interaction of three elements: sufficient heat to ignite the fire, combustible material (fuel), and oxygen to support the fire.

HOME HEALTH CARE

Preventing Fires and Burns

- Turn handles of pots and pans toward the center of the stove to prevent children from pulling them down and burning themselves
- Keep matches in a metal can and in a place where children cannot reach them
- Be aware of loose, flowing clothing when cooking, especially over an open flame
- Avoid using candles for light or heat and never leave a burning candle unattended
- Install smoke alarms near bedrooms and check batteries twice a year
- Do not place portable heaters near curtains, which can easily catch on fire
- Allow only certified electricians to work on wiring in the home
- Do not place electrical cords under carpeting
- Do not use multiple plug outlets
- Do not stick anything into appliances that are plugged in (e.g., a fork in the toaster)
- Teach family members routes of escape from the house, pick a place to meet outside to verify that everyone is safe, and conduct practice fire drills.
- Teach *stop*, *drop*, and *roll* to extinguish fire on clothing

Immobilized or incapacitated clients are at increased risk during a fire. Common causes of fire are smoking in bed, discarding of cigarette butts in trash cans, and faulty electrical equipment. Because smoking is a health hazard, many facilities are now smoke free.

Nursing goals are twofold: fire prevention and client protection during a fire. Nursing interventions aimed at preventing or reducing the risk of fire include the following:

- Clearly marking fire exits
- Knowing the locations and operation of fire extinguishers
- Practicing fire evacuation procedures
- Posting emergency phone numbers near all telephones
- Keeping open spaces and hallways clear of clutter
- Checking electrical cords and outlets for exposed or damaged wires
- Educating clients about fire hazards

In the event of a fire, the nurse should follow institutional policy and procedures for fire containment and evacuation (Figure 20-9). Nursing interventions during a fire are directed at protecting the client from injury and containing the fire. If a fire occurs, the nurse should ensure client safety, immediately report the type of fire and its exact location, and evacuate the premises if necessary. Nurses should know the locations and operation of fire extinguishers (Figure 20-10). The four types of fire extinguishers are water, carbon dioxide, regular dry chemical, and multipurpose dry chemical. Each type of fire extinguisher is used for a specific class of fire, as outlined in Table 20-6.

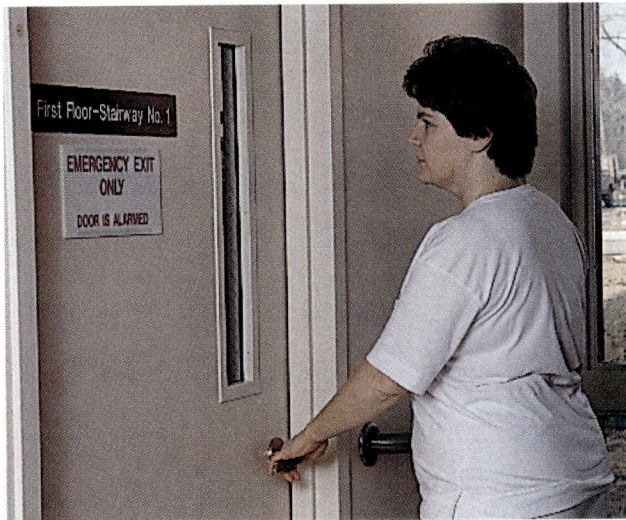

Figure 20-9 All personnel should be familiar with the evacuation plan and emergency exits.

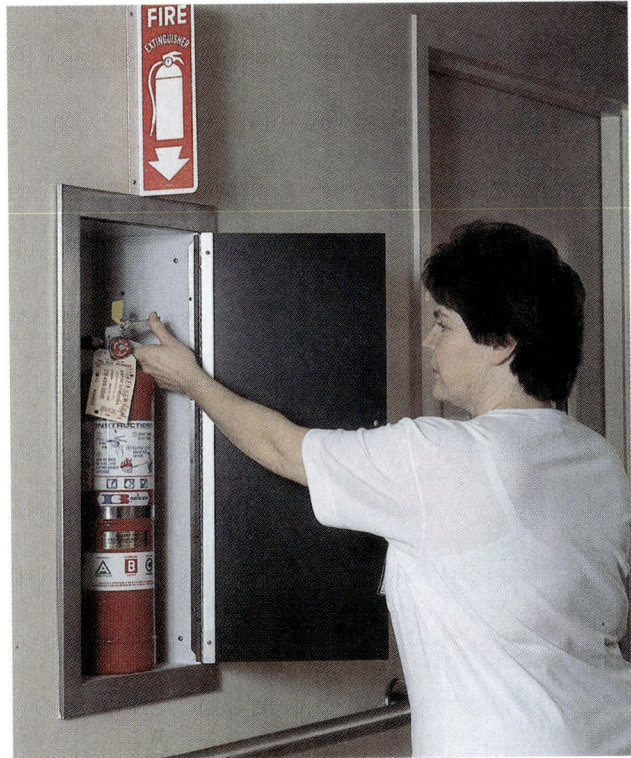

Figure 20-10 Know the location and use of fire extinguishers.

Table 20-6 FIRE EXTINGUISHERS

TYPE	CLASS OF FIRE
Water (type A)	Paper, wood, draperies, upholstery, or rubbish
Carbon dioxide or regular dry chemical (types B and C)	Flammable liquids, flammable gases, or electrical fires
Multipurpose dry chemical (types A, B, and C)	Any type of fire

From Fundamentals of Nursing: Standards & Practice, by S. Delaune and P. Ladner, 1998, Albany, NY: Delmar Publishers. Copyright 1998 by Delmar Publishers. Reprinted with permission.

Ensure the Safety of Equipment

Checking all equipment and supplies carefully before use and refusing to use any damaged goods or equipment can prevent many accidents. A good rule to follow is to never use any piece of equipment that is in any way damaged or not working properly. If a wheel comes off an overbed table, the nurse should not attempt to prop the table up but, rather, should remove it from the room and send it to the appropriate area for repair. The same holds true for smaller supplies given to or used on clients. The safety of clients must always come first.

Glass and Plastic Glass and plastic equipment and supplies should be inspected for cracks and chips before use. The nurse should also check that there are no rough edges that may injure clients.

Disposable Sterile Supplies When using disposable sterile supplies, the nurse should first always check that the package is intact. Any break in or wetness of the wrapper renders it unsterile. Expiration dates should also be verified prior to use.

Electrical Equipment Clients have contact with a variety of electrical equipment in the hospital environment, such as bed controls and intravenous and patient-controlled analgesia (PCA) pumps. Each piece of electrical equipment should have a three-pronged electrical plug that is grounded. A grounded plug transmits any stray electrical current from equipment to ground. To protect the client from electrical injury, the nurse should read the warning labels on all equipment, use only grounded electrical equipment, check for frayed electrical cords, avoid overloading circuits, and report to the biomedical department any shocks received from equipment (Figure 20-11).

Personal electrical appliances that the client is allowed to keep at the bedside, such as shavers, hair dryers, or curling irons, should be safety checked by the biomedical department before being used.

 PROFESSIONAL TIP

Oxygen Use

Special precautions must always be taken when oxygen is in use. Because one of the three elements essential to starting a fire is oxygen, the presence of pure oxygen can transform the tiniest spark into a tremendous hazard.

When oxygen is being used, "No Smoking" signs must be posted in the room and on the outside of the door to the room. It is vital that all visitors and other clients understand that the rule applies to everyone in the room, not just to the person receiving the oxygen. Because many critically ill clients use oxygen, it is also necessary for the nurse to caution clergy not to use open flames or candles in any religious rites.

Woolen and nylon blankets should not be used, as they can cause static electricity and thus pose a fire risk in an atmosphere of pure oxygen. Cotton blankets are recommended.

Electrical appliances such as radios and razors are generally not used in the presence of oxygen. Because it is flammable, oil should not be used on oxygen equipment. Hospital policy, as well as equipment itself, must be checked to determine what is safe to be used in a room where oxygen is being used and what is not.

Whenever tank oxygen is used, the cylinders must be securely strapped to a holder or cart to prevent the tank from tipping over and knocking off the valve, which could in turn cause a spark that would quickly ignite in the presence of oxygen.

If a client receives an electrical shock, the nurse should turn off the electricity before touching the client. Then, the client's pulse should be checked. If the client has no pulse, CPR should be initiated. If the client has a pulse, the nurse should assess vital signs, mental status, and skin integrity for burns. A physician

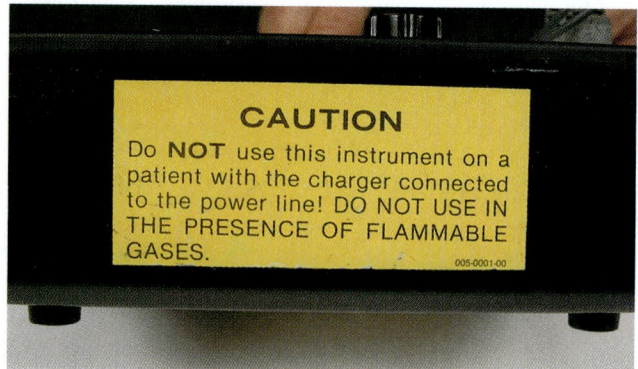

Figure 20-11 Heed warning labels on electrical equipment.

should then be notified of the event, and an incident report should be completed.

Reduce Exposure to Radiation

Clients are exposed to radiation during diagnostic testing and therapeutic interventions. Injury can occur from radiation if overexposure or exposure to untargeted tissues occurs. Exposure to untargeted tissues can result from the dislodgment of radiation implants. General principles of radiation exposure and protection are based on time, distance, and shielding. Protection from radiation therapy involves the following:

- Minimizing the time spent in contact with the radiation source (implant or client)
- Maximizing the distance from the radiation source (implant or client)
- Using appropriate radiation shields
- Monitoring radiation exposure with a film badge
- Labeling all potentially radioactive material
- Never touching dislodged implants or body fluids of a client receiving radiation therapy (Eriksson, 1994)

Both the client and the nurse are at risk for radiation injury. The client's risk for injury can be reduced by educating the client about radiation treatment and necessary precautions, placing the client in a private room, and providing a lead apron, when necessary, to protect nontargeted body tissues. The nurse's risk for injury can be reduced by observing all radioactive labels, wearing gloves when handling radioactive body discharges, washing hands, wearing lead aprons, disposing of radioactive substances in special containers, reducing the time of client contact, and wearing badges that measure the amount of radiation exposure.

Prevent Poisoning

A **poison** is any substance that when taken into the body interferes with normal physiologic functioning. Poisons may be inhaled, injected, ingested, or absorbed into the body. It is important to realize that many substances can be poisonous if taken in sufficient quantity.

 ### Safety: Aspirin
Aspirin can be poisonous when taken in sufficient quantity.

Dangerous chemicals may be found in any workplace, but some are specific to the health care industry, such as radioactive isotopes, laboratory dyes, antiseptics, irrigating solutions, disinfectants, and therapeutic drugs. To guard against accidental poisoning in health care facilities, the nurse must be aware of the client's mental and physical condition. The nurse must also ensure that potentially dangerous materials are never left unattended in clients' rooms. Alcohol and other

 LIFE CYCLE CONSIDERATIONS

Vitamins and Minerals
Adult iron preparations are especially poisonous to young children.

antiseptics or medications used for dressing changes or other procedures must be removed from the client's room after use.

 ### Safety: Medications and Cleaning Carts
- Medication trays and cleaning and supply carts should never be left unattended.
- Confused, visually impaired, or very young clients may help themselves to something harmful or something that they may use in a harmful way.
- Medication cupboards and carts must be kept locked when not in use.

On admission, clients are asked whether they have brought any medications to the facility. If so, these medications must be either removed to a safe place or sent home with the client's family. Because family members, in an effort to be helpful, sometimes bring in remedies that the client uses at home, the nurse should check bedside stands periodically to ensure medications or other potentially harmful substances are not being stored there.

The poison control center should be notified when poisoning is suspected. The number can generally be found on the inside cover or first few pages of the telephone book. The person reporting the poisoning should be prepared to state the amount and type of poison ingested, inhaled, or injected and the client's age and symptoms. Clients who have ingested poison should be turned on the side to prevent aspiration while awaiting further treatment. Client education about safety measures can prevent some accidental poisonings (Stanhope & Knollnueller, 1996).

 HOME HEALTH CARE

Proper Storage and Use of Medications

Teach clients about:

- Childproofing cupboards where medications are stored,
- The proper use and dosages of medications, and
- The use of special medication containers that are divided into days and times (to help prevent the client from duplicating a medication dose).

CLIENT TEACHING

Measures To Prevent Accidental Poisonings

- Store medications in child-resistant containers (Figure 20-12A).
- Do not take medications in front of children
- Never call medicine candy
- Place toxic substances in a locked cabinet out of the reach of children
- Never remove labels from containers
- Do not place poisonous substances in food or beverage containers
- Place poison stickers on toxic substances
- Keep syrup of ipecac available at all times (Figure 20-12B).
- Display poison control center phone numbers near telephones

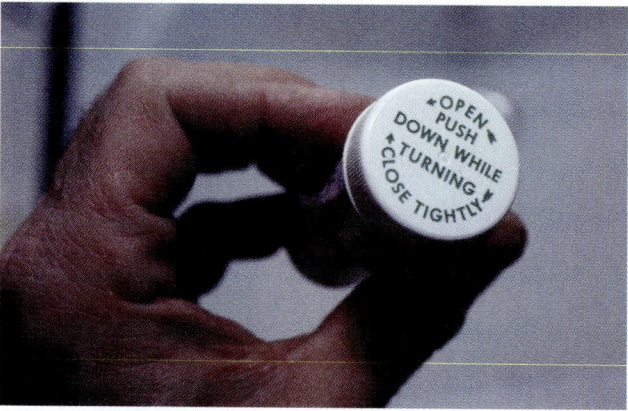

A.

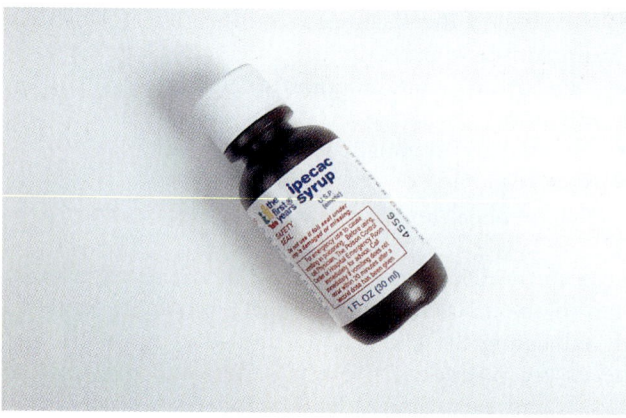

B.

Figure 20-12 Poison Prevention Methods: A. Medications stored in child-resistant containers, B. Syrup of Ipecac

Prevent Choking

To prevent choking on food, special techniques must be used when feeding clients in at-risk categories. Nothing should ever be given by mouth to an unconscious client, because the epiglottis does not function, and choking and suffocation are thus likely. Likewise, to prevent aspiration of vomitus, food and drink are usually withheld before the induction of general anesthesia. After some tests, such as a bronchoscopy, food and drink are withheld until the gag reflex returns.

Prevent Suffocation

Smothering can be prevented by proper nursing observation of at-risk clients such as infants, those who are impaired with regard to ADL, and paralyzed or unconscious clients. Such clients should be repositioned frequently and checked for a patent (open) airway. Soft pillows, mattresses, and comforters, in which they might bury their faces, should not be used. In the presence of oral secretions, the client's head should be turned to the side to prevent choking. Monitors that beep if breathing ceases should be used for at-risk clients.

Prevent Drowning

Infants, young children, and weak or confused clients are most at-risk for drowning. These clients should never be left alone in the bathtub. If the nurse must leave for any reason, either the client must be removed from the tub or another member of the health care team must stay with the client until the nurse returns or the bath is completed.

Clients should be instructed in the use of call systems installed in tub and shower rooms. Clients should also be instructed to first pull the plug in the tub and then call the nurse, should they feel weak or faint.

Reduce Noise Pollution

Noise pollution, or a noise level that is uncomfortable for the client or staff, frequently occurs in the health care setting because of visitor traffic, medical equipment, and personnel. It can result in an unorganized environment, hearing loss, and sensory overload. **Sensory overload** is an increased rate and intensity of auditory and visual stimuli. Sensory overload can alter a client's recovery by inducing or increasing anxiety, paranoia, hallucinations, and depression.

 Safety: Noise Pollution
- Maintain a quiet environment
- Control traffic
- Provide earplugs

Provide for the Client's Bathing Needs

Bathing of clients is an essential component of nursing care. Whether the nurse performs the bath or delegates the activity to another health care provider, the nurse retains the responsibility for ensuring that the hygiene needs of the client are met. The type of bath provided depends on the purpose of the bath and the client's self-care abilities. The two general categories of baths are cleansing and therapeutic.

Cleansing Baths Cleansing baths are provided as routine client care. The purpose of a cleansing bath is personal hygiene. The five types of cleansing baths are shower bath; tub bath; self-help, or assisted, bed bath; complete bed bath; and partial bath.

Shower Bath Most ambulatory clients are capable of taking a shower. Clients with limited physical ability can be accommodated by placing a waterproof chair in the shower. The nurse provides minimal assistance with the shower.

Tub Bath Clients frequently prefer and enjoy a tub bath. Tub baths can also be therapeutic. Clients with limited physical ability should be assisted when entering and exiting the tub.

Safety: Tub Bath

Check the temperature of the water in the bath tub before allowing the client to enter.

Self-Help Bath A self-help, or assisted, bed bath is used to provide hygiene care for clients who are confined to bed. In the self-help bed bath, the nurse prepares the bath equipment but provides minimal assistance. This assistance is usually limited to washing difficult-to-reach body areas such as the feet, legs, back, and perineal area.

Complete Bed Bath A complete bed bath is provided to clients who are dependent and confined to bed. The nurse washes the client's entire body during a complete bed bath.

Partial Bath In a partial, or abbreviated, bath, only those body areas that would cause discomfort or odor if not washed thoroughly are cleansed. These areas are the face, axillae, hands, and perineal area. The nurse or client may perform a partial bath, depending on the client's self-care abilities. Partial baths may be performed with the client lying in bed or standing at the sink.

Therapeutic Baths Therapeutic baths require a physician's order stating the type of bath, temperature of the water, body surface to be treated, and type of medicated solutions to be used. A therapeutic bath is usually performed in a tub and lasts approximately 20 to 30 minutes. Therapeutic baths are classified as

PROFESSIONAL TIP

Bathing

- Baths are an excellent time to perform a complete skin assessment.
- The bathing process provides time for the nurse to meet the client's psychosocial needs through assessment and counseling.
- Bathing provides time to educate the client on basic and special hygiene needs.

PROFESSIONAL TIP

Tub or Shower Bath

- Schedule use of tub or shower and provide necessary equipment
- Clean tub or shower according to agency policy
- Assist the client with ambulation to and from tub or shower
- Place bath mat in tub or shower; provide shower chair, if necessary
- Place "Occupied" sign on door
- Adjust room temperature and temperature of water
- Fill tub halfway with water; do not allow the client to soak longer than 20 minutes
- Assist the client with getting into and out of tub or shower; provide with a call system
- Assist with cleansing, as necessary
- Clean tub or shower after use, according to agency policy

hot, warm, cool, or tepid; soak or sitz; and oatmeal (Aveeno), cornstarch, or sodium bicarbonate, depending on the prescribed type of bath.

Hot- or warm-water tub baths are used to reduce muscle spasms, soreness, and tension. Hot- or warm-water baths, however, have the potential for causing skin burns. Cool or tepid baths are used to relieve tension or to lower body temperature. The nurse must prevent chilling and rapid temperature fluctuations during a cool or tepid bath by not leaving the client in the tub too long.

A soak can involve the entire body or be limited to only one body part. In a soak bath, water, with or without a medicated solution, is applied to reduce pain, swelling, or irritation or to soften or remove dead tissue.

Sitz baths cleanse and reduce inflammation in the perineal and anal areas. Sitz baths are commonly used for hemorrhoids or anal fissures and after perineal or rectal surgery. Skin irritations can be soothed with oatmeal (Aveeno), cornstarch, or sodium bicarbonate baths (Shaffer, 1997).

Provide Clean Bed Linen

After a bath, clean linens are placed on the bed to promote comfort. If the client is able to get out of the bed, the nurse can assist the client to a chair and proceed with making the bed.

If the client is unable to get out of the bed, the nurse will need to make an occupied bed. Assistance will be needed if the client is in traction or cannot be turned. Care must be taken to avoid disturbing the traction weights.

Provide Perineal Care

Perineal care is the cleansing of the external genitalia and the perineum and surrounding area. Perineal care is also referred to as *peri-care* or *perineal-genital* care. The purposes of perineal care are to prevent or eliminate infection and odor, promote healing, remove secretions, and provide comfort. Perineal care can be provided separately or as part of the bed bath.

Offer Back Rubs

Back rubs and massages stimulate the client's circulation, relax muscles, and relieve muscle tension as well as provide the nurse with an opportunity to assess the skin. Emollient creams and lotions are used to facilitate the rubbing and lubrication of the skin during a back rub or massage.

The client is positioned either prone or lying on the side. The nurse creates friction and pressure by rubbing the hands on the client's skin. The friction creates heat, which, in turn, dilates the peripheral circulation and increases the blood supply to the skin. The pressure manually stimulates the muscle fibers, which, in turn, relaxes the muscles. Prior to performing a back rub or massage, the nurse must assess for contraindications. Caution should be exercised when massaging limbs; especially the lower limbs, because a thrombus (blood clot) might be dislodged, resulting in an embolus (circulating blood clot). Bony prominences should be massaged lightly to prevent damage to underlying tissue (Shaffer, 1997).

Provide Foot and Toenail Care

Proper foot and toenail care are essential for ambulation and standing. Foot and toenail care are often ignored until problems occur. Common problems with the feet and toenails may directly result from abuse and neglect, such as inadequate foot and toenail hygiene, incorrect nail trimming, poorly fitted shoes, and exposure to harsh chemicals. These problems result in alterations of skin integrity and the potential for infection.

The first sign of foot and toenail problems is usually foot pain or tenderness. These symptoms affect a client's posture and may result in limping and in sub-

sequent strain to certain muscle groups. Clients with illnesses such as diabetes mellitus require special foot and toenail care, as these clients experience alterations in circulation that predispose them to foot problems.

The purposes of foot and toenail care are to prevent infection and soft tissue trauma from ingrown or jagged nails and to eliminate odor. Hygiene care of feet and toenails consists of regular trimming of the toenails; cleansing under the toenails; cleansing, rinsing, and drying the feet and toenails; and wearing properly fitted shoes.

If toenails are dirty or thickened, soaking facilitates cleansing. An orangewood stick is used to clean under the toenails, because a metal instrument can roughen the nail and cause it to harbor dirt. The safest instrument for trimming the toenails is the nail clipper; however, some clients feel that cutting the nails makes them brittle. If the client chooses not to cut the nails, they should instead be filed straight across with an emery board. Special attention should be given to drying the areas between the toes. An emollient, such as cold cream, helps to keep toenails and cuticles soft.

Callused areas should never be cut. Repeated soaking usually facilitates the removal of calluses. Lotion should be applied to the feet to maintain moisture and soften callused areas. If the client's feet maintain excessive moisture (sweat), water-absorbent powder should be applied between the toes.

The client should wear clean, properly fitted shoes. Shoes should not be extremely tight, but should be snug enough to provide support to the feet. Each shoe should have an arch support. Shoe size should be large enough so that the shoe is ½ inch longer than the longest toe. Common foot problems can often be alleviated by assessing footwear and providing proper education on footwear and foot and toenail care.

Provide Oral Care

The oral cavity functions in mastication, secretion of mucus to moisten and lubricate the digestive system, and secretion of digestive enzymes. Common problems occurring in the oral cavity include the following:

- Bad breath (**halitosis**)
- Cavities (**dental caries**)
- Plaque
- Periodontal disease (**pyorrhea**)
- Inflammation of the gums (**gingivitis**)
- Inflammation of the oral mucosa (**stomatitis**)

Poor oral hygiene and loss of teeth may affect a client's social interaction and body image as well as nutritional intake. Daily oral care is essential to maintain the integrity of the mucous membranes, teeth, gums, and lips. Through preventive measures, the oral cavity and teeth can be preserved. Preventive oral care consists of rinsing with fluoride; flossing; and brushing.

Fluoride Researchers have determined that fluoride can prevent dental caries. This finding has led to

PROFESSIONAL TIP

Foot and Toenail Care

- Soak feet in warm water and a detergent or in warm oil
- Use an orangewood stick to clean under the nails and release the cuticle growth from the nail
- File or cut the nails straight across to prevent in-grown nails
- Trim the cuticles as necessary
- Pat all areas dry using a clean towel
- Apply an emollient

PROFESSIONAL TIP

Oral Care for the Unconscious Client

Oral care for the unconscious client maintains a clean oral cavity and intact mucous membranes. Special care should be exercised when administering oral care to the unconscious client to prevent both client aspiration and injury to the nurse (from the client biting because of the gag reflex).

- Never use your fingers to hold a client's mouth open; a bite block or padded tongue blade can be used instead.
- Assess for gag reflex.
- Turn the client's head to one side and place a basin under the mouth.
- Use oral suctioning to facilitate removal of secretions; only a small amount of liquids should be used.
- Brush the teeth and tongue in the usual manner. Exercise caution to prevent aspiration.

the fluoridation of water supplies in many communities. Fluoride is a common component of mouthwashes and toothpastes. However, persons with excessively dry or with irritated mucous membranes should avoid commercial mouthwashes because of the alcohol content, which further dries the mucous membranes.

Infants can be given fluoride drops as early as 2 weeks of age to prevent dental caries. Nurses should inform clients that fluoride is an excellent preventive measure against dental caries, but that excessive fluoride usage can affect the color of tooth enamel. To prevent discoloration of the tooth enamel, fluoride should be administered with a dropper directed toward the back of the throat.

Flossing Flossing should be performed daily in conjunction with brushing of the teeth. Flossing prevents the formation of plaque, removes plaque between the teeth, and removes food debris. Dental caries and periodontal disease can be prevented by regular flossing.

Brushing Brushing removes plaque and food debris and promotes blood circulation in the gums. Brushing of the teeth should follow flossing. Teeth should be brushed after each meal. Brushing should be performed using a dentifrice (toothpaste) that contains fluoride to aid in preventing dental caries. An effective homemade dentifrice is the combination of two parts salt and one part baking soda. Dentures should be brushed using the same brushing motion used for brushing the teeth. The oral cavity of a client who wears dentures also must be cleansed.

Provide Hair Care

Hair affects a client's personal appearance and body image. Hair functions to maintain body temperature and as a receptor for the sense of touch. Assessment of hair texture, growth, and distribution provides information on a client's general health status. Common hair problems include dandruff, hair loss, tangled or matted hair, and infestations such as pediculosis and lice. Hair problems can be reduced with daily hair care, which helps to promote hair growth, prevent hair loss, prevent infections or infestations, promote circulation to the scalp, evenly distribute oils along hair shafts, and maintain the client's physical appearance. Hair care consists of brushing and combing, shampooing, shaving, and mustache and beard care.

Brushing and Combing Hair should be brushed or combed daily in accordance with the client's preferred hairstyle. Brushing and combing stimulate circulation to the scalp, distribute oils along hair shafts, and style the hair. A clean brush or comb should be used. Hair should be brushed from the scalp toward the hair ends. Sensitive scalps should be gently brushed or combed.

Clients who are immobilized may have tangled or matted hair. Care should be taken to prevent pain when combing tangled or matted hair by holding the tangled hair near the scalp while combing. If the client permits, the hair can be braided to prevent tangling or matting, but braiding the hair tightly should be avoided because tight braids may cause pain and hair loss. A nurse must receive written informed consent in order to cut a client's hair.

Shampooing When soiled, the hair should be shampooed according to the client's usual routine. The purposes of shampooing are to stimulate scalp circulation, remove soil from the hair, and facilitate brushing and combing. Hair can be shampooed in the tub, in the shower, at the sink, or in the bed, depending on the client's abilities and preferences.

Clients confined to bed can have their hair shampooed with water or with shampoos that do not require water. Hair is shampooed by thoroughly wetting all hair, applying approximately 1 teaspoon of shampoo, lathering the shampoo, and using the pads of the fingertips to gently massage the scalp. After shampooing, hair should be rinsed thoroughly, dried with an absorbent towel, combed, and styled as desired by the client.

Shaving Shaving is the removal of hair from the skin surface. Males often shave to remove facial hair, and women may shave to remove leg and/or axillary hair. Operative procedures may also require shaving of an area of the body.

Shaving may be performed before, during, or after the bath. Care should be taken to avoid cutting the skin. Prior to shaving, the area should be washed with soap and warm water to soften the hair. A warm washcloth may be placed over the area for several minutes to facilitate softening of the hair. A shaving cream or mild soap is then applied to the area to ease hair removal. The skin should be pulled taut, and the razor should be held at a 45-degree angle and moved over the skin in short, firm strokes in the direction of hair growth. After the skin is shaved, it should be washed, rinsed, and patted dry.

Safety: Shaving
- Review the client's medical record and the facility's policy regarding the use of razors for shaving.
- Clients prone to bleeding should be instructed to use only electrical razors for shaving.
- The nurse should wear gloves unless using an electric razor.

Mustache and Beard Care Mustaches and beards require daily care. Mustache and beard care consists of keeping the hair clean, trimmed, and combed. Mustaches and beards can be washed with soap or shampoo. Frequently, mustaches and beards require only gentle wiping with a moist washcloth. A mustache or beard should never be shaved off by the nurse without written informed consent from the client.

Provide Eye, Ear, and Nose Care

Eye, ear, and nose care should be included in routine hygiene care.

Eye Care Eyes are continually cleansed by tears and the movement of the eyelids over the eyes. Eyelids should be washed daily with a warm washcloth and from the inner to the outer canthus.

Infection Control: Eye Care
In order to prevent the transfer of pathogens, a new, clean corner of the washcloth should be used for each eye and with each stroke.

Eyelashes function to prevent foreign material from entering the eyes and conjunctival sacs. Eyelashes and eyebrows should be washed as necessary.

Although some artificial eyes (prosthetics) are permanently implanted, others may require daily removal and cleaning: The eye is removed from the eye socket and washed.

Comatose clients have special eye care needs because they lack a blink reflex. These clients require frequent instillations of lubricants or eyedrops to prevent corneal abrasions.

The nursing history should indicate whether the client wears contact lenses, and the routine care and level of assistance required should be recorded on the client's care plan. Clients who can insert, remove, and manage the care of their lenses require minimal assistance from the nurse. If the client is unable to assist with lens care and also has corrective eyeglasses, the nurse can suggest that the client wear the eyeglasses during hospitalization. There are two types of contact lenses: hard and soft. Each type requires different cleansing and care. During emergency situations, the nurse should remove the lenses and place them in the appropriate solution.

Ear Care Hearing can be affected by foreign material or wax in the external ear canal. Cleansing of the ears involves cleansing the external ear canal and auricles. Objects should not be inserted into the ear canal. Excess wax or foreign material should be removed by using a warm washcloth to gently wash the external ear and auricles while pulling the ear downward, in the adult client. In children, the ear is pulled up and back. Irrigation of the ear may be necessary to remove dried wax; this will require a physician's order.

Hearing aids amplify sound. The health history should indicate whether the client wears a hearing aid, and the plan of care should discuss the cleaning schedule of the aid. Clients with hearing aids should cleanse the ear mold regularly to ensure proper functioning.

If the hearing aid is not functioning properly, the nurse should check the on–off switch and volume control; the battery (and replace as necessary); the plastic tubing, for cracks and loose connections; and the telephone switch, which should be in the off position unless the client is using the phone. Hearing aids should be handled carefully, because dropping or bumping the hearing aid can damage the delicate mechanisms of the aid. When not in use, the hearing aid should be stored in a container, because dust and dirt can damage the mechanism.

Nose Care The nose provides the sense of smell, prevents entrance of foreign material into the respiratory tract, humidifies inhaled air, and facilitates breathing. Excessive or dried secretions may impair nasal function. Excessive nasal secretions are removed by inserting a cotton-tip applicator moistened with water or saline into the nostrils. The applicator should not be inserted beyond the cotton tip. Excessive nasal secretions in infants may be removed by a suction bulb. The client with a nasogastric tube should receive meticulous skin care to the nose area to prevent skin breakdown.

Evaluation

Evaluation is based on the achievement of goals and expected outcomes, regardless of the setting. Clients with alterations in health-perception–health-management pattern or activity–exercise pattern are at risk for injury and self-care deficits. Keeping the client free from injury requires both frequent reassessment through the use of risk appraisals and timely adjustments to the plan of care in order to facilitate effectiveness of nursing interventions.

It is imperative that the client not only be kept free of injury during hospitalization, but also be helped in developing a true awareness of the internal and external factors that increase the risk for injury. Achievement of this outcome measure is directly related both to the behaviors the client observes while in the hospital and to client teaching. In the home, modifications to ensure a safe environment serve as evidence for the home health nurse that learning has taken place.

The therapeutic value of hygiene is maximized when the client can participate and is kept free from infection and alterations in skin integrity. Evaluation should identify the client's level of functioning in self-care activities. At the time of discharge from the hospital, appropriate referrals should be made to home health care agencies to assist the client in achieving optimal function with regard to safety and hygiene practices.

SAMPLE NURSING CARE PLAN

THE CLIENT AT RISK FOR INJURY

Mr. Simon, age 75 years, presents with coronary heart disease (CHD) upon being admitted to the hospital. He has a family history of CHD. He smokes two packs of cigarettes per day, has diabetes mellitus, and is obese. He has gained 7 pounds in the past month, and exhibits diminished visual acuity, decreased bladder tone, weakness, and syncope. His blood cholesterol is 320 mg/dL, and his high-density lipoprotein (HDL) level is 28 mg/dL. On the GCS, he received a score of 12 (15 is fully oriented; 7 is comatose). His blood pressure is 186/116.

Nursing Diagnosis *Injury, Risk for, related to failure to adapt to sensory dysfunctions as evidenced by diminished visual acuity and a GCS score of 12*

PLANNING/GOALS	NURSING INTERVENTIONS	RATIONALE	EVALUATION
Mr. Simon will be protected from injury during hospitalization.	Initiate fall-prevention protocol.	Identifies and reduces the risk for injury.	The fall prevention protocol was implemented.
	Place Mr. Simon in a room as close as possible to the nurses' station.	Facilitates faster response time to the client's needs.	When discharged on the third day of hospitalization, Mr. Simon was free of injury.

continued

Place fall-alert signs on Mr. Simon's door and head of bed.	Alerts other health care workers to the client's risk status.
Put the bed alarm on.	Helps monitor client status and facilitates prompt response if the client tries to get out of bed unassisted.
Monitor Mr. Simon and the environment every 2 hours and whenever a caregiver passes by his room.	Provides information on status, progress, and needs of the client; encourages team approach to client care.
Reassess Mr. Simon's injury status every 4 hours.	Identifies changes and, thus, the need to modify the plan of care.
Instruct all caregivers to respond promptly to the call light.	Ensures rapid response to the client's needs.
Teach Mr. Simon to use the call light; reinforce teaching each time before leaving him alone.	Ensures that the client has the means and knowledge to call for assistance if necessary.

CASE STUDY

Manuela, age 30 years, received a broken right arm and a broken right leg in a car accident. The arm and leg are each in a cast.

The following questions will guide your development of a nursing care plan for the case study.

1. What assessment information should be gathered?
2. Identify three nursing diagnoses for Manuela.
3. Formulate possible goals for each nursing diagnosis.
4. Plan nursing interventions for each nursing diagnosis.

SUMMARY

- Maintaining a safe environment for clients must be the highest priority for nurses.
- The best way to ensure safety is to recognize hazards and eliminate them. Prevention is the best safety measure.
- Clients having a high risk factor for injury must be provided extra protection measures.

- Factors influencing client safety are age, lifestyle, sensory and perceptual alterations, mobility, and emotional state.
- The accidents that occur in health care settings relate to client behavior, therapeutic procedures, and equipment.
- Assessment of a safe environment involves performing an injury risk appraisal.

- Nurses can help clients in maintaining a safe environment by resolving or alleviating hazards related to falls, lighting, obstacles, the bathroom, fire, electricity, radiation, poisoning, and noise pollution.
- Safety precautions should be explained thoroughly to clients and/or families.
- Hygiene practices are influenced by body image, social and cultural practices, personal preference, socioeconomic status, and knowledge.
- Basic hygiene practices include bathing, skin care, perineal care, back rubs, foot and nail care, oral care, hair care, and eye, ear, and nose care.

Review Questions

1. Mingo, a 60-year-old diabetic, had his left leg amputated. He is in a semiprivate room with another client who is receiving oxygen. What sign should be posted on the door?

    a. "Amputee"
    b. "No Visitors"
    c. "No Smoking"
    d. "Regular Diet"

2. Felicita, just admitted to the hospital, is overweight, unsteady on her feet, and visually impaired. Her two daughters enter the room as the nurse puts the side rails up on the bed. Felicita begins to cry. The daughters accuse her of being a baby. The best nursing intervention would be to:

    a. tell the daughters to leave until Felicita has calmed down.
    b. explain to the daughters that they are making their mother feel worse.
    c. explain to Felicita that side rails must be used to protect her from falling out of bed.
    d. explain to Felicita and her daughters both the purpose of the side rails and the facility's alternate policy.

3. The priority for nursing care is:

    a. safety.
    b. timeliness.
    c. one-to-one care.
    d. the execution of procedures exactly as written.

4. The use of side rails:

    a. is only needed at night.
    b. is required for all clients.
    c. has caused injury to clients.
    d. relieves the nurse from checking on the client as frequently.

5. Hygiene is considered a safety measure because:

    a. it changes a person's self-image.
    b. the same thing is done for all clients.
    c. it rids the body of all microorganisms.
    d. it promotes the health of the body's first line of defense.

6. The water (type A) fire extinguisher is to be used on:

    a. paper.
    b. flammable gases.
    c. electrical fires.
    d. flammable liquids.

7. If a client receives an electrical shock, the first thing the nurse should do is:

    a. call for help.
    b. unplug the equipment.
    c. check the client's pulse.
    d. move the client out of the room.

Critical Thinking Questions

1. Gloria Hernandez is an 83-year-old widow who fractured her hip when she fell in the bathtub. She had hip replacement surgery yesterday. Tonight she is very confused and is trying to dislodge the bandage and stitches. Mrs. Hernandez is now being restrained for her protection. What other nursing activities could have been implemented prior to the use of restraints? Do you think that restraints will affect Mrs. Hernandez's mental status? If so, in what way(s)? What are some other effects Mrs. Hernandez may experience as a result of being restrained?

2. How is noise a safety factor?

3. How would you approach providing perineal care to someone of the opposite sex or of similar age?

⚡ WEB FLASH!

- What Internet sources can you locate that relate to safety and hygiene? What types of information are available?
- Which of the resources listed for this chapter have Web sites? What kind of information is provided?

UNIT

8
Infection Control

INFECTION CONTROL/ ASEPSIS

MAKING THE CONNECTION

Refer to the following chapters to increase your understanding of infection control/asepsis:

- **Chapter 18, Basic Nutrition**
- **Chapter 20, Safety/Hygiene**
- **Chapter 22, Standard Precautions and Isolation**
- **Chapter 23, Fluid, Electrolyte, and Acid–Base Balance**
- **Chapter 39, Nursing Care of the Client: Immune System**

- **Chapter 40, Nursing Care of the Client: Integumentary System**
- **Procedures:** B1, Handwashing; B2, Use of Protective Equipment; I1, Surgical Asepsis: Preparing and Maintaining a Sterile Field; I2, Performing Open Gloving and Removal of Soiled Gloves; I17, Applying a Dry Sterile Dressing

LEARNING OBJECTIVES

Upon completion of this chapter, you should be able to:
- *Define key terms.*
- *Describe the chain of infection.*
- *Discuss the body's nonspecific and specific immune defenses.*
- *Describe the stages of the inflammatory process.*
- *Discuss the stages of the infectious process.*
- *Identify the signs and symptoms of inflammation and infection.*
- *Explain the principles of medical and surgical asepsis.*
- *Provide client care maintaining the principles of medical and/or surgical asepsis.*

KEY TERMS

acquired immunity	aseptic technique
agent	bactericide
airborne transmission	biological agent
anthropogenic	carrier
antibody	chain of infection
antigen	chemical agent
asepsis	clean object

cleansing	medical asepsis
colonization	mode of trans-
communicable agent	mission
communicable disease	nosocomial infection
compromised host	pathogen
contact transmission	pathogenicity
convalescent stage	physical agent
dirty object	portal of entry
disinfectant	portal of exit
disinfection	prodromal stage
edema	reservoir
erythema	resident flora
flora	risk for infection
fomite	sebum
germicide	spore
handwashing	sterilization
host	surgical asepsis
humoral immunity	susceptible host
illness stage	systemic infection
immunization	transient flora
incubation period	vaccination
infection	vectorborne trans-
infectious agent	mission
inflammation	vehicle transmission
localized infection	virulence
lymphokine	

INTRODUCTION

Nurses are responsible for providing quality care that incorporates infection-control principles. These principles are a major component of a safe environment. This chapter discusses infection-control principles including naturally occurring microorganisms, pathogens, infection and colonization, chain of infection, normal defense mechanisms, stages of the infectious process, and nosocomial infections. Discussion of the nurse's role in controlling infections is also included.

FLORA

Flora are microorganisms which occur or have adapted to live in a specific environment, such as intestinal, skin, vaginal, or oral flora. There are two types of flora: resident and transient. **Resident (normal) flora** are microorganisms that are always present, usually without altering the client's health; an example would be *proprionibacterium* on the skin. Handwashing with soap and water alone is not sufficient to remove resident flora; there must be considerable friction, which is created by rubbing the hands and scrubbing the nails. Resident flora prevent the overgrowth of harmful microroganisms; only when the balance is upset does disease result. **Transient flora** are microorganisms that are episodic (of limited duration); an example would be *staphylococcus aureus*. They attach to the skin for a brief period of time but do not continually live on the skin. Transient flora are usually acquired from direct contact with the microorganisms on environmental surfaces. Handwashing with soap and water is an effective means of removing transient flora (Ellner & Neu, 1992).

PATHOGENICITY AND VIRULENCE

Although most microorganisms found in the environment do not cause disease and infection, there are some that do. Disease-producing microorganisms are called **pathogens**; **pathogenicity** refers to the ability of a microorganism to produce disease. **Virulence** refers to the frequency with which a pathogen causes disease. The factors affecting virulence are the strength of the pathogen to adhere to healthy cells; the ability of a pathogen to damage cells or interfere with the body's normal regulating systems; and the ability of a pathogen to evade the attack of white blood cells (WBCs).

Five types of microorganisms can be pathogenic: bacteria, viruses, fungi, protozoa, and *Rickettsia*.

Bacteria

Bacteria are small, one-celled microorganisms that lack a true nucleus or mechanism to provide metabolism. Therefore, bacteria need an environment that will provide food for survival. Bacteria can be spherical, rodlike, spiral, or curving in shape, usually appearing as single cells, pairs, chains, or groups. Although most bacteria multiply by simple cell division, some forms of bacteria produce **spores**, a resistant stage that withstands unfavorable environments. When proper environmental conditions return, spores germinate and form new cells. Spores are difficult to kill because of their resistance to heat, drying, and disinfectant. The growth rate of bacteria is affected by environmental factors such as changes in temperature and nutrition. The optimal temperature for pathogenic bacteria is 98.6°F.

Bacteria can be found in all environments, yet not all bacteria are harmful or cause disease. Only a small percentage of bacteria are actually pathogenic. Common bacterial infections include diarrhea, pneumonia, sinusitis, urinary tract infections, cellulitis, meningitis, gonorrhea (Figure 21-1), otitis media, and impetigo.

Viruses

Viruses are organisms that can live only inside cells. They cannot get nourishment or reproduce outside cells. Viruses contain a core of deoxyribonucleic acid (DNA) or ribonucleic acid (RNA) surrounded by a protein coating. Some viruses have the ability to create an additional coating called an envelope. This envelope helps protect the cell from attack by the immune system. Viruses damage the cells they inhabit by blocking the normal protein synthesis of the cells and by using the cell's mechanism for metabolism to reproduce.

The same viral infection may cause different symptoms in different individuals, based on the individual's immune response to the invading virus. Some viruses will immediately trigger a disease response whereas others may remain latent for many years. Common viral

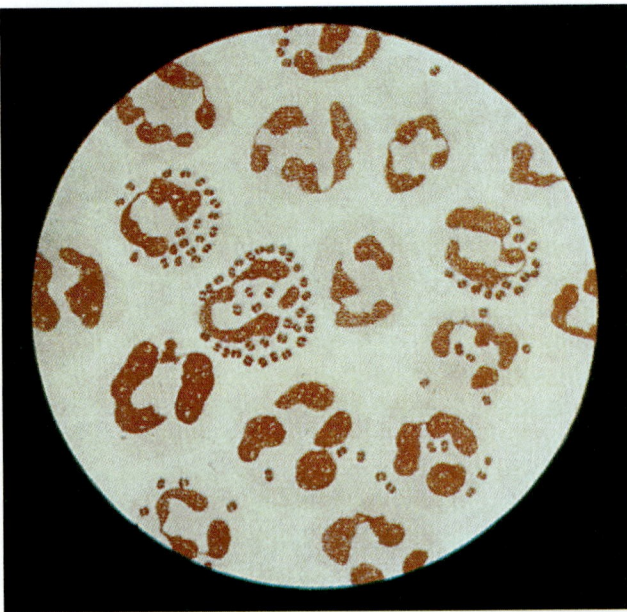

Figure 21-1 Neisseria Gonorrhea *(Courtesy of the Centers for Disease Control and Prevention, Atlanta, GA)*

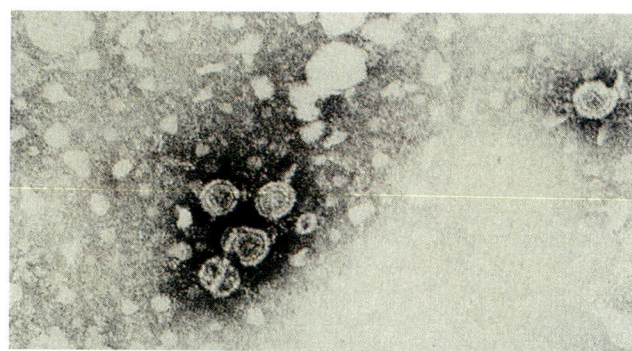

Figure 21-2 Electron Micrograph of Hepatitis B Virus *(Courtesy of the Centers for Disease Control and Prevention, Atlanta, GA)*

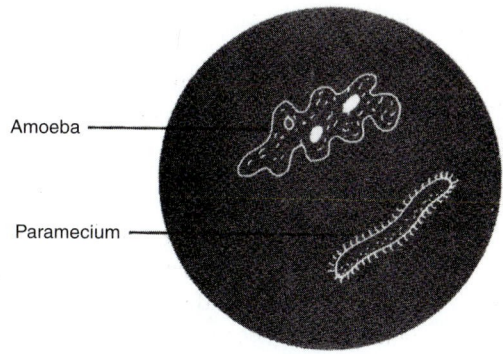

Figure 21-4 Protozoa

infections include influenza, measles, common cold, chickenpox, hepatitis B (Figure 21-2), genital herpes, and HIV.

Fungi

Fungi grow in single cells, as in yeast, or in colonies, as in molds (Figure 21-3). Fungi obtain food from dead organic matter or from living organisms. Most fungi are not pathogenic and make up many of the body's normal flora. Disease from fungi is found mainly in individuals who are immunologically impaired. Fungi can cause infections of the hair, skin, nails, and mucous membranes.

Protozoa

Protozoa are single-celled parasitic organisms with the ability to move (Figure 21-4). Most protozoa obtain their nourishment from dead or decaying organic matter. Infection is spread through ingestion of contaminated food or water or through insect bites. Common protozoan infections include malaria, gastroenteritis, and vaginal infections.

Rickettsia

Rickettisa are intracellular parasites that need to be in living cells to reproduce. Infection from *rickettsia* is

spread through fleas, ticks, mites, and lice. Common *rickettsia* infections include typhus, Rocky Mountain spotted fever, and Lyme disease.

INFECTION AND COLONIZATION

Infection and colonization are not synonymous. **Infection** is an invasion and multiplication of pathogenic microorganisms that occurs in body tissue and results in cellular injury; an example is strep throat. These microorganisms are called **infectious agents**. Infectious agents that are capable of being transmitted to a client by direct or indirect contact, through a vehicle (or vector) or airborne route are also called **communicable agents**. Diseases produced by these agents are referred to as **communicable diseases**.

Colonization is the multiplication of microorganisms that occurs on or within a host but does not result in cellular injury; an example of colonization is the normal flora (microorganisms) in the intestines. However, microorganisms that are colonized on a host may be a potential source of infection, especially if host susceptibility increases or the microorganism's virulence increases.

CHAIN OF INFECTION

Neither a susceptible host nor the presence of a pathogen means that an infectious process will occur. The **chain of infection** describes the phenomenon of the development of an infectious process. An interactive process that involves the agent, host, and environment is required. This interactive process must involve several essential elements, or "links in the chain," for transmission of microorganisms to occur. Figure 21-5 identifies the six essential links (elements) in the chain of infection. Without the transmission of microorganisms, an infectious process cannot occur. Therefore, knowledge about the chain of infection for an infectious process facilitates control or elimination of

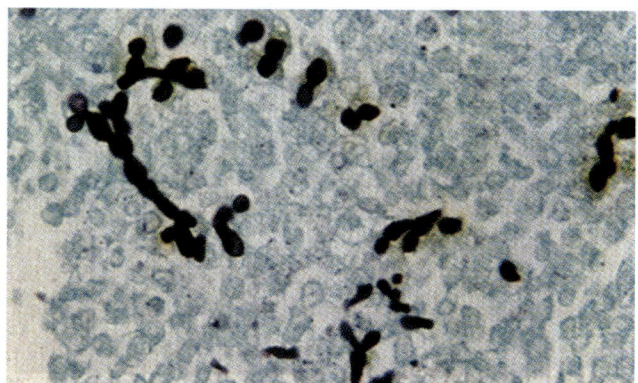

Figure 21-3 Candida Albicans *(Courtesy of the Centers for Disease Control and Prevention, Atlanta, GA)*

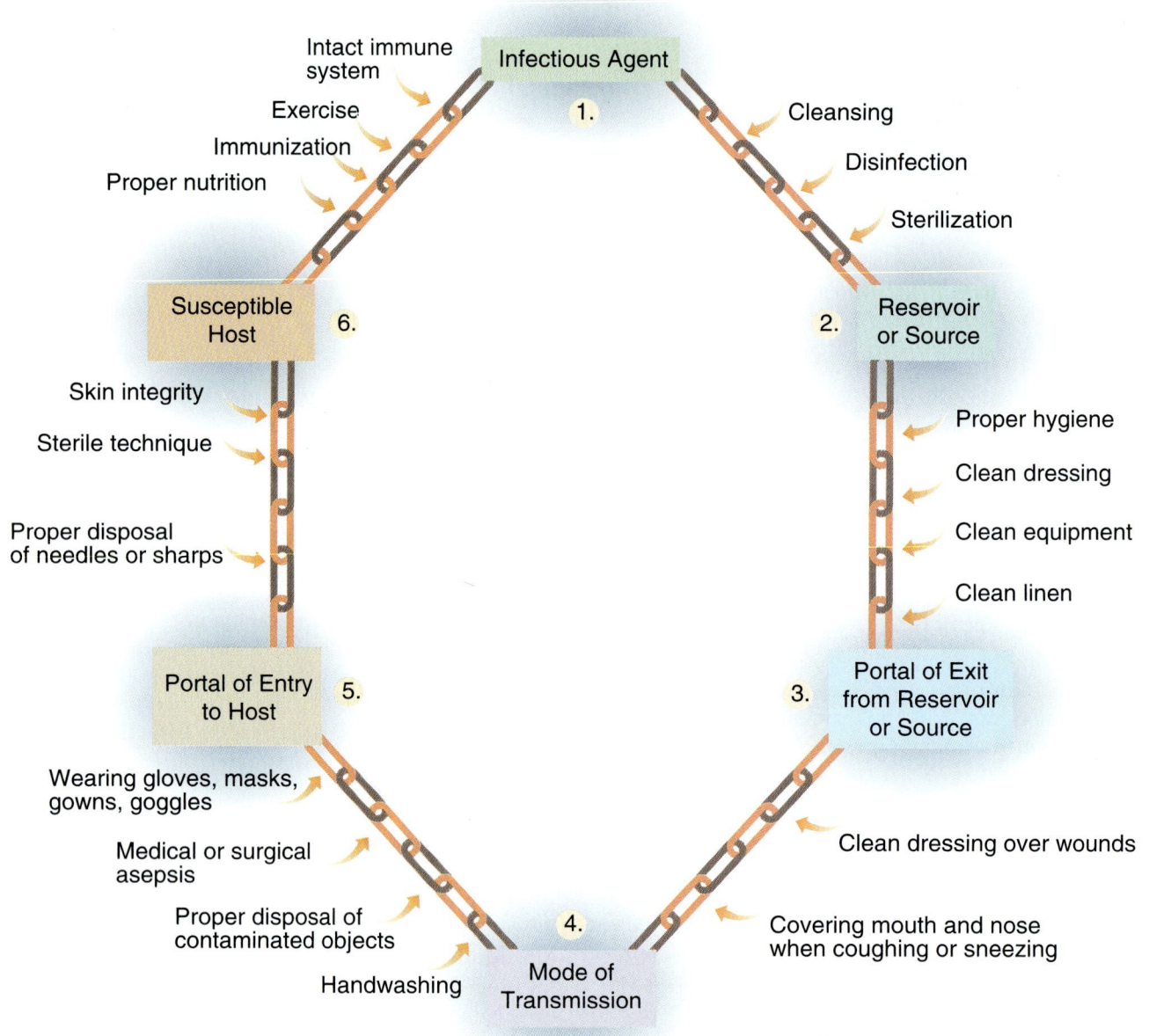

Figure 21-5 The Chain of Infection: Preventive Measures Follow Each Link of the Chain (*Adapted from* Fundamentals of Nursing: Standards & Practice, *by S. DeLaune and P. Ladner, 1998, Albany, NY: Delmar Publishers. Copyright 1998 by Delmar Publishers.)

microorganism transmission by breaking the links in the chain of infection. Breaking the chain of infection is achieved by altering the interactive process of agent, host, and environment. Each of the six links in the chain of infection is discussed following.

Agent

An **agent** is an entity that is capable of causing disease. Agents that cause disease may be as follows:

- **Biological agents**: living organisms that invade the host, causing disease, such as bacteria, viruses, fungi, protozoa, and *Rickettsia*

- **Chemical agents**: substances that can interact with the body, causing disease, such as pesticides, food additives, medications, and industrial chemicals
- **Physical agents**: factors in the environment that are capable of causing disease, such as heat, light, noise, radiation, and machinery

In the chain of infection, the main concern is biological agents and their effect on the host.

Reservoir

The **reservoir** is a place where the agent can survive. Colonization and reproduction take place while the agent is in the reservoir. A reservoir that promotes growth of pathogens must contain the proper nutrients (such as oxygen and organic matter), maintain proper temperature, contain moisture, maintain a compatible pH level (neither too acidic nor too alkaline), and maintain the proper amount of light exposure. The most common reservoirs are:

- Humans,
- Animals,
- Environment, and
- **Fomites** (objects contaminated with an infectious agent, such as bed pans, urinals, bed linens, instruments, dressings, specimen containers, and other equipment).

Humans and animals can have symptoms of the infectious agents or can be strictly carriers of the agent. **Carriers** have the infectious agent but are symptom free. The agent can be spread to others in both instances.

Portal of Exit

The **portal of exit** is the route by which an infectious agent leaves the reservoir to be transferred to a susceptible host. The agent leaves the reservoir through body secretions including:

- Sputum, from the respiratory tract;
- Semen, vaginal secretions, or urine, from the genitourinary tract;
- Saliva and feces, from the gastrointestinal tract;
- Blood;
- Draining wounds; and
- Tears.

Modes of Transmission

The **mode of transmission** is the process that bridges the gap between the portal of exit of the infectious agent from the reservoir or source and the portal of entry of the susceptible "new" host. Most infectious agents have a primary or usual mode of transmission; however, some microorganisms may be transmitted by more than one mode (Table 21-1). Almost anything in the environment can become a potential means of transmitting infection, depending on the agent.

Contact Transmission

The most important and frequent mode of transmission is **contact transmission**, which involves the physical transfer of an agent from an infected person to a host through direct contact with the infected person, indirect contact with the infected person through a fomite, or close contact with contaminated secretions (Figure 21-6). Sexually transmitted diseases are examples of diseases spread by direct contact. Common viral infections (cold, measles, flu) are spread by close contact with contaminated secretions.

Table 21-1 MODES OF TRANSMISSION

MODE	EXAMPLES
Contact	Direct contact of health care provider with client: • Touching • Bathing • Rubbing • Toileting (urine and feces) • Secretions from client Indirect contact with fomites: • Clothing • Bed linens • Dressings • Health care equipment • Instruments used in treatments • Specimen containers used for laboratory analysis • Personal belongings • Personal care equipment • Diagnostic equipment
Airborne	Inhaling microorganisms carried by moisture or dust particles in air: • Coughing • Talking • Sneezing
Vehicle	Contact with contaminated inanimate objects: • Water • Blood • Drugs • Food • Urine
Vectorborne	Contact with contaminated animate hosts: • Animals • Insects

Airborne Transmission

Airborne transmission occurs when a susceptible host contacts droplet nuclei or dust particles that are suspended in the air. Particle size influences the length of time that the organism can remain airborne. The longer the particle is suspended, the greater the chance it will find an available port of entry to the human host. An example of an organism that relies on airborne transmission is measles. Contaminated droplets containing the measles virus are contained in the spray from sneezing (Figure 21-7). The droplet can find a portal of entry through the mucous membranes or conjunctiva. Droplets that do not remain airborne or settle out are excluded from this category (Benenson, 1995).

Vehicle Transmission

Vehicle transmission occurs when an agent is transferred to a susceptible host by contaminated inanimate

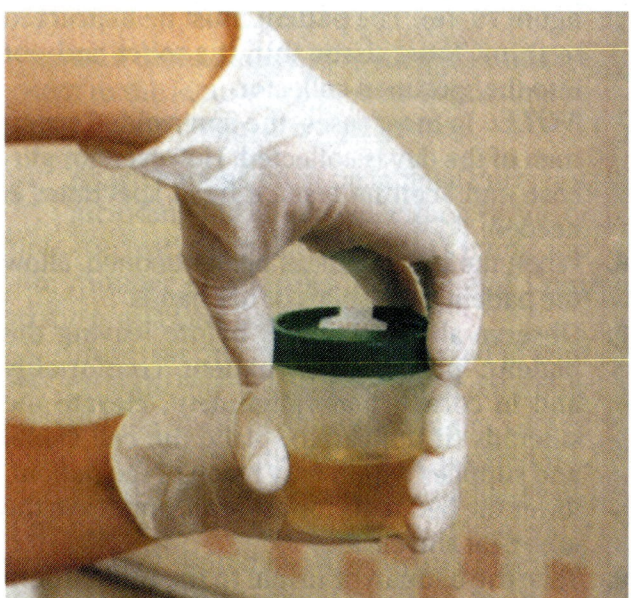

Figure 21-6 Care must be taken in the handling of bodily fluids to prevent the transfer of infectious agents through contact with secretions.

objects such as water, food, milk (Figure 21-8), drugs, and blood. Cholera, which is transmitted through contaminated drinking water, and salmonellosis, which is transmitted through contaminated meat, are examples of vehicle transmission.

Vectorborne transmission

Vectorborne transmission occurs when an agent is transferred to a susceptible host by animate means such as mosquitoes, fleas, ticks, lice, and other animals (Figure 21-9). Lyme disease and malaria are examples of diseases spread by vectors.

Portal of Entry

A **portal of entry** is the route by which an infectious agent enters the host. Portals of entry include the following:

- Integumentary system, through a break in the integrity of the skin or mucous membranes (for instance, infections of surgical wounds)
- Respiratory tract, by inhaling contaminated droplets (such as cold, influenza, measles)
- Genitourinary tract, through contact with infected vaginal secretions or semen (as in sexually transmitted diseases)
- Gastrointestinal tract, by ingesting contaminated food or water (for example, typhoid, hepatitis A)
- Circulatory system, through the bite of insects (such as mosquito bites resulting in malaria)
- Transplacental, through transfer of microorganisms from mother to fetus via the placenta and umbilical cord (including HIV, hepatitis B)

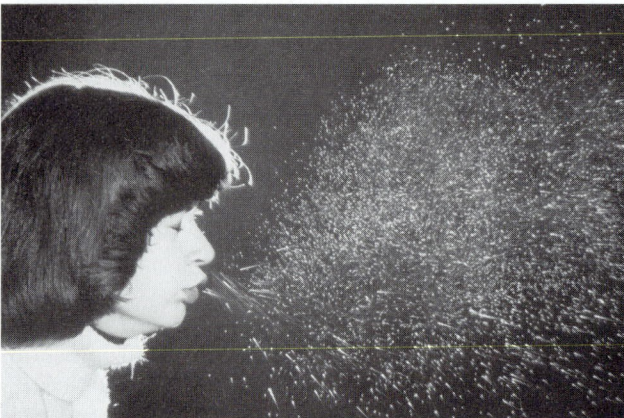

Figure 21-7 This photo illustrates the width of the area that droplet nuclei from a sneeze can encompass. *(Courtesy of Lester V. Bergman/Corbis)*

Host

A **host** is a simple or complex organism that can be affected by an agent. Generally, a human being is considered a host. A **susceptible host** is a person who lacks resistance to an agent and is thus vulnerable to disease. For example, an individual who has not received the measles vaccine is more likely to contract the infection due to the lack of immunity to the infectious agent. A **compromised host** is a person whose normal defense mechanisms are impaired and who is therefore susceptible to infection. For example, a person with a common cold or superficial burns is at greater risk for infection due to the impaired state of the body system mechanisms.

Characteristics of the host influence the susceptibility to and severity of infections. These include:

- Age: As a person ages, immunity declines, thus increasing susceptibility to infection.
- Concurrent diseases: The existence of comorbid diseases indicates an environment susceptible to infection.

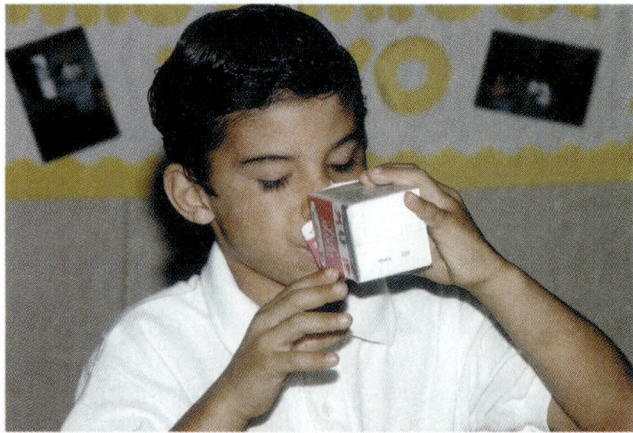

Figure 21-8 Vehicle transmission occurs through contamination of inanimate objects, such as milk.

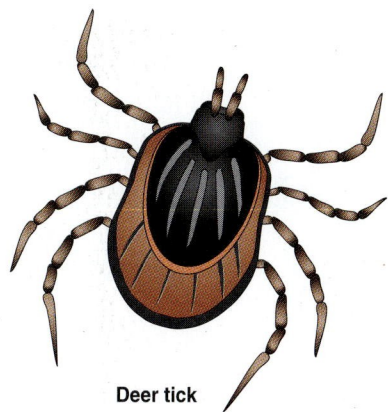

Deer tick

Figure 21-9 Lyme disease and other infections are caused by the bite of a tick.

- Stress: An individual experiencing a compromised emotional state may have altered or decreased immune system response.
- Immunization/vaccination status: Individuals who are not fully immunized are at greater risk for infection.
- Lifestyle: Lifestyle practices such as having multiple sex partners or sharing intravenous drug needles increase an individual's potential for illness.
- Occupation: Forms of employment that involve an increased exposure to pathogens might include dealing with chemical agents (such as asbestos) or handling sharp instruments (such as scalpels).
- Nutritional status: Individuals who maintain targeted weight for height and body frame are less prone to illness.
- Heredity: Some individuals are naturally more susceptible to infection than others (Black & Matassarin-Jacobs, 1997).

Interaction between agent and host occurs in the environment; the environment consists of everything other than the agent and host. Environmental factors that affect the chain of infection are water, food, plants, animals, housing conditions, noise, meteorological conditions, and environmental chemicals. Many of the conditions that promote the transmission of microorganisms are **anthropogenic**, reflecting changes in the relationship between humans and their environments.

BREAKING THE CHAIN OF INFECTION

Nurses focus on breaking the chain of infection by applying proper infection-control practices to interrupt the transmission of microorganisms. Specific strategies can be directed at breaking or blocking the transmission of infection from one link in the chain to the next. A discussion regarding each of the six links follows (refer back to Figure 21-5).

PROFESSIONAL TIP

Infectious Diseases

Berlinguer (1992) notes that the causes of most emerging infectious diseases are the same today as throughout recorded history: the transfer and dissemination of existing agents to new host populations (a process called "global microbial traffic"). For instance, cholera probably originated in Asia in ancient times; in the 19th century, it spread to Europe and the New World because of increased global travel. Cholera entered South America for the first time in 1992, through the possible contaminated bilge water released from a Chinese freighter. The causes of emerging infectious diseases and outbreaks require careful consideration of environmental changes and especially of anthropogenic factors.

Infection Control: First Line of Defense
Handwashing is the first line of defense against infection and is the single most important practice in preventing the spread of infection.

Between Agent and Reservoir

The first link in the chain of infection is between the agent and the reservoir. The keys to eliminating infection at this point in the chain are cleansing, disinfection, and sterilization. These tactics serve to prevent the formation of a reservoir or environment within which infectious agents can live and multiply.

Cleansing

Cleansing is the removal of soil or organic material from instruments and equipment used in providing client care. Nurses are involved in cleansing instruments after assisting or performing invasive procedures. To reduce the amount of contamination and loosen the material on reusable objects, the objects are cleansed prior to sterilization and disinfection. Cleansing involves the use of water, mechanical action, and, sometimes, a detergent. Contaminated objects are cleansed using a soft-bristled brush to scrub the surface. The steps for proper cleansing are:

1. Rinsing the object under *cold* water, because warm water causes proteins in organic material to coagulate and stick.
2. Applying detergent and scrubbing the object under running water using soft-bristled brush.
3. Rinsing the object under warm water.
4. Drying the object prior to sterilization or disinfection.

Infection Control: Cleansing
Cleansing presents a potential hazard to the nurse in the form of the splashing of contaminated material onto the body. Nurses should wear gloves, masks, and goggles during cleansing.

Disinfection

Disinfection is the elimination of pathogens, except spores, from inanimate objects. **Disinfectants** are chemical solutions used to clean inanimate objects. Bed pans, blood pressure cuffs, linens, stethoscopes, thermometers, and some types of endoscopes are disinfected in the hospital setting. The U.S. Environmental Protection Agency (EPA) licenses (registers) disinfection products and monitors the products to ensure that they work as claimed on the label (Pugliese, 1994). Common disinfectants are alcohol, sodium hypochlorite, quaternary ammonium, phenolic solutions, and glutaraldehyde.

A **germicide** is a chemical that can be applied to both animate (living) and inanimate objects for the purpose of eliminating pathogens. Antiseptic preparations such as alcohol and silver sulfadiazine are germicides.

Sterilization

Sterilization is the total elimination of all microorganisms including spores. Instruments that are used for invasive procedures must be sterilized. Methods of achieving sterilization are moist heat or steam, radiation, chemicals, and ethylene oxide gas. The method of sterilization depends on the type and amount of contamination and the object to be sterilized.

Autoclaving sterilization, which uses moist heat or steam, is the most common sterilization technique used in the hospital setting (Figure 21-10). Boiling water is not an effective sterilization measure, because some viruses and spores can survive boiling water. Objects that have been boiled in water for 15 to 20 minutes at 121°C (249.8°F) are considered clean but not sterile (Department of Labor, 1991).

Between Reservoir and Portal of Exit

Promoting proper hygiene, maintaining clean dressings and linens, and ensuring the use of clean equip-

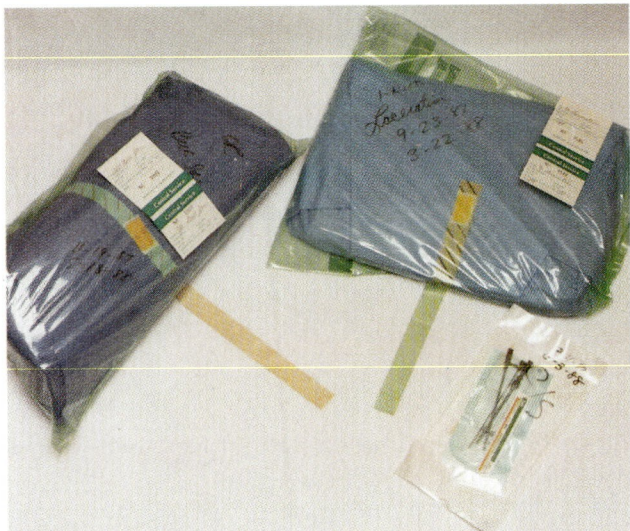

Figure 21-10 Sterilized packages. The strips below each package show the way they looked before sterilization. The strips on the packages have changed color because they have been sterilized.

ment in client care are the methods used to break the chain of infection between the reservoir and the portal of exit. The aim at this juncture is to eliminate the reservoir for the microorganism before the pathogen can escape to a susceptible host.

Proper Hygiene

The nurse must teach the client the importance of maintaining the cleanliness and the integrity of the skin and the mucous membranes. Clean skin, hair, and nails will maintain the body's normal flora and eliminate transient flora or infectious agents from the client's system. Bathing and handwashing are important means of eliminating the potential for infection. Clients should be encouraged to practice daily routines of bathing and teeth brushing. The nurse should assist clients who are unable to perform these activities independently.

Clean Dressings

Any open injury or other break in skin integrity represents a potential reservoir for infectious agents or portal of exit for a pathogen to be transferred to another individual. Dressings on open or oozing wounds must be changed and cleaned regularly. To protect both themselves and the client from infection, nurses must follow proper aseptic technique when changing dressings. This technique is discussed in detail later in this chapter.

Clean Linen

Bed linens, dressing gowns, and towels are catchalls for bodily secretions. Infectious agents can be easily transferred from one individual to the next through contact with a client's linens. Linens must be changed

HOME HEALTH CARE

Disinfection
In the home, Lysol and bleach are common disinfectants capable of eliminating several pathogens.

HOME HEALTH CARE

Sterilization at Home
Boiling water is still the best and most common sterilization measure used in the home. For example, boiling baby bottles and nipples makes them safe for use.

PROFESSIONAL TIP

The Client Who Is Bedridden
You should be alert to the formation of pressure ulcers in clients who are bedridden. Open ulcers are a possible source for infection if left untreated.

regularly, and soiled linens must be properly disposed. When changing linens, the nurse should take care to keep the soiled articles from coming into contact with the nursing uniform. This will prevent the nurse from contracting an infection from the soiled linens or passing the infection on to other clients in her care.

Clean Equipment

All equipment used in the care of a client must be cleansed and disinfected after each use. Although many items such as disposable gowns can be discarded after use, items such as beds and bed pans must be thoroughly cleansed after each use. Clients should be instructed never to share care items. Any nondisposable equipment used in an invasive procedure (such as equipment used in the operating room [OR]) must be sterilized before being used again. To protect themselves, nurses should wear gloves and masks when cleansing equipment to avoid being splashed with contaminated waste products or secretions.

Between Portal of Exit and Mode of Transmission

The goal in breaking the chain of infection between the portal of exit and the mode of transmission is to prevent the exit of the infectious agents. The nurse must maintain clean dressings on all injuries. Clients should be encouraged to cover the mouth and nose when sneezing or coughing, and the nurse must do so as well. Gloves must be worn whenever caring for a client who may have infectious secretions, and care must be taken to properly dispose of any article contaminated with secretions.

Between Mode of Transmission and Portal of Entry

To break the chain of infection between the mode of transmission and the portal of entry, nurses must ensure asepsis and wear barrier protection whenever the care of clients involves contact with body secretions. Gloves, masks, gowns, and goggles are all forms of barrier protection that can be used. Proper handwashing and the proper disposal of contaminated equipment and linens are also keys to preventing the transmission of microorganisms to other clients and health care workers. A thorough discussion of asepsis

and disposal of contaminated items is included later in this chapter.

Between Portal of Entry and Host

Maintaining skin integrity and using sterile technique for client contacts are methods of breaking the chain of infection between portal of entry and host. Avoiding needle sticks by properly disposing of sharps also reduces the potential for infection by denying a portal of entry. The goal at this point in the chain is to prevent the transmission of infection to a client or health care worker who has not yet been infected.

Between Host and Agent

Breaking the chain of infection between host and agent means eliminating infection before it begins. There are many ways whereby individuals can reduce their risk of acquiring infection. Proper nutrition, exercise, and immunizations allow an individual to maintain an intact immune system, thus preventing infection.

Proper Nutrition

Proper nutrition assists the body's immune system to function properly. Clients need adequate amounts of protein in their diets to maintain and repair tissue as well as to produce the antibodies needed to fight infection. A balanced diet also allows the body to maintain appropriate acid–base balance.

Exercise

Exercise maintains the body's metabolic rate and, therefore, allows the body to maintain the antibodies and energy necessary to ward off infection.

Immunization

Immunization is the process of creating immunity, or resistance to infection, in an individual. Most immunizations or vaccinations are given in early childhood; examples include vaccinations for measles, mumps, and rubella.

NORMAL DEFENSE MECHANISMS

A host's immune system serves as a normal defense mechanism against the transmission of infectious agents.

A unique feature of the immune system is its ability to recognize "self" and "nonself"; that is, the immune system recognizes which agents are not consistent with the genetic composition of the host (self). These agents are usually referred to as antigens (nonself). **Antigens** are foreign proteins that cause the formation of an antibody and react specifically with that antibody. An immune response is mounted against an antigen, which is recognized as nonself, to protect the body from infection. The immune defenses are categorized as nonspecific and specific immune defenses. Nonspecific and specific immune defenses work in harmony to defend the host from pathogens (Bouman, 1998; Porche, 1998).

Nonspecific Immune Defense

The nonspecific immune defense mounts a response to protect the host from all microorganisms; it is not dependent on prior exposure to the antigen. Nonspecific immune defenses are skin and normal flora; mucous membranes; sneezing, coughing, and tearing reflexes; elimination and acidic environment; and inflammation.

Skin and Normal Flora

The skin is the first line of defense against infection, serving as a physical barrier to infectious agents. Skin cells are shed daily, removing potentially harmful microorganisms. **Sebum** is a substance that is produced by the skin and contains fatty acids that kill some bacteria. The normal flora that reside on the skin and in the body compete with pathogenic flora for food and inhibit the multiplication of pathogens. The balance of normal flora may become disrupted, which allows pathogenic organisms to proliferate and cause infection or superinfection.

Mucous Membranes

Mucous membranes also function as a physical barrier to infectious agents. Mucus produced by these membranes entraps infectious agents and contains substances such as antibodies, lactoferrin, and lysozyme, which inhibit bacterial growth. For example, the cilia of the respiratory tract trap and propel mucus and microorganisms away from the lungs, thereby reducing the potential for infection.

Sneezing, Coughing, and Tearing Reflexes

The sneeze and cough reflexes physically expel mucus and microorganisms from the respiratory tract and oral cavity with force. Tears protect the eyes by continually flushing away microorganisms. Tears also contain **bactericides**, which are bacteria-killing chemicals.

Elimination and Acidic Environment

Elimination patterns and an acidic environment normally prevent microbial growth of pathogenic organ-

CLIENT TEACHING

Inappropriate Use of Antibiotics
- Do not pressure the physician to prescribe antibiotics for every illness. Antibiotics are not always appropriate, for instance antibiotics are not effective against viruses.
- When antibiotics are prescribed, instruct client to take *all* of the medication as directed.
- Antibiotics taken only until the client feels better, allows the microorganisms to become resistant to the antibiotic and the antibiotic will no longer be effective.
- Antibiotics also destroy normal flora microorganisms, and other illnesses may ensue.

isms. Resident flora of the large intestines prevent the growth of pathogens. The mechanical process of defecation evacuates the bowel of feces and microorganisms. Acidity of the urine prevents microbial growth. The flushing action of urination cleanses the bladder neck and urethra of microorganisms and prevents microorganisms from ascending into the urinary tract.

Normal vaginal flora prevent growth of several pathogens. At puberty, lactobacilli ferment and produce sugars in the vagina that lower the pH to an acidic range. The acidic environment of the vagina prevents pathogenic growth.

Inflammation

Inflammation is a nonspecific cellular response to tissue injury. Tissue injury caused by bacteria, trauma, chemicals, heat, or any other phenomenon releases multiple substances that produce dramatic secondary changes in the injured tissue (Figure 21-11). This entire complex of tissue changes and response to injury is referred to as the *inflammatory process* (Table 21-2). The inflammatory process has five stages, which facilitate the localization, neutralization, and resolution of the offending agent within the damaged tissue. The body's response to injury produces the characteristic local and systemic signs of inflammation.

Inflammation is not necessarily the result of invading microorganisms but does have signs and symptoms similar to those of an infection. The primary signs of inflammation and infection are as follows:

- Redness (erythema), the result of increased blood flow to the area
- Heat, the result of increased blood flow and metabolism in the area
- Pain, the result of increased pressure on pain sensors in the area
- Swelling (**edema**, a detectable accumulation of increased interstitial fluid), the result of fluid and

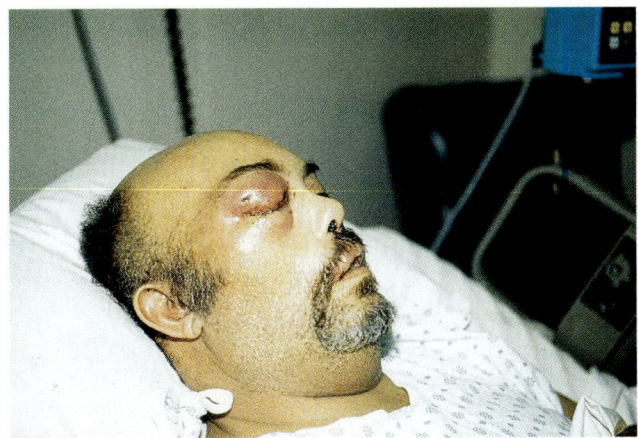

Figure 21-11 Cellulitis, an example of a bacterial infection, is marked by redness, swelling, and pain. *(Courtesy of Dr. Mark Dougherty, Lexington, KY)*

leukocytes entering the tissues from the circulatory system

- Loss of function, the result of both pain and swelling and the body's way of resting the injured part
- Pus (**purulent exudate**), the result of an infection, a secretion made up of white blood cells, dead cells, bacteria, and other debris

The intensity of the inflammatory process is usually in proportion to the degree of tissue injury. For example, when staphylococci invade the tissues, they release lethal cellular toxins that cause the inflammatory process to develop quickly; the staphylococcal infec-tion is characteristically walled off rapidly before the organism can multiply and spread. Streptococci, on the other hand, do not cause such intense local tissue de-struction, and the walling-off process develops slowly, allowing the organism to reproduce and migrate. Therefore, the streptococci have a far greater tendency than do staphylococci to spread throughout the body and cause death, even though staphylococci are far more destructive to the tissue (Guyton & Hall, 1995).

Specific Immune Defense

The specific immune defense mounts an immune response that is specific to the invading antigen. The specific immune defense is activated by the failure of phagocytes to completely destroy the antigen; this causes the production of T lymphocytes (T cells), which regulate the immune response by activating other cells. Stimulated T-cells are referred to as sensitized T cells. These T cells migrate to the area of injury and release chemical substances called **lymphokines**. Lympho-kines attract other phagocytes and lymphocytes to the area of injury and assist in antigen destruction.

The T cells also stimulate the production of B cells, which differentiate into plasma cells, producing anti-bodies specific to the antigen. **Antibodies** are protein substances that counteract and neutralize the effects of antigenic toxins and destroy bacteria and other cells. Antibodies destroy the antigen. The stimulation of B cells and the production of antibodies are collectively referred to as **humoral immunity**.

The B cell activation causes formation of memory B cells. Memory B cells remember the antigen and

Table 21-2 STAGES OF THE INFLAMMATORY PROCESS

STAGE	DESCRIPTION	RESULT
1	Initial injury precipitates release of chemicals: histamine, bradykinin, serotonin, prostaglandins (reaction products of the complement and blood-clotting systems), and lymphokines (hormonal substances released by sensitized T-cells).	Activates the inflammation process
2	Blood flow increases to the inflamed area (**erythema**).	Produces characteristic signs of redness and increased warmth
3	Increased capillary permeability with leakage of large quantities of plasma out of the capillaries and into the damaged tissue; tissue spaces and lymphatics are blocked by fibrinogen clots.	Initiates the inflammation process; "walls off" infection; results in nonpitting edema
4	Damaged tissue infiltrated by leukocytes, which engulf the bacteria and necrotic tissue. After several days, these leukocytes eventually die and form a cavity of necrotic tissue and dead leukocytes (mainly neutrophils and some macrophages).	Produces purulent exudate (pus)
5	Destroyed tissue cells are replaced by identical or similar structural and functioning cells and/or fibrous tissue.	Promotes tissue healing or the formation of fibrous (scar) tissue, which may reduce the functional capacity of the tissue.

From Fundamentals of Nursing: Standards & Practice, *by S. DeLaune and P. Ladner, 1998, Albany, NY: Delmar Publishers. Copy-right 1998 by Delmar Publishers. Reprinted with permission.*

prepare the host for future antigen invasion. Thus, when the antigen enters the body again, the immune response will occur more rapidly by producing antibodies faster. The formation of these antibodies is referred to as **acquired immunity**, which protects the individual against future invasions of already experienced antigens such as lethal bacteria, viruses, toxins, and even foreign tissues.

The process of **vaccination** (inoculation with a vaccine to produce immunity against specific diseases) provides acquired immunity. There are three ways an individual can be vaccinated:

- By the introduction of dead organisms that are no longer capable of causing disease but still have their chemical antigens, such as in the cases of typhoid fever, whooping cough, and diphtheria.
- By the introduction of toxins that have been treated with chemicals so that their toxic nature has been destroyed even though their antigens for causing immunity are still intact, such as for tetanus and botulism.
- By the introduction of live organisms that have been attenuated (grown in a special culture media or passed through a series of animals for mutation, rendering the organisms incapable of causing the disease yet still carrying the specific antigen), such as for poliomyelitis, yellow fever, measles, smallpox, and many other viral diseases (Guyton & Hall, 1995).

STAGES OF THE INFECTIOUS PROCESS

Activation of the immune response indicates the occurrence of infection. Infection results from tissue invasion and damage by an infectious agent. There are two types of infectious responses:

- **Localized infections**, which are limited to a defined area or single organ with symptoms that resemble inflammation (redness, tenderness, and swelling), such as a cold sore
- **Systemic infections**, which affect the entire body and involve multiple organs, such as AIDs

Localized and systemic infections progress through four stages: incubation, prodromal, illness, and convalescence.

Incubation Stage

The **incubation period** is the time interval between entry of an infectious agent in the host and the onset of symptoms. During this time period, the infectious agent invades the tissue and begins to multiply to produce an infection; the client is typically infectious to others during the latter part of this stage. For example, the incubation period for varicella (chickenpox) is 2 to 3 weeks; the infected person is contagious from 5 days before any skin eruptions to no more than 6 days after the skin eruptions appear.

Safety: Incubation Period

Always verify the incubation period of a suspected infection. Keep in mind that, depending on the infectious agent, a client may be able to transmit the infection to another person, even prior to the onset of symptoms.

Prodromal Stage

The **prodromal stage** is the time interval from the onset of nonspecific symptoms until specific symptoms of the infectious process begin to manifest. During this period, the infectious agent continues to invade and multiply in the host. A client may also be infectious to other persons during this time period. In the client with chickenpox, a slight elevation in temperature will occur during this stage, followed within 24 hours by eruptions of the skin.

Illness Stage

The **illness stage** is the time period when the client is manifesting specific signs and symptoms of an infectious process. The client with chickenpox will experience a further rise in temperature and continued outbreaks of skin eruptions for at least 2 to 3 more days.

Convalescent Stage

The period of time from the beginning of the disappearance of acute symptoms until the client returns to the previous state of health is referred to as the **convalescent stage**. The client with chickenpox will see the skin eruptions and irritation begin to resolve during this stage.

NOSOCOMIAL INFECTIONS

A **nosocomial infection** is an infection that was acquired in a hospital or other health care facility and was not present or incubating at the time of the client's admission. Nosocomial infections are also referred to as *hospital-acquired infections*. These types of infections typically fall into four categories: urinary tract, surgical wounds, pneumonia, and septicemia.

Nosocomial infections also include those infections that become symptomatic after the client is discharged, as well as infections passed among medical personnel. Most nosocomial infections are transmitted by health care personnel who fail to practice proper handwashing procedures or who fail to change gloves between client contacts (Compliance Control Center, 1998).

Hospitalized clients are at risk for nosocomial infections because the environment provides exposure to a variety of virulent organisms to which the client has not typically been exposed in the past; therefore, the

Nosocomial Infections

Each year more than 2,400,000 nosocomial infections occur in the United States. Annually, nosocomial infections directly cause 30,000 deaths and contribute to 70,000 more deaths. Further, the client's length of stay is increased, costing $2,300 per incident and $4.5 billion annually for the associated extended care and treatment (Compliance Control Center, 1998).

client has not developed any resistance to these organisms. In addition, illness, often the reason for hospital admission, impairs the body's normal defense mechanisms.

Nicolle and Garibaldi (1995) discuss the increased risk of infections in long-term care facilities. The most common endemic infections in this setting affect the urinary tract, upper and lower respiratory tracts, gastrointestinal tract, conjunctiva, and skin. The CDC estimates that 1.5 million cases of nosocomial infection occur annually in long-term care facilities and nursing homes. That is an average of one infection per year per client (Compliance Control Center, 1998).

Clients in long-term care facilities and hospitals often have multiple comorbidities (illnesses), which increases their risk of infection. For example, urologic abnormalities are associated with increased risk for urinary tract infections. Chronic obstructive lung disease and congestive heart failure increase a client's risk of developing pneumonia. Diabetes or vascular insufficiency may lead to more frequent and severe skin infections (pressure ulcers, cellulitis, and vascular ulcers). Because these high-risk clients are housed together, the transmission of pathogens is increased among residents. For instance, organisms may be transmitted through the air (e.g., tuberculosis, influenza), on the

Drug-Resistant Organisms

Nosocomial infections are receiving increased attention because of the development of drug-resistant organisms. The common drug-resistant nosocomial infections that occur in acute and long-term care facilities are vancomycin-resistant enterococci (VRE) (Hospital Infection Control Practices Advisory Committee [HICPAC], 1995), methicillin-resistant *S. aureus* (MRSA) (Hartstein, 1995), and multidrug-resistant (MDR) tuberculosis (TB) (Ikeda et al., 1995).

hands of staff members (e.g., *Staphylococcus aureus* or uropathogens), and by contaminated items (e.g., *E. coli*).

NURSING PROCESS

Quality nursing care requires the reduction of microorganism transmission in the health care environment. Infection-control practices are directed at controlling or eliminating sources of infection in the health care agency or home. Nurses are responsible for protecting clients and themselves by using infection-control practices.

Assessment

The nursing process facilitates an understanding of the scope of challenges inherent in the nursing care of clients at risk for infection. The assessment data guides the prioritization of the client's problem and the appropriate nursing diagnoses. Clients at risk for infection require frequent reassessment of status followed by appropriate changes in the plan of care, goals, and nursing interventions.

The health history and physical examination data are correlated with the laboratory indicators to identify those clients who are at risk for problems related to infection. Appropriate risk appraisals may be incorporated into the nursing health history interview.

Subjective Data

Key elements of relevant data regarding the client at risk for infection are obtained in the health history. During the nursing health history interview, the client's general health perception and management status are assessed to ascertain the ways and degree to which the client manages self-care. This information provides data regarding the client's routine self-care and health-promotion needs. Questions that relate specifically to habits that foster safe, healthy patterns of behavior are appropriate for home health and ambulatory care settings, as well as for inpatient settings.

A comprehensive nursing assessment also involves appraising the client's environment to detect potential hazards and the client's self-care abilities. The analysis of such factors as work environment, immunization status, and other health related issues alerts the nurse to actual or possible infection risks.

Objective Data

Objective data is gathered through the physical examination and the diagnostic and laboratory findings.

Physical Examination A complete health assessment includes a systematic physical examination, generally conducted from head to toe, in order to obtain objective data relative to the client's health status and presenting problems. When assessing the client to determine the level of risk for infection, the nurse should

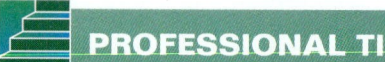

Questions Related to Infection Control

- What do you do to stay healthy?
- Do you have any health care concerns?
- Have you recently come in contact with some-one who has an infectious disease?
- Do you wash your hands before preparing food? After using the toilet?
- Do you keep meats and dairy products refriger-ated until ready to use?
- Have you traveled out of the country, especially to Third World countries, in the past 6 months?

focus the physical examination on the following areas and signs:

- Range of motion or total immobilization of an ex-tremity. (A client with limited mobility is at risk for developing joint contractures, skin breakdown, and muscle atrophy.)
- Localized infection as manifested by redness, swel-ling, warmth, tenderness, pain, and loss of move-ment in a specific body part.
- Systemic infection as manifested by fever with a corresponding increase in pulse and respirations; weakness; anorexia, with possible accompanying findings of nausea, vomiting, and diarrhea; enlarged and/or tender lymph nodes.
- Secretions or exudate of the skin or mucous mem-branes; crackles or wheezes in the lungs on auscul-tation.
- Condition of the skin. (Assessment of skin integrity provides data concerning a client's nutritional and hydration status, continuity of intact skin, hygienic practices, and overall physical abilities.)

Diagnostic and Laboratory Data The labora-tory indicators for an infection are:

- An elevated leukocyte (white blood cell [WBC]) and WBC differential:

  Neutrophils: increased in acute, severe inflammation

  Lymphocytes: increased in chronic bacterial and viral infections

  Monocytes: increased in some protozoan and rick-ettsial infections and TB

  Eosinophils and basophils: unaltered in an infec-tious process

- An elevated erythrocyte sedimentation rate (ESR): increased in the presence of inflammation
- An elevated pH of involved body fluids (gastric, urine, or vaginal secretions): indicative of microor-ganism presence

- Positive cultures of involved body fluids (blood, sputum, urine, or other drainage): indicative of mi-croorganism growth (Guyton & Hall, 1995).

Nursing Diagnosis

After data collection and analysis, the nurse is able to formulate a nursing diagnosis. The North American Nursing Diagnosis Association (NANDA) identifies one nursing diagnosis related to infection: *Infection, Risk for*.

Risk for infection is the state wherein an individ-ual is at increased risk for being invaded by patho-genic organisms (NANDA, 1999). The risk factors that increase a client's susceptibility to infections are as follows:

- Inadequate primary defenses (broken skin, trauma-tized tissue, decrease in ciliary action, stasis of body fluids, change in pH of secretions, and altered peri-stalsis)
- Inadequate secondary defenses (decreased hemoglo-bin, leukopenia, suppressed inflammatory response)
- Inadequate acquired immunity
- Immunosuppression
- Tissue destruction and increased environmental ex-posure
- Chronic disease
- Malnutrition
- Invasive procedures
- Pharmaceutical agents
- Trauma
- Rupture of amniotic membranes
- Insufficient knowledge to avoid exposure to patho-gens (NANDA, 1999)

Clients who are at risk for infection may have other associated physiologic and psychological concerns. The common nursing diagnoses that often accompany *Infection, Risk for* are:

- *Nutrition, Altered* (specify *Less than Body Require-ments or More than Body Requirements*)
- *Protection, Altered*
- *Tissue Integrity, Impaired*
- *Oral Mucous Membrane, Altered*
- *Skin Integrity, Impaired*
- *Knowledge Deficit* (specify)

This list indicates a number of related problems that must be considered when planning care for the client at risk for infection.

Planning/Outcome Identification

During the planning phase, the nurse collaborates with the client and other health care providers to de-termine the goals, outcomes, and interventions to re-duce the risk of infection. Identified outcomes provide direction for the nursing care that is implemented to reduce the risk of infection. Another critical element of the care plan is client and caregiver education related to the identification of potential hazards and health-promotion practices.

Implementation

Nurses are responsible for providing the client with a safe environment, which includes preventing the transmission of nosocomial infections. Nursing interventions to reduce the risk of infection center around ensuring asepsis and properly disposing of infectious materials to reduce or eliminate infectious agents. **Asepsis** refers to the absence of microorganisms. Providing nursing care using aseptic technique decreases the risk and spread of nosocomial infections. **Aseptic technique** is the infection-control practice used to prevent the transmission of pathogens. There are two types of asepsis: medical and surgical.

Medical Asepsis

The term **medical asepsis** refers to those practices used to reduce the number, growth, and spread of microorganisms. Medical asepsis is also referred to as *clean technique*. Objects are generally referred to as "clean" or "dirty" in medical asepsis. **Clean objects** are considered to have the presence of some microorganisms that are usually not pathogenic. **Dirty** (soiled) **objects** are considered to have a high number of microorganisms, some being potentially pathogenic. Common medical aseptic measures used for clean or dirty objects are handwashing, daily changing of linens, and daily cleansing of floors and hospital furniture.

Handwashing Handwashing is the rubbing together of all surfaces and crevices of the hands using a soap or chemical and water, followed by rinsing in a flowing stream of water. Handwashing is the most basic and effective infection-control measure to prevent and control the transmission of infectious agents. It is the single most important procedure for preventing nosocomial infections (Association for Professionals in Infection Control and Epidemiology [APIC], 1996).

The three essential elements of handwashing are soap or chemical, water, and friction. Soaps that contain antimicrobial agents are frequently used in high-risk areas such as emergency departments and nurseries. Friction physically removes soil and transient flora, and a flowing stream of water rinses it all away.

Infection Control: Handwashing

- Wash hands before and after every client contact.
- The most common cause of nosocomial infections is contaminated hands of health care providers.
- When in doubt, *wash your hands.*

Handwashing should be performed after arriving at work, before leaving work, before and after each client contact, after removing gloves, when hands are visibly soiled, before eating, after excretion of body waste (urination and defecation), after contact with body fluids, before and after performing invasive procedures, and after handling contaminated equipment. A washing time of 10 to 15 seconds is recommended to remove transient flora from the hands. High-risk areas such as nurseries usually require a handwash of approximately 2 minutes duration. Soiled hands usually require more time (APIC, 1996; CDC, 1991; Department of Labor, 1991).

Surgical Asepsis

Surgical asepsis, or sterile technique, consists of those practices that eliminate all microorganisms and spores from an object or area. Surgical asepsis refers to surgical handwashing, establishing and maintaining sterile fields, donning surgical attire (caps, masks, and eyewear), and sterile gloves, gowning, and closed gloving.

Surgical asepsis is practiced by the nurse in the OR, in labor and delivery, and for many diagnostic and therapeutic interventions at the client's bedside. Common nursing procedures that require sterile technique are as follows:

- All invasive procedures, either intentional perforation of the skin (injections, insertion of intravenous needles or catheters) or entry into a bodily orifice (tracheobronchial suctioning, insertion of a urinary catheter)
- Nursing measures for clients with disruption of skin surfaces (changing a surgical wound or intravenous site dressing) or destruction of skin layers (trauma and burns)

Surgical Handwashing Surgical handwashing or scrub is used to remove soil and microorganisms from the skin. Nurses working in the OR perform surgical handwashing to minimize the client's risk for infection. The skin on the nurse's hands and arms should be intact (free of lesions). Agency policy determines the way to perform the scrub with regard to method and timing.

Sterile Field and Equipment The nurse must establish and maintain a sterile field when performing those procedures that require sterile technique, such as inserting a urinary catheter or changing wound dressings. Agency policy and supplies vary in different health care settings; the nurse should review the agency's policy and gather all the necessary supplies before preparing the sterile field.

Donning Surgical Attire Surgical nurses are required to wear a surgical mask (Figure 21-12) and a clean cloth or paper cap that covers all of the hair. Protective eyewear (glasses or goggles) is worn during

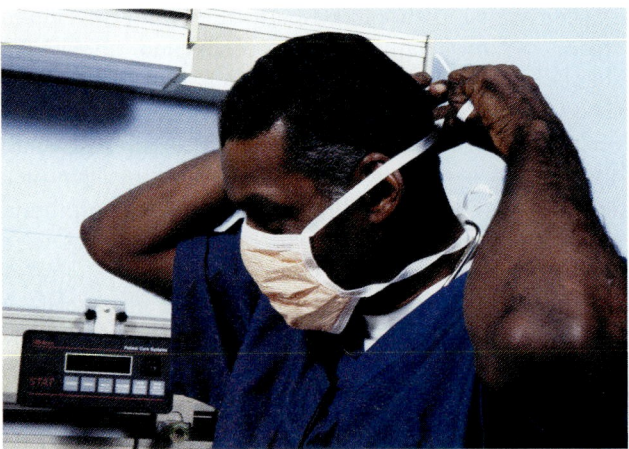

Figure 21-12 Putting on a Surgical Mask

all procedures that pose a threat of body fluids splashing into the eyes. Masks, caps, eyewear, gowns, and gloves are considered barrier precautions because they present a physical impediment to the spread of microorganisms.

Donning Sterile Gloves There are two methods of applying sterile gloves: open and closed. The open method is used most frequently when performing procedures that require the sterile technique, such as dressing changes. The closed method is used when the nurse wears a sterile gown.

Gowning and Closed Gloving Nurses in the OR and special procedure areas such as cardiac catheter labs use the closed gloved method when donning a sterile gown. After the surgical scrub, the nurse proceeds to don the sterile gown and gloves using the closed method. The sterile gown serves as a barrier to decrease the risk of wound contamination. The sterile gown also allows the nurse to move freely in the environment with sterile drapes and objects.

Disposal of Infectious Materials All health care facilities must have guidelines for the disposal of infectious-waste materials as required by the OSHA Act of 1991. The types of materials included are:

- Laboratory wastes
- Blood, blood products, and all other body fluids
- Client care items (soiled bed linen and protection pads, urinals, and bed pans)
- Disposable instruments
- Medication and soiled treatment items
- Surgical wastes

All health care workers must be diligent in observing the biological hazard symbol and handling all infectious materials as hazardous.

When disposing of infectious waste, all personnel must be careful to:

- Wear gloves;
- Use the proper containers (red or one labeled with the biological hazard symbol as required by the fa-

cility), leakproof plastic bags for waste from client areas (soiled dressings, gloves, linen), and sharps containers for needles, scalpels, and other sharp instruments or devices;
- Ensure that all infectious waste is properly labeled;
- Use care when handling plastic bags to avoid punctures and tearing;
- Disinfect carts used to carry infectious waste;
- Dispose of waste in designated areas only; and
- Wash hands after disposing of hazardous materials.

Containers for contaminated sharps should be readily accessible to personnel and maintained in an upright position.

Infection Control: Needle Disposal
- Used needles should not be recapped, bent, or broken.
- Needles should be placed in a puncture-resistant marked or color-coded container close to the work site.
- Correct disposal decreases the risk of needle punctures to caregivers.

Weltman, Short, and Mendelson (1995) studied disposal-related sharps injuries in a teaching hospital. Of the 361 persons in the study who reported sharps injuries, 72 of the injuries were related to sharps disposal. The majority of exposures to HBV and human immunodeficiency virus (HIV) were due to sharp objects.

Finkelstein and Mendelson (1998) report that results from multicenter studies estimate the transmission rate for HIV as being 0.36% after percutaneous exposure and for hepatitis C virus (HCV) as being 1.8% when injured by hollow-bore needles. Most health care workers acutely infected with HBV will eventually clear the virus, but 5% to 10% percent may develop chronic infection.

Evaluation

Evaluation of the effectiveness of nursing care is based on the achievement of goals and expected outcomes, regardless of the setting. Keeping the client free from infection requires frequent reassessment followed by timely adjustments made in the plan of care in order for nursing interventions to be effective.

It is imperative that the client be not only free of infection during hospitalization, but also helped in de-

HOME HEALTH CARE

Clients at Risk for Infection

Clients at risk for infection should have follow-up visits by the home health nurse to measure the effectiveness of client teaching and assess resources in the home to prevent the transmission of infections.

veloping a true awareness of the factors that increase the risk for infection. Adherence to barrier precautions is critical in preventing the spread of infectious agents, especially nosocomial infections to clients, self, and other health care workers. The nurse must correlate the client's diagnostic laboratory results and temperature in evaluating the expected outcome of remaining free of signs and symptoms of infection. If the nurse is caring for a client with an infection, the evaluation should indicate the stage of the inflammatory process.

SAMPLE NURSING CARE PLAN

THE CLIENT AT RISK FOR INFECTION

Mr. Filar, a 38-year-old homeless person, was struck and dragged by a speeding car as he crossed the street. He was taken to the hospital by ambulance. His left leg is broken, and there are lacerations and abrasions on his right side, arm, and leg. The left leg is in a cast and the lacerations have been sutured. Mr. Filar grimaces when he tries to move his legs, but he does not verbalize pain. Mr. Filar is very thin and says that he has not eaten for 2 days.

Nursing Diagnosis 1 *Infection, Risk for, related to inadequate primary defenses as evidenced by lacerations and abrasions*

PLANNING/GOALS	NURSING INTERVENTIONS	RATIONALE	EVALUATION
Mr. Filar will not have developed an infection in the lacerations and abrasions at discharge.	Thoroughly wash hands using antimicrobial soap before and after caring for Mr. Filar.	Antimicrobial soap is more effective in reducing microorganisms on hands.	Mr. Filar has some redness around one laceration.
	Use sterile technique when caring for lacerations and abrasions.	Prevents introduction of microorganisms into lacerations and abrasions.	
	Apply antibiotic ointment on abrasions, as ordered.	Promotes healing of abrasions.	
	Keep bed linens clean and dry.	Removes any drainage that may harbor microorganisms.	
	Administer oral antibiotics, as ordered.	Prevents or cures infection.	

Nursing Diagnosis 2 *Pain, related to physical injury as evidenced by facial grimacing*

PLANNING/GOALS	NURSING INTERVENTIONS	RATIONALE	EVALUATION
Mr. Filar will experience increased comfort and will verbalize that pain is under control within 24 hours.	Use pain scale to determine level of discomfort.	Provides objective measure of pain.	Mr. Filar states that he is experiencing less discomfort by 16 hours but that he still desires pain medication.
	Assist client to a position of comfort and elevate extremities.	Reduces pain and swelling by increasing blood return to the heart.	
	Administer analgesics, as ordered.	Provides comfort.	

continued

Nursing Diagnosis 3 *Nutrition, Altered, Less than Body Requirements, related to economic factors as evidenced by extreme thinness and not having eaten for 2 days*

PLANNING/GOALS	NURSING INTERVENTIONS	RATIONALE	EVALUATION
Mr. Filar will eat balanced meals while hospitalized.	Assist Mr. Filar to select foods high in protein, vitamins A and C, calcium, zinc, and copper. Provide between-meal snacks, especially milk or milk products.	Wound healing depends on the availability of protein, vitamins, and minerals. Snacks will increase overall caloric intake; increased protein will promote wound healing; increased calcium will promote bone healing.	Mr. Filar eats both everything on his meal trays and the between-meal snacks.

CASE STUDY

Mrs. Glassel has an open-wound ulcer on her right lower leg.

The following questions will guide your development of a nursing care plan for the case study.

1. What other assessment data should be gathered?
2. What nursing diagnosis is appropriate?
3. Identify two goals for Mrs. Glassel.
4. Identify appropriate nursing interventions.

SUMMARY

- Flora are microorganisms that occur or have adapted to live in a specific environment.
- Pathogens are microorganisms that cause disease; they include bacteria, viruses, fungi, protozoa, and *Rickettsia*.
- The elements of the chain of infection include the agent, the reservoir, the portal of exit, the modes of transmission, the portal of entry, and the host.
- The body has two primary defense mechanisms: the nonspecific immune defense, which protects the host from all microorganisms regardless of previous exposure, and the specific immune defense, which is a reaction to a specific antigen that the body has previously experienced.

- Infections progress through four stages: incubation, prodromal, illness, and convalescence.
- Handwashing must be done before and after every client contact and after removing gloves. It is the most important procedure for preventing nosocomial infections.
- Other means of preventing the spread of infection include cleansing equipment, cleansing soiled linen, changing dressings over wounds, practicing barrier precautions, maintaining skin integrity, and receiving all appropriate immunizations.
- The OSHA regulations mandate that sharps be properly disposed of immediately after use.

Review Questions

1. With regard to the chain of infection, the main focus of attention in infection control in a health care facility is the:

   a. portal of exit.
   b. infectious agent.
   c. susceptible host.
   d. mode of transmission.

2. The microorganisms that are always present on a person are called:

   a. resident flora.
   b. colonized flora.
   c. transient flora.
   d. communicable flora.

3. The most important procedure for preventing nosocomial infection is:

   a. sterilizing.
   b. handwashing.
   c. disinfecting.
   d. the use of bactericides.

4. A client with the flu is vulnerable to infection and is called a:

   a. susceptible host.
   b. infectious agent.
   c. compromised host.
   d. anthropogenic agent.

5. Living organisms that invade a host are called:

   a. animated agents.
   b. physical agents.
   c. chemical agents.
   d. biological agents.

6. Fomites are an example of which type of transmission?

   a. Contact
   b. Vehicle
   c. Airborne
   d. Vectorborne

7. Lyme disease and malaria are examples of diseases spread by:

   a. contact transmission.
   b. vehicle transmission.
   c. airborne transmission.
   d. vectorborne transmission.

8. The redness noted during the inflammation process is the result of:

   a. fluid entering the tissues.
   b. increased pressure in the area.
   c. increased blood flow to the area.
   d. increased metabolism in the area.

9. Vaccination provides which type of immunity?

   a. Humoral
   b. Acquired
   c. Antibody
   d. Lymphokine

10. A client is infectious to other persons during the:

    a. illness stage.
    b. prodromal stage.
    c. incubation period.
    d. convalescent stage.

Critical Thinking Questions

1. How are medical asepsis and surgical asepsis the same? How are they different?

2. How is the chain of infection applicable in everyday life in a person's home?

3. Why are nosocomial infections such a huge problem?

WEB FLASH!

- What resources can be found on the Internet about infection control and asepsis?
- Visit the Websites of the resources listed for this chapter at the end of the book. What type of information do they provide?

MAKING THE CONNECTION

Refer to the following chapters to increase your understanding of Standard Precautions and isolation:

- **Chapter 21, Infection Control/Asepsis**
- **Chapter 31, Nursing Care of the Client: Respiratory System**

- **Procedures:** B1, Handwashing; I2, Performing Open Gloving and Removal of Soiled Gloves; A1, Initiating Strict Isolation Precautions

LEARNING OBJECTIVES

Upon completion of this chapter, you should be able to:
- *Define key terms.*
- *Describe each of the eleven aspects of Standard Precautions.*
- *Identify the three transmission-based precautions and when each is to be used.*
- *Apply Standard Precautions in providing appropriate client care.*

KEY TERMS

Airborne Precautions
aseptic technique
barrier precautions
Contact Precautions
Droplet Precautions
endemic
epidemic
isolation
nosocomial infection
reverse isolation
Standard Precautions
Transmission-Based Precautions

INTRODUCTION

For over 120 years, health care facilities and their personnel have struggled to prevent the spread of infections among their clients. This chapter describes some of the historical methods as well as the current methods used to prevent the spread of infections.

HISTORICAL PERSPECTIVE

A hospital handbook published in 1877 recommended placing clients with infectious diseases in a separate facility (Lynch, 1949). These facilities became known as infectious-disease hospitals. Yet, **nosocomial infections** (infections acquired in the hospital that were not present or incubating at the time of the client's admission) continued in these facilities because the infected clients were not separated according to disease, and **aseptic technique** (infection-control practices used to prevent the transmission of pathogens) was seldom, if ever, practiced. To combat the

continuing problem of nosocomial infections in the infectious-disease hospitals, personnel began to set aside a floor or ward for clients with similar diseases (Gage, Landon, & Sider, 1959).

Nursing has always been at the forefront of preventing the spread of infections among clients and personnel. Infectious-disease hospital personnel began practicing aseptic technique as recommended in nursing textbooks published from 1890 to 1900 (Lynch, 1949). Isolation practices and the use of infectious disease hospitals were altered in 1910 when the cubicle system of isolation was introduced in U.S. hospitals (Gage et al., 1959). The cubicle system of **isolation** (separation from other persons, especially those with infectious diseases) placed clients in multiple-bed wards, with hospital personnel using a separate gown when caring for each client, washing their hands in an antiseptic solution after contact with each client, and disinfecting objects contaminated by any client. These nursing procedures were known as *barrier nursing*. Barrier nursing was aimed at preventing transmission of pathogenic organisms to other clients and to health care personnel. The cubicle system of isolation, including the barrier nursing procedures, gave the clients the alternative of receiving care in general hospitals instead of the infectious-disease hospitals (Centers for Disease Control and Prevention [CDC]/Hospital Infection Control Practices Advisory Committee [HICPAC], 1997a).

During the 1950s, infectious-disease hospitals closed, with the exception of the tuberculosis (TB) hospitals, which closed in the 1960s. Thus, by the end of the 1960s, clients with infectious diseases were cared for in general hospitals.

In 1970, the Centers for Disease Control and Prevention (CDC) published *Isolation Technique for Use in Hospitals* (National Communicable Disease Center, 1970), a revised edition of which was released in 1975 (CDC, 1975). This manual introduced and recommended seven categories of isolation: Strict Isolation, Respiratory Isolation, Protective Isolation, Enteric Precautions, Wound and Skin Precautions, Discharge Precautions, and Blood Precautions. By the mid 1970s, 93% of U.S. hospitals had adopted the recommendations of this book (Haley & Schactman, 1980).

By 1980, **endemic** (occuring continuously in a particular population and having low mortality) and **epidemic** (infecting many people at the same time, in the same geographic area) nosocomial infections were surfacing. Some of these infections were caused by multidrug-resistant (MDR) microorganisms, others by newly identified pathogens. Both types required isolation precautions different from those specified in any of the seven isolation categories. As Schaffner (1980) describes, isolation precautions needed to be directed more specifically at nosocomial transmission in special-care units rather than at community-acquired infectious diseases being spread within the hospital.

In 1983, the CDC replaced the 1975 isolation manual with the *Guideline for Isolation Precautions in Hospitals* (Garner & Simmons, 1983). One of the most important changes was the emphasis on decision making by the users as to which guideline was appropriate in a particular situation (Garner, 1984; Haley, Garner, & Simmons, 1985).

Another change was to rename Blood Precautions, primarily used for clients who were chronic carriers of hepatitis B virus (HBV), to Blood and Body Fluid Precautions, which now were to apply to clients with acquired immunodeficiency syndrome (AIDS); body fluids other than blood, such as semen and vaginal secretions; amniotic, cerebrospinal, pericardial, peritoneal, pleural, and synovial fluids; and any other body fluid visibly contaminated with blood. It did not apply to feces, nasal secretions, sputum, sweat, tears, urine, or vomitus unless blood was visible in them.

Until 1985, clients placed in isolation either had a confirmed diagnosis or were suspected of having an infectious disease. Mainly because of the human immunodeficiency virus (HIV) epidemic and those other bloodborne infections often yet unrecognized in a client, it was decided that Blood and Body Fluid Precautions were to be applied universally to all clients, regardless of their presumed infection status (CDC, 1985). Thus, the new name became Universal Precautions.

A new system of isolation called Body Substance Isolation (BSI) was proposed in 1987 as an alternative to the diagnosis-driven isolation system of the 1983 *Guideline for Isolation Precautions in Hospitals*. Body Substance Isolation focused on isolating all moist and potentially infectious body substances (blood, feces, urine, sputum, saliva, wound drainage, and other body fluids) from *all* clients. The use of gloves was the primary method of isolating infectious agents. However, BSI did not contain adequate provisions to prevent droplet transmission, direct or indirect contact transmission, or true airborne transmission of infections. Also, BSI recommended handwashing after removal of gloves only if the hands were soiled (Lynch, Jackson, Cummings, & Stamm, 1987), whereas Universal Precautions recommended handwashing after every removal of gloves (CDC, 1987; CDC, 1988).

In 1991, the Hospital Infection Control Practices Advisory Committee (HICPAC) was established to provide advice and guidance to the Secretary and Assistant Secretary of the U.S. Department of Health and Human Services (USDHHS), the Director of the CDC, and the Director of the National Center for Infectious Diseases (CDC/HICPAC, 1997a). The committee also provides advice to the CDC about updating guidelines and other policy statements related to the prevention of nosocomial infections.

The CDC, with the assistance of HICPAC, revised the *Guideline for Isolation Precautions in Hospitals* in 1996. The new guideline combined the major features of Universal Precautions and Body Substance Isolation into a single set of Standard Precautions, and the specific isolation categories into three Transmission-based Precautions (CDC/HICPAC, 1997b) (Figure 22-1).

The CDC recommendations are not subject to legal enforcement. However, regulations of the Occupational Safety and Health Administration (OSHA) must be followed by all health care facilities. These regulations, laws enforced through the Department of Labor (OSHA, 1991), ensure that Standard Precautions and Transmission-based Precautions are followed. According to OSHA regulations, all health care facilities must:

• Determine which employees have occupational exposure.

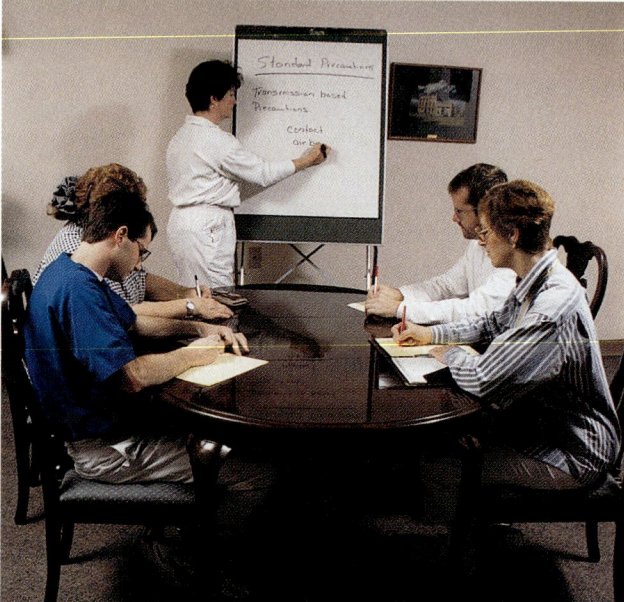

Figure 22-1 Hospital Personnel Reviewing Standard Precautions and Transmission-Based Precautions

- Provide hepatitis B vaccine free of charge to all employees with occupational exposure.
- Provide personal protective equipment (e.g., gowns, gloves, masks, goggles) for all employees with occupational exposure.
- Provide adequate handwashing facilities and supplies.
- Provide training regarding these rules to all employees with occupational exposure, both at hire and, then, annually.
- Provide evaluation and follow-up for any employee who experiences an exposure incident.
- Provide appropriate, properly labeled containers for contaminated sharps.
- Provide and prominently display an exposure control plan for staff to follow.

STANDARD PRECAUTIONS

Standard Precautions, listed on the inside back cover of this book, are preventive practices to be used in the care of all clients in hospitals regardless of diagnosis or presumed infection status. These guidelines

PROFESSIONAL TIP

Exposure Incident
- Immediately report all exposure incidents to the proper person in the health care facility.
- The OSHA regulations require initial screening and follow-up care.

CLIENT TEACHING

Standard Precautions
- Assist the client to understand that the techniques and procedures associated with Standard Precautions are designed to prevent the transmission of microorganisms and not to isolate the client.
- Explain why each technique and procedure is used.

are designed to reduce the risk of microorganism transmission from both recognized and unrecognized sources of infection in hospitals (CDC/HICPAC, 1997b).

Standard Precautions apply to:

- Blood
- All body fluids, secretions, and excretions *except* sweat, regardless of whether those fluids contain visible blood
- Nonintact skin
- Mucous membranes

Infection Control: Standard Precautions
- Standard Precautions must be practiced with all clients.
- Standard Precautions represent the most effective means of decreasing the risk of infection among clients and caregivers.

Barrier precautions, used to minimize the risk of exposure to blood and body fluids, involve the use of personal protective equipment, such as masks, gowns, and gloves, to create a barrier between the person and the microorganism and thus prevent transmission of the microorganism. Handwashing, however, is the most basic aspect of Standard Precautions. The other aspects of Standard Precautions are gloves; mask, eye protection, face shield; gown; client-care equipment; environmental control; linen; occupational health and bloodborne pathogens; and client placement.

Handwashing

Hands are to be washed after touching blood, body fluids, secretions, excretions, and contaminated items, regardless of whether gloves were worn. Hands must be washed, immediately after gloves are removed, between client contacts, and any other time when transfer of microorganisms to other clients or environments is possible. To prevent cross-contamination of different body sites on one client, it may be necessary to wash hands between tasks and procedures on that client.

Plain, nonantimicrobial soap is adequate for routine handwashing. An antimicrobial agent or waterless antiseptic agent is needed only for specific circumstances as defined by the facility's infection-control program.

Gloves

Clean, nonsterile gloves are to be worn when touching blood, body fluids, secretions, excretions, and contaminated items. Clean gloves should be put on just before touching mucous membranes and non-intact skin. Gloves must be changed between tasks and procedures being performed on one client if material that may contain microorganisms in high concentrations is touched. Gloves must be removed promptly after use and hands must be washed immediately before touching uncontaminated items or providing care to another client.

Safety: Latex Allergies
- Standard Precautions include the use of gloves when there is a possibility of contact with client body fluids.
- Be alert that health care personnel or the client may be allergic to the latex gloves. Reactions range from an eczematous contact dermatitis to anaphylactic shock.
- Prior to touching clients when wearing latex gloves, ask whether they have a known allergy to latex products. If they do, use non-latex gloves for those clients.

Mask, Eye Protection, Face Shield

A mask and eye protection or a face shield should be worn to protect the mucous membranes of the eyes, nose, and mouth when procedures and client–care activities are likely to generate splashes or sprays of blood, body fluids, secretions, or excretions.

Gown

A clean, nonsterile gown should be worn to protect the skin and prevent soiling of clothing during procedures and client-care activities that are likely to generate splashes or sprays of blood, body fluids, secretions, or excretions. A gown that is appropriate for the activity and potential amount of fluids should be selected. A soiled gown should be removed as promptly as possible, and the hands should be washed to prevent transfer of microorganisms to other clients or environments.

Client-Care Equipment

Client-care equipment soiled with blood, body fluids, secretions, or excretions must be handled in a manner to prevent skin and mucous membrane exposure, clothing contamination, and microorganism transfer to other clients or environments. Reusable equipment must not be used in the care of another client until it has been cleaned and sterilized appropriately. All single-use items must be properly discarded.

Environmental Control

The hospital must have adequate procedures for the routine care, cleaning, and disinfection of environmental surfaces, beds, bed rails, bedside equipment, and other frequently touched surfaces. All personnel must ensure that these procedures are followed.

Linen

Linen that is soiled with blood, body fluids, secretions, or excretions must be handled, transported, and processed in a manner to prevent skin and mucous membrane exposure, clothing contamination, and microorganism transfer to other clients and environments.

Occupational Health and Bloodborne Pathogens

Care must be taken to prevent injury when using needles, scalpels, and other sharp instruments and when handling, cleaning, and disposing of such items after use. The OSHA regulations state that "contaminated (used) sharps shall be discarded immediately or as soon as feasible in containers that are closable, puncture-resistant, leakproof on the sides and bottom and are labeled or color coded" (OSHA, 1996) (Figure 22-2).

Used needles should never be recapped by using both hands. A one-handed "scoop" method is acceptable. Used needles should never be removed from disposable syringes by hand, nor should they be bent,

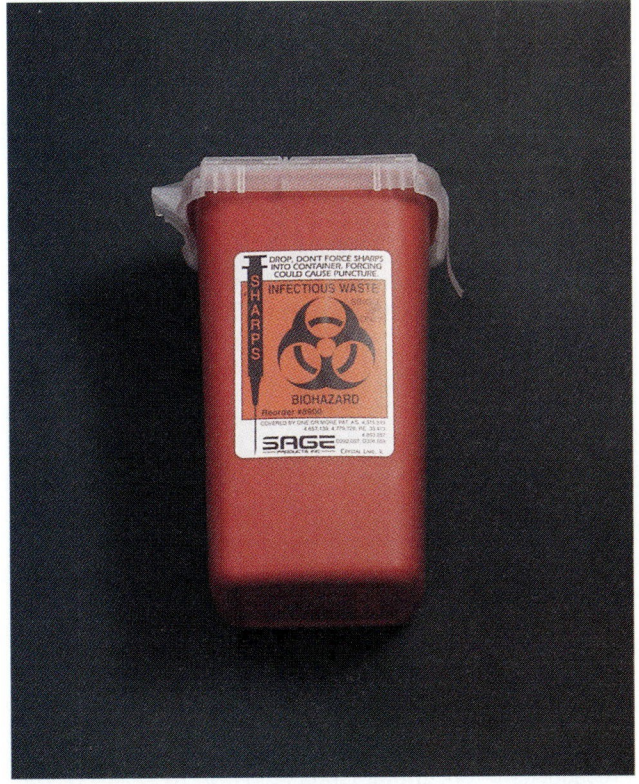

Figure 22-2 Sharps-Disposal Container

broken, or otherwise manipulated by hand. Disposable syringes and needles, scalpel blades, and other sharp items should be placed in designated puncture-resistant containers. Reusable syringes and needles should be placed in a separate puncture-resistant container and transported to the appropriate area for cleaning and sterilizing.

In areas where the need for resuscitation is predictable, mouth pieces, resuscitation bags, or other ventilation devices should be used instead of the direct mouth-to-mouth resuscitation method.

Client Placement

Any client who contaminates the environment or who does not or cannot be expected to assist with maintaining appropriate hygiene or environment control should be placed in a private room. When a private room in unavailable, infection-control professionals must be consulted.

ISOLATION

The 1996 CDC guideline eliminated the previous category-specific isolation precautions and condensed the former disease-specific precautions into three sets of precautions based on the route of transmission: airborne (Figure 22-3), contact (Figure 22-4), or droplet (Figure 22-5). These new, Transmission-Based Precautions are to be used *in addition to* the Standard Precautions. **Transmission-based Precautions** are practices designed for clients documented as or suspected of being infected with highly transmissible or epidemiologically important pathogens for which additional precautions beyond the Standard Precautions are required to interrupt transmission in hospitals (CDC/HICPAC, 1997b) (see Table 22-1).

The Transmission-based Precautions are also to be used in addition to the Standard Precautions in the

---

AIRBORNE PRECAUTIONS
(In addition to Standard Precautions)

VISITORS: Report to nurse before entering

Patient Placement
Private room that has:
  Monitored negative air pressure,
  6 to 12 air changes per hour,
  Discharge of air outdoors or HEPA filtration if recirculated.
Keep room door closed and patient in room.

Respiratory Protection
Wear an **N95 respirator** when entering the room of a patient with known or suspected infectious pulmonary **tuberculosis**.
Susceptible persons should not enter the room of patients known or suspected to have **measles** (rubeola) or **varicella** (chickenpox) if other immune caregivers are available. If susceptible persons must enter, they should wear an **N95 respirator**.(Respirator or surgical mask not required if immune to measles and varicella.)

Patient Transport
Limit transport of patient from room to essential purposes only.
Use **surgical mask** on patient during transport.

Figure 22-3 Transmission-Based Precautions: Airborne Precautions *(From Brevis Corporation, 3310 S. 2700, Salt Lake City, UT 84109. Copyright 1996 by Brevis Corporation. Reprinted with permission.)*

CONTACT PRECAUTIONS
(In addition to Standard Precautions)

VISITORS: Report to nurse before entering

Patient Placement
Private room, if possible. Cohort if private room is not available.

Gloves
Wear gloves when entering patient room.
Change gloves after having contact with infective material that may contain high concentrations of microorganisms (**fecal material** and **wound drainage**).
Remove gloves before leaving patient room.

Wash
Wash hands with an **antimicrobial** agent immediately after glove removal. After glove removal and handwashing, ensure that hands do not touch potentially contaminated environmental surfaces or items in the patient's room to avoid transfer of microorganisms to other patients or environments.

Gown
Wear gown when **entering** patient room if you anticipate that your clothing will have substantial contact with the patient, environmental surfaces, or items in the patient's room, or if the patient is **incontinent**, or has **diarrhea**, an **ileostomy**, a **colostomy**, or **wound drainage** not contained by a dressing. **Remove** gown before leaving the patient's environment and ensure that clothing does not contact potentially contaminated environmental surfaces to avoid transfer of microorganisms to other patients or environments.

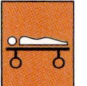

Patient Transport
Limit transport of patient to essential purposes only. During transport, ensure that precautions are maintained to minimize the risk of transmission of microorganisms to other patients and contamination of environmental surfaces and equipment.

Patient-Care Equipment
Dedicate the use of noncritical patient-care equipment to a single patient. If common equipment is used, clean and disinfect between patients.

Figure 22-4 Transmission-Based Precautions: Contact Precautions *(From Brevis Corporation, 3310 S. 2700, Salt Lake City, UT 84109. Copyright 1996 by Brevis Corporation. Reprinted with permission.)*

DROPLET PRECAUTIONS
(In addition to Standard Precautions)

VISITORS: Report to nurse before entering

Patient Placement
Private room, if possible. Cohort or maintain spatial separation of **3 feet** from other patients or visitors if private room is not available.

Mask
Wear mask when working within **3 feet** of patient (or upon entering room).

Patient Transport
Limit transport of patient to essential purposes only.
Use **surgical mask** on patient during transport.

Figure 22-5 Transmission-Based Precautions: Droplet Precautions *(From Brevis Corporation, 3310 S. 2700, Salt Lake City, UT 84109. Copyright 1996 by Brevis Corporation. Reprinted with permission.)*

Table 22-1 PRECAUTIONS RELATED TO TYPE OF DISEASE

PRECAUTION	TYPE OF DISEASE
Standard Precautions	All clients, regardless of disease or condition
Airborne Precautions	In addition to Standard Precautions, used for clients known to have or suspected of having serious illnesses spread by airborne droplet nuclei, including: • Measles • Varicella • Tuberculosis

Contact Precautions	In addition to Standard Precautions, used for clients known to have or suspected of having serious illnesses easily spread by direct client contact or contact with fomites, including:
	• Wound infections
	• Gastrointestinal infections
	• Respiratory infections
	• Skin infections including:
	   Herpes simplex
	   Impetigo
	   Major abscesses, cellulitis, or pressure ulcers
	   Pediculosis
	   Scabies
	   Varicella (Zoster)
	• Viral hemorrhagic infections (Ebola)

Droplet Precautions	In addition to Standard Precautions, used for clients known to have or suspected of having illnesses spread by large particle droplets, including: • Meningitis • Adenovirus • Pneumonia • Influenza • Diphtheria • Mumps • Pertussis • Rubella • Scarlet fever • Parvovirus 19

From Table I Synopsis of Types of Precautions and Patients Requiring Precautions *[On-line], by Centers for Disease Control and Prevention (CDC)/Hospital Infection Control Practices Advisory Committee (HICPAC), 1997c, Available: www.cdc.gov/ncidod/hip/isolat/isotab_1.htm*

event of suspicious infections and with clients who are immunosuppressed either from disease or chemotherapy. More than one of the transmission-based precautions is used at the same time for clients with certain infections or conditions.

Isolation precautions are usually ordered by the physician; however, nurses may initiate these precautions whenever a nursing diagnosis related to the infectious process is identified, for example, *Infection, Risk for, related to decreased resistance of immune system.* Most agencies require nurses to obtain a culture from a draining body area and to initiate isolation precautions when positive cultures are reported. After isolation precautions have been instituted, visitors and all personnel should comply with the agency's policy regarding isolation precautions. Signs should be posted in a prominent location outside the client's room. The signs should indicate the type of isolation precautions and preparation required prior to entering the room (Figure 22-6). The necessary supplies should be readily available.

Clients requiring isolation should be placed in a private room with adequate ventilation and should have their own supplies. Personal belongings should be kept to a minimum, and health care providers

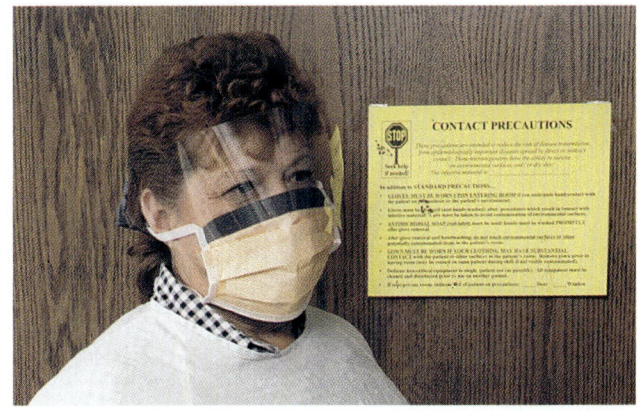

Figure 22-6 Sign on Door to Client's Room Indicating Type of Isolation Precaution and Preparation Needed Prior to Entering Room

should use disposable supplies and equipment whenever possible. All articles leaving the room, such as soiled linen and collected specimens, should be labeled and either placed in impermeable bags or double bagged.

Reverse isolation, also known as protective isolation, is a barrier protection designed to prevent infection in clients who are severely compromised and highly susceptible to infection. This includes clients who:

- are taking immunosuppressive medications
- are receiving chemotherapy or radiation therapy
- have diseases such as leukemia, which depress resistance to infectious organisms
- have extensive burns, dermatitis, or other skin impairments that prevent adequate coverage with dressings

These clients are at increased risk for infection from their own microorganisms, contact with health care workers whose hands have not been properly washed, and exposure to improperly disinfected and nonsterile items such as air, food, water, and equipment. Nursing responsibilities toward these clients include ensuring that everyone entering the client's room has completed a meticulous handwashing and is properly attired in

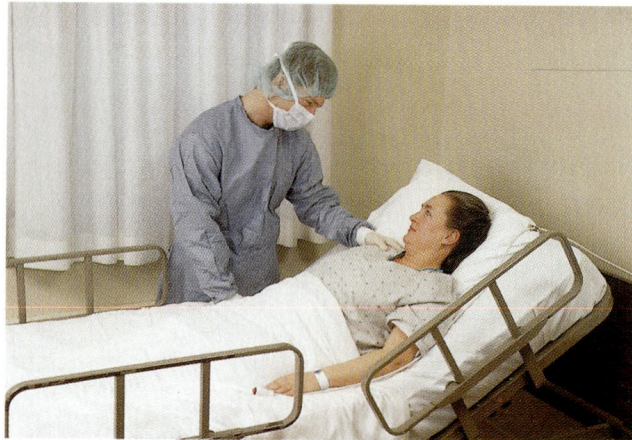
Figure 22-7 Nurse Interacting with Client Requiring Isolation Precautions

gown, gloves, and mask; ensuring that the client's environment is as clear of pathogens as possible; and knowing the institutional policy regarding caring for clients requiring reverse isolation.

CLIENT RESPONSES TO ISOLATION

Isolation precautions are for the client's protection; however, clients who are placed on isolation precautions may experience psychological discomfort (Figure 22-7). Nurses should be alert to symptoms of anxiety, depression, rejection, guilt, or loneliness. Clients should be educated on those isolation precautions that will be practiced and their purposes. Nurses should encourage clients to verbalize their feelings regarding the isolation precautions and should provide the client with intellectual stimulation and diversional activities such as paperback books, crossword puzzles, music, radio, or television. Visitors should be encouraged as a method to alleviate the client's feelings of isolation and loneliness. Wearing appropriate barrier precautions, visitors can safely enter an isolated client's room.

SUMMARY

- Standard Precautions are to be used when caring for *every* client.
- Airborne Precautions are to be used when caring for clients who have or may have serious illnesses spread by airborne droplet nuclei.
- Droplet Precautions are to be used when caring for clients who have or may have serious illnesses spread by large-particle droplets.
- Contact Precautions are to be used when caring for clients who have or may have serious illnesses spread by direct client contact or fomite contact.

PROFESSIONAL TIP

Psychological Interventions for Clients in Isolation

- Explain the pertinent isolation procedures and rationales
- Discuss the client's feelings about the isolation procedures
- Convey a sense of empathy and understanding
- Permit visitors in accordance with isolation precautions
- Support existing coping mechanisms
- Visit the client

CASE STUDY

Joe Spanutius is admitted with a diagnosis of influenza. After 24 hours, the nurses question whether he may also have pediculosis. The physician is out of town for the day.

The following questions will guide your development of a nursing care plan for this case study.

1. On admission, what precautions should be followed for Mr. Spanutius?
2. What additional precautions, if any, should the nurses follow until the physician sees Mr. Spanutius again?
3. What equipment is required and should be available for persons entering Mr. Spanutius' room right after admission?
4. What equipment is required and should be available for persons entering Mr. Spanutius' room after 24 hours?

Review Questions

1. In 1996, the revised *Guideline for Isolation Precautions in Hospitals* combined Universal Precautions and Body Substance Isolation into:
   a. Barrier Precautions.
   b. Contact Precautions.
   c. Standard Precautions.
   d. Transmission-Based Precautions.

2. The use of masks, gowns, and gloves is termed:
   a. Droplet Precautions.
   b. Barrier Precautions.
   c. Contact Precautions.
   d. Standard Precautions.

3. The nursing action most basic to Standard Precautions is:
   a. gloving.
   b. gowning.
   c. handwashing.
   d. wearing a face mask.

4. Airborne Precautions require:
   a. paper masks.
   b. a private room.
   c. the wearing of gloves.
   d. the wearing of a gown.

5. Contact Precautions require:
   a. a private room.
   b. the wearing of a mask.
   c. the wearing of a gown.
   d. the wearing of gloves.

6. Those precautions to be used in the care of all clients in hospitals regardless of diagnosis or presumed infection status are called:
   a. Standard Precautions.
   b. Airborne Precautions.
   c. Universal Precautions.
   d. Body Substance Isolation.

Critical Thinking Questions

1. How are the three Transmission-Based Precautions the same? How are they different?

2. When, where, and why are Standard Precautions to be implemented?

 ## WEB FLASH!

- What type of information is available on the Web about Standard Precautions?
- What Web site might you recommend to a client or family for information about Transmission-Based Precautions?

FLUID, ELECTROLYTE, AND ACID–BASE BALANCE

MAKING THE CONNECTION

Refer to the following chapters to increase your understanding of fluid, electrolyte, and acid–base balance:

- **Chapter 18, Basic Nutrition**
- **Chapter 21, Infection Control/Asepsis**
- **Chapter 22, Standard Precautions and Isolation**
- **Chapter 24, Medication Administration**
- **Chapter 25, Assessment**
- **Chapter 30, Nursing Care of the Oncology Client**
- **Chapter 31, Nursing Care of the Client: Respiratory System**
- **Chapter 32, Nursing Care of the Client: Cardiovascular System**
- **Chapter 33, Nursing Care of the Client: Blood and Lymph Systems**
- **Chapter 34, Nursing Care of the Client: Gastrointestinal System**
- **Chapter 37, Nursing Care of the Client: Endocrine System**
- **Chapter 42, Nursing Care of the Client: Urinary System**

LEARNING OBJECTIVES

Upon completion of this chapter, you should be able to:
- *Define key terms.*
- *Discuss the importance of pH regulation in the body.*
- *Describe the three buffer systems of the body.*
- *Describe and give examples in the body of diffusion, osmosis, and filtration.*
- *Name the fluid compartments, the fluids contained in them, and the function of those fluids.*
- *Describe the way the kidneys work to maintain fluid and electrolyte balance.*
- *Describe the way the lungs work to maintain pH in the body.*
- *Detail causes, assessment data, nursing interventions, and criteria for evaluating effectiveness of care for clients with a nursing diagnosis of* Fluid Volume Deficit *or* Fluid Volume Excess.
- *Detail causes, assessment data, nursing diagnoses, nursing interventions, and criteria for evaluating the effectiveness of nursing care for clients with sodium, potassium, calcium, and magnesium imbalances.*
- *Relate principles of nursing management for clients receiving fluids and electrolytes via oral supplements, intravenous solutions, enteral feedings, and total parenteral nutrition.*
- *Differentiate the causes, assessment data, and nursing management of metabolic and respiratory acidosis and alkalosis.*
- *Use the nursing process to plan care for a client experiencing a fluid, electrolyte, and/or acid–base imbalance.*

KEY TERMS

acid	crenation
acidosis	decomposition
alkalosis	dehydration
anion	dialysis
arterial blood gases	diffusion
atom	edema
base	electrolyte
buffers	elements
cation	extracellular fluid
compound	filtration

KEY TERMS *(continued)*

hemolysis	matter
homeostasis	mixture
hydrostatic pressure	molecule
hypertonic solution	osmolality
hypotonic solution	osmolarity
hypoxemia	osmosis
infiltration	osmotic pressure
interstitial fluid	oxidized
intracellular fluid	permeability
intravascular fluid	salt
intravenous therapy	semipermeable
ion	membrane
isotonic solution	synthesis
isotope	turgor

INTRODUCTION

The external environment within which we live undergoes continual changes, both small and large. For example, the daily and seasonal temperatures may fluctuate over a wide range. The light intensity may be bright on sunny days and less so on cloudy days. The humidity may be either high or low. These are just a few of the many factors that may change constantly in the external environment. Our bodies must continually adjust to such changes in the external environment. In order for life to continue, however, our internal environment—the one inside our bodies—must remain relatively constant, varying only slightly within narrow ranges. This internal environment consists of the various body fluids such as the fluid inside cells, the blood, tissue fluids that bathe the cells, and other fluids. Constant maintenance of the internal environment within very narrow limits—in equilibrium—is termed **homeostasis**.

HOMEOSTASIS

Homeostasis is an ongoing process; that is, the body simply does not reach a state of equilibrium and remain there. Small changes constantly occur in response to the physiologic processes, which take place at all times. As a result, changes occur in the internal environment. The body must therefore continuously make subtle adjustments to maintain the constancy of the internal environment within a range of normal values.

Homeostasis is accomplished by various physiologic processes and the coordinated activities of the organ systems. Some examples are as follows:

- The gastrointestinal (GI) system changes large, complex molecules of ingested food to simpler, less-complex molecules that can be utilized by the cells of the body to produce the energy necessary for life.
- The respiratory system supplies the cells with the constant source of oxygen required to release the energy from the products of digestion.
- The respiratory system also eliminates carbon dioxide, the waste product produced by the cells as a result of energy production.
- The blood acts as a transport mechanism, carrying the products of digestion along with hormones and oxygen to the cells, where these substances are utilized.
- The blood also transports carbon dioxide from the energy-releasing processes of the cells to the lungs, where it will be eliminated.
- All of the activities of the various organ systems are integrated and coordinated through the nervous system and the endocrine system.

When the body loses the ability to maintain homeostasis, and the internal environment changes, the physiologic processes can be interrupted or changed, leading to disease, disorder, or death. In essence, then, maintaining homeostasis is essential to life. Because the processes of homeostasis involve many chemical and physical processes, it is necessary to examine some of these before studying homeostasis in more detail.

CHEMICAL ORGANIZATION

The human body is highly organized. This organization exists in increasing levels of complexity. Most basic is the chemical level. To understand the higher levels of organization, it is necessary to know something about basic chemical and physical principles.

Elements

The cell consists of living matter. **Matter** is anything that occupies space and possesses mass. All matter has certain physical properties such as color, odor, hardness, and density. Matter also has extensive properties such as size, shape, and weight. Matter is composed of basic substances called **elements**. Elements are made of tiny units called atoms. Atoms of each element are alike. Different elements have different kinds of atoms. Presently, 108 elements are recognized. Some examples are iron, gold, carbon, hydrogen, oxygen, nitrogen, and copper. Many of the elements occur in the human body in varying amounts. Some are present in large amounts, and others are found in only trace amounts. The four elements oxygen, carbon, hydrogen and nitrogen constitute more than 95% of the total body weight of the elements. Some of the elements and their function in the body are presented in Table 23-1.

Atoms

An **atom** is the smallest unit of chemical structure, and no chemical change can alter it. Atoms are made

Table 23-1   ELEMENTS OCCURRING IN THE HUMAN BODY

ELEMENT	APPROXIMATE % OF BODY WEIGHT	FUNCTION
Major Elements		
Oxygen	65.0	Found in both organic and inorganic compounds; as a gas, is necessary in metabolizing glucose and other chemical compounds into energy
Carbon	18.5	Found in all organic compounds such as carbohydrates, protein, lipids, and nucleic acids; necessary for cellular respiration
Hydrogen	9.5	Found in many organic and inorganic compounds; in ionic form, involved in pH; component of water; necessary for life
Nitrogen	3.2	Important in proteins, which are the body building blocks, an energy source, and a component of hormones
Calcium	1.5	Important element in bone and tooth composition; involved in nerve conduction, muscle contraction, and blood clotting
Phosphorus	1.0	Found in bones, teeth, the high-energy carrying compound adenosine triphosphatase (ATP), some proteins, and nucleic acid
Potassium	0.4	Major electrolyte in intracellular fluid; important in muscle contraction and transmission of nerve impulses; activates enzymes; influences cellular osmotic pressure; involved in kidney function and acid–base balance
Sulfur	0.3	Found in some proteins, nucleic acids, and some vitamins and hormones
Sodium	0.2	Constitutes major electrolyte in extracellular fluid; important in osmoregulation and acid–base balance; necessary for nerve transmission and muscle contraction
Chlorine	0.2	Found in extracellular fluid; important in water balance, acid–base balance, and production of hydrochloric acid in the stomach
Magnesium	0.1	Important to muscle and nerve function and bone formation and in some coenzymes
Essential Trace Elements		
Present in the human body in minimal amounts, constituting approximately 0.1% of body weight; have known functions		
Cobalt		Important component of vitamin B_{12}
Copper		Necessary for formation of hemoglobin and for bone development
Chromium		A cofactor involved with enzymes for fat, cholesterol, and glucose metabolism
Flourine		Gives hardness to teeth and bones
Iodine		Necessary for synthesis of thyroid hormone
Iron		Necessary for transportation of oxygen by hemoglobin
Manganese		Necessary in activating some enzymes
Selenium		Acts with vitamin E as an antioxidant; component of teeth
Zinc		Found in some enzymes; needed for protein metabolism and carbon dioxide transport
Other Trace Elements		
Have probable, but as yet undetected, functions		
Aluminum Nickel Arsenic Tin Boron Silicon Cadmium Vanadium		

up of three basic particles: protons, neutrons, and electrons. Protons and neutrons are similar in size, but whereas protons have a positive electrical charge, neutrons have no charge. Together, they form the nucleus of the atom. Because the protons have a positive charge and the neutrons are neutral, the nucleus of an atom has a positive charge. The electrons have a negative charge and move in an orbit around the nucleus. There are as many electrons as protons, rendering the overall atom neutral. The number of protons in an atom is called its atomic number. The simplest element is hydrogen. It has an atomic number of 1. One proton with a positive charge forms the nucleus, and one electron moves in an orbit around the nucleus. Hydro-

gen atoms may or may not have a neutron. A hydrogen atom is illustrated in Figure 23-1.

Depending on the element, other atoms may have more than one proton and one electron shell and may have neutrons. The number of protons and neutrons in the nucleus is approximately equal to the atomic weight. Thus, hydrogen has an atomic weight of 1.

Isotopes

The number of protons in the nucleus is the same for all atoms of a given element, but the number of neutrons may vary in atoms of the same element. For instance, all hydrogen atoms have one proton and one electron. However, whereas some hydrogen atoms

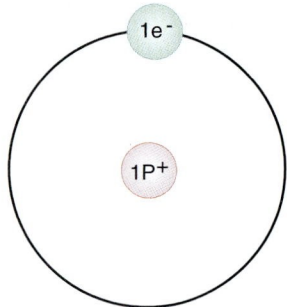

Figure 23-1 Hydrogen Atom Showing Positively Charged Proton in the Nucleus and Negatively Charged Electron in Orbit

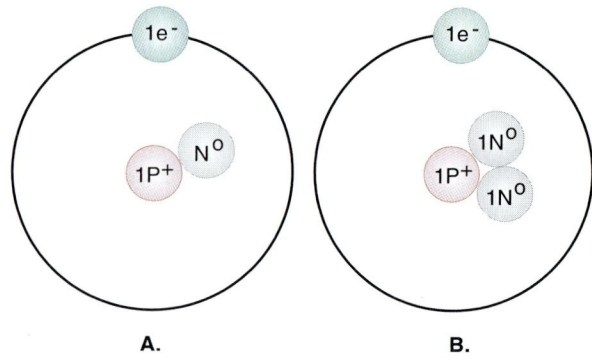

A.　　　　　　　　　　**B.**

Figure 23-2 Isotopes of Hydrogen: A. Deuteridium has one positively charged proton and one neutron in the nucleus and one electron in orbit; B. Tritium has one positively charged proton and two neutrons in the nucleus and one electron in orbit.

have one neutron in the nucleus, others have two (Figure 23-2). Atoms of the same element that have different atomic weights (i.e., have a different number of neutrons) are called **isotopes**. All of the isotopes of a given element react chemically in the same way.

Some isotopes, called radioactive isotopes, have an unstable nucleus, which decomposes and gives off energy in the form of radiation. This radiation can be in the form of alpha, beta, or gamma rays. All are damaging to cells. Alpha radiation is the least harmful, and gamma radiation is the most harmful. Iodine, oxygen, and cobalt are examples of elements having radioactive isotopes. Some of the radioactive isotopes are useful as biological markers and can be used to track metabolic pathways of food. Others such as iodine[131] can be injected in the body and used to track the circulation of blood. Still others such as cobalt[60] are used in cancer treatment.

Molecules and Compounds

Atoms of the same element can unite with each other to form a **molecule**. For example, atoms of hydrogen unite to form a hydrogen molecule. This can be expressed in a chemical equation using the chemical symbol for hydrogen:

$$H + H \rightarrow H_2$$

In this reaction, the atoms on the left are the reactants; the arrow is read as "yield"; and the last symbol is the product—a molecule of hydrogen. A chemical equation uses the chemical symbols of elements and shows the ratios by which they combine. Because atoms of elements always combine in the same ratio under similar conditions, it is possible to predict the nature of a chemical change.

When atoms of two or more different elements combine (react) they form a **compound**. For example, if one atom of sodium (Na) and one atom of chlorine (Cl) react, they form a molecule of the compound called sodium chloride. This is expressed in the following equation:

$$Na + Cl \rightarrow NaCl$$

Compounds can be divided into two groups. Those without carbon are inorganic compounds, and those with carbon are organic compounds. By using chemical equations, chemical changes, called chemical reactions, can be shown. Sometimes, different substances are combined in no specific way, and the components do not have a definite ratio every time. For instance, water, sugar, and table salt mixed without being measured will yield different results depending on the ratio of each substance. Such a combination is called a **mixture**. Its composition may vary each time the components are mixed.

Chemical reactions occur whenever atoms join together or separate. They join together by forming bonds, and they separate by breaking bonds. Either way, new combinations result. When two or more atoms (reactants) bond and form a more complex molecular product, the reaction is called **synthesis**. A sample equation would be as follows:

$$2H + O \rightarrow H_2O$$
hydrogen and oxygen yields water

When the bonding between the atoms in a molecule is broken and simpler products are formed, the reaction is called **decomposition**. If a molecule of sodium chloride is decomposed it forms sodium and chlorine. This can be expressed as follows:

$$NaCl \rightarrow Na + Cl$$
sodium chloride yields sodium and chloride

(decomposition)

It is important to understand that when synthesis occurs, energy is tied up in the bonds formed during the reaction. When decomposition occurs, energy is released. In the cells of the body, these kinds of chemical reactions are repeatedly occurring: Molecules form and decompose. Body cells can utilize these reactions to form energy sources and to free energy to drive the various metabolic processes of the cells.

Ions

When some compounds are placed in water, they decompose, or ionize. The result is an **ion**, an atom bearing an electrical charge. An ion with a positive charge is called a **cation**; an ion with a negative charge is termed an **anion**. For example, sodium chloride in water dissociates to form sodium ions bearing a positive charge and chloride ions bearing a negative charge (Figure 23-3). Because the atoms in this combination are charged, they will conduct electricity. The reaction can be shown as follows:

$$NaCl \rightarrow Na^+ + Cl^-$$

sodium chloride yields sodium and chloride
                                (cation)   (anion)

A compound that dissociates into ions in water is called an **electrolyte**. Many electrolytes are extremely important in body chemistry; some of these are listed in Table 23-2.

WATER

Water constitutes approximately 60% of the total body weight of an adult and is involved in many of the physical and physiological processes of the body. Because water is so integral to the body's processes, fluctuations in the amount of water in the body can have harmful or even fatal consequences.

Water is the major component of blood. Approximately 92% of the body's organic and inorganic compounds dissolve in this water into less-complex molecules and atoms and then are transported throughout the body. Necessary substances such as oxygen and nutrients from the GI system are carried to the cells, where they are utilized. Cellular waste products such as carbon dioxide, urea, and excessive minerals are carried by water to sites of elimination: carbon dioxide to the lungs, urea and minerals to the kidneys.

Table 23-2 IMPORTANT ELECTROLYTES IN BODY FLUIDS

FORMULA	CHEMICAL NAME
NaCl	Sodium chloride
Na_2SO_4	Sodium sulfate
Na_2HPO_4	Disodium phosphate
$NaHCO_3$	Sodium bicarbonate
MgCl	Magnesium chloride
$CaCl_2$	Calcium chloride
KCl	Potassium chloride

LIFE CYCLE CONSIDERATIONS

Body Water and Body Size

The amount of body water is inversely proportional to body size. The smaller the body, the higher the water content:

Embryo:	97%
Infant:	77%
Child:	60% to 77%
Adult:	60%
Elders:	45% to 50%

Body water diminishment in elderly persons is related to tissue loss.

Water also absorbs heat resulting from muscle contractions and distributes this heat over the body. Water in the form of perspiration released from sweat glands in the skin can cool the body by evaporation. Water also can break apart the bonds in large molecules such as starches to form smaller molecules in the digestive process. This type of reaction is called *hydration*.

GASES

Two important gases in the body are oxygen (O_2) and carbon dioxide (CO_2). Because these elements are gases, their molecules are free and can move swiftly in all directions. Oxygen enters the body through the lungs and is transported by the red blood cells throughout the body to the cells. The cells use oxygen in the release of energy from glucose and other molecules. This energy is needed by the cells to carry out their activities. As a result of the energy-releasing processes, carbon dioxide is produced by the cells and transported in the blood to the lungs, where it is eliminated.

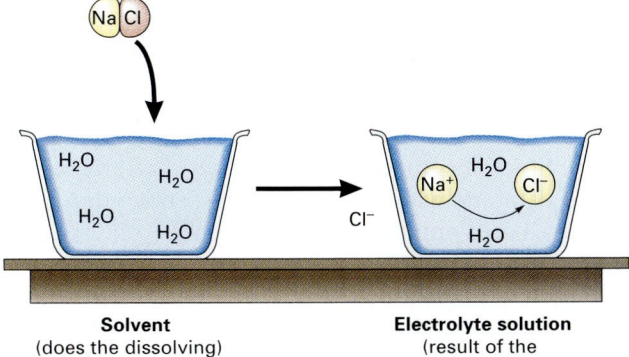

Solute
(the thing being dissolved)

Solvent
(does the dissolving)

Electrolyte solution
(result of the dissolving process)

Figure 23-3 Dissociation of Electrolytes

ACIDS, BASES, SALTS, AND PH

Other chemical substances important for life are acids, bases, and salts; pH is the measure of acid and base strength.

Acids

An **acid** is any substance that in solution yields hydrogen ions bearing a positive charge. As an example, hydrochloric acid (HCl) in water dissociates as shown following:

$$HCl \rightarrow H^+ + Cl^-$$
hydrochloric acid yields hydrogen and chlorine

The hydrogen ion characterizes this as an acid. Important acids in the body are hydrochloric acid, produced in the stomach, and carbonic acid, formed when the carbon dioxide released from cells reacts with some of the water in the extracellular fluid (all body fluids except for those contained within the cells).

Bases

A **base** is a substance that when dissociated produces ions that will combine with hydrogen ions. For example, when sodium hydroxide dissociates in water, it forms a sodium ion bearing a positive charge and a hydroxyl ion bearing a negative charge as shown following:

$$NaOH \rightarrow Na^+ + OH^-$$
sodium hydroxide yields sodium and hydroxyl

The hydroxyl ion is capable of combining with a hydrogen ion to form water. Sodium bicarbonate is an example of a base found in the body.

Salts

A **salt** is formed when an acid and a base react with each other. Salts result from the neutralization of an acid by a base, as illustrated by the following reaction:

$$HCl + NaOH \rightarrow H_2O + NaCl$$
hydrochloric and sodium yields water and sodium
acid hydroxide chloride

The hydrochloric acid reacts with the sodium hydroxide to form a molecule of water and a molecule of a salt—sodium chloride. When salts are placed in water, they dissociate into a cation and an anion. For instance, in water, the sodium chloride would dissociate into Na^+ and Cl^-. One reason salts are of great biological importance is that many of the compounds that dissociate into ions in living cells are salts. For example, sodium and chlorine ions are present in great amounts in body fluids. Many other salts occur in lesser amounts.

pH

Acid and bases are classified as either strong or weak by the number of hydrogen ions or hydroxyl ions they produce when they dissociate. Strong acids release many hydrogen ions; weak acids release relatively few. The same is true of hydroxyl ions in strong and weak bases. The acidity or alkalinity of a solution is determined by the concentration of hydrogen ions in the solution. Potential hydrogen (pH) indicates the hydrogen ion concentration in a solution, expressed as a number from 0 to 14. A solution with a pH of 7 is neutral, that is, it is neither an acid or a base. A solution with a pH greater than 7 is a base, or alkaline. A solution with a pH below 7 is an acid. The higher above 7 the pH, the more alkaline the solution; the lower below 7 the pH, the more acid the solution. pH is of great biological importance. The human body can tolerate only very slight changes in pH. For example, the pH of human blood ranges from 7.35 to 7.45. Blood pH above or below this range can cause severe or even fatal physiological problems.

Although small amounts of acids may enter the body through food intake, the greatest source of acids—and thus H^+ ions—is cellular metabolism, resulting in products including lactic acid, phosphoric acid, pyruvic acid, and many fatty acids. When blood pH falls below 7.35 as a result of an elevated concentration of H^+ ions, **acidosis** occurs. Rarely does blood pH fall to 7 or become acidic, because death will usually occur first. As acidosis increases, the central nervous system (CNS) becomes involved, and the client may become unconscious. The heartbeat may become weak and irregular, and blood pressure may decrease or even disappear.

When blood pH increases above 7.45, **alkalosis** occurs. Alkalosis is a condition characterized by an excessive loss of hydrogen ions. This happens less often than does acidosis. Symptoms of alkalosis include a heightened state of nervous system activity, resulting in spasmodic muscle contractions, convulsions, and even death.

BUFFERS

Buffers are substances that attempt to maintain pH range, or H^+ ion concentration, in the presence of added acids or bases. Buffers usually occur in pairs in the body fluids. They act to keep the pH of body fluids within normal range. If body fluids become acidic, buffers in the body fluids combine with the excess hydrogen ions and restore normal pH. Likewise, if the body fluids become alkaline, other buffers in the blood combine with the strong bases, converting them to weak bases and restoring normal pH.

Three important buffer systems occur in body fluids: the bicarbonate buffer system, the phosphate buffer system, and the protein buffer system. Because a change in pH of one fluid may bring corresponding changes in the pH of other fluids, an interplay between buffer systems acts to maintain the body's pH. The buffer systems react quickly to prevent excessive changes in the hydrogen ion concentration.

Bicarbonate Buffer System

The bicarbonate buffer system is found in both the extracellular and intracellular fluids and is the body's primary buffer system. It has two components: carbonic acid (H_2CO_3) and sodium bicarbonate ($NaHCO_3$). When a strong acid such as hydrochloric acid is added to this buffer system, the acid will react with the sodium bicarbonate and form a weaker acid (carbonic acid) and a salt (sodium chloride).

$$HCl \quad + \quad NaHCO_3 \quad \rightarrow \quad H_2CO_3 \quad + \quad NaCl$$
hydrochloric and   sodium   yields carbonic and sodium
acid   bicarbonate   acid   chloride

The strong acid is converted into a weak acid, and the pH is raised toward normal.

If a strong base such as sodium hydroxide is added to this buffer system, the carbonic acid will react with it to form a weak base (sodium bicarbonate) and water.

$$NaOH \quad + \quad H_2CO_3 \quad \rightarrow \quad NaHCO_3 \quad + \quad H_2O$$
sodium and carbonic yields   sodium   and water
hydroxide   acid   bicarbonate

The strong base, which initially raised the pH, is converted to a weak base, which will lower the pH toward normal. It is vital to note that hydrochloric acid and sodium hydroxide are substances not normally added to the blood. They are used here only as good examples of the way buffers work. This buffer system normally buffers organic acids found in body fluids.

In the body, bicarbonate helps to stabilize pH by combining reversibly with hydrogen ions. Most of the body's bicarbonate is produced in red blood cells, where the enzyme carbonic anhydrase accelerates the conversion of carbon dioxide to carbonic acid. The production of bicarbonate is illustrated in the following reversible equation:

$$CO_2 \quad + \quad H_2O \leftrightarrow H_2CO_3 \leftrightarrow \quad H^+ \quad + \quad HCO_3^-$$
carbon   water   carbonic   hydrogen   bicarbonate
dioxide   acid

When the hydrogen ion concentration increases in the extracellular (outside of the cell) space, the reaction shifts toward the left. A decreased concentration of hydrogen ions drives the reaction to the right.

Phosphate Buffer System

The phosphate buffer system is involved in regulating the pH of intracellular fluid and the fluid of the kidney tubules. It has two phosphate compounds: sodium monohydrogen phosphate ($NaHPO_4$) and sodium dihydrogen phosphate (NaH_2PO_4). In the presence of a strong acid such as hydrochloric acid, the sodium monohydrogen phosphate reacts with the acid to form a weak acid (sodium dihydrogen phosphate) and a salt (sodium chloride), thus raising the pH.

$$HCl \quad + \quad NaHPO_4 \quad \rightarrow \quad NaH_2PO_4 \quad + \quad NaCl$$
hydro- and   sodium   yields   sodium   and sodium
chloric   monohydrogen   dihydrogen   chloride
acid   phosphate   phosphate

When sodium dihydrogen phosphate encounters a strong base such as sodium hydroxide, a weak base (sodium monohydrogen phosphate) and water are formed.

$$NaOH \quad + \quad NaH_2PO_4 \quad \rightarrow \quad NaHPO_4 \quad + \quad H_2O$$
sodium and   sodium   yields   sodium   and water
hydroxide   dihydrogen   monohydrogen
phosphate   phosphate

Protein Buffers

Proteins are complex substances formed when amino acids bond. Each amino acid contains a carboxyl group (COOH) and an amino group (NH_2). The carboxyl group can ionize and release hydrogen, thus acting as an acid. The amino group can accept hydrogen, thus acting as a base. This ability allows proteins to act as a buffer system. The protein buffer system is found inside cells, especially in the hemoglobin of red blood cells, where the proteins can act to maintain the pH inside the cell. They are also found in the plasma.

SUBSTANCE MOVEMENT

Substances must be able to both enter and leave cells. For example, oxygen and various end products of digestion must enter a cell through the cell membrane for use by the cell. Waste products from cellular processes must be eliminated from the cell. Various ions must also both enter and leave cells. Everything that enters and leaves the cell must pass through the cell membrane. Thus, the cell membrane serves not only as an envelope around the cell, but also as a gatekeeper, regulating which substances can enter and leave the cell. The cell membrane is a very thin and delicate, but complex and living, elastic covering around each cell. It consists of an inner and outer layer of phospholipids in which protein molecules are embedded. Many small channels pass through the membrane. These channels allow some water molecules and some water-soluble substances to pass through the membrane. The ability of a membrane to permit substances to pass through it is called **permeability**. Because a cell membrane allows passage of only certain substances, it is called a selective permeable membrane, or **semipermeable membrane**.

Some substances can pass through the cell membrane without energy expenditure on the part of the cell. This is called passive transport. The passage of other substances requires an expenditure of energy by the cell. This is called active transport.

Passive Transport

There are several types of passive transport: diffusion, osmosis, and filtration.

Diffusion

Diffusion is the tendency of molecules of either gases, liquids, or solids to move from a region of higher molecular concentration to a region of lower molecular concentration until an equilibrium is reached. This movement is due to the kinetic energy in molecules. Kinetic energy causes the molecules to move constantly, colliding with one another and knocking each other about, thus causing them to move farther apart. An example is a drop of black ink placed in a glass of water; over a period of time, the glass of water will turn a uniform black color because of diffusion, as shown in Figure 23-4.

In the body, oxygen moves by diffusion from the lungs to the bloodstream because the oxygen concentration is higher in the lungs and lower in the blood. Carbon dioxide moves by diffusion from the bloodstream, where the concentration of carbon dioxide is higher, to the lungs, for elimination. The size of the channels in the cell membrane can prevent large molecules from passing through the membrane. Some substances, such as glucose molecules, combine with carrier molecules, which carry them into the interior of the cell, where they are released.

The term **dialysis** is used when diffusion is employed to separate molecules out of a solution by passing them through a semipermeable membrane. Dialysis is the process used in the artificial kidney. Blood from a client is circulated through a long, coiled tube. Small, toxic waste molecules such as urea leave the blood and pass through the pores of the tubing by diffusion and out into the fluid surrounding the tubing. The blood, thus cleaned, is then returned to the body.

Osmosis

Osmosis is the diffusion of water through a semipermeable membrane from a region of higher water concentration to a region of lower water concentration. In a solution undergoing osmosis, only the water (solvent) molecules move through the membrane; the dissolved molecules do not (Figure 23-5).

If a cell, having both a membrane that will not allow sodium chloride to pass through and a molecular concentration of 10% sodium chloride, were placed in a container with a 5% sodium chloride solution, the cell would contain 10% sodium chloride and 90% water, and the 5% solution in which it was placed would contain 5% dissolved sodium chloride and 95% water. There would be more water outside than inside the cell; thus, water would pass through the membrane into the cell. Because the cell membrane is elastic, the cell would increase in size as a result of the water accumulation within it facilitated by the process of osmosis. The pressure exerted against the cell membrane by the water inside the cell is called **osmotic pressure**.

A solution that has the same molecular concentration as does the cell is called an **isotonic solution**. It neither increases nor decreases the size of the cell. A solution that has a lower molecular concentration than does the cell is called a **hypotonic solution**. Placing cells in a hypotonic solution causes them to swell, possibly to the point of eventual rupture. The rupture of red blood cells due to osmosis is called **hemolysis**. As red blood cells swell, the hemoglobin contained within passes to the outside of the cell and into the solution surrounding the cell, rendering the blood cells no longer capable of carrying oxygen. A solution that has a higher molecular concentration than does the cell is called a **hypertonic solution**. When placed in such a solution, water leaves the cell, and the cell decreases in size. In the case of red blood cells, they shrivel and become wrinkled. This shrinkage, called **crenation**, leaves the cells incapable of functioning.

In persons who have lost large volumes of blood, it is sometimes necessary to administer additional fluids to maintain blood pressure. Generally, normal saline can be used. This 0.9% sodium chloride solution has approximately the same osmotic concentration as does blood. Because it is isotonic, it will not damage the cells. Figure 23-6 shows osmosis in cells with different solution concentrations.

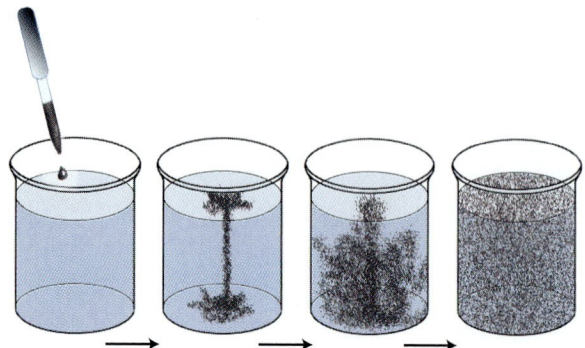

Figure 23-4 Diffusion is the spreading of particles from an area of greater concentration to an area of lesser concentration. Dye put into a beaker of water gradually spreads throughout the water.

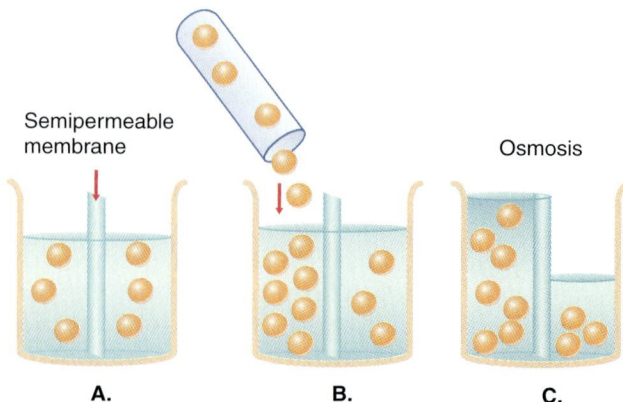

Semipermeable membrane

Osmosis

A.　　B.　　C.

Figure 23-5 The Process of Osmosis (*From* Fundamentals of Nursing: Standards & Practice, *by S. DeLaune and P. Ladner, 1998, Albany, NY: Delmar Publishers. Copyright 1998 by Delmar Publishers. Adapted with permission.*)

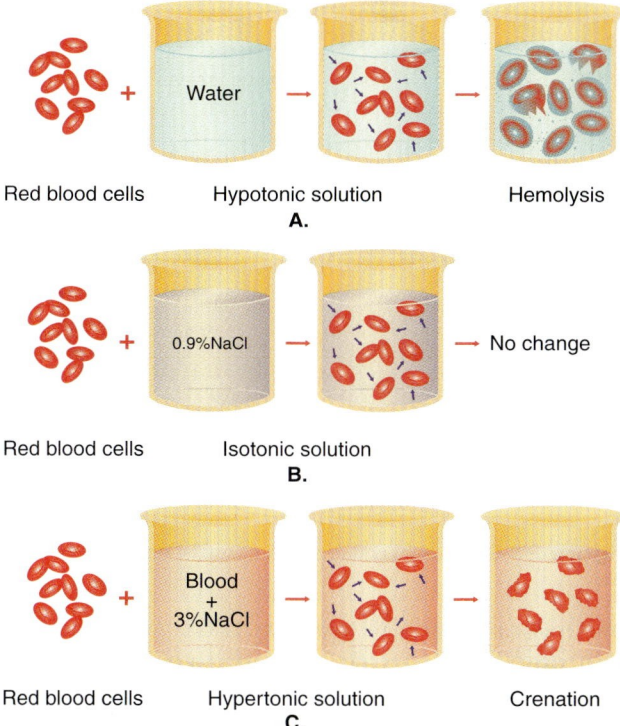

Figure 23-6 Osmosis is the movement of water through a membrane from an area of lower concentration to one of higher concentration. A. In a hypotonic solution, the water moves into the cells, causing them to swell and burst. B. In an isotonic solution, cells are normal in size and shape because the same amount of water is entering and leaving the cells. C. In a hypertonic solution, cells are losing water because water moves from an area of lower concentration (inside the cell) to an area of higher concentration (outside the cell).

Filtration

In **filtration**, fluids and the substances dissolved in them are forced through cell membranes by hydrostatic pressure. **Hydrostatic pressure** is the pressure that the fluid exerts against the membrane. The molecules passing through the membrane are determined by the size of the pores in the membrane. Tissue fluids are formed by filtration. As blood passes through the capillaries, hydrostatic pressure exerted by the pumping action of the heart causes some of the liquid fraction of the blood (but not the cells) to pass out of the capillaries, resulting in the formation of the tissue fluid (Figure 23-7). As the blood circulates through the capillaries of the kidneys, the hydrostatic pressure of the blood causes many materials to leave the blood through the filtration process. These materials pass into the tubules of the kidneys, where the toxic waste products are removed to form urine. The urine is then eliminated from the body.

Active Transport

In the processes discussed thus far, the movement of molecules depends on the concentration of mole-

cules or on pressure. In other words, the cells do not have to expend energy to move the molecules in or out of the cell. In active transport, the cell must use energy to move the molecules. For instance, in the body, sodium ions are in higher concentration in the fluids surrounding the cell than inside the cell. Though some sodium ions can diffuse into the cell, the cell actively transports them through the membrane to the outside. Active transport is accomplished by means of carrier molecules, which can latch onto specific molecules and transport them in or out of the cell. This process requires an expenditure of cellular energy (Figure 23-8). Examples of important ions transported by this process are calcium, sodium, potassium, and magnesium.

FLUID AND ELECTROLYTE BALANCE

Human life is suspended in a saline solution having a salt concentration of 0.9%. This solution, which both surrounds the cells and is contained within them, constitutes the body fluids. The water and electrolytes composing these body fluids come from ingested water and nutrients, and from the water that results from metabolism.

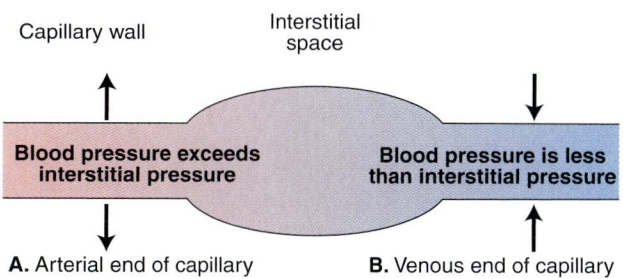

Figure 23-7 Filtration: A. Pressure in the arteriole is greater than interstitial (between the cells) pressure, causing fluid with dissolved substances to move out of capillaries: B. Pressure in venules is less than interstitial fluid pressure, causing fluid and waste products to move back into the capillaries.

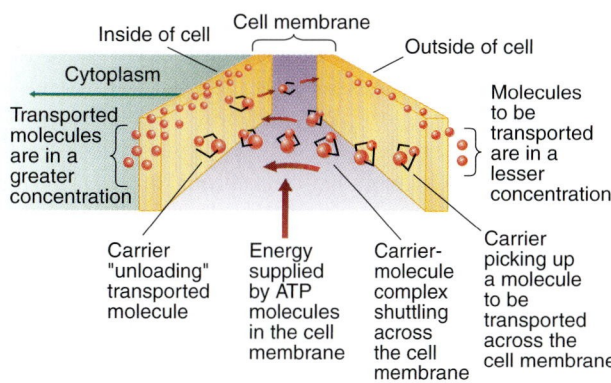

Figure 23-8 Active Transport of Molecules from an Area of Lesser Concentration to an Area of Greater Concentration.

For life to continue and the cells to properly function, the body fluids must remain fairly constant with regard to the amount of water and the specific electrolytes of which they are composed. Water is essential because it is the basic component of all the body fluids. Water is involved in many of the metabolic processes in the body and is a by–product of some of these reactions. The various electrolytes all have essential roles in cellular physiological processes. If some of either is lost, it must be replaced, and if either water or an electrolyte is in excess, it must be removed. Maintaining the consistency of this fluid environment is homeostasis.

For cells to survive and carry out their multitude of physiologic functions, they need both a continuing source of water, nutrients, and oxygen and a mechanism to remove cellular wastes. These physiologic processes affect the amount of water, the pH, and the ions both inside and outside the cells. A balance must be maintained between the components of the fluids inside and outside the cell. Because the ions are dissolved in water, these two components are tied together: Anything affecting the amount of water in the body will affect the ion concentration.

Body Fluids

Much of the body weight of an average adult is due to the water in the body fluids surrounding the cells and contained within them. The fluid around the cells cushions them and serves as the medium of exchange. Everything that enters or leaves the cells must pass through this fluid layer.

There are two kinds of body fluids. They can be thought of as being contained within two separate containers, called compartments. The **intracellular fluid** (ICF) compartment contains all of the water and ions inside the cells. By far the largest amount of water in the body, approximately 65%, is found within this compartment.

The extracellular fluid compartment contains the remaining body fluids, called **extracellular fluid** (ECF), or fluid outside the cells. These can be further subdivided into interstitial, intravascular, and other fluids. **Interstitial fluid** is the fluid in the tissue spaces around each cell. The **intravascular fluid** is the plasma in the blood vessels and the lymph in the lymphatic system (Figure 23-9). There are also small amounts of other specialized body fluids such as synovial fluid, cerebrospinal fluid, serous fluid, aqueous and vitreous humor, and the endolymph and perilymph. The proportions of extracellular fluid and intracellular fluid vary with age.

Generally speaking, the major ions in the extracellular fluid are sodium (Na^+), chloride (Cl^-), and bicarbonate (HCO_3^-), although other ions do occur. In the intracellular fluid, the major ions are potassium (K^+), phosphate (PO_4^{--}), and magnesium (Mg^{++}), with lesser

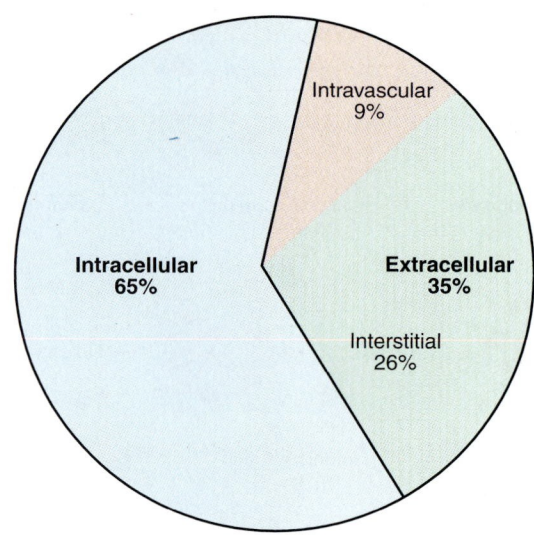

Figure 23-9 Body Fluid Compartments of an Adult

amounts of other ions present. There are also large numbers of protein molecules bearing a negative charge.

Exchange between the Extracellular and Intracellular Fluids

Water and ions moving between the extracellular and intracellular fluids must first pass through the selectively permeable cell membrane. This movement is governed primarily by osmosis. Diffusion and active transport also play a role.

The difference in the ion concentration inside the cell and outside the cell is due primarily to the cell's ability to pump some ions inside and pump others out. If the intracellular fluid becomes hypertonic to the extracellular fluid, water from the extracellular fluid will move by osmosis into the cell to restore the balance, and vice versa.

A fluid balance also occurs between the interstitial fluid and the plasma. This balance is regulated primarily by hydrostatic pressure (blood pressure) and osmotic pressure. When the circulating blood passes from the arterioles into the capillaries, the pressure in the capillaries is higher than that in the interstitial fluid. This forces some of the water from the plasma out of the capillaries and into the interstitial fluid. Due to osmotic pressure, some of the water in the interstitial fluid is forced back into the capillaries in the area where they join the venules. Some water is also returned to the bloodstream through the lymphatic system. If the amount of interstitial fluid returned to the circulatory system lessens and the fluid accumulates in the tissue spaces, the tissues become swollen. This condition is called **edema**. A number of conditions can cause edema, including kidney or liver disease and heart disorders. Many of these conditions can have serious consequences.

When more water is lost from the body than is replaced, **dehydration** occurs. Among the various causes of dehydration are water deprivation, excessive urine production, profuse sweating, diarrhea, and extended periods of vomiting. As water is lost, the amount of water in the interstitial fluid decreases. Water then moves from the cells to the tissue spaces by osmosis, causing an electrolyte imbalance. Circulatory impairment occurs, which in turn affects the kidney's ability to function normally. This condition is corrected by supplying water and the appropriate electrolytes.

Regulators of Fluid and Electrolyte Balances

There must be a balance in the amounts of fluids and electrolytes consumed and lost daily. Under typical conditions, the average adult loses some water through the skin, lungs, and GI tract and loses the largest amount of water through urine production. This can amount to a per-day fluid loss of approximately 2500 mL, depending on conditions.

Skin

In the average adult, an estimated water loss of 300 to 400 mL per day occurs by diffusion through the skin. Because the person is not aware of this water loss, it is called *insensible loss.* Water is also lost through the skin by perspiration. The total amount of water lost through perspiration varies depending on environmental factors and body temperature.

Lungs

In the average adult, an estimated insensible water loss of 300 to 400 mL per day occurs with expired air, which is saturated with water vapor. This amount varies with the rate and depth of respirations.

Gastrointestinal Tract

Although a large amount of fluid—approximately 8,000 mL per day in the average adult—is secreted into the gastrointestinal tract, almost all of this fluid is reabsorbed by the body. In adults, approximately 200 mL of water is lost per day in feces. Severe diarrhea can cause a fluid and electrolyte deficit because the GI fluids contain a large amount of electrolytes.

Kidneys

The kidneys play a major role in maintaining fluid balance by excreting 1,200 to 1,500 mL of water per day in the average adult. The excretion of water by healthy kidneys is proportional to the fluid ingested and the amount of waste or solutes excreted.

When an extracellular fluid volume deficit occurs, hormones play a key role in restoring the extracellular fluid volume. The release of the following hormones into circulation causes the kidneys to conserve water:

- Antidiuretic hormone (ADH): released by the posterior pituitary gland; acts on the distal tubules of the kidneys to reabsorb water
- Aldosterone: produced in the adrenal cortex; causes the reabsoption of sodium from the renal tubules, leading to water retention in the extracellular fluid, thereby increasing its volume
- Renin: released by the juxtaglomerular cells of the kidneys; promotes vasoconstriction and the release of aldosterone

The interaction of these hormones with regard to renal functions serves as the body's compensatory mechanism to maintain homeostasis.

Sodium is the main electrolyte that promotes the retention of water. An intravascular water deficit causes the renal tubules to reabsorb more sodium into circulation. Because water molecules go with the sodium ions, the intravascular water deficit is corrected by this action of the renal tubules.

Fluid and Food Intake

Fluids must be replaced in the amounts lost. The primary source of fluid replacement is water consumption. Approximately 60% may be obtained in this way, with an additional 30% being obtained from foods and 8% to 10% being a product of metabolism (metabolic water) for a total of 2,500 mL. Figure 23-10 illustrates fluid balance.

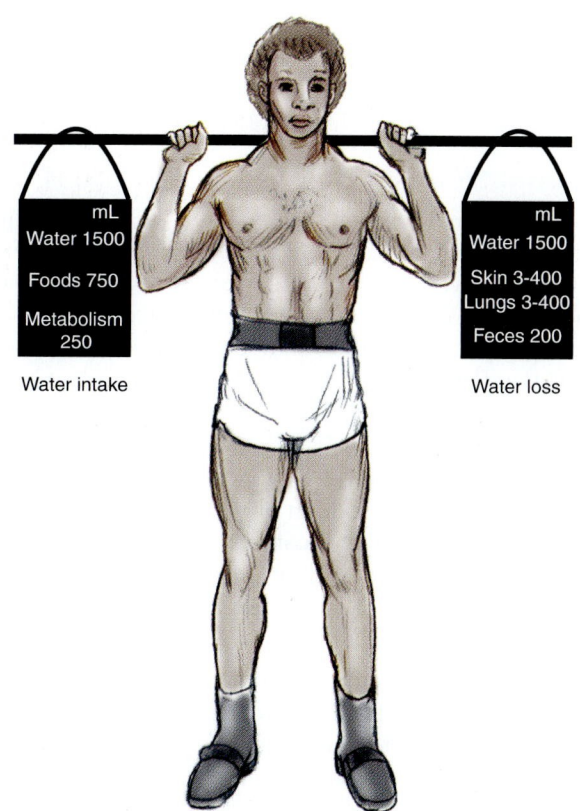

Figure 23-10 Water Balance

Thirst

Water consumption usually occurs in response to the sensation of thirst. This mechanism is poorly understood. It is generally believed to be brought about by the loss of body fluids, which in turn causes a dryness in the mouth and the thirst sensation. Replacing the lost fluids by water consumption causes the sensation to diminish. The thirst mechanism appears to be regulated by the hypothalamus in the brain.

Dehydration is one of the most common and most serious fluid imbalances that can result from poor monitoring of fluid intake. One nursing goal is to ensure that all clients understand both the role that water plays in health and the way to maintain adequate hydration.

DISTURBANCES IN ELECTROLYTE BALANCE

In health, normal homeostatic mechanisms function to maintain electrolyte balance. In illness, one or more of the regulating mechanisms may be affected, or an imbalance may become too great for the body to correct without treatment. Electrolytes are measured by laboratory analysis of a blood sample.

Sodium

Sodium (Na^+) is the major electrolyte in extracellular fluid. It regulates fluid balance through osmotic pressure that results from water following sodium in the body. Sodium stimulates conduction of nerve impulses and helps maintain neuromuscular activity. Excretion occurs primarily via the kidneys. The normal serum sodium for an adult is 136 to 145 mEq/L.

Hyponatremia

A subnormal serum sodium value (< 136 mEq/L) indicates hyponatremia. The cause is either a sodium deficit or a water excess. A hypo-osmotic state exists: The water moves out of the vascular space, into the interstitial space, and then into the intracellular space, causing edema.

Hypernatremia

A serum sodium level of > 145 mEq/L indicates hypernatremia. Excess sodium or a loss of water causes a rise in the extracellular osmotic pressure and pulls water out of the cells and into the extracellular space.

Potassium

Potassium (K^+) is the major electrolyte in intracellular fluid. Its concentration inside cells is approximately 150 mEq/L. The normal value range of extracellular (serum) potassium is narrow: 3.5 to 5.0 mEq/L. Consequently, the slightest changes can dramatically affect physiological functions. Potassium maintains normal

PROFESSIONAL TIP

Hypokalemia

Hypokalemia can cause cardiac arrest when:

- The potassium level is < 2.5 mEq/L.
- The client is taking digitalis (a drug that strengthens the contraction of the myocardium and slows down the heart rate). *Hypokalemia enhances the action of digitalis, causing toxicity.*

nerve and muscle activity, especially of the heart, and osmotic pressure within the cells. It also assists in the cellular metabolism of carbohydrates and proteins. The kidneys prefer to retain sodium and excrete potassium, even when both electrolytes are depleted. When potassium is lost from cells, sodium and hydrogen move into the cells. This aids in regulating acid–base balance. Intracellular potassium deficit may coexist with an excess of extracellular potassium.

Hypokalemia

A serum potassium level < 3.5 mEq/L indicates hypokalemia. Gastrointestinal tract disturbances and the use of diuretics can place the client at risk for hypokalemia and an acid–base imbalance (metabolic alkalosis). Potassium-wasting diuretics, such as furosemide (Lasix) or chlorothiazide (Diuril) can cause hypokalemia.

 Safety: Potassium Chloride
- Use IV route only when hypokalemia is life threatening or when oral replacement is not feasible
- Always dilute potassium chloride in a large amount of IV solution
- Never administer more than 10 mEq/L of IV potassium chloride (KCl) per hour; the normal dose of IV KCl is 20 to 40 mEq/L infused over an 8-hour period
- Never give KCl intramuscularly (IM) or as an IV bolus; potentially fatal hyperkalemia may result
- Monitor the IV site frequently for early signs of infiltration, as potassium is caustic to the tissues

Hyperkalemia

A serum potassium level > 5.0 mEq/L indicates hyperkalemia. Clients with renal disease develop hyperkalemia, because potassium cannot be excreted adequately by the kidneys. Extensive trauma causes potassium to be released from the cells and enter the bloodstream, leading to hyperkalemia. Hyperkalemia inhibits the action of digitalis. This condition is much more critical than is hypokalemia.

PROFESSIONAL TIP

Serum Calcium

Approximately 50% of serum calcium is bound to protein. Correlate the serum calcium level with the serum albumin level when evaluating laboratory results. *Any change in serum protein will result in a change in the total serum calcium.*

CLIENT TEACHING

Calcium and Vitamin D

Vitamin D is necessary for the absorption of calcium from the GI tract. Clients who do not get adequate exposure to the sun or who use sunscreen (which is needed to prevent skin cancer) may not make enough vitamin D to support adequate calcium absorption. Advise these clients to consult their physicians regarding a vitamin D supplement.

Calcium

Calcium (Ca^{++}) plays an essential role in bone and teeth integrity, blood clotting, muscle functioning, and nerve impulse transmission. Vitamin D is required for absorption of calcium from the GI tract. Only 1% of the body's calcium is found in the blood plasma (serum). Normally, 50% of the serum calcium is ionized (physiologically active), with the remaining 50% being bound to protein. Free, ionized calcium is needed for cell membrane permeability. The calcium that is bound to plasma protein cannot pass through the capillary wall and, therefore, cannot leave the intravascular compartment. The normal ionized serum calcium range for an adult is 4.5 to 5.6 mEq/L. Total serum calcium concentration measures both the ionized calcium and the calcium bound to albumin. The normal value range of total serum calcium concentration for an adult is 9.0 to 10.5 mg/dL, with values for the older adult being slightly lower.

Hypocalcemia

Hypocalcemia is indicated by a total serum calcium concentration of < 9.0 mg/dL or an ionized serum calcium level of < 4.5 mEq/L. An ionized serum calcium level of < 3.0 mEq/L is related to tetany. Alkalosis, elevated serum albumin, and the rapid administration of citrated blood increase the activity of calcium binders, thereby decreasing the amount of free calcium.

Hypercalcemia

A total serum calcium level of > 10.5 mg/dL or an ionized serum calcium level of > 5.6 mEq/L indicates

hypercalcemia. Generally, three separate evaluations of either total serum calcium or ionized serum calcium are performed before a diagnosis of hypercalcemia is made. Often, hypercalcemia is a symptom of an underlying disease such as metastatic bone tumors, Paget's disease, acromegaly, and hyperparathyroidism, which all increase bone reabsorption and, thereby, foster the release of calcium into circulating blood. Calcium-containing antacids and excess calcium from the diet may also cause hypercalcemia.

Magnesium

Most magnesium (Mg^{++}) is found in intracellular fluid and in combination with calcium and phosphorus in bone, muscle, and soft tissue. Blood serum contains only approximately 1%. Magnesium plays an important role as a coenzyme, in the metabolism of carbohydrates and proteins, and as a mediator, in neuromuscular activity. It is the only cation that is found in higher concentration in cererospinal fluid than in extracellular fluid. When a magnesium deficiency develops, the body conserves magnesium at the expense of excreting potassium. A close relationship exists between magnesium, calcium, and potassium in the intracellular fluid: A low level of one results in low levels of the other two. The normal serum magnesium level for an adult is 1.5 to 2.5 mEq/L.

Hypomagnesemia

A serum magnesium level of < 1.5 mEq/L indicates hypomagnesemia, which most commonly results from chronic alcoholism. Increased renal excretion is associated with prolonged diuretic therapy or use of gentamicin (Garamycin), cyclosporin (Sandimmune), or cisplatin (Platinol).

Hypermagnesemia

A serum magnesium level of > 2.5 mEq/L indicates hypermagnesemia. This condition rarely occurs if kidney function is normal. An increased magnesium level is associated with uncontrolled diabetes (ketoacidosis), renal failure, and ingestion of magnesium antacids (Maalox, Mylanta) or laxatives (milk of magnesia [MOM], magnesium citrate [Citromal]).

PROFESSIONAL TIP

Hypercalcemic Crisis

A rapid increase in the extracellular level of calcium (above 8 to 9 mEq/L) can trigger a hypercalcemic crisis (coma and cardiac arrest). To prevent a hypercalcemic crisis, provide adequate hydration and administer loop diuretics, phosphate, or both, as prescribed by the physician.

PROFESSIONAL TIP

Hyperalimentation

Total parenteral nutrition (TPN) provided continuously (hyperalimentation) and without a magnesium supplement can cause hypomagnesemia.

Safety: Magnesium Level
When the serum magnesium level reaches 10 to 15 mEq/L, respiratory paralysis may occur.

Phosphate

Phosphate (PO_4^{--}) is the main intracellular anion. It appears as phosphorus in the serum, where the normal value range is 1.7 to 2.6 mEq/L. Phosphorus is critical for normal cell functioning. Most phosphorus is found combined with calcium in teeth and bones. Phosphate and calcium exist in an inverse relationship; that is, as one increases the other decreases.

Hypophosphatemia

A client with a serum phosphorus level < 1.7 mEq/L has hypophosphatemia. Rarely does this condition result from decreased dietary intake. More commonly, is stems from respiratory alkalosis. Intense, prolonged hyperventilation can cause severe hypophosphatemia.

Hyperphosphatemia

A client with a serum phosphorus level > 2.6 mEq/L has hyperphosphatemia. This condition most commonly results from renal failure with resultant decreased renal phosphorus excretion. Excessive use of phosphate-containing laxatives or phosphate enemas may cause hyperphosphatemia.

Chloride

Chloride (Cl^-) is the major anion in extracellular fluid. Chloride functions in combination with sodium to maintain osmotic pressure. It also assists in maintaining acid–base balance. When the carbon dioxide level increases, bicarbonate shifts from the intracellular compartment to the extracellular compartment. Chlo-

PROFESSIONAL TIP

Hyperphosphatemia

A client with hyperphosphatemia generally remains asymptomatic unless hypocalcemia results, in which case the client may describe both tingling sensations around the mouth and in the fingertips and muscle cramps.

ride, in an effort to maintain homeostasis, then moves into the intracellular compartment. The kidneys selectively excrete chloride or bicarbonate ions depending on the acid–base balance. The normal serum chloride range is 95 to 106 mEq/L.

Hypochloremia

A serum chloride level < 95 mEq/L indicates hypochloremia. Excess losses of chloride may result from prolonged diarrhea or diaphoresis. Loss of hydrochloric acid related to vomiting, gastric suctioning, or gastric surgery may cause hypochloremia.

Hyperchloremia

A serum chloride level > 106 mEq/L indicates hyperchloremia, which usually occurs in conjunction with dehydration, hypernatremia, or metabolic acidosis.

ACID–BASE BALANCE

As described earlier, the body maintains a normal pH within the relatively narrow range of 7.35 to 7.45. Body pH is maintained by the buffer systems, the respiratory system, and the kidneys. A pH below 7.35 is termed acidosis, and a pH above 7.45 is termed alkalosis. Either of these conditions can be brought about by respiratory or metabolic changes.

Regulators of Acid–Base Balance

The body has three main control systems that regulate acid–base balance to counter acidosis or alkalosis: the buffer systems, respirations, and renal control of hydrogen ion concentration. These systems vary in their reaction times in regulating and restoring balance to the hydrogen ion concentration.

Buffer Systems

The buffer systems—bicarbonate, phosphate, and protein—were previously discussed. They react quickly to prevent excessive changes in the hydrogen ion concentration.

Respiratory Regulation of Acid–Base Balance

The respiratory buffering system helps to maintain acid–base balance by controlling the content of carbon dioxide in extracellular fluid. The *rate of metabolism* determines the formation of carbon dioxide. Various intracellular metabolic processes continuously form carbon dioxide in the body. The carbon in foods is **oxidized** (joined with oxygen) to form carbon dioxide.

It takes the respiratory regulatory mechanism several minutes to respond to changes in the carbon dioxide concentration of extracellular fluid. With the increase of carbon dioxide in extracellular fluid, respiration increases in rate and depth so that more carbon dioxide is exhaled. As the respiratory system removes carbon dioxide, less carbon dioxide is present in the blood to combine with water to form carbonic acid. Likewise, if the blood level of carbon dioxide is low, respirations decrease to maintain a normal ratio between carbonic acid and basic bicarbonate.

Renal Control of Hydrogen Ion Concentration

The kidneys control extracellular fluid pH by eliminating either hydrogen ions or bicarbonate ions from body fluids. If the bicarbonate concentration in the extracellular fluid is greater than normal, the kidneys excrete more bicarbonate ions, making the urine more alkaline. Conversely, if more hydrogen ions are excreted in the urine, the urine becomes more acidic. The renal mechanism for regulating acid–base balance cannot readjust the pH within seconds, as can the extracellular fluid buffer system, nor within minutes, as can the respiratory compensatory mechanism; but it can function over a period of several hours or days to correct acid–base imbalance.

Diagnostic and Laboratory Data

The biochemical indicators of acid–base balance are assessed by measuring the **arterial blood gases (ABGs)**. The arterial blood gas test measures the levels of oxygen and carbon dioxide in arterial blood. The test assesses pH, partial pressure of oxygen (PO_2 or PaO_2), partial pressure of carbon dioxide (PCO_2 or $PaCO_2$), saturation of oxygen (SaO_2), and bicarbonate (HCO_3). pH has already been discussed.

The PO_2 or PaO_2 expresses the amount of oxygen that can combine with hemoglobin to form oxyhemoglobin, the form in which oxygen is transported through the body. At sea level, the normal range is 80 to 100 millimeters of mercury (mm Hg). The rate at which the oxygen/hemoglobin reaction occurs is influenced by pH. The rate decreases as the pH value decreases.

The PCO_2 or $PaCO_2$ in the blood is a reflection of the efficiency of gaseous exchange in the lungs. At sea level, the normal range is 35 to 45 mm Hg. If the alveoli are obstructed or damaged by disease, carbon dioxide cannot be eliminated and will combine with water to form carbonic acid, which in turn causes acidosis. Conversely, in a person who is hyperventilating, too much carbon dioxide is eliminated, which may trigger alkalosis.

The SaO_2 is the percent of oxygen that combines with hemoglobin in the blood. The normal range is 95% to 100% saturation. This value along with the PO_2 and hemoglobin levels indicates the degree to which the tissues are receiving oxygen. Oxygen saturation can also be measured with an oximeter, a noninvasive technique.

Determining the amount of bicarbonate (HCO_3) in the blood is important because, along with carbonic acid, bicarbonate is a major buffer in the blood. The two substances occur in a ratio of 20 parts bicarbonate to 1 part carbonic acid. Regardless of the carbonic acid and bicarbonate values, the pH of the blood will remain in the normal range as long as the ratio remains 20:1. The normal range for HCO_3 at sea level is 24 to 28 mEq/L. The carbonic acid level is always 3% of the PCO_2 level.

DISTURBANCES IN ACID–BASE BALANCE

The acid–base imbalances are respiratory acidosis and alkalosis and metabolic acidosis and alkalosis. In determining whether the acid–base imbalance is caused by a respiratory or a metabolic alteration, the key indicators are bicarbonate and carbonic acid levels (Figure 23-11). Table 23-3 lists those changes in laboratory values that indicate the various acid–base imbalances.

Respiratory Acidosis

When carbon dioxide is not eliminated by the lungs as fast as it is produced by cellular metabolism, the

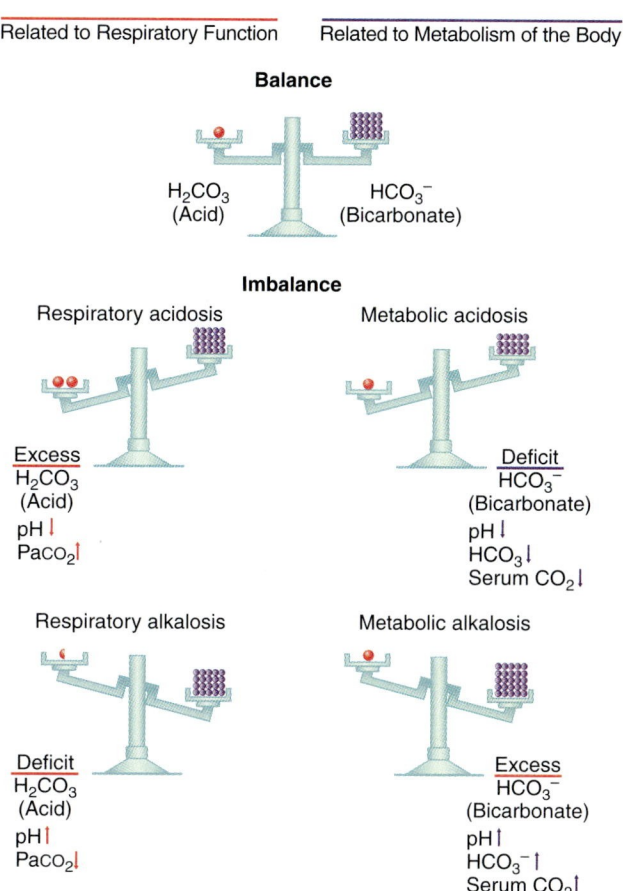

Figure 23-11 Acid–Base Balance and Imbalance (*From Fundamentals of Nursing: Standards & Practice, by S. DeLaune and P. Ladner, 1998, Albany, NY: Delmar Publishers. Copyright 1998 by Delmar Publishers. Adapted with permission.*)

Table 23-3 LABORATORY VALUES IN ACID–BASE IMBALANCES

SITUATION	PH	PCO$_2$	HCO$_3$
Normal parameters	7.35 to 7.45	35 to 45 mm Hg	24 to 28 mEq/L
Respiratory acidosis			
Acute	< 7.35	> 45 mm Hg	Normal
Chronic	< 7.35	> 45 mm Hg	> 28 mEq/L
Respiratory alkalosis	> 7.45	< 35 mm Hg	Normal
Metabolic acidosis	< 7.35	Normal	< 24 mEq/L
Metabolic alkalosis	> 7.45	Normal	> 28 mEq/L

amount of carbon dioxide increases in the blood. It then reacts with water and forms excess hydrogen ions, as shown in the following reaction:

$$CO_2 + H_2O \rightarrow H^+ + HCO_3$$

Respiratory acidosis is characterized by an increased hydrogen ion concentration (a blood pH below 7.35), an increased PCO$_2$ level (greater than 45 mm Hg), and an excess of carbonic acid. It is caused by hypoventilation or any condition that depresses ventilation. When the respiratory rate and the amount of oxygen supplied to the lungs suddenly lessen, acute respiratory acidosis can occur. This condition can be life threatening, and it must be recognized and corrected quickly. Chronic respiratory acidosis occurs when the respiratory rate is continually depressed.

Clients with respiratory acidosis experience neurological changes resulting from the acidity of the cerebrospinal fluid and brain cells. Hypoventilation causes **hypoxemia** (decreased oxygen in the blood), which in turn causes further neurological impairment. Hyperkalemia may accompany acidosis.

Respiratory Alkalosis

Respiratory alkalosis is characterized by a decreased hydrogen ion concentration (a blood pH above 7.45) and a below normal PCO$_2$ level (lower than 35 mm Hg). It is caused by hyperventilation (excessive exhalation of carbon dioxide) resulting in hypocapnia (decreased arterial carbon dioxide concentration). As the breathing rate increases, the amount of carbon dioxide in the blood decreases. This in turn increases the pH of the blood.

Hyperventilation can be triggered by anxiety, fear, pain, fever, rapid mechanical ventilation, and hypoxia at high altitudes. This condition is usually self-correcting.

PROFESSIONAL TIP

Electrolyte Shift

Metabolic acidosis causes an electrolyte shift: Hydrogen and sodium ions move into the cells, and potassium moves into the extracellular fluid. Hyperkalemia may cause ventricular fibrillation and death.

As the breathing returns to normal, the carbon dioxide level in the blood increases, and the normal pH is restored. Other causes of hyperventilation, which involves overstimulation of the respiratory center, include salicylate poisoning, brain tumors, meningitis, encephalitis, and pulmonary embolus.

Metabolic Acidosis

Metabolic acidosis is characterized by an increase in hydrogen ion concentration (blood pH below 7.35) or a decrease in bicarbonate concentration. Such a change may be brought about by kidney disease when the mechanism to excrete excess hydrogen ions is compromised. Vomiting, diarrhea, diabetes mellitus, and, sometimes, diuretics may also be responsible. The lungs eliminate more carbon dioxide but are usually ineffective in decreasing acids. The kidneys try to increase the pH and the excretion of hydrogen by exchanging sodium ions for hydrogen ions. Metabolic acidosis is most common in individuals with kidney disease or diabetes mellitus.

Metabolic Alkalosis

Metabolic alkalosis is characterized by a loss of acid from the body or a gain in base (increased level of bicarbonate). Blood pH is above 7.45. A gain in base may result from excessive ingestion of antacids and milk. These substances neutralize acids, resulting in alkalosis and hypercalcemia. Excessive oral or parenteral administration of sodium bicarbonate or other alkaline salts (e.g., sodium or potassium acetate, lactate, or citrate) increases the amount of base in extracellular fluid.

The respiratory and renal compensatory mechanisms respond to an increased bicarbonate/carbonic acid ratio. The rate and depth of respirations decreases in an effort to retain carbon dioxide. To counter the pH imbalance of metabolic alkalosis, the arterial carbon dioxide concentration rises, creating respiratory acidosis.

A normal serum potassium level is a prerequisite for renal compensation. In alkalosis, potassium ions enter the cells in exchange for hydrogen ions, causing hypokalemia. Hypokalemia further potentiates metabolic alkalosis because the kidneys conserve hydrogen ions

Metabolic Alkalosis

The following clinical conditions can place clients at risk for metabolic alkalosis:

- Vomiting and nasogastric suctioning or lavage cause a loss of hydrochloric acid and chloride. With the loss of the hydrogen and chloride ions, bicarbonate ions are absorbed, unneutralized, into the bloodstream, and the pH of the extracellular fluid rises (alkalosis).
- Diarrhea and steroid or diuretic therapy can cause excessive loss of potassium, chloride, and other electrolytes. The potassium deficit causes the kidneys to exchange hydrogen ions (instead of potassium ions) for sodium ions, which promotes the loss of hydrogen, thereby increasing bicarbonate level.

by excreting potassium ions in exchange for sodium ions. When hypokalemia is present, the kidneys cannot function as a compensatory mechanism; they continue to excrete hydrogen, and bicarbonate excess continues.

NURSING PROCESS

The nursing process assists the nurse in planning client care.

Assessment

Assessment data are used to identify clients who have potential or actual alterations in fluid volume. Electrolyte and acid–base imbalances are identified primarily with laboratory data, while fluid balances are identified primarily with the health history and physical examination.

Health History

The nursing history should elicit data in the following areas:

- Lifestyle (sociocultural and economic factors, stress, exercise)
- Dietary intake (recent changes in the amount and types of fluid and food, increased thirst)
- Weight (sudden gain or loss)
- Fluid output (recent changes in the frequency or amount of urine output)
- Gastrointestinal disturbances (prolonged vomiting, diarrhea, anorexia, ulcer, hemmorrhage)
- Fever and diaphoresis
- Burns, trauma, draining wounds
- Disease conditions that can upset homeostasis (renal disease, endocrine disorders, neural malfunction, pulmonary disease)

- Therapeutic programs that can produce imbalances (special diets, medications, chemotherapy, IV fluid or TPN administration, gastric or intestinal suction)

Physical Examination

Because fluid alterations may affect any body system, the nurse performs a complete physical examination and identifies all abnormalities.

Daily Weight Changes in the body's total fluid volume are reflected in body weight. For instance, each liter (1,000 mL) of fluid gained or lost is equivalent to 1 kilogram (2.2 lb) of weight.

Vital Signs Measurement of vital signs provides the nurse with information regarding the client's fluid, electrolyte, and acid–base statuses and the body's compensatory response for maintaining balance. An elevated temperature places the client at risk for dehydration related to an increased loss of body fluid.

Changes in the pulse rate, strength, and rhythm are indicative of fluid alterations. Fluid volume alterations may cause the following pulse changes:

- Fluid volume deficit: increased pulse rate and weak pulse volume
- Fluid volume excess: increased pulse volume and third heart sound

Respiratory changes are assessed by inspecting the movement of the chest wall, counting the respiratory rate, and asculating the lungs. Changes in the rate and depth may cause respiratory acid–base imbalances or may be indicative of a compensatory response to metabolic acidosis or alkalosis, as previously discussed.

Blood pressure measurements can be used to assess the degree of fluid volume deficit. Fluid volume deficit can lower the blood pressure. A narrow pulse pressure (lower than 20 mm Hg) may indicate fluid volume deficit that occurs with severe hypovolemia.

Intake and Output The client's I&O should be measured and recorded for a 24-hour period to assess for an actual or potential imbalance. A minimum intake of 1,500 mL is essential in balancing urinary output and the body's insensible water loss. Intake includes all liquids taken by mouth (e.g., ice cream, soup, gelatin, juice, and water) and liquids administered through tube feedings (nasogastric or jejunostomy) and parenterally (IV fluids and blood or its components). Output includes urine, diarrhea, vomitus, and drainage from tubes such as gastric suction or surgical drains.

Safety: Fluid Measurements
To protect both the nurse and the client from transfer of microorganisms, Standard Precautions are always instituted during fluid administration and output measurement.

Thirst The most common indicator of fluid volume deficit is thirst. With a decrease in extracellular fluid volume or an increase in plasma osmolality, the hypothalamus triggers a thirst response.

Food Intake The intake of food also contributes to maintaining extracellular fluid volume. One-third of the body's fluid needs are met with ingested food. Food also provides the body with necessary electrolytes.

Skin Edema and skin turgor are two important indicators related to fluid, electrolyte, and acid–base balances.

Edema Edema is the main symptom of fluid volume excess. Edema may be localized (confined to a specific area) or generalized (occurring throughout the body's tissue). Localized edema is characterized by taut, smooth, shiny, pale skin. The body may retain 5 to 10 pounds of fluid before edema is noticeable (Bulechek & McCloskey, 1992). The dependent body parts—sacrum, back, and legs—should be assessed for peripheral edema. Pitting edema is rated on a four-point scale, as follows:

+0: no pitting

+1, 0 to ¼ inch pitting (mild)

+2: ¼ to ½ inch pitting (moderate)

+3: ½ to 1 inch pitting (severe)

+4: greater than 1 inch pitting (severe)

Turgor Skin **turgor** refers to the normal resiliency of the skin, a reflection of hydration status. When the skin is pinched and released, it springs back to a normal position because of the outward pressure exerted by the cells and interstitial fluid. To measure the client's skin turgor, the nurse uses the thumb and forefinger to grasp and raise and then release a small section of the client's skin. Dehydration is the main cause of decreased skin turgor, which manifests as lax skin that returns slowly to the normal position. Increased skin turgor, which occurs in conjunction with edema, manifests as smooth, taut, shiny skin that cannot be grasped and raised.

Buccal (Oral) Cavity The nurse should inspect the buccal cavity. With fluid volume deficit, saliva decreases, causing sticky, dry mucous membranes and dry, cracked lips. The tongue displays longitudinal furrows.

LIFE CYCLE CONSIDERATION

Assessing Skin Turgor
- In adults, the anterior chest under the clavicle; the abdomen; or the back of the hand are the preferred sites for assessing skin turgor.
- In children, the abdomen or the medial aspect of the thigh are the preferred sites.

LIFE CYCLE CONSIDERATIONS

Skin Turgor in Elderly Clients
With aging, the skin loses elasticity, resulting in reduced skin turgor. Assess the tongue for creases or furrows to monitor dehydration in elderly clients (Hogstel, 1994).

Eyes The nurse should inspect the eyes for sunkenness, dry conjunctiva, and decreased or absent tearing all signs of fluid volume deficit. Puffy eyelids (periorbital edema, or papilledema) are characteristic of fluid volume excess. The client may also have a history of blurred vision.

Jugular and Hand Veins Circulatory volume is assessed by measuring venous filling of the jugular and hand veins. The nurse places the client in a low Fowler's position and then:

1. Palpates the jugular (neck) veins. Fluid volume excess causes a distention in the jugular veins (Figure 23-12).
2. Places the client's hand below heart level and palpates the hand veins. Fluid volume deficit causes decreased venous filling (flat hand veins).

Neuromuscular System Fluid and electrolyte imbalances may cause neuromuscular alterations. The muscles lose their tone and become soft and flabby, and reflexes diminish. Calcium and magnesium imbalances cause an increase in neuromuscular irritability. To assess for neuromuscular irritability, the tests for Chvostek's sign and Trousseau's sign are performed. Other neurological signs of fluid, electrolyte, and acid–base imbalances include inability to concentrate, confusion, and emotional lability.

Diagnostic and Laboratory Data
Laboratory tests can reveal imbalances before clinical symptoms are evident in the client. However, un-

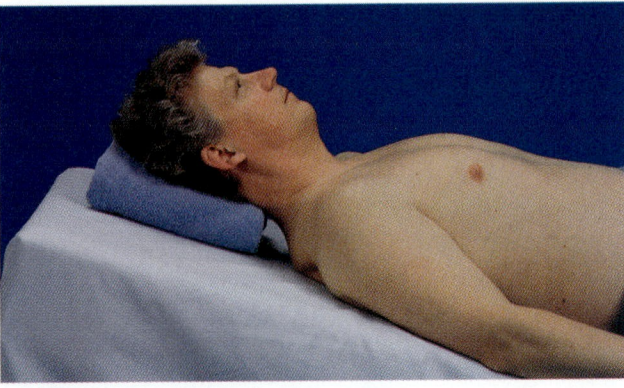

Figure 23-12 Client Position When Assessing Jugular Vein Distention

less clients are having the tests for some other reason, symptoms are detected first.

Hemoglobin and Hematocrit Indices Hematocrit (Hct) is affected by changes in plasma volume. For instance, with severe dehydration and hypovolemic shock, hematocrit increases. Conversely, overhydration decreases hematocrit. The hemoglobin (Hgb) level decreases in the event of severe hemorrhage.

Osmolality Osmolality is a measurement of the total concentration of dissolved particles (solutes) per kilogram of water. Osmolality measurements are performed on both serum and urine samples to determine alterations in fluid and electrolyte balance. Osmolality can also be explained in relation to the specific gravity of body fluids. Specific gravity expresses the weight of the solution when compared to an equal volume of distilled water. The osmolality of a solution can be estimated by the specific gravity.

Serum Osmolality Serum osmolality is a measurement of the total concentration of dissolved particles per kilogram of water in serum, recorded in milliosmoles per kilogram (mOsm/kg). The particles measured in serum osmolality include electrolyte ions, such as sodium and potassium, and electrically inactive substances dissolved in serum, such as glucose and urea. Water and sodium are the main entities that control the osmolality of body fluids. Serum sodium is responsible for 85% to 90% of the serum osmolality (McFarland & Grant, 1994).

The normal range of serum osmolality is 280 to 295 mOsm/Kg (Noe & Rock, 1994). The value increases with dehydration and decreases with water excess.

In clinical practice, the terms *osmolality* and **osmolarity** (the concentration of solutes per liter of cellular fluid) are often used interchangeably to refer to the concentration of body fluid. However, these terms actually have different meanings, in that *osmolality* refers to the concentration of solutes in the total body water rather than in cellular fluid. The appropriate term to use in conjunction with IV fluid therapy is *osmolarity* (Bulechek & McCloskey, 1992).

Urine Osmolality Urine osmolality is a measurement of the total concentration of dissolved particles per kilogram of water in urine. The particles measured in urine osmolality come from nitrogenous waste (cre-

atinine, urea, and uric acid), with urea being predominant. Urine osmolality varies greatly with diet and fluid intake and reflects the ability of the kidney to adjust the concentration of urine in order to maintain fluid balance. The dehydrated client with normal kidney function will have elevated urine osmolality, whereas the client with shock, hyperglycemia, hemoconcentration, or acidosis will have elevations in both urine and serum osmolalities.

Urine pH The measurement of urine pH reveals the hydrogen ion concentration in the urine, indicating the urine's acidity or alkalinity. When the kidney buffering system is compensating for either metabolic acidosis or alkalosis, the pH of the urine should be within normal range (4.6 to 8.0). This is considered a sign of normal function. However, when the renal compensatory function fails to respond to the blood pH, the urine pH will either increase, with acidosis, or decrease, with alkalosis.

Serum Albumin Albumin is synthesized in the liver from amino acids. Serum albumin plays an important role in fluid and electrolyte balance by maintaining the colloid osmotic pressure of blood, which in turn prevents fluid accumulation (edema) in the tissues. However, serum albumin has a half-life of 21 days and fluctuates according to the level of hydration. Therefore, it is not a good indicator of acute protein depletion. Clinically, this blood test is used to measure prolonged protein depletion, which occurs in chronic malnutrition.

Nursing Diagnosis

NANDA (1999) identifies the primary nursing diagnoses for clients with fluid imbalances as *Fluid Volume Excess, Fluid Volume Deficit,* and *Fluid Volume Deficit, Risk For.* Numerous secondary nursing diagnoses may also apply.

Fluid Volume Excess

Fluid Volume Excess exists when the client has edema and increased interstitial and intravascular fluid retention. Fluid volume excess is related to excess fluid in either the tissues of the extremities (peripheral edema) or the lung tissues (pulmonary edema). Factors that put the client at risk for fluid volume excess are:

- Excessive fluid intake (e.g., IV therapy, sodium);
- Excessive loss or decreased intake of protein (chronic diarrhea, burns, kidney disease, malnutrition);
- Compromised regulatory mechanisms (kidney failure);
- Decreased intravascular movement (impaired myocardial contractility);
- Lymphatic obstruction (cancer, surgical removal of lymph nodes, obesity);
- Medications (steroid excess); and
- Allergic reactions.

PROFESSIONAL TIP

Urine Osmolality

Urine osmolality is a more accurate indicator of hydration than is the specific gravity of urine. Some medications and the presence of protein and glucose solutes in the urine can give a false high specific gravity reading.

Table 23-4 CLINICAL MANIFESTATIONS OF EDEMA	
PULMONARY EDEMA	**PERIPHERAL EDEMA**
Constant cough	Pitting edema in extremities
Dyspnea	Edematous area: tight, smooth
Engorged neck and hand veins	Shiny, pale, cool skin
Moist rales in lungs	Puffy eyelids
Bounding pulse	Weight gain

(From Fundamentals of Nursing: Standards & Practice, *by S. DeLaune and P. Ladner, 1998, Albany, NY: Delmar Publishers. Copyright 1998 by Delmar Publishers. Reprinted with permission.)*

Assessment findings in the client with fluid volume excess include acute weight gain; decreased serum osmolality (lower than 275 mOsm/Kg), protein and albumin, blood urea nitrogen (BUN), Hgb, Hct; increased central venous pressure (greater than 12 to 15 cm H_2O); and signs and symptoms of edema. The clinical manifestation of edema are relative to the area of involvement, either pulmonary or peripheral (Table 23-4).

Fluid Volume Deficit

Fluid Volume Deficit exists when the client experiences vascular, interstitial, or intracellular dehydration. The degree of dehydration is classified as mild, marked, severe, or fatal on the basis of the percentage of body weight lost. The multiple causes of fluid volume deficit include:

- Excessive fluid loss resulting from diaphoresis, vomiting, diarrhea, hemorrhage, burns, ascites, wound drainage, indwelling tubes, or suction;
- Diabetes insipidus;
- Diabetes mellitus;
- Addison's disease (adrenal insufficiency);
- Gastrointestinal fistula or draining abscess; and
- Intestinal obstruction.

 PROFESSIONAL TIP

Loss of Gastric Juices

Clients who lose excessive amounts of gastric juices, either through vomiting or suctioning, are prone to not only fluid volume deficit, but also metabolic alkalosis, hypokalemia, and hyponatremia. Gastric juices contain hydrochloric acid, pepsinogen, potassium, and sodium.

 LIFE CYCLE CONSIDERATIONS

Infants and Respiratory Problems

Assessment findings for infants experiencing respiratory problems may include nasal flaring, sternal and costal retractions, and expiratory grunting.

Assessment findings in the client with fluid volume deficit include thirst and weight loss of an amount consistent with the degree of dehydration. Marked dehydration manifests as dry mucous membranes and skin; poor skin turgor; low-grade temperature elevation; tachycardia; respirations of 28 or greater; decreased (10 to 15 mm Hg) systolic blood pressure; slowed venous filling; decreased urine output (fewer than 25 mL/hr); concentrated urine; elevated Hct, Hgb, and BUN; and acidic blood pH (less than 7.4).

Severe dehydration is characterized by the symptoms of marked dehydration plus a flushing of the skin. Systolic blood pressure continues to drop (to 60 mm Hg or below), and behavioral changes (restlessness, irritability, disorientation, and delirium) occur. The signs of fatal dehydration are anuria and coma leading to death.

Fluid Volume Deficit, Risk for

Fluid Volume Deficit, Risk for exists when the client is at risk of developing vascular, interstitial, or intracellular dehydration resulting from active or regulatory loss of body water in excess of needs. The multiple factors that can place the client at risk for fluid volume deficit were listed previously.

Other Nursing Diagnoses

In clients with a fluid imbalance, the relationship between the primary nursing diagnoses previously discussed and the secondary nursing diagnoses is reciprocal: The primary nursing diagnoses influence and are influenced by the secondary nursing diagnoses. Some commonly identified secondary nursing diagnoses include.

- *Gas Exchange, Impaired*
- *Cardiac Output, Decreased*
- *Breathing Pattern, Ineffective*
- *Anxiety*
- *Thought Processes, Altered*
- *Injury, Risk for*
- *Infection, Risk for*
- *Oral Mucous Membrane, Altered*
- *Knowledge Deficit*

Planning/Outcome Identification

Holistic nursing care for clients experiencing a fluid imbalance requires that the nurse, in collaboration with each client, identify specific goals for each nursing diagnosis. These goals should be individualized to reflect the client's capabilities and limitations and should be appropriate to the diagnosis and the assessment data.

During the planning phase, the nurse also selects and prioritizes nursing interventions to support the client's achievement of expected outcomes based on the goals. For example, if vomiting and diarrhea along with a 5% weight loss and dry mucous membranes led to a nursing diagnosis of *Fluid Volume Deficit,* the goals might include relief from vomiting and diarrhea and achievement of the proper balance of intake and output.

Expected outcomes for the client with a fluid imbalance are not only specific to the primary diagnosis, but also must be relative to the interventions. For example, an expected outcome for clients receiving IV therapy might be: "IV site remains free of erythema, edema, and purulent drainage" (because these clients are at risk for infection). Achievement of the goals and the client's expected outcomes indicates resolution of the problem.

Implementation

The nurse has a responsibility to collaborate with and advocate for clients to ensure receipt of care that is appropriate, ethical, and based on practice standards. The data obtained from the history serve as the basis for formulating expected outcomes and selecting nursing interventions appropriate to the client's natural patterns as revealed in their history.

The rationale for interventions related to alterations in either fluid, electrolyte, or acid–base balance is based on the goal of maintaining homeostasis and regulating and maintaining essential fluids and nutrients. Clients' adaptive capabilities are kept in mind when selecting interventions based on the clients' perceptions of their support systems, strengths, and options.

Bulechek and McCloskey (1992) address the importance of the nursing interventions relative to fluid therapy by identifying the nurse's responsibilities to:

- Understand the client's metabolic needs and make judgments concerning the outcomes of therapy,
- Perform frequent assessment and monitoring to recognize the adverse effects of fluid and electrolyte therapy and prevent complications, and
- Prevent the rapid depletion of the body's protein and energy reserves.

The nursing activities relative to assessment and implementation often require the same measurements: for example, weight and vital signs. Common interventions that promote attainment of expected outcomes relative to restoring and maintaining homeostasis are discussed following.

Monitor Daily Weight

Daily weight is one of the main indicators of fluid and electrolyte balance. The nurse is responsible for the accurate measurement and recording of the client's daily weight. The physician uses this data along with other clinical findings to determine fluid therapy for the client.

Measure Vital Signs

The frequency with which vital signs are measured depends on the client's acuity level and clinical situation. For example, the vital signs of the typical postoperative client might be taken every 15 minutes until stable, whereas vital signs should be monitored continuously for the client experiencing shock or hemorrhage. Vital sign measurements and other clinical data are used to determine the type and amount of fluid therapy.

Measure Intake and Output

Intake and output measurements are initiated to monitor the client's fluid status over a 24-hour period. Agency policy relative to I&O may vary with regard to:

- Time frames for charting (e.g., every 8 hours versus every 12 hours),
- Time at which the 24-hour totals are calculated, and
- Definition of "strict" I&O.

 Safety: Removing Gloves Before Charting
To prevent the transfer of microorganisms when the I&O form is removed from the client's room, remove gloves and wash hands before recording the amount of drainage on the form.

The nurse should review the client's 24-hour I&O calculations to evaluate fluid status. Intake should exceed output by 500 mL to offset insensible fluid loss. Intake and output and daily weight are critical components of intervention, because these measurements are also used to evaluate the effectiveness of diuretic or rehydration therapy.

Securing an accurate I&O requires the full support of the client and family. The client and family members

 PROFESSIONAL TIP

"Strict" I&O
- "Strict" I&O measurement usually involves accounting for incontinent urine, emesis, and diaphoresis and might require weighing soiled bed linens.
- *Gloves should always be worn when handling soiled linen.*

HOME HEALTH CARE

Considerations for Measuring I&O

- Elicit client and family member input when selecting household items to be used for intake measurement
- Provide containers for measuring output, adapting the urinary container to home facilities, and teach client and family about proper washing and storage
- Teach handwashing technique
- Provide written instructions on what is to be measured
- Provide sufficient I&O forms to last between the nurse's visits
- Identify the parameters for evaluating a discrepancy between the intake and the output and for notifying the nurse or physician

should be taught the way to measure and record the I&O.

Provide Oral Hygiene

The nurse is responsible for providing oral hygiene to promote both client comfort and the integrity of the buccal cavity. The frequency of oral hygiene depends on the condition of the client's buccal cavity and the type of fluid imbalance. A client who is dehydrated or permitted no oral fluids for more than 24 hours may have decreased or absent salivation, coated tongue, and furrows on the tongue. Such clients are at risk for developing oral diseases such as stomatitis, oral lesions or ulcers, and gingivitis.

Initiate Oral Fluid Therapy

Oral fluids may be totally restricted—a situation commonly referred to as *nothing by mouth* (NPO, which is from the Latin *non per os*)—or they may be restricted or forced, depending on the client's clinical situation.

Nothing by Mouth Clients are placed on NPO status as prescribed by the physician. On the basis of agency policy and clarification from the physician, the client may be allowed small amounts of ice chips

when designated NPO. Common clinical situations that may require NPO status include the need to:

- Avoid aspiration in unconscious, perioperative, and preprocedural clients who will receive anesthesia or conscious sedation;
- Rest and heal the GI tract in clients with severe vomiting or diarrhea or a GI disorder (inflammation or obstruction);
- Prevent the further loss of gastric juices in clients on nasogastric suctioning.

Clients designated NPO should receive oral hygiene every 1 to 2 hours or as needed for comfort and to prevent alterations of the mucous membranes.

Restricted Fluids Fluid intake is commonly restricted in the treatment of fluid volume excess related to heart and renal failure. Intake may be restricted to 200 mL in a 24-hour period. Client and family teaching and collaboration are the main nursing interventions in implementing this measure.

The way fluids are limited should be determined in collaboration with the client. For example:

- Half of the allowed fluid might be divided between breakfast and lunch and
- The remaining half might be divided between the evening meal and before bedtime, unless the client must be awakened during the night for medication.

Forced Fluids "Forcing" or encouraging the intake of oral fluids, mainly water, is sometimes done when treating clients who are at risk for dehydration or who have renal and urinary problems (kidney stones). Compliance is obtained through client education and honoring client preference relative to timing and the type of liquids. A client might, for example, be requested to consume 2,000 mL over a 24-hour period. If the client is intimidated at hearing this amount, which may sound very large, the nurse might explain that the number of glasses to which this volume equates is only eight. This would roughly translate into one glass every 2 hours. The nurse could also tell the client that ice, gelatin, soups, and ice cream all count as liquid.

Maintain Tube Feeding

When the client cannot ingest oral fluids but has a normal GI tract, fluids and nutrients can be administered through a feeding tube as prescribed by a physician.

PROFESSIONAL TIP

Mouthwashes

Avoid using mouthwashes with alcohol or glycerin, and swabs with lemon or glycerin. Although they may feel refreshing, these ingredients dry the mucous membranes.

PROFESSIONAL TIP

Temperature of Fluids

Advise clients to drink room-temperature fluids. Hot or cold fluids may increase peristalsis and abdominal cramping.

Fluid Replacement

Fluid replacement is based on weight loss. A 2.2 pound (1 kg) weight loss is equivalent to 1 liter (1,000 mL) of fluid loss.

Monitor Intravenous Therapy

When fluid loss is severe or the client cannot tolerate oral or tube feedings, fluid volume is replaced parenterally through the IV route. **Intravenous** (IV) **therapy** is the administration of fluids, electrolytes, nutrients, or medications by the venous route. The physician prescribes IV therapy to treat or prevent fluid, electrolyte, or nutritional imbalances. The nurse has specific responsibilities relative to IV therapy. Specifically, the nurse must:

- Know why the therapy is prescribed;
- Document client understanding;
- Select the appropriate equipment according to agency policy;

- Obtain the correct solution as prescribed;
- Assess the client for allergies relative to tape, iodine, ointment, or antibiotic preparations to be used for skin preparation of the venipuncture site;
- Administer the fluid at the prescribed rate;
- Observe for signs of **infiltration** (seepage of the fluid into the interstitial tissue as a result of accidental dislodgement of the needle from the vein) and other complications that are fluid specific; and
- Document in the client's medical record the implementation of the prescribed IV therapy.

Evaluation

Evaluation is an ongoing process for clients with fluid, electrolyte, or acid–base imbalances. When evaluating whether the time frames and expected outcomes are realistic (such as whether the intake and output are within 200 to 300 mL of each other), the focus should be on the client's responses. The client's vital signs should be within normal limits. The IV infusion rate should be accurately calculated and reassessed throughout therapy to maintain the client's hydration. The IV site should remain free from erythema, edema, and purulent drainage. The nursing care plan should be modified as necessary to support the client's expected outcomes.

SAMPLE NURSING CARE PLAN

THE CLIENT WITH FLUID VOLUME EXCESS

When brought to the emergency department by his granddaughter, Mr. Gomez, a 68-year-old widower, stated, "I can't breathe." Mr. Gomez has a history of hypertension and heart disease, and he is obese. The practitioner ordered a stat chest x-ray, CBC, and electrolytes, which revealed pulmonary congestion (x-ray), decreased Hct, and decreased Hgb. The physical assessment results were as follows: Wt 162; TPR 97.6, 98, 30 (labored); BP 186/114; shortness of breath, crackles; constant cough; pitting edema (ankles); and engorged neck veins. Mr. Gomez stated, "I thought I could stop taking the heart medication and eat what I wanted when I felt good again."

Nursing Diagnosis 1 *Fluid Volume Excess related to a compromised regulatory mechanism as evidenced by edema, shortness of breath, crackles, decreased Hgb and Hct, and jugular vein distention*

PLANNING/GOALS	NURSING INTERVENTIONS	RATIONALE	EVALUATION
Mr. Gomez will have a balanced I&O for 2 days.	Measure and document hourly I&O; restrict fluids as ordered	Monitors fluid status	Output for the first 3 hours was 2,020 mL; on day two, I&O was indicative of fluid balance.
	Administer diuretics as ordered and document response	Increases excretion of fluids and electrolytes	

continued

Mr. Gomez will identify a specific amount of weight to lose over the next 6 months.	Weigh daily at the same time, with the same scale, and with Mr. Gomez wearing the same clothing	Allows weight to be compared from one day to another	Mr. Gomez identified the need to lose 30 pounds over the next 6 months.
	Discuss with Mr. Gomez the need for weight loss	Allows Mr. Gomez to voice his thoughts about weight loss and provides an avenue to determine number of pounds to be lost	
Mr. Gomez will show normal hydration status prior to discharge.	Measure and document vital signs every hour until shortness of breath subsides, then every 2 hours	Monitors Mr. Gomez's response to therapy	Mr. Gomez demonstrated normal hydration status, as shown by normal levels of Hct and Hgb; BP 156/92; normal breath sounds; and absence of shortness of breath, jugular engorgement, and peripheral edema.
	Hourly assess heart sounds; breath sounds; rate, rhythm, and depth of respirations; and the position Mr. Gomez takes to relieve the shortness of breath	Provides information for use in modifying the plan of care	

Nursing Diagnosis 2 *Knowledge Deficit related to information misinterpretation as evidenced by Mr. Gomez's statement "I thought I could stop taking the heart medication and eat what I wanted when I felt good again."*

PLANNING/GOALS	**NURSING INTERVENTIONS**	**RATIONALE**	**EVALUATION**
Mr. Gomez will demonstrate an understanding of the causes of fluid excess and the role of heart medications, foods, and exercise in assisting with weight reduction.	Assess Mr. Gomez's knowledge of hypertension; decreased cardiac output; digitalis; the effects of a large abdominal girth on breathing; and foods low in sodium, fats, and carbohydrates.	Provides a basis for educating Mr. Gomez about causes, aggravating and alleviating factors, and effects of fluid excess	Mr. Gomez was unable to verbalize understanding of the way that weight, high-sodium diet, and failure to take his heart medications caused the fluid excess. He was referred to home health for client teaching.

CASE STUDY

Mrs. Meisenbach is a 75-year-old woman with diabetes who has been experiencing flu-like symptoms of vomiting and diarrhea for 5 days. She lives alone and does not like to cook. When she got up this morning, she felt weak and dizzy. She called 911 to take her to the clinic. The emergency medical technicians called the practitioner en route, and Mrs. Meisenbach was taken directly to the infusion center, where 1,000 mL of lactated Ringer's solution was started. Later, she was given Gatorade to drink.

Assessment data revealed:

- *Marked thirst*
- *Temperature 99°F*
- *BP 94/74, Resp. 30*
- *Wt 157 lb (loss from 165)*
- *Dry mucous membranes*
- *Apical pulse 108/min*
- *Increased Hct, Hgb, and BUN*

The following questions will guide your development of a nursing care plan for the case study.

1. What other data would you collect?
2. What is the primary nursing diagnosis for Mrs. Meisenbach?
3. What goals would be appropriate for this nursing diagnosis?
4. Identify the nursing interventions and rationale to meet the goals.
5. Ascertain the fluid intake replacement needed. Include the IV and oral fluids.
6. On the basis of the intake, what should have been her output prior to discharge?

SUMMARY

- Homeostasis is the maintenance of the body's internal environment within a narrow range of normal values. It is an ongoing process, with changes constantly occurring in the body.
- Many chemical and physical processes are necessary for homeostasis.
- Ions are electrically charged atoms.
- Compounds that ionize in water are called electrolytes.
- The normal range of blood pH is 7.35 to 7.45. A decrease or increase beyond this range can cause severe or even fatal physiologic problems.
- The bicarbonate buffer system works to regulate pH in both intracellular and extracellular fluids.
- The phosphate buffer system works to regulate the pH of intracellular fluid and fluid in kidney tubules.
- Protein buffers work to regulate pH inside cells, especially red blood cells.
- Substances move in and out of cells by the passive transport methods of diffusion, osmosis, and filtration and by active transport.
- The kidneys regulate fluid and electrolyte balance.
- Sodium is the main electrolyte that promotes the retention of water.

- The slightest decrease or increase in electrolyte levels can cause serious, adverse, or life-threatening effects on physiologic functions.
- Hospitalized clients, especially elderly clients, are at risk for developing dehydration.
- Clients receiving IV therapy require constant monitoring for complications.

Review Questions

1. The basic unit of an element is:
   a. an atom.
   b. the nucleus.
   c. an electron.
   d. small groups of atoms called molecules.

2. The phosphate buffer system is involved in regulating the pH of the:
   a. carbonic acid in the lungs.
   b. carbon dioxide in the lungs.
   c. bicarbonate ions in the lungs.
   d. intracellular fluid and the fluid in the kidney tubules.

3. Diffusion is:
   a. the movement of molecules from a region of high concentration to a region of low concentration.
   b. the movement of molecules from a region of low concentration to a region of high concentration.
   c. the movement of a liquid from a region of high concentration through a membrane to a region of low concentration.
   d. the movement of a liquid from a region of low concentration through a membrane to a region of high concentration.

4. When gas is exchanged in the lungs:
   a. carbon dioxide concentration is equal in the alveoli and lungs.
   b. oxygen concentration is higher in the alveoli than in the blood.
   c. oxygen concentration is higher in the blood than in the alveoli.
   d. carbon dioxide has a higher concentration in the alveoli than in the blood.

5. When blood flows into a capillary bed, the pressure of the blood is:
   a. high in the venule.
   b. low in the arteriole.
   c. high in the arteriole.
   d. low but increases to high.

6. Acidosis and alkalosis are identified by changes in the pH. Which of the following statements is true?
   a. A pH above 7.45 is called acidosis.
   b. A pH above 7.45 is called alkalosis.
   c. A pH increase caused by an increase of bicarbonate in the blood is metabolic acidosis.
   d. A pH decrease caused by an accumulation of carbonic acid results in respiratory alkalosis.

7. The maximum amount of IV potassium chloride that can be infused per hour is:
   a. 5 mEq.
   b. 10 mEq.
   c. 15 mEq.
   d. 20 mEq.

Critical Thinking Questions

1. A client has been vomiting for 3 days and is unable to keep anything down. Besides fluid volume deficit, what other alterations would you expect to find?

2. Because half of serum calcium is bound to another solute in the blood, which other serum level must be considered when monitoring the serum level of calcium?

 WEB FLASH!

- Visit the Intravenous Nurses Society site for standards for IV therapy; certification information; and education.
- Look on the Web for information about IV therapy.

MEDICATION ADMINISTRATION

MAKING THE CONNECTION

Refer to the following chapters to increase your understanding of medication administration:

- **Chapter 6, Legal Responsibilities**
- **Chapter 10, Documentation**
- **Chapter 18, Basic Nutrition**
- **Chapter 21, Infection Control/Asepsis**
- **Chapter 22, Standard Precautions and Isolation**
- **Chapter 27, Diagnostic Tests**
- **Chapter 33, Nursing Care of the Client: Blood and Lymph Systems**
- **Chapter 34, Nursing Care of the Client: Gastrointestinal System**
- **Chapter 41, Nursing Care of the Client: Nervous System**

- **Chapter 43, Nursing Care of the Client: Sensory System**

Procedures: B28, Administering a Large Enema/Small (Mini) Enema; B29, Measuring Intake and Output; I9, Administering an Oral Medication; I10, Withdrawing Medication from an Ampule; I11, Withdrawing Medication from a Vial; I12, Administering an Intradermal Injection; I13, Administering a Subcutaneous Injection; I14, Administering an Intramuscular Injection; I15, Administering an Eye Medication; I16, Instilling an Ear Medication; A6, Administering Medications by IV Piggyback to an Existing IV

LEARNING OBJECTIVES

Upon completion of this chapter, you should be able to:
- *Define key terms.*
- *Describe the influence of drug standards and legislation on medication administration.*
- *Explain the principles of pharmacokinetics, including absorption, distribution, metabolism, and excretion of drugs.*
- *Describe factors that can affect a drug's action.*
- *Explain the different types of medication orders, when each is used, and the nurse's responsibilities for each type.*
- *Discuss principles of safe medication administration.*
- *Discuss potential liabilities for the nurse administering medications.*
- *Develop teaching guidelines for clients regarding medication administration in the home.*
- *Explain procedures for the different methods of medication administration, including the choice of route and site.*

KEY TERMS

absorption	intracath
angiocatheter	intradermal (ID)
aspiration	intramuscular (IM)
bioavailability	intravenous (IV)
butterfly needle	IV push (bolus)
chemical name	metabolism
distribution	onset of action
drug allergy	parenteral
drug incompatibility	patency
drug interaction	peak plasma level
drug tolerance	pharmacokinetics
enteral instillation	phlebitis
excretion	piggyback
flashback	plateau
flow rate	stock supply
generic name	subcutaneous (SC/SQ)
half-life	toxic effect
hypervolemia	trade (brand) name
idiosyncratic reaction	unit dose form
implantable port	vesicant
infiltration	

INTRODUCTION

Medication management requires the collaborative efforts of many health care providers. Medications may be prescribed by a physician, dentist, or other authorized prescriber such as advanced practice registered nurses as determined by individual state licensing bodies. Pharmacists are licensed to prepare and dispense medications. Nurses are responsible for administering medications. Dietitians are often involved in identifying possible food and drug interactions.

Medication administration requires specialized knowledge, judgment, and nursing skills based on the principles of pharmacology. The focus of this chapter is to assist the student in applying knowledge of pharmacology and in acquiring skills in the safe administration of medications. The nursing process is used to direct nursing decisions relative to safe drug administration and to ensure compliance with standards of practice.

DRUG STANDARDS AND LEGISLATION

A drug is a chemical substance intended to elicit a specific effect. An assumption made by nurses before administration of any medication is that the drug will be safe for the client to consume if the dose, frequency, and route are within the therapeutic range for that drug. This assumption is implied in accord with standards that are set to ensure drug uniformity in strength, purity, efficacy, safety, and **bioavailability** (readiness to produce a drug effect).

Standards

Standards have been developed to ensure drug uniformity so that effects are predictable. The *United States Pharmacopeia* and the *National Formulary* (USP and NF) are books of drug standards for use in the United States. The USP and NF list drugs that have been recognized as being in compliance with legal standards of purity, quality, and strength.

The USP has been providing standards for pharmaceutical preparations since its first edition was published in 1851. The NF was first published in 1898 by the American Pharmaceutical Association to provide a listing of drugs that complied with established standards.

Legislation

The Pure Food and Drug Act of 1906 designated the USP and the NF as the official bodies to establish drug standards. It also gave the federal government the authority to enforce these standards. The federal Food, Drug, and Cosmetic Act of 1938 empowered the Food and Drug Administration (FDA) to test all new drugs for toxicity before granting the pharmaceutical company the approval to market a drug. The federal Food, Drug, and Cosmetic Act of 1938 was amended in 1952 to distinguish prescription (legend) drugs from nonprescription (over-the-counter) drugs and to regulate the dispensing of prescriptions. Testing for drug effectiveness materialized with the Kefauver-Harris Act of 1962 (Lehne, 1998).

The Harrison Narcotic Act of 1914 classified habit-forming drugs as narcotics and began regulating these substances. This law and other drug abuse laws have been replaced with the Comprehensive Drug Abuse Prevention and Control Act (Controlled Substance Act) of 1970. This act defines a *drug-dependent person* in terms of physical and psychological dependence and provides for strict regulation of narcotics and other controlled drugs such as barbiturates through the establishment of five categories of scheduled drugs (see Table 24-1). Any controlled substance must be recorded by the dispensing pharmacist. The Drug Enforcement Agency (DEA) employs pharmacists to inspect all types of records, including prescriptions, to detect the illicit distribution of these substances.

The scheduling of controlled substances must be adhered to by all states as minimum standards; however, an individual state can enact stricter control of these substances. For example, the Controlled Substance Act has codeine in antitussives as a schedule V

Table 24-1 CONTROLLED SUBSTANCES

Schedule (C-I): Includes substances for which there is a high abuse potential and no current approved medical use (e.g., heroin, marijuana, LSD, other hallucinogens, certain opiates and opium derivatives).

Schedule (C-II): Includes drugs that have a high abuse potential and a high ability to produce physical and/or psychological dependence and for which there is a current approved or acceptable medical use.

Schedule (C-III): Includes drugs for which there is less potential for abuse than drugs in Schedule II and for which there is a current approved medical use. Certain drugs in this category are preparations containing limited quantities of codeine. Also, anabolic steroids are classified in Schedule III.

Schedule (C-IV): Includes drugs for which there is a relatively low abuse potential and for which there is a current approved medical use.

Schedule (C-V): Drugs in this category consist mainly of preparations containing limited amounts of certain narcotic drugs for use as antitussives and antidiarrheals. Federal law provides that limited quantities of these drugs (e.g., codeine) may be bought without a prescription by an individual at least 18 years of age. The product must be purchased from a pharmacist, who must keep appropriate records. However, state laws vary, and in many states such products require a prescription.

From PDR Nurse's Handbook 2000 by G. Spratto & A. Woods, 2000, Albany, NY: Delmar Publishers. Copyright 2000 by Delmar Publishers.

drug, but an individual state that identifies abuse of antitussives with codeine may place this drug in the schedule II category, which is more restrictive.

DRUG NOMENCLATURE

A drug may be used as an aid in the diagnosis, treatment, or prevention of disease or under other conditions for the relief of pain or suffering or to improve any physiologic or pathological condition. The terms *drug, medication,* and *medicine* are often used interchangeably by health care providers and laypersons.

Drugs can be identified by their chemical, generic, official, or trade name. The **chemical name** is a precise description of the drug's composition (chemical formula). The *nonproprietary,* or **generic**, **name** in the United States is the name assigned by the U.S. Adopted Names Council to the manufacturer who first develops the drug. When the drug is approved, it is given an *official name,* which may be the same as the nonproprietary name (Lehne, 1998). Drugs with a proven therapeutic value are listed in the USP and NF by their official name. When pharmaceutical companies market the drug, they assign a *proprietary name,* also called a **trade (brand) name**; therefore, one generic drug may have several trade names based on the number of companies marketing the drug. For example, ibuprofen is a generic name; common trade names for this drug are Advil, Excedrin IB, Motrin, and Nuprin. Generic names are not capitalized, but trade names are always capitalized.

DRUG ACTION

Drug action refers to a drug's ability to combine with a cellular drug receptor. Depending on the location of different cellular receptors affected by a given drug, a drug can have a local effect, a systemic effect, or both local and systemic effects. For example, when diphenhydramine hydrochloride (Benadryl) cream is applied to the skin, it elicits only a local effect; however, when this drug is administered in a tablet or injectable form, it causes both systemic and local effects.

Pharmacology

Pharmacology is the study of the effects of drugs on living organisms. This section discusses the pharmacological activities of drug action as it is related to medication management, drug classification, drug preparation, and routes of administration.

Medication Management

The purpose of medication management is to produce the desired drug action by maintaining a constant drug level. Drug action is based on the half-life of a drug. A drug's **half-life** refers to the time it takes the body to eliminate half of the blood concentration level of the original drug dose. For example, if a drug has a half-life of 6 hours, 50% of the drug's original dose is present in the blood 6 hours after administration; in 12 hours after administration, 25% of the drug is present. Because of a drug's half-life, repeated doses are often required to maintain the drug level over a 24-hour interval.

The nurse should understand other terms used to describe drug action: onset, peak plasma level, and plateau. **Onset of action** is the time it takes the body to respond to a drug after administration. A **peak plasma level** is the highest blood concentration of a single drug dose before the elimination rate equals the rate of absorption. Once the peak plasma level is achieved, the blood concentration level will decrease steadily unless another drug dose is given. If a series of scheduled drug doses is administered, the blood concentration level is maintained; maintenance of a certain level is called a **plateau**.

Classification

Drugs are commonly classified by the body system with which they interact (e.g., cardiovascular) or in accord with the drug's approved therapeutic usage (e.g., antihypertensive). Drugs with multiple therapeutic uses are usually classified in accordance with their most common usage.

Preparation and Route

Drugs are available in many forms for administration by a specific route (see Table 24-2). The route refers to how the drug is absorbed: oral, buccal, sublingual, rectal, parenteral, topical, and respiratory.

 Safety: Do Not Substitute Drug Forms
Drugs prepared for administration by one route should not be substituted by administering the drug prepared for another route. For example, when a client has difficulty swallowing a large tablet or capsule, the nurse should not administer an oral solution or elixir of the same drug without first consulting the physician because a liquid may be more easily and completely absorbed, producing a higher blood level than would a tablet.

Oral Route Most drugs are administered by the oral route because it is the safest, most convenient, and least expensive method. The disadvantage of the oral route is that it acts more slowly than the other routes, such as injectables. Drugs may not be given orally to clients with gastrointestinal intolerance or those on NPO (nothing by mouth) status. Oral administration is also precluded by coma.

Table 24-2 TYPES OF DRUG PREPARATIONS

TYPE	DESCRIPTION
Oral Solids	• Tablets: compressed or molded substances, to be swallowed whole, chewed before swallowing, or placed in the buccal pocket or under the tongue (sublingual) • Capsules: substances encased in either a hard or a soft soluble container or gelatin shell that dissolves in the stomach • Caplets: gelatin-coated tablets that dissolve in the stomach • Powders and granules: finely ground substances • Troches, lozenges, and pastilles: preparations designed to dissolve in the mouth • Enteric-coated tablets: coated tablets that dissolve in the intestines • Time-release capsules: encased substances that are further enclosed in smaller casings that deliver a drug dose over an extended period of time • Sustained-release: compounded substances designed to release a drug slowly to maintain a steady blood medication level
Topicals	• Liniments: substances mixed with an alcohol, oil, or soapy emollient that is applied to the skin • Ointments: semisolid substances for topical use • Pastes: semisolid substances, thicker than ointments, absorbed slowly through the skin • Suppositories: gelatin substances designed to dissolve when inserted in the rectum, urethra, or vagina
Inhalants	• Inhalations: drugs or dilutions of drugs administered by the nasal or oral respiratory route for a local or systemic effect
Solutions	• Solutions: contain one or more soluble chemical substances dissolved in water • Enemas: aqueous solutions for rectal instillation • Douches: aqueous solutions that function as a cleansing or antiseptic agent that may be dispensed in the form of a powder with directions for dissolving in a specific quantity of warm water • Suspensions: particles or powder substances that must be mixed with, not dissolved in, a liquid by shaking vigorously before administration • Emulsions: two-phase systems in which one liquid is dispersed in the form of small droplets throughout another liquid • Syrups: substances dissolved in a sugar liquid • Gargles: aqueous solutions • Mouthwashes: aqueous solutions that may contain alcohol, glycerin, and synthetic sweeteners and surface-active flavoring and coloring agents • Nasal solutions: aqueous solutions in the form of drops or sprays • Optic (eye) and otic (ear) solutions: aqueous solutions that are instilled as drops • Elixirs: solutions that contain water, varying amounts of alcohol, and sweeteners

From Fundamentals of Nursing: Standards & Practice *by S. DeLaune and P. Ladner, 1998, Albany, NY: Delmar Publishers. Copyright 1998 by Delmar Publishers. Adapted with permission.*

PROFESSIONAL TIP

Special Considerations Regarding Medication Administration

- Chewable tablets are designed to be chewed before swallowing because chewing enhances gastric absorption.
- Buccal and sublingual medications must be allowed to dissolve completely before the client can drink or eat.
- Suspensions and emulsions should be administered immediately after shaking and pouring from the bottle.

When small amounts of drugs are required, the buccal or sublingual route is used. Drugs administered through these routes act quickly because of the oral mucosa's thin epithelium and large vascular system, which allows the drug to quickly be absorbed by the blood.

Certain oral drugs are prepared for sublingual or buccal administration to prevent their destruction or transformation in the stomach or small intestines. Buccal drugs are designed to be placed in the buccal pocket (superior-posterior aspect of the internal cheek next to the molars) for absorption by the mucous membrane of the mouth. Sublingual medications are designed to dissolve quickly when placed under the tongue. For example nitroglycerin (Nitrostat), an anti-anginal drug, can be given either sublingually or buccally as prescribed, whereas isoproterenol hydrochloride (Isuprel), a bronchodilator, is given sublingually and methyltesterone (Testred), an androgen, is given only buccally.

Parenteral Route Parenteral drugs are administered with sterile technique by injectable routes. By definition, **parenteral** route refers to any route other than the oral-gastrointestinal tract; however, the medical usage of the term excludes topical administration. There are four routes that nurses routinely use to administer parenteral medications:

- **Intradermal** (ID) is an injection into the dermis.
- **Subcutaneous** (SC or SQ) is an injection into the subcutaneous tissue.
- **Intramuscular** (IM) is an injection into the muscle.
- **Intravenous** (IV) is an injection into a vein.

Other parenteral routes, such as intrathecal or intraspinal, intracardiac, intrapleural, intra-arterial, and intra-articular, are used by physicians and in some cases by advanced practice registered nurses for medication administration.

Topical Route Most topical drugs are given to deliver a drug at, or immediately beneath, the point of application. Although a large number of topical drugs are applied to the skin, other topical drugs include eye, nose and throat, ear, rectal, and vaginal preparations. Drugs directly applied to the skin are absorbed through the epidermal layer into the dermis, where they create local effects or are absorbed into the bloodstream. Drug action varies with the vascularity of the skin, usually requiring several applications over a 24-hour period to cause the desired therapeutic effect.

Transdermal patches, another type of topical preparation, are used to deliver medications such as nitroglycerin (Transdermal-NTG), an antianginal, and certain supplemental hormone replacements for absorption by the blood to produce systemic effects. Some topical drugs, such as eye and nasal drops and vaginal and rectal suppositories, can be applied directly to the mucous membranes. These drugs are absorbed quickly into the bloodstream, and, depending on the drug's dose (strength and quantity), may cause systemic effects.

Inhalants Inhalants such as oxygen and most general anesthetics deliver gaseous or volatile substances that are almost immediately absorbed into the systemic circulation. The inhalants are delivered into the alveoli of the lungs, which promote fast absorption due to:

- Permeability of the alveolar and vascular epithelium
- Abundant blood flow
- Very large surface area for absorption

Oropharyngeal hand-held inhalers deliver topical drugs to the respiratory tract to create local and systemic effects. There are three types of inhalers: the metered-dose inhaler, or nebulizer; the turbo-inhaler; and the nasal inhaler. They are explained later in this chapter.

Pharmacokinetics

Pharmacokinetics refers to the study of the absorption, distribution, metabolism, and excretion of drugs to determine the relationship between the dose of a drug and the drug's concentration in biological fluids. The knowledge of pharmacokinetics is used by health care providers in medication management.

The physician, when ordering a drug, is concerned mainly with determining the dose and route that will produce the most therapeutic effects; physicians, pharmacists, and nurses are all involved in identifying appropriate times for drug administration and for avoiding interactions with other substances that could alter the drug's actions. Physicians and nurses monitor the client's response to the drug's action. Drug actions are dependent on four properties: absorption, distribution, metabolism, and excretion.

Absorption

The degree and rate of **absorption**, or passage of a drug from the site of administration into the bloodstream, depend on several factors: the drug's physicochemical effects, its dosage form, its route of administration, its interactions with other substances in the digestive system, and various client characteristics such as age (Springhouse, 2000). Oral preparations, such as tablets and capsules, must first disintegrate into smaller particles for gastric juices to dissolve and prepare the drug for absorption in the small intestines.

Drugs administered intramuscularly are absorbed through the muscle into the bloodstream. Suppositories are absorbed through the mucous membranes into the blood. Intravenous drugs are immediately bioavailable because of their direct injection into the blood.

Distribution

Distribution refers to the movement of drugs from the blood into various body fluids and tissues. The degree of binding between blood proteins and chemical substances can limit the drug's distribution in the body. The actual volume of distribution of any drug can be altered by the client's health condition.

Metabolism

Metabolism refers to the physical and chemical processing of a drug by the body. Most drugs are metabolized in the liver. The rate of metabolism is determined by the presence of enzymes in the liver cells that detoxify the drugs. Certain drugs can also increase the rate of metabolism.

Excretion

Excretion is the elimination of drugs from the body. This occurs mainly through hepatic metabolism and renal excretion. Other organs such as the lungs, exocrine glands, skin, and intestinal tract can eliminate some drugs.

Drug Interaction

Drug interaction refers to the effect one drug can have on another drug. Drug interactions may occur when one drug is administered in combination with a second drug or a short time interval exists between the administration of two different drugs. Drugs can be combined deliberately to produce a positive effect; for example, hydrochlorothiazide (HydroDIURIL), a potassium-depleting diuretic, and spironolactone (Aldactone), a potassium-sparing diuretic, can be combined to maintain a normal blood level of potassium. A positive drug combination can also occur when one drug is deliberately given to potentiate the action of another drug, as in preoperative medications.

Not all drug combinations are therapeutic. Some drug combinations can interfere with the absorption, effect, or excretion of other drugs. For example, calcium products and magnesium-containing antacids can cause inadequate absorption of tetracycline (Tetracyn), an antibiotic, in the digestive tract.

Side Effects and Adverse Reactions

Drug effects other than those that are therapeutically intended and expected are called *adverse reactions*. A nontherapeutic effect may be mild and predictable (side effect) or unexpected and potentially hazardous (adverse effect). There are several types of adverse reactions: drug allergy, drug tolerance, toxic effect, and idiosyncratic reactions.

A **drug allergy** (hypersensitivity to a drug) is an antigen-antibody immune reaction that occurs when an individual who has been previously exposed to a drug has developed antibodies against the drug. The type of reaction may be mild (skin rash, urticaria, headache, nausea, or vomiting) or severe (anaphylaxis). Drug reactions are often manifested in the skin because of its abundant blood supply.

Anaphylaxis is an immediate, life-threatening reaction to a drug, such as penicillin, characterized by respiratory distress, sudden severe bronchospasm, and cardiovascular collapse. If emergency measures are not instituted immediately (administration of epinephrine, bronchodilators, and antihistamines), anaphylaxis can be fatal.

Drug tolerance occurs when the body becomes so accustomed to a specific drug that larger doses are needed to produce the desired therapeutic effect. For example, clients with cancer who experience severe pain may require larger and larger doses of morphine (a narcotic analgesic) to control the pain as the body builds up a tolerance to the morphine.

A **toxic effect** occurs when the body cannot metabolize a drug, causing the drug to accumulate in the blood. Toxic reactions can result after prolonged intake of high doses of medication or after only one dose.

An **idiosyncratic reaction** is a highly unpredictable response that may be manifested by an overresponse, an underresponse, or an atypical response. For example, 1 of 40,000 clients will develop aplastic anemia after receiving chloramphenicol (an antibiotic) (Springhouse, 2000).

Food and Drug Interactions

Medication management requires avoidance of possible food and drug interactions. There are three primary types of food and drug interactions:

1. Certain drugs may interfere with the absorption, excretion, or use in the body of one or more nutrients.
2. Certain foods may increase or decrease the absorption of a drug into the body.
3. Other foods may alter the chemical actions of drugs, preventing their therapeutic effect on the body.

Most interaction problems occur with the use of diuretics, oral antibiotics, and anticoagulant and antihypertensive drugs. Clients on sodium-restricted diets should be advised to consult with a pharmacist regarding the sodium content in prescription and over-the-counter drugs. Some drugs can contain almost half the total daily allowance of sodium. Alcohol is also considered a drug. Small amounts of alcohol interact with many drugs, such as antibiotics, antihistamines, anticoagulants, and sleeping pills. Food and drug interactions can vary depending on the dose and the form in which the drug is taken and the client's age, gender, body weight, nutritional status, and specific medical condition.

FACTORS INFLUENCING DRUG ACTION

Individual client characteristics such as genetic factors, age, height and weight, and physical and mental conditions can influence the action of drugs on the body. Sometimes mistaken for drug allergies, genetic factors can interfere with drug metabolism and produce an abnormal sensitivity to certain drugs.

The physician often correlates the client's age, height, and weight when determining the dosage for

LIFE CYCLE CONSIDERATIONS

Age-Related Factors Influence Drug Action and Dosing

- Neonates and infants have underdeveloped gastrointestinal systems, muscle mass, and metabolic enzyme systems and inadequate renal function.
- Elderly clients often experience decreased hepatic or renal function and diminished muscle mass.

many drugs. The nurse should make sure that this information is accurately recorded in the client's medical record. The amount of body fat may also alter drug distribution because some drugs such as digoxin (Digoxin), an inotropic drug, are poorly distributed to fatty tissues.

The client's physical condition can also alter the effects of drugs. For example, the drug must be distributed to a larger volume of body fluids in an edematous client than in a nonedematous client; therefore, the edematous client may require a larger drug dose to produce the drug action, whereas a dehydrated client would require a smaller dosage. Diseases that affect liver and renal functions can alter the metabolism and elimination of most drugs.

MEDICATION ORDERS

In health care settings (long-term care facilities and hospitals), medication orders are written on a physician's order form in each client's medical record. When a client is admitted to an inpatient health care facility, the drug order form is stamped with the client's name, room number, age, and weight. The client's weight will be used by the pharmacist in compounding and dispensing drugs.

All orders should be written clearly and legibly, and the drug order should contain seven parts:

1. The name of the client
2. The date and time when the order is written
3. The name of the drug to be administered
4. The dosage
5. The route by which it is to be administered and special directives about its administration
6. The time of administration and frequency
7. The signature of the person writing the order, such as the physician or advanced practice registered nurse

Drug prescriptions written in settings other than acute care facilities may also specify whether the generic or trade name of the drug is to be dispensed, the quantity

to be dispensed, and how many times the prescription can be refilled.

The nurse is responsible and held accountable for questioning any medication order if, in the nurse's judgment, the order is in error. The nature of the error may be in any part of the drug order, and the nurse should seek clarification from the physician as necessary. A drug error has serious legal implications if the nurse involved could have been expected, on the basis of knowledge and experience, to have noted the error.

Most agencies have policies relative to medication administration, such as stop dates for certain types of drugs, regularly scheduled times to administer medications as specified in the drug order, and a listing of abbreviations officially accepted for use in the agency. The agency's medical records department maintains the official listing of abbreviations adopted by the medical staff of that agency. Only abbreviations from the official list can be used in any part of the client's medical record at that agency (see Appendix B).

Types of Orders

Medications are prescribed in different ways, depending on their purpose. Medications can be prescribed as stat, single-dose, scheduled, and prn orders.

Stat Orders

Stat medication orders are those that should be administered immediately, not an hour or two later. Stat drugs are often prescribed in emergency situations to modify a serious physiologic response such as a stat dose of nitroglycerin for a client experiencing chest pain. The nurse should assess and document the client's response to all stat medications.

Single-Dose Orders

Single-dose orders are one-time medications. The nurse should administer single-dose orders either at a time specified by the physician or at the earliest convenient time. These drugs are often prescribed in preparation for a diagnostic or therapeutic procedure; for example, a laxative may be administered in preparation for a lower GI x-ray.

Scheduled Orders

Scheduled orders are administered routinely as specified until the order is canceled by another order. The scheduled orders stay in effect until the physician discontinues or modifies the dosage or frequency with another order or until a prescribed number of days have elapsed as determined by agency policy. The purpose of a scheduled medication order is to maintain the desired blood level of the medication.

Agency policy determines the actual times for administering medications over a 24-hour time interval. For example, t.i.d. drugs may be administered at 0800, 1400, and 2000 or at 0900, 1500, and 2100. Medications ordered qd may have a specified time identified in the order, such as Isophane (NPH) Insulin 10 U SC qd at 0600, or they may be given at the agency's designated time, for example, Lanoxin 0.25 mg po qd would be given at 0900.

When the order specifies the number of days or dosages of the drug the client is to receive, the order has an automatic stop date to discontinue the drug. For example, the order may read tetracycline 250 mg po q6h for 5 days. The nurse should execute this order by administering 250 mg tetracycline orally every 6 hours for 5 days for a total of 20 doses. Day one begins with the administration of the drug and the time the first dose is given.

PRN Orders

A drug may be ordered on a prn (as needed) basis as circumstances indicate. The drug is administered when, in the nurse's judgment, the client's condition requires it. This type of order is commonly written for analgesics, antiemetics, and laxatives. For example, a client may have an order for meperidine (Demerol), a narcotic analgesic, 75 mg IM q3–4h prn. The nurse administers the pain medication on the basis of the assessment of the client's pain and as specified in the order.

SYSTEMS OF WEIGHT AND MEASURE

Medication administration requires the nurse to have a knowledge of weight and volume measurement systems. In the United States there are three different systems of measurement used in medication management: metric, apothecary, and household.

Metric System

The metric system of weights and measures was adopted by the USP in 1890 to the exclusion of all other systems except for equivalent dosages. The Council on Pharmacy and Chemistry of the American Medical Association adopted the metric system exclusively in 1944. Resistance to changing established customs interfered with the exclusive adoption of the metric system. Today, however, the metric system is used in every major country of the world and is used almost exclusively in health care facilities in the United States (*Remington: The Science and Practice of Pharmacology,* 1995).

The metric or decimal system is a simple system of measurement based on units of 10. The basic units can be multiplied or divided by 10 to form secondary units. The decimal point is moved to the right when changing from a larger unit to a smaller unit, and the decimal point is moved to the left when changing from a smaller unit to a larger unit. For example:

5 g	=	5,000 mg	0.5 mg	=	500 mcg
5 mcg	=	0.005 mg	1.25 L	=	1,250 mL
0.25 g	=	250 mg	2.45 kg	=	2,450 g

The basic units of measurement in the metric system are the meter (linear), the liter (volume), and the gram (mass, or weight). Important metric equivalents and abbreviations to remember are:

- Volume (liquid)

  1 milliliter (mL) = 1 cubic centimeter (cc)

  1,000 milliliters = 1 liter (L)

- Weight

  1,000 micrograms (mcg or µg) = 1 milligram (mg)

  1,000 milligrams = 1 gram (g)

  1,000 grams = 1 kilogram (kg)

The metric system uses prefixes derived from Latin to designate subdivisions of the basic units, and prefixes derived from Greek to designate multiples of the basic units (see Table 24-3).

 Safety: Metric System

A zero is *always* placed in front of the decimal for values less than 1 (0.5) to prevent error.

Apothecary System

The apothecary system, which originated in England, is based on the weight of one grain of wheat. Therefore, the basic unit of weight is the grain (gr) and the basic unit of volume is the minim (the approximate volume of water that weighs a grain). Important apothecary equivalents and abbreviations are:

- Volume (liquid)

  60 minums (ɱ) = 1 fluid dram (fl dr, or ʒ)

  8 fluid drams = 1 fluid ounce (fl oz, or ℥)

  16 fluid ounces = 1 pint (pt)

- Weight

  60 grains (gr) = 1 dram (dr, or ʒ)

  8 drams = 1 ounce (oz, or ℥)

  12 ounces = 1 pound (lb)

Table 24-3 METRIC SYSTEM PREFIXES

PREFIX	EXAMPLE
Latin Prefixes— subdivisions of the basic unit	deci (1/10, or 0.1) centi (1/100, or 0.01) milli (1/1,000, or 0.001) micro (1/1,000,000, or 0.000001)
Greek Prefixes— multiples of the basic unit	deka (10) hecto (100) kilo (1,000)

Household System

The household system of measurement is similar to the apothecary system of liquid measures and is the least accurate of the three systems. It is not ordinarily used in dose calculations, but is used as a reference standard to help the client. The units of liquid measure are drop (gtt), teaspoon (tsp), tablespoon (Tbsp), ounce (oz), and cup (Figure 24-1). The 16-ounce pound of the household system *is* used in dose calculations, with 2.2 lb equal to 1 kg.

The USP recognizes the use of the teaspoon as the ordinary practice for household medication administration and states that the teaspoon may be regarded as representing 5 mL (American Hospital Formulary Service, 1996). Household spoons are not appropriate when accurate measurement of a liquid dose is required; therefore, the USP recommends that a calibrated oral syringe or dropper be used for accurate measurement of liquid drug doses.

Household units are often used to inform clients of the size of a liquid dose and are generally used in the calculation of a client's intake and output. Important household equivalents and abbreviations to remember are:

- Volume (liquid)

60 drops (gtt)	=	1 teaspoon (tsp)
3 tsp	=	1 tablespoon (Tbsp)
2 Tbsp	=	1 ounce (oz)
8 oz	=	1 cup (c)
2 cup	=	1 pint (pt)
2 pints	=	1 quart (qt)

- Weight

16 ounces	=	1 pound (lb)

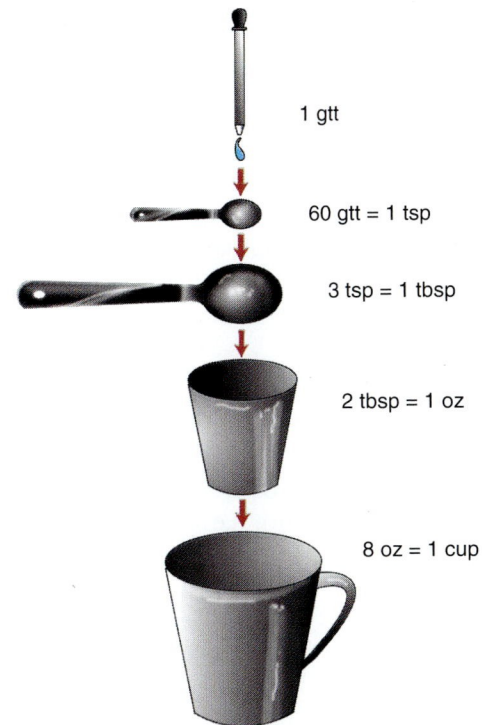

Figure 24-1 Relationship between Household Measures (*From* Medications & Mathematics for the Nurse *[8th ed.] by J. Rice, 1998, Albany, NY: Delmar Publishers. Copyright 1998 by Delmar Publishers. Reprinted with permission.*)

1 gtt

60 gtt = 1 tsp

3 tsp = 1 tbsp

2 tbsp = 1 oz

8 oz = 1 cup

APPROXIMATE DOSE EQUIVALENTS

The conversion of metric doses with the apothecary and household systems are *approximate dose equivalents* (see Table 24-4). The approximate dose equivalents represent the quantities usually ordered by physicians when using either the metric or apothecary system of

Table 24-4 APPROXIMATE EQUIVALENTS TO THE METRIC SYSTEM

METRIC		APOTHECARY		HOUSEHOLD	Weight	
Liquid (Volume)					0.4 mg (400 mcg or μg)	= 1/150 gr
Liquid	Weight	Liquid	Weight		1 mg (1,000 mcg)	= 1/60 gr
0.06 mL	= 60 mg	= 1 *m*	= 1 gr	= 1 gtt	4 mg	= 1/15 gr
1 mL	= 1 g	= 15–16 *m*	= 15 gr	= 15 gtt	10 mg	= 1/6 gr
5 mL	= 5 g	= 1 fl dr	= 1 dr	= 1 tsp	15 mg	= 1/4 gr
15 mL	= 15 g	= 4 fl dr	= 4 dr	= 1 Tbsp	30 mg	= 1/2 gr
30 mL	= 30 g	= 1 fl oz	= 1 oz	= 1 oz	1000 g (1 kg)	= 2.2 lb
240 mL	= 240 g	= 8 fl oz	= 8 oz	= 8 oz		
380 mL	= 380 g	= 12 fl oz	= 1 lb	= 16 oz		
500 mL	= 500 g	= 1 pt	= 16 oz	= 1 pt		
1,000 mL	= 1,000g	= 1 qt	= 32 oz	= 1 qt		

Adapted from Fundamentals of Nursing: Standards & Practice *by S. DeLaune and P. Ladner, 1998, Albany, NY: Delmar Publishers. Copyright 1998 by Delmar Publishers. Adapted with permission.*

weights and volumes for drug doses (American Hospital Formulary Service, 1996). If the prepared dosage form is prescribed in the metric system, the pharmacist may dispense the corresponding approximate equivalent in the apothecary system and vice versa. For example, if the physician prescribes morphine gr ¼, the pharmacist may dispense morphine 15 mg. The USP and NF reference *exact equivalents* that must be used to calculate quantities in pharmaceutical formularies and prescription compounding.

Converting Units of Weight and Volume

The nurse has to apply the knowledge of measurement systems and their conversions when the physician prescribes a drug dosage in one system and the pharmacy dispenses the equivalent dose in another. The conversions may be completed with either a proportion or a ratio. For example:

Proportion

$$\underset{\text{Extremes}}{\overset{\text{Means}}{2 : 4 \ = \ 6 : 12}}$$

Ratio

$$\frac{2}{4} = \frac{6}{12}$$

In a proportion, the product (multiplication) of the means equals the product of the extremes. In a ratio, the products of cross-multiplication are equal.

$$4 \times 6 = 24 \qquad 2 \times 12 = 24$$
$$2 \times 12 = 24 \qquad 4 \times 6 = 24$$

If one of the terms is unknown, it can be determined by substituting x for the number. The term with the x (unknown) is always put on the left.

$$2 : x = 6 : 12 \qquad \frac{2}{x} = \frac{6}{12}$$
$$6x = 24 \qquad\qquad 6x = 24$$
$$x = 4 \qquad\qquad x = 24$$

Proof that the answer is correct can be determined by substituting the answer for the x and multiplying.

Proportion can be used when converting units of weight and volume, conversions within the metric system, conversions between systems, and in drug dosage calculations. When the physician orders morphine gr ¼ and the pharmacist dispenses morphine 15 mg, the nurse is responsible for ensuring the correct dose. The nurse knows that 1 grain equals 60 milligrams; to convert the ordered dose to milligrams, the nurse should use the following calculation:

$$1 \text{ gr} : 60 \text{ mg} = 1/4 \text{ gr} : x$$
(the grains cancel out)
$$1 \, x = (60 \text{ mg})(1/4)$$
(divide 60 by 4)
$$x = 15 \text{ mg}$$

 Safety: Know What Is Being Calculated
All terms must be labeled (gr, mg, mL, and so on) to avoid errors.

Measurement Conversions within the Metric System

Because the metric system is based on units of 10, dose equivalents within the system are computed by simple arithmetic, either dividing or multiplying. For example, to change milligrams to grams (1,000 mg equals 1 g) or milliliters to liters (1,000 mL equals 1 L), divide the number by 1,000:

$$250 \text{ mg} = x \text{ g}$$
(move the decimal point three places to the left)
$$x = 0.25 \text{ g}$$
or
$$500 \text{ mL} = x \text{ L}$$
(move the decimal point three places to the left)
$$x = 0.5 \text{ L}$$

To convert grams to milligrams or liters to milliliters, the nurse multiplies the number by 1000:

$$0.005 \text{ g} = x \text{ mg}$$
(move the decimal point three places to the right)
$$x = 5 \text{ mg}$$
or
$$0.725 \text{ L} = x \text{ mL}$$
(move the decimal point three places to the right)
$$x = 725 \text{ mL}$$

The nurse may need to convert the volume of liters and milliliters for enemas and irrigating solutions as might be prescribed for bladder and wound irrigations. Intravenous solutions are sterile, prepackaged solutions dispensed in volumes as ordered by the physician, such as 50 mL, 100 mL, 250 mL, 500 mL, or 1,000 mL (1 liter).

Measurement Conversions between Systems

The nurse would have to convert between systems when, for example, the physician orders nitroglycerin (an antianginal drug) gr 1/150 po for chest pain and the dispensed dose is 0.4 mg:

$$1 \text{ gr} : 60 \text{ mg} = 1/150 \text{ gr}: x$$
$$1 \text{ gr} \, x = (60 \text{ mg})(1/150 \text{ gr})$$
(the grains cancel out)
$$1 \, x = 60/150 \text{ mg}$$
(divide by 60 by 150)
$$x = 0.4 \text{ mg}$$

The nurse can use proportion when converting pounds to kilograms (2.2 lb = 1 kg). For example, if the client weighs 154 lb, what is the weight in kilograms?

$$2.2 \text{ lb} : 1 \text{ kg} = 154 \text{ lb} : x$$

(the pounds cancel out)

$$2.2 x = 154$$

(divide 154 by 2.2)

$$x = 70 \text{ kg}$$

Drug Dose Calculations

Several formulas may be used by the nurse when calculating drug doses. One formula uses ratios based on the *desired dose* and the *dose on hand*. For example, cephalexin hydrochloride (Keftab), an anti-infective cephalosporin, 500 mg po q.i.d. (dose desired) is ordered by the physician; the dose on hand is 250 mg/5 mL. The formula is as follows:

$$\frac{500 \text{ mg (desired dose)}}{250 \text{ mg (dose on hand)}} \times \frac{x \text{ (quantity desired)}}{5 \text{ mL (quantity on hand)}}$$

(cross-multiply)

(milligrams cancel out)

$$250 x = 500 \times 5$$

$$x = \frac{500 \times 5}{250}$$

$$x = 10 \text{ mL}$$

In another example, the physician orders heparin (an anticoagulant) 10,000 units SC; the dose on hand is 40,000 units/mL:

$$\frac{10,000 \text{ units}}{40,000 \text{ units}} \times \frac{x}{1 \text{ mL}}$$

(cross-multiply)

(units cancel out)

$$40,000 x = 10,000$$

(zeros cancel out)

$$x = ¼ \text{ mL}$$

Because ¼ mL would be difficult to measure, it is best converted to minums. It is known that 1 mL = 15–16m. It will be best to use 16 so it will come out with a whole number for the answer.

$$1 \text{ mL} : 16m = ¼ \text{ mL} : x$$

(mL cancel out)

$$1 x = (16)(¼)$$

$$x = 4m$$

Pediatric Dosages

"Children are sometimes more susceptible than adults to certain drugs" (*Remington: The Science and Practice of Pharmacology*, 1995, p. 91). Several rules have been devised to calculate infants' and childrens' dosages, such as *Young's Rule, Clark's Rule,* and *Fried's Rule,* but these rules give only approximate dosages. Even when pediatric drug dosages are calculated on body surface area (BSA), they are based on a proportion of the usual adult dose (approximate). Body surface area is considered to be one of the most accurate methods of calculating medication dosages for infants and children up to 12 years of age (Rice, 1998). Regardless of the method used in calculating pediatric drug dosages, the nurse should realize that dosages are approximate and often need adjustment based on the child's response.

Body surface area refers to the square meter surface area method of relating the surface area of individuals to drug dosage. The BSA is based on weight and height and gives an approximate dose by using the following formula:

$$\frac{\text{Body surface area of child}}{\text{Body surface area of adult}} \times \frac{\text{Usual}}{\text{adult}} = \frac{\text{Child's}}{\text{dose}}$$
$$\text{dose}$$

The BSA of an adult is 1.73 square meters (m²); the 1.73 m² is based on an adult weighing 150 pounds.

A nomogram is used to compute the child's BSA (Figure 24-2). A straight line is drawn from the child's height in the left column to the child's weight in the right column. The point at which this line intersects the body surface area column (designated SA) indicates the child's BSA. For example: A 3-year-old child is 38

PROFESSIONAL TIP

Reasonable Answer

- The final step in figuring a dose is to ask whether the answer is reasonable.
- Seldom are more than 2 or 3 tablets or capsules given of one medication or more than 2 or 3 ounces of a liquid medication.
- Seldom is a parenteral injection, except for IV, given of more than 3 mL.
- If your calculations are outside these parameters, recheck your calculations and have a colleague check the calculations too.

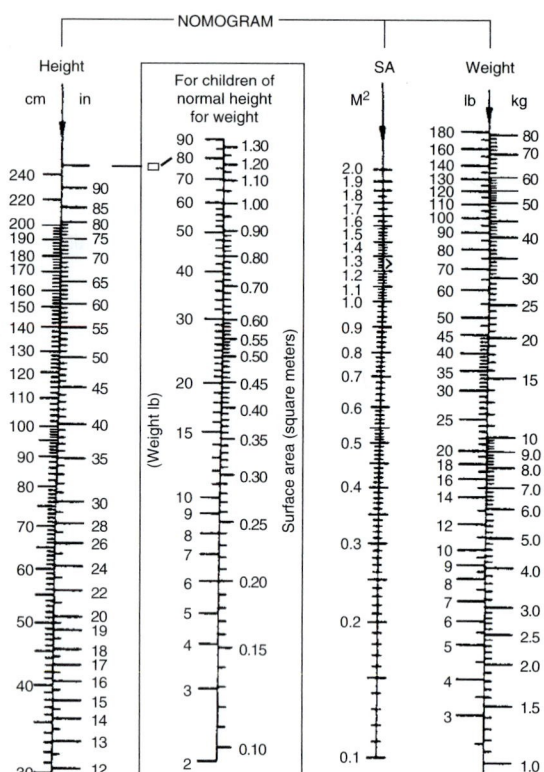

Directions for use: (1) Determine client height. (2) Determine client weight. (3) Draw a straight line to connect the height and weight. Where the line intersects on the SA line is the derived body surface area (M²).

Reprinted with permission from Behrman, R.E., Kliegman, R. and Arvin, A.M., editors. *Nelson Textbook of Pediatrics*, 15th ed. (Philadelphia: W.B. Saunders Company, 1996.)

Figure 24-2 Nomogram for Estimating Body Surface Area (*From* Nelson Textbook of Pediatrics *[15th ed.] by R.E. Behrman, R. Kliegman, & A.M. Arvin, 1996, Philadelphia: Saunders. Copyright 1996 by Saunders. Reprinted with permission.*)

inches tall and weighs 36 pounds. The physician orders meperidine (Demerol) for pain. The average adult dose is 50 mg. How much Demerol should the child receive? From the nomogram the child's BSA is 0.66 m².

$$\frac{0.66 \ (m^2)}{1.73 \ (m^2)} \quad \times \quad 50 \ mg$$
(square meters cancel out)
$$\frac{33}{1.73}$$
(divide 33 by 1.73)
$$= 19.07 \ mg \quad = \quad 19 \ mg$$

Now use the desired dose/dose on hand formula to determine how much to give.

$$\frac{19 \ mg}{50 \ mg} = \frac{x}{1 \ mL}$$
(milligrams cancel out)
(cross-multiply)
$$50x = 19 \ mL$$
$$x = 0.32 \ mL$$

This will have to be given in a tuberculin syringe. Nomograms are used primarily in calculating pediatric drug dosages; however, they are also used when calculating some adult drug dosages such as aminoglycosides and antineoplastic agents.

SAFE DRUG ADMINISTRATION

Nurses must administer numerous drugs daily in a safe and efficient manner. The nurse should administer drugs in accord with nursing standards of practice and agency policy. The safe storage and maintenance of an adequate supply of drugs are other responsibilities of the nurse.

The nurse should document the actual administration of medications on the MAR. The MAR is a medication administration record that contains the drug's name, dose, route, and frequency of administration. Drug data are entered either by the nurse when transcribing the order (hand-written onto the form) or by the pharmacist when dispensing the order (computer-generated form; Figure 24-3).

Guidelines for Medication Administration

To protect the client from medication errors, nurses have traditionally used as a guideline the "five rights" of drug administration as follows:

1. Right drug
2. Right dose
3. Right client
4. Right route
5. Right time

The nurse is legally responsible for knowing the usual dose, the expected action, the side effects, the adverse reactions, and any interactions with other drugs or food of every drug administered. Without this knowledge, the nurse should not administer any medication.

Right Drug

Before administering any medication the nurse compares the medications listed on the MAR or, less frequently, on a medication card against the physician's order. When administering a medication, the nurse should check the label written on the container against the MAR at least three times before giving the drug. The nurse should:

1. Check the label when removing the drug container from the client's medication drawer.
2. Check the drug when removing it from the container.
3. Check the drug before returning it to the client's medication drawer.

PHARMACY MAR

START	STOP	MEDICATION	SCHEDULED TIMES	OK'D BY	0001 HRS. to 1200 HRS.	1201 HRS. to 2400 HRS.
08/31/xx 1800 SCH		PROCAN SR 500 MG TAB-SR 500 MG Q6H PO	0600 1200 1800 2400	JD	0600 LW 1200 LW	1800 MS 2400 JD
09/03/xx 0900 SCH		DIGOXIN (LANOXIN) 0.125 MG TAB 1 TAB QOD PO ODD DAYS-SEPT.	0900	JD	0900 LW	
09/03/xx 0900 SCH		FUROSEMIDE (LASIX) 40 MG TAB 1 TAB QD PO	0900	JD	0900 LW	
09/03/xx 0845 SCH		REGLAN 10 MG TAB 10 MG AC&HS PO GIVE ONE NOW!	0730 1130 1630 2100	JD	0730 LW 1130 LW	1630 MS 2100 MS
09/04/xx 0900 SCH		K-LYTE EFFERVESCENT 25 MEQ TAB 1 EFF. TAB BID PO DISSOLVE AS DIR. START 9-4	0900 1700	JD	0900 LW	1700 GP
09/03/xx 1507 PRN		NITROGLYCERIN 1/50 GR 0.4 MG TAB-SL 1 TABLET PRN* SL PRN CHEST PAIN		JD		
09/03/xx 1700 PRN		DARVOCET-N 100* 1 TAB Q4-6H PO PRN MILD-MODERATE PAIN		JD		
09/03/xx 2100 PRN		MEPERIDINE*(DEMEROL) INJ 50 MG Q4H IM PRN SEVERE PAIN W PHENERGAN		JD		2200 (H) MS
09/03/xx 2100 PRN		PROMETHAZINE (PHENERGAN) INJ 50 MG Q4H IM PRN SEVERE PAIN W DEMEROL		JD		2200 (H) MS

Gluteus	Thigh	Nurse's Signature	Initial	Allergies: NKA	Patient:	Patient, John D.
A. Right	H. Right				Patient #:	3-81512-3
B. Left	I. Left	7-3 L. White, R.N.	LW			
Ventro Gluteal		3-11 M. Smith, R.N.	MS		Admitted:	08/31/xx
C. Right	J. Right			Diagnosis: CHF	Physician:	J. Physician, MD
D. Left	K. Left	11-7 J. Doe, R.N.	JD			
E. Abdomen 1|2 3|4					Room:	PCU-14 PCU

Figure 24-3 Computerized Medication Administration Record (*Adapted from* Fundamentals of Nursing: Standards & Practice *by* S. DeLaune *and* P. Ladner, *1998, Albany, NY: Delmar Publishers. Copyright 1998 by Delmar Publishers. Adapted with permission.*)

Right Dose

The nurse must know how to reduce the risk of error by correctly calculating doses and having them double-checked before administration. Policy in some agencies, for instance, mandates that two nurses check insulin dosages to ensure accuracy.

To prepare scored or crushed medications the nurse should make sure scored tablets are broken evenly. This practice will prevent overdosage or underdosage of a medication. If the medication has to be crushed with a mortar and pestle, the nurse should thoroughly cleanse the pestle after each use. Cleansing the pestle will avoid mixing of different medications and will prevent the client from receiving minute amounts of a medication that may cause serious adverse effects.

Right Client

The nurse should correctly identify the client by asking the client to state his or her full name and by checking the client's identification armband. The nurse should never identify a client solely by calling the person's name because some clients may be confused and will answer to any name.

Right Route

The route of the medication is specified in the written order. The nurse should consult the physician whenever a route is not identified in the prescription, when the route indicated differs from the recommended one, or when the nurse questions the choice of route prescribed. For example, the nurse should not substitute an oral medication for an intramuscular medication simply because the oral medication is available.

Right Time

Medications are generally ordered on a schedule. A drug should not be given more than an hour before or after the scheduled time, or as per agency policy, without first checking with the physician. For the drug's effect to be maintained, the medication has to been given in a timely manner.

Safety: Guidelines for Safe Administration of Medications

- *Never administer medications that are prepared by another nurse.* You are responsible for a medication error if you administer a medication that was inaccurately prepared by another nurse.
- Nurses should listen carefully to the client who questions the addition or deletion of a medication. If a client questions the drug or dose you are preparing to administer, recheck the order.
- If a medication is withheld, indicate the exact reason in the client's record. Legally you are responsible for giving prescribed medications to the client; however, circumstances may prevent you from giving them, and these must be documented.
- Do not leave medications at the client's bedside. The client may forget to take the medication, medications can accumulate, and the client could take two or more of the same medication, causing an overdose.
- Initial the MAR only for those medications you actually have administered. This practice ensures accurate charting by clearly indicating which actions you have performed.
- Advise clients not to take medications belonging to others and not to offer their medications to others. Medications are ordered for each client on the basis of the history, physical examination, and effectiveness of the medication.

In the home health and community care settings, such as a retirement home, the nurse has different responsibilities regarding drug safety (Figure 24-4). The nurse should promote drug safety measures that are appropriate to the environment and inherent risk factors.

Documentation of Drug Administration

A critical element of drug administration is documentation. The standard is *"if it was not documented it was not done."* Many drug errors can be avoided with appropriate documentation. The nurse responsible for

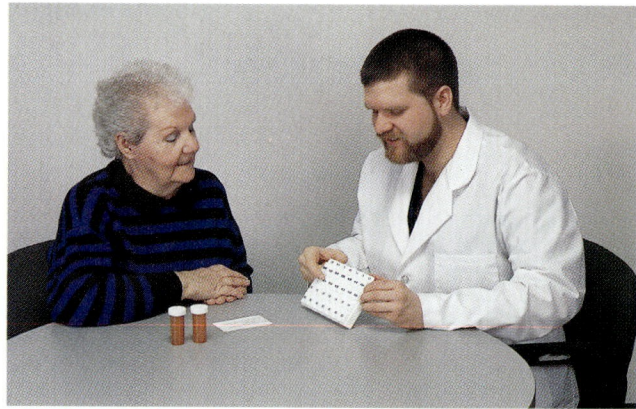

Figure 24-4 Assisting Client at Home with a Pillbox Correlated to the Days of the Month

administering the medication must initial the medication on the MAR for the time the drug was given. Usually there is a space available for a full signature on the record. The nurse should document that a drug has been given *after* the client has received the drug.

If the client refuses to take a medication once it has been prepared, the nurse must indicate that a dose was missed. The nurse should write in the record why the dose was missed and should notify the physician. The client may have refused because the tablet was too large. The medication may be supplied as a liquid so an alternate form of the medication can be given if the physician changes the order to the liquid form. Clients do have the right to refuse medication, but if they understand the actions of a medication, most will be willing to take it. Clients who are scheduled for various diagnostic tests or treatments at the time the medication is to be administered will need to have the medication time rescheduled, and the change will have to be documented.

HOME HEALTH CARE

Drug Safety Considerations

- Assist the client in removing outdated prescriptions and over-the-counter drugs from medication cabinets. The chemical composition may change over time, causing a different drug action. Over-the-counter drugs can interact with prescription drugs, either by decreasing or potentiating the effects of the prescription medication.
- Encourage the client or caregivers to maintain drug refills to decrease the risk of missing scheduled medications.
- Use a mechanism such as a paper clock, reminder calendar, or pillbox to help the client or caregiver remember to take or administer prescribed medications as scheduled.

Drug Supply and Storage

Drugs are dispensed by the pharmacy to nursing units through various methods to accommodate the agency's medication system. Once the pharmacy delivers the drugs to a nursing unit, the nurse is responsible for their safe storage.

Scheduled drugs for each client are usually dispensed in a **unit dose form**. Unit dose is a system of packaging and labeling each dose of medication by the pharmacy, often to supply the scheduled drugs for a 24-hour time period. The pharmacy usually delivers the drugs and stores the drugs in the designated area for each client. Unit dose drugs are usually stored in a medication cart that contains individual drawers for each client's medication supply or in the medication room in a separate, organized container for each client. The unit dose system makes it easy for nurses to administer the correct dose, thereby minimizing the number of medication errors.

The nurse, usually at the beginning of each shift, checks the medications in each client's drawer. Some medication carts are locked and the nurse keeps the key. Medication drawers should be removed one at a time from the cart when the nurse is preparing the medication for administration. The client's drawer should never be left unattended on top of the cart. Drugs should not be removed from one client's supply for administration to another client.

Certain drugs may be **stock supplied** (dispensed and labeled in large quantities) and stored in the medication room or other area on the nursing unit. Stock supplies are kept together in a secured area. Certain intravenous fluids and medications must be stored in the medication refrigerator to preserve the integrity of the drug. The Public Health Department and accrediting agencies mandate that only drugs can be stored in the medication refrigerator.

Narcotics and Controlled Substances

Health care agencies have forms to record the supply on hand and the administration of narcotics and controlled substances in accord with federal regulations. These forms usually require the recording of the following information for each drug administered:

- Name of the client receiving the drug
- Amount of the drug used
- Time the drug was administered
- Name of the prescribing physician
- Name of the nurse administering the drug

Nursing practice usually requires that nurses count the narcotics and controlled substances at specified intervals. For example, at the change of shifts, one nurse who is going off duty counts the drugs with a nurse coming on duty. Each drug used must be accounted for on the narcotic record. When the narcotic count does not check, the nurse must report the discrepancy immediately. Narcotics and controlled substances are kept in a double-locked drawer, box, room, or medication-dispensing cart, such as a computer-controlled dispensing system as shown in Figure 24-5. The law requires these safety precautions in the use of narcotics and controlled substances.

MEDICATION COMPLIANCE

Medication compliance can be associated with the client's understanding of why a medication was ordered and how a medication can decrease the likelihood of getting a disease or how it can lessen the effects of an existing disease. When clients do not consistently take their prescribed medications, or when they adjust the scheduling or dose of the medication, they are *noncompliant*.

There are several reasons why clients choose not to take ordered medications. It may be difficult for a hypertensive client who is asymptomatic (without distress) to understand the need to take prescribed medications. If medications are taken, the dose may be altered at the discretion of the client. Medications are costly, and the client may be on a fixed income or unemployed. If the medication does not provide prompt relief, the client may consider the medication useless and discontinue it. The medication may be discontinued if the client experiences undesirable side effects, such as impotence or weight gain.

Compliance can be enhanced if the client is given information on the medication to take home when discharged from the hospital. If the client is elderly, large-type print or illustrations should be used. Caregivers should be included when educating the client. Scheduling the medications around certain activities of daily living may serve as a reminder to the client that the medication must be taken. Providing the client with a telephone number and a name of a nurse to call if questions arise can foster compliance.

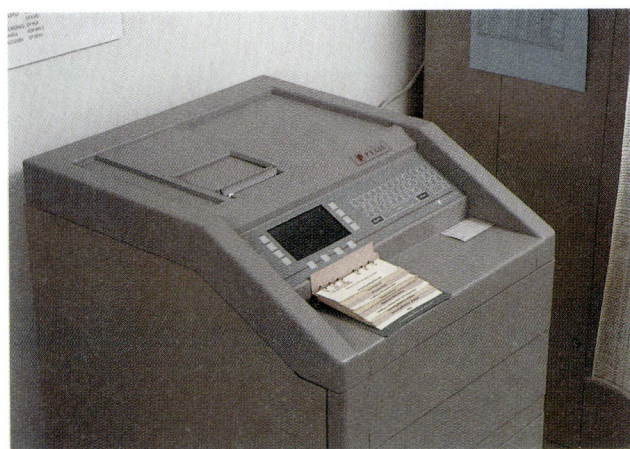

Figure 24-5 Computer-Controlled Dispensing System

The nurse in the community has an opportunity to see how medications are arranged in the client's home. Outdated medications must be discarded. After consulting with the client and caregiver, the nurse can make suggestions that may improve compliance.

Nurses have to remember that many elderly clients take a multitude of drugs. Some drugs actually cancel each other out when taken together, thus eliminating the therapeutic response. A client taking buspirone hydrochloride (BuSpar) and digoxin (Lanoxin) may experience digoxin toxicity. The BuSpar may displace the serum binding of digoxin and increase the toxic levels of that drug (Shannon, Wilson, & Stang, 1999). Nurses must sort through the medications with the client and report back to the physician any drugs taken in addition to those ordered by that physician.

LEGAL ASPECTS OF ADMINISTERING MEDICATIONS

Nurses have learned the "five rights" as a guideline to safe administration of medications. If the nurse gives the wrong medicine to the wrong person, an error has occurred. If the nurse has the right medicine but wrong dose or wrong route, a medication error has occurred. If the nurse gives the medication at the wrong time, an error has occurred. Nurses must inform the physician of the error made. If an antidote must be given, the physician needs accurate information to make appropriate care decisions.

Medication errors must be reported in a timely manner. Knowing the actions and the side effects of drugs will aid the nurse in assessing the client's response and health status. Incident reports are required in some agencies to document medication errors. A report of a medication error must include the name of the medication, dose given, route, time administered, specific error, time the physician was contacted about the error, and what countermeasures were taken.

Sometimes nurses discover errors made by other nurses. These must also be documented and reported.

NURSING PROCESS

The nursing process is vital in planning client care and in ensuring safe and accurate medication administration.

Assessment

Drug administration is based on assessment data obtained from eliciting a drug history, reviewing the client's medical history, performing a physical examination, and obtaining and interpreting relevant laboratory results.

Drug History

A drug history is obtained when a client is admitted to a health care facility. The drug history should contain specific questions about the client's medication background, including allergies, and use of prescription and over-the-counter drugs.

Allergies The nurse should inquire about all food and drug allergies. If the client has had an allergic reaction to a drug, the nurse should have the client describe the details of the reaction: name of the drug; dosage, route, and number of times the drug was taken before the reaction; onset of the reaction; and manifestations of the reaction. The nurse should question the client about possible contributing factors to the allergic reaction, such as concurrent use of stimulants or depressants (tobacco, alcohol, or illegal drugs) or significant changes in nutritional status.

Allergies to foods should also be queried by the nurse because drugs may contain the same elements or nutrients that cause allergic reactions to some foods. For example, clients who are allergic to shellfish may also experience a reaction to drugs that contain iodine. Vaccines are commonly derived from chick embryos and would be contraindicated in clients with allergies to eggs.

Prescription Drugs The nurse should have the client identify all current prescription drugs and describe:

- Why the drug was prescribed and by whom
- The drug's dosage, route, and frequency
- The client's knowledge of the drug's action: side and adverse effects, when to notify the physician, and special administration considerations such as with or without foods

If the client is receiving any drug that requires monitoring before administration, such as insulin (antidiabetic hormone), the nurse needs to make sure the client is checking blood sugar and that the results are within normal limits.

Over-the-Counter Drugs Clients usually have to be questioned separately about nonprescription drugs because they often fail to identify these drugs when asked to list all the medications they take routinely. For example, the nurse must determine if the client takes aspirin, antacids, or laxatives routinely. The client should describe the dosage, route, and frequency of these drugs. Because many drugs are available in topical form, the nurse should also inquire about the use of creams, ointments, patches, or sprays. Clients admitted to inpatient facilities should be asked if they have any over-the-counter drugs with them.

Medical History

The nurse should identify all chronic diseases and disorders and correlate these data with the drugs prescribed by the physician. Preexisting conditions such as liver and kidney dysfunction may require drug alteration because they prolong drug action, thereby increasing the potential for toxicity. The nurse needs to elicit this type of information during the medical history so that these clients can be closely monitored for signs of adverse reactions to drugs.

Biographical Data The client's biographical data, including age, education, occupation, and insurance coverage, may influence the nursing care plan and teaching plan. These data are also used by the nurse when assisting the client in the development of a drug regimen that complements the client's daily routine.

Lifestyle and Beliefs The client's lifestyle and beliefs affect attitudes toward health, use of the health care system, and daily activity patterns. These factors often determine the client's dietary habits and use of illegal drugs or other substances such as tobacco and alcohol.

Sensory and Cognitive Status The nurse should assess for and inquire about sensory deficits such as vision or hearing impairments, weakness or paralysis, or loss of sensation in one or more extremities. These deficits may impair a client's ability to comply with a prescribed drug plan, administer a subcutaneous injection, break a scored tablet, or open a medication container.

The nurse should assess the client's cognitive abilities throughout the drug history interview by noting if the client is alert and oriented and interacts appropriately. Clients who are not able to express their thoughts coherently or who exhibit impaired memory function will require special consideration by the nurse.

Physical Examination

The nurse assesses the client's condition before administering any drug to establish the client's baseline, or normal, health status. For example, the nurse assesses the client's apical pulse before administering digoxin (Lanoxin), an inotropic, so that the heart rate after receiving the drug can be compared with the baseline measurement.

Diagnostic and Laboratory Data

Common laboratory values, such as electrolytes, blood urea nitrogen, creatinine, glucose, complete blood count, and a white blood cell count, are usually monitored over a period of time to identify trends and to measure the body's response to infection.

Nursing Diagnosis

Once the nurse identifies the actual or potential problems, relevant nursing diagnoses can be formulated. The NANDA (1999) nursing diagnoses commonly related to medication administration include:

- *Health Maintenance, Altered*
- *Knowledge Deficit*
- *Management of Therapeutic Regimen, Ineffective*
- *Physical Mobility, Impaired*
- *Sensory/Perceptual Alterations*
- *Swallowing, Impaired*

Planning/Outcome Identification

The nurse develops the care plan and goals on the basis of the nursing diagnoses. For example, the client with a knowledge deficit related to a newly prescribed drug, insulin, may have the following expected outcomes:

Before discharge the client will:

- Correctly state the actions of insulin in the body.
- Prepare the correct dose of insulin in a syringe three times.
- State the reasons for rotating the injection sites and demonstrate by self-administering insulin to three different sites.
- Correctly identify the onset of action, peak plasma level, and half-life of the insulin preparation prescribed.
- Correctly perform glucometer testing to ensure a normal range of blood sugar before administering the insulin injection.
- Correctly describe the signs of hyperglycemia and hypoglycemia and the appropriate actions to take.

Nursing Interventions

The primary nursing interventions related to medication management are assessment, administration, and teaching. The nurse should use the time spent during medication administration to assess the client's knowledge and response to the drug's action.

The administration of medication requires the implementation of safety guidelines, following the five rights. Medications are administered in accordance with set procedures based on the prescribed route. This section presents procedures and guidelines for medication administration by the following routes: oral, including sublingual and buccal; parenteral; site-specific topical applications; and inhalation.

Drug teaching usually occurs in two phases. The first phase involves a formal teaching session. The nurse explains the drug's action, route, side and adverse effects, and the specific signs of a drug reaction that require physician notification. Clients often need assistance in developing a drug schedule that promotes compliance and complements their lifestyle. Self-administration may require the nurse to teach the client and/or support person specific procedural techniques, such as subcutaneous injection.

Written Medication Information

The American Nurses Association and various governing bodies support written medication information for clients that is "scientifically accurate, unbiased in content and tone, sufficiently specific and comprehensive, presented in an understandable and legible format, timely, up to date, and useful." Written medication information should:

- Be appropriate to client literacy level
- Reflect print size appropriate to client's visual abilities
- Give straightforward instructions
- Include generic and trade names
- Prominently display drug warnings
- Outline indications for use, contraindications, and precautions
- List possible adverse reactions and risks, storage, and use

(From American Nurses Association, 1997, American Nurse, 29[2], p. 11.)

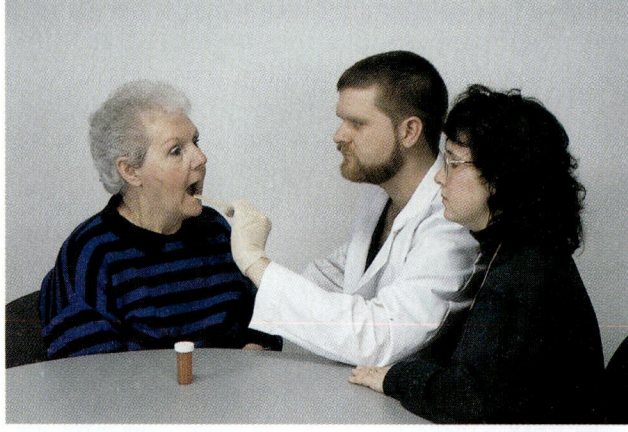

Figure 24-6 Check the client's mouth if unsure that medications have been swallowed.

The second phase of client teaching is ongoing, occurring whenever the nurse administers a drug. The nurse should assess and reinforce the client's knowledge of drugs at each interaction. If the client is being taught self-administration, the drug teaching plan should identify the dates for teaching, and expected outcomes should identify a date for client achievement of targeted goals.

Oral Drugs

Oral administration of drugs is the most common route; however, there are potential risk factors that the nurse must consider. Before administering oral drugs, the nurse should assess the client's ability to take the medication as prescribed. This assessment includes the client's gag reflex, state of consciousness, and presence of nausea and vomiting.

The nurse should protect the client against aspiration when administering any form of oral drugs. **Aspiration** refers to the inhalation of regurgitated gastric contents into the pulmonary system. To prevent aspiration, the nurse checks the client's gag reflex and ability to swallow.

Liquid medications are measured out in a medicine cup that is calibrated, usually in at least two of the three measuring systems. Doses smaller than 1 dr, 1 tsp, or 5 mL are measured in a syringe for acuracy. Solid oral medications are put into a medicine cup or small paper (soufflé) cup, depending on agency policy. Individually wrapped medications should be opened at the bedside.

When administering an oral drug, the nurse should remain with the client until all of the medications have been swallowed. If there is doubt that the client has swallowed a pill, the nurse should don a nonsterile glove and visually inspect the client's mouth with a tongue depressor (Figure 24-6).

Sublingual and Buccal Prior to administering sublingual and buccal drugs, the nurse should assess the integrity of the mucous membranes by inspecting under the client's tongue and in the buccal cavity. If the membranes are excoriated or painful, the nurse should withhold the medication and notify the physician. Some buccal drugs may irritate the mucosa, requiring the nurse to use alternate sides of the mouth to prevent irritation of the mucosa. Drugs given by these

Sublingual and Buccal Drug Administration

Sublingual Drugs:

- Keep the medication under the tongue until it dissolves completely to ensure absorption.
- Avoid chewing the tablet or manipulating it with the tongue to prevent accidental swallowing.
- Do not smoke before the drug has completely dissolved because nicotine has a vasoconstriction effect that slows absorption.

Buccal Drugs:

- Keep the medication in place until it dissolves completely to ensure absorption.
- Do not drink liquids for an hour because some tablets take up to an hour to dissolve.
- Do not smoke before the drug has completely dissolved because nicotine has a vasoconstriction effect that slows absorption.

routes are quickly absorbed by the mucosa's thin epithelium and the abundant blood supply.

Enteral **Enteral instillation** refers to the delivery of drugs through a gastrointestinal tube. Enteral tubes provide a means of direct instillation of medications into the gastrointestinal system of clients who cannot ingest them orally.

There are several types of enteral tubes. A nasogastric tube (NG) is a soft rubber or plastic tube that is inserted through a nostril and into the stomach. The gastrostomy tube is surgically inserted into the stomach through the creation of an artificial fistula. The physician uses an endoscope to insert a percutaneous endoscopic gastrostomy (PEG) tube into the stomach.

The nurse should assess the client for the presence of bowel sounds and check the tube for **patency** and placement before administering a medication. Patency refers to being freely opened. The instillation of drugs is contraindicated when the tube is obstructed or improperly placed, when the client is vomiting, or if bowel sounds are absent.

Safety: Verifying Placement of an Enteral Tube

The usual check for patency and placement of a nasogastric tube is performed as follows:

- Wash hands and don nonsterile gloves.
- Unclamp the tube.
- Create a 20-mL air space in a 50- or 60-mL syringe.
- Attach the syringe to the free end of the tube.
- Place the stethoscope on the left upper quadrant, 3 inches (7.5 cm) below the sternum.
- Gently instill 20 mL of air into the tube while simultaneously listening for a gastric bubble. (The gastric bubble is the "swish" sound heard as the air moves into the stomach.)
- When sound is heard, draw back on the piston of the syringe. (The appearance of gastric contents in the syringe may imply that the tube is in the stomach.) If the nurse fails to hear the swish sound and aspirates gastric contents, the tube may have risen into the client's esophagus. If this occurs, notify the nursing supervisor; do not administer the medication until placement in the stomach is verified. The nursing supervisor may elect to advance the tube into the stomach and check its placement by instilling air and aspirating or by obtaining a physician's order to confirm the tube's placement with an x-ray.

Once the patency and placement of the tube have been determined, the nurse prepares the medication for instillation as prescribed by the physician. When the physician orders a drug in the tablet or capsule form, the nurse should crush the tablet into minute particles and dissolve the crushed tablet in 15 to 30 mL of warm water before instillation. The instillation of cold solution may cause abdominal cramps. Capsules are prepared for administration by opening the capsule and emptying the contents into a liquid. When the drug has been prepared, the nurse is ready to instill the medication.

PROFESSIONAL TIP

Instilling Drugs into Enteral Tubes

- Wash hands and don nonsterile gloves.
- Place the client in a high or semi-Fowler's position, as the client's condition allows; for an NG tube, unpin the tube from the client's gown to allow manipulation of the tube's free end. Place a linen saver over the bed linens to prevent soilage during administration of the medication.
- Attach the syringe to the free end of the tube, pour 30 ml of medication into the syringe barrel, and open the clamp; for NG tube instillation, hold the NG tube at the client's nose level.
- Hold the syringe barrel at a slight angle and allow the medication to flow at a steady, slow rate; add more medication before the syringe empties to prevent air from entering the stomach. If necessary, adjust the height of the NG tube to achieve a steady flow rate.
- Observe the client while instilling the medication. If the client experiences any discomfort, slow the rate by lowering the height of the syringe.
- When instilling more than one medication, give each separately, with a 5-mL water rinse between medications.
- As the syringe barrel begins to empty with the last of the medication, slowly add 30 to 50 mL of room-temperature water into the syringe to clear the medication from the sides and distal end of the tube to prevent clogging.
- Before the syringe empties of water, clamp the tube, and detach and dispose of the syringe.
- Position the client as appropriate; clients with an NG tube should be placed on the right side with the head of the bed slightly elevated for at least 30 minutes after the instillation.
- Clean area, remove and dispose of gloves in the proper receptacle, and wash hands.
- Document the instillation of the medication on the MAR and record the total amount of fluid instilled on the intake and output sheet.

Parenteral Drugs

Parenteral medications are given through a route other than the alimentary canal; these routes are intradermal, subcutaneous, intramuscular, or intravenous. The angle of insertion of the syringe or needle and the depth of penetration will indicate the type of injection (Figure 24-7).

Equipment Nurses use special equipment such as syringes, needles, ampules, and vials when administering parenteral medications.

Syringes A syringe has three basic parts: the hub, which connects with the needle; the barrel, or outside part, which contains measurement calibrations; and the plunger, which fits inside the barrel and has a rubber tip (Figure 24-8). The nurse must ensure that the hub, the inside of the barrel, and the shaft and rubber plunger tip are kept sterile. When handling the syringe, the nurse should touch only the outside of the barrel and the plunger's handle.

Most syringes are disposable, made of plastic, and individually packaged for sterility. There are several types of syringes, such as the hypodermic, insulin, and tuberculin (Figure 24-9). When a medication is incompatible with plastic, it is usually prefilled into a single-dose glass syringe. Syringes are often prepackaged with the commonly used needle size and gauge.

The *hypodermic syringe* comes in 2-, 2.5-, and 3-mL sizes. The measurement calibrations (scales) are usu-

ally printed in milliliters and minims. Most syringes are marked in cubic centimeters (cc), and most drugs are ordered in milliters; these are equivalent measurements (1 cc = 1 mL). The hypodermic syringe is used most often when a medication is ordered in milliliters. When the order is written in minims, it is safer to prepare the drug in a tuberculin syringe.

The *insulin syringe* is designed especially for use with the ordered dose of insulin. For example, if the physician writes the order for 30 units of U-100 insulin, the nurse will use an insulin syringe that is calibrated on the 100-unit scale. The nurse should always compare the size of insulin syringe and the dose indicated on the insulin bottle with the physician's order; all three unit doses must be the same.

The *tuberculin syringe* is a narrow syringe, calibrated in tenths and hundredths of a milliliter (up to 1 mL) on one scale and in sixteenths of a minim (up to 1 minim) on the other scale. This syringe is commonly used today to administer small or precise doses, such as pediatric dosages. The tuberculin syringe should be used for doses 0.5 mL or less.

Prefilled single-dose syringes should not be confused with a unit dose. The nurse must be careful to check the prescribed dose against that in the prefilled syringe and discard excess medication. For example, if the physician orders diazepam (Valium) 5 mg IM as a preoperative sedative and the prefilled single-dose contains 10 mg/2 mL, the nurse must calculate dosage

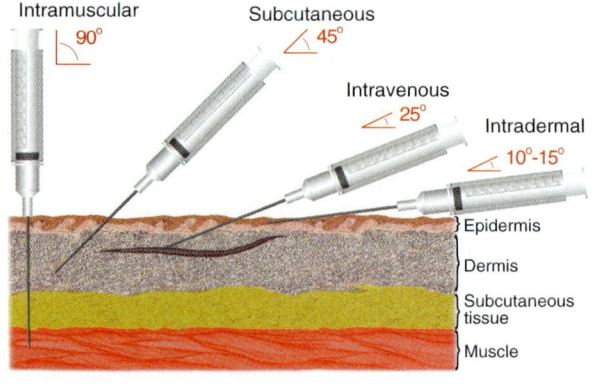

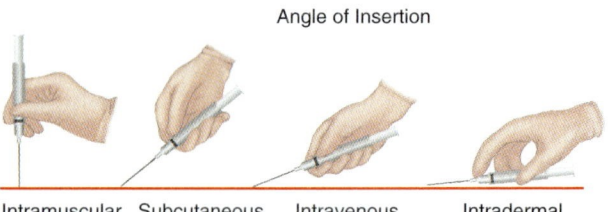

Figure 24-7 Angle of Insertion for Parenteral Injections (*From* Fundamentals of Nursing: Standards & Practice *by* S. DeLaune and P. Ladner, 1998, Albany, NY: Delmar Publishers. Copyright 1998 by Delmar Publishers. Adapted with permission.)

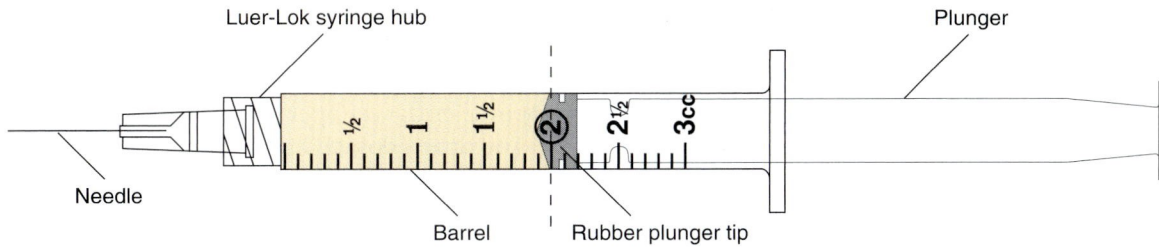

Figure 24-8 The Parts of a Syringe

(5 mg/1 mL) and destroy 1 mL from the syringe before administration.

Needles Most needles today are disposable, made of stainless steel, and individually packaged for sterility. Reusable needles are seldom used today, except in certain areas such as surgery and special procedure rooms; these needles require frequent inspection to ensure that the needle is sharp, and resterilization is necessary between uses.

The needle has three basic parts: the hub, which fits onto the syringe; the cannula, or shaft, which is attached to the hub; and the bevel, which is the slanted part at the tip of the shaft (Figure 24-10). Needles come in various sizes, from ¼ to 5 inches long, and with gauges that range from 28 to 14. The *gauge* of the needle refers to the diameter of the shaft; the larger the gauge number the smaller the diameter of the shaft. Smaller needles (larger gauge) produce less trauma to the body's tissue; however, the nurse has to consider the viscosity of a solution when selecting the gauge.

The *shaft* of the needle indicates its length. The nurse selects the length of the needle on the basis of the client's muscle development and weight and the type of injection, such as intradermal versus intramuscular.

The needle may have a short or a long *bevel*. The length of bevel selected is based on the type of injection. Long bevels are sharp and produce less pain when injected into the subcutaneous or muscle tissues. A short-bevel needle must be used for intradermal and intravenous injections to prevent occlusion of the bevel either by the tissue or by a blood vessel wall.

When the nurse removes a needle from its sterile wrapper, the hub of the needle should be immediately attached to the hub of the syringe to prevent contamination. Likewise, the protective cover should remain on the needle's shaft until the nurse is ready to use the needle.

After an injection, used needles should be disposed of in the proper receptacles, such as a sharps container, to prevent needlesticks. Most agencies have sharps containers in all client care areas. Discussion of the needleless system is found under IV therapy later in this chapter.

Ampules and Vials Drugs for parenteral injections are sterile preparations. Drugs that deteriorate in solution are dispensed as tablets or powders and are dissolved in a solution immediately before injection.

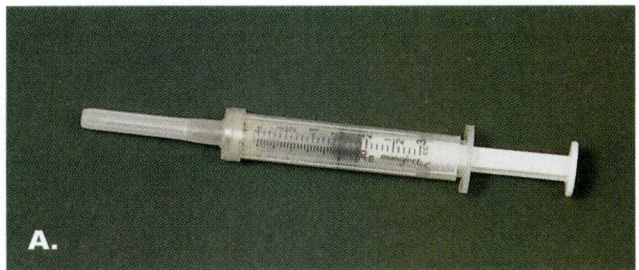

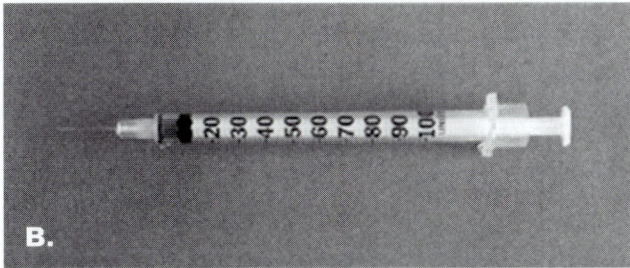

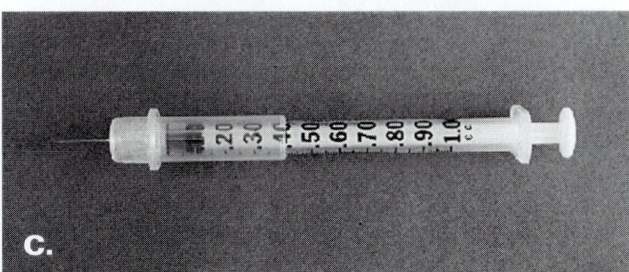

Figure 24-9 Types of Syringes: A. Hypodermic; B. Standard U-100 insulin (*Courtesy of Becton Dickinson Consumer Products*); C. 1-mL tuberculin (*Courtesy of Becton Dickinson and Company*)

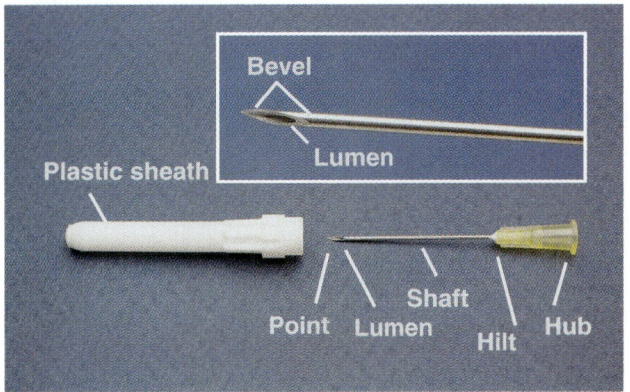

Figure 24-10 Parts of a needle

Drugs that remain stable in a solution are dispensed in ampules and vials in an aqueous or an oily solution or suspension.

Ampules are glass containers of single-dose drugs (Figure 24-11). The glass container has a constriction in the stem to facilitate opening the ampule. Because many drugs are irritating to the subcutaneous tissue, the needle on the syringe should be changed after withdrawing a drug from an ampule. The nurse should consider the use of a needle filter when withdrawing medication from an ampule or vial.

Glass, single- or multiple-dose rubber-capped drug containers are called vials (Figure 24-12). The vial is usually covered with a soft metal cap that can be easily removed. The needle on the syringe should be changed after withdrawing a drug from a vial.

Intradermal Injection Intradermal (ID) or intracutaneous injections are typically used to diagnose tuberculosis, identify allergens, and administer local anesthetics. The site below the epidermis is the loca-

tion for administering ID injections; drugs are absorbed slowly from this site. The sites commonly used for ID injection are the inner aspect of the forearm, upper chest, and upper back (Figure 24-13).

The drug's dosage for an ID injection is usually contained in a small quantity of solution (0.01 to 0.1 mL). A 1-mL tuberculin syringe with a short bevel, 25 to 27 gauge, ⅜- to ½-inch needle is used to provide accurate measurement. If repeated doses are ordered, the site should be rotated. Intradermal injections are administered into the epidermis layer by angling the needle 10° to 15° perpendicular to the skin.

Subcutaneous Injection Subcutaneous (SC or SQ) injections are commonly used in the administration of medications such as insulin and heparin because drugs are absorbed slowly, producing a sustained effect. Subcutaneous injections place the medication into the subcutaneous tissue, between the dermis and the muscle. The amount of medication given varies but should not exceed 1.5 mL. If repeated drug doses are to be given, the sites should be rotated.

Common sites for SC injections are the abdomen, the lateral and anterior aspects of upper arm or thigh, the scapular area on the back, and the upper ventrodorsal gluteal area (Figure 24-14). The nurse should

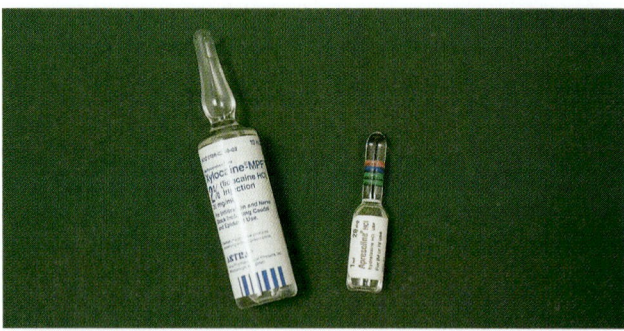

Figure 24-11 Ampules

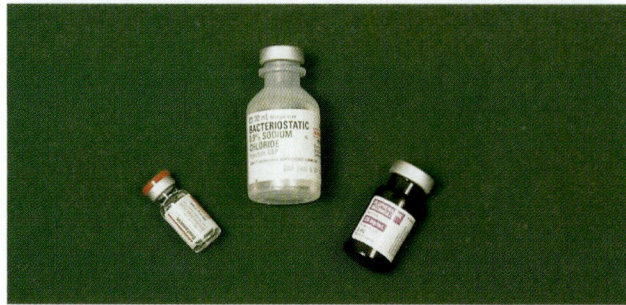

Figure 24-12 Vials

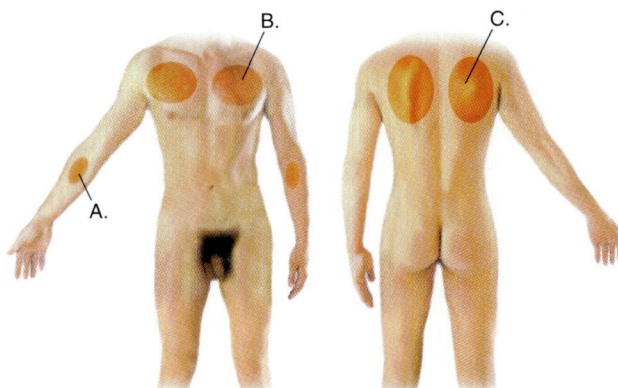

Figure 24-13 Intradermal Injection Sites: A. Inner aspect of the forearm; B. Upper chest; C. Upper back

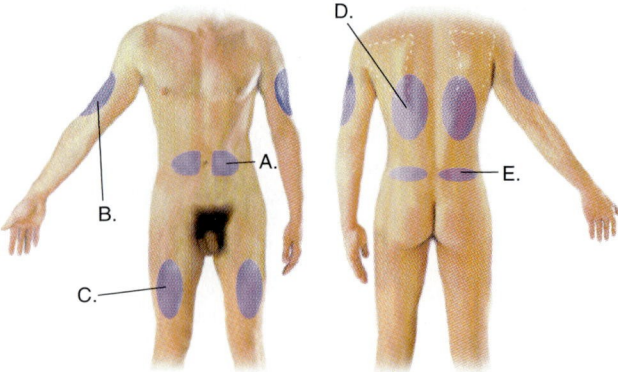

Figure 24-14 Subcutaneous Injection Sites: A. Abdomen; B. Lateral aspect of upper arm; C. Anterior aspect of upper thigh; D. Scapular area on back; E. Upper ventrodorsal gluteal area

select a sterile 0.5- to 3-mL syringe with a 25 to 29 gauge and a ⅜- to ½-inch needle. The medication is administered by angling the needle 45° to 90° perpendicular to the skin.

Intramuscular Injection Intramuscular (IM) injections are used to promote rapid drug absorption and to provide an alternate route when the drug is irritating to subcutaneous tissue. The IM route enhances the absorption rate because there are more blood vessels in the muscles than in subcutaneous tissue. However, the absorption rate may be affected by the client's circulatory status.

There are four common sites for administering IM injections: dorsogluteal and ventrogluteal (gluteus maximus muscle); anterolateral aspect of thigh (vastus lateralis muscle); and upper arm (deltoid muscle). Injection sites are identified by using appropriate anatomic landmarks (Figure 24-15). An IM injection is administered at a 90° angle.

Z-Track Injection The Z-track (zig-zag) technique refers to a method used in administering IM injections, most commonly for administering ventrogluteal and dorsogluteal injections.

A.

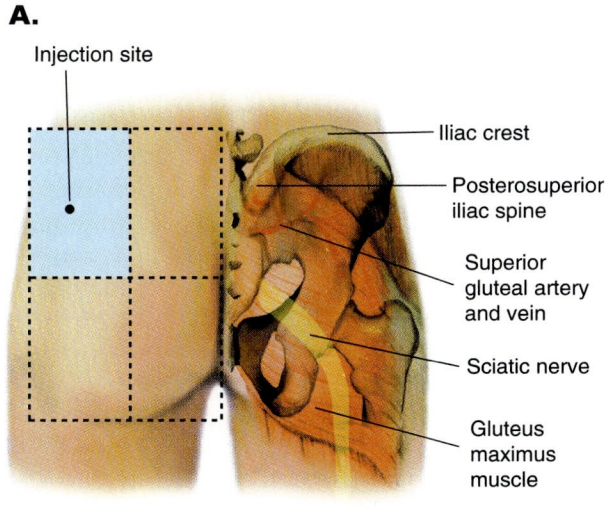

B.

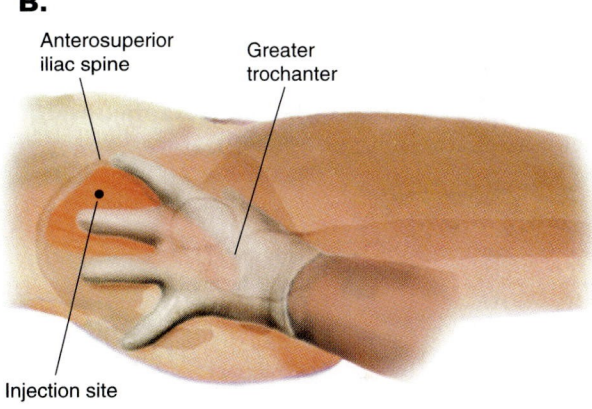

C.

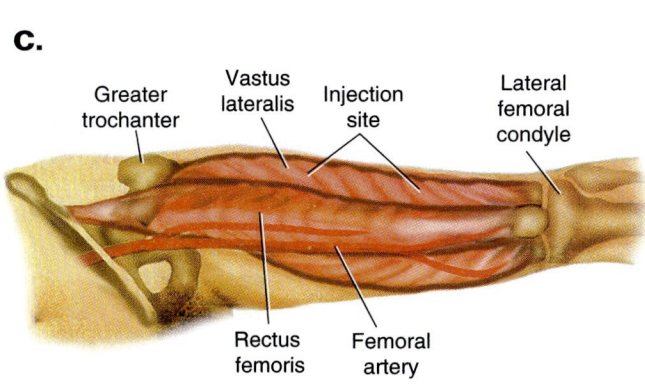

D.

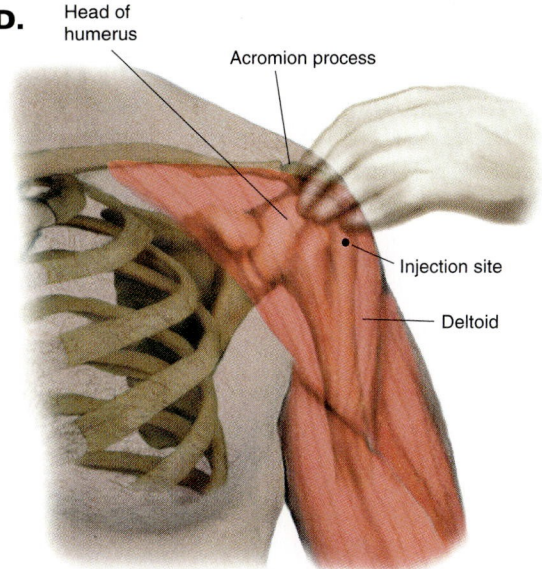

Figure 24-15 Intramuscular Injection Sites: A. Dorsogluteal: Place hand on iliac crest and locate the posterosuperior iliac spine. Draw an imaginary line between the trochanter and the iliac spine; injection site is the outer quadrant. B. Ventrogluteal: Place palm of left hand on right greater trochanter so that the index finger points toward the anteriosuperior iliac spine. Move middle finger to form a V between index and middle fingers; injection site is the middle of the V. C. Vastus lateralis: Identify the greater trochanter. Place hand at the lateral femoral condyle; injection site is middle third and anterior lateral aspect. D. Deltoid: Locate the lateral side of the humerus from two to three fingerwidths below the acromion process in adults or one fingerwidth below the acromion process in children. (*From* Fundamentals of Nursing: Standards & Practice *by S. DeLaune and P. Ladner, 1998, Albany, NY: Delmar Publishers. Copyright 1998 by Delmar Publishers. Adapted with permission.*)

For administration of a Z-track injection, the client is placed in the prone position; the skin is pulled to one side, the needle inserted at a 90° angle and the medication administered (Figure 24-16). The nurse waits 10 seconds, withdraws the needle, and then releases the skin. The site should not be massaged because massaging could cause tissue irritation. Spreading the skin, a common method formerly used for IM injections, increases the risk that medication will leak into the needle track and the subcutaneous tissue; this risk is virtually eliminated in the Z-track technique, making it the technique of choice (Beyea & Nicoll, 1996).

Intravenous Therapy Intravenous (IV) therapy requires parenteral fluids (solutions) and special equipment: administration set, IV pole, filter, regulators to control IV flow rate, and an established venous route.

Parenteral Fluids The nurse should confirm the type and amount of IV solution by reading the physician's order in the client's medical record. Intravenous solutions are sterile and are packaged in plastic bags or glass containers. Solutions that are incompatible with plastic are dispensed in glass containers.

Plastic IV solution bags collapse under atmospheric pressure to allow the solution to enter the infusion set. Plastic solution bags are packaged with an outer plastic bag, which should remain intact until the nurse prepares the solution for administration. When the plastic solution bag is removed from its outer wrapper, the solution bag should be dry. If the solution bag is wet, the nurse should not use the solution. The moisture on the bag indicates that the integrity of the bag has been compromised and that the solution cannot be considered sterile. The bag should be returned to the dispensing department that issued the solution. Glass containers are discussed in the section on equipment.

The three types of parenteral fluids are classified based on the tonicity of the fluid relative to normal blood plasma. A solution may be hypotonic, isotonic, or hypertonic. The type of solution is prescribed on the basis of the client's diagnosis and the goal of therapy. The desired effect of the solution is determined as follows:

- Hypotonic fluid: lowers the osmotic pressure and causes fluid to move into the cells. If fluid is infused beyond the client's tolerance, water intoxication may result.
- Isotonic fluid: increases only extracellular fluid volume. If fluid is infused beyond the client's tolerance, cardiac overload may result.

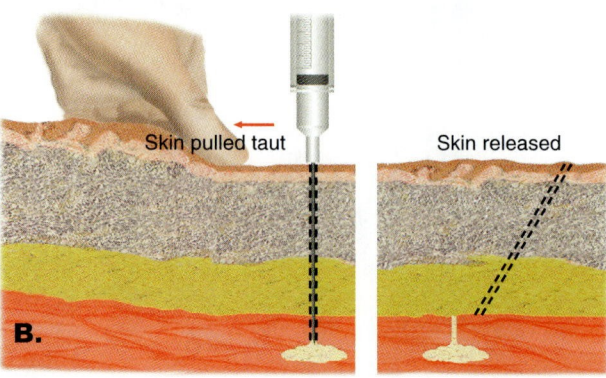

Figure 24-16 Z-Track Technique for IM injection: A. With client supine, grasp and pull the muscle laterally before injecting medication. B. Inject medication; keep skin pulled taut for 10 seconds; quickly withdraw the needle and release the skin to seal the site. (*Adapted from* Fundamentals of Nursing: Standards & Practice *by S. DeLaune and P. Ladner, 1998, Albany, NY: Delmar Publishers. Copyright 1998 by Delmar Publishers. Adapted with permission.*)

Skin pulled taut   Skin released

A.

B.

- Hypertonic fluid: increases the osmotic pressure of the blood plasma, drawing fluid from the cells. If fluid is infused beyond the client's tolerance, cellular dehydration may result (Bulechek & McCloskey, 2000).

Equipment Intravenous equipment is sterile, disposable, and prepackaged with user instructions. The user instructions are usually placed on the outside of the package and include a schematic that labels the parts, allowing the user to read the package before opening. The syringe tip and port require sterile technique during handling because they are in direct contact with fluids to be infused into the bloodstream.

The administration (infusion) set includes the plastic tubing used to infuse solutions. It contains an insertion spike with a protective cap, a drip chamber, tubing with a slide clamp and regulating (roller) clamp, a rubber injection port, and a protective cap over the needle adapter (Figure 24-17). The protective caps keep both ends of the infusion set sterile and are removed only just before use. The insertion spike is inserted into the port of the IV solution container.

Infusion sets can be vented or nonvented. The nonvented type is used with plastic bags of IV solutions and vented bottles. The vented set is used for glass containers that are not vented (Figure 24-18).

The drip chamber is calibrated to allow a predictable amount of fluid to be delivered. There are two types of drip chambers: a macrodrip, which delivers 10 to 20 drops per milliliter of solution, and a microdrip, which delivers 60 drops per milliliter. The drip rate, which is indicated on the package, varies with the manufacturer.

The IV tubing has a roller clamp that is used to compress the plastic tubing to control the rate of flow. The end of the IV tubing contains a needle adapter that attaches to the sterile injection device inserted into

LIFE CYCLE CONSIDERATIONS

Choosing IV Equipment

Neonates, infants, and children are at risk for *Fluid volume excess, related to rehydration.* Intravenous tubing with a microdrip and special volume control chamber is used to regulate the amount of fluid to be administered over a specific time interval.

the client's vein. Extension tubing may be used to lengthen the primary tubing or to provide additional Y-injection ports for the administration of additional solutions.

Intravenous Filters Intravenous filters remove from the solution particulate matter that may cause irritation and **phlebitis** (inflammation of a vein). Intravenous filters come in various sizes; the finer the filter, the greater is the degree of solution filtration. Although studies have shown that IV filters reduce the risk of bacteremia and phlebitis as much as 40%, some agencies do not use IV filters because of cost. Many IV catheters contain an in-line filter. If the catheter has an in-line filter, it is not necessary to add a filter to the tubing.

Needles and Catheters Needles and catheters provide access to the venous system. A variety of devices is available in different sizes to complement the age of

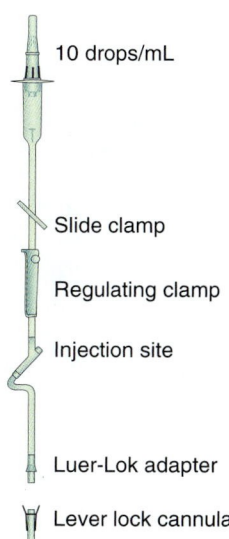

Figure 24-17 Sample Basic Administration Set

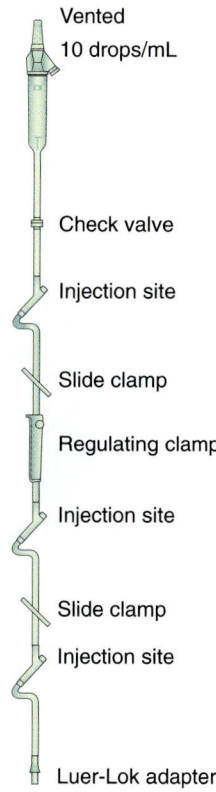

Figure 24-18 Sample Vented Administration Set

![sunrise icon]
LIFE CYCLE CONSIDERATIONS

Selecting Needle Gauge
Consider the client's age and body size and the type of solution to be administered when selecting the gauge of the needle or catheter.

- Infants and small children, 24 gauge
- Preschool through preteen, 24 or 22 gauge
- Teenagers and adults, 22 or 20 gauge
- Elderly, 22 or 24 gauge

the client and the type and duration of the therapy (Figure 24-19). The larger the number, the smaller the lumen of the needle or catheter.

Butterfly (scalp vein or wing-tipped) **needles** are short, beveled needles with plastic flaps attached to the shaft. The flaps (which are flexible) are held tightly together to facilitate ease of insertion and then are flattened against the skin to prevent dislodgment during infusion. These needles are commonly used for short-term or intermittent therapy and for infants and children.

There are several types of catheters used to access peripheral veins. During insertion, some of these catheters are threaded over a needle, and others are threaded inside a needle. **Intracath** is a term used to refer to a plastic tube inserted into a vein. An **angiocatheter** (angiocath, for short) is a type of intracath with a metal stylet to pierce the skin and vein, after which the plastic catheter is threaded into the vein and the metal stylet is removed, leaving only the plastic catheter in the vein.

Peripheral Intravenous and Heparin Locks Peripheral intravenous (PI) and heparin locks are devices that establish a venous route as a precautionary measure for clients whose condition may change rapidly or who may require intermittent infusion therapy. A butterfly needle or peripheral catheter is inserted into a vein and the hub is capped with a lock port, also called a Luer-Lok. The patency of the device is maintained with the injection of either normal saline or heparin (an anticoagulant drug) in accord with the agency's protocol.

Needle-Free System Safety is a concern with IV therapy. Accidental needlestick injuries and puncture wounds with contaminated devices increase the employee's risk for infectious diseases such as AIDS, hepatitis (B and C), and other viral, rickettsial, bacterial, fungal, and parasitic infections (Wolfrum, 1994). Most health care agencies now use totally needle-free IV systems (Figure 24-20) to decrease the risk of employee injuries.

Vascular Access Devices Vascular access devices (VADs) include various catheters, cannulas, and infusion ports that allow for long-term IV therapy or repeated access to the central venous system. The kind of VAD used depends on the client's diagnosis and the type and length of treatment. Central venous catheters (CVCs) are inserted by a physician.

Another type of VAD is an **implantable port** (a device made of a radiopaque silicone catheter and a plastic or stainless steel injection port with a self-sealing silicone-rubber septum). *Only nurses who have been specially trained are allowed to access an implanted port because of the risk of infiltration into the tissue if needle placement is incorrect.*

Preparing an Intravenous Solution To prepare an IV solution, the nurse should first read the agency's protocol and gather the necessary equipment. Because IV equipment and solutions are sterile, the expiration date on the package should be checked before use. The solution can be prepared at the nurses' work area or in the client's room.

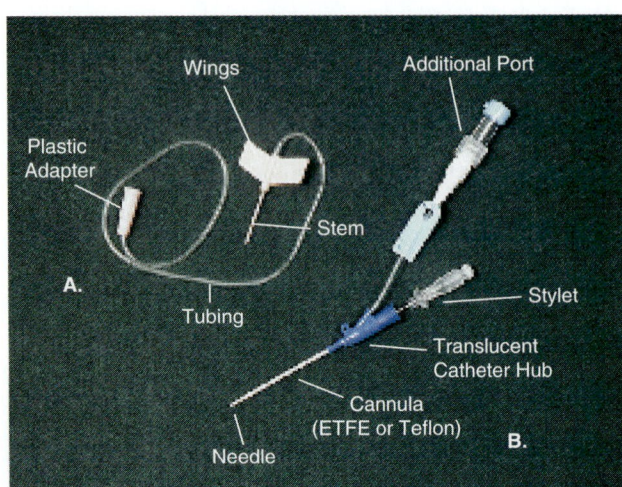

Figure 24-19 Peripheral IV Devices: A. Butterfly; B. Angiocatheter

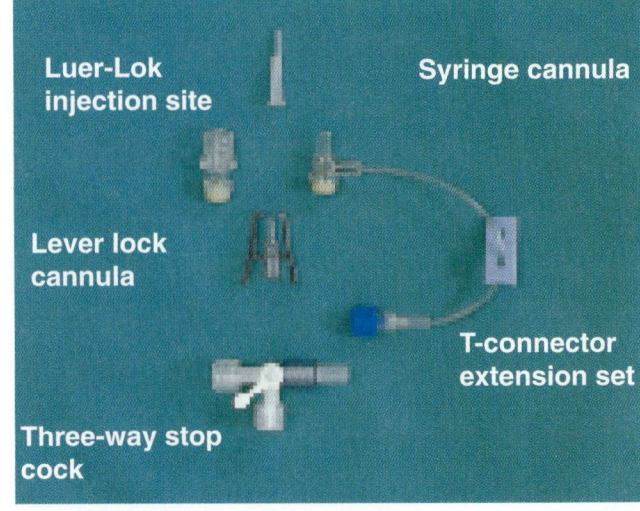

Figure 24-20 Needle-Free System

PROFESSIONAL TIP

Inserting a CVC

When assisting with the insertion of a long-line central catheter, observe the client for symptoms of a pneumothorax: sudden shortness of breath or sharp chest pain; increased anxiety; a weak, rapid pulse; hypotension; pallor or cyanosis. These symptoms indicate accidental puncture of the pleural membrane.

The nurse will prepare and apply a time strip to the IV solution bag to facilitate monitoring of the infusion rate as prescribed by the physician (Figure 24-21). The IV tubing is tagged with the date and time to indicate when the tubing replacement is necessary. Intravenous tubing is changed every 24 to 48 hours according to agency policy. The nurse initials the time strip and the IV tubing tag.

Safety: Marking an IV Bag

Do not use a felt-tip pen to mark an IV bag. The ink from the pen can leak through the plastic and contaminate the solution.

Initiating IV Therapy When initiating IV therapy, the nurse should assess for a venipuncture site. Figure 24-22 presents the common peripheral sites for starting IV therapy.

When assessing a client for potential sites, the nurse should consider age, body size, clinical status and impairments, and skin condition. Venipuncture site contraindications are:

- Signs of infection, infiltration, or thrombosis
- Affected arm of a postmastectomy client
- Arm with a functioning arteriovenous fistula (dialysis)

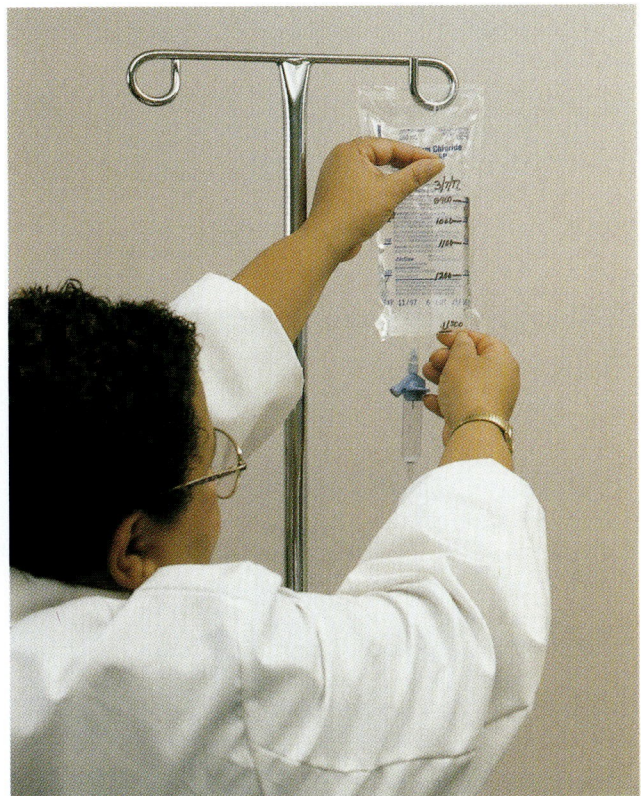

Figure 24-21 Applying a Time Strip to the IV Container

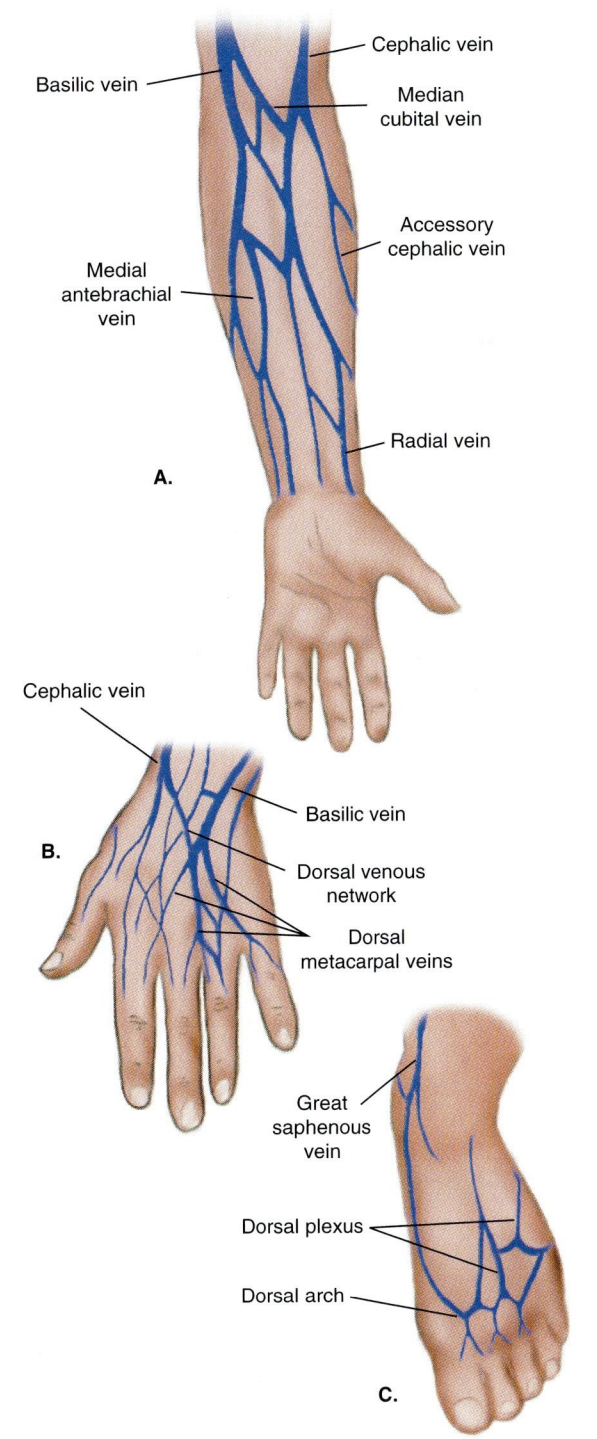

Figure 24-22 Peripheral Veins Used in Intravenous Therapy: A. Forearm; B. Dorsum of the hand; C. Dorsal plexus of the foot

- Affected arm of a paralyzed client
- Any arm that has circulatory or neurological impairments

Venous blood flows with an upward movement toward the heart, a vein should be selected for puncture at its most distal end to maintain the integrity of the vein. When a vein is punctured with an instrument, such as a needle, fluids can infiltrate (leak from the vein into the tissue at the site of puncture). If IV therapy has to be discontinued for any reason, such as infiltration, it can be restarted above the initial puncture site only.

Safety: Prepping Skin for Venipuncture

When prepping the client's skin for a venipuncture, cleanse the skin with Betadine and wait for it to dry. Do not apply alcohol after the skin has been prepped with Betadine. If these substances are combined, they form a toxic material that may be absorbed through the skin.

Administering IV Therapy Once the solution has been prepared for administration, the nurse calculates the rate and explains the procedure to the client. Fluid administration can be continuous, ongoing over a 24-hour period, or intermittent, 1,000 mL ordered once in a 24-hour period. Although fluids may be continuous, the type of fluids can alternate over a 24-hour period. For example, an order might be *add 40 mEq of KCl to first bag of 1,000 mL of normal saline.*

Intravenous medications may be **piggybacked**, connected to an existing IV to infuse concurrently. Intravenous solutions and medications that have been refrigerated should be warmed to room temperature before administration (usually for 30 minutes) to increase the client's comfort.

Regulating IV Solution Flow Rate The flow rate for IV solutions can be regulated by calculating the drops per minute and adjusting the drip rate to that number or by the use of volume controllers and pumps.

Calculating Flow Rate The **flow rate** is the volume of fluid to infuse over a set period of time as prescribed by the physician. The physician will identify the amount to infuse per time period such as: 125 mL per hour or 1,000 mL over an 8-hour period. The hourly infusion rate is calculated as follows:

$$\frac{\text{Total volume}}{\text{Number of hours to infuse}} = \text{mL/hour infusion rate}$$

For example, if 1,000 mL is to be infused over 8 hours:

$$\frac{1,000}{8} = 125 \text{ mL/hour}$$

Calculate the actual infusion rate (drops per minute) as follows:

$$\frac{\text{Total fluid volume}}{\text{Total time (minutes)}} \times \text{Drop factor} = \text{Drops per minute}$$

For example, if 1,000 mL is to be infused over 8 hours with a tubing drop factor of 10 drops per milliliter:

$$\frac{1,000 \text{ mL}}{8 \ (60) \text{ min}} \times 10 \text{ drops/mL} = \frac{10,000 \text{ drops}}{480 \text{ min}} = \begin{array}{c} 20.8, \text{ or } 21, \\ \text{drops/min} \end{array}$$

Another way to calculate the actual infusion rate is to use the hourly infusion rate; for the first example:

$$\frac{125 \text{ mL} \times 10 \text{ drops/mL}}{60 \text{ min}} = 20.8 \text{ or } 21 \text{ drops/min}$$

Volume Controllers and Pumps Controllers are devices that depend on gravity to maintain a preselected flow without adding pressure to IV systems to overcome resistance (for example, Dial-a-Flo or Buretrol). Resistance may develop from the use of a large catheter in a small vein, infusion of a viscous solution, high venous pressure, or a decrease in the height of the container from the IV site. Resistance may cause a decrease in the flow and sound the controller alarm. Volumetric controllers permit flow rates to be set in milliliters per hour.

Pumps are devices that maintain preselected volume delivery by adding pressure to the system when needed. They do not depend on gravity. Pumps may be used for viscous fluids and when large volumes must be delivered in a short period of time. Pumps have maximum pressure limits that, when reached, sound an alarm. Clients are at a greater risk for complications when a drug or solution is administered under high pressure.

Managing IV Therapy Intravenous therapy requires frequent client monitoring by the nurse to ensure an accurate flow rate and other critical nursing actions. These other actions include ensuring client comfort and positioning; checking the IV solution to ensure that the solution, amount, and timing are correct; monitoring expiration dates of the IV system (tubing, venipuncture site, dressing) and changing as necessary; and being aware of safety factors.

PROFESSIONAL TIP

Setting Volume to Be Infused

When setting the volume to be infused (e.g., 1,000 mL), set the volume to be infused slightly lower (e.g., 950 mL) so that the alarm will go off before the fluids are completely gone. This practice will give you time to have the next bag of fluids ready when all 1,000 mL has be absorbed. Having the extra time is especially helpful when dealing with refrigerated fluids that must be warmed to room temperature before being administered. If you will be off duty when the volume will be absorbed and the alarm is set to go off early, tell the oncoming nurse during report.

Catheter Sepsis

If a client complains of chills and fever, check the length of time that this IV solution has been hanging and the needle or catheter has been in place. Assess the client's vital signs, and assess for other symptoms of pyrogenic reactions, such as backache, headache, malaise, nausea, and vomiting. Unexplained fever may be related to catheter sepsis. Pulse rate increases, and temperature is usually above 100°F if IV-related sepsis occurs. Stop the infusion, notify the physician, and obtain blood specimens if ordered.

The nurse must coordinate client care with the maintenance of IV lines. Clients with IV therapy usually require assistance with hygienic measures, including changing the gown. Changing IV tubing when doing site care to decrease the number of times the access device is manipulated will thereby decrease the risk for infiltration and phlebitis. Peripherally inserted devices are changed every 72 hours as directed by the Centers for Disease Control and Prevention (CDC) guidelines.

Hypervolemia **Hypervolemia** (increased circulating fluid volume) may result from rapid IV infusion of solutions. This causes cardiac overload, which may lead to pulmonary edema and cardiac failure. The infusion rate must be monitored hourly to prevent this complication.

If a solution infuses at a rate greater than prescribed, the rate must be decreased to *keep vein open* (KVO) and the physician notified immediately. The nurse must report the amount and type of solution that is infused over the exact time period and the client's response.

Infiltration **Infiltration** (seepage of foreign substances into the interstitial tissue, causing swelling and discomfort at the IV site) may result from inserting the wrong type of device, using the wrong-gauge needle, or dislodgment of the device from the vein. Administration of a drug or solution under high pressure by a pump may also cause infiltration or vein irritation. The client usually complains of discomfort at the IV site. The nurse should inspect the site by palpating for swelling, and feel the temperature of the skin (coolness and paleness of skin are indications of infiltration).

The nurse should also confirm that the needle is still in the vein by pinching the IV tubing. This action should cause **flashback** (blood will rush into the tubing if the needle is still in the vein). If flashback does not occur, the injection port nearest the device should be aspirated. The needle or catheter should be discontinued if it cannot be aspirated and a sterile dressing applied to the puncture site.

After the IV has been removed, the puncture site may ooze or bleed (especially in clients receiving anticoagulants). If oozing or bleeding occurs, pressure is applied and a sterile dressing reapplied until it stops. The degree of edema must be accurately assessed and documented.

Clients may be injured by infiltration. If the IV site becomes grossly infiltrated, the edema in the soft tissue may cause a nerve compression injury with permanent loss of function to the extremity. If a **vesicant** (medication that causes blistering and tissue injury when it escapes into surrounding tissue) infiltrates, it may cause significant tissue loss with permanent disfigurement and loss of function (Masoorli, 1995).

Phlebitis Phlebitis may result from either mechanical or chemical trauma. Mechanical trauma may be caused by inserting a device with too large a gauge, using a vein that is too small or fragile, or leaving the device in place for too long. Chemical trauma may result from infusing too rapidly or from an acidic solution, hypertonic solution, a solution that contains electrolytes (especially potassium and magnesium), or other medications.

Phlebitis may be a precursor of sepsis. Client descriptions of tenderness are usually the first indication of an inflammation. The IV site must be inspected for changes in skin color and temperature (a reddened area or a pink or red stripe along the vein, warmth, and swelling are indications of phlebitis).

If phlebitis is present, the IV infusion must be discontinued. Before removing and discarding the venous device, the nurse should check the agency's protocol to see whether the tip of the device is to be cultured. If so, it must be sent to the laboratory for a culture and sensitivity test. After removing the device, a sterile dressing should be applied to the site and wet, warm compresses to the affected area. Documentation in the nurse's notes must reflect the time, symptoms, and nursing interventions.

Intravenous Dressing Change Intravenous dressing changes require the use of Standard Precautions and aseptic technique. Institutional protocol and the type of intravenous access device and dressing determine the frequency of care. Persistent drainage at the IV site may require dressing changes more frequently or may necessitate changing the IV site.

Intravenous Drug Therapy The intravenous (IV) route is used when a rapid drug effect is desired or when the medication is irritating to tissue. Intravenous administration provides immediate release of medication into the bloodstream; consequently it can be dangerous. Intravenous medications are administered by one of the following methods:

- Intravenous fluid container
- Volume-control administration set
- Intermittent infusion by piggyback or partial fill
- Intravenous push (IVP or bolus)

Adding Drugs to an Intravenous Fluid Container When administering IV medications, regardless of the method used, the nurse should assess the patency of the infusion system and the condition of the injection site for signs of complications such as infiltration and phlebitis. Some IV medications or solutions with high or low pH or high osmolarity are irritating to veins and can cause phlebitis.

Before administering any IV medication, the nurse should note the client's allergies, drug or solution incompatibilities, the amount and type of diluent needed to mix the medication, and the client's general condition to establish a baseline for administering medication. The nurse should check for drug compatibilities of drug additives before injecting a medication into an infusion bag. **Drug incompatibilities** cause an undesired chemical or physical reaction between a drug and a solution, between two drugs, or between a drug and the container or tubing. For example, diazapam (Valium) and chlordiazepoxide hydrochloride (Librium) must not come into contact with a saline solution; insulin should not be added to an infusion bag because the insulin adheres to the inside of the solution bag.

Adding Drugs to a Volume-Control Administration Set A volume-control set is used to administer small volumes of IV solution. These devices have various names as determined by the manufacturer, such as Soluset, Metriset, VoluTrol, or Buretrol. To administer a drug by this method, the nurse should:

- Withdraw the prescribed amount of medication into a syringe that is to be injected into the volume-control set.
- Cleanse the injection port of a partially filled volume-control set with an alcohol swab.
- Inject the prepared medication into the port of the volume-control set.
- Gently mix the solution in the volume-control chamber.

After injecting the medication into the volume-control chamber, the nurse should check the infusion rate and adjust as necessary to the prescribed rate of infusion.

Administering Medications by Intermittent Infusion A common method of administering IV medications is by using a secondary, or partial-fill additive bag, often referred to as an IV piggyback (IVPB). A secondary line is a complete IV set (fluid container and tubing with either a microdrip or a macrodrip system) connected to a Y-port of a primary line. The primary line maintains venous access. The IVPB is used for medication administration (Figure 24-23). When the IVPB medication is incompatible with the primary IV solution, the nurse must flush the primary IV tubing with normal saline before and after administering the medication.

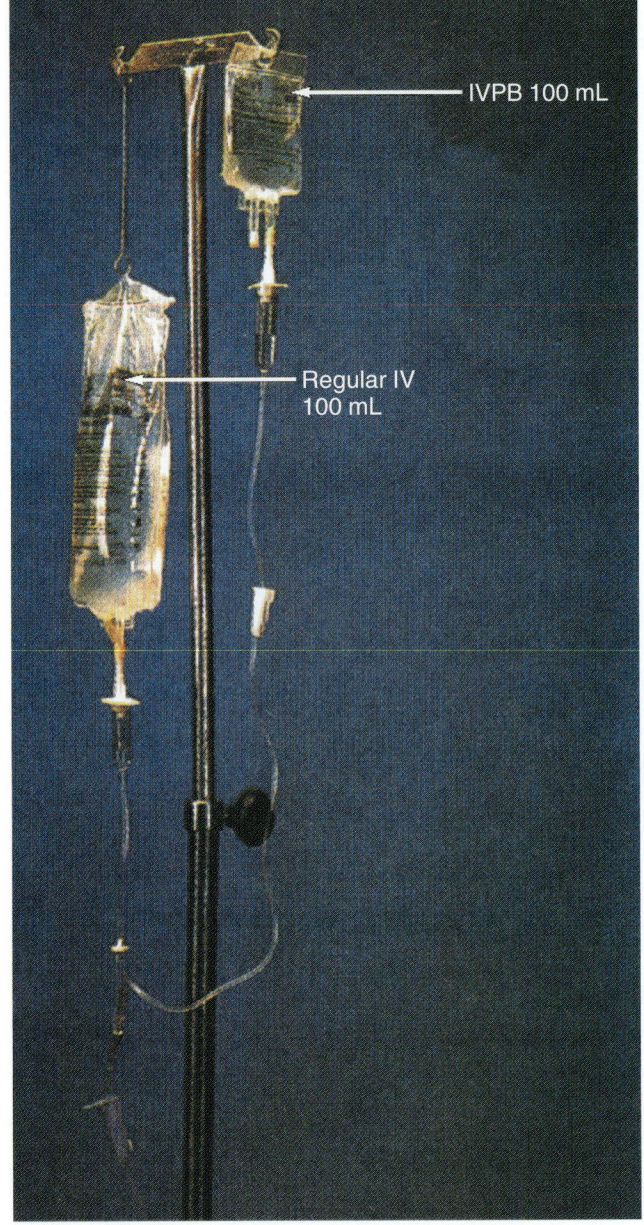

Figure 24-23 Intravenous with Piggyback (IVPB)

Intermittent Infusion Devices When the client requires only the administration of IV medications without the infusion of solutions, an intermittent infusion device is attached to a peripheral needle or catheter in the client's vein. This device is commonly referred to as a heparin or saline lock (Figure 24-24) depending on the agency's policy regarding the device's maintenance. A lock provides continuous access to venous circulation, eliminating the need for a continuous IV, and it increases the client's mobility.

The device can be used to infuse intermittent IVPB or IV push (also called bolus) medications, or it can be converted to a primary IV. An **IV push (bolus)** is a method of administering a large dose of medication in a relatively short time, usually 1 to 30 minutes. A major

The photo label reads: IVPB 100 mL / Regular IV 100 mL

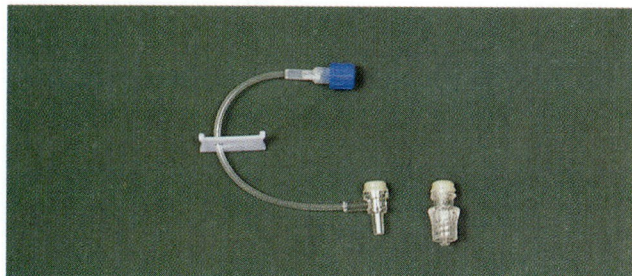

Figure 24-24 Heparin-Locking Device

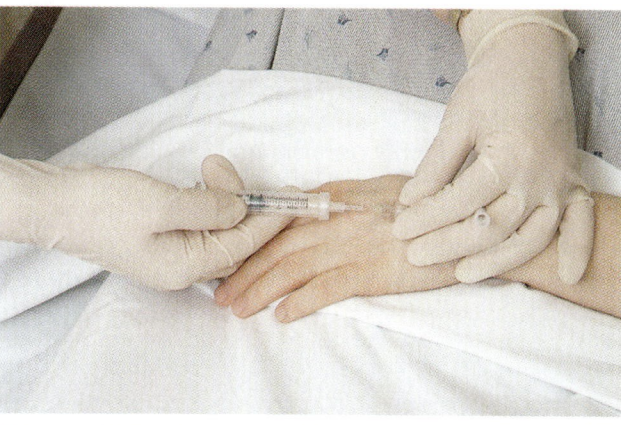

Figure 24-26 Injecting an IV Push (Bolus) Medication into a Primary Infusion Line. The IV tubing must be pinched closed first.

consideration for inserting a heparin lock device is that it provides venous access in case of an emergency. Lock devices are routinely used with cardiac clients.

Administering IV Push Medications The method of medication administration by IV push (bolus) injection is determined by the type of IV system. For example, an IV push medication can be injected into a saline or a heparin lock (Figure 24-25) or into a continuous infusion line. When giving an IV push medication into a continuous infusion line, the nurse must stop the fluids in the primary line by pinching the IV tubing closed while injecting the drug (Figure 24-26). This technique is safe and prevents the nurse from having to recalculate the drip rate of the primary infusion line.

Blood Transfusion

The purpose of a blood transfusion is to replace blood loss (deficit) with whole blood or blood components. On the basis of the client's unique needs, the physician determines the type of transfusion to administer, either whole blood or a component of whole blood.

Whole Blood and Blood Products Clients with a demonstrated deficiency in either whole blood or a specific component of blood are given a blood transfusion. Whole blood contains red blood cells (RBCs) and plasma components of blood. It is used when the client needs all the components of blood to restore blood volume after severe hemorrhage and to restore the capacity of the blood to carry oxygen.

When the physician prescribes the administration of whole blood or a blood product, the client's blood is typed and crossmatched. Check with the family for donors if time and the client's condition permit. The blood is stored in the blood bank after typing and crossmatching.

Although whole blood has a refrigerated shelf life of 35 days, platelets must be administered within 3 days after they have been extracted from whole blood. If the RBCs and plasma are frozen, their shelf life can be extended up to 3 years (Kee & Paulanka, 1999).

Initial Assessment and Preparation The nurse must perform an initial assessment before administering blood. The nurse should:

- Verify that the client has signed a blood administration consent form and that this consent matches what the physician has prescribed.
- Verify whether the client has an 18- or a 19-gauge needle or catheter in a vein. The viscosity of whole blood usually requires this gauge needle or catheter to prevent damage to the red blood cells. If blood is to be infused quickly, a 14- or 15-gauge device must be used.

 HOME HEALTH CARE

Blood Temperature

Blood is transported to the client in a container that maintains proper storage temperature for 6 hours. Because the container does not have thermometers and alarms, it is not considered "monitored" storage, and the blood cannot be returned to inventory if the transfusion is canceled (Fitzpatrick & Fitzpatrick, 1997).

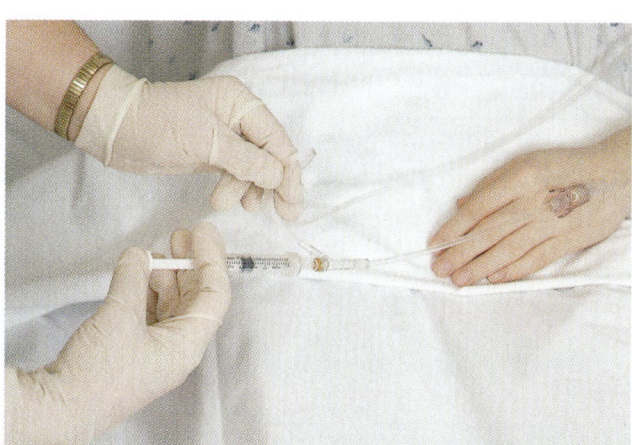

Figure 24-25 Injecting an IV Push (Bolus) Medication into a Peripheral Saline Lock

LIFE CYCLE CONSIDERATIONS

Initial Assessment

If pediatric, elderly, or malnourished clients are at risk for circulatory overload, notify the blood bank to divide the 500-mL bag of blood into two 250-mL bags or discuss with the physician other alternatives, such as packed RBCs rather than whole blood.

- Ensure patency of the existing IV site.
- Establish baseline data for vital signs, especially temperature, and assess skin for eruptions or rashes.
- Check client's blood type against the label on the whole blood or blood component before administration, to ensure compatibility.
- Assess the client's age and state of nutrition.

Scheduled IV medications should be infused before blood administration. This sequence prevents a reaction to a medication while blood is infusing. If a reaction were to occur, the nurse would not be able to discern whether the medication or the blood was causing the reaction.

Administering Whole Blood or a Blood Component The agency's blood protocol may require that a licensed person sign a form to release the blood from the blood bank and that a blood product be checked by two licensed personnel before infusion. The following information must be on the blood bag label and verified for accuracy: the client's name and identification number, ABO group and Rh factor, donor number, type of product ordered by the practitioner, and expiration date.

Blood should be administered within 30 minutes after it has been received from the bank, to maintain RBC integrity and to decrease the chance of infection. Whole blood should not go unrefrigerated for more than 4 hours. Room temperature will cause RBC lysis, releasing potassium and causing hyperkalemia.

Safety Measures The client should be observed for the initial 15 minutes for a transfusion reaction. Vital signs are usually taken every 15 minutes for the first hour, then every hour while the blood is transfusing.

PROFESSIONAL TIP

Transfusion Reaction

The severity of a transfusion reaction is relative to its onset. Severe reactions may occur shortly after the blood starts to infuse. At the first sign of a reaction, stop the blood infusion immediately.

Safety: Blood Transfusion Incompatibilities

Only normal saline should be used with a blood product. Blood transfusions are incompatible with dextrose and with Ringer's solution.

There are three basic types of transfusion reactions: allergic, febrile, and hemolytic. Other complications include sepsis, hypervolemia, and hypothermia. An allergic reaction may be mild or severe, depending on the cause. Hemolytic reactions may be immediate or delayed up to 96 hours, depending on the cause of the reaction. The classic symptoms of a reaction and sepsis are fever and chills.

The nursing actions for all types of reactions and complications are given in Table 24-5.

Topical Medications

Topical medications may be administered to the skin, eyes, ears, nose, throat, ear, rectum, and vagina. The medication generally provides a local effect but can also cause systemic effects. Drugs applied directly to the skin to produce a local effect include lotions, pastes, ointments, creams, powders, and aerosol sprays. The rate and degree of the drug's absorption are determined by the vascularity of the area.

Topical drugs are usually given to provide continuous absorption to produce different effects: to relieve pruritus (itching), to protect the skin, to prevent or treat an infection, to provide local anesthesia, or to create a systemic effect. Topical medications are usually ordered two or three times a day to achieve their therapeutic effect.

Before applying a topical preparation, the nurse should assess the condition of the skin for any open lesions, rashes, or areas of erythema and skin breakdown. The nurse should check with the client and the medical record for any known allergies.

Table 24-5 NURSING ACTIONS FOR BLOOD REACTIONS

IMMEDIATE NURSING ACTION	OTHER MEASURES
• Stop transfusion. • Keep vein open with normal saline. • Notify the physician.	• Monitor client's vital signs every 15 minutes for 4 hours or until stable. • Monitor I&O. • Send IV tubing and bag of blood back to the blood bank. • Obtain a blood and urine specimen. • Label specimen "Blood Transfusion Reaction." • Process a transfusion reaction report.

Body oils may interfere with the adhesive properties of the patch, disk, or tape. The skin harbors microorganisms, and lesions can cause encrustation. The nurse should cleanse the area by washing it with soap and warm water, unless contraindicated by a specific order. The skin should be thoroughly dry before applying a topical medication. Open wounds require the nurse to use surgical asepsis.

When the skin is dry, the nurse can apply the medication. When applying a paste, cream, or an ointment, the nurse should follow Standard Precautions and use a sterile tongue depressor to remove the medication from the container; this method prevents cross-contamination. The medication is transferred from the tongue blade to a gloved hand for application. The medication should be applied in long, smooth strokes in the direction of the hair follicles to prevent the medication from entering the hair follicles. A new sterile tongue depressor should be used whenever more medication is removed from the container. Two to 4 hours after the application, the nurse should assess the area for signs of an allergic reaction.

Eye Medications Eye medications refer to drops, ointments, and disks. These drugs are used for diagnostic and therapeutic purposes, to lubricate the eye or socket for a prosthetic eye, and to prevent or treat eye conditions such as glaucoma (elevated pressure within the eye) and infection. Diagnostically, eyedrops can be used to anesthetize the eye, to dilate the pupil, or to stain the cornea to identify abrasions and scars.

Safety: Prevent Cross-Contamination
- Each client should have his or her own bottle of eyedrops.
- Check the expiration date before administering eyedrops.
- Discard any solution remaining in the dropper after instillation.
- Discard the dropper if the tip is accidentally contaminated, as by touching the bottle or any part of the client's eye.

The nurse should insert medication disks at bedtime because they usually cause blurring of the eyes on in-

PROFESSIONAL TIP

Systemic Effects of Eyedrops
- Apply pressure to the inner canthus when instilling eyedrops that have potential systemic effects such as atropine and timolol maleate (Timoptic).
- Gentle pressure over the inner canthus prevents the medication from flowing into the tear duct, thereby decreasing the absorption rate of the drug.

sertion. Standard Precautions are used when administering eye care and medications because of the potential contact with bodily secretions.

Ear Medications Solutions ordered to treat the ear are often referred to as *otic* (pertaining to the ear) drops or irrigations. Eardrops may be instilled to soften ear wax, to produce anesthesia, to treat infection or inflammation, or to facilitate removal of a foreign body, such as an insect. External auditory canal irrigations are usually performed for cleaning purposes and less frequently for applying heat and antiseptic solutions.

Before instilling a solution into the ear, the nurse should inspect the ear for signs of drainage, an indication of a perforated tympanic membrane. Eardrops are usually contraindicated when the tympanic membrane is perforated. If the tympanic membrane is damaged, all procedures must be performed using sterile aseptic technique; otherwise, medical asepsis is used when instilling medications into the ear.

Nasal Instillations Nasal instillations can be performed with different preparations: drops or nebulizers (atomizer or aerosol). Nasal drugs are administered to produce one or more of the following effects: to shrink swollen mucous membranes, to loosen secretions and facilitate drainage, or to treat infections of the nasal cavity or sinuses. Because many of these products are nonprescription drugs, clients should be taught their correct usage. For example, nasal decongestants are common over-the-counter drugs used to shrink swollen mucous membranes. However, when

HOME HEALTH CARE

Considerations for Use of Nasal Inhalers
- Provide the client with the manufacturer's directions for the specific type of inhaler, such as how to replace a medication cartridge for a nasal aerosol.
- Store inhalers at room temperature.
- Do not puncture or place aerosols in an incinerator because they are prepared under pressure.
- Instruct the client not to allow other people to use the inhaler.
- Caution the client about overuse that could cause a rebound effect, making the condition worse.
- Ensure that the client is knowledgeable about the expected and adverse effects of the drug. Some of these drugs do not produce therapeutic effects for severals days, and some require 2 weeks of continuous use before the drug's effects appear.
- Provide the client with a telephone number to call if assistance is needed.

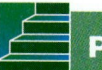

PROFESSIONAL TIP

Administering Nose Drops

- Gather equipment: MAR; prescribed medication with dropper; emesis basin; and tissues.
- Check the MAR against the written orders and the chart for allergies.
- Wash hands, and follow the five "rights" of drug administration.
- Check the client's identification armband, explain the procedure to the client, and provide for privacy.
- Don nonsterile gloves.
- Instruct the client to blow the nose to facilitate the removal of mucus and secretions.
- Place the client in a supine position and hyperextend the neck. Position the head so that the drops will reach the expected site, as shown in Figure 24-27.
- Squeeze some medication into the dropper.
- Insert the nasal drops about ⅜ inch into the nostril, keeping the tip of the dropper away from the sides of the nares.
- Instill the prescribed dosage of medication and observe the client for any signs of discomfort.
- Instruct the client to remain supine for 5 minutes to prevent the medication from leaking out of the nose.
- Discard any unused medication remaining in the dropper.
- Return the client to a comfortable position and provide the client with the emesis basin and tissues to expectorate any medication that flows into the oropharynx and mouth.
- Remove gloves and wash hands.
- Record on the MAR the drug given, number of drops instilled, and nostril medicated.

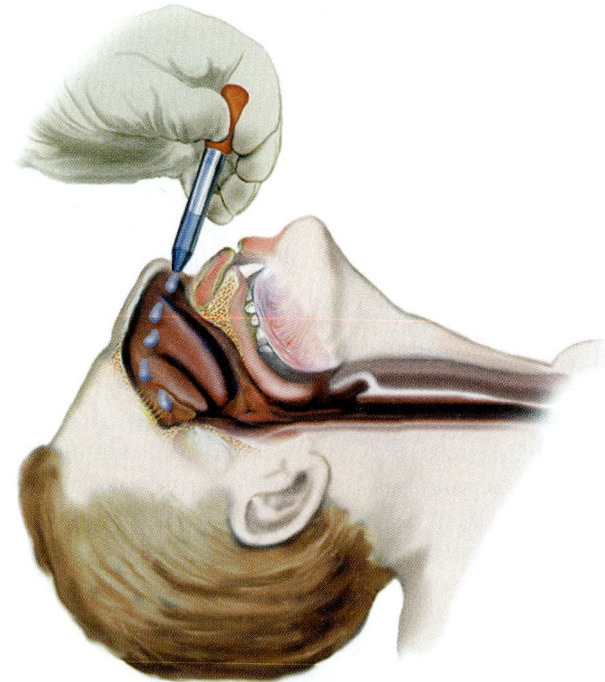

Figure 24-27 Positioning a Client for Nose Drop Instillation

For atomizers:
- Occlude one nostril to prevent air from entering the nasal cavity and to allow the medication to flow freely in the open nostril.
- Insert the atomizer tip into the open nostril and instruct the client to inhale, then squeeze the atomizer once, and instruct the client to exhale.

For aerosols:
- Shake the aerosol well before each use.
- Grasp between thumb and index finger and insert the adapter tip into one nostril while occluding the other nostril with a finger, then press the adapter cartridge firmly to release one measured dose of medication.
- Repeat the above steps as ordered for the other nostril.
- Instruct the client to keep the head tilted backward for 2 to 3 minutes and to breathe through the nose while the medication is being absorbed.

Respiratory Inhalants Respiratory inhalants are delivered by devices that produce fine droplets that are inhaled deep into the respiratory tract. These medication droplets are absorbed almost immediately through the alveolar epithelium into the bloodstream. This section addresses only oropharyngeal hand-held inhalers.

Oropharyngeal hand-held inhalers deliver medications, such as bronchodilators and mucolytics, that produce both local and systemic effects. Bronchodilators (drugs that dilate the bronchi) improve airway patency and are used to prevent or treat bronchospasms, asthma, and allergic reactions. Mucolytics are used to liquify tenacious (thick) bronchial secretions.

these drugs are used in excess, they may have a reverse or rebound effect by increasing nasal congestion.

Although the nose is considered a clean (not sterile) cavity, because of its connection with the sinuses, the nurse uses medical asepsis when performing nasal instillations.

Nebulizers (inhalers) are used to deliver a fine mist containing medication droplets. When the client is discharged with a nasal inhaler, the nurse should teach the client how to store and use the device. The nurse should administer or assist clients with the use of atomizers and aerosols:

- Instruct the client to clear the nostrils by blowing the nose.
- Client should be in an upright position with head tilted back slightly.

CLIENT TEACHING

Self-Administration with a Metered-Dose Inhaler

- Review with the client the purpose of each prescribed medication. Some clients are ordered several inhalant medications and need to be taught the correct sequencing. For example, fast-acting bronchodilators such as albuterol sulfate (Ventolin) are taken before slower-acting bronchodilators such as salmeterol xinafoate (Serevent).
- Explain that the inhaler must be shaken before each use to mix the medication and the aerosol propellant.
- Remove the mouthpiece and cap from the bottle and insert the metal stem of the bottle into the small hole on the flattened portion of the mouthpiece.
- Instruct the client to exhale, place the mouthpiece into the mouth, and ensure that the lips form a tight seal around the mouthpiece.
- Instruct the client to firmly push the cylinder down against the mouthpiece only once (Figure 24-28) and to inhale slowly until the lungs feel full.
- Ask the client to remove the mouthpiece while holding the breath for several seconds to allow the medication to reach the alveoli, and then to exhale slowly through pursed lips.
- Inform the client that a mouthwash can be used to remove the taste of medication.
- Show the client how to wash the mouthpiece under tepid running water to remove secretions.

Clients must be able to form an airtight seal around the inhaling devices and must be able to assemble the turbo-inhaler. This requirement prevents some clients, such as clients with visual or coordination impairments,

from using these devices. Bronchodilators are contraindicated in clients who have a history of tachycardia.

Rectal Instillations Rectal instillations can be in the form of enemas, suppositories, or ointments. Rectal ointments are used to treat local conditions and symptoms such as pain, inflammation, and itching caused from hemorrhoids. Rectal suppositories are

PROFESSIONAL TIP

Administering a Rectal Suppository

- Gather equipment: MAR; prescribed rectal suppository; water-soluble lubricant, such as K-Y jelly; nonsterile gloves; tissues; bedpan (optional).
- Check the MAR against the written orders and the chart for allergies.
- Wash hands, and follow the five "rights."
- Check the client's identification armband, and explain the procedure to the client.
- Ask the client if he or she needs to void because the client will have to remain in bed after insertion of the suppository. Provide for privacy.
- Don nonsterile gloves.
- Place the client in the Sims', left lateral, position, with the upper leg flexed.
- Fold back the bed linen to expose the rectum.
- Open the package of lubricant and remove the foil wrapper from the suppository. Read the manufacturer's instructions on the wrapper for the recommended time interval the client should retain the suppository after insertion.
- Apply a small amount of lubricant to the smooth rounded end of the suppository to reduce mucosal irritation.
- Lubricate the gloved index finger.
- Instruct the client to breathe through the mouth to relax.
- Insert the suppository into the rectal canal beyond the internal anal sphincter, about 4 inches (10 cm) for an adult and 2 inches (5 cm) for a child to prevent the suppository from slipping out (Figure 24-29). Avoid inserting the suppository into feces.
- Withdraw the finger and wipe the anal area with tissues to provide comfort.
- Instruct the client to remain in the left lateral or supine position for at least 15 minutes until the medication is absorbed and to avoid the urge to defecate for 30 to 40 minutes, or as directed by the manufacturer's instructions.
- Remove gloves, turning them inside out, dispose, and wash hands.
- Record the drug on the MAR: name, dosage, route, and time of administration.

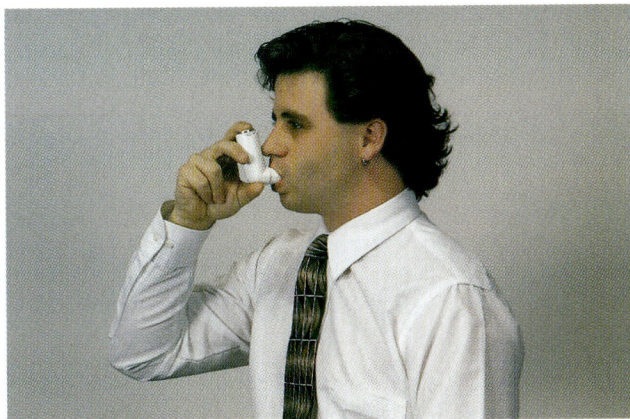

Figure 24-28 Self-Administration with a Metered-Dose Inhaler

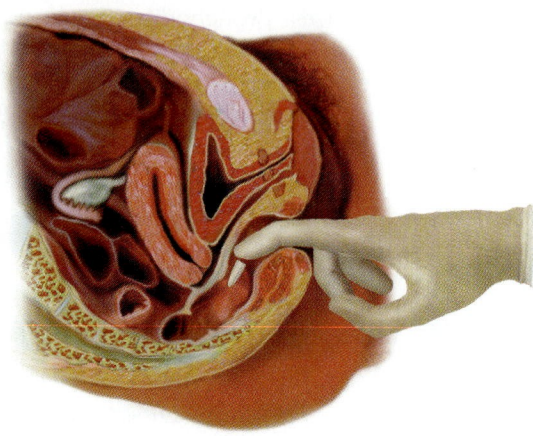

Figure 24-29 Inserting a Rectal Suppository

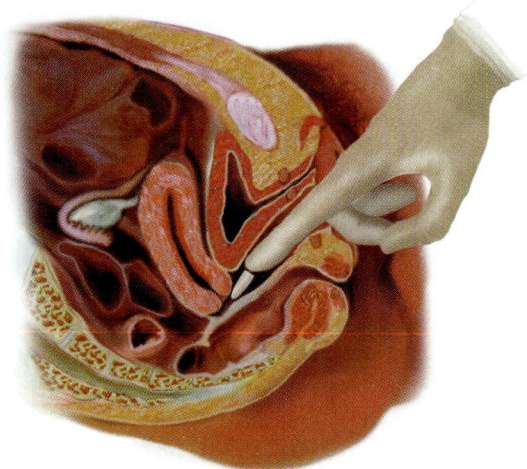

Figure 24-30 Inserting a Vaginal Suppository Along the Posterior Wall of the Vagina

cone-shaped masses of substances designed to melt at body temperature and to produce the intended effect at a slow and steady rate of absorption.

Suppositories provide a safe and convenient route for administering drugs that interact poorly with digestive enzymes or have a bad taste or odor. They are also used to provide temporary relief for clients who cannot tolerate oral preparations: for example, to relieve nausea and vomiting. Suppositories are also used to relieve pain and local irritation, reduce fever, and stimulate peristalsis and defecation in clients who are constipated.

The nurse should assess the rectum for irritation or bleeding and check sphincter control. Some clients may experience problems in retaining the suppository. The nurse should instruct those clients to remain in the Sims' position for at least 15 minutes or should place the client on the abdomen, if the condition allows, and hold the buttocks closed. The physician should be notified when the client is unable to retain a suppository so that another route can be ordered.

Vaginal Instillations Medications inserted into the vagina are in the form of suppositories, creams, gels, ointments, foams, or douches. These medications may be used to treat inflammation, infections, and discomfort or as a contraceptive measure.

Vaginal creams, gels, or ointments usually come with a disposable tubular applicator with a plunger to insert the drug. Suppositories are usually inserted with the index finger of a gloved hand; however, small suppositories may come with an applicator and the suppository is placed in the applicator's tip. After insertion of these preparations, the client may notice drainage and should be informed that this is expected. The nurse should advise the client to wear a perineal pad to prevent soiling of the underpants.

Sterile technique is usually required by agency policy, especially if there is an open wound when administering a vaginal douche (irrigation). The nurse should ensure that the client does not have an allergy to iodine because many vaginal preparations contain povidone-iodine.

Evaluation

Inherent in safe drug administration is the nursing responsibility to follow the five "rights." Administering medications in accord with these guidelines requires the nurse to verify that safe nursing care was provided to the client. For example, a client receiving a sublingual medication knows not to drink water until the tablet has dissolved completely; the client receiving medications through an NG tube did not aspirate; or the diabetic client can safely self-administer insulin by withdrawing the prescribed dose and administering the injection in the subcutaneous tissues while maintaining sterile technique.

PROFESSIONAL TIP

Contraindications for Rectal Suppositories
- Contraindicated for cardiac clients because insertion may stimulate the vagus nerve, causing cardiac dysrhythmias (abnormal heart patterns).
- Contraindicated for clients recovering from rectal or prostate surgery because suppositories may cause pain on insertion and trauma to the tissues.

CLIENT TEACHING

Tampon Use

Clients should not use tampons after the insertion of vaginal medications because the tampon can absorb the medication and decrease the drug's effect.

PROFESSIONAL TIP

Administering a Vaginal Suppository

- Gather equipment: MAR; prescribed vaginal suppository; disposable applicator if indicated; water-soluble lubricant; nonsterile gloves; tissues.
- Check the MAR against the written orders and the chart for allergies.
- Wash hands, and follow the five "rights" of drug administration.
- Check the client's identification armband, and explain the procedure to the client.
- Ask the client to void because a full bladder may cause discomfort and injury to the vaginal lining when the suppository is inserted. Provide for privacy.
- Don nonsterile glove.
- Place the client in a dorsal recumbent, back-lying position with knees flexed and hips rotated laterally or in a Sim's position if the client cannot maintain the dorsal recumbent position.
- Assess the perineal area, inspect the vaginal orifice, note any odor or discharge from the vagina, and inquire about any problems, such as discomfort or itching.
- If secretion or discharge is present, cleanse the perineal area with soap and warm water to prevent the introduction of microorganisms into the vagina.
- Remove the suppository from the foil wrapper, and if applicable, insert the suppository into the applicator's tip.

- Apply a small amount of lubricant to the smooth rounded end of the suppository to reduce mucosal irritation.
- If not using an applicator, apply a small amount of lubricant to gloved index finger.
- Insert the suppository into the vaginal canal at least 2 inches (5 cm) along the posterior wall of the vagina or as far as it will go to prevent the suppository from slipping out (Figure 24-30). If using an applicator, insert as described above and depress the plunger to release the suppository. Wipe the perineum with clean, dry tissues.
- Instruct the client to remain in bed for 15 minutes until the suppository is absorbed.
- Wash the applicator under cool running water to clean (warm or hot water produces coagulation of protein secretions) and return to appropriate storage in the client's room.
- Remove the gloves, turning them inside out, and dispose of the gloves in the proper receptacle.
- Record on the MAR the drug's name, dosage, route, and date and time of administration; document any evidence of discharge or odor from the vagina.
- Check on the client in 15 minutes to ensure that the suppository did not slip out and to allow the client the opportunity to verbalize any problems or concerns.

The nurse who identifies a potential medication risk and initiates actions to prevent client injury is performing another form of evaluation. For example, if the client in the home setting cannot remember if the prescribed medications have been taken, providing the client with a daily or weekly pillbox that is filled when the nurse is present prevents the client from taking too much medication or failing to take the dose as ordered.

SUMMARY

- The *United States Pharmacopeia* and the *National Formulary* outline drug standards for use in the United States.
- The Food and Drug Administration tests all drugs for toxicity before granting a company the right to market a drug.
- Drugs are usually referred to by their generic name, not capitalized, or by their trade name, always capitalized.
- The oral administration route is the safest and least expensive administration route, although it is also the slowest to act.

- Parenteral drugs are injected through intradermal (ID), subcutaneous (SC or SQ), intramuscular (IM), or intravenous (IV) routes and are typically fast-acting.
- The pharmacokinetics of drugs includes absorption, distribution, metabolism, and excretion.
- Safe drug administration is facilitated by following the five "rights": right drug, right dose, right client, right route, and right time.
- Nurses are both morally and legally responsible for correct administration of medications; this includes following institutional policy, considering clients' desires and abilities, fostering compliance, and correctly documenting all actions related to medication administration and medication errors.
- Before administering medications, the nurse must thoroughly assess the client's drug history, medical history, and psychosocial factors that may affect drug acceptance and compliance.
- Oral medications should be poured and measured at eye level to ensure accuracy.
- Although the physician will determine the dose and route of a parenteral drug, the nurse is responsible for choosing the correct gauge and length of the needle to be used.

SAMPLE NURSING CARE PLAN

THE CLIENT WITH DEEP VEIN THROMBOSIS

Mrs. Landry, a 45-year-old, was admitted to your floor with a diagnosis of deep vein thrombosis. She noticed swelling of her left leg about a week ago but decided to treat it at home. Four days later the lower leg was very edematous, warm, and painful to move. After an office visit, Mrs. Landry was admitted to the hospital. This is her first hospitalization. On examination the left leg is warmer than the right. The left thigh circumference is 3 inches larger than the right. The physician ordered a heparin IV drip after a loading dose bolus was given. The drip contained 10,000 units heparin in 500 mL of D_5W at 10 mL/h (200 units/h). The physician anticipates that Mrs. Landry will be weaned off of the heparin drip and started on subcutaneous heparin within 5 days. At the time of discharge she will be given Coumadin.

Nursing Diagnosis 1 *Tissue Perfusion, Altered, related to the development of venous thrombi in the deep femoral vein as evidenced by left leg being warmer than right leg and left thigh circumference being 3 inches larger than right thigh circumference.*

PLANNING/GOALS	NURSING INTERVENTIONS	RATIONALE	EVALUATION
Mrs. Landry will: Report an absence of pain.	Maintain on bed rest.	Reduces the possibility of embolus; may decrease the pain and swelling.	Mrs. Landry is able to ambulate without difficulty or pain.
	Apply moist heat to the affected extremity.	Heat provides an analgesic effect; it decreases venospasms and pain.	
Demonstrate an absence of edema.	Elevate the legs above the heart.	Elevation facilitates venous return and decreases the edema.	Mrs. Landry's left thigh is only ½ inch larger than her right thigh.
	Measure the circumference of the left thigh and compare with that of the right thigh.	Measuring the circumference provides a quantitative reference point that can be used to evaluate the swelling.	
Experience the same degree of skin temperature in both legs.	Administer the heparin drip at 200 units/h.	Heparin prevents the conversion of fibrinogen to fibrin and prothrombin to thrombin, thereby limiting the extension of the thrombus.	Mrs. Landry has no temperature difference between her legs.
	Monitor the partial thromboplastin time (PTT).	The partial thromboplastin time is used to monitor heparin therapy because heparin, a short-acting anticoagulant, increases the PTT.	

continued

Nursing Diagnosis 2 *Injury, Risk for, bleeding related to the administration of an anticoagulant.*

PLANNING/GOALS	NURSING INTERVENTIONS	RATIONALE	EVALUATION
Mrs. Landry will: Not demonstrate evidence of bleeding from gums or nose, in urine or stool, or under the skin.	Advise Mrs. Landry to withhold the medication in the event that bleeding occurs and to notify the physician immediately.	The dose may need to be adjusted.	Mrs. Landry has had no bleeding episodes.
	Encourage the client to discontinue smoking.	Smoking has a tendency to increase the metabolism of the medication, necessitating an increase in the dose.	
Maintain her prothrombin time (PT) or international normalized ratio (INR) within therapeutic range.	Advise the client to watch food intake.	Foods high in fat and foods rich in vitamin K can interfere with the PT.	Mrs. Landry still has many questions about taking the oral anticoagulant on discharge. Discharge follow-up will be needed to monitor the client's progress on the oral anticoagulant.
	Warn against taking oral contraceptive medication.	There may be a decrease in anticoagulant effect due to the increased production of clotting factors with oral contraceptives.	
	Warn against taking aspirin and other over-the-counter medications.	Aspirin may increase the risk of bleeding; it inhibits platelet formation.	

CASE STUDY

Mrs. Cheng is a 76-year-old client who was discharged from the hospital with cancer of the lungs. Mrs. Cheng elected not to have surgery and was given her first chemotherapy before discharge. She is not accustomed to taking medications. Before the onset of symptoms that necessitated her admission to the hospital, Mrs. Cheng considered herself in good health, only bothered with the discomfort of arthritis in her hands. She is being discharged on the following medications:

- sulfamethoxazole (Gantanol), a sulfonamide anti-infective, 500 mg/5 mL susp po b.i.d.
- granisetron (Kytril), an antiemetic, 1 mg po q12h
- morphine sulfate 30 mg po q4h, prn for pain

The following questions will guide your development of a nursing care plan for the case study.

1. What other assessments would you make about Mrs. Cheng?
2. What two nursing diagnoses with a goal for each might be appropriate for Mrs. Cheng?
3. What nursing interventions might help Mrs. Cheng meet the goals?

- The nurse must always carefully monitor client reactions to medications and ensure that clients are appropriately educated as to the actions, side effects, and contraindications of all medications they are receiving.
- Clients receiving intravenous therapy or blood transfusions require constant monitoring for complications.

Review Questions

1. The law that began the regulation of habit-forming drugs is called the:

   a. Kefauver-Harris Act.
   b. Harrison Narcotic Act.
   c. Controlled Substance Act.
   d. Food, Drug, and Cosmetic Act.

2. A client is unable to swallow the pills ordered by the physician. The best action for the nurse is to:

   a. tell the client to chew the pills.
   b. crush the pills and give them to the client.
   c. call the physician for a change in the orders.
   d. ask the pharmacy to send the medications in liquid form.

3. The only household measure used in calculating dosages is the:

   a. drop.
   b. pound.
   c. ounce.
   d. teaspoon.

4. The method considered to be one of the most accurate for calculating medication dosages for infants and children up to 12 years of age is:

   a. Clark's rule.
   b. Young's rule.
   c. weight and height.
   d. body surface area.

5. The client is in the bathroom when the nurse brings the medications. The best action for the nurse is to:

   a. return with the medications when the client is finished in the bathroom.
   b. leave the medications for the client to take when finished in the bathroom.
   c. knock on the bathroom door and give the medications to the client at this time.
   d. ask the nursing assistant to see that the client takes the medications when finished in the bathroom.

6. The best time for the nurse to document medication administration is:

   a. whenever the nurse has time.
   b. before the client receives the medication.
   c. only after the client has received the medication.
   d. toward the end of the shift so all medications can be charted at one time.

7. Sublingual medications are to be:

   a. chewed.
   b. placed under the tongue.
   c. placed between the cheek and teeth.
   d. swallowed with 8 ounces of water.

8. Standard Precautions are required with:

   a. venipuncture.
   b. IM injections.
   c. oral medications.
   d. nasal instillation.

9. An intravenous solution of sodium chloride (0.45%) is:

   a. isotonic.
   b. iso-osmolar.
   c. hypertonic.
   d. hypotonic.

10. A client receiving a blood transfusion tells the nurse, who is taking the first set of 15-minute vital signs, that she is cold (chills) and her chest hurts. The first thing the nurse should do is:

    a. stop the transfusion.
    b. get a warm blanket for the client.
    c. call the blood bank to come and check the blood.
    d. stay with the client and talk quietly to her help her relax.

Critical Thinking Questions

1. You discover that a similar but incorrect drug (not the drug ordered) is being given IV to a client. What is the first thing you should do? What is your next course of action? How do you feel about the nurse who made the medication error but did not recognize it?

2. How can the different transfusion reactions be differentiated?

⚡ WEB FLASH!

- Visit the Web for sites related to IV therapy, medication administration, and medication errors. What type of information is available?
- Are there any organizations on the Web related to medication administration?

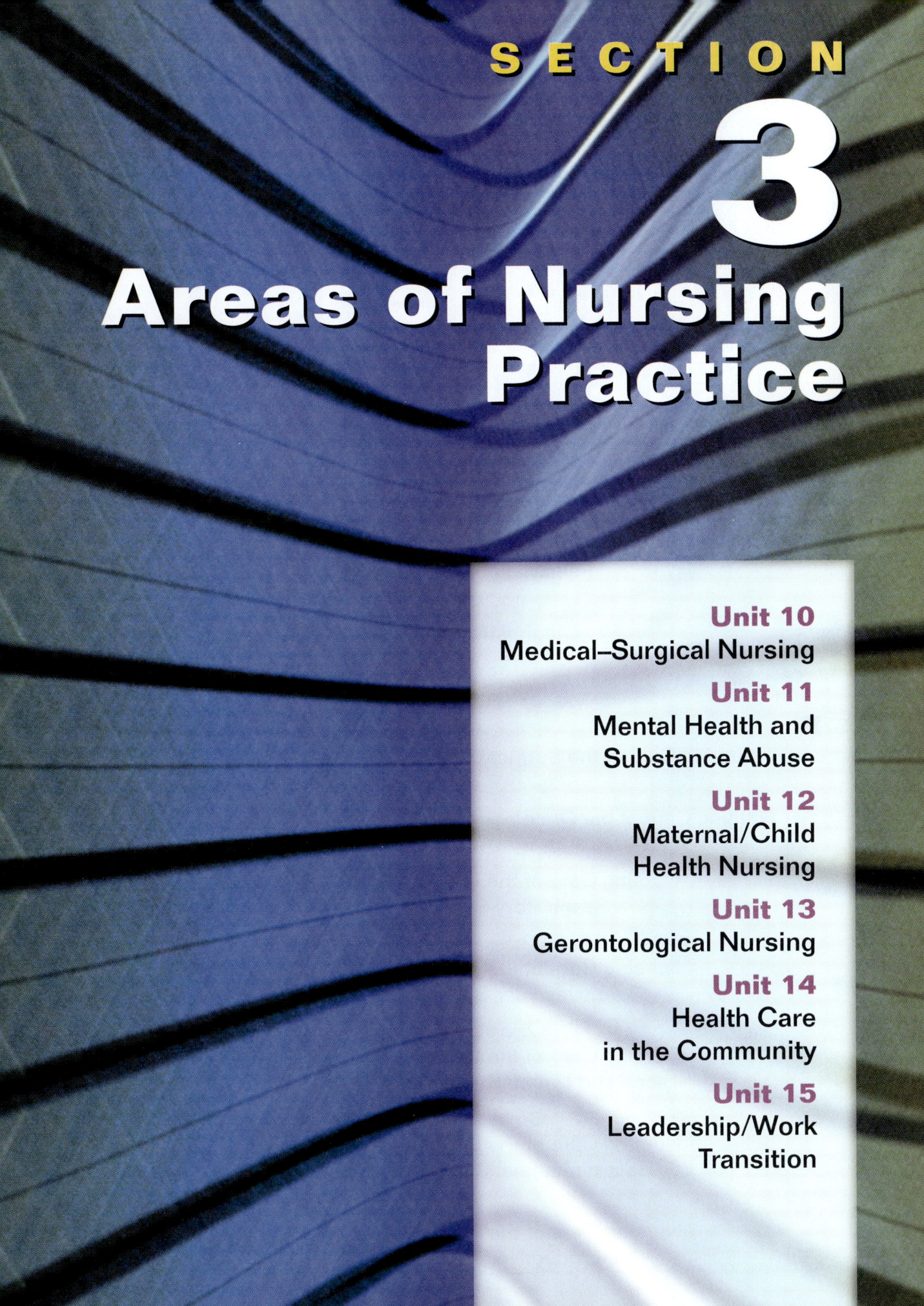

UNIT

10
Medical–Surgical
Nursing

ASSESSMENT

MAKING THE CONNECTION

Refer to the following chapters to increase your understanding of assessment:

- **Chapter 8, Communication**
- **Chapter 9, Nursing Process**
- **Chapter 12, Cultural Diversity and Nursing**
- **Chapter 17, Loss, Grief, and Death**
- **Chapter 23, Fluid, Electrolyte, and Acid-Base Balance**
- **Chapter 29, Nursing Care of the Surgical Client**
- **Chapter 30, Nursing Care of the Oncology Client**
- **Chapter 31, Nursing Care of the Client: Respiratory System**
- **Chapter 32, Nursing Care of the Client: Cardiovascular System**
- **Chapter 33, Nursing Care of the Client: Blood and Lymph Systems**
- **Chapter 34, Nursing Care of the Client: Gastrointestinal System**
- **Chapter 35, Nursing Care of the Client: Reproductive System**

- **Chapter 36, Nursing Care of the Client: Sexually Transmitted Diseases**
- **Chapter 37, Nursing Care of the Client: Endocrine System**
- **Chapter 38, Nursing Care of the Client: Musculoskeletal System**
- **Chapter 39, Nursing Care of the Client: Immune System**
- **Chapter 40, Nursing Care of the Client: Integumentary System**
- **Chapter 41, Nursing Care of the Client: Nervous System**
- **Chapter 42, Nursing Care of the Client: Urinary System**
- **Chapter 55, Nursing Care of the Older Client**
- **Procedures:** B1, Handwashing; B3, Measuring Body Temperature; B4, Assessing Pulse Rate; B5, Assessing Respirations; B6, Assessing Blood Pressure; B7, Weighing Client, Mobile and Immobile

LEARNING OBJECTIVES

Upon completion of this chapter, you should be able to:
- *Define key terms.*
- *Identify the components of functional health patterns.*
- *Utilize the framework of functional health to facilitate a holistic assessment process.*
- *Analyze the components of the head-to-toe assessment.*
- *Incorporate the four assessment techniques within the head-to-toe assessment.*
- *Utilize the head-to-toe assessment in clinical situations.*

KEY TERMS

adventitious breath sound	dyspnea
affect	eupnea
auscultation	health history
borborygmi	hyperventilation
bradycardia	hypoventilation
bradypnea	inspection
bronchial sound	orthostatic hypotension
bronchovesicular sound	palpation
crackle	percussion
cyanosis	pleural friction rub
	pulse amplitude
	pulse deficit

KEY TERMS (*continued*)

pulse rate
pulse rhythm
review of systems
sibilant wheeze
Snellen chart

sonorous wheeze
stridor
tachycardia
tachypnea
vesicular sound

INTRODUCTION

Within the scope of the nursing profession, a complete nursing assessment is necessary to analyze each client's needs in a holistic manner. Nursing assessment includes both physical and psychosocial aspects to evaluate a client's condition. A nurse demonstrates caring, respect, and concern for each client when doing a nursing assessment.

A thorough nursing assessment includes both a health history and a physical examination. To perform a health history, the nurse interviews the client to identify how the client adjusts to or lives within the environment. This data is subjective data, or information based on client self-report. During the physical examination the nurse collects objective data, which includes observations made by the nurse while utilizing the assessment techniques of inspection, palpation,

percussion, and auscultation. Other sources of objective data are laboratory tests, x-rays, and measurements of the client's vital signs, height, and weight.

The health history and the physical examination assist the nurse in focusing on the client as a whole. The initial nursing assessment generally occurs within 8 hours of a client's admission to a health care facility, and continues throughout the stay. In a physician's office or health care clinic, the nursing assessment would be completed immediately. Most institutions have a standard asessment form (Figure 25-1).

Usually a health history is completed prior to the physical examination. However, in emergency situations or when performing care in a health care facility after the initial admitting assessment, it will be necessary to incorporate history-taking within the physical examination. When incorporating a health history within the head-to-toe assessment, the nurse must remember to incorporate questions about the client's habits or usual patterns along with the physical data collected in the head-to-toe assessment. Functional assessment is best done within the framework of the physical assessment since the environment in which each client resides and participates becomes a part of the physical assessment. The functional assessment brings the environment in which the client lives and the physical needs of that client together to establish a holistic picture.

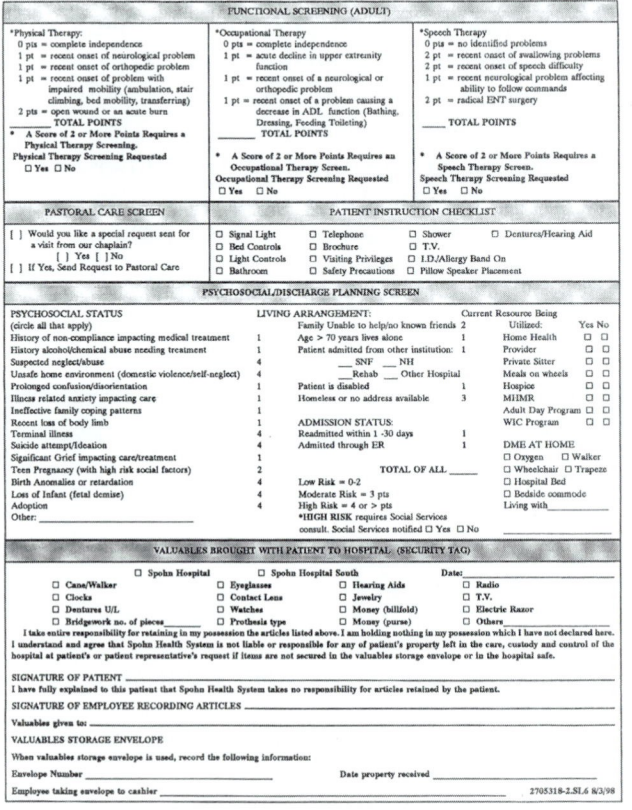

Figure 25-1 Patient Admission Data Base (*Courtesy of Spohn Health System, Corpus Christi, TX*)

continued

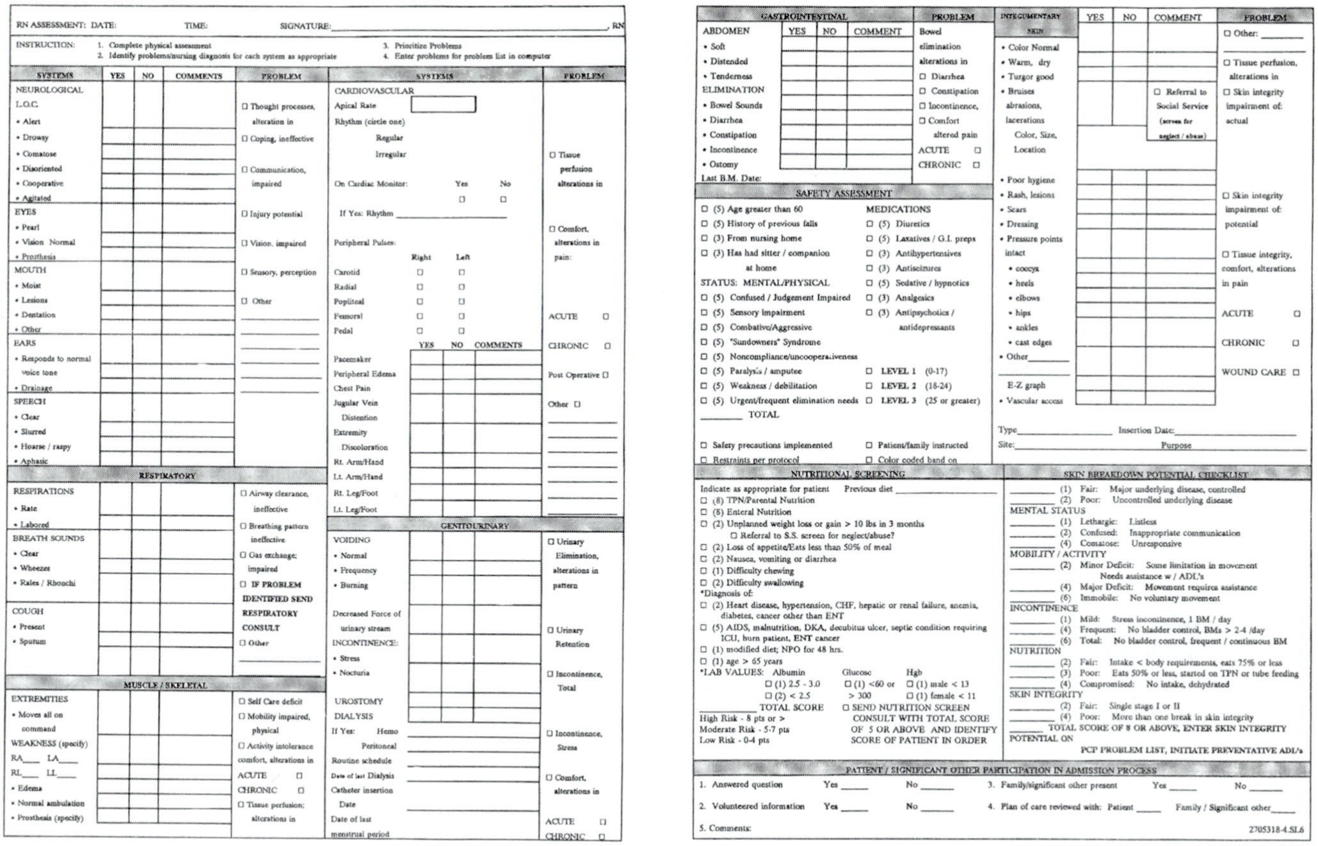

Figure 25-1 (continued)

HEALTH HISTORY

A primary focus of the data collection interview is the health history. The **health history** is a review of the client's functional health patterns prior to the current contact with a health care agency. While the medical history concentrates on symptoms and the progression of disease, the nursing health history focuses on the client's functional health patterns, responses to changes in health status, and alterations in lifestyle. The health history is also used in developing the plan of care and formulating nursing interventions.

Demographic Information

Personal data including name, address, date of birth, gender, religion, race/ethnic origin, occupation, and type of health plan/insurance should be included. Factors that are derived from this information may be useful in helping to foster understanding of a client's perspective.

Reason for Seeking Health Care

The client's reason for seeking health care should be described in the client's own words. For example, the statement "fell off four-foot ladder and landed on right shoulder; unable to move right arm" is the client's actual report of the event that precipitated his or her need for health care. The client's perspective is important because it explains what is significant about the event from the client's point of view. It is also important to determine the time of the onset of symptoms as well as a complete symptom analysis.

Perception of Health Status

Perception of health status refers to the client's opinion of his or her general health. It may be useful to ask clients to rate their health on a scale of 1 to 10 (with 10 being ideal and 1 being poor), together with the client's rationale for their rating score. For example, the nurse may record a statement such as the following to represent the client's perception of health: "Rates health a 7 on a scale of 1 (poor) to 10 (ideal) because he must take medication regularly in order to maintain mobility, but the medication sometimes upsets his stomach."

Previous Illnesses, Hospitalizations, and Surgeries

The history and timing of any previous experiences with illness, surgery, or hospitalization are helpful in order to assess recurrent conditions and to anticipate responses to illness, since prior experiences often have an impact on current responses.

Client/Family Medical History

The nurse needs to determine any family history of acute and chronic illnesses that tend to be familial. Health history forms will frequently include checklists of various illnesses that the nurse can use as the basis of the questions about this aspect. The client should be instructed that family history refers to blood relatives. It is also helpful to indicate the relative's relationship to the client (e.g., mother, father, sister).

Immunizations/Exposure to Communicable Diseases

Any history of childhood or other communicable diseases should be noted. In addition, a record of current immunizations should be obtained. This is particularly important with children; however, records of immunizations for tetanus, influenza, and hepatitis B can also be important for adults. If the client has traveled out of the country, the time frame should be indicated in order to determine incubation periods for relevant diseases. The client should also be asked about potential exposure to communicable diseases such as tuberculosis or human immunodeficiency virus (HIV).

Allergies

Any drug, food, or environmental allergies should be noted in the health history. In addition to the name of the allergen, the type of reaction to the substance should be noted. For example, a client may report that he or she developed a rash or became short of breath after taking penicillin. This reaction should be recorded. Clients may report an "allergy" to a medication because they developed an upset stomach after ingesting it, which the nurse will recognize as a side effect that would not preclude administration of the drug in the future.

Safety: Assessment for Allergies

It is essential that the nurse explore possible allergies prior to administering any medications. Allergic reactions can be life-threatening and can occur even with very low dosages of medications. A client's sensitivity to a drug can also change over time, resulting in severe reactions even though the client has successfully taken the drug during prior illnesses or experienced only mild reactions to the drug in the past.

Current Medications

All medications currently taken, both prescription and over-the-counter, should be recorded by name, frequency, and dosage. Clients should be reminded that this information should include medications such as birth control pills, laxatives, and nonprescription pain relief medications.

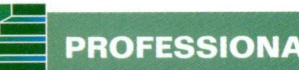
PROFESSIONAL TIP

Expired Medications
Remind clients to check all medications for expiration dates prior to use.

Developmental Level

Knowledge of developmental level is essential for considering appropriate norms of behavior and for appraising the achievement of relevant developmental tasks. Any recognized theory of growth and development can be applied in order to determine if clients are functioning within the parameters expected for their age group. For example, if the nurse uses Erikson's stages of psychosocial development, validation of an adult client's attainment of the developmental task of generativity versus stagnation can be made by the nurse's statement, such as "client prefers to spend time with his family; very involved in children's school activities."

Psychosocial History

Psychosocial history refers to assessment of dimensions such as self-concept and self-esteem as well as usual sources of stress and the client's ability to cope. Sources of support for clients in crisis, such as family, significant others, religion, or support groups, should be explored.

Sociocultural History

In exploring the client's sociocultural history, it is important to inquire about the home environment, family situation, and client's role in the family. For example, the client could be the parent of three children and the sole provider in a single-parent family. The responsibilities of the client are important data through which the nurse can determine the impact of changes in health status and thus plan the most beneficial care for the client. Patterns related to caffeine and alcohol intake and use of tobacco or recreational drugs should also be explored.

Activities of Daily Living

The activities of daily living is a description of the client's lifestyle and capacity for self-care and is useful both as baseline information and as a source of insight into usual health behaviors. This baseline should include information on nutritional intake and eating habits, elimination patterns, rest/sleep patterns, and activity/exercise.

Review of Systems

The **review of systems** (ROS) is a brief account from the client of any recent signs or symptoms associated with any of the body systems. This can most effectively be obtained as the physical examination is being performed. The review of systems relies on subjective information provided by the client rather than on the nurse's own physical examination. When a symptom is encountered, either while eliciting the health history or during the physical examination of the client, the nurse should obtain as much information as possible about the symptom. Relevant data include:

- *Location:* The area of the body in which the symptom (such as pain) is felt.
- *Character:* The quality of the feeling or sensation (e.g., sharp, dull, stabbing).
- *Intensity:* The severity or quantity of the feeling or sensation and its interference with functional abilities. The sensation can be rated on a scale of 1 (very little) to 10 (very intense).
- *Timing:* The onset, duration, frequency, and precipitating factors of the symptom.
- *Aggravating/alleviating factors:* The activities or actions that make the symptom worse or better.

PHYSICAL EXAMINATION

The physical examination is performed in all health care settings (home, outpatient facilities, extended care institutions, and acute care facilities) for all age groups to gather comprehensive, pertinent assessment data. The physical examination provides a complete picture of the client's physiological functioning. When combined with a health and psychosocial assessment, it forms a database to direct decision making. The examination should be performed according to the agency's policy. Policy may vary from one agency to another.

The physical examination is done in a sequential, head-to-toe fashion to ensure a thorough assessment of each system. This method not only prevents the nurse from forgetting to examine an area, it also decreases the number of times the nurse and the client have to change positions.

The nurse performs the physical or the head-to-toe assessment by using specific assessment techniques. These techniques include: inspection, palpation, percussion, and auscultation.

Inspection

Inspection consists of a thorough visual observation of the client. This visual assessment gives the nurse a description of the body's outward response to its internal functioning. Inspection of the skin, for example, can assist the nurse in identifying signs of a fever through the client's flushed facial cheeks. The skin can also be an indicator of a decreased oxygen supply when **cyanosis**, a bluish or dark purple coloration, is noted in the client's lips, skin, or nail beds. Sharing observations with the client during inspection

enhances the holistic data collected. For example, when the nurse mentions the observation of visible scars, the client may discuss previous surgeries or hospitalizations. Instruments such as a penlight and otoscope are often used to enhance visualization.

Effective inspection requires adequate lighting and exposure of the body parts being observed. Beginning nurses often feel self-conscious or embarrassed using the technique of inspection; however, most become comfortable with the technique over time. Nurses must also be sensitive to the client's feelings of embarrassment with the use of inspection and respond to this situation by discussing the technique with the client and using measures such as draping in order to increase the client's comfort level.

Palpation

In **palpation**, the nurse uses the sense of touch to assess texture, temperature, moisture, organ location and size, vibrations, pulsations, swelling, masses, and tenderness. The nurse's finger pads are placed flat against the client's skin, exerting slight pressure for light palpation, as seen in Figure 25-2. Assessment of the kidneys, liver, spleen, bowel, and fundal height may be accomplished through deep palpation, in which more pressure is exerted. Pulses are also palpated. The abdomen is palpated for distention, softness, firmness, rigidity, or tenderness.

Palpation requires a calm, gentle approach and is used systematically, with light palpation preceding deep palpation and palpation of tender areas performed last.

 Safety: Palpation

Deep palpation is a technique requiring significant expertise and should not be employed by beginning nursing students without supervision.

Percussion

Percussion uses short, tapping strokes on the surface of the skin to create vibrations of underlying organs.

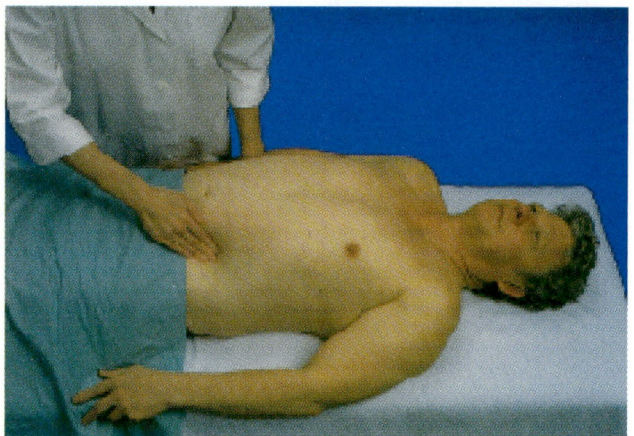

Figure 25-2 Light Palpation

It is used for assessing the density of structures or de-termining the location and size of organs in the body. The nurse uses the fingertips to tap the client's body to produce sounds and vibrations. The nurse places the middle finger of the nondominant hand on the cli-ent's skin in the area to be percussed, then taps lightly with the middle finger of the dominant hand on the distal phalanx of the middle finger positioned on the body surface (Figure 25-3). The nurse taps twice in one place before moving to a new area. Percussion should not be painful to the client. If it is painful, the percussion should be discontinued and the response documented.

Percussion is a skill that requires much practice to master, and it is important to be familiar with the sounds produced when percussion is used. Table 25-1 de-scribes the various percussion tones.

Auscultation

Auscultation involves listening to sounds in the body that are created by movement of air or fluid. Areas most often auscultated include the lungs, heart, abdomen, and blood vessels. Although direct ausculta-tion is sometimes possible, a stethoscope is usually employed in order to channel the sound (Figure 25-4).

HEAD-TO-TOE ASSESSMENT

Prior to beginning the examination, the nurse should keep in mind some important concepts to be utilized throughout the examination. The client's pri-vacy should be respected by pulling the curtain, clos-ing the door, and providing appropriate draping of the client. When possible, distracting noises such as radio or television and people talking should be eliminated. Assessment should be performed under natural light because fluorescent light can change the color tones of the skin. All procedures should be explained to the client and confidentiality of data acquired during the examination maintained.

Infection Control: Standard Precautions
Remember to utilize standard precautions when in contact with any body fluids by using gloves, gown, or mask when appropriate.

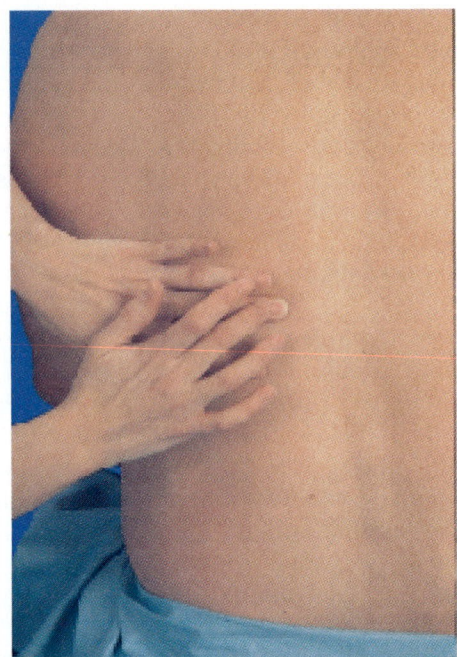

Figure 25-3 Percussion

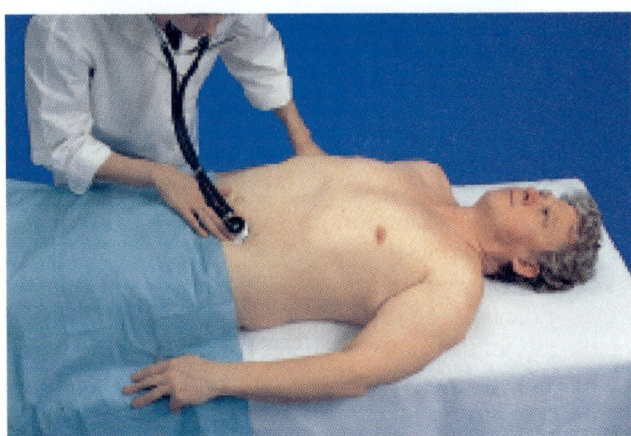

Figure 25-4 Auscultation

The nurse should position the client to ensure ac-cessibility to the body part being assessed. Figure 25-5 presents the positions used in conducting a physical examination.

The primary purpose of draping the client is to pre-vent unnecessary exposure during the examination.

Table 25-1	DESCRIPTION OF PERCUSSION TONES				
TONE	**INTENSITY**	**PITCH**	**DURATION**	**QUALITY**	**NORMAL LOCATION**
Dullness	Medium	High	Medium	Thudlike	Liver
Flatness	Soft	High	Short	Extreme dullness	Muscle
Hyperresonance	Very loud	Very low	Long	Booming	Child's lung
Resonance	Loud	Low	Long	Hollow	Peripheral lung
Tympany	Loud	High	Medium	Drumlike	Stomach

Sitting

To examine head, neck, back, posterior thorax and lungs, anterior thorax and lungs, breast, axillae, heart, extremities.

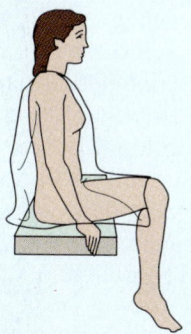

Client can expand lungs; nurse can inspect symmetry. *Institute risk precautions for elderly and debilitated clients.*

Dorsal recumbent

To examine head, neck, anterior thorax and lungs, breast, axillae, heart.

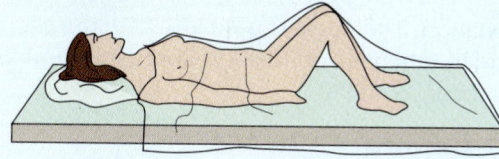

Client comfortable; increases abdominal muscle tension. *Contraindicated in abdominal assessment.*

Prone

To examine posterior thorax and lungs, hip

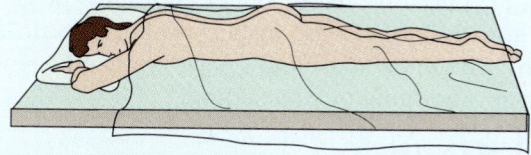

Assessment of hip extension. *Contraindicated in clients with cardiopulmonary alterations.*

Supine

To examine head, neck, anterior thorax and lungs, breasts, axillae, heart, abdomen, extremities.

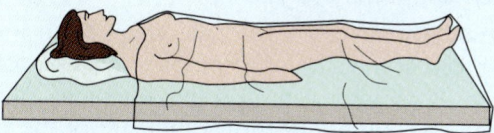

Client relaxed; decreases abdominal muscle tension; nurse can palpate all peripheral pulses. *Contraindicated in clients with cardiopulmonary alterations.*

Sims'

To examine rectum and vagina.

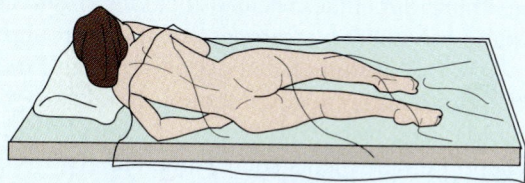

Relaxes rectal muscles. Painful for clients with joint deformities.

Knee-chest

To examine rectum

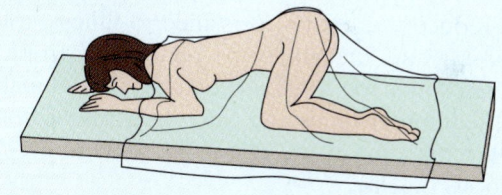

Maximal rectal exposure. *Contraindicated in clients with respiratory alterations.*

Lithotomy

To examine female genitalia, rectum, genital tract.

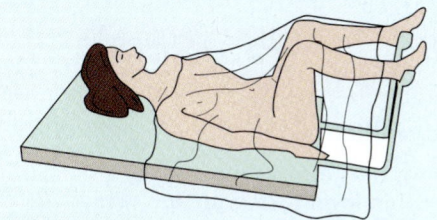

Maximal genitalia exposure; embarrassing and uncomfortable for client. *Contraindicated in clients with joint disorders.*

Figure 25-5 Various Positions for Physical Examination (*Adapted from* Health Assessment and Physical Examination, *by M.E.Z. Estes, 1998, Albany, NY: Delmar Publishers. Copyright 1998 by Delmar Publishers. Adapted with permission.)*

Feelings of embarrassment elicit tension and restlessness and will decrease the client's ability to cooperate. The drapes also prevent the client from being chilled.

General Survey

The nurse's introduction to the client is an important first step at the start of a complete head-to-toe assessment. It is important for the nurse to identify herself and to express intent for the care of the client and the time frame involved. During this introductory time, it is appropriate for the nurse to utilize inspection to make a general assessment of the client. This overview is the first impression the nurse will have of the client and is the beginning point of the head-to-toe assessment. It includes such aspects as the general state of health and any signs of distress, such as pain or breathing difficulties. It also includes observations regarding the client's awareness of the surroundings, body type and posture, facial expressions, and mood.

The nurse should document the general survey data in an organized fashion to portray a clinical picture of the client. Certain clients such as the elderly, disabled, and abused will require special consideration during the physical examination.

Elderly

When nurses assess elderly clients, it is important to know the normal changes that result from aging. Aging may reduce the body's resistance to illness, tolerance of stress, and the ability to recuperate from illness (Firth & Watanabe, 1996). The nurse should make sure the client understands and can follow instructions, and allow extra time if the client has difficulty changing positions quickly.

Disabled Clients

When assessing disabled clients, nurses should adapt their interactions to the client's ability; for example,

LIFE CYCLE CONSIDERATIONS

The Older Client

- All senses are less acute.
- Endorphin level rises with age, which decreases awareness of painful events.
- Temperature normal range is 96°F to 98.9°F.
- Strength and endurance decline.
- Height decreases.
- Digestive and urinary functions slow down.
- Older clients are prone to constipation and nocturia.
- Respirations are slowed.
- Older clients are prone to fatigue, dizziness, and falls (Andresen, 1998).

CULTURAL CONSIDERATIONS

Cultural Values and Assessment

Cleanliness is highly valued by mainstream American society. However, in some cultures, a daily bath is not perceived as necessary or desirable. In fact, some cultures do not define natural body odors as offensive. It is important to consider the client in the context of cultural beliefs before labeling a client. Think of the terms *dirty, unkempt,* or *foul-smelling.* These value-laden terms can certainly cloud the assessment process and subsequently the care provided to a client.

a hearing-impaired client should be given a written questionnaire. An intellectually impaired client might require simple, direct sentences and questions or use of pictures. It is best to determine the client's ability to participate before conducting the examination. To allay the disabled client's fears and anxiety, a family member may be allowed to remain with the client during the examination. The nurse should ascertain the client's level of independence and feelings about the disability (Firth & Watanabe, 1996).

Abused Clients

Nurses must be observant for signs of abuse, especially in children and the elderly. The symptoms may be psychological as well as physical; for example, refusal to be touched, inability to maintain eye contact, or unwillingness to talk about bruises, burns, or other injuries may indicate abuse. Bruises or lacerations most typically appear on breasts, buttocks, thighs, or genitalia. The nurse should also inspect for healed scarring or burns. The nurse must know state laws and agency policies for reporting possible abuse.

Vital Signs

Once the nurse has established rapport with the client through introductions, measurement of vital signs is the next step in a head-to-toe assessment. Vital signs are the "signs of life" of an individual. They provide a way of connecting the external inspection of each client with the internal functioning of the client's organs. When checking vital signs, the nurse obtains the temperature, pulse, respirations, and blood pressure of the client. See Table 25-2 for normal values and variations. Equipment used for vital sign measurement is shown in Figure 25-6.

Temperature

When assessing the client's temperature (T), the nurse can use an electronic, chemical, or mercury thermometer. Body temperature can be taken by 5 routes: oral, rectal, axillary, skin, or tympanic membrane. The

Thermometer

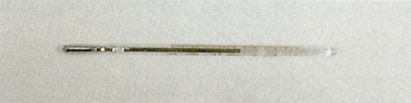

Oral   Slim tip

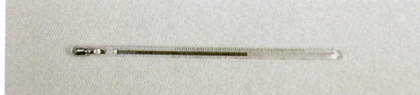

Rectal   Stubby, pear-shaped tip

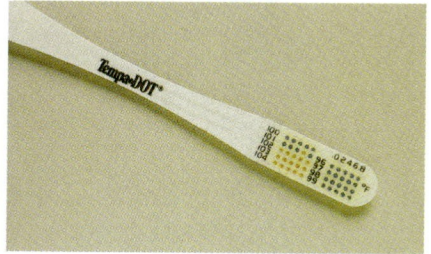

Disposable (chemical), single-use   Thin strips of plastic with chemically impregnated dots that change color to reflect temperature

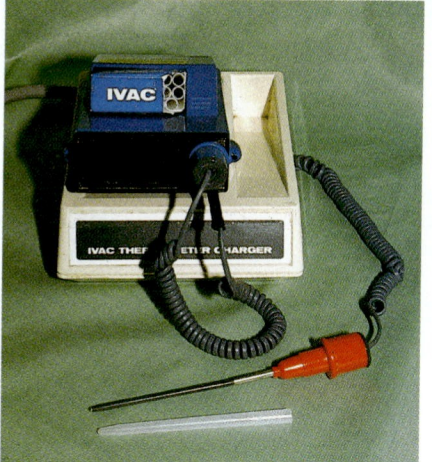

Electronic   Battery-powered display unit with a sensitive probe (blue for oral and red for rectal) covered with a disposable plastic sheath for individual use

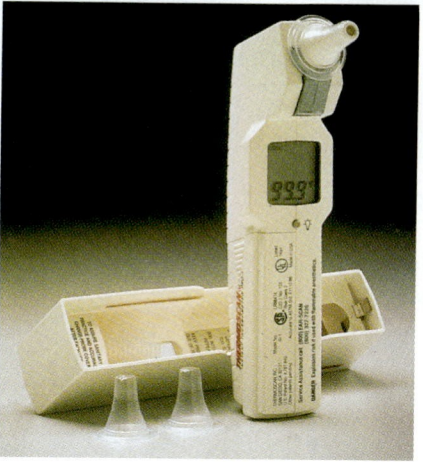

Tympanic   Battery-powered display unit with disposable probe covers and infrared-sensing electronics. (Courtesy The Gillette Company)

Stethoscope

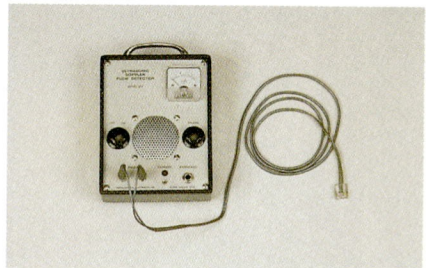

Acoustical   Closed cylinder that prevents dissipation of sound waves and amplifies the sound through a diaphragm. Flat-disc diaphragm transmits high-pitched sounds, and the bell-shaped diaphragm transmits low-pitched sounds.

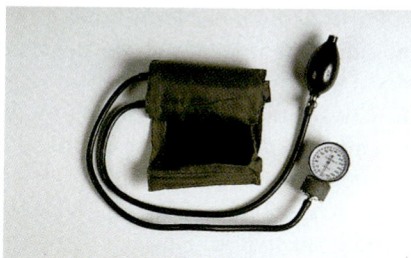

Ultrasound (Doppler)   Battery-operated headset with earpieces attached to a volume-controlled audio unit and ultrasound transducer that detects movement of red blood cells through a vessel.

Sphygmomanometer

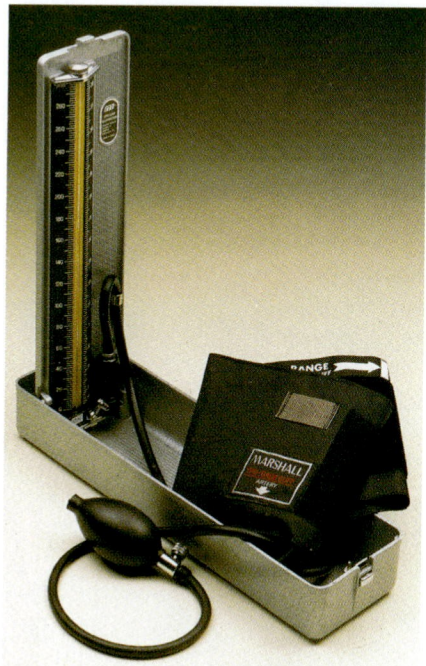

Mercury manometer   Wall or portable unit that contains a mercury-filled glass column, calibrated in millimeters; the mercury rises and falls in response to pressure created when the cuff is inflated.

Aneroid manometer   Portable unit with a glass-enclosed gauge containing a needle to register millimeter calibration and a metal bellows within the gauge that expands and collapses in response to pressure variations from the inflated cuff.

Figure 25-6 Equipment Used for Vital Sign Assessment (*From* Fundamentals of Nursing: Standards and Practice, *by S. DeLaune & P. Ladner, 1998, Albany, NY: Delmar Publishers. Copyright 1998 by Delmar Publishers. Reprinted with permission.*)

Table 25-2 VITAL SIGNS AND VARIATIONS

VITAL SIGN	NORMAL READING		VARIATIONS
Temperature	Axillary	36.5°C or 97.6°F	<36°C or 96.8°F Hypothermia
	Tympanic	37°C or 98.6°F	> 38°C or 100.4°F Pyrexia
	Oral	37°C or 98.6°F	
	Rectal	37.5°C or 99.6°F	
Pulse	60–100 beats/min.		< 60 Bradycardia
			> 100 Tachycardia
Respirations	16–20 resp./min.		< 16 Bradypnea
			> 20 Tachypnea
Blood Pressure	90/60–140/90		< 90/60 Hypotension
			> 140/90 Hypertension

route is chosen depending upon the client's age and physical condition. Factors such as age, gender, physical activity, and environment can affect a person's temperature. Consumption of hot or cold food or beverage and smoking 15 to 30 minutes before taking an oral temperature can also affect the result.

Pulse

Pulse assessment is the measurement of a pressure pulsation created when the heart contracts and ejects blood into the aorta. Assessment of pulse characteristics provides clinical data regarding the heart's pumping action and the adequacy of peripheral artery blood flow.

There are multiple pulse points (Figure 25-7). The most accessible peripheral pulses are the radial and carotid sites. Because the body shunts blood to the brain whenever a cardiac emergency such as hemorrhage occurs, the carotid site should always be used to assess the pulse in these situations. Pulse point assessments are described in Table 25-3.

Assessment of the client's pulse (P) includes the rate, rhythm, and amplitude.

Pulse rate is an indirect measurement of cardiac output obtained by counting the number of peripheral pulse waves over a pulse point. A normal pulse rate for adults is between 60 and 100 beats per minute. **Bradycardia** is a heart rate less than 60 beats per minute in an adult. **Tachycardia** is a heart rate in excess of 100 beats per minute in an adult.

Pulse rhythm is the regularity of the heartbeat. It describes how evenly the heart is beating: regular (the beats are evenly spaced) or irregular (the beats are not evenly spaced). Dysrhythmia (arrhythmia) is an irregular rhythm caused by an early, late, or missed heartbeat.

Pulse amplitude is a measurement of the strength or force exerted by the ejected blood against the arterial wall with each contraction. It is described as normal

---

PROFESSIONAL TIP

Temperature Conversion

To convert Fahrenheit to Celsius (centigrade):

$$(\text{Temperature }°F - 32) \times \tfrac{5}{9} = °C$$

Example:

$$98.6°F - 32 = 66.6 \times \tfrac{5}{9} = 37°C$$

To convert Celsius to Fahrenheit:

$$\tfrac{9}{5} \times \text{temperature}°C + 32 = °F$$

Example:

$$\tfrac{9}{5} \times 40°C = 72 + 32 = 104°F$$

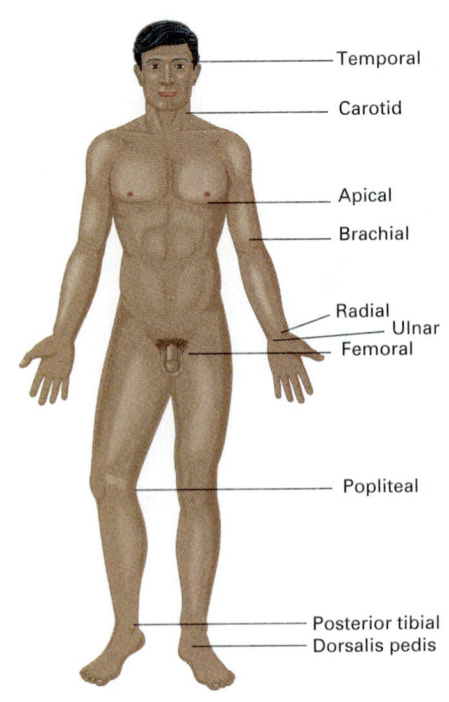

Temporal
Carotid
Apical
Brachial
Radial
Ulnar
Femoral
Popliteal
Posterior tibial
Dorsalis pedis

Figure 25-7 Pulse Points

Table 25-3 PULSE POINT ASSESSMENT

PULSE POINT	ASSESSMENT CRITERIA
Temporal: over temporal bone, superior and lateral to eye	Accessible; used routinely for infants and when radial is inaccessible
Carotid: bilateral, under lower jaw in neck along medial edge of sterno-cleidomastoid muscle	Accessible; used routinely for infants and during shock or cardiac arrest when other peripheral pulses are too weak to palpate; also used to assess cranial circulation
Apical: left midclavicular line at fourth to fifth intercostal space	Used to auscultate heart sounds and assess apical-radial deficit
Brachial: inner aspect between groove of biceps and triceps muscles at antecubital fossa	Used in cardiac arrest for infants, to assess lower arm circulation, and to auscultate blood pressure
Radial: inner aspect of forearm on thumb side of wrist	Accessible; used routinely in adults to assess character of peripheral pulse
Ulnar: outer aspect of forearm on finger side of wrist	Used to assess circulation to ulnar side of hand and to perform the Allen's test
Femoral: in groin, below inguinal ligament (midpoint between symphysis pubis and anterosuperior iliac spine)	Used to assess circulation to legs and during cardiac arrest
Popliteal: behind knee, at center in popliteal fossa	Used to assess circulation to legs and to auscultate leg blood pressure
Posterior tibial: inner aspect of ankle between Achilles tendon and tibia (below medial malleolus)	Used to assess circulation to feet
Dorsalis pedis: over instep, midpoint between extension tendons of great and second toe	Used to assess circulation to feet

From Fundamentals of Nursing: Standards and Practice, by S. DeLaune & P. Ladner, 1998, Albany, NY: Delmar Publishers. Copyright 1998 by Delmar Publishers. Reprinted with permission.

PROFESSIONAL TIP

Carotid Pulse Assessment

When assessing a carotid pulse, apply light pressure to only one carotid artery to avoid disruption of cerebral blood flow.

During the pulse assessment, the nurse should integrate questions about endurance, fatigue, and any possible episodes of palpitations, "feeling the heart beating," over the chest area.

Respirations

Respiratory assessment is the measurement of the breathing pattern. Assessment of respirations provides clinical data regarding the pH of arterial blood. Normal breathing is slightly observable, effortless, quiet, automatic, and regular. It can be assessed by observing chest wall expansion and bilateral symmetrical movement of the thorax. Another method the nurse can use to assess breathing is to place the back of the hand next to the client's nose and mouth to feel the expired air.

Assessment of external respirations (R) should include specific characteristics of respirations as well as the use of any type of oxygen equipment. Each respiration includes one complete inhalation (breathing in) and exhalation (breathing out) by the client. When identifying the characteristics of respirations, the rate, depth, and rhythm of each breath should be determined.

Eupnea refers to easy respirations with a rate of breaths per minute that is age-appropriate. **Bradypnea** is a respiratory rate of 10 or fewer breaths per minute. **Hypoventilation** is characterized by shallow respirations. **Tachypnea** is a respiratory rate greater than 24 breaths per minute. **Hyperventilation** is characterized by deep, rapid respirations. **Dyspnea** refers to difficulty in breathing as observed by labored or forced respirations through the use of accessory muscles in the chest and neck. Dyspneic clients are acutely aware of their respirations and complain of shortness of breath.

PROFESSIONAL TIP

Positioning for Dyspneic Clients

Dyspneic clients should never be placed flat in bed; maintain them in a semi-Fowler's or Fowler's position. To facilitate maximal lung expansion, place the client in a forward-leaning position over a padded, raised overbed table with arms and head resting on the table.

(full, easily palpable), weak (thready and usually rapid), or strong (bounding).

Usual assessment of the radial pulse occurs for 30 seconds and the number of beats is doubled for documentation. If the pulse rhythm is irregular, assessment must occur for 60 seconds. In addition, the nurse must assess for a **pulse deficit** (condition in which the apical pulse rate is greater than the radial pulse rate). A pulse deficit results from the ejection of a volume of blood that is too small to initiate a peripheral pulse wave.

It is also important to observe for nasal flaring and the use of accessory muscles for breathing as evidenced by sternal, costal, and subclavicular retractions. The nurse should be aware that children and males typically utilize abdominal muscles to breathe, whereas women use thoracic muscles (Fuller & Shaller-Ayers, 1999). If a client is receiving oxygen, the route and flow rate must be identified.

During the assessment of respirations, the nurse may determine functional ability by asking about any periods of shortness of breath, any difficulty in breathing with increased exercise, or problems following through with activities of daily living.

Blood Pressure

After checking a client's respirations, the nurse assesses the client's blood pressure (BP). The most common site for indirect blood pressure measurement is the client's arm over the brachial artery.

When pressure measurements in the upper extremities are not accessible, the popliteal artery, located behind the knee, becomes the site of choice. The nurse can also assess the blood pressure in other sites, such as the radial artery in the forearm and the posterior tibial or dorsalis pedis artery in the lower leg. Because it is difficult to auscultate sounds over the radial, tibial, and dorsalis pedis arteries, these sites are usually palpated to obtain a systolic reading.

A person's blood pressure is the result of the interaction of cardiac output and peripheral resistance, and will be dependent on the speed with which the arterial blood flows, the volume of blood supplied, and the elasticity of the walls of the artery. The force exerted by the blood against the wall of the artery as the heart contracts and relaxes is called the *arterial pressure.* When the ventricles contract and blood is forced into the aorta and pulmonary arteries, the systolic arterial pressure is measured. This is the first sound heard. When the heart is in the filling or relaxed stage, the force is described as the *diastolic blood pressure.* This is when the last sound is heard. The difference be-

tween the systolic and diastolic blood pressures is called the *pulse pressure.* A pulse pressure is usually between 30 and 40 mm Hg.

An accurate reading also requires the correct width of the blood pressure cuff as determined by the circumference of the client's extremity. The bladder cuff must encircle the width and length of the site. According to the American Heart Association (1987), the bladder width should be approximately 40% of the circumference or 20% wider than the diameter of the midpoint of the extremity. To measure the width of the bladder, the nurse should place the cuff lengthwise on the client's extremity and extend the width to cover 40% of the extremity's circumference (Figure 25-8). Table 25-4 recommends bladder sizes based on different arm circumferences. A falsely elevated reading will result if the bladder is too narrow, and a falsely low reading will result if it is too wide.

This is an appropriate time to ask if the client ever becomes lightheaded or dizzy when moving from a reclining position to a sitting or standing position. This may occur as a result of an abnormally low blood pressure caused by the inability of the peripheral blood vessels to compensate quickly for the change in position and is referred to as **orthostatic hypotension.**

PROFESSIONAL TIP

Contraindications for Brachial Artery Blood Pressure Measurement

When the client has any of the following, *do not* measure blood pressure on the involved side:
- Venous access devices, such as an intravenous infusion or arteriovenous fistula for renal dialysis
- Surgery involving the breast, axilla, shoulder, arm, or hand
- Injury or disease to the shoulder, arm, or hand, such as trauma, burns, or application of a cast or bandage

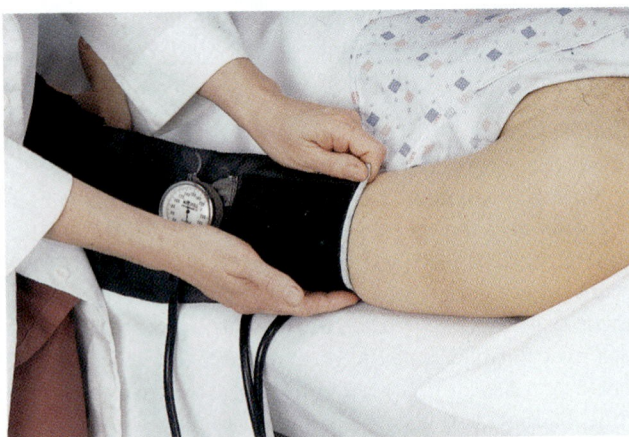

Figure 25-8 Measure width of arm by holding cuff against client's upper arm.

Table 25-4 GUIDELINES FOR SPHYGMOMANOMETER CUFF SELECTION		
MIDPOINT* ARM CIRCUMFERENCE**	**BLADDER CUFF WIDTH****	**LENGTH****
5–7.5 (newborn)	3	5
7.5–13 (infant)	5	8
13–20 (child)	8	13
24–32 (average adult)	13	24
32–42 (large adult)	17	32

*Distance between the acromion and olecranon processes.
**Measurement in centimeters (cm).

From Fundamentals of Nursing: Standards and Practice, *by S. DeLaune & P. Ladner, 1998, Albany, NY: Delmar Publishers. Copyright 1998 by Delmar Publishers. Reprinted with permission.*

Height and Weight Measurement

Measuring height and weight is as important as assessing the client's vital signs. Routine measurement provides data related to growth and development in infants and children and signals the possible onset of alterations that may indicate illness in all age groups. The client's height and weight are routinely taken on admission to acute care facilities and on visits to physicians' offices, clinics, and in other health care settings.

Height

A scale for measuring height, calibrated in either inches or centimeters, is usually attached to a standing weight scale. This type of scale is used for measuring the height of children and adults. The nurse should ask the client to stand erect on the scale's platform. The metal rod attached to the back of the scale should be extended to gently rest on the top of the client's head, and the measurement should be read at eye level.

Weight

When a client has an order for "daily weight," the weight should be obtained at the same time of day on the same scale, with the client wearing the same type of clothing.

Infection Control: Measuring Weight
When standing on a scale, the client should wear some type of light foot covering, such as socks or disposable operating room slippers, to prevent the transmission of infection and to enhance comfort.

Head and Neck Assessment

The nurse will assess the head and neck and determine the client's mental and neurological status, and

the client's overall **affect** (outward expression of mood or emotion).

Hair and Scalp

The hair and scalp of a client should be inspected. The hair distribution, quantity, texture, and color should be noted. The scalp should be smooth and free of any debris or infestations.

Eyes

The eyes should be examined to determine if they are symmetrical. The nurse should look at the eyebrows and eyelids to determine if there is any drooping, which may be a sign of muscle weakness or neurological impairment. The color of the sclera and conjunctiva, as well as the presence of any drainage, should be noted.

The pupils should be assessed to determine their size, shape, and reaction to light. This is accomplished by darkening the room and asking the client to gaze into the distance. The nurse will move a light in from the side and notice if the pupil constricts; this is called the *direct light reflex.* The pupil size in millimeters both before and after the light response (Figure 25-9) is noted. Accommodation is tested by asking the client to focus on an object in the distance; this will dilate the pupils. The client is then asked move his or her gaze to a near object such as a pen or finger held approximately 3 inches from the nose. The pupils should constrict as they focus on the near object and the eyes will converge or move in toward midline. This normal response is documented as PERRLA or Pupils Equal, Round, Reactive to Light and Accommodation.

The nurse should determine if the client utilizes glasses and for what reason, and ask if any eye problems such as blurry vision, diplopia (double vision), or difficulty seeing at night are being experienced.

The assessment of visual acuity is a simple, noninvasive procedure that is performed with the use of a **Snellen chart** (a chart that contains various-sized letters with standardized numbers at the end of each line of letters). The standardized numbers (called the denominator) indicate the degree of visual acuity when the client is able to read that line of letters at a distance of 20 feet.

Nose

The nose should be symmetrical, midline, and in proportion to other features. Any deformity, inflammation,

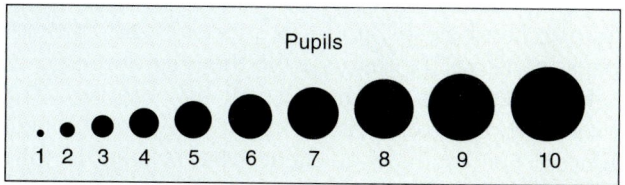

Figure 25-9 Scale Used to Measure Pupil Size, in Millimeters

or prior trauma should be noted. The patency of the nostrils can be tested by asking the client to sniff inward while closing off each nostril. The nurse should ask the client if the following are ever experienced: nosebleeds, dryness, or decrease in sense of smell.

Lips and Mouth

The lips and mucous membranes of the mouth are observed for color, symmetry, moisture, or lesions. If the client has dentures or partial plates, the nurse should ask them to be removed for a more thorough inspection of the mouth. Unusual breath odors should be noted. The oral mucosa can be inspected by inserting a tongue depressor between the teeth and the cheek. The mucous membranes and gums should be pink, moist, smooth, and free of lesions. Inspection of the tongue assists in determining the client's hydration. The tongue should be pink with a slightly rough texture. During the examination the nurse can determine if the client is able to enunciate words appropriately and if there have been any voice changes such as hoarseness. Usual dental hygiene practices should be discussed and the client's history of tobacco usage obtained.

Neck

The neck should be assessed to determine if there is full range of motion. The accessory neck muscles should be symmetrical. As the client moves the head, any enlargement of the lymph nodes or thyroid gland should be noted. The nurse should observe for any pulsations in the neck. The carotid pulsation is seen just below the angle of the jaw. Normally there are no other visible pulsations while the client is in the sitting position.

Mental and Neurological Status and Affect

All head-to-toe assessments must incorporate an assessment of the client's mental and neurological status and affect. A client's mental status includes identification of the level of orientation to person, place, and time. Also included within the mental status is the client's responsiveness to the environment. When assessing for responsiveness, the client's ability to follow directions and to respond appropriately to comments and to his or her name when called is observed.

Neurological assessment of the client focuses on the following: level of consciousness (LOC), pupil response, hand grasps, and foot pushes. Each of these assessments will be discussed in the area of the head-to-toe assessment in which it will be observed. The level of consciousness is the client's degree of wakefulness. For example, a client who is alert is fully awake with eyes open and responds to environmental stimuli. The client who is less awake will be drowsy and slow in response to environmental stimuli.

PROFESSIONAL TIP

Common Abnormal Breath Odors

- Acetone breath ("fruity" smell) is common in malnourished or diabetic clients with ketoacidosis.
- Musty smell is caused by the breakdown of nitrogen and presence of liver disease.
- Ammonia smell occurs during the end stage of renal failure from a buildup of urea.

When documenting the client's affect, words such as *pleasant, happy, cooperative, uncooperative, angry, depressed,* or *hostile* should not be used. Instead, the description of affect should focus specifically upon the behaviors exhibited by the client such as facial expression and verbal and nonverbal behaviors. In doing this, the nurse not only maintains the accuracy of the conversation or the behaviors observed, but also maintains the legal appropriateness of the assessment.

Skin Assessment

Assessment of the skin should be performed as each area of the body is assessed. The color of the skin as well as its moisture or dryness should be noted. The nurse should inspect and palpate the client's skin, assessing temperature, turgor, edema, and integrity. Palpation of the skin with the dorsal aspect of the hand on the right and left sides of the body provides a comparison of the client's skin temperature. The client should also be asked if any pain or discomfort in relation to the skin and/or mucous membranes has occurred. Identification of the skin's turgor is best accomplished by pinching the skin of the anterior chest and observing the speed of return of the skin to its previous position. If the skin stays pinched during assessment, it may indicate dehydration, and further assessment should occur.

Palpate dependent areas (sacrum, legs, ankles, feet) for edema. Firmly apply pressure with a finger for 5 seconds. The degree of edema is based on the depth of indentation in centimeters:

1+	equals an indentation of 1 cm or less
2+	equals an indentation of 2 cm
3+	equals an indentation of 3 cm
4+	equals an indentation of 4 cm
5+	equals an indentation of 5 cm or more

The location, size, distribution, and appearance of skin lesions throughout the body should be determined. Documentation of any breaks in or changes in the skin integrity is an important aspect of nursing assessment. Scratches, bruises, skin tears, cuts, and scars from previous injuries or surgeries are examples of skin characteristics that should be noted. The general

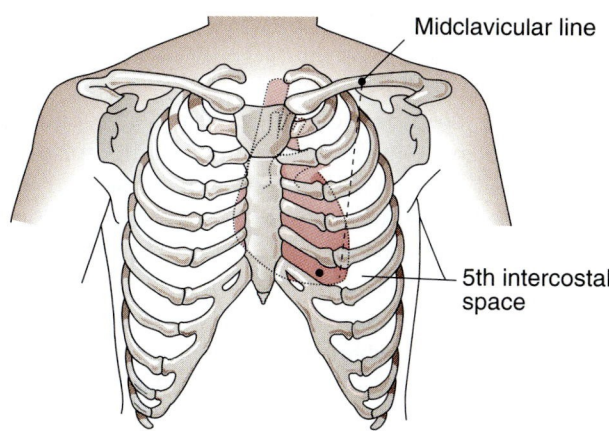

Figure 25-10 Assessing the Apical Pulse

hygiene of the skin should be noted, and the client asked about usual skin care routines.

Thoracic Assessment

During thoracic assessment, the nurse will determine the condition of the client's cardiovascular and respiratory systems along with assessment of the breasts.

Cardiovascular Status

Assessment of the client's cardiovascular status by the LP/VN focuses specifically on listening to the apical pulse, identifying heart tones, and checking the nail beds. The apical pulse is determined by using auscultation and palpation. To assess the apical pulse, the nurse must palpate over the apex of the heart at the fourth or fifth left intercostal space at the midclavicular line. A slight, short duration tap against the fingers will be felt, and this is where the apical pulse will be auscultated (Figure 25-10). Listening to the apical pulse is the most accurate assessment of the heart rate, and should occur for 60 seconds. The apical pulse is assessed first with the diaphragm of the stethoscope for the regularity or irregularity of its rhythm. Second, the bell of the stethoscope is used to differentiate the loudness or tones of the heart. Along with the apical pulse, the other pulse points may be assessed now or when the extremities are asessed.

To assess blood perfusion of peripheral vessels and skin, the nurse should note changes in skin temperature, color, and sensation, and changes in the pulses. Feeling the toes for warmth and color provides important information relative to peripheral circulation and tissue perfusion. Because the position of the extremities can affect the skin temperature and appearance, extremities must always be assessed at heart level and at normal room and body temperature. Peripheral pulses should be compared bilaterally, and changes in strength and quality should be noted (Bosley, 1995).

The focus of the functional assessment includes personal habits contributing to or preventing cardiovascular disease. The nurse should determine the client's personal exercise habits and elicit information regarding past chest pain or shortness of breath. The client should describe any pain, its location, duration, precipitating factors, and what is done to alleviate the pain. The nurse should also ask if the client has ever fainted or felt dizzy. Any lower leg swelling and its cause should also be noted.

Respiratory Status

Breath sound assessment is performed after determination of the apical pulse rate. Respiratory auscultation reveals the presence of normal and abnormal breath sounds. During auscultation, the client should be instructed to breathe only through the mouth because mouth breathing decreases air turbulence that could interfere with an accurate assessment.

There are three distinct types of normal breath sounds with their own unique pitch, intensity, quality, location, and relative duration in the inspiratory and expiratory phases of respiration:

- **Bronchial sounds:** loud and high-pitched sounds with a hollow quality heard longer on expiration than inspiration from air moving through the trachea
- **Bronchovesicular sounds:** medium-pitched and blowing sounds heard equally on inspiration and expiration from air moving through the large airways,

posteriorly between the scapula and anteriorly over bronchioles lateral to the sternum at the first and second intercostal spaces

- **Vesicular sounds:** soft, breezy, and low-pitched sounds heard longer on inspiration than expiration that result from air moving through the smaller airways over the lung's periphery, with the exception of the scapular area

Breath sounds that are not normal are described as either abnormal or **adventitious breath sounds**. Adventitious breath sounds include sibilant wheeze (formerly wheeze), sonorous wheeze (formerly rhonchi), fine and coarse crackle (formerly rales), pleural friction rub, and stridor. **Sibilant wheezes** are high-pitched, whistling sounds heard during inhalation and exhalation. A **sonorous wheeze** is a low-pitched snoring sound that is louder on exhalation. Coughing may alter the sound if caused by mucous. **Crackles** are popping sounds heard on inhalation or exhalation, not cleared by coughing. A **pleural friction rub** is a low-pitched grating sound on inhalation and exhalation. **Stridor** is a high-pitched, harsh sound heard on inspiration when the trachea or larynx is obstructed. Breath sounds of the anterior, posterior, and lateral chest wall must be assessed for normal as well as adventitious breath sounds. Adventitious breath sounds must be monitored on a consistent basis. The lungs are assessed from side to side so the two sides can be compared as shown in Figure 25-11.

The functional assessment information to be obtained when assessing the respiratory status of the client includes any difficulty breathing or the presence of a cough. The client should be asked if the cough is nonproductive or productive, and to describe the secretions produced. Terms used to describe secretions expectorated would be *thick, thin, yellow, green*. The client's occupational or home environment may affect breathing patterns; exposure to dust, chemicals, vapors, tobacco, smoke, or paint fumes, and irritants such as asbestos should be noted.

Wounds, Scars, Drains, Tubes, Dressings

When assessing the thorax, the nurse should note any type of wounds, scars, drains, tubes, or dressings the client may have. Assessment of these must include the location, size, and amount of drainage or discharge, and if present, signs of inflammation.

Breasts

Assessment of the breast tissue should be done for both male and female clients. The nurse can begin by inspecting the breasts for size and symmetry. It is common to have a slight difference in size of breasts. Any obvious masses, dimpling (a depression in the surface skin), or inflammation should be noted. The skin nor-

mally is smooth and even in color. The nurse should determine if the nipples and areola are symmetrical in size, shape, and color, and note any discharge from the nipples.

Any abnormal area should be palpated for size, consistency, mobility, tenderness, and location of the lesion. Another area to include in breast assessment is the axillary lymph nodes that drain the breasts. The nurse should palpate the axilla for enlarged or inflamed lymph nodes, ask if there is any tenderness, and also determine if and when the client performs self-breast exams. The nurse can note if the client has had mammography and when the last x-ray was taken.

Abdominal Assessment

During abdominal assessment, the nurse determines the status of the client's gastrointestinal and genitourinary systems. The nurse should also note any type of wounds, scars, drains, tubes, dressings, or ostomies the client may have. Assessment of these must include the location, size, and amount of drainage or discharge, and if present, any signs of inflammation.

Gastrointestinal Status

The abdomen is first inspected for rashes and scars. The nurse should determine if the abdomen is flat, rounded, or distended, and should observe the abdomen for symmetry and visible signs of peristalsis or pulsations. If the abdomen is distended, the client should be asked questions pertaining to bowel movements and urinary status.

Auscultation is the second component of the abdominal assessment of a client's bowel status. A "bubbly-gurgly" sound, caused by peristalsis and movement of the intestinal contents, can be heard by placing the stethoscope on each quadrant of the abdomen and listening for approximately 1 minute. These sounds should be present in all four quadrants of the abdomen, beginning in the right lower quadrant (RLQ) and moving clockwise around the four quadrants as

PROFESSIONAL TIP

Assessment of the Abdomen

Although the usual sequence for implementing assessment techniques is inspection, palpation, percussion, and auscultation, assessment of the abdomen entails a different sequence. Because palpation can affect sounds heard on auscultation, the sequence for abdominal assessment is as follows:

- Inspection
- Auscultation
- Percussion
- Palpation

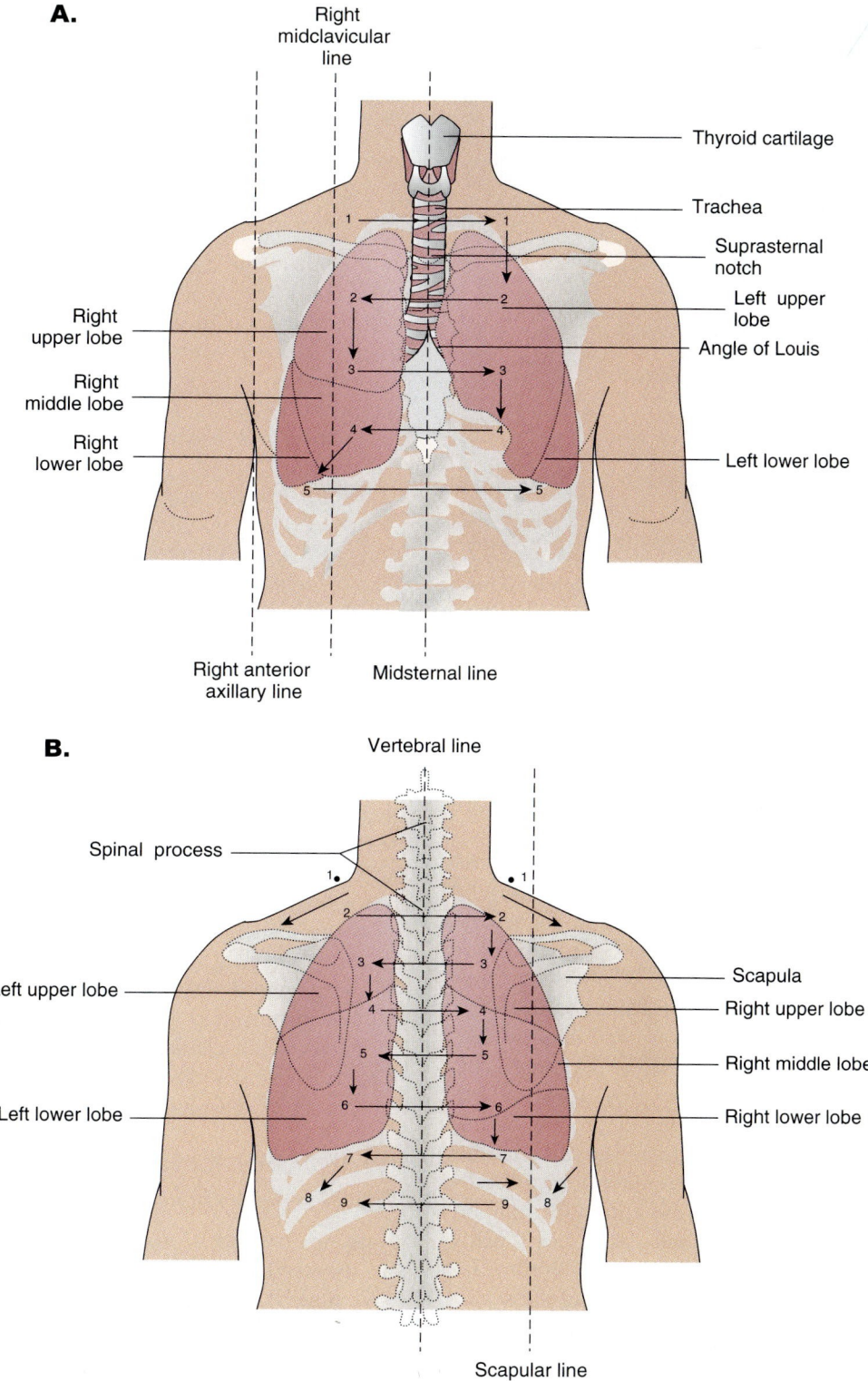

A.

Right
midclavicular
line

Thyroid cartilage

Trachea

Suprasternal
notch

Right
upper lobe

Left upper
lobe

Angle of Louis

Right
middle lobe

Right
lower lobe

Left lower lobe

Right anterior
axillary line

Midsternal line

B.

Vertebral line

Spinal process

Left upper lobe

Scapula

Right upper lobe

Right middle lobe

Left lower lobe

Right lower lobe

Scapular line

Figure 25-11 Symmetrical Assessment of Breath Sounds: A. Anterior; B. Posterior

shown in Figure 25-12. When approximately 5 to 20 bowel sounds are heard per minute, or 1 at least every 5 to 15 seconds, the bowel sounds are considered active.

The absence of bowel sounds during 1 minute of auscultation in each quadrant is documented as absent bowel sounds. Bowel sounds of less than 5 "bubbly-gurgly" sounds per minute are described as hypoactive, while an excess of 20 or more bowel sounds per minute is defined as hyperactive. High-pitched, loud, rushing sounds heard with or without a stethoscope are termed **borborygmi**. This is caused by the passage of gas through the liquid contents of the intestine.

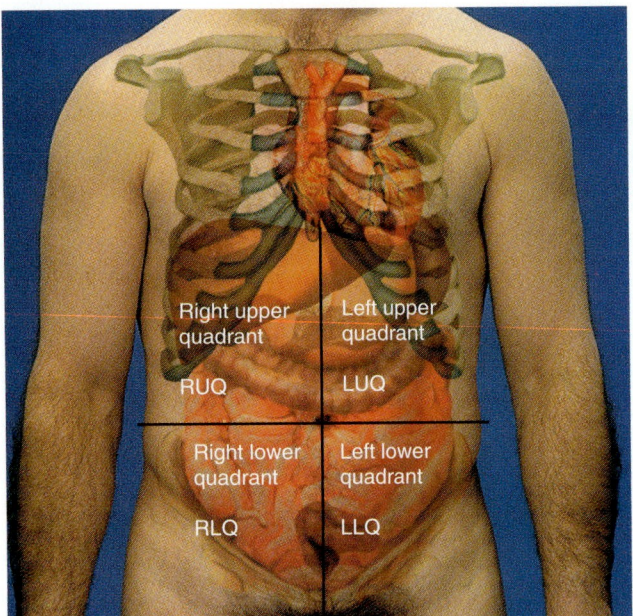

Figure 25-12 The Four Quadrants of the Abdomen *(From Health Assessment and Physical Examination, by M.E.Z. Estes, 1998, Albany, NY: Delmar Publishers. Copyright 1998 by Delmar Publishers. Reprinted with permission.)*

Percussion of the abdomen should occur in all four quadrants. The predominant abdominal percussion sound is tympany caused by percussing over the air-filled stomach and intestines.

Light palpation of the abdomen is done to assess for muscle tone, masses, pulsations, or any signs of tenderness or discomfort. Abdominal muscles may be palpated and should feel relaxed on light palpation, not tightly contracted or spastic. If the client is anxious, muscle contraction may be evident. Palpation of a separation of the rectus abdominous muscle may be felt, especially in clients who are obese or pregnant. The rectus abdominous muscle includes two large, midline muscles that extend from the xiphoid process to the symphysis pubis, and can be palpated midline as the client raises his or her head. Rebound tenderness, indicating possible inflammation of the appendix, may be elicited by depressing the abdomen and quickly withdrawing the fingers. This examination is done at the end of the abdominal assessment because of the possibility of increasing the client's level of pain. If any of the abdominal organs can be felt with light palpation, it is abnormal and should be reported to the nursing supervisor. After assessment of bowel sounds, the nurse should question the client about diet, usual bowel patterns, appetite, weight changes, indigestion, heartburn, nausea, pain, and use of enemas or laxatives.

Genitourinary Status

Assessment of the client's urinary and reproductive status is accomplished mainly by inspection and use of interview skills. Genitourinary assessment includes ex-

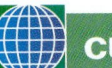

amination of the abdomen, urinary meatus and genitalia, and assessment of the client's urine.

The abdomen should be inspected for any enlargement or fullness. In the normal adult, the abdomen is smooth, flat, and symmetrical. The urinary meatus should be inspected for any abnormalities such as inflammation and discharge, which may signal a urethral infection.

In females, the appearance of the genitalia (labia, clitoris, vaginal opening) should be observed. Questions to ask the client that focus on the reproductive history include: pregnancies, use of birth control, menstrual cycle history, present sexual activity, use of protection during intercourse, date of the last Pap test, and determination of how any present illness has or will affect sexual activity.

In males, assessment of the genitalia includes inspection of the penis, urethral meatus, foreskin (if uncircumcized), and scrotum. Questions to ask the client that focus on the reproductive history include: present sexual activity, use of protection during intercourse, and also how the present illness has or will affect sexual activity. The nurse should determine if the client performs testicular self-examinations.

Any lesions or ulcerations that may indicate sexually transmitted disease should be noted. The usual voiding pattern and any recent changes should be determined if the client has had any history of urinary tract infections, kidney stones, change in the urinary stream, or painful urination or nocturia.

Musculoskeletal and Extremity Assessment

Symmetry and strength of major muscle groups can be assessed throughout the head-to-toe assessment. Any time during the assessment when the client is repositioned, the range of movement the client utilizes to make that position change can be observed. Asking the client to walk across the room and noting the client's movements and stance when sitting up in bed are observations made to assess gross motor movement and posture. Assessment of the client's handshake gives an estimate of muscle strength. Palpating muscles lightly determines swelling, tone, or any specific changes in shape of the muscles.

Hand grasps and foot pushes assess the strength and equality of the client's extremities. Upper extremity strength is assessed by having the client grasp the nurse's index and middle fingers of each hand. The grasp should be equal in both hands. Foot pushes assess the lower extremities. The nurse's hands should be placed on the soles of the client's feet. The client is asked to push both feet against the nurse's hands. The push should be equal in both feet. Asking the client to touch the tip of her nose with a finger and then the tip of the nurse's finger as it is moved to different locations tests the client's coordination skills.

Strength and symmetry of some of the major muscle groups can be assessed by watching gait and postural movements. Any aids to ambulation must be noted. Symmetrical examination of muscles should occur in pairs, first one extremity and then the other; equality of size, contour, tone, and strength should be assessed.

The skin of the lower extremities should be carefully assessed to determine color changes, loss of feeling or hair, change in temperature within the extremity and from one extremity to the other, and presence of varicose veins, ulcers, and edema. The nurse should determine if the client experiences any leg pain or cramps.

The nurse should ask the client if muscle weakness is experienced or if difficulty or pain when walking or performing routine daily activities occurs. The functional assessment should also include asking the client about routine activities such as cooking, shopping, exercise, yard work, and hobbies. Tolerance limitations can be observed by assessing for stiffness, crepitus, or fatigue during ambulation. Safe and appropriate performance of functions essential for home life and activities of daily living must be determined.

SUMMARY

- Psychosocial needs of clients are identified within the scope of a functional assessment.
- The health history and the physical examination used together present a holistic view of client needs.
- The four techniques used in a head-to-toe assessment include: inspection, palpation, percussion, and auscultation.

CASE STUDY

Tom Turner, age 40, has been admitted to the hospital with pneumonia. He has never been hospitalized before. His wife and three children are at home. Because his wife has just given birth to their third child, Tom's wife cannot drive the other two children to school. Tom provides the sole income for the family, and he has only three more sick days to use at work before he will be off without pay.

Tom's vital signs are BP 120/72, P 100, R 34, T 100.6°F. His breath sounds show sonorous wheezes throughout, cleared by coughing. His cough is frequent and productive of foamy, cloudy, yellow secretions. His apical pulse is 102 and regular, but distant heart tones were noted. The abdomen is firm and distended with hypoactive bowel sounds noted in all four quadrants. He moves all extremities slowly but per self and with purpose.

Tom is oriented to person, place, and time. His pupils are PERRLA. Hand grips are strong and equal bilaterally, as are foot pushes. He speaks only when spoken to, and his eye contact with staff is minimal. Whenever his wife visits, his voice raises and his heart rate increases about 2–5 beats. At one point, Tom stated, "How much more of this can we take?" Tom's wife mentions that their church would love to help, but Tom refuses to take charity. Tom states, "Any income for this family has to come from me."

Other added information acquired during the assessment includes the fact that Tom has a history of drinking 1 to 2 beers daily, and has not performed testicular self-exams. He eats and drinks what he likes, and he states he really "hates seafood." Usually he bathes daily in the early morning and helps to bathe two of their children each evening. He works 9–5:30 P.M., five days per week, and also some Saturday mornings. Tom pays all of the household bills, and is the sole decision maker of the family.

The following questions will guide your development of a nursing care plan for the case study.

1. List the functional assessment data collected from Mr. Turner that identify psychosocial concerns.

2. What are two possible reasons for identifying the added information about Mr. Turner in the last paragraph?

3. Write two nursing diagnoses that are supported by the health history and physical assessments documented about Mr. Turner.

4. Write goals and nursing interventions for each nursing diagnosis.

- Introduction of the nurse at the beginning of a physical assessment enhances the ability to accomplish the complete assessment.
- Collection of vital signs is the foundation to each head-to-toe assessment and includes: temperature, pulse, respirations, and blood pressure.
- Assessment of a client's mental and neurological status is performed when the nurse obtains information about the client's level of consciousness, pupil response, as well as hand grip and foot push capabilities.
- When describing a client's affect, the nurse must utilize terms that are descriptive of the specific behavior observed, not the nurse's judgment about the behavior.
- Assessing the cardiovascular status of each client includes palpation of specific pulse points.
- Auscultation of lung fields assists in collection of data regarding the breath sounds of the client.
- An abdominal assessment includes use of inspection, auscultation, percussion, and palpation within the four quadrants of the abdomen to establish bowel status and function.
- Through observation of client gait and overall range of movement, the nurse is able to obtain some knowledge of the symmetry and strength of muscles.
- During the assessment of wounds, drains, dressings, and other external devices, the nurse must maintain accurate documentation of the amount of drainage, color, or other changes.

Review Questions

1. Jim's apical pulse is 102. He states to the nurse that he can feel his heart pounding. Which of the following charting terms would accurately describe Jim's statement of concern regarding his heart rate?

    a. Bradycardia
    b. Changing of rhythm
    c. Palpitation
    d. Tachycardia

2. Mrs. Jones is 54 years old. While performing the assessment overview, Mrs. Jones states, "I just get so lightheaded when I first get up in the morning." Mrs. Jones most likely has:

    a. cyanosis.
    b. hypertension.
    c. orthostatic hypertension.
    d. orthostatic hypotension.

3. During the physical head-to-toe assessment of the client, the nurse checks the pulse and blood pressure. Which of the four assessment techniques did the nurse utilize?

    a. Auscultation, palpation, and inspection
    b. Auscultation, percussion, and inspection
    c. Auscultation and palpation
    d. Palpation and inspection

4. Upon admission to your unit, the client verbalizes an increased pain in her left leg. What would be the pertinent assessment information to collect about this client?

    a. Listen to the client's bowel sounds.
    b. Check circulation in the right leg.
    c. Assess both of the client's legs.
    d. Ask the client about her current diet.

5. Which of the pulses should be palpated when assessing circulation to the lower extremities?

    a. Dorsalis pedis
    b. Femoral
    c. Temporal
    d. Popliteal

6. How often a nurse assesses a client's vital signs depends upon the:

    a. availability of personnel.
    b. doctor's orders.
    c. nurse's discretion.
    d. client's condition.

7. The nurse checks the radial pulse for 30 seconds and multiplies by 2. She notices an irregularity in the beat. What is the next action the nurse should take?

    a. Check the radial pulse for 60 seconds.
    b. Listen to the apical pulse for 60 seconds.
    c. Listen to the apical for 30 seconds and multiply by 2.
    d. Continue with the rest of the assessment.

Critical Thinking Questions

1. How do you feel about performing a complete physical assessment on a client?

2. How do you feel when you receive a complete physical assessment?

 WEB FLASH!

- Search the Internet for information regarding physical examination (assessment). What type of information is available?
- Are there any organizations on the Internet that focus on physical examination (assessment)? Are they specific by age group (pediatrics, adolescents, elderly)?

PAIN MANAGEMENT

MAKING THE CONNECTION

Refer to the following chapters to increase your understanding of pain management:

- Chapter 8, Communication
- Chapter 9, Nursing Process
- Chapter 11, Client Teaching
- Chapter 12, Cultural Diversity and Nursing
- Chapter 13, Alternative/Complementary Therapies
- Chapter 16, Stress, Adaptation, and Anxiety
- Chapter 29, Nursing Care of the Surgical Client
- Chapter 30, Nursing Care of the Oncology Client

LEARNING OBJECTIVES

Upon completion of this chapter, you should be able to:
- *Define key terms.*
- *Identify the four components of pain conduction.*
- *Discuss the gate control theory of pain.*
- *Describe the types of pain.*
- *List three guidelines that should be included in a thorough pain assessment.*
- *Identify three general principles of pain management.*
- *List the nurse's responsibilities in administration of analgesics.*
- *Identify site of action of both nonopioid and opioid analgesics.*
- *Describe three examples of nonpharmacological measures for pain relief.*
- *Discuss nursing interventions that promote comfort.*

KEY TERMS

acupuncture
acute pain
adjuvant medication
afferent pain pathway
analgesia
analgesic
ceiling effect
chronic acute pain
chronic nonmalignant pain
chronic pain
colic
cryotherapy
cutaneous pain
distraction
efferent pain pathway
endorphin
epidural analgesia
gate control pain theory
hypnosis
intrathecal analgesia
ischemic pain
mixed agonist-antagonist
modulation
myofascial pain syndromes
neuralgia
nociceptor
noxious stimulus
pain
pain threshold
pain tolerance
patient-controlled-analgesia
perception
phantom limb pain
progressive muscle relaxation
recurrent acute pain
referred pain
reframing
relaxation technique
somatic pain
tolerance
transcutaneous electrical nerve stimulation
transduction
transmission
visceral pain

INTRODUCTION

Pain is a phenomenon that crosses all specialties of nursing. No matter the setting a nurse practices in, including neonatal intensive care, intraoperative, home care, or clinics, the nurse will be exposed to challenges in pain management. While other health care team members address pain management with clients, it is the nurse who spends the most time with the client experiencing pain. For example, in an acute care setting, the physician orders the **analgesics** (substances that relieve pain) for the client, but may only spend 10 to 15 minutes each day with that client. The nurses are the ones who are present 24 hours a day, administer the medications, assess the client's response, and report the response to the physician. It is for this reason the nurse is often called the "backbone" or "cornerstone" of pain management. The nurse's role can be pivotal in relieving the client's pain.

Studies have documented undertreatment of pain of all types and in all age groups (Liebeskind & Melzack, 1987). In one such study, the researchers interviewed medical and surgical clients, finding that 58% had experienced excruciating pain in the previous 72 hours. Fifty-five percent of these clients could not recall a nurse asking about their pain (Donovan, Dillon, & McGuire, 1987). Another study examined pain management in metastatic cancer clients in an outpatient setting. Forty-two percent of the clients with pain were not given adequate analgesic therapy (Cleeland, Gonin, Hatfield, Edmonson, Blum, Stewart, & Pandya, 1994).

It is generally thought that this undertreatment of pain is partially due to the lack of knowledge in both physicians and nurses. It is, therefore, important for the nurse to understand not only the psychological and physiological components that add up to the pain experience, but also the wide range of interventions available to provide relief. Another reason for undertreatment may be the health care workers' own biases regarding pain. Consequently, nurses should also recognize their own responses to pain and how they respond to others' expressions of pain.

The experience of pain is a factor that can have a significant impact on a client's health. It is a personal experience that can affect all other aspects of an individual's health, including physical well-being, mental status, and effectiveness of coping mechanisms. This chapter provides an overview of the complex phenomenon of pain, including: pain definitions, pain physiology, and pain assessment. Strategies to control pain will also be discussed, including pharmacological, noninvasive, and invasive techniques.

DEFINITIONS OF PAIN

The phenomenon of pain is evidenced in ancient history with references being made as far back as the Babylonian clay tablets. Aristotle (4th century B.C.) described pain as an emotion, being the opposite of pleasure. While emotions certainly play an important role in pain perception, we now know there is much more to the experience than the feelings involved.

In the Middle Ages, pain was viewed with religious connotations. Pain was seen as God's punishment for sins, or as evidence that an individual was possessed by demons. This definition of pain is still embraced by some clients, who might tell the nurse that the suffering is their "cross to bear." Pain relief may not be the goal for those individuals who believe in this definition of pain. Spiritual counseling may need to be implemented before this person is willing to work toward relief.

Currently, the most widely accepted definition of **pain** is that developed by the International Association for the Study of Pain (IASP). This organization defines pain as "an unpleasant sensory and emotional experience associated with actual or potential tissue damage or described in terms of such damage" (Merskey & Bogduk, 1994). This definition incorporates both the sensory and emotional components of pain. It also acknowledges that evidence of actual tissue damage is not required in order for the pain to be considered real.

Many pain experts emphasize the subjective nature of pain. Unlike a blood pressure or a blood glucose measurement, the intensity of discomfort the client is feeling cannot be measured with an instrument. McCaffery and Pasero (1999) say it best by defining pain as "whatever the person experiencing it says it is, existing whenever [he or she] says it does." This philosophy is emphasized in professional pain management guidelines. For example, the Agency for Health Care Policy and Research (AHCPR) (1994) guideline for cancer pain states, "Health professionals should ask about pain, and the patient's self-report should be the primary source of assessment." The American Pain Society (APS) also stresses the importance of self-report: "Pain is always subjective. . . . The clinician must accept the patient's report of pain" (1992).

Though pain has had many definitions throughout humankind's history, research in pain physiology has shown that pain is a complex phenomenon. Pain is often difficult for clients to describe and nurses to understand; yet it is among the most common complaints that cause individuals to seek health care. Until recently, pain was viewed as a symptom that required diagnosis and treatment of the underlying cause. It is now clear that pain itself can be detrimental to the health and healing of clients. McCaffery and Pasero (1999) write that pain control, not just relief from pain once it occurs, must be recognized as a priority in the care of clients in all settings.

NATURE OF PAIN

A major function of the pain experience is to signal ongoing or potential tissue damage (Schecter, Berde, & Yaster, 1993), as is seen in the pain of cancer and chronic illness. Pain can also be a protective mechanism to prevent further injury, as is seen in clients who guard or protect an injured body part. The sensation of pain as the warning of potential tissue damage may be absent in people with hereditary sensory neuropathies, congenital nerve or spinal cord abnormalities, diabetic neuropathy, multiple sclerosis, leprosy, alcoholism, and nerve or spinal cord injury (Brand & Yancey, 1993).

COMMON MYTHS ABOUT PAIN

Because pain is subjective (dependent on the client's perception) and cannot be objectively measured by another individual through a laboratory test or diagnostic data, pain is often misunderstood and misjudged. A client's report of level of pain will vary on the basis of cultural and experiential backgrounds, and the nurse's interpretations of a client's pain will be filtered through the nurse's own biases and expectations. Misalignment of the nurse's view and the client's perception of pain can often lead to undermedication and unnecessary suffering on the client's part. Some common myths related to pain are discussed in Table 26-1.

TYPES OF PAIN

Pain can be qualified or described in two basic ways: by its cause or origin and by its description or nature. Pain categorized by its origin is either cutaneous, somatic, or visceral. Pain categorized by its nature is either acute or chronic.

Pain Categorized by Origin

Cutaneous pain is caused by stimulation of the cutaneous nerve endings in the skin and results in a well-localized "burning" or "prickling" sensation; getting a knot in the hair that is pulled out during combing may cause cutaneous pain. **Somatic pain** is nonlocalized and originates in support structures such as tendons, ligaments, and nerves; jamming a knee or finger will result in somatic pain. **Visceral pain** is discomfort in the internal organs and is less localized and more slowly transmitted than cutaneous pain. Visceral pain is often difficult to assess because the location may not be directly related to the cause. Pain originating from the abdominal organs is often called **referred pain** because the sensation of pain is not felt in the organ itself but instead is perceived at the spot where the organs were located during fetal development (Figure 26-1).

Pain Categorized by Nature

It is important to understand the difference between acute and chronic pain, as they each present a different clinical picture.

Acute Pain

Acute pain is most frequently identified by its sudden onset and relatively short duration, mild to severe intensity, and a steady decrease in intensity over a period of days to weeks. Some forms of acute pain may have a slower onset. Once the **noxious stimulus** (underlying pathology) is resolved, the unpleasant sensation usually disappears (Stevens, 1994) (see Table 26-2). It can usually be associated with a specific injury, condition, or disease that has caused tissue damage. Acute pain should diminish as healing occurs. Everyone has experienced acute pain, for example:

Table 26-1 COMMON MYTHS ABOUT PAIN

MYTH	FACT
• The nurse is the best judge of a client's pain.	• Pain is a subjective experience; only the client can judge the level and severity of pain.
• If pain is ignored, it will go away.	• Pain is a real experience that is appropriately treated with nursing and medical intervention.
• Clients should not take any measures to relieve their pain until the pain is unbearable.	• Pain control and relief measures are effective in lowering the pain level, which will help clients function more normally and comfortably.
• Most complaints of pain are purely psychological (e.g., "it's all in your head"); only "real" pain manifests in obvious physical signs such as moaning or grimacing.	• Most clients report honestly on their perception of pain, both physical and emotional, and need effective intervention and teaching; physical responses to pain vary greatly depending on experience and cultural norms, and visible expressions of pain are not always reliable indicators of its severity.
• Clients taking pain medications will become addicted to the drug.	• Addiction is unlikely when analgesics are carefully administered and closely monitored.
• Clients with severe tissue damage will experience significant pain; those with lesser damage will feel less pain.	• Individuals' perceptions of pain are subjective; the extent of tissue damage is not necessarily proportional to the extent of pain experienced.
• Clients ask for pain medication when they need it.	• Many clients do not ask for medication because they are afraid of side effects, do not want to bother the nurse, have cultural norms and beliefs against it, or believe pain is inevitable and untreatable.

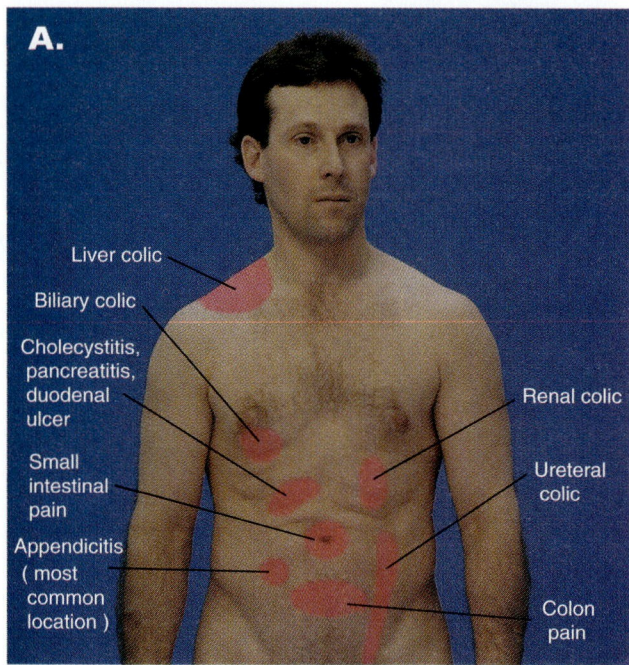

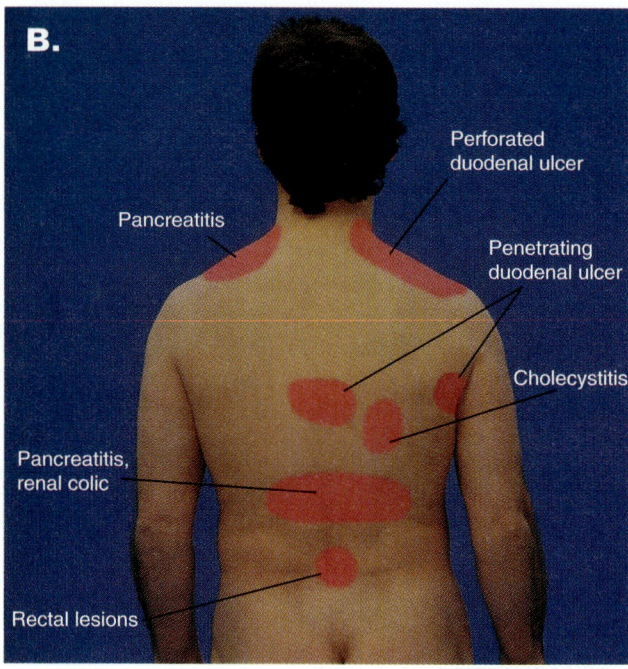

Figure 26-1 Areas of Referred Pain: A. Anterior view; B. Posterior view

Table 26-2 **ACUTE VERSUS CHRONIC PAIN**		
	ACUTE	**CHRONIC**
Time Span	Less than 6 months	More than 6 months
Location	Localized, associated with a specific injury, condition, or disease	Difficult to pinpoint
Characteristics	Often described as sharp, diminishes as healing occurs	Often described as dull, diffuse, and aching
Physiologic Signs	• Elevated heart rate • Elevated BP • Elevated respirations • May be diaphoretic • Dilated pupils	• Normal vital signs • Normal pupils • No diaphoresis • May have loss of weight
Behavioral Signs	• Crying and moaning • Rubbing site • Guarding • Frowning • Grimacing • Complains of pain	• Physical immobility • Hopelessness • Listlessness • Loss of libido • Exhaustion and fatigue • Complains of pain only when asked

headaches, toothaches, needle sticks, burns, skinned knees, muscle pain, childbirth, postoperative pain, fractures, and a sprained ankle. The client will describe the pain as highly localized and is usually able to pinpoint the hurt. Acute pain is often described as sharp, although if the pain is deep, it may be described as dull and aching. Accompanying signs will be those of the activation of the sympathetic nervous system, that is, the fight-or-flight response. Therefore, the client will exhibit elevated heart rate, respiratory rate, and blood pressure. The client may become diaphoretic and have

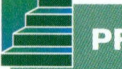 **PROFESSIONAL TIP**

Effect of Acute Pain

Page, Ben-Eliyahu, Yirmiya, and Liebeskind (1993) studied the effect of acute surgical pain on tumor metastasis in the rat model. Stress response to surgery includes increases in serum epinephrine, norepinephrine, cortisol, growth hormone, and prolactin; several of these hormones can affect immune system function. The study findings suggest that the experience of postoperative pain can increase metastatic growth in laboratory animals, and that "If a similar relationship between pain and metastasis occurs in humans, then pain control must be considered a vital component of postoperative care" (p. 23).

dilated pupils. These signs resemble those of anxiety, which often accompanies acute pain. Behaviors may include crying and moaning, rubbing the site of pain, guarding, frowning, and grimacing. The client will often verbally complain of the discomfort.

Recurrent acute pain is identified by repetitive painful episodes that may recur over a prolonged period or throughout the client's lifetime. These painful episodes alternate with pain-free intervals. Examples of recurrent pain often seen in children include recurrent abdominal, chest, or limb pain that occurs in 5% to 10% of school-age children; headaches; and sickle cell pain crises with vaso-occlusion that leads to ischemia or infarction (Schecter, Berde, & Yaster, 1993). Examples of recurrent pain experienced by adults include migraine headaches, sickle cell pain crises, and the pain of angina pectoris due to hypoxia of the myocardium.

Chronic Pain

Chronic pain is generally identified as long-term (lasting 6 months or longer), persistent, nearly constant, or recurrent pain that produces significant negative changes in the client's life. Unlike acute pain, chronic pain may last long after the pathology is resolved. Although severe chronic persistent pain is experienced by some infants, children, and adolescents, it is much more common in the adult population (Schecter et al., 1993). More than 30% of all persons in the U.S. experience chronic pain, with the most common chronic pain in adults being back pain (Vasudevan, 1993).

Chronic acute pain occurs almost daily over a long period, has the potential for lasting months or years, and has a high probability of ending. Severe burn injuries and cancer are examples of pathophysiology that leads to chronic acute pain, which may last for long periods before the condition is cured or controlled. In some cases, the pain ends only with the death of the client, as in the case of those terminally ill with cancer (McCaffery & Pasero, 1999). This type of pain is also known as *progressive pain.*

Chronic nonmalignant pain, also called *chronic benign pain,* occurs almost daily and lasts for at least 6 months, with intensity ranging from mild to severe. McCaffery and Pasero (1999) identify three critical characteristics of chronic nonmalignant pain in that it:

- is due to non–life-threatening causes.
- is not responsive to currently available methods of pain relief.
- may continue for the remainder of the client's life.

Examples of pathophysiology leading to chronic nonmalignant pain include:

- Many forms of **neuralgia** (paroxysmal pain that extends along the course of one or more nerves)
- Low back pain
- Rheumatoid arthritis
- Ankylosing spondylitis
- **Phantom limb pain** (a form of neuropathic pain that occurs after amputation with pain sensations referred to an area in the missing portion of the limb)
- **Myofascial pain syndromes** (a group of muscle disorders characterized by pain, muscle spasm, tenderness, stiffness, and limited motion)

When chronic nonmalignant pain is severe enough to disable the client, it is identified as *chronic intractable nonmalignant pain syndrome.*

The signs and symptoms of chronic pain can look very different from those of acute pain. The body cannot tolerate the sympathetic nervous system signs for such a long period of time and, therefore, adapts. The vital signs will often be normal, with no accompanying pupil dilatation or perspiration. Lack of these signs may prompt some health care workers to question the client's description of pain.

The signs and symptoms of chronic pain, such as hopelessness, listlessness, and loss of libido and weight, are similar to those of depression. The client will often complain of exhaustion and fatigue. Behaviors include no complaints of pain unless asked and physical inactivity or immobility that can lead to functional disability. The crying, moaning, guarding, and grimacing that most clinicians associate with pain are absent. Treatment of chronic pain is more complex than that of acute pain. Chronic pain is viewed by pain experts as a disease state, rather than a symptom (Bonica, 1990). Management includes identifying the cause of pain, recognizing emotional and environmental factors that may be contributing to the pain, and rehabilitation to improve the client's functional abilities.

PURPOSE OF PAIN

Pain serves an important purpose as a protective mechanism. For example, if a person touches a hot stove, the pain signal will cause the person to pull the hand away immediately. The skin would be seriously burned if this did not happen. Pain not only protects, but it prompts clients to seek out medical care.

Pain is also useful as a diagnostic tool. Characteristics of the pain, such as the quality and duration, can give important clues in determining a client's medical diagnosis. For example, in acute appendicitis, the clinician looks for rebound tenderness (the pain increases when pressure is released) when palpating the abdomen. This particular type of pain helps to confirm the diagnosis of appendicitis rather than other gastrointestinal disorders.

PHYSIOLOGY OF PAIN

There are two known endogenous (developing within) analgesia systems in humans: the opioid system and the nonopioid system. The opioid system is best known and is mediated by a family of chemicals known as **endorphins** (endogenous neuropeptides that have morphinelike effects). The nonopioid system is mediated by monoamine substances such as norepinephrine and serotonin.

When pain occurs, sensory input from injured tissue causes peripheral **nociceptors** (receptive neurons for painful sensations) and central nervous system (CNS) pain pathways to enhance subsequent responses to pain stimuli (Dubner, 1991). Thus, long-lasting changes in cells within the spinal cord **afferent** (ascending) and **efferent** (descending) **pain pathways** may occur after a brief noxious stimulus.

Physiological responses (such as elevated blood pressure, pulse rate, and respiratory rate; dilated pupils; pallor; and perspiration) to even a brief acute pain episode will begin showing adaptation within a short period, possibly minutes to a few hours. Physiologically, the body cannot sustain the extreme stress response for other than short periods of time. The body conserves its resources by physiological adaptation: returning to normal or near normal blood pressure, pulse rate, and respiratory rate; normal pupil size, and dry skin with little evidence of poor perfusion, *even in the face of continuing pain of the same intensity.*

Stimulation of Pain

The specific action of pain varies depending on the type of pain. In cutaneous pain, cutaneous nerve transmissions travel through a reflex arc from the nerve ending (point of pain) to the brain at a speed of approximately 300 feet per second, with a reflex response causing an almost immediate reaction. This explains why, when a hot stove is touched, the person's hand jerks back *before* there is conscious awareness that damage is occurring (Figure 26-2). After a hot stove is touched, a sensory nerve ending in the skin of the finger initiates nerve transmission that travels through the dorsal root ganglion to the dorsal horn in the gray matter of the spinal cord. From there, the impulse travels though an interneuron that synapses with a motor neuron, which exits the spinal cord at the same level. This motor neuron, and the stimulation of the muscle it innervates, is responsible for the swift movement of the hand away from the hot stove.

In the case of the hot stove, the sensory neuron

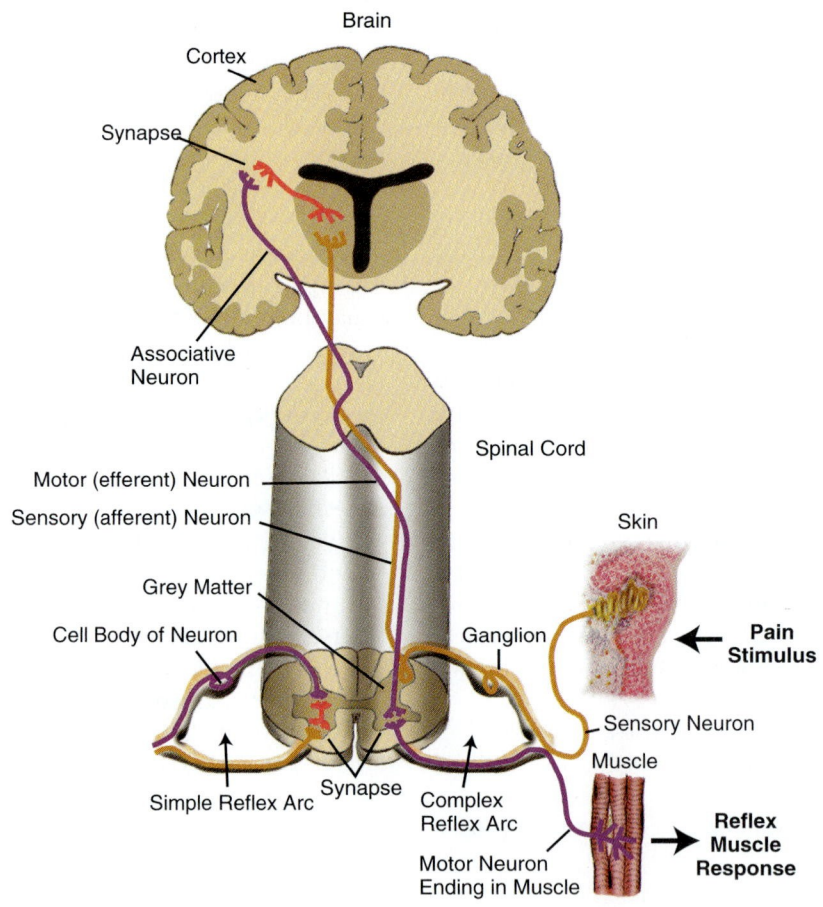

Figure 26-2 Reflex Arcs (*From* Fundamentals of Nursing: Standards and Practice, *by S. DeLaune and P. Ladner, 1998, Albany, NY: Delmar Publishers. Copyright 1998 by Delmar Publishers. Reprinted with permission.*)

synapses not only with an interneuron but also with an afferent sensory neuron. The impulse travels up the spinal cord to the thalamus, where a final synapse conducts the impulse to the cortex of the brain. Once the signal reaches the cortex and is interpreted by the brain, the information is available on a conscious level. It is then that the person becomes aware of the intensity, location, and quality of pain. This information is interpreted in light of previous experience, adding the affective component to the pain experience. Efferent or descending motor neuron response is conducted from the brain through the spinal cord, where it synapses with a motor neuron that exits the spinal cord and innervates the muscle.

In visceral pain, transmission of pain impulses is slower and less localized than in cutaneous pain. The internal organs (including the gastrointestinal tract) have a minimal number of nociceptors, which explains why visceral pain is poorly localized and is felt as a dull aching or throbbing sensation. However, internal organs have extreme sensitivity to distension. The cramping pain of **colic** (acute abdominal pain), for example, results when:

- Flatus or constipation causes distension of the stomach or intestines
- There is hyperperistalsis, as in gastroenteritis
- Something tries to pass through an opening that is too small

The physiology of **ischemic pain**, or pain occurring when the blood supply of an area is restricted or cut off completely, also differs from that of cutaneous pain. The restriction of blood flow causes inadequate oxygenation of the tissue supplied by those vessels, as well as inadequate metabolic waste product removal. Ischemic pain has the most rapid onset in an active muscle and a much slower onset in a passive muscle. Examples of ischemic pain are muscle cramps, sickle cell pain crisis, angina pectoris, and myocardial infarction. When ischemic pain occurs in a muscle that continues to work, a muscle spasm (cramp) is the outcome. If the blood supply to the heart is severely restricted or completely cut off and is not restored quickly, a myocardial infarction will occur.

PROFESSIONAL TIP

Sensation of Pain

It takes 0.2 grams of pressure per square millimeter for the cornea of the eye to feel pain, as opposed to 20 grams on the forearm, 200 grams on the sole of the foot, and 300 grams on the fingertips (Brand & Yancey, 1993).

Safety: Ischemic Pain

Supplemental oxygen and pain medication must be administered quickly to clients with ischemic pain to minimize oxygen deprivation and prevent infarction (tissue death).

In acute pain episodes, substances released from injured tissue lead to stress hormone responses in the client. This causes an increased metabolic rate, enhanced breakdown of body tissue, impaired immune function, increased blood clotting, and water retention. It triggers the fight-or-flight reaction leading to tachycardia and negative emotions.

The Gate Control Theory

Theories of pain transmission and interpretation attempt to describe and explain the pain experience. Early pain theorists focused on the neuroanatomical and neurophysiological mechanisms while failing to consider the psychological, social, cultural, and developmental factors involved (Stevens, 1994).

In 1965, Melzack and Wall proposed the **gate control pain theory**, which was the first to recognize that the psychological aspects of pain are as important as the physiological aspects. The gate control theory combines cognitive, sensory, and emotional components—in addition to the physiological aspects—and proposes that they can act on a gate control system to block the individual's perception of pain. The basic premise of this theory is that transmission of potentially painful nerve impulses to the cortex is modulated by a gating mechanism in the spinal cord and by CNS activity. As a result, the level of conscious awareness of painful sensation is altered.

The theory suggests that nerve fibers that contribute to pain transmission converge at a site in the dorsal horn of the spinal cord. This site is thought to act as a gating mechanism that determines which impulses will be blocked and which will be transmitted to the thalamus. The image of a gate can be useful in teaching clients and their families about pain relief measures. If the "gate" is closed, the signal is stopped before it reaches the brain, where **perception** (being aware of) of pain occurs. If the gate is open, the signal will continue on through the spinothalamic tract to the cortex, and the client will feel the pain. Whether the gate is opened or closed is influenced by the impulses from peripheral nerves (the sensory components) and nerve signals that descend from the brain (motivational-affective and cognitive components). For example, stimulation of some types of peripheral nerves by cutaneous stimulation such as massage can close the gate, whereas stimulation of the nociceptors will open the gate.

If a person is anxious, the gate can be opened by signals sent from the brain down to the mechanism in the dorsal horn of the spinal cord. On the other hand, if the person has had positive experiences with pain control in the past, the cognitive influence can send signals down to the gating mechanism and close it. The gate theory offered a great benefit by suggesting new approaches to relieving both acute and chronic pain. Pain could be relieved by blocking the transmission of pain impulses to the brain by both physical modalities and by altering the individual's thought processes, emotions, or other behaviors.

Conduction of Pain Impulses

Conduction of pain impulses refers to the physiologic processes that occur from the initiation of the pain signal to the realization of pain by the individual. There are four processes involved in the conduction of this signal. The first of these, **transduction**, is the step where a noxious stimulus triggers electrical activity in the endings of afferent nerve fibers (nociceptors). Once the signal is triggered, **transmission** occurs. The impulse travels from the receiving nociceptors to the spinal cord. Projection neurons then carry the message to the thalamus, and the message continues to the somatosensory cortex. This is where the third step, perception of pain, occurs. It is here that neural messages are converted into the subjective experience. The fourth process, **modulation**, is a central nervous system pathway that selectively inhibits pain transmission by sending blocking signals back down to the dorsal horn of the spinal cord.

FACTORS AFFECTING THE PAIN EXPERIENCE

McCaffery and Pasero (1999) point out that *the client is the only authority about the existence and nature of his or her pain.* Many factors account for the differences in clients' individual responses to pain, including age, previous experience with pain, and cultural norms.

Age

Age can greatly influence a client's perception of the pain experience. Infants are sensitive to pain and typically exhibit discomfort through crying or physical movement. Toddlers also use crying and physical movement to indicate pain, and they begin to develop the skills needed to verbally describe pain or point to the area that is hurting. Children of all ages often do not understand why pain occurs and can therefore be frightened or resentful of the pain experience; in some cases, children will revert to habits of their younger years (regression) as a coping mechanism when faced with pain they cannot otherwise manage.

Adolescents often sense great peer pressure and may be reluctant to admit to pain for fear of being called

weak or sensitive. Adults may continue pain behaviors they learned as children and may also be reluctant to admit pain or seek medical care because of fear of the unknown or fear of the impact that treatment may have on their lifestyle. Older adults may often ignore their pain, viewing it as an unavoidable consequence of aging; family and health care members may inadvertently support this stereotype and be less than responsive to an older client's complaints of pain.

Previous Experience with Pain

Clients' previous exposures to pain will often influence their reactions. Coping mechanisms that were used in the past may affect clients' judgments about how the pain will affect their lives and what measures are within their control to successfully manage the pain on their own. Client teaching about pain expectations and management methods can often allay client fears and lead to more successful pain management, especially in those clients who do not have previous pain experience or who have memories of a previous devastating pain experience that they do not wish to repeat.

Cultural Norms

Cultural diversity in pain responses can easily lead to problems in pain management. Laboratory studies on subjects of various cultures found no significant difference among the groups in the level of intensity at which pain becomes appreciable or perceptible. However, the same studies showed that the subjects differed significantly in the level of intensity or duration of pain the client was willing to endure. Expression of pain is also governed by cultural values. In some cultures, tolerance to pain, and therefore "suffering in silence," is expected; in others, full expression of pain may include animated physical and emotional responses. The nurse must be careful not to equate the level of expression of pain with the level of actual pain experienced, but to instead consider cultural and other influences that affect the expression of pain.

NURSING PROCESS

The nursing process will provide the correct framework for managing a client's pain.

Assessment

Assessment of the client's pain is a crucial function of the nurse. During the assessment process, nurses need to be aware of their own values and expectations about pain behaviors. Just as the client's experience and cultural background help determine how pain is demonstrated, nurses' cultures and experiences help determine which pain behaviors are viewed as acceptable. Nurses need to be aware of these values and avoid biases when assessing client pain and planning client care. Once a self-assessment about pain has been conducted, the nurse is ready to assess the client.

Pain assessment tools are the single most effective method of identifying the presence and intensity of pain in clients. *These tools must be used, and the results must be believed.* Figure 26-3 shows the Initial Pain Assessment Tool developed by McCaffery and Beebe and found in AHCPR's acute pain management guideline (AHCPR, 1992). This tool is particularly effective when clients have complex pain problems because it assesses location, intensity, quality, precipitating and alleviating factors, and how the pain affects function and quality of life. Once this tool is completed, another less detailed tool can be used for ongoing monitoring of the client's pain level.

Subjective Data

Gathering subjective information regarding the client's pain is the first step in pain assessment. The nurse should determine a client's pain threshold and pain tolerance level. **Pain threshold** is the level of intensity at which pain becomes appreciable or perceptible and will vary with each individual and with each different type of pain. **Pain tolerance** is the level of intensity or duration of pain the client is willing or able to endure.

The client's description of the pain should cover several qualifiers, including its location, onset and duration, quality, intensity, aggravating factors (variables that worsen the pain, such as exercise, certain foods, or stress), alleviating factors (measures the client can take that lessen the effect of the pain, such as lying down, avoiding certain foods, or taking medication), associated manifestations (factors that often accompany the pain, such as nausea, constipation, or dizziness), and what pain means to the client.

Whenever subjective and objective data conflict, the subjective reports of pain are to be considered the primary source.

Date__________
Patient's Name__________ Age______ Room______
Diagnosis__________ Physician__________
Nurse__________

I. Location: Patient or nurse marks drawing.

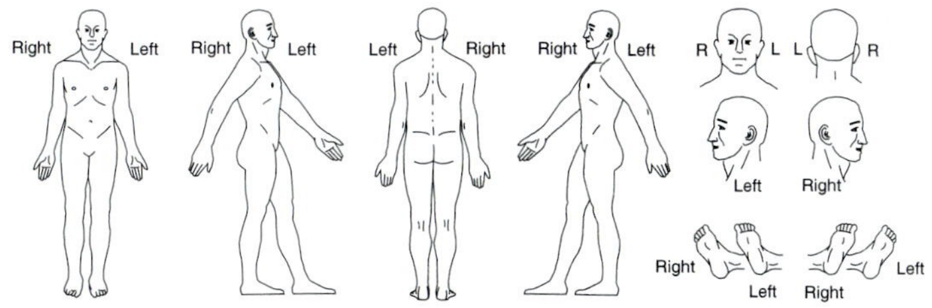

II. Intensity: Patient rates the pain. Scale used__________

Present: __________

Worst pain gets:__________

Best pain gets:__________

Acceptable level of pain:__________

III. Quality: (Use patient's own words, eg., prick, ache, burn, throb, pull, sharp)__________

IV. Onset, duration, variations, rhythms:__________

V. Manner of expressing pain: __________

VI. What relieves the pain?__________

VII. What causes or increases the pain?__________

VIII. Effects of pain: (Note decreased function, decreased quality of life.)

Accompanying symptoms (e.g., nausea)__________

Sleep__________

Appetite__________

Physical activity__________

Relationship with others (e.g., irritability)__________

Emotions (e.g., anger, suicidal, crying)__________

Concentration__________

Other__________

IX. Other comments:__________

X. Plan:__________

Figure 26-3 Initial Pain Assessment Tool (*From* Pain: Clinical Manual for Nursing Practice, *by M. McCaffery and A. Beebe, 1989, St. Louis, MO: Mosby. Copyright 1989 by Mosby. Reprinted with permission.*)

PROFESSIONAL TIP

Location of Pain

During intershift report on a postoperative client recovering from abdominal surgery, the nurse reported that the client had stated she had pain and had been medicated with IM Demerol. When greeting her client, the nurse asked the client about the pain she had experienced during the night. The client replied, "Oh, it is fine now, I only had a headache." The night nurse had assumed the client's pain was in her surgical site and chose the medication accordingly. The headache probably could have been relieved with a milder medication. All reports of pain must be thoroughly asessed prior to any interventions being implemented.

Location The client can point to the location of the pain on the client's own body or locate it on a body diagram on a pain assessment tool. The client should be asked if there is more than one site of pain; if the pain radiates, and if so to where; and ask if the pain is deep or superficial.

Onset and Duration The nurse should ask the client how long the pain has existed; what, if anything, triggers its onset; and if there are any patterns to the pain; for example, whether it is worse at certain times of the day or night.

Quality The nurse should ask the client what the pain feels like, and record the words used to describe the pain. Clients may use sensory-type words, such as "pricking," "radiating," "burning," or "throbbing." However, some clients use words that have an affective connotation, such as "fearful," "sickening," or "punishing." Other words used may be evaluative, such as "miserable" or "unbearable." The quality of pain provides information that may be useful in diagnosing the cause of the pain. For example, pain described as "burning" or "freezing" is usually neuropathic in origin.

Intensity The client may have difficulty in judging the intensity of pain. However, it is important to obtain an estimate of the severity of the pain. This information allows the clinician to evaluate the effectiveness of pain relief measures tried by comparing intensity before and after the interventions.

Pain intensity scales are an effective method for clients to rate the intensity of their pain (Figure 26-4). The simple descriptive pain-intensity scale and the visual analog scale (VAS) are best used by showing the scale to the client and asking the client to point to the spot on the scale that corresponds to the present pain. The pain scale most frequently used with adolescent and adult clients is the verbal 0 to 10 scale. No equipment or supplies are needed, and it requires only enough time to ask one question: "On a scale of 0 to

CLIENT TEACHING

Pain at Night

- It is common for pain to be worse at night when there are fewer distractions. Knowing that this is normal can be reassuring because the client may attribute the increased pain to complications.

10, with 0 being no pain at all and 10 being the worst pain you could ever have, how much do you hurt right now?" If there are multiple painful areas, this question can be asked regarding each area.

Aggravating and Alleviating Factors The nurse should question the client about what makes the pain worse and what makes the pain better, including behaviors or activities that influence the pain. This information provides input into developing the plan of care for the client in pain. If there are specific activities that relieve the pain, the nurse can incorporate them into the care plan. Being aware of activities that increase the pain can allow for interventions that may prevent the pain. For example, if physical therapy exercises trigger an increase in pain, the nurse can administer an analgesic as ordered prior to treatment.

Associated Manifestations The initial pain assessment should include the impact of pain on the activities of daily living. Pain may cause changes in sleep patterns or the ability to work and carry out the many

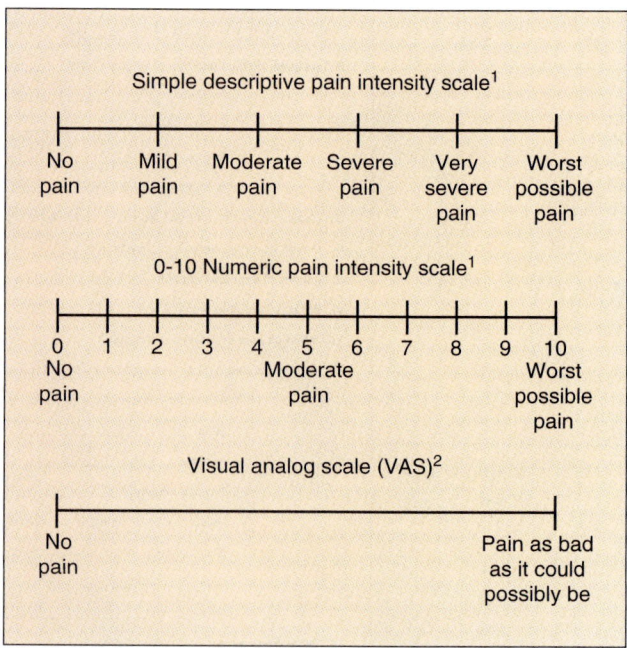

[1] If used as a graphic rating scale, a 10-cm baseline is recommended.
[2] A 10-cm baseline is recommended for VAS scales.

Figure 26-4 Pain Intensity Scales: Three Commonly Used Self-Report Intensity Scales (*Courtesy of Agency for Health Care Policy and Research, 1992.*)

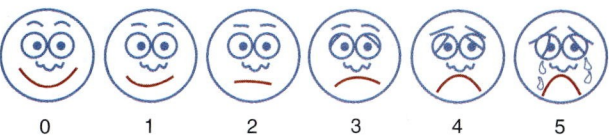

Figure 26-5 Wong/Baker Faces Pain Rating Scale *(From Whaley & Wong's Nursing Care of Infants and Children [6th ed.], by D. L. Wong, 1999, St. Louis, MO: Mosby. Copyright 1999 by Mosby. Reprinted with permission.)*

LIFE CYCLE CONSIDERATIONS

Children and Pain Assessment

Children provide a special challenge in pain assessment. Three useful tools for assessing pain in children are the Wong/Baker Faces Pain Rating Scale, the Oucher scale, and the Poker Chip Tool.

- The Wong/Baker Faces Pain Rating Scale can be used with children as young as 3 years. It helps children express their level of pain by pointing to a cartoon face that most closely resembles how they are feeling (Figure 26-5).
- The Oucher pediatric pain intensity scale (Figure 26-6) consists of two scales: a 0 to 100 numeric scale and a 6-point facial scale. If the child can count from 1 to 100 by ones or by tens, the numeric scale can be used; if not, the facial scale can be used. The facial scale has been successfully used in children as young as 3 to 4 years.
- The Poker Chip Tool uses of four red poker chips. The chips are aligned horizontally on a hard surface in front of the child, and they are described as "pieces of hurt." The chips are described from left to right as just a little bit of hurt, a little more hurt, more hurt, and the most hurt you could ever have. The child is then asked, "How many pieces of hurt do you have right now?" This tool can be used with children 4 to 13 years old.

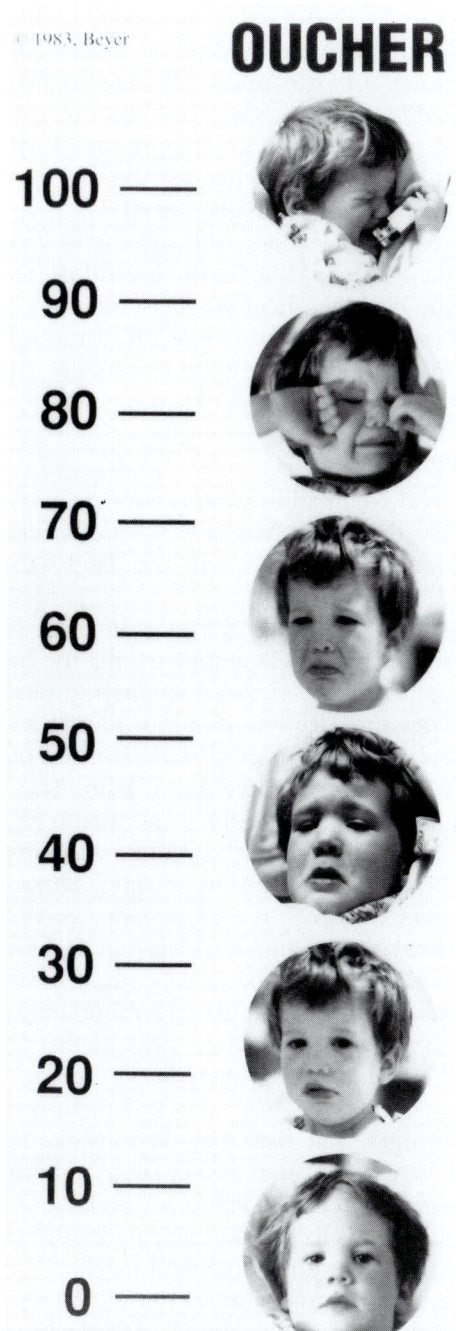

Figure 26-6 The Oucher Pain Assessment Tool: For Use with Children 3–12 Years of Age. Caucasian, Hispanic and African American versions are available. *(The Caucasian version of the Oucher, developed and copyrighted by Judith E. Beyer, RN, PhD, 1983.)*

roles in a client's life. Pain may affect appetite, mood, sexual functioning, or the ability to participate in recreational activities. If pain is interfering with daily life, the client's quality of life can be greatly affected.

Pain is fatiguing. It requires a significant amount of energy to deal with pain. The longer a person suffers from pain, the greater the level of fatigue. Although there is no conscious awareness of pain during sleep, there may be a dream-state awareness (McCaffery & Pasero, 1999). The stress response (which can be seen even in clients under general anesthesia) continues, and the body physiologically pays the price. Clients also wake up with considerably more pain than they had going to sleep, thereby requiring even more intervention (pharmacologic and nonpharmacologic) to reduce the pain.

Meaning of Pain Due to the motivational-affective components of the pain experience, the meaning of pain can have a great impact on how the client perceives the pain. A frequently cited classic study on this phenomenon was conducted by Beecher (1956), who compared the pain perceived by soldiers wounded in battle to pain perceived by civilians with similar surgical

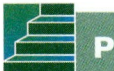

wounds. He found that only 32% of the soldiers required narcotics for pain relief, whereas 85% of the civilians needed the narcotics. This was interpreted that for the soldiers, the wound represented a ticket away from the battlefield, while for the civilians, the surgical wound was a depressing event.

The nurse should explore with the client what implications the pain may have for the individual. Does it mean that the client's cancer is metastasizing? Or that the client's condition is worsening? All of these interpretations may influence the pain experience for the client.

Objective Data

As discussed when addressing acute versus chronic pain, the objective data often presents a different picture depending on the type of pain the client is experiencing.

Physiologic Acute pain activates the sympathetic nervous system, and the client may exhibit the following: elevated heart rate, elevated respiratory rate, elevated blood pressure, diaphoresis, pallor, muscle tension, and dilated pupils. These signs resemble those of anxiety, which often accompanies acute pain. The signs and symptoms of chronic pain show adaption, and, therefore, are different from those of acute pain, with vital signs being normal and no accompanying pupil dilation or perspiration.

Behavioral Acute pain behaviors may include crying and moaning, rubbing the site of pain, restlessness, a distorted posture, clenched fists, guarding the painful area, frowning, and grimacing. The client usually speaks of the discomfort and may be restless or afraid to move.

The client in chronic pain may demonstrate behaviors similar to those of depression such as hopelessness, listlessness, and loss of libido and weight. Chronic pain also often leads to physical inactivity or immobility, which can lead to functional disability.

Clients' behavioral adaptation may yield no report of pain unless questioned specifically. **Distraction** (focusing attention on stimuli other than pain) may also be used by clients. McCaffery and Pasero (1999) recognize that clients often minimize the pain behaviors they are able to control for a number of reasons including:

- To be a "good" client and avoid making demands
- To maintain a positive self-image by not becoming a "sissy"
- By using distraction as a method of making pain more bearable (young children are particularly adept at this)
- Exhaustion

Occasionally, there is a discrepancy between pain behaviors observed by the nurse (objective data) and the client's self-report of pain. Client pain behaviors (AHCPR, 1992) include splinting of the painful area, distorted posture, impaired mobility, insomnia, anxiety, attention seeking, and depression. Discrepancies between behaviors and the client's self-report can be due to good coping skills (e.g., relaxation techniques or distraction), stoicism, anxiety, or cultural differences in expected pain behaviors. Whenever these discrepancies occur, they should be addressed with the client, and the pain management plan must be renegotiated accordingly.

Ongoing Assessment

The initial assessment obtains a baseline of information regarding the client's pain. Subsequent assessments provide information regarding the effectiveness of the interventions. Physiologic and behavioral signs, and most important, the client's subjective pain ratings of the intensity will all help the health care team determine whether the interventions should be continued or changed. Pain assessments should be performed to coincide with when the intervention should be providing the most relief. For example, the onset of intravenous morphine is rapid, peaking approximately 20 minutes after administration. If the client has not obtained relief by 20 minutes, the intravenous morphine

CULTURAL CONSIDERATIONS

Perception of Pain

Culture determines the way persons derive meaning from their lives and also determines appropriate behaviors. One's cultural upbringing teaches behaviors, including those that are exhibited when in pain. People from different cultures use different types of words to describe pain (for example, in sensory or emotional terms). These differences should not be ignored, but the nurse also needs to be careful not to prejudge a client based on cultural background or ethnicity. Due to the unique experience of pain, the person will exhibit individualized behaviors even though they are influenced by cultural upbringing.

was ineffective, and the plan of care would need to be changed.

Recording Pain Assessment Findings

No matter which pain assessment tool is chosen, it will be of little effect unless the pain rating and related information are recorded in a manner easily understood by the health care team. Figure 26-7 is a flow sheet (McCaffery & Beebe, 1989) that is an excellent record in an acute care setting. It provides one place to document the majority of information used to make pain management decisions, including pain rating, vital signs, analgesic administered, and level of arousal.

Nursing Diagnoses

The two primary nursing diagnoses used to describe pain are *Pain* and *Chronic Pain*. According to the North American Nursing Diagnosis Association (NANDA, 1999), *Pain* is defined as "an unpleasant sensory and emotional experience arising from actual or potential tissue damage or described in terms of such damage . . . [with] sudden or slow onset of any intensity from mild to severe, with an anticipated or predictable end and a duration of less than 6 months" (p. 122). *Chronic Pain* is defined as *Pain,* with the last phrase replaced by "constant or recurring without an anticipated or predictable end and a duration of greater than 6 months."

Pain may be the etiology (cause) of other problems, for example: Physical Mobility, Impaired, related to arthritic hip pain. Whether the pain is addressed in the problem statement or the etiology will be determined by the client's primary problem. There are many diagnoses that can be related to the client in pain depending on the effects of the pain:

- *Activity Intolerance*
- *Anxiety*
- *Body Image Disturbance*
- *Breathing Pattern, Ineffective*
- *Constipation*
- *Coping, Individual, Ineffective*
- *Fatigue*
- *Fear*
- *Hopelessness*
- *Knowledge Deficit*

Patient _____ Date _____
Pain rating scale used* _____
Purpose: To evaluate the safety and effectiveness of the analgesic(s)
Analgesic(s) prescribed: _____

Time	Pain rating	Analgesic	R	P	BP	Level of arousal	Other**	Plan and comments

May be duplicated for use in clinical practice.
*Pain rating: A number of different scales may be used. Indicate which scale is used and use the same scale each time.
**Possibilities for other columns: bowel function, activities, nausea and vomiting, and other pain relief measures. Identify the side effects of greatest concern to patient, family, physician, and nurse.

Figure 26-7 Flow Sheet for Pain Management Documentation. *(From* Pain: Clinical Manual for Nursing Practice, *by M. McCaffery and A. Beebe, 1989, St. Louis, MO: Mosby. Copyright 1989 by Mosby. Reprinted with permission.)*

- *Mobility, Impaired, Physical*
- *Powerlessness*
- *Role Performance, Altered*
- *Sleep pattern disturbance*
- *Social Interaction, Impaired*
- *Management of Therapeutic Regimen (individual), Ineffective*
- *Thought Processes, Altered*

Planning/Outcome Identification

When planning care for the client experiencing pain, mutual goal setting is of utmost importance. After assessing the client's perception of the problem, the nurse and client can work together in developing realistic outcomes. Both nonpharmacologic and pharmacologic interventions should be considered in planning strategies to return clients to control or to maintain them at desired levels of functioning and pain.

When asking about the client's goal for pain relief, the nurse often has to state, "We can't usually get rid of all your pain, but if we could get it down to a place that it didn't bother you so much, what would that be?" That way the client, the family, and health care professionals involved will all be aware of the goal for pain relief and can adjust the plan of care accordingly.

Often several approaches must be combined for adequate relief to be obtained. No matter which type of intervention is being utilized, there are general principles that apply: individualization, prevention, and utilization of a multidisciplinary approach.

Individualize the Approach

A variety of pain relief measures can be tried in many combinations until the goal of pain relief is reached. This often means some trial-and-error of interventions until the right combination is found. It is important to include measures that the client believes will be effective. The cognitive component of pain perception can have a powerful influence on the effectiveness of interventions. This may mean including folk remedies or nonscientific relief measures. It is important to keep an open mind. This comes with the caution that the nurse needs to avoid those remedies that may harm the client.

Use a Preventive Approach

Pain is much easier to control if it is treated before it gets severe. Interventions should be implemented when pain is mild, or when it is anticipated. For example, medicate a client prior to a painful dressing change or treatment rather than waiting for the pain to occur.

Use a Multidisciplinary Approach

Pain relief is a complex phenomenon requiring input from various members of the health care team. The nurse's role is pivotal in managing a client's pain. The physician also plays a key role, diagnosing and treating the medical cause of the pain, which includes prescribing appropriate medications. In complex cases, other professionals, such as physical therapists, psychologists, social workers, or chaplains may be needed. The multidisciplinary team approach is the most successful way to manage chronic pain and improve the quality of a client's life.

Nursing Interventions

Nonpharmacologic and pharmacologic interventions can both be effective in caring for clients with pain. In some cases of mild pain, nonpharmacologic techniques may be the primary intervention, with medication available as "backup." In cases of moderate to severe pain, nonpharmacologic techniques can be an effective adjunctive, or complementary, treatment.

There are three categories of pain control interventions: (1) pharmacological, (2) noninvasive, and (3) invasive. Each category will be discussed separately, but these methods are often used in combination.

Pharmacological Interventions

Drug therapy is the mainstay of treatment for pain control. The American Pain Society (1992) and AHCPR (1992, 1994) have published guidelines that provide specific recommendations for the use of drug therapy in pain control. These guidelines were developed by panels of experts who analyzed current research available on pain control and represent concise information that can help nurses, physicians, and other health care workers to effectively administer medications for pain relief.

The World Health Organization (WHO) has made worldwide relief of cancer pain one of their primary goals (1990). In order to help meet this goal, it developed an analgesic ladder to help the clinician determine which analgesic to prescribe (Figure 26-8). Combining analgesics and the use of adjuvant medication provides effective pharmacologic intervention for clients with pain. **Adjuvant medications** are those drugs used to enhance the analgesic efficacy of opioids, to treat concurrent symptoms that exacerbate pain, and to provide independent analgesia for specific types of pain. The ladder recommends that the analgesic, plus or minus an adjuvant, is chosen based on the level of pain the client is experiencing. For mild pain, the ladder recommends a nonopioid. If the pain persists or if the client has moderate pain to begin with, WHO recommends a weak opioid, plus or minus the nonopioid, plus or minus an adjuvant. If pain persists, a strong opioid is used. The *nonopioid should be continued,* and an adjuvant medication should be considered (AHCPR, 1994). This ladder gives health care workers guidelines in determining if the drug regimen is appropriate for the client with cancer pain.

Nurses' Role in Administration of Analgesics The nurse is the health care professional who

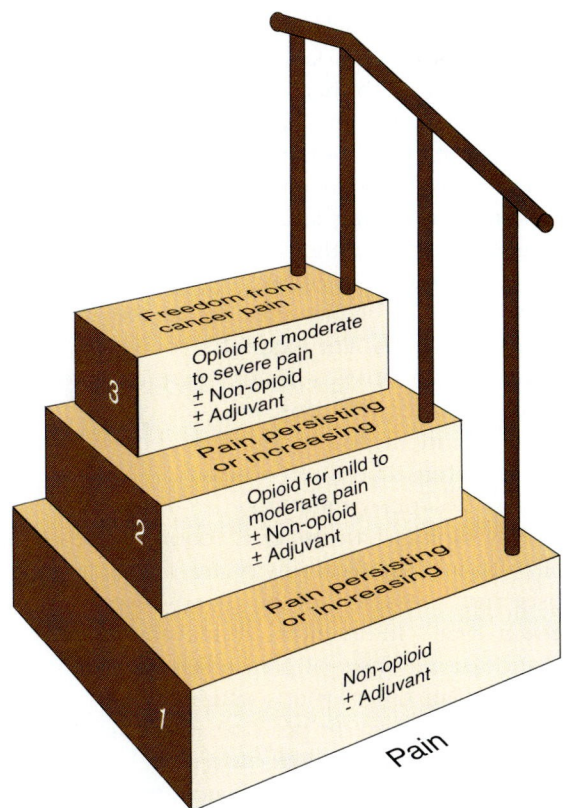

Figure 26-8 WHO Analgesic Ladder. Gives guidelines for choosing analgesic therapy for cancer pain, based on the level of pain the client is experiencing. (*Courtesy of World Health Organization, 1990. Used with permission.*)

spends the most time with the client in pain and is the team member who is most often able to assess the effectiveness of pain control interventions. When analgesics are prescribed, the nurse is often given choices of drug, route, and interval. For example, the postop client may have the following orders:

- Morphine 10–15 mg IM or IV q2–4h prn severe pain
- Vicodin i–ii tabs q3–4h prn moderate pain

When this client complains of pain, which analgesic should the nurse administer? Which route? Which dose? How frequently? The nurse in this situation carries a large responsibility in making these decisions. The nurse also has autonomy in making these decisions. The client may not be aware of all the available choices. Each nurse may make a different decision, often based on the nurse's own biases.

These choices and autonomy require responsibility on the part of the nurse. McCaffery and Pasero (1999) identify the following as the responsibilities of the nurse in administering analgesics. The nurse must:

- Determine whether or not to give the analgesic, and if more than one is ordered, which one

CLIENT TEACHING

Pain Management

Clients and their families must be educated regarding:

- The importance of taking or requesting pain medication before the pain becomes severe and more difficult to control
- The numerous nonpharmacologic approaches that clients can use to augment their pharmacologic pain management
- The individualization of pain management (The client may be taking different medications or different dosages than other individuals.)

- Assess the client's response to the analgesic, including assessing the effectiveness in pain relief and occurrence of any side effects
- Report to the physician when a change is needed, including making suggestions for changes based on the nurse's knowledge of the client and pharmacology
- Teach the client and family regarding the use of analgesics

Principles of Administering Analgesics "How an analgesic is used is probably more important than which one is used" (McCaffery & Pasero, 1999). There are principles that should be applied in the administration of analgesics, no matter which one is given.

Establishing and maintaining a therapeutic serum level is important. Figure 26-9 illustrates the peaks and valleys that often occur when analgesics are administered in the traditional prn (as needed) manner. When the dose is administered on an intermittent schedule, a larger dose is often required, causing the client to have a peak serum drug level in the sedation range. The

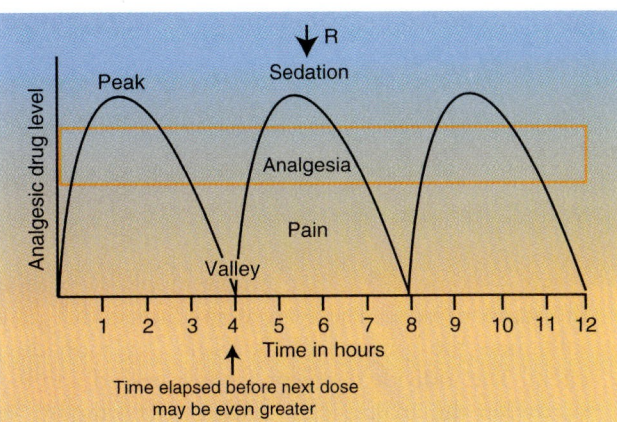

Figure 26-9 Peaks and Valleys of Analgesic Administration. (*From* Pain: Clinical Manual for Nursing Practice, *by* M. McCaffery and A. Beebe, 1989, St. Louis, MO: Mosby. Copyright 1989 by Mosby. Reprinted with permission.)

client must wait for the return of pain before requesting the next dose of analgesic. Depending on the length of time it takes to obtain the medication and, once taken, to reestablish an adequate blood level, there could be a period of up to an hour or so with inadequate pain control.

Preventive Approach Pain is much easier to control if treated when it is anticipated or at a mild intensity. Once pain becomes severe, the analgesics ordered may not be effective enough to relieve it. Many clinicians still teach their clients to wait to take medication until they are sure they really need it. This practice leads to uncontrolled pain. There are two ways the preventive approach may be implemented:

- ATC (around the clock)—When pain is predictable, for example, the first few days following surgery or with chronic cancer pain, the medication is administered on a scheduled basis. This prevents the peaks and valleys of serum drug level that can lead to oversedation or toxicity and recurrence of pain, respectively. If the analgesics are ordered by the physician to be given PRN, it can still be a nursing measure to administer the drugs ATC, as long as they are given within the time constraints of the order.
- PRN (Latin for *pro re nata,* which means "as required")—Pain cannot always be predictable, therefore PRN dosing may be required. For some clients this may be used in addition to scheduled dosing for "breakthrough" pain (pain that surpasses the level of **analgesia**, or pain relief, that the steady level of analgesics is providing). Examples of this include a cancer client on prolonged-release morphine who needs extra analgesics to participate in activities such as shopping or receiving visitors. Another example would be the orthopedic client who is receiving regularly scheduled analgesics for postop pain who needs additional pain relief for therapy sessions. In order to implement the preventive approach with PRN dosing, the medications should be given as soon as the pain appears, or when it is anticipated to begin.

Titrate to Effect Due to the unique nature of the pain experience, the analgesic regimen needs to be titrated until the desired effect is achieved. This involves adjusting the following:

- *Dosage*—Some clients may require more or less than the standard dose. There are many factors that may influence the pharmacokinetics in an individual client. The individual's response is assessed and the dosage of the analgesic is regulated accordingly. In clients with chronic cancer pain, opioid analgesics are recommended to be increased until pain relief is obtained or unacceptable side effects occur. This may be done due to the lack of a **ceiling effect** (the

dosage beyond which no further analgesia occurs) in pure opioids. The lack of a ceiling effect means there is no limit to the dose that can be given. For example, cancer clients have been known to receive over 1 gram per hour intravenously. Because the dosage is gradually increased, the client develops a **tolerance** (requiring larger and larger doses of an analgesic to achieve the same level of pain relief) to the side effects of the opioid.

- *Interval*—Some clients metabolize the analgesics faster than others. For example, young adults tend to metabolize opioids faster, therefore they may need more frequent doses. Older clients tend to metabolize them slower, therefore they will require a longer interval between doses.
- *Route*—The appropriate route is chosen depending on how rapidly pain relief is required, the client's ability to take medications orally, the client's diagnosis, and assessment of the client's response to the current route. Intravenous administration provides the most rapid onset of pain relief. All other routes require a lag time for absorption of the analgesic into the circulation. In postoperative pain, IV is the preferred route for opioids when the oral route is not appropriate. If IV access is not available, sublingual, rectal, or transdermal routes should be considered (AHCPR, 1992).

    With cancer pain, the oral route is preferred. If these clients are unable to take oral medications, rectal and transdermal routes are preferred since they are less invasive than other routes (AHCPR, 1994). In addition, tolerance develops at a slower rate with the oral route compared to the more invasive routes.
- *Choice of drug*—If one drug is not providing relief or has unacceptable side effects, another analgesic may be tried.

The key to administering an analgesic is to monitor the client's response to it. This includes assessing the effectiveness of pain relief and the occurrence of side effects.

Classes of Analgesics There are three classes of drugs used for pain relief: (1) nonopioid analgesics; (2) opioid analgesics; and (3) analgesic adjuvants already discussed (WHO, 1986). Nonopioid and opioid analgesics will be addressed separately, as indications and side effects are different for each one.

Nonopioids The medications in this category are useful for a variety of painful conditions, including surgery, trauma, and cancer (American Pain Society, 1992). The indications include mild to moderate pain, and they are used in conjunction with opioids. These drugs differ from opioids in several ways in that they:

- Are subject to the ceiling effect
- Do not produce the effect of tolerance or physical dependence
- Are antipyretic, and should not be given in cases where they may mask an infection

Ketorolac

Ketorolac should not be used in a client with any history of renal dysfunction, gastric irritation, bleeding problems, low platelet count, or allergy to aspirin or other NSAIDs.

Ketorolac is the only NSAID available in parenteral form and has proven useful in clients on NPO status who would benefit from a NSAID. Even when administered intramuscularly or intravenously, ketorolac produces significant gastric irritation and the potential for gastric bleeding. The most frequent use of ketorolac is orally or intramuscularly in adults, but some pediatric centers have used it intravenously under strict supervision for a limited course (less than 5 days) in children and adolescents with great success.

Action Action of these drugs is thought to inhibit prostaglandin formation. If prostaglandins are inhibited, the sensory neurons are less likely to receive the pain signal. Thus, this class of analgesics works in the peripheral nervous system.

Opioids The opioid analgesics fall into three classes: pure opioid agonists, partial agonists, and **mixed agonist-antagonists** (a compound that blocks opioid effects on one receptor type while producing opioid effects on a second receptor type). Pure agonists are those that produce a maximal response from cells when they bind to the cells' opioid receptor sites. Morphine (the gold standard against which all other opioids are measured), fentanyl (Duragesic), methadone (Dolophine), hydromorphone hydrochloride (Dilaudid), and codeine are pure agonists. Meperidine (Demerol), although classified as a pure agonist, is not recommended except in clients with a true allergy to all other narcotics, because of its neurotoxicity. Meperidine produces clinical analgesia for only 2.5 to 3.5 hours when given intramuscularly in adults.

Unlike the NSAIDs, pure agonist opioids are not subject to the ceiling effect. As the dosage is increased, there is increasing pain relief.

Action Opioids act in the central nervous system by binding to opiate receptor sites on afferent neurons. The pain signal is stopped at the spinal cord level, and does not reach the cortex where pain is perceived.

Side Effects The only limiting factor in the use of pure agonist opioids is the degree of side effects, particularly respiratory depression and constipation. Other side effects include pruritus and nausea, but the degree to which they are present from each medication varies among individuals. Clients must be instructed regarding these normal responses to opioids and informed that it does not mean that they are allergic to them. A true allergy to opioids would be indicated by a rash or hives that starts after receiving the opioid, a local histamine release at the site of infusion, or anaphylaxis. Clients also need to know that the pruritus and nausea generally subside after 4 to 5 days of opioid therapy. In the meantime, an antihistamine such as diphenhydramine hydrochloride (Benadryl) or hydroxyzine hydrochloride (Atarax, Vistaril) may be used for pruritus, and an antiemetic such as metoclopromide hydrochloride (Clopra) or trimethobenzamide hydrochloride (Tigan) can be used to treat the nausea.

Almost all medications used to treat side effects have their own side effect of sedation. Thus, there is the possibility of a cumulative effect of severe sedation. These medications must be used with caution and appropriate monitoring until the client's response is determined. Ondansetron hydrochloride (Zofran) is

Types of Nonopioid Drugs

- *Salicylates*—These include aspirin and other salicylate salts. Common side effects of aspirin include gastric disturbances and bleeding due to the antiplatelet effect. Some of the salicylate salts, such as choline magnesium trisalicylate (Trilisate) and salsalate (Salgesic) have fewer gastrointestinal and bleeding effects than aspirin.
- *Acetaminophen*—This is a nonsalicylate that is similar to aspirin in its analgesic action, but has no anti-inflammatory effect. Its mechanism of action for pain relief is not known.
- *NSAIDs*—The effectiveness of these drugs varies, with some being close to the effectiveness of aspirin and acetaminophen, while others are much stronger. Clients tend to vary in response, so once the maximum recommended dose has been tried with ineffective results, it would be worth trying another NSAID. The drugs in this group inhibit platelet aggregation, and are contraindicated in clients with coagulation disorders or on anticoagulation therapy.

Effects of Meperidine (Demerol)

- In pediatric clients receiving intravenous meperidine, analgesia may last for only 1.5 to 2.0 hours.
- In the elderly, most of whom show decreased glomerular filtration rates, there is generally a higher peak and longer duration of action as it takes longer to excrete the opioid as well as its toxic metabolite, normeperidine.

one antiemetic on the market with little, if any, sedative effect. It has recently received Food and Drug Administration (FDA) approval for use with postoperative nausea and has been effective in clients with refractory nausea and vomiting unresponsive to other antiemetics. The current cost per dose, close to $100 in many hospitals, limits its use to the extreme nausea associated with cancer chemotherapy or to clients with refractory nausea and vomiting.

Mixed agonist-antagonist opioids are believed to be subject to the ceiling effect for pain relief, as well as a ceiling effect for respiratory depression. Mixed agonist-antagonist opioids activate one opioid receptor type while simultaneously blocking another type. Butorphanol tartrate (Stadol), pentazocine hydrochloride (Talwin), and nalbuphine hydrochloride (Nubain) are the most frequently used in pain management.

Opioid antagonists include naloxone (Narcan) and naltrexone (Trexal), with the most commonly used being naloxone (Narcan). They work by blocking opioid stimulation of receptor sites. Naloxone effectively reverses opioid side effects of sedation, respiratory depression, and nausea *while it completely reverses any pain control.*

Alternative Delivery Systems Opioids are administered in more than just the traditional oral, subcutaneous, intramuscular, intravenous, and rectal routes.

Patient-Controlled Analgesia Patient-controlled analgesia (PCA) is a device that allows the client to control the delivery of intravenous or subcutaneous pain medication in a safe, effective manner through a programmable pump (Figure 26-10). This system helps to eliminate the time required for the nurse to draw up the medication, and allows the client to feel some control over the pain. The pump has the safety feature of locking out once a maximum dose has been reached. This prevents the client from overdosing. Requirements for the use of PCA are the cognitive ability to understand how to use the pump and the physical ability to push the button. The PCA has been successfully used with many types of pain and in many settings, including pediatrics and home health.

Epidural/Intrathecal Analgesia Epidural analgesia refers to administering the opioid via a catheter

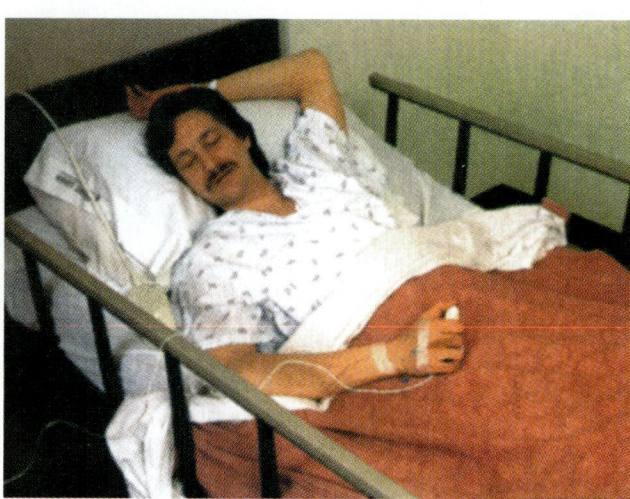

Figure 26-10 Client on Patient-Controlled Analgesia (PCA)

that terminates in the epidural space, the space outside the dura mater that protects the spinal cord. **Intrathecal analgesia** refers to administering the drug directly into the subarachnoid space. These may be administered as a one-time injection by the anesthesiologist, or via a catheter that has been placed. Both of these routes are occasionally referred to as *intraspinal anesthesia*. Because the opioid is delivered close to the site of action, these routes require much lower doses of opioid (usually morphine [Duramorph] or fentanyl [Sublimaze] are used) for pain relief. The incidence of systemic side effects is also much lower with these routes. Duration is longer than systemic routes, for example, the duration of one dose of intrathecal morphine can last 24 hours.

Transdermal Analgesia Another route of opioid administration is the transdermal patch. The only opioid drug currently available via this route is fentanyl (Duragesic). This medication is on an adhesive patch that attaches to the skin. It is available in 25, 50, 75, and 100 mcg/hour dosages. The fentanyl transdermal patch allows slow infusion of the drug through the skin. The fentanyl patch is indicated for continuous pain with high dosage requirements. The advantage of this route is that it is simple to apply and it is effective for 72 hours. The disadvantage is that dosage adjustments are difficult to make due to the slow infusion rate. In addition, side effects may not be reversed as rapidly as when opiates are administered via the oral route.

PROFESSIONAL TIP

Constipation and Opioids
Clients who are expected to require opioid analgesics for more than 1 or 2 days should be administered a stool softener as soon as they are taking fluids orally. While they are still NPO, a glycerin or bisacodyl (Dulcolax) suppository should be administered if the client has not had a bowel movement in 1 or 2 days.

LIFE CYCLE CONSIDERATIONS

Injections and Children
Because children lack the cognitive ability to weigh the pain of an injection against the pain relief from the medication, oral and rectal routes are preferred over injections.

Local Anesthesia Local anesthetics are effective for pain management in a variety of settings. Topical anesthetics are available for teething, sore throats, denture pain, laceration repair, and intravenous catheter insertions. One topical anesthetic, EMLA cream, is a mixture of local anesthetics, combining prilocaine and lidocaine (Xylocaine). It produces complete anesthesia for at least 60 minutes when topically applied on intact skin. Another topical anesthetic, TAC, is available for anesthesia during closure of lacerations. It is a combination of tetracaine hydrochloride (Pontocaine) 0.5%, adrenaline (epinephrine) 1:2000, and cocaine 11.8% in a normal saline solution that can be applied directly to the open wound surface in place of local anesthetic infiltration with a needle. This allows pain-free cleansing of the laceration as well as suturing. Because both adrenaline (epinephrine) and cocaine cause vasoconstriction, TAC cannot be used in areas supplied by end-arteriolar blood supply such as digits, the ear, or the nose. It also is contraindicated on burned or abraded skin because this could lead to increased systemic absorption of cocaine and tetracaine, thus placing the client at risk for seizures.

Noninvasive Interventions

Noninvasive relief measures consist of cognitive-behavioral strategies and physical modalities that use cutaneous stimulation. These treatments can be used to supplement pharmacological therapy and other modalities to control pain. Clients and their families can also be instructed to utilize these treatments at home and in inpatient settings.

Cognitive-Behavioral Interventions
The cognitive-behavioral interventions influence the cognitive and the motivational-affective components of pain perception. These methods can not only help influence the level of pain, but also help the client gain a sense of self-control.

Trusting Nurse–Client Relationship Establishment of a therapeutic relationship is the foundation for effective nursing care of the client experiencing pain. Clients who trust their nurses to be there, to listen, and to act are the clients who are most likely to be comfortable.

Relaxation Relaxation techniques (a variety of methods used to decrease anxiety and muscle tension)

CLIENT TEACHING

Timed-Release Tablets

Teach clients and families the difference between extended-release and immediate-release tablets. Emphasize that the extended-release tablets become immediate-release if crushed (e.g., for a client who has difficulty swallowing the tablet).

LIFE CYCLE CONSIDERATIONS

Opioid Analgesia in the Elderly

- Cheyne-Stokes respiratory patterns are not unusual during sleep in the elderly and should not be used as a reason to restrict appropriate opioid pain relief unless accompanied by unacceptable degrees of arterial desaturation (less than 85%).
- The elderly experience a higher peak and longer duration of effect of opioid medications and are more sensitive to sedation and respiratory depressant effects.
- Opioid dose titration must be based on analgesic effects and degree of side effects such as sedation, urinary retention, constipation, respiratory depression, or exacerbation of Parkinson's disease (AHCPR, 1992).

result in decreased heart rate and respiratory rate, and decreased muscle tension. These signs and symptoms are opposite of the effects of sympathetic nervous system activation that occurs with acute pain. The body's response to pain is almost "tricked" into reversing itself when relaxation exercises are implemented.

Relaxation exercises help reduce pain by decreasing anxiety and decreasing reflex muscular contraction. There are a wide variety of relaxation techniques, including focused breathing, progressive muscle relaxation, and meditation. Simple techniques should be used during episodes of brief pain (for example, during procedures) or when pain is so severe that the client is unable to concentrate on complicated instructions.

To teach simple relaxation techniques, the nurse can instruct the client to: (1) take a deep breath and hold it; (2) exhale slowly and concentrate on going limp; and (3) start yawning (McCaffery & Pasero, 1999). The yawning triggers a conditioned response in the client, that is, the body associates yawning with relaxation and will relax when the client yawns. The technique can be enhanced if the nurse starts yawning. It is so contagious that even the client compromised by severe pain will usually start yawning with the nurse.

A more complex technique is **progressive muscle relaxation**, a strategy in which muscles are alternately tensed and relaxed. This type of technique is especially useful for clients who do not know what muscle relaxation feels like. By purposely contracting and releasing the muscle groups, the client is able to compare the difference and identify feelings of relaxation. Meditative relaxation techniques are also available, including audiotapes sold in most bookstores.

Relaxation is a learned response. The more frequently the client practices these techniques, the more skilled the body will be in learning to relax. Ideally, the best time to teach the client these methods is when

Cognitive–Behavioral Interventions

Cognitive–behavioral interventions should be introduced as early as possible so that clients can learn and practice the techniques before experiencing intense pain, which impairs learning.

pain is controlled, or before the pain occurs (for example, in the preoperative period).

Reframing **Reframing** is a technique that teaches clients to monitor their negative thoughts and replace them with ones that are more positive. Teaching a client to view pain by replacing an expression such as, "I can't stand this pain, it's never going away," with one such as, "I've had similar pain before, and it's gotten better," is an example of effective reframing.

Distraction Distraction focuses one's attention on something other than the pain, therefore placing pain on the periphery of awareness (McCaffery & Pasero, 1999). Successful use of distraction does not eliminate the pain; it makes it less troublesome to the client. The main disadvantage of distraction is that as soon as the distractive stimuli stop, the pain returns in full force. For this reason, the most appropriate use of distraction techniques is for the relief of brief, episodic pain. For example, it can be effective for procedural pain or the period of time between administration of an analgesic and the onset of the drug. Examples of distraction include:

- Active listening to recorded music (have the client tap fingers in rhythm to the beat)
- Reciting a poem or rhyme (children do this well)
- Describe a plot of a novel or movie
- Describe a series of pictures

Guided Imagery Guided imagery is using one's imagination to provide a pleasant substitute for the pain. This modality incorporates features of both relaxation and distraction. The client imagines a pleasant experience, such as going to the beach or the mountains. The experience should include use of all five senses in order to fully involve the client in the image.

The images chosen need to be ones that are pleasant for the client. Describing an ocean cruise would not be appropriate for a person who becomes seasick.

Using Distraction

Distraction should never be used as the *only* pain management intervention, but it can be extremely helpful while waiting for other techniques to take effect.

Humor The old saying, "Laughter is the best medicine," carries some truth to it. While there is nothing very funny about pain, laughing has been shown to provide pain relief. The act of laughing can cause distraction from the pain, induce relaxation by taking deep breaths and releasing tension, release endorphins, and provide a pleasant substitute for pain. Norman Cousins (1979) relates obtaining 2 hours of pain relief from watching episodes of the Candid Camera television show and Marx Brothers films. The nurse can implement this technique by encouraging the client to watch humorous movies, read funny books, or listen to comedy routines. Because different people see humor in different types of situations, the nurse needs to be sensitive to what the client views as funny.

Biofeedback Biofeedback training is another method that may be helpful for the client in pain, especially one who has difficulty relaxing muscle tension. **Biofeedback** is a process through which individuals learn to influence their physiological responses to stimuli. Through the use of biofeedback, clients can alter their pain experience.

Cutaneous Stimulation The technique of cutaneous stimulation involves stimulating the skin to control pain. It is theorized that this technique provides relief by stimulating nerve fibers that send signals to the dorsal horn of the spinal cord to "close the gate." The main advantage of these therapies is that many techniques are easy for the nurse to implement, and easy to teach the client and family to perform. They are not usually meant to replace analgesic therapy, but to complement it.

The site chosen on which to apply the skin stimulation will depend on the client's diagnosis, treatments or procedures being performed, and client preference. There are several options to choose from:

- *Site of pain*—Apply stimulation directly to the site.
- *Around the pain*—Apply stimulation in circular motion around the site.
- *Proximal*—Apply between site of pain and the center of the body (McCaffery & Pasero refer to this as "between pain and the brain").
- *Contralateral*—Apply stimulation to the opposite side of the body. (This is effective due to the crossing over of the nerves in the spinal cord.)
- *Acupuncture points*—Stimulation is applied to specific sites defined by Oriental medicine that is based on a system of meridians.
- *Trigger points*—Apply stimulation to areas that cause referred pain, pain felt in a point other than the point of origin.

Heat and Cold Application In addition to stimulating nerves that can block pain transmission, superficial heat application serves to increase the circulation to the area, which can promote oxygenation and nutrient delivery to the injured tissues. It can also decrease

Hot or Cold Applications

Teach the client or family that hot or cold applications:

- Must have at least one layer of towel between the heating or cooling device and the skin
- Should be placed on the skin only for short periods of time
- Should not be applied to tissue that has been exposed to radiation therapy (AHCPR, 1994)

joint and muscle stiffness. Heat is contraindicated in cases of acute injury because it can increase the initial response of edema. It is also contraindicated in rheumatoid arthritis flare-ups, and over topical applications of mentholated ointments. Heat treatments should be limited to 20- to 30-minute intervals because maximum vasodilatation occurs in that time.

Cryotherapy (cold applications) induces local vasoconstriction and numbness, therefore altering the pain sensations. It is contraindicated in any condition where vasoconstriction might increase symptoms, for example, peripheral vascular disease. For best results, cold therapy should be limited to 20- to 30-minute intervals. Either heat or cold can be used as cutaneous stimulation unless one is specifically contraindicated. Cold often provides faster relief (McCaffery & Pasero, 1999). If the client has used heat or cold before, the nurse should incorporate the modality that the client believes will be the most effective. Combining the two might provide better relief. An example of this would be to apply a hot pack for 4 minutes, followed by an ice pack for 2 minutes, repeated 4 times. In a hospital setting, a physician order is required for this therapy.

Acupressure and Massage One of the first responses to pain is to rub the painful part. Instinctively people seem to understand the pain-relieving aspects of this intervention. In addition to blocking the pain transmission through nerve stimulation, massage can also promote relaxation. Acupressure is a type of massage that consists of continuous pressure on or the rubbing of acupuncture points. It is based on the same principles as acupuncture, but needles are not used. Massage also provides a form of nonverbal communication that can be therapeutic on its own.

Mentholated Rubs Ointments or lotions containing menthol are thought to provide relief by providing a counterirritation to the skin. The menthol gives the client the perception that the temperature of the skin has changed (becoming either warmer or cooler). This alters the sensation of pain or provides a distraction from the pain. Client response varies to mentholated rubs; some gain effective relief, while others have poor results. Their use is contraindicated on broken skin, on mucous membranes, or if pain increases.

Transcutaneous Electrical Nerve Stimulation Transcutaneous electrical nerve stimulation (TENS) is the process of applying a low-voltage electrical current to the skin through cutaneous electrodes. This modality modulates the pain transmission as do other cutaneous stimulation methods but also distracts the client from pain. Research supports the effectiveness of using TENS for the relief of postoperative pain (AHCPR, 1992). It has also been used successfully in many pain syndromes, for example: chronic low back pain, menstrual cramps, temporomandibular joint (TMJ) syndrome, phantom limb pain, and others. It is administered by health professionals especially trained in its use, usually a physical therapist. Other modalities of pain management should *not* be abandoned while a trial of TENS occurs.

 Safety: TENS Contraindications
- No electrodes should be placed in the area over or surrounding demand cardiac pacemakers.
- No electrodes can be placed over the uterus of a pregnant woman.

Exercise Exercise is an important treatment for chronic pain because it strengthens weak muscles, helps mobilize joints, and helps restore balance and coordination. Passive range of motion should not be used if it increases pain or discomfort. Immobilization is frequently used for clients with episodes of acute pain or to stabilize fractures; however, prolonged immobilization should be avoided whenever possible because it can lead to muscle atrophy and cardiovascular deconditioning.

Psychotherapy Psychotherapy may be beneficial to many clients, particularly those:

- In whom the pain is difficult to control
- Who are clinically depressed
- Who have a history of psychiatric problems

Some psychotherapists use **hypnosis** (a state of heightened awareness and focused concentration) to help clients alter their perception of pain. Hypnosis can be effective in modifying the pain response, but it should be used only by specially trained professionals.

Positioning The final noninvasive technique is proper positioning and body alignment. Moving the client with the least possible stress on joints and skin will minimize exposure to painful stimuli. This includes supporting joints appropriately and maintaining wrinkle-free sheets.

Invasive Interventions

Invasive interventions are meant to complement behavioral, physical, and pharmacological therapies in those clients who do not obtain relief from those measures alone (AHCPR, 1994). Invasive measures are indicated primarily for chronic cancer pain and in some cases of chronic benign pain. These procedures are usually tried only when noninvasive measures have been attempted first with poor results.

Nerve Block Neural blockade is the process of injecting a local anesthetic or neurolytic agent into the nerve. An anesthetic agent may be injected to act as a diagnostic tool in order to identify the nerves involved in a pain syndrome. A neurolytic agent is a chemical agent that causes destruction of the nerve and, therefore, creates an interruption in the pain signal.

Neurosurgery Neurosurgical measures for pain control include neurostimulation procedures and destructive or ablative procedures. Neurostimulation procedures involve the implantation of electrical stimulation devices that send impulses to different parts of the nervous system. Some of these devices stimulate areas of the brain; others stimulate the spinal cord. Relief is thought to be provided by blocking the afferent fiber input at the spinal cord level, or by stimulating release of endorphins using the body's ability to modulate pain.

Destructive or ablative procedures are used to destroy part of the nervous system that conducts pain. By interrupting the pain signal, it is prevented from reaching the cortex where realization of pain occurs. These procedures are reserved for clients with terminal illness.

Radiation Therapy Radiation can be used as a palliative measure for pain relief in clients with cancer. It can relieve both metastatic pain and pain caused by tumors at the primary cancer site. It enhances other pain management strategies such as analgesic therapy because it is aimed specifically at the cause of the client's pain. When administered for pain relief, the smallest dose of radiation is utilized to minimize the side effects that accompany radiation therapy.

Acupuncture Acupuncture is the insertion of small needles into the skin at selected (or hoku) sites. The specific sites will be chosen after the practitioner takes a detailed history and uses traditional Oriental diagnostic techniques. The needles used for acupuncture have rounded ends that enter the skin without cutting the tissue. The practitioner may twirl or vibrate the needles manually or electrically. It is important that the nurse keep an open mind when the client chooses this therapy, or the client may be reluctant to discuss its use.

The advantages and disadvantages of selected pain therapies are outlined in Table 26-3.

Table 26-3 ADVANTAGES AND DISADVANTAGES OF SELECTED PAIN THERAPIES

INTERVENTION	ADVANTAGES	DISADVANTAGES
Relaxation, Imagery, Biofeedback, Distraction, and Reframing	• May decrease pain and anxiety without drug-related side effects. • Can be used as adjuvant therapy with most other modalities. • Can increase client's sense of control. • Most are inexpensive, require no special equipment, and are easily administered.	• Patient must be motivated to use self-management strategies. • Requires professional time to teach interventions.
Psychotherapy, Structured Support, and Hypnosis	• May decrease pain and anxiety for clients who have pain that is difficult to manage. • May increase client's coping skills.	• Requires skilled therapist.
Cutaneous Stimulation (Superficial Heat, Cold, Massage)	• May reduce pain, inflammation, or muscle spasm. • Can be used as adjuvant therapy with most other modalities. • Relatively easy to use. • Can be administered by clients or families. • Relatively low cost.	• Heat may increase bleeding and edema after acute injury. • Cold is contraindicated for use over ischemic tissues.
Transcutaneous Electrical Nerve Stimulation (TENS)	• May provide pain relief without drug-related side effects. • Can be used as adjuvant therapy with most other modalities. • Gives patient sense of control over pain.	• Requires skilled therapist to initiate therapy. • Potential risk of infection, bleeding.
Acupuncture	• May provide pain relief. • Can be used as adjuvant therapy with most other therapies.	• Requires skilled therapist.

Adapted from Agency for Health Care Policy and Research, Clinical Practice Guideline. Acute Pain Management: Operative or Medical Procedures and Trauma, *1992 [AHCPR Publication No. 92-0032], Rockville, MD: Author.*

SAMPLE NURSING CARE PLAN

THE CLIENT WITH CHRONIC PAIN

Sally Jeffries, a 48-year-old woman, injured her back 3 years ago while lifting some boxes of paper at work. Since that time, she has had 4 epidural steroidal injections for the pain associated with 2 ruptured discs. Her pain has been intermittent with some alleviation from the epidural injections. Her last epidural was 3 months ago. She arrives at the clinic stating, "I just don't know how I can go on like this. The pain has been tolerable until last night. I'm hurting so bad!" She is tearful and pacing, saying, "It hurts too much when I sit down." Verbalizes pain is "9" on a 1 to 10 pain intensity scale. Blood pressure is 148/90. Pulse is strong and regular at 92. She has guarded movements.

Nursing Diagnosis 1 *Chronic Pain, related to muscle spasm and ruptured discs as evidenced by back injury 3 years ago and client statement "I just don't know how I can go on like this. The pain has been tolerable until last night. I'm hurting so bad!"*

PLANNING/GOALS	NURSING INTERVENTIONS	RATIONALE	EVALUATION
Ms. Jeffries will verbalize a decrease in pain.	Assess Ms. Jeffries's level of pain, determining the intensity at its best and worst.	Determines a baseline for future assessment.	After practicing relaxation techniques, Ms. Jeffries rates her pain as a 2 to 3 on the pain intensity scale.
	Listen to Ms. Jeffries while she discusses the pain; acknowledge the presence of pain.	Acknowledging Ms. Jeffries pain decreases anxiety by communicating acceptance and validating her perceptions.	
	Discuss reasons why pain may be increased or decreased.	Helps the Ms. Jeffries determine a cause-and-effect relationship between pain and specific activities.	
Ms. Jeffries will practice selected noninvasive pain relief measures.	Teach relaxation techniques such as deep breathing, progressive muscle relaxation, and imagery.	Reduces skeletal muscle tension and anxiety, which potentiates the perception of pain.	Ms. Jeffries demonstrates the use of deep breathing and progressive muscle relaxation.
	Teach Ms. Jeffries and her family about treatment approaches (biofeedback, hypnosis, massage therapy, physical therapy, acupuncture, and exercise).	Makes the Ms. Jeffries and her family aware of the availability of treatment options.	
	Teach Ms. Jeffries about the use of medication for pain relief. Provide accurate information to reduce fear of addiction.	Lack of knowledge and fear may prohibit Ms. Jeffries from taking analgesic medications as prescribed.	
	Encourage Ms. Jeffries to rest at intervals during the day.	Fatigue increases the perception of pain.	

continued

Nursing Diagnosis 2 *Anxiety related to chronic pain as evidenced by pacing and tears*

PLANNING/GOALS	NURSING INTERVENTIONS	RATIONALE	EVALUATION
Ms. Jeffries will verbalize an increase in psychological and physiological comfort level.	Assess Ms. Jeffries's level of anxiety.	To collect baseline data to be used in measuring a decrease or increase in anxiety level.	After practicing relaxation techniques, Ms. Jeffries rates her pain as a 2 to 3 on the pain intensity scale. She voices concern that the pain will soon come back.
	Encourage Ms. Jeffries to verbalize angry feeling.	Anger is often a component of chronic conditions because of the prolonged sense of powerlessness.	
Ms. Jeffries will demonstrate ability to cope with anxiety as evidenced by normal vital signs and a verbalized reduction in pain intensity.	Speak slowly and calmly.	Avoids escalating Ms. Jeffries's anxiety level and increases the likelihood of her comprehension.	After a relaxation session, her vital signs returned to normal limits. Ms. Jeffries denies feeling angry.

CASE STUDY

Johnny Prince, a 27-year-old male, is admitted to the medical unit diagnosed with hemophilia and septic arthritis in his left ankle. He has a history of epilepsy, arthritis, artificial knee joints (bilateral), and two hip surgeries. Medications taken at home include: factor VIII, phenobarbital 100 mg hs, and Naprosyn 5 mg tid. His chief complaint is swelling and severe pain in his left ankle.

Current RX: Colace, Milk of Magnesia, ceftriaxone sodium (Rocephin) IV piggy-back, phenobarbital 100 mg qhs, FeSO$_4$, multivitamins, vitamin C, oxacillin (Bactocill), factor VIII 20,000 IVP q12h, hydromorphone HCl (Dilaudid) 8 mg po q8h (hold SBP < 90, resp. < 12), MS 4 mg IVP q4h prn, flurazepam HCl (Dalmane) 30 mg po qhs prn.

The following questions will guide your development of a nursing care plan for the case study.

1. What will you include in assessing Mr. Prince's pain?

2. What factors in his history will influence his pain perception?

Your pain assessment gives you the following information:
- Location—through center of ankle.
- Intensity—pain at time of assessment is 5 (medicated 30 minutes prior to interview) on scale of 0 to 10; worst is 25, best is 3.
- Quality—describes pain as throbbing at times, a jabbing pain. It hurts worse between 9 and 10 A.M., and 9 and 12 at night. Mainly worse when medicine wears off.
- Effects of pain—only gets 2 or 3 hours of sleep, often dreaming about it. Pain makes him avoid activity, get grumpy and snappy. Concentration turns totally to pain.
- Behaviors—he yells at times, but doesn't like to. He'd prefer to "sweat it out." Also grimaces, grips hands, and tries repositioning.

CASE STUDY (continued)

3. Why did the physician order the analgesics on that schedule?
4. Mr. Prince requests a dose of morphine. The narcotic drawer has the following available in prefilled syringe cartridges: 2 mg per cc, and 8 mg per cc. Which cartridge(s) should the nurse select?
5. Why is the morphine ordered IVP, not IM?
6. Why did the physician order colace and Milk of Magnesia?
7. What are some noninvasive relief measures that might be tried with Mr. Prince?
8. Write two individualized nursing diagnoses and goals for Mr. Prince.
9. What teaching will Mr. Prince need before discharge?

Evaluation

Evaluating the efficacy of the pain management interventions is ongoing, with client input throughout the process. Evaluation focuses primarily on the client's subjective reports. Objective data used to evaluate pain management efficacy include:

- Client's facial expression and posture
- Presence (or absence) of restlessness
- Vital sign monitoring
- Ongoing use of pain assessment tools

SUMMARY

- *Pain* may be defined as "an unpleasant sensory and emotional experience associated with actual or potential tissue damage," and "whatever the client says it is, existing whenever the client says it does."
- The gate control theory proposes that several processes (sensory, motivational-affective, and cognitive) combine to determine how a person perceives pain.
- Assessment of pain helps establish a baseline of data, and helps to evaluate the effectiveness of interventions.
- Several factors influence the perception of pain, including age, previous experience with pain, and cultural norms.
- The subjective data to gather includes: location of pain, onset and duration, quality, intensity (on a scale of 0 to 10), aggravating and relieving factors, and how pain affects the activities of daily living.
- The three general principles to follow with pain relief measures are: (1) individualize the approach; (2) use a preventive approach; and (3) use a multidisciplinary approach.

- The nurse carries a great deal of autonomy in administering analgesics, which leads to specific responsibilities for which the nurse is accountable.
- Pharmacologic agents can be therapeutic for clients experiencing pain. However, the medications should not be the only interventions used.
- Noninvasive treatments for pain relief are measures that can supplement pharmacological and invasive treatments for pain relief.
- Invasive techniques are interventions used when the noninvasive and pharmacological measures do not provide adequate relief. Methods include nerve blocks, neurosurgery, radiation therapy, and acupuncture.

Review Questions

1. According to McCaffery and Pasero, pain may be defined as:

   a. discomfort resulting from identifiable physiologic or iatrogenic sources.
   b. a syndrome of behavioral and physical manifestations that can be objectively identified by the nurse.
   c. whatever the patient says it is, existing whenever and wherever the patient says it does.
   d. a sensory response to noxious stimuli.

2. Which of the following is a useful tool for assessing the intensity of pain that is easy to use?

   a. The gate control scale
   b. Acute pain monitor
   c. Numeric pain scale
   d. Pressure pain monitor

3. Mr. Levy, 45, has experienced chronic low back pain since a fall 8 years ago. He describes his pain as "a gnawing, constant dull pain" that makes him feel tired. The nurse caring for him recognizes that one of the differences between acute and chronic pain characteristics is:

   a. acute pain is more severe.
   b. chronic pain is often described as dull and is difficult to localize.
   c. chronic back pain is often not real.
   d. acute pain is more diffuse and difficult to describe.

4. Nancy Johnson, 84 years old, is recuperating from a total hip replacement. Morphine, 8 mg IV q4h prn, is prescribed for Ms. Johnson. Her respiratory rate is 18, her pulse rate is 96 beats per minute, and her blood pressure is elevated slightly above her normal level. She is complaining of severe pain, 8 on a scale of 0 to 10. The most appropriate initial nursing intervention is:

   a. question the physician regarding the dosage amount for a client this age.
   b. turn her and then reevaluate her need for opioid analgesia.
   c. administer the medication as ordered.
   d. advise Ms. Johnson to cough and breathe deeply since you are unable to give her anything for pain until her respiratory rate is 20.

5. Ms. Redgrave, 55 years old, is hospitalized with an exacerbation of rheumatoid arthritis. She has a favorite television show she watches every afternoon. She reports feeling comfortable during this show and seldom requests pain medication when she is watching it. The nurse's assessment of this phenomenon is that:

   a. the assessment of pain that prompted hospitalization is inaccurate.
   b. Ms. Redgrave is bored and the boredom usually makes her pain seem worse.
   c. inactivity is the best approach to Ms. Redgrave's pain.
   d. distraction is an effective modifier of the pain experience for Ms. Redgrave.

6. One of the general principles of pain management is:

   a. anticipated or mild pain is easier to relieve than severe pain.
   b. the more experience a person has with pain, the better that person will be able to tolerate it.
   c. no pain, no gain.
   d. the cause of pain must be identified in order to relieve it.

Critical Thinking Questions

1. What are the differences between somatic, cutaneous, visceral, referred, ischemic, acute, and chronic pain?

2. How would you decide which noninvasive technique to use with a client?

 WEB FLASH!

- Search the Internet for the organizations listed in the Resources for this chapter at the end of the book. What kind of information is available for clients, families, and health care professionals?
- Search the word *pain* on the Internet. What information is available?

DIAGNOSTIC TESTS

CHAPTER

27

MAKING THE CONNECTION

Refer to the following chapters to increase your understanding of diagnostic tests:

- **Chapter 13, Alternative/Complementary Therapies**
- **Chapter 21, Infection Control/Asepsis**
- **Chapter 22, Standard Precautions and Isolation**
- **Chapter 25, Assessment**
- **Chapter 28, Anesthesia**

- **Procedures:** B30, Urine Collection: Closed Drainage System; B31, Urine Collection: Clean Catch, Female, Male; I3, Performing Urinary Catheterization: Male Client; I4, Performing Urinary Catheterization: Female Client; I26, Skin Puncture; A3, Venipuncture

LEARNING OBJECTIVES

Upon completion of this chapter, you should be able to:
- *Define key terms.*
- *Discuss the relevant client teaching guidelines for the care of the client before, during, and after diagnostic testing.*
- *Describe the common specimen collection methods.*
- *Describe common invasive and noninvasive diagnostic procedures.*
- *Discuss nursing responsibilities for the common diagnostic procedures.*

KEY TERMS

agglutination	ascites
agglutinin	aspiration
agglutinogen	bacteremia
amniocentesis	barium
analyte	biopsy
aneurysm	cation
angiography	central line
anion	computed
antibody	tomography
antigen	conscious sedation
arteriography	contrast medium

culture	Papanicolaou test
cytology	paracentesis
electrocardiogram	phlebotomist
electroencephalogram	pneumothorax
electrolyte	port-a-cath
endoscopy	radiography
enzyme	sensitivity
fluoroscopy	stable
hematuria	stress test
invasive	thoracentesis
ketone	transducer
lipoprotein	trocar
lumbar puncture	type and cross-
magnetic resonance	match
imaging	ultrasound
necrosis	urobilinogen
noninvasive	venipuncture
occult blood	void
oliguria	

INTRODUCTION

Health care providers use the findings from a thorough history and physical examination to determine the need for diagnostic testing. The client's history and presenting symptoms determine those diagnostic procedures that are necessary to formulate a medical diagnosis and course of treatment. The challenge of cost-effective health care pushes practitioners to rely on basic assessment and to be selective with regard to expensive diagnostic tests. To reflect the emphasis on cost containment, the nurse's role has changed from doing for the client to teaching clients to do for themselves. The role of the nurse is to teach the client, family, and significant others about the procedures involved in diagnostic testing, the steps to be taken in preparation for the specific test(s) in question, and the care that will follow the procedure. Although the primary focus is on teaching, the nurse may assist in performing various noninvasive and invasive procedures. Nurses must be aware of the implications of diagnostic testing so as to deliver appropriate nursing care to the client.

To understand the nature of diagnostic tests, nurses must review anatomy and physiology. Knowing the anatomic and physiologic functions of the body will assist nurses in relating certain diagnostic tests to specific disease processes and in understanding the meaning of test results.

This chapter discusses common diagnostic tests. The terms *test* and *procedure* are used interchangeably throughout the chapter. The term *practitioner* is used in this chapter to refer to either the physician or an advanced practice registered nurse. Most state boards of nursing allow advanced practice registered nurses to order and perform certain diagnostic tests.

DIAGNOSTIC TESTING

Diagnostic tests are either noninvasive or invasive. **Noninvasive** means that the body is not entered with any type of instrument; the skin and other body tissues, organs, and cavities remain intact. **Invasive** means that the body's tissues, organs, or cavities are accessed through some type of procedure making use of instruments.

Nursing Care of the Client

Diagnostic testing is a critical element of assessment. In collaboration with feedback from the client, assessment data are used to formulate nursing diagnoses, a plan of care, and outcome measures. Ongoing client assessment and evaluation of the client's expected outcomes require the incorporation of diagnostic findings.

 Safety: Diagnostic Testing
To protect your health and safety, as well as that of other health care providers and the client, use Standard Precautions whenever performing invasive or noninvasive procedures.

Preparing the Client for Diagnostic Testing

The nurse plays a key role in scheduling and preparing the client for diagnostic testing. When tests are not scheduled correctly, not only is the client inconve-

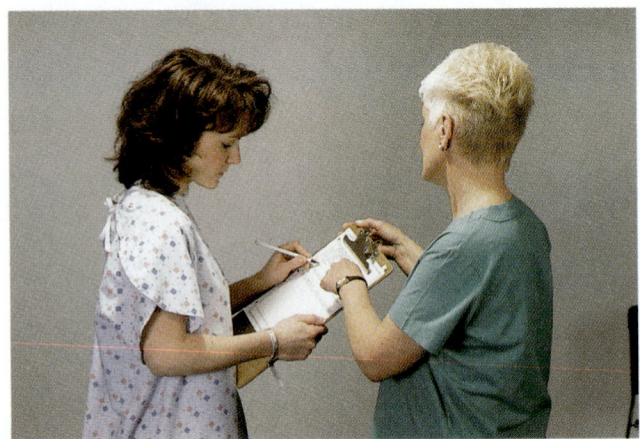
Figure 27-1 Preparing a Client for Diagnostic Testing

nienced, but interventions may be delayed, which may place the client's health at risk. The institution is also at risk to lose money. Table 27-1 outlines a sample protocol of the nursing care to prepare a client for diagnostic testing.

During the assessment of the client, the nurse must ensure that the client is wearing an identification band and understands those things to be done. It is also the nurse's responsibility to see that needed consent forms have been signed (Figure 27-1).

Other key nursing measures in ensuring client safety are to establish baseline vital signs, identify known allergies, and assess the effectiveness of teaching. In ambulatory and outpatient centers, the nurse might have only one opportunity to assess and record vital signs. It is important for the nurse to confirm that the vital signs are normal values *for the client*. To accurately assess the client's response to anesthetic agents and the procedure performed, the nurse must compare the vital signs taken during and after the procedure to those obtained before as baseline data.

The client must be made aware of those things to expect during the procedure. Such teaching can both increase the level of cooperation and decrease the degree of anxiety. The client's family should also be informed of what will happen during the procedure and approximately how long the procedure should last. Nurses must also know the institution's specific protocols and procedures, because these are not standardized in all practice settings.

Care of the Client during Diagnostic Testing

Although client care must be individualized according to the specific procedure, general guidelines for client care during a procedure are outlined in Table 27-2. Protocols are used to assist the nurse with client care.

Standard Precautions are initiated when exposure to body fluids presents a threat to the safety of the caregiver or client. Protective barriers, such as gloves and a gown, should be used during invasive procedures.

Table 27-1 PROTOCOL: PREPARING THE CLIENT FOR DIAGNOSTIC TESTING

Purpose	To increase the reliability of the test by providing client teaching on the reason the test is being performed, those things the client can expect during the test, and the outcomes and side effects of the test To decrease the client's anxiety about the test and the associated risks
Supportive Data	Increase the client's knowledge, thereby promoting cooperation and enhancing the quality of the testing Decrease the time required to perform the tests, thereby increasing cost effectiveness Prevent delays by ensuring proper physical preparation
Assessment	Ensure that the client is wearing an identification band Review the medical record for allergies and previous adverse reactions to dyes and other contrast media; a signed consent form; and the recorded findings of diagnostic tests relative to the procedure Assess for the presence, location, and characteristics of physical and communicative limitations or pre-existing conditions Monitor the client's knowledge of both the reasons for the test and those things to expect during and after testing Monitor vital signs of the client who is scheduled for invasive testing, to establish baseline data Assess client outcome measures relative to the practitioner's preferences for preprocedure preparations Monitor level of hydration and weakness for clients who are designated nothing by mouth (NPO)
Report to Practitioner	Notify practitioner of allergy, previous adverse reaction, or suspected adverse reaction following the administration of drugs Notify practitioner of any client or family concerns not alleviated by discussions with nurse
Interventions	Clarify with practitioner whether regularly scheduled medications are to be administered Implement NPO status, as determined by the type of test Administer cathartics or laxatives as denoted by the test's protocol except for children and infants, for whom a specific practitioner's order is needed before administration of a laxative; instruct clients who are weak to call for assistance to the bathroom Teach relaxation techniques, such as deep breathing and imagery Establish intravenous (IV) access if necessary for the procedure
Evaluation	Evaluate the client's knowledge of those things to expect Evaluate the client's anxiety level Evaluate the client's level of safety and comfort

Client Teaching	Discuss the following with the client and family, as appropriate to the specific test:
	• The reason for the test and those things to expect
	• An estimation of how long the test will take
	• Specifics of NPO status, including amount of water to drink if oral medication is to be taken
	• Cathartics or laxative: amount, frequency
	• Sputum: cough deeply, do not clear throat
	• Urine: voided, clean-catch specimen; timing of collection
	• Removal of objects (e.g., jewelry or hair clips) that will obscure x-ray film
	• Contrast medium:
	    Barium: taste, consistency, after effects (lightly colored stools for 24 to 72 hours; possibly, obstruction/impaction)
	    Iodine: metallic taste, delayed allergic reaction (itching, rashes, hives, wheezing and breathing difficulties)
	• Positioning during the test
	• Positioning posttest (e.g., immobilize limb after angiography)
	• Posttest (encourage fluid intake if not contraindicated)

Documentation	Record in the client's medical record: • Practitioner notification of allergies or suspected adverse reaction to contrast media • Presence, location, and characteristics of symptoms • Teaching and the client's response to teaching • Responses to interventions (client outcomes)

Table 27-2 PROTOCOL: CARE OF THE CLIENT DURING DIAGNOSTIC TESTING

Purpose	To increase cooperation and participation by allaying the client's anxiety To provide the maximum level of safety and comfort during a procedure
Supportive Data	Encourage relaxation of the muscles and thus facilitation of instrumentation by increasing the client's participation and comfort Ensure both efficient use of time during the test and reliable results from the test with proper preparation of the client
Assessment	Check the client's identification band to ensure the correct client Review the medical record for allergies Assess the client's reaction to the preprocedure sedatives administered prior to the induction of anesthesia during the procedure Assess airway maintenance and gag reflex, if a local anesthetic is sprayed into the client's throat Assess vital signs throughout the procedure and compare to baseline data Assess the client's ability to maintain and tolerate the prescribed position Assess the client's comfort level to ensure the effectiveness of the anesthetic agent Assess for related symptoms indicating complications specific to the procedure (e.g., accidental perforation of an organ)
Report to Practitioner	Notify the practitioner of any client concerns or questions not answered in discussions with the nurse Notify the practitioner of any family members present and their location during the procedure Notify the practitioner when the client is positioned properly and the anesthetic agent has been administered to the client
Interventions	Institute Standard Precautions or appropriate aseptic technique for the specific test Report to all personnel involved in the test any known client allergies Place the client in the correct position, drape, and monitor to ensure that breathing is not compromised Remain with the client during induction and maintenance of anesthesia If the procedure requires the administration of a dye, ensure that the client is not allergic to the dye; if the client has not received the dye before, perform the skin allergy test according to the manufacturer's instructions that accompany the medication Maintain the client's airway and keep resuscitative equipment available Assist the client to relax during insertion of the instrument by telling the client to breathe through the mouth and to concentrate on relaxing the involved muscles Explain what the practitioner is doing so that the client knows what to expect Label and handle the specimen according to the type of materials obtained and the testing to be done Report to the practitioner any symptoms of complications Secure client transport from the diagnostic area Posttest in the diagnostic area: • Assist the client to a comfortable, safe position • Provide oral hygiene and water to clients who were designated NPO for the test, if they are alert and able to swallow • Remain with the client awaiting transport to another area
Evaluation	Evaluate the client's ventilatory status and tolerance to the procedure Evaluate the client's need for assistance Evaluate the client's understanding of what was performed during the procedure Evaluate the client's understanding of findings identified during the procedure Evaluate the client's knowledge of what to expect after the procedure
Client Teaching	Discuss the following with the client and family, as appropriate to the specific test: • Those things that occurred during the procedure • Questions and concerns of the client or family member • Those things to expect during the immediate recovery phase • Those things to report to the nurse during the immediate recovery phase
Documentation	Record in the client's medical record: • Person who performed the procedure • Reason for the procedure • Type of anesthesic, dye, or other medications administered • Type of specimen obtained and where it was delivered • Vital signs and other assessment data such as client's tolerance of the procedure or pain/discomfort level • Any symptoms of complications • Person who transported the client to another area (designate the names of persons who provided transport and the destination)

The nurse is responsible for labeling any specimen with the client's name and room number (for hospitalized clients), and the date, time, and source of the specimen. Some specimens may need to be taken immediately to the laboratory or placed on ice (e.g., arterial blood gases [ABGs]).

Ongoing assessment of the client's status is required during the procedure. The patency of the client's airway should be continuously assessed, as it may be compromised by the client's position, by anesthesia, or by the procedure itself. During an invasive procedure, the nurse also must monitor for signs and symptoms of accidental perforation of an organ (e.g., sudden changes in vital signs).

The nurse has the following additional responsibilities:

- Preparing the procedure room (e.g., ensuring adequate lighting)
- Gathering and charging for supplies to be used during the procedure
- Testing the equipment to ensure it is functional and safe
- Securing proper containers for specimen collection

Practitioners usually have preference cards within the diagnostic testing area that specify the type of equipment to be used, the position in which to place the client, and the type of sedative or anesthesic agent to be used.

Some diagnostic tests are performed with the registered nurse administering IV sedation, also called conscious sedation. **Conscious sedation** is a minimally depressed level of consciousness during which the client retains the ability to maintain a continuously patent airway and respond appropriately to physical stimulation or verbal commands (Somerson, Husted, & Sicilia, 1995). The nurse managing conscious sedation is usually functioning in an expanded role that requires additional education and demonstrated ability beyond that afforded by basic education.

Care of the Client after Diagnostic Testing

Postprocedure nursing care is directed toward restoring the client's prediagnostic level of functioning (Table 27-3). Nursing assessment and interventions are based mainly on the nature of the test and whether the client received anesthesia.

The client is monitored closely for signs of respiratory distress and bleeding. Some diagnostic procedures require that vital signs be measured every 15 minutes for the first hour, and then at gradually longer intervals until the client is **stable** (alert and with vital signs within the client's normal range).

Some diagnostic tests require the use of medications that are excreted through the kidneys. The client's intake and output (I&O) is monitored by the nurses for 24 hours. The client is taught to monitor I&O and to report **hematuria** (presence of blood in the urine).

 Safety: Radioactive Iodine and Urine Collection

Clients receiving radioactive iodine must have their urine collected and properly discarded in a special container, according to agency policy for handling radioactive medical wastes.

When clients are discharged after diagnostic testing, they should receive written instructions. Most agencies have discharge forms on which the nurse documents teaching regarding medications, dietary and activity restrictions, and signs and symptoms to be reported immediately to the practitioner. Clients may also need to have follow-up appointments made for them.

LABORATORY TESTS

Common laboratory studies are usually simple measurements to determine the amount or number of **analytes** (i.e., measured substances) present in a specimen. Laboratory tests are ordered by the practitioner to:

- Detect and quantify the risk of future disease,
- Establish or exclude diagnoses,
- Assess the severity of the disease process and formulate a prognosis,
- Guide the selection of interventions,
- Monitor the progress of the disorder, or
- Monitor the effectiveness of the treatment.

Specimen Collection

The scheduling and sequencing of laboratory tests are important functions of the nurse. All tests requiring **venipuncture** (the use of a needle to puncture a vein to aspirate blood) are grouped together so that the client is subjected to only one venipuncture. Fasting laboratory and radiological studies are scheduled on the same day so that the client is required to fast for only 1 day. Appropriate scheduling increases the client's comfort level and satisfaction.

 PROFESSIONAL TIP

Documentation of Specimen-Collection Difficulties

Document on the laboratory requisition slip and in the nurses' notes any difficulty experienced during collection of a specimen. Such problems may indicate adverse effects related to the nature of the test and thus must be reported and treated immediately.

Table 27-3 PROTOCOL: CARE OF THE CLIENT AFTER DIAGNOSTIC TESTING

Purpose	To restore the client's prediagnostic level of functioning by providing care and teaching relative to both those things the client can expect after a test and the outcomes or side effects of the test
Supportive Data	Decrease client anxiety by increasing the client's participation and knowledge of expected outcome measures after a diagnostic test
	Through proper postprocedure care and client teaching, alert the client to those signs and symptoms that must to be reported to the practitioner
Assessment	Check the identification band and call the client by name
	Assess the client closely for signs of airway distress, adverse reactions to anesthesic or other medications, and other signs that may indicate accidental perforation of an organ
	Assess for bleeding those areas where a biopsy was performed
	Assess the client's color and skin temperature
	Assess vascular access lines or other invasive monitoring devices
	Assess the client's ability to expel air, if air was instilled during a gastrointestinal test
	Assess the client's knowledge of those things to expect during the recovery phase
Report to Practitioner	Notify the practitioner of any signs of respiratory distress, bleeding, or changes in vital signs; adverse reactions to anesthetic, sedative, or dye; and other signs of complications
	Notify the practitioner of any client or family concerns or questions not answered in discussions with the nurse
	Notify the practitioner when any results are obtained from the diagnostic test
	Notify the practitioner when the client is fully alert and recovered (for an order to discharge)
Interventions	Implement the practitioner's orders regarding the postprocedure care of the client
	Institute Standard Precautions or surgical asepsis as appropriate to the client's care needs
	Position the client for comfort and accessibility so as to facilitate performance of nursing measures
	Monitor vital signs according to the frequency required for the specific test
	Observe the insertion site for hematoma or blood loss; replace pressure dressing, as needed
	Monitor the client's urinary output and drainage from other devices
	Enforce activity restrictions appropriate to the test
	Schedule client appointments as directed by the practitioner
Evaluation	Evaluate the client's respiratory status, especially if an anesthetic agent was used
	Evaluate the client's tolerance of oral liquids
	Evaluate the client's understanding of the procedural findings of when the practitioner expects to receive written results
	Evaluate the client's knowledge of those things to expect after discharge
Client Teaching	Based on client assessment and evaluation of knowledge, teach the client or family about the following:
	• Dietary or activity restrictions
	• Signs and symptoms that should be reported immediately to the practitioner
	• Medications
Documentation	Record in the client's medical record on the appropriate forms:
	• Assessment data, nursing interventions, and achievement of expected outcomes
	• Client or family teaching and demonstrated level of understanding
	• Written instructions given to the client or family members

Accuracy in laboratory testing requires that:

- The practitioner's order be transcribed onto the correct requisition form,
- All requested information be written on the form (e.g., the client's full name and medical number),
- Pertinent data that could influence the test's results, such as medications taken, be included,
- Collection of the specimen from the correct client be confirmed by checking the identification band, and
- Laboratory results be placed in the correct medical record.

Venipuncture

Venipuncture can be performed by various members of the health care team. Although laboratories employ **phlebotomists** (individuals who perform venipuncture) to collect blood specimens, the nurse must know how to perform venipuncture, because nurses routinely perform venipuncture in the home, long-term care settings, and hospital critical care units.

Venipuncture can be performed by using either a sterile needle and syringe or a vacuum tube holder with a sterile two-ended needle. Test tubes are used to collect blood specimens. Test tubes have different colored stoppers to indicate the type of additive in the test tube. Collection tubes are universally color coded as follows:

- Red: no additive
- Lavender: ethylenediaminotetraacetic acid (EDTA)
- Light blue: sodium citrate
- Green: sodium heparin
- Gray: potassium oxalate
- Black: sodium oxalate

Arterial Puncture

Assessment of ABGs reveals the ability of the lungs to exchange gases by measuring the partial pressures of oxygen (PaO_2) and carbon dioxide ($PaCO_2$) and evaluates the potential of hydrogen (pH) of arterial blood. Blood gases are ordered to evaluate:

- Oxygenation,
- Ventilation and the effectiveness of respiratory therapy, and
- Acid–base balance in the blood.

Arterial blood samples are drawn from a peripheral artery (e.g., radial or femoral) or from an arterial line. The arterial blood sample is collected in a 5 mL heparinized syringe. To prevent clotting, the syringe is then rotated to mix the blood with the heparin. The blood sample is then placed on ice to reduce the rate of oxygen metabolism.

In some agencies, it is within the scope of nursing practice to perform radial artery puncture; however, femoral artery puncture is usually performed only by an advanced practitioner, because of the associated increased risk of hemorrhage. Although it is not common practice for student nurses to draw ABG samples, students often assist with the procedure and care for the client after the procedure.

Regardless of who performs the arterial puncture, the nurse is responsible for assessing the client for symptoms of postpuncture bleeding or occlusion. Direct pressure must be applied to the puncture site until all bleeding has stopped (for a minimum of 5 minutes). Symptoms of impaired circulation include the following:

PROFESSIONAL TIP

Arterial Blood Gases

To ensure an accurate determination of the client's actual blood gases, ABGs should not be drawn within 30 minutes after any respiratory treatment.

CLIENT TEACHING

Postarterial Puncture

The client should *immediately* notify the nurse if any pain or numbness occurs in the arm or leg after an arterial puncture. These symptoms indicate impaired circulation.

- Numbness and tingling
- Bluish color
- Absence of a peripheral pulse

Capillary Puncture

Skin punctures are performed when small quantities of capillary blood are needed for analysis or when the client has poor veins. Capillary puncture is also commonly performed for blood glucose analysis. Figure 27-2 illustrates a capillary puncture of a fingertip.

Central Lines

Blood samples can also be collected from central lines. A **central line** refers to a venous catheter inserted into the superior vena cava through the subclavian or internal or external jugular vein. Central lines are used in the treatment of alterations in fluid or electrolyte balance, such as severe dehydration due to vomiting. Insertion is necessary when a peripheral route cannot be obtained. Central lines can be used for treatment and to withdraw blood for analysis.

The first sample of blood drawn from the central line cannot be used for diagnostic testing; it must be discarded, with the volume of discard being directly related to the dead space (catheter size) (Laxson & Titler, 1994). The agency's protocol should indicate the volume to discard relative to the type and size of catheter.

The care of central lines requires strict sterile technique. The practitioner must write an order to allow a blood sample to be obtained from a central line.

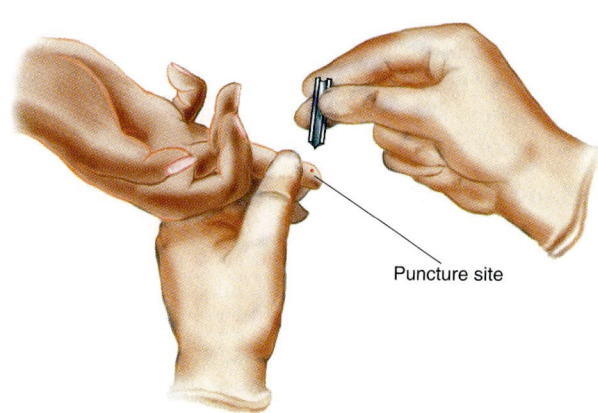

Puncture site

Figure 27-2 Capillary Puncture of Fingertip

Common Sites for Capillary Puncture
- Heel: most commonly used site in neonates and infants
- Inner aspect of a palmar fingertip: most commonly used site in children and adults
- Earlobe: used when the client is in shock or the extremities are edematous

Implanted Port

Some clients have a **port-a-cath** (a port that has been implanted under the skin) over the third or fourth rib. The port has a catheter that is inserted into the superior vena cava or right atrium through the subclavian or internal jugular vein. The implanted port is used for the same purpose as is a central line. Blood can be withdrawn for sampling by accessing the port while using strict sterile technique. Accessing a port should be performed only by a nurse who has the education to be able to properly do so. Students are not usually taught how to access an implanted port.

Urine Collection

Urine can be collected for various studies. The type of testing determines the method of collection. The different methods of urine collection are as follows:

- Random collection (routine analysis)
- Timed collection (24-hour urine)
- Collection from a closed urinary drainage system
- Sterile specimen (catheterized)
- Clean-voided specimen

Client teaching depends on the client's age and the method of collection. The method of collection should be written on the laboratory requisition.

 Safety: Standard Precautions and Urine Collection
All urine collection requires the use of Standard Precautions to prevent the transmission of microorganisms among nurses, clients, and other health care providers. All specimen containers should be sealed in a biohazard bag prior to transport to the laboratory.

Random Collection The practitioner usually writes the order for a UA (routine urine analysis), which is also called a random collection. The specimen can be collected at any time using a clean cup. The container does not have to be sterile. The specimen should be taken immediately to the laboratory to prevent both bacteria growth and changes in the urine's analytes.

Timed Collection Timed collection is done over a 24-hour period. The urine is collected in a plastic gal-

Central Line
Clients receiving prolonged therapy in the home environment usually have a central line in place. Because one of the primary complications of central venous catheter insertion is infection, the nurse must be alert for signs of infection (e.g., fever).

lon container that contains preservative(s), some of which are caustic.

For a timed collection, the client is told to **void** (eliminate urine) and discard the specimen at the beginning of the collection. Timing for a 24-hour urine collection begins after the first voiding has been discarded. For example, if the client voids at 1000 hours (24-hour [military] time), that urine should be discarded, but all other urine specimens until 1000 hours the following day saved. The client can void throughout the test into a clean container, then pour the urine into the collection bottle. Toilet tissue should not be dropped into the container used to catch the urine. The collection container should be refrigerated or kept on ice throughout the 24 hours to retard bacterial growth and stabilize the analytes.

Collection from a Closed-Drainage System
A sterile specimen can be collected from a client with an indwelling Foley catheter and closed drainage system. A sterile specimen is used for urine culture. The urine specimen should *not* be obtained from the drainage bag, because the analytes in the urine drainage bag change, leading to inaccurate results, and bacteria grows quickly in the drainage bag. The catheter's closed drainage tubing has an aspiration port that is used for sterile specimen collection.

Sterile Specimen Sometimes a sterile urine specimen is required when the client does not have an indwelling catheter and closed drainage system. In such cases, the client is catheterized. A small amount of urine is allowed to run out of the catheter into a basin, then the urine is allowed to run into a sterile specimen bottle.

Urine Collection in the Home
Clients in the home should place the urine container in a reclosable ("zipper") plastic bag and refrigerate until delivering to a laboratory. Doing so prevents bacteria growth and promotes accuracy of results.

LIFE CYCLE CONSIDERATIONS

Clean-Voided Specimen: Infant and Child

Explain the procedure to the family member accompanying the infant or child. If the child can cooperate, tell the child what to do before having someone hold the child in position.

1. Have the child lie in the supine position, with the hips externally rotated
2. Flex and abduct the child's knees and hold the knees throughout the procedure
3. Cleanse the perineal area as for an adult
4. Place a sterile collection bag over the perineum or penis and scrotum, then apply a diaper
5. Remove the collection bag immediately after voiding occurs

Clean-Voided Specimen Clean-voided (clean-catch, or midstream) specimen collection is done to secure a specimen uncontaminated by skin flora. Different aseptic techniques are used for women and men. The female client is instructed to cleanse from the front to the back and then void into the specimen bottle; the male client is instructed to cleanse from the tip of the penis downward and then void into the specimen bottle.

Stool Collection

The nurse should first explain to the client the reason for collection of the stool specimen. The client can then be instructed to defecate into a clean bed pan or container, discarding used tissue in the toilet. Stools can be collected for a one-time defecation or over 24, 48, or 72 hours. If stools are to be collected over a prolonged period of time, all must be placed into a container and refrigerated. Once all stools have been collected, the container should be labeled with the client's name, the date and time, and the test to be performed on the specimen. All stool specimens are placed in a biohazard bag before being transported to the laboratory.

Safety: Collecting Stool from a Client with Hepatitis

When collecting a stool specimen from a client with hepatitis, write on the requisition form that the client has hepatitis. Doing so alerts laboratory personnel to be especially careful when handling the specimen.

Specific Tests

Many tests can be performed on the blood. Tests specific to the hematological system are described in Table 27-4.

Type and Crossmatch

A **type and crossmatch** is a laboratory test that identifies the client's blood type and determines the compatibility of blood between a potential donor and recipient (client). There are four basic blood types: A, B, AB, and O. The blood types are determined by the presence or absence of A or B antigens. **Antigens** are substances, usually proteins, that cause the formation of and react specifically with antibodies. **Antibodies** are immunoglobulins produced by the body in response to bacteria, viruses, or other antigenic substances. Type A and type B are antigens that are classified as **agglutinogens**, or substances that cause **agglutination** (clumping of RBCs). **Agglutinins** are specific kinds of antibodies whose interaction with antigens manifests as agglutination.

Blood types are also designated as either positive or negative, depending on the presence or absence of the Rh factor. The Rh factor is an antigen that may be found on the RBC. The designation *Rh positive* means the antigen is present; *Rh negative* means the antigen is absent. An individual's blood type and Rh are determined genetically.

Crossmatch determines the compatibility of the donor's blood with that of the recipient. In the laboratory, a sample of the recipient's blood is mixed with the blood of a possible donor. If the blood sample is compatible, the mixed sample does not agglutinate.

Blood Chemistry

Blood chemistry tests are often grouped together into profiles, or panels, requiring one requisition and a single venous specimen. Tests performed include glucose, electrolytes, enzymes, lipids, creatinine, and protein values. Other tests that may be performed on a blood specimen are listed in Table 27-5.

Blood Glucose Blood for glucose measurement is obtained by either skin puncture or venipuncture; glucose is measured as either fasting (FBS) or nonfasting (usually 2 hours postprandial) blood sugar. This test is used to screen for diabetes mellitus. If the results are abnormal, the practitioner may order a glucose tolerance test, the most accurate test for diagnosing hypoglycemia and hyperglycemia (diabetes mellitus).

Serum Electrolytes An **electrolyte** is a substance that, when in solution, separates into ions and conducts electricity. Some electrolytes act on the cell membrane, allowing for the transmission of electrochemical impulses in nerve and muscle fibers. Other electrolytes determine the activity of different enzymatically catalyzed reactions necessary for cellular metabolism (Guyton & Hall, 1996).

Cations are ions that have a positive charge, such as sodium (Na^+), potassium (K^+), calcium (Ca^{++}), and magnesium (Mg^{++}). **Anions** are ions that have a negative charge, including chloride (Cl^-), bicarbonate (HCO_3^-), and phosphate (HPO_4^{--}).

Table 27-4 TESTS SPECIFIC TO THE HEMATOLOGIC SYSTEM

TEST	EXPLANATION/NORMAL VALUES	NURSING RESPONSIBILITIES
Red blood cells (RBCs)	Number of RBCs per mm^3 of blood. May be low in clients with rheumatoid arthritis. Clients living in high altitudes may have an elevated RBC level. Normal: Male: 4.6–5.9 million/mm^3 Female: 4.2–5.4 million/mm^3	The client is not required to fast for the test.
White blood cells (WBCs)	Number of WBCs per mm^3 of blood. Elevation is associated with infectious processes. Normal: 4300–10,800 mm^3	The client is not required to fast for the test. Exercise, stress, last month of pregnancy, labor, previous splenectomy, and eating may increase level and alter differential values. Note medications taken that may affect test; aspirin, heparin, and steroids may increase WBC level, whereas antibiotics and diuretics may decrease WBC level.
Differential count Neutrophils Segs (mature neutrophils) Bands (immature neutrophils)	Percentage of types of WBCs in 1 mm of blood. Increase in bacterial infections and trauma. Normal: Segs: 50%–65% Bands: 0%–5%	The client is not required to fast for the test.
Eosinophils	Increased in allergic reactions or parasitic infestation. Normal: 1%–3%	Corticosteroid therapy causes a decreased level.
Basophils	Increased in allergic reactions and during healing periods. Normal: 0.4%–1.0%	Steroids cause a decreased level.
Lymphocytes	Increased in viral infections and other diseases, such as pertussis and tuberculosis (TB). Decreased in acquired immunodeficiency syndrome (AIDS). Normal: 25%–35%	Steroids cause a decreased level.
Monocytes	Increased in chronic diseases, such as malaria, TB, Rocky Mountain spotted fever. May be low in clients with rheumatoid arthritis. Normal: 4%–6%	
Hemoglobin (Hgb)	Measures the oxygen-carrying capacity of the blood. Normal: Male: 14–18 g/dL Female: 12–16 g/dL Critical value: < 5 g/dL	The client is not required to fast for the test. Sample may be drawn from a finger of a child or the heel of an infant.
Hemoglobin electrophoresis	Detects abnormal forms of hemoglobin. Performed after positive sickle cell test. If the hemoglobin electrophoresis is negative, the client has the sickle cell trait. If the hemoglobin electrophoresis is positive, the client has sickle cell anemia. Normal: Hgb S: 0% Hgb F: < 2% Hgb Ca: 0%	If the client has had a blood transfusion within the last 12 weeks, the results of the test may be altered.
Hematocrit (Hct)	Measures the percentage of blood cells in a volume of blood. Clients living in high altitudes may have an increased level. Normal: Male: 42%–52% Female: 37%–47% Critical value: < 15%	The client is not required to fast for the test.

continued

Table 27-4 TESTS SPECIFIC TO THE HEMATOLOGIC SYSTEM *continued*

TEST	EXPLANATION/NORMAL VALUES	NURSING RESPONSIBILITIES
Platelet count	Measures the number of platelets per cubic milliliter of blood. Normal: 150,000–400,000/mm^3 Critical level: < 50,000 and > 1 million/mm^3	Instruct the client that strenuous exercise and oral contraceptives increase platelet level. Instruct the client that aspirin, acetaminophen, and sulfonamides decrease platelet level. If the client has a low platelet count, maintain digital pressure to the puncture site.
Bleeding time	Measures the length of time for a platelet plug to occlude a small puncture wound. Normal: 1–9 minutes (Ivy method) Critical value: > 12 minutes	Notify the laboratory if the client is taking aspirin, anticoagulants, or other medications that may affect the clotting process.
Prothrombin time (PT, protime)	Measures the effectiveness of several blood-clotting factors. Normal: 11–12.5 seconds INR: 2.0–3.0 In the presence of anticoagulant therapy, the values should be 1½–2 times the normal value. Critical value: > 20 seconds In the presence of anticoagulant therapy, the critical value should be > 3 times the normal critical value.	Ensure that the blood specimen is drawn before the daily dose of warfarin (Coumadin) is administered. Instruct the client that alcohol intake may increase PT and that a diet high in fat may decrease PT. Note those medications taken that may affect results; salicylates, sulfonamides, and methyl-dopa (Aldomet), as these may increase PT, whereas digitalis and oral contraceptives decrease the level. Instruct the client not to take any medication without notifying the physician, as medications may affect the PT level.
International normalized ratio (INR)	Normal: 2–3 (2.5–3.5 for the client with a mechanical prosthetic heart valve). The INR is more accurate than PT in monitoring warfarin (Coumadin) therapy.	The daily warfarin (Coumadin) dose should be given after blood has been drawn for the INR.

Partial thromboplastin time (PTT), also called activated partial thromboplastin time (APTT)	Normal:
	   PTT: 60–70 sec
	   APTT: 30–40 sec
	In the presence of anticoagulant therapy, the normal value is 1.5–2.5 times the control value.
	Critical value:
	   APTT: > 70 seconds
	   PTT: > 100 seconds
		If the client is receiving intermittent heparin doses, schedule the APTT to be drawn 30–60 minutes before the next heparin dose.
		
		If heparin is given continuously, the blood specimen can be drawn at any time.
		
		If APTT is greater than 100 seconds, the client is at risk for bleeding, and the physician is notified.
		
		The antidote for heparin is protamine sulfate.
		
		Note whether the client is taking antihistamines, vitamin C, or salicylates, as these prolong PTT time.

D dimer test (fragment D dimer, fibrin degradation fragment)	Measures a fibrin split product that is released when a clot breaks. Confirms the diagnosis of disseminated intra-vascular coagulation (DIC). Normal: negative for D-dimer fragments	Note whether the client is on thrombolytic therapy, as the results of this test would be increased from negative to positive.

Blood Enzymes **Enzymes** are globular proteins produced in the body that catalyze chemical reactions within the cells by promoting the oxidative reactions and synthesis of various chemicals, such as lipids, glycogen, and adenosine triphosphate (ATP). Enzyme tests play a key role in diagnosing the degree of tissue damage, mainly to the myocardium and, to a lesser degree, to the brain.

Elevations in plasma levels of intracellular enzymes occur in the presence of myocardial **necrosis** (tissue death as the result of disease or injury). Enzymes are released into the bloodstream in proportion to the degree of cellular damage. The enzymes are not used as single diagnostic values in determining a diagnosis but, rather, are reviewed in relation to other diagnostic studies.

Blood Lipids An elevated serum lipid level is one of the controllable contributing risk factors to CHD. **Lipoproteins** (blood lipids bound to protein) are measured along with cholesterol.

Table 27-5 ADDITIONAL TESTS PERFORMED ON BLOOD SPECIMEN

TEST	EXPLANATION/NORMAL VALUES	NURSING RESPONSIBILITIES
Acid phosphatase	Acid phosphatase is an enzyme found in highest concentrations in the prostate gland. An elevated level is seen in clients with prostatic cancer that has metastasized to other body parts. If tumors are treated successfully, the level will decrease. A rising level may indicate a poor prognosis. Normal: 0.11–0.60 U/L	Tell the client that no food or drink restrictions are associated with this test. Apply pressure to the venipuncture site. Observe the site for bleeding.
Adrenocorticotropic hormone (ACTH), corticotropin	Determines the function of the anterior pituitary. Because of diurnal variation, specimens should be drawn in both morning and evening. Normal: A.M.: 15–100 pg/mL, or 10–80 ng/L P.M.: < 50 pg/mL, or < 50 ng/L	Emotional or physical stress or recent radio-isotope scans can interfere with test results. Drugs that may increase ACTH level include corticosteroids, estrogens, ethanol, and spironolactone. Explain the procedure to the client. This is especially important to decrease the client's stress level. Evaluate the client for increased stress level. Initiate NPO status after midnight. The blood specimen must be drawn with a heparinized syringe, chilled by placing the specimen on ice, and immediately transported to the lab.
ACTH stimulation test, cortisol stimulation test, cosyntropin test	Monitors plasma cortisol level to indicate adrenal gland response to ACTH. Normal: Rapid: ↑ 7 μg/dL above baseline 24 hours: > 40 μg/dL 3 days: > 40 μg/dL	Note those medications taken that may affect results: cortisone, estrogens, hydrocortisone, and spironolactone may increase plasma cortisol level. Explain the procedure to the client. Initiate NPO status after midnight. For all tests, obtain baseline serum cortisol level. Rapid test: Administer IV injection of cosyntropin over 2 minutes. Draw blood specimen at 30 and 60 minutes after injection. 24-hour test: Start an IV infusion of cosyntropin in 1 liter normal saline and run at 2 U/h for 24 hours. Draw plasma cortisol level after 24 hours. 3-day test: Administer 25 units cosyntropin IV over 8 hours for 2 or 3 days. At the end of 3 days, draw plasma cortisol level.
Alanine aminotransferase (ALT, formerly serum glutamic pyruvic transiminase [SGRT])	ALT is an enzyme released in response to liver injury. Normal: 5–35 U/L	Note those medications taken that affect results: many medications may increase level, including antibiotics, narcotics, oral contraceptives, and many others.
Albumin	Albumin, a protein formed by the liver, is responsible for maintaining colloidal osmotic pressure. Indicates how well the liver is functioning. Normal: 3.5–5.0 g/dL	Note those medications taken that may affect results; steroids and hormones such as insulin, and growth hormones may increase level, whereas oral contraceptives and liver toxic drugs may decrease level.
Alkaline phosphatase	Alkaline phosphatase is an enzyme found in many tissues. The highest concentrations are found in the liver, biliary tract, and bone. Detection is important for determining possible liver and bone cancers. Normal: 30–85 lmU/mL	Fasting may be required. Apply pressure to the venipuncture site. Observe the site for bleeding.
Alpha-fetoprotein	Test for tumor marker; elevated in nonseminomatous testicular cancer. Performed between 16 and 18 weeks of pregnancy. A high level is suggestive of neural tube defects, whereas a low level may suggest Down syndrome. Normal: 0.9 ng/mL	Apply pressure to site and watch for bleeding or hematoma. First sample must be drawn between 15–20 weeks of gestation.

continued

Table 27-5 ADDITIONAL TESTS PERFORMED ON BLOOD SPECIMEN *continued*

TEST	EXPLANATION/NORMAL VALUES	NURSING RESPONSIBILITIES
Amylase	Amylase is an enzyme secreted by the pancreas. Elevation indicates pancreatitis. Normal: 56–190 IU/L	Note those medications taken that affect test results; steroids, aspirin, alcohol, some narcotics, some diuretics, and other drugs may increase level, whereas citrate, glucose, and oxalates may decrease level.
Antidiuretic hormone (ADH), vasopressin	Determines the production of ADH by the posterior pituitary. Normal: 1–5 pg/mL, or < 1.5 ng/L	Explain the procedure to the client. The blood specimen should be collected in a plastic, not glass, container. Note those medications taken that may interfere with test results. Drugs that elevate ADH level include acetaminophen, barbiturates, cholinergic agents, estrogen, nicotine, oral hypoglycemic agents, some diuretics such as thiazides, and tricyclic antidepressants. Drugs that decrease ADH level include alcohol, beta-adrenergic agents, morphine antagonists, and phenytoin (Dilantin). Client should fast for 12 hours before the test. Evaluate the client for high level of physical or emotional stress.
Antinuclear antibodies (ANAs)	ANA attack cell nuclei. The result is positive in 95% of clients with systemic lupus erythematosis. Levels are low in clients with mononucleosis, rheumatic fever, and liver diseases. Normal: negative	Fasting is not required. Hydralazine (Apresoline) and procainamide (Pronestyl) may increase level. A radioactive scan in the past week may alter results; inform the lab, if applicable.

Antistreptolysin O (ASO)	High titer indicates presence of *beta-hemolytic streptococcus*, which may cause rheumatic fever or acute glomerulonephritis. Upper limit of normal varies with age, season, and geographic area.
	Normal:
	  Adult: < 1 : 100
	  12–19 years: < 1 : 200
	  2–5 years: < 1 : 100
		There are no food or fluid restrictions.
		Antibiotics decrease ASO level.
		Check urine output if ASO is elevated.
		Urine output of less than 600 mL/24 h is associated with acute glomerulonephritis.

Antithyroid microsomal antibody, antimicrosomal antibody, microsomal antibody, thyroid autoantibody, thyroid antimicrosomal antibody	Used to detect thyroid microsomal antibodies found in clients with Hashimoto's thyroiditis. Normal: titer < 1 : 100	Explain the procedure to the client.

Aspartate aminotransferase (AST, formerly serum glutamic oxaloacetic transiminase [SGOT])	AST is an enzyme that indicates inflammation of heart, liver, skeletal muscle, pancreas, or kidneys.
	Normal:
	  Male: 7–21 U/L
	  Female: 6–18 U/L
		Avoid intramuscular (IM) injections; record date and time of any injections. Avoid hemolysis. Withhold medications that affect results, for 12 hours if possible; several medications, such as antihypertensives, cholinergic agents, anticoagulants, digitalis, and others, may increase level, as may exercise.

Arterial blood gases (ABGs)	Direct measurement of the pH, PaO_2, and $PaCO_2$, and calculated measurement of HCO_3^- and SaO_2 from samples of arterial blood. pH = expresses the acidity or alkalinity of the blood. PaO_2 = partial pressure of oxygen in the blood. $PaCO_2$ = partial pressure of carbon dioxide in the blood. SaO_2 = arterial oxygen saturation. HCO_3^- = bicarbonate ion concentration in the blood. The oxygen content of the blood expressed as a percentage of the oxygen carrying capacity of the blood.	Explain that an arterial sample of blood is required. Arterial punctures cause more discomfort than venous. Instruct the client not to move. Assess the adequacy of collateral circulation. The blood sample is drawn in a syringe containing heparin. After the specimen has been obtained, rotate the syringe to mix the blood and heparin. The blood sample is placed on ice and taken immediately to the lab. Apply pressure to the arterial site for 3 to 5 minutes or 15 minutes if client is on an anticoagulant. Assess site for bleeding.

continued

Table 27-5 ADDITIONAL TESTS PERFORMED ON BLOOD SPECIMEN *continued*

TEST	EXPLANATION/NORMAL VALUES	NURSING RESPONSIBILITIES
Arterial blood gases (ABGs) (*continued*)	Normal: 　pH: 7.35–7.45 　PaO_2: 80–100 mm Hg 　$PaCO_2$: 35–45 mm Hg 　HCO_3^-: 22–26 mEq 　SaO_2: > 95% (at sea level)	
Bilirubin	Measures bilirubin in the blood. Indicates how well the liver is functioning. Normal: 0.1–1.0 mg/dL	Note those medications taken that affect results; steroids, antibiotics, oral hypoglycemics, narcotics, as well as others may cause increased level, whereas barbiturates, caffeine, penicillins, and salicylates may cause decreased level. Fasting may be required. Do not shake the tube; protect the tube from light.
Blood glucose, fasting blood sugar, (FBS)	Measures blood level of glucose (serum values). Results depend on method used by laboratory. Normal: 70–115 mg/dL Diabetic: ≥ 126 mg/dL Critical values: 　> 400 mg/dL 　< 50 mg/dL	Client must fast (except for water) for 6–8 hours before test. Withhold insulin or oral antidiabetic medications until blood is drawn. Be certain client receives medications and meal after fasting specimen drawn. Cortisone, thiazide, and loop diuretics cause increase.
2 hour post prandial glucose (2h PPG) or 2 hour post prandial blood sugar (2h PPBS)	Measures blood glucose 2 hours after a meal. Normal: 70–140 mg/dL Diabetic: > 140 mg/dL	Instruct the client to eat entire meal and then to not eat anything else until blood is drawn. Notify the laboratory of the time meal was completed.
Blood urea nitrogen (BUN)	Measures urea, end product of protein metabolism. Normal: 5–25 mg/dL	Initiate NPO status 8 hours prior to test, if possible. Note the client's hydration status. Note those medications taken that may affect results, including phenothiazines, nephrotoxic drugs, diuretics (hydrochlorthiazide [Hydro-Diuril], ethacrynic acid [Edecrin], furosemide [Lasix]); antibiotics (bacitracin, gentamicin, kanamycin, methicillin, neomycin); antihypertensives (methyldopa [Aldomet], guanethidine [Ismelin]), sulfonamides, propranolol, morphine, lithium, carbonate, salicylates.
CA-15-3	CA-15-3 (cancer antigen) is a tumor marker for monitoring breast cancer. Because benign breast or ovarian disease can also cause elevations, it has limited use in diagnosis. Normal: < 22 U/mL	Fasting is not required. Apply pressure to the venipuncture site. Observe the site for bleeding.
CA-19-9	CA-19-9 (cancer antigen) is a tumor marker used primarily in the diagnosis of pancreatic carcinoma. Normal: < 37 U/mL	Fasting is not required. Apply pressure to the venipuncture site. Observe the site for bleeding.
CA-125	CA-125 (cancer antigen) is a tumor marker especially helpful in making the diagnosis of ovarian cancer. Normal: 0–35 U/mL	Fasting is not required. Apply pressure to the venipuncture site. Observe the site for bleeding.
Calcitonin, HCT, thyrocalcitonin	Determines thyroid and parathyroid activity. Also used as a tumor marker to detect thyroid cancer and several other cancers. Normal: basal 　Male: ≤ 19 pg/mL, or ≤ 19 ng/L 　Female: ≤ 14 pg/mL, or ≤ 14 ng/L	Note those medications taken that may increase calcitonin level, including calcium, cholecystokinin, epinephrine, glucagon, pentagastrin, and oral contraceptives. Explain the procedure to the client. The client should fast overnight but may have water.

continued

Table 27-5 ADDITIONAL TESTS PERFORMED ON BLOOD SPECIMEN *continued*

TEST	EXPLANATION/NORMAL VALUES	NURSING RESPONSIBILITIES
Carcinoembryonic antigen (CEA, carcinoembryonic antigen)	CEA was thought to be a specific indicator of the presence of colorectal cancer, but has been found in clients with a variety of carcinomas. It is especially useful in monitoring treatment response in breast and gastrointestinal cancers and is occasionally the first sign of tumor recurrence. Normal: < 5 ng/mL	Fasting is not required. Apply pressure to the venipuncture site. Observe the site for bleeding. Note whether the client smokes or has a disease that will alter results, such as hepatitis, cirrhosis, or colitis.

Cardiac enzymes
  Serum AST
	Indicates possible tissue damage if elevated.
	Normal:
	  Male: 7–21 U/L
	  Female: 6–18 U/L
		Neither fasting nor NPO status is necessary.
		Pattern of elevated levels of AST, CPK, and LDH is indicative of myocardial infarction (MI).

Creatine kinase CPK (CK)	Normal:
	  Male: 55–170 U/L
	  Female: 30–135 U/L
		CPK is the first enzyme elevated after MI, and peaks within the first 24 hours.

CK isoenzymes	Present in skeletal muscle, brain, lungs, and heart muscle. Normal:	Elevation of an isoenzyme indicates damage to tissue in a specific organ; CK-MB is specific for myocardial cells.

CK-MM (muscle)
    CK-BB (brain)
    CK-MB (heart)
	95%–100%
	0%–1%
	< 3%–4% (> 5% in MI)	

Lactic dehydrogenase (LDH) LDH isoenzymes	Normal: 70–180 mg/dL, or 95–200 U/L	LDH_1 value greater than LDH_2 value is indicative of an acute MI. LDH_5 is elevated with congestive heart failure (CHF).

LDH_1 (heart and erythrocytes)
    LDH_2 (reticuloendothelial system)
    LDH_3 (lungs and other tissues)
    LDH_4 (kidney, placenta, pancreas)
    LDH_5 (liver and striated muscles)
	*17.5%–28.3%
	*30.4%–36.4%
	*18.8%–26.0%
	*9.2%–16.5%
	*5.3%–13.4%	

CD4 T-cell count	Predictor of HIV progression; baseline taken after positive HIV test. Normal: 500–1000/mm^3 Critical value: < 200/mm^3	Explain the meaning of the test. Provide follow-up explanation of test results.
Cholesterol (lipid profile)	Lipid necessary for steroid, bile, and cell membrane production. Normal: < 200 mg/dL (total)	Have client fast 12 to 14 hours prior to test. No alcohol 24 hours prior to test. Diet intake 2 weeks prior to test will affect results. Note those medications taken that may affect results; steroids, phenytoin, diuretics, and others may elevate level, whereas MAO inhibitors, some antibiotics, lovastatin, and others may decrease level. If elevated, increased risk of coronary artery disease (CAD), hypertension, and MI.

High density lipoprotein (HDL)
  Low density lipoprotein (LDL)
  Very low density lipoprotein (VLDL)
  Triglycerides
	Normal: 30–70 mg/dL
	Normal: 60–160 mg/dL
	Normal: 25%–50%
	Normal: 40–150 mg/dL
		
		Elevated level in CAD; level increases when LDL level increases.

Complement assay (total complement, C3 and C4)	Decreased levels in autoimmune diseases due to depletion of complement by antibody–antigen complexes.
	Normal:
	  C3: Male: 80–180 mg/dL
	      Female: 76–120 mg/dL
	  C4: 15–45 mg/dL
		Fasting is not required.

Coombs' test (direct antiglobulin test)	Detects whether immunoglobulins are attached to RBCs. Normal: negative	Note whether the client is taking ampicillin (Unasyn), captopril (Capoten), indomethacin (Indocin), or insulin, as these cause false-positive results.

*% of total LDH

continued

Table 27-5 ADDITIONAL TESTS PERFORMED ON BLOOD SPECIMEN *continued*

TEST	EXPLANATION/NORMAL VALUES	NURSING RESPONSIBILITIES
Cortisol, hydrocortisone	Determines adrenal cortex function. There is normally a diurnal variation, with higher level around 6 to 8 A.M. and lowest levels around midnight. Normal: 8 A.M.: 6–28 μg/dL, or 170–625 nmol/L 4 P.M.: 2–12 μg/dL, or 80–413 nmol/L	Note whether the client has been under physical or emotional stress as either can artificially elevate plasma cortisol level. Likewise, recent use of radioisotopes can interfere with test results. Note those medications taken that may affect results. Drugs that may increase plasma cortisol level include estrogen, oral contraceptives, and spironolactone (Aldactone). Drugs that may decrease plasma cortisol level include androgens and phenytoin (Dilantin) Explain the procedure to the client. Two specimens are drawn—one at 8 A.M. and another at 4 P.M. Assess the client for physical or emotional stress and report to the physician. Indicate times of collection on laboratory requisitions.
C-reactive protein test (CRP)	An abnormal protein appears in the blood of clients with an acute inflammatory process. Used to monitor the progress of clients with auto-immune disorders such as rheumatoid arthritis. Negative except in pregnancy. More sensitive than erythrocyte sedimentation rate (ESR).	Some labs may require clients to fast, except for water, for 4 to 12 hours prior. Note those mediations that may affect results: nonsteroidal anti-inflammatory drugs (NSAIDs), steroids, and salicylates may decrease level, whereas oral contraceptives and intrauterine devices (IUDs) may increase level. Inform laboratory, if applicable.
Dexamethasone suppression test (DST), prolonged/rapid DST, cortisol suppression test (ACTH suppression test)	Monitors plasma cortisol level to measure adrenal gland function. Normal: nearly 0 cortisol level	Stress can interfere with test results. Note those medications taken that may affect results, including barbiturates, estrogens, oral contraceptives, phenytoin (Dilantin) spironolactone, steroids, and tetracyclines. Explain the procedure to the client. Weigh the client for baseline weight. Rapid test: Administer dexamethasone 1 mg orally at 11 P.M. with milk or antacid. Administer sedative, if ordered. At 8 A.M. before client rises, draw plasma cortisol level. Overnight 8-mg dexamethasone suppression test: If no cortisol suppression occurs, repeat test using 8 mg dexamethasone. If there is still no cortisol suppression, a prolonged test over 6 days involving six 24-hour urine collections should be done.
Electrolytes	Determines blood electrolyte levels. First four are the most commonly measured.	Sodium and potassium are necessary for cardiac electrical conduction.
Sodium (Na⁺)	Measures level of serum sodium. Function in the body: Major electrolyte in extracellular fluid, regulates fluid balance, stimulates conduction of nerve impulses, helps maintain neuromuscular activity. Normal: 135–145 mEq/L	There are no food or fluid restrictions.
Potassium (K⁺)	Measures level of serum potassium. Function in the body: Major electrolyte in intracellular fluid, maintains normal nerve and muscle activity, assists in cellular metabolism of carbohydrates and proteins Normal: 3.5–5.0 mEq/L	There are no food or fluid restrictions. If the client has hypokalemia or hyperkalemia, evaluate the client for cardiac dysrhythmias.
Chloride (Cl⁻)	Measures level of serum chloride Function in the body: Major electrolyte in extracellular fluid, functions in combination with sodium to maintain osmotic pressure, assists in maintaining acid–base balance Normal: 100–110 mEq/L	There are no food or fluid restrictions.

continued

Table 27-5 ADDITIONAL TESTS PERFORMED ON BLOOD SPECIMEN *continued*

TEST	EXPLANATION/NORMAL VALUES	NURSING RESPONSIBILITIES
Electrolytes (*continued*)		
Calcium, total/ionized Ca^{++}	Indicates parathyroid gland function and calcium metabolism. Because ionized calcium is unaffected by serum albumin, it can give more accurate results; however, most laboratories do not have the equipment to perform the test. Normal: Total: 9.0–10.5 mg/dL, or 2.25–2.75 nmol/L Ionized: 4.5–5.6 ng/dL, or 1.05–1.30 nmol/L	Note those medications taken that may affect results. Drugs that may increase serum calcium level include calcium salts, hydralazine, lithium, thiazide diuretics, parathyroid hormone (PTH), thyroid hormone, and vitamin D. Drugs that may decrease serum calcium level include acetazolamide, anticonvulsants, asparaginase, aspirin, calcitonin, cisplatin, corticosteroids, heparin, laxatives, loop diuretics, magnesium salts, and oral contraceptives. Vitamin D and excessive milk ingestion can also interfere with test results. Explain the procedure to the client. Fasting is not required for serum calcium, but might be required if other blood chemistry tests are to be drawn.
Magnesium (Mg^{++})	Measures level of serum magnesium Function in the body: Combines with calcium and phosphorous in intracellular bone tissue, essential for neuromuscular contraction, synthesis of protein, and body temperature regulation Normal: 1.5–2.5 mEq/L	There are no food or fluid restrictions.
Phosphate (PO_4^{--})	Measures level of serum phosphate Function in the body: An essential intracellular electrolyte, exists in an inverse relationship with calcium Normal: 1.8–2.6 mEq/L	Initiate NPO status after midnight. Intravenous fluids containing glucose are sometimes discontinued several hours before the test.
Bicarbonate (HCO_3^-) (total carbon dioxide content or carbon dioxide capacity)	Always in a 20 : 1 ratio with carbonic acid. Normal: 24–30 mEq/L	There are no food or fluid restrictions. Loss of gastric contents is the most common reason for increased level.
ELISA	Screening test used to indicate the presence of HIV Normal: negative	Inform the client that if the first ELISA test is positive, a second ELISA will be drawn before confirmation is done with Western blot. Provide pretest counseling. Obtain informed consent. Provide or arrange for post-test counseling.
Erythrocyte sedimentation rate (ESR or sed rate test)	Measures, in mm, RBC descent in a normal saline solution after 1 hour. Level is increased in inflammatory, infectious, necrotic, or cancerous conditions, due to increased protein content in plasma. Used to monitor the course of therapy for clients with autoimmune diseases, such as rheumatoid arthritis. Normal: Male: 1–13 mm/h Female: 1–20 mm/h	The test should be performed within 3 hours after the blood is drawn. Menstruation or pregnancy may increase level. Ethanbutal, quinine, aspirin, cortisone, and prednisone may alter results.
Folic acid (Folate level)	Measures folic acid level in the blood. Normal: 5–20 ug/mL, or 14–34 mmol/L	Fasting is not required. Instruct the client not to drink any alcoholic beverages before the test. The test is drawn before folic acid medications are administered. Note whether the client is taking phenytoin (Dilantin), primidone (Mysoline), methotrexate, antimalarial agents, or oral contraceptives, as these cause decreased level.

continued

Table 27-5 ADDITIONAL TESTS PERFORMED ON BLOOD SPECIMEN *continued*

TEST	EXPLANATION/NORMAL VALUES	NURSING RESPONSIBILITIES

Follicle-stimulating hormone (FSH)	Determines anterior pituitary function. Usually measured with luteinizing hormone level.
	
	Normal: varies with phase of menstrual cycle
	  Follicular: 5–20 mU/mL
	  Midcycle peak: 15–30 mU/mL
	  Luteal: 5–15 mU/mL
	  Postmenopause: 50–100 mU/mL
	  Male: 5–20 mU/mL
		Note whether client is taking estrogen or progesterone, as these may decrease FSH level. Recent use of radioisotopes can also interfere with test results.
		
		Explain the procedure to the client.
		
		Indicate on the laboratory requisition the date of the last menstrual period (LMP) or that the client is postmenopausal. Indicate use of estrogen or progesterone on laboratory requisition.
		
		The client should be relaxed and recumbent for 30 minutes before the test.

Gamma-glutamyl transpeptidase (GGT or GGTP)	Enzyme that detects liver cell dysfunction.
	Normal:
	
	  Female, < 45 years: 5–27 U/L
	  Female, > 45 years; male: 8–38 U/L
		The client must fast for 8 hours prior to test.
		
		Note those medications taken that interfere with results; alcohol, dilantin, and phenobarbital may elevate results, whereas oral contraceptives and clofibrate may decrease results.

Globulin	Key for antibody production. Indicates how well the liver is functioning. Normal: 2.3–3.3 g/dL	Note those medications taken that affect results (see albumin).
Glucose tolerance test (GTT)	Evaluates blood and urine glucose 30 minutes before, and 1, 2, 3, and 4 hours after a standard glucose load. Normal: blood glucose ≤ 140 mg/dL within 2 h. urine negative for glucose Diabetic: blood glucose 200 mg/dL or greater, 2 hr after a load of 75 g anhydrous glucose	The client must fast (except for water) for 6–8 hours prior to the test. Withhold drugs that interfere with results. After administration of glucose load, withhold all food. The client should drink water, however. Collect urine specimens at hourly periods. Administer meal and medications after test is completed.

Glycosylated hemoglobin (GHb)	Measures glycohemoglobin, evaluating average blood glucose level over 120 days.
	Normal: 4%–8%
	
	  Good control: 7.5% or less
	  Fair control: 7.6%–8.9%
	  Poor control: ≥ 9% or more
		Fasting is not required.
		
		Blood can be drawn at any time.

Growth hormone (GH), human growth hormone (HGH), somatotropin hormone (SH)	Determines the function of the anterior pituitary, although other tests such as the growth stimulation test are more accurate.
	Normal:
	
	  Males: < 5 ng/mL, or < 5 μg/L
	  Female: < 10 ng/mL, or < 10 μg/L
		The client should fast but may have water.
		
		Random measurement of growth hormone is not adequate because the hormone is not secreted constantly.
		
		A radioactive scan within the week; stress; exercise; or decreased blood glucose level can interfere with test results.
		
		Drugs that may increase GH level include amphetamines, arginine, dopamine, estrogens, glucagon, histamine, insulin, levodopa, methyldopa, and nicotinic acid.
		
		Drugs that may decrease GH levels include corticosteroids and phenothiazines.
		
		Explain the procedure to the client.
		
		The client should be well rested and not emotionally or physically stressed.
		
		Additional blood specimens should be obtained during sleeping hours.
		
		Additional information for the laboratory requisition includes fasting time, time of specimen collection, and the client's recent activity.
		
		Because GH half-life is only 20–25 minutes, the specimen should be taken to the laboratory immediately.

continued

Table 27-5 ADDITIONAL TESTS PERFORMED ON BLOOD SPECIMEN *continued*

TEST	EXPLANATION/NORMAL VALUES	NURSING RESPONSIBILITIES
GH stimulation test, GH provocation test, insulin tolerance test (ITT), arginine test	Indicates growth hormone deficiency Normal: > 10 ng/mL, or 10 µg/L	This test is not to be done on a client with epilepsy, cerebrovascular disease, MI, or decreased basal plasma cortisol levels. Explain the procedure to the client and parents. Initiate NPO status after midnight, except for water. To prevent multiple puncture, a heparin lock should be inserted. Baseline GH, cortisol, and glucose levels are done. An injection of insulin or arginine is given. Blood specimens for growth hormone are drawn at 0, 60, and 90 minutes after injection. Blood glucose level is monitored every 15 to 30 minutes. Blood glucose must drop to 40 mg/dL for effectiveness. Monitor client for signs and symptoms of hypoglycemia. This test takes approximately 2 hours. Although the test can be performed by a nurse, a physician should be readily available. If vigorous exercise is used instead of medication, the client should run or stair-climb for 20 minutes. Blood specimens are drawn at 0, 20, and 40 minutes. At the conclusion of the test, the client is given cookies and punch or IV glucose. Blood specimens should be taken to the laboratory immediately after being drawn.
Hepatitis B surface antigen (HB$_s$AG)	A positive result indicates presence of hepatitis or that the person is a carrier. Normal: negative	
Human chorionic gonado-tropin (HCG)	Test for tumor marker; elevated in germ cell testicular cancer. Normal: Male: 0 Female, pregnant: < 5.0 mIU/mL Female, abnormal pregnancy or chorio-carcinoma: > 25 mIU/mL	Apply pressure to the site and observe for bleeding or hematoma.
Human leukocyte antigen DW4 (HLA-DW4)	Positive (present in 50% of clients with rheumatoid arthritis. Normal: negative	Fasting is not required.
Lupus erythematosus test (LE prep)	Positive in 70%–80% of clients with systemic lupus erythematosus. May be positive in clients with rheumatoid arthritis. Used to diagnose and monitor the course of treatment for clients with systemic lupus erythematosus. Normal: negative	Fasting is not required. May be ordered daily for 3 days. Note whether the client is taking Apresoline, Pronestyl, oral contraceptives, quinidine, penicillin, Aldomet, tetracycline, isoniazid, or reserpine, as these may cause false-positive results.
Luteinizing hormone (LH) assay	Determines anterior pituitary function. It can be used to determine whether ovulation has occurred. Can also determine whether gonadal insufficiency is primary or secondary. Normal: Males: 7–24 mU/mL Females: 6–30 mU/mL	Note whether the client is taking estrogen or progesterone, as these may decrease LH level. Recent use of radioisotopes can also interfere with test results. Explain the procedure to the client. Indicate on the laboratory requisition the date of the LMP or that the client is postmenopausal.
Parathyroid hormone (PTH), parathormone	Measures the quantity of PTH to determine hyperparathyroidism or whether hypercalcemia is caused by parathyroid glands. Normal: < 2,000 pg/mL	Recent use of radioisotope can interfere with test results. Explain the procedure to the client. Initiate NPO status after midnight, except for water. Obtain morning blood specimen and indicate time of collection.

continued

Table 27-5 ADDITIONAL TESTS PERFORMED ON BLOOD SPECIMEN *continued*

TEST	EXPLANATION/NORMAL VALUES	NURSING RESPONSIBILITIES
Phosphorus	Determines the level of phosphorus in the blood. Normal: 3.0–4.5 ng/dL, or 0.97–1.45 nmol/L	Laxatives or enemas containing sodium phosphate can increase serum phosphorus level. Note those medications taken that may affect results. Drugs that may increase serum phosphorus level include methicillin and excessive vitamin D. Recent carbohydrate ingestion including IV administration causes decreased serum phosphorus level, as do antacids and mannitol. Explain the procedure to the client. Initiate NPO status after midnight. Discontinue IV fluids containing glucose for several hours before test, if possible.

Plasma renin assay, plasma renin activity (PRA)	Measures the amount of renin and is used as a screening procedure to detect essential or renal hypertension. When combined with plasma aldosterone level, determines adrenal cortex activity.
	Normal:
	  Upright position, sodium depleted or restricted diet:
	    20–39 years: 2.9–24 ng/mL/h
	    > 40 years: 2.9–10.8 ng/mL/h
	  Upright position, sodium repleted or normal diet:
	    20–39 years: 0.1–4.3 ng/mL/h
	    > 40 years: 0.1–3.0 ng/mL/h
		Pregnancy, salt intake, or licorice ingestion can interfere with test results. Time of day (early in the day), a low-salt diet, or an upright position increases renin value.
		Note those medications taken that may interfere with test results, including antihypertensives, diuretics, estrogens, oral contraceptives, and vasodilators.
		Explain the procedure to the client. The client should maintain a normal diet with sodium restricted to 3 grams per day for 3 days before the test. Drugs and licorice should be discontinued for 2 to 4 weeks before the test. The client should stand or sit upright for 2 hours before blood is drawn. Client position, dietary status, time of day, and drugs should be recorded on the laboratory requisition. Blood specimen should be placed in ice and taken immediately to the laboratory. After blood specimen is obtained, the client may resume a normal diet and restart medications.

Polymerase chain reaction (PCR)	Detects HIV-specific DNA (virus). Normal: negative	Explain the meaning of the test. Provide follow-up explanation of test results.
Progesterone assay	Determines ovulation and function of corpus luteum. Adrenal tumors can elevate level. Normal, midcycle: 300–2,400 ng/dL	Recent use of radioisotopes or hemolysis resulting from rough handling of blood specimen can interfere with test results. Note those medications taken that may interfere with test results, including estrogen and progesterone. Explain the procedure to the client. Indicate the date of LMP on the laboratory requisition.

Prolactin level (PRL)	Determines anterior pituitary secretion. Among the problems indicated by an elevated level are pituitary tumors or primary hypothyroidism.
	Normal:
	  Female, or male: 0–20 ng/mL
	  Pregnant: 20–400 ng/mL
		Note those medications taken that may affect results. Drugs that may increase prolactin level include phenothiazines, oral contraceptives, reserpine, opiates, verapamil, histamine antagonists, monoamine oxidase (MAO) inhibitors, and antihistamines. Drugs that may decrease prolactin level include ergot alkaloid derivatives, clonidine, levodopa, and dopamine.
		Explain the procedure to the client.
		The blood specimen should be obtained in the morning and placed on ice if not taken immediately to the laboratory

Prostate-specific antigen (PSA)	PSA is an antigen detected in all males; level increases with prostatic cancer. It is more sensitive and specific than the acid phosphatase. Normal: < 4 ng/mL	Fasting is not required. Apply pressure to the venipuncture site. Observe the site for bleeding.

continued

Table 27-5 ADDITIONAL TESTS PERFORMED ON BLOOD SPECIMEN *continued*

TEST	EXPLANATION/NORMAL VALUES	NURSING RESPONSIBILITIES
Rheumatoid factor (RF)	Abnormal protein in serum of approximately 80% of clients with rheumatoid arthritis. Formed as a result of the reaction of IgM to an abnormal IgG. Also elevated in clients with other autoimmune diseases such as systemic lupus erythematosus. Normal: < 60 IU/mL	Fasting is preferred.
Schilling test	Determines vitamin B_{12} absorption by the intestine. Differentiates between pernicious anemia and gastrointestinal malabsorption problems. Normal: 8%–40% of the radioactive vitamin B_{12} is excreted in the urine within 24 hours.	Collect the urine for a 24- to 48-hour period. Laxatives are not given during the test, as they decrease the absorption of vitamin B_{12}.
Serum acid phosphatase (prostatic)	Serum measurement of prostatic acid phosphatase, elevated in malignancy; because it detects cancer in the later stages, no longer commonly used. Normal: 0.0–0.8 U/L	Apply pressure to the site. Observe the site for bleeding or hematoma.
Serum alkaline phosphatase	Serum measurement of alkaline phosphates, elevated in malignancy. Normal: 30–120 U/L	Apply pressure to the site. Observe the site for bleeding or hematoma.

Serum creatinine	Specific indicator of renal disease.
	Normal:
	    Male: 0.6–1.5 mg/dL
	    Female: 0.6–1.1 mg/dL
		Note those medications taken that may affect results, including amphotericin B, cephalosporins (cepfazolin [Ancef], cephalothin [Keflin]), methicillin, ascorbic acid, barbiturates, lithium carbonate, methyldopa (Aldomet), triamterene (Dyrenium).

Sickledex (sickle-cell test)	Screening test to determine the presence of Hgb S. Normal: no Hbg S If results are positive, a hemoglobin electrophoresis test is done.	There are no food or fluid restrictions. Note on the laboratory requisition whether the client had a blood transfusion in the past 3 to 4 months.
Thyroid-stimulating hormone (TSH), thyrotropin	Determines thyroid function as well as monitors exogenous thyroid replacement. Normal: 2–10 μU/mL, or 2–10 mU/L	Recent use of radioisotopes may affect test results. Severe illness may decrease TSH level. Note those medications taken that may affect results. Drugs that may increase TSH level include antithyroid drugs, lithium, potassium iodide, and TSH injection. Drugs that may decrease TSH level include aspirin, dopamine, heparin, steroids, and T_3. Explain the procedure to the client. The client should be relaxed and recumbent for 30 minutes before the test.
TSH stimulation test	Differentiates between primary and secondary hypothyroidism. Normal: none given	Explain the procedure to the client. Obtain baseline level of radioactive iodine intake or serum T_4. Administer 5–10 units of TSH intramuscularly for 3 days. Repeat radioactive iodine intake or T_4 as indicated for comparison studies.
Thyrotropin-releasing hormone (TRH) test, thyrotropin-releasing factor (TRF) test	Assesses the responsiveness of the anterior pituitary by its secretion of TSH in response to an IV injection of TRH. Also tests the function of the thyroid gland. Normal: undetectable to 15 μU/mL	Pregnancy may increase TSH response to TRH. Note those medications taken that may modify TSH response, including antithyroid drugs, aspirin, corticosteroids, estrogens, levodopa, and T_4. Explain the procedure to the client. Any thyroid preparations should be discontinued for 3–4 weeks before the test.

continued

Table 27-5 ADDITIONAL TESTS PERFORMED ON BLOOD SPECIMEN *continued*

TEST	EXPLANATION/NORMAL VALUES	NURSING RESPONSIBILITIES
Triiodothyronine (T_3) radio-immunoassay (T_3 by RIA)	Determines thyroid gland function Normal: 110–230 ng/dL, or 1.2–1.5 nmol/L	Radioisotope administration may interfere with test results. Pregnancy increases T_3 results. Note those medications taken that may affect results. Drugs that may increase T_3 level include: estrogen, methadone, and oral contraceptives. Drugs that may decrease T_4 level include anabolic steroids, androgens, phenytoin (Dilantin), propranolol (Inderal), reserpine, and salicylates (high dose). Explain the procedure to the client. Determine whether exogenous T_3 is being taken. With physician's approval, withhold those drugs that would interfere with test results.
Triiodothyronine (T_3) serum free	Measures the amount of free T_3 that actually enters the cells and is active in metabolism. A true indicator of thyroid activity. Can be used to diagnose thyroid status in pregnant females or clients on drugs that can interfere with results of other tests. Normal: 0.2–0.6 ng/dL	Explain the procedure to the client. Blood specimens for T_3 and T_4 uptake must be obtained to calculate T_3.
Thyroxine (T_4) Screen	Directly measures the amount of T_4 present. Normal: radioimmunoassay: 5–12 μg/dL, or 65–155 nmol/L	X-ray iodinated contrast studies may increase T_4 levels. Pregnancy will increase T_4 level. Note those medications taken that may affect results. Drugs that may increase T_4 level include clofibrate, estrogens, heroin, methadone, and oral contraceptives. Drugs that may decrease T_4 level include anabolic steroids, androgens, antithyroid drugs, lithium, phenytoin (Dilantin), and propranolol (Inderal). Explain the procedure to the client. Evaluate the client's drug history. If needed, instruct the client to stop exogenous T_4 medications for 1 month prior to test.
Thyroxine index free, FTI, FT_4 Index	Measures the amount of free T_4 that actually enters the cells and is active in metabolism. A true indicator of thyroid activity. Can be used to diagnose thyroid status in pregnant females or clients on drugs that can interfere with results of other tests. Normal: 0.8–2.4 ng/dL, or 10–31 pmol/L	Recent radionuclear scans can interfere with test results. Explain the procedure to the client. Blood specimens for T_4 and T_3 uptake must be obtained to calculate T_4.
Total iron-binding capacity (TIBC)	Determines the ability of iron to bind to a protein called transferrin. Normal: 250–420 ug/dL, or 45–73 umol/L	If possible, initiate NPO status 8 hours prior to the test. A recent blood transfusion or a diet high in iron may affect test results. Note whether the client is taking oral contraceptives, as these increase TIBC level.

Triglycerides	Form of fat produced in the liver.
	Normal:
	  Male: 40–160 mg/dL
	  Female: 35–135 mg/dL
		Instruct the client to fast for 12–14 hours prior to the test, and to have no alcohol for 24 hours before. Dietary intake for 2 weeks prior to the test affects results.

Total protein	Total measure of albumin and globulin. Normal: 6.4–8.3 g/dL	Note medications taken that affect results (see Albumin, this table). Instruct the client to avoid eating foods high in fat for 24 hours before the test.

Uric acid (serum, urine)	Elevated in gout.
	Normal, serum:
	  Male: 2.1–8.5 mg/dL
	  Female: 2.0–6.6 mg/dL
		There are no food or drink restrictions. Note those medications and other substances taken that may affect results, including ascorbic acid, diuretics, levadopa, allopurinol, and Coumadin.

continued

Table 27-5 ADDITIONAL TESTS PERFORMED ON BLOOD SPECIMEN *continued*

TEST	EXPLANATION/NORMAL VALUES	NURSING RESPONSIBILITIES
Uric acid (serum, urine) (*continued*)	Normal, urine: 250–750 mg/24 h	Label container with client's name and date/times of collection. Note those medications and other substances taken that may affect results, including corticosteroids and cytotoxic agents.
VDRL (Venereal Disease Research Laboratories), RPR (rapid plasma reagin), FTA-ABS (fluorescent treponemal antibody-absorption test), Reiter test, fluorescent antibody Treponema pallidum immobilization (TPI) test (performed only at Centers for Disease Control [CDC] in Atlanta)	Blood tests for presence of syphilis. Normal: negative or nonreactive	Explain the test to the client, including amount of blood to be drawn.
Western blot	Confirmatory test for the presence of antibodies to HIV. Normal: negative	Provide pretest counseling. Obtain informed consent. Provide or arrange post-test counseling.

Urine Tests

Urinalysis is performed to assist in the diagnosis of various conditions. Urine specimens are obtained to measure substances such as amylase, catecholamines, chloride, and certain hormones. Substances not normally found in the urine include RBCs, white blood cells (WBCs), protein, glucose, ketones, and casts. Tests often performed on a urine specimen are found in Table 27-6.

Urine pH

The pH is governed by the hydrogen ion concentration in the urine. Disorders such as diabetes mellitus, dehydration, diarrhea, emphysema, and starvation make the urine acidic. Chronic renal failure, renal tubular acidosis, urinary tract infections, and salicylate poisoning cause the urine to be alkaline.

Specific Gravity

Specific gravity measures the number of solutes in a solution. Urea and uric acid (the by–products of nitrogen metabolism) have the greatest influence on the specific gravity of urine. A urinometer and cylinder are used to measure specific gravity (Figure 27-3). The urinometer has a specific gravity scale and a weighted mercury bulb. A fresh urine specimen is poured into the cylinder, then the urinometer is twirled into the cylinder. When the urinometer stops spinning, the urinometer is read at eye level.

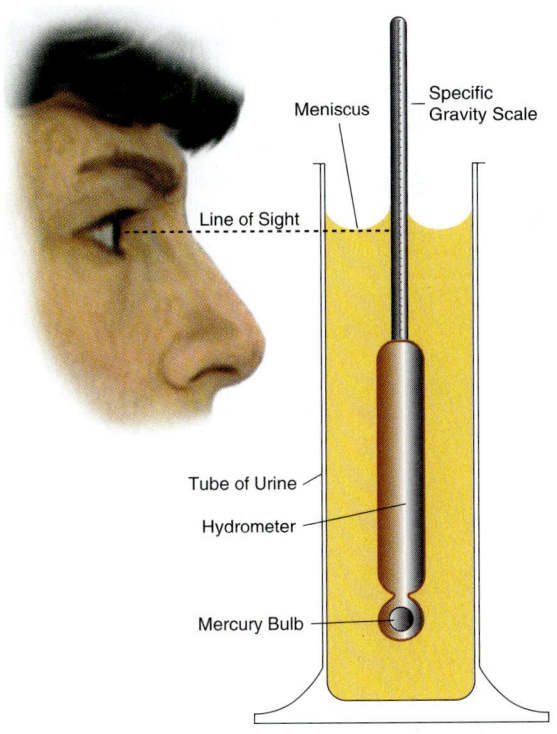

Figure 27-3 Urinometer measures specific gravity.

PROFESSIONAL TIP

Drugs and Laboratory Tests

Note drugs the client is taking when those drugs may influence the results of laboratory tests.

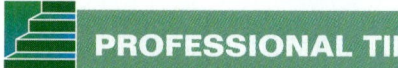

PROFESSIONAL TIP

Testing for Blood Lipid Level
To allow for the proper balance between the vascular and extravascular compartment and ensure valid test results, the blood should always be drawn after the client has been sitting quietly for 5 minutes.

Specific gravity increases with conditions that increase fluid loss from the body. Decreases in specific gravity result from renal disease. When the amount of urine increases and the specific gravity decreases, there is an absence of the antidiuretic hormone (ADH), usually triggered by diabetes insipidus (a disorder of the posterior pituitary gland).

Urine Glucose

When the blood level of glucose exceeds the renal threshold (180 mg/dL), glucose spills into the urine. Many agents are available for measuring the glucose content of urine, although these agents are not as accurate as is measuring the blood glucose level.

Urine Ketones

Ketones, products of incomplete fat metabolism, are completely metabolized by the liver under normal conditions. The most common cause of ketonuria (excessive ketones in the urine) is diabetes.

Urine Cells and Casts

Normally, the urine is free of blood cells and casts. When the renal system is impaired, as in cases of renal damage or failure, nephritis, and urinary stones or infections, the following can occur:

Table 27-6 TESTS PERFORMED ON URINE

TEST	EXPLANATION/NORMAL VALUES	NURSING RESPONSIBILITIES
Urinalysis		Explain the procedure and purpose to the client and assist with specimen collection, if needed.
Color	Clear amber	Ensure that specimen is taken to the laboratory in a timely manner.
Odor	Pleasantly aromatic until left standing; offensive and unpleasant in kidney infection.	
pH	4.6–8.0	
Specific gravity	1.005–1.030	
Glucose	Negative	
Acetone (ketone)	Negative	
Casts	Rare	
Albumin (protein)	Negative	
RBCs	2–3/HPF	
WBCs	4–5/HPF	
Bilirubin	Negative	
Bacteria	Negative	
Aldosterone Assay	A blood test or 24-hour urine collection to evaluate the adrenal cortex, especially for tumors. The 24-hour urine is more reliable, but the blood specimen is more convenient. Normal, blood: Supine: 3–10 ng/dL, or 0.08–0.30 nmol/L Upright: Male: 6–22 ng/dL, or 0.17–0.61 nmol/L Female: 5–30 ng/dL, or 0.14–0.80 nmol/L Normal, urine: 2–80 µg/24 h, or 5.5–72.0 nmol/24 h	Strenuous exercise and stress can increase aldosterone level. Excessive licorice ingestion can decrease aldosterone level. Posture, dietary sodium, and pregnancy can interfere with test results. Note those medications taken that may affect results. Drugs that may increase aldosterone level include diazoxide, hydralazine, and nitroprusside. Drugs that may decrease aldosterone level include fludrocortisone and propranolol (Inderal). Explain the procedure to the client. The client should follow a normal diet with 3 grams of sodium/day and no licorice for at least 2 weeks before the test. Medications should be stopped for at least 2 weeks before the test, if possible. Blood: Blood should be drawn before the client gets out of bed. A second blood specimen might be obtained 4 hours later. Indicate on laboratory requisition time and client position. Transport blood specimen on ice to the laboratory.

continued

Table 27-6 TESTS PERFORMED ON URINE *continued*

TEST	EXPLANATION/NORMAL VALUES	NURSING RESPONSIBILITIES
Aldosterone Assay (*continued*)		24-hour urine: Initiate 24-hour urine collection after discarding first specimen. Post signs with times of collection. Each voiding does not have to be measured. Instruct the client not to contaminate urine with feces or toilet tissue. Force fluids unless medically contraindicated. Collection must be preserved and refrigerated. Indicate times of collection and any drugs that might interfere with results on laboratory requisition. Send collection to laboratory immediately upon conclusion.
Bence Jones Protein	Bence Jones proteins are immunoglobulins typically found in the urine of clients with multiple myeloma. They may also be associated with tumor metastases to the bone and chronic lymphocytic leukemia. Normal: no Bence Jones proteins present in urine.	Instruct the client to collect an early morning urine specimen of at least 50 mL. Instruct the client not to contaminate specimen with toilet paper or stool.

Creatinine clearance	Normal:
	   Male: 95–135 mL/min
	   Female: 85–125 mL/min
	   Minimum: 10 mL/min to maintain life
		Instruct the client about the 24-hour urine test. Encourage hourly water intake. Keep urine on ice or in special refrigerator. Drugs that affect results include phenacetin, anabolic steroids, thiazides, ascorbic acid, levodopa, methyldopa (Aldomet), phenolsulfonphthalein (PSP) (test).

17-hydroxycorticosteroids (17-OHCS)	24-hour urine test that measures adrenal cortex function.
	Normal:
	   Male: 4.5–10.0 mg/24 h
	   Female: 2.5–10.0 mg/24 h
		Emotional or physical stress or licorice ingestion may increase adrenal activity.
		
		Note those medications taken that may affect results. Drugs that may increase 17-OHCS level include acetazolamide, chloral hydrate, chlorpromazine, colchicine, erythromycin, meprobamate, paraldehyde, quinidine, quinine, and spironolactone. Drugs that may decrease 17-OHCS level include estrogens, oral contraceptives, phenothiazines, and reserpine.
		
		Explain the procedure to the client.
		
		Initiate 24-hour urine collection after discarding first specimen. Post signs with times of collection. Each voiding does not have to be measured. Instruct the client not to contaminate urine with feces or toilet tissue. Force fluids unless medically contraindicated. Collection must be refrigerated. Indicate on laboratory requisition times of collection and any drugs that might interfere with results. Send collection to laboratory immediately upon conclusion.

17-ketosteroids (17-KS)	24-hour urine test that measures adrenal cortex function.
	Normal:
	   Male: 7–25 mg/24 h, or 24–88 μmol/24 h
	   Female: 4–15 mg/24 h, or 14–52 μmol/24 h
		Stress may increase adrenal activity.
		
		Note medications taken that may affect results. Drugs that increase 17-KS level include antibiotics, chloramphenicol, chlorpromazine, dexamethasone, meprobamate, phenothiazines, quinidine, secobarbital, and spironolactone. Drugs that may decrease 17-KS level include estrogen, oral contraceptives, probenecid, promazine, reserpine, salicylates (prolonged use), and thiazide diuretics.
		
		Explain the procedure to the client. With physician's approval, withhold all drugs for several days before test. Monitor client for stress and report to physician.
		
		Initiate 24-hour urine collection after discarding first specimen. Post signs with times of collection. Each voiding does not have to be measured. Instruct the client not to contaminate urine with feces or toilet tissue. Force fluids

continued

Table 27-6 TESTS PERFORMED ON URINE *continued*

TEST	EXPLANATION/NORMAL VALUES	NURSING RESPONSIBILITIES
17-ketosteroids (17-KS) (*continued*)		unless medically contraindicated. Collection must be preserved and refrigerated. Indicate on laboratory requisition times of collection and any drugs that might interfere with results. Send collection to laboratory immediately upon conclusion.
Urine cortisol, hydrocortisone	24-hour urine test that measures adrenal cortex function. Normal: 10–100 μg/24 h, or 27–276 nmol/24 h	Pregnancy or stress increases cortisol level. Recent radioisotope scans can interfere with test result. Note medications taken that may interfere with test result, including oral contraceptives and spironolactone. Explain the procedure to the client. Assess for stress and report to physician. Initiate 24-hour urine collection after discarding first specimen. Post signs with times of collection. Each voiding does not have to be measured. Instruct the client not to contaminate urine with feces or toilet tissue. Force fluids unless medically contraindicated. Collection must be preserved and refrigerated. Indicate on laboratory requisition times of collection and any drugs that might interfere with results. Send collection to laboratory immediately upon conclusion.
Vanillylmandelic acid (VMA) and catecholamines (epinephrine, norepinephrine, metanephrine, normetanephrine, dopamine)	24-hour urine test that diagnoses pheochromocytoma and other adrenal tumors. Normal: VMA: 2–7 mg/24 h, or 10–35 μmol/24 h Epinephrine: 0.5–20.0 μg/24 h, or < 275 nmol/24 h Norepinephrine: 15–80 μg/24 h Metanephrine: 24–96 μg/24 h Normetanephrine: 75–375 μg/24 h Dopamine: 65–400 μg/24 h	Certain foods (e.g., tea, coffee, cocoa, vanilla, chocolate), vigorous exercise, stress, or starvation may increase VMA level. Uremia, alkaline urine, or iodinated contrast dyes may falsely decrease VMA level. Note those medications taken that may affect results. Drugs that may increase VMA level include caffeine, epinephrine, levodopa, lithium, and nitroglycerine. Drugs that may decrease VMA level include clonidine, disulfiram (Antabuse), guanethidine, imipramine, MAO inhibitors, phenothiazines, and reserpine. Drugs that may increase catecholamine level include ethyl alcohol, aminophylline, caffeine, chloral hydrate, clonidine (chronic therapy), contrast media (iodine containing), disulfiram (Antabuse), epinephrine, erythromycin, insulin, methenamine, methyldopa, nicotinic acid (large doses), nitroglycerin, quinidine, riboflavin, and tetracyclines. Drugs that may decrease catecholamine level include guanethidine, reserpine, and salicylates. Explain the procedure to the client. The client should be on a VMA-restricted diet for 2–3 days before the test. Items restricted include coffee, tea, bananas, chocolate, cocoa, licorice, citrus fruit, anything with vanilla, and aspirin. Client should not take antihypertensive drugs before the test. Initiate 24-hour urine collection after discarding first specimen. Post signs with times of collection. Each voiding does not have to be measured. Instruct the client not to contaminate urine with feces or toilet tissue. Collection may need to be preserved (consult laboratory) and is to be refrigerated. Indicate times of collection and any drugs that might interfere with results.

- Bleeding, resulting in RBCs in the urine
- Accumulation of epithelial cells accompanied by cast formation
- WBCs in the urine, which indicate infection

Stool Tests

Stool specimens are collected for examination of both normal substances (such as urobilinogen) and blood, bacteria, and parasites (Table 27-7).

Urobilinogen

Urobilinogen is a colorless derivative of bilirubin formed by the normal bacterial action of intestinal flora on bilirubin. It increases in the presence of severe hemolysis and decreases in the presence of most biliary obstructions.

Occult Blood

Occult blood is invisible on inspection; it is blood in the stool that can be detected only with a microscope or by chemical means. In the gastrointestinal tract, the digestive process acts on blood, making it occult. Random sampling for occult blood is done to diagnose gastrointestinal bleeding, ulcers, and malignant tumors.

To decrease the possibility of a false-positive result when occult blood is to be used to confirm suspicions of a gastrointestinal disorder, the client is placed on a 3-day diet free of meat, poultry, and fish. Common drugs that can cause a false-positive test for occult blood are salicylate, steroids, and indomethacin.

Parasites

The gastrointestinal tract can harbor parasites and their eggs (ova). Whereas some of these parasites are harmless, others cause clinical symptoms. With the exception of pinworms (which can enter the body through both the oral and anal routes), most common parasites enter the body through the mouth when contaminated water or food is ingested.

PROFESSIONAL TIP

Cultures

All culture tests should be performed before initiating antibiotic therapy so as to identify the type of pathogen and its sensitivity to specific antibiotics.

Culture and Sensitivity Tests

Culture refers to the growing of microorganisms to identify the pathogen. Culture and **sensitivity** (C&S) tests are performed to identify both the nature of the invading organism and its susceptibility to commonly used antibiotics. Sensitivity allows the practitioner to select the appropriate antibiotic therapy. All C&S specimens should be taken immediately to the laboratory.

Blood Culture

Bacteremia is bacteria in the blood. The blood culture should be obtained while the client is experiencing chills and fever. A series of three venipuncture collections are performed using strict sterile technique. The needle should be changed after the specimen is collected and before injecting the blood sample into the test tube.

Throat (Swab) Culture

The throat normally hosts many organisms. Throat cultures serve to isolate and identify such pathogens as beta-hemolytic streptococci, *Staphylococcus aureus,* meningococci, gonococci, *Bordetella pertussis,* and *Corynebacterium diphtheria.* A throat swab is commonly done to identify streptococcal infections, which, if left untreated, can cause rheumatic fever or glomerulonephritis.

To obtain a throat swab, the nurse uses a wooden blade to depress the tongue and swabs the white patches, exudate, or ulcerations of the throat using a

Table 27-7 TESTS PERFORMED ON STOOL

TEST	EXPLANATION/NORMAL VALUES	NURSING RESPONSIBILITIES
Stool occult blood (guaiac) Fecal occult blood test (FOBT) Hemocult	Fecal occult blood screening studies may be utilized as possible indicators of colorectal cancer. Normal: negative for blood	Place a smear of stool on a card. Medications such as anticoagulants, aspirin, iron preparations, NSAIDs, and steroids may cause a false-positive result, whereas vitamin C may cause a false negative. Red meat should not be ingested for 3 days prior to the test. Wear gloves when obtaining and handling the specimen.
Stool O & P (ova & parasite)	A positive result indicates infection. Normal: negative	Place the stool specimen in a container and take warm to the laboratory.

sterile applicator. The applicator should not touch any other parts of the mouth. Once the swab is obtained, the applicator should be placed in a sterile container.

Sputum Culture

Sputum tests performed include culture, smear, and cytology. Sputum is created by the mucous glands and goblet cells of the tracheobronchial tree and is raised by coughing. Sputum is sterile until it reaches the throat and mouth, where it comes in contact with normal flora. To yield a more accurate identification of pulmonary organisms, sputum can be obtained by tracheobronchial suctioning and transtracheal aspiration.

In addition to the same organism(s) found in a culture, a sputum smear identifies eosinophils, epithelial cells, and other substances. Smears are helpful in diagnosing asthma (eosinophils) and fungal infections. The specimen must be refrigerated if it cannot be taken immediately to the laboratory.

Sputum **cytology** (the study of cells) is performed to diagnose cancer of the lungs. The specimen should be collected early in the morning and after a deep cough.

Urine Culture

Urinary C&S tests are performed whenever a urinary tract infection is suspected.

Stool Culture

Stool C&S is performed to identify bacterial infections. If the client has diarrhea, a rectal swab can be taken and used as a specimen. Fecal material must be visible on the swab in order for the laboratory to perform the test.

Papanicolaou Test

The **Papanicolaou test** (a smear method of examining stained exfoliative cells), commonly called a Pap smear, is performed to evaluate the cellular maturity, metabolic activity, and morphological variations of cervical tissue. Papanicolaou testing can also be done on specimens from other organs, such as bronchial aspirations and gastric secretions.

LIFE CYCLE CONSIDERATIONS

Pap Smear

Cervical Pap smear testing is recommended every 2 to 3 years after the onset of sexual activity. Annual testing is indicated for those women who:

- Are over 40 years of age,
- Have a family history of cervical cancer, and/or
- Previously had a positive Pap smear.

CLIENT TEACHING

Pap Smear

Advise female clients to prepare for a Pap smear by:

- Avoiding intercourse, douches, and vaginal creams for 24 hours before the test and
- Informing the practitioners if they are menstruating, as the test will need to be delayed.

RADIOLOGICAL STUDIES

Radiography (the study of film exposed to x-rays or gamma rays through the action of ionizing radiation) is used by the practitioner to study internal organ structure. When used in conjunction with a **contrast medium** (a radiopaque substance that facilitates roentgen imaging of the body's internal structures), **fluoroscopy** (immediate, serial images of the body's structure and function) reveals the motion of organs. X-rays are valuable to the practitioner in either formulating a diagnosis or helping to determine the necessity for other studies (e.g., a lung lesion requiring biopsy to differentiate between a benign or malignant tumor).

Certain radiological tests require a contrast medium that might interfere with other diagnostic studies. Barium and iodine are commonly used contrast media. Laboratory blood samples measuring thyroid function should be drawn before initiating an intravenous pyelogram (IVP), where radioactive iodine dye is administered. If the client needs both an IVP and a barium enema, the IVP is performed first because the barium is likely to decrease visualization of the kidneys. Commonly performed radiological studies are described in Table 27-8.

Safety: X-rays
- Prior to scheduling x-rays, question the client about the possibility of pregnancy, asthma, and allergic reactions to contrast media (iodine) as well as to other foods and drugs.
- If the client has not previously received iodine, note this on the requisition to indicate that allergic status is unknown.

PROFESSIONAL TIP

Contrast Media

Carefully monitor those clients who are scheduled for dye injection studies and have a history of allergies to any foods or drugs (particularly fish or iodine), because such allergies may predispose these clients to allergic reactions to contrast media.

Table 27-8 RADIOLOGIC STUDIES

TEST	EXPLANATION/NORMAL VALUES	NURSING RESPONSIBILITIES
Radiograph (x-ray)	Most common diagnostic study. Identifies traumatic disorders, i.e., fractures, dislocations, tumors, bone disorders, joint deformities, bone density, and changes in bone relationships. Performed by a technician.	Explain the procedure to the client. Prepare the client as ordered. No specific post procedure care is required. Administer an analgesic, especially for the arthritic client.
Abdominal x-rays	Determines diaphragm position and gas and fluid distribution in the abdomen.	No preparation is required.
Adrenal angiography, Adrenal arteriogram	Study of adrenal glands and arterial system after injection of radiopaque dye to detect benign or malignant tumors or hyperplasia of the adrenal glands. Normal: no growth or enlargement	Assess for allergy to shellfish or iodine; arteriosclerosis; pregnancy; or blood disorders, as they preclude the test. Explain the procedure to the client. Assess for allergies. Informed and written consent must be obtained before the procedure. Note whether client has been taking anticoagulants. Initiate NPO status after midnight. Mark peripheral pulses with a pen before the procedure. Inform the client that a warm flush may be felt when the dye is injected. Observe the puncture site. Monitor vital signs. Monitor peripheral pulses, color, and temperature of extremities. Institute bed rest for 12–24 hours. Apply cold compresses to puncture site, if needed. Force fluids to prevent possible dehydration from the dye.
Adrenal venography	Involves insertion of a catheter through the femoral vein and into the adrenal vein to withdraw a blood specimen to detect the function of each adrenal gland. A contrast dye is injected to visualize size and position of the adrenal glands. Normal: no growth or enlargement	Explain the procedure to the client. Assess for allergies. Obtain informed and written consent. Inform the client that a burning sensation may be experienced when the dye is injected. Although this study involves the venous system, monitor vital signs and injection site as well as pulses, temperature, and color of extremities.
Arthrogram (-graphy)	Visualization of a joint. Radiopaque dye or air is injected into the joint cavity to outline soft tissue, usually on knee/shoulder joints. Local anesthetic and sterile technique are used. Performed by a physician; takes approximately 30 minutes.	Explain the procedure to the client. Obtain informed consent. Client wears an elastic bandage for several days; check for edema. Administer a mild analgesic for pain. Monitor for increased pain. Neither fasting nor sedation is required.
Barium enema	An enema of barium is given while x-rays are taken of the large intestine.	Initiate NPO status the night before. Administer the ordered medication to clean the bowel. Observe the results of the laxatives, and inform the x-ray department if there have been no results. After the test, force oral fluids and administer a cleansing enema, as ordered. Document status of abdomen and stools.
Barium swallow	The client drinks a glass of barium while x-rays are taken of the esophagus and cardiac sphincter.	Initiate NPO status the evening before. Explain the procedure and the time frame for results. Encourage the client to drink fluids and eat fiber after the test. A laxative is sometimes given after the test. The client should be instructed that bowel movements will be white for 1–2 days. During the test, the client will be tilted on the x-ray table in various positions. There may be repeated pictures taken at ½-hour intervals as the barium moves through the bowel. Document the client's tolerance of the procedure and passage of the barium. Because the procedure can be lengthy, encourage the client to take reading material.
Cardiac catheterization (cardiac angiogram, coronary arteriogram)	A catheter is passed into the right and/or left side of the heart to determine oxygen level, cardiac output, and pressure within the heart chambers.	Assess the client for allergy to iodine or shellfish. The client is to fast for 6 hours prior to the test, but medications can be taken with sips of water. Inform the client of the possibility of feeling warm or flushed during the test. *continued*

Table 27-8 RADIOLOGIC STUDIES *continued*

TEST	EXPLANATION/NORMAL VALUES	NURSING RESPONSIBILITIES
Cardiac catheterization (*continued*)		After the procedure, assess the peripheral pulses every 15 minutes for 2–4 hours, or according to physician's orders. Assess color, temperature, and pulse in the extremity below the catheter insertion site. Instruct the client to keep the involved extremity straight for 6–8 hours.
Chest x-ray	Provides a two-dimensional image of the lungs without using contrast media. Used to detect the presence of fluid within the interstitial lung tissue or the alveoli; tumors or foreign bodies; and the presence and size of a pneumothorax. The size of the heart can also be determined by chest x-ray.	Explain the test to the client. If appropriate, inquire whether the client may be pregnant, to prevent exposure of the fetus to x-ray. The client is generally required to stand for various views; if the client is unable to stand, views may be obtained with the client in a sitting position, or a portable x-ray may be obtained. Instruct the client to inspire deeply and hold the breath. Instruct the client to remove all metal objects from the chest and neck area and to don a hospital gown that does not have snap closures.
Conduitogram	Radiopaque dye is injected through a catheter into either the conduit or a piece of ileum to assess by means of x-ray the length and emptying ability of the conduit as well as the presence of stricture or obstruction.	A conduit is a connection between the bladder or pouch and the outside of the body. Explain the procedure to the client. Assess the client for allergies to iodine-based dye.
Fistula gram	Radiopaque dye or barium is given to drink, and x-rays are taken as the dye or barium passes through the gastrointestinal tract. The dye shows the location of the fistula and how it is connected to the gastrointestinal tract.	Initiate NPO status as ordered. Explain the procedure and the time frame for the results and identify the person who will give the client the results.
Fluoresce in angiography	Following IV injection of sodium fluorescein, rapid-sequence photographs of the fundus are taken with a special camera. Visualization of microvascular structures of the retina and choroid are enhanced, allowing evaluation of the entire retinal vascular bed.	Instill eye drops to dilate the pupils. Start an IV so the sodium fluorescein can be injected. Remove the IV following completion of the test. Inform the client that skin and urine may be yellow for 24–48 hours.
Gallbladder series	X-ray visualization of the gallbladder.	Administer dye tablets the evening before the test. Provide a low-fat or fat-free meal the evening before. Initiate NPO status except for water after taking the dye.
Hysterosalpingogram	Radiopaque dye is instilled through the cervix. Used to diagnose uterine cavity and tubal abnormalities. Performed as a part of an infertility workup.	Explain the procedure and prepare the client in the lithotomy position. The test is done in the radiology department. Inquire about allergies to iodine or other dyes. Assist the physician.
Intravenous pyelogram (IVP)	Infusion of radiopaque dye into a vein, allowing visualization of the urinary system. The renal pelvis, ureters, and bladder can be seen.	Explain the procedure to the client. Explain that client will experience a warm feeling during dye injection. Ask the client about allergy to iodine or shellfish. Serve a light supper, then initiate NPO status overnight. Administer a laxative or enema. Schedule test before barium studies. Post-test, observe for untoward reaction to dye. Encourage fluids for 24 hours to eliminate dye.
Kidney-ureter-bladder x-ray (KUB)	Shows abnormalities such as calculi, tumors, or changes in anatomic position.	Explain the procedure to the client. No preparation is required.
Long bone x-rays	Serial x-rays of the long bones to determine bone growth.	Explain the procedure to the client. Instruct the client to keep extremities still while the x-ray is being taken. Shield ovaries, testes, or pregnant uterus. Remove all metallic objects from area being x-rayed.

continued

Table 27-8 RADIOLOGIC STUDIES *continued*

TEST	EXPLANATION/NORMAL VALUES	NURSING RESPONSIBILITIES
Lymphangiogram	A contrast dye is injected into the lymph vessels in the hands or feet to examine the lymph vessels and nodes. Used to stage lymphomas and evaluate the effectiveness of chemotherapy and radiation therapy. Normal: Normal-sized lymph nodes with no malignant cells	The dye remains in the lymph nodes for 6 months to 1 year, so disease progress can be evaluated with an x-ray. Obtain informed consent. Inform the client that if a blue-colored dye is used, the skin and urine may have a bluish discoloration. Assess the client's breath sounds after the procedure, as lipoid pneumonia is a possible complication if the dye gets into the thoracic duct.
Mammography	Used to diagnose benign and malignant disorders of the breast.	Explain the procedure to the client. The breast will be compressed, possibly causing discomfort for several seconds. Explain that it is important to have a baseline mammogram done between the ages of 35 and 40 and a breast examination done by a physician or nurse practitioner every 3–4 years. For women ages 40–49, a mammogram should be performed every 1–2 years; for those over 50, an annual mammogram is recommended along with an annual breast examination by physician or nurse practitioner.
Myelogram	X-ray of spinal subarachnoid space following injection of an opaque medium.	Follow nursing responsibilities for lumbar puncture in Table 27-14. Inform the client that the table may be tilted during the procedure. Obtain informed consent according to facility guidelines. Withhold the meal prior to procedure. Administer a light sedative, if ordered. Postprocedure care is determined by the type of medium used; follow physician's orders for activity and fluids.
Pouchogram	Installation of radiopaque dye into the Kock or Indiana pouch. Done with the continent ostomies to determine the state of healing and size of the pouch created.	Assess the client for allergy to iodine. Explain the procedure to the client.
Pulmonary angiography	Assesses the arterial circulation of the lungs. Most often used to detect pulmonary emboli.	Explain the procedure to the client. Assess for allergy to iodine or shellfish. Inform the client that an arterial puncture is required, usually of the femoral artery, and that injection of the dye may cause a flushing or warm sensation due to vasodilation. After the study, assess the arterial puncture site frequently for evidence of bleeding. Assess vital signs and respiratory status. The client may be required to lie flat for up to 6 hours if the femoral artery is used for access. Obtain informed consent per facility policy.
Renal angiography	A catheter is inserted into the femoral artery and threaded into the renal artery. Dye is injected to show blood vessels in the kidney.	Initiate NPO status; administer enema. Assess client for allergy to iodine or shellfish. Check vital signs and peripheral pulses. Institute post-test bedrest, with leg straight. Monitor vital signs, peripheral pulses, urine output, and puncture site.
Voiding cystrourethrography	The bladder is filled with dye, and x-rays are taken to observe bladder filling and emptying. Detects structural abnormalities of the bladder and urethra and reflux into the ureters.	Administer enema. Insert a Foley catheter and inject dye into bladder while x-rays are taken. Remove catheter and ask the client to void while more x-rays are taken. Allow the client to express feelings, as this test may be embarrassing.

continued

Table 27-8 RADIOLOGIC STUDIES *continued*

TEST	EXPLANATION/NORMAL VALUES	NURSING RESPONSIBILITIES
Computed tomography (CT) scan	Provides a three-dimensional cross sectional view of tissues. Computer-constructed picture interprets densities of various tissues. Most useful for viewing tumors in the chest, abdominal cavity, and brain.	Explain the procedure to the client. Obtain informed consent. Remove wigs and hairpins and clips for head CT. Initiate NPO status 8 hours prior to scan. Assess for iodine allergy. Observe for signs of anaphylaxis, if dye is used. Check for claustrophobia. Inform the client that the test will take approximately 45 minutes to 1 hour. The client must lie still on a hard, flat table and will be put through a large machine. Because barium will interfere with the test, schedule tests using barium either after or 4 or more days before the scan.
Cardiac positron emission tomography (PET) scan	Radioactive tracers are injected intravenously prior to the test. Nuclear imaging is used to confirm tissue that has adequate blood supply and tissue that has become impaired due to a lack of blood.	Instruct the client not to have caffeine for 18 hours and not to smoke for 4 hours prior to the test. Initiate NPO status from 10 P.M. the evening before the test, except for medications and water. Obtain informed written consent. Encourage the client to drink fluids after the procedure to facilitate faster excretion of the radioactive material.
Orbital CT scan	Allows visualization of abnormalities not readily seen on standard x-rays, delineating size, position, and relationship to adjoining structures. The orbital CT is a series of images reconstructed by a computer and displayed as anatomic slices on an oscilloscope. It identifies space-occupying lesions earlier and more accurately than do other x-ray techniques. It also provides three-dimensional images of orbital structures, especially the ocular muscles and optic nerve. Enhancement with a contrast agent may help define ocular tissue and circulation abnormalities.	Explain the test and the procedure to the client: that the client is positioned on an x-ray table; that the head of the table is moved into the scanner; that the scanner rotates during the test and may make loud, crackling sounds; that if an IV contrast agent is required, the client may feel flushed and warm or experience a transient headache; and that salty taste, nausea, and vomiting may occur following injection of the IV contrast dye. Reassure the client that the reaction is common and she may signal the technician if she is unable to tolerate the test.

Chest X-Ray

The most common radiological study is the noninvasive, noncontrasted chest x-ray. Radiographic projections of chest x-ray films are taken from various views (Figure 27-4), because the practitioner needs multiple views of the chest to assess the entire lung field. To prepare for a chest x-ray, the client should remove all clothing from the waist up and don a gown. The client should also remove all metal objects (jewelry), as metal will appear on the x-ray film, thereby obscuring visualization of parts of the chest. Pregnant women are advised against x-rays; however if x-ray is absolutely necessary, the woman should be draped with a lead apron to protect the fetus.

Computed Tomography

Computed tomography (CT) is the radiological scanning of the body. X-ray beams and radiation detectors transmit data to a computer that transcribes the data into quantitative measurement and multidimensional images of the internal structures. Figure 27-5 illustrates the sagittal, transverse, and coronal planes used in CT scanning.

The procedure requires the client's informed consent. Because the client will be positioned on the scanning table and told to remain motionless, the client's cooperation is essential during the CT scanning. The nurse should prepare the client by providing an explanation and pictures of what to expect.

Safety: Contrast Media

If a contrast medium is used, observe the client for indicators of allergic reaction to the dye, such as respiratory distress, urticaria, hives, nausea, vomiting, decreased production of urine (**oliguria**), and decreased blood pressure.

PROFESSIONAL TIP

Computed Tomography

Assess the client's ability to relax, and review imagery relaxation. Sedation can be administered with an order from the practitioner.

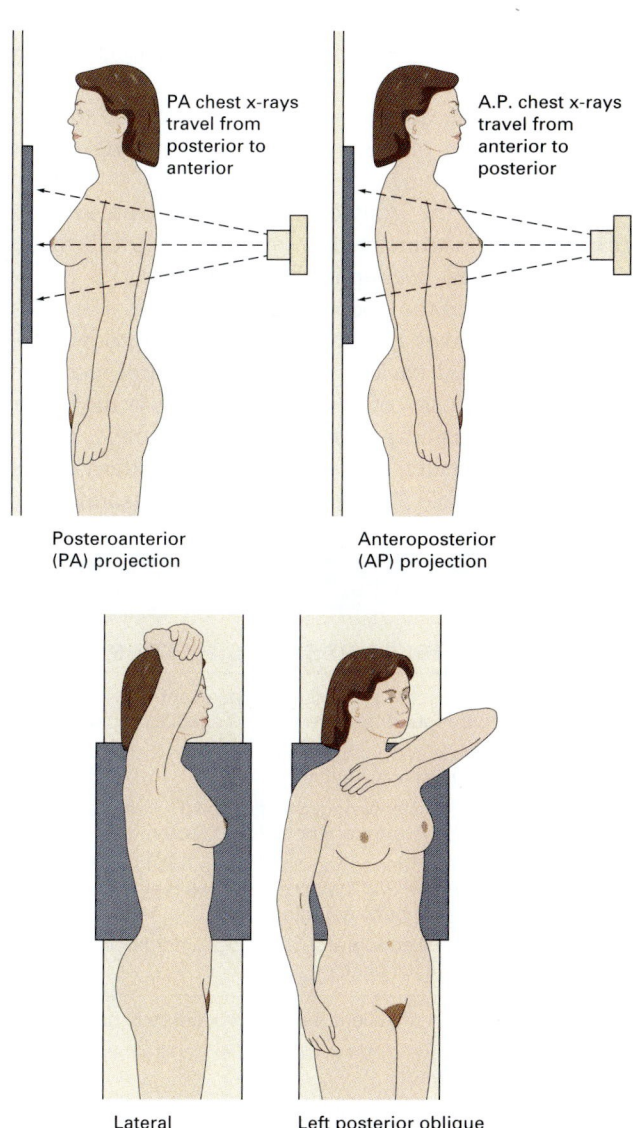

Figure 27-4 Radiographic Projection Positions

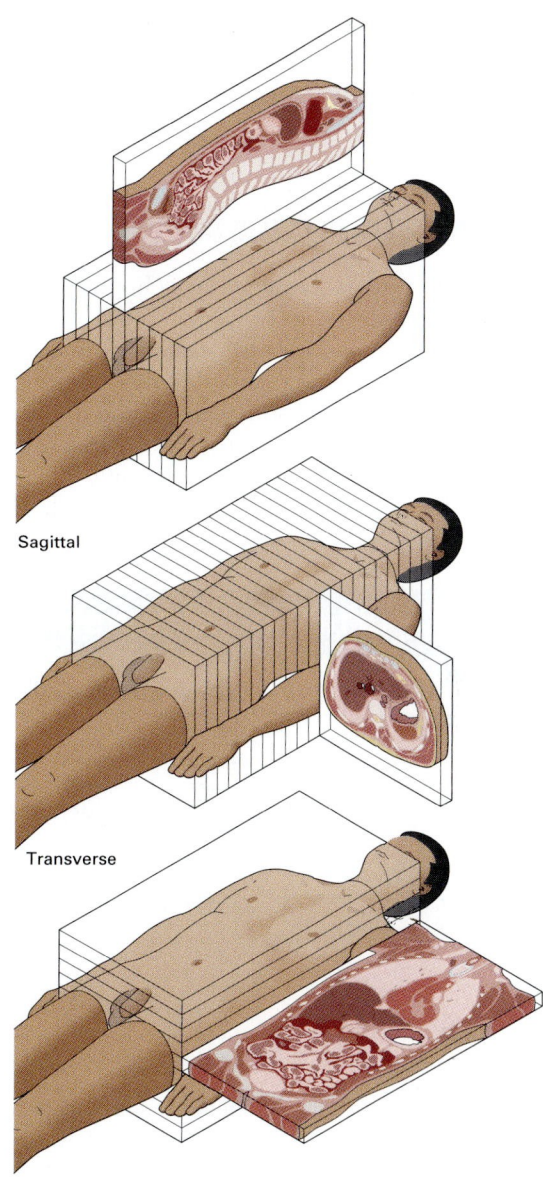

Figure 27-5 Computed Tomography

Barium Studies

Barium (a chalky white contrast medium) is a preparation that permits roentgenographic visualization of the internal structures of the digestive tract. The results of barium studies can reveal congenital abnormalities, lesions, spasm, reflux, stricture, obstruction, inflammation, ulceration, varices, and fistula.

Angiography

Angiography allows visualization of the vascular structures through the use of fluoroscopy in conjunction with a contrast medium. The test reveals the blood flow to the heart, lungs, brain, kidneys, and lower extremities. It is also useful in diagnosing an **aneurysm** (weakness in the wall of a blood vessel).

Arteriography

Arteriography is the radiographic study of the vascular system following injection of a radiopaque dye through a catheter. The practitioner uses fluoroscopy to thread the catheter through a peripheral artery and into the area to be studied, such as the aorta or the cerebral, coronary, pulmonary, renal, iliac, femoral, or popliteal artery. The client is placed on a cardiac monitor. Dye is injected through the vascular catheter, and a rapid sequence of films is taken to visualize the vasculature.

Dye Injection Studies

Iodine is a common dye used in radiographic studies. Iodine injection might cause the client to experience the following temporary symptoms: shortness of breath; nausea; and a warm to hot flushed sensation. Most dye injections studies are invasive and thus require written consent.

ULTRASONOGRAPHY

An **ultrasound,** also called an echogram or sonogram, is a noninvasive procedure that uses high-frequency sound waves to visualize deep body structures. To ensure accuracy, this procedure should be scheduled before any studies requiring the use of a contrast medium or air, because the contrast medium would reflect the sound waves differently than body structures do. The client is instructed to lie still during the procedure.

Ultrasound is used to evaluate the brain, thyroid gland, heart, vascular structures, abdominal aorta, spleen, liver, gallbladder, pancreas, and pelvis. An ultrasound is commonly done during pregnancy to evaluate the size of the fetus and placenta. A full bladder is needed to ensure visualization.

To increase the contact between the skin and the **transducer** (instrument that converts electrical energy to sound waves), a coupling agent (lubricant) is placed on the surface of the body area to be studied. The transducer emits waves that travel through the body tissue and are reflected back to the transducer and recorded. The varying density of body tissues deflects the waves into a differentiated pattern on an oscilloscope. Photographs can be taken of the sound wave pattern on the oscilloscope. Table 27-9 describes some ultrasound tests.

Table 27-9 ULTRASOUND TESTS

TEST	EXPLANATION/NORMAL VALUES	NURSING RESPONSIBILITIES
Ultrasound	High-frequency ultrasound waves are sent into the body, and echoes are recorded as they strike tissues of different densities, producing an image or photograph. Useful in distinguishing between cystic and solid masses. Most often used to assess the pelvis, heart, and abdomen. Diagnostic for cysts, tumors, pregnancy, fetal gestational age, and multiple gestation.	Explain the procedure to the client. Most ultrasound tests require no special preparation: Pelvic sonogram: Instruct the client to have a full bladder. Abdominal sonogram: Initiate NPO status at bedtime; prepare bowel as directed. Gallbladder sonogram: Initiate NPO status for 12 hours and institute a fat-free diet the evening before the test. Vaginal sonogram: Client does not need to have a full bladder.
Doppler ultrasound	Determines patency of veins and arteries in conditions such as arterial occlusive disease, arteriosclerotic disease, or Raynaud's disease. Normal: audible "swishing" sound of the Doppler when placed over vessel A Doppler unit with blood pressure cuffs can measure the pulse volume of arteries and veins. An AB index is obtained by dividing the blood pressure reading in the ankle by the blood pressure reading in the arm (brachial artery). This is known as the ankle-to-brachial arterial blood pressure. There should be a less than 20 mm Hg difference between the pressure in the lower extremity as compared to the pressure in the upper extremity. Normal, AB index: 0.85 or greater	Inform the client that the procedure is painless. Remove clothing from the extremity being evaluated. Instruct the client not to smoke for 30 minutes prior to the test, because nicotine causes vasoconstriction of the vessels. Remove conductive or acoustic gel from the skin after the test is completed.
Echocardiogram	An ultrasound of the heart to determine hypertrophies, cardiomyopathies, or congenital defects. Very helpful in diagnosing valve abnormalities and pericardial effusion.	Explain the procedure to the client and assure the client that there is no discomfort during the procedure, although some pressure may be felt on the chest wall from the transducer.
Thyroid ultrasound	Detects the size, shape, and position of the thyroid gland.	Explain the procedure to the client: that the client will lie supine, with the neck hyperextended; that breathing or swallowing will not be affected by the sound transducer; that a liberal amount of lubricating gel will be placed on the neck for the transducer; and that a series of photos will be taken over a 15-minute period. Assist the client in removing the lubricant.
Transrectal bladder ultrasound	Produces an image of the prostate or bladder and surrounding tissue.	Explain the procedure to the client.

Table 27-10 MAGNETIC RESONANCE IMAGING

TEST	EXPLANATION/NORMAL VALUES	NURSING RESPONSIBILITIES
Magnetic resonance imaging (MRI)	Uses magnetic field and radio waves to detect edema, hemorrhage, blood flow, infarcts, tumors, infections, aneurysms, demyelinating disease, muscular disease, skeletal abnormalities, intervertebral disk problems, and causes of spinal cord compression. Provides greater tissue discrimination than do chest x-ray or CT scans. Performed by qualified technologist. Takes approximately 1 hour.	Assess the client for the presence of metal objects within the body (i.e., shrapnel, cochlear implants, pacemakers). Explain the procedure to the client: that the client will be required to lie still for up to 20 minutes at a time; that the client will be placed within a scanning tunnel; that sedation may be required if the client has claustrophobic tendencies; that the magnet will make a loud thumping noise as images are obtained (provide earplugs as necessary). As the test may require up to 2 hours to perform, have the client void prior to entering the scanning tunnel. Obtain informed written consent, per facility policy.

MAGNETIC RESONANCE IMAGING

Magnetic resonance imaging (MRI) uses radiowaves and a strong magnetic field to make continuous cross-sectional images of the body. A noniodine IV paramagnetic contrast agent may be used during the study. The study reveals lesions and changes in the body's organs, tissues, and vascular and skeletal structures (Table 27-10).

RADIOACTIVE STUDIES

Radionuclide imaging (nuclear scanning) uses radionuclides (or radiopharmaceuticals) to image the morphological and functional changes in the body's structure. A scintigraphic scanner is placed over the area of study to detect emitted radiation and produce a visual image of the structure on film. Radiopharmaceutical agents are administered by various routes, with consideration given to time delays of absorption. The results reveal congenital abnormalities, lesions, skeletal changes, infections, and glandular and organ enlargement (Table 27-11).

Table 27-11 RADIOACTIVE STUDIES

TEST	EXPLANATION/NORMAL VALUES	NURSING RESPONSIBILITIES
Scan (radioisotope test)	A radioactive substance or isotope is taken up by the part of the body being examined. Organ sites most frequently studied are the liver, spleen, lungs, heart, urinary tract, thyroid, and brain. The radioactive substance is given orally or intravenously by nuclear medicine personnel.	Explain the procedure to the client: that the client must lie still for 30–60 minutes and that the machine makes clicking noise at times. For liver, spleen, lung, thyroid, and brain scans, no special preparation is required. For a heart scan, initiate NPO status the evening before. For a kidney scan, hydrate as ordered.
Brain scan	A radioactive agent is injected into a vein and allowed to circulate to the brain; the brain is then scanned in successive layers and a picture composite of the structures developed. Useful in identifying structural lesions, whether vascular or tumors.	No food or fluid restrictions. The test takes approximately 2 hours. Obtain informed consent according to facility guidelines. Explain that the client may experience a hot feeling when dye is injected. Assess for allergies, especially to iodine or shellfish. Administer a light sedative, if ordered.
Radioactive iodine uptake, (RAIU), iodine uptake test, ^{131}I uptake	Uses oral radioactive iodine to determine thyroid function by the thyroid's ability to trap and retain iodine. Normal: 2 hours: 4%–12% absorbed 6 hours: 6%–15% absorbed 24 hours: 8%–30% absorbed	The client who is allergic to iodine or shellfish or is pregnant should not have the test. Exogenous iodine preparations or recent x-ray studies using iodinated contrast material will decrease thyroid gland uptake. *continued*

Table 27-11 RADIOACTIVE STUDIES continued

TEST	EXPLANATION/NORMAL VALUES	NURSING RESPONSIBILITIES
Radioactive iodine uptake, (continued)		Note those medications taken that may affect results. Drugs that may increase RAIU level include barbiturates, estrogen, lithium, phenothiazines, and TSH. Drugs that may decrease RAIU level include ACTH, antihistamines, saturated solution of potassium iodine, thyroid drugs, antithyroid drugs, and tolbutamide.
Radionuclide angiography (multiplegated radioisotope scan, multigated acquisition scanning, MUGA)	A radioisotope is injected to evaluate the function of the left ventricle. The ejection fraction (a comparison of the volume of blood pumped by the left ventricle to the total volume of blood left in the ventricle) is measured.	Obtain informed written consent per agency policy.
Renal scan	Uses radioactive material (gallium 67) to show blood flow in the kidneys.	Check policy on disposal of client's urine for first 24 hours. Pregnant nurses should not care for clients undergoing this test because of the associated radiation.
Technetium pyrophosphate scanning	Important in diagnosing acute MIs, with the best accuracy obtained at 48 hours after the client experiences symptoms suggestive of an infarct. A tracer or radioisotope, which is injected intravenously, accumulates in the damaged or infarcted tissue areas, called hot spots.	Instruct the client not to smoke or consume caffeine or alcohol for 3 hours before the test. Inform the client that the test will take 45–60 minutes.
Thyroid scan, thyroid scintiscan	Uses a radioactive substance to visualize the size, shape, position, and function of the thyroid gland. Normal: no growth or enlargement	Assess for allergy to iodine or shellfish and for pregnant. Recent exposure to iodine-containing foods or x-ray iodinated contrast agents can interfere with test results. Drugs that can interfere with test results include cough medicines, multiple vitamins, some oral contraceptives, and thyroid drugs. Explain the procedure to the client. Certain drugs may have to be restricted for weeks before the test. Obtain a history concerning previous contrast x-ray studies, nuclear scans, or intake of thyroid-suppressive or antithyroid drugs. Fasting is usually not required. The scan may be taken 2 hours or 24 hours after oral ingestion of the radioactive substance. The client should be instructed to remove all jewelry, metal objects, and dentures before the scan. The scan takes approximately 30 minutes. Neither isolation nor specific urine precautions are necessary.
Ventilation-perfusion scan	Assesses ventilation and perfusion of the lungs. Most often used to detect the presence of pulmonary emboli.	Assess for allergy to iodine and shellfish. Explain the procedure to the client: that a radioactive contrast media will be introduced via an IV access and inhalation of radioactive gas and that the client will be required to hold the breath for short periods as images are obtained. Obtain informed written consent per facility policy.

ELECTRODIAGNOSTIC STUDIES

Electrodiagnostic tests use devices to measure the electrical activity of the heart, brain, and skeletal muscles. Electrical sensors (electrodes) are placed at certain anatomic points to measure the tone, velocity, and direction of the impulses. The impulses are then transmitted to an oscilloscope or printed on graphic paper. Table 27-12 describes the various electrodiagnostic studies.

Electrocardiography

An **electrocardiogram** (ECG or EKG) is a graphic recording of the heart's electrical activity. The client may be asked not to smoke or drink caffeinated beverages

Table 27-12 ELECTRODIAGNOSTIC STUDIES

TEST	EXPLANATION/NORMAL VALUES	NURSING RESPONSIBILITIES
Electrocardiogram (ECG or EKG)	Electrodes are placed on the skin to record wave patterns of the electrical conduction of the heart. Detects myocardial damage, rhythmic disturbances, and hyperkalemia.	Explain the procedure to the client. Inform the client that the test is painless.
Electroencephalogram (EEG)	Record of electrical activity generated in the brain and obtained through electrodes applied to the scalp or microelectrodes placed in brain tissue during surgery.	Withhold caffeine due to stimulant effect. Serve meal so that blood sugar will not be altered. Explain the procedure to the client: that the test takes approximately 45 minutes to 2 hours; that electrical shock will not occur; that the procedure is painless and that there are no after effects; that the client may be asked to open and close the eyes during the test and that there may be flashing lights or small electrical stimulations.
Electromyography (EMG)	Detects primary muscular disorders. A needle electrode is inserted into the muscle being examined. Measures electrical activity of skeletal muscle at rest and during voluntary muscle contraction.	Explain the procedure to the client. Obtain informed written consent. Instruct the client to refrain from consuming caffeine and smoking for 3 hours before the test. Assure client that the needle will not cause electrocution. Inform the client that there will be temporary discomfort when the needle electrode is inserted. Observe the site for hematoma or inflammation after the test. The procedure takes approximately 1 hour.
Electroretinogram (ERG)	A record of the changes in the retina's electric potential following stimulation by light. Clinically useful in some clients with retinal disease. Performed by placing a contact lens electrode on the anesthetized cornea. The electrical potential recorded on the cornea is identical to the response that would be obtained if the electrodes were placed directly on the surface of the retina.	Explain the test and procedure to the client.
Esophageal motility studies (manometry)	Evaluates muscle contractions and coordination by using a tube with transducers. Used as a diagnostic tool for disorders of the esophagus and lower esophageal sphincter (LES).	Initiate NPO status 6–8 hours prior to the test.
Holter monitor	A portable EKG monitors and records the electrical conduction of the heart for a period of 24 hours. The heart rhythm is compared to client activities.	Instruct the client to engage in normal daily activities and to keep a journal of symptoms experienced in performing these activities.
Stress test	An EKG taken as the client exercises. Evaluates the effects of exercise on the heart. Often, the client is asked to walk on a treadmill, the incline of which is elevated at various times throughout the test. Used frequently on clients who have CAD.	Explain the procedure to the client. Encourage the client to wear good walking shoes during the test.
Thallium test (myocardial perfusion scan)	A radioactive tracer (Thallium[201]) is injected and accumulates in myocardial tissue that is well perfused. Accumulation is lessened in areas of myocardial tissue that are not well perfused, areas called "cold spots." The client may be asked to perform exercise, such as riding a bike, during the test to evaluate the perfusion of myocardial tissue during exercise.	Instruct the client to refrain from eating and drinking for 3 hours prior to the test.

for 24 hours before the test, as nicotine and caffeine can affect heart rate.

Electrodes are applied to the chest wall and extremities. A lubricating gel applied to the electrodes increases the conduction of electrical activity between the skin and electrodes. The client is instructed to lie still during the pain-free test. The test can reveal abnormal transmission of impulses and electrical position of the heart's axis.

A portable cardiac monitor (Holter monitor) is a device that records the heart's electrical activity. It produces a continuous recording over a specified time (e.g., 24 hours). The portable unit allows the client to ambulate and perform regular activities. Clients are instructed to maintain a log of those activities that result in the heart beating faster or irregularly. The practitioner reviews the ECG tracing in relation to the client's log to determine whether certain activities, such as walking, are associated with abnormal transmission of impulses.

Stress Test

A **stress test** measures the client's cardiovascular fitness. It demonstrates the ability of the myocardium to respond to increased oxygen requirements (the result of exercise) by increasing the blood flow to the coronary arteries.

The client is connected to an ECG machine and asked to walk on a treadmill. Continuous ECG recordings are made of the client's heart response (rate, electrical activity, and cardiac recovery time) to frequent changes in the treadmill's speed and slope. The test is stopped immediately if the client experiences any symptoms of decreased cardiac output (chest pain, dyspnea, fatigue, or ischemic changes revealed by the ECG monitor).

Thallium Test

Thallium[201] is a radioactive isotope that emits gamma rays and closely resembles potassium. Although a radioactive study, the thallium test is discussed here because it is often performed in conjunction with an ECG. Thallium is rapidly absorbed by normal myocardial tissue but is slowly absorbed by areas with poor blood flow and damaged cells. During the test, thallium is administered intravenously and the scanner detects the radiation and makes a visual image. The light areas on the image represent heavy isotope uptake (normal myocardial tissue), whereas the dark areas represent poor isotope uptake (poor blood flow and damaged cells).

There are two types of thallium test: resting imaging and stress imaging. Resting imaging can detect a myocardial infarction within its first few hours. Stress imaging (thallium stress test) is performed while the client is on a treadmill and being monitored with an ECG. At peak stress, the IV thallium is injected. Scanning is performed 3 to 5 minutes postinjection and again in 2 to 3 hours. The test is stopped immediately if the client becomes symptomatic for ischemia.

Electroencephalography

An **electroencephalogram** (EEG) is the graphic recording of the brain's electrical activity. During the procedure, electrodes are placed on the client's scalp. The electrodes transmit impulses from the brain to an EEG machine. The machine amplifies the brain's impulses and makes a recording of the waves on strips of paper. An EEG can reveal not only the presence of a seizure disorder or intracranial lesion, but also the type. The absence of the brain's electrical activity is used to confirm death.

ENDOSCOPY

Endoscopy is the visualization of a body organ or cavity through a scope. An endoscope (a metal or fiberoptic tube) is inserted directly into the body structure to be studied (Figure 27-6). A light and, in some studies, a camera at the end of the scope allow the practitioner to assess, via direct visualization or television picture, for lesions and structural problems. The endoscope has an opening at the distant tip that allows the practitioner to administer an anesthetic agent and to lavage, suction, and biopsy tissue. Common endoscopic procedures are listed in Table 27-13.

After the procedure, the nurse must monitor vital signs, observe for bleeding, and assess for procedural risks (e.g., return of the gag and swallowing reflexes following a bronchoscopy performed under local anesthesia).

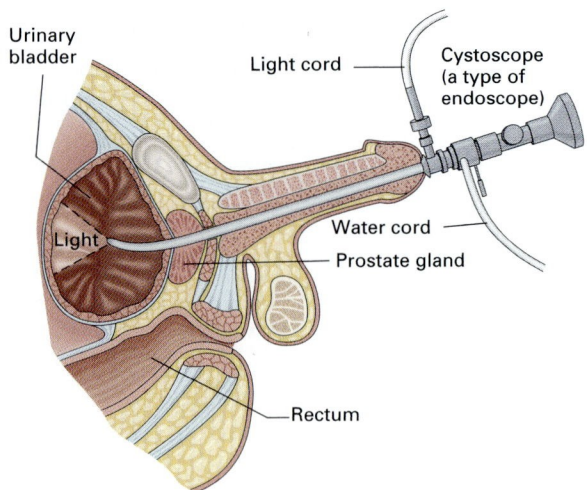

Figure 27-6 Cystoscope

Table 27-13 ENDOSCOPIC PROCEDURES

TEST	EXPLANATION/NORMAL VALUES	NURSING RESPONSIBILITIES
Endoscopy	Permits visual examination of internal structures of the body using specially designed instruments. The observation may be done through a natural body opening or through a small incision. A biopsy of suspicious areas may then be done for further study.	Explain the procedure to the client. Initiate NPO status 8–10 hours before test, except for sigmoidoscopy, before which a liquid diet should be followed for several days prior to the examination. Administer a laxative and then a cleansing enema.
Arthroscopy	Endoscopic procedure for direct visualization of a joint. Done in an operating room under sterile conditions and local or general anesthesia.	Perform frequent neurovascular checks. Elevate the client's leg. Apply compression dressing. Administer analgesic for discomfort.
Bronchoscopy	Direct visual examination of the bronchi through a fiber optic scope. Used to remove foreign bodies, for aggressive pulmonary cleansing, and to obtain sputum and tissue specimens.	Explain the procedure to the client: that the client must be NPO for at least 6 hours prior to the test; that, if ordered, preprocedure sedation is administered; that an IV access will be obtained and sedation given during the procedure via this route. Following the procedure, frequently assess vital signs and respiratory status. Assess the client for unusual amounts of bleeding. Inform the client that sputum may be blood tinged initially following the procedure. Maintain the client in a side-lying position until the gag reflex returns. Withhold all food and fluids until the client is fully awake and has a gag reflex. Obtain written informed consent per facility policy.
Colonoscopy	Examination of the rectum, colon, cecum, and ileocecal valve.	Initiate sedation. Cleanse the bowel. Offer only clear liquids after cleansing. Initiate NPO status for 6–8 hours prior to the test. Inform the client that flatulence and cramping will be experienced after the test.
Cystoscopy	A cystoscope is passed through the urethra and into the bladder to examine the interior of the bladder for inflammation, stones, tumors, or congenital abnormalities. A biopsy may be performed, and small stones may be removed. Ureteral catheters may be inserted to obtain urine from each kidney. May require topical, spinal or general anaesthesia.	Explain the procedure to the client. Obtain informed written consent. Check vital signs. Instruct in deep breathing, if general anesthesia is to be used. Allow a full liquid diet if topical anesthetic is to be used. Monitor I&O.
Endoscopic retrograde cholangiopancreatogram (ERCP)	Examination of the common bile duct (CBD) and biliary and pancreatic systems following injection of dye. Sphincterotomy, stone crushing, and stone removal can be done.	Initiate sedation. X-ray is used in conjunction. Initiate NPO status 6–8 hours prior to examination. Schedule PT, PTT, and bleeding time tests prior to this examination. Inform the client that the test can last up to 2 hours.
Esophagogastro-duodenoscopy (EGD)	Examination of the esophagus, stomach, and duodenum. Biopsies can be taken, and dilations done.	Initiate sedation. Initiate NPO status 6–8 hours prior to the examination.
Flexible sigmoidoscopy	Examination of the sigmoid colon and rectum.	Sedation is optional. Administer enemas prior to examination. Inform the client to expect some flatulence and cramping after the examination.
Laparoscopy	Examination of the internal pelvic structures by direct visualization with a laparoscope. Usually performed under general anesthesia. Diagnostic for pelvic disorders and infertility problems.	Explain the procedure to the client. Prepare the client, conduct pre- and postoperative assessment, and institute interventions. Provide discharge instructions on activity and follow-up.

ASPIRATION/BIOPSY

Aspiration is performed to withdraw fluid that has abnormally collected or to obtain a specimen. To minimize client discomfort when the skin is pierced by the needle, a local anesthetic is administered in the area to be studied.

A stylet with an outer, hollow-bore needle is used to pierce the skin. Once the needle is in place, the stylet is withdrawn, leaving only the outer needle to aspirate the fluid. A **biopsy** (excision of a small amount of tissue) can be obtained during aspiration or in conjunction with other diagnostic tests (e.g., bronchoscopy).

Table 27-14 outlines various aspiration/biopsy procedures.

Amniocentesis

Amniocentesis is the withdrawal of amniotic fluid to obtain a sample for examination. This test is indicated when:

- Maternal age exceeds 35,
- A spontaneous abortion has occurred with a previous pregnancy, and/or
- There is a family history of genetic, chromosomal, or neural tube defects.

Amniocentesis is performed when the amniotic fluid volume reaches 150 mL, usually at approximately the 16th week of pregnancy.

There are no fluid or food restrictions. The procedure usually lasts 10 to 15 minutes. The woman should be instructed to void to eliminate the risk of puncturing a full bladder. An ultrasound is performed first to identify the positions of the fetus and placenta.

The client is positioned supine, and the fetal heart tones are assessed. The abdomen is prepped and injected with lidocaine hydrochloride (a local anesthetic agent). The practitioner withdraws 10 to 20 mL of amniotic fluid by transabdominal needle aspiration and puts the fluid in a sterile, brown bottle. The nurse monitors the client's vital signs and the fetal heart tones and assesses for signs of labor. The client is instructed to notify the practitioner of any signs of labor or infection.

Bone Marrow Aspiration/Biopsy

The sternum and iliac crest are common sites for bone marrow puncture. During a bone marrow puncture, a fluid specimen (aspiration) or a core of marrow cells (biopsy) can be obtained. Both tests are commonly done concurrently to obtain the best possible marrow specimen. The test can reveal anemias; cancers such as leukemia, multiple myeloma, or Hodgkin's disease; or the client's response to chemotherapy.

Client positioning is determined by the site to be used, supine for the sternum and side lying for the iliac crest. The site is prepped to decrease the skin's normal flora in the area to be punctured. The nurse should explain to the client that pressure may be experienced as the specimen is withdrawn. The client should not move when the specimen is being withdrawn, as a sudden movement may dislodge the needle.

After the procedure, the client should be kept on bed rest for 1 hour. The nurse should monitor vital signs to assess for bleeding (rapid pulse rate, low blood pressure), and the client instructed to report to the practitioner any bleeding or signs of inflammation.

LIFE CYCLE CONSIDERATIONS

Aspiration

Restrain infants and small children during aspiration by holding them throughout the procedure.

Paracentesis

Paracentesis is the aspiration of fluid from the abdominal cavity. This test can be diagnostic, therapeutic, or both. With end-stage liver or renal disease, for instance, **ascites** (an accumulation of fluid in the abdomen) occurs. Pressure caused by the ascites can interfere with breathing and gastrointestinal functioning. Aspiration in this instance is therapeutic. If a culture specimen is taken, it is also diagnostic.

The client should be instructed to void and the nurse should weigh the client before the procedure. The client should be placed in a high-Fowler's position in a chair or sitting on the side of the bed. The skin is prepped, anesthetized, and punctured with a **trocar** (a sharply pointed surgical instrument contained in a cannula). The trocar is held perpendicular to the abdominal wall and advanced into the peritoneal cavity. When fluid appears, the trocar is removed, leaving the inner catheter in place to drain the fluid. The client's vital signs are observed for changes resulting from the rapid removal of fluid.

After the procedure, a sterile dressing is applied to the puncture site, and the client monitored for changes in vital signs and electrolytes. The nurse should instruct the client to record the color, amount, and consistency of drainage on the dressing after discharge.

Thoracentesis

Thoracentesis is the aspiration of fluids from the pleural cavity. The pleural cavity normally contains a small amount of fluid to lubricate the lining between the lungs and pleura. Infection, inflammation, and trauma may cause an increased production of fluid, which can impair ventilation.

To facilitate access to the rib cage, the client should be positioned with the arms crossed and resting on a bedside table (Figure 27-7). The nurse should instruct the client not to cough during insertion of the trocar. The practitioner selects, preps, and anesthetizes the puncture site. The trocar is usually inserted into the intercostal space at the location of maximum dullness to percussion. The site should be above the ninth rib posteriorly and above the seventh rib laterally.

During the procedure the client must be carefully monitored for symptoms of a **pneumothorax** (collection of air or gas in the pleural space, causing the lungs to collapse), such as dyspnea, pallor, tachycardia,

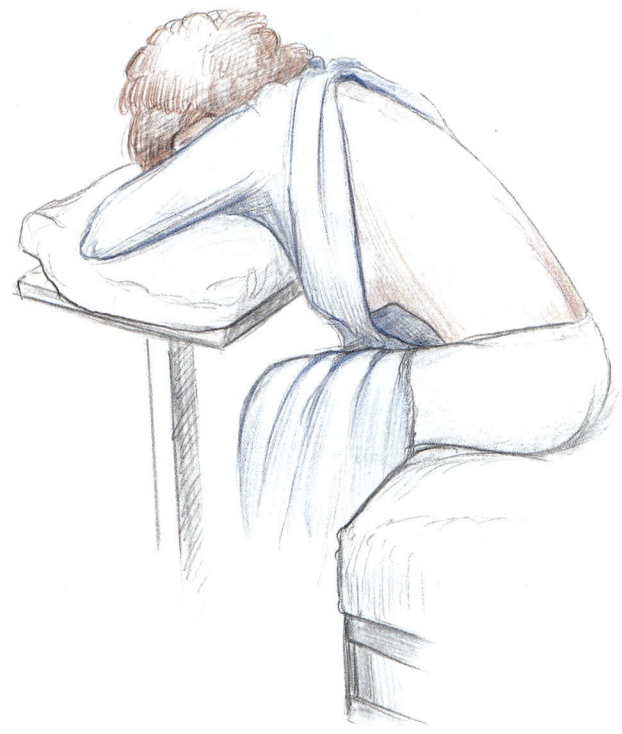

Figure 27-7 Client Position for Thoracentesis

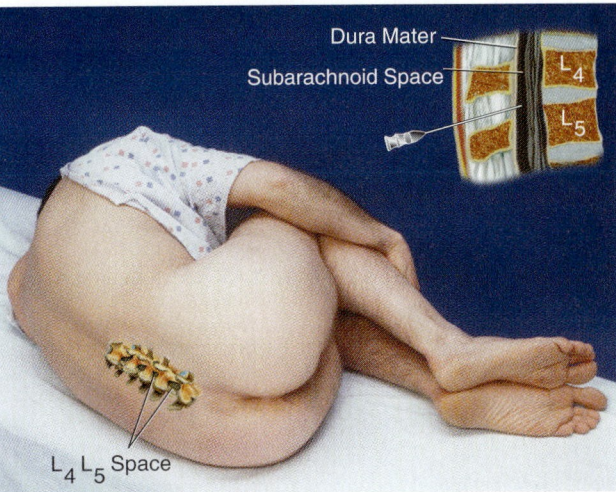

Figure 27-8 Lumbar puncture: Position of client and insertion of the needle into the subarachnoid space are shown.

vertigo, and chest pain. After the procedure, the nurse assesses for signs of cardiopulmonary changes and a mediastinum shift, as indicated by bloody sputum and changes in vital signs.

Cerebrospinal Fluid Aspiration

Lumbar puncture ("spinal tap") is the aspiration of cerebrospinal fluid (CSF) from the subarachnoid space. The specimen is examined for organisms, blood, and tumor cells. A spinal tap is also performed:

- To obtain a pressure measurement when blockage is suspected,
- During a myelogram, or
- To instill medications (anesthetics, antibiotics, or chemotherapeutic agents).

The client assumes a lateral recumbent position, with the craniospinal axis parallel to the floor, the flat of the back perpendicular to the procedure table. The client should assume a flexed knee–chest position to bow the back, thereby separating the vertebrae. Most clients require assistance in maintaining this position throughout the procedure. To do so, the nurse stands facing the client and places one hand across the client's shoulder blades and the other hand over the client's buttocks.

The practitioner selects, preps, and anesthetizes the puncture site (usually interspace L3–L4, L4–L5, or

L5–S1). The needle and stylet are inserted into the midsagittal space and advanced through the longitudinal subarachnoid space (Figure 27-8).

Once in the subarachnoid space, the stylet is removed, leaving the needle in place. An initial CSF pressure reading is taken. If the pressure reading is greater than 200 mm H_2O or falls quickly, only 1 or 2 mL of CSF is withdrawn for analysis. If the pressure is less than 200 mm H_2O, an adequate specimen is withdrawn slowly.

After the pressure reading is taken, the stopcock is turned to allow the CSF to slowly flow into a sterile test tube. A sterile cap is placed on the test tube, and the sample is taken to the laboratory for analysis. Rapid withdrawal of CSF can cause a transient postural headache. The client's cardiorespiratory status is monitored throughout the procedure (Noe & Rock, 1994).

OTHER TESTS

Other diagnostic tests are described in Table 27-15.

PROFESSIONAL TIP

CSF Pressure

The client should remain relaxed and quiet during the initial pressure reading, because straining increases CSF pressure.

After the procedure, pressure is applied to the puncture site, followed by a sterile bandage to prevent leakage of CSF. The client's neurological and cardiorespiratory statuses are then assessed. A postural headache is the most common complication of a lumbar puncture.

Table 27-14 ASPIRATION/BIOPSY PROCEDURES

TEST	EXPLANATION/NORMAL VALUES	NURSING RESPONSIBILITIES
Aspiration Procedures		
Arthrocentesis	Procedure to obtain fluid from a joint using strict sterile technique. The knee is anesthetized, the sterile needle is inserted into joint space, and synovial fluid is aspirated. Used to diagnose infections, crystal-induced arthritis, and synovitis, and to inject anti-inflammatory medications. Performed by physician. Takes approximately 10 minutes.	Explain the procedure to the client. Obtain informed consent. Assess site for edema, pain. The client should fast if possible. Apply pressure dressing and ice.
Bone marrow aspiration	Evaluates how well the bone marrow is producing RBCs, WBCs, and platelets. Normal: adequate numbers of RBCs, WBCs, and platelets.	Inform the client that pressure will be felt when the physician aspirates the bone marrow. Assess the site for bleeding after the procedure is completed. Institute bed rest for at least 30 minutes after the test.
Gastric analysis, tube and tubeless test	Determines the amount of hydrochloric (HCl) acid in the stomach. If no HCl acid is present, that indicates parietal cells are malfunctioning. Parietal cells secrete the intrinsic factor that is essential for vitamin B_{12} absorption. Used to diagnose pernicious anemia. Normal tube test: Basal acid output: 2–5 mEq/h Maximal acid output 10–20 mEq/h Normal, tubeless test: presence of dye in urine (usually blue or blue-green in color)	If the client is having the tube test, initiate NPO status after midnight and instruct the client not to smoke prior to the test. Inform the client that a nasogastric tube is inserted prior to the test so that gastric contents can be aspirated after the administration of pentagastrin. If the client is having the tubeless test, inform the client of the possibility of a blue or blue-green discoloration of urine. Note any medications taken that affect results; antacids, anticholinergics, and cimetidine (Tagamet) decrease HCl level, whereas adrenergic-blocking agents, cholinergics, steroids, and alcohol elevate HCl level.
Lumbar puncture (LP)	A needle is inserted into the subarachnoid space to measure CSF pressure and/or to obtain a specimen. Normal pressure: 60–180 mm water pressure Normal specific gravity: 1.007 Normal glucose: 60–80 mg/100 mL Normal complete blood count (CBC): 0 Normal WBC: 0–5 cells/mm^3	Obtain informed written consent. Have the client empty the bowel and bladder prior to procedure. Position the client in the dorsal recumbent position on the side of bed of physician's choice. Place the hips at the edge of the bed, client's back to the physician. Assist in setting up a sterile field and pouring solutions, if not included in the tray. Assist the client to maintain the position. Postprocedure, deliver the specimen to the lab for testing, keep the client flat in bed for 3–24 hours or as ordered by physician; encourage fluid intake to replace fluids lost; and monitor vital and neurological signs.
Peritoneal aspiration	Fluid is withdrawn from the abdominal cavity by inserting a needle into the abdomen. The specimen in analyzed for infection or bleeding.	Have the client empty the bladder prior to the procedure. Prepare the abdomen by scrubbing it with a surgical prep solution and draping it with a sterile drape. Post procedure, dress the site with a sterile dressing and monitor the site for further drainage. Assess vital signs one time post procedure.
Perciardiocentesis	Fluid is removed from the pericardial sac for analysis or to relieve pressure.	Inform the client that the procedure will be done under a local anesthetic and that pressure may be felt when the needle is inserted. Position the client in the semi-Fowler's position during the procedure and attach to an EKG monitor. Postprocedure, take vital signs every 15 minutes and monitor EKG rhythm.
Thoracentesis	Removal of fluid for diagnostic purposes. May also obtain biopsy, instill medications, and remove fluid for client comfort and safety.	Explain the procedure to the client. Obtain informed consent. Position the client in an upright sitting position, leaning forward.

continued

Table 27-14 ASPIRATION/BIOPSY PROCEDURES *continued*

TEST	EXPLANATION/NORMAL VALUES	NURSING RESPONSIBILITIES
Thoracentesis (*continued*)		Have client rest the arms on an overbed table to facilitate this position. Explain to the client that the area will be anesthetized prior to the procedure. Instruct the client to hold as still as possible during the insertion of the thoracentesis needle. Assist the physician during the procedure. Deliver the specimen to the laboratory as soon as possible. Observe the thoracentesis site for bleeding following the procedure. Assess breath sounds before and after the procedure. Report absent breath sounds immediately.
Biopsy	Removal of sample tissue for microscopic study. Tissue may be quickly frozen or placed in formalin before it is chemically stained and thinly sliced for analysis. Frozen section analysis takes only a few minutes and is often completed while a client is still in surgery. The full biopsy analysis takes 24–48 hours to complete but is the most accurate means of establishing a cancer diagnosis. Tissue biopsy is essential to confirming the type of cancer, the amount of lymph node involvement, and whether the cancer was successfully removed.	Explain the procedure to the client. Follow the physician's orders and/or agency protocol for client preparation. Obtain informed written consent.
Breast biopsy	Performed with or without local or general anesthesia and by aspiration, needle biopsy, excision, or incision. Tissue or fluid is obtained and sent to pathology for examination and identification of abnormal cells. New method of obtaining breast biopsies may be done with the stereotactic mammography studies.	Explain the procedure to the client. Have the client undress down to the waist. Cleanse the biopsy region and shave the area, if needed. Drape the breast and adjacent skin. Provide emotional support prior to, during, and following the procedure. Monitor vital signs. Apply a sterile dressing or bandage. Instruct the client in post-biopsy wound care.
Cardiac biopsy	Done during a cardiac catheterization. The tissue sample is taken from the apex or septum to determine toxicity related to drugs; inflammation; or rejection of a transplanted heart.	Preparation is the same as for Cardiac Catheterization (refer back to Table 27-8). After the procedure, observe the client for symptoms of a perforation, such as chest pain, decreased blood pressure, or dyspnea.
Endometrial biopsy	Obtained with special biopsy instruments and used to diagnose endometrial tissue abnormalities.	Explain the procedure to the client. Prepare the tissue preservation agent and label and send the sample to pathology. Assist the client in relaxing during the procedure, to offset the discomfort/cramping she may experience.
Liver biopsy	Obtained by inserting a needle into the liver. May be done with ultrasound or CT scan to guide needle placement. Evaluates cirrhosis, cancer, and hepatitis.	Schedule H&H, PT, PTT, and platelet tests prior to the procedure. Instruct the client to refrain from using NSAIDs including aspirin for 1 week prior to the procedure. Prepare the site by scrubbing it with a surgical prep solution and draping with a sterile towel. Monitor for signs of hemorrhage post procedure by frequently monitoring vital signs and pain. Have the client lie on the right side. Support the biopsy site with a towel or bath blanket for 2 hours. Monitor the site for ecchymosis.
Prostatic biopsy	Removal of a small piece of tissue for microscopic examination.	Monitor for and educate the client about signs and symptoms of hemorrhage, infection, and post-procedure pain.
Testicular biopsy	Determines presence of sperm and rules out vas deferens obstruction.	Monitor for and educate the client about signs and symptoms of infection or hemorrhage.
Thyroid biopsy	Excision of thyroid tissue for histological examination after noninvasive tests prove abnormal or inconclusive. Can be obtained through needle biopsy or open surgical biopsy under general anesthesia.	Explain the procedure to the client. Obtain informed written consent. Assess for allergies. Have coagulation blood studies done. Assess for bleeding and respiratory and swallowing difficulties after the test. To prevent undue strain on the biopsy site, instruct the client to put both hands behind the neck when sitting up. Warn the client that a sore throat is possible after the biopsy.

Table 27-15 OTHER TESTS

TEST	EXPLANATION/NORMAL VALUES	NURSING RESPONSIBILITIES
Arterial plethysmography (pulse volume recorder)	Determines arteriosclerotic disease in the upper extremities and occlusive disease in the lower extremities. Done by applying three blood pressure cuffs to an extremity. The cuffs are connected to a pulse volume recorder, which records the amplitude of each pulse wave. If there is a decrease in the amplitude of the pulse wave, an occlusion is in the artery proximal to the cuff. A decrease of 20 mm Hg of pressure indicates arterial occlusion. The test is not as reliable as arteriography but also does not have the risks associated with an arteriogram. Normal: normal arterial pulse waves	Explain to the client that the test is painless. Instruct the client to lie still during the test. Instruct the client not to smoke for 30 minutes prior to the test. Instruct the client to remove clothing from the extremity on which the test is to be done.
Audiometric testing	Evaluates both bone and air conduction and determines the degree of hearing loss. The client wears headphones, through which a series of tones is delivered at different frequencies. The client signals to the audiologist when the tones are audible. The results are recorded on an audiogram. The client is kept in a sound proof booth during the test.	Explain the procedure and its purpose to the client. Ensure that the client is not claustrophobic.
Brainstem auditory-evoked response (ErA and BAER)	Detects hearing dysfunctions of the central nervous system and cochlear nerve (cranial nerve VII). Valuable for testing comatose clients, clients with neurological damage, and children. An altered appearance of the brainstem waveforms or a delay or loss of a waveform indicates an abnormality including a possible cochlear lesion or acoustic neuroma.	Explain the procedure and its purpose to the client particularly that the client will be in a darkened room and will have both electrodes attached to the head and earphones in place.
Caloric test	Assesses alteration in vestibular function. The client is placed in a supine or Fowler's position and each ear is irrigated with cold and then warm water. A decreased response or failure to respond within 3 minutes indicates that an abnormality may be present. Most commonly done on comatose clients. A punctured eardrum or Meniere's disease may contraindicate the test. Normal: vertigo, nystagmus, nausea, vomiting, and unsteady gait.	Explain the procedure and its purpose to the client. Tell the client that nystagmus, vertigo, nausea, vomiting, and an unsteady gait represent a normal response. Stay with the client and have an emesis basin and tissues available.
Color vision tests	Most common color vision tests use pseudoisochromatic (seemingly the same color) plates comprising patterns of dots of the primary colors superimposed on backgrounds of randomly mixed colors. A client with normal vision can identify the patterns; a client with a color deficiency cannot distinguish between pattern and background.	Explain the test and procedure to the client.
Colposcopy	Direct visualization of the vagina and cervix through a high-powered microscope. Acetic acid or other solution is applied to the tissue to dehydrate the cells for improved visualization. Used to diagnose cervical dysplasia or carcinoma in situ of the cervix. Biopsies may be obtained as needed.	Explain the procedure and prepare the client in the dorsal lithotomy position. Assist with the procedure. Prepare biopsy specimens for pathological examination.
Culture and sensitivity (C&S)	Determines presence of microorganism and identifies the antibiotic that will kill or inhibit growth of microorganism. Drainage from infected lesions is obtained with a sterile swab and is incubated in order to identify the causative organism and to determine antibiotic sensitivity. Normal: negative for microorganism growth.	Ensure that the specimen has been obtained before initiating antibiotic therapy. Specimens should be taken to the laboratory within 30 minutes of being obtained.
Cytology	The study of cells and fluids obtained from various organs by scrapings, brushings, or needle aspiration. Cytologic smears, such as the Pap	Explain the procedure to be used for obtaining cells and fluids for study. Follow agency protocol for client preparation. *continued*

Table 27-15 OTHER TESTS *continued*

TEST	EXPLANATION/NORMAL VALUES	NURSING RESPONSIBILITIES
Cytology (*continued*)	smear, are routinely done to study cells from the female genital tract. A cytological smear showing evidence of malignancy is followed by a biopsy to facilitate a more comprehensive diagnosis.	
Dark field examination of wart scrapings	Microscopic examination to differentiate genital warts from syphilis condylomata.	Take a careful client history. Examine the genital area carefully and provide scalpel and slide, if specimen is to be obtained. Explain the procedure thoroughly to the client.
Dilatation and curettage (D&C)	Surgical scraping of the endometrial lining, performed under general, epidural, or paracervical anesthesia and on an outpatient basis. Diagnostic or therapeutic for uterine bleeding disorders.	Explain the procedure to the client. Perform pre- and postoperative assessment and provide care. Provide discharge instructions related to activities and follow-up appointments.
Dynamic infusion cavernosometry and cavernosography (DICC)	Group of diagnostic tests that measure neuro-vascular events of penile erection.	Perform baseline assessment, monitor during the procedure, and assess for postoperative complications; advise the client of possible discomfort related to the injection.
		Explain the procedure to the client. Assess for allergies. If preferred by the laboratory, initiate NPO status after midnight. Restrict iodine and thyroid preparations a week before test.
		Inform the client that radioactive iodine may be given orally or intravenously. Withhold food for 45 to 60 minutes after the iodine is given. Provide the client with a list of times to report to radiology. Tell the client that he will lie supine for test, which takes about 30 minutes, and that neither isolation nor specific urine precautions are necessary.
Huhner test (post-coital test)	Performed in the office. The couple has intercourse 2 hours before the appointment. A sample of secretions is removed from the vagina and placed on a microscopic slide. The sperm are observed for number and motility in the cervical mucous. Normal: a minimum of 20 sperm per field that demonstrate good motility	Explain the procedure to the client and schedule it near client's normal ovulation. Prepare the client in the lithotomy position. Assist the physician or nurse practitioner with the procedure. Perform microscopic observations as directed.
Nocturnal tumescence penile monitoring	Various devices are attached to the penis at night to monitor swelling (tumescence).	Explain to the client that the test will require application of a device to the penis and that the device is to be worn while sleeping. Show the client the device and explain how to apply it.
Ophthalmoscopic examination	Examination of the fundus (posterior eye) using an ophthalmoscope. Magnifies vascular and nerve tissue of the fundus, including the optic disk, retinal vessels, macula, and retina. Used to diagnose diseases of the eye and aberrations in the refractive mechanism.	Explain the test and procedure to the client.
Otoscopic examination	Visual examination of the ear canal using an otoscope. The examiner looks for signs of inflammation, discharge, or foreign bodies. The tympanic membrane is normally pearly gray. The position and color of the membrane are noted as is any unusual appearance.	Explain the procedure and its purpose to the client. The ear should be clear of cerumen. Tilt the head away from the examiner and pull the earlobe up, back, and out to straighten the auditory canal. In children, pull the earlobe down and out to straighten the canal.
Papanicolaou (Pap) smear	Cells are obtained from the external and internal cervical canal. Used to diagnose cervical dysplasia or cancer.	Explain the procedure. Have client empty bladder and undress. Position client in dorsal lithotomy position. Help client relax during procedure. Prepare microscopic slides for pathology. Instruct the client on the importance of having an annual Pap smear.
Past-point testing	Measures the ability or inability to accurately place a finger on some part of the body, usually the client's or examiner's face and fingers. For example, the examiner will instruct the client to close her eyes and touch her nose, then, with eyes open, touch the examiner's nose or the examiner's index finger.	Explain the test and procedure to the client. Explain that it is painless and represents a helpful measure of vestibular function (coordination).

continued

Table 27-15 OTHER TESTS *continued*

TEST	EXPLANATION/NORMAL VALUES	NURSING RESPONSIBILITIES
Patch testing	Allergens within occlusive patches are applied to normal skin (usually the upper back) for 48 hours. If the client is allergic to a specific allergen, an erythematous skin reaction will occur.	Clean and dry the skin where the patches are to be applied. Tell the client that the patches must be left in place for the full 48 hours.
Pelvic examination (recommended annually for women over 18 through menopause)	Performed by a physician or nurse practitioner. The external and internal pelvic structures are visualized, the pelvic organs are palpated via bi-manual examination, and the cervix is examined via a speculum. A Pap smear and rectovaginal exam are also performed, and cultures and wet smears may be obtained.	Explain the procedures to the client; prepare the client by having her void and undress; position the client on the examination table in a dorsal lithotomy position; help the client to relax during the examination, prepare slides and culture medium; obtain other supplies; and assist with the procedure.
Prostatic smears	Microscopic examination of prostatic secretions obtained via rectal massage performed by a physician.	Explain to the client that to obtain the specimen, the prostate must be massaged via the rectum and that this will cause some discomfort.
Pulmonary function tests (PFTs)	A group of studies used to evaluate ventilatory function. Measurements are obtained directly via spirometer or calculated from the results of spirometer measurements. Bronchodilators may be used during the study. Measurements included are: Tidal volume: the amount of air inhaled and exhaled during a normal respiration. Inspiratory reserve volume: the amount of air inspired at the end of a normal inspiration. Expiratory reserve volume: the amount of air expired following a normal expiration. Residual volume: the amount of air left in lungs after maximal expiration. Vital capacity: the total volume of air that can be expired after maximal inspiration. Total lung capacity: the total volume of air in the lungs when maximally inflated. Inspiratory capacity: the maximum amount of air that can be inspired after normal expiration. Forced vital capacity: the capacity of air exhaled forcefully and rapidly following maximal inspiration. Minute volume: the amount of air breathed per minute.	Explain the procedure to the client, PFTs should not be done within 1–2 hours after a meal. After the test, monitor respiratory status. Advise the client to avoid activity and to rest following the test, as fatigue may result.
Pulse oximetry	A noninvasive procedure. A transdermal clip is placed on a finger or earlobe to detect the arterial oxygen saturation (SaO_2). Normal: > 95% (at sea level)	Explain the procedure to the client. Assess peripheral circulation, as this may alter results. Place the sensor on the earlobe, fingertip, or pinna of the ear. Keep the sensor intact until a consistent reading is obtained. Observe and record readings. Report to the physician measurements below 95%.
Rinne test (tuning fork)	Detects loss of hearing in one or both ears. Tuning fork is struck and placed against the mastoid bone to measure the sound conduction through the bone. The tuning fork is then placed beside and parallel to the ear to test conduction through the air. If the sound is louder when the tines are placed beside the ear, hearing is normal or the hearing loss is sensorineural. If the sound is louder when conducted through the bone, the hearing loss is conductive.	Explain the procedure and its purpose to the client.
Romberg test	Assesses vestibular (balance) function. The client stands with the eyes closed, arms extended in front, and feet together. Normal: slight swaying.	Explain the procedure and its purpose to the client. Stand close and reassure the client that someone will catch him if he begins to fall.
Schiller test	Performed during colposcopy. An iodine solution is applied to the cells of the cervix. Abnormal cells turn white or yellow. Aids in visualization of abnormal tissue and indicates areas for biopsy. Normal: cells turn brown	Explain the reason for the application of the solution. Assist with the biopsy procedure as necessary. Label tissue specimens and send to histology.

continued

Table 27-15 OTHER TESTS *continued*

TEST	EXPLANATION/NORMAL VALUES	NURSING RESPONSIBILITIES
Segmented bacteriologic localization cultures	The first 5–10 mL of urine is collected, the next 200 mL is discarded, then 5–10 mL is collected midstream. The prostate is then massaged until prostatic secretions can be collected. Finally, 5–10 mL urine is collected before the bladder is emptied. Four samples are needed in sterile culture tubes.	Ensure that the client is well hydrated and has a full bladder.
Semen analysis	Determines the presence, number, and motility of sperm.	Teach the client about proper collection of sperm.
Skin scrapings	A lesion is scraped with an oiled scalpel blade. The cells are then examined under a microscope. Used to diagnose fungal lesions.	Explain the procedure and its purpose to the client.
Slit-lamp examination	The cornea is examined with the aid of a slit lamp. A slit-like beam facilitates visualization of the layers of the cornea and lens, facilitating evaluation of the thickness of these structures and the location of disease processes. Useful in detecting and evaluating abnormalities of anterior segment tissues and structures. May reveal disorders such as iritis, corneal abrasions, conjunctivitis, and lens opacities (cataracts).	Explain the procedure and its purpose to the client.
Speech audiometry (Spondee threshold)	Evaluates ability to hear and understand the spoken word. A series of two-syllable words commonly recognized by their vowel sounds (like *toothbrush* and *baseball*) are delivered through earphones. When the client correctly repeats the word, the sound intensity is recorded in decibels. The test is normally conducted in a soundproof booth.	Explain the procedure and its purpose to the client. Ensure that the client is not claustrophobic.
Sputum analysis	Sputum samples are examined for the presence of bacteria, fungi, molds, yeasts, and malignant cells. Appropriate antibiotic therapy is determined via C&S studies.	Explain the procedure and its purpose to the client. Obtain specimens early in the morning to prevent contamination via ingested food or fluids. Instruct the client to breathe deeply and cough, so as to facilitate collection of a specimen originating from the lower respiratory tract. If necessary, pulmonary suctioning may be used to induce such a specimen. Instruct the client to expectorate sputum into the appropriate container. Deliver specimens to the laboratory as soon as possible.
Tonometry	Used to measure intraocular pressure and to aid in the diagnosis and follow-up evaluation of glaucoma. Two types of tonometric devices are used for assessment: applanation and indentation. An applanation tonometer is the most accurate and commonly used device and measures the force (delineated by the reading on the tension dial on the tonometer) required to flatten a small, standard area of the cornea. An indentation tonometer measures the deformation of the globe in response to a standard weight placed on the cornea. Before use of either apparatus, the eyes are anesthetized with a local ophthalmic solution, such as benoxinate with fluorescein or tetracaine, so that the pressure from the tonometer will not be felt. Normal: 12–22 mm Hg	Explain the procedure and its purpose to the client. Explain to the client that this test measures the pressure within the eyes and that although the test requires the client's eyes to be anesthetized, the anesthesia will wear off shortly after the examination is complete. Reassure the client that the procedure is painless.
Typanometry	Measures the movement of the eardrum in response to air pressure in the ear canal. Evaluates the presence of fluid in the middle ear and is commonly used to evaluate otitis media in children or adults.	Explain the procedure and its purpose to the client. Inform the client a small burst of air is introduced through the otoscope, which may produce an uncomfortable sensation.
Tzanck smear	Fluid from the base of a vesicle is applied to a glass slide, stained, and examined under a	Describe to the client how the laboratory technician will obtain the specimen and that

continued

Table 27-15 OTHER TESTS continued

TEST	EXPLANATION/NORMAL VALUES	NURSING RESPONSIBILITIES
Tzanck smear (continued)	microscope. Used to diagnose herpes zoster, herpes simplex, varicella, or pemphigus. Normal: negative	although the procedure will likely not be painful, the client must remain still to prevent injury. Provide scalpel blade, glass slide, and stain for collection.

Urethra pressure profile (UPP)	Assesses functional urethral length and general competency of the urethra and sphincter, either at rest or during coughing, straining, or voiding. Functional profile length is the length from bladder outlet to the point in the urethra where urethral pressure equals intravesical pressure. Used to diagnose stress or overflow incontinence or urethral obstruction.
	
	Normal:
	
	  Male: bladder outlet through membranous urethra
	
	  Female: bladder outlet through mid-urethra
		Explain the procedure and its purpose to the client: that it is often performed when the bladder is empty and the client is at rest; that it may be performed simultaneously with CMG; and that the client may be asked to cough or void. Provide privacy, as the test can be embarrassing.

Uroflowmetry	Noninvasive assessment of urination. An electronic device connected to a funneled commode calculates the rate of urine flow, volume voided, and time taken to void.	Explain the procedure and its purpose to the client. Instruct the client to void as usual, leaving client alone to do so, if possible.
Venous plethysmography (cuff pressure test)	Assists in determining patency of veins. Two blood pressure cuffs are placed on the extremity, one proximally (occlusion cuff) and one distally (recording cuff). The cuffs are attached to pulse volume recorders. The occlusion cuff is inflated to 50 mm Hg pressure to occlude the venous flow of blood; the recording cuff is inflated to 10 mm Hg pressure. The pulse volumes are recorded and then the occlusion cuff is rapidly deflated. The pulse volume of the extremity should return to the preocclusion volume within 1 second if there is no occlusion in the venous system. A delay in the return of volume pressure is indicative of a thrombus. Normal: return of volume pressure to preocclusion value within 1 second after deflation of occlusion cuff The test is often done in conjunction with a doppler ultrasound. The test is not as reliable as a venogram.	Nursing responsibilities are the same as for Arterial Plethysmography (see beginning of table).
Visual acuity	Used to test distant and near visual acuity and to identify refractive errors in vision. Distant visual acuity is measured with a standardized visual acuity chart, e.g., a Snellen chart. Near visual acuity is measured with a Jaeger card (a card with print in graded sizes). Visual acuity is recorded as a fraction, with the numerator representing the distance to the chart and the denominator representing the distance at which a normal eye can read the line. Thus, the larger the denominator, the poorer the client's visual acuity. For example, if the client's vision is normal, results are expressed as 20/20, which means that the smallest symbol one can identify at 20 feet is the same symbol the normal eye can identify from the same distance.	Explain the procedure and its purpose to the client. Have the client stand the specified distance from the eye chart, usually 10 feet. Instruct the client to first cover one eye and then the other. If the client wears glasses, perform the test first with the client's glasses on and then with the client's glasses off.
Weber test (tuning fork)	Detects loss of hearing in one or both ears. Tuning fork is struck and the handle is placed in the middle of the forehead. Clients with normal hearing or bilateral deafness will hear or not hear the sound equally in both ears. Clients with unilateral hearing loss will hear the sound only in the unaffected ear.	Explain the procedure and its purpose to the client.
Wood's light examination	Skin and hair are examined under ultraviolet light (black light) in a darkened room. Used to diagnose fungal infections (tinea) of hair and skin.	Explain the procedure and its purpose to the client. Reassure the client that the rays are not harmful.

SUMMARY

- Most invasive procedures require that the client give informed consent.
- Nurses prepare clients for diagnostic testing by ensuring client understanding and compliance with preprocedural requirements.
- Clients, families, and significant others must be involved in the testing process. The nurse must advise them of the estimated time required to perform the procedure.
- To help offset the discomfort and anxiety experienced during procedures, the nurse teaches the client how to perform relaxation techniques such as imagery.
- After a diagnostic test, the nurse provides care and teaches the client those things to expect, including the outcomes or side effects of the test.
- The role of the nurse in diagnostic testing is to facilitate the scheduling of diagnostic tests, perform client teaching, perform or assist with procedures, and assess clients for adverse responses to procedures.
- Nurses should schedule diagnostic procedures to promote both client comfort and cost containment.
- Standard Precautions are used when obtaining a specimen for diagnostic examination or when assisting with an invasive procedure.
- Before the procedure, the nurse is responsible for obtaining baseline vital signs and assessing the client's preparation for testing.
- After the procedure, the nurse assesses the client for secondary procedural complications and performs any necessary nursing interventions.

Review Questions

1. Scheduling and sequencing of laboratory tests are important functions of the:

   a. nurse.
   b. physician.
   c. phlebotomist.
   d. laboratory supervisor.

2. The most commonly used site for capillary puncture in neonates and infants is the:

   a. heel.
   b. toetip.
   c. earlobe.
   d. fingertip.

3. When collecting a 24-hour urine specimen, the nurse knows:

   a. to put a large bottle at the client's bedside.
   b. the collection begins at the time of the first discarded voiding.
   c. that the client must urinate at a specific start time.

   d. to teach the client how to void in the large collection bottle.

4. The nurse knows that glucose spills into the urine when the blood glucose level exceeds the renal threshold of:

   a. 120 mg/mL.
   b. 140 mg/mL.
   c. 160 mg/mL.
   d. 180 mg/mL.

5. Occult blood may be found in which type of specimen?

   a. Blood
   b. Stool
   c. Urine
   d. Sputum

6. When scheduling a series of tests, the nurse knows to schedule:

   a. a barium enema before an upper GI.
   b. an ultrasound after all other tests.
   c. an upper GI before a gallbladder x-ray.
   d. a gallbladder x-ray before any barium studies.

7. A test that combines a radioactive scan with an electrodiagnostic study is a:

   a. MUGA.
   b. brain scan.
   c. thallium stress test.
   d. radioactive iodine uptake test.

Critical Thinking Questions

1. If a client's blood type is AB positive, what are the possible blood types of the client's parents? Can the client receive Rh-negative blood? Explain your answer.

2. The physician orders gallbladder x-rays, a barium swallow, an upper GI, and a barium enema. In which order should these tests be scheduled? Why?

⚡ WEB FLASH!

- Search the Web for "diagnostic tests." How many sites can you find? What type of information is available?
- Search the Web for the specific diagnostic tests discussed in this chapter. How many tests have sites devoted to them? Is the information for health professionals or the general public?

CHAPTER

28

ANESTHESIA

MAKING THE CONNECTION

Refer to the following chapters to increase your understanding of anesthesia:

- **Chapter 6, Legal Responsibilities**
- **Chapter 23, Fluid, Electrolyte, and Acid–Base Balance**

- **Chapter 26, Pain Management**
- **Chapter 29, Nursing Care of the Surgical Client**

LEARNING OBJECTIVES

Upon completion of this chapter, you should be able to:
- *Define key terms.*
- *Describe the difference between regional and general anesthesia.*
- *List the purposes of sedation.*
- *Describe the effects of sedation or general anesthesia on memory and cognitive function.*
- *Describe the types of monitoring necessary to ensure client safety during sedation.*
- *Describe the signs and symptoms and risks of oversedation.*
- *Describe the dangers involved in aspiration of gastric contents and how gastric aspiration is prevented during anesthesia.*
- *List the medications that are typically given on the day of surgery.*
- *List and describe the different types of regional anesthesia.*
- *Describe the risks involved with regional and general anesthesia.*
- *Describe the residual effects of anesthesia on the client.*
- *List three methods of postoperative pain management and explain briefly how each is administered.*

KEY TERMS

amnesia
analgesia
anesthesia
anesthesiologist
anesthetist

general anesthesia
orthostatic hypotension
regional anesthesia
sedation
synergism

purpose of preventing pain during surgery began in the United States in the 1800s. When surgeons began using anesthesia routinely, they soon realized the need for someone trained in its administration and turned to the nurses with whom they worked daily. Early nurse anesthetists were trained on the job by the surgeons with whom they worked.

Anesthesia is now a specialty of both nursing and medicine. Experienced registered nurses (RNs) with a baccalaureate degree can become certified registered nurse anesthetists (CRNAs) after completing two or more years of graduate education in nurse anesthesia. There are currently approximately 25,000 CRNAs in the United States. Certified registered nurse anesthetists administer the majority of all anesthetics given in the United States every year, often working in groups with or under the supervision of anesthesiologists. An **anesthesiologist** is a licensed physician educated and skilled in the delivery of anesthesia who also adds to the knowledge of anesthesia through research or other scholarly pursuits. An **anesthetist** is a qualified RN, dentist, or physician who administers anesthetics under the direct supervision of an anesthesiologist or a surgeon.

INTRODUCTION

Anesthesia refers to the absence of normal sensation. **Analgesia** refers to pain relief without producing anesthesia. The delivery of general anesthesia for the

Prior to administering an anesthetic, the anesthesia provider will assess a client's health status, discuss anesthesia with the client, and plan an anesthetic appropriate for the client and the surgical procedure. The surgical nurse can help prepare clients to talk with their anesthesia providers by encouraging them to ask any questions they have about anesthesia and the care they will receive.

The delivery of an anesthetic is essential to the health and well-being of clients undergoing surgery. Yet, while anesthesia prevents the sensation of what would be extreme pain, it also temporarily eliminates or diminishes the client's ability to control many essential physiologic functions such as respiration, heart rate, and temperature regulation. In addition to ensuring adequate levels of anesthesia throughout a surgical procedure, the anesthesia provider monitors and, when necessary, controls physiologic functions such as respiratory rate and blood pressure. Prior to the end of the surgery, the anesthesia provider administers appropriate medications to ensure that the client is comfortable when emerging from the anesthetic. Pain relief may be accomplished with local anesthetic infiltration, opioid analgesics, or nonopioid analgesics.

PREANESTHETIC PREPARATION

Preparing a client for anesthesia and surgery is a cooperative effort involving the surgeon, the anesthesia provider, and the nursing staff who will care for the client both before and after surgery. The client may be having general (total body) anesthesia, where the control of body functions is temporarily lost; regional anesthesia, where a region of the body is made insensible to pain; or local anesthesia, where only a small area of the body is made insensible to pain.

Oral Intake

Normally, only air should enter the trachea and lungs. The body prevents foreign material from entering the trachea by coughing forcefully when something other than air enters or by tightly closing the vocal cords to prevent entry of the foreign substance. Anyone who has ever been drinking something and

LIFE CYCLE CONSIDERATIONS

Anesthesia for Pediatric Clients

- Explain the anesthesia procedure at the child's level of understanding. For instance, say, "This mask will help you go to sleep for a while."
- Allow the child to play with a mask that will be used.

CLIENT TEACHING

Oral Intake Prior to Surgery

- Clearly explain to clients those things that they will or will not be allowed to eat or drink before surgery.
- Emphasize the need to exactly follow the instructions related to the time at which eating or drinking must cease before surgery.

had it go down the wrong "pipe" knows how uncomfortable it is and how hard the body works to cough up the foreign substance.

General anesthesia removes a person's ability to guard the airway by coughing or closing the vocal cords. Passive regurgitation of stomach contents into the back of the throat can occur at any time during the delivery of general anesthesia. Aspiration of gastric contents into the lungs can cause significant illness or death. An important step in preventing aspiration of gastric contents is ensuring that the stomach is as empty as possible. In the past, adults have been instructed not to eat or drink anything for at least 8 hours prior to surgery, and usually nothing past midnight the night before surgery. More recent information, however, strongly indicates that adults need not go without water for 8 or more hours prior to surgery (Phillips, Hutchinson, & Davidson, 1993; Soreide, Holst-Larsen, Reite, Mikkelsen, Sorejde, & Steen, 1993). In fact, the amount of liquid in a person's stomach at the time of surgery may actually be decreased if water is taken a couple of hours before surgery. Some anesthesia providers still prefer that their clients not have anything to eat or drink for at least 8 hours prior to surgery; others may allow water up to 2 hours before.

Preoperative Medication

Most scheduled medications that a person receives while in the hospital or takes at home every day will be continued up until the time of surgery. Most oral medications should be given with just enough water to swallow them, even when a client is going to have surgery first thing in the morning. The anesthesia provider will usually write orders to specify how the morning medication should be managed. Cardiovascular medications such as antihypertensives and heart medications are especially important for the client to receive.

Exceptions to the practice of continuing scheduled medications prior to surgery include administration of drugs such as insulin and oral antihyperglycemics, nonsteroidal anti-inflammatory drugs (NSAIDs) like aspirin, and anticoagulants like heparin or coumadin. Because food is being withheld, giving insulin or oral antihyperglycemic drugs is likely to result in a dangerously low blood sugar level. The way insulin and glucose administration is handled will depend on the severity of the client's disease and the preference of the physician and anesthesia provider. Anticoagulants and NSAIDs affect clotting. With some types of surgery, the bleeding caused by aspirin-like drugs or low-dose heparin is more likely. In some cases, no NSAIDs are allowed for 10 days to 2 weeks prior to surgery. In other circumstances, they may be taken right up until surgery. Low-dose heparin or heparinoids may be given preoperatively to prevent postoperative thromboembolism, but higher doses of heparin and any dose of coumadin will almost certainly be stopped

prior to surgery to allow the return of normal coagulation time.

Additional medications may be ordered to prepare the client for surgery or anesthesia. Surgeons often order prophylactic antibiotics. The anesthesia provider may order a sedative to help the client sleep the night before surgery or to ease the client's anxiety while waiting for surgery. Opioids like morphine or meperidine (Demerol) may also be used for pain relief or to ease the induction of anesthesia. Some anesthesia providers prefer to give preoperative medications in the operating room to precisely control the medication's effect on the client. This is especially true for very sick clients.

Consent

Consent for anesthesia is usually obtained on the same form as is surgical consent. The anesthesia department may have a separate consent form instead of or in addition to the combined consent. In either case, for an informed consent to be obtained, the anesthetic must be discussed with the client by someone with expert knowledge of anesthesia, usually an anesthesia provider or the surgeon.

SEDATION

Sedation refers to a reduction of stress, excitement, or irritability, and involves some degree of central nervous system (CNS) depression. Sedation is used to decrease awareness of events, relieve anxiety, control the physiologic changes that often accompany anxiety, and ease the induction of general anesthesia. This is welcome news to many clients who fear local or regional anesthesia because they do not want to be awake and see and hear everything during surgery or a diagnostic procedure.

Some drugs are better sedatives than others, although many drugs have sedative properties. Oftentimes, different sedatives given in combination have a greater effect on the client than does any one of the sedatives given alone. This phenomenon is called **synergism**. The synergistic effect that occurs when different sedative drugs are administered together, however, makes respiratory depression and unconsciousness more likely. In general, benzodiazepines (diazepam [Valium] and midazolam hydrochloride [Versed]) are better sedatives than are opioids (morphine and fentanyl [Sublimaze]). Even so, if a client's anxiety is due to pain, an opioid is a better choice of sedative than a benzodiazepine because the opioid will relieve the pain that caused the anxiety.

There is a great deal of variability in the dose of drugs needed to sedate different clients. Whereas many drugs given for specific effects are administered according to a set "mg per kg" dose alone, this is not possible with drugs used for sedation. Sedative medications should be administered based on the client's physical condition, weight, mental state, and the procedure being performed, with close observation of the effects of the drugs on the client.

The amount of sedation required by a client for comfort is always in balance with the amount of stimulation experienced due to pain or anxiety. A client who is only mildly stimulated (i.e., experiencing little anxiety) will be sufficiently sedated with a relatively small dose of sedative medication. A client who is greatly stimulated (i.e., undergoing a painful procedure or very frightened) will require a much larger dose of sedative to be comfortable. Sedation and general anesthesia both involve CNS depression; thus sedation and anesthesia exist on a continuum. As sedation becomes deeper and deeper, it eventually becomes general anesthesia. Sometimes, the line between sedation and general anesthesia is very difficult to distinguish. When sedation becomes general anesthesia, all the risks of general anesthesia are present, including airway obstruction, respiratory arrest, and aspiration of gastric contents. For this reason, all but the lightest sedation should be administered by an anesthetist or another provider skilled and experienced in airway assessment, protection, and management, as well as assessment of oxygenation and ventilation.

Sedation and Monitoring

Sedation is often used to alleviate client anxiety and discomfort during procedures performed under local anesthesia. Properly administered, local anesthetic injection blocks the painful stimulus of small incisions and minor surgical procedures. However, the injections necessary for local anesthetic administration can cause significant discomfort in some people due to tissue irritation caused by the acidity of the local anesthetic solution. Additionally, most clients are uncomfortable knowing that they are undergoing surgery and thus prefer to be less alert during the procedure. Sedation decreases the client's perception of these physical and mental discomforts.

During local anesthesia and sedation, the client must remain conscious and in control of his own airway and breathing reflexes. Oversedation is likely to result in airway obstruction and places the client at risk for aspiration of gastric contents. Because sedatives are CNS depressants and, thus, respiratory depressants, supplemental oxygen should be given to clients during sedation. Monitoring during sedation is done through observation by an individual knowledgeable and experienced in the assessment of respiratory volume and airway patency. Monitoring should also include an electrocardiogram (EKG), blood pressure, pulse rate, respiratory rate, and continuous oxygen saturation monitoring (pulse oximetry). The individual monitoring the client's breathing and vital signs should be devoted to that task to the exclusion of any other duties.

Residual Effects of Sedation

Sedation usually persists beyond the duration of the surgical procedure itself. The length of time it takes to recover from sedation depends on the health of the client, the properties of the drugs used, other drugs the client may be taking, and the amount of sedative drugs administered.

Amnesia (inability to remember things) produced by sedatives commonly lasts longer than the procedure itself, even in clients who appear to be completely recovered. Such clients will probably not remember any instructions given to them during or soon after the procedure. Given that minor procedures and surgery are commonly performed on an outpatient basis, some clients may be discharged prior to regaining the ability to remember verbal instructions. All instructions should thus be given in writing and explained to the person responsible for taking the client home.

If heavy sedation has been used or the procedure ends suddenly, the client may remain significantly sedated after the procedure is over, because the CNS stimulation has ended while the CNS depressant effect of the sedative remains. In such an instance, the client should be closely monitored until the effects of the sedative medications have worn off enough for the client to wake and become oriented.

REGIONAL ANESTHESIA

In **regional anesthesia** a region of the body is temporarily rendered insensible to pain by injection of a local anesthetic. Local anesthetics are a class of drugs that temporarily block the transmission of small electrical impulses through nerves. The duration of anesthesia produced by a local anesthetic depends on the drug used, the amount injected, and into which part of the body the drug is injected. In general, nerves carry either sensory information to the brain or instructions from the brain to muscles, telling them how and when to contract. Both types of nerves can be blocked by local anesthetics. Sensory nerves are highly subspecialized to carry specific types of information to the brain. One type carries information about the pain we experience when stuck with a needle; another carries information about joint position that tells us, without looking, whether our arm is down by our side or elevated over our head. There are many different types of nerves, and not all of them are blocked to the same degree or at the same time when a local anesthetic is injected. The amount of insulation surrounding a nerve fiber, the anatomic location of the fiber, and the diameter of the fiber all influence the ease with which nerve impulses are blocked by local anesthetics.

Types of Regional Anesthesia

There are three types of regional anesthesia: local anesthesia, nerve blocks, and spinal and epidural blocks.

Local Anesthesia

Clinically, the use of local anesthetics to block nerves is identified by different names depending on the amount of local anesthetic used and where it is injected. When a small amount of local anesthetic drug is injected either into the skin and subcutaneous tissues around a cut or at the site of a needle puncture for a central line placement, it is called *local anesthesia*. When a local anesthetic is injected in this way, it is not aimed at a specific nerve, rather it is meant to anesthetize whatever small superficial nerves are in the target area. Local anesthesia is most commonly performed using lidocaine (Xylocaine) and lasts approximately 1 hour. Occasionally, for some types of plastic surgery, this type of anesthesia is used over a large area of the body. When this is the case, longer acting local anesthetics may be used. Local anesthesia is technically easy to administer and presents little risk of bleeding or nerve damage. Because very small amounts of local anesthetics are generally used, the risk of local anesthetic toxicity is also small.

Topical anesthesia, achieved with direct application of a local anesthetic to tissue, may be desired in some situations. The anesthetic may take the form of an ointment, lotion, solution, or spray.

Safety: Preventing Choking and Aspiration

In order to prevent choking and aspiration after the use of an oral anesthetic solution (e.g., viscous lidocaine) or spray, fluids and foods must be withheld until the gag reflex returns.

Nerve Blocks

When a local anesthetic is injected more deeply into the body and/or is directed at a specific nerve or nerves, it is called a *nerve block*. Nerve blocks are often called by the name of the specific nerve or nerves they block. Examples include an ulnar nerve block in the arm or a brachial plexus block of all the nerves in the arm. Nerve blocks are technically more difficult to administer than are local anesthetics, and because the needle is usually directed into deeper structures that are often close to major veins or arteries, involve a variable risk of bleeding or nerve damage. Nerve blocks are often performed using lidocaine (Xylocaine), mepivacaine (Carbocaine), or bupivacaine (Marcaine) and may last from 1 to 12 hours. Larger volumes of drug are needed than are used for local anesthesia, and local anesthetic toxicity is a rare but known complication of these types of blocks.

Spinal and Epidural Blocks

Blocks may also be identified according to where the local anesthetic is injected. One example is an *epidural block,* for which local anesthetic is injected into the epidural space near the spinal cord to anesthetize a number of spinal nerves at once. With *spinal blocks* (also called subarachnoid blocks), the local anesthetic is injected into the cerebrospinal fluid, where it can bathe uninsulated spinal nerves as they exit the spinal cord to the periphery of the body (see Figure 28-1).

Spinal and epidural blocks are generally used to anesthetize a significant area of the body. They are capable of safely producing anesthesia sufficient for surgery in the abdomen, pelvis, perineum, or lower extremities. When an epidural block is performed, a catheter is usually inserted into the epidural space, making it possible to inject additional doses of drug.

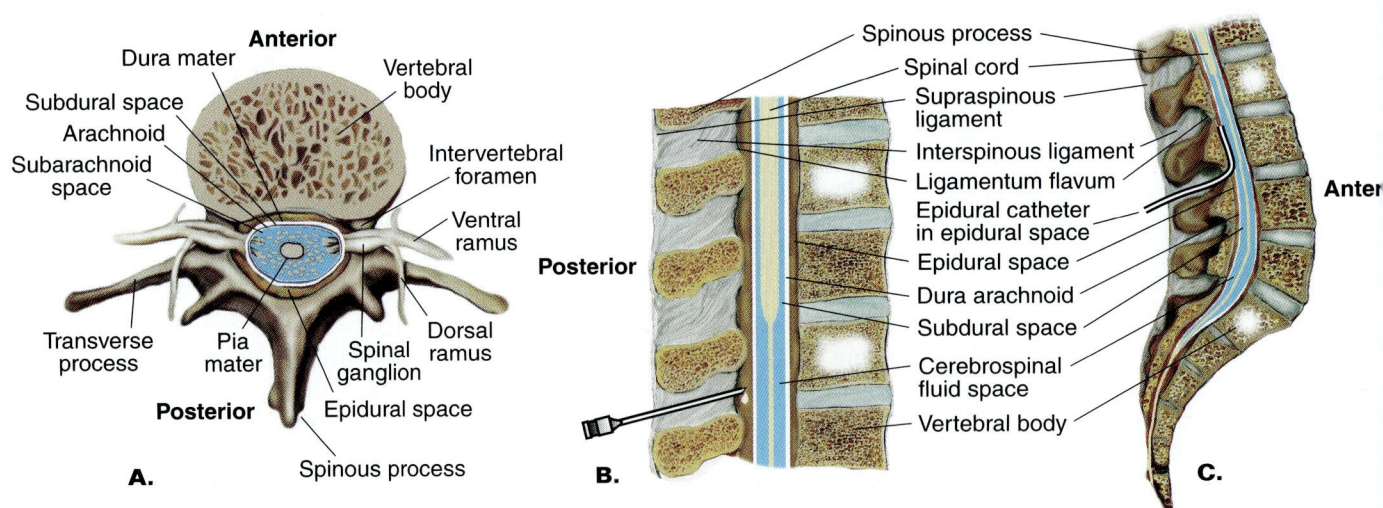

Figure 28-1 A. Cross sectional anatomy of the spine. B. Side view of the anatomy of the spine with the tip of an epidural needle placed in the epidural space. C. Side view of the anatomy of the spine with the tip of an epidural catheter placed in the epidural space.

The client must either be sitting in a bent-over position or lying on the side with head and knees as close together as possible. Either position separates the vertebra, making insertion of the needle or catheter possible. Epidural blocks have an added advantage in that by varying the way the anesthetic is used, the block can produce analgesia (pain relief without producing anesthesia), complete anesthesia, and even profound muscular relaxation (needed for some types of surgery). This allows epidural anesthesia to be used not only for surgical procedures, but also for analgesia during labor and for postoperative pain relief.

Spinal blocks are most often performed using lidocaine (Xylocaine) or bupivacaine (Marcaine) and last from 1 to 3 hours. Epidural blocks are most commonly performed using bupivacaine (Marcaine), and the block can be continued as long as local anesthetic is injected through the catheter into the epidural space (Figure 28-2).

Opioids such as morphine and fentanyl citrate (Sublimaze) may be added to the local anesthetic in either of these blocks to intensify the analgesic or anesthetic effect, or to provide postoperative pain relief after the block has worn off (Abouleish, Rawal, & Rashad, 1991; Liu et al., 1995).

One type of complication is peculiar to spinal and epidural regional anesthetics. When cerebrospinal fluid (CSF) leaks out through a hole made in the dural membrane during performance of a subarachnoid

block or an accidental dural puncture during the attempted performance of an epidural block, a postdural puncture headache (PDPH) may result. The headache is caused by the loss of CSF from around the brain. The headache is relieved by lying down and returns when the individual sits up or stands. Pain commonly occurs in both the front and the back of the head and is sometimes accompanied by neck and shoulder stiffness. Photophobia or double vision may be present with severe headache. The onset of the headache is usually not immediate and may take 1 to 2 days to become bothersome. Treatment involves adequate hydration to allow the normal production of CSF; analgesics; and bed rest in a supine position. Oral caffeine (Camann, Murray, Mushlin, & Lambert, 1990) and sumatriptan succinate (Imitrex) (Carp, Singh, Vadhera, & Jayaram, 1994) are effective in preventing and treating PDPH in some people. The definitive treatment for significant or persistent PDPH, however, is a procedure called an epidural blood patch, which involves injecting 15 to 20 mL of the client's own blood into the epidural space. Once the blood clots, it plugs the hole in the dural membrane.

A local anesthetic drug will always block the sympathetic nerves that control the dilation or constriction of blood vessels before it blocks sensory or motor nerves. This results in vascular dilation. With most blocks, the resultant vascular dilation is not sufficient to change blood pressure. With widespread spinal or epidural blocks, however, blood pressure may decrease due to sympathetic nerve block. To prevent this, the anesthesia provider will often infuse an extra volume of intravenous (IV) fluid or administer a vasoconstrictor such as ephedrine before the sympathetic block sets up. Client harm from hypotension is rare.

Spinal and epidural blocks, like other nerve blocks, carry some risk of bleeding (Dickman, Shedd, Spetzler, Shetter, & Sonntag, 1990; Horlocker, Wedel, & Offord, 1990; Horlocker et al., 1995; Onishchuk & Carlsson, 1992) and nerve damage (Ben-David, Vaida, Collins, Naum, & Gaitini, 1994; Bromage, 1993; Kroll, Caplan, Posner, Ward, & Cheney, 1990), but the high degree of expertise that many anesthesia providers have in delivering these blocks minimizes the risk. Only a small dose of local anesthetic is needed for a spinal block, so local anesthetic toxicity is very unlikely. Variable amounts of local anesthetic are used for epidural blocks, and some doses can approach the upper limits of safety. Anesthesia providers are careful to avoid overdoses of local anesthetics when delivering this block, and toxicity is exceedingly rare. If opioids, like morphine, are added to the local anesthetic solution, there is a risk of the drug migrating to the brain and causing respiratory depression (Abouleish et al., 1991), but this risk is small in light of careful dosing and is easily detected in time to prevent client harm.

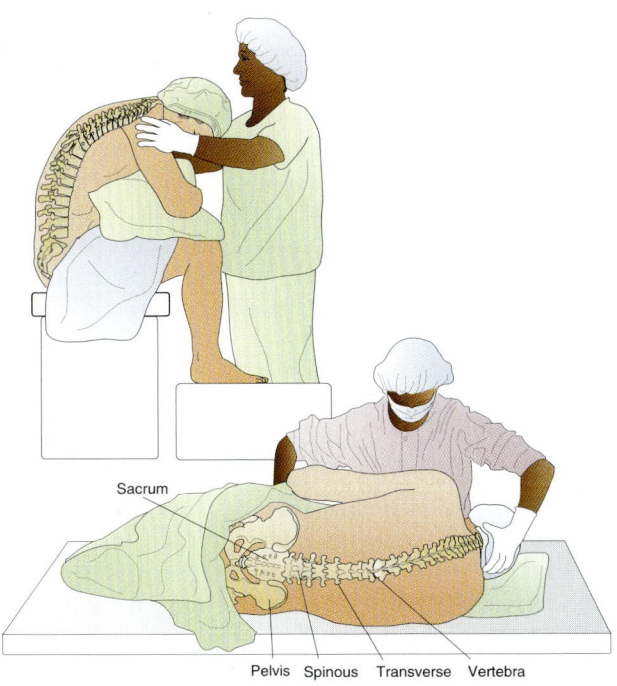

Sacrum

Pelvis Spinous Transverse Vertebra
        process process

Figure 28-2 Correct positions for performing a spinal block or inserting an epidural catheter in the lumbar area. The assistance of trained personnel is crucial to the proper positioning, reassurance, and safety of the client.

Residual Effects of Regional Anesthesia

All anesthetics must wear off as the drug responsible for causing the anesthesia is removed from its site of action within the body and is metabolized, and eliminated. Some anesthetic effects wear off faster than others, and important residual effects may not be detected by casual observation. This is especially true of a regional anesthetic because the client may be wide awake and able to carry on a conversation as if nothing has happened. Three common residual effects are discussed following.

Residual Motor Block

A motor block is a temporary condition caused when local anesthetic blocks nerves that carry instructions to skeletal muscles telling them to contract. Motor block results in the inability to move a body part and is usually the last effect to develop and the first to wear off. It results only when the regional block is very dense and complete.

A complete motor block results in a temporary paralysis, with the client being incapable of moving the blocked part despite tremendous effort. In the presence of a complete motor block, there is usually no function in any other type of nerve in the same area. A client experiencing a complete motor block of any part of the body would not likely be released from the recovery area because there would be no evidence that the block was wearing off. Clients experiencing residual (incomplete) motor block may be released from recovery, however; thus any client who has had any type of block involving the legs should never be allowed to get out of bed without assistance until it can be demonstrated that a complete recovery of motor strength in the legs has been regained. Even a small amount of residual motor block greatly increases the possibility that a client will fall.

As a regional block begins to wear off, motor function begins to return first, sensation begins to return next, and sympathetic nervous function returns last. Motor function and sensation can be detected easily by asking the client to move the blocked part or by touching the skin and asking the client whether it feels normal. The return of sympathetic function is more difficult to detect. Because sympathetic nervous function returns last, orthostatic hypotension may still occur even after motor and sensory function have completely returned and the regional block appears to have worn off. To prevent fainting, clients should not be allowed to get out of bed without the presence of a nurse until after they have been able to do so without any dizziness or significant decrease in blood pressure.

Residual Sensory Block

The effects of any regional anesthetic used for surgery is the loss of pain sensation. Normal sensation may not have returned completely upon client discharge from the recovery area. As the regional block wears off, sensation will return gradually. Not all types of sensation return at the same time, however. For example, as sensation begins to return, the client may experience a "pins and needles" feeling in an arm or leg that has been blocked and may feel touch or pressure before recovering complete sensation. Until complete recovery of normal sensation, any blocked areas of the client's body must be frequently checked and carefully protected, as the client may be unaware that a finger or hand, for example, is being pinched or denied blood supply.

Residual Sympathetic Block

The first types of nerve fibers to be blocked when a local anesthetic begins to work, and the last to recover as a local anesthetic wears off, are those responsible for carrying instructions to the muscles that surround blood vessels. When these sympathetic nerves are blocked, veins and arteries dilate, lowering the blood pressure. The venous system has a large capacity, and venous dilation results in the pooling of a large amount of blood. This decreases the amount of blood that returns to the heart, and the blood pressure falls. The amount of blood that pools is greatest in parts of the body that are farthest below the level of the heart. Even in a client who has had a spinal or epidural block and is lying supine, a significant amount of venous pooling occurs, resulting in lower-than-normal blood pressure. If the same client is allowed to sit up, even more venous pooling will occur, less blood will return to the heart, and blood pressure will fall substantially. This phenomenon of having a large drop in blood pressure when sitting up or standing is called **orthostatic hypotension**. Orthostatic signifies that it involves body position, and hypotension means low blood pressure. Clients who have had a spinal or epidural block are more likely to have orthostatic hypotension the higher in the spinal column the level of their block.

GENERAL ANESTHESIA

General anesthesia involves unconsciousness; complete insensibility to pain; amnesia; motionlessness; and muscle relaxation. With general anesthesia, the body also loses the ability to control many important functions, including the abilities to maintain an airway, control vital functions like breathing and heart rate, and regulate temperature. These functions are controlled by the anesthesia provider during administration of general anesthesia.

General anesthesia involves four overlapping stages: induction (going to sleep), maintenance, emergence (waking up), and recovery.

Induction and Airway Management

The induction of general anesthesia is a short but critical period of time during which the client is rendered unconscious, vital functions are controlled, and enough anesthetic drug is introduced into the body to keep the client asleep during surgery. In adults, drugs are usually injected into an IV line to quickly produce unconsciousness, and additional anesthetic is then inhaled.

Immediately after the induction of general anesthesia, the anesthesia provider will usually secure the airway using a cuffed endotracheal tube (ETT). The ETT is usually inserted under direct visualization with the aid of a laryngoscope, an instrument designed to provide visualization and illumination of the trachea, as shown in Figure 28-3. An ETT provides a breathing passage from outside the client to within the client's trachea. The ETT cuff seals the space between the ETT and the trachea, making it difficult, though not impossible, for air to escape from or gastric contents to enter into the lungs. An ETT also offers a dependable way to provide oxygen and ventilation to the client's lungs. Breaths given through a properly positioned cuffed ETT go directly into the lungs and prevent any gas from entering the stomach.

Maintenance

General anesthesia is maintained with some combination of IV and inhaled drugs. Some of these drugs are used only as general anesthetics, and others are used for other purposes but are also useful as anesthetics. Isoflurane (Forane) is an example of a drug used only for anesthesia. It produces all the compo-

LIFE CYCLE CONSIDERATIONS

Induction of Anesthesia in Small Children

- Inhalation of an anesthetic vapor, which produces unconsciousness a little more slowly than does IV administration, is used first.
- An IV line is then started, and additional IV drugs are administered.

nents of a general anesthetic by itself. Figure 28-4 shows a client connected to an anesthesia machine by a breathing circuit. Benzodiazepines and opioids (sometimes called narcotics), used for many other purposes, are sometimes used as part of a general anesthetic. Neither produces all the components of a general anesthetic by itself. In healthy clients undergoing simple surgeries, anesthetic drugs may be all that are needed. In critically ill clients and those undergoing complicated types of surgery other drugs may be needed to strengthen heart contraction, control blood pressure, or produce complete paralysis of skeletal muscles.

Skeletal Muscle Relaxation

Some types of surgery require complete relaxation of skeletal muscles. In these cases, the anesthesia provider administers a skeletal muscle relaxant like pancuronium bromide (Pavulon) or vecuronium bromide (Norcuron) to completely paralyze the client. These types of drugs prevent clients from breathing on

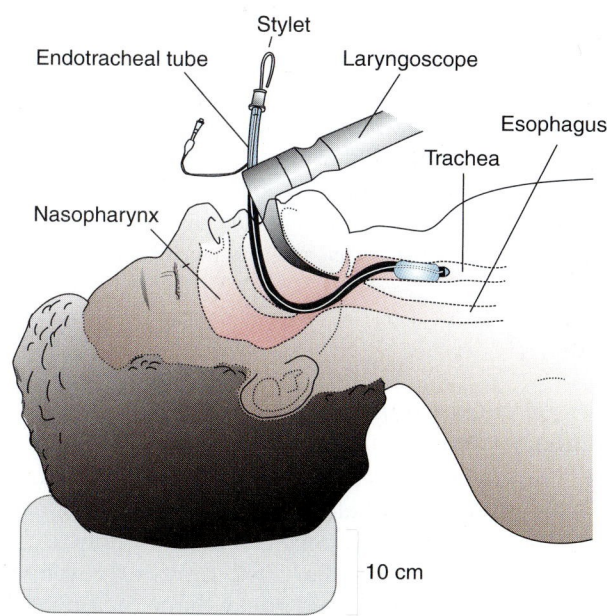

Figure 28-3 Placing an Endotracheal Tube in the Trachea with Direct Visualization by Laryngoscopy.

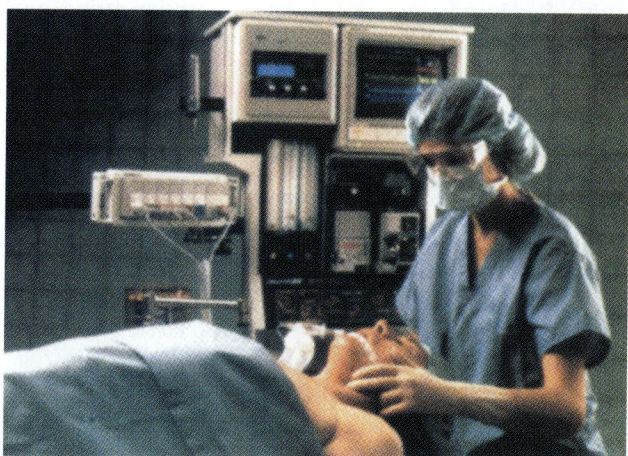

Figure 28-4 A typical anesthesia machine is a complex equipment set. This machine has anesthetic vaporizors and flowmeters to deliver oxygen, nitrous oxide, and air, and also contains a small ventilator and equipment to monitor ventilation, oxygen content of inspired gas, client oxygen saturation, blood pressure, heart rate, and respiration. (*Pictured above is the Ohmeda Excel 210 SE Anesthesia Delivery System equipped with the Hewlett Packard OmniCare Anesthesia Component Monitoring System [A-CMS] and the Anesthesia Gas Module [AGM]. Reprinted with permission of Ohmeda, Inc.*)

their own, requiring the anesthesia provider to ventilate clients during surgery. Usually, a mechanical ventilator is used. Paralysis must be eliminated prior to emergence from anesthesia in order for the client to be able to breathe independently again. As soon as the skeletal muscle relaxant has begun to wear off, an anticholinesterase drug such as neostigmine methylsulfate (Prostigmin), or pyridostigmine bromide (Regonol) is used to reverse the remaining paralysis. When the paralyzing effect of an anesthetic muscle relaxant has begun to wear off on its own, the anesthesia provider can administer an anticholinesterase drug to reverse the remaining paralysis. This normally results in a quick return of muscle strength and the ability to breathe.

Inadequate reversal of paralysis may present as anything from total skeletal muscle paralysis to the inability of the client to cough and clear the airway. Typically, a client with partial paralysis has uncoordinated large muscle movements and is weak. If only small levels of paralysis remain, the client may complain of difficulty swallowing or difficulty breathing deeply. Any detectable paralysis in a postoperative client should immediately be brought to the attention of the anesthesia service for evaluation. If the client is having difficulty breathing, basic life support should be provided until the arrival of an anesthesia provider.

Emergence

Emergence from general anesthesia occurs when anesthetic drugs are allowed to wear off. The anesthesia provider must carefully control the timing and amount of anesthetic drug given in order for the client to emerge from general anesthesia at the desired time. This takes experience and a detailed understanding of both the drugs used and the client's response to those drugs. The initial phase of emergence is usually quite quick, allowing the client to awaken enough to respond to verbal directions and maintain an airway. After this time, the client's breathing tube can usually be removed, and the client can be taken to the post-anesthesia care unit (recovery room). If, for some reason, the client must be left on a ventilator and with a breathing tube in place, the anesthesia provider may take the client to an intensive care unit asleep instead of waking the client up from the anesthetic.

Recovery

Recovery from general anesthesia is not complete simply because the client has regained consciousness. The client may not remember what has happened for minutes or even hours after having received an anesthetic. The ability to think clearly often takes longer to return, with some residual thinking difficulty persisting for several days or even weeks. Inhalation anesthetics are eliminated from the body through the lungs, and very small amounts of anesthetic are still being exhaled for several weeks. (Yasuda, Lockhart, & Eger,

1991). Many anesthetic drugs are stored in body fat and released back into the bloodstream very slowly after anesthetic administration has ended. The speed of this release depends on the amount of anesthetic given during the surgery, the length of the surgery, and how deeply the client is breathing.

Oxygenation and Ventilation

Almost all anesthetics are respiratory depressants. Benzodiazepines, opioids, and inhalation anesthetic agents have significant respiratory depressant effects. Any one of these drugs may be used in a dose that causes apnea, or lack of respirations for more than 10 seconds, during a general anesthesia. When used in combination their effect on respiration is at least additive. When the rate or depth of respirations decrease, the elimination of carbon dioxide is retarded, and carbon dioxide builds up in the blood and in the lungs. The buildup of carbon dioxide actually blocks the entry of oxygen into the bloodstream and makes it harder to keep the client adequately oxygenated. Oxygen saturation is monitored by pulse oximetry. Even small amounts of supplemental oxygen given to a client whose rate or depth of breathing is decreased adds significantly to the amount of oxygen in the bloodstream. This is the most important reason that oxygen is given to even healthy clients when they are recovering from general anesthesia.

Heart Rate and Blood Pressure

Few direct effects on heart rate (HR) and blood pressure (BP) regulation are seen during recovery from general anesthesia. Some anesthetic techniques that are heavily based on opioids, like fentanyl (Sublimaze) or sufentanil citrate (Sufenta), can cause a slow HR; but as long as BP is maintained, no specific treatment is necessary. Although most general anesthetics are myocardial depressants, the depressive effects of current agents are mild, especially after anesthetic administration is ended. Some individuals become sympathetically activated during the initial period after regaining consciousness. This occurs most commonly in clients with cardiac or vascular disease (hypertension, coronary artery disease, or peripheral vascular

LIFE CYCLE CONSIDERATIONS

Oxygenation and Ventilation in the Elderly Client

- Impaired mobility allows secretions to pool in the lungs. Therefore, elderly clients must be monitored more closely, and secretions suctioned.
- Most anesthetic agents cause decreased respiratory rate and decreased tidal volume, putting elderly clients at greater risk for hypoventilation.

occlusive disease). If the increase in HR or BP is a danger to the client, it can usually be successfully treated using a combined alpha and beta blocker like labetalol hydrochloride (Normodyne) or a calcium channel blocker such as nifedipine (Procardia).

Most HR and BP changes seen during recovery result from factors related indirectly to the anesthetic. Both HR and BP increase due to sympathetic stimulation. Pain, hypoxia, and fear can all result in sympathetic stimulation with an increase in HR and BP. Pain results when inadequate analgesia has been provided as the client emerges from anesthesia. An opioid such as morphine or meperidine (Demerol) will relieve the pain. The residual effects of anesthesia on respiratory centers or airway muscles in the throat may result in hypoventilation or airway obstruction. Provision of supplemental oxygen, proper airway management, and mechanical ventilation, if necessary, will ensure adequate oxygenation. Discovering and addressing the source of the client's fear often reduces the anxiety. When the causes of sympathetic stimulation are addressed, HR and BP should normalize.

Temperature Regulation and Shivering

With general anesthesia, the body loses its natural ability to regulate temperature. General anesthetic agents dilate the blood vessels close to the surface of the body, exposing the client's warm blood to the cool exterior. During anesthetization, the client is mostly uncovered in a cold operating room, and the area of the body to be operated on is cleaned with cold solutions. After this is done, the client's insulating covering (skin and subcutaneous fat) is cut open to expose the warm interior of the body and allow its heat to escape. Room temperature intravenous fluids are infused into the veins, and the client breathes cool gases. Surgical clients lose a great amount of heat at a time when the body is least able to respond to warm the tissues. Hypothermia adds to the CNS depression resulting from any residual anesthetics. Surface warming with a forced-air warming blanket is an effective way to increase the temperature of a client recovering from general anesthesia; cloth blankets or heating lamps may also be useful. Forced-air warming blankets are also used to prevent or limit the development of hypothermia intraoperatively. Figure 28-5 shows use of a forced-air warming blanket.

All potent inhalation agents are associated with shivering during emergence from general anesthesia when the blood level of the anesthetic agent is very low. This phenomenon was first associated with halothane and was thus called the "halothane shakes"; but it can occur following the administration of any inhalation anesthetic. The cause of the shivering is not clear but does not appear to be related to the client's body temperature. (Of course, postoperative clients also shiver when they are cold.) The key to eliminating

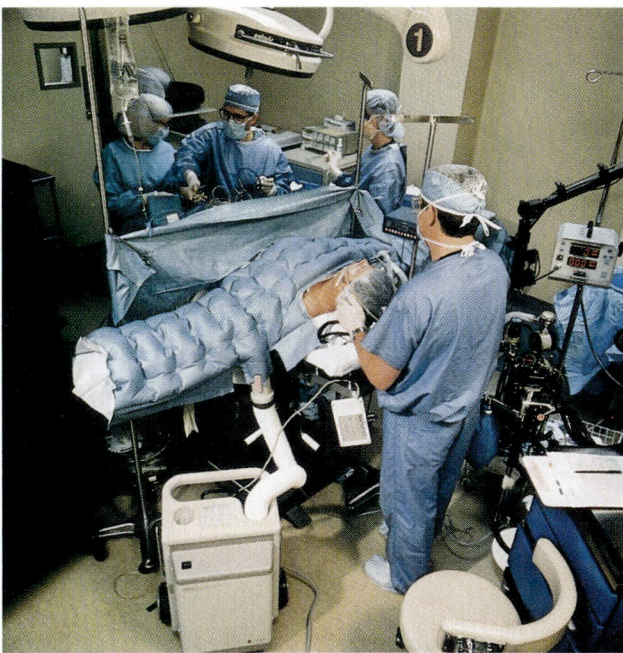

Figure 28-5 A forced-air warming blanket applied to the upper abdomen, chest, and arms of a client during surgery. The unit on the floor to the left of the anesthesia provider (foreground) is the heating unit, which contains a fan that pushes warm air through the hose and into the blanket much like a furnace pushes warm air through heating ducts and into a house. Warm air exits hundreds of pinholes on the surface of the blanket and next to the client. (*Courtesy of Mallinckrodt Medical, Inc.*)

shivering postoperatively is to ensure client warmth and encourage deep breathing so that the anesthetic is eliminated as quickly as possible.

Fluid Balance

Surgical procedures and the injuries that necessitate them have major effects on the body's distribution of fluid. Appropriate care during anesthesia sometimes necessitates the delivery of a large volume of IV fluid. This IV fluid does not stay in the vascular system long, moving out of the vascular space to replace losses from the interstitial and intracellular spaces.

Trauma, whether due to an accidental injury or a surgical incision, results in fluid losses or shifts in three general areas as follows: direct blood loss, evaporation through the surgical wound, and fluid shifts. Large volumes of fluid can be lost to the air through the surgical wound, especially during abdominal procedures. A major abdominal procedure, for example, can result in the loss of up to 10 cc/kg/hour of fluid by evaporation.

POSTOPERATIVE PAIN MANAGEMENT

Pain has many causes. Postoperative pain results from tissue injury, release of local and hormonal substances, inflammation, mental outlook, and, perhaps, neural hyperexcitability related to excessive noxious input. As such, baseline postoperative pain, pain from pressure placed on an incision, and pain from client movement may each respond best to different pain relieving strategies.

The amount of medication needed to relieve pain depends on the intensity and type of pain, the size of the client, and the client's age. The dose requirement for most opioids is dramatically lower for clients who are elderly as compared to younger clients. An 89-year-old needs 50% less opioid analgesic than does a 20-year-old (Scott & Stanski, 1987).

Patient-Controlled Analgesia

Patient-controlled analgesia (PCA) allows clients to self-administer pain medication by pushing a button when they experience pain. After an IV catheter is in place, a client-controlled analgesia pump is connected "piggyback" to the IV line. The pump is programmed to deliver a predetermined dose of morphine or meperidine (Demerol) when the client pushes a button. It will not, however, deliver unlimited amounts. A set time must pass between each successive dose, and when the total dose of opioid delivered in any hour reaches a preset limit, the pump will not deliver any more medicine until the next hour. This is referred to as lockout.

Properly programmed, PCA allows the client a great deal of control over when pain medicine is received, which is likely to help decrease anxiety. Patient-controlled analgesia also results in a shorter interval between the need for pain medicine and its administration; better pain relief than that obtained with intermittent IM injections; and a reduction in nursing time necessary for the delivery of pain medicine. It does not, however, decrease the need for client assessment while the PCA machine is in use.

Regional Analgesia

Regional analgesia and anesthesia have many applications in the relief of postoperative pain. Regional anesthetics do not cease working when the surgery ends and provide pain relief for a variable period of

time afterwards. The duration of postoperative pain relief can be extended by continuing the infusion of pain medication into the epidural space or by adding opioids to either epidural or spinal anesthetics.

Local Anesthetics

Local anesthetics, either alone or in combination with opioids, can be administered into the epidural space at low concentrations that do not cause complete anesthesia. This type of pain relief is most commonly used for women in labor who receive epidural analgesia. Local anesthetic in low concentrations is a powerful analgesic. If local anesthetic is administered in a way to relieve pain in the lower extremities, clients are usually confined to bed, because even dilute concentrations of local anesthetic may affect the strength of leg muscles enough to increase the risk of falling. Clients receiving analgesia via an epidural block should be watched carefully to ensure that they do not develop pressure necrosis in the blocked areas.

PROFESSIONAL TIP

Nursing Postanesthetic Care
- Immediately report to the anesthesia provider or surgeon any breathing difficulty.
- Immediately report to the surgeon or the anesthesia department a fall in the client's BP or increase in HR.
- Verify client's ability to stand or walk with normal motor strength and coordination and without any dizziness while in your direct care before allowing the client to get up without assistance.
- Do not allow clients to rub their eyes. Clients who are still drowsy may try to rub out protective eye moisturizer and, in the process, cause painful corneal abrasions.
- Observe clients immediately for bladder distention. Both regional and general anesthesia can sometimes cause temporary urinary retention.
- If clients have an epidural catheter for postoperative pain management, ensure that they change positions from time to time to prevent pressure necrosis. Do not allow the lateral aspect of the leg to rest on the side rails.
- Report to the anesthesia department as soon as possible any headache that gets worse when the client sits up or stands.
- Before giving discharge instructions, verify that the client's ability to remember instructions has returned. Always share discharge instructions with the individual responsible for taking the client home and provide the client with a written copy of the instructions.

CLIENT TEACHING

Patient-Controlled Analgesia (PCA)
- Only the client should push the button to administer more analgesic.
- The client should not ask visitors to push the button because doing so may result in an overdose of the medication.

Local anesthetic pain relief can occasionally do such an effective job of relieving pain that the client may be unaware that pressure necrosis is occurring (Cohen, Van Duker, Siegel, & Keon, 1993).

Opioids

The spinal cord has receptors for opioids, and when opioids are added to a spinal or epidural anesthetic, they provide pain relief even after the anesthetic block has worn off. Morphine added to a spinal or epidural anesthetic can provide hours of postoperative pain relief, often enough so that no other pain medication is needed (Abouleish, et al., 1991); it may even provide better pain relief than do IM injections or intravenous PCA (Kilbride, Senagore, Mazier, Ferguson, & Ufkes, 1992). Opioids may be added to spinal or epidural anesthetics as a single dose or be infused into the epidural space postoperatively. Although spinal and epidural morphine provide excellent pain relief, they may also produce significant respiratory depression. Respiratory depression is exceedingly rare in association with properly dosed epidural or spinal fentanyl (Sublimaze), however (Brockway, Noble, Sharwood-Smith, & McClure, 1990). Fortunately, the respiratory depression following spinal or epidural morphine administration is rarely rapid in onset. With current client selection and dosing protocols, life-threatening respiratory depression is a rare event. When it does occur, it can be detected long before it causes harm, by observing the client frequently, noting respiratory rate and depth, and periodically measuring oxygen saturation by pulse oximetry.

CASE STUDY

Mrs. Pinkerton is in the recovery room following outpatient surgery. She received a general anesthetic and is now awake, breathing deeply, and talking to the staff. She has received meperidine (Demerol) intravenously and is quite comfortable. Before being discharged home from the surgery center, Mrs. Pinkerton rests in an easy chair in the transitional recovery area. The nurse taking care of her notices that she asks questions about things that have already been discussed and has even asked one question three times.

The following questions will guide your development of a nursing care plan for the case study.

1. After making these observations what nursing diagnoses and goals might the nurse identify for Mrs. Pinkerton?
2. List the nursing interventions to be performed in caring for Mrs. Pinkerton.
3. Identify teaching approaches.

SUMMARY

- In addition to ensuring an adequate level of anesthesia throughout a surgical procedure, the anesthesia provider monitors and controls physiologic functions.
- Some anesthesia providers prefer that clients not have anything to eat or drink for at least 8 hours prior to surgery. Others allow water up to 2 hours before surgery.
- Most scheduled medications that a client takes every day will be continued up to and including the morning of surgery.
- Sedation depresses brain activity, decreasing awareness, reducing anxiety, and easing the induction of general anesthesia.

- Oversedation results in respiratory depression, which can cause airway obstruction, and places the client at risk for aspiration of gastric contents.
- Regional anesthesia by the injection of a local anesthetic temporarily renders a "region" of the body insensible to pain.
- General anesthesia produces unconsciousness, complete insensibility to pain, amnesia, motionlessness, and muscle relaxation.
- A person is unlikely to remember what has happened for minutes to hours after sedation or a general anesthetic.
- Intravenous patient-controlled analgesia (PCA) allows clients to self-administer pain medication by pushing a button on the PCA machine. Limits are programmed into the machine to prevent overdose.

- Local anesthetics, alone or in combination with opioids, can be injected into the epidural space at low concentrations to provide postoperative analgesia.
- Spinal and epidural morphine can produce dangerous respiratory depression. This can be detected by frequent observations of the client's respiratory rate and depth and by periodic measurement of oxygen saturation via pulse oximetry.

Review Questions

1. Who is qualified to explain anesthesia and its risks and benefits in a manner sufficient to secure an informed consent from a client or legal guardian?

   a. A medical–surgical staff nurse
   b. An anesthesia provider or surgeon
   c. An operating room nurse
   d. A nursing supervisor

2. Why are clients at risk for aspiration of gastric contents into the lungs when receiving a general anesthetic?

   a. General anesthesia causes stomach distention.
   b. General anesthesia eliminates protective airway reflexes.
   c. Gastric peristalsis is reversed during general anesthesia.
   d. Vomiting normally occurs during general anesthesia.

3. What is the most dangerous result of oversedation?

   a. Lack of response to verbal directions
   b. Longer recovery time and resultant delayed discharge
   c. Prolonged amnesia
   d. Inability to breathe adequately

4. What is a sign that a client has a postdural puncture headache following a spinal or epidural regional block?

   a. The headache subsides after intake of plenty of liquids.
   b. The headache begins after the surgical procedure.
   c. The headache worsens when the client sits up or stands.
   d. The client is confused in addition to having a headache.

5. In addition to keeping the client unconscious, preventing the sensation of pain, and relaxing muscles to hold the client still and allow for surgical exposure, what does an anesthesia provider do to ensure a safe anesthetic?

   a. Controls vital functions like breathing and heart rate
   b. Records the amount of anesthetic drug used
   c. Monitors the length of surgery
   d. Administers prophylactic antibiotics

6. How long after cessation of a general anesthetic might it be before the client can think as clearly as before the client received the anesthetic?

   a. Before being discharged from the recovery room
   b. Within 2 hours
   c. Six hours
   d. Several days

7. What effect might a spinal or epidural anesthetic block still have after normal sensation and motor function have returned?

   a. Decrease in pulse rate when the client is lying in bed
   b. Decrease in blood pressure when the client stands up
   c. Inhibition of protective airway reflexes
   d. Sore muscles

Critical Thinking Questions

1. Why is physical assessment important relative to anesthesia?

2. Why must clients be monitored very closely after receiving an anesthetic?

 WEB FLASH!

- What organizations are identified from which a person could get information about anesthesia?
- How many types of anesthesia can you find discussed on the Web?

NURSING CARE OF THE SURGICAL CLIENT

MAKING THE CONNECTION

Refer to the following chapters to increase your understanding of perioperative nursing:

- **Chapter 6, Legal Responsibilities**
- **Chapter 7, Ethical Responsibilities**
- **Chapter 8, Communication**
- **Chapter 12, Cultural Diversity and Nursing**
- **Chapter 16, Stress, Adaptation, and Anxiety**
- **Chapter 21, Infection Control/Asepsis**
- **Chapter 23, Fluid, Electrolyte, and Acid–Base Balance**
- **Chapter 25, Assessment**
- **Chapter 26, Pain Management**

- **Chapter 28, Anesthesia**
- **Chapter 31, Nursing Care of the Client: Respiratory System**
- **Chapter 32, Nursing Care of the Client: Cardiovascular System**
- **Chapter 40, Nursing Care of the Client: Integumentary System**
- **Procedures:** B1, Handwashing; B14, Transferring a Client from Bed to Stretcher; B25, Applying Antiembolism Stockings; I25, Postoperative Exercise Instruction

LEARNING OBJECTIVES

Upon completion of this chapter, you should be able to:
- *Define key terms.*
- *List risk factors to be identified in a preoperative nursing assessment.*
- *List information to include in a general teaching plan for a preoperative client.*
- *Identify common nursing care for the preoperative, intraoperative, and postoperative phases.*
- *Identify members of the surgical team and describe their functions.*
- *Describe the principles of asepsis and their application to nursing practice.*
- *Identify nursing interventions to prevent or treat postoperative complications.*
- *Identify information needed by the postoperative client prior to discharge.*
- *Discuss the physiologic changes of aging that may affect the elderly client's response to surgery.*

KEY TERMS

Aldrete Score	intraoperative phase
ambulatory surgery	perioperative
asepsis	postoperative phase
aseptic technique	preoperative phase
circulating nurse	scrub nurse
dehiscence	sterile
evisceration	sterile conscience
first assistant	sterile field
informed consent	surgery

INTRODUCTION

Surgery refers to the treatment of injury, disease, or deformity through invasive operative methods. Surgery is a unique experience, with no two clients responding alike to similar operations. Even the same client may respond differently to two separate surgical situations or to the same surgery performed at a later time. Each client has a unique socioeconomic background and fills different family and community roles. Regardless of background or roles, however, surgery is a major stressor for all clients. To a client, there is no such thing as minor surgery; anxiety and fear are normal. Surgery, even when planned well in advance, is a stressor that produces both psychological (anxiety, fear) and physiologic (neuroendocrine) stress reactions. Surgery is a stressful experience because it involves entry into the human body and is sometimes a threat to life itself.

Surgeries are classified as minor (presenting little risk to life) or major (possibly involving risk to life) and may be performed for a variety of reasons. Table 29-1 lists indications for surgery.

The term **perioperative** encompasses the **preoperative** (before surgery), **intraoperative** (during surgery), and **postoperative** (after surgery) phases of surgery. Each phase refers to a particular time during the surgical experience, and each requires a wide range of specific nursing behaviors and functions. Perioperative nursing has one continuous goal: to provide a standard of excellence in the care of the client before, during, and after surgery. Perioperative nursing is client oriented; therefore, the nursing activities must be geared to meet the client's psychosocial needs as well as immediate physical needs.

Surgical intervention is a distinctive event for clients. Individuals face this particular event with their own values. Every client not only has specific expectations of the surgical experience, but also has distinct hopes for the outcome of the surgery. The nurse must take an active part in the entire perioperative process in order to ensure quality and continuity of client care.

PREOPERATIVE PHASE

The **preoperative phase** is that time during the surgical experience that begins with the client's decision to have surgery and ends with the transfer of the client to the operating table.

The outcome of surgical treatment is tremendously enhanced by accurate preoperative nursing assessment and careful preoperative preparation. The client must be assessed by the nurse both physiologically and psychologically. Assessment of the client involves the integration of factors relating to the client's illness, physical condition, related medical conditions, and current surgical diagnosis. Regardless of how minor the surgical procedure, a thorough health history is essential and should be available to the perioperative team throughout the client's surgical experience.

The psychological well-being of the client may have an impact on the surgical outcome. The surgical client is at high risk for anxiety related to the surgical experience and the outcome of surgery. Fear and anxiety can affect the client's ability to cope with the proposed plan of care. Anxiety is a normal adaptive response to the stress of surgery. Because individuals differ in their perceptions of the meaning of surgery, the degree of anxiety and fear experienced will vary. If fear and anxiety become excessive, however, these emotions can interfere with recovery by magnifying the normal physiologic stress response. The nurse, by assessing and being aware of the fears and anxieties of the surgical client, can provide support and information so that stress does not become overwhelming. The most common fears related to surgery are as follows:

- Fear of the unknown
- Fear of pain and discomfort
- Fear of mutilation and disfigurement
- Fear of anesthesia
- Fear of disruption of life patterns
    Separation from family/significant others
    Sexuality
    Financial
    Permanent/temporary limitations
- Fear of death/not waking up
- Fear of not being in control

Fear of the unknown is the most prevalent fear prior to surgery and is the fear that the nurse can most easily help control through client education and preoperative teaching.

Preoperative Physiologic Assessment

Physiologic assessment should include a physical examination and a review of the client's laboratory values and diagnostic studies. Laboratory and diagnostic studies may be divided into those that are routine and those that are done specifically to evaluate the client's primary disease process or coexisting condition. The following summarizes common preoperative laboratory tests:

Table 29-1 INDICATIONS FOR SURGERY

TYPE OF SURGERY	PURPOSE	EXAMPLE
Diagnostic	Determine cause of symptoms	Biopsy
		Exploratory laparotomy
Curative	Remove a diseased body part or replace a body part to restore function	Colecystectomy
		Total knee arthroplasty
Palliative	Relieve symptoms without curing disease	Tumor resection associated with cancer
Restorative	Strengthen a weakened area	Herniorrhaphy
Cosmetic	Improve appearance	Face lift
	Change shape	Mammoplasty

- Hemoglobin and hematocrit (Hgb and Hct)
- White blood cell count (WBC)
- Blood typing and cross matching (screening)
- Serum electrolytes
- Prothrombin time (PT) and partial thromboplastin time (PTT)
- Bilirubin
- Liver enzymes: alanine aminotransferase (ALT) and aspartate aminotransferase (AST)
- Urinalysis
- Blood urea nitrogen (BUN) and creatinine

Although it is common practice to obtain a chest x-ray for many clients admitted to the hospital, this study is increasingly omitted for healthy children and healthy adults under the age of 40 years in whom the physical examination is normal and there is no reason to suspect pulmonary or cardiac disease. Additional radiographic or fluoroscopic examinations, sonograms, radioisotopic scans, magnetic resonance imaging, and computerized tomography scans give useful information as to the nature of the disease process and its anatomic location and extent. Any organ that is undergoing major surgery should be adequately evaluated with these techniques prior to the operation.

Electrocardiograms (EKGs) are routinely performed in middle-age and elderly clients undergoing surgery, because of the prevalence of ischemic heart disease in these age groups. It is also of value to have a baseline study for comparison should subsequent EKGs be needed.

Preoperative testing may be done several days be-fore the date of surgery. The type and amount of screening will depend on the age and condition of the client, the nature of the surgery, and the surgeon's preference. Surgeons (doctors who perform surgery) are coming under increasing economic pressure to minimize routine testing procedures. The current trend is based on cost versus benefits, moving away from extensive testing in the absence of indicative/warranting data from the health history and physical examination.

The nurse's role in preoperative testing is to ensure that the tests are ordered and performed and that the results are placed in the client's chart. Abnormal results are reported to the physician immediately.

The physiologic nursing assessment is completed prior to surgery. Preoperative assessment can take place in the surgeon's office, in the hospital during hospitalization, or in the hospital or ambulatory surgery unit on the day of surgery. The nurse collects client health data by interviewing the client, the family, significant others, and health care providers. Data collection can also be accomplished through review of the client's records; assessment; and/or consultation. Assessment is essential to establishing nursing diagnoses and predicting outcomes (Association of Operating Room Nurses [AORN], 1995a). When performing the nursing assessment, the nurse screens the client for risks that may contribute to complications in the perioperative period. Table 29-2 lists risk factors and possible complications of each. The nurse's role in the preoperative phase ensures client safety, understanding, and compliance with health care treatment.

Table 29-2 VARIABLES AFFECTING SURGICAL STATUS

VARIABLE	RELATED RISK FACTORS		POSSIBLE COMPLICATIONS
Age	Infancy	• Dehydration • Fluid overload • Hypothermia	• Infection • Respiratory obstruction
	Old age	• Decreased metabolism and elimination of anesthetics and medications • Hypothermia • Hypervolemia • Hypovolemia and shock • Deep vein thrombosis, thrombo-phlebitis, pulmonary embolus • Decreased urinary output/renal function • Urinary incontinence/retention	• Urinary tract infections • Poor or delayed wound healing • Pressure sores • Atelectasis/pneumonia • Constipation/fecal impaction • Infection • Physical injury (falls or joint overextension)
Nutritional status	Malnutrition	• Fluid and electrolyte imbalance • Delayed wound healing • Wound infection	• Poor tolerance to anesthetics • Bleeding/hemorrhage
	Obesity	• Retention of anesthetics and medications • Wound infection • Delayed wound healing	• Deep vein thrombosis, thrombophlebitis, pulmonary embolus • Atelectasis • Pneumonia *continued*

Table 29-2 *continued*

VARIABLE	RELATED RISK FACTORS	POSSIBLE COMPLICATIONS	
Fluid and electrolyte status	Deficits and excesses of fluids and electrolytes	• Anorexia, nausea, vomiting • Diarrhea and cramps • Constipation • Paralytic ileus • Hypotension • Hypertension • Edema (including pulmonary edema) • Confusion • Lethargy • Tetany • Weakness	• Parathesias • Paralysis • Restlessness • Delusions and hallucinations • Seizures • Laryngospasm • Respiratory arrest • Tachycardia • Dysrhythmias • Cardiac arrest • Renal failure
Respiratory status	Acute respiratory infections History of chronic respiratory diseases/ smoking	• Bronchospasm • Laryngospasm • Hypoxemia • Atelectasis • Pneumonia	• Atelectasis • Pneumonia
Cardiovascular status	History of preexisting cardiac disease	• Dysrhythmias • Hypotension/syncope • Myocardial infarction • Congestive heart failure	• Cardiac arrest • Stroke • Shock • Deep vein thrombosis, thrombophlebitis, or pulmonary embolism
Renal and hepatic status	History of pre-existing renal or hepatic diseases	• Fluid and electrolyte imbalances • Bleeding/hemorrhage • Infection	• Impaired wound healing • Hyperglycemia/hypoglycemia • Decreased metabolism and elimination of anesthetics and medications
Neurological, musculoskeletal, and integumentary status	Surgical positioning or prolonged immobility	• Pressure alopecia • Pressure point compression • Pressure sores • Nerve injury to axillary neurovascular bundle, subclavian neurovascular bundle, brachial plexus, and facial, peroneal, radial, and ulnar nerves • Neck pain, lower back pain, joint damage	• Postural hypotension • Eye abrasion • Ear compression • Atelectasis on dependent side • Air embolism • Facial and airway edema
Endocrine and immunological status	Diabetes Immunocompromised	• Fluid and electrolyte imbalances • Deep vein thrombosis, thrombophlebitis, and pulmonary embolism • Infection of respiratory and urinary tract • Infection • Respiratory infections	• Neurogenic bladder • Impaired wound healing • Hyperglycemia/hypoglycemia • Ketoacidosis • Pressure sores • Impaired wound healing
Medications	Chemical dependency	• Increased or decreased effectiveness of anesthetic agents, narcotics, and/or sedatives	• Drug interactions • Symptoms of withdrawal (hallucinations, disorientation, convulsions)

Age

Surgery can be performed on individuals of any age, although persons at both extremes of age (infants and elders) may be at greater risk for complications. Infants can easily become dehydrated or fluid overloaded and suffer resultant electrolyte imbalances. Because their metabolic rate is two to three times that of an adult, infants can have formula up to 6 hours before surgery, and breastfed infants may be nursed up to 4 hours before surgery. Infants may then have clear liquids for up to 2 hours before surgery.

Body temperature regulation and the renal, immune, and respiratory systems are different in infants than in adults. Renal function in the infant is comparatively less efficient due to a lower glomerular filtration rate and less efficient renal tubular function (Atkinson & Fortunato, 1996). This may lead to retention of anesthesia and medications and to fluid overload. Due to a comparatively larger ratio of body surface area to body mass, infants are also more prone to hypothermia when placed in a cool environment or when large areas of their body surface is exposed. Further, an immature immune system renders the infant more susceptible to infections. Because of a smaller and less developed anatomic structure and enlarged tongue and lymphoid tissue, the infant is also more prone to respiratory obstruction. The nursing process and nursing care must be tailored to meet the unique needs of the infant client.

Elderly clients experience many physiologic changes associated with aging and are more likely to have degenerative disease in many organs. Elders are more likely to become dehydrated and are thus less able to adapt to fluid loss during surgery. The elderly client is also more sensitive to central nervous system depressants used during the perioperative period. However, even elderly clients can favorably tolerate extensive surgery when carefully assessed and managed.

Nutritional Status

Nutritional assessment includes evaluation of individual deficiencies or excesses that can place the client at greater risk for complications during surgery. Surgery increases the body's need for nutrients necessary for tissue healing and resistance to infection.

Nutritional deficiencies place the client at higher risk for fluid and electrolyte imbalance, delayed wound healing, and wound infections. The malnourished individual may have diminished stores of carbohydrates and fats; in such an instance, proteins are utilized for energy instead of tissue building and restoration. In addition to carbohydrates and fats, vitamins B complex and C are also significant, because these vitamins are essential to healing. Poor nutritional status can also adversely affect liver and kidney function, leaving the client with a poor tolerance for anesthetic agents and a tendency for bleeding.

LIFE CYCLE CONSIDERATIONS

Surgery in the Elderly Client

Morbidity and mortality rates for surgical clients over the age of 90 years are much higher than for those age 70 to 75 years (Hogstel, 1994). Elderly clients do not tolerate emergency or long, complicated surgery as well as do younger clients because of a lesser ability to adapt to physical and psychological stress.

Nutritional excesses or obesity increase the risk for respiratory, cardiovascular, and gastrointestinal complications. Obesity makes access to the surgical site more difficult, which prolongs surgical time and increases the amount of anesthetic agents required. Because inhalation anesthetics are absorbed and stored by adipose tissue and released postoperatively, recovery time from anesthesia is slower in the overweight client. Adipose tissue is less vascular and more difficult to suture, which predisposes the client to wound infection, delayed wound healing, and increased incidence of wound complications including postoperative incisional hernias. Failure to exercise and ambulate increases the chances of decreased respiratory function accompanied by atelectasis and pneumonia, and also may lead to decreased wound healing and an increased risk of thrombus formation. Often, obese clients also have other chronic conditions, such as hypertension or diabetes mellitus, that increase the likelihood of surgical complications. In some surgical situations, such as joint replacement, surgery may be delayed until nutritional status improves and the client loses weight.

Fluid and Electrolyte Status

Dehydration and hypovolemia, with correlating electrolyte disturbances, predispose a client to complications during and after surgery. Both may be caused by diarrhea, excessive nasogastric suctioning, inadequate oral intake, vomiting, and/or bleeding. As outlined in Table 29-2, the complications of fluid and electrolyte imbalances are numerous and varied, ranging from minor (delayed recovery) to major (death). Changes in fluid and electrolyte balance affect cellular metabolism, renal function, and oxygen concentration in the circulation. Nursing care focuses on administering parenteral fluids or blood products as prescribed, keeping a detailed intake and output record, and evaluating results of laboratory studies.

Respiratory Status

Respiratory assessment should include detection of acute and chronic problems. Because acute respiratory

CLIENT TEACHING

Postoperative Deep Breathing, Incentive Spirometry, Coughing, and Turning

Activity	Description	Instruction
Deep breathing	• Mode of breathing during which the diaphragm expands fully, allowing expansion of the thorax, upper abdomen, and alveoli as air enters and followed by abdominal and diaphragmatic contraction during expansion	• Sit in semi-Fowler's position with hands placed over lower ribs and upper abdomen • Inhale deeply through the mouth and nose • Hold the breath for 5 seconds • Exhale fully through mouth and nose • Repeat 15 times with short rest periods as needed • Perform twice daily
Incentive spirometry (Figure 29-1)	• Method of using a commercial cylinder that measures deep breaths, with a float that rises during inhalation	• Sit as upright as possible • Seal lips around mouthpiece • Inhale and watch float rise • Hold deep breath for 5 seconds • Remove mouthpiece and exhale slowly • Repeat 10 to 12 times per hour • Cough after the last breath
Coughing (Figure 29-2)	• Method of moving lung secretions from smaller airways to larger airways	• Sit as upright as possible • Splint incision with hands or pillow • Inhale deeply using deep breathing technique • Cough several times until it feels as if no air is left in the lungs • May continue with another deep inhalation followed by one or two strong coughs • Repeat one time per hour
Turning	• Method of alternating position from back to either side to promote circulation, lung expansion and drainage, and relief from pressure areas	• Change position every 1 to 2 hours (assistance and support pillows may be required)

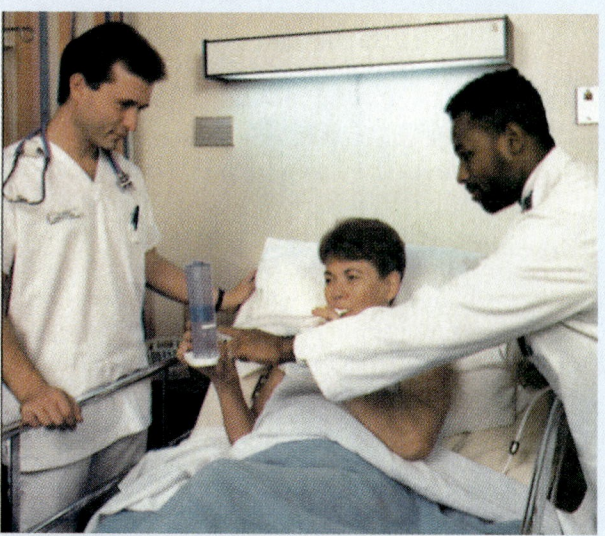

Figure 29-1 Using an Incentive Spirometer

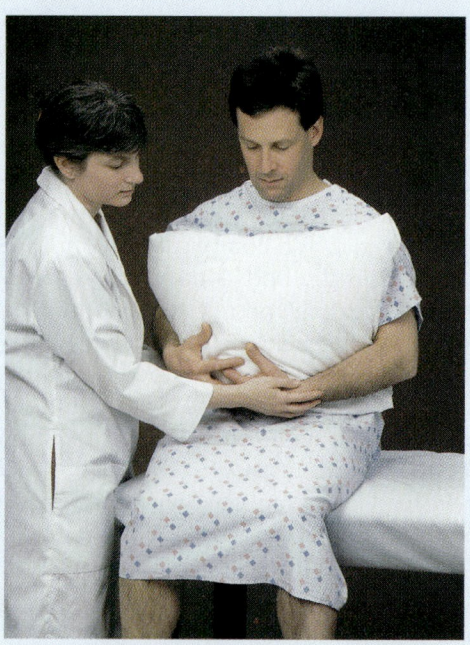

Figure 29-2 Splinting to Cough

infections may lead to bronchospasms or laryngospasms, surgery for clients with these conditions may be delayed or contraindicated. Chronic respiratory problems, such as asthma and chronic obstructive pulmonary disease, impair the client's gas exchange and increase the risk associated with inhalation anesthetic agents. Clients with chronic respiratory problems are more likely to develop atelectasis and pneumonia.

Respiratory assessment as performed by the nurse includes assessing breath sounds and color of the skin and mucous membranes. It also involves assessing for shortness of breath (dyspnea), clubbed fingers, and coughing. In addition to a chest x-ray, arterial blood gases or an oxygen saturation baseline may be ordered. Restriction of smoking should be encouraged at least 4 to 6 weeks before a scheduled surgery, when possible. All clients, and especially those clients who smoke and have chronic lung disease, should be taught deep breathing, use of incentive spirometry, coughing, and preoperative turning.

Cardiovascular Status

Cardiovascular assessment focuses on diseases that would require close observation by the nurse and make necessary the avoidance of sudden changes of position, overhydration with intravenous fluids, and prolonged immobilization. Examples of such diseases include angina, recent myocardial infarction or cardiac surgery, hemophilia, hypertension, and congestive heart failure. Clients with a history of cardiac disease are prone to developing complications such as dysrhythmias, hypotension, myocardial infarction, congestive heart failure, cardiac arrest, stroke, shock, deep vein thrombosis, thrombophlebitis, or pulmonary embolism.

The nurse also assesses for anxiety; elevated blood pressure; slow, rapid, or irregular pulse; chest pain; edema; coolness or cyanosis/discoloration of extremities; weakness; and shortness of breath (dyspnea). All clients must be taught postoperative leg exercises to prevent thrombophlebitis (Figure 29-3 and the accompanying display). The goal of nursing care is to improve the client's cardiovascular condition to the highest degree possible by promoting rest alternated with activity; encouraging a low-sodium and low-cholesterol diet; administering heart medications; and judiciously administering parenteral fluids and recording intake and output.

Renal and Hepatic Status

Because many medications and anesthetic agents are detoxified by the liver and excreted by the kidneys, renal and hepatic sufficiency constitute a major concern. Renal disease affects fluid and electrolyte balance and protein equilibrium. Liver disease may be accompanied by bleeding tendencies or carbohydrate, fat, and amino acid imbalances that impair wound healing and increase the risk of infection. The nurse assesses for symptoms of urinary frequency, dysuria, and anuria, and records the color and amount of the urine. The nurse also assesses for a history of bleeding tendencies, easy bruising, nosebleeds, and use of anticoagulants. The most commonly ordered preoperative tests to assess renal function are urinalysis, blood urea nitrogen (BUN), and creatinine. The most common liver tests are prothrombin time (PT), partial thromboplastin time (PTT), bilirubin, and the liver enzymes alanine aminotransferase (ALT) and aspartate aminotransferase

PROFESSIONAL TIP

Client's Psychological Condition

The client "who fears dying while under anesthesia runs a greater risk of cardiac arrest on the operating table than [do] clients with known cardiac disease" (Atkinson & Fortunato, 1996).

- The psychological condition of the client can have a stronger influence than does the physical condition.
- Encourage clients to express their feelings and fears about receiving anesthetic and having surgery.
- Observe the client for nonverbal clues indicative of anxiety.
- To reduce client anxiety, explain to the client what will be happening throughout the surgical experience.

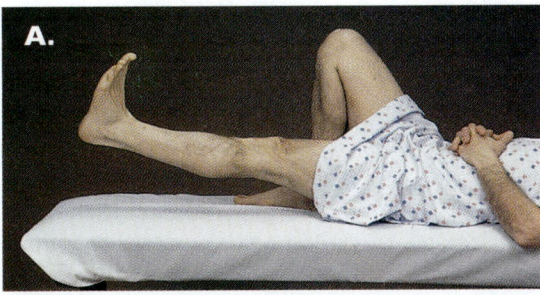

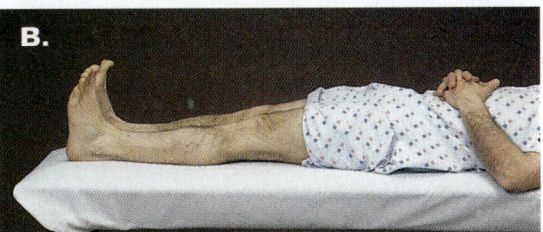

Figure 29-3 Leg Exercises: A. Lift leg and circle ankle, first to the right and then to the left. Repeat three times; relax. Repeat with other leg. B. With heels on the bed, push toes of both feet toward the foot of the bed until the calf muscles tighten; relax. Pull toes up toward chin until calf muscles tighten; relax feet.

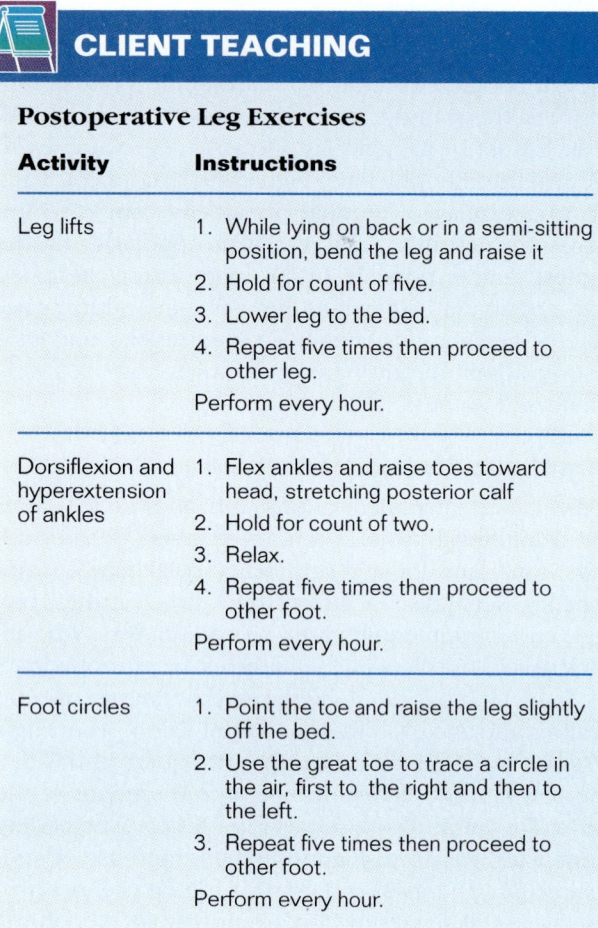

CLIENT TEACHING

Postoperative Leg Exercises

Activity	Instructions
Leg lifts	1. While lying on back or in a semi-sitting position, bend the leg and raise it 2. Hold for count of five. 3. Lower leg to the bed. 4. Repeat five times then proceed to other leg. Perform every hour.
Dorsiflexion and hyperextension of ankles	1. Flex ankles and raise toes toward head, stretching posterior calf 2. Hold for count of two. 3. Relax. 4. Repeat five times then proceed to other foot. Perform every hour.
Foot circles	1. Point the toe and raise the leg slightly off the bed. 2. Use the great toe to trace a circle in the air, first to the right and then to the left. 3. Repeat five times then proceed to other foot. Perform every hour.

(AST). Nursing care focuses on administering fluids and adequate nutrition, monitoring fluid intake and output, and evaluating results of laboratory tests.

Neurological, Musculoskeletal, and Integumentary Status

The nurse assesses the client's overall mental status including level of consciousness; orientation to person, place, and time; and the ability to understand and follow instructions. The nurse assesses the condition of the skin, including turgor; and notes any rashes, bruises, lesions, or previous incisions. Client mobility and sensation are also assessed through observation of both range of motion and ability to ambulate and through client statements. The nurse notes any abnormalities, injuries, or previous surgery and assesses the risk for falls. The presence of internal or external prostheses or implants such as pacemakers, heart valves, or joint prosthesis is also noted, because the presence of these may necessitate preoperative antibiotics.

Thin clients, clients undergoing long surgical procedures or vascular procedures, and elderly clients are the most vulnerable to neurological, musculoskeletal, or integumentary injuries. Some underlying disease processes, such as edema, infection, cancer, osteoporosis, arthritic joints, or neck or back problems, also place a client at higher risk for injury. Clients who are

malnourished, anemic, obese, hypovolemic, paralyzed, or diabetic are also prone to skin breakdown. Information gathered about the neurological, musculoskeletal, and integumentary systems is used for preparation of the surgical site, for surgical positioning, and as a comparative basis for postoperative assessments and complication screening. Table 29-2 lists potential complications of surgical positioning and prolonged immobility after surgery.

Endocrine and Immunological Status

Clients with diabetes who are undergoing surgery require special consideration. They should be scheduled as early in the morning as possible, and a fasting glucose should be drawn immediately prior to surgery. Surgery is a stressor, and stress raises the serum glucose level in the client with diabetes. Thus, the morning dose of insulin may need to be adjusted.

When anesthetized during surgery, the diabetic client exhibits very few symptoms of glucose imbalance. Serum glucose must therefore be checked frequently during surgery, usually by the anesthesia provider. Stability is attained by the administration of insulin, glucose, or both. Besides hyperglycemia and hypoglycemia, a diabetic client is more prone to fluid and electrolyte imbalances; infection including respiratory and urinary tract infections; neurogenic bladder; impaired wound healing; ketoacidosis; deep vein thrombosis; thrombophlebitis; and pulmonary embolism.

Because the immunological system protects the client from infections, the immunocompromised surgical client is very prone to infection. Clients receiving steroids or chemotherapy, or who have systemic lupus erythematosus, Addison's disease, or acquired immunodeficiency syndrome (AIDS) are considered to be immunocompromised. The immune response in these clients is weakened or deficient, resulting in an increased incidence of infection. Because surgery breaks the integrity of the skin and the normal inflammatory response is suppressed, wound healing may be impaired. Strict adherence to aseptic technique, covered later in this chapter, is thus even more imperative. Prevention of infection is crucial in these clients. The role of the nurse is to communicate the presence of potential immunosuppression to other health care team members involved in the client's care, and to help prevent infection by practicing aseptic technique.

Medications

Knowledge of the client's use of drugs for recreational or therapeutic purposes is essential to preoperative assessment. The history of medication usage by the client should include type and frequency of use for over-the-counter, prescription, and street drugs. The use of certain drugs can affect the client's reaction to anesthetic agents and surgery (Table 29-3). Some drugs increase surgical risks; these medications usually are

Table 29-3 MEDICATION CLASSIFICATIONS AND POSSIBLE EFFECTS WITH ANESTHETIC AGENTS AND SURGERY	
CLASSIFICATION	**POSSIBLE EFFECTS**
Antibiotics	• Respiratory paralysis when combined with certain muscle relaxants
Anticoagulants	• Hemorrhage
Anti-Parkinson drugs	• Increase hypotensive effects of anesthetic agents
Diuretics	• Electrolyte imbalance
Hypoglycemics	• Hypoglycemia or hyperglycemia
Monoamine oxidase (MAO) inhibitors	• Hypertensive crisis when combined with certain anesthetics
Steroids	• Cardiovascular collapse if abruptly withdrawn • Impaired physiologic response to stress • Delayed wound healing • Increased risk of infection
Street drugs and alcohol abuse	• Tolerance to narcotics
Tranquilizers	• Potentiation of narcotics and barbiturates

PROFESSIONAL TIP

Questions To Assess Psychosocial Status

• Why are you having surgery?
• When did this problem start?
• What do you think caused this problem?
• Has this caused any problems in your relationships with others?
• Has your problem prevented you from working?
• Are you able to take care of your own needs?
• Are you experiencing any discomfort or pain?
• What are you expecting from this surgery?
• Is there anything that you do not understand regarding your surgery?
• Are you worried about anything?
• Will someone be available to assist you when you return home?

temporarily discontinued when a client goes to surgery. Other medications, such as heart or hypoglycemic medications may still be given even though the client is to undergo surgery; the surgeon or anesthesia provider will write specific orders in such instances. Dosages of medications may also be adjusted during the perioperative period.

Chronic alcohol use increases surgical risk because it is often accompanied by impaired nutrition and liver disease. Postoperatively, the client may exhibit delirium tremens or acute withdrawal syndrome. Furthermore, pain medication may be less effective.

Psychosocial Health Assessment

The psychosocial health status of the client is also assessed. The nurse elicits the client's perceptions of surgery and the expected outcome. The nurse also ascertains the client's coping mechanisms and the client's knowledge level and ability to understand. The data collected are incorporated into nursing care throughout the perioperative experience.

Cultural beliefs can influence a client's perception of surgery. For example, some cultures believe that surgery is a "final effort" performed only when all other possible treatments have been of no avail. Furthermore, surgeries that cause changes in the appearance of the body can alter body image and self-esteem; the client may worry about being sexually attractive or active after surgery.

Clients should be provided the opportunity to express their spiritual values and beliefs. Many clients wish to see a member of the clergy before having surgery.

Surgical Consent

An **informed consent** is a legal form signed by the client and witnessed by another person that grants permission to the client's physician to perform the procedure described by the physician. An informed consent is needed whenever:

• Anesthesia is used,
• The procedure is considered invasive,
• The procedure is nonsurgical but has more than a slight risk of complications (such as with an arteriogram), or
• Radiation or cobalt therapy is used.

Informed consent protects both the client (against unauthorized procedures) and the physician and the health care institution and its employees (against claims that an unauthorized procedure was performed). Although the ultimate responsibility for obtaining the informed consent lies with the physician, it is often the nurse who obtains and witnesses the client's signature and ensures that the client signs the consent form

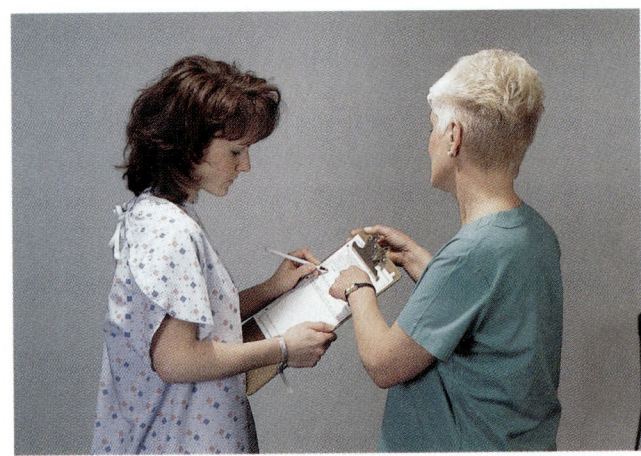

Figure 29-4 Nurse Obtaining a Signature on a Consent Form

voluntarily and is alert and comprehending of the action (Figure 29-4).

Most hospitals use a standard preprinted form. The information written by the health care personnel must be specific to the individual client. The client's signature on the consent form indicates the information has been read and is correct. The client has the right to refuse treatment even after the consent has been signed. When this occurs, the nurse must inform the physician immediately of the client's decision.

Preoperative Teaching

The client about to undergo surgery is at high risk for knowledge deficit related to preoperative procedures and protocols and to postoperative expectations. Preoperative teaching is the giving of information to the client prior to a surgical procedure. The potential benefits of preoperative teaching include reduced anxiety and more rapid recovery with fewer complications and shorter hospitalization. Reduction in anxiety has a secondary benefit: The client usually requires less medication for pain. The purpose of preoperative teaching is to (1) answer questions and concerns about surgery; (2) ascertain the client's present knowledge of the intended surgery; (3) ascertain the need or desire for additional information; and (4) provide information in a manner most conducive to learning.

One-on-one sessions constitute the most personal method of instruction. The nurse should also try to include the family or significant other when possible. The level of learning increases when more than one teaching medium is used. For example, using materials such as videotapes, charts, tours, anatomic models, pictures, and brochures reinforces both visual and auditory learning. Demonstration followed by return demonstration is helpful. Written instructions serve as a reference for later use. Instructions should be simple, using terms the client can understand. Any unfamiliar words or concepts should be thoroughly explained.

Clients are often interested in any information that describes the sights, sounds, tastes, feelings, odors, and temperature of what they are about to experience. For example, the feeling of relaxation from preoperative medications; the sounds of instruments or equipment in the operating room (OR); the pressure from the automatic blood pressure cuff; the warmth or coolness of skin-preparation solutions; or the brightness of the operating room lights are all sensations the client may experience. Analogies or stories of real or fictitious situations of sensory experiences help the client understand concepts being presented. The teaching methods used by the nurse strongly influence the client's degree of learning and retention of information.

Preoperative teaching should begin as soon as surgery is agreed upon. Instructions given over the phone and/or mailed to the client during the time leading up to surgery are beneficial. Just prior to surgery, a brief review with additional information tailored to the needs of the client may be given. The client should be given an opportunity to ask questions.

Information should always be targeted to the client's needs. Teaching plans should be tailored according to the client's level of knowledge and anxiety. Mild to moderate anxiety actually heightens a person's alertness and motivates learning. Mildly anxious clients should receive the most complete instructions. Moderately anxious clients should receive less information but more attention to specific areas of concern. Severely anxious clients should receive only basic information but should be encouraged to verbalize their concerns. Clients in a state of panic are unable to learn; in such cases no instruction shall be given, and the surgeon should be notified.

Physical Preparation

Extremely close attention must be given to identifying the proper client both verbally and by reading the identification name band. The nurse then begins the important task of verifying the operative procedure. This must be completed through client statements, surgeon verification, and the signed surgical consent form. Particular attention should be given to differentiating between right and left operative sites.

In order to lessen the chance of infection, special care is given to the preparation of the operative site.

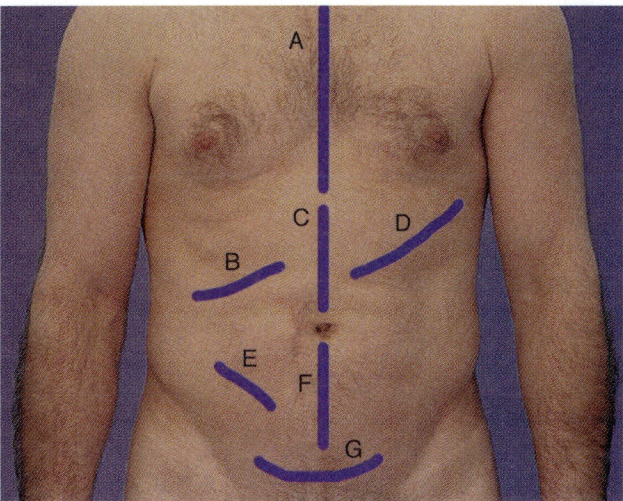

Figure 29-5 Common Surgical Incisions: A. Sternal split; B. Oblique subcostal; C. Upper vertical midline; D. Thoraco-abdominal; E. McBurney; F. Lower vertical midline; G. Pfannenstiel

CLIENT TEACHING

Preoperative Teaching

- Introduce self
  Identify role in client's care
- Determine client's knowledge level and need or desire for additional information
- Explain the routine for the day of surgery
  Restricted food or fluid intake
  Intravenous fluids
  Premedication
  Time of surgery
  Anticipated length of surgery
  Transportation to the operating room
  Special skin preparations
  Type of surgical incision (Figure 29-5)
- Familiarize the client with the operating room environment
  Operating room lights and table
  Accessory equipment
  Monitoring equipment
  Anesthesia induction
- Include significant others
  Time to arrive at the hospital
  Location of surgical waiting area
  What to expect when client returns to the unit
- Explain postanesthesia care unit (PACU)
  Location of recovery room
  Purpose of recovery room
  Routine of postanesthesia care
- Identify anticipated dressings, drains, catheters, casts, etc.
- Demonstrate and evaluate client's proficiency with:
  Coughing and deep breathing exercises
  Turning
  Incentive spirometry
  Extremity exercises
  Any special transfer procedures or aids required after surgery
- Describe pain management strategies appropriate for the specific surgical procedure

To reduce the number of microorganisms on the skin, the operative site is thoroughly cleansed with an antiseptic soap such as povidone-iodine. Typically, the operative site is not shaved; but if shaving is to be performed, it is done in the operating room immediately prior to surgery. To reduce the number of bacteria in the gastrointestinal tract for gastrointestinal, peritoneal, perianal, or pelvic surgery, an enema is ordered. Enemas prevent contamination of the peritoneal area by fecal content passed during surgery. The reduction in colon size related to the loss of bulk also helps prevent colon injury and increases visualization of the opera-

tive site. Enemas are usually given the night before surgery. If the enema is to be done at home, the client must be given detailed instructions. Many types of surgery require special preparations. The specific protocol for each surgical procedure is available from the health care facility or the physician.

 Safety: Iodine Allergy

- Each client must be asked about allergy to iodine.

- If a client is allergic to iodine, document the allergy on the client's record and inform the surgeon and OR personnel so that an iodine-free solution can be used for skin preparation and for other procedures for which iodine is routinely used.

The nurse checks the client's vital signs including blood pressure, temperature, pulse and respirations. Due to anxiety, some changes in vital signs are normal. If marked differences exist from the baseline data, however, the surgeon must be notified.

The nurse assists the client in putting on a hospital gown, hair cap, and, if ordered, antiembolic hose. Institutional policy requires that jewelry be removed; however wedding rings may be taped on and left in place. Hairpins, wigs, and prostheses must also be removed. The nurse is responsible for recording the disposition of any personal items removed for surgery. If policy requires, nail polish (from at least one nail, if dark polish) is removed so that oxygen saturation may be read via pulse oximetry, although some pulse oximeters may be able to read oxygen saturation through nail polish. Makeup is also removed so that skin color can be observed.

Allergies to medication, food, and chemicals (including contrast agents) are verified, as are previous blood reactions. The nurse must differentiate between a medication intolerance and a true allergic reaction. With a medication intolerance, the client may suffer side effects that are unpleasant. For example, many clients experience nausea when given meperidine (Demerol); although unpleasant, this is not a drug allergy. A true allergy produces a skin reaction or anaphylactic reaction, where the client experiences cardiorespiratory reactions that may be life threatening, such as hypotension and pulmonary edema. A client with multiple food allergies is also prone to hypersensitivities to medications. When allergies are identified, the client's chart is marked accordingly, and an allergy wrist band is applied. By being aware of and alerting other team members to the client's allergies, client safety and comfort are maintained.

The nurse verifies the NPO (nothing by mouth) status of the client for the amount of time specified by the surgeon's order. Restricting oral intake reduces the possibility of aspiration pneumonia. Typically, the client is designated NPO after midnight. If surgery takes place in the afternoon, the client may have a clear liquid breakfast if ordered by the surgeon. Careful client instruction is required because surgery may need to be postponed if the client consumes food or fluid.

In addition to the previously outlined preparations, dentures and bridgework are removed to prevent loss, damage, and possible dislodgement and airway obstruction during the surgery. The nurse also ensures that the client has an empty bladder by allowing time for the client to void prior to transfer to surgery.

The nurse should identify any sensory deficits in the client and communicate this information to other health care team members. Glasses, contact lenses, and hearing aids are usually removed to prevent loss or damage; if policy allows, however, it is best to leave these items in place so that the client is better able to see and hear. The nurse would then be responsible for communicating the presence of these aids to other health care team members.

The surgeon or anesthesiologist (a doctor trained in providing anesthesia) may order preoperative medication. Table 29-4 lists medications that may be given alone or in combination to elicit the desired effects. The nurse gives the medication by the prescribed route (intramuscular, intravenous, or oral) at the specified time (typically 1 hour prior to surgery). Often, preoperative medications are ordered "on call," this means that the nurse is notified by a member of the surgical team when the preoperative medication needs to be given. Prior to administering the medication, the nurse should ask the client to void. After administering the preoperative medication, the nurse should raise the side rails of the gurney or bed, put the bed in the lowest position, and instruct the client not to get up without assistance.

When the surgical team is ready, the client is transported on a gurney by a member of the OR team, typically an orderly. The client is always transported feet first and with the side rails up to ensure safety and minimize the likelihood of dizziness and nausea. If on a clinical nursing unit, the client may be taken to a preoperative holding area first (Figure 29-6). The nurse instructs the family or significant others where to wait.

The information collected as part of preoperative preparation is documented in the client record, usually on a preoperative checklist. Figure 29-7 illustrates a typical preoperative checklist. This checklist is completed

Table 29-4 PREOPERATIVE MEDICATIONS: COMMON CLASSIFICATIONS, EXAMPLES, AND DESIRED EFFECTS

CLASSIFICATION	EXAMPLE	DESIRED EFFECTS
Tranquilizers	diazepam (Valium) lorazepam (Ativan)	Reduce anxiety Decrease motor activity Promote rapid induction of anesthesia
Sedatives	phenobarbitol sodium (Luminal sodium) secobarbital (Seconal) midazolam hydrochloride (Versed)	Promote sleep Decrease anxiety Reduce amount of anesthesia required
Narcotics	morphine sulfate meperidine (Demerol)	Reduce pain Relax the client Reduce anxiety
Vagolytic agents (anticholinergics)	atropine sulfate scopolamine hydrobromide glycopyrrolate (Robinul)	Reduce tracheobronchial secretions Drying of mucous membranes Interrupt vagal stimulation Produce sedative and amnesia effects
Antinausea agents	droperidol (Inapsine) promethazine hydrochloride (Phenergan)	Reduce nausea Prevent vomiting Provide mild relaxation
H_2 receptor antagonists	cimetidine (Tagamet) ranitidine hydrochloride (Zantac) famotidine (Pepcid)	Decrease gastric secretions

prior to the client leaving the clinical unit or upon the client's admission to ambulatory surgery. The nurse must also verbally communicate to other health care members any necessary information collected.

INTRAOPERATIVE PHASE

The **intraoperative phase** is the time during the surgical experience that begins when the client is transferred to the operating room table and ends when the client is admitted to the postanesthesia care unit (PACU).

Physical Description of the Operating Room Environment

For the purposes of preventing wound infections, the surgical suite is environmentally controlled. Personnel restriction and geographic isolation from other areas of the hospital or clinic constitute part of this control. Constant filtered airflow and positive air pressure in the operating rooms also aid in environmental control. Furthermore, clean areas and contaminated areas are separated within the suite. Finally, equipment and supplies needed for each client are centralized in the surgical suite so that members of the surgical team do not have to leave the area.

Operating rooms vary in size depending on the amount of equipment needed for each particular type of operation, with open-heart surgery operating rooms

usually being the largest. Supplies and furniture are limited to prevent dust collection and are usually made of stainless steel to withstand corrosive disinfectants. Furniture and equipment are easily movable on wheels. In addition to general illumination from ceiling lights, the operative site is illuminated by overhead operating lights. Figure 29-8 shows a typical operating room. The temperature of the room can be adjusted but usually is maintained at a cool 66°F to 68°F. This range provides comfort for the surgical team (the members of which are wearing gowns, gloves, and masks under hot lights), and for the client (who is beneath layers of

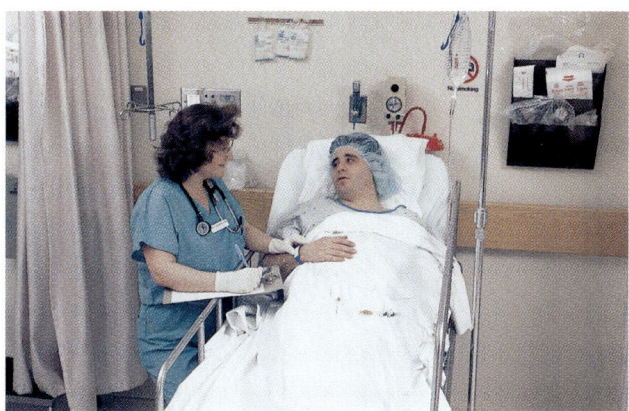

Figure 29-6 The holding area is used for clients who are waiting to have surgery

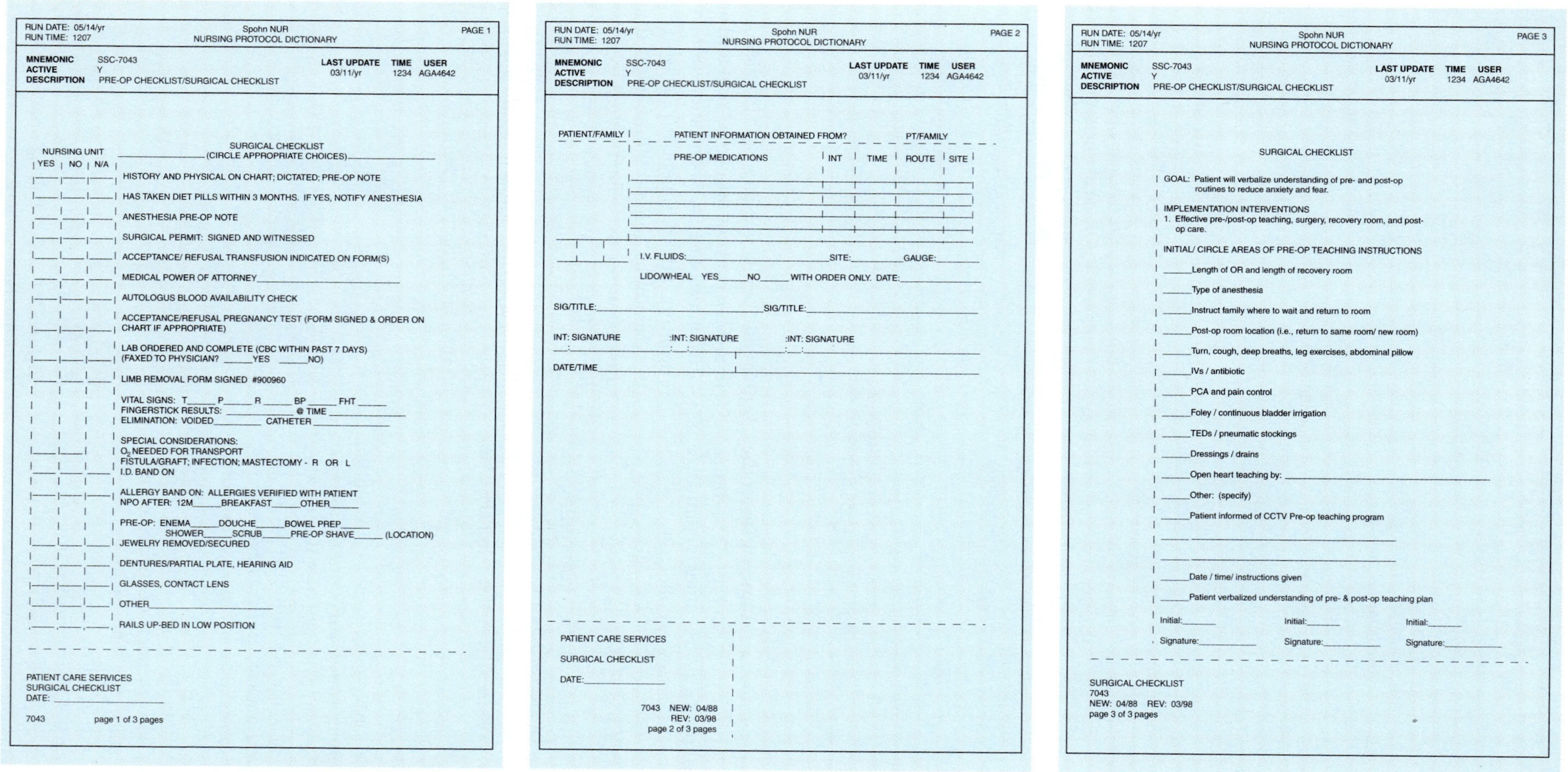

PAGE 3

RUN DATE: 05/14/yr
RUN TIME: 1207

Spohn NUR
NURSING PROTOCOL DICTIONARY

	LAST UPDATE	TIME	USER
	03/11/yr	1234	AGA4642

MNEMONIC   SSC-7043
ACTIVE   Y
DESCRIPTION   PRE-OP CHECKLIST/SURGICAL CHECKLIST

SURGICAL CHECKLIST

I GOAL: Patient will verbalize understanding of pre- and post-op
      routines to reduce anxiety and fear.

IMPLEMENTATION INTERVENTIONS
1. Effective pre-/post-op teaching, surgery, recovery room, and post-
   op care.

INITIAL/ CIRCLE AREAS OF PRE-OP TEACHING INSTRUCTIONS
____ Length of OR and length of recovery room
____ Type of anesthesia
____ Instruct family where to wait and return to room
____ Post-op room location (i.e., return to same room/ new room)
____ Turn, cough, deep breaths, leg exercises, abdominal pillow
____ IVs / antibiotic
____ PCA and pain control
____ Foley / continuous bladder irrigation
____ TEDs / pneumatic stockings
____ Dressings / drains
____ Open heart teaching by:
____ Other: (specify)
____ Patient informed of CCTV Pre-op teaching program
____ Date / time/ instructions given
____ Patient verbalized understanding of pre- & post-op teaching plan

Initial: _____   Initial: _____
Signature: _____   Signature: _____

SURGICAL CHECKLIST
7043
NEW: 04/88 REV: 03/98
page 3 of 3 pages

PAGE 2

RUN DATE: 05/14/yr
RUN TIME: 1207

Spohn NUR
NURSING PROTOCOL DICTIONARY

	LAST UPDATE	TIME	USER
	03/11/yr	1234	AGA4642

MNEMONIC   SSC-7043
ACTIVE   Y
DESCRIPTION   PRE-OP CHECKLIST/SURGICAL CHECKLIST

PATIENT/FAMILY	PATIENT INFORMATION OBTAINED FROM?		PT/FAMILY		
	PRE-OP MEDICATIONS	INT	TIME	ROUTE	SITE

I.V. FLUIDS: _____   SITE: _____   GAUGE: _____
LIDO/WHEAL   YES ____   NO ____   WITH ORDER ONLY. DATE: _____

SIG/TITLE: _____   SIG/TITLE: _____

INT: SIGNATURE _____   INT: SIGNATURE _____

DATE/TIME: _____

PATIENT CARE SERVICES
SURGICAL CHECKLIST
DATE: _____
7043   NEW: 04/88
       REV: 03/98
       page 2 of 3 pages

PAGE 1

RUN DATE: 05/14/yr
RUN TIME: 1207

Spohn NUR
NURSING PROTOCOL DICTIONARY

	LAST UPDATE	TIME	USER
	03/11/yr	1234	AGA4642

MNEMONIC   SSC-7043
ACTIVE   Y
DESCRIPTION   PRE-OP CHECKLIST/SURGICAL CHECKLIST

SURGICAL CHECKLIST
(CIRCLE APPROPRIATE CHOICES)

NURSING UNIT _____
| YES | NO | N/A |
____ HISTORY AND PHYSICAL ON CHART; DICTATED; PRE-OP NOTE
____ HAS TAKEN DIET PILLS WITHIN 3 MONTHS. IF YES, NOTIFY ANESTHESIA
____ ANESTHESIA PRE-OP NOTE
____ SURGICAL PERMIT: SIGNED AND WITNESSED
____ ACCEPTANCE/ REFUSAL TRANSFUSION INDICATED ON FORM(S)
____ MEDICAL POWER OF ATTORNEY
____ AUTOLOGUS BLOOD AVAILABILITY CHECK
____ ACCEPTANCE/REFUSAL PREGNANCY TEST (FORM SIGNED & ORDER ON
      CHART IF APPROPRIATE)
____ LAB ORDERED AND COMPLETE (CBC WITHIN PAST 7 DAYS)
      (FAXED TO PHYSICIAN?   YES ____   NO ____)
____ LIMB REMOVAL FORM SIGNED #900960
____ VITAL SIGNS: T ____ P ____ R ____ BP ____ FHT ____
____ FINGERSTICK RESULTS: ____ @ TIME ____
____ ELIMINATION: VOIDED ____ CATHETER ____
SPECIAL CONSIDERATIONS:
____ O₂ NEEDED FOR TRANSPORT
____ FISTULA/GRAFT; INFECTION; MASTECTOMY - R OR L
____ I.D. BAND ON
____ ALLERGY BAND ON: ALLERGIES VERIFIED WITH PATIENT
      NPO AFTER: 12M ____ BREAKFAST ____ OTHER ____
____ PRE-OP: ENEMA ____ DOUCHE ____ BOWEL PREP ____
      SHOWER ____ SCRUB ____ PRE-OP SHAVE ____ (LOCATION)
____ JEWELRY REMOVED/SECURED
____ DENTURES/PARTIAL PLATE, HEARING AID
____ GLASSES, CONTACT LENS
____ OTHER
____ RAILS UP-BED IN LOW POSITION

PATIENT CARE SERVICES
SURGICAL CHECKLIST
DATE: _____
7043   page 1 of 3 pages

Figure 29-7 Sample Preoperative Checklist (*Courtesy Spohn Health System, Corpus Christi, TX*)

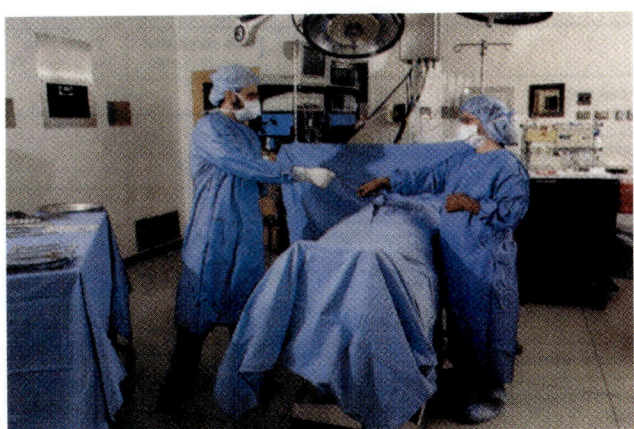

Figure 29-8 A Typical Operating Room and Proper Surgical Attire (*Photo courtesy of the U.S. Army*)

sterile drapes). This atmospheric temperature also provides an unfavorable environment for bacterial incubation and growth.

The client entering the operating room is confronted with an environment that is most likely unfamiliar. The operating room is cold. The surgical team members dress in characteristic surgical scrubs, and have their hair covered by caps and their faces covered by surgical masks, making them appear impersonal and distant. Furthermore, the sounds of equipment being prepared can be unfamiliar and alarming. Finally, the terminology used in conversations among OR personnel may be foreign. These elements in combination with the sight of ominous overhead lights and the feel of the hard operating room table may serve to increase the client's fear, anxiety, and feelings of powerlessness.

Members of the Surgical Team

The surgical team is a group of hospital personnel assigned to successfully see a client through an operative procedure. At no other time during hospitalization will the ratio of personnel to client be higher than when the client is undergoing surgery. The surgical team includes **sterile** (without microorganisms) team members: the surgeon, the **first assistant** (a physician or RN who assists the surgeon in performing hemostasis, tissue retraction, and wound closure), and the **scrub nurse** (an LP/VN, RN, or surgical technologist who, under the direction of the circulating nurse, prepares and maintains the integrity, safety, and efficiency of the sterile field throughout the operation). Sterile team members scrub their arms and hands, don sterile gowns and gloves, and then perform their duties in the sterile field. The **sterile field** is that area surrounding the client and the surgical site that is free from all microorganisms. It is created by using sterile drapes to drape the work area and the client. Nonsterile team members include the anesthesia provider (an **anesthesiologist** or **anesthetist**) and **circulating nurse** (an RN responsible for management of personnel, equipment, supplies, environment, and communica-

tion throughout a surgical procedure). The nonsterile team members perform their duties outside of the sterile field. Each team member has a clearly defined role and duties. Clear communication among team members and coordination of their activities improve the chances of the most favorable outcome for the client. Table 29-5 provides descriptions of surgical team members and their duties.

Asepsis

Prevention of infection is the responsibility of the entire surgical team. The environment of the surgical client contains both pathogenic (disease producing) and nonpathogenic microorganisms. When the skin, a prime barrier to infection, is broken, as during surgery, the susceptibility of the client to a bacterial invasion increases. Bacteria carried by dust or nose and throat droplets are easily transported by air currents. When unnecessary activity occurs in the room, such as when a team member pulls off his mask for any reason, the environment of the operating room is affected, and a wound can easily be invaded by undesirable microorganisms.

Asepsis is the absence of pathogenic microorganisms. **Aseptic technique** is a collection of principles used to control and/or prevent the transfer of pathogenic microorganisms from sources within (endogenous) and outside (exogenous) the client. For example, scrubbed persons wear sterile gowns and gloves; sterile drapes are used to create a sterile field; items used in a sterile field are sterilized; and those working within a sterile field maintain the integrity of the sterile field. Aseptic technique is applicable to other nursing functions such as changing dressings, inserting a foley catheter, or preparing for an obstetrical delivery. Thus, the practice of aseptic technique is not confined to the OR, but applies to other clinical nursing units and other procedures as well.

The practice of aseptic technique requires the development of **sterile conscience**, an individual's personal sense of honesty and integrity with regard to adherence to the principles of aseptic technique. Aseptic technique must be strictly followed. Doing so requires constant assessment and monitoring of self and others. It is sometimes easier or less expensive for surgical team members to overlook an infraction of aseptic technique rather than to correct that infraction. This must *never* be allowed. Compromising the principles of aseptic technique may increase the likelihood of infection and, thus, harm to the client.

Surgical Hand Scrub

An item is considered sterile when all microorganisms are removed. The skin, however, cannot be sterilized. For this reason, the sterile team members wear gloves as barriers between the sterile field and the skin. Because accidental tearing or puncturing of the

Table 29-5 MEMBERS OF THE SURGICAL TEAM: QUALIFICATIONS AND RESPONSIBILITIES

TYPE OF TEAM MEMBER	NAME OF TEAM MEMBER	TYPICAL QUALIFICATIONS AND RESPONSIBILITIES
Sterile team members	Surgeon	• May be a doctor of medicine (MD) or osteopathy (DO); oral surgeon; or podiatrist who is specially trained and qualified • Has completed a residency program approved by the American Board of Surgery and may or may not be board certified • Identifies need for surgery • Determines and plans appropriate treatment • Discusses surgical risks, benefits, possible complications, and treatment alternatives with the client • Obtains informed consent • Performs the surgery
	First assistant	• May be an associate physician in practice, referring physician, or surgical resident • May be a registered nurse first assistant (RNFA) who has been approved by the Association of Operating Room Nurses (AORN) and endorsed by the American College of Surgeons • Assists the surgeon • Retracts tissue and aids in the removal of blood and fluids at the operative site • Assists with hemostasis and wound closure
	Second or third assistants	• May be a qualified registered nurse, licensed practical/vocational nurse, or surgical technologist who is qualified by way of training or experience • Usually holds retractors
	Scrub nurse	• May be a registered nurse, licensed practical/vocational nurse, or surgical technologist • Provides services under the direction of the circulating nurse • Opens sterile supplies • Assists in gowning and gloving other sterile team members • Prepares instrument tables • Maintains integrity, safety, and efficiency of sterile field • Assists with sterile draping of client's operative site • Passes instruments, sutures, and the like to the surgeon • Performs instrument, sponge, and sharp counts • Aids in cleaning room after procedure
Nonsterile team members	Anesthesiologist or anesthetist	• Anesthesiologist: may be a doctor of medicine (MD) who has completed a 2-year residency in anesthesia and is preferably board certified by the American Board of Anesthesiology; may also be a doctor of osteopathy (DO) who specializes in anesthesia • Anesthetist: may be a qualified registered nurse, a dentist, or an MD who administers anesthetics • Certified registered nurse anesthetist (CRNA): a registered nurse with critical care nursing experience who has completed an accredited program of nurse anesthesia and has passed a certifying examination • Anesthetist: works under the direct supervision of an anesthesiologist or a surgeon • Assesses client during a preoperative visit • Chooses, induces, and maintains anesthesia • Monitors oxygenation and gas exchange • Manages untoward effects of anesthesia during surgery and postoperatively • Monitors and maintains fluid and electrolyte balance
	Circulating nurse	• Always a registered nurse • Responsible and accountable for all activities during a surgical procedure • Manages personnel, equipment, supplies, the environment, and communication throughout the operation • Arranges furniture and equipment in room • Opens sterile supplies • Ties gowns of sterile team members • Attends to needs and supplies of sterile team members

continued

Table 29-5 *continued*

TYPE OF TEAM MEMBER	NAME OF TEAM MEMBER	TYPICAL QUALIFICATIONS AND RESPONSIBILITIES
		<ul><li>Identifies and assesses client</li><li>Brings client to operating room and transfers to operating room table</li><li>Applies and assists in insertion of monitoring devices</li><li>Assists anesthesiologist in the induction of anesthesia</li><li>Positions client for surgery</li><li>Performs designated surgical skin preparation</li><li>Assists with sterile draping and setup of sterile field around operative site</li><li>Monitors sterile technique of surgical team</li><li>Collects, labels, and distributes specimens</li><li>Completes intraoperative record</li><li>Monitors blood and fluid loss</li><li>Counts sponges, instruments, and sharps with scrub nurse and reports results to surgeon</li><li>Communicates with surgical team members and others such as client's family, pathologist</li><li>Applies dressings</li><li>Assists in transferring client to cart and, possibly, in transporting client to postanesthesia care unit</li><li>Aids in cleaning room after procedure</li></ul>

surgical glove and resultant introduction of microorganisms into the surgical wound are possible, however, the sterile team members must take measures to lower the number of microorganisms on their hands and arms. The surgical hand scrub, performed before gowning and gloving, removes soil and transient (not always present and easily removed) microorganisms from the hands and forearms. The antimicrobial soap used lowers the count of resident (almost always present and not easily removed) microorganisms and continues to prevent sudden bacterial rebound or regrowth after the scrub is completed. The surgical scrub thus reduces the possibility of transmission of microorganisms from the surgical team to the client.

Watches, rings, and bracelets are removed before the surgical hand scrub. Fingernails must be short, clean, and healthy. Artificial nails cannot be worn, although unchipped fingernail polish that has been applied within the last 4 days may be worn (AORN, 1995b). The hands and forearms should be free of breaks in skin integrity.

To perform the surgical scrub, an antimicrobial soap, usually iodophor or chlorhexidine, is applied to moistened hands and arms, making a lather. The subungual (under the nails) areas are cleaned first. A sterile brush with the same antimicrobial soap is then used to scrub all four sides of each finger, the hands, and the forearms for a minimum of 5 minutes or for the time designated by the institutional policy. Hands are always held higher than the elbows, allowing the fluid to run from the cleanest area (the fingers and hands) to the dirtiest area (the forearms and elbows).

Surgical Skin Preparation

Like the skin of the surgical team members, the skin surface at the client's incision site also cannot be sterilized. As with the surgical hand scrub, the goal of surgical skin preparation at the client's incision site is to lower the number of microorganisms on and near the incision site, thereby reducing the possibility of postoperative wound infections from microorganisms on the client's own skin. Surgical skin preparation removes soil and transient microorganisms from the incision site. The antimicrobial soap used lowers the count of resident microorganisms and continues to prevent sudden bacterial rebound after the scrub is completed.

Typically, the client is asked to shower or to wash the operative site either before arriving at the surgical facility or immediately prior to surgery. The client is then transferred to the operating room. After general anesthesia induction or regional block completion or before local infiltration of the operative site, the circulating nurse performs the surgical skin preparation. Using aseptic technique, the circulating nurse scrubs the area with an antimicrobial soap. Typically the soap used is povidone iodine (containing iodine) or chlorhexidine, thus, potential allergies to iodine must be verified. The circulating nurse scrubs a generous area surrounding the operative site to allow for extension of the surgical incision if the need arises. The scrub is completed in an ever-widening circular motion from the incision site, which is considered clean, to the periphery, which is considered dirty (Figure 29-9). Once the periphery is reached, the same sponge is never brought back toward the center of the area. The concept

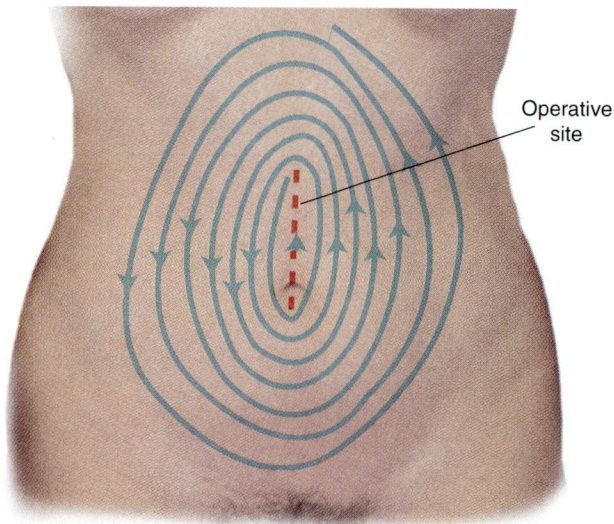

Operative
site

Figure 2-9 Skin Preparation at Operative Site

of cleansing from the center (incision site) to the periphery also applies to skin preparation for other procedures such as intravenous (IV) insertion, chest tube insertion, thoracentesis, or subclavian catheter placement. Surgical skin preparation lasts 5 to 10 minutes. After the scrub is completed, the area is blotted dry with sterile towels. An antiseptic solution, often also iodine based, is then applied in the same manner.

Intraoperative Nursing Care

The success of nursing care in the operating room is measured by client outcomes. The AORN has established client outcome standards for evaluating perioperative clients upon completion of surgery. These outcomes state that the client is to be free from infection and injury related to positioning, foreign objects, or chemical, physical, and electrical hazards. In addition, skin integrity and fluid and electrolyte balance are to be maintained. Consequently, nursing care in the operating room strives to provide these standards to all clients undergoing surgery.

Although the responsibilities of the circulating nurse and scrub nurse may seem to be a series of tasks or duties, these same tasks and duties provide quality nursing care to the client. The nurse planning for surgery is involved in selection of equipment and supplies, room preparation, and formation of the sterile field prior to the delivery of actual nursing care. There are six areas of risk that nurses are responsible for managing.

1. *Clients undergoing surgery are at high risk for infection related to the invasive procedure undertaken and the exposure to pathogens from the environment, personnel, and client.* Some clients are at a higher risk for developing nosocomial infections. Clients undergoing surgery lasting longer

than 2 hours or surgeries of the abdomen or thorax are more prone to infection. Poor nutritional status, the presence of an underlying disease process, obesity, and smoking or substance abuse also place a client at higher risk for infection. In addition, the very young (under 1 year of age) and those who are elderly (over 65 years of age) are at increased risk. Regardless of risk factors, nursing care for all clients requires strict aseptic technique to prevent nosocomial surgical wound infections.

2. *Clients undergoing surgery are at high risk for injury related to positioning during surgery.* Positional injuries may include postural hypotension, pressure alopecia, lower back or neck pain, facial and airway edema, eye abrasion, ear compression, joint damage, and nerve injury to the brachial plexus, suprascapular nerve, subclavian neurovascular bundle, axillary neurovascular bundle, or peroneal, radial, or ulnar nerve. The client's position during surgery is usually determined by the surgical approach, the surgeon's preference, and individual considerations. The ideal surgical position does not interfere with respiration and circulation, and should not cause pressure on any nerve. Proper positioning provides access to the operative site and allows easy access for the administration of anesthesia. Proper body alignment to prevent postoperative discomfort is maintained as much as possible.

    Because positioning usually occurs after initiation of anesthesia, the client is never moved without the anesthesia provider's guidance. The circulating nurse ensures availability of positioning devices and adequate personnel for lifting or turning.

3. *The client is at high risk for injury related to retention of foreign objects inadvertently left in the wound.* The placement of some foreign objects is deliberate and recorded. For example, vascular replacement grafts or orthopedic implants are designed to be left in the surgical wound as part of the surgical procedure. A wound occasionally may be packed with gauze or sponges for a physiological purpose such as hemostasis. Retention of a foreign object inadvertently left in the wound, however, constitutes a significant risk. Nursing interventions to prevent this type of injury include using only x-ray detectable sponges on the operative field and counting sponges, instruments, and sharps according to institutional policy. The circulating nurse both reports the results of the various counts to the surgeon and documents the counts on the operative record.

4. *The client undergoing surgery is at high risk for injury related to chemical, physical, and electrical hazards.* Clients are exposed to numerous chemicals used to clean the environment, prepare the skin, and sterilize instruments. Because anesthetized

clients do not have the reflexes to protect themselves, bodily injury is more likely to occur during positioning, transfers, or falls. Physical hazards may also include the use of both ionizing (x-ray) and nonionizing (laser) radiation, when the surgical procedure warrants their use. The majority of equipment used during surgery requires electricity, thus exposing the client to electrical hazards. A frequently used piece of equipment is the electrical surgical unit (ESU), or cautery, which stops bleeding through electrical coagulation of blood vessels.

Safety: Electrical Equipment

- Electrical equipment must be plugged into grounded outlets.
- Electrical equipment must be regularly checked by a bioelectronic technician.
- A grounding pad must be placed under the client and in direct contact with the client's skin.

Nursing care focuses on minimizing and documenting the exposure to these hazards. Skin integrity is assessed prior to and after completion of the surgical procedure. Allergies to antimicrobial soaps are verified. Pooling of preparation solutions beneath the client is prevented. Institutional protocols are followed for radiation and laser safety. In addition, after surgery the area around the dressing site is cleansed to remove any residual antibacterial soap and antiseptic solution. Equipment is set up, checked prior to use, and operated according to the manufacturers' recommendations.

5. *The client undergoing surgery is at high risk for impaired tissue integrity related to positioning, electrical hazards, and chemical hazards.* Nursing actions are geared toward ensuring no bruising, areas of skin breakdown, reddened areas, discolored skin, open skin lesions, excoriation, or itching after surgery. Nursing care to prevent skin breakdown is similar to that prevent injury related to positioning and chemical, physical, or electrical hazards.

6. *The client undergoing surgery is at high risk for alteration in fluid and electrolyte balance related to abnormal blood loss and NPO status.* The goal of nursing care is to maintain fluid and electrolyte balance. Application of hemodynamic monitoring devices by the circulating nurse and anesthesia provider allows the physiologic monitoring of fluid and electrolyte parameters. Intravenous patency is protected and maintained. Nursing care is aimed at monitoring and replacing fluid loss. The circulating nurse accomplishes this by assisting the anesthesia provider in estimating blood loss as evidenced in sponges and suctioning and monitoring urine output. Intravenous fluids and blood products are administered according to the anesthesia provider's instructions. Fluid and electrolyte values and vital signs should be consistent with preoperative measurements.

After completion of surgery, the circulating nurse applies and secures the dressing. When the anesthesia provider is ready, the client is transferred to a stretcher or a gurney. The unconscious or semiconscious client is placed in a side-lying or semiprone position unless contraindicated by the surgical procedure. If the client is supine, the client's head is turned to the side in case the client vomits. The client is then taken to the PACU, accompanied by the anesthesia provider and another surgical team member.

POSTOPERATIVE PHASE

The **postoperative phase** is the time during the surgical experience that begins with the end of the surgical procedure and lasts until the client is discharged not just from the hospital or institution, but from medical care by the surgeon. Upon transfer from the operating room, the client usually goes to the PACU (Figure 29-10). All clients who receive general anesthesia, spinal anesthesia, or regional anesthesia are admitted to the PACU. Occasionally, clients who have undergone surgery with local anesthesia or no anesthesia or who have received only IV sedation are placed in the PACU for a short period to be monitored closely until their conditions stabilize. The PACU is usually located next to the operating room. Typically, it is one large room with individual units for clients along the perimeter of the room. Each of these units has an oxygen delivery system, suction, various other supplies, and cardiac, respiratory, and blood pressure monitoring devices. Curtains can be pulled to provide privacy if needed, but an open view allows continual assessment of all clients.

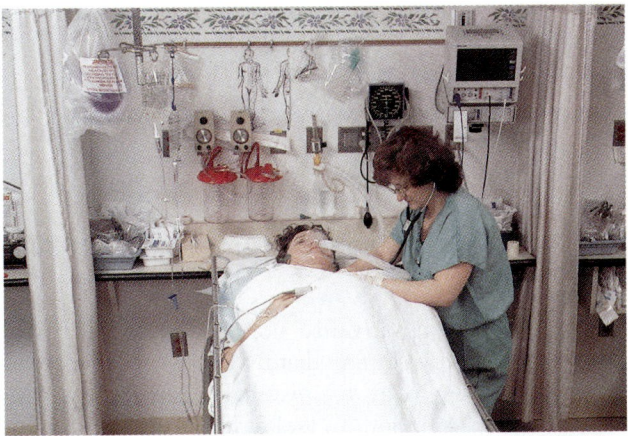

Figure 29-10 Postanesthesia Care Unit (PACU)

Postoperative Nursing Care

The postanesthesia care nurse is an RN specially trained in caring for immediate postoperative clients. The goal of postanesthesia nursing care is to promote recovery from anesthesia and the immediate effects of surgery. The postanesthesia nurse has knowledge and skill in recognizing and treating anesthetic and surgical complications very quickly. The postanesthesia nurse is empathetic and is able to assess and manage pain for the client who may not be able to express himself.

Upon the client's arrival in the PACU, the anesthesia provider verbally reviews the client's anesthesia and operative procedure with the postanesthesia nurse. The postanesthesia nurse begins the following nursing assessment and care in the immediate postoperative period:

- Time of arrival in recovery room
- Patency of airway
- Respirations
- Presence of artificial airway devices
    Oral airway
    Nasopharyngeal airway
    Endotracheal airway
- Oxygen saturation
- Need for supplemental oxygen
    Mode of administration
    Flow rate
- Breath sounds
- Color of skin, nail beds, and lips
- Presence of cardiac dysrhythmias
- Other vital signs
    Blood pressure, pulse
- Skin condition (moist or dry, warm or cool) and skin temperature
- Initiate Aldrete Score
- Intravenous infusion
    Type of solution
    Amount in bottle or bag
    Flow rate
    Appearance and location of IV site
- Dressings
    Amount and character of drainage
- Drains and tubes
    Intactness and function
    Connection to drainage and/or suction
    Amount and character of drainage
- Level of consciousness
- Activity level
- Other assessments according to surgical procedure
- Pain

The postanesthesia nurse notes the client's arrival time to the unit and immediately begins to assess the patency of the airway by placing a hand above the client's nose and mouth to feel exhalation. The quality and quantity of respirations are then immediately ob-

served, as is the presence of an artificial airway. The client is attached to a pulse oximeter, and breath sounds are auscultated. The color and condition of the skin are noted as part of the respiratory assessment. Peripheral cyanosis may be an indication of hypothermia rather than respiratory distress. Thus, correlating with the "A-B-Cs" of *a*irway, *b*reathing, and *c*irculation, the respiratory system is assessed first.

Because the vast majority of clients admitted are in an unconscious state and have received muscle relaxants during surgery, respiratory exchange is often affected. Snoring, stridor, labored chest movement, sternal retractions, cyanosis, and apnea are all signs of respiratory distress. Respiratory distress is the gravest of all complications because respiratory crisis and subsequent death can occur in a matter of minutes if distress is not observed and treated quickly. In the event of any signs of respiratory distress, the postanesthesia nurse must be alert to the possibility of respiratory arrest and be ready to initiate cardiopulmonary resuscitation. There are seven areas of risk that postoperative nurses are responsible for managing:

1. *The postoperative client is at high risk for ineffective airway clearance.* Respiratory complications can occur with any anesthetized client. Often airway obstruction occurs from the tongue falling backward over the pharynx. Nursing interventions include manually lifting the jaw forward to raise the tongue from the pharynx and open the airway (see Figure 29-11). Because of airway obstruction, clients will often arrive in the PACU with an artificial airway inserted (Figure 29-12).

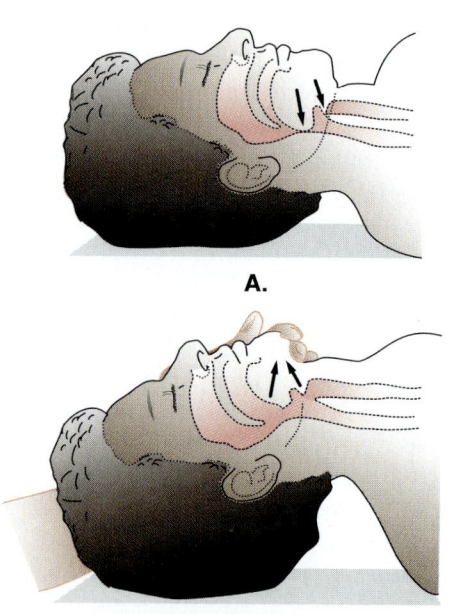

A.

B.

Figure 29-11 A. An Obstructed Airway (tongue against pharynx); B. Manual Jaw Lift (anterior displacement)

Laryngospasm is the spastic contraction of the larynx that effectively causes airway obstruction. It is often caused by larynx irritation from the ET tube or may be a side effect of some anesthetic gases. Laryngospasm is most likely to occur after removal of the ET tube and when the client develops an acute inspiratory stridor with sternal retractions. The postanesthesia nurse starts oxygen via a mask, reassures the client, and immediately notifies the anesthesia provider.

2. *The postoperative client is at high risk for ineffective breathing pattern.* Hypoventilation is most likely due to the depressant effects of anesthesia. In hypoventilation, oxygen and carbon dioxide are not exchanging adequately in the alveoli of the lung.

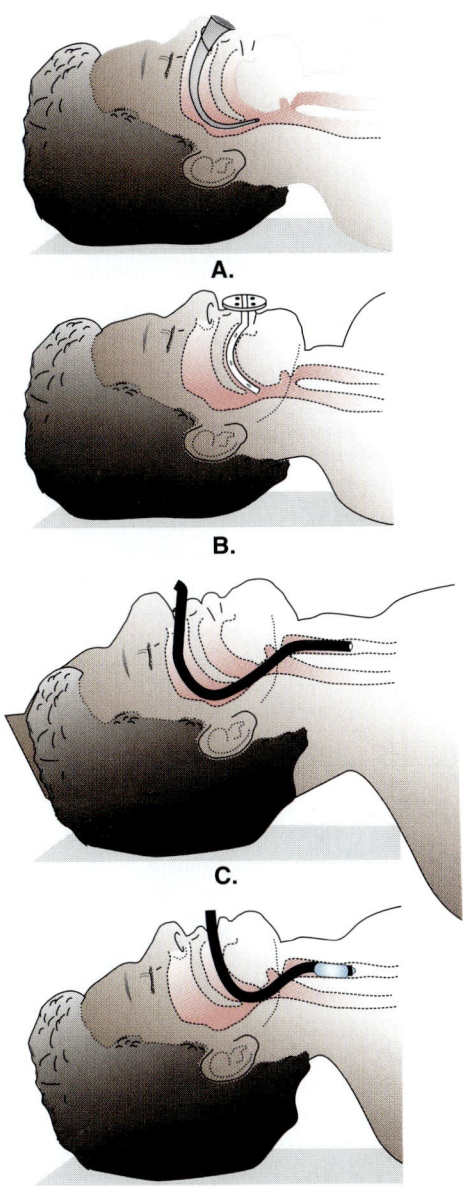

Figure 29-12 Four Types of Artificial Airways: A. Nasal trumpet; B. Oral airway; C. Nasal endotracheal tube; and D. Oral endotracheal tube with cuff inflated

Additional oxygen is provided to the client, as needed, through the oral airway or a nasal catheter or mask, if indicated. The client's oxygen saturation is monitored via a pulse oximeter (Figure 29-13). It is desirable to maintain oxygen saturation above 90%, with the aid of additional oxygen, if necessary. Pallor, hypotension, tachycardia, and respiratory distress are other indications for oxygen administration. Oxygen may be provided prophylactically to clients who have undergone prolonged or traumatic surgery.

3. *The postoperative client is at high risk for aspiration.* With certain anesthesias, the client temporarily loses the gag and cough reflexes necessary to protect the lungs, increasing the risk of aspiration of stomach contents, oral secretions, bloody secretions, and foreign bodies into the lungs. Aspiration later causes pneumonia and atelectasis. The postanesthesia nurse intervenes by having suction ready and using it frequently to prevent aspiration. Antiemetics are given as needed to prevent nausea and vomiting. Coughing and deep breathing are initiated as soon as the client is able to follow directions. If not contraindicated, the client may be positioned on the side to prevent aspiration. When the client must be supine, the head is turned to the side so that any secretions will drain out of the mouth.

4. *The postoperative client is at high risk for decreased cardiac output.* The cardiovascular system is assessed next, according to the A-B-Cs of airway, breathing, and circulation. The client is attached to an EKG monitor. Then blood pressure and pulse are taken and, along with respirations, are reported to the anesthesia provider, if still present in the PACU. If a client does not already have a skin thermometer or other means of obtaining temperature, one is applied and the temperature noted. Skin condition is observed for the presence

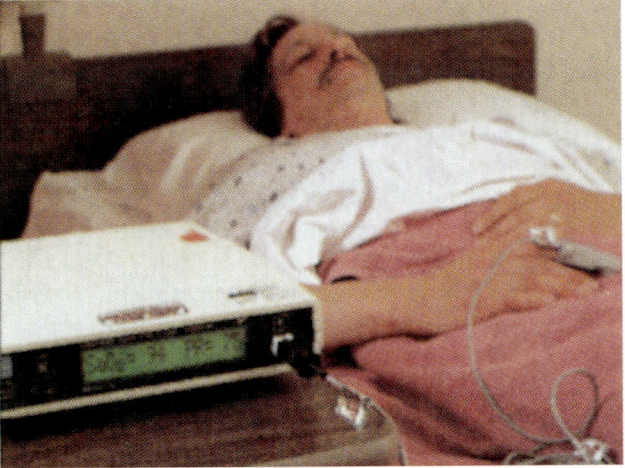

Figure 29-13 Client with Pulse Oximeter

of diaphoresis. The initial Aldrete Score is then determined.

The **Aldrete Score**, also known as the Post-anesthetic Recovery Score, is used in PACUs to objectively assess the physical status of clients recovering from anesthesia, and serves as a basis for discharge from the PACU (Table 29-6). The Aldrete Score was recently adapted to also assess the readiness of clients for discharge from ambulatory surgery. The first five indexes are used for discharge from the PACU. Clients are assessed at the time of admission to the PACU and every 15 minutes until discharge. The first five indexes include assessing activity, respiration, consciousness, circulation, and color (oxygen saturation). Each of the five indexes is scored from 0 to 2, according to the degree of functional disturbance. The score is expressed as a total score, with 10 being the maximum. Typically, a minimum score of 8 is required for discharge from the PACU.

As complete as the Aldrete Score may seem, it does not consider some problems that may warrant either continued stay in the PACU or admission to a critical care unit. Cardiac dysrhythmias that do not affect blood pressure, bleeding at the incision site, uncontrollable severe pain, and persistent nausea and vomiting may be present even if the client has an Aldrete Score of 10. Any such problems indicate a need to stay in the PACU or to be transferred to a critical care unit until the problem is resolved.

Hypotension is frequently encountered during the immediate postoperative period. Hypotension can be caused by blood loss, residual effects of anesthesia, narcotics or tranquilizers, position changes, and even pain. If hypotension is due to the residual effects of anesthesia, the effects are usually mild, and the client's blood pressure gradually returns to the preoperative level. Narcotics may potentiate the effects of residual anesthesia and may contribute to hypotension. Sympathetic nerve blockages in the spinal cord that occur during spinal and epidural blocks may result in arterial dilation and decreased venous return, producing hypotension. Whereas mild to moderate pain may cause an increase in blood pressure, severe pain may cause hypotension resulting from the release of norepinephrine, which, in turn, decreases heart rate and cardiac output. Hypotension may even have existed preoperatively.

The cardiovascular assessment includes comparing the present blood pressure to the preoperative blood pressure and to the blood pressures during surgery. In addition to reduced blood pressure, the postanesthesia nurse assesses other symptoms of hypotension, such as pallor, clammy skin, diaphoresis, rapid weak pulse, rapid shallow res-

Table 29-6 ALDRETE SCORE/POSTANESTHETIC RECOVERY SCORE

Activity	Able to move 4 extremities voluntarily or on command	2
	Able to move 2 extremities voluntarily or on command	1
	Able to move 0 extremities voluntarily or on command	0
Respiration	Able to breathe deeply and cough freely	2
	Dyspnea or limited breathing	1
	Apneic	0
Consciousness	Fully awake	2
	Arousable on calling	1
	Not responding	0
Circulation	B/P ± 20% of preanesthetic level	2
	B/P ± 20% to 50% of preanesthetic level	1
	B/P ± 50% of preanesthetic level	0
Color	Normal	2
	Pale, dusky, blotchy, jaundiced, other	1
	Cyanotic	0

Additional Assessments: Aldrete Score/Postanesthetic Recovery Score for Clients Having Anesthesia on an Ambulatory Basis

Dressing	Dry and clean	2
	Wet but stationary or marked	1
	Growing area of wetness	0
Pain	Pain free	2
	Mild pain handled by oral medication	1
	Severe pain requiring parenteral medication	0
Ambulation	Able to stand up and walk straight	2
	Vertigo when erect	1
	Dizziness when supine	0
Fasting/feeding	Able to drink fluids	2
	Nauseated	1
	Nausea and vomiting	0
Urine output	Has voided	2
	Unable to void but comfortable	1
	Unable to void and uncomfortable	0

Courtesy J. Antonio Aldrete, M.D., M.S., Defuniak Springs, FL.

pirations, and restlessness. An imperceptible blood pressure and weak pulse are reported to the surgeon and anesthesia provider immediately. Oxygen is begun, the intravenous rate is increased, and the client is placed in the Trendelenburg position while evidence of bleeding is sought. If blood pressure is low but all other signs are normal, the client is watched closely until the client has a chance to awaken; he may be merely depressed from anesthesia. If pulse is slow (under 50 and not comparable to the preoperative range) or irregular but other signs are normal, the anesthesia provider should be notified. Again, in the event of cardiac arrest, the postanesthesia nurse is ready to initiate cardiopulmonary resuscitation.

5. *The postoperative client is at high risk for fluid volume deficit.* Blood loss usually ranges from 100 mL to 500 mL in an average surgery. Blood transfusions are usually not given unless more than one unit of blood is needed and blood loss is greater than 500 mL. Hypovolemic shock usually does not occur until the client has lost more than 1.5 L to 2.0 L of blood, or 20% to 25% of the blood volume (Lewis, Collier, & Heitkemper 1996).

Fluid intake and output are assessed. The amounts and types of IV solutions hanging are identified, as are any added medications. The IV fluids are infused according to the surgeon's order and are run at a specified rate. The IV site is assessed for patency, redness, and swelling. The client is restrained as necessary to maintain patency of the IV site. All other infusions and irrigations are also assessed.

The postanesthesia nurse checks dressings and/or peripads for any evidence of bloody drainage and notes the amount so that any subsequent appearance of blood may be accurately evaluated. All drainage tubes are then connected, and the type of drain and the drainage amount are recorded according to physicians' orders. Table 29-7 outlines common types of drains placed in surgery. Urinary output is also monitored. Scanty urinary drainage (less than 50 cc/hour or as ordered) is noted and reported to the surgeon.

Surgical drains are placed so that the wound can drain freely of blood clots, body fluids, pus, and necrotic material that otherwise would collect in the wound and provide a rich medium for bacterial growth. Figure 29-14 illustrates common drainage devices. All drains are inserted at the operative site and exit through the incision or a separate stab wound adjacent to the incision. The type of drain is chosen according to the location of wound, size of wound, and type of drainage anticipated. The use of drains decreases pain and infection while aiding wound healing. However, if the wound is draining, the skin is not closed, and a

pathway exists for the entrance of microorganisms. Drain sites can thus also be a source of infection. Potential complications of drains include hemorrhage, sepsis, drain loss, and bowel herniation. Thus, nursing care of all drains includes assessing the color, character, and odor of drainage, ensuring the patency of the drain (making sure there are no kinks in the tubing), and ensuring that the drain does not accidentally become dislodged. Table 29-8 lists additional nursing care according to surgical procedure.

Hypertension may also be assessed in the postoperative period. Because the client may have preexisting hypertension, blood pressure is compared to the client's normal and admitting blood pressure. Hypertension can be due to pain, the anesthesia or medication used, or restlessness or apprehension. Increased intracranial pressure, increased or rapid fluid intake, hypoxia, and fighting the artificial airway may also increase blood pressure. The postanesthesia nurse uses judgment and then proceeds to treat the probable cause by medicating for pain, slowing the IV rate, removing the artificial airway, administering oxygen, or raising the head of the bed. If these measures fail or if blood pressure is dangerously high, the surgeon or anesthesia provider is notified.

6. *The postoperative client is at high risk for sensory/perceptual alterations.* The next system to be assessed, therefore, is the neurological system. In the Aldrete Score, level of consciousness and activity level are assessed. With regard to level of consciousness, the client is typically labeled as able to answer questions clearly, demonstrates arousal only when called, or unresponsive to verbal stimulation. The neurological assessment does not include orientation to person, place, and time. A surgical client is usually oriented to person. Due to the amnesic effects of some medications, however,

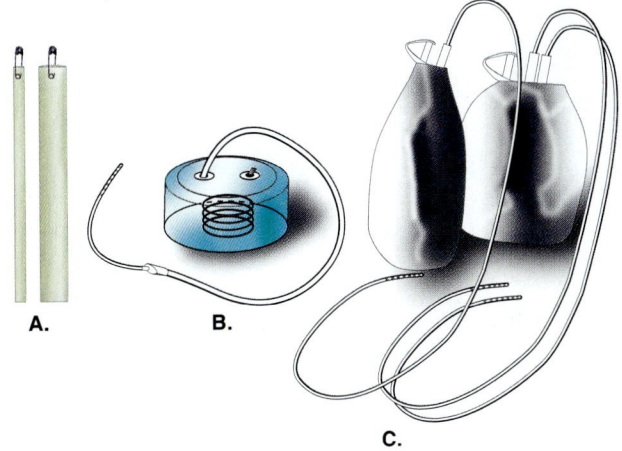

Figure 29-14 ▶ Common Drainage Devices: A. Penrose drains; B. Hemovac; and C. Jackson-Pratt

Table 29-7 DESCRIPTION, USES, AND NURSING CARE OF COMMON DRAINAGE DEVICES PLACED DURING SURGERY

TYPE	EXAMPLE	DESCRIPTION	USES	NURSING CARE
Passive	Penrose	A single-lumen, soft latex tube that works with gravity directly from the surgical incision	To remove drainage when more than a minimal amount of drainage is expected	• Inspect dressing • Check underneath client to ensure drainage has not leaked from the side of the dressing • Always keep a dressing over drain • Check safety pin through end of drain
	T-tube	A single-lumen tube shaped like a T and made of latex	Used after common bile duct exploration to drain bile from the duct as suture lines heal and swelling decreases	• Attach to a drainage bottle or to a T-tube bag
Active	Hemovac Jackson Pratt J-Vac Relia Vac Surgivac	Closed wound drainage system with drain and reservoir having self-suction when reservoir is compressed	Used after multiple types of procedures; provides continuous gentle suction of the operative site to increase drainage of serosanguinous fluid and collapse tissue to facilitate healing	• Assess the drainage system as appropriate to client's condition for: 　1. Continued drainage 　2. Maintained decompression 　3. Air-tight tubings 　4. Need for emptying • To reactivate suction, wash hands and wear gloves and eye/face protection • Empty reservoirs every 8 hours, when drainage nears the full line, or as ordered by the physician
Passive or active	Davol Sump Axiom Sump	Large, multilumen tube with a larger main port for drainage and/or suction and with smaller side port(s) for irrigation and/or air venting to help prevent tissue from being suctioned against catheter and damaged	To drain intra-abdominal fluids from abscesses, cysts, or hematomas	• Use one of the smaller or sump ports for continuous irrigation • Calculate intake and output carefully with irrigations • Place impervious pads underneath client • Change dressings frequently when saturated • Attach to catheter drainage bag if not attached to suction • Do not plug sump ports
	Chest tube ThoraKlex Pleure Vac	Large single-lumen drain attached to closed water-seal drainage system	To drain fluid or air from pleural cavity	• Assess breath sounds and respirations, including depth, rate, symmetry of chest expansion, color of mucous membranes, and presence of crepitus with suction off or tubing clamped • If present, assess amount and type of suction • Ensure that connections are tight and sealed with tape • Keep chest tube drainage reservoir lower than client's chest • Observe for air leaks in air leak indicator or drainage chamber of drainage reservoir • Place petroleum jelly gauze nearby for quick access should the tube become dislodged • Measure drainage at least every 8 hours (more frequently if in a critical care unit or client's condition warrants it) • Clamp or milk the chest tube only if ordered by surgeon • Notify surgeon if drainage is greater than 100 cc/hour • Change drainage system when ⅔ full

Table 29-8 ADDITIONAL NURSING CARE ACCORDING TO CLASSIFICATION OR TYPE OF SURGICAL PROCEDURE

CLASSIFICATION OR TYPE OF SURGICAL PROCEDURE	NURSING CARE	
Orthopedic	• Expose wet casts to the air. • Check surgeon's orders for positioning of client; operated extremities typically are elevated. • Check for digital warmth, color, mobility, circulaton (pulses), and sensation in affected extremity.	
Urologic	• Attach all catheters to drainage. • Closely monitor continuous irrigation to ensure that flow in and flow out are equal; if obstructed, the bladder could rupture. • Increase or decrease irrigation flow rate according to amount of bleeding. • Assess for chills or elevated pulse, possibly indicative of hemolysis or bacterial infection. • Assess abdomen for signs of distension and rigidity and report, especially if client complains.	
Oral	• Suction frequently and carefully around sutures. • Observe breathing; ensure that drainage or packing does not obstruct airway. • Apply ice bag, when ordered. • Remove dental packs as ordered and assess every 15 minutes for further bleeding.	
Eye, ears, nose, & throat (EENT)	*Eye surgery*	• Assess for facial paralysis • Minimize head movement, coughing, vomiting, and restlessness.
	Ear surgery	• Assess edema and tracheal patency (listening for stridor and observing for restlessness).
	Nose surgery	• Maintain open airway; suction orally; and apply ice.
	Tonsillectomy	• Place on side to facilitate drainage: elevate head of bed; have suction available; and observe closely for bleeding, vomiting, and obstruction.
Neurologic	• Assess level of consciousness; be alert to drowsiness, slurred speech, disorientation, or irritability that differs from that exhibited in the preoperative state. • Observe for pupil changes: inequality, constriction, and nonreactivity to light. • Assess for respiratory changes such as snoring, retraction of cheeks and trachea, shallowness, and slowed rate. • Monitor blood pressure and pulse; an elevated blood pressure coupled with a lowered pulse leads to shock. • Observe extremity movement for weakness, paralysis, and rigidity; observe for unilateral drooping of facial features. • Use caution when medicating.	
	Laminectomy or discectomy	• Move only as ordered. • Assess sensation, circulation, and motion of extremities distal to incision site.
	Craniotomy	• Position as ordered. • Complete a neurological check. • Use Trendelenburg position only with permission of the surgeon.
Vascular (all grafts, carotid endarterectomy, femoral-popliteal bypass)	• Assess color, sensation, warmth, and mobility of extremity. • Observe presence and strength of pedal and post-tibial pulses. • Complete a neurological check for carotid endarterectomy. • Frequently check all dressings and the area directly beneath the client.	
Thoracic	• Closely observe chest tube for patency, amount of bleeding, and air leaks. Tape all connections. Mark drainage container upon client's admission and discharge. Assess fluctuation of drainage in tubing. Attach suction as ordered. • Observe respirations closely with regard to color change, restlessness, apprehension, dyspnea, or mediastinal shift.	

continued

Table 29-8 ADDITIONAL NURSING CARE ACCORDING TO CLASSIFICATION OR TYPE OF SURGICAL PROCEDURE *continued*

CLASSIFICATION OR TYPE OF SURGICAL PROCEDURE	NURSING CARE
	• Elevate head of bed 30°, unless contraindicated. • Encourage coughing and deep breathing. • Use caution in administering narcotics, especially morphine sulfate, as client cannot afford respiratory depression.
Pneumonectomy	• Do not turn on nonoperative side. Alternately turn from back to operated side.
Lobectomy and resection	• May turn client to either side.
Gynecologic	• Assess vaginal drainage.

the client may be oriented to the facility yet may not be oriented to the specific area of the facility even after being told. Because the postoperative client loses the ability to track time while undergoing some types of anesthesia and has no way of knowing how long the surgical procedure has taken, the client may be oriented to year and month but is rarely oriented to the specific time of the day. For these reasons, assessing orientation to person, place, and time is not part of the neurological assessment. Level of consciousness affects the ability to breathe, maintain oxygen saturation without assistance, and move on command.

Part of the neurological assessment involves assessing the activity level, or the ability to move extremities voluntarily. The ability to move extremities on command indicates voluntary movement. Hearing is the first sensation to return to the client after having been anesthetized. Clients in the PACU are asked to squeeze the postanesthesia nurse's hands and to plantarflex and dorsiflex the feet. Due to a regional block or previous condition, however, the client may be unable to move more than two extremities.

7. *The postoperative client is at high risk for injury and for altered thought processes.* Some clients are in a state of delirium, wherein uncontrollable physical movements occur. Thus, all clients are restrained: The side rails are put up, the stretcher safety strap is applied across the torso, and the stretcher wheel brakes are locked. Clients showing signs of restlessness may need additional physical restraint. Safety is the utmost concern, but when placing restraints, the postanesthesia nurse must first determine that the restlessness is related to the state of anesthesia rather than pain or anoxia.

Continuing Nursing Care in the PACU

After the client has been admitted and assessed in PACU, the postanesthesia nurse checks the surgeon's and the anesthesia provider's orders and initiates any therapy designated for the PACU. All stat IV or intramuscular (IM) medications are given, and inhalation therapy and specific equipment are initiated as ordered. The clinical unit is notified of any specialized equipment that will be needed in the client's room.

Narcotics are given in the PACU in reduced amounts and according to the client's state of consciousness, vital signs, and the type of anesthesia administered during surgery. A typical dosage is one-half or less of a regular dose, which may be repeated in ½ hour if the client continues to experience pain. Some anesthesia providers write specific orders for the administration of narcotics during the client's stay in the PACU. Clients who are medicated typically stay in the PACU for at least ½ hour after administration of the first dose and for 15 minutes after administration of the second dose. The postanesthesia nurse considers the client's need for medication and dosage based on the length of time it takes to arouse the client, the type of anesthetic agent used during surgery, the type of surgery performed, and the client's general condition, vital signs, and age.

The postanesthesia nurse charts on a separate nursing record for the PACU. Anything unusual must be adequately documented. If vital signs are in the normal range, the postanesthesia nurse checks them every 15 minutes. If vital signs are unstable, they are checked every 5 minutes or as often as necessary until stable. If vital signs fail to stabilize, the surgeon and anesthesia provider are notified. The surgical site is checked at least every 30 minutes. If any initial bleeding has not subsided, the surgeon is notified. Routine checks are continued until the client is discharged from the PACU.

The Aldrete Score is assessed every 15 minutes, as is skin temperature. Temperature may be checked with a thermometer if there is any question. If temperature is abnormal, the surgeon and/or anesthesia provider is notified. A significantly elevated temperature can be indicative of malignant hyperthermia, a potentially fatal complication of some anesthetics in sensitive individuals that is characterized by a hypermetabolic crisis.

The postanesthesia nurse determines whether the client meets the criteria for discharge from the PACU. Typically, the client's vital signs must be stable and within the client's normal limits. The Aldrete Score must be 8 to 10. If 7 or less, a surgeon's or anesthesia provider's order is required for discharge. Also prior to client discharge, the dressing must be checked, changed, or reinforced according to orders. All other parameters are reassessed and charted. Institutional protocol dictates minimum stay in the PACU. Adults are typically kept in the PACU for a minimum of 1 hour, except outpatients, who go to ambulatory surgery when they are awake and when postmedication time has been fulfilled. Children are typically kept in the PACU until they are awake, stable, and have an Aldrete Score of 8 to 10. When criteria for discharge are met, the postanesthesia nurse calls the clinical unit or ambulatory surgery unit and reports the client's name, vitals, surgery, and any other pertinent information. The client is then transferred to the appropriate unit.

Later Postoperative Nursing Care

Prior to the client's arrival in the clinical unit, the nurse has prepared for the client. The linen has been changed, the bed clothing folded down, and the room cleared of clutter. Special required equipment, as directed by the postanesthesia nurse, has been gathered. An emesis basin and tissue are available. The nurse is ready to assess the client in an organized manner, focusing on the body system affected by surgery.

Upon the client's arrival in the clinical unit, the nurse assists in the transfer of the client to the bed. Nursing assessment and care of the client upon admission to the clinical unit includes the following:

- Time of arrival in unit
- Transfer from cart to bed
  Place bed in lowest, locked position, with side rails up
  Place client in position of comfort, or as ordered
- Vital signs including airway assessment and breath sounds
- Color of skin, nail beds, and lips
- Skin condition (moist or dry, warm or cool)

- Level of consciousness
- Activity level
- Intravenous infusion
  Type of solution
  Amount in bottle or bag
  Flow rate
  Appearance and location of IV site
- Dressings
  Amount and character of drainage
- Drains and tubes
  Intactness and function
  Connection to drainage and/or suction
  Amount and character of drainage
- Urinary output
  Need to void or time of voiding
  Presence of patency and catheter; output/hour
- Pain
  Last dose of analgesia
  Current pain location, intensity, quality
- Compare assessment with PACU report
- Call light within reach
  Reorient client to usage
- Location of family or significant others
- Postoperative orders

A brief assessment including vital signs is completed every 15 minutes for 1 hour; every ½ hour for 2 hours; and every hour for 4 hours, or as prescribed by physician. The possibilities of postanesthetic complications continue, but as time passes, different postsurgical complications may develop; the nurse is responsible for managing these.

1. *The client is at risk for ineffective airway clearance caused by atelectasis and hypostatic pneumonia.* Respiratory complications can still occur with any anesthetized client. As in the PACU, the postoperative client is at high risk for ineffective airway clearance, ineffective breathing patterns, and aspiration. Now, however, nursing measures are directed toward preventing ineffective airway clearance caused by atelectasis and hypostatic pneumonia, both of which usually occur within the first 48 hours postoperatively. In postoperative atelectasis, the bronchioles of the lungs become plugged with mucus so that air cannot reach the alveoli. The alveoli then collapse. The client develops dyspnea, fever, tachypnea, tachycardia, and cyanosis. In postoperative hypostatic pneumonia, stagnant mucus promotes the growth of bacteria, and atelectasis then develops into a secondary infection. To prevent these complications, the client is actively encouraged by the nurse to cough, deep breathe (with and without incentive spirometry), and turn as instructed preoperatively. In addition, the client is encouraged to sit up and ambulate as soon and as often as possible. The nurse must ensure adequate pain relief measures so that mobility is well tolerated.

2. *The client is at high risk for peripheral neurovascular dysfunction, fluid volume excess/deficit, and activity intolerance.* The client continues to be at high risk for decreased cardiac output and fluid volume deficit; but as the postoperative period progresses, the client becomes at risk for additional complications. The nurse implements measures to prevent deep vein thrombosis; thrombophlebitis; pulmonary embolism; complications of fluid overload; fluid deficit; hypokalemia; and syncope.

The stress response to surgery; inactivity; pressure related to body position; obesity; and injury to pelvic veins during surgery may contribute to the formation of deep vein thrombosis, thrombophlebitis, or pulmonary embolism. These complications may appear immediately following surgery or 1 to 2 weeks later. The nurse routinely assesses for a positive Homan's sign and for warm, tender, reddened, hardened areas in the calves. To assess for Homan's sign, the client is asked to forcefully dorsiflex the foot. If pain is felt in the calf of the leg, it is considered a positive finding for Homan's sign; if no pain is felt, it is considered a negative finding. A positive finding for Homan's sign may indicate thrombophlebitis and should be reported to the surgeon. Deep vein thrombosis and thrombophlebitis may lead to a pulmonary embolus, although there may be no warning of pulmonary embolism. When pulmonary embolism occurs, the client may experience dyspnea, chest pain, cyanosis, cough, hemoptysis, tachycardia, and fever coupled with an elevated white blood cell count. If the embolism is large enough, shock may develop rapidly. Pulmonary embolism may be fatal.

To prevent the formation of deep vein thrombosis, thrombophlebitis, and pulmonary embolism, the nurse should encourage the client to ambulate to the extent that the client is able. When in bed, the client should perform postoperative leg exercises each hour. Antiembolism stockings are usually ordered, as is a sequential compression device, which is a sleeve applied to the legs to simulate walking by repetitive pumping. The sleeves and antiembolism stockings should be removed every day so that the skin can be cleansed. It is very important to note that antiembolism stockings and the sequential compression device are not substitutes for leg exercises. Leg exercises must still be performed.

When it is ordered, the nurse also administers low-dose heparin therapy to hemostatically stable clients who are more than 40 years of age and have undergone pelvic, abdominal, or thoracic surgery. Heparin is usually given subcutaneously every 12 hours until discharge. If the drug is administered at low dosage and if preoperative pro-

thrombin time, partial thromboplastin time, and platelet count were within the normal range, no laboratory test is necessary to determine the drug's effect. This regimen is followed and ordered at the discretion of the surgeon.

The nurse measures intake and output and monitors laboratory findings (e.g., electrolytes, hematocrit, hemoglobin, and serum osmolality) and signs and symptoms of hemorrhage by assessing vital signs, skin color and condition, dressings, drains, and tubes, as in the PACU.

Clients often experience syncope when changing from a lying position to a sitting or standing position. The nurse can prevent syncope by assisting the client to change positions slowly, proceeding in steps and allowing time for the client's internal equilibrium to adjust. The nurse checks the radial pulse frequently and asks the client for subjective statements of dizziness or nausea. If syncope occurs during ambulation, the nurse can ask for assistance in obtaining a wheelchair for the client, use a nearby chair, or lower the client to the floor until the client recovers. Although frightening for the client, syncope is not physiologically threatening unless the client is injured in a fall.

3. *The client may be at high risk for altered nutrition—less than body requirements related to nausea and vomiting, hiccoughs, abdominal distension, constipation, and NPO status.* Gastrointestinal complications become more prevalent after immediate postoperative recovery. The client also may experience pain related to hiccoughs and slowed gastrointestinal function.

Nausea and vomiting are caused by anesthetic agents, narcotics, hypotension, and the manipulation of the bowel during surgery. Handling of the bowel during pelvic and abdominal surgery causes peristalsis to stop or severely slow. Bowel function normally returns 2 to 5 days following surgery. If bowel inactivity persists, a paralytic ileus may develop. As bowel function resumes, the nurse continues to assess the client for bowel sounds and, if a nasogastric tube is present, a reduction in drainage. As peristalsis returns in a discontinuous fashion, the client may experience distention along with flatulence and gas pains. After bowel sounds resume in all quadrants, the client may be removed from NPO status according to the surgeon's orders. The nurse also provides good oral hygiene when the client is designated NPO and administers antiemetics as needed for nausea and vomiting.

Hiccoughs are caused by irritation of the phrenic nerve. Impulses then cause the diaphragm to contract rhythmically and violently. Abdominal distention, gastric distention, and the presence of a nasogastric tube are common causes, but electrolyte and acid–base disturbances, intestinal obstruction, and intra-abdominal bleeding may also initiate hiccoughs. The nurse may need to notify the surgeon when hiccoughs are prolonged.

Gas pains and signs and symptoms of abdominal distention may be minimized by early and frequent ambulation and resumption of oral intake. Gas pains might also be helped by frequently repositioning the client to encourage movement of air through the intestines. As air rises and peristalsis moves from right to left, the client can be moved from lying on the left side (where air will rise on the right), to lying supine, to lying on the right side (where air will rise on the left). If the client can tolerate it and there are no contraindications, lying prone with the head turned to the side places pressure on the abdomen, forcing air to rise and move out through the rectum. Other nursing care measures to relieve abdominal distention might include irrigation of the nasogastric tube, if present. Irrigating the nasogastric tube may also relieve hiccoughs.

Constipation is a major source of discomfort for the client. Analgesics combined with decreased activity and NPO status are very constipating. Oral fluids and activity should be encouraged. If ordered, the medical regimen of stool softeners and suppositories may be indicated.

4. *The client is at high risk for developing urinary retention related to anesthesia, immobility, and pain. The client is also at high risk for infection related to Foley catheter placement.* The quantity and quality of urine are more directly related to cardiac output and the perfusion of the kidneys than to anesthesia, immobility, and pain; although a stress response following surgery causes the body to retain fluids for 24 to 48 hours following surgery. Urine output should be at least 30 cc per hour if a catheter is in place. The catheter must be assessed for patency. If not catheterized, the client should void at least 200 cc at the first postoperative voiding. Most clients void within 6 to 8 hours after surgery. However, urinary retention occurs frequently in the postoperative period, especially following abdominal or pelvic surgery. Anesthesia depresses the urge to void. Narcotics, vagolytic agents (anticholinergics), and spinal anesthesia also interfere with the ability to initiate voiding. The nurse can facilitate voiding by encouraging fluid intake and assisting the client to void in an anatomically correct position depending on the client's condition. Privacy, running water, indirect bladder pressure (placing a firm hand over the bladder), and warm water over the perineum may also encourage voiding.

If the client has not voided, the nurse should palpate, inspect, and percuss the bladder. Often, the surgeon orders a Foley catheter to be inserted if the client has not voided after 8 to 10 hours.

5. *The client may become at high risk for sensory perceptual alterations related to anesthesia, narcotics, change of environment, fluid and electrolyte imbalances, sleep deprivation, hypoxia, and sensory deprivation or overload. The client may also experience pain related to the surgical incision; hypothermia related to anesthesia and surgical environment; and hyperthermia related to infection.* Alterations in neurological function vary and may manifest as pain, fever, or delirium. Assessing the level of consciousness is a priority. A change in level of consciousness may be the first indication of a stroke and/or increased intracranial pressure. Determining the level of consciousness may be difficult, especially in the elderly client or at night, when clients may be groggy from being awakened. Often, thoughts will clear if the client is given the opportunity to thoroughly awaken. Encouraging the presence of loved ones, offering explanations, and listening to the client may decrease sensory perceptual alterations. Encouraging previous sleep patterns, providing uninterrupted sleep, and alternating rest and activity may also be beneficial.

Pain assessment is essential. Subjective data regarding pain location, intensity on a scale of 0 to 10, quality, and duration as well as factors contributing to pain are assessed and recorded. Objective data such as grimacing and crying are also recorded. Analgesics are usually ordered to be administered via patient-controlled analgesia (PCA) or epidural analgesia or intravenously, intramuscularly, or orally, all on a prn (as needed) basis. The client must be encouraged to ask for the medication before the pain becomes severe. The nurse should offer medication before activity or painful procedures such as wound irrigation. The nurse must attend to analgesic requests promptly. Ensuring comfort encourages the client's full participation in coughing, deep breathing, turning, and ambulation.

Hypothermia is common in the first few hours following surgery. The nurse can offer blankets as needed. Because of the normal inflammatory response, temperature may later elevate to a low-grade fever. If temperature rises higher than 101°F, the surgeon must be notified. Atelectasis and dehydration may cause elevated temperature (higher than 101°F) in the first 24 to 48 hours following surgery. After 48 hours, temperature higher than 101°F may be indicative of a wound, respiratory, or urinary tract infection; thrombophlebitis; or pulmonary embolism.

The nurse's primary role is to prevent infection by using aseptic technique. Once a fever has occurred, the nurse follows orders to ascertain the cause of the elevation by taking urine, wound, blood, or sputum cultures. The nurse also administers antipyretics as ordered. Providing light covers and clothing, performing frequent linen changes, offering cool washcloths, and ensuring a cool environment are nursing measures that may increase comfort.

6. *The surgical client is at risk for impaired skin integrity related to surgical incision and at high risk for infection related to surgical incision.* The nurse generally does not remove the primary dressing without an order to do so. Bleeding may be monitored by circling the drainage on the dressing and then reassessing later to ascertain whether the drainage area has increased in size. The dressing may also be reinforced with additional absorbent dressings as needed. In some institutions, the nurse may change the dressing as necessary after the first dressing change. Dressings may not be necessary if there is no drainage or drains, but this is usually the surgeon's preference.

Drainage on dressings and in drains typically changes from sanguinous to serosanguinous to serous over several hours to several days, depending on the type of surgery. The amount should also decrease over the same time period. Purulent, odorous drainage may be a sign of infection. A sudden increase in drainage may be a sign of impending wound separation. The surgeon should always be notified of any excessive or abnormal drainage.

All wounds heal by primary, secondary, or tertiary intention. In primary intention, the wound layers are sutured together and have no gaping edges. The wound generally heals in 8 to 10 days, but may take up to 3 months. There is minimal scar formation. Most surgical wounds are of this type.

In secondary intention, the wound heals by filling in with granulation tissue and by contracting where the skin edges are not approximated. This method is used for ulcers when there is not enough tissue to approximate the edges or for infected wounds when drainage is desirable. Wounds healing by secondary intention are assessed according to the presence of granulation tissue having a red, granular appearance. Wound healing is slow, possibly taking many months or years. Thus, wound healing by primary intention is preferable.

In tertiary intention, the approximation of tissue edges is delayed. This allows an infection to drain or an area of extensive tissue removal to begin healing. The edges of the wound are closed 4 to 6 days later. Because areas of granulation tissue are brought together at this time, the scar is usually much wider (Figure 29-15).

Wound dehiscence and evisceration are serious complications of wound healing. **Dehiscence** occurs when the wound edges separate. **Evisceration** occurs when the wound separates completely and the viscera protrude from the wound

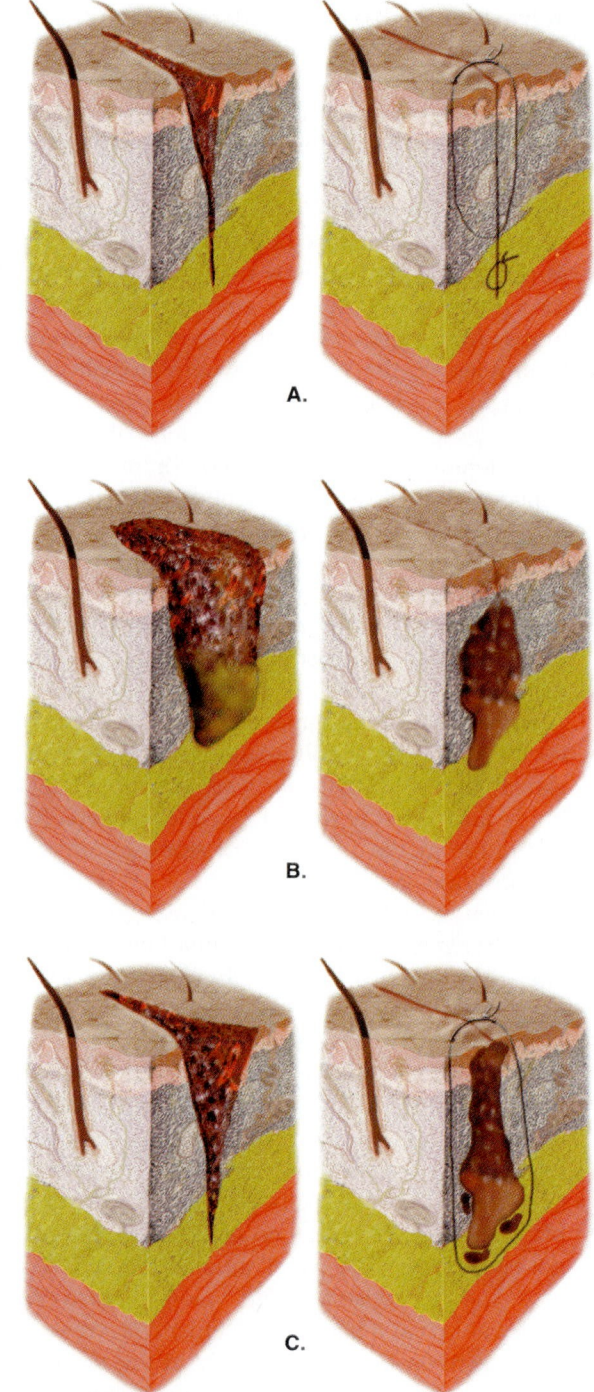

Figure 29-15 Wound Healing: A. Primary intention; B. Secondary intention; and C. Tertiary intention

(Figure 29-16). Both are more likely to occur 7 to 10 days following surgery and are preceded by a sudden spillage of serosanguinous drainage. Dehiscence and evisceration are more likely to occur in the very elderly client, the malnourished client, the client with an infection, or the client with abdominal distention who is straining severely. If evisceration occurs, the viscera should be immediately covered with sterile saline dressings and the surgeon notified of the wound disruption.

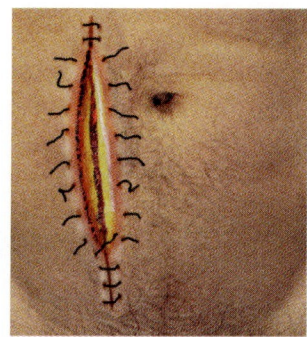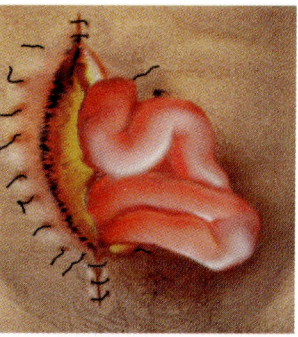

Figure 29-16 A. Dehiscence; B. Evisceration

When dressings are changed, the surgical incision is cleansed to remove debris and bacteria from the incision. The choice of cleansing agent depends on the physician's prescription as well as institutional protocol. It is recommended that isotonic solutions such as normal saline or lactated ringers be used.

The major principles to keep in mind when cleansing a surgical incision are:

- Use Standard Precautions at all times.
- Use a sterile swab or gauze and work from the clean area out toward the dirtier area. Begin over the incision line and swab downward from top to bottom. Change the swab and proceed

again on either side of the incision, using a new swab each time (see Figure 29-17).

The surface closures, staples, or sutures must be removed as the incision heals. Continuous sutures are made with one thread and tied at the beginning and end of the suture line. Intermittent sutures are each tied individually. In blanket continuous sutures, the single thread is grounded again in the last suture exit (Figure 29-18).

The incisional dressing keeps the incision clean and protects it from physical trauma and bacterial invasion. Generally, the same kind of dressing can be put on as was taken off. As the incision heals and drainage lessens, a small, thinner dressing can usually be applied. Bandages and binders may be applied over the incision dressing to secure, immobilize, or support a body part; to hold the dressing in place; or to prevent or minimize swelling of a body part. Bandages are long rolls of material, such as gauze, webbing, or muslin, designed to be wrapped around body parts. Figure 29-19 illustrates several different methods of bandaging. Binders are bandages made for specific body parts, usually the abdomen, perineal area, or arm (sling) (Figure 29-20). Abdominal binders support the abdomen and are used following abdominal surgery or childbirth. Perineal binders, called T-binders, are used

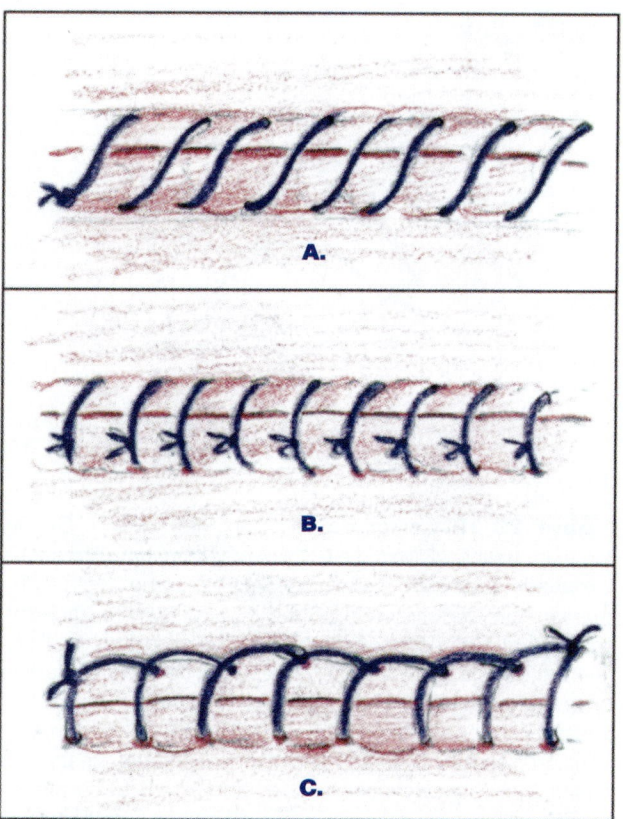

Figure 29-18 Selected Suturing Methods: A. Continuous; B. Intermittent; and C. Blanket continuous

Figure 29-17 Use a clean, sterile swab for each stroke when cleansing a surgical incision. A. Gently clean the incision, then each side alternately. B. Gently wipe swab outward, away from the incision. C. Clean around a drain site in a circular motion.

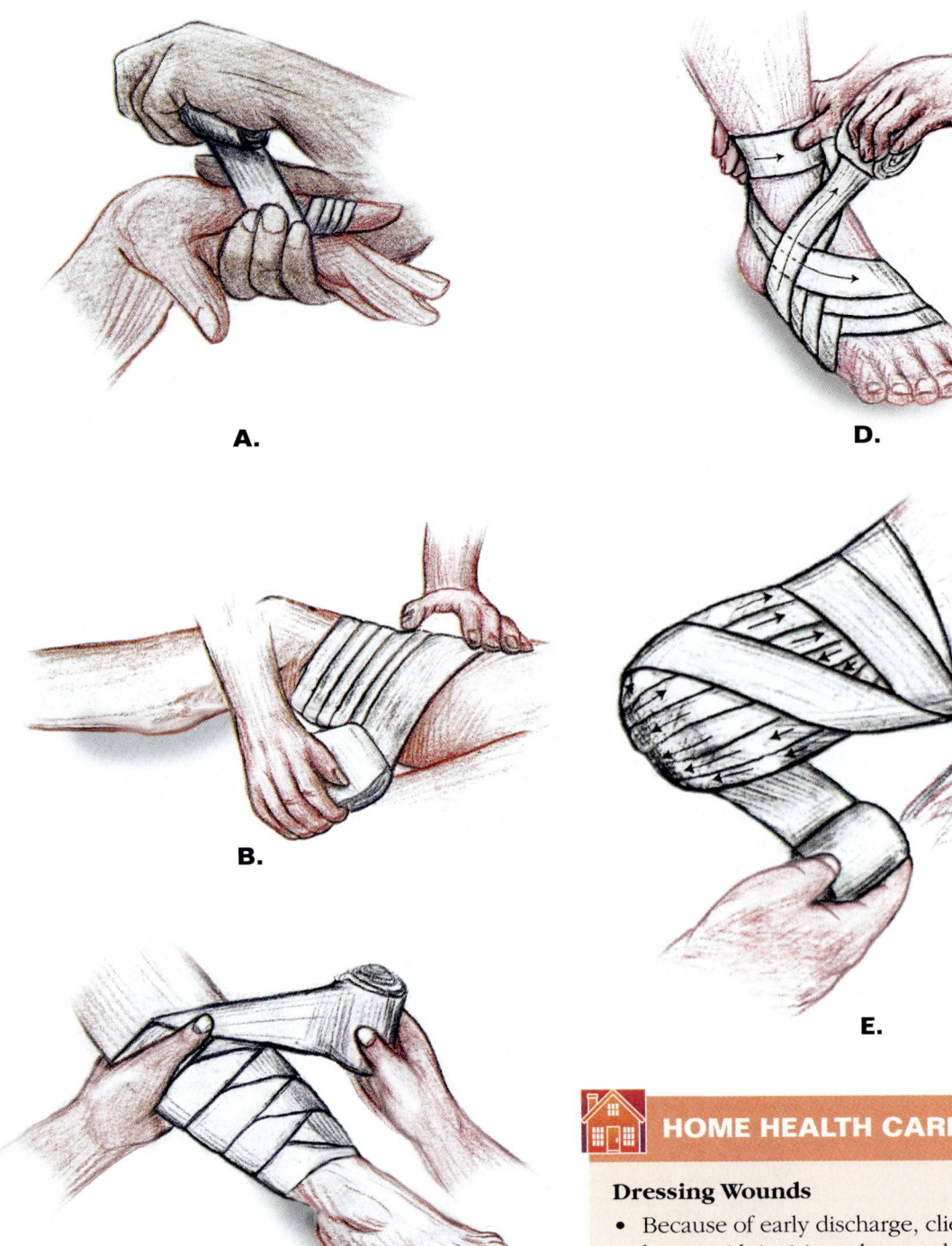

A.

B.

C.

D.

E.

Figure 29-19 Common Bandaging Methods: A. Circular turns are wrapped around a body part several times to anchor the bandage or supply support. B. Spiral turns begin with a circular turn then proceed up the body part, with each turn covering two-thirds the width of the preceding turn. C. Spiral reverse turns begin with a circular turn. The bandage is then reversed, or twisted, once each turn to accommodate a limb that gets larger as the bandaging progresses. D. Figure-eight turns crisscross in the shape of a figure eight and are used on a joint that requires movement. E. Recurrent turns are anchored with circular turns, follow a back-and-forth motion, and are completed with circular turns; they are used to cover a fingertip, head, or amputated stump.

HOME HEALTH CARE

Dressing Wounds

- Because of early discharge, clients are often sent home with incisions that need dressing changes.
- Ascertain the client's support system, including caregivers, the home environment, and available resources.
- Teach the client and/or home caregiver the correct method of changing the dressing.
- Have the client and/or home caregiver actually change the dressing before the client is discharged.
- Provide a list of signs and symptoms of complications of wound healing.
- At times, a referral for home care nursing is necessary.

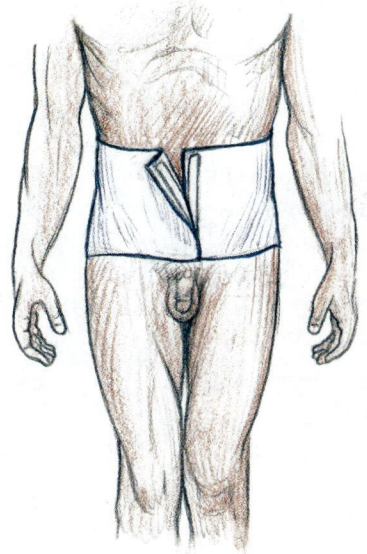

A.

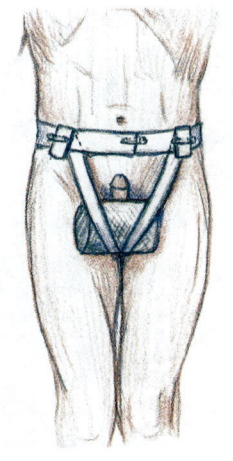

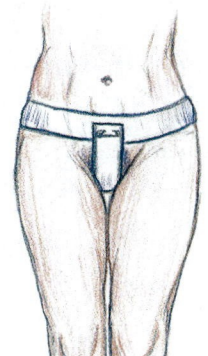

B.

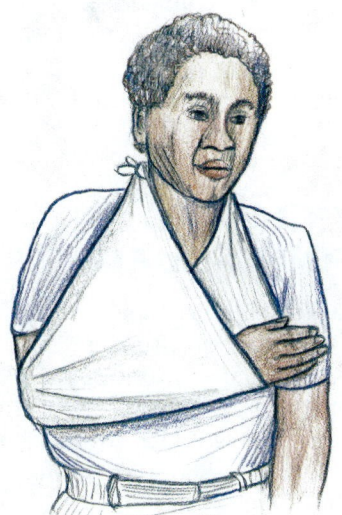

C.

Figure 29-20 Common Binders: A. Abdominal; B. T-binders; female and male; and C. Arm sling

to hold pads or dressings in the perineal area. Because of the urination and defecation needs of clients, T-binders must be changed regularly. A sling is a cloth support for an injured arm; it wraps around the back of the neck to maintain the arm in a set position.

During dressing changes and after the dressing has been removed, the surgical wound is assessed for the skin edge approximation, edema, and bleeding. The skin edges may be slightly reddened and swollen from the normal inflammatory response. Possible signs of a wound infection include increased suture tension, warmth, erythema, drainage, odor, pain, and induration around the incision site. The nurse can enhance wound healing by promoting nutrition, discouraging smoking, and performing proper wound cleansing. The practice of aseptic technique cannot be emphasized enough in preventing nosocomial infections in a surgical incision.

7. *Clients are at high risk for anxiety or ineffective individual coping related to disturbance in body image, change in lifestyle, financial strain, or a poor prognosis.* Many clients undergo a psychological adjustment to surgery. Taking time to talk and listen to the client as well as offering simple explanations and reassurances may be all the support the client needs to combat anxiety.

As the client recovers and is discharged from the hospital, the client is at high risk for knowledge deficit related to home care. Ideally, the client has been instructed routinely about home care since admission. Adequate teaching about home care results in a quicker recovery, fewer complications, and greater independence.

AMBULATORY SURGERY

Ambulatory surgery is defined as surgical care performed under general, regional, or local anesthesia and involving fewer than 24 hours of hospitalization. Other names for ambulatory surgery include same-day, one-day, outpatient, in and out, or short-stay surgery.

A trend in health care is to promote a philosophy of wellness. Clients are encouraged to accept more personal responsibility for their state of health. In the past, the message sent to clients was that the client is sick, and the medical community will provide all care. Today, ambulatory surgery clients are being sent a totally different message: that the postoperative client is not sick and, except for a few minor limitations, can often resume normal daily activities soon after undergoing anesthesia and surgery.

Ambulatory surgery provides the longest period of time for the client to receive skilled postoperative care or monitoring without being formally admitted to the hospital. The practice of ambulatory surgery attempts

HOME HEALTH CARE

Postoperative Care

For proper home care, the client and family must be given information about the following topics:

- Medication regimen
- Diet
- Activity restrictions
- Follow-up appointments
- Wound care
- Special instructions

The specifics for each topic will vary with each client and will depend on the surgical procedure and the client's age and physical condition.

PROFESSIONAL TIP

Ambulatory Surgery

- Precertification documents are approved before the preadmission visit.
- Preadmission diagnostic tests, preoperative nursing assessment, and initial teaching are usually performed the day before the scheduled surgery.
- On the day of surgery, care is focused on the immediate needs of the client.

to overcome the risk of premature dismissal while at the same time meeting fiscal requirements. The emphasis on cost containment coupled with government reductions in Medicare and Medicaid payments has further promoted the concept of ambulatory surgery.

To further reduce health care costs, few clients are admitted to the hospital prior to the day of surgery. Most surgical clients are processed through the ambulatory surgery unit. These clients are called "day of surgery" or "A.M. admit" clients. Necessary laboratory work, radiology tests, or other examinations are completed on an outpatient basis prior to the day of surgery. Even clients undergoing extensive surgeries such as open-heart surgery (a coronary artery bypass), craniotomy, or total joint replacement, can be admitted the day of surgery. Then, after discharge from the perioperative suite, the client may either be admitted to the hospital as an inpatient or may be sent home from the ambulatory surgery unit.

In addition to fiscal considerations, the growth of ambulatory surgery can also be traced to technological advances. Clients now require shorter recovery periods due to new procedural technology, such as laporoscopic cholecystectomy. The introduction of shorter-acting anesthetic agents also decreases the immediate postoperative recovery time, facilitating the client's ability to function independently upon discharge from the ambulatory surgery setting.

The benefits of ambulatory surgery are many. Ambulatory surgery decreases cost to the client, institution, insurance carriers, and governmental agencies. Because clients are hospitalized for such a short period of time, the risk of acquiring a nosocomial infection during the perioperative period is also decreased. The client experiences less disruption to personal life and less psychological distress related to hospitalization. With ambulatory surgery, the client especially benefits from early postoperative ambulation.

Ambulatory surgery is performed in several different settings. Hospital-based integrated facilities are formal ambulatory surgery programs incorporated into existing inpatient surgery programs. Clients are cared for preoperatively and postoperatively in the ambulatory surgery unit, but are mixed with inpatients on the operating room schedule. This type of facility also allows preoperative processing of day-of-surgery clients. Hospital-affiliated facilities consist of a separate department with designated preoperative, intraoperative, and postoperative areas. Such a facility may be located within the hospital, adjacent to the hospital, or at a satellite location. Free-standing facilities are independently owned and operated and are not affiliated with a hospital or medical center. In the past, physicians generally owned such facilities, but today the trend is for health care corporations to own these facilities. Some doctors' offices also have facilities for performing minor ambulatory surgery.

The Aldrete Score has been modified for use with clients having anesthesia on an ambulatory basis. Five assessments were added to the Aldrete Score for this purpose (Table 29-6). Attainment of these criteria indicates that clients should be able to care for themselves at home and accomplish activities of daily living independently and safely. The points are totaled at regular intervals (usually every ½ hour), and clients may be discharged home when their total score is 18 or higher.

ELDERLY CLIENTS UNDERGOING SURGERY

Elderly clients (over 65 years of age) are at high risk for developing complications from surgery or anesthesia. Unfortunately, because an increased incidence of disease correlates with increasing age, more elderly clients require surgery than does any other age group. As the percentage of elderly persons in the whole population rises, the number of surgeries on elders will also rise. Because of the complex needs of the elderly client undergoing surgery, the nurse must be knowledgeable in promoting health and rehabilitation in the elderly client.

Surgery is a stressor. Because of depleted energy sources, the elderly client may not have sufficient resilience to react defensively to this stressor. The risk of complications from surgery further rises in elderly clients who have one or more chronic diseases. In these clients, surgery then can be the source of a downward spiraling effect toward debilitation or possibly death.

Elderly clients vary in their abilities to respond to the stress of surgery. Physiologic changes related to the aging process may inhibit the elderly client from readily coping with surgery. The number of physio-

logic changes in the very elderly client (over 80 years of age) is markedly greater than that in those in their 60s and 70s. Breathing capacity, renal blood flow, cardiac output, and conduction velocity of the nervous system all diminish. Table 29-9 lists the physiologic changes in the elderly client along with correlating nursing interventions for postoperative care. Aging affects all body systems, and the nurse must be familiar with these changes and the interventions geared toward each to prevent and detect complications of surgery.

Table 29-9 PHYSIOLOGIC CHANGES OF AGING AND RELATED POSTOPERATIVE NURSING INTERVENTIONS

BODY SYSTEM	CHANGES	NURSING INTERVENTIONS
Cardiovascular	• Decreased elasticity of the vascular system • Decreased cardiac output • Decreased peripheral circulation	• Closely monitor vital signs and peripheral pulses • Encourage early ambulation • Use antiembolism stockings • Monitor intake and output, including blood loss • Monitor preoperative response to activity and compare to postoperative response
Respiratory	• Decreased vital capacity • Decreased alveolar volume • Decreased movement of cilia	• Closely monitor respirations • Auscultate breath sounds frequently • Encourage coughing and deep breathing • Turn frequently • Monitor oxygen saturation
Urinary	• Decreased glomerular filtration rate • Decreased bladder muscle tone • Weakened perineal muscles	• Monitor intake and output every 1 to 2 hours • Assist frequently with toileting • Monitor fluid and electrolyte status
Gastrointestinal	• Decreased gastric and intestinal motility • Altered digestion and absorption • Decreased food consumption	• Assess for obesity and malnutrition • Encourage fluids and activity • Encourage high-protein foods and supplements • Assist with meals as needed • Provide companionship during mealtime
Immunological	• Decreased level of gamma globulin • Decreased plasma proteins	• Follow strict aseptic technique • Monitor temperature • Assess incision site
Neurological	• Decreased conduction velocity • Decreased visual acuity • Loss of hearing • Decreased sensation	• Allow use of glasses and hearing aids • Orient to environment • Provide for safe environment • Repeat information as needed • Use medications sparingly • Provide written instructions • Allow for extra education time
Integumentary	• Lack of elasticity • Loss of collagen • Decreased subcutaneous fat	• To prevent shearing forces on skin when positioning client, lift rather than slide client • Pad bony prominences • Use tape that is easy to remove • Use warm prepping solutions, irrigating solutions, and IV solutions intraoperatively • Provide extra blankets • Ensure warm room temperature • Turn frequently • Encourage early ambulation

In the cardiovascular system, the elderly client experiences decreased elasticity of the blood vessels and decreased pumping action of the heart, resulting in less blood reaching the peripheral circulation. Ultimately, blood flow is slower, and less blood reaches vital organs such as the brain, heart, lungs, liver, and kidneys. In the older adult, decreased blood flow to vital organs delays elimination of anesthetics and medications through the lungs, liver, and kidneys. Decreased elasticity of the blood vessels does not allow vasoconstriction and vasodilation to compensate for hypovolemia and hypervolemia; thus the elderly client is more prone to hypotension and shock or, conversely, fluid overload. Slower blood flow combined with an increased incidence of atherosclerosis, the presence of other cardiovascular diseases, and decreased mobility increases the elderly client's risk for developing deep vein thrombosis, thrombophlebitis, and accompanying pulmonary embolism. Decreased blood flow to vital organs may also cause confusion, decreased urinary output, and drug retention or overdose. Decreased peripheral circulation may contribute to poor or delayed wound healing as well. The effects of aging on the cardiovascular system increase the likelihood of multiple surgical complications in the elderly client.

As with the cardiovascular system, the respiratory system in elderly clients demonstrates less elasticity, and expansion of the chest wall and lungs is adversely affected. As a result, elderly clients are unable to exhale fully, causing increased air retention in the lung (residual lung volume) and decreased ability to forcefully exhale air (forced expiratory volume). The amount of air inhaled and exhaled (vital capacity) also decreases. Less air reaches the alveoli, causing decreased alveolar volume. Decreased vital capacity and alveolar volume result in reduced exchange of carbon dioxide and oxygen in the lungs. The cilia lining the passageways of the lungs do not move as efficiently, resulting in a decreased cough reflex in the elderly client. All of these changes may lead to atelectasis, pneumonia, and postoperative confusion.

The urinary system is affected by age as well. Kidney function deteriorates as blood flow to the kidneys decreases. Waste products are not excreted as quickly and urine output decreases. Reduced blood flow also decreases the glomerular filtration rate. Decreased bladder muscle tone results in urinary retention, and weakened perineal muscles can lead to urinary incontinence. The effects of aging also increase the likelihood of renal failure.

A combination of age-related changes in renal and liver function, related to decreased perfusion rate, results in slower drug metabolism. To prevent side effects of postoperative analgesics, the elderly client may need either a reduced dosage, given less frequently, or smaller, more frequent doses. Decreased peripheral circulation may reduce or delay the absorption of intramuscular

analgesics. Oral analgesics may also be poorly absorbed due to decreased gastrointestinal motility and decreased mesenteric blood flow. Intravenous analgesia may be preferred for the elderly client to provide careful dosing according to individual response and need.

In the gastrointestinal system, decreased gastric and intestinal motility result in constipation and fecal impaction. Decreased activity stemming from loss of muscle strength and range of motion further contributes to constipation. Because elderly clients are often less mobile after surgery, constipation and fecal impaction are very common.

The nutritional status of the elderly client prior to surgery may also have a profound effect on wound healing, susceptibility to infection, degree of postoperative recovery, and length of hospital stay (Talabiska, 1995). Nutritional status can be affected by the presence of a chronic illness, resulting in the client expending more energy to maintain metabolism and activities of daily living. Dementia, depression, and altered mental status may also affect nutritional status. Because the elderly client may take multiple medications, drug–food interactions are common. Food consumption, gastric motility, and digestion and absorption all decrease. The financial situation and social status of the elderly client may also affect nutritional status, as may poorly fitting dentures and decreased sense of taste. The nutritional status of the elderly client must be carefully assessed both preoperatively and postoperatively to facilitate optimal recovery from surgery.

Elderly clients are prone to infections such as wound infections, pneumonia, and urinary tract infections. Delayed wound healing, including wound dehiscence or evisceration, are also common in the elderly client. Changes in the metabolism and the immune system of the elderly client may contribute to these effects. The levels of gamma globulin and plasma proteins fall, causing inadequate inflammatory responses. Fewer killer T-cells and a decreased response to foreign proteins render the body less able to protect itself from pathogenic microorganisms. An increased production of leukocytes and an elevated temperature for 48 hours postoperatively is a normal inflammatory response. If temperature elevates markedly and continues longer than 48 hours, however, an infectious process may be occurring. In the elderly client, a reduction in the basal metabolic rate results in a lower normal temperature. Thus, fever in the elderly client is even more significant.

The conduction velocity of the nervous system diminishes in the elderly client, slowing movements and impairing equilibrium. These and other sensory changes increase the risk of injury in the elderly surgical client. Dimished vision, hearing, and sensation contribute to falls, burns, and other injuries. Overstimulation and the lack of a familiar environment often cause confusion, another factor in injury. Chronic conditions that limit mobility, such as arthritis or previous stroke, may also

CASE STUDY

Mr. Glen Stone, a 74-year-old retired schoolteacher who is married and the father of four and the grand-father of sixteen, weighs 275 lbs. He has undergone a right hemicolectomy, wherein the right side of his colon was removed because of cancer. He has a history of smoking, but has no other health problems. The surgery was uncomplicated, and he is in the PACU. He has a midline incision with a Penrose drain; a stab wound with a Jackson Pratt drain is adjacent to the incision. He also has a nasogastric tube attached to low intermittent suction. He is alert and oriented, and he can move all four extremities. His blood pressure is normal for him in comparison to his preoperative levels. He is breathing regularly and easily at a rate of 16 breaths per minute, and his skin color is normal. His oxygen saturation, however, is 86% with additional oxygen being given via mask.

The following questions will guide your development of a nursing care plan for the case study.

1. What risk factors for developing postoperative complications can you identify for Mr. Stone?
2. What is his Aldrete Score at this point?
3. What nursing measures can you institute to promote oxygenation?
4. What type of drainage is expected from the incision and the drains during the first 1 to 2 days?
5. What nursing observations can be made and reported to indicate to the surgeon that the nasogastric tube can be removed?
6. What nursing measures can be implemented to prevent deep vein thrombosis, thrombophlebitis, and pulmonary embolism?
7. Write and prioritize three individualized nursing diagnoses and goals for Mr. Stone.
8. What information will Mr. Stone need prior to discharge?

contribute to the incidence of injury. The physiologic changes in the nervous system may lead to integumentary complications as mobility and sensation decrease.

Due to lack of elasticity and loss of collagen, the skin of the elderly client is often dry, flaky, and itchy. It thins and is easily bruised and abraded. Lack of subcutaneous fat and decreased circulation render the older adult prone to hypothermia and pressure sores.

The elderly client has a lifetime of experiences that affects the response to surgery. A lifetime of watching family and friends experience surgery, illness, and death particularly influences personal reactions to impending surgery. Due to the variation in such experiences, each client reacts differently to similar situations. Simply talking with the client to provide information or listening to the client's fears helps the client prepare for upcoming surgery.

Third-party reimbursement policies often require elderly clients to undergo surgical procedures on an outpatient basis. Because many elderly clients have neurological deficits and other chronic disease processes, the elderly outpatient poses a particular challenge to the nurse. Additional postoperative self-care deficits may result from the surgical procedure and the effects of anesthesia. Elderly clients often live alone and lack the support systems necessary for home care. In order to provide realistic discharge planning, the nurse must

assess the ability of the client, family, and friends to provide care at home.

SUMMARY

- Surgery is a major stressor for all clients. Anxiety and fear are normal. Fear of the unknown is both the most prevalent fear prior to surgery and the fear easiest for the nurse to help the client overcome.
- The outcome of surgical treatment is tremendously enhanced by accurate preoperative nursing assessment and careful preoperative preparation. Information gathered through preoperative assessment and risk screening is later used for preparation of the surgical site, for surgical positioning, and as a comparative basis for postoperative assessments and complication screening.
- The teaching methods used by the nurse strongly influence the degree of learning and the retention of information.
- Aseptic technique is a collection of principles used to control and/or prevent the transfer of microorganisms from sources within (endogenous) and outside (exogenous) the client. These principles are practiced in all clinical nursing units. The sterile conscience governs personal behavior with regard to adherence to aseptic technique.

- Nursing care in the operating room focuses on the safety and protection of the client.
- Postoperative nursing assessments are completed in an organized manner, focusing first on the priorities of airway, breathing, and circulation, and then on the body system affected by surgery.
- The nurse can help prevent the formation of deep vein thrombosis, thrombophlebitis, and pulmonary embolism through encouraging early ambulation and postoperative leg exercises and by providing antiembolism stockings and/or sequential stockings, if ordered.
- Ambulatory surgery is defined as surgical care performed under general, regional, or local anesthesia and involving fewer than 24 hours of hospitalization. Cost containment, governmental changes, and technological advances have all promoted the concept of ambulatory surgery.
- Because of the physiologic changes and complex needs of the elderly client undergoing surgery, the nurse must be knowledgeable in promoting health and rehabilitation in the elderly surgical client.

Review Questions

1. When performing client teaching, the nurse does which one of the following?
   a. Assesses barriers to learning
   b. Completes teaching in a single time frame
   c. Provides information in one mode of learning
   d. Allows little time for questions

2. Client education is:
   a. completed when time allows.
   b. started when discharge is scheduled.
   c. always more beneficial when completed in a structured group setting.
   d. directed toward the client's family when the client is unable to learn.

3. The role of the nurse in obtaining consent includes which of the following?
   a. Judging the quality of the explanation and ascertaining the client's understanding of the consent form
   b. Acting as a witness to the signature of the client
   c. Administering the preoperative medication before the client signs the consent
   d. Ensuring that coercion was used to obtain the client's signature on the consent

4. The use of drains will:
   a. increase postoperative pain.
   b. prevent tissue healing.
   c. increase scarring.
   d. eliminate fluid accumulation.

5. Upon the client's admission to the PACU, the nurse must first:
   a. take the client's blood pressure.
   b. assess the airway.
   c. assess the client's level of consciousness.
   d. check the incision site.

6. The nurse is making a preoperative assessment on a client. Which of these findings is the most important to know for a client who is having general anesthesia?
   a. Hearing impaired
   b. A right-leg amputee
   c. Color blind
   d. A smoker

7. Which of the following persons is responsible and accountable for all activities during a surgical procedure?
   a. Surgeon
   b. Anesthesia provider
   c. Circulating nurse
   d. Scrub nurse

8. The surgical skin preparation will:
   a. sterilize the skin.
   b. cleanse the skin and inhibit bacterial growth.
   c. prevent fingernails from growing.
   d. remove the dermis.

9. The nursing intervention that has the greatest impact on reducing overall surgical risk is:
   a. encouraging activity and early ambulation.
   b. assessing blood pressure.
   c. ensuring adequate nutrition.
   d. monitoring intake and output.

10. Surgical risk increases in the elderly client due to:
    a. type of surgery.
    b. physiologic changes of aging.
    c. exposure to infectious processes.
    d. number of children.

Critical Thinking Questions

1. How can you use a sterile conscience when providing nursing care?

 WEB FLASH!

- Research "incision glue" on the Web. What information is available on this topic?
- What sites could a client access for information on a particular surgery (e.g., coronary bypass)?

NURSING CARE OF THE ONCOLOGY CLIENT

MAKING THE CONNECTION

Refer to the following chapters to increase your understanding of oncology nursing:

- **Chapter 7, Ethical Responsibilities**
- **Chapter 17, Loss, Grief, and Death**
- **Chapter 26, Pain Management**
- **Chapter 27, Diagnostic Tests**
- **Chapter 29, Nursing Care of the Surgical Client**
- **Chapter 33, Nursing Care of the Client: Blood and Lymph Systems**
- **Chapter 35, Nursing Care of the Client: Reproductive System**
- **Chapter 39, Nursing Care of the Client: Immune System**
- **Chapter 40, Nursing Care of the Client: Integumentary System**
- **Chapter 55, Nursing Care of the Elderly Client**

LEARNING OBJECTIVES

Upon completion of this chapter, you should be able to:
- *Define key terms.*
- *Explain how the behavior of cancer cells differs from that of normal cells.*
- *Describe the role of the nurse in cancer detection.*
- *Discuss three medical treatments for cancer.*
- *Describe four complications that can occur in advanced cancer.*
- *Discuss ways the licensed practical/vocational nurse can aid the client in coping with cancer.*

KEY TERMS

alopecia	extravasation
anorexia	leukemia
antineoplastic	lymphoma
benign	malignant
biologic response	metastasis
modifiers	neoplasm
cachexia	oncology
cancer	palliative
carcinogen	radiotherapy
carcinoma	reconstructive
chemotherapy	sarcoma
curative	tumor markers
differentiation	vesicant

INTRODUCTION

Cancer is a disease resulting from the uncontrolled growth of cells, which causes malignant cellular tumors. One in three Americans will develop some type of cancer during their lifetime. Cancer is the second leading cause of death in the United States and can develop in individuals of any race, gender, age, socioeconomic status, or culture. It is not a single disease but, rather, a group of more than 200 different diseases that can attack any tissue or organ of the body.

According to the American Cancer Society (ACS), in the 1930s fewer than one in five cancer clients was alive 5 years after diagnosis. In the 1940s one in four survived 5 years. Today, four of ten people diagnosed with cancer will be alive in 5 years (American Cancer Society, 1998). Survival rates are influenced by the type of cancer, the progression of the disease at diagnosis, and the client's response to the treatment.

INCIDENCE

Women develop cancer more often than do men, although a greater number of men actually die from the disease. Incidence and mortality rates are usually higher for African Americans than for Anglo Americans. The incidence of cancer is higher in the elderly population than in any other age group. In men, the most common cancers are skin, prostate, lung, and colorectal; in women, they are skin, breast, colorectal, lung, and uterine cancer (see Figure 30-1).

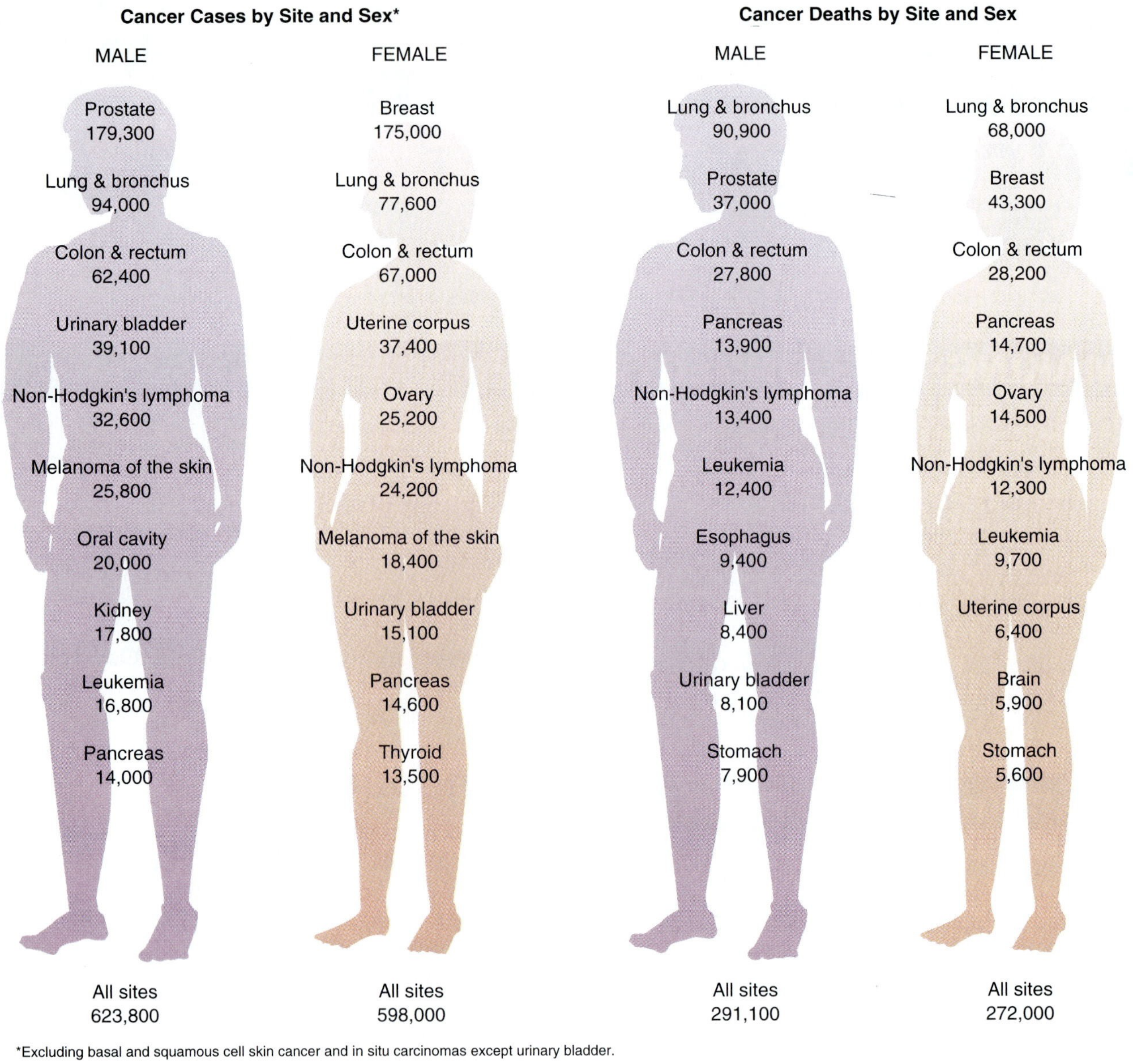

Cancer Cases by Site and Sex*

MALE	FEMALE

Prostate 179,300	Breast 175,000
Lung & bronchus 94,000	Lung & bronchus 77,600
Colon & rectum 62,400	Colon & rectum 67,000
Urinary bladder 39,100	Uterine corpus 37,400
Non-Hodgkin's lymphoma 32,600	Ovary 25,200
Melanoma of the skin 25,800	Non-Hodgkin's lymphoma 24,200
Oral cavity 20,000	Melanoma of the skin 18,400
Kidney 17,800	Urinary bladder 15,100
Leukemia 16,800	Pancreas 14,600
Pancreas 14,000	Thyroid 13,500
All sites 623,800	All sites 598,000

Cancer Deaths by Site and Sex

MALE	FEMALE

Lung & bronchus 90,900	Lung & bronchus 68,000
Prostate 37,000	Breast 43,300
Colon & rectum 27,800	Colon & rectum 28,200
Pancreas 13,900	Pancreas 14,700
Non-Hodgkin's lymphoma 13,400	Ovary 14,500
Leukemia 12,400	Non-Hodgkin's lymphoma 12,300
Esophagus 9,400	Leukemia 9,700
Liver 8,400	Uterine corpus 6,400
Urinary bladder 8,100	Brain 5,900
Stomach 7,900	Stomach 5,600
All sites 291,100	All sites 272,000

*Excluding basal and squamous cell skin cancer and in situ carcinomas except urinary bladder.

Figure 30-1 Leading Sites of New Cancer Cases and Deaths—1999 Estimates (*Reprinted from American Cancer Society Cancer Facts and Figures, 1998*)

The ACS estimates that 1,228,600 new cancer cases were diagnosed in the United States in 1998. Not included in this estimate were basal- and squamous-cell skin cancers and noninvasive cancers except for urinary bladder cancer. There are over 1,000,000 cases each year of highly curable basal- and squamous-cell skin cancers (American Cancer Society, 1998).

In 1998, approximately 175,000 cancer deaths were estimated to be caused by tobacco, with an additional 19,000 cancer deaths related to excessive alcohol use. Up to one-third of the 564,800 cancer deaths estimated for 1998 are related to dietary choices such as types of food; food preparation methods; portion sizes; and food variety.

PATHOPHYSIOLOGY

Cancer is a disease characterized by neoplasia, an uncontrolled growth of abnormal cells. Unlike normal cells, which reproduce in an orderly manner and grow for a purpose, cancer cells develop rapidly, undiscriminatingly, and serve no useful function as they grow at the expense of healthy tissue. **Neoplasms**, or any abnormal growth of new tissue, can be found in any body tissue. Neoplasms may be **benign** (not progressive, and thus, favorable for recovery) or **malignant** (becoming progressively worse and often resulting in death).

Benign neoplasms are not cancerous and are usually

harmless. They grow slowly, are encapsulated and well-defined, and do not spread to neighboring tissues. Unless their location interferes with vital functions, benign neoplasms are associated with a favorable prognosis.

Malignant neoplasms form irregularly-shaped masses with fingerlike projections. They usually multiply quickly and spread to distant body parts through the bloodstream or the lymph system. This process is called **metastasis**. Patterns of metastasis will differ depending on the type of cancer.

Cancers are usually named according to the site of the primary tumor or to the type of tissue involved. There are four main classifications of cancer according to tissue type:

- **lymphomas** (cancers occurring in infection-fighting organs, such as lymphatic tissue)
- **leukemias** (cancers occurring in blood-forming organs, such as the spleen, and in bone marrow)
- **sarcomas** (cancers occurring in connective tissue, such as bone)
- **carcinomas** (cancers occurring in epithelial tissue, such as the skin)

The exact mechanism that causes cancer is unknown, but most authorities believe that cancer develops from a combination of factors rather than from a single factor. Environmental, genetic, and viral factors have been implicated in the development of cancer. Chemical substances that initiate or promote the development of cancer are known as **carcinogens**. These agents are thought to alter the DNA in the cell nucleus.

RISK FACTORS

A number of risk factors, such as environmental/lifestyle, genetic, and viral, may increase an individual's chances of developing cancer. These factors are discussed following.

Environmental Factors

The first environmental carcinogen was discovered in 1760 when Percival Pott noted that chimney sweeps had a very high rate of what is now known to be scrotal cancer because they were exposed to cancer-causing oils in the soot that was rubbed into their clothing. Since that time, hundreds of chemical carcinogens have been identified.

Many individuals come into contact with cancer-causing agents through occupational exposure. Many industrial chemicals, such as asbestos or vinyl chlorides, have been found to be carcinogenic. For workers who handle these chemicals, the risk of developing cancers is greatly increased if occupational exposure is combined with cigarette smoking. Tobacco may act synergistically with other substances to promote cancer development. Occupational exposure to coal tar,

creosote, arsenic compounds, or radium constitutes a risk factor for development of skin cancer. The effects of carcinogenic agents are usually dose dependent. The larger the dose or the longer the duration of exposure, the greater the risk of cancer development. It is estimated that 80% of all cancers may be associated with environmental exposures and might be prevented if exposure is avoided. For those likely to be exposed to chemical carcinogens at work, safety standards and levels of exposure have been established by the Occupational Safety and Health Administration (OSHA).

In 1993, the U.S. Environmental Protection Agency (EPA) declared secondhand smoke a human carcinogen. Approximately 3,000 nonsmoking adults die each year of lung cancer from breathing secondhand smoke (ACS, 1998).

Lifestyle Factors

Other agents include exposures determined by individual lifestyle choices such as the use of tobacco, sun exposure, alcohol consumption, and diet. Tobacco accounts for nearly one in five deaths in the United States (ACS, 1998). Tobacco use includes cigarettes, cigars, pipes, and smokeless forms (snuff and chewing tobacco). The same carcinogens are found in all forms of tobacco, causing cancer of the oral cavity, esophagus, pharynx, and larynx. When tobacco is smoked, it can also cause cancer of the lung, pancreas, uterus, cervix, kidney, and bladder.

Overexposure to the sun's ultraviolet rays over long periods of time is the cause of many skin cancers. The most serious form of skin cancer is melanoma. The ACS (1998) estimates 41,600 newly diagnosed cases of melanoma in 1998. Other factors predisposing a person to skin cancer are family history, multiple nevi, and atypical nevi.

Heavy alcohol consumption has also been implicated in mouth, throat, esophageal, and liver cancers. Alcohol is hypothesized to cause 5% of cancer deaths. Alcohol and tobacco used together greatly increase the risk of oral and esophageal cancers. The combined effect of alcohol and tobacco is greater than the sum of their individual effects (ACS, 1998). The association between alcohol consumption and breast cancer has also been noted in some studies. Despite the epidemiological evidence linking alcohol to cancer, the exact carcinogen in alcohol is yet to be determined. Table 30-1 lists some risk factors for cancer.

Although findings from studies of the link between cancer and diet are controversial, current research suggests an increase in dietary fiber may help prevent colon cancer (Hansen, 1995). Some studies have suggested that obesity is a significant risk factor for breast, colon, endometrial, and prostate cancers. Studies have also shown that diets high in salt-cured, smoked, and nitrite-cured foods increase an individual's risk for cancer of the stomach and esophagus. Food substances

Table 30-1	RISK FACTORS FOR CANCER
Breast Cancer	• Family history (immediate female relatives) • High-fat diet • Obesity • Early menarche • Late menopause • Long-term estrogen therapy • First child after age 30
Cervical Cancer	• Multiple sexual partners • Exposure to genital herpes • Exposure to human papillomavirus • Smoking
Colorectal Cancer	• Family history (immediate relatives) • Low-fiber diet • History of rectal polyps
Esophageal Cancer	• Heavy alcohol consumption • Smoking
Lung Cancer	• Smoking • Asbestos exposure • Air pollution • Tuberculosis
Skin Cancer	• Extensive exposure to ultraviolet sunlight • Fair complexion • Work with coal, tar, pitch, or creosote
Stomach Cancer	• Family history • Diet heavy in smoked, pickled, or salted foods
Testicular Cancer	• Undescended testicles • Consumption of hormones by mother during pregnancy
Prostate Cancer	• Increasing age • Family history • Diet high in animal fat

Genetic Factors

Some families have a high incidence of certain types of cancer. Breast cancer, for example, occurs more frequently in women whose mothers, grandmothers, or sisters have had the disease. Leukemia and cancers of the colon, stomach, prostate, lung, and ovary, may also run in families. Therefore, relatives of persons with these cancers should be carefully monitored.

Viral Factors

Although viruses have been linked to a number of cancers, their exact role is unclear. It has been theorized that they incorporate themselves into the genetic structure of the cell. Herpes simplex II virus and some of the human papillomaviruses that are transmitted sexually are known to predispose women to cervical cancer. Reducing the number of sexual partners can reduce the risk of contracting these viruses.

DETECTION

When cancer does develop, the earlier it is detected the more likely it is to be controlled. In some cases, diagnosis can be made before symptoms become apparent. Cancer is usually found by the affected individual, who notices a warning sign, or a health care provider

CLIENT TEACHING

Dietary Guidelines To Reduce the Risk of Cancer

• Choose most foods from plant sources.
  – Eat five or more servings of fruits and vegetables each day, especially green and dark-yellow vegetables and those in the cabbage family.
  – Consume other foods from plant sources including breads, cereals, pastas, beans (legumes), and soy products.

• Limit intake of high-fat foods, particularly from animal sources.
  – Choose foods low in fat.
  – Limit consumption of meats, especially red meats and high-fat meats.

• Be physically active and achieve and maintain a healthy weight.
  – Physical activity can help by balancing caloric intake with energy expenditures or by other mechanisms.

• Limit or eliminate consumption of alcoholic beverages.

(ACS, 1998)

that may reduce cancer risk include cruciferous vegetables (cabbage, broccoli, cauliflower, brussels sprouts, kohlrabi); possibly vitamins A, E, and C; and selenium. Some foods have been found to contain carcinogens in the forms of additives or as byproducts of storage. On the basis of current knowledge, the ACS has offered dietary guidelines to reduce cancer risk (see the accompanying display).

CLIENT TEACHING

Lifestyle Guidelines to Reduce the Risk of Cancer

- Do not smoke or use tobacco in any form.
- Avoid overexposure to the sun.
- Eat a healthy diet.
- Get plenty of exercise.
- Have a physical examination on a routine basis, including a mammogram, Pap smear, testicular, and colon examinations.
- Get plenty of sleep (6 to 8 hours per night).
- Keep weight within normal limits.
- Practice regular self-examinations and see your physician if any changes are noted.
- Know and follow health and safety rules at the workplace.

during a checkup. A cancer checkup is recommended every 3 years for persons ages 20 to 39 years and annually for those ages 40 years and over. Risk assessment is the first step in cancer prevention. The cancer examination should include both a medical history of exposures to environmental agents and a comprehensive family history.

If cancer is suspected, diagnostic studies are ordered. The diagnostic studies performed depend on the suspected primary or metastatic site of the cancer and include laboratory studies or blood tests, radiologic studies, endoscopy, cytology, and biopsy. Nurses must be able to give brief descriptions of such tests as well as assist in client preparation.

Although no one blood test can confirm a cancer diagnosis, some malignancies do alter the chemical composition of the blood. Specialized laboratory tests have been developed to detect **tumor markers**, substances such as specific proteins, antigens, genes, hormones, or enzymes that are found in the serum and indicate the possible presence of malignancy. Tumor markers are not 100% accurate, as benign processes can also cause elevations; they are, however, useful in monitoring response to treatment or detecting a relapse.

COMMON DIAGNOSTIC TESTS

Commonly used diagnostic tests for clients who present with symptoms of cancer are listed in Table 30-2. See Chapter 27, Diagnostic Tests, for explanation/normal values and nursing responsibilities related to each test.

STAGING OF TUMORS

Staging determines the extent of the spread of cancer. The TNM classification proposed by the American Joint Commission on Cancer is one of the most frequently used systems. The *T* refers to the anatomical size of the primary tumor; *N*, the extent of lymph node involvement; and *M*, the presence or absence of metastasis (see Table 30-3). Use of this internationally recognized staging system for tumors ensures a reliable comparison of clients in many different hospitals. Staging is important because it influences decisions about treatment modalities and helps predict overall prognosis.

GRADING OF TUMORS

Normal body cells have individual characteristics that allow them to perform different body functions. This process is called **differentiation**. Tumor cells that retain many of the identifiable tissue characteristics of the original cell are termed *well differentiated*. Tumor cells having little similarity to the tissue of origin are termed *undifferentiated*. Tumor grading is based primarily on the degree of differentiation of malignant cells. Grading evaluates tumor cells in comparison to normal cells. Pathologists indicate tumor cell grades by using the Roman numerals I through IV; the higher the grade, the higher the number and the worse the prognosis. Thus, a grade I tumor is the most differentiated, and a grade IV tumor is the most undifferentiated (or least differentiated). Tumors containing poorly differentiated cells are more aggressive in growth and

Table 30-2 COMMON DIAGNOSTIC TESTS FOR CANCER DETECTION

Laboratory Tests
- Acid phosphatase
- Alkaline phosphatase
- Bence Jones protein
- CA-15-3
- CA-19-9
- CA-125
- CEA (carcinoembryonic antigen)
- PSA (prostate-specific antigen)
- Stool for occult blood (Guaiac)
- Serum calcitonin

Radiologic Studies
- X-ray studies
- Computerized axial tomography (CT scan or CAT scan)
- Magnetic resonance imaging (MRI)
- Scans (radioisotope test)
- Ultrasound

Invasive Diagnostic Techniques
- Endoscopy
- Cytology
- Biopsy

Table 30-3 STAGING OF TUMORS: TNM CLASSIFICATION

STAGE	TUMOR	LYMPH NODE	METASTASIS
I	< 2 cm diameter Mobile Often superficial Confined to organ of origin	No involvement	No evidence
II	2 to 5 cm diameter Not as mobile Extension into adjacent tissue	Palpable, mobile > 2 to 3 cm diameter Firmer than normal	No evidence
III a	> 5 cm diameter Not mobile Regional involvement	No involvement	No evidence
III b	< 2 to > 5 cm diameter Mobile or not mobile Localized or extended	> 2 to 3 cm diameter Firmer than normal	No evidence
IV a	> 10 cm diameter Extension into another organ; major arteries, veins, or nerves; or bone	No involvement or > 2 to 3 cm diameter Firmer than normal	No evidence
IV b	No evidence to > 10 cm diameter	3 to 5 cm diameter Partially mobile Firm to hard; or > 5 cm diameter Extended and fixed to bone, large blood vessels, skin, or nerves	No evidence
IV c	No evidence to > 10 cm diameter	No evidence to > 10 cm diameter Fixed and destructive Extension to second or distant stations	Solitary or multiple

may display uncharacteristic behaviors, leading to a poorer prognosis. Grading criteria vary for different neoplasms.

TREATMENT MODALITIES

After cancer is diagnosed, staged, and graded, a medical treatment plan is developed. The most common treatment methods used today are surgery, radiation therapy, and **chemotherapy** (use of drugs to treat illness); biotherapy and bone marrow transplantation may also be used. These methods may be used alone or in combination.

Surgery

Surgery is the oldest form of cancer treatment and remains the most common method of treatment today. Surgery can be classified as **curative**, **palliative**, or **reconstructive**.

The goal of **curative** surgery is to heal or restore to health; this involves excising all of the tumor, the involved surrounding tissue, and the regional lymph nodes. Surgery most often has curative results when performed in the early stages of such diseases as cervical, breast, or skin cancer. The first commonly used surgical procedure for treating cancer was the radical mastectomy for breast cancer, which removed the breast, the lymph nodes from the axilla, and the pectoral muscles. This radical approach to operable tumors is no longer routinely used because results are just as good with less radical surgery combined with radiation and/or chemotherapy.

Because 70% of clients unfortunately show evidence of metastasis at diagnosis, cure is not always possible, and **palliative** surgery may be necessary. This surgery is effective in relieving symptoms in more advanced stages of cancer, although it does not alter the course of the disease. It is usually performed in an attempt to relieve complications such as obstructions or to surgically interrupt nerve pathways for intractable pain. It may also be used to insert special access devices or to place tubes for enteral nutrition.

Reconstructive surgery may follow curative or radical surgery. The goal is to reestablish function or rebuild for a better cosmetic effect. Reconstructive surgery to areas such as the head, neck, breast, and extremities can minimize deformity. The surgery may be completed all at once or done in stages.

Radiation Therapy

Radiation therapy is the second most common method of treating cancer. Radiation therapy, or **radiotherapy**, uses high-energy ionizing radiation to kill cancer. Ionizing radiation has the ability to penetrate tissue cells and deposit energy within them. This intense energy causes breakage in chromosomes within the cell, thus preventing the ability of the cell to replicate. Cell death may occur hours, days, or even years after treatment, depending on the rate of mitosis.

The goal of radiation therapy is to eradicate malignant cells without causing harm to healthy tissues. Some cells are more sensitive to radiation than others. Better vascularized, better oxygenated cells and those that divide rapidly are the most sensitive.

It is estimated that radiation therapy is used to treat more than one-half of all people with cancer, at some point during their illnesses. It may be used alone or as an adjunct to other therapies. As a single treatment modality, it is most often used when the disease is localized. Preoperative radiation is frequently used to reduce the tumor mass before surgery. Postoperative radiation therapy is frequently used to decrease the risk of local recurrence following surgery. Some chemotherapeutic drugs increase the sensitivity of cancer cells to radiation and thus are used together with radiation. Radiation therapy can be classified as curative or palliative. It is frequently used to alleviate symptoms of metastasis, such as pain.

There are two types of radiation therapy: external radiation and internal radiation.

PROFESSIONAL TIP

Drug To Enhance Radiation's Effect

The drug diamine metronidazole may enhance radiation's effects on cancer by 500 times. If clinical trials demonstrate this degree of effectiveness, radiation dose could be reduced by 60% to 70%, thereby resulting in fewer side effects from radiation. ("Researchers Say New Drug," 1998)

CLIENT TEACHING

External Radiation
- Do not wash off the skin markings used to designate reference points for treatment.
- Client is alone in the room during treatment.
- Client must lie absolutely still.
- Treatment typically lasts 1 to 3 minutes.
- Treatment is usually painless.

External Radiation

External radiation, or teletherapy, is performed with special equipment that can deliver high-energy radiation. Treatments are usually administered on an outpatient basis, divided over many days or weeks. Customized shielding blocks may be created to protect healthy tissues, and immobilization devices may be used to maintain the exact position for each treatment. Dyes or tattoos may be used to designate reference points on the skin.

Nursing care should be directed toward client teaching, safety, and carrying out interventions that provide relief from side effects. Undesirable side effects that are most likely to occur include varying degrees of skin reactions and gastrointestinal discomfort such as abdominal cramping, diarrhea, loss of appetite, and fatigue. Treatments have a cumulative effect and may thus produce symptoms after the therapy has been completed.

Internal Radiation

Internal radiation delivers radioactive isotopes directly within the body. Clients treated with internal sources of radiation can be a source of radioactivity. Isotopes may be introduced into the body by sealed or unsealed sources.

With sealed sources, radioactive elements are encapsulated in special containers such as tubes, wires, needles, seeds, or capsules. These containers are implanted close to the cancer cells in the hope that they will deliver a highly concentrated dose of radiation to the cancer cells. Radioactive implants are commonly used in the treatment of cancers of the tongue, lip, breast, vagina, cervix, endometrium, rectum, bladder, and brain.

Because sources are sealed, body fluids are not radioactive. Personnel caring for clients who have sealed sources must still be familiar with the hazards of radiation, however. Generally, the degree of exposure is dependent on three factors:

- The distance between the individual and the source (Figure 30-2)
- The amount of time an individual is exposed
- The type of shielding provided

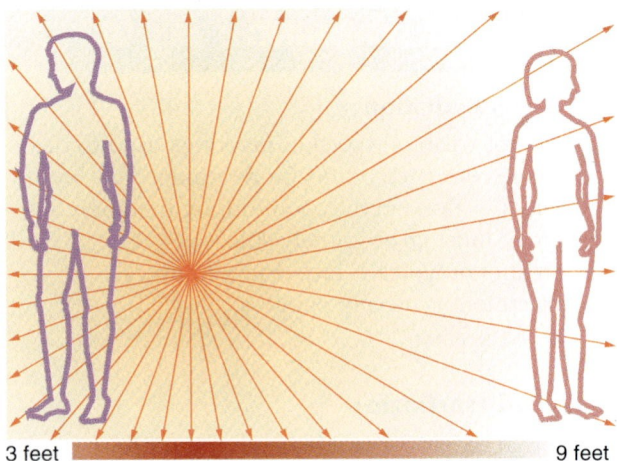

Figure 30-2 Radiation dose decreases with distance. (*Courtesy of the U.S. Nuclear Regulatory Commission*)

Safety: Internal Radiation

Client care should be modified based on the three factors related to the degree of exposure to sealed-source radiation by:

- Preparing everything outside of the room so that as little time as possible is spent close to the client;
- Having several nurses assigned to care for the client so that the time of exposure of each nurse is lessened; and
- Wearing a lead apron or other shielding device, as provided.

Radioactive isotopes can also be placed in suspensions or solutions as unsealed sources of radiation. They may be given orally or parenterally or be instilled into intrapleural or peritoneal spaces.

Some radioactive elements used in unsealed radiation sources are eliminated in body secretions, including urine and stool; thus special precautions should be taken by health care workers to avoid exposure. Agency policies and procedures as well as Standard Precautions must be followed closely. Unsealed sources are not usually radioactive as long as they are sealed sources.

Chemotherapy

Chemotherapy may be used to cure, prevent, or relieve cancer symptoms. The term *chemotherapy* means using chemical therapy or drugs to treat illness, especially cancer. Drugs used in chemotherapy are called **antineoplastics** because they inhibit the growth and reproduction of malignant cells. To understand how anticancer drugs work, one must have a basic understanding of the cell cycle.

Almost all anticancer drugs kill cancer cells by affecting DNA synthesis or function, but they vary in how they exert their activity within the cell-cycle. Most chemotherapeutic drugs are classified as cell-cycle specific (CCS) or cell-cycle nonspecific (CCNS).

Cell-cycle specific drugs attack cancer cells when the cells enter a certain phase of reproduction. These agents are most effective against rapidly growing tumors. Many of the drugs are "schedule dependent" because they produce a greater cell kill when given in multiple, repeated doses.

Cell-cycle nonspecific drugs can destroy cancer cells in any phase of the cell cycle and are used for large tumors that have fewer actively dividing cells. These drugs are not schedule dependent, but, rather, dose dependent. This means that the number of cells destroyed is determined by the amount of drug given.

Anticancer agents are cytotoxic (toxic to cells) and destroy both normal and abnormal cells. They are most effective against cells that reproduce rapidly, such as those in bone marrow, gastrointestinal lining, hair follicles, and the ova and sperm. Because cells multiply at their most rapid rate at the beginning of the disease, the drugs work best against cancer in its earliest stages.

Classifications of drugs commonly used in chemotherapy include:

- Alkylating agents (CCNS): act by causing breaks in DNA strands, preventing mitosis.
- Antimetabolites (CCS): block essential enzymes necessary for DNA synthesis or become incorporated into the DNA and RNA so that a false message is transmitted.
- Antibiotics (CCNS): disrupt DNA transcription and inhibit DNA and RNA synthesis. Antitumor antibiotics are not used for infections because they are highly toxic.
- Nitrosureas (CCNS): inhibit DNA and RNA synthesis.
- Vinca alkaloids (CCS): bind to proteins during M phase, causing the cell to lose the ability to divide.
- Hormones (CCNS): alter the environment of the cell by affecting the cell membrane's permeability, thereby reducing tumor growth.
- Antihormones (CCNS): inhibit natural hormones used by hormone-dependent tumors.
- Miscellaneous agents (CCS or CCNS): act by a variety of mechanisms. (For example, L-asparaginase [Elspar] acts by inhibiting protein synthesis.)
- Corticosteroids: reduce inflammation.

Many of these drugs are given in combination with or after radiation or surgery to achieve maximum effect. They are usually given intermittently over an extended period of time. Drug resistance can occur.

The most common routes of administration are oral and intravenous. A few drugs may be given topically, subcutaneously, or intramuscularly. Recently, other methods have been introduced to increase the local concentration of the drug at the tumor site, including intrathecal injection and intracavity instillation. Table 30-4 lists some commonly used drugs.

Careful attention must be given to intravenous administration. Leakage of chemotherapeutic drugs from the vein into the surrounding tissues during infusion is called **extravasation**. Because most of these drugs are irritating to the tissues, extravasation is a potentially serious problem, especially if the drugs being administered are **vesicants**. These agents are so irritating that they can cause blistering and even necrosis. All sites must be monitored carefully. Pain, swelling, redness, and the presence of vesicles are all signs of extravasation. Additional signs include the following:

- Pain or burning at the site or along the vein
- Absent or sluggish blood return
- Redness 6 to 12 hours later
- Swelling
- Diffuse hardening

PROFESSIONAL TIP

Chemotherapy and Protective Equipment

- Because many chemotherapy drugs are carcinogenic, the nurse preparing and administering the chemotherapy must wear protective equipment.
- All personnel involved in any aspect of handling chemotherapeutic agents must receive instructions about the known risks of the drugs, the proper use of protective equipment, the applicable skill procedures, and the policies regarding pregnant personnel.

Table 30-4 DRUGS COMMONLY USED IN CHEMOTHERAPY

Antimetabolites (CCS)	**Antibiotics (CCNS)**	**Antihormonal Agents (CCNS)**
cytarabine (Cytosar)	dactinomycin (Cosmegan)*	flutamide (Eulexin)
fluorouracil (Adrucil)	daunorubicin (Cerubidine)*	goserelin acetate (Zoladex)
methotrexate (Mexate)	doxorubicin hydrochloride (Adriamycin)*	tamoxifen (Nolvadex)
6-mercaptopurine (Purinethol)	mitomycin (Mutamycin)*	
	mithramycin (Mithracin)	
	bleomycin (Blenoxane)	

Vinca Plant Alkaloids (CCS)	**Hormones (CCNS)**	**Nitrosureas (CCNS)**
vinblastine sulfate (Velban)*	diethylstilbestrol (DES)	carmustine (BiCNU)
vincristine sulfate (Oncovin)*	megestrol acetate (Megace)	lomustine (CeeNU)
	medroxyprogesterone acetate (Depo-Provera)	
	testosterone (Histerone, Testoderm)	

Alkylating Agents (CCNS)	**Corticosteroids**	**Miscellaneous Agents**
busulfan (Myleran)	dexamethasone (Decadron)	etoposide (VePesid)
chlorambucil (Leukeran)	hydrocortisone sodium succinate	L-asparaginase (Elspar)
cisplatin (Platinol)	(Solu-Cortef)	procarbazine hydrochloride
cyclophosphamide (Cytoxan)	prednisone (Deltasone)	(Matulane)
mechlorethamine hydrochloride (Mustargen)*		
melphalan (Alkeran)		
thiotepa (Thiotepa)		

Frequently Used Combinations

CMF±P	cyclophosphamide, methotrexate, 5-fluorouracil, and prednisone
CAMP	cyclophosphamide, doxorubicin (Adriamycin), methotrexate, and procarbazine
CAE	cyclophosphamide, doxorubicin (Adriamycin), and etoposide
CVP	cyclophosphamide, vincristine, and prednisone
FAC	5-fluorouracil, Adriamycin, and Cytoxan
MOPP	mechlorethamine hydrochloride (Mustargen), vincristine (Oncovin), procarbazine, and prednisone

*=vesicant drug

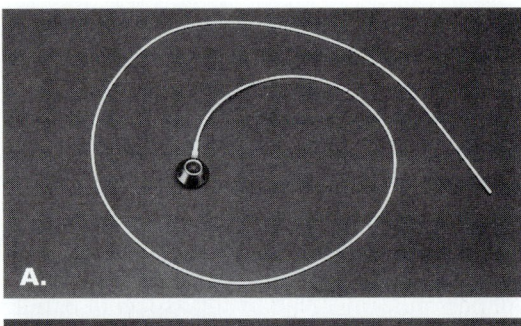

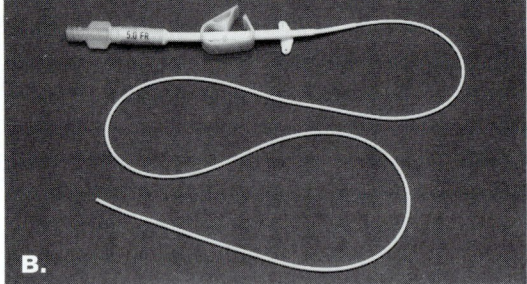

Figure 30-3 Explantable/Implantable Devices: A. Mini-vital port; B. Peripherally inserted central venous catheter (*Courtesy of Cook Incorporated, Bloomington, IN*)

If extravasation does occur, the drug must be stopped immediately and protocols for treatment initiated.

Chemotherapy may also be administered with explantable venous access devices (EVADs) or implantable vascular access devices (IVADs) (Figure 30-3).

Explantable devices are special catheters that may be used for short- or long-term periods. They may be inserted peripherally or centrally into the subclavian or jugular vein, and they terminate in the superior vena cava or right atrium. Long-term central venous catheters are used when a prolonged course of therapy is expected. They are surgically threaded to an exit site in the chest and are sutured in place.

Implantable devices consist of a self-sealing silicone rubber septum enclosed in a metal or plastic port that is attached to a silicone catheter. The port is implanted under the skin. The catheter is surgically threaded subcutaneously into the right atrium. The system is accessed by a needle puncture through the skin and into the port's septum.

Implantable devices are especially useful in clients who have poor quality veins or require multiple venipunctures or long-term therapy. These devices can also be used to administer blood products, total parenteral nutrition, and other medications.

 Safety: Chemotherapy and Contamination
- Any personnel handling blood, vomitus, or excreta from clients who have received chemotherapy within the previous 48 hours should wear disposable latex gloves and a disposable gown.
- Place contaminated linen in specially marked laundry bags according to agency procedures.

 HOME HEALTH CARE

Home Care Following Chemotherapy
Teach clients receiving chemotherapy to monitor the side effects of therapy at home.

- Inspect the skin daily for any signs of rash or dermatitis, which may signal hypersensitivity to a drug.
- Report taste loss and tingling in the face, fingers, or toes, which may signal peripheral neuropathy.
- Report signs of dizziness, headache, confusion, slurred speech, or convulsions, which may be signs of central nervous system (CNS) toxicity.
- Report signs of unusual bleeding or bruising; fever; sore throat; or mouth sores, which may signal developing myelosuppression.
- Report signs of jaundice; yellowing of the eyes; clay-colored stools; or dark urine, which may signal developing hepatic dysfunction.
- Report a continued cough or shortness of breath, which may signal developing pulmonary fibrosis.

Improved infusion techniques, control of symptoms such as nausea and vomiting, and cost-containment restrictions have reduced the length of hospitalizations for clients undergoing chemotherapy. Teaching clients and family members to monitor side effects in the home setting is thus an essential function of the **oncology** (study of tumors) nurse. Some important points to emphasize are outlined in the accompanying display.

Clients should also be advised that lifestyle may need to be adjusted to accommodate the side effects of chemotherapy. Clients should be instructed to pace themselves according to their energy levels and allow time for rest throughout the day. It is also important to inform clients that even between treatments they may not have the same amount of energy as before the initiation of treatment. Whereas many clients do not experience any adverse effects, others experience life-threatening toxicity. Nursing care of the client receiving chemotherapy requires not only a thorough understanding of the drugs used to destroy the cancer,

 PROFESSIONAL TIP

Drugs to Eradicate Cancer
A combination of the drugs angiostatin and endostatin cuts off the blood supply to all forms of cancer in mice. Clinical trials in humans are to begin soon (Noonan, 1998).

but also skills in helping clients and families cope with the side effects of the therapy.

Biotherapy

Biotherapy is performed with **biologic response modifiers** (BRMs), which are agents that stimulate the body's natural immune system to control and destroy malignant cells. Most BRMs are still being evaluated in trial studies. Biotherapy is used after surgery, radiation, and chemotherapy have removed the bulk of the tumor. Some agents currently being investigated include interferons, monoclonal antibodies, interleukin-2, tumor necrosis factor, *bacillus Calmette-Guérin* (BCG), and colony-stimulating factors. Side effects are usually less severe than those seen in chemotherapy and may include fever, malaise, myalgia, and headache. Because an anaphylactic reaction can occur, the client must be closely monitored.

Bone Marrow Transplantation

Bone marrow transplantation (BMT) is used for cancers that respond to high doses of chemotherapy or radiation therapy. Treatment involves aspirating and storing a fraction of bone marrow, exposing the client to high-dose drug therapy or total body irradiation, and then reinfusing the bone marrow after the treatment is complete.

The bone marrow used in transplantation can be the client's own marrow (autologous), marrow taken from an identical twin (syngeneic), or marrow taken from a histocompatibly matched donor, preferably a sibling (allogeneic).

According to Otto (1997), the cost of BMT is high. Client expenses may range from $100,000 to $200,000 unless covered or partially covered by insurance. The average length of hospital stay is 35 to 40 days. Complications can be life threatening and include infection, bleeding, gastrointestinal effects, renal insufficiency, veno-occlusive disease (deposits of fibrin obstruct venules of liver), and graft-versus-host disease (new bone marrow cells recognize environment as foreign and try to destroy the host). Clients who undergo autologous BMT do not experience graft-versus-host disease.

SYMPTOM MANAGEMENT

Cancer clients undergoing treatment experience a variety of secondary problems. One of the most important responsibilities of the oncology nurse is to formulate nursing interventions to manage these problems.

Bone Marrow Dysfunction

Cancer treatments kill both malignant cells and normal cells in bone marrow. Blood counts should thus be monitored carefully during and after treatment.

A low white-cell count increases the risk of infection. A decreased neutrophil count (below 500/mm^3), is an indicator that special infection prevention measures should be initiated. Scrupulous handwashing is the most effective method of controlling bacterial infection. Personnel should maintain strict asepsis when changing dressings or performing invasive procedures. Clients should avoid contact with anyone who is ill. Antimicrobial soaps should be used for bathing clients. The skin and mucous membranes should be inspected daily for signs of infection. Vital signs should be taken every 4 hours, and the client observed for fever and chilling.

Clients with a platelet count below 50,000/mm^3 should be monitored for bleeding. Their skin should be inspected daily for bruises or petechiae. Shaving should be done with an electric razor to minimize the chance of cutting the skin. Stool and urine should be monitored for occult blood. The nurse should observe the client for bleeding from the vagina, rectum, nose, mouth, and venipuncture sites. If bleeding does occur, pressure should be applied to the site for 5 minutes. Any bleeding that does not stop in 5 minutes should be reported. A soft toothbrush may be recommended for oral care. Aspirin or any medication containing acetylsalicylic acid should not be given.

Nutritional Alterations

Blackburn (1998) describes cytokines, substances that are secreted by the tumor in an attempt to cannibalize the body and by the immune system to fight the tumor. Cytokines make the body digest muscle for energy instead of using stored fat for this purpose. This state of malnutrition and protein (muscle) wasting is called **cachexia**. It occurs in conjunction with lung, pancreatic, stomach, bowel, and prostate cancers but rarely with breast cancer.

In some cases, untreated cachexia, rather than the cancer itself, is the cause of death. Untreated cachexia also can decrease the effectiveness of cancer treatments and may increase the side effects of these treatments. Treating cachexia with drugs has met with little success. Some drugs such as megesterol acetate (Megace) improve appetite but do not add muscle mass.

Blackburn (1998) suggests that nurses can help the cachexic client find a registered dietitian who understands cancer cachexia and can identify appetizing foods that are nutrient and calorie dense. Foods that appeal to the client should be eaten anytime. Use of canned or powdered nutritional supplements such as Ensure, Sustacal, or Carnation Instant Breakfast is most appropriate.

Hallmarks of malnutrition are a weight loss of 10% or more or a serum albumin level below 3.4 g/dL. Clients unable to maintain sufficient oral intake for long periods of time may be given enteral or total parenteral nutrition (TPN). Nutritional problems associated

CLIENT TEACHING

Increasing Nutritional Intake

- Drink 4 ounces of a nutritional supplement before breakfast.
- Eat breakfast (if desired), then take a walk. Doing so will help to build muscle and increase appetite.
- Drink another 4 ounces of nutritional supplement 1 hour before having a lunch consisting of whatever foods are appealing.
- Have another 4 ounces of nutritional supplement at mid-afternoon and at bedtime.
- If not hungry for dinner, take another walk.

with cachexia include anorexia, nausea and vomiting, altered taste sensation, mucosal inflammation, and dysphagia.

Anorexia

Anorexia, or loss of appetite, is a common complaint among individuals with cancer. It is generally best for these clients to eat small, frequent, high-calorie (carbohydrate and fat-rich) meals. Nurses should try to ascertain the client's likes and dislikes. Highly seasoned foods help increase taste. Clients should be encouraged to eat when they are feeling best. Weight should be monitored weekly.

Nausea and Vomiting

Nausea and vomiting usually occur within 3 to 4 hours after chemotherapy is administered and may last up to 72 hours. According to Held-Warmkessel (1998), antiemetics should be given before chemotherapy and continued afterward as needed (Table 30-5). Small, frequent feedings of complex carbohydrates may be beneficial. Liquids should be given 30 to 60 minutes before meals. Although highly seasoned foods may increase taste, they often also increase nausea and vomiting. Cool, bland foods are more easily tolerated. Foods with strong odors should be avoided. Frequent mouth care can help remove the taste of chemotherapy and thus increase the likelihood of the client's wanting to eat. The client should be monitored for dehydration and electrolyte imbalances.

CLIENT TEACHING

Enhancing Taste Sensation

- Tart food usually enhances taste sensation.
- Many foods taste better if they are cold or at room temperature.
- Using plastic utensils reduces metallic taste.

Table 30-5   COMMONLY USED ANTIEMETICS

prochlorperazine (Compazine)
metoclopramide (Reglan)
trimethobenzamide hydrochloride (Tigan)
ondansetron hydrochloride (Zofron)
lorazepam (Ativan)

Altered Taste Sensation

Taste sensation can be altered because cancer cells release substances that stimulate bitter taste buds, causing a bitter or metallic taste in the mouths of some clients. Some find they no longer enjoy the taste of red meat and others say they have an aversion to sweets.

Mucosal Inflammation

Stomatitis, or inflammation of the mucous membrane of the oral cavity, occurs in one-half of cancer clients receiving treatment. It usually occurs 7 to 14 days after chemotherapy administration and lasts 2 to 3 weeks. To minimize stomatitis, assess for early signs and symptoms such as edema, ulceration, erythema, excessive saliva, and infection. If the client is receiving a chemotherapy drug that is known to cause stomatitis (methotrexate, for example) oral care should be administered at least 4 times a day.

Rough, chewy foods and acidic foods should be avoided. Straws are beneficial because food can be taken in the back of the mouth and swallowed. Popsicles and frozen fruit bars sometimes help numb and lessen pain. Commercial mouthwashes containing alcohol should be avoided. A saline rinse may be helpful after meals. If the client has dentures, they should be removed at night. Viscous Xylocaine rinses can be ordered for pain. Lemon and glycerine swabs should not be used because lemon may be irritating to mouth lesions.

PROFESSIONAL TIP

Mucosal Inflammation

- The condition of the client's mouth provides a clue to the appearance and integrity of other areas of the gastrointestinal tract because mucosal inflammation caused by cancer treatments affects all mucosa.
- Mucositis (inflammation of the mucous membrane) in the esophagus, also called esophagitis, may cause painful swallowing.
- In female clients, mucosal inflammation may be found in the vagina, causing pain, itching, and discharge.

CLIENT TEACHING

Stomatitis

- Use soft bristle toothbrush.
- Avoid flossing if bleeding or discomfort occurs.
- Avoid tobacco products and alcohol because of their drying effects.

Dysphagia

Dysphagia, or difficulty in swallowing, often occurs in clients with esophageal cancers, or in those receiving radiotherapy.

Artificial saliva may be ordered for severe dryness. A softer diet along with nutritional supplements may be prescribed. Dry foods such as toast can scratch the delicate tissues of the throat. Food pureed in a blender may be easier to tolerate. Clients should take plenty of time to chew and swallow.

Pain

Approximately 60% to 90% of all individuals with progressive malignancy will experience pain. The pain may be acute, but it is more likely to be chronic (greater than 3 months in duration). Pain usually does not occur until the advanced stages of the disease. The most common causes of pain are metastatic bone disease, venous or lymphatic obstruction, or nerve compression.

Pain can have profound effects on a cancer client, possibly causing anxiety, depression, and feelings of helplessness in addition to physical discomfort. It can affect the client's sleeping habits, eating patterns, work, family, and social relationships. Ultimately, pain can affect the client's quality of life.

Noninvasive pain-relief techniques may be useful in pain management. They include cutaneous stimulation (heat, cold, massage), transcutaneous electrical nerve stimulation (TENS), relaxation techniques, imagery, and hypnosis. Most of these techniques are inexpensive and easy to perform. They have few side effects and can usually be done in any environment. They also give the client some control over the treatment of

PROFESSIONAL TIP

Inadequate Pain Control in the Cancer Client

A major reason given for inadequate pain control in the cancer client is the fear of inducing respiratory depression. This, however, is a rare occurrence in the cancer client.

pain. Although not every client will respond successfully to these measures, it is worthwhile to attempt them before using invasive techniques.

The federal government has taken steps toward ensuring that cancer pain can be treated. The Agency for Health Care Policy and Research (AHCPR, 1994) has developed Cancer Pain Guidelines for clients, family members, and health care professionals. Some points emphasized by the guidelines include the following:

- Cancer pain can be managed effectively through relatively simple means in up to 90% of cancer clients in the United States. Skin patches, slow-release tablets, and client-controlled pumps are now available to complement standard drugs.
- The mainstay of pain assessment is the client self-report. Because there is no standard test for pain, the nurse must respect the client's report of pain and regard it as the single most reliable indicator. Kohr (1995) recommends using both a verbal assessment measurement tool based on a scale from 0 to 5, where each number represents a precise description of pain; and a pain intensity flow sheet. For example:

  0 no pain
  1 mild pain
  2 moderate pain or discomfort
  3 severe or distressing pain
  4 horrible or incapacitating pain
  5 excruciating or unbearable pain

- The simplest dosage schedules and least invasive pain management modalities should be used first. Nonnarcotics are the first step in the analgesic ladder. They should be tried first for mild to moderate pain. Because much of cancer pain is due to inflammation, many of the nonnarcotics used are potent, anti-inflammatory drugs. These drugs are helpful in pain relief because they inhibit the release of prostaglandins, which cause pain, edema, and inflammation.
- Morphine is the most commonly used opioid for moderate to severe pain because it is available in a wide variety of dosage forms, it has well-characterized pharmacokinetics and pharmacodynamics, and it is relatively low in cost. Morphine can be given orally, subcutaneously, intramuscularly, intravenously, rectally, and intraspinally. It can also be given in sustained-release preparations. Because needs vary with cancer pain, there is no limit to the dosing of morphine.
- Health care providers should work to prevent pain in the first place rather than try to treat pain after it has occurred. Analgesics work better when given regularly around the clock before pain becomes severe. A major nursing responsibility is to teach the client to request pain medication before the pain becomes severe. When medication is ordered

around the clock, the nurse should not hesitate to wake the client to administer analgesics.

If pain control cannot be achieved with noninvasive techniques or medications, neurosurgical procedures such as nerve blocks may be performed.

Fatigue

Fatigue may occur as a direct result of the cancer or because of anemia, chronic pain, stress, depression, insufficient rest, or inadequate nutritional intake. Although the etiology is not well understood, fatigue is often related to side effects of medications and treatments such as radiation therapy. Fatigue may contribute to client non-compliance with the treatment regimen.

Frequent rest periods should be provided for the client. The nurse should assess for the presence and pattern of fatigue. Proper planning allows for the client to be active during times when energy levels are higher, which may in turn restore a greater sense of control. The nurse should evaluate factors that increase or decrease fatigue, such as nutritional intake. Blood count should be monitored for anemia.

Alopecia

Alopecia, the thinning or loss of hair, may be induced by chemotherapy or radiation treatments. The extent of hair loss depends on the dose and duration of the therapy. Scalp hair is most commonly affected, but pubic, axillary, and facial hair, even eyebrows and eyelashes, may also be affected. The treatments cause hair loss by interfering with the growth processes in the hair follicle. This results in weakening of the hair shaft, thereby causing the hair to break off at the surface of the scalp. Hair loss usually begins 2 to 3 weeks after the initial treatment. Drug induced alopecia is not permanent. Hair usually begins to grow back within 8 weeks after treatment is completed. The color and consistency of the hair may change.

CLIENT TEACHING

Alopecia, Threat to Body Image
Encourage client to:

- Buy a wig or hairpiece before treatment actually begins so that it will match the client's normal hair;
- Wear hats, scarves, or bandanas to cope with the change in body image due to hair loss; and
- Focus on other positive aspects rather than on just physical appearance.

Odors

Unpleasant odors emanating from the cancer client may be a source of embarrassment. These odors are usually associated with drainage, exudates, or incontinence. Fortunately, meticulous nursing care can eliminate most offending odors. Soiled linens, drainage pads, and dressings should be changed immediately and washed or discarded. The client's skin should be washed gently with soap and warm water. Protective creams may be used if the areas are not receiving radiation. Room deodorizers can be helpful but should be used cautiously as many clients experience nausea when exposed to the odors from room fresheners. Placing a drop of oil of wintergreen or oil of cloves on a cotton ball near the ventilation system can sometimes lend a light freshness to the environment.

Dyspnea

One-half of all clients with terminal cancer experience dyspnea, or difficulty in breathing. Possible causes include fluid development in the chest, infection such as pneumonia, fibrosis due to radiation, and anemia. Lungs should be auscultated every 4 hours. Oxygen may be ordered. Fluid may be drained by an invasive procedure called a thoracentesis. High-Fowler positioning helps maximize ventilation. The nurse should plan care to keep activity to a minimum so as to balance oxygen requirements and oxygen supply. Oxygen status can be monitored with a pulse oximeter. The nurse should report a sustained reading of less than 90%. The nurse should avoid pulling the privacy curtain or shutting the client's door unless absolutely necessary, because either of these actions may reduce air flow and create more anxiety.

Bowel Dysfunctions

Cancer clients frequently exhibit changes in bowel patterns. Constipation, diarrhea and subsequent perineal skin breakdown, and bowel obstructions are common elimination disorders.

Constipation results from decreased motility of the colon. It is frequently caused by chemotherapy, narcotic analgesic, or inactivity. Nurses should monitor and record the frequency of the client's bowel movements. Constipation can be an early sign of vincristine toxicity. Fluid consumption may be encouraged and a stool softener given daily. Clients at risk for constipation should be started on a high-fiber diet, with increased intake of bran and prune juice.

Common causes of diarrhea include radiation therapy, chemotherapy, antibiotics, tube feedings, hyperosmolar dietary supplements, stress, and fecal impactions. Clients can develop fluid and electrolyte imbalances from constant diarrhea. If the client is receiving a chemotherapy drug known to cause diarrhea (such as fluorouracil [Adrucil] or doxorubicin hydrochloride

[Adriamycin]), a low-residue and lactose-free diet should be encouraged. The nurse should instruct the client to avoid foods that stimulate the gastrointestinal tract, such as warm liquids and coffee.

Bananas (which are high in potassium) and sports drinks (which contain sodium and potassium) can help replace lost fluids and electrolytes without irritating the gastrointestinal tract.

The perineum should be kept clean and dry after each loose stool. Anal irritations should be treated cautiously with agents such as heat lamps, ointments, and cornstarch, although these may be contraindicated in clients receiving radiation therapy. Signs of fluid and electrolyte imbalances such as thirst, dry mucous membranes, and decreased skin turgor, should be noted. The potassium level should be monitored. The nurse should measure and record the amount, frequency, and characteristics of all client bowel movements. Antidiarrheal medications such as Lomotil or Imodium should be given for every loose stool. Sitz baths will help soothe sore or broken-down tissues.

Bowel obstructions occur more commonly in conjunction with advanced abdominal malignancies and should always be suspected if the client has received radiation or has adhesions from prior surgeries. Symptoms include nausea, vomiting, and abdominal pain. Surgery may be required to relieve the obstruction.

Pathological Fractures

Pathological fractures are a major problem in cancers that metastasize to bone. These cancers weaken the bone to the point that normal activities can cause painful breaks. Thus, limbs should be supported and handled gently and extreme care should be taken when moving clients. Special devices such as splints may be used for extra protection. Weight-bearing restrictions may be ordered.

Ascites

Abdominal cancers may cause ascites, or fluid accumulation in the abdomen. Clients may experience abdominal swelling and difficult breathing. Symptoms may be treated temporarily with an invasive procedure called a paracentesis, wherein a small, plastic tube is advanced through the abdominal wall and excess fluid is withdrawn. Chemotherapy drugs sometimes are instilled in an attempt to prevent the fluid from returning. The nurse should visually assess the abdomen. A protruding abdomen may be indicative of ascites as well as intestinal distention and enlarged organs. Abdominal girth at the umbilicus should be measured daily with a tape measure to monitor changes. The abdomen should then be auscultated in all four quadrants. Gurgling bowel sounds heard every 5 to 15 seconds indicate normal peristalsis. Decreased or absent bowel sounds may indicate peritonitis or paralytic ileus. Fluid accumulation can be confirmed by percussing for shifting dullness. When a large amount of fluid is present, the nurse may see fluid waves. Gentle palpation is used to detect pain and tenderness as well as abdominal masses. The nurse should carefully document any abnormal findings.

The nurse should weigh the client daily to monitor weight gain. Fluid consumption may be restricted. Good skin care, especially to the abdomen, is essential. Fowler positioning helps maximize ventilation. Clients should be observed closely for electrolyte imbalance if large amounts of fluids are withdrawn via paracentesis.

Sexual Alterations

Many chemotherapy drugs can interfere with sexual functioning and reproduction. Premenopausal women may become infertile. Those under age 35 may regain their fertility after therapy is completed. Men may experience impotence, decreased libido, interrupted sperm production, and ejaculation problems. Women may experience vaginal dryness.

The nurse should encourage clients and their partners to express their feelings and concerns to each other and to explore other avenues of sexual expression, such as cuddling, kissing, and stroking. Birth control should be practiced during therapy and for 1 or 2 years after therapy (depending on physician recommendation) to ensure that all chemotherapy drugs have been eliminated and, thus, will have no ill effects on a pregnancy.

MEDICAL EMERGENCIES

Medical emergencies occur in approximately 20% of clients with advanced-stage cancer. Early recognition and treatment can prevent irreversible complications and improve the quality of life. Four complications with which nurses should become familiar are hypercalcemia, spinal cord compression, superior vena cava syndrome, and cardiac tamponade.

HYPERCALCEMIA

Hypercalcemia occurs commonly and can be a potentially fatal complication if not detected early. It is found most often in clients with malignant tumors that have metastasized to bone, such as breast cancer tumors. The condition occurs when the tumor destroys bone and the serum calcium level rises higher than 10.5 mg/dL, rendering the kidneys unable to eliminate excess calcium.

Early symptoms of hypercalcemia, such as nausea, vomiting, constipation, and weakness, may be overlooked because these are common side effects of many cancer therapies. Later symptoms such as dehydration, renal failure, coma, and cardiac arrest may develop swiftly.

Hypercalcemia is treated aggressively with intravenous normal saline and furosemide (Lasix), which increase calcium excretion. Clients may also be given drugs to decrease bone reabsorption. Serum calcium level should be monitored when Lasix is being administered. Clients should be taught early symptoms of hypercalcemia so that they can recognize a recurrence. These clients are also at increased risk for pathological fractures because calcium has been released from the bones, leaving them very fragile.

SPINAL CORD COMPRESSION

Spinal cord compression can result in permanent paralysis if not treated promptly. Cancer of the lung, breast, and prostate carry the greatest risk of metastasizing to the spinal cord.

The chief symptom of metastasis to the spinal cord is back pain. The discomfort is aggravated by lying down, coughing, or moving, and may be relieved by sitting upright.

Treatment is aimed at reducing tumor size to decrease pressure on the spinal cord. Radiation, surgery, and steroid therapy may be initiated. Pain medications should be given frequently, and clients should be supported carefully during transfers.

SUPERIOR VENA CAVA SYNDROME

Superior vena cava syndrome is a collection of symptoms caused by an obstruction of the superior vena cava. It occurs more frequently in conjunction with lung cancer and lymphomas. Typically, clients experience dyspnea and swelling of the face and neck. Edema in the upper extremities, chest pain, and coughing are other possible symptoms. Central nervous system symptoms such as headache, visual disturbances, and alteration in consciousness rarely occur.

The goal of treatment is to reduce tumor size. Radiation along with diuretics is usually ordered. The nurse should administer oxygen as ordered and provide a calm, restful environment. The client should be encouraged to limit activities and lie in Fowler's position. Respirations should be carefully monitored, and lower extremities should not be elevated, as doing so will increase venous return to an already engorged area.

CARDIAC TAMPONADE

Cardiac tamponade is caused by the formation of pericardial fluid, which reduces cardiac output by compressing the heart. Tumor metastasis to the pericardium is associated with lung cancer, breast cancer, Hodgkin's disease, lymphoma, melanoma, gastrointestinal tumors, and sarcoma. Common symptoms of cardiac tamponade include a rapid, weak pulse; distended neck veins during inspiration; ankle or sacral edema; pleural effusion; ascites; enlarged spleen; lethargy; and altered consciousness.

Treatment is aimed at aspirating the fluid constricting the heart (pericardiocentesis). The nurse should reassure the client, explain the procedure, and administer medication for pain.

PSYCHOSOCIAL ALTERATIONS

Perhaps of all the problems that clients with cancer experience, none is more challenging than the associated psychosocial alterations. The mere diagnosis of cancer invokes fear and misunderstanding. A myriad of emotions may surface initially. These may range from deep depression to denial and total refusal of treatment. Anxiety, sadness, and withdrawal are common. Some clients may feel that the disease is a punishment for some misguided deed. Every client will respond differently to the diagnosis, depending on individual coping mechanisms and support systems.

Research has identified effective and ineffective coping mechanisms. Clients who seek information or share feelings tend to cope more effectively than do those who submit to treatment and procedures without asking questions or who use small talk to avoid discussing threatening issues.

Cancer affects not only the client, but the client's family as well. Responses of family members to the disease will have a significant impact on the client's coping. The client and family must face issues such as loss of control, changes in body image, and financial burdens.

The nurse has several roles in this context. The client needs time and space to adjust to the diagnosis. Nurses should be available to offer support and reassurance. They should answer questions but not bombard the client with information. They may interpret information given by the physician and may help the client formulate questions to ask the physician. The nurse should also encourage the client to express feelings and fears about the illness.

The initial treatment is very frightening for most cancer clients, many of whom have heard the myth that "the treatment is worse than the cure." Nurses can allay anxiety by giving information about the treatment's purpose; adverse reactions; and signs and symptoms to report to the physician. Explaining procedures and answering questions in simple language can help the client and family regain a feeling of some control. Treatment modalities cause many discomforts, but if the client knows what to expect, the distress can generally be handled. Symptom management is critical in preventing lifestyle disruptions.

HOME HEALTH CARE

Psychosocial Aspects of Cancer

- Clients may see themselves as burdens to their families.
- Family caregivers may be angry that their own needs must go unmet.
- Family caregivers may feel inadequate with regard to caring for the client.
- Medical equipment such as a hospital bed, commode chair, or wheelchair may need to be brought into the home. These may have an impact on family member state of mind and disposition with regard to the family member with cancer.

Families and clients facing the terminal phase of cancer are confronted with a complex set of problems. The client and family must face separation and impending death. Some families will demand that extraordinary measures be taken to keep the client alive. Some will search for meaning in life and will experience a genuine closeness. Nurses should give the client and family privacy and time to share feelings. Sometimes, the only psychosocial support the client needs is to have someone sitting by the bedside. Touch, especially at times when words are hard to find, can often be the most comforting intervention.

As the client's condition deteriorates, physical needs become more pronounced. The nurse should focus on keeping the client comfortable and free of pain. Hospice care is designed to provide spiritual, emotional, and physical support during the final days of illness. The goal of hospice is to keep the client as comfortable as possible. Pain relief and symptom management are stressed. The focus is shifted from cure to care. Care may be given in an institution, but most hospice care is given in the home. Hospice care is medically managed and nurse coordinated. Members of the hospice team typically include a chaplain, physician, nurse, social worker, physical therapist, and home health aide, as well as various volunteers. The team functions to ensure that the client's plan of care is carried out and that family members receive adequate support. The family is instructed in the area of care to be given. Bereavement counseling is offered to help family members deal with their loss.

▶ NURSING PROCESS

▶ Assessment

▶ Subjective Data

The client interview serves as a forum for ascertaining the client's perception of the illness, treatment, and prognosis; health practices; and health concerns. The client's significant other may also be interviewed to ascertain support systems.

▶ Objective Data

Vital signs are measured, and a head-to-toe assessment is performed. Past hospital records are reviewed along with the current record. Laboratory reports, biopsy results, treatment modalities, and comments from other health care professionals are studied.

Nursing diagnoses for a client with cancer may include the following:

Nursing Diagnoses	Planning/Goals	Nursing Interventions
▶ *Fear related to cancer diagnosis*	The client will express anxieties and fears to family and/or health care providers.	Review the client's previous experience with cancer to ascertain any current misconceptions based on past beliefs.
		Encourage the client to share feelings regarding the diagnosis to facilitate identification of coping strategies.
		Explain hospital routines and focus on the recommended treatment, including its purpose and potential side effects. Accurate descriptions that convey what the client can expect help ease fears associated with the unknown. A calm, reassuring environment can also enhance coping abilities.
▶ *Grieving, Anticipatory, related to potential loss of body function*	The client will express grief to family and/or health care providers.	Open, honest discussions can help the client cope with the situation. Be aware that mood swings, hostility, and other negative behaviors often occur. Discuss the loss of body function with the client. Ask what the loss of body function means to the client.
		Encourage the client to seek help and support from close family members.

continued

Nursing Diagnoses	Planning/Goals	Nursing Interventions
▶ *Nutrition: Altered, Less than Body Requirements, related to side effects of chemotherapy*	The client will maintain body weight.	Encourage the client to eat a high-calorie, nutrient-rich diet. Supplements may be useful. Some clients may benefit from frequent, small meals and snacks. Foods high in protein, such as cheese, fish, and poultry, are also recommended.
		Provide oral hygiene before and after meals so foods will taste better.
		Administer antiemetics approximately 30 minutes before meals. Mints, hard candies, and saltine crackers may help if the client complains of metallic taste.
		Nondietary interventions may include varying the surroundings, using small plates, eating at a table with friends, and minimizing food odors.
		Monitor intake and output along with daily weight to assess nutritional status.
▶ *Skin Integrity, Impaired, Risk for, related to chemotherapy and radiation*	The client will maintain skin integrity.	Assess skin frequently for side effects of cancer therapy. (A reddening or tanning effect may develop with radiation. Skin reactions such as rashes, pruritus, and alopecia develop with chemotherapy.)
		Use lukewarm water and soap to gently wash the client's skin. Skin often becomes sensitive during radiation treatments.
▶ *Infection, Risk for, related to side effects of chemotherapy*	The client will remain free of infection.	Monitor vital signs at least every shift. White blood count should be monitored and protective isolation should be instituted if the count falls below 500/mm³.
		Educate the client, staff, and visitors in all aspects of infection prophylaxis. Thorough handwashing is the most important means of preventing and controlling the transmission of organisms. Because fresh flowers and raw fruits and vegetables can transmit microbes, they should be eliminated. The client should not be exposed to anyone who has an infection or who has been recently vaccinated against or exposed to a communicable disease. Visitors should be limited.
▶ *Injury, Risk for, related to altered clotting factors secondary to side effects of chemotherapy*	The client will remain free of injury related to bleeding.	Every shift, assess the client for signs of bleeding (petechiae, ecchymoses, hematomas, bleeding gums, epistaxis, tarry stools, hematuria, frank or prolonged bleeding from puncture sites) because transfusions may be indicated.
		Monitor platelet count, which is an indicator of clotting ability. Institute special precautions if the count falls below 50,000/mm³.
		Apply pressure to all puncture sites for 3 to 5 minutes. Doing so prevents prolonged bleeding, which can cause damage to underlying tissues such as nerves.
		Instruct the client to use a soft toothbrush or sponge for oral hygiene to prevent damage to oral mucosa, which is particularly susceptible to bleeding. Instruct the client to use an electric razor when shaving.
▶ *Fatigue related to analgesics, anemia, stress, increased metabolism, and chemotherapy*	The client will experience less fatigue.	Plan frequent rest periods for the client to restore energy, and schedule activities when the client has the most energy.
		Monitor nutritional intake, as adequate nutrients are necessary to meet energy needs.
		Recognize that weakness places the client at increased risk for injury. Because fatigue may make activities of daily living difficult to complete, assistance may need to be provided.

Evaluation Each goal must be evaluated to determine how it has been met by the client.

SAMPLE NURSING CARE PLAN

THE CLIENT WITH LUNG CANCER

Mr. Sanez is a 54-year-old carpenter. He is admitted with pain over his left scapula and radiating to his left arm. He describes having dyspnea and admits that he does have a productive cough. He denies any recent weight loss but does acknowledge experiencing extreme fatigue for the last 2 months. Mr. Sanez has been a chronic smoker for 20 years. A chest x-ray reveals an area of density in the left lung. A needle biopsy confirms small-cell lung cancer. A computerized tomography (CT) scan confirms extrathoracic involvement. His physician referred Mr. Sanez to an oncologist for palliative chemotherapy. Mr. Sanez is to receive his first treatment of cisplatin (Platinol) and etoposide (VePesid). Mr. Sanez states that he is not sure about this treatment given that it will not cure him and he does not know how he will keep breathing. He has never before been hospitalized.

Nursing Diagnosis 1 *Anxiety related to unfamiliar surroundings and uncertainty regarding change in health status as evidenced by Mr. Sanez's statement that he does not know how he will keep breathing and the fact that he has never before been hospitalized*

PLANNING/GOALS	NURSING INTERVENTIONS	RATIONALE	EVALUATION
Mr. Sanez will share his feelings regarding his dyspnea.	Ascertain what the physician has told Mr. Sanez and what conclusions Mr. Sanez has reached. Encourage Mr. Sanez to share his feelings concerning cancer.	Accurate description of the treatment regimen can help decrease fear of the unknown. Verbalization can identify the source of any misconception that is serving to increase anxiety.	Mr. Sanez shares his feelings about his diagnosis and treatment regimen.
Mr. Sanez will express less anxiety about being in the hospital.	Maintain frequent contact with Mr. Sanez. Explain the hospital routine and what Mr. Sanez should anticipate in terms of his care.	Maintenance of contact helps to reassure Mr. Sanez that he is not alone. An unfamiliar environment increases anxiety.	Mr. Sanez exhibits less anxiety about the change in his health status and being in the hospital.

Nursing Diagnosis 2 *Gas exchange, Impaired, related to decreased lung capacity and increased secretions as evidenced by dyspnea, productive cough, and dense area in left lung*

PLANNING/GOALS	NURSING INTERVENTIONS	RATIONALE	EVALUATION
Mr. Sanez will report less dyspnea with oxygen saturation > 90%.	Monitor pulmonary status by ascultating breath sounds; checking rate, depth, and pattern of respirations; evaluating skin color for cyanosis; and monitoring pulse oximetry.	Provides information regarding pulmonary status changes indicating either improvement or onset of complications.	Adequate ventilation with oxygen saturation > 90% is maintained.
	Position Mr. Sanez in Fowler's position.	Promotes expansion of lungs and respiratory muscles.	

continued

	Administer oxygen at prescribed level.	Supplemental oxygen corrects hypoxemia and provides oxygen for metabolic needs.	
	Administer narcotics with caution.	Narcotics can depress the respiratory center.	
	Monitor amount, color, and consistency of sputum.	Changes in sputum suggest infection or change in pulmonary status.	
	Plan care and treatments within Mr. Sanez's tolerance.	Oxygen demands increase with activity.	

Nursing Diagnosis 3 *Pain related to tumor growth and tissue destruction as evidenced by verbal report of pain over left scapula radiating to left arm*

PLANNING/GOALS	NURSING INTERVENTIONS	RATIONALE	EVALUATION
Mr. Sanez will report less pain following pain-relief measures.	Provide routine comfort measures such as repositioning and backrub.	Noninvasive pain-relief techniques may be helpful in pain management.	Mr. Sanez reports less pain; < 4 on a scale of 0 to 10.
	Teach Mr. Sanez to request pain medication prior to onset of severe pain.	To keep pain under control, medication should be administered as soon as pain begins.	
	Have Mr. Sanez rate pain on a scale of 0 to 10 (0 = no pain and 10 = worst pain).	The scale provides a method of evaluating the subjective experience of pain.	
	Teach Mr. Sanez relaxation techniques.	Relaxation may decrease the perception of pain.	
	Document Mr. Sanez's response to the pain-control regimen and adjust as needed.	Ongoing assessment of the effectiveness of pain-relief techniques is essential for optimal comfort.	

Nursing Diagnosis 4 *Fatigue related to chronic pain and dyspnea as evidenced by client's description of dyspnea and extreme fatigue for 2 months*

PLANNING/GOALS	NURSING INTERVENTIONS	RATIONALE	EVALUATION
Mr. Sanez will report feeling less fatigued.	Plan care to allow for rest periods.	Frequent rest periods help conserve energy.	Mr. Santez exhibits less fatigue in light of having frequent rest periods daily.
	Assess for related factors such as nutritional imbalances, lack of sleep, and causes of stress.	Identification of contributing factors may reduce fatigue.	

continued

| Have Mr. Sanez rate fatigue on a scale of 0 to 10 (0 = not tired, 10 = total exhaustion) throughout a 24 hour period. | Identifies peak energy and exhaustion times and plan activities to minimize energy output. |

| Teach energy-conservation strategies such as planning ahead, setting priorities, scheduling rest periods, and resting before a difficult task. | Conserving energy will decrease physical and psychological stress. |

Nursing Diagnosis 5 *Grieving, Anticipatory, related to loss of body function as evidenced by Mr. Sanez's statement that he does not know how he will keep breathing*

PLANNING/GOALS	NURSING INTERVENTIONS	RATIONALE	EVALUATION
Mr. Sanez will verbalize his loss and develop coping skills as he acknowledges his illness as terminal.	Provide opportunities for Mr. Sanez to express his feelings.	Such information helps the nurse detect Mr. Sanez's coping strategies for moving through the stages of grief.	Mr. Sanez comes to terms with the reality of his diagnosis and prognosis.
	Answer all of Mr. Sanez's questions honestly.	Open, honest discussions can help Mr. Sanez cope with the situation.	
	Encourage Mr. Sanez's participation in his care.	Gives Mr. Sanez a greater sense of control over his life.	
	Encourage family support and visits from friends.	Assures Mr. Sanez that he is not alone and provides time to discuss concerns openly.	
	Utilize appropriate referrals to professionals such as clergy, as needed.	Facilitates the grief process and spiritual care.	

CASE STUDY

Mr. John Dalton is a 70-year-old male with a history of cancer of the prostate, which was treated with palliative hormones and radiation. His admitting diagnosis is adenocarcinoma of the prostate with widespread bone metastasis. Mr. Dalton is married and has one grown daughter, who often helps with his care. His chief complaint is severe back pain. The physician has ordered intrathecal morphine sulfate and aspirin 10 gr for pain relief.

CASE STUDY *continued*

The following questions will guide your development of a nursing care plan for the case study.

1. List symptoms typically seen in clients diagnosed with prostate cancer.
2. Identify the population most at risk for developing prostate cancer.
3. List three possible risk factors for prostate cancer.
4. Discuss why the physician's orders include aspirin along with morphine sulfate.
5. Discuss why benzodiazepines should not be used for pain relief.
6. List the subjective and objective data the nurse would want to obtain.
7. When you walk into Mr. Dalton's room he greets you with a smile and continues talking and joking with his daughter. While assessing him, you note that his vital signs are normal. You ask him to rate his pain on a scale of 0 to 10. He pauses to think about it, then rates the pain at 8. In the chart, you must record your nursing assessment by circling the appropriate number on the scale. Which number do you think you should circle?
8. Write three individualized nursing diagnoses and goals for Mr. Dalton.
9. Discuss which oncological emergency Mr. Dalton is most likely to develop.

SUMMARY

- Cancer is the second most common cause of death in the United States.
- Most cancers are curable if treated early.
- Benign neoplasms are localized and encapsulated and do not spread.
- Malignant neoplasms spread to neighboring tissues via blood and lymph.
- Biopsy is the most accurate diagnostic test for cancer.
- The most common medical treatments for cancer are surgery, radiation, and chemotherapy. They may be used alone or in combination.
- Surgery is the treatment of choice for early cancers.
- Chemotherapy is the treatment of choice for metastatic cancers. It is also the treatment most responsible for increasing cancer cure rates in recent years.
- Lung cancer is the leading cause of cancer death among men and women. Eighty percent of all cases are related to smoking.
- Quality of life, not quantity of life, is the ultimate goal for clients living with cancer.

Review Questions

1. The nurse carefully monitors the client's intravenous chemotherapy. Which is an early indicator that extravasation may be occurring?
    a. The fluid stops infusing.
    b. Edema is noted at the site.
    c. Blood returns when the bottle is lowered.
    d. Burning occurs at the site.

2. A breast cancer client states that the doctor says he is going to prescribe hormone therapy. Which of the following hormones would probably be ordered?
    a. Thyroxin
    b. Parathormone
    c. Progesterone
    d. Testosterone

3. A cancer client develops a low white-cell count. She is placed on neutropenic precautions. Which of the following menu selections would be best?
    a. Meat loaf, mashed potatoes, green beans, and fruit gelatin
    b. Meat loaf, mashed potatoes, marinated carrots, and a garden salad
    c. Meat loaf, mashed potatoes, chef salad, and tapioca
    d. Meat loaf, mashed potatoes, green beans, fruit salad, and a cookie

4. As stomatitis develops, which would be best to encourage in the client?
    a. Drinking plenty of orange juice
    b. Using lemon and glycerine swabs frequently
    c. Brushing teeth before and after eating
    d. Rinsing with commercial mouthwash as needed

5. Which should be encouraged in clients receiving radiation?

   a. Washing and drying the skin carefully and applying lotion

   b. Not bathing

   c. Not applying deodorants or lotions

   d. Washing the skin with soap and applying baby powder

6. The cancer that causes the most deaths each year is:

   a. skin

   b. lung

   c. prostate

   d. colorectal

Critical Thinking Questions

1. What diagnostic tests should a person have as part of a routine physical to detect cancer?

2. What methods can a person use to detect a tumor in oneself?

3. What is the rationale for each nursing intervention given for the possible nursing diagnoses in this chapter?

WEB FLASH!

- Research the clinical trial results of diamine metronidazole (Florida State University). Is the drug working as predicted?
- What new treatments for cancer can you find on the Web?
- What resources are available on the Web for cancer clients and their families?

NURSING CARE OF THE CLIENT: RESPIRATORY SYSTEM

MAKING THE CONNECTION

Refer to the the following chapters to increase your understanding of respiratory disorders:

- **Chapter 22, Standard Precautions and Isolation**
- **Chapter 25, Assessment**
- **Chapter 27, Diagnostic Tests**
- **Chapter 30, Nursing Care of the Oncology Client**
- **Chapter 32, Nursing Care of the Client: Cardiovascular System**

- **Chapter 33, Nursing Care of the Client: Blood and Lymph Systems**
- **Procedures:** B36, Clearing an Obstructed Airway; I21, Administering Oxygen; I22, Performing Nasopharyngeal and Oropharyngeal Suctioning; I23, Performing Tracheostomy Care

LEARNING OBJECTIVES

Upon completion of this chapter, you should be able to:
- *Define key terms.*
- *Describe components of a complete respiratory assessment.*
- *Describe assessment of the client with a chest tube.*
- *Identify normal parameters for common respiratory diagnostic studies.*
- *Discuss the etiology, medical–surgical management, and nursing care for clients with respiratory disorders.*
- *Prepare a nursing care plan for a client with a respiratory disorder.*

INTRODUCTION

Respiratory disorders account for millions of the dollars spent in the U.S. health care arena. From loss of time on the job due to the common cold to care for those with chronic respiratory disorders, the cost of respiratory disease is staggering. This chapter explores the various respiratory disorders, with a focus on the nursing process.

KEY TERMS

adventitious breath sounds
asthma
atelectasis
audible wheezes
bronchial breath sounds
bronchiectasis
bronchitis
bronchovesicular breath sounds
caseation
cavitation
chemoreceptors
coarse crackles
diffusion
emphysema
epistaxis
external respiration

fine crackles
hemothorax
internal respiration
liquefaction necrosis
lung stretch receptors
perfusion
pleural effusion
pleural friction rub
pleurisy
pneumonia
pneumothorax
primary tubercle
respiration
sibilant wheezes
sonorous wheezes
status asthmaticus
surfactant
ventilation
vesicular breath sounds

ANATOMY AND PHYSIOLOGY REVIEW

The primary function of the respiratory system is delivery of oxygen to the lungs and removal of carbon dioxide from the lungs.

Thoracic Cavity

The chest cage is a closed compartment bounded on the top by the neck muscles and at the bottom by the diaphragm. The walls of the chest cage are formed by the ribs and intercostal muscles laterally, the thoracic vertebrae posteriorly, and the sternum anteriorly. The inside of the chest cage is called the *thoracic cavity*. Contained within the thoracic cavity are the lungs. The lungs are cone-shaped, porous organs separated from the other chest organs by the mediastinum. The lungs lie free, except for their attachment to the heart

and trachea, and are encased in the pleura, a thin, transparent double-layered serous membrane lining the thoracic cavity. The layers of the pleura are the parietal pleura, which lies adjacent to the chest wall, and the visceral pleura, which adheres to the surface of the lungs. The area between the two pleura is known as the *pleural space.*

The pleural space contains approximately 5 to 20 cubic centimeters of serous fluid (pleural fluid), which allows the layers of the pleura to slide on each other yet hold together. The pressure within the pleural space is less than that of outside air. This difference in pressure creates a suction that prevents the lungs from collapsing on exhalation.

The right lung is larger than the left and is divided into three sections, or lobes: upper, middle, and lower. The left lung is divided into two lobes: upper and lower (Figure 31-1). The upper portion of the lung is

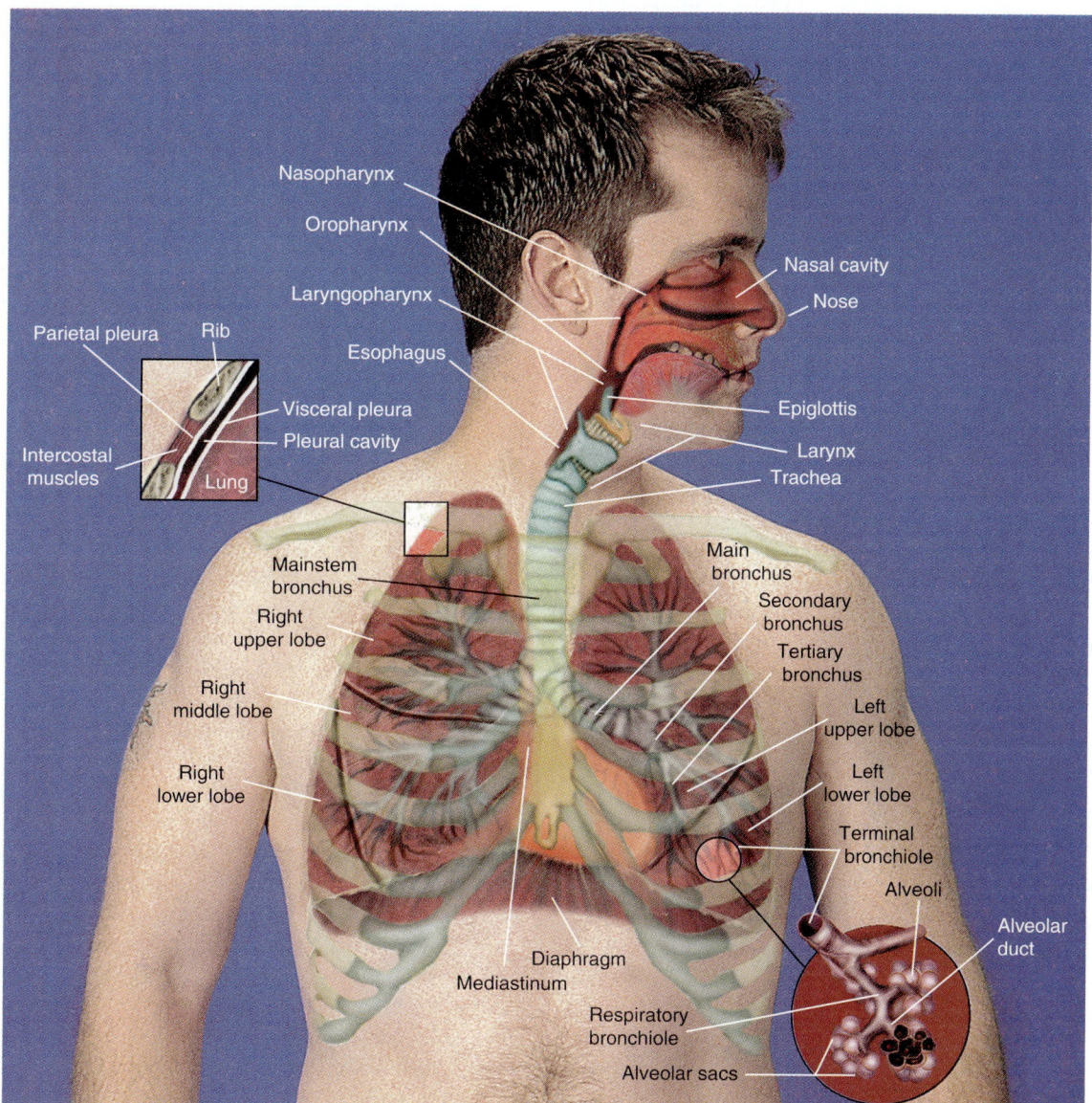

Figure 31-1 Structures of the Respiratory Tract (*Adapted from* Health Assessment & Physical Examination, *by M. E. Z. Estes, 1998, Albany, NY: Delmar Publishers. Copyright 1998 by Delmar Publishers. Adapted with permission.)*

referred to as the *apex* (plural, apices). The lower portion is called the *base*. The lungs possess a dual blood supply: bronchial circulation and pulmonary circulation. Bronchial circulation begins with the bronchial artery, which provides the passageways of the lungs with blood to meet nutritional needs. Bronchial circulation terminates when the venous blood enters the pulmonary veins, which slightly dilutes the oxygen content in the pulmonary vein. Pulmonary circulation is the route by which blood is delivered to the alveoli for gas exchange.

Conducting Airways

The conducting airways are tubelike structures that provide a passageway for air as it travels to the lungs. These are the nasal passages, mouth, pharynx, larynx, trachea, bronchi, and bronchioles (refer again to Figure 31-1). The conducting airways are lined with epithelial tissue containing serous glands, mucus-secreting Goblet cells, and hairlike projections called *cilia*. The mucus of the Goblet cells together with the cilia form a mucociliary blanket that serves to protect the respiratory system from invasion by foreign particles. The constant upward motion of the cilia propels the mucociliary blanket toward the pharynx, where any foreign matter may be expectorated.

The nasal passages are the preferred route for air to enter the respiratory tract. In addition to the function of filtering inspired air, the nasal passages are richly supplied with blood vessels that warm and moisten the air. An alternate route for air to enter is the mouth. Breathing through the mouth, however, reduces the ability to filter, warm, and moisten inspired air, because the mouth lacks cilia and abundant blood supply.

Connecting the nasal passages and mouth to the lower parts of the respiratory tract is the pharynx. The pharynx, located behind the oral cavity, serves as a passageway for both inspired air into the larynx and ingested food passing into the digestive system. At the distal portion of the pharynx is the larynx, also known as the voice box.

The larynx is the passageway for air entering and leaving the trachea, and contains the vocal cords. The larynx is composed of four structures: the uppermost thyroid cartilage (Adam's apple), the cricoid cartilage (which lies at the lower edge), the epiglottis (a leaf-shaped structure that covers the larynx during swallowing), and the glottis (the triangular space between the vocal cords when they are relaxed).

The trachea, commonly known as the windpipe, is a tube composed of connective tissue mucosa and smooth muscle supported by C-shaped rings of cartilage, extending into the bronchi. The trachea is 2.0 to 2.5 centimeters in diameter (approximately 1 inch) and 10 to 12 centimeters in length (4 to 6 inches). The trachea terminates by branching into two tubes: the right and left primary bronchi. The bronchi are somewhat smaller in diameter than the trachea and each passes into its respective lung. Within the lungs, the bronchi branch off into increasingly smaller diameter tubes until they become the terminal bronchioles. These branch further, forming alveolar ducts that end in numerous saclike, thin-walled structures called the *alveoli*. Collectively the alveoli and the alveolar ducts within resemble a cluster of grapes. The branching makes this portion of the respiratory tract resemble an inverted tree, giving rise to the term *bronchial tree* (see Figure 31-1).

Respiratory Tissues

The respiratory tissues perform the function of gas exchange. These structures are the alveolar ducts and the alveoli. Although each is supplied with a means for gas exchange, the alveoli constitute the primary site of gas exchange. The alveolar ducts are smooth, muscular tubes containing abundant alveolar macrophages to remove foreign particles (e.g., bacteria). The alveoli, into which the alveolar ducts terminate, consist of interconnected spaces with thin walls, or septa, occupied by a network of capillaries called the *alveolar capillary membrane*.

The alveoli contain two specialized types of cells. Type I alveolar cells are flat, squamous, epithelial cells across which gas exchange occurs. Type II alveolar cells produce a phospholipid substance called **surfactant**. Surfactant coats the inner surfaces of the alveoli, which reduces the surface tension of pulmonary fluids, allows gas exchange, and prevents the collapse of the airways. Each lung contains approximately 300 million alveoli.

Respiration

Respiration is a process of gas exchange. This process is necessary to supply cells with oxygen for carrying on metabolism, and to remove the carbon dioxide produced as a waste by-product. There are two types of respiration: external respiration and internal respiration. **External respiration** is the exchange of gases between the inhaled air, now in the alveoli, and the blood in the pulmonary capillaries. **Internal respiration** is the exchange of gases at the cellular level (Figure 31-2). These functions are dependent on the adequacy of ventilation, perfusion, and diffusion. **Ventilation** is the movement of air into and out of the lung. **Perfusion** refers to the flow of blood through the vessels of a specific organ or body part. **Diffusion** is the movement of a substance (in this case, gases) from areas of high concentration to areas of lower concentration. Factors that affect ventilation, perfusion, and diffusion will affect respiration. These factors are described in Table 31-1.

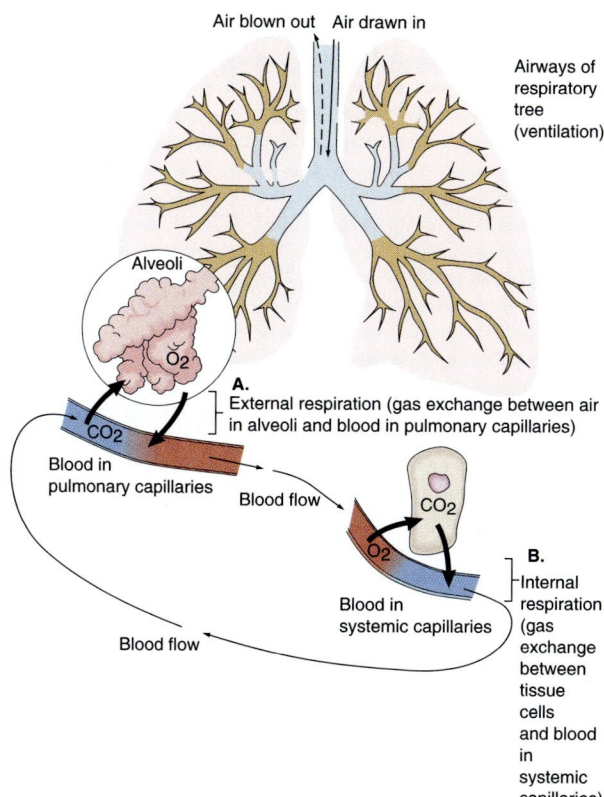

Air blown out   Air drawn in

Airways of respiratory tree (ventilation)

Alveoli

O₂

A.
External respiration (gas exchange between air in alveoli and blood in pulmonary capillaries)

CO₂

Blood in pulmonary capillaries

Blood flow

CO₂

O₂

B.
Internal respiration (gas exchange between tissue cells and blood in systemic capillaries)

Blood in systemic capillaries

Blood flow

Figure 31-2 A. External Respiration; B. Internal Respiration

Table 31-1	FACTORS AFFECTING VENTILATION, PERFUSION, AND DIFFUSION
Ventilation	Position: Dependent areas receive majority of air.
	Lung volume: Low volume results in shunting air to lung apices.
	Disease: Bronchial constriction and airway collapse decrease ventilation.
Perfusion	Position: Dependent areas receive majority of blood.
	Hypoxia: Results in vasoconstriction and decreased perfusion.
	Blockage: Results in decreased or absent perfusion to distal areas.
Diffusion	Alveolar capillary membrane: Alterations may occur in thickness and permeability of membrane.

Neuromuscular Control of Respiration

Unlike the heart muscles, the respiratory muscles must receive continuous neural stimuli to function. Regulation of respiration is integrated by neurons located in the pons and medulla of the brain. The control of respiration is influenced by involuntary (automatic) and voluntary components. Involuntary components include chemoreceptors, lung stretch receptors, and impulses from other sources. **Chemoreceptors** monitor the levels of carbon dioxide and oxygen and the acidity/alkalinity (pH) of the blood. Normally, chemoreceptors initiate respiration in response to rising levels of carbon dioxide in the blood. With certain chronic pulmonary disorders, such as emphysema, chemoreceptors become more responsive to low levels of oxygen. This becomes significant when administering oxygen to persons whose drive to breathe is dependent on low levels of oxygen in the blood. **Lung stretch receptors** monitor the patterns of breathing and prevent overexpansion of the tissues. Many other sources involuntarily send impulses to the respiratory center. For example, if a person becomes frightened or angry, the respiratory rate increases in response to stimuli from the autonomic nervous system. Voluntary components of respiratory control integrate breathing with acts such as talking and speaking.

The diaphragm acts as the primary muscle of respiration. During inspiration, the diaphragm contracts and flattens out in response to stimuli from the respiratory center, increasing the length of the thoracic cavity. At the same time, the intercostal muscles contract, elevating the ribs and increasing the diameter of the thoracic cavity. The total thoracic space increases, reducing the pressure within the thoracic cavity. The pressure within the thoracic cavity then becomes negative in relation to that of atmospheric pressure, and air moves into the thoracic cavity. Upon expiration, the respiratory center signals the diaphragm and intercostal muscles to relax. The thoracic cavity returns to its original size. Aided by the elastic recoil of the lungs, the decrease in size of the thoracic cavity increases pressure, and air moves out of the lungs.

Gas Exchange

Gas exchange occurs at the alveolar capillary membrane. Venous blood from the right ventricle is pumped into the pulmonary arteries and travels to the alveolar capillary network. Here, blood in the alveolar capillaries is exposed to the inhaled air. Due to the higher concentration of oxygen in the alveoli, oxygen diffuses into the blood within the alveolar capillary network. The majority of oxygen binds to the iron atoms of the hemoglobin molecule in the red blood cells. Approximately 1% to 3% of oxygen dissolves into the blood plasma. The exchange of carbon dioxide also occurs within the alveoli. Most of the carbon dioxide formed as a by-product of cellular metabolism diffuses into the red blood cells. There, due to the presence of carbonic anhydrase, carbon dioxide (CO_2) is hydrated and changed into carbonic acid (H_2CO_3). The carbonic acid dissociates into hydrogen ions (H^+) and bicarbonate ions (HCO_3^-). The hydrogen ions combine with hemoglobin, and the bicarbonate ions enter the blood plasma. Hemoglobin that has been reduced (by removal of the oxygen) combines with approximately 15% to 25% of the carbon dioxide. Within the alveolar capillary network, the carbon dioxide detaches from hemoglobin and diffuses into the alveolar space. Carbon dioxide is removed from the alveolar space when exhalation occurs. The blood within the pulmonary capillary network is now oxygenated and travels to the heart via the pulmonary veins. From this point, oxygenated blood is sent to the body via the aorta and the arterial network (Figure 31-3).

ASSESSMENT

Refer to Chapter 25 for detailed information regarding physical assessment.

To understand the assessment of the respiratory system, the student must be familiar with related terminology, outlined in Table 31-2.

Health History

Nursing assessment begins with a complete history. The client should be questioned regarding allergies,

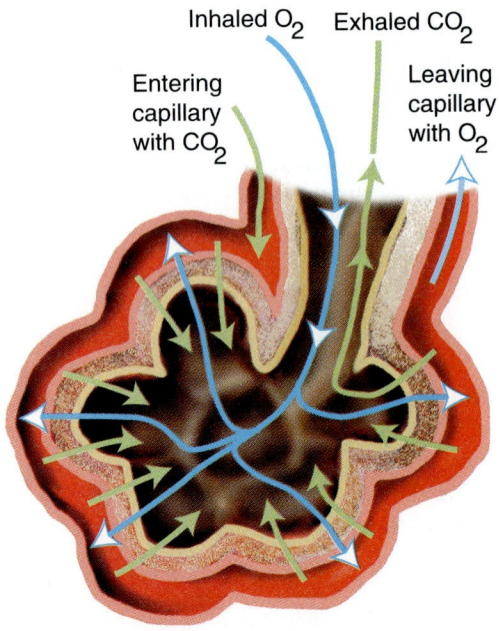

Figure 31-3 Alveolar Gas Exchange

Inhaled O_2 Exhaled CO_2

Entering capillary with CO_2 Leaving capillary with O_2

Table 31-2 RESPIRATORY TERMS

TERM	DEFINITION
Eupnea	Normal breathing
Apnea	Cessation of breathing, possibly temporary in nature
Dyspnea	Labored or difficult breathing, possibly normal if associated with exercise
Bradypnea	Abnormally slow breathing
Tachypnea	Abnormally rapid breathing
Orthopnea	Discomfort or difficulty with breathing in any but an upright sitting or standing position
Kussmaul's respirations	Abnormal respiratory pattern characterized by irregular periods of increased rate and depth of respiration; most often seen with diabetic ketoacidosis
Biot's respirations	Abnormal respiratory pattern characterized by irregular periods of apnea alternating with short periods of respiration of equal depth; most commonly seen with increased intracranial pressure
Cheyne-Stokes respirations	Abnormal respiratory pattern characterized by initially slow, shallow respirations that increase in rapidity and depth and then gradually decrease until respiration stops for 10 to 60 seconds; pattern then repeats itself in the same manner
Anoxia	Without oxygen
Hypoxia	Lack of adequate oxygen in inspired air such as occurs at high altitude
Hypoxemia	Insufficient amount of oxygen in the blood possibly due to respiratory, cardiovascular, or anemia-related disorders
Cyanosis	Bluish, grayish, or purplish discoloration of the skin due to abnormal amounts of reduced (oxygen-poor) hemoglobin in the blood; not always a reliable indicator of hypoxia
Acrocyanosis	Cyanosis of the fingertips and toes; often due to vasomotor disturbances associated with vasoconstriction
Circumoral cyanosis	Bluish discoloration encircling the mouth
Oxygen saturation	Amount of oxygen combined with hemoglobin

occupation, lifestyle, and health habits such as smoking. The client who smokes must be evaluated for the amount of tobacco smoked daily and length of time the client has smoked. Symptoms such as dyspnea, decreased exercise tolerance, and cough must be explored in depth. Following a complete history, the nurse completes a physical assessment of the client.

Inspection

Physical assessment of the respiratory system starts with inspection. The nurse notes the client's color, level of consciousness, and emotional state. Respirations are observed as to their rate, depth, quality, rhythm, and the effort required to breathe. Symmetry of chest wall movement is also noted. The nurse observes for use of accessory muscles to aid breathing. The position the client assumes provides information as to respiratory status. Individuals having trouble breathing often lean forward.

Palpation and Percussion

The next steps in the respiratory assessment are palpation and percussion. These are normally done by the registered nurse or physician. Through the use of palpation and percussion, areas of varying densities in the lung can be detected. The density of lung tissues changes with disease states such as pneumonia, pneumothorax, and pleural effusion.

Auscultation

Auscultation provides information about respiratory status. The listener assesses breath sounds at each location for the length of a complete inspiration and expiration. Breath sounds are assessed for duration, pitch, and intensity.

Normal Breath Sounds

Under normal circumstances, **bronchial breath sounds** are heard over the sternum. These loud, tubular, hollow-like sounds last longer during expiration than during inspiration. When heard in areas other than the sternum, bronchial breath sounds indicate fluid, exudate, or lung tissue compression. **Bronchovesicular breath sounds** are heard over the anterior one-third of the chest near the sternum and also around the scapula posteriorly. Bronchovesicular breath sounds have a medium pitch and intensity with inspiration and expiration being equal in duration. Bronchovesicular breath sounds may be heard in the periphery of the lung when consolidation and fluid are present.

Vesicular breath sounds are heard over the majority of the lungs. These breath sounds are soft and low in pitch. Vesicular breath sounds are best heard during inspiration and may be inaudible during expiration.

Adventitious Breath Sounds

Abnormal breath sounds are called **adventitious breath sounds**. Adventitious breath sounds include: **fine crackles, coarse crackles, sonorous wheezes, sibilant wheezes, pleural friction rub**, and **stridor**. Table 31-3 describes the general characteristics of these adventitious breath sounds.

Table 31-3 CHARACTERISTICS OF ADVENTITIOUS BREATH SOUNDS

BREATH SOUND	RESPIRATORY PHASE	TIMING	DESCRIPTION	CLEAR WITH COUGH	ETIOLOGY	CONDITIONS
Fine crackle	Predominantly inspiration	Discontinuous	Dry, high-pitched crackling and popping of short duration; sounds like hair rolled between fingers when held near ears	Possibly	Air passing through moisture in small airways that suddenly reinflate	Chronic obstructive pulmonary disease (COPD), congestive heart failure (CHF), pneumonia, pulmonary fibrosis, atelectasis
Coarse crackle	Predominantly inspiration	Discontinuous	Moist, low-pitched crackling and gurgling of long duration	Possibly	Air passing through moisture in large airways that suddenly reinflate	Pneumonia, pulmonary edema, bronchitis, atelectasis
Sonorous wheeze	Predominantly expiration	Continuous	Low-pitched snoring	Possibly	Narrowing of large airways or obstruction of bronchus	Asthma, bronchitis, airway edema, tumor, bronchiolar spasm, foreign body obstruction
Sibilant wheeze	Predominantly expiration	Continuous	High-pitched and musical	Possibly	Narrowing of large airways or obstruction of bronchus	Asthma, chronic bronchitis, emphysema, tumor, foreign body obstruction
Pleural friction rub	Inspiration and expiration	Continuous	Creaking, grating	Never	Inflamed parietal and visceral pleura; can occasionally be felt on thoracic wall as two pieces of dry leather rubbing against each other	Pleurisy, tuberculosis, pulmonary infarction, pneumonia, lung abscess
Stridor	Predominantly inspiration	Continuous	Crowing	Never	Partial obstruction of the larynx, trachea	Croup, foreign body obstruction, large airway tumor

Adapted from Health Assessment & Physical Examination, *by M. E. Z. Estes, 1998, Albany, NY: Delmar Publishers. Copyright 1998 by Delmar Publishers. Adapted with permission.*

Table 31-4 COMMON DIAGNOSTIC TESTS FOR RESPIRATORY DISORDERS

Laboratory Tests
- Hemoglobin
- Arterial blood gases (ABGs)
- Pulmonary function tests (PFTs)
- Sputum analysis

Radiologic Studies
- Chest x-ray
- Ventilation-perfusion scan
- Computerized axial tomography (CAT scan)
- Pulmonary angiography

Other
- Pulse oximetry
- Bronchoscopy
- Thoracentesis
- Magnetic resonance imaging (MRI)

Table 31-5 ARTERIAL BLOOD GASES: NORMAL VALUES

MEASUREMENT IN BLOOD	NORMAL VALUE
Acidity or alkalinity (pH)	7.3 to 7.45
Partial pressure of oxygen (PaO_2)	80 to 100 mm Hg
Partial pressure of carbon dioxide ($PaCO_2$)	35 to 45 mm Hg
Bicarbonate ion (HCO_3^-)	22 to 26 mm Hg
Arterial oxygen saturation (SaO_2)	95% (at sea level)

COMMON DIAGNOSTIC TESTS

Commonly used diagnostic tests for clients with respiratory disorders are listed in Table 31-4. See Chapter 27, Diagnostic Tests, for explanation/normal values and nursing responsibilities. Table 31-5 lists normal values for arterial blood gases.

INFECTIOUS/INFLAMMATORY DISORDERS

Infectious/inflammatory disorders of the upper respiratory tract, pneumonia, tuberculosis, and pleurisy/pleural effusion are discussed in the sections following.

INFECTIOUS/INFLAMMATORY DISORDERS OF THE UPPER RESPIRATORY TRACT

Infectious and inflammatory disorders of the upper respiratory tract are common and usually self-limiting. Table 31-6 summarizes the various types of disorders associated with infection and inflammation of the upper respiratory tract. Among the causal factors of infectious and inflammatory disorders are various viruses and bacteria such as rhino viruses, influenza viruses, streptococci, and pneumococci. Group A *beta-hemolytic streptococci* infections of the upper respiratory system are associated with serious sequelae such as rheumatic fever. Allergic reactions frequently play a role in the development of sinusitis and pharyngitis. Laryngitis is associated with irritation due to factors such as pollution, smoking, and excessive use of the voice. Breathing cold air decreases local immune responses of the respiratory tract. This fact coupled with closer and prolonged contact with others indoors during the colder months leads to an increased incidence of acute upper respiratory tract inflammatory disorders.

The signs and symptoms that occur with acute upper respiratory tract infection or inflammation are a result of the inflammatory process. Early signs and symptoms include general malaise, low-grade fever, localized redness, and edema of affected tissues. With viral disorders, symptoms such as joint pain are common. Furthermore, the client may complain of nasal or sinus congestion and headache. Drying of the mucous membranes coupled with edema cause local discomfort such as sore throat. Cough and nasal or sinus discharge may occur. Nasal secretions that are thick and purulent indicate bacterial infection.

Table 31-6 UPPER RESPIRATORY TRACT INFECTIONS OR INFLAMMATORY DISORDERS

DISORDER	ETIOLOGY
Rhinitis (coryza, common cold)	Viral
Allergic rhinitis	Exposure to allergens
Sinusitis	Bacterial (streptococci, pneumococci) or viral
Pharyngitis	Bacterial or viral
Tonsillitis	Bacterial (streptococci, most commonly)
Laryngitis	Irritation due to excessive use of voice or exposure to irritants (e.g., cigarette smoke); extension of rhinitis

Medical–Surgical Management

Medical

The majority of clients with acute upper respiratory tract infectious or inflammatory disorders are treated in a clinic or office setting. Unless the disorder becomes chronic or bacterial infection occurs, treatment is symptomatic. When infection is suspected, specimens for culture and sensitivity are obtained, and appropriate antibiotic therapy is initiated.

Surgical

Disorders that develop into chronic conditions (e.g., tonsillitis and sinusitis) may require surgical intervention to remove or drain affected tissues.

Pharmacological

Nonprescription antipyretic, analgesic, anti-inflammatory medications may be used to reduce discomfort, fever, and inflammation. Examples of such medications are acetaminophen (Tylenol), ibuprofen (Advil), and acetylsalicylic acid (aspirin). Antitussives such as dextromethorphan hydrobromide combinations (Comtrex, Dimetane-DM, Rondec-DM) or hydrocodone bitartrate (Hycodan) preparations may be used to suppress cough and allow for rest. To aid in removal of secretions, expectorants such as guaifenesin (Robitussin, Humibid L.A.) are used. Bacterial infections are treated with various antibiotics according to culture and sensitivity studies. Some of the more common antibiotics used are erythromycin base (E-mycin, PCE Disperstab), ampicillin (Omnipen), amoxicillin (Amoxil), cefaclor (Ceclor), and cephalexin monohydrate (Keflex). Comfort measures such as saline gargles may be useful.

Diet

Clear fluids are advocated to liquefy secretions and hydrate dry mucous membranes. Nausea may occur if secretions are swallowed as opposed to expectorated. The client should be encouraged to cough up all secretions and dispose of them properly (in a tissue). With severe coughing, emesis may occur. The client should be encouraged to rest prior to meals and may require an antitussive to reduce coughing.

LIFE CYCLE CONSIDERATIONS

Respiratory Status in Children
- The majority of common childhood diseases are respiratory in nature or have a respiratory component.
- Standard Precautions should be used when dealing with discharges from the eyes, nose, ears, and throat.

Activity

Normally, activity does not need to be restricted, but energy level may decrease. The client who is infectious should be encouraged to avoid contact with others. Strenuous activity should be avoided to reduce oxygen requirements and coughing.

▶ NURSING PROCESS

▶ Assessment

▶ Subjective Data

Subjective data include information about present signs and symptoms, onset of symptoms, exposure to allergens or infected individuals, and frequency of the disorder. Common symptoms include sore throat, dyspnea, and headache.

▶ Objective Data

Objective data include fever and inflammation, redness, edema, and drying of the mucous membranes of the oropharynx. Secretions are evaluated for their color, viscosity, amount, and odor, which will help in identifying the specific illness. The client may have hoarseness and a cough. Culture and sensitivity studies may reveal a causative organism and, thus, serve to guide antibiotic therapy. If infection with group A *beta-hemolytic streptococci* is suspected, an ASO (antistreptolysin O) titer may be done to reveal the presence of antibodies formed in reaction to this bacteria. Nonspecific diagnostic studies include elevated white blood cell counts and erythrocyte sedimentation rates.

Nursing diagnoses for a client with an upper respiratory infection or inflammatory disorder may include the following:

Nursing Diagnoses	Planning/Goals	Nursing Interventions
▶ *Knowledge Deficit, related to signs and symptoms of respiratory bacterial infection, potential allergens, and antibiotic therapy*	The client will be able to state the signs and symptoms of bacterial infection. The client will be able to identify individual potential allergens.	Educate the client regarding signs and symptoms indicating a respiratory bacterial infection, such as purulent or green secretions, fever. Assist the physician in allergy testing. Teach the client to avoid those things that precipitate an allergic response.

continued

Nursing Diagnoses	Planning/Goals	Nursing Interventions
	The client will complete entire course of antibiotic therapy.	Instruct client to complete the entire course of antibiotics.
▶ *Airway Clearance, Ineffective, related to nasal secretions.*	The client will verbalize a decrease or absence of nasal congestion.	Teach client to blow nose and not "snuffle" secretions back up into nose.

Evaluation Each goal must be evaluated to determine how it has been met by the client.

PNEUMONIA

Pneumonia is inflammation of the bronchioles and alveoli accompanied by consolidation, or solidification of exudate, in the lungs. It can result from bacteria, viruses, mycoplasms, fungi, chemical exposures, or parasite invasions. Pneumonia can also be caused by aspiration, oversedation, or inadequate ventilation. Pneumonia remains a common cause of hospitalization and is often a cause of death, particularly among elderly persons. Under normal circumstances, the alveolar macrophages are able to remove foreign matter. When confronted with overwhelming numbers of virulent microorganisms, however, this protective mechanism fails. The invading organism irritates the walls of the alveoli. In response to this irritation, the alveolar walls secrete exudate (an accumulation of fluid in the pulmonary passageways). Eventually, the alveoli fill with the exudate, resulting in consolidation. The presence of the exudate within the alveoli also interferes with gas exchange.

Risk factors for the development of pneumonia include immobility, depressed cough reflex (due to anesthesia or cerebrovascular accident [CVA]), alterations in respiratory function (e.g., chronic obstructive pulmonary disease [COPD]), advanced age, and numerous other chronic debilitating conditions (e.g., congestive heart failure [CHF], diabetes mellitus). Common bacterial causes of pneumonia are *Streptococcus pneumoniae, Pneumococcus, Staphylococcus aureus, Klebsiella pneumoniae,* and *Pseudomonas aeruginosa.* Chemical pneumonia is due to entry of irritating substances into the pulmonary passageways. A common source of chemical pneumonia is the aspiration of gastric contents. Inhalation of irritating substances can also result in a chemical pneumonia. A common, serious viral source of pneumonia is the *Cytomegalovirus.* The *Cytomegalovirus* affects those clients with compromised immune status, such as those taking immunosuppressant medications or those infected with human immunodeficiency virus (HIV) or acquired immunodeficiency syndrome (AIDS). *Pneumocystis carinii* pneumonia can also occur in the immunosupressed client. The invading organism associated with *Pneumocystis carinii* pneumonia is thought to be a protozoan. The infecting microorganisms that cause pneumonia

are spread by airborne droplets or direct contact with infected individuals or carriers. Pneumonia is now classified according to the causative factor rather than the area of the lung affected, as was done in the past.

A high fever of sudden onset is often the presenting complaint of the client. The elderly client, however, may be seriously ill and have only a low-grade fever. A productive cough yielding abnormally thick and discolored sputum may be present. Associated respiratory symptoms include dyspnea, coarse crackles, and diminished breath sounds. The majority of clients complain of pleuritic chest pain. This type of pain is stabbing in nature and increases on inspiration. Pain occurs due to irritation of the pleura lying adjacent to the affected alveoli.

In the case of bacterial pneumonia, white blood cell count increases and may go as high as 40,000/mm³. Pneumonia caused by viruses or mycoplasms may produce normal or lowered white blood cell count. Chest x-ray will reveal consolidation in the affected areas. Arterial blood gases (ABGs) may reveal a decrease in PaO_2 or oxygen saturation due to interference with gas exchange. Pulmonary function tests (PFTs) are usually within normal limits unless the client has an underlying pulmonary disorder such as emphysema.

Medical–Surgical Management

Medical

Clearing the airways of exudate and maintaining adequate oxygenation are the goals of treatment for clients with pneumonia. Postural drainage and percussion may be ordered to aid the client in mobilizing secretions (see Figure 31-4). Aerosol or nebulization treatments may also be utilized. Medications are often added to aerosol or nebulization treatments, as discussed in the subsequent section on pharmacological management of pneumonia. The client is encouraged to cough and deep breathe, particularly following respiratory treatments. Incentive spirometry, which measures the amount of air inspired in one inhalation, may be ordered to aid the client when coughing and deep breathing are inadequate (Figure 31-5). If the client is unable to mobilize secretions, suctioning of the respiratory tract is indicated. When secretions are overwhelming, the physician may perform a bronchoscopy

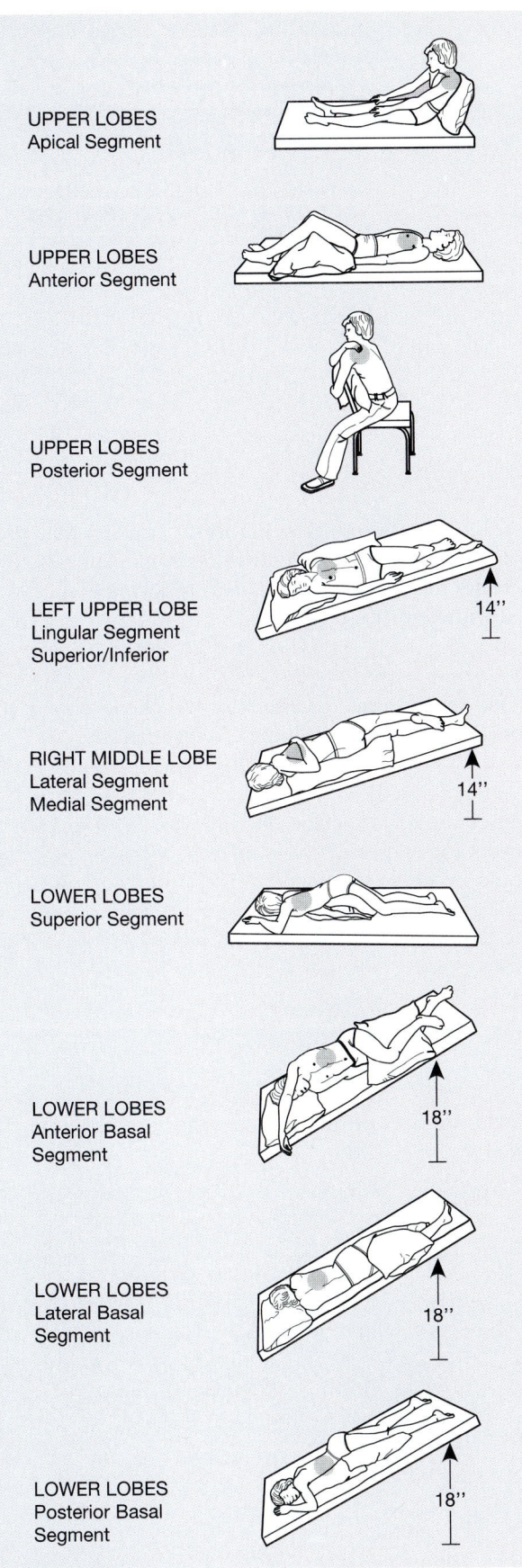

UPPER LOBES
Apical Segment

UPPER LOBES
Anterior Segment

UPPER LOBES
Posterior Segment

LEFT UPPER LOBE
Lingular Segment
Superior/Inferior

14"

RIGHT MIDDLE LOBE
Lateral Segment
Medial Segment

14"

LOWER LOBES
Superior Segment

LOWER LOBES
Anterior Basal
Segment

18"

LOWER LOBES
Lateral Basal
Segment

18"

LOWER LOBES
Posterior Basal
Segment

18"

Figure 31-4 Postural drainage positions that facilitate drainage of exudate from the lobes of the lungs. May be used with percussion.

LIFE CYCLE CONSIDERATIONS

Respiratory Status in the Elderly Client

- Respiratory effort increases because muscles atrophy, the diaphragm flattens out, costochondral cartilage calcifies, ligaments and joints stiffen, and intervertebral discs degenerate.
- Alveolar gas exchange diminishes due to a decrease in the lung's elastic recoil, which causes air to be trapped, especially in the lower lobes, for a portion of the respiratory cycle.
- The medulla becomes less sensitive to changes in carbon dioxide and oxygen levels, thereby rendering the respiration triggering mechanism less active.
- Ciliary activity diminishes, thereby increasing susceptibility to infection.
- Cough reflex decreases.
- Aspiration risk increases due to the decrease in the cough reflex.

in order to remove them. Intravenous fluids may be utilized to maintain adequate hydration, especially in the presence of fever. Adequate hydration promotes liquefaction of respiratory secretions and thus aids in their removal. Pulse oximetry or ABGs are done to assess the level of oxygenation. Supplemental oxygen is used when oxygenation is inadequate (refer to Figure 31-6 and Table 31-7).

Pharmacological

The treatment of choice for bacterial pneumonia is specific pharmacological therapy. A sputum specimen for culture and sensitivity should be obtained prior to initiating antibiotic therapy. After a specimen has been obtained, the physician may start therapy with a broad-spectrum antibiotic. If laboratory data indicate resistant microorganisms, a specific antibiotic will be

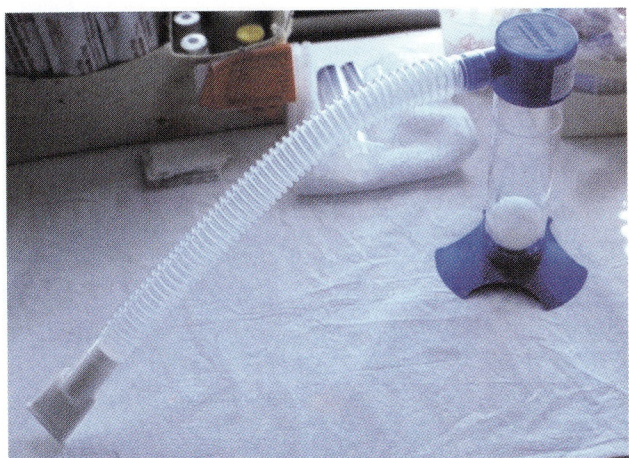

Figure 31-5 An incentive spirometer

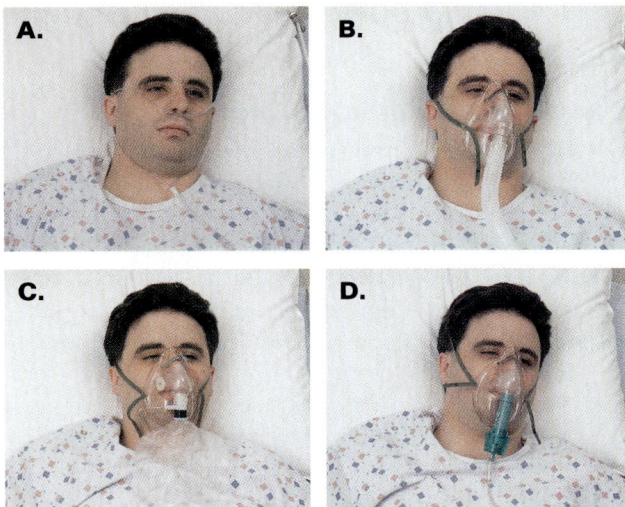

Figure 31-6 Oxygen Delivery Systems: A. Nasal cannula; B. Simple face mask; C. Reservoir mask; D. Venturi mask

Table 31-7	**SUPPLEMENTAL OXYGEN DEVICES AND OXYGEN CONCENTRATIONS PROVIDED**	
DEVICE	**FLOW RATE**	**OXYGEN CONCENTRATION**
Nasal cannula	1 to 6 L/min	20% to 40%
Simple mask	8 to 10 L/min	40% to 60%
Reservoir masks	6 to 10 L/min	60% to 100%
Venturi mask (used to control oxygen concentrations for the COPD patient)	4 to 8 L/min	24% to 40%

started. Antiviral agents, such as acyclovir sodium (Zovirax), are utilized for clients with chronic respiratory problems related to viral pneumonia. Prophylactic antibiotic therapy is often utilized for viral pneumonia to prevent a secondary bacterial infection. To promote opening and clearing of the airways, bronchodilators, such as albuterol (Ventolin), and mucolytic agents, such as acetylcysteine (Mucomyst), are administered via aerosol or nebulization by the respiratory therapist or nurse. Expectorants such as guaifenisin (Robitussin) may be given orally. Cough suppressants and pain relievers, especially those containing narcotics such as codeine sulfate, are administered only with discretion, because they may further inhibit the client's ability to clear the airways.

Diet

The client with pneumonia is encouraged to force fluids, as doing so aids in the liquefaction of respiratory secretions. Small, frequent, nutritionally balanced meals are preferred. Respiratory treatments that promote coughing should be avoided immediately before and after meals to prevent nausea and vomiting associated with vigorous coughing.

Activity

Bed rest or limited activity for the client with pneumonia promotes optimal tissue oxygenation.

Health Promotion

Pneumococcal vaccine (Pneumovax 23), a vaccine to prevent infection caused by *Streptococcus pneumonia*, should be given to clients at risk of developing pneumonia, such as those with chronic respiratory or cardiac conditions. The vaccine is recommended for all elderly persons.

LIFE CYCLE CONSIDERATIONS

Oxygen Therapy in Children

- Any child receiving oxygen therapy should not play with friction toys or use a nylon or wool blanket.
- For the child receiving oxygen, the oxygen concentration in the air surrounding the child's head must be measured with an oxygen analyzer because prolonged exposure to a high oxygen concentration can be toxic to certain tissues (the retina in preterm babies, the lungs in all children), especially in children with asthma or cystic fibrosis.

PROFESSIONAL TIP

Assessment and Respiratory Assistive Devices

When caring for clients with respiratory assistive devices in place, the following must be assessed:

- Oxygen
  - Mode of delivery (e.g., nasal cannula, face mask)
  - Percentage of oxygen that is being delivered (e.g., 25%, 40%)
  - Flow rate of the oxygen (e.g., 2 liters per minute, 4 liters per minute)
  - Humidification provided and oxygen warmed
- Incentive Spirometer
  - Frequency of use
  - Volume achieved
  - Number of times client reaches goal with each use

▶ NURSING PROCESS

▶ Assessment

▶ Subjective Data

Data gathered in the history include the onset, duration, and severity of cough; the color, amount, and odor of sputum, if present; the onset and duration of elevated temperature; and the presence or absence of night sweats.

▶ Objective Data

The client's level of consciousness should be noted. Evidence of dyspnea, orthopnea, tachypnea, and cyanosis may be present. On auscultation of the lung fields, moist crackles or diminished breath sounds are heard. In the event of obstruction of the airways, sibilant wheezes occur. Vital signs including temperature are taken prior to and following drug therapy so as to

CLIENT TEACHING

Pneumonia

- Discuss pertinent information about medications being taken
- Instruct in measures to prevent spread of infection (covering the mouth and nose with a tissue when coughing or sneezing)
- Encourage disposal of tissues in a closed paper sack
- Outline individual's specific risk factors (age, chronic respiratory condition, cardiac condition)
- Instruct in methods to prevent future infection (avoiding crowds and obtaining vaccine)

provide information regarding the severity of the illness and the efficacy of treatment. The color, amount, viscosity, and odor of sputum are noted.

Nursing diagnoses for a client with pneumonia may include the following:

Nursing Diagnoses	Planning/Goals	Nursing Interventions
▶ *Airway Clearance, Ineffective, related to inability to remove airway secretions.*	The client will have clear breath sounds upon auscultation.	Encourage the client to breathe deeply and cough a minimum of every 2 hours.
		Teach use of the incentive spirometer to encourage lung expansion.
		Administer aerosol and nebulizer treatments as ordered.
		Assess breath sounds and respiratory rate prior to and following respiratory procedures to evaluate their effectiveness.
		Encourage fluids to liquefy thickened secretions.
		For clients who are able, assist in sitting up or ambulating three to four times daily.
		For the client who is on bed rest, turn every 2 hours.
		Administer medications as ordered.
		Provide oral care several times a day.
▶ *Gas Exchange, Impaired, related to inflammatory changes in alveolar capillary membrane*	The client will have an oxygen saturation of 95% or greater.	Monitor pulse oximetry and/or ABGs.
		Administer supplemental oxygen as ordered.
▶ *Activity Intolerance related to hypoxia secondary to pneumonia*	The client will be able to complete activities of daily living (ADL) and activity as ordered and without complaints of fatigue.	Encourage the client to complete ADL according to ability and the physician's orders.
		To prevent client fatigue, alternate periods of activity and care with periods of rest.

Evaluation Each goal must be evaluated to determine how it has been met by the client.

TUBERCULOSIS

Pulmonary tuberculosis (TB) is an infection of the lung tissue by *Mycobacterium tuberculosis*. Infection by the tubercle bacillus can occur in other parts of the body, but with less frequency. Other parts of the body that may be affected include bones, joints, gastroin-

testinal and genitourinary tracts, nervous system, skin, and lymph nodes. In the case of pulmonary tuberculosis, the tubercle bacilli are inhaled into the lungs. Whether infection occurs depends on the host's susceptibility, the virulence of the tubercle bacilli, and the number of bacilli inhaled. Tuberculosis is not as highly contagious as once thought. Prolonged exposure to the bacilli is required to produce infection. In addition, persons with uncompromised immune systems are able to combat the bacilli and do not develop the disease itself.

Once inhaled in sufficient numbers, the tubercle bacilli cause an inflammatory response within the alveoli of the lung. A small nodule called a **primary tubercle**, which contains tubercle bacilli, forms within the lung tissue. In an attempt to isolate these primary tubercles, the body forms a fibrous outer coating around each tubercle. This fibrous surface interferes with the blood and nutritional supplies to the primary tubercle. In time, the interior of the tubercle becomes soft and cheese-like due to decreased perfusion, a process known as **caseation**. At this point, the tubercles may become calcified. **Liquefaction necrosis** may occur, wherein the tissue dies and changes to a liquid or semi-liquid state; this fluid may then be coughed up. A cavity is formed at the site where the primary tubercle liquefied and ruptured. This condition is known as **cavitation** or cavitary disease.

Following the advent of antitubercular medications in the 1950s, the incidence of TB decreased dramatically. In recent years, however, TB has been occurring with increased frequency. In addition, new forms of TB that are resistant to conventional drug therapy have surfaced. Some of the factors that may be responsible for the increase in TB cases are: increased numbers of persons with compromised immune systems (e.g., many AIDS clients suffer from TB); increased mobility of the world's population (persons from areas of high TB incidence moving to areas of low incidence); widespread IV drug abuse; increased numbers of those with poor access to health care; and increased numbers of those living in impoverished conditions.

Symptoms of TB develop gradually following infection. The nurse should suspect TB if the following symptoms are present: low-grade fevers that recur in a specific pattern, persistent cough, hemoptysis, hoarseness, dyspnea on exertion, night sweats, fatigue, and weight loss. Due to the body's attempt to fight the infection, lymph nodes also may be enlarged.

The Mantoux skin test is the preferred method of screening for TB. For the Mantoux test, 0.1cc of purified protein derivative (PPD) of killed tubercle bacilli is injected intradermally in the inner forearm. The test is evaluated by measuring the area of induration (palpable swelling) that occurs 48 and 72 hours following injection. Whether an induration area of a given size is considered indicative of a positive reaction depends on the client's risk factors for TB (Table 31-8). Those at highest risk, such as persons infected with the HIV virus or those with recent close contact with a person infectious with TB, are considered to have a positive reaction if the area of induration is 5 mm or more. Individuals with no risk factors for TB are considered to have a positive reaction if the area of induration is 15 mm or greater. A positive skin test, however, indicates

only that the client has been infected with and developed antibodies against the tubercle bacillus. Most people are able to fight the bacteria and stop them from growing. The bacteria remain alive but inactive in the body, often for a lifetime. Many people who have TB infection never develop TB disease. In persons with weak immune systems, the bacteria become active and cause TB disease. Some individuals may develop TB disease soon after infection; some develop TB disease at a later date when their immune systems become weak for some reason; and others never develop TB disease.

Table 31-8 POSITIVE RESULTS OF MANTOUX TUBERCULIN SKIN TEST	
CONSIDERED POSITIVE	**POPULATION**
Induration of 5mm or more	*High-risk groups:* • Persons with HIV infection • Persons in close contact with someone who has infectious TB • Persons who have chest x-rays consistent with old, healed TB • Intravenous drug users whose HIV status is unknown
Induration of 10 mm or more	*Moderate-risk groups:* • Intravenous drug users known to be HIV seronegative • Foreign-born persons from high-prevalence areas (Asia, Africa, Latin America) • Residents of long-term care facilities (prisons, nursing homes, mental institutions) • Medically underserved low-income populations, including high-risk racial or ethnic minority populations (Blacks, Hispanics, Native Americans) • Persons with medical conditions that have been shown to increase the risk of TB, such as silicosis; persons who are 10% or more below ideal body weight; persons receiving high-dose corticosteroid or other immunosuppressive therapy; and persons with some hematologic disorders (leukemias and lymphomas) and other malignancies • Locally identified high-risk populations • Health care workers who provide services to any of the high-risk groups
Induration of 15 mm or more	*Persons having low risk*

From Core Curriculum on Tuberculosis, *1984, Centers for Disease Control and Prevention, Atlanta: U. S. Department of Health and Human Services.*

A negative reaction does not rule out the possibility of TB exposure. Individuals at high risk, such as those who are infected with HIV or who have compromised immune status, may have a negative reaction because they are unable to develop antibodies. Immediately following exposure to TB, a skin test may read falsely negative because it can take up to 10 weeks for an infected individual to develop antibodies to react to the killed tubercle bacilli. An additional skin test may be done in 10 to 12 weeks. If the second TB test is positive, the client's history is reviewed for the presence of symptoms suggesting TB, and further evaluation is indicated.

Chest x-ray and sputum specimens are utilized to confirm a diagnosis of TB. Sputum is tested for the presence of acid-fast bacilli, or AFB. The sputum specimen is collected when the client arises in the morning to prevent specimen contamination with ingested food and liquids. In most instances, three specimens collected on consecutive days and testing positive for AFB indicate a positive diagnosis of TB. The TB diagnosis is confirmed if the TB bacilli grow in a culture. Individuals who are unable to produce sputum, including children and elderly persons, may have stomach contents aspirated for the purpose of AFB testing. Chest x-ray may reveal the presence of primary tubercles in the lung. Areas of calcified lesions and cavitation are also revealed on x-ray.

Medical–Surgical Management

Medical

The majority of clients are treated briefly in the hospital, with long-term treatment continuing at home. In the hospital Airborne Precautions must be followed in addition to Standard Precautions. The precautions include placing the client in an isolation room with negative air pressure (where air inflow is controlled through one vent and air outflow is exhausted through another vent directly to the outside and is not recirculated to other rooms.). The doors and windows of the client's room must be kept closed to maintain control of air flow. Furthermore, caregivers should wear N95 particulate respirator masks, as standard isolation masks do not prevent *Mycobacterium tuberculosis* from passing through to the wearer (Figure 31-7).

Infection Control: Use of a Particulate Respirator

- Follow facility's procedure for fit-testing
- Use the correct size mask
- Put on respirator before entering client's room and remove after leaving client's room
- Ensure that the respirator is free of holes
- Check that the seal between face and respirator is intact
- Discard soiled or damaged respirators

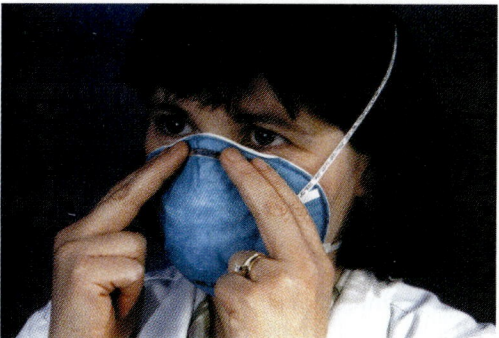

Figure 31-7 A particulate respirator must be tightly fitted around the nose and face. *(Photo courtesy of Donna Hannum, RN, BSN)*

The Centers for Disease Control and Prevention recommend periodic TB skin testing for health care personnel. Health care workers with low risk for developing TB, including those who have contact with fewer than five TB clients per year, should be tested yearly. Health care workers who have had contact with five or more TB clients within the past year should be tested every 6 months. Any health care worker who is exposed to clients in a variety of settings (e.g., ambulance personnel) or who deals with a transitory client population should be tested every 3 months.

Infection Control: Tuberculosis

- Instruct client to cover mouth and nose when coughing or sneezing
- Double-bag secretions and dispose of them as infectious waste
- Use disposable items for care when possible
- Thoroughly clean and disinfect nondisposable items

Safety: Caregivers in Health Care Institutions

- Be aware of risks when caring for a client with TB
- Follow Standard Precautions and Airborne Precautions
- Use face and/or eye shield in addition to particulate mask when performing sputum-induction procedure
- Plan care to limit prolonged exposure to client

Surgical

In the past, surgical intervention involving the removal of affected lung tissues was common. With the advent of effective chemotherapy (treatment with drugs), however, surgical intervention is now rarely utilized.

Pharmacological

Active TB is treated with a combination of medications. Three medications, rifampin (Rifadin), isoniazid

(Laniazid), and pyrazinamide (Pyrazinamide), are given for a period of 2 months. This is followed by a regimen of rifampin and isoniazid for 4 additional months. The combination of three drugs is given initially to rapidly decrease the number of active bacilli and prevent the development of drug resistance. After 3 weeks on medication, the client is usually no longer contagious. Long-term therapy is required because TB bacilli have long periods of metabolic inactivity. Those clients with bone and joint infections, meningitis, or resistant forms of TB must be treated with isoniazid and pyrazinamide for longer periods. Clients who are HIV positive require a 7-month regimen of isoniazid and pyrazinamide; prophylactic treatment with isoniazid is indicated from then on. Ethambutol hydrochloride (Myambutol) and streptomycin sulfate are added to the treatment regimen if the infecting organism is resistant to one of the three medications normally used to treat TB. Infection with a multidrug resistant form of TB requires the use of medications such as kanmycin (Kantrex), capreomycin sulfate (Capastat Sulfate), and cycloserine (Seromycin). The client is considered noninfectious following three negative AFB sputum specimens. At that point, the client may return to work and other normal activities. Prophylactic treatment of high-risk individuals is recommended to reduce their chances of developing the disease following their exposure.

Diet

The client with TB often also suffers from nutritional deficits. Correction of these deficits is necessary to assist the client in overcoming the disease process. Dietary management is based on the type of deficiency present. A well-balanced diet is encouraged for all clients with TB. Fluids are encouraged to aid in the liquefaction of respiratory secretions.

Activity

Activity is restricted based on the client's tolerance. The client who is severely compromised from a respiratory standpoint may be placed on bed rest. If the client's condition allows, activity should be encouraged, as it promotes lung expansion and aids in the re-

moval of static secretions. The client in isolation whose condition permits it may ambulate in the hallways, as long as a particulate respirator mask is worn by the client while outside of the room.

Health Promotion

Prevention of TB is by far preferred to treatment of the infection. In areas where the disease remains endemic (seldom in the United States), a vaccine containing attenuated tubercle bacilli, BCG (*bacillus Calmette-Guérin*), is recommended. One disadvantage of the vaccine is that individuals receiving it will test positive to the tuberculin skin test. Also, lifelong immunity to the disease has not been proven. It is currently indicated that any person who has had close contact with a client with TB without practicing appropriate protective measures should be tested. Other measures that decrease the likelihood of TB include adequate nutrition, housing, and health care access, and treatment of individuals who have or are at risk for developing TB.

▶ NURSING PROCESS

▶ Assessment

▶ Subjective Data

The history includes questions about the presence of signs and symptoms of TB, such as night sweats, dyspnea on exertion or at rest in late disease, anorexia, loss of muscle strength, and fatigue. Pleuritic pain occurs when the pleura is involved.

▶ Objective Data

Objective data include weight loss; persistent, low-grade fever; and persistent cough. The cough may be nonproductive early in the disease. Later, the cough is

---

CLIENT TEACHING

Rifampin Side Effects

- Urine, saliva, or tears may turn orange.
- Skin becomes more sensitive to the sun.
- Birth control pills and implants become less effective.
- In the presence of methadone, withdrawal symptoms may occur.

(CDC, 1994b)

HOME HEALTH CARE

The Client with Tuberculosis

Advise the client of the following:

- Keep all clinic appointments.
- Continue medications for 6 to 12 months.
- Take all medications exactly as directed.
- After 3 weeks on medication, daily routine (e.g., work, school) may be resumed. Until that time:
  - Put used tissues in a closed paper sack and throw away;
  - Avoid close contact with anyone;
  - Sleep alone in bedroom;
  - Air out bedroom often, using a fan in the window to blow air outside; and
  - Thoroughly clean articles such as eating utensils.

productive and yields thick, purulent sputum. Eventually, hemoptysis (blood spitting) occurs. Auscultation of breath sounds reveals coarse crackles. In the presence of cavitary disease, breath sounds are diminished or absent in the affected areas. Sputum is observed as to amount, color, odor, and consistency.

Nursing diagnoses for a client with TB may include the following:

Nursing Diagnoses	Planning/Goals	Nursing Interventions
▶ *Breathing Pattern, Ineffective, related to pulmonary infectious process*	The client will have color and respiratory rate within normal limits and will not complain of dyspnea.	Assess the client's color, respiratory rate, and respiratory effort. Auscultate the breath sounds. Obtain sputum specimens for AFB; note the amount, color, and viscosity of the sputum. Plan care activities to allow the client uninterrupted periods of rest. Assist the client in assuming the position that most aids respiratory effort. Administer medications as ordered. Encourage fluids if not otherwise contraindicated.
▶ *Knowledge Deficit related to disease process and its treatment*	The client will verbalize an understanding of the disease process and its treatment.	Teach client and family about the basic pathophysiology of TB, how the infection is contracted, who is at risk of developing an infection, the signs and symptoms of TB infection, and complications that may arise. Present information regarding the actions, side effects, and untoward effects of the drugs being administered. Teach the client signs and symptoms of adverse drug reactions to report to the physician. Emphasize the necessity of long-term therapy to cure TB. Inform the client and family that symptoms decrease and are often gone long before the organism is eliminated from the body.
▶ *Management of Therapeutic Regimen: Individual, Ineffective, related to client value system*	The client will continue medication regimen for the prescribed length of time.	Include the client and family in making decisions about the care, when appropriate. Allow the client to be an active participant in care decisions, to increase personal responsibility and accountability. Visits from public health or home care nurses may be necessary to monitor the client for compliance. Explore the reasons for noncompliance with the client and family. Based on information obtained, identify strategies to increase compliance. Refer the client who is unable to afford the cost of medications to agencies such as the local health department for assistance. Begin directly observed therapy if the client continues to be noncompliant. Directly observed therapy involves sending the nurse or another health care worker to the client to administer the medications and verify that they are taken.

Evaluation Each goal must be evaluated to determine how it has been met by the client.

SAMPLE NURSING CARE PLAN

THE CLIENT WITH TUBERCULOSIS

Mr. Stuart is an 87-year-old male admitted to the hospital with a chief complaint of productive cough and fatigue. Four months ago, Mr. Stuart was placed in a long-term care facility due to his inability to care for himself at home following his wife's death 1 year previously. Since admission to the long-term care facility, Mr. Stuart has lost 15 pounds. The nurses at the facility report that Mr. Stuart has experienced progressive

continued

fatigue, dyspnea on exertion, cough, night sweats, and anorexia. Initially, his cough was nonproductive, but it is now productive of moderate amounts of thick, purulent sputum that is occasionally streaked with blood. Vital signs are: temperature 99.8°F, pulse 108, respirations 26, and blood pressure 138/86. A TB skin test done at the long-term care facility 1 week ago was evaluated as negative at 6 mm. Sputum specimens for AFB reveal the presence of active tubercle bacilli, and chest x-ray is positive for TB. Auscultation of breath sounds reveals crackles in the right lower half of the lung. Mr. Stuart says, "I don't understand why I can't breathe good and what all this fuss is about."

Nursing Diagnosis 1 *Breathing Pattern, Ineffective, related to infectious pulmonary process as evidenced by dyspnea on exertion and productive cough*

PLANNING/GOALS	NURSING INTERVENTIONS	RATIONALE	EVALUATION
Mr. Stuart will have respiratory rate, oxygen saturation, and color within normal limits and will not complain of dyspnea.	Initially and periodically assess Mr. Stuart's respiratory status including color, respiratory rate, respiratory effort, oxygen saturation, breath sounds, level of consciousness, cough, and sputum.	The initial assessment provides a database from which the plan of care can be formulated and against which the effectiveness of treatment can be evaluated. Subsequent assessments provide a means of detecting changes in Mr. Stuart's condition, allowing for the evaluation of the effectiveness of interventions and the modification of the care plan.	Mr. Stuart verbalizes a decrease in dyspnea and cough. Mr. Stuart's color, respiratory rate, and oxygen saturation are within normal limits.
	Assist Mr. Stuart in assuming the position which most aids respiratory effort.	An upright, high or semi-Fowler's position allows for greater ease of respiration and lung expansion.	
	Alternate care activities with periods of rest.	Alternating care with periods of rest allows Mr. Stuart to compensate for the increased oxygen demand required by activity.	
	Encourage activity within Mr. Stuart's tolerance and per physician's orders.	Activity promotes expansion of the lungs.	
	Encourage fluids.	Fluids promote the liquefaction of respiratory secretions, thus aiding in their removal.	
	Administer medications for fever as ordered.	Fever increases cellular metabolism, which requires water. Thus, fever	

continued

that persists can lead to dehydration, which will hinder the removal of respiratory secretions.

Administer oxygen as ordered to maintain an SaO$_2$ of 95% or greater.

Oxygen saturation of 95% or greater is necessary for optimal cellular function.

Administer antitubercular drugs as ordered.

Antitubercular drugs decrease the number of viable tubercle bacilli and, thus, decrease respiratory secretions.

Nursing Diagnosis 2 *Infection, Risk for, spread related to viable bacilli in secretions as evidenced by AFB in sputum*

PLANNING/GOALS	NURSING INTERVENTIONS	RATIONALE	EVALUATION
Mr. Stuart will verbalize both those situations that allow for the transmission of the tubercle bacilli and the means to prevent their transmission.	Place Mr. Stuart in a negative air pressure, private room; keep door closed at all times. On the door, place Airborne Precaution signs indicating that Mr. Stuart has an infectious process and asking visitors to see nursing personnel prior to visiting. Instruct visitors to wear N95 respirators when in Mr. Stuart's room, to limit the length of their visits, to avoid intimate contact, such as kissing, with Mr. Stuart, and to wash their hands when leaving the room.	A negative air pressure, private room is required to prevent the transmission of the tubercle bacilli in air that has been circulated into and out of Mr. Stuart's room. Informing the public of the infectious disease process is necessary to prevent inadvertent contact and exposure. The nature of the infection is not revealed publicly to maintain client confidentiality. Visitors are informed of precautions to take to prevent exposure to the tubercle bacilli.	Persons exposed to Mr. Stuart have been tested for TB. Those with TB are being treated. No further unprotected exposures to Mr. Stuart will occur.
	Instruct Mr. Stuart to cover his mouth and nose when coughing and sneezing.	Covering the nose and mouth aids in the containment of the tubercle bacilli.	
	Instruct Mr. Stuart to cough up secretions in tissues and to place the tissues in a plastic bag. Dispose of contained secretions as infectious waste.	Containment and proper disposal of infectious secretions aids in preventing the spread of the tubercle bacilli.	

continued

Inform the long-term care facility and family/significant others of the positive results of the AFB studies. Instruct those persons who have been exposed to Mr. Stuart to have a TB skin test.

Known exposure to active tubercle bacilli necessitates testing to identify individuals who may have become infected.

Observe Standard Precautions and Airborne Precautions.

Compliance with Standard Precautions and Airborne Precautions decreases the likelihood of transmitting the tubercle bacilli (and other infectious diseases) to staff and other clients.

Wear a fitted N95 respirator when in Mr. Stuart's room.

A fitted N95 respirator is necessary to prevent the inhalation of tubercle bacilli, which are able to pass through a simple surgical mask.

Plan care activities to limit the time spent in close contact with Mr. Stuart.

Prolonged exposure to the tubercle bacilli, even when taking precautions, increases the likelihood of infection.

Nursing Diagnosis 3 *Knowledge Deficit related to disease process and its treatment as evidenced by client statement: "I don't understand why I can't breathe good and what all this fuss is about."*

PLANNING/GOALS	NURSING INTERVENTIONS	RATIONALE	EVALUATION
Mr. Stuart will verbalize an understanding of the disease process and the required medication regimen.	Assess Mr. Stuart's present level of knowledge regarding TB and its treatment.	Provides a database regarding Mr. Stuart's present level of knowledge regarding TB and its treatment. Client education can then be individualized to build and expand on that knowledge base. Misinformation can also be corrected.	Mr. Stuart verbalizes his individual treatment regimen and the purpose of the regimen. Mr. Stuart accurately demonstrates medication administration. Mr. Stuart reports adverse effects of medication to health care personnel to allow for early intervention.
	Provide information in small amounts and use a variety of approaches (e.g., verbal, written, video).	Providing information in small amounts increases the likelihood of learning by not overwhelming Mr. Stuart with information. Pro-	

continued

viding information in a variety of media increases the likelihood of learning by supplying stimuli to the various senses (sight, sound, and touch).

Encourage and allow time for Mr. Stuart to ask questions.	Provides a means for Mr. Stuart to clarify information as well as for the nurse to evaluate learning and to correct misconceptions.
Have Mr. Stuart demonstrate medication administration regimen by setting up a day's dose of medications as ordered.	Demonstration on the part of Mr. Stuart reinforces learning and provides the nurse with a means to evaluate the effectiveness of teaching.
Have Mr. Stuart verbalize signs and symptoms of adverse medication effects that should be reported to the staff of the long-term care facility and/or the physician.	Verbalization provides a means of evaluating the effectiveness of teaching. Mr. Stuart needs to be informed of those signs and symptoms that require further evaluation and follow-up by health care personnel.

PLEURISY/PLEURAL EFFUSION

Pleurisy is a painful condition that arises from inflammation of the pleura, or sac that encases the lung. This pleuritic pain is sharp and stabbing in nature. Pain increases on inspiration as the irritated pleura rub over each other. Inflammation of the pleura occurs with many disorders, such as viral infections, cancer of the lung, trauma, tuberculosis, congestive heart failure, and pulmonary embolism. The inflamed pleura secretes increased amounts of pleural fluid into the pleural cavity, creating a **pleural effusion**. As fluid accumulates within the pleural space, it compresses the lung tissue (Figure 31-8). Collapse, or atelectasis, results if the effusion is left untreated. Those areas of collapsed lung tissue are unable to take part in gas exchange, thereby decreasing oxygenation. Empyema is a condition wherein the pleural exudate becomes infected.

The primary manifestation of pleurisy is pain on inspiration. Signs and symptoms of pleural effusion depend on the amount of lung tissue compressed and the source of the effusion. With large pleural effusions, the mediastinum (heart, great vessels, and trachea) shifts toward the unaffected side; this can be detected by inspection, and heart sounds will move toward unaffected side. Magnetic resonance imaging (MRI) or computerized tomography (CT) studies are useful in detecting pleural effusions, particularly small ones. A chest x-ray will show pleural effusions of 250 cc of fluid or more. Culture and sensitivity studies will identify the presence and type of infection, if empyema is suspected. The client with empyema will also have an elevated temperature and white blood cell count.

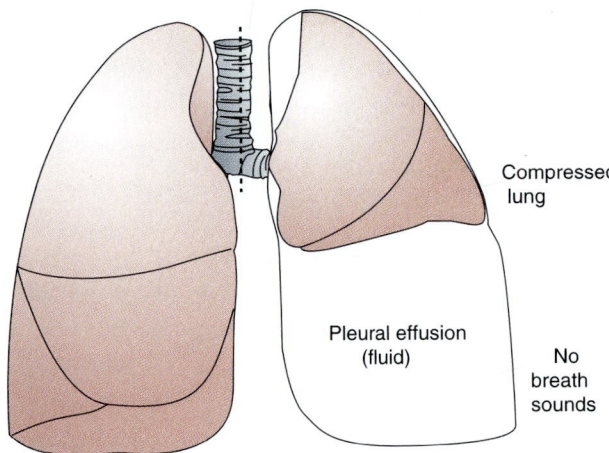

Contralateral mediastinal shift

Compressed lung

Pleural effusion (fluid)

No breath sounds

Figure 31-8 Pleural Effusion

Medical–Surgical Management

Medical

Treatment of pleurisy is aimed at eliminating the underlying cause, maintaining adequate oxygenation to the tissues, and preventing complications such as atelectasis and pneumonia. Adequacy of oxygenation is evaluated by means of arterial blood gases and/or pulse oximetry. Supplemental oxygen is given to maintain an oxygen saturation of 95% or greater. Respiratory treatments to aid lung expansion such as incentive spirometry are used.

Surgical

Larger pleural effusions require a thoracentesis be performed by the physician to remove accumulated fluid. After the overlying tissues are anesthetized, a large bore needle is placed into the pleural space. Fluid is removed and may be sent to the laboratory for diagnostic purposes (i.e., culture, cytology). If fluid accumulation continues to present a problem, as with empyema, the physician will place a thoracotomy tube into the pleural space to drain fluid continuously. Following administration of local anesthetics, the physician places a large bore catheter into the pleural space. This catheter is attached to an underwater seal drainage device (refer to Figure 31-9). The underwater seal drainage device prevents the negative pressure within the pleural space from pulling air into the pleural space, and allows for the drainage of accumulated fluid or air. In addition, most devices also include a chamber to which suction may be applied to assist in the removal of fluid or air from the pleural space. Following insertion of a chest tube, a chest x-ray is done to evaluate its placement and effectiveness.

Pharmacological

If a pleural effusion is small and does not interfere greatly with respiratory function, diuretics are used to promote removal of fluid from the pleural space. Furosemide (Lasix) and bumetanide (Bumex) may be given for this purpose. If empyema is present, specific therapy is used once the causative agent is identified. Relief of pain is a high priority. Analgesia that also decreases inflammation is preferred. Ketorolac trometha-

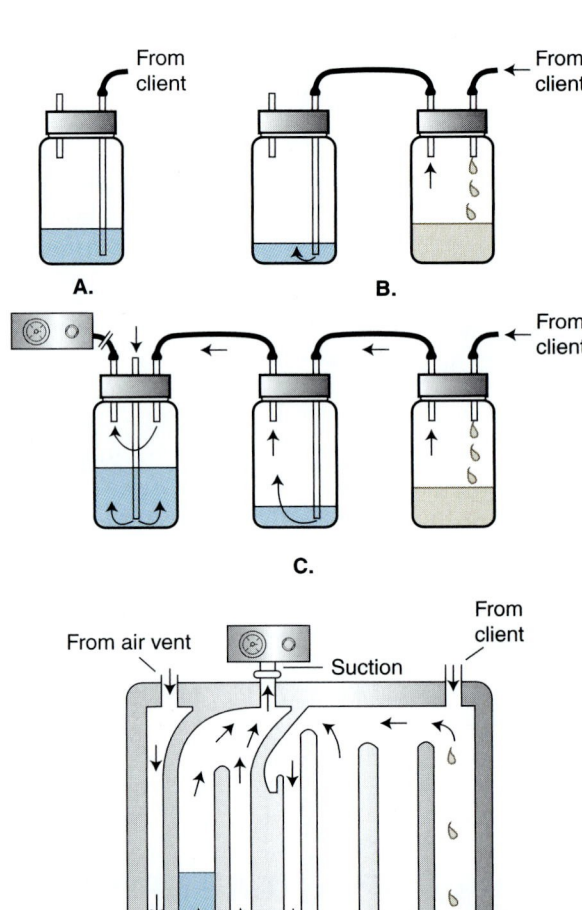

From client

A.

From client

B.

From client

C.

From air vent

Suction

From client

Water seal

Suction control

Drainage collection chambers

Chest drainage

D.

Figure 31-9 Underwater Seal Chest Drainage Devices: A. One-bottle system drains by gravity. B. Two-bottle system uses the first bottle for drainage and water seal and the second bottle for suction. C. Three-bottle system uses the first bottle for drainage, the second bottle for a water seal, and the third bottle for suction. D. One-piece, disposable plastic system combines three-bottle system into one device.

mine (Toradol) and other NSAIDs are often used. Severe pain will require narcotics such as morphine sulfate or meperidine (Demerol). If inflammation is extensive, corticosteroids such as hydrocortisone sodium succinate (Solu-Cortef) may be utilized.

Activity

The client's activity is limited to prevent fatigue. The client on bed rest is placed in a high Fowler's position to assist respirations.

▶ NURSING PROCESS

▶ Assessment

▶ Subjective Data

A nursing history is obtained from the client regarding onset, duration, and severity of symptoms. The client usually describes both chest pain that increases with each inspiration and difficulty breathing.

▶ Objective Data

The client's level of consciousness should be assessed, and the client's color, respiratory rate, and effort evaluated. Abnormalities in vital signs are noted. Breath sounds over the areas of involvement are diminished or absent. A pleural friction rub may be audible. Dysp-

PROFESSIONAL TIP

Assessment of Client with a Chest Tube

- Obtain vital signs as ordered.
- Be alert for dyspnea.
- On an intake and output (I&O) sheet, describe and record amount of drainage.
- Look for loops of tubing containing drainage.
- Monitor water level in the water seal. Fluctuation (called tidaling) should occur with respirations and will stop when lung is reexpanded, tubing is kinked, connections are not tight, or chest tube becomes dislodged.
- Keep chest drainage system below the level of the client's chest.
- Every 2 hours, monitor client's response to coughing and deep breathing.
- If chest tube is accidentally dislodged, cover opening and petrolatum gauze and apply pressure to prevent air from being sucked back into chest.

nea, cyanosis, and hypoxia occur proportional to the severity of the condition. If a chest tube is in place, the amount and color of drainage are assessed.

Nursing diagnoses for a client with a pleural effusion may include the following:

Nursing Diagnoses	Planning/Goals	Nursing Interventions
Pain related to inflammation of the pleura	Using a scale of 1 to 10, the client will verbalize a decrease in the level of pain.	Administer pain medications as ordered. Assist the client in attaining the position that allows for greatest comfort. Elevate the head of the bed. Provide diversional activities.
Gas Exchange, Impaired, related to compressed lung	The client will maintain an oxygen saturation of 95% or greater and a respiratory rate of 14 to 22 and will have clear breath sounds.	Monitor vital signs. Provide supplemental oxygen as ordered. Encourage the client to breathe deeply or use the incentive spirometer as ordered. Administer diuretics and anti-inflammatory medications as ordered. Assist the physician with the thoracentesis or the placement of a thoracotomy tube. Provide aseptic chest tube care. Collect specimen for culture and sensitivity and other studies.
Self-care Deficit related to mobility restriction	The client will increase self-care activities as mobility increases.	Assist the client with hygiene and self-care needs. Encourage participation in self-care activities within the limits of the physician's orders.
Activity Intolerance related to hypoxia secondary to pleural effusion	The client will increase activity without complaining of fatigue.	Stagger periods of activity with periods of rest. To prevent fatigue, plan activities around therapies.

Evaluation Each goal must be evaluated to determine how it has been met by the client.

ACUTE RESPIRATORY TRACT DISORDERS

Acute respiratory tract disorders include atelectasis, pulmonary embolism, pulmonary edema, adult respiratory distress syndrome, and acute respiratory failure.

ATELECTASIS

Atelectasis refers to the collapse of a lung or a portion of a lung. The most common cause of atelectasis is airway obstruction. A bronchiole becomes blocked with secretions, and the alveoli distal to it collapse (Figure 31-10). Airway obstruction of this nature is common after surgery and with immobility problems. Anesthesia, pain, narcotics, and immobility can cause hypoventilation and retention of secretions. Hypoventilation can cause atelectasis, and atelectasis increases hypoventilation. Atelectasis also occurs with compression of lung tissue, as is the case with pleural effusion or pneumothorax. An insufficient level of surfactant results in increased recoil properties of the lungs, leading to atelectasis.

Signs of respiratory distress are proportional to the amount of lung tissue involved. When large areas of the lung are involved, orthopnea or cyanosis may develop. Breath sounds are diminished or absent over collapsed areas. Late in the disease process, chest wall movement decreases on the affected side. Oxygenation decreases as demonstrated by ABGs or pulse oximetry. Pulse and respiratory rate increase as the heart and lungs work harder to meet the body's oxygen needs. Trapped secretions are a growth medium for microorganisms. An elevated temperature indicates secondary infection (pneumonia). Chest x-ray studies reveal the areas of collapse. Bronchoscopy (insertion of a bronchoscope through the nasal passages into the trachea) is used to directly visualize the area of obstruction and obtain a specimen for diagnostic purposes.

Medical–Surgical Management

Medical

The physician will order various measures to promote expansion of the lungs. Incentive spirometry and deep breathing and coughing exercises are ordered. Postural drainage along with percussion aids in the removal of any static secretions. If the client is unable to cough up secretions, suctioning of the respiratory tract is performed. Bronchoscopy may be done by the physician. Arterial blood gases and pulse oximetry are utilized to evaluate the need for supplemental oxygen. Oxygen is administered to maintain an oxygen saturation of 95% or greater.

Surgical

Clients with pneumothorax or pleural effusion as the underlying cause of atelectasis require removal of trapped air or fluid via thoracentesis or placement of a thoracotomy tube (refer to the sections on pleural effusion and pneumothorax). Atelectasis resulting from the growth of a tumor requires treatment of the tumor.

Pharmacological

Adequate pain control aids the client, particularly the surgical client, in being able to breathe deeply and cough. Client-controlled analgesia or a routine schedule of pain medications may be used to provide effective pain management. Aminophylline (Aminophyllin) and other bronchodilators may be used to open the airways. Mucolytic agents such as guaifenisin (Humibid) are used to liquefy respiratory tract secretions. Bronchodilators, such as albuterol sulfate (Ventolin), and mucolytics, such as acetylcysteine (Mucomyst), may also be administered via updraft or nebulizer treatments. The client with an infection requires treatment with an appropriate antibiotic such as ciprofloxacin hydrochloride (Cipro).

Diet

Unless otherwise contraindicated, fluids are encouraged to promote liquefaction of trapped respiratory secretions.

Activity

Activity promotes lung expansion. Immobile clients are turned a minimum of every 2 hours and are assisted in doing range-of-motion exercises. Surgical clients may do leg exercises as well as deep breathing and coughing. Ambulation is recommended if the client's condi-

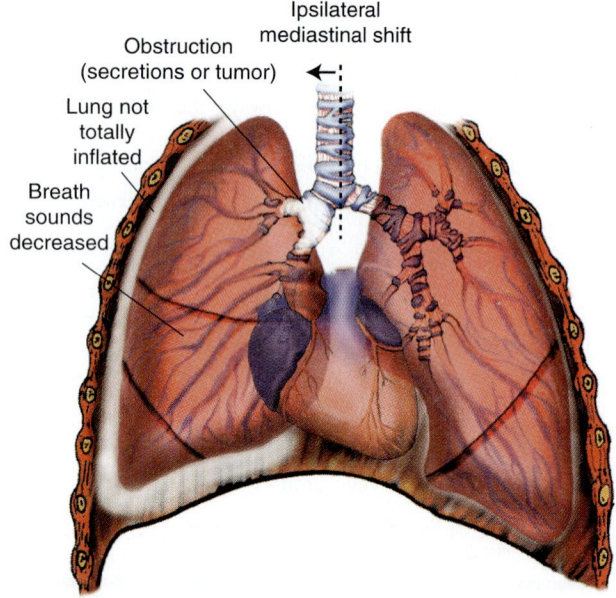

Figure 31-10 Atelectasis (collapsed lung)

tion allows. If the client is unable to walk, sitting up in a chair is encouraged. To prevent fatigue, rest periods are planned between activities.

▸ NURSING PROCESS

▸ Assessment

▸ Subjective Data

Clients who smoke or those who are immunocompromised or have known chronic respiratory or cardiovascular diseases are at increased risk of developing atelectasis. The client should be questioned about the onset, duration, and severity of symptoms such as pain, cough, and dyspnea. The client may complain or show signs of air hunger, shortness of breath, fatigue, and anxiety.

▸ Objective Data

The client must be assessed for changes in level of consciousness, an early sign of decreased oxygenation. The client should be periodically evaluated for dyspnea, tachypnea, cyanosis, and restlessness. Vital signs should be measured frequently, with particular attention to respiratory rate and effort. Auscultation reveals diminished or absent breath sounds over the areas of atelectasis. Crackles or sonorous wheezes may be heard if pneumonia develops. Objective indicators

of pain such as facial grimacing should be noted, and can be validated by subjective questioning. The effectiveness of the client's cough is assessed. A productive cough is evaluated for amount, color, consistency, and odor of secretions (Table 31-9).

Table 31-9 PATHOLOGIES ASSOCIATED WITH DIFFERENT TYPES OF SPUTUM

SPUTUM	PATHOLOGY
Color	
Mucoid	Tracheobronchitis, asthma
Yellow or green	Bacterial infection
Rust or blood tinged	Pneumonia, pulmonary infarction, TB
Black	Black lung disease
Pink, thin frothy	Pulmonary edema
Odor	
Foul smelling	Anaerobic infection

Adapted from Health Assessment & Physical Examination, by M. E. Z. Estes, 1998, Albany, NY: Delmar Publishers. Copyright 1998 by Delmar Publishers. Adapted with permission.

Nursing diagnoses for a client with atelectasis may include the following:

Nursing Diagnoses	Planning/Goals	Nursing Interventions
▸ *Knowledge Deficit related to the complications of surgery and/or immobility*	The client will verbalize the purpose of deep breathing, coughing, and activity following surgery and will demonstrate deep breathing and coughing.	Teach all preoperative and immobile clients to cough and breathe deeply at least every 2 hours. Have the client demonstrate coughing and deep breathing to ensure that learning has occurred. Teach the surgical client to splint the surgical incision to minimize discomfort that might occur with coughing and deep breathing. Instruct clients at risk for developing atelectasis in the use of incentive spirometry. Emphasize the importance of early ambulation and activity to promote lung expansion.
▸ *Gas Exchange, Impaired, related to decreased alveolar–capillary surface*	The client will have an oxygen saturation of 95% or greater, a respiratory rate of 14 to 22, and clear breath sounds.	Establish a schedule for coughing and deep breathing. Encourage clients to ambulate and/or sit up in a chair three to four times daily. Turn the immobile client every 2 hours or more frequently. Assess the client's vital signs and breath sounds every 4 hours or more frequently as situation warrants. Encourage fluids if the client's condition allows. Administer respiratory treatments as ordered. Administer medications as ordered. Assess secretions (sputum) for color, amount, consistency, and odor.

continued

Nursing Diagnoses	Planning/Goals	Nursing Interventions
▶ *Activity Intolerance related to hypoxia secondary to atelectasis*	The client will complete activity without complaints of shortness of breath, dyspnea, or fatigue.	Encourage some activity, such as walking, to promote lung expansion.
		Alternate periods of activity with periods of rest. Avoid client fatigue.
		Provide assistance with ADL as the client's condition requires.
		Place the client in a high or semi-Fowler's position to aid lung expansion.
		Position client on the unaffected side.

Evaluation Each goal must be evaluated to determine how it has been met by the client.

PULMONARY EMBOLISM

Pulmonary embolism develops when a bloodborne substance lodges in a branch of a pulmonary artery and obstructs flow. A common source of pulmonary embolism is a deep vein thrombus. Other sources are air from intravenous infusions; fat from long bone fractures; and amniotic fluid. The size and location of the emboli determine the severity and outcome of the condition.

Pulmonary emboli rarely develop before adulthood. As age increases, the risk for pulmonary embolism becomes greater due to the development of arteriosclerosis and other vascular changes associated with aging. Other factors that increase the risk for pulmonary embolism are heredity, smoking, peripheral vascular disease, diabetes mellitus, and oral contraceptive use.

Emboli interfere with gas exchange to the pulmonary circulation distal to the emboli, resulting in hypoxemia. The client complains of breathlessness and dyspnea. Pulse oximetry or ABGs will demonstrate the degree to which oxygenation has been affected. Obstruction of a main branch of a pulmonary artery can result in lung infarction and necrosis.

All clients at risk for pulmonary embolism should be observed for signs and symptoms of deep vein thrombosis, such as localized calf tenderness or swelling. Measures to prevent thrombus formation should be taken for these individuals. Any signs of thrombophlebitis should be immediately reported to the physician.

Signs and symptoms of pulmonary embolism are abrupt in onset. The client becomes anxious and restless. Sudden, sharp chest pains of a pleuritic nature (worse on inspiration) develop. Dyspnea and cough along with hemoptysis occur. Venous return is diminished, resulting in jugular venous distention. The client becomes diaphoretic. A low-grade fever develops in response to inflammation. A high temperature is indicative of lung infarction. Diagnosis of pulmonary embolism is accomplished by a ventilation/perfusion lung scan. Arterial blood gases show hypoxia and respiratory alkalosis. In severe cases, pulmonary angiography is performed to find the exact location of the clot.

Medical–Surgical Management

Medical

Preventive measures are instituted for the client at risk of developing deep vein thrombosis. Following surgery, antiembolism stockings and early ambulation are indicated. When hypoxia occurs, supplemental oxygen is given to increase oxygenation. The underlying cause of the pulmonary emboli is treated when identified.

Surgical

In severe cases, the physician may elect to remove the clot via an embolectomy. This procedure is usually done at the time of angiography. Clients who experience successive episodes of pulmonary embolism may require a venacaval plication. This surgical procedure involves placing a sieve-like device in the inferior vena cava to catch emboli before they enter the pulmonary circulation (see Figure 32-00 in Chapter 32).

Pharmacological

The client at risk of developing deep vein thrombosis and/or pulmonary embolism may be treated with enoxaparin sodium (Lovenox). Lovenox is often used in the postoperative client to prevent clot formation. After pulmonary emboli have developed, anticoagulation is ordered to prevent the formation of further clots. Heparin (Hep-Lock) is initially used to establish anticoagulation and is administered parenterally by either the intravenous or subcutaneous route. After adequate anticoagulation has been established, warfarin sodium (Coumadin) therapy is initiated. Coumadin is given orally and may be used long term on an outpatient basis. If the clot is large or lies in a branch of a main pulmonary artery, fibrinolytic therapy may be used. Fibrinolytics lyse, or dissolve, the clot versus inhibiting the formation of new clots. Examples of fibrinolytic agents are alteplase (Activase) and strepto-

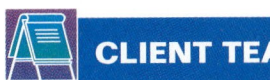

CLIENT TEACHING

Anticoagulant Therapy (Coumadin)

Stress the importance of the following:

- Follow-up laboratory testing
- Using a soft toothbrush to prevent trauma to the gums (bleeding)
- Inspecting the skin for bruises or petechiae
- Using an electric razor to avoid scratching skin
- Reporting nosebleeds, tarry stool, hematuria, or hematemesis to the physician
- Eating a consistent amount of green, leafy vegetables daily (differing amounts alter anticoagulant effects)
- Avoiding other medications (including aspirin) without approval from physician

LIFE CYCLE CONSIDERATIONS

Anticoagulant Therapy (Coumadin)

- In the female client, monitor menstrual flow for excessive amount
- For clients who are breastfeeding infants, observe infants for unexpected bleeding
- Monitor elderly clients closely, as they are especially sensitive to effects

kinase (Streptase). These agents may be administered intra-arterially at the site of the clot or intravenously to achieve a systemic effect. Narcotic analgesics such as morphine are ordered to control pain.

Diet

To prevent hemoconcentration leading to clot formation, fluids are encouraged. Unless contraindicated, fluids should be encouraged for the client at risk of developing pulmonary embolism.

Activity

To prevent the formation of clots, activity is encouraged. After a clot has formed, however, the client's activity is restricted to prevent the clot from moving and becoming an embolus. Activities such as sitting, crossing the knees, or prolonged bending at the hips are to be avoided, because these promote venous stasis.

▶ NURSING PROCESS

▶ Assessment

▶ Subjective Data

The client's history is obtained to identify potential risk factors for the development of pulmonary emboli. The client is asked about the onset, duration, and severity of symptoms. Shortness of breath, dyspnea, and severe pleuritic chest pain are abrupt in onset. Pain is evaluated as to onset, location, duration, severity, and character.

▶ Objective Data

Pulse oximetery measurements should be monitored. The client's respirations are rapid and shallow. Pallor progressing to cyanosis develops as oxygenation decreases. The client becomes diaphoretic. Increased anxiety or a change in level of consciousness may be the first indication of a pulmonary embolism. The pulse increases in response to anxiety and in an attempt to supply oxygen to the body's cells. Blood pressure may increase or decrease in response to hypoxia, anxiety, and pain. Temperature may elevate in response to inflammation and tissue necrosis. On auscultation, breath sounds may or may not be decreased. The jugular veins are distended.

Nursing diagnoses for a client with pulmonary embolism may include the following:

Nursing Diagnoses	Planning/Goals	Nursing Interventions
▶ *Gas Exchange, Impaired, related to alteration in pulmonary circulation*	The client will maintain an oxygen saturation of 95% or greater, have a respiratory rate of 14 to 22, and have color within normal limits.	Assess the client for indications of decreasing oxygenation.
		Auscultate breath sounds every 4 hours or more often.
		Assess peripheral pulses and capillary refill.
		Encourage deep breathing and coughing.
		Provide supplemental oxygen to maintain oxygen saturation at greater than 95% or as ordered.
		Administer subcutaneous heparin as ordered.
		After anticoagulation is established, administer Coumadin as ordered.
		Encourage fluids, unless contraindicated, to prevent hemoconcentration.

continued

Nursing Diagnoses	Planning/Goals	Nursing Interventions
▶ *Pain related to decreased perfusion of lung tissue*	Using a scale of 1 to 10, the client will indicate decreased pain.	Administer pain medication as ordered. Assist the client in assuming a position of comfort. If possible, place the client in a high Fowler's position to aid respiratory effort.
▶ *Injury, Risk for, related to anticoagulation/fibrinolytic therapy*	The client will be free of abnormal bleeding and maintain hemoglobin and hematocrit within normal limits.	Assess for evidence of bleeding. Monitor lab reports for activated partial thromboplastin time (APTT), international normalized ratio (INR), prothrombin time (PT), and hemoglobin and hematocrit levels. Evaluate blood pressure and pulse for signs of bleeding, i.e., rapid pulse and low blood pressure. Check stool for occult blood. Assess gums for bleeding.

Evaluation Each goal must be evaluated to determine how it has been met by the client.

PULMONARY EDEMA

Acute pulmonary edema is a life-threatening condition characterized by a rapid shift of fluid from plasma into the pulmonary interstitial tissue and the alveoli (Figure 31-11). As a result, gas exchange is markedly impaired. Pulmonary edema can occur as a result of severe left ventricular failure (i.e., following myocardial infarction), rapid administration of i.v. fluids, inhalation of noxious gases, or opiate or barbiturate overdose.

The hallmark of acute pulmonary edema is a cough producing a copious amount of frothy, blood-tinged sputum, often appearing pinkish. The client rapidly becomes dyspneic, orthopneic, and cyanotic. Anxiety ranging from restlessness to panic occurs. Heart and respiratory rate increase. Progressive crackles are heard in the lung fields on auscultation. Initially, fine crackles are present in the posterior bases of the lung. As pulmonary edema progresses, the crackles become increasingly coarser, louder, and more diffuse. Wheezes are heard in the presence of significant airway obstruction by fluid. Left untreated, the client deteriorates rapidly as oxygenation decreases.

Medical–Surgical Management

Medical

The goals of medical management are to remove fluid from the alveoli and pulmonary interstitial space, prevent further influx of fluid, and improve oxygenation. Arterial blood gases and pulse oximetry values are used to assess oxygenation. Oxygen is administered per physician's order when hypoxia is present.

Pharmacological

A diuretic such as furosemide (Lasix) is given to remove fluid, resulting in increased urinary output. When the pumping force of the left ventricle is impaired, a digitalis preparation, (i.e., digoxin [Lanoxin]) is given to improve the contractile force of the my-

ocardium. To prevent further influx of fluid into the lungs, venous pooling is enhanced. This also decreases the workload on the heart by limiting venous return. Morphine is used to promote vasodilatation and, thus, venous pooling and to relieve anxiety. Bronchodilators such as aminophylline (Aminophyllin) are administered to dilate airways obstructed with fluid.

Diet

To prevent fluid retention, the physician may order a diet restricted in sodium. Intake and output as well as daily weight are measured to monitor fluid balance.

Activity

The client is placed on bed rest to reduce the workload on the heart and lungs. High Fowler's position aids respiratory effort and enhances venous pooling. Activities are increased slowly according to the physician's orders and the client's ability to tolerate activity.

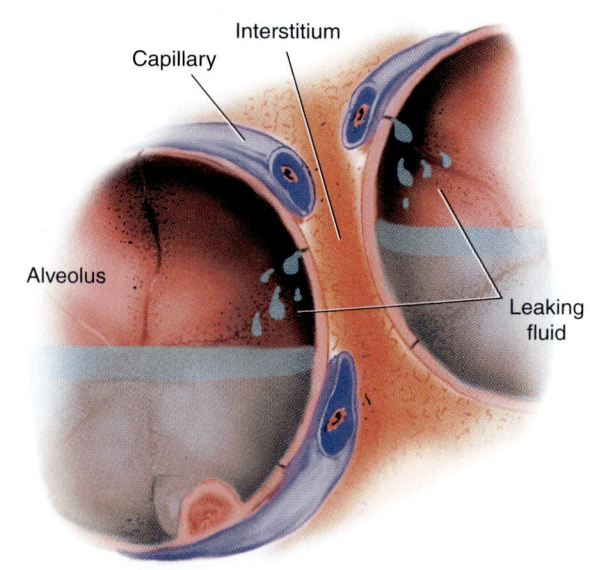

Figure 31-11 Pulmonary Edema

▶ NURSING PROCESS

▶ Assessment

▶ Subjective Data

The nurse must be aware of those conditions that predispose the client to pulmonary edema. The client may describe feeling anxious, breathless, and fatigued.

▶ Objective Data

Breath sounds are auscultated for the presence of crackles. Increasingly coarse and diffuse crackles are reported to the physician. The client's level of consciousness, respiratory rate and effort, and color should be assessed. Dyspnea, tachypnea, cyanosis and/or pallor may be present. Oxygenation is assessed via pulse oximetry or ABGs. A productive cough may be present, as may symptoms of CHF, such as rapid weight gain and peripheral edema. Pulse may be rapid and weak. Blood pressure may increase in response to anxiety and decreased oxygenation.

Nursing diagnoses for a client with pulmonary edema may include the following:

Nursing Diagnoses	Planning/Goals	Nursing Interventions
▶ *Gas Exchange, Impaired, related to fluid in the lung tissue*	The client will maintain an oxygen saturation of 95% or greater and will have respiratory rate and color and blood gases within normal limits and clear breath sounds.	Place the client in high Fowler's or orthopneic position (sitting upright).
		Continually assess oxygenation with ABG or pulse oximetry measurements and provide supplemental oxygen to maintain an oxygen saturation of 95% or greater or per physician's order.
		Frequently assess respiratory rate, breath sounds, apical heart rate, and blood pressure. Administer respiratory treatments as ordered.
		Assist the client with activities to reduce the workload on the heart and lungs, and alternate periods of activity with periods of rest to prevent client fatigue. Administer medications as ordered and evaluate the effectiveness of each. Monitor lab reports for electrolyte values.
▶ *Fluid Volume Excess related to altered tissue permeability*	The client's weight will return to normal.	Weigh client daily.
		Monitor I&O.
		Frequently assess the client for peripheral edema.
		Provide the client with a low-salt diet as ordered.
		Administer diuretics per order and evaluate their effectiveness.
		Monitor lab reports for electrolyte values.
		Monitor the rate at which intravenous fluids are given.

Evaluation Each goal must be evaluated to determine how it has been met by the client.

ADULT RESPIRATORY DISTRESS SYNDROME

Adult respiratory distress syndrome (ARDS) is a life-threatening condition characterized by severe dyspnea, hypoxemia, and diffuse pulmonary edema. The condition usually follows a major assault on multiple body systems or severe lung trauma. Underlying causes include trauma, sepsis, coronary artery bypass surgery, major thoracic or vascular surgery, renal failure, severe pulmonary infections, inhalation lung injuries, and acute drug poisoning. Adult respiratory distress syndrome is also called noncardiogenic pulmonary edema, shock lung, progressive pulmonary congestion, or traumatic wet lung. The term *adult respiratory distress syndrome* more accurately describes the pathophysiology underlying this condition.

During the initial assault on the body, the pulmonary capillary membrane is damaged; this allows fluid to leak from the vascular system into the pulmonary interstitial tissue and the alveoli themselves. Gas exchange is severely impaired due to the damage to the pulmonary capillary membrane and the presence of fluid in the alveoli. The surfactant is rendered inactive, resulting in the collapse of the alveoli, further reducing gas exchange. Hypoxemia that is resistant to conventional oxygen therapy then develops.

The client with ARDS is critically ill, as reflected by severe dyspnea, tachypnea, and cyanosis. Arterial blood gases will show PaO_2 less than 70 mm Hg, $PaCO_2$ more than 35 mm Hg, bicarbonate ion less than 22 mEq/L, and initially elevated then steadily decreasing pH. The ABGs and pulse oximetry reveal severe hypoxemia and progressive respiratory and metabolic acidosis. On auscultation, the lung fields are filled with diffuse coarse crackles and sonorous wheezes. The client will have a productive cough yielding blood-tinged sputum. Chest x-ray will show widely scattered infiltrates, often referred to as a "white out."

Medical–Surgical Management

Medical

The client with ARDS is cared for in the intensive care unit. The underlying cause of ARDS is ascertained and treated; until that time, supportive care is given. Mechanical ventilatory support is necessary, with multiple other systems often also being supported. A mechanical ventilator allows the oxygen percentage, pulmonary pressure, and lung volume to be controlled. Oxygenation is monitored with ABGs and pulse oximetry. Respiratory secretions are removed by frequent bronchial suctioning.

Pharmacological

Pharmacological therapy includes high doses of corticosteriods such as hydrocortisone sodium succinate (Solu-Cortef) or methylprednisolone sodium succinate (Solu-Medrol). Furosemide (Lasix) and other diuretics are given to remove fluids and increase uri-

PROFESSIONAL TIP

Client on a Mechanical Ventilator

Check the following:
- Type of ventilator (e.g., Servo, Bear)
- FiO$_2$ setting
- Mode being used (e.g., assist, intermittent mandatory)
- Amount of positive end-expiratory pressure
- Rate and tidal volume
- Peak inspiratory pressure
- Temperature of the humidification
- Alarm set

nary output. Aminophylline (Aminophyllin) is administered to open the bronchi. While the client is on the mechanical ventilator, pancuronium bromide (Pavulon) is given to suppress the client's own respiratory effort. Blood pressure can fall dangerously low, and vasopressors such as dopamine hydrochloride (Intropin) may be required to maintain the blood pressure within an acceptable range.

Diet

Total parenteral nutrition (TPN) may be given to the client, especially during the acute phase of the illness. When possible, enteral feedings are preferred.

Activity

The client with ARDS will be on bed rest. Special beds that provide movement and pressure adjustment prevent the complications associated with immobility.

▶ NURSING PROCESS

▶ Assessment

▶ Subjective Data

The client history is typically gathered from family members or significant others, as the client is usually too ill to communicate.

▶ Objective Data

The client's level of consciousness and response to stimuli are assessed, and the client is observed for restlessness and anxiety. Vital signs should be measured every 15 minutes or more often if the client is critically ill. Heart rate is increased, and arrhythmias may be present. Blood pressure is usually low. Respiratory rate, rhythm, and effort are assessed for signs of dyspnea, nasal flaring, cyanosis, tachypnea, and other indications of respiratory distress. Arterial blood gas and pulse oximetry values are assessed to evaluate oxygenation and acid–base balance. Diffuse, coarse crackles and wheezes are heard throughout the lung fields.

Nursing diagnoses for a client with ARDS may include the following:

Nursing Diagnoses	Planning/Goals	Nursing Interventions
▶ Gas Exchange, Impaired, related to pulmonary capillary membrane damage	The client will have an oxygen saturation of 95% or greater, ABGs within normal limits, and respiratory rate and effort within normal limits.	Provide adequate oxygenation and ventilation as ordered.
		Monitor ABGs and pulse oximetry to evaluate oxygenation and acid–base balance.
		Assess the client's respiratory rate and effort and auscultate the lungs frequently.
		Suction the respiratory tract as necessary to remove excess secretions.
		Provide oral care frequently.

continued

Nursing Diagnoses	Planning/Goals	Nursing Interventions
▶ *Anxiety related to the condition and mechanical ventilation*	The client, if able, will verbalize a decrease in anxiety or will exhibit fewer objective signs of anxiety, such as restlessness and facial grimacing.	Describe care and purposes to the client.
		Allow rest periods between periods of activity to avoid overwhelming the client with stimuli.
		Plan care to allow for uninterrupted rest.
		Allow family and significant others to visit and participate in care, as appropriate.
		Assess the client for signs of sensory overload/deprivation.

Evaluation Each goal must be evaluated to determine how it has been met by the client.

ACUTE RESPIRATORY FAILURE

Acute respiratory failure is not a disease entity in and of itself; rather, the term is used to refer to conditions wherein there is a failure of the respiratory system as a whole. This condition occurs as a result of the client's literally becoming too tired to continue the "work" of breathing. Mechanical ventilatory support is required during the acute phase. Clients with preexisting pulmonary conditions coupled with acute respiratory tract infections are at risk of developing acute respiratory failure.

CHRONIC RESPIRATORY TRACT DISORDERS

Chronic obstructive pulmonary disease (COPD), asthma, chronic bronchitis, emphysema, and bronchiectasis are discussed following.

CHRONIC OBSTRUCTIVE PULMONARY DISEASE

Chronic obstructive pulmonary disease, also called chronic obstructive lung disease (COLD), describes a broad category of respiratory conditions with a variety of etiologic factors. Chronic obstructive pulmonary disease is characterized by chronic airflow limitation. Changes within the lungs lead to a narrowing of the bronchial airways, excessive mucous secretions within the airways, and an increase in the size of the airways distal to the terminal bronchioles (the alveoli) and resultant trapping of air. The conditions most often associated with COPD are: asthma, chronic bronchitis, emphysema, and bronchiectasis.

ASTHMA

Asthma is a condition characterized by intermittent airway obstruction in response to a variety of stimuli.

The epithelial lining of the airways responds by becoming inflamed and edematous. Bronchospasm occurs in the smooth muscles of the bronchi and bronchioles. Secretions increase in viscosity. Elastic recoil decreases. All of these changes result in a reduction of the diameter of the airways and in breathing difficulty on inspiration. Over time, the changes may become chronic, and COPD results. Some clients who develop asthma in childhood experience spontaneous recovery.

Asthma may be classified as extrinsic or intrinsic. Extrinsic asthma is caused by substances outside the body that precipitate the asthma response, such as pollen, house dust, or food additives. Intrinsic asthma is diagnosed when no extrinsic factor can be identified and the asthma is the result of internal factors such as emotional stress, exercise, or fatigue. Allergies; environmental factors such as air pollution; heredity; exercise; and psychological factors have been indicated in predisposing an individual to asthma. An asthma attack that does not respond to treatment and persists is known as **status asthmaticus**.

LIFE CYCLE CONSIDERATIONS

Asthma and Age

In children:

- Asthma attacks often become less severe and less frequent as the child ages;
- Asthma attacks are usually associated with definite allergens; and
- Oral bronchodilators should be taken 30 to 60 minutes before exercise, inhaled bronchodilators, 15 to 20 minutes before exercise.

In adults:

- Asthma attacks usually become more severe and more frequent as the individual ages, and
- Asthma attacks are usually not associated with definite allergens.

The hallmark of an asthma attack is sudden onset of wheezing, increasing dyspnea, and chest tightness. Mild asthma can usually be controlled by routine medication. Severe asthma attacks usually occur at night and require extra medication. With severe attacks, wheezing may be audible to the unaided ear. Expiratory wheezes are common as air attempts to escape through the narrowed airways. Both inspiratory and expiratory wheezes may be heard. The respiratory rate rises initially, but as the client tires, the rate may decrease. Nasal flaring and costal and sternal retractions may be present, particularly in the young client. The client uses accessory muscles to assist respiratory effort. Cough occurs as the respiratory secretions become thick and block the airways. Cyanosis and a decrease in oxygen saturation occur. Heart rate elevates, as may blood pressure. The client becomes anxious and may complain of a sense of impending doom. These responses are thought to be caused by a release of catecholamines. Values of ABGs indicate hypoxia and respiratory acidosis. Chest x-ray shows hyperinflation of the lungs. Pulmonary function tests reveal an abnormal flow rate and lung volume. With a severe asthma attack, apnea and sudden death can occur in minutes.

Medical–Surgical Management

Medical

In addition to medications, treatment for asthma may include manipulating known triggers. The client with allergies should avoid specific antigens, such as animal hair, pollens, and dietary factors, that might bring on an attack. Some clients with asthma are aided by control of psychological stressors. Routine physical exercise is beneficial in treating exercise-induced asthma. The client with asthma should be told to avoid other respiratory irritants such as cigarette smoke and air pollution.

Pharmacological

The primary treatment for an acute asthma attack is pharmacological. A combination of medications is used to open the narrowed airways. Medications used to dilate the bronchi include bronchodilators such as

HOME HEALTH CARE

Asthma
- Prohibit smoking in the home, especially if a child has asthma
- Use a humidifier, especially in the bedroom of the person with asthma
- Use fans to circulate air

CLIENT TEACHING

Use of Nebulizer
Advise clients to:
- Keep nebulizer with them at all times,
- Take only two to three whiffs every 4 hours
- Call physician if nebulizer is needed more frequently.

aminophylline (Aminophyllin) and terbutaline sulfate (Brethine, Bricanyl); beta agonists such as epinephrine (Primatene Mist) and albuterol sulfate (Ventolin); and anticholinergics such as atropine sulfate and ipratropium bromide (Atrovent). Corticosteroids such as prednisone (Delatsone) are utilized to decrease inflammation. Mucolytic agents such as acetylcysteine (Mucomyst) aid in liquefying secretions. Supplemental oxygen may also be given.

Diet

Adequate fluid intake should be maintained to promote liquefaction of secretions.

Activity

The nurse should incorporate several rest periods into the day. Relaxation techniques can be used to manage anxiety. The client should not overexert to the point of dyspnea, wheezing, or fatigue. If overexertion occurs, the client should sit down and sip warm water. Doing so promotes slower, regular breathing, as well as bronchodilation, and loosens secretions.

▶ NURSING PROCESS

▶ Assessment

▶ Subjective Data

A detailed history is taken regarding exposure to triggering stimuli prior to past asthma attacks. Also ascertained are the onset, duration, and severity of symptoms such as dyspnea.

▶ Objective Data

The effectiveness of ventilation should be noted. Wheezes are evaluated as to their duration, location, and the phase of respiration during which they occur (e.g., inspiration). Wheezes heard without the aid of a stethoscope are called **audible wheezes**. Respiratory rate, depth, rhythm and effort; position assumed; and client color are evaluated. Monitoring of pulse oximetry or lab reports of ABG values is done to determine oxygenation and acid–base balance. If sputum is produced, its color, amount, viscosity, and odor are noted.

Nursing diagnoses for a client with asthma may include the following:

Nursing Diagnoses	Planning/Goals	Nursing Interventions
▶ *Breathing Pattern, Ineffective, related to narrowed airways*	The client will have respiratory rate and color within normal limits, clear breath sounds on auscultation, and ABG or pulse oximetry values within normal limits.	Assist the client in assuming a position that facilitates ventilation. Administer medication as ordered. Assist the client in the use of inhalers and aerosol treatments. Assess oxygenation by ABG or pulse oximetry values, as ordered. Administer supplemental oxygen, as ordered. Frequently assess respiratory rate and effort as well as color as client's condition dictates. Auscultate the lung fields for presence of wheezes. If sputum is produced, note its color, amount, viscosity, and odor. Frequently assess vital signs as client's condition dictates. Unless otherwise contraindicated, encourage fluid intake to promote liquefaction of respiratory secretions.
▶ *Knowledge Deficit related to asthma, asthma treatment, and individual triggers for asthma attacks*	The client will verbalize an understanding of both the pathophysiology and treatment of asthma, including the medications taken and their purposes and side effects. The client will also identify individual triggers and means of avoiding these triggers.	Teach client about the disease process. Teach client and family the purpose, effect, adverse effects, side effects, and use of all prescribed medications, especially inhalers and respiratory aerosol equipment. Assist client in establishing a medication schedule that will facilitate regular and timely taking of medications. Instruct the client to use the inhaler prior to meals to aid in breathing while eating. If the client is taking steroids, teach to rinse mouth after using the inhaler so as to prevent fungal infection. Encourage exercise because it increases respiratory reserve and improves overall physical condition. Assist client in identifying triggering stimuli and ways to avoid them. Teach client and family signs and symptoms of asthma attacks and respiratory tract infections. Teach client to avoid crowded areas and close contact with persons with infections.
▶ *Anxiety related to perceived threat of dying*	The client will verbalize a decrease in anxiety.	Provide the client with explanations for all care. Provide care in a calm, unhurried manner. Plan care to allow the client uninterrupted periods of rest. Allow the client to make decisions regarding care, if possible. Provide the client with opportunities to discuss anxiety with staff, family, or significant others.

Evaluation Each goal must be evaluated to determine how it has been met by the client.

CHRONIC BRONCHITIS

Bronchitis is an inflammation of the bronchial tree accompanied by hypersecretion of mucus. The condition becomes chronic if an individual has an infection with a productive cough at least 3 months a year for two consecutive years. Constant irritation of the bronchi results in hypertrophy of the mucus-secreting glands. The bronchioles fill with exudate, and subsequent infections are common. The alveoli adjacent to the bronchioles eventually become damaged and fibrosed. Environmental factors, especially cigarette smoke, play an important role in the development of chronic bronchitis. Certain individuals may have a hereditary predisposition to developing chronic bronchitis. Exposure to cold, damp air coupled with repeated respiratory infections has been identified as a cause of chronic bronchitis.

The client usually has a history of recurrent respiratory infections, dyspnea, cyanosis, and chronic or recurrent cough yielding copious amounts of sputum. Often, the sputum is purulent or green in color. Over the course of time, the chest wall configuration becomes slightly distended. There are coarse crackles present throughout the lung fields. Breath sounds may be diminished or absent over the periphery of the lung fields. Elevation of pulmonary artery pressure results in increased workload for the right ventricle and in signs and symptoms of right-sided CHF, such as peripheral edema and fatigue. Arterial blood gases reveal increased $PaCO_2$ and decreased PaO_2. The red blood cell count elevates, as do hemoglobin and hematocrit. The increases in the amounts of red blood cells and hemoglobin represent an attempt by the body to compensate for the lower oxygen level. Chest x-ray shows hyperexpansion of the lungs. When CHF occurs, the chest x-ray also shows an enlarged heart.

Medical–Surgical Management

Medical

The goals of medical treatment are to decrease symptoms of airway irritation, decrease airway obstruction related to secretions and inflammation, prevent infection, maintain oxygenation, and increase the client's exercise tolerance. Respiratory therapy includes the use of updraft (nebulizer) and aerosol treatments along with percussion and postural drainage. Humidification of inspired air helps liquefy secretions. Supplemental oxygen is administered based on ABG or pulse oximetry measurements.

Pharmacological

Bronchodilators such as theophylline (Theo-Dur), oxtriphylline (Choledyl), terbutaline sulfate (Brethine), and ipratropium bromide (Atrovent) are given to open the airways. Inhalation or aerosol treatments with bronchodilators such as albuterol (Ventolin) or metaproterenol sulfate (Alupent) are often used in conjunction with oral medications to control symptoms. Prednisone (Meticorten), a corticosteroid, is given as short-term therapy for acute exacerbations. If steroids are required on a long-term basis, they may be given by inhalation to prevent some adverse systemic effects. Examples of inhalation forms of steroids are beclomethasone dipropionate (Beclovent) and triamcinolone acetonide (Azmacort). In addition to agents that open the airways, medications that liquefy respiratory secretions are administered. Acetylcysteine (Mucomyst) may be given by inhalation. Mucolytic medications such as guaifenesin (Humibid LA) may be given orally. If infection occurs, broad spectrum antibiotics such as cephalexin monohydrate (Keflex), cefaclor (Ceclor), erythromycin base (E-Mycin), or penicillin V potassium (Pen-Vee K) are given. Immunization against influenza viruses and *Streptococcus pneumoniae* are recommended.

The client with chronic bronchitis who also suffers from CHF will receive medications to aid the function of the weakened heart. Digoxin (Lanoxin) is given to strengthen the force of the contraction of the heart muscle. Diuretics such as furosemide (Lasix) are given to remove fluid by increasing urinary output. Supplemental potassium chloride (K-Dur, Kay-Ciel elixir) is administered if the client's level of potassium decreases due to the effect of the diuretic.

Diet

The client is encouraged to eat a well-balanced diet. If the client also has CHF, sodium intake is restricted. Unless contraindicated, fluids are encouraged.

Activity

Activity is restricted to decrease the workload on the heart and lungs. With acute exacerbations, the client is placed on bed rest. The level of activity is then slowly increased based on the client's ability to tolerate activity.

Programs consisting of breathing exercises and graded (easy to difficult) exercise regimes are utilized to assist the client in achieving the maximum level of activity tolerance. The client is taught breath-retaining exercises such as coughing techniques, pursed-lip breathing, and diaphragmatic or abdominal breathing. Graded exercise regimens are similar to those used for cardiac rehabilitation, except that the client is monitored from a respiratory standpoint while exercising. The goal is to increase the client's capacity for all ADL.

▶ NURSING PROCESS

▶ Assessment

▶ Subjective Data

A thorough past medical history is obtained, including informaton about the onset, duration, and severity of symptoms. The client may describe fatigue and difficult breathing.

▶ Objective Data

Changes in level of consciousness or mental status should be noted, as should the client's color and respiratory rate and effort. The position the client assumes to aid respiratory effort and the use of accessory muscles must be noted. Arterial blood gases or pulse oximetry values are reviewed. Lung fields should be auscultated for crackles and diminished breath sounds. Color, amount, viscosity, and odor of sputum are noted. Specimens are obtained for culture and sensitivity, if indicated. Vital signs must be frequently measured. The pulse may be elevated and irregular. Blood pressure may be elevated or low. An elevated temperature may indicate infection. Assessment of the client for peripheral edema, neck vein distention, and rapid weight gain should be performed.

Nursing diagnoses for a client with chronic bronchitis may include the following:

Nursing Diagnoses	Planning/Goals	Nursing Interventions
▶ *Airway Clearance, Ineffective, related to thicker and increased amounts of respiratory secretions*	The client's color, respiratory rate, and ABG values will be within normal limits.	Frequently assess level of consciousness, mental status, vital signs, respiratory effort, and color.
		Auscultate breath sounds at least every 4 hours.
		Obtain sputum specimens as ordered, and assess sputum for amount, viscosity, color, and odor.
		Assist the client in assuming the position that most aids respiratory effort, usually an upright position.
		Administer oxygen and respiratory treatments as ordered and assess their effectiveness.
		Evaluate the results of diagnostic and laboratory tests (ABGs) and notify the physician of abnormalities.
		Alternate care with periods of uninterrupted rest.
		Administer antibiotics and bronchodilators as ordered.
		Provide the client with a well-balanced diet.
		Unless otherwise contraindicated, encourage fluids.
		Assess the client for signs and symptoms of CHF, i.e., fine crackles heard on auscultation, peripheral edema, weight gain, and fatigue.
		Report any signs and symptoms of CHF to the physician.
▶ *Knowledge Deficit related to chronic bronchitis and its treatment and prevention*	The client will verbalize signs and symptoms to report to the physician, safety precautions to take with medication and equipment, medication and respiratory treatment regimen, and techniques for facilitating breathing.	Teach the client to avoid respiratory infections, maintain adequate nutrition, increase fluid intake, and obtain adequate rest.
		Instruct the client in the purpose, expected effects, and side effects of medications.
		Teach the client to administer respiratory treatments and medications prior to eating to aid in breathing.
		If the client is taking steroids, instruct to rinse mouth following administration of inhalers.
		Teach the client to self-administer oxygen.
		Provide information regarding both the use of equipment and safety measures for the equipment.
		Refer the client to an established respiratory rehabilitation program. If such a program is not available, instruct the client in breathing techniques.
		Encourage regular exercise within the client's limitations.
		Encourage the client to obtain immunization against influenza viruses and *Streptococcus pneumoniae*.

Evaluation Each goal must be evaluated to determine how it has been met by the client.

EMPHYSEMA

Emphysema is a complex and destructive lung disease wherein air accumulates in the tissues of the lungs. The airways become fibrotic and lose their elasticity, resulting in narrower lumens. Airflow is impeded as it leaves the lungs (i.e., during expiration). The alveoli distal to these airways become overdistended with trapped air (Figure 31-12). Rupture of the alveolar wall may occur. The alveolar capillary membrane is destroyed, resulting in a loss of available area for gas exchange. Emphysema is the leading cause of respiratory death in the United States. Cigarette smoking is the most common cause of emphysema. Other factors such as air pollution and exposure to occupational respiratory irritants have been identified as contributing to the development of emphysema. Deficiency in alpha-1-antitrypsin is a familial disorder that leads to the development of emphysema.

Emphysema develops slowly over a period of years. The client first notes increasing dyspnea in response to activity. The degree of dyspnea corresponds to the degree of hypoxia, which is usually mild at rest but becomes increasingly severe in response to activity. In advanced stages of the disease, hypoxia is evident even at rest. Sputum produced is scant and mucoid in nature, unless an infection is present. When infection is present, a cough yielding purulent sputum occurs.

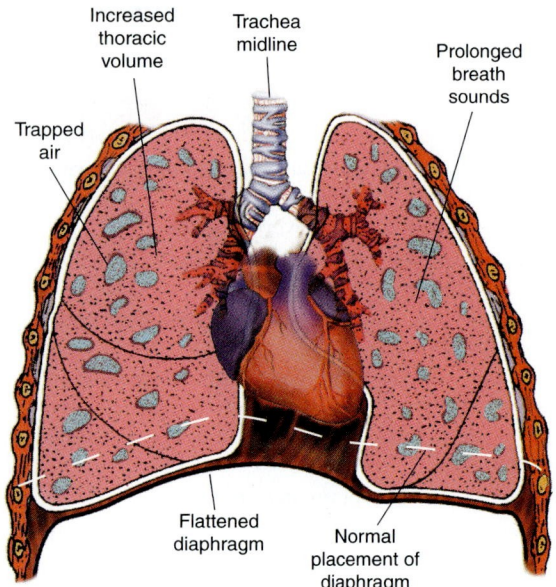

Figure 31-12 Emphysema

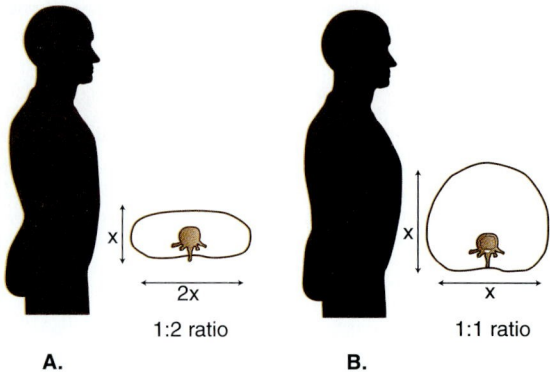

Figure 31-13 Changes in Chest Configuration and Posture: A. The normal ratio of the anterior posterior diameter to the lateral diameter is 1:2. B. With a barrel chest, the ratio between the diameters is 1:1.

The client's complexion appears ruddy, or reddish in color. The chest becomes barrel shaped (Figure 31-13) as the chest cage enlarges to accommodate distended lung tissues. The respiratory rate elevates. The expiratory phase of respiration becomes increasingly difficult. Accessory muscles are used to aid respiratory effort. Due to destruction of the alveoli, bronchial breath sounds are heard in the periphery of the lungs. As the disease progresses, breath sounds diminish and eventually disappear over the periphery of the lungs. Arterial blood gases reveal varying degrees of hypoxia depending on the severity of the disease. Hypercapnia, or retention of carbon dioxide, is not as likely as with chronic bronchitis. The extra effort required to breathe increases metabolic need, resulting in weight loss. Chest x-ray reveals hyperinflated lung tissue and a flattened diaphragm, which has been displaced by distended lung tissues. Pulmonary function studies reveal a decrease in expiratory volume. Polycythemia and elevation of hemoglobin and hematocrit occur in response to prolonged hypoxia.

Medical–Surgical Management

Medical

The goals of treatment are to prevent further damage to the lung tissues, maintain adequate oxygenation, prevent infection, and improve the client's activity tolerance. The client who smokes should stop or, at least, decrease the number of cigarettes smoked daily. Supplemental oxygen is given to maintain oxygenation. The client with advanced emphysema and severe, chronic hypoxia may be maintained at PaO_2 of 55 to 59 mm Hg and/or oxygen saturation of 90% or greater. As with chronic bronchitis, the client with em-physema is given supplemental oxygen at the lowest possible flow rate, usually 2 to 3 L, to prevent respiratory and CNS depression.

Pharmacological

The client with emphysema receives many of the same medications used to treat chronic bronchitis. To open airways that have become fibrotic, theophylline and similar preparations are used. Steroids may be required for exacerbations. The client with emphysema usually does not need mucolytic agents, unless infection is present. Antibiotics are used to treat and prevent respiratory tract infections. The client should receive immunizations against influenza and *Streptococcus pneumoniae*. The client who smokes may use nicotine polacrilex gum (Nicorette [gum]) or nicotine transdermal system (Nicoderm) to aid in smoking cessation.

Diet

The client with emphysema requires a diet high in carbohydrates to supply the energy necessary for breathing. If a negative nitrogen balance exists due to the client's using muscle tissue to provide energy, a diet high in protein is ordered. Dietary supplements, such as Ensure may be needed to supply the necessary calories and nutrients. Unless contraindicated, fluids are encouraged.

 CULTURAL CONSIDERATIONS

Skin Color

- For a client with highly pigmented skin, establish a baseline skin color
- Observe skin surfaces that have the least amount of pigmentation, such as the palms, the soles of the feet, the abdomen, or the inner aspect of forearms

Activity

The client is placed on bed rest. Level of activity is increased based on the client's oxygenation. Oxygen saturation is evaluated periodically as the activity level is increased to determine the effect of activity on oxygenation.

Health Promotion

The client with emphysema benefits from a respiratory rehabilitation program. The client is taught breathing exercises similar to those taught to the client with chronic bronchitis. A graded exercise program is also used for the client with emphysema. Group programs that aid in smoking cessation are useful for the client who smokes.

▶ NURSING PROCESS

▶ Assessment

▶ Subjective Data

Included in the history is information regarding the timing of dyspnea, those factors that exacerbate dyspnea, and those factors that relieve dyspnea.

▶ Objective Data

If cough is present, the client is assessed for other indications of infection, such as elevated white blood cell count and fever. The cough is evaluated as to onset, duration, and severity. Any sputum produced is assessed for color, amount, viscosity, and odor. Vital signs are assessed frequently. An elevated pulse may indicate hypoxia and/or infection. Auscultation of the lungs will reveal the presence of adventitious, diminished, or absent breath sounds. The position the client assumes to aid respiratory effort, and the client's color, respiratory rate and effort, and use of accessory muscles to aid breathing should be noted. Evaluation of the client's nutritional status includes weighing the client and measuring nutrient and caloric intake. The results of laboratory and diagnostic tests should also be reviewed.

Nursing diagnoses for a client with emphysema may include the following:

Nursing Diagnoses	Planning/Goals	Nursing Interventions
▶ Gas Exchange, impaired, related to destruction of the alveoli	The client's respiratory rate, color, and ABG values will be within normal limits.	Assess the client's level of consciousness and mental status.
		Frequently evaluate the client's respiratory rate, respiratory effort, and color.
		Evaluate oxygenation with ABG and/or pulse oximetry measurement.
		Assess the effect of activity on oxygenation, particularly when activity is being increased.
		Provide supplemental oxygen as ordered.
		Auscultate the lungs and report abnormalities to the physician.
		Assess the client's vital signs: Heart rate and temperature elevations may indicate infection. An elevated pulse can also indicate hypoxia.
		Review the results of diagnostic and laboratory tests and report abnormalities.
		Administer medications and respiratory treatments as ordered.
		Assist the client in assuming the position that offers the most comfort and that most aids respiratory effort.
		Instruct the client in breathing techniques, such as pursed-lip breathing.
▶ Activity Intolerance related to hypoxia	The client will complete activity without experiencing fatigue or dyspnea.	Assist the client with ADL and hygiene needs.
		Plan care and treatments to allow the client uninterrupted periods of rest.
		As activity increases, assess the effects on oxygenation.
		Allow the client to rest prior to and after meals.

continued

Nursing Diagnoses	Planning/Goals	Nursing Interventions
▶ *Nutrition: Altered, Less than body requirements, related to increased energy requirements to maintain respiration*	The client will achieve or maintain a weight within normal limits for height.	Assess the client's weight and evaluate in relation to the client's height.
		Evaluate the client's diet for nutritional adequacy.
		Review the client's food likes and dislikes.
		Provide a well-balanced diet based on the client's likes and dislikes.
		Provide nutritional supplements as ordered.
		Avoid activities or procedures prior to meals that might reduce appetite (e.g., enemas).
		Administer medications and respiratory treatments prior to meals to aid in breathing.

Evaluation Each goal must be evaluated to determine how it has been met by the client.

BRONCHIECTASIS

Bronchiectasis is chronic dilation of the bronchi. The main causes of this disorder are pulmonary TB infection, chronic upper respiratory tract infections, and complications of other respiratory disorders of childhood, particularly cystic fibrosis. The bronchi become distended and eventually lose their elastic recoil property. The mucociliary blanket's function becomes impaired, and secretions thicken. Secretions accumulate in the bronchi, resulting in a medium for infection. As with chronic bronchitis and emphysema, airflow is hindered, reducing gas exchange.

The client with bronchiectasis complains of a frequent or chronic productive cough. Other complaints include dyspnea, weight loss, and fatigue. Sputum is thick. When infection is present, the sputum is purulent. Crackles, which clear with coughing, are heard scattered throughout the lung fields and are more prominent on the client's arising in the morning. Accessory muscles are used to aid respiration. Over a period of time, right-sided CHF develops, and symptoms such as peripheral edema occur. Arterial blood gases reveal elevated $PaCO_2$, decreased PaO_2, and respiratory acidosis. Sputum analysis reveals whether infection is present, the causative organism, and the organism's resistance or sensitivity to specific antibiotics. Polycythemia and elevated hemoglobin and hematocrit levels are revealed in the complete blood count. Chest x-ray shows slight hyperinflation of lung tissue and, in the presence of CHF, cardiomegaly. Respiratory flow rate decreases, and lung volume increases, as demonstrated by pulmonary function studies. Table 31-10 compares asthma, chronic bronchitis, emphysema, and bronchiectasis.

Medical–Surgical Management

Medical

Medical treatment is aimed at removing respiratory secretions, eliminating and preventing infection, and maintaining adequate oxygenation. Percussion and postural drainage are used to aid in the removal of secretions. Aerosol and updraft respiratory treatments may be ordered prior to percussion and drainage. If the client is unable to expectorate secretions, bronchial suctioning is performed. The physician may perform a bronchoscopy to remove especially tenacious and copious secretions. Arterial blood gases and/or pulse oximetry values are evaluated to assess the need for supplemental oxygen. Daily weight and I&O are performed to detect signs of CHF. Pulmonary function studies are performed to evaluate the severity of lung damage. Genetic studies and genetic counseling are indicated for the family and client with cystic fibrosis.

Pharmacological

Acetylcysteine (Mucomyst) and other mucolytic agents are given to promote liquefaction of respiratory secretions. Antibiotics are ordered to treat and prevent infection. The client is immunized against influenza and against *Streptococcus pneumoniae* with the pneumococcal vaccine (Pneumovax 23). Bronchodilators are indicated to open the fibrotic airways. Inflammation is treated with oral steroids such as prednisone (Meticorten), and/or by inhalation with beclomethasone dipropionate (Beclovent). The client with cystic fibrosis is required to take pancreatic enzymes, pancrelipase (Pancrease capsules, Cotazym capsules) to replace those that are missing with this disorder. If CHF occurs, the client is treated with digoxin (Lanoxin), furosemide (Lasix), and potassium supplements, as indicated.

Diet

To provide energy for breathing, the diet should be high in carbohydrates and calories. Protein is supplemented if necessary. Dietary supplements such as Ensure may be required. Fluids are encouraged, unless otherwise contraindicated. Sodium is restricted in the diet of the client with CHF. The diet for the client with cystic fibrosis is restricted in fats.

Table 31-10 SIGNS AND SYMPTOMS OF ASTHMA, CHRONIC BRONCHITIS, EMPHYSEMA, AND BRONCHIECTASIS

	ASTHMA	CHRONIC BRONCHITIS	EMPHYSEMA	BRONCHIECTASIS
History	Intermittent attacks of dyspnea and wheezing	Recurrent respiratory infections, chronic cough	Insidious onset, dyspnea on exertion to dyspnea at rest	Cystic fibrosis, recurrent respiratory infections
Cough	Present during attack	Chronic or recurrent productive cough	Present with infections	Frequent or chronic productive cough
Sputum	Thick	Copious, purulent, green	Scanty mucoid, unless infection present	Thick, tenacious, sometimes purulent secretions
Weight	No weight loss	Slight or no weight loss	Weight loss common	Commonly, weight loss or failure to gain
Appearance	Flushed then cyanotic	Commonly cyanosis ("blue bloater")	Ruddy complexion ("pink puffer")	Clubbing of fingernails
Chest Configuration	Slight overdistention	Slight overdistention	Overdistention prominent ("barrel chest")	Slight overdistention
Breath Sounds	Audible wheezing Prolonged expiration	Coarse crackles	Bronchial breath sounds in peripheral lung fields Diminished or absent in late disease	Crackles
Edema	Infrequent	Peripheral edema common, especially in ankles	Infrequent	Peripheral edema in late disease
Right-sided CHF (Cor Pulmonale)	Infrequent	Frequent	Infrequent	Frequent late in disease
CO Retention (Hypercapnia)	Sometimes	Common	Unlikely	Common in late disease
Hypoxemia	Depends on severity of attack	Possibly severe	Usually mild, especially at rest	Possibly severe in late disease and with infection
Dyspnea	Increases during attack	Progressive	Dyspnea on exertion to dyspnea at rest usually presenting symptom	With respiratory infection and late disease
Accessory Muscles Used for Respiration	Yes	Yes	Yes	Yes
Polycythemia	Uncommon	Late in disease	Yes	In late disease
Respiratory Failure	Possible	Common	Possible	Common

Activity

During acute exacerbations or in the presence of serious infection, activity is limited. The client is placed on bed rest. Activity is progressively increased depending on the client's tolerance. Respiratory rehabilitation and graded exercise programs are useful in the treatment of bronchiectasis. Regular exercise is encouraged, particularly for the pediatric client with cystic fibrosis.

▶ NURSING PROCESS

▶ Assessment

▶ Subjective Data

In gathering the history, the following information should be obtained: history of recent and past respiratory tract infections, history of or exposure to TB or other respiratory infections, and family or client history of cystic fibrosis. The onset, duration, and severity of symptoms such as dyspnea and cough are noted.

▶ Objective Data

The client may display a change in level of consciousness. Dyspnea, tachypnea, and cyanosis may be present. To aid respiratory effort, the client may assume the orthopneic position and use accessory muscles. Heart rate may elevate in response to hypoxia and/or infection. Elevated temperature and purulent sputum indicate infection. Subnormal weight and muscle wasting are seen in the client with chronic disease. Secretions within the airways create crackles heard on auscultation. The results of diagnostic and laboratory data should be evaluated. Signs and symptoms of CHF (e.g., peripheral edema, weight gain) should be noted.

Nursing diagnoses for a client with bronchiectasis may include the following:

Nursing Diagnoses	Planning/Goals	Nursing Interventions
▶ *Airway Clearance, Ineffective, related to increased and viscous respiratory tract secretions*	The client's breath sounds will be clear and respiratory rate, color, and ABGs will be within normal limits.	Observe the client's level of consciousness, color, respiratory effort, and use of accessory muscles, as well as the position the client assumes to ease respiration.
		Assist the client in assuming the position that most aids respiratory effort.
		Assess vital signs.
		Auscultate the lung fields.
		Alternate care with periods of rest.
		Evaluate sputum for amount, color, viscosity, and odor.
		Administer medications and respiratory treatments as ordered.
		Obtain ABG or pulse oximetry measurements as ordered.
		Supply supplemental oxygen as indicated.
		Provide the client with prescribed diet, including supplements.
		Unless contraindicated, encourage fluids to aid in the liquefication of secretions.
▶ *Nutrition: Altered, Less than Body Requirements, related to increased energy requirements for maintaining respiration*	The client will achieve or maintain a weight within the ideal range for height.	Provide an environment conducive to eating.
		Prior to meals, avoid treatments and therapies that fatigue the client or are painful.
		Assess the client's food likes and dislikes.
		Provide the prescribed diet based on the client's likes and dislikes.
		Prior to meals, administer medications and respiratory therapies that aid breathing.
		Assess the client's weight and compare to the ideal weight for the client's height.
		Assess the client's nutritional intake and evaluate for adequacy.
		Provide dietary supplements as ordered.

Evaluation Each goal must be evaluated to determine how it has been met by the client.

CHEST TRAUMA

Pneumothorax/hemothorax is discussed following.

PNEUMOTHORAX/HEMOTHORAX

Normally, there is no space between the visceral and parietal pleura. They are held together by surface tension. Thus, the pleural space is a closed compartment with a pressure that is negative in comparison to that within the lungs or of the atmosphere. When the integrity of the pleura is interrupted, air from the atmosphere or from the lungs moves between the pleura, creating a space. This condition of accumulated air or gas in the pleural space is known as a **pneumothorax** (Figure 31-14). The lung tissue underlying the pneumothorax is compressed and thus unable to fully expand. If the pneumothorax is large enough, the underlying lung tissue collapses as a result of the compression. A pneumothorax may occur spontaneously following blunt chest trauma, as in a

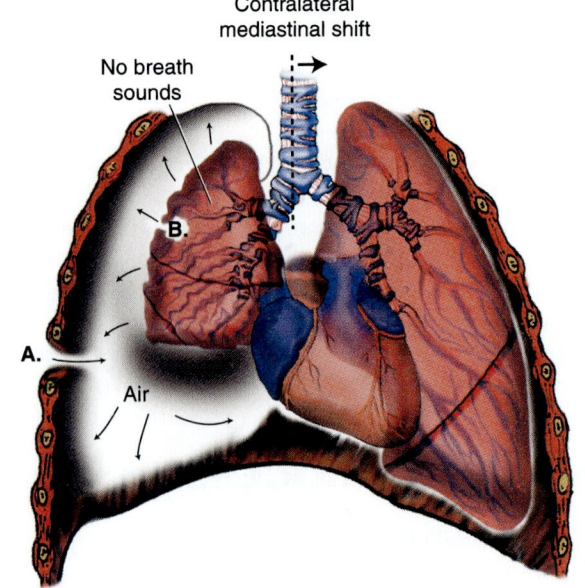

Figure 31-14 Pneumothorax: A. Penetrating wound; B. Ruptured bleb on the lung

motor vehicle accident; penetrating chest trauma, as in knife or gunshot wounds; or surgery involving the thoracic cavity.

A pneumothorax may be referred to as closed, open, spontaneous, or tension. A closed pneumothorax occurs when there is no communication between the pleura and the external environment. One example of a closed pneumothorax would be that associated with blunt trauma to the chest. In this instance, a broken rib may pierce the pleura and lung, allowing air to enter between the pleura. Conversely, an open pneumothorax exists when there is direct communication between the external environment and the pleural space. A spontaneous pneumothorax occurs without an obvious underlying cause. A tension pneumothorax is a life-threatening condition wherein air enters the pleural space on inspiration but is unable to exit on expiration. The air thus continues to accumulate in the pleural space, compressing the underlying structures. If left untreated, a tension pneumothorax will collapse the lung and encroach on the structures on the opposite side. All of the structures within the mediastinum—including the heart, aorta, and vena cava—are affected. Without intervention, tension pneumothorax will result in cardiopulmonary arrest. Tension pneumothorax is often associated with mechanical ventilation. The pressure exerted by the ventilator on compromised lung tissue interrupts the integrity of the pleura. Air continues to enter the pleural space but is unable to exit as mechanical ventilation continues. In the case of a pneumothorax associated with trauma or surgery, bleeding of adjacent vessels into the pleural cavity often occurs. Blood within the pleural space is referred to as a **hemothorax**. When accompanied by air, the condition is called a **hemopneumothorax**.

The severity of injury and the amount of lung tissue affected determine the signs and symptoms the client exhibits. The client with a small pneumothorax may be asymptomatic or may complain of minor dyspnea, whereas the client with a significant pneumothorax may exhibit signs of severe respiratory distress. Dyspnea, tachypnea, orthopnea, and cyanosis may be present. Oxygenation is impaired. Pleuritic pain is common. Breath sounds are absent in the area of the pneumothorax. In the case of a tension pneumothorax, the structures of the mediastinum will shift to the unaffected side as more and more air accumulates in the pleural space. The client with an accompanying hemothorax will exhibit signs and symptoms of shock associated with blood loss.

Medical–Surgical Management

Medical

In order for the affected lung to reexpand, the air and/or blood must be removed from the pleural space.

When the blood loss associated with a hemothorax is significant, fluid and blood replacement may be necessary.

Surgical

A thoracotomy tube, or chest tube, is inserted by the physician into the pleural space to drain fluid and air and allow the lung to reexpand. To drain fluid and air, the tube is placed in the midaxillary line at approximately the fifth intercostal space. To drain air alone, the tube is placed in the anterior chest at the midclavicular line and the fourth intercostal space. The thoracotomy tube is connected to an underwater seal drainage device (refer back to Figure 31-9). The underwater seal is necessary to prevent the negative pressure within the pleural space from pulling more air in through the chest tube itself. A drainage chamber allows for removal of any fluid or blood within the pleural space. In addition, most devices also have a chamber to which suction can be applied to assist in the removal of air and fluid from the pleural space. Following insertion of the chest tube, a chest x-ray is done to confirm proper placement of the tube and to assess reexpansion of the lungs. The underlying cause of the hemopneumothorax then must be treated.

Spontaneous pneumothorax that recurs may require a pleural cortication to prevent further episodes. This surgical procedure involves roughing the adjacent surfaces of the visceral and parietal pleura in the hopes that resulting scar tissue will improve adhesion between the two surfaces. To render emergency treatment for a tension pneumothorax that is severely compromising the function of the heart and lungs, a large bore needle is placed into the anterior chest at the fourth intercostal space. A thoracotomy tube is then inserted until the lung(s) are fully reexpanded and to prevent a recurrence.

Pharmacological

To control pleuritic pain, narcotic analgesics such as morphine sulfate or meperidine (Demerol) are prescribed. Analgesics may be given orally or parenterally depending on the severity of the pain. Prior to insertion of a thoracotomy tube, intravenous narcotics may be given prophylactically. Tissues adjacent to the area of the pneumothorax are injected with local anesthetics prior to insertion of a thoracotomy tube.

Diet

A well-balanced diet with sufficient amounts of protein is encouraged for healing. The client with other injuries and conditions may require TPN or enteral feedings.

Activity

The presence of a pneumothorax or a thoracotomy tube does not in itself call for restricting the client's activity. If hypoxia results from compromised breathing, activity restrictions are necessary. The presence of other injuries or conditions may also necessitate activity restrictions. After the client is adequately oxygenated and stable, activity is encouraged to promote expansion of the lungs.

▶ NURSING PROCESS
▶ Assessment
▶ Subjective Data

Information about the source of the pneumothorax should be gathered, and the client asked about previous pneumothoraces, recent chest injury, falls, and severe coughing. The client often describes being very anxious.

▶ Objective Data

The client's level of consciousness and mental status must be assessed and the client's color, respiratory effort, and chest wall movement must be observed. Chest wall movement is decreased on the affected side. When a large pneumothorax is present, the trachea shifts toward the unaffected side. Dyspnea and cyanosis may occur. The cough is forceful and nonproductive. Respiratory rate and heart rate are elevated. Blood pressure may be elevated due to the presence of pain and anxiety or may be low due to blood loss. Breath sounds are diminished or absent over the affected areas. The location, duration, and severity of pain should be noted. Once inserted, chest tubes are assessed for their function, patency, and amount and character of drainage.

Nursing diagnoses for a client with a pneumothorax may include the following:

Nursing Diagnoses	Planning/Goals	Nursing Interventions
▶ *Breathing Pattern, Ineffective, related to decreased lung expansion*	The client's respiratory rate and color will be within normal limits, and the client will have clear breath sounds in affected area.	Monitor the amount and character of drainage from the chest tube. Note any drainage from the chest tube as output. Observe fluctuations (tidaling) in the water seal chamber, which indicates that the tube has been placed in the pleural space. Investigate the absence of tidaling, as this may indicate that the lung is fully reexpanded or that the tube itself is occluded or kinked. Observe for the presence of bubbling in the water seal chamber, which is indicative of an air leak. Assess the connections and chest tube to determine whether leaks are present. If no air leaks are present, notify the physician as to the possibility of an air leak within the client's lungs. Encourage the client to cough and deep breathe to prevent further respiratory complications.
▶ *Pain, related to pleural space irritation*	The client will verbalize a decrease in pain on a scale of 1 to 10.	Assist the client in assuming the position that most aids respiration. The majority of clients find this to be the orthopneic position. Assess vital signs and respiratory status. Administer pain medications as ordered. Be aware that respiratory depression is possible with narcotic medications. Provide diversional activities.

Evaluation Each goal must be evaluated to determine how it has been met by the client.

NEOPLASMS OF THE RESPIRATORY TRACT

Neoplasms discussed following include benign neoplasms, lung cancer, and cancer of the larynx.

BENIGN NEOPLASMS

A benign tumor or cyst in the lung has sharply defined edges, as revealed on an x-ray. Peripheral tumors usually have no symptoms. Bronchial tumors may cause obstruction, infection, or atelectasis.

LUNG CANCER

Malignant tumors (carcinomas) of the lung may originate within the lung itself or may result from metastasis from other tumor sites (e.g., breast, colon, or kidney). Men, especially those over 40 years of age, are more likely to suffer from lung cancer than are women. However, the incidence of lung cancer is rising among women and declining among men (American Cancer Society [ACS], 1998). Tobacco smoking is one of the most common causal factors of lung cancer. Air pollution and exposure to carcinogens such as asbestos are also risk factors for developing lung cancer. Prognosis depends on the size of the tumor when diagnosed and the specific cell type (see Figure 31-15).

Most lung cancers are relatively silent, meaning that symptoms develop late in the course of the disease. Peripheral lesions generally have few symptoms. Initially, the client may complain of a chronic cough or wheezing. Central lesions cause obstruction and erosion of the bronchi. As the tumor grows and occludes the air passages, the client may experience shortness of breath, dyspnea, and blood-tinged sputum. Pain oc-

CLIENT TEACHING

Tips for Preventing Lung Cancer
- Do not smoke
- Avoid secondhand smoke
- Avoid exposure to air with high concentrations of pollutants
- Support efforts to decrease air pollution
- Protect self from carcinogens in the workplace, such as asbestos

curs relatively late in the course of the disease and indicates that the tumor has grown to a significant size to put pressure on adjacent nerves and other structures. Although some tumors can be seen on chest x-ray, many cannot. Computerized axial tomography (CAT) and MRI scans are more reliable studies when assessing soft-tissue structures. To confirm diagnosis, the physician orders cytology studies on specimens collected via bronchoscopy, needle biopsy, or mediastinoscopy. Lung scans are occasionally useful for diagnosis. Prior to initiating treatment, the client is evaluated for metastatic disease using bone and total body scans.

Family members and significant others often need assistance in coping with their feelings related to the person with lung cancer.

Medical–Surgical Management

Medical

Treatment of lung cancer depends on the type and stage of the cancer.

Surgical

Surgical intervention involves the removal of the tumor and adjacent lung tissue. Pneumonectomy is the removal of an entire lung. Lobectomy is the removal of a lobe of a lung. Segmental resection is the removal of a segment of a lung. The client will have a thoracotomy tube on the operative side. Radiation and chemotherapy are often used in conjunction with surgery. The incidence of lung tumor recurrence following surgery is high. Surgery is often indicated for early non–small-cell carcinomas.

Pharmacological

The specific type of chemotherapy used depends on the cell type and the extent of tumor growth.

Health Promotion

The foremost method of preventing lung cancer is to avoid smoking or to cease smoking. The second-hand smoke of others should also be avoided.

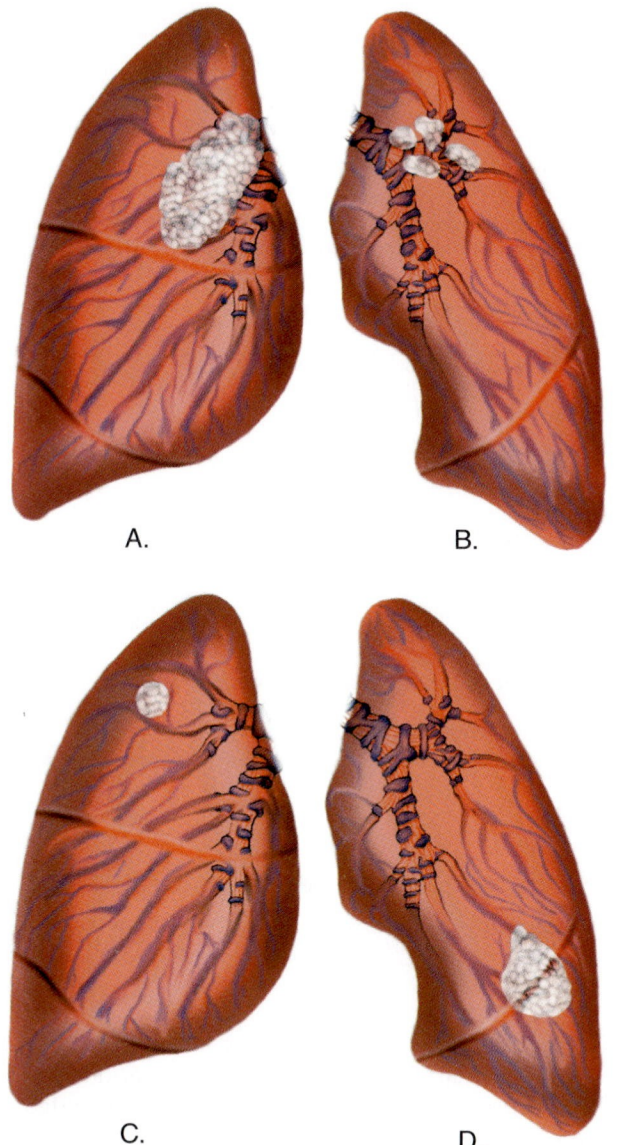

Figure 31-15 Lung Cancers: A. Small-cell carcinoma; B. Epidermoid (squamous-cell) carcinoma; C. Adenocarcinoma; D. Large cell (undifferentiated) carcinoma

▶ NURSING PROCESS

▶ Assessment

▶ Subjective Data

The client's history is reviewed for history of smoking, exposure to carcinogens, and other causative factors. Information should be gathered regarding the onset, duration, and severity of symptoms. The client may report hoarseness, chronic cough, pain, and shortness of breath. Pain is assessed as to its location, character, duration, and severity.

▶ Objective Data

The color, amount, consistency, and odor of sputum are noted. Prior to surgery, the nurse may hear wheezing or decreased breath sounds on the affected side. Following surgery, breath sounds are diminished or absent on the affected side. The amount and color of drainage from the thoracotomy tube are monitored. The wound is assessed for hemorrhage and infection. Respiratory rate and effort may be increased. Pulse rate may be elevated due to a variety of factors including decreased oxygenation, hemorrhage, and infection. Hypotension occurs with significant blood loss. High blood pressure may indicate pain, anxiety, or other underlying pathology such as essential hypertension.

Nursing diagnoses for a client with lung cancer may include the following:

Nursing Diagnoses	Planning/Goals	Nursing Interventions
▶ *Breathing Pattern, Ineffective, related to disease process*	The client's respiratory rate and color will be within normal limits.	Frequently monitor the client's level of consciousness, vital signs, color, and respiratory effort.
		Auscultate breath sounds.
		Stagger activities with periods of rest to prevent overtaxing the client's reserves.
		Assist the client in assuming the position that maximizes respiratory effort by positioning the client in semi-Fowler's position or lying on the affected side.
		Assess oxygenation and provide supplemental oxygen as indicated.
		Monitor lab reports for blood gas levels.
▶ *Pain related to lung cancer*	The client will state pain is decreased on a scale of 1 to 10.	Administer pain medication as ordered.
		Monitor for respiratory depression.
		Provide diversional activities.
		Assist the client in assuming a position of comfort.
▶ *Grieving, Anticipatory, related to prognosis and perceived separation from significant others*	The client will be able to express to significant others and/or staff feelings related to diagnosis and prognosis.	Aid the client in expressing feelings of grief related to the diagnosis.
		Hope should not be eliminated, but false hope should not be encouraged.
		Allow the client and family time to express their feelings.

Evaluation Each goal must be evaluated to determine how it has been met by the client.

LARYNGEAL CANCER

Cancer of the larynx is more common among men than women. Risk factors for cancer of the larynx include smoking, chronic alcohol abuse, chronic laryngitis, and overuse of the voice. Laryngeal cancer is relatively asymptomatic. The client may experience hoarseness or difficulty speaking above a whisper. If either persists for more than 2 weeks, medical care should be sought. Difficulty swallowing is sometimes present. Laryngeal pain radiating to the ear or a lump in the throat are often signs of metastasis.

Medical–Surgical Management

Treatment is determined by the extent of tumor growth.

Surgical

Surgical removal of the larynx, a laryngectomy, is used to treat laryngeal cancer. If the cancer has spread to surrounding tissues, a simple or radical neck dissection may be required. Radiation may be used as an adjunct to surgery or as primary treatment if the tumor is detected in the early stages. Following surgery, a permanent tracheostomy is necessary to allow air to enter

CLIENT TEACHING

Daily Stoma Care

After the stoma has healed:
- Use warm water to clean around the stoma;
- Do not use tissues, linty cotton, or soap for cleansing; and
- Wear a bib or dressing over the stoma to filter and warm incoming air.

HOME HEALTH CARE

Client with Laryngeal Stoma
- The client's home should be humidified, especially in winter.
- The client and family must know how to suction the respiratory tract, care for the stoma, and care for the respiratory equipment.
- The client should not swim or splash water in the stoma when showering or bathing.
- The client should notify the physician if any signs of respiratory infection develop, such as fever, cough, yellow or green mucus, or redness around the stoma.
- The client must keep follow-up appointments with the physician.

the respiratory tract. A small incision is made into the trachea and below the Adam's apple, and a plastic tracheostomy tube is inserted.

▶ NURSING PROCESS

▶ Assessment

▶ Subjective Data

Assessment of the client with laryngeal cancer includes taking a history as to the onset, duration, and severity of symptoms, such as hoarseness or laryngitis and alcohol and tobacco use. The client may describe ear pain and difficulty breathing and swallowing.

▶ Objective Data

The client's respiratory status is evaluated for other respiratory problems that may accompany laryngeal cancer, such as COPD. Sputum is examined for the presence of blood.

Nursing diagnoses for a client with laryngeal cancer may include the following:

Nursing Diagnoses	Planning/Goals	Nursing Interventions
▶ Communication, Impaired Verbal, related to removal of the larynx	The client will be able to communicate needs.	Before surgery, establish a means of communication to be used afterwards. If available, a manual or computer word/picture board works well.
		Keep call light by client's bed.
		Avoid mouthing communications, as this is frustrating to the client and is time consuming.
		As possible, ask questions that require only a "yes" or "no" answer.
		Refer the client to the local support group (Lost Chord Club) or the American Cancer Society.
▶ Airway Clearance, Ineffective, related to tracheostomy tube	The client's respiratory rate and color will be within normal limits, and the client will have clear breath sounds to auscultation.	Suction frequently following surgery to remove static secretions.
		Provide routine tracheostomy care.
		Provide small, frequent feedings of liquid or pureed food to prevent choking.
		Assist client to turn, cough, and deep breathe two to four times an hour.
		Teach client stoma protection.
		Auscultate lung sounds.
		Assess respirations two to four times an hour, if secretions are copious.
		Keep head of bed elevated.
		Provide extra humidity.

continued

Nursing Diagnoses	Planning/Goals	Nursing Interventions
▶ *Knowledge Deficit related to tracheostomy care*	The client will verbalize precautions and safety measures for a tracheostomy; how to use equipment; how to suction the respiratory tract; how to change a tracheostomy tube; and actions to take in an emergency.	Teach the client and family how to suction the respiratory tract, care for the tracheostomy, and use respiratory equipment.
		Instruct the client and family in what to do in case of an emergency, such as clogging of the tracheostomy tube with secretions.
		Advise client not to swim and to avoid aspirating water when showering or bathing.
		Suggest that the client avoid extremely cold temperatures. If the tracheostomy site is covered for warming or cosmetic purposes, the covering must be of a porous material without frayed or loose threads.

Evaluation Each goal must be evaluated to determine how it has been met by the client.

DISORDERS OF THE NOSE

The most common disorder of the nose is epistaxis, or nose bleed.

EPISTAXIS

Epistaxis is hemorrhage of the nares or nostrils. It may be either unilateral, which is most common, or bilateral. Epistaxis may be primary in nature, stemming from drying of the nasal mucosa, local irritation, or trauma, or may occur secondary to uncontrolled hypertension or coagulopathies (e.g., thrombocytopenia, anticoagulant therapy). The diffuse vascularity and proximity of blood vessels to the surface of the nasal mucosa make the nares a susceptible avenue for hemorrhage. Blood loss can be minimal to severe. With significant blood loss, hypovolemic shock occurs.

Medical–Surgical Management

Medical

The client with epistaxis usually arrives at an urgent care facility or emergency room following unsuccessful attempts to stop the bleeding. Signs of airway obstruction or aspiration require immediate attention. The goals of treatment are to maintain airway, stop bleeding, identify the cause, and prevent recurrence. Nosebleeds are usually responsive to compression of the nares. Firm pressure should be maintained for 5 minutes. If bleeding persists, the client is instructed to blow the nose and clear the nasal passages. Pressure is then resumed for a full 10 minutes. Epistaxis that continues following these measures requires more aggressive treatment. Bleeding sites that cannot be visualized require packing. Sterile nasal packing is inserted following application of a local anesthetic. In severe cases, a nasostat is inserted. This device resembles a Foley catheter and provides direct compression to the site of bleeding via a balloon. Clients with severe nose-

bleeds may require fluid and blood replacement to prevent hypovolemic shock. Persistent or recurrent epistaxis may require surgical ligation of the artery supplying the area.

 Infection Control: Epistaxis
Wear gloves, goggles or a face mask, and a gown when caring for a client with epistaxis. A cough or sneeze can splatter blood.

Pharmacological

Sites of bleeding that can be visualized are cauterized by the physician. Silver nitrate sticks are used for this purpose. Hemostasis may also be accomplished by packing the affected nostril with epinephrine 1:1000 on cotton packing.

▶ NURSING PROCESS

▶ Assessment

▶ Subjective Data

The client should be questioned about the onset, precipitating events, duration, and frequency of epistaxis, as well as associated symptoms such as nausea, vomiting, headache, and lightheadedness. The client with an occult, or hidden, bleed may complain of needing to swallow frequently.

 LIFE CYCLE CONSIDERATIONS

Child with Epistaxis
- Assess for presence of foreign objects in the nares
- Assess for local trauma resulting from insertion of objects into the nares

▸ Objective Data

Blood flow is evaluated for amount, consistency, color, and rate (or severity). Overt bleeding from the nose may be present. This bleeding can vary in flow, from a continuous drip to a pulsating stream of blood. The client who has an occult epistaxis should have the posterior oropharynx visually examined by the nurse or physician to assess blood flow. Vomiting may be present. Lowered blood pressure and rapid heart rate are signs of hypovolemic shock. Conversely, the client with uncontrolled hypertension has an abnormally high systolic blood pressure. Prothrombin time (PT), APTT, INR, and other clotting studies will be abnormal with underlying coagulopathies. Decreased red blood cell count, hemoglobin, and hematocrit are evidence of significant bleeding.

Nursing diagnoses for a client with epistaxis may include the following:

Nursing Diagnoses	Planning/Goals	Nursing Interventions
Gas Exchange, Impaired, related to airway obstruction	The client's respiratory rate, color, and blood gases will be within normal limits.	Place the client in a high Fowler's position, with the head bent slightly forward. Instruct the client to breathe through the mouth and allow the blood to escape freely from the nose and into a container. This aids in preventing obstruction of the airway and swallowing of blood. Monitor the client for signs and symptoms of airway obstruction. Assess the client's color and respiratory rate and effort. Auscultate breath sounds. Administer supplemental oxygen as indicated by pulse oximetry or ABG values. Monitor pulse oximetry and lab reports of ABGs.
Aspiration, Risk for, related to epistaxis	The client will develop no complications related to aspiration.	Place the client in the position previously described to aid in preventing aspiration of blood. Assess the client for signs of aspiration, such as choking, coarse crackles on auscultation, or elevated temperature. Suction the respiratory tract through the mouth to remove secretions and blood.
Fluid Volume Deficit related to blood loss.	The client will maintain adequate fluid volume.	With a gloved hand, compress the nares for 5 minutes. If bleeding persists, have client blow nose to clear passages, then compress nares for 10 minutes. If bleeding continues following compression attempts, prepare to assist the physician with procedures such as cautery or insertion of nasal packing. Administer medications to control blood pressure, as ordered. After hemostasis has been established, the clots formed should not be removed or dislodged, as this will lead to recurrence of bleeding. Every 30 minutes, evaluate the blood pressure and pulse of the client who shows signs of volume depletion. Assess for orthostatic hypotension as a means of measuring volume depletion. A decrease in systolic blood pressure of greater than 10 mm Hg when the position is changed from lying to sitting or standing indicates hypovolemia. Administer intravenous fluids, as ordered.

Evaluation Each goal must be evaluated to determine how it has been met by the client.

CASE STUDY

Mrs. White is a 77-year-old female with a history of smoking two to three packs of cigarettes a day for the past 60 years. Mrs. White has been diagnosed with COPD for the past 4 years. She has required supplemental oxygen at 2 L/min for the last 18 months. Three days ago, Mrs. White was admitted with chief complaints of increasing dyspnea on exertion and a productive cough yielding thick, green-yellow sputum. She states that she does "not know why she is coughing up this awful stuff."

Physical examination of Mrs. White this morning revealed vital signs of T = 101.5°F, P = 124, R = 38, BP = 168/74; and sonorous and sibilant wheezes on expiration and in the posterior lung fields, with superimposed coarse crackles heard in the right posterior lower lung field. She is unable to ambulate to the bathroom or complete other ADL due to the dyspnea. Chest x-ray showed a large area of consolidation in the right lower lobe. Sputum culture is still pending.

The following questions will guide your development of a nursing care plan for the case study.

1. List the clinical manifestations that indicate Mrs. White is experiencing an infection concomitant with her COPD.
2. Explain why COPD predisposes a client to respiratory infection.
3. Explain why the physician will increase Mrs. White's oxygen flow to 3 to 4 L/min.
4. List the subjective and objective data the nurse should obtain during the nursing assessment.
5. Identify three nursing diagnoses and client goals that would be pertinent to Mrs. White's care.
6. List the above diagnoses in order of priority, with number one being the highest.
7. Describe client outcomes indicating that Mrs. White's treatment and nursing care regimen have been successful.

SUMMARY

- The primary function of the respiratory system is delivery of oxygen to the lungs and removal of carbon dioxide from the lungs.
- Pneumonia is a lung infection wherein infectious secretions accumulate in the air passages and interfere with gas exchange. Clients with chronic pulmonary disorders or problems of immobility are at increased risk of developing pneumonia.
- Pulmonary TB is an infection of the lung tissue caused by the *Mycobacterium tuberculosis*. Treatment of TB requires the long-term administration of pharmacological agents.
- A common respiratory tract disorder associated with immobility and the administration of anesthetic agents is atelectasis. Clients at risk are encouraged to cough and breathe deeply to aid in preventing atelectasis.
- Obstruction of a pulmonary artery by a bloodborne substance is known as pulmonary embolism. Deep vein thrombosis is a common cause of pulmonary emboli.
- Chronic pulmonary obstructive disease is a collective term used to refer to chronic lung disorders

wherein air flow into or out of the lungs is limited. Disorders associated with COPD are asthma, chronic bronchitis, emphysema, and bronchiectasis.
- Traumatic disorders of the respiratory tract include pneumothorax and hemothorax, wherein the underlying lung tissue is compressed and eventually collapses.
- Cigarette smoking is indicated as a major causative factor in the development of respiratory disorders, such as lung cancer, cancer of the larynx, emphysema, and chronic bronchitis.

Review Questions

1. The physician orders 2 to 3 L of oxygen to be delivered to the client with COPD because:

   a. no client ever requires more than 2 to 3 L of oxygen.
   b. the client requests it.
   c. a higher flow rate may suppress the client's drive to breathe.
   d. 2 to 3 L is the maximum flow that a nasal cannula can effectively deliver.

2. A particulate respirator mask is used by the nurse caring for a client with TB because:

   a. regular masks allow the tubercle bacilli to pass through.
   b. this mask is more comfortable for long-term use.
   c. this type of masks allows the nurse to be in close contact with the client for prolonged periods of time.
   d. there is no need for this type of mask when caring for clients with TB.

3. Bronchodilators are used to treat bronchiectasis in order to:

   a. dilate airways that are in bronchospasm due to an antigen–antibody reaction.
   b. dilate airways that have lost their elasticity.
   c. dilate airways that are clogged with secretions.
   d. dilate airways that are chronically narrowed.

4. Incentive spirometry is used to measure the amount of air that:

   a. is exhaled in 1 minute.
   b. is inspired in 1 minute.
   c. is inspired with one inhalation.
   d. is exhaled with one exhalation.

5. Asthma is characterized by:

   a. chronic narrowing of the airways.
   b. intermittent airflow obstruction.
   c. chronic dilation of the airways.
   d. fibrosis of the alveoli.

6. The client with a pneumothorax experiences hypoxia due to:

   a. the entry of air into the thoracic cavity.
   b. compression of the lung tissue underlying the pneumothorax.
   c. impairment of gas exchange.
   d. a lack of surfactant.

Critical Thinking Questions

1. Why is TB becoming more prevalent?

2. What are the differences and similarities of the disorders classified as COPD?

3. What is the rationale for each nursing intervention given for the possible nursing diagnoses in this chapter?

WEB FLASH!

- Search *tuberculosis* on the Internet. What type of information is available? How can this information be used by clients and families?
- Do the resources listed for this chapter at the end of the book have Web sites? If so, what type of information do they provide?

CHAPTER 32

NURSING CARE OF THE CLIENT: CARDIO-VASCULAR SYSTEM

MAKING THE CONNECTION

Refer to the following chapters to increase your understanding of cardiovascular disorders:

- **Chapter 15, Wellness Concepts**
- **Chapter 23, Fluid, Electrolyte, and Acid-Base Balance**
- **Chapter 25, Assessment**
- **Chapter 26, Pain Management**
- **Chapter 27, Diagnostic Tests**
- **Chapter 31, Nursing Care of the Client: Respiratory System**
- **Chapter 33, Nursing Care of the Client: Blood and Lymph Systems**

- **Chapter 37, Nursing Care of the Client: Endocrine System**
- **Procedures:** B1, Handwashing; B2, Use of Protective Equipment; B4, Assessing Pulse Rate; B6, Assessing Blood Pressure; B7, Weighing Client, Mobile and Immobile; B10, Assisting a Client with Ambulation; B25, Applying Antiemboli Stockings

LEARNING OBJECTIVES

Upon completion of this chapter, you should be able to:
- *Define key terms.*
- *Describe the anatomy and physiology of the cardiovascular system.*
- *Relate laboratory results to each disorder.*
- *Describe basic heart dysrhythmias.*
- *Explain the pathophysiology of each disorder.*
- *Describe nursing interventions in caring for clients with cardiovascular conditions.*

KEY TERMS

aneurysm
angina pectoris
annulus
arteriosclerosis
ascites
atherosclerosis
automatic implant-
  able cardioverter-
  defibrillator
  (AICD)
baseline level
bradycardia
cardiac output
cardiac tamponade
depolarization
dyspnea
dysrhythmia
embolus
heart sound
hemolysis
Homans' sign
hypertrophies
myocardial infarction
myocarditis
necrosis
orthopnea
palpitation
paroxysmal nocturnal
  dyspnea
percutaneous balloon
  valvuloplasty
pericardial friction rub
pericardiocentesis
pericarditis
peripheral
  resistance
phlebitis
phlebothrombosis
primary hyper-
  tension
repolarization
sclerotherapy
secondary hyper-
  tension
stasis dermatitis
stent
stroke volume
tachycardia
thrombectomy
thrombophlebitis
thrombosis
thrombus
transesophageal
  echocardiography
  (TEE)
varicosities
vasoconstriction
vasodilation
vein ligation
vein stripping
Virchow's triad

INTRODUCTION

Since 1900, heart disease has been the leading cause of death in the United States every year except in 1918 (American Heart Association, 1999a). Approximately 1.1 million Americans experience a myocardial infarction each year with 367,000 of the occurrences ending in death (American Heart Association, 1999b). Congestive heart failure is a contributing factor in approximately 250,000 deaths each year (American Heart Association, 1999a).

Even though these facts are astounding, the death rate for cardiovascular disease has been declining in the last fifteen years. This is due to public education in modifying and decreasing risk factors such as smoking, high-fat diets, and minimal exercise.

This chapter reviews the anatomy and physiology of the cardiovascular system. Pathophysiology, medical management, and nursing interventions related to cardiovascular conditions are discussed with an emphasis on decreasing risk factors and improving lifestyles.

ANATOMY AND PHYSIOLOGY REVIEW

The cardiovascular system consists of the heart and its vasculature and the peripheral vascular system. The heart is located in the lower anterior area of the mediastinum with the apex near the diaphragm. In an average lifetime, the heart will pump 80 million gallons of blood.

The peripheral vascular system consists of arteries, arterioles, capillaries, venules, and veins. The arteries carry oxygenated blood away from the left side of the heart to the body tissues and the veins carry deoxygenated blood back to the right side of the heart. The capillaries connect the arterioles to the venules. In the capillaries, oxygen, nutrients, minerals, and hormones move from the blood to the body cells, and carbon dioxide and waste products move from the body cells into the blood. The venules and veins contain 60% to 70% of the body's total blood volume.

The function of the cardiovascular system is to provide oxygen, nutrients, and hormones to the cells of the body and remove carbon dioxide and waste products of cellular metabolism from body cells. Body temperature is maintained by the distribution of heat throughout the body that has been produced by the metabolic activity of muscles and other body organs.

Structure of the Heart

The heart consists of three layers; endocardium, myocardium, and epicardium. The endocardium is the inner endothelial lining of heart chambers and valves. The myocardium is the thickest part of the heart and consists of cardiac muscle. The epicardium consists of a visceral layer and a parietal layer. The visceral epicardium attaches to the myocardium and is the outer layer of the heart. The parietal epicardium forms the inner layer of a double walled sac called the pericardium that surrounds the heart.

The heart is a hollow muscular organ containing four chambers that fill and empty of blood with each contraction (**depolarization**) and recovery phase (**repolarization**) of the cardiac muscle. The upper chambers are the atria and the lower chambers are the ventricles (Figure 32-1). When the atria contract, blood is forced into the ventricles. Contraction of the right ventricle pumps blood into the pulmonary arteries and on to the lungs (pulmonary circulatory system). Contraction of the left ventricle pumps blood into the aorta and out to the entire body (systemic circulatory system). The myocardium of the left ventricle is thicker than the right ventricle as more force is needed to pump blood throughout the body.

There are four sets of valves in the heart; tricuspid, bicuspid (mitral), pulmonary, and aortic. One end of fibrous cords called *chordae tendineae* is attached to the cusps of the tricuspid and mitral valves and the other end is attached to papillary muscles on the walls of the ventricles. The chordae tendineae keep the valves from inverting when the ventricles contract, thus preventing blood from flowing back into the atrium. The pulmonary and aortic valves prevent blood from flowing back into the ventricles from the pulmonary artery and aorta during repolarization.

Circulation of Blood

Blood enters the heart through veins and leaves the heart through arteries. With the contraction of the right ventricle, blood is forced through the pulmonary valve

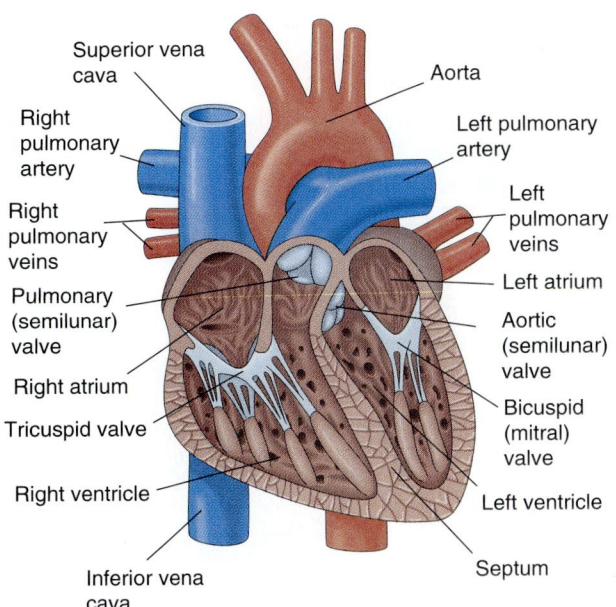

Figure 32-1 Internal View of the Heart with Aorta, Vena Cava, and Pulmonary Arteries and Veins

into the pulmonary artery. Blood circulates through the pulmonary circulatory system where carbon dioxide is exchanged for oxygen in the lungs. The blood then returns to the left atrium through the pulmonary veins providing oxygenated blood for systemic circulation. When the left ventricle contracts, blood is forced through the aortic valve into the aorta beginning systemic circulation. Blood is then distributed throughout the body and returns to the right atrium of the heart through the inferior and superior vena cava.

Each time the heart beats, the ventricle pumps 60 to 80 cc of blood. The volume of blood pumped by the ventricle with each contraction is called **stroke volume**. The volume of blood pumped by the left ventricle per minute is known as **cardiac output** and averages 5 liters for an adult at rest. Stroke volume multiplied by the pulse rate yields the cardiac output. If the heart has a strong ventricular contraction, more blood will be pumped by the heart into the systemic circulatory system. Therefore, cardiac output has a direct effect upon the volume of arterial blood being circulated.

Coronary Arteries

Coronary arteries supply nutrients and oxygen to the muscle tissue of the heart. The two coronary arteries are the right coronary artery and the left coronary artery, which branch off the aorta (Figure 32-2). The right coronary artery divides into the posterior descending artery (interventricular artery) and the marginal artery and supplies blood to the anterior area of the right and left ventricles, the posterior area of the right ventricle, the AV node, and the posterior section of the interventricular septum. The left coronary artery divides into the anterior descending artery and the cir-

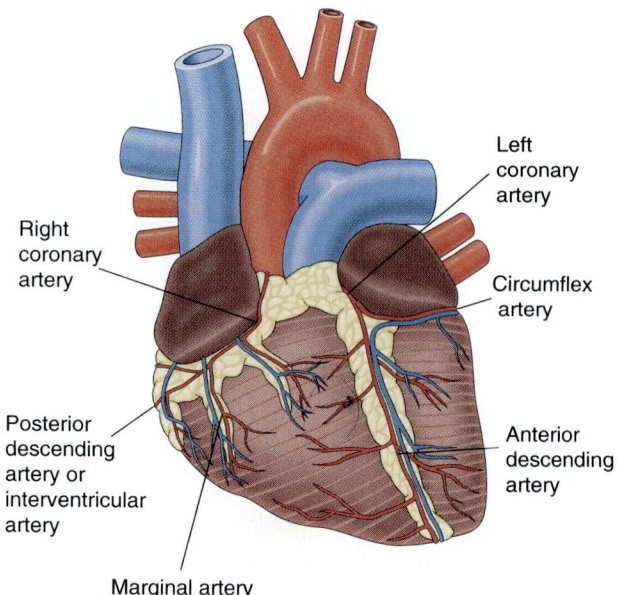

Figure 32-2 Coronary Arteries that Supply Blood to the Heart Tissue

Right coronary artery

Left coronary artery

Circumflex artery

Posterior descending artery or interventricular artery

Anterior descending artery

Marginal artery

cumflex artery. The left anterior descending (LAD) artery supplies blood to the anterior section of the interventricular septum, anterior area of the left ventricle, and the lateral aspect of the left ventricle. The circumflex artery nourishes the left atrium and ventricle.

Conduction System

The specialized cardiac muscle cells are capable of conducting electrical impulses from one part of the heart to another. For the heart to beat regularly in a rhythmic sequence, electrical impulses follow a set pattern through the conduction system of the heart. The conduction system consisting of the sinoatrial node (SA node), atrioventricular node (AV node), bundle of His, bundle branches, and Purkinje fibers controls the heartbeat (Figure 32-3).

Heart Sounds

There are two normal **heart sounds** called S_1 and S_2, heard on auscultation. They yield a sound like "lubb-dubb." S_1, or the "lubb," is the sound of the mitral and tricuspid valves closing simultaneously. It is heard on the left fifth intercostal space. S_2, or the "dubb," is the simultaneous closing of the pulmonary and aortic valves. S_2 is heard on the right second intercostal space. There is a slight pause after the "lubb-dubb" is heard. Clients with congestive heart failure may have a third sound known as S_3. This low-pitched sound occurs after the S_2 sound, or the "dubb," making the heart sound like the word Kentucky ("lubb-dubb-by"). The S_3 sound has also been described as a gallop.

Arterioles and Arteries

The arteries are thick-walled tubes consisting of three layers or tunics as illustrated in Figure 32-4. The inner layer is called the *tunica intima* and consists of a single layer of smooth endothelial cells. The middle layer is the *tunica media* and is composed of smooth muscle cells. The smooth muscle layer of the artery receives nerve stimulation from the sympathetic nervous system. The suppleness of the smooth muscle allows the vessel to **vasoconstrict** (decrease in diameter) and **vasodilate** (increase in diameter). The outer layer, the *tunica adventitia* or *tunica externa,* consists of a connective tissue sheath with some of its collagen fibers fusing with those of the surrounding tissue to

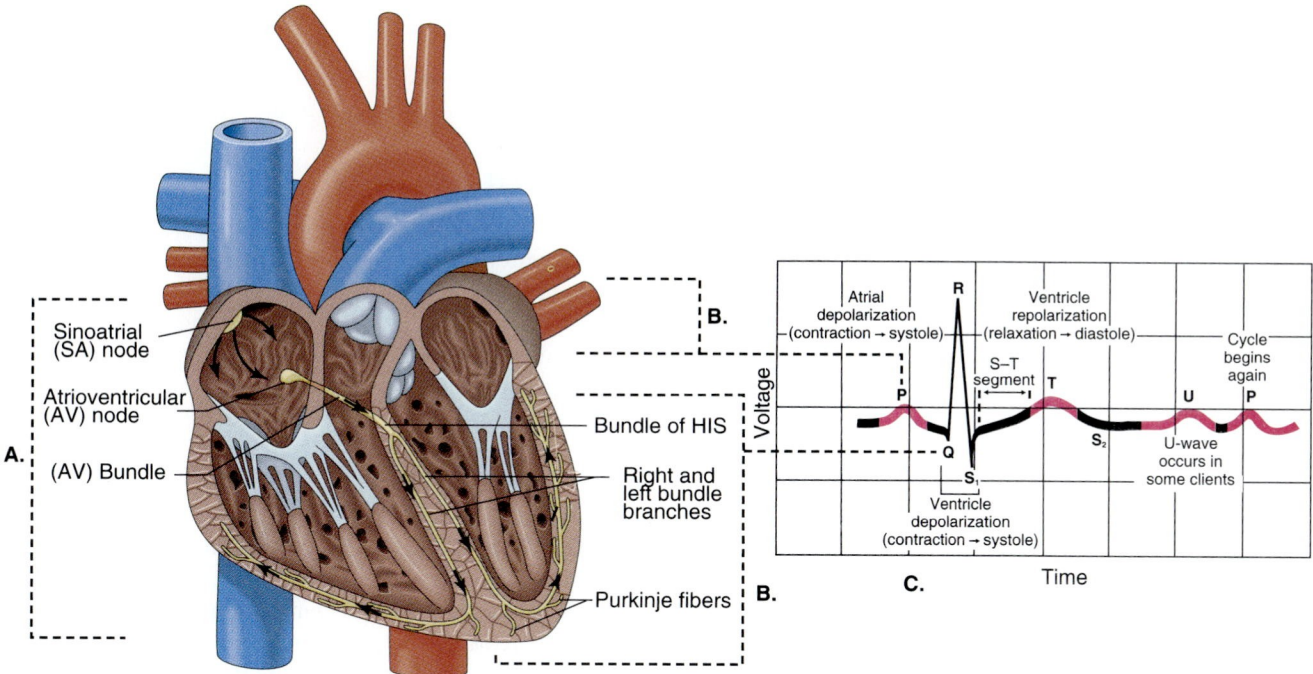

Figure 32-3 A. Conduction System of the Heart; B. Relationship of the Conduction System to an EKG Strip; C. Relationship of S_1 and S_2 Heart Sounds to an EKG Strip

hold the vessels in place. The elastic connective tissue allows the artery to expand and recoil with each contraction of the ventricle as an increased volume of blood is pumped through the vessel. The arteries have thick walls so they can withstand the increased pressure from the left ventricle pumping blood through the body.

The arteries divide and branch into smaller vessels called *arterioles* which are smaller arteries. The same three layers are present in the walls, but as the arterioles approach the capillaries their walls become thinner. The outer layer is reduced to a very thin layer of connective tissue.

Capillaries

Capillaries are very tiny thin vessels that connect the smallest arterioles with the smallest venules. They have only one layer of endothelial cells whose cell membranes are the semipermeable membrane that allows oxygen, nutrients, carbon dioxide, and waste products to be exchanged between the tissues of the body and the blood.

Venules and Veins

Venules are small vessels that emerge from the capillaries and gradually increase in size. As the venules increase in size, they eventually form veins.

Veins have three layers or tunics like the arteries, but the middle layer of a vein is thinner, having less smooth muscle and elastic tissue. This allows the walls of the veins to dilate more easily. Endothelial flaps, called *valves,* are on the inside lining of veins. The valves open and close with each contraction of the surrounding muscles. The purpose of the valves is to assist the blood in returning to the heart. Blood is held by the valves at a certain level until the skeletal muscle contractions cause the blood to move higher in the vein (Figure 32-5).

HEALTH HISTORY

The nurse has three goals when obtaining a health history from a client. The goals are to identify present and potential health problems, identify possible familial and lifestyle risk factors, and involve the client in planning long-term health care.

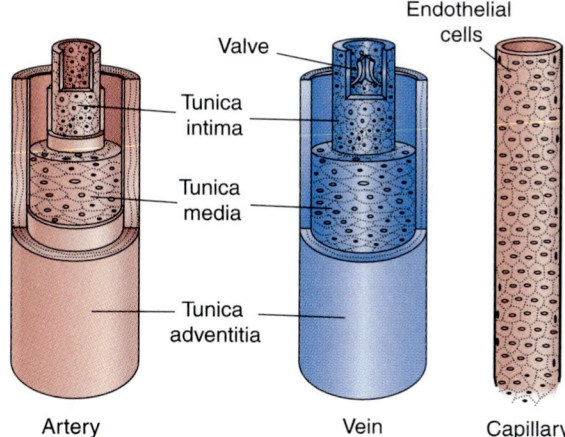

Figure 32-4 Tunic Layers of Each Type of Vessel

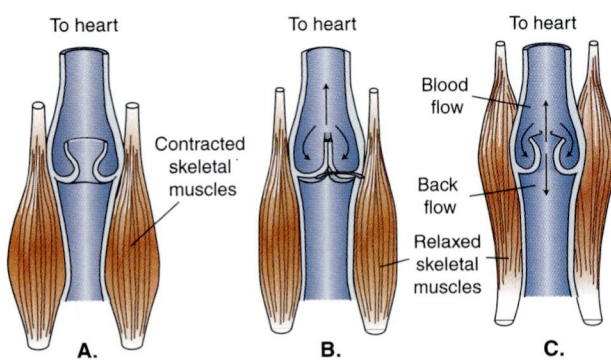

Figure 32-5 Valves in the veins hold the blood at a certain level in the vein. A. Contracted skeletal muscles apply pressure to veins and assist with the circulation of blood; B. Valves prevent the backflow of blood; C. Incompetent valves allow a backflow of blood

The nurse should ascertain the onset of the symptoms, the predisposing factors that cause the symptoms, and the client's treatment of the symptoms. The nurse should ask if the client has noticed any other bodily changes that occur or have occurred at the same time as the main symptoms. Special attention should be given to the client's activity level or limitations in activity. When asking about dietary habits, the nurse should determine if there has been an increase or decrease in appetite. Asking about sleeping habits will help evaluate the client's ability to sleep, the need for the trunk of the body to be supported with pillows when sleeping, or the need to sleep in a chair.

Major risk factors associated with cardiovascular diseases are age, gender, heredity (including race), smoking, dyslipidemia (presence of increased total serum cholesterol and low-density lipoprotein [LDL]), high blood pressure, physical inactivity, obesity and overweight, and diabetes mellitus. An individual's response to stress may be a contributing factor. Additional contributing factors for women may include menopause, use of birth control pills, and high triglyceride level (American Heart Association, 1999f and 1999g; Mosca, Manson, Sutherland, Langer, Manolio, & Barrett-Connor, 1997).

Advancing age, male gender, diabetes, heredity, and familial history of chest pain or myocardial infarctions are risk factors that cannot be altered. Alterable risk factors are physical inactivity, smoking, contraceptive method, dyslipidemia, obesity and overweight, and triglyceride level. A change in diet may alter the last three factors.

The nurse has a two-fold objective in directing the client toward a healthier lifestyle. The first objective is to educate the client about the risk factors. The second objective is to determine what risk factors the client would like to modify. Once this has been determined, the nurse can assist the client in establishing goals and determining actions to achieve the goals.

ASSESSMENT

Assessment includes clients' self-report of symptoms as well as physical findings and confirming lab data.

Subjective Data

The typical concerns expressed by a client with a cardiac disorder are chest pain, **dyspnea** (difficulty breathing), edema, fainting, palpitations, diaphoresis, and fatigue. When a client talks about having chest pain, it is important to ascertain the onset of the pain, situation occurring at the onset of pain, location and radiation of pain, severity of chest pain, duration, past episodes of chest pain, and methods used to alleviate pain. Women are more likely to express having abdominal pain, dyspnea, nausea, and fatigue (Mosca et al., 1997).

There are several types of dyspnea the client may be experiencing. Exertional dyspnea occurs when a person participates in moderate activity and becomes short of breath. This occurs in the early stages of heart failure and indicates that the heart is not able to meet the demands of the body during moderate activity. **Orthopnea** is when a client has difficulty breathing while lying down and must sit upright or stand to relieve the dyspnea. This occurs in a more advanced stage of heart failure. **Paroxysmal nocturnal dyspnea** is when a person suddenly awakens, is sweating, and is having difficulty breathing. This usually occurs 2 to 5 hours after the person has fallen asleep.

A client may have fainting spells for various physical and psychological reasons. In cardiac clients, fainting occurs because of decreased cardiac output that causes a decreased blood flow to the brain.

A client may describe a "fluttering" or "pounding" sensation in the chest. This is known as **palpitations**. If these sensations occur during exercise, it is a sign that the heart is having to work harder to meet the demands of the body. Palpitations may also be caused by anxiety, ingestion of a large meal, lack of adequate rest, or a large intake of caffeine.

A cardiac client usually will experience fatigue because the heart is not able to keep up with the daily demands of the body. Often the fatigue will increase throughout the day. Frequent rest periods will help alleviate some of the fatigue.

The typical concerns expressed by the client with a peripheral vascular disorder are pain, paresthesia, and/or paralysis in the hands, thigh, calf, ankles, foot, abdomen, or lower back. The quality of the pain (aching, cramping, sharp, or throbbing) and any numbness or tingling should be noted.

Objective Data

In a head-to-toe assessment on a cardiac client, the skin, neck veins, respirations, heart sounds, abdomen, and extremities are carefully assessed. The skin should be observed for cyanosis in the earlobes, lips, fingers, and feet. Assessment of skin turgor could give an indication of fluid volume. If the skin is dry and has poor turgor, the client may be dehydrated from diuretics. If a client has distended neck veins when the head of the bed is at a 45° angle or higher, he or she may be experiencing right-sided heart failure. The nurse should assess the quality of respirations for rate and ease of breathing and also observe for dyspnea and coughing. Heart sounds are assessed for the normal S_1 and S_2 sounds. If the typical lubb-dubb is heard, the valves are closing properly. A pericardial friction rub may be heard if the client has pericarditis. This is an extra sound heard as the heart rubs against the pericardial sac. The sound will be a short, high-pitched squeak.

While listening to the heart, the radial pulse should be palpated to account for every heartbeat. If a heartbeat is heard through the stethoscope but not felt in the radial pulse, the heart has decreased cardiac output to the extremities. If the abdomen is distended, the client may have **ascites**, which is excess fluid in the abdomen. After the heart and lung sounds have been assessed, the peripheral pulses should be checked. Pulses on both sides of the body should be checked at the same time to determine adequate bilateral perfusion. It is important to check pedal pulses in both feet to determine blood flow to each foot.

If the hands and feet are cold or have mottling, this could indicate decreased cardiac output. Capillary refill should be assessed in the fingers and toes.

It should be noted if the feet, ankles, or legs are edematous (Figure 32-6). A client may gain 10 pounds before edema can be detected. It is important that fluid volume be assessed daily on cardiac clients with edema by having the client weighed daily. The weight must be taken on the same scale, at the same time of day, with the client wearing the same amount of clothing.

Assessment of the peripheral vascular system includes assessment of rate, rhythm, and quality of peripheral pulses to give an indication as to the perfusion of the extremities. It is important to compare the two extremities to determine that the pulses are the same in both extremities.

If an artery in the leg is occluded, the foot and/or leg becomes reddish in color when the leg is in a dependent position, and pale when elevated. As the ischemia progresses, the leg and/or foot becomes mottled. The skin is smooth and shiny. If the veins are occluded, the foot and/or leg becomes cyanotic when in a dependent position, and has a normal coloration when elevated. Often the anterior area of the lower leg and ankle have a brown pigmentation with venous involvement.

Clients with decreased circulation to the extremities have hardened and brittle nails. The leg will be cool if there is an arterial circulatory problem but warm if there is a venous circulatory problem. Skin ulcerations around the ankles and toes should be assessed.

The client's ankles should be observed for **stasis dermatitis**, an inflammation of the skin due to de-

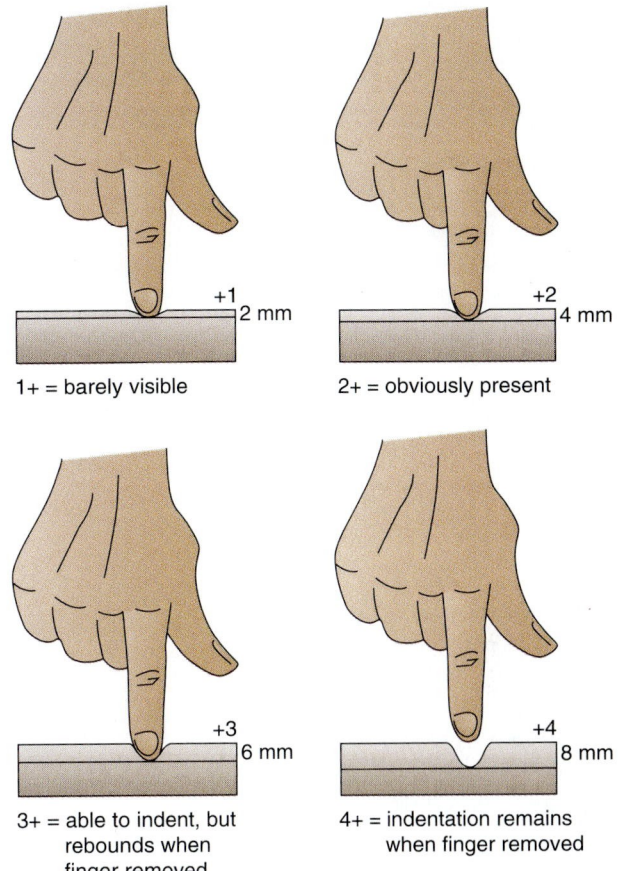

1+ = barely visible

2+ = obviously present

3+ = able to indent, but rebounds when finger removed

4+ = indentation remains when finger removed

Figure 32-6 Edema Rating Scale

creased circulation. Waste products that normally are carried away in the circulatory system remain in the tissues, causing pruritus and irritation of the skin. At first, the ankle area is reddened and edematous, then vesicles form and start oozing. The skin becomes crusted, thickened, and brown in color.

A positive Homans' sign is present in 10% to 20% of deep vein thrombosis (DVT) cases (Hickey, 1994). To test for the **Homans' sign**, the nurse dorsiflexes the client's foot. If there is pain in the calf of the leg or behind the knee, the Homans' sign is positive and may indicate the presence of a venous clot.

COMMON DIAGNOSTIC TESTS

Commonly used diagnostic tests for clients with symptoms of cardiovascular system disorders are listed in Table 32-1. See Chapter 27, Diagnostic Tests, for explanation/normal values and nursing responsibilities.

CARDIAC RHYTHM/ DYSRHYTHMIA

As a basis for understanding cardiac dysrhythmias, the normal sinus rhythm must first be understood.

Table 32-1 COMMON DIAGNOSTIC TESTS FOR CARDIOVASCULAR SYSTEM DISORDERS

Laboratory Tests

Arterial blood gasses (ABGs)
Complete blood count (CBC)
Platelet count
Hemoglobin (Hgb)
Hematocrit (Hct)
Electrolytes
Cardiac enzymes
   Serum aspartate aminotransferase (AST)
   Creatine kinase CPK (CK)
   Lactic dehydrogenase (LDH)
Erythrocyte sedimentation rate (ESR)
Glucose
Prothrombin time (PT)
Partial thromboplastin time (PTT)
International Normalized Ratio (INR)
Serum lipids (lipid profile)
   Cholesterol
   High-density lipoprotein (HDL)
   Low-density lipoprotein (LDL)
   Very low-density lipoprotein (VLDL)
   Triglycerides

Radiologic Tests

Chest x-ray
Cardiac positron emission tomography scan
Radionuclide angiography (multiplegated radioisotope scan, multi-gated aquisition scanning, MUGA)
Technetium pyrophosphate scanning
Thalium scan

Other Diagnostic Tests

Cardiac biopsy
Cardiac catheterization
Echocardiogram
Electrocardiogram (EKG or ECG)
Holter monitor
Magnetic resonance imaging (MRI)
Pericardiocentesis
Pulse oximetry
Stress test
Arterial plethysmography (pulse volume recorder)
Venous plethysmography (cuff pressure test)

NORMAL SINUS RHYTHM

The electrical conduction of the heart begins with the sinoatrial (SA) node located in the superior section of the right atrium. From the SA node, the electrical impulse spreads in wave fashion through the atria similar to the ripples from a pebble dropped in water. The fir-

ing of the SA node and the electrical impulse spreading across both atria yields a P wave on the EKG. Thus the P wave represents the electrical activity causing the contraction of both atria.

After the atria contract, the electrical impulse then reaches the atrioventricular (AV) node where it pauses for approximately one-tenth second allowing blood to enter both ventricles. The electrical impulse then starts down the AV bundle, also called the *bundle of His,* which divides into right and left bundle branches in the interventricular septum. The electrical impulse continues from the right and the left bundle branches to the Purkinje fibers. The Purkinje fibers transmit the electrical impulse to the myocardial cells causing contractions of the ventricles. On an EKG the QRS complex represents the electrical impulse as it travels through the AV node, bundle of His, bundle branches, Purkinje fibers, and myocardial cells terminating with the ventricles contracting.

There is a pause after the QRS complex. The pause is called the ST segment. The ST segment represents the period between the contraction and the beginning of the recovery or repolarization of the ventricular muscles. The T wave represents the repolarization of the ventricles.

After the repolarization of the ventricles, the entire cycle begins all over again at the SA node. In this way the P wave, QRS complex, and T waves are repeated with each heartbeat. Figure 32-7 shows an EKG strip of normal sinus rhythm.

DYSRHYTHMIAS

A **dysrhythmia** is an irregularity in the rate, rhythm, or conduction of the electrical system of the heart. The dysrhythmia can occur in the atria, ventricles, or any part of the conduction system. Specialized cells in the heart muscle have the ability to generate an electrical impulse. Under certain conditions these cells start sending impulses to other cells in the heart causing irregular beats called *ectopic beats.* The most common causes of dysrhythmias are coronary artery disease (CAD) and myocardial infarction (MI). Other causes of dysrhythmias are electrolyte imbalances and drug toxicity.

Symptoms of a client experiencing a dysrhythmia can vary from asymptomatic to cardiac arrest. The

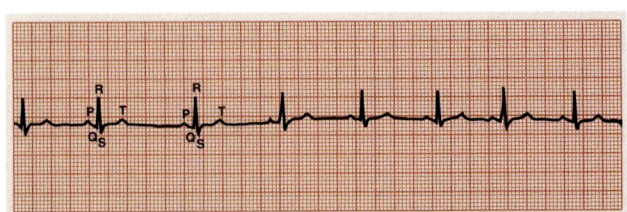

Figure 32-7 An EKG Strip Showing a Normal Sinus Rhythm with the P Wave, QRS Complex, and T Wave Identified

client may experience fainting, seizures, fatigue, decreased energy level, exertional dyspnea, chest pain, and palpitations.

BRADYCARDIA

Sinus **bradycardia** is a heart rate of 60 beats/minute or less (Figure 32-8). Causes of sinus bradycardia are myocardial ischemia, electrolyte imbalances, vagal stimulation, heart block, drug toxicity, intracranial tumors, sleep, and vomiting. The treatment for bradycardia is the administration of atropine. Some clients with bradycardia may require a permanent pacemaker.

TACHYCARDIA

Tachycardia is a sinus rhythm with a heart rate ranging from 100 to 150 beats/minute; the EKG pattern is much closer together. Causes of tachycardia are exercise, emotional stress, fever, medications, pain, anemia, thyrotoxicosis, pericarditis, heart failure, excessive caffeine intake, and tobacco use. When the heart is beating at this rate, there is limited time for the ventricles to fill with blood. This causes a decreased amount of blood to be pumped to the coronary arteries and throughout the body. If the cause is stress or anxiety, the client is treated for anxiety. Sometimes the heart rate will slow spontaneously. At other times, medications such as beta blockers, calcium channel blockers, and digitalis are needed.

ATRIAL DYSRHYTHMIAS

Atrial dysrhythmias occur from disturbances in the electrical conduction in the atria resulting in premature beats or abnormal atrial rhythms. Common causes for atrial dysrhythmias are myocardial infarction, congestive heart failure, electrolyte imbalances, emotional stress, and drugs.

Premature Atrial Contractions

A premature atrial contraction (PAC) is an ectopic impulse not originating in the sinoatrial node, but rather in the atrial tissue. This causes an atrial depolarization to occur earlier in the cycle than expected, thus the term *premature atrial contraction.*

PACs often do not cause the client to experience physical symptoms depending on how often they occur. Generally they are benign and occur several times a day in healthy individuals. If their occurrence causes an increase or decrease in the pulse rate, they should be evaluated. PACs can be a symptom of myocardial ischemia, developing congestive heart failure, digitalis toxicity, hypokalemia, or an inflammatory condition. Stress, caffeine, and smoking can also cause PACs. PACs can be the first indication that more serious atrial dysrhythmias could occur if not treated properly.

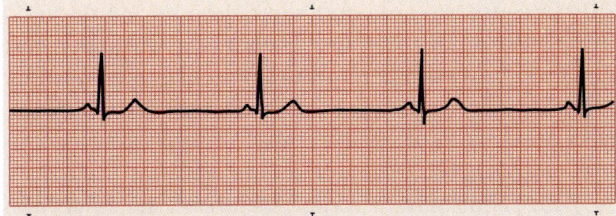

Figure 32-8 Sinus Bradycardia

Atrial Tachycardia

Atrial tachycardia is an ectopic impulse that causes the atria to contract at the rate of 140 to 250 beats/minute. This is sometimes referred to as a *supraventricular dysrhythmia,* meaning the impulse causing the dysrhythmia is occurring above the ventricles. This dysrhythmia can occur as a continuous rhythm or as short, sudden eruptions that start and end spontaneously.

Atrial tachycardia occurs with hypokalemia, digitalis toxicity, and ischemia. Potassium supplements are given if the cause of the dysrhythmia is hypokalemia. If an increased level of serum digitalis is the cause, digitalis is withheld until the level returns to normal. An artificial pacemaker may be surgically inserted to regulate the atrial tachycardia dysrhythmia.

Paroxysmal Supraventricular Tachycardia

Paroxysmal supraventricular tachycardia (PSVT) was previously called paroxysmal atrial tachycardia (PAT). PSVT is a rapid atrial beat accompanied by an abnormal conduction in the AV node. The dysrhythmia occurs suddenly (paroxysmally) and is usually initiated by a premature beat. PSVT can stop as abruptly as it begins. It can be caused by myocarditis, caffeine, alcohol ingestion, smoking, and stress. PSVT may also be present in clients with coronary artery disease, mitral valve prolapse, and acute pericarditis.

Atrial Flutter

Atrial flutter, a rapid contraction of the atria, yields a heart rate of 250 to 350 beats/minute. The EKG displays a sawtooth wave pattern. The AV node attempts to block some of the atrial impulses, but usually the ventricles are also contracting at a rate of 300 beats/minute. This causes a decreased blood supply to the

 LIFE CYCLE CONSIDERATIONS

Paroxysmal Supraventricular Tachycardia
PSVT is a common dysrhythmia in children and young adults and may not be indicative of heart disease.

body because the atria and ventricles are unable to fill with blood when they are contracting at such a fast rate. This dysrhythmia requires immediate intervention.

Underlying causes of atrial flutter are coronary artery disease, pulmonary embolism, mitral valve disease, acute myocardial infarction, and cardiomyopathy. The client may experience palpitations or go into cardiac shock depending on the underlying cause. If atrial flutter occurs during an MI or with congestive heart failure, it is a sign of poor prognosis.

Atrial Fibrillation

Atrial fibrillation is an erratic electrical activity of the atria, resulting in a rate of 350 to 600 beats/minute. Atrial depolarization is so uncoordinated during the dysrhythmia that the atria quiver rather than contract. The AV node is bombarded with impulses and randomly transmits the impulses to the ventricles causing varied irregular contractions of the ventricles with a ventricular rate of 100 to 180 beats/minute. The underlying cause of the dysrhythmia is of an organic nature such as mitral conditions, CAD, acute MI, hypertensive heart disease, and hyperthyroidism. Since the atria are not contracting properly, blood pools in the atria predisposing the person to thrombi forming on the walls of the atria. The clots can dislodge and travel to the brain, lungs, and other parts of the body.

Once the underlying condition is treated, atrial fibrillation may stop. However, it is usually treated with quinidine or procainamide hydrochloride (Procan SR) and digoxin (Lanoxin). A calcium channel blocker, verapamil (Calan) or nifedipine (Procardia), or a beta blocker, atenolol (Tenormin) or timolol maleate (Blocadren), is used for a short time to slow the heart rate. If the dysrhythmia cannot be controlled with medication, cardioversion may be necessary. Cardioversion should be done with caution if the client has been digitalized. Digitalization causes the heart to be sensitive to cardioversion and the heart may fibrillate from the cardioversion. Anticoagulants should be used before the client undergoes cardioversion so a thrombus is not released into the system.

VENTRICULAR DYSRHYTHMIAS

Ventricular dysrhythmias originate in the ventricles. They are more life threatening than atrial dysrhythmias because the ventricles supply blood to the lungs and the body. These dysrhythmias must be treated promptly.

Premature Ventricular Contractions

Premature ventricular contractions (PVCs) arise from ectopic beats in the ventricles and are the most common ectopic beats. PVCs can easily be identified on the

EKG because of the wide, bizarre QRS complexes. There are no P waves preceding the QRS complex.

Coronary artery disease is the most common cause of PVCs. Other causes of PVCs are myocardial ischemia, CHF, electrolyte imbalances, digitalis toxicity, anxiety, exercise, hypoxia, caffeine, and excessive alcohol consumption.

The most common pharmacological treatment for PVCs is lidocaine hydrochloride (Xylocaine HCl). Initially lidocaine is given as an IV bolus and then titrated according to the client's response.

Other medications used to treat PVCs are procainamide hydrochloride (Procan SR), quinidine, disopyramide phosphate (Norpace), bretylium tosylate (Bretylol), and magnesium sulfate.

Administering oxygen may increase the oxygen perfusion to the myocardial tissue and decrease the frequency of premature beats.

Ventricular Tachycardia

Ventricular tachycardia (VT) is the occurrence of 3 or more consecutive PVCs. The ventricular rate is 100 beats/minute and may go as high as 140 to 240 beats/minute. The EKG reveals a wide, abnormally shaped QRS complex. Underlying conditions in which VT occurs are cardiomyopathy, hypoxemia, digitalis toxicity, and electrolyte imbalance.

During VT, the client will have a low blood pressure, weak or absent peripheral pulses, body weakness, and may become unconscious. The ventricle is beating so rapidly that it is unable to fill with blood or eject blood properly. This causes blood to back up in the pulmonary circulation leading to pulmonary congestion.

It is important that VT be treated promptly because a ventricular tachycardia rhythm may lead into ventricular fibrillation, a life-threatening dysrhythmia. The client is given oxygen and an intravenous line is inserted if one is not already in place. The drug of choice is procainamide hydrochloride (Procan SR) given intravenously because it slows the electrical conduction in the ventricle. Lidocaine hydrochloride (Xylocaine HCl) is given if PVCs occur with myocardial ischemia or infarct. If the VT is not controlled with medications, the client may be cardioverted if peripheral pulses are present, or defibrillated if peripheral pulses are absent.

Cardioversion

Cardioversion is the delivery of a synchronized electrical shock to change a dysrhythmia to a rhythm that will circulate more blood to the body tissues and improve oxygenation of the tissues. The electrical shock is set to be delivered on the R wave, as a shock during ventricular depolarization may cause ventricular fibrillation. Cardioversion is done as an elective or emergency treatment. Electrodes are placed to the right of the sternum below the clavicle and at the apex of the heart. The electrodes are lubricated with a special gel or placed on normal saline pads. The electrical current delivered through the electrodes depolarizes the myocardium and allows the heart's pacemaker to reestablish a sinus rhythm.

The client is NPO for 8 hours prior to an elective cardioversion. Diuretics and digitalis preparations are withheld 24 to 72 hours before the cardioversion since the myocardium cells are less responsive to convert to a normal rhythm or may develop a serious dysrhythmia after the cardioversion. Anticoagulants and oral antiarrhythmics are still given before cardioversion. Anticoagulants are given so a thrombus is not released into the system. The client is given a sedative such as diazepam (Valium) or midazolam hydrochloride (Versed) intravenously before the procedure. The client's vital signs and EKG strip are monitored closely for the first hour after the cardioversion and then as ordered by the physician.

Defibrillation

Defibrillation is the delivery of an unsynchronized, high-energy electrical shock during an emergency situation such as a cardiac arrest or pulseless VT to convert the life-threatening dysrhythmia or arrhythmia to a sinus rhythm. Defibrillation is done by a physician or a nurse who has had special education to handle emergency situations. Paddles are lubricated with a special gel or normal saline pads are applied to the skin where the paddles will be placed. The paddles are placed to the right of the sternum below the clavicle and at the apex of the heart. When the electrical shock is delivered to the client, everyone stands clear of the bed to prevent them from also receiving the electrical shock. More than one electrical shock may be delivered in an attempt to convert the rhythm.

If conservative measures do not control the VT and the client has periodic episodes of VT, an **automatic implantable cardioverter-defibrillator (AICD)** is implanted in the client (Figure 32-9). This device senses the dysrhythmia and automatically sends an electrical shock directly to the heart to defibrillate it.

One type of AICD has leads that are attached to the heart muscle. The pulse generator that initiates the shock is placed in a pocket of subcutaneous tissue in the abdominal wall. The pulse generator is powered by lithium batteries. Another type of AICD has an endocardial lead that is guided through a vein into the right side of the heart. The pulse generator may be placed under the skin below the collarbone or in the abdomen.

The AICD detects VT and ventricular fibrillation (VF) through the leads attached to the heart muscle. Once VT or VF are detected, an electrical shock is sent from the pulse generator. The AICD is capable of

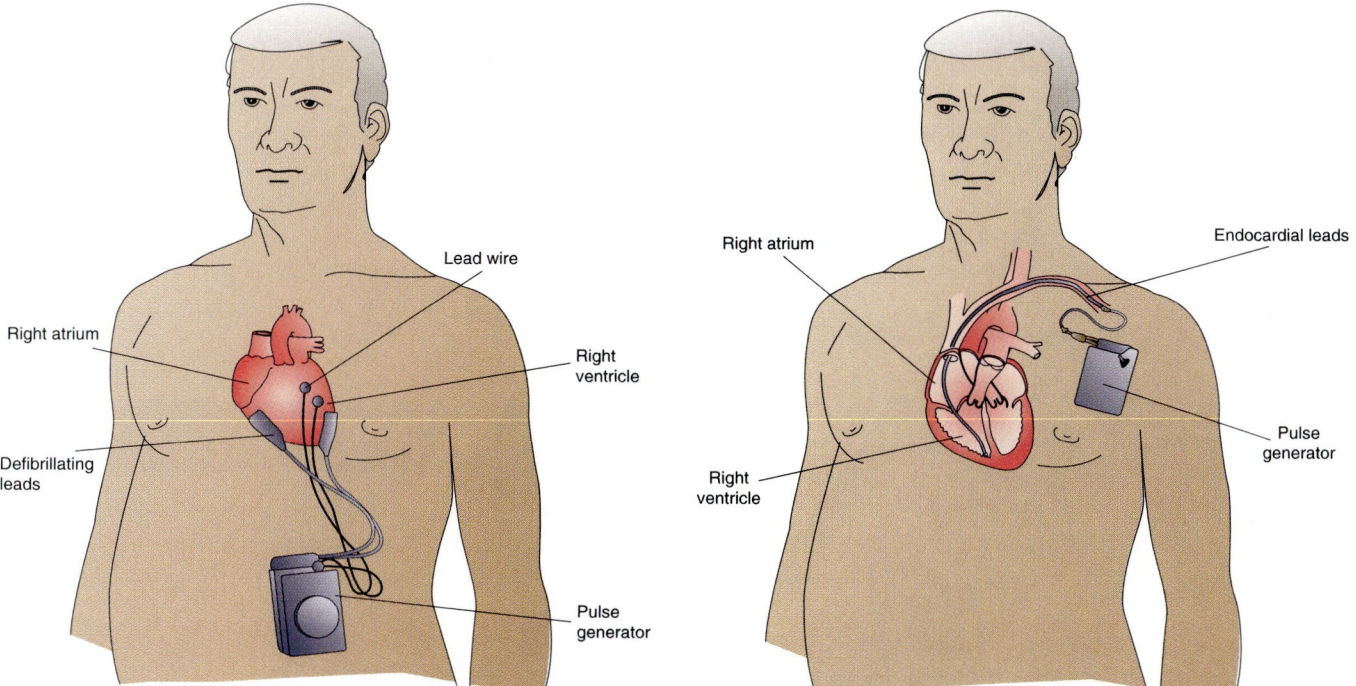

Figure 32-9 Two Different Types of Automatic Implantable Cardioverter-Defibrillators (AICD): A. Pulse generator implanted in the subcutaneous tissue of the abdomen with lead wires and defibrillating leads going to the heart; B. Pulse generator implanted below the collar bone with endocardial leads positioned in the heart through a vein.

delivering three more shocks to the heart muscle if the heart does not return to normal sinus rhythm (NSR). Usually clients are converted to NSR with the first shock. Complications following the insertion of a AICD are atelectasis, pneumonia, pneumothorax, thrombus, and a seroma at the generator site.

Ventricular Fibrillation

The most common cause for VF is CAD. VF is a disorganized, chaotic quivering of the ventricles. The ventricles are unable to contract and no blood is ejected into the circulatory system. The EKG reading is a series of jagged, unidentifiable waves. The client will not have a pulse, blood pressure, or respirations. This dysrhythmia is serious. Aggressive measures must be taken to initiate CPR and defibrillate the client immediately.

Ventricular Asystole

Ventricular asystole is represented only by a P wave or by a straight line on the EKG. The ventricles are not contracting and the client is in cardiac arrest. The client loses consciousness and has no pulse or respirations. Aggressive treatment should be initiated within 1 minute to prevent chemical changes within the body that jeopardize recovery. CPR is started and the client is defibrillated. Atropine sulfate and epinephrine are given intravenously.

ATRIOVENTRICULAR BLOCKS

In atrioventricular blocks the electrical conduction is interrupted to some degree between the atria and ventricles at the AV node. The extent of interruption is classified as first degree, second degree, or third degree.

First Degree AV Block

In first degree block the impulse is delayed in traveling through the AV node. The impulse eventually reaches the ventricles, but is delayed. There are no physical symptoms or treatment for first degree block.

Second Degree AV Block

In second degree block some of the impulses pass through the AV node to the ventricles and others are blocked. Symptoms include irregular pulse, vertigo, and weakness. A temporary pacemaker may be inserted until the conduction pattern is stabilized. If the dysrhythmia persists, a permanent pacemaker may be implanted.

Third Degree AV Block

Third degree heart block is when no impulses are able to pass from the atria through the AV node to the ventricles. The atria and ventricles beat independently

of each other. The causes of third degree block are myocardial ischemia, drug toxicity, and electrolyte imbalances. Atropine sulfate may be given to improve conduction through the AV node. A permanent pacemaker is usually required to control the dysrhythmia.

Safety: Pacemaker
The client should wear a medical identification tag indicating the presence of a pacemaker.

Medical–Surgical Management

Pharmacological

Dysrhythmias originating in the atria are treated with a digitalis preparation while dysrhythmias originating in the ventricles are treated with lidocaine hydrochloride (Xylocaine HCl) or other antiarrhythmic agents.

Diet

The client is usually placed on a low-fat, low-cholesterol diet. Caffeine consumption is restricted.

▶ NURSING PROCESS

▶ Assessment

▶ Subjective Data

The nurse should inquire if the client has experienced palpitations, lightheadness, nausea, dyspnea, anxiety, fatigue, or chest discomfort.

▶ Objective Data

If a client is experiencing dysrhythmias, the heart rate, blood pressure, and respirations should be checked. While listening to the apical pulse and respirations, abnormal heart sounds should be noted and breath sounds monitored for crackles. The presence of crackles indicates the lungs are filling with fluid. Observe the skin for pallor and cyanosis. Urine output may decrease.

CLIENT TEACHING

Pacemaker
- High-tension wires, high-voltage electrical generators, or MRIs may cause pacemaker malfunction.
- Contact sports should be avoided.
- Pacemakers may activate airport security alarms.

Nursing diagnoses for a client with dysrhythmias may include the following:

Nursing Diagnoses	Planning/Goals	Nursing Interventions
▶ *Cardiac Output, Decreased, related to inadequate electrical conduction*	The client will have increased cardiac output.	Apply electrodes for telemetry monitoring. Balance activity with rest periods. Monitor the vital signs during activity and at rest. Listen to the apical pulse, especially noting rate and rhythm. Elevate the extremities so they are not in a dependent position. Perform cardiac resuscitation as needed.
▶ *Anxiety, related to fear of potential diagnosis, treatment regimen, and death*	The client will relate fears of potential cardiac problems.	Care for the client in a calm, confident, and efficient manner. Remain with the client and explain procedures and treatments. Encourage client input regarding the care. Encourage the client to verbalize concerns about the dysrhythmia and potential future complications. Teach the client relaxation activities.
▶ *Knowledge Deficit, related to electrical conduction of the heart and treatment methods*	The client will describe electrical disorder and treatment methods.	Explain medication administration times, action, side effects, and symptoms that need reporting. Provide written instructions to the client and family. Explain symptoms of dysrhythmias such as fatigue, edema, palpitations, lightheadness, nausea, dyspnea, and anxiety. If a pacemaker is needed, explain the purpose, insertion procedures, and home care. Include the family in all the teaching sessions.

Evaluation Each goal must be evaluated to determine how it has been met by the client.

INFLAMMATORY DISORDERS

Inflammatory disorders include rheumatic heart disease, infective endocarditis, myocarditis, pericarditis, and valvular heart disease.

RHEUMATIC HEART DISEASE

Rheumatic heart disease is a complication of rheumatic fever. Rheumatic fever and rheumatic heart disease affect about 1.8 million persons in the United States (American Heart Association, 1999e). Rheumatic fever is a systemic inflammatory disease that occurs 2 to 3 weeks after an inadequately treated pharyngitis caused by the group A *beta-hemolytic streptococcus*. Symptoms of rheumatic fever are a mild fever, polyarthritis, carditis, chorea, and a rash. The endocardium, myocardium, and epicardium can become inflamed with the most damage occurring to the mitral valve. The mitral valve becomes incompetent because of thickening and stenosis of the valve leaflets. Mitral prolapse (valve leaflets fall into the left atrium during systole) may result.

Once afflicted with rheumatic fever, a person is more prone to having it again. It is treated with intravenous antibiotics, anti-inflammatory agents, corticosteroids, and strict bed rest. The main goal is to treat the inflammation, prevent cardiac complications, and prevent the recurrence of the disease. These clients must be placed on prophylactic antibiotic therapy prior to dental procedures or invasive surgery. Antibiotic therapy has reduced the mortality from 15,000 in 1950 to 5,000 in 1996 (American Heart Association, 1999e).

INFECTIVE ENDOCARDITIS

Infective endocarditis is an inflammation or infection of the inside lining of the heart, particularly the heart valves. The etiology of inflammatory endocarditis is a collagen-vascular disease or rheumatic fever. Infective endocarditis is caused by bacteria, fungi, or rickettsia. As the microorganisms invade the valves, they form fibrinous substances called *vegetations*. Vegetations cause scar tissue on the valves so they become hard and brittle and do not close properly. When the valve is incapable of holding the blood in the appropriate chamber, blood seeps into the next chamber. The valve is said to be insufficient. Sometimes the vegetations cause the valve flaps to grow together resulting in a narrowing of the opening. This is called a *valvular stenosis*. The mitral valve is more frequently affected than the other valves. When the mitral valve is affected, it is termed *mitral insufficiency* or *mitral stenosis.*

Historically, rheumatic fever was the common cause of endocarditis. More recently, endocarditis is a risk factor for IV drug users, immunosuppressed clients, and clients with valvular heart disease.

The client with endocarditis will have a fever, heart murmur, splenomegaly, and petechiae on the conjunctiva, palate, buccal mucosa, and distal extremities. There are two forms of endocarditis: acute and subacute. Symptoms of acute endocarditis are elevated temperature, tachycardia, pallor, diaphoresis, and symptoms of a systemic infection, such as temperature of 103°F and shaking chills. Clients with subacute endocarditis have low-grade fever, malaise, weight loss, and anemia. Clients with both types of endocarditis may have murmurs and symptoms of congestive heart failure, such as dyspnea, peripheral edema, and pulmonary congestion.

Endocarditis is diagnosed by the client's history and symptoms. A **transesophageal echocardiography (TEE)** can confirm the diagnosis of endocarditis by allowing ultrasonic imaging of the cardiac structures through the esophagus. The erythrocyte sedimentation rate (ESR) and WBC are elevated. A blood culture and sensitivity is done to determine the causative organism and to determine the most effective antibiotic.

Medical–Surgical Management

Surgical

Surgical repair or replacement of a valve is done in severe cases.

Pharmacological

Clients are treated with intravenous antibiotics. The antibiotics are usually continued for 2 to 6 weeks. The most commonly used antibiotics are penicillin V potassium (V-Cillin K), vancomycin hydrochloride (Vancocin), and gentamicin sulfate (Garamycin).

Diet

The client is provided a well-balanced nutritious diet with between-meal snacks.

Activity

The client is placed on bed rest to decrease the workload of the heart. A calm, quiet environment should be provided.

Health Promotion

Clients who have previously had endocarditis or have a mitral valve prolapse are more prone to develop endocarditis. They should take antibiotics prophylactically before having dental work and genitourinary or gastrointestinal invasive procedures. Clients prone to developing endocarditis should take amoxicillin trihydrate (Amoxil) 1 hour before the procedure and again after the procedure.

Nursing Management

Oxygen should be administered as needed, and blood pressure and pulse measured before and after activity to monitor toleration. Apical pulse rate and rhythm should be noted, and breath sounds assessed for adventitious sounds. Activity should be balanced with rest periods. If a client is on vancomycin hydrochloride (Vancocin) or gentamicin sulfate (Garamycin), BUN and creatinine levels must be monitored as both of these drugs are nephrotoxic.

MYOCARDITIS

Myocarditis is an inflammation of the myocardium of the heart. Lymphocytes and leukocytes invade the muscle fibers of the heart causing the chambers to enlarge and the muscle to weaken. This can lead to congestive heart failure. Myocarditis is caused by bacteria, viruses, fungi, or parasites. It can also be an autoimmune reaction such as in the conditions of rheumatic fever or lupus erythematosus. Usually the cause is a virus. Recently myocarditis has been more prevalent in clients with AIDS.

Acute myocarditis presents itself with flulike symptoms of fever, pharyngitis, myalgias, and gastrointestinal complications. The client will also have chest pain and should be monitored for signs of congestive heart failure. A **pericardial friction rub** is often heard if the pericardium becomes involved. The friction rub is a "squeaky" sound heard through the stethoscope when the two inflamed pericardial surfaces rub together with the contraction of the heart.

Myocarditis diagnostic symptoms are nonspecific. They include elevated ESR and elevated LDH, CK, and SGOT levels. The diagnosis of myocarditis can be confirmed with an endomyocardial biopsy.

Medical–Surgical Management

Pharmacological

Digitalis preparations are given to try to prevent congestive heart failure. Broad spectrum antibiotics are also given to treat the infection. Anti-inflammatory agents may be given to reduce the inflammation. Oxygen is administered as needed.

Activity

The client is placed on bed rest. This decreases the workload of the heart.

Nursing Management

The client should be monitored for symptoms of congestive heart failure or pericarditis. The client is placed in a semi-Fowler's position. A quiet environment and frequent rest periods are important for the client. A pulse oximeter is applied to monitor oxygen saturation.

PERICARDITIS

When the membranous sac surrounding the heart becomes inflamed, the condition is called **pericarditis**. Causative organisms are viral, bacterial, fungal, or parasitic. Inflammation can also occur from rheumatic or collagen-vascular conditions like systemic lupus erythematosus. The most common cause of pericarditis is idiopathic, meaning no known cause. Symptoms of pericarditis are severe precordial pain (pain on the anterior surface of the chest over the heart) and a pericardial friction rub. The pain may radiate to the neck, back, or abdomen and become worse when the client coughs or lies on his left side. If the client sits erect and leans forward, the pain is relieved. Pericardial effusion (excess fluid in pericardial space) may develop. **Cardiac tamponade** will result if the fluid rapidly increases and hinders the functioning of the ventricle. The S_1 and S_2 sounds are often muffled and hard to hear with fluid accumulation.

With inflammation, scar tissue develops in the pericardial sac. Heart movement is limited by the scar tissue and cardiac failure results.

Medical–Surgical Management

Medical

A **pericardiocentesis** is done to aspirate the excess fluid from the pericardial sac. A needle is inserted through the chest wall into the pericardial space.

Surgical

If fibrotic scar tissue in the pericardium hinders heart performance, a pericardiectomy or pericardial window may be done. Pericardiectomy is removal of the pericardium. When a pericardial window is done, a section of the parietal pericardium is cut and tacked back onto itself allowing fluid to escape from the pericardial sac.

Pharmacological

Clients are given antipyretics, analgesics, and anti-inflammatory agents. The infection is combated with antibiotics. Clients may also be given a digitalis preparation and diuretics to improve the pumping action of the heart and decrease fluid retention.

Nursing Management

The client's apical pulse and blood pressure should be assessed, and the EKG monitored for dysrhythmias. Assessment for signs of cardiac tamponade such as decreased pulse and blood pressure, muffled heart sounds, increased respirations, restlessness, and oliguria is critical. Oxygen can be administered as needed, and the client assisted to a position of comfort. Analgesics, antibiotics, and anti-inflammatory agents should be administered as ordered and the client's responses

monitored. The nurse should encourage the client to verbalize concerns and fears.

VALVULAR HEART DISEASES

Valvular heart disease occurs when the valves do not open and close properly. A thickening of the valve tissue, causing the valve opening to be narrow, is called *valvular stenosis*. Valvular insufficiency is the inability of the valve to close completely. When the valve does not close completely, blood leaks back into the chamber from which it was just pumped. This is called regurgitation (Figure 32-10). The client with valvular heart disease often has a history of rheumatic fever.

STENOSIS AND INSUFFICIENCY

The definitions, symptoms, diagnostic findings, medical–surgical management, and nursing interventions for mitral and aorta valve conditions are covered in Table 32-2.

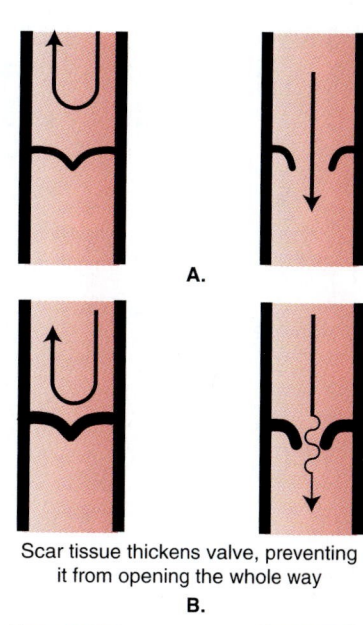

Scar tissue thickens valve, preventing it from opening the whole way

B.

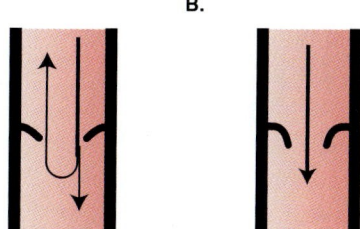

Scar tissue causes the valve to harden and pull apart, preventing it from closing completely and allowing blood to leak backwards

C.

Figure 32-10 A. Normal Valve; B. Stenosed Valve; C. Insufficient Valve

Table 32-2 MITRAL AND AORTIC VALVE STENOSIS AND INSUFFICIENCY

VALVE CONDITION	DEFINITION	SYMPTOMS	DIAGNOSTIC FINDINGS	MEDICAL–SURGICAL MANAGEMENT	NURSING INTERVENTIONS
Mitral stenosis	The diseased valve becomes narrowed and the leaflets thickened, preventing blood from freely flowing from the left atrium into the left ventricle.	Gradual onset of symptoms: exertional dyspnea, fatigue, orthopnea, paroxysmal nocturnal dyspnea, murmur. **Later symptoms:** peripheral edema, atrial fibrillation, jugular venous distention, hepatomegaly, abdominal distention, hypotension, thrombus from blood pooling in the left atrium.	**Chest x-ray:** hypertrophy and enlargement of left atrium and right ventricle. **EKG:** atrial fibrillation. **Echocardiogram:** fusion of valve leaflets, enlarged left atrium, decreased blood flow through valve.	**Medical management:** diuretics, digitalis, anticoagulants, antidysrhythmics, prophylactic antibiotics for invasive procedures, low-sodium diet, semi-Fowler's position, activity restrictions as needed. **Surgical management:** commissurotomy, percutaneous balloon mitral valvuloplasty, mitral valve replacement.	Encourage rest periods, administer oxygen, elevate head of bed, reposition frequently to decrease pressure points, elevate legs, low-sodium diet, monitor for signs of right and left-sided heart failure, teach stress reduction techniques, daily weight.
Mitral Insufficiency	The valve leaflets become hard and do not close completely. Blood backs up in both the left atria and ventricle, causing both chambers to hypertrophy.	Gradual onset of symptoms: exertional dyspnea, palpitations, fatigue, atrial fibrillation, loud murmur and gallop.	**Chest x-ray:** hypertrophy and enlargement of left atrium and left ventricle. **EKG:** atrial fibrillation.	**Medical management:** same as mitral stenosis. **Surgical management:** valvuloplasty, mitral valve replacement.	Same as mitral stenosis, teach exercise modification.
Aortic Stenosis	The valve cusps become hard and calcify due to rheumatic fever, syphilis, a congenital anomaly, or the aging process.	Syncope, exertional dyspnea, arrhythmias, angina, murmur, and gallop; sudden death may occur. **Later symptoms as the disease progresses:** paroxysmal atrial tachycardia, orthopnea.	**Chest x-ray:** enlargement of left ventricle, calcification of aortic valve. **EKG:** hypertrophy of left ventricle inverted T wave echocardiogram fusion of valve leaflets, regurgitation.	**Medical management:** same as mitral stenosis. **Surgical management:** percutaneous balloon aortic valvuloplasty, aortic valve replacement.	Same as mitral stenosis.
Aortic Insufficiency	The valve cusps become so hardened they do not close completely. The blood no longer flows through the vessel but backs up into the left ventricle.	Palpitations, chest pain, exertional dyspnea, nocturnal angina, dizziness, fatigue, decreased activity, intolerance, paroxysmal nocturnal dyspnea, visible pulsation of the neck veins, murmur, lung congestion.	**Chest x-ray:** hypertrophy and enlargement of left ventricle.	**Medical management:** same as mitral stenosis. **Surgical management:** aortic valve replacement.	Same as mitral stenosis, teach exercise modification.

MITRAL VALVE PROLAPSE

Mitral valve prolapse is an extension of mitral insufficiency in which the valve leaflets, chordae tendineae, and papillary muscle become damaged. The valve leaflets flip back into the left atrium when the left ventricle contracts. This condition affects more women then men. Often the client remains asymptomatic. The symptoms that a client may experience depend on how seriously the mitral valve is affected. Sometimes clients experience palpitations and fatigue due to a decreased cardiac output. They also may experience angina, dizziness, and syncope. Some clients have panic attacks. Often a click or murmur can be heard.

Medical–Surgical Management

Medical

Clients with valvular heart disease are to take antibiotics prophylactically before any dental procedures and genitourinary or gastrointestinal invasive procedures.

Surgical

When the activities of a client with valvular heart disease become curtailed because of decreased cardiac output and the symptoms can no longer be controlled by medical means, surgery may be done. The type of surgery performed will depend on the client's overall condition and on the involved valve.

For the mitral valve, surgery alleviates the symptoms, but it does not cure the condition. Surgeries frequently have to be repeated. A commissurotomy is done for mitral stenosis. In this surgery the valve leaflets are surgically separated. For mitral regurgitation or insufficiency, a valvuloplasty is becoming the treatment of choice. A percutaneous mitral valvuloplasty is a repair of perforated cusps or torn chordae tendineae. The risk of a thrombus is less with valvuloplasty than with grafts or prosthetic valves. An annuloplasty, a repair of an **annulus** or valvular ring, can also be done. The annulus is tightened with a purse-string suture or an annular ring. The mitral valve is replaced when other repair measures are not feasible.

The aortic valve is not repaired, only replaced, if the symptoms cannot be controlled by medical means. The preferred treatment for a client with an aortic stenosis is percutaneous aortic valvuloplasty. This treatment is often used in elderly or high-risk surgical clients. A **percutaneous balloon valvuloplasty** can be done in the cardiac catheterization laboratory and no anesthesia is required. A catheter is advanced to the affected valve and a balloon is inflated in the stenosed valve. The narrowed valvular space is expanded by the balloon leaving a wider opening. Later, larger balloons may be used to expand the opening as needed.

There are two types of replacement valves: mechanical and biological. The mechanical valves are the caged-ball valve or the tilting-disk valve (Figure 32-11). There is a higher risk of a thromboembolism with a caged-ball valve. Clients remain on anticoagulant therapy with both types of valves. The biological valves come from calves, pigs, or humans. The disadvantage of the biological valves is tissue degeneration and calcification of the valve.

▶ NURSING PROCESS

▶ Assessment

▶ Subjective Data

Review past medical history for conditions such as rheumatic fever or streptococcal infections. Inquire if the client has experienced any dyspnea, palpitations, fatigue, cough, lightheadness, or numbness and tingling in the extremities.

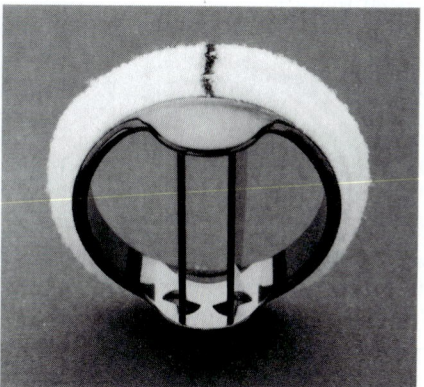 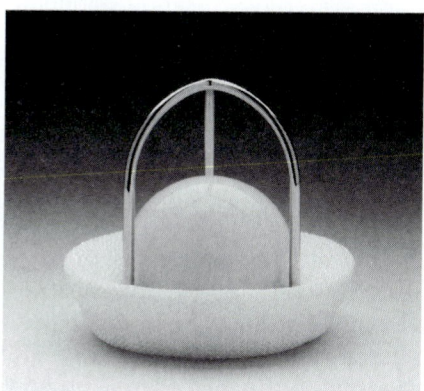 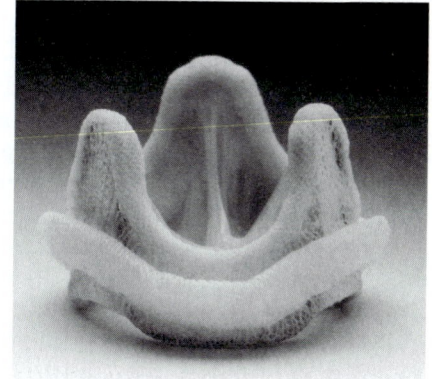

Figure 32-11 Types of Artificial Valves: A. St. Jude Medical® Mechanical Heart Valve (St. Jude Medical® is a registered trademark of St. Jude Medical, Inc.); B. Starr-Edwards Silastic Ball Valve, Model 1260 Aortic; C. Carpentier-Edwards® Bioprosthesis, Model 2625 Aortic (A. Courtesy of St. Jude Medical, Inc. All rights reserved; B. and C. Courtesy of Baxter Healthcare Corporation, Edwards CVS Division.)

▶ **Objective Data**

Take the vitals signs and listen to the apical pulse for rate, rhythm, murmurs, and S_3 sound. Listen to the breath sound for adventitious sounds. Check for edema, jugular distention, cyanosis, and equality of peripheral pulses.

Nursing diagnoses for a client with cardiac valvular disorders may include the following:

Nursing Diagnoses	Planning/Goals	Nursing Interventions
▶ *Cardiac Output, Decreased, related to structural changes in valves*	The client will have increased cardiac output.	Administer oxygen as needed.
		Help the client balance activities with rest periods. The pulse should return to the baseline within 10 minutes of activity; if not, activity has been excessive.
		Discourage smoking and refer clients to support groups to assist them to stop smoking. Encourage clients to use Nicoderm or Nicorette gum while attempting to stop smoking if ordered by the physician.
▶ *Fluid Volume Excess, related to decreased cardiac output*	The client will have a decrease in edema.	Administer diuretics as needed.
		Support the extremities and do not let them be in a dependent position.
		Encourage the client to maintain a low-sodium diet.
▶ *Anxiety, related to threat to or change in health status*	The client will list ways to cope with stressors.	Calmly explain the procedures before doing them.
		Encourage the client's input to decisions regarding care.
		Assist the client and the client's family in identifying ways to cope with stressors.
		Teach relaxation techniques.
▶ *Knowledge Deficit, related to disease process and treatment*	The client will relate the disease process and needed self-care management.	Explain the valvular disease process, medication actions, dosage times, and medication side effects to report.
		Refer the client and family members to the dietitian for low-sodium diet instructions.
		Encourage the client to begin an appropriate exercise program.

Evaluation Each goal must be evaluated to determine how it has been met by the client.

OCCLUSIVE DISORDERS

Occlusive disorders include arteriosclerosis, angina pectoris, and myocardial infarction.

ARTERIOSCLEROSIS

Arteriosclerosis is a narrowing and hardening of arteries. A buildup of lipids, collagen, and smooth muscle cells narrows the inner lining of the vessel (Sommers, 1994). Blood flow through the vessel is decreased causing decreased perfusion to body cells beyond the narrowed or hardened area.

There are three types of arteriosclerosis: atherosclerosis, calcific sclerosis, and arteriolar sclerosis (Sommers, 1994). **Atherosclerosis** is fatty deposits on the inner lining, the tunica intima, of vessel walls. The fat deposit is called *plaque*. In calcific sclerosis, calcium deposits are on the middle layer of the wall of the arteries, the tunica media. Hypertension causes a thickening of the arterioles and is called *arteriolar sclerosis*. With these conditions, vessels lose their elasticity resulting in various conditions, such as arteriosclerotic heart disease, angina, myocardial infarction, stroke, and peripheral vascular disease.

ANGINA PECTORIS

When coronary arteries lose elasticity or become narrow due to plaque collection, the heart muscle receives less blood and oxygen. Physical exertion, emotional stress, smoking, exposure to extreme cold, heavy meals, or an arterial spasm may cause a temporary inadequate blood and oxygen supply to the heart. Myocardial ischemia and angina pectoris result. Myocardial ischemia is a temporary inadequate blood and oxygen supply to the myocardial tissues. When this temporary condition occurs, the person experiences chest pain or **angina pectoris**.

At first, the person may experience a squeezing

pain under the sternum, which radiates to the left shoulder. For some, the pain may radiate to the right shoulder, jaw, or ear. The discomfort may vary from a mild discomfort to an immobilizing pain. Anginal attacks usually increase in frequency and severity over time. The severity of the condition depends on the amount of collateral circulation that has developed.

Collateral circulation develops as larger vessels gradually narrow or harden. Blood that normally passes through the larger vessels is shunted into surrounding smaller vessels. These vessels enlarge in an attempt to supply blood to the affected area. Collateral circulation increases the blood supply to tissues that suffer from an inadequate blood supply. There is a high incidence of angina pectoris in clients with hypertension and diabetes mellitus.

Many people experiencing ischemic attacks do not experience angina. These people may be having a silent myocardial infarct or ischemia. Symptoms indicative of silent ischemia are chest pressure or heaviness, restlessness, shortness of breath with increased respiratory rate, a sensation of epigastric fullness with noisy belching, numbness or tingling in both arms or shoulders, physical or mental fatigue, and dizziness. The person may also experience a change in sleep patterns and mental alertness. The person may state that he or she "feels funny."

Two other types of angina are unstable angina and Prinzmetal's angina. Unstable angina occurs at rest or with minimal exertion and is not relieved with nitroglycerin. This client is more susceptible to myocardial infarction and sudden death. Prinzmetal's angina is caused by a coronary artery spasm and occurs at rest.

The diagnosis of angina is made after reviewing the client's history, lifestyle, laboratory tests, and stress tests. Cholesterol, low-density lipoprotein (LDL), and high-density lipoprotein (HDL) levels are evaluated. Angina pectoris can be diagnosed by a stress test, thallium scan, or a coronary arteriogram. During a stress test, the heart is placed under stress through increasing physical activity on a treadmill or exercise bicycle. The increased oxygen demand of the body puts an extra load on the heart causing electrocardiogram changes and sometimes pain. Thallium and multigated acquisition (MUGA) scans evaluate the blood supply to the myocardial tissue and determine how well the left ventricle is functioning. A coronary arteriogram shows a narrowing or occlusion of the vessels of the heart.

Medical–Surgical Management

Medical

Treatment for angina includes measures to increase the blood supply to the affected area. This can be accomplished by rest and vasodilation medications.

Silent ischemia is treated in the same way symptomatic ischemia is treated. The client needs to be edu-

cated about cardiac risk factors, the importance of following the prescribed medical regimen, and maintaining regular physical checkups.

Surgical

A percutaneous transluminal coronary angioplasty (PTCA) may be done if only one coronary artery is involved and if the atherosclerotic material is small and has not hardened. When a PTCA is done, atherosclerotic matter is pressed against the walls of the coronary vessels to improve circulation to myocardial tissue supplied by that coronary artery (Figure 32-12). A guide wire is inserted to the stenosed area and a special balloon-tipped catheter is placed in the narrowed sclerotic area. When the balloon is inflated, the atherosclerotic material is pressed against the wall of the vessel. The vessel, now open, allows more blood to flow to the myocardial tissue. During this procedure, a piece of the atherosclerotic material may break off and occlude the vessel. If this occurs, the client would have to undergo immediate coronary artery bypass graft (CABG) surgery. Other complications of the procedure are occlusion of the vessel because of a vascular spasm or vessel rupture.

An intracoronary **stent** may be implanted into a stenosed vessel to prevent the vessel from collapsing and to keep the atherosclerotic plaque pressed against

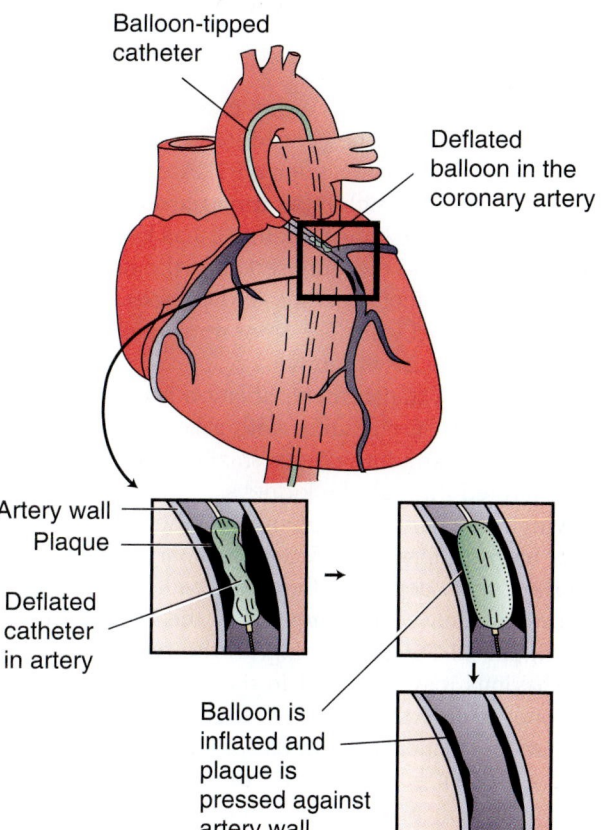

Figure 32-12 Demonstration of the Function of a Balloon-Tipped Catheter during a PTCA Procedure

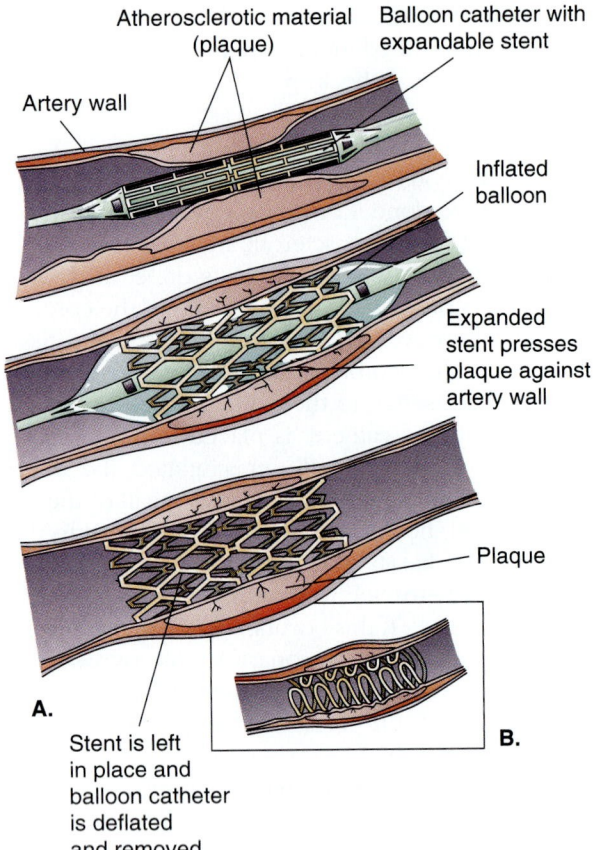

Figure 32-13 Placement of a Stent in a Coronary Artery. A. Palmaz-Schatz Stent; B. Gianturco-Roubin Ex-Stent

Labels on figure: Atherosclerotic material (plaque); Balloon catheter with expandable stent; Artery wall; Inflated balloon; Expanded stent presses plaque against artery wall; Plaque; Stent is left in place and balloon catheter is deflated and removed; A.; B.

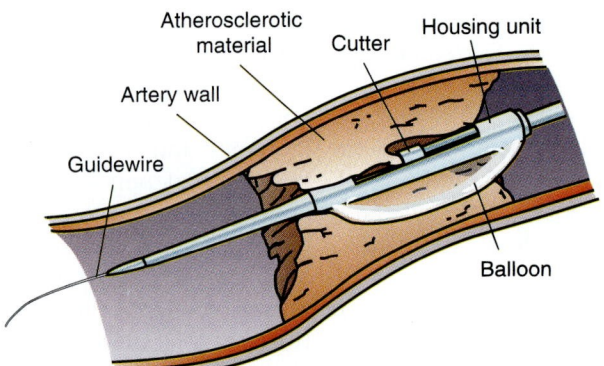

Figure 32-14 A Simpson Coronary AtheroCath cuts the atherosclerotic material (plaque) away from the artery wall.

Labels on figure: Atherosclerotic material; Cutter; Housing unit; Artery wall; Guidewire; Balloon

the vessel wall. A stent is a tiny metal tube with holes in it (Figure 32-13). The procedure is sometimes done when a vessel collapses after a PTCA or in place of a PTCA. The stent is tightly wrapped around a balloon catheter. When the balloon catheter has been threaded through a vessel to the stenosed area, the balloon is inflated and the stent expands and presses the plaque against the vessel wall. The stent remains in the vessel and the catheter is withdrawn.

Sometimes a transcatheter ablation is done to break up the atherosclerotic areas with a laser. The sclerotic material is broken into pieces smaller than blood cells and excreted through the kidneys.

With a coronary atherectomy, an atherectomy catheter is inserted into the affected coronary vessel to the atheroma (fatty deposit in the vessel wall). The cutter on the catheter shaves the plaque from the wall of the vessel (Figure 32-14). Depending on the type of catheter, the shavings may be saved in the end of the catheter, suctioned out, or shaved so small they pass through the capillary circulation without damage to the body.

If a CABG is performed, the internal mammary artery, the saphenous vein, or an accordion type of synthetic graft material is used. The vein or synthetic material is grafted to the aorta and passed beyond the obstruction in the coronary vessel (Figure 32-15). The

graft provides an increased blood supply to the affected myocardium. The client then experiences reduced angina and has an increased tolerance for activities.

Pharmacological

Vasodilators, such as nitroglycerin tablets, cause the blood vessels to dilate, thus providing an increased blood supply to body tissues. The client may not need as much analgesic medication if beta blockers are given. Beta-adrenergic blockers and calcium channel blockers slow the heart rate and decrease the oxygen demand of the heart. Calcium channel blockers also dilate vessels and decrease spasms of the coronary vessels. All these measures provide an increased blood supply to the myocardium.

Diet

The client is placed on a low-fat, low-cholesterol, salt-restricted diet. Sodium restriction may vary from no salt to 4 grams daily depending on the ability of the client's kidneys to excrete excess sodium.

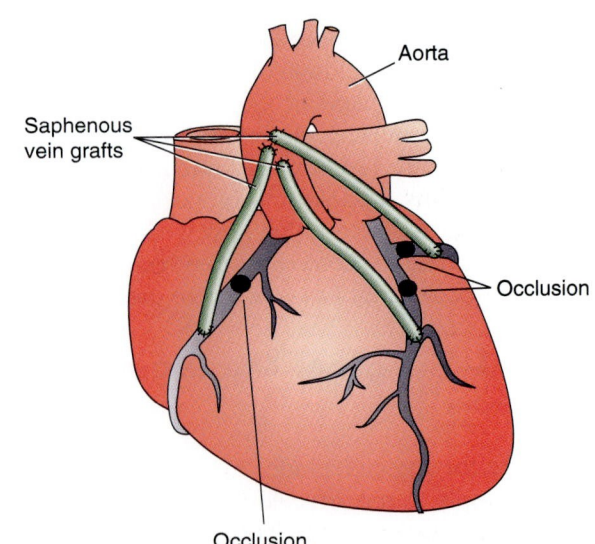

Figure 32-15 Coronary Artery Bypass Graft (CABG) with the Saphenous Vein

Labels on figure: Aorta; Saphenous vein grafts; Occlusion; Occlusion

Activity

Activity should be slower and for shorter periods of time with more rest periods.

Health Promotion

To prevent coronary artery disease resulting in angina, it is recommended that a person limit fat intake to 30 grams or less per day and exercise 3 to 5 times a week for at least 20 minutes. Simple activities such as parking a car further from an entrance to increase walking distance and taking stairs instead of an elevator improve circulation and help decrease cholesterol levels. Activities such as gardening or housework are also good.

▶ NURSING PROCESS

▶ Assessment

▶ Subjective Data

The client should be asked to describe the pain as to type, radiation, onset, duration, and precipitating factors.

▶ Objective Data

The client's actions during the anginal attack should be observed and documented. Vital signs should be measured, and the client attached to an EKG monitor and observed for any dysrhythmias.

Nursing diagnoses for a client with angina may include the following:

Nursing Diagnoses	Planning/Goals	Nursing Interventions
▶ *Pain related to decreased oxygen supply to the myocardium*	The client will experience decreased episodes of angina.	Administer nitroglycerin tablets sublingually. The pain should be relieved within 1 to 2 minutes. If the pain has not stopped after 3 doses 5 minutes apart, notify the emergency personnel.
		Once the acute situation is over, administer nitroglycerin as ordered. It is supplied in ointment, transdermal patch, extended-release capsules, and sprays.
		Administer other medication such as beta blockers or calcium channel blockers as ordered and monitor client's response.
▶ *Anxiety related to perceived threat of death or change in lifestyle*	The client will relate concerns and practice stress reduction techniques.	Assist the client in learning to decrease personal expectations and to live within personal activity limitations.
		Emphasize the importance of getting adequate rest and stopping before becoming too exhausted.
▶ *Knowledge Deficit related to disease process, medications, and treatment regimen*	The client will explain the disease process, medication actions, dosage times and side effects, and self-care practices.	Explain the cause of angina. Teach the client to avoid stressful situations that may produce angina. Other ways to prevent angina are to sleep in a warm room, eat smaller proportions at mealtimes, and not exercise outside in cold weather.
		Inform the client to carry nitroglycerin at all times in a tightly closed container.
		Nitroglycerin may cause orthostatic hypotension, so inform the client to sit after taking it and to change position slowly after taking the medication.
		Encourage the client to start and maintain a regular exercise program as recommended by the physician.

Evaluation Each goal must be evaluated to determine how it has been met by the client.

MYOCARDIAL INFARCTION

A myocardial infarction (MI) is the leading cause of sudden death in men and women, and in 57% of the men and 64% of the women there were no previous symptoms. Of the 367,000 persons who died in 1996 from an MI, 250,000 died within 1 hour of symptom onset and before reaching the hospital (American Heart Association, 1999c). In the United States, 24% of men and 42% of women die within 1 year after having

an MI. The most common cause for myocardial infarction is atherosclerosis.

A **myocardial infarction** is caused by an obstruction in a coronary artery resulting in necrosis (death) to the tissues supplied by the artery. The obstruction is usually due to atherosclerotic plaque, a thrombus, or an embolism. The area most commonly affected is the left ventricle.

Obstruction of a large coronary artery damages the myocardial tissue and affects the pumping efficiency of the heart. A client's prognosis is better if a small coronary artery or arteriole is obstructed and there is good collateral circulation to the heart. If a large vessel is obstructed and the client does not have sufficient collateral circulation, the client may die immediately.

The typical symptoms of an MI in men are feelings of chest heaviness or tightness that progresses to a severe gripping pain in the lower sternal area. The pain is not relieved by rest or nitroglycerin. The client becomes short of breath (dyspneic), diaphoretic, and anxious. Women are more likely to have upper abdominal pain, dyspnea, nausea, and fatigue as well as chest pain (Kudenchuk, Maynard, Martin, Wirkus, & Weaver, 1996). The client frequently becomes nauseated and vomits. The pulse will be irregular, rapid, and weak and the blood pressure will be low. The skin will be pale and then turn cyanotic. Even though a person may not experience the typical MI symptoms, the condition can still be serious or fatal. Complications such as heart failure and stroke may also occur.

A myocardial infarction can be diagnosed by client symptoms, electrocardiogram tracings, cardiac enzyme values, and a radioactive isotope scan. However, in women the electrocardiographic stress test has less diagnostic value than in men because women are less likely to achieve an adequate heart rate response and more likely to have repolarization abnormalities (Roger, Pellikka, Bell, Chow, Bailey, & Seward, 1997). The pattern of the rising and falling values of CK, LDH, and AST are significant in diagnosing a myocardial infarction. The CK level rises within 3 to 6 hours of the infarct, peaks within 12 to 18 hours, and returns to normal in 3 days. The higher the CK level rises the greater the damage to the heart, and the longer the level peaks the more serious the prognosis. AST value increases in 6 hours, peaks in 12 to 14 hours, and returns to normal in 3 to 4 days. LDH level peaks in 72 hours and slowly returns to normal in 11 to 14 days.

During the first 3 days after the infarction, the client may have a low-grade fever and an increased white cell count. The infarcted heart tissue is soft and necrotic and incapable of responding to electrical stimuli. Life-threatening dysrhythmias are most likely to occur at this time. Four to 7 days after the infarction, the infarcted tissue is the softest and weakest. An aneurysm, or ballooning effect, can occur on the wall of the ventricle with the potential of rupturing. There is a possibility of the ventricle rupturing from the time of the infarct to 2 weeks after the infarct. Collateral circulation begins forming around the edges of the infarct, but it will be 2 to 3 weeks before the collateral circulation will function effectively. Two to 3 months will pass before the heart muscle will regain maximum strength.

Medical–Surgical Management

Medical

Medical–surgical management focuses on reducing the workload of the heart, relieving pain, improving tissue perfusion, and preventing complications and further tissue damage. Immediately after an MI, a client is admitted into a coronary care unit. The client's heart is constantly monitored for dysrhythmias and vital signs are monitored for any changes.

Three dysrhythmias that may occur following an MI are ventricular fibrillation, bradycardias, and tachycardias. Ventricular fibrillation is treated by defibrillation. Atropine and, if needed, a temporary pacer may be inserted for bradycardias. Two tachycardias that may occur are atrial fibrillation and ventricular tachycardia. Atrial fibrillation is treated with digoxin (Lanoxin) or amiodarone hydrochloride (Cordarone). Ventricular tachycardia is treated with lidocaine or cardioversion. If dysrhythmias continue, magnesium may be given.

Medical complications that can occur following an MI are acute left ventricular failure, cardiogenic shock, pericarditis, embolism and/or thrombosis, and cardiac rupture. The health care team must closely monitor the client for signs of these complications. Women have a worse prognosis and die more often than men after a heart attack or bypass surgery (Mosca et al., 1997).

Surgical

Primary treatment may be PTCA instead of thrombolytic therapy. Along with balloon compression, a stent(s) may be inserted.

Clients with multiple vessels occluded, or for whom thrombolytic therapy and PTCA have not been effective, may have the CABG procedure performed.

Pharmacological

Oxygen will be given by a Venturi mask or nasal cannula. Morphine sulfate is given intravenously to control the pain. Nitrates are also given intravenously or sublingually to relieve pain and dilate coronary arteries. Sedatives may be given to help calm and relax the client. A stool softener is given to prevent rectal straining.

Thrombolytic therapy is sometimes used within 3 to 6 hours of the myocardial infarction to dissolve a clot blocking an artery and reperfuse the area. Medications such as streptokinase (Streptase), anistreplase (Eminase), and alteplase recombinant (Activase) are used. A possible complication from thrombolytic therapy is bleeding. Bleeding problems are rare but the nurse should be alert for symptoms of hemorrhaging in the gastrointestinal tract (hematemesis and tarry stools), retroperitoneum (low back pain and numbness in lower extremities), or cerebrum (headache, vomiting, and confusion). Heparin therapy inhibits further clotting. Aspirin or ticlopidine (Ticlid) is given to prevent vasoconstriction and platelet aggregation.

Diet

Until the client is stabilized, a diet is withheld in case a PTCA or CABG procedure is required. Fluids may be offered during the acute stage. A liquid diet is progressed to a regular low-fat, low-cholesterol, low-salt diet. The client may tolerate small frequent feedings better than three large meals. Caffeine and extreme hot and cold foods are avoided.

Activity

It is vital the client receive physical, mental, and emotional rest. The less stimuli the client receives, the less demand is placed upon the heart. Procedures must be explained in simple terms so the client will understand the care being provided.

The client is usually limited to bed rest during the first 24 hours and progressed to sitting in a chair by the second day. If pain returns or other complications occur, the client should be confined to bed rest. Early ambulation is encouraged to prevent thrombosis. During and after each activity, the client's tolerance is assessed by monitoring the heart rate for an increase of 20 beats/minute, checking for a decrease in systolic blood pressure, and observing for dyspnea and dysrhythmias. Verbal and nonverbal statements of fatigue and chest pain are assessed.

Before the client is dismissed, low-intensity exercise tests may be done to determine types of activities in which the client may engage at home. When the client is able to climb two flights of stairs, sexual activity may be resumed.

Health Promotion

A diet of less than 30 grams of fat a day helps prevent atherosclerosis. Regular exercise, 30 minutes at least 5 days a week, and smoking cessation help prevent an MI.

Participation in a cardiac rehabilitation program provides the client with monitored exercise sessions as well as education and counseling about reducing the risk of future heart problems and coping with a new lifestyle. Because women have a worse prognosis than men, it is critical for women to participate in a cardiac rehabilitation program.

▶ NURSING PROCESS

▶ Assessment

▶ Subjective Data

The nurse should note the medications the client has taken including over-the-counter medications, anticoagulants, and thrombolytic medications. The client's pain should be assessed as to onset, duration, intensity, location, radiation, and precipitating factors; the client can be asked to describe the symptoms. Not all persons having angina or an MI will experience or state having pain. Some may describe feelings of chest heaviness, indigestion, or "something not right." These statements should be explored with the client so the client can explain them in more detail. Dizziness, weakness, and shortness of breath may be expressed. The nurse should ask about how the client tried to relieve pain.

▶ Objective Data

The nurse's assessment will include vital signs, skin changes, breath sounds, and EKG rhythm strips. Vital signs are monitored for an irregular or increased pulse, hypotension, or slight temperature elevation. The client may have pallor, cyanosis, diaphoresis, vomiting, cool clammy skin, or confusion. Breath sounds should be assessed for lung congestion, and the EKG monitored for dysrhythmias. Any client clenching of hands or clutching at the chest should be noted.

Nursing diagnoses for a client with myocardial infarction may include the following:

Nursing Diagnoses	Planning/Goals	Nursing Interventions
▶ *Cardiac Output, Decreased, related to damaged heart tissue*	The client will have increased cardiac output.	Maintain bed rest with head of bed elevated 30° until the condition is stabilized.
		Auscultate breath sounds every 4 hours.
		Administer oxygen per mask or nasal cannula at 2 to 4 liters per minute.
		Palpate pedal pulses every 4 hours.
		Start an IV so medications such as morphine and antidysrhythmics can be administered.
		If beta-blockers are administered, monitor closely for a drop in heart rate and blood pressure.
		Constantly monitor the client for dysrhythmias. Place a rhythm strip on the chart at least once a shift.
		Monitor I&O.
		Administer medications as prescribed by the physician. *continued*

Nursing Diagnoses	Planning/Goals	Nursing Interventions
▶ *Pain, Acute, Chest, related to decreased oxygenation of myocardial tissue*	The client will verbalize decrease in frequency and intensity of chest pain.	Maintain client on bed rest. Observe for verbal and nonverbal signs of pain such as grimacing, diaphoresis, or increased heart rate. Ask the client to rate the pain on a scale of 0 to 10, 0 being no pain and 10 extreme pain. Administer analgesic, usually morphine, as ordered. Administer oxygen as ordered.
▶ *Activity Intolerance related to decreased circulation to body tissues*	The client will increase activities with decreased symptoms of angina, dyspnea, cyanosis, and dysrhythmia.	Place objects within reach of the client. Balance activity with rest periods. Assist the client and partner to discuss their fears and feelings candidly about resuming sexual activity.
▶ *Anxiety, Moderate, related to change in health status and threat of death*	The client will verbalize situations that are causing stress.	Encourage the family and client to verbalize their feelings. Provide a quiet, calm environment to relax the client and family. Provide the client with periods of uninterrupted rest. Administer sedatives to help the client relax. Since the myocardial client may be in denial, be aware of denial symptoms such as attempting to conduct business over the phone while hospitalized or statements that the pain is really nothing.

Evaluation Each goal must be evaluated to determine how it has been met by the client.

CONGESTIVE HEART FAILURE

Congestive heart failure (CHF) is often the final stage of many other heart conditions. A weakened muscle wall from a myocardial infarction or a heart that has been stressed over a period of time to meet metabolic needs of the body can cause congestive heart failure. Congestive heart failure develops when the heart is no longer capable of pumping enough blood to meet the needs of the body. The heart is literally failing. The muscle of the left ventricle **hypertrophies** (increases in muscle mass) and often the ventricular chamber enlarges in an attempt to meet the oxygen needs of the body.

Both the right and left ventricles act as pumps. Each of these pumps can fail separately resulting in two types of heart failure: right-sided heart failure and left-sided heart failure. Heart failure usually begins on the left side. Left-sided failure is caused by left ventricular myocardial infarction, aortic valve stenosis, prolapsed valve complications, and hypertension. Some of the causes of right-sided failure are untreated left ventricular failure, right ventricular myocardial infarction, chronic obstructive pulmonary disease, cor pulmonale, and pulmonary valve stenosis. Notice that right- and left-sided failure are caused by a defect of the ventricle or an increased resistance ahead of the ventricle in the blood flow, causing an increased workload for the involved ventricle.

When left-sided heart failure occurs, the left ventricle is not able to completely empty of blood or effec-

tively pump blood out through the aorta to the body systems. Usually the right ventricle continues to pump adequate quantities of blood. This causes blood to back up in the left ventricle, left atrium, and pulmonary veins. The lungs become congested with fluid as fluid leaks through the capillaries and fills air spaces in the lungs. The client becomes cyanotic, dyspneic, restless, and coughs up blood-tinged sputum. The breath sounds have moist crackles. Often the client has tachycardia with low blood pressure because the heart is not able to pump sufficient blood to meet the body's demands. The client may have decreased urinary output because enough blood is not being pumped through the kidneys. As the blood oxygen level decreases, the client becomes confused.

As the right side of the heart fails, blood becomes congested in the inferior vena cava causing edema first in the extremities and then in the trunk of the body. As the condition progresses, the client experiences edema of the ankles, lower legs, thighs, and finally in the abdomen. The excess abdominal fluid causes the client to be anorectic. Hepatomegaly (enlargement of the liver) and splenomegaly (enlargement of the spleen) develop. The jugular veins in the neck become distended when the client is sitting or standing and pitting edema occurs in the lower extremities. Refer back to Figure 32-6. Oliguria occurs as decreased amounts of blood are pumped through the kidneys.

In the early stages of congestive heart failure, the client experiences fatigue, dyspnea with slight exertion, pedal edema, and a slight cough with a small amount of expectoration. The client may also have paroxysmal nocturnal dyspnea.

Medical–Surgical Management

Medical

Goals for treating congestive heart failure are to improve circulation to the coronary arteries and decrease the workload of the left ventricle. To meet these goals, cardiac efficiency is increased with medication; oxygen requirements of the body are decreased through bed rest with head elevated 45°; edema and pulmonary congestion are treated with medications, diet, and restricted fluid intake; and fluid retention is monitored by weighing the client daily. A chest x-ray is done to directly visualize the ventricles and check for evidence of lung congestion. An EKG is done and arterial blood gases are evaluated. The client's oxygen saturation level is also monitored by pulse oximetry. Depending on the seriousness of the client's condition, a pulmonary artery catheter may be inserted to determine left ventricular function.

In right-sided failure, the symptoms of edema, hepatomegaly, and neck vein distention are significant diagnostic evidence.

Surgical

Two mechanical devices are available: an intra-aortic balloon pump and a ventricular assist device (VAD). An intra-aortic balloon is threaded through the femoral artery to the descending aorta (Figure 32-16). The pump is synchronized with the contractions of the left ventricle so the balloon inflates during diastole and deflates during systole. Inflation of the balloon increases the blood flow to the coronary arteries, thus increasing oxygenation of the myocardium. Deflation of the balloon allows the left ventricle to pump blood to the body tissues with less peripheral resistance.

The left ventricular assist device has a cannula that takes blood from the left atrium to the aorta bypassing the ineffective left ventricle (Figure 32-17). This gives

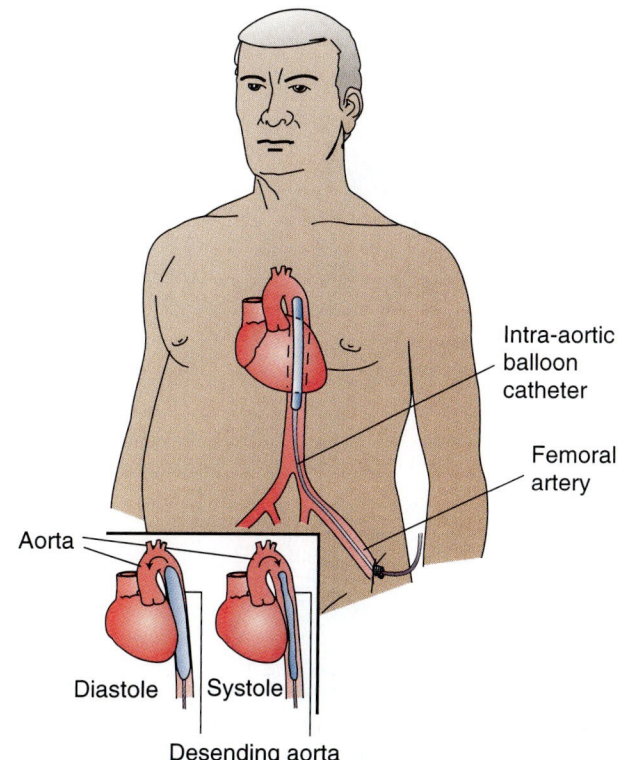

Figure 32-16 An intra-aortic balloon pump increases circulation to the coronary arteries and decreases the workload of the left ventricle.

the left ventricle time to rest and heal. The same process can be done for the right ventricle or both ventricles.

A cardiomyoplasty may be performed to assist the heart's functioning and improve circulation (Figure 32-18). The latissimus dorsi muscle is wrapped around the heart and a cardiomyostimulator and leads are implanted to stimulate contractions of the muscle. The stimulator is programmed to begin functioning 2 weeks after the surgery. After 4 months, the muscle stimulation is at either a 1 : 1 or 1 : 2 heartbeat ratio.

Pharmacological

The client with CHF will receive diuretics such as chlorothiazide (Diuril), furosemide (Lasix), or spironolactone (Aldactone) to decrease fluid retention and a digitalis preparation to increase the strength and contractility of the heart muscle. Vasodilators such as nitroglycerine (Cardabid) are given so the blood will stay in the peripheral vessels and not return to the heart, thereby decreasing the possibility of an overload on the heart. To reduce blood pressure and peripheral arterial resistance and improve cardiac output, ACE (argioteroin-converting enzyme) inhibitors such as captopril (Capoten) or enalopril (Vasotec) may be given. Morphine sulfate is given in the acute phase to control pain and decrease anxiety.

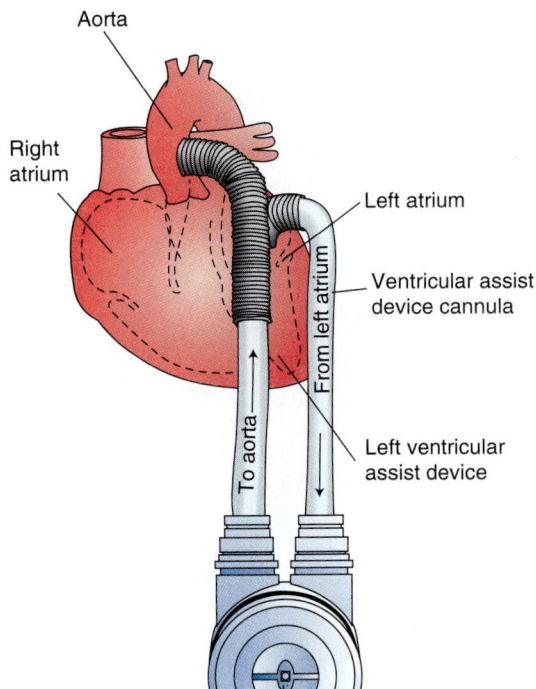

Figure 32-17 The cannula of the ventricular assist device (VAD) takes blood from the left atrium to the aorta, bypassing the ineffective left ventricle.

Diet

A daily weight and strict intake and output are necessary to assess fluid retention. Sometimes fluid intake is limited. The client is generally on a low-sodium diet.

Activity

Activity orders will depend on the client's activity tolerance. The client's activity may vary from strict bed rest to ambulation depending on the severity of the condition. When in bed, the head of the bed should be elevated 45°. Visitation privileges may be monitored to provide rest periods.

Health Promotion

To prevent CHF following coronary artery disease, a diet low in fat, high in fiber, and balanced in caloric intake to maintain optimum weight is recommended. Stress reduction and a regular exercise program will also decrease the risk of developing CHF. Clients developing CHF from congenital heart defects may not be able to prevent the prognosis of CHF, but following the prescribed medical regimen may prevent the early development of CHF.

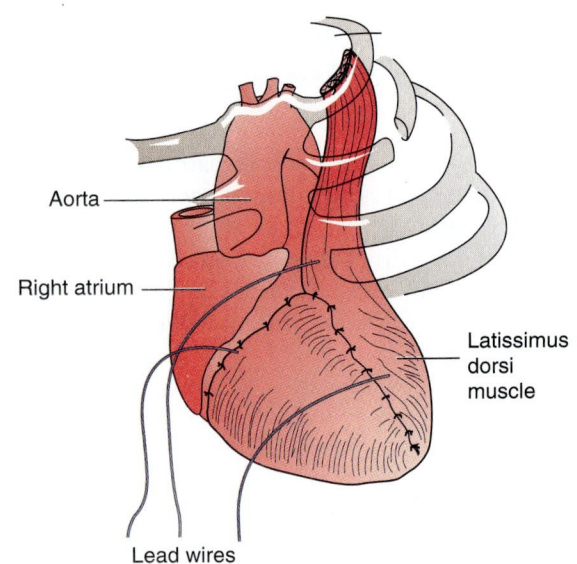

Figure 32-18 Cardiomyoplasty: The latissimus dorsi muscle is wrapped around the heart and stimulated by electrical impulses.

▶ NURSING PROCESS

▶ Assessment

▶ Subjective Data

The nurse should inquire if the client has recently experienced more dyspnea, orthopnea, fatigue, anxiety, weight gain, edema, or pain. Any difficulty in performing activities of daily living should be noted.

▶ Objective Data

The client's level of consciousness should be assessed to determine circulation of blood to the brain and skin color checked for cyanosis or pallor. Assessment of skin turgor will help determine the level of hydration. Jugular distention will give an indication of the functioning level of the right ventricle. Breath sounds should be assessed for adventitious sounds, and heart sounds for gallop or murmurs. Bowel sounds may be hypoactive depending on the amount of fluid retention in the abdomen. Quality of peripheral pulses and capillary refill must be checked to assess the level of circulation to the extremities. Edema in the extremities and abdomen should be documented according to the edema rating scale. The client's daily weight is monitored for possible increase from fluid retention. The physician should be notified if there is a gain of more than 2 pounds in one day. I & O must be monitored and assessment made for oliguria.

Nursing diagnoses for a client with congestive heart failure may include the following:

Nursing Diagnoses	Planning/Goals	Nursing Interventions
▶ *Cardiac Output, Decreased, related to mechanical failure of heart muscle*	The client's vital signs will remain stable. The client will have decreased adventitious breath sounds.	Take an apical pulse on all cardiac clients, especially checking the rate and rhythm. Monitor the client's heart rate and rhythm by telemetry. Auscultate breath sounds every 4 hours. Administer diuretics, digitalis, and vasodilators as prescribed. Closely monitor the electrolytes, especially the potassium level, as diuretics can deplete the potassium level. Administer potassium supplements as ordered to keep the potassium serum level within the normal level. Take the apical pulse before giving a digitalis preparation. If the heart rate is below 60, withhold the medication and notify the physician. In some institutions the heart rate can drop to 50 before the physician is notified if the client is taking a calcium channel blocker or beta-blocker along with digitalis.
▶ *Gas Exchange, Impaired, related to decreased cardiac output and pulmonary edema*	The client will have increased gas exchange.	Provide oxygen by mask or nasal cannula at 2 to 6 liters/minute to assist in the oxygen needs of the body. Elevate the head of the bed to a semi-Fowler's or Fowler's position to relieve pressure on the diaphragm. Apply a pulse oximeter and monitor the oxygenation status. If the pulse oximeter is ≤90%, notify the physician.
▶ *Fluid Volume Excess related to decreased cardiac output and decreased renal output*	The client will have less edema of the extremities.	Encourage elevation of the client's legs, not letting them hang in a dependent position. Monitor daily fluids by obtaining an accurate intake and output. Take a daily weight at the same time each day, on the same scales, and with the client wearing the same type of clothing. If the client is on a fluid-restricted diet, offer hard candies to quench the thirst.
▶ *Activity Intolerance related to edema, dyspnea, and fatigue*	The client will have an increased tolerance for activity.	Schedule nursing care so the client is given frequent rest periods with minimal interruptions at night. Teach the client to take frequent rest periods and to stop activities before becoming tired. Monitor the client's vital signs for an increase or decrease in heart rate or blood pressure, especially after periods of activity.
▶ *Anxiety, Moderate, related to change in health status, lifestyle changes, or fear of death*	The client will be able to verbalize anxieties.	Explain procedures to the client and family members. Assist the family in identifying stress factors. Refer the client to a local support group such as American Heart Association or Mended Hearts, Inc.

Evaluation Each goal must be evaluated to determine how it has been met by the client.

COR PULMONALE

With this condition, the heart is affected because of a lung condition that interferes with the exchange of carbon dioxide and oxygen in the alveoli. The carbon dioxide level increases in the blood. For some unknown reason, the pulmonary arteries vasoconstrict causing pulmonary hypertension. The right ventricle is forced to pump against increased pulmonary pressure. The right ventricle enlarges and finally weakens in the attempt to pump blood into the lungs. The symptoms the client experiences and medical and nursing care are the same as for right-sided heart failure.

CARDIAC TRANSPLANTATION

Cardiac transplantations are done for cardiomyopathy, end-stage coronary artery disease, and valvular disease. Recipients are evaluated for emotional stability, minimal disease involvement, and a good support system. The heart donor and the recipient's tissues are matched.

The transplant is performed by removing the recipient's heart except for posterior sections of the atria. The posterior sections of the atria are removed from the donor's heart and then the heart is sutured to the recipient's posterior atria.

The recipient must remain on an immunosuppressant medication for the remainder of life so the donor heart will not be rejected. Some immunosuppressant medications are azathioprine (Imuran), cyclosporine (Sandimmune), antithymocytic globulin, ATG (Atgam), antilymphocytic globulin (ALG), rapamycin, and FK 506 (Prograf).

PERIPHERAL VASCULAR DISORDERS

Disorders in this category include: venous thrombosis/thrombophlebitis; varicose veins; Buerger's disease; Raynaud's disease; aneurysm; and hypertension.

VENOUS THROMBOSIS/ THROMBOPHLEBITIS

The terms *phlebitis, thrombosis, phlebothrombosis* and *thrombophlebitis* are often used interchangeably even though each word has a separate meaning and etiology. **Phlebitis** is an inflammation in the wall of a vein without clot formation. The formation of a clot in a vessel is a **thrombosis** and a formed clot that remains at the site where it formed is a **thrombus**. If the thrombus moves, it would become an **embolus**, a mass such as a blood clot or an air bubble, that circulates in the bloodstream. **Phlebothrombosis** is the formation of a clot because of blood pooling in the vessel, trauma to the vessel's endothelial lining, or a coagulation problem. With phlebothrombosis, there is little or no inflammation in the vessel. **Thrombophlebitis** is the formation of a clot due to an inflammation in the wall of the vessel.

In 1846, Virchow listed three factors leading to the formation of a clot. These are known as **Virchow's triad**. The three factors are pooling of blood, vessel trauma, and a coagulation problem. Risk factors for thrombi formation are prolonged bed rest, leg trauma, oral contraceptives, obesity, varicose veins, hip fractures, and total hip and knee replacement.

There are two types of thrombi, a superficial thrombus and a deep vein thrombus (DVT). A superficial vein thrombus is a clot in a superficial vein such as the saphenous vein in the leg. A DVT can form in the deep veins of the arms, pelvic area, or legs, but the legs are the most common site. Leg veins in which clots form are the femoral, popliteal, iliac, and deep veins of the calf.

Phlebitis can either form spontaneously or as a result of trauma. IV catheters or cannulas, IV medications such as potassium or antibiotics, or direct trauma to a vein can cause phlebitis. A clot may then form as red blood cells pass over the damaged area, rupture, and start the clotting process.

A phlebitis may manifest as a reddened streak over a vein. If a clot is in a superficial vein, the site becomes reddened, warm, tender, and swollen. The nurse may be able to palpate a hardening in a section of the vein. There may be no symptoms with a deep vein thrombus, or there may be warmth and tenderness at the site, unilateral edema of the affected extremity, positive Homans' sign, dilation of superficial veins, and cyanosis of the foot. The client may say the leg feels "tight" or "heavy." If the clot is in the calf of the leg, the calf may feel tender. If the swelling restricts the arterial blood flow, the leg may be cool and pale. If there are obvious clinical signs of a thrombosis, Homans' sign should not be assessed as the clot may be dislodged and become an embolus.

A complication of a DVT is a pulmonary embolus that results in approximately 50,000 to 60,000 deaths each year in the United States (Beare & Myers, 1998). Symptoms of a pulmonary embolus are sudden and severe chest pain, dyspnea, and tachypnea. Emboli may travel and block other vessels in the heart, brain, or peripheral vessels.

Medical–Surgical Management

Medical

A superficial phlebitis or thrombus should be assessed and may need no further treatment. Warm soaks may be applied to the affected area. Acetaminophen or a nonsteroidal anti-inflammatory drug is given for pain. Elevating the extremity decreases swelling and improves venous return. Some doctors recommend the application of an elastic support hose. If a DVT has been diagnosed, the client is placed on bed rest.

Surgical

If a clot has formed in a large vein and all conservative methods have failed, the clot may be removed surgically. This procedure is called a **thrombectomy** and is performed only if the tissue in the area becomes ischemic or gangrenous or if the client has a history of thromboemboli.

Another surgical procedure is a vena cava interruption surgery (venacaval plication) in which a Greenfield vena cava filter or umbrella filter is placed in the inferior vena cava to prevent thromboemboli from traveling from the lower extremities to the lungs, heart, or brain. Figure 32-19 shows these filters and their placement in the vena cava. The procedure is done on clients with a history of pulmonary emboli.

Pharmacological

If a client is at risk for a thrombus or phlebitis, anticoagulant therapy can be initiated. A prophylactic heparin dose is given. Enoxaparin injection (Lovenox), a low-molecular-weight heparin, is used prophylactically

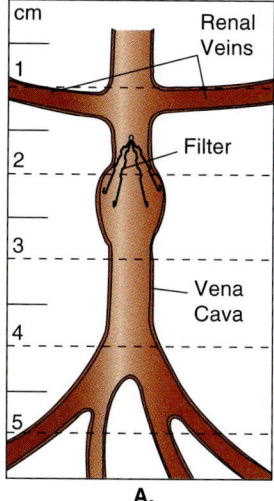

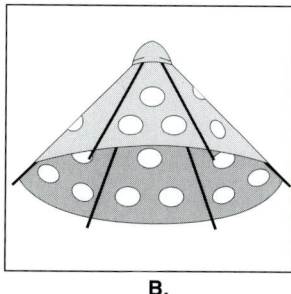

Figure 32-19 A filter in the vena cava prevents an embolus from traveling to the heart, lungs, or brain: A. Greenfield Filter in Place; B. Umbrella Filter

after hip replacement surgery. Lovenox is started within 24 hours after surgery and is given subcutaneously twice daily for 7 to 10 days. Lovenox should be used cautiously with clients on oral anticoagulants.

If a clot forms, the client is immediately started on heparin as an IV bolus and then followed with a continuous IV drip of heparin. Before heparin is started, a partial thromboplastin time (PTT) or activated partial thromboplastin time (APTT) and a platelet count are drawn by the laboratory to establish a baseline level. The heparin dose is regulated by the PTT or the APTT. For effective heparin therapy, the client's PTT or APTT level should be two and one-half times the baseline. A **baseline level** is a value at a particular time that will serve as a reference point for future value levels.

Clients are generally given heparin subcutaneously or intravenously in an acute setting. Since warfarin sodium (Coumadin) is taken orally, a client may be discharged on Coumadin. Because of rapid hospital discharges, clients are often started on Coumadin the next day after heparin has been initiated. Once the Coumadin dose is regulated, heparin is stopped.

After the initial Coumadin dose, the daily Coumadin dose is regulated by the prothrombin time (PT) or the International Normalized Ratio (INR). A PT level of 1.3 to 1.6 times the hospital laboratory control value indi-

CLIENT TEACHING

Use of Warfarin Sodium (Coumadin)

- Eat a consistent amount of foods high in vitamin K each day to maintain a consistent therapeutic effect of Coumadin.
- Avoid eating kale or parsley.
- Eat one serving each day of spinach, turnip or other greens, broccoli, or Brussels sprouts.

cates effective Coumadin therapy. For a client on Coumadin, an INR of 2 to 3 indicates a therapeutic level. The client generally remains on Coumadin for 3 to 6 months.

Thrombolytic drugs, urokinase (Abbokinase), streptokinase (Streptase) and tissue plasminogen activator, t-PA (Alteplase), are used locally and systemically if there is a massive DVT. Streptokinase should only be used on the same client once every 6 months. If the client has had a recent streptococcal infection, urokinase is given rather than streptokinase because antibodies are present in the blood that will make the streptokinase ineffective (Beare & Myers, 1998). The main complication in a client receiving thrombolytic drugs is bleeding. Heparin and Coumadin are given after the thrombolytic drugs to prevent thrombi formation.

CLIENT TEACHING

Thrombophlebitis

- Drink 2 to 3 quarts of water per day.
- Do not to sit with legs crossed.
- Elevate both legs when sitting.
- Avoid sitting or standing for extended periods.
- Wear support hose.
- When standing, shift weight frequently and occasionally stand on tiptoes to stimulate the calf muscle to pump blood.
- Notify the physician immediately if leg pain, tenderness or swelling, difficulty breathing, or chest pain is experienced.
- Take the medication at the same time each day.
- Maintain appointments to have the PT or INR level checked.
- Watch for signs of bleeding and avoid aspirin or drugs containing aspirin because it increases the clotting time.
- Notify physician if abdominal pain occurs as this could indicate internal bleeding.

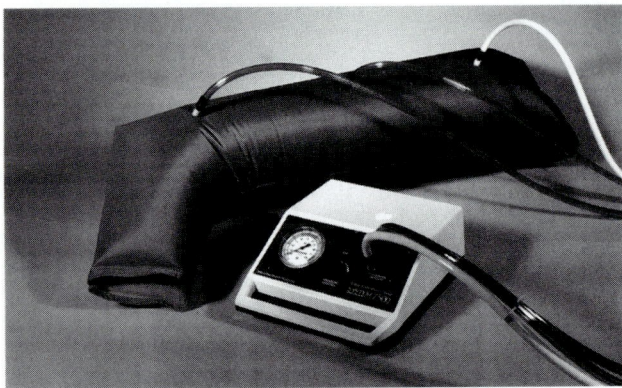

Figure 32-20 Alternating pneumatic compression device helps prevent thrombi formation. (*Courtesy of Beiersdorf-Jobst, Inc. Charlotte, North Carolina.*)

Diet

Adequate hydration is important for clients at risk for thrombi. This can be accomplished orally or intravenously.

Activity

During the acute stage, the client is placed on bed rest to prevent the clot from dislodging and embolizing. Later the leg is elevated periodically to improve venous return and decrease swelling. The client's leg should never be massaged as a clot could be dislodged and become an embolus.

Health Promotion

Prevention is the best way to treat a DVT. Early ambulation, adequate hydration, alternating pneumatic compression devices, prophylactic anticoagulants, elevation of legs, leg exercises, and deep breathing exercises all contribute to the prevention of thrombi. Figure 32-20 shows an alternating pneumatic compression device.

▶ NURSING PROCESS

▶ Assessment

▶ Subjective Data

The nurse should ask the client if there has been any recent injury to the extremity, if the affected area is tender to the touch, or if there have been clots previously. Any chest pain, dyspnea, tachycardia, or hemoptysis must be noted.

▶ Objective Data

IV sites are checked at least once a shift to see if a phlebitis or reddened area is developing at the insertion site. If a positive Homan's sign is detected during an assessment, the nurse should notify the physician and not perform another Homan's sign until a clot has been ruled out. The skin should be assessed for redness, tenderness, hardness, or warmth, and both legs are measured to determine baseline measurements. The circumference of the affected leg is measured every shift to determine an increase or decrease in swelling. Peripheral pulses are obtained as baseline data and charted according to the acceptable institutional scale. Peripheral pulses should be checked every 4 hours and more frequently if the client experiences increased pain in the leg, cyanosis of the foot or extremity, or increased swelling. These are signs of an occlusion.

Nursing diagnoses for a client with a venous thrombosis may include the following:

Nursing Diagnoses	Planning/Goals	Nursing Interventions
▶ *Tissue Perfusion, Altered Peripheral, related to decreased venous blood flow and/or clot formation*	The client will have adequate tissue perfusion.	Elevate the client's entire affected leg when on bed rest to improve venous return. When elevated, the leg should be slightly flexed at the knee with a pillow under the thigh and calf.
		Apply elastic support or intermittent pneumatic compression stockings on the client.
		If the client has received thrombolytic or anticoagulant drugs, assess for signs of bleeding which include hematuria, bruising, bleeding from the gums, and blood in the stool.
		Monitor pedal pulses and capillary refill.
		Measure thigh or calf circumference daily.
▶ *Pain related to inflammatory process*	The client will state absence of pain.	If the client has a phlebitis, apply warm moist soaks to the affected area.
		Administer acetaminophen or a nonsteroidal anti-inflammatory as ordered for discomfort.
▶ *Anxiety related to possibility of the clot becoming an embolus*	The client will express anxiety about possible embolus.	Encourage client to discuss the possibility of embolus formation.

Evaluation Each goal must be evaluated to determine how it has been met by the client.

VARICOSE VEINS

Varicose veins, also called **varicosities**, are visibly prominent, dilated, and twisted veins. Veins in the lower extremities are more frequently involved, but the veins in the esophagus (esophageal varices) and anus (hemorrhoids) can also be affected. Usually it is the saphenous vein that is affected in the leg. Women are more prone to varicose veins than men (Beare & Myers, 1998). Risk factors for developing varicose veins are a familial tendency, congenital abnormalities, pregnancy, obesity, constrictive clothing, and occupations that require periods of prolonged standing. Pregnancy and obesity cause more pressure in the veins of the legs.

The causes of varicose veins are incompetent or absent valves and veins that have lost their elasticity. The wall of the vessel is weakened from a lack of elastin or collagen and is unable to support the normal pressure of the blood in the vessel. The vein dilates as the blood in it flows backward. As the walls of the vein dilate, the valves become incapable of holding the blood and allow blood to leak backward through the space between the valves. Refer to Figure 32-5C.

Medical–Surgical Management

Medical

Varicose veins are usually treated with conservative measures such as elastic support hose, elevation of the legs when sitting, not crossing legs, and ankle and leg exercises.

Sclerotherapy involves injecting a chemical into the vein, causing the vein to become sclerosed (hardened) so blood no longer flows through it. A compression bandage or elastic stocking is applied to the extremity for 4 to 5 days. The client wears support hose for 5 more weeks. Complications of the procedure are **necrosis** (tissue death) at the injection site, vasospasm, allergic responses, and **hemolysis** (destruction of red blood cells).

Surgical

In more severe cases, varicose veins can be ligated (tied off) or stripped. **Vein stripping** involves introducing a wire into a vein. The wire has collapsible claws on the end. As the wire is withdrawn, the claws expand and strip the walls of the vein. This measure is used when there is a threat of thrombus or leg ulcers. **Vein ligation** is tying off an involved section of a vein with suture.

Pharmacological

Analgesics are given for leg discomfort. Anticoagulants may be given to prevent clot formation.

Activity

The client is encouraged to exercise regularly. Walking is a very good exercise to improve circulation because the blood circulates faster in response to an increased heartbeat. Muscles in the legs also apply pressure to the veins forcing the blood upward toward the heart. Ankle exercises such as rotating the ankle in circular motions also improves circulation.

Health Promotion

Clients with a familial tendency for varicose veins are encouraged to elevate their legs 6 to 10 inches on a small stool when sitting in a chair. Frequent position changes and not standing in one spot for extended times also improve circulation.

Nursing Management

The nurse should assist the client in elevating the legs above the heart when in bed or elevating the feet 6 to 10 inches on a pillow or stool when sitting in a chair.

After a vein stripping, the client is on bed rest for the first 24 hours. Elastic hose are worn continuously for 5 days to compress the blood into the deeper veins. The client continues to wear compression or support hose for 5 weeks after the surgery. Pain medication should be administered 30 minutes before the client ambulates until walking is tolerated without discomfort. Walking and leg exercises are encouraged after the vein stripping.

After sclerotherapy the affected area may be tender and discolored. Most discoloration will disappear in a few weeks, but a darkened pigmentation may last for 6 to 8 months. Repeated sclerotherapy may be needed. The client should be encouraged to maintain a walking exercise program to improve circulation to the legs.

CLIENT TEACHING

Varicose Veins

Apply support hose after the legs have been elevated for an extended time, 10 to 15 minutes, so the venous blood drains from the legs. Application before getting out of bed in the morning is ideal. Do not fold or roll hose down from the top as this would act like a tourniquet causing pooling of blood. Smooth the hose on the legs as wrinkles or creases may cause extra pressure leading to stasis or pooling of blood or pressure ulcers. Remove hose daily so the leg can be washed and dried before reapplication.

BUERGER'S DISEASE (THROMBOANGIITIS OBLITERANS)

Buerger's disease is an inflammatory disease of small and medium arteries and veins that leads to vascular obstruction. Inflammation occurs in the adventitia and media layers of the vessels and may affect only a portion of the vessel or the entire vessel. Hands and feet are mainly involved, but the wrists and lower extremities may also be affected. The distal tips of the hands and feet are pale, but as the disease progresses, the hands and feet become reddened when held in a dependent position. At first, pain in the palm of the hand and arch of the foot is the main symptom. Pain becomes more severe with disease progression, and as ischemia affects the nerves, the client may experience numbness, burning, pain when at rest, and decreased sensation in the hands and lower extremities. The dorsalis pedis, posterior tibia, and ulnar and radial pulses are weak or absent. Skin color changes, cold sensitivity, ulcers, and gangrene may occur in the later stages.

Buerger's disease occurs primarily in men between the ages of 20 and 40 of Israeli, Indian, and Oriental descent. There is a correlation between smoking and Buerger's disease.

Medical–Surgical Management

Medical

The client is encouraged to stop smoking and may be referred to a smoking clinic or seminar. Buerger-Allen exercises are recommended and explained. Buerger-Allen exercises consist of elevating the legs until they blanch and supporting them at that angle for 2 to 3 minutes. The legs are then lowered to a dependent position until they become red and supported at that level for 5 to 10 minutes. The legs are then placed flat on the bed with the client in a supine position for 10 minutes. The exercises are repeated as tolerated by the client.

Surgical

A sympathectomy may be done to relieve pain and prevent vasospasm in the affected area. Digits and toes may have to be amputated in the later stages of the disease if gangrene occurs.

Pharmacological

Analgesics are given to control pain. Vasodilators are given to increase circulation to the affected area.

Nursing Management

Nursing diagnoses and interventions are the same as for other obstructive vascular conditions and are described under Raynaud's disease.

RAYNAUD'S DISEASE/PHENOMENON

Raynaud's disease or primary Raynaud's disease is an intermittent spasm of the digital arteries and arterioles resulting in decreased circulation to the fingers and toes. Sometimes the tip of the nose and ears can also be affected. The cause of the condition is unknown but seems to be related to vasospastic disorders, a disturbance with the innervation of the sympathetic nervous system, and angiography complications. During a spasm that lasts approximately 15 minutes, the fingers become pale, and then cyanotic. As the circulation returns to the fingers, the fingertips become reddened and the person experiences a tingling or throbbing pain in the fingers. Some people experience only pallor and cyanosis. The episode may last 1 to 2 hours. Symptoms usually occur when the person is exposed to cold or experiences emotional stress. Gangrene is not common but can occur in the fingertips if the disease has been longstanding. Ulcerations can also occur and are difficult to heal because of decreased circulation in the fingers.

The condition is called Raynaud's phenomenon or secondary Raynaud's phenomenon when it is associated with a connective tissue or collagen vascular disease, medications, or occupational trauma. Raynaud symptoms may occur 10 years before the related disease is diagnosed. A 2-year history of signs and symptoms with no evidence of underlying disease, especially an autoimmune disease, is necessary for a diagnosis of Raynaud's disease.

Raynaud's is more prevalent in cool, damp climates. It occurs more frequently in women between the ages of 16 and 40 (Linton et al., 1995). Persons who use vibrating hand tools such as air hammers or grinding wheels or whose hands perform repetitive movements such as typing or playing the piano are also affected. Researchers have also found Raynaud's phenomenon in persons exposed to vinyl chloride which is used in the manufacturing of plastics (Stephenson, 1992).

Diagnostic examinations include a complete blood count, digital blood pressure measurement, digital plethysmography waveforms, and a cold-challenge test. A digital blood pressure of 30 mm Hg below the brachial pressure is indicative of a digital artery obstruction. A sedimentation rate, antinuclear antibody, and rheumatoid factor are done to determine the presence of autoimmune diseases. During a cold challenge test, thermistors are placed on the fingers and a baseline temperature is taken. The hands are submerged into ice water for 20 seconds, then removed. The temperature of the hands is then taken every 5 minutes until it returns to the baseline level. Hand x-rays determine the presence of subcutaneous calcium deposits and narrowing of bone in the digits. The diagnostic tests distinguish between Raynaud's phenomenon and

Raynaud's disease. If a client has unilateral or single digit Raynaud's, an obstruction or emboli is suspected.

Medical–Surgical Management

Medical

Raynaud's phenomenon is treated conservatively. The client is assessed regularly for symptoms of autoimmune diseases. If the symptoms of Raynaud's are due to a vasospastic disease, relief is best achieved with medications. Biofeedback allows clients to voluntarily control the temperature of their hands (Stephenson, 1992).

Surgical

In previous years, a sympathectomy (excision of a nerve, plexus, or ganglion of the sympathetic portion of the autonomic nervous system) was sometimes done to alleviate the client's symptoms. However, clients with connective tissue diseases generally do not receive long-term relief from a sympathectomy, and, therefore, a sympathectomy is no longer recommended.

Pharmacological

Clients may be given nifedipine (Adalat, Procardia) at night for severe cases of Raynaud's phenomenon. Clients may also take the medication 1 to 2 hours before engaging in an outdoor activity during cold weather. They may not need to take the medication during warmer months. Other medications used to improve symptoms in severe Raynaud's phenomenon are diltiazem hydrochloride (Cardizem), verapamil (Calan), nicardipine hydrochloride (Cardene), and captopril (Capoten). Drug therapy improves the symptoms in about two-thirds of the clients (Stephenson, 1992).

Medications that aid in healing finger ulcers are iloprost, a prostaglandin which is given intravenously and ciprofloxacin (Cipro), an antibiotic. In clinical research at Oregon Health Sciences University, clients with digital ulcers were given pentoxifylline (Trental),

which decreases the viscosity of blood and improves the blood flow to peripheral arteries (Whitaker & Kelleher, 1994).

Beta blockers, birth control pills, cold medications, and diet pills cause some clients to have Raynaud's phenomenon. These medications should be substituted or discontinued if they are the source of the symptoms. Chemotherapy drugs such as bleomycin sulfate (Blenoxane) and cisplatin, CDDP (Platinol), also cause secondary Raynaud's.

Health Promotion

The client is encouraged to avoid exposure to cold, repetitive hand movements, and stressful situations. The client is encouraged to quit smoking and avoid secondary smoke as nicotine is a potent vasoconstrictor. Stress management techniques, e.g., biofeedback, may assist in alleviating some distress from the condition.

▶ NURSING PROCESS

▶ Assessment

▶ Subjective Data

A history must be obtained from the client as to how frequently the vasospastic episodes occur, what symptoms the client experiences, what triggers the episodes, which digits are affected during an episode, and how long the incident lasts. The nurse should inquire about daily activities that the client finds difficult such as tying shoes, washing dishes, or handling frozen foods and should obtain a history of occupational activities.

▶ Objective Data

Pallor, blanching, cyanosis, coldness, and appearance of the digits should be assessed. If the disease is long-standing, the digits may be tapered and the skin shiny in appearance. There may be ulcerated or gangrenous areas on the fingertips.

Nursing diagnoses for a client with Raynaud's disease may include the following:

Nursing Diagnoses	Planning/Goals	Nursing Interventions
▶ Tissue Perfusion, Altered, Peripheral, related to vasospasm of peripheral arteries	The client will have fewer vasospastic episodes and increased circulation in digits.	Encourage the client to use caution when engaging in activities that may cause a cut or scratch as healing may be impaired because of decreased circulation.
		If a client has ulcers, wash the areas with soap and water and administer prescribed medications such as ciprofloxacin (Cipro) and intravenous iloprost.
▶ Pain, Acute, related to decreased circulation in digits	The client will experience decreased pain as vasospasms are controlled.	Teach client to keep the indoor temperature at a comfortable level to avoid ischemic attacks.

continued

Nursing Diagnoses	Planning/Goals	Nursing Interventions
		Encourage client to avoid dramatic changes in environmental temperatures, e.g., entering a cold air-conditioned room during hot summer months. Encourage the client to wear woolen or wind-proof gloves or mittens and layered clothes when exposed to colder temperatures. Mittens may be better than gloves so the fingers can obtain warmth from each other. Chemical warming devices may be used inside gloves and shoes.
		Encourage the client to stop smoking and make a referral to a smoking cessation clinic.
		Teach the client relaxation exercises that may decrease the number of ischemic attacks.
▶ *Self-esteem Disturbance related to inability of hands to perform activities of daily living*	The client will learn ways to handle activities of daily living.	Encourage client to use mitts or pot holders when removing items from the freezer or handling cold food to decrease the risk of a Raynaud's episode. Clients can wear mittens or socks to bed. Use of insulated mugs, foam rubber holders, or stemware glasses may reduce ischemic attacks.
		Instruct client to wash vegetables under tepid water instead of cold, to bathe in lukewarm water, and to apply lotion regularly to prevent dry and chapped skin.
		Encourage client to use gloves when pushing shopping carts or operating some vibrating machines as this may decrease the cold sensation and soften the vibration.

Evaluation Each goal must be evaluated to determine how it has been met by the client.

ANEURYSM

An **aneurysm** is a localized dilation occurring in a weakened section of an artery's medial layer. The main cause for aneurysms has previously been attributed to atherosclerosis. Recent research indicates a hereditary lack of elastin in the arterial wall as the most common cause of an aneurysm (Beare & Myers, 1998). Another factor indicating a hereditary component is if a person has an abdominal aortic aneurysm (AAA), the risk ratio is 6:1 that a first-degree relative may also develop an aneurysm compared to the general population (Beare & Myers, 1998). Some aneurysms occur because of congenital conditions such as Marfan's syndrome. Others are acquired because of trauma to the vessel wall, infection and/or inflammation, syphilis, or arteritis. Two other possible causes of an aneurysm are an increased turbulence in a section of the vessel and a slower production of smooth muscle cells. Clients have a higher tendency to develop an aneurysm if they smoke cigarettes and have hypertension.

Aneurysms can occur in any artery or peripheral vessel, but occur most often in the abdominal aorta. Abdominal aneurysms occur more frequently in men between the ages of 60 and 70 than in women (Beare & Myers, 1998). Other involved vessels are the ascending, transverse, and descending aorta, thoracic aorta, popliteal arteries, and femoral arteries.

Deposits of atherosclerotic plaque on the tunica intima cause a hardening of the vessel, and the media layer of the vessel loses elasticity. Atherosclerosis and a lack of elastin in the vessel wall predisposes the vessel to a weakened area which develops into an aneurysm.

Symptoms of an aneurysm depend upon the location of the aneurysm in the body. Aneurysms are often asymptomatic until they start leaking or pressing on other structures. A thoracic aneurysm may press on surrounding structures causing dull upper back pain or deep, scattered chest pain. Pressure on the trachea and bronchus may cause dyspnea, coughing, wheezing, and hoarseness. The client experiences dysphagia from pressure on the esophagus.

An aneurysm is usually diagnosed when a client has an x-ray or ultrasound done for other conditions/symptoms.

Medical–Surgical Management

Medical

If the client has hypertension, control of the hypertension is the focus of care. Aneurysms are monitored for enlargement. Thrombi formation and ischemia may also result. Rupture of an aneurysm is an emergency situation. Signs of rupture may include hypotension, tachycardia, paleness, weakness, and abdominal, back, or groin pain.

Surgical

Before elective surgery, the status of the client's carotid arteries and peripheral vessels are checked with a Doppler flow analysis (Doppler ultrasound).

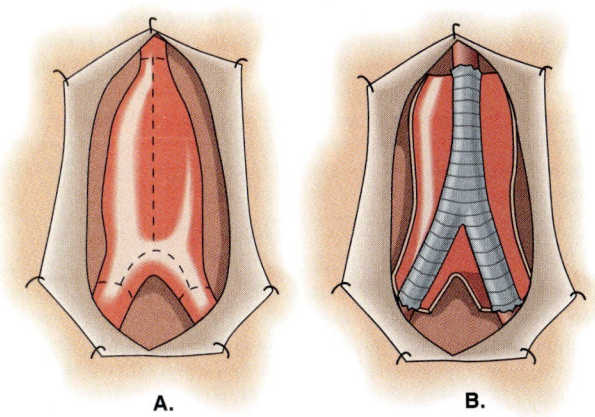

Figure 32-21 A. Aortoiliac Aneurysm; B. Bifurcated Synthetic Graft

The client's cardiac status is usually evaluated by a stress test or cardiac catheterization before surgery is scheduled. The surgeon often orders an angiogram, ultrasound, or CT scan of the affected vessel prior to surgery in order to assess the blood supply to the area surrounding the aneurysm. Prior to surgery, it is common to place 4 to 8 units of blood on hold since hemorrhage is a possibility. The surgeon clamps the aorta, removes the section of the vessel involving the aneurysm, and replaces it with a section of the client's saphenous vein or a synthetic graft (Figure 32-21). Complications that can occur from clamping the aorta are myocardial infarctions, strokes, and renal damage. Vessels below the repaired aneurysm may become occluded because of decreased blood flow during surgery or from plaque that has broken off from the wall of the vessel. A nasogastric tube may be inserted to decrease pressure on the aneurysm repair site and incision. After surgery, the client may be in ICU with mechanical ventilator assistance in breathing.

Pharmacological

Clients with aortic aneurysms may be given propranolol hydrochloride (Inderal) to decrease the pressure of the blood coming from the heart to the affected vessel. Clients with hypertension will be placed on antihypertensive medications and diuretics. Analgesics are given to control pain.

Activity

Any activity that increases blood pressure, especially exercise and lifting, can increase pressure in the arteries and should be avoided.

Health Promotion

Clients are encouraged not to smoke. Education for the hypertensive client includes the importance of closely monitoring the blood pressure and taking antihypertensive medication as prescribed.

▶ NURSING PROCESS

▶ Assessment

▶ Subjective Data

Preoperatively, the client may be concerned about an abdominal pulsation when reclining. The client may also have chest, back, abdominal, or flank pain depending on the location of the aneurysm. Postoperatively the nurse listens for statements of pain and assesses the level of pain according to a scale of 1 to 10, or the appropriate scale used in the facility.

▶ Objective Data

If the client has an AAA, the abdomen should be palpated for a pulsating mass, and vital signs checked. Immediate intervention is needed if symptoms of bleeding or a rupturing aneurysm occur. The peripheral pulses should be checked prior to surgery and the level documented. Pulses can then be compared preoperatively and postoperatively. Postoperatively, the extremities are assessed for color, temperature, peripheral pulses, and sensation.

 CLIENT TEACHING

Aneurysms

- The client and significant others must know the symptoms of a rupturing aneurysm: sudden pain, the sensation of a tearing or ripping, pallor, diaphoresis, and loss of consciousness. If these symptoms occur, the client will need immediate medical attention.
- First-degree relatives of a person with an aneurysm are encouraged to share this information with their physician.

Nursing diagnoses for a client with an aneurysm may include the following:

Nursing Diagnoses	Planning/Goals	Nursing Interventions
▸ *Tissue Perfusion, Altered Peripheral, Risk for, related to decreased arterial blood flow*	The client will have well-oxygenated tissues as manifested by strong pulses and the skin remaining baseline color and warm.	Monitor for symptoms of an occluded vessel (pain, paleness, cyanosis, and coldness). Monitor the temperature, color, and fullness of the peripheral pulses in both extremities and compare them to the preoperative pulses. Assess capillary refill. Assess client's feet for mottling and darkened areas on the toes and soles of the feet. Notify physician immediately if any of these symptoms occur.
▸ *Tissue Perfusion, Altered Renal, Risk for, related to interruption of blood flow during surgery*	The client will have a urine output above 25 cc/hour.	Measure hourly output to make sure the client has at least 25 to 30 cc of urine per hour. Provide fluids as ordered. Assess for edema which could indicate fluid overload or a vessel occlusion.

Evaluation Each goal must be evaluated to determine how it has been met by the client.

HYPERTENSION

Hypertension (HTN), also known as high blood pressure, is defined as an elevated arterial blood pressure. A systolic blood pressure above 140 or a diastolic blood pressure above 90 is indicative of hypertension. As many as 50 million (1 in 5) people in the United States age 6 and older have hypertension. Of those who have hypertension, 14.8% are not on medication, 26.2% are on medication but blood pressure is not controlled, 27.4% are controlled with medication, and 31.6% are unaware that they have hypertension (American Heart Association, 1999d). In 1996, hypertension was the primary cause of death of 41,634 persons and

contributed to the deaths of 202,000 persons in the U.S. (American Heart Association, 1999d)

Prior to age 55, more men than women have hypertension, but after age 55 more women have hypertension (American Heart Association, 1999d). Risk factors include family history of hypertension, smoking, dyslipidemia, obesity, lack of exercise, diabetes mellitus, poor education, and low socioeconomic status (Woods, 1999) (Figure 32-22).

When the cause of hypertension is unknown, it is called **primary hypertension** or "essential hypertension." Ninety-five percent of the clients with hypertension have primary hypertension (Woods, 1999). In 5 percent of the cases, the cause of hypertension is due

CULTURAL CONSIDERATIONS

Hypertension

African Americans develop hypertension earlier in life, and it is more severe at any decade of life. The estimated prevalence of individuals with hypertension in the population at large is as follows:

POPULATION	MALES	FEMALES
American Indians	26.8%	27.5%
African Americans	35.0%	34.2%
Anglo-Americans	24.4%	19.3%
Asian/Pacific Islanders	9.7%	8.4%
Cuban Americans	22.8%	15.5%
Mexican Americans	25.2%	22.0%
Puerto Ricans	15.6%	11.5%

(American Heart Association, 1999d)

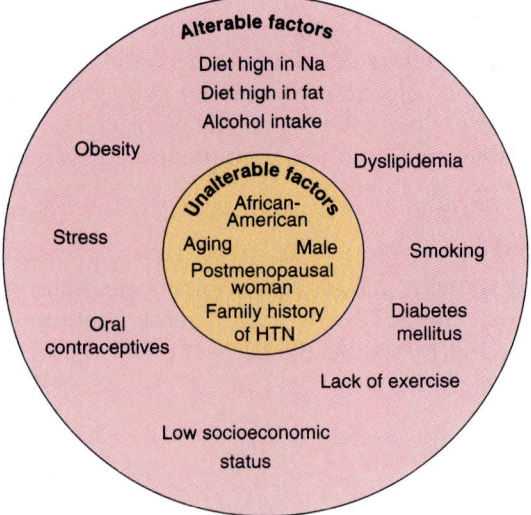

Figure 32-22 Risk Factors for Hypertension (*Adapted from Beare and Myers,* Factors Contributing to Hypertension.)

to another condition within the body such as renovascular disease, polycystic kidney disease, coarctation of the aorta, Cushing's syndrome, or pheochromocytoma (Woods, 1999). Arteriosclerosis, atherosclerosis, hypernatremia (increased sodium in the blood) or prolonged stress may also cause hypertension.

Renal diseases may interfere with the flow of blood to the kidneys causing them to release an enzyme called *renin*. When renin is released, it interacts with plasma proteins forming a vasopressor called *angiotensin*. Vasoconstriction caused by angiotensin increases the blood pressure because more force is required to get the blood through the vessel. Vasodilation decreases vascular or **peripheral resistance** (pressure within a vessel that resists the flow of blood. Figure 32-23 depicts how renal disease causes hypertension.

Arteriosclerosis causes the vessel walls to have less elasticity, decreasing their ability to expand and recoil. Since the vessel is not able to expand, more pressure is needed to force the blood through the vessel. Atherosclerosis narrows the vessel lumen, or opening, because of plaque buildup along the wall of the vessel. The plaque buildup causes resistance to the flow of blood through the vessel and more pressure is needed to get the blood through the vessel. Hypernatremia (increased blood sodium) causes vasocongestion. With vasocongestion, the heart must pump with more force, increasing the pressure in the arteries, thus causing HTN.

Stress stimulates the sympathetic nervous system which supplies nerves to the smooth muscles of the arteries, arterioles, veins, and venules. Stimulation of smooth muscles by the sympathetic nervous system causes the vessel to vasoconstrict leading to HTN.

Some complications of HTN are cerebral vascular accident (stroke), myocardial infarction, and congestive heart failure. Table 32-3 lists the recognized classification of blood pressure and the recommended time frame for follow-up care.

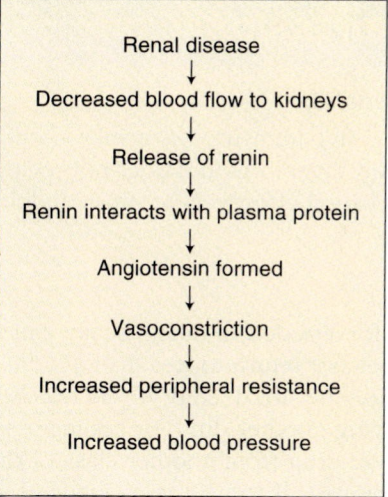

Figure 32-23 Pathophysiology of Renal Diseases and Hypertension

Medical–Surgical Management

Medical

The physician's main goal in caring for a client with HTN is keeping the blood pressure within normal limits. The regimen is referred to as a stepped-care approach. The first step is to encourage the client to try some diet and lifestyle changes. These include losing weight if the client is more than 15% over the optimum weight; limiting sodium, saturated fat, cholesterol, and alcohol intake; exercising on a regular basis; stopping the use of nicotine; and maintaining an adequate intake of calcium, magnesium, and potassium. This step is tried for 3 to 6 months, and if the BP then is less than 140/90, these steps would be continued. If the BP still remains high, the second step would be implemented which would be adding a diuretic or a beta blocker to the client's care regimen. The client would again be

Table 32-3 **CLASSIFICATION OF BLOOD PRESSURE AND RECOMMENDED FOLLOW-UP**				
CATEGORY	**SYSTOLIC (MM HG)**		**DIASTOLIC (MM HG)**	**RECOMMENDED FOLLOW-UP**
Optimal	< 120	and	<80	Recheck 2 years
Normal	< 130	and	< 85	Recheck 2 years
High normal	130–139	or	85–89	Recheck 1 year
Hypertension				
Stage 1 (mild)	140–159	or	90–99	Recheck within 2 months
Stage 2 (moderate)	160–179	or	100–109	Recheck within 1 month
Stage 3 (severe)	> 180	or	> 110	Immediate care

From The Sixth Report of the Joint National Committee on Prevention, Detection, Evaluation, and Treatment of High Blood Pressure, *1997, Bethesda, MD: National Institutes of Health.)*

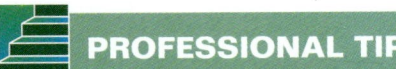

Hypertension
Often the hypertensive client may not be experiencing any symptoms and does not see the importance of caring effectively for this condition.

evaluated for a period of time, usually 2 months. If the BP still does not return to less than 140/90 within that time frame, the third step of increasing the drug dosage, trying another drug, or adding a second antihypertensive drug from another class of drugs would be implemented. If the BP is maintained at less than 140/90, the regimen would be continued. If the BP is still high, the last step would be implemented by adding a second or third antihypertensive drug.

Pharmacological

Diuretics are usually the first pharmacological step in treating HTN. Diuretics increase the renal excretion of sodium and water from the body decreasing the total fluid volume. When less fluid is in the body, less pressure or force is needed to pump the blood through the body.

Beta-adrenergic blocking agents are given to block the epinephrine and norepinephrine receptor sites. With these receptor sites blocked, the vessels will not constrict and the blood will have less resistance flowing through the vessel. Diuretics and antihypertensive medications may cause impotence.

Other medications used to lower blood pressure are alpha$_1$-receptor blockers, angiotensin-converting enzyme (ACE) inhibitors, calcium channel blockers, centrally acting alpha$_2$-agonists, peripherally acting adrenergic antagonists, and direct vasodilators. Refer to Table 32-4 for a list of antihypertensive medications.

Diet

The hypertensive client is encouraged to have a low-fat, low-cholesterol, and low-sodium diet. Restricting sodium intake to 2.3 grams of sodium or 6 grams of sodium chloride a day assists in decreasing blood pressure. Slight lifestyle changes such as avoiding processed foods, carbonated drinks, and most cereals help decrease sodium intake. The client should have an adequate intake of potassium, magnesium, and calcium. These minerals can be obtained by eating fresh oranges, bananas, broccoli, and collards. Fresh foods are better sources for minerals than frozen foods. Yogurt is a good calcium supplement. The National

Table 32-4 ANTIHYPERTENSIVE MEDICATIONS

Alpha-adrenergic Blockers
clonidine hydrochloride (Catapres)
doxazosin mesylate (Cardura)
methyldopa (Aldomet)
phentolamine mesylate (Regitine)
prazosin hydrochloride (Minipress)
terazosin hydrochloride (Vasocard, Hytrin)

Angiotensin-converting Enzyme (ACE) Inhibitors
captopril (Capoten)
enalapril maleate (Vasotec)

Beta-andrenergic Blockers
propranolol hydrochloride (Inderal)
timolol maleate (Blocardren)
atenolol (Tenormin)

Calcium Channel Blockers
diltiazem hydrochloride (Cardizem)
nifedipine (Procardia)
verapamil (Calan, Isoptin)

Ganglionic Blockers
trimethaphan camsylate (Arfonad)

Loop Diuretics
bumetanide (Bumex)
furosemide (Lasix)

Potassium-sparing Diuretics
amiloride hydrochloride (Midamor)
spironolactone (Aldactone)
spironolactone with HCTZ (Aldactazide)
triamterene (Dyrenium)

Thiazide Diuretics
chlorothiazide (Diuril)
hydrochlorothiazide (Esidrex, HydroDIURIL)
methyclothiazide (Enduron)
metolazone (Zaroxolyn)

Thiazide-like Diuretics
chlorthalidone (Hygroton)
indapamide (Lozol)

Peripherally Acting Adrenergic Antagonists
reserpine (Serpasil)

Direct Vasodilators
diazoxide (Hyperstat)
hydrolazine hydrochloride (Apresoline)
nitroprusside sodium (Nipride)

Committee on Prevention, Detection, Evaluation, and Treatment of High Blood Pressure recommends that clients with hypertension not consume more than 2 ounces of alcohol at a time and no more than twice a week.

Activity

A regular aerobic exercise regimen assists in lowering blood pressure. The client is to gradually increase the exercise period to 30 to 45 minutes 3 to 5 times per week with a pulse rate at 75% of the target heart rate (target heart rate = $220 - \text{age} \times 0.75$). Walking, swimming, and jogging are excellent aerobic exercises.

Health Promotion

Measures to prevent hypertension are exercising regularly; reducing sodium in the diet; maintaining an optimum weight; reducing and managing stress; maintaining intake of potassium, calcium, and magnesium; decreasing alcohol consumption; and ceasing smoking.

▶ NURSING PROCESS

▶ Assessment

▶ Subjective Data

The hypertensive client should be asked about general lifestyle habits such as smoking, alcohol consumption, exercise routine, dietary intake, and family history of hypertension. Any dizziness, blurred vision, and headache in the occipital region upon rising in the morning should be noted.

▶ Objective Data

The basic assessment for HTN is taking the blood pressure in both arms in supine and sitting positions. Before taking the blood pressure, the client should rest quietly for 5 minutes. If the client has an elevated BP, a repeat blood pressure should be taken 15 minutes later and compared to previous readings. Client height and weight should be recorded, and heart sounds and peripheral pulses measured.

Nursing diagnoses for a client with hypertension may include the following:

Nursing Diagnoses	Planning/Goals	Nursing Interventions
Health Maintenance, Altered, related to lack of knowledge about lifestyle habits contributing to hypertension	The client will relate needed changes in lifestyle habits to decrease blood pressure.	Make referrals to the appropriate personnel to teach the client lifestyle changes. These may include a dietitian, smoking cessation clinic, fitness center, or stress management seminars. Explain the pathophysiology, risk factors, lifestyle changes, medication actions and side effects, and complications of hypertension.
Noncompliance related to individual's value system (lack of physical symptoms and expense of medication)	The client will keep appointments for regular check-ups and take medications as prescribed.	Regularly inquire about the client's satisfaction in regard to the prescribed regimen of diet, exercise, and prescribed medication(s). If the client cannot afford needed medications, refer the client to financial assistance programs. Encourage the client to become an active participant in the treatment as this will give the client a sense of control over the condition. Encourage the client to record BP readings, weekly weight, exercise activities, and dietary intake as a way of giving a sense of control and encouraging compliance.
Nutrition, Altered, more than body requirements, related to excess caloric intake and excess sodium intake	The client will maintain weight at no more than 15 percent over optimum weight and have no more than 2.3 grams of sodium per day.	Give basic dietary instructions as stated under medical management or make a referral to a dietitian. Weigh the client at scheduled appointments.
Sexual Dysfunction, related to altered body structure or function (antihypertensive medications)	The client will state satisfaction with sexual function while taking antihypertensive medications.	Since diuretics and antihypertensive medications may cause impotence, discuss this effect in an open and candid manner, so the client and spouse will be more open to discuss difficulties in this area.

Evaluation Each goal must be evaluated to determine how it has been met by the client.

SAMPLE NURSING CARE PLAN

THE CLIENT WITH HYPERTENSION

Thomas Liggins, a 28-year-old African American, is in his last year of law school and is clerking for a prestigious law firm. He and his fiancé are planning to be married as soon as he graduates. During the last week he has had 4 dizzy spells and has had a headache at the base of his skull upon awakening for the last 2 days. His father has a history of hypertension, so Thomas is aware that his symptoms may be indicative of high blood pressure. Thomas stops by the clinic on his way home from work and asks to have his blood pressure checked. The nursing assessment has the following data.

Subjective data: States he has had 4 dizzy spells and has awakened with a headache in the occipital lobe the last 2 mornings. Thomas has been having 1 glass of wine at lunch and 2–3 beers in the evening to relax from the tension of school and work. Most of his meals have been at fast-food establishments and have a high fat content. Thomas does not smoke. He used to jog 4 mornings a week but quit when he starting clerking. He has been getting up twice in the night to urinate for the last 3 weeks. He is not taking any medication. Thomas states he is concerned about having hypertension because he does not want to take medication.

Objective data: T 98.6 P 78 R 16 BP 142/92 Wt 190 (optimum weight 160). No edema noted in hands, feet, or legs.

Nursing Diagnosis 1 *Health Maintenance, Altered, related to ineffective individual coping as evidenced by high-fat diet, lack of exercise, stressful job, and alcohol intake*

PLANNING/GOALS	NURSING INTERVENTIONS	RATIONALE	EVALUATION
Thomas will change lifestyle habits by engaging in aerobic exercises at least 3 times a week for 30 to 45 minutes, stating three ways to reduce stress, and limiting alcohol consumption to 2 ounces twice a week.	Refer Thomas to a dietitian to learn ways to cut fat and sodium in his diet.	Knowledge of a low-sodium, low-fat diet will encourage compliance.	Thomas starts exercising with his fiancé 3 times a week. Thomas uses breathing techniques and a hot shower to reduce daily stress. Thomas limits alcohol consumption to 1 beer a day.
	Discuss ways Thomas can exercise and still meet responsibilities of work, school, and personal and social life.	Thomas will be more willing to exercise if he sees ways that he can still meet responsibilities of life.	
	Explain that alcohol consumption should be limited to 2 ounces of alcohol twice a week.	Knowledge of alcohol content in alcoholic beverages will encourage compliance.	

Nursing Diagnosis 2 *Nutrition, Altered, more than body requirements, related to excessive caloric intake as evidenced by 30 pounds overweight and high-fat diet*

PLANNING/GOALS	NURSING INTERVENTIONS	RATIONALE	EVALUATION
Thomas will lose 30 pounds and maintain a low-fat, low-sodium diet.	Refer Thomas to a weight support group.	It will be easier for Thomas to change life habits if others are encouraging him.	Thomas and his fiancé are maintaining a diet low in sodium and no

continued

	Encourage Thomas to maintain a weekly weight record and to monitor daily intake of fat grams.	Monitoring personal diet and recording weight weekly promotes self-care and personal involvement in health maintenance.	more than 30 grams of fat per day. Thomas keeps a weekly record of his weight.

Nursing Diagnosis 3 *Anxiety related to threat to or change in health status and stress as evidenced by alcohol consumption to relax and statement of not wanting to take medications*

PLANNING/GOALS	NURSING INTERVENTIONS	RATIONALE	EVALUATION
Thomas will state preventive measures to reduce blood pressure.	Have Thomas identify stress factors in life.	Thomas may not be aware of some stressors in his life. Action to cope with stressors can be taken only if stressors are identified.	Thomas states 4 ways to reduce blood pressure.
	Discuss stress reduction techniques with Thomas.	Knowledge of ways to reduce stress will promote compliance.	
	Discuss risk factors of hypertension and ways to reduce blood pressure.	Knowledge of risk factors will promote identification of risk factors in personal life.	
	Explain to Thomas and his fiancé that hypertension is a chronic condition, possibly without symptoms, and with some potentially serious complications.	Knowledge of disease process promotes compliance. It is important for client and client's support system to understand disease process so lifestyle changes can be made more easily.	

CASE STUDY

Mr. Lance Jeffers, a 55-year-old truck driver, is admitted to the emergency room with a feeling of heavy squeezing pressure in his sternal area. The pain is radiating to his left shoulder. He is diaphoretic, short of breath, and nauseated. He states the sternal pain came on suddenly while watching a football game. He had been mowing his yard and decided to rest. The emergency physician gives Mr. Jeffers a nitroglycerin tablet and connects him to an EKG monitor. Cardiac enzymes with isoenzyme fractions and a chest x-ray are requested STAT. Morphine sulfate 2 mg is given intravenously. Oxygen is given by mask at 4 liters/ minute. Mr. Jeffers's apical pulse is 102 and his blood pressure is 130/88. A cardiac catheterization with flu-oroscopy is ordered to determine the patency of the coronary blood vessels and functioning of the heart mus-cle. Three hours after admission, crackles are heard in the lungs.

The following questions will guide your development of a nursing care plan for the case study.

1. List symptoms/clinical manifestations, other than Mr. Jeffers's, a client may experience when having a myocardial infarction.
2. List two reasons morphine sulfate was given to Mr. Jeffers.
3. List two other diagnostic tests that may have been ordered for Mr. Jeffers.
4. List subjective and objective data a nurse would want to obtain about Mr. Jeffers.
5. Write three individualized nursing diagnoses and goals for Mr. Jeffers.
6. Mr. Jeffers is moved from the critical care unit. List pertinent nursing actions a nurse would do in car-ing for Mr. Jeffers related to:

   oxygenation

   cardiac output

   comfort/rest

   activity

   medications

   teaching
7. List teachings that Mr. Jeffers will need before his discharge.
8. List at least three successful client outcomes for Mr. Jeffers.

SUMMARY

- The coronary arteries supply blood to the heart. If the blood flow through these vessels becomes di-minished or occluded, ischemia to the heart tissue occurs resulting in angina or a myocardial infarction.
- Typical symptoms experienced by a person with car-diac problems include chest pain, dyspnea, edema, fainting, palpitations, diaphoresis, and fatigue.
- Cardiac catheterization provides information on the patency of the heart vessels, pressure in the cham-bers, oxygen saturation in the chambers and ves-sels, and cardiac output.
- A dysrhythmia is an irregularity in the rate, rhythm, or conduction of the electrical system of the heart.
- Inflammatory or infectious conditions of the heart include endocarditis, myocarditis, and pericarditis.

- Endocarditis may cause valvular heart disease with the possibility of the valve needing to be surgically repaired (valvuloplasty) or replaced with a mechan-ical (caged-ball valve or tilting-disk valve) or biolog-ical valve from a calf, pig, or human.
- Surgical treatment for angina includes a PTCA, intra-coronary stent, transcatheter ablation, or a coronary artery bypass graft.
- Nursing interventions for CHF are monitoring vital signs with each client activity; administering digitalis, diuretics, and vasodilators as ordered; administering and observing the effects of oxygen; weighing the client daily; obtaining accurate I & O; and teaching healthy lifestyle changes.
- To assess the peripheral vascular system, the nurse as-sesses pain, pulse, pallor, paresthesia, and paralysis.

- Three factors leading to the formation of a clot—pooling of blood, vessel trauma, and a coagulation problem—are called Virchow's triad.
- A client with a DVT may be asymptomatic or may have warmth and tenderness at the site, edema of the extremity, a positive Homans' sign, cyanosis of the foot, and a sensation of heaviness or tightness in the extremity.
- Treatment for a thrombus includes bed rest, warm soaks, elevation of the extremity, and application of elastic stockings or intermittent pneumatic compression. It is important for the nurse to measure the leg circumference every shift and check peripheral pulses.
- The cause of varicose veins is incompetent valves and veins that have lost their elasticity.
- Primary Raynaud's disease is an intermittent spasm of the digital arteries and arterioles resulting in decreased circulation to the digits.
- An aneurysm is a localized dilation of a weakened section of the medial layer of an artery.
- Hypertension is an elevated arterial blood pressure of 140/90.

Review Questions

1. The nurse may assist in relieving the chest pain of a client with pericarditis by having the client:
   a. lie flat and turn on the right side.
   b. lie flat and turn on the left side.
   c. sit in a semi-Fowler's position.
   d. sit erect and lean forward.

2. To assess a client with right-sided heart failure, the nurse would:
   a. listen for a pericardial friction rub.
   b. listen for a muffled S_1 and S_2 heart sound.
   c. check for distended neck veins with the bed at a 45° angle.
   d. assess for radiation of the squeezing sensation under the sternum.

3. A diagnostic test for a myocardial infarction is:
   a. cardiac enzymes.
   b. arterial blood gases.
   c. cardiac biopsy.
   d. pulse oximetry.

4. It would be important to teach a client with angina to:
   a. take antibiotics before having dental work.
   b. carry nitroglycerin tablets at all times.
   c. perform the Valsalva maneuver daily.
   d. massage the carotid sinuses in the neck.

5. A client with the diagnosis of a myocardial infarction has just been admitted to the ER. To relieve chest pain, the physician orders:
   a. amoxicillin (Amoxil).
   b. ibuprofen (Motrin).
   c. digoxin (Lanoxin).
   d. morphine sulfate.

6. A cardiac dysrhythmia that has an erratic electrical activity of the atria resulting in a rate of 350 beats/minute to 600 beats/minute is:
   a. atrial fibrillation.
   b. bradycardia.
   c. ventricular asystole.
   d. third degree AV block.

7. A nursing intervention to improve cardiac output is:
   a. encouraging the client to verbalize fears.
   b. teaching the side effects of new medications.
   c. a referral to a dietitian for low-sodium diet instructions.
   d. administer oxygen per physician orders.

8. The most appropriate nursing diagnosis for a client with coronary artery disease is:
   a. decreased cardiac output.
   b. social isolation.
   c. fatigue.
   d. altered nutrition.

9. Instructions to a client on anticoagulant therapy include:
   a. taking Coumadin twice a day.
   b. watching for symptoms of bleeding.
   c. taking over-the-counter medications as needed.
   d. no dietary or activity limitations.

10. When assessing a client with a possible DVT, the nurse:
    a. routinely does a Homans' sign.
    b. massages the calf of the leg.
    c. gently touches the affected area and checks for warmth.
    d. calls the physician immediately.

11. A nurse is assigned to care for a client who has just had a hysterectomy. To prevent the formation of a thrombus, the nurse:
    a. encourages the client to lie in bed with the knee gatch activated.
    b. encourages the client to ambulate with assistance according to the physician's orders.
    c. assesses Homans' sign as part of the routine postop assessment.
    d. checks peripheral pulses every 4 hours.

12. A client, admitted with the diagnosis of AAA, states he can feel a pulsation when he lies flat in bed. To assess the pulsation, the nurse would palpate:

   a. the epigastric area.
   b. the right lower quadrant.
   c. one inch above the symphysis pubis.
   d. left of umbilicus.

13. The symptoms a client with an aneurysm pressing on the inferior vena cava would most likely experience are:

   a. low dull back pain and a pulsating mass in the abdomen.
   b. dyspnea, wheezing, and hoarseness.
   c. bloating, nausea, and vomiting.
   d. edema in the extremities and possible cyanosis.

14. The first step of the stepped-care approach in treating hypertension is:

   a. changes in lifestyle.
   b. diuretics.
   c. beta-blockers.
   d. adding a second or third antihypertensive.

Critical Thinking Questions

1. What lifestyle changes could a person take to decrease the risk factors for a myocardial infarction? Prepare a teaching strategy to teach the hypertensive client ways to modify the present lifestyle.

2. What is the rationale for each nursing intervention given for the nursing diagnoses in this chapter?

 WEB FLASH!

- Search the Internet for information about the disorders covered in this chapter. What information is available? For whom is the information suitable?
- Do the resources for this chapter at the end of the book have information on the Internet? What information do they provide?

NURSING CARE OF THE CLIENT: BLOOD AND LYMPH SYSTEMS

MAKING THE CONNECTION

Refer to the following chapters to increase your understanding of blood and lymph systems:

- **Chapter 23, Fluid, Electrolyte, and Acid-Base Balance**
- **Chapter 25, Assessment**
- **Chapter 26, Pain Management**
- **Chapter 30, Nursing Care of the Oncology Client**
- **Chapter 31, Nursing Care of the Client: Respiratory System**

- **Chapter 32, Nursing Care of the Client: Cardiovascular System**
- **Chapter 37, Nursing Care of the Client: Endocrine System**
- **Chapter 39, Nursing Care of the Client: Immune System**
- **Procedures:** B1, Handwashing; A1, Initiating Strict Isolation Precautions

LEARNING OBJECTIVES

Upon completion of this chapter, you should be able to:
- *Define key terms.*
- *Relate anatomy and physiology of the blood and lymph systems to disease processes.*
- *Relate diagnostic test results to the blood and lymph disorders.*
- *Describe nursing interventions in caring for clients with blood and lymph disorders.*
- *Assist in developing a nursing care plan for clients with blood and lymph disorders.*

INTRODUCTION

The hematological system of the body comprises blood and blood-forming organs. Blood consists of formed elements (red blood cells, white blood cells, and platelets) and plasma. As blood is pumped through the body, it carries essential substances to the tissues and removes waste products from the tissues. Disorders of the hematological system usually result from abnormal production or functioning of the cells. Some of these disorders are the result of genetics, environment, or pathogenic organisms.

The lymph system consists of lymph vessels, nodes, and organs. Lymph vessels collect and return lymph

KEY TERMS

agranulocytosis	induction dose
apheresis	leukocytosis
bands	leukopenia
blastic phase	lymphoma
combination	maintenance therapy
chemotherapy	median survival time
erythrocytapheresis	microthrombi
fibrinolysis	phlebotomy
hemarthrosis	purpura
hematocrit	reticulocyte
hematopoiesis	secondary malignancy
hemolysis	sickled
hyperuricemia	thrombocytopenia
idiopathic	

fluid to the blood vessels through the right and left lymphatic ducts at the right and left subclavian veins. The functions of the lymph system are to assist with immunity, control edema, and absorb digested fats.

Medical management and nursing diagnoses, goals, and interventions are given for each blood and lymph disorder. It is important for the nurse to have a complete understanding of the blood and lymph disorders when providing nursing care to clients.

ANATOMY AND PHYSIOLOGY REVIEW

The blood and lymphatic systems are discussed following.

Blood

The heart pumps 5–6 liters of blood per minute through the circulatory system of an adult. Blood is an aqueous mixture consisting of plasma and cells (Figure 33-1).

Plasma

Blood plasma is a straw-colored liquid consisting of water, proteins, electrolytes, lipids, carbohydrates, and various other organic and inorganic substances. The formed elements in plasma are red blood cells (RBCs), white blood cells (WBCs), and platelets. The proteins in the plasma—including albumin, fibrinogen, and globulins, RBCs, WBCs, platelets, and immunoglobulins (gamma globulins)—are transported by the plasma throughout the circulatory system.

Red Blood Cells

Red blood cells, also called erythrocytes, are the most numerous blood cells in the body, generally 4.5 to 6.1 million/mm^3 in an adult. RBCs are biconcave disks that do not have a nucleus. They are about the

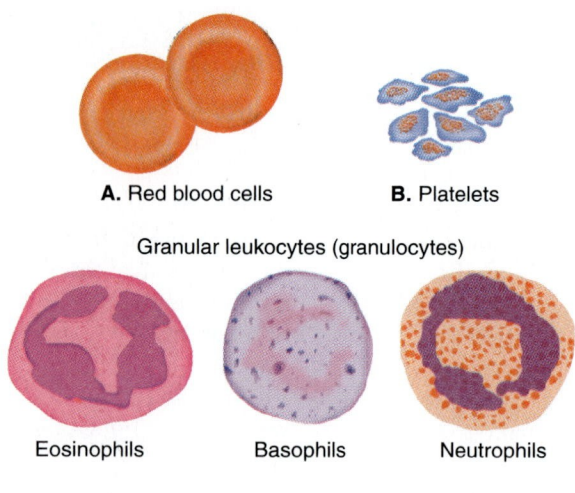

A. Red blood cells   **B.** Platelets

Granular leukocytes (granulocytes)

Eosinophils   Basophils   Neutrophils

Nongranular leukocytes (agranulocytes)

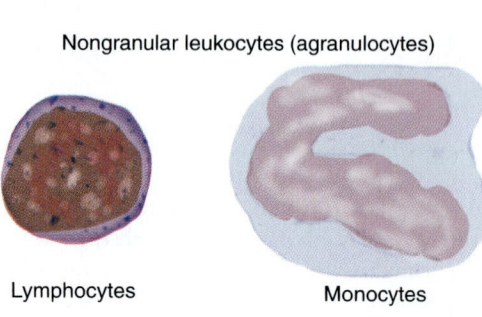

Lymphocytes   Monocytes

C. Granular and nongranular white blood cells

Figure 33-1 The Cells in Blood: A. Red blood cells (erythrocytes); B. Platelets (thrombocytes); C. White blood cells (leukocytes).

size of the smallest capillary but are flexible and capable of changing shape so they can squeeze through the capillaries.

RBCs in conjunction with the respiratory and circulatory systems oxygenate body tissues. In the capillary bed of the alveoli, blood receives oxygen (O_2), and carbon dioxide (CO_2) is eliminated. The O_2-enriched RBCs (oxyhemoglobin) carry O_2 to systemic capillaries, where O_2 is exchanged for CO_2. The carbon dioxide–laden blood then returns the CO_2 to the alveoli in the lungs, where it is again exchanged for oxygen. The CO_2 is exhaled from the body with each breath. Hemoglobin is a protein in the RBC that carries O_2 and is responsible for the exchange of O_2 and CO_2.

The average life span for an RBC is 120 days. Blood cells originate from a single stem cell that proliferates and differentiates into lymphoid stem cells or blood stem cells (Figure 33-2). The lymphoid stem cells further divide and differentiate into T cells and B cells. The blood stem cells divide and differentiate into RBCs, WBCs, and platelets. The process of blood cell production and development is called **hematopoiesis**. RBCs are produced daily by the bone marrow according to the demand of the body. When the partial pressure of O_2 drops, a renal hormone, erythropoietin, stimulates the bone marrow to produce more immature RBCs (**reticulocytes**), which are released into the bloodstream. These reticulocytes develop into mature red blood cells. The number of circulating reticulocytes can be used as a diagnostic tool for RBC disorders.

As RBCs age, their outer membrane deteriorates and they are destroyed by large macrophages in the liver and are filtered out of the body by the spleen. The iron from heme in the old RBCs is used in the production of new RBCs.

Hematocrit is the percentage of blood cells in a volume of blood. A normal hematocrit is 42% to 45% of blood volume; that is, 42% to 45% of a certain amount of blood consists of cells.

White Blood Cells

White blood cells, also called leukocytes, fight infection and assist with immunity. The life span of a

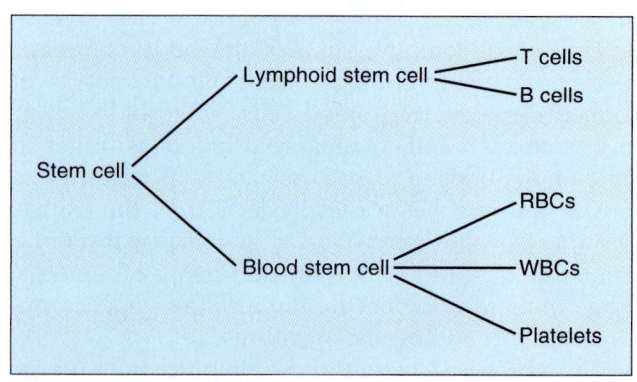

Figure 33-2 Origin of T cells, B cells, RBCs, WBCs, and Platelets

WBC varies from hours to years, depending on the type of WBC. Neutrophils, basophils, and eosinophils live from a few hours to days, whereas lymphocytes and monocytes live from days to years. The normal WBC count is 5,000 to 10,000/mm³ of blood (Pagana & Pagana, 1999). An increased number of WBCs (**leukocytosis**) may signify the presence of an infection, inflammation, tissue necrosis, or leukemia. A decreased number of WBCs (**leukopenia**) may indicate bone marrow failure, a massive infection, dietary deficiencies, a drug toxicity, or an autoimmune disease.

WBCs are classified as granulocytes or polymorphonuclear leukocytes (PMNs, or polys), and agranulocytes. The granulocytes have granules (grainy substances) in their cytoplasm, and the agranulocytes do not have granules. Granulocytes are divided into three types: the neutrophils, eosinophils, and basophils. Agranulocytes are classified into two groups, monocytes and lymphocytes. Neutrophils are the most numerous WBCs, making up approximately 60% of the total number of WBCs. The main function of neutrophils is to digest and kill microorganisms. If a client has an acute infection, the bone marrow is stimulated to produce more neutrophils, resulting in an increased circulation of immature neutrophils called **bands**. An increased production of neutrophils indicates the presence of an acute infection. An increased number of basophils and especially of eosinophils indicates an allergic response.

Monocytes become macrophages, cells that destroy dead and injured cells and bacteria. There are two types of lymphocytes, T cells and B cells, which are involved in the body's immune response.

Platelets

Platelets (thrombocytes) are not typical cells but nonnucleated, granular ovoid, or spindle-shaped cell fragments. The normal life span of a platelet is approximately 10 days. Platelets are active in the clotting mechanism of the body. When platelets flow over a rough or damaged area in a vessel, they adhere to the area and release thromboplastin and clotting factors that start the blood-clotting process. They also secrete prostaglandins and serotonin, which cause the vessel to constrict, thereby decreasing the blood flow through the area. Prothrombin, thromboplastin, and calcium ions form thrombin which joins with fibrinogen to form fibrin. The fibrin strands seal the opening or area and a clot is formed (Figure 33-3).

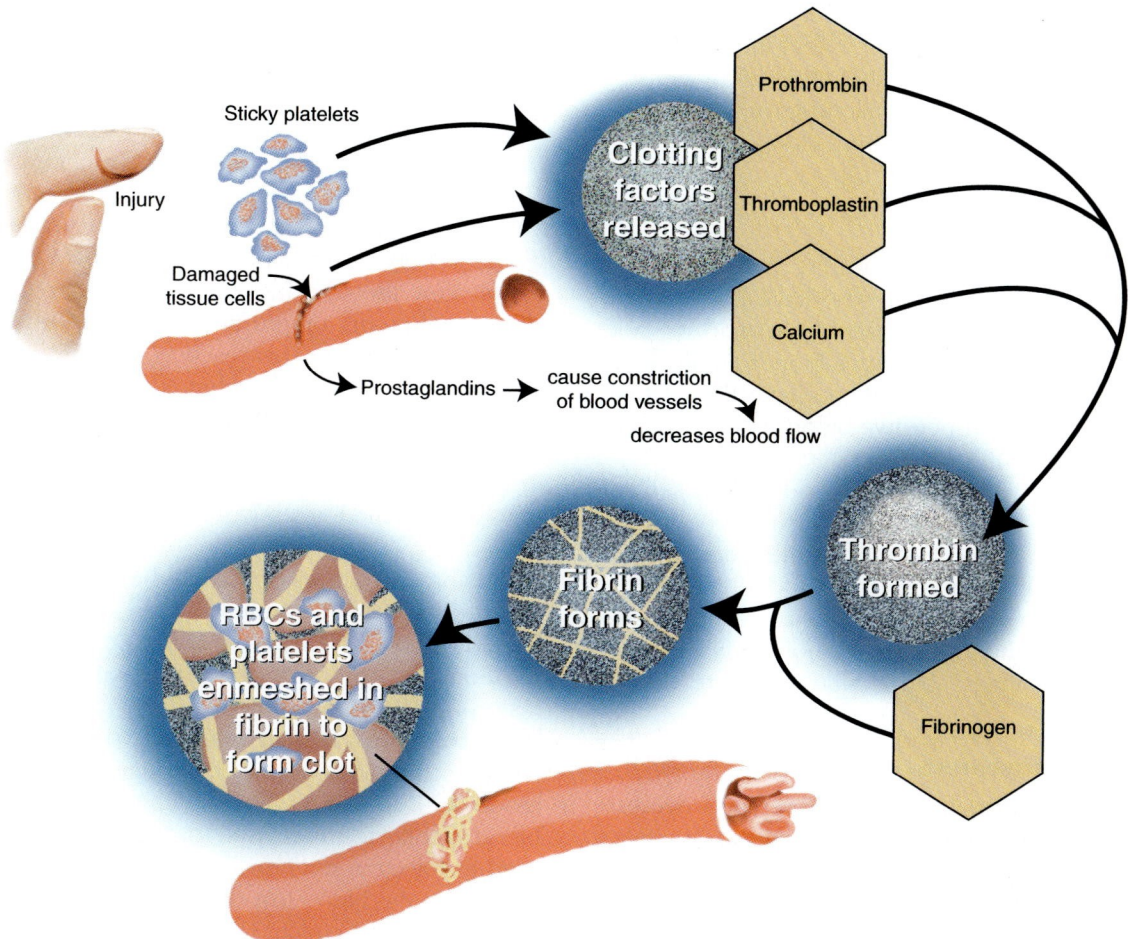

Figure 33-3 The Process of Clot Formation

Blood Types

On the surface of RBC membranes are genetically determined antigens called agglutinogens. The A and B antigens constitute the ABO blood group. If the A antigen is on the RBC membrane, the client has type A blood. If the B antigen is on the RBC membrane, the client has type B blood. If both an A and a B antigen are present, the client has type AB blood, and if no antigen is present, the client has type O blood.

Anti-A or anti-B antibodies are present in the serum of every person with type A and type B blood. Type A blood has anti-B antibodies in the serum, and type B blood has anti-A antibodies. If a person with type A blood receives type B blood during a transfusion, the anti-B antibodies will attack the infused RBCs and hemolyze (destroy) them. The hemoglobin released when these cells are hemolyzed can lead to kidney damage.

A person with AB blood does not have anti-A or anti-B antibodies. People with AB blood are theoretically universal recipients because they can receive blood from all blood types. Type O blood does not have any antigens that the antibodies can attack. Persons with type O blood can theoretically give blood to persons having any type of blood. Persons with type O blood are called universal donors. The terms *universal recipient* and *universal donor* are only theoretical because during blood transfusions, blood incompatibilities can occur because of the other types of antigens.

There are fourteen different blood groups and over 100 different antigens. The different blood groups vary in number with different ethnic groups.

Rh Factor

Another factor to consider during blood transfusions is the Rh factor. Persons who have Rh antigens (the D antigen) are Rh positive. Those who do not have Rh antigens on their RBC membranes are Rh negative. Approximately 85% of people have Rh-positive blood and 15% have Rh-negative blood (Lewis, Collier, & Heitkemper, 1996).

If a person with Rh-negative blood is exposed to Rh-positive blood during a blood transfusion or during childbirth, anti-Rh antibodies form in the blood serum. When a person with Rh-negative blood is exposed a second time to Rh-positive blood, the anti-Rh antibodies will react with the Rh-positive blood and cause hemolysis of the infused blood and a severe blood reaction.

Blood Transfusions

Blood transfusions are given to replace needed blood components because of hemorrhage, anemia, clotting disorders, or blood deficiencies. Transfusable blood products are whole blood, packed red cells, platelets, fresh frozen plasma, and cryoprecipitate. Whole blood is given to increase blood volume and the various blood components. Packed red cells are given for anemia. Platelets assist in controlling bleeding. Fresh frozen plasma is administered for clotting disorders. Cryoprecipitate corrects fibrinogen deficiencies.

Before blood products are given, the lab does a type- and crossmatch to check compatibility between the donor blood type and Rh factor and the client's blood type and Rh factor. The lab also checks all blood products for HIV and hepatitis B and C viruses. Blood must be handled gently so as not to damage the cells. Administration of the blood should begin within 30 minutes of obtaining it from the laboratory refrigerator.

The nurse takes baseline vital signs—temperature, pulse, and blood pressure—before administering the blood product. Once the transfusion is started, temperature and pulse are measured after 15 minutes, 30 minutes, and then hourly; blood pressure is measured hourly during the transfusion. Blood is generally administered through a peripheral vein using an 18- or 19-gauge cannula. A large cannula is used so the blood cells do not break when passing through the cannula.

Before the transfusion, two nurses check the compatibility of the blood product and the client's blood. The first 50 cc is given within 5 to 10 minutes. The client is observed closely for a hemolytic blood reaction during this time.

There are three types of blood reactions: hemolytic, febrile, and allergic. Symptoms of a hemolytic reaction include chest pain, dyspnea, flushing, oliguria, hypotension, and shock. It is usually a severe reaction occuring within 15 minutes. The transfusion should be stopped immediately and the physician notified. A client with a febrile reaction has a temperature above 101.4°F, often with severe shaking, sweating, and tachycardia. This is usually a mild reaction occuring within 30–90 minutes but may occur up to several hours after the transfusion. An allergic reaction includes symptoms of pruritus, urticaria, and possibly anaphylactic shock. This reaction may be mild or severe and usually occurs within 30 minutes, but it may occur up to several hours after the transfusion.

If a client experiences any symptoms of a reaction, the infusion must be stopped immediately and the physician notified. Institutional protocol should be followed.

The blood transfusion should be completed within 4 hours of the start of administration. No medications should be given at the blood administration site during infusion. The only solution given during a blood transfusion is 0.9% sodium chloride.

Autologous Blood Transfusion If time and the client's condition permit, autologous ("from self") blood as opposed to homologous ("from a donor") blood is collected and saved for the client. This may be used for elective surgeries. An alternative procedure is to recover the blood lost during surgery and transfuse it back into the client. The use of autologous blood eliminates the possibility of a transfusion reaction and prevents the transmission of disease.

Lymphatic System

The lymphatic, or lymph, system is a separate vessel system. The two main functions of the lymph system are to transport excess fluid from the interstitial spaces to the circulatory system and to protect the body against infectious organisms.

Lymph Fluid and Vessels

Lymph fluid is a pale yellow fluid. Fluid and substances move from the plasma through the capillary walls and become interstitial fluid. As fluid accumulates in the interstitial space, pressure within the interstitial space increases. The interstitial fluid then diffuses through the lymphatic vessel wall into the lymph vessel. The flow of fluid is illustrated in Figure 33-4.

Semilunar valves in the lymphatic vessels assist the lymph system in returning the interstitial fluid, which is now called lymph, to the venous system. When the valves do not work properly or the vessels become obstructed, edema occurs. The pumping action or contractions of the skeletal muscles and the rhythmic action of the respiratory muscles assist in the movement of the lymph toward the subclavian veins. The right lymphatic duct drains lymph from the right side of the head, neck, thorax, and arm into the right subclavian vein. The lymph from the rest of the body drains into the left subclavian vein through the thoracic duct.

Lymph Nodes

Lymph nodes are scattered throughout the body along the lymph vessels (Figure 33-5). They contain dense patches of lymphocytes and macrophages. Lymphocytes act against such foreign particles as viruses and bacteria. Macrophages ingest and destroy foreign substances, damaged cells, and cellular debris. Lymph nodes can be superficial or deep. Those located superficially such as in the neck, axilla, and groin can be palpated, especially if they become infected and swollen. The tonsils in the pharynx and Peyer's patch in the mucosal lining of the ileum are located deeper within the body and cannot be palpated.

As lymph is collected from body tissues, cancer cells may enter the lymphatic system and escape into the circulation or to other body tissues, such as the lungs. Wherever the cancer cells collect, more cancer cells may be produced. In this way cancer can spread to other body parts. Lymph nodes are biopsied to check for the spread of cancer.

Lymph Organs

The spleen and thymus are lymph organs. The spleen removes old RBCs, platelets, and microorganisms from the blood. Approximately 350 mL of blood are stored in the spleen and approximately 200 mL can be pumped out within a minute into the body as needed (Thibodeau & Patton, 1995). During an infection, the spleen enlarges to produce and release monocytes and lymphocytes. Lymphocytes in the lymph tissue differentiate into T lymphocytes (T cells) and B lymphocytes (B cells).

In infancy and childhood, the thymus gland is large but decreases in size with age. In advanced age, it is replaced with fat and connective tissue. The thymus performs an important role in the special processing and proper functioning of the thymus-derived T lymphocytes (T cells). The T cells are actively involved in immunity.

ASSESSMENT

Information is based on client report, physical examination, and diagnostic tests.

Subjective Data

Biological and demographic data including age, sex, ethnic background, and race are important for

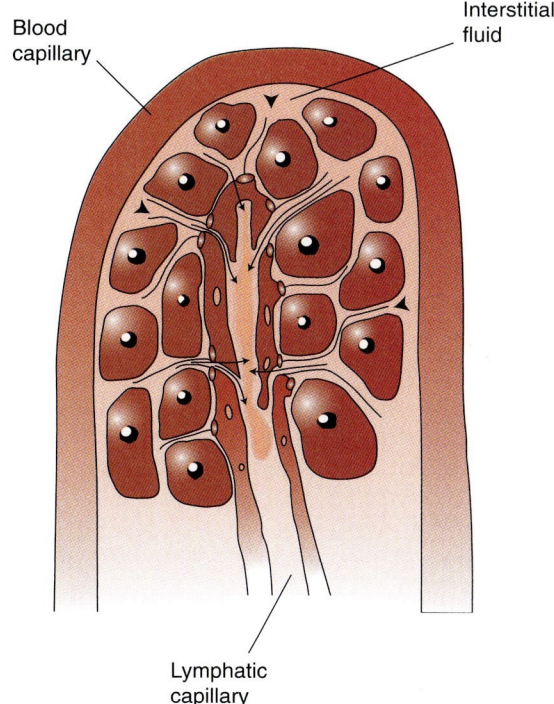

Figure 33-4 Flow of Fluid from the Blood into the Lymphatic System

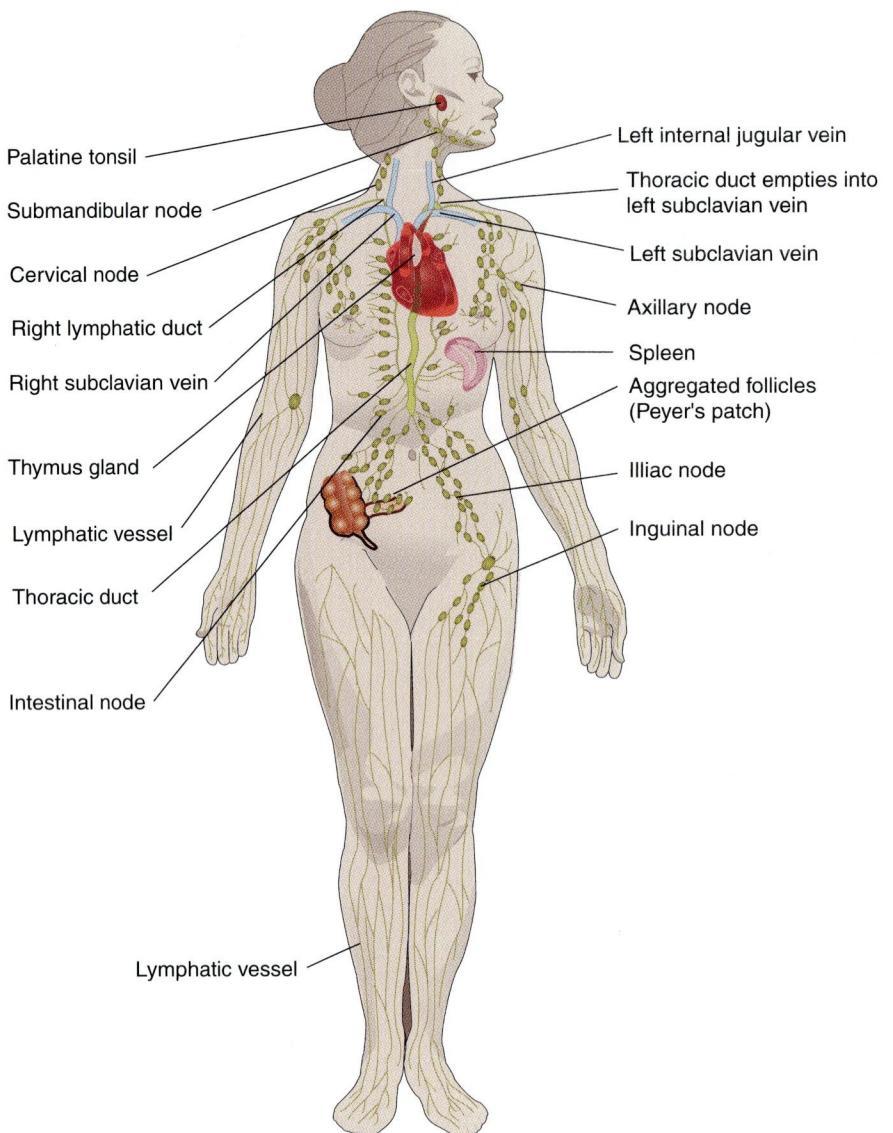

Figure 33-5 The Lymphatic System

many hematological problems. The nurse should inquire about the client's occupation and hobbies as there may be exposure to radiation or chemicals. Past military experience is also important, as some military personnel have been exposed to toxic chemicals. A medication history should be obtained from the client, including prescription and over-the-counter medications. Recent or recurring infections, night sweats, palpitations, bleeding problems, previous blood transfusions and any complications should be noted.

Neurological functioning is assessed by asking if the client has experienced any cognitive or mental difficulties or numbness and tingling of the extremities. A headache may be indicative of a low erythrocyte count or intracranial bleeding. Hearing or vision difficulties must also be noted.

The nurse should ask the client about past surgeries and any complications from surgeries; if the client has had a duodenal, gastric, or ileal resection, the absorp-

tion of iron and vitamin B_{12} may be affected. Alcohol use may be important because alcohol may affect vitamin intake and is caustic to the GI tract. The client should be asked about the presence of blood in the stool or urine and any anorexia, nausea, vomiting, oral discomfort, or problems with taste perception. A history of dietary intake is helpful when reviewing the erythrocyte level. The nurse must inquire if the client has difficulty accomplishing ADLs because of decreased energy.

Objective Data

The assessment begins by obtaining the client's height, weight, and vital signs. An elevated temperature may indicate an infection. Recent weight gains or losses should be noted.

Laboratory tests are very important when assessing the hematological and lymphatic systems. Past laboratory tests and present laboratory results must be compared.

The lymph nodes in the neck, axillae, and groin are palpated; normal findings include small (0.5–1.0 cm) nodes that are freely movable, firm, and nontender. Tender nodes are indicative of inflammation. Hard, fixed nodes may be malignant.

Next, the skin and extremities are inspected for petechiae, bruises, lesions, and brittle nails. Urine and stool should be checked for blood. Dyspnea, an enlarged abdomen, or swollen joints should be documented.

COMMON DIAGNOSTIC TESTS

Commonly used diagnostic tests for clients with symptoms of blood and lymph system disorders are listed in Table 33-1. See Chapter 27, Diagnostic Tests, for explanations, normal values, and nursing responsibilities.

Table 33-1 COMMON DIAGNOSTIC TESTS FOR BLOOD AND LYMPHATIC SYSTEM DISORDERS

Partial thromboplastin time (PTT)
Activated partial thromboplastin time (APTT)
Bleeding time
Blood culture and sensitivity
Coombs' test (direct antiglobulin test)
D dimer test
(Fragment D-dimer, Fibrin degradation fragment)
Erythrocyte sedimentation rate (sed rate, ESR)
Folic acid (Folate level)
Hematocrit (Hct)
Hemoglobin (Hgb)
Hemoglobin electrophoresis
Platelet count
Prothrombin time (PT, Protime)
Red blood cells (RBCs)
Schilling test
Sickledex (Sickle cell test)
Total iron binding capacity (TIBC)
White blood cells (WBCs)
Differential count (WBCs)
Granulocytes
  Basophils
  Eosinophils
  Neutrophils
  Bands
Agranulocytes
  Lymphocytes
  Monocytes
Radiologic lymphangiogram
Bone marrow aspiration
Gastric analysis, tube and tubeless test

RED BLOOD CELL DISORDERS: ANEMIAS AND POLYCYTHEMIA

Red blood cell disorders discussed in this section are the anemias and polycythemia vera. The nursing process for anemias is presented after the discussion of sickle-cell anemia because the nursing diagnoses, goals, and interventions are similar for all anemias.

Anemia is a common hematopoietic disorder in which the client has a decreased number of RBCs and a low hemoglobin level. The causes for anemia are a decreased production of RBCs, an increased destruction of RBCs, or a loss of blood. The types of anemia discussed in this section are iron deficiency anemia, hypoplastic (aplastic) anemia, pernicious anemia, acquired hemolytic anemia, and sickle-cell anemia.

IRON DEFICIENCY ANEMIA

Iron deficiency anemia is the most common type of anemia and occurs when the body does not have enough iron to synthesize functional Hgb. The decrease in iron may be due to a decreased dietary intake, a decreased iron absorption from the gastrointestinal tract, chronic intestinal or uterine blood loss, or an increased bodily need for iron such as during growth periods or pregnancy. Iron deficiency anemia is more frequently found in premature or low-birthweight infants, adolescent girls, alcoholics, and the elderly. The symptoms are fatigue, loss of appetite, decreased ability to concentrate, and pallor. Clients with chronic anemia may have tachycardia, exertional dyspnea, hypotension, dysphagia, stomatitis, glossitis, and brittle nails. Diagnostic tests of a client with iron deficiency anemia would reveal decreased RBCs, a low Hgb level, a low Hct, a low serum iron, and a high total iron binding capacity (TIBC).

Medical–Surgical Management

Pharmacological

Oral iron preparations are ferrous gluconate (Fergon) and ferrous sulfate (Feosol). These preparations are not given with milk because milk interferes with iron absorption. The administration of iron with meals, with orange juice, or vitamin C–rich drinks increases iron absorption. Iron dextran (Imferon), an intramuscular iron preparation, is given by Z-track technique.

Diet

The treatment for iron deficiency anemia is iron supplements and a diet high in iron. Foods rich in iron are red meats, fish, raisins, apricots, dried fruits, dark green vegetables, dried beans, eggs, and iron-enriched whole grain breads. An increase of vitamin C in the diet assists in the absorption of iron. If the client has a loss of appetite, small frequent snacks may be tolerated better than three large meals.

Activity

Daily activities should be spaced to provide rest periods between times of exercise.

HYPOPLASTIC (APLASTIC) ANEMIA

The bone marrow decreases or stops functioning in a client with aplastic anemia. The client with aplastic anemia has pancytopenia, a drop in the number of red blood cells, white blood cells, and platelets. It develops without a known cause and is thought to be congenital. Secondary aplastic anemia is caused by exposure to viruses, chemicals (benzene or airplane glue), radiation, or medications. Some medications that cause aplastic anemia are chloramphenicol (Chloromycetin), mephenytoin (Mesantoin), trimethadione (Tridione), mechlorethamine or nitrogen mustard (Mustargen), methotrexate (Folex PFS), 6-mercaptopurine or 6-MP (Purinethol), and phenylbutazone (Butazolidin). Symptoms include fatigue, weakness, tachycardia, dyspnea, susceptibility to infection, petechiae, gingival bleeding, and epistaxis. Clients with aplastic anemia are extremely ill. Diagnosis is confirmed by a bone marrow aspiration.

Medical–Surgical Management

Medical

The cause of aplastic anemia is removed if possible. Another treatment is antithymocyte globulin or ATG (Atgam) immunosuppressive therapy, which is given to suppress the reaction causing the aplastic anemia and to allow the client's bone marrow to recover. ATG is given daily through a central venous catheter for 7 to 10 days. A client who has a good response to ATG will improve in 3 to 6 months. The sooner the diagnosis is made and ATG started, the better the prognosis. Transfusions of packed red cells and platelets may be given.

Surgical

Bone marrow transplants are done if the client's bone marrow fails to start functioning. Cyclosporine (Sandimmune), an immunosuppressant, is given for a bone marrow transplant to decrease the graft rejection. The best response occurs in a young client who has not previously had a transfusion because transfusions increase bone marrow graft rejection. Bone marrow transplants from a human leukocyte antigen- (HLA-) matched sibling donor is the treatment of choice for clients less than 45 years of age. The treatment of

PROFESSIONAL TIP

Bone Marrow–Depressing Medication
When a client is taking medications that cause bone marrow depression. Monitor the blood cell count closely.

choice for an older adult or a client who does not have a HLA-matched sibling donor is immunosuppression with ATG or cyclosporine. (Bone marrow transplants are discussed in the section on acute myelocytic leukemia.)

Pharmacological

Infections are treated with antibiotics. Steroids and androgens are also sometimes used to stimulate the bone marrow.

PERNICIOUS ANEMIA

The parietal cells of the gastric mucosa secrete a protein intrinsic factor that is essential for the proper absorption of vitamin B_{12}. Pernicious anemia is an autoimmune disease in which the parietal cells are destroyed and the gastric mucosa atrophies. Without the secretion of the intrinsic factor, vitamin B_{12} cannot be absorbed in the distal portion of the ileum.

The onset of the disease occurs between 50 and 60 years of age. Pernicious anemia occurs most frequently in those of Northern European and African American descent. African American women are especially affected with the disease and often severely. Pernicious anemia can occur in clients who have had a gastrectomy with the section of the stomach removed that secretes the intrinsic factor. A gastric analysis and Schilling test are confirming diagnostic tests.

Pernicious anemia has an insidious onset, and it may take several months for the symptoms to be fully manifested. Symptoms include extreme weakness, a sore tongue, numbness and tingling of the extremities, edema of the legs, ataxia, dizziness, dyspnea, headache, fever, blurred vision, tinnitus, jaundice with pallor, poor memory, irritability, and loss of bladder and bowel control. The client may have decreased sensitivity to heat and pain because of neurological involvement. Clients with pernicious anemia are highly susceptible to gastric carcinoma and should be monitored closely for symptoms.

Medical–Surgical Management

Pharmacological

Topical anesthetics are given to relieve oral discomfort during the acute phase of the disease. Cyanocobalamin or vitamin B_{12} (Rubramin PC) is given IM daily for 2 weeks and then weekly until the Hct returns to a normal level. Then cyanocobalamin is usually administered monthly for the rest of the client's life. The frequency of administration will depend on the client's symptoms and response to the medication. Oral administration of vitamin B_{12} is not effective because vitamin B_{12} cannot be absorbed without the intrinsic factor. Folic acid or folate (Folvite) is prescribed. The client is encouraged to increase folic acid in the diet by eating green leafy vegetables, meat, fish, legumes, and whole grains. Iron is usually not prescribed because once the condition is corrected with regular administration of cyanocobalamin, erythrocytes are produced and the Hgb and Hct return to normal.

ACQUIRED HEMOLYTIC ANEMIA

In hemolytic anemias, **hemolysis**, or destruction of RBCs, occurs and iron and hemoglobin are released. Several causes for acquired hemolytic anemia are an autoimmune reaction, radiation, blood transfusion, chemicals, arsenic, lead, or medications. Sulfisoxazole (Gantrisin), penicillin, and methyldopa (Aldomet) are medications that can cause hemolysis. A substance produced by the bacterium *Clostridium perfringens* can also cause hemolysis. Symptoms may go unnoticed, or there may be a severe reaction. Symptoms are mild fatigue and pallor. More severe symptoms include jaundice, palpitations, hypotension, dyspnea, and back and joint pain. Diagnostic tests would reveal a low Hgb and Hct and an elevated LDH. LDH is an enzyme in the heart, liver, kidneys, skeletal muscle, brain, red blood cells, and lungs. As these tissues are damaged, LDH is released into the bloodstream, causing an elevated LDH.

Medical–Surgical Management

Medical

Treatment is aimed at removing the cause of the hemolytic anemia, if possible. The client may be given blood transfusions or **erythrocytapheresis** (a procedure that removes abnormal RBCs and replaces them with healthy RBCs).

Surgical

The function of the spleen is to destroy RBCs. In severe cases of hemolytic anemia, a splenectomy may be done in an attempt to stop the destruction of RBCs.

Pharmacological

Corticosteroids are administered to decrease the autoimmune response. Folic acid may also be given to increase the production of RBCs.

SICKLE CELL ANEMIA (INHERITED HEMOLYTIC ANEMIA)

Sickle cell anemia is also known as either inherited hemolytic anemia or sickle cell disease. It is a genetic disorder in which there is abnormal hemoglobin S rather than hemoglobin A in the RBCs. Sickle cell anemia is caused by a recessive gene that is passed through the generations (Figure 33-6). The client with one s gene has sickle cell trait (Hb sA) and is asymptomatic but is a carrier of the disease. The client with sickle cell anemia has two s genes (Hb ss) and manifests symptoms.

The condition occurs most frequently in African Americans, with an estimated 1 of 12 persons being sickle cell carriers (Phipps, Cassmeyer, Sands, and Lehman, 1999). It also occurs in persons from Asia Minor, India, and the Mediterranean and Caribbean areas.

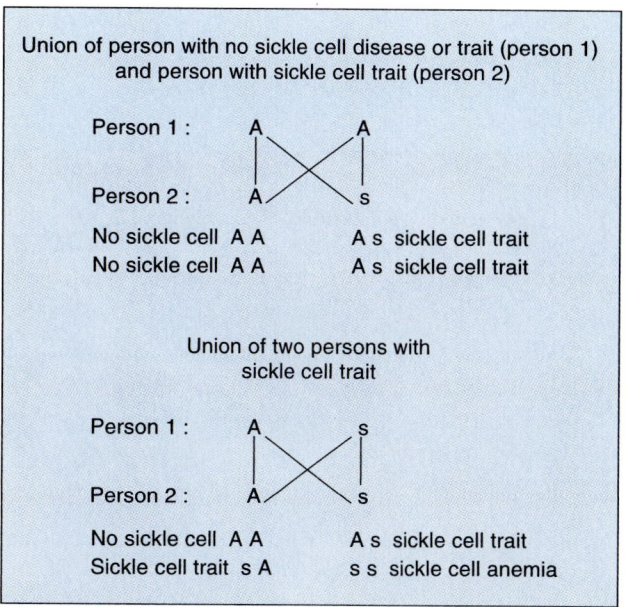

Figure 33-6 Inheritance of the Sickle Cell Trait and Sickle Cell Anemia

LIFE CYCLE CONSIDERATIONS

Sickle Cell Anemia

In infants, symptoms do not appear until after 6 months of age. Up to that age the infant still has fetal hemoglobin, which does not become sickled.

CLIENT TEACHING

Sickle Cell Anemia

- Encourage client to avoid high altitudes and nonpressurized airplanes.
- It is important for the client to have adequate fluid intake as dehydration causes a sickle cell crisis.
- All infections should be promptly treated.
- Client should avoid tight-fitting, restrictive clothing, and strenuous exercise, smoking, and cold temperatures.
- Encourage client to receive yearly flu vaccine and pneumococcal vaccine.

Situations that precipitate sickle cell crisis are dehydration, fatigue, infection, emotional stress, and alcohol consumption. When oxygenation is compromised, the RBCs become **sickled** (crescent-shaped and elongated) and obstruct capillaries and larger vessels (see Figure 33-7). The sickled cells cause circulatory problems by obstructing vessels and rupturing. When the cells obstruct vessels, the area normally supplied by these vessels becomes ischemic and infarcted. The sickled cells are much more fragile than normal cells and rupture more easily. The rupturing of sickled RBCs causes chronic anemia, causing the heart to enlarge in an attempt to circulate more blood for adequate oxygenation of body tissues. Symptoms include fatigue, jaundice, chronic leg ulcers, tachypnea, dyspnea, and arrhythmias. Any situation that decreases oxygenation can cause a sickle cell crisis. The client experiencing a sickle cell crisis has symptoms of fever, severe pain, and loss of blood supply to various organs because of obstructed vessels. Areas most frequently affected are the joints, bone, brain, lungs, liver, kidneys, and penis. Joints become painful, swollen, and immobile. The client may experience cerebrovascular accidents, renal failure, pulmonary infarction, shock, and priapism (a continuous, painful erection). Anesthesia also may cause a sickle cell crisis.

A hemoglobin S blood test (Sickledex) or sickle cell test is done to detect the presence of Hgb S. If Hgb S is present, a hemoglobin electrophoresis is done to distinguish between sickle cell trait and sickle cell disease.

Medical–Surgical Management

Medical

Medical management of sickle cell disease is still evolving in administration of medications and treatments. Infections are treated promptly with antibiotics. Large amounts of oral and intravenous fluids (3–5 L/day) are given to remove the by-products of broken RBCs. Skin grafting may be necessary for chronic leg ulcers.

Genetic counseling is recommended for clients with sickle cell trait and sickle cell anemia. There may be more openness to counseling if the counselor is from the same community as the client.

Pharmacological

Folic acid or folate (Folvite) is administered daily to assist in the production of RBCs. Cetiedil citrate has an antisickling effect by changing the RBC membrane. Pentoxifylline (Trental) reduces blood viscosity, increases RBC flexibility, and lengthens the time between sickle cell crises. Blood transfusions may be given during a crisis.

Patient-controlled analgesia (PCA) with morphine is effective during a crisis. The client is progressed from narcotics to nonnarcotic analgesics as indicated.

▶ NURSING PROCESS

▶ Assessment

▶ Subjective Data

A history of the client's medical problems is obtained, including a history of familial hematopoietic

Normal red
blood cell   Sickle-shaped
                  red blood cell

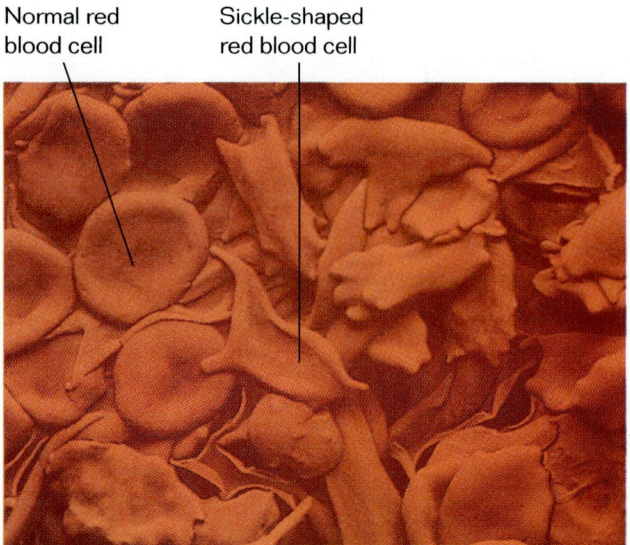

Figure 33-7 Blood cells magnified through a scanning electron microscope show normal and sickle-shaped red blood cells. *(Courtesy of Philips Electronic Instruments Company.)*

illnesses. Some anemias may be caused by drugs and environmental conditions, so gather information about medications taken and about environmental situations at work and in recreational settings. The client should be asked about fatigue, dyspnea with exertion, palpitations, dizziness, pain, petechiae, tingling and numbness in the extremities, blurred vision, and oral discomfort.

▶ Objective Data

The client's weight and vital signs; apical pulse and peripheral pulses; breath sounds; sensation and movement in the extremities; abdominal tenderness; and edema, pallor, and signs of bruising or jaundice must all be assessed. A thorough assessment of the cardiac system is completed because severe anemia can cause cardiac enlargement and arrhythmias.

Nursing diagnoses for a client with decreased erythrocytes and hemoglobin may include the following:

Nursing Diagnoses	Planning/Goals	Nursing Interventions
▶ *Knowledge deficit related to prescribed treatment regimen*	The client will relate the prescribed treatment regimen.	Teach the cause of the particular type of anemia and, if possible, ways to avoid the occurrence of that anemia in the future.
		For iron deficiency anemia, teach the importance of taking iron and increasing iron in the diet.
		Instruct clients with pernicious anemia to obtain a vitamin B_{12} injection at regularly scheduled times.
		Teach clients with hemolytic anemias the significance of following the prescribed regimens.
▶ *Activity intolerance related to imbalance between oxygen supply and demand.*	The client will increasingly tolerate activity.	Assist the client as needed with activities of daily living.
		Teach the client the importance of alternating periods of rest with activity.
▶ *Tissue perfusion, altered, related to a decreased hemoglobin concentration in the blood.*	The client will have increased tissue perfusion.	Administer oxygen as needed to relieve symptoms of dyspnea.
		Monitor Hgb, Hct, RBCs, ABGs, and electrolytes.
		Monitor vital signs and mental alertness.
		Monitor for symptoms of obstructed vessels such as pain, leg ulcerations, abdominal tenderness, dyspnea, confusion, and blurred vision.
		Administer blood products as ordered.
		Monitor the client closely after blood transfusions for possible reactions such as chills, fever, dyspnea, pruritus, wheezing, and pain in the lumbar region.

Evaluation Each goal must be evaluated to determine how it has been met by the client.

SAMPLE NURSING CARE PLAN

THE CLIENT WITH SICKLE CELL ANEMIA

Reggie Thompson, a 19-year-old African American, was diagnosed with sickle cell anemia 5 years ago. Reggie works for a computer company and has been working 12-hour days to get a system installed. He has felt fatigued lately and decided to relax by playing golf on a warm Saturday morning. After the seventh hole, Reggie experienced dyspnea and tingling and numbness in his legs. After the next hole, he experienced severe pain in his ankles and knees. He was taken to the local medical center, where he was admitted. The physician ordered oxygen by nasal cannula, IV fluids, and a PCA pump with morphine sulfate.

continued

Nursing Diagnosis 1 *Pain related to occlusion of small vessels by sickled cells as evidenced by severe pain in the knees and ankles*

PLANNING/GOALS	NURSING INTERVENTIONS	RATIONALE	EVALUATION
Reggie will state pain has been relieved as the analgesic becomes effective.	Assess pain type, location, and intensity.	Other vessels to the brain, heart, lungs, spleen, gallbladder, kidney, and penis may become occluded, causing pain.	The morphine in the PCA pump relieved Reggie's pain, and oral analgesics were ordered.
	Monitor analgesic administration by PCA pump.	Analgesic administration is monitored to assess relief from pain.	
	Support joints and lower extremities with pillows.	Support of joints and lower extremities relieves joint pain.	
	Keep bed linens off knees and ankles with a bed cradle.	Use of a bed cradle keeps linen from putting pressure on painful areas.	

Nursing Diagnosis 2 *Tissue perfusion altered, related to a decreased number of RBCs and decreased oxygenation as evidenced by dyspnea and tingling and numbness in his ankles and knees*

PLANNING/GOALS	NURSING INTERVENTIONS	RATIONALE	EVALUATION
Reggie will experience improved circulation in his extremities as RBCs increase in number.	Elevate the head of the bed and administer oxygen as needed to relieve symptoms of dyspnea.	Lungs can expand more fully if the head of the bed is elevated, and oxygen administration increases blood oxygen level.	Circulation in lower extremities has improved as manifested by prompt capillary refill and strong pedal and popliteal pulses. Extremities are warm to touch.
	Administer IV fluids as ordered.	Adequate hydration decreases the possibility of RBCs' sickling.	
	Encourage Reggie to drink eight to ten glasses of water daily.	Dehydration causes RBCs to sickle.	
	Monitor for symptoms of obstructed vessels such as pain, leg ulcerations, abdominal tenderness, dyspnea, confusion, and blurred vision.	Since RBCs are sickling, vessels supplying blood to other vital organs can become obstructed.	

continued

| | Administer blood products as ordered. | Administration of blood products increases the number of normal RBCs, which improves the blood oxygen concentration. | |
| | Closely monitor for possible blood transfusion reactions such as chills, fever, dyspnea, pruritus, wheezing, and pain in the lumbar region. | Administration of blood products may cause adverse reactions. | |

Nursing Diagnosis 3 *Activity intolerance related to imbalance between oxygen supply and demand, as evidenced by weakness, fatigue, dyspnea, tingling, and numbness*

PLANNING/GOALS	NURSING INTERVENTIONS	RATIONALE	EVALUATION
Reggie will tolerate some activity.	Assist Reggie as needed with activities of daily living.	Assistance with daily activities would conserve energy resources.	Reggie takes periods of rest after each period of activity. He acknowledges that he had been working too hard and not getting enough rest before hospitalization.
	Teach Reggie the importance of alternating periods of rest with activity.	Conservation of energy is important. Impaired circulation to the brain may cause dizziness when ambulating.	

Nursing Diagnosis 4 *Knowledge deficit related to prescribed treatment regimen as evidenced by a lack of rest and working long hours*

PLANNING/GOALS	NURSING INTERVENTIONS	RATIONALE	EVALUATION
Reggie will relate the prescribed treatment regimen before discharge.	Teach Reggie the pathophysiology related to sickle cell disease.	An understanding of the disease process improves compliance with the medical regimen.	Reggie states his RBCs have Hgb S rather than Hgb A, and a lack of oxygen causes his RBCs to sickle. Situations that may cause sickling are fatigue, lack of oral fluids, emotional and physical stress, infection, and anesthesia. He knows the purpose and side effects of each of his medications and the times he is to take them.
	Encourage Reggie to take medications as ordered.	Medications will improve circulation and postpone sickle cell crisis situations.	
	Explain the importance of avoiding stressful situations and the symptoms of infection.	Clients with sickle cell disease should avoid situations that increase oxygen demands. Lack of oxygen can precipitate a sickle cell crisis.	
	Explain the importance of adequate rest on a routine basis.	Allows adequate oxygenation and reduces stress.	Reggie states that he will try to routinely have enough rest.

POLYCYTHEMIA

Polycythemia is a disease in which there is an increased production of red blood cells. Usually the numbers of white blood cells and platelets are also increased. The increased production of cells increases the blood volume and viscosity and decreases the ability of the blood to circulate freely. There are two types of polycythemia: polycythemia vera (primary polycythemia) and secondary polycythemia. Polycythemia vera occurs most frequently in the middle-aged and in Jewish men. The etiology of the disease is unknown. Secondary polycythemia results from long-term hypoxia, as from chronic obstructive pulmonary disease, chronic heart failure, smoking, or living in a high altitude. It is a compensatory mechanism as the body makes more red blood cells as a response to the low oxygenation caused by the previously mentioned situations.

Symptoms of the two types are the same. As the blood viscosity and volume increase the client experiences headaches, epistaxis, dizziness, tinnitus, blurred vision, fatigue, weakness, pruritus, exertional dyspnea, angina, and increased blood pressure and pulse. The client's complexion becomes ruddy (reddish), and the lips become reddish purple. The client may have petechiae and bruise easily because of a platelet dysfunction. The client is susceptible to thrombi formation because of the increased viscosity of the blood. The increased destruction of RBCs causes **hyperuricemia** (increased uric acid blood level). The Hgb is over 18 mg/dL, and the Hct is over 55%.

Medical–Surgical Management

Medical

The treatment for polycythemia is **phlebotomy**, which is the removal of blood from a vein. Generally 350 mL to 500 mL of blood is withdrawn every other day until the Hct level is 40% to 50%. Radioactive phosphorus (^{32}P) and radiation therapy may be used to decrease the production of blood cells in the bone marrow.

Complications that can occur from the disease process are cerebral vascular accident, thrombosis, myocardial infarction, and hemorrhage.

Pharmacological

Antineoplastic drugs such as busulfan (Myleran), chlorambucil (Leukeran), cyclophosphamide (Cytoxan), and mechlorethamine or nitrogen mustard (Mustargen) are also used to decrease bone marrow production. Allopurinol (Zyloprim) is given to decrease the

CLIENT TEACHING

Polycythemia
- Drink at least 3 L of water daily.
- Elevate feet when resting.
- Avoid tight or restrictive clothing.
- Wear support hose.
- Take medications as ordered.
- Report chest pain, joint pain, fever, or activity intolerance to physician.
- Keep appointments for laboratory testing and physician checks.

production of uric acid. Pruritus can be relieved with the administration of antihistamines.

Diet

The client is placed on a diet that has increased calories and protein. A diet low in sodium decreases fluid volume. Iron-containing foods should be avoided.

Activity

Activities of daily living may need to be adjusted so the client can have regular periods of rest to relieve fatigue.

▶ NURSING PROCESS

▶ Assessment

▶ Subjective Data

The client should be asked about the history of symptoms, especially difficulty breathing, chest pain, dizziness, headache, pruritus, tinnitis, blurred vision, and sensitivity to hot and cold. Nutritional status of the client must be assessed as there may be an inadequate dietary intake due to GI symptoms of fullness and dyspepsia.

▶ Objective Data

The nurse should observe the skin for bruises and changes in skin color. The cardiovascular system can be assessed by checking for distention of neck vessels, listening to the apical pulse, taking radial and pedal pulses, and checking for Homans' sign and edema. The respiratory system can be assessed by observing for epistaxis and dyspnea and listening to the breath sounds. The central nervous system is checked through pupil response and presence of numbness or tingling.

Nursing diagnoses for a client with polycythemia may include the following:

Nursing Diagnoses	Planning/Goals	Nursing Interventions
▶ *Knowledge deficit related to disease process and treatment*	The client will relate disease process and treatment.	Explain the cause of the disease, possible symptoms, side effects of medications, and possible future complications to report.
		Teach client to report headache, chest pain, dyspnea, or redness, swelling, or tenderness in the arms or legs to the physician or nurse practitioner immediately.
▶ *Tissue perfusion, altered, related to decreased blood circulation*	The client will have increased circulation.	Administer oxygen as needed for dyspnea.
		Check vital signs frequently.
		Assess Homans' sign and signs of thrombi formation.
		Explain process of phlebotomy.
▶ *Injury, risk for, related to dizziness*	The client will relate measures to avoid injury.	Encourage the client to change positions slowly to prevent dizziness.
		Encourage activities of daily living when the client is feeling well.
		Teach client to avoid activities in which bruising or trauma may occur.

Evaluation Each goal must be evaluated to determine how it has been met by the client.

WHITE BLOOD CELL DISORDERS

White blood cell disorders include leukemia and agranulocytosis.

LEUKEMIA

Leukemia is a malignancy of blood-forming tissues in which the bone marrow produces increased numbers of immature white blood cells that are incapable of protecting the body from infections. The increased number of WBCs crowds out the other cells in the bone marrow, causing a decreased production of RBCs and platelets. Anemia and bleeding result from the decreased number of RBCs and platelets.

Leukemia has two classifications: acute and chronic. The acute leukemias are subclassified into acute myelocytic leukemia (AML) and acute lymphocytic leukemia (ALL). Chronic leukemias are subclassified into chronic myelocytic leukemia (CML) and chronic lymphocytic leukemia (CLL).

Research conducted with the survivors of the Japanese A-bomb indicates a connection between radiation and AML (Campbell, 1995). Other suspected etiological causes of AML are rheumatoid arthritis treated with drugs that suppress the immune system and cancer treated with cytotoxic drugs and radiation therapy (Campbell, 1995). This later condition is known as **secondary malignancy**, which means the client had a malignancy, was treated with chemotherapy or radiation therapy, had a period of time with no malignancy, and then developed a second malignant condition. There is a high risk of ALL occurring in clients with Down syndrome (Campbell, 1995).

Because of the increased production of immature WBCs, clients with acute leukemia generally are fighting persistent infections and have a fever and chills. The decreased number of RBCs causes symptoms of anemia such as fatigue, pallor, malaise, tachycardia, and tachypnea. The decreased platelet production causes bleeding tendencies, and the client will experience petechiae, bruising, epistaxis, melena, gingival bleeding, and increased menstrual bleeding. The client may also experience weight loss, night sweats, and swollen lymph nodes. As the malignant cells invade the central nervous system, the client will experience headaches and visual disturbances. Some clients experience bone pain because the rapid production of WBCs causes cells to become crowded in the bone marrow. Refer to Table 33-2 to see the relationship of leukemia symptoms to laboratory results.

ACUTE LEUKEMIA

Acute leukemias have a rapid onset and must be treated quickly for a good prognosis. ALL usually occurs in children between the ages of 2 and 6 and has a more rapid onset than AML. Left untreated, clients with ALL have a **median survival time** (average length of life) of 4 to 6 months. Children with ALL have a good prognosis rate with chemotherapy. Approximately 90% of children have complete remissions, but only 50% to 70% of adults have complete remission (Monahan, Drake, & Neighbors, 1994; Phipps et al., 1999).

Table 33-2 RELATIONSHIP OF LABORATORY TESTS TO LEUKEMIA SYMPTOMS

LAB RESULT	OVERALL SYMPTOM	SYMPTOM MANIFESTATION
Immature WBCs	Persistent infections	Fever Chills
Decreased RBCs	Anemia	Fatigue Pallor Malaise Tachycardia Tachypnea
Decreased platelets	Bleeding	Petechiae Bruising Epistaxis Melena Gingival bleeding Increased menstrual bleeding

AML occurs most frequently in adolescence and after 55 years of age (Phipps et al., 1999). The median survival time for clients with untreated AML is approximately 2 to 3 months (Phipps et al., 1995). With chemotherapy, complete remission occurs in approximately 50% to 75% of AML clients, with a median survival time of 2 to 3 years (Phipps et al., 1999).

Medical–Surgical Management

Medical

Diagnosis of acute leukemia is confirmed with a CBC and a bone marrow biopsy. A lumbar puncture determines the presence of malignant cells in the central nervous system. An x-ray, MRI, or CT scan of the chest and skeleton determine the presence of infection and bone marrow tissue involvement.

Surgical

Bone marrow transplants are used with relapsed ALL clients and AML clients under age 55. AML clients who have a bone marrow transplant have a 50% to 70% cure rate (Campbell, 1995). High doses of chemotherapy and radiation therapy are given to the client to destroy the bone marrow. Leukemic white blood cells and healthy bone marrow cells are both destroyed, placing the client at a high risk for infection and death. Identical human leukocyte antigen (HLA) bone marrow from a sibling, the client, or an antigen-matched donor is given intravenously in a manner similar to a blood transfusion. The transfused bone marrow finds its way to the client's bone marrow and starts producing WBCs, RBCs, and platelets. The bone marrow is matched in a process very similar to the process of crossmatching

blood. If the client's own bone marrow is used, it is removed from the client, treated with chemotherapy, and then reinfused into the client.

Pharmacological

Initial doses of chemotherapy are called **induction doses**. Small doses of chemotherapy given every 3 to 4 weeks to maintain remission are called **maintenance therapy**. Induction doses of chemotherapy for ALL consists of vincristine (Oncovin) and prednisone (Deltasone). Maintenance therapy consists of giving 6-mercaptopurine or 6-MP (Purinethol) and methotrexate or amethopterin (Methotrexate). Usually vincristine (Oncovin) and prednisone (Deltasone) are given periodically with the maintenance therapy.

Leukemic cells can lie dormant in the brain and spinal area because the chemotherapeutic drugs are unable to pass through the blood-brain barrier. Intrathecal (within the spinal canal) administration of methotrexate has decreased recurrences of ALL. Methotrexate is given by a lumbar puncture into the cerebrospinal fluid or through a subcutaneous cerebrospinal reservoir. Sometimes radiation therapy is also used on the brain and spinal area.

AML is treated with chemotherapeutic agents, blood products, and antibiotics. Refer to Table 33-3 for a review of chemotherapeutic agents used in treating acute leukemia.

Diet

Extremely hot or cold foods and drinks should be avoided. A bland, high-protein, high-carbohydrate diet is usually ordered. Drinking alcohol should be avoided.

Table 33-3 CHEMOTHERAPEUTIC AGENTS TO TREAT LEUKEMIA

LEUKEMIA	CHEMOTHERAPEUTIC AGENTS
Acute lymphocytic leukemia (ALL)	vincristine (Oncovin) prednisone (Deltasone) 6-mercaptopurine or 6-MP (Purinethol) methotrexate (Methotrexate)
Acute myelocytic leukemia (AML)	daunorubicin HCl (Cerubidine) cytarabine or ara-C (Cytosar-U) 6-thioguanine (Thioguanine) doxorubicin HCl (Adriamycin)
Chronic myelocytic leukemia (CLL)	chlorambucil (Leukeran) COP (Cytoxan, Oncovin, and prednisone)
Chronic lymphocytic leukemia (CML)	busulfan (Myleran) hydroxyurea (Hydrea) DAT (daunorubicin, ara-C, thioguanine)

Activity

Clients should alternate periods of rest with activity. They should keep frequently used items nearby to conserve energy.

CHRONIC LEUKEMIA

Chronic leukemia generally occurs in adults with a gradual increase in the white cell count over months or years. Clients treated with oral chemotherapy have a life expectancy of 2 to 10 years with CLL and 3 to 4 years with CML (Phipps et al., 1999). The prognosis depends on the severity of the disease at the time of diagnosis.

CLL clients have increased abnormal B lymphocytes, with a WBC count between 20,000 and 100,000 (Phipps et al., 1999). CLL can develop at any age but occurs most frequently between the ages of 50 to 70 and has an incident rate three times higher in men than in women (Phipps et al., 1999).

CML occurs most frequently in clients between 35 and 50 years of age with a higher incidence of CML in males (Campbell, 1995). The WBC count ranges from 15,000 to 500,000 (Phipps et al., 1999). Most clients feel good and maintain a relatively normal life until later in the disease process when the chronic recessed phase changes into an intensified stage that resembles an acute phase of leukemia. This acute phase is called a **blastic phase** in which there is an increased production of WBCs. Approximately 50% to 60% of CML cases develop a later blastic phase. When this occurs, the general condition spirals downhill and the client soon dies. The most common cause of death in the leukemic client is viral and fungal pneumonia (Black & Mastassarin-Jacobs, 1997).

Medical–Surgical Management

Medical

Diagnosis of chronic leukemia is confirmed with a CBC and a bone marrow biopsy.

Surgical

In the CML chronic phase, the HLA-identical allogenic bone marrow is given, and the client's own treated bone marrow is given in the blastic phase.

Pharmacological

Refer to Table 33-3 for a review of chemotherapeutic agents used in treating CLL and CML. Chemotherapy does not extend the length of life but seems to give a better quality of life by prolonging the chronic phase. In a recent clinical trial, interferon increased the survival time to 61 months as opposed to 41 months (Campbell, 1995).

Diet

The client is on a diet high in protein, carbohydrates, and vitamins. A bland, nonirritating diet prevents oral mucosal irritation. Alcohol should be avoided.

Activity

The decreased RBC level causes the client to have symptoms of anemia that include weakness and increased respirations. It is important for the client to learn methods to conserve energy, such as placing frequently used items nearby.

▶ NURSING PROCESS

▶ Assessment

▶ Subjective Data

A thorough history of the symptoms the client has experienced is needed. The nurse should ask the client or family about chromosomal abnormalities, exposure to chemicals, viral infections, and previous chemotherapy or radiation therapy. The client should describe the location, type, and duration of pain, especially in bones or joints. Symptoms of infection such as the presence of a cough or pain or burning on urination should be noted. A history of bleeding such as epistaxis, gingival bleeding, melena, or hematuria should be documented. Fatigue, malaise, and irritability are often described.

▶ Objective Data

Signs of infection, bleeding, and chemotherapy complications must be noted. Common sites for infection include the mouth, pharynx, lungs, skin, bladder, and perianal area. During chemotherapy the reduced white cell count may stop the formation of pus, so infection may manifest as redness, swelling, and pain.

Assessment for bleeding includes monitoring the platelet count as bleeding occurs easily if the platelet count falls below 50,000. Clients can bleed from any orifice, so it is important for the nurse to inspect any discharge from the body. Occult blood may be present in the urine and stool.

Chemotherapy complications are nausea, vomiting, and stomatitis. Alopecia occurs 1 to 2 weeks after treatments are initiated.

Nursing diagnoses for a client with leukemia may include the following:

Nursing Diagnoses	Planning/Goals	Nursing Interventions
▶ *Infection, risk for, related to increased production of immature white blood cells*	The client will describe ways to prevent infection.	Follow good handwashing techniques.
		Teach proper handwashing to the family and friends who come into contact with the leukemic client.
		Use antimicrobial soaps for the client's daily bath.
		Provide frequent oral care with a soft toothbrush and nonirritating mouthwash to prevent open sores and stomatitis.
		Wash the perianal area after each bowel movement to decrease bacterial contamination and prevent rectal fissures.
		Avoid taking a rectal temperature.
		Monitor the temperature every 4 hours for signs of infection.
		Report any temperature over 100°F to the physician.
		Administer antibiotics and antifungals as ordered.
		Closely monitor respiration rate and breath sounds as the client is prone to respiratory infections.
▶ *Injury, risk for, related to decreased production of platelets*	The client will identify ways to avoid injury and prevent bleeding.	Frequently observe the client for signs of bleeding such as epistaxis, gingival bleeding, petechiae, ecchymoses, hematemesis, enlarged abdomen, hematuria, melena, and confusion, which can occur from intracranial hemorrhage.
		Administer stool softeners frequently to prevent anal irritation from hard stools.
		Use cotton swabs instead of a toothbrush for oral care.
		Encourage the client to use an electric razor.
		Avoid giving injections as much as possible.
		If a catheter is needed, lubricate it well to avoid trauma to the mucosal lining of the urethra.
▶ *Nutrition, altered, less than body requirements related to effects of disease process and chemotherapy on gastrointestinal tract*	The client will choose nonirritating, high-protein, high-carbohydrate meals and snacks.	Administer antiemetics as ordered to relieve nausea and vomiting.
		Suggest that the client may tolerate small frequent feedings better than three large meals.
		Provide the client with a high-protein, high-carbohydrate diet to prevent infection and provide needed energy.
		Administer vitamin supplements as ordered.
		Teach the client to avoid raw fruits and vegetables as these foods may contain more bacteria than cooked foods.
▶ *Coping, individual, ineffective, related to uncertainty about treatment of disease and prognosis*	The client will identify ways to cope with concerns about disease process.	Inform the client of the possibility of alopecia from therapy treatments.
		Encourage the client to voice concerns and fears related to having leukemia.
		Teach the client, family members, and significant others to monitor and report signs of infection and bleeding.
		Refer to support groups, social workers, and clergy as needed.

Evaluation Each goal must be evaluated to determine how it has been met by the client.

AGRANULOCYTOSIS

A severely reduced number of granulocytes (basophils, eosinophils, and neutrophils) is called **agranulocytosis**. The primary cause is an adverse reaction to medication or medication toxicity, especially with administration of phenylbutazone (Butazolidin), chloramphenical (Chloromycetin), penicillin derivatives, cephalosporins, phenytoin (Dilantin), antihistamines, vincristine (Oncovin), propythiouracil, diuretics, chlorpromazine hydrochloride (Thorazine), fluphenazene (Prolixin), promazene hydrochloride (Sparine), and sulfonamides and its derivatives. Other causes of agranulocytosis are neoplastic disease, chemotherapy, radiation therapy, and bacterial and viral infection. The causative agent suppresses the bone marrow, reducing the production of leukocytes.

The client exhibits the symptoms of infection: headache, fever, chills, and fatigue as well as mucous membrane ulcerations of the nose, mouth, pharynx, vagina, and rectum. The white blood count and neutrophils will be low.

Medical–Surgical Management

Medical

The main goals of treatment are to remove the cause of the bone marrow suppression and either prevent or treat any infection. When the client's temperature is elevated, blood cultures may be performed; if mucosal ulcerations occur, they may be cultured. Blood transfusions are given to provide mature leukocytes. Protective isolation may be instituted.

Pharmacological

Antibiotics specific for cultured microorganisms are given.

Diet

A soft, bland diet that is high in calories, protein, and vitamins is ordered.

Activity

Periods of activity must be balanced with periods of rest to prevent weakness and fatigue.

Infection Control: The Client with Agranulocytosis

- Caregivers must thoroughly wash their hands and follow aseptic technique when caring for the client.
- The client's environment must be kept very clean.
- The client should avoid crowds.
- Visitors must be screened so no one with a cold or any type of infection is allowed to see the client.
- Teach client to avoid hot or cold environments.
- Ensure that the client reports any signs or symptoms of infection.

▶ NURSING PROCESS

▶ Assessment

▶ Subjective Data

The client may describe having extreme fatigue, weakness, headache, chills, and fever. Inquire about all medications taken, including over-the-counter and prescription drugs.

▶ Objective Data

Assess vital signs especially for a temperature over 100.6°F. Mucosal ulcerations may be reddened. Auscultate the lungs for crackles and wheezes.

Nursing diagnoses for a client with agranulocytosis may include the following:

Nursing Diagnoses	Planning/Goals	Nursing Interventions
▶ *Infection, risk for, related to decreased leukocyte production*	The client will not have signs and symptoms of infection.	Thoroughly wash hands before caring for the client.
		Screen all persons for signs of infection before allowing them near the client.
		Monitor vital signs for signs of infection.
		Use strict asepsis for all procedures.
		Encourage the client to drink an adequate amount of fluids.
		Monitor WBC count.
		Provide personal hygiene to prevent infection.
		Provide client with periods of rest between activities.

Evaluation Each goal must be evaluated to determine how it has been met by the client.

COAGULATION DISORDERS

Coagulation disorders include disseminated intravascular coagulation, hemophilia, and thrombocytoperia.

DISSEMINATED INTRA-VASCULAR COAGULATION

Disseminated intravascular coagulation (DIC) is not a disease in itself but a syndrome that occurs because of a primary disease process or condition. A few of the conditions in which DIC may occur are burns, acute leukemia, metastatic cancer, polycythemia vera, pheochromocytoma, shock, acute infections, septic abortion, abruptio placenta, blood transfusion reactions, and trauma.

DIC is a condition in which there is alternating clotting and hemorrhaging. The primary disease stimulates the clotting mechanism, causing many **microthrombi** (very small clots) to form and block the circulation in the arterioles and capillaries. With the formation of the numerous small clots, the body's fibrinolytic process responds in an attempt to stop the clot formation, thus causing hemorrhaging (Figure 33-8). This can be a very serious and potentially fatal condition.

The occlusion of blood vessels with the clots causes infarcts and necrosis of organs and tissues. The kidneys are the most commonly affected organ.

If a client with a predisposing condition develops **purpura** (reddish purple patches on the skin indicative of hemorrhage), bleeding tendencies, or renal impairment, the nurse should assess for DIC. Symptoms of DIC may present as oozing from a venipuncture, mucus membrane, or surgical wound. The oozing may progress rapidly into a hemorrhage within a few hours to a day. The client may have decreased urine output from decreased blood flow or renal infarction.

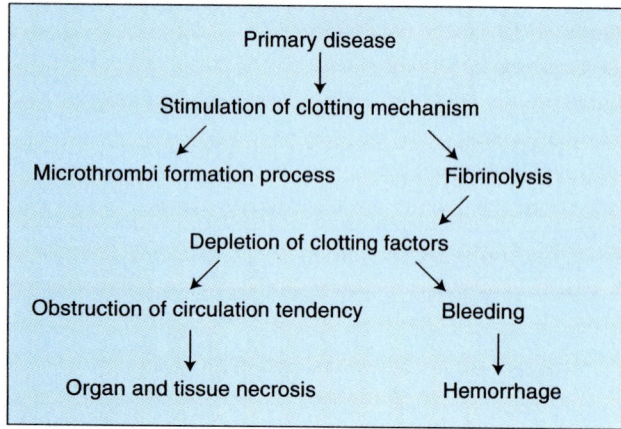

Figure 33-8 Pathophysiology of DIC

Medical–Surgical Management

Medical

DIC is diagnosed by the client's symptoms and laboratory tests. With DIC there is an increased prothrombin time, partial thromboplastin time, thrombin time, and a decreased fibrinogen and platelet count. A laboratory test that confirms the diagnosis is the D dimer, which measures a fibrin split product that is released when a clot breaks.

The primary disease or condition must be treated. For example, if the primary disease is an infection, an antibiotic is given. If cancer is the primary disease, chemotherapy is given.

DIC is treated by administering whole blood or blood products to normalize the clotting factor levels. Platelets and packed red cells are given to replace those lost during hemorrhage. Cryoprecipitate or fresh-frozen plasma is given to normalize clotting factor levels.

Pharmacological

Heparin has no effect on the thrombi that are already formed but may be given to prevent the formation of more microthrombi. The administration of heparin is controversial because of the risk of hemorrhage. After thrombi formation has been controlled with heparin, aminocaproic acid (Amicar) can be given to stop the bleeding because it stops the fibrinolytic process. **Fibrinolysis** is the process of breaking fibrin apart.

▶ NURSING PROCESS

▶ Assessment

▶ Subjective Data

The client should be asked about previous conditions such as infectious processes, trauma, or cancer. Client statements of joint pain may indicate bleeding into the joint. Recent visual changes should also be documented.

▶ Objective Data

The nurse should observe and record the amount of bleeding from any wound or body orifice. I&O is monitored closely. Purpura on the chest and abdomen is a common first sign. Abdominal tenderness is often present. Presence of pulmonary edema, hypotension, tachycardia, absence of peripheral pulses, confusion, restlessness, convulsions, and coma must all be noted.

Nursing diagnosis for a client with DIC may include the following:

Nursing Diagnoses	Planning/Goals	Nursing Interventions
▶ *Injury, risk for, related to altered clotting factors*	The client will experience a minimal amount of injury.	Monitor vitals signs, peripheral pulses, neurological checks, and urine output.
		Check urine and stool for the presence of blood. Assess for abdominal bleeding by checking for abdominal firmness or rigidity.
		If abdominal bleeding is suspected, measure the abdominal girth every 4 hours.
		Assess surgical wounds and all body orifices for bleeding.
		Assess color, warmth, sensation, and movement of extremities.
		Observe for changes in mental status.
		Apply pressure to any oozing site.
		Avoid giving injections and venipunctures as much as possible.
		Observe for signs of orthostatic hypotension.

Evaluation Each goal must be evaluated to determine how it has been met by the client.

HEMOPHILIA

Hemophilia is an inherited bleeding disorder in which there is a lack of clotting factors. Approximately 20,000 persons in the United States have hemophilia (Beare & Myers, 1998). There are two types of hemophilia: hemophilia A is lacking clotting factor VIII, and hemophilia B (Christmas disease) is lacking clotting factor IX. The hemophilia trait is carried on the recessive X chromosome, so a mother is asymptomatic but can pass the trait to the son, who then manifests the symptoms of hemophilia (Figure 33-9). In the male population, hemophilia A occurs at the rate of 1 : 10,000 and hemophilia B occurs at the rate of 1 : 100,000 (Phipps et al., 1999). Genetic counseling is often advantageous for clients who are carriers or who have hemophilia.

There are three classifications of hemophilia: severe (factor level less than 1% of normal), moderate (factor level 1% to 5% normal), and mild (factor level 40% of

normal). The main symptom of hemophilia is bleeding. The client with severe hemophilia bleeds when there is minor trauma to an area but can also bleed spontaneously. **Hemarthrosis** (bleeding into the joints) occurs most frequently, causing pain, swelling, redness, and fever. The client can have spontaneous ecchymoses and bleed from the mouth and gastrointestinal and urinary tracts. The most common cause of death is intracranial hemorrhage. Clients with mild hemophilia will not have spontaneous muscle and joint bleeding but will bleed after minor or major surgery. This condition could prove fatal if the diagnosis is not determined promptly.

Medical–Surgical Management

Medical

Hemophilia is diagnosed by a deficient or absent blood level of factors VIII or IX. The prothrombin time (PT), thrombin time, platelet count, and bleeding time are normal, but the partial thromboplastin time (PTT) is usually prolonged.

The treatment for hemophilia is the administration of clotting factors VIII and IX. Clients with hemophilia A are given fresh frozen plasma and cryoprecipitate that has factor VIII. Clients with hemophilia B are given fresh frozen plasma that contains factor IX. Hemophiliacs who received blood products before 1984 later often tested seropositive for HIV (Beare & Myers, 1998). This risk has been greatly reduced by heat-treating human-derived factor VIII. The heat treatment inactivates viruses. Factor IX can also be treated in a similar manner. A genetically engineered product called *recombinant factor VIII* is viral safe and relatively economical.

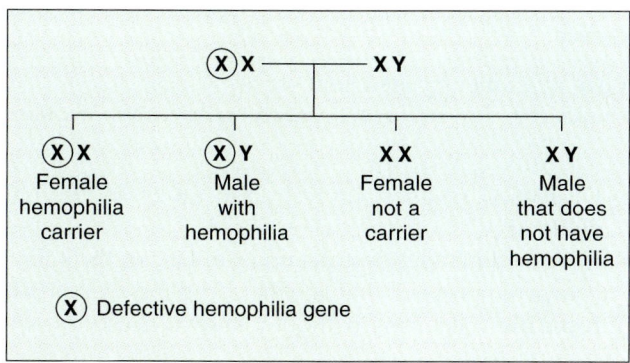

Figure 33-9 Hemophilia Inheritance Pattern between a Female Hemophilia Carrier and a Male without Hemophilia

HOME HEALTH CARE

Hemophilia

The client and family must understand the disease process, learn how to recognize signs and symptoms of bleeding, and be able to administer treatments at home. The client should:

- Obtain medical care for trauma, cuts, edema, or pain in muscles and joints.
- Wear a Medic-Alert tag.
- Not take aspirin.
- Use soft-bristled toothbrush and carefully perform oral hygiene.
- Prevent injuries: wear gloves and long-sleeved clothing when doing household chores, participate in noncontact sports and activities.

Pharmacological

Desmopressin acetate (DDAVP) and aminocaproic acid (Amicar) can be given to mild hemophiliacs to decrease the fibrinolytic process.

▶ NURSING PROCESS

▶ Assessment

▶ Subjective Data

The client should be assessed for pain and asked what measures had been used in the past to relieve pain and bleeding.

▶ Objective Data

The nurse should assess the client for bleeding by checking for petechiae, ecchymoses, hematuria, hematemesis, melena, epistaxis, hemarthrosis, abdominal firmness and rigidity, and frank bleeding. Edematous or immobile joints should be noted.

Nursing diagnoses for a client with hemophilia may include the following:

Nursing Diagnoses	Planning/Goals	Nursing Interventions
▶ *Knowledge deficit related to disease process*	The client will relate symptoms to report and treatment methods if bleeding occurs.	Discuss ways to improve the safety of the client's home environment.
		Advise client not to take aspirin.
		Encourage the client to use an electric razor and soft-bristled toothbrush.
		Teach family members or significant others administration of clotting factors for prophylactic purposes and if injury occurs.
		Encourage client to wear Medic-Alert bracelet.
		Refer for genetic counseling.
▶ *Pain related to bleeding into tissues and joints*	The client will have minimal pain.	Assess the client for bruising, swelling, and joint discomfort.
		Apply ice and pressure to bleeding sites.
		When a joint is hurting, immobilize it in a flexed position with a supportive device.
		Give analgesics as needed. Aspirin is not given because of the anticoagulant effect.
▶ *Injury, risk for, related to altered clotting factors*	The client will take precautions to avoid injury.	Transfuse clotting factors as ordered.
		Encourage the client to avoid activities that may cause trauma.
		Post emergency medical numbers in convenient places in case of future need.

Evaluation Each goal must be evaluated to determine how it has been met by the client.

THROMBOCYTOPENIA

Thrombocytopenia is a decrease in the number of platelets in the blood. The decrease may be related to:

- Decreased platelet production as in aplastic anemia, tumors, leukemia, and chemotherapy

- Decreased platelet survival as in infection or viral illnesses
- Increased platelet destruction as in DIC or thrombocytopenic purpura that is either drug induced or **idiopathic** (occurring without a known cause)

Withdrawal of the causative drug will usually allow the platelet count to return to normal in 1 to 2 weeks.

The acute form of idiopathic thrombocytopenic purpura (ITP) is an autoimmune process caused by an autoantibody destroying platelet antigen.

Petechiae, ecchymoses, and bleeding from mucous membranes are observed. Bleeding may occur in internal organs. The platelet count is very low; the bleeding time is prolonged; Hgb and Hct may be low; and bone marrow aspiration shows mostly immature platelets.

Medical/Surgical Management

Medical

Transfusions of platelet concentrates may be given, or **apheresis** (removal of unwanted components) may be performed on the client's blood to remove the autoantibodies.

Surgical

A splenectomy may be performed because the spleen is the primary site of platelet destruction. This treatment is usually reserved until all other treatments have been unsuccessful.

Pharmacological

Corticosteroids are given to prolong platelet life and strengthen the capillaries. Immunosuppressive drugs, gamma globulin, and vitamin K may be given.

Diet

A high-fiber diet is used to prevent constipation and the need to strain when having a bowel movement.

CLIENT TEACHING

Thrombocytopenic Purpura
- Use electric razor for shaving.
- Use soft toothbrush.
- Wear shoes or slippers at all times.
- Do not take aspirin.
- Eat high-fiber diet.
- Blow nose gently, if at all.

Activity

Activity should be undertaken thoughtfully and carefully to prevent any trauma.

▶ NURSING PROCESS

▶ Assessment

▶ Subjective Data

The client should be asked about medications being taken and any recent infection.

▶ Objective Data

Observe for petechiae, ecchymoses, and any signs of blood or internal bleeding.

Nursing diagnoses for a client with thrombocytopenia may include the following:

Nursing Diagnoses	Planning/Goals	Nursing Interventions
▶ *Pain, related to hemorrhage*	The client will verbalize having less pain.	Assess client's pain on 0 (least) to 10 (most) pain scale. Assess client's ability to cope with pain. Administer analgesic as ordered. Note client's response to analgesic.
▶ *Injury, risk for, related to thrombocytopenia*	The client will have minimal injury.	Monitor client's vital signs and neurological and mental status. Assess client's skin and excretions for signs of bleeding. Handle client very carefully when turning, assisting out of bed, and in all other care situations.

Evaluation Each goal must be evaluated to determine how it has been met by the client.

LYMPH DISORDERS

A **lymphoma** is a tumor of the lymphatic system. Two malignant lymphomas discussed in this chapter are Hodgkin's disease (HD) and non-Hodgkin's lymphoma (NHL). The overview and medical management of each disease will be presented separately. The nursing process for both diseases will be presented together since the nursing diagnoses, goals, and interventions are the same for HD and NHL.

HODGKIN'S DISEASE

Hodgkin's disease is a rare lymphoma that usually arises as a painless swelling in a lymph node. The diagnosis is confirmed when Reed-Sternberg cells are biopsied from the swollen lymph node. The incidence is highest in adolescents and young adults (Leukemia Society of America, 1998a). The 5-year survival rate has doubled from 40% in 1960 to 81% in 1998 (Leukemia Society of America, 1998b). In children, the 5-year survival rate is 94% (Leukemia Society of America, 1998b).

The cause of Hodgkin's disease is unknown. Researchers are investigating genetic factors. Some researchers suspect an infectious origin especially in connection with infectious mononucleosis. Other researchers suspect a viral origin associated with the oncovirus and Epstein-Barr virus (Beare & Myers, 1998).

Clients with Hodgkin's disease most commonly have painless enlarged lymph nodes in the neck, in the area above the clavicles, and in the groin. Lymph nodes in the mediastinum may also be enlarged but are not usually diagnosed until the nodes enlarge and press on the mediastinal structures causing dyspnea and a cough. A chest x-ray or a computed tomography (CT) scan confirms the involvement of the mediastinal lymph nodes. Other symptoms are weight loss, anorexia, fatigue, pruritis, fever, chills, night sweats, anemia, thrombocytopenia, and lowered resistance to infections.

If a client has painless, enlarged lymph nodes and the symptoms of an elevated temperature, night sweats, pruritus, and weight loss of more than 10% of the body weight in a 6-month period, the prognosis is worse than if only enlarged lymph nodes are present. Hodgkin's disease spreads throughout the body in a predictable pattern. From the site of the original swollen gland, the disease spreads to nearby lymph nodes then to other lymphatic tissue in the body such as the liver, spleen, and bone marrow.

The invasion of other nodes and lymphatic tissue determines the prognosis of the disease. As more tissue is invaded, the disease process moves through different phases which is known as staging. The Ann Arbor Staging Classification is used to classify the progression of HD and NHL within the body (Figure 33-10). A classification of A or B is added to each stage depending on whether the client has symptoms other than swollen lymph nodes. A client who has lymph node enlargement only is asymptomatic (A). A client

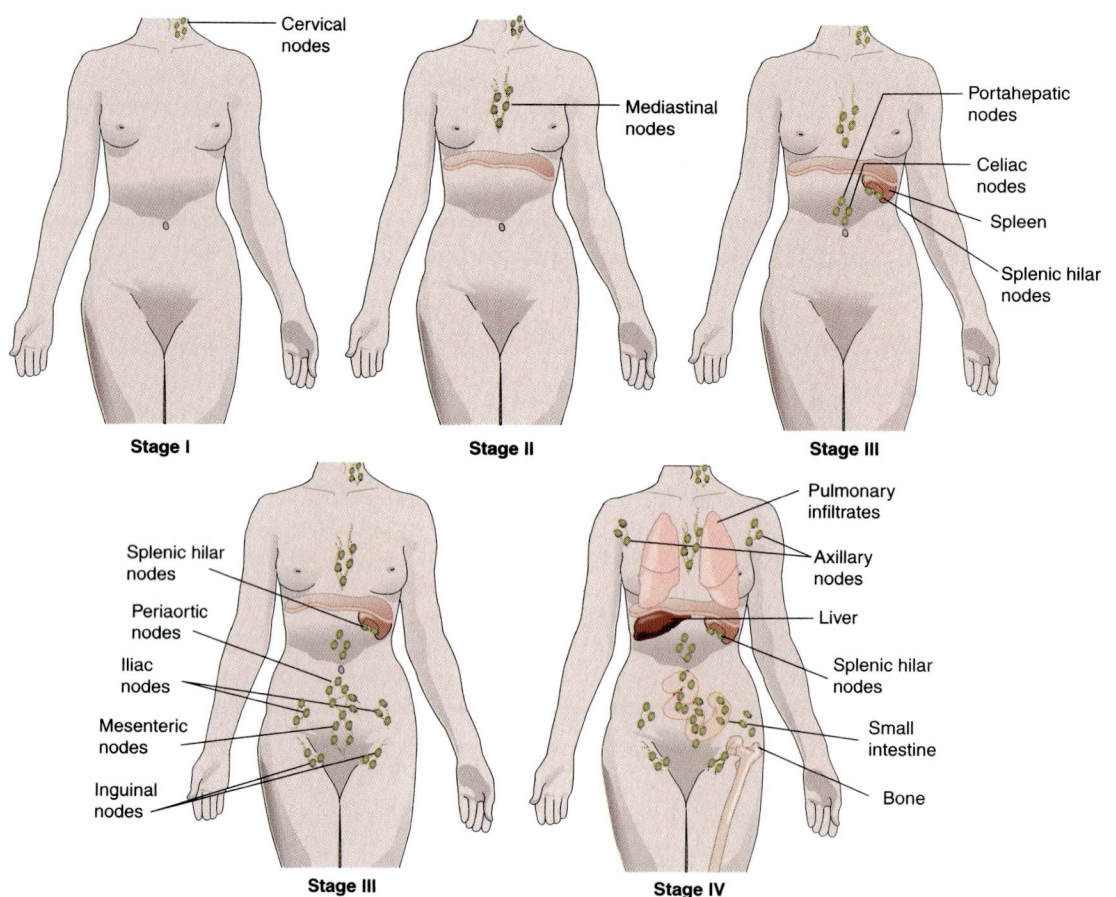

Figure 33-10 Staging of Hodgkin's Disease and Non-Hodgkin's Lymphoma *(From Medical-Surgical Nursing: Assessment and Management of Clinical Problems (4th ed.), by S. Lewis, I. Collier, and M. Heitkemper, 1996, St. Louis: Mosby-Year Book. Reprinted with permission.)*

who has symptoms other than lymph node enlargement is symptomatic (B).

Medical–Surgical Management

Medical

Based on the history and physical examination, diagnostic tests to determine the staging of the disease include CBC, platelet count, bone marrow aspiration, chest x-ray, abdominal CT scan, lymphangiogram, and lymph node biopsy.

Localized Hodgkin's disease stages I and II are treated with radiation therapy over a 4-week period. Clients with massive mediastinal involvement and those who have relapsed after radiation therapy alone are treated with radiation therapy and chemotherapy.

During radiation therapy the client may experience symptoms of toxicity, which are weight loss, nausea and vomiting, skin reactions, esophagitis, fatigue, and bone marrow suppression. The client's blood count is monitored closely during the therapy treatments to check for infections and bleeding tendencies. If the WBC level drops too low, the client will be more susceptible to infections. A decrease in RBCs and platelets causes a bleeding tendency. Long-term complications from radiation therapy include hypothyroidism, radiation pneumonitis, immune system impairment, herpes zoster, and the development of a second cancer.

Generalized Hodgkin's disease, stages III_1, III_2, and IV, are treated with **combination chemotherapy**, which is administering a series of combined drugs over a set period of time. Serious late complications of chemotherapy are infertility and a secondary malignancy or cancer.

Surgical

Sometimes a laparotomy is done to see if the liver and spleen are involved. The rationale of performing the procedure is being questioned since the overall treatment plan is not altered.

Pharmacological

During radiation therapy antiemetics, such as ondansetron HCl (Zofran), are given for nausea and vomiting. Analgesics can be given for esophagitis discomfort.

Chemotherapy drugs are often given in combinations such as MOPP and ABVD. MOPP combines mechlorethamine or nitrogen mustard (Mustargen), vincristine sulfate (Oncovin), procarbazine HCl (Matulane), and prednisone (Deltasone). ABVD combines doxorubicin HCl (Adriamycin PFS), bleomycin sulfate (Blenoxane), vinblastine sulfate (Velban), and dacarbazine (DTIC-Dome). These drugs are usually administered through an implanted venous port. Allopurinol (Zyloprim) is given to prevent uric acid renal stones caused by the rapid destruction of cells during therapy.

Diet

During therapy the client is on a high-calorie, high-protein diet. An intake of 2,500 mL of fluid per day is encouraged to prevent the formation of renal stones.

Activity

Extra rest periods may be necessary to cope with fatigue that occurs with Hodgkin's disease.

NON-HODGKIN'S LYMPHOMA

Non-Hodgkin's lymphoma (NHL) is more common than Hodgkin's disease and is the seventh most common cause of cancer-related deaths in the United States. Approximately 55,700 new cases occurred in 1998 (Leukemia Society of America, 1998a). The 5-year survival rate has increased from 31% in 1960 to 51% in 1998; in children, the 5-year survival rate has increased from 18% in 1960 to 73% in 1998 (Leukemia Society of America, 1998c).

NHL originates from the B lymphocytes and the T lymphocytes. NHL arising from the B lymphocyte occurs in the older adult population; NHL arising from the T lymphocytes manifests in malignant skin diseases such as mycosis fungoides or Sezary syndrome. More men are affected than women. NHL does not have the Reed-Sternberg cell present. The incidence for non-Hodgkin's lymphoma has nearly doubled since 1970 probably because of exposure to certain infectious agents and chemicals.

Symptoms of NHL are enlarged tonsils and adenoids and diffuse enlarged painless, rubbery lymph nodes in the cervical, axillary, and inguinal areas. Symptoms include fever, night sweats, weight loss, excessive tiredness, indigestion, abdominal pain, loss of appetite, and bone pain.

Medical–Surgical Management

Medical

The diagnosis of NHL is confirmed by a lymph node biopsy. Physicians use a staging system to define the progression of the disease within the body and to determine the appropriate treatment and prognosis of the disease. (Refer to Figure 33-10.)

Pharmacological

There are three different chemotherapy regimens, CHOP, CVP, and COPP: CHOP combines cyclophosphamide (Cytoxan), doxorubicin HCl (Adriamycin), vincristine sulfate (Oncovin), and prednisone (Deltasone); CVP combines cyclophosphamide (Cytoxan), vincristine sulfate (Oncovin), and prednisone (Deltasone); COPP combines cyclophosphamide (Cytoxan), vincristine sulfate (Oncovin), procarbazine HCl (Matulane), and prednisone (Deltasone).

▶ NURSING PROCESS

▶ Assessment

▶ Subjective Data

Ask if the client is experiencing pruritus, night sweats, weight loss, decreased appetite, fever, fatigue, weakness, or chest pain.

▶ Objective Data

The nursing physical assessment consists of weighing the client, taking the vital signs, and assessing for skin infections; dyspnea; cough; voice changes; enlarged lymph nodes in the neck, axilla, and groin; and edema in the extremities. Bone scan shows fractures and tumor infiltration. Review blood tests. Blood tests show hypercalcemia if bone lesions are present, and a CBC often indicates anemia.

When the client is having radiation or chemotherapy treatments, the assessment includes observing for dysphagia, nausea and vomiting, skin rashes, and alopecia.

Nursing diagnoses for a client with Hodgkin's disease or non-Hodgkin's disease may include the following:

Nursing Diagnoses	Planning/Goals	Nursing Interventions
▶ Breathing pattern, ineffective, related to tracheobronchial obstruction from enlarged mediastinal nodes	The client will complete activities of daily living without dyspnea.	Elevate the head of the bed to assist the client's breathing.
		Encourage the client to take frequent deep breaths to expand the lungs and prevent infection.
		Assess the client's breathing pattern every shift and as needed for dyspnea.
▶ Infection, risk for, related to radiation/chemotherapy treatments, decreased WBCs and pruritus	The client will remain free of infection.	Monitor the lab results.
		Teach the client the importance of avoiding situations where there is exposure to infections.
		Provide cool sponge baths or oral medication to relieve pruritus.
		Assess the radiated skin areas for redness or breaks in the skin.
		Encourage the client to report symptoms of dyspnea, sore throat, and burning or frequency of urination.
▶ Nutrition, altered, less than body requirements related to decreased appetite	The client will consume an adequate amount of a nutritional diet.	Serve attractive high-calorie, high-protein meals in a pleasant environment.
		Offer six to eight smaller meals throughout the day to decrease a feeling of fullness.
		Offer a soft, bland diet, which may be more palatable during radiation or chemotherapy treatments.
		Avoid hot, spicy foods as they are caustic to mucous membranes and may lead to infection.
		Encourage an adequate intake of fluids to prevent constipation and renal stones.
		Weigh the client biweekly or more frequently if needed.

Evaluation Each goal must be evaluated to determine how it has been met by the client.

PLASMA CELL DISORDER

The main plasma cell disorder is multiple myeloma.

MULTIPLE MYELOMA

There were an estimated 13,800 new cases of multiple myeloma diagnosed in 1998, and an estimated 11,300 persons died from it (Leukemia Society of America, 1998d). Most cases occur in men over age 60.

The plasma cells, mainly in bone marrow, become malignant, crowd out normal cell production, destroy normal bone tissue, and thereby cause pain. The normal production of antibodies is changed, making the client susceptible to infections. The first sign of multiple myeloma is often bone pain, especially in the ribs, spine, and pelvis. The long bones ache; joints are swollen and tender; and a low-grade fever and general malaise are present. The client tires easily and has weakness from anemia. The weakened bones fracture easily. The cause of multiple myeloma is not known.

Diagnosis is made with bone marrow biopsy showing large numbers of immature plasma cells and x-rays showing demineralization and osteoporosis. Bence Jones protein is found in the urine of many clients with multiple myeloma. The client will also have hypercalcemia, hyperuricemia, anemia, and hypercalciuria.

Medical–Surgical Management

Medical

Multiple myeloma is not curable, so treatment is symptomatic. Both radiation and chemotherapy are used to reduce tumor size and slow tumor growth.

Surgical

A laminectomy may be required if any vertebrae collapse. If the client gets kidney stones from the large amount of calcium in the blood and urine, surgery may be required.

Pharmacological

Steroids such as prednisone (Metcorten) along with antineoplastic drugs such as cyclophosphamide (Cytoxan), chlorambucil (Leukeran), or melphalan (Alkeran) are given. An analgesic is given for pain relief.

Diet

Six small meals a day are often tolerated better than the usual three meals a day; nutritious meals based on the client's food preferences are recommended. A fluid intake of 3 to 4 L/day is essential to minimize the complications of excessive calcium in the blood and urine.

Activity

It is important to keep the client mobile as much as possible. Walking stimulates calcium resorption and decreases demineralization. When the client is in bed, it is important to reposition the client frequently using a lift sheet to decrease the risk of pathological fractures.

▶ NURSING PROCESS

▶ Assessment

▶ Subjective

The client describes constant pain that increases with movement. The pain is usually in the back, ribs, or pelvis. Achiness in the long bones and joints and general malaise may also be described.

▶ Objective

Pain should be assessed using a 0 (none) to 10 (most) pain scale. Temperature may be elevated. The client's ability to perform activities of daily living should be evaluated.

Nursing diagnoses for a client with multiple myeloma may include the following:

Nursing Diagnoses	Planning/Goals	Nursing Interventions
▶ *Pain, related to disease process*	The client will express a decrease in pain level.	Administer analgesic as ordered. Monitor the client's response to the analgesic. Assess the client's pain level with pain scale.
▶ *Injury, risk for, related to bone demineralization*	The client will have minimal injuries.	Handle client gently. Reposition the client using a lift sheet. Keep the client's personal items within easy reach.
▶ *Infection, risk for, related to disease process and pharmaceutical agents*	The client will have few infections.	Thoroughly wash hands before caring for the client. Teach the client and family proper handwashing. Assist the client with personal hygiene as needed. Screen visitors for signs of infections before allowing them to visit the client.

Evaluation Each goal must be evaluated to determine how it has been met by the client.

CASE STUDY

James Johns, 46, owns a hobby shop. He has had a cold for 3 weeks that has recently settled in his chest. He has been tired lately and takes naps each evening before the evening meal. His wife noticed several bruises on his arms and legs, but James could not recall any particular injury. James has gradually lost 10 pounds over the last 3 months but has not been concerned about it. When James went to the clinic for some antibiotics for his cold, a physical assessment was completed, and a chest x-ray and CBC were ordered. WBCs were 250,000/mm³; RBCs, 4.2 million/mm³ and platelets, 100,000/mm³. After several other tests were performed over the next few days, a diagnosis of chronic myelocytic leukemia (CML) was confirmed.

The following questions will guide your development of a nursing care plan for the case study.

1. List the symptoms occurring in James Johns that are typical of CML.
2. List five other typical symptoms of CML that were not stated in the case study.
3. List other diagnostic tests that could be done to confirm the diagnosis of CML.
4. List subjective and objective data the nurse would obtain about James Johns.
5. Write three individualized nursing diagnoses and goals for James Johns.
6. List nursing interventions for James Johns.
7. List community resources specific to locale that could assist James and his family during his illness with CML.
8. List discharge teaching the nurse would give to James and his family.
9. List successful client outcomes for James Johns.
10. List chemotherapeutic agents and side effects of the agents that may be prescribed for James.
11. List other medical treatments that may be ordered for James.
12. What measures could the nurse take to meet the emotional needs of James and his family?

SUMMARY

:• The main formed components of the blood are red blood cells, white blood cells, and platelets.
• The lymphatic system is composed of lymph vessels that drain lymph into the venous system and lymph nodes that filter microorganisms in the body.
• Sickledex and hemoglobin electrophoresis are diagnostic tests for sickle cell anemia.
• A client with anemia has a decreased number of RBCs and low hemoglobin and hematocrit levels.
• Some of the symptoms of anemia are fatigue, pallor, exertional dyspnea, and tachycardia.
• Symptoms of polycythemia vera are headache, epistaxis, dizziness, tinnitus, blurred vision, fatigue, weakness, pruritus, exertional dyspnea, angina, and increased blood pressure and pulse.
• Polycythemia vera is treated with chemotherapeutic agents.
• DIC is not a disease but a syndrome that occurs because of a client's having a primary disease or condition. The primary disease causes the client to alternate between forming many small clots and hemorrhaging.

• Hemophilia is a recessive X chromosome inherited bleeding disorder in which the client is lacking clotting factors. The main symptom is spontaneous bleeding or bleeding due to trauma.
• The two types of malignant lymphomas are Hodgkin's disease and non-Hodgkin's lymphoma. Clients with both types of lymphoma have enlarged lymph nodes.
• Hodgkin's disease is diagnosed by the presence of the Reed Sternberg cell in the swollen lymph nodes. Non-Hodgkin's lymphoma arises from the B lymphocytes and T lymphocytes and does not have the Reed Sternberg cell in the lymph system.

Review Questions

1. The diagnostic test for sickle cell anemia is the:
   a. D dimer.
   b. sickledex.
   c. hemoglobin electrophoresis.
   d. Schilling test.

2. For improved iron absorption, a client with iron deficiency anemia takes Feosol with:

   a. milk.
   b. an orange.
   c. water.
   d. processed cheese.

3. A thorough assessment of the cardiac system on a client with sickle cell anemia is important because:

   a. the heart enlarges in an attempt to provide the oxygen needs to the body tissues.
   b. cells sickle more easily in the heart chambers.
   c. more cardiac force is needed to pump RBCs with Hbg S.
   d. people with sickle cell anemia are prone to bradycardia.

4. Clients with leukemia are prone to infections because:

   a. there are too many WBCs.
   b. the bone marrow is not producing WBCs.
   c. the bone marrow is producing too many cells.
   d. the WBCs are incapable of fighting infections.

5. A nursing action for a client with pernicious anemia is to:

   a. inquire about exposure to radiation and chemicals.
   b. administer cyanocobalamin (vitamin B_{12}) as ordered.
   c. teach the importance of increasing iron in the diet.
   d. administer oral vitamin B_{12} as ordered.

6. Nursing care for a client with polycythemia vera includes:

   a. doing a Homans' sign to check for blood clots.
   b. administering folic acid as ordered.
   c. observing for blood in the stool and urine.
   d. observing for petechiae and ecchymotic spots.

7. Symptoms that alert a nurse that a client may have DIC are:

   a. tinnitus and numbness and tingling in the extremities.
   b. jaundice, palpitations, and dyspnea.
   c. purpura, bruising, and decreased urine output.
   d. ruddy complexion, epistaxis, and tinnitus.

8. A client with hemophilia is taught to:

   a. administer clotting factors as needed.
   b. administer cyanocobalamin (vitamin B_{12}) as needed.
   c. maintain a high-calorie, high-protein diet.
   d. report night sweats.

9. Encourage a client with non-Hodgkin's lymphoma to:

   a. use an electric razor.
   b. take folic acid as prescribed.
   c. apply ice and pressure to bleeding sites.
   d. avoid exposure to infections.

Critical Thinking Questions

1. Explain how the symptoms of iron deficiency anemia are related to a decreased red blood cell count and a decreased hemoglobin.

2. Compare the etiologies and symptoms of iron deficiency anemia, hypoplastic (aplastic) anemia, pernicious anemia, acquired hemolytic anemia, and sickle cell anemia.

WEB FLASH!

- Search the Internet for the various disorders discussed in this chapter. What new or experimental treatments are discussed?
- What information do the resources for this chapter at the end of the book provide on the Internet? For whom is this material intended?

NURSING CARE OF THE CLIENT: GASTRO-INTESTINAL SYSTEM

MAKING THE CONNECTION

Refer to the following chapters to increase your understanding of digestive disorders:

- **Chapter 15, Wellness Concepts**
- **Chapter 17, Loss, Grief, and Death**
- **Chapter 23, Fluid, Electrolyte, and Acid-Base Balance**
- **Chapter 25, Assessment**
- **Chapter 26, Pain Management**
- **Chapter 30, Nursing Care of the Oncology Client**
- **Chapter 39, Nursing Care of the Client: Immune System**

- **Chapter 45, Nursing Care of the Client: Mental Illness**
- **Chapter 55, Nursing Care of the Older Client**
- **Procedures:** B33, Collecting Stool Specimen; B34, Applying Abdominal, T-, Breast, or Sculteatus Binders; I7, Changing a Colostomy Pouch; I20, Irrigating a Wound; A2, Inserting a Nasogastric or Nasointestinal Tube for Suctioning or Enteral Feedings

LEARNING OBJECTIVES

Upon completion of this chapter, you should be able to:

- *Define key terms.*
- *Discuss diagnostic tests associated with the digestive system.*
- *Discuss components necessary for a complete assessment of the digestive system.*
- *List medical and surgical management for clients with digestive disorders.*
- *Describe nursing interventions for clients with digestive disorders.*
- *Assist with the formulation of nursing care plans for clients with digestive disorders.*

INTRODUCTION

Disorders and diseases of the gastrointestinal system and accessory organs can affect not only the digestive process and nutrient absorption, but the lifestyle of the individual as well.

KEY TERMS

adhesion	hematemesis
appendicitis	hemorrhoid
ascites	hepatitis
calculi (calculus, sing.)	ileostomy
cholecystitis	intussusception
cholelithiasis	jaundice
chyme	ligation
cirrhosis	melena
colostomy	occult blood test
constipation	(guaiac)
digestion	pancreatitis
diverticula	peptic ulcer
diverticulitis	peritonitis
diverticulosis	peristalsis
effluent	polyp
gastric ulcer	postprandial
gastritis	steatorrhea
glycogenesis	stoma
glycogenolysis	stomatitis
haustra	volvulus

ANATOMY AND PHYSIOLOGY REVIEW

The digestive system, also known as the *gastrointestinal (GI) tract* or the *alimentary system,* is responsible for breaking down the complex food into simple nutrients the body can absorb and convert into energy (see Figure 34-1). This process is known as **digestion**.

Mouth/Esophagus

Digestion begins in the mouth where the teeth mechanically break food down into smaller pieces by chewing and mixing it with saliva. The chemical breakdown of cooked starches is begun by the enzyme salivary amylase in the mouth. The food is then swallowed as a small ball or bolus and transported down the esophagus, a hollow, muscular tube approximately 10 inches long. **Peristalsis**, coordinated rhythmic contractions of the muscles, pushes the bolus through the esophagus. The cardiac sphincter, also called the *lower esophageal sphincter (LES),* located at the distal end of the esophagus relaxes and allows the food to pass into the stomach.

Stomach

Further mechanical and chemical breakdown of the food occurs in the stomach, a J-shaped muscular organ located beneath the diaphragm. The stomach secretes gastric juices that contain hydrochloric acid (HCl) and pepsinogen, a nonactive form of the enzyme pepsin. HCl and pepsin are responsible for beginning the breakdown of protein and continuing the breakdown of starches. Starch digestion in the stomach gradually stops due to the acid environment. Mucous is secreted to protect the lining of the stomach. The stomach also secretes an intrinsic factor, which is necessary for vitamin B_{12} absorption, and gastrin, which stimulates HCl release.

The peristaltic movement of the stomach mixes the partially digested food and digestive enzymes into a semiliquid mass called **chyme**. The chyme will not pass into the small intestine until it is the proper consistency and particles are 1 millimeter or less. On average, the stomach empties in 3 to 4 hours. Carbohydrates are digested most readily, followed by proteins, with fats taking the longest to pass from the stomach. When the chyme has reached the proper consistency, the pyloric sphincter relaxes, releasing a portion at a time of the chyme into the small intestine.

Small Intestine

The small intestine is approximately 20 to 25 feet long and is responsible for absorbing nutrients from the chyme. The small intestine also secretes digestive

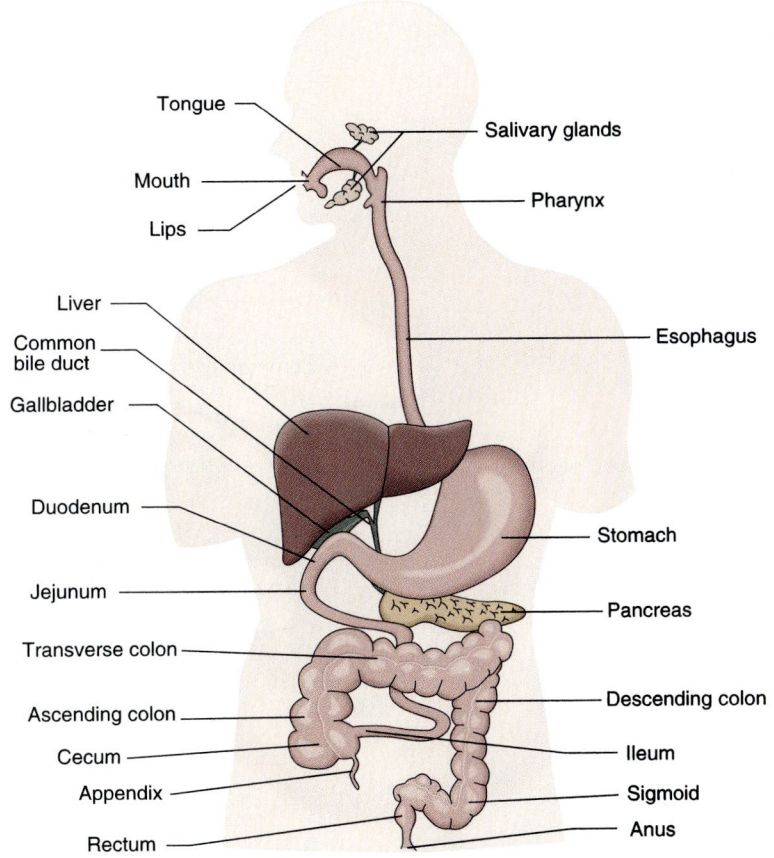

Figure 34-1 The Digestive System

enzymes, mucous to protect the mucosa, and hormones to aid in the absorption of nutrients.

The chyme enters the duodenum, the first 10 to 12 inches of the small intestine. The duodenum is responsible for absorbing calcium and iron as well as neutralizing the acids in the chyme. Enzymes from the pancreas and bile from the liver enter the duodenum from the common bile duct by way of the ampulla of vater; it is here that fats are digested.

The jejunum, the middle of the small intestine, is 8 to 10 feet long. It is responsible for absorption of fats, proteins, and carbohydrates. Vitamin B_{12} and bile salts are absorbed in the ileum, which is the distal 12 feet of the small bowel.

Large Intestine

The chyme enters the large intestine, also known as the *colon*, through the ileocecal valve into the cecum, a small pouch to which the appendix is attached. The colon is approximately 4 to 5 feet long and consists of the ascending or right colon, the transverse colon, the descending or left colon, and the sigmoid colon, an S-shaped segment before the rectum. The colon is responsible for absorbing water, electrolytes, and bile salts.

The last 5 inches of the large intestine comprise the rectum. The distal end of the rectum forms the anal canal composed of muscles that control defecation. The opening to the anal canal is called the *anus*.

Accessory Organs

The digestive system is also comprised of accessory organs that aid in the digestion of food. The accessory organs include the pancreas, liver, and gallbladder (Figure 34-2).

Pancreas

The pancreas is a fish-shaped glandular organ 6 to 8 inches long extending from the duodenum across the abdomen behind the stomach. The pancreas has both endocrine and exocrine functions. The endocrine functions, which include the production of glucagon and insulin to regulate the blood sugar level, are presented in Chapter 37.

The pancreas produces 3 main groups of enzymes in pancreatic juice for its exocrine function. The enzymes are:

amylase—converts carbohydrates into glucose

lipase—aids in fat digestion

protease—breaks down protein

Liver

The liver is the largest glandular organ of the body. It is located in the right upper quadrant of the abdomen. The liver is one of the most vascular organs, filtering 1,500 cc of blood per minute. Some of the many functions of the liver are to:

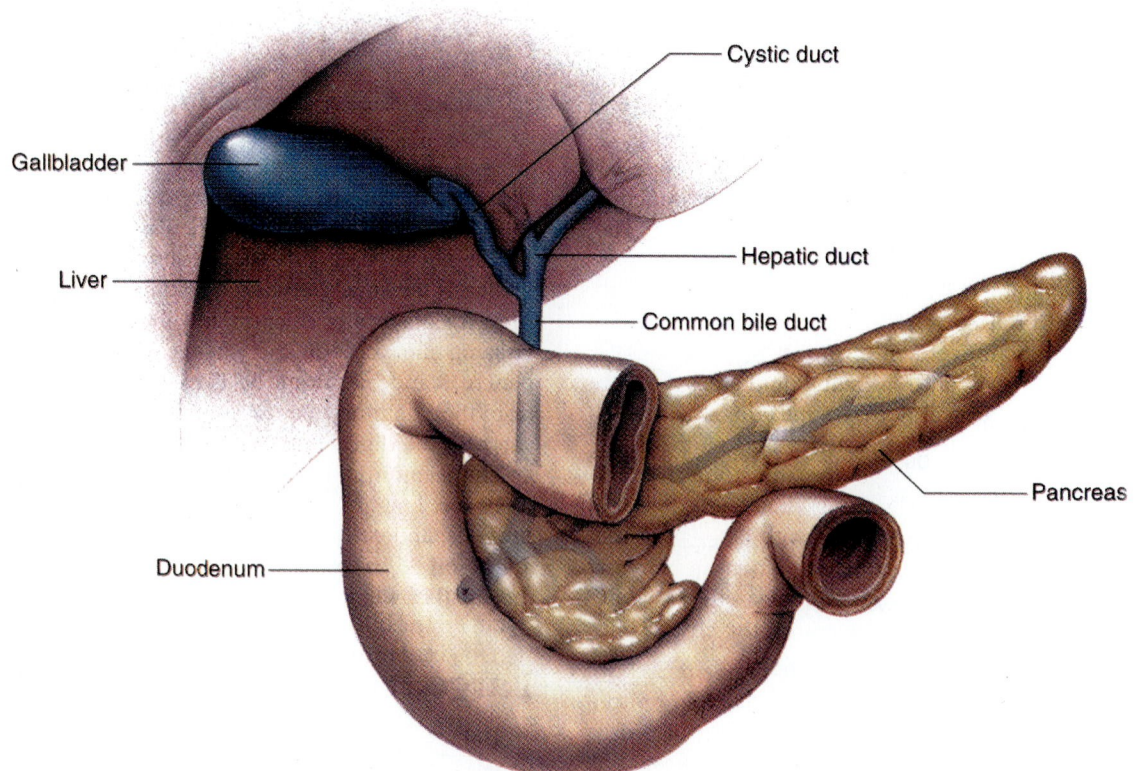

Figure 34-2 Accessory Organs. Bile travels from the liver to the gallbladder via the hepatic and cystic ducts. The bile is released into the duodenum via the common bile duct. The pancreas releases its digestive juice into the duodenum.

- Produce and secrete bile, which emulsifies fats
- Convert glucose into glycogen for storage (**glycogenesis**)
- Convert glycogen to glucose when blood sugar level drops (**glycogenolysis**)
- Metabolize hormones
- Break down nitrogenous wastes to urea
- Incorporate amino acids into proteins
- Filter blood and destroy bacteria
- Produce prothrombin and fibrinogen, which are necessary for blood clotting
- Manufacture cholesterol
- Produce heparin
- Store vitamin B_{12} and fat soluble vitamins A, D, E, and K
- Detoxify poisonous substances

Gallbladder

The gallbladder is a pear-shaped sac attached to the undersurface of the liver. The liver produces bile and transports the bile to the gallbladder by way of the hepatic and cystic ducts. The gallbladder stores and concentrates the bile until it is needed in the small intestine. When fats enter the small intestine, the gallbladder releases the bile through the cystic duct into the common bile duct and finally into the small intestine. The cystic duct, hepatic duct, and pancreatic duct combine to form the common bile duct.

Effects of Aging

As the body ages, several changes may occur in the digestive system (Table 34-1). It is important to educate clients about these changes and ways they can adapt their lifestyles.

ASSESSMENT

As discussed in Chapter 25, a thorough assessment is necessary to collect data on which to formulate an accurate nursing diagnosis. For clients complaining of GI symptoms, the assessment should include:

1. History of the present complaint including length and frequency of symptoms, when symptoms occur, as well as aggravating factors.
2. Medication history including prescribed and over-the-counter (OTC) medications, and their effectiveness. Clients with GI symptoms frequently self-medicate with antacids, laxatives, suppositories, and enemas.
3. A complete nutritional history; a note should be made of any foods that increase or decrease symptoms. Also, assess if meals aggravate symptoms or if symptoms occur within a specific time period after a meal. Note the fiber and fat content

LIFE CYCLE CONSIDERATIONS

Hernias in Children
- Inguinal hernias become strangulated more frequently during the first 6 months of life, therefore timely assessment and intervention are recommended.
- Surgery is not advised for an umbilical hernia unless it enlarges or persists until 5 years of age.

Table 34-1 CHANGES IN DIGESTIVE SYSTEM WITH AGING

COMMON CHANGES	RESULT	IMPLICATIONS FOR NURSES
Decrease in peristalsis	Food moves more slowly through digestive system. Bowel movements more infrequent. Increase in constipation. Feeling full and bloated and may eat less.	Increase fiber and fluid intake. Encourage smaller, frequent meals. Offer fiber supplements.
Oral changes	Dentures are common. Chewing is more difficult. Eating and drinking time may be prolonged. Number of taste buds decreases.	Make sure dentures fit. Cut food into small bites. Teach that softer foods may be better tolerated. Some clients may start using more salt and seasonings to compensate for less flavor; monitor salt usage.
Decrease in enzyme secretion	Food is harder to digest. Increase in indigestion. Intolerance to some food and seasonings.	Encourage water between meals. Avoid foods that are not tolerated while ensuring adequate nutrient intake.
Decrease in saliva	Food is more difficult to chew. Swallowing becomes difficult.	Encourage fluid intake with meals. Have clients chew food well and do two swallows with each bite of food. Have clients sit up to eat.

LIFE CYCLE CONSIDERATIONS

The Aging GI Tract

- Loss of elasticity and slowed motility of the GI tract, accompanied by lack of exercise, make the elderly prone to constipation.
- As the intestinal wall weakens, diverticuli, or scars on the intestinal wall, can develop.
- Decreased liver mass and blood flow alter the pharmacokinetics of various drugs.

of the diet as well as the amount of fluids typically consumed.

4. Psychosocial factors including compliance and noncompliance with health status. Meal patterns should be evaluated: note if the client eats alone, eats large meals at regular intervals, or snacks all day.

5. Physical examination including inspection, auscultation, percussion, and palpation of the abdomen. An evaluation of the client's ability to chew and swallow is also important.

6. Bowel elimination patterns including frequency, consistency, and amounts of bowel movements.

7. Evaluation of diagnostic data including laboratory analysis and radiologic and endoscopic examinations.

COMMON DIAGNOSTIC TESTS

Commonly used diagnostic tests for clients with digestive disorders are listed in Table 34-2. See Chapter 27, Diagnostic Tests, for explanation/normal values and nursing responsibilities.

DISORDERS OF THE GASTROINTESTINAL TRACT

Disorders of the gastrointestinal tract include: stomatitis, esophageal varices, gastritis, ulcers, appendicitis, diverticulosis and diverticulitis, inflammatory bowel disease, intestinal obstruction, hernias, peritonitis, hemorrhoids, and constipation.

STOMATITIS

Stomatitis is a painful condition characterized by inflammation and ulcerations in the mouth. Stomatitis can be caused by infections, damage to the mucous membranes by irritants, or chemotherapy.

Medical–Surgical Management

Medical

Cultures may be done to determine if an infectious process is present.

Table 34-2 COMMON DIAGNOSTIC TESTS FOR GASTROINTESTINAL DISORDERS

Laboratory Tests
- Complete blood count (CBC)
- Prothrombin time (PT)
- Partial thromboplastin time (PTT)
- Bilirubin
- Albumin
- Globulin
- Total protein
- Alkaline phosphatase
- Lactate hydrogenase (LDH-5)
- Gamma-glutamyl transpeptidase (GGT or GGTP)
- Aspartate aminotransferase (AST/SGOT)
- Alanine aminotransferase (ALT/SGPT)
- Cholesterol
- Triglycerides
- Amylase
- Carcinoembryonic antigen (CEA)
- HAA, now called hepatitis B surface antigen (HB_5AG)
- Stool O & P
- Stool occult blood (guaiac)
  Fecal occult blood Test (fOBT)
  Hemocult

Radiologic Studies
- Barium swallow
- Upper gastrointestinal tract (UGI) with small bowel follow-through
- Abdominal x-rays
- CT scans
- Ultrasound
- Barium enema
- Gallbladder series

Other
- Flexible sigmoidoscopy
- Esophagogastro-duodenoscopy (EGD)
- Endoscopic retrograde cholangiopancreatogram (ERCP)
- Colonoscopy
- Esophageal motility studies (manometry)
- Gastric secretion analysis
- Liver biopsy
- Peritoneal aspiration

Pharmacological

Because the client's mouth can be sore, topical anesthetics such as xylocaine may be used. Analgesics may also be ordered. If an infection is present, the appropriate medication will be ordered.

Diet

Dietary restrictions are based on what the client is able to tolerate. Bland, soft foods or liquids are usually tolerated best. As the sores heal, the diet may be advanced as tolerated. It is important to monitor dietary intake as caloric and fluid intake may be poor due to discomfort.

▶ NURSING PROCESS

▶ Assessment

▶ Subjective Data

Clients usually complain of pain in the mouth and difficulty swallowing.

▶ Objective Data

Observations include inflamed mucosa of the mouth with ulcerations frequently present.

Nursing diagnoses for a client with stomatitis may include the following:

Nursing Diagnoses	Planning/Goals	Nursing Interventions
▶ Pain, Acute, related to stomatitis	The client will verbalize increase in comfort within 1 hour of initiation of treatment.	Assess the client frequently for discomfort. Administer medications such as topical xylocaine and analgesics as ordered. Allow for rest periods as indicated.
▶ Nutrition, Altered, less than body requirements, related to inadequate caloric and fluid intake	The client will be able to maintain caloric intake of 1,500 calories per day by 48 hours after initiation of treatment. The client will be able to maintain fluid intake at 2,000 cc per day by 48 hours after initiation of treatment.	Monitor daily caloric intake and consult with the dietitian to assist with food selection. Administer IV fluids as ordered and monitor I & O.
▶ Oral Mucous Membranes, Altered, related to stomatitis	The client will have less inflammation and a decrease in the size of the ulcers by 36 hours after initiation of treatment.	Monitor the stomatitis every shift to assess status of condition. Provide oral care every 4 hours. Administer medications as ordered to combat the infection.

Evaluation Each goal must be evaluated to determine how it has been met by the client.

ESOPHAGEAL VARICES

A varix is an enlarged, tortuous vein or, occasionally, an artery. Although varices can occur in any part of the digestive system, they occur most frequently in the distal veins of the esophagus. The varices are often associated with cirrhosis of the liver or any other condition that causes chronic obstruction of drainage from the esophageal veins into the portal veins. Swelling of the veins causes the walls to weaken, making them prone to ulceration and bleeding. Anything that causes increased abdominal venous pressure such as sneezing, coughing, vomiting, the Valsalva maneuver, swallowing large, poorly chewed pieces of food, and the erosion of vessel walls by gastric acid can cause the varices to rupture.

Varices have no symptoms so clients may not be aware of them until they start bleeding. Death may ensue rapidly if the hemorrhaging varix is not treated immediately.

Medical–Surgical Management

Medical

The varices may be treated with sclerotherapy, ligation, or balloon tamponade. Sclerotherapy is a procedure in which a caustic substance is injected into the varix. An EGD is performed and a sclerosing agent is injected through a special needle. Several treatments are necessary to cause formation of scar tissue and to stop the bleeding. After the bleeding has stopped and the client has stabilized, the remaining treatments may be done on an outpatient basis.

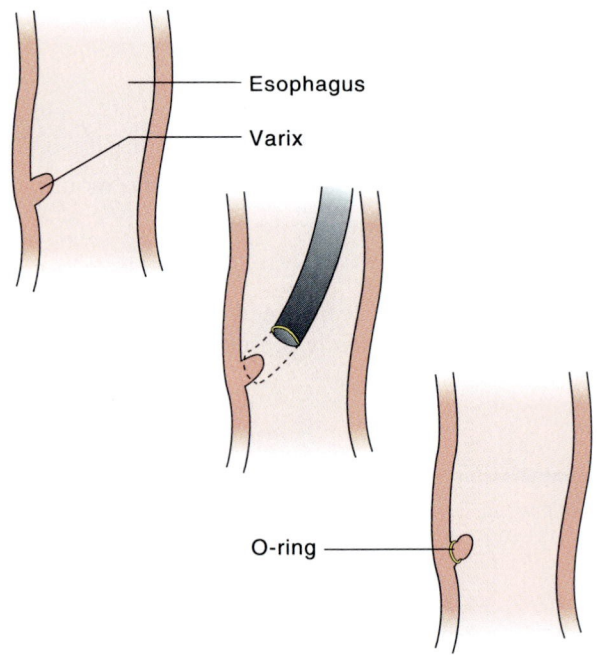

Figure 34-3 Banding of an Esophageal Varix: A. Varix; B. Insertion of tube with O-ring; C. O-ring is placed around the varix.

Complications to sclerotherapy include mediastinal inflammation secondary to extra esophageal injection, perforation, ulceration, stricture secondary to scar formation, and rebleeding.

Esophageal **ligation**, also called *banding,* involves placing a rubber band, tie, or O-ring on the varix (Figure 34-3). An EGD is performed to guide the placement of the bands. The complications include rebleeding and stricture formation.

In a case where varices are actively bleeding, a 3 or 4 lumen balloon tamponade, known as a Minnesota or Sengstaken-Blakemore tube, is passed into the esophagus. The balloon is then inflated in the esophagus to put direct pressure onto the bleeding varices. The balloon is periodically deflated to prevent necrosis of the esophageal tissue. Iced isotonic saline lavages may also be done through the tube. During the procedure, the client must be kept NPO with the head of the bed elevated 30 to 45 degrees. Complications include perforation of the esophagus from pressure from the balloon and necrosis of the surrounding tissue.

Surgical

A portosystemic shunt eventually must be placed in clients with end-stage liver disease. The shunt relieves the pressure on the esophageal veins by redirecting blood from the portal vein to the inferior mesenteric vein. Some of the blood bypasses the liver and reenters the circulatory system (Figure 34-4).

A nonsurgical but invasive procedure, transjugular intrahepatic portosystemic shunt (TIPS), may also be performed. With this procedure, the right internal jugular vein is used to place a cannula into the hepatic

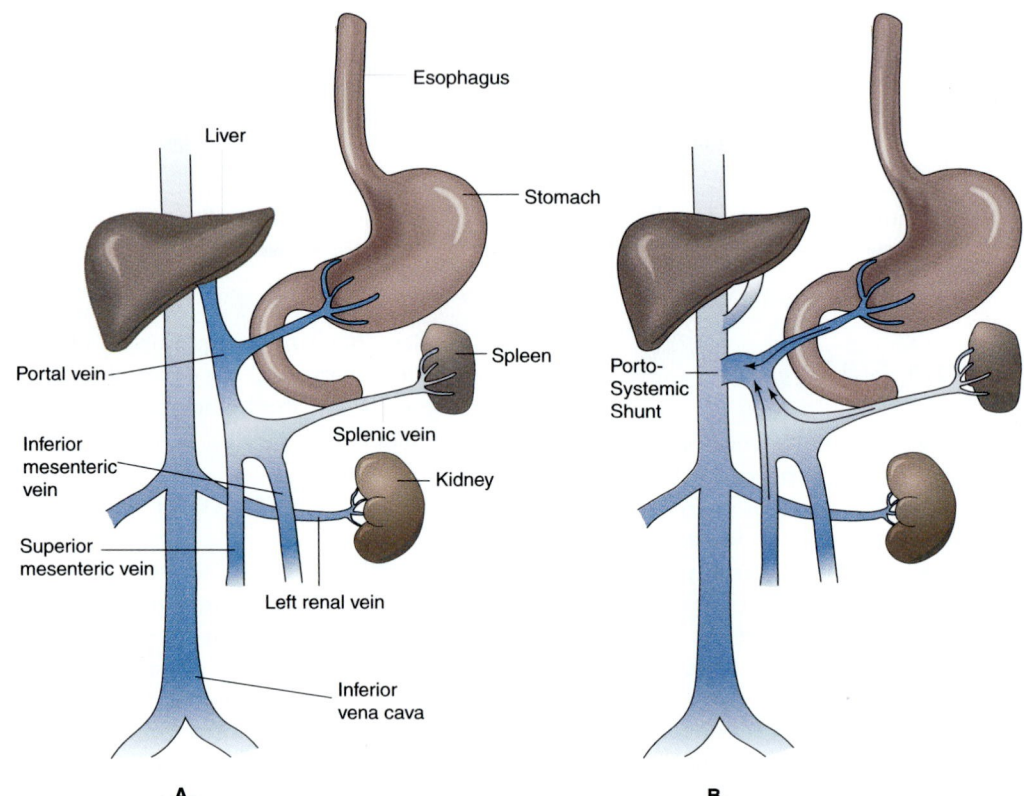

Figure 34-4 A. Normal Circulation of the Liver; B. An Example of a Portosystemic Shunt (may be performed in clients with elevated portal vein pressure that is resistant to medical management).

and portal veins. A connection is made through the liver tissue between the hepatic and portal veins. A stent is placed in the connection. This allows some of the blood to bypass the liver and relieve pressure in the portal vein. This procedure is done in x-ray and is used with clients who are too unstable for surgery (also refer to Figure 34-11.)

Pharmacological

Octreotide (Sandostatin) may be given by IV to help control the bleeding by decreasing blood flow to the gut, thus lowering pressure in the portal system. Analgesics may be necessary following sclerotherapy if clients complain of chest discomfort. Clients should avoid NSAIDs, aspirin, and all anticoagulants. Sucralfate (Carafate) liquid may be given to coat the esophagus, protecting it from erosion by gastric acid. IV rehydration as well as blood transfusions may be necessary for clients with active bleeding.

Activity

If varices are bleeding or have recently bled, the client should remain on bed rest. If no active bleeding is present, the client may be ambulatory but should avoid strenuous exercise.

▶ NURSING PROCESS

▶ Assessment

▶ Subjective Data

Assessment includes history of liver disease or alcohol abuse and nausea. There is no abdominal pain. This is a classic pertinent negative that helps distinguish esophageal varices from bleeding ulcers, which generally do cause pain (Giacchino & Houdek, 1998).

▶ Objective Data

Assessment includes testing stools for **occult blood** (**guaiac**) and **melena** (black, sticky, tar-like stools containing partially broken down blood), and assessing for **hematemesis**, or vomiting blood. The nurse should review hemoglobin and hematocrit (H & H) to evaluate anemia and liver profile for elevated bilirubin and globulin levels and a decrease in albumin.

If cirrhosis of the liver is present, **jaundice**, a yellowing of the skin, mucous membranes, and sclerae of the eyes, is present. Jaundice results when the liver is unable to fully remove bilirubin from the blood. If the client abuses alcohol, nutritional status is usually poor.

Nursing diagnoses for a client with esophageal varices may include the following:

Nursing Diagnoses	Planning/Goals	Nursing Interventions
▶ *Fluid Volume Deficit, High risk for, related to bleeding esophageal varices (if the varices are not actively bleeding)*	The client will maintain adequate fluid volume.	Monitor vital signs every 4 hours including orthostatic blood pressures. Orthostatic blood pressure is obtained by taking the blood pressure when the client is lying down and then when standing up. A 20 mm Hg difference in blood pressures from lying to standing would indicate a change in fluid volume, possibly indicating varix bleeding. Monitor for nausea and dizziness. Monitor H & H every 4 to 8 hours as ordered. A decrease in H & H values would indicate bleeding.
▶ *Fluid Volume Deficit related to bleeding esophageal varices and gastric loss from vomiting*	The client will maintain an H & H within normal limits. The client's blood pressure will be within 20 mm Hg of baseline with no orthostatic changes.	Monitor H & H. Frequently monitor vital signs. Administer IV fluids, electrolyte replacement, and blood transfusions as ordered.
▶ *Anxiety (Moderate-severe), related to change in health status, threat of death*	The client will discuss concerns about health status.	Explain all tests and procedures to decrease anxiety. Allow client to express fears and concerns regarding condition.

Evaluation Each goal must be evaluated to determine how it has been met by the client.

GASTRITIS

Gastritis is an inflammation of the stomach mucosa occurring when the stomach has been exposed to irritating substances such as medications, smoke, food allergens, or toxic chemicals. Another contributing factor to gastritis may be impaired mucosal defenses, which occur when the epithelial cells of the stomach are not able to secrete adequate quantity or quality of mucous to protect the stomach. The presence of the bacteria *Helicobactor pylori* (*H. pylori*) has also been associated with gastritis.

Medical–Surgical Management

Medical

Diagnosis of gastritis is based on history and symptoms. An UGI or an EGD may be done to help diagnose the condition. If *H. pylori* is suspected, a biopsy is obtained during an EGD and a culture is performed.

Pharmacological

Treatment for gastritis is primarily pharmacological involving antacids and histamine (H_2) receptor antagonists (also call H_2 blockers). Occasionally, a proton pump inhibitor such as omeprazole (Prilosec) or prostaglandins may be used. If *H. pylori* is present, the use of bismuth preparations to inhibit *H. pylori* growth and antibiotics to eliminate the bacteria may be used (Table 34-3).

NSAIDs such as ibuprofen (Motrin) and indomethacin (Indocin) have been shown to compromise mucosal defenses and increase acid secretion. Clients who are on NSAIDs chronically, such as clients with arthritis, may need to be evaluated to determine if other analgesics would be effective or if a prostaglandin should be taken with the NSAIDs.

Diet

Although studies have shown that dietary modifications have little impact on the rate of gastritis healing, some modifications are indicated. Any foods that aggravate symptoms should be eliminated. Also, foods that increase acid secretions such as milk, coffee, decaffeinated coffee, tea, colas, and chocolate should be consumed only in small amounts or eliminated if possible. Bedtime eating should be avoided as it increases nocturnal acid secretions.

Health Promotion

Smoking and alcohol aggravate the mucosal lining of the stomach and significantly impair gastritis healing. Smoking and alcohol consumption should be minimized or eliminated if possible.

▶ NURSING PROCESS

▶ Assessment

▶ Subjective Data

Clients with gastritis may have no symptoms or may describe epigastric pain or burning, or nausea. They may also state that certain foods aggravate symptoms.

▶ Objective Data

Stools may test positive for blood.

Table 34-3 MEDICATIONS USED FOR ULCERS AND GASTRITIS

MEDICATION	PURPOSE	NURSING IMPLICATIONS
Antacids • aluminum hydroxide (Amphogel) • aluminum hydroxide and magnesium hydroxide (Maalox) • dihydroxyaluminum sodium carbonate (Rolaids)	Seal impaired mucosa. Neutralize acids.	Antacids containing aluminum hydroxide may cause constipation. Antacids containing magnesium hydroxide may cause diarrhea; monitor serum electrolytes; do not give with other meds.
H_2 Receptor Antagonists • ranitadine HCl (Zantac) • cimetidine (Tagamet)	Decrease gastric acid secretion.	Do not give within 1 hour of antacids.
Proton Pump Inhibitor • omeprazole (Prilosec)	Stop gastric acid secretion.	Give with food. Suspend granules in an acid liquid. Takes 4 days to achieve blood level.
Prostaglandins • misoprostol (Cytotec)	Decrease gastric acid secretion. Enhance mucosal defenses.	Give when NSAIDs need to be continued.
Bismuth Compounds • bismuth subsalicylate (Pepto-Bismol)	Enhance mucosal barriers. Inhibit *H. pylori* growth.	Do not give within 1 hour of H_2 blockers.
Antibiotics • ampicillin (Omnipen) • metronidazole (Flagyl)	Eliminate *H. pylori*.	Some antibiotics will cause N/V if taken with alcohol. Do not give with antacids or meals with the exception of Flagyl, which must be taken with food. Clients usually placed on two different antibiotics simultaneously.

Nursing diagnoses for a client with gastritis may include the following:

Nursing Diagnoses	Planning/Goals	Nursing Interventions
▶ *Pain, related to gastric acid on inflammation*	The client will experience less pain within 24 hours of onset of treatment as identified by pain scale.	Administer medications as ordered. Assess client for improvement of symptoms. Provide diet as ordered. Implement education about lifestyle changes.
▶ *Knowledge Deficit, related to condition, therapy, and symptoms of potential complications*	The client will verbalize understanding of factors related to condition and symptoms of complications and comply with treatment regimen.	Educate regarding medication regimen and lifestyle changes. If the client smokes or drinks alcohol, provide information on smoking and drinking cessation. Discuss dietary modifications.

Evaluation Each goal must be evaluated to determine how it has been met by the client.

ULCERS

Peptic ulcers are erosions that form in the esophagus, stomach, or duodenum resulting from acid/pepsin imbalance. **Gastric ulcers** refer to erosions in the stomach and are correlated to exposure to irritants such as NSAIDs, smoking, alcohol, food allergens, toxic chemicals, *H. pylori* infections, and impaired mucosal defenses. Impaired mucosal defenses occur when the epithelial cells of the stomach are not able to secrete adequate quantity or quality of mucous to protect the stomach.

Clients with gastric ulcers frequently complain of pain 1 to 2 hours after eating. Eating may not relieve pain or may even increase pain. Weight loss is common. Risk factors include alcohol use, stress, and NSAID use.

Stress ulcers are a type of gastric ulcer that form when gastritis becomes erosive and starts bleeding. As the name implies, stress ulcers occur in clients whose bodies are experiencing stress, such as clients who have experienced major surgery, trauma, burns, chemotherapy, or radiation therapy. Clients with chronic respiratory disorders may also experience stress ulcers as hypoxia can lead to impaired mucosa. Bleeding may be massive resulting in significant blood loss or can be slow and insidious. Because of the multiple sites of bleeding, stress ulcers may be difficult to manage.

Duodenal ulcers refer to ulcers in the duodenum. Incidents of duodenal ulcers have been correlated to a high secretion of HCl. Clients with duodenal ulcers frequently complain of pain 2 to 4 hours after eating. Nocturnal pain may be present, occurring between midnight and 3:00 A.M. Eating frequently relieves symptoms. Weight gain is common. Risk factors include a history of pulmonary disease, cirrhosis, chronic pancreatitis, and/or chronic renal failure.

If an ulcer erodes through a blood vessel, the client may experience a life-threatening hemorrhage. A perforation occurs if the ulcer erodes through the wall of the stomach or small intestine resulting in gastric or intestinal contents entering the abdominal cavity and causing peritonitis.

Diagnosis of ulcers is based on symptoms, history, and an UGI or an EGD performed to visualize the ulcer. If an *H. pylori* infection is suspected, a biopsy is obtained during an EGD and a culture is performed.

Medical–Surgical Management

Medical

If an ulcer bleeds, an EGD may be performed and the ulcer is either injected with epinephrine to cause vasoconstriction or a special electrical probe is used to cauterize or burn the tissue that is bleeding. A nasogastric (NG) tube may be inserted to remove gastric contents and blood, and iced isotonic saline may be instilled to help cause vasoconstriction and stop the bleeding.

Surgical

If the ulcer continues to bleed or if the ulcer has perforated, the client is taken to surgery and a gastrectomy is performed, in which the portion of the stomach or duodenum that is perforated is removed and the bowel is reconnected with an anastomosis (see Figure 34-5). A vagotomy may also be performed. A vagotomy is a procedure in which the vagal innervation to the fundus of the stomach is removed, thereby decreasing acid production in the stomach.

Complications from gastrectomies include gastric dumping in which the stomach experiences **postprandial** (after eating) rapid gastric emptying. Clients experience abdominal pain, nausea, vomiting, explosive diarrhea, weakness, and dizziness. Clients with gastric dumping have malabsorption of nutrients

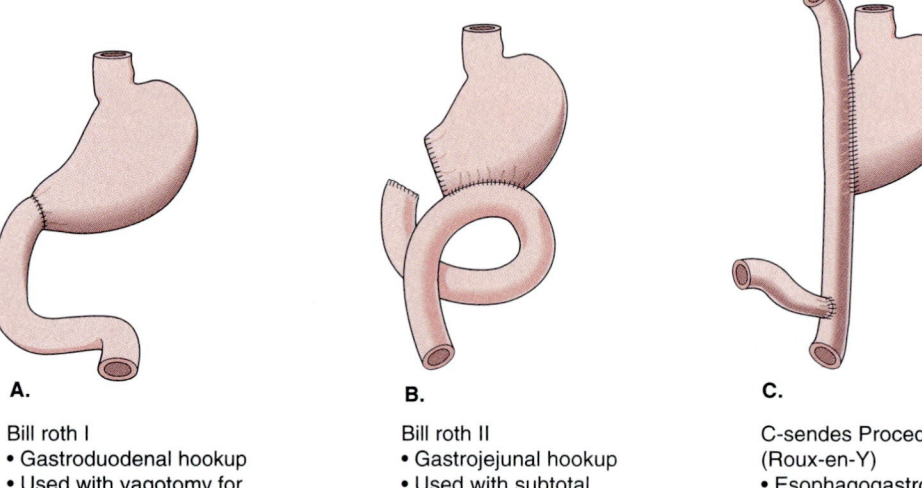

A.

Bill roth I
• Gastroduodenal hookup
• Used with vagotomy for
  duodenal ulcer

B.

Bill roth II
• Gastrojejunal hookup
• Used with subtotal
  gastrectomy

C.

C-sendes Procedure
(Roux-en-Y)
• Esophagogastrojejunostony
• Used in ulcers high in
  the stomach

Figure 34-5 Gastric resections are necessary when an ulcer perforates. The type of gastrectomy depends on the location of the ulcer.

because the food passes too quickly to permit absorption, thus leading to malnutrition. In addition, many clients with significant symptoms may limit dietary intake to avoid symptoms, compounding the malnutrition and weight loss issues.

Management of gastric dumping includes small, frequent meals of high fiber and high protein and avoidance of simple carbohydrates.

Pharmacological

Treatment of ulcers is primarily pharmacological involving antacids, histamine (H₂) receptor antagonists (also called *H₂ blockers*), proton pump inhibitor, or prostaglandins. If *H. pylori* is present, the use of bismuth preparations to inhibit its growth and antibiotics to eliminate the bacteria are generally used (refer back to Table 34-3).

NSAIDs such as ibuprofen (Motrin) and indomethacin (Indocin) have been shown to compromise mucosal defenses and increase acid secretion. Clients who are on NSAIDs chronically, such as clients with arthritis, may need to evaluate if other analgesics would be effective or if a prostaglandin should be taken with the NSAIDs.

Diet

Although studies have shown that dietary modifications have little impact on the rate of ulcer healing, some modifications are indicated. Foods that aggravate symptoms should be eliminated. Also, foods that increase acid secretions such as milk, coffee, decaffeinated coffee, tea, colas, and chocolate should be consumed only in small amounts or eliminated if possible. Bedtime eating should also be avoided as it increases nocturnal acid secretions.

Health Promotion

Smoking and alcohol aggravate the mucosal lining of the stomach and duodenum and significantly impair ulcer healing. Smokers also experience a higher ulcer recurrence rate. Stress has been shown to increase the rate of peptic ulcers. Although the type or severity of stress may not be significant, the client's interpretation of the events as stressful is. Clients need to develop mechanisms for reducing stress such as exercise, biofeedback, and relaxation.

▶ NURSING PROCESS

▶ Assessment

▶ Subjective Data

Clients with gastric ulcers are often asymptomatic or may describe epigastric pain or burning one to two hours after eating, and nausea or bloating. Clients may experience an increase of symptoms when they eat and therefore may decrease dietary intake. When questioned about lifestyle, NSAID usage, stress, smoking, and alcohol use may be discovered.

Clients with duodenal ulcers may exhibit no symptoms or may complain of pain 2 to 4 hours after eating. Eating will frequently decrease symptoms so clients will often eat more frequently. When questioned about lifestyle, stress, smoking, and alcohol consumption may be discovered. The client may also have a history of pulmonary disease, cirrhosis, chronic pancreatitis, and/or chronic renal failure.

A client who is actively bleeding from an ulcer will experience an acute onset of epigastric pain, shortness of breath, and nausea.

▶ Objective Data

Clients with gastric ulcers may show a weight loss and stools may test positive for blood. An H & H may show anemia.

Clients with duodenal ulcers may show a weight gain and stools may test positive for blood. An H & H may show anemia.

The client who is actively bleeding from an ulcer will show signs of shock: pale clammy skin, an elevated pulse rate, and a drop in blood pressure. The client may also have hematemesis. Laboratory tests may show a low H & H. Stools may test positive for blood.

Nursing diagnoses for a client with ulcers may include the following:

Nursing Diagnoses	Planning/Goals	Nursing Interventions
▶ *Pain, related to gastric acid on ulcerated mucosa*	The client will experience less pain within 24 hours of onset of treatment as identified on pain scale.	Assess clients for decrease of pain. Administer medications as ordered. Assess for elevated BP.
▶ *Knowledge Deficit, related to condition, therapy, and symptoms of complications*	The client will verbalize understanding of factors related to condition and symptoms of complications. Client will comply with treatment regimen.	Identify client's learning style and provide information in a manner compatible with the learning style. Educate regarding medication regimen and lifestyle changes. If indicated, provide client with smoking cessation information and stress reduction techniques such as exercise and biofeedback. Include signs and symptoms of possible complications.
▶ *Fluid Volume Deficit, related to bleeding ulcer*	The client will exhibit normal fluid volume as evidenced by stable H & H and blood pressure within 20 mm Hg of baseline.	Check vital signs every 4 hours and PRN including orthostatic blood pressure. Administer IV fluids, electrolyte replacement, and blood transfusions as ordered. Monitor for dizziness and nausea. Check stool for blood.

Evaluation Each goal must be evaluated to determine how it has been met by the client.

APPENDICITIS

Appendicitis is the inflammation of the vermiform appendix, a 10-cm small, slender tube attached to the cecum. The appendix may be inflamed, gangrenous, or ruptured. If the opening to the appendix becomes blocked with feces, the *E. coli* multiply in the appendix and infection develops with pus formation. If it ruptures, fecal content spills into the abdominal cavity causing peritonitis. Peritonitis may be fatal.

A barium enema or an ultrasound may be ordered to confirm inflammation in the appendiceal area.

Medical–Surgical Management

Early diagnosis and treatment are necessary for the best client outcome. A white blood count and differential are usually ordered. Most clients will have a WBC above 10,000/mm^3, neutrophils over 75%, and an elevated temperature, which indicates infection. Sometimes an appendectomy may be performed along with other abdominal surgeries as a preventive measure.

Surgical

A surgical procedure called an *appendectomy* is necessary before the appendix ruptures. Appendectomies are the most common emergency surgery and require a hospital stay of 2 to 7 days. If no rupture has occurred, a laparoscopic appendectomy, in which the appendix is removed through a scope, may be done. A laparoscopic appendectomy requires only a small incision and allows the client to be discharged 24 hours after the surgery.

Pharmacological

Preoperatively, no analgesics are given so that symptoms will not be masked by the medication. Fluids and electrolytes may need to be replaced prior to surgery. Antibiotics are usually given preoperatively. Postoperatively, analgesics are administered for the relief of incisional discomfort. Antibiotics are usually given postoperatively, especially if a perforation is present.

Diet

Preoperatively, the client is to be NPO. Initially postoperatively, the client is again NPO. If a perforation with peritonitis has occurred, the client will be kept NPO longer and an NG tube may be inserted until bowel sounds have returned. The client is first started on clear liquids and advanced to full liquids and finally, to a regular diet as normal bowel function returns.

Activity

Initially postoperatively, the client is encouraged to turn, cough and deep breathe every 2 hours. Next, the client should be encouraged to leave bed and increase ambulation gradually. Activity restrictions will depend on the severity of the appendicitis. Driving, exercise, and lifting will be limited for a few weeks to allow for incisional healing.

▶ NURSING PROCESS

▶ Assessment

▶ Subjective Data

Clients with appendicitis describe abdominal pain, typically located in the right lower quadrant around McBurney's point (halfway between the umbilicus and the right iliac crest). Clients also complain of anorexia (a loss of appetite) and nausea.

▶ Objective Data

Clients may have vomiting and a fever. Bowel sounds may be diminished or absent. Rebound tenderness, or pain that occurs when fingers are pressed into the right lower quadrant and then released suddenly, may also be present. A CBC will be done and WBCs will be elevated above $10,000/mm^3$ with neutrophils over 75%.

Nursing diagnoses for the client with appendicitis may include the following:

Nursing Diagnoses	Planning/Goals	Nursing Interventions
▶ *Pain, Acute, related to appendicitis/appendectomy*	The client will experience a decrease in pain as evidenced by improved mobility and as identified on pain scale.	Preoperatively, monitor client's pain. Check abdomen for rigidity. Provide an ice pack to help relieve pain as ordered; never use heat. Postoperatively, give analgesics as ordered and medicate prior to activities such as ambulation. Teach client to use a pillow to splint the incision when coughing. If client is having difficulty passing flatus, administer enemas or a rectal tube as ordered, and encourage ambulation.
▶ *Skin Integrity, Impaired, related to the abdominal incision*	The client will verbalize signs and symptoms of infection and factors that enhance wound healing, by discharge.	Administer antibiotics as ordered. Educate the client that incision may be left open to the air after 24 hours and that showers may be taken, per physician instruction. If adhesive strips are present, leave in place until they no longer cover the incision (approximately 10 days to 2 weeks). Educate client regarding signs and symptoms of infection and activity restrictions.

Evaluation Each goal must be evaluated to determine how it has been met by the client.

DIVERTICULOSIS AND DIVERTICULITIS

Diverticula are saclike protrusions of the intestinal wall. **Diverticulosis** refers to a condition of the colon in which multiple diverticula are present (see Figure 34-6). The exact cause of diverticulosis is not known. However, a diet low in fiber is felt to contribute to the formation of the pouches. Diverticulosis affects 30% to 40% of the elderly population (Cameron, 1998). It is asymptomatic unless perforation or hemorrhage occur.

Diverticulitis refers to the inflammation of one or more diverticula generally in the sigmoid colon. It is a

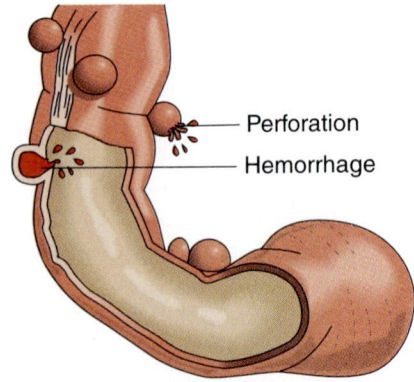

Perforation

Hemorrhage

Figure 34-6 Diverticula in the Sigmoid Colon. Diverticulosis is almost always located in the descending or sigmoid colon.

complication of diverticulosis and is thought to be caused by stool impacted in the diverticula.

Medical–Surgical Management

Medical

Diverticulosis is typically asymptomatic and needs no intervention. Most cases of diverticulitis are treated with analgesics, antibiotics, bed rest, NPO to rest the bowel, and IV fluid hydration.

A barium enema or abdominal ultrasound is usually ordered when diverticulitis is suspected. A flexible sigmoidoscopy may also be performed.

Surgical

If bleeding or perforation of the diverticula has occurred, or if an abscess has formed, surgery is required to remove the portion of the bowel affected. A colon resection is performed. A colostomy may also be required. A **colostomy** is a surgically created opening to relieve either a disease or functional problem in the large intestine.

Stool consistency depends on the placement of the **stoma** in the colon. A colostomy (opening from colon through the skin) is named for the part of the colon where it is located. An ascending colostomy takes its name from the ascending colon and would be on the right side of the abdomen. It has a liquid output. A transverse colostomy would be more toward the midline of the abdomen, and the output would be a pasty liquid. A descending colostomy or sigmoid colostomy would have solid output. Figure 34-7 shows the different colostomy sites.

If a large amount of inflammation is present, a temporary colostomy may be performed to allow the colon to heal. The colon will be reconnected at a later time. In rare cases, a permanent colostomy may need to be performed.

Pharmacological

Clients who have been identified as having diverticulosis are usually placed on fiber supplements or stool softeners. Clients with diverticulitis will be treated with sulfa antibiotics and other antimicrobial agents. Analgesics may also be ordered for discomfort.

Diet

A diet high in fiber is believed to help reduce the occurrence of diverticulosis and diverticulitis.

Clients experiencing diverticulitis will be NPO to rest the bowel. Once the diverticulitis begins healing, the client will be placed on clear liquids and then advanced to a bland, low-residue diet while the diverticulitis heals.

The client will be NPO, if surgery is performed, until bowel sounds return. The client will then be started on clear liquids, advanced to full liquids as

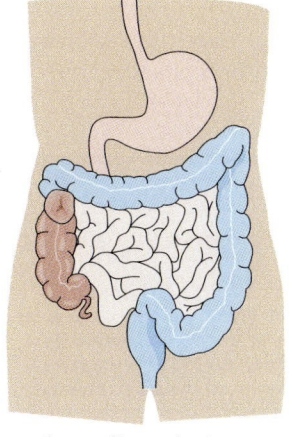
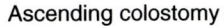
Ascending colostomy

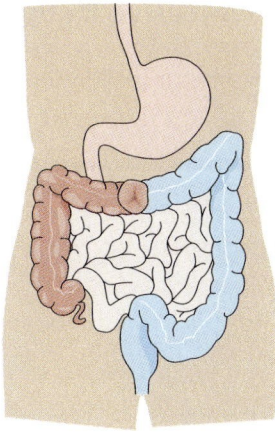
Transverse colostomy

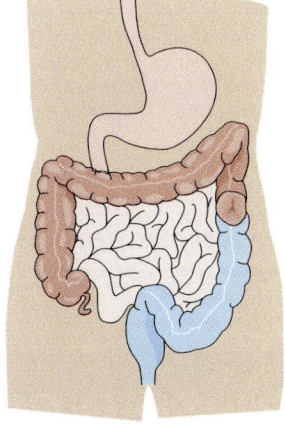
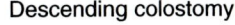
Descending colostomy

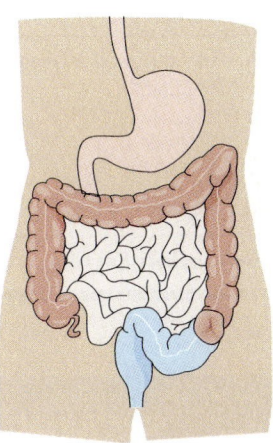
Sigmoid colostomy

Figure 34-7 Colostomy Sites

more bowel function returns, and then finally advanced to a regular diet. A high-fiber diet should be encouraged for clients once the diverticulitis episode has resolved.

Activity

For clients experiencing diverticulitis, bed rest and decreased mobility are encouraged to allow the bowel to rest. In clients who have had a bowel resection, activity will gradually be progressed postoperatively.

▶ NURSING PROCESS

▶ Assessment

Diverticulosis often has no symptoms, and therefore, clients may not be aware they have it.

▶ Subjective Data

Clients with diverticulitis frequently complain of left lower abdominal pain, constipation or diarrhea, bloating, anorexia, and nausea.

▶ Objective Data

Assessment shows abdominal distention with tenderness on palpation, decreased bowel sounds, fever, vomiting, and stools that test positive for blood. A CBC will show an elevated WBC and, if bleeding is present, a low H & H.

Nursing diagnoses for clients with diverticulosis or diverticulitis may include the following:

Nursing Diagnoses	Planning/Goals	Nursing Interventions
▶ *Pain, Acute, related to diverticulitis*	The client will verbalize a decrease in pain within 24 hours after intervention as measured by the pain scale.	Encourage bed rest to allow healing. Maintain client as NPO. Administer analgesics and antibiotics as ordered.
▶ *Infection, Risk for, related to abscess formation or perforation*	The client will verbalize understanding of signs and symptoms of possible complications.	Monitor vital signs and pain level every 4 hours. Assess abdomen every 4 hours for increased tenderness and distention. Educate the client to notify staff of chills, shortness of breath, or increasing pain.
▶ *Anxiety, related to possible surgery*	The client will verbalize fears related to surgery and exhibit decreased anxiety regarding the procedure and follow-up treatment.	Explain all tests and treatments to decrease the client's anxiety level. Allow the client to verbalize fears and concerns. Answer all concerns and questions. If a colostomy is planned, arrange a consult with an enterostomal therapist to help answer concerns.

Evaluation Each goal must be evaluated to determine how it has been met by the client.

SAMPLE NURSING CARE PLAN

THE CLIENT WITH DIVERTICULITIS

Mr. W. is a 67-year-old male admitted to the hospital with abdominal pain that started 2 days ago. The pain has been increasing in intensity and is now accompanied by nausea and anorexia. A physical assessment includes temperature 101.7, pulse 96, respirations 24, and blood pressure of 162/90. Mr. W.'s abdomen is tender on palpation. Mr. W. is in obvious discomfort and is unable to lie on his back. Mr. W. states he has not been eating any food or drinking adequate fluids for 24 hours. Skin turgor is poor. An abdominal ultrasound is ordered and demonstrates diverticulitis. An IV of D5 1/2 NS with 20 mEq KCl, droperidol (Inapsine) IV for nausea, meperidine (Demerol) IM for pain, and IV antibiotics are ordered. Mr. W. is placed on I & O, bed rest with bathroom privileges, and is made NPO. Mr. W. states that he does not understand why all this is being done. His first two voidings are 50 cc each and very concentrated (dark gold colored).

Nursing Diagnosis 1 *Knowledge Deficit related to diagnosis and treatment regimen as evidenced by statement that he does not understand why all this is being done*

PLANNING/GOALS	NURSING INTERVENTIONS	RATIONALE	EVALUATION
Mr. W. will verbalize understanding of treatment plan.	Assess Mr. W.'s knowledge level of diverticulosis/diverticulitis.	Building on present knowledge helps client relate new information and integrate it into his behavior.	Mr. W. verbalizes understanding of the disease process and treatment regimen.

continued

	Assess Mr. W.'s learning style and present information in a manner compatible with his style.	Presenting information in a learning style compatible with the client's increases understanding and retention.	
	Monitor for signs of pain and fatigue.	Pain and fatigue impair learning.	
	Answer questions and reinforce information.	Following up and clarifying information reinforces the new information learned.	

Nursing Diagnosis 2 *Pain, Acute, related to diverticulitis as evidenced by tender abdomen*

PLANNING/GOALS	NURSING INTERVENTIONS	RATIONALE	EVALUATION
Mr. W. will verbalize a decrease in pain within 24 hours of pain intervention.	Assess pain utilizing a scale of 1 (no pain) to 10 (extreme pain).	Using the pain scale to assess pain is an objective measure of the client's perceived discomfort and the effectiveness of the analgesics.	Mr. W. demonstrates adequate pain relief as demonstrated by a decrease in pain scale.
	Medicate with analgesics as ordered.	Provides pain relief.	
	Encourage Mr. W. to request analgesics when pain is increasing rather than waiting for pain to get intense.	Provides better control of pain.	
	Monitor effectiveness of pain medication by reassessing pain utilizing the pain scale 45 minutes after administration of medication.	Provides a measure of effectiveness of analgesic.	

Nursing Diagnosis 3 *Fluid Volume Deficit, as evidenced by low urine output and poor skin turgor*

PLANNING/GOALS	NURSING INTERVENTIONS	RATIONALE	EVALUATION
Mr. W. will demonstrate adequate hydration by I & O being nearly equal, normal skin turgor, and electrolytes within normal limits by 24 hours after intervention.	Monitor I & O every shift.	Provides information on the hydration level of Mr. W.	Mr. W. demonstrates adequate hydration by nearly equal I & O, normal skin turgor, and electrolytes within normal limits.
	Administer IV fluids as ordered.	Provides needed hydration.	
	Assess skin turgor every shift.	Provides information on Mr. W.'s hydration.	
	Monitor laboratory reports for electrolyte levels.	Provides information on electrolyte balance.	

INFLAMMATORY BOWEL DISEASE

Inflammatory bowel disease (IBD) is the term used to describe Crohn's disease and ulcerative colitis (UC). Crohn's disease and UC are diseases characterized by inflammation and ulcerations of the bowel (Table 34-4).

Crohn's disease is characterized by lesions that affect the entire thickness of the bowel and can occur anywhere throughout the colon and small intestine. Symptoms include abdominal pain, diarrhea that usually does not contain blood, fever, anorexia, weight loss, and **steatorrhea** (fatty stools). Electrolyte imbalances, iron deficiency anemia, and amino acid malabsorption may occur when the disease involves the jejunum and the ileum. Long-term complications of Crohn's disease include bowel obstructions, fistulas, abscesses, and perforation. The risk for colorectal cancer, while not as high as in UC, is still elevated. There is malabsorption of fat and fat-soluble vitamins.

UC is characterized by mucosal lesions occurring typically in the rectal area and sigmoid colon and progressing throughout the colon. The lesions may progress from pinpoint hemorrhages to abscesses, ulceration, and necrosis (Martin, 1997). Symptoms include fever, anorexia, weight loss, cramping, spasms, abdominal pain, and bloody diarrhea. Long-term complications include fissures, abscesses, and an increased risk for colorectal cancer. Toxic megacolon, a severe, acute dilation of the colon, may occur in severe cases.

Tests to diagnose Crohn's disease and UC include barium enema with small bowel follow-through, and colonoscopy with biopsies. Early symptoms for Crohn's disease and UC are similar and can make early diagnosis difficult.

Medical–Surgical Management

Medical

Treatment for Crohn's disease and UC is similar. Crohn's disease, however, is more debilitating since it involves more of the GI tract. UC is more limited, but can still produce significant symptoms.

A sigmoidoscopy done on a UC client will reveal continuous mucosal inflammation and ulceration, loss of mucosal vascularity, diffuse erythema, and often purulent exudate. A barium enema and x-rays may show stricture, pseudopolyps, and loss of **haustra** (the saclike pouches of the colon) (Martin, 1997).

The goals of treatment are to control inflammation, relieve symptoms, maintain fluid and electrolyte balance, provide adequate nutrition, and prevent complications (Martin, 1997).

Surgical

In severe cases of UC resistant to medical management, the colon is removed and an ileostomy is performed, curing the disease. An **ileostomy** is an opening created in the small intestine (ileum). The output from an ileostomy is a thin liquid, usually of a yellowish-green color. This thin output is called **effluent**. It generally has no odor, and may get thicker in time as the body adapts to the need to retain moisture. Many ileostomies have almost constant effluent output. The Kock continent ileostomy has a pouch made inside the abdomen to hold the effluent until the client is ready to empty the pouch. Figure 34-8 illustrates a Kock continent ileostomy.

Most clients with Crohn's disease need surgery at some point to repair the structural damage caused by scarring. Intestinal obstructions and perforations may also occur in Crohn's disease, necessitating further surgery. Surgical intervention, however, does not cure the disease.

Table 34-4 COMPARISON OF CROHN'S DISEASE AND ULCERATIVE COLITIS

PARAMETER	CROHN'S DISEASE	ULCERATIVE COLITIS (UC)
Involvement	Patchy areas. Can involve small and large intestine.	Starts in lower colon and spreads progressively throughout colon.
Tissue affected	Affects entire thickness of bowel.	Affects mucosal lining of bowel.
Major complication	Malabsorption.	Toxic megacolon.
Long-term complications	Intestinal obstruction, fistulas, abscesses, perforations; cancer risk increases with age.	Fissures, abscesses, increased risk for colorectal cancer.
Surgical intervention	Usually needed at some point to repair structural damage. Does not cure or limit the progress of the disease.	Ileostomy performed in approximately 20% of cases to remove the colon. Cures the disease.
Cause	Unknown: possibly altered immune state.	Unknown: possibly enteric bacterium *E. coli*.
Stools	3 to 4 semisoft/day; rarely bloody; steatorrhea and mucus present.	15 to 20 liquid/day; blood present; no steatorrhea.

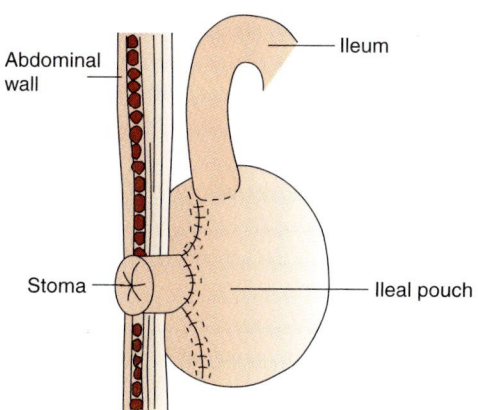

Figure 34-8 A Kock Continent Ileostomy

Pharmacological

Treatment for both UC and Crohn's disease includes 5-ASA compounds such as sulfasalazine (Azulfidine) or salicylates such as mesalamine (Rowasa) or olsalazine sodium (Dipentum). If inflammation is severe, corticosteroids may also be administered. In cases resistant to the 5-ASA compounds and corticosteroids, immunosuppressors may be used. If an infection is present, antibiotics will be administered. According to Martin (1997), clients are seldom given antidiarrheal medications since they may precipitate colonic dilation.

Clients may need IV fluid and electrolyte replacement during severe flare-ups. In the most severe cases, clients may be placed on total parenteral nutrition (TPN) to allow for complete bowel rest and to improve nutritional status.

Diet

Malnutrition is a particular concern in clients with IBD. Because of the severe cramping, pain, and diarrhea brought on by foods, these clients typically put themselves on a very restrictive diet that is not nutritionally balanced. Clients with Crohn's disease may also have malabsorption of iron, vitamin B_{12}, and amino acids, and may develop lactose intolerance.

Nutritional support includes modifying the diet to eliminate foods that exacerbate symptoms while maintaining a balanced diet. A high-calorie, low-residue, nonspicy, caffeine-free diet that uses few milk products is recommended (Martin, 1997).

Health Promotion

Although stress has not been shown to exacerbate the symptoms of Crohn's disease or UC, the impact on the client's lifestyle can be significant, especially with Crohn's disease. Support groups can be beneficial. Clients should be encouraged to develop mechanisms to help them cope with the disease process and reduce stress. Exercise, meditation, and biofeedback are often helpful.

▶ NURSING PROCESS

▶ Assessment

▶ Subjective Data

Clients may complain of mild abdominal spasms and cramping, which may increase to severe abdominal pain, nausea, and anorexia. Clients with UC may have an urge to defecate with the cramping.

▶ Objective Data

Clients show abdominal tenderness on palpation, guarding, distention, weight loss, diarrhea, an elevated WBC count, and fever. In clients with Crohn's disease, steatorrhea and iron deficient anemia may be present. In clients with UC, stools may be positive for blood and the H & H may be low. The serum potassium, magnesium, and albumin levels are usually low. Because Crohn's disease is so debilitating, clients may also look and act depressed or exhibit a flat affect.

CLIENT TEACHING

IBD

- Schedule a colon cancer screening regularly.
- If taking oral corticosteroids, strictly adhere to the prescribed schedule for taking medication.

Nursing diagnoses for clients with Crohn's disease or UC may include the following:

Nursing Diagnoses	Planning/Goals	Nursing Interventions
▶ *Nutrition, Altered, less than body requirements, related to postprandial pain, bowel hypermobility, and decreased absorption*	The client will demonstrate adequate nutritional status as exhibited by maintaining weight within range for height and body type.	Monitor I & O every shift; caloric count and weight daily.
		Administer IV fluid and electrolyte replacement as ordered.
		Provide high-calorie, high-protein supplements as ordered along with small, frequent meals.
		Administer TPN, a high-calorie and nutrient-dense IV solution, as ordered.
		If TPN is administered, closely monitor lab reports for electrolytes and glucose level.

continued

Nursing Diagnoses	Planning/Goals	Nursing Interventions
▶ *Fluid Volume Deficit, Risk for, related to diarrhea and altered intake*	The client will exhibit adequate hydration as evidenced by electrolytes within normal range, moist mucous membranes, and I & O nearly equal within 48 hours of start of intervention. The frequency and amount of diarrhea will decrease within 48 hours of start of intervention.	Administer 5-ASA compounds, corticosteroids, and immunosuppressors as ordered. Monitor I & O every shift. Administer IV fluid and electrolyte rehydration as ordered.
▶ *Powerlessness, related to impairment in lifestyle secondary to disease process*	The client will verbalize a plan to seek support, by discharge.	Provide client with information on national organizations and local support groups. Allow client to verbalize feelings. Arrange social work consult if needed.

Evaluation Each goal must be evaluated to determine how it has been met by the client.

INTESTINAL OBSTRUCTION

An intestinal obstruction, sometimes called an *ileus,* occurs when the contents cannot pass through the intestine. Obstructions may occur in the large or the small intestine, with most occurring in the ileum. Obstructions may be mechanical, neurogenic, or vascular in origin.

A mechanical obstruction may be a partial or complete obstruction caused by a tumor; fecal impaction; hernia; **volvulus,** a twisting of the bowel on itself; **intussusception,** a telescoping of the bowel where the bowel slides inside itself; (Figure 34-9); or **adhesions,** scar tissue in the abdomen from previous surgeries or disease process such as Crohn's disease.

A neurogenic obstruction, known as a *paralytic ileus,* occurs when nerve transmission to the bowel is interrupted by trauma, infection, or medications, resulting in a portion of the bowel being paralyzed.

A vascular obstruction occurs when blood flow to a portion of the bowel is interrupted, as in atherosclerosis, and that portion of the bowel becomes necrotic.

When the small intestine becomes obstructed, large amounts of fluid, bacteria, and swallowed air build up in the bowel proximal to the obstruction. The normal process of secretion and absorption of the electrolyte-rich fluid is interrupted. Distention and poor absorption occur when water and salts move from the circulatory system to the lumen of the intestine.

An abdominal x-ray and a barium enema or UGI with small bowel follow-through may be ordered when a bowel obstruction is suspected.

Medical–Surgical Management

Medical

Treatment of the obstruction is dependent on the cause and location. Some can be treated medically by inserting an NG tube for decompression, providing IV fluids for rehydration, and treating the cause, such as the use of enemas for fecal impaction.

Surgical

Most bowel obstructions require surgery. A bowel resection is performed to remove the portion of the bowel affected by the obstruction.

Pharmacological

Nonnarcotic analgesics are used to avoid the intestinal motility decrease caused by narcotic analgesics. Antibiotics may also be ordered.

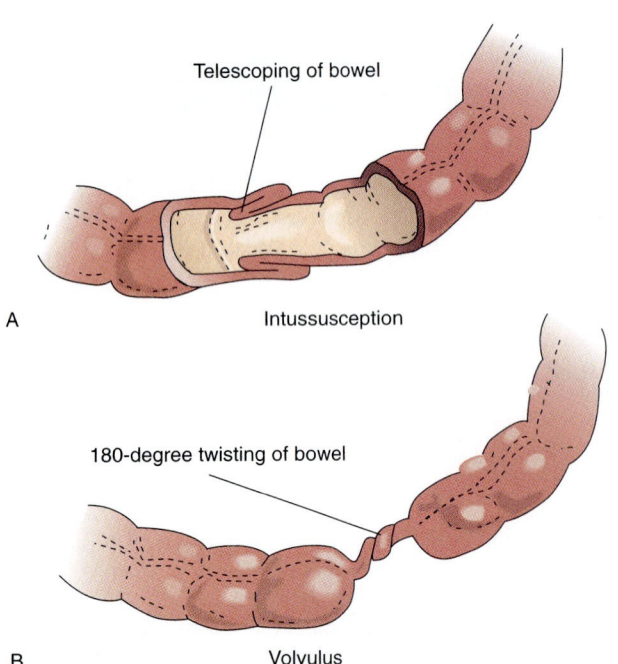

Telescoping of bowel

A   Intussusception

180-degree twisting of bowel

B   Volvulus

Figure 34-9 Bowel Obstructions. Can be caused by: A. An intussusception; or B. A volvulus

Activity

In cases of paralytic ileus, ambulation should be encouraged to help bowel function return. Clients who have had a bowel resection should be encouraged to turn, cough, and deep breathe every 2 hours initially postoperatively. Activity should be progressed the next day.

▶ NURSING PROCESS

▶ Assessment

▶ Subjective Data

Clients may complain of colicky abdominal pain, nausea, constipation, and bloating.

▶ Objective Data

Objective assessment includes abdominal distention and tenderness on palpation. Vomiting temporarily relieves the abdominal pain. The vomitus may include fecal material.

Laboratory analysis demonstrates decreased levels of sodium and potassium on electrolytes, elevated BUN, elevated amylase, and elevated H & H due to hemoconcentration.

Nursing diagnoses for a client with an intestinal obstruction may include the following:

Nursing Diagnoses	Planning/Goals	Nursing Interventions
▶ Fluid Volume Deficit, related to vomiting, shift in fluids, and NPO status	The client will exhibit adequate hydration within 48 hours of initiation of treatment as evidenced by moist mucous membranes, electrolytes within normal limits, and I & O approximately equal.	Monitor I & O every shift. Administer IV fluid and electrolyte replacements as ordered. Assess weight daily.
▶ Pain, Acute, related to distention, edema, or ischemia	The client will verbalize increased comfort within 1 hour of analgesic administration as measured on pain scale.	Administer nonnarcotic analgesics as ordered. In clients with a paralytic ileus, encourage ambulation to encourage return of bowel function. Maintain and monitor NG tube as ordered for abdominal decompression. Check bowel sounds every 4 hours or PRN.
▶ Knowledge Deficit, related to disease process, treatment regimen, and possible surgery	The client will verbalize treatment course, possible complications, and possible need for surgery.	Identify client's learning style and present information in a manner compatible with learning style. Include intestinal decompression, need for ambulation, need for good oral care due to fecal drainage, and surgery.

Evaluation Each goal must be evaluated to determine how it has been met by the client.

HERNIAS

A hernia occurs when the wall of a muscle weakens and the intestine protrudes through the muscle wall (Figure 34-10). Hernias that do not return to the abdominal cavity with rest or manipulation and cause complete bowel obstruction are said to be *incarcerated*. If the blood supply to the hernia is cut off, the hernia is said to be *strangulated*. Immediate surgery is required to restore the blood supply. If this is not done, gangrene will develop and the situation may be fatal.

Several types of hernias exist. In an umbilical hernia, a portion of the bowel protrudes through the umbilicus. In children, these generally resolve on their own once the child begins to walk. Umbilical hernias

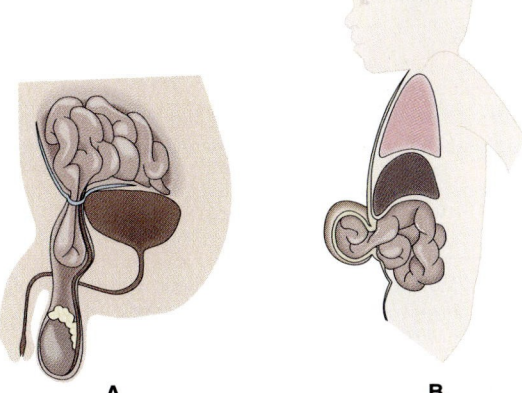

A.   **B.**

Figure 34-10 Two Types of Hernias: A. Inguinal; B. Umbilical. If the blood flow to the bowel is cut off, the hernia is said to be strangulated.

most commonly occur in a multiparous female or in adults having cirrhosis with **ascites** (abnormal accumulation of fluid in the peritoneal cavity). Due to a high risk for strangulation in adults with umbilical hernias, surgery is usually performed.

Abdominal hernias occur in the midline of the abdomen between the umbilicus and the xyphoid process. Most are asymptomatic with a few causing pain on exertion that resolves with reclining and rest.

Inguinal hernias, the most common hernia, occur in the groin area. Inguinal hernias frequently occur after activities, such as lifting, that increase intraabdominal pressure; they subside with relaxation. Pain is located lower than in the abdominal hernia.

Femoral hernias occur when the intestine pushes into the passageway carrying blood vessels and nerves to the legs, and are more common in women than in men.

A hiatal hernia occurs when a portion of the stomach protrudes into the mediastinal cavity through the diaphragm. Symptoms of hiatal hernias include indigestion and heartburn, especially after eating a large meal.

Upon evaluation and recommendation of a physician, some hernias can be reduced or pushed back into place. This can be accomplished by having the client recline, applying direct pressure to the hernia and, in some cases, having the client exhale to decrease intraabdominal pressure. The nurse should never try to reduce a hernia.

Medical–Surgical Management

Medical

Because some hernias have no symptoms or have minimal symptoms, clients may not be aware they have one or may simply learn to live with it by reducing it when needed. Clients who are a poor surgical risk may use a truss, a device that applies pressure to the hernia, thus keeping it in the abdominal cavity.

Surgical

Hernias can be repaired with a surgery called a herniorrhaphy. The surgery is typically performed on an outpatient basis with clients going home the same day. If the surgery is more complicated because the hernia is incarcerated, the client may stay overnight.

If the hernia is strangulated, surgery is required to restore the blood flow; a bowel resection may even be required.

Surgical repair of a hiatal hernia involves reinforcing the esophagus with a portion of the stomach. The surgery is performed laparoscopically with the client remaining in the hospital 3 to 5 days postoperatively. Initially, the client will have an NG tube. The NG tube is removed 24 to 48 hours later and the diet gradually progressed to a soft diet.

Diet

Clients with hiatal hernias may need to modify their dietary patterns to include small frequent meals, and to avoid eating after supper, lying down for 2 hours after eating, and aggravating foods.

▶ NURSING PROCESS

▶ Assessment

▶ Subjective Data

Clients may complain of pain at the site of the hernia.

▶ Objective Data

Assessment may show a bulge through the abdominal wall. If the hernia is strangulated, the client will have the symptoms of a bowel obstruction.

Nursing diagnoses for a client with a hernia may include the following:

Nursing Diagnoses	Planning/Goals	Nursing Interventions
▶ *Pain, Acute, related to tissue edema*	The client will experience less pain within 1 hour of intervention as measured on the pain scale.	Administer analgesics as ordered. Evaluate aggravating activities (e.g., straining to have a bowel movement) and provide information on modification if indicated. Educate regarding signs of complications and when to notify staff of symptoms.
▶ *Tissue Perfusion (gastrointestinal), Altered, related to strangulation*	The client will have minimal tissue necrosis.	Assess abdomen for bowel sounds every 4 hours. Insert NG tube to decrease abdominal distention as ordered. Prepare client for surgery as ordered. Keep client NPO. Administer IV hydration as ordered.

Evaluation Each goal must be evaluated to determine how it has been met by the client.

PERITONITIS

Peritonitis is the inflammation of the peritoneum, the membranous covering of the abdomen. Peritonitis is caused by irritating substances such as feces, gastric acids, bacteria, or blood in the abdominal cavity. A ruptured portion of the digestive system (such as a the appendix) a ruptured tubal pregnancy, or invasion of tumors through the gastric wall, can lead to peritonitis. Peritonitis can be a serious, life-threatening condition. Complications following peritonitis include adhesions (scar tissue), ileus, and pneumonia.

Medical–Surgical Management

Surgical

Treatment is primarily surgical with repair of the cause and irrigation of the abdominal cavity with saline and antibiotic solutions. Drains may be left in the abdomen for several days postoperatively to allow any remaining fluid to drain. Since bowel function usually stops due to the irritating substances, an NG tube is placed to decompress the abdomen and relieve nausea.

Pharmacological

Analgesics will be ordered postoperatively for discomfort. If an ileus develops, nonnarcotic analgesics will be ordered. Antibiotics will also be ordered preoperatively and postoperatively.

Diet

Clients will be NPO preoperatively and postoperatively until bowel sounds return. Clients will then be placed on a clear liquid diet and slowly progressed to a regular diet as more bowel function returns.

Activity

Preoperatively, clients will be placed on bed rest. Postoperatively, clients need to be encouraged to turn, cough, and deep breathe. Because clients tend to breathe shallowly with peritoneal inflammation, pulmonary hygiene is important. Activity should be progressed postoperatively, as soon as tolerated, to increase lung expansion and to encourage bowel function return. Exercise, lifting, and driving will be restricted until the incision heals.

▶ NURSING PROCESS

▶ Assessment

▶ Subjective Data

Clients may describe abdominal pain, nausea, and constipation.

▶ Objective Data

Assessment may reveal vomiting, absent bowel sounds, a tense or distended abdomen with tenderness on palpation, shallow and rapid respirations, weak and rapid pulse, dry mucous membranes, low urine output, fever, and limited mobility because of pain.

Laboratory analysis will include a CBC, which will show an elevated WBC. If bleeding is occurring, the H & H will be low. Electrolytes may show low sodium, potassium, and chloride.

Nursing diagnoses for a client with peritonitis may include the following:

Nursing Diagnoses	Planning/Goals	Nursing Interventions
▶ *Fluid Volume Deficit (Active Loss), related to gastric losses and restricted intake*	The client will maintain hydration as indicated by an I & O that is nearly equal and electrolytes within normal limits.	Monitor I & O every shift. Monitor for signs of dehydration: dry mucous membranes, poor skin turgor, and low urine output. Monitor electrolytes as ordered. Administer IV rehydration and electrolyte replacement as ordered.
▶ *Hyperthermia, related to inflammatory process and dehydration*	The client will maintain temperature within normal limits.	Assess VS including temperature every 4 hours. Administer antipyretics as ordered; probably rectal suppositories due to NPO status. Monitor for dehydration: decrease in urine output, dry mucous membranes, and poor skin turgor. Provide comfort measures: cool cloth to the head or neck, assistance to turn, and a back rub with cooling lotion.
▶ *Pain, Acute, related to abdominal distention*	The client will have less pain and improved mobility within 1 hour of receiving analgesics as measured on the pain scale.	Administer analgesics as ordered. Encourage activity such as coughing and deep breathing after analgesics. Monitor NG tube to decompress abdomen. Maintain patency of NG tube. Teach splinting of incision for cough and deep breathing.

Evaluation Each goal must be evaluated to determine how it has been met by the client.

HEMORRHOIDS

Hemorrhoids are swollen vascular tissues in the rectal area. The hemorrhoids may be internal or external. Hemorrhoids may be caused by straining with constipation. Sitting on the toilet (reading) for an extended time may also be a cause. Hemorrhoids frequently occur with pregnancy. Hemorrhoids can cause burning, pruritis, and pain with defecation. At times, hemorrhoids can bleed, leading to anemia.

Medical–Surgical Management

Medical

Sitz baths or warm compresses on the rectal area for 20 minutes, 4 times a day, often helps decrease swelling.

Surgical

If bleeding continues despite medical intervention, or if discomfort is significant, the hemorrhoids can be surgically removed by a hemorrhoidectomy. If hemorrhoids are external, surgery is performed on an outpatient basis by placing a rubber band around the hemorrhoid, allowing it to necrose and fall off on its own. If hemorrhoids are internal, surgery can be done using sclerotherapy, cryotherapy, or laser. This usually requires an overnight stay in the hospital. Hemorrhoids can recur after surgical removal if the cause is not eliminated.

Pharmacological

Treatment includes creams and suppositories to decrease inflammation, some with cortisone to decrease swelling. Fiber supplements and stool softeners may be ordered to keep bowel movements soft.

Diet

Bowel movements can be kept soft with a high-fiber diet of 20 to 30 grams of fiber a day and at least 2,500 cc of fluid intake daily.

▶ NURSING PROCESS

▶ Assessment

▶ Subjective Data

Clients may complain of rectal burning, pain, and pruritis with bowel movements; constipation; and, occasionally, bright red bleeding. A dietary history should be obtained to determine fiber and fluid intake.

▶ Objective Data

If hemorrhoids are external, they can be visualized during a physical examination. If chronic bleeding is present, laboratory analysis may show a low H & H.

Nursing diagnoses for a client with hemorrhoids may include the following:

Nursing Diagnoses	Planning/Goals	Nursing Interventions
▶ *Pain, Acute, related to edema and inflammation of swollen vascular tissues*	The client will verbalize a decrease in discomfort within 48 hours of initiation of treatment.	Provide sitz baths or warm compresses for 20 minutes, 4 times a day. Administer creams and suppositories as ordered. Increase fiber and fluids in diet to keep stools soft to avoid straining.
▶ *Knowledge Deficit, related to diet, causes of condition, treatment, and potential complications*	The client will be able to verbalize treatment regimen and long-term management of hemorrhoids.	Determine client's learning style and present information in a manner compatible with learning style. Educate client about increasing fiber in diet to 20 to 30 grams per day, increasing fluid intake to 2,500 cc per day, causes of hemorrhoids, possible complications such as anemia, and modification of bowel habits (such as not sitting on the toilet for long periods).

Evaluation Each goal must be evaluated to determine how it has been met by the client.

CONSTIPATION

Constipation is characterized by hard, infrequent stools that are difficult and/or painful to pass. Constipation can be caused by tumors, low-fiber diet, inactivity, some diseases that interfere with the mechanical functioning of the bowel (such as multiple sclerosis), or some medications (such as narcotics, antidepressants, or anti-Parkinson drugs).

Medical–Surgical Management

Pharmacological

Fiber supplements and stool softeners may be ordered. Laxatives and enemas may be ordered, but long-term use should be avoided as they interrupt normal bowel function. If constipation is caused by medications the client is taking, the client should discuss with the physician other options such as modifying the dosage or changing medications.

Diet

Fiber should be increased to 20 to 30 grams a day. Fluid intake should be increased to 2,500 cc a day.

Activity

Activity level should be increased if possible as exercise, such as walking, increases motility in the colon.

LIFE CYCLE CONSIDERATIONS

Constipation in the Older Client

The slowing of peristalsis, which is part of the aging process, may lead to constipation in the older client. An increase in dietary fiber and fluid intake (water) will help prevent constipation. A regular schedule for bowel evacuation is also helpful.

▸ NURSING PROCESS

▸ Assessment

▸ Subjective Data

Clients complain of infrequent, difficult to pass stools. Dietary assessment of fiber and fluids usually reveals inadequate intake. Activity/exercise levels should also be assessed.

▸ Objective Data

Bowel movements will be hard-formed.

Nursing diagnoses for a client with constipation may include the following:

Nursing Diagnoses	Planning/Goals	Nursing Interventions
▸ Constipation related to inadequate intake of fiber and fluids	The client will have soft stools every other day by one week from start of intervention.	Encourage client to increase fiber in the diet to 20 to 30 grams a day and fluid intake to 2,500 cc a day. Administer fiber supplements and stool softeners as ordered. Determine fluid preferences of client and always have fluids at client's bedside within reach. Help the client establish a regular schedule for bowel movements, usually 30 minutes after a meal.
▸ Knowledge Deficit related to dietary sources of fiber and the importance of adequate fluid intake and exercise	The client will be able to select a menu high in fiber and fluids utilizing nutrients from the food pyramid within 48 hours and verbalize the need for adequate exercise.	Assess client's learning style and present information in a manner compatible with learning style. Teach client about foods that are high in fiber (fruits, vegetables, whole grains) as well as importance of fluid intake. Discuss with client importance of exercise in maintaining bowel function.

Evaluation Each goal must be evaluated to determine how it has been met by the client.

DISORDERS OF THE ACCESSORY ORGANS

Disorders of the accessory organs include: cirrhosis, hepatitis, pancreatitis, and cholecystitis/cholelithiasis.

CIRRHOSIS

Cirrhosis refers to the chronic, degenerative changes in the liver cells and thickening of surrounding tissue that result from the liver repairing itself after chronic inflammation. Causes of cirrhosis include chronic hepatitis, repeated exposure to toxic substances, disease processes (such as sclerosing cholangitis and hemochromatosis), cancer, and chronic alcohol abuse. Alcohol abuse accounts for most cases of cirrhosis.

Because the liver is responsible for so many functions, complications can be significant. Complications include: malnutrition, hypoglycemia, clotting disorders, jaundice, portal hypertension, ascites, hepatic encephalopathy, and hepatorenal syndrome.

Liver dysfunction causes several organ-related complications. Malnutrition results from the liver's inability to absorb fat and fat soluble vitamins, and leads to muscle wasting, weight loss, and fatigue. Hypoglycemia occurs when the liver is unable to perform glycogenolysis efficiently. Clotting disorders result when the liver is not able to produce sufficient amounts of prothrombin and fibrinogen.

Portal hypertension results when blood flow through the cirrhotic liver is inhibited, resulting in blood backflowing in the portal vein. Portal hypertension leads to distention of the esophageal veins, resulting in esophageal varices.

Because the liver is responsible for metabolizing medications, clients frequently become intolerant to some medications. Jaundice, a yellow discoloration of the skin, is usually present. Jaundice occurs when the liver is unable to convert bilirubin, an end product of red blood cell breakdown, into a water soluble form that can be excreted in the bile. The extra bilirubin collects in areas that contain elastin such as the sclera of the eyes, the skin, and the nail beds.

When blood flow through the cirrhotic liver is inhibited, blood backs up into the portal system. Congestion of blood in the portal system causes distention of the esophageal, gastric, mesenteric, splenic, and portal veins. The backflow of blood in these vessels increases the pressure in the vessels, causing portal hypertension. The distended esophageal veins cause esophageal varices (see the earlier section on esophageal varices in this chapter), and the distended rectal veins result in hemorrhoids. The distended splenic vein causes splenomegaly.

Fluid may accumulate in the pleural cavity in the form of pleural effusions. Fluid may also accumulate in the peritoneal cavity. This condition is called ascites. The cause of ascites is the congestion of blood in the portal system.

Hepatic encephalopathy is a condition in which too much ammonia accumulates in the bloodstream from the liver's inability to filter proteins and protein by-products. Confusion, lethargy, and/or coma may occur. Symptoms of impending hepatic encephalopathy are disorientation and asterixis (liver flap), a flapping tremor of the hands. When the client extends the arms and hands in front of the body, the hands rapidly flex and extend.

Hepatorenal syndrome is a complication of cirrhosis in which the client goes into renal failure. Symptoms include oliguria (diminished production of urine), azotemia (excess nitrogen in the blood), anorexia, fatigue, and weakness.

Cirrhosis is a form of end-stage liver disease for which there is no cure. The process of cirrhosis can be slowed by removing the cause (i.e., abstaining from alcohol), but the damage cannot be reversed. Clients in end-stage liver disease may be evaluated to determine if they qualify for a liver transplant.

Medical–Surgical Management

Medical

The physician may perform a paracentesis to remove the fluid from the abdomen and relieve pressure on the diaphragm and lungs. A paracentesis is done by making a small incision and inserting a trochar into the abdomen to drain the fluid. Albumin may be infused at the same time to pull excess fluid back into the vascular system.

Surgical

If the client continues to develop ascites after medical treatment, a LeVeen or Denver peritoneal venous shunt may be used. The pressure-regulated shunt is implanted in the peritoneal cavity and threaded through the subcutaneous tissue into the superior vena cava, returning the fluid back to the vascular system. As fluid pressure builds in the peritoneal cavity, a valve opens and drains the fluid into the superior vena cava.

If esophageal varices are present, an EGD with sclerotherapy or banding will be done to prevent hemorrhage (refer back to Figure 34-3).

If portal hypertension cannot be controlled with medications, a portosystemic shunt or a transjugular intrahepatic portosystemic shunt (TIPS) may be performed. The purpose of the shunt is to redirect the blood flow, thereby relieving the portal hypertension and decreasing the risk of rupturing distended veins in the esophagus (Figure 34-11).

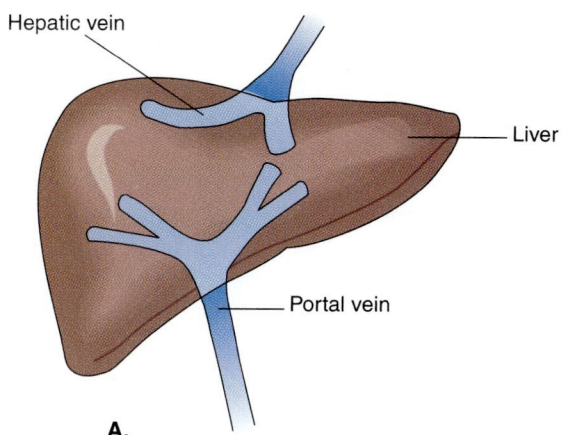

A.

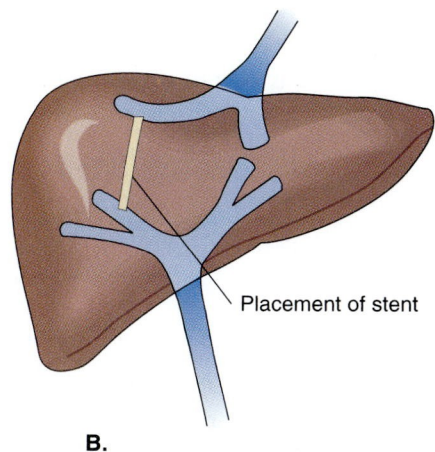

B.

Figure 34-11 A. Blood flow prior to TIPS; B. TIPS is performed in radiology on clients deemed too unstable for the surgery necessary for a portosystemic shunt. A stent is placed to redirect the blood flow.

Pharmacological

A potassium sparing diuretic, such as spironolactone (Aldactone) is used to decrease ascites and pleural effusion. Lactulose (Cholac) is used to eliminate the ammonia from the blood into the bowel. The lactulose acts as a laxative and causes the body to excrete the stool containing ammonia. Tap water enemas may also be ordered to help the body eliminate the ammonia.

Propranolol hydrochloride (Inderal), an antihypertensive medication, may be ordered to lower portal hypertension. All unnecessary medications should be avoided since the liver cannot metabolize them.

Diet

Clients with cirrhosis are placed on a low-protein diet, usually 40 grams per day. If ascites is present, sodium will also be restricted to 2 grams or less a day to decrease the amount of fluid retained by the body. Fluids may also be restricted to 1,000 cc to 2,000 cc a day depending on the severity of fluid accumulation.

Activity

 Safety: Cirrhosis

If hepatic encephalopathy is present, precautions should be taken to ensure the client's safety, such as elevating bedrails and allowing the client to ambulate only with assistance, especially if the client's gait is unsteady.

Because fatigue is such a common symptom of cirrhosis, the client's tolerance for activity will be diminished. Rest periods should be planned during the day, and activities should be scheduled between rests.

▶ NURSING PROCESS

▶ Assessment

▶ Subjective Data

Clients describe fatigue, nausea, anorexia, weakness, and indigestion.

▶ Objective Data

Assessment shows ascites, jaundice, enlarged liver and spleen, petechiae (small bruises on the skin), vomiting, weight loss, fever, epistaxis, and decreased breath sounds. Lethargy, confusion, or coma may be present if encephalopathy has occurred.

Laboratory analysis includes a CBC, which will demonstrate low WBCs, RBCs, Hgb, and platelets. A liver panel will show an elevated bilirubin, alkaline phosphatase, GGT, ALT, and AST. Albumin will be low. PT, PTT, and clotting times will be delayed.

Nursing diagnoses for a client with cirrhosis may include the following:

Nursing Diagnoses	Planning/Goals	Nursing Interventions
▶ *Fluid Volume Excess, related to ascites*	The client will have less ascites by discharge.	Weigh daily. Measure abdominal girth daily. Restrict fluid to 1,000 to 2,000 cc per day depending on the severity of the ascites.

continued

Nursing Diagnoses	Planning/Goals	Nursing Interventions
		Educate client to notify physician of weight gain of 1½ lbs or more in 1 week.
		Provide low-sodium diet of 500 to 2,000 mg a day depending on severity of the ascites.
		Teach client how to measure fluids and calculate sodium in diet.
		If a paracentesis is done, check vital signs every 15 minutes during the procedure and after the procedure until the vitals are stable. The amount of fluid removed from the abdomen should be measured and sent to the laboratory.
▶ *Skin Integrity, Impaired, High risk for, related to accumulation of bile salts in skin, poor skin turgor, ascites, and edema*	The client will not experience skin breakdown while hospitalized.	Provide egg crate mattress.
		Turn client every 2 hours.
		Monitor skin closely for redness and skin breakdown.
		Apply lotion to skin frequently, especially to pressure areas. Assist with ADLs to promote good hygiene and conserve client's energy.
▶ *Nutrition, Altered, Less than body requirements, related to inadequate diet, anorexia, or vomiting*	The client will eat a balanced diet of 1,500 calories a day.	Offer small, high-calorie meals frequently.
		Assist and encourage client to eat.
		Offer high-nutrient supplements if client is unable to maintain adequate caloric intake.
		Provide frequent oral hygiene.
		Observe for changes in mental status that would interfere with caloric intake (e.g., increased lethargy).

Evaluation Each goal must be evaluated to determine how it has been met by the client.

HEPATITIS

Hepatitis is a chronic or acute inflammation of the liver caused by a virus, bacteria, drugs, alcohol abuse, or other toxic substances. There is a diffuse inflammatory reaction with liver cells degenerating and dying. The functions of the liver slow down. Since viral infections are the most common cause of hepatitis, emphasis will be placed on viral hepatitis.

Researchers are still learning about the viruses that cause hepatitis. Five viruses are known to cause hepatitis: A, B, C, D, and E. The viruses are similar and have almost identical signs and symptoms. Incubation period, mode of transmission, and prognosis vary. See Table 34-5 for a summary of the hepatitis viruses.

Medical–Surgical Management

Treatment is focused on resting the liver and early detection of complications. The liver is rested by modifying the diet so that less bile is needed to digest the food. Treatment is related to the signs and symptoms present and the prevention of transmission.

Pharmacological

Antiemetics such as hydroxyzine hydrochloride (Atarax, also Vistaril) or trimethobenzamide hydrochloride (Tigan) may be given before meals if nausea is present. IV hydration with vitamin C for healing may be ordered. Vitamin B complex may also be ordered to help client absorb fat-soluble vitamins. Vitamin K may be ordered if clotting time is prolonged. All unnecessary medications, especially sedatives, should be avoided.

Those exposed to hepatitis B by needle puncture or sexual contact should have hepatitis B immunoglobin (HBIG). A vaccine for hepatitis A (HAV) is available and provides protection for up to 10 years or more. HAV is recommended for people at risk for exposure to hepatitis A such as homosexuals, IV drug users, travelers to countries with poor sanitation conditions, and laboratory workers who handle live hepatitis A virus.

 LIFE CYCLE CONSIDERATIONS

Hepatitis B Vaccine

Newborns whose mothers test positive for hepatitis B are given the vaccine immediately after birth. For other infants, the hepatitis B vaccine has been added to the vaccine schedule.

Table 34-5 COMPARISON OF DIFFERENT TYPES OF VIRAL HEPATITIS

FACTORS	HEPATITIS VIRUS				
	A	**B**	**C**	**D**	**E**
Other Names	Infectious hepatitis	Serum hepatitis	Post transfusion non-A, non-B hepatitis	Delta virus	Enteric non-A hepatitis
Routes of Transmission	Fecal-oral: Spread by feces, saliva, and contaminated food and water.	Parenteral or sexual: Spread by blood and blood products (via transfusion, needle stick, or IV drug use); body fluids such as saliva, semen, and vaginal secretions; maternal-fetal transmission; and unknown exposures.	Parenteral: Spread by blood and blood products (via transfusion, needle stick, or IV drug use) and unknown exposures.	Appears as a co-infection with hepatitis B; transmitted the same way as hepatitis B.	Fecal-oral: Spread through contaminated water.
Incubation Period	15–50 days	45–160 days	14–180 days	15–64 days	15–50 days
Infectivity Period	Latter half of incubation period until 1–2 weeks after symptoms start.	Begins before symptoms appear and may continue for client's lifetime if client becomes a carrier.	Begins before onset of symptoms and may continue for client's lifetime if client becomes a carrier.	Not known.	Not known.
Diagnostic Tests	Anti-HAV igM	HBsAG, HBeAG, anti-HBs, and anti-HBc (numerous other blood tests can also be used)	Anti-HCV	Anti-HDV	No test available
Preventive Measures and Post-exposure Treatment	Standard and enteric precautions indicated; vaccine available; vaccine and immune globulin therapy indicated for postexposure prophylaxis.	Standard precautions indicated; vaccine available; vaccine and hepatitis B immune globulin therapy indicated for postexposure prophylaxis; recombinant interferon alfa-2b injections indicated for chronic state.	Standard precautions indicated; no vaccine available; recombinant interferon alfa-2b injections indicated for chronic state.	Standard precautions indicated; vaccine and hepatitis B immune globulin therapy indicated for postexposure prophylaxis; experimental use of recombinant interferon alfa-2b injections still being studied.	Standard and enteric precautions indicated; no vaccine available; no postexposure prophylaxis available.
Prognosis	Rarely fatal; no carrier state or chronicity; lifelong immunity.	High mortality rate; client can become immune or can become chronic carrier; 5–10% of cases progress to chronic hepatitis; chronic hepatitis B associated with liver cancer.	Client can become chronic carrier; 50% of all cases progress to chronic hepatitis, and 20% of chronic cases progress to cirrhosis; possibly associated with liver cancer.	Frequently leads to chronic, active hepatitis and death; client can become carrier, immunity to B gives client immunity to D.	Does not progress to chronic hepatitis but has a 10% mortality rate in pregnant women.

Diet

Diet modifications may include decreasing fat intake to decrease the amount of bile needed in the digestive tract. A low-protein diet may be needed if the liver is no longer able to metabolize the protein. Anorexia is a common symptom that can be treated with small, frequent, high-calorie meals. Fluids may be restricted if the client is starting to retain fluids. No alcoholic beverages are recommended for at least 1 year or longer.

Activity

Bed rest is usually recommended for the first several weeks, generally at home unless the serum bilirubin is greater than 10 mg/dL or the PT is prolonged. If either occurs, hospitalization is usually recommended.

Once bed rest is no longer necessary, activity should be increased gradually as fatigue will be present for up to several months. Rest periods should be included throughout the day.

▶ NURSING PROCESS

▶ Assessment

▶ Subjective Data

Symptoms may include fatigue, anorexia, photo-phobia, nausea, headaches, abdominal pain, general-ized muscle aches, chills, pruritis, and bloating.

▶ Objective Data

The client may have weight loss, hepatomegaly, fever, jaundice, dark amber urine, and clay-colored stools.

Laboratory analysis will show an elevated bilirubin, GGT, AST, ALT, LDH, and alkaline phosphatase. Clot-ting time and PT will be prolonged. Specific hepatitis test will be elevated (refer back to Table 34-5).

Nursing diagnoses for the client with hepatitis may include the following:

Nursing Diagnoses	Planning/Goals	Nursing Interventions
▶ *Knowledge Deficit re-lated to disease process, treatment regimen, and mode of transmission*	The client will be able to explain disease process, incubation period, and mode of transmission, by discharge. The client will practice pre-cautions to prevent spread of disease. The client will be able to select a menu using foods from the food guide pyramid and maintain a low-fat, low-protein diet.	Assess client's learning style and present information in a manner compatible with learning style.
		Educate about disease process and incubation period.
		Teach proper handwashing technique and emphasize importance of washing hands after using the bathroom.
		Emphasize that client cannot donate blood.
		Emphasize importance of follow-up laboratory analysis.
		Instruct in selection of low-fat, low-protein diet.
		For clients with hepatitis A, teach client to disinfect articles contam-inated with feces (such as the toilet), not to prepare food for oth-ers, and not to share articles such as eating utensils or toothbrushes.
		For clients with hepatitis B, teach to avoid sexual contact until they test negative for HBsAg or their partners are immunized with the HBV vaccine.
		For clients with hepatitis C, teach that it is unknown whether it can be transmitted through sexual contact, so precautions are recom-mended until more is known.
▶ *Nutrition, Altered, Less than Body Requirements, related to inadequate caloric intake, fat intol-erance, nausea, and vomiting*	The client will maintain a caloric intake of 2,000 calo-ries/day.	Monitor daily calorie count.
		Monitor I & O every shift.
		Weigh daily.
		Offer small, frequent, high-calorie, low-fat meals. Encourage low-protein diet of 40 gm of protein.
		Offer largest meal in morning, as food tends to be tolerated better in the morning.
		Note color and consistency of stools and color of urine.
		Encourage fluid intake of 2,500 to 3,000 cc daily.
		Administer antiemetic 30 minutes before meals as ordered.
▶ *Fatigue, related to de-creased energy produc-tion and altered body chemistry*	The client will verbalize plan to modify activity, by discharge.	Educate client regarding reasons for fatigue and that fatigue may be present for several months.
		Encourage client to maintain bed rest for several weeks. Advise client that when resuming normal activity, rest periods should be included until stamina returns.

Evaluation Each goal must be evaluated to determine how it has been met by the client.

PANCREATITIS

Pancreatitis is an acute or chronic inflammation of the pancreas caused when pancreatic enzymes digest the lining of the pancreas. Pancreatitis occurs when obstruction of the pancreatic duct occurs as a result of gallstones, tumors, exposure to chemicals or alcohol, or injury to the pancreas. In severe cases, the pancreas can hemorrhage resulting in a life-threatening condition.

Medical–Surgical Management

Medical

Treatment is dependent upon the cause of the pan-creatitis. If the pancreatitis results from exposure to chemical or alcohol abuse, treatment is primarily med-ical. An NG tube is inserted to rest the bowel and re-lieve abdominal distention.

Surgical

If the pancreatitis is caused by structural changes such as gallstones, an ERCP with stone removal may be performed. Surgery to relieve the pancreatic duct obstruction may be necessary in cases where tumors or injury are the causes of the pancreatitis.

Pharmacological

Insulin may be given if the pancreas is unable to secrete enough to maintain normal blood sugar level. If nausea and vomiting are present, antiemetics may be ordered. Meperidine (Demerol) will be ordered for analgesia as morphine sulfate may cause spasms of the sphincter of Oddi. Atropine sulfate or propantheline bromide (Pro-Banthine) may be ordered to decrease pancreatic activity. Antacids or an H_2 receptor antagonist may be ordered to prevent stress ulcers.

Diet

Clients are kept NPO while the serum amylase level is elevated to decrease the demand for digestive enzymes in the bowel. An NG tube may be inserted to decrease pancreatic activity, and to prevent nausea, vomiting, and abdominal distention. As the serum amylase level begins to decrease, clients will be started on clear liquids and slowly advanced to a bland, low-fat, high-protein, high-carbohydrate diet. No coffee or alcohol is allowed.

IV rehydration is necessary while the client is NPO. If the pancreatitis is severe and the client must be NPO for a prolonged period, TPN, a high-calorie, high-nutrient IV solution, may be administered.

Activity

Clients are frequently placed on bed rest to decrease metabolic rate. Activity can be increased as the serum amylase decreases.

▶ NURSING PROCESS

▶ Assessment

▶ Subjective Data

Clients complain of excruciating epigastric pain that radiates to the back. Pain may decrease by leaning forward or lying in a fetal position. Nausea and anorexia are also present.

▶ Objective Data

Assessment includes steatorrhea, vomiting, low-grade fever, tachycardia, and jaundice. Laboratory analysis includes an elevated serum amylase followed by an elevated urine amylase and serum lipase, leukocytosis, and an elevated Hct. Glucose, alkaline phosphatase, and bilirubin may also be elevated.

Nursing diagnoses for a client with pancreatitis may include the following:

Nursing Diagnoses	Planning/Goals	Nursing Interventions
▶ Pain, Acute, related to inflammation and edema of the pancreas	The client will verbalize a decrease in pain as evidenced by pain scale by 1 hour after initiation of interventions.	Monitor NG tube to decompress the abdomen. Administer analgesics as ordered and monitor for relief. Position client in most comfortable position. Assess pain for increasing severity that would indicate worsening pancreatitis. Monitor serum amylase, WBCs, and H & H for signs of increasing severity of pancreatitis or hemorrhage.
▶ Nutrition, Altered, less than body requirements, related to NPO status, nausea, vomiting, and altered ability to digest nutrients	The client will experience no further weight loss during hospitalization.	Monitor I & O every shift. Weigh client daily. Maintain bed rest to decrease the metabolic rate. Insert NG tube to decompress the abdomen as ordered. Administer IV rehydration or TPN as ordered.
▶ Fluid Volume Deficit, Risk for, related to vomiting, NG tube, or hemorrhage	The client will maintain adequate hydration as evidenced by I & O that is nearly equal, electrolytes within normal limits, and moist mucous membranes.	Monitor I & O every shift. Administer IV hydration or TPN as ordered. Monitor electrolyte levels and H & H as ordered.

Evaluation Each goal must be evaluated to determine how it has been met by the client.

CHOLECYSTITIS AND CHOLELITHIASIS

Cholecystitis is an inflammation of the gallbladder. In more than 90% of the cases, gallstones are present. **Cholelithiasis** is the presence of gallstones or **calculi** (concentration of mineral salts) in the gallbladder. Not all gallstones cause cholecystitis. Some gallstones may pass out of the gallbladder and into the duodenum with the client being unaware of the stones. Sometimes gallstones migrate into the cystic or common bile duct causing an obstruction that, in turn, leads to cholecystitis. The exact cause of the formation of these stones is not known.

These two diseases are more common in multiparous women, age 45 and older; obese people; those who use birth control pills or control cholesterol with gemfibrozil (Lopid); and people with a history of a disease of the small intestine such as Crohn's disease. Also, clients on sudden weight reduction diets that are low in fat will cause the bile to pool in the gallbladder, increasing the risk for gallstone formation.

Ultrasound of the gallbladder is ordered if gallstones are suspected.

Medical–Surgical Management

In asymptomatic clients, no intervention is necessary.

Medical

If stones are lodged in the common bile duct, an ERCP may be performed.

Surgical

A sphincterotomy, an incision in the ampulla of vater, may be performed to enlarge the opening of the common bile duct. Stones may then be removed or crushed. If the stones are too large or for clients with repeated episodes of cholelithiasis, a cholecystectomy, the surgical removal of the gallbladder, may be performed. The cholecystectomy may be performed laparoscopically or by making a large abdominal incision.

Laparoscopic cholecystectomies, while having been performed for less than 10 years, have become the surgery of choice for cholelithiasis and cholecystitis. The gallbladder is removed by making 4 small incisions and extracting the gallbladder through an endoscope. If the cholecystectomy is performed laparoscopically, it is more difficult to perform an exploration of the common bile duct, especially in clients with cholecystitis. An ERCP may need to be performed if stones remain in the common bile duct (CBD). Clients are ready for discharge 24 hours after the surgery.

The cholecystectomy can also be performed by making a large abdominal incision. A cholangiogram can be performed easily and therefore this type of procedure is more common in clients with much inflammation of the gallbladder. If damage has occurred to the CBD due to severe inflammation or from a stone, a T-tube will be left in place to allow the bile to drain into a collection bag. This allows the CBD to heal. Clients are typically ready for discharge 3 to 7 days after surgery. Exercise, lifting, and driving will be restricted to allow for incisional healing.

Pharmacological

In acute cholecystitis, analgesics will be ordered to relieve the discomfort. Meperidine (Demerol) is preferred over morphine sulfate as morphine sulfate is believed to increase sphincter spasms. IV hydration may also be ordered if clients are unable to maintain hydration. Antiemetics will also be ordered if nausea and vomiting are present.

In clients who have surgery, analgesics will be ordered after surgery to control discomfort.

Diet

In clients with mild or moderate symptoms, a clear liquid diet to rest the bowel, followed by small frequent meals low in fat, may resolve the symptoms.

If clients are to have surgery, they will be NPO before surgery and initially after surgery until bowel sounds return. They will then be started on clear liquids first and then advanced, as tolerated, to a regular diet.

Activity

In acute cases of cholecystitis, bed rest is recommended to decrease metabolic rate. If surgery is performed, the client will be encouraged to turn, cough, and deep breathe every 2 hours initially after surgery. On the day following surgery, the client should be helped out of bed and encouraged to gradually increase activity. Clients who have had a laparoscopic cholecystectomy may be ambulated the evening of surgery. Clients can typically return to previous activity level 2 weeks after surgery. Clients who have an incision must restrict lifting, driving, and exercise until incisional healing is complete, usually 4 to 6 weeks.

▶ NURSING PROCESS

▶ Assessment

▶ Subjective Data

Clients describe pain in the right upper quadrant radiating to the right scapular area that occurs 2 to 4 hours after a meal containing significant amounts of fat; nausea; flatulence; and indigestion.

▶ Objective Data

Assessment may show vomiting, occasionally a fever, jaundice, steatorrhea, clay-colored stools, and dark amber urine. Laboratory analysis may show elevated alkaline phosphatase, GGT, WBCs, and bilirubin.

Nursing diagnoses for a client with cholecystitis and cholelithiasis may include the following:

Nursing Diagnoses	Planning/Goals	Nursing Interventions
▶ *Pain, Acute, related to inflammation or blocked bile duct*	The client will experience less pain as evidenced by pain scale within 1 hour of initiation of treatment.	Keep client NPO or on a clear liquid diet as ordered. Administer analgesics as ordered. Monitor NG tube to decompress the abdomen as ordered. Observe for jaundice and bile flow obstruction.
▶ *Breathing Pattern, Ineffective, related to decreased lung expansion because of pain*	The client will demonstrate appropriate breathing pattern and will not have respiratory complications while hospitalized.	Assist client to cough and breathe deeply every 2 hours. Teach splinting techniques for comfort and to facilitate breathing. Turn client every 2 hours and ambulate as soon as indicated. Teach use of incentive spirometer.
▶ *Fluid Volume Deficit, Risk for, related to nausea, NG tube, NPO, or bile drainage*	The client will maintain adequate hydration as evidenced by I & O that is nearly equal and moist mucous membranes.	Monitor I & O every shift including NG drainage and T-tube drainage if present. Administer IV hydration as ordered. Maintain patency of NG tube.

Evaluation Each goal must be evaluated to determine how it has been met by the client.

NEOPLASMS OF THE GASTROINTESTINAL SYSTEM

Neoplasms of the gastrointestinal system include oral cancer, colorectal cancer, and liver cancer.

ORAL CANCER

Oral cancer refers to cancers of the lips, tongue, oral cavity, and pharynx. According to the American Cancer Society, the occurrence of oral cancer is several times more frequent in people who use tobacco. The 5-year survival rate is low, primarily because the early symptoms are ignored. Symptoms include a mouth sore that does not heal, a sore throat, or difficulty swallowing. On the lips, the cancer may be a growth.

Medical–Surgical Management

Surgical

Treatment is primarily surgical and involves removal of the cancer with excision of tissue and lymph nodes surrounding the cancer. In cases of cancer involving the pharynx, a radical neck dissection is performed, which requires reconstruction of the pharynx. Clients undergoing radical neck dissection frequently have a tracheostomy.

Pharmacological

Chemotherapy is not effective against most oral cancers and is, therefore, used only in the most severe cases with metastases. Medications ordered will be based on the client's symptoms. If the client is experiencing side effects from the radiation such as nausea, antiemetics will be ordered.

If a client has surgery, analgesics will be ordered postoperatively. Analgesics may also be ordered if the cancer has progressed and is causing discomfort.

Diet

Because the surgery is in the oral area, it may be difficult to maintain adequate nutrition. Depending on the extent of the surgery, clients may require a soft diet or, in some cases, nutritional supplements to allow the surgical area to heal. Tube feedings, either by a feeding tube or by a gastrostomy tube (a special tube inserted through the abdomen into the stomach), are frequently needed in clients who have undergone a radical neck dissection.

Activity

If the surgery is minor, no activity restrictions will be necessary. If surgery is extensive, postoperatively, the client will need to turn, cough, and deep breathe. Activity will need to be progressed postoperatively. Clients receiving radiation treatments frequently experience fatigue and must have scheduled rest periods.

Other Therapies

In cases where the lesion cannot be surgically removed, radiation or radium implants may be used. High-energy radiation is used to destroy cancer cells. Clients may experience irritated skin, swallowing difficulties, dry mouth, nausea, diarrhea, hair loss, or fatigue. If radiation is done, the client will receive radiation daily for a specified period of time. If radium implants are used, the client will have a radioactive capsule implanted into the area.

▶ NURSING PROCESS

▶ Assessment

▶ Subjective Data

Clients may complain of a sore throat, difficulty swallowing, or a painful area in the mouth.

▶ Objective Data

Assessment may include a sore or lesion of the lips or in the oral cavity, and hoarseness.

Nursing diagnoses for a client with oral cancer may include the following:

Nursing Diagnoses	Planning/Goals	Nursing Interventions
▶ *Fear, related to diagnosis and long-term prognosis*	The client will verbalize fear and express plan to cope with diagnosis.	Allow client time alone and with significant others.
		Answer questions.
		Allow client and family to express fears and concerns.
		Encourage contact with support system (e.g., clergy).
		Discuss past experiences with stress and individual responses to those situations.
▶ *Nutrition, Altered, Less than Body Requirements, related to oral surgery or radical neck dissection*	The client will maintain weight while hospitalized.	Monitor I & O every shift.
		Weigh client daily.
		Administer tube feedings and IV rehydration as ordered.
		When indicated, introduce fluids.
		Monitor for aspiration.
▶ *Body Image Disturbance, related to disfiguring surgery*	The client will verbalize feelings regarding surgery and altered body image.	Allow client time to verbalize feelings.
		Discuss options (e.g., plastic surgery or makeup).
		Answer questions.
		Provide information on support groups.

Evaluation Each goal must be evaluated to determine how it has been met by the client.

COLORECTAL CANCER

Colorectal cancer is the third most common cancer in the United States. Almost all colorectal cancers arise from **polyps**, an abnormal growth of tissue that protrudes into the colon. Risk factors for colorectal cancer include age 45 or older, history of polyps, family history of polyps and/or colorectal cancer, a history of ulcerative colitis, and a diet high in fat and low in fiber.

Prognosis is very good if caught in the early stages. Recommended routine screenings for early detection are outlined in Table 34-6.

A colonoscopy or barium enema may demonstrate the disease. A CBC may show anemia if the cancer is bleeding. A CEA may be effective in detecting recurrent cancer, but is not a valid screening test. Signs and symptoms include a change in bowel habits, guaiac positive stools, and abdominal pain.

Medical–Surgical Management

Surgical

Treatment is surgical to remove the cancer (see Table 34-7). In class A tumors, a colonoscopy is performed with a polypectomy, the removal of the polyp. In class B or C tumors, a colon resection will be done (Figure 34-12). In some cases a colostomy, either temporary or permanent, may be performed. In class D tumors, surgery will be done only to relieve symptoms (e.g., bowel obstruction).

Follow-up colonoscopies must be done throughout the client's life to monitor for recurrence of the disease.

Pharmacological

In cases of class B, C, and D tumors, chemotherapy will be given following the surgery. Side effects of chemotherapy include nausea, vomiting, weight loss,

Table 34-6 RECOMMENDED SCREENINGS FOR COLORECTAL CANCER

RISK	DEFINITION	RECOMMENDATIONS
Average Risk	No personal or family history of colorectal cancer or polyps.	Fecal occult blood testing (FOBT) age 40. Sigmoidoscopy every 3 to 5 years after age 50.
Mild Risk	Blood relative with colorectal cancer.	Begin above testing 5 to 10 years prior to age relative diagnosed or, at minimum, the above guidelines.
Moderate Risk	Client with previous colorectal cancer.	Colonoscopy at 6 months, 1 year, and 2 years after diagnosis, then every 1 to 3 years.
High Risk	Familial polyposis syndrome.	FOBT age 10 with sigmoidoscopy. Colonoscopy every 1 to 3 years.
Ulcerative Colitis	UC 8 years throughout colon or 14 years in sigmoid colon.	Colonoscopy every 2 years with biopsies.

Table 34-7 COLORECTAL CANCER CLASSIFICATION AND TREATMENT

CLASS	INVOLVEMENT	TREATMENT
Class A	Limited to the inner lining of the colon.	Polypectomy during colonoscopy removes cancer.
Class B	Involves from 2 layers to entire thickness of colon wall.	Colon resection, chemotherapy.
Class C	Class B with invasion to lymph nodes.	Colon resection, chemotherapy, and immunotherapy.
Class D	Metastases to other organs (lung and liver most common).	Colon resection as a palliative measure only. Chemotherapy, radiation, and immunotherapy.

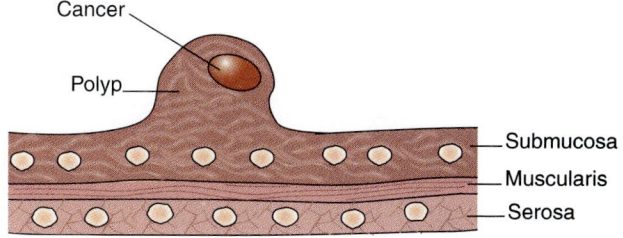

Class A colorectal cancer

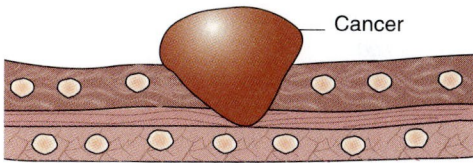

Class B colorectal cancer

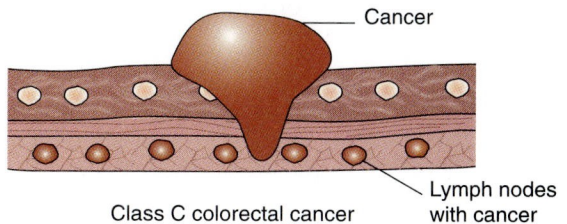

Class C colorectal cancer

Figure 34-12 Classes of Colorectal Cancer

hair loss, fatigue, and dry skin. Medications to combat some of the side effects of the chemotherapy will be ordered.

Immunotherapy as an adjunct therapy for class C and D tumors may also be ordered to boost the immune system.

Diet

Preoperatively, the client will be NPO. Postoperatively, the client will be NPO and an NG tube will be in place until bowel sounds return. The client will then be started on a clear liquid diet and progressed to a high-fiber, low-fat diet.

Activity

Postoperatively, the client will need to be encouraged to turn, cough, and deep breathe every 2 hours. The client will be ambulated the next day and activity will need to be progressed.

Other Therapies

No significant benefits have been found with the use of radiation on colorectal cancer. However, radiation may be used on metastatic sites in class D tumors.

▶ NURSING PROCESS

▶ Assessment

▶ Subjective Data

Clients may complain of a change in bowel habits and possibly abdominal pain.

▶ Objective Data

Stools may be guaiac positive for blood. An H & H may show anemia.

Nursing diagnoses for a client with colorectal cancer may include the following:

Nursing Diagnoses	Planning/Goals	Nursing Interventions
▶ *Fear related to diagnosis and long-term prognosis*	The client will verbalize fear and express plan to cope with diagnosis.	Allow client time alone and with significant others. Allow client and family to express fears and concerns. Answer questions. Encourage contact with support system (e.g., clergy). Discuss past experiences with stress and identify individual responses to those situations.
▶ *Knowledge Deficit regarding disease process, treatment options, and follow-up*	The client will be able to explain disease process, treatment, and follow-up care.	Determine client's learning style and present information in a manner compatible with the learning style. Educate client regarding disease process. Discuss treatment options. Recognize that information may need to be presented more than once.

Evaluation Each goal must be evaluated to determine how it has been met by the client.

LIVER CANCER

Primary liver cancer is rare. Most liver tumors are metastatic from other sites in the body. Most cases of primary liver cancer are asymptomatic until later stages. Risk factors for primary liver cancer include a history of cirrhosis, hepatitis B, and exposure to toxic chemicals.

A primary liver tumor can be removed surgically if the disease is not extensive. Metastases cannot be surgically removed and are usually treated with chemotherapy and radiation.

CASE STUDY

Ms. R. is a 52-year-old female admitted to the hospital with acute abdominal pain. Ms. R. complains of right upper quadrant pain radiating to the back. She has had prior episodes, usually occurring about two hours after eating. This episode, however, is not resolving. Ms. R. also complains of nausea. Her vital signs are BP 152/88, pulse 92, and respirations 24 and shallow. Ms. R. is a slightly obese female who states she has recently been dieting to lose weight. Laboratory analysis includes a CBC with slightly elevated WBCs; elevated bilirubin; and elevated alkaline phosphatase. An IV is started and Ms. R. is given meperidine (Demerol) IM for pain. Ms. R. has been made NPO. An ultrasound of the gallbladder is ordered.

The following questions will guide your development of a nursing care plan for this case study.

1. List subjective and objective data a nurse would want to obtain about Ms. R.
2. List risk factors other than those Ms. R. has that would put a client at risk for developing cholecystitis.
3. List two nursing diagnoses and goals for Ms. R.
4. The ERCP is successful in removing the CBD stone. The decision is made to perform a laparoscopic cholecystectomy. What teaching will Ms. R. need?
5. Why is meperidine (Demerol) the medication of choice for pain control?
6. List at least 3 successful outcomes for Ms. R.

SUMMARY

- The gastrointestinal system is a complex system composed of the digestive tract as well as accessory organs.
- Disorders of the GI tract affect the breakdown and absorption of nutrients, breakdown of wastes and by-products, and the lifestyle of the individual.
- Because the liver is responsible for so many functions in the body, disorders of the liver can affect other systems significantly.
- Peptic ulcers may be either gastric or duodenal. *H. pylori* is a common cause of ulcers and can be treated with antibiotics.
- Diverticulosis is a commonly occurring disorder in the United States and is believed to be caused by a low-fiber diet.
- Inflammatory bowel disease includes both Crohn's disease and ulcerative colitis. IBD can lead to nutritional imbalances, bowel obstructions, alterations in the structure of the intestine, and affected lifestyle.
- Bowel obstructions have multiple causes and can lead to electrolyte imbalances, dehydration, and possibly sepsis.
- Viral hepatitis is a concern for health care professionals at risk for exposure. Standard precautions must be used to prevent the transmission of the virus.
- Colorectal cancer is one of the most preventable forms of cancer if routine screenings are performed.

Review Questions

1. A client with a bleeding esophageal varix:

   a. should be encouraged to vomit the blood so as to decrease abdominal distention and pressure.
   b. should have an NG tube placed to suction blood from the stomach.
   c. should have the Minnesota tube deflated every 4 hours.
   d. will not need follow-up once the bleeding has stopped.

2. A client with a perforated duodenal ulcer:

   a. requires an EGD to repair the perforation.
   b. may need to modify his or her diet after surgery.
   c. will have a vagotomy performed.
   d. may experience an increased risk for cholecystitis.

3. Clients with hepatitis C:

   a. should be instructed that all the mechanisms of transmission are not known.
   b. will have a negative HCV if they are a carrier.
   c. should be instructed that recombinant interferon alpha-2b will cure the hepatitis C.
   d. are not contagious until symptoms develop.

4. Changes in the gastrointestinal system caused by aging:

   a. are minimal and have little impact on clients.
   b. include an increase in digestive enzymes leading to an increase in the occurrence of ulcers.
   c. require clients to eat larger, fewer meals.
   d. may require the client to swallow 2 to 3 times with each bite.

5. Crohn's disease:

   a. can be cured by removing the colon.
   b. usually causes clients to gain weight from the slower metabolism of nutrients.
   c. can be a debilitating disease leading to depression.
   d. is cured as long as the clients remain on 5-ASA compounds.

6. Hernias are a protrusion through the muscle wall and:

   a. can be easily reduced by the nurse applying gentle pressure.
   b. are benign occurrences that do not need any intervention.
   c. can lead to bowel obstructions.
   d. are caused by a lack of exercise.

Critical Thinking Questions

1. What lifestyle changes are needed with a diagnosis of hepatitis A, B, C, and D?

2. What nursing interventions would be effective for a client with an NG tube in place?

3. Compare and contrast the symptoms, treatments, and nursing interventions of Crohn's disease and ulcerative colitis.

4. Identify and discuss the rationale for each nursing intervention given for the nursing diagnoses in this chapter.

WEB FLASH!

- Can you locate support groups or resources on the Web for clients with GI disorders and their families? What resources are available for purchase?
- Visit the CDC's Web site. Do they offer information on the infectious disease hepatitis?
- What sites can you locate that specialize in GI cancer?

CHAPTER 35

NURSING CARE OF THE CLIENT: REPRODUCTIVE SYSTEM

MAKING THE CONNECTION

Refer to the following chapters to increase your understanding of the female and male reproductive systems:

- **Chapter 15, Wellness Concepts**
- **Chapter 23, Fluid, Electrolyte, and Acid-Base Balance**
- **Chapter 25, Assessment**
- **Chapter 30, Nursing Care of the Oncology Client**
- **Chapter 32, Nursing Care of the Client: Cardiovascular System**
- **Chapter 36, Nursing Care of the Client: Sexually Transmitted Diseases**

- **Chapter 37, Nursing Care of the Client: Endocrine System**
- **Chapter 42, Nursing Care of the Client: Urinary System**
- **Chapter 55, Nursing Care of the Older Client**
- **Procedures:** B30, Urine Collection—Closed Drainage System; I5, Irrigating an Open Catheter; I6, Irrigating a Closed Catheter

LEARNING OBJECTIVES

Upon completion of this chapter, you should be able to:
- *Define key terms.*
- *Identify the components of the reproductive systems.*
- *Describe the hormonal mechanisms that regulate the reproductive functions, including the menstrual cycle.*
- *Describe diagnostic tests for disorders of the reproductive systems.*
- *Describe the changes in the reproductive systems that occur with aging.*
- *Differentiate between impotence and infertility.*
- *Discuss contraceptive methods, including actions, side effects, and client teaching.*
- *Utilize the nursing process to develop a care plan for a client with a reproductive system disorder.*

KEY TERMS

abortion	nocturia
amenorrhea	oligomenorrhea
contraception	orchiectomy
cystocele	polymenorrhea
dysmenorrhea	post void residual
dyspareunia	priapism
endometriosis	prolapsed uterus
hematuria	rectocele
hesitancy	spermatogenesis
impotence	stent
infertility	tenesmus
menopause	urethrocele
menorrhagia	urethrostomy
metrorrhagia	vasectomy

INTRODUCTION

Because of modern technology, current medical and nursing knowledge, and health education programs, laypersons have access to much information about their bodies and their reproductive systems.

However, individuals continue to be seriously affected by health disorders. In some instances they may lack knowledge of how to detect signs and symptoms of these disorders. Often they simply delay routine medical examinations or avoid seeking medical treatment. In addition, individuals may have difficulty discussing symptoms related to their reproductive system.

Routine health care must be maintained and early diagnosis made in order to reduce the incidence and seriousness of reproductive health disorders. These goals can be facilitated with skilled nursing assessment and client education.

A member of a holistic health care team in health care settings, the nurse actively participates in prevention, maintenance, and restoration for women and men experiencing reproductive system disorders.

For the majority, the reproductive system functions without problems throughout life. For others, minor and major disorders require treatment. Some of the problems are related to alterations in structure; others are related more to altered physiology of the reproductive system. This chapter discusses disorders of the reproductive systems by applying the steps of the nursing process.

ANATOMY AND PHYSIOLOGY REVIEW

The female and male reproductive systems consist of external and internal structures and organs.

External Female Structures

The area known as the vulva includes the external female structures, such as the mons pubis, labia majora, labia minora, and clitoris. The Bartholin glands and Skene's glands, located proximal to the vaginal opening, produce and secrete lubricating fluids. The labia majora and minora serve as protective barriers for the softer internal structures. The clitoris, located proximal to the mons pubis, and superior to the urinary meatus, plays a role in sexual arousal in the female and is considered analogous to the male penis. During foreplay, the clitoris engorges and stimulates orgasm or climax in the female. It is covered by a small hood called the prepuce. The perineum is the distal portion of the vulva, located below the vaginal opening and superior to the anus.

The breasts are also a part of the external female reproductive system (Figure 35-1). Their external structures include the nipple, areola, and Montgomery tubercles. The nipples have several openings, or ducts, that lead from the lactiferous glands inside the breast. Milk is ejected through the ducts when the infant sucks on the breast. The areola, or the darker area around the nipple, becomes darker in response to the increased hormone levels during pregnancy. Small, mole-like, raised areas around the areola are the Montgomery tubercles. These glands produce a lubricant that keeps the nipple soft and supple.

Internal Female Structures

The vagina is an elastic, tubelike structure leading from the outside of the female body to the cervix. Ap-

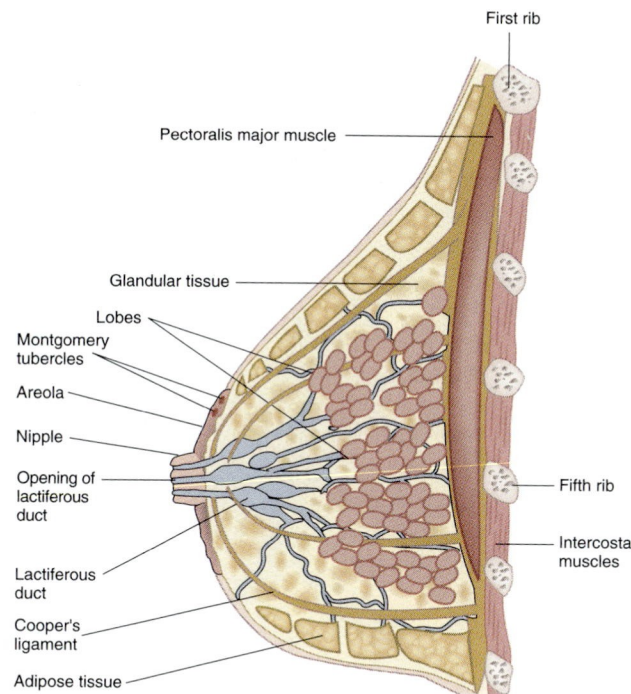

Figure 35-1 The Female Breast

proximately 2 to 3 inches long, it contains many rugae that allow it to stretch during intercourse and also permit the passage of the baby during delivery. The pH environment of the vagina is normally acidic, providing protection from microorganisms that could cause infections.

The uterus is a 3-inch long, 2-inch wide, 1-inch thick hollow, muscular structure as seen in Figure 35-2. The top is the fundus, the middle is the body (corpus), and the lower portion is the cervix. Four sets of ligaments hold the uterus in its normal anteverted (forward) position and permit it the freedom to grow and move during pregnancy. The uterus has three distinct layers. The innermost layer is the endometrium, which sloughs with menstruation each month. The middle layer is the myometrium, which is constructed of many muscle fibers that are interwoven for strength, stretch, and contractility. The outer layer is the perimetrium, which is an external serous membrane covering.

The fallopian tubes are connected to the uterus on either side. They are continuous with the mucous membrane lining of the endometrium on the inside. Billions of cilia line each fallopian tube and make a sweeping motion toward the uterus, especially at the time of ovulation. This sweeping action moves the ovum along the path toward the uterus. The movement may also impede the progress of the sperm, which must swim upstream against the downward current produced by the cilia.

The cervix is the lower portion of the uterus and extends into the vaginal vault. Like the vagina, the cervix has muscle layers that allow it to stretch to a diameter of at least 10 cm (about 4 inches) during delivery.

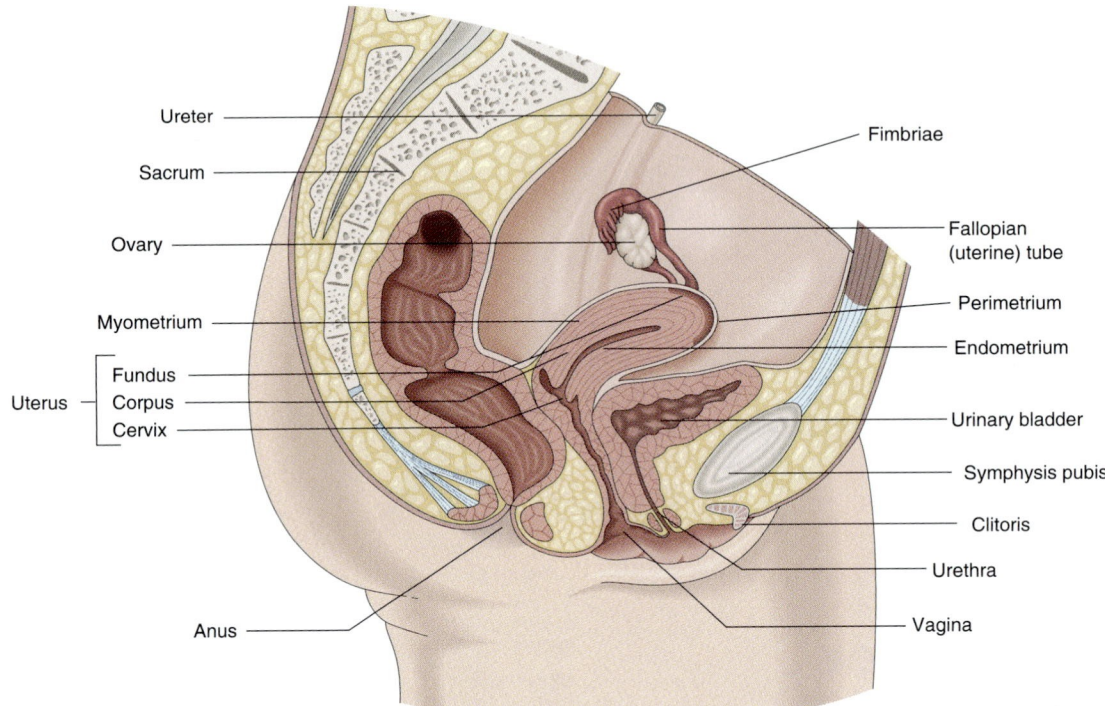

Figure 35-2 The Female Reproductive System

An almond-shaped ovary, about 2 inches long and 1 inch wide, is located within the broad ligament on either side of the uterus, just below the fimbriae, the fingerlike projections at the distal end of the fallopian tubes. The ovaries contain all of the ova (eggs) that a woman will have from puberty until menopause. Each month, the ovary responds to hormonal signals from the anterior pituitary gland to ripen one or more ova. Follicle-stimulating hormone (FSH) is released by the anterior pituitary and sends a message to the ovary to release estrogen, which causes the ovum to ripen and enlarge. The entire first part of the cycle is known as the proliferative phase.

Luteinizing hormone (LH) is then released. LH triggers a chain of events that stimulates the ovary to release the ovum. This point in the menstrual cycle is called ovulation. Another hormone, progesterone, causes the glands and blood vessels of the endometrial lining to grow and thicken as they prepare for the implantation of a fertilized ovum. If fertilization does not occur, the progesterone level will decrease, the endometrium will be sloughed off, and the woman experiences menstruation. If fertilization does occur, the progesterone level remains elevated to ensure the optimal environment for implantation of the zygote about 6 to 8 days after fertilization. Figure 35-3 illustrates the menstrual cycle.

Male Reproductive Structures

The male reproductive organs and associated structures are illustrated in Figure 35-4. The scrotum is a fleshy structure that is suspended below the perineum, anterior to the anus. It is divided into two parts, each of which contains a testis, an epididymis, and a portion of the spermatic cord (vas deferens). The left side of the scrotum is usually lower than the right because the left spermatic cord is often longer.

The testes, two smooth, oval endocrine glands, are suspended in the scrotum. This location helps to maintain proper temperature and also protects the testes

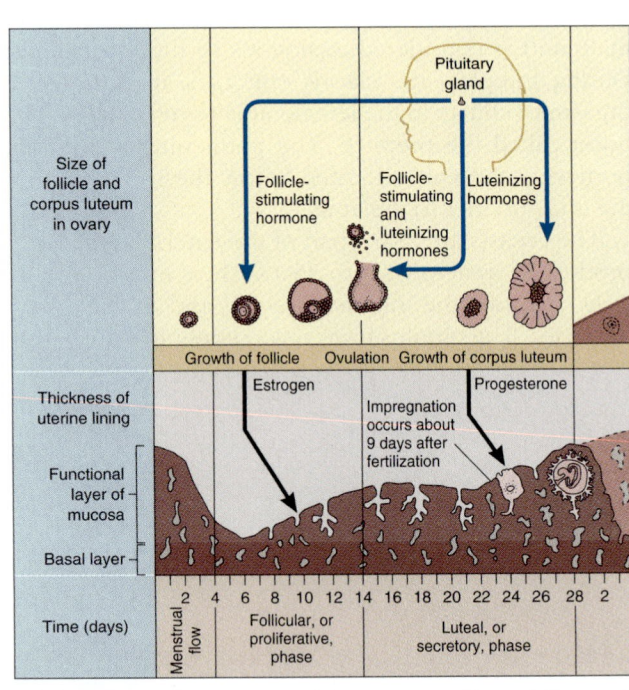

Figure 35-3 Sequence and Approximate Time of Events in the Menstrual Cycle

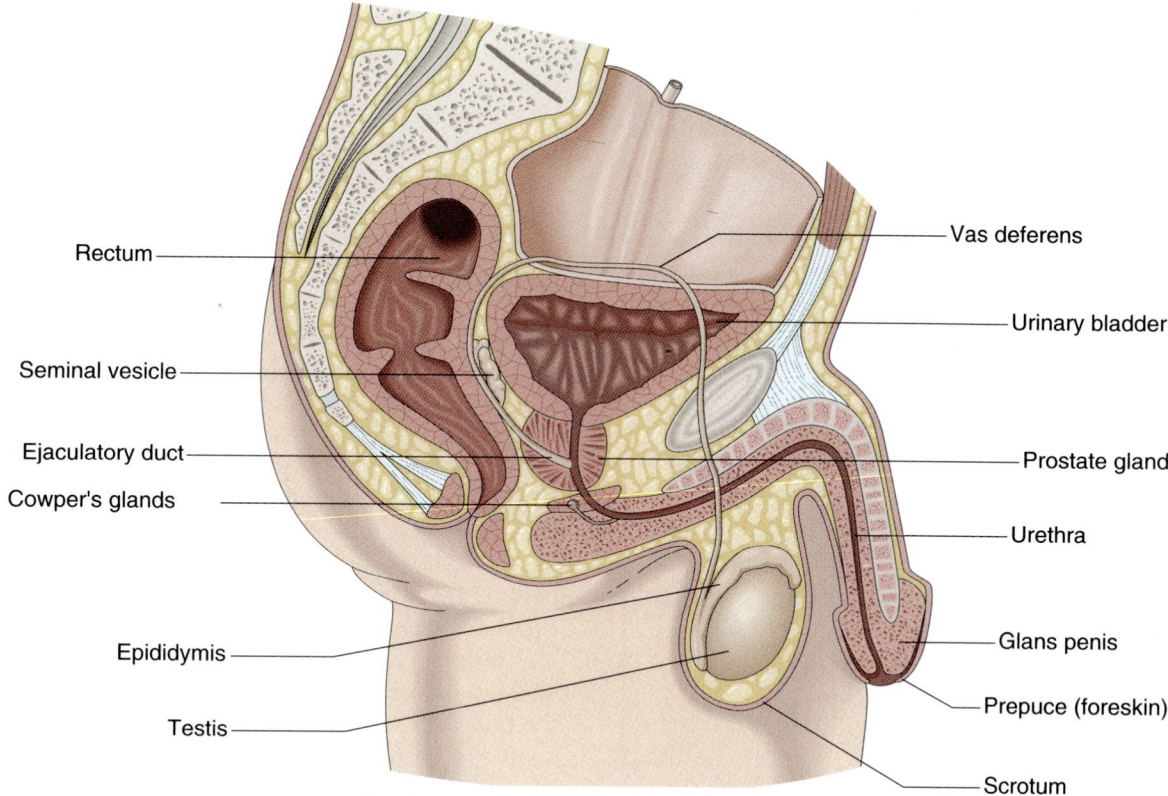

Figure 35-4 The Male Reproductive System

from trauma. Certain cells of the epithelium lining the seminiferous tubules of the testes produce half a billion sperm each day (**spermatogenesis**). They also secrete the androgenic (causing masculinization) hormone testosterone. Spermatogenesis is regulated by the follicle-stimulating hormone (FSH), which is produced by the anterior pituitary gland. The production of testosterone is regulated by luteinizing hormone (LH), which is also produced by the anterior pituitary gland. After the sperm mature in the epididymis, they travel through the vas (ductus) deferens, a long tube that is attached to the epididymis. The vas deferens, along with associated nerves and blood vessels, forms the spermatic cord.

LIFE CYCLE CONSIDERATIONS

Circumcision
Circumcision is performed on many Western society infants to remove the prepuce, or foreskin. In 1975 the American Academy of Pediatrics (AAP) did not support any medical need for routine circumcision. In 1988 they reversed their position on the basis of increased evidence that circumcision reduces the incidence of urinary tract infections. Circumcision is also performed for cultural or religious reasons.

The vas deferens travels up and around the bladder and carries sperm from the epididymis to the seminal vesicle. The seminal vesicle is a small pouch that produces secretions that, when mixed with sperm and prostatic fluid, form semen.

The prostate is an encapsulated gland that encircles the proximal portion of the urethra. The prostatic fossa, a depression on the cranial border of the prostate, allows entry of the ejaculatory ducts. Within the prostate is a cluster of 30 to 50 tubuloalveolar glands that secrete prostatic fluid. The prostate gland is of clinical significance because as men age, it is a common site for malignant disease or benign enlargement that can cause urethral obstruction.

The penis is a cylindrical organ through which urine is passed and semen is ejaculated. Half of the penis is located within the body. The external half of the penis is flaccid, unless the male is sexually aroused, at which time it becomes erect owing to engorgement with blood. A fold of skin, the prepuce, surrounds the tip of the penis in the uncircumcised male.

COMMON DIAGNOSTIC TESTS

Commonly used diagnostic tests for clients with symptoms of reproductive system disorders are listed in Table 35-1. See Chapter 27, Diagnostic Tests, for explanation/normal values and nursing responsibilities.

Table 35-1 COMMON DIAGNOSTIC TESTS FOR REPRODUCTIVE SYSTEM DISORDERS

Laboratory Tests
- Alpha-fetoprotein (AFP)
- Cultures
- Human chorionic gonadatropin (HCG)
- Pap smear
- Prostate-specific antigen (PSA)
- Prostatic smear
- Serum alkaline phosphatase
- Serum calcium
- Semen analysis
- Segmented bacteriologic localization culture

Radiologic Tests
- Dynamic infusion cavernosometry and cavernosography (DICC)
- Hysterosalpingogram
- Mammography

Surgical Tests
- Breast biopsy
- Dilatation & curettage (D&C)
- Endometrial biopsy
- Laparoscopy
- Prostatic biopsy
- Testicular biopsy

Other Tests
- Colposcopy
- Nocturnal tumescence penile monitoring
- Pelvic examination
- Schiller test
- Ultrasound

INFLAMMATORY DISORDERS

Inflammatory disorders discussed include pelvic inflammatory disease, endometriosis, vaginitis, toxic shock syndrome, and epididymitis/orchitis/prostatitis.

PELVIC INFLAMMATORY DISEASE

Pelvic inflammatory disease (PID) is an inflammatory process involving pathogenic invasion of the fallopian tubes (salpingitis) or ovaries (oophoritis), or both, as well as any vascular or supporting structures within the pelvis, except the uterus. Pathogenic microorganisms such as gonococcus, streptococcus, and staphylococcus are frequent causes of PID. Infections are usually ascending by nature; that is, the pathogens are introduced into the reproductive system from outside and travel upward from the vagina to the fallopian tubes and then out into the pelvis. Risk factors associated with the incidence of PID include multiple sexual partners, frequent intercourse, IUDs (intrauterine contraceptive devices), and childbirth.

The symptoms of PID include a low-grade fever, pelvic pain, abdominal pain, a "bearing down" backache, a foul-smelling vaginal discharge, nausea and vomiting, **dysmenorrhea** (painful menstruation), **dyspareunia** (painful intercourse), and intense pelvic tenderness upon examination. Peritonitis or pelvic abscesses may develop as complications of PID if the pathogens spread into the pelvic cavity. Future **infertility** (inability or diminished ability to produce offspring) can be related to scarring and strictures of the fallopian tubes, which have developed as a result of a chronic inflammatory process within the pelvis. These problems have been associated with ectopic pregnancies because the fertilized ovum becomes trapped inside the fallopian tube before it can complete its trip to the uterus.

PID is often diagnosed during a pelvic examination. The nurse usually obtains a history of the client's symptoms. Frequently, vaginal and cervical cultures are obtained at the time of the exam to determine the causative agent. A pelvic ultrasound may be ordered to rule out other causes of pelvic pain. The nurse needs to instruct the client in the purpose of these procedures and any special preparations that may be required, such as having a full bladder.

Medical–Surgical Management

Medical

The client who is not acutely ill from PID may be treated as an outpatient at home with oral antibiotics and bed rest, unless the infection is herpes simplex virus II. Clients with herpes simplex II infections may require more intensive care in the hospital with IV antibiotic therapy. The physician may also order medicated vaginal suppositories for the vaginal discharge. The acutely ill client may require hospitalization for IV antibiotic therapy.

Surgical

If the inflammation is extensive, or if medical treatment is not successful, the client may require a hysterectomy.

Pharmacological

Antibiotics used may include doxycycline monohydrate (Vibramycin) or metronidazole (Flagyl). IV fluids are frequently administered to promote adequate hydration. A 5% dextrose in lactated Ringer's solution or a plain lactated Ringer's solution is often used.

CLIENT TEACHING

Inserting Vaginal Suppositories
- Have the client wash her hands, then cleanse the vulva with a mild soap and warm water to remove any external discharge.
- Client should lie down in a supine position with her knees flexed.
- With one hand, the client can separate the labia and gently insert the suppository high inside the vagina.
- The client should remain supine for a minimum of 30 minutes to ensure adequate absorption of the medication through the vaginal mucosa.

Activity

During hospitalization, the client is placed on bed rest with bathroom privileges. A semi-Fowler's position is preferred because it will facilitate drainage of the pelvis. If vaginal suppositories are used, the client should lie in a supine position for 30 minutes.

▶ NURSING PROCESS

▶ Assessment

▶ Subjective Data

On the initial assessment, the nurse should inquire about the client's sexual activity, including the number of partners. Unprotected intercourse is the most frequent method of entry for the microorganisms that cause PID. The nurse should also include the client's history of **contraception** (measures taken to prevent pregnancy), previous vaginal infections and treatments, obstetrical history, and normal hygiene practices such as douching and tampon use. Complaints of nagging pelvic pain and a low-grade fever are often expressed.

▶ Objective Data

The nurse may note an elevated temperature, flushed, dry skin, the presence of a malodorous vaginal discharge, and positive vaginal or cervical cultures.

Nursing diagnoses for a client with pelvic inflammatory disease may include the following:

Nursing Diagnoses	Planning/Goals	Nursing Interventions
▶ *Pain, related to inflammation of the pelvic structures caused by invasion of pathogens*	Using a pain rating scale of 0 to 10, the client will report that her pain has decreased.	Assess client's pain level every 4 hours, noting the location, duration, sensation, intensity, and factors that increase or decrease the pain.
		Administer analegesics as ordered.
▶ *Knowledge Deficit, related to the etiology of the pelvic inflammatory process, treatment regimen, self-care, and preventive measures*	The client will follow prescribed treatment regimen, self-care, and preventive measures.	If suppositories are ordered, instruct the client in the proper method of insertion. Provide instructions to the client and partner (if available) about the causes of PID and ways to prevent the inflammation.
		Teach proper pericare and hygiene, especially handwashing before and after changing sanitary pads.
		Instruct client to change sanitary pads every 3 to 4 hours.
		Encourage client to make time for rest periods during the acute phase of the inflammation.
		Instruct client about pelvic rest, which includes no douching, tampons, or intercourse.
		Advise client to avoid strenuous activities such as straining or heavy lifting.
		Advise client to wear underpants with a cotton crotch.
		Teach client to cleanse the perineal area from front to back after each voiding or bowel movement.
		Discuss and encourage the use of safe sexual practices and the use of barrier contraceptives to prevent recurrence of PID symptoms.
		Make follow-up appointment.
	The client will contact her health care provider for follow-up and if her symptoms persist, worsen, or return.	Encourage client to notify the NP or physician at the first sign of PID symptoms. Advise client to monitor her own temperature, upon discharge, twice daily for 2 weeks and notify the physician or NP if the temperature increases or remains elevated.

continued

Nursing Diagnoses	Planning/Goals	Nursing Interventions
▶ *Hyperthermia, related to physiologic responses to the inflammatory or infectious process*	The client's temperature will return to normal range after the initiation of therapy.	Monitor client's vital signs every 4 hours. Administer antipyretic and antibiotic as ordered by the physician.

Evaluation Each goal must be evaluated to determine how it has been met by the client.

ENDOMETRIOSIS

Endometriosis is the growth of endometrial tissue, the normal lining of the uterus, outside of the uterus within the pelvic cavity. The disease occurs most frequently in women 30 years and older and tends to be familial. It predominantly affects Caucasian females who have not given birth and is most common among the higher socioeconomic population. Endometriosis has been called the "career woman's disorder," because it is often diagnosed in the late twenties or thirties when the working woman makes plans for childbearing.

The endometrial tissue implants itself on other pelvic structures (Figure 35-5). Two of the most common areas for endometrial implants are the pouch of Douglas and the ovaries. The tissue implants respond to the monthly hormonal changes in the same way as the endometrial tissue inside the uterus does. Bleeding of the implants during the menses results in the formation of adhesions and scar tissue. The endometriosis appears as brownish or black "powder burns" or larger lesions. If the endometriosis becomes encapsulated in an ovarian cyst it is called a "chocolate cyst."

The disease appears to be progressive and has a tendency to be recurrent. Some women with minimal endometriosis experience severe monthly symptoms, such as lower backache, painful intercourse, a feeling of heaviness on the pelvis, and spotting. Other women have a more extensive disease but have minimal symptoms. Thus, the amount of endometriosis present may or may not be correlated with the severity of the symptoms experienced by the client.

Endometriosis is one cause of female infertility. Pregnancy inhibits the growth and bleeding of the endometrial implants because ovulation and menstruation are suppressed. Often it is difficult for the client to become pregnant because of the amount of scar tissue and adhesions around the pelvic organs, ligaments, and fallopian tubes.

Medical–Surgical Management

Medical

Endometriosis may be tentatively diagnosed by palpation of endometrial implants within the pelvis, but this method is inconclusive for treatment. Further investigation is required to confirm the diagnosis. Laparoscopy, performed under general anesthesia, is the best method of diagnosis by direct visualization of the pelvic structures. Consideration for treatment is dependent upon the client's age and desire for future childbearing. Sometimes pregnancy relieves the symptoms even after delivery.

Surgical

The older multigravida who is experiencing severe, debilitating symptoms that affect her lifestyle and normal functions, role, or activity, may desire a hysterectomy. If the lesions are large or extensive, a laparotomy may be performed for adequate removal. However, if the implants are small and scattered, cauterization or laser vaporization may be most desirable. Lysis of pelvic adhesions would be done at the same time.

Pharmacological

The goals of pharmacological therapy are to suppress ovulation and menstruation, reduce symptoms, and cause the implants to shrink. Medications used in the treatment of endometriosis must effectively suppress the monthly hypothalamic-pituitary-ovarian hormonal stimulation of ovulation. Some medications act on the body as "pseudopregnancy" agents that produce anovulation, breast tenderness, nausea, weight

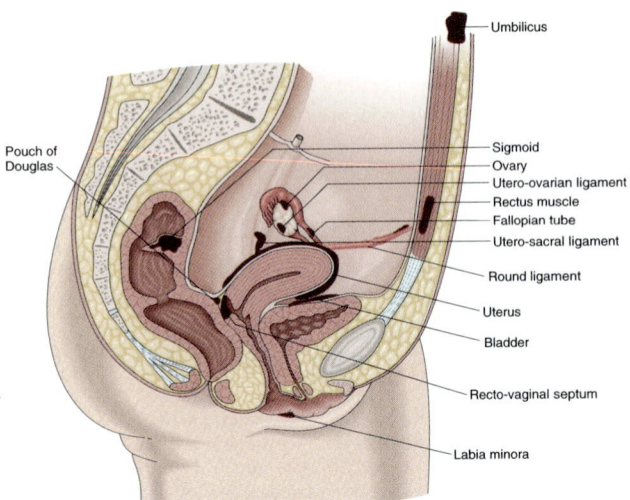

Figure 35-5 Common Sites of Endometriosis

gain, and hirsutism. Other hormonal therapies cause a temporary medically induced menopause state. Oral contraceptives may be administered continuously. Nafarelin acetate (Synarel) is a nasally administered gonadatropin analog that inhibits cyclic hormone release. Danazol (Danocrine) is another androgen hormone that must be taken continuously for 6 to 8 months or longer. This medication inhibits the release of gonadotropin. The resulting **amenorrhea** (absence of menstruation) will suppress the growth of the endometrial tissue. This medication is used in moderate to severe cases of endometriosis. Occasionally, Danocrine is given after surgical removal or cauterization of the endometriosis to relieve symptoms from residual disease.

All medications used to treat endometriosis cause mild to moderate side effects that may affect the client's desire to take them or her compliance with continuous usage. Examples of problems that may be experienced include oily skin, fluid retention, weight gain, acne, hot flashes, metrorrhagia, mastalgia, and depression.

▶ NURSING PROCESS

▶ Assessment

▶ Subjective Data

The data to be gathered include a description of pelvic pain, which is especially worse around the time of menstruation. The client may also voice concerns about pelvic discomfort with intercourse. The nurse should be alert to what the client says as well as what is left unsaid. Dyspareunia may result in marital tension if the client avoids sexual intimacy to reduce her pain. Equally important to the client's pain is the occurrence of prolonged, excessive menstrual periods. The client may report that she is experiencing periods that are getting closer and closer together. Another sign, although not as significant, is pain with defecation during the menstrual period.

In obtaining a client history, the nurse should note the onset of menses, regularity of cycles, and any changes the client has noted in the frequency, comfort, duration, and amount of menstrual flow. It is important to note the onset of the client's symptoms in relationship to the menstrual cycle, the severity as reported by the client, any alterations in lifestyle related to the pain or other symptoms, and the client's future plans for childbearing.

▶ Objective Data

The nurse's role in caring for this client is usually focused on collecting subjective data from the client interview and assisting the physician during actual procedures.

Nursing Management

Nursing diagnoses for a client with endometriosis may include the following:

- *Pain, related to bleeding from endometrial implants in the pelvic cavity*
- *Anxiety, related to treatment options, possible side effects, and infertility*
- *Sexuality Patterns, Altered, or Sexual Dysfunction, related to altered body function or structure (painful intercourse)*
- *Self-Esteem Disturbance, related to the inability to conceive*

VAGINITIS

Several common types of vaginitis are caused by bacteria, protozoa, viruses, and yeasts. The vaginal mucosa is normally protected by an acid mantle. The acidic (pH less than 5.0) environment inhibits the growth of many pathogenic microorganisms. Because the vaginal opening is close to the external environment, microorganisms have an opportunity to invade the reproductive tract. Some organisms that cause vaginitis are transmitted to the female from the male partner during sexual contact. Natural protective barriers may vary with the fluctuating hormonal levels during the woman's monthly cycle because the hormones affect the vaginal pH. At ovulation, the vaginal pH becomes slightly less acidic owing to the high level of estrogen. Periods when the woman's system has lower estrogen levels, such as immediately after the menses and after menopause, are also times when there is a higher risk for infection because the epithelium is less active, no glycogen is present, and the pH may reach as high as 7.0.

Diagnosis is made after performing a vaginal examination and obtaining a sample of the vaginal discharge. When the client contacts the physician or nurse practitioner to report symptoms of vaginitis, the nurse should instruct her to avoid douching or using tampons before being examined because douching will wash away the discharge needed to be examined and tampons will absorb it.

Common types of vaginitis include candidiasis caused by *Candida albicans* (a fungus), trichomoniasis caused by *Trichomonas vaginalis* (a protozoan), *Gardnerella vaginalis* (a bacterium), and *Chlamydia trachomatis* (a parasite). Other causes of vaginitis symptoms may include streptococcus, staphylococcus, gonococcus, and herpes simplex II. Usually the symptoms depend upon the causative agent. The client's description of her symptoms along with the examination of the discharge help confirm the diagnosis. Most infections have a characteristic discharge and irritation with burning or itching that may be internal, external, or both.

Predisposing factors for candidiasis, also called monilia, may include obesity, diabetes, pregnancy, oral contraceptives, antibiotics, and frequent douching. Many of these factors alter the pH of the vagina. Symptoms of this fungal infection include a thick, white, cheesy or curdlike discharge with a musty, sweet odor, accompanied by vaginal or vulvar itching and irritation. Upon examination. the vaginal mucosa will have patches of white discharge present. If the patches are scraped off, the tissue underneath will appear reddened and may bleed. Externally, the vulva may be reddened and edematous. The client may have scratches from attempting to ease the itching.

The preferred treatment is vaginal application of antifungal creams or suppositories such as miconazole (Monistat), clotrimazole (Mycelex-G, Gyne-Lotrimin), or nystatin (Mycostatin). The length of treatment is usually 7 days. Alternative therapies include douching with white vinegar solution (1 tablespoon/1 pint of water) twice a day for a week. This treatment restores the acid balance of the vagina and washes away the *Candida albicans.* Eating cultured yogurt with active acidophilus or applying the yogurt directly to the labia helps restore the normal bacteria and protective mechanisms in the vagina.

Trichomonasis is frequently passed from partner to partner during intercourse. A copious green-yellow, foul-smelling, frothy vaginal discharge is characteristic of this type of vaginal infection. It may produce itching or external burning and irritation. Metronidazole (Flagyl) is taken orally by both partners as a treatment of choice for this infection.

Flagyl is normally contraindicated in the first trimester of pregnancy, so obtaining a menstrual history or a pregnancy test may be needed before administration of this medication. It is also essential to inform the client and her partner to avoid any alcohol intake during therapy. Flagyl causes a strong antabuse-like effect which results in severe nausea and vomiting. Clients should read labels on over-the-counter medications being taken concurrently with the Flagyl because many preparations contain alcohol bases.

The nurse should instruct the client and her partner to abstain from intercourse during therapy and to finish all of the medication.

Gardnerella vaginalis often produces a gray-white vaginal discharge with a strong fishy odor or is asymptomatic. If itching or burning is present, it may suggest another microorganism. For the treatment of *Gardnerella,* and other bacterial vaginitis, the physician may order Flagyl or an oral antibiotic such as tetracycline hydrochloride (Achromycin) or ampicillin (Omnipen). Sulfa-based creams such as Sultrin, Triple Sulfa, and AVC may be used vaginally in conjunction with the oral medications once or twice a day for 6 to 14 days to completely treat this type of infection.

Chlamydial vaginitis infections are often asymptomatic but have been associated with infertility prob-

CLIENT TEACHING

Ways to Decrease Risk of Vaginitis
- Wear cotton-crotch underwear.
- Avoid sitting in a wet bathing suit in warm weather for long periods.
- Seek prompt medical attention at the first signs of infection.
- Eat an 8-oz container of yogurt with active cultures daily while taking antibiotics.

lems. A culture of vaginal secretions is necessary to specifically identify the organism. The treatment is usually oral antibiotics for at least 7 days. A repeat culture is recommended following treatment to ensure that the parasites have been eradicated.

Postmenopausal vaginitis (atrophic) is caused by a decreased level of estrogen in the vaginal tissue. The client may complain of painful intercourse (dyspareunia), itching, burning, or irritation. Estrogen replacement therapy often relieves the symptoms of this type of vaginitis. The medication may be administered orally, vaginally, or by transdermal patch.

▶ NURSING PROCESS

▶ Assessment

▶ Subjective Data

The nurse should obtain information from the client regarding the nature of her symptoms, the onset, menstrual history, contraceptive methods, recent or current use of antibiotics or other medications, recent illness, diabetes mellitus, sexual history, pregnancy history, usual hygiene practices such as douching, deodorant sprays, bubble baths, wearing of panty hose, type of underwear, and use of deodorized tampons or pads.

▶ Objective Data

The vaginal discharge is observed and any odor noted. Vaginal or vulvar irritation and possible scratches may be seen.

Nursing Management

Nursing diagnoses for a client with vaginitis, regardless of the etiology, may include the following:

- *Knowledge Deficit, related to the origin of the infection, prevention, and treatment options*
- *Tissue Integrity, Impaired, related to the presence of vaginal discharge, itching, or irritation*
- *Sexual Dysfunction, related to discomfort during intercourse or fear of transmitting the infection to the sexual partner*
- *Skin Integrity, Impaired, Risk for, related to internal and external irritation from discharge and itching*

TOXIC SHOCK SYNDROME

Toxic shock syndrome (TSS) is a condition most often associated with *Staphylococcus aureus,* which enters the bloodstream. A strong relationship has been found between the use of tampons (especially super-absorbent) during menstruation and the onset of TSS symptoms. It has been hypothesized that the fibers from the tampon lower the level of magnesium in the woman's body and, therefore, produce a favorable environment for the growth of pathogenic micro-organisms. The condition was first diagnosed in the mid-1970s and the incidence increased throughout the 1980s. A high percentage of women who are affected by toxic shock syndrome are under 30. TSS can also occur in nonmenstruating women and men.

The client may present with a temperature of 102°F or greater, vomiting, diarrhea, and progressive hypotension. The client may also experience flulike symptoms of malaise, muscle soreness, sore throat, and headache. There may be a macular erythematous (flat, red) rash that is followed in 1 to 2 weeks by the peeling of the palms and soles. Disorientation may occur from the release of toxins and dehydration.

Medical–Surgical Management

Medical

Blood, urine, genitourinary, and throat cultures may be obtained and are usually negative except for *Staphylococcus aureus.* The goals of treatment are focused on the control of the falling blood pressure, fluid volume replacement, halting the infectious process, and maintaining adequate ventilation efforts. IV fluids are administered per the physician's order. The client may require mechanical ventilation and CPAP (continuous positive airway pressure).

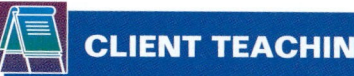

CLIENT TEACHING

TSS and Tampon Use

Instruct client to avoid tampon use for several cycles. If she chooses to use tampons in the future, they should be changed every 2 to 3 hours, especially the superabsorbent types.

Pharmacological

Broad-spectrum antibiotic therapy is recommended. Culture and sensitivity tests will indicate which type of antibiotic is best against the staphylococcus organism. Examples may include dicloxacillin sodium (Dynapen), clexacillin sodium (Tegopen), nafcillin sodium (Nafcil), and methicillin sodium (Staphcillin). The medication regimen is continued for at least 2 weeks to ensure control of the pathogens.

Activity

Bed rest is usually prescribed.

▶ NURSING PROCESS

▶ Assessment

▶ Subjective Data

Data to be obtained include recent use of tampons, length of time tampon is left in before changing, sore throat, headache, myalgia, and fatigue.

▶ Objective Data

Erythematous rash, edema, peeling of palms and soles, hypotension, level of consciousness, nonpurulent conjunctivitis, and hyperemia of vagina and oropharynx are all assessed.

Nursing diagnoses for a client with toxic shock syndrome may include the following:

Nursing Diagnoses	Planning/Goals	Nursing Interventions
▶ *Hyperthermia, related to inflammatory process*	The client will have normal-range temperature within 48 hours.	Administer antipyretics as ordered. Give cooling sponge bath. Encourage oral fluids as tolerated.
▶ *Fluid Volume Deficit, related to diarrhea, vomiting, fever, and decreased intake*	The client will have fluid and electrolyte balance within 24 hours.	Administer intravenous fluids as ordered. Encourage oral fluids if client is not vomiting. Administer antiemetic and antidiarrheal medications as ordered. Assess skin turgor and mucous membranes. Monitor I & O.
▶ *Skin Integrity, Impaired, Risk for, related to dehydration and effects of circulating toxins*	The client will maintain skin integrity.	Encourage or assist with position change every 2 hours. Provide or assist with personal hygiene, especially after diarrhea. Assess bony prominences for reddened areas.

Evaluation Each goal must be evaluated to determine how it has been met by the client.

EPIDYMITIS/ORCHITIS/ PROSTATITIS

Epididymitis can be a sterile or nonsterile inflammation of the epididymis. A sterile inflammation may be caused by direct injury or reflux of urine down the vas deferens. Urinary reflux that is related to strain exerted by a male while his bladder is full can be caused by lifting heavy objects or doing strenuous exercises. Nonsterile inflammation may occur as a complication of gonorrhea, chlamydia, mumps, tuberculosis, prostatitis, or urethritis. Prolonged use of an indwelling catheter or an invasive procedure can also lead to non-sterile inflammation.

Signs and symptoms of epididymitis include sudden, severe pain in the scrotum, scrotal swelling, fever, dysuria, and pyuria. Treatment includes bed rest, antibiotics, scrotal support (Figure 35-6), and ice compresses to the area. Bilateral epididymitis can cause sterility. Untreated epididymitis leads quickly to testicular tissue necrosis, septicemia, and death.

Orchitis is an inflammation of the testes that most often occurs as a complication of a bloodborne infection originating in the epididymis. Other causes of orchitis include gonorrhea, trauma, surgical manipulation, and tuberculosis and mumps that occur after puberty. In most instances, both testes are involved, and often sterility results. In orchitis, unilateral involvement does not cause sterility. Orchitis signs and symptoms include sudden scrotal pain with pain radiating to the inguinal canal, scrotal edema, chills, fever, nausea, and vomiting. Treatment includes bed rest, scrotal support, and ice to the area.

Prostatitis, an inflammation of the prostate, is a common complication of urethritis caused by chlamydia or gonorrhea. Infecting organisms may reach the genital tract by direct spread through the urethra or may be borne by blood or lymph. The condition may be acute or chronic, with the chronic form leading to development of fibrotic tissue. This fibrotic tissue causes the prostate to harden, so prostatitis may be difficult to differentiate from prostate cancer. It may take 3 to 6 months for the granulomatous form to resolve. Signs and symptoms of prostatitis include perineal pain, fever, dysuria, and urethral discharge.

Medical–Surgical Management

Medical

When it is suspected that the client currently has urethritis, he should not be catheterized. The infection spreads rapidly to the genital organs because of the trauma of catheterization and the possible spread of bacteria from the nonsterile distal part of the urethra. The physician may order that segmented bacteriologic localization cultures be obtained.

Pharmacological

Treatment of epididymitis and orchitis includes antibiotics and injection of procaine around the spermatic cord. Pharmacological treatment of prostatitis includes antibiotics, analgesics, and stool softeners.

Activity

Treatment of prostatitis includes bed rest. While the client is in bed, his scrotum should be elevated and cold packs applied to the area. The client should be encouraged to drink a large amount of fluids and use sitz baths for comfort. These interventions are used to reduce inflammation, swelling, and discomfort. Periodic digital massage of the prostate by the physician increases the flow of infected prostatic secretions.

▶ NURSING PROCESS

▶ Assessment

▶ Subjective Data

The nurse should question the client about the presence of urethral discharge or dysuria as well as the nature and location of the pain. A description of pain may include arthralgia, low-back pain, and myalgia. In addition, a careful medical history should be obtained. A positive history of recent bacterial or viral infection is of special significance. Ongoing nursing assessment should include monitoring for pain, using a pain scale to objectify data. The nurse should ask the client if he is experiencing nausea, as this could be a sign that his condition is deteriorating. The client also needs an assessment of his educational and emotional needs as he may be worrying needlessly about possible sterility or impotence.

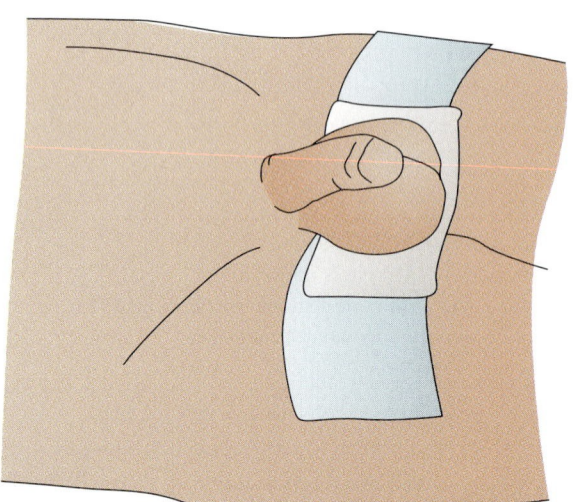

Figure 35-6 A Bellevue Bridge for Scrotal Support

▶ Objective Data

The client's vital signs, especially his temperature, should be monitored. An increase in temperature may be an indicator that the client's condition is worsening.

Scrotal edema and purulent urethral discharge may be present. Intake and output need to be monitored. The client also needs to be monitored for constipation.

Nursing diagnoses for the male client with an inflammatory disorder may include the following:

Nursing Diagnoses	Planning/Goals	Nursing Interventions
▶ *Injury, Risk for, related to worsening of the inflammatory process*	The client will not experience worsening of his condition.	Monitor the client's vital signs, especially his temperature. Report hyperthermia, hypotension, nausea, and tachycardia to the physician immediately.
▶ *Fluid Volume Deficit, related to nausea and vomiting*	The client will maintain fluid balance.	Monitor the client's intake and output. Encourage him to drink plenty of fluids when not nauseated.
▶ *Pain, Acute, related to inflammation*	Using a pain scale of 0 to 10, the client will report pain has decreased to 2 or less within 48 hours after treatment initiation.	Assess client's pain level every 4 hours. Administer analgesics as ordered. Encourage the client to maintain bed rest. Provide diversional activities to increase compliance. Encourage the client with prostatitis to take a sitz bath, but never the client with epididymitis or orchitis as local heat may increase destruction of sperm cells. Fill a plastic glove with crushed ice and place it under the scrotum when heat is contraindicated. Remove the ice for short intervals every hour to prevent ice burns.
▶ *Anxiety, related to concerns about possible sterility or impotence*	The client will verbalize decreased anxiety.	Reassure the client that with proper treatment, sterility and impotence are not likely complications of prostatitis.

Evaluation Each goal must be evaluated to determine how it has been met by the client.

BENIGN NEOPLASMS

Benign neoplasms include fibrocystic breast disease, fibroid tumors, and benign prostatic hyperplasia.

FIBROCYSTIC BREAST DISEASE

Fibrocystic breast disease (FBD) is also called chronic cystic mastitis or lumpy breast syndrome. It is the most common breast lesion in females and usually occurs between 35 and 50 years of age. Many cases will subside after menopause. The incidence of the potential for developing breast cancer is increased 3 to 4 times with fibrocystic breast disease. There appears to be a familial tendency toward the development of breast cancer.

Lumps may occur as single or multiple cysts that are frequently fluid-filled. It is difficult to differentiate fibrocystic tissue changes from other breast lesions because the dense fibrocystic areas may mask areas of breast cancer. Figure 35-7 shows the differences among cysts, fibroadenomas, and carcinomas of the breast.

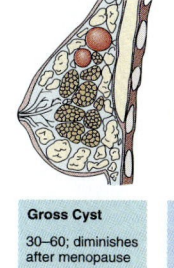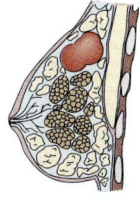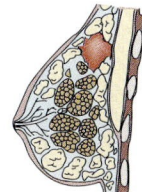

	Gross Cyst	Fibroadenoma	Carcinoma
Age	30–60; diminishes after menopause	puberty to menopause	most common after 50 years of age
Shape	round	round, lobular, or ovoid	irregular, stellar, or crab-like
Consistency	soft to firm	usually firm	firm to hard
Discreteness	well defined	well defined	not clearly defined
Number	single or grouped	most often single	usually singular
Mobility	mobile	very mobile	may be mobile or fixed to skin, underlying tissue or chest wall
Tenderness	tender	nontender	usually nontender
Erythema	no erythema	no erythema	may be present
Retraction/dimpling	not present	not present	often present

Figure 35-7 Comparison of Breast Neoplasms *(From Health Assessment & Physical Examination, by M. E. Z. Estes, 1998 Albany, NY: Delmar Publishers. Copyright 1998 by Delmar Publishers. Reprinted with permission.)*

The pathophysiology of fibrocystic breast disease is found in the formation of fibrous tissue caused by hyperplasia of the epithelial cells in the breast lobules and ducts. The proliferation of the fibrous tissue deviates from the expected normal cyclic response to female hormone shifts during the menstrual cycle.

Routine mammograms may be ordered to provide baseline information and to differentiate the palpable breast lumps between benign and malignant types. A computer-directed biopsy may also be performed.

Women should be taught breast self-examination (BSE) as adolescents and encouraged to practice it at the end of each menstrual cycle, when it is easier to palpate the breast tissue. Figure 35-8 provides specific information on how to perform a breast self-examination.

A yellow-greenish, sticky discharge from the nipple is occasionally present with fibrocystic breast disease. A Pap smear may be done on the discharge to rule out the presence of malignant cells. The presence of any breast discharge should be noted and reported to the

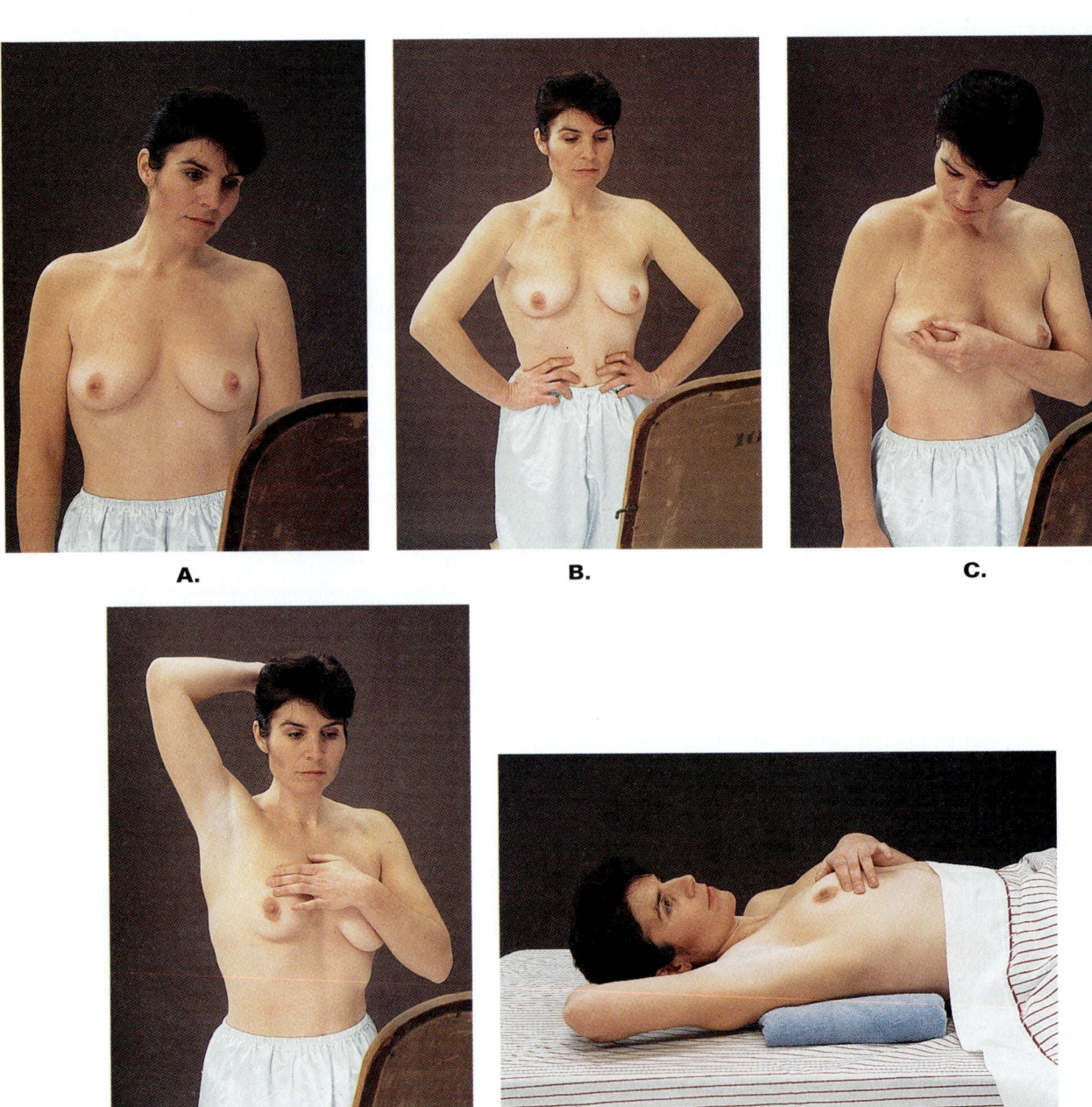

A.   **B.**   **C.**   **D.**   **E.**

Figure 35-8 Performing a Breast Self-Examination: A. Standing in front of mirror, check breasts for puckering, dimpling, scaliness, or discharge from nipples. B. Clasp hands behind head and press hands forward, watching for changes in the shape or contour of breasts. Press hands on hips and bend toward mirror while pulling shoulders and elbows forward (shown). C. Gently squeeze each nipple, looking for discharge. D. Raise one arm and use fingers of other hand to check breast for lumps or masses under skin. Use a pattern of motion (circular, up-and-down, etc.) to cover entire breast. E. Repeat "D" while lying flat on back with one arm over head and a towel under the shoulder.

health care provider as soon as possible. The physician or nurse practitioner (NP) may perform a biopsy or aspiration of the abnormal areas in the office. If fluid is obtained from the area, it is sent to pathology for examination. If no fluid is obtained, it may be a solid cyst or tumor, and biopsy may be required.

In the office, a breast biopsy may be performed with a local anesthetic. If there is any question of malignancy, or if the physician suspects that the lesion will be malignant on the basis of the mammography report, the biopsy may be performed in the hospital under general anesthetic so that additional tissue may be removed if necessary. A frozen section may be obtained and sent to the laboratory for a preliminary examination to rule out a malignant lesion.

Medical–Surgical Management

Surgical

Aspiration or surgical excision may be indicated for diagnostic or therapeutic reasons. The cystic tissue may be aspirated with a small-gauge needle and syringe. The nurse prepares the client for the procedure and assists the doctor or NP with the procedure. The nurse assists the client into a supine position on the examination table and sets up the equipment and instruments needed. The area to be biopsied is cleansed. Upon completion of the aspiration or biopsy, the nurse labels the specimen and sends it to the pathology department.

If the areas of fibrocystic tissue are extensive and have not responded to conservative treatments and methods, or if the risk of cancer is high, the tissue may be excised completely. Removal of fibrocystic tissue does not guarantee that the client will not develop breast cancer in the remaining tissue, and she must continue to perform monthly BSE.

Pharmacological

Some physicians recommend up to 600 units of vitamin E daily. It is believed that the vitamin supplement helps to break down the fibrocystic tissue because it reacts with the polyunsaturated fats in the membrane of the cell. It may also have some effect on the balance of female hormones.

Diet

Most health care providers recommend limiting or completely eliminating caffeine-containing products from the woman's diet. This would include teas, colas, coffee, and chocolate. These products are all available in caffeine-free forms.

▶ NURSING PROCESS

▶ Assessment

▶ Subjective Data

The client may report that the lumps are more tender as she approaches her menstrual period and that there is a greenish, sticky discharge from one or both breasts. The nurse should inquire about the client's dietary habits, especially caffeine intake, frequency of BSE, and the date of the most recent mammogram, if applicable. Since FBD lumps are more tender near the menses, the client should be seen for an exam the week after her menstrual period. The tissue contains less fluid during that time and palpation is easier and less uncomfortable.

▶ Objective Data

When examined, single or multiple lumps may be palpated in one or both breasts. The lumps are not always discrete but should be freely movable.

Nursing diagnoses for a client with fibrocystic breast disease may include the following:

Nursing Diagnoses	Planning/Goals	Nursing Interventions
▶ *Knowledge Deficit, related to the cause of fibrocystic breast disease and method of breast self-examination*	The client will verbalize and demonstrate her understanding of the cause of FBD and her role in treatment.	Demonstrate BSE for the client either in person or by video with a follow-up return demonstration by the client.
		Observe the client as she performs the BSE so that immediate feedback can be given. Explain the best timing for the BSE and the rationale for performing the procedure after the menses.
		Assist client with mammogram. Encourage mammography at regular intervals dependent upon the client's age and risk factors.
		Teach the client about dietary modifications, such as limiting caffeine.
▶ *Anxiety, related to the underlying potential and risk of breast cancer*	The client will display behaviors of decreased anxiety related to the potential for breast cancer.	Explain the differences between malignant breast lesions and FBD to help alleviate the client's anxiety.

Evaluation Each goal must be evaluated to determine how it has been met by the client.

FIBROID TUMORS

Fibroids (leiomyomas) are benign tumors that grow in or on the uterus. A higher incidence is seen with nulliparous women and those who are over 30 years old. The fibroids may appear below the serosal membrane or the mucosa. An early symptom is often **menorrhagia**, an excessively heavy menstrual flow. Later, the client may experience increasing pelvic pressure as the tumors grow, along with dysmenorrhea, abdominal enlargement, and constipation. Growth of the fibroids is usually slow but can be stimulated by estrogen. During pregnancy, when the estrogen and progesterone levels dramatically increase, the tumors grow much faster. Concern arises for the fetus when the fibroids begin to enlarge and crowd the uterus. Overcrowding may compress the fetus or initiate the onset of preterm labor. With either situation, the pregnancy must be monitored carefully.

A medical diagnosis of uterine fibroids may initially be based upon the client's symptoms and the findings of the pelvic examination. If on palpation the uterus feels like an irregular mass or several masses, a pelvic ultrasound will be ordered to confirm the diagnosis.

Medical–Surgical Management

Medical

The physician may opt to wait and observe the growth pattern of the fibroids before advising the client to have surgery. This "wait and see" attitude may be swayed by the significance of the client's symptoms, size of the fibroids, amount of discomfort the

CULTURAL CONSIDERATIONS

Fibroid Tumors

Fibroid tumors are most prevalent in African Americans and Mediterraneans with dark skin.

client is experiencing, and amount of menorrhagia and/or **metrorrhagia**, vaginal bleeding between menstrual periods. Reexamination is encouraged at least every 6 months.

Surgical

If the menorrhagia is significant with each menstrual cycle, a dilatation and curettage (D&C) may be performed to determine the exact etiology of the bleeding. A myomectomy, a surgical procedure to remove the tumor, may be performed if the client desires future pregnancies. In the case of severe menorrhagia, with a dropping hemoglobin level or multiple tumors, the physician may recommend a hysterectomy as the option of choice.

Diet

A diet with many sources of iron helps prevent iron deficiency anemia, which may result from the extra blood loss.

▶ NURSING PROCESS

▶ Assessment

▶ Subjective Data

These would include the client's description of excessive menstrual flow, dysmenorrhea, and/or pelvic pain and pressure. The client may also report difficulty fitting into clothes because of abdominal enlargement, constipation, or urinary frequency or urgency.

▶ Objective Data

These would include counting the number of sanitary pads the client saturates in an hour; observing the presence or absence of clots in the blood, and a hemoglobin level of less than 12 mg/dL. The nurse may observe that the client's skin color is pale. Her blood pressure may be slightly lower than normal and her pulse may be increased as a compensatory mechanism. When the pelvic examination is performed, irregularities in or on the uterus may be palpated.

Nursing diagnoses for a client with fibroids may include the following:

Nursing Diagnoses	Planning/Goals	Nursing Interventions
▶ *Fluid Volume Deficit, Risk for, related to excessive blood losses*	The client will have a hemoglobin above 12 mg/dL and will maintain fluid balance.	Assess client's blood loss for amount, color, and clots.
		Provide an accurate count of the saturated sanitary pads, along with the length of time taken to saturate a pad.
		Monitor vital signs at least every 4 hours, or more frequently if the client is having active blood loss.
		Monitor laboratory report for Hgb level.

continued

Nursing Diagnoses	Planning/Goals	Nursing Interventions
▸ *Pain, related to pressure on pelvic structures caused by growing tumors and cramping during the menses*	The client will verbalize less discomfort and pelvic pressure.	Administer analgesics as ordered. Assess pain on 0 (least) to 10 (most) pain scale and note location, onset, and duration.

Evaluation Each goal must be evaluated to determine how it has been met by the client.

BENIGN PROSTATIC HYPERPLASIA

Benign prostatic hyperplasia (BPH) is a progressive adenomatous enlargement of the prostate gland that occurs with aging. More than 50% of men over the age of 50 and 75% of men over the age of 70 demonstrate some increase in the size of the prostate gland (Martini, 1995). Although this disorder is not harmful, the urinary outlet obstruction that may be associated with the disorder is a problem.

Because the urethra is encircled by the prostate, common early symptoms of BPH are related to partial or complete obstruction of the urethra. Early symptoms include **hesitancy** (difficulty initiating the urinary stream), decreased force of stream, urinary frequency, and **nocturia** (awakening at night to void). However, a temporary reduction of these symptoms may occur as the bladder muscles hypertrophy in response to the increased work they must do to force the urinary stream past the obstruction.

Although this bladder muscle compensatory response may temporarily reduce symptoms, eventually the muscle decompensates, becoming noncompliant and hypotonic. This decompensation leads to atony of the mucous membranes between the muscle bands that causes stagnant urine to collect in the small compartments (cellules) of the membranes. In addition, the man is unable to completely empty the bladder when voiding (**post void residual**). Because these changes in urinary function promote urinary alkalosis by increasing the urine pH, a perfect environment for bacterial growth is created. This bacterial growth can cause a urinary tract infection (UTI), which may eventually lead to kidney damage.

Medical–Surgical Management

Medical

The physician will perform a digital rectal examination in order to identify any enlargement of the lateral lobes or nodular lumps on the surface of the prostate gland. Diagnostic tests will be ordered to learn more about the client's condition; these may include a prostate-specific antigen (PSA), measurement of residual urine, cystoscopy, intravenous pyelogram, and ultrasonography. The physician will also carefully monitor the client's condition to detect any exacerbation of symptoms such as increased hesitancy, urgency, hematuria, or repeated urinary tract infections.

Many alternatives to surgical treatment of BPH have been introduced over the past several years. Medical treatment methods have ranged from balloon dilation of the prostate to a prostate urethral **stent**, as shown in Figure 35-9, to thermotherapy. Balloon dilation of the prostate during an endoscopic examination is done to break the prostatic capsule and facilitate decompression of the prostate. A stent is material that is used to hold tissue in place or, in this instance, to provide support to the urethra, which is being compressed by the prostate. Various types of thermotherapy that may be used are microwave thermotherapy and hyperthermia. Although these minimally invasive treatments are safe, they do not remove the urinary obstruction.

Surgical

The traditional surgical intervention for enlargement of the portion of the prostate that surrounds the urethra has been transurethral resection of the prostate (TURP). This surgery is performed via a resectoscope, an instrument that includes a cutting and cauterization device (Figure 35-10). The client receives either a general or a spinal anesthetic, and the resectoscope is passed through the urethra for the purpose of removing small pieces of prostate tissue while controlling

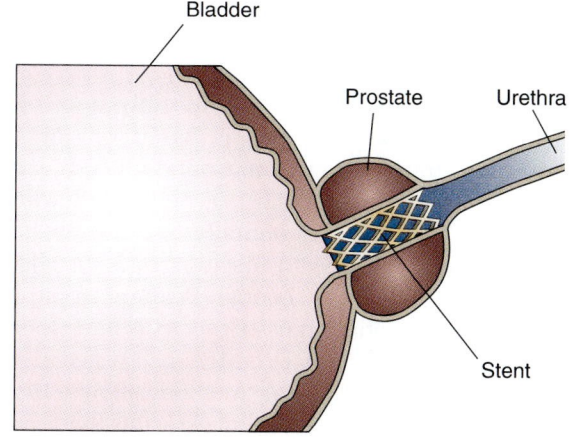

Figure 35-9 Urethral Stent

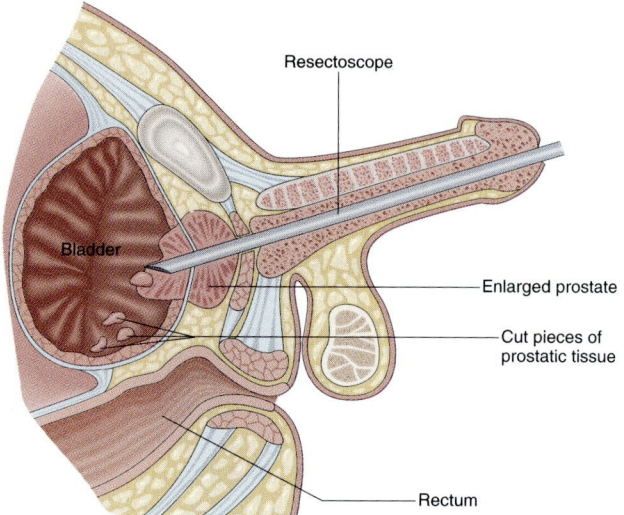

Figure 35-10 Transurethral Resection of the Prostate Gland via Resectoscope

bleeding. The bladder is continuously irrigated with normal saline or another solution during the procedure. This irrigation is continued during the postoperative period to reduce clot formation that would interfere with urinary drainage.

The traditional surgical alternatives to a TURP are open operations. A suprapubic resection, in which the prostate is removed from around the urethra via the bladder, is performed when the prostate mass is large. In a retropubic prostatectomy, the bladder is not opened but instead is retracted and prostatic tissue is removed through an incision in the anterior prostatic capsule. Both of these alternatives involve an abdominal incision. In a perineal prostatectomy, a perineal incision is made and the prostatic tissue is removed through an incision in the posterior prostatic capsule.

Although these traditional surgeries successfully relieve bladder obstruction, they are costly, and postoperative complications can endanger or seriously affect the quality of a man's life. These complications include hemorrhage, water intoxication, infection, thrombosis, damage to surrounding structures, sexual dysfunction, and urinary incontinence.

Laser prostatectomy, the most recently developed surgical intervention for BPH, is based on thermal action. The transurethral ultrasound-guided laser-induced prostatectomy (TULIP) is performed with a probe that is passed transurethrally into the prostatic urethra. While the adjacent prostate area is visualized by ultrasound, the laser energy is directed at the prostate tissue, resulting in tissue necrosis and sloughing. The client is less likely to experience water intoxication because this surgical method allows blood vessels to seal rapidly, keeping irrigant fluid from being forced into the circulation.

Pharmacological

A pharmacological intervention that has been successfully used to treat BPH is the use of alpha blockers. These drugs relax the smooth muscles along the urinary tract without compromising normal urinary control reflexes. Because alpha blockers such as terazosin hydrochloride (Hytrin) and doxazosin mesylate (Cardura) are also used to treat hypertension, the side effect of orthostatic hypotension is possible. Belladonna and opium (B & O) suppositories are used to reduce postoperative bladder spasms, and narcotic analgesics are used to relieve postoperative pain.

▶ NURSING PROCESS

▶ Assessment

▶ Subjective Data

Urinary patterns are the primary focus of a preoperative nursing assessment of a client with BPH. The nurse should ask the client about the presence of urinary frequency, hesitancy, dribbling, number of times he gets up at night to void, and the force of the urinary stream. In addition to a careful general medical history, any information pertaining to a history of chronic urinary tract infections needs to be noted.

Postoperative nursing assessment should include assessing for pain (on a 0 to 10 scale) related to bladder spasms. The client's emotional needs should also be assessed as he may be experiencing anticipatory grieving, body image disturbance, anxiety, or concerns about alteration in sexuality patterns or possible sexual dysfunction. Behavioral or verbal cues from the client may indicate a need for further information or reassurance regarding his condition and related treatment.

▶ Objective Data

When assessing for hemorrhagic shock or postoperative infection, the nurse should monitor vital signs and avoid the use of a rectal thermometer. A bright red urine color persisting for more than a few hours after surgery may be a sign of hemorrhage. Hemorrhage, hyperthermia, hypotension (low blood pressure), and tachycardia should be reported to the physician immediately.

After a TURP, the client will have a three-way Foley catheter and continuous bladder irrigation for at least 24 hours. Intake and output will need to be recorded to ensure that the client has adequate oral intake to promote urinary flow and reduce the infection risk. In measuring output, the amount of irrigant must be subtracted from the total output in order to determine the actual urinary output. After the catheter is removed, the client should be assessed for post void residual and incontinence. Palpating the abdomen for bladder distention, checking the bed linens and clothing for signs of incontinence, or asking the client if he is experiencing loss of urinary control are also assessments to be performed.

It is important for the nurse to assess for water intoxication, which may be the result of absorbing irrigating fluid in addition to the IV fluids. The most common early symptoms of water intoxication are changes in the client's mental status. These may be manifested by agitation, confusion, and, later, convulsions. The client may also have a slow bounding pulse with an increase in systolic and decrease in diastolic blood pressure.

A suprapubic or retropubic prostatectomy does not require a three-way Foley. Instead the client will have a urethral catheter, a tissue drain from the prostatic fossa, and an abdominal dressing. The nurse needs to assess for incisional pain and do a dressing check, being careful to also check the linens underneath the client's back for drainage.

Nursing diagnoses for a postoperative client having a TURP for benign prostatic hyperplasia may include the following:

Nursing Diagnoses	Planning/Goals	Nursing Interventions
▶ *Pain, Acute, related to bladder spasms or incision*	The client will state that pain has decreased.	Assess for pain using a pain scale every 2 to 4 hours.
		Maintain traction on the urethral catheter by anchoring the catheter to the leg with tape, taking care that accidental additional traction will not occur with leg movement.
		Monitor for signs of bladder spasm pain such as facial grimacing, nonflow of irrigating solution into bladder, and urinating around the catheter. Administer analgesics and antispasmodics as ordered.
		Teach deep breathing, relaxation techniques.
▶ *Fluid Volume Excess, Risk for, related to post-operative irrigation*	The client will not experience water intoxication.	Accurately record I&O including irrigation fluid.
		Monitor for changes in the client's behavior, especially confusion and agitation, which may be the first signs of cerebral edema.
		Monitor for hypertension, bradycardia, weakness, and seizures.
▶ *Incontinence, Stress or Urge, related to poor sphincter control after catheter removal after surgery*	The client will achieve urinary control after removal of the catheter.	Advise the client that temporary urinary incontinence frequently occurs after surgery, and reassure him that this is normal.
		Teach the client perineal exercises that will help him regain urinary control. These exercises consist of tightening and relaxing gluteal muscles and are to be used each time the client urinates.
▶ *Knowledge Deficit, related to surgery and postoperative care*	The client will demonstrate understanding of postoperative activity restrictions and medical follow-up.	Encourage the client to maintain a fluid intake of 2,500 to 3,000 mL/day.
		Teach the client that vigorous exercise, driving, stair climbing, sexual activity, and lifting more than 10 pounds should be avoided until approved by the physician.
		Instruct the client to avoid straining at stool and to use stool softeners or mild cathartics as ordered.
		Instruct the client to report any bleeding or diminished urinary stream to the physician.
▶ *Sexual Dysfunction, related to surgery*	The client will regain sexual function postoperatively.	Monitor the client's statements to determine if he has any misunderstanding of the surgery and sexual function.
		Instruct the client to avoid sexual intercourse until physician approval is given and that it may take time for his previous level of sexual function to return.
		Encourage the client to use a variety of forms of sexual expression, such as kissing, stroking, and cuddling.
		Provide the client with opportunities to voice his feelings and ask questions.
		Advise the client that it is normal and not harmful if his urine has a milky appearance due to retrograde ejaculation.

Evaluation Each goal must be evaluated to determine how it has been met by the client.

MALIGNANT NEOPLASMS

Malignant neoplasms include breast, cervical, endometrial, ovarian, prostate, testicular, and penile cancers.

BREAST CANCER

Breast cancer is the second major cause of cancer death among women. Statistics indicate that 1 woman in 10 will develop breast cancer sometime during her life. The American Cancer Society (ACS) estimates that 180,300 new cases were diagnosed in the United States in 1998. The 5-year survival rate is 97% for localized cancer, 76% for cancer that has spread regionally, and 21% for cancers having distant metastases (ACS, 1998). Elderly women (those over 65) have twice the incidence of breast cancer as do younger women. Less than 1% of all breast cancers occur in men; in 1998, approximately 1,600 new cases of breast cancer were diagnosed in men.

The key to cure is early detection by physical examination, mammography, and breast self-examination. A painless mass or thickening is the most common presenting symptom.

Because it is so uncommon, breast cancer in men is all the more dangerous since it is not considered a threat. Late diagnosis is quite common; therefore, males need to be educated in the technique of and encouraged to do breast self-examination (BSE). Signs and symptoms of breast cancer include breast lumps, pain, or discharge from the nipple.

Women at greatest risk for developing breast cancer are those who:

- Had a mother or sibling with breast cancer
- Never had children or had their first child after the age of 30
- Never breast fed
- Have a history of fibrocystic breast disease
- Started menstruating before age 10
- Are obese
- Consume a high-fat diet and a moderate amount of alcohol
- Smoke
- Experienced a late menopause

A woman generally presents at the health care office after the discovery of a lump in her breast. If she has been performing BSE routinely each month, she is likely to be familiar with even minute changes in the breast tissue. Breast cancers often occur in the upper, outer quadrant of the breast and may extend into the tail of the breast and spread upward into the axilla. It is important to teach clients to examine the axillary region as well as the breast during BSE (refer to Figure

35-8). Approximately 96% of women know about the importance of performing BSE monthly; however, only 33% actually perform it on a regular basis (Baron & Walsh, 1995).

Women also seek medical advice because they notice a discharge from the breast, dimpling of the skin, retraction of the nipple, pain, a unilateral change in breast size (Figure 35-11), or an orange-peel appearance (peau d'orange) of the skin. Dimpling and puckering are usually associated with the breast tissue or tumor attaching to the skin or the underlying muscle mass, which does not permit movement. The nurse should not be misled by the client's report of a tender lump or mass and assume it is fibrocystic breast disease (FBD). All new or enlarged lumps or masses in the breast require immediate assessment.

The presence of tiny, palpable clusters of calcium, or "microclusters," may be an early sign of breast cancer. These should be followed closely with mammography every 6 to 12 months to detect subtle changes in shape or size.

The American Cancer Society (1998) recommends that women ages 20 to 40 perform BSE each month and have a clinical breast examination every 3 to 4 years. For women 41 to 49 years of age, BSE should also be performed monthly, a clinical examination every 1 to 2 years, and a mammogram every 1 to 2 years. Women 50 and older should follow the monthly routine for BSE and have a clinical examination and mammogram every year.

Mammography may be performed by the stereotactic computer guided technique. This advanced method allows needle biopsies to be taken at the same time if necessary. Often, the physician or nurse practitioner will recommend this method after an initial mammogram has shown suspicious areas. This technique is less costly than excisional biopsy and can be performed with little discomfort to the client. The client is placed in a prone position on the special examination

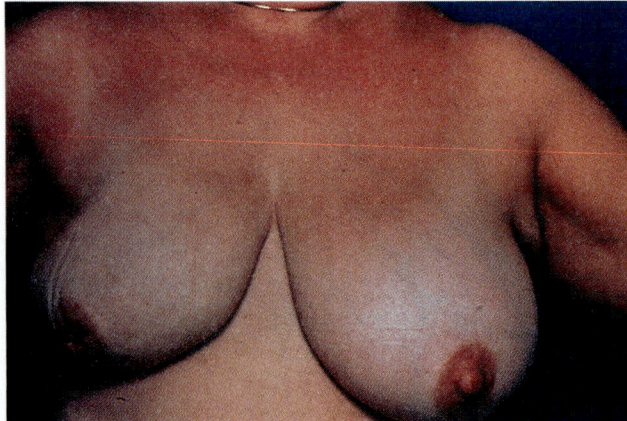

Figure 35-11 Asymmetry of Breasts Due to Cancer *(Courtesy of Dr. S. Eva Singletary, University of Texas, M. D. Anderson Cancer Center)*

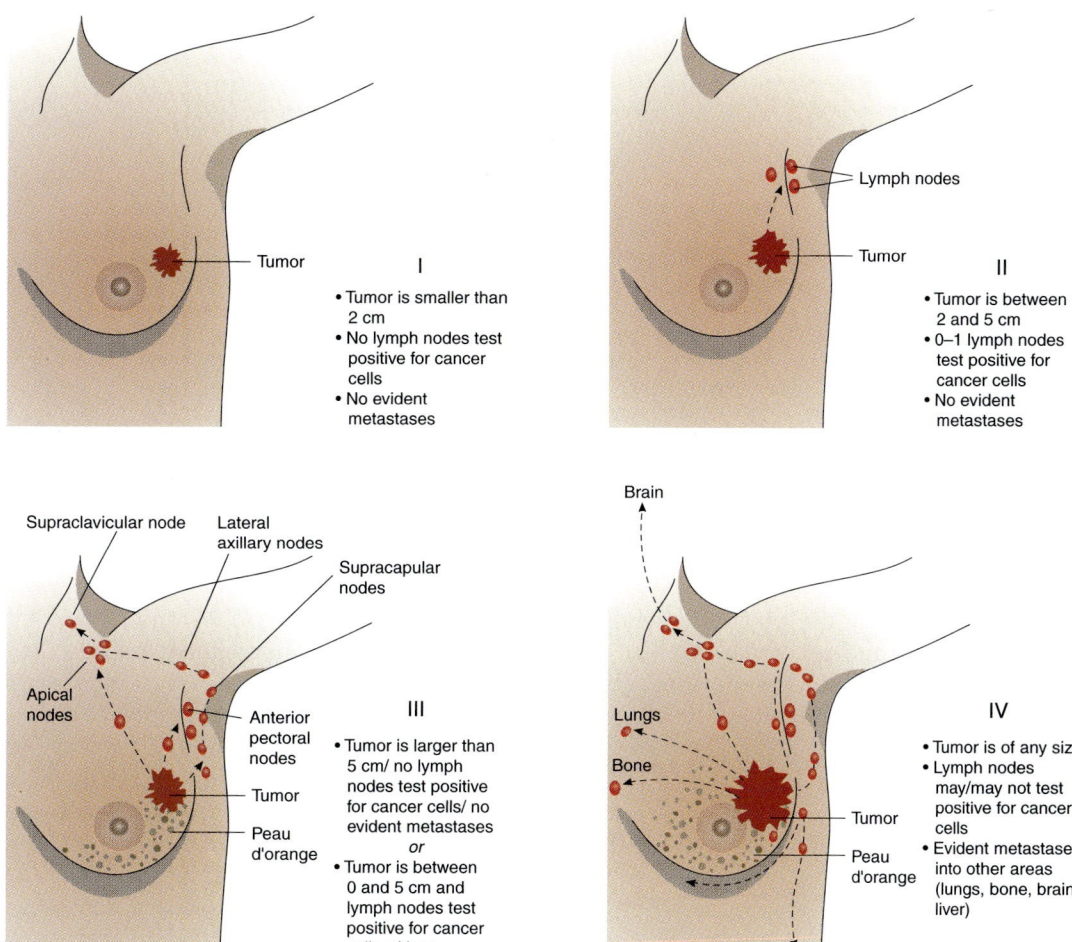

Figure 35-12 Breast Cancer Staging

table with the breast hanging down through the opening in the table. The operator moves the position of the table to visualize the entire breast area via computerized guidance.

After the breast has been biopsied and the tissue has been examined by the pathologist, if a malignancy is confirmed, the client may be advised to proceed with surgical removal of the affected tissue. This procedure is referred to as a lumpectomy or mastectomy. Figure 35-12 shows the staging of breast cancer.

Medical–Surgical Management

Medical

Radiation and chemotherapy may be used as adjuvant therapy, but surgery is the primary form of treatment.

Surgical

There is an abundance of lymphatic vessels proximal to the breast. Malignant cells can thus escape into the general lymphatic system and be spread throughout the body. A lumpectomy is surgical removal of the cancerous mass. A simple mastectomy removes the

tumor mass and only a small portion of the adjacent tissue. In the modified mastectomy, the entire breast tissue and nearby lymph nodes are removed; the muscles of the chest wall are left relatively intact. With the radical mastectomy, the entire breast, lymph nodes, and underlying pectoralis muscle are removed. Figure 35-13 shows the various options in the surgical management of breast cancer. The greater the extent of the surgical removal, the longer the client's recovery process and the greater the need for rehabilitation in the use of the upper extremity on the affected side.

Reconstructive surgery after a mastectomy may be determined by the amount of breast tissue and muscle remaining after the initial procedure, the position of the mastectomy scar, and the probability of recurrent breast cancer. Breast reconstruction can help the client deal with the disfigurement that results from the mastectomy.

The client's desire for reconstruction and her psychological status play an important role in determining the personal value of additional surgery. In the United States particularly, the breast is associated with childbearing and female sexuality. It may be difficult for the client to express her concerns to her partner regarding her sexuality and desirability after the mastectomy.

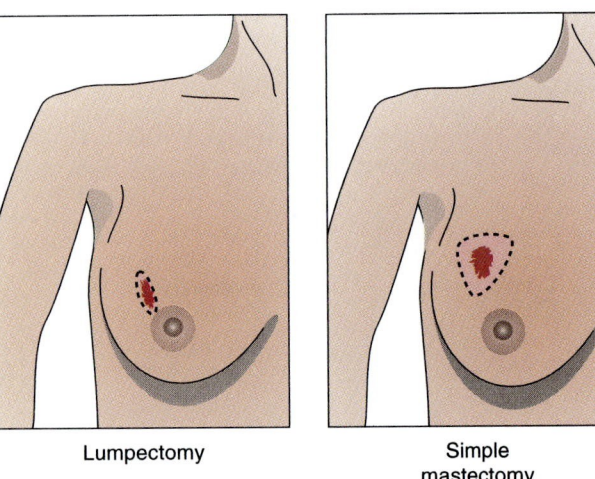
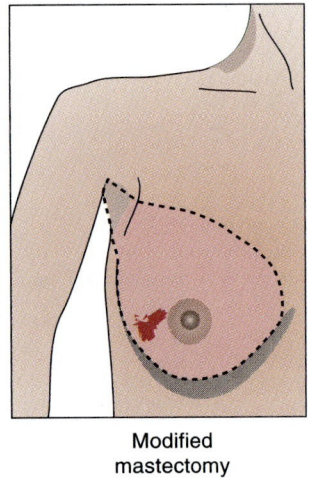
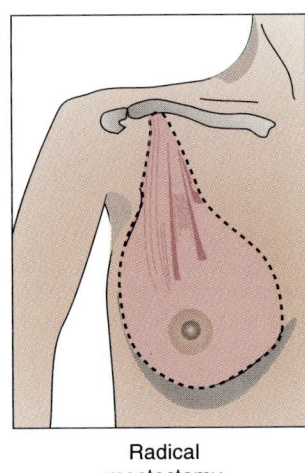

| Lumpectomy | Simple mastectomy | Modified mastectomy | Radical mastectomy |

Figure 35-13 Surgical Options for Breast Cancer

She may have difficulty facing the physical alteration immediately after surgery and for some time in the future. The caring nurse with good interpersonal communication skills can help the client identify and verbalize her feelings of loss and thus promote the psychological healing process and acceptance of the altered body image.

Breast prostheses constructed to look and feel like real breast tissue are available. The prosthesis fits into a special pocket inside the brassiere. Some types are available for swim suits and strapless tops. The construction of the prosthesis varies from sponge rubber to fluid- or air-filled.

Volunteers from the local cancer society often visit new mastectomy clients to assist them in the physical and psychological transition and adjustment after breast surgery. The American Cancer Society publishes a pamphlet entitled *Help Yourself to Recovery,* which includes simple postmastectomy exercises to perform as a part of the rehabilitation process.

Pharmacological

Some of the agents used in the treatment of breast cancer include antineoplastic drugs such as antiestrogens: megestrol acetate (Megace), medroxyproges-

terone acetate (Depo-Provera), tamoxifen citrate (Nolvadex), and aminoglutethamide (Cytadren). Androgens for postmenopausal clients include testolactone (Teslac); methyltestosterone (Testred), or rotating combinations of chemotherapy agents such as cyclophosphamide (Cytoxan), an alkalating agent, doxorubicin hydrochloride (Adriamycin), an antitumor antibiotic; 5-fluorouracil (Adrucil) and methotrexate sodium (Rheumatrex); antimetabolites; and prednisone (Orasone), a glucocorticoid via intravenous or oral routes. These drugs may be initiated before or after surgery. These antineoplastic agents act in several ways to either inhibit cellular growth or interfere with DNA replication. A laboratory test called tissue assay determines if estrogen or progesterone stimulates the cancer cells to grow. If the cancerous growth is stimulated by estrogen, antiestrogen drugs are used to treat the breast cancer. When the tumors are not estrogen-dependent, estrogen is used as a chemotherapy agent to treat breast cancers. Examples of two estrogen medications are diethylstilbestrol diphosphate (Stilphostrol) and ethinyl estradiol (Estinyl).

Paclitaxel (Taxol) has demonstrated positive results in clinical trials with breast cancer therapies. It acts by prohibiting cell replication. One of the benefits of this agent is that it causes milder nausea than many of the other chemotherapy agents that are used. It has the potential to cause severe anaphylactic reactions due to a histamine release. To avoid this problem, the client should be medicated with the following medications before Taxol infusion therapy: a corticosteroid such as dexamethasone (Decadron), a histamine blocker such as cimetidine (Tagamet), and an antihistamine diphenhydramine hydrochloride (Benadryl).

Other Therapies

Breast tissue and lymphatic regions may be radiated before or after surgical excision of the tumor. This treatment may be done prophylactically to prevent the

HOME HEALTH CARE

After a Mastectomy
- Avoid carrying items in the affected arm or wearing purse straps over the affected shoulder.
- Have vaccinations and lab tests or blood draws done on the unaffected side only.
- Obtain immediate medical attention for all injuries and infections of the affected side to prevent complications.

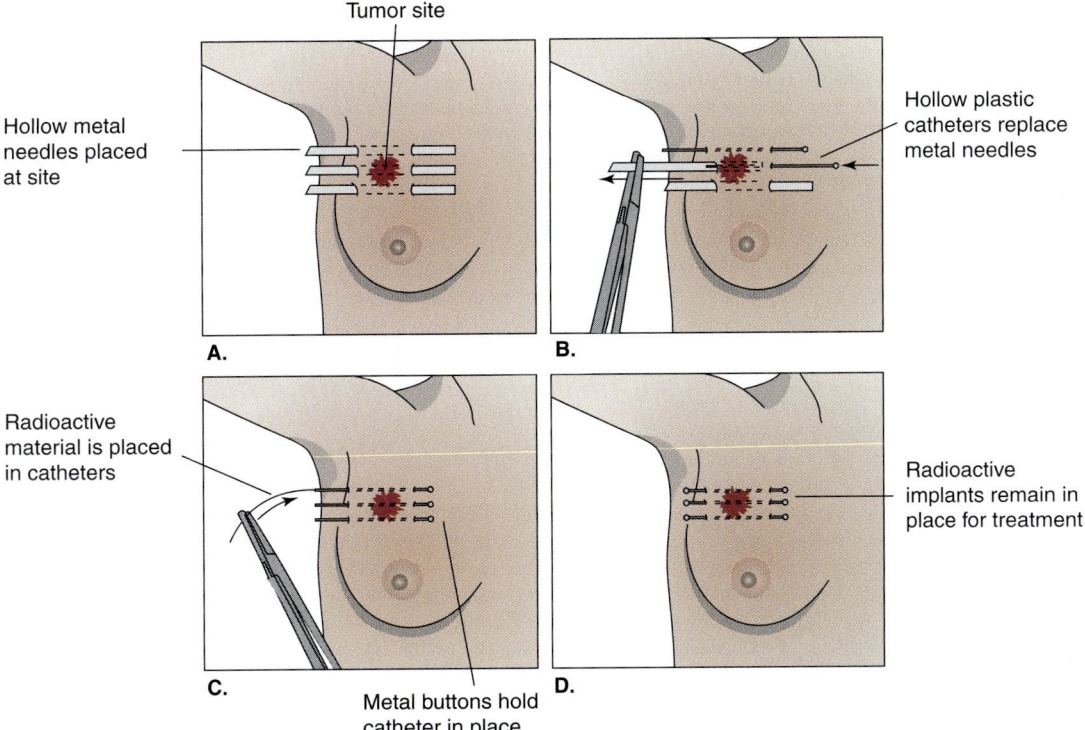

Tumor site

Hollow metal needles placed at site

Hollow plastic catheters replace metal needles

A.

B.

Radioactive material is placed in catheters

Radioactive implants remain in place for treatment

C.

D.

Metal buttons hold catheter in place

Figure 35-14 Brachytherapy for Treatment of Breast Cancer

metastasis of malignant cells to other areas, or it may be done as a palliative measure to maintain the client's comfort. Figure 35-14 illustrates brachytherapy, the use of radioactive implants at the site of breast cancer.

▶ NURSING PROCESS

▶ Assessment

▶ Subjective Data

The client may come to the office concerned about a newly discovered breast lump and other changes in the breast, such as dimpling, puckering, or discharge. The nurse should ask how long the lump has been present, whether it is movable, whether it is tender, the frequency that BSE is performed, the date of the most recent mammogram, and current medications being taken. Pain should be assessed, using a pain scale to objectify data. Other questions should include the risk factors.

PROFESSIONAL TIP

Tamoxifen

In October 1998, tamoxifen (Nolvadex) was approved to be used for prevention of breast cancer in healthy women who have a higher-than-normal risk factor for breast cancer ("Tamoxifen for breast cancer prevention," 1998).

▶ Objective Data

The nurse should assess vital signs and weight and review the report of the last mammogram. Breasts should be examined for lumps and discharge from the nipples. During the postoperative phase, the client's vital signs and incisional site must be assessed, and the client's statements and behaviors monitored to determine emotional status.

Nursing diagnoses for a client with breast cancer may include the following:

Nursing Diagnoses	Planning/Goals	Nursing Interventions
▶ *Fear, related to breast cancer, possible metastasis, surgery, and disfigurement*	The client will express fears. The client will state one positive method of coping.	Encourage client to express specific feelings of fear. Take extra time to clarify or explain procedures and treatments. Provide written information along with verbal information. Encourage support of family members and significant others. Encourage a preoperative visit by a member of the cancer society or Reach to Recovery.

continued

Nursing Diagnoses	Planning/Goals	Nursing Interventions
▶ *Body Image Disturbance, related to removal of the breast*	The client will discuss her feelings related to the loss of her breast and demonstrate acceptance of the change in physical appearance.	Remain attentive to signals from the client indicating readiness to look at the surgical site and encourage doing so when readiness is displayed.
		Be alert for client's comments regarding body changes.
		Encourage client recommended for chemotherapy to obtain a wig before therapy begins. Approximately 80% of clients undergoing chemotherapy will experience hair loss, and, if the client becomes accustomed to wearing a wig before hair begins to fall out, the client may feel more comfortable later.
		Inform client that she may have decreased sensation and lymphatic fluid retention in the arm on the affected side.
		Teach client to keep arm on affected side elevated above the level of the heart to promote lymph drainage.
		Encourage client to wear a properly fitting elastic compression sleeve on the affected arm that will help reduce the lymphedema.
		Anticipate the client's need to grieve the loss of her breast.
		Encourage use of rehabilitation services (Reach to Recovery).
▶ *Breathing Pattern, Ineffective, related to the proximity of the surgical incision to respiratory muscles and pain with respiratory effort*	The client's breath sounds will remain clear to auscultation. The client will effectively cough and deep breathe every 2 hours.	Preoperatively, teach the client how to turn, cough, and deep breathe.
		Postoperatively, assess the client's breath sounds, rate, and quality of respirations every 4 hours.
		Monitor O_2 saturation with pulse oximeter.
		Encourage deep breathing or the use of incentive spirometry every hour.
		Provide O_2 as needed.
		Medicate the client or encourage use of the PCA pump before performing exercises or deep breathing.
▶ *Self-Care Deficit, related to limited use and range of motion on the affected side and postoperative discomforts*	The client will gradually regain ROM and provide self-care.	Begin passive range-of-motion exercises on the first or second postop day as ordered.
		Demonstrate postoperative exercises for the affected arm or request a consult from the physical therapy department.
		Observe the client as exercises are performed and reinforce correct performance.
		Encourage active ROM as soon as ordered by the physician to strengthen the operative side. This may be difficult at first due to tissue soreness from surgery.
		Encourage client to provide self-care as much as able.

Evaluation Each goal must be evaluated to determine how it has been met by the client.

SAMPLE NURSING CARE PLAN

THE CLIENT WITH BREAST CANCER

Claire Wilder, age 57, is married, with two children ages 24 and 22. During a bath, she noted a small, movable lump in her right breast, grew concerned, and went to see her health care provider. Family history is significant for fibrocystic breast disease and breast cancer on the maternal side (mother, aunt, sister). Personal history: onset of menses at age 10 with regular 28-day cycle, 5-day flow. She is 5 feet 5 inches tall and weighs 175 pounds. Her history is negative for alcohol use, but she smokes one to one-and-a-half packs of cigarettes daily. She did not breastfeed the children. Her last mammogram was 15 years ago. BSE is not practiced routinely. States: "I'm not sure just how to do the exam anyway."

Physical examination reveals a pea-sized lump in the upper right quadrant of the right breast and multiple clusters of lumps throughout each breast. Dimpling is present superior to the nipple. No nipple

continued

discharge was noted. The remainder of the exam was unremarkable. Vital signs were within normal limits. A mammogram revealed a suspicious mass, and a biopsy performed using stereotactic visualization was positive for cancer cells. A modified mastectomy was performed the next day with biopsies of adjacent lymph nodes. Six of ten nodes were also positive.

The morning after surgery, Claire displayed behaviors that the nurse interpreted as anxiety. She confided in the nurse that she was afraid she was going to die, as her mother had, from the cancer. Claire had a large chest pressure dressing with two Jackson-Pratt drains in place. She stated that she was glad she had the PCA pump to take care of the pain.

Nursing Diagnosis 1 *Self-Care Deficit, bathing/dressing, related to temporary altered function of arm as evidenced by large chest pressure dressing and two drains in place*

PLANNING/GOALS	NURSING INTERVENTIONS	RATIONALE	EVALUATION
Claire will meet her daily hygiene needs before discharge.	Assess Claire's ability to use affected arm to perform ADLs.	Assessment provides the nurse with baseline information related to Claire's abilities and limitations.	Claire's hygiene needs were met.
	Provide assistance as needed to complete hygiene tasks, such as bathing and grooming.	Assisting with tasks and encouraging Claire to participate will facilitate the return of function and self-esteem.	
	Encourage gradual resumption of activities as Claire indicates readiness.	By gradually increasing the use of the affected arm, Claire will regain strength and maintain the mobility of the extremity. Claire is empowered to help perform her own care, which validates her self-image and worth.	

Nursing Diagnosis 2 *Fear, related to removal of the breast as evidenced by her fear of dying as her mother had*

PLANNING/GOALS	NURSING INTERVENTIONS	RATIONALE	EVALUATION
Claire will have less fear about breast removal.	Encourage Claire and family to verbalize their feelings and concerns related to the diagnosis and treatment.	Sharing feelings and concerns often relieves fear. Claire's and family's perceptions may differ from health care worker's and should be identified.	Claire verbalized having less fear about the removal of her breast.

continued

	Assess Claire's normal or previously used coping behaviors	Identification of previous coping patterns enables the nurse to help the client use or change coping behaviors.	
	Involve Claire and her family in care planning.	Involving the client and the family in the planning of the care makes them more likely to feel a part of the team rather than simply accepting a passive "client role."	

Nursing Diagnosis 3 *Pain, related to surgical manipulation of tissues and excision of tissue as evidenced by client statement that she was glad she had the PCA pump to take care of the pain*

PLANNING/GOALS	NURSING INTERVENTIONS	RATIONALE	EVALUATION
Claire will verbalize that pain is controlled.	Assess Claire's pain level and response to analgesia every 2 hours.	The nurse must be alert to increasing pain and how the client is tolerating the pain medication.	Claire reports pain is controlled at less than 2 on a 1–10 scale.
	Instruct Claire how to use the PCA pump.	Use of the PCA pump allows the client greater control over analgesia and provides consistent relief from pain.	
	Evaluate the effectiveness of analgesia q 2 hours.	Evaluating the client's response to medication allows the nurse to identify any untoward effects and effectiveness of the medication.	
	Reposition Claire q 2 hours.	Changing positions helps to improve vascular flow and relieves pressure on bony prominences.	
	Elevate the arm on the right side on pillows.	Increased venous flow decreases edema and discomfort due to pressure on nerves in the area.	

CERVICAL CANCER

An abnormal condition of the cervix known as dysplasia may be an early sign of developing cervical cancer. Dysplasia is a change in the size and shape of the cervical cells, and it is classified as mild, moderate, or severe. An abnormal Papanicolaou (Pap) smear may be the first indication of a problem. Pap smears are classified from 1 through 5. A 1 is considered a normal cervix, and a 5 would indicate a malignant condition.

Cervical cancer is the most preventable gynecological cancer. Sexual habits constitute a major factor in the development of cancer of the cervix. Sexually transmitted disease, particularly the human papillomavirus (HPV), is a particularly significant factor. According to Otto (1997), some 15% of all women who have genital herpes will develop dysplasia or cancer *in situ*. Other factors associated with cervical cancer include a history of multiple sexual partners and maternal use of diethylstilbestrol (DES) during pregnancy. The most common sign of cervical cancer is abnormal bleeding, which progresses from a thin, watery, blood-tinged discharge to frank bleeding. Contact bleeding may also occur after intercourse. Advanced disease is indicated by odor, pain in the lower back and groin, difficulty in voiding, hematuria, and rectal bleeding. The Pap smear is the key to early detection. Promotion of regular pelvic exams and education regarding risk are essential.

Although cervical cancer can occur at any age, it occurs most frequently in women between 35 and 55 years of age. It is usually insidious in its onset because it is asymptomatic. Cervical cancer has a high cure rate in the early stages, and it is easily detected by the routine annual Pap smear. The overall 5-year survival rate is 69% (ACS, 1998).

The nurse should immediately bring any abnormal Pap smear results to the attention of the physician or nurse practitioner so the client can be notified and the appropriate follow-up treatment initiated. A repeat Pap smear may be indicated after treatment with a vaginal antibiotic cream, or a colposcopy may be performed.

Staging of the cancer progresses from I to IV (Figure 35-15). Carcinoma *in situ* (CIS) means that the cancerous cells remain within the cervix and have not yet spread to adjacent areas. The higher the number on the staging table, the more the cancer has metastasized to other structures. Stages II through IV indicate that the cancer cells have invaded the bladder, vagina, or other pelvic organs.

STAGING SYSTEM FOR CANCER OF THE CERVIX	
Stage	Characteristics
I	• Carcinoma is strictly confined to cervix (extension to corpus should be disregarded)
IA	• Preclinical carcinoma
IA1	• Minimal microscopically evident stromal invasion
IA2	• Microscopic lesions no more than 5 mm depth measured from base of epithelium surface or glandular from which it originates, and horizontal spread not to exceed 7 mm
IB	• All other cases of stage I; occult cancer should be marked "occ"
II	• Carcinoma extends beyond cervix but has not extended to pelvic wall; it involves vagina, but not as far as lower third
IIA	• No obvious parametrical involvement
IIB	• Obvious parametrical involvement
III	• Carcinoma has extended to pelvic wall; on rectal examination, there is no cancer-free space between tumor and pelvic wall; tumor involves lower third of vagina; all cases with hydronephrosis or nonfunctioning kidney should be included, unless they are known to be due to another cause
IIIA	• No extension to pelvic wall, but involvement of lower third of vagina
IIIB	• Extension to pelvic wall, or hydronephrosis or nonfunctioning kidney due to tumor
IV	• Carcinoma has extended beyond true pelvis or has clinically involved mucosa of bladder or rectum
IVA	• Spread of growth to adjacent pelvic organs
IVB	• Spread to distant organs

Figure 35-15 Cervical Cancer Staging

Medical–Surgical Management

Surgical

Treatment modalities may include conization, a surgical excision of a cone-shaped section of the abnormal cervical tissues. This procedure is desirable if the client is of childbearing age and wants to bear children in the future.

Laser surgery, cryosurgery (freezing of the cells with liquid nitrogen), or cauterization (burning) may be performed as alternative methods of treatment if the cervical lesions are easily visible for the procedure. A total hysterectomy or radical pelvic surgery may be required to eradicate the cancer. If the spread of the disease has become too extensive, treatment will be directed toward palliative measures.

Other Therapies

The physician may recommend the use of radium implants or radiation therapy before the surgical excision of the cervix. The nurse must be cautious in providing nursing care for the client with radium implants. Pregnant nurses or female nurses of childbearing age should not care for this client or spend extended periods of time at the bedside. Direct client care should be organized to optimize time spent at the bedside. A sign should be hung on the door to indicate that radiation is being used in the room and provide a warning for visitors to limit their visit time. With the implants in place, the client will remain on complete bed rest.

In addition, chemotherapy may be utilized as an adjunct therapy to help shrink the tumor or slow its growth.

▶ NURSING PROCESS

▶ Assessment

▶ Subjective Data

The client may complain of postcoital bleeding (bleeding after intercourse) or spotting between menstrual periods or after menopause and, occasionally, a foul-smelling vaginal discharge. Later, as the disease progresses, she may complain of increased or bloody discharge, weight loss, and pain that radiates down the lower back and legs.

▶ Objective Data

Objective data may include the presence and appearance of a vaginal discharge. The cervix may appear eroded or raw and may bleed easily when touched with a cotton-tipped applicator or Pap scraper. Necrotic tissue may be present and cause the foul odor. Pap smear results will probably indicate dysplasia or Class II through Class IV cell changes. Tissue samples obtained through colposcopic examination will also demonstrate cellular changes. In advanced disease, weight loss and anemia may be present. Laparotomy may be performed to stage the disease along with other laboratory and diagnostic testing to identify metastases. Areas most likely to be investigated will be proximal to the cervix, including the rectum, vagina, bladder, and pelvis.

Nursing diagnoses for a client with cervical cancer may include the following:

Nursing Diagnoses	Planning/Goals	Nursing Interventions
▶ *Anxiety-related to unknown outcome and possible treatments*	The client will verbalize having less anxiety about treatment and possible outcome.	Be aware of the client's emotional state throughout the course of care and use effective interpersonal communication to facilitate the client's acceptance of her condition and the treatments.
		Explain diagnostic tests and procedures to client to decrease her anxiety.
		Provide therapeutic emotional support to client to help her cope with feelings.
▶ *Sexuality Patterns, Altered, related to vaginal bleeding, discomfort, and procedures*	The client will return to normal pattern of sexuality after recovery from treatment for cervical cancer.	Inform client that she may experience dyspareunia related to vaginal dryness after radiation therapy.
		Listen to client's concerns.
		Instruct client to use a water-soluble lubricant during intercourse or to use lubricated condoms to decrease irritation.
▶ *Urinary Elimination, Altered related to sensory motor impairment from radiation effects*	The client will regain normal urinary elimination.	Assess the function of the Foley catheter to ensure patency and drainage.
		Provide careful catheter care.
		Record I&O, including color of urine.
		Encourage the client to drink many fluids to flush the kidneys and decrease risk of UTI.
		Promote urination when catheter is removed.

Evaluation Each goal must be evaluated to determine how it has been met by the client.

ENDOMETRIAL CANCER

Postmenopausal women are at the greatest risk for endometrial cancer, especially if they have taken estrogen replacement therapy for several years (usually more than 5 years). Research has shown that unopposed estrogen stimulation of the endometrial lining has a strong relationship with the development of endometrial cancer. During the normal menstrual cycle, estrogen and progesterone rise and fall. These hormonal fluctuations affect the stimulation of the endometrial tissue to grow or to be sloughed off, in a sense in opposition to each other. Without the progesterone effects, the endometrial tissue is not sloughed off at regular intervals and may undergo cellular changes leading to a high risk for endometrial dysplasia or cancer. For this reason, many physicians and nurse practitioners recommend estrogen-progesterone therapy for clients who experience menopausal symptoms. The combination of the two hormones stimulates the normal menstrual hormonal cycle and causes monthly sloughing of the endometrium. Clients may resist this combination therapy because they are reluctant to continue having menstrual periods in their fifties and sixties.

Other risk factors associated with endometrial cancer may include never having borne a child, being Caucasian, being middle class, never having had sexual intercourse, or being of Jewish descent.

Cancer of the endometrium usually does not produce symptoms until it becomes relatively advanced. Routine Pap smear and pelvic examinations are inadequate for early diagnosis. An endometrial biopsy, which examines the tissue from the uterine lining under a microscope, is the best diagnostic tool to identify cellular changes. This may be done on an annual basis when the client has a routine examination. The medical follow-up treatment plan is dependent upon the biopsy results. D&C has a potential for spreading the cancer cells to adjacent tissues because the malignant cells may escape into the bloodstream at the time of the procedure. This is not usually a problem with the biopsy because the amount of tissue removed is so small and blood loss is minimal. A D&C is also more expensive, higher risk, and requires some type of anesthesia. The 5-year survival rate for endometrial cancer is 84% (ACS, 1998).

Medical–Surgical Management

Treatments for endometrial cancer may range from radiation, radium implants, chemotherapy, or surgery to a combination of any of the above. The choices of treatment are related to the staging of the cancer.

Medical

Intravenous fluid administration will be implemented to replace fluids lost by the excessive bleeding. A blood transfusion may also be ordered because of a low hemoglobin. A hemoglobin above 10 gm/dL is preferred before surgical intervention. The physician may order whole blood or packed red blood cells to increase the hemoglobin rapidly.

Surgical

Surgery for endometrial or cervical cancer includes hysterectomy. A total hysterectomy is the removal of the cervix and the uterus. In a subtotal hysterectomy, only the uterus is removed and the cervix remains. A radical or pan hysterectomy includes the removal of the ovaries, cervix, uterus, fallopian tubes, pelvic lymph nodes, and part of the vagina. Vaginal hysterectomy procedures have been refined with the laparoscopic approach so that many clients are released from the hospital within 24 to 36 hours postoperatively. If the cancer has spread beyond the uterus into the pelvic region, an abdominal hysterectomy may be the best approach for visualization and maneuvering room during the surgical procedure. The physician may recommend a course of radiation therapy after surgery.

Pharmacological

Hormonal therapy with megestrol acetate (Megace), medroxyprogesterone acetate (Depo-Provera), or hydroxyprogesterone caproate (Prodrox) may be administered to suppress tumor growth when the cancer is considered inoperable or has metastasized, especially if the tumor receptors are estrogen-stimulated.

Other Therapies

There is a tendency for endometrial cancer to confine itself to the uterus, which increases the client's 5-year survival prognosis. Endometrial cancer is also one that usually responds well to the therapies available at this time, including radiation. Radiation may be delivered to the pelvic region via external sources, or it may be delivered via intracavitary devices or implants with radium or cesium. There is a potential danger for injury to adjacent pelvic structures during radiation therapy. The nurse should be alert for signs of complications, such as bleeding from the rectum, moderate to severe abdominal pain, constipation, or diarrhea. New therapies are being developed using protons that are capable of more direct application of radiation, which decreases the chance of injury to other organs or structures.

PROFESSIONAL TIP

Radiation Exposure Risk

Owing to the risk of radiation exposure to the caregiver from the radiation implant device, keep procedures that require exposure to the client's perineal area at a minimum.

Nursing Management

One of the earliest symptoms reported by many clients is vaginal bleeding. If the client is postmenopausal, it is imperative that all bleeding be investigated as soon as possible unless it is from hormonally induced periods. Late in the progression of the cancer, the client may experience symptoms similar to those discussed with cervical cancer. Pain is often associated with the spread of cancer to adjacent organs and is considered a late sign.

Objective data may be collected from the client's physical exam findings, biopsy reports, and a history of hormone replacement therapy with or without the estrogen-progesterone combination.

OVARIAN CANCER

Ovarian cancer most often originates in the epithelial tissue of the ovary, and, like cervical and endometrial cancer, does not produce symptoms until it is in an advanced, inoperable stage and is sometimes called "the silent killer." Its symptoms are vague and may be ignored for a long time before the client seeks medical attention.

Ovarian cancer causes more deaths than does any other gynecological cancer, an estimated 14,500 in 1998 (ACS, 1998). The incidence is greatest in women between 45 and 65 years of age. Nulliparity (never having borne a child), smoking, alcohol, infertility, and a high-fat diet are factors that place the client at higher risk for developing ovarian cancer. Metastasis occurs in over 75% of cases before diagnosis, and often the cancer has spread beyond the pelvis. The colon is the most frequent site of ovarian cancer metastasis, then the stomach, and diaphragm.

Unfortunately, medical research has not yet developed an early diagnostic or screening tool to detect ovarian cancer. It is believed, however, that there is an increased risk of ovarian cancer for clients with breast cancer and vice versa. A family history of two or more female relatives with breast or ovarian cancer provides a sound rationale for more frequent breast and pelvic examinations. Often the physician or NP palpates an ovarian mass on a routine bimanual examination. This finding is cause for further investigation by pelvic ultrasound or CT scan to determine the size, character, and consistency (solid or fluid-filled) of the mass and whether other pelvic structures are involved. Some experts believe that there is a link between the occurrence of ovarian cysts and the development of ovarian cancers in certain women.

General diagnostic studies, such as a lower GI series, chest x-ray, intravenous pyelogram (IVP), and laparoscopy may be useful in determining the extent of the primary and secondary lesions. A substance called

CA-125 may be measured in the blood if ovarian cancer is suspected because this type of malignancy produces the CA-125. Used alone, this is not diagnostic of ovarian cancer because the CA-125 marker in the blood may be present in some benign conditions of the ovary, such as benign ovarian cysts (National Cancer Institute, 1991). If the client develops peritoneal fluid or ascites as the cancer progresses, it may be removed by paracentesis for cytologic examination.

Recurrent disease is common and may occur in 2 years or less. Continued medical surveillance is recommended every 2 months for a period of 2 years for the earliest possible detection of new lesions. The 5-year survival rate is 46% (ACS, 1998).

Medical–Surgical Management

Surgical

Surgical excision of the ovary is rarely successful because of the extensiveness of the disease. A total abdominal hysterectomy with a bilateral salpingo-oophorectomy is performed for most stages of the disease. Most often a combination of radiation, chemotherapy, immunotherapy, and surgery produces the best results, even if they are only palliative for the client. The client must be actively involved and informed of her treatment options as well as her prognosis to enable her to make sound choices in the treatments chosen.

Pharmacological

Chemotherapy drugs that have been used with ovarian cancer treatment include cyclophosphamide (Cytoxan), doxorubicin hydrochloride (Adriamycin), mitomycin (Mutamycin), and paclitaxel (Taxol). These may be administered by regional or intraarterial perfusion techniques. These percutaneous modes direct the drugs to the lesion's vascular supply. If the cancer has not metastasized, a regimen of chemotherapy using a single drug, such as Cytoxan, may be administered over the course of 5 days and repeated again at regular intervals over the course of a year. A combination of the chemotherapy agents, used in a rotating series, is often more effective for reproductive cancers in the advanced stages. For example, the client would receive one drug over the course of 5 days, then switch to another drug for 5 days, and then a third drug for 5 days. This series may be repeated over the year in a similar pattern to that used with a single agent.

Sometimes two or three different medications are necessary to achieve pain control. Intravenous medications are often given by a PCA pump with continuous low-dose narcotics. This method seems more effective for the client than IV bolus doses every 4 hours. Medications may also be given slow IV push (an RN procedure), orally in tablets or liquids, intramuscularly, or by transdermal patches (Duragesic). A liquid mixture of syrup, cocaine, morphine, alcohol, flavoring, and water called "Brompton's mixture or elixir" may be ordered. The client may drink up to 20 cc every 3 to 4 hours for pain relief. Most of these methods of narcotic administration are equally effective and may be used in the home care or hospice setting. Other types of medication that may be given include tranquilizers, antiemetics, and laxatives.

▶ NURSING PROCESS

▶ Assessment

▶ Subjective Data

The client may describe fatigue, malaise, diarrhea or constipation, pelvic pressure, frequency of urination, loss of appetite, nausea, weight gain or loss, vaginal bleeding or spotting with intercourse, a foul-smelling vaginal discharge, and pain in the lower back. The list of symptoms is very vague and could be related to many reproductive and nonreproductive disorders.

▶ Objective Data

Objective data pertinent to all cancers of the pelvic reproductive organs may include information from the client's previous health history, reproductive history (onset of menses, pregnancies, contraceptives methods, infections, hormonal replacement therapy, and surgeries), the discovery of a palpable mass during a bimanual examination, an abnormal appearance of the cervix or adjacent tissues, abnormal Pap smear results greater than Class II dysplasia, abnormal cervical or endometrial biopsies, increased abdominal girth, or the presence of ascites and pleural effusion.

Diagnostic tests and laboratory studies may include all or some of the following: Pap smear, pelvic ultrasound, chest x-ray, IVP (intravenous pyelogram), kidney/ureters/bladder x-ray (KUB), CBC with differential, blood chemistry studies, bleeding and clotting time, endometrial biopsy, cervical biopsy, D&C tissue specimens, Schiller's test and colposcopy, laparoscopy, barium enema, and bone scan.

Nursing diagnoses for a client with endometrial or ovarian cancer may include the following:

Nursing Diagnoses,	Planning/Goals,	Nursing Interventions,
Preoperative		
▶ *Fear related to tentative diagnoses, pending surgical procedures, cancer treatment and its side effects, incapacitating or extended illness with resulting dependence, and possible death*	The client will verbalize fears and have behaviors consistent with reduced fear before and after surgery.	Facilitate the client's expression of fear by encouraging the client's open discussion of her concerns. Be alert for nonverbal cues as well. Arrange a consultation with a social worker or chaplain, if appropriate.
▶ *Pain, related to the spread of cancer throughout the pelvis and adjacent structures*	The client will have pain controlled at a level that allows the client to continue to function in her activities of daily living as long as possible.	Administer analgesics as ordered. Provide comfort measures, such as position changes and back rub.

Nursing Diagnoses,	Planning/Goals,	Nursing Interventions,
Postoperative		
▶ *Skin Integrity, Impaired, related to surgical interventions, radiation, and chemotherapy side effects*	The client's skin integrity will be maintained.	Provide the client with proper skin care instructions during and after radiation therapy that may include avoiding soaps, creams, powder, deodorants, and other substances around the incision that may irritate the skin; not washing off the radiation markings; and avoiding tight clothing around the area. Teach the client to look for signs of reactions to radiation therapy, such as tenderness, flushed color (like a sunburn), delayed wound healing, and itching. Perform daily cleansing of the incisional area with water only. If the client is on complete bed rest due to radium implant therapy, provide a complete bedbath as well as morning and bedtime skin care.

continued

Nursing Diagnoses,	Planning/Goals,	Nursing Interventions,
		Organize time near the client's bedside to brief periods to avoid overexposure to radiation.
		Wear rubber gloves when disposing of soiled materials.
		Put soiled dressings in a biohazard waste container.
▶ *Urinary Elimination, Altered, Incontinence, Bowel or Constipation, related to the proximity of surgical site to bowel and bladder, spread of cancer to adjacent structures, manipulation of organs during surgery, administration of narcotic analgesics, lack of activity, and changes in dietary intake*	The client will have adequate bowel and bladder function during the postoperative period.	Explain dietary modifications designed to reduce residue. The diet should be limited in dairy products, raw fruits, grains, and vegetables. Meats must be well cooked and possibly ground.
		If the client is not receiving radium implant therapy, weigh her daily on the same scale at the same time of the day.
		Review the client's normal elimination patterns from the baseline assessment data to help identify early changes in bowel or bladder elimination.
		Forewarn the client of radiation enteritis and cystitis, and common tissue responses to radiation therapy. Instruct her to report symptoms, such as diarrhea, cramping, frequency, urgency, and dysuria.
		Assess bowel sounds and abdominal distention at least every 4 to 8 hours.
		Carefully monitor the client's urinary pattern and maintain an accurate intake and output record.
		Observe urine and stool for color, consistency, amount, and the presence of blood.
		Monitor the client for other gastrointestinal problems, such as nausea, vomiting, and **tenesmus** (spasmodic contraction of the anal or bladder sphincter, causing pain and a persistent urge to empty the bowel or bladder).
▶ *Physical Mobility, Impaired, related to intracavity radiation*	The client will not develop deep vein thrombosis.	Accurately measure the client's legs to ensure the proper fit of the hose.
		Apply thigh-high antiembolitic stockings (TEDS) as ordered.
		Assist client to ambulate when allowed.

Evaluation Each goal must be evaluated to determine how it has been met by the client.

PROSTATE CANCER

Prostate cancer is the second leading cause of cancer deaths in men. According to 1998 estimates by the ACS, 184,500 new cases were diagnosed. Unfortunately, incidence and mortality are currently increasing. Incidence increases with age, as 80% of all prostate cancers are diagnosed in men over age 65, but it is much more lethal in younger men. Improved detection methods have greatly increased the number of individuals having positive outcomes. Diagnostic tests that may be performed are measurement of serum prostate specific antigen (PSA), transrectal ultrasonic examination, and prostatic biopsy. Studies indicate that the use of the PSA for routine screening is not necessarily useful because of the number of false-positive levels reported in men with benign prostatic hyperplasia (BPH) and the false-negative levels in men with prostate cancer. Therefore, the most useful screening method continues to be a rectal examination, which all men over the age of 40 should have annually.

Most prostatic cancers are adenocarcinomas, slow-growing tumors that spread through the lymphatics (Figure 35-16). Early symptoms include dysuria, a weak urinary stream, and increased urinary frequency. Later symptoms are related to complete urethral obstruction or hematuria. Blood in the urine (**hematuria**),

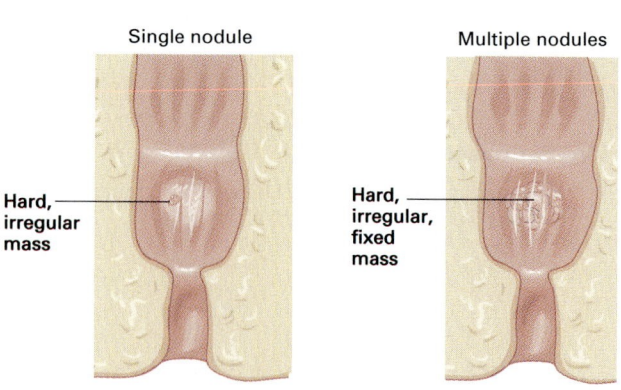

Single nodule   Multiple nodules

Hard, irregular mass

Hard, irregular, fixed mass

Figure 35-16 Cancer of the Prostate *(From Health Assessment & Physical Examination, by M. E. Z. Estes, 1998 Albany, NY: Delmar Publishers. Copyright 1998 by Delmar Publishers. Reprinted with permission.)*

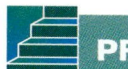

which can lead to anemia, occurs because of the rupture of blood vessels that have been overstretched.

Medical–Surgical Management

Treatment depends on the extent of the disease and the age of the client.

Medical

Radiation is the traditional alternative to surgical removal of the malignant prostate gland. However, radiation may fail to eradicate the tumor or may lead to diarrhea, bowel obstruction, lymphocele formation, edema of the extremities, pulmonary embolism, wound infections, infection, impotence, incontinence, or radiation cystitis. An alternative successful radiation treatment option for early stage prostate cancer is transrectal assisted radioactive seed implant. With the use of ultrasound, the physician is able to precisely position the rice-sized radioactive seeds inside the malignant prostate gland. During the first 5 years of clinical trials, 91% of the men remained disease-free and their PSA level remained normal (Wolcott, 1995). In addition, the men have reported no incontinence, and the impotency rate is less than half that reported with traditional surgical treatment.

Surgical

Surgical treatment of prostatic cancer involves removal of the entire prostate gland, including the capsule and adjacent tissue. The urethra is then anastomosed to the bladder neck. Sometimes the retropubic approach is used, but the usual approach is perineal with the incision made between the scrotum and the rectum. Because of the proximity of the bladder sphincters to the prostate gland, urinary incontinence may be a complication. Other complications include sexual dysfunction and the universal surgical risks of hemorrhage, infection, thrombosis, and strictures. Removal of the testes (**orchiectomy**) may also be done as a palliative measure to help eliminate the androgenic effect that promotes tumor growth.

Another surgical alternative is cryosurgical ablation. This method was used in the 1960s but abandoned owing to the complications of tissue sloughing and fistula development. With the advent of the transrectal ultrasound and the transurethral warming device, cryosurgery has become a more viable alternative. The ultrasound allows the surgeon to selectively freeze prostate gland tissue while the temperature of the prostatic urethra is kept at 44°C by irrigation with heated water. This surgical approach is an option for those who cannot tolerate more extensive surgery, have a localized tumor, or do not have successful radiation treatment. It can be performed more than once, involves a shorter hospital stay, and produces fewer side effects.

Pharmacological

Hormonal agents such as diethylstilbestrol (DES), goserelin acetate (Zoladex), or leuprolide acetate (Lupron) may be used to counteract the production of androgen-dependent hormones. Although systemic chemotherapy has not proved very effective in the treatment of prostate cancer, it may be used for clients who fail to respond to hormone manipulation. Unfortunately, response is limited. Overall, the 5-year survival rate is 89% (ACS, 1998).

▶ NURSING PROCESS

▶ Assessment

▶ Subjective Data

The client may seek care for BPH, which often accompanies cancer of the prostate. The client may describe back pain or sciatica, frequency, dysuria, or nocturia.

▶ Objective Data

The client needs a complete physical assessment that includes palpation of the abdomen and skin assessment. The abdomen is palpated to determine if there is any bladder distention. Skin assessment is important because the client is at risk for skin breakdown. There may or may not be hematuria present. Vital signs, the incisional site, and intake and output must all be assessed. Hyperthermia, hypotension, tachycardia, or increased incisional drainage should be reported to the physician immediately.

Because a catheter is used postoperatively to maintain urinary drainage and as a splint for the urethral anastomosis rather than for hemostasis, there are minimal bladder spasms. Patency of the catheter can be monitored by assessing the drainage for color, amount, and presence of clots. If the tubing is not draining freely, it should be repositioned or milked. The nurse should call the physician if these measures fail to restore patency. During the first week of the postoperative period the client also needs to be monitored for fecal incontinence related to relaxation of the perineal sphincter. This is a complication that occurs when a perineal surgical approach is used because the incision is made between the scrotum and the rectum.

Nursing diagnoses for a client (postoperative) with prostate cancer may include the following:

Nursing Diagnoses	Planning/Goals	Nursing Interventions
▶ *Urinary Retention, related to urethral obstruction, secondary to urethral anastomosis*	The client will not experience urinary retention.	Monitor the client's urinary output, noting the amount, color, and presence of clots. The urine should not appear bright red for more than a few hours postoperatively, after which time it should be dark red.
		Reposition or milk the catheter tubing if not patent. If these interventions fail, notify the physician.
		Monitor the client's intake, encouraging a fluid intake of 2,500 to 3,000 mL/day.
▶ *Incontinence, Bowel, related to loss of rectal sphincter control because of perineal incision*	The client will achieve rectal sphincter control.	Advise the client that temporary fecal incontinence frequently occurs after a perineal incision.
		Teach the client perineal exercises that will help him regain bowel control.
		Avoid the use of rectal thermometers, rectal examinations, and enemas.
▶ *Skin Integrity, Impaired, Risk for, related to incontinence*	The client will not experience skin breakdown.	Keep the client clean and dry, especially if he is experiencing fecal or urinary incontinence.
		Reposition client every 2 hours.

Evaluation Each goal must be evaluated to determine how it has been met by the client.

TESTICULAR CANCER

Although testicular cancer accounts for only 1% of all cancer in men, it is the most common cancer in young men between the ages of 15 and 35. According to the ACS (1998), advances in treatment have made the 5-year survival rate 95%. The etiology is unknown, but the incidence is highest in men with undescended testicles and those whose mothers had taken hormones during pregnancy. A small, hard, painless lump is usually the first symptom noted (Figure 35-17).

Because early diagnosis of testicular cancer is so essential for a positive surgical outcome, men need to be taught how to perform a testicular self-examination (TSE) and be encouraged to routinely perform that examination (Figure 35-18).

TSE is performed as follows:

- Perform TSE after a bath or shower when scrotum is warm and most relaxed.
- Grasp testis with both hands and palpate gently between thumbs and forefingers.
- The testis should feel smooth, egg-shaped, and firm to the touch.
- The epididymis, located behind the testis, should feel like a soft tube.
- Any abnormal lumps or changes in the testes should be reported to a physician.

Medical–Surgical Management

Medical

Testicular ultrasound is used to study the testes for enlargement or lesions. In addition to a testicular ultrasound, the client may have a serum acid or alkaline phosphatase test done. They are both elevated in malignancies.

Surgical

Biopsy of the testis is contraindicated because of the increased potential for metastases. Surgical removal of the testis, spermatic cord, and inguinal canal contents, with examination of the nodes, is indicated

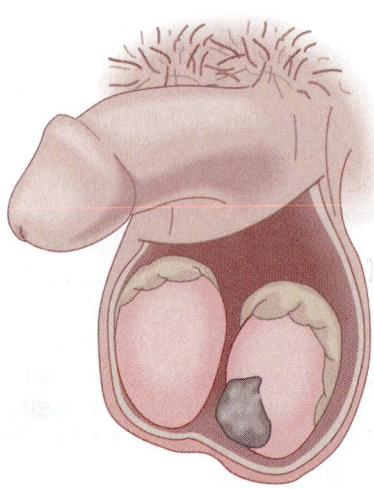

Figure 35-17 Testicular Tumor. (*From* Health Assessment & Physical Examination, *by M. E. Z. Estes, 1998 Albany, NY: Delmar Publishers. Copyright 1998 by Delmar Publishers. Reprinted with permission.*)

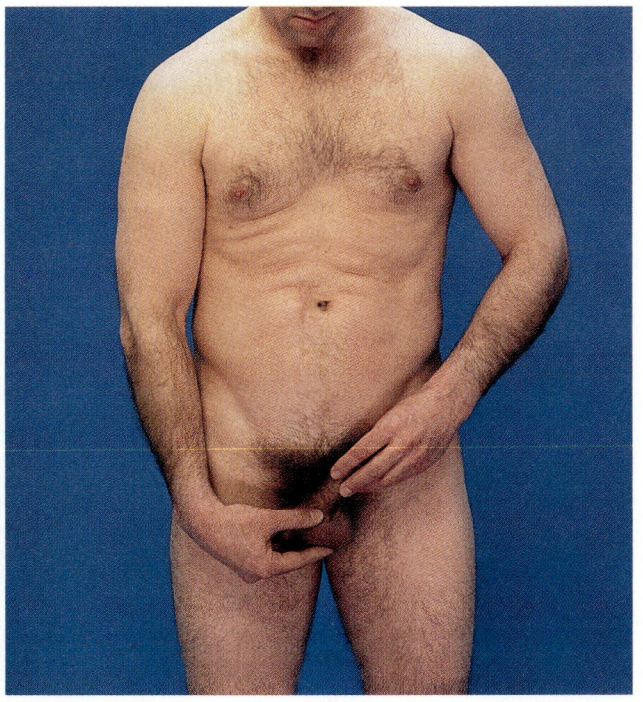
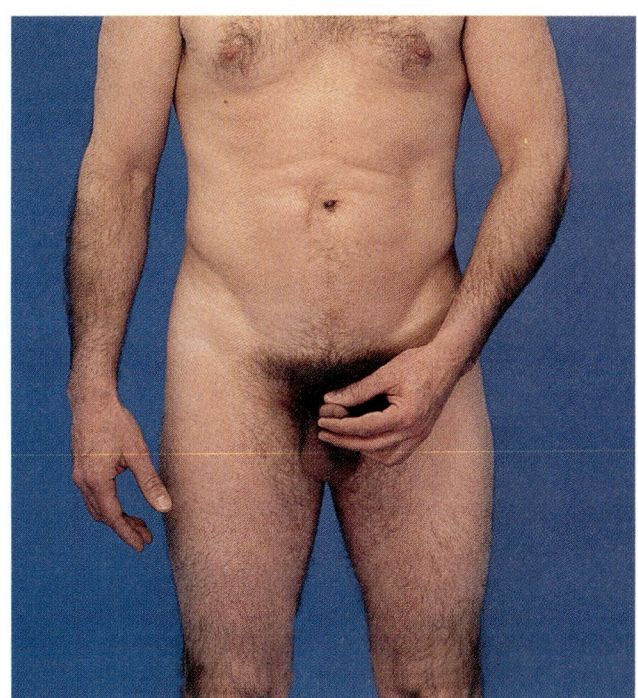
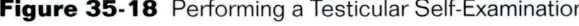

Figure 35-18 Performing a Testicular Self-Examination

for testicular cancers. If unilateral removal of a testis is indicated, the remaining healthy testis will continue to maintain sperm and androgen production.

Pharmacological

Although chemotherapy and radiation are used as adjuvant treatments, radical inguinal orchiectomy remains the primary intervention. Combination chemotherapy with cisplatin (Platinol), vinblastine sulfate (Velban), and bleomycin sulfate (Blenoxane) is effective.

▶ NURSING PROCESS

▶ Assessment

▶ Subjective Data

The client may describe a feeling of heaviness in the scrotum, and may mention weight loss. During the postoperative phase, the client needs to be assessed for pain, using a pain scale to objectify data. He also needs to have emotional and educational needs assessed. For example, the client should be able to accurately describe his activity restrictions and how to provide scrotal support postoperatively. His behaviors and statements need to be monitored for signs of anxiety or depression.

▶ Objective Data

Physical examination should include palpation of the abdomen and assessment of the scrotum. Positive findings in the scrotum include a firm, painless mass in the testis and an enlarged scrotum. As gynecomastia (breast enlargement) is another symptom of testicular cancer, the client's breast tissue should be assessed for enlargement. Postoperative assessment includes monitoring vital signs to detect signs of hemorrhage or infection. Also, the incisional site should be monitored for excess drainage, swelling, or redness.

Nursing diagnoses for the client with testicular cancer may include the following:

Nursing Diagnoses	Planning/Goals	Nursing Interventions
▶ *Injury, Risk for,* due to infection and hemorrhage related to surgery	The client will experience minimal bleeding and avoid infection.	Monitor the client's vital signs and incisional drainage.
		Report hyperthermia, tachycardia, hypotension, increased incisional drainage, and swelling or redness around the incision to the physician immediately.
		Maintain strict asepsis when handling wound dressings.

continued

Nursing Diagnoses	Planning/Goals	Nursing Interventions
▸ *Body Image Disturbance, related to surgery*	The client will maintain or regain a positive body image.	Provide the client with opportunities to voice concerns and ask questions.
		Monitor the client for statements and behaviors that indicate concern about loss of masculinity.
		Suggest sexual counseling if he does not appear to be resolving these issues.
		Advise the client that unilateral removal of a testis will not cause him to be sterile or demasculinized.
▸ *Knowledge Deficit, related to surgery and postoperative care*	The client will demonstrate understanding of postoperative activity restrictions and medical follow-up.	Advise the client that he needs to be on bed rest for 12 to 24 hours postoperatively.
		Instruct the client to wear tight-fitting underwear or an athletic supporter when ambulating and to avoid heavy lifting for 4 to 6 weeks.

Evaluation Each goal must be evaluated to determine how it has been met by the client.

PENILE CANCER

Penile cancer is rare and has a high correlation with poor hygiene and delayed or no circumcision. The bacteria harbored in the foreskin of the uncircumcised male are irritants to the glans penis and the prepuce. The chronic nature of this irritation is thought to be carcinogenic. Males with a history of STDs are also predisposed to developing penile cancer. Symptoms of penile cancer include a painless, nodular growth on the foreskin, fatigue, and weight loss. Metastases are common in the inguinal nodes and adjacent organs.

Medical–Surgical Management

Medical

The primary penile cancer treatment is surgery. Treatment with radiation alone is ineffective, and chemotherapy alone is used only for palliative treatment of penile cancer with deep distant metastases. However, the client may receive adjuvant therapy with either radiation or chemotherapy.

Surgical

If the tumor is not extensive and no metastases are involved, the remaining penis should be long enough for the client to void standing and avoid soiling himself. If a penectomy is necessary, a permanent fistula opening into the urethra will be made between the scrotum and the anus (**urethrostomy**).

▶ NURSING PROCESS

▶ Assessment

▶ Subjective Data

Although the tumor is painless, the client should be asked if he is experiencing any pain, to rule out other possible diagnoses. The client also needs to be asked if he is experiencing fatigue or weight loss. Preoperatively, the client needs an assessment of his emotional and educational needs. He needs to be asked questions that can be used to determine his understanding of the surgical procedure and the need for counseling. Postoperative assessment also includes monitoring for pain and using a pain scale to objectify data.

▶ Objective Data

The client needs a physical assessment that includes inspection of the penis for the presence of painless, nodular growths. During the postoperative phase, monitoring of vital signs, incisional site, and intake and output must be done. Hypotension, tachycardia, excessive incisional drainage, redness or swelling around the incision, or bright red or low urinary output, could be signs of complications.

Nursing diagnoses for a client with penile cancer may include the following:

Nursing Diagnoses	Planning/Goals	Nursing Interventions
▸ *Injury, Risk for, due to infection and hemorrhage related to surgery*	The client will experience minimal bleeding and avoid infection.	Monitor the client's vital signs and incisional drainage.
		Report hyperthermia, tachycardia, hypotension, increased incisional drainage, and swelling or redness around the incision to the physician immediately.
		Maintain strict asepsis when handling wound dressings.

continued

Nursing Diagnoses	Planning/Goals	Nursing Interventions
◗ *Anxiety, related to surgery*	The client will discuss anxieties.	Provide the client with information about the operative procedure, postoperative and discharge care.
		When available, a video may be used to present this information, with the nurse being available to answer the client's questions.
◗ *Sexuality Patterns, Altered, related to the altered body function or structure*	The client will maintain satisfactory sexuality patterns postoperatively.	Advise the client to seek sexual counseling for both himself and his partner if he is unable to maintain normal sexuality patterns.

Evaluation Each goal must be evaluated to determine how it has been met by the client.

MENSTRUAL DISORDERS

Abnormalities of menstruation may be associated with an increase or decrease in secretion from any of the following glands: hypothalamus, pituitary, ovaries, adrenals, and thyroid. The normal menstrual pattern is controlled by a series of hormonal negative feedback mechanisms. The average menstrual cycle occurs every 28 to 30 days when the endometrial lining of the uterus sloughs off in the absence of a fertilized ovum.

DYSMENORRHEA

Painful menstruation, dysmenorrhea, also called "menstrual cramps," is more common in nulliparous women and in women who are not having intercourse. The exact pathophysiology is unknown, but it may be related to endocrine secretions such as prostaglandin F, which causes uterine cramping, irritation, and contractions. Other causes may include uterine anatomical anomalies, chronic illness, or psychological factors.

The primary symptom is pelvic pain before or at the onset of the menses that may be due to spasms of the uterus, narrowing of the cervical canal, emotional factors, endometriosis, pelvic inflammatory disease, or the presence of an intrauterine contraceptive device (IUD). The client may also state that the pain radiates across the lower back and downward into the legs.

The condition is diagnosed on the basis of the client's complaints and description of the timing of the onset of symptoms. The nurse should obtain information pertaining to the menstrual history and general health status of the client. A thorough physical exam will be performed by the physician, including a bimanual exam to rule out other possible causes. A pelvic ultrasound may be ordered.

One effective preventive intervention may begin before the young woman begins menstruation. A positive parental attitude toward the onset of menstruation can aid the young girl in adjusting to the physiologic and psychological changes that occur with puberty.

Certain medications have been used over the last

10 to 15 years that are effective in the treatment of dysmenorrhea. Analgesics such as acetaminophen (Tylenol) and ibuprofen (Motrin) are useful in relieving pain. Oral contraceptives have been used for some clients to inhibit ovulation, which appears to be an associated cause. Prostaglandin inhibitors such as naproxen sodium (Anaprox) and mefenamic acid (Ponstel) are useful if taken at the earliest sign of discomfort.

AMENORRHEA

Amenorrhea, the absence of menstruation, may be primary or secondary. Primary amenorrhea is defined as the absence of menstruation by the age of 17. Possible causes are related to anatomical or genetic abnormalities (Turner's syndrome). The treatment is dependent upon the cause. Secondary amenorrhea is defined as the absence of menstruation after 6 months of regular periods or after 12 months of irregular periods. Several etiologies are possible for secondary amenorrhea, including anatomic abnormalities, nutritional deficits (anorexia nervosa), excessive exercise with significant decreases in body fat, endocrine dysfunction, emotional disturbances, side effects of medications, pregnancy, and lactation.

This condition is diagnosed based upon the length of absence of menstruation. A complete physical examination should be performed, including a pelvic examination to rule out many factors discussed earlier. A progesterone challenge test may be administered in an attempt to force the body to respond hormonally. Medroxyprogesterone acetate (Depo-Provera) is taken orally for 5 to 10 days as ordered by the physician. When the medication is finished, the client should have a menstrual period within 3 or 4 days. A menstrual flow after taking the medication may be an indicator that the client has not been ovulating. If no bleeding occurs, further investigation may be necessary to uncover other causes. Hormonal imbalances, microscopic pituitary tumors, and nutritional deficits are common etiologies of secondary amenorrhea. A microscopic pituitary tumor will cause an elevation in the prolactin level and result in anovulation and amenorrhea. A serum prolactin level should be ordered, especially if the client has noticed any breast discharge. Normal prolactin level should not exceed 15 ng/dL. With pituitary tumors, the prolactin level may exceed 400 ng/dL. In these cases, the drug of choice is bromocriptine mesylate (Parlodel), which had been used in the past to suppress lactation in mothers who did not breastfeed their newborns. A careful examination of the client is needed before administration of Parlodel, because of an increased potential for cardiovascular problems recently associated with this medication. Because of this risk, the medication is no longer used for the postpartum client to suppress milk production. Other medical or surgical interventions will be dependent upon the cause of the amenorrhea.

OTHER DISORDERS

Other menstrual disorders include menorrhagia and metrorrhagia. Both types of abnormal bleeding can be problematic for the client and require further investigation. **Polymenorrhea** is a term used to describe short menstrual cycles of less than 21 days in length. The causes are similar to those of the other menstrual disorders. **Oligomenorrhea** is a diminished menstrual flow, but it is not classified as amenorrhea. It may be associated with low-dose oral contraceptives that inhibit the growth of the endometrium and result in minimal tissue sloughing at the end of the cycle. Other causes may be metabolic or hormonal. Again, treatment is specific to the etiology.

For conditions associated with heavy bleeding or bleeding between periods, a dilatation and curettage (D&C) may be performed. In this case, the procedure may be diagnostic and therapeutic. Tissue removed from the uterus will be examined microscopically and histologically to evaluate its stage in the menstrual cycle. A hysterectomy may be indicated if abnormalities are discovered or if the bleeding is so excessive that the client is significantly compromised. The client may require a blood transfusion to correct low hemoglobin and hematocrit levels before any other procedures. Supplemental iron generally is prescribed by the physician to also help correct the deficiency.

▶ NURSING PROCESS

▶ Assessment

▶ Subjective Data

The nurse should ask the client about the onset of the bleeding and its relationship to the timing of her normal menstruation, the color of the bleeding, amount, number of pads saturated, presence of clots, and presence of pain with the bleeding. A history of current medications, contraception, and the possibility of pregnancy are additional assessment data. Any preexisting health problems that could affect bleeding and clotting times, as well as life stressors, should be explored by the nurse during the data-gathering process.

▶ Objective Data

Assessment of vital signs may indicate hypertension and tachycardia. Laboratory test results must be monitored.

Nursing Management

Possible nursing diagnoses for a client with any of the menstrual disorders discussed in this section may include:

- *Pain, related to uterine cramping or heavy bleeding*
- *Cardiac Output, Decreased, related to excessive blood loss*
- *Fatigue, related to decreased hemoglobin and hematocrit levels*
- *Body Image Disturbance, related to the absence of menstruation*

PREMENSTRUAL SYNDROME

One-third to one-half of women between 20 and 50 years of age experience some of the symptoms known as premenstrual syndrome (PMS). Once, this condition was thought by many physicians to be a psychological problem of women; however, recent research has supported data that there are many physiologic as well as psychological factors involved. PMS often occurs during the secretory phase of the menstrual cycle, after ovulation. Risk factors associated with the development of PMS include age (over 30), multiple life stressors, inappropriate nutritional status, a previous reaction to or side effects from oral contraceptive use, a sedentary lifestyle, marital status, a history of preeclampsia in pregnancy, and multiparity.

Over 150 symptoms have been reported that have been related to PMS. These include weight gain, bloating, irritability, edema, headache, mood swings, inability to concentrate, food cravings, acne, and numerous others. For many women, the PMS symptoms are merely a monthly nuisance, but for others, the symptoms are so incapacitating that they cannot function in their normal roles or responsibilities. The onset of symptoms is usually 7 to 10 days before the menstrual period starts; symptoms end after the menstrual flow begins.

Research has correlated hormonal imbalances of estrogen, progesterone, ACTH, and androgens with the symptoms of PMS. The presence of prostaglandin F in the tissue may also be a cause of some of the symptoms. Prostaglandins are associated with many inflammatory responses in the tissues.

The first step in identifying PMS is a physical examination to rule out other possible disorders of the reproductive system. The client may be asked to keep a monthly calendar of symptoms to see if there are patterns in severity, type, or onset. Blood tests may be ordered to assess estrogen and progesterone levels, as well as checking the glucose level. Low blood glucose level has been associated with irritability that sometimes accompanies PMS symptoms. The client should receive counseling, if needed, to facilitate coping with life stressors that may be complicating the complexity of the PMS symptoms.

Medical–Surgical Management

Pharmacological

Some physicians and NPs recommend medication such as acetaminophen (Tylenol), naproxen (Naprosyn), mefenamic acid (Ponstel), and ibuprofen (Advil) for the relief of minor discomforts of PMS. Tranquilizers and antidepressants have not proved to be effective for short-term use in PMS; however, in severe cases, they may be a last resort. Several PMS symptoms are thought to be related to a low progesterone level. For some clients, the use of progesterone suppositories or oral progesterone to supplement their own production during the secretory phase of the menstrual cycle has been useful.

Diet

A thorough diet history should be included in the assessment data collected. Certain nutritional deficits or cravings have been linked to the worsening of PMS. Items such as sugar, salt, caffeine, and chocolate are in this category. Many studies have shown that limiting intake of these substances may be helpful. Caffeinated beverages may increase anxiety, irritability, and deplete vitamin B stores in the body. Dairy products interfere with the absorption of magnesium, which helps stabilize the mood. Chocolates have been related to increased sugar cravings, mood swings, fluid retention,

and increased vitamin B demands. Oranges and other fruits or vegetables that are highly acidic may worsen PMS. Foods that are recommended are whole grains, nuts, pasta, legumes, root vegetables, fruits like apples and pears, poultry, and seafood. A good vitamin supplement rich in vitamin B-complex, calcium, magnesium, and zinc should be taken daily, especially during the PMS period. Herbal tea formulas have shown some promise as alternative methods of relieving PMS.

Activity

As mentioned previously, a sedentary lifestyle and lack of exercise are associated with PMS. A regular exercise routine, coupled with the use of stress-management techniques such as deep breathing and relaxation exercises help the client cope with the increased sense of anxiety or irritability that may accompany the PMS. Meditation, positive affirmation, visualization, and imagery may be helpful. Other alternative therapies may include acupressure, neurolymphatic or neurovascular massage, and yoga.

▶ NURSING PROCESS

▶ Assessment

▶ Subjective Data

The client should describe her symptoms and the impact on her lifestyle. Many times, clients will seek medical attention for their PMS symptoms when the emotional impact has caused friction in the home, marriage, work, or family environment. Symptoms described may include weight gain, bloating, irritability, headache, mood swings, inability to concentrate, or food cravings. The client should be asked to relate symptoms to time of menstrual cycle.

▶ Objective Data

The client should be assessed for weight gain and edema. Results of all laboratory tests should be reviewed.

Nursing diagnoses for a client with premenstrual syndrome may include the following:

Nursing Diagnoses	Planning/Goals	Nursing Interventions
▶ *Fluid Volume Excess, related to hormonal imbalance and increased sodium or sugar intake*	The client's intake and output will be balanced, and edema will be decreased.	Advise client that a certain amount of fluid retention is normal before the onset of the menstrual period and cannot be avoided, but by limiting sodium and sugar intake, she may be able to influence the amount of fluid retained.
▶ *Health-Seeking Behaviors, related to finding methods to cope with symptoms of PMS*	The client will develop effective health-promotion skills to increase coping with PMS symptoms or to decrease symptom severity or frequency.	Teach client how to keep a monthly PMS calendar of events. Discuss prescribed medications with the client, including the dosage, expected effects, and side effects. Discuss relationship of foods to PMS.

Evaluation Each goal must be evaluated to determine how it has been met by the client.

COMPLICATIONS OF MENOPAUSE

Menopause, or climacteric, is the cessation of menstruation. It may occur as a natural hormonal decline or it may be surgically induced by removal of the uterus and ovaries. Some people may think of menopause as the "change of life." Many women will begin to experience signs and symptoms of approaching menopause around 50 years of age; however, the range of onset is from 45 to 60 years old. Menstrual cycles become further apart and the flow decreases. The onset is usually gradual, and it may take over a year before the woman has completely ceased menstruation. Reproductive capability is also lost with menopause. For some women this is a sad time perceived as the loss of womanhood; for others it is a welcome relief.

The decreasing level of ovarian hormone production affects women in a variety of ways, more than just the end of menstruation. There may be a relaxation of the pelvic support structures, loss of skin turgor and elasticity, and thinning of the hair on the head, axilla, and pubic regions. Other signs of decreasing hormones (estrogen and progesterone) are vaginal dryness, thinning of the vaginal mucosa, weight gain, dry skin, and stress incontinence. The estrogen level plays an important protective role in maintaining an adequate calcium balance in the bones and preventing coronary artery disease. Without calcium, bones become brittle, and there is an increased risk of fractures and osteoporosis. A baseline bone density study may be recommended before menopause.

Some women experience psychological responses to menopause, such as mild to moderate depression, nervousness, and insomnia. Consultation with a psychologist, minister, or counselor may be useful in facilitating the transition through this period for some women.

Women may also experience mild to moderate periods of profuse perspiration called hot flashes. These usually move from the waist upward. They are caused by the decreased estrogen level and its effect on the hypothalamus. The sensation may last from a few seconds to 2 to 3 minutes. It appears that many different things can trigger a hot flash—drinking hot beverages, eating spicy foods, smoking, and consuming caffeine and alcohol.

Medical–Surgical Management

Pharmacological

For some women, estrogen replacement therapy is recommended, especially if they are experiencing moderately uncomfortable symptoms. Estrogen replacement therapy (ERT) may help decrease some symptoms, such as insomnia, hot flashes, mood swings, and lack of concentration. Another positive benefit of taking estrogen is its protective nature against osteoporosis and cardiovascular disease. Estrogen elevates the high-density lipoproteins (healthy ones) and lowers the low-density lipoproteins (unhealthy) in the circulation. Estrogen may be administered orally, as a transdermal patch, or as a vaginal cream. The transdermal patch releases the hormone into the bloodstream percutaneously. This results in a bypass of the stomach and liver, which means less gastrointestinal tract irritation for the client. The patch is a good option of estrogen administration for clients with liver disease. Occasionally, the client may complain of a rash or skin irritation from the patch that is usually related to the adhesive.

Conjugated estrogen (Premarin), estradiol (Estrace), and estropipate (Ogen) are examples of oral estrogens available. Estrogen creams or water-soluble gels such as Lubrifax or K-Y, may be used to combat the vaginal dryness and resulting dyspareunia.

Many health care providers are concerned about the possible effects of unopposed estrogen's causing endometrial cancer. To alleviate some of this concern, a progesterone supplement may be added to the hormone regimen if the client still has a uterus. Progesterone, along with the estrogen replacement, will cause the woman to have some amount of endometrial sloughing every month, a menstrual period. This prevents the buildup of tissue inside the uterus, which has the potential to undergo cellular changes or mutation into cancerous cells. Some studies have suggested that a woman should be on ERT for approximately 10 to 15 years after menopause to reach the maximum benefits of the therapy.

Diet

The nurse should provide the client with instructions regarding the importance of an adequate daily intake of calcium-rich products, such as dairy products. Many low-fat, high-calcium products are available if the client has a concern about weight gain. Calcium supplements may also be taken in a tablet form. The woman should consult her health care provider before

CLIENT TEACHING

Estrogen Transdermal Patch

- Rotate the application sites of the patch every 3 to 4 days.
- Hold the patch to the open air for 10 to 15 seconds before application to decrease the potential for skin irritation.
- The estrogen patch may provide less protection against bone and heart problems than oral estrogen does.

adding a calcium supplement because too much calcium increases the risk for other health problems. Herbal teas, vitamin E, magnesium, and primrose oil have been used as alternative methods to alleviate or decrease hot flashes and promote relaxation for some women.

Activity

One important way that the client can decrease the potential for calcium loss from weight-bearing bones is to exercise. A planned 30-minute program performed at least 3 times a week is adequate to maintain bone density. Exercises such as walking or swimming are excellent. Swimming provides good non-weight-bearing activity and promotes active movement of all extremities. Biking is a good exercise to maintain joint mobility in the lower extremities, but it does not require the use of the same muscle groups as walking.

▶ NURSING PROCESS

▶ Assessment

▶ Subjective Data

The client may present with concerns about decreasing regularity of menstruation or hot flashes. The nurse should obtain information from the client about gynecological and obstetrical history, including menstruation. It is helpful to know when the client began experiencing symptoms in predicting the length of time they may continue.

▶ Objective Data

These include a physical examination and Pap smear. The results of the Pap smear can indicate if there is less estrogen present in the cervical tissue than normal.

Nursing diagnoses for a client experiencing menopausal symptoms may include the following:

Nursing Diagnoses	Planning/Goals	Nursing Interventions
▶ *Health-Seeking Behaviors, related to perceived physiological and psychologic impact of decreased estrogen*	The client will develop effective health promotion skills to increase coping with menopausal symptoms or to decrease symptom severity or frequency.	Encourage the client to continue to see her health care provider for annual Pap smears and breast examinations.
		Explain nutritional requirements for vitamins and calcium that increase with menopause.
		Encourage the client to begin a regular exercise program that includes weight-bearing activities such as walking to prevent loss of calcium from the bones.
▶ *Tissue Integrity, Impaired, related to vaginal dryness and dry skin*	The client will maintain skin integrity, and vagina will not be dry.	Advise the client to try estrogen creams or water-soluble gels such as Lubrifax or K-Y, to combat the vaginal dryness and resulting dyspareunia.
		Encourage the client to use body lotion to prevent dry skin.
▶ *Decisional Conflict, related to taking supplemental estrogen therapy*	The client will make informed decisons about taking supplemental estrogen.	Discuss the advantages and disadvantages of estrogen replacement therapy with the client.
		Remind the client that if she has a uterus and takes hormonal replacements, she will continue to have monthly menstrual cycles.

Evaluation Each goal must be evaluated to determine how it has been met by the client.

STRUCTURAL DISORDERS

Structural anomalies are separated into female and male disorders

CYSTOCELE, URETHROCELE, RECTOCELE, PROLAPSED UTERUS

Cystocele, urethrocele, rectocele, and prolapsed uterus are often associated with relaxation of the pelvic muscles that support the uterus, bladder, and rectum. A **cystocele** is a downward displacement of the bladder into the anterior vaginal wall. A **urethro**cele is a downward displacement of the urethra into the vagina, and a **rectocele** is an anterior displacement of the rectum into the posterior vaginal wall. **Prolapsed uterus** is a downward displacement of the uterus into the vagina (Figure 35-19). Possible causes for the four conditions are multiple pregnancies, third- or fourth-degree perineal lacerations with childbirth, and weakening of the pelvic muscles as an aging process.

A prolapsed uterus is often accompanied by a cystocele and/or rectocele. Variations in the severity of uterine prolapse are described as first-, second-, and third-degree. With a first-degree prolapse, the cervix is visible at the vaginal introitus, or opening, without straining. With a second-degree prolapse, the cervix extends beyond the vaginal opening to the perineum.

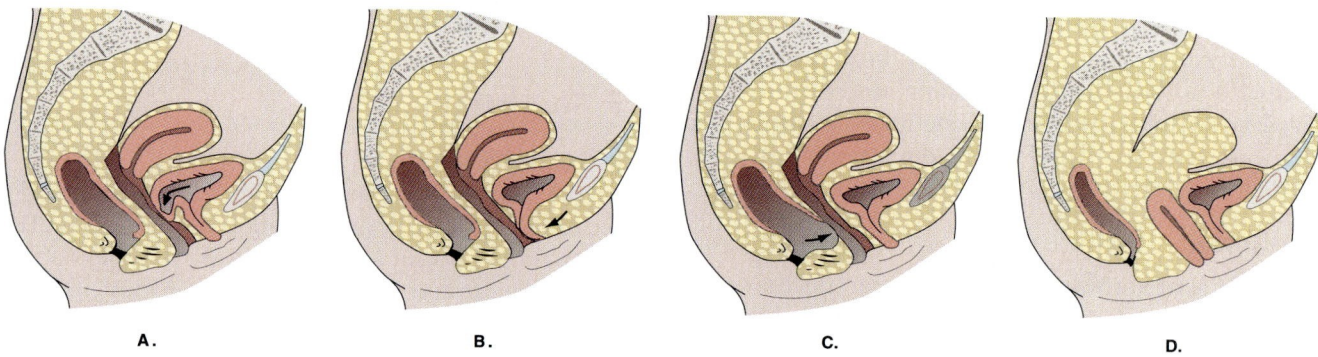

Figure 35-19 A. Cystocele; B. Urethrocele; C. Rectocele; D. Uterine prolapse

With a third-degree prolapse, the uterus protrudes outside of the vagina. This severe condition is called *procidentia uteri.*

Medical–Surgical Management

Medical and surgical interventions for the treatment of each of these conditions are focused on relief of the discomforts and restoration of the structure and function of the pelvic organs.

Medical

The pessary is a small molded plastic or rubber apparatus that fits into the vagina behind the pubic bone and in front of the rectum. Its function is to provide an artificial or mechanical support for the uterus. Pessaries are not uncomfortable and should not be felt by the client if properly fitted and in the correct position. The client should be taught how to insert and remove the pessary so it can be cleaned. The pessary may be washed in warm, soapy water once every 1 to 2 weeks. Prolonged use of a mechanical device such as a pessary may result in vaginal necrosis and ulceration. Periodic examination by a health care professional is recommended, especially with weight gain or loss of greater than 10 to 15 pounds.

Surgical

Surgery for a prolapsed uterus may require a hysterectomy. If the prolapse is accompanied by a cystocele or rectocele, an A&P repair may also be performed. An A&P repair (anterior/posterior colporrhaphy) may be performed vaginally to replace the bladder, urethra, or rectum in the correct anatomic position. Another procedure, the Marshall-Marchette-Krantz, may be performed to attach the bladder to the inferior surface of the pubic bone. Postoperatively, the client may be sent home with an indwelling Foley catheter because of the potential inability to void. This is a common postoperative situation that usually resolves itself spontaneously within 1 or 2 weeks after discharge.

Activity

Clients should be taught the Kegel exercise before childbearing. This exercise is performed by tightening and releasing the perineal muscles. An important muscle group, called the "levators," helps lift and support the organs inside the pelvis.

▶ NURSING PROCESS

▶ Assessment

▶ Subjective Data

The client often describes stress incontinence, which is a loss of urine when she coughs, sneezes, laughs, or jumps. She may describe it as "a leaky bladder." She may notice that her panties are damp or that she dribbles urine. Many women complain of frequent urination in small quantities with a feeling of urgency without burning or dysuria. The client may notice that she has been experiencing more constipation or a sense of bearing down pressure in the pelvis with a rectocele. Many of these symptoms will decrease or subside completely when she is lying down. The nurse should obtain information about the client's childbearing history, onset of current symptoms, and any other pertinent gynecological data.

 CLIENT TEACHING

Kegel Exercises

- Suggest that the client practice when she has a full bladder. If she can successfully start and stop the flow of urine from the bladder, she is identifying and using the correct muscle groups.
- The muscles should be tightened and held for 5 to 10 seconds and then released slowly.
- Repeat the exercises at least 10 times.
- Kegel exercise can be practiced anytime and anyplace.
- A secondary benefit of increasing the strength and contractility of the pelvic and perineal muscles is seen in an improvement in pelvic sensations for both partners during intercourse.

▶ Objective Data

These include the visualization of a bulging of the bladder, urethra, or rectum into the vagina. The bulging increases when the client is asked to bear down. Urinalysis results should be evaluated.

Nursing diagnoses for a female client with a structural disorder of the reproductive system may include the following:

Nursing Diagnoses	Planning/Goals	Nursing Interventions
▶ *Incontinence, Stress, related to relaxation of the pelvic muscles*	The client will have less stress incontinence.	Teach the client Kegel exercise and encourage routine practice daily. Encourage client to empty bladder frequently.
▶ *Constipation, related to relaxation of the anterior rectal wall into the vagina and decreased function*	The client will not have constipation.	Encourage client to defecate at same time each day. Encourage regular exercise. Encourage client to eat high-fiber foods and to drink plenty of fluids.
▶ *Infection, Risk for, related to exposure of internal tissues to external environmental factors*	The client will be free of signs and symptoms of infection.	Monitor the client's vital signs. Encourage client to practice proper personal hygiene and wear clean undergarments daily.
▶ *Sexual Dysfunction, related to discomforts with intercourse*	The client will have a fulfilling sexual relationship without discomfort.	Be sensitive to client cues related to her sexual concerns. Encourage the client to openly discuss her feelings with her partner. Help the client set realistic goals during her recovery period to facilitate a new outlook on her relationship.

Evaluation Each goal must be evaluated to determine how it has been met by the client.

CRYPTORCHIDISM, HYDRO-CELE, HYPOSPADIAS AND EPISPADIAS, SPERMATOCELE, VARICOCELE, TORSION OF THE SPERMATIC CORD

Cryptorchidism is a condition in which one or both testicles fail to descend into the scrotum by the time of birth. The cause is usually unknown. Decrease or loss of sperm production may occur because of the damage that occurs to the seminiferous epithelium. When the testes are within the normal path and do not descend or cannot be pulled into the scrotum, surgery (orchiopexy) is usually done between 5 and 7 years of age. Even with the corrective surgery, as adults, these males have a 10 to 30 times higher incidence of testicular cancer.

A hydrocele is a benign, nontender collection of clear, amber fluid within the space of the testes and the tunica vaginalis or along the spermatic cord. This collection of fluid may result in scrotal swelling, which can be painful if it develops suddenly. Inflammation of the epididymis or testis or a lymphatic or venous obstruction may cause this condition. Congenital hydrocele in the newborn occurs when the canal between the peritoneal cavity and the scrotum does not close completely during fetal development. Aspiration of the fluid serves only as a temporary measure and can lead to secondary infection. Therefore, treatment for the condition is surgery.

Hypospadias is an abnormal placement of the urethral opening on the ventral surface of the penis. Epispadias is the opening of the urethra on the dorsal surface of the penis. The treatment is determined by the position of the urethra on the penis. Infants with either condition should not be circumcised before a urology consultation is obtained, because the foreskin is used in the repair.

A spermatocele is a benign nontender cyst of either the epididymis or the rete testis. It contains milky fluid and sperm. Usually this condition is painless and does not require medical treatment.

A varicocele is dilation of the veins of the scrotum that occurs when the venous system that drains the testicle lengthens and enlarges. This dilation occurs when incompetent or absent valves in the spermatic venous system permit blood to accumulate, resulting in increased hydrostatic pressure. This condition is most commonly found on the left side because of the increased retrograde pressure of the renal vein, the length, and fewer competent valves. It is theorized that the hyperthermia that occurs with this condition decreases spermatogenesis, resulting in decreased fertility. Symptoms may include a bluish discoloration of the scrotal skin or palpation of a wormlike mass when the male bears down. This condition seldom requires treatment.

Torsion of the spermatic cord occurs when the vascular pedicle of the testis twists, resulting in partial or complete venous occlusion. The three forms of this disorder are (1) rotation of the spermatic cord, (2) torsion of a testicular appendage, or (3) torsion of the spermatic cord and epididymis. Testicular torsion may be related to recent trauma, and the onset of symptoms often occurs quite suddenly. Symptoms of testicular torsion may include abdominal and scrotal pain, scrotal edema, nausea and vomiting and, possibly, a slight fever. The pain caused by testicular torsion is not relieved by bed rest or scrotal support.

Medical–Surgical Management

Medical/surgical management of male structural disorders is specific to the condition. Cryptorchidism may be treated with hormonal therapy. If this is not successful, surgery should be done within the first 18 months of life, in order to avoid possible sterility. In some newborns a hydrocele may resolve without medical intervention. Clients of all ages may have aspiration performed to reduce the swelling caused by fluid or a hematoma. However, this solution is usually only temporary, and surgical removal of the sac provides the only permanent solution to the problem. Although a spermatocele usually does not require treatment, sometimes surgical aspiration or excision is necessary.

Hypospadias and epispadias are surgically repaired (urethroplasty) before the child is 1 year of age. Usually, successful repair requires more than one surgery and often results in scarring of the penis.

Because a common complication of a varicocele is male infertility, ligation of the spermatic vein may be performed if infertility is a concern. Sometimes this does not resolve infertility problems because varicoceles may recur after surgery. When fertility is not a concern, the varicocele may be treated simply with scrotal support.

Torsion of the spermatic cord is one disorder that does require immediate surgery to perform surgical detorsion (untwisting) and suturing of the testicle to the scrotum.

▶ NURSING PROCESS

▶ Assessment

▶ Subjective Data

Diagnostic assessment for all structural disorders should include asking the client about the type and location of his pain. He should also be asked about related symptoms such as alteration in urinary patterns, warmth, fatigue, nausea, or vomiting. Postoperative assessments include monitoring for pain and using a pain scale to objectify data. The client's knowledge of his condition, treatment, and follow-up care also need to be assessed, as do the implications of sterility and impotence to the client's life.

▶ Objective Data

Physical assessment should include inspection and palpation of the genitals to detect the presence of scrotal swelling, testicular enlargement, scrotal immobility, redness, and warmth of the scrotum. Large varicoceles may be visible through the scrotal skin as a bluish discoloration. Bilateral palpation of the newborn's scrotum will determine the bilateral presence of testes.

Nursing diagnoses for a male client with a structural disorder of the reproductive system may include the following:

Nursing Diagnoses	Planning/Goals	Nursing Interventions
▶ *Injury, Risk for, related to inflammation and hemorrhage*	The client will experience minimal bleeding and avoid infection.	Monitor the client's vital signs and incisional drainage.
		Report hyperthermia, tachycardia, hypotension, increased incisional drainage, and swelling or redness around the incision to the physician immediately.
		Maintain strict asepsis when handling wound dressings.
▶ *Knowledge Deficit, related to the condition and possible complications*	The client will demonstrate understanding of the possible complications of his condition.	Monitor statements made by the client to determine if there is any misunderstanding about how the surgery will affect his masculinity and fertility.
		Provide the client with opportunities to voice his feelings and ask questions.

Evaluation Each goal must be evaluated to determine how it has been met by the client.

FUNCTIONAL DISORDERS AND CONCERNS

Included in this category are impotence, infertility, and contraception.

IMPOTENCE

Impotence is defined as the inability of an adult male to have an erection firm enough or to maintain it long enough to complete sexual intercourse. There are three types of impotence: functional, atonic, and anatomic. Psychological factors that lead to concerns about sexual performance may contribute to functional impotence. These factors include aging and difficulty with communication or relationships.

Atonic impotence may be the result of medications such as antihypertensives, sedatives, antidepressants, or tranquilizers. For example, antihypertensives lower blood pressure in all arteries of the body, and reduction of the blood pressure to penile arteries may lead to failure of the penis to fill sufficiently to achieve erection. The use of alcohol, cocaine, and nicotine can also decrease potency. Disease processes leading to atonic impotence include diabetes and vascular and neurological disorders. Diabetic clients are at increased risk for impotence owing to their tendency to develop atherosclerosis and autonomic neuropathy. Vascular and neurological disorders include atherosclerosis, hypertension, spinal cord injuries, and multiple sclerosis. End-stage renal disease and chronic obstructive pulmonary disorders can also decrease potency.

Peyronie's disease causes development of nonelastic, fibrous tissue just beneath the penile skin, leading to anatomic impotence. The resulting loss of elasticity leads to a decreased ability of the penis to fill with and store blood during an erection. Peyronie's disease often causes the penis to bend upward, possibly leading to pain and an inability to penetrate the vagina (Figure 35-20).

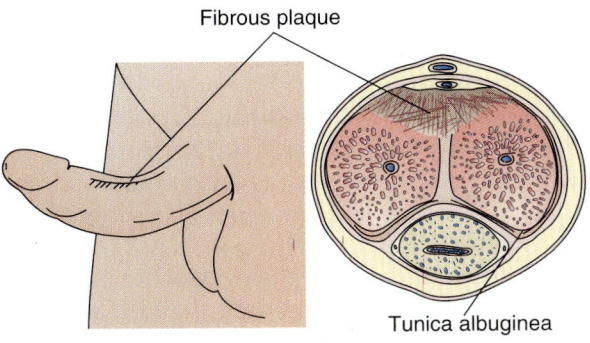

Fibrous plaque

Tunica albuginea

A. External view   **B.** Internal view

Figure 35-20 Peyronie's Disease: A. Fibrous plaque causes a curvature of the penis; B. Cross section of the penis showing plaque.

Medical–Surgical Management

Medical

The first step in treating impotence is to determine whether the client's lifestyle is a factor. Further assessment may include nocturnal penile tumescence monitoring or dynamic infusion cavernosometry and cavernosography (DICC). Treatment will be based on the assessment findings and test results. Treatment may include changes in lifestyle to reduce the need for medications, manage stress, lose weight, and exercise. These changes often help to improve the client's physical health, self-image, and attitude about his ability to function sexually.

External devices can be used to promote an erection. A vacuum constriction device (VCD) may be used to increase the blood supply to the penis, causing engorgement and rigidity. The client inserts his penis into a plastic cylinder and squeezes a pump to withdraw the air from the cylinder, creating a vacuum that draws blood into the penis. Once an erection has been achieved in this manner, a rubber ring is moved from the bottom of the cylinder to the base of the penis. This permits the blood to be safely trapped in the penis for up to one-half hour. Advantages of the VCD over surgical intervention are decreased expense and fewer complications.

Surgical

Surgical interventions for impotency include revascularization and penile implants. For clients with impotence related to blocked arteries, revascularization is done to bypass blocked arteries and remove veins that are causing excessive drainage. For clients who are not candidates for revascularization, penile prostheses are another option. One type is a semirigid implant, which is a silicone cylinder that may be flexible or inflexible. Another type is a hydraulic implant that has a cylinder that can be inflated by squeezing a pump located in the scrotum or at the end of the penis. Because of its ability to fill and empty, the hydraulic implant, unlike the silicone implant, which is always semirigid, most closely mimics flaccidity and erection. The disadvantages of surgical interventions are expense and postoperative complications, the most serious being postoperative infection.

Pharmacological

Medications that promote erections are available. The one most widely used is sildenafil citrate (Viagra). One side effect of drug therapy is prolonged erection that does not occur in response to sexual stimulation (**priapism**). Oral neurotransmitters have been used with variable success, and sublingual apomorphine shows some promise as an erectogenic agent. When administered sublingually rather than subcutaneously, as was done in the past, there are fewer side effects.

Self-injections of vasodilators or other drugs may result in serious complications.

▶ NURSING PROCESS

▶ Assessment

▶ Subjective Data

A complete assessment includes a history of illicit and prescribed drug use, alcohol consumption, previous diagnoses, lifestyle, sexual functioning, and family disorders. The client's emotional and educational needs must be assessed to determine whether anxiety about sexual performance or lack of knowledge are contributing factors to impotence.

▶ Objective Data

If the client has surgery, the nurse needs to monitor vital signs, incisional site, and intake and output.

Nursing Management

Nursing diagnoses for a client who is impotent may include the following:

- *Sexual Dysfunction, related to altered body function or structure*
- *Sexuality Patterns, Altered, related to altered body function or structure*
- *Body Image Disturbance, related to impotence*
- *Knowledge Deficit, related to impotence*

INFERTILITY

Approximately one in every six couples experiences infertility, the inability to produce offspring. Infertility may be primary or secondary. In primary infertility, the couple have never achieved a pregnancy or have never carried a pregnancy to viability. Secondary infertility involves problems that arise after the couple has had a successful pregnancy. Many factors may be investigated as causes of infertility in both female and male clients. Forty percent of infertility factors are female-related, 40% are male-related, and 20% are a combination of multiple factors that involve both partners. The more factors that are involved, the more difficult the infertility resolution.

The etiology of infertility may be related to anatomic or endocrine problems. The female anatomic or structural abnormalities may include blocked passages through the cervix or fallopian tubes caused by failed development or by past infections, such as PID, or STDs. Uterine and cervical abnormalities may also occur. The cervix may be too narrow or closed and sperm are unable to navigate through the passage. The uterus may have a partial or complete septum inside

that limits the internal cavity space. Immune problems involve the development of antibodies by the woman's system to the male's sperm. These antibodies may be present in the cervical mucus and kill the sperm on contact. Hyposecretion or hypersecretion of FSH, LH, estrogen, or progesterone have been associated with infertility.

The causes of infertility in males include varicoceles, cryptorchidism, impaired sperm, insufficient number of sperm, and hormonal imbalance. The use of hot tubs or saunas may decrease the sperm count.

The first step in treating an infertile couple is to obtain a history of sexual practices. In addition, a detailed health history needs to be obtained and physical examination performed.

A basic infertility workup may be initiated when the client has been unable to conceive after 6 to 12 months of unprotected intercourse. One simple, noninvasive procedure is the use of a basal body temperature chart. The chart is kept for a minimum of 3 months and then reviewed for normal ovulatory fluctuations in the basal temperature. During the first half of the menstrual cycle, the body temperature may remain below 98°F. At ovulation, there is often a slight decrease in the temperature for a 24-hour period. This is the optimal period of fertility. After ovulation, the woman's basal body temperature should go above 98°F and remain in that range for a period of 14 days. The length of the luteal phase (secretory phase) of the cycle following ovulation is a critical factor in some infertility disorders. Variations in the temperature chart may indicate that the client has had an anovulatory cycle or has a shortened luteal phase. Since the fertilized ovum does not implant in the endometrium until 6 to 8 days after conception, the luteal phase is critical to maintain the blood-rich lining long enough for implantation to occur. A low progesterone level during the luteal phase may result in spontaneous **abortion** (ending a pregnancy before the age of viability) of the fertilized ovum before implantation. Diagnostic tests that may be ordered include the following:

- Endometrial biopsy to detect tissue responses during both phases of the menstrual cycle
- Semen analysis, including sperm count, motility, and morphology
- Testicular biopsy (done when sperm are absent from the semen) to ascertain the presence of sperm
- Endocrine imbalance testing which measures pituitary, gonadotropin, testosterone, estrogen, and progesterone levels
- Male-female interaction studies (Huhner test) to determine motility and number of sperm 2 to 4 hours after intercourse
- Laparoscopy to discover conditions such as endometriosis, adhesions, or scar tissue that potentially immobilize the fimbriae or polycystic ovarian disease (Stein-Leventhal syndrome)

Medical–Surgical Management

There is no one treatment for infertility problems. The goal of treatment is successful achievement of a pregnancy that is carried to full term and produces a healthy offspring.

Medical

Infertility treatment may include artificial insemination with either the partner's sperm or donor sperm. This method is particularly useful if the male partner has a low sperm count, abnormal sperm, or no sperm production. With the procedure, the semen is placed directly into the cervix or uterus with a small flexible catheter and a syringe.

Surgical

Several methods can be used to accomplish a pregnancy, but each one is directed toward a different underlying cause of the infertility. One method is *in vitro* fertilization. This may be by GIFT (gamete-intra-fallopian transfer), or ZIFT (zygote-intra-fallopian transfer). With the GIFT technique, the female partner receives monthly cyclic hormone injections that cause ova to ripen. The hormones may cause more than one ovum to ripen during each cycle, which enhances the possibility that more than one ovum will be fertilized and implanted in the uterus. A semen specimen is collected from the male partner 1 to 2 hours before the GIFT procedure and the sperm placed into a special catheter. The ripened ovum is obtained from the female via laparoscopy or ultrasound aspiration and is loaded into the catheter in a sequential manner with the sperm and then injected through the fimbrial end of the fallopian tube, also by laparoscopy. This procedure takes approximately 1 hour to complete. Pregnancy is confirmed within 7 to 10 days with a blood hormonal test (Beta HCG) or an ultrasound, or both.

The ZIFT procedure is similar to GIFT. However, several ova are obtained just before ovulation and are placed in a special fluid for several hours while the sperm are prepared. The ova and sperm are then carefully mixed and closely observed for 2 to 3 days. The fertilized ova (now zygotes) are transferred into the fallopian tube or into the uterine cavity. Another name for the ZIFT procedure is IVF-ER (*in vitro* fertilization and embryo replacement), which more clearly defines what actually occurs.

Both GIFT and ZIFT are relatively expensive procedures (approximately $5,000 or more per cycle) and may or may not be covered by health insurance. For many couples, these are final efforts to conceive.

Pharmacological

Several medications are used in the treatment of infertility disorders, and most are focused on hormone imbalances or deficiencies. Clomiphene citrate (Clomid) stimulates release of follicle-stimulating hormone (FSH) and luteinizing hormone (LH) and is used to induce ovulation. Clomid is administered orally beginning on the fifth day of the menstrual cycle. If ovulation does not occur, the dosage will be increased for 5 days in the next cycle. If ovulation does not occur by the time the dose has been increased 4 or 5 times, it may be considered a Clomid failure. There is some chance of multiple gestation while the client is taking Clomid, and she should be informed of the potential. Most often it is a twin pregnancy, but occasionally triplets may be conceived.

Menotropins (Pergonal) mimics FSH and LH, causing follicular growth and maturation. It is administered by intramuscular injection. Although Pergonal is an expensive drug, it has been shown to increase the possibility for ovulation in clients who have not responded to other medications.

Human chorionic gonadotropin (Pregnyl) may also be administered with the Clomid or Pergonal therapy to help maintain the endometrial lining for implantation. It stimulates the production of progesterone from the ovary until the fertilized ovum implants and the placenta begins to function. Progesterone suppositories may be used vaginally 2 times a day to help correct a luteal phase defect by lengthening the time from ovulation until the onset of the menses or through implantation and pregnancy. Some clients continue with the progesterone suppositories throughout the first few weeks of the pregnancy to ensure that the endometrium remains intact. If the sperm count or motility is low, testosterone or thyroid extracts may be prescribed.

Health Promotion

Seeking prompt medical treatment for infections that involve the reproductive system is an essential means of preventing infertility problems, especially with STDs and PID. PID causes scarring of the outside of the fallopian tubes, and gonorrhea can result in scarring or strictures of the internal fallopian tube. Either cause can result in an ectopic pregnancy when the fertilized ovum cannot pass through the tube.

Other considerations may include wise choices in contraceptive methods. The use of oral contraceptives has been associated with primary and secondary infertility due to decreased pituitary function. This condition may resolve spontaneously, or medications may be required to stimulate ovulation in order to conceive.

Multiple sexual partners have also been associated with an increased risk of sexually transmitted disease, infections, and cervical cancer.

CONTRACEPTION

Contraception, or prevention of pregnancy, has been accomplished by many methods over the centuries. In weighing the options, safety, ease of use, effectiveness, and cost should be considered. Both partners' wishes should be considered in this decision-making process.

Contraception may be accomplished by natural means or medical interventions. This section of the chapter will discuss a basic overview of the types of contraceptive methods currently available, the advantages and disadvantages, the effectiveness of each kind, the mechanisms by which they work, and the client education that should accompany the methods (Table 35-2).

NATURAL METHOD

Natural methods of contraception may include what is called the "rhythm method." During the woman's fertile period of the month, usually lasting 7 days (3 days before ovulation to 3 days after), the couple should abstain from intercourse. The determination of the fertile period is based on the time of ovulation. Sperm can live up to 72 hours after ejaculation, and it is possible for sperm to still be in the cervix or uterus if the couple had intercourse 3 days before ovulation. The couple may also decide to maintain a basal body temperature chart to more accurately pinpoint ovulation each month. Another method to determine the approaching ovulation is to monitor the stretchiness of the cervical mucus. This is called "spinnbarkeit." As the woman nears ovulation, the hormones (estrogen) cause the cervical mucus to become clear, thin, and stretchy. This type of mucus provides a favorable environment for the sperm and helps their motility toward the ova. Immediately after ovulation, the cervical mucus becomes hostile to sperm. It becomes thick, cloudy, and more acidic. It also loses its stretchiness. Kits are available for purchase from the local drug store or pharmacy that react to chemicals in the cervical mucus and predict the time of ovulation. The kits are inexpensive and simple to use, much like home pregnancy tests.

Table 35-2 CONTRACEPTION: METHODS, EFFECTIVENESS, AND CONCERNS

METHOD	EFFECTIVE-NESS RATE	RISKS	SIDE EFFECTS	OTHER ADVANTAGES
Abstinence	100%	None known	Psychological reactions	Prevents infections including HIV
Barriers diaphragm cervical cap spermicide	84% 73–92% 79%	Mechanical irritation, vaginal infections, toxic shock syndrome	Pelvic pressure, cervical erosion, vaginal discharges if left in too long	Protects to some degree against sexually transmitted diseases
Condoms	86%	None known	Decreased sensation, allergy to latex, less spontaneity in lovemaking	Protects against sexually transmitted disease, including AIDS; delays premature ejaculation
Oral contraceptives	97%	Cardiovascular complications such as stroke, blood clots, high blood pressure, and heart attacks with the higher-dose combined oral contraceptive	Possible nausea, headaches, dizziness, spotting, weight gain, breast tenderness, chloasma, cramping	Protects against PID, decreases risk of ovarian and endometrial cancer, decreases menstrual blood loss and dysmenorrhea (cramps), decreases benign breast disease, regulates irregular menses, protects bone density, decreases risk of atherosclerosis, lessens the risk of rheumatoid arthritis, decreases uterine fibroids, and decreases ovarian cysts
Norplant implants	99%	Infection at implant site	Menstrual changes, weight gain, headaches	May protect against PID, may decrease menstrual cramps and blood loss
Depo-Provera	98%	Pulmonary embolism	Headache, depression, hypertension, edema, nausea	Effective to treat obstructive sleep apnea
IUD	94%	Pelvic inflammatory disease, uterine perforation, anemia	Menstrual cramping, spotting, increased bleeding	None known except with progestin-releasing IUD, which may decrease menstrual pain and blood loss
Sterilization female male	99.6% 99.8%	Infection	Pain at surgical site, psychological reaction with subsequent regret	None known

BARRIER AND SPERMICIDE METHODS

Methods of barrier contraception include male and female condoms, the diaphragm, and the cervical cap. Barrier devices work by blocking the pathway of the sperm through the cervix into the uterus. Spermicides kill sperm before they can enter the cervix. This type of contraceptive requires some preplanning on the part of one or both of the partners and may reduce the spontaneity of the sex act.

Spermicides contain a chemical, nonoxynol-9, that kills sperm on contact. If used alone, spermicidal agents have a lower efficacy rate than if used with a condom. The nurse should advise the couple to use a spermicidal gel, foam suppository, or film in addition to another barrier method for the greatest effectiveness. Foam should not be used with the diaphragm because it can result in deterioration of the latex. These agents must be placed in the vagina at least 15 minutes before intercourse to promote the spermicidal reaction. This method is safe and inexpensive but requires a high level of compliance each time or the effectiveness of the method drops significantly.

HORMONAL METHODS

Oral contraceptives, Norplant, and Depo-Provera are discussed following.

Oral Contraceptives

The "pill" has been available as a contraceptive method for many years. Since its earliest form, it has been refined and the level of hormones reduced. Oral contraceptives work by suppressing ovulation. In a sense, the body thinks it is pregnant when the pill is used. Some oral contraceptives contain estrogen and progesterone; others contain only progestins.

In response to the pseudopregnancy state, the client may experience mild side effects and discomforts often associated with pregnancy such as, nausea, headache, breast tenderness, or weight gain. Major side effects from oral contraceptives may include cardiovascular accidents or thrombophlebitis.

There is approximately a 1 in 200 chance of becoming pregnant while taking the oral contraceptive. If the woman thinks that she might be pregnant, she should stop the pill immediately and contact her physician. When the woman and her partner decide that it is time for a pregnancy, she should discontinue the oral contraceptive for at least 2 to 3 cycles before having unprotected intercourse. This "rest period" will lessen the possibility that pill effects will remain in her system and will allow her body to return to its own natural rhythm. Some women will find that they experience primary or secondary infertility problems after being on the pill for several years owing to pituitary suppression. The remedy is often fertility drugs such as clomiphene citrate (Clomid). Women who have never established a regular pattern of menstruation may not be good candidates for oral contraceptives, except as being used to regulate the cycle by artificial means. Other clients who should not take oral contraceptives include women with a history of hypertension, diabetes, cardiovascular disease, or thrombophlebitis. Some physicians may consider oral contraceptives in the newer low-dose combinations for clients who were previously in this high-risk group.

Norplant

Levonorgestrel (Norplant System) consists of six small progestin-filled pellets that are inserted under the skin of the upper arm under a local anesthetic. Theoretically, Norplant is effective for up to 5 years. Some clients will experience mild breakthrough bleeding during the first few months after the Norplant is in place. This usually subsides or lessens with time, but for some clients it is an inconvenience. This is a good option for the woman who is sure she does not desire a pregnancy for at least 5 years, although the pellets may be removed before the end of that time. Because of the expense of the Norplant and placement procedure, the nurse or physician should make sure the client has a clear understanding of the method before proceeding.

Depo-Provera

The medroxyprogesterone acetate (Depo-Provera) injection is administered intramuscularly every 12 weeks. It works like oral contraceptives to suppress ovulation. The client may experience breakthrough bleeding after the first injection, but this is not an indication that the hormone is not working. It usually requires about 3 weeks after the first injection before the contraceptive is effective, so the client should be advised to use a barrier contraceptive method during that period. The client must receive the injections at regular intervals to ensure effectiveness. Norplant and Depo-Provera are good options for the client who is approaching her forties or who smokes because they contain only progestins, which decreases the risk of cardiovascular problems.

INTRAUTERINE DEVICE METHOD

The intrauterine device (IUD) has been used for many years and has undergone several changes. The Dalcon shield, which was used in the 1960s and 1970s, caused many problems from infection to infertility. The IUD works by causing an irritation inside the uterine cavity that results in a hostile environment for the fertilized ovum that causes it not to implant. It is then sloughed off with the menstrual flow. The intrauterine device is recommended for women who have had children because the cervix has been dilated. This allows for easier insertion of the device. The IUD is inserted or removed while the client is having her period because there is slight dilatation of the cervix at that time. A string attached to the distal end of the device hangs out of the cervix into the vagina. The client is instructed to check the string each month after the menstrual period to make sure the device has not been expelled. Some women experience more dysmenorrhea with the IUD in place and a heavier menstrual flow. Because there is an increased risk of infection with the IUD, a monogamous relationship is advisable for the client. The intrauterine devices that are currently available are effective for 1 year or 7 years.

STERILIZATION METHOD

Sterilization is considered a permanent and very effective method of contraception. In a rare incident, a woman will become pregnant after a tubal ligation or after her partner has had a vasectomy. The procedure interrupts the pathway through the fallopian tube. Sterilization may be performed on an outpatient basis in a surgical clinic or the outpatient department at the hospital. The tubal ligation is done under a general or epidural anesthetic with laparoscopy. The procedure takes about 30 to 60 minutes. The abdomen is distended with a gas to permit better visualization of the pelvic structures during the procedure.

The male sterilization, **vasectomy** (surgical resection of the vas deferens), is usually performed with local anesthesia on an outpatient basis. Rest, with ice to the scrotum, for 4 hours should follow. The client should not engage in strenuous activity or exercise for 1 week.

It may take up to 6 weeks for the semen to be clear of sperm. The client is instructed to return to the clinic for a sperm count after 20 ejaculations. If he is sexually active, during those ejaculations he should use a condom or some other form of contraception. At 6 months a sperm count should be repeated and then monitored annually thereafter.

The female sterilization is more expensive and, because it requires more anesthesia, carries a slightly higher risk than the male procedure.

Refined microsurgical techniques have made it possible to reverse sterilization procedures. The reversals are not always successful, and the couple need to consider the odds of success before venturing into the expense of this type of surgery.

CASE STUDY

Mr. Able is a 70-year-old Caucasian male with a diagnosis of benign prostatic hyperplasia. Before his hospital admission for a TURP he had been in good health. He returned from surgery 3 hours ago with a three-way Foley catheter and continuous bladder irrigation. His vital signs 1 hour ago were as follows: temperature 98.9°F, apical pulse 68, blood pressure 130/84, and respirations 18. When the nurse enters his room to take another set of vitals, Mr. Able is restless and moaning and has cool, moist skin; his catheter is not draining properly. His pulse is now 120 and blood pressure is 88/50. The nurse calls the physician to report the change in Mr. Able's condition. The physician orders a STAT hematocrit and a bleeding and clotting time. An increase in the IV fluid drip rate is also ordered. The doctor is planning to arrive at the hospital within the next hour.

The following questions will guide your development of a nursing care plan for the case study.

1. List symptoms and clinical manifestations, other than Mr. Able's, that a client may experience after a TURP.

2. List reasons why the doctor has ordered the STAT blood work and the IV changes.

3. List other diagnostic tests that may have been ordered for Mr. Able.

4. Mentally do a head-to-toe or functional assessment on Mr. Able. List subjective and objective data a nurse would want to obtain.

5. Write three individualized nursing diagnoses and goals for Mr. Able.

continued

CASE STUDY *continued*

6. Upon assessing Mr. Able, the doctor decides to inject additional fluid into the balloon that anchors the indwelling catheter and apply increased traction to the catheter. List pertinent nursing actions a nurse would do following these medical interventions:

   • Medications

   • Comfort/rest

   • Cardiac output

   • Intake and output

   • Activity

   • Teaching

7. List resources within the medical center and the local area that could assist Mr. Able with his postoperative recovery.

8. List teaching that Mr. Able will need before his discharge.

9. List at least three successful outcomes for Mr. Able.

SUMMARY

• Potential complications from PID may include sterility or infertility from scarring of fallopian tubes.

• Toxic shock syndrome (TSS) occurs during the menses, and a strong correlation exists between the onset and use of super-absorbent tampons.

• Common male reproductive system inflammatory disorders include epididymitis, orchitis, and prostatitis. Bilateral epididymitis and orchitis can lead to sterility. Treatment includes antibiotic therapy.

• A BSE is an important method for detecting breast changes and should be practiced each month. Breast cancer is the most common female cancer in the United States.

• Benign prostatic hyperplasia is a common disorder in males over age 50. Early symptoms include hesitancy, decreased force of stream, urinary frequency, and nocturia.

• Cervical cancer is most common in women with multiple sexual partners.

• Endometrial cancer often produces symptoms only after it is widespread. Any unusual vaginal bleeding should be investigated, especially if it occurs after menopause.

• Male cancers related to the reproductive system involve the prostate, testes, breast, and penis. Emphasis should be placed on testicular self-examination and regular physical examinations in order to facilitate early diagnosis and treatment.

• Menstrual disorders are often associated with hormonal imbalances, increased or decreased function of the endocrine glands, or neoplasms.

• Menopause is a normal, gradual decline in the ovarian production of female hormones that occurs around age 50. Estrogen replacement therapy is recommended by many health care providers to decrease the symptoms of menopause and as a preventive measure against cardiovascular disease and osteoporosis.

• Infertility affects at least 1 in every 4 couples in the United States and is caused by hormonal imbalances, and structural or physiologic abnormalities in both male and female clients.

• Women who smoke and are over age 40 are at greater risk for major complications while using oral contraceptives. Major health risks include cardiovascular accidents and deep vein thrombosis.

• Impotence may be caused by emotional or physical factors. Treatment includes counseling, medications, circulatory aids, and surgery.

Review Questions

1. The best method of screening for cervical cancer is:

   a. genitourinary cultures.

   b. cervical biopsy.

   c. Pap smear.

   d. ultrasound.

2. The female client should perform BSE (breast self-examination):

   a. just before the menstrual period.

   b. just after the menstrual period.

   c. at ovulation.

   d. any time of the month.

3. Bowel and bladder complications that may follow pelvic radiation therapy for uterine cancer are often caused by:

   a. dehydration.
   b. lack of mobility.
   c. damage to the tissue from radiation effects.
   d. damage to tissues during surgery.

4. The most common cancer of the female reproductive system is:

   a. breast.
   b. ovarian.
   c. cervical.
   d. uterine.

5. The primary microorganism associated with the occurrence of toxic shock syndrome is:

   a. *Escherichia coli*.
   b. *Streptococcus aureus*.
   c. *Staphylococcus aureus*.
   d. *Pseudomonas*.

6. A dietary element frequently associated with fibrocystic breast disease is:

   a. fats.
   b. protein.
   c. sodium.
   d. caffeine.

7. Which of the following are characteristic signs of a trichomonas vaginitis?

   a. Thick, white, "cheesy" discharge with itching
   b. Frothy, foul-smelling, yellow discharge with itching and irritation
   c. Creamy, thin, vaginal discharge with a musty or fishy odor
   d. Painful intercourse due to decreased lubrication

8. Which of the following factors predisposes males to penile cancer?

   a. Alcohol consumption
   b. Not being circumcised
   c. Advanced age
   d. Circumcision

9. Which of the following self-examinations should a young man be taught to do?

   a. Rectal
   b. Scrotal
   c. Prostate
   d. Testicular

10. Which of the following complications may occur after a TURP?

    a. Water intoxication
    b. Difficulty voiding
    c. Constipation
    d. Hypertension

11. The purpose of post-TURP continuous bladder irrigation is to:

    a. decrease urinary output.
    b. reduce clot formation.
    c. decrease bleeding.
    d. increase urinary output.

12. Which of the following nursing interventions can help alleviate bladder spasms post-TURP?

    a. Increasing fluid intake
    b. Maintaining traction on the urethral catheter
    c. Administering B&O suppositories
    d. Applying ice to and elevating the scrotum

13. Which of the following is a method that can be used to assess the client's level of knowledge related to his inflammatory disorder of the reproductive system?

    a. Asking the client if he has any questions
    b. Asking the client to describe "safe sex" practices
    c. Asking the client if he has read the pamphlets about his disorder
    d. Asking the client to describe the symptoms of his disorder

Critical Thinking Questions

1. Prepare a teaching plan for a breast self-examination.

2. Prepare a teaching plan for testicular self-examination.

3. What is the rationale for each nursing intervention given for the nursing diagnoses in this chapter?

WEB FLASH!

- Search the Internet for the disorders discussed in this chapter. Are there any new treatments discussed for any of the disorders?
- Visit the Web sites for the Resources listed at the end of the book for the reproductive systems. What type of information do these organizations have available for the client and family? For health care providers?

NURSING CARE OF THE CLIENT: SEXUALLY TRANSMITTED DISEASES

LEARNING OBJECTIVES

Upon completion of this chapter, you should be able to:
- *Define key terms.*
- *List the most prevalent STDs, including causative agents.*
- *Describe currently used methods of prevention of STDs.*
- *Describe signs and symptoms, diagnostic aids, and treatment of the common STDs.*
- *Utilize the nursing process to plan the care of a client with an STD.*
- *Demonstrate the ability to teach self-care and reinfection prevention measures to the client with an STD.*

KEY TERMS

antibiotic resistance	incidence
chancre	incubation period
chlamydia	syphilis
cytomegalovirus	trichomoniasis
exposure	venereal disease
gonorrhea	

INTRODUCTION

Sexually transmitted diseases (STDs) can be defined as those diseases that are transmitted or passed from one person to another primarily through sexual contact. Another term that was used for STDs is **venereal disease**. Today the term *sexually transmitted disease* is preferred. The STDs covered in this chapter are chlamydia, gonorrhea, syphilis, genital herpes, cytomegalovirus, genital warts, trichomoniasis, and hepatitis B. Acquired immunodeficiency syndrome (AIDS) is not solely a sexually transmitted disease, although sexual activity is one of the primary modes of transmission (ways through which it is spread): AIDS is discussed in detail in Chapter 39.

The **incidence** (frequency of disease occurence) of STDs has been increasing worldwide, with trichomoniasis, chlamydia, and gonorrhea being the most widespread STDs today. Some diseases, such as syphilis, have been described as sexually transmitted diseases for centuries. Currently over 13 million Americans annually are diagnosed with an STD. Chlamydia, for example, affects over 3 million Americans every year, making it more than twice as common as gonorrhea (National Institute of Allergy and Infectious Diseases [NIAID] and National Institutes of Health [NIH], December 1998). Syphilis, although less common than either chlamydia or gonorrhea, still affects about 9,000 people each year in the United States (NIAID and NIH, December 1998).

The development of antibiotic treatment for STDs in the 1940s caused a dramatic decrease in the prevalence of STDs, and for a while it was predicted that STDs would be eradicated completely. But a variety of factors have contributed to the dramatic increase of STDs such as: casual sex, asymptomatic carriers of the disease, the use of nonbarrier methods of birth control, and lack of knowledge of methods of preventing STDs.

Another factor that has contributed to the vast increase in STDs in recent years is the increased consumption of alcohol and the use of illegal drugs. Not only is the sharing of needles among intravenous drug abusers a factor in the increased incidence of STDs, but so also is the lessening of inhibitions that occurs with drug and alcohol abuse. The trading of sex for drugs is also a factor in the spread of STDs.

Inadequate reporting of STDs may also cause statistics to be inaccurate. There is no great uniformity in the reporting requirements for STDs. Reporting regulations differ from state to state and from disease to disease. All states in the United States require that cases of gonorrhea and syphilis be reported to a health officer in that state. Only 35 states have mandatory HIV reporting (Sharts-Hopko, 1997). The Centers for Disease Control and Prevention (CDC) keep statistics on reportable diseases.

Public education regarding the causes, methods of transmission, and methods of prevention of STDs is the most important weapon in the battle against STDs. Although many STDs caused by bacterial infection are curable with modern antibiotics, the viruses are not.

Since sexual activity is beginning at earlier ages today, sex education, including information about STDs, is being presented in elementary schools. Many schools have comprehensive education programs already in place to teach about STDs and recommendations to prevent the spread of STDs. Television, especially educational programs, also has been helpful in informing the public of the dangers of having sex without protection against STDs.

Many messages have been disseminated to the general public regarding the best methods of prevention of STDs. The only 100% effective method of prevention of STDs is abstinence (refraining from sexual intercourse or mucous membrane to mucous membrane contact altogether). Couples who are mutually monogamous are also not at risk, unless one of them was pre-

LIFE CYCLE CONSIDERATIONS

Young Adults and STDs

Eighty-six percent of STD cases occur in adolescents and young adults age 15 to 29. One in 5 have been treated for an STD by age 21 (Sharts-Hopko, 1997).

viously infected. The popularity of the pill has decreased consistent condom use. Most current methods of birth control are not effective in preventing the transmission of STDs. Only a barrier method, the latex condom, has been effective in preventing the spread of STDs, although even this method only provides safer sex, not totally safe sex.

Once the diagnosis of an STD is made, identification of all sexual contacts is also important. Many people are reluctant to be candid regarding sexual activity and sexual contacts, since this is an area of life considered to be extremely private. One of the most difficult aspects in dealing with STDs is that many of the diseases are totally asymptomatic, especially in women. These asymptomatic partners can both transmit the disease to new partners and/or reinfect a treated partner, if they are not identified and treated.

An overview of the STDs covered in this chapter is presented in Table 36-1.

ANATOMY AND PHYSIOLOGY REVIEW

The major system affected by the sexually transmitted diseases is the reproductive system. Males are generally more symptomatic than females and will seek

Table 36-1 SEXUALLY TRANSMITTED DISEASES: AN OVERVIEW

DISEASE	CHARACTERISTICS	NURSING IMPLICATIONS
Chlamydia	*Male:* Painful urination Urethral discharge *Female:* Asymptomatic or may experience purulent discharge *Note:* If untreated, pelvic inflammatory disease (PID) can develop.	Instruct client to notify sexual partner(s) of past 2 months of their need for treatment. Instruct client to avoid sexual activity or to use condoms until both client and partner(s) are symptom free. Provide instruction regarding medications prescribed.
Cytomegalovirus (CMV)	Often asymptomatic, occasionally fever, fatigue, and weakness Generally acquired during childhood or adolescence 80% to 100% of adults have antibodies to CVM.	Implicated in some spontaneous abortions or mental retardation. Congenital infection produces cytomegalic inclusion disease. May be life threatening in a client with a poorly functioning immune system. *continued*

Table 36-1 SEXUALLY TRANSMITTED DISEASES: AN OVERVIEW

DISEASE	CHARACTERISTICS	NURSING IMPLICATIONS
Genital Herpes: Herpes Simplex Virus 2 (HSV-2)	Vesicles on penis, vagina, labia, perineum, or anus Can progress to painful ulceration Lesions may last up to 6 weeks Recurrence common *Note:* May be asymptomatic	Refer sexual partner(s) for examination. Teach that virus can be transmitted even when the person experiences no symptoms. Instruct in use of condoms. Teach females of need for annual Pap smear. Provide instruction regarding medications prescribed.
Gonorrhea	*Male:* Urethritis (inflammation of the urethra) Purulent discharge Urinary frequency Epididymitis (inflammation of the epididymis) *Female:* Often asymptomatic May lead to PID or salpingitis (inflammation of the fallopian tube) Can occlude the fallopian tubes, resulting in sterility	Instruct client to return if symptoms persist. Sexual partner(s) of past 60 days must be assessed. Instruct client to avoid sexual activity until symptoms subside in both client and partner(s). Provide instruction regarding medications prescribed.
Hepatitis B Virus (HBV)	Varies greatly from asymptomatic state to severe hepatitis to cancer	Partner(s) should receive medical prophylaxis within 14 days after exposure. For client and partner(s), recommend three-dose immunization series when this episode has abated.
Genital Warts (Human Papillomavirus)	Fleshy, cauliflowerlike growth on genitalia	Inform and treat sexual partner(s). Provide instruction regarding medications prescribed.
Syphilis	Disease consists of 4 stages with distinct manifestations as follows: *Primary:* A painless papule on penis, vagina, or cervix (chancre) Usually negative serologic blood test Highly infectious during this stage *Secondary:* Rash, especially prevalent on palms and soles Low-grade fever Sore throat Headache *Early latency:* Possible infectious lesions, otherwise asymptomatic Reactive serologic tests *Late latency:* Possible lesions in central nervous and cardiovascular systems Noninfectious except to fetus of pregnant woman	Interview client to identify sexual contacts. All those exposed to the disease should be given penicillin. Educate client and sexual contacts about the disease. Provide instruction regarding medications prescribed. Counsel and educate client. Counsel and educate client.
Trichomoniasis	Petechial lesions Profuse urethral or vaginal discharge that is foul smelling, yellow, and foamy	Treat sexual partners simultaneously with metronidazole (Flagyl). Provide instruction regarding medication prescribed.

health care more readily since the signs of disease on the external genitalia are more visible. In females, the sex organs are internal; females, therefore, are more likely to suffer complications and increased severity of symptoms by the time the disease is identified.

In addition to the reproductive system, any area of sexual contact, such as oral and rectal areas, may also exhibit signs and symptoms of the disease process.

COMMON DIAGNOSTIC TESTS

Commonly used diagnostic tests for clients with symptoms of sexually transmitted diseases are listed in Table 36-2. See Chapter 27, Diagnostic Tests, for explanation/normal values and nursing responsibilities.

CHLAMYDIA

Chlamydia is caused by a spherical bacterial organism known as *Chlamydia trachomatis*. Outside the body, the organism has difficulty surviving, but inside the body, chlamydia reproduces rapidly inside host cells. The mode of transmission in chlamydia must be through intimate body contact, since the organism is so fragile that it cannot survive long when outside of the body.

Most chlamydia infections are asymptomatic. Chlamydia is known as the "silent STD" for this reason. If left untreated, chlamydial infections cause tissue inflammation, ulceration, and scar tissue formation in both women and men. Salpingitis (inflammation of the fallopian tubes) or pelvic inflammatory disease (PID)

LIFE CYCLE CONSIDERATIONS

Chlamydial Infection

- The highest rates are in 15- to 19-year-old adolescents regardless of demographics or location.
- Infection during pregnancy can lead to complications such as preterm labor, premature rupture of membranes, and low birth weight babies.
- A newborn exposed to *Chlamydia trachomatis* during the birth process may develop conjunctivitis within 10 days and pneumonia within 3 to 6 weeks.

---

can lead to scarring of the delicate fallopian tubes, ectopic pregnancy, or even infertility.

When symptoms of chlamydia appear in males, they are dysuria and genital discharge. Females may have a grayish white mucopurulent vaginal discharge, itching, and dysuria, although as many as 85% of women will be asymptomatic (NIAID and NIH, June 1998b).

Medical–Surgical Management

Pharmacological

The treatment of choice is doxycycline (Vibramycin). If compliance with an extended period of drug therapy is thought to be a problem, azithromycin (Zithromax) can be given orally in a single dose. Pregnant women may be treated with erythromycin estolate (Ilosone) or amoxicillin (Amoxil), but they should be cultured again after treatment is completed to confirm the absence of chlamydial infection. Retesting is not required after treatment with doxycycline or azithromycin. It is important that all sexual partners be tested and treated for chlamydia since reinfection is probable if only one partner is treated.

Health Promotion

Persons who have more than one sexual partner, especially women less than 25 years old, should regularly be tested for chlamydial infection even when there are no symptoms. The use of male or female condoms or diaphragms during sexual intercourse may help reduce transmission (NIAID and NIH, June 1998b).

GONORRHEA

Gonorrheal infections are often seen in combination with chlamydia. **Gonorrhea** is a serious bacterial infection, caused by the gram-negative bacterial organism *Neisseria gonorrhea*. An estimated 800,000 cases occur annually in the United States (NIAID and NIH, June 1998c). The organism multiplies quickly in warm,

---

Table 36-2 COMMON DIAGNOSTIC TESTS FOR SEXUALLY TRANSMITTED DISEASES

Blood Tests
- Enzyme-linked immunosorbent assay (ELISA)
- Western blot
- Venereal Disease Research Laboratories (VDRL)
- Rapid plasma reagin (RPR)
- Fluorescent treponemal antibody-absorption test (FTA-ABS)
- Reiter test

Culture
- Tissue: Male urethra, female endocervix
- Discharge
- Tzanck

Urine
- Urine specimen

Other
- Dark field examination of wart scrapings
- Microscopic examination

moist areas of the body including the oral cavity, reproductive tract, and the rectum. Mouth-to-mouth kissing does not transmit gonorrhea. It is spread during sexual intercourse—vaginal, oral, and anal. The cervix is the usual site of infection in women. The disease progresses in much the same manner as chlamydia and can cause many of the same complications, such as infertility from salpingitis and PID.

Symptoms of infection may occur within 2 to 10 days after **exposure** (contact with an infected person or agent). Again, men are more likely to exhibit symptoms such as burning on urination and a purulent discharge from the penis. Many women are asymptomatic, but the remainder may have pain or burning on urination and/or a yellow or bloody vaginal discharge.

If a woman is infected with gonorrhea when she gives birth, the infection may be transmitted to the newborn's eyes as the baby travels through the birth canal. In the United States, all infants are treated with silver nitrate drops or an antibiotic opthalmic ointment within 1 to 2 hours of birth to prevent the gonorrheal-induced eye infection known as opthalmia neonatorum.

Medical–Surgical Management

Once the presence of gonorrhea has been confirmed, both partners should be treated with a course of antibiotic therapy. One of the problems in treating gonorrhea is that new strains of gonorrhea have developed **antibiotic resistance** (resistance to a previously effective antimicrobial agent). Penicillin used to be the drug of choice when treating gonorrhea, but since penicillin has been so widely used against many types of infection, some strains of *Neisseria gonorrhea* have adapted and are no longer affected by penicillin. The current practice is to treat all cases of gonorrhea as though they were resistant to the traditional drug therapies.

Pharmacological

A variety of antibiotics are effective against gonorrhea. One of the most effective therapies includes a single dose of ciprofloxacin (Cipro), followed by a 7-day course of oral doxycycline (Vibramycin). Because almost half of all clients with gonorrhea also have chlamydia, doxycycline (Vibramycin) is an appropriate choice of drug therapy since it combats both infections effectively. For pregnant clients, or those under 16

years of age, an injection of ceftriaxone sodium (Rocephlin), followed by oral erythromycin estolate (Ilosone), is recommended. Follow-up cultures to determine the success of the course of treatment are recommended when the treatment has been completed.

SYPHILIS

Syphilis, an STD almost eradicated after the discovery of antibiotic therapy in the 1940s, is on the upswing again, with 8,550 cases reported in 1997 (NIAID and NIH, December 1998). The causative organism of syphilis is a spirochete, a spiral-shaped bacteria known as *Treponema pallidum*, which was first identified in 1905. Transmission of syphilis is either through sexual contact or congenitally (mother to child). Syphilis is often seen with human immunodeficiency virus (HIV) infection, just as chlamydia is often seen with gonorrhea.

Syphilis has 4 stages. In primary stage syphilis, the **incubation period**, or interval between exposure to an infectious disease and the first appearance of symptoms, can be 10 to 90 days, with the development of a **chancre** usually occurring within 2 to 6 weeks. A chancre is a clean, painless ulcer, which usually is present at the site of body contact (Figure 36-1). There is usually just one chancre present, but multiple chancres have been known to occur. Chancres may occur on the internal genitalia of women (for example, the cervix) and thus not be noticed. The chancre will heal within a few weeks, even without treatment, and either leave a thin scar or none at all. If not identified and treated, about one-third will progress to secondary syphilis.

In secondary syphilis, the client has a skin rash of penny-sized brown sores that appear approximately 3 to 6 weeks after the chancre. The rash may be on all or any part of the body, but almost always involves the palms of the hands and the soles of the feet. Active bacteria are in the sores so any contact, sexual or nonsexual, with the broken skin of the infected person

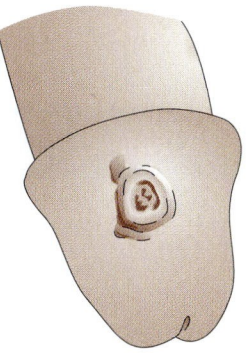

Figure 36-1 The chancre usually occurs at the point where the organism contacted the body.

may spread the infection. The rash heals within several months. Other symptoms such as low-grade fever, fatigue, headache, sore throat, and generalized lymph node swelling may occur. Occasionally a wartlike growth known as condyloma latum may be present in the genital area of both men and women (Figure 36-2). Since this is so close in appearance to the condylomata acuminata of human papillomavirus infection, it may be confused with genital warts. Symptoms of secondary syphilis may come and go for 1 or 2 years. Since many of these symptoms are also common to many other diseases, syphilis has often been called "the great imitator."

When not treated, syphilis enters into a latent period when no symptoms are present and the disease is no longer contagious. Only about one-third of those clients with secondary syphilis will develop the symptoms of tertiary syphilis; that is, when the bacteria damages the heart, eyes, brain, nervous system, bones, joints, or any other part of the body. Tertiary syphilis can last for years or decades and may result in heart disease, blindness, neurologic problems, and death.

Approximately 3% to 7% of untreated persons will develop neurosyphilis (NIAID and NIH, July 1998c). Symptoms may range from none to headache, fever, seizures, and stroke symptoms. Sometimes it may take 20 years for this to occur.

Medical–Surgical Management

Pharmacological

Since the time that syphilis was first treated with antibiotic therapy, penicillin has remained the drug of choice, since no cases of penicillin-resistant syphilis have been identified. All types of penicillin are effective, but penicillin G benzathine (Bicillin L-A) is often preferred. Antimicrobial therapy will destroy *Treponema pallidum* at any stage, but any damage done to body organs is irreversible. If the client has a demonstrated allergy to penicillin, alternative medications may be administered, such as doxycycline (Vibramycin), tetracycline HCl (Achromycin V), or erythromycin estolate (Ilosone). For pregnant women who are allergic to penicillin, erythromycin is recommended as the best alternative therapy.

Clients being treated for syphilis must have periodic

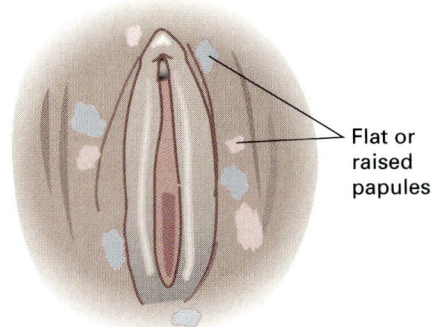

Figure 36-2 Condyloma latum, a wartlike growth, may be present in the genital area of males and females in secondary syphilis.

blood tests to ensure that the infecting agent has been completely destroyed.

GENITAL HERPES

Genital herpes affects an estimated 45 million persons in the United States with an estimated 500,000 new cases each year (NIAID and NIH, July 1998a). It is caused by the herpes simplex virus (HSV). There are two types of HSV. HSV type 1 commonly causes sores on the lips (fever blisters, cold sores). HSV type 2 causes genital sores. Either can infect the other area following oral-genital sex. Genital herpes is usually acquired through sexual contact with an infected person. That person may or may not be aware of having genital herpes. In fact, 80% of persons infected with genital herpes are unaware of their disease (NIAID and NIH, July 1998a).

When symptoms occur in the first episode, they usually appear in 2 to 10 days after infection and last an average of 2 to 3 weeks. Itching or burning sensations; pain in genital area, legs, or buttocks; vaginal discharge; or abdominal pressure are the early symptoms. Within a few days lesions (sores) appear at the infection site (perianal area), in the vagina or on the cervix of females, or in the urethra of females and males.

 LIFE CYCLE CONSIDERATIONS

Syphilis

- Approximately 40% to 70% of untreated pregnant women will have a syphilis-infected infant.
- Approximately 25% of these pregnancies end in stillbirth or neonatal death.
- Some infants with congenital syphilis may have symptoms at birth; most develop symptoms in 2 to 12 weeks.
- Any moist sores on the infant are infectious (NIAID and NIH, July 1998c).

 CLIENT TEACHING

Testing for Syphilis

- Sexually active individuals with a suspicious rash or sore in the genital area should see a health care provider.
- If treated for another STD, the client should also be tested for syphilis.

Flat or raised papules

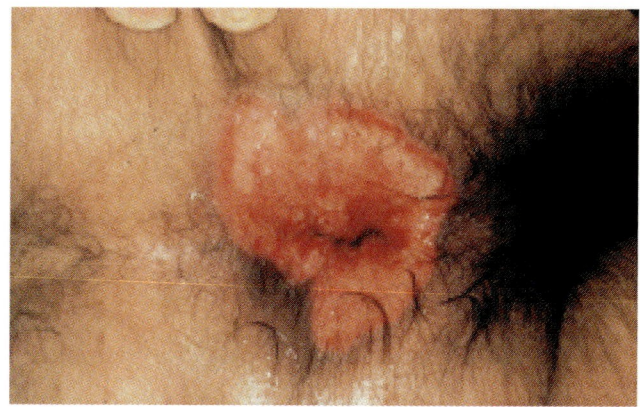

Figure 36-3 Chronic Mucocutaneous Perianal Herpes Infection *(Courtesy of Centers for Disease Control and Prevention, Atlanta; GA 30333.)*

Small red bumps appear first, change into blisters (Figure 36-3), and then become open sores that crust over in a few days. Other symptoms with the first episode may include fever, muscle aches, headache, dysuria, vaginal discharge, and swollen glands in the groin.

With the first episode, the virus travels through the sensory nerves and remains inactive in nerve cells (Figure 36-4) until the virus travels back to the skin, causing a recurrence. Most people will have monthly recurrences (some only 1 or 2 a year), but new sores may or may not be apparent. Symptoms are usually milder than the first episode and last approximately 1 week.

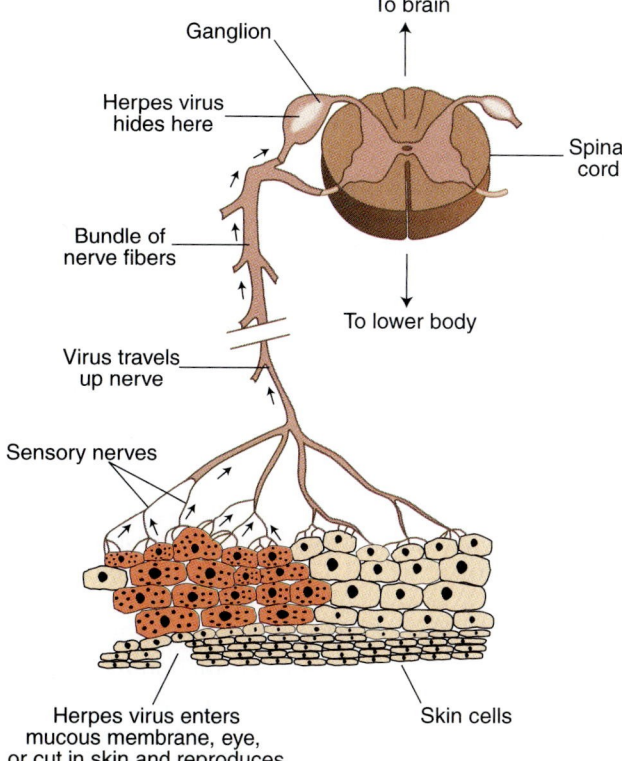

Figure 36-4 Herpes virus invades the nervous system from its portal of entry. *(Adapted from National Foundation March of Dimes, White Plains, NY.)*

The most accurate method of diagnosis is a viral culture, which takes several days. A blood test detecting HSV antibodies only indicates that the person has been infected at some time.

Medical–Surgical Management

Pharmacological

There is no known cure for the herpes simplex virus at this time. Treatment has been geared toward alleviating symptoms of the disease. Acyclovir (Zovirax) has been utilized in the treatment of herpes. A topical form may be applied to the lesions; the drug may also be taken orally to shorten the duration of the lesions in a primary outbreak. When taken daily, it prevents most recurrences. Famciclovir (Famvir) and valacyclovir (Valtrex) suppress viral activity and also prevent recurrences.

Cleansing the area of the lesions with mild soap and water, hydrogen peroxide, or Burow's solution often helps reduce the discomfort of the lesions and decrease the chance of secondary infections. The area should be blown dry with a hairdryer and then the dry skin may be dusted with a cornstarch powder, which aids in decreasing client discomfort.

CYTOMEGALOVIRUS

Another virus in the herpesvirus family is **cytomegalovirus** (CMV), which is found in saliva, urine, and often in semen and vaginal secretions. Figure 36-5 shows an electron micrograph of CMV. Unlike the more commonly recognized herpes viruses, CMV rarely produces noticeable clinical symptoms.

CMV is primarily transmitted from person to person through contact with body fluids like saliva, urine, and blood. The virus has been identified in semen and cervical mucus, so it can be spread by sexual contact. CMV is incurable. People are infected for life. The inactive virus may reactivate from time to time.

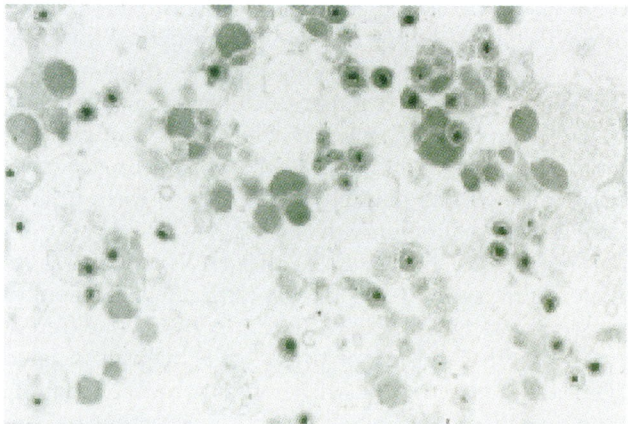

Figure 36-5 Electron Micrograph of CMV *(Courtesy of Centers for Disease Control and Prevention, Atlanta, GA 30333.)*

Most people acquire CMV during childhood or adolescence through contact with saliva and respiratory secretions, and by adulthood somewhere between 80% and 100% of adults will have developed antibodies to CMV. Most of these people will not notice any symptoms, but occasionally a client will present with fever, fatigue, and weakness. These symptoms may persist for several weeks and may lead to a tentative diagnosis of infectious mononucleosis, although the sore throat and swollen lymph nodes of "mono" are not present with CMV.

CMV has been implicated in some complications of pregnancy such as spontaneous abortion or mental retardation of the neonate. Congenital infection of an infant produces cytomegalic inclusion disease that ranges from an asymptomatic condition to a severely debilitating condition that may even result in death. The central nervous system damage to the infant may be profound, although it occurs rarely. An estimated 6,000 babies each year develop life-threatening complications of congenital CMV at birth or have mental retardation, blindness, or epilepsy (NIAID and NIH, June 1998c). CMV can also become a life-threatening illness in a client who has a poorly functioning immune system, such as a client with AIDS.

There is no antiviral agent specifically utilized for this disorder, since most of the population will not have any symptoms.

GENITAL WARTS

Another virus that is sexually transmitted is the human papillomavirus (HPV), which causes genital warts, also called condylomata acuminata. These genital warts may occur in the urogenital, perineal, or anal areas, and may be either external or internal. The population at risk seems to be teenage girls or young women in their twenties. In the United States, it is estimated that there are approximately 1 million new cases of genital warts identified every year, and as many as 24 million already infected with HPV (NIAID and NIH, July 1998b). The incubation period for genital warts appears to be approximately 1 to 2 months, but may be up to 6 months. Unlike genital herpes, genital warts are usually painless, soft fleshy growths appearing most commonly in the genital area. Sometimes many warts may grow together to form a large cauliflower-shaped growth (Figure 36-6).

The greatest health threat that HPV poses to a female client is the predisposition to the development of cervical cancer. Although there are over 60 different types of HPV, only 6 of those have been associated with the development of cervical cancer. Cigarette smoking has been linked to the development of cancerous cervical changes in women with HPV. Women who have HPV should be advised not to smoke. HPV

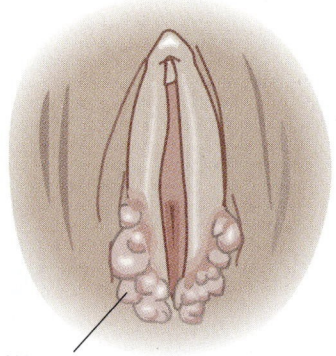

Warts caused by
human papillomavirus (HPV)

Figure 36-6 Genital Warts (Condyloma acuminatum)

appears to play a role in the development of cervical cancer, along with many other factors. An abnormal Pap test may be the first indication of HPV.

Genital warts are less common in men. If seen, they are usually on the tip of the penis.

Medical–Surgical Management

Since genital warts are caused by a virus, there is no cure for the disease. The focus is on preventing the spread of the disease to sexual partners, and reducing the possibility of cancer. Use of a condom during sexual intercourse may provide some protection. Once the genital warts disappear, the disease may lie dormant for many years until there is a recurrence of the outbreak.

Surgical

The warts may be removed under local anesthesia. This is especially recommended if the warts have formed a large fleshy cauliflowerlike growth. Freezing the warts off with cryosurgery, or surgical use of extreme cold, is the treatment of choice for small warts. The warts may also be removed with laser surgery, or cauterized. Whatever treatment is recommended, it must be remembered that the treatment will not cure HPV, but only provide a palliative effect. The warts may recur after any treatment.

Pharmacological

A topical solution of podophyllum resin (Poddoen) may be applied to the genital warts. It is only recommended for treatment of 1 or 2 lesions at a time, since it can be toxic if applied to too large an area at one time. Most people report experiencing a good deal of pain from the treatment. After the solution has been in contact with the genital warts for a period of 4 to 6 hours, it is then washed off with soap and water. If not thoroughly washed off, podophyllum may cause chemical burns that heal very slowly and are very painful. This therapy must not be used on a diabetic client, a client with poor circulation, or a pregnant client.

A cream, imiquimod (Aldara), is applied before bedtime and washed off in the morning. It can be used 3 times a week for 16 weeks or less.

AIDS

AIDS, or acquired immunodeficiency syndrome, is not truly a sexually transmitted disease, but needs to be discussed briefly here since sexual contact remains one of the primary modes of transmission of this disease. AIDS is the end stage of the disease process caused by the human immunodeficiency virus (Chapter 39). Similar to the viruses previously discussed in this chapter, AIDS is not curable. Unlike the other viruses, herpes genitalis and genital warts, AIDS is ultimately fatal. AIDS results in a severe disorder of the body's immune system functioning, leading to an inability of the body to fight off disease. The client's failing immune system makes him vulnerable to opportunistic infections, such as *Pneumocystis carinii* pneumonia.

Persons at risk are those who have multiple sexual partners, IV drug users who share needles, and persons with hemophilia. There are three basic modes of transmission—sexual, bloodborne, and from mother to baby either prenatally, during the birth process, or when breast-feeding. When first identified in 1981, HIV infection was primarily found among homosexual men, but by 1990 the disease was moving into heterosexual populations with great rapidity. By the mid-1990s, cases of AIDS were occurring more frequently among women than among men. The greatest growth in AIDS rates among women occurred in African American and Hispanic women. Teenagers also have one of the fastest growing rates of HIV infection.

TRICHOMONIASIS

Trichomoniasis is caused by a parasitic protozoan called *Trichomonas vaginalis*. Trichomoniasis is a very common STD, with an incidence of approximately 3 million new cases every year (NIAID and NIH, June 1998d). It is seen frequently in combination with gonorrhea. The most common method of transmission is sexual, although the protozoa can survive for a period of time in water so other modes of transmission are possible.

The incubation period after initial exposure to trichomoniasis ranges from approximately 4 to 20 days. About 25% of women infected with trichomoniasis will have no symptoms, and men almost never have symptoms. In these clients, the *Trichomonas* organisms may remain dormant for years, without becoming an active infection. Precipitating factors that may encourage the growth of *Trichomonas* include pregnancy, sexual intercourse, menstruation, or illness. Vulval and vaginal

CLIENT TEACHING

Metronidazole (Flagyl)
No alcohol should be consumed as it causes severe nausea and vomiting, flushing, palpitations, abdominal cramps, and headache.

pruritus is the most common symptom, with a vaginal discharge of a frothy, copious yellow-green mucus. Only 10% of women will present with the classic symptoms of a *Trichomonas* infection: severe itching of the vulva, redness, swelling of the vulva, pain on intercourse and urination, urinary frequency, and a grayish, malodorous discharge. Males most often have a watery, whitish discharge and difficult or painful urination, but may also have urethritis and an accompanying inflammation. In men, *Trichomonas* in the dormant state are usually harbored in the prostate or urethra.

Medical–Surgical Management

Pharmacological

Both partners should be treated with metronidazole (Flagyl) either given orally in a single dose or for a period of approximately 1 week. Metronidazole is effective against both protozoal and bacterial infections. If given vaginally, metronidazole (Flagyl) is not as effective. Pregnant women are usually treated after the first trimester to avoid the possibility of birth defects, since metronidazole is known to cross the placenta.

Adverse effects occur in about 10% of clients taking metronidazole (Flagyl) and usually affect the gastrointestinal system in the form of nausea, vomiting, diarrhea, and abdominal cramping. CNS effects, such as headache or dizziness, may also be seen.

HEPATITIS B

Hepatitis B, caused by the hepatitis B virus, is now recognized as an STD. Today it is primarily transmitted through sexual contact, as opposed to the oral-fecal or blood contact routes that were far more prevalent 20 years ago (Sharts-Hopko, 1997). An estimated 77,000 cases of sexually transmitted hepatitis B occur each year in the United States (NIAID and NIH, December 1998).

Clients with hepatitis B experience anorexia, vague abdominal discomfort, nausea, vomiting, fatigue, and jaundice. Fever may be mild or absent. Symptoms may progress to chronic liver disease, hepatic cancer, hepatic failure, and death.

Medical–Surgical Management

Medical

There is no specific therapy. Treatment is based on relieving symptoms.

Health Promotion

Hepatitis B is the only STD for which a vaccine is available. It is recommended that all newborn infants, 11- to 12-year-old children, and high-risk groups of all ages receive the vaccine (CDC, July 1999a).

▸ NURSING PROCESS

The following is a general nursing process for the client with an STD.

▸ Assessment

▸ Subjective Data

Data to be gathered from a client who presents with a suspected STD are very similar, regardless of the actual STD. Either the nurse or physician must take a thorough history. A relaxed, nonjudgmental attitude will help to elicit accurate information from the client, since pertinent questioning will deal with very private areas of the client's life. Confidentiality and privacy are extremely important when dealing with both the history and physical examination for STDs. Pertinent information must be gathered regarding the client's sexual orientation (homosexual, heterosexual, bisexual), any prior treatment for an STD, and the number of sexual partners that the client has had in the last 6 months.

Women will be asked about symptoms such as vulval or vaginal itching, vaginal discharge, pain or discomfort, skin rashes or pruritus, and any changes in the menstrual periods or other abnormal bleeding. Men will be questioned regarding the presence of symptoms such as pain or burning on urination, abnormal penile discharges, skin rashes or itching, or lesions on external genitalia. Both men and women will be questioned regarding urinary frequency or discomfort and systemic symptoms such as fatigue, malaise, or sore throat. Homosexual men need to be questioned regarding rectal symptoms such as abnormal discharge, itching, lesions, or pain on defecation.

▸ Objective Data

The systems that need to be carefully evaluated include the reproductive, gastrointestinal, and integumentary systems. The presence or absence of skin rashes or lesions and abnormal discharges must be determined. Females need a speculum examination of the vagina and cervix to closely observe internal organs for changes consistent with STDs. The rectal area is examined to look for any abnormal discharge, lesions, or tenderness. Inguinal lymph nodes should be palpated to look for signs of infection.

Nursing diagnoses for the client with an STD may include the following:

Nursing Diagnoses	Planning/Goals	Nursing Interventions
▸ Anxiety related to unknown procedures, embarrassment, or other factors (relates to nearly every client who presents with an STD)	The client will admit lack of knowledge and embarrassment.	Provide a relaxed, nonjudgmental attitude which will aid in reducing client anxiety. The nurse must examine own attitudes toward STDs and the clients who suffer from them. Listen actively to both the spoken and unspoken concerns of the client.
▸ Knowledge Deficit related to mode of transmission of the STD, prevention methods, and risk for spread of the STD	The client will accurately discuss the mode of transmission of an STD and list appropriate measures to avoid reinfection or future infection.	Teach mode of transmission, prevention of further infection, and risk for spread. Take time to make sure the client has a thorough understanding of all necessary aspects of the disease.
▸ Infection, Risk for, related to incomplete treatment or lack of precautions with untreated, infected partners	The client will state the need for having all sexual partners notified and treated. The client will state understanding of the treatment regimen and of the importance of completing treatment. The client will explain appropriate use of latex condoms, including how and when to apply and remove the device.	Discuss the need for all sexual partners to be notified and treated. Discuss the importance of completing treatment regimen. Teach the importance of abstaining from sexual intercourse until the infection is resolved, or of using appropriate measures, such as latex condoms, to prevent reinfection.

Evaluation Each goal must be evaluated to determine how it has been met by the client.

SAMPLE NURSING CARE PLAN

THE CLIENT WITH GENITAL HERPES

Julie Blackwell is a single woman in her middle twenties who has been coming to the clinic for annual Pap smears and birth control for several years. She is a well-nourished, healthy-appearing young woman of medium height. She rescheduled her annual Pap smear to come into the clinic early because she noticed a cluster of small blisters on the inside of her left thigh that also involves the labia majora. She also reports that she has just gotten the flu as evidenced by headache, fever, and general achiness.

Ms. Blackwell has used birth control pills in the past, and reports satisfaction with this method of birth control. She reports that she and her new boyfriend became intimate about 2 weeks ago, so she wants to renew her birth control pill prescription. She also states that intercourse has been uncomfortable since the appearance of the lesions and that she does not feel comfortable with sexual activity while the lesions are present, since they make her feel "ugly."

The assessment determines the presence of a cluster of small blisters as well as swollen, tender inguinal lymph nodes. A Tzanck smear test is obtained.

Nursing Diagnosis 1 *Sexuality Patterns, Altered, related to lesions as evidenced by her comment that intercourse has been uncomfortable since the appearance of the lesions.*

PLANNING/GOALS	NURSING INTERVENTIONS	RATIONALE	EVALUATION
Ms. Blackwell will express her feelings about potential changes in her sexual behavior before leaving the clinic.	Provide a nonjudgmental atmosphere to encourage Ms. Blackwell to express her feelings about this perceived change in her sexual identity.	This demonstrates the caregiver's positive feelings toward Ms. Blackwell, and any concerns she may have regarding her future sexuality.	Ms. Blackwell states that she is still in shock, but thinks that she will be able to deal with her diagnosis. She also states that she will call back to the clinic in a few days with more questions after she has assimilated some of the information.
	Provide privacy and an uninterrupted amount of time to talk with Ms. Blackwell.	This demonstrates respect for Ms. Blackwell, and conveys reassurance that the caregiver will be comfortable discussing sexuality issues and concerns with her.	
	Provide accurate information to Ms. Blackwell about genital herpes, and include literature or videos that she can share with her boyfriend later.	This helps Ms. Blackwell focus on specific, necessary information and encourages her to ask questions.	
	Offer the names of local support groups such as HELP (Herpetics Engaged in Living Productively) or other support persons who will be able to provide information and group support to Ms. Blackwell.	This provides Ms. Blackwell with resources for support once she has returned home and the reality of her diagnosis has set in.	

continued

Nursing Diagnosis 2 *Anxiety related to threatened sexual identity as evidenced by her comment that she is not comfortable with sexual activity while the lesions are present since they make her feel "ugly."*

PLANNING/GOALS	NURSING INTERVENTIONS	RATIONALE	EVALUATION
Ms. Blackwell will be able to express feelings of anxiety and identify support systems to help her cope with these feelings before leaving the clinic.	Explain any procedures clearly and concisely before performing them. Listen attentively to any concerns or expressions of anxiety that Ms. Blackwell may offer. Include Ms. Blackwell in as many decisions related to her care and follow-up as is possible.	This will help alleviate anxiety. This will identify any anxious behaviors that she may be exhibiting and the source of her anxiety. Involving Ms. Blackwell in decision making regarding her care may reduce her feelings of anxiety and make her feel like she has regained some control.	Ms. Blackwell expresses feelings of anxiety about the diagnosis of herpes. She states that she has a cousin with herpes whom she will use as a resource person. She states that she has a secure relationship with her boyfriend and will talk to him about herpes also. She states that she will continue to call the clinic for any further support or information that she may need.

Nursing Diagnosis 3 *Infection, Risk for, related to break in skin integrity as evidenced by the presence of blisters.*

PLANNING/GOALS	NURSING INTERVENTIONS	RATIONALE	EVALUATION
Ms. Blackwell's herpes blisters will heal without secondary infection within 10 days.	Wear gloves when examining perineal area and when handling exudate from herpes lesions. Teach Ms. Blackwell how to wash hands very thoroughly after using the toilet or handling the area around the herpes lesions. Instruct Ms. Blackwell in the importance of keeping the herpes lesions clean and dry until they heal.	Gloves prevent secondary infection in herpes blisters from caregiver's hands and offer protection to the caregiver when dealing with wound exudate as part of a standard precautions policy. Handwashing prevents the spread of herpes infection in the genital area to other areas of Ms. Blackwell's body or to another person. Keeping the herpes lesions clean and dry until they heal will help prevent the occurrence of a secondary infection that may delay healing for up to 6 weeks.	Ms. Blackwell has been taught to keep blisters clean and dry and states that she will contact the clinic if the lesions develop any signs of a secondary infection. She makes an appointment to return to the clinic in 10 days for a follow-up evaluation.

continued

Instruct Ms. Blackwell to wear cotton underwear and loose-fitting clothing during occasions of herpes outbreaks.	These measures will provide for air circulation to promote healing and reduce further local irritation.

CASE STUDY

Noelle Landers, a 17-year-old student, has come to your clinic seeking treatment. Noelle is complaining of pain and burning on urination, as well as pain during intercourse. She states that she is infrequently sexually active with her 17-year-old boyfriend, and is also seeking a form of birth control. She has not used any form of birth control in the past and neither has her boyfriend. She also complains of a yellowish vaginal discharge, and has been wearing a panty liner to deal with this. Upon examination, Noelle complains of some abdominal tenderness, but denies that she has had any tenderness prior to this time. Noelle is screened for chlamydia and gonorrhea. She denies having had sex with any other partners, but does admit that she and her boyfriend had a fight and broke up temporarily about a month ago. They went back together about a week later. She does not know if he had any other sexual contacts during their period of separation. Noelle is concerned that she has contracted an STD, and states, "I'll die of embarrassment!"

The following questions will guide your development of a nursing care plan for the case study.

1. What other information should be elicited from Noelle?
2. What other sexually transmitted diseases will Noelle most likely be tested for in addition to chlamydia and gonorrhea?
3. Write 3 nursing diagnoses and goals for Noelle.
4. List the medications that Noelle will be most likely to receive to treat a chlamydial infection.
5. List some complications that Noelle may experience if she does not receive treatment for an active chlamydial or gonorrheal infection.
6. What information will you include when you counsel Noelle regarding sexual activity and forms of birth control? (See Chapter 35, Nursing Care of the Client: Reproductive System, for additional information.)

SUMMARY

- Sexually transmitted diseases are among the most common infections occurring in the United States today.
- Despite massive education efforts, the number of new STD cases identified each year continues to grow.
- Early, intensive education regarding STDs is being utilized to help combat the high incidence of STDs,

virtually an epidemic among young, urban-dwelling populations.
- Many STDs, such as gonorrhea, syphilis, and chlamydia, are treatable with antibiotics, but many others are caused by viruses and are not curable.
- Identification of groups at risk for STDs and appropriate prevention teaching are the most effective weapons in the ongoing battle against STDs.

Review Questions

1. The two most effective medications commonly used to treat chlamydia are:

   a. doxycycline and azithromycin.
   b. penicillin and podophyllum.
   c. erythromycin and acyclovir.
   d. doxycycline and penicillin.

2. If a female client with chlamydia fails to complete treatment, complications that may arise in the future include:

   a. fever and headache.
   b. nausea, vomiting, and diarrhea.
   c. infertility and ectopic pregnancy.
   d. urinary retention.

3. When instructing a client with gonorrhea regarding medication, the nurse will be sure to tell the client:

   a. to take the medication until it is gone.
   b. to take the medication until symptoms subside.
   c. to take the medication at bedtime.
   d. to avoid sunlight while taking the medication.

4. When obtaining a health history from a client, the nurse asks the client to report on the presence of which of the following common symptoms of syphilis?

   a. Nausea and vomiting
   b. Fever, cellulitis, and diarrhea
   c. Dysuria and mucopurulent discharge
   d. Painless sore or ulcer in the genital area

Critical Thinking Questions

1. Develop a teaching plan for a client with multiple sexual partners. Consider the sensitivity of the information to be shared and the client's receptivity.

2. What is the rationale for each nursing intervention given for the nursing diagnoses in this chapter?

 WEB FLASH!

- Search the Internet for information about sexually transmitted diseases. What type of information is available? For whom is it intended?
- What information do you find about syphilis and gonorrhea specifically? How can a client become part of a clinical trial?

NURSING CARE OF THE CLIENT: ENDOCRINE SYSTEM

MAKING THE CONNECTION

Refer to the following chapters to increase your understanding of endocrine disorders:

- **Chapter 15, Wellness Concepts**
- **Chapter 23, Fluid, Electrolyte, and Acid-Base Balance**
- **Chapter 25, Assessment**
- **Chapter 30, Nursing Care of the Oncology Client**
- **Chapter 32, Nursing Care of the Client: Cardiovascular System**
- **Chapter 33, Nursing Care of the Client: Blood and Lymph Systems**
- **Chapter 35, Nursing Care of the Client: Reproductive System**
- **Chapter 38, Nursing Care of the Client: Musculoskeletal System**

- **Chapter 39, Nursing Care of the Client: Immune System**
- **Chapter 40, Nursing Care of the Client: Integumentary System**
- **Chapter 41, Nursing Care of the Client: Nervous System**
- **Chapter 42, Nursing Care of the Client: Urinary System**
- **Chapter 43, Nursing Care of the Client: Sensory System**
- **Chapter 55, Nursing Care of the Older Client**
- **Procedures:** B29, Measuring Intake and Output; I11, Withdrawing Medication from a Vial; I13, Administering a Subcutaneous Injection; I26, Skin Puncture

LEARNING OBJECTIVES

Upon completion of this chapter, you should be able to:
- *Define key terms.*
- *Identify and locate the endocrine glands and list function(s) and hormone(s) secreted by each.*
- *Differentiate between type 1 and type 2 diabetes in terms of pathophysiology, presenting symptoms and treatment.*
- *Discuss the roles of diet and exercise in the management of diabetes mellitus.*
- *Identify signs, causes, and treatment of complications of hypoglycemia, diabetic ketoacidosis, and hyperosmolar hyperglycemic nonketotic syndrome.*
- *Discuss the major long-term complications of diabetes.*
- *Discuss rationale for the pituitary gland being traditionally called the "master" gland.*
- *Compare symptoms of the disease process resulting from a hyper- or hyposecretion of an endocrine gland.*
- *Discuss assessment techniques for a client suspected of having an endocrine disorder.*
- *Formulate a nursing care plan for the client with an endocrine disorder.*

KEY TERMS

agranulocytosis	hypovolemia
autosomal	iatrogenic
Chvostek's sign	insulin
cretinism	ketone
dawn phenomenon	ketonuria
endocrine	lipodystrophy
exophthalmos	myxedema
glucagon	paroxysmal
glycosuria	polydipsia
goiter	polyphagia
gynecomastia	polyuria
hirsutism	Somogyi phenom-
hormone	enon
hyperglycemia	tetany
hypoglycemia	Trousseau's sign

INTRODUCTION

The endocrine system is unique in that the components are not in direct physical contact but scattered throughout the body. The endocrine system provides the same general functions as the nervous system: communication and control; however, the endocrine system is generally slower and has longer lasting control over the various body activities and functions. It exerts this control through the secretion of hormones that circulate through the blood. A malfunction of any part of the endocrine system can result in a shift of homeostasis with far-reaching systemic reactions.

Assessment of the endocrine system is difficult. Not only are the components not in direct contact, but only the thyroid gland is close enough to the body surface for direct physical assessment. Still the nurse needs to be familiar with the normal functioning of the endocrine system. In assessing the client for endocrine dysfunction, the nurse must take note of negative findings as well as positive ones. Assessment includes results of diagnostic tests as well as any precipitating or aggravating factors.

ANATOMY AND PHYSIOLOGY REVIEW

The endocrine system is composed of a group of various glands scattered throughout the body. The term **endocrine** (endo-within, crin-secrete) indicates that the secretions formed by these glands directly enter the blood or lymph circulation, rather than being transported via tubes or ducts. These secretions, called **hormones**, are chemical substances that initiate or regulate activity of another organ, system, or gland in another part of the body. The level of hormone in the blood is regulated by the homeostasis mechanism called negative feedback. If the blood level for a specific hormone falls below normal, negative feedback causes the specific endocrine gland to produce more of the hormone, which when increased to the normal level causes a decrease in production.

The glands discussed in this chapter that comprise the endocrine system are: the pancreas, pituitary, hypothalamus, thyroid, parathyroid, and adrenals (Figure 37-1). Several endocrine glands such as the pineal, thymus, ovaries, and testes are of great importance; however, they will be discussed in other chapters in connection with the organ system in which they function.

The pancreas lies horizontally behind the stomach at the level of the first and second lumbar vertebrae. The head of the pancreas is attached to the duodenum with the tail reaching to the spleen. It has both exocrine and endocrine functions.

The pituitary gland consists of an anterior and a posterior lobe. It has traditionally been called the "master" gland because so many of its secretions influence other endocrine glands and body systems. It is

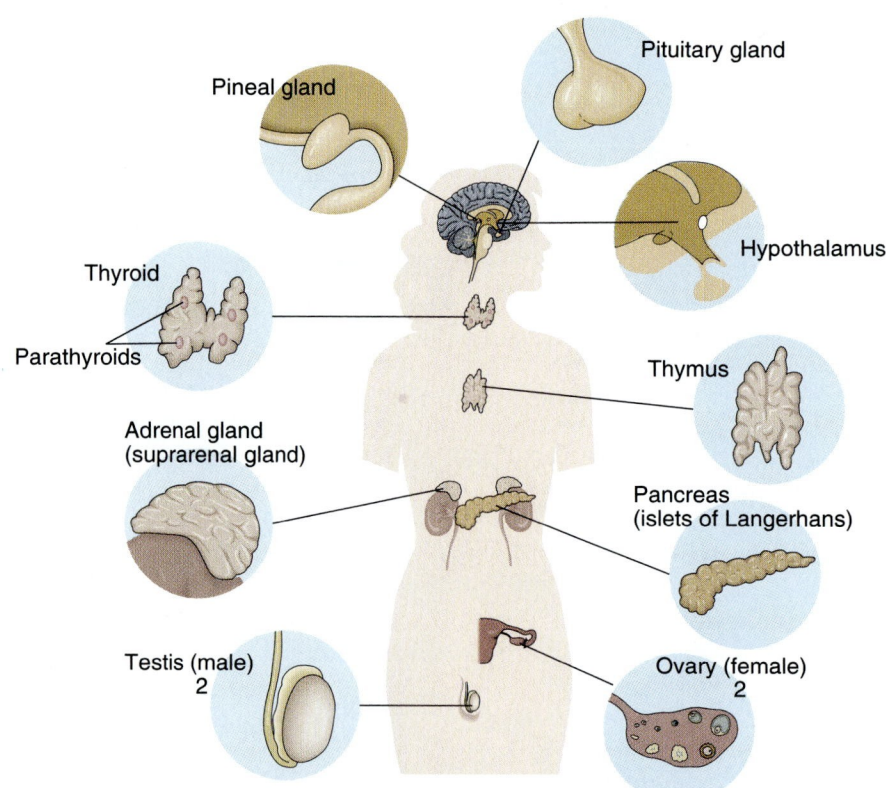

Figure 37-1 Structures of the Endocrine System

attached to the hypothalamus by a stalk called the *infundibulum*. The hypothalamus is located in the lower portion of the brain and produces secretions influencing the production and release of the anterior pituitary hormones as well as the production of the posterior pituitary hormones. Both the pituitary and hypothalamus are located in the head. The pituitary, about the size of a pea, is located in the sella turcica, a small depression in the sphenoid bone. The anterior pituitary, or adenohypophysis, produces and secretes the following 7 hormones:

- Thyroid-stimulating hormone (TSH)
- Adrenocorticotropic hormone (ACTH)
- Follicle-stimulating hormone (FSH)
- Luteinizing hormone (LH)
- Melanocyte-stimulating hormone (MSH)
- Growth hormone (GH)
- Prolactin or lactogenic hormone

The posterior pituitary, or neurohypophysis, releases two hormones—antidiuretic hormone (ADH) and oxytocin. The pituitary hormones have a variety of functions. Refer to Table 37-1 for specific endocrine hormones and functions.

The thyroid gland is butterfly-shaped and lies in the neck. It consists of two lobes—one on each side of the trachea connected by an isthmus. The gland sits saddlelike starting on the anterior surface of the trachea just below the larynx and surrounds it partway. The thyroid gland stores iodine. The thyroid gland produces thyroid hormones including thyroxine, which is the most abundant, and triiodothyronine. It regulates the metabolic rate for carbohydrates, protein, and fats.

Table 37-1 ENDOCRINE GLAND HORMONES

HORMONE	FUNCTION
Pancreas	
Glucagon	Raises blood glucose
Insulin	Lowers blood glucose
Somatostatin	Inhibits secretion of insulin, glucagon, and growth hormone from the anterior pituitary and gastrin from the stomach
Anterior Pituitary	
Thyroid-stimulating hormone (TSH)	Stimulates thyroid growth and secretion of the thyroid hormone
Adrenocorticotropic hormone (ACTH)	Stimulates adrenal cortex growth and secretion of glucocorticoids
Follicle-stimulating hormone (FSH)	Stimulates ovarian follicle to mature and produce estrogen; in the male, stimulates sperm production
Luteinizing hormone (LH)	Acts with FSH to stimulate estrogen production; causes ovulation; stimulates progesterone production by corpus luteum; in male, stimulates testes to produce testosterone
Melanocyte-stimulating hormone (MSH)	Causes increase in synthesis and spread of melanin (pigment) in skin
Growth hormone (GH)	Stimulates growth
Prolacting or lactogenic hormone	Stimulates breast development during pregnancy and milk secretion after delivery of baby
Posterior Pituitary	
Antidiuretic hormone (ADH)	Stimulates water retention by kidneys to decrease urine secretion
Oxytocin	Stimulates uterine contractions; causes breast to release milk into ducts
Thyroid Gland	
Thyroid hormone (thyroxine T_4 and triiodothyronine T_3)	Increases metabolic rate
Calcitonin	Decreases blood calcium concentration
Parathyroid Gland	
Parathyroid hormone	Increases blood calcium concentration
Adrenal Cortex	
Glucocorticoids (cortisol, hydrocortisone)	Stimulates gluconeogenesis and increases blood glucose; antiinflammatory; antiimmunity; antiallergy
Mineralocorticoids	Regulates electrolyte and fluid homeostasis
Sex hormones (androgen)	Stimulate sexual drive in females; in males, negligible effect
Adrenal Medulla	
Epinephrine (adrenalin)	Prolongs and intensifies sympathetic nervous response to stress
Norepinephine	Prolongs and intensifies sympathetic nervous response to stress

There are 4 parathyroid glands, although some individuals may have as many as 6. Two glands are embedded in the posterior portion of each thyroid lobe. They produce parathyroid hormone, parathormone, which regulates the concentration of blood calcium and phosphorus.

The adrenal, or suprarenal, glands are located on top of each kidney. The adrenal cortex secretes mineralocorticoids including aldosterone, glucocorticoids including cortisol, and androgens which are sex hormones. The adrenal medulla secretes epinephrine or adrenalin and norepinephrine or noradrenalin which help the body to function under stress.

It is important to understand the normal function of the endocrine glands and hormones. Most endocrine disorders are a result of either overactivity or underactivity of these glands.

COMMON DIAGNOSTIC TESTS

Commonly used diagnostic tests for clients with symptoms of endocrine system disorders are listed in Table 37-2. See Chapter 27, Diagnostic Tests, for explanation/normal values and nursing responsibilities.

DIABETES MELLITUS

Diabetes mellitus is a disorder of metabolism. When we eat, most of the food we eat is broken down by digestive juices into chemicals, including a simple sugar called *glucose*. Of the food we eat, 100% of carbohydrate and approximately 58% of protein and 10% of fat is broken down to glucose. For the glucose to get into the cells, insulin must be present (Figure 37-2).

Insulin is a hormone produced and secreted by the beta cells in the islets of Langerhans of the pancreas. Insulin stimulates the active transport of glucose into muscle and adipose tissue cells, making it available for cell use. For glucose to cross the cell membrane, insulin must connect with a receptor on the cell membrane. Some clients with diabetes mellitus have enough insulin, but too few functioning receptor sites. Others have inadequate or no insulin production. Blood glu-

---

Table 37-2 COMMON DIAGNOSTIC TESTS FOR ENDOCRINE SYSTEM DISORDERS

Pancreas Diagnostic Tests

Blood glucose, Fasting blood sugar (FBS)

2-hour postprandial glucose (2hPPG) or 2-hour postprandial blood sugar (2hPPBS)

Glucose tolerance test (GTT)

Pituitary Gland Diagnostic Tests

Adrenocorticotropic hormone (ACTH), Corticotropin

Antidiuretic hormone (ADH), Vasopressin

Follicle-stimulating hormone (FSH)

Growth hormone (GH), Human GH (HGH), Somatotropin hormone (SH)

Growth hormone (GH) stimulation test, GH provocation test, Insulin tolerance test (ITT), Arginine test

Luteinizing hormone (LH) assay

Prolactin levels (PRL)

Thyrotropin-releasing hormone (TRH) test, Thyrotropin-releasing factor (TRF) test

Urine specific gravity

Long bone x-rays

Sella turcica x-ray

Computed tomography of head (CT scan of head), Computerized axial transverse tomography (CATT)

Thyroid Gland Diagnostic Tests

Antithyroid microsomal antibody, Antimicrosomal antibody, Microsomal antibody, Thyroid autoantibody, Thyroid antimicrosomal antibody

Calcitonin, HCT, Thyrocalcitonin

Serum free triiodothyronine (T_3)

Thyroid-stimulating hormone (TSH), Thyrotropin

Thyroid-stimulating hormone (TSH) stimulation test

Thyroxine index free, FTI, FT_4 Index

Thyroxine, T_4, Thyroxine screen

Triiodothyronine, T_3 radioimmunoassay, T_3 by RIA

Radioactive iodine uptake, (RAIU), Iodine uptake test, ^{131}I uptake

Thyroid scan, Thyroid scintiscan

Thyroid ultrasound, Thyroid echogram, Thyroid sonogram

Thyroid biopsy

Parathyroid Gland Diagnostic Tests

Parathyroid hormone (PTH), Parathormone

Calcium, total/ionized Ca^{++}

Phosphorus

Adrenal Glands Diagnostic Tests

Adrenocorticotropic hormone (ACTH) stimulation test, Cortisol stimulation test, Cosyntropin test

Cortisol, Hydrocortisone

Dexamethasone suppression test (DST), Prolonged/rapid DST, Cortisol suppression test, ACTH suppression test

Plasma renin assay, Plasma renin activity (PRA)

Progesterone assay

Aldosterone assay

17-Hydroxycorticosteroids (17-OHCS)

17-Ketosteroids (17-KS)

Urine cortisol, Hydrocortisone

Vanillylmandelic acid (VMA) & catecholamines, VMA & epinephrine, Norepinephrine, Metanephrine, Normetanephrine, Dopamine

Adrenal angiography, Adrenal arteriogram

Adrenal venography

Computed tomography of adrenals (CAT scan of adrenals), CT scan of adrenals

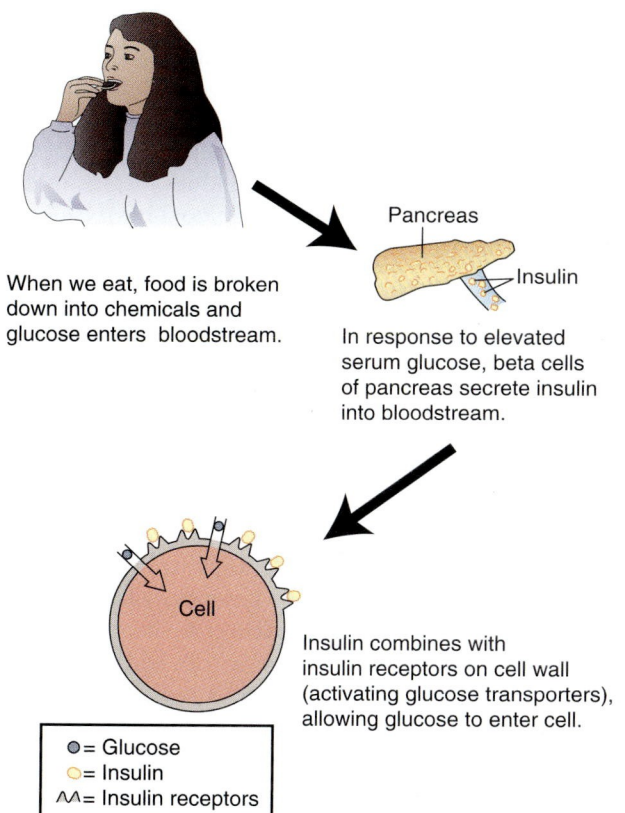

When we eat, food is broken down into chemicals and glucose enters bloodstream.

Pancreas

Insulin

In response to elevated serum glucose, beta cells of pancreas secrete insulin into bloodstream.

Cell

Insulin combines with insulin receptors on cell wall (activating glucose transporters), allowing glucose to enter cell.

○ = Glucose
○ = Insulin
ᴧᴧ = Insulin receptors

Figure 37-2 How Insulin Works

cose can always be used by the brain and kidneys. Insulin is not needed for glucose to enter brain cells or cells of the glomeruli.

The amount of glucose in the blood regulates the rate of insulin secretion. When a meal is eaten, the blood glucose elevates and the beta cells of the islets of Langerhans release insulin. As the blood glucose level drops, insulin secretion diminishes. It is important to note that during times of fasting (overnight or between meals) a low level of insulin continues to be secreted along with **glucagon**. Glucagon secreted by the alpha cells of the pancreas stimulates release of glucose by the liver. The balance and interactions of insulin and glucagon serve to maintain a constant serum glucose level.

Other functions of insulin include:

- Promoting conversion of glucose to glycogen for storage in the liver and inhibiting conversion of glycogen to glucose
- Promoting the conversion of fatty acids into fat that can be stored as adipose tissue and preventing breakdown of adipose tissue and conversion of fat to ketone bodies
- Stimulating protein synthesis within tissues and inhibiting the breakdown of protein into amino acids

In summary, insulin actively promotes those processes that lower the blood glucose level and inhibits

those processes that raise the blood glucose level. A deficiency of insulin results in **hyperglycemia**, or elevated blood glucose. Excess insulin results in **hypoglycemia** (low blood glucose). Diabetes mellitus is actually a group of disorders characterized by chronic hyperglycemia.

DIAGNOSIS AND CLASSIFICATION

The Expert Committee on the Diagnosis and Classification of Diabetes Mellitus (1997) presented to the American Diabetes Association (ADA) new criteria for diagnosis and new classifications for diabetes which the ADA approved.

Diagnosis

The Committee identified two precursors to diabetes, new screening criteria, and new diagnostic criteria, and it eliminated one diagnostic test.

The two precursors identified are:

1. Impaired glucose tolerance (IGT)—a glucose level of 140 to 199 mg/dL 2 hours after a glucose load
2. Impaired fasting glucose (IFG)—a fasting glucose of 110 to 125 mg/dL

The new criteria for who should be screened for diabetes include:

PROFESSIONAL TIP

Diabetes

According to the Centers for Disease Control and Prevention (CDC) (1998), there are 10.3 million Americans diagnosed as having diabetes mellitus. This is an increase from 8 million in 1995. Another 5 million are estimated to be undiagnosed. Diabetes was the seventh leading cause of death in the United States and is associated with many serious complications (CDC, 1999). Diabetes is the leading cause of new blindness among adults, the leading cause of new cases of renal failure, and is present in more than half of persons experiencing non-traumatic lower extremity amputations. Diabetes and its complications shorten a person's life span, create disability, and impose an economic burden on persons who have the disease (CDC, 1999).

Diabetes is seen in all age groups and races. One-third of clients with diabetes are over age 60. African American, Hispanic, and some Native American populations have a higher incidence of diabetes than the white population.

1. Anyone age 45 and older
2. Anyone, regardless of age, with one of the following risk factors:
   - Obesity (body mass index of 27 or greater)
   - Immediate family member with diabetes
   - Member of high-risk ethnic group (African American, Hispanic American, some Native American groups)
   - Having a baby weighing more than 9 pounds
   - History of gestational diabetes mellitus (GDM)
   - Hypertension
   - High-density lipoprotein level of 35 mg/dL or less, or a triglyceride level of 250 mg/dL or more
   - Have either of the two precursors of diabetes

The new diagnostic criteria identify when a physician can make a diagnosis of diabetes. The situations are:

- A random blood glucose of 200 mg/dL or greater with the classic symptoms of polyuria, polydipsia, and unexplained weight loss
  or
- A fasting blood sugar of 126 mg/dL or greater
  or
- The 2-hour sample of the oral glucose tolerance test is 200 mg/dL or greater using a load of 75 grams of anhydrous glucose

The committee also recommended not using glycosylated hemoglobin to diagnose diabetes. Terminology is confusing, and there are many methods of measuring glycosylated hemoglobin.

Classification

The new system uses etiology, not insulin use, to classify diabetes into four categories: type 1 diabetes, type 2 diabetes, other specific types, and gestational diabetes mellitus.

Type 1 Diabetes

There are two forms of diabetes resulting from pancreatic beta-cell destruction or a primary defect in beta-cell function resulting in no release of insulin and ineffective glucose transport. There is usually an absolute insulin deficiency so the clients are insulin-dependent. The two subdivisions of type 1 diabetes are:

- Immune-mediated—islet cell or insulin antibodies destroy beta cells. The rate of this destruction is usually higher in children than in adults. Children and adolescents may rapidly develop ketoacidosis. Adults seldom develop ketoacidosis unless they have an infection or other stressor. This is what used to be called type I, insulin-dependent diabetes mellitus (IDDM), or juvenile-onset diabetes.
- Idiopathic—no evidence of autoimmunity; the individual just does not produce insulin and is prone to ketoacidosis.

In the absence of insulin, glucose from food eaten cannot be used or stored and remains in the bloodstream, resulting in hyperglycemia. In addition, glucose production from the liver goes unchecked, further elevating the blood glucose level.

As the blood glucose rises, the kidney begins to excrete excess glucose in the urine (**glycosuria**). Glucose eliminated in the urine pulls excessive amounts of water with it (osmotic diuresis), resulting in fluid volume deficit and producing symptoms of excessive thirst (**polydipsia**) and increased urination (**polyuria**).

Insulin deficiency also results in impaired metabolism of fats and proteins. Because of the impaired glucose, fat, and protein metabolism and the inability to store glucose, clients frequently experience protein wasting, weight loss, and increased hunger (**polyphagia**).

Metabolism of fat stores for energy leads to production of acid by-products called ketones, which can be detected in the urine (**ketonuria**). As ketones accumulate, the associated decrease in pH leads to metabolic acidosis, or more specifically a condition known as *diabetic ketoacidosis,* discussed later in this chapter.

Type 2 Diabetes

These clients have insulin resistance with relative insulin deficiency. Most of these clients are obese. When weight is lost, insulin resistance diminishes but reappears if the client regains weight. Age, lack of exercise, history of GDM, hypertension, dyslipidemia, and being of African American, Hispanic American, or Native American origin are all risk factors. A strong family history of diabetes is often evident. Many clients do not require insulin, but eventually one-third will need insulin to maintain a normal glucose level. This is what used to be called type II, noninsulin-dependent diabetes mellitus (NIDDM), or adult-onset diabetes.

Hyperglycemia results when the pancreas cannot match the body's need for insulin and/or when the number of insulin receptor sites are decreased or altered. Although available insulin may be insufficient to meet the body's metabolic needs and prevent hyperglycemia, there is a sufficient amount of insulin to prevent fat breakdown for energy and the resulting ketoacidosis. Extremely elevated glucose in the type 2 diabetic will result in development of hyperosmolar hyperglycemic nonketotic syndrome (HHNK), discussed later in this chapter. Table 37-3 compares the clinical manifestations of type 1 and type 2 diabetes.

Other Specific Types

This includes conditions such as beta-cell genetic defects, endocrinopathies, and drug- or chemical-induced diabetes. These are in a separate category because there are different disease etiologies.

Table 37-3 COMPARISON OF THE CLINICAL MANIFESTATIONS OF TYPE 1 DIABETES AND TYPE 2 DIABETES

	TYPE 1 DIABETES (Type I, IDDM, Juvenile, Brittle/labile)	TYPE 2 DIABETES (Type II, NIDDM, Adult Onset)
Etiology	Autoimmune	Genetic susceptibility associated. Usually associated with long duration obesity.
Age of onset	Rare before age 1	Incidence increases with age
Percent of diabetics	5–10%	85–90%
Onset	Abrupt, rapid	Gradual, over years
Body weight at onset	Normal or thin	80% are overweight
Insulin production	None	Less than normal, normal, or greater than normal
Insulin injection	Always	Necessary for approximately 30%
Ketosis	Occurs mainly in children and adolescents	Unlikely
Management	Insulin, diet, exercise	Diet and weight loss, exercise, possibly oral hypoglycemics or insulin

Gestational Diabetes Mellitus

Occurring during pregnancy, this may be controlled either with or without insulin. Generally the client's glucose tolerance returns to normal after the infant's birth. The client should be rechecked 6 weeks after the birth to see if the diabetes persists.

Contributing Factors

Persons with a family history of diabetes are at greater risk for developing diabetes. In addition to family history, factors associated with diabetes include obesity, aging, and ethnic group. The most powerful risk factor for type 2 diabetes is obesity. For persons with a family history of type 2 diabetes, maintenance of an ideal body weight may delay or prevent the onset of diabetes.

Aging can also be considered a contributing factor.

It is known that members of certain racial groups are more likely to develop diabetes. In the United States, there is a greater chance of developing type 2 diabetes for Hispanics, certain Native American populations, and African Americans.

Other groups at risk for development of diabetes include those with a history of gestational diabetes or impaired glucose tolerance (IGT).

Medical–Surgical Management

Medical

There is no known cure for diabetes. The goal of therapeutic management is aimed at the control of blood sugar, and the prevention and early detection of the complications associated with diabetes. Diabetes is considered under control if the client maintains ideal body weight and enjoys good health, preprandial glucose levels are less than 140 mg/dL, postprandial glucose levels do not rise above 180 mg/dL.

Treatment plans vary and are individualized for each client. Control of blood glucose generally involves a balance of a dietary prescription, an exercise plan, and medications. Ultimately, the client is the manager of the treatment plan and, therefore, must be very well informed about diabetes and involved in all aspects of care planning and decision making.

Since the advent of home glucose monitoring devices, urine testing for glucose is rarely used for the estimation of serum glucose levels in the management of diabetes. Testing urine for ketone (product of fatty acid oxidation) production, however, continues to be recommended when the blood glucose level is consistently ≥ 240 mg/dL or when any symptoms of ketoacidosis are present.

The client with type 1 diabetes will always require administration of insulin to lower the glucose level and prevent complications of diabetes. Diet and exercise regimens are also important for the control of the glucose level and maintenance of health.

Dietary management is the cornerstone of treatment for the person with type 2 diabetes. As the obese person loses weight, the body's insulin requirements decrease, resulting in improved glucose tolerance. Exercise can also play a valuable role in losing weight and lowering the blood glucose level. Type 2 diabetes not controlled by diet and exercise may necessitate administration of medications. Oral hypoglycemic agents or parenteral administration of insulin may be required for optimal control.

HOME HEALTH CARE

Glucose Monitoring

The availability and use of home glucose monitoring equipment to evaluate serum (blood) glucose has revolutionized self-care for the diabetic client (Figure 37-3). Also called "finger stick blood glucose" (FSBG), self-monitoring of blood glucose (SMBG) can be done quickly using capillary blood that provides fairly accurate reading of the current blood glucose. Most often, the glucose level is checked before meals and at bedtime, thus allowing the client to adjust the treatment plan accordingly. Self-monitoring of blood glucose is recommended for all clients requiring insulin and for clients with widely fluctuating glucose levels. Symptoms of hypoglycemia at any time warrant immediate evaluation of the blood glucose level.

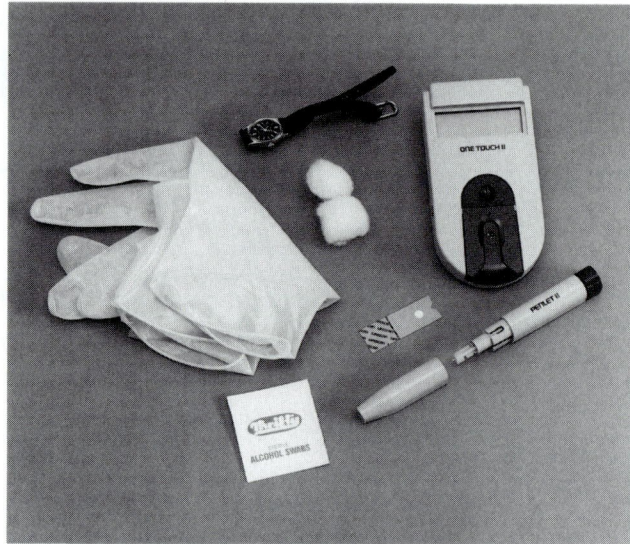

Figure 37-3 Diabetic Blood Testing Equipment: Glucose Meter, Cotton Balls, Lancet, Alcohol, Blood Testing Strip, and Watch

Surgical

Pancreas transplantations have been performed and have successfully eliminated the need for exogenous insulin in some clients. At present pancreas transplants are being performed primarily on clients with type 1 diabetes who also need kidney or other organ transplants. This is because the serious side effects of the antirejection medications do not justify a pancreas transplant alone. Pancreatic islet cell transplants are also being done experimentally with limited success, but hold much promise for the future.

Pharmacological

Various pharmacological treatments that are used in the management of type 1 and type 2 diabetes are discussed in the following text.

Insulin Persons with type 1 diabetes always require insulin administration. Persons with type 2 diabetes often do not require insulin when initially diagnosed, but insulin therapy may become necessary over time, as endogenous insulin production decreases, or during times of stress or illness.

Historically, insulin has been obtained from beef or pork pancreas. Today, biosynthetic human insulin is used almost exclusively, but there are some clients still using pork or beef insulin. Human insulin is purer, more effective, and has a much lower incidence of causing insulin allergies and resistance. Insulin is available in short-, intermediate-, and long-acting forms that can be injected separately or mixed in the same syringe. Premixed insulins are also available. See Table 37-4 for descriptions of types of insulins and their actions. Insulin is routinely administered subcutaneously. Regular insulin (short-acting) may be administered intravenously when immediate response is desired, as in

treatment of greatly elevated glucose levels occurring with diabetic ketoacidosis (DKA) or hyperosmolar hyperglycemic nonketotic syndrome (HHNK). Regular insulin, which is the only clear insulin, is the *only* insulin that can be given intravenously (IV).

The strength of insulin correlates to the number of units of insulin per cubic centimeter. The most common concentrations of insulin used today are U-50 and U-100 insulin (50 and 100 units of insulin per 1 cc respectively). U-500 insulin is also available for clients who have developed insulin resistance and require very high doses.

Insulin should always be measured in an insulin syringe which is marked in units. When mixing two types of insulin in the same syringe, it is important that the regular (clear, short-acting) insulin be drawn up first. The policy of many health care institutions requires that 2 nurses check insulin dosages prior to administration. Even if the facility does not have such a policy, checking the insulin dosage with another nurse will help protect against an adverse reaction due to error.

Insulin dosages are individually determined, usually requiring 2 or more injections per day and involving a combination of a short-acting and a longer-acting insulin. Various regimens of insulin administration can be used, each with its own advantages and disadvantages. In general, the more complex the regimen, the more normal the blood glucose level throughout the day. Clients can be taught to use the results of their self monitoring blood glucose to adjust their insulin doses, allowing more flexibility in their meals and schedules. Recent studies strongly support the theory that intensive insulin regimens that tightly control the blood glucose level delay the onset and progression of complications of diabetic retinopathy, nephropathy, and neuropathy.

Sliding Scale Insulin During times of surgery, illness, or stress, clients may have their glucose level managed with an insulin sliding scale in lieu of their regular regimen of insulin or oral hypoglycemics. A sliding scale determines insulin dosage based on fingerstick blood glucose level. Regular (short-acting) insulin is used and a dose is administered every 4 or 6 hours based on the blood glucose level. The sliding scale allows for much flexibility and ensures frequent monitoring of and response to changes in the client's glucose level. An example sliding scale might be:

- 4u Humulin R Insulin for glucose 151–200 mg/dL
- 6u Humulin R Insulin for glucose 201–250 mg/dL
- 8u Humulin R Insulin for glucose 251–300 mg/dL
- 10u Humulin R Insulin for glucose 301–350 mg/dL
- Call physician for glucose > 350 mg/dL

Insulin Injections Insulin injections are administered into the subcutaneous tissue. If an inch of skin can be pinched, the needle is injected at a 90-degree angle, otherwise, at a 45 degree angle. The 4 main areas for injection are the abdomen, arms, thighs, and hips (Figure 37-4). Factors affecting absorption should be considered when selecting an injection site. Absorption occurs most quickly in the abdomen, followed by the arms, thighs, and hips.

Rotation of sites for injection has traditionally been recommended to prevent **lipodystrophy** (atrophy or hypertrophy in the subcutaneous fat). More recently, some authorities are recommending that the abdomen, which provides the most predictable absorption of insulin, be used exclusively for insulin administration.

If sites other than the abdomen are used, site rotation needs to be done in a systematic manner to pre-

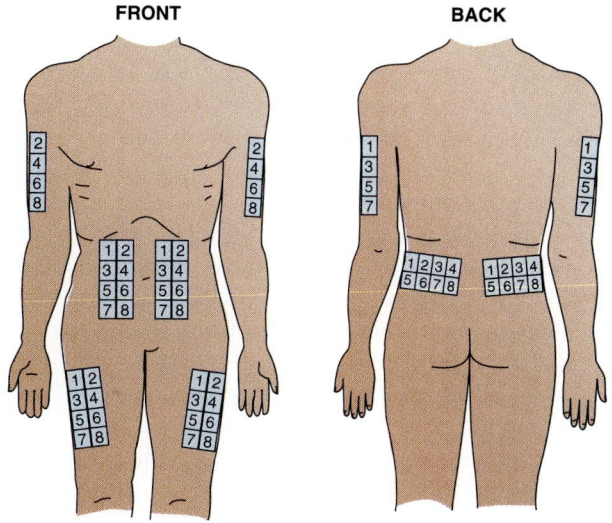

Figure 37-4 Possible Sites and Rotation for Insulin Administration

vent erratic absorption. One system of rotation is to always use the same area of injection the same time each day, e.g., always using the abdomen in the morning and the thigh in the afternoon. Another system of rotation is to use all available injection sites in one area before moving to another.

Areas of lipodystrophy should not be used for injection, as absorption may be diminished. Exercise will increase the rate of absorption, so diabetics planning to exercise should not inject insulin into the areas to be exercised.

Vials of insulin not being used should be refrigerated to prevent loss of potency. Vials in use may be kept at room temperature to decrease local irritation at the injection site, which can occur when cold insulin is

Table 37-4 TYPES OF INSULIN AND THEIR ACTIONS

TYPES OF INULSIN	APPEARANCE	ACTION IN HOURS		
		ONSET	**PEAK**	**DURATION**
Very short-acting insulin				
Lispro (Humalog)	clear	¼	1–1½	5 or less
Short-acting				
Humulin R	clear	½–1	2–4	6–8
Intermediate-acting				
Humulin U	cloudy	1–1½	4–12	up to 24
Humulin L	cloudy	1–2-½	7–15	22
Long-acting				
Humulin U	cloudy	4–8	10–30	36+
Premixed				
Reg/Humulin N				
Humulin 70/30	cloudy	½–1	4–8	24
Humulin 50/50				

used. When mixing a short-acting and a longer-acting insulin in the same syringe, the regular (clear) should always be drawn up into the syringe first, followed by the longer-acting (cloudy) insulin. Figure 37-5 illustrates mixing and administering insulin.

It is recommended that insulin syringes be used only once and then discarded.

The visually and/or neurologically impaired diabetic client may benefit from assistive devices available to facilitate drawing up the insulin and administering it. Clients dependent on others for drawing up their insulin may benefit from prefilled syringes, which are considered stable for up to 3 weeks when stored in the refrigerator.

The nurse should keep in mind that the most important factor in the administration of insulin is consistency in technique. Also, simplification of the procedure may have a major impact on a client's ability to comply and to maintain independence. It is important that the nurse understand the basic principles of insulin administration and thereby remain flexible when teaching new clients or assessing the skills of experienced clients.

HOME HEALTH CARE

Insulin Injections

Some clients are able to safely reuse insulin syringes to decrease expense. Discard the syringe when the needle becomes dull, has been bent, or has come into contact with any surface other than the skin. Recap the needle after each use if syringes are reused. Syringe reuse is not advisable for clients with poor hygiene, open wounds, or decreased resistance to infection. It is safe to inject insulin through clothing (Fleming, 1999).

Insulin Pumps A portable insulin infusion pump delivers insulin continuously through a subcutaneous needle, usually anchored in the abdomen (see Figure 37-6). A continuous, or basal rate, of regular (rapid-acting) insulin is programmed and delivered to closely imitate the body's natural insulin secretion. Additional boluses can be manually administered to coordinate with meal times. The injection site is changed every

---

The client may withdraw two different types of insulin into the same syringe. In this series of diagrams, a rapid-acting insulin (R vial) is combined with an intermediate-acting insulin (N vial).

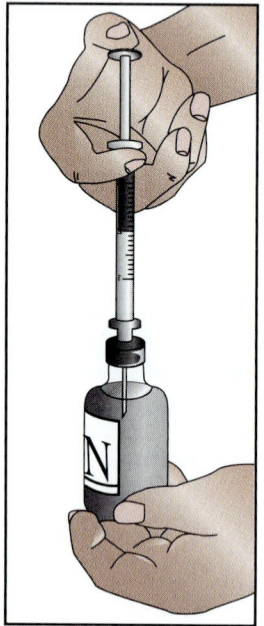

1 After cleaning the rubber stopper on both vials with an alcohol wipe, inject the amount of air equal to the dose of the intermediate-acting insulin into the N vial.

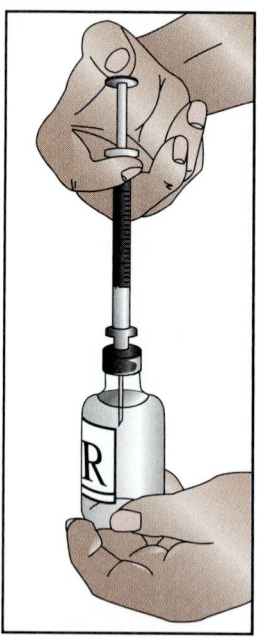

2 Inject the amount of air equal to the dose of the rapid-acting insulin into the R vial.

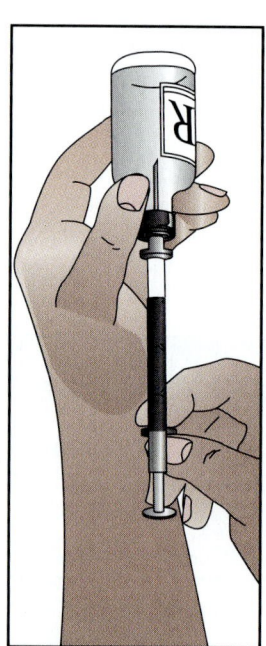

3 Withdraw the correct amount of rapid-acting insulin.

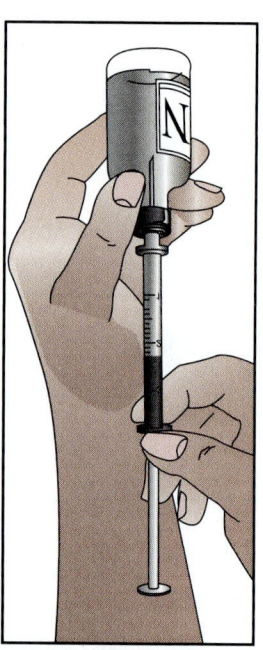

4 Withdraw the correct amount of intermediate-acting insulin. (Note: Pull the plunger down to the unit mark that equals the dose of rapid-acting insulin plus the dose of intermediate-acting insulin. The insulins will mix immediately in the syringe. If too large an amount of intermediate-acting insulin is withdrawn, the entire contents of the syringe must be discarded.)

Figure 37-5 How to Mix Insulin (*Adapted from* Clinical Pharmacology and Nursing, *3rd ed., by C. L. Baer & B. R. Williams, 1996,* Springhouse, PA: Springhouse Corporation.)

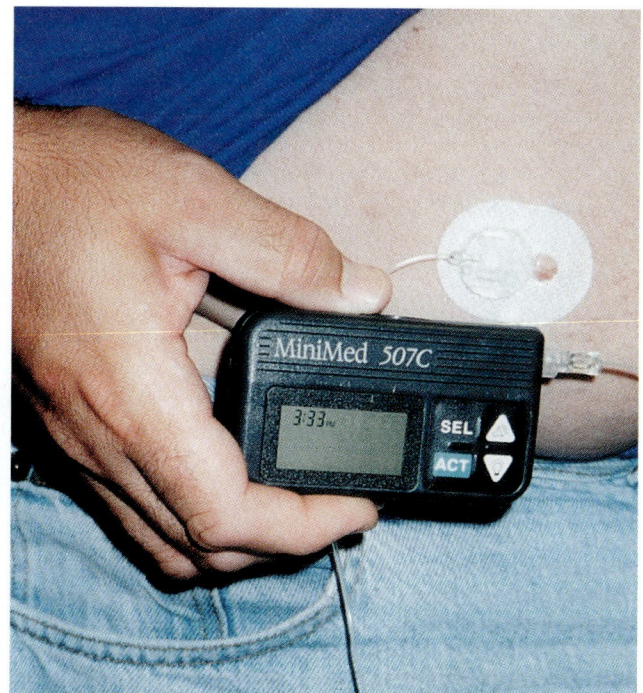

Figure 37-6 The Insulin Pump

24 to 48 hours. The use of the insulin pump prevents multiple injections and allows flexibility in meal size and time. Use of the pump requires a motivated and educated client, because intensive self-monitoring of blood glucose is essential.

Complications of Insulin Therapy Complications of insulin therapy include hypoglycemia (discussed later in this chapter), insulin resistance (requiring more than 200 units/day), lipodystrophy, Somogyi phenomenon, and the dawn phenomenon. Lipodystrophy can be minimized by using human insulin, using room temperature insulin, and by rotating sites of insulin injection.

The **Somogyi phenomenon** occurs when a rapid decrease in blood glucose (hypoglycemia) generates the release of glucose-elevating hormones (epinephrine, cortisol, glucagon). The hypoglycemia usually occurs during the night, but manifests as an elevated glucose in the morning and may be inadvertently treated with an increase in insulin dosage. The Somogyi phenomenon can be diagnosed by checking the blood glucose during the night about 3 A.M. Adjusting the insulin regimen to avoid the peaking of insulin during the night will correct this effect.

The **dawn phenomenon** is an early morning glucose elevation produced by the release of growth hormone. Administering the evening insulin dose at a later time will coordinate the insulin peak with the hormone release.

Oral Hypoglycemic Agents Oral hypoglycemic agents are used in the treatment of persons with type 2 diabetes who are not controlled with exercise and diet. These agents are meant to supplement diet and exer-

cise, not replace them. Oral hypoglycemics are not insulin and work by other mechanisms.

Sulfonylurea is the class of oral hypoglycemic medications most commonly used for diabetes therapy. The sulfonylureas work primarily by increasing the ability of the islet cells of the pancreas to excrete insulin. It is also believed that they have some effect by increasing the cells' sensitivity to insulin and decreasing glucose production by the liver.

All sulfonylureas can be taken with food, except for glipizide (Glucotrol) which should be taken 30 minutes before eating (Chase, 1997). Hypoglycemia can occur in any client taking a sulfonyluric oral hypoglycemic, but hypoglycemia is more common and more dangerous in the elderly. Recognition of hypoglycemia may be more difficult for the older adult because aging decreases the adrenergic mediated hypoglycemic responses of shaking, sweating, and nervousness. Older adults are also more likely to be taking medications for other chronic illnesses that may interact with the oral hypoglycemic. Various medications have the potential to interfere with or enhance the action of oral hypoglycemics.

Other side effects of sulfonyluric oral hypoglycemic agents are rare, but can include skin rashes and gastrointestinal disturbances. Clients should be warned that the oral hypoglycemics, especially chlorpropamide (Diabinese), are known to produce a disulfiram (Antabuse)-like effect in some clients when alcohol is ingested. Reaction may be severe and include symptoms of flushing, sweating, nausea and vomiting, palpitations, and hyperventilation.

Metformin (Glucophage), a biguanide, does not increase insulin release but works by making existing insulin more effective at the cellular level. Metformin may be given alone or in combination with other oral hypoglycemics. In some clients, Glucophage works more effectively if given with some dose of Diabeta. Because it does not stimulate increased insulin release, metformin is not associated with episodes of hypoglycemia. The major side effects of metformin are

PROFESSIONAL TIP

Insulin Injection Practices

Fleming (1999) suggests:
- Rolling the insulin vial does not adequately mix lente or NPH insulins; the vial should be shaken vigorously.
- Skin preparation with alcohol is unnecessary.
- The angle of injection may vary from 45° to 90°, depending on the client's weight.
- Aspiration before injection, for needle placement, has never been proven in clinical studies.
- Unrefrigerated insulin is effective for 1 month.

gastrointestinal and include anorexia, nausea, abdominal discomfort, and diarrhea.

Oral hypoglycemics require some production of insulin by the pancreas and, therefore, are not useful in the treatment of type 1 diabetes. See Table 37-5 for a description of oral hypoglycemic agents available in the United States.

Diet

Nutritional therapy continues to be considered the cornerstone of diabetic management. Dietary prescriptions are individualized to meet client and family needs. Consideration must be given to usual eating habits and other lifestyle factors such as dietary likes and dislikes, cultural influences, who prepares the meals, and family finances. It is important that meals remain a social experience, and the diabetic person does not feel isolated or different.

The goals of nutrition are to maintain as near-normal blood glucose level as possible, achieve optimal serum lipid levels, provide adequate energy for maintaining or attaining a reasonable weight, prevent complications of diabetes, and improve overall health. Because of the complexity of nutrition issues, it is recommended that clients be referred early to a registered dietician for nutritional education.

Diabetes is a strong risk factor for atherosclerosis and cardiovascular disease. Therefore, reducing the serum lipid level is a goal of diabetic nutrition therapy. To reduce the risk of cardiovascular disease, the ADA recommendations incorporate a reduction in saturated fat and cholesterol consumption.

It is recommended that individuals taking insulin or oral hypoglycemic agents eat at consistent times synchronized with the actions of the medications used. Distribution of calories over 24 hours, with regular meals and snacks, helps to prevent extreme highs and lows in blood glucose.

Exchange System The diabetic exchange system, developed by the American Diabetes Association and the American Dietetic Association, is the most frequently used system for ensuring that the diabetic integrates all aspects of the dietary prescription. This system divides food into 4 categories according to the amount of protein, carbohydrate, fat, and calories supplied by the food. Clients are given meal plans or prescriptions, specifying the number of exchanges from each list that should be eaten at each meal. With the exchange group system, any food in the proper amount may be substituted for another food in the same exchange list. Table 37-6 shows a sample menu based on the exchange system. The diabetic exchange system continues to be widely used. Once it is learned, it is simple, flexible, and provides wide variety.

Other Diet Systems Many tools and plans for dietary compliance are available to diabetics. Another system gaining more popularity is one that monitors the amount of carbohydrate available in each meal. Insulin doses are then regulated according to total available carbohydrate.

Position Statement: American Diabetes Association According to *Nutrition Recommendations and Principles for People with Diabetes Mellitus, 1996,* there are five goals of nutrition therapy besides improved metabolic control. They are:

1. Maintain as near-normal blood glucose level.
2. Achieve optimal serum lipid levels.
3. Provide adequate calories to maintain or attain a reasonable weight (reasonable weight is determined by client and health care provider).
4. Prevent and treat acute complications of insulin-treated diabetes.

Table 37-5 ORAL HYPOGLYCEMICS

GENERIC (BRAND)	USUAL DOSE	ONSET TIME (HOURS)	DURATION (HOURS)
First-Generation Sulfonylureas			
tobutamide (Orinase)	500–2,000 mg divided dose	1	6–12
acetohexamide (Dymelor)	250–1,500 mg single or divided dose	1	12–24
tolazamide (Tolinase)	100–1,000 mg single or divided dose	4–6	12–24
chlorpropamide (Diabanese)	100–750 mg single dose	1	60
Second-Generation Sulfonylureas			
glipizide (Glucatrol)	2.5–40 mg single or divided dose	1–1½	10–16
glimepride (Amaryl)	1–4 mg single dose	1	24
glyburide (Diabeta, Micronase)	1.25–20 mg single or divided dose	2–4	24
Biguanides			
metformin hydrochloride (Glucophage)	500–2,500 mg two or three divided doses	24–48	6–12
Alpha-Glucosidase Inhibitors			
acarbose (Precose)	25–100 mg with meals (tid)	1	No data
miglitol (Glyset)	25–100 mg with meals (tid)	2–3	4–6
Thiazolidenediones			
troglitazone (Rezulin)	200–600 mg with a meal (qd)	2–3	No data

Table 37-6 SAMPLE DIET, USING EXCHANGE SYSTEM (2,200 CAL)

FOOD GROUP	TOTAL EXCHANGES	BREAKFAST	LUNCH	DINNER	SNACKS P.M.	SNACKS HS
Carbohydrates						
Milk and milk products	3	1	1	—	—	1
Vegetable	4	—	2	2	—	—
Fruit	4	1	1	1	1	—
Starch/bread	9	3	2	2	1	1
Other carbohydrates	1	—	—	1	—	—
Meat and Meat Substitutes	7	1	2	3	—	1
Fat	5	2	2	—	1	—
Free Foods	—	1	1	2	—	—

Breakfast	Lunch	P.M. Snack	Dinner	Hour of Sleep (H/S) Snack
1 medium peach	½ c summer squash	5 crackers	3 oz pork chop	3 c popcorn, plain
½ c oatmeal	½ c broccoli	2 tsp peanut butter	⅓ c brown rice	1 oz cheese
1 poached egg on slice wheat toast	tuna sandwich (2 breads, 1 oz tuna, 2 tsp mayo)	1 orange	½ c green beans	1 c skim milk
1 bran muffin	1 medium pear		Tossed green salad with Italian dressing (¼ cup)	
1 tsp margarine	Diet soda		½ c applesauce	
1 c skim milk	1 c yogurt, nonfat		1 dinner roll	
coffee			½ c fat-free ice cream	
			iced tea	

5. Improve overall health through optimal nutrition (Dietary Guidelines for Americans and Food Guide Pyramid are examples to follow).

Protein intake of both animal and vegetable sources should make up 10% to 20% of the daily calorie intake. If nephropathy is present, protein should be 10% of the daily calorie intake.

Total fat intake depends on the goals set by the client and health care provider for desired levels of glucose, lipid, and weight. If lipid level is normal, 30% or less of calories should come from fat with less than 10% from saturated fat. If weight loss is a primary issue, reduction in fat intake is an efficient way to reduce calorie intake. When lipid level is a problem, a decrease of saturated fat intake to < 7% of the total calories, total fat to < 30% of total calories, and cholesterol to < 200 mg/day is recommended.

The remainder of the calorie intake comes from carbohydrates. The amount consumed is more important than the source of the carbohydrate.

Persons with diabetes should follow the same precautions regarding the use of alcohol as applied to the general public. Alcohol may increase the risk for hypoglycemia in people treated with insulin or sul-fonylureas such as acetohexamide (Dymelor), chlorpropamide (Diabinese), or tolazamide (Tolinase).

Activity

The beneficial effects of regular exercise for the diabetic are multiple. Exercise decreases the blood glucose by increasing the uptake of glucose by body muscles and improving insulin usage. Exercise also increases circulation, improves cardiovascular status, decreases stress, and assists with weight loss.

Before starting an exercise program, the diabetic individual should have a complete physical and review the exercise plan with the physician or primary health care provider. Regular daily exercise rather than sporadic exercise should be encouraged.

Diabetics need to correlate exercise with their blood glucose, taking care to avoid periods of hypoglycemia or exercising when blood glucose is too high. Exercise potentiates the action of insulin, resulting in lower insulin requirements and an increased risk of hypoglycemia during and after exercise. On the other hand, in the diabetic who is insulin-deficient, exercise may cause a further rise in blood glucose and rapid development of ketosis. Diabetics must know they should not exercise at the peak of insulin activity,

CLIENT TEACHING

Guidelines for Exercising

- Try to exercise at the same time and in the same amount each day.
- Test blood glucose level before, during, and after exercise.
- Do not inject insulin into a limb that you will be exercising.
- Do not exercise at the peak of insulin activity.
- Do not exercise before meals unless trying to lower blood glucose level.
- Do not exercise with a blood glucose level over 250 mg/dL or with ketones in the urine. This indicates severe insulin deficiency and may predispose to hyperglycemia.
- Eat a snack (15 gm carbohydrates) prior to or during exercise if appropriate, based on blood glucose level.
- Always carry a source of carbohydrates and emergency cash, if away from home, in case hypoglycemia occurs while exercising.
- Always carry personal and medical alert identification.
- Watch for postexercise hypoglycemia. Individuals who have more than usual exercise during the day should increase their carbohydrate intake and test their glucose during the night to detect nocturnal hypoglycemia. (Hypoglycemia can occur 8 to 15 hours following exercise.)

when blood glucose is greater than 250 mg/dL, or if they have ketones in their urine.

Health Promotion

The diabetic educator plays a pivotal role in assisting the diabetic client/family to understand diabetes and the necessary lifestyle changes. Some teaching is unique to an individual client and is done one-to-one, while some teaching applies to all clients with diabetes and is often done in a class setting. This also allows clients with diabetes to meet each other and share concerns, information, and ideas that have worked for them.

The diabetic educator nurse is part of a team including the client/family, physician, dietitian, and pharmacist who all work together to help the client understand and comply with the treatment plan.

Sick Day Management It is important that diabetics have a plan for managing their diabetes in the event of illness. They should know that it is important that they continue to receive their insulin or oral hypoglycemic medication when they are experiencing illness, as illness and fever can increase blood glucose and the need for insulin. Some diabetics who do not normally take short-acting insulin may require insulin

CLIENT TEACHING

Fingersticks

- Use shallow skin penetration, just to get enough blood for the meter.
- Rotate sites; use sides of fingertips and thumb.
- Use alcohol sparingly or wash hands with warm soapy water before fingerstick *instead* of using alcohol. The warm water brings more blood into the fingers.
- Apply firm pressure *directly* over the puncture for 10 to 15 seconds; if area is still bleeding, apply pressure until it stops.

coverage during times of fever or illness. Blood glucose should be monitored 4 to 6 times per day and urine should be checked for ketones. Blood glucose greater than 300 mg/dL or ketones in the urine should be reported to the physician.

If the client cannot ingest the planned meal, carbohydrates in the form of soft foods and liquids can be substituted. Extreme nausea and vomiting or diarrhea should be reported to the physician because extreme fluid loss can be dangerous. Clients with type 1 diabetes who are unable to retain fluids may need to be hospitalized to avoid ketoacidosis.

Acute Complications of Diabetes

There are three major acute complications of diabetes related to blood glucose imbalance: hypoglycemia, diabetic ketoacidosis (DKA), and hyperglycemic hyperosmolar nonketotic syndrome (HHNK).

Hypoglycemia (Insulin Reaction)

Hypoglycemia (low blood glucose) occurs when a client's glucose level drops below 70 mg/dL with the most severe reactions occurring when it drops below 50 mg/dL. Hypoglycemia can occur any time of the day, but most often will occur before meals or when insulin action is peaking. Factors that can contribute to the development of a hypoglycemic reaction are skipping meals or eating late, unplanned exercise, and administration of excess insulin.

Hypoglycemic symptoms can occur suddenly and unexpectedly, and vary from client to client (Table 37-7). The cardinal rule is: *Always believe clients who tell you they are having an insulin reaction.* Most diabetics have had hypoglycemic reactions before, so they know the symptoms that precede an insulin reaction.

When a hypoglycemic reaction is suspected, the nurse must respond immediately according to the institution's protocol. Treatment involves assessing the client, checking blood glucose level, and administering glucose in the most appropriate form. Hutchison and Peppard (1998) suggest using glucose tablets or gel for hypoglycemia. The client taking acarbose (Pre-

Table 37-7 SYMPTOMS OF ACUTE COMPLICATIONS OF DIABETES

Symptoms of Hypoglycemia (Insulin Reaction)

Mild hypoglycemia
- Diaphoresis
- Pallor
- Paresthesias
- Excess hunger
- Palpitations
- Tremors
- Anxiety

Moderate hypoglycemia
- Confusion, disorientation
- Slurred speech
- Behavior changes
- Irritability

Severe hypoglycemia
- Seizures
- Loss of consciousness
- Shallow respirations
- Nursing Alert: Severe hypoglycemia is a medical emergency. Administer some form of glucose immediately.

Symptoms of Diabetic Ketoacidosis (DKA)
- Same as HHNK plus symptoms of acidosis:
- "Fruity" odor to breath
- Kussmaul's respirations (deep, nonlabored)

Symptoms of Hyperglycemic Hyperosmolar Nonketotic (HHNK) Syndrome
- Polyuria
- Polydipsia
- Skin hot, dry, decreased turgor
- Dehydration—hypotension, increased pulse
- Blurred vision
- Weakness
- Mental status changes, confusion to coma

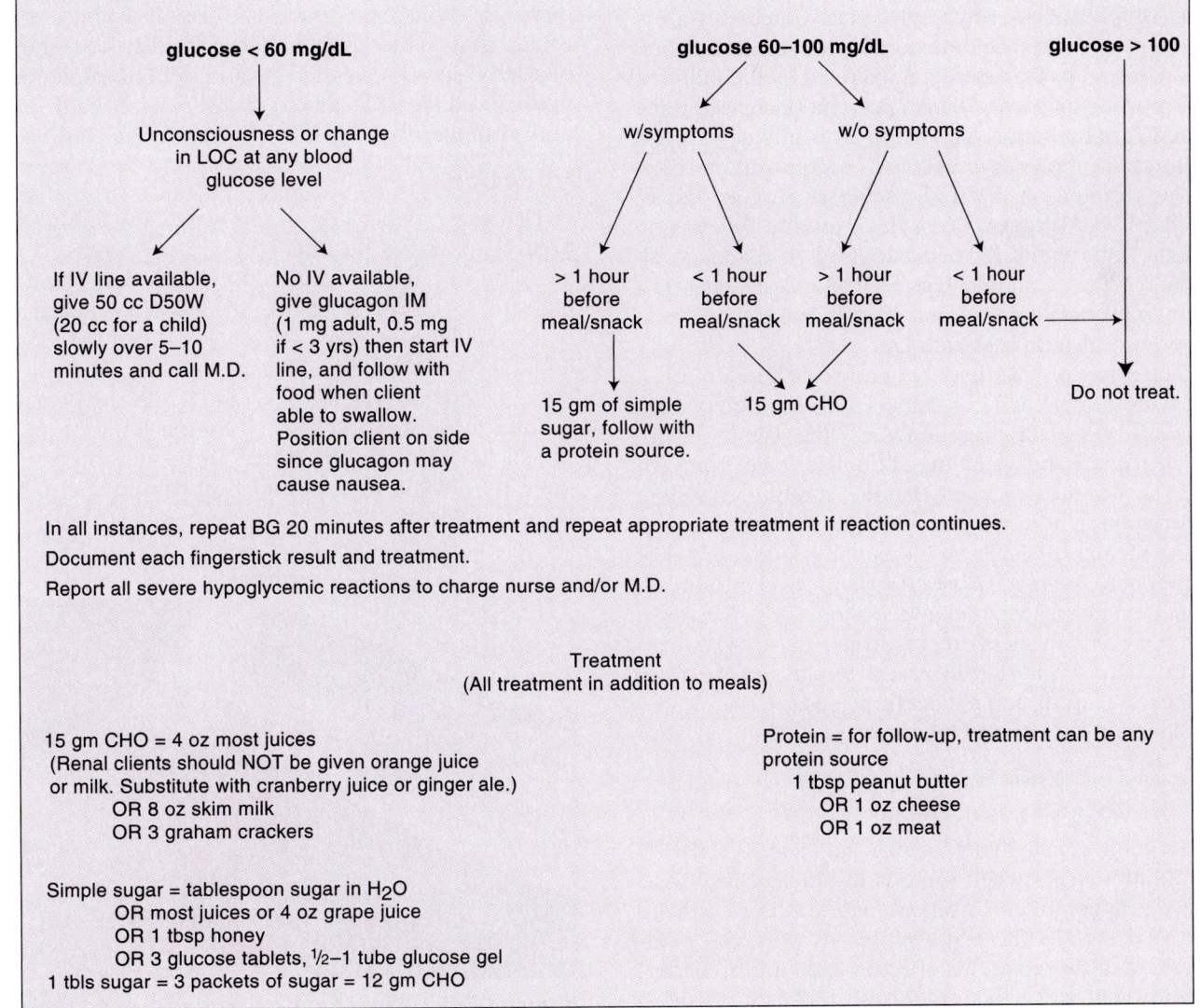

Figure 37-7 Sample Hypoglycemic Protocol

cose), which slows digestion and absorption of most carbohydrates—including hard candies and many fruit juices—but not gluocse, will not have the rapid response to fruit juice or sugar that other clients will have. Hypoglycemic reactions can be fatal, so *leaving the client untreated is more dangerous than causing mild hyperglycemia with overtreatment.* Figure 37-7 provides a sample hypoglycemic protocol.

Diabetics and their families must be instructed about the symptoms and treatment for hypoglycemia. Hypoglycemic episodes can be prevented by following a regular pattern of eating, exercise, and insulin administration. Between meals and bedtime snacks can be used to cover times of peak insulin action. Additional food should be eaten when engaging in greater than usual exercise. Blood glucose level should be checked at the first suspicion of hypoglycemia. All diabetics should wear an identification bracelet or tag indicating that they have diabetes, as hypoglycemic reactions can occur unexpectedly.

Diabetic Ketoacidosis

Diabetic ketoacidosis (DKA) is one of the most serious complications of hyperglycemia. Glucose is a hyperosmolar substance drawing fluid out of the cell and into the circulation where it is excreted by the kidneys. This oncotic diuresis results in polyuria (increased urine output), dehydration, and electrolyte imbalances. Increased fat metabolism results in accumulation of ketones, resulting in metabolic acidosis. Surgery, stress, or illness may trigger DKA, which usually develops in clients with immune mediated type 1 diabetes, although it can occur in clients with type 2 diabetes. The client with undiagnosed immune mediated type 1 diabetes may also present with DKA.

The onset of DKA may be gradual or sudden. Classic symptoms of hyperglycemia (polyuria, polyphagia, polydipsia) usually precede DKA. Other symptoms include nausea and vomiting, abdominal pain from acidosis, headache, weakness, fatigue, and blurred vision. Assessment may reveal hot, flushed skin and signs of hypovolemia or shock. Acidosis will produce signs of hyperpnea (Kussmaul's breathing), fruity odor to breath from respiratory elimination of acetone, and decreased level of consciousness ranging from lethargy to coma.

Laboratory values will reveal blood glucose from 300 to 800 mg/dL and metabolic acidosis. Urine will be positive for glucose and ketones.

Hyperglycemic Hyperosmolar Nonketotic Syndrome

Hyperglycemic hyperosmolar nonketotic (HHNK) syndrome occurs when there is insufficient insulin to prevent hyperglycemia, but enough insulin to prevent ketoacidosis. HHNK occurs in persons with type 2 diabetes. Because symptoms of acidosis do not occur, hyperglycemia and oncotic diuresis can be much more severe.

HHNK occurs most often in the elderly client with undiagnosed type 2 diabetes. HHNK can also occur in the poorly controlled client and is usually precipitated by illness or other stressor.

Clinical manifestations of HHNK reflect dehydration and shock. Hyperosmolality eventually results in lethargy, seizures, and coma (refer back to Table 37-7). Blood glucose level ranges from 600 to 2,000 mg/dL and serum osmolality > 350 mOsm/L.

Medical management of DKA and HHNK involves fluid and electrolyte replacement (particularly potassium), insulin, and treatment of any precipitating factors. DKA and HHNK are associated with significant mortality rates, and the client is usually acutely ill. Treatment will occur in the intensive care setting until the client is stabilized.

Chronic Complications of Diabetes

Long-term complications of diabetes occur 5 to 10 years after diagnosis in both type 1 and type 2 diabetes. The exact pathophysiology is not completely understood but is known to be related to effects of elevated blood glucose level. Recent studies have shown that intensive insulin therapy and tight glycemic control can reduce or delay the occurrence of many long-term complications associated with diabetes.

Infections

Diabetics, particularly clients who are poorly controlled, appear to be more prone than others to developing certain infections. Infections of particular concern to diabetics include diabetic foot infections, boils, cellulitis, necrotizing fasciitis, urinary tract infections, and yeast infections. Small cuts on the feet can become gangrenous (Figure 37-8) and require amputation.

Infections increase the need for insulin and can result in ketoacidosis. Infections, once they occur, can often be difficult to treat and heal slowly due to impaired circulation.

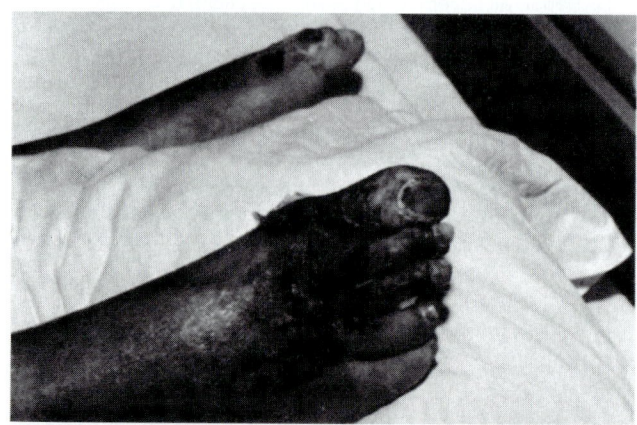

Figure 37-8 Gangrene of the toes and foot as a result of an infection often means eventual amputation.

CLIENT TEACHING

Guidelines to Healthy Feet

- Wash feet daily and dry them carefully, especially between the toes.
- Inspect feet and between toes for blisters, cuts, and infections. Use a mirror to see the bottoms of the feet. If your vision is impaired, have a family member examine your feet. Remember, because of decreased feeling in your feet, you may have an infection and not know it.
- Avoid activities that will restrict blood flow to the feet, especially smoking. Do not sit with legs crossed.
- Wear shoes that are comfortable, well-fitting, and closed toed. Wear new shoes for short intervals until broken in. Do not walk barefoot.
- Prevent cuts and irritations. Always wear stockings. Look inside shoes for rough edges, nail points, foreign objects.
- Avoid temperature extremes. Test bath water with hands before getting in. Do not use water bottles or heating pads on feet.
- See your physician regularly and make sure that your feet are examined each visit.
- When toe nails are trimmed, cut them straight across. When corns or calluses are present, see a physician or podiatrist. Do not cut them yourself.

Diabetic Neuropathies

Neuropathies are the most common chronic complication associated with diabetes. The incidence of peripheral neuropathies increases with age and duration of disease and is related to elevated blood glucose level. Neuropathies can affect all types of nerves but the two most common types of diabetic neuropathy are sensorimotor polyneuropathy and autonomic neuropathy.

Sensorimotor polyneuropathy, also called *peripheral neuropathy,* causes paresthesias and burning sensations, primarily in the lower extremities. Decreased sensations of pain and temperature coupled with decreased peripheral circulation place the client at high risk for injury and undetected foot injury.

Autonomic neuropathy can affect almost any organ system including: gastrointestinal (delayed gastric emptying,

LIFE CYCLE CONSIDERATIONS

Diabetic Neuropathy

Advancing age is the strongest risk factor regardless of disease duration and blood sugar control.

constipation, diarrhea), urinary (retention, neurogenic bladder), and reproductive (male impotence).

Nephropathy (Chronic Renal Failure)

Diabetic nephropathy develops slowly over many years, progressing eventually to kidney failure. Controlling hypertension and blood glucose level is the key to delaying renal damage. Good hydration before and diuresis following any dye study is valuable in preventing renal damage. Urinary tract infections can be prevented by encouraging the client to use the bathroom "by the clock" to reduce stagnant, residual urine (Hernandez, 1998).

Retinopathy

Changes in the small vessels of the retina result in diabetic retinopathy, which is a major cause of blindness among diabetics. Because of the insidious onset of type 2 diabetes, retinopathy is often present at diagnosis. The severity and progression of retinopathy appear to be closely related to glucose and blood pressure control. Diabetics also develop cataracts at an earlier age. Although the majority of clients develop some degree of retinopathy, most do not develop visual impairment. To facilitate early detection, diabetics should have ophthalmologic evaluations every 6 to 12 months.

Vascular Changes

Diabetes is an independent risk factor for atherosclerotic vessel disease. Atherosclerotic changes that occur in diabetics are similar to those that occur in nondiabetics, but they occur at earlier ages and progress at a more rapid rate.

Cardiovascular Hypertension is twice as common in diabetics and is an important factor in the progression of retinopathy, nephropathy, and vascular (large vessel) disease. The incidence of coronary artery disease, angina, and myocardial infarction is higher when compared to the nondiabetic population. Cerebral vascular disease and cerebral vascular accident are also more common in persons with diabetes.

Therapies aimed at lowering risk factors and effects of atherosclerosis are recommended for the diabetic client. These management techniques include weight control, low-fat diet, treatment of hypertension and hyperlipidemia, regular exercise, and control of blood glucose level.

CLIENT TEACHING

Retinopathy Prevention

- Refrain from straining to have a bowel movement.
- Use stool softener or laxative.
- Avoid postures that lower the head.
- Avoid lifting weight above shoulders.

Peripheral Vascular Disease Peripheral vascular disease (PVD) occurs most commonly in diabetics with hypertension or hyperlipidemia and in diabetics who smoke. Diabetics have 2 to 3 times the incidence of occlusive peripheral arterial disease when compared to the nondiabetic population. Diabetes is present in more than half of persons experiencing nontraumatic lower extremity amputations.

▶ NURSING PROCESS

▶ Assessment

▶ Subjective Data

This includes assessment of the health history, family history, diet, activity regimen, and the understanding of the disease and medical therapies. The client may describe fatigue, weakness, weight changes, mental status changes, polyuria, polyphagia, polydipsia, numbness or tingling of the extremities, blurred vision, and increased appetite.

▶ Objective Data

Objective data should focus on the symptoms of diabetes, the common acute and chronic complications, and the results of diagnostic tests. There may be dependent redness or cyanosis of the lower extremities as well as the absence of hair. A fasting glucose level greater than 126 mg/dL or a nonfasting (random) level greater than 200 mg/dL, on two separate occasions, suggests a diagnosis of diabetes (The Expert Committee on the Diagnosis and Classification of Diabetes Mellitus, 1997).

Nursing diagnoses, based on the assessment findings, may be varied and extensive due to the multiple problems and complications caused by diabetes mellitus. Nursing diagnoses may include the following:

Nursing Diagnoses	Planning/Goals	Nursing Interventions
▶ *Knowledge Deficit, diabetes, medical regimen, diet, exercise, self-care management skills (insulin injection, SMBG) related to new diagnosis or changes in treatment*	The client will relate basic understanding of pathophysiology of diabetes, and relationship between insulin and hyper-/hypoglycemia.	Teach client about diabetes and the use of insulin to prevent hyper-/hypoglycemia or assist client to enroll in a formal diabetic education program.
	The client will verbalize how/when to take oral hypoglycemics and the side effects to report or will correctly demonstrate how to administer insulin and rotate sites.	Teach client about oral hypoglycemics or insulin, whichever the client will be using.
	The client will relate importance of an exercise program.	Discuss how exercise is related to diabetes management.
	The client will describe the relationship between dietary management and glycemic control; choose foods that comply with diet prescription.	Discuss how dietary management is related to the control of blood glucose and provide an exchange list of foods.
	The client will correctly demonstrate how to use SMBG to determine blood glucose level.	Teach client how to perform SMBG and have client return demonstration.
	The client will verbalize symptoms and treatment of hypoglycemia.	Provide client with a list of symptoms and treatment for hypoglycemia.
▶ *Fluid Volume Deficit, Risk for, related to hyperglycemia, polyuria, and dehydration*	The client will exhibit normal skin turgor, moist mucous membranes, and maintain oral fluid intake of 2,500–3,000 mL/day.	Measure client's intake and output, administer intravenous fluids as ordered, and encourage oral fluids.
	The client will have vital signs within normal limits.	Monitor vital signs and serum electrolytes.
▶ *Nutrition, Altered, less than body requirements, related to imbalance between insulin, diet, and activity*	The client will have weight within normal range for height and age.	Assist client to adjust dietary intake in order to maintain weight in normal range.

Evaluation Each goal must be evaluated to determine how it has been met by the client.

PITUITARY DISORDERS

Hyperpituitarism and hypopituitarism are discussed following.

HYPERPITUITARISM

Hyperpituitarism is most commonly diagnosed between the second and fourth decade of life but can appear in infancy and childhood. Although other pituitary hormones may be affected, the most common are the growth hormone and antidiuretic hormone.

Excess secretion of growth hormone (GH) produces different changes depending on the client's age when it occurs. When the excess secretion occurs in childhood before the epiphyses close, gigantism is the result; in adults, acromegaly is the result.

Syndrome of inappropriate antidiuretic hormone and pituitary tumors are also discussed.

GIGANTISM

Gigantism affects infants and children, causing proportional overgrowth of all body tissues. By the time these children reach adulthood, they may be more than 8 feet tall.

Hyperplasia of the anterior pituitary is usually the cause of GH oversecretion. This tissue may develop into a tumor causing other symptoms. Clients with gigantism do not have the strength their size implies.

Medical–Surgical Management

Medical

Irradiation of the anterior pituitary may be the treatment chosen. The child must then be observed for heart failure, hypertension, thickened bones, osteoporosis, and delayed sexual development.

Surgical

If the cause is a tumor, surgery may be performed to remove the tumor (explained under "Acromegaly").

Pharmacological

When the pituitary is either destroyed by irradiation or removed by surgery, pituitary hormone replacement is necessary.

▶ NURSING PROCESS

▶ Assessment

▶ Subjective Data

Listening to the child's description of the disease process may provide insight into the child's emotional responses.

▶ Objective Data

Frequent measurements of growth indicate a more rapid rate of growth than expected.

ACROMEGALY

Since acromegaly occurs after epiphyseal closure of bones, there is bone thickening with transverse growth and tissue enlargement. This occurs between 30 and 50 years of age. Photographs over years will reveal a progressive enlargement of the face and hands.

Acromegaly involves a gradual onset of clinical manifestations including: visual defects from pressure of the pituitary tumor on the optic nerve, soft tissue swelling, or hypertrophy of the face and extremities. The cartilaginous and connective tissue overgrowths result in a characteristic hulking appearance with thickened ears and nose, and marked projection of the jaw. The jaw can appear enlarged and the tongue may also thicken. The paranasal sinuses can become enlarged. Also laryngeal hypertrophy can occur. The client has thick fingers with tips that appear "tufted" (shaped like arrowheads on x-rays). The client exhibits a characteristic moist, weak, doughy handshake. The heart, liver, and spleen may enlarge. Some other characteristics are: diaphoresis (profuse perspiration), oily or leathery skin, fatigue, heat intolerance, weight gain, headache, joint pain, hirsutism (excessive hairiness especially in females), and sleep disturbance. The client may experience decreased libido or impotence, oligomenorrhea (scanty or infrequent menstruation), and infertility.

The client's history and clinical manifestations along with cranial x-rays and a CT scan make a diagnosis of acromegaly. Serum growth hormone levels are elevated.

Prognosis depends upon the causative factor, hyperplasia or a tumor; however, there is generally a reduced life span. Diabetes mellitus is a possible complication of hyperpituitarism because of glucose intolerance caused by the insulin-antagonistic character of the growth hormone.

Medical–Surgical Management

Medical

Medical treatment consists of either medication that affects the growth hormone or irradiation of the pituitary gland. Proton beam therapy uses a very low dose of radiation and is much less destructive to nearby tissue than conventional radiation therapy.

Surgical

Surgical treatment for hyperpituitarism is to remove the pituitary gland. Two surgical approaches to remove the pituitary are transfrontal or transsphenoid hypophysectomy. The transfrontal approach is rarely used because it has a high risk of mortality as well as permanent loss of smell and taste and causes severe diabetes insipidus. The transsphenoid approach

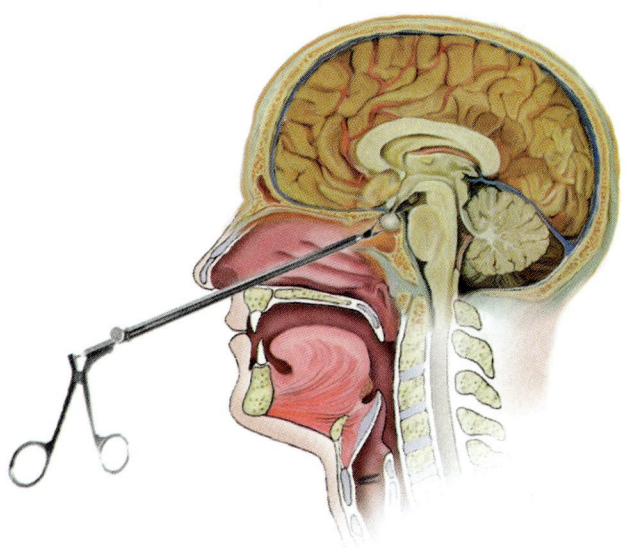

Figure 37-9 Transsphenoidal Approach to Hypophysectomy

(Figure 37-9) involves an incision in the superior maxillary gingiva. Surgery may be the treatment of choice or used after attempting medical treatment.

Postoperatively, nasal packing should be checked for clear colorless drainage. If it occurs, the drainage must be documented and reported to the physician. If this drainage is suspected of being cerebrospinal fluid, it should be checked for glucose, which is found in cerebrospinal fluid. The nurse should observe for infection which includes elevated leukocytes, sudden temperature elevation, or complaint of headache or nuchal rigidity. Analgesics are administered as needed. The client should avoid activities such as coughing, straining, vomiting, or sneezing. The client should be encouraged to use an incentive spirometer instead of coughing. The client should not brush teeth for 2 weeks to avoid problems with the incision. Mouthwash can be used. The client should be instructed to avoid lifting and bending at the waist for 2 to 3 months after surgery.

Pharmacological

Two drugs may be prescribed for acromegaly. Bromocriptine mesylate (Parlodel) is a nonhormonal drug that activates dopamine receptors to inhibit the release of the growth hormone and prolactin. Bromocriptine mesylate (Parlodel) should be given with food to decrease gastric upset. Since it can cause drowsiness or dizziness, the client should be instructed to avoid activities that require mental alertness. If the client is on oral contraceptives, alternate contraceptive measures should also be used because bromocriptine can stimulate ovulation.

The other drug, octreotide acetate (Sandostatin), inhibits the growth hormone. Although octreotide is given by injection, it can still cause gastric distress. The injections should be given between meals and at bedtime. Clients with diabetes mellitus should closely monitor their blood sugar level.

▶ NURSING PROCESS

▶ Assessment

▶ Subjective Data

The nurse should obtain a thorough nursing history and ask about vision impairment, headache, muscular weakness, and psychological disturbances.

▶ Objective Data

Objective data includes gait changes, vital sign changes (tachycardia or hypotension which may indicate congestive heart failure), and dyspnea. The jaw is enlarged and projected, so the client may have difficulty in chewing.

Nursing diagnoses for a client with gigantism or acromegaly may include the following:

Nursing Diagnoses	Planning/Goals	Nursing Interventions
▶ *Altered Growth, Risk for, related to increased level of growth hormone*	The client will comply with treatment to minimize hyperpituitarism and stop excessive growth with treatment.	Assist client with activities of daily living. Administer medications as ordered. Assist client with range of motion exercises. Remind client to carry medications on person.
▶ *Self-Esteem, Chronic Low, related to irreversible physical changes*	The client will acknowledge physical changes, express positive feelings about self, and exhibit ability to cope with altered body.	Encourage client to verbalize feelings. Offer emotional support and help client to develop coping strategies. Show respect and acceptance of the client as a person. Refer to professional counseling as needed. Assist client in setting achievable short-term goals. Provide a positive but realistic assessment of the situation.

Evaluation Each goal must be evaluated to determine how it has been met by the client.

SYNDROME OF INAPPROPRIATE ANTIDIURETIC HORMONE

Syndrome of inappropriate antidiuretic hormone (SIADH) results from an excess of ADH. This causes the kidneys to reabsorb excess water, which decreases urine output and increases fluid volume. The most common cause is bronchogenic lung cancer (Heater, 1999b). Other causes are lymphoid pancreatic, duodenal, thymus, and prostate cancer; lupus erythematosis; central nervous system trauma, infection, hemorrhage, or neoplasm; chronic obstructive pulmonary disease; acute respiratory failure; mechanical ventilation; and medications such as antineoplastic agents, tricyclic antidepressants, and anesthetics.

The client will have hyponatremia (< 130 mEq/L), water retention, weight gain, concentrated urine (urine osmolality > 1,200 mOsm/L; specific gravity > 1.020), muscle cramps, and weakness. The low osmolality of the blood allows fluid to leak out of vessels and causes brain swelling. If untreated, lethargy, seizures, coma, and death will result.

Medical–Surgical Management

Medical

The underlying disorder must be treated or medications stopped that may be contributing to SIADH. Water restriction will be implemented to prevent further hemodilution. Serious hyponatremia (< 120 mEq/L) will usually be treated with intravenous administration of 5% NaCl. The serum sodium level should be increased by 12 mEq/L or less per day.

Pharmacological

Furosemide (Lasix) is given to increase urine output, while demeclocycline hydrochloride (Declomycin) and fludrocortisone (Florinef) are given to enhance sodium retention.

Diet

Fluid restriction will be determined by the serum sodium level.

▶ NURSING PROCESS

▶ Assessment

▶ Subjective Data

The client may describe muscle cramps, weakness, anorexia, nausea, and headache.

▶ Objective Data

The client will have weight gain and fluid intake greater than output. The client may be irritable and disoriented, become progressively lethargic, and have seizures and diminished or absent deep tendon reflexes. Serum sodium and osmolality will be decreased. Urine osmolality and specific gravity will be increased.

Nursing diagnoses for a client with SIADH may include the following:

Nursing Diagnoses	Planning/Goals	Nursing Interventions
▶ *Fluid Volume Excess related to decreased urine output*	The client will have increased urine output.	Assess client's weight daily on same scale at same time.
		Assess vital signs.
		Accurately record I & O.
		Monitor laboratory reports.
		Administer medications as ordered.
		Maintain fluid restrictions.
▶ *Oral Mucous Membrane, Altered, related to restriction of fluid intake*	The client will have moist, intact oral mucous membranes.	Provide frequent oral care, avoiding alcohol-based mouth washes and lemon-glycerine swabs.
		Allow client to rinse mouth with water, but not swallow any.
		Provide lubricant for client's lips.
		Allow client to choose fluids and times to drink them.

Evaluation Each goal must be evaluated to determine how it has been met by the client.

PITUITARY TUMORS

Pituitary tumors more often affect the anterior pituitary rather than the posterior portion. Adenomas of the pituitary, which are rarely malignant, replace glandular tissue and enlarge the sella turcica. The cause is unknown, but there may be a predisposition toward tumor formation from an inherited **autosomal** dominant trait, meaning it is a dominant characteristic carried on any chromosome other than the one determining sex.

Clinical manifestations frequently start with a headache unrelated to stress or other factors. The next obvious manifestation is visual problems caused by the tumor putting pressure on the optic nerve. Others include personality changes, dementia, amenorrhea, impotence, lethargy, and weakness. The client may complain of cold intolerance, increased fatigue, and constipation. The client may have seizures. Although the tumor is not malignant, damage is done by tumor invasion of normal tissue.

Treatment is removal of the tumor. Complications of pituitary tumors are endocrine abnormalities if there is no replacement therapy after removal of the tumor. If the hypothalamus is compressed, diabetes insipidus can result. If the tumor has eroded the base of the skull, the client may have rhinorrhea (thin watery nasal discharge). Prognosis depends upon the extent of invasion. In most cases, the tumor causes excessive secretion of the anterior pituitary hormones.

Medical–Surgical Management

Medical

Medical treatment of a pituitary tumor would be radiation therapy. This can be used for small tumors or if the client is a poor surgical risk. Radiation can also be used after surgery to shrink tissue remaining after surgical excision. Another alternative to surgery is cryo-

hypophysectomy. This involves freezing the area with a probe inserted via the transsphenoidal approach.

Surgical

Large tumors, especially those impinging on the optic nerve, are generally removed by using the transfrontal approach. Smaller tumors can be resected via the transsphenoidal approach.

Pharmacological

After surgery, the client will need hormone replacement therapy.

▶ NURSING PROCESS

▶ Assessment

▶ Subjective Data

The nurse will obtain a thorough client history and assess for manifestations of a tumor such as visual problems, headache, impotence, lethargy, cold intolerance, fatigue, or constipation. The family may also provide insight into any personality changes.

▶ Objective Data

The client is assessed for tilting of the head to compensate for visual disturbances, axillary and pubic hair loss, a waxy appearance to the skin, and few wrinkles.

Nursing diagnoses for a client with a pituitary tumor may include the following:

Nursing Diagnoses	Planning/Goals	Nursing Interventions
▶ *Fatigue, related to decreased ACTH and TSH levels*	The client will verbalize an understanding of the relationship between fatigue, the disease, and activity level, and express feeling of increasing energy as treatment progresses.	Explain relationship between pituitary tumor, fatigue, and activity level. Suggest alternating periods of activity with periods of rest. Administer medications as ordered. Encourage completion of all treatments.
▶ *Sensory/Perceptual Alterations (Vision), related to altered sensory reception, transmission, and/or integration due to pressure on optic nerve by the pituitary tumor*	The client will use adaptive devices and appropriate resources to compensate for visual changes, and regain normal vision with treatment.	Provide information about adaptive devices and resources for visual changes. Provide a safe clutter-free environment. Make certain that the bed is in the low position and the call signal in reach of the client. Use side rails as needed.

Evaluation Each goal must be evaluated to determine how it has been met by the client.

HYPOPITUITARISM

Hypopituitarism is a complex syndrome marked by metabolic dysfunction, sexual immaturity, and growth retardation when it occurs in childhood; Simmonds' disease and diabetes insipidus are examples of hypopituitarism. The most common cause of hypopituitarism is a tumor. Other causes are: congenital defects

(hypoplasia or aplasia), pituitary infarction (from postpartum hemorrhage), pituitary surgery or irradiation, or chemical agents. Hypopituitarism can be primary (meaning there is no known cause) or secondary. Secondary hypopituitarism can be a result of a deficiency of hypothalamic releasing hormones. This deficiency can be idiopathic (without a known cause) or a result of infection, trauma, or tumor.

Clinical manifestations develop slowly and generally are not apparent until 75% of the pituitary is destroyed. Specific manifestations will vary with the specific hormone that is deficient.

Deficiency of the growth hormone results in dwarfism, which becomes apparent by 6 months of age as the infant exhibits growth retardation, with chubbiness in the lower trunk and a short stature. As it progresses, secondary tooth eruption is delayed and later there is a delay in puberty. Growth continues at about half the normal rate until the child reaches about 4 feet in height. Body proportions are normal as is mental development. Frequently in adulthood, sex organs may not develop normally unless treated with hormones. Clients experience an accelerated pattern of aging, resulting in the life span being shortened by as much as 20 years. If the deficiency occurs in adults, manifestations are not as apparent. There are subtle signs such as wrinkles near the mouth and eyes.

Deficiencies of follicle-stimulating hormone (FSH) and luteinizing hormone (LH) cause differences in clinical manifestations between female and male clients. In the female, symptoms include: amenorrhea, dyspareunia, infertility, decreased libido, breast atrophy, sparse or absent axillary and pubic hair, and dry skin. In the male, symptoms include: weakness, impotence, decreased libido, decreased muscle strength, testicular softening and shrinkage, and retarded secondary sexual hair growth.

In a child a deficiency of thyroid-stimulating hormone (TSH) will result in severe growth retardation even with treatment. Other deficiency manifestations include: cold intolerance; constipation; increased or decreased menstrual flow; lethargy; dry pale puffy skin, and bradycardia. Thought processes may also be slowed.

A deficiency of adrenocorticotrophic hormone (ACTH) results in fatigue, nausea, vomiting, anorexia, weight loss, and depigmentation of the skin and nipples. Vital signs taken during periods of stress would show fever and hypotension.

Prolactin deficiency results in absent postpartum lactation, amenorrhea, and sparse or absent axillary and pubic hair. There may also be manifestations of thyroid or adrenal cortex failure.

Findings of hypopituitarism depend upon the specific hormone, client's age, and severity of condition when detected. X-rays of the wrist determine bone age, and a skull series will rule out a pituitary tumor. Total failure of the pituitary without treatment is fatal; however, prognosis is good with treatment by the appropriate hormone(s). Treatment is primarily replacement therapy for the deficient hormone(s).

SIMMONDS' DISEASE

Simmonds' disease is defined as a total absence of all pituitary secretions. This is also called *panhypopitu-*
itarism. This disease results from surgery, infection, injury, or tumor. It may also occur after a difficult labor in childbirth due to thrombosis formation during or after delivery.

Clinical manifestations, which vary in intensity, include: extreme weight loss, general debility, lethargy, pallor, and dry yellowish skin. There is also a loss of libido, amenorrhea, and intolerance to cold. The disease leads to loss of axillary and pubic hair, and atrophy of genitalia and breasts. It progresses to bradycardia (slow pulse), hypotension, premature wrinkling of the skin, and atrophy of the thyroid and adrenal glands.

Treatment consists of administration of ACTH, TSH, or thyroid, adrenal, and sex hormones for a lifetime.

DIABETES INSIPIDUS

Diabetes insipidus is a deficiency of ADH, causing a metabolic disorder characterized by severe polyuria and polydipsia. Diabetes insipidus generally starts in childhood or early adulthood with a median onset of 21 years. It affects males more often than females. Although a deficiency of ADH is the most common cause (neurogenic), diabetes insipidus can also be caused by failure of the kidneys to respond to ADH (nephrogenic).

Neurogenic diabetes insipidus may be caused by injury or ischemia to the hypothalamus or pituitary gland, CNS infections, pregnancy, sickle cell disease, or medications such as lithium carbonate (Carbolith), amphotereicin B (Fungizone), furosemide (Lasix) or ethycrynic acid (Edecrin). Nephrogenic diabetes insipidus may be caused by pyelonephritis, chronic renal failure, polycystic disease, or renal transplantation (Heater, 1999).

Clinical manifestations have an abrupt onset. The client experiences extreme polyuria of 4 to 16 L of dilute urine daily. In some cases, there can be up to 30 L of urine per day. Serum osmolality is > 295 mOsm/L and urine osmolality is < 150 mOsm/L. Urine specific gravity is < 1.005 and serum sodium is > 145 mEq/L. The client also has extreme thirst, preferring cold beverages. Even though there is an extraordinary volume of fluid intake, weight is lost. Other manifestations include dizziness, weakness, constipation, slight to moderate nocturia, and fatigue that could be a result of inadequate rest due to frequent nighttime voiding and excess thirst.

Complications of untreated diabetes insipidus are **hypovolemia** (abnormally low circulatory blood volume), circulatory collapse, unconsciousness, and central nervous system damage. Prolonged urine flow can cause chronic urinary system conditions such as bladder distension, enlarged calyces, and hydronephrosis.

Prognosis is generally good with fluid replacement in uncomplicated cases. Prognosis also depends upon the underlying cause of diabetes insipidus.

Medical–Surgical Management

Pharmacological

In addition to intravenous fluids, several medications can be used to treat diabetes insipidus. For neurogenic diabetes insipidus, desmopressin acetate (Stimate), a synthetic antidiuretic hormone which can be given parenterally or nasally, is the drug of choice. Also vasopressin (Pitressin) may be given parenterally or nasally. The nurse needs to make certain that the nasal passage is clear before administering the medication. The nurse must also monitor intake and output and assess for hypovolemia and electrolyte imbalance.

For nephrogenic diabetes insipidus, a diuretic such as hydrochlorothiazide (Hydrodiuril) increases sodium excretion which increases fluid reabsorption in the kidneys.

▶ NURSING PROCESS

▶ Assessment

▶ Subjective Data

A thorough client history is needed, including severity of thirst, weakness, fatigue, and lethargy.

▶ Objective Data

The client must be assessed for weight loss, constipation, and signs of fluid volume deficit such as dry skin and mucous membranes, fever, dyspnea, and poor skin turgor. Urine is checked for color, amount, and specific gravity, and weight is assessed daily.

Nursing diagnoses for a client with diabetes insipidus may include the following:

Nursing Diagnoses	Planning/Goals	Nursing Interventions
▶ *Fluid Volume Deficit, Risk for, related to polyuria*	The client will have sufficient fluid intake to prevent dehydration.	Provide easy access to bedpan/bathroom. Answer call signal promptly.
		Monitor the client for dizziness and weakness. Record client intake and output.
		Provide fluids as ordered to cover output.
		Teach client and family how to record intake and output.
		Monitor weight daily.
		Provide oral care. Use a soft toothbrush, mild mouthwash, and lubricant for the lips.
		Assess condition of oral mucous membranes.
▶ *Skin Integrity, Impaired, Risk for, related to altered hydration*	The client will maintain skin integrity.	Assess skin, especially pressure points, 3 times a day.
		Apply moisturizing lotion to skin.
		Prevent pressure on skin by turning or ambulating client.
		Use eggcrate mattress or sheepskin.
		Encourage adequate intake of fluids, protein, vitamin C, and calories.

Evaluation Each goal must be evaluated to determine how it has been met by the client.

THYROID DISORDERS

Worldwide, a deficiency of iodine is the most likely cause of thyroid disorders. However, in countries where idoine in food is plentiful, autoimmune thyroid disease is the most common thyroid disorder (Walpert, 1998). Thyroid disorders are classified as hyperthyroidism, hypothyroidism, tumors, cancer, or goiter.

HYPERTHYROIDISM

Hyperthyroidism is a collective term for a condition marked by increased thyroid activity and overproduction of thyroid hormones thyroxine (T_4) and tri-

iodothyronine (T_3). The thyroid gland itself may be enlarged. Variations of hyperthyroidism are Grave's disease, Basedow's disease, Parry's disease, or thyrotoxicosis. Although these are different forms of hyperthyroidism, Grave's disease is the most common. It generally affects females more often than males; however, it tends to affect males more severely. The highest incidence is in the 20- to 40-year-old group (Walpert, 1998).

In this autoimmune disorder, the immune system triggers the formation of thyroid-stimulating immunoglobulins (TSIs). The TSIs bind with thyroid-stimulating hormone (TSH) receptors and abnormally stimulate thyroid functioning.

Clinical manifestations include two obvious physi-

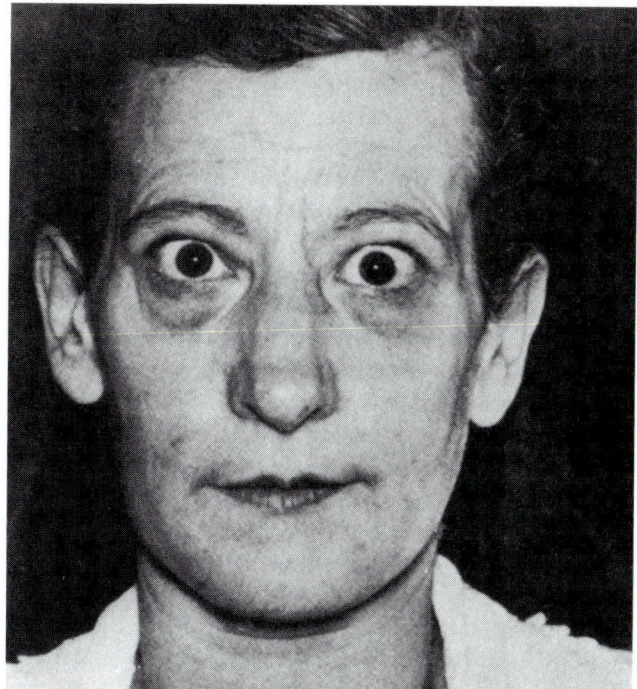

Figure 37-10 Hyperthyroidism with Exophthalmia *(From The Thyroid and Its Diseases, 4th ed., by DeGroot, 1975, John Wiley & Sons, Inc.)*

cal changes. The thyroid can be palpated for asymmetry and size. It may enlarge 3 to 4 times its normal size. The enlargement of the thyroid gland is called **goiter**. This is generally a result of overactivity of the thyroid gland. If there is an accumulation of orbital fluid behind the eyeball forcing it to protrude, this is called **exophthalmos** (Figure 37-10). This occurs in about half the cases of hyperthyroidism. It produces a characteristic stare.

As a result of increased thyroid hormone production, the client has an increased metabolic rate. This leads to weight loss despite increased appetite, fatigue, poor tolerance to heat, and profuse perspiration. The client is very nervous, leading to restlessness, irritability, difficulty concentrating, emotional lability, mood swings, possible personality changes, and sleep disturbances. The client may have fine tremors of the fingers and tongue, shaky handwriting, clumsiness, trouble climbing stairs, or dyspnea on exertion and possibly at rest. The skin is warm and moist with a velvety texture. The skin may be a characteristic salmon color. The hair is fine and soft with premature graying and increased hair loss. The nails appear fragile with distal nail separation from the nail bed (onycholysis). There may be general or local muscle atrophy and acropachy (soft tissue swelling with underlying bone changes where new bone forms). There is a tachycardia with bounding pulse up to 160 beats per minute and down to 80 beats per minute during sleep. Pulse pressure is widened. There can be muscular weakness and atrophy, osteoporosis, and paralysis. There may be vi-

tiligo, which is characterized by milky-white patches on the skin surrounded by areas of normal pigmentation. There is decreased libido, impaired fertility, and **gynecomastia** (abnormal enlargement of one or both breasts in males).

Diagnostic tests generally include TSH, T_3, T_4, radioactive iodine uptake, and a thyroid scan.

One major complication is thyrotoxic crisis, also called *thyroid storm*. This is a medical emergency that can lead to cardiac, hepatic, or renal failure. Thyroid storm can be precipitated by stressful situations such as surgery, infection, or trauma. Less common causes are cerebrovascular accident (CVA), myocardial infarction, sudden discontinuing of antithyroid medications, subtotal thyroidectomy with excess intake of synthetic thyroid hormone, toxemia, or diabetic ketoacidosis. Any of these events can lead to overproduction of thyroid hormone which, in turn, causes an increase in systemic adrenergic activity. This causes an overproduction of epinephrine and severe hypermetabolism leading to rapid cardiac, gastrointestinal, and sympathetic nervous system decompensation. The client will exhibit severe and rapid clinical manifestations of hyperthyroidism.

If the nurse suspects that the client is experiencing thyrotoxic crisis, the physician must be informed immediately. The client will be transferred to intensive care for closer monitoring of vital signs, EKG pattern, and cardiopulmonary status. Antithyroid therapy will be initiated immediately. The client's temperature is monitored and cooling measures initiated as needed. Acetaminophen may be administered to lower the temperature, but aspirin will not be given since it could cause a further increase in the client's metabolic rate. Supportive care would be given until the client is out of the thyrotoxic crisis.

Medical–Surgical Management

Medical

The goal of managing hyperthyroidism is to decrease excessive thyroid hormone production. With treatment to decrease the thyroid production of its hormone, the prognosis is good. The client can live a normal life. There can be a combination of treatment methods. The first method is to administer antithyroid medications. This is usually a temporary solution.

LIFE CYCLE CONSIDERATIONS

Hyperthyroid Complications
The older client particularly develops cardiovascular problems such as arrhythmias (atrial fibrillation), cardiac insufficiency leading to cardiac decompensation, and resistance to the usual dose of digoxin.

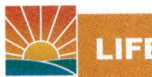

LIFE CYCLE CONSIDERATIONS

Radioactive Iodine

Pregnant females should not have this method of treatment since the radioactive iodine crosses the placenta to the fetus. Use with caution in children and adolescents because of the potential to develop cancer or leukemia in later years.

Radiation therapy of the thyroid gland could consist of external radiation to the neck; however, the more accepted method is the oral administration of a radioactive iodine, either liquid or capsule, that targets the thyroid tissue. It is most commonly used for the woman past the reproductive years or clients who do not plan to have children. If the client is of reproductive age, the client must sign an informed consent form since small amounts of the radioactive iodine could lodge in the gonads.

The client should stop taking antithyroid medications 4 to 7 days prior to treatment. The physician needs to be informed if the client is receiving amiodarone hydrochloride (Cordarone), an antiarrhythmic, because it contains large amounts of iodine. The oral ^{131}I should not be given to the client with severe vomiting or diarrhea.

This method involves a single dose of ^{131}I orally. It will destroy some iodine concentrating cells that produce the thyroxine. Clinical manifestations decrease in about 3 weeks with the full effect in about 3 months. Some clients may require a second or third dose.

Safety: Radioactive Iodine

No pregnant nurse should care for the client. The client should expectorate carefully for the first day since the saliva is radioactive. The client should drink plenty of fluids for 2 days to help circulate and eliminate the radioactive iodine. The toilet should be flushed twice after each use for at least 2 days or throughout the hospitalization. Disposable eating utensils should be used by the client. Close contact with children or pregnant females should be avoided for a week after the administration. Females should avoid pregnancy for 6 months after treatment.

The client usually resumes the thyroid hormone antagonist 3 to 5 days after ^{131}I therapy until the physician determines the thyroid to be atrophic (decreased in size). The physician may have the client continue to take propranolol hydrochloride (Inderal) for tachycardia, tremor, and diaphoresis. The client requires continued monitoring of thyroid hormone blood levels and physical condition.

The most common complication is hypothyroidism, which occurs about 2 to 4 months after treatment. The client is placed on thyroid replacement therapy, generally for life.

Surgical

Generally just a portion of the thyroid gland is removed, but a total thyroidectomy may be performed. This is the most expensive option and has the most risks. A thyroidectomy may also be done for respiratory obstruction by a goiter or thyroid cancer. If a partial thyroidectomy is done, the remaining thyroid tissue should provide adequate amounts of thyroid hormones. If a complete thyroidectomy is done, the client will require thyroid hormone replacement for a lifetime.

Preoperatively, the client should be given explanations concerning activities after surgery. There will be a neck incision generally with some type of drain. The client may experience a sore throat and hoarseness. The client probably has taken propylthiouracil PTU for 4 to 6 weeks prior to surgery. Iodine preparations may have been prescribed 10 to 14 days before surgery to decrease thyroid vascularity and decrease bleeding. Depending upon the symptoms of hyperthyroidism, the client may also be taking propranolol hydrochloride (Inderal). Thyroid function tests and an EKG would be performed before surgery to provide baseline information. Informed consent must be obtained.

After surgery, the client is placed in high-Fowler's position to promote venous drainage. The client should support the head with a hand when moving the head to prevent strain on the incision. Respiratory problems may occur. Respiratory obstruction can be a result of tracheal collapse, tracheal mucous accumulation, or laryngeal or local tissue edema. A tracheotomy tray or endotracheal tubes and insertion tray must be kept readily available at the client's bedside in case of a respiratory emergency.

Since the thyroid is so vascular, the dressing must be checked frequently for drainage, especially at the back of the neck for bleeding. If there is a drain, approximately 50 cc of drainage is expected the first day. If there is no drainage, the drain must be checked for kinks or obstruction of the tubing. The nurse should encourage voice rest for 48 hours with voice checks every 2 to 4 hours as ordered to make certain there is no laryngeal nerve damage.

Because the parathyroid glands could be accidentally removed during the thyroidectomy, the client's blood calcium level must be monitored. The client is checked for Chvostek's sign or Trousseau's sign. (These will be discussed more fully in hypoparathyroidism.) Analgesics are administered as needed.

Complications of thyroidectomy are respiratory distress and hemorrhage. There can be damage to the laryngeal nerves affecting the voice. Manipulation of the thyroid gland during surgery can cause a release of large amounts of thyroid hormone causing thyroid storm, which is rare but may occur. Thyroid crisis usually occurs within the first 12 hours postoperative. Hyperthyroid signs and symptoms are exaggerated plus the client may vomit, have severe hypertenison and tachycardia, and sometimes have hyperthermia up to 106°F (41°C). The client may develop congestive heart failure and die. The client must be advised that tetany can occur up to ten days after surgery. **Tetany** is sharp flexion of the wrist and ankle joints, muscle twitchings, or cramps caused by decreased blood calcium level.

Pharmacological

Antithyroid therapy is used for children, younger adults, pregnant females, the client who refuses surgery, or clients following surgery. There are several drugs that can be used for antithyroid therapy. Propylthiouracil (PTU) is used frequently, especially in cases of thyroid storm. It reduces the production of the thyroid hormones. It should be given with food. The client must be instructed to avoid foods high in iodine such as shellfish and iodized salt. Over-the-counter preparations must be checked to see if they contain iodine. This drug requires several weeks to exert the full effect and it may be administered up to 2 years. This drug may cause **agranulocytosis** (a decreased number of granulocytes) so it is important to report signs and symptoms of infection immediately to the physician.

Methimazole (Tapazole) is another antithyroid preparation that interferes with thyroid hormone synthesis. It has a more rapid onset than PTU; however, it does not have as much consistency in effect. It should be administered at evenly spaced intervals with food to prevent gastric upset. This drug can also cause agranulocytosis, particularly in the client over the age of 40.

Iodide preparations may be given to the client with hyperthyroidism. Because iodides inhibit the release of thyroid hormones rather than the synthesis, they take effect in 2 days. Two common preparations are potassium iodide saturated solution, SSKI, and a solution of iodine and potassium iodide that is called Lugol's solution. When iodide preparations are administered orally, they should be mixed with milk, juice, or water and given after meals to decrease gastric upset. Drinking the preparations through a straw will decrease discoloration of the teeth. These drugs are contraindicated

LIFE CYCLE CONSIDERATIONS

Pregnancy and Antithyroid Therapy Propylthiouracil and methimazole:

The minimum dosage should be prescribed to avoid fetal hypothyroidism. The drugs should not be given to a lactating mother.

PROFESSIONAL TIP

Hypersensitivity to Iodides
The first signs of hypersensitivity reactions caused by iodides are irritation and swollen eyelids.

in the client with acute bronchitis or a known hypersensitivity to iodine.

Clients may be prescribed propranolol hydrochloride (Inderal) to counteract tachycardia and peripheral effects of hyperthyroidism. Clients should not smoke while taking this medication. Abrupt withdrawal of the drug can cause hypertension, myocardial ischemia, or cardiac arrhythmias. Clients should rise slowly from a sitting or lying position in order to prevent orthostatic hypotension.

Topical medications such as isotonic eye drops may be ordered to protect the eyes of the client with exophthalmos. Care must be taken that the eyes are not injured or infected. Some physicians may order high doses of corticosteroids to help reduce exophthalmos.

During a thyrotoxic crisis, antithyroid drugs are given. Other medications that may be used are propranolol, corticosteroids, and iodine preparations. Individual client needs could indicate a need for vitamins, nutrients, fluids, or sedation.

Diet

Since the client has a greatly increased metabolic rate as well as weight loss, diet is a consideration. The client may require between 4,000 to 5,000 calories per day. There is a need for increased protein, vitamins (especially vitamins B and C), and minerals. In addition to 3 meals a day, the client will need additional meals or snacks. Fluids should be encouraged, but caffeine should be avoided.

▶ NURSING PROCESS

▶ Assessment

▶ Subjective Data

The nurse must obtain a thorough client history and ask about the ability to concentrate, nervousness, insomnia, jitteriness, excitability, emotional lability, or dysphagia.

▶ Objective Data

The nurse will assess for rapid pulse, elevated blood pressure, warm skin, elevated temperature, diaphoresis, or hand tremors. Female clients may cease to menstruate. Hair is fine and soft.

Nursing diagnoses for a client with hyperthyroidism may include the following:

Nursing Diagnoses	Planning/Goals	Nursing Interventions
Preoperative		
▶ *Nutrition, Altered, less than body requirements related to increased metabolism*	The client will eat a nutritionally balanced diet with enough calories to prevent weight loss.	Arrange a consultation with the dietitian to assist in determining the client's increased nutritional needs. Provide snacks throughout the day. Encourage client to eat a well-balanced diet.
▶ *Injury, Risk for, related to exophthalmos*	The client's eyes will not be injured from exophthalmos.	Administer isotonic solutions or eye lubricants to keep the eye moist. At night, elevate head of the bed which may assist in keeping the eyelids closed, or the eyes may be taped shut to prevent drying. Suggest to client that dark or tinted wraparound glasses may protect the eyes from wind and airborne particles.
Postoperative		
▶ *Swallowing, Impaired, related to mechanical obstruction (edema)*	The client will have diminished problems with swallowing.	Ensure gag, cough, and swallowing reflexes are present before offering oral fluids. Encourage client to drink slowly and chew thoroughly. Maintain client in Fowler's position when drinking or eating.
▶ *Airway Clearance, Ineffective, related to edema and pain*	The client will be able to clear airway.	Keep suctioning equipment ready. Administer analgesic as ordered.

Evaluation Each goal must be evaluated to determine how it has been met by the client.

SAMPLE NURSING CARE PLAN

THE CLIENT WITH HYPERTHYROIDISM

Janey Jackson, 33 years old, has returned to her physician's office to find out results of her tests for hyperthyroidism. She continues to have multiple complaints. "I have lost fifteen pounds in the last month despite eating all the time. I am restless and can't sleep. I feel jittery and irritable. My family says my moods change so rapidly they don't know what to expect from me. I feel so hot most of the time and sweat a lot."

The office nurse notes Mrs. Jackson appears flushed and her eyes protrude slightly. Her vital signs, T.-100.6 orally, P.-120, R.-26, and B/P.-140/88, are slightly elevated from her previous office visit. Her test results confirm that she has hyperthyroidism.

Nursing Diagnosis 1 *Nutrition, Altered, less than body requirements related to increased metabolism as evidenced by weight loss despite eating*

PLANNING/GOALS	NURSING INTERVENTIONS	RATIONALE	EVALUATION
Mrs. Jackson will eat a nutritionally balanced diet with enough calories to prevent weight loss.	Monitor amount of food ingested and caloric intake.	Provides data to determine if diet is adequate to prevent weight loss.	Mrs. Jackson gained or maintained weight.
	Monitor weight daily.	Determines weight gains or losses.	
	Provide a diet high in calories, protein, and carbohydrates.	Maintains or increases weight while preventing muscle mass break-	

continued

Advise Mrs. Jackson to avoid highly seasoned or fibrous foods or foods causing flatulence.

Provide small frequent meals spread over waking hours.

Obtain nutritional consult as needed.

down, yet providing adequate energy.

Gas accumulation is common and could cause increased peristalsis resulting in diarrhea.

Provides adequate calories without extremely large meals.

Assists with meal planning to ensure nutritional status while considering personal food preferences.

Nursing Diagnosis 2 *Hyperthermia related to increased metabolic rate as evidenced by complaints of feeling hot, flushing, and elevated temperature*

PLANNING/GOALS	NURSING INTERVENTIONS	RATIONALE	EVALUATION
Mrs. Jackson's body temperature will be within normal range.	Assess for elevated temperature, heat intolerance, and diaphoresis.	Indicates increased heat production from increased metabolic rate.	Mrs. Jackson maintained her temperature in a normal range.
	Provide a well-ventilated room with temperature controlled to coolness for comfort.	Promotes comfort if heat intolerant.	
	Suggest wearing cool loose-fitting lightweight clothing.	Provides comfort and prevents overheating.	
	Provide frequent bathing and changes in linens or clothing.	Promotes comfort if diaphoretic.	
	Provide fluids up to 3 liters per day.	Replaces fluid if diaphoretic.	

Nursing Diagnosis 3 *Skin Integrity, Impaired, Risk for, related to diaphoresis as evidenced by excessive sweating*

PLANNING/GOALS	NURSING INTERVENTIONS	RATIONALE	EVALUATION
Mrs. Jackson's skin will remain intact and free of injury.	Assess skin for flushing and moisture.	Indicates heat intolerance.	Mrs. Jackson maintained an intact skin without impairment.
	Monitor skin for redness or breakdown, especially bony prominences.	Indicates potential for breakdown.	
	Keep Mrs. Jackson clean and dry.	Prevents skin breakdown.	

HYPOTHYROIDISM

Hypothyroidism is a condition in which the metabolic processes are decreased because of a deficiency of the thyroid hormone. It is termed primary if the problem arises from a dysfunction solely of the thyroid. It is secondary if the thyroid gland is not stimulated to produce normally or if the target cells fail to respond to normal thyroid functioning. This condition is more common in females than males. There is a significant increase in incidence between the ages of 30 to 60. Hypothyroid conditions include cretinism, myxedema, and Hashimoto's thyroiditis.

CRETINISM

A congenital condition due to a lack of thyroid hormones causes defective physical development and mental retardation. This is called **cretinism**. This occurs in about 1 of 4,000 live births. The child generally has a large head, short limbs, puffy eyes, thick and protruding tongue, excessively dry skin, and a lack of coordination. If untreated, the child will be permanently dwarfed, mentally retarded, and sterile. This condition is rare in the United States and is tested by the T_4.

MYXEDEMA

Myxedema is the term for severe hypothyroidism in adults. There are a variety of abnormalities that lead to decreased thyroid hormone production. The obvious ones are thyroid gland surgery such as thyroidectomy or irradiation of the thyroid gland. Some other causes are chronic autoimmune Hashimoto's thyroiditis, inflammatory conditions (sarcoidosis), pituitary failure to produce TSH, or hypothalamus failure to produce thyrotropin-releasing hormone. There may be an inability to synthesize thyroid hormones related to iodine deficiency (rarely from general diet deficiency) or as a result of taking antithyroid medications.

Clinical manifestations are vague and varied, developing slowly over a period of time, but are primarily related to the reduced metabolic rate. These include an energy loss, fatigue, forgetfulness, sensitivity to cold, unexplained weight gain, hypoventilation, and constipation. As the condition progresses, manifestations include reduced libido, menorrhagia, paresthesias, joint stiffness, and muscle cramping. There is a characteristic alteration in overall appearance and behavior including decreased mental stability and a thick and dry tongue, causing hoarseness and slow, slurred speech. The skin is flaky and inelastic, feels cool, dry, rough, and doughy. There is edema of the face, hands, and feet. The hair is dry and sparse, with patchy hair loss including loss of outer third of the eyebrow. The nails are thick and brittle with visible transverse and longitudinal grooves. The pulse is weak and bradycardic due to the decreased pumping strength of the heart. The thyroid gland may be so small that it may not be palpated unless there is a goiter. The blood pressure is generally lower than normal for the client.

Diagnostic tests generally include: TSH, T_3, T_4, radioactive iodine uptake, and a thyroid scan.

Complications affect almost every system. Cardiovascular complications include ischemic heart disease, poor peripheral circulation, enlarged heart, or pleural or pericardial effusion. Gastrointestinal complications include adynamic colon (decreased functioning of the colon), megacolon (massive and abnormal dilation of the colon), or intestinal obstruction. Other complications include conductive or sensorineural deafness, psychiatric disorders, carpal tunnel syndrome, or impotence or infertility. Prognosis depends upon the organs involved, duration, and severity of condition.

Myxedema coma or hypothyroid crisis is a serious complication of extreme hypothyroidism. It is life threatening. It is characterized by severe metabolic disorders, hypothermia, and cardiovascular collapse leading to coma. It has a gradual onset but is triggered by severe stress such as infection, exposure to cold, or trauma. Abrupt withdrawal of thyroid medication or the use of narcotics, sedatives, or anesthetics can also cause myxedema coma. If myxedema coma occurs, it must be reported to the physician immediately. The client would be moved to the intensive care unit. Intubation and mechanical ventilation are instituted (Young, 1999). The client will be monitored closely for vital signs, EKG changes, and cardiopulmonary status. Wrapping the client in blankets will warm the client, but a warming blanket should not be used as it could cause peripheral vasodilation and shock. Thyroid medications and possibly corticosteroids would be administered. Supportive care would be given until the client comes out of the myxedema coma. Myxedema coma is often fatal.

Medical–Surgical Management

Pharmacological

Thyroid replacement therapy lasts a lifetime. Thyroid (Armour Thyroid) is a natural form while levothyroxine sodium (Levothroid, Synthroid) is a synthetic. The physician will order thyroid hormone to begin slowly and increase the dosage every 2 to 3 weeks until the desired response is achieved. The medication should be given in 1 dose in the morning to prevent insomnia.

If the client has diabetes mellitus, insulin or oral hypoglycemic dosage might have to be adjusted. The blood sugar level must be monitored closely. If the client is on anticoagulant therapy, thyroid hormones potentiate the anticoagulant action. The client needs to be informed to watch for excessive bleeding or bruising. Digitalis preparations are also potentiated by thyroid hormone.

Because hypothyroidism impairs the metabolic rate, the client may have difficulty metabolizing medications. The client may have an increased sensitivity to hypnotics, sedatives, or opiates. Dosage may have to be adjusted appropriately. Synthesis of the thyroid hormone can be impaired by drugs such as lithium carbonate (Lithotabs) or aminoglutethimide (Cytadren).

Diet

The client should be instructed to avoid foods high in iodine and foods that interfere with thyroid hormone replacement. These include dried kelp, shellfish, iodized salt, saltwater fish, cabbage, turnips, pears, and peaches. The diet is designed to increase weight loss and combat constipation. A high-fiber, high-protein, low-calorie diet is given. Sodium should be decreased to prevent fluid retention. A dietary consultation for meal planning and a list of foods to avoid should be provided to the client.

▶ NURSING PROCESS

▶ Assessment

▶ Subjective Data

Obtain a thorough client history and ask about lethargy, depression, irritability, impaired memory, and slowing of thought processes. The client may describe speech and hearing problems, anorexia, decreased libido, and constipation.

▶ Objective Data

Assess for hearing and speech deficits, thin hair, dry and thickened skin, enlarged facial features, masklike expression, low and hoarse voice, bradycardia, decreased blood pressure and respirations, and exercise intolerance.

Nursing diagnoses for the client with myxedema may include the following:

Nursing Diagnoses	Planning/Goals	Nursing Interventions
▶ *Activity Intolerance related to decreased metabolic and energy level*	The client will express understanding for the need to increase activity level gradually.	Assist the client to gradually increase activity level but encourage rest between activities to avoid fatigue and decrease cardiac oxygen demands.
	The client will maintain blood pressure, pulse, and respirations within normal limits when active.	Measure the client's legs correctly so antiembolic hose, which help venous return, will fit properly when worn.
	The client will regain and maintain normal activity levels.	Reposition client every 2 hours and encourage client to continue activity when normal activity level is achieved.
▶ *Tissue Perfusion, Altered, cardiopulmonary related to decreased cardiac output*	The client will not have chest pain at rest.	Assess for chest pain and advise client to report any episodes of angina immediately.
	The client will have a normal heart rate and rhythm.	Monitor the client's vital signs.
	The client will avoid ischemic EKG changes.	Monitor cardiac status through EKG and assessment of heart and lung sounds plus checking for edema.
	The client will maintain adequate cardiopulmonary perfusion.	Restrict fluid and sodium during the time of cardiac decompensation as ordered. Monitor intake and output and weight.
▶ *Constipation related to decreased motility of the gastrointestinal tract*	The client will have a regular bowel movement.	Provide high-fiber diet.
		Encourage intake of oral fluids.
		Assess frequency and character of stool.
		Administer stool softener, bulk laxative, or enema as ordered.

Evaluation Each goal must be evaluated to determine how it has been met by the client.

HASHIMOTO'S THYROIDITIS

Hashimoto's thyroiditis is an autoimmune disease characterized by the production of antiperoxidase antibodies which destroy an essential enzyme necessary for production of T_3 and T_4. The disease occurs more often in females than in males, between the ages of 30 and 50, and shows a marked hereditary pattern. There is an increased incidence in clients with Down syndrome and Turner's syndrome.

Clinical manifestations include a thyroid that is enlarged and has a lumpy surface. Generally the goiter is asymptomatic, but it could cause dysphagia and a feeling of local pressure. The thymus gland is also enlarged. Other clinical manifestations are similar to hypothyroidism.

Treatment of Hashimoto's thyroiditis is also similar to that of hypothyroidism. Thyroid hormone replacement is used. This is a chronic disorder that can be treated, but not cured. The client will be on lifetime thyroid hormone replacement.

THYROID TUMORS

There are several neoplasms of the thyroid gland. The benign thyroid cyst and adenoma are firm, encapsulated, noninvasive, slowly growing neoplasms of unknown etiology. Diagnosis of benign neoplasms is done by needle biopsy. These growths tend to be nonfunctioning (not affecting the functioning of the thyroid gland) so there is no treatment other than continued monitoring. If the adenoma is functioning (increasing the functioning of the thyroid gland), then it is treated by radioactive iodine or surgery.

CANCER OF THE THYROID

Cancer of the thyroid is rare and occurs in all age groups. Individuals who have had radiation therapy to the neck are more susceptible. There are 4 major types of thyroid cancer:

- Papillary carcinoma is the most common type. It can affect any age but is more common in females of childbearing age. It is well-differentiated, grows slowly, is usually contained and does not spread beyond the adjacent lymph nodes. Cure rate after thyroidectomy is excellent.
- Follicular carcinoma metastasizes to the regional lymph nodes and spreads through the blood vessels to the bone, liver, and lungs. It has a very low cure rate.
- Medullary carcinoma is a solid carcinoma associated with pheochromocytoma. It is curable if detected before signs and symptoms occur. Without treat-

ment, it grows rapidly, metastasizing to the bones, liver, and kidneys.
- Anaplastic or undifferentiated carcinoma resists radiation. It is almost never curable by resection. It metastasizes rapidly, generally causing death by invasion of the trachea and adjacent structures. It generally affects individuals over the age of 60.

Since there is no known cause of cancer, there are several risk factors. They are radiation exposure, especially in those children and adolescents who received radiation therapy to treat severe cases of acne vulgaris, or to shrink enlarged tonsils, adenoids, and thymus tissue; prolonged secretion of TSH resulting from radiation or heredity; familial disposition; or chronic goiter.

The first clinical manifestation is a painless lump. As it enlarges, it destroys the thyroid which leads to clinical manifestations of hypothyroidism. Although rare, the tumor could trigger excessive thyroid hormone production causing the client to display the clinical manifestations of hyperthyroidism. There can be dysphagia, hoarseness, and vocal stridor. There may be a detectable, disfiguring thyroid mass with a firm nodule on palpation.

The thyroid scan shows a "cold" nodule (decreased uptake of ^{131}I) for papillary carcinoma. Follicular carcinoma and benign adenomas show a "hot" nodule. Thyroid function tests are usually normal. A needle biopsy may be done to confirm diagnosis.

Medical–Surgical Management

Surgical

All carcinomas can be treated with surgery (discussed previously). Radioactive iodine or external radiation therapy may also be used. Response of the tumor will depend upon early diagnosis and treatment. These methods of treatment may be used individually or in combination. Client care is the same as for hyperthyroidism.

Pharmacological

Exogenous thyroid hormone may suppress thyroid activity. To increase tolerance to surgery or radiation therapy, the physician may prescribe simultaneous exogenous thyroid hormone and adrenergic blocker such as propranolol hydrochloride (Inderal). If there is widespread metastasis, the cancers will be treated with neoplastic chemotherapy.

Nursing Management

The nurse will monitor the client's level of anxiety and encourage the client to discuss feelings about the diagnosis and possible surgery. The nurse will also assist the client in identifying previously successful coping methods, and teach new coping methods if needed.

GOITER

A goiter is an enlargement of the thyroid unrelated to inflammation or neoplasm. There are three types of goiter. One type is a diffuse toxic goiter found in hyperthyroidism. This type of goiter may be moderate to massively enlarged. The consistency varies from soft to firm and rubbery. It generally feels smooth. Frequently it is associated with exophthalmos.

Another type of goiter is a simple nontoxic goiter. It develops when the thyroid is unable to utilize iodine properly or in response to a low iodine level in the blood. These goiters are more common in females. They develop during times of great metabolic demands such as adolescence or pregnancy. A deficiency of iodine can cause goiter formation. Clinical manifestations depend upon the size of the goiter. There is an obvious enlargement of the thyroid gland. A large goiter can compress the esophagus or trachea causing dysphagia, a choking sensation, or respiratory difficulty. If the goiter impairs venous return from the head and neck, the client may experience dizziness and syncope.

Diagnosis is based on history, clinical manifestations, and results of thyroid function tests. T_3 is generally very low. Treatment concentrates on the underlying cause. This may involve thyroid hormone replacement therapy or prescribing iodine supplements or increasing dietary iodine sources. Surgery is done when respiration or swallowing is impaired or for cosmetic effect.

The third type of goiter is the nodular goiter. It is similar to the simple goiter except that palpation reveals multiple nodules causing the enlargement. It is found frequently in females over 40. It usually is asymptomatic. Treatment varies with the client's age and clinical manifestations.

PARATHYROID DISORDERS

Disorders discussed include hyperparathyroidism and hypoparathyroidism.

HYPERPARATHYROIDISM

Hyperparathyroidism is a condition resulting from overactivity of one or more of the parathyroid glands. It results in increased secretion of parathyroid hormone (PTH), which causes calcium to leave the bones and accumulate in the blood. This cannot be compensated by renal excretion or uptake into the soft tissues. It occurs twice as often in postmenopausal females than males. It occurs frequently between the ages of 35 and 65. Hypercalcemia may also be caused by excessive intake of thiazide diuretics, vitamin D, or calcium supplements.

X-rays will show skeletal decalcification. Blood PTH and alkaline phosphate levels are increased. Serum calcium level is elevated.

It is termed primary if there is an enlargement of one or more of the parathyroid glands increasing secretion of PTH and thus increasing the blood calcium level. The most common cause is adenoma, but other primary causes include genetics or multiple endocrine neoplasms.

The condition is termed secondary if there is excess compensatory production of PTH stemming from a hypocalcemia-producing abnormality other than the parathyroid gland. Some of these abnormalities are rickets, chronic renal failure, vitamin D deficiency, or osteomalacia due to laxative abuse or phenytoin (Dilantin).

Many clients are asymptomatic; however, there are several clinical manifestations. The client may have polyuria, chronic low back pain, bone tenderness, or renal calculi. The client may also experience nausea, vomiting, anorexia, constipation, lethargy, or drowsiness. There can be changes in level of consciousness, disorientation, stupor, coma, or personality changes with a loss of initiative and memory. There may be marked muscle weakness and atrophy especially of the legs, joint hyperextensibility, long bone skeletal deformity, or hyporeflexia.

Without treatment, there can be permanent damage to the skeleton or kidneys. There can be bone and articular problems including pathologic fractures. Renal complications include colic, nephrolithiasis, urinary tract infection, and renal insufficiency leading to chronic renal failure. Other complications may be stone formation in various organs, cardiac or vascular problems, or central nervous system changes.

Medical–Surgical Management

Medical

Medical management is aimed at decreasing overactivity of the parathyroid glands. This may be accomplished by medication therapy or surgery. If there is severe renal involvement, the client may require dialysis.

Surgical

Primary hyperparathyroidism can be treated by surgical removal of three and one-half of the four parathyroid glands. Surgery can relieve bone pain in 3 days but may not reverse renal damage.

Preoperative care includes explanations, encouraging fluids, limiting calcium intake, and administering medications to lower the blood calcium level.

Postoperative care involves administration of magnesium or phosphate. The client may receive calcium supplements for several days. The nursing care is similar to that provided to the client with thyroidectomy (refer to hyperthyroidism). A major complication is airway obstruction.

Pharmacological

Pharmacological treatment is aimed toward correcting secondary hyperparathyroidism. This involves treating the underlying cause. Since hypercalcemia is a major manifestation, medications are geared to decrease the calcium level in the blood. This includes the use of diuretics such as furosemide (Lasix) and ethacrynic acid (Edecrin).

Other drugs that decrease the calcium level in the blood are calcitonin-human (Cibacalcin), plicamycin (Mithracin), and magnesium- or phosphate-based drugs. Phosphate-based drugs lower the calcium level based on the inverse relationship between phosphorus and calcium.

▶ NURSING PROCESS

▶ Assessment
▶ Subjective Data

The nurse should obtain a thorough client history and ask about muscle weakness, apathy, nausea, mental status, and pain (low back or renal). The client is assessed for increased calcium intake, either dietary or supplements.

▶ Objective Data

Fatigue, drowsiness, anorexia, constipation, personality changes, renal colic, skeletal deformity, output, hematuria, vomiting, weight loss, hypertension, bradycardia, or dysrhythmias should all be noted.

Nursing diagnoses for the client with hyperparathyroidism may include the following:

Nursing Diagnoses	Planning/Goals	Nursing Interventions
▶ Activity Intolerance related to generalized weakness caused by neuromuscular dysfunction	The client will regain and maintain normal muscle mass and strength, maintain maximum joint range of motion, and perform self-care activity as tolerated.	Alternate rest and activity periods. Assist client with prescribed, individualized activities. Assist client to identify factors that increase or decrease activity intolerance. Encourage client to perform self-care.
▶ Pain related to musculoskeletal changes resulting from persistently increased serum calcium level	The client will express relief after analgesics, use comfort measures to decrease pain, and be pain-free when serum calcium level reaches normal.	Administer analgesics as ordered. Provide comfort measures for bone pain, and include turning and repositioning every 2 hours. Assess pain level and compare to serum calcium level. Assess environment for hazards and eliminate them. Assist the client to ambulate. Maintain the bed in a low position with siderails up and call light in reach. Lift and move the client gently to prevent pathologic fractures.

Evaluation Each goal must be evaluated to determine how it has been met by the client.

HYPOPARATHYROIDISM

Hypoparathyroidism is a condition resulting from a deficiency of parathyroid hormone (PTH) secretion by the parathyroids or the decreased action of peripheral PTH. Since the parathyroids normally regulate the serum calcium level, hypoparathyroidism will result in a decreased serum calcium level. PTH normally maintains the serum calcium level by increasing bone resorption and gastric reabsorption. It also maintains the inverse relationship between calcium and phosphorus levels. Hypoparathyroidism can be acute or chronic.

If hypoparathyroidism is idiopathic, it may be the result of an autoimmune disorder or congenital absence of parathyroid glands. Acquired hypoparathyroidism is generally irreversible. The most common cause is accidental removal during thyroid or other neck surgery. It could also be a result of ischemic infarction during surgery, sarcoidosis, tuberculosis, neoplasms, trauma, or massive thyroid irradiation. Reversible hypoparathyroidism can result from hypomagnesemia-induced impairment of hormone synthesis, suppression of normal gland function because of hypercalcemia, or delayed maturation of the parathyroid glands.

The characteristic sign of hypoparathyroidism is tetany, which is muscle spasms and tremors caused by a lack of calcium. Other clinical manifestations include dry skin, brittle hair, alopecia (loss of hair or baldness), and loss of eyelashes and fingernails. The teeth are stained, cracked, and decayed due to weak enamel. The client may have altered neuromuscular irritability, tingling and twitching of the face and hands, and increased deep tendon reflexes. There may be personality changes or EKG changes.

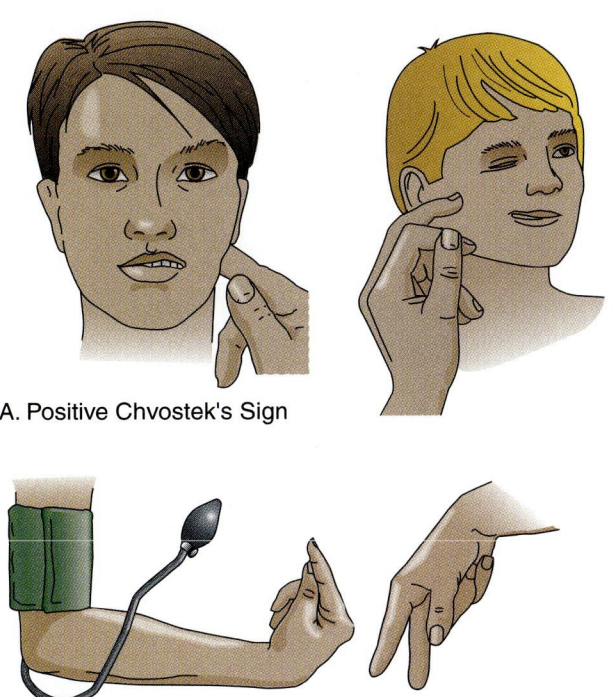

A. Positive Chvostek's Sign

B. Positive Trousseau's Sign

Figure 37-11 Signs of Hypocalcemia and Hypoparathyroidism: A. Chvostek's sign; B. Trousseau's sign

There are two diagnostic assessment tests that can be performed. One is the **Chvostek's sign**, which is an abnormal spasm of the facial muscles in response to a light tapping of the facial nerve. The other test is **Trousseau's sign**, which is a carpal spasm caused by inflating a blood pressure cuff above the client's systolic pressure and leaving it in place for 3 minutes (Figure 37-11).

Expected test results include: decreased serum calcium, increased urinary calcium, increased serum phosphorus, and decreased urinary phosphorus.

Complications are related to long-standing hypocalcemia. This leads to decreased heart contractility leading to cardiac failure. There can be cataract formation or papillary edema from increased intracranial pressure. There may be bone deformity. In cases of severe tetany, the client can experience laryngospasm, respiratory stridor, anoxia, paralysis of vocal cords, and death.

Medical–Surgical Management

Pharmacological

Calcium gluconate or calcium chloride may be given intravenously. Give very slowly since it is very irritating to the vessel wall. Too rapid IV calcium infu-

LIFE-CYCLE CONSIDERATIONS

Hypoparathyroidism
A child may have mental retardation, stunted growth, and malformed teeth.

sion can cause cardiac arrest. After the initial IV dose, calcium may be given orally.

Unless the hypoparathyroidism is reversible, the client will require lifelong calcium replacement. Vitamin D may also be given to assist in the absorption of calcium. The calcium supplements should be given 1 to 1½ hours after meals to increase absorption. If the client cannot swallow the large tablets, they can be dissolved in hot water and the suspension cooled before administering to the client. The best sources of calcium are from the diet. The client needs to take calcium as ordered and not abruptly stop taking the drug. The client must be advised that calcium may cause digitalis toxicity. Cimetidine (Tagamet) interferes with normal parathyroid functioning.

Diet

The diet should be high in calcium and low in phosphorus containing foods. Since many foods that are high in calcium are also high in phosphorus, the client should be given a list of foods that are high in calcium but lower in phosphorus. Foods on this list include vegetables such as asparagus, broccoli, collards, and tomatoes; fruits such as apricots, bananas, cantaloupe, and many berries; and other foods such as kidney beans, lima beans, and brown sugar. Foods that have a high phosphorus content and should be avoided include: most legumes, nuts, cheeses, and seafood.

▸ NURSING PROCESS

▸ Assessment

▸ Subjective Data

The nurse will obtain a thorough client history and ask the client about recent surgery or irradiation, use of alcohol, numbness or tingling of the skin, anxiety, headache, irritability, depression, or nausea.

▸ Objective Data

The nurse will assess for dysphagia, laryngeal spasm, stridor, cyanosis, or dysrhythmias, and also check for Chvostek's sign and Trousseau's sign.

Nursing diagnoses for the client with hypoparathyroidism may include the following:

Nursing Diagnoses	Planning/Goals	Nursing Interventions
▶ *Injury, Risk for, related to calcium deficiency*	The client will not exhibit signs and symptoms of tetany, and will prevent injury from hypocalcemia.	Monitor Chvostek's and Trousseau's signs, serum calcium and phosphorus levels, as well as EKG changes.
		Keep tracheotomy tray readily available and maintain seizure precautions.
		Support the client while walking to prevent injury.
		Monitor the client taking digoxin for toxicity.
▶ *Nutrition, Altered, less than body requirements, related to calcium intake*	The client will have adequate calcium intake.	Provide diet with calcium-rich foods.
		Give calcium replacement as ordered. The client who is taking digoxin must be monitored for toxicity.

Evaluation Each goal must be evaluated to determine how it has been met by the client.

ADRENAL DISORDERS

Disorders in this category include Cushing's disease/syndrome, Addison's disease, and pheochromocytoma.

CUSHING'S DISEASE/SYNDROME (ADRENAL HYPERFUNCTION)

Cushing's *disease,* primary adrenal hyperfunction, is the result of increased pituitary secretion of ACTH which causes an increased production of cortisol by the adrenal cortex. Cushing's *syndrome* refers to symptoms of cortisol excess caused by other factors. One cause is a corticotropin producing tumor in another organ such as oat-cell carcinoma of the lung (secondary adrenal hyperfunction). The most common cause of Cushing's syndrome is prolonged used of glucocorticoid or corticotropin medications for chronic inflammatory disorders such as chronic obstructive pulmonary disease, Crohn's disease, and rheumatoid arthritis. This is **iatrogenic** (caused by treatment or diagnostic procedures) adrenal hyperfunction.

Cushing's syndrome occurs in females more than males, generally between 30 and 50 years of age.

Classic clinical manifestations are adiposity of the face, neck, and trunk which give rise to the moon-shaped face and buffalo hump (Figure 37-12). Others include purple striae on the abdomen, hirsutism, and thin extremities due to muscle wasting. Boys exhibit an early onset of puberty, while girls exhibit development of masculine characteristics. The client may complain of fatigue, muscle weakness, sleep disturbances, water retention, amenorrhea, decreased libido, irritability, and emotional lability. There could be petechiae, ecchymoses, decreased wound healing, or swollen ankles.

There are multiple complications of Cushing's syndrome, most of which are produced by the stimulating and catabolic effects of cortisol. There can be increased calcium resorption from the bone leading to osteoporosis and pathologic fractures. It can cause increased hepatic gluconeogenesis and insulin resistance causing glucose intolerance and diabetes mellitus. The client may have frequent infections and slowed wound healing. There is a suppressed inflammatory response that can mask severe infections. The client may have decreased ability to handle stress, which can lead to psychological problems from mood swings to psychosis. Other complications include hypertension, ischemic heart disease, congestive heart failure, menstrual disturbances, and sexual dysfunction.

Plasma cortisol level is elevated. Plasma ACTH level may be elevated or low. Adrenalangiography is done for adrenal tumor. Twenty-four-hour urine tests for 17-ketosteroids and 17-hydroxysteroids are elevated.

Prognosis depends upon early diagnosis, identifying the underlying cause, and effective treatment. Without treatment, about half of these clients will die within 5 years.

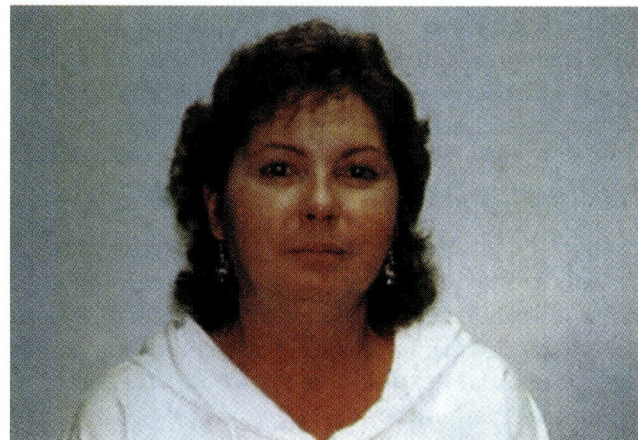

Figure 37-12 A Client with Cushing's Syndrome: Untreated *(Photo courtesy of Dr. Matthew Leinuing, Acting Head, Division of Endocrinology, Albany Medical College, Albany, NY)*

Medical–Surgical Management

Medical

The major goal is to restore hormone balance. Treatment is based on the causative factor. This is accomplished primarily by medications. If there is adrenal cancer, the client may either have radiation therapy to the adrenal gland or surgery on either the pituitary gland or the adrenal glands, or all three treatments.

Surgical

If the underlying cause of Cushing's syndrome is related to the pituitary gland, the client may have a hypophysectomy done. (Refer to hypophysectomy in the section on hyperpituitarism.)

For an adrenal tumor, an adrenalectomy is performed. This could be unilateral or bilateral. During the first 24 to 48 hours after surgery, the client is observed closely for hemorrhage and shock. Vital signs and urine output must be monitored. Glucocorticoids are administered with changing dosage until a maintenance dose is established. The client's blood glucose level must be monitored, especially for hypoglycemia.

Pharmacological

Aminoglutethimide (Cytadren) inhibits synthesis of adrenal steroids. It can cause dizziness or drowsiness. The client should be instructed to avoid activities requiring mental alertness or manual dexterity.

Ketoconazole (Nizoral), while classified as an antifungal, inhibits adrenal steroidogenesis and is used in Cushing's syndrome.

Mitotane (Lysodren) directly suppresses the activity of the adrenal cortex. This cytotoxic agent is generally used for inoperable adrenal cortex cancer. It is given for at least 3 months. The client should avoid situations that cause injury or exposure to infections.

If the client had pituitary or adrenal surgery, cortisol therapy may be given before and after surgery to decrease physical stress. Steroid therapy could be a lifetime situation. The client should take the drug with food or antacids to decrease gastric distress. Two-thirds dose of the steroids should be taken in the morning with the remaining one-third in the early evening to mimic the body's diurnal schedule. Steroids can lead to osteoporosis and the possibility of pathologic fractures.

LIFE CYCLE CONSIDERATIONS

Steroids

Females should be warned that steroid use can interfere with oral contraceptive effectiveness. There may be an adverse effect on the male's sperm production and count.

HOME HEALTH CARE

Cushing's Syndrome

- Carry Medic Alert medal indicating Cushing's syndrome.
- Avoid extreme temperature changes, activities that could result in trauma, and people with infections.
- Wash hands often.
- Protect skin with good care.
- Maintain medication regimen.
- Notify physician if weakness, fainting, fever, nausea, or vomiting occur.

The client with diabetes mellitus may have to adjust insulin dosage because the steroids can affect the glucose levels. Steroids can mask severe infections and cause some immunosuppression. Wounds are slower to heal. The client should be instructed to contact a physician before using over-the-counter preparations. The client should not abruptly discontinue the steroid drug; dosage should be tapered before discontinuing.

Diet

The diet should be high in protein and potassium but low in sodium. Foods high in protein include: eggs, milk, whole grains, legumes, and meat; however, milk, cheeses, and whole grains are also high in sodium, depending upon processing. Many foods high in potassium are also low in sodium. These foods are: legumes; fruits such as figs, oranges, bananas, prunes, and raisins; and vegetables such as avocado, potato, and spinach. The client should be advised to read labels for sodium content. Processed foods and many preservatives have high sodium content and should be avoided. Reduced carbohydrates and calories help control hyperglycemia.

▶ NURSING PROCESS

▶ Assessment

▶ Subjective Data

The nurse should obtain a thorough client history and ask about the use of steroids, stress, methods of coping with stress, irritability, depression, mood swings, loss of libido, and the possibility of suicide.

▶ Objective Data

The client is assessed for thin and fragile skin, petechiae, ecchymoses, delayed wound healing, weight gain, increased abdominal girth, purple striae, hyperglycemia, and hypokalemia. Women may have **hirsutism** (excessive body hair in a masculine distribution), deepening of the voice, and menstrual irregularities.

Nursing diagnoses for the client with Cushing's syndrome may include the following:

Nursing Diagnoses	Planning/Goals	Nursing Interventions
▶ *Body Image Disturbance related to changes in physical appearance*	The client will verbalize feelings about changed appearance.	Encourage the client to verbalize feelings about changed body image. Offer emotional support and a positive realistic assessment of the condition.
▶ *Infection, Risk for, related to suppressed inflammatory response from excessive corticosteroid production*	The client will take precautions to avoid or decrease exposure to infection.	Advise client to avoid people with infections. Provide a private room with reverse or protective isolation as indicated. Monitor the client's vital signs, intake and output, and weight.

Evaluation Each goal must be evaluated to determine how it has been met by the client.

ADDISON'S DISEASE (ADRENAL HYPOFUNCTION)

Addison's disease, primary hypofunctioning of the adrenals, involves decreased functioning of the adrenal cortex and its secretions—mineralocorticoids, glucocorticoids, and androgens. It can also be called *adrenal hypofunction* or *insufficiency*. It is fairly uncommon, occurring in one per 100,000 people in the United States. Although it affects all ages and both sexes, it is less common among the elderly.

Addison's disease occurs when more than 90% of the adrenal gland is destroyed. It is an autoimmune disease in response to conditions such as tuberculosis, histoplasmosis, HIV, and meningococcal pneumonia. It can be caused by bilateral adrenalectomy, hemorrhage into the adrenal gland related to anticoagulant therapy, or cancer of the adrenal gland. It is termed secondary if it results from decreased pituitary or hypothalamus function or abrupt withdrawal of long-term steroid therapy.

A classical clinical manifestation of Addison's disease is a bronze coloration of the skin resembling a deep suntan, especially in the creases on the hands, elbows, and knees. There may be some areas of vitiglio. The client may complain of fatigue, muscle weakness, lightheadedness upon rising, weight loss, and craving for salty foods. The client may have decreased tolerance even to minor stress. The client is anxious, irritable, and may become confused. The pulse may be weak and irregular. There is hypotension and a variety of GI complaints.

The acute form is called adrenal crisis. It may occur when there is trauma, surgery, other physiologic stress, or abrupt withdrawal of steroids. The clinical manifestations are the same only more severe with a rapid onset. The crisis requires immediate treatment. The client will be placed on intravenous therapy and IV administration of hydrocortisone (Cortef, Hydrocortone). Measures to maintain a stable blood pressure and normal water and sodium levels are instituted. After the crisis, the client will be placed on a maintenance dose of hydrocortisone.

Expected test results include: low serum sodium, high serum potassium, low serum glucose, low cortisol and aldosterone serum levels, and decreased urinary 17-ketosteroid and 17-hydroxysteroid levels.

Medical–Surgical Management

Medical

Treatment is geared toward prompt restoration of fluid and electrolyte balance and replacement of deficient adrenal hormones.

Pharmacological

The client will require lifetime maintenance of steroids. Administration of glucocorticoids such as hydrocortisone (Hydrocortone) and mineralocorticoids such as fludrocortisone acetate (Florinef) are given two-thirds of the daily dose in the morning and one-third in the evening. In times of stress the dose may need to be doubled or tripled.

Diet

The diet should be high in sodium and low in potassium. It should contain adequate calories and protein. If the client is anorexic, six small meals may increase caloric intake. A late afternoon or evening snack should be available if there is a drop in the client's blood glucose level.

▶ NURSING PROCESS

▶ Assessment

▶ Subjective Data

The nurse should obtain a thorough client history and ask about recent synthetic steroid use, adrenal surgery, infection, salt craving, nausea, weakness, vertigo, headache, disorientation, emotional status, anxiety, and apprehension.

▶ Objective Data

Assess for postural hypotension, inability to perform normal activities, syncope, dark pigmented areas on skin and mucous membrane, weight loss, vomiting, diarrhea, and very low or very high temperature.

Nursing diagnoses for the client with Addison's disease may include the following:

Nursing Diagnoses	Planning/Goals	Nursing Interventions
▶ *Fluid Volume Deficit, related to low sodium level, vomiting, diarrhea, and increased renal losses*	The client will regain normal fluid and electrolyte balance.	Monitor the client's vital signs, level of consciousness, intake and output, and weight. Administer IV fluids as ordered and encourage fluid intake.
▶ *Infection, Risk for, related to suppressed inflammatory response*	The client will maintain normal temperature and leukocyte count and differential and use precautions to avoid or reduce risks of infection.	Monitor temperature every 4 hours unless elevated, then every 2 hours. Provide a private room with reverse or protective isolation as needed. Screen personnel and visitors for infection. Teach proper handwashing. Monitor laboratory test results for WBC and differential.

Evaluation Each goal must be evaluated to determine how it has been met by the client.

PHEOCHROMOCYTOMA

Pheochromocytoma, sometimes known as *chromaffin cell tumor,* is a rare disease characterized by **paroxysmal** (a symptom that begins and ends abruptly) or sustained hypertension due to excessive secretion of epinephrine and norepinephrine. Some medical experts estimate that about one-half percent of clients newly diagnosed with hypertension have pheochromocytoma. Although the tumor is generally benign, it can be malignant in 5% to 10% of the cases. It affects all races and both sexes. It is most common in females ages 20 to 50 years.

It is caused by a chromaffin cell tumor of the adrenal medulla, more commonly on the right side. Extraadrenal pheochromocytomas can also occur. Epinephrine overproduction occurs with the adrenal pheochromocytoma; however, norepinephrine overproduction is associated with both adrenal and extraadrenal pheochromocytoma. It is associated with a familial history of pheochromocytoma or endocrine gland cancer. It is considered to be inherited on the autosomal dominant gene in about 5% of the cases.

The classic triad of clinical manifestations is hypertension with diastolic pressure above 115 mm Hg, unrelenting headache, and profuse diaphoresis. Other clinical manifestations include palpitations, visual disturbances, nausea, or vomiting. These attacks may be triggered by activities or conditions that displace the abdominal contents such as heavy lifting, exercise, bladder distention, or pregnancy. Severe attacks can be precipitated by administration of opiates, histamine, glucagon, and corticotropin. Some attacks may have no precipitating factor. Some other clinical manifestations are mild to moderate weight loss due to increased metabolism or orthostatic hypotension when arising to an upright position. The client will have tachycardia. The actual tumor is rarely palpable; however, palpation could trigger a hypertensive attack.

The complications are similar to those of severe and persistent hypertension. These complications are stroke, retinopathy, heart disease, or irreversible kidney disease. The client with pheochromocytoma has an increased risk of severe complications or death during invasive diagnostic tests or surgery.

Although pheochromocytoma can be potentially fatal, the prognosis is good with treatment. About 90% of the clients are cured.

 LIFE CYCLE CONSIDERATIONS

Pheochromocytoma

Pheochromocytoma is frequently diagnosed during pregnancy when the enlarged uterus puts pressure on the tumor causing more frequent attacks. The attacks could prove fatal to both mother and fetus. Although there is an increased risk of spontaneous abortion, most fetal deaths occur during labor or immediately after delivery.

Medical–Surgical Management

Surgical

The treatment of choice is surgical removal of the tumor. Sometimes the adrenal gland is also removed. The blood pressure is monitored closely during the immediate postoperative period. The client may have hypotension, but hypertension is more common. About 10% of the cases are not surgical candidates. These would be treated with medications to lower the blood pressure. Some may be given neoplastic chemotherapy.

Pharmacological

During acute hypertensive attacks, the drugs of choice are phentolamine mesylate (Regitine) or nitroprusside sodium (Nipride). Phentolamine mesylate (Regitine) and phenoxybenzamine HCl (Dibenzyline) are alpha-adrenergic blocking agents. They are used to control hypertension before surgery or when surgery is contraindicated. The client's blood pressure and pulse should be monitored. The client should be warned about orthostatic hypotension and rise slowly from a supine position to an upright position. The client should not take over-the-counter drugs or alcohol.

Nitroprusside sodium (Nipride, Nitropress) acts on the vascular smooth muscle to cause peripheral vasodilation. The drug is given in an intravenous infusion. An electronic infusion device must be used to monitor the infusion rate. The client's blood pressure is used to titrate the infusion rate per the physician's orders.

Metyrosine (Demser) is used to block catecholamine synthesis. This drug must be continued for life if the tumor is inoperable. Ongoing medications include adrenergic blockers such as propranolol hydrochloride (Inderal), atenolol (Tenormin), prazosin HCl (Minipress), labetalol HCl (Normodyne), or nifedipine (Procardia), a calcium channel blocker. The client's blood pressure must be monitored frequently to determine the effectiveness of the medication.

Propranolol hydrochloride (Inderal) should not be stopped abruptly. The client should not smoke while taking this medication. Atenolol (Tenormin) may enhance the client's sensitivity to cold. Prazosin HCl (Minipress) should be taken on an empty stomach. The initial dose should be given at bedtime. The client should not use cough, cold, or allergy medications without the physician's knowledge. If the client is given parenteral labetalol HCl (Normodyne, Trandate), the client should remain supine for 3 hours to decrease the possibility of orthostatic hypotension. Nifedipine (Adalat, Procardia) should be protected from light and moisture and stored at room temperature. Over-the-counter medications should not be taken.

Diet

The diet should be high in protein with adequate calories. Stimulating foods such as aged cheeses and yogurt; caffeine-containing beverages such as coffee, tea, and soft drinks; and beer and red wine should be avoided (Smeltzer & Bare, 1996).

Nursing Management

The nurse will ask about heat intolerance, severe headaches during hypertensive crisis, anxiety, trouble sleeping, palpitations, nervousness, dizziness, paresthesias, and nausea. The client is assessed for dyspnea, tremors, diaphoresis, glycosuria, hyperglycemia, or dilated pupils. The nurse must frequently assess blood pressure, pulse, and respirations for elevations, and observe for signs of anxiety to prevent it from triggering a hypertensive crisis.

CASE STUDY

Mr. Carnes, a 44-year-old African American male, is admitted to the medical unit from his physician's office. He reports that he has lost 18 pounds over the last month and has been very tired. He also reports symptoms of thirst, frequent urination, and blurred vision. His vital signs are: BP 166/92, P 88, R 16, T 99.2°F. Physical assessment reveals hot, dry, flushed skin. Laboratory exams reveal a blood glucose 490 mg/dL and urine negative for ketones. Mr. Carnes is a truck driver and leads a fairly sedentary lifestyle. History reveals that he is usually 30 to 35 pounds overweight, but has otherwise been in good health. He reports that his mother died from diabetes and renal failure, and an older brother was diagnosed as having type 2 diabetes three years ago.

The following questions will guide your development of a nursing care plan for this case study:

1. List physical symptoms that Mr. Carnes is experiencing that are suggestive of diabetes.

2. Based on history and laboratory values, would you expect Mr. Carnes to be diagnosed with type 1 or type 2 diabetes?

3. Which nursing diagnoses would you identify as priority for Mr. Carnes right now? List two.

continued

CASE STUDY (continued)

4. Mr. Carnes is treated with IV fluids and insulin sliding scale until his blood glucose is stabilized. Describe what an insulin sliding scale is, and when it is used.

5. A 2,000 calorie ADA diet is ordered for Mr. Carnes. Mr. Carnes does not care to eat the apple that came on his breakfast tray and asks if he can exchange it for another serving of scrambled eggs. How would you respond to Mr. Carnes?

6. Mr. Carnes is being discharged and will continue to attend diabetic education classes at a local diabetic treatment center. Assuming Mr. Carnes is to continue on a diabetic diet and will be receiving mixed insulin injections, list the pertinent information Mr. Carnes will need to know about his disease and therapies related to:

- Diabetes and symptoms of hyperglycemia
- Role of exercise
- Effects of diet
- Self-monitoring blood glucose
- Insulin injections/technique
- Symptoms of hypoglycemia
- Sick day care
- Long-term complications

SUMMARY

- The endocrine system is composed of glands at various body locations producing secretions (hormones) that directly enter the blood or lymph circulation.
- The endocrine system provides slower and longer lasting control over various body activities and functions.
- A malfunction of any part of the endocrine system can result in a shift of homeostasis with far-reaching systemic reactions.
- Assessment of the endocrine system can be challenging since the glands are scattered. Negative findings are as important as positive findings.
- Diabetes is a complex chronic disease with multiple acute and chronic complications. It is a systemic disease caused by an imbalance between insulin supply and demand.
- A coordinated program of exercise, diet, and medications is used to achieve diabetic control. Persons with type 1 diabetes always require insulin therapy in addition to dietary control and an exercise program. Persons with type 2 diabetes are managed through diet and exercise, and may or may not require oral hypoglycemic agents or insulin.
- The goal of diabetes management is enabling the diabetic to manage the disease by maintaining a blood glucose level within an acceptable range and thereby minimizing the incidence of acute and chronic complications.

- Regardless of disorder, the client should wear a Medic Alert bracelet and be aware that the treatment generally lasts a lifetime.

Review Questions

1. Mrs. Gavin tells the nurse that she is surprised that she developed diabetes at 40 years of age. The nurse knows that the development of diabetes in middle-aged people is most directly the result of:
   a. atherosclerosis.
   b. eating too much sugar.
   c. obesity.
   d. viral infection.

2. When teaching the diabetic client about mixing short- and longer-acting (NPH) insulin in the same syringe, the nurse should teach that:
   a. regular insulin should be drawn up first.
   b. the NPH insulin should be drawn up first.
   c. it does not matter which insulin is drawn up first since they will be mixed anyway.
   d. the two insulins do not mix and should be drawn up and administered separately.

3. Which of the following principles is used when planning for a diabetic who is to undergo surgery?
   a. All insulin is withheld until surgery is over and the client is eating.

b. Insulin or oral hypoglycemics are given as usual.

c. Sliding scale insulin is used to regulate glucose levels during the operative period.

d. Hyperglycemia poses the most serious danger to the client during surgery.

4. Mr. Schultz and the nurse collaborate to establish a meal plan for his 1,800 calorie ADA diet. The principle used in the exchange system is based on the fact that Mr. Schultz:

a. may eat any food as long as he has 3 meals and limits his calories to 1,800 calories.

b. may substitute any food in the correct amount for another on the same exchange list.

c. can eat any food any time as long as it is on an exchange list.

d. must weigh all food before determining serving size.

5. Ms. Perez, who has type 1 diabetes, complains of weakness and shakiness. She is pale, diaphoretic, and her pulse rate is increased. The nurse should recognize these symptoms as indications of:

a. hyperglycemia.

b. hypoglycemia.

c. ketoacidosis.

d. potassium excess.

6. Mrs. Lally, age 24, is newly diagnosed with type 1 diabetes. If Mrs. Lally's husband comes home and finds her unconscious, what is the first thing he should do?

a. Place some easily absorbed glucose under her tongue (e.g., monogel) or give glucagon SC or IM

b. Call the doctor

c. Administer 20U regular insulin

d. Add sugar to orange juice and administer orally

7. Explanations prior to diagnostic tests for an endocrine disorder are most important to:

a. enable the client to collect a 24-hour urine specimen.

b. ensure client compliance with test instructions.

c. prevent taking medications that interfere with test results.

d. reduce stress that can interfere with test results.

8. Which of the following nursing diagnoses would be most appropriate for the client with diabetes insipidus?

a. Alteration in growth and development related to increased growth hormone production

b. Alteration in thought processes related to decreased neurologic function

c. Fluid volume deficit related to polyuria

d. Hypothermia related to decreased metabolic rate

9. Meticulous skin care is especially important for the client with hyperthyroidism because of:

a. diaphoresis from heat intolerance.

b. edema from sodium and water retention.

c. poor nutrition due to nausea and vomiting.

d. pressure from immobility due to paralysis.

10. The nurse would assess for which of the following clinical manifestations in the client with hypothyroidism?

a. Hypertension, diaphoresis, nausea, and vomiting

b. Tetany, irritability, dry skin, and brittle nails

c. Unexplained weight gain, energy loss, and cold intolerance

d. Water retention, moon-faced, hirsutism, and purple striae

11. The client with hyperparathyroidism should have extremities handled gently because:

a. decreased calcium bone deposits can lead to pathologic fractures.

b. edema causes stretched tissue to tear easily.

c. hypertension can lead to a stroke with residual paralysis.

d. polyuria leads to dry skin and mucous membranes that can break down.

12. Which of the following assessments would the nurse expect to observe in the client with pheochromocytoma?

a. Bradycardia and tetany

b. Nausea, vomiting, and diarrhea

c. Personality changes

d. Systolic pressure up to 300 mm Hg

Critical Thinking Questions

1. What kind of lifestyle changes are necessary for each endocrine disorder?

2. Prepare a teaching plan for a client with type 2 diabetes.

⚡ WEB FLASH!

- Search the Internet for information about the various endocrine disorders. What kind of information is available? Is it helpful in planning nursing care for a client?

- What information is available on the Internet from the various resources listed for the endocrine system at the end of the book?

- What electronic resources and information can you locate for clients with diabetes? Is the information grouped by type of diabetes?

NURSING CARE OF THE CLIENT: MUSCULO-SKELETAL SYSTEM

MAKING THE CONNECTION

Refer to the following chapters to increase your understanding of musculoskeletal disorders:

- **Chapter 15, Wellness Concepts**
- **Chapter 25, Assessment**
- **Chapter 26, Pain Management**
- **Chapter 30, Nursing Care of the Oncology Client**
- **Chapter 32, Nursing Care of the Client: Cardiovascular System**
- **Chapter 39, Nursing Care of the Client: Immune System**

- **Chapter 55, Nursing Care of the Older Client**
- **Procedures:** B9, Performing Passive Range-of-Motion Exercises; B10, Assisting a Client with Ambulation; B11, Positioning a Client in Bed; B12, Moving a Client in Bed; B13, Transferring a Client from Bed to Wheelchair; B14, Transferring a Client from Bed to Stretcher; B15, Logrolling a Client with a Turn Sheet; I27, Assisting a Client with Crutch Walking

LEARNING OBJECTIVES

Upon completion of this chapter, you should be able to:
- *Define key terms.*
- *List the diagnostic tests used in the evaluation of orthopedic disorders and diseases.*
- *Describe preventive nursing care of the orthopedic client, i.e., positioning, mobility, and so on.*
- *Identify the various types of casts used in the treatment of orthopedic disorders.*
- *Describe nursing care of clients with these devices.*
- *List four types of fractures and their related treatment.*
- *Discuss the nursing care of the client undergoing a total hip replacement.*
- *Utilize the nursing process to plan nursing care including physical and emotional needs of the orthopedic client.*

KEY TERMS

amphiarthrosis	lordosis
amputation	open reduction
arthroplasty	orthopedics
bruxism	osteoporosis
closed reduction	paresthesia
contracture	phantom limb pain
crepitus	scoliosis
diarthrosis	sprain
dislocation	strain
fracture	subluxation
Heberden's nodes	synarthrosis
kyphosis	tophi
locomotor	windowing

INTRODUCTION

Orthopedics, also spelled orthopaedics, is the branch of medicine that deals with the prevention or correction of the disorders and diseases of the musculoskeletal system. It involves the muscles, skeleton, joints, and supporting structures such as ligaments and tendons.

The prime concern of the nurse caring for a client with **locomotor** (pertaining to movement or the ability to move) disorders is the prevention of **contractures** (permanent shortening of a muscle) or deformities. The objective of all caregivers is to maintain good body position, preserve muscle tone, and continue joint motion for the client with acute or long-term therapeutic or rehabilitative needs. Caring for orthopedic clients also requires an understanding of basic principles that apply to all of these clients whether they are in traction, casts, or recovering from surgery.

ANATOMY AND PHYSIOLOGY REVIEW

The musculoskeletal system consists of bones, muscles, tendons, ligaments, cartilage, and joints. When it is functioning properly, the musculoskeletal system allows an individual to stand erect and ambulate. Figure 38-1 identifies the bones of the skeleton.

The skeletal system consists of bones attached to each other by cartilage and strong ligaments. The functions of the skeleton are to:

- provide the body with structural framework.
- act as a protective casing for internal organs such as the brain, heart, and lungs.
- allow movement by muscles attached to the skeleton.
- store calcium, phosphorus and magnesium and release these minerals when the body requires them.
- manufacture blood cells in the red bone marrow.

Bones in the skeletal system are classified as long, short, flat, or irregular. Examples include the humerus, a long bone; the phalanges of the finger, short bone; occiput, flat bone; and the vertebrae, irregular bone. Figure 38-2 illustrates these bones.

There are two types of bone. One type of bone is cancellous, which resembles a sponge with spaces and is found in the epiphysis or end of the long bones as well as in all other bones. The other type is cortical bone, which is compact bone and is found in the diaphysis or shaft of the long bones. Short bones consist of cancellous bone covered by a layer of compact bone. Flat bones are made of cancellous bone layered between compact bone. Generally, the makeup of irregular bones is similar to that of flat bones.

The muscular system is composed of muscle fibers and tendons innervated by nerves (Figure 38-3). The muscle fibers vary in size and shape and are arranged according to a muscle's function. The muscles act as motors controlled by nerve impulses from the cerebral cortex. The muscles and the skeleton work together to permit body movement. Muscles are attached to bones by tendons.

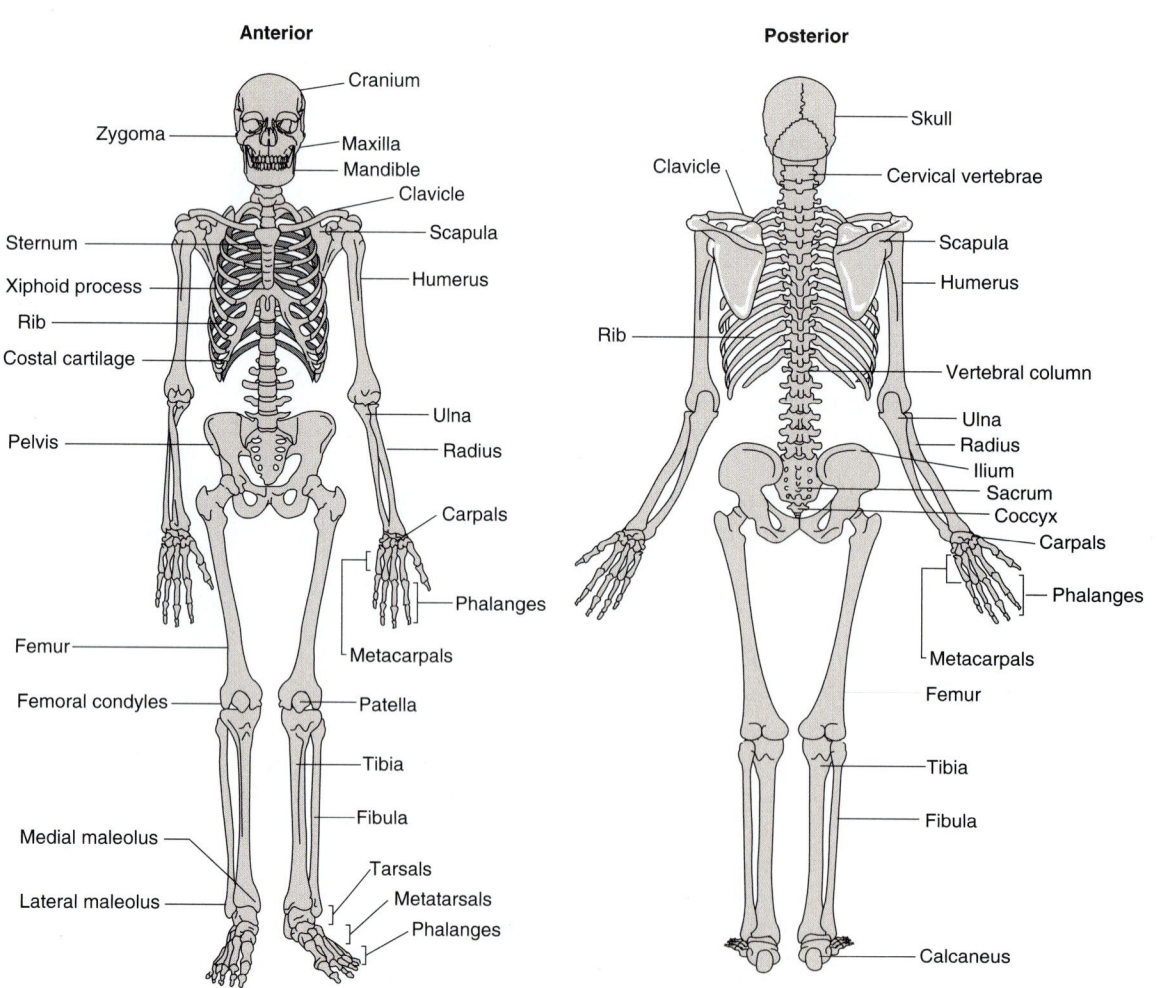

Figure 38-1 Anterior and Posterior Views of the Adult Human Skeleton

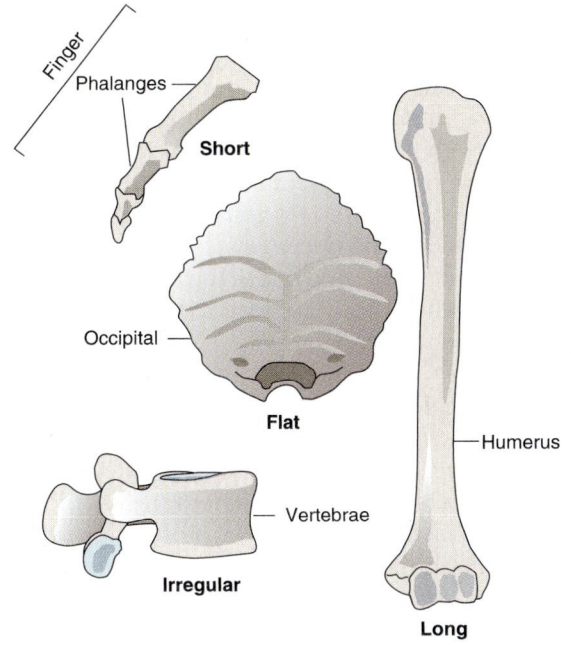

Figure 38-2 Bone Shapes

Muscles are surrounded and divided by fibrous envelopes called *fascia*. In the extremities, the muscles surround and give support to main blood vessels and nerves. Muscles also give support to and keep the body erect as well as give shape to the body.

Movement of the muscles may be either voluntary or involuntary. Muscles attached to bone can function at the will of the person (voluntary). Involuntary muscles are found within body organs and the actions are not under the person's control. They regulate the physical activity of the organs so the organs can perform their functions. Involuntary muscles are located in the intestinal tract, the pupil of the eye, and in the heart and blood vessels.

A joint is a junction of two or more bones. There are three types of joints: diarthrosis, synarthrosis, and amphiarthrosis. **Diarthrosis** joints are freely movable joints such as the hinge (elbow, knee), ball and socket (hip and shoulder), pivot (skull and first vertebrae), gliding (wrist), and saddle (thumb). **Synarthrosis** joints are immovable, such as the suture line between the temporal and occipital bones of the skull. **Amphiarthrosis** joints are slightly movable, such as the vertebrae and pelvic bones separated by fibrous cartilage. Figure 38-4 illustrates types of joints.

The ends of articulating joints are covered with a smooth articular cartilage. The joint capsule is composed of an outer fibrous layer and an inner synovial

The action of muscles is to contract or shorten. Muscles are arranged within the body as opposing pairs to act as antagonists to each other. For example, the biceps flex the forearm and the triceps extend it.

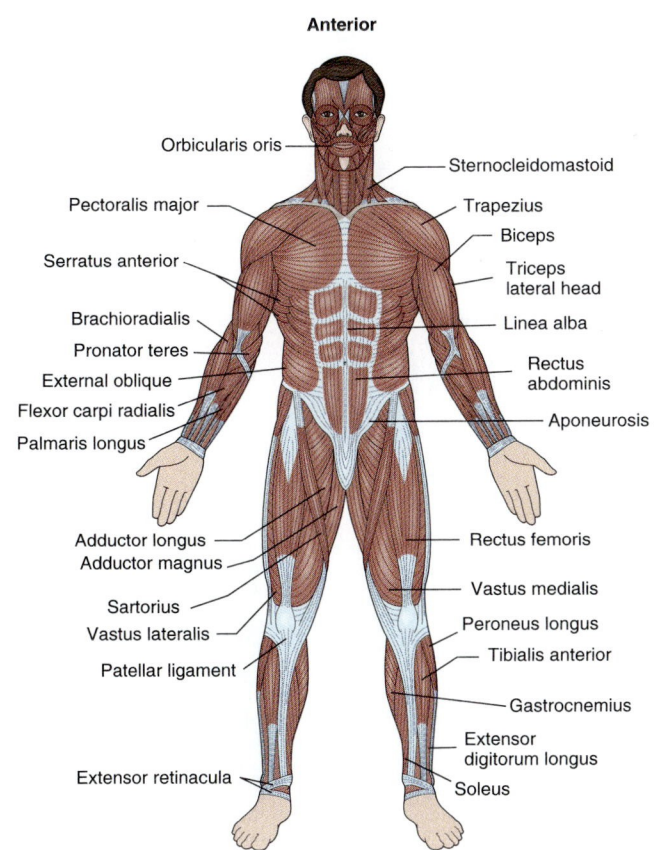

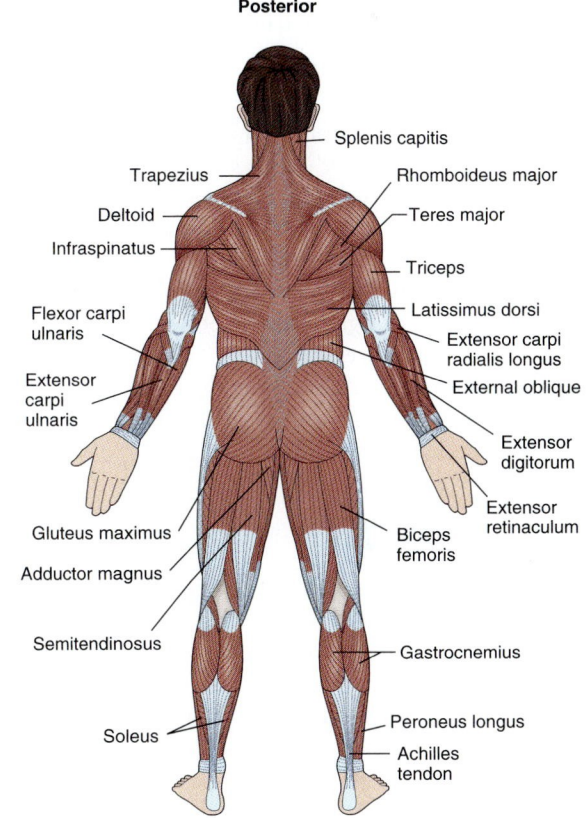

Figure 38-3 Muscular System: Anterior and Posterior Views

Diarthrosis

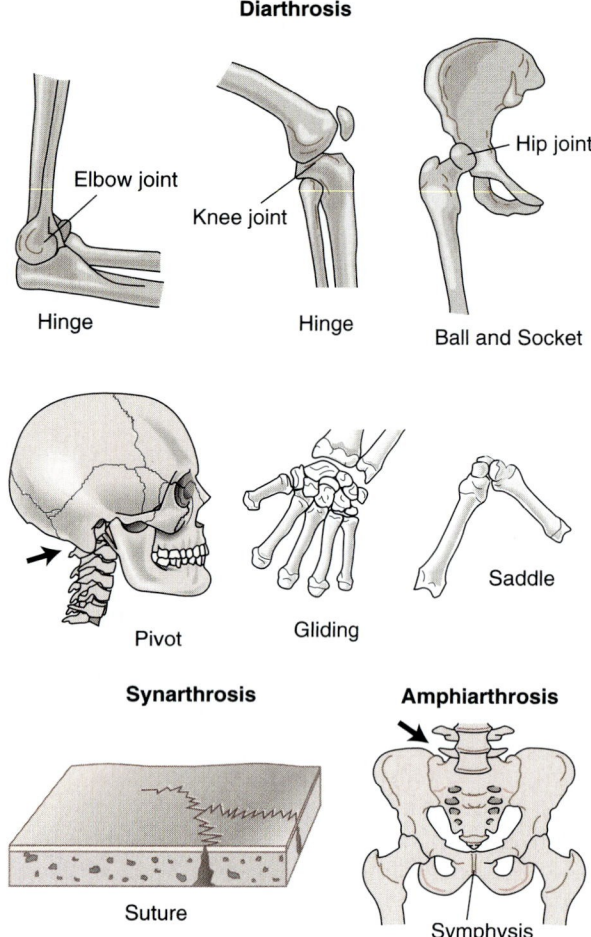

Figure 38-4 Joints Classified by the Degree of Movement Permitted

layer that secretes synovial fluid. This clear fluid acts as a lubricating fluid for the joints.

Other structures related to the musculoskeletal system include bursa, fascia, tendons, and ligaments. Bursae are sacs filled with fluid that facilitate joint movement by making it possible for muscles and tendons to move or glide over ligaments or bones. Fascia is connective tissue that covers a muscle. Tendons are strong fibrous tissue attaching muscle to bones, providing mobility. Ligaments grow out of the periosteum and lash bones together more firmly.

ASSESSMENT

Assessment of the musculoskeletal system ranges from a basic assessment of functional abilities done by the nurse to a complete physical exam by the physician for diagnosis of specific muscle and joint disorders. The extent of the physical exam will depend on the client's complaints, the health history, and any other physical signs or symptoms.

The nurse, in making an assessment, will inspect and palpate to evaluate bone integrity, posture, joint function, muscle strength, and gait. An assessment is

also made of the client's ability to perform basic activities of daily living.

The medical history includes information on any past medical or surgical disorders. It also includes any symptoms with relation to onset, duration, or location of discomfort or pain. The nurse should ask if activity makes symptoms better or worse. A family medical history should also be obtained.

Assessment of the bony skeleton includes notation of any deformities, body alignment, abnormal growths due to bone tumors, shortened extremities, amputations, abnormal angulation other than at the joints, and **crepitus,** a grating or crackling sensation or sound.

Assessment of the spine will necessitate exposure of the client's back, buttocks, and legs for adequate visualization. Differences in the height of the shoulders or iliac crests should be noted. Gluteal folds should appear symmetrical. The vertebral column should be straight and perpendicular to the floor with the spine convex through the thoracic portion and concave through the cervical/lumbar portion.

Three common spinal curvatures are: scoliosis, kyphosis, and lordosis. A lateral curving deviation is known as **scoliosis**. Scoliosis (crooked back) is seen most frequently in schoolage children and adolescents. **Kyphosis** (hump back) is seen as an increased roundness of the thoracic spinal curve. This condition is frequently seen in the older person with osteoporosis. **Lordosis** (sway back) is an exaggeration of the lumbar spine curvature as seen in pregnancy as a woman's body adjusts to the center of gravity. These three curvatures are illustrated in Figure 38-5.

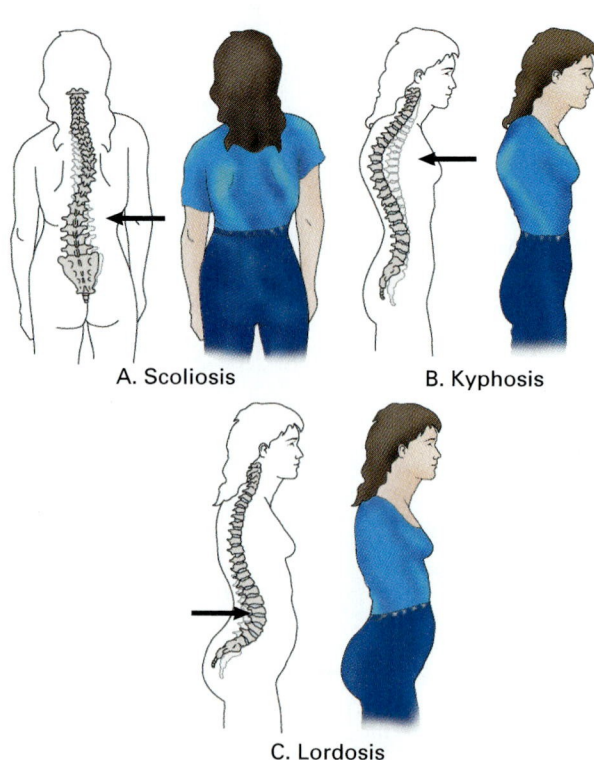

Figure 38-5 Curvatures of the Spine

Assessment of the articular system includes: range of motion (limited, active, and passive), stability of joints, deformities and any nodular formation, and pulses in the extremities.

Range of motion (ROM) includes assessment of the client's ability to change position, muscle strength and coordination, and the size of individual muscles. When assessing passive range of motion, the nurse should remember to keep the motion steady and avoid causing any pain.

Joints are examined for excessive fluid. The knee is the most common site for fluid accumulation. Edema and an elevated temperature may be signs of active inflammation in the joint. Normal joint movement is stable and smooth. If there is a snap or crack sound when a joint is passively moved, it may be indicative of a ligament slipping over a bony prominence.

Deformities may be due to several factors including contractures, dislocations, and **subluxation** (a partial separation of an articular surface). Nodular formations are produced by musculoskeletal diseases such as gout, rheumatoid arthritis, and osteoarthritis.

Pulse points in the extremities are palpated to assess for weak or absent pulses. The strength of the pulse in affected extremities is compared with that of nonaffected extremities. Skin color and temperature are noted, and capillary refill is checked by pressing down on the client's fingernail or toenail for a few seconds, then releasing and noting the time it takes for the client's nail to return to normal color. The color should return immediately (less than 2 seconds); if a client has an arterial disorder, the color will take longer than 2 seconds to return to normal.

COMMON DIAGNOSTIC TESTS

Commonly used diagnostic tests for clients with symptoms of musculoskeletal system disorders are listed in Table 38-1. See Chapter 27, Diagnostic Tests, for explanation/normal values and nursing responsibilities.

MUSCULOSKELETAL TRAUMA

Trauma to the musculoskeletal system may cause a variety of injuries to clients of all ages. Such injuries include strains, sprains, dislocations, fractures, and compartment syndrome.

STRAIN

A **strain** is an injury to a muscle or tendon due to overuse or overstretching. A strain may be either acute or chronic. An acute strain may be caused when an individual performs unaccustomed exercises vigorously.

Table 38-1 COMMON DIAGNOSTIC TESTS FOR CLIENTS WITH MUSCULOSKELETAL DISORDERS
Laboratory Tests
Antinuclear antibodies (ANA)
Complete blood count (CBC)
• WBC
• Hg
C-reactive protein (CRP)
Erythrocyte sedimentation rate (ESR)
Rheumatoid factor (RF)
Serum calcium
Uric acid
• serum
• urine
Radiologic Studies
Arthrogram/graphy
Computed tomography (CT scan)
Electromyography (EMG)
Magnetic resonance imaging (MRI)
Radiograph (x-ray)
Other Tests
Arthrocentesis
Arthroscopy

A chronic strain may develop after repeated overuse of certain muscles. Individuals suffering acute strains experience sudden severe pain while the onset is gradual in chronic strains, with the affected part feeling only stiff and sore.

Chronic strains require no specific treatment, but acute strains will require rest and possibly immobilization. Immediately following injury cold packs may be applied for 20- to 30-minute periods, then removed for 1 hour during a 24-hour period to reduce any edema. Heat may then be applied for the client's comfort. In the case of a severe strain when the muscle may be completely ruptured, surgical repair may be necessary.

SPRAIN

A **sprain** is an injury to ligaments surrounding a joint caused by a sudden twist, wrench, or fall. Symptoms include pain, edema, loss of motion, and ecchymosis. X-ray will reveal soft tissue edema but no evidence of joint or bone injury. Immediate treatment is RICE (rest, ice, compression, and elevation). The client rests and ice is applied to the injured area. The part may then be immobilized with an elastic compression bandage or a brace, and elevated. After the edema has decreased significantly, a cast may be applied.

DISLOCATION

Dislocation occurs when articular surfaces of a joint are no longer in contact. The bones are literally "out of joint." The displaced bone may hinder the blood supply, damage nerves, tear ligaments, or rupture muscle attachments. Traumatic dislocations are considered orthopedic emergencies. Congenital dislocations are present at birth, while spontaneous or pathologic dislocations are caused by diseases affecting joints.

Symptoms of a dislocation include localized joint pain, loss of function of the joint, and a change in the length of the extremity and contour of the joint. Diagnosis is based on the symptoms, physical exam, and x-rays. X-rays reveal either a complete or partial separation of the articulating surfaces.

FRACTURE

A **fracture** is a break in the continuity of a bone. Fractures occur when the forces from outside the body become greater than the strength of the bone, causing the bone to break. Fractures usually involve soft tissue (edema and bleeding), damaged nerves, and tendons. Most fractures are caused by accidents. These may be the result of direct force, torsion or twisting, or violent contractions of highly developed muscles. Other fractures may be the result of a disease process that weakens the bone. This type of fracture is known as pathologic or spontaneous. Individuals considered at high risk for fractures include those who have predisposing bone conditions such as metastatic or primary bone tumors or osteoporosis, poor coordination, diminished vision, dizzy spells, or general weakness.

There are more than 90 different classifications of fractures. Some of the more common types include: greenstick or incomplete, simple or closed, compound or open, impacted or telescoped, spiral, and comminuted.

In a greenstick fracture, the continuity of the bone is not completely disrupted but has splintering on one side and bending on the other. This fracture is seen most frequently in children. An uncomplicated (clean) fracture in which the skin remains intact is called a closed or simple fracture; the fractured surfaces are not contaminated by outside air. In a compound or open fracture, the bone is broken and the skin is also broken, allowing the bone to protrude and be susceptible to a greater chance for infection. An impacted fracture is also called a telescoped fracture; one portion of a bone fragment is forcibly driven into another. A spiral fracture twists around the shaft of the bone. This type of fracture may occur from a twisting force. In a comminuted fracture, the bone is splintered into many unaligned fragments. Various types of fractures are shown in Figure 38-6.

Healing time for fractures is affected by the age of the client and the type of injury or any underlying disease process, and may take weeks, months, or even years before the healing is complete. The sequence of healing takes place beginning with the formation of a hematoma, then granulation tissue formation, callus formation, callus ossification, and ultimately remodeling.

Hematoma formation begins with the formation of a clot that serves as a fibrin network. Bleeding comes from ruptured vessels within the bone as well as from tears in the periosteum and adjacent tissues. The hematoma is not absorbed but develops into granulation tissue. Granulation tissue forms a soft tissue callus that surrounds the fracture site and serves as a temporary splint. Callus ossification is the result of deposits of calcium salts in the callus forming rigid bone in excess as a protective measure. The formation of bone binds the bone ends together. Remodeling is completed by osteoclastic activity, whereby excess bone is

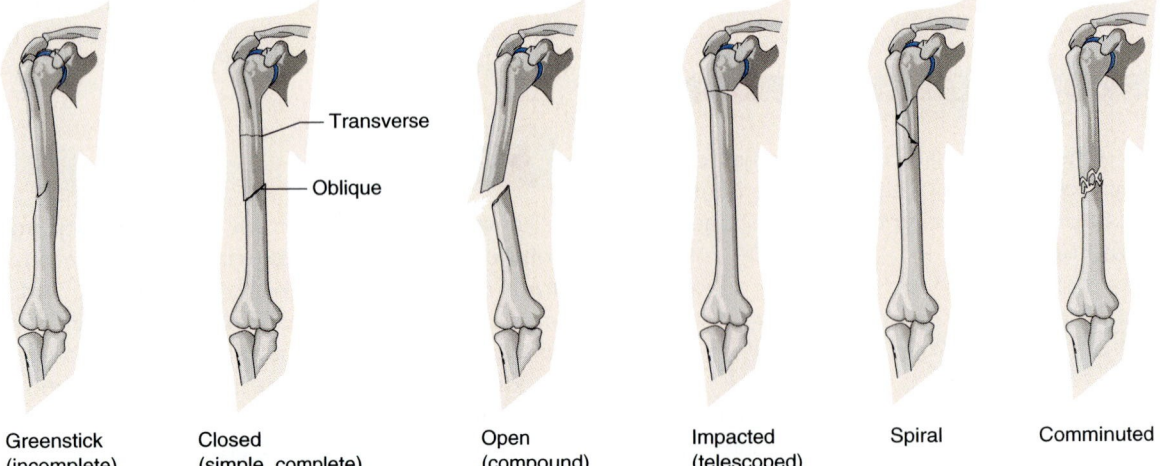

Greenstick   Closed   Open   Impacted   Spiral   Comminuted
(incomplete)   (simple, complete) (compound)   (telescoped)

Figure 38-6 Types of Bone Fractures

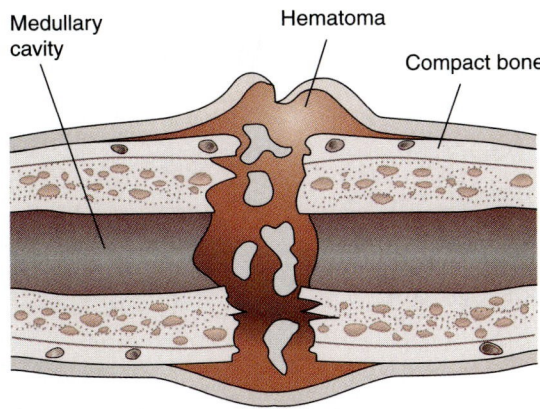

Medullary cavity   Hematoma   Compact bone

A. A hematoma forms from blood from ruptured vessels.

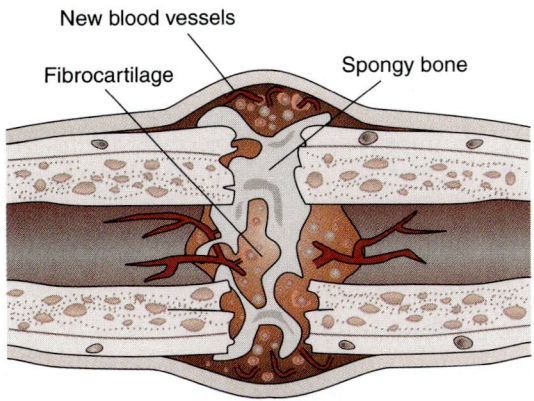

New blood vessels   Fibrocartilage   Spongy bone

B. Spongy bone forms close to developing blood vessels; fibrocartilage forms away from new blood vessels.

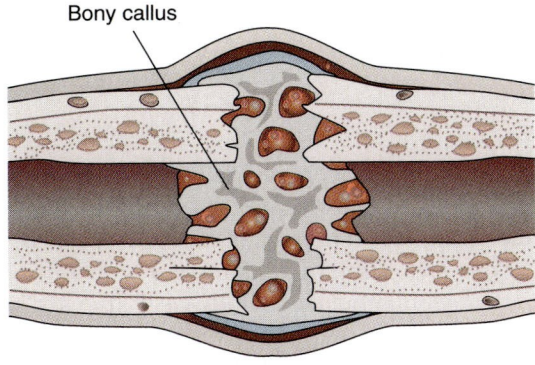

Bony callus

C. Bony callus replaces fibrocartilage.

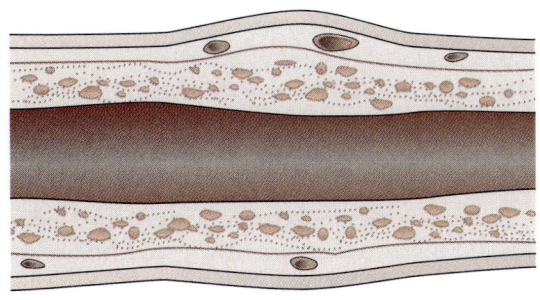

D. Excess bony tissue is removed by osteoclasts.

Figure 38-7 Steps of Bone Repair

gradually reduced and removed by absorption until the original shape and outline of the fractured bone is reestablished. Figure 38-7 outlines the healing sequence.

Complications of a fracture include infection, fat embolism, and compartment syndrome. Complications may delay healing or be life threatening.

Infections may result from an open fracture in which the bone extends through the skin, allowing contamination from the outside. They may also occur following surgical repair of a fracture using an internal fixation device. Any infection may lead to a delayed union of the bone.

A fat embolism occurs when a particle of fat from the marrow of a broken bone travels in the bloodstream toward the heart and lungs. It is usually associated with fractures of the long bones, multiple fractures, or crushing injuries. An embolus usually occurs within 24 to 72 hours following a fracture but may occur up to a week after injury. When a small area of the lungs is involved, the symptoms are pain, tachycardia, and dyspnea. Larger areas of lung involvement produce more pronounced symptoms, including severe pain, dyspnea, cyanosis, restlessness, and shock. Petechiae may appear over the neck, upper arms,

chest, or abdomen. Treatment consists of bed rest, gentle handling, oxygen, and IV fluids.

COMPARTMENT SYNDROME

Compartment syndrome is a form of neurovascular impairment that may lead to permanent injury of an affected limb caused by the progressive constriction of blood vessels and nerves. It can occur with any orthopedic injury as a result of bleeding into the tissue, tissue edema, or pressure from a cast or tight dressing. If untreated, in 4 to 6 hours it may lead to irreversible damage to nerves and muscles and within 24 to 48 hours permanent loss of normal limb function. A neurovascular assessment that reveals pain which is not relieved by narcotic analgesics, diminished capillary refill, weak or unequal pulses, **paresthesia** (numbness or tingling), and paralysis is indicative of this orthopedic emergency. Treatment consists of relieving pressure by removing the cast or dressing or by performing a fasciotomy. A surgical fasciotomy is an incision into the fascia to relieve pressure on the nerves and blood vessels.

Medical–Surgical Management

Medical

The treatment of a fracture requires immediate attention. The most important objectives are to: (1) realign the fracture, (2) maintain the alignment, and (3) regain the function of the injured part. The method of treatment will depend on the first aid given; the site, severity, and type of the fracture; and the age and condition of the client.

Closed Reduction Repair of a fracture accomplished without surgical intervention is called *closed reduction*. External manipulation is used to correct bone position. This manipulation requires three maneuvers: traction and countertraction, angulation, and rotation. Following the reduction, x-rays are taken to visualize the fracture alignment. The part is then immobilized by using a cast, bandage, or traction. Local or general anesthesia may be used to make the reduction easier and less painful to the client.

Casts A well-made and applied cast is as perfect a fixation apparatus as can be devised for the human body. Casts are made either from plaster bandages or synthetic materials such as fiberglass. Synthetic casts are used for non-weight bearing parts of the body. The cast should include the joint above and below the affected part. The major purposes of casts are: immobilization, support and protection of the affected part, prevention of deformities that may be the result of conditions such as arthritis, and the correction of deformities like scoliosis.

A dry cast should be odorless, shiny in appearance, resonant when percussed, and have a temperature similar to the room air. Moisture occurring from any underlying drainage will give the cast a musty smell, dullness on percussion, a lusterless color, and cool temperature.

Numerous types of casts exist. Long and short arm casts allow the fingers to be visible; long and short leg

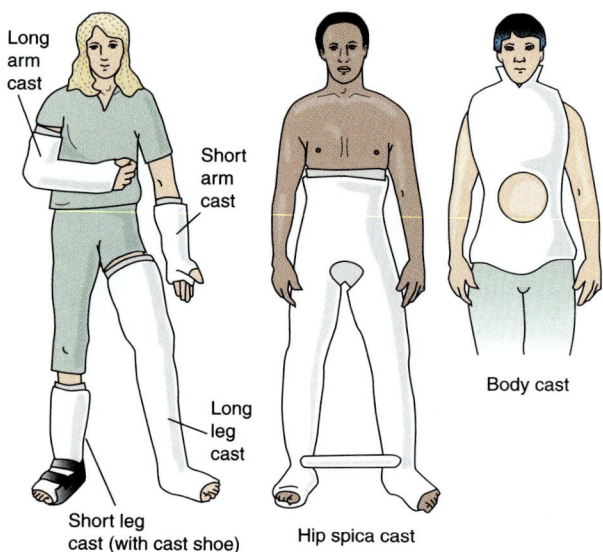

Figure 38-8 Casts Used to Correct Musculoskeletal Disorders

casts allow the toes to be visible. A spica cast is used for hip, shoulder, and thumb dislocations or injuries. The hip spica has an abduction bar that keeps the cast in the correct position. A walking cast with a cast shoe facilitates client ambulation. Body casts are used to immobilize the spine following surgical spinal fusions, unstable spinal injuries, or for degenerative disorders. Figure 38-8 shows different types of casts.

After the application and drying of a cast, it may be necessary for the doctor to order a cast cut to allow visualization of a body area or to relieve pressure. This procedure is known as **windowing**. An arm cast may be cut in order to take a radial pulse or to dress a wound. Abdominal distention may be a reason to window a hip spica.

When a cast is removed, the client may become conscious of aches and discomforts caused by the constricted joint structures and immobilized muscles. The client's discomfort may be minimized by supporting the joint and maintaining the part in the same position as it was in the cast. The skin will be cool and pale with mottling and edema present. A yellow exudate, which is part dead skin and part secretions from oil sacs, will be on the skin. This exudate should not be rubbed or forced off.

Traction The principle of traction is to have two forces pulling in opposite directions. Traction consists of weights and counterweights. Countertraction forces can be provided by the weight of the client's body or other weight such as elevating the foot of the bed. Traction may be used to reduce a fracture, immobilize an extremity, lessen muscle spasms, or correct or prevent a deformity.

Types of traction are skeletal, skin, and manual. Skeletal traction requires the surgical insertion of pins (Steinmann) or wires (Kirschner) through the bones.

CLIENT TEACHING

Casts

Since plaster casts dry from the inside out, they should not be covered or dried with a hairdryer or heat lamp. Moisture and heat from the drying cast should be allowed to evaporate naturally. Clients should be informed that the heat they feel during the application, drying, and setting process is normal and should subside after 10 to 15 minutes. To avoid indentation, a drying cast should be placed on pillows and not on a hard surface. For the same reason, when handling the cast, only the palms of the hands should be used. Synthetic casts dry in minutes.

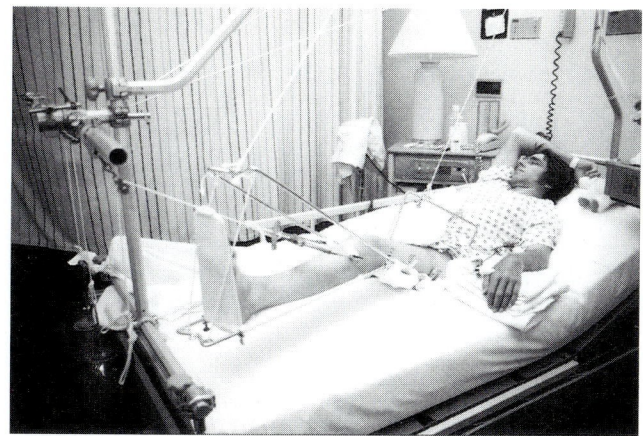

A.

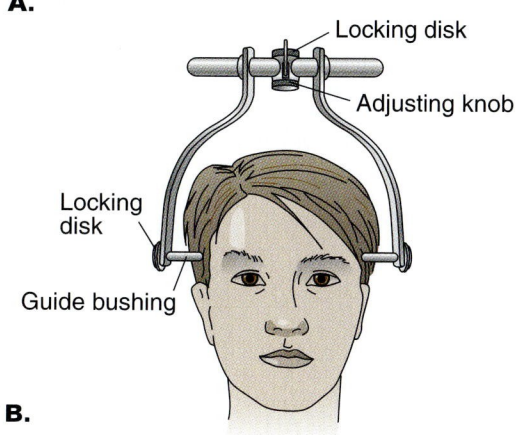

Locking disk

Adjusting knob

Locking disk

Guide bushing

B.

Figure 38-9 Types of Traction Devices: A. Skeletal traction; B. Head tongs

Skeletal traction is continuous and is used most frequently for fractures of the femur, tibia, and cervical spine. Head tongs (e.g., Gardner-Wells tongs) are fixed in the skull to apply traction that immobilizes cervical fractures. Figure 38-9 shows examples of traction devices.

Skin traction is a nonsurgical method of providing necessary pull for shorter periods of time, such as Buck's traction (Figure 38-10). Materials used include tapes, traction strips, cervical halters, and pelvic belts. Skin traction is frequently used to temporarily immobilize a part or stabilize a fracture. The disadvantage of skin traction for adult use is that it does not adequately control rotation and cannot be maintained for the length of time necessary for adult healing. Tapes and bandages should be applied smoothly to prevent any pressure areas.

A nurse caring for a client in traction should know the purpose of the traction, how it accomplishes its purpose, and any complications associated with the use of the traction. It is also important to know the extent of the injury and the movements and positions allowed. Care of the client should include maintenance of the injured part, general body alignment, the alignment of the traction apparatus, and range of motion in as many joints as possible.

Rehabilitation The physician will determine when the bone has healed sufficiently for rehabilitation. Healing is monitored by periodic x-rays and physical examinations. The major objective of rehabilitation is to assist the client to return to the former level of functioning. Rehabilitation programs vary depending on the injury and the client.

Physical therapy may be started with the use of parallel bars or other exercise equipment before the client is allowed to exercise independently. The nurse has a major role in client education reinforcing the directions of both the physician and the physical therapist. Patience and encouragement are extremely important in assisting the client to feel comfortable in learning self-care techniques. The client should be taught to report any unusual signs or symptoms to the physician.

The client will also need to learn the proper use of equipment such as crutches, canes, or walkers. Crutches allow ambulation with limited or no weight bearing on the affected extremity. Walkers allow limited weight bearing and provide stability while the client ambulates. Canes allow the client to walk with balance and support.

The tripod position is the basic stance for crutch walking. Tips of the crutches are placed approximately 8 to 10 inches in front of and beside the client's feet. The client must place his weight on the handpiece of the crutches and not on the axilla. Crutch gaits depend on the client's disability and are prescribed by the physician. See Figure 38-11 for basic crutch walking gaits.

Canes are held in the hand opposite the affected extremity. In normal walking, the opposite arm and leg move together. This same action should be done when walking with a cane. Walkers provide more support than canes or crutches. They are especially useful for clients who have poor balance. The client should

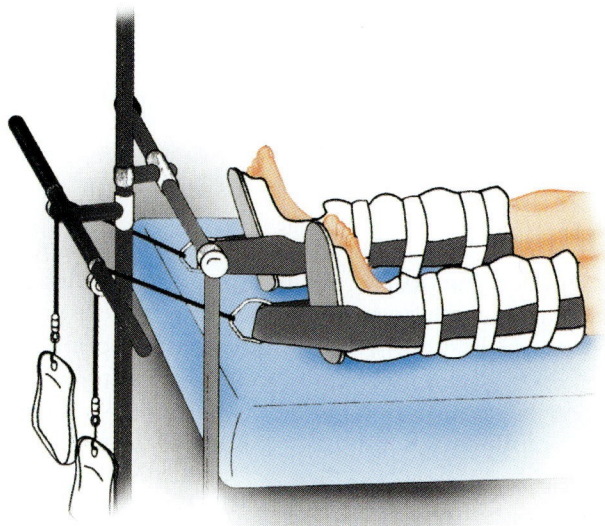

Figure 38-10 Buck's Traction, a Type of Skin Traction

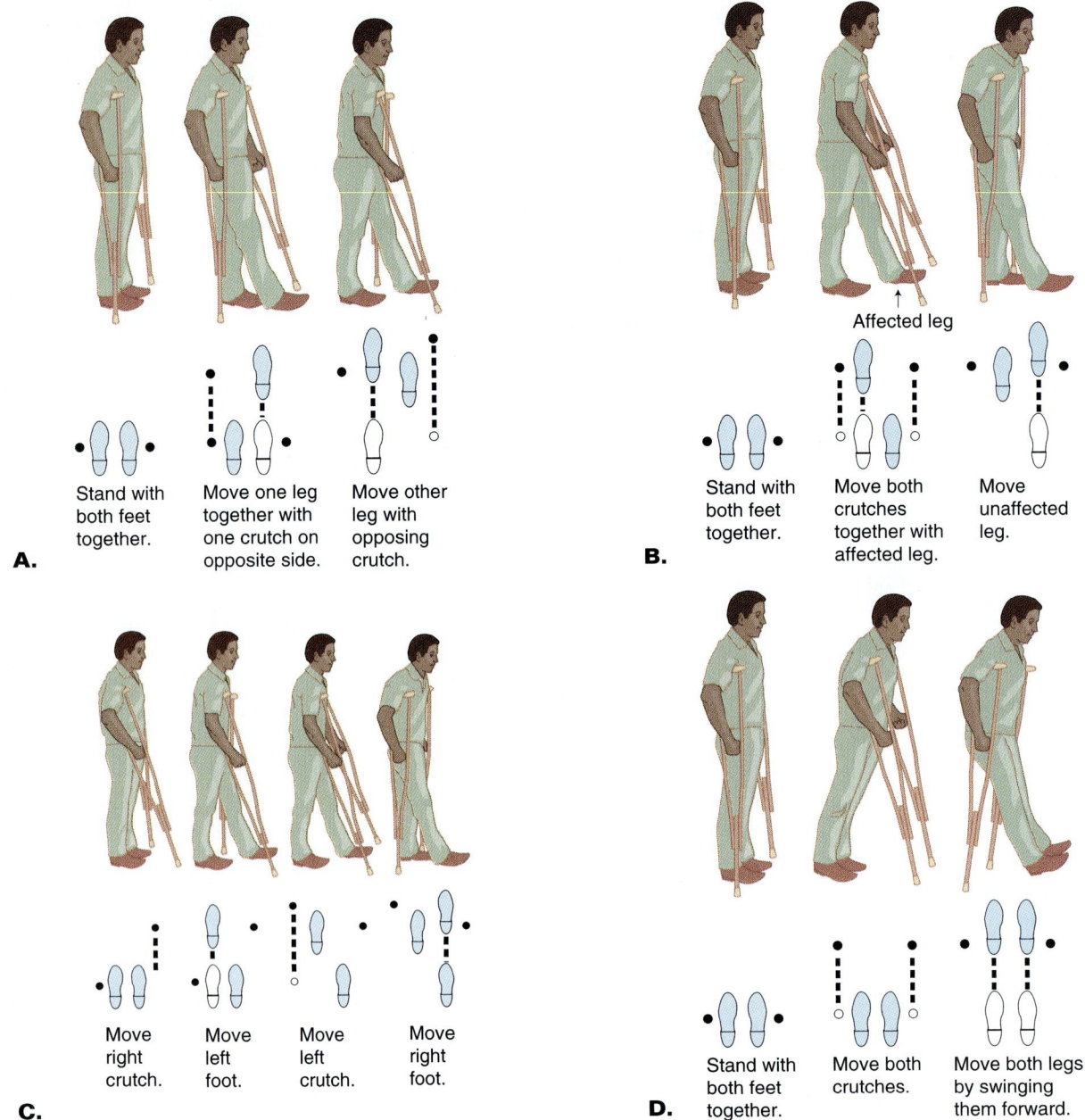

Figure 38-11 Various Crutch Gaits: A Two-point gait (partial weight bearing); B. Three-point gait (partial or non-weight bearing); C. Four-point alternate crutch gait (partial or full weight bearing); D. Swing through gait (non-weight bearing)

place the walker 12 to 18 inches in front and walk toward the walker holding onto the hand grips.

Surgical

Open reduction is a surgical procedure that enables the surgeon to reduce (repair) the fracture under direct visualization. When an open reduction/internal fixation (ORIF) is done, orthopedic devices are used to maintain the reduction. Some of the devices used include pins, screws, nails, plates, wires, and rods. These internal fixation devices may be inserted through bone fragments or fixed to the sides of the bones.

The major disadvantage of the open reduction is the possibility of introducing infection into the bone.

Other disadvantages include impaired circulation and accidental injury to major nerves, blood vessels, and bone caused by the fixation devices. X-rays may be taken during and after the open reduction to evaluate the alignment of the fracture.

Pharmacological

Analgesics may be given to relieve pain. Muscle relaxants, such as cyclobenzaprine hydrochloride (Flexeril), may also be prescribed for muscle spasms. Severe or continued pain may indicate complications and should be given immediate attention. Stool softeners, such as docusate sodium (Colace), may be given to prevent constipation in the immobilized client.

Diet

The client should be encouraged to eat regular meals. The meals should include foods that provide fiber, protein, calcium, phosphorus, and fluids. For the client whose dietary intake is inadequate, vitamin and mineral supplements, especially calcium and phosphorus, may be included. Consultation with a dietitian regarding food preferences of the client may be necessary.

Activity

Client activity and exercise are important in maintaining muscle strength and tone, and minimizing cardiovascular problems. Joints that are not immobilized should be exercised either actively or passively to maintain function. Isometric (maintaining constant resistive force) exercises help to maintain muscle strength of immobilized muscles.

▶ NURSING PROCESS

▶ Assessment

▶ Subjective Data

The neurovascular assessment of a client with a fracture may reveal subjective data of pain, especially on movement; muscle spasms; and paresthesia.

▶ Objective Data

Edema, shortening and deformity of the affected limb, and pallor may be found. Pulses in the affected and unaffected extremity must be checked and compared. The client's vital signs should be taken routinely, and the general physical and mental condition of the client should be noted. The skin, especially over

PROFESSIONAL TIP

Neurovascular Assessment

- Circulation, movement, and sensation (CMS) assessments are performed on clients following musculoskeletal trauma; after surgery, if nerve or blood vessel damage is possible; and following casting, splinting, and bandaging.
- The CMS assessment is performed every 15 to 30 minutes for several hours, and then every 3 to 4 hours.
- All findings must be documented.
- Tingling and numbness may be relieved by flexing fingers or toes or repositioning extremity.
- The nurse should remember 5 Ps when performing a CMS assessment:
  1. Pain
  2. Pallor (slow capillary return)
  3. Paresthesia (unrelieved tingling or numbness)
  4. Puffiness (edema)
  5. Pulselessness

bony prominences, should be checked for color and temperature.

The client who has a cast applied must have all cast edges checked for smoothness. The cast should also be checked for spots indicating wound drainage including the color and amount. Extremities including fingers, toes, hands, and feet should be assessed for changes in skin color, pulse, or temperature. All traction wires, pulleys, and weights should be checked. Weights should hang free.

Nursing diagnoses for a client with musculoskeletal trauma may include the following:

Nursing Diagnoses	Planning/Goals	Nursing Interventions
▶ *Pain, Acute, related to fracture*	The client will have relief of pain with medication.	Provide comfort measures.
		Administer medications for pain as ordered.
▶ *Skin Integrity, Impaired, Risk for, related to immobility*	The client will experience no skin breakdown.	Change client position, if allowed, maintaining correct body alignment.
		Check bony prominences and keep the client's skin clean and dry.
		For the client in a cast, check the edges of the cast for roughness, keep the exposed skin next to the cast clean and dry.
		Inspect all body pressure points including the head, ears, and heels; turn the client as orders direct; and check for friction rubs.
		Instruct clients not to poke anything under the cast or use objects to scratch, causing skin breakdown or infections.
		Avoid getting the cast wet.

continued

Nursing Diagnoses	Planning/Goals	Nursing Interventions
▶ *Mobility, Impaired, Physical, related to loss of integrity of bone structures*	The client will perform range of motion exercises in unaffected joints. The client will demonstrate use of adaptive devices to improve mobility.	If the client in a cast is allowed to turn, use an overhead trapeze. Assist client in performing ROM exercises. Assist client in use of adaptive devices.

Evaluation Each goal must be evaluated to determine how it has been met by the client.

INFLAMMATORY DISORDERS

Inflammatory disorders involve inflammation of the joints and include conditions such as rheumatoid arthritis, bursitis, polymyositis, and osteomyelitis.

RHEUMATOID ARTHRITIS

Rheumatoid arthritis is a chronic systemic disease of unknown etiology, with recurring inflammation involving the synovium or lining of the joints. It can also affect the lungs, heart, blood vessels, muscles, eyes, and skin. Rheumatoid arthritis is a potentially destructive and disabling disease. The course is variable with either slow or rapid progress and/or periods of remissions. Women are affected more often than men. Rheumatoid arthritis can occur at any age; however, it most commonly affects young adults. In children it occurs in a form known as juvenile rheumatoid arthritis (Still's disease). See Chapter 39 for more information on rheumatoid arthritis.

BURSITIS

Bursitis is inflammation of the bursa, a sac filled with synovial fluid that facilitates joint movement. Major bursae are found in the shoulder, knee, hip, and elbow. The inflammation is usually the result of trauma or repetitive movements. The client experiences painful joint movement. Diagnosis is made from the client's symptoms and x-ray which shows a calcified bursa. Treatment includes rest of the joint and the administration of anti-inflammatory drugs including salicylates and NSAIDs. For some clients, corticosteroids may be injected into the bursa.

POLYMYOSITIS

Polymyositis is an inflammatory disease involving striated muscle. The etiology of this disease is unknown, but probably is an autoimmune mechanism. It is primarily a disease of skeletal muscle; however, the heart, gastrointestinal tract, and lungs are also frequently involved. Symptoms include muscle weakness with activities like climbing the stairs, getting out of a chair, or combing the hair. The muscles of swallowing may also become involved. This weakness is the result of degeneration and necrosis of parts or entire groups of muscle fibers. Some individuals have arthralgia and Raynaud's phenomenon.

Medical–Surgical Management
Pharmacological

Treatment is symptomatic and begins initially with high doses of prednisone (Deltasone). The doses are then modified in response to muscle enzymes. Reduction of the muscle enzymes may take several months, thus requiring long-term maintenance treatment.

Diet

If the neck flexor muscles are involved, the client may need frequent small meals and antacids for reflux esophagitis.

Activity

Physical therapy is begun to preserve muscle strength and prevent contractures. Complete bed rest with the head of the bed elevated is eventually required.

▶ NURSING PROCESS

▶ Assessment

▶ Subjective Data
Questions regarding muscle or joint pain, appetite, dyspnea, and gastrointestinal symptoms are appropriate.

▶ Objective Data
Objective data is gathered from observations of the client's ability to complete activities of daily living and any evidence of respiratory difficulty. Muscles and joints should be palpated for tenderness or pain.

Nursing diagnoses for a client with polymyositis may include the following:

Nursing Diagnoses	Planning/Goals	Nursing Interventions
▶ Mobility, Impaired, Physical, related to muscle weakness	The client will perform physical activity as tolerated.	Assist client and encourage physical mobility, provide rest periods before and after activity.
▶ Self-Care Deficit related to muscle weakness	The client will perform ADLs as able.	Assist the client in activities whenever necessary. Provide frequent position change and ROM exercises to prevent contractures.
▶ Nutrition, Altered, less than body requirements, related to difficulty in swallowing	The client will maintain adequate nutritional status.	Provide small, frequent, high-caloric feedings.

Evaluation Each goal must be evaluated to determine how it has been met by the client.

OSTEOMYELITIS

Osteomyelitis is the inflammation of the bone and bone marrow. The most common cause of osteomyelitis is the introduction of pathogenic bacteria into a penetrating injury such as an open fracture. Bone infections may also result from the spread of infection from another site such as infected teeth, tonsils, or an upper respiratory infection. The most common pathogen causing osteomyelitis is *Staphylococcus aureus*. Other organisms found in osteomyelitis are *Pseudomonas* and *Escherichia coli*. Osteomyelitis may become a chronic disabling problem affecting the quality of life. The affected bone may have spontaneous fractures.

Local symptoms of an acute infection are sudden pain and tenderness of the affected bone, warmth, redness, edema, and pain on movement. General symptoms with acute severe bone infections may include chills, elevated temperature, rapid pulse, and marked leukocytosis.

Medical–Surgical Management

Medical

The client is placed on bed rest and the infected bone is kept at rest with the use of sandbags or casts. Antibiotics are given as soon as osteomyelitis is suspected. Unless the infective process is controlled early, a bone abscess forms (Figure 38-12). Cultures of the abscess may indicate a need for change in the antibiotic therapy. The abscess may drain naturally; however, it usually requires an incision allowing it to drain. The abscess cavity of dead bone tissue does not liquefy easily, drain, and heal as in soft tissue abscesses.

A bone sheath forms around the sequestrum (dead bone) giving the appearance of healing. However, chronically infected sequestrum has the tendency to produce recurrent abscesses throughout the life of the individual.

Surgical

A sequestrectomy to remove the dead bone tissue may need to be performed. Strict aseptic technique must be maintained when changing any dressings. Because infected bone may be extremely painful, unnecessary movement should be avoided and the affected extremity should be handled very gently.

Pharmacological

Vigorous antibiotic therapy and analgesics are the medications used for the treatment of osteomyelitis. Wound irrigations with antiseptics or antibiotics are often prescribed by the physician. Specific drugs given are determined by the causative organism.

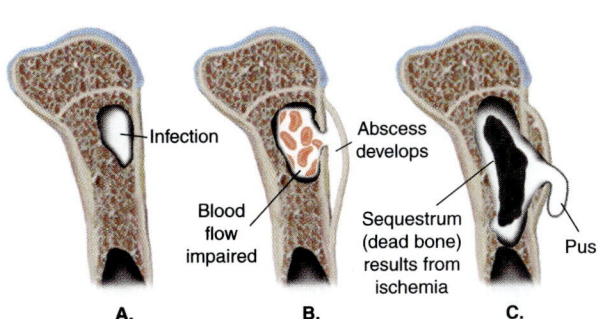

Figure 38-12 A. Osteomyelitis; B. Without early treatment, an abscess forms; C. Bone dies (sequestrum) and pus forms.

Diet

A high-caloric, high-protein diet is generally ordered for the client with osteomyelitis. Dietary supplements of vitamins and calcium are also given. Fluids should be increased as tolerated.

Activity

There should be absolute rest of the affected extremity. Excessive handling of the extremity is very painful and should be avoided. The extremity should be handled in a smooth unhurried manner, supporting the joints above and below the affected area.

▶ NURSING PROCESS

▶ Assessment

▶ Subjective Data

Inquire about pain, muscle spasms, and tenderness in the bone. Ask about any traumas, surgeries, and other diseases.

▶ Objective Data

Observe the client for signs of infection, including chills, elevated temperature, pain, redness, and edema of the affected extremity. The client may also experience headaches, restlessness, and irritability.

Nursing diagnoses for a client with osteomyelitis may include the following:

Nursing Diagnoses	Planning/Goals	Nursing Interventions
▶ *Mobility, Impaired, Physical, related to pain*	The client will maintain movement of unaffected extremities.	Encourage and assist client to maintain active ROM or perform passive ROM to unaffected extremities.
▶ *Skin Integrity, Impaired, Risk for, related to immobility*	The client will maintain skin integrity.	Handle the affected extremity gently, protect it from injury, keep it in good body alignment and level with the body.
		Irrigate wound as ordered.
		Use aseptic technique when irrigating the affected area and when changing the dressing.
		Assess skin and bony prominences for reddened areas.
		Encourage adequate fluid intake.
▶ *Pain related to inflammation*	The client will verbalize reduction of pain.	Protect client from jerky movements and falls.
		Assess wound appearance and new sites of pain.
		Provide diet high in protein and vitamin C.
		Administer pain medications as ordered.

Evaluation Each goal must be evaluated to determine how it has been met by the client.

DEGENERATIVE DISORDERS

Conditions discussed following include osteoporosis, degenerative joint disease, and total joint arthroplasty.

OSTEOPOROSIS

Osteoporosis is an increase in the porosity of bone. It is a common disorder in bone metabolism in which both mineral and protein matrix components are diminished and the bone becomes brittle and fragile. There is an increased susceptibility to fractures of the hip, spine, and wrist.

Ten million individuals in the United States have osteoporosis and another 18 million have low bone mineral density which places them at risk for osteoporosis (Dowd & Cavalieri, 1999; National Osteoporosis Foundation [NOF], 1999b; National Institute of Arthritis and Musculoskeletal and Skin Diseases [NIAMS], October

1998). Of those affected by osteoporosis, 80% are women (NOF, 1999c). More than 1.5 million fractures occur annually related to osteoporosis, including 300,000 hip fractures, 700,000 vertebral fractures, 250,000 wrist fractures, and more than 300,000 fractures of other types (NOF, 1999c).

Osteoporosis has been called the "silent disease" because there are no symptoms of bone loss. Bone loss may be 50% before pain or a fracture occurs (Darovic, 1997). Because the bone tissue loses its density, fractures and kyphosis may occur. Very slight trauma may fracture the brittle bones. With multiple vertebral fractures, the individual may experience a loss of height.

The only way to determine if an individual has osteoporosis is to measure bone mineral density (BMD). There are several methods of measuring BMD; all are painless, noninvasive, and safe. They include:

- DXA or DEXA (dual energy X-ray absorptiometry) measures spine, hip, or total body.

- SXA (single energy X-ray absorptiometry) measures wrist or heel.
- DPA (dual photon absorptiometry) measures spine, hip, or total body.
- Ultrasound measures heel, shin bone, and kneecap (NOF, 1999b).

Medical–Surgical Management

There is no cure for osteoporosis. Prevention through diet, regular exercise, and eliminating tobacco and alcohol use is the best defense against osteoporosis (Dowd and Cavalieri, 1999).

Pharmacological

Four medications are approved for postmenopausal women to prevent and/or treat osteoporosis; no medications are as yet approved for men (NOF, 1999c). Estrogen is used both for prevention and treatment. It is the primary choice for prevention in postmenopausal women. Alendronate sodium (Fosamax) is used for prevention and treatment. Calcitonin (Miacalcin) for treatment of osteoporosis is available as a nasal spray. To obtain its full therapeutic effect, the client should also take calcium and vitamin D supplements. To pre-vent osteoporosis, raloxifene (Evista) may be used. It prevents bone loss throughout the body, but may cause venous thrombosis.

Testosterone replacement therapy may be used for men with low testosterone levels.

Nonnarcotic analgesics may be prescribed for relief of pain. The client may also be advised to take supplemental calcium.

Diet

The client is encouraged to maintain an adequate balanced diet rich in calcium and vitamin D. A reduction in the consumption of caffeine, alcohol, excess protein, and the use of cigarettes is recommended.

Activity

The client is encouraged to practice good body mechanics and posture. Walking, preferably outdoors for the benefits of sunshine (vitamin D), is also encouraged. This is effective in preventing further bone loss and stimulating new bone formation.

▶ NURSING PROCESS

▶ Assessment

▶ Subjective Data

This includes the client's gender, age, and family health history. Any symptoms the client expresses regarding altered body image or back or neck pain that worsens when coughing, sneezing, straining, or standing should be noted. A nutritional history should be taken. Lifestyle patterns such as smoking, inactivity, or immobilization should be noted. A medical history regarding any medications is also important.

▶ Objective Data

This includes a dowager's hump, gait impairment, and posture.

Nursing diagnoses for a client with osteoporosis may include the following:

Nursing Diagnoses	Planning/Goals	Nursing Interventions
▶ *Pain, Chronic, related to disease process*	The client will express minimal discomfort.	Administer analgesics as ordered; teach the client about the medications.
		Handle the client carefully; instruct the client to avoid any twisting movements.
		The bed should have a firm mattress or bed board for support.
▶ *Injury, High Risk for, related to disease process*	The client will practice correct body mechanics.	Teach client correct body mechanics.
▶ *Mobility, Impaired, Physical, related to disease process*	The client will maintain physical activity.	Teach client about types of exercises and physical activities that will help maintain bone mass and isometric exercises to strengthen muscles.
		Encourage ambulation with the client using a walker or cane if necessary.

Evaluation Each goal must be evaluated to determine how it has been met by the client.

DEGENERATIVE JOINT DISEASE (OSTEOARTHRITIS)

Since osteoarthritis is not an inflammatory disorder, as the name implies, the term *degenerative joint disease* (DJD) is often used to better reflect the pathophysiology. Osteoarthritis is considered a "wear and tear" disease and is characterized by the slow and steady progressive destructive changes of the joint. It is a nonsystemic, noninflammatory disorder causing bones and joints to degenerate. It is the most common type of arthritis. The etiology is unknown but predisposing factors include obesity, an injury to a joint, poor posture, or occupations that put strain on joints. Recent studies suggest that there may also be a genetic cause of osteoarthritis (NIAMS, May 1998). The weight bearing joints of the lower extremities as well as the hands and cervical and lumbar vertebrae are the joints most frequently affected. The cartilage covering the bone becomes thin and then wears off. The synovial membrane thickens and fibrous tissue around the joint ossifies. The effects of degenerative changes on the knee joint are shown in Figure 38-13.

The onset of osteoarthritis begins during middle age, and by age 60 most people have some degeneration. Symptoms include early morning stiffness and pain after physical activity. There is joint enlargement and characteristic hypertrophic spurs, called **Heberden's nodes,** in the terminal interphalangeal finger joints. More women are affected with DJD, especially in the hands. The hips are more affected in men.

Diagnosis is made from the client's symptoms and examination of the joints that are enlarged and tender. X-ray shows a narrowing of joint spaces and gross irregularities of joint structure. A CT scan or MRI may be used to show vertebral joint involvement.

Medical–Surgical Management

Medical

No treatment exists to stop the degenerative process; therefore, treatment focuses on the relief of the client's discomfort. Medical management includes local heat and rest for the affected joint, weight reduction for obese clients to relieve strain on affected joints, and orthotic devices (braces, canes, crutches) to support the inflamed joints. Physical therapy can provide exercises to strengthen muscles and teach self-management skills.

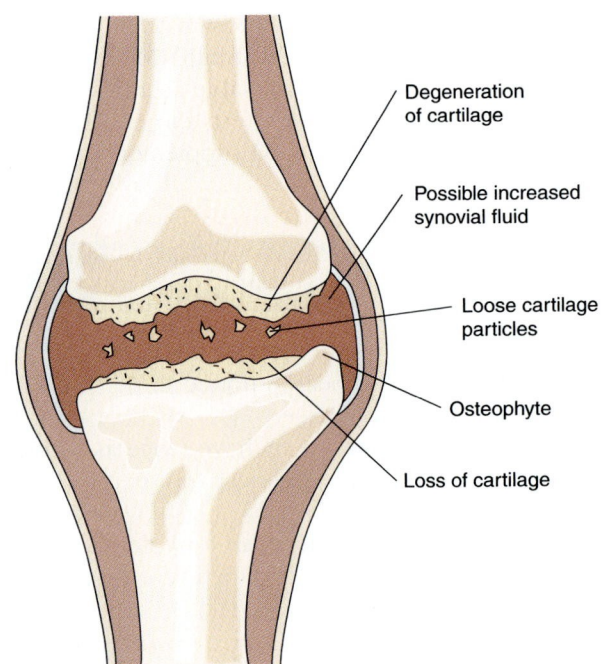

Figure 38-13 Degenerative Changes in the Cartilage of the Knee Due to Osteoarthritis

Surgical

Surgical procedures such as total hip or knee replacement may be recommended for clients with severe osteoarthritis. Osteotomy may help correct malalignment situations. Refer to the section on total joint arthroplasty in this chapter.

Pharmacological

Pharmacological treatment includes the use of aspirin or NSAIDs. Narcotics should be avoided because of the chronic nature of the disease. Steroids may be used and are sometimes injected into a joint to provide immediate relief of pain and to stop the degenerative process temporarily. If the client has vertebral involvement with muscle spasms, cyclobenzaprine hydrochloride (Flexeril) may be given to relax the muscles.

▶ NURSING PROCESS

▶ Assessment

▶ Subjective Data

The client may describe nonspecific symptoms such as general musculoskeletal pain, joint stiffness especially on rising, and joint pain or tenderness. Weight gain and occupation and any conditions or situations that may exacerbate the client's joint pain should be noted. Some of these situations may include cold weather, overexercising, or extreme fatigue. The client's understanding of the disease and its effect on lifestyle and ability to perform activities of daily and social living should also be assessed.

▶ Objective Data

This includes edema and tenderness around the joints and bony enlargements of distal interphalangeal joints (Heberden's nodes).

Nursing diagnoses for a client with osteoarthritis may include the following:

Nursing Diagnoses	Planning/Goals	Nursing Interventions
▶ *Pain, Chronic, related to joint tenderness and edema*	The client will express minimal discomfort.	Handle the affected extremity gently and apply heat as ordered. Administer prescribed analgesic and evaluate its effectiveness.
▶ *Mobility, Impaired, Physical, related to joint deterioration*	The client will maintain mobility within the parameters of the disease process.	Coordinate with physical therapy and assist in a planned exercise program as ordered. Advise the client to plan rest periods during the day.

Evaluation Each goal must be evaluated to determine how it has been met by the client.

TOTAL JOINT ARTHROPLASTY

Joint replacement or **arthroplasty** is the replacement of both articular surfaces within a joint capsule. The hip, knee, shoulder, and fingers are the joints most frequently replaced in this procedure. Replacements consist of metal and polyethylene and may be cemented in the prepared bone with methyl methacrylate which has properties similar to bone. See Figure 38-14 for knee and hip replacement components.

Newer techniques use porous-coated cementless artificial joint components. These allow bone to grow into the joint component and securely fix the prosthesis. This reduces the incidence of prosthesis failure.

Joint replacement is usually an elective procedure and clients may wish to have autologous blood transfusions whereby they pre-donate their own blood in case a blood transfusion is needed.

TOTAL HIP REPLACEMENT

Total hip replacement is the replacement of a severely damaged hip with an artificial joint. This procedure is usually reserved for clients over 60 with severe pain or irreversibly damaged hip joints. However, with improved prosthetic materials and operative techniques, younger clients with severely damaged hips are being considered for total hip replacement surgery. Potential problems with the hip replacement include

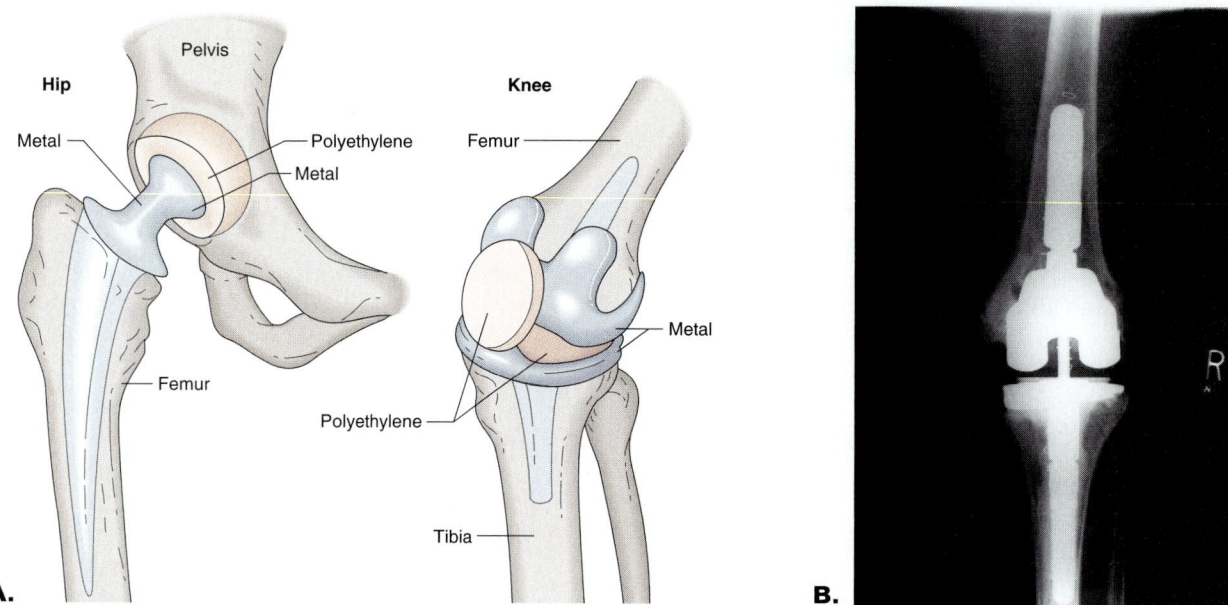

Figure 38-14 A. Total hip and knee replacement; B. Radiograph of a total knee replacement (anterior-posterior view). Because the patella is plastic, it is not visible here.

dislocation of the prosthesis, excessive wound drainage, and infection.

Following a total hip replacement the client's hip and leg should be kept in a position of abduction and extension. The knees are kept apart by using foam wedges, several pillows, or an abductor pillow. The client may lie on the unaffected side. When the client turns from the back to a side-lying position, the entire leg should be supported with pillows to keep the hip abducted. The client should be instructed to avoid acute flexion of the hip. The legs should not be crossed nor the hips flexed to pull up a blanket or sheet. A fracture bedpan should be used until the client can ambulate to the bathroom. In the bathroom a raised toilet seat should be used. Any specific client turning, movement, and positioning will be ordered by the physician. Vital signs and circulation, movement, and sensation (CMS) checks should be done routinely.

Dressings should be inspected frequently. If the surgical site is drained with a portable suction device, it should be monitored for patency, and the type and amount of drainage. Initially drainage might be 200 to 500 cc. Within 48 hours the drainage should decrease to 30 cc or less and the suction device can be removed.

The goal for clients who have total hip or knee joint replacement is to ambulate independently. Ambulatory activity progresses rapidly for clients with joint replacement. Clients who have total hip replacement are usually out of bed the night of surgery or early the next day. Gait training may begin with the use of a walker and progress to the use of crutches or a cane.

The client should avoid hip flexion of more than 90 degrees. Stair climbing should be avoided for at least 3 months.

TOTAL KNEE REPLACEMENT

Total knee replacement, like the hip replacement, is considered for clients experiencing severe pain and functional disability related to joint destruction. The prosthesis chosen for the replacement provides the client with a painless, stable, and functional joint. Following total knee replacement surgery, clients may use a continuous passive motion (CPM) machine. This machine helps to increase circulation to the operative area and promotes flexibility within the knee joint. The surgeon orders the frequency of use and the amount of tension, flexion, and extension produced by the machine.

Following knee arthroplasty, the client's knee may be immobilized with a firm compression dressing and an adjustable soft knee immobilizer. The client may transfer out of bed to a wheelchair with the immobilizer in place. No weight bearing is allowed on the knee until it is prescribed by the surgeon. If ordered, a sequential compression device (SCD) may be used or antiembolism stockings worn to minimize the development of thrombophlebitis.

Rehabilitation generally starts the second day for clients who have total knee arthroplasty. When the client sits in a chair, the knee should be elevated. Ambulation with assistive aids and weight bearing limits is usually started 1 to 2 days after surgery.

▶ NURSING PROCESS

▶ Assessment

▶ Subjective Data

This involves assessing for irritability, restlessness, orientation, and neurovascular assessment of the affected extremity for pain, numbness, tingling, and paresthesia.

▶ Objective Data

This involves assessing the incision for approximation, redness, and drainage. Assessment of skin over all bony prominences should also be made, as well as assessment for tachypnea, dyspnea, hypoxemia, and crackles and wheezes in the lungs (signs of fat embolism). Vital signs, pedal pulses, and I & O are also assessed.

The client with a total hip replacement should be assessed for position of the affected hip. The hip should be maintained in a position of abduction and extension. The most prominent symptom of a dislocation is a clicking, popping sound. Other symptoms are a sudden sharp pain that is unrelieved by narcotic analgesics, loss of leg motion, and edema of the affected hip. The client should not be moved and the physician should be notified immediately.

Assessment of the client with a total knee replacement includes the neurovascular status of the leg, the dressing and drainage device, keeping the knee elevated, and monitoring the CPM machine. Vital signs, intake and output, and the color and temperature of the extremity are also assessed.

Nursing diagnoses for the client undergoing arthroplasty surgery may include the following:

Nursing Diagnoses	Planning/Goals	Nursing Interventions
▶ *Skin Integrity, Impaired, related to immobility and surgical incision*	The client's skin will remain free from redness or any other signs of breakdown.	Maintain a clean and dry dressing. If a drainage device is used, assess functioning.
		Keep client's skin and bed clean and dry.
		Assess bony prominences for redness.
		Provide high-protein diet with dairy products and vitamin C.
▶ *Mobility, Impaired, Physical, related to surgery*	The client will ambulate following physician's direction.	Keep client in a position of abduction. Use an abductor pillow or wedge to maintain the position when turning the client.
		Assist the client in accomplishing activities of daily living.
		Encourage client to use the trapeze to raise hips off the bed to use the bedpan.
▶ *Tissue Perfusion, Altered Peripheral, related to surgery and immobility*	The client will have adequate circulation of extremity.	Encourage the client to cough and deep breathe.
		Monitor vital signs until stable.
		Assess pedal pulses and capillary refill in both extremities.

Evaluation Each goal must be evaluated to determine how it has been met by the client.

MUSCULOSKELETAL DISORDERS

Musculoskeletal disorders discussed include amputations, temporomandibular joint disease/disorder, and carpal tunnel syndrome.

AMPUTATIONS

An **amputation** is the removal of all or part of an extremity. Amputations are done in response to injuries resulting in extensive laceration of arteries or nerves, or diseases such as malignant tumors, infections, and peripheral vascular disorders. Other disease conditions that may require amputation include extensive osteomyelitis, or congenital disorders. In severe trauma situations, an amputation may be done to save the client's life.

Recent advances in microsurgical techniques have allowed replantation (limb reattachment) in some injuries. These procedures involve the use of microscopes and highly specialized instruments to reconnect severed nerves and blood vessels. Amputations involving the hand or wrist are more likely to be considered for replantation rather than an injury involving a large muscle mass because of extensive tissue, bone, and muscle damage. Any amputation creates a major physical and psychological adjustment for the client.

Medical–Surgical Management

Medical

Rehabilitation for the client with an amputation requires the effort of the entire rehabilitation team. The client's physical and psychological responses to the amputation are monitored by all members of the team. If appropriate, counseling and job training will enable many clients to return to their jobs.

Surgical

Before surgery the surgeon must evaluate the client and make several decisions. These decisions include: necessity of an amputation, type of amputation (open or closed), level of amputation, potential for rehabilitation, and type of prosthesis and rehabilitation program.

The surgeon will try to save as much of the limb as possible. A closed amputation is done by using skin flaps to cover the bone end of the extremity. This type of amputation is done when there is no evidence of infection. Sometimes a Guillotine (open) amputation is necessary. This amputation requires a straight cut and allows for free drainage of infectious material. Tissue, bone, and vessels are severed at the same level without skin flaps. The major indication for doing an open amputation is infection.

The level of an amputation is determined by the vascular supply and is never higher than absolutely necessary. If the blood flow at the site of the incision is normal, the amputation is performed at that level. If the bleeding is scant, a higher level of amputation is performed to ensure adequate postoperative healing.

Pharmacological

Narcotic analgesics may be required immediately following surgery. After several days pain may be controlled with nonnarcotic analgesics. If infection exists, appropriate antibiotic therapy will be ordered.

Diet

A balanced diet with adequate vitamins and protein is essential for adequate wound healing. Many elderly clients are poorly nourished or require special diets. Nutritional care plans should be discussed with the physician and a dietitian.

Activity

Postoperative positioning of the stump will be determined by the surgeon. The stump may be placed in an extended position or elevated on pillows for short periods. The client should also be encouraged to spend some time in the prone position. This position helps to stretch the flexor muscles and to prevent contractions of the hip. One to 2 days following surgery the client may begin bed exercises. These exercises, taught by the physical therapist, are done to prevent contractures and increase muscle strength. Ambulation begins in physical therapy after transfer techniques are learned by the client. Ambulation progresses according to whether the client is to be fitted with a prosthesis immediately or at a later time.

▶ NURSING PROCESS

▶ Assessment

▶ Subjective Data

This should include pain, sensations felt on extremity to be amputated, and the emotional status of the client. If a client has experienced chronic pain prior to the amputation, pain may seem mild following the surgery. Severe pain may indicate a hematoma or excessive pressure from a cast or elastic bandage on a bony prominence. The client may confuse **phantom limb pain** with the incisional pain. Phantom limb pain is the sensation that there is pain, soreness, and stiffness in the amputated limb. Phantom pain will decrease as inflammation subsides at the incisional site.

▶ Objective Data

This includes the color and temperature of the skin, pulse, and responses to limb movement. The unaffected extremity should also be assessed for function and circulation.

Nursing diagnoses for the client who has an amputation may include the following:

Nursing Diagnoses	Planning/Goals	Nursing Interventions
▶ *Skin Integrity, Impaired, related to amputation*	The client will remain free from infection.	Inspect the incision for any inflammation, excessive drainage, edema, increased pain, and hypersensitivity to touch.
		Use aseptic technique for all dressing changes.
		Monitor vital signs.

continued

Nursing Diagnoses	Planning/Goals	Nursing Interventions
▸ *Body Image Disturbance related to loss of limb*	The client will participate in the care of the residual limb.	Handle the residual limb gently and treat it as though a prosthesis will be worn.
		Encourage client to watch dressing change and eventually assist with and do the dressing changes.
		Encourage the client to express feelings and concerns about the amputation.
▸ *Mobility, Impaired, Physical, related to loss of limb*	The client will demonstrate improved physical mobility.	Encourage the client to participate in physical therapy.
		Assist the client when ambulating with assistive devices.
		Encourage client to perform ROM exercises.

Evaluation Each goal must be evaluated to determine how it has been met by the client.

SAMPLE NURSING CARE PLAN

THE CLIENT WITH A BELOW THE KNEE AMPUTATION

Mrs. Spencer is a 76-year-old resident in a retirement home. She has remained active since her retirement from the secretarial job she held for 20 years. Her health history indicates she has had circulatory problems with inadequate peripheral circulation resulting from atherosclerosis. Her physician has hospitalized her for a planned below the knee amputation on the left leg and has ordered an arteriogram to assist in determining the site for the amputation. The arteriogram will help determine the circulatory status of her leg necessary to promote wound healing.

The nurse's assessment of Mrs. Spencer's vital signs indicated B/P 120/68, pulse 72, and respirations 18. Femoral pulses were present in both extremities; however, the pedal pulse in her left foot was barely palpable, and the skin was cool and pale. She stated that lately her left foot is always cold and is a "bluish-black" color. Mrs. Spencer has expressed concern about her ability to take care of herself after she loses her foot.

Nursing Diagnosis 1 *Body Image Disturbance, related to scheduled amputation as evidenced by statement of concern over losing foot*

PLANNING/GOALS	NURSING INTERVENTIONS	RATIONALE	EVALUATION
Mrs. Spencer will communicate her concerns and feelings about the changes in her body image.	Involve Mrs. Spencer in participating in her daily care.	Gives sense of independence.	Mrs. Spencer has demonstrated beginning acceptance of body changes by taking an active interest in her appearance.
	Encourage Mrs. Spencer to voice her concerns.	Helps resolve concerns.	
	Provide positive reinforcement when Mrs. Spencer attempts to adapt to body changes.	Encourages her to continue adapting.	

Nursing Diagnosis 2 *Self-Esteem, Situational Low, related to loss of body part as evidenced by expression of concern about ability to care for self*

PLANNING/GOALS	NURSING INTERVENTIONS	RATIONALE	EVALUATION
Mrs. Spencer will identify at least two positive qualities about herself.	Encourage Mrs. Spencer to express her feelings about herself.	Listening helps Mrs. Spencer identify positive qualities.	Mrs. Spencer has voiced two positive qualities about herself.

continued

| | Involve Mrs. Spencer in the decision-making process regarding her care. | Helps Mrs. Spencer maintain a sense of control over her life. | |
| | Provide Mrs. Spencer with positive feedback. | Gives Mrs. Spencer a feeling of approval. | |

Nursing Diagnosis 3 *Grieving, Anticipatory, related to loss associated with amputation as evidenced by her expression of concern*

PLANNING/GOALS	NURSING INTERVENTIONS	RATIONALE	EVALUATION
Mrs. Spencer will express her feelings about the loss of her foot.	Encourage Mrs. Spencer to express her feelings by talking, crying, writing.	Some people are uncomfortable expressing their feelings; gives several options for expression.	Mrs. Spencer expresses feelings about her potential loss.
	Spend a specific amount of nonnursing time each shift with Mrs. Spencer to allow for uninterrupted conversation.	Allows expression of feelings and shows concern and understanding.	
	Inform Mrs. Spencer and her family about support groups and organizations in the community.	May help Mrs. Spencer find new ways of adapting to loss.	

Nursing Diagnosis 4 *Knowledge Deficit related to postoperative care and activity as evidenced by concern about ability to care for self*

PLANNING/GOALS	NURSING INTERVENTIONS	RATIONALE	EVALUATION
Mrs. Spencer will perform stump wrapping correctly.	Encourage Mrs. Spencer to participate in the care of the residual limb.	Encouraging participation helps client adjust to body changes.	Mrs. Spencer demonstrated the ability to care for the residual limb by wrapping the stump correctly.
	Demonstrate how to wrap her stump, then allow her to do it several times.	Discharge instructions help clients to know how to take care of themselves.	

TEMPOROMANDIBULAR JOINT DISEASE/DISORDER

Temporomandibular joint disease/disorder (TMD) is commonly referred to as TMJ by the general public. It is a collection of conditions affecting the temporomandibular joint and/or the muscles of mastication.

Over 10 million people in the United States have TMD. It affects both males and females, but 90% of those seeking treatment are females between puberty and menopause (The TMJ Association, 1998). The majority of clients will get better with or without treatment (The TMJ Association, 1998).

The temporomandibular joint is the articular surface

between the mandible and temporal bone of the skull. It is a combined hinge and gliding joint. Normally, the mandible moves smoothly, appears symmetrical, and is without deformity. Causes for TMD include: trauma, stress, teeth clenching or grinding (**bruxism**), and joint diseases such as rheumatoid arthritis or osteoarthritis. Common symptoms of TMD include limited jaw movement, clicking or crepitus when the jaw moves, popping when chewing or talking, and radiating pain in the face, neck, or shoulders. The clicking is caused by displaced cartilage. The jaw may lock as a result of muscle spasms.

Diagnosis of TMD may include an x-ray to evaluate the bony structure, a CT scan, to evaluate any degenerative changes, an MRI or arthrography, and an evaluation of the teeth and jaw in a bite position. Nursing assessment of the joint includes movement and appearance. If the mandible protrudes, it may indicate a mandibular dislocation.

Medical management consists of moist heat to promote muscle relaxation, cold therapy to reduce muscle spasms, and analgesics or nonsteroidal anti-inflammatory drugs. Clients may be fitted with a dental retainer or bite plate to prevent teeth clenching or grinding, or splints to help realign malocclusions. Procedures such as arthroscopy or surgery to reshape the joint may be done in some cases that do not respond to medical treatment.

A soft diet allows the jaw and muscles to relax. Clients should be advised against chewing gum.

CARPAL TUNNEL SYNDROME

Carpal tunnel syndrome occurs when the median nerve in the wrist is compressed by inflamed, edematous flexor tendons and tenosynovium (Figure 38-15). Symptoms include pain, paresthesia, and weakness of the thumb, index, middle and part of ring fingers but never the little finger. Persons working in occupations requiring repetitive movement of hands and fingers, such as computers, typing, intense quilting, or crocheting, have a higher incidence of this syndrome. Arthritis or fractures may also be a cause. Diagnosis is based on a physical examination and the subjective symptoms of the client and may be confirmed by motor nerve velocity studies.

Medical–Surgical Management

Medical

Treatment consists of rest for the hands. Splints to immobilize the hand and wrist may also be used to help relieve some of the discomfort.

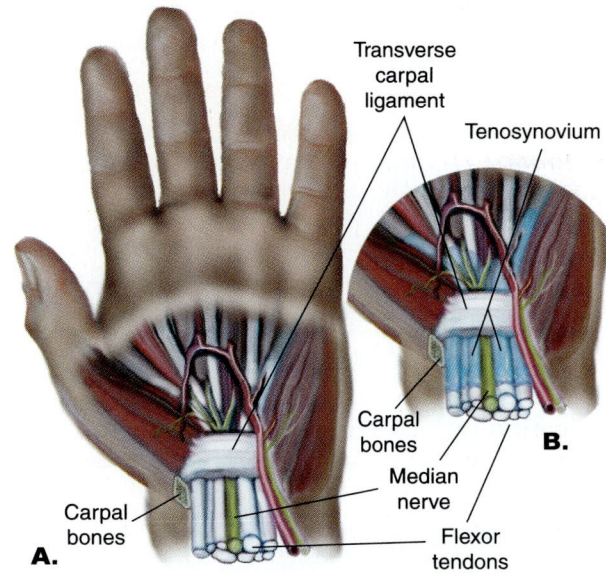

Figure 38-15 Carpal Tunnel Syndrome: A. Cross-section of carpal tunnel showing nerves and tendons; B. Inflamed flexor tendons and tenosynovium put pressure on the median nerve.

Surgical

If conservative treatment does not control the symptoms, surgery may be necessary to relieve the pressure on the median nerve. After surgery, the hand is elevated and may be in a splint for up to 2 weeks. Lifting is restricted for several weeks.

Pharmacological

Anti-inflammatory drugs may decrease inflammation and edema and reduce symptoms. NSAIDs may provide pain relief. If symptoms are not controlled with these measures, cortisone may injected into the carpal tunnel.

▶ NURSING PROCESS

▶ Assessment

▶ Subjective Data

This consists of the client's description of tingling in the hands, and numbness in the thumb, index, middle and part of the ring fingers. The client may also state that there is a feeling of "puffiness" in the affected hand and that the client is unable to grasp or hold small objects. Waking in the middle of the night with pain and a feeling that the entire hand is asleep is very common.

▶ Objective Data

This may include atrophy of the padded area at the base of the thumb.

Nursing diagnoses for a client with carpal tunnel syndrome may include the following:

Nursing Diagnoses	Planning/Goals	Nursing Interventions
▶ *Pain related to inflammation and swelling causing pressure on the median nerve*	The client will have less discomfort.	Administer analgesics as ordered and teach client about use, side effects, and dosage.
		Encourage client to wear wrist brace.
		Encourage client to refrain from repetitive hand movements.
▶ *Disuse Syndrome, Hand, Risk for, related to tingling and numbness of hand and wrist*	The client will use fingers and hand.	Teach client to do ROM exercises, and to prevent twisting and turning of wrist.

Evaluation Each goal must be evaluated to determine how it has been met by the client.

SYSTEMIC DISORDERS WITH MUSCULOSKELETAL MANIFESTATIONS

Disorders discussed following include gout and lyme disease.

GOUT

Gout is a metabolic disease of ineffective purine metabolism resulting from deposits of needlelike crystals of uric acid in connective tissue, joint spaces, or both. It affects 2.1 million individuals in the United States (Arthritis Foundation, 1998). Middle-aged men are most commonly affected, but it may occur in women after menopause. Gout may be primary (an inherited problem with purine metabolism), secondary (complication from another disease or from use of certain drugs), or idiopathic (unknown cause). Up to 18% of clients with gout have a family history of the disease (NIAMS, January 1999). The excessive use of alcohol interferes with uric acid removal from the body and may contribute to or exacerbate symptoms.

The attack generally begins abruptly with severe constant pain. The joint becomes swollen, red, and tender. The great toe is the joint most frequently involved; however, any joint may be affected. The course of gout is variable with 1 to 2 attacks being severe. If the disease is untreated, the attacks may occur with increasing frequency. Clients with symptoms of gout may develop **tophi** which are subcutaneous nodular deposits of sodium urate crystals appearing in various parts of the body including the rim of the ears, the knuckles, and great toe. Diagnosis is made from the client's health history and an examination of the affected joint. Aspiration of the joint synovial fluid will show urate crystals. The client should be instructed to avoid foods high in purine. These foods include liver, sardines, sweetbreads, anchovies, gravies, and asparagus. Oral fluid intake should be increased to 3,000 mL/day to reduce the possibility of urate stone formation in the kidneys.

To reduce inflammation, NSAIDs are given, especially indomethacin (Indocin) and naproxen (Anaprox, Naprosyn). Colchicine may be used if NSAIDs are ineffective. When tophi develop, medicine to reduce hyperuricemia may be used, such as allopurinol (Zyloprim) and probenecid (Benemid).

LYME DISEASE

Lyme disease is caused by a spirochete *Borrelia burgdorferi* carried by deer ticks. In the United States it has been reported in nearly all states, but most cases are in the coastal northeast, mid-Altantic states, Minnesota, and northern California (National Institute of Allergies and Infectious Diseases [NIAID], 1999).

These ticks should be removed by using a tweezers. Early manifestations occur from spring through late fall. People living in states with a high incidence of Lyme disease should wear protective clothing and check for ticks frequently. Insect repellent containing DEET should be applied to exposed parts of the body and to clothing. Household pets should wear a flea and tick collar and also be checked frequently for ticks.

For most individuals, the first symptom is a red rash called erythema migrans. It starts as a red spot at the site of the tick bite and expands resembling a bull's eye. Other symptoms are headache, neck stiffness, fever, and pain. For those individuals untreated with antibiotics, arthritis (joint swelling and pain), fatigue, and neurological abnormalities like facial palsy, meningitis, and encephalitis become evident. The antibody test ELISA is used to identify antibodies to *B. burgdorferi* in blood or spinal fluid specimens. Antibiotics such as doxycycline (Vibramycin), cefuroxime exetil (Ceftin), or amoxicillin (Amoxil) speed healing of the rash and prevents arthritis and neurological symptoms.

CASE STUDY

George Ellis, a 40-year-old truck driver, was getting ready to help unload his cargo. He was climbing into the truck when he lost his balance and fell to the ground, twisting his left leg. He stated he was in severe pain and was unable to stand. His coworkers called the emergency ambulance service to transport him to the hospital. Upon arrival in the emergency room, the nurse immediately took Mr. Ellis's vital signs. His vital signs were temperature 98.6°F, pulse 92, respirations 24, and blood pressure 158/90. The nurse also noted that Mr. Ellis's face was flushed and his left leg was shorter than his right.

The following questions will guide your development of a nursing care plan for the case study.

1. List five types of fractures.
2. Based on the action of the fall, what type of fracture do you think Mr. Ellis may have received?
3. What diagnostic measures will determine whether or not Mr. Ellis has a fracture of his left leg?
4. What immediate care should have been given to Mr. Ellis?
5. List four nursing interventions for clients in traction.
6. What options may be considered for treatment of Mr. Ellis's injury?
7. List objective and subjective information the nurse would obtain regarding Mr. Ellis's injury.

SUMMARY

- When assessing the client with a musculoskeletal disorder, the nurse should evaluate any changes in appearance including alignment, loss of motion, and any signs of circulatory impairment.
- Treatment of a fracture may include any one or more of the following methods: closed reduction, open reduction that may include internal fixation, casts, and traction.
- Complications of a fracture include infection, fat embolism, and compartment syndrome.
- Compartment syndrome is a serious form of neurovascular impairment. Symptoms include severe pain that is not relieved with narcotic analgesics, sluggish capillary refill, weak pulses, numbness, and paralysis.
- When a client is in traction it is important to remember to preserve body alignment, maintain continuous pull and countertraction, keep the ropes moving freely through the pulleys, use the prescribed amount of weights, and keep the weights hanging freely.
- Osteoarthritis is characterized by slow progressive degeneration of joint articular cartilage.
- Hips, knees, and fingers are the joints most frequently considered for replacement.
- Following total hip replacement, the hip should be kept in a position of abduction and extension.
- Following total knee replacement surgery, some clients may use a CPM machine that promotes knee joint flexibility and increased circulation to the operative area.

- Individuals at greatest risk for developing osteoporosis are postmenopausal women and older adults who are generally inactive.
- Carpal tunnel syndrome occurs in individuals who perform jobs requiring repetitive wrist and hand movements. The resulting trauma causes inflammation and edema that compresses the median nerve, causing numbness, pain, and impaired mobility to the hand and fingers.

Review Questions

1. A fracture caused by forceful twisting is known as a:
   a. comminuted fracture.
   b. spiral fracture.
   c. transverse fracture.
   d. greenstick fracture.

2. The primary goal in the treatment of a fracture is to:
   a. aid in the formation of osteoclasts.
   b. aid in the formation of granulation tissue.
   c. establish a callus between the broken ends of bone.
   d. prevent further injury to the fractured limb.

3. A closed reduction of a fracture:
   a. always requires surgery.
   b. is completed by manual manipulation.
   c. never requires a cast.
   d. requires the use of immobilizing plates.

4. The nurse knows that proper body positioning and alignment of an immobilized client is always maintained to prevent:
   a. scoliosis.
   b. lordosis.
   c. contractures.
   d. atony.

5. One of the first symptoms a client with arthritis may complain of is:
   a. nausea after each meal.
   b. joint stiffness especially on arising.
   c. an increased appetite.
   d. muscle spasms after exercising.

6. Traction is frequently used to treat clients with a musculoskeletal problem. One of the primary reasons for traction is to:
   a. heal a fracture.
   b. maintain a corrected position.
   c. stop muscle spasms.
   d. prevent infection.

7. Osteomyelitis:
   a. affects mainly the hip bone.
   b. is a bacterial infection of the bone.
   c. occurs most often in adults.
   d. causes a great deal of deformity.

Critical Thinking Questions

1. Prepare a teaching plan for a client to learn how to use crutches.

2. How would you explain "phantom limb pain" to a client?

3. What is the rationale for each nursing intervention for the nursing diagnoses given in this chapter?

 WEB FLASH!

- Search the Internet for information about the disorders in this chapter. What new diagnostic tests or treatments are being tested?
- Is there information focused for clients' use? What type of information is this?

NURSING CARE OF THE CLIENT: IMMUNE SYSTEM

CHAPTER 39

MAKING THE CONNECTION

Refer to the following chapters to increase your understanding of immune system disorders:

- **Chapter 6, Legal Responsibilities**
- **Chapter 8, Communication**
- **Chapter 15, Wellness Concepts**
- **Chapter 21, Infection Control/Asepsis**
- **Chapter 22, Standard Precautions and Isolation**
- **Chapter 23, Fluid, Electrolyte, and Acid-Base Balance**
- **Chapter 25, Assessment**
- **Chapter 26, Pain Management**
- **Chapter 30, Nursing Care of the Oncology Client**
- **Chapter 31, Nursing Care of the Client: Respiratory System**
- **Chapter 32, Nursing Care of the Client: Cardiovascular System**
- **Chapter 33, Nursing Care of the Client: Blood and Lymph Systems**
- **Chapter 34, Nursing Care of the Client: Gastrointestinal System**
- **Chapter 36, Nursing Care of the Client: Sexually Transmitted Diseases**
- **Chapter 38, Nursing Care of the Client: Musculoskeletal System**
- **Chapter 40, Nursing Care of the Client: Integumentary System**
- **Chapter 41, Nursing Care of the Client: Nervous System**
- **Chapter 46, Nursing Care of the Client: Substance Abuse**
- **Procedures:** B1, Handwashing; B2, Use of Protective Equipment; A1, Initiating Strict Isolation Precautions

LEARNING OBJECTIVES

Upon completion of this chapter, you should be able to:
- *Define key terms.*
- *Identify three allergic reactions with a systemic response.*
- *Describe symptoms of anaphylaxis and appropriate first aid.*
- *Recall common diagnostic tests used to evaluate immunological functioning.*
- *Discuss the medical/surgical management of clients with immunological disorders.*
- *Relate signs and symptoms of complications clients with immunological disorders could experience.*
- *Explain the modes of transmission of HIV.*
- *Identify methods of risk reduction of HIV for health care workers.*
- *Use the nursing process to plan the care of clients with immune system disorders.*

KEY TERMS

acquired immuno-deficiency syndrome
allergen
anaphylaxis
angioedema
antibodies
antigen
autoimmune disorder
autologous
cellular immunity
cytomegalovirus
diplopia
enzyme-linked immuno-sorbent assay
exacerbation
histamine
HIV-wasting syndrome
homologous
human immuno-deficiency virus
human leukocyte antigen
humoral immunity
hypersensitivity
immune response
immunity
immunotherapy
Kaposi's sarcoma
myasthenia gravis
Mycobacterium avium complex

INTRODUCTION

Immunity is the body's ability to protect itself from foreign agents or organisms. This occurs through the complex interaction of the tissues within the immune system. Constant surveillance of cells within the body occurs to differentiate self from nonself. Those identified as nonself are then neutralized or destroyed. Dead or damaged cells are eliminated and homeostasis is maintained. When alterations in the system develop, immunological conditions develop. They may be hypersensitivity responses such as allergies, immunological deficiencies, such as those associated with corticosteroid medications; or **autoimmune disorders**, where the body identifies its own cells as foreign and activates mechanisms to destroy them. Rheumatoid arthritis, systemic lupus erythematosus, and myasthenia gravis are examples of autoimmune disorders. Immunosuppressive disorders suppress the body's natural immune response to an antigen. Kaposi's sarcoma and non-Hodgkin's lymphoma are examples of immunosuppressive disorders.

ANATOMY AND PHYSIOLOGY REVIEW

The human body has a variety of natural physical and chemical mechanisms that enhance immunological functioning. The skin, eyelashes, cilia in the nose and respiratory system, gastric acidity, intestinal mucosa, and pH of vaginal mucosa all act to protect against invading organisms. In addition, all body tissues are linked together via lymphatic ducts and blood vessels to the organs and cells of the immune system.

Organs of the Immune System

The organs of the immune system are classified as primary or peripheral lymphoid organs. Primary lymphoid organs are bone marrow and the thymus gland. Within bone marrow, stem cells, the parent cells for all blood cells, are produced. Peripheral lymphoid organs are lymph nodes, spleen, tonsils, appendix, Peyer's patches of the small intestines, and the liver. Lymph nodes, located throughout the body, connected by an elaborate ductal system, filter lymphatic fluid, remov-ing destroyed matter. Enlargement of lymphoid organs indicates an infectious or malignant process is occurring. The spleen serves as a reservoir for macrophages, lymphocytes, and plasma cells. The tonsils, appendix, and Peyer's patches also contain plasma cells and lymphocytes. The Kupffer cells of the liver house monocytes that ingest and destroy foreign organisms in hepatic circulation.

Cells of the Immune System

Leukocytes, white blood cells (WBCs), are vital components of the immune system. They are formed mostly in the bone marrow and partially in the lymph tissue. After formation, they are transported to different parts of the body where they fight infectious organisms. There are 6 types of WBCs normally found in the blood. They are neutrophils, eosinophils, basophils, monocytes, lymphocytes, and plasma cells (Guyton & Hall, 1996). Adults have about 7,000 WBCs/mm^3 of blood. Each type is a percentage of the total number of WBCs (Table 39-1).

Those cells with granules in the cytoplasm are called *granulocytes,* while those lacking them are called *agranulocytes* (Figure 39-1). Eosinophils, neutrophils, and basophils are granular leukocytes. Monocytes and lymphocytes are agranular leukocytes. Each has its own unique function. Eosinophils come into play during allergic reactions or parasitic invasions. Neutrophils are useful in ingesting bacteria. Basophils secrete **histamine**, a substance released during allergic reactions, and heparin. Monocytes travel to the sites of invading organisms and transform into macrophages, capable of ingesting large quantities of microorganisms and damaged cells, a process known as *phagocytosis.* They also secrete Interleuken-1, which stimulates the activation of specific lymphocytes. Granulocytes, also called *polymorphonuclear leukocytes,* make up the greatest number of WBCs.

B-lymphocytes, or B-cells, and T-lymphocytes, or T-cells, play a vital role in the immune response. B-cells are responsible for **humoral immunity**, or immunity dominated by antibodies (Table 39-2). They stimulate plasma cells to secrete **antibodies** (proteins that react with antigens to neutralize or destroy them) in response to **antigens** (any substance identified by the body as nonself). Antibodies are also called *im-

Table 39-1	PERCENTAGES OF DIFFERENT WBC TYPES
Neutrophils	55%–70%
Eosinophils	1%–4%
Basophils	0.5%–1.0%
Monocytes	2%–8%
Lymphocytes	20%–40%

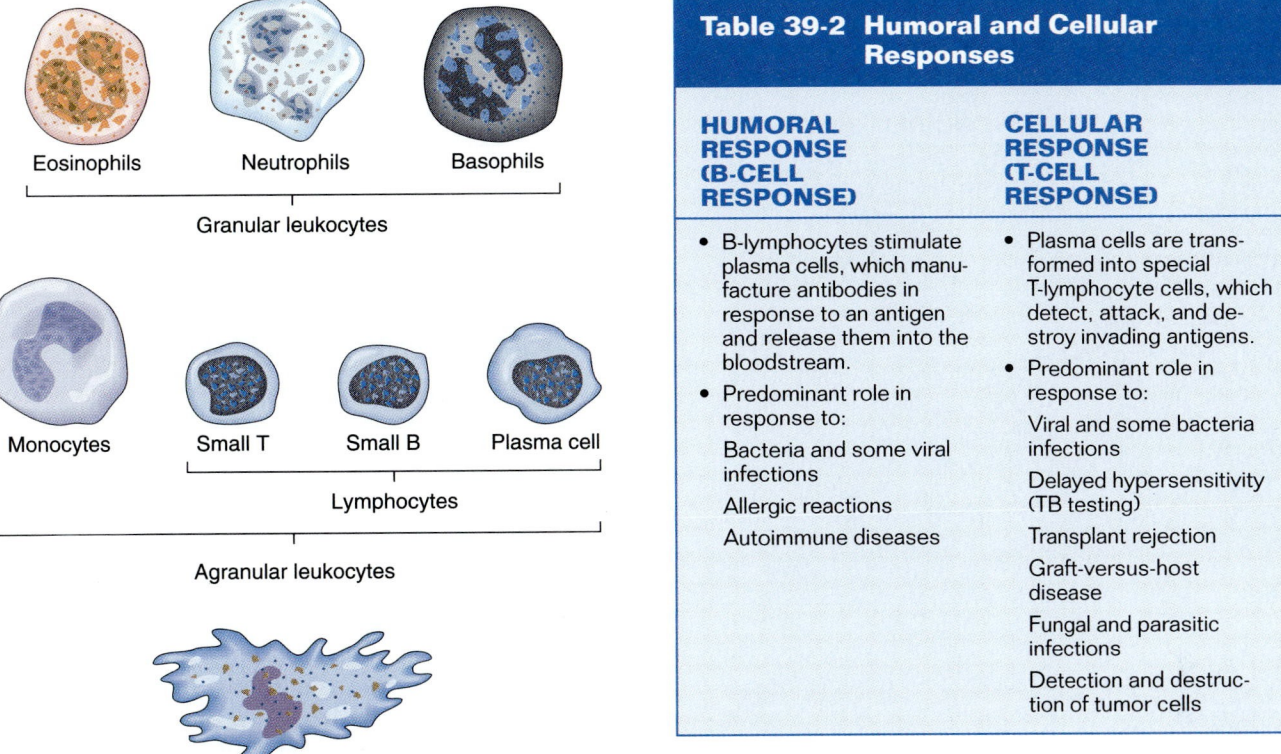

Figure 39-1 Cells of the Immune System

HUMORAL RESPONSE (B-CELL RESPONSE)	CELLULAR RESPONSE (T-CELL RESPONSE)
Table 39-2 Humoral and Cellular Responses	
• B-lymphocytes stimulate plasma cells, which manufacture antibodies in response to an antigen and release them into the bloodstream.	• Plasma cells are transformed into special T-lymphocyte cells, which detect, attack, and destroy invading antigens.
• Predominant role in response to:	• Predominant role in response to:
Bacteria and some viral infections	Viral and some bacteria infections
Allergic reactions	Delayed hypersensitivity (TB testing)
Autoimmune diseases	Transplant rejection
	Graft-versus-host disease
	Fungal and parasitic infections
	Detection and destruction of tumor cells

munoglobulins. IgA, IgD, IgE, IgG, and IgM are common antibodies found in plasma. When an antibody-antigen reaction occurs, the complement system, a complex sequential immunological process, is activated. This system is composed of plasma proteins made in the liver. They alter cell membranes in the antibody-antigen reaction, facilitating the cellular breakdown of the invading antigen, and attract macrophages and granulocytes to the antibody-antigen reaction site. When a B-cell identifies an antigen, it places the characteristics of that antigen in a memory bank. B-cells also produce "memory cells" capable of identifying the antigen, if and when it is introduced to the body again.

T-cells are responsible for **cellular immunity**, a type of acquired immunity involving T-cell lymphocytes. (again, see Table 39-2). With T-cell mediated immunity, there is a formation of large numbers of activated lymphocytes that are specifically designed to destroy the foreign agent. T-cells include helper cells (CD4), suppressor cells (CD8), and killer (cytotoxic) cells. CD4 and CD8 are molecules on the T-helper and T-suppressor cells and are important in understanding how HIV attacks the immune system.

Human immunodeficiency virus (HIV) infection affects the immune system and the brain. In the immune system, the main characteristic of HIV infection is progressive depletion of the CD4 T-helper cells. The normal ratio of T-helper cells to T-suppressor cells (CD4:CD8 ratio) is 2:1. As immunodeficiency worsens, it is not uncommon for the CD4:CD8 ratio to fall to as low as 0:1. The altered T-helper cells cause malfunction of the B-cells and macrophages, which leads to collapse of the immune system. HIV also affects the CD4 molecule present on microglial cells in the brain, causing memory loss and other brain dysfunctions.

HIV is a retrovirus. Retroviruses use RNA to make DNA copies that then become part of the genetic material of the human cell. It is because this is a reversal of the usual DNA-to-RNA transcription of genetic information that these viruses are called retroviruses.

Types of Immunity

There are 2 types of immunity: natural (innate) and acquired (adaptive) (Table 39-3). One is born with natural immunity. It is species specific. For example, humans have an innate resistance to distemper while dogs never develop measles or syphilis. Acquired immunity develops after birth and may be active or passive. Active acquired immunity is the result of exposure to the disease itself or its vaccine. As a result, the body develops antibodies and memory cells for the causative microorganism. A repeated exposure results in rapid activation of these components of the immune system and annihilation of the invading agent. Passive acquired immunity utilizes antibodies produced by another human being or an animal. Injection of these immunoglobulins temporarily prevents development of the disease once exposed. Transmission of antibodies through fetal circulation is an example of passive acquired immunity.

Table 39-3 COMPARISON OF NATURAL AND ACQUIRED IMMUNITY

NATURAL IMMUNITY	ACQUIRED IMMUNITY	
	ACTIVE ACQUIRED IMMUNITY	**PASSIVE ACQUIRED IMMUNITY**
• Innate immunity • Present at birth • Includes physical and chemical barriers to invading antigens	• Long-term immunity • Antibodies develop as a result of exposure to a disease or vaccine • Antibodies neutralize future invasions of the same antigen	• Temporary immunity • Antibodies obtained from an animal or another human who has been exposed to an antigen • Examples are gamma-globulin or antiserum

Factors Influencing Immunity

Although the exact physiological mechanisms involved are unknown, it has been well documented that a number of factors influence the **immune response** (body's reaction to substances identified as nonself, neutralization of antigen). These include age, sex, nutritional status, stress, and treatment modalities. As one ages, the immune system becomes less effective. Sex hormones affect immunity; estrogen enhances immunological functioning, while androgen suppresses it. Therefore, women are especially prone to autoimmune diseases, while men are more prone to immunosuppressive disorders. Poor nutritional status and emotional stress lead to increased susceptibility to infections. Radiation therapy and a variety of medications, such as corticosteroids and chemotherapeutic agents, suppress the immune system.

ASSESSMENT

Physical assessment of the immune system involves the entire body. The skin and mucous membranes are evaluated for urticaria, inflammation, or bleeding. Superficial head, neck, supraclavicular, axilla, and inguinal lymph nodes are inspected and palpated for redness, tenderness, or swelling. Elevated temperature may indicate infection. Joints must be evaluated for possible tenderness, swelling, or limited range of motion. Changes in the rate and rhythm of respirations, presence of a cough, or abnormal lung sounds may indicate immunological conditions. Cardiovascular status, including rate, rhythm, arrhythmias, and peripheral vascular circulation, must be assessed. Enlarged liver or spleen and gastrointestinal conditions, such as nausea, vomiting, or diarrhea, may have an immuno-

logical basis. Alterations in vision, hearing, urinary habits, and neurological function may occur.

COMMON DIAGNOSTIC TESTS

Commonly used diagnostic tests for clients with symptoms of immune system disorders are listed in Table 39-4. See Chapter 27, Diagnostic Tests, for explanation/normal values and nursing responsibilities.

HYPERSENSITIVE IMMUNE RESPONSE

Hypersensitive immune responses include allergies, anaphylaxis, transfusion reactions, transplant rejection, and latex allergy.

ALLERGIES

Allergic disorders are the result of a **hypersensitivity** (excessive reaction to a stimulus) of the immune system to **allergens** (a type of antigen commonly found in the environment). Allergens may be inhaled, injected, ingested, or contacted. There are four types of hypersensitivity reactions based on how tissue is injured.

Type I reactions occur immediately upon exposure

Table 39-4 COMMON DIAGNOSTIC TESTS FOR IMMUNE SYSTEM DISORDERS

- Antinuclear antibodies (ANA)
- Complement assay (Total complement, C3 and C4)
- C-reactive protein test (CRP)
- CD4 T-cells
- Enzyme-linked immunosorbent assay (ELISA)
- Erythrocyte sedimentation rate (ESR or Sed Rate Test)
- Human leukocyte antigen DW4 (HLA-DW4)
- Lupus erythematosus test (LE Prep)
- Polymerase chain reaction (PCR)
- Red blood cell count (RBC count)
- Rheumatoid factor (RF)
- Total white blood cell count
  Differential count
  Neutrophils
  – Segs (mature neutrophils)
  – Bands (immature neutrophils)
  Eosinophils
  Basophils
  Lymphocytes
  Monocytes
- Western blot

Allergic response

First exposure

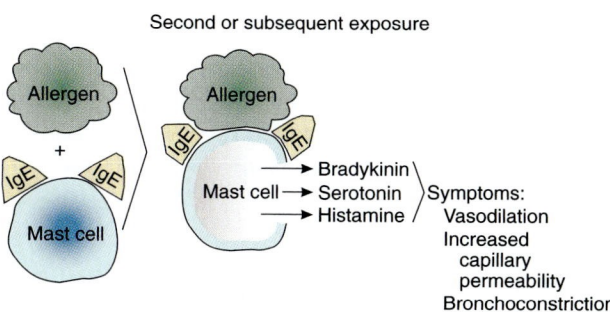

Second or subsequent exposure

Figure 39-2 Allergic Response

to a specific antigen. Upon first exposure to an allergen, IgE antibodies are produced. They adhere to mast cells. When a subsequent exposure occurs, these cells attach to the antigen and activate the release of chemical mediators, such as histamine, bradykinin, and serotonin. These chemicals cause vasodilation, enhanced capillary permeability, and bronchoconstriction (Figure 39-2).

The most common Type I reactions include allergic rhinitis, urticaria, and angioedema. Anaphylaxis is the most severe and is covered separately.

Allergic rhinitis, also known as *hay fever* or *pollinosis,* is a common allergy in our society caused by airborne allergens such as pollen, mold, animal dander, dust, and ragweed. Symptoms include nasal congestion, thin, clear, watery discharge, sneezing, itching, swelling, and redness of the eyes. Headaches and ear infections may also develop. An estimated 10% or 26 million persons in the United States are affected by allergic rhinitis (National Institute of Allergy and Infectious Diseases [NIAID], July 1999a).

Urticaria (hives) are raised pruritic, red, nontender wheals on the skin. They are usually on the trunk and on the areas of the extremities closest to the trunk.

LIFE CYCLE CONSIDERATIONS

Allergy to Foods

- 8% of children under 6 years of age have food intolerance(s).
- 2% to 4% of children under age 6 are estimated to have food allergies (NIAID, July 1999a).

Angioedema, edema of subcutaneous layers and mucous membranes, is painless and only slightly pruritic. Urticaria and angioedema together affect approximately 15% of the United States population each year (NIAID, July 1999a).

Drug and food allergies are also Type I hypersensitivity.

Any drug potentially may cause a drug reaction, but common ones include penicillin, cephalosporins, insulin, vaccines, and local anesthetics. Reactions vary from mild to severe. Usually symptoms do not occur until the client has taken several doses of the medication, although they can occur at first exposure. The most common reaction is the sudden development of a bright red, itchy rash, often appearing initially on the trunk or arms. Occasionally, a client may develop an anaphylactic reaction. Approximately 2% to 3% of hospitalized clients have an allergic reaction to drugs, especially penicillin and cephalosporins (NIAID, July 1999a).

Although individuals may be allergic to any edible substance, certain foods, such as milk, fish, chocolate, and nuts, are common allergens that cause diarrhea as a result of immunological reaction in the intestinal mucosa. Headache, nausea, vomiting, rash, itching, and wheezing may also develop.

Type II reactions are the destruction of cells or substances with antigens attached that either immunoglobulin G (IgG) or immunoglobulin M (IgM) senses as being foreign. Antibodies cause either lysis of the cells or accelerated phagocytosis. Hemolytic transfusion reactions are this type of reaction. Transfusion reactions are discussed in further detail later.

Type III reaction involves IgG immune antigen-antibody complexes. It is a local reaction evident after several hours that may change from red skin to hemorrhage and tissue necrosis. Occasionally this is noted after penicillin or sulfonamide use.

Type IV is a delayed reaction involving sensitized T-lymphocytes coming in contact with the allergen. Contact dermatitis and transplant rejection are examples of this type of reaction. Poison ivy and poison oak are the most common causes of contact dermatitis. Latex rubber is a more recently discovered cause of contact dermatitis or occasionally a Type I (anaphylactic) reaction. Transplant rejection and latex allergy are covered separately.

Medical–Surgical Management

Medical

Medical management of clients experiencing an allergic response (reaction to allergen) includes drug therapy to treat symptoms and identification of precipitating agents. Once the allergen(s) have been identified, **immunotherapy** (treatment to suppress or enhance immunological functioning) is begun. This involves repeated injections of the diluted allergen. Subsequently, decreased levels of histamine are released upon exposure to the allergen.

Pharmacological

A number of medications are employed to treat the symptoms of an allergic response. Antihistamines counteract the effects of histamine. They may be taken orally, topically, or intravenously, depending upon the type of allergic response and urgency for treatment. Nasal decongestants help relieve respiratory symptoms. Topical corticosteroids effectively relieve inflammation associated with contact dermatitis and dermatitis medicamentosa. Oral or injectable forms of corticosteroids may be used either alone or in combination with antihistamines and nasal decongestants.

Skin testing by a physician can determine the specific causative allergen.

Diet

Individuals allergic to certain foods should be taught to check food labels carefully, be aware of how food is prepared, and not eat any product that could lead to a reaction. This includes restaurant foods and foods prepared in another person's home.

Activity

Avoidance of the causative allergen prevents allergic reactions. Activities should be centered around doing this, if at all possible. For instance, individuals who are allergic to pollen may need to stay in air-conditioned environments on those days when the pollen count is extremely high.

▶ NURSING PROCESS

▶ Assessment

▶ Subjective Data

A detailed, comprehensive client history should include information about previous allergic reactions, foods eaten or medications taken recently, and contact with environmental pollutants or anything not normally encountered.

▶ Objective Data

Physical assessment includes gastrointestinal and respiratory functioning, and cardiovascular and neurological status. It is also important to assess for the presence of urticaria and angioedema.

Nursing diagnoses for clients with allergies may include the following:

Nursing Diagnoses	Planning/Goals	Nursing Interventions
▶ *Injury, Risk for, related to an allergic reaction*	The client will identify factors that increase the potential of a reaction.	Assist client in identifying those factors that increase the potential for a reaction.
▶ *Health Seeking Behaviors related to causative allergen, therapeutic modalities, and/or preventive measures*	The client will relate methods to avoid exposure to allergens.	Assist client in planning lifestyle changes that will help in avoiding exposure to allergens.
▶ *Knowledge Deficit related to lack of information about allergens, treatment, or preventive measures*	The client will demonstrate an understanding of and compliance with therapeutic modalities if a reaction occurs. The client will demonstrate an understanding of and compliance with preventive measures to avoid subsequent allergic reactions.	Teach client about allergy treatments and what to do if a reaction occurs.

Evaluation Each goal must be evaluated to determine how it has been met by the client.

ANAPHYLACTIC REACTION

Anaphylaxis is a type I systemic reaction to allergens and is the most serious type of allergic reaction. It occurs in individuals who are extremely sensitive to an allergen. Symptoms develop suddenly and can progress to severe levels within minutes. Foods, drugs, hormones, insect bites, blood, and vaccines all are as-

sociated with anaphylactic reactions. Shellfish, eggs, nuts, berries, and chocolates are the most common foods involved. Any medication has the potential of causing a reaction, but antibiotics (especially penicillin), insulin, muscle relaxants, and x-ray dyes are the most frequent precipitating agents. Bee, wasp, hornet, and snake bites may also cause anaphylactic reactions. At least 40 deaths in the United States each year are the result of insect sting anaphylaxis (NIAID, July 1999a).

Anaphylactic reactions may be life-threatening. Symptoms involve the skin, GI tract, and cardiovascular and respiratory systems. Clients experience peripheral tingling, flushing, fullness in the mouth, throat/nasal congestion, tearing and swelling around the eyes, itching, cough, laryngeal edema, bronchospasms, severe dyspnea, vasodilation, and cyanosis. If untreated, these catastrophic effects lead to respiratory failure, severe hypotension, anaphylactic shock, and death. Therefore, it is crucial that symptoms be identified early and treatment initiated immediately, as death can occur in minutes.

Medical–Surgical Management

Medical

Medical management centers around establishing an intravenous line, administering fluids and emergency drugs, and maintaining an airway. Oxygen is provided via nasal cannula or face mask. In severe cases, endotracheal intubation or a tracheotomy may be required.

Pharmacological

Epinephrine is administered subcutaneously as soon as symptoms develop to dilate bronchioles, increase heart contractions, and constrict blood vessels. Antihistamines, such as diphenhydramine hydrochloride (Benadryl), block the effects of histamine in bronchioles, blood vessels, and the GI tract. Corticosteroids are given for their anti-inflammatory effect. Vasopressors, such as norepinephrine bitartrate (Levophed) or dopamine hydrochloride (Intropin) may be needed to increase blood pressure. If bronchoconstriction and spasms are severe, albuterol (Proventil), metaproterenol sulfate (Alupent), and/or aminophylline (Aminophyllin) may be administered.

Diet

Clients will be NPO until normal respiratory and circulatory function have been restored.

CLIENT TEACHING

Severe Allergies
- Advise clients with severe allergies wear a Medic Alert tag.
- Encourage clients allergic to insect stings to carry an emergency anaphylactic kit containing epinephrine at all times.

Activity

Clients will remain on bedrest until vital signs are stable and normal breathing patterns have been restored. Those experiencing severe anaphylactic responses are generally transferred to intensive care units for continued treatment and observation.

▶ NURSING PROCESS

▶ Assessment

▶ Subjective Data

Client history may reveal a previous anaphylaxis reaction. The client may describe feelings of uneasiness, anxiety, weakness, itching, dizziness, nausea, peripheral tingling, and a generalized warm sensation throughout the body.

▶ Objective Data

Since anaphylaxis is a sudden, unexpected event, nurses must be aware that variations in a client's cardiovascular and respiratory status may be signs of an impending anaphylactic reaction. The first symptoms are sweating, sneezing, tachycardia, hypotension, dysrhythmias, cyanosis, edema of tongue and larynx, wheezing, bronchospasms, vascular collapse, and cardiac arrest. Regularly assessing client's vital signs and cardiovascular, respiratory, and neurological status will detect changes before the severe signs of respiratory distress and impending shock develop.

Nursing diagnoses for clients with anaphylaxis may include the following:

Nursing Diagnoses	Planning/Goals	Nursing Interventions
▶ *Tissue Perfusion, Altered, related to increased capillary permeability and vasodilation*	The client will have adequate tissue perfusion.	Monitor vital signs frequently. Monitor I & O. Place client in Trendelenburg position for hypotension. Administer IV fluids and medications as ordered.
▶ *Breathing Patterns, Ineffective, related to bronchoconstriction, laryngeal edema, and increased secretions*	The client will have effective breathing patterns.	Monitor vital signs. Suction secretions as needed. Maintain patent airway. Administer oxygen and medications as ordered.

continued

Nursing Diagnoses	Planning/Goals	Nursing Interventions
▶ *Knowledge Deficit related to causative allergen, therapeutic modalities, and/or preventive measures*	The client will relate causative allergen, therapeutic modalities, and preventive measures.	Teach client importance of avoiding allergen. Advise client to provide the name of the causative agent and a description of reaction experienced when asked about allergies. Document allergy on all medical records. Teach client and family symptoms of anaphylactic reactions.

Evaluation Each goal must be evaluated to determine how it has been met by the client.

TRANSFUSION REACTIONS

Blood components, such as whole blood, packed or frozen RBCs, leukocytes, platelets, and plasma, may be administered to clients when their own bodies are incapable of manufacturing them at a rate required to maintain vascular homeostasis. Any client receiving blood products that are **homologous** or from a donor of the same species may develop a transfusion reaction. For this reason, some clients are arranging to have their own blood collected, saved, and available for infusion, if needed, during or following elective surgeries. This is known as an **autologous** blood transfusion. Immunological reactions do not develop with this type of blood transfusion.

There are 5 types of transfusion reactions: febrile nonhemolytic, allergic urticarial, delayed hemolytic, acute hemolytic, and anaphylactic. Febrile nonhemolytic reactions are the most common and occur in clients who have had previous blood transfusions. It is the result of an antibody-antigen reaction to WBCs. Symptoms may develop soon after the infusion has started or up to 5 to 6 hours after completion. Fever is the classic symptom and may be accompanied by chills, nausea, headache, hypotension, and respiratory problems. Clients who have allergic urticarial reactions develop a skin rash during or within 1 hour following the transfusion. A delayed hemolytic reaction may occur days to weeks following the transfusion. The client's hemoglobin level falls due to incompatibility of RBC antigens. This type of reaction is often misdiagnosed and thought to be related to the condition that created the need for blood replacement rather than a transfusion reaction. An acute hemolytic reaction is potentially a life-threatening situation. Symptoms, resulting from the incompatibility of ABO groups usually occur during the first 15 minutes of administration, but can develop anytime during the transfusion. Clients complain of chills, nausea, and back pain. Fever, drop in blood pressure (hypotension), vomiting, hematuria, or oliguria may be observed. As the condition progresses, chest pain, dyspnea, anuria, and shock develop. Anaphylactic reactions, although rare, are also life-threatening. Symptoms of acute gastrointestinal malfunctioning and cardiovascular and respiratory collapse develop moments after the transfusion has started.

Medical–Surgical Management

Medical

Medical management of clients experiencing a blood transfusion reaction depends on the type of reaction. Treatment of a febrile nonhemolytic reaction includes stopping the blood, infusing normal saline, and treating the symptoms. For clients experiencing an allergic urticarial reaction, the transfusion should be slowed and an antihistamine administered. Delayed hemolytic reactions often go undetected and untreated. Both an acute hemolytic reaction and anaphylactic reactions are medical emergencies. The transfusion must be stopped immediately. Normal saline and emergency drugs are given intravenously.

Pharmacological

If a febrile nonhemolytic or allergic urticarial reaction occurs, diphenhydramine (Benadryl) and a corticosteroid (hydrocortisone or prednisone) are administered to counteract the immunological response. Antipyretics are ordered to control fever. For life-threatening conditions, emergency medications are employed. (Refer back to Anaphylactic Reaction.)

Diet

Clients should not be fed if a reaction is occurring, especially if respiratory symptoms have developed, as aspiration could occur.

Activity

Clients should remain in bed until symptoms of the reaction have subsided.

▶ NURSING PROCESS

▶ Assessment

▶ Subjective Data

Occasionally, clients verbalize the feeling of something "not being right" or "something strange is going on in my body" before actual symptoms become apparent. They may have itching, headache, or low back pain.

▶ Objective Data

Clients receiving blood components need to be carefully assessed for any signs of a transfusion reaction, such as fever, chills, or respiratory problems.

A nursing diagnosis for clients with transfusion reactions may be:

Nursing Diagnoses	Planning/Goals	Nursing Interventions
▶ *Injury, Risk for, related to infusion of homologous blood components*	The client will not have injury from infusion of homologous blood products.	Follow protocol for blood products and administration.
		Check client's identification and blood product with another nurse.
		If a reaction occurs, stop transfusion immediately, then call the physician.
		Administer medications as ordered.
		Send blood tubing and a urine specimen to the lab for analysis.
		Monitor and document client's condition.
		Teach client who has a blood transfusion reaction to inform health care providers whenever questioned about allergies.

Evaluation Each goal must be evaluated to determine how it has been met by the client.

TRANSPLANT REJECTION

In 1995, more than 20,000 organ transplants were performed in the United States (NIAID, July 1999b). The success of these procedures is directly related to matching antibodies and antigens of the donor and recipient and to the effectiveness of immunosuppressive medications in preventing rejection. Even with the use of immunosuppressive drugs, 10% to 15% of transplanted organs fail (NIAID, July 1999b). Immunosuppressive medications make the client prone to the development of infections and cancers. Clients must have a regular medical check-up, including cancer screening tests.

Medical–Surgical Management

Medical

Although blood components are the most common type of tissue transplants, today it is possible to transplant bone marrow, corneal tissue, skin, kidneys, pancreas, hearts, livers, and lungs. Bone marrow and blood components often employ autologous donations. Homologous donations may be from living related donors or living nonrelated donors. Cadaveric donations are harvested from individuals after they are pronounced clinically dead. It is important to match ABO blood groups and **human leukocyte antigen** (antigens present in human blood), to prevent rejection when homologous and cadaveric donors are used.

Pharmacological

A combination of immunosuppressive medications is used to hinder rejection. Steroids such as prednisone (Deltasone) and methylprednisolone sodium succinate (Solu-Medrol) decrease the inflammatory response. Cyclosporine (Sandimmune), antithymocyte globulin (equine), ATG (Atgam), and tacrolimus (Prograf) inhibit T-cells. Azathioprine (Imuran) inhibits purine synthesis. Muromonab-CD3 (Orthoclone, OKT 3) prevents acute rejection in kidney transplant clients. Clients taking immunosuppressive medications are especially prone to developing infections. Antibiotics may be prescribed prophylactically.

Steroids cause fluid and sodium retention, low potassium level, elevated blood pressure, moon face, muscle wasting, elevated glucose level, impaired wound healing, mood swings, and masculinization in women. Cyclosporine may be toxic to the kidneys and liver. Imuran may cause hair loss and lower platelet level. OKT 3 also causes fluid retention.

Activity

Activity is dependent upon the type of transplant. Clients who receive a major organ, such as a heart, lung, pancreas, or liver, are placed in reverse isolation in the hospital setting for at least 2 weeks. They are carefully observed for signs of rejection. Exposure to others is limited. Prior to discharge, they are taught to avoid contact with any one who may have an infection and to wear a mask whenever out in public.

▶ NURSING PROCESS

▶ Assessment

▶ Subjective Data

Client history may reveal fear of possible transplant rejection. The client generally describes tenderness at the transplant site.

▶ Objective Data

Following transplantation, clients' vital signs, nutritional status, fluid balance, urinary output, mental status, and respiratory and cardiovascular functioning need to be carefully monitored. Daily weight should be taken. Wound sites should be checked frequently. Signs of rejection include fever, weight gain, and swelling or tenderness at the transplant site.

Nursing diagnoses for clients with organ transplants may include the following:

Nursing Diagnoses	Planning/Goals	Nursing Interventions
▶ *Fear related to possible transplant rejection.*	The client will relate less fear regarding rejection.	Allow client to verbalize concerns and develop realistic expectations. Set aside time to sit down and talk to client.
▶ *Knowledge Deficit related to home care following transplantation*	The client will discuss signs and symptoms of rejection. The client will demonstrate an understanding of the side effects of immunosuppressive drugs and lifestyle changes to adapt to their effects.	Teach client and family about signs of rejection and infection. Teach client and family ramifications of taking immunosuppressive medications. Teach client to watch for side effects and report them to physician.
▶ *Infection, Risk for, related to immunosuppressive medications*	The client will demonstrate appropriate wound care. The client will be free of infection.	Teach client and family appropriate wound care and proper handwashing. Teach client importance of taking antibiotics as ordered. Teach the client to wear a mask whenever out in public. Teach client importance of regular checkups, including cancer screening tests.

Evaluation Each goal must be evaluated to determine how it has been met by the client

LATEX ALLERGY

Since 1987, when universal precautions (now called Standard Precautions) were mandated, exposure to latex by health care workers has dramatically increased. Between 1988 and 1992, more than 1,000 systemic allergic reactions to natural rubber latex were reported (NIAID, July 1999a). By June 1996, 28 latex-related deaths had been reported to the Food and Drug Administration (FDA) (Burt, 1998).

The latex proteins can enter the body through the skin and mucous membranes, intravascularly, and by inhalation. The cornstarch powder on gloves absorbs the latex proteins and becomes airborne when the gloves are put on or taken off. From the air, the latex proteins may be inhaled or may be in contact with the skin and mucous membranes. Anyone, client or health care worker, who after exposure to latex develops red, watery, itchy eyes; sinus or nasal irritation; hives; shortness of breath; dry cough; wheezing; chest tightness; or flushing, tachycardia, and hypotension should be suspected of latex allergy.

There are more than 20,000 medical products containing latex (Burt, 1998). Synthetic versions of products are often available. An individual product may be "latex free," but an environment is "latex safe" only when all items of latex that might come in contact with the allergic individual are removed.

 Safety: Latex Allergy
A MedicAlert tag stating "latex allergy" should be worn by any individual with a latex allergy.

AUTOIMMUNE DISEASES

Disorders in this category include rheumatoid arthritis, systemic lupus erythematosus, and myasthenia gravis.

RHEUMATOID ARTHRITIS

Rheumatoid arthritis (RA) is a chronic, systemic autoimmune disease characterized by joint stiffness. It affects 2.1 million people in the United States, including 1.5 million women and 600,000 men (Arthritis Foundation, 1999a). It affects people of all races, usually beginning between the ages of 25 and 50, but RA is reported in persons of all ages (Arthritis Foundation, 1999b).

The cause of RA is unknown, but there seems to be a genetic predisposition (susceptibility) in many, but not all, persons affected. It is believed that something must trigger the disease process such as a virus, bacterium, hormonal factors, or stress. The person's immune system attacks the cells inside the joint(s), producing substances that act as antigens. Immune complexes are formed within the joint, causing inflammation, swelling, and increased synovial fluid. As this chronic, systemic condition progresses, surrounding cartilage, tendons, and ligaments become involved. Thickening of synovial tissue eventually leads to calcification of the joint, joint pain, limited mobility, and deformity.

It is believed that the damage to the bones begins within the first two years of the onset of RA. Early diagnosis and aggressive treatment are important to control the disease. Usually, the joints of the hand and wrist are affected initially. As the disease progresses, shoulder, elbow, hip, knee, ankle, and cervical spine joints become affected. The pattern of joint involvement is symmetrical, that is, if a joint is affected on the right side of the body, the same joint will also be affected on the left side (Arthritis Foundation, 1999c). Other areas of the body where connective tissue is present may also be involved, such as blood vessels, lining of the lungs, and pericordial sac.

Clients experience periods of **remission**, a decrease or absence of symptoms, and **exacerbations**, an increase in symptoms. Both physical and emotional stressors lead to increased symptomatology. This means that simple tasks such as answering the telephone or buttoning clothes may become very challenging.

Medical–Surgical Management

Medical

Medical management centers around reducing inflammation, relieving pain, maintaining normal joint function, and promoting general health. Therapeutic regimen includes medications, exercise, rest, hot and cold applications, and stress management.

Surgical

Hip, knee, and finger joints may be surgically replaced. Refer to Chapter 38, Nursing Care of the Client: Musculoskeletal System, for a discussion of joint replacement.

Pharmacological

Nonsteroidal anti-inflammatory drugs (NSAIDs) and salicylates have the potential to relieve symptoms such as joint pain, stiffness, and swelling but do not control the disease. Disease-modifying anti-rheumatic drugs (DMARDs) have the potential for modifying the disease and should be given early in the disease to control progression. The commonly used DMARDs include prednisone (Deltasone), gold salts, and sulfasalazine (Azulfidine EN-Tabs) (Table 39-5). Because of the large doses required to control inflammation and the long-term use due to the chronicity of this condition, side effects often develop. In severe cases, azathioprine (Imuran), hydroxychloroquine sulfate (Plaquenil Sulfate), D-penicillamine (Depen), or methotrexate sodium (Rheumatrex) may be used. These medications also have serious side effects.

Table 39-5 MEDICATIONS USED TO TREAT RHEUMATOID ARTHRITIS

DRUG	USE/ACTIONS	SIDE EFFECTS	NURSING CONSIDERATIONS
Salicylates • aspirin	Inhibit prostaglandin synthesis resulting in decreased pain. (Analgesia) antipyretic and anti-inflammatory effects.	GI upset, tinnitus, easy bruising, nausea, prolonged bleeding time.	Instruct client to take with food or take enteric coated aspirin and to report ringing in ears. Do not give to clients on oral anticoagulants. Assess for bleeding/bruising.
Nonsteroidal Anti-inflammatory Drugs (NSAIDs) • ibuprofen (Motrin, Rufen) • naproxen (Naprosyn) • phenylbutazone (Butazolidin) • nambumetone (Relafen)	Inhibit prostaglandin synthesis. Reduce joint swelling stiffness. Analgesic and antipyretic properties.	GI irritation, nausea, vomiting, heartburn. GI bleeding and ulceration, dizziness, headache, liver toxicity.	Administer with food. May prolong bleeding time, may require frequent blood count.
Indole Analogues • indomethacin (Indocin) • sulindac (Clinoril)	Analgesic anti-inflammatory effect.	Gastric bleeding, headaches, dizziness, psychiatric disturbances.	Administer with food. Instruct client to report any bleeding (tarry stools, hematemesis). Avoid giving aspirin.
Corticosteroids • prednisone (Deltasone)	Decreases inflammation.	GI irritation, muscle weakness, fluid retention, moon face, muscle wasting, impaired wound healing.	Administer with food. Weigh daily. Monitor BP, sleep pattern, and serum potassium.
Antimalarials • hydroxychloroquine sulfate (Plaquenil Sulfate)	Not a drug of choice.	Visual disturbances, nightmares, skin lesions, nausea, diarrhea, low blood count.	Monitor CBC and liver function tests. Discontinue after 6 months if no beneficial effects noted.

continued

Table 39-5 MEDICATIONS USED TO TREAT RHEUMATOID ARTHRITIS *continued*

DRUG	USE/ACTIONS	SIDE EFFECTS	NURSING CONSIDERATIONS
Gold Salts • auranofin (Ridaura)	Anti-inflammatory effect.	Diarrhea, nausea, vomiting, jaundice.	Remind client to keep all physician appointments. Beneficial effects may take 3 months to appear.
Chelating Agent • penicillamine (Depen)	Palliative when other medications have failed.	Bone marrow depression, fever, rashes, blood dyscrasias, liver toxicity.	Give on empty stomach. Have epinephrine 1:1,000 handy for anaphylaxis. Fluids to 3,000 mL/day to prevent renal failure.
Sulfonamide • sulfasalazine (Azulfidine EN-TABS)	For clients who do not respond well to NSAIDs.	Anorexia, headache, nausea, vomiting, gastric distress, reversible oligospermia.	Give with food. May discolor urine or skin yellow-orange. Take at least 2–3 L/day of water. May increase sensitivity to sun.

Diet

Clients need to be taught to eat a nutritious, well-balanced diet. Poorly nourished individuals are prone to infections. For clients with RA, an infection results in exacerbation of symptoms. Foods high in iron are encouraged when RBCs are low.

Activity

Since joint mobility is a major problem, occupational and physical therapists are part of the therapeutic team. Range of motion exercises, resting splints, and assistive devices such as canes and hand rails are often employed to promote mobility.

▶ NURSING PROCESS

▶ Assessment

▶ Subjective Data

Client history frequently reveals a gradual development of symptoms, beginning initially with early morning stiffness and pain in finger joints. Eventually, other joints become involved. Fatigue, weight loss, temperature elevation, and anemia develop. Subjective data often include malaise, loss of appetite, fatigue, and muscle weakness. Information about periods of remissions and exacerbations should be obtained, as well as the clients' understanding of and compliance with the treatment regimen.

▶ Objective Data

Assessment of the hands may reveal the classic deformities associated with RA: boutonniere deformity (fixed flexion of the proximal interphalangeal joint and hyperextension of the distal interphalangeal joint), ulnar drift (deviation of the fingers to the ulnar side of the hand), and swan-neck deformity (fixed flexion of the distal interphalangeal joint and hyperextension of the proximal interphalangeal joint). Figure 39-3 illustrates these changes in the hands.

Skin may show the presence of ulcers, due to vasculitis, and moveable, subcutaneous skin nodes, known as *rheumatoid nodules*. Eye tissue may be inflamed. Reduction in tear and saliva production can occur, causing dryness of the eyes, mouth, and mucous membranes. This is known as Sjogren's syndrome. The client may have weight loss and an elevated temperature.

X-rays demonstrate the amount and degree of deformity. There is no specific laboratory test that confirms a diagnosis of RA, though alterations in the following may occur: RBCs decrease (anemia) as the disease progresses, elevation of WBCs, erythrocyte sedimentation rate (ESR), antinuclear antibodies (ANAs), C-reactive proteins, and platelet count. The rheumatoid factor (RF) is present in about 80% of adult clients with RA (Arthritis Foundation, 1999d).

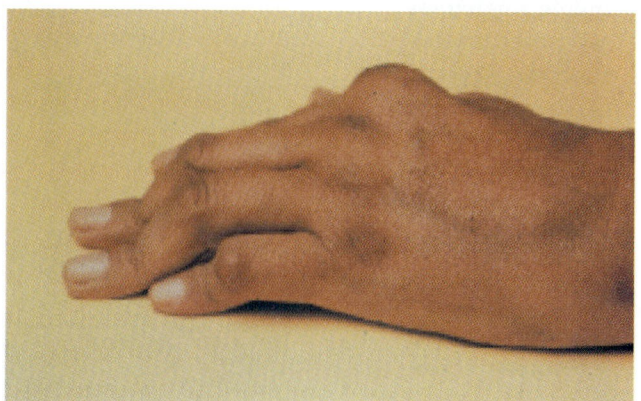

Figure 39-3 Arthritic Hands

Nursing diagnoses for clients with rheumatoid arthritis may include the following:

Nursing Diagnoses	Planning/Goals	Nursing Interventions
▶ *Pain, Chronic, related to swollen, inflamed joints*	The client will relate appropriate use of anti-inflammatory medications. The client will relate methods to decrease pain.	Teach client about prescribed analgesics and anti-inflammatory medications. Encourage client to practice relaxation techniques and take warm shower to relieve early morning joint stiffness and pain. Use hot and cold packs to decrease muscle spasms. Teach client proper body alignment and to avoid using pillows under the knees, which leads to pooling of blood in the feet.
▶ *Mobility, Impaired, Physical, related to edema, and joint immobility*	The client will demonstrate measures to maintain joint mobility. The client will demonstrate use of adaptive devices.	Teach hospitalized clients to use the overhead trapeze when moving in bed and to change position frequently. Assist with ROM exercises. Maintain planned rest periods. Teach client use of assistive devices, such as handrests, tools to pick up objects, or three-legged canes, as needed. Check with occupational and physical therapists for available equipment. Assist client to use handrails in tub, shower, and toilet; raised toilet seat; and rubber-tipped walker or cane.
▶ *Self-care Deficit: Bathing/ Dressing/Grooming related to joint inflammation or deformity*	The client will bathe, dress, and groom to abilities.	Recommend shoes with Velcro® closures. Encourage client to stop and rest when getting tired. Teach self-care using assistive devices, as required. Assist with routine plan for ADLs.
▶ *Fatigue related to chronic inflammatory process*	The client will state less fatigue. The client will establish priorities for daily activities. The client will balance daily activities with periods of rest.	Explain that fatigue is a common symptom of autoimmune disorders. Allow the client to express feelings about altered lifestyle. Inform client of community services such as Meals on Wheels. Plan rest periods between activities. Help identify activities client should perform and what can be delegated. Instruct client to record level of fatigue and activities performed on an hourly basis for 24 hours. One method uses 0 to 10 scale (0 = not tired, peppy; 10 = totally exhausted). Help plan important tasks during high-energy periods and distribute difficult ones throughout the week.

Evaluation Each goal must be evaluated to determine how it has been met by the client.

SYSTEMIC LUPUS ERYTHEMATOSUS

Systemic lupus erythematous (SLE) is a chronic, progressive, incurable autoimmune disease affecting multiple body organs. It is characterized by periods of exacerbation and remission. SLE occurs most commonly in women during their childbearing years and develops 3 times more frequently in African Americans and is more common in Hispanic, Asian, and Native Americans than in the white population (National Institute of Arthritis, Musculoskeletal, and Skin Diseases [NIAMS], 1999). More people have lupus than AIDS, cerebral palsy, multiple sclerosis, sickle-cell anemia, and cystic fibrosis combined (Lupus Foundation of America, 1995). In clients with SLE, abnormal B-lymphocyte cells produce autoantibodies that destroy body cells. Immune complexes are formed and circulate in serum, causing inflammation and tissue damage in the skin, brain, kidney, lung, heart, or joints. Production of these autoantibodies is influenced by genetic predisposition, medications, infections, stress, and sunlight (ultraviolet light rays).

No single test is conclusive for a diagnosis. The American Rheumatism Association has established criteria for SLE. If 4 or more of these criteria are present, a diagnosis of SLE is confirmed (Table 39-6).

Medical–Surgical Management

Medical

Medical treatment is aimed at decreasing tissue inflammation and destruction. A knowledgeable client

Table 39-6   THE ELEVEN CRITERIA USED FOR THE DIAGNOSIS OF LUPUS ERYTHEMATOSUS

CRITERION	DEFINITION
Malar Rash	Rash over the cheeks
Discoid Rash	Red raised patches
Photosensitivity	Reaction to sunlight, resulting in the development of or increase in skin rash
Oral Ulcers	Ulcers in the nose or mouth, usually painless
Arthritis	Nonerosive arthritis involving 2 or more peripheral joints (arthritis in which the bones around the joints do not become destroyed)
Serositis	Pleuritis or pericarditis (inflammation of the lining of the lung or heart)
Renal Disorder	Excessive protein in the urine (greater than 0.5 gm/day or 3+ on test sticks) and/or cellular casts (abnormal elements in the urine, derived from red and/or white cells and/or kidney tubule cells)
Neurologic Disorder	Seizures (convulsions) and/or psychosis in the absence of drugs or metabolic disturbances which are known to cause such effects
Hematologic Disorder	Hemolytic anemia or leukopenia (white blood count below 4,000 cells per cubic millimeter) or lymphopenia (less than 1,500 lymphocytes per cubic millimeter) or thrombocytopenia (less than 100,000 platelets per cubic millimeter). The leukopenia and lymphopenia must be detected on two or more occasions. The thrombocytopenia must be detected in the absence of drugs known to induce it.
Antinuclear Antibody	Positive test for antinuclear antibodies (ANA) in the absence of drugs known to induce it.
Immunologic Disorder	Positive anti-double stranded anti-DNA test, positive anti-Sm test, positive antiphospholipid antibody such as anticardiolipin, or false-positive syphilis test (VDRL).

To assist the physician in the diagnosis of lupus, the American College of Rheumatology (ACR) in 1982 issued a list of 11 symptoms, or signs, that help distinguish lupus from other diseases. This was revised in 1998.

Adapted from "The 1982 revised criteria for the classification of SLE," by E. M. Tan et al., 1982, Arth. Rheum., 25, pp. 1271–1277. Used with permission.

can assist in controlling the disease process through stress management, rest, exercise, taking medications as prescribed, and immediately reporting symptoms to the health care provider. During acute exacerbations, plasmapheresis may be used. This treatment modality involves removal of the client's plasma, processing it through a special machine to eliminate various cellular elements, and reinfusing the cleansed plasma. In SLE, autoantibodies are removed.

CLIENT TEACHING

Systemic Lupus Erythematosus
- Get adequate rest.
- Use stress-reduction techniques such as visualization, guided imagery, meditation, or yoga.
- Avoid exposure to sunlight; use sunscreen.
- Involve family and friends in care.
- Report fever, chills, anorexia, or symptom worsening to health care provider immediately.
- Never just stop taking medications.
- Contact the Lupus Foundation of America, Inc., for information and support (see Resources at the end of the book).

Since clients with SLE are prone to a variety of complications, they are carefully monitored for renal, cardiac, pulmonary, hematological, and neurological damage. A large percentage of SLE clients eventually develop renal failure, requiring dialysis to maintain life.

Pharmacological

NSAIDs are used for muscle and joint pain. The lowest possible dose of corticosteroid is used to suppress immune system activity. During periods of exacerbations, higher doses may be required. Prolonged use of these medications leads to multiple side effects. Hydroxychloroquine sulfate (Plaquenil sulfate), an antimalarial agent, is used. Although the exact mechanism involved is unknown, it does work effectively in decreasing joint and skin problems. It can lead to the development of retinal toxicity; therefore, clients should have yearly eye exams. Cyclophosphamide (Cytoxan) or azathioprine (Imuran) may be used for severe SLE or for those clients who are steroid-resistant (Johnson, 1999).

Diet

Clients on corticosteroids are prone to developing hypernatremia, hyperglycemia, hypokalemia, and fluid retention. Diet should be low in sodium and glucose and high in potassium. Excessive fluid intake should be discouraged.

PROFESSIONAL TIP

RA and SLE

Clients with RA and SLE have common nursing diagnoses of fatigue and impaired mobility. Clients with SLE have an additional risk for infection if WBC count is low.

Activity

Clients should be encouraged to sleep at least 8 hours a night and rest periodically during the day. Regular exercise helps prevent muscle weakness and fatigue.

▶ NURSING PROCESS

▶ Assessment

▶ Subjective Data

The client should be asked when the disease began, what symptoms have developed, and how they have been treated. Information about medications the client is taking and side effects should be elicited, and activity level and degree of fatigue noted. The nurse should determine client's understanding of the disease process, how lifestyle has changed, and how effectively client is coping. The client may describe having malaise, photosensitivity, pain in joints, irregular menses, irritability, confusion, or hallucinations.

▶ Objective Data

A complete head-to-toe assessment is needed. Most common findings include joint swelling and pain, fever, swollen glands, nausea, vomiting, anorexia, hypertension, respiratory and cardiac infections, renal involvement, enlarged liver and spleen, and skin lesions, especially the classic "butterfly" rash. Figure 39-4 shows an individual with a "butterfly rash." If exposed to the cold, Raynaud's phenomenon, intermittent attacks of diminished blood supply to fingers, toes, ears, and nose, may develop.

Laboratory tests frequently reveal serum antinuclear antibodies (ANA) and anti-DNA antibodies. Lupus erythematosus cells (LE cells) are present in most clients. Anemia, leukopenia, and thrombocytopenia are evident.

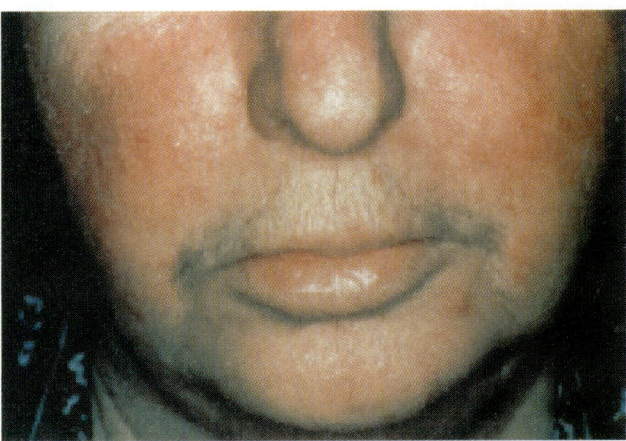

Figure 39-4 Butterfly Rash *(Courtesy of the American Academy of Dermatology)*

Nursing diagnoses for a client with SLE may include the following:

Nursing Diagnoses	Planning/Goals	Nursing Interventions
▶ *Skin Integrity, Impaired, related to presence of butterfly rash, skin lesions, Raynaud's phenomenon, and/or oral ulcers*	The client will participate in a plan to promote wound healing.	Teach client to clean and dry area prior to application of topical corticosteroids. Warn client that sunlight and ultraviolet rays increase symptoms and tanning sessions are contraindicated. Encourage client to wear protective clothing, sunscreen of at least SPF 15, and sunglasses. In cold weather, client should wear a hat and gloves. Encourage client in regular oral care to promote healing of mouth sores.
▶ *Knowledge Deficit related to adapting lifestyle with treatment and prevention of complications*	The client will describe disease process, factors contributing to symptoms, and regimen for control.	Teach client effects of disease and methods to control complications. Teach stress management techniques. Allow client to vent feelings. Help client plan methods to adapt lifestyle. Encourage client to visit the physician on a regular basis to monitor for early symptoms of major organ involvement. Advise client to have regular eye exam if taking Plaquenil Sulfate. Inform client of community support groups available through the Lupus Foundation of America, Inc. (see Resources).

Evaluation Each goal must be evaluated to determine how it has been met by the client.

MYASTHENIA GRAVIS

Myasthenia gravis (MG) is an autoimmune disease characterized by extreme muscle weakness and fatigue due to the body's inability to transmit nerve impulses to voluntary muscles. It is thought that clients with MG develop antibodies that act to decrease the number and effectiveness of acetylcholine receptor sites at neuromuscular junctions. Voluntary muscles are most commonly involved, especially those innervated by cranial nerves. Muscle weakness increases during periods of activity and improves after a period of rest.

Severity of symptoms varies. In mild conditions known as Group I ocular myasthenia, only the eye muscles are involved. As severity increases, symptoms of Group II generalized myasthenia develop. Facial, neck, skeletal, and respiratory muscles become affected. The thymus gland is enlarged in most clients. It is in this organ that anti-ACh receptor antibodies are produced. MG affects men more frequently than women with the onset of symptoms after age 50. Periods of remission and exacerbation occur, usually during the first few years.

There are 3 possible complications: respiratory distress, myasthenic crisis, and cholinergic crisis. Clients need to be carefully monitored for early signs of respiratory distress, such as dyspnea, tachypnea, tachycardia, and diaphoresis.

Myasthenia crisis is an acute emergency characterized by increased muscle weakness; difficulty swallowing, chewing, or talking; and respiratory distress. It occurs in newly diagnosed clients who are not responding to anticholinesterase medications following infections, surgery, or delivery of a child.

Cholinergic crisis is the result of an overdose of anticholinesterase medications. Physical symptoms of both myasthenia crisis and cholinergic crisis are the same. An edrophonium chloride (Tensilon) test is used to differentiate between the two. Tensilon is administered intravenously; symptoms of clients experiencing a myasthenia crisis will be relieved within seconds, while clients in cholinergic crisis will show no response. Atropine is administered to counteract the effects of excessive amounts of anticholinesterase drugs. The treatment goal for both is restoration of normal respiratory functioning and alleviation of symptoms.

Medical–Surgical Management

Medical

Medical management involves the use of anticholinesterase medications and plasmapheresis. Plasmapheresis removes anti-ACh receptor antibodies. Since it affords only temporary relief of symptoms, it is used primarily for clients in acute crisis who are not responding to drug therapy or prior to a thymectomy. A client's relief of symptoms is a good indicator of how successful surgery might be.

Surgical

Surgical removal of the thymus gland has shown the best results in young people early in the course of the disease. Clients with disease onset after the age of 60 seldom show substantial improvement after thymectomy (Howard, 1997).

Pharmacological

Anticholinesterase medications, such as pyridostigmine bromide (Mestinon), neostigmine bromide (Prostigmin), and ambenonium chloride (Mytelase), are prescribed early in the course of the disease and act to increase acetylcholine at the neuromuscular junction. Dosages need to be individually determined. Early side effects of overdosage include nausea, abdominal cramping, vomiting, diarrhea, increased saliva, diaphoresis, and low pulse rate. Variation may occur in muscle group responses for the same client. Steroids are also prescribed to slow down the immunological response.

Diet

Clients need to be encouraged to eat a snack prior to taking anticholinesterase medications to avoid GI irritation. If the client's ability to chew and swallow is affected, the diet may need adjustment.

Activity

Symptoms of MG increase with exercise. Clients should avoid excessive muscular activity and should rest periodically throughout the day. ROM exercises, braces, splints, and walkers assist in keeping the client independent.

▶ NURSING PROCESS

▶ Assessment

▶ Subjective Data

Client describes muscle weakness, fatigue, and possibly difficulty chewing or swallowing.

PROFESSIONAL TIP

Myasthenia Gravis

Clients with myasthenia gravis experience problems similar to those with RA and SLE, i.e., fatigue and impaired physical mobility. Although the cause, in this case, is due to weakness of voluntary muscles, client goals and nursing interventions are the same.

▶ Objective Data

The nurse must assess level of muscle groups affecting the eyes, face, neck, and chest, looking for **diplopia** (double vision), **ptosis** (drooping upper eyelids) and facial symmetry. Chewing or swallowing problems should be noted. Vocal tones and breath sounds should be assessed. Level of weakness in arm and legs muscles as well as muscles used for breathing should all be noted.

ACh receptor antibody and LE cell tests are often positive. X-rays and CT scans of the thymus gland are used to detect enlargement. Electromyogram (EMG) determines the extent of muscle damage.

Nursing diagnoses for a client with MG may include the following:

Nursing Diagnoses	Planning/Goals	Nursing Interventions
▶ *Breathing Pattern, Ineffective, related to muscle weakness*	The client will have normal respiratory rate and rhythm and normal breath sounds bilaterally.	Monitor client's respiratory rate and rhythm and breath sounds frequently. Administer oxygen as ordered. Elevate head of client's bed. Notify physician immediately if respiratory problem develops.
▶ *Aspiration, Risk for, related to impaired swallowing*	The client will not experience aspiration.	Have client eat in a sitting position or with head of the bed elevated. Teach client to chew food well and swallow only small bites. Request a special diet of thickened, soft foods. Suction oral secretions as required. Teach client to suction secretions as needed.
▶ *Knowledge Deficit related to disease process and understanding of methods to control disease and prevent complications*	The client will describe disease process, factors contributing to symptoms, and regimen for control. The client will practice health behaviors needed to manage the effects of MG and methods to prevent complications.	Teach client stress management techniques and methods to avoid infections. Teach clients to take medications at regularly scheduled times to maintain appropriate level. Encourage client to wear a MedicAlert bracelet indicating the name and dosage of medications being taken. Refer to the Myasthenia Gravis Foundation for information and support groups (see Resources).

Evaluation Each goal must be evaluated to determine how it has been met by the client.

SAMPLE NURSING CARE PLAN

THE CLIENT WITH MYASTHENIA GRAVIS

Mrs. Henry, a 29-year-old mother of two preschool children, was diagnosed with myasthenia gravis 2 years ago. Initially, she had double vision and drooping eyelids, but after beginning a course of pyridostigmine bromide (Mestinon), she went into remission. Recently, she has been experiencing facial, neck, and chest muscle weakness and is now admitted to the hospital for evaluation. Occasionally, she has difficulty swallowing and breathing. Her thymus gland is enlarged. She has asked the nurse to teach her some strategies for managing this chronic illness.

Nursing Diagnosis 1 *Breathing Pattern, Ineffective, related to respiratory muscle fatigue as evidenced by facial, neck, and chest weakness*

PLANNING/GOALS	NURSING INTERVENTIONS	RATIONALE	EVALUATION
Mrs. Henry's respiratory rate and rhythm and	Assess Mrs. Henry's breathing patterns q2h.	Frequent client assessment detects early signs of respiratory distress.	Mrs. Henry's respiratory rate and rhythm have

continued

breath sounds will remain within normal limits.	Inform Mrs. Henry to notify the nurse immediately if she begins to develop any breathing difficulties.	Some clients are reluctant to call the nurse and need to be encouraged to do so.	remained within normal limits.
	Notify physician immediately if respiratory problems develop.	When respiratory problems develop, the physician needs to determine the exact cause and if a tracheostomy is needed.	

Nursing Diagnosis 2 *Aspiration, Risk for, related to impaired swallowing as evidenced by difficulty swallowing*

PLANNING/GOALS	**NURSING INTERVENTIONS**	**RATIONALE**	**EVALUATION**
Mrs. Henry will not experience aspiration.	Position Mrs. Henry to eat in a sitting position.	Eating in a sitting position promotes the passage of food into the stomach.	Mrs. Henry has not aspirated. She makes a point of always sitting up when eating.
	Teach Mrs. Henry the importance of thoroughly chewing food, and swallowing only small bites.	Swallowing big bites of food can cause aspiration.	
	Have oral suctioning available at the bedside.	If food or secretions become caught in the mouth or throat, suctioning may be required.	

Nursing Diagnosis 3 *Knowledge Deficit, related to disease process and understanding of methods to control effects of myasthenia gravis and prevent complications as evidenced by verbalization of need for future teaching*

PLANNING/GOALS	**NURSING INTERVENTIONS**	**RATIONALE**	**EVALUATION**
Mrs. Henry will practice health behaviors needed to manage the effects of MG and prevent complications.	Assess Mrs. Henry's prior knowledge of MG and methods of controlling the effects of prescribed medications and preventing complications.	Assessing a client's prior knowledge provides a basis for planning teaching.	Mrs. Henry and her husband related information about MG, action and side effects of Mestinon, signs and symptoms to watch for, and when to notify the physician. She has obtained a MedicAlert bracelet and has con-
	Include Mrs. Henry's family members in teaching sessions.	Including family members in the teaching session fosters imple-	

continued

Teach Mrs. Henry and family members basic information about MG, the actions of anticholinesterase medication, the need to take it on a regular basis with a snack, side effects of overdose, and the importance of notifying the physician of any signs of respiratory problems or infection.

Encourage Mrs. Henry to wear a MedicAlert bracelet, which lists her name, diagnoses, and dosage of prescribed medications.

Provide Mrs. Henry with the address and telephone number of the Myasthenia Gravis Foundation and encourage her to contact them for additional information and support.

mentation of the teaching in the home setting.

Information about one's disease, medications, and when to notify the physician is essential knowledge the client and family members need in order to effectively manage this chronic illness.

A MedicAlert bracelet provides accurate information to medical personnel in case of an emergency.

Providing a resource for additional information facilitates future attainment of knowledge and possible involvement with a support group.

tacted the MG Foundation. She plans to attend the next local chapter meeting.

INADEQUATE IMMUNOLOGICAL RESPONSE

This category includes HIV/AIDS; pulmonary, gastrointestinal, oral, gynecological, and central nervous system opportunistic infections; and opportunistic malignancies.

HIV/AIDS

While allergies are hypersensitive immune responses, and autoimmune diseases literally have the body attacking itself, acquired immunodeficiency syndrome (AIDS) is a disease that causes an inadequate immunological response by the body. The human immunodeficiency virus (HIV) may be acquired anytime after conception.

The **human immunodeficiency virus** (HIV), a retrovirus that causes **acquired immunodeficiency syndrome** (AIDS), was first reported in the United States in 1981. AIDS is a progressively fatal disease that

destroys the immune system and the body's ability to fight infection. By the end of 1998, it was estimated that 33.4 million people in the world were living with HIV/AIDS (National Institute of Allergy and Infectious Diseases [NIAID] and National Institutes of Health [NIH], May 1999). In the United States, 688,200 cases of AIDS had been reported by the end of 1998, and as many as 900,000 may be infected with HIV (NIAID and NIH, March 1999).

Following exposure to HIV and an incubation period of 2 to 4 weeks, some individuals, but not all, will experience flulike symptoms such as fever, sweats, headache, myalgia, neuralgia, sore throat, GI distress, and photophobia (Figure 39-5). Many persons, if tested at this time, will test negative because antibodies may not yet be present in the blood. In 2 or 3 weeks, these symptoms disappear. Infected individuals are very infectious during this period with large quantities of HIV present in genital secretions.

Most individuals will remain symptom free for years (10 or more), but some may begin to have symptoms in a few months. During this "asymptomatic"

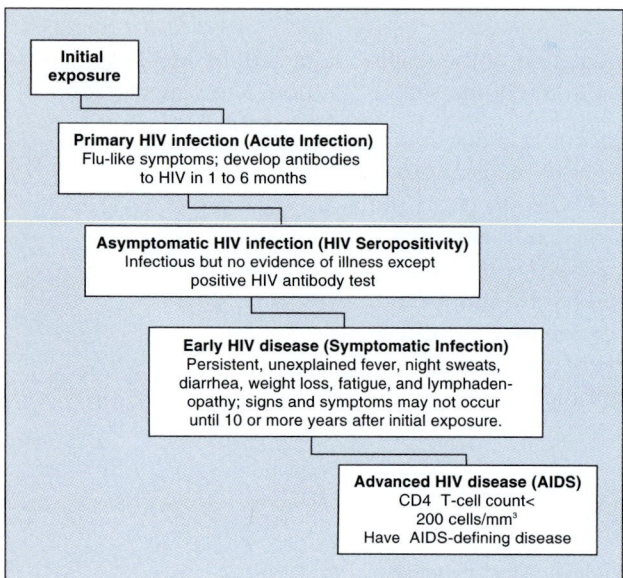

Figure 39-5 Continuum of HIV Disease

period, HIV is multiplying, infecting, and killing the CD4 T-cells of the immune system.

A variety of symptoms become evident as the CD4 T-cells disappear. Lymph nodes enlarged for more than 3 months are one of the first symptoms. Others may include weight loss, lack of energy, fevers and sweats, persistent skin rashes or flaky skin, persistent or frequent oral or vaginal yeast infections, PID that does not respond to treatment, and short-term memory loss. Oral, genital, or anal herpes infection or shingles may also develop.

When the CD4 T-cell count is less than 200 cells/mm^3 (healthy persons have 1,000 or more CD4 cells/mm^3) and the individual has 1 or more of the 26 clinical conditions that affect persons with advanced HIV disease, the individual is considered to have AIDS. Most of the AIDS-defining conditions are **opportunistic infections** (infections in persons with a defective immune system that rarely cause harm in healthy individuals). *Pneumoncystis carinii* pneumonia is the most frequent AIDS-defining diagnosis in the United States and Europe (Lisanti & Zwolski, 1997).

The **enzyme-linked immunosorbent assay** (ELISA) is the basic screening test to detect antibodies to HIV. A positive test result is always retested to rule out false-positive results and/or technician error. A confirmatory test, the **Western blot** test, is always employed when the ELISA test is positive. Results of both the ELISA and Western blot taken together have an extremely high accuracy rate.

Obtaining a signed informed consent for testing is often a nursing responsibility. Most states mandate a consent form solely for HIV testing. Some states allow verbal consent and a statement of the client's consent signed by the health care provider.

Demographics of AIDS in the United States

Demographics are viewed in terms of clients' age, gender, and race.

Age

AIDS mainly affects people during the most productive years of their life. As of December 1998, AIDS is now the fifth leading cause of death among persons ages 25 to 44 (NIAID and NIH, May 1999). Children under the age of 13 made up 1% (8,461) of cases reported to the CDC by the end of 1998 (NIAID and NIH, May 1999).

Gender

Trends in HIV-related mortality reflect changes in the demographic patterns of the HIV epidemic. Although more men than women are infected with HIV, the number of AIDS cases in women in the United States has increased from 7% in 1985 to 16% in 1998. Of 688,200 cases of AIDS that had been reported to the CDC by the end of 1998, 570,425 (83%) were males 13 years old and older, and 109,311 (16%) were females 13 years old and older (NIAID and NIH, May 1999).

Race

Of the new AIDS cases reported in the United States in 1998:

- African Americans accounted for 66.4/100,000 population.
- Hispanic Americans accounted for 28.1/100,000 population.
- Whites accounted for 8.2/100,000 population.
- American Indian/Alaska Natives accounted for 7.4/100,000 population.
- Asian American/Pacific Islanders accounted for 3.8/100,000 population (NIAID and NIH, May, 1999)

The HIV/AIDS epidemic is growing most rapidly among some minority populations and is a leading cause of death of African American males. The CDC reports that the prevalence for AIDS is 6 times higher in African Americans and 3 times higher in Hispanic Americans than among whites (NIAID and NIH, March 1999).

Modes of Transmission

There are many ways to become infected with HIV. The virus may be found in blood, semen, vaginal secretions, and breast milk of infected individuals. There is no evidence that HIV is spread through sweat, tears, urine, or feces. The saliva of infected individuals has the virus, but there is no evidence that it is spread to others through kissing. The risk of infection from "deep kissing" and oral sex is unknown. Tissue transplantation (including artificial insemination), blood transfusion, and needle sticks are high-risk situations but are relatively rare methods of transmission in the

United States today. Having another sexually transmitted disease such as chlamydia, genital herpes, syphilis, or gonorrhea seems to make an individual more susceptible to becoming infected with HIV during sexual intercourse with an infected partner. Theoretically, HIV is present in sufficient quantities in amniotic fluid, cerebrospinal fluid, pleural fluid, peritoneal fluid, and pericardial fluid whereby infection could occur with exchange of these body fluids, particularly in health care settings where contact with these fluids may occur. Behaviors associated with increased risk of sexual transmission of HIV by infected persons include unprotected sexual intercourse, multiple sex partners, failure to disclose HIV status, and trading sex for money or drugs (CDC, 1996b). Transmission of HIV can also take place by having contact with infected blood or sharing needles or syringes; it may also transmit from mother to fetus during pregnancy or birth.

Sexual intercourse (anal, oral, vaginal) without using a condom is the most frequently reported risk behavior for infection with HIV. Among individuals reported with AIDS in the United States in 1998, 45% of the men and 38% of the women had unprotected sex (NIAID and NIH, May 1999). Injection-drug use is the second most frequently reported risk behavior for infection with HIV. Among individuals reported with AIDS in the United States in 1998, 21% of the men and 29% of the women reported injection-drug use. When HIV seropositive women take zidovudine (AZT) during pregnancy and labor and zidovudine is given to the newborn, perinatal transmission is significantly reduced.

Medical–Surgical Management

Medical

The goal of care is to keep the disease from progressing for as long as possible. The client's chance of disease progression can now be monitored by a **viral load test** that measures copies of HIV RNA. The approved viral load test is the Amplicor HIV-1 Monitor test, better known as the *polymerease chain reaction (PCR) test* (AIDS Treatment Data Network, May 1999). It can be used to see if individuals with HIV are at risk for getting sick, for checking the effects of drugs taken by individuals with HIV to see if they are working against the virus, and to distinguish the difference between actual HIV infection in a newborn and maternally acquired antibodies. The "ultra-sensitive" PCR test can measure as few as 50 copies/mL of HIV RNA.

Pharmacological

The goal of anti-HIV treatment is to keep the viral load as low as possible for as long as possible, ideally below what the viral load test can detect (AIDS Treatment Data Network, May 1999). Currently available antiretroviral drugs do not cure HIV/AIDS. Treatment is usually begun at the time of **seroconversion** (evidence of antibody formation in response to disease or vaccine). In high-risk occupational exposures, treatment may be started immediately.

One group of drugs, called *nucleoside analog reverse transcriptase inhibitors (NRTIs),* interrupt HIV's life cycle at an early stage. The spread of HIV in the body may be slowed and the onset of opportunistic infections may be delayed by NRTIs, but these drugs *do not* prevent HIV transmission to other individuals. This group includes zidovudine (Retrovir), formerly known as AZT, zalcitabine (Hivid), didanosine (Videx), stavudine (Zerit), lamivudine (Epivir), and abacavir (Ziagen). A combination of zidovudine and lamivudine

PROFESSIONAL TIP

HIV Testing

Although physicians are responsible for client counseling, the nurse must know the information to be able to answer questions and clarify the client's knowledge. Pretest counseling should include the following:

- Ask why the client believes the test should be done.
- Explain the meaning of a positive or negative test result and the possibility of a false-negative result.
- Discuss risk reduction and ways to modify behavior.
- Share state reporting requirements.
- Ensure confidentiality of test results.
- Explain that there is often stress related to test results and possible reactions to learning the results, such as depression or anxiety.
- Discuss the potential negative social consequences of positive results.
- Assist the client in making a decision about testing.
- Arrange a return appointment for the client to receive test results.

Posttest counseling should include the following:

- Review the test results with the client.
- Assess the client's understanding of the test results.
- Allow the client to express feelings about the test results.
- Review routes of HIV transmission.
- Assess the client's psychological condition including the risk for suicide.
- Assess the client's risk behavior and strategies for reducing risk.
- Provide information about support groups and national/local resources.

(Combivir) is now available. Zidovudine (Retrovir) may cause depletion of red or white blood cells. If this depletion is severe, the drug must be discontinued. Painful nerve damage and pancreatitis may be caused by didanosine (Videx).

Non-nucleoside reverse transcriptase inhibitors (NNRTIs) are available to be used only in combination with other antiretroviral drugs. These include delavirdine (Rescriptor), nevirapine (Viramune), and efavirenz (Sustiva).

The protease inhibitors interrupt HIV's life cycle at a later step. These include ritonavir (Norvir), saquinavir mesylate (Fortovase, Invirase), indinavir sulfate (Crixivan), and nelfinavir mesylate (Viracept). Nausea, diarrhea, and other GI symptoms are common side effects of protease inhibitors. Some individuals have an abnormal redistribution of body fat (NIAID and NIH, March 1999).

HIV can become resistant to each type of drug, so combination treatments are necessary to effectively suppress the virus. Current guidelines recommend drug therapy for any client with symptomatic HIV disease (evidence of opportunistic infections or tumors). For asymptomatic HIV-positive clients, drug therapy is recommended if:

- Viral load test results are greater than 500 copies/mL, or
- The client's CD4 T-cell count is under 500 cells/mm^3 (Kirsten & Whipple, 1998).

Health Promotion

The CDC and the Occupational Safety and Health Administration (OSHA) have developed recommendations to reduce the risk of health care personnel exposure to blood and body fluids. These recommendations are called Standard Precautions. Personal protective equipment should be worn while caring for all clients when there is a reasonable likelihood of contact with any blood or body fluids.

PULMONARY OPPORTUNISTIC INFECTIONS

Conditions discussed following include *pneumocystis carinii* pneumonia, histoplasmosis, and tuberculosis.

PNEUMOCYSTIS CARINII PNEUMONIA

***Pneumocystis carinii* pneumonia** (PCP) is the most common opportunistic infection associated with advanced HIV disease (CDC, 1995b). A marked decrease in the number of AIDS clients diagnosed with PCP is due to initiation of prophylactic treatment when the CD4 T-cell count is 200 or less/mm^3. Although *Pneumocystis carinii* is found primarily in the lungs, it has also been reported in the adrenal glands, bone marrow, skin, thyroid, kidneys, and spleen of persons with AIDS.

Clinical signs and symptoms include fever, shortness of breath, nonproductive cough, and crackles. Initial diagnosis is made by chest x-ray, which shows diffuse infiltrates. Fiberoptic bronchoscopy is the procedure of choice to obtain a definitive diagnosis. During the bronchoscopy, sputum is obtained to demonstrate the presence of the organism.

Current standard treatment for PCP includes either intravenous pentamidine isethionate (Pneumopent, Pentam 300) or sulfamethoxazole-trimethoprim (Bactrim, Septra), given orally or intravenously. Oral sulfamethoxazole-trimethoprim is the treatment of choice; however, approximately one-third of people with AIDS eventually develop hypersensitivity reactions and must switch to pentamidine for primary therapy. Prophylaxis against PCP is a therapeutic necessity for all persons infected with HIV when the CD4 T-cell count is 200 or less. Primary prophylaxis refers to therapy for those considered at risk for PCP based on the CD4 count to prevent infection with PCP. Secondary prophylaxis refers to therapy to prevent recurrences in clients who have already had PCP. Current guidelines recommend either oral sulfamethoxazole-trimethoprim or aerosolized pentamidine for prophylaxis. For those allergic to sulfamethoxazole-trimethoprim, pentamidine diluted in sterile water administered by a Respigard II nebulizer can be used.

HISTOPLASMOSIS

Histoplasmosis is an infection caused by the fungus *Histoplasma capsulatum*. The fungus has been isolated in bird droppings, dirt from chicken coops, and caves. The spores from the fungus are introduced into the body by inhalation. Histoplasmosis is not specific to the lung. In most clients with HIV disease, histoplasmosis is disseminated (spread out). Histoplasmosis should be suspected if the person presents with fever of uncertain origin, cough, and malaise.

The diagnosis is confirmed by culture or biopsy of the bone marrow, blood, lymph nodes, lungs, or skin. Initial treatment of histoplasmosis consists of IV amphotericin B (Amphotericin B) (Muma, Lyons, Borucki, & Pollard, 1994). Oral ketoconazole (Nizoral) can be used for maintenance therapy. The CDC has recommended prophylaxis against reoccurrence of histoplasmosis with itraconazole (Sporanox) (CDC, 1995b).

TUBERCULOSIS

Mycobacterium tuberculosis, an acid-fast aerobic bacterium, is the cause of tuberculosis (TB). It is spread through airborne particles and enters the body by inhalation. The particles usually lodge in the apex of the lungs; however, one-half to two-thirds of cases of HIV-associated or AIDS-associated TB involve organs outside the lungs as well. Tuberculosis is more prevalent in medically underserved populations, foreign-born persons from areas of the world with a high prevalence, homeless persons, correctional-facility inmates, alcoholics, injection-drug users, the elderly, and people with compromised immune systems (CDC, 1994).

Clinical manifestations include fever, night sweats, cough, and weight loss. People with AIDS will commonly present with a productive cough and pleuritic pain. Diagnosis is made by a combination of tests: skin testing with purified protein derivative (PPD); examination and culture of sputum, urine, and other fluids; x-rays; and other tests such as IVP.

The most common test for exposure to TB is the Mantoux skin test, which consists of injecting 0.1 ml of (PPD) intradermally. A negative reaction does not rule out infection. HIV-positive clients with a CD4 count lower than $200/mm^3$ may no longer have an immune response to the PPD. The chest x-ray may reveal middle and lower lobe infiltrates. A sputum specimen is smeared and stained with an acid-fast stain, then examined under the microscope for acid-fast bacillus (AFB). Other body fluids such as urine, blood, and stool may also be tested for AFB.

The risk of transmission of TB to health care workers is highest during and immediately after procedures that induce coughing. In the home and health care setting, cough-inducing procedures should be performed only in well-ventilated areas.

Infection Control: TB

A densely woven, snug-fitting mask (particulate respirator) should be worn by all persons in contact with the person who has TB until the person has received treatment for 2 to 3 weeks. Persons with TB should also be taught to cover their mouths while coughing and should wear a particulate respirator when they are out of their room for tests.

Due to the upsurge of multidrug-resistant TB (MDR-TB), the CDC recommends treating with multiple medications (CDC, 1994). Treatment is provided in two phases. In the initial treatment phase, the client receives isoniazid (Laniazid), rifampin (Rifadin), pyrazinamide, and ethambutol HCl (Myambutol) or streptomycin sulfate for 2 to 6 months, depending on whether *Mycobacterium tuberculosis* is identified outside the lungs. In the continuation phase, treatment with 2 to 4 of the medications used in the initial phase is indicated for 4 to 6 months longer.

▶ NURSING PROCESS

▶ Assessment

▶ Subjective Data

The nurse must assess the client's ability to dress, bathe, ambulate, and so on. The client's perception of breathlessness should be noted.

▶ Objective Data

The client's respiratory rate, depth, and breath sounds should be assessed. Cough (productive or nonproductive), cyanosis, dyspnea, use of accessory muscles, and fever must be noted. Arterial blood gas (ABG) results are monitored for decreased PaO_2, increased $PaCO_2$, and decreased pH.

Nursing diagnoses for the HIV-positive client with pulmonary disorders may include the following:

Nursing Diagnoses	Planning/Goals	Nursing Interventions
▶ *Airway Clearance, Ineffective, related to chronic, unrelieved cough, pain, or viscous secretions*	The client will mobilize secretions effectively.	Administer 2.5–3 L of fluid per day (oral or IV) to decrease thick secretions. Administer medications as ordered to suppress cough and decrease pain. Reposition client every 2 hours and PRN.
▶ *Gas Exchange, Impaired, related to inadequate ventilation/oxygenation*	The client will maintain an SaO_2 > 90%.	Administer oxygen as ordered. Encourage use of incentive spirometer, if not contraindicated.
▶ *Breathing Pattern, Ineffective, related to fatigue*	The client will pace activities to minimize fatigue.	Plan care to allow rest periods.

Evaluation Each goal must be evaluated to determine how it has been met by the client.

GASTROINTESTINAL OPPORTUNISTIC INFECTIONS

Disorders discussed following include: *Mycobacterium avium* complex, cytomegalovirus, cryptosporidiosis, hepatitis, and HIV-wasting syndrome.

MYCOBACTERIUM AVIUM COMPLEX

Mycobacterium avium and *Mycobacterium intracellulare* are two closely related mycobacteria that are grouped together and called **Mycobacterium avium complex** (MAC). For humans, the source of exposure to MAC is contaminated water although it has been isolated from soil, dust, sediments, and aerosols (Muma, Lyons, Borucki, & Pollard, 1994). In persons with AIDS, MAC involvement of the bowel is usually extensive, suggesting that the gastrointestinal tract may be the site of initial infection, with spread to other organs after that. The microorganism can fill the bone marrow and lymph nodes.

The most common symptoms of MAC include chronic fever, malaise, anemia, weight loss, diarrhea, and abdominal pain. Often the client will appear cachectic due to malabsorption. Because the symptoms are nonspecific, MAC is often difficult to distinguish from other AIDS-related infections. MAC is usually disseminated at the time of diagnosis. Diagnosis is made by tissue biopsy and cultures of the lung, bone marrow, lymph nodes, liver, or blood.

Treatment for MAC infection may include one or more of the following medications: clarithromycin (Biaxin Filmtabs) to treat disseminated MAC; and a combination of amikacin sulfate (Amikin), azithromycin (Zithromax), ciprofloxacin hydrochloride (Cipro), cycloserine (Seromycin), and ethionamide (Trecator-SC). For persons with AIDS who have a CD4 count of less than $75/mm^3$, rifabutin (Mycobutin) is recommended for prevention of disseminated MAC (CDC, 1995b).

CYTOMEGALOVIRUS

Cytomegalovirus (CMV) belongs to the herpes virus group. Thus, it shares the same phenomena of latency and reactivation. The virus lies dormant in tissues waiting to be reactivated in the immunocompromised client. The potential for infection with CMV is increased during two periods: the perinatal period through the preschool years, and later during the sexually active years.

CMV causes disease by destroying the brain, lung, retina, and liver. CMV infection has been identified in all parts of the gastrointestinal tract from the oral cavity to the perianal area. CMV can be life-threatening for persons with suppressed immune systems. Persons with HIV infection or AIDS may develop severe infections including CMV retinitis that can lead to blindness.

Signs and symptoms of CMV include weight loss, fever, diarrhea, and malaise. The diagnosis of CMV is based on microscopic identification of CMV from specific organs such as the brain, lung, liver, or adrenal gland. Ganciclovir sodium (Cytovene) is the drug of choice for treating individuals infected with CMV. Maintenance therapy is required to prevent relapse. Intravenous foscarnet sodium (Foscavir) has been approved as an alternative therapy.

CRYPTOSPORIDIOSIS

Cryptosporidium, a protozoan causing cryptosporidiosis, usually infects the epithelial cells that line the digestive tract. Transmission is often by the fecal-oral route, but can be spread from animal to person as well as person to person. *Cryptosporidium* can also be spread by ingesting contaminated food and water.

Clinical signs and symptoms include profuse watery diarrhea, up to 20 liters per day (Lisant & Zwolski, 1997). Abdominal pain, serious weight loss, abdominal cramping, anorexia, low-grade fever, dehydration, electrolyte imbalance, and malaise may also be present. Diagnosis is made by identifying the organism in fresh stool specimens.

There is no effective treatment for cryptosporidiosis. Antidiarrheals such as diphenoxylate hydrochloride with atropine sulfate (Lomotil), loperamide hydrochloride (Imodium), and opium tincture (Paregoric) should be given on a programmed schedule rather than PRN. Treatment is palliative and focused toward the symptoms. This includes fluid and electrolyte replacement (orally if possible), analgesics, and occasionally the use of total parenteral nutrition. Anticryptosporidial agents are under investigation. Protecting the integrity of the client's perianal skin is extremely important. A low-residue, high-protein, high-calorie diet helps maintain nutritional status.

HEPATITIS

Only 3 of the 5 hepatitis viruses are commonly seen with HIV infection (Paar, 1994). They are hepatitis B virus (HBV), hepatitis C virus (HCV), and hepatitis D virus (HDV). All 3 viruses have been associated with chronic infection and have similar transmission and risk factors. Risk factors include exposure to blood or blood products, exposure to contaminated needles and syringes, and multiple sexual contacts.

Signs and symptoms include malaise, weakness, anorexia, nausea, vomiting, and right upper quadrant pain. Abnormalities in bilirubin and hepatic enzymes may also occur. Diagnosis is made by serologic assays identifying antigens and antibodies.

Interferon has been approved for treatment of chronic HBV and HCV and is being investigated for the treatment of HDV. Response to therapy varies but is decreased with HIV infection. Clients with a CD4 count greater than 400 mm^3 respond best to this therapy (Parr, 1994).

HIV-WASTING SYNDROME

HIV-wasting syndrome is defined as unexplained weight loss of more than 10% of body weight accompanied by weakness, chronic diarrhea, and fever in those infected with HIV (NIAID and NIH, May 1997). Weight loss and malnutrition are related to reduced food intake, malabsorption of nutrients, and altered metabolism of nutrients. Some of the factors related to reduced intake include anorexia, oral or esophageal lesions, nausea, neurologic or psychiatric conditions, fatigue, inadequate finances, and side effects of medications. Nutritional malabsorption is related to injury of the small intestine caused by opportunistic infections or by HIV infection of the cells in the gastrointestinal tract. Opportunistic infections produce fever that depletes the body's energy stores and causes weight loss.

Signs and symptoms of HIV-wasting syndrome are anorexia, diarrhea, nausea, vomiting, changes in taste and smell, aphthous ulcers of mouth and esophagus, and abdominal pain.

Symptom control is the major focus for HIV-wasting syndrome. Medications to control nausea and vomiting should be given routinely and not PRN. Treatment of anorexia includes megestrol acetate (Megace) or dronabinol (Marinol). Antimotility drugs such as loperamide hydrochloride (Imodium), luminal acting agents such as kaolin and pectin mixture (Kaopectate), and hormonal agents such as octreotide acetate (Sandostatin) are used to treat diarrhea. The aphthous ulcers are safely and effectively healed with the drug thalidomide (NIAID and NIH, May 1997). This makes eating much easier. Oral nutritional supplements are most frequently used for weight loss. Total parenteral nutrition (TPN) is usually considered a final option except in cases of severe malnutrition, because of the risk and expense involved.

▶ NURSING PROCESS

▶ Assessment

▶ Subjective Data

The client should be asked about bowel habits, and what causes and relieves diarrhea. The nurse should inquire about alcohol consumption since excessive alcohol intake depletes B vitamins and provides no nutrition. Activities that cause fatigue are noted. Food likes/dislikes, food intolerances, and food intake for the previous 3 days should be discussed.

▶ Objective Data

The nurse should assess the client's skin integrity including temperature, moisture, color, vascularity, texture, lesions, areas of excoriation, and poor wound healing. Fever, weight, and daily nutritional intake must be noted. Laboratory values of nutritional status including serum albumin, total protein, hemoglobin, and hematocrit, as well as stool specimens for ova and parasites, should all be assessed.

Nursing diagnoses for the HIV-positive client with gastrointestinal disorders may include the following:

Nursing Diagnoses	Planning/Goals	Nursing Interventions
▶ *Fluid Volume Deficit related to nausea, vomiting, diarrhea, or inadequate oral intake*	The client will have normal skin turgor and decreased frequency and amount of stools.	Suggest client use hard candy or chewing gum to stimulate saliva production if mouth is dry.
		Encourage client to drink liquids between (not with) meals.
		Monitor and record intake and output.
		Monitor client for evidence of electrolyte imbalance (hypokalemia, hypochloremia, confusion, muscle weakness).
▶ *Nutrition, Altered, Less than Body Requirements, related to anorexia, dysphagia, malabsorption, or side effects of medications*	The client will eat 75% of prescribed diet and maintain current weight.	Provide the prescribed diet (usually low-residue, high-caloric, high-protein) in small frequent meals at room temperature.
		Offer commercially prepared nutritional supplements between meals.
		Administer supplemental vitamins and minerals as prescribed.
		Provide oral hygiene before and after meals to enhance taste sensation.
		Administer antiemetics and antidiarrheals as ordered.
		Weigh client daily.
		Advise client to keep a food diary and a log of exacerbation and remission of signs and symptoms.

continued

Nursing Diagnoses	Planning/Goals	Nursing Interventions
▸ *Skin Integrity, Impaired, Risk for, related to diarrhea, malnutrition, decreased mobility*	The client will maintain skin integrity.	Monitor stool for presence of blood, fat, undigested food.
		Monitor stool cultures for evidence of new infections.
		Protect the perirectal area by keeping it clean and using compounds such as Aloe Vesta cream.
		Avoid prolonged pressure on bony prominences by a scheduled turning plan.
		If nonambulatory, provide client with a pressure relief mattress.
		Teach client to use nondrying soaps and to pat skin dry.
		Use soft sheets on the bed and avoid wrinkles.

Evaluation Each goal must be evaluated to determine how it has been met by the client.

ORAL OPPORTUNISTIC INFECTIONS

Candidiasis and leukoplakia are discussed following.

ORAL AND ESOPHAGEAL CANDIDIASIS

Oral candidiasis (thrush) is a fungal infection caused by *Candida albicans* (Figure 39-6), which occurs in more than 90% of AIDS clients (Lisanti & Zwolski, 1997). Many clients complain of an unpleasant taste or mouth dryness. Other clinical signs and symptoms include creamy, white oral plaques and mucosal tenderness. When the white oral plaques are wiped off, they leave an erythematous or even bleeding mucosal lesion (Lisanti & Zwolski, 1997). Esophageal candidiasis, an AIDS-defining disease, causes dysphagia and painful swallowing.

These symptoms may interfere with the client's eating, nutrition, and weight. Diagnosis is established by the presence of the characteristic lesions in the oral cavity. Microscopic examination of oral or esophageal lesions reveals budding yeast cells.

Treatment for esophageal candidiasis is oral fluconazole (Diflucan). Oral candidiasis is treated with nystatin suspension (Mycostatin) and clotrimazole (Mycelex Troches). Another medication used to treat candidiasis is ketoconazole (Nizoral). Amphotericin B (Amphotericin B) is used to treat disseminated candida infection. The antiulcer drug sucralfate (Carafate) may be used in a slurry form to relieve mouth pain prior to eating.

ORAL HAIRY LEUKOPLAKIA

Oral hairy leukoplakia (OHL) usually appears as a white patch on the lateral borders of the tongue as shown in Figure 39-7. It is caused by the Epstein-Barr virus. The lesions are rarely in other areas of the mouth and are different in appearance from candidia-

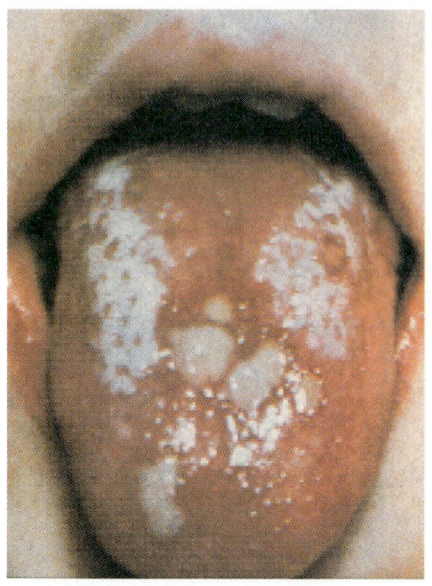

Figure 39-6 Oral Candidiasis (Thrush)

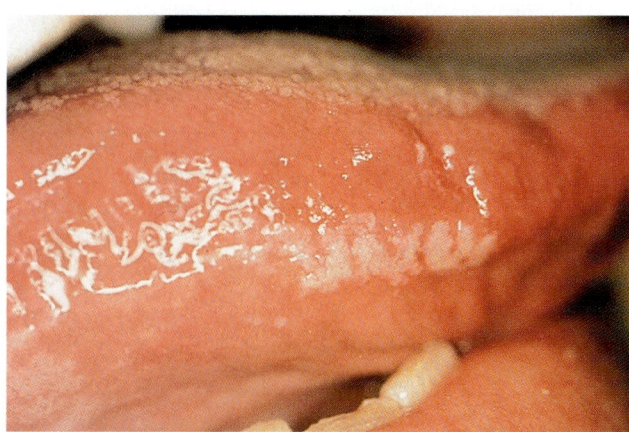

Figure 39-7 Oral Hairy Leukoplakia (*Courtesy of Dr. Joseph Konzelman, School of Dentistry, Medical College of Georgia.*)

sis. The irregular surface of the lesion appears as projections that resemble hairs and cannot be scraped off. Diagnosis is made by visual inspection of the lesion. OHL is not usually bothersome to the client and may regress spontaneously. No treatment is necessary for most cases of OHL; however, oral acyclovir (Zovirax) may be given to selected clients. More than 50% of clients with OHL develop AIDS within 30 months (Lisanti & Zwolski, 1997).

▶ NURSING PROCESS

▶ Assessment

▶ Subjective Data

The client's history of symptoms and oral hygiene habits should be assessed, and the client asked about recent nutritional intake, use of alcohol and tobacco, and current medications.

▶ Objective Data

The client's lips, tongue, and buccal mucosal surfaces are assessed for lesions, white cheesey patches, and bleeding. Any difficulty swallowing should be noted.

A nursing diagnosis for an HIV-positive client with oral manifestations may be:

Nursing Diagnosis	Planning/Goals	Nursing Interventions
▶ *Oral Mucous Membrane, Altered,* related to oral lesions	The client will be free from oral lesions.	Administer prescribed medications. Frequently assess the oral cavity. Instruct client to avoid commercial mouthwashes containing alcohol or glycerine. Provide oral hygiene with a small soft toothbrush before and after meals.

Evaluation Each goal must be evaluated to determine how it has been met by the client.

GYNECOLOGICAL OPPORTUNISTIC INFECTIONS

Gynecological infections discussed include vaginal candidiasis and cervical intraepithelial neoplasia.

VAGINAL CANDIDIASIS

Vaginal candidiasis is a fungal infection caused by *Candida albicans*. It is the most common initial infection occurring in HIV-infected women. Clinical manifestations include a white, clumped-appearing vaginal discharge, vaginal wall inflammation, and vaginal itching. Diagnosis is made by microscopic identification of yeast.

Most cases of vaginal candidiasis are treated with topical antifungal agents such as clotrimazole (Gyne-Lotrimin). For clients who do not respond to treatment with clotrimazole, ketoconazole (Nizoral) or fluconazole (Diflucan) is recommended.

CERVICAL INTRAEPITHELIAL NEOPLASIA

Women infected with HIV have a much higher incidence of cervical intraepithelial neoplasia (CIN) than women who are not infected. CIN and cancer of the cervix are considered to be on a continuum of abnormal cervical cells, ranging from mild abnormality (Grade I) to severe abnormality and cancer (Grade III). CIN in HIV-infected women progresses more rapidly and is less responsive to standard treatments than in noninfected women. Factors related to increased risk of CIN in HIV-positive women include a decreased number of CD4 T-cells and infection with human papilloma virus (HPV). It is thought that HIV activates HPV, causing cellular abnormalities.

The early stages of CIN have no symptoms. Clinical manifestations of cervical cancer include painless postcoital bleeding and blood-tinged vaginal discharge. As CIN progresses, back pain, abdominal or pelvic pain, weight loss, anorexia, and leg edema caused by obstruction of lymph nodes may occur. Initial diagnosis is made by Pap smear to determine the presence of abnormal cells. Clients with abnormal Pap smears are referred for cervical biopsy and colposcopy.

Treatment for CIN includes laser therapy, conization, and hysterectomy. Treatment for invasive cervical cancer depends on the stage of the disease and may include chemotherapy, surgery, and radiation.

▶ NURSING PROCESS

▶ Assessment

▶ Subjective Data

Assess the client's history of symptoms, and ask the client about bleeding after intercourse, abdominal and pelvic pain, and vaginal itching or discharge.

▶ Objective Data

Vaginal discharge is assessed for white or blood-tinged secretions. Weight loss and edema are noted.

Nursing diagnoses for a female HIV-positive client with gynecological manifestations may include the following:

Nursing Diagnoses	Planning/Goals	Nursing Interventions
▶ *Tissue Integrity, Impaired, related to vaginal mucosal lesions*	The client will be free of vaginal infections.	Teach the client to have Pap smears every 6 months. Assess the frequency and consistency of vaginal discharge. Teach client to keep the vaginal area clean and dry and to wear loose fitting cotton underwear to prevent irritation.
▶ *Body Image Disturbance related to chronic vaginal infections or surgery, radiation, or removal of cervix*	The client will verbalize feelings and concerns about body image.	Encourage client to verbalize feelings and concerns about body image. Refer client to a support group for women with HIV.

Evaluation Each goal must be evaluated to determine how it has been met by the client.

CENTRAL NERVOUS SYSTEM OPPORTUNISTIC INFECTIONS

Disorders covered include AIDS dementia complex, toxoplasmosis, and cryptococcosis.

AIDS DEMENTIA COMPLEX

The most common central nervous system complication in persons with AIDS is AIDS dementia complex (ADC). Without early treatment with zidovudine (Retrovir), the chance of developing ADC is approximately 33% (Lisanti & Zwolski, 1997). This disorder is chronic and progressive with cognitive, motor, and behavioral dysfunction. ADC is caused by infection of glial cells in the brain with HIV. Signs and symptoms are sometimes vague during the initial stages of ADC. Early signs include poor concentration, forgetfulness, loss of balance, leg weakness, apathy, and social withdrawal. Clients with advanced ADC may exhibit psychotic behaviors and delirium and progress to a catatonic-like state with minimal responsiveness to the environment.

Diagnosis is made by neurological testing of cognitive, motor, and behavioral functioning. Other diagnostic tests include brain imaging to look for cerebral atrophy. Cerebrospinal fluid analysis can show elevated proteins and will exclude other pathogens. Clients treated with zidovudine (Retrovir) have shown improvement in cognitive and motor skills, but the effect only lasts about 12 months (Lisanti & Zwolski, 1997).

TOXOPLASMOSIS

Toxoplasmosis is caused by the protozoan *Toxoplasma gondii*. Cats and other animals serve as a reservoir for this organism. It is spread to humans by ingestion of oocytes found in contaminated water, soil, or food, especially raw or undercooked meat. After entering the body, *Toxoplasma gondii* reproduces and spreads via the blood or lymph system. A person with an intact immune system may have no symptoms or mild symptoms, and the organism may remain dormant for years. In the immunocompromised person, the infection may be reactivated (secondary) or occur with the ingestion of oocytes from contaminated sources. Clinical signs and symptoms may be vague and nonspecific, or range from a mild headache, fever, and lethargy to poor coordination, seizures, and coma. Diagnosis is made by identification of a lesion through brain imaging (computerized tomography or magnetic resonance imaging), presence of serum antibodies to *Toxoplasma gondii,* and recent onset of a neurologic abnormality.

The treatment of choice is oral pyrimethamine (Daraprim) and sulfadiazine (Microsulfon). Lifelong suppressive therapy of pyrimethamine plus sulfadiazine and leukovorin calcium (Wellcovorin) is required (CDC, 1995b).

CRYPTOCOCCOSIS

Cryptococcosis is a fungal infection caused by *Cryptococcus neoformans*. Cryptococcosis is the most life-threatening fungal infection associated with AIDS (Lisanti & Zwolski, 1997). The organism is acquired in the environment, usually from bird droppings. In the noncompromised host, the fungus is inhaled and contained in the lungs. In the immunocompromised host with AIDS, *Cryptococcus neoformans* can be disseminated, remain in the lungs, or infect the brain and meninges. Clinical manifestations include fever, headache, nausea and vomiting, dizziness, photophobia, mental status changes, seizures, and a stiff neck. Detection of cryptococcal antigen in cerebrospinal fluid, urine, or blood can be used for diagnosis. If untreated, this is a fatal condition.

Treatment for acute cryptococcal infections includes intravenous amphotericin B (Fungizone Intravenous) to be given for at least 2 weeks, followed by fluconazole (Diflucan) for 10 to 12 weeks. Once treatment for acute infection is complete, lifelong suppressive therapy with oral fluconazole daily is recommended (Lisanti & Zwolski, 1997).

▶ NURSING PROCESS

▶ Assessment

▶ Subjective Data

Ask the client about forgetfulness, missing appointments, ability to complete activities of daily living, and if there have been any recent falls or accidents. Ask the client's family and significant others about behavior changes such as social withdrawal or unusual behavior.

▶ Objective Data

Assess the client for subtle mental status changes such as poor concentration and inability to remember instructions or previous conversations. Assess the client for motor impairment such as dropping things, poor coordination, or changes in writing ability. Assess the client's ability to remember usual medication schedule. Observe the environment for safety.

Nursing diagnoses for an HIV-positive client with central nervous system manifestations include the following:

Nursing Diagnoses	Planning/Goals	Nursing Interventions
▶ *Thought Processes, Altered, related to mental status changes*	The client will maintain cognitive functioning.	Assess mental and neurologic status. Evaluate client's emotional, cognitive, and motor skills. Provide cues for reorientation (clock, calendar). Monitor client for adherence to medical regimen.
▶ *Social Isolation related to alteration in mental status*	The client will have contact and interact with significant others.	Encourage family and significant others to visit client. Provide structured activities and environment for social interaction. Encourage client to verbalize feelings and concerns.

Evaluation Each goal must be evaluated to determine how it has been met by the client.

OPPORTUNISTIC MALIGNANCIES

Kaposi's sarcoma and non-Hodgkin's lymphoma are discussed.

KAPOSI'S SARCOMA

Kaposi's sarcoma (KS) is a vascular malignancy that can occur any place in the body, including internal organs. The first lesions often appear subtly on the face or in the oral cavity. The more immunosuppressed the person is, the more aggressive the spread of KS. Clinical manifestations of KS are red to purple lesions, which are painless, nonblanching, and palpable (Figure 39-8). These lesions are sometimes mistaken for bruises. Edema in the face, penis, scrotum, and legs can occur as a result of blockages in the lymphatic system. KS can also be found in the GI tract and lungs. Diagnosis is made by tissue biopsy.

Treatment involves a variety of options depending on whether the lesions are local or systemic. Radiation therapy, intralesional therapy with interferon alpha 2a or 2b (Roferon A, Intron A) or vinblastine sulfate (Velban), laser therapy, and cryotherapy are used on single or isolated KS lesions. For clients with advanced widespread symptomatic disease, single or combination chemotherapeutic regimens include vinblastine sulfate (Velban), vincristine sulfate (Oncovin), etoposide

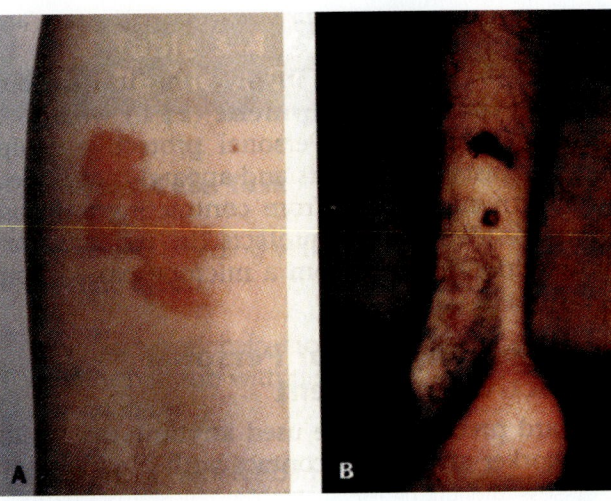

Figure 39-8 Kaposi's Sarcoma (*Courtesy of Daniel J. Barbaro, MD, Fort Worth, Texas.*)

(VePesid), bleomycin sulfate (Blenoxane), doxorubicin HCl (Rubex), and mitoxantrone HCl (Novantrone).

NON-HODGKIN'S LYMPHOMA

Lymphomas are malignant tumors of the immune system. B-cells are the origin of malignancy for the majority of clients with AIDS-related non-Hodgkin's lymphoma (NHL). Clinical manifestations are nonspecific and may include fever, night sweats, and weight loss. Confusion, lethargy, and memory loss may be present in persons with CNS involvement.

Diagnosis of NHL is complicated because of the nonspecific symptoms. Examination of tissue is the recommended diagnostic procedure. There is no standard treatment of NHL. Individualized treatment may include a combination of chemotherapy, antiretroviral agents, prophylaxis against opportunistic infections, and colony-stimulating factors to enhance bone marrow production of blood cells. However, in many clients with advanced HIV disease, treatment of NHL is withheld because it is not tolerated well and may even lead to earlier death.

▶ NURSING PROCESS

▶ Assessment

▶ Subjective Data
The client must be asked about frequency, onset, and persistence of current symptoms. The effect of current symptoms on ability to perform activities of daily living and relationships with others should be noted, as well as the effect of treatment plan on quality of life.

▶ Objective Data
Skin lesions should be assessed. Increased frequency, intensity, or recurrence of nonspecific symptoms including fever, night sweats, and weight loss should be documented.

Nursing diagnoses for an HIV-positive client with a malignancy may include the following:

Nursing Diagnoses	Planning/Goals	Nursing Interventions
▶ *Skin Integrity, Impaired, Risk for, related to lesions or treatment*	The client will maintain skin integrity.	Teach client to avoid scratching skin lesions, to avoid drying soaps, and to make sure clothing and linen have been thoroughly rinsed of detergent.
▶ *Social Isolation related to change in appearance*	The client will maintain usual social interactions and identify factors that enhance quality of life.	Facilitate the client's interaction with others. Keep client and significant others aware of treatment plan. Encourage significant others to participate in the care of client. Encourage physical closeness between the client and significant others. Provide client with access to clergy, social worker, or HIV counselor. Encourage the client to join a support group or obtain peer support. Assist client in identifying positive coping strategies.

Evaluation Each goal must be evaluated to determine how it has been met by the client.

CASE STUDY

Jim Hayes, a 37-year-old male, suspects that he is HIV positive. He enters the medical unit with chronic symptoms such as fever, night sweats, diarrhea, weight loss, shortness of breath, and a nonproductive cough. On the initial assessment, he is alert and oriented, color is pale, temperature 100.6°F, pulse 92, respirations 36, and blood pressure 140/70. He has generalized lymphadenopathy. His height is 5'11", and his weight is 125 pounds. Jim states that he is not currently taking any medications although he is "familiar" with the drug zidovudine (Retrovir).

The following questions will guide your development of a nursing care plan for the case study.

1. List symptoms/clinical manifestations, other than Mr. Hayes's, that a client may experience when HIV positive.

2. List 2 reasons zidovudine (Retrovir) may be initiated for Mr. Hayes.

3. List 2 diagnostic tests that will confirm the diagnosis of HIV.

4. List subjective and objective data the nurse would want to obtain about Mr. Hayes.

5. Write 3 individual nursing diagnoses and goals for Mr. Hayes.

6. List pertinent nursing actions the nurse would perform in caring for Mr. Hayes related to:

   hydration

   fatigue

   nutrition

   oxygenation

   medications

7. List resources that could assist Mr. Hayes with his diagnosis.

8. List teaching Mr. Hayes will need before leaving the medical unit.

SUMMARY

- The immune system identifies substances as self or nonself and protects the body by neutralizing or destroying foreign organisms.
- Immunity to a disease is either natural or acquired.
- Age, sex, nutritional status, medications, and stress influence the immune response.
- Clients receiving blood transfusions must be carefully monitored, especially during the first half hour, for signs of a reaction.
- Anaphylactic reactions, which may occur as a result of exposure to foods, medications, blood, or insect bites, can potentially be life-threatening.
- Organ transplant clients must understand the implications of taking immunosuppressive medications.
- Clients with rheumatoid arthritis must be taught methods of adapting to the effects of synovial joint inflammation, immobility, and deformity.
- Systemic lupus erythematosus affects multiple body systems.
- Clients with myasthenia gravis experience extreme muscle weakness and fatigue and must be carefully monitored for signs of respiratory distress, and myasthenic or cholinergic crisis.

- Diagnosis of HIV/AIDS is made by the ELISA and Western blot test. These tests determine the presence of antibodies to HIV, not the virus itself.
- *Pneumocystis carinii* pneumonia is the most common opportunistic infection associated with HIV.
- Oral candidiasis can be painful and interfere with the client's nutritional status.
- AIDS dementia complex is a progressive disorder with cognitive, motor, and behavioral dysfunction.

Review Questions

1. Ms. Caldwell has just been diagnosed with syphilis and has an order for 1,000,000 units of penicillin I.M. She has no history of allergies to medications. She has never had penicillin. When giving her the injection in the right upper outer quadrant of her buttocks, you note a tattoo. Several minutes after receiving the injection, she tells you she feels anxious and weak. You note she is diaphoretic, scratching her forearm, and is breathing faster than normal. Based upon this assessment data, you would conclude:

a. she is embarrassed because you saw her tattoo.

b. she is probably anxious since you know she has a sexually transmitted disease.

c. her syphilis is getting worse.

d. these are early signs of an anaphylactic reaction.

2. Which of the following is a potentially life-threatening transfusion reaction?

a. Acute hemolytic reaction

b. Allergic urticarial reaction

c. Delayed hemolytic reaction

d. Febrile nonhemolytic reaction

3. Sensitivity to sunlight, a butterfly rash, and renal failure are symptoms of which of the following conditions?

a. Anaphylaxis

b. Myasthenia gravis

c. Rheumatoid arthritis

d. Systemic lupus erythematosus

4. Rheumatoid arthritis is:

a. an autoimmune disease characterized by abnormal IgG antibodies.

b. associated with abnormal B-cell lymphocytes.

c. curable if the client takes large doses of Plaquenil Sulfate.

d. the results of a hypersensitivity reaction.

5. Increased muscle weakness, difficulty chewing or swallowing, and shortness of breath in clients with myasthenia gravis are signs of:

a. cholinergic crisis.

b. myasthenia crisis.

c. both cholinergic crisis and myasthenic crisis.

d. reaction to plasmapheresis.

6. Which of the following statements shows that the client understands a diagnosis of HIV positive?

a. "Being HIV positive means that I have AIDS."

b. "Since I am only HIV positive I cannot infect others."

c. "Because I am HIV positive I have the virus that causes AIDS."

d. "I became infected by donating blood."

7. The drug of choice for treating *Pneumocystis carinii* pneumonia (PCP) is:

a. co-trimoxazole (Septra).

b. ganciclovir (Cytovene).

c. megestrol acetate (Megace).

d. fluconazole (Diflucan).

8. The nurse is caring for a client who is experiencing diarrhea and weight loss. Which of the following nursing interventions is appropriate for him?

a. Encourage fluids with meals

b. Substitute a milk shake for lunch

c. Offer small, frequent meals

d. Suggest he eat more sweets

9. The nurse is caring for a client who asks when zidovudine (Retrovir) is normally started. Which of the following would be the nurse's correct response?

a. When the client becomes symptomatic

b. When CD4 level reaches 500/mm³

c. After the client's first opportunistic infection

d. As soon as the client is diagnosed as HIV positive

10. The nurse is discussing transmission of HIV with a client. Which of the following statements indicates that the client needs more education?

a. "I should not share needles with anyone."

b. "I can spread the virus through sexual contact."

c. "I can no longer donate blood."

d. "I should not hug or kiss anyone."

Critical Thinking Questions

1. What are the lifestyle implications of being diagnosed with a chronic disease such as rheumatoid arthritis or systemic lupus erythematosus?

2. What are the pros and cons about receiving a blood transfusion from a donor?

3. How might a person's lifestyle change after receiving a diagnosis of HIV positive?

WEB FLASH!

- Search the Internet for the disorders discussed in this chapter. Can information be found for all of them? What type of research is being performed for these disorders? What type of drugs are available? Diagnostic tests? Other treatments?

- Search the Web for the resources listed for this chapter at the end of this text. How many of them have a Web page? What other information is provided?

NURSING CARE OF THE CLIENT: INTEGU-MENTARY SYSTEM

MAKING THE CONNECTION

Refer to the following chapters to increase your understanding of integumentary disorders:

- **Chapter 23, Fluid, Electrolyte, and Acid-Base Balance**
- **Chapter 25, Assessment**
- **Chapter 27, Diagnostic Tests**
- **Chapter 30, Nursing Care of the Oncology Client**
- **Chapter 39, Nursing Care of the Client: Immune System**
- **Chapter 55, Nursing Care of the Older Client**

- **Procedures:** B9, Performing Passive Range-of-Motion Exercises; B11, Positioning a Client in Bed; B12, Moving a Client in Bed; B14, Transferring a Client from Bed to Stretcher with Minimum Assistance/Maximum Assistance; I8, Application of Heat and Cold; I17, Applying a Dry Sterile Dressing; I18, Applying a Wet to Dry Dressing; I19, Culturing a Wound; I20, Irrigating a Wound

LEARNING OBJECTIVES

Upon completion of this chapter, you should be able to:
- *Define key terms.*
- *Describe common disorders of the integumentary system.*
- *Relate the pathophysiology of each skin disorder.*
- *Discuss the common diagnostic tests used to differentiate skin disorders.*
- *State the usual treatment for each skin disorder.*
- *Assess the nursing care needs of a client with a disorder of the integument.*
- *Plan and implement effective nursing care.*

KEY TERMS

alopecia	jaundice
angiogenesis	keloid
angioma	keratin
blanching	lipoma
cyanosis	melanin
debride	nevi
ecchymosis	pallor
erythema	petechiae
eschar	purulent exudate
friction	sebaceous cyst
granulation tissue	sebum
hemorrhagic exudate	serosanguineous
hemostasis	exudate
hyperthermia	serous exudate
hypothermia	telangiectasia
inflammation	vitiligo
ischemia	wound

INTRODUCTION

As an old adage asserts, the health of the skin mirrors the health of the body. Many systemic diseases have skin manifestations. Psychological stress can affect the condition of the skin, and skin rashes can be a complication of drug therapy. As the largest and the most visible system in the body, the integumentary system (skin, hair, scalp, nails, and mucous membranes) is vulnerable to injury and is susceptible to a number of primary diseases. It is estimated that skin-related problems account for 5% to 10% of all ambulatory client visits in the United States (Deters, 1996).

While the outward appearance of the skin is important for psychological well-being, the healthy, intact status of the skin also is essential for physiologic well-being. Maintaining this status of the integumentary system is, therefore, an important independent nursing function. The focus of this chapter will be to describe common skin disorders, identify the usual treatment modalities for these disorders, and discuss measures that nurses can implement to provide effective nursing care for clients with disorders of the integument.

ANATOMY AND PHYSIOLOGY REVIEW

As the external covering of the body, the skin performs the vital function of protecting internal body structures from harmful microorganisms and substances. The skin is continuous with mucous membranes at external body openings of the respiratory tract, the digestive system, and the urogenital tract. As appendages of the skin, the hair and nails also have protective functions. In addition to its vital protective role, the skin also plays other roles in the normal functioning of the human organism. These roles include participating in the regulation of body temperature, functioning as a sensory organ, helping to maintain fluid and electrolyte balance, producing vitamin D, and excreting certain waste products from the body.

Structure of the Skin

The skin is composed of three layers: the epidermis, the dermis, and the subcutaneous fatty tissue (Figure 40-1).

Epidermis

The epidermis is a layer of squamous epithelial cells. Most of the cells are keratinocytes that produce a tough, fibrous protein called **keratin**. As new cells are produced in the deep layers of the epidermis, old cells are pushed to the surface of the skin. As these cells move from the deeper epidermal layers to the surface, they undergo a process of keratinization in which they become filled with keratin, thus hardening the outer layer of epidermal cells. The keratin creates a barrier that repels bacteria and foreign matter and is impermeable to most substances. The epidermal cells on the palms of the hands and soles of the feet, areas of the body subjected to increased friction and pressure, contain larger amounts of keratin, resulting in thickened skin and callouses.

The epidermis also contains specialized cells called melanocytes. These cells produce **melanin**, the pigment that gives the skin its color. The more melanin present, the darker the skin color. Moles and birthmarks (**nevi**), pigmented areas in the skin, are aggregations of melanocytes. In **vitiligo**, melanocytes are destroyed, causing milk-white patches of depigmented skin surrounded by normal skin. Exposure to ultraviolet light (sun) causes an increase in the production of melanin, which darkens (tans) the skin and provides some protection against the harmful effects of suntanning.

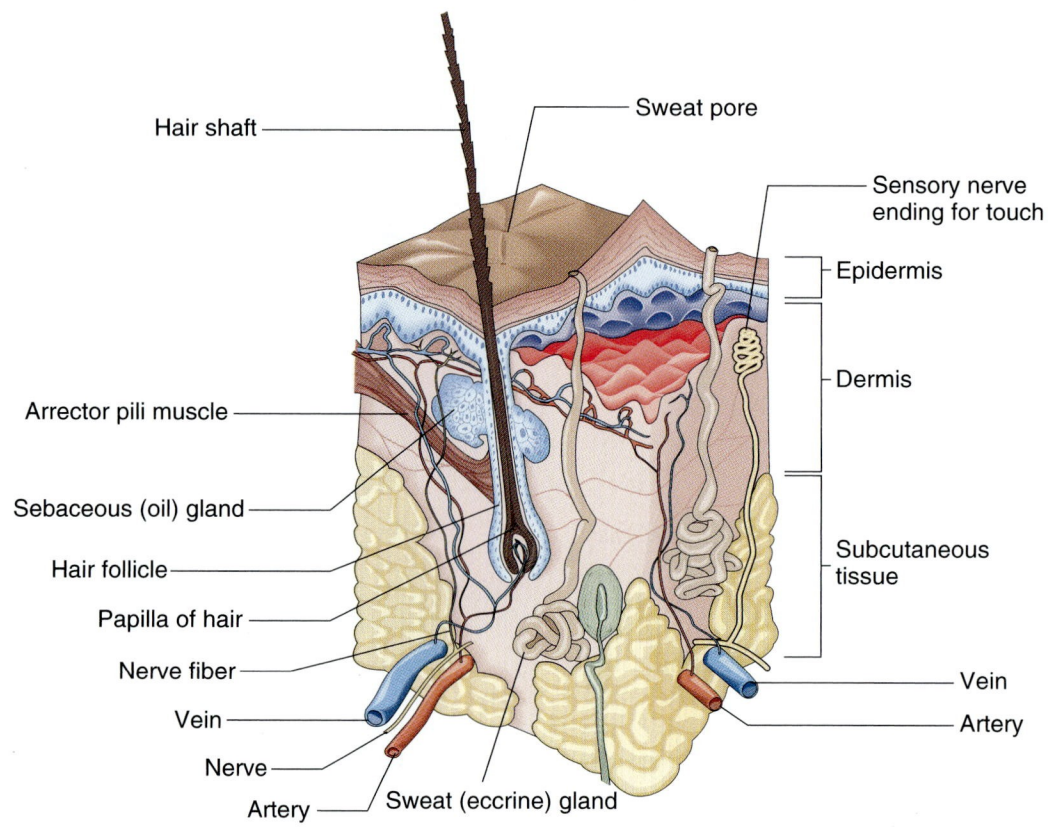

Figure 40-1 Cross Section of the Skin

Dermis

The dermis is dense, irregular connective tissue composed of collagen and elastic fibers, blood and lymph vessels, nerves, sweat and sebaceous glands, and hair roots. The sebaceous glands secrete an oily substance called **sebum** that lubricates the skin, helping to keep it soft and pliable. Sweat (eccrine) glands are found in the skin over most of the body surface. Another type of sweat gland, apocrine glands, is concentrated in the axillae, anal region, scrotum, and labia majora. These glands secrete an organic substance that is odorless at first but is quickly metabolized by skin bacteria causing the characteristic odor commonly referred to as body odor (Seeley, Stephens, & Tate, 1995). Intradermal injections, such as the TB skin test, are given in the dermis.

Subcutaneous Tissue

The subcutaneous tissue is primarily connective and adipose (fatty) tissue. Here the skin is anchored to muscles and bones. An individual's nutritional status and genetic makeup dictate the amount of subcutaneous tissue present. Emaciated persons have very little subcutaneous tissue while obese persons may have several inches of subcutaneous tissue. The amount of subcutaneous tissue is an important factor in body temperature regulation.

Functions of the Skin

Understanding the functions of the skin and contiguous mucous membranes guides the nurse in planning and implementing appropriate nursing care. Because intact, healthy skin and mucous membranes serve as the first line of defense against harmful agents, maintaining skin integrity is one of the most important independent functions of the nurse. Nursing interventions such as providing daily hygiene care and regularly turning and repositioning dependent clients are aimed at preventing skin breakdown.

Protection

The first and most important function of the skin is protection. As long as the skin is intact and healthy, it is a barrier against microorganisms and numerous substances that could be harmful to the individual. Not only is the skin a barrier to keep harmful substances out, it is also a barrier to keep essential substances such as water and electrolytes inside the body.

Temperature Regulation

The body produces heat as a result of metabolism of food. Exercise, fever, or a hot environment can raise body temperature. Through several mechanisms, the skin can either release or conserve body heat to maintain normal body temperature. Radiation is the primary means of heat loss. As body heat increases, arterioles in the dermis dilate, bringing body heat to the skin surface. By the process of radiation, waves of heat from uncovered body surfaces are released to the environment. Layering clothes in winter, for example, helps to prevent excess loss of body heat by radiation. Heat is also lost by conduction. In conduction, heat is transferred from warmer surfaces to cooler ones. Placing a cool washcloth on a client's forehead is an example of using the principle of conduction. The washcloth becomes warmer, the forehead cooler. Evaporation is another way in which excess body heat is lost. As moisture on the skin, either from perspiration or from a tepid sponge bath, dries the body is cooled. To conserve (prevent excess loss) body heat, arterioles in the dermis contract to decrease the flow of blood to the skin surface, thus decreasing heat lost by radiation. The phenomenon of "goose flesh" is another method of conserving body heat. Tiny hairs standing on end create a layer of air insulation decreasing loss of body heat to the environment.

Sensory Perception

The skin contains receptors for pain, touch, pressure, and temperature. The sensory receptors help protect the body from environmental dangers as well as provide sensations of comfort and pleasure.

Fluid and Electrolyte Balance

The skin helps to maintain the stability of the internal environment by preventing loss of body fluids and electrolytes and by preventing subcutaneous tissues from drying out. Skin damage, such as that occurring with severe burns, results in rapid loss of large quantities of fluid and electrolytes. This can lead to shock, circulatory collapse, and death.

Structure of Hair

Hair is composed of dead epidermal cells that begin to grow and divide in the base of the hair follicle. As the cells are pushed toward the skin surface, they become keratinized and die. Hair color is genetically determined.

Hair Growth and Replacement

Scalp hair grows for 2 to 5 years, then the follicle becomes inactive. When the growth cycle begins again, a new hair is produced and the old hair is pushed out. Approximately 50 hairs are lost each day. Sustained hair loss of more than 100 hairs each day usually indicates that something is wrong (Martini, 1992).

Function of Hair

There are 5 million hairs covering the entire human body except for the lips, palmar and plantar surfaces, nipples, and the glans penis. The amount and texture of hair vary with age, gender, race, and body part.

- Vellus hair: Fine "peach fuzz" hair that covers most of the body
- Terminal hair: Coarser, darker, sometimes curly hair on the head, eyebrows, and eyelashes; axillary and pubic hair become terminal with the onset of puberty
- Intermediate hair: Have intermediate characteristics such as the hairs on the arms and legs

Hair on the head protects the scalp from the ultraviolet rays from the sun and cushions blows to the head. Eyelashes help prevent foreign particles from entering the eyes just as the hairs in the nostrils and external ear canals help keep particles from entering the nose and ears.

Structure and Function of Nails

Nail production occurs in the nail root, an epithelial fold that cannot be seen from the surface (Figure 40-2). The nail plate covers the nail bed. The blood vessels under the nail bed give the nails their pink color.

The nails protect the ends of the fingers and toes.

Structure and Function of Mucous Membranes

Mucous membranes have epithelium overlying a layer of loose connective tissue. Specialized cells within the mucous membrane secrete mucus.

The cavities and tubes that open to the outside of the body are lined with mucous membranes. These include the oral and nasal cavities and the tubes of the respiratory, gastrointestinal, urinary, and reproductive systems. Mucous membranes perform absorptive or secretory functions depending on their placement.

Effects of Aging

With advancing years, the blood flow to the skin is reduced. The skin becomes thinner and is more easily injured. Older skin breaks down easily from prolonged pressure. The long accepted rule of thumb is to turn

LIFE CYCLE CONSIDERATIONS

Effects of Aging on the Skin

- Skin vascularity and the number of sweat and sebaceous glands decrease, affecting thermoregulation.
- Inflammatory response and pain perception diminish, increasing the risk of adverse effects from noxious stimuli.
- A thinning epidermis and prolonged wound healing make the elderly more prone to injury and skin infections.
- Skin cancer is more common among the elderly.
- Use of skin lotions containing alcohol can cause drying of the skin, increasing the risk of injury. Moisture-enhancing products should be used instead.

clients every 2 hours, but for the ill elderly client, every 2 hours may not be often enough. Significant skin damage can occur in just 1 hour of unrelieved pressure. Preventing skin breakdown in the elderly client depends on an accurate assessment of both the client's skin condition and mobility status.

Loss of subcutaneous tissue causes skin sagging and wrinkling. The activity of sebaceous and sweat glands diminishes, resulting in dry skin and a decreased ability to adapt to changes in environmental temperature. Extremes in temperature pose hazards for older adults. In very hot weather they are susceptible to **hyperthermia**, a condition in which the core body temperature reaches 106°F. In hyperthermia, the hypothalamus no longer functions appropriately. Sweating stops, the skin becomes dry and flushed, and the person becomes confused and eventually comatose. Each summer many elderly persons die from the effects of hyperthermia. Winter puts older adults at risk for **hypothermia**, a condition in which the core body temperature drops below 95°F. The hypothermic client may become confused and disoriented. As the core body temperature continues to drop, the person becomes comatose. Each winter some older adults die from severe hypothermia (Seeley et al., 1995).

On the hands and face, melanocytes increase in number, causing the age spots commonly seen in older adults. Gray hair occurs from a lack of melanin production. Skin exposed to sunlight ages faster.

ASSESSMENT

Assessing clients with disorders of the integument includes obtaining a health history and performing a physical assessment of the skin, hair, nails, and mu-

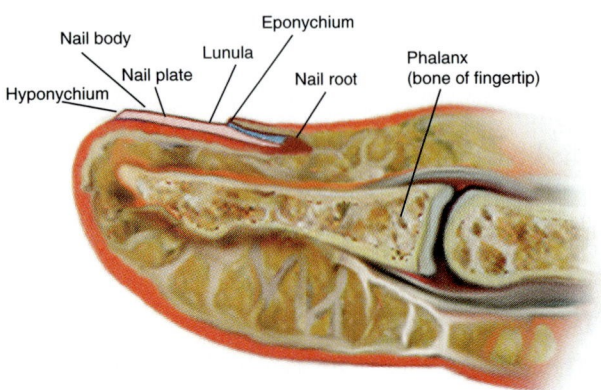

Figure 40-2 Structure of the Fingernail

Table 40-1 OBTAINING A CLIENT HISTORY OF SKIN PROBLEMS

- When did you first notice this problem?
- Where did the first symptom appear?
- What did the rash/lesion look like when it first appeared?
- Describe what happened in the days/weeks after the first symptom appeared.
- Are the symptoms worse at any particular time? Season?
- Have you experienced any itching or burning sensations?
- Are the lesions painful?
- What do you think might have caused this problem?
- Have you ever had a skin problem like this before?
- Has anyone in your family ever had a problem like this?
- What have you been doing to treat this problem?
- What kind of skin care products do you normally use?
- Have you changed any of your usual products/habits/routines?
- Is there anything else you would like to tell me about this problem?

cous membranes. The nurse's assessment skills along with an understanding of the anatomy and physiology of the integumentary system ensure a complete, factual database from which to plan and implement appropriate nursing care. Table 40-1 contains a list of questions to use in obtaining a health history.

Assessment of Skin

There are 7 parameters that should be examined when performing a physical assessment of the skin. They are integrity, color, temperature and moisture, texture, turgor and mobility, sensation, and vascularity. Inspection and palpation are the two assessment techniques used when examining the skin. Good lighting is essential for accurate assessment. Table 40-2 outlines these parameters with the normal and abnormal findings.

Any skin lesions should be identified according to type and described as to color, size, and location. The nurse should describe the amount, color, odor, and appearance of any drainage that might be present. Assessment findings must be documented clearly, concisely, and completely. The intent of nursing care is to maintain the integrity of intact skin and to restore damaged skin or mucous membranes to an intact state. Aging changes skin texture, moisture, and mobility requiring increased nursing vigilance to maintain

Table 40-2 SKIN ASSESSMENT PARAMETERS

PARAMETER	NORMAL	ABNORMAL
Integrity	Skin intact; no diseased or injured tissue.	Broken skin; open areas such as fissures, ulcers, excoriations. Rash or lesions such as papules, nodules, vesicles, pustules, wheals, scales (Figures 40-3 and 40-4).
Color	Varies with skin type and race: pink, tanned, olive, brown.	**Pallor**—pale skin, especially in face, conjunctiva, nail beds, and oral mucous membranes. **Cyanosis**—bluish discoloration noticed in lips, earlobes, and nail beds. **Jaundice**—a yellowing of the skin, mucous membranes, and sclera. **Erythema**—reddish hue to the skin as in sunburn and inflammation.
Temperature and moisture	Usually warm and dry, depending on environmental temperature.	Cool, cold, moist, clammy, or warmer than normal.
Texture	Smooth, soft. Thickness varies in different areas.	Loose, wrinkled, rough, thickened, thin, oily, flaking, scaling.
Turgor and mobility	An assessment of skin hydration. Normally skin moves freely. A pinched fold of skin returns immediately to normal position (Figure 40-5, page 0000).	Taut with edema; slack with dehydration. Rigid in some diseases such as scleroderma.
Sensation	Distinguishes hot and cold, sharp and dull.	Numbness, tingling, insensitive to pressure and sharp objects.
Vascularity	Clear; no discoloration.	**Telangiectasia** (permanent dilation of groups of superficial capillaries and venules); **Petechiae** (pinpoint hemorrhagic spots); **Ecchymosis** (large, irregular, hemorrhagic areas) (Figure 40-6, page 1010).

NONPALPABLE

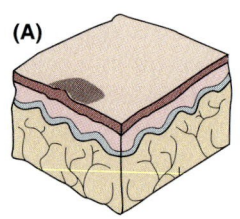

(A)

Macule:
Localized changes in skin color of less than 1 cm in diameter
Example:
Freckle

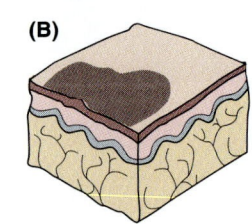

(B)

Patch:
Localized changes in skin color of greater than 1 cm in diameter
Example:
Vitiligo, stage 1 of pressure ulcer

PALPABLE

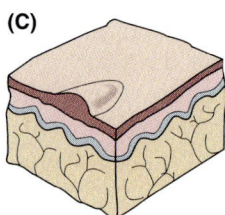

(C)

Papule:
Solid, elevated lesion less than 0.5 cm in diameter
Example:
Warts, elevated nevi

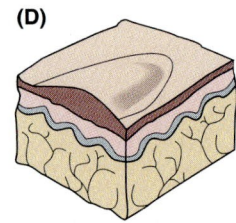

(D)

Plaque:
Solid, elevated lesion greater than 0.5 cm in diameter
Example:
Psoriasis

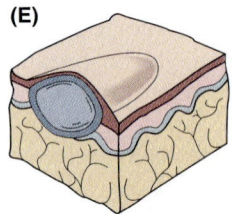

(E)

Nodules:
Solid and elevated; however, they extend deeper than papules into the dermis or subcutaneous tissues, 0.5–2 cm
Example:
Lipoma, erythema nodosum, cyst

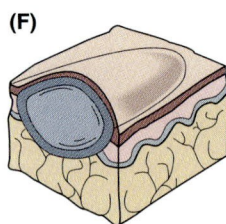

(F)

Tumor:
The same as a nodule only greater than 2 cm

Example:
Carcinoma (such as advanced breast carcinoma); not basal cell or squamous cell of the skin

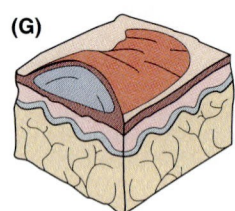

(G)

Wheal:
Localized edema in the epidermis causing irregular elevation that may be red or pale
Example:
Insect bite or a hive

FLUID-FILLED CAVITIES WITHIN THE SKIN

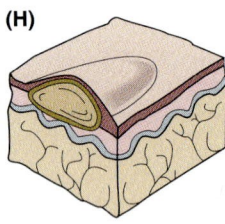

(H)

Vesicle:
Accumulation of fluid between the upper layers of the skin; elevated mass containing serous fluid; less than 0.5 cm
Example:
Herpes simplex, herpes zoster, chickenpox

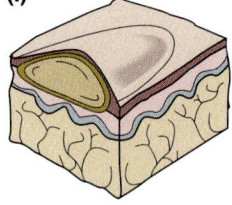

(I)

Bullae:
Same as a vesicle only greater than 0.5 cm
Example:
Contact dermatitis, large second-degree burns, bullous impetigo, pemphigus

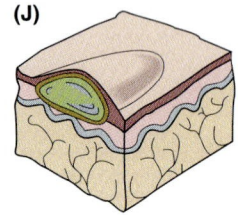

(J)

Pustule:
Vesicles or bullae that become filled with pus, usually described as less than 0.5 cm in diameter
Example:
Acne, impetigo, furuncles, carbuncles, folliculitis

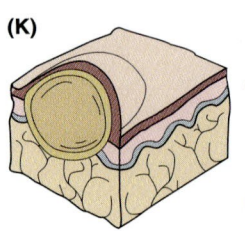

(K)

Cyst:
Encapsulated fluid-filled or a semi-solid mass in the subcutaneous tissue or dermis
Example:
Sebaceous cyst, epidermoid cyst

Figure 40-3 Types of Primary Skin Lesions (*From* Health Assessment & Physical Examination, *by M. E. Z. Estes, 1998, Albany, NY: Delmar Publishers. Copyright 1998 by Delmar Publishers. Reprinted with permission.*)

ABOVE THE SKIN SURFACE

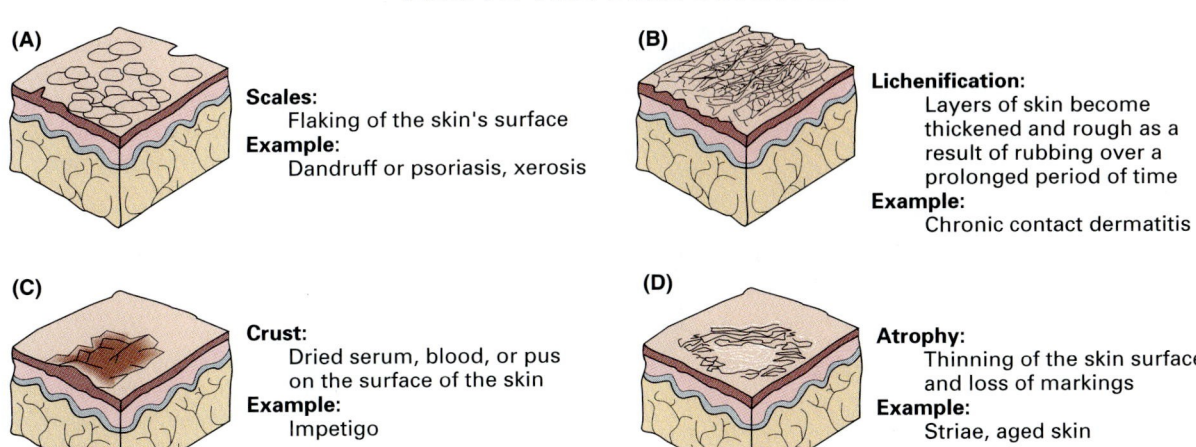

(A)

Scales:
    Flaking of the skin's surface
Example:
    Dandruff or psoriasis, xerosis

(B)

Lichenification:
    Layers of skin become
    thickened and rough as a
    result of rubbing over a
    prolonged period of time
Example:
    Chronic contact dermatitis

(C)

Crust:
    Dried serum, blood, or pus
    on the surface of the skin
Example:
    Impetigo

(D)

Atrophy:
    Thinning of the skin surface
    and loss of markings
Example:
    Striae, aged skin

BELOW THE SKIN SURFACE

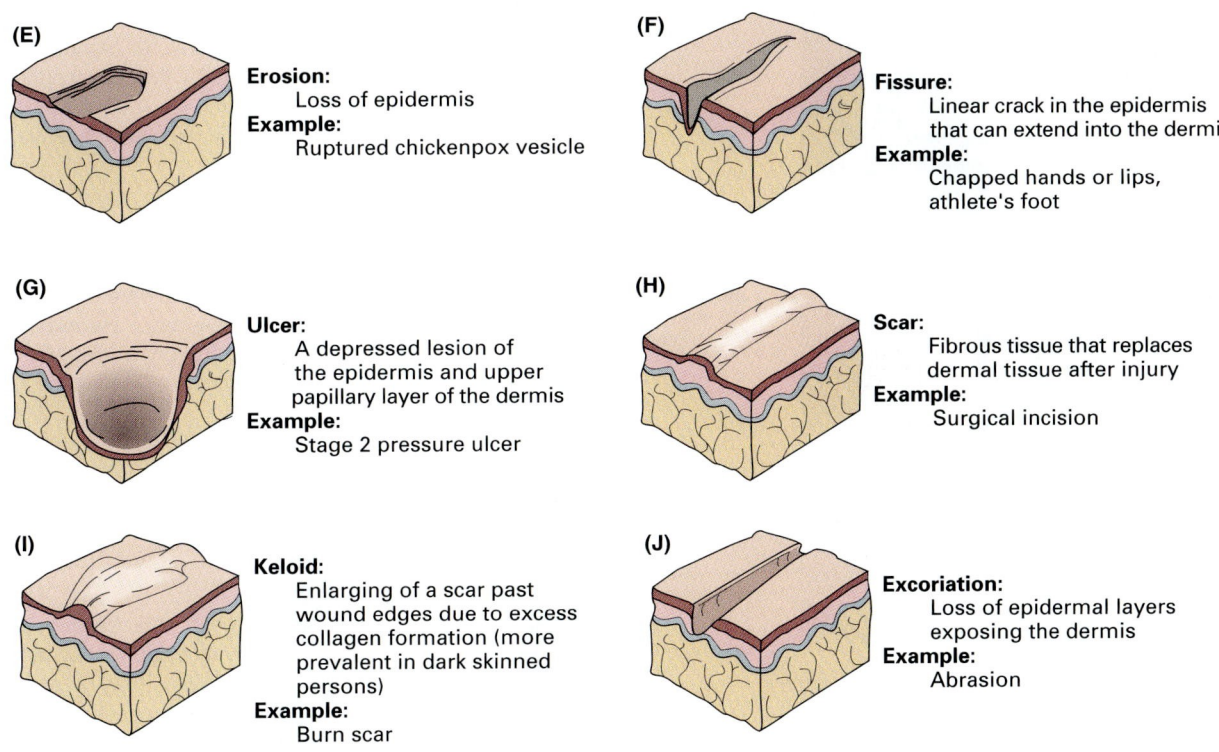

(E)

Erosion:
    Loss of epidermis
Example:
    Ruptured chickenpox vesicle

(F)

Fissure:
    Linear crack in the epidermis
    that can extend into the dermis
Example:
    Chapped hands or lips,
    athlete's foot

(G)

Ulcer:
    A depressed lesion of
    the epidermis and upper
    papillary layer of the dermis
Example:
    Stage 2 pressure ulcer

(H)

Scar:
    Fibrous tissue that replaces
    dermal tissue after injury
Example:
    Surgical incision

(I)

Keloid:
    Enlarging of a scar past
    wound edges due to excess
    collagen formation (more
    prevalent in dark skinned
    persons)
Example:
    Burn scar

(J)

Excoriation:
    Loss of epidermal layers
    exposing the dermis
Example:
    Abrasion

Figure 40-4 Types of Secondary Skin Lesions (*From* Health Assessment & Physical Examination, *by M. E. Z. Estes, 1998, Albany, NY: Delmar Publishers. Copyright 1998 by Delmar Publishers. Reprinted with permission.*)

skin integrity. Daily hygiene products should be selected to meet the client's individual skin care needs.

Assessment of Hair, Nails, and Mucous Membranes

Hair should be smooth, shiny, and resilient. Excess hair loss can result from drugs, radiation, dietary or hormonal factors, stress, and high fever.

Nails should be pink, smooth, and shiny and feel firm yet flexible when palpated. An angle of approximately 160° should be present between the nail body and the eponychium (Figure 40-7).

Mucous membranes normally appear pink and moist.

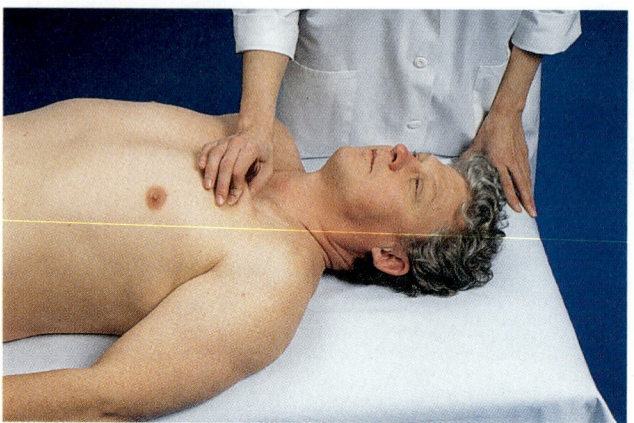

Figure 40-5 Assessment of Skin Turgor

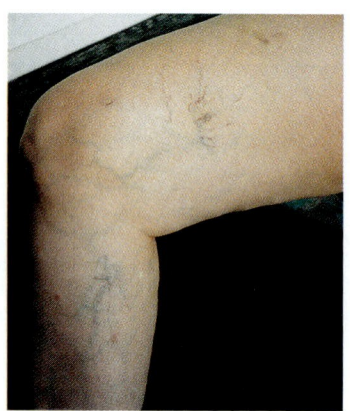

A.

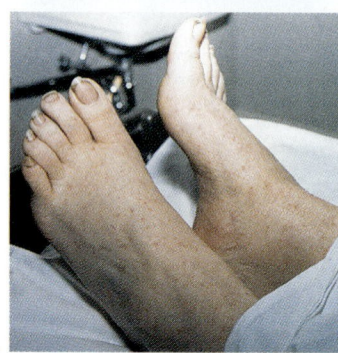

B.

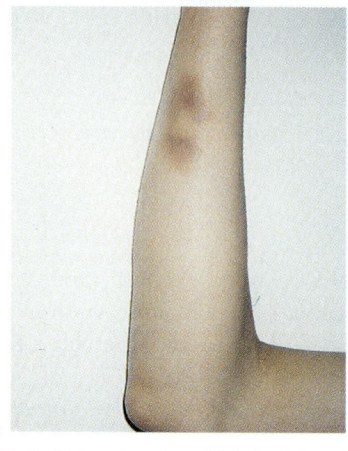

C.

Figure 40-6 A. Telangiectasia (Spider Veins); B. Petechiae (*Courtesy of Dr. Mark Dougherty, Lexington, KY*); C. Ecchymosis (bruise)

Normal nail angle

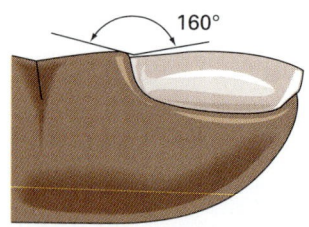

Normal nail: Has an angle of approximately 160° between the fingernail and nail base; nail feels firm when palpated.

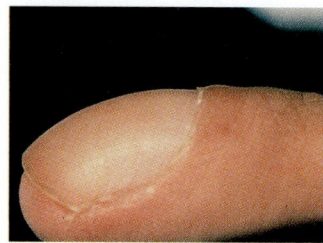

Clubbing: Hypoxia causes an angle greater than 180° between the fingernail and nail base; nail feels springy when palpated.

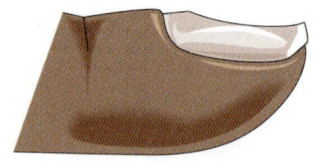

Koilonychia (spoon nail): Characterized by concave curves; associated with iron deficiency anemia.

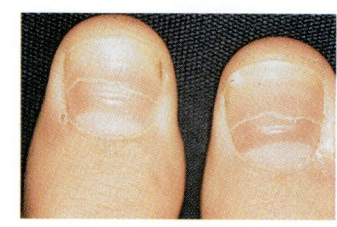

Beau's line: Characterized by transverse depression in the nails; associated with injury and severe systemic infections.

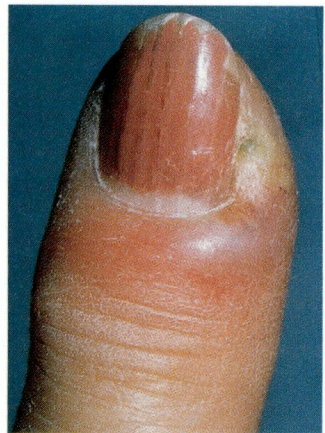

Paronychia: Characterized by an inflammation at the nail base (may be swollen, red, or tender); associated with trauma and local infection.

Figure 40-7 Nail Variations (*Photos of clubbing and Beau's line courtesy of Robert A. Silverman, MD, Clinical Associate Professor, Department of Pediatrics, Georgetown University*)

PROFESSIONAL TIP

Possible Signs of Physical Abuse

Areas of ecchymosis are one sign of trauma that could be the result of physical abuse. Injuries noted at the base of the skull or on the face, buttocks, breasts, abdomen, or any area such as the top of the back that the client could not reach, are suspicious for abuse. Unusual marks on the skin such as cigarette burns and belt buckle or bite marks may also be signs of abuse. Injuries that are inconsistent with the client's story may also be the result of abuse.

Institutional policies generally relate to reporting and to whom to report when the situation of possible physical abuse is encountered. This is usually based on state laws about reporting physical abuse. Nurses must know the reporting laws of the state in which they are employed.

COMMON DIAGNOSTIC TESTS

Commonly used diagnostic tests for clients with integumentary disorders are listed in Table 40-3. Refer to Chapter 27, Diagnostic Tests, for explanation/normal values and nursing responsibilities.

WOUNDS

A disruption in the integrity of body tissue is called a **wound**.

Physiology of Wound Healing

When an injury is sustained, a complex set of responses is set into motion, and the body begins a three-phase process of wound healing. Understanding these physiological responses will assist the nurse in caring for clients with impaired skin integrity and promoting optimal wound healing.

Defensive (Inflammatory) Phase

The defensive phase occurs immediately after injury and lasts about 3 to 4 days. The major events that

Table 40-3 COMMON DIAGNOSTIC TESTS FOR INTEGUMENTARY DISORDERS

Biopsy
Patch testing
Tzanck smear
Immunofluorescence (IF testing)
Wood's light examination
Skin scrapings
Culture and sensitivity

occur in this phase are hemostasis and inflammation. **Hemostasis**, or cessation of bleeding, occurs by vasoconstriction of large blood vessels in the affected area. Platelets, activated by the injury, aggregate to form a platelet plug and stop the bleeding. Activation of the clotting cascade results in the eventual formation of fibrin and a fibrinous meshwork, which further entraps platelets and other cells. The result is fibrin clot formation, which provides initial wound closure, prevents excessive loss of blood and body fluids, and inhibits contamination of the wound by microorganisms.

Inflammation is the body's defensive adaptation to tissue injury and involves both vascular and cellular responses. During the vascular response, tissue injury and activation of plasma protein systems stimulate the release of various chemical mediators, such as histamine (from mast cells), serotonin (from platelets), complement, and kinins. These vasoactive substances cause blood vessels to dilate and become more permeable, resulting in increased blood flow and leakage of serous fluid into the surrounding tissues. The increased blood supply carries nutrients and oxygen, which are essential for wound healing, and transports leukocytes to the area to participate in phagocytosis, or the envelopment and disposal of microorganisms. The increased blood supply also removes the "debris of battle," which includes dead cells, bacteria, and exudate, or material and cells discharged from blood vessels. The area is red, edematous, and warm to touch, and it has varying amounts of exudate.

During the cellular response, leukocytes move out of the blood vessel into the interstitial space. Neutrophils are the first cells to arrive at the injured site and begin phagocytosis. They subsequently die and are replaced by macrophages, which arise from blood monocytes. Macrophages perform the same function as neutrophils but remain for a longer time. In addition to being the primary phagocyte of debridement, macrophages are important cells in wound healing because they secrete several factors, including fibroblast activating factor (FAF) and angiogenesis factor (AGF). FAF attracts fibroblasts, which form collagen or collagen precursors. AGF stimulates the formation of new blood vessels. The development of this new microcirculation supports and sustains the wound and the healing process.

Reconstructive (Proliferative) Phase

The reconstructive phase begins on the third or fourth day after injury and lasts for 2 to 3 weeks. This phase contains the process of collagen deposition, angiogenesis, granulation tissue development, and wound contraction.

Fibroblasts, normally found in connective tissue, migrate into the wound because of various cellular mediators. They are the most important cells in this phase because they synthesize and secrete collagen. Collagen is the most abundant protein in the body and is the material of tissue repair. Initially, collagen is gel-like, but within several months it cross-links to form collagen fibrils and adds tensile strength to the wound. As the wound gains strength, the risk of wound separation or rupture is less likely. The wound can resist normal stress such as tension or twisting after 15 to 20 days. During this time, a raised "healing ridge" may be visible under the injury or suture line.

Angiogenesis (formation of new blood vessels) begins within hours after the injury. The endothelial cells in preexisting vessels begin to produce enzymes that break down the basement membrane. The membrane opens, and new endothelial cells build a new vessel. These capillaries grow across the wound, increasing blood flow, which increases the supply of nutrients and oxygen needed for wound healing.

Repair begins as granulation tissue, or new tissue, grows inward from surrounding healthy connective tissue. Granulation tissue is filled with new capillaries that are fragile and bleed easily, thus giving the healing area a red, translucent, granular appearance. As granulation tissue is formed, epithelialization, or growth of epithelial tissue, begins. Epithelial cells migrate into the wound from the wound margins. Eventually, the migrating cells contact similar cells that have migrated from the outer edges. Contact stops migration. The cells then begin to differentiate into the various cells that comprise the different layers of epidermis.

Wound contraction is the final step of the reconstructive phase of wound healing. Contraction is noticeable 6 to 12 days after injury and is necessary for closure of all wounds. The edges of the wound are drawn together by the action of myofibroblasts, specialized cells that contain bundles of parallel fibers in their cytoplasm. These myofibroblasts bridge across a wound and then contract to pull the wound closed.

Maturation Phase

Maturation, the final stage of healing, begins about the 21st day and may continue for up to 2 years or more, depending on the depth and extent of the wound. During this phase, the scar tissue is remodeled (reshaped or reconstructed by collagen deposition and lysis and debridement of wound edges). Although the scar tissue continues to gain strength, it remains weaker than the tissue it replaces. Capillaries eventually disappear, leaving an avascular scar (a scar that is white because it lacks a blood supply).

Types of Healing

Tissue may heal by one of three methods, which are characterized by the degree of tissue loss. Primary intention healing occurs in wounds that have minimal tissue loss and edges that are well-approximated (closed). If there are no complications, such as infection, necrosis, or abnormal scar formation, wound healing occurs with minimal granulation tissue and scarring.

Secondary intention healing is seen in wounds with extensive tissue loss and wounds in which the edges cannot be approximated. The wound is left open, and granulation tissue gradually fills in the deficit. Repair time is longer, tissue replacement and scarring are greater, and the susceptibility to infection is increased because of the lack of an epidermal barrier to microorganisms.

Tertiary intention healing, also known as delayed or secondary closure, is indicated when primary closure of a wound is undesirable. Conditions in which healing by tertiary intention may occur include poor circulation or infection. Suturing of the wound is delayed until the problems resolve and more favorable conditions exist for wound healing.

Kinds of Wound Drainage

Chemical mediators released during the inflammatory response cause vascular changes and exudation of fluid and cells from blood vessels into tissues. Exudates may vary in composition, but all have similar functions. These functions include the following:

- Dilution of toxins produced by bacteria and dying cells
- Transport of leukocytes and plasma proteins, including antibodies, to the site
- Transport of bacterial toxins, dead cells, debris, and other products of inflammation away from the site

The nature and amount of exudate vary depending on the tissue involved, the intensity and duration of the inflammation, and the presence of microorganisms.

Serous exudate is composed primarily of serum (the clear portion of blood), is watery in appearance, and has a low protein level. This type of exudate is seen with mild inflammation resulting in minimal capillary permeability changes and minimal protein molecule escape (e.g., seen in blister formation after a burn).

Purulent exudate is also called pus. It generally occurs with severe inflammation accompanied by infection. Purulent exudate is thicker than serous exudate because of the presence of leukocytes (particularly neutrophils), liquefied dead tissue debris, and dead and living bacteria. The process of pus formation is called suppuration, and bacteria that produce pus are referred to as pyogenic bacteria. Purulent exudates may vary in color (e.g., yellow, green, brown) depending on the causative organism.

Hemorrhagic exudate has a large component of red blood cells (RBCs) due to capillary damage, which allows RBCs to escape. This type of exudate is usually present with severe inflammation. The color of the exudate (bright red versus dark red) reflects whether the bleeding is fresh or old.

Mixed types of exudates may also be seen, depending on the type of wound. For example, a **serosanguineous exudate** is clear with some blood tinge and is seen with surgical incisions.

Factors Affecting Wound Healing

Wound healing is dependent on multiple influences, both intrinsic and extrinsic. Wounds may fail to heal or may require a longer healing period when unfavorable conditions exist. Factors that may negatively influence healing include age, oxygenation, smoking, drug therapy, and diseases such as diabetes. Such factors reduce local blood supply and, therefore, impair wound healing. Nutrition and diet can also affect the healing process.

Hemorrhage

Some bleeding from a wound is normal during and immediately after initial trauma and surgery, but hemostasis usually occurs within a few minutes. Hemorrhage (persistent bleeding) is abnormal and may indicate a slipped surgical suture, a dislodged clot, or erosion of a blood vessel. Swelling in the area around the wound or affected body part and the presence of sanguineous drainage from the surgical drain may indicate internal bleeding. Other evidence of bleeding may include the signs and symptoms seen in hypovolemic shock (decreased blood pressure, rapid thready pulse, increased respiratory rate, diaphoresis, restlessness, and cool clammy skin). A hematoma (localized collection of blood underneath the tissues) may also be seen and appears as a reddish-blue swelling or mass. External hemorrhaging is detected when the surgical dressing becomes saturated with sanguineous drainage. It is also important to assess the linen under the client's wound site because it is possible for the blood to seep out from under the sides of the dressing and pool under the client. The risk for hemorrhage is greatest during the first 24 to 48 hours after surgery.

Infection

Bacterial wound contamination is one of the most common causes of altered wound healing. A wound can become infected with microorganisms preoperatively, intraoperatively, or postoperatively. During the preoperative period, the wound may become exposed to pathogens because of the manner in which the wound was inflicted, such as in traumatic injuries. Nicks or abrasions created during preoperative shaving may also be a source of pathogens. The risk for intraoperative exposure to pathogens increases when the respiratory, gastrointestinal, genitourinary, and oropharyngeal tracts are opened.

If the amount of bacteria in the wound is sufficient or the client's immune defenses are compromised, clinical infection may result and become apparent 2 to 11 days postoperatively. Infection slows healing by prolonging the inflammatory phase of healing, competing for nutrients, and producing chemicals and enzymes that are damaging to the tissues.

Wound Classification

Many different classification systems are used to describe wounds. These systems describe either how the wound was acquired, how clean it is, or which tissue layers are involved. A classification system will assist the nurse in planning wound care management. The following are commonly used classification systems.

Cause of Wound

Intentional wounds occur during treatment or therapy. These wounds are usually made under aseptic conditions. Examples include surgical incisions and venipunctures.

Unintentional wounds are unanticipated and are often the result of trauma or an accident. These wounds are created in an unsterile environment and therefore pose a greater risk of infection.

Cleanliness of Wound

This classification system ranks the wound according to its contamination by bacteria and risk for infection (Schwartz, Shires, & Spencer, 1994).

- *Clean wounds* are intentional wounds that were created under conditions in which no inflammation was encountered and the respiratory, alimentary, genitourinary, and oropharyngeal tracts were not entered.
- *Clean-contaminated wounds* are intentional wounds that were created by entry into the alimentary, respiratory, genitourinary, or oropharyngeal tract under controlled conditions.
- *Contaminated wounds* are open, traumatic wounds or intentional wounds in which there was a major break in aseptic technique, spillage from the gastrointestinal tract, or incision into infected urinary or biliary tracts. These wounds have acute nonpurulent inflammation present.
- *Dirty and infected wounds* are traumatic wounds with retained dead tissue or foreign material or intentional wounds created in situations where purulent drainage was present.

Depth of Wound

The third classification system is based on the depth of the wound, taking into account the skin layers involved.

- *Superficial wounds* are confined to the epidermis layer, which comprises the four outermost layers of skin.
- *Partial-thickness wounds* involve the epidermis and part of the dermis, which is the layer of skin beneath the epidermis.
- *Full-thickness wounds* involve the entire epidermis and dermis. Deeper structures such as fascia, muscle, and bone may be involved.

Assessment

Nurses are confronted with wounds that are extremely diverse. The wound may have occurred traumatically just before the client presents to the emergency room, or the wound may be a slow-healing chronic ulcer. Despite all this diversity, the nurse should approach assessment of the wound in a systematic manner, evaluating the wound's stage in the healing process. The nurse also needs to show sensitivity to the client's pain and tolerance levels during assessment and must always follow Standard Precautions to prevent transfer of pathogens. Following are some basic criteria for wound assessment.

Location

Assessment begins with a description of the anatomical location of the wound, for example, "5-inch suture line on the right lower quadrant of the abdomen." This task often becomes difficult if the client has multiple wounds close to each other, as is common in burn or multiple trauma victims. Use of a skin documentation form that incorporates drawings of the body (Figure 40-8) allows the nurse to draw circles and write numbers to depict the location of the various wounds.

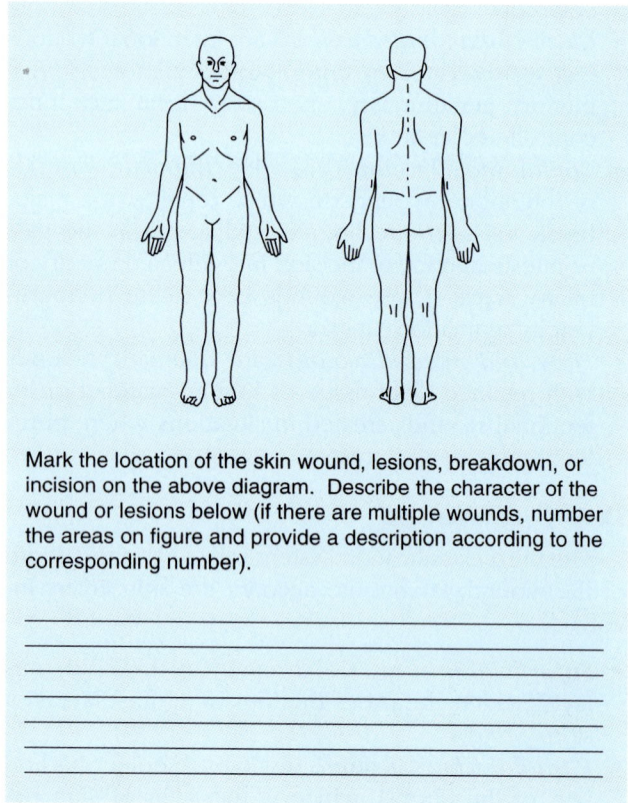

Mark the location of the skin wound, lesions, breakdown, or incision on the above diagram. Describe the character of the wound or lesions below (if there are multiple wounds, number the areas on figure and provide a description according to the corresponding number).

Figure 40-8 Documenting Location and Character of Wounds *(From* Fundamentals of Nursing: Standards & Practice, *by S. DeLaune and P. Ladner, 1998, Albany, NY: Delmar Publishers. Copyright 1998 by Delmar Publishers. Reprinted with permission.)*

Size

The length (head to toe), width (side to side), and depth of a wound are measured in centimeters. Single-use measurement guides (tape measures) often come with dressing supplies. To determine the depth of a wound, a sterile cotton swab is inserted into the deepest point of the wound and marked at the skin surface level. Then the swab can be measured and the wound depth in centimeters documented. Tunneling, also called undermining, can be measured by using a cotton swab to gently probe the wound margins. If tunneling is noted, the location and depth are documented. For clarity in describing the location of the tunneling, the hands of the clock can be used as a guide, with 12 o'clock pointing at the client's head. Example: "Tunneling occurs at 1 o'clock and its depth is 2 cm."

For extremely irregularly shaped wounds, the wound edges can be traced on a plastic surface. A plastic bag or piece of plastic sheeting folded in half is placed on the wound, and the wound margins are traced. The side of the plastic that has been placed against the skin is cut off and discarded. The rest of the plastic can be placed in the chart.

General Appearance and Drainage

A general description of the color of the wound and surrounding area helps to determine the wound's present phase of healing. The edges of the wound should be gently palpated for swelling, and the amount, color, location, odor, and consistency of any drainage documented.

Pain

The nurse should document and notify the physician of any pain or tenderness at the wound site. Pain may indicate infection or bleeding. It is normal to experience pain at the incision site of a surgical wound for approximately 3 days. If there is any sudden increase in pain accompanied by changes in the appearance of the wound, the physician must be notified immediately.

Laboratory Data

Cultures of the wound drainage are used to determine the presence of infection and the identity of the causative organism. The sensitivity results list the antibiotics that will effectively treat the infection. An elevated WBC count is indicative of an infectious process. A decreased leukocyte count may indicate that the client is at increased risk for developing an infection related to decreased defense mechanisms. Albumin is a measure of the client's protein reserves; if the albumin is decreased, the client will have decreased resources of protein for wound healing.

Nursing Diagnoses

Nursing diagnoses for clients with wounds focus on prevention of complications and promotion of the healing process through proper wound care and client teaching. Following are NANDA-approved nursing diagnoses with a partial list of related factors:

- *Tissue Integrity, Impaired related to surgical incision, pressure, shearing forces, decreased blood flow, immobility, mechanical irritants*
- *Infection, Risk for, related to malnutrition, decreased defense mechanisms*
- *Pain related to inflammation, infection*
- *Body Image Disturbance related to changes in body appearance secondary to scars, drains, removal of body parts*
- *Knowledge Deficit (wound care) related to lack of exposure to information, misinterpretation, lack of interest in learning*

Planning/Outcome Identification

After identifying the nursing diagnoses, the nurse establishes targeted outcomes for wound healing based on the client's identified needs and individualized to the client's condition. Changes in the health care delivery system have brought about early discharge from the hospital, so clients are often sent home with wounds that need continued care; the goals for clients with wounds generally focus on promoting wound healing, preventing infection, and educating the client.

Implementation

Nursing interventions to promote wound healing and prevent infection include emergency measures to maintain homeostasis (state of internal constancy of the body), and cleansing and dressing of the wound.

Emergency Measures

The nurse assesses the type and extent of injury that the client has sustained. If hemorrhage is detected, sterile dressings and pressure should be applied to stop the bleeding, and the physician notified immediately. Standard Precautions are always implemented. The client's vital signs should be monitored frequently.

When dehiscence or evisceration occurs, the client should be instructed to remain quiet and to avoid coughing or straining. The client should be positioned to prevent further stress on the wound. Sterile dressings, such as ABD pads soaked with sterile normal saline, should be used to cover the wound and internal contents. This will reduce the risk of bacterial contamination and drying of the viscera. The surgeon should be notified immediately and the client prepared for surgical repair of the area.

Cleansing the Wound

The goal of cleansing the wound is to remove debris and bacteria from the wound bed with as little trauma to the healthy granulation tissue as possible.

PROFESSIONAL TIP

Wound Cleansing

Following are the major principles to keep in mind when cleansing a wound:

- Use Standard Precautions at all times.
- When using a swab or gauze to cleanse a wound, work from the clean area out toward the dirtier area. For example, when cleaning a surgical incision, start over the incision line, and swab downward from top to bottom. Change the swab and proceed again on either side of the incision, using a new swab each time.
- When irrigating a wound, warm the solution to room temperature, preferably to body temperature, to prevent lowering of the tissue temperature. Be sure to allow the irrigant to flow from the cleanest area to the contaminated area to avoid spreading pathogens.

Choice of cleansing agent depends on the physician's prescription as well as agency protocol. It is recommended that isotonic solutions such as normal saline or lactated Ringer's be used to preserve healthy tissue.

Dressing the Wound

Following are the three purposes of a wound dressing:

1. To keep the wound moist and therefore enhance epithelialization
2. To clean the wound or keep it clean
3. To protect the wound from physical trauma or bacterial invasion

Keeping these three purposes in mind, an appropriate dressing for the client's wound is determined. There are thousands of different wound care products on the market. The physician may prescribe a specific dressing, or agency policy is followed. It is important to remember that the dressing plans must be modified as the wound changes.

Monitoring Drainage of Wounds

During the inflammatory response, exudates develop within a wound. When excessive drainage accumulates in the wound bed, tissue healing is delayed. If the outer surface is allowed to heal while the drainage remains entrapped within the wound, infection and abscess formation may occur. To facilitate drainage of any excess fluid, the physician may insert a tube or drain.

Evaluation

The nurse needs to evaluate the client's achievement of the goals established during the planning phase to achieve or maintain skin integrity. Goals for clients with wounds generally focus on wound healing, prevention of infection, and client education. If the goals are not achieved, the nurse will need to examine the nursing interventions and strategies that were employed and revise the nursing care plan accordingly. Reviewing techniques and procedures, especially those performed by the client or other caregivers in the client's support system, is especially important.

BURNS

Burns are among the most devastating injuries that an individual can suffer. Burns can be painful and disfiguring, requiring long hospitalizations. Many are fatal. Most accidental burns occur in the home and are preventable. Frequently, the burn injury is the result of the individual's own action. Feelings of anger and guilt can complicate recovery. Often the individual suffers self-image disturbances, and family relationships can be strained.

Major Causes

There are many different causes for burns to the skin. A major source of burn injury for all ages is overexposure to the sun. The greatest number of burn injuries to adults are associated with cigarette smoking and cooking. The elderly are more likely to suffer burns by spilling hot liquid on themselves or by catching their clothes on fire as they cook or smoke. Young children are especially prone to burn injuries from spilling scalding liquids on themselves and playing with matches or cigarette lighters. Industrial accidents account for a significant number of burn injuries in young adults.

Severity

Burns are classified according to the depth of the burn and the extent of skin surface involved. First- and second-degree burns are partial-thickness (within the epidermis/dermis) burns. First-degree burns involve only the epidermis. The skin is hot, red, and painful. A sunburn is an example of a first-degree burn. First-degree burns heal in about a week without scarring. Second-degree burns damage the dermis and the epidermis. The skin is red, hot, and painful; blisters form and tissue around the burn is edematous, or swollen, with an excessive amount of fluid. An example of a second-degree burn is spilling boiling water on the skin. Usually, second-degree burns heal in about 2 weeks without scarring. However, if deep layers of the dermis are involved, healing might take months and scarring can occur. Second-degree burns involving deep layers of the dermis may appear white, tan, or red in color.

When the dermis and epidermis are completely destroyed and deeper tissues are involved, burns are classified as full-thickness burns. Third-degree and fourth-degree burns are full-thickness burns. In third-degree burns all dermal structures are destroyed and cannot be regenerated. Subcutaneous tissue is also damaged. Full-thickness burns can be white, tan, brown, black, charred, or bright red in color. Fourth-degree burns, which extend to the underlying muscles and bones, appear white to black or charred with dark networks of thrombosed capillaries visible inside the wound. Fourth-degree burns result from fires, explosions, and nuclear radiation. Figure 40-9 depicts the various layers of skin involved in burn injuries.

Severely burned individuals generally have both partial-thickness and full-thickness burns. While first- and second-degree burns are painful, third- and fourth-degree burns themselves are not painful because of the destruction of sensory nerve endings. The client, however, will still be in severe pain. Body movement causes pain in areas of first- and second-degree burns that often surround the full-thickness burns. Skin can regenerate only from the edges of full-thickness burns. Scarring is inevitable. Skin grafting is necessary to promote healing because the section of skin destroyed by the burn cannot regenerate itself.

Prognosis in burn cases depends upon the severity of the burn, the surface area of the body burned, and the preinjury health status of the individual. If the client's health status before the burn was good, a burn covering 40% of the body will require a minimum of 40 days to heal (Fritsch & Yurko, 1995). Elderly burn victims whose physiologic reserves are already reduced as an effect of aging will have an extended recovery period and a greater risk of complications.

Documenting the extent of the burn injury can be done by using a burn assessment chart such as the Rule-of-Nines method (Ogden, 1998). The Rule-of-Nines method of estimating the body surface area burned is used for adults. The body is divided into areas that are about 9% (or multiples of 9%). The head comprises 9% (4.5% anterior and 4.5% posterior). Each arm is 9% (4.5% anterior and 4.5% posterior). The anterior trunk and posterior trunk are each 18%. Each leg is 18% (9% anterior and 9% posterior). The genitalia comprise the remaining 1% (Figure 40-10).

Complications

Destruction of the skin renders it unable to fulfill its functions. Vast amounts of internal fluids and electrolytes are lost. The ability to maintain body temperature is altered, and the individual is susceptible to serious infections. Initially the complications that are the most life threatening are respiratory failure and massive loss of body fluids.

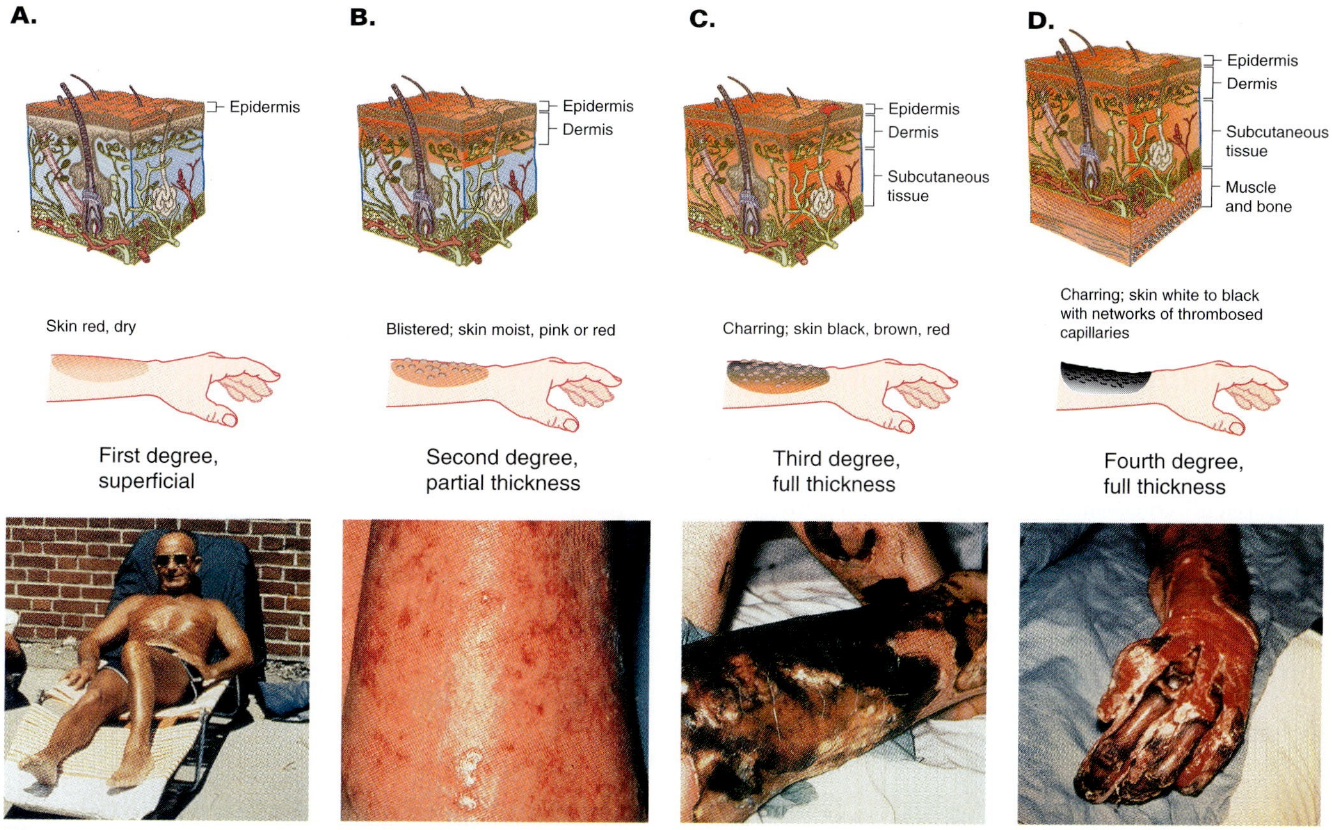

A.

┌ Epidermis

Skin red, dry

First degree,
superficial

B.

┌ Epidermis
└ Dermis

Blistered; skin moist, pink or red

Second degree,
partial thickness

C.

┌ Epidermis
├ Dermis
└ Subcutaneous
  tissue

Charring; skin black, brown, red

Third degree,
full thickness

D.

┌ Epidermis
├ Dermis
├ Subcutaneous
│ tissue
└ Muscle
  and bone

Charring; skin white to black
with networks of thrombosed
capillaries

Fourth degree,
full thickness

Figure 40-9 Skin Layers Involved in Burn Injuries: A. First-degree burn; B. Second-degree burn; C. Third-degree burn; D. Fourth-degree burn (*Photos courtesy of the Phoenix Society for Burn Survivors, Inc.*)

Smoke Inhalation and Carbon Monoxide Poisoning

Heat and smoke can cause serious damage to the respiratory tract. Facial burns, singed nasal hairs, and carbon-tinged sputum are signs that the client may have suffered respiratory tract damage (Ogden, 1998).

Inhaling heat and smoke in a closed-space fire causes airway inflammation and edema of the respiratory mucosa. The carbon monoxide that is inhaled along with the heat and smoke attaches to hemoglobin, forming the compound, carboxyhemoglobin. A high level of carboxyhemoglobin in the blood means that oxygen is not being delivered to vital body tissues. The client may be stuporous because of cerebral anoxia. Keeping an open airway and administering 100% humidified oxygen are essential for treating these two conditions. Intubation is often necessary.

Shock

Severely burned clients may suffer both hypovolemic shock (a life-threatening condition caused by massive loss of blood and circulating fluids) and neurogenic shock (a form of shock that occurs when peripheral vascular dilation occurs causing hypotension). Fluids and electrolytes must be replaced as fast as they are being lost. Tremendous amounts of fluids are lost through the burn wounds themselves as well as into surrounding tissues in the form of edema. The fluid loss shock that results can lead to circulatory collapse and renal shutdown. Using the Rule-of-Nines to assess the extent of the burn can be helpful in guiding fluid replacement. Expect at least two large-bore venous catheters to give large volumes of fluid rapidly.

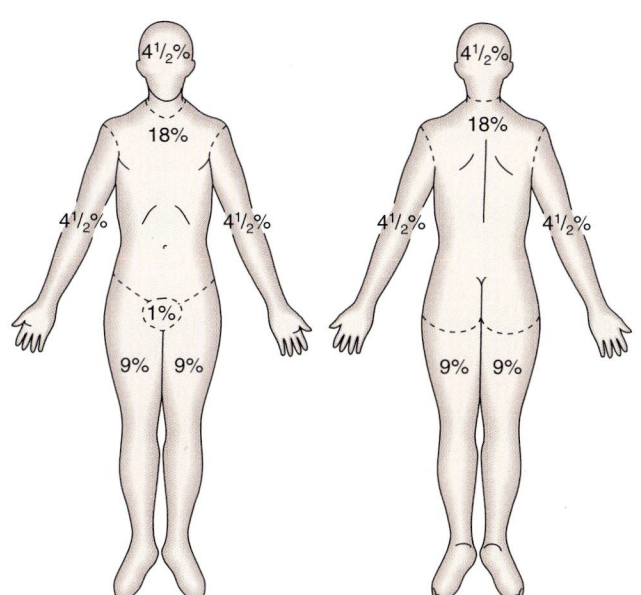

Figure 40-10 Rule-of-Nines

Infection

Once the client has been stabilized, infection poses a serious risk. *Staphylococcus aureus,* an ever-present organism in the environment, is a common cause of infections. Of grave concern is an infection caused by methicillin-resistant *Staphylococcus aureus* (MRSA) because this strain of staphylococcus is resistant to all antibiotics except vancomycin hydrochloride (Vancocin). This antibiotic has serious side effects, especially to the otic nerve and to the liver, and is used only when other antibiotics fail.

All persons coming into contact with the burn client must wear gowns, gloves, masks, and caps to help prevent the introduction of organisms such as *Staphylococcus aureus, Pseudomonas aeruginosa,* or coliform bacilli into burn wounds. Sterile technique is used for wound care and dressing changes. Care of severely burned clients in special burn units reduces the chance of infection because of stringent infection control precautions and a carefully controlled environment.

Medical–Surgical Management

Medical

Immediate Care Initially, medical management of the client involves keeping an open airway, maintaining an adequate level of oxygenation, replacing body fluids and electrolytes, monitoring kidney function, controlling pain, and protecting the burns with sterile dressings to minimize the loss of body temperature and the risk of infection. In cases of severe burns, the client usually requires endotracheal intubation and administration of 100% humidified oxygen. A multiport central venous catheter or two large-bore peripheral venous catheters are needed for fluid and electrolyte replacement. A Foley catheter is used and urine output measured hourly to help monitor kidney function.

Pain can be controlled with small intravenous doses of narcotics. Emotional and psychological trauma can intensify pain perception. The client will be anxious, not only for his survival but also about his physical appearance and the effect this injury will have on his family. Prophylactically the client receives tetanus toxoid.

Stabilized Care Once the client's condition has been stabilized, care focuses on promoting healing, preventing complications, controlling pain, and restoring function. During the recovery phase, preventing infection is an important priority. Burn wounds may require daily cleansing and dressing changes. Because of the nature of the injury, burn wounds contain a large amount of dead tissue along with fluids and proteins, making them highly susceptible to infection even with the best of care. Antibiotics and strict aseptic technique are essential. The dead tissue of full-thickness burns forms a dry, dark leathery **eschar** (a scab of denatured protein) within 48 to 72 hours. Infection

can often begin under the eschar, causing tissue sloughing. Loose eschar must be **debrided** before skin grafting can occur. Debriding, removing dead and damaged tissue or foreign material within the burn wound, can sometimes be done mechanically by hydrotherapy, either by submersion in a whirlpool bath or by placing the client on a spray table and directly spraying the wound with a hose system that controls both the force and the temperature of the solution (Fritsch & Yurko, 1995). Burn wounds may require surgical debridement. The base of the wound must be free of infection and necrotic tissue before it can be covered with skin grafts.

Infection Control: Debridement
Strict aseptic techniques must be followed during burn debridement procedures.

Use of specialty beds such as fluidized or alternating air-filled mattresses minimizes pressure on skin surfaces, thus promoting comfort. Limiting movement and maintaining normal body alignment with the use of splints can also help alleviate client discomfort.

Surgical

Skin grafts cover the burn wound to promote healing. Four types of skin grafts might be used:

1. Autograft—the client's own skin that is removed from an unburned area and applied to the wound
2. Homograft—skin obtained from a cadaver within 6 to 24 hours after death
3. Heterograft—skin obtained from an animal, such as a pig
4. Synthetic skin substitute—a man-made product that has properties similar to skin (Fritsch & Yurko, 1995)

Homografts, heterografts, and synthetic skin substitutes are temporary grafts that facilitate healing. These grafts prevent water, electrolyte, and protein loss. They decrease pain and allow more freedom of movement for the client. When the client's condition is stable and the wound beds have healthy **granulation tissue** (delicate connective tissue consisting of fibroblasts, collagen, and capillaries), permanent closure of the burn wounds is done with autographs. Granulation tissue is red in color and provides a base for healing (Seeley et al., 1995).

Autografts are taken from areas of healthy skin. They may be either split-thickness grafts or full-thickness grafts. Split-thickness grafts include the epidermis and part of the dermis. They are not so deep as to prevent regeneration of skin at the donor site.

Infection Control: Skin Grafts
Follow strict aseptic care of both the donor sites and the newly grafted burn wounds to prevent infection.

The application of pressure dressings during the rehabilitative phase reduces the development of hypertrophic scarring, a condition in which the scar becomes elevated and has a "Swiss cheese" appearance (Beare & Myers, 1998). Pressure dressings, which may be elastic wraps, stockinettes, or custom-made pressure garments, must be worn constantly and are to be removed only for daily hygiene care. Full maturation of the burn scar may take 1 to 2 years. As the physical wounds heal, so do the emotional and psychological wounds. The client's ability to cope with daily stresses and resume social and work activities typically coincides with the physical healing process.

Pharmacological

Dressing changes, wound debridement, as well as any movement or manipulation are extremely painful for clients. Many clients become extremely anxious, fearing pain as well as permanent disfiguration and loss of function. Intravenous narcotics, usually morphine, may be administered 10 to 15 minutes prior to procedures. By decreasing anxiety and fear, daily doses of psychotropic drugs can enhance the effectiveness of pain medications and help the client cope with the prospect of long-term rehabilitation.

Treatment of the burn wound with topical agents can decrease infection and promote healing. Common topical agents used are mafenide acetate (Sulfamylon); silver sulfadiazine (Silvadene); povidone-iodine (Betadine); nitrofurazone (Furacin); and antibiotic agents such as neomycin sulfate (Myciguent), bacitracin (Baciguent), and gentamicin sulfate (Garamycin). Mafenide acetate (Sulfamylon) can penetrate thick eschar and is effective against gram-negative and gram-positive organisms, including *Pseudomonas aeruginosa*. Silver sulfadiazine (Silvadene) is effective against many gram-positive and gram-negative organisms as well as *Candida* organisms. It is painless and somewhat soothing but may cause a skin rash. Povidone-iodine (Betadine) has broad-spectrum microbial action against a wide variety of bacteria, fungi, yeasts, viruses, and protozoa. Application of povidone-iodine to large open areas could lead to elevated serum iodine levels. Nitrofurazone (Furacin) has broad-spectrum activity and is effective against *Staphylococcus aureus*. It is not absorbed systemically and has a low incidence of sensitivity.

Antibiotic ointments are used to decrease infection. Neomycin sulfate (Myciguent) and gentamicin sulfate (Garamycin) can be absorbed systemically and have serious side effects of ototoxicity and nephrotoxicity. Bacitracin (Baciguent) has minimal antimicrobial activity, but it is especially useful to prevent drying of the wound. Topical agents must be applied in a thin layer with a sterile glove. The wound may be left open to air or covered with a gauze dressing, depending on the properties of the medication and the physician's orders. Application of these medications can be painful

PROFESSIONAL TIP

Silver Nitrate Therapy

Silver nitrate therapy, commonly used in the past, is prescribed less often now. Silver nitrate has bacteriostatic effects, lessens pain, and reduces odor, but the dressings must be kept constantly wet. The procedure for dressing changes is involved and painful. Silver nitrate also stains dark purple everything it touches (Fritsch & Yurko, 1995).

because of manipulation of the burned tissue. Administration of pain medication may be necessary before providing wound care. The surrounding skin should be assessed for any allergic rashes.

Diet

Following a moderate to severe burn, the need for calories and protein increases. Actual protein loss occurs with the burn injury itself. Additionally, some protein is metabolized to meet the increased energy requirements brought on by stress. For tissue repair and healing to occur, daily protein needs may increase by 2 to 4 times the normal daily protein requirement (Fritsch & Yurko, 1995). Twice the normal caloric requirement may be needed to meet the body's energy needs. Supplemental vitamins and minerals are also given.

Initially, the client's daily nutritional needs may be met with total parenteral nutrition (TPN) because of a paralytic ileus and gastric dilation. Following a severe burn, decreased enteric circulation leads to slowed or stopped peristalsis. Food and fluids cannot be given orally or by tube feeding until peristalsis is restored. Hearing active bowel sounds is one indication of peristaltic activity in the bowel. Immobility, stress, and the negative nitrogen balance brought on by protein catabolism depress appetite. Meeting the client's nutritional needs can be a challenge. Six to 8 small feedings daily and high-protein milk shakes or protein supplements can help meet daily nutritional needs. Involving the family in bringing in favorite foods can also stimulate the client's appetite.

PROFESSIONAL TIP

Serving Meals

Serve foods attractively and put an occasional small "surprise" on the tray (e.g., a flower, a small, brightly colored seasonal decoration, a funny card) so that the client will look forward to meals.

Activity

Contractures are among the most serious complications of severe burns. They can be prevented with a program of positioning, splinting, exercising, and ambulating. When repositioning, the client's body must be kept in correct alignment. Pillows can be used to keep limbs in alignment. Splints can be used on limbs to prevent contractures or to immobilize joints following skin grafting. Range-of-motion exercises maintain joint mobility. Whenever possible, active rather than passive range-of-motion exercises should be encouraged. Active exercise increases circulation, maintains joint flexibility, and improves muscle tone. As the client recovers, activities of daily living can be increased and ambulation can be initiated.

▶ NURSING PROCESS

▶ Assessment

▶ Subjective Data

Emotional status needs to be assessed. Clients with burns are likely to be frightened and anxious. Feelings of guilt, anger, and depression are also common following burns. Nonverbal behavior such as grimacing should be noted. The client should be asked to describe the pain according to location, intensity, and duration, and also to rate the pain on a scale of 0 to 10. Hypoxia or fluid and electrolyte imbalances can cause confusion, disorientation, and decreased level of consciousness. The client may be nauseated.

▶ Objective Data

Vital signs, level of consciousness, and breath sounds should be assessed. If the client has a productive cough, the amount and color of sputum should be noted. Black/gray sputum indicates smoke inhalation. Clients suffering from smoke inhalation may also have crackles, wheezing, or diminished breath sounds. Burn wounds should be observed for signs of infection such as redness, swelling, purulent drainage, and a foul odor. Urine output must be measured hourly. Intake and output and daily weight must be monitored. Bowel sounds and vomiting should be checked. As rehabilitation progresses, the nurse must continue to assess wounds for signs of healing such as a moist, clean, red wound base and decrease in the size of the wound. The client's mobility status and degree of involvement in care should be noted. Daily dietary intake should be assessed. Laboratory test results need to be monitored:

LIFE CYCLE CONSIDERATIONS

Burn Injuries in the Elderly

- Normal physiologic changes that occur with aging delay recovery and put the older adult at greater risk for complications following a burn injury.
- As a person ages, the physiologic reserves of organ systems decrease.
- While the older person may have adequate pulmonary and cardiac functions at rest, the stress of a severe burn can leave the body unable to cope with demands for increased oxygen and increased cardiac output.
- Renal changes that occur with aging, such as decreased renal blood flow, fewer nephrons, and a decreased glomerular filtration rate, put the older adult at higher risk for kidney failure following a severe burn.
- With loss of subcutaneous tissue and decreased secretion of sebum, the older person's skin is normally more fragile.
- Circulation, especially in the lower extremities, may already be compromised, so healing will be delayed.
- Skin grafting procedures may not be successful because of impaired circulation and impaired tissue nutrition.

- Red blood cell count and hemoglobin level give information about the body's ability to meet oxygen demands of body tissues and organs.
- Creatinine and blood urea nitrogen as well as the specific gravity of the urine give information about kidney function.
- Total protein and albumin levels yield information about the ability to maintain the volume of circulating fluid as well as information about nutritional status.
- White blood cell count indicates the presence of infection and the body's ability to fight it.
- Wound culture and sensitivity data indicate the specific organisms causing infection and the specific antibiotics that are effective against these organisms.
- Electrolytes yield information about the homeostasis of body fluids. Alterations in pH and electrolyte levels affect cell function in every body tissue, particularly vital body organs such as the heart and cerebrum.

Nursing diagnoses for a client with a burn injury may include the following. Initially, the greatest dangers to the client will be:

Nursing Diagnoses	Planning/Goals	Nursing Interventions
▶ *Gas Exchange, Impaired, related to edema and inflammation of the respiratory tract*	The client will achieve a regular respiratory pattern and oxygen saturation level >90%.	Monitor the client's vital signs every 4 hours if stable; otherwise, every 1 to 2 hours.
		Listen to breath sounds, especially noting respiratory pattern and effort.
		If the client is on continuous oximetry, note the oxygen saturation reading each time vital signs are assessed.
		Assess the client's color and level of consciousness.
		Document assessments and keep the physician informed about the client's condition.
		Elevate the head of the bed 30° to facilitate full chest expansion with each breath.
▶ *Fluid Volume Deficit, related to increased capillary permeability with loss of large amounts of fluid through open burn wounds*	The client will maintain electrolytes within normal limits and an hourly urine output >30 mL per hour.	Administer intravenous fluids at the ordered rate.
		Monitor for signs and symptoms of fluid overload such as shortness of breath, crackles auscultated in lung bases, changes in heart rate and/or heart sounds, changes in blood pressure, increased anxiety, or changes in mental status.
		Measure urine output hourly, report outputs below 30 mL to the physician.
		Record intake and output. Involve the client and family in keeping a bedside record of fluid intake.
		Weigh client daily, preferably before breakfast, and in the same type of clothing each day.
		When the client can tolerate oral fluids, set a fluid intake goal for each shift (e.g., 1,200 mL during the day; 800 mL during the evening; 500 mL during the night).
		Explain to the client and family the reasons for a high fluid intake.
		Involve family members in helping the client achieve the fluid maintenance goal.
		Keep fluids available at the bedside, including within dietary restrictions, the client's favorite fluids.
		Monitor for signs and symptoms of electrolyte imbalances such as increased muscle weakness, muscle cramps, cardiac arrhythmias, fatigue, nausea, dizziness.
		Monitor the client's laboratory results.

During the stabilization and recovery period following a burn, the nursing diagnoses may include the following:

Nursing Diagnoses	Planning/Goals	Nursing Interventions
▶ *Infection, Risk for, related to risk factors of tissue destruction and inadequate primary defenses*	The client's burn wounds will exhibit signs of healing without serious or life-threatening infections.	Wear clean gloves when giving client care.
		Wash hands with an antibacterial skin cleanser before and after gloving.
		Wear an isolation gown over your uniform when giving client care.
		Whenever the client's wounds are exposed, wear gown, cap, mask, and sterile gloves.
		Use sterile technique for wound care and dressing changes.
		Monitor wound daily for signs of infection: redness, swelling, purulent drainage, pain.
		Assess for signs of systemic infections.
		Observe for increased pulse and respirations, decreased blood pressure, and fever.
		Observe for any changes in mentation such as disorientation and delirium.
		Note urinary output.
		Assess for hypoactive bowel sounds.

continued

Nursing Diagnoses	Planning/Goals	Nursing Interventions
		Monitor the client's white blood cell count.
		Assist client with personal hygiene, and keep noninjured areas of the body clean.

Other nursing diagnoses common to most burn clients include the following:

Nursing Diagnoses	Planning/Goals	Nursing Interventions
▶ *Pain related to physical injury*	The client will verbalize that pain is controlled at a tolerable level.	Assess for pain every 2 to 4 hours by asking client to rate pain level on a scale of 0 to 10.
		Observe for nonverbal signs of pain such as grimacing or crying.
		Administer pain medications as ordered, especially prior to wound care or exercise and mobilization activities.
		Monitor and document response to medications.
		Implement comfort and diversional measures:
		a. Reposition client; use pillows or foam supports to keep all body parts in good alignment.
		b. Teach client to use progressive relaxation exercises or to use guided imagery.
		c. Encourage the client to use diversionary activities of his choice such as television or music, or place him so that he can see into the hallway.
▶ *Nutrition, Altered, Less Than Body Requirements, related to increased caloric requirements and difficulty ingesting sufficient quantities of food*	The client will ingest sufficient calories daily to meet increased metabolic needs.	If the client is currently on TPN or enteral tube feedings, administer the ordered nutrients at the correct rate and closely monitor the client's reaction.
		When oral intake is tolerated, encourage the client to eat 90% to 100% of daily diet.
		Provide oral hygiene before meals to stimulate salivation and eliminate any bad taste in the client's mouth.
		Give 6 to 8 small feedings daily of the client's favorite foods within dietary restrictions and encourage family members to bring in home-prepared foods and eat with the client.
		When permitted, encourage the client to sit up in a chair for each meal.
		Plan care so that painful procedures are not done immediately before meals. A rest period of 20 to 30 minutes before meals helps the client feel more like eating.
		Determine the time of day when the client feels most like eating and does indeed eat most of the meal, and serve the highest calorie/protein nutrients at that time.
▶ *Physical Mobility, Impaired, related to pain and decreased muscle strength*	The client will participate in daily activity to maintain joint mobility and prevent contractures.	Perform passive ROM exercises 4 times a day by supporting the limb above and below the joint and performing exercises slowly and smoothly.
		As the client is able, instruct him to perform active ROM exercises every 3 to 4 hours.
		Use small pillows and foam supports to keep the client's body in good alignment.
		Turn and reposition the client every 2 hours.
		Use splints as ordered by the physician to keep hands, wrists, feet, and ankles in natural alignment and explain the reason for these activities to the client.
		As healing and rehabilitation progress, encourage progressive ambulation and self-care activities.
		Gradually guide and assist the client to resume activities of daily living (ADL).
		Encourage family members to participate in ADLs and provide positive reinforcement as the client becomes involved in his care.

continued

Nursing Diagnoses	Planning/Goals	Nursing Interventions
▶ *Body Image Disturbance related to change in physical appearance with loss of body tissues or body parts*	The client will state realistic expectations for recovery and participate in rehabilitation.	Provide time for the client to express feelings (fear, anger, frustration, regret, and depression are commonly expressed by clients with burns) and practice active listening.
		Explain the healing process to the client.
		Give the client daily updates on the degree of wound healing and on his progress in rehabilitation.
		Encourage the client to look at the wounds, to show evidence of healing. Stress that wound healing following serious burn injuries proceeds slowly and that complete healing with improved skin appearance may take a year or more.
▶ *Family Processes, Altered, related to the shift in health status of a family member*	The client and family members will verbalize feelings to nurses and each other and will participate in client care.	Involve family members in the client's care and encourage daily visits.
		Encourage family members to express their fears and concerns, especially any feelings of anger, blame, or guilt.
		Guide family members in recognizing and reflecting to the client small, step-by-step progress that is made.
		Maintain an honest, open approach with the client and family but do not give false reassurance.
		Collaborate with counselor, social worker, and chaplain to help the client and family cope with the condition.
		Assist the family to appraise the situation and plan for discharge. What is at stake? What is realistic for the future? What can they expect during the rehabilitation phase? What are their choices? Where can they get help?

Evaluation Each goal must be evaluated to determine how it has been met by the client.

NEOPLASMS: MALIGNANT

Skin cancer is one of the most common malignant neoplasms in the United States and is the most preventable cancer. Basal cell carcinoma, squamous cell carcinoma, and malignant melanoma are the three most common skin cancers; mycosis fungoides is another type of malignancy. Exposure to the sun is the leading cause of skin cancer. Skin damage from sun exposure is cumulative. The ability of skin to tan is not fully developed until the teenage years, meaning that most of the long-term skin damage from sun exposure occurs during childhood (Morton, 1993). By age 20, most adults have already experienced significant skin damage; however, it takes 10 to 20 years before unprotected sunbathing results in skin cancer.

BASAL CELL CARCINOMA

Basal cell carcinoma, the most frequent type of skin cancer, arises from the epidermis. Prolonged sun exposure, poor tanning ability, and previous therapy with x-rays for facial acne are associated with basal cell carcinoma (Figure 40-11).

As the disease develops, it extends into the dermis and may form an open ulcer. Surgical removal cures this type of cancer.

SQUAMOUS CELL CARCINOMA

Squamous cell carcinoma appears as a nodular lesion in the epidermis. It is much less common than basal cell carcinoma. Risk factors include prolonged sun exposure and exposure to gamma radiation and x-rays. The sun-exposed lower lip is a common site for squamous cell carcinoma. Without treatment it can extend into the dermis and ultimately metastasize to other body tissues, causing death (Figure 40-12). The

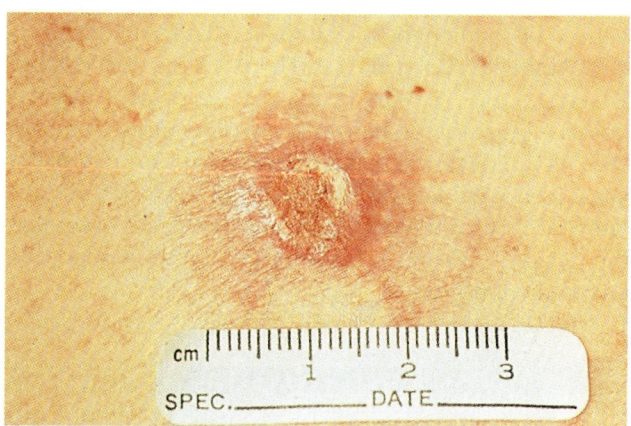

Figure 40-11 Basal Cell Carcinoma *(Courtesy of Robert A. Silverman, MD, Clinical Associate Professor, Department of Pediatrics, Georgetown University)*

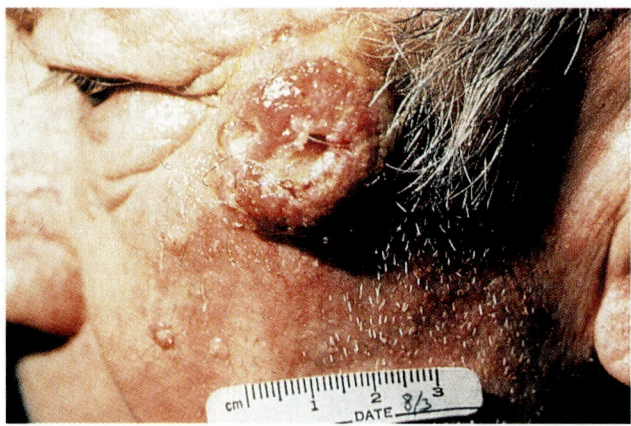

Figure 40-12 Squamous Cell Carcinoma *(Courtesy of Robert A. Silverman, MD, Clinical Associate Professor, Department of Pediatrics, Georgetown University)*

lesion may be excised surgically or it may be treated with chemosurgery, which involves application of a dressing with a fixative paste such as zinc chloride. When the dressing is removed, tumor cells trapped in the dressing are removed also. Dressings are reapplied and removed in this fashion until all malignant tissue has been removed (Weaver, 1995).

MALIGNANT MELANOMA

In malignant melanoma, atypical melanocytes are present in both the dermis and epidermis. Malignant melanoma is the most serious of the three types of skin cancers and may begin in a preexisting mole (nevus). These moles have an irregular shape. Contrasted to normal moles, they are larger than 6 mm in diameter and do not have a uniform color. Malignant melanoma can metastasize to every organ in the body through the bloodstream and lymphatic system.

The incidence of malignant melanoma is increasing in the United States as a result of increased sun exposure. Deters (1996) succinctly summarizes the incidence of malignant melanoma: "The incidence is doubling every 10 years. . . . The peak incidence is between 21 and 45 years of age. . . . At present there is no cure." Clearly the best hope of preventing skin cancer lies in education. Limiting sun exposure and using sunscreen products on exposed skin markedly reduce damage from ultraviolet rays and ultimately decrease the risk of skin cancer. Figure 40-13 shows lentigo malignant melanoma.

MYCOSIS FUNGOIDES

Mycosis fungoides, also known as cutaneous T-cell lymphoma, is a malignant disease involving T-helper cells that have both skin manifestations and multiple organ system manifestations. In the early stages it re-

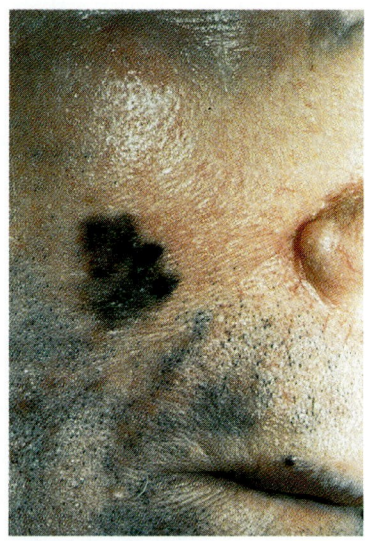

Figure 40-13 Lentigo Malignant Melanoma *(Courtesy of Robert A. Silverman, MD, Clinical Associate Professor, Department of Pediatrics, Georgetown University)*

sembles psoriasis or seborrheic dermatitis. Later, fissures and skin ulcers develop. Pruritus can be severe. Even if the skin condition can be improved with topical steroids and chemotherapeutic agents, the disease is ultimately fatal because of the involvement of vital organ systems (Nicol, 1997). Clients with AIDS can develop mycosis fungoides.

Medical–Surgical Management

Surgical

Electrosurgery, cryosurgery, and surgical excision are the primary methods of treatment for malignant neoplasms. Electrosurgery uses electric current to destroy and remove malignant tissue. It is best used for small lesions 1 to 2 cm in diameter. Cryosurgery destroys tumor tissue by freezing it. A special type of needle apparatus directs liquid nitrogen through the tumor until a temperature of −40° to −60°C is reached at the base of the tumor (Deters, 1996). In addition, regional perfusion chemotherapy can be used to treat malignant melanomas of the extremities. The circulation of the involved extremity is isolated and a high dose of a cytotoxic drug is perfused directly into the tumor area (Deters, 1996). This method of treating just the area of the malignancy minimizes systemic effects of cytotoxic drugs. Because most skin cancers are treated by excision, client teaching and follow-up care focus on proper wound care to promote healing and prevent infection.

Nursing Management

Careful assessment of the client's skin condition can reveal suspicious skin lesions. Clients who have had one skin cancer are likely to have more. Early referral and prompt care can ensure a good prognosis. Clients who have just had skin cancers removed need to be taught good wound care to prevent infection and facilitate healing. Many clients will experience body image disturbance; the nurse will need to help the client cope with this. All other nursing care should be focused on prevention.

NEOPLASMS: NONMALIGNANT

Benign tumors of the skin include a variety of lesions such as skin tags, lipomas, keloids, sebaceous cysts, nevi (moles), and angiomas. In general, they do not require medical or nursing intervention except for cosmetic reasons or unless they are subject to continual irritation that might predispose to a break in skin integrity and infection. **Lipomas** (benign, fatty tumors) or **sebaceous cysts** (distended sebaceous glands filled with sebum) might cause pressure on surrounding nerves or interfere with normal body function. In these instances they would be surgically removed. A **keloid** is abnormal growth of scar tissue that is elevated, rounded, and firm with irregular, clawlike margins. Surgical removal is not always successful; healing following surgery can again result in a keloid. Steroids or radiation have been helpful in some conditions. **Angiomas**, commonly known as birthmarks, are vascular tumors involving skin and subcutaneous tissue. They can be raised, bright red nodular lesions (strawberry birthmarks) or dark red/purple patches (port-wine angiomas). Cosmetics can be used to camouflage them. According to Deters (1996), the argon laser is being used on some angiomas with some success.

INFECTIOUS DISORDERS OF THE SKIN

Given an accessible portal of entry and decreased host resistance, virulent organisms can invade the skin, causing inflammation, infection, itching, and pain. Bacteria, viruses, fungi, or parasites can cause infectious disorders of the skin (Figure 40-14). Treating the client's disease is only one aspect of the treatment plan; preventing the spread of infection is the other. Table 40-4 outlines several disease conditions and identifies the organism responsible, clinical manifestations, and the medical management for each disorder.

▶ NURSING PROCESS

▶ Assessment

▶ Subjective Data

The client should be asked how long the problem has existed, if there is any itching or pain, and what

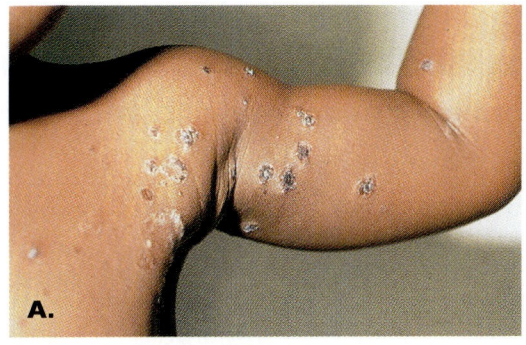
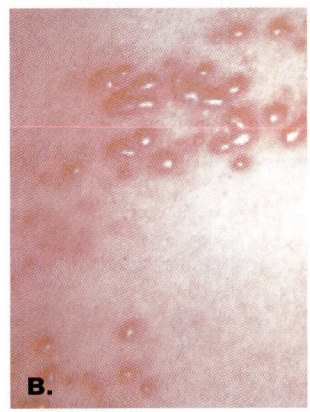
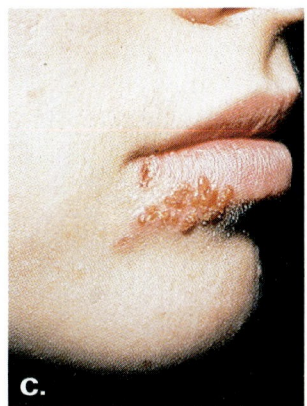
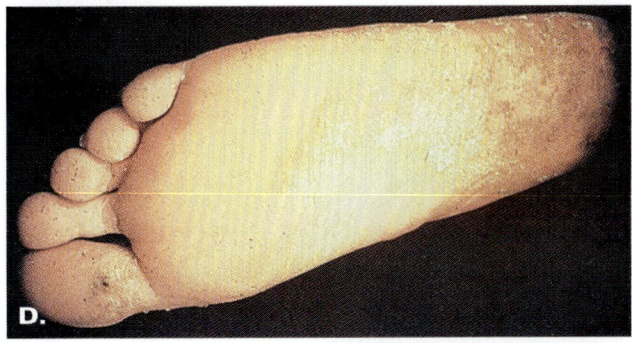
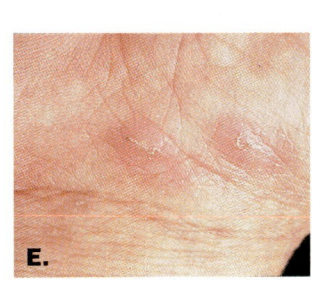
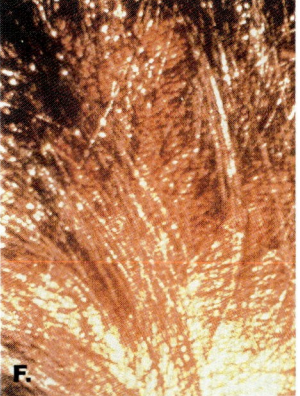

Figure 40-14 Infectious Disorders of the Skin: A. Impetigo contagiosa; B. Herpes zoster (shingles); C. Herpes simplex type 1; D. Tinea (ringworm); E. Scabies; F. Pediculosis (lice) (A, C, and E courtesy of Robert A. Silverman, MD, Clinical Associate Professor, Department of Pediatrics, Georgetown University; B and D courtesy of the Centers for Disease Control and Prevention, Atlanta, GA; F courtesy of Reed and Carnrick Pharmaceuticals)

Table 40-4 INFECTIOUS DISORDERS OF THE SKIN

DISEASE	ORGANISM	CLINICAL MANIFESTATIONS	MEDICAL MANAGEMENT
Bacterial Infections			
Impetigo contagiosa	*Staphylococcus aureus*	Begins as a small vesicle; becomes a weeping lesion; forms a light brown crust. Usually on the face and upper trunk (Figure 40-14A). More common in children. More common in spring and fall. Poor hygiene coupled with warm weather facilitates the spread of the disease.	Cleanse the affected area at least 3 times a day. Apply an antibiotic ointment. Occasionally, systemic antibiotics are needed.
Carbuncle	*Staphylococcus aureus*	Begins as infected hair follicles in the dermis. Symptoms are redness, swelling, pain. Yellow cores of pus develop. Carbuncles usually occur on the nape of the neck and upper back. Obese or malnourished persons with poor hygiene as well as diabetics are most susceptible to carbuncles.	Warm, moist soaks may help "bring the boil to a head." Once the carbuncle ruptures or is incised and drained, pain subsides. Carbuncles tend to recur. The staphylococcus organism may be resistant to topical antibiotics. Systemic antibiotics may be needed.
Viral Infections			
Herpes zoster (shingles)	V-Z (varicella-zoster)	Clusters of small vesicles over the course of a peripheral sensory nerve. Two-thirds of clients have lesions just in the thoracic region. Lesions can occur over the trigeminal nerve, affecting the face, scalp, and eyes (Figure 40-14B). Crusts develop in several days. Symptoms are mild to severe pain, itching, fever, malaise. In older adults, pain can last for months or years. Persons who have not had chickenpox risk contracting the disease if they care for herpes zoster clients with open lesions. Persons who previously had chickenpox, but developed only partial immunity to it, may still be susceptible to herpes zoster.	Acyclovir (Zovirax) is given to clients in severe pain or to immunosuppressed clients. Analgesics help control the pain. Narcotic analgesics are prescribed for severe pain. Antipruritic topical medications decrease the itching.
Herpes simplex, type 1 and 2 (fever blisters, cold sores) Type 2 (genital)	*Herpes simplex virus*	Type 1—a cluster of vesicles on an erythematous base occurring most commonly at the corners of the mouth (Figure 40-14C) or at the edge of the nostrils. Type 2—lesions in the vagina or cervix of a woman or on the penis of a man. The lesions itch, burn, and frequently break open, forming a crust. Healing occurs in about 10 days.	Topical use of antiviral agents such as acyclovir decreases discomfort. Even with treatment cold sores and fever blisters tend to recur, especially with fever, upper respiratory infections, and stress. Oral administration of acyclovir helps to prevent recurrence of genital herpes.
Warts	Human papillomavirus	Seen as small, painless round papules on hands, face, and neck. On the bottom of the feet, warts grow inward from the pressure and are painful (plantar warts). Warts in the anogenital region itch. Genital warts increase the risk of cervical cancer.	No treatment is indicated for painless warts; they tend to disappear eventually. Plantar warts may be removed by cryosurgery or with locally applied chemicals such as nitric acid. Warts are not highly contagious from person to person but may be spread on the person's own body by rubbing or scratching. Genital warts are spread by sexual intercourse.
Fungal Infections			
Tinea (ringworm) Tinea capitis (ringworm of the scalp) Tinea corporis (ringworm of the body) Tinea cruris ("jock itch") Tinea pedis (athlete's foot)	*microscorim audouini*	Tinea is a superficial infection of the skin, called ringworm because of its circumscribed appearance, typically round, and reddened with slight scaling (Figure 40-14D). Lesions of tinea corporis have a pale center. Itching is common with tinea cruris. Itching and burning occur with tinea pedis. Tinea is spread easily. Jock itch and athlete's foot are more common among men than women.	Treat mild infections with a topical antifungal drug such as miconazole nitrate (Micatin) or tolnaftate (Aftate). Severe infections are treated with oral administration of griseofulvin microsize (Grisactin).

continued

Table 40-3 INFECTIOUS DISORDERS OF THE SKIN (*continued*)

DISEASE	ORGANISM	CLINICAL MANIFESTATIONS	MEDICAL MANAGEMENT
Parasitic Infections			
Scabies	*Sarcoptes scabiei* (female itch mite)	The itch mite burrows under the skin, lays eggs, and deposits fecal material. Short, dark-red wavy lines may be seen on hands, wrists, elbows, axillary folds, nipples, waistline, and gluteal folds (Figure 40-14E). Pruritis is severe and can persist for up to 3 months after treatment. Scratching leads to secondary infection. Scabies is spread by prolonged contact and is frequently seen in several members of a family.	Apply the scabicide, lindane (Kwell), topically to the entire body at bedtime so that the medication remains on the skin 8 to 12 hours. Treat all family members even if they do not have symptoms. Wash all underclothing and bed and bath linens in hot water. Change linens daily.
Pediculosis (lice)	*Pediculus capitis* (head lice) *Pediculus corporis* (body lice) *Phthirus Pubis* (pubic lice)	Eggs, or nits, of pediculosis capitis attach themselves firmly to a hair shaft on the head or in a beard (Figure 40-14F). Nits have a gray, pearly appearance. The pubic louse resembles a tiny crab that attaches itself to pubic hair. Body lice live in the seams of clothing. The bite of the louse causes severe pruritis. Scratching leads to secondary infection.	Lindane (Kwell) is applied topically to the hair as a shampoo or to the body as a cream or lotion. Repeat the treatment again in 8 to 10 days. Wash or dry-clean clothing and linens. Disinfect combs and brushes. Vacuum carpets and furniture; then spray with a pediculicide.

treatment has been used. Clients with infectious disorders of the skin may feel shame or embarrassment because of stigmas attached to some of these conditions, so the client's mood should also be noted.

▶ Objective Data

A complete skin assessment is in order, describing the size, appearance, and distribution of any lesions, as well as any drainage present.

CLIENT TEACHING

Herpes Zoster
- Take full course of prescribed medications.
- Use topical measures along with NSAIDs for pain management.
- Avoid persons who have not had chickenpox, especially pregnant women, so they do not get chickenpox.
- When dark crusts form over pustules, the client is no longer contagious.
- In older adults, pain may last for months or years.

Nursing diagnoses for a client with an infectious disorder of the skin may include the following:

Nursing Diagnoses	Planning/Goals	Nursing Interventions
▶ *Skin Integrity, Impaired, related to invasion of skin structures by pathogenic organisms*	The client will regain skin integrity.	Wear gloves when caring for the client with skin lesions.
		Cleanse the skin thoroughly, but gently. In the case of bacterial infections or lesions with secondary infections, use an antibacterial soap.
		Gently remove crusts, scales, and traces of old medication before applying fresh creams or lotions.
		Administer prescribed medications; apply creams and lotions; then monitor their effectiveness.
		Explain what you are doing and why.
▶ *Pain, related to itching, burning, and infection*	The client will report less pain.	Instruct the client to keep the environmental temperature cool because warmth increases itching.
		Cleanse skin lesions with tepid water, not hot.
		Stress the importance of not scratching the lesions.

continued

Nursing Diagnoses	Planning/Goals	Nursing Interventions
▶ *Body Image Disturbance, related to unsightly skin lesions and embarrassment*	The client will verbalize a positive body image.	Encourage the client to ask questions and to talk about feelings.
		Provide positive reinforcement as the client learns to care for the skin lesions.
		When possible, suggest ways to camouflage the lesions or minimize their appearance.
		When there is no danger of spreading the infection, encourage the client to participate in social and work activities.

Evaluation Each goal must be evaluated to determine how it has been met by the client.

SAMPLE NURSING CARE PLAN

THE CLIENT WITH SCABIES

Emma Evans, 68, has had a skin rash for the past 2 weeks. The dark red lesions occur mainly on her hands, wrists, and elbows, around her nipples, at her waistline, and in her gluteal folds. The itching has become increasingly intense. She states that she has been scratching the lesions, sometimes until they are open and bleeding. Upon examination, some of the lesions are open with small amounts of serosanguineous drainage. Other lesions are scabbed. She lives with her daughter and 2 teenaged granddaughters. Because the lesions were getting steadily worse, her daughter finally convinced her to seek medical attention. She was horrified when the doctor told her that she had scabies. She had always associated "the itch" with "dirty people who didn't take care of themselves."

Nursing Diagnosis 1 *Skin Integrity, Impaired, related to scratching scabies lesions as evidenced by open lesions draining serosanguineous fluid, scabbed lesions, and client statements of scratching the lesions until they bleed*

PLANNING/GOALS	NURSING INTERVENTIONS	RATIONALE	EVALUATION
Mrs. Evans will follow the prescribed treatment protocol to promote healing of skin lesions and regain skin integrity.	Instruct Mrs. Evans to cleanse lesions carefully using an antibacterial soap and tepid water. Depending upon the condition of the lesions and the severity of the itching, the lesions will need to be cleaned 1 to 3 times daily.	Maintaining cleanliness of the skin reduces the number of microorganisms present and decreases the risk of infection. Tepid water does not intensify itching as hot water does.	Mrs. Evans's lesions are still red, but none are open and draining. Some lesions are still scabbed. No new open lesions have developed. Mrs. Evans states that the recommended measures "help," but that the itching is still "pretty bad." Goal of promoting healing of skin lesions is being met. Encourage Mrs. Evans to continue outlined protocols. Reassure her that itching will gradually subside as healing progresses.
	Teach Mrs. Evans to apply antipruritic lotions as prescribed by the doctor after cleansing the skin.	Cleansing removes dirt, oils, and microorganisms. Lotion applied to clean skin is more effective. Lotions applied just after bathing help to retain skin moisture.	
	Instruct Mrs. Evans to keep fingernails short with smooth edges.	Short fingernails with smooth edges are less likely to break the skin if	

continued

Teach Mrs. Evans to press itching lesions, and not to scratch them.	the client does scratch the scabies lesions.
	Pressing the skin stimulates nerve endings and can reduce the sensation of itching. Pressing itching skin areas rather than scratching them prevents breaks in the skin, which would be portals of entry for microorganisms.
Explain that itching can persist up to 3 months following treatment with the scabicide and that persistent itching does not mean that treatment to kill the itch mite was ineffective.	Skin reaction to the toxins and secretions of the itch mite can persist for up to 3 months after the itch mites are killed by the scabicide.
Keep room temperature between 68° and 72°F and humidity constant at 30% to 35%.	Itching is intensified in hot, humid environments. Maintaining room humidity at a constant level decreases drying of the skin and increases comfort.

Nursing Diagnosis 2 *Knowledge Deficit (infection control measures), related to lack of familiarity with treatment and prevention protocols as evidenced by client's inability to recognize the skin lesions as infectious and by statements about scabies happening only to people with poor hygiene*

PLANNING/GOALS	NURSING INTERVENTIONS	RATIONALE	EVALUATION
Mrs. Evans will apply the scabicide correctly and state ways to avoid spreading infection to others.	Assess Mrs. Evans' knowledge of scabies, its treatment regimen and infection control measures. Ask specific questions.	Building on knowledge that Mrs. Evans already has provides a frame of reference for the client, which helps her relate new information and integrate it into her behavior.	Mrs. Evans and her family did apply the scabicide as prescribed. The client can describe how scabies are transmitted, but continues to express fear that she will give "this awful thing to somebody." Goal of correctly applying scabicide met. Although Mrs. Evans can state how scabies are transmitted, she still has doubts; hence, the goal of stating ways to avoid spreading the infection to others
	Explain that scabies is transmitted by skin-to-skin contact or by contact with articles freshly contaminated by infected persons and in the United States, infection with scabies affects persons of all social, economic, and age levels.	Teaching that does not "talk down" to the client communicates respect.	
	Stress the importance of following treatment protocol exactly. Review salient	Failure to apply the scabicide as directed and/or failure to leave the lotion	

continued

points such as (1) Shower before applying the scabicide; (2) apply the scabicide to the entire body surface, including skin without scabies lesions; and (3) apply the scabicide at bedtime so that the medication remains on the skin 8 to 12 hours.

Give Mrs. Evans step-by-step written instructions.

Instruct Mrs. Evans to wash hands under warm running water with plenty of soap (preferably an antibacterial soap) for at least 10 seconds after touching lesions and clean carefully under fingernails while washing hands.

Advise to not share washcloths, towels, clothing, pillows, or bed linens with other family members.

Instruct to wash underclothing and bed and bath linens in detergent and hot water and dry outside in sunlight or in a dryer on the hot setting.

Advise to shower daily, use an antibacterial soap, rinse thoroughly, and dry carefully, especially in skin folds and between toes, using a towel and washcloth only once before laundering it.

on the skin for the prescribed length of time will not kill the itch mite.

Giving the client written step-by-step instructions enhances compliance with the treatment regimen.

Thorough handwashing is the single most effective means of preventing the spread of infection. Large numbers of bacteria reside under the fingernails.

Disease-causing microorganisms can be spread to well individuals indirectly when their skin comes into contact with contaminated items.

Soap reduces surface tension. When fat or protein substances that shield organisms are broken down, the organisms are exposed to the killing effects of heat. Prolonged exposure to heat or ultraviolet rays from direct sunlight kills microorganisms.

Regular cleansing reduces the number of microorganisms on the skin. Antibacterial soap further decreases the number of microorganisms on the skin. Moisture in skin folds and between toes encourages the growth of microorganisms. Laundering the towel and washcloth after only one use prevents the indirect transfer of the itch mite.

has only been partially met. Reinforce that even though red skin lesions are still visible, the itch mites were killed by treatment and cannot be transmitted to others even if the client does shake hands, hug, or touch someone else.

continued

Assess lesions daily for signs of healing. Report any signs and symptoms of infection in secondary lesions such as redness, swelling, pain, drainage (describe characteristics of the drainage) to the physician or clinic.	Early recognition of signs of infection increases the probability of effective treatment with fewer complications.
Teach Mrs. Evans and family members the early signs and symptoms of scabies infection, such as any reddened papules with wavy, threadlike lines visible on the skin around the papules and severe itching, especially at night.	Early recognition and treatment of scabies can minimize the severity of the infection.
Instruct them to assess their skin daily.	A daily examination allows treatment to begin as soon as the problem is identified.

Nursing Diagnosis 3 *Body Image Disturbance related to unsightly lesions and embarrassment as evidenced by distribution of lesions on exposed skin areas and client statements of being horrified about the diagnosis and associating scabies with "dirty people"*

PLANNING/GOALS	NURSING INTERVENTIONS	RATIONALE	EVALUATION
Mrs. Evans will assume self-care of lesions and maintain relationships with family and friends.	Encourage Mrs. Evans to express her feelings about herself and her opinions about scabies.	Allowing the client to express feelings and opinions brings them out into the open where they can be dealt with appropriately.	The client has assumed self-care responsibilities. She does interact with her family but emphasizes that she "doesn't want to get too close to them until these things are completely gone." She has refused to go to church, social gatherings, or activities outside of the house.
	Provide information to correct any misconceptions she might have.	If the client has any misconceptions, accurate information can dispel them and lead to an improved self-image.	
	Encourage Mrs. Evans to verbalize the perceptions she has about her family's and friends' feelings about persons with scabies.	If the client perceives that her friends have derogatory opinions of her, she is likely to socially isolate herself from them.	Goal has been partially met in that the client does follow proper procedures when caring for her skin lesions, but goal has not been met in so far as maintaining relationships is concerned. Encourage the
	Be alert to verbal and nonverbal messages.	Nonverbal behavior gives insight into the client's real feelings. Identifying and discussing feelings can lead to behavioral changes.	
	Reassure her that she will not infect friends and fam-	The client will be unlikely to avoid friends or make	*continued*

ily members by going places with them, sitting beside them, or being in the same room with them for prolonged periods.

Share with Mrs. Evans that wearing long-sleeved cotton blouses or dresses will hide most of the visible lesions.

Explain that by using the scabicide, lindane (Kwell), as directed and by following measures to prevent secondary infection of the scabies lesions, she can expect complete healing of the lesions without any visible scars within a few weeks.

disparaging remarks about herself when she realizes that she is not a danger to them.

Covering unsightly skin lesions makes the client less self-conscious and embarrassed. Cotton fabric allows good air circulation. When the skin feels cooler, itching is less intense.

Reassurance that scabies can be cured enhances the client's self-image.

client to talk about her feelings, particularly feelings of embarrassment. Point out to her the evidence that her lesions are healing. Emphasize that symptoms of intense itching, worsening of present skin lesions, and signs of more skin lesions would be present if the itch mites were alive and still spreading. Encourage her to go on at least 1 outing with her family during the coming week. Reevaluate in 1 week.

INFLAMMATORY DISORDERS OF THE SKIN

Included in this category are dermatitis and psoriasis.

DERMATITIS

By definition, dermatitis is an inflammatory condition of the skin. In current usage, eczema has almost become synonymous with dermatitis, although eczema tends to be used most often to refer to chronic forms of dermatitis. Other types of this inflammatory disorder include contact dermatitis and exfoliative dermatitis.

ECZEMA

Eczema is an atopic dermatitis often associated with allergic rhinitis and asthma. It is a chronic superficial

LIFE CYCLE CONSIDERATIONS

Skin Integrity in the Elderly
With thinning and drying of the skin secondary to aging, elderly clients are more susceptible to irritants that cause dermatitis. Restoring skin integrity in elderly clients takes longer and requires persistent nursing effort.

inflammation that evolves into pruritic, red, weeping, crusted lesions (Estes, 1998). See Figure 40-15.

CONTACT DERMATITIS

In contact dermatitis the skin reacts to external irritants such as (1) allergens like poison ivy or cosmetics, (2) harsh chemical substances like detergents or insec-

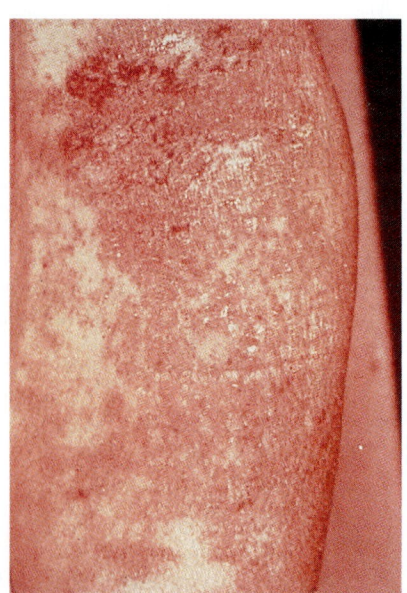
Figure 40-15 Eczema *(Courtesy of the Centers for Disease Control and Prevention, Atlanta, GA)*

Exfoliative Dermatitis

Elderly clients have a greater risk of fatal complications from exfoliative dermatitis. As body systems age, they are less able to respond quickly and effectively to the stress of illness.

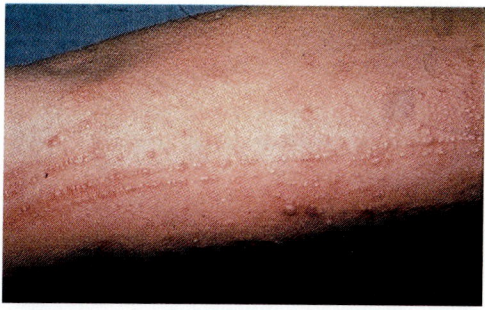

Figure 40-16 Allergic Contact Dermatitis from Poison Oak: Note Linear Pattern to Lesions (*Courtesy of the Centers for Disease Control and Prevention, Atlanta, GA*)

ticides, (3) metals such as nickel, (4) mechanical irritation from wool or glass fibers, and (5) body substances like urine or feces. Symptoms include pruritus, burning, and erythema. Often a maculopapular rash or a combination of papules and vesicles develops. Scratching the lesions may spread the dermatitis as well as lead to secondary infections of the skin (Figure 40-16).

EXFOLIATIVE DERMATITIS

In exfoliative dermatitis, inflammation of the skin gradually worsens. Localized symptoms include erythema, severe pruritus, extensive scaling, and loss of skin surface. Exfoliative dermatitis affects the entire body, not just the skin. Systemic symptoms include chills, fever, and malaise. With the loss of large areas of skin surface, the individual has difficulty maintaining body temperature, loses body fluids and electrolytes, and is susceptible to infection.

In most cases, the cause of exfoliative dermatitis is unknown. Severe reactions to drugs such as penicillin may sometimes cause exfoliative dermatitis. It may also be associated with other types of dermatitis or lymphoma. Exfoliative dermatitis can be fatal, primarily because of overwhelming systemic infections and/or massive loss of body fluids and electrolytes.

Medical–Surgical Management

Medical

Clients with contact dermatitis can be treated as outpatients. Patch testing may identify a specific allergen that is causing the dermatitis. Taking precautions to avoid the allergenic substance may prevent future cases of contact dermatitis. In some cases, application of topical corticosteroids may be all that is needed. When weeping lesions are present, treatment with Burow's solution (1:40 dilution of aluminum acetate) for 20 minutes 4 times a day relieves symptoms and promotes healing (Weaver, 1995).

When clients are hospitalized with exfoliative dermatitis, medical management is directed toward maintaining fluid balance, preventing infection, decreasing inflammation, and promoting comfort. The client requires intravenous fluids to maintain the volume of circulating fluid, corticosteroids to decrease inflamma-

tion, and antibiotics to treat infection. Medicated baths, topical steroids, and mild analgesics may be prescribed to ease the pruritus.

Nursing Management

As with other skin disorders, nursing management is directed toward promoting healing, providing comfort, preventing infection, and fostering a positive attitude to help the client cope with an altered body image. Nursing diagnoses may include *Skin Integrity, Impaired; Infection, Risk for; Pain;* and *Body Image Disturbance.* These clients will need to know how to care for the lesions, how to prevent infection, how to cope with conditions that alter their physical appearance and psychological well-being, and how to keep their physical discomfort at a tolerable level. Client teaching focuses on identifying and avoiding substances that cause dermatitis.

PSORIASIS

Psoriasis, a chronic, inflammatory, noninfectious disease of the skin, affects a fairly large segment of the population, especially young adults. The parts of the body most commonly affected are the scalp, hands, arms, knees, lower back, and genitalia (Weaver, 1995) (Figure 40-17). The exact cause of psoriasis is unknown, although a genetic component may be involved. Emotional stress, infections, trauma, and seasonal and hormonal changes trigger exacerbations of psoriasis. It may improve for a while only to recur. This process of subsiding and recurring continues to occur throughout the client's life. Psoriasis is not curable. In psoriasis the process of keratinization has gone awry. Instead of producing cells that provide a natural barrier against harmful substances and microorganisms, abnormal keratinization causes large, red patches covered with thick silvery scales in the outermost layer of the epidermis (Seeley et al., 1995). If these scales are scraped away, bleeding occurs. When fingernails are affected, pitting and yellow discoloration will be seen.

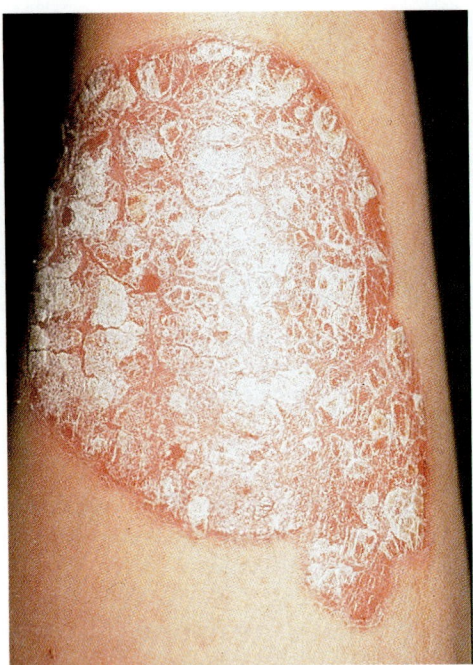

Figure 40-17 Psoriasis *(Courtesy of Robert A. Silverman, MD, Clinical Associate Professor, Department of Pediatrics, Georgetown University)*

Medical–Surgical Management

Medical

Treatment is directed toward slowing down the rate of cell formation in the epidermis or toward altering the abnormal process of keratinization. Treatment regimens can be effective in reducing the scaling and itching; however, the client must recognize that psoriasis can only be controlled, not cured. Further, the client must be committed to lifetime therapy.

Pharmacological

Keratolytic agents such as salicylic acid preparations and coal tar preparations are applied topically to the lesions. Corticosteroids may also be used to reduce inflammation. Ultraviolet light and methotrexate (Mexate) inhibit DNA synthesis in the epidermal cells, thus slowing down the rate of cell division and the process of abnormal keratinization. Because of its toxicity to the liver, methotrexate is used only in severe cases of psoriasis that do not respond to any other form of treatment. The Goeckerman regimen, which combines the use of coal tar and ultraviolet light, is one of the oldest treatments available but is effective and is still widely used (Weaver, 1995).

Photochemotherapy is used for severe psoriasis. Photochemotherapy (psorafen ultraviolet A-range, or PUVA) combines the use of methoxsalen (Oxsoralen) with ultraviolet A light waves. The dose of Oxsoralen is based on body weight and must be taken 2 hours before exposure to ultraviolet A light waves. Oxsoralen is a photosensitizing agent that reacts with ultraviolet A light waves to markedly reduce DNA synthesis, thereby slowing cell division in psoriasis lesions and relieving symptoms. While the treatment is generally effective, the results are not seen immediately (Hill, 1998).

Etretinate (Tegison), a compound related to retinoic acid vitamin A, is used in severe psoriasis not amenable to other therapies. It may be used alone or in combination with ultraviolet A light waves. Etretinate has numerous adverse effects, including liver damage and severe birth defects. The client must be monitored closely. Women of childbearing age must use effective contraception during treatment and for at least 1 month after treatment.

▶ NURSING PROCESS

▶ Assessment

▶ Subjective Data

Psoriasis lesions are generally very visible and likely to make the client feel quite self-conscious as well as very uncomfortable. These clients also tend to suffer self-esteem and body image disturbances, and sometimes depression, because psoriasis requires lifelong treatment. The treatment can be time-consuming, bothersome and, from the client's point of view, not completely effective. The client should be encouraged to verbalize feelings. Itching, burning, and discomfort, as well as the client's mood, should all be assessed.

▶ Objective Data

A careful skin assessment, noting the distribution, size, and appearance of lesions, should be performed. Signs of infection such as redness, swelling, pain, or drainage must be noted.

Nursing diagnoses for a client with psoriasis may include the following:

Nursing Diagnoses	Planning/Goals	Nursing Interventions
▶ *Knowledge Deficit related to psoriasis and its treatment*	The client will discuss condition and adhere to treatment.	Help the client gain an understanding of psoriasis and comply with the treatment regimen.
		Support and encourage the client.
		Explain the purpose of each medication.

continued

Nursing Diagnoses	Planning/Goals	Nursing Interventions
▶ *Infection, Risk for, related to open lesions*	The client will not get an infection.	Teach the client how to prevent infections by proper handwashing and not scratching the lesions.
▶ *Body Image Disturbance related to scaly lesions*	The client will identify positive attributes about self.	Listen actively and encourage the client to express feelings and frustrations. Reinforce positive behavior.
▶ *Self-Esteem Disturbance related to appearance*	The client will demonstrate behaviors that promote self-esteem.	Guide the client in identifying effective coping techniques. Help the client focus on personal attributes that contribute to effective functioning and a positive self-image. Encourage work and social interactions.

Evaluation Each goal must be evaluated to determine how it has been met by the client.

ULCERS

The two most common types of ulcers of the skin are stasis ulcers and pressure ulcers.

STASIS ULCERS

Poor venous circulation, especially in lower extremities, can lead to a condition known as stasis dermatitis (Figure 40-18). The skin changes in texture, turgor, and color. The skin develops a brownish discoloration and a brawny induration, that is, skin in the affected area becomes dry and looks rough; subcutaneous tissue atrophies; and the texture loses its usual resiliency and feels hard to the touch. Body hair is lost in this area of the skin. Pruritus is common. Scratching or small injuries can lead to ulcer formation because of the poor circulation.

Venous stasis ulcers begin as small, tender, inflamed areas above the ankle. Any slight trauma to the area causes an open area that develops into an ulcer. Some edema surrounds the ulcer, which can easily become infected, most often with staphylococcus or streptococcus. Healing is very slow. In an effort to decrease venous congestion and improve circulation, varicose veins, if present, may be removed. Ulcers that do not heal may require surgery. If diagnostic testing reveals adequate circulation, skin grafting will result in the healing of large venous stasis ulcers. In severe cases that do not respond to treatment, the affected leg has to be amputated.

Medical–Surgical Management

Medical

Vacuum-assisted closure (VAC) therapy may be used for chronic open wounds such as stasis ulcers. Applying negative pressure to the wound is painless for the client. The negative pressure stretches or distorts the cells, causing the epithelial cells to multiply rapidly and form granulation tissue. As the vacuum pulls fluid from the surrounding tissues, reducing edema that compressed blood vessels, blood flow to the wound is improved.

A sterile foam sponge is fitted into the wound, the vented end of pliable vacuum tubing is placed on the sponge, and an occlusive adhesive dressing applied over all. The occlusive adhesive dressing keeps the wound moist, prevents bacteria from entering, and

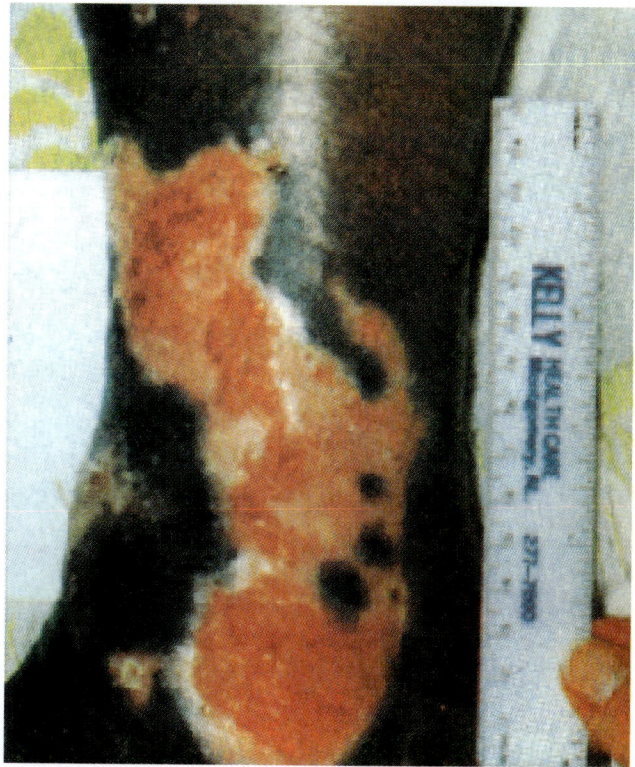

Figure 40-18 Venous Stasis Ulcer *(Courtesy of Carrington Laboratories, Inc., Irving, TX)*

maintains the vacuum pressure. The amount of internal negative pressure and suction (continuous or intermittent) is set on the pump. Dressings are usually changed 3 times a week.

Enzyme preparations such as fibrinolysin and dexsoxyribonucleas (ELASE) or wet-to-dry dressings may be used to debride the ulcer. Normal saline is the solution most often used in wet-to-dry dressings because it is not irritating to healthy tissue.

Pharmacological

For healing to occur, the ulcer must have adequate circulation and be free of infection and necrotic tissue. Usually antibiotics are prescribed. For small ulcers, especially in ambulatory clients, an Unna's boot may be ordered. The "boot" is a special type of gauze impregnated with gelatin, glycerin, and zinc oxide paste that is applied in a spiral fashion around the leg. It hardens around the client's leg, providing even, constant support during ambulation. Unna's boot can achieve a 70% healing rate (Dennison & Black, 1997).

Diet

A diet high in protein and vitamin C is needed for tissue regeneration. If the client is anemic, lean meats, whole grains, and green, leafy vegetables should be encouraged.

▶ NURSING PROCESS

▶ Assessment

▶ Subjective Data

The client should be asked to describe any pain and rate its severity on a scale of 1 to 10. It should be noted whether the pain is worse with the leg in a dependent position or when the client is standing. Measures used to relieve the pain should be documented. If the skin around the ulcer itches, this must be noted. The length of time the client had the ulcer prior to seeking care, and any palliative measures tried, should also be noted.

▶ Objective Data

The size and location of the ulcer must be described, as well as the appearance of the ulcer and surrounding skin. The nurse should observe for necrotic tissue inside the ulcer. It may be yellow and look like thin strands of fibers. The base of the ulcer may have a dark red, "beefy" appearance. The color and appearance of the extremity in both a dependent and an elevated position should be assessed. Any drainage needs to be noted, including its odor and characteristics. Edema may be present, and the lower extremity may appear swollen. Hardened and indurated tissue surrounds the ulcer. Tissue farther away from the ulcer may "pit" with firm pressure. Peripheral pulses must be assessed.

Nursing diagnoses for a client with a stasis ulcer may include the following:

Nursing Diagnoses	Planning/Goals	Nursing Interventions
▶ *Tissue Perfusion, Altered, Peripheral, related to edema and pooling of venous blood*	Client will follow prescribed measures to improve peripheral circulation.	Encourage the client to elevate legs while sitting or when in bed.
		Advise the client to avoid standing for more than a few minutes at a time.
		Advise client to wear elastic stockings when walking and that new stockings should be purchased every few months because continual wear and laundering tend to decrease the elasticity of the stockings. Instruct not to wear garters, tight girdles, or sit with legs crossed.
		Note the client's hemoglobin level since anemic clients will have difficulty meeting tissue demands for oxygen.
▶ *Pain, Chronic, related to exposed sensory nerve endings and edema*	Client will report decreased pain after implementing recommended measures.	Encourage client to elevate legs.
		Cleanse ulcer with prescribed solutions.
		Keep ulcer covered with prescribed medications and dressings.
▶ *Infection, Risk for, related to poorly nourished tissue in and around the ulcer and to nonintact skin*	Client will describe and implement measures to minimize the risk of infection.	Assess the ulcer daily for signs of healing.
		Assess the client's ability to care for the ulcer physically and financially.
		Review diet with the client and instruct in food choices as needed. Encourage foods high in iron such as fortified cereal, lean meats, whole grains, and leafy green vegetables.

Evaluation Each goal must be evaluated to determine how it has been met by the client.

PRESSURE ULCERS

Pressure ulcers, also known as bedsores or decubitus ulcers, are localized areas of tissue necrosis that tend to develop when soft tissue is compressed between a bony prominence and an external surface such as a mattress or chair seat for a prolonged period of time. Pressure ulcers are due to **ischemia**, local and temporary decrease in blood supply, and commonly occur in areas subject to high pressure from body weight on bony prominences.

Physiology of Pressure Ulcers

A pressure ulcer occurs when pressure on the skin is sufficient to cause collapse of blood vessels in the area. Ischemia and redness can occur at the site within 1 hour; when pressure continues for more than 2 hours, necrosis (tissue death) may occur in the involved area. Bony prominences such as the occipital skull, pinna of ears, sacrum, ischial tuberosities, trochanter area of hips, ankles, and heels are the areas most likely to develop a pressure ulcer. By far the most common location is the sacrum (Barczak, Barnett, Childs, & Bosley, 1997).

Other forces acting in conjunction with pressure contribute to pressure ulcer formation. **Shearing** is the force exerted against the skin by movement or repositioning. The skin and subcutaneous tissue tend to adhere to the bed surface and remain stationary while deeper underlying tissues pull away and slide in the direction of movement. This action results in stretching and tearing of blood vessels, reduced blood flow, and necrosis.

Friction is the force of two surfaces moving across one another. When a client moves or is pulled up in bed, rubbing of the skin against the sheets creates friction. Friction can remove the superficial layers of the skin, making it more prone to breakdown.

The reduction of blood flow causes **blanching** (white color) of the skin when pressure is applied. When pressure is relieved, the skin takes on a brighter color (reactive hyperemia) due to vasodilation, the body's normal compensatory response to the absence of blood flow. If this area blanches with fingertip pressure or if the redness disappears within an hour, no tissue damage is anticipated. If, however, the redness persists and no blanching occurs, then tissue damage is present.

Pressure ulcers are staged to classify the degree of tissue damage (Figure 40-19). The National Pressure Ulcer Advisory Panel (NPUAP) (United States Department of Health and Human Services [USDHHS], 1992) recommends the following staging system:

- Stage I: Nonblanchable erythema of intact skin; the heralding lesion of skin ulceration.

- Stage II: Partial-thickness skin loss involving epidermis, dermis, or both. The ulcer is superficial and presents clinically as an abrasion, blister, or shallow crater.
- Stage III: Full-thickness skin loss involving damage or necrosis of subcutaneous tissue that may extend down to, but not through, underlying fascia. The ulcer presents clinically as a deep crater with or without undermining of adjacent tissue.
- Stage IV: Full-thickness skin loss with extensive destruction, tissue necrosis, or damage to muscle, bone, or supporting structures. Undermining and sinus tracts may also be associated with stage IV pressure ulcers.

The National Pressure Ulcer Advisory Panel (1999) has developed an assessment tool, Pressure Ulcer Scale for Healing (PUSH Tool). It uses three parameters: the surface area of the wound, amount of exudate, and type of tissue present in the wound. The scores for each are added together and plotted to show wound healing or worsening. This PUSH Tool is available on the Internet.

Risk Factors for Pressure Ulcers

Pressure ulcers can be prevented if at-risk individuals are identified and the specific factors placing them at risk are reduced or eliminated. More than 1 million clients each year have pressure ulcers, and most of these clients are in their 70s and 80s (National Decubitus Foundation, 1998). Both intrinsic and extrinsic factors may influence tissue response to pressure. Intrinsic factors include impaired immobility, incontinence, nutritional status, and altered level of consciousness. Extrinsic factors include pressure, shearing, friction, and moisture. Any condition that decreases tissue per-

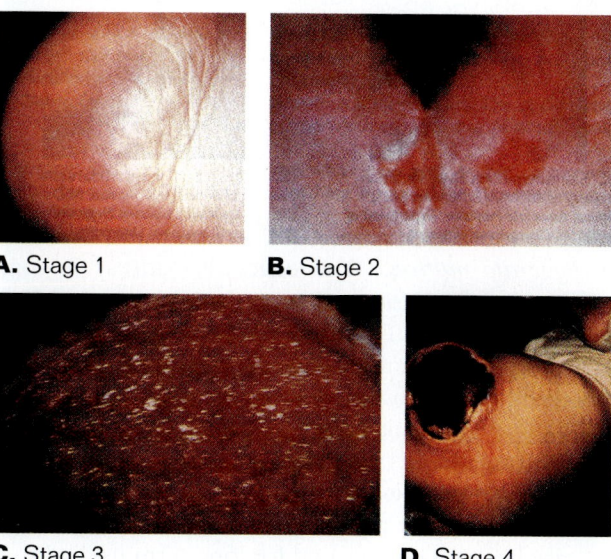

A. Stage 1   **B.** Stage 2

C. Stage 3   **D.** Stage 4

Figure 40-19 Pressure Ulcers *(Courtesy of Emory University Hospital, Atlanta, GA)*

fusion, such as edema, anemia, or atherosclerosis, also increases the risk. Other factors are decreased mental status, diminished sensation, and age-related changes.

Individuals should be assessed for pressure ulcer risk on admission to acute care hospitals, nursing homes, and other health care facilities and at least weekly thereafter.

Medical–Surgical Management

Medical

Sterile technique is followed in the care of all pressure ulcers to prevent secondary infection. The wound should be cleansed with normal saline or a noncytotoxic wound cleaner at each dressing change. Such agents as povodine-iodine, iodophor, sodium hypochlorite, hydrogen peroxide, or acetic acid should not be used because they can damage the cells. A 35 mL syringe with a 19 gauge needle or angiocatheter provides enough pressure to cleanse the wound and enhance wound healing without causing trauma to the tissue.

Debridement must be done as needed. Topical enzyme agents may be applied or a mechanical method of wet-to-dry dressings, or hydrotherapy may be used. Refer to the discussion of VAC therapy in the section on stasis ulcers; this therapy can also be used for pressure ulcers.

There are many commercial products available for treatment and dressing of pressure ulcers. Whichever products the physician prescribes, everyone should be taught how to use them and have a commitment to use them properly.

Support Surfaces and Beds A variety of support surfaces and beds is available to support the entire body and evenly distribute pressure. These devices are used to help reduce pressure and prevent ulcers, but they are no substitute for frequent positioning. There is no scientific evidence that any one support surface works consistently better than any other (USDHHS, 1992).

In addition to pressure reduction or relief, many support surfaces reduce shear and friction and control moisture. Pressure-reducing support surfaces include overlays filled with foam, gel, or water.

- *Eggcrate mattress:* The eggcrate mattress is composed of thick foam with a unique, eggcrate design (Figure 40-20). The purposes of the eggcrate mattress include minimizing pressure and shearing force. The open design of the mattress surface allows air to circulate to dissipate heat and moisture. Eggcrate foam is also used as wheelchair cushions, heel-ankle protectors, wrist restraint cushioning pads, and ulnar protectors. They are used in acute care hospital settings and for long-term use.
- *Air-filled mattresses:* The air-filled mattress is placed over the mattress of the hospital bed. The purpose

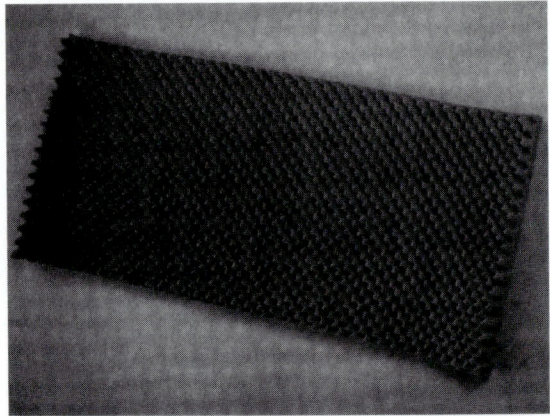
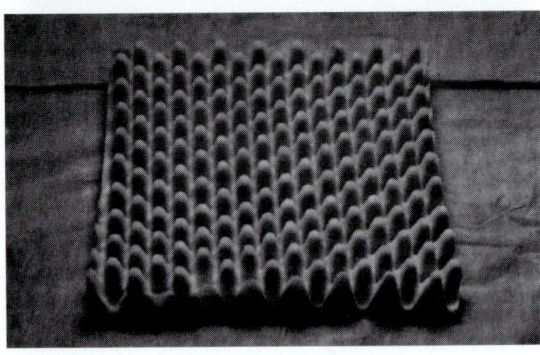

Figure 40-20 Eggcrate Pressure Relief Aids: A. Mattress; B. Wheelchair cushion (*Courtesy of Graham-Field, Inc., Hauppauge, NY*)

of the air-filled mattress is weight redistribution. Varieties of air-filled mattresses include some with a pump and alternating bands of inflation and deflation and some that are inflated continuously with air. Mattresses are covered with a sheet for client comfort. These types of mattresses are frequently used in long-term care situations.

- *Clinitron® bed:* A Clinitron® bed is a specialized bed that has a mattress filled with small glass sand particles. Moisture from urine, stool, or drainage flows through the mattress, preventing moisture exposure to the skin. Because warm air is circulating through the mattress, the accumulation of moisture next to the skin is inhibited. The mattress aids in positioning the client because it is constructed to mold against the client's body. Figure 40-21 shows a Clinitron® bed.
- *Kin Air bed:* A Kin Air bed, another type of specialized bed, has a mattress of air-inflated pillows divided in sections for the head, back, seat, legs, and feet. The pressure can be adjusted in each of the sections for the client's specific needs. Air flows from the mattress to eliminate moisture. The bed frame can be adjusted for various positions such as Fowler's, Trendelenburg, prone, or supine. A trapeze can be connected to the bed frame (Figure 40-22).

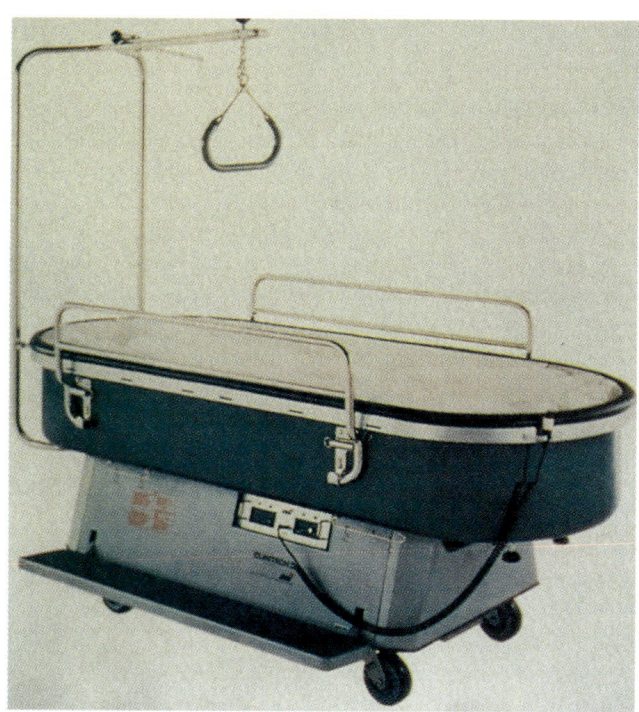

Figure 40-21 Clinitron® Air Fluidized Therapy Unit Model CII *(Courtesy of Support Systems International, Inc., Charleston, SC)*

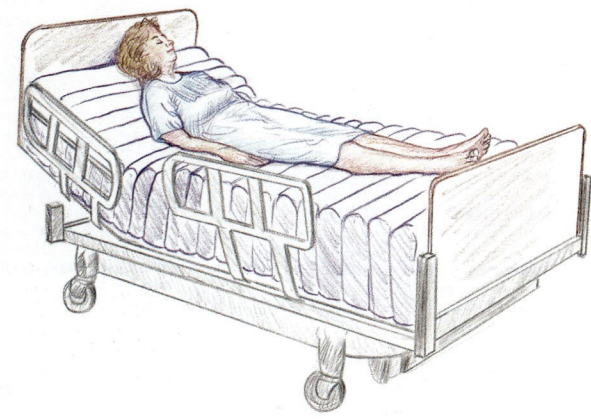

Figure 40-22 Kin Air Bed

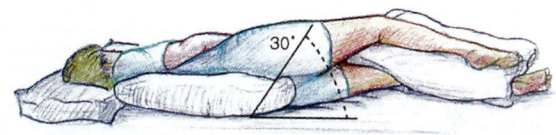

Figure 40-23 Avoiding Pressure Points with the 30° Lateral Position

- *Roto Kinetic bed:* A Roto Kinetic bed is a specialized bed that rocks slowly from side to side, thus relieving pressure areas and countering the effects of immobility. The client is placed on the mattress, with dividers between the legs and dividers between the trunk and arms. Clients can be maintained in traction while on this bed.

Regardless of the type of surface or bed on which the client is lying, the 30° side-lying position prevents pressure on the sacrum and trochanters. This position is illustrated in Figure 40-23.

Surgical

Occasionally, surgical debridement may be necessary.

Pharmacological

Vitamin and mineral supplements may be ordered. Antibiotics may also be ordered.

Diet

Eating a well-balanced diet should be encouraged, including 2 half-cup servings of orange juice or other juice high in vitamin C and 6 ounces of a high-protein drink.

Activity

Active ROM exercises should be performed, if possible. If not, passive ROM exercises should be performed with the client several times a day.

PROFESSIONAL TIP

Preventing Pressure Ulcers
- Establish written repositioning/turning schedule for clients, including those on pressure-reducing support surfaces.
- Use 30° position when side-lying position is used.
- Prevent direct contact between bony prominences by using pillows and foam wedges.
- Use a lifting sheet.
- Encourage clients in wheelchairs to shift their weight every 15 minutes.
- Raise heels off the bed with pillow lengthwise to support legs.
- Use knee gatch when head of bed is elevated.
- Keep head of bed elevated to less than 30° except at mealtimes.
- Limit sitting time to 1 hour at a time whether in bed, chair, or wheelchair.
- Use proper positioning, transferring, and turning techniques.
- Inspect skin at least once a day.
- Use mild cleansing agent, but avoid hot water for bathing.
- Avoid massage over bony prominences.
- Use moisturizer on skin.
- Use protective barrier on skin if client is incontinent.
- Cleanse skin at time of soiling and at routine intervals.

▶ NURSING PROCESS

▶ Assessment

▶ Subjective Data

Statements such as, "I'm tired of lying on my side"; "I wish I could move more"; or "my hips (back, heels, and so on) are sore" may be expressed.

▶ Objective Data

Symptoms may include any of the risk factors already mentioned; shiny, erythematous area; small blisters or erosions or ulcerations. The nurse should check for reddened areas and blanching of those areas.

Nursing diagnoses for a client at risk for pressure ulcers or who has a pressure ulcer may include the following:

Nursing Diagnoses	Planning/Goals	Nursing Interventions
▶ *Skin Integrity, Impaired, Risk for, related to immobility*	The client will maintain skin integrity.	Assess skin 3 times a day for pressure areas.
		Provide daily bath and skin care as needed for incontinence of urine or stool.
		Use mild cleansing agents with warm water.
		Use moisturizing lotion and minimize exposure to cold and low humidity.
		Avoid massage over bony prominences.
		Keep bed linen clean, dry, and free from wrinkles.
		Encourage adequate fluid intake and a well-balanced diet, including 2 half-cup servings of orange juice or other juice high in vitamin C and 6 ounces of a high-protein drink.
		Encourage active ROM exercises or provide passive ROM exercises.
		Turn and reposition client at least every 2 hours. If reddened area does not blanch when you press it, turn the client more often.
		Use the 30° lateral position to avoid pressure on the sacrum and trochanters.
		Use pressure-reducing surfaces. Do not use donut-shaped cushions because they just put pressure around the pressure ulcer.
▶ *Skin Integrity, Impaired, related to pressure ulcer formation*	The client will show healing of pressure ulcer.	Assess skin daily, identifying the stage of pressure ulcer development (size, color, odor, and exudate).
		Continue all preventive nursing interventions.
		Position client on unaffected areas.
		Protect skin surface and affected area as per facility protocol or as ordered.
		Monitor temperature.
		Administer antibiotics as ordered.
▶ *Body Image Disturbance, related to trauma or injury (pressure ulcer)*	The client will make a positive statement about body image.	Encourage client to discuss meaning of pressure ulcer to the client.
		Provide information as requested by client.
▶ *Anxiety related to threat to or change in health status (pressure ulcer)*	The client will discuss concerns about pressure ulcer with caregivers.	Schedule time to be with client, other than care times.
		Provide information as requested by client.
		Encourage client to discuss fears and concerns.

Evaluation Each goal must be evaluated to determine how it has been met by the client.

ALOPECIA

Alopecia, which is partial or complete baldness or loss of hair, can be caused by illness, malnutrition, effects of certain drugs such as those used in cancer therapy, hormonal imbalances, or diseases that affect the scalp.

There are many types of alopecia, ranging from head or beard hair loss to loss of all hair over the entire body. Treatment depends on the cause. Hair transplants may be performed on the head, but this is very expensive. In some clients, minoxidil (Rogaine) can promote hair growth, but hair growth stops when the drug is stopped. This also is very expensive.

CASE STUDY

Maude Murphy, age 68, noticed that the skin on the outside of her left lower leg just above the ankle was changing in color and texture. The skin felt rigid and did not move as easily as skin on the upper part of her leg did. Itching was becoming a problem. Inadvertently she would scratch the area, sometimes causing small excoriations. One day she bumped her leg against the rough edge of the outside steps as she was going into the house. The cut was only an inch long and was not very deep. Over the next few weeks, she noticed that instead of healing, it was getting bigger and was becoming quite painful. The skin around the wound was red and swollen. The yellow drainage coming from the wound had a bad smell. She had never had this kind of problem before. She did have varicose veins in that leg, and while she knew that she was uncomfortable if she was standing for long periods, she did not think the problem was serious. When she went to the doctor, he diagnosed a venous stasis ulcer and cultured the drainage. He ordered the following treatment:

1. *Cefaclor (Ceclor) 500 mg p.o. every 8 hours for 2 weeks (culture of the wound identified Staphylococcus aureus).*
2. *Wet-to-dry dressings with normal saline solution. Change every 8 hours.*
3. *Bed rest with left leg elevated. May have bathroom privileges and be up for meals.*

The doctor explained that he would be ordering an Unna's boot after the wound was debrided and the infection controlled so that she could be ambulatory, but that even after the Unna's boot was applied, he would want her to have rest periods during the day with her leg elevated. Mrs. Murphy thought she could learn to change the dressings, but she expressed doubt that she could stay in bed most of the time. She was used to being up and active and getting her work done each day.

The following questions will guide your development of a nursing care plan for the case study.

1. List the clinical manifestations of a venous stasis ulcer.
2. What is the usual medical treatment?
3. List the subjective and objective assessment data that the nurse should obtain from Maude Murphy.
4. Write 2 to 4 individualized nursing diagnoses to address these problems.
5. What will be the goals (expected outcomes) of nursing treatment?
6. List appropriate nursing actions for each diagnosis. Include basic nursing care measures. Be specific about client education needs. Address nutrition and pharmacologic implications. Give a rationale for each action.
7. Describe how to evaluate goal achievement for Maude Murphy.

SUMMARY

- Maintaining intact skin and mucous membranes to protect internal body structures from harmful substances and from invasion by microorganisms is an important independent nursing responsibility.
- Burns are devastating, traumatic injuries that can often be prevented.
- In general, skin cancers can be prevented by avoiding excessive sun exposure.
- Treatment of benign skin tumors such as nevi, lipomas, keloids, sebaceous cysts, and angiomas depends on the kind of tumor and its location.
- Psoriasis is a chronic skin condition that can be treated, but not cured.

- Skin infections caused by bacteria, viruses, fungi, or parasites can be effectively treated with medications and supportive nursing care.
- Dermatitis, an inflammation of the skin, can be a contact dermatitis or an exfoliative dermatitis.
- Eczema is a term that is often used for chronic forms of dermatitis.
- Venous stasis ulcers are more common in older persons, heal slowly, and often recur following a slight injury.
- Alopecia, or baldness, can be caused by illness, drugs, hormonal imbalances, or heredity.

Review Questions

1. The skin has a vital role in the normal functioning of the human organism. That role is:

   a. production of antibodies.
   b. protection from invasion by microorganisms.
   c. support for internal organs.
   d. regulation of cellular oxygenation.

2. The nurse charted that the client's skin was loose, wrinkled, and thin with mild scaling. The nurse was describing:

   a. integrity.
   b. texture.
   c. turgor and mobility.
   d. vascularity.

3. An effective nursing intervention related to the care of open burn wounds that require daily dressing changes would be:

   a. keep the head of the bed elevated 30° with all four side rails up.
   b. set a fluid intake goal of 2,500 mL/24 hours (1,200 mL during the day; 950 mL during the evening; 350 mL during the night).
   c. wear a cap, gown, mask, and sterile gloves when providing wound care.
   d. weigh daily, preferably before breakfast, and in the same type of clothing each day.

4. The client has lesions on his scalp and on his arms near his elbows. The lesions appear as red patches covered with thick silvery scales. The most likely cause of these lesions is:

   a. herpes zoster (shingles).
   b. pemphigus vulgaris.
   c. psoriasis.
   d. tinea (ringworm).

5. A nursing care plan for a client with an infectious disorder of the skin would include interventions to teach the client:

   a. how to avoid spreading the infection to others.
   b. how to do range-of-motion exercises to maintain joint flexibility.
   c. ways to conserve energy.
   d. which foods are most likely to cause allergic reactions.

6. Which of the following is a malignant tumor?

   a. Angioma
   b. Lipoma
   c. Melanoma
   d. Sebaceous cyst

Critical Thinking Questions

1. How might a person's self-image be affected when the person has a skin disorder on the face or hands?

2. Prepare a teaching plan related to preventing the spread of skin infections.

3. Identify the rationale for each nursing intervention given for the possible nursing diagnoses in this chapter.

 WEB FLASH!

- Search the Internet for information about the disorders discussed in this chapter. What type of information do you find? Will it be helpful to you in client care?
- What type of information do the resources for this chapter have on the Internet? Is it for the client, family, or professional caregivers?

NURSING CARE OF THE CLIENT: NERVOUS SYSTEM

MAKING THE CONNECTION

Refer to the following chapters to increase your understanding of nervous system disorders:

- **Chapter 25, Assessment**
- **Chapter 30, Nursing Care of the Oncology Client**
- **Chapter 32, Nursing Care of the Client: Cardiovascular System**
- **Chapter 37, Nursing Care of the Client: Endocrine System**
- **Chapter 38, Nursing Care of the Client: Musculoskeletal System**

- **Chapter 55, Care of the Older Client**
- **Chapter 56, Rehabilitation, Home Health, Long-Term Care, and Hospice**
- **Procedures:** B9, Performing Passive Range of Motion Exercises; B10, Assisting a Client with Ambulation; B11, Positioning a Client in Bed; B13, Transferring a Client from Bed to Wheelchair; B15, Logrolling a Client with a Turn Sheet

LEARNING OBJECTIVES

Upon completion of this chapter you should be able to:
- *Define key terms.*
- *Identify basic functional areas of the human nervous system.*
- *Perform a neurological screening and a basic neurological examination.*
- *Prepare a client for common neurological diagnostic examinations.*
- *Derive a Glasgow Coma Scale score for a client.*
- *Recognize common symptoms of neurological disorders.*
- *Plan interventions for a client with a neurological disorder.*

INTRODUCTION

The human nervous system is highly complex, controlling and integrating all other body systems. The purpose of the nervous system is to control motor, sensory, and autonomic functions of the body. This is accomplished by coordination and initiation of cellular activity through the transmission of electrical impulses and various hormones.

KEY TERMS

affect
agnosia
anosognosia
aphasia
areflexia
ataxia
aura
automatism
autonomic nervous
  system
bradykinesia
central nervous system
cephalalgia
chorea
dysarthria
dysphagia
emotional lability
encephalitis
fasciculations
functional area
Glasgow Coma Scale
graphesthesia
hemiparesis
hemiplegia

homonymous
  hemianopia
Kernig's sign
meningitis
mentation
neuralgia
neurogenic shock
neurotransmitters
nuchal rigidity
nystagmus
orientation
paraplegia
peripheral nervous
  system
quadriplegia
responsiveness
sclerotic
somatic nervous
  system
spinal shock
status epilepticus
stereognosis
unilateral neglect
vertigo

ANATOMY AND PHYSIOLOGY REVIEW

The nervous system is divided into the **central nervous system**, consisting of the brain and spinal cord; the **peripheral nervous system**, which consists of the cranial nerves and spinal nerves; and the **autonomic nervous system**, which is part of the peripheral nervous system and consists of the sympathetic and parasympathetic systems.

Central Nervous System

The central nervous system (CNS) comprises the brain and the spinal cord (Figure 41-1).

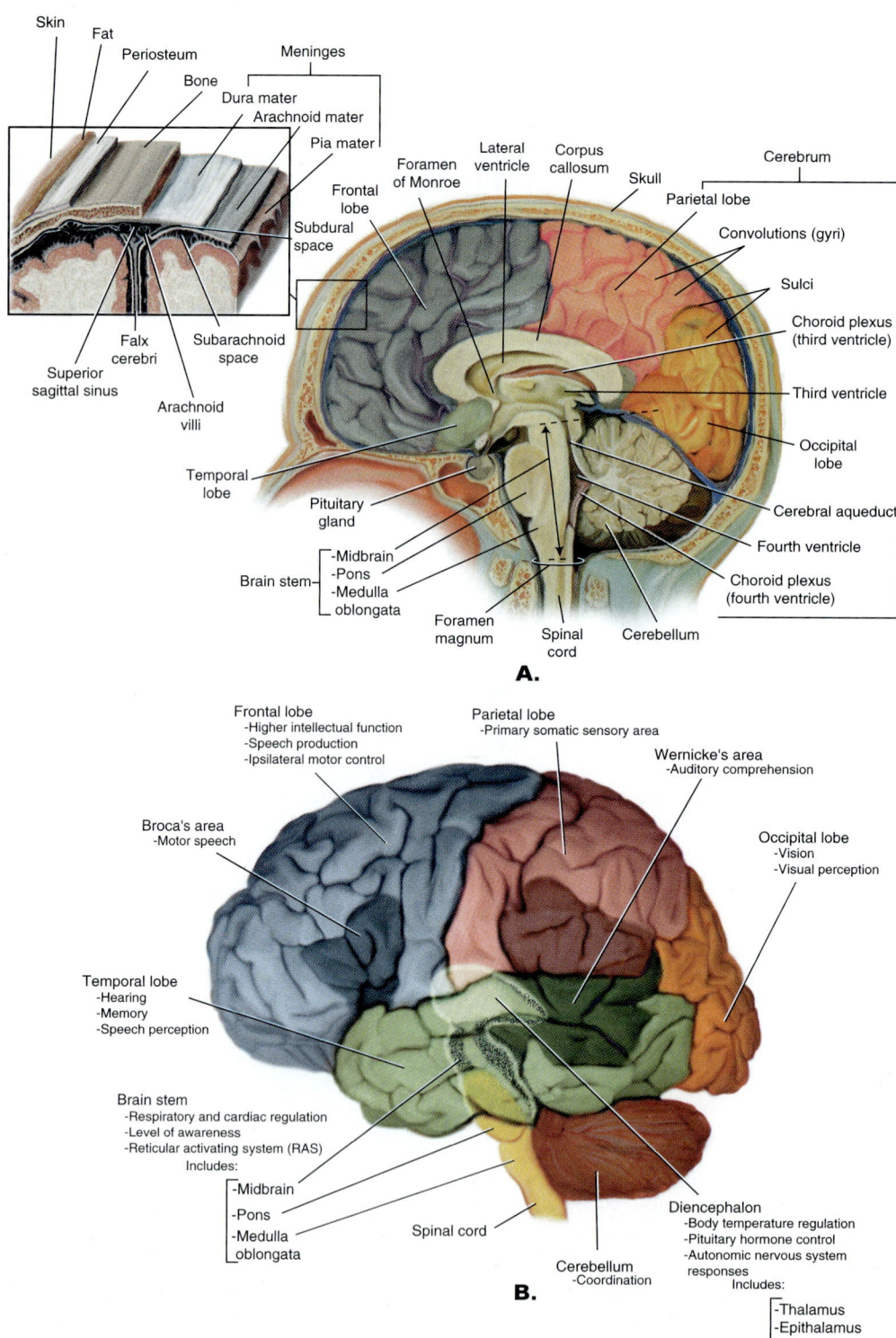

Figure 41-1 The central nervous system includes the brain, spinal cord, and meninges. A. Structures of the brain; B. Functional areas of the brain. (*From* Health Assessment & Physical Examination, *by M. E. Z. Estes, 1998, Albany, NY: Delmar Publishers. Copyright 1998 by Delmar Publishers.)*

The Brain

The brain, composed of gray matter and white matter, controls, initiates, and integrates body functions through the use of electrical impulses and complex molecules. The gray matter, on the outer part of the brain, contains billions of neurons. Neurons, the basic cells of the nervous system, have three major components: the cell body, the axon, and the dendrites (Figure 41-2). The axon carries impulses away from the cell body, and the dendrites carry impulses toward the cell body. The cell body controls the function of the neuron. Functions include the conduction of impulses and the release of neurotransmitters. **Neurotransmitters** are chemical substances that excite, inhibit, or modify the response of another neuron (Hickey, 1997).

The white matter of the inner structures of the brain contains association and projection pathways that transmit nerve impulses to communicate information to the different areas of the brain. These communication pathways are necessary for integration of brain activity (Hickey, 1997).

The brain is contained within the skull, or cranium, which is a bony, rigid box that protects the brain tissue. There are three coverings of the brain, called meninges. They are the dura mater, arachnoid mater, and pia mater. The purpose of these coverings is to provide protection, support, and small amounts of nourishment. The meninges are separated by spaces.

The brain is divided into two hemispheres. The right side of the brain receives information from and controls the left side of the body. The left hemisphere receives information from and controls the right side of the body. Both hemispheres of the brain communicate through nerve fibers in the corpus callosum. A predominate hemisphere exists for special tasks so that confusion does not occur. The right side specializes in the perception of physical environment, art, nonverbal communication, music, and spiritual aspects. The left hemisphere generally specializes in analysis, calculation, problem solving, verbal communication, interpretation, language, reading, and writing.

The Spinal Cord

The spinal cord is a continuation of the brain stem. It exits the skull through the foramen magnum, an opening in the base of the skull. The spinal cord is approximately 45 centimeters, or 18 inches, in length and is the thickness of one finger. The cord is divided into right and left halves and has a shallow groove, called the posterior median sulcus, on the dorsal side and a deep groove, called the anterior median fissure, on the ventral side. The cord tapers to a thin tip, called the conus medullaris, at the first lumbar vertebrae, and terminates as a thin cord of connective tissue, called the filum terminale, which continues as far as the second sacral vertebrae (Figure 41-3). The vertebral column provides vertical support for the cord. The meninges

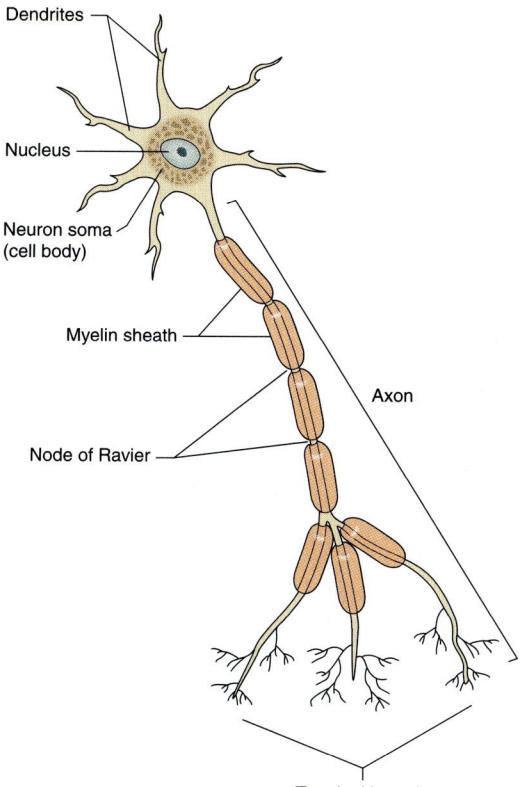

Figure 41-2 Neuron (Nerve Cell) Structure

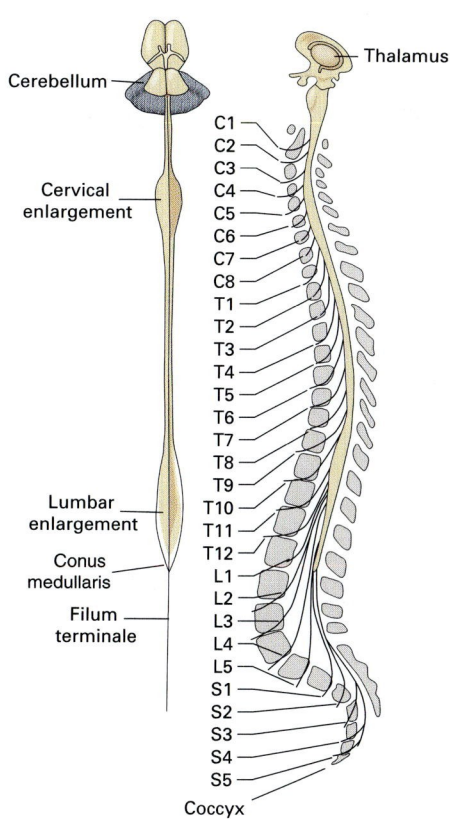

Figure 41-3 The Spinal Cord (*Adapted from* Health Assessment & Physical Examination, *by M. E. Z. Estes, 1998, Albany, NY: Delmar Publishers. Copyright 1998 by Delmar Publishers.*)

cover the spinal cord, providing protection. Reflex activity is initiated within the spinal cord.

There are 31 pairs of spinal nerves originating from the spinal cord. Each pair contains a dorsal, or posterior, nerve root and a ventral, or anterior, nerve root. The dorsal nerve roots carry sensory impulses from the body to the brain; the ventral nerve roots carry motor impulses from the spinal cord to the body. The spinal cord has an **H**-shaped appearance of gray matter within the white matter. The horns forming the **H** shape are referred to as the anterior (ventral) horns, the posterior (dorsal) horns, and the lateral horns. These horns contain the cell bodies of neurons that innervate the skeletal muscles.

Cerebrospinal Fluid

Cerebrospinal fluid (CSF) is produced primarily in the choroid plexus. Five hundred milliliters of CSF are produced daily, with excess being reabsorbed by the arachnoid villi in the subarachnoid space. The circulation of CSF is from the lateral ventricles to the third and fourth ventricles. From there, it enters the subarachnoid space to flow around the spinal cord and the brain.

Cerebrospinal fluid provides for shock absorption and bathes the brain and spinal cord. It contains glucose, protein, urea, and salts. These nutritive substances are delivered to the CNS cells, and the waste and toxic substances are removed.

Peripheral Nervous System

All of the nerve tissue outside of the CNS is part of the peripheral nervous system (PNS). The PNS consists of the cranial nerves and the spinal nerves and has both sensory and motor components. The PNS can be divided into the **somatic nervous system** and the autonomic nervous system. The somatic portion connects the CNS to the skin and skeletal muscles. It is involved in conscious activities such as walking. The autonomic portion connects the CNS to visceral organs such as the heart, stomach, intestines, and various glands. It is involved in unconscious activities, such as breathing.

Cranial Nerves

The twelve pairs of cranial nerves have sensory, motor, or mixed functions. Table 41-1 lists functions and describes assessment of cranial nerves. The cranial nerves originate from the brain or brain stem, with most originating from the brain stem. Although always identified by Roman numerals, the cranial nerves also have names.

Table 41-1 CRANIAL NERVES

CRANIAL NERVE	FUNCTION	ASSESSMENT	EXPECTED FINDINGS
Olfactory (I)	Sensory: smell	Have client identify smells such as coffee or alcohol, with one nostril occluded; repeat for opposite nostril.	Correct identification of smell or ability to choose smell from a list of choices.
Optic (II)	Sensory: vision	Ask client to read printed material, identify number of fingers held in front of client, or read from Snellen eye chart. Test visual fields by having client identify when the examiner's finger enters visual field.	Vision intact or correctable with lenses. Visual field intact.
Oculomotor (III)	Motor: pupil constriction	Cranial nerves III, IV, and VI are tested together. Inspect for ptosis, or drooping of eyelid. Assess extraocular eye muscles by having client follow the examiner's finger to each quadrant of the visual field. Assess for accommodation by asking the client to look at the examiner's finger held 4 to 6 inches from the client's nose, and then to follow the finger to 18 inches from the client's nose. Ask client about double vision.	Pupils are equal and round and react equally to light. No ptosis or double vision. Eyes move smoothly and consensually inward and downward. As the examiner's finger moves away from the client, the pupil will accommodate by dilating; as the finger moves closer; the pupil will normally constrict.
Trochlear (IV)	Motor: upper eyelid elevation, extraocular eye movement	See oculomotor (III).	Eyes should move smoothly and consensually upward and outward without nystagmus or diplopia.
Trigeminal (V)	Sensory: cornea, nose, and oral mucosa Motor: mastication	Test corneal reflex by lightly touching cornea with a small piece of cotton. Check sensation of face by touching lightly with a cotton ball while the client's eyes are closed and asking the client whether sensation is pres-	Corneal reflex as evidenced by rapid blinking when cotton swept across cornea. Feeling cotton ball on face indicates that facial sensation is intact. Jaw movement symmetrical and able to overcome resistance.

continued

Table 41-1 CRANIAL NERVES *continued*

CRANIAL NERVE	FUNCTION	ASSESSMENT	EXPECTED FINDINGS
		ent. Check motor function by having client clench jaws shut while the examiner palpates the contraction of the temporalis and masseter muscles.	
Abducens (VI)	Motor: extraocular eye movement	See oculomotor (III)	Eyes move outward.
Facial (VII)	Motor: facial muscles; Sensory: taste (anterior two-thirds of tongue)	Ask client to smile, show teeth, wrinkle forehead, or whistle. Have client close eyes lightly and keep them closed against the examiner's trying to open them. Have client identify salt and sugar when dabbed on tongue.	Facial movement symmetrical; sense of taste intact.
Acoustic (VIII)	Sensory: hearing, equilibrium	Assess ability to hear ticking watch or whispered voice. Observe gait for swaying. Perform Romberg test (refer to assessment of motor function).	Sense of hearing intact; no swaying or loss of balance.
Glossopharyngeal (IX)	Sensory: sensation to throat and taste (posterior one-third of tongue) Motor: swallowing	Have client identify taste of salt and sugar on back of tongue. Have client say "ah" and assess for symmetrical position of uvula. Test gag reflex by touching back of pharynx with tongue depressor. Observe swallowing ability and speech patterns.	Taste sensation intact; uvula raises symmetrically; gag reflex intact; swallowing and speech intact.
Vagus (X)	Motor and sensory	Test along with glossopharyngeal nerve.	
Spinal accessory (XI)	Motor: movement of uvula, soft palate, sternocleidomastoid muscle, trapezius muscle	Place examiner's hand on side of client's face and ask client to turn head against resistance; have client shrug shoulders against resistance of the examiner's hand.	Ability to move shoulder and head against resistance.
Hypoglossal (XII)	Motor: tongue movement	Ask client to stick out tongue and observe for symmetry, deviation to side; have client push tongue against tongue depressor and move tongue from side to side.	Tongue should be centrally aligned, able to push against resistance of tongue depressor; no **fasciculations** (involuntary twitching of muscle fibers) should be present.

Spinal Nerves

Thirty-one pairs of spinal nerves exit from the spinal cord through the vertebral column (Table 41-2). The dorsal, or posterior, nerve roots carry sensory impulses to the brain. The ventral, or anterior, nerve roots carry motor impulses from the spinal cord and brain to the muscles. Motor and sensory impulses are transmitted from the body and internal organs.

Reflex activity is a stereotypical response to a stimulus that is initiated by the nervous system (Hickey, 1997). The three classifications of reflexes are: muscle stretch, or deep tendon; superficial, or cutaneous; and pathological (see section on assessment of reflexes). Reflex activity requires the function of five areas in the nervous system: the sensory fibers, the neuron relaying the impulse, the association center in the brain, the neuron relaying the motor impulse from the brain to the body, and the specific organ involved. Disease processes at any of these areas can cause an abnormal reflex response.

Autonomic Nervous System

The main function of the autonomic nervous system (ANS) is to maintain internal homeostasis. There are two subdivisions of the ANS: the sympathetic system

Table 41-2 SPINAL NERVES

NERVES	NUMBER OF PAIRS
Cervical	8
Thoracic	12
Lumbar	5
Sacral	5
Coccyx	1

and the parasympathetic system. The sympathetic system, activated by stress, prepares the body for the "fight or flight" response. The activity of the sympathetic system causes increased heart rate, increased blood pressure, vasoconstriction, decreased peristalsis, dilated pupils, increased secretions of epinephrine and sweat, and decreased secretions of digestive juices and saliva (Table 41-3).

The parasympathetic system conserves, restores, and maintains vital body functions (Hickey, 1997), slowing heart rate, increasing gastrointestinal activity, and activating bowel and bladder evacuation.

The sympathetic and parasympathetic systems work antagonistically to regulate the smooth muscles, the heart, and the glands of the body. When one system increases an action, the other system decreases the action. Thus, when one stimulates, the other inhibits; when one dilates, the other one constricts, and so forth. The purpose is to maintain a stable internal environment (Hickey, 1997). Both systems function simultaneously, but one can dominate the other as needed.

NEUROLOGICAL NURSING ASSESSMENT

A complete health history and a neurological screening assessment allow the nurse to identify areas of dysfunction in order to focus the neurological assessment. Observation (inspection) is necessary for the majority of the assessment; palpation, auscultation, and percussion are also used.

Health History

A baseline assessment is essential to ascertaining changes in neurological functioning. Any change from the baseline assessment must be identified and early intervention initiated. A thorough health history includes asking the client about headaches; clumsiness; loss of or change in function of an extremity; seizure activity; numbness or tingling; change in vision; pain; extreme fatigue; personality changes; and mood swings.

Neurological Assessment

The neurological screening involves assessment of level of consciousness and verbal responses to specific questions; selected cranial nerves for eye movement and visual acuity; muscle strength; movement; gait for motor function; and tactile and pain sensation of extremities for sensory screening (Fitzgerald, 1994).

A complete nursing assessment of neurological function includes assessment of the following areas: cerebral function, cranial nerve function, motor function, sensory function, and reflexes. Neurological nursing assessment is discussed in more detail following.

Cerebral Function

Areas of assessment of cerebral function include level of consciousness, mental status, intellectual function, emotional status, pupil reaction, and communication.

Level of Consciousness Level of consciousness is assessed by determining the client's responsiveness and orientation and is the most important indicator of

Table 41-3 SYMPATHETIC AND PARASYMPATHETIC RESPONSES

SYSTEM	SYMPATHETIC RESPONSE	PARASYMPATHETIC RESPONSE
Neurological	Pupils dilated Heightened awareness	Pupils normal size
Cardiovascular	Increased heart rate Increased myocardial contractility Increased blood pressure	Decreased heart rate Decreased myocardial contractility Vasodilation
Respiratory	Increased respiratory rate Increased respiratory depth Bronchial constriction	Bronchial relaxation
Gastrointestinal	Decreased gastric motility Decreased gastric secretions Increased glycogenolysis Decreased insulin production Sphincter contraction	Increased gastric motility Increased gastric secretions Sphincter dilatation
Genitourinary	Decreased urine output Decreased renal blood flow	Normal urine output

LIFE CYCLE CONSIDERATIONS

Neurological Changes with Aging

Remember the following with regard to the elderly client:

- Nerve impulse transmission slows.
- Cardiovascular system changes that lead to a decreased oxygen supply to the brain affect mental acuity, sensory interpretation, and motor ability.
- The amount of neurotransmitters produced diminishes, and the enzyme activity that degrades neurotransmitters increases.
- Changes in neurotransmitters affect sleep, temperature control, and mood.
- The brain tends to atrophy, leaving the cortical bridging veins, which connect the brain to the meninges, vulnerable to trauma and bleeding.

Table 41-4 LEVELS OF CONSCIOUSNESS

Alert	Oriented, opens eyes spontaneously, responds appropriately.
Lethargic	Sleepy; slow to respond, but responds appropriately; oriented; opens eyes in response to verbal stimuli.
Stuporous	Aroused only in response to painful stimuli; never fully awake; conversation, if present, is confused or unclear; opens eyes to painful stimuli.
Semicomatose	May move in response to painful stimuli; does not converse; protective blink, swallowing, and pupil reflexes are present.
Comatose	Unresponsive except to severe pain; protective reflexes are absent; pupils are fixed; no voluntary movement.

change in neurological status. **Responsiveness** is the person's ability to perceive environmental stimuli and body reactions and then respond with thought and action. The client's responsiveness state can be described in terms of consciousness, such as alert, lethargic, stuporous, semicomatose, or comatose (see Table 41-4).

A more objective assessment is made using the **Glasgow Coma Scale**, an objective tool for assessing consciousness in clients, most frequently in clients with head injuries. With the Glasgow Coma Scale, eye opening, verbal response, and motor response are scored using measurable criteria (Table 41-5). The scores are then totalled to indicate severity of coma. A score of 15 indicates a fully oriented person. A score of 3 is the lowest possible score and is indicative of deep coma. A score of 7 or less is considered a state of coma.

Changes in the Glasgow Coma Scale indicate changes in client condition. To prevent further damage to the brain in instances of decreasing scores, the nurse must act quickly. The physician must be notified immediately and measures must be taken to decrease intracranial pressure (see section on increased intracranial pressure).

Orientation is the person's awareness of self in relation to person, place, and time. In some instances, awareness of situation is also a necessary measure. Using open-ended communication techniques, the nurse will instruct the client to "tell me who you are," "tell me what day of the week it is," "tell me where you are," and so on in order to ascertain the client's level of orientation.

Mental Status Assessment of mental status requires observation of the client's appearance, behavior, posture, mood, gestures, movements, and facial expressions. The nurse compares these behaviors to expected behaviors based on the client's age, health status, educational level, and social position. Mood is assessed by observation and asking the client about moods and feelings.

Intellectual Function Intellectual function is the ability of the brain to perform thought processes. Ability

Table 41-5 GLASGOW COMA SCALE

BEHAVIOR	RESPONSE	SCORE
Eye opening response	Spontaneous	4
	To verbal command	3
	To pain	2
	No response	1
Best verbal response	Oriented, conversing	5
	Disoriented, conversing	4
	Use of inappropriate words	3
	Incomprehensible sounds	2
	No response	1
Best motor response	Obeys verbal commands	6
	Moves to localized pain	5
	Flexion withdrawal to pain	4
	Abnormal posturing— decorticate	3
	Abnormal posturing— decerebrate	2
	No response	1
Total		3 to 15

to concentrate, memory function (both long-term and short-term), recall, calculation activities, and abstract reasoning are all aspects of intellectual function.

Nursing assessment of intellectual function involves asking individuals to perform certain tasks, such as the following:

- Repeating a series of numbers, such as 1, 3, 7, 1
- Telling what the individual ate for breakfast
- Adding a couple of numbers, for example, 2 + 6
- Explaining a proverb such as "the early bird gets the worm"

The nurse will determine the client's ability to process thoughts by evaluating the responses to questions such as these. For purposes of comparison, the client's ability to perform these tasks prior to assessment should be ascertained by asking the family. For example, if the client was math illiterate prior to the nursing assessment, the client will still not be able to add or subtract.

Emotional Status Emotional status is assessed by observation of the client's **affect** (emotional response or mood). Is affect appropriate for the situation? Is affect labile (prone to rapid change)? Is affect consistent with verbal communication?

Pupil Reaction Size, equality, and roundness of pupils are assessed (Figure 41-4). Size is measured in millimeters. Pupils are evaluated for symmetry of size and for reaction to light. The nurse should briefly shine a penlight into the client's eye by passing the light from the outer edge of the eye toward the center of the eye (Figure 41-5). Reaction is assessed as being brisk, sluggish, or nonreactive; consensual reaction (the opposite pupil responding at the same time) is also noted. Accommodation is assessed as described in Table 41-1.

The abbreviation PERRLA is used for documenting pupils that are equal, round, and reactive to light and that demonstrate accommodation. This abbreviation can be used only when pupil reaction is normal. If any part of the assessment is abnormal in one or both eyes, the assessment findings must be written out for clarity.

Communication Both written and oral communication are assessed. Various specialized areas of the

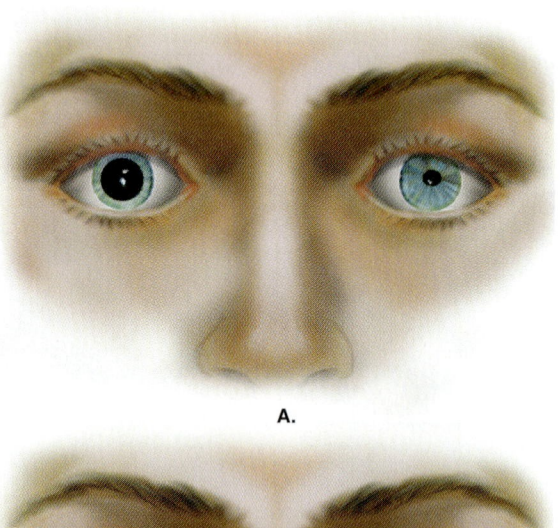

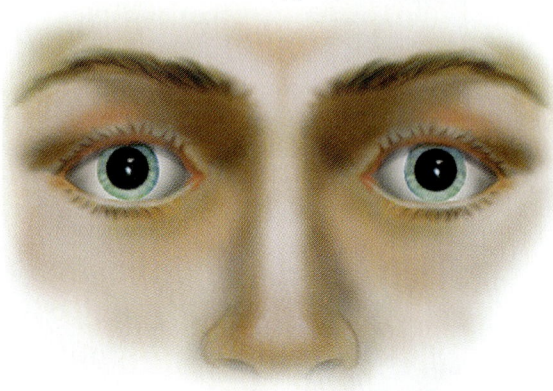

B.

Figure 41-4 A. Unequal pupils; B. Dilated, fixed pupils

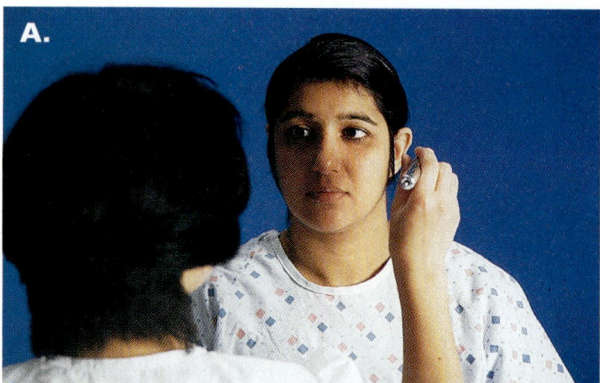

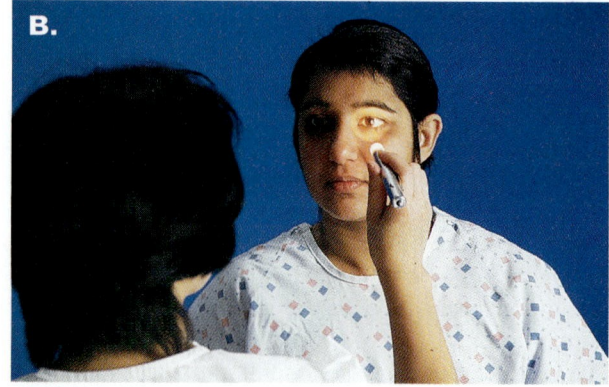

Figure 41-5 Pupil Assessment: A. Starting position, with penlight to side of pupil; B. Moving penlight directly in front of pupil

Table 41-6 MUSCLE STRENGTH	
SCORE	**DEFINITION**
5/5	Full power of contraction
4/5	Fair or moderate power of contraction
3/5	Just able to overcome force of gravity
2/5	Can move, but cannot overcome power of gravity
1/5	Minimal contractile power
0/5	No movement

nervous system are involved in communication. The inability to communicate, termed **aphasia**, can be caused by the inability to form words or the inability to understand written or spoken words. To assess communication function, various approaches are necessary. The client is asked to follow a simple command such as "Close your eyes." A written card instructing the client to complete a simple task such as "Touch your nose" should also be used. The ability to form words; appropriate use of words; speech patterns, clarity, rate, and flow; and voice modulation are all noted. The client's ability for verbal and written expression of self is noted during the health history by asking the client about expectations of health care. The ability to write is evaluated by having the client write his name and address on paper.

Cranial Nerve Function

Cranial nerve function essentially reflects brain stem activity. A complete cranial nerve examination, if required, is usually performed by the physician or advanced practice nurse.

Motor Function

The neurological screening includes assessment of muscle strength, arm and leg movement, and gait (Fitzgerald, 1994). A complete motor function assessment is performed if a deficit is identified. A complete motor function assessment includes evaluating muscle size, symmetry, tone, and strength; coordination; balance; and posturing.

Muscle Size and Symmetry Muscle size and symmetry are assessed by palpating major muscle groups of the arms and legs and then comparing them to the muscle groups of the opposite side of the body. Unilateral atrophy may indicate a nervous system problem.

Muscle Tone Muscle tone is assessed during palpation of major muscle groups for size and symmetry, while at rest and during passive movement. Muscle tone is described as normal, flaccid, spastic, or rigid. Flaccid muscles are hypotonic, or soft and flabby. Spastic muscles are at first resistant to passive movement, but then release resistance. Rigid muscles may have tremors but are constantly rigid. Rigidity is a more constant state of spasticity, with fewer periods of release of resistance.

Muscle Strength To assess muscle strength, each extremity is placed through passive movement. The client is then asked to move the extremity, first against gravity, by lifting the extremity off the bed, then against resistance, by lifting against slight resistance exerted by the nurse's hand pushing on the extremity. Strength is graded on a scale of 0 to 5 (Table 41-6).

Coordination Coordination, a function of the cerebellum, is assessed by asking the client to perform repetitious movement. The client should close her eyes and repeatedly, rapidly touch her own nose with alternate index fingers (Figure 41-6). Lower extremity coordination is assessed by asking the client to run the heel of one foot down the opposite shin, and then repeat with the other heel (Figure 14-7). Inability to perform these movements is termed **ataxia**, incoordination of voluntary muscle action.

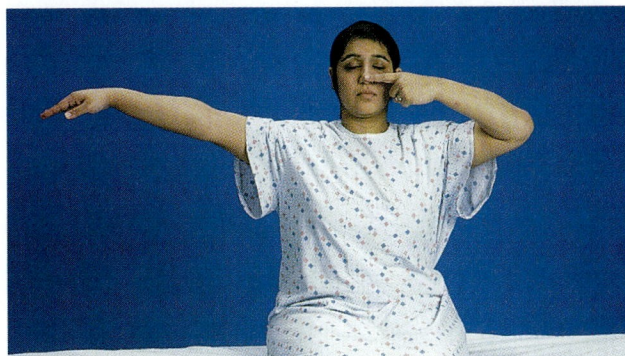

Figure 41-6 Assessment of Coordination: Fingertip-to-Nose Touch

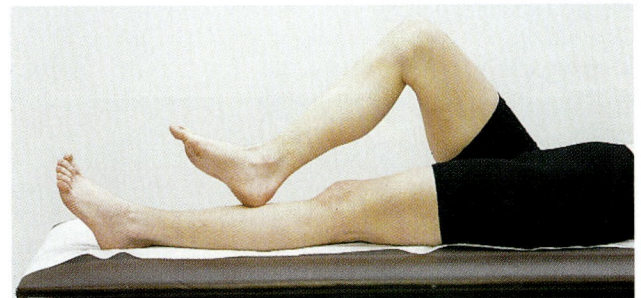

Figure 41-7 Assessment of Coordination: Heel Slide

Balance Balance is evaluated by using the Romberg test. The client stands with the feet together, arms extended in front, and eyes closed. Balance is observed; a slight swaying is normal.

Safety: Romberg Test
Always stand in front of the client during the Romberg test, anticipating that the client might fall.

Posturing Abnormal posturing occurs with injury to the motor tract. Two types for which to observe are decorticate and decerebrate posturing. Decorticate posturing is characterized by flexion of the arms, adduction of the upper extremities, and extension of the lower extremities. Lesions of the cerebral hemispheres or internal structures of the brain cause decorticate posturing. Decerebrate posturing is caused by brain stem injury and is characterized by an arcing of the back, backward flexion of the head, adduction and hyperpronation of the arms, and extension of the feet (Figure 41-8).

Abnormal posturing may be present either at all times or in response to stimuli such as loud noises, bright lights, or painful stimuli. The nurse must note whether bilateral or unilateral posturing is present, and, if intermittent, the cause of the posturing. The presence of either type of posturing should be reported at once, because either represents an ominous sign of cerebral dysfunction. Decerebrate posturing represents greater dysfunction than does decorticate

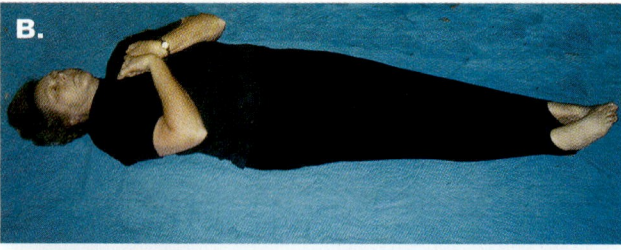
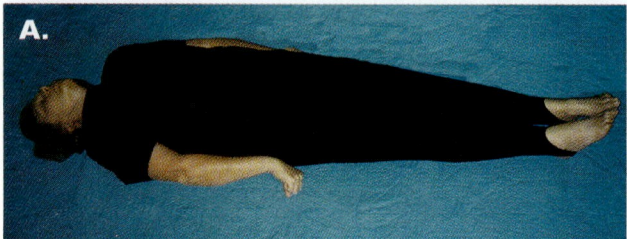

Figure 41-8 Abnormal Posturing: A. Decorticate posturing; B. Decerebrate posturing *(Courtesy John White, Corpus Christi, TX)*

PROFESSIONAL TIP

Assessing Coordination
Ensure that clients who wear eyeglasses have their glasses on prior to the assessment being performed.

PROFESSIONAL TIP

Assessing Pain and Temperature Sensory Function
- Test upper and lower extremities
- Begin with the upper arms, moving down to the hands; then work from thighs to feet (proximo–distal)

posturing, and any change from decorticate to decerebrate posturing indicates a worsening of condition.

Sensory Function

A subjective examination of sensory function, performed with the client's eyes closed, is generally done only when a dysfunction is suspected. Different pathways are used to transmit different sensory impulses. To evaluate all pathways, the examiner must test tactile sensation, pain and temperature, vibration, proprioception, stereognosis, graphesthesia, and integration of sensations.

Tactile Sensation Tactile sensation is tested by using a cotton ball to lightly touch the client's arms, hands, upper legs, and feet. Comparison is done side to side. The client, with eyes closed, indicates whether the cotton ball is felt.

Pain and Temperature Sensations of pain and temperature are transmitted along the same pathways and are evaluated using a sharp and dull touch. A paper clip or cotton-tipped applicator is used.

Safety: Assessing Pain Sensation
Do not use a safety pin to test pain because skin integrity may be compromised.

The nurse touches the client with the rounded end of a paper clip or cotton-tipped applicator to test for dull sensation, and the pointed end of paper clip or uncovered end of the applicator to test for sharp sensation. The client's ability to distinguish sharp and dull is noted, again comparing both sides of the body.

Vibration Vibration is tested using a tuning fork. The nurse strikes the tuning fork on the palm, holding only the handle, then places the end of the handle first on the client's wrists and then on the ankles and asks whether the vibrations are felt (Figure 41-9). The client's eyes should be closed during the test.

Proprioception Proprioception is the sense of joint position in space. With the client's eyes remaining closed, the nurse moves a joint of the client's finger or extremity up or down in space and asks the client to distinguish the direction of movement of the digit or extremity as being either up or down.

Stereognosis Stereognosis is the ability to recognize an object by feel. Placing a familiar object such as a coin or key in the client's hand and asking that the

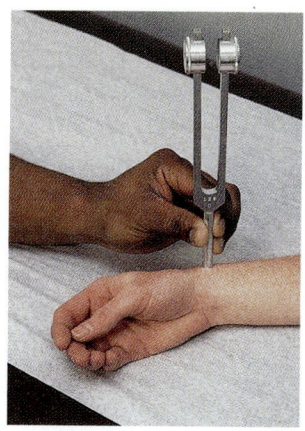

Figure 41-9 Assessment of Vibration

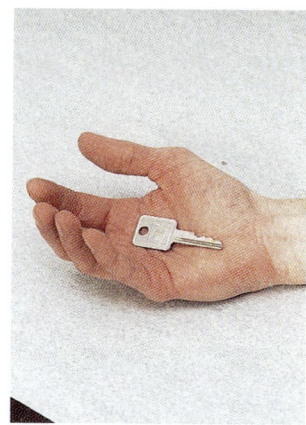

Figure 41-10 Assessment of Stereognosis

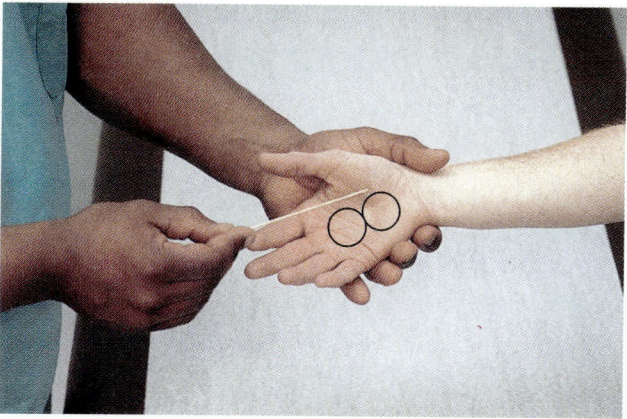

Figure 41-11 Assessment of Graphesthesia

object be identified is a test of stereognosis. This sensation is a function of the brain, not of the spinal pathways (Figure 41-10).

Graphesthesia Graphesthesia is the ability to identify letters, numbers, or shapes drawn on the skin. The nurse holds the client's hand and, with the stick end of a cotton-tipped applicator or a closed pen, traces an outline on the open palm, ensuring that the letter, number, or shape is right side up for the client (Figure 41-11).

Integration of Sensation Integration of sensation is a higher cortical function. A two-point discrimination test is performed by touching the client simultaneously on opposite sides of the body with a sharp object and asking the client to ascertain the number of objects felt. The normal response is two. If only one is felt, the brain function of integration is abnormal.

Reflexes

Both deep tendon reflexes and superficial reflexes are assessed. Deep tendon reflexes are involuntary contractions of muscles or muscle groups responding to brisk stretching near the insertion site of the muscle (Smeltzer & Bare, 1996). Testing of these reflexes is generally the responsibility of the physician or registered nurse, although the licensed practical/vocational nurse should be familiar with these assessments, as abnormal reflex responses may be an early indicator of motor or sensory dysfunction.

Superficial, or cutaneous, reflexes are elicited by irritating the skin on the area being assessed. They are diminished or absent with dysfunction of the reflex arc.

Examination A reflex hammer held loosely between the thumb and index finger is used to examine deep tendon reflexes. The insertion site of the muscle is directly struck with the hammer or indirectly struck by placing the thumb of the examiner over the insertion site and then striking the thumb. The muscle must be relaxed and the joint in midposition. Deep tendon reflexes commonly tested are the Achilles, patellar, biceps, and triceps (Figure 41-12).

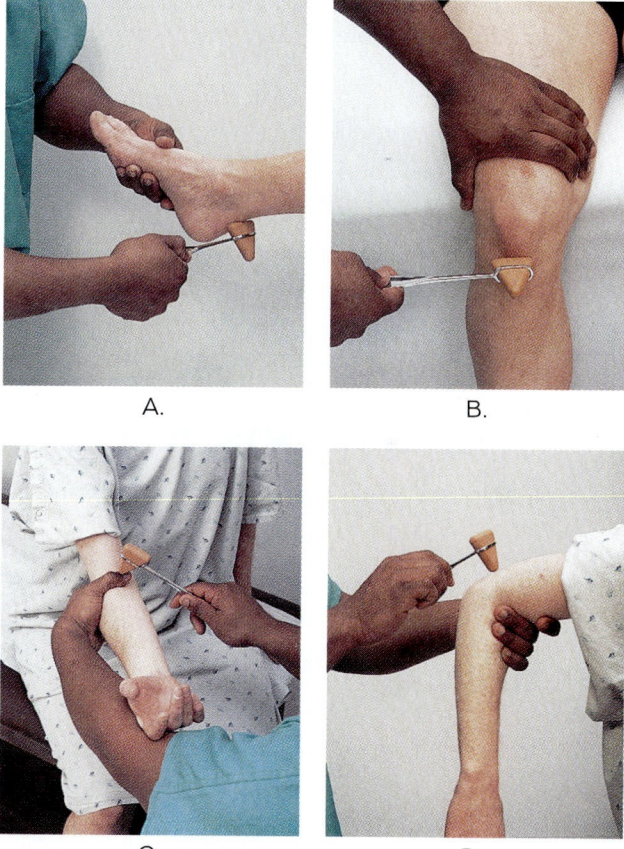

A.   B.

C.   D.

Figure 41-12 Assessment of Deep Tendon Reflexes: A. Achilles; B. Patellar; C. Biceps; D. Triceps

The superficial reflexes generally assessed are the plantar and abdominal. To assess the plantar reflex, the handle of the reflex hammer is used. The outer aspect of the sole of the foot is stroked from the heel and across the ball of the foot to just below the big toe. Plantar flexion, or curling under of the toes, should occur.

To assess the abdominal reflex, the stick end of a cotton-tipped applicator is used to stroke the skin of the abdomen. An upward and outward contraction of the upper abdominal muscles and a contraction of the lower abdomen muscles should occur.

Table 41-7 REFLEX GRADING SCALE

GRADE	DEFINITION
4	Hyperactive with clonus (alternating muscle contractions between antagonistic muscles)
3	Hyperactive
2	Normal
1	Hypoactive
0	Absent

Description or Grading of Response Reflexes are generally described as present, absent, or diminished. If a grading scale is used, it is important to note whether a four-point or five-point scale is used. The description of each number varies between agencies, but a typical scale is presented in Table 41-7.

Abnormal Reflexes The absence of deep tendon reflexes in clients is considered an abnormal finding. A fanning of the toes and dorsiflexion of the big toe in response to the assessment of the plantar reflex is called a positive Babinksi's reflex (Figure 41-13). This abnormal response is indicative of corticospinal disease and is the most important abnormal superficial reflex.

COMMON DIAGNOSTIC TESTS

Commonly used diagnostic tests for clients with symptoms of nervous system disorders are listed in Table 41-8. See Chapter 27, Diagnostic Tests, for explanation/normal values and nursing responsibilities.

HEAD INJURY

Head injuries involve trauma to the scalp, skull, or brain.

Table 41-8 COMMON DIAGNOSTIC TESTS FOR NERVOUS SYSTEM DISORDERS

- Lumbar puncture (LP)
- Electroencephalogram (EEG)
- Electromyogram (EMG)
- Imaging procedures: computerized tomography (CT), positron emission tomography (PET), single photon emission computed tomography (SPECT), magnetic resonance imaging (MRI)
- Cerebral angiography
- Brain scan
- Myelogram

LIFE CYCLE CONSIDERATIONS

Reflexes
- Babinski's reflex is normally present in infants under the age of 6 months
- The absence of the Achilles reflex in the elderly client is not considered abnormal.

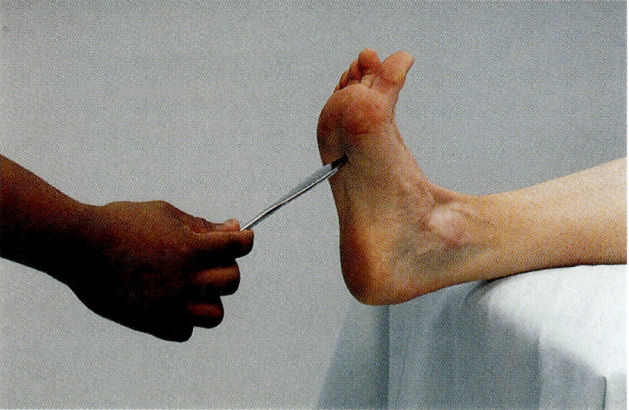

Figure 41-13 Pathologic Reflex: Babinski

SCALP

Scalp injuries bleed profusely because of the abundance of blood vessels in the scalp. As with any break in skin integrity, infection is of major concern. The wound is cleansed and irrigated to remove foreign matter before closing the wound with sutures or butterfly dressings.

SKULL

Skull injuries and fractures of the skull may occur with or without brain injury. A fracture is usually caused by extreme force. Skull fractures are considered closed if the dura mater is intact, and open if the dura mater is torn. The clinical manifestation of skull fracture is localized pain. If the brain is injured, other symptoms may occur.

Types of skull fractures are linear fracture, comminuted fracture, depressed fracture, and basilar fracture. Linear fractures are nondisplaced cracks in the bone. Comminuted fractures occur when the bone is broken into fragments. Depressed fractures have bone fragments pressing into the intracranial cavity. Basilar skull fractures are of the bones in the base of the skull.

Basilar fractures are of particular concern because of the close proximity of the fragile sinus bones and the adhesion of the dura mater to this area. The dura mater can easily tear, and CSF can leak from the ears or nose. The internal carotid artery and cranial nerves can also be damaged easily with a basilar skull fracture.

BRAIN

Brain injuries are caused by primary injuries of acceleration–deceleration force, rotational force, or penetrating missile. Acceleration injuries are caused by moving objects striking the head, such as a baseball bat. Deceleration injuries result when the head is moving and strikes a solid object such as a car dashboard. Rotational injuries are hyperextension, hyperflexion, or lateral flexion of the head, which cause twisting of the cerebrum on the brain stem, such as a whiplash injury. Penetrating missile injuries are a direct penetration of an object, such as a bullet, into brain tissue (Thelan, Davie, & Urden, 1998).

Open Injury

Brain injuries from skull fractures and penetrating injuries are referred to as open head injuries. Hemorrhaging from the nose, pharynx, or ears; ecchymosis over the mastoid area (Battle's sign); or blood in the conjunctiva may occur in conjunction with open head injuries. Cerebrospinal fluid may leak from the ears or nose. A computed tomography (CT) scan or magnetic resonance imaging (MRI) is performed to determine the extent of injury. Neurological deficits depend on the extent and area of injury.

Closed Injury

Closed head injuries are caused by blunt force to the head. Coup injuries are caused by the impact of the head against an object. Contrecoup injuries are caused by the impact of the brain against the opposite side of the skull (Figure 41-14).

Types of closed head injuries are concussion, contusion, and laceration. Concussions are transient neurological deficits caused by the shaking of the brain. Clinical manifestations may include immediate loss of consciousness lasting from minutes to hours, momentary loss of reflexes, respiratory arrest for several seconds, and amnesia for the period immediately prior to and following the event. Headaches, drowsiness, confusion, dizziness, irritability, visual disturbances, and unsteady gait may also occur (Hickey, 1997).

Post-concussion syndrome may develop following the injury, as manifested by headache and dizziness. Nervousness, irritability, emotional lability, fatigue, insomnia, loss of **mentation** (ability to concentrate, remember, or think abstractly), and sometimes other neurological deficits occur. This syndrome may last from several weeks up to a year (Hickey, 1997).

Contusions are surface bruises of the brain. Symptoms depend on the area of injury. Frequently, the client is unconscious for a longer period of time than with a concussion. The client may become conscious only to drift back into unconsciousness. Pulse, blood pressure, and respirations are below normal. Skin is cool and pale. Cerebral edema may occur in conjunction with widespread injury (see section on cerebral edema).

Return of consciousness may be followed by cerebral irritability to stimuli. Headache and dizziness may be present for an indefinite period. Permanent damage may cause either changes in mental function or seizure disorders. Prognosis ranges from full recovery to death.

Cerebral laceration is the tearing of cortical tissue. Symptoms of brain stem injury include deep coma from time of impact, decerebrate posturing, autonomic dysfunction, nonreactive pupils, and respiratory difficulty. The ability to relay nerve impulses from high levels in the brain is lost. Diffuse axonal injury (DAI) usually occurs in conjunction with brain stem injuries. This widespread damage to nerve cells in the white matter of the brain causes immediate coma, decerebration, and increased intracranial pressure.

Hemorrhage

Intracranial hemorrhage is a common complication of any head injury. Bleeding may occur in the epidural space, subdural space, subarachnoid space, or ventricles or intracerebrally. Neurological change is caused by pressure on the brain resulting from the space-occupying hemorrhage. With epidural hematoma (bleeding in the epidural space), momentary unconsciousness is followed by a conscious state of a few hours to a week, depending on the rapidity of the bleeding. As the bleeding continues, neurological status begins to deteriorate, with decreasing level of consciousness; headache; seizures; hemiparesis; decerebration; and dilated, fixed pupils. Treatment is surgery to evacuate the hematoma, stop the bleeding, and relieve pressure on the brain.

Subdural hematomas (bleeding in the subdural space) cause immediate pressure on the brain. Classification of subdural hematomas is acute (within 48 hours of injury), subacute (from 2 to 14 days following injury), and chronic (from 2 weeks to months following injury). Common symptoms are headache, drowsiness, slow mentation, and confusion. The symptoms slowly progress as the size of the subdural clot increases, causing increased pressure on the brain. Small hematomas are usually reabsorbed. Large hematomas require surgical removal.

Subarachnoid (below the arachnoid) and intraventricular (within the ventricles of the brain) hemorrhages are common in severe head injury. The symptoms include those listed for hematoma, as well as **nuchal rigidity**, stiffness or inability to bend the neck. Blood in the subarachnoid space interferes with the reabsorption of CSF, further increasing intracranial pressure.

Intracranial hematomas from contusions usually occur in the temporal or frontal lobes; from shearing forces, they usually occur deep in the brain. The hematoma usually expands rapidly. The injury may cause immediate unconsciousness. Headache, deteriorating

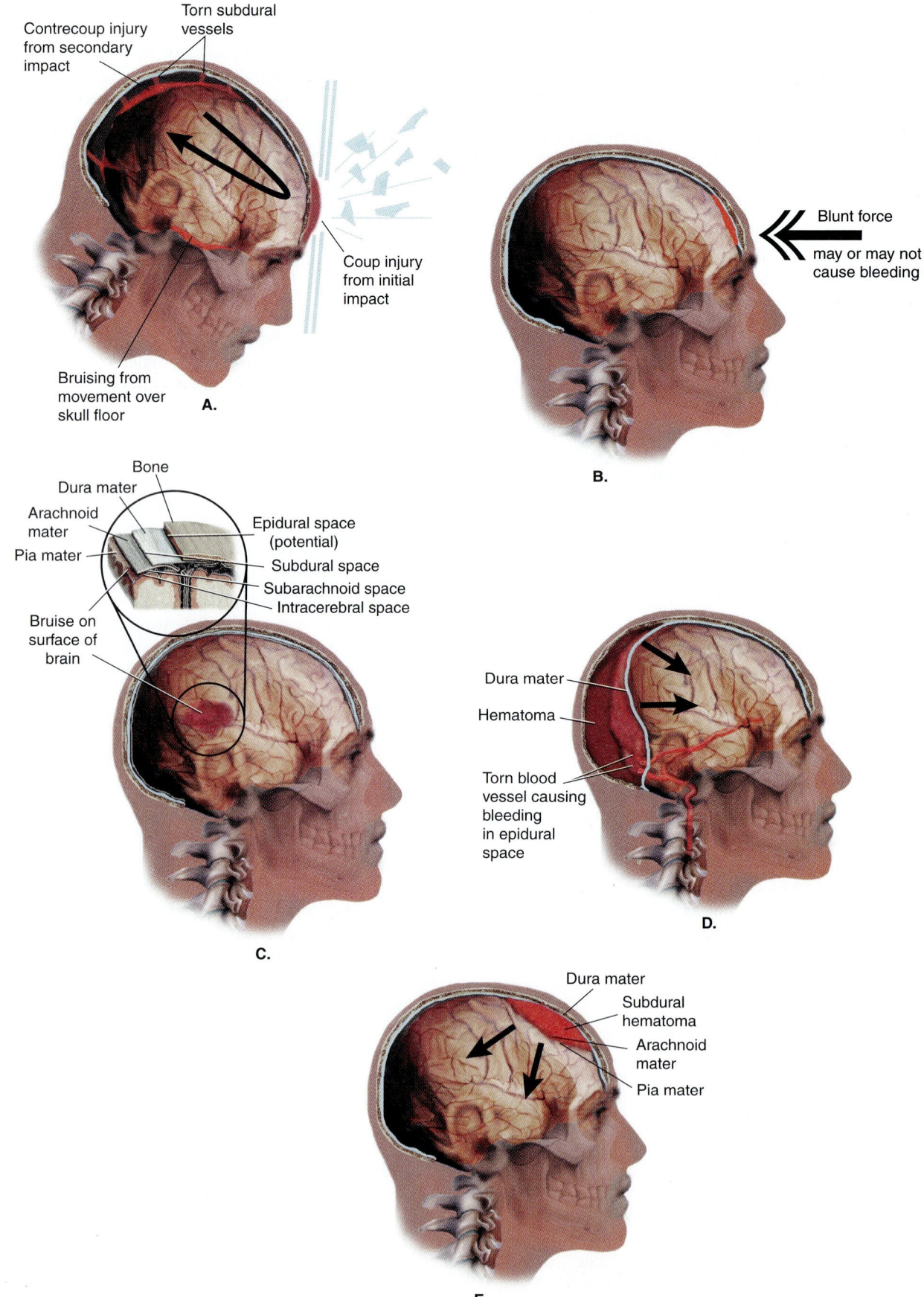

Figure 41-14 Brain Injuries: A. Coup/contrecoup; B. Concussion; C. Contusion; D. Epidural hematoma; E. Subdural hematoma

level of consciousness, hemiplegia, and dilated pupils are initial signs of an internal hematoma. As intracranial pressure increases, herniation of the brain stem occurs, causing changes in pupils, respirations, and vital signs. Craniotomy along with evacuation and control of bleeding may be performed depending on the condition of the client, extent of cerebral contusion, and accessibility of the bleeding site.

Signs and symptoms of increased intracranial pressure include a deterioration in level of consciousness; confusion; difficulty in rousing; and, initially, restlessness. Other signs and symptoms are changes in pupil size or reaction to light. The pupil gradually dilates and becomes less responsive to light. Muscle weakness progressing to **hemiplegia**, paralysis of one side of the body, or **paraplegia**, paralysis of lower extremities, and abnormal posturing may occur. Headache and vomiting are experienced by some clients. Vital sign changes generally do not occur until the increased intracranial pressure has progressed to the point of involving the brain stem. An increase in systolic blood pressure and a widening pulse pressure accompanied by a slowing pulse are the effects of pressure on the brain stem.

Cerebral Edema and Increased Intracranial Pressure

The brain is contained in a rigid container, the skull. The only normal opening to the adult skull is the foramen magnum at the base of the skull. Intracranial pressure is a result of the pressure exerted by the contents of the skull, which are the brain, blood, and CSF.

Regulatory mechanisms maintain intracranial pressure between 0 and 15 mm Hg. The Monroe-Kellie hypothesis states that when one component of the cranial contents increases in volume, the volumes of the other components decrease in order to compensate and maintain intracranial pressure between 0 and 15 mm Hg. As long as this ability to compensate remains effective, no neurological changes occur.

In decompensation, the volume increase is so excessive that intracranial pressure cannot be maintained below 15 mm Hg by decreasing the volume of the remaining components. Neurological changes are exhibited because of cellular hypoxia and displacement of the brain, which compresses neurons, especially in the brain stem. These changes include deteriorating level of consciousness; decreased motor response to commands; fixed, dilated pupils; and vital sign changes known as Cushing's triad or reflex. Cushing's triad refers to bradycardia, widening pulse pressure along with increasing systolic pressure, and respiratory irregularities. Respiratory changes include periods of apnea, decreased respiratory rate and depth, and irregular respirations.

Causes of increased intracranial pressure are increased blood volume resulting from vascular vasodilatation; increased volume of brain tissue resulting from edema, infection, tumor, or hemorrhage; or increased volume of CSF resulting from overproduction, decreased reabsorption, or interruption of CSF circulation. If intracranial pressure continues to increase, brain herniation will occur at the tentorial notch or through the foramen magnum, resulting in death.

Medical–Surgical Management

Management of head injury is focused on early recognition and treatment of increasing intracranial pressure and maintenance of normal body functions.

Medical

Suctioning may be necessary but is never done through the nose on a head injury client because of the possibility of CSF leakage. Oxygen is given to maintain cerebral perfusion. Arterial blood gases (ABGs) are checked.

If the client has an endotracheal tube in place, the $PaCO_2$ level can drop below normal. This causes a slightly alkaline pH, which decreases vasodilation and, thus, intracranial pressure.

Surgical

Decompression is performed surgically by removing a bone flap from the skull to allow room for the expansion of the brain. A space-occupying lesion such as a tumor, hematoma, or abscess may be surgically removed. Excess CSF may be drained from the ventricles.

LIFE CYCLE CONSIDERATIONS

Care of Infants with Head Injuries

- Measure the occipital–frontal circumference with a measuring tape every 8 hours. An increase indicates cerebral edema.
- Feel the tension of the fontanels. Increased intracranial pressure will cause increased tension and, eventually, bulging of the fontanels.
- An infant with CNS irritation will have a high-pitched cry.

CLIENT TEACHING

Surgery for Head Injury

Inform the client of the following:

- The head will be shaved in the area of the incision.
- Edema of the head and face may be present after surgery but will gradually disappear.
- A mechanical ventilator may be used for a day or two following surgery.

Pharmacological

Corticosteroids such as dexamethasone (Decadron) are given to reduce cerebral edema. Antacids, such as Mylanta or Maalox, or histamine receptor antagonists, such as cimetidine (Tagamet), are given to decrease both the side effects of corticosteroids and stress-induced gastric acidity. Osmotic diuretics such as mannitol (Osmitrol), are administered to rapidly reduce fluid in the brain tissue; muscle relaxants, sedatives, barbiturates, or muscle paralyzing agents are administered to decrease activity and reduce the oxygen need of the brain.

Antipyretic drugs are used to decrease body temperature and the metabolic needs of the brain, thereby reducing the volume of blood sent to the brain to supply oxygen and glucose. Anticonvulsants are given to prevent or treat seizure activity.

Activity

Activity is limited to keep the metabolic needs of the brain at a minimum. Increased metabolic needs require more oxygen and glucose supplied by increases in blood volume in the cranium, which, in turn, further increases intracranial pressure.

▶ NURSING PROCESS

▶ Assessment

Nursing assessment for any head injury is focused on neurological status.

▶ Subjective Data

Subjective data to be gathered includes a history of what happened, including type of trauma (accelera-tion, deceleration, or missile), site of blow, and any loss of consciousness, including timing, length, and ability to be roused.

▶ Objective Data

A neurological screening is done to obtain a base-line neurological status; then, a more in-depth neuro-logical exam is performed to identify any early signs of increasing intracranial pressure.

Frequent assessment of neurological status including level of consciousness, motor function, eye movement, pupil size and reaction, protective reflexes, and vital signs allows for early recognition of and intervention for increasing intracranial pressure. Nursing observation also includes assessing for double vision, headache, nausea, and bleeding from any orifice. Ipsi-lateral pupil reaction (reaction of the pupil on the same side as the injury or lesion), may occur as a result of pressure on the oculomotor nerve caused by increased intracranial pressure or cerebral edema. Recognition of factors that cause increased intracranial pressure is a necessary aspect of assessment.

For the client undergoing intracranial surgery, an assessment of teaching needs of the client and family must be performed. Emotional and psychosocial needs and support systems are also assessed.

Longer-term care involves assessment of bowel elimination status to prevent the need for straining; skin assessment to prevent skin breakdown, and assessment for complications of immobility.

Nursing diagnoses for a client with a head injury may include the following:

Nursing Diagnoses	Planning/Goals	Nursing Interventions
▶ *Tissue perfusion, Altered Cerebral, related to disruption in cerebral blood flow*	The client will demonstrate improvement or maintenance on Glasgow Coma Scale.	Assess neurological status of client every 15 to 60 minutes. Note findings on Glasgow Coma Scale. Compare findings to previous assessments to uncover changes in condition.
		Administer oxygen as ordered to supply a high concentration of oxygen to the brain.
		Position client with head of the bed up 30° to 40° and client's head at midline to promote venous drainage from the head.
		Minimize physical activity to prevent increasing metabolic demands. Maintain blood $PaCO_2$ between 25 and 30 mm Hg to prevent vasodilatation.
▶ *Breathing Pattern, Ineffective, related to neurological impairment of respiratory status or mechanical ventilation*	The client will have an effective breathing pattern.	Assess respiratory status every 15 to 60 minutes.
		Provide mechanical ventilation if necessary.
		Continually assess ABG levels or pulse oximeter readings to identify need for assisting respirations to prevent vasodilatation in the brain and increasing intracranial pressure.
		Administer oxygen as ordered to maintain blood oxygen concentration.

continued

Nursing Diagnoses	Planning/Goals	Nursing Interventions
▶ *Family Processes, Altered, related to sudden crisis*	The client and/or family will demonstrate effective coping mechanisms.	Assess family's coping mechanisms.
		Provide information about the client in an ongoing fashion. Provide teaching about the injury and pathophysiology involved.
		Prepare family for possible outcomes of the injury, such as paralysis or death.
		Collaborate with clergy, social services, mental health counselors, and support groups.
		Involve the family in client care as appropriate.
		Teach the family to report increased drowsiness, arm/leg weakness, muscle twitching, nausea or vomiting, visual or hearing disturbances, and so on.
		Inform the family that the client may not be aware of the symptoms and that signs and symptoms of the head injury may not be immediately apparent.

Evaluation Each goal must be evaluated to determine how it has been met by the client.

BRAIN TUMOR

Brain tumors are space-occupying intracranial lesions, either benign or malignant. Classification of brain tumors is by location or tissue type. Intracranial lesions may be primary lesions, which develop initially in brain tissue; extensions of tumors of the meninges, cranial nerves, or pituitary gland; or metastatic lesions from tumors originating in other body systems.

Pathophysiology of brain tumors depends on the increase in volume of brain tissue. The etiology is unknown. Clinical manifestations differ according to the area of the lesion and the rate of growth. Intracranial pressure increases as compensatory mechanisms are no longer able to balance tumor growth. Clinical manifestations commonly include alterations in consciousness, decreased mental functioning, headaches, seizures, or vomiting (sometimes sudden and projectile). Other signs and symptoms are relative to the functions of areas involved, such as visual problems resulting from occipital lobe tumors.

Diagnostic evaluation is by CT scan, MRI, or electroencephalogram (EEG). Total body scans, chest x-rays, and needle biopsies of the tumor may be performed to identify the type of tumor and, thus, serve as a basis for medical treatment.

Medical–Surgical Management

Medical

Medical management is based on tissue type, growth rate, and assessment of the client. Radiation therapy may be administered for treatment of specific tumor types or for inoperable tumors. The goal is to destroy the tumor cells, which are more susceptible to radiation than are normal cells. Radiation is also used in conjunction with surgery and chemotherapy.

Surgical

Surgical intervention, conventional or laser, includes resection of tumors (benign or malignant) to decrease the space occupied by the lesion or to obtain tissue for biopsy. Some CSF may be removed to relieve increased pressure.

Pharmacological

Pharmacological interventions are based on presenting symptoms. Dexamethasone (Decadron) is administered to decrease cerebral edema. Phenytoin (Dilantin) is given to prevent seizure activity. Antacids and H_2 blockers such as cimetidine (Tagamet) are given to prevent gastric irritation. Analgesics, NSAIDs, or codeine are used for headaches, and stool softeners are administered to prevent straining. Antineoplastic agents may be administered based on tumor type and whether the client meets the requirements for receiving the drug.

▶ NURSING PROCESS

▶ Assessment

▶ Subjective Data

Subjective assessment involves asking the client about fatigue, pain, headache, weakness, and ability to perform daily activities. Sensory alterations such as hearing, visual, or olfactory changes should be noted.

LIFE CYCLE CONSIDERATIONS

Brain Tumors
Metastatic tumors of the brain are rare in children.

The nurse must assess the client's pain and evaluate effectiveness of interventions. A thorough psychosocial assessment, including changes in personality or judgment, serves as the basis for providing emotional support.

▶ Objective Data

Included is assessment of functional ability, mobility, and mental status, including motor strength, gait, ability to perform activities of daily living (ADL), and level of consciousness. Signs of neurological changes, deficits, or increased intracranial pressure, such as restlessness, changes in logic, changes in vital signs, pupil responses, speech abnormalities, seizure activity, or changes in respiratory patterns, must all be noted.

Nursing diagnoses for a client with a brain tumor may include the following:

Nursing Diagnoses	Planning/Goals	Nursing Interventions
▶ *Anxiety related to fear of unknown and treatment plans*	The client will demonstrate effective use of coping mechanisms.	Allow client to verbalize feeling of anxiety and discuss coping patterns previously used.
		Observe for verbal and nonverbal cues of anxiety.
		Provide emotional support by listening and guiding client to explore feelings of helplessness, fear of the unknown, and potential impending death.
		Teach client and family about diagnostic tests, treatments, and expected outcomes.
		Collaborate with pastoral care, physician, social services, and family to provide emotional support.
		Maintain a calm demeanor.
		Teach relaxation exercises and techniques such as slow, deep breathing and progressive muscle relaxation.
		Administer tranquilizers and sedatives as ordered.
▶ *Fatigue related to effects of treatment*	The client will verbalize lessened fatigue with frequent rest periods.	Allow client to discuss feelings of fatigue.
		Involve client in planning daily schedule that includes frequent rest periods.
		Assess client's ability to perform ADL, need for assistance to conserve energy.
		Cluster care activities to provide frequent rest periods that coincide with peak effectiveness of analgesics.
▶ *Nutrition: Altered, Less than Body Requirements related to side effects of treatment and disease process*	The client will maintain weight within 5 pounds of initial weight.	Assess client's weight every other day.
		Provide frequent small feedings of high-calorie and high-protein foods.
		Offer foods of client's choice.
		Use nutritional supplements to maintain weight. Offer fluids frequently.

Evaluation Each goal must be evaluated to determine how it has been met by the client.

CEREBROVASCULAR ACCIDENT/TRANSIENT ISCHEMIC ATTACKS

Cerebrovascular accident (CVA), or stroke, is a sudden loss of brain function accompanied by neurological deficit. Stroke is the third highest cause of death in the United States. Death rates from stroke have steadily declined from 120 per 100,000 in 1970 to 26 per 100,000 in 1992 (National Stroke Association, 1998a). The first rise in death rates in 35 years occurred in 1993, with 26.5 per 100,000, and again in 1995, with 26.7 per 100,000. Deaths totaled 157,991 in 1995. The rise in deaths in two groups among this population is noteworthy: rates for African American women ages 45 to 60 increased by 15% and rates for African American men over age 65 increased by 10% (National Stroke Association, 1995). Reasons for this sharp rise have not

CLIENT TEACHING

Stroke-Prevention Guidelines

- Have an annual blood pressure check
- Be aware of cholesterol level
- Consume lesser amounts of sodium (salt) and fat

(National Stroke Association, 1998b)

PROFESSIONAL TIP

Risk Factors for Stroke

- The major risk factor for stroke is hypertension.
- Other risk factors are diabetes mellitus, atherosclerosis, aneurysm, cardiac disease, high blood cholesterol, obesity, sedentary lifestyle, smoking, stress, drug abuse (especially of cocaine), and use of oral contraceptives. Clients with more than one risk factor are at even greater risk.

been determined. A proposed cause is decreased mortality from other diseases such as heart disease.

Strokes are caused by ischemia (oxygen deprivation) resulting from a thrombus, embolus, severe vasospasm, or cerebral hemorrhage. Blood supply to the brain is interrupted, causing neurological deficits of sensation, movement, thought, memory, or speech. The loss of function can be temporary or permanent.

Transient ischemic attacks (TIAs) frequently precede a CVA. A TIA is a temporary or transient episode of neurological dysfunction caused by temporary impairment of blood flow to the brain. The loss of motor or sensory function may last from a few seconds to minutes to 24 hours. A classic symptom is fleeting blindness in one eye. A reversible ischemic neurological deficit (RIND) is a TIA that lasts 24 to 48 hours.

Clinical manifestations of TIA or CVA vary according to the location of interrupted blood supply in the brain. As with head injury, the specific functions of the involved area of the brain are interrupted, causing the symptoms. Common neurological deficits are motor deficits of hemiplegia (paralysis of one side of the body on the side opposite of the brain lesion), **hemiparesis** (weakness of one side of the body), **dysarthria** (impairment of speech due to muscle dysfunction), and dysphagia (impairment of swallowing muscles). **Emotional lability** (loss of emotional control), inability to control behavior, and inability to process multiple pieces of information are also common manifestations of a stroke.

Sensory deficits include visual deficits of double vision, decreased visual acuity, and **homonymous hemianopia**, the loss of vision in half of the visual field on the same side of both eyes. Other possible sensory deficits include decreased sensation to touch, pressure, pain, heat, and cold. The client also may be confused and disoriented.

Intellectual deficits include memory impairment, poor judgment, short attention span, difficulty organizing thoughts, and inability to reason or calculate. Emotional deficits include depression and decreased tolerance to stressors.

Most clients experience initial bowel and bladder dysfunction. With early recognition of the problem and use of bowel and bladder retraining programs,

however, most clients regain continence of bowel and bladder.

Differences in the affected side of the brain have been identified. Clients with left-side CVA tend to have communication deficits of aphasia, or inability to communicate. These clients tend to be slow and cautious in behavior and have intellectual impairments such as memory deficits or loss of problem solving skills. Defects in the right visual field occur, and hemiplegia occurs on the right side.

Clients with right-side CVA have left-sided paralysis and defects in the left visual field. Spatial–perceptual defects, called **agnosia**, cause the inability to recognize familiar objects such as a hairbrush. These clients demonstrate poor judgment and impulsive behavior and are unaware of the deficits. This is called **anosognosia**, which is gross or unconscious denial of the stroke or neurological deficit. Furthermore, these clients are easily distracted and usually show **unilateral neglect**, or the failure to recognize or care for the affected side of the body.

Cerebral edema and increased intracranial pressure may further complicate neurological status. Cerebral edema maximizes in 3 to 5 days following CVA. Neurological deficits begin to resolve within 2 days as cerebral edema decreases. Gradual progression in the return of various functions from proximal to distal can occur for 1 to 2 years.

Medical–Surgical Management

Medical

Medical management of the client with CVA is directed toward airway maintenance and supportive therapy during the first 24 to 48 hours. Early diagnosis of the cause and type of stroke is necessary to determine the appropriate treatment. Maintaining adequate cerebral perfusion and preventing cerebral edema reduce neurological deficit. Respiratory failure is treated with mechanical ventilation; temperature is regulated, with the help of a hypothermia blanket if necessary. (See the section on increased intracranial pressure for information on prevention and treatment.)

Medication and Cerebrovascular Accident

Calcium channel blockers should not be used for the client with CVA, as they dilate blood vessels and increase cerebral perfusion.

To prevent further loss of function, a focus on rehabilitation must begin on admission. Self-care and mobility that remain must be maintained.

Surgical

Surgical removal of the thrombus (thrombolectomy) or embolus (embolectomy) may be necessary to relieve pressure on the brain.

Pharmacological

Antihypertensive agents are used to control blood pressure. To prevent further clot formation in cases of stroke caused by thrombi, anticoagulants, aspirin, heparin, or coumadin are used. To dissolve the clot, thrombolytic agents such as alteplase (Activase), anistreplase (Eminase), streptokinase (Streptase), or urokinase (Abbokinase) may be ordered. A stroke caused by bleeding would not be treated with thrombolytic agents. Dexamethasone (Decadron) may be used to reduce intracranial pressure. Anticonvulsants such as phenytoin (Dilantin) may be used if convulsions are present.

Diet

Fluids may be restricted for a few days following a CVA. The client will, however, be given intravenous fluids or tube feedings. The gag reflex must be assessed to identify choking risk, and food restrictions implemented accordingly.

Caregivers for Client with CVA

To provide consistency in understanding of the CVA client's needs, assign the same caregiver to the client whenever possible.

Activity

In cases of an embolic or thrombolic stroke, the client's bed is kept flat to increase cerebral perfusion. In the event of a hemorrhagic stroke, the head of the bed is elevated to decrease cerebral perfusion. The type of CVA and the physician's judgment determines the length of time the client stays in bed.

Other Therapies

Both following the initial acute phase and during rehabilitation, physical, occupational, and speech therapy are vital for the client to reach the optimal functional level of recovery.

▸ NURSING PROCESS

▸ Assessment

▸ Subjective Data

Subjective data collected include client statements regarding how the client is feeling, frustration level with limitations, reports of pain, numbness, tingling, and sensory deficits of vision or hearing

▸ Objective Data

Specific attention must be paid to objective findings of assessment of level of consciousness, respiratory status, hemiparesis, hemiplegia, mobility, and cognitive perceptual functioning including the inability to think clearly and the ability to understand the condition.

Post-CVA Care
*   Consult with the family to evaluate the home for safety and use of wheelchair or walker, if needed
*   Evaluate the client's ability to perform self-care so that assistive devices or personal assistance can be obtained
*   Determine whether a hospital bed or other medical equipment will need to be rented

Nursing diagnoses for a client with a CVA may include the following:

Nursing Diagnoses	Planning/Goals	Nursing Interventions
▸ *Knowledge Deficit related to home care*	The client and/or family will verbalize or demonstrate home health care management.	Assess client's and family's needs for discharge teaching, knowledge level about necessary home care.
		Develop a multidisciplinary plan for client and family teaching.
		Provide education in verbal, written, and picture forms to accommodate the varying possible impairments from the stroke.

continued

Nursing Diagnoses	Planning/Goals	Nursing Interventions
		Teach small segments of information at a time and reinforce teaching, then, to ascertain effectiveness of teaching, have client and family return demonstrate or verbalize knowledge. Primary areas of teaching are medication administration; dosages, actions, and side effects to report to the physician; mobility needs; self-care needs; safety factors; communication; swallowing; elimination; and skin care.
▶ *Communication, Impaired Verbal, related to neuromuscular impairment*	The client will communicate needs to the caregiver.	Assess communication deficits and consult a speech therapist to determine a method of communication, if deficits are apparent.
		Allow time for the client to attempt to communicate needs; anticipate needs to prevent client frustration in trying to communicate.
		Use gestures, pictures, and closed questions (those requiring only a "yes" or "no" answer). Provide paper and pencil if dominant side is unaffected.
▶ *Unilateral Neglect related to neuromuscular impairment*	The client will move paralyzed extremities with assistance from functioning extremities.	Adapt environment to prevent injury of the client with unilateral neglect by positioning water and personal items on the unaffected or unneglected side. Approach the client from the unneglected side.
		Gradually cue client to remind to tend to the neglected side.
		Remind client of safety factors such as arm trailing over edge of wheelchair or close proximity of a wall on the neglected side.
		Teach client and family to place small bites of food on unaffected side and to check for food in the cheek on the affected side after meals.
		Instruct client to scan environment for safety factors at all times.
		Teach client how to dress and tend to neglected side.
		Place arm either in a sling, if client is ambulatory, or on a wheelchair tray, if client is in a wheelchair.

Evaluation Each goal must be evaluated to determine how it has been met by the client.

EPILEPSY/SEIZURE DISORDER

Epilepsy is a disorder of cerebral function in which the client experiences sudden attacks of altered consciousness, motor activity, or sensory phenomenon. Convulsive seizures are the most common type of attack. Most recurrent seizure patterns are due to epilepsy. Most clinicians and authors use the term "seizure disorder" for epilepsy or seizures (Hickey, 1997).

A seizure is initiated by an electrical disturbance in the neurons, which, in turn, causes an aberrant discharge of electrical activity from any part of the cerebral cortex and possibly from other areas of the brain (Samuels, 1995). This electrical discharge may cause involuntary episodes of loss of consciousness, excessive muscular movement or loss of muscle tone, and changes in behavior, mood, sensation, and/or perception (Smeltzer & Bare, 1996).

The etiology of the electrical disturbance may be birth trauma, hypoxia, infection, tumor, alcohol toxicity, drugs, drug withdrawal, carbon monoxide or lead poisoning, vascular abnormalities such as CVA, hypoglycemia electrolyte imbalance, or fever. Often, the cause is idiopathic, or unknown.

Seizures are classified as generalized or partial. In generalized seizures, the entire brain is affected simultaneously, causing bilateral, symmetrical reactions. Generalized seizures are classified as tonic and/or clonic (grand mal), absence (petit mal), or myoclonic.

Tonic–clonic seizures involve rigid tonic contractions of muscles and loss of postural control followed by a clonic stage of intermittent contraction and relaxation. Loss of continence of stool or urine is common. Absence seizures involve loss of conscious activity without the muscular involvement of tonic–clonic seizures. Myoclonic seizures may be very mild, sudden, involuntary contractions of a muscle group or may be rapid, forceful movements. They usually occur in the trunk or extremities and involve no loss of consciousness.

Partial seizures initiate in a focal point in the brain and involve the function of those specific neurons. Partial seizures are either simple or complex. In simple partial seizures, the area affected may be a hand, a finger, the ability to talk, or a sense such as smell. Consciousness is not lost.

Complex partial seizures generally involve loss of consciousness and may produce cognitive, affective, psychosensory, or psychomotor symptoms (Chipps, Clanin, & Campbell, 1992). The client may perform inappropriate purposive behaviors, called **automatisms**, or mechanical, repetitive motor behaviors performed unconsciously, such as lip-smacking. **Auras**, peculiar sensations that precede the seizure and may take the form of a taste, smell, sight, or sound; dizziness; or a "funny" feeling. After the seizure, the client typically cannot remember the episode.

Diagnostic testing to determine the type of seizure activity includes the EEG to identify abnormal electrical activity and/or the focal point of the seizure. Sleep and video EEGs are performed to document changes in electrical activity of the brain. Computerized tomography scans are used to identify or rule out lesions, degenerative changes, or vascular abnormalities.

Medical–Surgical Management

Surgical

Surgical intervention may be indicated for a very small percentage of clients. Microsurgery may be utilized to irradiate focal points of abnormal electrical discharge caused by tumor, vascular abnormality, or abscess.

Pharmacological

The primary method of controlling seizure activity is pharmacological. Seizure activity in 75% of clients is controlled with an anticonvulsant agent or a combination of anticonvulsants (Hickey, 1997). Phenytoin (Dilantin), phenobarbital (Phenobarbital), carbamazepine (Tegretol), valproic acid (Depakene), and primidone (Mysoline) are often used. Anticonvulsant agents are started one at a time in gradually increasing doses. The client's blood level is monitored for therapeutic range, and the client is assessed for side effects of the drug and signs of drug toxicity, such as drowsiness, dizziness, gastric distress, rash, blood dyscrasias, and ataxia.

The goal is to obtain seizure control with minimal side effects. Any anticonvulsant should be gradually discontinued. Abrupt withdrawal can cause **status epilepticus,** an acute prolonged episode of seizure activity lasting at least 30 minutes with or without loss of consciousness (Smeltzer & Bare, 1996). Status epilepticus is a medical emergency that can result in respiratory arrest and irreversible brain damage.

Diet

Nutritionally balanced meals are required. The client should never consume alcohol.

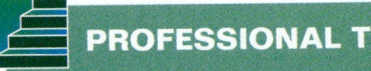

PROFESSIONAL TIP

Long-Term Use of Dilantin
The client on Dilantin requires good oral hygiene because of hyperplasia of the gums, which become edematous and enlarged.

Activity

Adequate rest is required. Driving, operating machinery, and swimming are not allowed until seizures are controlled.

Safety: Precautions During a Seizure

If the client is in bed:
- Be sure the side rails are up, and
- Put padding (blankets) on the side rails to prevent injury.

If the client is out of bed:
- Carefully ease the client to the floor,
- Move nearby objects so that the client will not be injured, and
- Place a soft item beneath the client's head.

Whether the client is in or out of bed:
- Never leave the client alone,
- Do not restrain the client,
- Do not attempt to put anything in the client's mouth after the seizure has begun,
- Loosen any restrictive clothing around the client's neck,
- Turn the client's head to the side, and
- Monitor seizure activity carefully, noting the exact time that the seizure began and ended.

After the seizure:
- Call the client by name and ask to perform a simple command,
- Test the client's memory by asking to remember two words,
- Ask the client whether an aura was experienced before the seizure,
- Check the oral cavity—especially the tongue—for injury,
- Offer comfort and reassurance, as the client may be frightened and embarrassed, and
- Document everything observed.

▶ NURSING PROCESS

▶ Assessment

▶ Subjective Data

This includes client statements of experiences prior to the seizure and what activity the client was performing when the seizure occurred. The nurse must determine whether an aura was experienced and the sensations that were manifested, and ascertain if the client has a prior history of seizure disorder.

▶ Objective Data

Assessment of the nature of the seizure and sequencing of events is important in determining cause and management of seizure activity. During the seizure, the nurse assesses the client's respiratory status and observes for muscular stiffness or flaccidity, the position of the eyes and head, the size and equality of the pupils, automatism, any cry or sounds made, and incontinence of urine or stool. The duration of the phases of the seizure, total duration, and whether unconsciousness occurred are noted. If the onset of seizure activity was observed, this should be noted along with what the client was doing when the seizure began.

Following the seizure the client should be observed for postictal signs of paralysis of arms or legs, inability to speak, sleep following seizure, difficulty in awakening from sleep, confusion, or general dazed affect (Smeltzer & Bare, 1996; Hickey, 1997). The postictal phase can last from several minutes to hours. The client should be assessed for signs of injury and vital signs. Clients on anticonvulsant therapy need a thorough nursing assessment because of the wide variety of side effects involving multiple body systems.

Nursing diagnoses for a client with a seizure may include the following:

Nursing Diagnoses	Planning/Goals	Nursing Interventions
▶ *Airway Clearance, Ineffective, related to mucus accumulation during the seizure and uncontrollable tonic–clonic muscle contractions involving the respiratory muscles*	The client will maintain an effective airway during seizure activity.	Following tonic–clonic activity, turn client to the side to allow secretions to drain from the airway.
		Prepare to suction oropharynx if necessary to clear airway.
		Assess skin color and respiratory rate and depth during and following seizure.
		Administer oxygen as needed.
		Insert oral airway or epistick if client's jaw is not clenched. Never insert an object if the jaw is already clenched. Do not place fingers between client's teeth. Loosen restrictive clothing.
▶ *Injury, Risk for, related to seizure activity*	The client will be free of injury related to seizure activity.	During seizures in bed, use blankets or protective pads to pad side rails.
		If client is standing or sitting, ease client to the floor when seizure activity begins. Place client in a supine position, but do not physically restrain client.
		Remove objects from around client so that he or she will not hit them.
		Following the seizure, turn client to the side to allow secretions to drain from the mouth.
		Maintain a low-stimulus environment to prevent further seizure activity.
		Observe client for injuries, i.e., tongue lacerations; broken bones; body lacerations or bruising.
		Teach client about ways of maintaining a safe environment, including driving restrictions; lying down in a safe area if an aura is experienced; showering instead of tub bathing; either avoiding swimming or swimming with a partner if the physician allows; and wearing a medical identification tag.
▶ *Coping, Ineffective Individual, related to anxiety secondary to seizure disorder and altered self-concept*	The client will verbalize fears and concerns about seizure activity; and will use effective coping methods.	Allow client to verbalize fears and concerns.
		Explore coping mechanisms with client.
		Collaborate with mental health counselor or clergy to assist client in development of coping mechanisms.

Evaluation Each goal must be evaluated to determine how it has been met by the client.

HERNIATED INTERVERTEBRAL DISK

Herniated intervertebral disks are a major cause of chronic back pain. Most clients with herniated disks are 30 to 50 years of age. The majority of herniated disks occur in the lumbar or cervical spine because of the flexibility of these regions (Hickey, 1997). This can occur either suddenly from trauma, lifting, or twisting or gradually from aging, osteoporosis, or degenerative changes. Most herniated disks are caused by trauma, such as falls, accidents, or repeated lifting. Degenerative

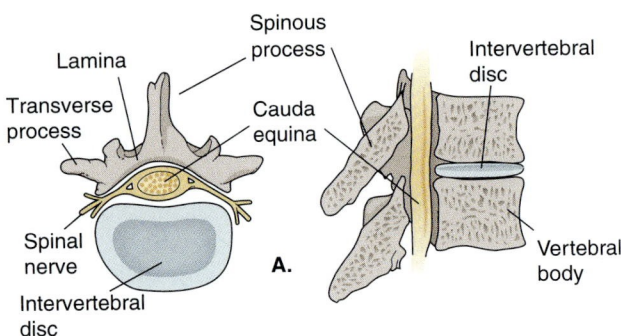

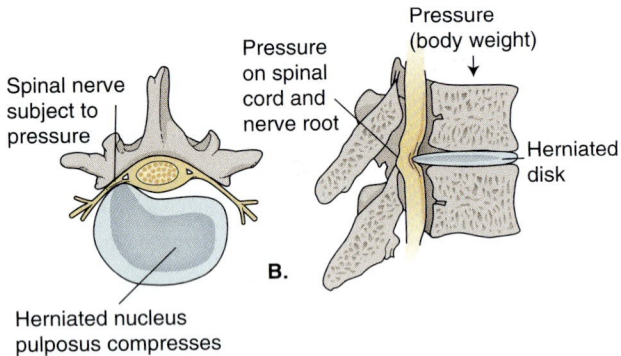

Figure 41-15 A. Normal Intervertebral Disc, B. Herniated Disc

changes related to arthritis, aging, or repeated minor injuries predispose the client to herniated intervertebral disks.

The intervertebral disk is a cartilaginous cushion between vertebral bodies (Figure 41-15). In herniation, or rupture of the disk, the nucleus pulposus protrudes into the fibrous ring, the annulus fibrosus. This protrusion presses on the spinal cord and nerve roots, causing pain, motor changes, sensory changes, and alterations in reflexes.

The nerve root affected and the degree of compression lead to specific symptoms. Ninety percent to 95% of lumbar herniations occur at the L-4 to L-5 and S-1 levels (Hickey, 1997). Low-back pain that radiates across the buttock and down the leg along the path of the sciatic nerve is the most common symptom. The affected leg tingles and is numb. Sneezing, straining, stooping, standing, sitting, blowing the nose, and jarring movements aggravate the pain. Positions of comfort are lying on the back, with knees flexed and a small pillow under the head, or lying on the unaffected side, with the affected knee flexed.

Motor weakness may be experienced. Paresthesia and numbness of the leg and foot occur. Knee and ankle reflexes are diminished or absent. Lasegue's sign, pain experienced upon gentle raising of the fully extended leg of the supine-positioned client to 20° to 60°, stems from stretching of the inflamed sciatic nerve. Inflammation in the nerve roots may also be

present as indicated by a positive finding for **Kernig's sign**. To test for Kernig's sign, the client is placed in a dorsal recumbent position and attempts to flex the hip and knee and then extend the knee. Normally, the client should be able to extend the knee to 90°. With a low-back herniated disk, however, the client will be unable to extend the knee because of severe pain radiating down the hip and leg. Symptoms vary with the area and degree of nerve root compression.

Cervical herniation commonly occurs at levels C-5 to C-6 or C-6 to C-7. Symptoms of lateral herniation include pain and paresthesia in the neck, arms, and shoulders. Loss of muscle strength and reflexes may also occur, as may muscle atrophy.

Because of anatomic position, cervical disks may herniate centrally more frequently than do lumbar disks, thereby compressing the spinal cord. Symptoms are weakness of the lower extremities and unsteady gait. Spasticity and hyperactive reflexes may develop in the lower extremities. Difficulty in voiding and sexual dysfunction may occur.

Degenerative spinal cord disease can follow compression from a herniated disk. Spinal cord tumors and herniated lumbar disk are differential diagnoses that are ruled out through the use of MRI or CT scans.

Medical–Surgical Management

Medical

Conservative medical treatment, providing rest, stress reduction and immobility of the spine, and pain relief, is often tried for several weeks.

Surgical

Surgery to remove the herniated disk is done when neurological deficit or pain are not responsive to conservative treatment or when symptoms require immediate surgical intervention.

Pharmacological

Narcotic analgesics, such as hydrocodone bitartrate with acetaminophen (Vicodin), and nonnarcotic analgesics, such as tramadol hydrochloride (Ultram), are ordered for pain control. Antiinflammatory drugs, steroids, or NSAIDs such as ibuprofen (Motrin) or naproxen (Anaprox) are prescribed to reduce the inflammatory response. Muscle relaxants such as methocarbamol (Robaxin) are given to reduce spasms of surrounding muscles, which decreases the pain. Antianxiety medications such as diazepam (Valium) are given to decrease muscle tension and promote rest.

Diet

To decrease the workload on the involved muscles, weight reduction is advocated if the client is overweight. A high-protein diet with calcium, vitamin D, and phosphorus is necessary for bone repair and prevention of osteoporosis. Fiber is necessary for bowel function, because constipation is a common side effect of analgesics.

Activity

Bed rest, a support garment (back brace) or cervical collar, a firm mattress, and traction may be used to decrease stress on the affected vertebrae. Postoperatively, log-roll turning is used to prevent injury to the vertebrae and spine.

The client may not lift or carry more than 5 pounds for at least 8 weeks. Twisting movements are to be avoided. The client cannot drive a car until the surgeon permits. Sitting should be limited during the early postoperative period; the client should either stand or lie down. Physical therapy is focused on muscle strengthening and client comfort. Heat therapy, ultrasound, and exercises are often used to promote comfort and healing.

▶ NURSING PROCESS

▶ Assessment

▶ Subjective Data

Assessment includes eliciting client statements about motor and sensory function, pain, and effectiveness of comfort measures.

▶ Objective Data

Assessment entails a neurological evaluation of motor and sensory function of the extremities innervated below the herniated area. Reflex testing may be a part of the nursing assessment in some facilities. Range of motion (ROM) of the affected extremity is assessed. The nurse assesses the client's knowledge about the disease process, the planned treatment including pain management and surgery, and the postsurgical care. Status of bowel and bladder elimination is assessed for potential nerve involvement or effects of immobility. Gait alteration and limited bending should also be noted.

Nursing diagnoses for a client with a herniated intervertebral disk may include the following:

Nursing Diagnoses	Planning/Goals	Nursing Interventions
▶ *Pain related to nerve compression or surgical intervention*	The client will experience increased comfort.	Assess pain intensity and location, as well as activities or position when pain began. Have the client rate pain on a scale of 1 to 10.
		Maintain activity level as ordered by physician.
		Place client in position of comfort, usually on back, with knees slightly flexed and a small pillow beneath head, or on unaffected side, with affected extremity flexed and a pillow between the legs.
		Maintain immobility of vertebrae with corset, brace, or traction.
		Apply moist heat as prescribed and administer medications to relieve pain, relax muscles, and relieve inflammation and anxiety, as ordered. Document effectiveness.
		Provide diversional activities.
▶ *Physical Mobility, Impaired, related to nerve compression or surgical intervention*	The client will have no complications of immobility.	Assess for complications of immobility.
		Turn client every 1 to 2 hours. The client will tend to limit position to one of comfort.
		Assist the client to log roll, that is, move the body as a unit without twisting the back.
		Ambulate as ordered by the physician.

Evaluation Each goal must be evaluated to determine how it has been met by the client.

SPINAL CORD INJURY

Spinal cord injury (SCI) occurs from trauma to the spinal cord or from compression of the spinal cord due to injury to the supporting structures. Each year, almost 10,000 new spinal cord injuries occur. Most of the victims are males between the ages of 16 and 30 years. Leading causes of injury are motor vehicle acci-

dents; acts of violence; falls; and sporting accidents (Beare & Meyers, 1998; Hickey, 1997; National Spinal Cord Injury Statistical Center, 1998).

Numerous classification systems exist for SCIs. Spinal cord injuries may be classified by level of injury, mechanism of injury, or neurological or functional level (Figure 41-16). The injury may be considered complete or incomplete. When injury is complete, no

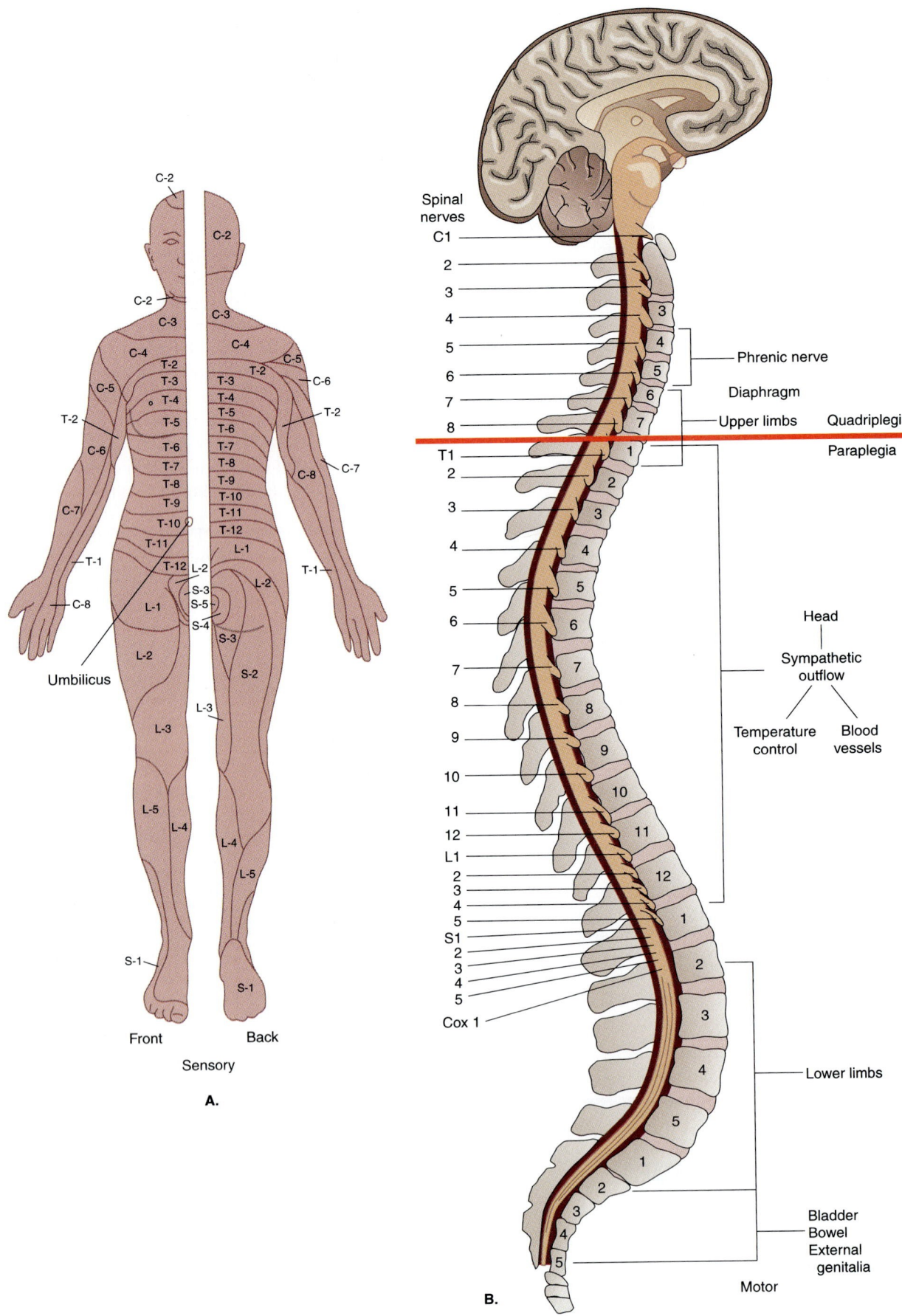

Figure 41-16 Spinal Cord—Levels of Injury: A. Areas of sensory function; B. Areas of motor function

impulses are carried below the level of injury. There is complete disruption of the spinal cord functions including motor (voluntary) movement, sensation, and reflexes to areas innervated by the spinal nerves at and below the level of the injury. In an incomplete injury, some of the spinal cord tracts are affected while others are able to carry impulses normally.

The mechanism of injury is usually an acceleration–deceleration event that causes hyperflexion, hyperextension, axial loading, or excessive rotation injury (Hickey, 1997). Hyperflexion is the extreme forward movement of the head, which causes compression of the vertebral bodies and damage to the posterior ligaments and intervertebral disks. Hyperextension is the extreme backward movement of the head, causing injury to the posterior vertebral structures and the anterior ligaments. Axial loading or compression occurs when extreme pressure is placed on the spinal column, such as in diving accidents or falls landed on feet or buttocks. Compression of the vertebrae causes shattering of the vertebral body. Compression fractures and posterior ligament injury can also be caused by excessive rotation, or turning the head beyond the normal range.

Classification of injury by cause includes concussion, contusion, laceration, transection, hemorrhage, or damage to blood vessels supplying the spinal cord. Immediately following injury to the spinal cord, an autodestructive process begins, with chemical and vascular changes that lead to ischemia and necrosis of the spinal cord.

Spinal shock (cessation of motor, sensory, autonomic, and reflex impulses) and **areflexia** (the absence of reflexes) occur immediately upon transection of the spinal cord or upon injury to the spinal cord. Flaccid paralysis of all skeletal muscles; loss of spinal reflexes; loss of sensation; and absence of autonomic function below the level of injury also occur. The diaphragm is innervated at levels C3 through C5. Injuries in this area cause partial or complete disruption of respiratory function. The client does not perspire below the level of the injury. Bowel and bladder function may be lost either for a few days to months, or permanently, though this loss generally lasts from 1 to 6 weeks.

As spinal shock resolves, reflex activity returns below the level of injury. The client with a lower motor neuron injury continues to experience flaccid paralysis, areflexia, hypotonic bowel and bladder function, and sexual dysfunction. Lower motor neuron injury causes paraplegia, or paralysis of lower extremities.

Neurogenic shock, a hypotensive situation resulting from the loss of sympathetic control of vital functions from the brain, may occur during spinal shock. This happens in clients with injury above the sixth thoracic vertebra. The client develops orthostatic hypotension, bradycardia, decreased cardiac output, loss of ability to sweat below the level of injury, and subnormal temperature.

Upper motor neuron injury results in spastic paralysis, loss of voluntary skeletal muscle movement, and reflexive bowel, bladder, and sexual responses. Complete upper motor neuron injury results in **quadriplegia**, or dysfunction or paralysis of both arms, both legs, bowel, and bladder. Injuries above C5 affect respiratory function because of innervation of the diaphragm and accessory respiratory muscles. Mechanical ventilation is required to keep the client alive. Fractures below the cervical vertebrae result in diaphragmatic breathing, if the phrenic nerve is functioning.

The client with an injury above the sixth thoracic vertebra is at risk for developing autonomic dysreflexia or autonomic hyperreflexia. Autonomic dysreflexia is an emergency situation resulting in a hypertensive crisis and possibly stroke or seizure activity. The cause is noxious stimuli such as a full bladder, a fecal impaction, a wrinkle in clothing, menstrual cramps, an erection, an ingrown toenail, a bladder infection, or sitting on catheter tubing. Autonomic reflexes below the level of the injury cause vasoconstriction in this area. The controlling impulses from the higher cortical levels do not transmit past the level of injury but cause bradycardia and vasodilatation above the level of injury. Skin above the level of injury is warm and moist, but skin below the level of injury is cold, with goose flesh (Beare & Meyers, 1998; Hickey, 1997; Latham, 1994).

The noxious stimuli must be removed, if possible, and the client placed in a sitting position immediately. Blood pressure must be assessed immediately and monitored every few minutes until within normal limits (Huston & Boelman, 1995). The drug of choice, nitroprusside sodium (Nipride), may be given if the conservative measure does not work. Autonomic dysreflexia must be prevented when possible, recognized when it develops, and treated immediately. Once autonomic dysreflexia is relieved, the client may develop hypotension from the decreased sympathetic response and the residual effects of medication and positioning changes. A pattern of individual response to stimuli and of sympathetic response is soon identified for the client. However, the client with an upper motor neuron injury above T-6 is always at risk for developing autonomic dysreflexia. Some clients experience the first episode years after the injury.

The extent of permanent injury cannot be determined immediately, because of necrosis, edema, and spinal shock. Functional loss depends on the level, degree, and type of injury.

Medical–Surgical Management

Medical

Medical management of the client with spinal cord injury begins prior to reaching the hospital. Further damage to the spinal cord is prevented by immobilizing the head, neck, and vertebral column with devices such as rigid cervical collars and splinting backboards. All trauma clients are treated as potential spinal cord injuries. When the client reaches the emergency room, x-rays of the spine are taken prior to removing the immobilizing devices.

Respiratory function is continuously assessed, and ventilatory support is provided as necessary. The client may have multiple injuries, necessitating astute diagnostic skills by the emergency room physician. Assessment of the trauma client must involve evaluating for internal hemorrhaging, cardiac contusion, head injury, hemorrhagic shock, and spinal shock resulting from the spinal cord injury. A thorough assessment is done to specifically evaluate the degree of deficit and to establish the level or degree of injury.

Immobilization of the spinal cord continues to be the focus of care during early medical management of the client. Traction may be used to maintain alignment of the spinal column. Cervical tongs and halo devices are used to apply traction and to immobilize the cervical spine. Under local anesthesia, cervical tongs and halo rings are applied with spring-loaded pins that are embedded into the scalp. Antiseptic solution is used to cleanse the scalp, and a local anesthetic is injected into the insertion sites. Traction weights are applied to the cervical tongs or halo rings after the insertion pins are firmly embedded (Figure 41-17). Body casts, jackets, or braces are used to immobilize thoracic and lumbar fractures.

Surgical

Surgical interventions are performed for decompression, realignment, and stabilization of the vertebral column, depending on the nature of the injury. A laminectomy may be performed to decompress the spinal cord with fusion or placement of Harrington rods to stabilize the vertebral column. Realignment is maintained by surgical manipulation of the vertebral column.

If the client has respiratory involvement, an endotracheal tube is put in place to provide mechanical ventilatory support. Following urgent treatment, a tracheostomy will be performed to continue ventilation.

Pharmacological

Steroid therapy with dexamethasone (Decadron) is administered to prevent and reduce edema in the injured spinal cord (Drucker & Zeidman, 1994). To decrease and prevent edema and to improve blood flow, high loading doses of the steroid methylprednisolone sodium succinate (Solu-Medrol) are given immediately, with tapering dosages being given over the next 1 to 2 weeks. Mannitol, an osmotic diuretic, may be administered to decrease and prevent cord edema (Laskowski-Jones, 1993). Hydralazine hydrochloride

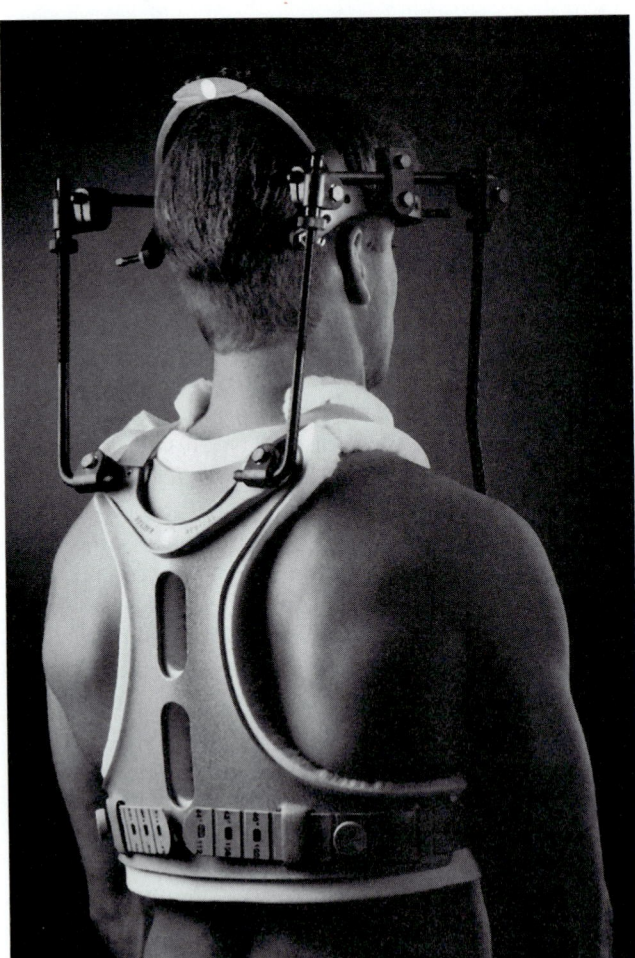

Figure 41-17 Halo Vest *(Courtesy of Depuy AcroMed)*

(Apresoline) or nifedipine (Procardia) is frequently ordered to reduce blood pressure in cases of autonomic dysreflexia.

Activity

Initially, immobilization of the spinal column is necessary. In the acute phase, ROM for all joints is performed to prevent mobility loss and muscle contracture. As the spine is stabilized, the client's activity progresses to sitting up in a chair, performing strengthening exercises, and increasing endurance. The nurse must observe for the complication of orthostatic hypotension.

Orthostatic hypotension is caused by the venous pooling of blood in the lower body and extremities resulting from impairment of the sympathetic nervous system. The client becomes hypotensive and develops bradycardia and syncope. Asystole may even occur (Laskowski-Jones, 1993). To maintain mean arterial pressure (MAP) between 80 and 90 mm Hg and to improve spinal cord perfusion during the acute phase, vasopressor agents such as dopamine hydrochloride (Intropin) are given. Prevention of orthostatic hypotension also requires the application of full leg support stockings and pneumatic boots and the gradual lowering of the lower extremities. The client's vital signs are monitored throughout the mobilization process to ascertain tolerance to the procedure.

After spinal shock has subsided, active rehabilitation begins, with the interdisciplinary team optimizing the functional capabilities of the client. The physical therapist plays a major role in the activity level; the occupational therapist, in ADL; and the speech therapist, in swallowing ability and communications.

Other Therapies

An interdisciplinary approach is used for rehabilitation. Rehabilitation begins immediately, with a focus on preventing disabilities and maximizing and strengthening remaining functional ability. Neurological function can be regained for up to 1 year.

▶ NURSING PROCESS

▶ Assessment

▶ Subjective Data

Subjective assessment involves eliciting input from the client regarding sensation, pain, and history of the accident. How the client is coping with the injury, the resulting disability, and the major lifestyle changes that have occurred should all be noted. How the family or support system is coping with the changes is also evaluated.

▶ Objective Data

In the acute phase of care of the client with a spinal cord injury, nursing assessment focuses on the critical factors of airway, breathing, circulation, disability, and exposure (Laskowski-Jones, 1993).

Assessment of circulatory status involves monitoring vital signs and observing for complications of neurogenic shock; orthostatic hypotension; hypertensive episodes of autonomic dysreflexia; and hemorrhaging.

Disability is assessed by performing a baseline neurological assessment (as described under the Components of Neurological Assessment section in this chapter).

Exposure refers to removing the client's clothing to perform a thorough assessment of the client's body for skin condition and for entrance and exit wounds. Body temperature must be monitored because of the neurological deficit in temperature regulation as caused by dysfunction of the autonomic nervous system.

Subacute assessment is based on the level of injury and neurological functioning of the client. With upper motor neuron injuries, the client is at higher risk of developing autonomic dysreflexia; thus, assessment includes monitoring for these signs.

All clients with spinal cord injury are assessed for skin condition, bowel and bladder function, respiratory status, and signs and symptoms of complications of immobility. Psychosocial assessment is also very important to the well-being of the client.

Nursing diagnoses for the client with a spinal cord injury in the subacute phase of care may include the following:

Nursing Diagnoses	Planning/Goals	Nursing Interventions
▶ *Injury, Risk for, related to motor and sensory deficits secondary to spinal fractures*	The client will not experience additional injury.	Assess the client's risk factors for additional injury.
		Monitor skin condition for pressure areas or shearing injuries from sliding across sheets or the mats in physical therapy.
		Turn client frequently to prevent pressure areas.
		Use enough personnel to turn client correctly to maintain alignment of client's spinal column.
		Provide call light that client can operate; teach to call nurse for assistance as necessary.
		Reinforce wheelchair safety factors and observe client for use of wheelchair.
		Prevent falls when transferring client to wheelchair.
		Prevent foot drop.
		Provide passive and active ROM exercises.
		Maintain adequate fluid intake and nutrition.
		Provide routine care for halo device by opening vest on one side to cleanse skin under vest at least daily and to assess for skin breakdown. Repeat procedure on the other side.
		Monitor pin sites of halo device every shift for placement.
		Perform pin site care using facility protocol.

continued

Nursing Diagnoses	Planning/Goals	Nursing Interventions
▶ *Powerlessness related to changes in motor and sensory function and in lifestyle*	The client will make decisions regarding care, treatment, and future.	Explain all procedures and care options.
		Establish an open, trusting relationship with client to foster therapeutic communication.
		Allow time for client to express concerns, anger, and fears.
		Foster a positive environment for client to explore feelings and accept disability.
		Allow client to participate in care decisions.
		Assess for signs and symptoms of depression.
		Collaborate with mental health professional to provide assistance in coping with lifestyle changes.
		Collaborate with family and support people to include them in the plan of care.
▶ *Dysreflexia related to noxious stimulation secondary to overstimulation of autonomic nervous system*	The client will state factors that cause autonomic dysreflexia, describe treatment, and notify the nurse if experiencing symptoms of dysreflexia.	Teach client causes and symptoms of autonomic dysreflexia: increased blood pressure, sudden throbbing headache, chills, pallor, goose flesh, nausea, and/or metallic taste in mouth.
		Prevent bladder distention and fecal impaction by implementing a bowel and bladder training program.
		Observe for bradycardia, vasodilatation, flushing, and diaphoresis above the level of spinal cord injury. If these symptoms occur, immediately notify the physician and administer medications as ordered to decrease blood pressure. Raise head of bed and lower legs to reduce blood pressure. Then, remove the noxious stimuli, which may include constrictive clothing, shoes, splints, or linens.
		Assess client for a distended bladder and empty the bladder if distended.
		Observe urine for signs of infection and obtain a urine specimen for culture, if needed to identify the cause of the reaction.
		Check for fecal impaction using xylocaine viscous per physician's order to decrease stimulation.
		Monitor blood pressure every few minutes.

Evaluation Each goal must be evaluated to determine how it has been met by the client.

PARKINSON'S DISEASE

Parkinson's disease is a chronic, progressive, degenerative disease affecting the area of the brain controlling movement. The cause is unknown in most cases, but toxicity, hypoxia, or encephalitis may precede the onset of Parkinson's disease. Vascular and genetic factors have been implicated. Drugs such as cocaine, reserpine (Serpasil), haloperidol (Haldol), and chlorpromazine (Thorazine) may cause a parkinsonian syndrome. The theory is that these drugs interfere with the synthesis or storage of dopamine.

Typical signs and symptoms of Parkinson's Disease are muscular rigidity, **bradykinesia** (slowness of voluntary movement and speech), resting tremors, muscular weakness, and loss of postural reflexes. Muscular rigidity along with bradykinesia impairs the person's ability to perform daily activities and speech.

Rigidity is noted along with increased muscle tone when the client is at rest. Stiffness of the trunk, head, and shoulders is present. The rigidity causes loss of arm swing when walking. A cogwheel phenomenon results from the muscle contractions breaking through the muscular rigidity. The alternating rigidity and rhythmic contractions causes a jerking-like movement. Motor impairment progressively affects facial expressions, eye blink, and voice, causing a typical presentation of a mask-like face and a monotone voice.

Resting tremors, usually in the upper extremities, are present when the hand is motionless. The hand moves in a "pill-rolling" motion. When the client is moving or sleeping, the tremors are usually absent. Tremors also occur in other areas including the feet, lip, tongue, or jaw. The tremors usually begin unilaterally in one area and progress to other areas and then to the opposite side of the body. Anxiety and concentration tend to increase the degree of tremors.

The posture and gait of people with Parkinson's disease is characterized by bowed head, forward-bent trunk, drooped shoulders, and flexed arms. The gait is characterized by shuffling movement and small steps. Balance is affected, resulting in a tendency to fall forward. Figure 41-18 shows the classic posture of a client with Parkinson's disease.

Autonomic dysfunction includes drooling, **dysphagia** (difficulty swallowing), excessive sweating, hyperactivity of oil glands, and constipation. Orthostatic hypotension may occur from loss of the peripheral autonomic response. Urinary incontinence and frequency occur.

Mental changes may also occur. Intelligence is not impaired, but problems with judgment and emotional stability may occur. Dementia is present 10% to 15% of the time. Depression frequently accompanies Parkinson's disease. Depression may occur from the chemical changes in dopamine level or in reaction to the disorder. Cognitive, perceptual, or memory deficits may occur. The major cause of death is from the complications of immobility or injury. Fatigue increases all signs and symptoms. Since there is no diagnostic test specific for Parkinson's disease, diagnosis is made from clinical signs and symptoms. In cases of early onset, it is important to differentiate from Wilson's disease, which is an increased absorption of copper, for which testing is available.

Medical–Surgical Management

Medical

The goals of medical management are to control the symptoms, provide supportive therapy and maintenance, maintain function via physiotherapy, and provide psychotherapy as necessary.

Surgical

Stereotactic thalamotomy, a surgical procedure to disrupt the transmission of motor impulses, is occasionally used to treat the tremors and muscular rigidity. This invasive procedure does not treat the disease, but, rather, alleviates the tremors.

Pharmacological

Drug therapy is used to control the symptoms of Parkinson's disease. L-dihydroxyphenylalanine (L-Dopa) is converted into dopamine in the basal ganglia to replace the deficit of dopamine. Dopamine itself is not given orally because it is metabolized before reaching the brain. L-Dopa, a precursor to dopamine, is given orally and reaches the brain to be converted into dopamine.

Dopadecarboxylase inhibitors such as carbidopa-levodopa (Sinemet) prevent the conversion of L-Dopa to dopamine in peripheral tissue. Dopamine in the peripheral tissue can cause numerous side effects as well as decrease the amount of L-dopa available to the brain. Dopadecarboxylase inhibitors that do not cross the blood–brain barrier are used to inhibit the enzyme that changes L-dopa to dopamine so that the conversion in the brain is not inhibited.

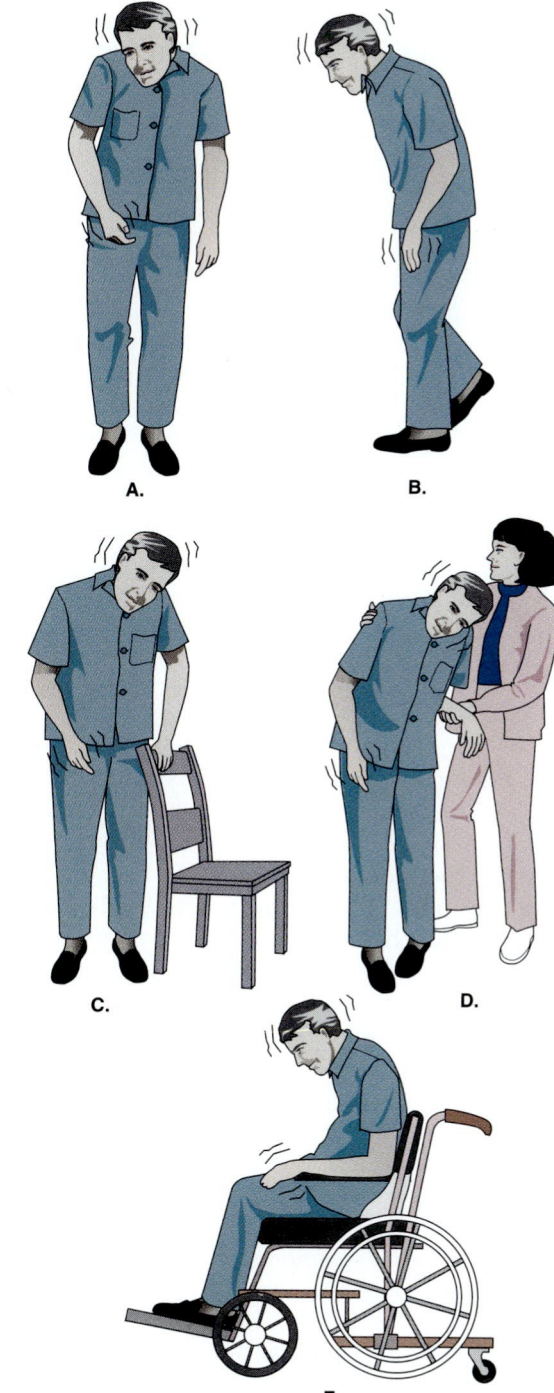

Figure 41-18 Progression of Parkinson's Disease: A. Flexion of affected arm; B. Shuffling gait; C. Need for sources of support to prevent falling; D. Progression of weakness to point of needing assistance for ambulation; E. Profound weakness

Anticholinergic drugs such as trihexyphenidyl hydrochloride (Artane), cycrimine hydrochloride (Pagitane hydrochloride), and benztropine mesylate (Cogentin), are administered to control tremors and rigidity. Anticholinergics are used alone for mild symptoms or if L-dopa is contraindicated. In other instances, they may be administered in conjunction with L-dopa.

PROFESSIONAL TIP

Pallidotomy

Pallidotomy, an operation of the 1950s for Parkinson's disease, is being used again. Improved surgical equipment and clients who no longer benefit from medications are causing a resurgence in the use of pallidotomy.

Using MRI and stereotactic equipment, the physician can pinpoint the area of the brain that is causing the unwanted symptoms. A probe is then inserted into the brain through a small hole in the client's head. A small lesion is made deep in the brain to interrupt the electrical pathways that cause the rigidity and tremors. The surgery relieves symptoms but does not cure Parkinson's disease. Furthermore, associated risks such as paralysis and bleeding must be considered (Raine, 1997).

Amantadine hydrochloride (Symmetrel), an antiviral agent, is effective in treating Parkinsonian symptoms. The mechanism by which the drug works is not known, but the theory is that it either releases dopamine storage areas or delays the reuptake of dopamine

Ethopropazine hydrochloride (Parsidol), a phenothiazine derivative, is used in combination with other anti-Parkinson drugs to alleviate symptoms. Dopamine agonist-ergot derivatives, such as pergolide mesylate (Permax), directly stimulate the dopamine receptors to improve the use of available dopamine. The monoamine oxidase (MAO) inhibitor selegiline hydrochloride (Eldepryl) inhibits dopamine breakdown. The tricyclic antidepressants amitriptyline hydrochloride (Elavil) and imipramine hydrochloride (Tofranil) alleviate depression as well as other symptoms.

Diet

Pureed foods or tube feedings may be required because of dysphagia. Maintenance of weight may require high- or low-calorie diets. A diet that discourages formation of free radicals is being researched as a deterrent to progression of the disease. Free-radical formation is thought to be discouraged by diets high in complex carbohydrates (such as those found in whole grain breads and lentils), low in fat, and high in vitamins A and E. Large doses of supplemental vitamins A and E are also given. A high-fiber diet will help in preventing constipation.

PROFESSIONAL TIP

Drug Therapy for Parkinson's Disease

- Numerous side effects, such as blurred vision, drowsiness, disorientation, and delirium may be noted.
- Dosage requirements vary greatly among individuals.
- Symptom control varies in the same individual from day to day.
- To maintain a constant therapeutic level for better symptom control, Sinemet solution may be ordered hourly while the client is awake.

Safety: Mealtime

The client with Parkinson's disease must be monitored for choking while eating because of dysphagia.

Activity

Ambulation with assistance is necessary to maintain joint mobility and to prevent injury. The client should not be hurried, as the bradykinesia becomes worse when the client is attempting to hurry.

Other Therapies

Physical therapy is directed toward the maintenance of joint mobility, posture, and gait. Occupational therapy focuses on maintaining optimal functioning in achieving ADL. Speech therapy is used to promote

HOME HEALTH CARE

Adaptations for the Client with Parkinson's Disease

- Arrange for bathroom facilities and bedroom on first floor
- Remove crepe- or rubber-soled shoes from the client, as they may drag on the floor, especially on carpeting
- Remove throw rugs or other obstacles over which the client may trip
- Install handrails at steps and in hallways and the bathrom
- Have no highly waxed floors
- Provide assistance to client as needed

communication and maintain swallowing function. Psychotherapy addresses the implications of living with a chronic disease; depression; and the possible psychiatric side effects of the medication regimen.

▶ NURSING PROCESS

▶ Assessment

▶ Subjective Data

Nursing assessment focuses on functional ability and activities. It includes eliciting client statements about symptom control and emotional status. Bowel and bladder elimination patterns are ascertained.

▶ Objective Data

Objective assessment involves evaluation of tremors, muscular rigidity, movement, posture, and gait for degree of impairment. Assessment of swallowing ability is necessary to maintain adequate nutrition and prevent aspiration. Mental/emotional status is evaluated for signs and symptoms of depression or dementia.

Skin is assessed for diaphoresis, or excessive oil production; skin integrity; and signs of injury from falls. Supine, sitting, and standing blood pressures are obtained to assess for orthostatic hypotension.

CLIENT TEACHING

Parkinson's Disease

Advise caregivers to:

- Encourage the client to be as independent as possible,
- Protect the client from injury, and
- Protect the client from unnecessary stress and fatigue.

Advise the client to:

- Use adaptive devices (cane, walker, feeding utensils),
- Take medications at scheduled times to maintain level in the body,
- Avoid taking multivitamins, foods high in vitamin B₆, and high-protein foods when taking L-dopa,
- Prevent constipation by drinking plenty of water and, possibly, using a stool softener, and
- Have intraocular pressure measured frequently if client has glaucoma.

Nursing diagnoses for a client with Parkinson's disease may include the following:

Nursing Diagnoses	Planning/Goals	Nursing Interventions
▶ *Physical Mobility, Impaired, related to muscle rigidity, gait disturbance, and bradykinesia*	The client will maintain optimal mobility.	Assess degree of muscle involvement by testing ROM, muscular rigidity, tremors, and gait.
		Administer medications within the time window that provides a constant therapeutic level for symptom control.
		Perform passive and active ROM exercises to maintain function.
		Ambulate, as client is able to tolerate.
		Frequently turn client in bed.
▶ *Self-care Deficit related to immobility, tremors, and bradykinesia*	The client will maintain optimal independence in self-care.	Assess client's ability to perform self-care.
		Encourage client to perform as much self-care as possible.
		Consult with occupational therapy for methods to increase the ability to perform self-care.
		Assist with daily care that the client is unable to perform alone.
▶ *Swallowing, Impaired, related to neuromuscular impairment*	The client will swallow with minimal choking and coughing and no aspiration.	Position client sitting upright when eating.
		Position client's head slightly forward and never extended to facilitate swallowing.
		Encourage client to take small bites.
		Provide small bites of food or pureed foods to prevent client from choking.
		Have suction equipment available during meals.

Evaluation Each goal must be evaluated to determine how it has been met by the client.

MULTIPLE SCLEROSIS

Multiple sclerosis (MS) is a chronic, progressive, degenerative disease wherein scattered nerve cells of the brain and spinal cord are demyelinated. The cause of MS is unclear. Research suggests, however, that it is an immune-mediated process with a viral trigger. The disease is more prevalent in colder climates and in people who lived in colder climates before the age of 15 years. In 75% of the cases, onset of symptoms is in adults between the ages of 20 and 40 (Frozena, 1997). Women are affected slightly more often than are men.

The white matter of the brain and spinal cord consists of axons covered by a white, lipid substance called myelin. This myelin sheath is an insulator that is involved in the conduction of impulses.

Multiple sclerosis is a central nervous system disease characterized by a loss of myelin in the brain, spinal cord, or both and by the occurrence of **sclerotic** (hardened) patches (Figure 41-19). The disease interferes with the conduction of impulses. The neurological deficit that occurs depends on which nerve cells are affected (Frozena, 1997).

As sclerotic tissue replaces the myelin, neurological function returns. Nerve fibers begin to degenerate as periods of exacerbation become more frequent. Degeneration of the nerve fibers leads to permanent neurological deficits.

Signs and symptoms of MS vary according to the areas of demyelination. The client may have one symptom or a combination of symptoms. Periods of exacerbation and remission also make diagnosis difficult. Symptoms may vary from hour-to-hour or day-to-day. Medical diagnosis is generally based on history and on elimination of other possible diagnoses. Magnetic resonance imaging and CT scan can be used to identify lesions of sclerotic tissue as the disease progresses. Cerebrospinal fluid reveals increased white blood cells, protein, and immunoglobulin (IgG), a diagnostic indicator.

Frozena (1997) classifies client symptoms as sensory, motor, or other disturbances. Sensory symptoms

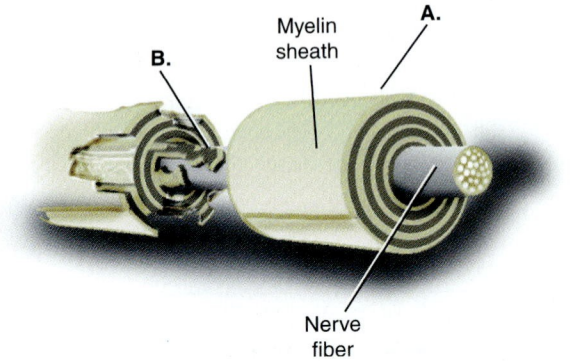

Figure 41-19 A. Normal Nerve Fiber and Myelin Sheath; B. Multiple Sclerosis Destruction of Myelin Sheath

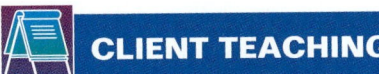

CLIENT TEACHING

Temperature Sensation

Because the client has a decreased sense of temperature, advise to:

- Be careful when cooking or otherwise around the kitchen stove,
- Use a bath thermometer to test bath or shower water so as to prevent burning, and
- Use only the low setting on a heating pad.

may include visual disturbances, numbness, paresthesia (burning, prickling, tingling), pain, and decreased sense of temperature. Motor symptoms may include decreased muscle strength, spasticity, paralysis, or bowel and bladder incontinence or retention.

Ataxia (loss of balance or coordination), **nystagmus** (constant, involuntary eye movements in any direction), speech disturbances, tremors, and **vertigo** (dizziness) may occur. Other possible symptoms are sexual dysfunction and mood changes ranging from depression to euphoria. Profound fatigue is common.

Exacerbations are frequently precipitated by periods of emotional or physical stress, such as infections, pregnancy, trauma, or fatigue. Hot baths or strenuous exercise may aggravate motor symptoms. Periods of exacerbation may last hours to months. Commonly, the periods of exacerbation become more frequent as the disease progresses. Complications such as urinary tract infection, pneumonia, pressure ulcers, contractures, and depression frequently occur. As the disease progresses and permanent neurological deficits occur, the client may become bedridden, have difficulty speaking and handling oral secretions, and/or develop emotional and intellectual disturbances.

Medical–Surgical Management

There is no cure or specific treatment for MS. Treatment goals are to limit exacerbations, prevent complications, and maintain functional level.

Pharmacological

According to Rudick (1997), the treatment of choice for relapsing–remitting MS is interferon beta (Avonex, Betaseron). For 2 or 3 months, clients usually experience flu-like symptoms after each injection. For clients who cannot take either of these two drugs, glatiramer acetate (Copaxone) is an option. The steroids adrenocorticotropic hormone (ACTH) or prednisone (Delasone) are used to decrease periods of exacerbation. Muscle relaxants such as dantrolene sodium (Dantrium) or baclofen (Lioresal) are used for muscle spasticity.

The immunosuppressive agents azathioprine (Imuran), cyclophosphamide (Cytoxan), or cyclosporine (Sandimmune) are administered to decrease immune response. Propantheline bromide (ProBanthine) is often used for urinary frequency and urgency. Bethanechol chloride (Urecholine) may be helpful for the client with a neurogenic bladder. Trimethoprim sulfamethoxazole (Bactrim or Septra) or nitrofurantoin macrocrystals (Macrodantin) is given prophylactically when urinary tract infections are a problem.

Diet

A well-balanced diet complete with roughage is necessary to promote bowel elimination. Plenty of fluids are also necessary. If the client is obese, a dietitian should be consulted for meal planning to help the client lose weight while maintaining adequate nutrition.

Activity

The goal of maintaining the highest possible functional level must be individualized to each client. Daily exercise is necessary for clients with limited motor involvement. Physical therapy may be necessary to prevent contractures, maintain muscle strength, or prevent loss of function from spasticity, or for gait training. Passive/active ROM exercises should be done several times per day. Occupational therapy may be used to maintain or attain self-care. Daily skills of cooking, doing laundry, or maintaining a job may also be encouraged.

▶ NURSING PROCESS

▶ Assessment

▶ Subjective Data

Subjective assessment includes eliciting client statements of symptoms and an historical accounting of exacerbations and remissions. Subjective data should

HOME HEALTH CARE

Adaptive Devices

To assist the client in self-care:

- Purchase a raised toilet seat,
- Use a long-handled comb and shoe horn, and
- Modify clothing so that the client can dress self.

CLIENT TEACHING

Risk of Falling

Advise the client to:

- Use assistive devices such as a walker or cane,
- Wear high-topped (above the ankles) shoes, with laces, and
- Watch feet when walking so as to know where they are.

include incidence of visual disturbances, hazy vision, loss of central vision, or diplopia (double vision). Symptoms of weakness, numbness, fatigue, bowel or bladder problems, sexual dysfunction, emotional instability, vertigo, changes in gait, urinary incontinence or retention, constipation, or difficulty swallowing must all be noted. Pain is not common.

▶ Objective Data

Objective assessment includes observation of gait for spastic or ataxic gait and a complete neurological examination.

Nursing diagnoses for a client with MS may include the following:

Nursing Diagnoses	Planning/Goals	Nursing Interventions
▶ *Physical Mobility, Impaired, related to muscle weakness, ataxia, spasticity, or perceptual impairment*	The client will maintain optimal mobility within physical limitations.	Assess motor status every 4 to 24 hours.
		Provide active and passive ROM every 8 hours.
		Turn bedridden clients every 2 hours.
		Use pillows, splints, high-topped (above the ankles) shoes with laces to maintain proper body alignment.
		Encourage client to perform daily activities as able given the limitations of the disease.
		Ambulate client four times daily with use of assistive devices as necessary.
▶ *Urinary Elimination, Altered, related to changes in innervation of the bladder*	The client will have adequate bladder elimination with minimal post-void residual, urinary tract infections, and episodes of incontinence.	Assess for bladder retention or incontinence.
		Maintain fluid intake of 1,000 cc/day.
		Catheterize as necessary for retention or post-void residual.

continued

Nursing Diagnoses	Planning/Goals	Nursing Interventions
		Develop bladder program to meet individual needs of client. Toilet client at scheduled times even if no urge to go.
		Assess for signs and symptoms of urinary tract infection, such as elevated temperature and burning on urination.
▶ *Self-esteem Disturbance related to neuromuscular and perceptual impairment*	The client will verbalize positive statements of self-esteem.	Assess client's concept of self in relation to changes brought about by the disease process.
		Allow client to verbalize feelings.
		Assist client in methods of adapting to change.
		Collaborate with other health care providers, such as mental health counselors and physicians.
		Teach client about the disease process.
		Refer client to local support groups (see Resources).
▶ *Sexual Dysfunction related to changes in sensation, genitalia, and musculature, and psychological response to diagnosis*	The client will seek counseling concerning sexual dysfunction.	Allow client to verbalize concerns.
		Suggest adaptations (planning time for sexual contact so as to conserve energy, alternatives to sexual intercourse, such as touching or holding).
		Refer client to appropriate health care providers.

Evaluation Each goal must be evaluated to determine how it has been met by the client.

SAMPLE NURSING CARE PLAN

THE CLIENT WITH MULTIPLE SCLEROSIS

Mrs. Donna Britton, a 37-year-old wife and the mother of two children, ages 3 years and 5 years, was diagnosed with MS two days ago. She presents with decreased sensation (paresthesia) in the lower extremities and muscle weakness of the right lower extremity. She has also experienced episodes of loss of central vision. Fatigue has affected her ability to care for her children and perform household tasks. She states, "I do not know what is going to happen to me." She is crying and states, "I do not know about multiple sclerosis or how I am going to take care of my children," and "I cannot get my housework done, and my children need more from me than I can give right now."

Her employer is concerned about her ability to perform her teaching responsibilities, but because he values her excellence as a teacher, he is willing to give her a few weeks off. She has bruises on her thigh, face, and arm from a fall that she experienced several days ago. The client presents in an outpatient clinic for follow-up care.

Nursing Diagnosis 1 *Knowledge Deficit related to disease process and lifestyle changes as evidenced by client statements, "I do not know what is going to happen to me, I do not know about multiple sclerosis or how I am going to take care of my children"*

PLANNING/GOALS	NURSING INTERVENTIONS	RATIONALE	EVALUATION
Mrs. Britton will verbalize knowledge of the disease process, pathophysiology, prognosis, and treatment, including the need to reduce stressors in her life, eat	Assess Mrs. Britton's knowledge of diagnosis, treatment regimen, and lifestyle changes. Ask specific questions.	Building on the knowledge base that Mrs. Britton already has provides a frame of reference for Mrs. Britton, helping her to relate new information and	Mrs. Britton verbalizes accurate information regarding the disease process, prognosis, and treatment. She states that by reducing

continued

a balanced diet, drink adequate fluids, and get adequate rest.

Begin teaching information about the pathophysiology and signs and symptoms of MS.

Discuss lifestyle changes that need to be made, such as planning rest periods, avoiding stressors, eating a balanced diet, and drinking plenty of fluids.

Emphasize the importance of keeping a diary of symptoms, activities, and overall feelings in order to identify stressors that exacerbate symptoms.

Provide information about the Multiple Sclerosis Society and offer available pamphlets. Provide the name and telephone number of a contact from the local MS support group or of another client who is willing to share.

integrate it into her behavior.

By keeping a diary of symptoms, activities, and overall feelings, Mrs. Britton can identify activities that exacerbate the symptoms.

Written material and contact with a national organization can provide more resources to strengthen Mrs. Britton's knowledge base.

Having an individual or support group with whom to discuss similar concerns can provide a great deal of emotional support as well as practical solutions to problems.

stressors, maintaining a balanced diet, taking in adequate fluids, and obtaining plenty of rest, she can prevent exacerbations of MS.

Nursing Diagnosis 2 *Home Maintenance Management, Impaired, related to fatigue, neuromuscular impairment, and difficulty in performing child care and household tasks as evidenced by client statements, "I cannot keep my housework done, my children need more from me than I can give right now" and by objective data including decreased sensation in lower extremities, muscle weakness, and fatigue*

PLANNING/GOALS	**NURSING INTERVENTIONS**	**RATIONALE**	**EVALUATION**
By the next appointment, Mrs. Britton will identify concerns and solutions to accomplishing home maintenance management.	Allow Mrs. Britton to verbalize concerns about home maintenance management.	By verbalizing fears and concerns, Mrs. Britton can begin to plan to organize tasks and responsibilities within her ability to perform home maintenance management.	Mrs. Britton identifies that she is able to care for her children with the assistance of her husband and her mother, but that she does not have the strength to maintain the housekeeping responsi-
	Assist Mrs. Britton in identifying areas of	Mrs. Britton can investigate methods of solving	

continued

concern, items that can be delegated, and possible solutions.

her home maintenance problems once she identifies concerns and explores possible solutions.

bilities. Following further discussion of family commitments and availability of social supports, Mrs. Britton agrees to request weekly assistance from the women's group at her church.

Assess the extended family's ability to assist with home maintenance management.

Assisting Mrs. Britton in assessment of extended family's ability to assist with home maintenance management may uncover opportunities that she had not considered.

Ask Mrs. Britton to start identifying ways to decrease workload and to set priorities in expending energy.

Setting priorities helps Mrs. Britton focus on needed changes.

Collaborate with social services to identify social agencies that can be of assistance.

Exploration of available resources gives Mrs. Britton other possible solutions to achieving home maintenance management.

Plan activities around rest periods.

Planned rest periods can conserve Mrs. Britton's strength and prevent fatigue.

Identify peak energy times and plan activities with peak energy in mind.

Mrs. Britton can accomplish more by using peak energy times to perform responsibilities.

Nursing Diagnosis 3 *Injury, Risk for, related to muscle weakness, decreased sensory perceptual deficits (vision, tactile, kinesthetic), and fatigue as evidenced by recent falls*

PLANNING/GOALS	NURSING INTERVENTIONS	RATIONALE	EVALUATION
Mrs. Britton will remain free of injury.	Teach Mrs. Britton to identify risk factors in the environment.	Mrs. Britton can avoid injury by recognizing and preventing environmental risk factors.	Injuries have been prevented by increasing Mrs. Britton's awareness of the risks involved with the disease process.
	Teach Mrs. Britton to identify risk factors of the disease process.	Mrs. Britton can reduce her risk of injury by identifying risk factors associated with the disease process, such as decreased sensation, weakness in the legs, and visual deficits.	

continued

Teach Mrs. Britton to avoid hot baths, hot tubs, saunas, and so on, because muscle weakness and paraesthesia can be exacerbated by the heat.	By avoiding hot baths, hot tubs, saunas, and so on, Mrs. Britton can prevent exacerbation of weakness and decreased sensation, thereby reducing her risk of injury.
Teach safety factors of wearing well-fitting, oxford-style shoes.	Wearing well-fitting tie shoes decreases the risk of falling by providing support for feet.

AMYOTROPHIC LATERAL SCLEROSIS (LOU GEHRIG'S DISEASE)

Amyotrophic lateral sclerosis (ALS) is a progressive, fatal disease characterized by the degeneration of motor neurons in the cortex, medulla, and spinal cord. The cause of the disease is not known, but a viral–immune response is suggested by current research. A genetic defect is also being researched. Age at onset is 40 to 70 years; men are affected two to three times more often than are women. Average time from onset to death is 3 years, but some have remained active 10 to 20 years after diagnosis.

The upper and lower motor neurons degenerate and deteriorate, causing atrophy of the muscles innervated by those neurons. The involved motor neurons are in the anterior horns of the spinal cord and lower brain stem. The muscles of the hands, forearms, and legs usually atrophy first. As the disease progresses most body muscles are affected. Muscle spasticity and reduced muscle strength result when upper motor neurons are involved. Lower motor neuron involvement causes muscle flaccidity, paralysis, and muscle atrophy. Sensory and intellectual function are not af-

fected. Respiratory function, ability to communicate, and emotional lability are affected as the disease progresses. Drooling, inability to handle oral secretions, and impaired swallowing occur.

Medical–Surgical Management

There is no known cure for ALS. The focus of medical management is to treat the symptoms and to promote independence for as long as possible.

Pharmacological

Muscle relaxants including diazepam (Valium), baclofen (Lioresal), and dantrolene sodium (Dantrium) are used to reduce spasticity. Quinidine is prescribed for muscle cramping. Increased salivation is treated with trihexyphenidyl hydrochloride (Artane), clonidine hydrochloride (Catapres), or amitriptyline hydrochloride (Elavil).

Diet

A regular diet adapted to provide soft, easily chewed food is maintained as long as the client can swallow. Tube feeding may be required to prevent aspiration as chewing and swallowing difficulties arise.

Activity

Ambulation and other activities are encouraged as long as possible.

Other Therapies

Physical and occupational therapy are used to maintain ROM and independence as much as possible. Speech therapy promotes maintenance of communication skills. Mental health counseling assists individual and family coping with the fatal disease.

PROFESSIONAL TIP

Advance Directives
Before the client with ALS becomes unable to communicate, suggest some advantages of drawing up a living will or giving someone power of attorney for health care.

▶ NURSING PROCESS

▶ Assessment

▶ Subjective Data

Subjective data gathered include the client's and family's emotional status and knowledge status. The client may also indicate chewing or swallowing difficulties as well as dyspnea and fatigue.

▶ Objective Data

Objective assessment includes evaluation of muscle weakness, muscle atrophy, spasticity of upper extremities, flaccid paralysis, difficulty chewing and swallowing, and respiratory status.

Nursing diagnoses for a client with ALS may include the following:

Nursing Diagnoses	Planning/Goals	Nursing Interventions
Physical Mobility, Impaired, related to muscle atrophy, weakness, and spasticity	The client will maintain the highest possible functional ability within limitations of the disease.	Provide active and passive ROM at least twice daily. Use assistive devices to prevent contractures, for ambulation, and for muscle strengthening. Assess breath sounds for presence of congestion; skin for pressure areas; and legs for thrombophlebitis. Turn every 2 hours.
Communication, Impaired Verbal, related to weakness of muscles used for speech	The client will communicate verbally or through an alternate communication method as speech muscles deteriorate.	Prolong verbal communication with speech therapy interventions consisting of voice projection and speech devices. Develop alternate methods of communicating prior to the loss of verbal skills. Eye-blinking for "yes" and "no"; communication boards, if any arm movement remains; and computer programs can be used.
Breathing Pattern, Ineffective, related to weakness of respiratory muscles and to fatigue	The client will maintain an adequate PaO₂ level.	Assess breathing patterns frequently and observe for aspiration and the loss of the swallow reflex. Assess breath sounds every 4 to 8 hours, depending on the progress of the disease. Provide good pulmonary hygiene to prevent aspiration and pneumonia by liquifying secretions and suctioning. Turn from side to side to allow oral secretions to drain from mouth; suction oral pharynx, as necessary. Provide ventilation support, as ordered.
Powerlessness related to loss of control over life; physical dependence; and presence of a fatal disease	The client will inform significant others of wishes while still able to communicate, so as to maintain some control over decisions.	Explore client and family emotional status and coping abilities. Allow client to verbalize feelings while still able to communicate and make decisions in daily care. Promote discussion of client's wishes with family, health care team, and legal representative while client is still able to speak. Provide client education about the disease process, support groups, and counseling to provide support.

Evaluation Each goal must be evaluated to determine how it has been met by the client.

ALZHEIMER'S DISEASE

Alzheimer's disease (AD) is a progressive, degenerative neurological disease wherein brain cells are destroyed. The cerebral cortex atrophies, and neuron loss and changes within the brain cells occur. Identified risk factors are advanced age, female gender, head injury, a history of thyroid disorders, and chromosomal abnormalities.

The cause of AD is unknown. Some hypothesized causes are genetic, viral, toxic, immunologic, traumatic, biochemical, or nutritional. The neurons of the frontal and medial temporal lobes are affected, with resultant biochemical and structural changes. Characteristic physiologic changes are neurofibrillary tangles and neuritic plaques (deposits of protein), which interfere with the cells' ability to transmit impulses (Figure 41-20). These changes are found in the association areas and scattered throughout the cortex. The hippocampus, that part of the limbic system responsible for learning, memory, and emotions, is affected (Selkoe, 1992). Those cells most affected are neurons that

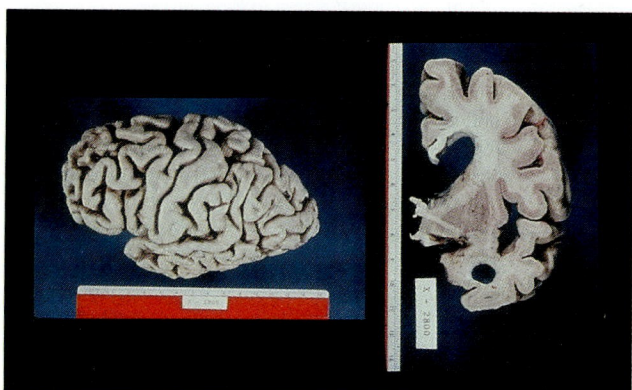

Figure 41-20 At autopsy, the cerebral cortex displays changes (white spots) caused by Alzheimer's disease. *(Photo courtesy of the Alzheimer's Association)*

use acetylcholine as the neurotransmitter. The size of the brain and the amount of acetylcholine both decrease. An increased amount of aluminum is found in the brain tissue on autopsy (Hickey, 1997; Smeltzer & Bare, 1996).

Diagnosis is difficult because of the variety in clinical manifestations and the lack of a test specific to AD. Diagnosis is thus based on the clinical picture and the exclusion of other conditions that can cause similar clinical patterns, such as overmedication, metabolic disorders, depression, thyroid imbalance, or brain tumors. Computerized tomography or MRI is used to both measure brain atrophy and rule out other conditions.

The stages of AD are scaled from early to late. Different authors identify from three to six stages of the disease. The time frame for each stage varies from person to person. Table 41-9 lists clinical manifestations of early, middle, and late stages of AD.

HOME HEALTH CARE

Safe Environment for the Client with Alzheimer's Disease

- Keep furniture in the same place
- Orient client to surroundings and reorient as necessary
- Keep floors free of clutter
- Provide adequate lighting
- Monitor temperature of hot water and food
- Maintain monitoring system to prevent outside wandering
- Prevent access to sharp items such as knives and razors; hot items such as coffee pot and heaters; poisonous solutions such as cleaning supplies, paints, medications, and insecticides; and hazardous items such as power tools, guns, and electric fans

Table 41-9 STAGES OF ALZHEIMER'S DISEASE	
STAGE	**CLINICAL MANIFESTATIONS**
Stage 1: Early	Forgetfulness, often subtle and masked by client
	Indecisiveness
	Increasing self-centeredness; decreasing interest in others, environment, social activities
	Difficulty in learning new information
	Slowed reaction time
	Beginnings of compromised performance at home and at work
Stage 2: Middle	Progressing forgetfulness, inability to remember names of family members or close friends
	Tendency to lose things
	Confusion
	Fearfulness
	Easily induced frustration and irritability; sometimes, angry outbursts
	Repetitive storytelling
	Beginnings of communication problems (inability to remember words, apparent aphasia)
	Inability to follow simple directions
	Difficulty in calculating numbers
	Beginnings of getting lost in familiar places
	Evasive or anxious interactions with others
	Physical activity (pacing, wandering)
	Changes in sleep–rest cycle (with frequent activity at night)
	Changes in eating patterns (possible constant hunger or none at all)
	Neglect of ADL and personal hygiene; changes in bowel and bladder continence; and dressing difficulties
	Inability to maintain safety without supervision
	Losses of social behaviors
	Paranoia
Stage 3: Late	Inability to communicate
	Inability to eat
	Incontinence (urine and feces)
	Inability to recognize family or friends
	Confinement to bed
	Total dependence relative to care

In late stages of the disease, EEG may indicate general slowing of brain waves. Definitive diagnosis is determined on autopsy with a brain biopsy. Though generally a disease of older people, AD does occur in people ages 40 to 50.

The family caring for a member who has Alzheimer's becomes more tied down as the disease progresses. Many clients with advanced Alzheimer's cannot be left alone. Respite care is important for the physical and mental health of the caregiver. With respite care, someone else (e.g., another family member, a friend, or a hired professional licensed practical/vocational nurse or registered nurse) comes in to care for the client with Alzheimer's while the primary caregiver gets away for a time. Respite care should be carried out on a routine basis, such as every 2 or 3 weeks or as often as is feasible.

Medical–Surgical Management

There is no curative treatment for AD. Management of the client is geared toward controlling undesirable symptoms. Other conditions such as drug reaction, depression, brain tumor, pernicious anemia, or hormonal imbalances must be ruled out.

Pharmacological

Antipsychotics, sedatives, antianxiety agents and antidepressants may be used to treat behavioral symptoms, though medications often make symptoms worse. Several medications that affect transmission of chemicals across synapses are under study. Tacrine hydrochloride (Cognex), an anticholinesterase, has demonstrated effectiveness in increasing cognitive function of clients with Alzheimer's, though there is a high incidence of liver toxicity, nausea, and vomiting with the use of this drug.

Diet

A high-fiber diet is used to prevent constipation. A high-calorie diet is needed for hyperactive clients. Frequent feedings of high nutritive value are preferable to three meals a day.

▶ NURSING PROCESS
▶ Assessment

▶ Subjective Data

Data about sleeping and eating habits must be collected. Each client must be assessed for individual signs and symptoms. The client is an expert at hiding these deficits in the early stages of the disease. A family interview may be helpful in ascertaining health and personal history.

▶ Objective Data

An objective neurological examination with particular attention to memory loss and gradual loss of thought processes and impaired judgment is important. Eating patterns, bowel and bladder control, aggressiveness, depression, ambulation, agitation, restlessness, sleep patterns, vision, and hearing should all be assessed. The client's ability to provide self-care, manage finances, drive, prepare meals, use the telephone, perform housekeeping, communicate needs, and perceive the environment also must be assessed. Attention must be directed to assessing the support system, the family caregiver, support groups, and availability of respite care for the caregiver. The care of the caregiver is often the focus of nursing care of the client with AD.

Nursing diagnoses for the client with Alzheimer's may include the following:

Nursing Diagnoses	Planning/Goals	Nursing Interventions
▶ *Injury, Risk for, related to inability to perceive danger in the environment, confusion, impaired judgment, and weakness*	The client will not experience injury.	Assess client's ability to perceive environmental hazards.
		Maintain a safe environment: eliminate clutter, position furniture/equipment in same place, monitor temperature of hot water and food, maintain monitoring system to prevent wandering into adverse climate or into traffic, provide adequate lighting, orient client and family to surroundings and reorient as necessary.
		Teach family to provide a safe home environment.
		Ensure that the client wears well-fitting tie shoes to reduce risk of falls.
▶ *Thought Processes, Altered, related to neuron degeneration, sleep deprivation*	The client will maintain optimal cognitive ability.	Assess for cognitive, memory, and communication deficits.
		Develop memory aids and cues to help client remember.
		Maintain a consistent environment and daily schedule.
		Approach client in a quiet, nonthreatening manner.
		Do not confront client with reality if it will only upset and agitate him. For example, do not tell a 90-year-old client who wants his mother that she is dead.
		Attend to nonverbal cues for unmet needs (e.g., pacing, grimacing, crying, agitation). The client may be hungry, have a full bladder, or be unable to ask to be repositioned.

continued

Nursing Diagnoses	Planning/Goals	Nursing Interventions
		Obtain a photo of client that can be recognized by the client. A current photo of client may appear as a stranger to the client, but a photo of the client at age 20 or 30 may be remembered.
		Give simple, single instructions.
▸ *Sleep Pattern Disturbance related to disorientation or irritability*	The client will sleep 4 to 5 hours each night.	Advise the client to avoid caffeine.
		Maintain a quiet environment.
		Provide a night light.
		Increase daytime activities to tolerance and use exercise to tire client.
		Provide comfort measures.

Evaluation Each goal must be evaluated to determine how it has been met by the client.

GUILLAIN-BARRÉ SYNDROME (POLYRADICULONEUROPATHY)

Guillain-Barré syndrome is an acute inflammatory process primarily involving the motor neurons of the peripheral nervous system. The cause of Guillain-Barré syndrome is not known, but most cases are preceded by a nonspecific infection. There may be an autoimmune or viral basis for this syndrome. Both spinal and cranial motor nerves can be involved. Sensory neurons may also be affected. The demyelination process begins in distal nerves and ascends symmetrically. Remyelination occurs from proximal to distal (Hickey, 1997).

Clinical manifestations occur in differing patterns, but include motor weakness and areflexia, or absence of reflexes. Characteristically, motor weakness begins in the legs and progresses up the body. Respiratory failure results from loss of respiratory muscle function. Cranial nerve involvement results in facial muscle deficits, difficulty in swallowing, and autonomic dysfunctions. Autonomic functions possibly affected are cardiac rhythm, blood pressure regulation, gastrointestinal mobility, and urine elimination.

Sensory involvement causes paresthesia and pain in the hands and feet. The pain progresses up the body and can interfere with sleep.

The three stages of Guillain-Barré syndrome are acute onset, lasting 1 to 3 weeks, the plateau period, lasting several days to 2 weeks, and the recovery phase, which involves remyelination and may last up to 2 years.

Diagnosis is based on the clinical picture of a recent viral infection and motor and possibly sensory deficits, along with characteristic diagnostic results. These results include both an elevated protein level in CSF without elevation of red blood cells or white blood cells and electromyelogram (EMG) showing slowed nerve conduction velocity of paralyzed muscles.

Medical–Surgical Management

Medical

The goal of medical management is prevention and treatment of complications such as immobility, infection, and respiratory failure.

Plasma exchanges have been found to decrease the severity and duration of symptoms. Plasmapheresis is performed in severe cases, this complete plasma exchange removes the antibodies affecting the myelin sheath. Three to four exchanges 1 to 2 days apart are initiated within the first 2 weeks of diagnosis of Guillain-Barré. Plasmapheresis may also be used late in the disease process for continued demyelination or lack of progress in remyelination. Mechanical ventilatory support will be initiated for decreased or lost respiratory function. Blood gas monitoring is used to assess respiratory function.

Surgical

Those who develop respiratory failure may require a tracheostomy along with mechanical ventilation.

Pharmacological

Steroids, such as adrenocorticotropic hormone (ACTH) and prednisone (Detasone) and immunosuppressive agents such as azathioprine (Imuran) or cyclophosphamide (Cytoxan), are prescribed to slow the demyelination process. Low doses of anticoagulants such as heparin are ordered to prevent thrombophlebitis.

Diet

A balanced diet is necessary to prevent tissue and muscle breakdown and to promote healing. If severe paralysis is present, a gastrostomy tube may be used to provide adequate nutrition.

Activity

Range of motion and muscle strength are maintained through physical therapy. Occupational therapy activities teach the client to maintain optional self-care within the limitation of the disease process. Pool therapy, or exercising in a swimming pool, is often used to maintain and strengthen muscles.

▶ NURSING PROCESS

▶ Assessment

▶ Subjective Data

Subjective data collected include client statements about return of sensation; pain; respiratory function; and knowledge.

▶ Objective Data

Assessment includes the status of motor and sensory functions which are monitored continuously in the acute phase of the illness. Progression of loss of function from distal to proximal is monitored, with particular emphasis on respiratory status. Decreased depth and quality of respirations and diminished breath sounds may be found. Status of autonomic functions is monitored by assessment of blood pressure, cardiac rhythm, urinary elimination, and bowel sounds. Assessment for complications of immobility includes breath sounds; signs of thrombophlebitis; loss of ROM; skin condition; and temperature.

Nursing diagnoses for a client with Guillain-Barré syndrome may include the following:

Nursing Diagnoses	Planning/Goals	Nursing Interventions
▶ *Breathing Pattern, Ineffective, related to loss of respiratory muscle function*	The client will be adequately ventilated.	Monitor respiratory status of client by assessing breath sounds, respiratory rate, and respiratory quality.
		Position client to facilitate maximal expansion of the chest wall for optimal breathing.
		Monitor oxygenation by assessing skin color, mental status, pulse oximeter readings, and blood gas values.
		Administer oxygen as ordered. Report failing respiratory status to the physician.
		Provide mechanical ventilation for respiratory failure.
▶ *Physical Mobility, Impaired, related to progressive loss of motor function*	The client will avoid complications of immobility (pneumonia, thrombophlebitis, pressure areas, and loss of ROM).	Monitor status of motor and sensory functions in an ongoing fashion.
		Have client turn, deep breathe, and cough every 2 hours.
		Suction client as necessary.
		Perform respiratory assessment for diminished breath sounds or congestion.
		Monitor vital signs (blood pressure, pulse, respiration, and temperature) every 4 to 8 hours.
		Assess for calf tenderness, redness, or increased warmth.
		Monitor for positive Homan's sign, indicative of deep vein thrombosis.
		Perform ROM to lower extremities every 2 to 4 hours.
		Use plexipulse boots, which are intermittent-pumping boots that promote return blood flow from the lower extremities.
		Administer low doses of heparin or other anticoagulants as prescribed.
		Apply antiembolism stockings.
		Assess condition of skin for pressure areas.
		Use specialty mattress.
		Massage client's back and pressure points with lotion three times a day.
		Assist client to sitting positions in wheelchair two to three times daily.
		Progress to ambulation as motor function returns.
		Apply high-topped shoes to keep feet in correct alignment.

continued

Nursing Diagnoses	Planning/Goals	Nursing Interventions
▶ *Self-care Deficit related to decreased motor function*	The client will have self-care needs met.	Encourage self-care within the limitations of the neurological deficits.
		Maintain muscle strength and ROM with physical therapy.
		Provide ROM to all extremities three to four times daily.
		Provide daily care needs that client is unable to perform.
		Initiate rehabilitation following acute phase of illness with strengthening exercises, occupational therapy, and getting client out of bed several times per day to build strength and endurance.

Evaluation Each goal must be evaluated to determine how it has been met by the client.

HEADACHE

Headache, or **cephalalgia**, the condition of pain in the head, is caused by stimulation of pain-sensitive structures in the cranium, head, or neck. Headaches are classified as symptoms rather than a disease.

The pain-sensitive areas of the intracranial structure include the peripheral nerves, cerebral vasculature, and parts of the dura mater. The external supporting structures of the skin, muscles, and nasal passages are also sensitive to pain. The skull, brain tissue, and most of the meninges are insensitive to pain.

More than 45 million people in the United States each year suffer from headaches that require treatment by a physician (American Academy of Neurology [AAN], 1997a). Headaches are generally classified as either primary or secondary.

PRIMARY HEADACHES

Primary headaches are not caused by an underlying medical condition. They include tension-type, migraine, and cluster headaches (AAN, 1997a) (Table 41-10).

Tension-Type Headache

The most common type of headache is the tension type, affecting 75% of the population each year. The ache is steady rather than throbbing, affects both sides of the head, and occurs frequently, sometimes daily.

Migraine Headaches

Up to 18% of women experience migraine headaches each year, compared to 6% of men. Migraine headaches are vascular and recurrent. The initial vasoconstriction can cause neurological symptoms or an aura prior to the vasodilatation that causes the headache. The aura is a visual disturbance typically consisting of brightly colored or blinking lights or a pattern moving across the field of vision. When only the aura occurs, and there is no pain in the head, the migraine

is termed "silent." Serotonin levels increase in the initial phase prior to the onset of the headache, indicating involvement of neurotransmitters in the pathophysiology. Recent studies demonstrate that migraine pain results from inflammatory changes in blood vessels induced by activation of certain nerves (AAN, 1997a). Some migraine headaches may be triggered by certain foods or chemicals.

Cluster Headaches

A cluster headache develops around or behind one eye and is very severe. Generally, it awakens the person from sleep. The affected eye may tear and the nose become congested on the same side. These headaches occur in clusters daily for weeks or months, then disappear for a year or more. Most cluster headaches occur in men.

SECONDARY HEADACHES

Secondary headaches are the result of pathological conditions such as aneurysm, brain tumor, or inflamed cranial nerves. The headache is caused by compression, inflammation, or hypoxia of pain-sensitive structures.

Medical–Surgical Management

Medical

Medical management is based on the underlying cause of the headache. A thorough history of headache pattern, dietary pattern, and coping pattern is essential. Underlying pathology of brain tumor, aneurysm, and infection must be ruled out. If pathology is identified, secondary headache is diagnosed and therefore treatment will be based on findings. If no cause is found, management of primary headache will be based on symptoms.

Surgical

Surgical management may include clipping of an aneurysm or resection of a brain tumor.

Table 41-10 PRIMARY HEADACHE PATTERNS

TYPE	AURA	PAIN	TYPICAL PATTERN	DURATION
Tension	None	Steady ache	Usually begins gradually in frontal or temporal areas; affects both sides of the head; occur frequently, maybe daily	Hours
Classic Migraine	Duration of 15 to 30 minutes; sensory, usually visual (bright spots, zig-zag lines), unilateral or bilateral numbness or tingling in lips, face, or hand; difficulty thinking; confusion or drowsiness; sometimes preceded by premonition 24 hours before	Throbbing, intense; unilateral; tenderness in scalp; muscle contractions in neck and scalp followed by feelings of exhaustion	Periodic, recurrent; usually begins on awakening; begins in childhood or early adolescence; tends to be familial; nausea and vomiting typical; sensitivity to light and sound	Hours to days
Cluster	None	Intense throbbing; unilateral pain in orbitotemporal area	Causes awakening two to three times during the night; accompanied by watering eyes, nasal congestion, runny nose, facial flushing over the throbbing area; after cluster headaches for days, weeks, or months may be free of symptoms for a year or more; same side of head usually involved; usually in men	30 minutes to 2 hours

Pharmacological

Management is either abortive, to stop the headache, or prophylactic, to prevent reccurrence or to decrease frequency of headaches. Abortive therapy for vascular headaches includes ergotamine tartrate (Ergostat), administered orally, sublingually, rectally, intramuscularly, or subcutaneously at the beginning of a migraine headache. Cafergot, containing ergotamine and caffeine, is also used for abortive therapy. These agents cause vasoconstriction and block serotonin uptake. Promethazine hydrochloride (Phenergan) is often used to control nausea and vomiting. Narcotic or non-narcotic analgesics are administered for pain relief.

Prophylactic treatment includes the beta blockers propranolol hydrochloride (Inderal) and methysergide maleate (Sansert), which prevent dilation of the blood vessels and interrupt the serotonin mechanism. Clonidine hydrochloride (Catapres) directly affects the ability of the blood vessels to constrict or dilate. Tricyclic antidepressants such as amitriptyline hydrochloride (Elavil), block the uptake of serotonin.

Diet

A strict food diary should be kept to identify precipitating foods. After all suspect foods have been eliminated from the diet, skin testing for allergies may be performed. Introduction of suspect foods may be done one at a time to identify triggering foods. Alcohol; cured meats containing nitrates; aged cheeses; monosodium glutamate (MSG); citrus fruits; chocolate; and red wines are common precipitating foods.

Activity

Activities that precipitate headaches must be identified and eliminated if possible. Stressful situations are frequently precipitating agents. Biofeedback, relaxation techniques, stress reduction, and development of coping mechanisms are useful in reducing the occurrence of headaches caused by stress and tension.

Nursing Management

Nursing interventions focus on relieving pain and assisting the client in managing the pain. Identifying methods of decreasing pain, such as effective use of medications and managing the environment to minimize stimulation from light, noise, activity, are also nursing priorities.

The client should be assisted in developing a plan for accomplishing daily activities when incapacitated

LIFE CYCLE CONSIDERATIONS

Pregnancy and Headache Medication

A pregnant woman must *not* take ergotamine, because the drug causes the uterus to contract.

CLIENT TEACHING

Headaches

Advise the client to:

- Keep a diary of headache history to ascertain pattern,
- Avoid foods that trigger headache,
- Reduce salt intake, and
- Practice relaxation techniques.

by a headache. Teaching the client to keep a diary of headache history to determine patterns in headache development is essential. The nurse must assist the client in changing lifestyle to decrease the incidence of headaches in ways such as minimizing stress, avoiding certain foods, reducing salt intake during premenstrual time frame, and using relaxation techniques.

TRIGEMINAL NEURALGIA (TIC DOULOUREUX)

Trigeminal neuralgia is a condition of cranial nerve V and is characterized by abrupt paroxysms of pain and facial muscle contractions. **Neuralgia** is nerve pain. The pain follows one of the three branches of the trigeminal nerve: the ophthalmic, maxillary, or mandibular. The last two branches are most commonly affected (Figure 41-21).

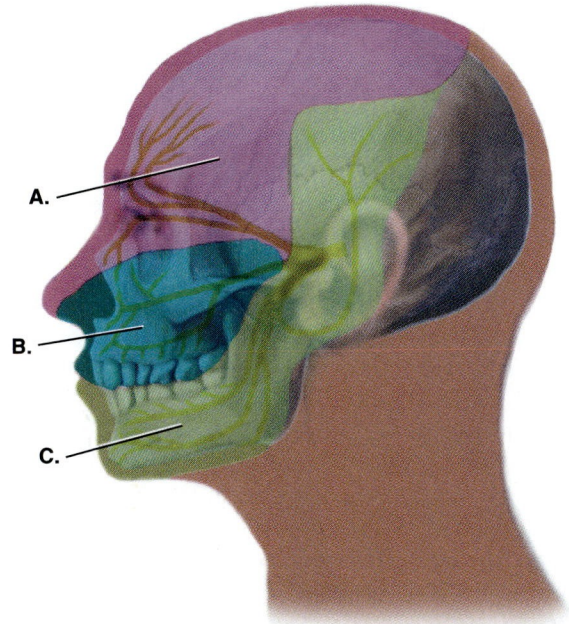

Figure 41-21 Areas of Face Innervated by the Trigeminal Nerve (CN-I): A. Opthalmic; B. Maxillary; C. Mandibular

The etiology of trigeminal neuralgia is not known, but injury, dental caries, dental work, and anatomic position of the nerves have been identified as possible causes. Pain is precipitated when trigger points are stimulated, causing periods of intense pain and facial twitching lasting from seconds to minutes. These periods may last several weeks to months. Periods of remission interspersed with exacerbations occur with increasing frequency with advancing age (Hickey, 1997).

Medical–Surgical Management

Drug therapy, nerve blocks, and surgery are treatment modalities for trigeminal neuralgia.

Surgical

Surgical approaches to relieve pain include percutaneous electrocoagulation with radio frequency. This procedure affects the pain-sensory fibers but causes little damage to the touch, proprioception, and motor fibers. Longer-term relief or permanent relief may be obtained.

Pharmacological

Phenytoin (Dilantin) and carbamazepine (Tegretol) are used to shorten the length of the paroxysmal pain. Nerve blocks using alcohol and phenol injections into the nerve provide temporary relief for 8 to 16 months.

Nursing Management

Goals of nursing interventions are relief of pain, prevention of injury, prevention of self-care deficits, and promotion of social interaction. The client with trigeminal neuralgia frequently experiences such severe pain that grooming, talking, and eating are avoided. It is especially important to provide good oral hygiene if the client is on phenytoin (Dilantin), because the medication causes hyperplasia of the gums. The client should be taught to identify both the trigger points that stimulate the pain and ways to avoid those areas without neglecting daily needs.

The client who has had surgery may have lost the mechanisms that protect the eye from injury, and will

CLIENT TEACHING

Dental Work in the Client with Trigeminal Neuralgia

The client with trigeminal neuralgia should:

- Plan to have dental work done during a period of remission,
- Inform the dentist of the condition, and
- Maintain good dental hygiene, especially during remission.

need to be taught not to touch his eye and to observe for redness of the eye and conjunctiva. Following surgery, the client may not feel pain caused by dental caries, so it is important to encourage routine visits to the dentist for oral examination.

ENCEPHALITIS, MENINGITIS

Encephalitis is inflammation of the brain. **Meningitis** is inflammation of the meninges. The most common cause of encephalitis or meningitis is a virus. Bacteria, fungi, or parasites can also be causative factors. The virus or other causative agent enters the brain either through the bloodstream as a direct extension of trauma or by nerve pathways.

The inflammatory process causes demyelination of white matter and degeneration of neurons. Cerebral edema, hemorrhage, and necrosis of brain tissue can also occur (Chipps, Clanin, & Campbell, 1992). Clinical manifestations vary depending on the causative agent, area of involvement, and degree of damage to nerve tissue. Fever, headache, nuchal rigidity, photophobia, irritability, lethargy, nausea, and vomiting are typical signs and symptoms. As the disease progresses, level of consciousness may decrease and other neurological dysfunctions occur, including motor weakness, aphasia, seizures, behavioral changes, or even death. A lumbar puncture is performed to test CSF for the causative agent, presence of white blood cells or red blood cells, and elevated protein level. A complete blood count is done to identify the presence of viral or bacterial infection.

Medical–Surgical Management

Medical

Treatment is supportive and based on presenting symptoms. The aim of treatment is to prevent or decrease intracranial pressure and to minimize neurological deficits. Intravenous fluids are given to rehydrate the client.

Pharmacological

Antibiotics or antiinfectives are administered in massive doses as appropriate for the causative agent. They may be given intravenously or intrathecally into the spinal canal. Most viral agents do not respond to antibiotics or antiinfectives. Glucocorticosteroids are administered to prevent cerebral edema. Osmotic diuretics may be used to reduce cerebral edema. To prevent seizures, anticonvulsants are often ordered. Antipyretics are often given to reduce fever.

Diet

Optimal nutritional status must be maintained to promote response to the infection.

Activity

A quiet environment with minimal stimulation from noise, light, or client activity is maintained. Routine turning, ROM exercises, pulmonary hygiene, and skin care are required to prevent the complications of immobility.

Nursing Management

In the acute stage, the client must be monitored for changes in neurological status, especially for changes in level of consciousness and for signs of increasing intracranial pressure. A quiet environment will decrease external stimulation. The client must be observed for seizure activity and protected from injury. Comfort measures such as oral hygiene, tepid baths, and administration of analgesics for relief of headaches should be offered.

HUNTINGTON'S DISEASE OR CHOREA

Huntington's disease is a chronic, progressive hereditary disease of the nervous system. It is characterized by a progressive involuntary choreiform movement and progressive dementia.

The cells of the basal ganglia, which control movement, die prematurely. Cells in the cerebral cortex also die, interfering with thought processes, memory, perception, and judgment. Age of onset is usually 35 to 45 years, with death occurring 10 to 15 years following onset of symptoms (Smeltzer & Bare, 1996). The theorized cause is lack of γ-aminobutyric acid (GABA), a neurotransmitter. Each child of a person with Huntington's disease has a 50% chance of developing the disease. A genetic marker has been discovered that indicates whether the person will develop the disease. However, there is no cure for this devastating progressive disease.

Clinical manifestations are **chorea**, abnormal involuntary, purposeless movements of all musculature of the body. Facial tic, grimacing, difficulty in chewing and swallowing, speech impairment, disorganized gait, and bowel and bladder incontinence also occur. Mental or intellectual impairment progresses to dementia. The client may experience paranoia, hallucinations, or delusions. Emotions are labile, from outbursts of anger to profound depression, apathy, or euphoria. A ravenous appetite is usually present, but because of the constant movement, the client is often emaciated and exhausted. Death usually results from heart failure, pneumonia, infection, or an accident (Smeltzer & Bare, 1996).

The entire family experiences this disease in an emotional, physical, social, and financial way. Supportive care is required as the family progresses through life with a loved one with Huntington's disease. Because of the hereditary factor, genetic counseling is necessary.

Medical–Surgical Management

Pharmacological

Medications used to decrease choreiform movement are dopamine receptor blockers, chlorpromazine (Thorazine), haloperidol (Haldol), thiothixene (Navane), and reserpine (Serpasil), which depletes presynaptic dopamine. Antidepressants, such as desipramine hydrochloride (Norpramin) and fluoxetine hydrochloride (Prozac), and antipsycotics, such as fluphenazine hydrochloride (Prolixin), are used for emotional disturbances.

Diet

The diet must be high in calories to provide for the high energy needs caused by the continuous movement. Chewing and swallowing difficulties necessitate foods that are easy to chew or foods cut into small pieces to prevent choking.

Activity

Ambulation is maintained as long as possible. A safe environment must be maintained to prevent injury from falls or from sharp objects. Driving is usually restricted when choreiform movement or impaired judgment interferes with the ability to drive safely.

Nursing Management

Nursing interventions include a holistic approach to the client's care. Collaboration with the social worker, the chaplain, the physician, and the mental health worker is necessary.

Teach the client and family about the disease process, the progress of the disease, and the genetic factors involved. Safety factors must be considered. Fall prevention measures, such as removing throw rugs and small objects from the floor, and injury prevention measures, such as removing sharp or dangerous objects such as guns and knives from the home, are implemented. The hazard of choking also must be addressed, by teaching the family to cut the client's food into small pieces and to serve soft foods and by teaching the Heimlich maneuver.

GILLES DE LA TOURETTE'S SYNDROME

Gilles de la Tourette's syndrome is a neurological movement disorder that also has prominent behavioral manifestations. Clinical manifestations include motor tics, and involuntary repetitive movements of the mouth,

face, head, or neck muscles. The trunk and extremities may also be involved. Motor tics may take the form of forceful eye blinking or toe touching. Vocal tics or repetitive involuntary vocalizations, may take the form of sniffing, grunting, throat clearing, or coprolalia (involuntary and inappropriate swearing). Other complex motor and vocal tics that may also be present include copropraxia, involuntary and effectively appropriate use of obscene gestures; echolalia, involuntary repetition of the speech of others; and palilia, involuntary repetition of the person's own speech (Hyde & Weinberger, 1995). The obsessive–compulsive symptoms of repetitive handwashing or checking rituals may also be exhibited.

Structural abnormalities in the basal ganglia and prefrontal cortex have been identified in research as the possible cause of Tourette's syndrome (Hyde & Weinberger, 1995). Attention deficit hyperactivity disorder and obsessive–compulsive disorders may also coexist with Tourette's syndrome.

Onset is prior to age 18 years, with males being more commonly affected than females. Estimates of prevalence range from 2.9 to 49.5 per 100,000 children. Tourette's is a genetic disorder, with the affected individual having a 50% chance of passing the gene on to children (AAN, 1997b).

Medical–Surgical Management

Pharmacological

Tics may be controlled with clonadine (Catapres), haloperidol (Haldol), or primozide (Orap). Coexisting attention deficit hyperactivity disorder may be controlled with clonidine (Catapres), methylphenidate (Ritalin), or pemoline (Cylert). Clomypramine (Anafranil) or fluoxetine (Prozac) can be used to keep obsessive–compulsive behaviors under control (Kurlan, 1998). Acetaminophen (Tylenol) may help the discomfort of muscle spasms.

Other Therapies

As they age, clients may learn to suppress tics in social situations. Psychotherapy and family counseling are beneficial in coping with social stigma and adjustment problems.

Nursing Management

The client and the family with Tourette's syndrome need a great deal of emotional support and will benefit from knowing about the availability of support groups for clients with Tourette's syndrome. The nurse should teach about the disease process and expectations for the client. Behavioral modification techniques are generally effective; the nurse must know which modification techniques are being used and must follow through with consistent responses.

CASE STUDY

Mr. Domingo Ochoa, a 76-year-old retired farmer, was admitted to the emergency room with left-sided hemiplegia, difficulty swallowing, and inability to speak. He was awake and watching the staff upon admission. He moved his right arm to indicate that Mrs. Ochoa was his wife, but was unable to speak or form sounds. Mrs. Ochoa stated that her husband was working in the garden, picking tomatoes and cucumbers, when he fell to the ground 30 minutes before admission. The emergency room nurse administered oxygen through nasal cannula at 2 liters per minute and obtained vital signs. His blood pressure was 182/98, pulse was 88, respirations were 20, and temperature was 100.5°F. The emergency room physician ordered an MRI scan of the head, a complete blood count, and prothrombin time (PT). The MRI indicated that Mr. Ochoa experienced a CVA caused by a bleeding into the brain.

The following questions will guide your development of a nursing care plan for the case study.

1. List clinical manifestations other than the ones Mr. Ochoa experienced that can occur with a CVA.
2. List subjective and objective data that a nurse would obtain.
3. Identify three individualized nursing diagnoses and goals for Mr. Ochoa.
4. Mr. Ochoa is transferred to a general medical unit for 3 days, then is transferred to a rehabilitation center for intensive therapy. What pertinent nursing actions should a nurse perform in caring for Mr. Ochoa in the acute setting and the rehabilitation setting related to:

   Mobility
   Safety
   Elimination
   Skin integrity
   Comfort and rest

5. What teaching will Mr. Ochoa need before discharge from the rehabilitation facility?
6. List at least three client outcomes for Mr. Ochoa.

SUMMARY

- The nervous system controls all bodily functions, from movement, to thinking, to processing information, to autonomic responses.
- Functional areas of the brain specialize in specific tasks.
- The frontal lobe of the cerebrum specializes in emotional attitudes and responses, formation of thought processes, motor function, judgment, personality, and inhibitions.
- The parietal lobe of the cerebrum is a purely sensory region for interpretation of all senses except smell; the purpose is to analyze sensations, including pain, touch, and temperature, from receptors in the skin.
- The temporal lobe of the cerebrum houses Wernicke's area, the primary auditory association area, where words that are heard are interpreted. Memory is also a function of the temporal lobe, espe-

cially memories that are highly detailed or involve multiple sensations.
- A special interpretive area located at the junction of the temporal, parietal, and occipital lobes integrates somatic, auditory, and visual sensory interpretations.
- The occipital lobe of the cerebrum is responsible for visual interpretation and visual association.
- Disorders of the nervous system cause complex dysfunctions; the nurse must use assessment skills and quickly recognize changes in condition.
- Teaching about injury prevention and the effects and prognosis of the disorder are required to meet the physical and psychosocial needs of the client and family.
- Many neurological disorders potentiate injury. Nursing care must include providing the client and family with necessary safety information.
- In order to maintain and restore functional ability, rehabilitation is initiated from the first contact with the client.

Review Questions

1. The most important indicator of change in neurological status is:

   a. level of consciousness.
   b. pupil reaction.
   c. vital signs.
   d. motor function.

2. Cranial nerves III, IV, and VI all have functions affecting:

   a. special senses.
   b. facial movement.
   c. eye movement.
   d. gag reflex.

3. Assessment of intellectual function requires that the nurse:

   a. have knowledge of the client's prior ability to function.
   b. administer a written test to determine the client's IQ level.
   c. utilize auscultation, percussion, and palpation skills.
   d. observe the client's behavior, posture, and facial expression.

4. Contusion of the brain is a (an):

   a. shaking of the brain.
   b. bleeding into the brain tissue.
   c. open head injury.
   d. bruising of the brain.

5. Benign brain tumors can be:

   a. more anxiety producing than are malignant tumors.
   b. more life threatening than are malignant tumors.
   c. treated with radiation therapy.
   d. the cause of increased intracranial pressure.

6. Miss Webster, a 24-year-old client with Guillain-Barré Syndrome, can be told which of the following?

   a. The nerve degeneration slowing continues to progress in this chronic degenerative nerve disease.
   b. The disease is an acute inflammatory process with most clients regaining complete function.
   c. Respiratory failure requiring chronic ventilatory support may occur.
   d. Motor function deficit will occur, but sensation will remain.

Critical Thinking Questions

1. What are the similarities between Parkinson's disease and Alzheimer's disease?

2. What are the most important things to teach a client with multiple sclerosis?

3. Identify the rationale for each nursing intervention given for the possible nursing diagnoses in this chapter.

WEB FLASH!

- Try to locate each of the disorders in this chapter on the Web. What type of information is available for each?
- What sites could you recommend to families and individuals coping with any of these disorders?
- Is there a listing on the Internet of books, videos, or other media on these disorders?

MAKING THE CONNECTION

Refer to the following chapters to increase your understanding of urinary disorders:

- **Chapter 15, Wellness Concepts**
- **Chapter 25, Assessment**
- **Chapter 32, Nursing Care of the Client: Cardiovascular System**
- **Chapter 35, Nursing Care of the Client: Reproductive System**
- **Chapter 55, Nursing Care of the Older Client**
- **Chapter 56, Rehabilitation, Home Health, Long-Term Care, and Hospice**

- **Procedures:** B1, Handwashing; B2, Use of Protective Equipment; B19, Perineal Care; B20, Catheter Care; B29, Measuring Intake and Output; B30, Urine Collection: Closed Drainage System; B31, Urine Collection: Clean Catch, Female, Male; I3 and I4, Performing Urinary Catheterization, Male Client, Female Client; I5, Irrigating an Open Cather; I6, Irrigating a Closed Catheter

LEARNING OBJECTIVES

Upon completion of this chapter, you should be able to:
- *Define key terms.*
- *Describe the anatomy and physiology of the urinary system.*
- *Relate diagnostic test results to urinary disorders.*
- *Discuss the pros and cons of peritoneal dialysis/hemodialysis and kidney transplantation, including lifestyle changes for the client receiving dialysis.*
- *List four drug classifications and two examples of each used in the treatment of urinary disorders.*
- *State two changes in the urinary system related to the normal aging process.*
- *Compare and contrast acute and chronic renal failure, including nursing care.*
- *Assist in formulating a nursing care plan for clients with urinary disorders.*

KEY TERMS

anasarca	micturition
azotemia	nephrotoxic
cachectic	nocturnal enuresis
calculus(i)	overflow incontinence
cystitis	pyelonephritis
dialysate	pyuria
dialysis	renal colic
dysuria	residual urine
erythropoiesis	retroperitoneal
fulguration	stress incontinence
ileal conduit	urge incontinence
intravesical	urinary incontinence
litholapaxy	urinary retention
lithotripsy	urolithiasis

INTRODUCTION

Urology is the study of disorders of the urinary system. The National Kidney Foundation estimates that approximately 20 million Americans have kidney or urinary tract related diseases and millions more are at risk (National Kidney Foundation [NKF], 1997). Disorders of the urinary system may seriously affect an individual's health and, thereby, affect the lives of family members. Clients are treated by a urologist, specialist in urinary tract disorders, or a nephrologist, specialist in structure, function, and diseases of the kidney.

According to the National Kidney Foundation (1999b), the following are warning signs of kidney disease:

- Burning or difficulty during urination
- Increase in the frequency of urination, especially at night
- Passage of bloody appearing urine
- Puffiness around the eyes, or swelling of the hands and feet, especially in children
- Pain in the small of the back just below the ribs (not aggravated by movement)
- High blood pressure

ANATOMY AND PHYSIOLOGY REVIEW

The urinary system consists of two kidneys, two ureters (upper urinary tract), a urinary bladder, and a urethra (lower urinary tract) (Figure 42-1). The kidneys manufacture urine. Urine normally consists of 95% water; the nitrogenous waste products of protein, which are urea, uric acid, and creatinine; the excessive electrolytes sodium, calcium, potassium, and phosphates; bile pigments; hormones; and metabolized drugs and toxins. Urine moves steadily by peristalsis through the ureters into the urinary bladder. The urine remains in the urinary bladder until capacity has been reached (about 500 mL) or until a desire to empty the urinary bladder (about 250 mL) is felt. The urine is then expelled from the bladder through the urethra, which is shorter in females than in males. **Micturition**, the process of expelling urine from the urinary bladder, is also called urination or voiding.

The kidneys are located beneath the false ribs, in the **retroperitoneal** space (behind the peritoneum outside the peritoneal cavity) of the abdominal cavity. The kidneys also assist in acid-base balance, raise blood pressure by secreting the enzyme renin, and produce the hormone erythropoietin which is responsible for **erythropoiesis** (the production of red blood cells and their release by the red bone marrow).

Within the kidneys are microscopic units called nephrons, which are responsible for urine formation. The nephron winds into the cortex and medulla of the kidney. Each nephron includes a renal corpuscle, which consists of a glomerulus, a ball-like network of capillaries formed from an arteriole and held within a cuplike Bowman's capsule. The Bowman's capsule is attached to a long, intricate, ultrathin looped and coiled tubular structure called the renal tubule. Continuing on from the glomerulus is an arteriole that forms a capillary network around the tubule. Blood flowing through this system is collected by venioles. The inset in Figure 42-1 illustrates a nephron.

Most of the contents of the blood, except for large molecules and blood cells, are forced out of the blood from the capillaries of the glomerulus and into the Bowman's capsule (glomerulofiltration). This occurs because of the high capillary blood pressure within the glomerulus. The glomerular basement membrane assists with the process of filtration. The material filtered from the blood is called glomerular filtrate, which contains water, electrolytes, glucose, various toxic substances, waste products (urea and creatinine), and just

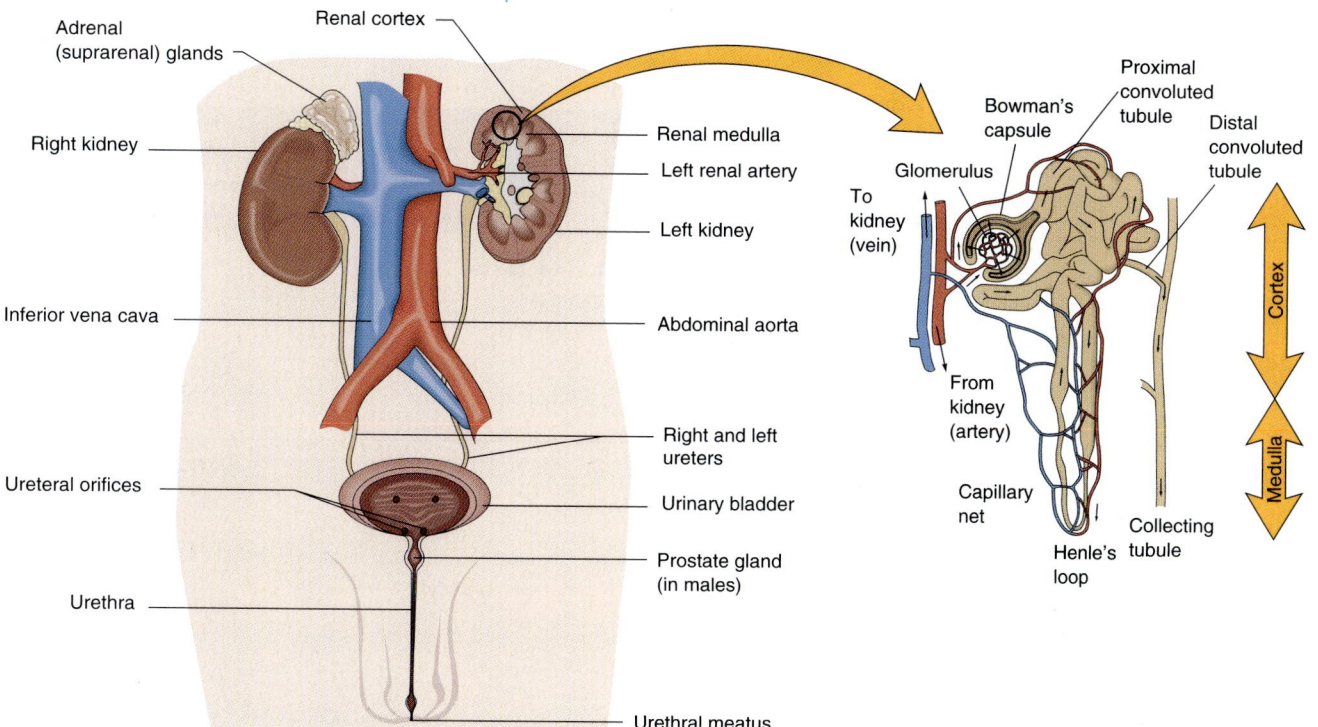

Figure 42-1 The Urinary System with Inset of a Nephron

about everything else in the blood except large protein molecules and blood cells. As the filtrate passes through the first parts of the tubular structure, various substances such as necessary amounts of electrolytes, glucose, and water are reabsorbed (tubular reabsorption) back into the circulatory system through the capillaries or into the interstitial fluid. Tubular secretion then removes certain ions, nitrogen waste products, and drugs from the blood in the capillaries and adds it to the filtrate. The remaining filtrate—water, urea, excess electrolytes, toxic substances, and wastes, all of which constitute urine—continues through the tubules into the collecting duct, which collects urine from many nephrons. The urine passes from the collecting duct into the pelvis of the kidney, then through the ureter into the bladder and out of the body through the urethra.

ASSESSMENT

Assessment of the urinary system is included in the baseline data for all clients. The client may be reluctant to discuss urinary problems. The nurse can assist the individual to relax by asking open-ended questions, using familiar terms, and making sure the client understands the medical terms.

A more in-depth assessment is performed when the client is at high risk for renal disease because of exposure to nephrotoxins; an altered health state such as diabetes mellitus, pregnancy, or hypertension; trauma, dehydration, or fluid retention, which can compromise renal function; and those with suspected or active renal disease.

Subjective Data

The client should be asked to describe how the symptoms developed and progressed. Is there pain? Is it sharp or a dull ache? Constant or intermittent? Does it radiate to the groin, genital area, or leg? Is the pain associated with urination? Have headaches been experienced?

Next, the client can describe the urine and urination pattern. Is there difficulty starting the stream? Is there urgency, frequency, incontinence, or hematuria? Does the bladder feel empty after voiding? Does the client have pruritis or dry skin?

Objective Data

If edema is present, the nurse should ask the client whether it is always present or whether it disappears during the night. Refer to Figure 32-3, Grading Edema. I & O and vital signs should be monitored, and the bladder palpated for retention. The client should be weighed. Mucous membranes are assessed for moisture and the skin for dryness—and uremic frost. Urine must be evaluated for color, clarity, and odor. Diagnostic tests should be assessed.

Changes with Aging

Needham (1993) identifies the following changes in the urinary system due to aging:

1. Nephrons decrease, resulting in decreased filtration and gradual decrease in excretory and reabsorptive functions of renal tubules.
2. Glomerular filtration rate decreases, resulting in decreased renal clearance of drugs.
3. Blood urea nitrogen (BUN) increases 20% by age 70. The creatinine clearance test is a better index than the BUN of renal function in the elderly.
4. Sodium-conserving ability is diminished.
5. Bladder capacity decreases, causing increased frequency of urination and nocturia.
6. Renal function increases when the client is lying down, sometimes causing a need to void shortly after going to bed.
7. Bladder and perineal muscles weaken, resulting in inability to empty the bladder. This results in residual urine and predisposes the elderly to cystitis.
8. Incidence of stress incontinence increases in females.
9. The prostate may enlarge, causing frequency or dribbling in males.

COMMON DIAGNOSTIC TESTS

Commonly used diagnostic tests for clients with symptoms of urinary system disorders are listed in Table 42-1. See Chapter 27, Diagnostic Tests, for explanation/normal values and nursing responsibilities.

Table 42-1 COMMON DIAGNOSTIC TESTS FOR URINARY SYSTEM DISORDERS

Urine Tests
Urinalysis
  Color
  Odor
  Albumin (protein)
  Acetone (ketone)
  RBCs
  WBCs
  Bilirubin
  Glucose
  Specific gravity
  Bacteria
  Casts
  pH
Culture and sensitivity (C & S)
Creatinine clearance   *continued*

Table 42-1 COMMON DIAGNOSTIC TESTS FOR URINARY SYSTEM DISORDERS *continued*

Blood Tests
Blood urea nitrogen (BUN)
Serum creatinine
Antistreptolysin O titer (ASO titer)
Serum electrolytes
    Sodium
    Potassium
    Chloride
    Calcium
    Phosphorus

Radiographic Tests
Voiding cystourethrography
Kidney-ureter-bladder (KUB) x-ray
Computed tomography (CT)
Magnetic resonance imaging (MRI)
Intravenous pyelogram (IVP)
Renal angiography
Renal scan
Ultrasound

Urodynamic Tests
Uroflowmetry
Cystometrogram (CMG)
Urethra pressure profile (UPP)

Endoscopic Exam
Cystoscopy

ALTERED URINARY ELIMINATION PATTERNS

Disorders in this category include urinary retention and urinary incontinence.

URINARY RETENTION

A person who is unable to void when there is an urge to void has **urinary retention**. This creates urinary stasis and increases the possibility of infection. The urine may overflow the bladder's capacity, causing incontinence.

There are a variety of causes such as a response to stress; obstruction of the urethra by **calculi** (concentration of mineral salts, known as stones), tumor, or infection; interference with the sphincter muscles during surgery; or as a side effect of medications or perineal trauma.

The client may experience discomfort and anxiety from urinary retention. Frequency of urination and voiding small amounts may also occur. The distended bladder can be palpated above the symphysis.

Treatment may include urinary analgesics and antispasmodics to help the client relax. A urinary catheter may be used to empty the bladder, or surgery may be performed to remove any obstruction.

When the client is able to void, a check for residual urine should be done. Immediately after the client voids, catheterization should be performed. The urine left in the bladder, **residual urine**, should be less than 50 mL.

URINARY INCONTINENCE

Urinary incontinence is the involuntary loss of urine from the bladder. The incontinence may be a complication of urinary tract problems or neurologic disorders and may be permanent or temporary. Medications such as sedatives, hypnotics, diuretics, anticholinergics, antipsychotics, and alpha antagonists may be associated with incontinence.

More than 13 million men and women in the United States experience incontinence, 11 million of whom are women (National Institute of Diabetes and Digestive and Kidney Diseases [NIDDK], 1998). This is not just a physiological problem but also affects the client's emotional, psychological, and social well-being. Incontinence can occur in clients of any age but is more common in the older adult. All types of incontinence can be treated at any age. At least 1 out of 10 persons age 65 or older has incontinence (National Institute on Aging, 1996). Incontinence is classified as stress, urge, overflow, total, or nocturnal enuresis.

STRESS INCONTINENCE

Stress incontinence is the most common type of incontinence. It is not a disease or a natural, inevitable effect of aging. Anyone can be affected; however, women are more likely to have this condition than men. In **stress incontinence** there is leakage of urine when a person does anything that strains the abdomen such as coughing, laughing, jogging, dancing, sneezing, lifting, making a quick movement, or even walking.

Medical management depends on the underlying cause. Stress incontinence often can be cured and nearly always can be substantially alleviated (Sasso, 1998). Treatment may include bladder retraining, medicines such as conjugated estrogens (Premarin Vaginal Cream), or surgery. Surgery may be necessary to restore the support of the pelvic floor muscles or to reconstruct the sphincter but is used after other treatments are unsuccessful. Another possible treatment is having collagen injected into the tissues surrounding the urethra. This closes the urethra enough to prevent urine from leaking out. The procedure is done in a nonsurgical outpatient setting. Several support prostheses and external barriers are now available (Sasso, 1998).

The client can be taught pelvic floor exercises (Kegel) to strengthen the muscles, thereby preventing or minimizing stress incontinence. Kegel exercises involve having the client tighten the pelvic floor muscles to stop the flow of urine when urinating, and then releasing the muscles to start the flow of urine again. Once the client can do this, the exercise may be done anytime, anyplace. Practicing the exercise 10 times, 7 or 8 times a day strengthens the muscles.

Bladder retraining begins with assessing the client's voiding pattern and encouraging the client to void 30 minutes before the projected time of incontinence. The schedule is extended until the client can stay dry for 2 hours, gradually increasing the time between voidings until a 3- to 4-hour schedule is achieved.

URGE INCONTINENCE

Urge incontinence occurs when a person is unable to suppress the sudden urge or need to urinate. Sometimes urine may leak without any warning. An irritated bladder is often the cause. Infection or very concentrated urine may irritate the bladder.

Treatment includes clearing up an infection, if present, and encouraging the client to have a fluid intake of 3,000 mL/day. This prevents the urine from becoming concentrated. Less fluid does not prevent incontinence but may promote infection.

OVERFLOW INCONTINENCE

When the bladder becomes so full and distended that urine leaks out, it is called **overflow incontinence**. This occurs when a blocked urethra or bladder weakness prevents normal emptying. The blockage may be an enlarged prostate. The distended bladder cannot contract with enough force to expel a stream of urine. Bladder weakness occurs most often in persons who have diabetes, drink a large quantity of alcohol, and have decreased nerve function. Bladder retraining may alleviate the situation.

TOTAL INCONTINENCE

When no urine can be retained in the bladder, it is termed total incontinence. The client may be able to manage with an indwelling catheter. A neurologic problem is usually the cause. Surgery to make a temporary or permanent urinary diversion may be required.

NOCTURNAL ENURESIS

Incontinence that occurs during sleep is called **nocturnal enuresis**. Limiting fluid intake after 6 P.M. will help the client remain continent during the night. However, the total fluid intake for the 24 hours should remain the same. The bladder should be emptied immediately before going to bed.

INFECTIOUS DISORDERS

Infectious disorders of the urinary system are called urinary tract infections (UTIs). There are two types: lower UTIs affect the bladder (cystitis) and urethra, while upper UTIs affect the kidneys (pyelonephritis, and acute and chronic glomerulonephritis) and ureters.

CYSTITIS

Cystitis is an inflammation of the urinary bladder. It is more common in females because of their short urethra, which allows bacteria to ascend through the urethra from the vagina or rectum to the urinary bladder. Also, bacteria from an infected kidney can descend through the ureter into the urinary bladder. The majority of urinary tract infections are caused by *Escherichia coli*. Other common causes of cystitis are coitus, prostatitis, and diabetes mellitus.

As women age, pelvic floor muscles relax, leading to a decreased ability to empty the bladder completely. This contributes to stasis of urine and promotion of bacterial growth, as in pregnancy or benign prostatic hypertrophy. In men, cystitis usually occurs secondary to another infection such as epididymitis or prostatitis.

Once bacteria enter the bladder, they multiply, causing redness and swelling of the wall of the bladder. These changes give rise to urinary frequency, dysuria, pyuria, hematuria, and sometimes burning and urgency with urination. These symptoms increase as the bladder distends with even a small volume of urine.

A clean-catch midstream urinalysis showing a bacteria count greater than 100,000 organisms/mL confirms

LIFE CYCLE CONSIDERATIONS

Elderly Clients and UTIs

- Ten percent to 20% of people over age 65 have bacteriuria (Marchiondo, 1998).
- Elderly clients are more prone to UTIs because of incomplete emptying of the bladder, fecal incontinence with perineal soiling, and a decrease in urine acidity.
- Incomplete emptying of the bladder in women is caused by bladder or uterine prolapse or loss of pelvic muscle tone; in men it is caused by an enlarged prostate gland.

the diagnosis. The microscopic examination of the urine will also show hematuria and pus.

Medical–Surgical Management

Medical

Treatment of cystitis includes medication and fluids. Recurrence of a urinary tract infection usually occurs when the bacteria are not effectively treated. Obtaining and sending a urine specimen for C & S before the administration of any urinary antimicrobial is necessary to determine the most effective medication. A repeat urinalysis after 2 or 3 days on medication will confirm its effectiveness. Chronic lower urinary tract infections are often a factor in the development of pyelonephritis.

Pharmacological

Cystitis treatment entails the use of antimicrobial medication in conjunction with urinary tract analgesics. Cystitis is generally treated with norfloxacin (Noroxin), nitrofurantoin (Furadantin), ciprofloxacin (Cipro), or sulfonamides such as sulfisoxazole (Gantrisin) or trimethoprim-sulfamethoxazole (Bactrim, Septra). It is necessary to determine whether the client is allergic to sulfonamides or penicillins before administering the medication. The antimicrobial ordered is determined by the results of the urine culture and sensitivity. The length of treatment is related to the type of cystitis, acute or chronic. Some physicians may order a single dose or short course (3 or 4 days) of antimicrobial therapy rather than the traditional 7- to 10-day course. A single-dose medication, fosfomycin (Monurol), is indicated exclusively for UTI treatment. Its antibacterial effect is sustained for up to 3½ days (Marchiondo, 1998). **Dysuria** (difficult or painful urination) related to a burning sensation when voiding can be alleviated with the use of the urinary tract analgesic phenazopyridine hydrochloride (Pyridium), which causes red-orange urine and stains clothing and toilets.

Diet

Fluids are to be encouraged. Clients are usually asked to drink between 3 and 4 liters of noncaffeinated fluid per day. The intake of meats and whole grains makes the urine more acid and may discourage the growth of bacteria in the urinary bladder. Drinking cranberry juice has been advised for years, but how it worked was not understood. It is now believed that the concentration of tannins in the juice prevents *E. coli* from sticking to cells lining the urinary tract (NKF, January, 1999).

Activity

Since cystitis causes frequency of urination, clients on bed rest or those in need of assistance to the bathroom must have the call light answered promptly. Clients on bed rest are generally not able to empty their bladder completely when using a bedpan. Orders for bathroom privileges or using a commode chair are encouraged. The nurse can help allay the client's fears of being incontinent with proper and timed bladder management.

▶ NURSING PROCESS

▶ Assessment

▶ Subjective Data

The client will usually describe having frequency or urgency of urination or nocturia. This becomes annoying and embarrassing, regardless of age or sex. Burning and pain when voiding are common reasons clients seek medical care. Even clients with an indwelling catheter may complain of dysuria, burning, and frequency. Clients often just do not feel well.

▶ Objective Data

Perineal irritation may be noticed when the client with a catheter pulls on it in hopes of alleviating the bladder pain. The urine will smell foul and appear cloudy. Hematuria may be present. The elderly population in particular may become anorexic and develop a low-grade fever. The urinalysis will indicate the presence of bacteria and the C & S will identify the specific microorganism causing the urinary tract infection and the medication to which the pathogen is most sensitive.

Nursing diagnoses for a client with cystitis may include the following:

Nursing Diagnoses	Planning/Goals	Nursing Interventions
▶ *Urinary Elimination, Altered, related to urinary tract infection*	The client will return to usual pattern of urinary elimination.	Encourage a large amount of fluid intake, at least 3,000 mL each day, especially water and cranberry juice.
		Administer urinary tract analgesics and antimicrobial medications as ordered.
		Alert the client, if Pyridium is being taken, that the urine will be red-orange and will stain clothing.

continued

Nursing Diagnoses	Planning/Goals	Nursing Interventions
▶ *Knowledge Deficit, related to treatment regimen and prevention of recurrence*	The client will comply with treatment regimen and practice preventive habits.	Discuss the importance of taking all medication ordered even after the symptoms are relieved.
		Teach or reinforce the following preventive measures.
		Clean the perineum from front to back.
		If nylon undergarments are worn, they should have a cotton crotch.
		Wearing tight-fitting jeans and taking long bike rides may be irritating to the perineum.
		Perfumed perineal products such as menstrual products, douches, powder, or bubble bath may also be contributing factors to bladder infections.
		Spermicidal contraceptive products can be irritating, thus encouraging a lower UTI.
		Advise the client to void more frequently and not keep urine in the bladder.
		Advise women to void after sexual intercourse.
		Teach the elderly person who uses incontinence control products, such as Attends®, to change the product frequently to prevent cystitis.
		When this client is hospitalized, plan time for frequent ambulation to the bathroom or commode chair.

Evaluation Each goal must be evaluated to determine how it has been met by the client.

PYELONEPHRITIS

Pyelonephritis is a bacterial infection of the renal pelvis, tubules, and interstitial tissue of one or both kidneys. This condition is also known as pyelitis or nephropyelitis. Bacteria generally ascend from the urinary bladder through the ureter and enter the kidney in the area known as the renal pelvis. The bacteria can also enter from the blood and lymph. Pyelonephritis can be secondary to ureterovesicular reflux (back flow of urine from the bladder into the ureters) or when urine cannot drain from the pelvis of the kidney because of an obstruction blocking the kidney or ureter. Pyelonephritis may also occur during pregnancy, with prostatitis, when bacteria are introduced during a cystoscopy or catheterization, or from trauma of the urinary tract. Pyelonephritis can be an acute illness or a chronic condition leading to the development of high blood pressure and/or chronic renal failure.

Escherichia coli is the microorganism most often cultured. The inflamed kidney becomes edematous and the renal blood vessels become congested. Sometimes abscesses form in the kidney. The urine is usually cloudy, containing mucus, blood, and pus.

Medical–Surgical Management

Medical

Diagnostic tests that may be ordered include an IVP, a urinalysis with a C & S, CBC, BUN, and serum creatinine. Urine specimens should be collected prior to the administration of the antimicrobial medication. Medical treatment and care are focused on preventing pyelonephritis from becoming chronic. Follow-up care and treatment may be necessary for up to 6 months.

Pharmacological

Pyelonephritis is generally treated with sulfonamides, such as trimethoprim-sulfamethoxazole (Bactrim) or the antimicrobial ciprofloxacin hydrochloride (Cipro). Cipro may not be indicated if the client has renal damage. Antipyretics are necessary for fever reduction and analgesics for pain management.

Diet

As with infections in general, the individual's diet should be light during the febrile stage. Fluids must be increased to 3,000 mL/day by mouth and supplemented intravenously when indicated.

Activity

The disease process will cause fatigue. Bed rest should be maintained during the acute phase of pyelonephritis. Diversionary activities are important while bed rest is ordered. When the client is allowed to be ambulatory, dizziness related to the analgesic medication taken for pain may be a problem.

▶ NURSING PROCESS

▶ Assessment

▶ Subjective Data

In acute pyelonephritis the client is acutely ill with malaise, urgency in urination, and pain during voiding and in the flank area. **Renal colic**, severe pain in the kidney that radiates to the groin, may occur, impairing urination. The client may complain of being hot, with or without chills. In chronic pyelonephritis, only a general symptom of nausea may be present. The client may be very anxious that this kidney infection will cause permanent kidney damage.

▶ Objective Data

Physical assessment may find the client tender on one or both sides of the lower back. Temperature, pulse, and respiratory rate may all be elevated. The urine is foul smelling and cloudy. The urinalysis results show bacteria and **pyuria** (pus in the urine), and the CBC indicates leukocytosis. The client with chronic disease will have the systemic signs of vomiting, diarrhea, and elevated blood pressure. Some clients with pyelonephritis may be asymptomatic.

Nursing diagnoses for a client with pyelonephritis may include the following:

Nursing Diagnoses	Planning/Goals	Nursing Interventions
▶ *Anxiety related to un-known prognosis*	The client will verbalize fears and concerns to family and health care team.	Encourage the client to verbalize fears and concerns. Use active listening and observe for behavioral signs of anxiety. Answer questions honestly.
▶ *Urinary Elimination, Altered, related to urinary tract infection*	The client will regain normal urinary pattern.	Encourage drinking cranberry juice. Encourage 3,000 mL fluid intake per day, especially water. Monitor intake and output. The intake of fluids is important to maintain function of the urinary system. Evaluate kidney function by measuring and observing urine output and monitoring the results of blood and urine tests.
▶ *Knowledge Deficit, related to disease process, treatment regimen, and prevention*	The client will verbalize understanding of disease process, treatment regimen, and preventive measures.	Teach or reinforce the hygiene measure of cleansing the perineum from front to back and practice this when doing perineal care on any client. Instruct the client on the importance of taking all the antimicrobial medication as prescribed in order to eliminate the bacteria. Teach the client to refrain from using perfumed perineal products such as menstrual pads, tampons, or douches, and avoid bubble baths and hot tubs because they can be irritating to the tissues of the genital area. Encourage the client to empty the bladder frequently to avoid distention. Promote rest periods, which aid the healing process. Inform the client to call the physician immediately if there is a decrease in urine output or signs of infection (elevated temperature, chills, flank pain, urgency, fatigue, nausea, and vomiting). Teach client to weigh daily and report sudden weight gain (2 pounds/week) to the physician. Emphasize the importance of keeping all appointments with the physician for follow-up care and when signs of infection appear. Teach the client the importance of long-term treatment and monitoring for chronic pyelonephritis.

Evaluation Each goal must be evaluated to determine how it has been met by the client.

ACUTE GLOMERULONEPHRITIS

Glomerulonephritis is a condition that can affect one or both kidneys. In both acute and chronic disease, the glomerulus within the nephron unit becomes inflamed. It is predominantly a disease of children and young adults when the cause is bacterial. The viral form can affect all ages. The prognosis for most clients

is a full recovery; however, some may develop chronic glomerulonephritis. Acute glomerulonephritis during childhood is known as Bright's disease.

Most clients develop symptoms 1 to 3 weeks after an upper respiratory infection (tonsillitis or pharyngitis with fever) or skin infection caused most commonly by group A β-*hemolytic streptococcus*. The infection triggers an autoimmune response and the glomeruli are attacked by antibodies at the site of the glomerular basement membrane, resulting in inflammation. Some clients are asymptomatic.

Immunologic effects on the body are not completely understood. Direct effects on the glomeruli result in the reduced ability of the glomeruli to function. The glomeruli become more permeable, resulting in the loss of red blood cells and protein from the blood. These substances escape from the body in the urine. The inflammatory process causes thickening of the membrane of the glomeruli and potential scarring.

Diagnostic tests on blood and urine as well as KUB x-rays will be performed. BUN, serum creatinine, potassium, erythrocyte sedimentation rate (ESR), and antistreptolysin O titer (ASO titer) will be elevated. Urinalysis will show protein and red blood cells.

Medical–Surgical Management

Medical

Medical treatment must start as soon as the client is diagnosed in order to restore the kidneys to normal functioning. Management includes drug therapy, diet, and rest. Treatment is correlated with the blood pressure and the results of urine testing for red blood cells and protein. The client is not considered to be free from the disease until the urine tests negative for protein and red blood cells for 6 months. Prevention of renal complications as well as complications to cardiac and cerebral functioning is the focus of care.

Pharmacological

Prophylactic antimicrobial therapy may be administered. The drug of choice is penicillin. Diuretic and antihypertensive medication furosemide (Lasix) may be ordered. Corticosteroids, chemotherapeutic drugs such as cyclophosphamide (Cytoxan), and/or immunosuppressive agents such as azathioprine (Imuran) may be ordered to control the inflammatory response.

Plasmapheresis may be indicated if there is no response from other treatments. Between 150 and 400 mL of blood is removed from the client and put in a cell separator. Here the blood is divided into plasma and formed elements. The formed elements are mixed with a plasma replacement and returned to the client through a vein. Another technique filters the client's own plasma to remove a specific disease mediator (antibody) and then returns the plasma to the client.

Diet

Fluid retention often requires fluid restriction. The restriction is adjusted according to the client's intake and output record and daily weight. Protein in the client's diet will be regulated according to the BUN and the creatinine blood levels. The kidneys need to rest; however, particularly in children, it may not be necessary to restrict protein. Potassium will need to be replaced if the diuretic promotes its excretion. Sodium may be restricted to prevent fluid retention. Strict intake and output are necessary to monitor kidney function.

Activity

Physical and emotional rest are essential. Compliance with bed rest may be difficult, especially for a child or the client who feels well. Bed rest is indicated until the inflammation subsides, urinary flow increases, and as long as the client has hematuria or proteinuria. During this time a strict turning schedule needs to be followed, as skin breakdown is more likely in the presence of edema. Once bed rest restrictions are lifted, the client may feel weakened from the effects of anemia and inactivity.

▶ NURSING PROCESS

▶ Assessment

▶ Subjective Data

The health history will likely reveal a recent sore throat, skin infection, flulike symptoms, and a headache. The client describes flank pain as the kidneys become congested. Other symptoms the client may describe are malaise, anorexia, cola-colored "smokey" urine (hematuria), and a marked decrease in the amount of urine (oliguria). Facial edema may have been the first sign noticed, may impair vision, and may cause the client to have negative feelings about body image.

▶ Objective Data

Vital signs will generally show an increase in body temperature and blood pressure. Facial (periorbital) edema is present. The edema will progress to dependent areas such as the sacral area and the legs. The location and degree of edema should be monitored daily. Ascites may also develop. The general condition of the skin and skin integrity should be assessed, and the client weighed to establish a baseline weight. Heart and lung sounds are assessed for signs of congestive heart failure and pulmonary edema (unusual heart sounds and crackles in the lungs). Neck veins

HOME HEALTH CARE

Sodium Restriction

Advise to use low-sodium bottled water in cooking and for the drinking allowance when water supplies are naturally high in sodium or if water is chemically softened.

may be distended. Dyspnea on exertion or when recumbent, and shortness of breath, may both be noted. Urine output is decreased and hematuria is present (cola-colored to red).

The nurse should monitor results of diagnostic tests: urine for red blood cells and protein (albumin) and blood for BUN, serum creatinine, potassium, ESR, ASO titer, and specific gravity, all of which will be elevated.

Nursing diagnoses for a client with acute glomerulonephritis may include the following:

Nursing Diagnoses	Planning/Goals	Nursing Interventions
▶ *Fluid Volume Excess related to compromised regulatory mechanism secondary to renal dysfunction*	The client will have decreased edema and adequate urinary output.	Fluids will be restricted with specific amounts designated throughout the day. For example, 900 mL of fluids for a day might be divided in the following manner: 7 A.M. to 3 P.M. 600 mL; 3 P.M. to 11 P.M. 200 mL; 11 P.M. to 7 A.M. 100 mL.
		Encourage compliance to the fluid amounts.
		Maintain accurate intake and output records hourly.
		Provide oral hygiene several times a day. This is extremely important when water intake is restricted.
		Advise that thirst may be relieved by sucking on hard candy or, if allowed, a few ice chips.
		Provide eye care with normal saline to promote comfort from the periorbital edema.
▶ *Social Interaction, Impaired, related to changes in body image*	The client will resume social interaction.	Encourage client to keep in contact with friends and relatives by telephone.
		Encourage keeping appointments with the physician and laboratory.
▶ *Nutrition, Altered, More than Body Requirements, related to the disease process*	The client will comply with nutritional restrictions.	Once the client's condition warrants solid foods, provide diet with complex carbohydrates instead of foods with concentrated sugar.
		If hematuria and/or proteinuria are still present, provide a diet with mild to moderate protein restriction to rest the kidney tissue. Protein foods that may be restricted include meats, fish, poultry, eggs, milk products, and whole grains.
		If edema persists, provide low-sodium diet. Processed, canned, or frozen foods will be substituted with foods made with fresh ingredients.
		If a restricted sodium and protein diet are ordered, arrange a dietary consultation to incorporate food preferences and religious and/or cultural needs. Finances may be an issue if the family has to incorporate foods that are not usually part of its budget.
		Teach client to plan menus and to read food labels in order to comply with the dietary restrictions.
		Before discharge, teach client and family about diet, fluids, and activity restrictions and measuring fluid intake and urine output.
		Provide client with guidelines listing reasons to call the physician.

Evaluation Each goal must be evaluated to determine how it has been met by the client.

CHRONIC GLOMERULONEPHRITIS

The prognosis for acute glomerulonephritis is often good when treatment is begun early; however, chronic glomerulonephritis generally leads to permanent kidney damage. Those who develop chronic glomerulonephritis may have neither symptoms nor a recent history of an infection. Chronic diseases, such as diabetes mellitus or systemic lupus erythematosus, often mask renal symptoms and the client does not seek medical care until kidney function is impaired. It may take up to 30 years for the signs of renal insufficiency to develop.

Chronic glomerulonephritis is a progressive but slow, destructive process affecting the glomeruli, causing loss of kidney function. The kidney will actually decrease in size as glomeruli are destroyed. If end-stage renal disease (ESRD) develops, the client may die quickly.

Nephrons lose their ability to filter nitrogenous wastes from the blood. Protein (albumin) and red blood cells escape into the urine and are present on a urinalysis. Nitrogenous waste remains in the blood, and the blood urea nitrogen (BUN) level increases. As glomeruli are destroyed, the serum level of creatinine also increases. BUN and serum creatinine are checked on a regular basis to monitor renal function and to assist with client care management. Serum electrolyte levels are also monitored. Anemia will be evaluated with a CBC.

Medical–Surgical Management

Medical

Medical treatment must begin immediately to limit further destruction of the glomerular tissue. Management includes drug therapy, diet, and bed rest. Exposure of the client to infection of any kind must be avoided. Blood transfusion may be required for severe anemia. The client may need to be transferred to a facility where dialysis and/or kidney transplantation can be performed. Prevention of further renal damage as well as heart or cerebral complications is the focus of care.

Pharmacological

Diuretic and antihypertensive medications are ordered. Antimicrobial therapy is generally given prophylactically. Side effects from all medications must be watched for and reported to the physician immediately.

Diet

Fluid intake is adjusted according to urinary output. Protein allowed in the diet will be regulated according to the BUN and the creatinine blood levels. As these levels increase, protein will be restricted to decrease the nitrogenous wastes. Sodium and potassium restrictions will be determined by the serum electrolyte levels. Carbohydrates are usually increased in the diet to provide adequate energy.

Activity

Bed rest is indicated when the client has hematuria or albuminuria.

▶ NURSING PROCESS

▶ Assessment

▶ Subjective Data

Clients may complain of a morning headache, pruritis, a decreased ability to concentrate, fatigue, and dyspnea making it difficult to perform ADLs. Facial edema and/or blurring of vision, due to retinal edema, may also be reported by clients.

▶ Objective Data

As chronic glomerulonephritis develops, fluid retention becomes evident, leading to shortness of breath, especially at night. Vital signs are monitored, and hypertension is usually present. Lung sounds need to be assessed every shift for crackles, a sign of fluid retention. Weight must be monitored daily, after the baseline weight is obtained, and the degree of edema, its location, and if it is pitting or nonpitting must be noted. **Anasarca** is generalized edema that appears as the client's condition deteriorates. The skin must be assessed for color, presence of ecchymosis or rash, dryness, and evidence of scratching. Mental functioning, irritability, tremors, ataxia, or slurred speech should be noted.

As nephrons lose their ability to concentrate urine, the urine becomes pale and dilute. Intake and output must be closely monitored because initially, polyuria develops giving the client a false sense that recovery will be soon. Results of blood and urine tests must be monitored.

Nursing diagnoses for a client with chronic glomerulonephritis may include the following:

Nursing Diagnoses	Planning/Goals	Nursing Interventions
▶ *Urinary Elimination, Altered, related to the failing kidney function*	The client will have adequate urine output.	Measure urine output hourly, or every 4 or 8 hours as ordered, to determine kidney function. Parameters will be set by the physician for immediate notification.
		Assess and document the color and consistency of the urine.
		Measure intake to determine compliance with the amount of fluids permitted.
		Weigh client daily at the same time each day, on the same scale and with the same clothes.
▶ *Fluid Volume Excess related to compromised regulatory mechanism*	The client will have decreased edema.	Assess and describe the location of the edema.
		Administer medications as ordered for treatment of the edema.
		Monitor electrolyte values.
		Maintain fluid intake at restricted amount.
		Document I & O.

continued

Nursing Diagnoses	Planning/Goals	Nursing Interventions
▶ *Anxiety related to threat to or change in health status (potential treatment with dialysis)*	The client will communicate less anxiety about possible treatment with dialysis.	Assist client to express concerns about possible treatment with dialysis. Arrange for a dialysis nurse to visit client.
▶ *Skin Integrity, Impaired, Risk for, related to immobility and edema*	The client will maintain skin integrity.	Assess skin every time the client is repositioned. Cleanse the skin frequently, especially when crystals of urea form on the skin, causing itching and dryness.

Evaluation Each goal must be evaluated to determine how it has been met by the client.

OBSTRUCTIVE DISORDERS

Disorders of this type include urolithiasis, urinary bladder tumors, renal tumors, and polycystic kidney.

UROLITHIASIS

Urolithiasis is a calculus, or stone, formed in the urinary tract. More than 1 million persons in the United States each year have kidney stones (NKF, 1998b). A calculus (plural–calculi) is a solid mass of mineral salts occurring within a hollow organ such as the renal pelvis, ureters, bladder, or urethra (Figure 42-2). A urinary calculus can range in size from microscopic to 10 to 20 mm in diameter.

Calculi are formed from minerals that precipitate out of solution and collect within hollow areas. The reason stones form has not yet been identified, but individuals who are immobile, hyperparathyroid, or have recurrent UTIs are predisposed. When a person is immobile for long periods, calcium is pulled from the bones into the blood. The nephrons filter the excess calcium out of the blood into the urine. Calculi can also lodge in and obstruct an indwelling catheter. The size and location of the stone within the urinary system greatly affects the degree of pain and other symptoms present. When the stone is in the kidney, the pain is dull and constant mainly in the back just below the ribs near the spine. Stones in the ureter often cause ureteral colic, an excruciating, intermittent pain that begins in the flank and radiates into the groin, inner thigh, or genitalia. It is caused by spasm of the ureter as the calculus moves down the ureter. The client often has nausea and vomiting also.

If a calculus becomes lodged any place along the ureter, the urine cannot pass and a condition called hydronephrosis and/or hydroureter occurs. The kidney and/or ureter become enlarged with the accumulated urine, as illustrated in Figure 42-3.

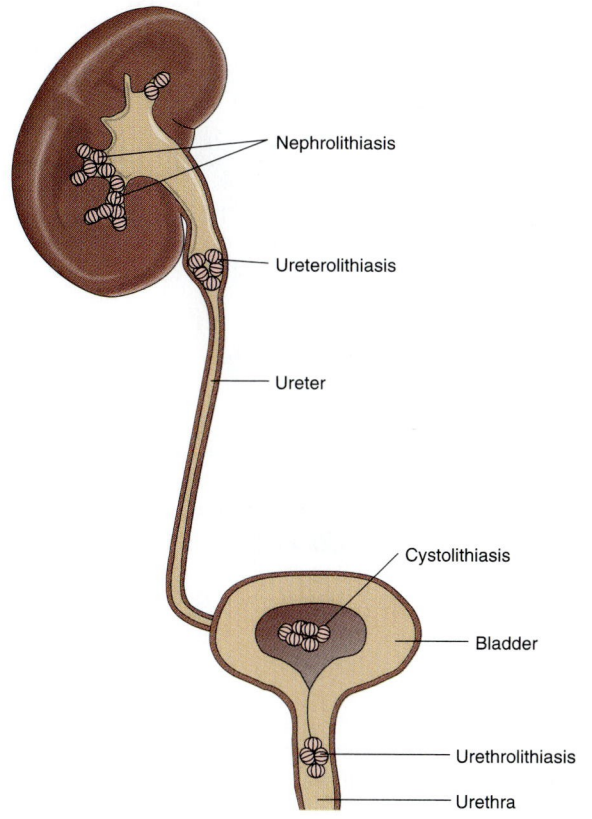

Figure 42-2 Common Locations of Urinary Calculi Formation

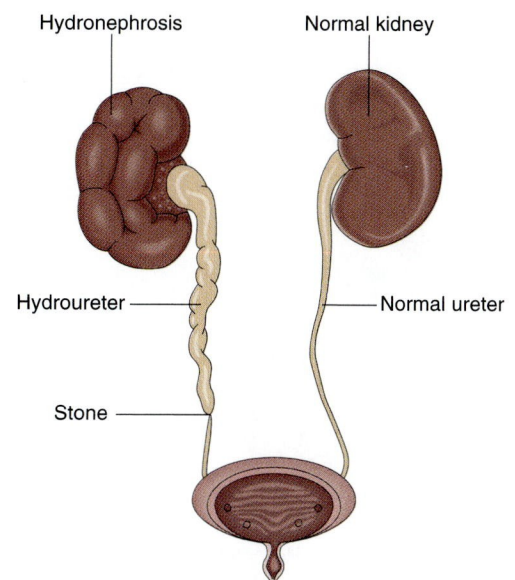

Figure 42-3 Hydronephrosis and Hydroureter Resulting from a Stone in the Ureter

Tests to confirm the diagnosis and determine the size and location of the stone include KUB, IVP, cystoscopy, and ultrasound. A BUN and serum creatinine indicate whether the calculus has damaged kidney function. A urinalysis with a culture and a CBC may be ordered to determine whether an infection is present. A 24-hour urine may be sent to the laboratory to determine whether there is abnormal excretion of calcium oxalate, phosphorus, and uric acid.

Medical–Surgical Management

Medical

All urine must be strained whether voided or from an indwelling catheter drainage bag. Urine from a catheter drainage bag must be drained and strained every 2 to 4 hours. All strained particles must be saved for the physician or sent to the laboratory.

A very small calculus may be flushed out by peristalsis and fluids. The client is encouraged to drink at least 4,000 mL of fluid/day, unless contraindicated by other health problems. The urologist may insert a small, pliable catheter into the ureter or urethra to allow temporary drainage of urine around the calculus.

Extracorporeal shock wave **lithotripsy** (ESWL) is a method of crushing a calculus any place in the urinary system with ultrasonic waves. The client is placed in a warm water bath and ultrasonic waves aimed at the stone break the stone into small pieces. An alternate method is to appropriately place a fluid-filled bag on the client's body and aim the ultrasonic waves at the stone through the bag. There is some discomfort and the client may be bruised where the ultrasonic waves hit the body. The urine will be slightly bloody for 24 to 48 hours and must be strained. The client should drink large amounts of fluids (3,000 mL to 4,000 mL/day) unless contraindicated. Clients should avoid taking aspirin and other drugs that affect blood clotting for several weeks before the procedure (NIDDK, 1998a).

Surgical

There are several surgical procedures, depending on the location and size of the calculus, from which the surgeon may choose. These include nephroscopic removal, pyelolithotomy, nephrolithotomy, or ureterolithotomy (Figure 42-4).

Percutaneous nephrolithotomy is the endoscopic procedure in which a small incision is made in the fleshy area on the client's side between the ribs and the hip. A catheter is inserted and an ultrasonic probe is inserted through the catheter. Ultrasound waves directed at the stone break it into small pieces that can be withdrawn through the catheter. The catheter is left in place until the edema subsides, usually 1 or 2 days.

A bladder calculus may be crushed with special surgical instruments and the fragments washed out through a catheter. This is called a **litholapaxy**.

Pharmacological

Narcotic analgesics are generally prescribed for the severe pain often called renal colic. Antispasmodics such as propantheline bromide (Pro-Banthine) or belladonna preparations may be ordered to relieve

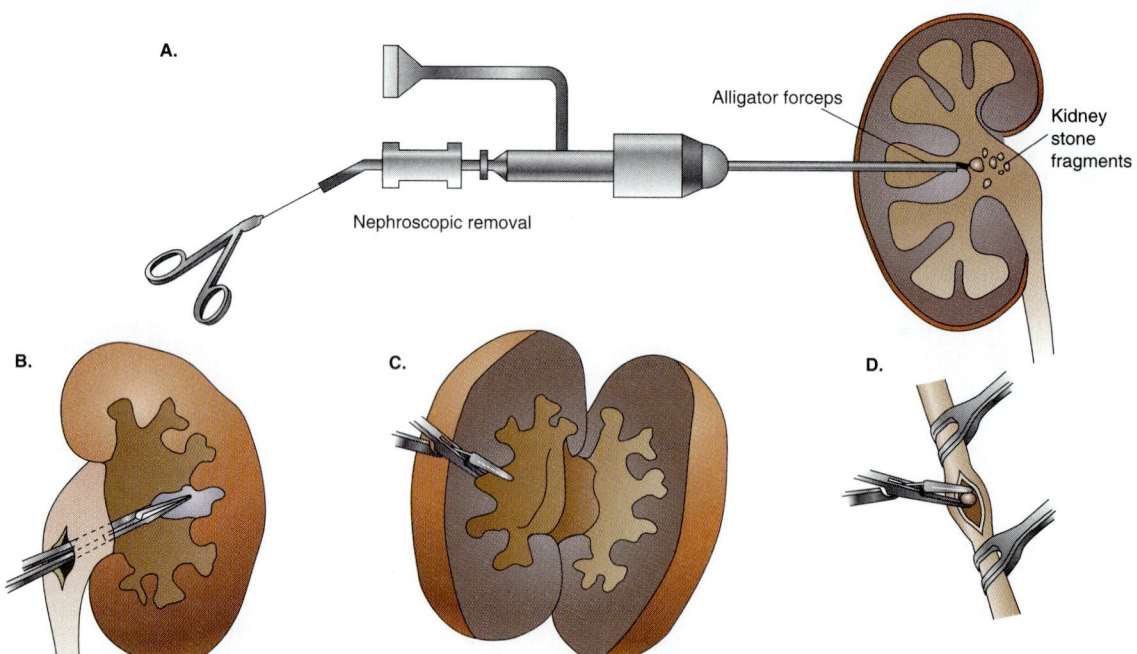

Figure 42-4 Methods of Removing Urinary Stones: A. Nephroscopic removal (percutaneous nephrolithotomy); B. Pyelolithotomy, removal through the renal pelvis; C. Nephrolithotomy, removal through incision into the kidney; D. Ureterolithotomy, removal through the ureter

ureteral spasms. Antibiotics may be ordered prophylactically.

Drug therapy is specific to stone composition. Allopurinol (Zyloprim) reduces the serum urate level, thus preventing calcium oxalate stones. Sodium cellulose phosphate (Calcibind) binds with calcium in the bowel and facilitates excretion of calcium. Aluminum hydroxide gel (Amphojel) binds with excess phosphates in the gastrointestinal tract. The phosphates are then excreted.

Diet

Individuals who form calcium calculi may need to reduce their intake of dietary calcium, mainly dairy products, to no more than 600 mg/day. When the stones contain uric acid, purine-rich foods (meat, fish, and poultry) are restricted, and organ meats, anchovies, and sardines avoided. Foods rich in oxalic acid (broccoli, asparagus, chocolate, tea, rhubarb, and spinach) are restricted when oxalate stones form. A deficiency of pyridoxine, thiamin, and magnesium may also contribute to the formation of oxalate stones.

Sometimes an effort is made to change the pH of the urine and thus prevent the formation of calculi. Acid-ash or alkaline-ash diets are used. Acid-ash foods are meats, fish, poultry, eggs, cereals, cranberries, and plums. Alkaline-ash foods are vegetables and all other fruits. These diets are often difficult for the client to maintain.

Drinking large amounts of fluid, at least half of it water, dilutes the urine and helps move any microscopic calculi through the system. Up to 4,000 mL/day of fluid is indicated for a client with renal calculi, unless contraindicated by another health problem such as congestive heart failure.

Activity

Exercising regularly helps reduce the formation of calculi and keeps calculi moving through the urinary tract. Clients on bed rest should perform active range-of-motion exercises daily in addition to frequent turning and positioning.

CLIENT TEACHING

Urinary System Calculi

A person with a family history of stones or who has had more than one stone is at risk to develop another stone. These clients can be instructed to:

- Drink plenty of fluids—water is best—to prevent stone formation,
- Avoid immobility,
- Take medications and modify diet as prescribed,
- Keep a record of intake and output, and
- Learn how to strain urine.

▶ NURSING PROCESS

▶ Assessment

▶ Subjective Data

Some individuals may be asymptomatic until the calculus begins to move or becomes too large. When the stone moves, the client usually describes intractable pain, that is, pain that is not relieved by ordinary measures. Nausea and vomiting are often reported also. The pain is often described as beginning in the flank and radiating down to the groin and inner thigh. Nonverbal client behaviors may indicate pain, such as tossing and turning when in bed or the inability to sit still when out of bed. If the calculus is not moving, the client may describe symptoms of infection such as lethargy, frequency of urination, dysuria, burning on urination, or feeling very warm. The client may express feelings of frustration related to the inability to complete daily tasks.

▶ Objective Data

Hematuria, vomiting, intake and output, and vital signs must be assessed. Elevated pulse and blood pressure may indicate pain. Urine should be checked for stones when it is strained.

Nursing diagnoses for a client with urolithiasis may include the following:

Nursing Diagnoses	Planning/Goals	Nursing Interventions
▶ Pain related to irritation of the urinary tract and the mobility of calculi	The client will verbalize a reduction in pain.	Develop a pain management plan.
		Inquire about intensity, location, duration, and alleviating factors of pain.
		Provide comfort measures and diversionary activities.
		Administer analgesics and antispasmodics as ordered.
		Observe for nonverbal signs of pain.

continued

Nursing Diagnoses	Planning/Goals	Nursing Interventions
▸ *Urinary Elimination, Altered, related to blockage of urine flow by the calculi*	The client will return to normal urine elimination.	Monitor urine for color and amount.
		Encourage fluids to dilute the urine and flush out the calculi.
		Assist client to ambulate, if able.
		Accurately monitor intake and output.
		If a ureteral catheter is in place, measure and record the urine output from it separately from the urine output from the bladder.

Evaluation Each goal must be evaluated to determine how it has been met by the client.

URINARY BLADDER TUMORS

According to the American Cancer Society estimates indicate approximately 54,200 new cases of urinary bladder cancer (ACS, 1999b). Men are affected 4 times more often than women. Bladder cancer occurs most frequently after the age of 50. The only early warning signs are increased urinary frequency and painless, intermittent hematuria. The main risk factor is cigarette smoking. Those individuals who smoke nicotine products have twice the risk of developing bladder cancer as do nonsmokers. Other risk factors are working with dyes, rubber, or leather products; caffeine intake; and the use of certain artificial sweeteners.

Benign papillomas are the most common urinary bladder tumor. Although the papillomas are quite small, they should be treated aggressively because they are considered to be premalignant. Cancer cells develop mainly in the area where the ureters enter the urinary bladder. The primary sites for metastasis are the liver, lungs, or bones. Symptoms resulting from obstruction of the ureters is a frequent reason for the client seeking medical care. Diagnostic studies done usually include a urinalysis, a cystoscopic visualization and biopsy of the lesions, an IVP, and CT scan.

Medical–Surgical Management

Surgical

Surgical removal of small tumors is generally done by **fulguration** (a procedure to destroy tissue with long, high-frequency electric sparks) to burn the lesions off the internal bladder wall. Other surgical procedures used are laser surgery or snaring of the lesion. These procedures are usually performed with cystoscopic visualization. Several times a year, the client who has had

bladder lesions should be monitored for recurrence of the lesions. A cytologic examination is done on any lesion(s) noted during a cystoscopic examination.

A cystoscopic examination is performed with either local anesthesia and sedation or general anesthesia. After the procedure, the client's legs may be sore as a lithotomy position is used. Analgesics will be prescribed for use as needed. After a cystoscopic procedure, the client may experience urinary frequency, burning on urination, and the presence of pink-tinged urine.

When the pathology of tissue specimens indicates a need for more extensive surgery, either a partial or total cystectomy may be performed. The surgery may be done in conjunction with radiation therapy or chemotherapy.

When the urinary bladder is completely removed, a urinary diversion is necessary. Consideration is made for age, extent of the disease, and the prognosis. One option is a bilateral cutaneous ureterostomy, in which the ureters are implanted directly into the abdominal wall. Another option is for the ureters to be implanted into a piece of the ileum, which is then attached to the abdominal wall as a stoma. This is known as an **ileal** ("wet") **conduit**.

Other methods of urinary diversion are the implantation of the ureters into the sigmoid colon (ureterosigmoidostomy) and the creation of a continent stoma with a pouch of bowel. This urinary diversion is known either as a Kock (Figure 42-5) or Mainz pouch

CULTURAL CONSIDERATIONS

Bladder Cancer
White persons are twice as likely to have bladder cancer as African Americans (ACS, 1999b).

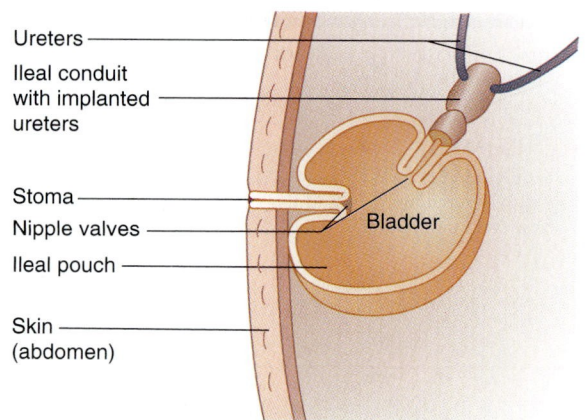

Ureters

Ileal conduit with implanted ureters

Stoma

Nipple valves

Ileal pouch

Bladder

Skin (abdomen)

Figure 42-5 Urinary Diversion—Kock Pouch

or a Gilchrist ileocecal reservoir, depending on which surgical procedure was used.

Pharmacological

One chemotherapy treatment is the instillation of an antineoplastic drug within the urinary bladder (**intravesical**). Systemic chemotherapy may also be used for cystectomy clients. Medications to relieve symptoms such as pain and nausea are important for the client's well-being.

Diet

If proctitis (inflammation of the rectum and anus) or diarrhea occurs, a low-residue diet is ordered to facilitate normal bowel elimination.

Activity

When the client is on bed rest, turning and positioning are important to maintain skin integrity because the client may be emaciated due to significant weight loss. Activity should be encouraged as the client's con-dition warrants. During the intravesical instillation of an antineoplastic drug, the client will have to change positions every 15 minutes, for a period of several hours, to evenly distribute the chemotherapeutic drug around the urinary bladder.

▶ NURSING PROCESS

▶ Assessment

▶ Subjective Data

The client will describe having painless, intermittent hematuria and changes in voiding patterns. Fatigue may also be mentioned.

▶ Objective Data

Weakness will be noted if the client has become anemic from the hematuria. The nurse should check urine specimen with a reagent strip for blood, review results of diagnostic tests, and assess the client's understanding of current health situation.

Nursing diagnoses for a client with urinary bladder tumors may include the following:

Nursing Diagnoses	Planning/Goals	Nursing Interventions
▶ *Knowledge Deficit, related to surgery and treatment regimen*	The client will describe surgical changes and treatment regimen.	If surgical removal of bladder lesions is done as an outpatient procedure, teach the client to observe for pink-tinged urine and to notify the physician if bright red urine is seen.
		Discuss the use of analgesics as ordered for pain of bladder spasms.
		Encourage adequate fluid intake.
		For urinary diversions: Refer the client with a stoma to the enterostomal therapist for specialized care and teaching. The therapist will assist the client with the appliance and skin care protocol.
		Monitor the color and integrity of the stoma daily to ensure that the tissue is receiving adequate circulation. The stoma is normally red and edematous for a time postoperatively. The stoma will remain red in color but will shrink in size during the healing process.
		If the stoma color changes, notify the physician.
		Refer to a local ostomy group for ongoing support and assistance or to the United Ostomy Association, which provides support and literature.
		Teach the signs and symptoms related to potential problems that should be reported to the physician.
		Encourage the intake of fluids, up to 3,000 mL per day, unless contraindicated.
		Teach about the medications to be taken at home.
		Encourage the client to attend all scheduled follow-up visits.
		Assist the client to plan the gradual return to the routines of driving, lifting, sexual activities, and work.
▶ *Urinary Elimination, Altered, related to surgical procedure*	The client will maintain adequate urinary elimination.	Accurately monitor urine output because this is the major postoperative concern.
		Assist client to discuss feelings about the altered urinary elimination method.
		Assist the client with a bilateral cutaneous ureterostomy to use leg bags for easier ambulation.
		Change the leg bag tubing back to straight bag drainage to promote uninterrupted sleep.
		Teach the client how to use both kinds of drainage systems.

Evaluation Each goal must be evaluated to determine how it has been met by the client.

RENAL TUMORS

The American Cancer Society estimates there will be approximately 30,000 new cases of kidney cancer in 1999 (ACS, 1999a). A unilateral renal adenocarcinoma is the most common tumor and is seen more often in men between the ages of 50 and 70. Risk factors include smoking, familial incidence, and preexisting renal disorders.

Intermittent, painless hematuria is often ignored by the client, and medical attention is not sought until the malignancy is quite advanced. By this time, the client usually has experienced weight loss, dull flank pain, gross hematuria, and a mass that may be palpable in the flank area. Lymph nodes in the area of the kidney, the renal vessels, and/or the inferior vena cava may become involved. The primary sites for metastases are the lungs, liver, brain, and bone. A pathological fracture may be the reason for admission of the client, resulting in the diagnosis of kidney cancer.

An IVP will detect a renal mass. Other diagnostic studies used to evaluate the kidney or the status of other body systems possibly involved are renal sonography or arteriogram, MRI, CT scan, or a needle biopsy. The painless hematuria contributes to a decreased hematocrit.

Medical–Surgical Management

Medical

The physician may insert a nephrostomy tube into the renal pelvis of each kidney to evaluate the function of each kidney. Chemotherapy and/or radiation therapy have proved to be of minimal benefit.

CULTURAL CONSIDERATIONS

Renal Cell Carcinoma

Those most at risk are:
- Hispanic men,
- Those exposed to leather, cadmium, asbestos, lead, and petrochemical products at their job, and
- Those with a family history of bilateral kidney disease (McKinney, 1996).

Surgical

Usually a radical nephrectomy is performed if the other kidney is healthy and the disease is localized. The surgeon may enter the thoracic as well as the abdominal cavity during this procedure. If the chest is opened, the client will have a closed chest drainage system postoperatively. A nasogastric drainage tube may be in place and attached to suction. Hemorrhage and compromised respiratory effort are the postoperative problems for which to observe.

Pharmacological

If the client is receiving radiation therapy treatments, antiemetics or antispasmodics may be ordered. Analgesics are ordered to control pain and facilitate respirations and client activity. An antiemetic will usually be ordered to promote comfort and to encourage eating.

Diet

The client having a nephrectomy will have intravenous fluids until food can be tolerated. A well-balanced diet is then ordered. Fluid intake of at least 2,000 mL/day is needed to maintain adequate hydration. The use of alcohol should be avoided. If the client is **cachectic** (in a state of malnutrition and wasting) because of the cancer's pathology, parenteral nutrition may be indicated.

Activity

Ambulation is to be encouraged during the client's recovery. Frequent rest periods are also necessary even after discharge.

▶ NURSING PROCESS

▶ Assessment

▶ Subjective Data

The client will mention having a dull pain in the flank area and noticing blood in the urine intermittently. However, the client often comments that there is no difficulty in urinating. Fatigue and weight loss are also described.

▶ Objective Data

Weight is compared with usual weight. Vital signs and diagnostic test results are monitored. The client's lung sounds are assessed for possible respiratory distress resulting from metastases. Hematuria may be seen. A mass may be palpated in the client's flank area.

Nursing diagnoses for a client with renal tumors may include the following:

Nursing Diagnoses	Planning/Goals	Nursing Interventions
▶ *Fatigue, related to disease process and treatment*	The client will understand reason for fatigue and not feel guilty for taking rest periods.	Discuss with client that fatigue is a result of blood loss in the urine and growth of the tumor.
		Because there is increased fatigue following any surgery, plan nursing care so the client will have several periods of uninterrupted rest each day.
▶ *Grieving, Anticipatory, related to diagnosis, treatment, and prognosis*	The client will maintain open communications with family and health care members.	Actively listen to what the client says.
		Encourage the client to express feelings about the diagnosis and treatment.
		Observe for signs of grieving such as crying, denial, anger, or withdrawal.
		Answer questions honestly.
		Assist client in identifying strengths and coping skills.
		Make referrals to other professionals as needed.
▶ *Knowledge Deficit, related to limited information of disease process and treatment regimen*	The client will verbalize understanding of information taught.	Inform the client of the assessments to be done: neurological status, lung sounds, the incision, Homans' sign, peripheral pulses, vital signs, and serum electrolyte values.
		Teach the importance of accurate intake and output records.
		Provide routine preoperative teaching.
		Encourage the client to eat a well-balanced diet to enhance healing.
		Instruct the client not to wash off the skin markings if radiation therapy is being used.
		Teach the name, purpose, dosage, schedule, and side effects of all medications and the importance of drinking plenty of fluids and ambulating as tolerated.
		Inform the client and family of community resources and support groups.
		Point out the importance of following the instructions for care when discharged and keeping physician appointments.

Evaluation Each goal must be evaluated to determine how it has been met by the client.

POLYCYSTIC KIDNEY

Polycystic kidney disease (PKD) may be inherited or acquired. Acquired cystic kidney disease (ACKD) is associated with dialysis and end-stage renal disease. Approximately 90% of clients on dialysis for 5 years develop ACKD (NIDDK, 1998a). In PKD, multiple grape-like clusters of fluid-filled cysts develop in and greatly enlarge both kidneys. They compress and eventually replace functioning kidney tissue. PKD has an insidious onset that becomes obvious between 30 and 50 years of age.

Early symptoms include hypertension, polyuria, and urinary tract infections. Flank pain and headache are common. Recurrent hematuria and proteinuria develop. Diagnosis is made by x-ray or sonogram showing the cysts. BUN and creatinine are used to monitor kidney function.

The goal of medical management is to preserve kidney function, prevent infections, and relieve pain. Hypertension is carefully managed with antihypertensive medications, diuretics, and fluid and dietary modifications. Eventually, dialysis or renal transplantation may be needed.

RENAL FAILURE

According to NIDDK (May, 1999), any acute or chronic loss of kidney function is called renal failure and is the term used when some kidney function remains. Total, or nearly total, and permanent kidney failure is called end-stage renal disease (ESRD). It may take only a few days or weeks to lose renal function or it may deteriorate slowly over decades. Disorders of renal failure are either acute or chronic.

ACUTE RENAL FAILURE

The rapid deterioration of renal function with rising blood levels of urea and other nitrogenous wastes (**azotemia**) is termed acute renal failure (ARF). The nephrons also are unable to regulate the fluid and electrolyte or the acid-base balance of the blood. Predisposing factors include acute glomerular disease; severe, acute kidney infection; decreased cardiac output; trauma; or hemorrhage.

There are three major forms depending on the location of the cause: postrenal ARF (disrupted urine flow), prerenal ARF (disrupted blood flow to the kidney), and intrarenal ARF (renal tissue damage). Both postrenal ARF and prerenal ARF are reversible situations if they are identified early and treatment is begun. Undiagnosed postrenal ARF and prerenal ARF lead to intrarenal ARF.

POSTRENAL ARF

Postrenal ARF is caused by an obstruction and makes up approximately 5% of all ARF cases (Kelley, 1997). It should be checked out first when a client has an unexplained decrease in urine output or has anuria. Kidney function can be easily restored by removing the obstruction. Urine volume will vary depending on the location and degree of obstruction. Catheterization, ultrasound, and retrograde pylogram are used to diagnose an obstruction. An obstruction may be caused by renal calculi, blood clots, edema, tumors, urethral strictures, benign prostatic hypertrophy (BPH), or pregnancy. Postrenal failure can be ruled out if there is no obstruction. If an obstruction is confirmed, relief of the obstruction is imperative to minimize renal damage and resolve azotemia. When postrenal failure is prolonged, both blood creatinine and BUN will rise.

PRERENAL ARF

Any abnormal decline in kidney perfusion that reduces glomerular perfusion can cause prerenal failure. Fluid volume status does not indicate perfusion. Effective arterial blood volume (EABV) is the amount of fluid in the vascular space that effectively perfuses the kidneys. Even in fluid volume excess situations, such as low cardiac output due to heart failure, the EABV falls, causing prerenal failure. The kidney interprets a fall in EABV as fluid volume deficit.

The glomeruli are then unable to filter waste from the blood. The renal tubules are structurally intact, and the kidneys can resume normal functioning if perfusion is restored fairly quickly. Ischemia results from prolonged inadequate perfusion, which can cause acute tubular necrosis (ATN).

The client generally has pale, cool skin; orthostatic hypotension; and oliguria. The BUN-to-creatinine ratio rises from 10:1 to more than 20:1. This rise is because there is greater reabsorption of urea when fluids flow slowly through the tubules. A urinalysis shows a low sodium level (less than 20 mEq/L), high osmolality (more than 500 mOsm/L), and high specific gravity (more than 1.020). This results because the kidneys are retaining sodium and water in an attempt to correct the perceived fluid volume deficit.

When the client truly has a fluid volume deficit, treatment consists of intravenous fluids and albumin, plasma, or blood to restore the EABV. When the cause is inadequate cardiac output, inotropic agents such as dobutamine hydrochloride (Dobutrex) or amrinone lactate (Inocor) are ordered.

INTRARENAL ARF

Tissue damage of the glomeruli and/or tubules causes a loss of renal function known as intrarenal ARF. Glomerulonephritis and ATN are the main reasons for renal tissue damage. The antigen/antibody complexes formed in glomerulonephritis become trapped in the basement membrane where they cause inflammation. The glomeruli then become more permeable so red blood cells and protein are allowed to enter the filtrate and ultimately the urine.

The majority of all intrarenal failure cases is caused by ATN, and is the most common cause of nosocomial acute renal failure. ATN is the result of ischemia or toxic insult to the renal tubules. Ischemia may result from untreated prerenal failure or severe hypoxemia. Radiographic contrast dye, pigments (myoglobin and hemoglobin), aminoglycoside and cephalosporin antibiotics, and NSAIDs are all **nephrotoxic** (substances that causes kidney tissue damage) and can cause acute tubular necrosis.

The BUN-to-creatinine ratio in acute tubular necrosis is usually normal between 10:1 and 15:1; however, both the BUN and creatinine are greatly elevated. For example, the BUN may be 70 mg/dL and the creatinine 7 mg/dL. Urine sodium is more than 40 mEq/L, urine osmolality less than 300 mOsm/L, and specific gravity less than 1.010.

There are three phases to the clinical course of ATN: oliguric/nonoliguric, diuretic, and recovery. The first phase is either oliguric or nonoliguric depending on the causative factor.

Oliguric/Nonoliguric Phase

A nonoliguric phase is usually seen when nephrotoxic agents are the causative factor. When adequate urine output is maintained, dialysis is needed less often and the morbidity and mortality rates are lower.

An oliguric phase, which may last 1 to 2 weeks, is seen more often when ischemia is the causative factor. Oliguria, voiding less than 400 mL/24 hours, can cause fluid volume overload; electrolyte imbalance, specifically high potassium and phosphorus, and low sodium and calcium; metabolic acidosis; and uremia.

Diuretic Phase

The diuretic phase is seldom seen because early dialysis keeps extracellular fluid volume at a fairly normal level. If it were seen, there would be a tremendous increase in urine output.

Recovery Phase

As renal function begins to improve, the client's urine output returns to normal and serum and urine laboratory test values move closer to normal. There is usually a short period of rapid improvement and then a period (may be several months) of slower improvement. Some clients will have residual renal insufficiency and a few will require long-term dialysis.

Medical–Surgical Management

Medical

Acute renal failure is often reversible, and complications can be prevented with early diagnosis and treatment. The goal is to have kidney function stabilized and returned to normal. Problems to be alert for are fluid volume overload, electrolyte imbalances, metabolic acidosis, high rate of catabolism, uremia, hematological abnormalities, and infection.

Dialysis is now an early treatment in ATN. Homeostasis is maintained while the cause of ATN is determined and treated. Permanent kidney damage may thus be averted. See the section on dialysis later in this chapter.

Surgical

The obstructions causing postrenal failure are often removed surgically. The exact procedure will depend on what type of obstruction is present and its location.

Pharmacological

Drugs used in the treatment of acute renal failure include antihypertensives, diuretics, cardiotonics (inotropics), phosphate-binding antacids, potassium-lowering agents, and electrolyte replacement. It is important to ensure that drugs used are not nephrotoxic. See Table 42-2 for drugs used in acute renal failure.

Diet

Restrictions generally include sodium, potassium, phosphorus, protein, and fluids. The amounts allowed are based on the laboratory tests results. Carbohydrates and fats are increased to be sure energy needs are met and protein will be spared as a source of energy. Clients with a high rate of catabolism often require total parenteral nutrition (TPN) to provide adequate nutrition.

Activity

Because the client is often weak and may also be confused, activity is restricted during the initial phase of acute renal failure. As recovery becomes evident, ambulation is begun.

Table 42-2 DRUGS USED IN ACUTE RENAL FAILURE	
DRUGS	**NURSING RESPONSIBILITIES**
Antihypertensives methyldopa (Aldomet) minoxidil (Loniten) clonidine HCl (Catapres) hydralazine HCl (Apresoline)	Monitor BP and pulse, weigh daily, monitor for postural hypotension and K, Na, Cl, and CO_2 levels, I & O.
Diuretics furosemide (Lasix) hydrochlorothiazide (HydroDiuril)	Monitor output, maintain fluid restrictions, weigh daily.
Cardiotonics/inotropics digoxin (Lanoxin) amrinone lactate (Inocor)	Assess apical pulse before giving, report blood level of digoxin, monitor BP and P, monitor blood level of potassium.
Phosphate-binding antacids aluminum hydroxide gel (Amphojel)	Administer wtih meals, assess for constipation.
Potassium exchange sodium polystyrene sulfonate (Kayexalate)	Monitor serum potassium, assess BP and P, and for constipation.
Electrolyte replacement calcitrol (Rocaltrol) calcifediol (Calderol)	Monitor blood calcium and phosphate levels, report metallic taste.

▶ NURSING PROCESS

▶ Assessment

▶ Subjective Data

The client may have various complaints, including diarrhea; nausea, possibly with vomiting; swelling; loss of appetite; headache; increasing fatigue; and/or

CLIENT TEACHING

Acute Renal Failure

Teach clients at risk for ARF (older clients; diabetic clients; and clients with renal, heart, or liver disease) to:

- Immediately report to health care provider signs of fluid retention, pain on urination, and changes in urine output (amount or appearance),
- Avoid chronic use of and high doses of NSAIDs,
- Follow sodium and fluid restrictions as prescribed, and
- Advise all health care providers of condition.

a change in mental alertness. Anxiety and fear related to "not knowing" what is happening is often expressed.

▶ Objective Data

Physical findings will depend on how far the disease process has progressed. Assess for hypertension, GI bleeding and/or bruising, reduction in urine output, anasarca, poor skin turgor, and dry mucous membranes because vomiting or diarrhea can cause dehydration. In a severe stage, the client may be drowsy and have muscle twitching and convulsions.

The BUN and serum creatinine will be elevated as are the serum electrolytes potassium and phosphorus. The serum electrolyte calcium will be low. Blood level of red blood cells will decrease as the production of erythropoietin decreases. Leukocyte level will increase in the presence of an infection.

Nursing diagnoses for a client with acute renal failure may include the following:

Nursing Diagnoses	Planning/Goals	Nursing Interventions
▶ *Fluid Volume Excess, related to sodium and water retention*	The client will maintain a stable fluid volume.	Monitor BUN, creatinine, and serum electrolyte and protein levels.
		Accurately measure urine output, often on an hourly basis. Parameters are often set for notification of the physician.
		Weigh daily to identify weight gain related to fluid retention. One pound of weight gain is equivalent to 500 mL of retained fluid.
		Assess skin turgor, edema, BP, lung sounds, jugular vein distention, pulse and respiratory rate and quality.
		Provide fluids within the prescribed limits.
		Teach client about importance of fluid restrictions.
▶ *Nutrition, Altered, Less than Body Requirements, related to anorexia, dietary restrictions, and increased catabolism*	The client will have stabilized weight within normal limits.	Arrange for a dietary consultation to provide food in keeping with the prescribed restrictions and client preferences, including cultural and religious factors.
		Suggest 6 small meals throughout the day.
		Offer antinausea medications before meals.
		Provide or assist with oral hygiene prior to meals.
		Monitor weight and serum albumin level weekly.

Evaluation Each goal must be evaluated to determine how it has been met by the client.

SAMPLE NURSING CARE PLAN

THE CLIENT WITH ACUTE RENAL FAILURE

Mr. Long, age 65, has had a history of heart trouble for several years. He is admitted because he has urinated very little for 2 days, he gets dizzy when he gets up from lying down, and he cannot get his shoes on because his feet are "fat." He states that he does not know what is happening to him. Results of laboratory tests are BUN 90 mg/dL, creatinine 4 mg/dL, urine sodium 15 mEq/L, and urine specific gravity 1.030.

Nursing Diagnosis 1 *Fluid Volume, Excess, related to sodium and water retention as evidenced by "fat feet," urine sodium 15 mEq/L, and urine specific gravity 1.030*

PLANNING/GOALS	NURSING INTERVENTIONS	RATIONALE	EVALUATION
Mr. Long will have reduced fluid volume excess.	Accurately measure and record intake and output.	Provides information about retention of intake.	Mr. Long's feet are no longer "fat." His urine sodium is 18 mEq/L

continued

Weigh Mr. Long daily—same time, scale, clothes.

Assess skin turgor, edema, BP, lung sounds for crackles.

Provides information related to presence of fluid in tissue, lungs, or vascular system.

Monitor BUN, creatinine, and serum electrolyte and protein levels.

Administer inotropics or cardiotonic medications as ordered.

Medications will strengthen heartbeat, which will give better perfusion to kidneys.

Provide fluids within prescribed limits.

and urine specific gravity is 1.027.

Nursing Diagnosis 2 *Anxiety related to disease process as evidenced by his statement that he does not know what is happening to him*

PLANNING/GOALS	NURSING INTERVENTIONS	RATIONALE	EVALUATION
Mr. Long will have less anxiety by understanding what is happening to him.	Establish rapport with Mr. Long.	Begins a nurse-client relationship.	Mr. Long says that he feels better knowing what is happening.
	Encourage him to express his fears and anxieties.	Some people need encouragement to express feelings.	
	Provide Mr. Long with information, at his level of understanding, about what is happening to his body, why I & O and weighing daily are important, and what the medications are supposed to do.	Understanding reduces anxieties.	

Nursing Diagnosis 3 *Urinary Elimination, Altered, as evidenced by his urinating very little for 2 days and BUN–creatinine ratio of 22.5:1*

PLANNING/GOALS	NURSING INTERVENTIONS	RATIONALE	EVALUATION
Mr. Long will increase amount of urination to 1,200 mL/day.	Administer diuretics as ordered.	Diuretics increase water elimination by enhancing the excretion of sodium by the kidneys.	Mr. Long is urinating 1,000 mL/day. His BUN is 50 mg/dL and creatinine is 3 mg/dL.
	Accurately measure and record intake and output.	Provides information about movement of fluid through the body.	

CHRONIC RENAL FAILURE (END-STAGE RENAL DISEASE)

Chronic renal failure is a slow, progressive condition in which the kidney's ability to function ultimately deteriorates. This condition is not reversible. The kidneys have an amazing capability to perform effectively, even though most of the nephrons are destroyed.

Renal erythropoietin decreases, causing anemia. Hypertension, acidosis, and glucose intolerance usually are also present. Urea in the blood is extremely elevated. As the disease progresses, uremia develops.

Kelly (1996) describes three stages of chronic renal failure: reduced renal reserve, renal insufficiency, and end-stage renal disease (ESRD). Symptoms of reduced renal reserve are not apparent until more than 40% of the nephrons fail. A prolonged urine concentration test or a decline in glomerular filtration rate (GFR) may be the only evidence of reduced renal reserve. When 75% of the nephrons stop functioning, renal insufficiency occurs. BUN and creatinine are above normal, and the client may have nocturia and polyuria. The onset of ESRD occurs when at least 90% of the nephrons fail. BUN and creatinine levels rise, polyuria changes to oliguria, and severe fluid and electrolyte imbalances are evident.

When the kidneys become unable to filter blood, an alternate method for filtration is necessary. Lifetime dialysis becomes inevitable unless kidney transplantation is performed and is successful. Life expectancy varies with the initial cause of chronic renal failure and the person's overall health at the time of diagnosis.

According to the American Society of Nephrology, 361,031 persons in the United States have ESRD, with the number increasing approximately 8% each year (American Society of Nephrology [ASN], 1999). There are numerous causes of chronic renal failure. The 4 leading causes are diabetes mellitus 34%, hypertension 25%, glomerulonephritis 16%, and cystic kidney 4% (ASN, 1999). Nephrotoxic drugs, including some over-the-counter drugs, aggravate the situation.

The diagnosis is confirmed when the BUN is at least 50 mg/dL and the serum creatinine level is greater than 5 mg/dL.

Medical–Surgical Management

Medical

Chronic renal failure is a multisystem disease process. See Table 42-3 for the effects of chronic renal failure on various body systems. Medical management

Table 42-3 EFFECTS OF CHRONIC RENAL FAILURE BY BODY SYSTEM	
SYSTEM	**EFFECT**
Urinary	Oliguria from renal insufficiency. Azotemia.
Blood	Anemia from decreased RBC production. Decreased platelet activity, causing bleeding tendency.
Cardiovascular	Hypervolemia and tachycardia. Hypertension and dysrhythmias from hyperkalemia.
Respiratory	Dyspnea, pulmonary edema. Hyperventilation from metabolic acidosis. Eventually Kussmaul respirations.
Gastrointestinal	Urea in the blood is converted to ammonia by the mouth, causing uremic halitosis. Hiccups, anorexia, and nausea from edema within the gastrointestinal tract.
Skin	Dry skin with pruritis from uremic frost (excretion of urea through the skin with an odor of urine). Pallor with anemia.
Nervous	Lethargy, headaches, confusion, impaired concentration with disorientation, depression, decreased level of consciousness, sleep disturbances, and uremic encephalopathy resulting in seizures and coma.
Sensory	Peripheral neuropathy with numbness and tingling of extremities with complaints of a prickly, crawling feeling in the feet and legs, especially at night.
Reproductive	Decrease in libido. Decreased sperm count. Amenorrhea. Impotence. Delayed puberty.
Musculoskeletal	Joint pain and muscle cramping. Bone demineralization from hypocalcemia.
Immune	Greater chance of infections from immunosupression. Decrease in antibody production.

CULTURAL CONSIDERATIONS

End-Stage Renal Disease

- African Americans account for 30% of clients with ESRD but make up only 12% of the U.S. population.
- The leading cause of ESRD in African Americans is high blood pressure, accounting for approximately 40% of new cases in that population (NKF, 1998a).
- End-stage renal disease is 4 times greater in African Americans than in whites.
- ESRD is increasing rapidly among Native Americans because of the significant increase in the incidence of diabetes in this population (NIAID, 1998).

focuses on preserving the remaining kidney function for as long as possible and preventing complications. This helps preserve the integrity of the person's life. Fluid retention increases the risk of complications such as edema (ascites), hypertension, and congestive heart failure. Electrolytes are monitored and regulated.

Pharmacological

Antihypertensives such as methyldopa (Aldomet) and propranolol hydrochloride (Inderal) are used to control hypertension. Diuretics such as furosemide (Lasix) are used for treatment of fluid retention; anticonvulsants, phenytoin (Dilantin) to control seizures; antiemetics, prochlorperazine (Compazine) to control vomiting; and antipruritics, cyproheptadine hydrochloride (Periactin) to control itching may also be used. Calcium acetate (Phos-Lo) is used to lower the phosphate level in the blood; however, it can be constipating. A low renal erythropoietin level causing anemia is often treated with epoetin alpha (Epogen). An iron supplement is used to decrease the anemia-related symptoms. Multivitamins with folic acid are used because dialysis promotes the loss of water-soluble vitamins.

Diet

Diet restrictions are similar to those in acute renal failure. Sodium, potassium, phosphorus, and protein are restricted. Fluids are also limited. Modifications are made as kidney function deteriorates. With consistent compliance, symptoms decrease, resulting in fewer complications. Resources are available for clients to obtain assistance with dietary restrictions. Meal ideas are published in newsletters like *NephroNotes*. Long-term dietary compliance is a challenge, and daily activities as well as special events during the year are a continual reminder of the client's dietary restrictions. As with other chronic diseases, those with renal failure need to have all members of their family and their friends encouraging them to adapt to their restrictions. Dietitians can assist the family to incorporate religious and cultural dietary practices. The person with chronic renal failure may also have to incorporate dietary guidelines for additional diagnoses such as diabetes mellitus and/or coronary artery disease.

With the progression of chronic renal disease, dialysis becomes necessary. Fluid restrictions must be adhered to and the amount allowed divided throughout the day. The greatest amount of fluid should be allowed during the day, incorporating enough fluids with oral medications. Some fluids should be planned for the evening meal, with a small amount to be allowed during the night; for example, days—500 cc, evenings—200 cc, and nights—100 cc. Protein restriction is closely monitored and regulated with the blood albumin level. The development of hyperkalemia will lead to a diet restricted in potassium. Foods high in potassium include dried fruits or dried beans and peas, peanuts, bananas, sweet potatoes, spinach, products with tomatoes, oranges, chocolate, artichokes, avocados, pumpkins, and mushrooms.

Activity

The client is encouraged to participate in activities of daily living. Safety becomes a significant factor during periods when the client has weakness, fatigue, or mental confusion. Confusion is seen in clients who have uremic encephalopathy. When bed rest is required, turning, ROM activities, and skin care are important. As symptoms continue to become more severe, the client will need total assistance for all the ADLs.

▶ NURSING PROCESS

▶ Assessment

▶ Subjective Data

The nurse must inquire about the client's past medical history including the treatments for maintenance of renal disease. A complete medication history should be taken, including the use of over-the-counter drugs. Description of fatigue, joint pain, severe headaches, nausea, anorexia, some chest pain, intractable singultus (hiccups), decreased libido, menstrual irregularities, and impaired concentration will be given by the client. The client may feel uncomfortable talking directly to the nurse if uremic halitosis is a problem.

▶ Objective Data

Changes in the client's neurological status such as reduced alertness and awareness should be noted. Kussmaul respirations appear as coma develops. Halitosis with a urine odor and "uremic frost," a white powder on the skin, result from the accumulation of urates.

Nursing diagnoses for a client with ESRD may include the following:

Nursing Diagnoses	Planning/Goals	Nursing Interventions
▶ *Fluid Volume Excess related to compromised renal mechanism*	The client will understand the importance of prescribed (restricted) fluid amounts.	Monitor daily weight, intake and output (maybe hourly), skin turgor, edema, blood pressure, respirations, and lung sounds. Provide prescribed amounts of fluids.

continued

Nursing Diagnoses	Planning/Goals	Nursing Interventions
		Teach client to plan nutritional and fluid intake within the prescribed amounts.
		Monitor laboratory reports for serum albumin level and serum electrolyte levels.
▶ *Nutrition, Altered, Less than Body Requirements, related to dietary restrictions, GI distress, anorexia*	The client will stabilize weight within normal limits and participate in dietary plan.	Provide or assist with complete mouth care before meals because uremic halitosis leaves a metallic taste in the client's mouth.
		Provide a clean, quiet, odor-free environment for meals.
		Suggest 6 small meals throughout the day.
		Arrange a consultation with the dietitian to plan alternate ways to prepare foods allowed on the diet.
		Ask the family to bring favorite foods, within the dietary restrictions, from home.
		Encourage self-feeding.
		Administer antiemetics 30 minutes before meals to control nausea.
		Suggest using herbs for flavoring instead of salt or salt substitutes, which often contain potassium.
▶ *Skin Integrity, Impaired, Risk for, related to altered metabolic state leading to pruritis from "uremic frost"*	The client will maintain skin integrity.	Bathe skin frequently to remove "uremic frost."
		Encourage the use of emollients and lotions on the skin.
		Administer antihistamines, as ordered, for the temporary relief of itching.
		Assist the client to change position every 2 hours.
		Provide an eggcrate mattress or Clinitron bed.
▶ *Coping, Ineffective Individual, related to uncertainty of long-term compliance of the treatment regimen*	The client will verbalize feelings and intention to comply with treatment.	Encourage the client to discuss feelings about long-term lifestyle changes.
		Refer client to the local office of the National Kidney Foundation for information about client services and treatments for diseases of the kidney.
		Include the client and family in rehabilitation and discharge planning to ensure compliance. Topics for these sessions include diet, rest, medications, fluid restrictions, intake and output, activities, dialysis, required lab tests, and frequent visits to the physician.
		Incorporate into the discharge planning and teaching the client's socioeconomic needs, cultural background, role in the family unit, accessibility to medical care, and anticipated follow-up care.
		Complete referrals prior to discharge in order to lessen client anxiety.
		Consider future needs of a newly diagnosed client with end-stage renal disease and include the availability of dialysis, vocational rehabilitation, home health care, financial assistance with medical needs, and psychological therapy for the client and family.

Evaluation Each goal must be evaluated to determine how it has been met by the client.

DIALYSIS

As the kidneys continue to deteriorate, nitrogenous waste products accumulate in the circulatory system. These waste products then need to be removed artificially with dialysis. **Dialysis** is a mechanical means of removing nitrogenous waste from the blood by imitating the function of the nephrons. It involves filtration and diffusion of wastes, drugs, and excess electrolytes and/or osmosis of water across a semipermeable membrane into a dialysate solution. The **dialysate**, a solution designed to approximate the normal electrolyte

 CLIENT TEACHING

Dialysis

Clients who are receiving dialysis need a significant amount of teaching. All clients should have the process thoroughly explained. Other teaching topics are the importance of doctor and laboratory visits, and observations for which the doctor needs to be notified. Clients undergoing dialysis should wear Medic Alert tags stating their condition.

structure of plasma and extracellular fluid, is prescribed specific to the individual client's needs.

There are two types of dialysis: hemodialysis and peritoneal dialysis.

Hemodialysis

Hemodialysis is performed by a machine with an artificial semipermeable membrane used for the filtration of the blood. This machine is often referred to as an artificial kidney. A graft or fistula is surgically prepared to access the client's circulatory system. Figure 42-6 illustrates several ways this can be done. Research and development is improving the quality of graft materials. With each hemodialysis treatment, a catheter is inserted into the graft or fistula. The client's blood is circulated through the semipermeable membrane. Excess fluids are removed by osmosis and by-products of protein metabolism, especially urea and uric acid, as well as creatinine, drugs, and excess electrolytes, are removed from the blood by diffusion or filtration. In return, the client receives fluids, electrolytes, and blood products, as necessary. The solution (dialysate) is especially prescribed to meet the client's metabolic needs.

For the entire process, Standard Precautions must be followed and strict asepsis maintained. The client should be weighed before and after each dialysis session to determine if fluid is being retained. It is important to keep the client comfortable and provide diversionary activities during the treatment. Hemodialysis is usually performed 3 times a week and takes 3 to 6 hours each time.

The graft or fistula site requires strict aseptic care and must be assessed daily for signs of infection: redness, swelling, or drainage. Circulation through the site is assessed by palpation or feeling the area and/or listening with a (Doppler) stethoscope. A thrill should be felt and/or a bruit should be heard. Lack of these may indicate a blood clot, which requires immediate surgical attention. Patency must be documented. Pulses peripheral to the graft site must also be assessed.

Blood pressure and blood draws should never be done on the extremity where the graft or fistula is placed. Also, restraints or intravenous solutions should never be applied to or inserted into that extremity. All health care personnel should be made aware of the location of the hemodialysis access site.

Since most medications are removed during dialysis, they are generally not administered until after the dialysis session. Vancomycin hydrochloride (Vancocin) is not removed during dialysis and so is often used. If the client is hypertensive before dialysis, nifedipine (Procardia) is given because of its fast action.

Possible complications include hemorrhage, infection, and emboli formation. Some factors for the client and family to consider about hemodialysis are the distance they must travel to the dialysis center, the expense, the time involved, and the presence of a permanent arteriovenous (AV) line. Clients can be taught to do their own hemodialysis at a center. Portable units are being developed to make hemodialysis more usable in the client's home. This is a growing trend with home health care.

Peritoneal Dialysis

Peritoneal dialysis uses the peritoneal lining of the abdominal cavity as the membrane through which diffusion and osmosis occur instead of the artificial kidney machine. It is usually performed 4 times a day 7 days a week. A catheter is placed by the physician, under aseptic conditions, into the client's peritoneal space.

The dialysate, held within a sterile soft container similar to an IV bag, is instilled aseptically through the catheter into the abdominal cavity. The container, still connected to the catheter, is then rolled up and the dialysate remains in the abdominal cavity for a specified length of time. The container is then unrolled and lowered below the abdominal cavity to allow the dialysate to drain, by gravity, back into the container. The dialysate now contains excess fluids, nitrogenous waste, and other impurities. The outflow of dialysate is inspected for color, sediments, and amount. The fluid should be light yellow and clear enough to read the printing on the bag when placed on a white towel.

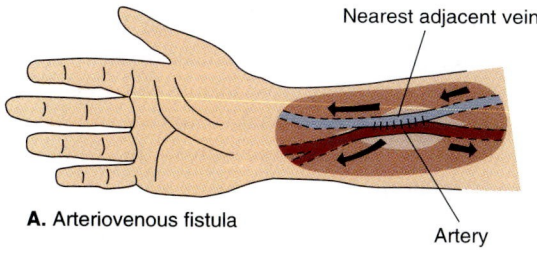

A. Arteriovenous fistula

Edges of incision in artery and vein are sutured together to form a common opening.

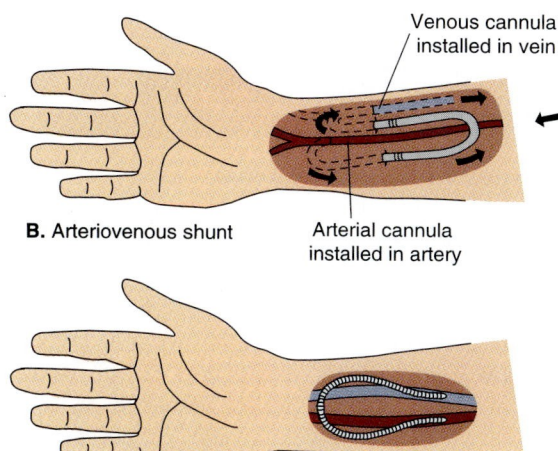

B. Arteriovenous shunt

C. Arteriovenous vein graft

Ends of natural or synthetic graft sutured into an artery and a vein.

Figure 42-6 Hemodialysis Access Sites

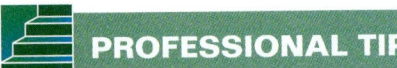

PROFESSIONAL TIP

Dialysate

To decrease client discomfort, the dialysate should be at body temperature and not instilled too rapidly.

Usually 2 liters of dialysate are exchanged each time. If the outflow does not at least equal the inflow, the client is asked to turn from side to side to increase the outflow.

Peritoneal dialysis is less expensive, easier to perform, less stressful for the client, and almost as effective as hemodialysis.

The main complication of peritoneal dialysis is infection. Strict aseptic care of the catheter site is necessary. Standard Precautions are essential in caring for the dialysis client. Figure 42-7 shows a peritoneal dialysis setup.

KIDNEY TRANSPLANTATION

According to the National Kidney Foundation (1998b) 11,460 kidney transplants were performed in 1997. Transplants are either from a live donor (usually a relative) or a cadaver. As of September 1998, there were

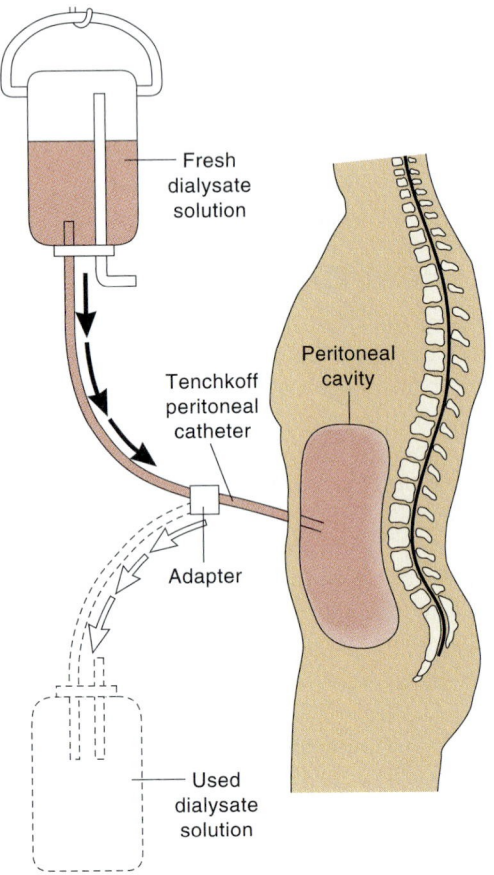

Figure 42-7 Peritoneal Dialysis Setup

80,000 persons on the waiting list for a kidney transplant.

Prior to being placed on the nationwide donor waiting list, the client with ESRD must be tissue- and blood-typed to determine a compatible donor. Insurance coverage varies for this procedure. Lack of funds does not exclude anyone from needed care. Since 1973, an amendment to the Social Security Act allows Medicare to pay 80% of the cost for treating ESRD clients, regardless of age, including dialysis and kidney transplantation.

At the time a donor kidney becomes available, the client must be transported to the transplant medical center. The donor kidney can be preserved for 36 hours in solution or up to 72 hours if it is attached to an irrigating pump with perfusion maintained while en route to the recipient. Through a lower abdominal incision, the surgeon attaches the donor kidney to the client's blood supply. The donor kidney is usually placed in the iliac fossa anterior to the iliac crest. The donor ureter is anastomosed (surgical connection of tubular structure) to the client's ureter or surgically implanted into the client's urinary bladder. Generally, the client's nonfunctioning kidney is left in place to reduce the postoperative risk of hemorrhage.

After a couple days of bed rest, the client will be allowed increasing activities and, if no complications occur, will be discharged in 1 to 3 weeks. Routine nursing care includes monitoring urine output, blood tests, vital signs, and level of consciousness. Turning, coughing, and deep breathing are encouraged. The incision is assessed to ensure that wound closures are intact. In addition to these measures, the nurse must assess for rejection.

Organ Rejection

Signs of rejection include generalized edema, tenderness over the graft site, fever, decreased urine out-

PROFESSIONAL TIP

Nutrition for Dialysis Clients
- Optimal protein intake for maintenance adult hemodialysis clients is 1.2g/kg body weight/day.
- Optimal protein intake for chronic peritoneal dialysis clients is 1.3g/kg body weight/day.
- Optimal energy intake (fats and carbohydrates) for adult dialysis clients 60 years old or less is 35 Kcal/kg body weight/day; clients over 60 years of age is 30–35 Kcal/kg body weight/day.
- Calories from peritoneal dialysis fluid must be taken into account when figuring the total energy intake for those clients (NKF, May 1999).

put, hematuria, edema (extremities or eyes), weight gain, oliguria or anuria, and/or an increase in feeling tired. The BUN and creatinine will be elevated.

Immunosuppressive drug therapy is begun to decrease the chance of organ rejection. These drugs include azathioprine (Imuran), cyclophosphamide (Cytoxan), cyclosporine (Sandimmune), and corticosteroids such as prednisone (Meticorten). The scheduling and dosage of these drugs vary with acceptance of the donor kidney and the side effects exhibited by the client. People continue to survive many years with a kidney transplant and maintain a quality life.

Complications

The greatest complication in renal transplantation is infection. The immunosuppressive therapy to prevent rejection of the kidney increases the risk and masks the usual signs of infection. The client and family must learn how to recognize these signs of infection. There will be only a slight increase in temperature, development of a cough, low back pain, cloudy urine, or wound drainage. The client must always monitor urine output.

CASE STUDY

Ruth Andrews, 56, is a client in the extended care facility. She has amyotrophic lateral sclerosis (ALS) with muscle weakness that has progressed and involves her legs and arms. A hydraulic lift is used to transfer her out of bed. A student nurse and a classmate enter with the lift to assist Ms. Andrews OOB, when she asks to use the bedpan. As they help her on the bedpan, they recall that the staff nurse gave Ms. Andrews the bedpan about a half hour ago. Returning in a few minutes, they help Ms. Andrews off the bedpan and notice the urine is cloudy with a foul odor. Ms. Andrews is not on I & O; however, they notice that there is a very small amount of urine. She tells them that she does not know why she is going to the bathroom so often and why her urine smells bad.

The following questions will guide your development of a nursing care plan for the case study.

1. What subjective data should be gathered? What objective data should be gathered?
2. List diagnostic tests that may be ordered.
3. Write two nursing diagnoses for Ms. Andrews, related to her cystitis/UTI.
4. Write a goal related to each of Ms. Andrews' nursing diagnoses.
5. List pertinent nursing actions for the care of Ms. Andrews for each of the following areas as they relate to the cystitis/UTI:

    elimination-bladder
    diet and fluids
    safety, comfort, and rest
    teaching (client and nursing staff)
6. List two classifications of medications used for the treatment of an UTI.
7. List two successful client outcomes for Ms. Andrews.

SUMMARY

- The functions of the urinary system are reflected in their relationship with nearly all the systems in the body.
- Accurate intake and output is imperative for every client with a urinary system disorder.
- Teach proper perineal care, especially to females of all ages, about cleansing from front to back.
- Diet management is important for clients with renal calculi, glomerulonephritis, and renal failure.
- Encourage an adequate intake of fluids for clients unless fluids are restricted.
- Monitor laboratory test results for BUN, creatinine, and electrolytes.
- Level of consciousness, vital signs, lung sounds, and urine characteristics are important to monitor.
- Strict aseptic care is mandatory for dialysis clients.

Review Questions

1. A client states she has had pain when urinating for 3 days. This would be documented as:

    a. polyuria.
    b. dysuria.
    c. hematuria.
    d. oliguria.

2. A client has been admitted for chronic pyelonephritis. She is jittery and states she is concerned. Which of the following signs would indicate potential kidney damage?

    a. Urine output is 100 mL on your shift.
    b. Blood pressure is decreased with a rapid pulse.
    c. Blood pressure is elevated with a decreased pulse.
    d. BUN and creatinine clearance are within normal limits.

3. Georgia Smithson has glomerulonephritis. This condition affects her:

    a. kidney.
    b. ureter.
    c. bladder.
    d. urethra.

4. Mr. Ronald Osborne, 76, has had hematuria for several years and has been diagnosed with cancer of the kidney. His prognosis is poor. He told the nurse that he was too dizzy to go to the bathroom alone. Which of the following shows Mr. Osborne needs further teaching?

    a. Putting his bathroom call light on for assistance
    b. Holding on to the nurse's arm while walking
    c. Refusal to wait for the nurse to lower the side rail
    d. Saving his urine to be measured and tested

5. Jake Jones, 64, has had hematuria for several years. He is admitted to your same-day surgical unit scheduled for cystoscopic fulguration. Post-operatively, which of the following would you anticipate?

    a. Blood in the urine
    b. An elevated temperature
    c. Hypotension
    d. Smoky urine

6. Lawrence Denny, 29, had impetigo two weeks prior to his noting a decrease in urine output and urine that "did not look right." His admission diagnosis is acute glomerulonephritis. He is on intake and output with fluid restriction. Which of the following comments indicates knowledge of his nursing care?

    a. "I had my wife empty my urinal."
    b. "My urine still looks pretty bad."
    c. "I put my call light on so you can empty my urinal."
    d. "My wife helped me out of bed, so I urinated in the bathroom."

7. Gael Dominich is a client with chronic glomerulonephritis. She is discharged home with home health care. As the LP/VN assigned to her case, you are planning Gael's A.M. care. While preparing the bath supplies, she says, "Please do not use any soap. My skin is so dry and flaky." The rationale for this would be:

    a. kidney failure leads to uremia.
    b. the bladder does not concentrate urine.
    c. her blood sugar is elevated.
    d. confusion leads to comments of this nature.

8. Mr. Diego Ochoa, in his 50s, is attending classes to be able to do his own peritoneal dialysis. He states he feels well and is eager to continue to learn. Mr. Ochoa asks if washing his hands before the procedure is important. The best response is:

    a. "Yes, only if you have not done so today."
    b. "Yes, as you want to keep the procedure as clean as possible."
    c. "No, since you just went to the bathroom."
    d. "No, because all the equipment is sterile."

Critical Thinking Questions

1. What are the pros and cons for peritoneal dialysis, hemodialysis, and kidney transplantation?

2. What can an individual do to prevent urinary disorders?

3. What are the differences between acute and chronic renal failure?

4. What is the rationale for each nursing intervention given for the nursing diagnoses in this chapter?

WEB FLASH!

- Search the Internet for information about the various diseases discussed in this chapter. What information would assist you in client care?
- Find the resources listed for this chapter in the back of this text on the Internet. What services do they have available for clients?

NURSING CARE OF THE CLIENT: SENSORY SYSTEM

MAKING THE CONNECTION

Refer to the following chapters to increase your understanding of sensory disorders:

- **Chapter 8, Communication**
- **Chapter 15, Wellness Concepts**
- **Chapter 17, Loss, Grief, and Death**
- **Chapter 25, Assessment**
- **Chapter 26, Pain Management**
- **Chapter 29, Nursing Care of the Surgical Client**

- **Chapter 41, Nursing Care of the Client: Nervous System**
- **Chapter 55, Nursing Care of the Older Client**
- **Procedures:** I15, Administering an Eye Medication; I16, Instilling an Ear Medication

LEARNING OBJECTIVES

Upon completion of this chapter, you should be able to:
- *Define key terms.*
- *Compare and differentiate common disorders of the special senses.*
- *Identify the structure and function of the major parts of the eye and ear.*
- *Explain the purpose of the common diagnostic tests for sensory problems.*
- *List the nursing assessments and common nursing diagnoses related to sensory impairment.*
- *Assist in planning nursing care for clients with sensory disorders.*
- *List some of the common sensory aids for the visual and hearing impaired.*

INTRODUCTION

From the moment we wake in the morning until we fall asleep at night, we are inundated with information from the outside world through our senses. Although most of us do not consider our senses as organs of protection, we depend on visual and auditory alarms to keep us from harm. This chapter reviews the structure and function, identifies appropriate nursing diagnoses, and presents the medical and nursing management of the five senses: hearing, vision, taste, smell, and touch.

KEY TERMS

acoustic neuroma
affect
afferent nerve
  pathways
arousal
astigmatism
awareness
cataract
cerumen
chalazion
cognition
conductive hearing
  loss
conjunctivitis
consciousness
disorientation
efferent nerve
  pathways
glaucoma
hallucination
hyperopia
illusion
judgment
keratitis

macular
  degeneration
Ménière's disease
myopia
nystagmus
orientation
otitis externa
otitis media
otosclerosis
perception
presbycusis
presbyopia
sensation
sensorineural hearing
  loss
sensory deficit
sensory deprivation
sensory overload
sensory perception
strabismus
stye
tinnitus
vertigo

SENSATION, PERCEPTION, AND COGNITION

Sensation is the ability to receive and process stimuli through the sensory organs. There are two types of stimuli; external and internal. External stimuli are received and processed through the senses of sight (visual), hearing (auditory), smell (olfactory), taste (gustatory), and touch (tactile). Internal stimuli are received and processed through kinesthetic (an awareness of the position of the body) and visceral (feelings originating from large organs within the body) modes.

Perception is the ability to experience, recognize, organize, and interpret sensory stimuli. **Sensory perception** is the ability to receive sensory impressions and, through cortical association, relate the stimuli to past experiences and form an impression of the nature of the stimulus.

Perception is closely associated with **cognition**, the intellectual ability to think. The processes of organizing and interpreting stimuli are dependent on a person's level of intellectual functioning. Cognition includes the elements of memory, judgment, and orientation. The well-being of an individual is dependent on the functions of sensation, perception, and cognition because it is through these mechanisms that the person fully experiences and interacts with the environment.

Sensory, perceptual, and cognitive alterations can be either temporary or progressive in their manifestations and can result from disease or trauma. Whatever the status or cause of the alterations, these conditions usually lead to social isolation and increased dependence on others. In addition, impairment in sensory, perceptual, and cognitive functions can place the individual at risk for injury to self or to others.

ANATOMY AND PHYSIOLOGY REVIEW

Sensation, perception, and cognition are neurological functions. The nervous system is composed of two major subsystems: the central nervous system (CNS) and the peripheral nervous system (PNS), which consists of the somatic and autonomic nervous systems (Figure 43-1). The CNS and PNS act in unison to accomplish three purposes: collection of stimuli from the receptors at the end of the peripheral nerves; transport of the stimuli to the brain for integration and cognition processing; and conduction of responses to the stimuli from the brain to responsive motor centers in the body. Refer to Chapter 41 for the anatomy of the nervous system.

Sensory perception involves the function of both the cranial and peripheral nerves. The cranial nerves arise from the brain and govern the movement and function of various muscles and nerves throughout the body. The peripheral nerves connect the CNS to other parts of the body (Figure 43-2).

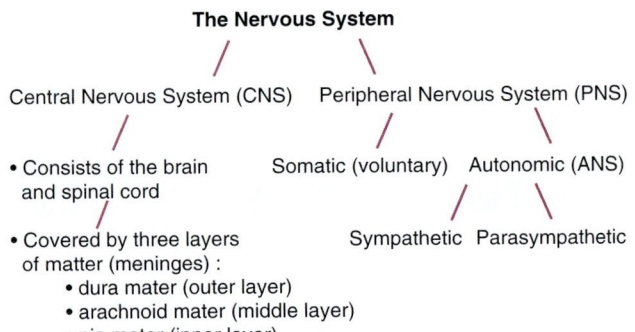

Figure 43-1 The Nervous System (*From* Fundamentals of Nursing Standards & Practice, *by S. DeLaune and P. Ladner, 1998, Albany, NY: Delmar Publishers. Reprinted with permission.*)

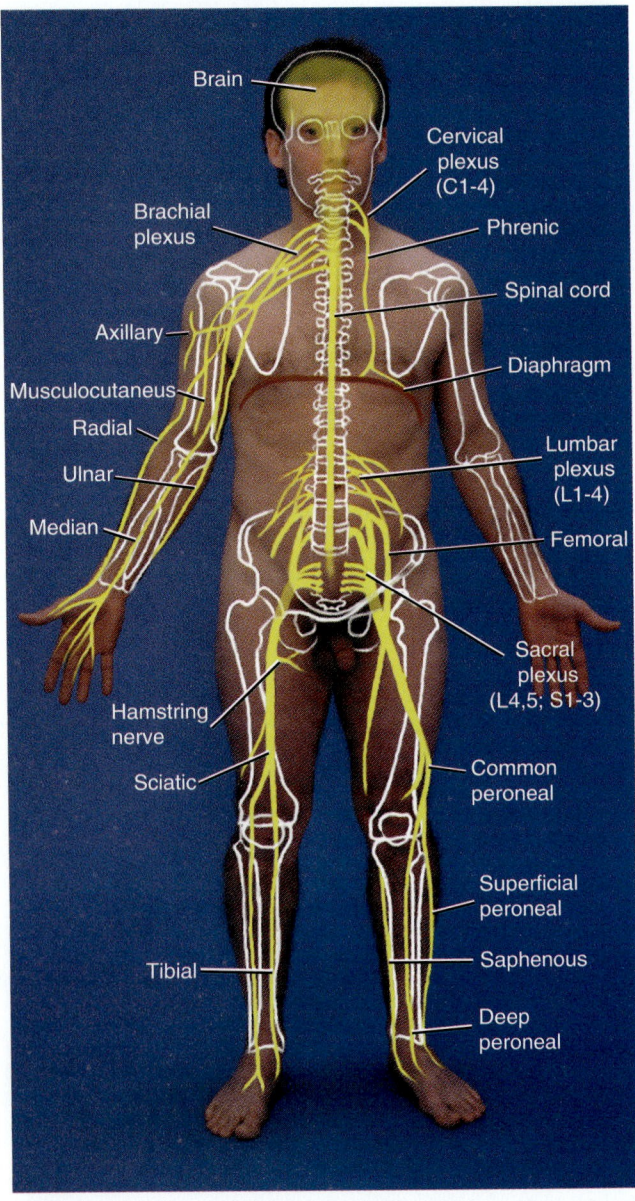

Figure 43-2 The Peripheral Nerves (*From* Fundamentals of Nursing Standards & Practice, *by S. DeLaune and P. Ladner, 1998, Albany, NY: Delmar Publishers. Reprinted with permission.*)

Components of Sensation and Perception

The sensory system is a complex network that consists of **afferent nerve pathways** (ascending pathways that transmit sensory impulses to the brain), **efferent nerve pathways** (descending pathways that send sensory impulses from the brain), the spinal cord, the brainstem, and the cerebrum.

Components of Cognition

Cognition includes the cerebral functions of memory, affect, judgment, perception, and language. In order for these higher functions to occur, consciousness must be present.

Consciousness

Consciousness is a state of awareness of self, others, and the surrounding environment. It affects both cognitive (intellectual) and affective (emotional) functions. An alert individual (one who is aware of self and stimuli) is able to perceive reality accurately and to base behavior on those perceptions. The components of consciousness provide a foundation for behavior and emotional expression, thereby contributing to the uniqueness of each individual's personality. Consciousness may be altered by various metabolic, traumatic, or other factors such as the pharmacological actions of drugs that affect mental status. The primary components of consciousness are arousal and awareness, both of which must be present before higher cognitive functioning occurs.

Arousal The degree of **arousal** (state of wakefulness and alertness) is indicated by a person's general response and reaction to the environment. People exhibit arousal by behaving in an alert and aware manner and by experiencing periods of wakefulness. The degree of an individual's arousal is indicated by the general response and reaction to the environment. Impaired arousal can exist when a sleep pattern deficit is experienced. There may be an inability to take advantage of opportunities for activity because of inadequate periods of rest.

Awareness **Awareness** is the capacity to perceive sensory impressions and react appropriately through thoughts and actions. An essential element in

PROFESSIONAL TIP

CNS Deficits and Illness
Specific conditions, such as diabetes mellitus and atherosclerosis, can impair neurosensory pathways and result in deficits in sensation, perception, and cognition. Diseases of the CNS can result in loss of sensory function and paralysis.

PROFESSIONAL TIP

Effects of Medications on Sensation
Certain medications have the potential to alter or depress the neurosensory system. For example, sedatives and narcotics can alter the perception of sensory stimuli. Medications such as analgesics can alter the level of consciousness.

awareness is **orientation** (perception of self in relation to the surrounding environment). When awareness is impaired, orientation to time is frequently the first area affected. The degree of disorientation is worse when the individual loses awareness of place and self (person).

Memory

There are three types of memory: immediate, recent, and remote. Immediate memory is the retention of information for a specified and usually short period of time. The recall of a telephone number long enough to dial it is an example of immediate memory. Recent memory is the ability to recall events that have occurred over the past 24 hours, such as remembering the foods eaten for dinner the previous night. Remote memory is the retention of experiences that occurred during earlier periods of life, such as an adult's memories of childhood or school days. The ability to learn is dependent on remote memory.

Affect

Affect (expression of mood or feeling) is an important component of cognition in that variations of mood can affect one's thinking ability. For example, a client with a flat affect due to depression may have difficulty sustaining concentration or attention.

Judgment

Judgment, the ability to compare or evaluate alternatives in order to arrive at an appropriate course of action, is closely related to reality testing and depends on effective cognitive functioning. Behaviors indicative of impaired judgment include impulsiveness, unrealistic decision making, and inadequate problem-solving ability.

Perception

Perceptions are considered in the context of the individual's awareness of reality. Misperceptions of reality can occur in the form of an **illusion** (an inaccurate perception or misinterpretation of sensory stimuli) or a **hallucination** (a sensory perception that occurs in the absence of external stimuli and is not based on reality).

Clients who are anxious and fearful or who are on therapeutic regimens involving the use of certain

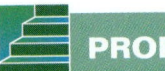

Remote Memory

Remote memory should be assessed only when client responses about past events can be validated, either by others or by written account.

medications may experience misperceptions of environmental stimuli. For example, a postoperative client, after receiving analgesic medication for pain, may see the belt from his bathrobe lying on the floor and become terrified because he thinks there is a snake in the room. Once the nurse determines that the client is experiencing an illusion, appropriate reassurance and reality orientation can be implemented to reduce the client's anxiety.

Language

Language is one of the most complex of cognitive functions, involving not only the spoken word but also reading, writing, and comprehension. Characteristics of speech are fluency (ability to talk in a steady manner), prosody (melody of speech that conveys meaning through changes in the tempo, rhythm, and intonation), and content.

ASSESSMENT

When caring for clients with sensory, perceptual, and cognitive alterations, the nurse must obtain a health history and perform a physical examination to identify existing or potential problems in this area of functioning. The physical examination focuses specifically on the client's ability to hear, see, taste, smell, and touch. Refer to Chapter 41 for assessment of cranial nerves. Table 43-1 provides some guidelines helpful in assessing sensory perceptual status.

When assessing clients for sensory, perceptual, and cognitive alterations, the level of consciousness (LOC)

LIFE CYCLE CONSIDERATIONS

Sensory Assessments for Children
- The eustachian tube is shorter, wider, and straighter in infants and small children, making them more prone to ear infections.
- If the Moro reflex persists past 4 months of age, impaired hearing should be investigated.
- By the age of 3 or 4, children should have a thorough ophthalmic examination.
- Between the ages of 6 and 10, children may become nearsighted and hold books very close to their eyes to read.

Table 43-1 ASSESSING SENSORY PERCEPTUAL STATUS

SENSATION BEING ASSESSED	ASSESSMENT FOCUS
Visual	• Presence of visual problems, including: —Decreased acuity —Blurred vision —Double vision —Blind spots —Rainbows or halos around objects —Photosensitivity —Loss of peripheral field (narrowing) • Difficulty seeing far or near • Family history of visual problems (such as glaucoma, cataracts) • Use of contact lenses or eyeglasses • Date of last eye examination
Auditory	• Presence of hearing problems • Recent changes in hearing ability • Ability to distinguish sounds (tone and pitch) • Presence of buzzing or ringing noises • Use of a hearing aid
Gustatory	• Changes in ability to taste • Difficulty in differentiating salty, sweet, sour, and bitter tastes • Changes in appetite
Olfactory	• Changes in ability to smell • Ability to distinguish common smells (such as food, perfume, flowers)
Tactile	• Difficulty in feeling temperature changes in extremities • Impairment of pain perception in extremities • Presence of unusual sensations in extremities (such as tingling or numbness)

From Fundamentals of Nursing Standards & Practice, by S. DeLaune and P. Ladner, 1998, Albany, NY: Delmar Publishers. Reprinted with permission.

must also be evaluated. Refer to Chapter 41 for the Glasgow Coma Scale, developed to assess LOC objectively.

 Safety: Sensory Impairments

Vision—Risk of tripping, falling

Hearing—Lack of awareness of warning sounds such as automobile horns, sirens, smoke alarms

Olfactory—Inability to perceive warning odors such as burning food, escaping gas

Gustatory—Inability to recognize spoiled or contaminated food or beverages

Tactile—Lack of awareness of excessive pressure on a body part; at risk for exposure to extreme temperatures (frostbite, burns)

Sensory Changes in the Elderly

- When the eye lens yellows and becomes cloudy, the ability to discern colors, especially greens and blues, is impaired.
- The elderly need more light to see because the pupils become smaller, letting in less light.
- It takes the elderly longer to accommodate (adjust) to darkness and glare.
- Tear production decreases with age, predisposing to dry eye syndrome and corneal irritation.
- The most common hearing loss is sensorineural, which can be helped by a hearing aid.
- Taste sensation may be dulled with age.

The Ear

The human ear can be divided into three main anatomical components: the outer ear, middle ear, and inner ear (Figure 43-3). Each part plays a major role in hearing. Similar to other paired organs in the body, dysfunction of part or all of one ear does not affect the function of the other.

Outer Ear

The outer ear is composed of the auricle (pinna), a cartilaginous flap on the temporal sides of the head, and the external ear canal, or external auditory meatus. The outer ear is responsible for collecting, conducting,

and amplifying sound waves. The auricle directs sounds through the external ear canal to the tympanic membrane (eardrum). This canal is lined with ceruminous glands that secrete **cerumen** (ear wax), a yellowish brown protective substance that guards against certain bacteria and small insects, and traps dust and debris that may damage the inner ear. Normally, the cerumen works its way out of the ear as we eat, chew, or speak. However, cerumen can build up and actually cause significant hearing loss in the affected ear.

The tympanic membrane (TM) serves as a boundary between the outer and middle ear. As sound waves vibrate against the membrane, the motion is transmitted to the bones of the inner ear. In an acute ear infection, fluid fills the middle ear, creating significant pressure on the tympanic membrane.

Middle Ear

The three bones of the middle ear are collectively referred to as the ossicles and include the malleus (hammer), incus (anvil), and stapes (stirrup), so named because they resemble the tools of a blacksmith's trade. The malleus is attached to the upper, inner portion of the tympanic membrane. The head of the malleus connects with the incus which then joins the stapes. The flat oval bone of the stapes, called the footplate, rests on the oval window (part of the inner ear). The vibration created by sound waves passes through the outer ear canal to the tympanic membrane and then to these three bones.

The eustachian tube opens into the pharynx from the middle ear. It is approximately 3 to 4 cm long, and

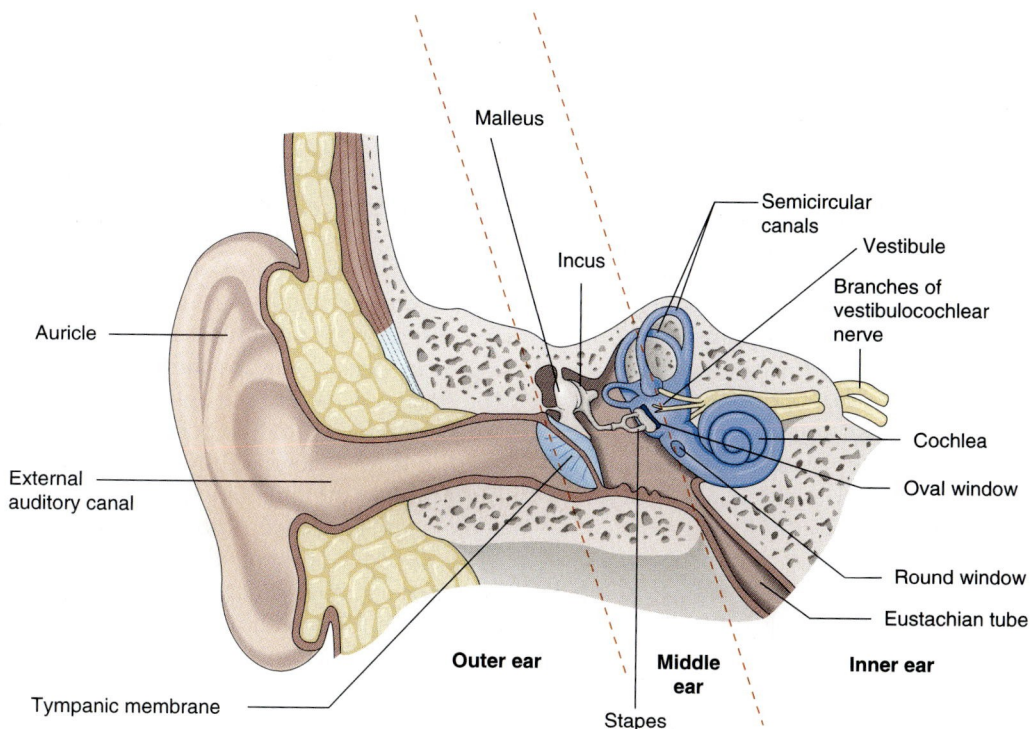

Figure 43-3 Structures of the Ear

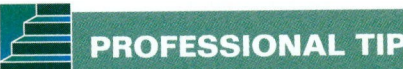

its primary function is to equalize pressure on both sides of the eardrum by providing a path (via the nasal passages) to relieve the pressure. In addition to pressure equalization, the functions of the middle ear include amplification of the sound waves and stimulation of the oval window to move the fluids of the inner ear.

Inner Ear

The inner ear has two main functions: hearing and equilibrium. It consists of a complex series of interconnected, fluid-filled chambers and tubes called the labyrinth. It can be divided into three main parts: the semicircular canals, the vestibule, and the cochlea, all located in the temporal bone. The semicircular canals, which function in providing the sense of balance, open into the vestibule. The vestibule is the central chamber of the inner ear. The cochlea is a snail-shaped structure that contains the auditory organ for the sense of hearing.

Vibration of the stapes creates pressure and causes the nerves to respond to different sounds and initiate neural responses that are sent along the auditory nerve (VIII cranial nerve) to the brain. Thus, mechanical information is translated into nerve impulses and sent to the brain, which translates the sound into meaningful impressions and language.

The Eye

The eyes are a pair of spherical organs located in bony orbital cavities in the front of the skull. They are the sensory receptor organs of the visual system that transduce light from the environment into electrical impulses, which the optic nerve then transmits to the brain where they are interpreted as the sensation of vision. The adult eyeball measures about 1 inch in diameter. Of its total surface area, only the anterior one-sixth is exposed. The remainder is recessed and protected by the bony orbit into which it fits. Anatomically, the eye can be divided into three separate coats, or "tunics": the outer fibrous tunic, the middle vascular tunic, and the inner nervous tunic.

Fibrous Tunic

The fibrous tunic is the outer coat of the eyeball and is composed posteriorly of the sclera, and anteriorly of the transparent cornea. The sclera, or "white of the eye," is leathery, white, and relatively thick, and is composed of connective tissue. The cornea, or "window of the eye," is a continuation of the sclera and forms a transparent rounded bulge through which light passes.

Vascular Tunic

The vascular tunic is the eye's middle layer and is composed of three portions: the posterior choroid, the anterior ciliary body, and the iris. Collectively, these three structures are called the uveal tract. The choroid carries the blood vessels for the eyeball and contains a large amount of pigment, thus preventing internal reflection of light. Around the edge of the cornea the choroid forms the ciliary body, a thickened structure containing smooth muscle. A thin diaphragm of mostly connective tissue and smooth muscle fibers with an opening in the center is attached around the anterior margin of the ciliary body. The muscles of the ciliary body serve to change the shape of the lens, allowing changes in the focal distance of the eye. The third portion of the vascular tunic is known as the iris, and contains the pigment responsible for the color of the eye. The hole in the iris is the pupil, which permits light to enter the eye. Some of the smooth muscle fibers in the iris encircle the pupil and others radiate from it. Contraction of the radial muscle dilates the pupil and contraction of the circular muscle constricts the pupil. By their control of pupil diameter, these muscles regulate the amount of light entering the eye.

Nervous Tunic

The third and innermost tunic of the eye, the retina, translates light waves into neural impulses. An extremely complex structure, the retina contains several layers of nerve cells and their processes, including two types of receptors, the rods for vision in dim light, and the cones for daytime or color vision. Cones are most densely concentrated in the central fovea, a small depression in the center of the macula lutea. The macula lutea, or yellow spot, is in the central part of the retina. The fovea is the area of sharpest vision because the highest concentration of cones are located there. Rods are absent from the fovea and macula, but they increase in density toward the periphery of the retina. The optic disk, where the optic nerve exits the eye, is a weak spot in the fundus (posterior wall) of the eye because it is not reinforced by the sclera. The optic disk is also called the blind spot, because it lacks photoreceptors and light focused on it will not be detected.

The interior of the eyeball contains an anterior and posterior chamber separated by the lens. The anterior chamber is filled with a watery fluid called the aqueous humor, which maintains intraocular pressure, provides nourishment, and helps maintain the shape of the eyeball. The posterior chamber is filled with a jelly-like substance called the vitreous humor, which main-

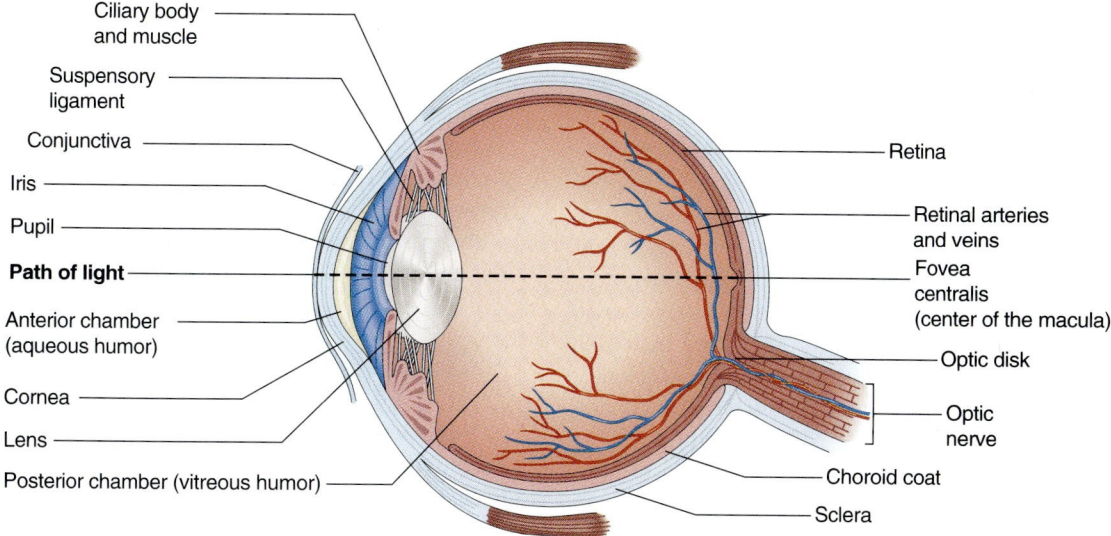

Figure 43-4 Lateral View of the Interior Eyeball

tains the spherical shape of the eye and supports the inner structures. Both substances are transparent, thus allowing light to pass through the eye to the retina (Figure 43-4).

The lens, located in the anterior chamber of the eye, is a transparent biconvex crystalline body enclosed in an elastic capsule held by suspensory ligaments. The shape of the lens changes to focus the image.

External Structures

The eyeball is protected from the external world by the eyelid, which contains a thin protective layer of epithelium, the conjunctiva (Figure 43-5). The conjunctiva covers the anterior portion of the eyeball and lines the eyelid. Projecting from the border of each eyelid is a row of eyelashes, which protect the eye from foreign particles. The lacrimal gland produces a secretion

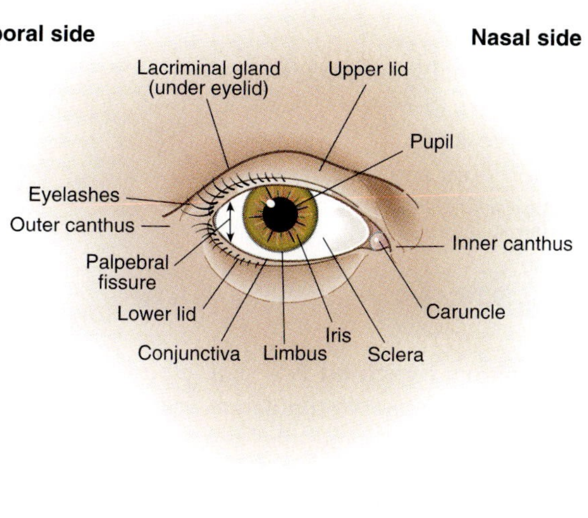

called tears, which contain a lysozyme, muramidase, to destroy pathogens.

COMMON DIAGNOSTIC TESTS

Commonly used diagnostic tests for clients with problems in hearing and vision are listed in Table 43-2. See Chapter 27, Diagnostic Tests, for explanation/normal values and nursing responsibilities.

Table 43-2 COMMON DIAGNOSTIC TESTS FOR SENSORY ALTERATIONS

- Weber test (tuning fork)
- Rinne test (tuning fork)
- Audiometric testing (audiogram)
- Speech audiometry (Spondee threshold)
- Caloric test
- Brainstem auditory evoked response (ErA and BAER)
- Tympanometry
- Computed tomography (CT)
- Magnetic resonance imaging (MRI)
- Romberg test
- Otoscopic exam
- Past-point testing
- Color vision tests
- Tonometry
- Slit lamp examination
- Perimetry
- Visual acuity
- Electroretinogram (ERG)
- Ocular ultrasonography
- Ophthalmoscopic examination
- Orbital computerized tomography
- Fluoresce in angiography

Figure 43-5 External View of the Right Eye

SENSORY, PERCEPTUAL, AND COGNITIVE ALTERATIONS

An individual usually experiences discomfort and/or anxiety when subjected to a change in the type or amount of incoming stimuli. A person can become confused as a result of either overstimulation or understimulation. According to the individual's ability to process the stimuli, confusion (or disorientation) may occur. **Disorientation** is a mentally confused state in which the person's awareness of time, place, self, and/or situation is impaired. When awareness of these four factors is accurate, a person is said to be "oriented × 4".

A person admitted to a health care agency experiences stimuli that are different from those usually encountered. A change in environment can overwhelm one's ability to perceive and interpret sensory input. As a result, the treatment setting itself can become a stressor that negatively affects sensory, perceptual, and cognitive functions. If one or more of the factors just discussed causes an alteration in sensation, perception, or cognition, the client may experience problems with perceiving and interpreting stimuli. These problems are manifested by three types of alterations: sensory deficit, sensory deprivation, and sensory overload.

SENSORY DEFICIT

A **sensory deficit** is a change in the perception of sensory stimuli. This deficit can affect all five senses. Examples of sensory deficit are vision and hearing losses such as those caused by cataracts, glaucoma, and presbycusis (steady loss of hearing acuity that occurs with aging).

The client's response to these losses usually depends on the time of onset and the severity of the condition. If the problem occurs suddenly and without warning, the client may have difficulty adjusting to the loss of sensory and perceptual function. If these alterations occur gradually, the client may be able to accommodate the change and actually compensate for it by strengthening one or more of the other senses.

 LIFE CYCLE CONSIDERATIONS

Neurosensory Pathways

Neurosensory pathways in infants and children are immature and do not allow for sophisticated discrimination among stimuli. As children mature, however, they learn to apply their perceptions of the environment to different situations and can thus modify their behaviors accordingly. This process continues throughout the life cycle.

The effects of hospitalization or intensive medical treatments can exacerbate the problems related to sensory deficit. For example, a client with acute hearing loss can feel alone and vulnerable when faced with an environment that does not provide an effective means, such as interpreters who sign, through which communication can occur. Because of these responses, clients with sensory deficit are at serious risk of experiencing either sensory deprivation or sensory overload.

SENSORY DEPRIVATION

Sensory deprivation is a state of reduced sensory input from the internal or external environment, manifested by alterations in sensory perception. Individuals can experience sensory deprivation as a result of illness, trauma, or isolation. A person experiencing sensory deprivation misinterprets the limited stimuli with a resultant impairment of thoughts and feelings. Factors that contribute to sensory deprivation include:

- Visual or auditory impairments that limit or prohibit perception of stimuli
- Drugs that produce a sedative effect on the CNS and interfere with the interpretation of stimuli
- Trauma that results in brain damage and decreased cognitive function
- Isolation (either physical or social) that results in the creation of a nonstimulating environment

Some contributing factors (such as brain damage or blindness) result in chronic sensory deprivation. Other factors lead to acute, transient states of deprivation (such as receiving analgesic medications).

Individuals who are sensory-deprived may exhibit any of the following characteristics:

- Inability to concentrate
- Poor memory
- Impaired problem-solving ability
- Confusion
- Irritability
- Emotional lability (mood swings)
- Hallucinations
- Depression
- Boredom and apathy
- Drowsiness

SENSORY OVERLOAD

Sensory overload is a state of excessive and sustained multisensory stimulation manifested by behavior change and perceptual distortion. The individual experiencing this alteration is unable to process the amount or intensity of stimuli being received. Factors contributing to sensory overload are:

LIFE CYCLE CONSIDERATIONS

Effects of Aging

Sensory, perceptual, and cognitive function begins to be diminished as the effects of aging, such as decreased visual or auditory senses or impairments in memory, are experienced. These changes can have a profound effect on a client's self-esteem and response to life.

- Pain originating from a heightened quality or quantity of internal stimuli
- Invasive procedures that result in an increased amount of external stimuli
- Activity-filled, busy environment that contributes to the amount of stimuli being perceived
- Medications that stimulate the CNS and prohibit the client from ignoring selective stimuli
- Presence of strangers (both health care professionals and others) who contribute to the quantity of stimuli
- Diseases that affect the CNS and maximize the perception of stimuli

DISORDERS OF THE EAR

Disorders of the ear include impaired hearing, Ménière's Disease, otosclerosis, acoustic neuroma, otitis media, otitis externa, and mastoiditis.

IMPAIRED HEARING

Hearing loss is the most common chronic disability in the United States, affecting nearly 30 million adults (Spencer, 1998). It can be seriously debilitating by limiting the ability to socialize and work, or respond to the telephone or alarms, yet relatively few individuals who experience impaired hearing actually seek help. Some may deny the problem and others may feel that a hearing aid is a sign of old age. Often family members are the first to be aware of a hearing deficit.

TYPES OF HEARING LOSS

Hearing loss is generally categorized in two ways, conductive and sensorineural. Mixed hearing loss, both conductive and sensorineural, is possible, but far less likely. Either may occur at birth (congenital), develop later in life, be genetic, or be caused by injury or trauma.

Conductive hearing loss indicates an inability of the sound waves to reach the inner ear. This may be due to cerumen buildup or blockage, perforated tympanic membrane, or fixation of one or all of the ossicles.

In **sensorineural hearing loss**, the inner ear or cochlear portion of cranial nerve VIII may be abnormal or diseased. A tumor, infection, trauma, or exposure to loud noises may cause destruction of the nerve and result in sensorineural hearing loss.

Sensorineural hearing loss associated with aging is termed **presbycusis**. Higher frequency sounds like women's voices become especially difficult to hear, and distinguishing words may be a problem. According to Spencer (1998), 95 percent of the people with sensorineural hearing loss can be helped by hearing aids.

BEHAVIORS INDICATING HEARING LOSS

A hearing impairment is a serious disorder that is often debilitating and embarrassing to the client. Hearing is part of the communication process, so the inability to hear may cause the person to do or say the wrong thing in response to a question or command. Persons with hearing impairment may withdraw from conversation or seem indifferent to their surroundings or to those around them.

Oftentimes alterations in hearing are manifested by changes in speech habits and patterns. Individuals with hearing impairments may not notice the changes in their own speech pattern until someone constantly asks them to repeat themselves or to speak clearly. Indifference and withdrawal are common behaviors in response to hearing loss. If left undiagnosed and untreated, the person may truly regress, become unhappy, lonely, and possibly even paranoid. Some individuals overcompensate for the hearing loss by becoming very loud and aggressive.

Research on hearing impairment has created many devices to aid speech and sound discrimination. Early diagnosis, treatment, and rehabilitation are essential to help hearing impaired persons enjoy and appreciate the world they live in.

PROFESSIONAL TIP

Hearing Specialists

An audiologist evaluates hearing and determines the extent and type of hearing loss, and also provides nonmedical treatment such as the fitting of hearing aids, advice about assistive listening devices, and communication/aural rehabilitative training. An otolaryngologist (ear, nose, and throat physician) provides medical evaluation of hearing disorders and medical and surgical interventions. A hearing aid specialist is licensed to dispense hearing aids but does not have a medical background or training.

LIFE CYCLE CONSIDERATIONS

Hearing Loss

Infants and toddlers with hearing loss may exhibit severely delayed or absent speech. In adults, speech can deteriorate as manifested by muttering, slurring words, and dropping consonants or syllables.

HEARING AIDS/ ASSISTIVE DEVICES

Hearing aids today come in a variety of designs and sizes. Some are quite small and tinted to a person's skin color so as to be virtually unnoticeable. Some are worn in the ear, behind the ear, or are part of eyeglasses frames. Persons with bilateral hearing loss may need binaural (worn in both ears) hearing aids.

A hearing aid converts environmental sound and speech into electronic signals that are amplified and converted to acoustic signals. It makes speech and sound louder, but not necessarily clearer. Depending on the extent of hearing impairment and preference, the client may need to experiment with several different types of hearing aids. In addition, speech therapy, lip reading, and auditory training may be necessary to help discriminate speech and develop better listening skills.

Many other assistive hearing devices are available for the hearing impaired. Numerous television programs are closed-caption. Advanced technology allows telecommunication through a device called Telecommunication Device for the Deaf (TDD), also called TTY Typewriter, which sends a printed message onto a small screen. Both sender and receiver must have the typewriter/telephone device. Many businesses offer this option to conduct transactions.

Alarm clocks offer strobe lights or vibrators to awaken clients. State of the art receivers give instant access to radio, television, computer, and stereos to enhance receiving and listening systems. For travelers, complete kits are available to provide ready access for smoke alarm, clock, TDD, and door knock alert in hotels or inns.

Hearing guide dogs are also available. The animals are specially trained to meet the needs of the hearing impaired. At home, the dog responds to alarms, knocking on doors, and babies crying. In public, the dog takes a position between owner and a potential threat. Special identifiers, such as a collar for the dog and ID card for the owner are available. The dogs are trained to go wherever their master goes including restaurants, grocery stores, and on public transportation.

Medical–Surgical Management

Medical

It is important to identify the type of hearing loss and underlying etiology to determine the best medical or surgical management. The client should undergo a complete physical examination as well as thorough diagnostic hearing tests. Once the etiology is determined, the client and doctor can decide upon the best course of therapy.

Surgical

Silverstein (1992) offers a technological advancement called the cochlear implant as a possible treatment for persons with profound deafness. Studies thus far indicate better success with the implant in children than in adults. In this procedure, a receiver/stimulator is implanted in the skull and a group of electrodes are planted in front of the round window in the inner ear. The client wears a microphone near the ear that picks up and translates sound into electrical signals. These signals are then transmitted to the brain via the cochlear implant and cranial nerve VIII.

▸ NURSING PROCESS

▸ Assessment

▸ Subjective Data

Subjective data may be obtained by asking the client to describe the initial onset of symptoms and possible familial traits. The nurse should ask the client about recent infections of the ears, nose, or upper respiratory system. Recent trauma and past surgery as well as medical history such as diabetes, heart disease, or cancer should be determined. The nurse should note allergies to food, drugs, or environmental factors. The client's work history may reveal exposure to loud noises. The client should be asked about associated symptoms such as **tinnitus** (ringing sound in the ear), **vertigo** (dizziness), nausea, and vomiting.

▸ Objective Data

Objective data may be obtained by listening closely to the client and noting any deterioration of speech, slurring, or dropping of word endings. Current and recent medication use should be documented.

The outer ear should be inspected for abnormalities, lesions, or cerumen. The mastoid process, neck, jaw, and temporal regions of the head should be palpated for swelling or tenderness to touch. The nurse should note the degree of hearing loss as reported by the client and compare it to the diagnostic tests such as the speech audiogram. The client's perception of hearing loss may be significantly different from the diagnostic findings.

A nursing diagnosis for a client with impaired hearing may be:

Nursing Diagnosis	Planning/Goals	Nursing Interventions
▶ *Social Isolation, related to hearing impairment*	The client will participate in conversations and other social situations.	Take time to engage client in conversation. Speak slowly and distinctly. Make sure you have the client's attention and be at eye level. Give the client time to respond. Provide the client and family members written information regarding the availability, variety, and quality of assistive hearing devices. Encourage client to participate in social situations.

Evaluation The goal must be evaluated to determine how it has been met by the client.

MÉNIÈRE'S DISEASE

Ménière's disease, also known as endolymphatic hydrops, is a state of hearing loss characterized by tinnitus and vertigo. Although the exact etiology is unknown, it is postulated that the cause is an excessive accumulation of endolymph in the cochlear duct and possible leakage of endolymph into the perilymph due to increased capillary permeability. Mixing of the two fluids chemically alters the homeostasis of the perilymph and endolymph and can be responsible for the symptoms associated with Ménière's disease.

The major symptoms are the classic triad of vertigo, tinnitus, and unilateral fluctuating hearing loss. The vertigo is often associated with nausea and vomiting. Tinnitus may either be a preceding aura or occur simultaneously with the vertigo. Initially, tinnitus is intermittent, but as the disease progresses, it may be a constant, low-pitched roaring sound. The fluctuating,

unilateral hearing loss becomes more profound with each attack.

The symptoms are frequently at their worst during the first attack, which may last from a few minutes to six hours. **Nystagmus**, repetitive and involuntary movement of the eyeballs, and diaphoresis may occur during an attack. Subsequent attacks are less severe, but over time may involve both ears and cause permanent bilateral hearing loss. Clients report many different precipitating events such as stress, weather changes, menstruation, or pregnancy, and various dietary influences including caffeine, alcohol, and salt. Smoking has also been implicated.

Medical–Surgical Management

Medical

Medical management is the preferred treatment and most helpful to about 80 to 85 percent of persons affected with this disease. Diagnosis is not difficult and is usually made based on the client's report of symptoms. Diagnosis may also be confirmed with caloric stimulation (though this test is primarily conducted on comatose clients) and an MRI to rule out a tumor. Medical management is symptomatic.

Surgical

Surgical intervention is usually needed only when the attacks are frequent and debilitating, or when the disease severely impacts the quality of life and the ability for self-care. Surgical treatment includes endolymphatic, subarachnoid shunt placement to drain excessive endolymph. With this procedure, hearing is preserved in 60% to 70% of the clients. With a vestibular neurectomy, the vestibular portion of cranial nerve VIII is severed; hearing is preserved in 90% of the clients having this procedure. In surgical destruction of the labyrinth, hearing is destroyed but the incapacitating vertigo is completely relieved.

Pharmacological

A number of medications are useful to help control the symptoms such as antihistamines, antiemetics, benzodiazepines, diuretics, tranquilizers, vasoactive

PROFESSIONAL TIP

Assisting the Hearing Impaired Client
- Speak slowly and distinctly after getting the client's attention.
- Face the client and sit or stand to be at eye level with the client.
- Use short, simple sentences and give the client time to respond. Repeat or rephrase if necessary.
- Use written materials when possible to communicate information.
- Keep a notepad and pen or pencil available to write down new or unfamiliar words and concepts.
- If sign language is the client's preferred method of communication, locate a person who understands sign language.
- If the client wears a hearing aid, make sure that the battery is functional, it is turned on, and adjusted to a comfortable level.

agents, and oral niacin. The medications may be prescribed for long-term use or at the onset of symptoms. Since the cause of Ménière's disease is unknown, there is no cure.

Diet

Dietary interventions include strict salt restriction and avoidance of those foods or beverages that precipitate or aggravate an attack. Examples are beer, wine, soda, salty food or snacks, chocolate, and caffeinated coffee and tea.

Activity

Activity is not limited in a normal daily routine. However, during or after an attack, clients may require prolonged bed rest and restriction of activities that may be unsafe, such as driving or operating heavy equipment.

▶ NURSING PROCESS

▶ Assessment

▶ Subjective Data

The history should begin with identifying significant contributory data. Subjective data may be obtained by asking the client to describe the initial onset of symptoms including, but not limited to, the classic triad of tinnitus, vertigo, and fluctuating unilateral hearing loss.

Questions should be related to recent viral illness; upper respiratory infections; past medical, surgical, and dental history; and any problems related to the neck and face. Food, drug, or environmental allergies should be documented. Current or recent long-term medications should be recorded. The client's occupation and hobbies that may contribute to hearing loss should be identified.

▶ Objective Data

Objective data may be obtained with a thorough physical examination that includes looking at the ear for abnormalities, lesions and cerumen blockage, or unusual drainage. The neck, jaw, and mastoid process should be palpated for possible lymph node enlargement and tenderness. The nurse may assist with the otologic examination as needed. Audiological testing determines unilateral or bilateral hearing loss.

Nursing diagnoses for a client with Ménière's disease may include the following:

Nursing Diagnoses	Planning/Goals	Nursing Interventions
▶ *Activity Intolerance, related to severe vertigo*	The client will be able to tolerate activities of daily living.	Provide adequate periods of bed rest. Keep the room dim and quiet when possible. Avoid jarring the bed and caution client to avoid sudden movements. Administer antiemetic before symptoms become too severe. Provide assistance with ambulation and encourage increased activity as tolerated.
▶ *Knowledge Deficit, related to abrupt onset and unknown progression of the disease*	The client will verbalize understanding of the disease process and potential precipitating factors and how to manage or control the symptoms.	Assess the client's current knowledge of the disease process. Review the disease process and underlying etiology of Ménière's disease with the client. Ask the client to identify possible precipitating factors such as stress or dietary habits. Discuss health promotion programs for stress management and healthy cooking classes. Suggest consultations with dietary and social services. Review follow-up appointments, medications, dietary management, activity, and rest parameters. Evaluate client's readiness to discuss progressive hearing loss and current assistive hearing devices available.
▶ *Injury, Risk for, related to vertigo*	The client will not fall or be injured because of vertigo.	Keep side rails up. Teach client to move or turn slowly. Reiterate need to call for assistance when ambulating. Keep call bell within client's reach. Administer medications for vertigo prior to worsening of symptoms. Avoid glaring, bright lights. Instruct client to sit or lie down when vertigo occurs.

Evaluation Each goal must be evaluated to determine how it has been met by the client.

OTOSCLEROSIS

Otosclerosis is a conductive hearing loss secondary to a pathologic change of the bones in the middle ear. The exact cause is unknown. The ossicles are normally hard, but over time and without warning, the bone becomes softened, spongy, highly vascular, and partially or totally fixed. This fixation reduces or prevents transmission of source waves to inner ear fluids. Although all three bones may be affected, the stapes, which must vibrate on the oval window in order to transmit sound waves, is most commonly afflicted.

Otosclerosis is more common in adults, women are affected more often than men, and it is familial in some cases. It is the most common cause of conductive hearing loss.

The primary clinical manifestations are subtle changes in hearing and low-pitched tinnitus. It becomes more difficult to distinguish a whisper, or to hear in crowded places or understand conversation. Individuals affected by otosclerosis often blame others for speaking too softly or mumbling. Frequently, rather than asking others to speak up or to repeat themselves, the person will be irritable and withdrawn.

Diagnostic testing begins with the Weber and Rinne tuning fork tests. In addition, audiometric testing should be performed. Schwartz's sign, a pink blush, is seen on otoscopic examination. Tympanometry shows stiffness in the sound conduction system.

Medical–Surgical Management

Medical

Treatment for otosclerosis is limited to three options. The individual may choose to do nothing and obtain periodic audiometry to evaluate progression of the disease. The second choice is to use a hearing aid and the third choice is surgical management with an outpatient procedure known as a stapedectomy.

Surgical

A stapedectomy is the preferred surgical technique for improving hearing loss due to otosclerosis. A stapedectomy may be done under local or general anesthesia and routinely requires a surgical incision in the posterior ear canal, removal of the stapes, and implantation of a plastic prosthesis. A new technique, laser stapedectomy, may be performed through the ear canal without an incision. The stapes tendon is vaporized, chards are removed with delicate micro instruments, and an opening is made allowing the surgeon to implant a prosthetic piston. This restores normal vibration against the inner ear.

▶ NURSING PROCESS

▶ Assessment

▶ Subjective Data

Subjective data will include a careful history to discover possible hereditary traits or acquired disease. The client should be asked about recent infections of the ears, nose, or upper respiratory system, and also about past surgery, trauma, or other illnesses such as diabetes, heart disease, or cancer. Associated symptoms such as dizziness, tinnitus, vertigo, and nausea should be identified.

The nurse should note allergies to foods, drugs, or any environmental factors. The client's work history may reveal exposure to loud noises. Current and recent medications should be recorded, especially those known to be ototoxic.

▶ Objective Data

Objective data includes a thorough physical examination. The nurse must inspect the outer ear for abnormalities, lesions, or impacted ear wax. The mastoid process, neck, jaw, and temporal regions of the head should be palpated for pain or swelling. The degree of hearing loss should be assessed. The client may be vomiting.

Nursing diagnoses for the client with otosclerosis may include the following:

Nursing Diagnoses	Planning/Goals	Nursing Interventions
▶ *Anxiety, related to decrease or loss in hearing*	The client will show evidence of reduced anxiety and verbalize understanding of the disease process and treatment regimen.	Encourage the client to explore feelings of anxiety and to ask questions to clarify concerns. Provide honest and realistic feedback. Collaborate with the physician to provide thorough and clear explanations of the disease process, treatment options, and anticipated results.
▶ *Injury, Risk for, related to vertigo*	The client will not fall or be injured because of vertigo.	Keep side rails up. Instruct the client to move or turn slowly. Reiterate need to call for assistance when ambulating and keep call bell within client's reach. Administer medications for vertigo prior to worsening of symptoms. Keep room well lit when client is ambulating.

continued

Nursing Diagnoses	Planning/Goals	Nursing Interventions
▶ *Knowledge Deficit, related to activities after surgery*	The client will demonstrate the ability to change dressing correctly and verbalize knowledge of self-care and follow-up.	Teach client how and when to perform dressing change and have client demonstrate the procedure.
		Instruct client to avoid pressure changes (such as flying in an unpressurized aircraft), avoid heavy lifting (60 lbs) for one month, avoid nose blowing for ten days and if sneezing occurs, keep mouth open.
		Advise client to keep water out of the ear and keep the ear exposed to air as much as possible for one month. There will be some drainage which is initially red, then pink, and then brownish.
		Tell client to report any greenish, yellowish, or foul smelling drainage.
		Instruct client to take all antibiotics as prescribed and complete the full course of treatment.
		Advise client there should be very little pain or discomfort but if there is, take prescribed analgesics and notify doctor if pain is prolonged or intense.
		Warn client that hearing may be decreased for three to four weeks after surgery until gel-foam packing dissolves.
		Inform client that audiometric testing will be conducted one month after surgery.
		Instruct client to schedule an appointment with the physician in one month but call physician if uncontrolled pain is experienced or a malodorous, greenish discharge comes from the ear.

Evaluation Each goal must be evaluated to determine how it has been met by the client.

ACOUSTIC NEUROMA

Acoustic neuroma is a slow-growing and usually benign tumor of the vestibular portion of the inner ear (cranial nerve VIII). Detection at the onset of symptoms is essential and may be accomplished with an MRI. Presenting symptoms of dizziness, tinnitus, and hearing loss are common to many dysfunctions of the ear and the possibility of acoustic neuroma must not be overlooked.

Clients who present with dizziness, tinnitus, and hearing loss should have a complete workup for auditory and vestibular (balance) function. Facial weakness may be caused by compression of the tumor on cranial nerve VII. The Vth cranial nerve may also be affected as the tumor grows, causing paresthesia of the face and loss of the corneal reflex. Large neuromas can cause increased intracranial pressure, papilledema, vomiting, and headache.

Medical–Surgical Management

Treatment is almost always surgical excision of the tumor. Although antihistamines may reduce the dizziness, the pharmacologic treatment is only temporary until diagnostic tests are completed and surgery is planned.

▶ NURSING PROCESS
▶ Assessment
▶ Subjective Data
Subjective data may be obtained through the client history of the chief complaint, reported signs and symptoms, and all contributing data.

▶ Objective Data
Objective data will be obtained with the physical examination and should include a complete cranial nerve evaluation performed by the physician or audiologist to determine the extent of cranial nerve involvement.

A nursing diagnosis for a client with acoustic neuroma may be:

Nursing Diagnosis	Planning/Goals	Nursing Interventions
▶ *Grieving, Anticipatory, related to diminished quality of life, loss of ability for self-care, or possible loss of life*	The client will express feelings of grief and demonstrate adaptive coping mechanisms.	Assist the client to express feelings about progressive hearing loss and changes in activities of daily living, employment, and quality of life issues.
		Collaborate with physician and other members of the health care team to provide thorough and clear explanations of the disease process, treatment options, and anticipated results.

continued

Nursing Diagnoses	Planning/Goals	Nursing Interventions
		Observe the client's coping styles. Support those that the client finds helpful and explore other coping mechanisms that may prove useful in time (e.g., hobbies and other diversional activities, prayer, reading, and so on).
		Include the family in all interventions that the client desires.
		Examine the family's feelings and ability to cope.
		Consult social services, pastoral care, or other hospital and community resources when appropriate.

Evaluation The goal must be evaluated to determine how it has been met by the client.

OTITIS MEDIA

Otitis media is an inflammation of the middle ear and a common cause of conductive hearing loss, though usually temporary. Presenting symptoms include ear pain, fever, redness of auricle and ear canal, and sometimes enlarged lymph nodes over the mastoid process, parotids, and upper neck. Otitis media occurs more frequently in children than in adults.

Fluid accumulates behind the eardrum due to blockage of the eustachian tube (Figure 43-6). This may be secondary to an upper respiratory infection, allergies, or acute bacterial infection. On physical examination the tympanic membrane may be retracted, normal, or bulging. A pneumatic otoscope allows the practitioner to blow soft puffs of air against the tympanic membrane to assess movement. A stiff, nonmoving, or bulging tympanic membrane may indicate inflammation or fluid accumulation in the middle ear. Visualization of the normal landmarks may be obscured. The Rinne tuning fork test and audiometry confirm a conductive hearing loss.

Medical–Surgical Management

Medical

Topical heat and systemic analgesics may be used to control pain. The client should lie on the affected side to facilitate drainage.

Surgical

Surgical management may be necessary for diagnostic or therapeutic reasons. A myringotomy may be performed, in which an incision is made in the eardrum and fluid is aspirated. A polyethylene tube may be placed in the eardrum to equalize pressure and allow drainage of fluid.

A tympanoplasty may be needed if the tympanic membrane is ruptured. If there is a large tympanic membrane perforation, the malleus, which is connected to the tympanic membrane, or other ossicles may be damaged. Ossicular chain reconstruction typically refers to the removal of the actual bones and replacement with a plastic prosthesis. Often the prosthesis and the tympanic membrane reconstruction result in a significant improvement in hearing.

Pharmacological

Medications used include decongestants such as pseudoephedrine hydrochloride (Sudafed), antihistamines such as diphenhydramine hydrochloride (Benadryl), and systemic antibiotics such as ampicillin (Omnipen).

Activity

Activity is not restricted unless surgical management is indicated.

▶ NURSING PROCESS

▶ Assessment

▶ Subjective Data

The nurse should ask about the onset, duration, and severity of pain and what home remedies have been used. Hearing loss and/or tinnitus and a deep throbbing pain in the ear may be reported.

▶ Objective Data

A watery or yellow discharge may be seen. It may have a foul odor. The client may have a fever.

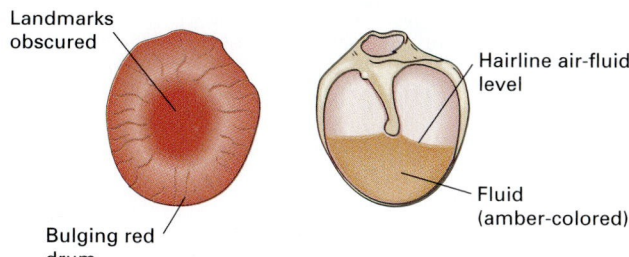

Figure 43-6 The Tympanic Membrane in the Presence of Otitis Media

A nursing diagnosis for a client with otitis media may be:

Nursing Diagnosis	Planning/Goals	Nursing Interventions
▶ *Pain, Acute, related to inflammation in the middle ear*	The client will experience pain relief.	Administer antibiotics as ordered.
		Teach client and family the importance of administering medications as ordered and to complete full course of prescription.
		Administer analgesics as ordered.
		Apply heating pad, set on low, for 20 minutes every 2 hours. Do not use on small children.
		Teach client if pain is unrelieved in 48 hours, to contact physician.

Evaluation The goal must be evaluated to determine how it has been met by the client.

OTITIS EXTERNA

Otitis externa or "swimmer's ear" typically involves a bacterial infection of the external ear canal skin. The canal skin becomes red and edematous. If the swelling is severe enough, it will block the ear passage and cause a mild conductive hearing loss. Also, in most cases there is a discharge. If the discharge is copious and the canal size is constricted, a mild conductive hearing loss may result.

MASTOIDITIS

Mastoiditis (inflammation of the mastoid) is most often the direct result of chronic or recurrent bacterial otitis media. The recurrent infection may find its way into the bone and structures surrounding the middle ear and, if left untreated, can cause severe damage, sensorineural deafness, facial weakness, brain abscess, and meningitis. Other symptoms include earache, fever, headache, and malaise. Antibiotics are given for a trial period. If symptoms do not resolve, surgical intervention such as mastoidectomy or meatoplasty may be necessary.

DISORDERS OF THE EYE

Disorders of the eye include cataracts, glaucoma, retinal detachment, infections, refractive errors, injuries, impaired vision, and macular degeneration.

CATARACTS

A **cataract** is a disorder that causes the lens or its capsule to lose its transparency and/or become opaque (Figure 43-7). The lens is normally clear and transparent and allows light to pass through to the retina. As clouding develops, visual impairment occurs. Cataracts usually affect both eyes; however the degree of visual impairment is often different in each eye.

Cataracts are typically associated with aging; however, they may be congenital, caused by severe eye injury, or secondary to certain systemic diseases characterized by metabolic problems (diabetes mellitus) and chronic eye disease (uveitis). Ophthalmoscopic examination is the primary method of evaluation.

Medical–Surgical Management

Surgical

The only treatment for a cataract is surgical removal of the lens. However, the mere finding of a cataract is not an indication for surgery. Surgery is indicated when significant vision loss has occurred. The lens may be removed by the intracapsular or extracapsular approach. During the intracapsular cataract extraction, the ophthalmologist removes the lens within its capsule. Extracapsular cataract extraction is the procedure most commonly used (Figure 43-8). The ophthalmologist removes the anterior portion of the capsule and then expresses, or removes, the lens. An intraocular

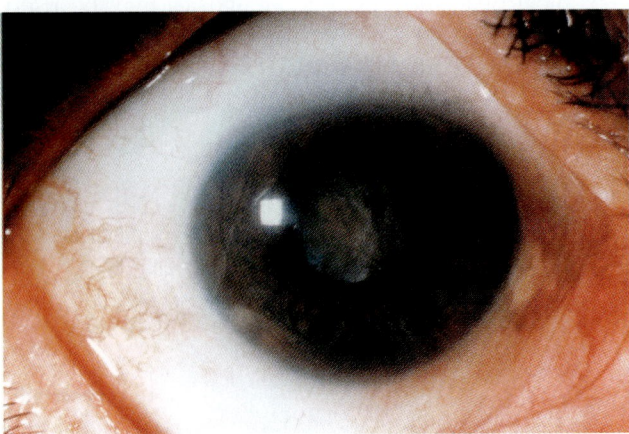

Figure 43-7 A cataract results in the loss of transparency of the lens of the eye. *(Courtesy of the National Eye Institute, Bethesda, MD)*

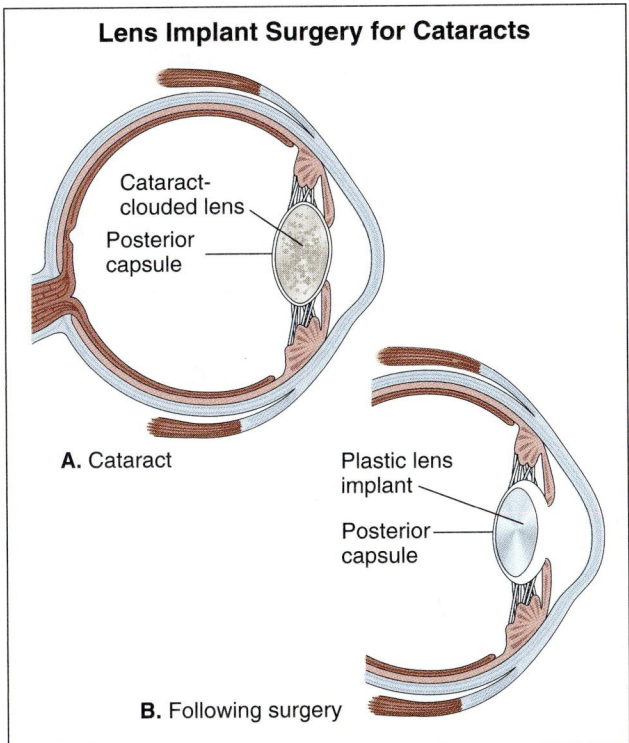

Lens Implant Surgery for Cataracts

Cataract-clouded lens
Posterior capsule

A. Cataract

Plastic lens implant
Posterior capsule

B. Following surgery

Figure 43-8 In extracapsular extraction to correct cataracts, the lens is removed, the posterior lens capsule is left intact, and a plastic intraocular lens (IOL) is placed.

lens (IOL) is generally implanted. Glasses or special contact lenses may also be used.

Most eye surgery is done on an outpatient basis under local anesthesia. General anesthesia can be used at the client's request and for clients who are extremely anxious, deaf, or mentally retarded. A tranquilizer such as diazepam (Valium) is often given to reduce anxiety when receiving injections on the face and around the eye.

Preoperatively, the client can receive several types of eye medications to prepare the eye for surgery: mydriatic (makes pupil dilate) and cycloplegic (paralyzes ciliary muscle) eye drops, antibiotic eye drops as a prophylaxis against infection, and an intravenous infusion of an agent to lower intraocular pressure (mannitol or a carbonic anhydrase inhibitor).

 PROFESSIONAL TIP

Eye Specialists

An ophthalmologist is a medical doctor who specializes in the diagnosis and treatment, both medical and surgical, of diseases of the eye, visual disorders, and eye injuries. An optometrist is a doctor of optometry and is licensed to examine, diagnose, manage and treat vision problems, diseases, and other abnormalities of the eyes and related structures.

The client is instructed to have a driver available to provide transportation postoperatively because driving is restricted for a few days. After the anesthesia wears off, the client is discharged.

Postoperatively, the client has a patch over the eye. The patch is removed and reapplied on the first postoperative day when miotic (makes pupil contract) eye drops are begun. Mild discomfort and scratchiness are expected. Atropine sulfate eye drops and cold compresses may be ordered to relieve these discomforts.

▶ NURSING PROCESS

▶ Assessment

▶ Subjective Data

A general medical history as well as a history of symptoms is needed. Symptoms may include: haziness, cloudiness, blurred vision, double vision, altered color perception, and glare when looking at lights, especially with night driving. Fear of losing one's eyesight can be very devastating. There is often a great deal of anxiety when the client seeks an eye examination.

▶ Objective Data

Upon inspection of the eye the usual black pupil appears clouded, progressing to a milky white appearance which is a characteristic finding of a mature cataract and indicates significant vision loss.

Nursing diagnoses for a client with cataracts may include the following:

Nursing Diagnoses	Planning/Goals	Nursing Interventions
▶ *Sensory/Perceptual Alterations, Visual, related to ocular lens opacity*	The client will demonstrate improved ability to process visual stimuli and communicate visual limitations.	Assess and document baseline visual acuity. Elicit functional description of what the client can and cannot see.
▶ *Injury, Risk for, related to difficulty in processing visual images and altered depth perception*	The client will avoid activities associated with increased potential for injury.	Teach the client to change position slowly. Teach the client to avoid reaching for objects to maintain stability when ambulating, as depth perception is altered.

continued

Nursing Diagnoses	Planning/Goals	Nursing Interventions
▶ *Home Maintenance Management, Impaired, related to age, limited vision or activity restrictions imposed by surgery*	The client will perform self-care activities in home environment.	Discuss the client's ability to meet self-care needs and activities of daily living.
		Evaluate how the client's current functional ability will be affected by activity restrictions and postoperative care needs.
		Help the client decide on a realistic site for postoperative care needs.

Evaluation Each goal must be evaluated to determine how it has been met by the client.

GLAUCOMA

Glaucoma is a disorder characterized by an abnormally high pressure of fluid inside the eyeball (intraocular pressure, IOP). The aqueous humor does not return into the bloodstream through the canal of Schlemm as quickly as it is formed. The fluid accumulates and, by compressing the lens into the vitreous humor, puts pressure on the neurons of the retina. If the pressure continues over a long period of time, it destroys the neurons and brings about blindness.

There are two primary forms of glaucoma: open-angle glaucoma and closed-angle glaucoma. Open-angle glaucoma (chronic simple glaucoma) is characterized by a gradual rise in IOP, a slowly progressive loss of peripheral vision, and, if not controlled, a late loss of central vision and ultimate blindness. This is the most prevalent form of glaucoma and is usually bilateral. Closed-angle glaucoma (acute glaucoma) is characterized by attacks of suddenly increased intraocular pressure, exhibited clinically by a bulging iris, which is an emergency situation. Closed-angle glaucoma is usually unilateral with severe pain and loss of vision caused by acute obstruction of aqueous humor drainage within the eye.

Secondary glaucoma results from ocular or systemic disorders that are responsible for the elevation in IOP. These disorders or conditions indirectly disrupt the activity of the structures involved in circulation and/or reabsorption of aqueous humor. This can happen suddenly and without warning.

CLIENT TEACHING

Glaucoma Care

- Continue the use of eye medications as ordered.
- Continue to receive medical supervision for observation of intraocular pressure to ensure control of the disorder.
- Avoid exertion, stooping, heavy lifting, or wearing constrictive clothing as these increase intraocular pressure.

Medical–Surgical Management

Medical

Medical management for glaucoma is focused on drug therapy and the main objective is to reduce intraocular pressure. Two mechanisms for reducing this pressure are: (1) physically constricting the pupil so that the ciliary muscle is contracted, which allows better circulation of the aqueous humor to the site of absorption, and (2) inhibiting the production of aqueous humor.

Surgical

Surgical intervention to facilitate drainage of the aqueous humor is called an iridectomy. A surgical incision is made through the cornea to remove a portion of the iris to facilitate aqueous drainage.

A laser may also be used to treat various eye disorders. In open-angle glaucoma, a laser is used to create multiple scars around the trabecular meshwork (a supporting or anchoring strand that allows increased outflow of aqueous humor) thereby reducing intraocular pressure. In closed-angle glaucoma, laser energy is used to create a hole in the periphery of the iris, creating an opening between the anterior and posterior chambers for aqueous drainage.

Pharmacological

Drugs that enhance pupillary constriction are commonly used to treat glaucoma. Miotics and cholinesterase inhibitors such as pilocarpine hydrochloride (Isopto Carpine), carbachol (Carbacel), and demecarium bromide (Humorsol) are frequently used.

Beta-adrenergics such as timolol maleate (Timoptic Solution) are the drugs of choice for decreasing IOP. When used as eye drops, beta-adrenergics reduce aqueous humor production without pupil constriction.

Carbonic anhydrase inhibitors, such as acetazolamide (Diamox), reduce production of aqueous humor to help maintain a lowered IOP. Side effects reported are numbness, weakness, tingling of extremities, and rashes. Adrenergics such as epinephrine bitartrate (Epitrate) also reduce aqueous humor production. Osmotic agents such as mannitol and glycerin (Osmoglyn) may be administered systemically to the client with closed-angle glaucoma in an emergency as an effort to decrease IOP. The high osmolarity of these agents is used to draw fluid into the intravascular space, which lowers the IOP.

▶ NURSING PROCESS

▶ Assessment

▶ Subjective Data

The nurse should obtain a history noting the presence of risk factors: positive family history (believed to be linked in open-angle glaucoma), eye tumor, intraocular hemorrhage, intraocular inflammation, or contusion of the eye from trauma during cataract surgery.

Symptoms of open-angle glaucoma include gradual loss of peripheral vision, eye pain, difficulty adjusting to darkness, halos around lights and an inability to detect color. For closed-angle glaucoma, symptoms include sudden onset of severe pain in the eye often accompanied by headache, nausea, vomiting, malaise, rainbow halos around lights, and blurred vision.

▶ Objective Data

Assessment reveals acute increased intraocular pressure (21 to 32 mm Hg) as measured with a tonometer (normal range is 12 to 22 mm Hg).

A nursing diagnosis for a client with glaucoma may be:

Nursing Diagnosis	Planning/Goals	Nursing Interventions
▶ *Pain, Acute, related to closed-angle glaucoma*	The client will verbalize relief from discomfort.	Administer prescribed ophthalmic agent for glaucoma.
		Notify physician of the following: hypotension, urinary output less than 240 mL for 8 hours, no relief in eye pain within 30 minutes of drug therapy, and continual diminishing visual acuity.
		Monitor blood pressure, pulse, and respiration every 4 hours if not receiving osmotic agent intravenously and every 2 hours if receiving intravenous osmotic agent.
		Monitor degree of eye pain every 30 minutes.
		Monitor intake and output every 8 hours while receiving intravenous osmotic agent.
		Monitor visual acuity prior to each instillation of prescribed ophthalmic agent by asking if objects are clear or blurred and if the client can read printed material held at arm's length.
		Remind the client that miotics may cause blurred vision for 1 to 2 hours after use and that adaptation to dark environments is difficult because of the pupillary constriction.

Evaluation The goal must be evaluated to determine how it has been met by the client.

RETINAL DETACHMENT

In retinal detachment, there is an actual separation of the retina from the choroid (Figure 43-9). Partial separation becomes complete, if untreated, with the subsequent total loss of vision. A tear or hole in the retina can extend the separation as vitreous humor seeps through the opening and separates the retina from the choroid. The cause of retinal detachment may be from severe trauma to the eye or from intraocular disorders such as cataract extraction, perforating injuries, or severe **myopia** (nearsightedness). This condition is painless since there are no pain receptors in the retina.

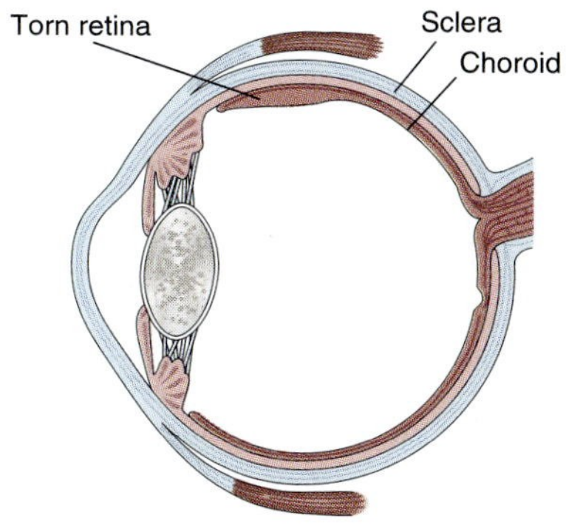

Medical–Surgical Management

Medical

Early corrective intervention to reattach the retina may use one of several techniques. Three procedures can be used to create an inflammatory reaction that, once healing and scarring occur, result in the retina reattaching to the choroid. One such technique is electrodiathermy (heat therapy) which uses an ultrasonic probe to burn (seal) the scleral surface directly over the retinal break. Another technique is cryotherapy which uses an intensely cold probe applied to the scleral surface

Figure 43-9 Retinal Detachment

directly over the hole in the retina. Laser photocoagulation is also used to seal tears or holes in the retina.

Surgical

A surgical procedure called scleral buckling is sometimes used. This operation reduces the scleral surface and allows contact between the choroid and retina.

Pharmacological

Cycloplegic-mydriatic and anti-infective eyedrops are often ordered following the attachment procedure.

Activity

Bed rest and a patch on one or both eyes restricts activity. If air is injected into the vitreous humor, the client either lies prone or sits forward with the unaffected eye upward.

▶ NURSING PROCESS

▶ Assessment

▶ Subjective Data

Obtain a medical history for presence of causative factors: trauma, recent cataract surgery, eye tumor, severe myopia, uveitis. The client may describe sudden flashes of light (photopsia), floating spots (caused by bleeding into the vitreous cavity), blurred vision that becomes progressively worse, or complaints of a sensation of a veil in the line of sight.

▶ Objective Data

Ophthalmoscopic examination visualizes the detachment.

Nursing diagnoses for a client with retinal detachment may include the following:

Nursing Diagnoses	Planning/Goals	Nursing Interventions
▶ *Anxiety, related to sensory visual impairment and lack of understanding about treatment*	The client will demonstrate reduction of emotional stress, fear, and depression; and an acceptance of surgery.	Assess degree and duration of visual impairment.
		Encourage conversation to determine client's concerns, feelings, and level of understanding.
		Answer questions, offer support, and assist client to devise methods for coping.
		Orient client to new surroundings.
		Explain surgery routines. Preoperative: Level of activity-ocular rest which includes bilateral eye patching and bed rest to facilitate settling of the retina and prevent detachment from worsening. The client will be NPO after midnight. The affected eye is maximally dilated before surgery to permit adequate visualization of the fundus. Intraoperative: Client must lie still during surgery or give surgeon warning if needs to cough or change position. Face covered with drapes. Air and oxygen provided. Monitoring, including frequent blood pressure measurements. Postoperative: Positioning (supine with a small pillow under the head), bilateral eye patches, activity restrictions, and need to call for assistance with ambulation until stable and vision is adequate.
		Explain interventions clearly.
		Announce yourself with each interaction; interpret unfamiliar sounds; use touch to assist with verbal communication.
		Encourage to carry out ADLs as ability allows.
		Order finger foods for those who cannot see well enough or do not have the coping skills to use implements.
		Encourage participation of family or significant others in client care.
		Encourage participation in social and diversional activities as allowed (visitor, radio, audio tapes, television, crafts, games).
▶ *Injury, Risk for, related to visual impairment or knowledge deficit*	The client will not have injury caused by visual impairment.	Assist client when able to ambulate postoperatively until stable and has adequate vision or coping skills (remember that clients with bilateral eye patches are unable to see).
		Assist client in arranging environment and do not rearrange furnishings without reorienting client.
		Discuss importance of wearing metal shield or glasses as ordered.
		Apply no pressure to the affected eye.
		Use proper procedure to administer eye medications.

Evaluation Each goal must be evaluated to determine how it has been met by the client.

INFECTIONS

Infections of the eye include keratitis, stye, chalazion, and conjunctivitis.

KERATITIS

Keratitis is inflammation of the cornea that may be caused by infection, irritation, injury, or allergies. Symptoms associated with keratitis include severe eye pain, red watering eye, photophobia, sometimes reduced vision, and sometimes rash (e.g., herpes simplex, herpes zoster, or rosacea).

Treatment of keratitis includes optical anesthetics to relieve pain and mydriatics to dilate the pupil. Dark glasses should be worn to relieve the photophobia. Antibiotic solutions are prescribed for the specific type of infection, since the microorganism may be bacterial, viral, or fungal.

STYE

A **stye** is also referred to as a hordeolum. It is a pustular inflammation of an eyelash follicle or sebaceous gland on the lid margin commonly caused by staphylococcal organisms. Symptoms include pain, redness, and swelling of a specific area of the eyelid. Treatment consists of warm compresses and topical antibiotic ointments. More severe cases may require incision and drainage. Once the pus drains, the pain is relieved and healing begins.

CHALAZION

A **chalazion** is a cyst of the meibomian glands, which are sebaceous glands located at the junction of the conjunctiva and inner eyelid margins. The hard cyst is filled with fatty material from the chronically obstructed meibomian glands. The inherent feature of a chalazion is painless localized swelling that develops over a period of weeks. Treatment usually involves surgical excision if the cyst is large, becomes infected, or interferes with vision or closure of the eyelids. The cyst remains when the inflammation subsides.

CONJUNCTIVITIS (PINK EYE)

Conjunctivitis is an inflammation of the conjunctiva (a membrane that lines the inside of the eyelids and covers the cornea) that results from invasion by bacterial, viral, or rickettsial organisms, allergens, or irritants. Symptoms include burning and itching of eyes, discharge, swelling, pain, and redness. Treatment consists of applying warm compresses using saline or boric acid solution and instilling antibiotic or antiviral ointments. When caused by allergens, treatment includes avoiding the allergen, taking antihistamines, or being desensitized.

Conjunctivitis is contagious. Proper handwashing must be done by nurse and client. Gloves should be worn when applying compresses or instilling ointment. The client's linen should be disinfected to prevent spread of the infection.

REFRACTIVE ERRORS

Refraction is the deflection or bending of light rays when they pass from a medium of one density to a medium of another density. In the case of the eye, light waves pass through the air (less dense) into the fluids of the eye (more dense) so that they can be brought to focus on the retina.

Refractive errors result in changes in visual acuity or vision that is not 20/20. Refractive errors include **myopia** (nearsightedness), **hyperopia** (farsightedness), **astigmatism** (asymmetric focus of light rays on the retina), **presbyopia** (inability of the lens to change curvature in order to focus on near objects), and **strabismus** (inability of the eyes to focus in the same direction). Figure 43-10 shows a child with strabismus.

With myopia, parallel light rays come to focus in front of the retina because the refractive system is too strong or the eyeball is elongated. Near vision is normal but distant vision is poor.

With hyperopia, parallel light rays come to focus behind the retina because the refractive system is too weak or the eyeball is flattened. Vision beyond 20 feet is normal, but near vision is poor. Figure 43-11 illustrates where light rays focus for myopia and hyperopia.

Astigmatism is a visual defect due to unequal curvatures of the refractive surfaces of the eye. Light rays from a point do not come to focus on the retina, resulting in visual distortion.

Presbyopia is the loss of elasticity of the lens of the eye caused by aging that causes the near point of

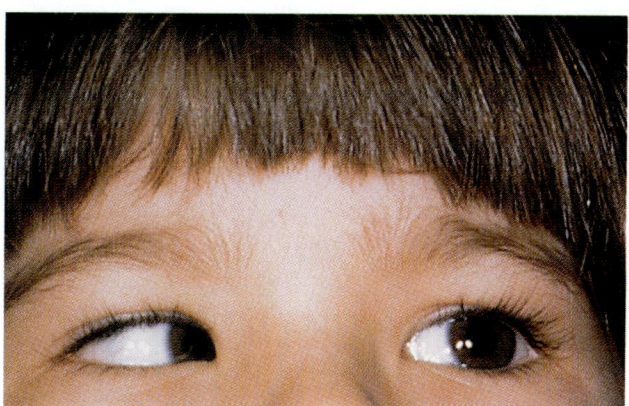

Figure 43-10 Strabismus *(Courtesy of the Armed Forces Institute of Pathology)*

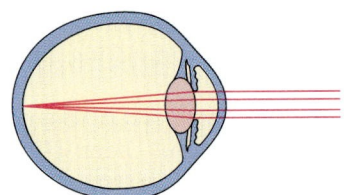

A. Normal eye
Light rays focus on the retina

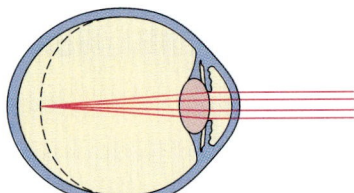

B. Myopia (nearsightedness)
Light rays focus in front
of the retina

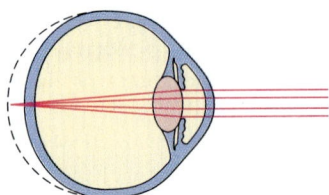

C. Hyperopia (farsightedness)
Light rays focus beyond
the retina

Figure 43-11 Refraction: A. Normal eye; B. Myopia; C. Hyperopia

vision to recede. The eye loses the ability to accommodate to near objects but remains accommodated for far objects.

Strabismus occurs when one eye is constantly deviated to the side.

Medical–Surgical Management

Medical

Refractory errors may be corrected by prescription glasses or contact lenses. The corrective lenses bend light rays to compensate for a client's refractive error.

Surgical

Radial keratotomy is a surgical procedure used to correct myopia and astigmatism. Under local anesthesia, incisions that resemble the spokes of a wheel are made in the cornea. These incisions start near the center of the cornea and extend outward to the edge. The incisions are made by a special knife that can be calibrated to cut at a predetermined depth. After the cuts are made, pressure in the anterior chamber of the eye reshapes the cornea to a normal or near-normal curvature.

▶ NURSING PROCESS

▶ Assessment

▶ Subjective Data

A general medical history should be obtained as well as a history of symptoms. Symptoms may include blurred vision, headache, or eye fatigue.

▶ Objective Data

The client is asked to view an eye chart while lenses of different strengths are systematically placed in front of the eye. The client is asked if the lenses sharpen or blur vision. The power or strength of the lens necessary to permit focusing of the image on the retina is expressed in measurements called diopters.

A nursing diagnosis for a client with refractive errors may be:

Nursing Diagnosis	Planning/Goals	Nursing Interventions
▶ *Anxiety, related to impaired vision and having to wear glasses or contact lenses*	The client will accept wearing glasses or contact lenses.	Allow client to discuss impact of wearing glasses or contact lenses. Encourage client to wear the glasses or contact lenses as prescribed.

Evaluation The goal must be evaluated to determine how it has been met by the client.

INJURY

Injury to the eye or periorbital area can result from a variety of things such as chemical sprays, tree branches, slingshots, BB guns, flying debris from lawn mowers, and fireworks. Both children and adults are susceptible to eye injuries and the importance of protecting the eyes cannot be overemphasized. Injuries to the eyes require immediate attention by an ophthalmologist. Even a few hours delay in treatment may lead to permanent damage.

Corneal abrasion is the disruption of cells and the loss of the superficial epithelium. The outer surface is easily separated from the underlying layers and can be injured or destroyed by exposure (lack of moisture), chemical irritants that dissolve in the protective tear film, and abrasion from foreign bodies.

 Safety: Avoiding Eye Injury
The eyes can be easily protected from injury by wearing protective goggles when performing tasks potentially hazardous to the eyes. Those who wear contact lenses should follow the manufacturer's recommendations for wearing them during certain activities such as swimming or when sleeping.

FOREIGN BODIES

Foreign bodies in the conjunctiva or on the cornea may cause excessive tearing, redness, and complaints of a foreign body sensation in the eye or under the eyelid, or just irritation in the eye. Foreign bodies often become embedded in the conjunctiva under the upper eyelid. The lid must be everted and the client instructed to look up to facilitate inspection and removal. If the particle is not located and removed, sterile fluorescein drops or strips should be instilled to visualize minute foreign bodies not readily visible with the naked eye.

CHEMICAL BURNS

Emergency treatment of chemical burns to the conjunctiva or cornea includes immediate lavage of the eye with tap water and referral to an emergency room or ophthalmologist. In the emergency room, a specially made lid speculum is placed directly on the eyeball and connected to a minimum of one liter of isotonic saline solution for irrigation. A topical anesthetic may be instilled to minimize pain during irrigation. No attempt should be made to neutralize the chemical, since the heat generated by the chemical reaction may cause further injury. Both eyes should then be patched to allow more comfort.

IMPAIRED VISION

The term blindness evokes an image of total darkness and is used for many legal purposes when central visual acuity is 20/200 or less with corrective lenses, in the better eye. Those who have visual acuity between 20/70 and 20/200 in the better eye, with the use of glasses, are often referred to as partially sighted.

The aids that follow are designed to make the most of the available vision (those in italics can also be used by persons who are blind): magnifying glasses; hand and stand magnifiers; telescopes; large print books, newspapers, magazines; talking books; *Braille* books; closed-circuit television which produces highly magnified images; *tactually marked watches and clocks; tactually modified table top games;* enlarged telephone dials, kitchen implements, tools, medication devices; talking clocks, timers, scales, calculators, computers; *text scanner which converts text to audio mode or Braille;* speech synthesizer; flashlight eye sonar devices; canes, laser canes, and seeing eye dogs.

MACULAR DEGENERATION

Macular degeneration is atrophy or deterioration of the macula, the point on the retina where light rays meet as they are focused by the cornea and lens of the eye. The person loses central vision, but still has peripheral vision.

The most common form of macular degeneration is associated with the aging process and is called age-related macular degeneration. Other forms of this disorder include exudative (wet) macular degeneration (sudden growth of new blood vessels in the area of the macula) and injury, infection, or inflammation that damages the macula.

Medical–Surgical Management

Medical

The treatment of age-related macular degeneration is geared toward assisting the client to maximize the use of the remaining vision. The loss of central vision may interfere with the client's ability to read, write, recognize safety hazards, and drive.

Management of clients with exudative macular degeneration is geared toward halting the initiating process and identifying further changes in visual perception. Fluid and blood may resorb in a small percentage of clients with exudative degeneration. Laser therapy to seal the leaking blood vessels in or near the macula may also limit the extent of the damage.

▶ NURSING PROCESS

▶ Assessment

▶ Subjective Data

A general medical history as well as a history of symptoms should be obtained. Symptoms would include blurred vision, disturbance in color vision (colors become dim), difficulty in reading or doing close work, distortion of objects (especially those with lines), and an empty area within the central field of vision.

▶ Objective Data

Coping mechanisms such as turning the head to use peripheral vision should be noted.

A nursing diagnosis for the client with macular degeneration may be:

Nursing Diagnosis	Planning/Goals	Nursing Interventions
▶ *Sensory/Perceptual Alterations, Visual, related to macular degeneration*	The client will discuss the impact of vision loss on lifestyle and use adaptive measures.	Allow client to express feelings about vision loss such as its impact on lifestyle. Convey a willingness to listen, but do not pressure client to talk.
		Provide a safe environment by removing excess furniture or equipment from client's surroundings.
		Orient client to surroundings and show how to use call light.
		Always introduce yourself or announce your presence upon entering the client's room; let client know when you are leaving.
		Provide sensory stimulation by using tactile, auditory, and gustatory stimuli to help compensate for vision loss.
		Suggest large print-books, talking books, audiotapes, or radio as preferred by client.
		Provide reality orientation if client is confused or disoriented.
		Give clear, concise explanations of treatments and procedures but avoid information overload.
		Make sure that health care personnel are aware of client's vision loss. Record information on the client's chart or post in room.
		Respond to call light quickly.
		Provide continuity by assigning same staff members to care for client when possible.
		Refer to appropriate community resources.

Evaluation The goal must be evaluated to determine how it has been met by the client.

SAMPLE NURSING CARE PLAN

THE CLIENT WITH MACULAR DEGENERATION

Mr. Datal is a 60-year-old high school Latin teacher. He describes having blurred vision in both eyes with a gradual loss of vision in only the right eye. He has trouble reading and is afraid to drive because he can no longer recognize safety hazards. He denies having pain. He also relates having fallen several times recently at home while going up and down the stairs. The family practitioner referred him to an ophthalmologist who diagnosed Mr. Datal as having macular degeneration in the right eye.

Nursing Diagnosis 1 *Sensory/Perceptual Alterations, Visual, Related to macular degeneration as evidenced by his inability to recognize safety hazards when driving*

PLANNING/GOALS	NURSING INTERVENTIONS	RATIONALE	EVALUATION
Mr. Datal will discuss impact of vision loss on lifestyle.	Encourage Mr. Datal to express feelings about vision loss, such as the impact on lifestyle.	Allowing Mr. Datal to discuss the impact of vision loss aids in the acceptance of it.	Mr. Datal discussed the effects of vision loss on his lifestyle and contacted a local agency that provides assistance to the visually impaired.
	Convey a willingness to listen, but do not pressure Mr. Datal to talk. Discuss Mr. Datal's current ability to meet	Discussion can determine needs for assistance which will, in part, be based on current functional level.	

continued

self-care needs and activities of daily living.

Determine Mr. Datal's awareness of his limitations.

Educate Mr. Datal in alternative ways of coping with vision loss; care of such adaptive devices as eyeglasses, magnifying glass, and contact lenses.

A knowledgeable client will be better able to cope with vision loss.

Refer to appropriate community resources to help Mr. Datal and his family adapt to his vision loss.

Support from outside resources will help Mr. Datal and his family cope better with his vision loss.

Nursing Diagnosis 2 *Injury, Risk for, related to difficulty in processing visual images and altered depth perception as evidenced by recent falls*

PLANNING/GOALS	NURSING INTERVENTIONS	RATIONALE	EVALUATION
Mr. Datal will not experience injury or visual compromise resulting from a fall.	Advise Mr. Datal that depth perception is changed with macular degeneration.	Information promotes understanding.	Mr. Datal has not fallen in two weeks.
	Teach Mr. Datal to avoid reaching for objects for stability when ambulating.	Objects may not be located where they are perceived. Excessive reaching alters the center of gravity which can precipitate a fall.	
	Advise Mr. Datal to go up and down steps one at a time.	Going up and down steps one at a time enhances the sense of balance.	

Nursing Diagnosis 3 *Home Maintenance Management, Impaired, related to limited vision, as evidenced by recent falls at home*

PLANNING/GOALS	NURSING INTERVENTIONS	RATIONALE	EVALUATION
Mr. Datal will develop a plan for self-care in the desired living environment.	Inform Mr. Datal about required self-care activities: personal care, eyedrop instillation, activities permitted, activity restrictions, medications, and how to monitor for complications.	Knowing what self-care activities are needed will help Mr. Datal plan for his care at home.	Mr. Datal is working on a plan so he can care for himself at home.

continued

Assist Mr. Datal to determine which activities will require assistance: personal care, meal preparation, eyedrop instillation, or shopping.	Helps Mr. Datal to plan for his care at home.
Evaluate sources of assistance: friends/family, home health care (skilled nursing care), or home care aids.	Determines availability of assistance.
Critique the safety of Mr. Datal's home: location of telephone, emergency plan, presence of loose rugs or carpets.	Changes can then be made to make Mr. Datal's home safer.

OTHER SENSES

Other senses include taste, smell, and touch.

TASTE

The sense of taste (gustation) serves as a protector from rotten or putrid food, and provides delightful sensations of creamy chocolate, crunchy carrots, chewy taffy, and fruitful pies. Taste sensors are most efficient at room temperature and respond only to substances in solution. The taste buds are located in four areas of the tongue that sense sweet, salt, bitter, and sour as shown in Figure 43-12.

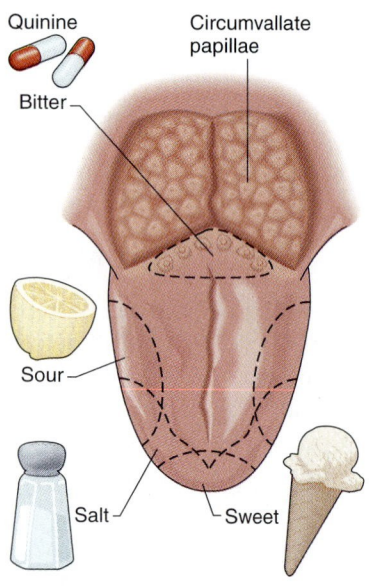

Figure 43-12 Taste Regions of the Tongue

LIFE CYCLE CONSIDERATIONS

Aging and Taste Sensation
The ability to taste sweetness remains as one ages, but the ability to taste bitterness declines.

Taste sensations can be altered secondary to neurological disorders or trauma. Clients who complain of food not "tasting good" should be evaluated for possible causes including dietary habits, medication use, smoking and caffeine use, as well as olfactory disturbances. The sense of taste works very closely with the sense of smell for identification of the taste sensations.

SMELL

The sense of smell (olfaction) also serves as a guardian from danger. Our nose warns us of impending danger from gas leaks, smoke, fires, rancid meat or fish, and sour dairy products. Body odors and halitosis are obvious clues regarding the need to maintain personal hygiene and dental care.

Disorders of the olfactory sense often go unnoticed. New tests such as the University of Pennsylvania Smell Identification Test (UPSIT) allow self-testing of smelling deficiencies. Early identification of the loss of the sense of smell may offer clues to alterations in dietary habits, weight loss or gain, anorexia, malnourishment, and changes in daily habits such as bathing and brushing teeth. The receptors for the sense of smell are located in the roof of the nasal cavity. If these cells are damaged, the sense of smell is impaired. The body cannot regenerate the olfactory cells.

TOUCH

The sense of touch (tactile) includes sensations pertaining to the skin. The tactile receptors are located throughout the integumentary system. Cutaneous sensations of touch, pressure, vibration, cold, heat, and pain are examples. Clients who are unable to sense temperature variations should be taught cautionary measures when applying heat or cold therapies, preparing bath water, cooking, or exposing self to hot or cold climates and environmental temperatures.

Clients with reduced or loss of tactile sensation risk injury when their condition confines them to bed. They are unable to sense pressure on bony prominences or the need to change position. The nurse's role in reducing or preventing impairment of skin integrity is crucial. Timely positioning, securing tubes or devices away from the client's body, and using products to minimize skin breakdown are a few of the interventions vital to excellent client care.

CASE STUDY

Katie Rollins is a 34-year-old nurse who was diagnosed with a right ear hearing impairment during a routine physical examination. She admitted to her doctor that she noticed she would only use her left ear to talk on the phone and that she had particular difficulty hearing her family or friends in a crowded restaurant or other public settings. She also noted that her husband asked her why she played the television so loud, yet if he turned it down to his normal hearing level, she could not hear it clearly. Her physician ordered an audiogram which showed a conductive hearing loss of 40% secondary to otosclerosis. Hearing in her left ear was normal.

Katie's doctor gave her three medical treatment options.
1. *Do nothing and monitor her hearing impairment by audiogram every six months. If it were to worsen, other options would be considered.*
2. *Be fitted with a hearing aid.*
3. *Have a surgical procedure to correct the hearing loss.*

Katie agreed to have surgery. She thought she would be too self-conscious to wear a hearing aid, after all she was only thirty-four, but she simply could not ignore the problem by doing nothing. Katie was scheduled for same-day surgery.

The following questions will guide your development of a nursing care plan for the case study.

1. How is a conductive hearing loss differentiated from a sensorineural hearing loss?
2. What does an audiogram tell you? What special things should Katie know before she has the audiogram?
3. Describe the surgical procedure that will most likely be used to correct the conductive hearing loss.
4. What will you teach Katie prior to her surgery about the procedure and expected postoperative course?
5. List four individualized nursing diagnoses and expected outcomes for Katie, and nursing interventions for each diagnosis.
6. Describe the expected discharge instructions that Katie must know related to diet, medications, activity restrictions, and follow-up care.

SUMMARY

- Hearing loss may be conductive, sensorineural, or a combination of the two. It may also be congenital.
- Ménière's disease is a result of excessive accumulation of endolymph causing severe vertigo, dizziness, and hearing loss. Treatment is primarily symptomatic.

- Otosclerosis is a conductive hearing loss resulting from fixation of the stapes, and may be treated medically with the use of a hearing aid, or surgically with a stapedectomy.
- Otitis media is inflammation of the middle ear. Treatment usually includes antibiotics, decongestants, and possibly a myringotomy.

- Cataract surgery is indicated when significant vision loss has occurred.
- Untreated retinal detachment results in total loss of vision.
- Many resources are available for the hearing impaired through community and national agencies.
- The senses of taste, smell, and touch are essential to our enjoyment of life and serve to protect us from danger or harm.

Review Questions

1. The three bones of the middle ear are:

   a. hammer, nail, and stirrup.
   b. malleus, incus, and cochlea.
   c. malleus, humorous, and stapes.
   d. malleus, incus, and stapes.

2. In a conductive hearing loss:

   a. the endolymph may cross the capillary membrane and mix with the perilymph resulting in severe vertigo.
   b. the ossicles of the middle ear fracture resulting in a tear of the eighth cranial nerve.
   c. sound waves are not transmitted through the ear canal to inner ear fluid.
   d. a tumor in the inner ear blocks the flow of fluid through the bony and membranous labyrinths.

3. A possible nursing diagnosis for a client with Ménière's disease is:

   a. activity intolerance related to impaired hearing.
   b. knowledge deficit related to surgical shunt placement to drain excessive endolymph.
   c. communication, impaired, verbal, related to tinnitus.
   d. injury, risk for, related to Ménière's disease.

4. Persons with hearing impairment or loss may benefit from:

   a. sitting in the middle of a crowded room so as to listen to all conversations at once.
   b. learning to lip read with family members.
   c. using a poorly fitted hearing aid with proper amplification.
   d. cupping the ear and turning the head toward the person speaking to them.

5. Chemical burns of the eye are initially treated with:

   a. local anesthetics and antibacterial drops for 24 to 36 hours.
   b. hot compresses applied at 15-minute intervals.
   c. flushing of the lids, conjunctiva, and cornea with water.
   d. cleansing of the conjunctiva with a small, cotton-tipped applicator.

6. Increased ocular pressure is indicated by a reading of:

   a. 0 to 5 mm Hg.
   b. 6 to 10 mm Hg.
   c. 11 to 20 mm Hg.
   d. 21 to 32 mm Hg.

7. A clinical symptom of a detached retina is:

   a. a sensation of floating particles.
   b. an area of vague vision.
   c. momentary flashes of light.
   d. pain in the eye.

8. Macular degeneration is characterized by:

   a. purulent periorbital drainage.
   b. pupil dilation.
   c. loss of central vision.
   d. ptosis (droopy lid).

Critical Thinking Questions

1. What would have to change in your life if you suddenly could not see?

2. What would change in your life if you suddenly could not hear?

3. Identify the rationale for each nursing intervention given for the possible nursing diagnoses in the chapter.

⚡ WEB FLASH!

- What sites can you locate on the Internet that provide resources for individuals with sensory alterations? Do they list self-help groups, books, media product, or other resources?
- Identify Web addresses that are specifically designed to help the elderly and their families manage the sensory alterations that are a normal part of aging.

NURSING CARE OF THE CLIENT: RESPONDING TO EMERGENCIES

CHAPTER 44

MAKING THE CONNECTION

Refer to the following chapters to increase your understanding of emergency situations:

- **Chapter 2, Critical Thinking**
- **Chapter 6, Legal Responsibilities**
- **Chapter 7, Ethical Responsibilities**
- **Chapter 20, Safety/Hygiene**
- **Chapter 31, Nursing Care of the Client: Respiratory System**
- **Chapter 32, Nursing Care of the Client: Cardiovascular System**
- **Chapter 34, Nursing Care of the Client: Gastrointestinal System**
- **Chapter 35, Nursing Care of the Client: Reproductive System**
- **Chapter 38, Nursing Care of the Client: Musculoskeletal System**
- **Chapter 40, Nursing Care of the Client: Integumentary System**

- **Chapter 41, Nursing Care of the Client: Nervous System**
- **Chapter 42, Nursing Care of the Client: Urinary System**
- **Chapter 43, Nursing Care of the Client: Sensory System**
- **Chapter 45, Nursing Care of the Client: Mental Illness**
- **Chapter 46, Nursing Care of the Client: Substance Abuse**
- **Chapter 53, Infants with Special Needs: Birth to 12 Months**
- **Chapter 54, Common Problems: 1–18 Years**
- **Procedures:** B36, Clearing an Obstructed Airway; B37, Performing Cardiopulmonary Resuscitation

LEARNING OBJECTIVES

Upon completion of this chapter, you should be able to:
- *Define key terms.*
- *Describe the emergency medical services.*
- *Explain the role of the nurse in emergency situations.*
- *List personnel needed to respond to an in-hospital emergency.*
- *Discuss the steps in assessing an emergency client.*
- *Cite the different levels of triage.*

KEY TERMS

chain of custody	Glasgow Coma Scale
emergency	paramedic
emergency medical technician (EMT)	shock
	trauma
emergency nursing	triage

INTRODUCTION

An **emergency** can be defined as a medical or surgical condition requiring immediate or timely intervention to prevent permanent disability or death. Emergency nursing has developed rapidly over the years in response to the changing environment and expectations of the community. Many advancements in emergency care can be attributed to the military. In order to manage vast numbers of injured soldiers, the military had to develop a systematic method of treating and responding to **trauma** (wound or injury). Casualties caused by wartime situations created the need for advancements in the care of large numbers of clients with injuries, wounds, and illness. Methods of caring for multiple clients were developed and implemented as a result of military influence.

Emergency nursing is the care of clients who require emergency intervention. The emergency nurse must be capable of rapid assessment and history taking and immediate intervention formulation and implementation utilizing the nursing process. This role carries great responsibility. Throughout the assessment and care of the client, the emergency nurse must plan and teach prevention and health promotion, as well as rapidly develop rapport with the client and family, including assisting with emotional needs. Clinical knowledge, communication, client teaching, and empathy skills are essential to effective emergency care. Although licensed practical/vocational nurses (LP/VNs) are seldom hired for emergency departments (EDs), they may at times be required to float or help during emergency situations; therefore, a brief overview of emergency nursing is justified.

APPROACHES TO EMERGENCY CARE

There are three general approaches to emergency care: hospital triage, disaster triage, and the emergency medical services. To care for the emergent client, one must first determine the severity of illness.

Hospital Triage

Each hospital with an ED has an established "triage" system in effect (Figure 44-1). **Triage** refers to classification of clients to determine priority of need and proper place of treatment. Triage is typically utilized in the ED to establish priorities and levels of care needed by the clients. Although clients and their families define emergency according to their perceptions, it is the triage nurse's responsibility to sort and prioritize the clients as they arrive in the ED.

The simplest method of triaging clients is to utilize the American Heart Association's basic life support principles: Airway, Breathing, and Circulation (ABCs).

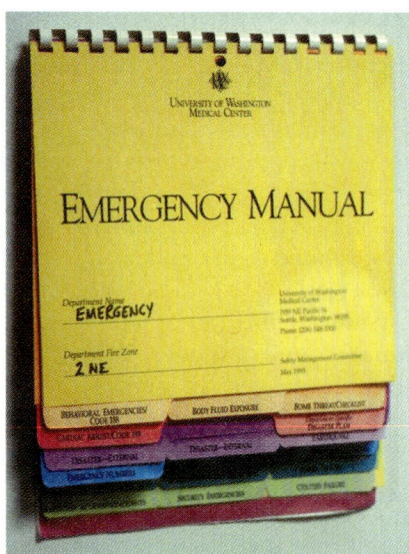

Figure 44-1 Hospitals have emergency manuals and procedures to guide personnel in caring for clients who present with emergent conditions.

PROFESSIONAL TIP

Golden Rules of Emergency Care
1. Establish the safety of the scene
2. Remove the client from danger
3. Establish airway, breathing, and circulation
4. Manage shock
5. Attend to eye injuries
6. Treat skin injuries
7. Call for help

By utilizing this method, those clients with airway problems would be immediately assessed and would become a top priority of care. If any of the ABCs were not functioning, either the Heimlich maneuver or cardiopulmonary resuscitation (CPR) would be initiated.

Infection Control: Mouth-to-Mouth Resuscitation
When delivering care to any client, the nurse should be careful to practice Standard Precautions. Direct mouth-to-mouth breathing should not be administered; instead, use of a bag-valve-mask for resuscitation is more effective in both protecting the health care worker and the client from possible infection and in administering respirations.

Most hospitals have a triage system established in order to provide expedient care to those requiring it first. Although the term *emergency department* implies emergency care, the client utilizing this department does not always require immediate care. The most commonly used triage classifications are emergent, urgent, and non-urgent (Table 44-1). Emergent clients re-

Table 44-1 TRIAGE CATEGORIES

CATEGORY/ PRIORITY	CLIENT NEEDS	EXAMPLES
Emergent	Immediate intervention is required to sustain life or limb.	Cardiac arrest Multiple trauma
Urgent	Care is required within 1 to 2 hours to prevent deterioration of condition.	Compound fractures Persistent vomiting and diarrhea
Non-urgent	Care may be delayed without risk of permanent sequelae.	Contusions Minor sprains and fractures

Developed from Military Standard Operating Procedure (SOP) for General Hospitals.

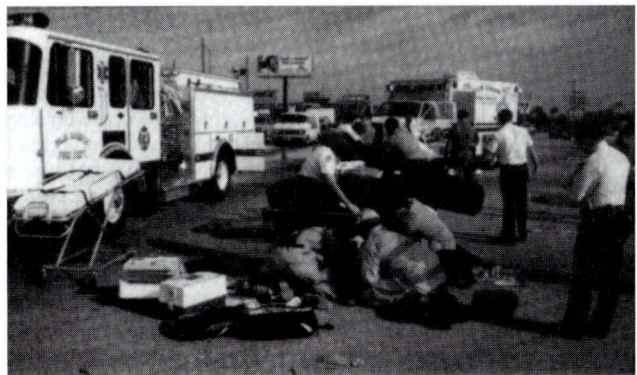

Figure 44-2 Establishing the safety of the scene is the first priority in emergency care, as in this scene of a motor vehicle accident, where rescue workers may be in danger from oncoming vehicles.

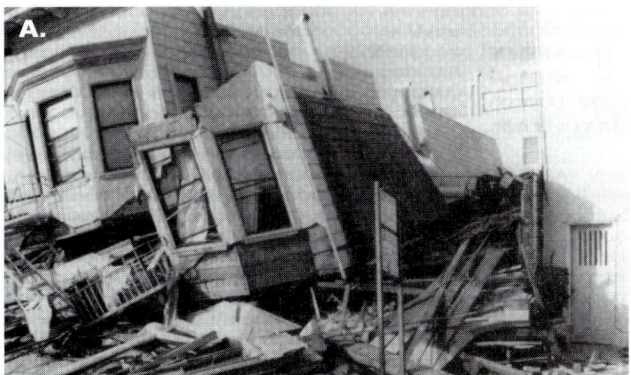

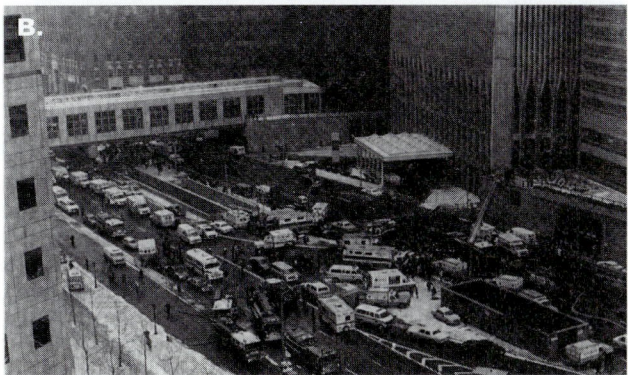

Figure 44-3 Disaster systems are designed for response to community emergencies: A. Structural collapse due to earthquake. (*Courtesy of Edwina Davis*); B. Terrorist bombing of the World Trade Center in New York City.

quire immediate care in order to sustain life or limb. Examples of emergent conditions include foreign bodies in the eye, shortness of breath, impending birth, and cardiopulmonary arrest. Urgent clients require care within 1 to 2 hours to prevent worsening of their conditions. Examples of urgent situations include acute abdominal pain and compound fractures. For non-urgent clients, care can be delayed without the risk of permanent consequences. Contusions and sprains are examples of non-urgent complaints.

Principles of first aid, developed for emergency medicine, are part of the triage process and include what are referred to as the golden rules of emergency care. The first of these rules cautions the health care worker to assess the physical environment for self protection. That is, safety at the scene must be established before rescue is attempted (Figure 44-2). The next rule is to remove the client from danger, such as that presented by passing vehicles. These first two rules typically apply to emergencies occurring outside of an institutional setting.

Once the safety at the scene and of the client have been established, assessment turns to the ABCs—*air*way, *b*reathing, and *c*irculation. When these functions have been stabilized, the client should be assessed for shock. Eye and skin injuries should be evaluated next. The last thing to do is to call for help.

Disaster Triage

Disaster triage systems represent a second approach to emergency care. These systems are utilized in the event of a community disaster, either natural or man made, such as a train accident, hurricane, or tornado (Figure 44-3). Given the possibility of large numbers of casualties as a result of disasters, a different approach to triaging from that of the hospital system is utilized (Table 44-2).

Most communities have disaster/mass casualty committees. These committees include all hospitals, the emergency medical services (EMS) system, and citizens needed to alert the community of an impending or real disaster.

Table 44-2 DISASTER TRIAGE

CATEGORY/ PRIORITY	CLIENT NEEDS	EXAMPLES
Immediate	Simple injuries requiring immediate care	Chest wounds Crush injuries Burns
Delayed	Multiple injuries requiring extensive care	Open fractures of the long bones
Minimal	Minor injuries (the walking wounded)	Sprains Contusions Minor cuts
Expectant	Severe injuries likely leading to death	Massive head trauma Spinal cord injuries

Developed from Military Standard Operating Procedure (SOP) for General Hospitals.

Emergency Medical Services

Prior to admission to the ED, the client may have been cared for by an **emergency medical technician** (EMT) or **paramedic** in the EMS (Figure 44-4). An EMT is a health care professional trained to provide basic lifesaving measures prior to arrival at the hospital. A paramedic is a more specialized health care professional trained to provide advanced life support to the client requiring emergency interventions. Both are part of the EMS and are essential to prehospital care of the emergency client.

SHOCK

Shock is a condition of profound hemodynamic and metabolic disturbance characterized by inadequate tissue perfusion and inadequate circulation to the vital organs (Table 44-3). Shock can result from trauma, injury, or insult. Recognizing and immediately treating shock are critical to the client's survival.

Hypovolemic shock is usually easily recognized. It results from severe fluid volume depletion through vomiting, dehydration, diarrhea, or blood loss. Severe external bleeding may be obvious, but internal bleeding, such as that from a gastric ulcer, is not readily observable.

Cardiogenic shock may be caused by several different heart conditions that result in loss of the contractile property of the heart muscle. The most common of these is acute myocardial infarction (heart attack). Severe heart failure and certain arrhythmias may also cause shock.

Septic shock is usually caused by overwhelming infection. Certain organisms may cause severe reactions resulting in collapse of the circulatory system. Toxic shock syndrome, gram-negative shock, and urogenic shock are types of septic shock.

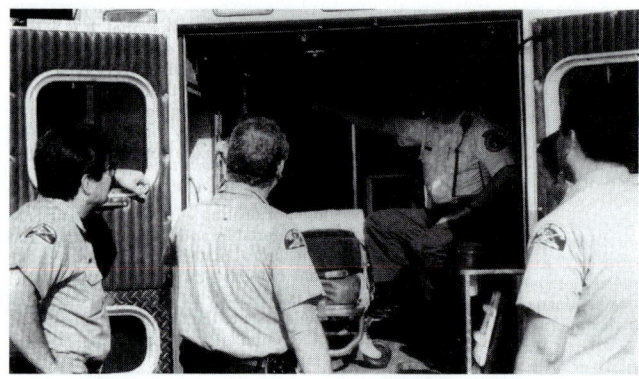

Figure 44-4 Emergency medical technicians (EMTs) and paramedics are often the first to arrive at an emergency scene.

Anaphylactic shock is a severe allergic reaction to a toxin to which a client has been exposed. Causes of anaphylactic reaction include insect bites and certain medications.

Neurogenic shock is the body's response to extreme pain or trauma to the spinal cord. As with the other forms of shock, it results in inadequate supply of oxygen, electrolytes, and other essential chemicals to the tissues.

Medical–Surgical Management

Medical

Management of shock is supportive in nature during initial resuscitation. The immediate priority is maintenance of the ABCs. Active bleeding should then be stopped. Blood may be administered in the event of major blood loss. After the client is stabilized, the underlying cause of shock must be identified and treated.

Pharmacological

Initial treatment involves the administration of oxygen and the insertion of two large-bore intravenous

Table 44-3 TYPES OF SHOCK			
TYPE	**CAUSES**	**SIGNS AND SYMPTOMS**	**EMERGENCY CARE**
Hypovolemic	Hemorrhage*, burns	Increased heart rate; hypotension; cold, clammy skin; profound thirst	Replace fluids
Cardiogenic	Myocardial infarction*	Increased heart rate; hypotension; cold, clammy skin	Initiate drug therapy for myocardial infarction; replace fluids; consider possible emergency coronary bypass surgery
Toxic	Overwhelming infection	Hot, dry, flushed skin; hypotension; increased heart rate	Locate source of infection and treat with broad-spectrum antibiotic; replace fluids
Anaphylactic	Medications*, insect bites or stings, foods	Throat edema in conjunction with increasing difficulty breathing; hypotension; increased heart rate	Manage ABCs; administer epinephrine (Adrenalin); administer diphenhydramine hydrochloride (Benadryl)
Neurogenic	Spinal cord injury	Slowed heart rate; hypotension	Replace fluids, administer drugs to increase blood pressure and heart rate

*Most common cause

(IV) lines. Intravenous lines must be instituted to establish lifelines through which life saving drugs and fluids may be administered. Fluid resuscitation and oxygen delivery are critical to management of the client in shock. Medications, including epinephrine, may be administered to improve circulation.

▶ NURSING PROCESS

▶ Assessment

▶ Subjective Data

Subjective assessment begins with determining whether the client is responsive and able to respond to questions, or is unconscious. After the client is alert and stabilized, assessment should include obtaining a history of the events leading to the injury or illness, including any food consumed or medication taken and any unusual event (such as a bee sting) that precipitated the shock state. The client should also be asked to describe any pain with regard to intensity, location, and duration.

▶ Objective Data

Immediate assessment involves evaluating the ABCs. Vital signs should be taken, because many clients in shock will present with hypotension, tachycardia, tachypnea, and pale, diaphoretic, clammy skin.

Nursing diagnoses for a client in shock may include the following:

Nursing Diagnoses	Planning/Goals	Nursing Interventions
Fluid Volume Deficit related to acute blood loss/vomiting/diarrhea	The client will maintain adequate fluid balance.	Initiate and maintain fluid replacement with two large-bore IV access lines. Administer blood as ordered.
Tissue Perfusion, Altered, related to decreased oxygen-carrying hemoglobin secondary to blood loss and fluid depletion	The client will maintain adequate tissue perfusion as manifested by stable vital signs.	Assess vital signs at least every 30 minutes. Administer oxygen per physician order.
Grieving, Anticipatory, related to grave nature of illness/injury	The client will cope with illness/injury by cooperating with care provided by health care workers and will discuss outcomes with nurse and family.	Communicate with client and family. Explain all interventions as they occur, to decrease acute anxiety. Allow client and family to express their fears and worries about the situation. Answer questions about care.

Evaluation Each goal must be evaluated to determine how it has been met by the client.

CARDIOPULMONARY EMERGENCIES

Cardiopulmonary emergencies are those emergencies that jeopardize the function of the heart and lungs. These emergencies can result from trauma or illness. Cardiopulmonary emergencies such as drowning, foreign body obstruction of the airway, chest trauma, and chest pain are grouped together, because the effects, medical management, and nursing priorities are similar.

Near-drowning episodes occur most frequently in the summer months. Many clients will suffer other related injuries associated with drowning, such as head and spinal cord injuries (Table 44-4).

Foreign body obstruction of the airway most commonly occurs in the larger, right main bronchus. The most common source of airway obstruction is the tongue. Other sources of airway obstruction include hot dogs, candy, steak, and coins (especially in children).

Penetrating or blunt trauma to the chest can cause multiple injuries. Penetrating injuries are insults that puncture the chest, such as gunshot or knife wounds. Blunt trauma is more likely caused by falls or by forceful contact with a blunt object such as a baseball bat or steering wheel. Injuries associated with pneumothorax include cardiac tamponade, fractured ribs, fractured sternum, and flail chest.

PROFESSIONAL TIP

Flail Chest

A flail chest is defined as instability in the chest wall. This condition is caused by fracture of three or more ribs in two or more places. With a flail chest, breathing is unique: The flail segment moves inward during inspiration and outward during expiration. This is called paradoxical breathing.

Table 44-4 FRESH-WATER VERSUS SALT-WATER NEAR-DROWNING

TYPE	CLIENT SYMPTOMS	PATHOPHYSIOLOGY	SIGNS
Fresh-water	Fatigue, anxiety, difficulty breathing, fear	Water in lungs causes changes in surfactant, which in turn causes alveolar collapse.	Hypoxia, collapsed alveoli
Salt-water	Fatigue, anxiety, difficulty breathing, fear, rales, rhonchi	Hypertonic salt water pulls fluid into the alveoli.	Hypoxia, pulmonary edema

One of the most common complaints evaluated in the ED is chest pain. Those clients presenting with the symptom of chest pain must be clearly and carefully evaluated. Chest pain has a multitude of potential causes and can be frightening to the client until the cause is confirmed.

Medical–Surgical Management

Medical

Management of all cardiopulmonary emergencies is directed at maintaining the ABCs. If indicated, intubation is part of resuscitation in cardiopulmonary emergencies. Establishment of an IV line is essential for medical management, because the line provides access for administration of lifesaving medications.

After resuscitation has been achieved, other treatment modalities must be instituted. Chest x-rays, electrocardiograms (ECGs), and blood tests must be obtained. Pain control must be initiated. Morphine sulfate is the drug of choice for clients with these types of emergencies, because morphine decreases both pain and anxiety in the client, which, in turn, leads to improved breathing.

Pharmacological

With the near-drowning client, mannitol (Osmitrol) and furosemide (Lasix) are occasionally indicated in the event of fluid overload. Pain medication is essential for the client with chest injury, because hypoventi-lation may occur due to the pain associated with deep breathing. Pain control is also essential for the client experiencing chest pain. Pain medications can vary from sublingual nitroglycerine to IV morphine sulfate.

Activity

Most clients with cardiopulmonary emergencies are initially confined to bed and must be frequently rolled from side to side. In addition, deep breathing and coughing should be encouraged to prevent stasis of fluid and development of pneumonia.

▶ NURSING PROCESS

▶ Assessment

▶ Subjective Data

The client should be evaluated for restlessness, an early sign of hypoxia. Description of pain should be noted. Other areas to include in assessment are fatigue, anxiety, and level of consciousness. Ability to give a brief history of events prior to the cardiopulmonary emergency should be evaluated.

▶ Objective Data

Airway and breathing must be immediately assessed. Any cough, stridor, cyanosis, or inability to talk should be noted. Initial vital signs are essential to developing a baseline.

Nursing diagnoses for a client with a cardiopulmonary emergency may include the following:

Nursing Diagnoses	Planning/Goals	Nursing Interventions
▶ *Breathing Pattern, Ineffective, related to injury to the chest and inability to fully expand the lungs*	Client will regain spontaneous respiration within normal rate and pattern.	Initiate CPR, if indicated.
		Keep client medicated to alleviate painful respirations.
		Administer pain medications as ordered to ease the work of breathing.
		Note response to pain medications.
		Remain with the client during episodes of respiratory distress, because being left alone at these times escalates both the anxiety and breathing problems.
		Explain all procedures.

continued

Nursing Diagnoses	Planning/Goals	Nursing Interventions
▶ *Airway Clearance, Ineffective, related to accumulation of fluid and blood in the airway and to the client's inability to cough*	Client's lungs will be clear bilaterally to auscultation.	Maintain airway and breathing with suctioning, if secretions accumulate. Turn client frequently to mobilize secretions. Encourage deep breathing and coughing. Suction client as needed. Listen to lungs hourly or more frequently to evaluate secretions and suctioning.

Evaluation Each goal must be evaluated to determine how it has been met by the client.

NEUROLOGICAL/ NEUROSURGICAL EMERGENCIES

Head injuries are the most common type of neurological trauma. Spinal cord trauma can also occur as a result of injuries sustained in a head injury. Head trauma most often results from motor vehicle collisions (MVCs) (Figure 44-5). Head injuries vary from very minor contusions to major head trauma.

Clients experiencing a cerebrovascular accident, or stroke, must be immediately admitted to the health care system for prompt evaluation and care. Strokes are now considered "brain attacks" requiring the same initial consideration given to myocardial infarctions, or "heart attacks."

Medical–Surgical Management

Medical

As with all trauma, management is aimed at maintaining the ABCs. In addition, if head, neck, or spinal cord trauma is suspected, the client should be placed on a backboard, with the head and neck immobilized. Blood alcohol level should be determined. Intravenous access should be initiated early in the resuscitation phase. Radiological examination is necessary to determine the extent of damage. If the client does not have spontaneous respirations, the injury has probably occurred at C-4 or above, meaning that the client will not be able to independently maintain respirations. The client should be continuously monitored for increased intracranial pressure. Early signs of increased intracranial pressure include a headache; later signs include widened pulse pressure, dilated pupils, and spontaneous emesis without warning. Hiccoughs are an ominous sign and should thus be reported immediately. Utilization of the **Glasgow Coma Scale**, a neurological screening test that measures a client's best verbal, motor, and eye response to stimuli, is indicated (Figure 44-6).

Pharmacological

Increased cranial pressure and buildup of carbon dioxide will complicate the client's condition; oxygen will most often alleviate the resultant complications. Thus, oxygen should be administered immediately. Pain management should be accomplished through IV access.

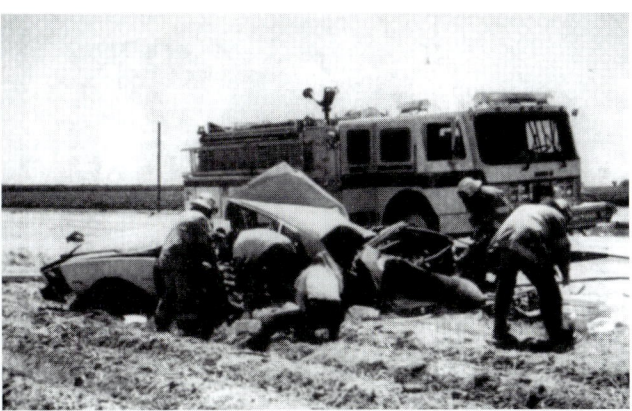

Figure 44-5 Motor vehicle collisions are the most common cause of head trauma.

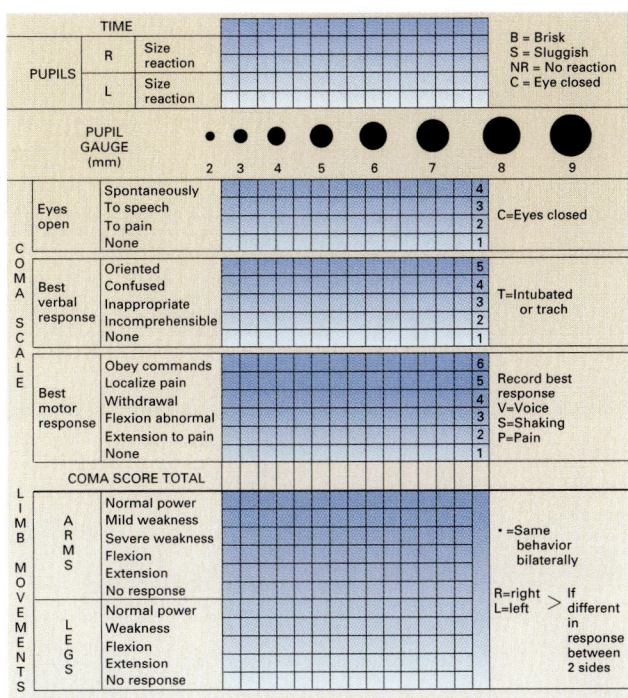

Figure 44-6 Neurological Flow Sheet, Including Glasgow Coma Scale

Activity

Clients with head injuries should be placed in semi-Fowler's position to decrease edema and intracranial pressure.

▶ NURSING PROCESS

▶ Assessment

▶ Subjective Data

Subjective assessment includes obtaining a history of the accident and the mechanism of injury. The client's perception of what has happened and the client's emotional response should also be evaluated. The client may describe having a headache and difficulty seeing.

▶ Objective Data

The client's vital signs and Glasgow Coma Scale level should be measured. Cerebrospinal fluid leaks, such as clear fluid coming from the nares or ear, should be noted. Unequal pupillary response, trouble making self understood, or difficulty swallowing should also be documented.

Nursing diagnoses for the client with a neurological/neurosurgical emergency may include the following:

Nursing Diagnoses	Planning/Goals	Nursing Interventions
▶ *Fluid Volume Excess, Cerebral, related to accumulation of fluid/blood in cranium*	The client will remain conscious, maintain a Glasgow Coma Scale score of 15, and experience no further increase in cranial fluid volume.	Monitor intracranial pressure. Maintain the client in semi-Fowler's position. Document vital signs hourly. Assess Glasgow Coma Scale score and record hourly. Administer oxygen.
▶ *Communication, Verbal, Impaired related to injury to speech center*	The client will be able to communicate with the nurse and family.	Orient the client frequently to date and time. Explain all nursing interventions. Modify communication methods, such as use of a message board, depending on the client needs. Allow the client choices about care when possible. Encourage client to verbalize feelings about condition; offer support.

Evaluation Each goal must be evaluated to determine how it has been met by the client.

ABDOMINAL EMERGENCIES

Abdominal emergencies can be diverse in nature. Trauma to the upper body and torso can result in multiple abdominal injuries, from a simple contusion and bruising to a ruptured spleen. Clients presenting to the ED with complaints of abdominal pain require careful evaluation. Illnesses causing abdominal pain range from gastroenteritis to gastrointestinal bleeding.

Abdominal injuries can result from blunt or penetrating trauma. It is important to determine the mechanism of injury, as certain causes, such as MVCs, often result in multi-system trauma. Blunt trauma, for instance from falling on the abdomen, usually results in injury to internal organs, such as the kidneys or spleen. Penetrating injuries such as gunshot wounds can affect any internal organ. Hemorrhage is a potential complication of both types of trauma.

Medical–Surgical Management

Medical

Initial management of abdominal emergencies is IV access with large-bore catheters. Oxygen should be administered immediately, and standard protocol calls for managing the ABCs. Blood products or plasma expanders may be administered in the event of large volume blood loss. Insertion of a nasogastric tube decompresses the stomach. A peritoneal lavage may be performed to check for blood in the abdominal cavity of clients with abdominal trauma. Presence of blood indicates a need for immediate surgical intervention. A computed tomography (CT) scan of the abdomen may be indicated as well. Blood work should be drawn, and a urinalysis should be done. Hematuria must be evaluated, and x-rays may be indicated.

Pharmacological

If the client is in severe pain and has been evaluated, narcotics may be indicated.

PROFESSIONAL TIP

Open Abdominal Wound

If loops of intestines are exposed to outside air, they should be covered with saline-soaked gauze.

▶ NURSING PROCESS

▶ Assessment

▶ Subjective Data

Assessment includes identifying the location, duration, severity, and radiation of pain. History of nausea, vomiting, and diarrhea must be obtained. In addition, the times of the client's last meal, bowel movement, and urination must be noted.

▶ Objective Data

Vital signs, active bleeding, abdominal girth, and weight should be assessed. The abdomen should be inspected for bruises, edema, and wounds.

Nursing diagnoses for the client with an abdominal emergency may include the following:

Nursing Diagnoses	Planning/Goals	Nursing Interventions
▶ *Fluid Volume Deficit related to active bleeding*	The client will stabilize, and vital signs and fluid balance will return to normal.	Establish IV access with at least two large-bore catheters. Monitor vital signs frequently, at least hourly. Evaluate abdominal girth and bowel sounds hourly.
▶ *Infection, Risk for, related to penetrating injury*	The client will not experience an elevated temperature or show signs and symptoms of infection.	Administer antibiotics as ordered to reduce the risk of infection. Monitor temperature at least every 2 hours. Change saturated dressings as needed. Note amount and quality of any drainage.
▶ *Activity Intolerance related to pain and bleeding*	The client will ambulate with assistance 1 day after surgical correction.	Turn client hourly from side to side. Assist client to ambulate when able to prevent stasis of fluid and to diminish the risk of infection.

Evaluation Each goal must be evaluated to determine how it has been met by the client.

GENITOURINARY EMERGENCIES

Rape is a legal term and is not considered a medical condition. It is defined as sexual penetration of a forceful and threatening nature with a nonconsenting person. Included under this legal term is penetration of persons who are unable to consent due to intoxication or mental illness. *Alleged sexual assault* is the terminology used by most centers for rape survivors. Due to the many legal implications and to the fact that there are not only physical symptoms, but also long-lasting psychological consequences of sexual assault, accurate and methodical care must be given to the survivors of sexual assault. Most communities have hospitals designated to care for rape survivors. These facilities are staffed with registered nurses and doctors familiar with the medical, psychological, and legal issues particular to caring for the client who has experienced a sexual assault.

Straddle injuries are another type of genitourinary emergency. These injuries occur when a client falls while straddling an object, such as a fence or metal bar, thereby injuring the perineum. Though not a very common injury, it is imperative to assess the client and promptly initiate treatment. These injuries can occur with multiple trauma or as a single injury.

PROFESSIONAL TIP

Chain of Custody

Care should be taken in handling the clothing and belongings of a survivor of sexual assault, as these items may become valuable in legal proceedings. For purposes of potential future litigation, it is thus imperative to maintain a strict chain of custody of evidence. The **chain of custody** is the documentation of the transfer of evidence from one worker to the next in a secure fashion. This means that to follow the rape protocol, each person handling the client's clothing or lab work must sign the document used by the facility to indicate receipt and release of items. The fewer the names on the chain, the more secure the integrity of evidence.

LIFE CYCLE CONSIDERATIONS

Suspected Abuse

Genitourinary trauma in any client under the age of consent (18 years), especially in an infant or young child, should raise suspicions of abuse. Learn your state and institutional requirements for reporting suspected child abuse and consider the ethical and legal responsibilities of caring for a sexually abused child.

Medical–Surgical Management

Medical

As with all emergencies, the ABCs must be managed first. Intravenous access should be established, and blood and urine specimens should be obtained. Rape crisis intervention is essential for the sexual assault victim. Those with straddle injuries must be evaluated for fractures. If blood is seen at the external urethral meatus, a urethral tear should be suspected, and catheterization should be avoided, as it will further damage the urethra. Radiological examination should be done to confirm injury.

Surgical

Certain injuries such as urethral or vaginal tears may require surgical repair.

Pharmacological

Douching and bathing for the sexual assault survivor should be delayed until all specimens are collected and all examinations are performed. For the sexual assault client, antibiotics are usually prescribed for possible sexually transmitted disease. Blood tests for baseline human immunodeficiency virus (HIV) and acquired immunodeficiency syndrome (AIDS) and a pregnancy test are usually part of the protocol. In addition, a "morning after" pill such as diethylstilbestrol diphosphate (DES) may be prescribed in the event of a possible pregnancy.

Diet

The client should be designated nothing by mouth (NPO) in case of the need to go to immediate surgery. Fluids can be given intravenously.

Activity

The sexual assault survivor may return to full activity as soon as able, though counseling may be needed before the client regains the desire to resume activities of daily living. Those with straddle injuries need bed rest and careful observation until testing is complete. Clients should be encouraged to resume sexual activities only when they feel physically and emotionally ready.

▶ NURSING PROCESS

▶ Assessment

▶ Subjective Data

Assessment of the sexual assault survivor includes obtaining a description of the rape or assault. A history of menstrual cycles, including date of last menstrual period, is vital in determining the potential for pregnancy.

▶ Objective Data

All bruises, scrapes, or abrasions caused by the assault must be assessed. A list of the client's clothing worn during the assault should be made, and the clothing should be kept for evidence in case of legal proceedings.

LIFE CYCLE CONSIDERATIONS

Sexually Abused Children

Children who are victims of rape need very special attention and should be evaluated by a pediatric specialist. An interdisciplinary team including a psychiatrist, social worker, and child welfare specialist may be brought in to care for the child's needs after the physical trauma and injuries have been addressed.

Nursing diagnoses for the client with genitourinary emergencies may include the following:

Nursing Diagnoses	Planning/Goals	Nursing Interventions
▶ *Urinary, Elimination, Altered, related to break in urethra*	Client will void clear urine before discharge and will regain normal pre-injury elimination patterns.	Closely monitor output. Test urine for blood using dipstick. Note and report hematuria. Offer bladder retraining and encourage client to resume pre-assault elimination patterns.
▶ *Infection, Risk for (Sexually Transmitted Disease), related to alleged sexual assault*	Client will have negative outcomes on all lab specimens obtained.	Obtain all specimens as ordered. Teach the client how and when to obtain further specimens, as needed. Keep the client informed about all test results.

continued

Nursing Diagnoses	Planning/Goals	Nursing Interventions
▶ *Rape-trauma Syndrome related to alleged sexual assault and violence of event*	Client will state awareness of help groups for therapy and follow-up care.	Maintain open and nonjudgmental communication with the client.
		Call rape crisis center for immediate referral and assistance for the client.
		Refer the client to crisis help per community offerings.
		Teach the client that the trauma does not resolve overnight and that help is available at all times.

Evaluation Each goal must be evaluated to determine how it has been met by the client.

OCULAR EMERGENCIES

Most eye emergencies are urgent to emergent in nature. Foreign bodies can cause damage to vision very rapidly and thus require immediate attention. Clients with objects impaled in the eye must be immediately evaluated by an ophthalmologist. An eyeball may be avulsed, or forcibly torn out of its socket, either by blunt or penetrating trauma; such an injury requires immediate referral to and treatment by an ophthalmologist. Retinal detachment is a surgical emergency, as it is one of the leading causes of accidental blindness.

Medical–Surgical Management

Medical

The primary goal of care is restoring the health of the eye. The foreign body or impaled object must be removed as soon as the client's condition allows and the effects on the eye of removal of the object have been determined. The client's eye must be protected until definitive treatment is provided. Protective dressings are needed. In the event of ocular avulsion, the eyeball must be protected with a warm saline dressing. Because both eyes move together, patching of the opposite eye will help decrease movement of the affected eye, allowing it to heal more quickly.

Surgical

Immediate surgical intervention is needed for retinal detachment.

Pharmacological

As a prophylactic measure, all eye trauma must be treated with an antibiotic eye medication.

Diet

There should be no modifications to the diet of the client with a foreign body in the eye. Clients with avulsed eyes must be kept NPO in case immediate surgical intervention is needed.

Activity

Because sensory and depth perceptions may be altered when one eye is patched, activity should be limited initially. Clients are maintained in semi-Fowler's position to prevent or alleviate intraocular edema.

▶ NURSING PROCESS

▶ Assessment

▶ Subjective Data

Assessment includes obtaining both the client's perception of what has happened to the eye and a history of the accident, including the time it occurred. Care that has been given to an avulsed eye, such as placement in a plastic bag with water, must be documented.

▶ Objective Data

Assessment includes visual acuity testing and observation of tearing and/or redness of the eye.

Nursing diagnoses for the client with an ocular emergency may include the following:

Nursing Diagnoses	Planning/Goals	Nursing Interventions
▶ *Sensory Perceptual Alterations (Visual) related to impaired vision*	The client will regain partial pre-injury vision.	Maintain the client in semi-Fowler's position in cases of ocular avulsion or retinal detachment.
		Assist the client to walk while wearing an eye patch and discuss problems that may be encountered and ways to accommodate decreased vision.
		Instruct the client to name one resource person to assist with decreased vision at home.

continued

Nursing Diagnoses	Planning/Goals	Nursing Interventions
▶ *Infection, Risk for, related to trauma caused by foreign body*	The client will not develop ocular infection.	Instill initial eye medication and apply initial eye patch for the client.
		Teach the client to instill eye medication.
		Teach the client to apply eye patch.
		Instruct the client to immediately report any visual changes or drainage.
		Be alert and listen to the client's concerns.

Evaluation Each goal must be evaluated to determine how it has been met by the client.

MUSCULOSKELETAL EMERGENCIES

Musculoskeletal emergencies can vary from simple muscle strains to major trauma. A muscle strain is the overstretching of a muscle. A sprain is defined as a twisting of the joint with partial rupture of ligaments, which can cause injury to surrounding tissue. Sprains often occur in the wrist and ankle. A dislocation is the displacement of a bone from its joint. The most common sits of dislocation are the fingers and toes. A fracture is a break in the continuity of a bone. In the event of a long bone fracture, care must also be given to the cardiopulmonary system: Fat emboli from the fracture site can develop and cause severe respiratory problems if they settle in the pulmonary system.

Medical–Surgical Management

Medical

Initial treatment of simple strains and sprains can be managed utilizing the "RICE" formula, meaning *r*est, *i*ce, *c*ompression, and *e*levation. Fractures must be immediately immobilized, with attention also being given to body areas proximal to the fracture. Radiological examination is indicated to validate the diagnosis. Dislocations must be immediately reduced. Many fractures and dislocations can be reduced in the ED using conscious IV sedation. Tetanus toxoid should be given to any client presenting with an open injury.

Surgical

Some fractures require immediate surgical intervention. Most open, compound fractures fall into this category. Debridement is often indicated, because most fractures are trauma related, and dirt and other matter may imbed in the wound.

Pharmacological

Pain control is a major consideration in relation to musculoskeletal system injuries. Reduction and immobilization often significantly decrease pain. Those clients with minor sprains and strains respond well to anti-inflammatory medications such as ibuprofen (Advil, Motrin) and other nonsteroidal anti-inflammatory drugs (NSAIDs). Those with major or multiple fractures may initially require narcotic relief.

Diet

Clients with sprains, strains, and simple fractures do not need special diets. Those with major fractures and trauma must be kept NPO pending surgical intervention.

Activity

Depending on the site of the fracture, activity may be limited due to casting or immobilization. To help strengthen the muscles and minimize atrophy in cases of immobilization, the client must be taught to contract and release those muscles immobilized in the casting.

▶ NURSING PROCESS

▶ Assessment

▶ Subjective Data

The client will initially verbalize intense pain, tingling, and loss of use of the injured part.

▶ Objective Data

Obvious deformities, edema, cool skin, and decreased capillary refill will be present on the affected part. A break in the skin and visual bone fragments may also be noted.

Nursing diagnoses for the client with a musculoskeletal emergency may include the following:

Nursing Diagnoses	Planning/Goals	Nursing Interventions
▶ *Pain related to traumatic fracture/dislocation*	The client's pain will decrease with immobilization and pain medications.	Administer pain medications as ordered. Immobilize affected body part. Elevate injured extremity. Apply ice packs, as directed. Listen attentively to the client's concerns and verbalizations of pain.
▶ *Tissue Perfusion, Altered, related to edema and fracture/dislocation*	The client's pulses will be equal bilaterally, and capillary refill will be less than 2 seconds at the affected site.	Assess the client's pulse, skin color, capillary refill, and ability to move the fingers and toes every 30 minutes. Ask the client about sensation in the injured body part. Instruct the client to move the toes and fingers. Apply an elastic bandage for compression in cases of a sprain.
▶ *Mobility, Impaired, Physical, related to limitations of pain and immobilization of fracture/dislocation*	The client will demonstrate the ability to mobilize with cast or other assistive devices.	Teach the client to care for the cast. Teach the client exercises to minimize muscle atrophy. Teach crutch walking, if needed.

Evaluation Each goal must be evaluated to determine how it has been met by the client.

SOFT-TISSUE EMERGENCIES

Most soft-tissue injuries are very common. Minor abrasions, lacerations, puncture wounds, contusions, bites of all varieties (human, insect, animal, and snake), and burn injuries fall into this category. Although most such injuries do not require emergency care, some are more severe than others and some are potentially fatal. Clients will seek medical attention for these injuries because of fear.

Medical–Surgical Management

Medical

Skin emergencies require prompt intervention. All injuries must be cleansed or debrided. Infection is a major consideration, and prophylactic treatment must therefore be initiated immediately. If a laceration is large, suturing may be necessary. Bites, unless extremely large, are usually not sutured due to the increased risk of infection presented by suturing these lacerations, which provide an excellent growth medium for bacteria. Burns can sometimes be treated in an ED, with follow-up care being provided at home. Cool water will decrease the pain associated with minor burns. Careful debridement using running cool water and antiseptic solution should follow. Because burns are painful, debridement should be performed after administration of pain medication. A silver sulfadiazine (Silvadene) dressing is usually applied after debridement.

Major burns may require client resuscitation with rapid EMS transport to a burn center. Initially, the ABCs must be established. "Packaging" the client for transport to a burn unit usually involves insertion of at least two large-bore IV lines, insertion of a nasogastric tube, intubation, Foley catheterization, sterile wrapping, and temperature regulation/monitoring.

Snakebites do not always result in envenomation (poisoning). A rubber band (not a tourniquet) above the site is the best intervention to control rapid spreading of the venom. Most snakebites occur in the foot, so a rubber band is easy to apply. In managing snake bites, it is best to establish the ABCs and, once the type of snake is identified, start antivenom treatment, as necessary.

Pharmacological

All clients with soft-tissue injuries, including those with burns, must be current with regard to immunizations, especially the diphtheria and tetanus (Td) immunizations. Pain medication should be given to alleviate pain related to lacerations, bites, and burns. Topical antibiotic agents must be applied to all injuries. Silver sulfadiazine (Silvadene) is the most widely used topical agent for burn injuries. Systemic antibiotics are often included in the treatment regimen.

PROFESSIONAL TIP

Animal Bites

Many states require that all instances of clients seeking treatment in an ED for animal bites be reported to animal control officials. Know your state reporting rules and regulations.

Activity

Movement may be somewhat limited depending on the location of injury. Because muscle weakness and atrophy can occur rapidly, physical therapy must be initiated immediately for clients who are immobilized.

▶ NURSING PROCESS

▶ Assessment

▶ Subjective Data

In obtaining the health history, the nurse should elicit the client's report of the injury. Pain should be evaluated, and the client's level of pain should be documented.

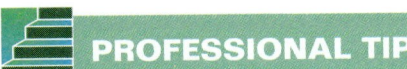

PROFESSIONAL TIP

Snake Bites

In the event of snakebite, it is essential to note the location of the fang marks and the distance (in centimeters) between the marks. Doing so helps determine the size of the snake and, thus, the likelihood of envenomation, as smaller, younger snakes typically have not yet learned to control the amount of venom.

▶ Objective Data

Vital signs must be measured. The wound or damaged area must be assessed with regard to depth, location, and size (in centimeters). In the event of a bite, the location and source of the bite must be noted.

Nursing diagnoses for the client with a soft-tissue injury may include the following:

Nursing Diagnoses	Planning/Goals	Nursing Interventions
▶ *Skin Integrity, Impaired, related to break/wound in skin*	The client's wound will heal.	Prepare client for cleansing and possible suturing of wound. Assist with possible suturing.
▶ *Infection, Risk for, related to imbedded dirt/bacteria in the wound*	The client's wound will heal without evidence of infection.	Cleanse wound thoroughly with soap and water. Administer tetanus intramuscularly (IM). Teach the client to keep the wound and sutures dry and clean. Apply a topical antibiotic and clean dressing, if indicated. Teach the client to remove and change the dressing if it becomes dirty or wet. Tell the client to return for additional care if wound becomes red, edematous, or painful or exhibits purulent discharge.

Evaluation Each goal must be evaluated to determine how it has been met by the client.

SAMPLE NURSING CARE PLAN

THE CLIENT WITH A SOFT-TISSUE INJURY

Mr. Perez, a 23-year-old Hispanic rancher, was brought to the ED after an accident at his ranch. He was riding his horse and fixing fences. The horse threw Mr. Perez over its head and stomped Mr. Perez's left upper abdomen with its right forefoot. Mr. Perez, who states that he has never been hurt or in the hospital before, presents with a large, 6-centimeter-by-3-centimeter-by-2 centimeter in depth, jagged laceration imbedded with dirt and other foreign material. There are no other associated injuries. A large pressure bandage that is saturated with bright-red blood is controlling the bleeding.

Nursing Diagnosis 1 *Fluid Volume Deficit related to active bleeding from traumatic abdominal laceration as evidenced by a large, jagged laceration measuring 6 centimeters by 3 centimeters and a large, bulky, saturated dressing.*

continued

PLANNING/GOALS	NURSING INTERVENTIONS	RATIONALE	EVALUATION
Mr. Perez will lose no more blood.	Control bleeding with a pressure dressing.	The amount of blood loss will increase if pressure to the laceration is not maintained.	Mr. Perez's wound was sutured. The dressing that was applied after suturing was clean and dry and showed no further evidence of bleeding at discharge.
	Prepare Mr. Perez for suturing of the laceration.	To effectively stop the bleeding, the laceration must be sutured as quickly as possible. The physician will also be able to visualize the arteries and ascertain whether any have been severed and, if so, repair them.	
	Monitor vital signs.	Frequent monitoring of vital signs is necessary in order to ensure that the client is not going into shock from the blood loss. Hypotension and increased pulse and respiration require immediate attention and intervention.	

Nursing Diagnosis 2 *Skin Integrity, Impaired, related to abdominal injury as evidenced by a jagged laceration measuring 6 centimeters by 3 centimeters and 2 centimeters in depth.*

PLANNING/GOALS	NURSING INTERVENTIONS	RATIONALE	EVALUATION
Mr. Perez will have regained skin integrity with sutures.	Prepare sterile environment for suturing.	The nurse is responsible for assisting the physician, who is suturing.	Mr. Perez had intact skin integrity, with 22 sutures in place.
	Assist physician with suturing of Mr. Perez's wound.	Maintaining a sterile field while suturing prevents additional bacteria from contaminating the wound.	

Nursing Diagnosis 3 *Infection, Risk for, related to laceration as evidenced by dirt and other foreign material imbedded in abdominal wound*

PLANNING/GOALS	NURSING INTERVENTIONS	RATIONALE	EVALUATION
Mr. Perez's wound will not become infected.	Administer tetanus booster.	All wounds require that the client be current with regard to tetanus booster.	Mr. Perez was given a tetanus booster because he remembered having

continued

Cleanse Mr. Perez's wound thoroughly after local anesthesia has been administered.	Because it has been exposed to an undetermined amount of dirt, including the horse's hoof, the wound should be thoroughly cleansed. This is done *after* the administration of anesthesia, because cleansing can cause the client a great deal of pain.	received his last at the age of 15. He verbalized the need to take the complete course of antibiotics when he went home.
Demonstrate wound cleansing to Mr. Perez.	Mr. Perez should actually see the way the wound is cleansed so that he has no fear or questions about doing it himself.	
Remove as much dirt and foreign material as possible.	All visible dirt should be removed because it can cause inflammation and infection at the wound site.	
Cleanse sutured wound and demonstrate care to Mr. Perez.	Once sutured, the wound must be cleansed to remove old blood and other debris from the suturing. If foreign matter is left in the wound, inflammation and infection could occur. Mr. Perez must be taught the cleansing procedure, as he will be responsible for home care of the wound.	
Give Mr. Perez explicit directions regarding taking oral antibiotics after discharge.	With the wound being very dirty, oral antibiotics will most likely be ordered by the physician. It is imperative that Mr. Perez takes the full course of the antibiotics in order to prevent infection.	
Teach Mr. Perez to care for wound.	Because Mr. Perez has no prior experience with injury, it is imperative that he be taught to care for his wound, including being told to remove the dressing when it becomes wet or dirty. Application of a new and clean dressing should be taught to alleviate any fear he may have about the process and thereby encourage	

continued

him to properly care for the wound and dressing.

Teach Mr. Perez the signs and symptoms that require a return visit to the doctor (redness, inflammation, increased pain, purulent drainage).

The signs and symptoms of infection should be taught, because Mr. Perez will need further care if the wound does become infected.

Nursing Diagnosis 4 *Anxiety related to reaction to fall and large laceration as evidenced by client's verbalizing that he had never been injured before*

PLANNING/GOALS	NURSING INTERVENTIONS	RATIONALE	EVALUATION
Mr. Perez will demonstrate decreased anxiety as evidenced by his talking about his injury and participating in his care.	Allow Mr. Perez to talk about injury.	Allowing Mr. Perez to talk about his injury gives him the ability to verbalize his fears and thoughts about the injury.	Mr. Perez viewed his injury with the use of a mirror before and after suturing. He was amazed to see that the laceration was completely closed following suturing. He was concerned about the bruising and edema to the area.
	Provide explanations for all procedures.	Explaining all procedures assists Mr. Perez in understanding why certain things are being done.	
	Give Mr. Perez simple choices to make.	Giving Mr. Perez simple choices allows him to participate in his care and gives him some sense of control.	Mr. Perez was not able to assist with the care of his sutures. His wife was taught how to clean and dress the wound.

POISONING AND OVERDOSES

Poisoning and overdoses can be accidental or intentional. Poison control centers are the best source of antidote information for the client suffering from poisoning or overdose.

There are many types of poisonings and overdoses and several different entry routes. Ingested poisonings are most common. It is important to obtain a clear history of the route of entry: inhalation, ingestion, topical, or injection. In addition, the client must be evaluated for any associated injuries, such as lacerations from a fall.

Medical–Surgical Management

Medical

In treating overdoses, the ABCs must be managed. Oxygen must be immediately initiated, and IV access

must be established. In addition, cardiac monitoring should be instituted. Blood and urine samples must be obtained for toxicology screening. After the client has been stabilized, efforts should be made to identify the substance so as to minimize or reverse the effects.

Pharmacological

If the substance has been ingested, and institutional protocol dictates, syrup of ipecac should be administered at 30 cc for a maximum of two doses in 20 minutes. Clients with caustic ingestions should not be given syrup of ipecac, as these products can damage the mucosal lining both from ingestion and emesis. Clients who have ingested caustic products should instead be given copious amounts of water to dilute the substance.

LIFE CYCLE CONSIDERATION

Syrup of Ipecac

Syrup of ipecac doses for children differ from those for adults only in amount. The usual dose is 15 cc initially followed by a second dose in 20 minutes. Vomiting is spontaneous and occurs without warning, so children and parents must be prepared.

Diet

The client who has overdosed is typically kept NPO except for the water needed following the administration of syrup of ipecac.

▸ NURSING PROCESS

▸ Assessment

▸ Subjective Data

The client must be asked about the timing and the route of overdose. Mental status must be evaluated to establish whether the exposure was intentional. Other incidences related to the overdose, such as an altercation with a loved one, must also be documented.

▸ Objective Data

The client's vital signs are critical for baseline data. The substance involved, as well as the amount, must be identified.

Nursing diagnoses for the client with an overdose may include the following:

Nursing Diagnoses	Planning/Goals	Nursing Interventions
▸ *Poisoning, Risk for, related to ingestion of toxin*	The client will recover with no residual effects of poisoning.	Manage the ABCs and stabilize the client. Monitor baseline laboratory work and ECG. Administer antidotes to toxins. Document the client's response.
▸ *Violence, Risk for, self-directed, related to harmful ingestion of toxic substance*	The client will not harm self and will participate in help groups to work through issues.	Encourage the client to share reasons for overdose. If overdose was accidental, discuss exposure to toxin and ways to avoid exposure in the future. Maintain a supportive, calm, reassuring environment for the client. Teach varying methods of coping. Refer to help groups.
▸ *Family Processes, Altered, related to ingestion of harmful toxin*	Client will begin to discuss problems with family.	Encourage client and family to discuss their problems openly and supportively. Assist the client in identifying different methods of coping. Encourage family counseling.

Evaluation Each goal must be evaluated to determine how it has been met by the client.

ENVIRONMENTAL/ TEMPERATURE EMERGENCIES

Exposure to extremes of heat and cold can be potentially life threatening. Severe cold, or hypothermia, can occur both in very cold weather and from pro-

longed submersion in cold water. Heart rate and metabolic rate fall, and cardiac arrest may follow. Frostbite is another potentially dangerous result of exposure to cold (Table 44-5). The most common sites of frostbite are the fingers, toes, ears, and nose. Initially, frostbite causes paleness and numbness to the affected areas. If

Table 44-5 DEGREES OF FROSTBITE SEVERITY		
DEGREE	**SYMPTOMS**	**TREATMENT**
Mild	Skin is cold to touch, pale, tingling, and numb, with a prickly sensation	Use blankets, warm clothing to warm cold flesh
Moderate	Affects deeper body tissue; skin appears waxy and is puffy to touch and itchy and burning with pain	Use gloves, blankets, warm clothing to warm cold flesh, observe closely for deeper injuries
Severe	Blistering, damage to all layers of soft tissue; flesh appears lifeless and is hard to the touch; no pain sensation in or ability to move frozen area	Initiate emergency rewarming in an ED using warm-water baths at 40.6° C (105°F); observe carefully for increased edema

Table 44-6 COMPARISON OF HEAT INJURIES

TYPE	SYMPTOMS	TREATMENT
Heat cramps	Muscle cramps in arms, legs, and abdomen	Move client to cool, shady area. Slowly administer copious amounts of water. Reevaluate.
Heat exhaustion	Diaphoresis, with pale, moist, cool skin, headache, weakness, dizziness; muscle cramps, nausea, chills, tachypnea, confusion, tingling of hands and feet	Move client to cool, shady area. Loosen/remove constrictive clothing. Pour water over client; place client near fan. Encourage client to slowly drink water. Elevate client's legs. Reevaluate.
Heat stroke (a medical emergency)	Red, flushed, hot, dry skin; no diaphoresis	Reduce client's body temperature by removing client's clothing and pouring cool water over client. Start two large-bore IV lines. Use fan to cool client. Place client on cardiac monitor. Elevate client's legs. Assess client's vital signs, especially core (rectal) temperature. Check for neurological signs (confused, combative, disoriented). Check client's core (rectal) temperature frequently.

Developed from U.S. Army Training Support Command Protocols.

exposure continues, frostbite can progress to blistering and loss of feeling. The client may lose voluntary control over the affected body part. Rewarming in an emergency setting is imperative.

Extreme heat can also cause potentially serious problems, especially in very young or elderly clients. As temperature rises, the body's ability to cool lessens. Table 44-6 compares heat injuries.

Medical–Surgical Management

Medical

For those exposed to extreme cold, rewarming is essential to resuscitation. The body's core (rectal) temperature must be taken. Gradual warming must be initiated using warm blankets, warmed oxygen, warmed IV fluids, warmed nasogastric tubes, and, in extreme instances, warmed enemas. Resuscitation should continue until the body has reached a core temperature of at least 34.4°C (94°F).

For frostbite, rewarming of the exposed body part is indicated. If the frostbite is severe, rapid rewarming is essential. This involves placing the frozen area in warm-water baths not exceeding 40.6°C (105°F). Teta-

nus should be administered. Acute pain should be treated with analgesics.

For heat injuries, rapidly reducing the body's temperature is vital. Supplemental oxygen may be administered. Pouring cool water over the client, chilling IV fluids, and fanning the client will accelerate the cooling process.

Pharmacological

For heat and cold injuries, establishment of at least two large-bore IV lines is essential. Supplemental oxygen should be administered. Replacement of fluid and electrolytes is essential.

Diet

In the event of heat injuries, fluids, especially water, should be encouraged, if the client is able.

▶ NURSING PROCESS

▶ Assessment

▶ Subjective Data

The client should be asked to give a history of both the heat/cold injury, if able, and any current medications.

▶ Objective Data

Core (rectal) body temperature and vital signs must be measured and documented. Skin color and temperature should be recorded. Cardiac monitoring should be initiated to track any cardiac response to the heat or cold stress to the body. Pupillary response must be evaluated because neurological problems may result from the heat/cold injury.

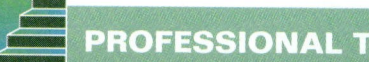

PROFESSIONAL TIP

Frostbite

Do not massage or rub frostbite injuries, as doing so can increase severity of damage to tissue. Caffeine, alcohol, and smoking should be avoided, as they decrease circulation to the damaged tissue.

Nursing diagnoses for the client with a temperature/environmental injury may include the following:

Nursing Diagnoses	Planning/Goals	Nursing Interventions
▶ *Hypothermia related to exposure to cold environment/long submersion in cold water*	The client will regain normal core body temperature.	Administer supplemental oxygen. Monitor cardiac response carefully. If CPR is in progress, continue until the client's core temperature reaches 94° F and cardiac status is evaluated. Administer warmed IV fluids. Place warmed blankets on the client.
▶ *Hyperthermia related to environmental exposure to heat*	The client will regain normal core body temperature.	Remove the client's clothing. Pour cool water over the client. Use large fan to cool the client. Administer chilled IV fluids. Administer supplemental oxygen. Initiate cardiac monitoring. Evaluate client's neurological status with reference to orientation to time, person, and place. Measure core temperature every 30 minutes to assess progress.

Evaluation Each goal must be evaluated to determine how it has been met by the client.

MULTIPLE-SYSTEM TRAUMA

Multiple-system trauma is injury sustained in more than one body system. During the initial care of the emergent client, the mechanism of injury is determined. Blunt injuries and penetrating trauma are most likely to result in multiple-system involvement.

Medical–Surgical Management

Medical

Immediate management of the ABCs is imperative. Bleeding must be stopped using pressure. Two to four large-bore IV lines should be started. All clothing must be removed for visualization of bleeding and injuries. Blood and urine specimens should be obtained. Radiographic studies must be done. Tetanus should also be administered.

▶ NURSING PROCESS

▶ Assessment

▶ Subjective Data

The client should be assessed for level of consciousness and orientation to time, person, and place. Verbalizations of pain should be evaluated. The client should be asked for an account of the accident.

▶ Objective Data

Airway, breathing, and circulation should be immediately assessed. Vital signs must be assessed, as must neurological status utilizing the Glasgow Coma Scale. Active bleeding must be assessed and controlled.

Nursing diagnoses for the client with multiple-system trauma may include the following:

Nursing Diagnoses	Planning/Goals	Nursing Intervention
▶ *Ventilation, Inability To Sustain Spontaneous, related to major trauma and severe hypotension*	The client will breathe without assistive devices.	Maintain open airway. Initiate rescue breathing. Assist with insertion of endotracheal tube. Ventilate per CPR protocol. Maintain pulse oximetry reading at 94% to 99%. Start multiple large-bore IV lines.

continued

Nursing Diagnoses	Planning/Goals	Nursing Intervention
▶ *Powerlessness related to the inability to sustain life without emergency interventions*	The client will survive emergency and within several hours will be able to indicate simple choices about care.	Explain all nursing/medical interventions to client. Provide emotional and physiological support to client and family as much as possible throughout resuscitation. Allow the client to make simple choices about care.

Evaluation Each goal must be evaluated to determine how it has been met by the client.

LEGAL ISSUES

Emergency medicine allows medical personnel to care for clients without obtaining informed consent. In life-threatening and emergency situations, consent is implied. In addition, the Good Samaritan Law, one of the laws and regulations enforced for the benefit of both the caregiver and the client, provides protection against malpractice to persons who stop at the scene of an accident and render care. It should be noted, however, that the Good Samaritan Law offers protection only to those who provide safe and appropriate care; it does not protect those charged with gross negligence or willful misconduct.

There are other legal issues specific to emergency care. Several injuries/illnesses must be reported to proper authorities. For instance, most states require that police be notified of MVCs, assaults, or rape. Likewise, animal control authorities require that animal bite reports be filed to facilitate follow-up on the possibility of rabies.

DEATH IN THE EMERGENCY DEPARTMENT

Death can occur in the ED at any time due to trauma, sudden illness, or even extended illness. This creates a delicate situation, as the death is usually unexpected. Family members may have a difficult time dealing with sudden death. If their loved one is being resuscitated in the ED, there is little time for health care personnel to comfort the family, as the personnel are very busy providing care to the client. In the event of sudden death, the family is usually in a state of shock and will need further assistance to cope with the death of their loved one. Special support groups are available for this assistance and should be contacted for the family.

CASE STUDY

Joe fell from a fishing boat into deep, cold water. He was wearing a life vest and was rescued within 10 minutes, at which time he was immediately dried, placed in a blanket, and brought to the ED. He is alert and oriented to person, time, and place, but is shivering uncontrollably and pale in color. His core temperature is 93°F.

The following questions will guide your development of a nursing care plan for the case study.

1. List the assessments in the order that they should be performed.
2. Identify the priority nursing diagnoses for Joe.
3. List nursing interventions in the order that they should be performed.
4. Identify the goal of treatment for Joe.

SUMMARY

- Clients in shock need immediate assessment and intervention.
- Rapid assessment and observation of ABCs is essential in treating all cardiovascular emergencies.
- Evaluation of abdominal emergencies should include taking a history of the onset of pain, as this is critical to outcome and survival.
- Ocular emergencies can be a threat to vision and thus require immediate assessment and treatment.
- Musculoskeletal and soft tissue injuries can be painful but manageable with rapid assessment and treatment.
- In cases of poisoning or overdoses, the ABCs must first be established, then the agent to which the client was exposed must be immediately identified so that prompt treatment can be initiated.

- Major trauma is a life-threatening and unexpected occurrence for both client and loved ones.
- Nurses must be aware of the legal issues related to emergency care, such as Good Samaritan Laws and mandated reporting.

Review Questions

1. Triage is a system of:
   a. identifying clients by disease.
   b. prioritizing client care.
   c. counting clients waiting for care.
   d. medical diagnosing.

2. A client with a small branch sticking out of the right mid-chest arrives at the ED during a hurricane. There is bubbling and oozing at the site. Medical personnel should first:
   a. remove the branch and save it.
   b. administer pain medication to the client.
   c. start the ABCs of CPR.
   d. stop the bleeding and take vital signs.

3. An example of a non-urgent client is:
   a. a client with CPR in progress.
   b. a client with fractures of both legs.
   c. a client with heat stroke.
   d. a client with a sprained ankle.

4. The ambulance brings a client with a large, bleeding laceration of the upper leg to the ED. Vital signs are as follows: blood pressure, 78/62; pulse, 112; and respirations, 26. A priority nursing diagnosis is:
   a. *Fluid Volume Deficit.*
   b. *Aspiration, Risk for.*
   c. *Infection, Risk for.*
   d. *Body Image Disturbance.*

5. Interventions for a client in shock include:
   a. pain control and assessment of vital signs.
   b. administration of oxygen and IV fluids.
   c. insertion of a nasogastric tube.
   d. calling the physician.

6. A client is brought to the ED after having run a marathon. His blood pressure is 128/78; pulse is 120; respirations are 26; and rectal temperature is 105°F. This is an example of:
   a. septic shock.
   b. runner's cramps.
   c. heat stroke.
   d. abdominal pain.

7. A method of assessing a client's neurological status is called:
   a. vital signs.
   b. pupillary response.
   c. Glasgow Coma Scale.
   d. cardiac monitor.

Critical Thinking Questions

1. On your way home from work, you come upon an MVC involving several vehicles. No emergency response vehicles have yet arrived on the scene. What steps can you take to secure the accident site and aid the victims until emergency services arrive?

2. Under what circumstances might a client present with multiple-system trauma? How would you proceed with the assessment of such a client? What immediate actions should be taken to maintain the stability of this client?

WEB FLASH!

- Visit the Web sites of various state boards of nursing to research available information on legal and ethical issues relating to emergency care.
- What information can you locate on the Internet about the Emergency Nurses Association? What coverage is offered regarding age-specific issues of emergency care across the life span?

Mental Health and Substance Abuse

MAKING THE CONNECTION

Refer to the following chapters to increase your understanding of mental illness:

- **Chapter 8, Communication**
- **Chapter 15, Wellness Concepts**
- **Chapter 16, Stress, Adaptation, and Anxiety**
- **Chapter 39, Nursing Care of the Client: Immune System**
- **Chapter 46, Nursing Care of the Client: Substance Abuse**
- **Chapter 52, Basics of Pediatric Care**
- **Chapter 54, Common Problems: 1–18 Years**
- **Chapter 55, Nursing Care of the Older Client**

LEARNING OBJECTIVES

Upon completion of this chapter, you should be able to:

- *Define key terms.*
- *Identify and describe the components of a therapeutic nurse–client relationship.*
- *Cite nursing interventions for working with clients who are angry, aggressive, homicidal, and/or suicidal.*
- *Detail nursing interventions for working with clients who are experiencing anxiety.*
- *Identify and explain the potential side effects associated with anti-anxiety medications.*
- *Recount nursing interventions for working with clients who are depressed.*
- *Identify and explain the potential side effects associated with antidepressant medications.*
- *Detail nursing interventions for working with clients who have schizophrenia.*
- *Identify and explain the potential side effects associated with antipsychotic medications.*
- *Detail nursing interventions for working with clients who have bipolar disorder.*
- *Identify and explain the potential side effects associated with mood stabilizers.*
- *Cite nursing interventions for working with clients who have attention-deficit/hyperactivity disorder.*
- *Recount nursing interventions for working with clients who have been neglected or abused or who have been exposed to domestic violence.*

KEY TERMS

abuse	hypomania
actively suicidal	insomnia
affect	lethargy
anger-control assistance	libido
anorexia nervosa	mania
anxiety	mental disorder
anxiolytic	mental illness
auditory hallucination	mood
brief dynamic therapy	neglect
bulimia nervosa	paradoxical reaction
cognitive behavior	physically aggressive
therapy	pressured speech
command hallucination	psychoanalysis
confidentiality	psychosis
crisis	psychotherapy
cycling	rapport
delusion	respect
depression	seclusion
domestic violence	serum lithium level
electroconvulsive	startle response
therapy	suicidal ideation
empathy	suicide
euphoric	tolerance
flashback	toxic
genuineness	trust
hallucination	verbally aggressive
hypersomnia	visual hallucination
hypervigilant	word salad

INTRODUCTION

Because they will encounter clients who are emotionally disturbed and/or mentally ill, it is imperative that nurses understand and feel comfortable working with such individuals—not just on psychiatric units, but in all types of circumstances and settings. This chapter is designed to give licensed practical/vocational nurses (LP/VNs) a beginning knowledge base regarding mental health and illness and to better prepare them for working with individuals who are in a state of crisis or who have emotional needs and/or psychiatric problems.

As the nurse becomes more knowledgeable about mental illness, opportunities arise to increase self-awareness and to examine any personal experiences, preconceived ideas, or prejudices that might negatively affect the nurse's ability to work effectively with clients. For example, the nurse who has some unresolved issues regarding sexuality or becomes embarrassed when discussing sexuality will probably be uncomfortable talking about the potential problems in sexual functioning secondary to antidepressant therapy (McEnany, 1998). Examining personal ideas and prejudices prior to working with clients will facilitate a positive nurse–client relationship.

MENTAL HEALTH AND ILLNESS

In general, a person is considered mentally healthy when he possesses knowledge of himself; meets his basic needs; assumes responsibility for his behavior; has learned to integrate thoughts, feelings, and actions; can successfully resolve conflicts; maintains relationships; communicates directly with others; respects others; and adapts to change. **Mental illness** occurs when an individual is not able to view self clearly or has a distorted view of self; is unable to maintain satisfying personal relationships; and is unable to adapt to the environment (Frisch & Frisch, 1998). The American Psychiatric Association defines **mental disorder** as "clinically significant behavior or psychological syndrome or pattern that occurs in an individual and is associated with present distress (i.e., negative response to stimuli that are perceived as threatening) or disability (i.e., impairment in one or more important areas of functioning) or with a significantly increased risk of suffering, death, pain, disability, or an important loss of freedom."

One of the ways to conceptualize psychiatric disorders is to think of a continuum, with mental health being situated at one end and mental illness at the other (Figure 45-1). Between these two extremes lie a variety of psychiatric disorders ranging in nature from mild to severe. The fourth edition of the *Diagnostic and Statistical Manual of Mental Disorders* (better

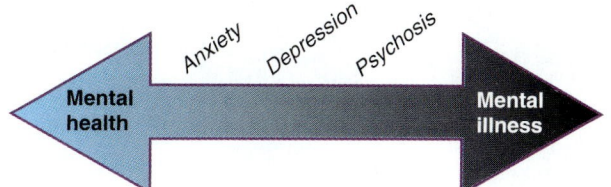

Figure 45-1 Mental Health Continuum

known as the *DSM-IV*) (American Psychiatric Association [APA], 1994) is the reference tool used to identify and establish psychiatric diagnoses. The psychiatrist is the individual most often involved in this process, although other mental health care practitioners may give input and make recommendations for diagnoses.

One of the primary roles of the nurse in working with clients who have mental illness is that of teaching. The nurse is responsible not only for teaching clients about their illnesses, including the probable courses of their given disorders, but also for adequately preparing and educating the client's family. The nurse is usually the first individual to have contact with the family and is most often the one with whom family members maintain consistent contact.

RELATIONSHIP DEVELOPMENT

Psychiatric nursing differs from some of the other fields of nursing in that the primary skill that the nurse employs is what is referred to as "the therapeutic use of self" (Sundeen, Stuart, Rankin, & Cohen, 1998). Many theorists such as Rogers and Peplau have been instrumental in identifying and exploring the factors that significantly influence the development of therapeutic relationships. Townsend (2000) identifies five components necessary to the development of a therapeutic working relationship and of particular importance in the therapeutic nurse–client relationship. These five components are trust, rapport, respect, genuineness, and empathy.

Trust

Trust is the ability to rely on an individual's character and ability. Trust must be present for help to be

PROFESSIONAL TIP

Confidentiality
Because of the highly personal and sensitive nature of mental disorders, the concept of **confidentiality**, which is the nondisclosure of the identity of or personal information about an individual, is vitally important in psychiatric nursing.

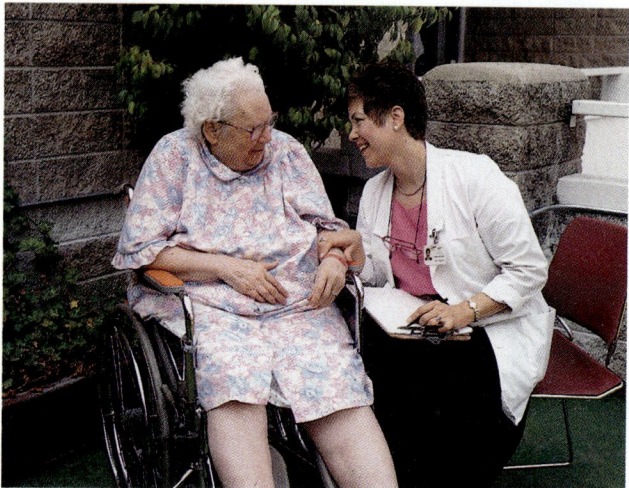

Figure 45-2 Spending time with the client one-on-one helps to promote a trusting relationship.

given and received. A therapeutic relationship is firmly rooted in trust. How does the nurse promote a trusting relationship? Three major activities facilitate the development of trust: consistency, respect, and honesty. Table 45-1 lists actions that facilitate the development of trust. Being consistently trustworthy is an expression of the nurse's personal integrity and builds the foundation for nursing effectiveness (Figure 45-2).

Many clients with emotional and/or psychiatric problems have great difficulty trusting and having confidence that others will be good to their word. They may have been lied to or hurt in the past, and this makes it difficult for them to trust again, even with health care professionals who are trying to help them. It is very important, therefore, that the nurse fulfill any promise made to the client.

Rapport

Rapport is a bond or connection between two people that is based on mutual trust. Such a bond does

not just happen spontaneously; it is planned by the nurse who purposefully implements behaviors that promote trust. The nurse sets the tone of the relationship by creating an atmosphere wherein the client feels free to express feelings. When seeking to develop trust, the nurse acts in a manner that indicates recognition of the client as a unique individual and reinforces that individuality. Such actions, which serve to humanize the client, are therapeutic. To establish rapport, the nurse must show that the client is considered important. Actions are implemented to boost the level of the client's self-esteem. Nonverbal interventions are of utmost importance in helping establish rapport. Interacting with family and significant others is also helpful in establishing rapport with the client. Recognizing the importance of the family and its influence on the healing process allows the nurse to bond with those who will encourage and support the client during recovery.

Respect

Respect is the acceptance of an individual as is and in a nonjudgmental manner. The concept of respect is an integral component of the nurse–client relationship. Respect means caring for clients whose value system may differ greatly from that of the nurse (Figure 45-3). To show respect, the nurse must not react with shock, surprise, or disapproval toward a client's lifestyle, dress, or behaviors. The nurse must respect the client's choices and actions while setting limits on unhealthy or undesirable behavior.

Genuineness

Genuineness (sincerity) is an attribute easily perceived by the client and can be the most significant as-

Table 45-1	ESSENTIAL FACTORS OF TRUST	
CONSISTENCY	**RESPECT**	**HONESTY**
Follow through on plans	Call client by name	Ask client about personal preferences
Adhere to schedule	Provide clear explanations	Keep any promises
Seek out client for extra time to interact	Recognize own strengths and limitations	Maintain confidentiality
Be straightforward/ no hidden motives	Listen to client	Be flexible in responding to requests

From Fundamentals of Nursing: Standards & Practice, *by S. DeLaune and P. Ladner, 1998, Albany, NY: Delmar Publishers. Copyright 1998 by Delmar Publishers.*

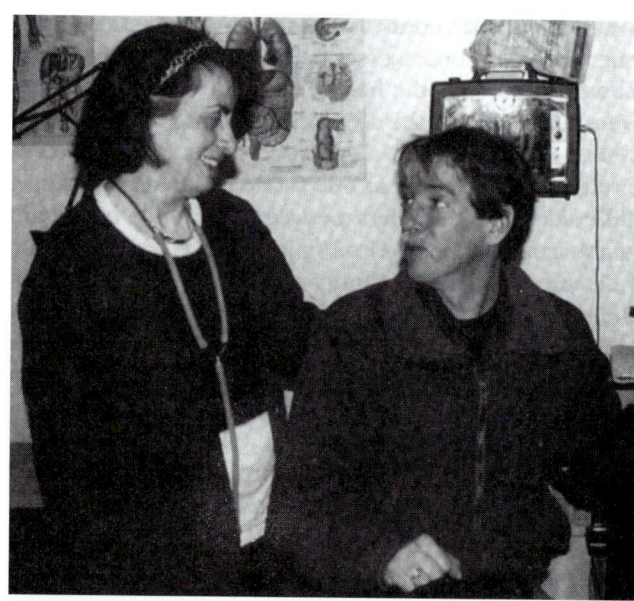

Figure 45-3 The nurse must show acceptance of the client, even if the client has values and beliefs that differ from her own. *(Photo courtesy of Pat O'Connor)*

pect of the nurse–client relationship. Nurses are often concerned about whether they will say the right thing to a client; though saying the right thing is important, more important is that the nurse be honest and genuine in communications with the client (Truax & Carkhuff, 1967).

Empathy

Empathy (the ability to perceive and relate to another's personal experience) is an important quality necessary to successful nurse–client interactions. The empathic nurse understands that the client's perception of the situation is real to him. By perceiving the client's understanding of his own needs, the nurse is better able to assist the client in determining what will work best. Empathy enables the nurse to assist the client to become a fully participating partner in treatment, rather than a passive recipient of care. Through empathy, the nurse validates the experiences of the client (Figure 45-4).

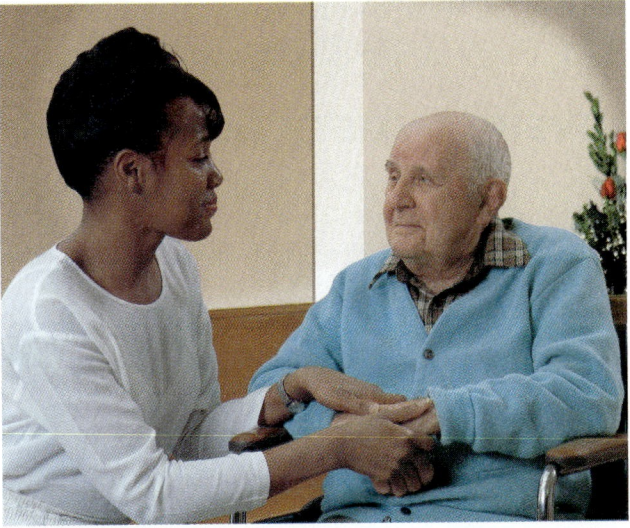

Figure 45-4 Through empathic listening, the nurse can reach an understanding of the client's experience and help the client see the positive aspects of the experience.

THE CLIENT EXPERIENCING A CRISIS

In psychological terms, a **crisis** is a stressor that forces an individual to respond and/or adapt in some way. Emotions may intensify during a crisis situation or serious illness, and any situation or illness can potentially become a crisis if the stressors are severe enough. The understanding of crisis is particularly important in psychiatric and mental health nursing. A crisis taxes the individual's coping resources, and each person responds differently to seemingly identical situations. Crisis requires that an individual call on all of her personal skills as well as on the outside social and familial supports that she has built through her life (Frisch & Frisch, 1998). Each individual has personality strengths, interpersonal networks, and socioeconomic resources that offer some protection against the threat of crisis. When any (or all) of these protections are weak, however, a person's response to crisis may be dysfunctional, and the result may be one or more symptoms of mental illness. While theories differ in their definitions of crisis and stress, it is generally accepted that most psychiatric problems result from or are strongly influenced by the interaction of stress and overwhelmed coping mechanisms (Frisch & Frisch, 1998). The client experiencing crisis may be anxious, angry, aggressive, homicidal, suicidal, psychotic, or any combination of these.

THE CLIENT WHO IS ANXIOUS

Anxiety is a state wherein a person feels a strong sense of dread frequently accompanied by physical symptoms of increased heart and respiratory rates and

elevated blood pressure in the absence of a specific source or reason for these emotions or responses. Nurses frequently encounter clients and family members who are anxious due to alterations in or threats to health and physical well-being. Peplau (1963) identifies four escalating stages of anxiety beginning with mild anxiety, moving to moderate anxiety, followed by severe anxiety, and, finally, to the stage of panic anxiety, if not effectively treated. Intervention can occur at any point along the continuum, preferably before the stages of severe or panic level anxiety are reached. Some of the most common psychiatric diagnoses related to anxiety are Generalized Anxiety Disorder, Panic Disorder, and post-traumatic Stress Disorder.

MILD ANXIETY

The mildly anxious client is beginning to experience some of the signs and symptoms of anxiety, such as irritability and restlessness; at this phase, however, the person is still able to concentrate and focus on the task at hand. In fact, *mild* anxiety can actually benefit an individual as far as enhancing performance ability (Townsend, 2000).

MODERATE ANXIETY

The individual with moderate anxiety experiences additional physiologic and cognitive symptoms. Blood pressure, pulse, and respirations increase, and the client becomes diaphoretic. The moderately anxious individual begins to have difficulty concentrating or learning new material. This is important to recognize before teaching a client about a medication or test, or performing a procedure. Before teaching can be effective, the client must be assisted in lowering the level of anxiety (Townsend, 2000).

SEVERE ANXIETY

Severely anxious clients are significantly impaired in a number of areas. Their ability to cognitively process material may drastically diminish, they may experience tunnel vision, their focus may become very limited, and the physiologic symptoms of anxiety become much more pronounced. Clients at this high level of anxiety are often very fearful and may be irrational in their thought processes (Townsend, 2000).

PANIC ANXIETY

The individual experiencing panic anxiety may begin to manifest symptoms of **psychosis** (losing touch with reality), such as **delusions** (false beliefs that misrepresent reality) and/or **hallucinations** (perceptions that something is present when it is not, e.g., hearing voices that are not really there). The individual with this level of anxiety requires constant reassurance, monitoring, and supervision to maintain safety (Townsend, 2000).

THE CLIENT WITH GENERALIZED ANXIETY DISORDER

The client with generalized anxiety disorder (GAD) exhibits symptoms of excessive anxiety or dread. Clients usually realize that their symptoms are out of proportion to any real threat. The symptoms include three or more of the following: restlessness, easy fatigue, difficulty concentrating, irritability, muscle tension, and sleep disturbance. For anxiety to be termed excessive, clients must experience symptoms frequently over a period of 6 months or more.

THE CLIENT WITH PANIC DISORDER

Panic disorder is a condition wherein the client experiences periods of intense anxiety that begin abruptly and peak within 10 minutes. These episodes are characterized by a set of any four of the following symptoms: palpitations or rapid heart rate, sweating, trembling, shortness of breath, sensation of choking, chest pain, nausea, dizziness, fear of losing control, fear of dying, numbness or tingling, chills or hot flushes, and some sense of altered reality. The client has a strong desire to run away or escape from the situation that triggered the attack. In some individuals,

the attack is brought about by specific stimuli or a particular setting, for example the dentist's office. In others, the attacks come on "out of the blue."

THE CLIENT WITH POST-TRAUMATIC STRESS DISORDER

Clients suffering from post-traumatic stress disorder (PTSD) have experienced a serious trauma. The client who has been severely beaten or emotionally, physically, or sexually abused or who has lived through or witnessed a catastrophic event or natural disaster such as a flood, earthquake, hurricane, or plane crash might be suffering from PTSD. "The traumas that cause the disorder range from a single loss of control over one's life ([such as] during a tornado, rape, mugging, or car accident) to repeated traumatization over time ([such as] in combat, abusive relationships, being held hostage, or [being] in a physically or psychologically unsafe work environment)" (Clark, 1997). The response to the trauma must have been one of fear or helplessness, and the event is persistently re-experienced through recurrent recollections, dreams, or hallucinatory-like flashbacks. Individuals with this disorder exhibit impairment of social functioning, the presence of specific anxiety symptoms, and "persistent avoidance of stimuli associated with the trauma, and numbing of general responsiveness" (American Psychiatric Association, 1994).

Medical–Surgical Management

Medical

Psychotherapy (the treatment of mental and emotional disorders through psychological rather than physical methods) continues to be widely used in the treatment of anxiety disorders. Psychotherapy can be viewed as falling into two general categories: those therapies based on helping individuals achieve insight into *why* they feel anxiety and those that emphasize behavioral means of controlling the anxiety.

Psychotherapy based on insight into symptoms may sometimes be valuable, especially for highly motivated individuals whose symptoms are not disabling. **Psychoanalysis** (therapy focused on uncovering unconscious memories and processes) is among the best known of the insight therapies and has been widely employed to assist persons with anxiety.

In contrast, there is strong empirical evidence that behaviorally based treatments are effective in treating at least some anxiety disorders. For example, studies consistently show that cognitive-behavior therapy results in significant benefit for persons suffering from panic attacks (Goldfried, Greenberg, & Marmar, 1990). **Cognitive-behavior therapy** assumes that clients can learn to identify the common stimuli that give rise to their anxiety, develop plans to respond to those stimuli with nonanxious responses, and problem solve when unanticipated anxiety-provoking situations arise. While insight is very much involved in this process, it is not insight into deep psychological causes, as in psychoanalysis, but, rather, practical, commonsense problem solving. Treatment appears both to be effective during the relatively brief course of therapy and to remain effective for some months after therapy finishes. It is still unclear, however, how long benefit from cognitive-behavior therapy truly lasts (Andrews, 1993). As a result, there may be an important need for medical and psychological follow-up to ensure satisfactory improvement.

Pharmacological

The drugs of choice for treating clients with anxiety are usually the **anxiolytics**, or antianxiety agents (Table 45-2). Some of the antianxiety medications such as alprazolam (Xanax) and lorazepam (Ativan) may also be helpful in alleviating the symptoms of anxiety, nervousness, and sleeplessness frequently associated with panic disorder and PTSD.

Most of these medications can be used on either a routine or as needed (PRN) basis, and the majority of these medications belong to the family of benzodiazepines. Onset of action for the benzodiazepines usually occurs within 30 minutes after oral administration, and most individuals respond favorably to these medications, that is, a reduction or cessation of the symptoms of anxiety is experienced.

Clients should be warned about the potential risk of addiction associated with the antianxiety medications. These particular medications should be used with extreme caution, as long-term use can lead to an increased **tolerance**, or acquired resistance to the effects of the drug. Tolerance results in the need to increase the frequency and amount of medication in

CLIENT TEACHING

Antianxiety Medications

Be sure to instruct each client taking an antianxiety medication in the following:

- Do not increase the dose or frequency of the medication without consulting your physician.
- Tolerance develops quickly with the medication and unsupervised use can lead to addiction.
- Do not drink alcohol while on the medication.
- Do not take any other medications unless prescribed by your physician.
- Do not stop taking the medication abruptly.
- Do not drive or operate heavy machinery while on the medication.

order to achieve the same benefit. Over time, this may cause a dependency on the medication, actually creating another serious problem for the client. Therefore, the antianxiety agents are usually indicated for short-term management of anxiety rather than for long-term use. The benefits of a particular medication for the client must always be weighed against the possible risk of addiction, particularly if long-term use is or may be indicated. The one exception is buspirone hydrochloride (BuSpar), a nonbenzodiazepine antianxiety medication, which does not appear to have any addictive potential. However, the therapeutic effectiveness of BuSpar is not reached for approximately 7 to 10 days; thus, although it can be given as a regularly scheduled antianxiety agent, BuSpar has absolutely no value as a PRN medication. When initiating therapy with BuSpar, another antianxiety medication such as alprazolam (Xanax) or lorazepam (Ativan) may be given concurrently until the therapeutic level is reached; the other medication can then be gradually decreased.

Table 45-2 ANTIANXIETY MEDICATIONS

GENERIC NAME	TRADE NAME	TYPE	POTENTIAL SIDE EFFECTS
alprazolam	Xanax	Benzodiazepine	Dizziness, drowsiness, lethargy, physical and psychological dependence, tolerance
buspirone hydrochloride	BuSpar	Nonbenzodiazepine	Blurred vision, chest pain, clamminess, dizziness, drowsiness, excitement, fatigue, headache, insomnia, nasal congestion, numbness, myalgia, nausea, nervousness, palpitations, paresthesia, rashes, sore throat, sweating, tachycardia, tinnitus, uncoordination, weakness
clonazepam	Klonopin	Benzodiazepine	Ataxia, behavioral changes, drowsiness, physical and psychological dependence, tolerance
diazepam	Valium	Benzodiazepine	Dizziness, drowsiness, lethargy, hypotension (when given intravenously [IV]), physical and psychological dependence, tolerance
lorazepam	Ativan	Benzodiazepine	Apnea and cardiac arrest (when given rapidly IV), dizziness, drowsiness, lethargy

Compiled from Davis's Drug Guide for Nurses *(6th ed.), by J. H. Deglin and A. H. Vallerand, 1999, Philadelphia: F. A. Davis.*

PROFESSIONAL TIP

Achieving a State of Relaxation

Clients who are anxious and feeling overwhelmed will often require assistance in achieving a state of relaxation. Nurses can help the client identify a number of activities that are relaxing, such as listening to favorite music, watching television, reading a book, playing a game, drawing a picture, working a puzzle, or whatever is calming to the client. Nurses can also teach the client a variety of stress-management techniques such as deep-breathing exercises, progressive deep-muscle relaxation, and guided imagery (Figure 45-5). All of these will assist the client in reaching a greater state of relaxation. Wilkinson (1996) states that becoming more centered or balanced is done by an "acquired ability to focus and channel emotional energy in a healthy and deliberate manner." The nurse can explore with the client the possibility of enrolling in a martial arts course such as Tai Chi, TaeKwondo, Karate, or Kung Fu as a means of stress reduction (Wilkinson, 1996). In addition to providing physical activity, the martial arts assist in achieving a state of balance and increasing one's ability to focus.

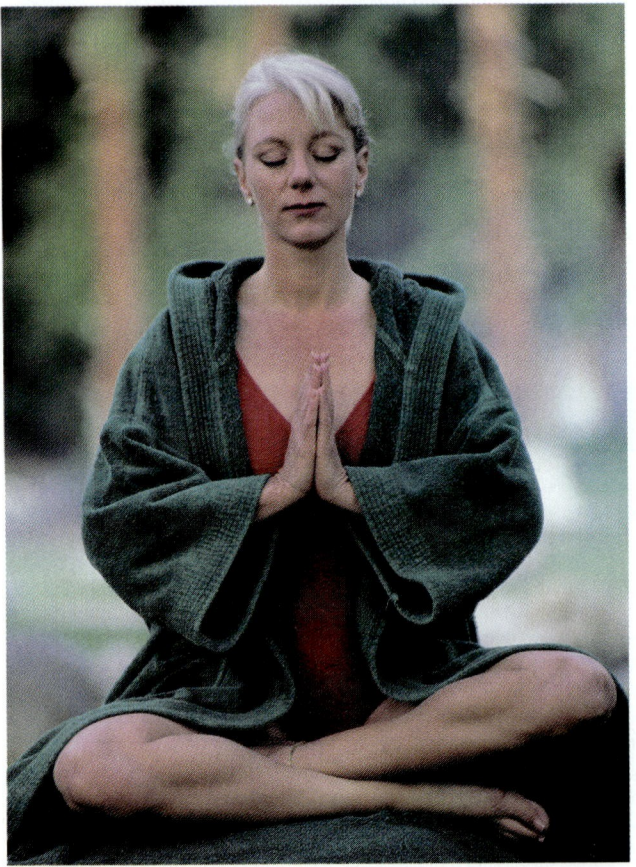

Figure 45-5 Clients may find relief from anxiety through meditation. *(Courtesy of Photo Disc)*

Activity

The anxious client's activity level may be negatively affected by both the anxiety disorder itself and the side effects of the prescribed medication. The side effects of sedation and drowsiness can pose safety hazards for certain activities and must be emphasized to the client.

▶ NURSING PROCESS

▶ Assessment

▶ Subjective Data

Clients experiencing anxiety report problems concentrating, and fear that something dreadful is about to happen. They may verbalize an overwhelming feeling of impending doom. They may also report that the anxiety is very frightening to them and that they are afraid of losing control. Table 45-3 lists questions that may help in identifying a client's anxiety.

Clients with PTSD "may complain of unwanted memories of an event, express suicidal ideation, or ex-

Table 45-3	ASKING CLIENTS ABOUT SYMPTOMS OF ANXIETY DISORDERS
Following are questions that have proven useful in eliciting information from clients about symptoms of anxiety disorders. You may find that you prefer to word these questions somewhat differently, but the important thing is to ask them. Many clients experience anxiety symptoms for years before a doctor, nurse, or psychologist takes the time to ask about these symptoms.	
Generalized anxiety disorder	Do you find yourself worrying frequently about a number of different things, such as the way things are going for you at home, work, or school?
	Do you find yourself feeling anxious or tense much of the time without any obvious reason?
Panic disorder	Have you ever experienced sudden, intense fear for no reason?
	Have you found yourself experiencing intense physical symptoms of chest pain, shortness of breath, dizziness, or sweating, along with a sense that something terrible or life threatening was happening to you?
Post-traumatic stress disorder	Have you ever had a particularly traumatic experience such as witnessing or experiencing violence or a catastrophic event (such as a flood or fire)?
	Have you ever found yourself re-experiencing a violent or catastrophic event through dreams or waking "flashbacks"?

From Psychiatric Mental Health Nursing, *by N. Frisch and L. Frisch, 1998, Albany, NY: Delmar Publishers. Copyright 1998 by Delmar Publishers.*

LIFE CYCLE CONSIDERATIONS

Children with PTSD

Children who have PTSD may manifest a variety of symptoms. Some children may exhibit "disorganized or agitated behavior," whereas others are "quiet, watchful, and immobile, avoiding any physical display of their inner agitation" (Clark, 1997).

PROFESSIONAL TIP

Flashbacks

The client experiencing a flashback is usually not aware of current surroundings and often does not recognize familiar individuals. For the duration of the flashback, the client is actually re-experiencing and reliving the original trauma once again. For this reason it is extremely important to never touch a client during a flashback, as the client may perceive you as dangerous and react to you as if you are trying to inflict harm. Talk to the client in a soft, calm voice and gently let the client know who you are, where the client is, and what is happening.

press fantasies of retaliation toward the identified source of trauma" (Clark, 1997). The client with PTSD may describe feeling extremely fearful and "on guard" at all times and may report having **flashbacks** (reliving of the original trauma as if currently experiencing it) along with recurrent dreams and/or nightmares.

▶ Objective Data

The anxious client may manifest changes in vital signs, such as an increase in blood pressure, pulse, and respirations. In addition, restlessness, irritability, pacing, and agitation may become more pronounced as anxiety level increases.

Clients with PTSD may exhibit an exaggerated **startle response** (overreaction to minor sounds or noises), or they may be **hypervigilant** (constantly scanning the environment for potentially dangerous situations). Clients with PTSD "may react under stress with survival responses appropriate for the trauma that they survived. For example, abused children may seek to placate adults, female incest victims may become flirtatious or seductive with men, and war veterans may become threatening or aggressive" (Clark, 1997).

Nursing diagnoses for the client with anxiety may include the following:

Nursing Diagnoses	Planning/Goals	Nursing Interventions
▶ *Anxiety related to a subjective sense of uneasiness and tension*	The client will learn how to demonstrate and utilize new and more effective methods of managing anxiety.	Teach the client relaxation exercises. Explore with the client those things that are calming and relaxing. Encourage physical movement or participation in some type of recreational or sporting activity to release excess energy.
▶ *Fear, related to a specific object (e.g., hospitals)*	The client will report feeling less fearful.	Remain with the client while level of fear is high. Talk to the client in a calm, soothing voice. Reassure the client that he is in a safe place.
▶ *Post-trauma syndrome, related to anxiety felt following a significant life-threatening event*	The client will experience a decrease in frequency and intensity of symptoms.	Orient the client to reality, if the client is confused, disoriented, or experiencing flashbacks. Do not touch the client without permission. Teach the client, family, and significant others about the symptoms of PTSD, including flashbacks, amnesia, memory loss, and nightmares.

Evaluation Each goal must be evaluated to determine how it has been met by the client.

THE CLIENT WHO IS DEPRESSED

Depression is the state wherein an individual experiences feelings of extreme sadness, hopelessness, and helplessness. A number of symptoms may be seen with depression, which can range anywhere from mild to severe and be manifested in many different ways. One of the first symptoms seen with depression is often a change in the usual pattern of sleeping. Individuals with depression experience symptoms uniquely, for example, a client may have **insomnia** (difficulty in falling asleep initially or returning to sleep once awakened) or **hypersomnia** (excessive sleeping). Other possible symptoms of depression include a change in the usual pattern of eating indicated by either an increase or decrease in appetite, **lethargy** (decreased energy level), decreased **libido** (sexual energy), frequent crying spells, racing thoughts, difficulty concentrating, forgetfulness, and **suicidal ideations** (thoughts of hurting or killing self). Clients can experience mild, moderate, or severe depression with varying degrees of symptomatology. Some of the psychiatric diagnoses associated with depression include Major Depressive Disorder and Dysthymic Disorder.

MILD DEPRESSION

Individuals with a mild depression may notice a difference in the way they are feeling and their ability to function in certain situations, but they may not be able to identify the problem at this point in time. Although they are still able to function and carry on their daily routines, doing so may put quite a strain on them both physically and mentally.

MODERATE DEPRESSION

Moderate depression interferes with the individual's life in a variety of ways. A decrease in the ability to perform on the job may be noticed. Relationships are affected as the individual becomes increasingly withdrawn and isolated and disinterested in things that previously were pleasurable, such as hobbies and leisure-time activities. Interventions performed at this stage are most effective in arresting the depression before the individual's mental health deteriorates any further.

SEVERE DEPRESSION

When depression progresses to a severe state, the individual becomes seriously impaired. The individual with severe depression may experience psychosis, or a loss of contact with reality, in addition to the symptoms of depression.

THE CLIENT WITH MAJOR DEPRESSIVE DISORDER

To qualify for the diagnosis of Major Depressive Disorder, DSM-IV requires the presence of at least one Major Depressive Episode. This episode must (1) last at least 2 weeks, (2) represent a change from previous functioning, and (3) cause some impairment in a person's social or occupational functioning. During an episode, it is also required that five or more symptoms be present. One of these symptoms *must* be either depressed mood or loss of interest in previously enjoyable activities. The individual must also experience at least four additional symptoms, which may include

changes in appetite or weight; sleep disturbance (usually trouble staying asleep); fatigue or loss of energy; feelings of worthlessness or guilt; difficulty concentrating, thinking, or making decisions; or recurrent thoughts of death or suicide.

A person experiencing a depressive episode may express feelings of sadness and hopelessness or may express the sense of feeling empty or having no feelings. Some persons express somatic symptoms such as bodily aches and pains rather than sadness. Also, some individuals, particularly adolescents, exhibit irritability or crankiness rather than sadness. Family members or close friends will notice a change in the individual, most commonly a social withdrawal and a neglect of activities that previously brought the person pleasure

Major depressive episodes frequently develop over a few days or weeks, and without treatment commonly last for longer than 6 months (Frisch & Frisch, 1998).

THE CLIENT WITH DYSTHYMIC DISORDER

Whereas the essence of Major Depressive Disorder is discrete episodes of depression, persons with Dysthymic Disorder feel depressed nearly all of the time. The DSM-IV criteria for Dysthymic Disorder include "depressed mood for most of the day, for more days than not . . . for at least 2 years." A person with Dysthymic Disorder must also have at least two of the following symptoms: appetite disturbance, sleep disturbance, fatigue, low self-esteem, poor concentration or difficulty making decisions, and feelings of hopelessness. As with Major Depressive Disorder, the symptoms must cause clinically significant distress or impairment in social or occupational functioning. Dysthymic Disorder is somewhat rarer than Major Depressive Disorder, occurring during a lifetime in approximately 6% of persons (Frisch & Frisch, 1998).

Medical–Surgical Management

Medical

Psychotherapy refers to any of over 250 types of largely verbal techniques designed to help individuals surmount psychological stresses including depression. Psychotherapy based on psychoanalytic interventions emphasizes helping clients gain insight into the causes of their depression. This approach is long term and requires much motivation on the part of the client to invest considerable time, effort, and money (Frisch & Frisch, 1998).

Brief dynamic therapy focuses on core conflicts that derive from personality and living situations. The goal is to resolve depressive symptoms by improving these conflicts and resolving stresses. The therapist in this approach takes an active role to direct sessions

PROFESSIONAL TIP

Journaling

Suggest to depressed clients that they keep personal journals in which they write down their thoughts and feelings. Putting thoughts and emotions down on paper may help clarify issues relating to depression and is an excellent way of venting or releasing pent-up feelings.

PROFESSIONAL TIP

Antidepressant Therapy

Prior to initiating antidepressant therapy, a baseline electrocardiogram (EKG) is needed to determine whether any pre-existing underlying cardiac problems are present. If the client develops cardiac difficulties during antidepressant therapy, another EKG can then be obtained and reviewed against the original to assist in ascertaining whether the administration of the antidepressant has exacerbated the cardiac condition.

toward resolution of conflicts. Techniques of confrontation and interpretation of behaviors and events are frequently used. Conflicts, their meanings, and individuals' choices are emphasized. This type of therapy can be done either with individuals or in a group format.

Cognitive therapy focuses on removing symptoms by identifying and correcting perceptual biases in clients' thinking and correcting unrecognized assumptions. The therapy concentrates on changing negative thoughts and behaviors into alternatives that do not sustain depression (Abraham, Neese, & Westerman, 1991).

Electroconvulsive therapy (ECT) is a procedure wherein the client is treated with pulses of electrical energy sufficient to cause a brief convulsion or seizure (Bolwig, 1993). Electroconvulsive therapy is carried out under anesthesia. Muscle-depolarizing agents are also given so that no actual convulsive movements occur; the primary effect of ECT is on the brain itself. Studies show that clients do not find the actual ECT treatment frightening, painful, or unpleasant. Although deaths have occurred from ECT, particularly in elderly clients or those with heart disease, the risk is quite low. Side effects depend on the specific technique used but are mostly limited to memory deficits (Frisch & Frisch, 1998).

Pharmacological

The main classification of medications usually prescribed for treatment of depression is the antidepres-

sants. Within this classification are several groups including the tetracyclic and atypical antidepressants (Table 45-4), the selective serotonin reuptake inhibitors (SSRIs) (Table 45-5), the tricyclic antidepressants (Table 45-6), and the monoamine oxidase inhibitors (MAOIs) (Table 45-7). These antidepressant families have unique properties, as do the individual medications within each. It is the responsibility of the nurse to adequately educate the client and family about the prescribed medications.

Diet

The client experiencing depression often has a disturbance in eating patterns. Some individuals will not be hungry and will eat very little or sometimes not at all, whereas others will overeat. A nutritional assessment should be done as part of the health history obtained by the nurse, and if any significant problem areas are identified, a dietary consult may be indicated.

When a client is started on antidepressant therapy, the client and family must be educated regarding any special dietary needs, depending on the type of medication prescribed. The client receiving SSRI therapy may experience an initial loss of appetite during the first part of therapy, because of the gastrointestinal (GI) side effects frequently associated with these medications

Table 45-4 TETRACYCLIC AND ATYPICAL ANTIDEPRESSANTS

GENERIC NAME	TRADE NAME	TYPE	POTENTIAL SIDE EFFECTS
mirtazapine	Remeron	Tetracyclic	Agranulocytosis, drowsiness, dry mouth, increased appetite, weight gain
nefazodone	Serzone	Atypical	Constipation, dizziness, dry mouth, insomnia, nausea, somnolence
venlafaxine hydrochloride	Effexor	Atypical	Abnormal dreams, altered taste, anorexia, chills, constipation, diarrhea, dizziness, dry mouth, dyspepsia, headache, nausea, nervousness, paresthesia, rhinitis, seizures, sexual dysfunction, visual disturbances, vomiting, weakness, weight loss

Compiled from Davis's Drug Guide for Nurses *(6th ed.), by J. H. Deglin and A. H. Vallerand, 1999, Philadelphia: F. A. Davis; and* "Depression and Your Patient," *by A. Isaacs, 1998,* American Journal of Nursing, 98(7), 26–31.

Table 45-5 SELECTIVE SEROTONIN REUPTAKE INHIBITORS (SSRIs)

GENERIC NAME	TRADE NAME	POTENTIAL SIDE EFFECTS
fluoxetine	Prozac	Abnormal dreams, anxiety, diarrhea, drowsiness, excessive sweating, headache, insomnia, nervousness, pruritus, seizures, tremors
fluvoxamine	Luvox	Constipation, diarrhea, dizziness, dry mouth, drowsiness, dyspepsia, headache, insomnia, nausea, nervousness, weakness
paroxetine	Paxil	Anxiety, constipation, diarrhea, dizziness, drowsiness, dry mouth, ejaculatory disturbance, headache, insomnia, nausea, sweating, weakness, tremors
sertraline	Zoloft	Diarrhea, dizziness, drowsiness, dry mouth, fatigue, headache, increased sweating, insomnia, nausea, sexual dysfunction, tremors

Compiled from Davis's Drug Guide for Nurses *(6th ed.), by J. H. Deglin and A. H. Vallerand, 1999, Philadelphia: F. A. Davis.*

Table 45-6 TRICYCLIC ANTIDEPRESSANTS

GENERIC NAME	TRADE NAME	POTENTIAL SIDE EFFECTS
amitriptyline hydrochloride	Elavil	Arrhythmia, blurred vision, constipation, dry eyes, dry mouth, hypotension, lethargy, sedation
clomipramine hydrochloride	Anafranil	Arrhythmia, blurred vision, constipation, dry eyes, dry mouth, lethargy, male sexual dysfunction, nausea, sedation, vomiting, weakness
imipramine hydrochloride	Tofranil	Arrhythmia, blurred vision, constipation, drowsiness, dry eyes, dry mouth, fatigue, hypotension, urinary retention

Compiled from Davis's Drug Guide for Nurses *(6th ed.), by J. H. Deglin and A. H. Vallerand, 1999, Philadelphia: F. A. Davis.*

Table 45-7 MONOAMINE OXIDASE INHIBITORS (MAOIs)

GENERIC NAME	TRADE NAME	POTENTIAL SIDE EFFECTS
isocarboxazid	Marplan	Arrhythmia, blurred vision, diarrhea, dizziness, headache, orthostatic hypotension, insomnia, restlessness, seizures, weakness; these medications usually have the side-effect of lowering blood pressure. A potentially fatal hypertensive crisis can result when MAOIs are taken in combination with certain foods and drugs such as broad beans, certain cheeses (e.g., brie, cheddar), liver, caffeine, figs, dry sausage (pepperoni), tea, yogurt, amphetamine, cocaine, dopa, and many OTC cold products, hay fever medications, and nasal decongestants.
phenelzine sulfate	Nardil	
tranylcypromine sulfate	Parnate	

Compiled from Davis's Drug Guide for Nurses *(6th ed.), by J. H. Deglin and A. H. Vallerand, 1999, Philadelphia: F. A. Davis; and* Lippincott's Need-to-know Psychotropic Drug Facts, *by K. P. Bailey, 1998, Philadelphia: Lippincott.*

(refer to Table 45-5). Anorectic clients or those at risk for weight loss must be closely monitored. The client receiving MAOI therapy must be especially alert to the dietary restrictions associated with this particular type of medication (refer to Table 45-7).

Activity

Clients suffering from depression often experience a significant decrease in level of activity and report feeling tired and lethargic. Clients experiencing depression will often require encouragement to engage in any type of physical activity (Figure 45-6).

CLIENT TEACHING

Potential Adverse Drug–Drug Reactions with MAOIs

A serious drug–drug reaction can occur when a MAOI is taken concurrently with certain other medications. The combination of a MAOI and some common prescription or OTC medications can result in a hypertensive crisis that is often fatal. Some of the most dangerous reactive medications include meperidine (Demerol), stimulants, decongestants, and weight-reduction aids.

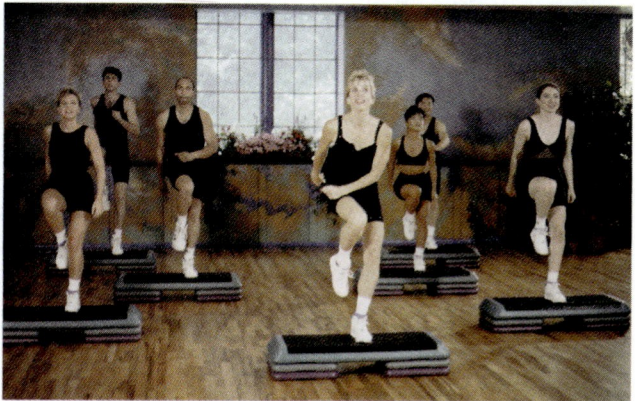

Figure 45-6 Exercise was found to be an effective antidepressant in a meta-analysis of 77 studies on exercise and depression (North, 1989). *(Courtesy of Photo Disc)*

CLIENT TEACHING

Tricyclic Antidepressants

Be sure to instruct each client taking a tricyclic antidepressant medication in the following:
- Do not drink alcohol while on the medication.
- Do not take any other medications unless prescribed by your physician.
- Drowsiness and sedation may impair the ability to drive and operate heavy machinery.
- Some of the side effects may diminish in intensity once your body adjusts to the medication.
- Do not stop taking the medications without physician approval.
- Increase fluid intake to assist in combating dry mouth and constipation.
- Sugarless candy and gum can help decrease the side effect of dry mouth.
- Increase dietary fiber to decrease the side effect of constipation.
- Rise slowly from a lying position to prevent dizziness and a sudden drop in blood pressure.

CLIENT TEACHING

Tetracyclic and SSRI Antidepressants

Be sure to instruct each client taking a tetracyclic, atypical, or SSRI antidepressant medication in the following:
- Take the medication *only* as directed by your physician.
- Do not take the medication unless prescribed by your physician.
- Do not take fluoxetine (Prozac), paroxetine (Paxil), or sertraline (Zoloft) on an empty stomach.
- Mirtazapine (Remeron) does not need to be taken with food.
- Ability to drive and/or operate heavy machinery may be impaired while taking the medication.
- Do not drink alcohol while taking the medication.
- If female, advise your physician if you are breastfeeding, suspect you are pregnant, or are planning a pregnancy while taking the medication.
- Wear sunscreen and protective clothing while outdoors, as fluoxetine (Prozac), paroxetine (Paxil), and sertraline (Zoloft) increase susceptibility to sunburn.

- The medications may cause drowsiness.
- If taking fluoxetine (Prozac), mirtazapine (Remeron), or nefazodone (Serzone), rise slowly from a lying position to prevent dizziness and a sudden drop in blood pressure.
- Utilize good oral hygiene in conjunction with sugarless candy or gum to minimize the discomforting side effect of dry mouth associated with fluoxetine (Prozac), mirtazapine (Remeron), nefazodone (Serzone), paroxetine (Paxil), and sertraline (Zoloft).
- Monitor weight, as mirtazapine (Remeron) may cause an increase in appetite.
- Do not take any over-the-counter (OTC) cold medications with mirtazapine (Remeron).
- If taking mirtazapine (Remeron), inform your physician of the medication regimen prior to surgery.
- If taking venlafaxine (Effexor), fluvoxamine (Luvox), or nefazodone (Serzone), inform your physician if signs of allergic reaction occur.

PROFESSIONAL TIP

MAOIs

MAOIs are most often used to treat depression that has proven resistant to other medications.

CLIENT TEACHING

MAOIs

Be sure to instruct each client taking an MAOI antidepressant medication in the following:

- *Do not take any other medications, including OTC medications,* unless prescribed by your physician.
- Take the medication exactly as prescribed.
- Do not drink alcohol while on the medication.
- Rise slowly from a lying position to prevent dizziness and a sudden drop in blood pressure.
- *Avoid all foods containing tyramine,* including alcoholic beverages, especially beer and wine; aged cheeses; avocados; bananas; caffeine; chocolate; and smoked or pickled meats (such as salami, pepperoni, smoked fish, and summer sausage).

▶ NURSING PROCESS

▶ Assessment

▶ Subjective Data

The client experiencing depression may verbalize any number of symptoms including overwhelming feelings of sadness, thoughts of suicide, a loss of interest and pleasure in activities that were previously enjoyable, and problems with memory, recall, and concentration. In addition, they may report a decreased libido, extreme lethargy, and having insufficient energy to complete activities of daily living (ADLs) and needed tasks. The depressed client who has become increasingly withdrawn and socially isolated may experience problems in intimate, personal, and social relationships.

▶ Objective Data

The client experiencing depression may manifest a noticeable decline in personal hygiene and grooming, possibly due to a lack of energy and an inability to perform even the simplest of tasks. Weight loss resulting from the client's failure to eat is also a symptom of depression.

Nursing diagnoses for the client with depression may include the following:

Nursing Diagnoses	Planning/Goals	Nursing Interventions
▶ *Social Isolation related to inability to engage in satisfying personal relationships*	The client will increase the number of interactions with other individuals.	Build rapport and develop therapeutic relationship with client. Spend time with client individually. Encourage client to interact with others. Encourage client to initiate conversation with others. Verbally praise client for increasing interactions and initiating conversation.
▶ *Self-care Deficit related to lack of concern or regard toward self*	The client will attend to own basic health care needs.	Encourage client to bathe and wear clean clothes. Teach client the importance of balanced nutrition. Praise client for each activity done on own.

Evaluation Each goal must be evaluated to determine how it has been met by the client.

THE CLIENT WHO IS POTENTIALLY VIOLENT

In today's society, violence has become increasingly common and widespread. The media routinely and graphically reports the numerous violent crimes and acts that occur on a daily basis (Aguilera, 1998). Upon occasion, nurses come face to face with angry clients and their families and significant others and, perhaps, even angry colleagues. When confronted by someone who is angry, the natural reaction is to respond in a like manner or, perhaps, to feel intimidated. In such difficult situations it is important to maintain objectivity and not get "hooked" into the client's anger and respond in an inappropriate manner.

Nurses may encounter clients who are **verbally aggressive** (prone to saying things in a loud and/or intimidating manner), **physically aggressive** (prone to threatening or actually harming someone), or a combination of the two. Mind-altering substances such as alcohol and phencyclidine (PCP) often increase the risk of aggression. **Anger-control assistance** is defined as a nursing intervention aimed at facilitation of the expression of anger in an adaptive and nonviolent manner (McCloskey & Bulechek, 1996). For the psychiatric nurse, anger control includes establishing a basic level of trust and rapport with the client and using a calm and reassuring manner. The nurse should use every means possible to learn from the client (or his family/friends) those situations that are likely to bring on anger. Further, the nurse should encourage the client to inform the nursing staff when he is feeling tension. While the nurse has a responsibility to help the client learn to deal with his anger, she also has a clear duty to assess for inappropriate aggression and to intervene before such aggression is expressed.

Some of the techniques used in anger control include limiting access to frustrating situations, providing physical outlets for expression of anger or tension (such as punching bags, large motor activities [sports], and anger journals), and ensuring that a client for whom anger is a problem is given enough personal space that he does not have to feel encroached upon by others when he is unable to tolerate environmental stimuli.

Two interventions commonly used in situations where the client is out of control are physical restraints and seclusion. These external controls may be used only when there is no other option for protecting the client and/or others.

THE CLIENT WHO IS HOMICIDAL

The client who is homicidal is planning or threatening to harm or kill another individual or individuals. It is the responsibility of health care personnel to attempt to ascertain the seriousness of the intent, that is, whether the individual is actually threatening someone else or just "blowing off steam." Once the nurse is aware of an individual's threat or intent to harm someone else, she must inform the individual(s) at risk of the potential for harm and/or notify the proper authorities and enlist their help. The first step in such a situation is to contact the supervisor and offer an accurate appraisal of the situation.

THE CLIENT WHO IS SUICIDAL

Purposefully taking one's own life, or **suicide**, is the ultimate form of self-destruction. Clients who are suicidal often feel overwhelmed by life events and decide that the only relief will come from ending their own lives. Intense feelings of fear, loss, anger, or despair can drive individuals to commit suicide, and the effects of an attempted or completed suicide can be devastating and long lasting. Nurses must learn to recognize the danger signs of clients at risk for suicide and know the appropriate interventions to help clients preserve their health and dignity.

"Suicide is the eighth leading cause of death in the United States, claiming some 30,000 lives each year" (Badger, 1995). The populations at greatest risk are individuals with diagnosed mood disorders such as Major Depressive Disorder, elders, and those with serious or life-threatening medical illnesses such as cancer or human immunodeficiency virus (Badger, 1995).

PROFESSIONAL TIP

Assessing for Risk of Violence
- Be aware of those clients with past history of violence and poor impulse control.
- Observe the client's body language: Notice changes in behavior, words, or dress.
- Assess for aggressive behaviors, increasing tension, clenched fists, loud or angry tone of voice, narrowed eyes, and pacing.
- Remember that hostility tends to be contagious. Do not reciprocate with anger and hostility!

LIFE CYCLE CONSIDERATIONS

Warning Signs of Potential Adolescent Suicide
- Drastic changes in behavior (e.g., sudden withdrawal in an otherwise socially active person or sudden gregariousness in an otherwise shy person)
- Stated feelings of sadness, loneliness, hopelessness, or despair
- Increased impulsive risk-taking behaviors (e.g., disregard for safety by not wearing seatbelt)
- Alienating behaviors (e.g., withdrawal or aggression)
- Giving away possessions (especially those with special meanings)
- Preoccupation with death or dying
- Sudden changes in personal appearance and hygiene
- Previous suicide attempt or gesture
- Direct suicidal comments such as "I wish I were dead"

From Psychiatric Mental Health Nursing, *by N. Frisch and L. Frisch, 1998, Albany, NY: Delmar Publishers.*

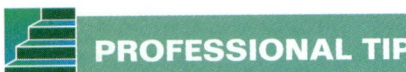

PROFESSIONAL TIP

Clues to Suicide

SYNDROMATIC CLUES

Depression

- Change in sleep patterns
- Loss of appetite and weight loss
- Complaints about illnesses, real or imaginary, or complaints about body aches and minor or major physical problems, real or imaginary
- Mood changes (sadness, lethargy)
- Loss of interest in usual activities
- Loss of energy and fatigue

Alcoholism

- Increased drinking
- Physical dependence on alcohol
- Loss of control over drinking
- Lying and denial
- Hiding liquor
- Sneaking drinks
- Drinking in spite of medical admonitions against it
- Blackouts
- Hangovers
- Cuts, scratches, bruises, cigarette burns

VERBAL CLUES

- "I am going to kill myself."
- "I am going to commit suicide."
- "I want to end it all."
- "I've had it."

- "I've lived long enough. No more."
- "I'm tired of life."
- "I'm tired of living."
- "My family would be better off without me."
- "Nobody cares about me."
- "Who cares if I'm dead anyway?"
- "I won't be around much longer."
- "Pretty soon you won't have to worry about me anyway."

BEHAVIORAL CLUES

- Previous suicide attempts
- Buying a gun
- Stockpiling pills
- Giving away money or possessions
- Loss of interest in favorite activities, church, or family
- Making or changing a will
- Making funeral plans
- Suspicious behavior

SITUATIONAL CLUES

- Death of a spouse, child, or close friend
- Death of a pet
- Major move
- Diagnosis of a terminal illness
- Retirement
- Flare-up with a friend or relative

THE CLIENT WITH SUICIDAL IDEATIONS

The client experiencing suicidal ideations has thoughts of hurting or killing himself but may or may not be planning to act on these thoughts. It is important to understand the difference between thoughts and actions; that is, having a thought does not necessarily mean that the behavior will follow. When confronted with a client's verbalization of possible suicide, however, it is always wise to take the client's expression of intent seriously. Because suicide is a leading cause of death in the United States, nurses must know how to evaluate a client for the likelihood of a completed suicide. It is critical that the nurse thoroughly assess the client and attempt to accurately ascertain the degree of danger the client is experiencing. Once this is done, the nurse must then take the precautions necessary to maintain the client's safety (Table 45-8).

THE CLIENT WHO IS ACTIVELY SUICIDAL

The **actively suicidal** client is intent upon hurting or killing himself and is in imminent danger of doing so. This situation requires immediate and appropriate action on the part of the nurse to protect the client from potentially fatal self-destructive behavior. If the client is in a supervised setting, it is the responsibility of the nurse to maintain the safety of the client and to inform other staff members of the client's suicidal intentions. The client at high risk for self-inflicted injury must be monitored closely (per institutional policy and the frequency as ordered by the physician). All pertinent observations such as verbalizations and behaviors that are indicative of self-harm potential should be documented in the client record. Any changes in the client's condition should be reported immediately to the physician. The conversation with the doctor as

Table 45-8 ASSESSMENT OF RISK FOR SUICIDE

The following areas are to be assessed in all potentially suicidal clients:

1. Does the client have a *plan* to commit suicide?

Example: Client plans to "end it all" after wife leaves for work on a Monday.	***Rationale***: Some clients may be experiencing thoughts of wishing they were dead or killing themselves, but may not have a plan for doing so. *The client who has a plan for committing suicide is at increased risk.*

2. How *specific* is the plan to commit suicide?

Example: Client states he plans to overdose on sleeping pills.	***Rationale***: *A specific plan increases the risk of completing a suicide.*

3. Does the client have access to the *means* to commit suicide?

Example: Client states he will use his spouse's sleeping pills to overdose.	***Rationale***: *Easy availability of the means to kill oneself increases the risk of suicide.*

4. How *lethal* is the intended means to commit suicide?

Example: Client states he will "blow his brains out" with a gun.	***Rationale***: Some means of suicide are more likely to result in a completed suicide. *Gunshots are the most common cause of completed suicide.* The lethality of guns makes the potential for a successful intervention very slim. Intervention in light of means that are less lethal may yield a more favorable outcome (e.g., overdose, cutting of wrists).

PROFESSIONAL TIP

Providing a Safe Environment

When a client verbalizes an intention to inflict self-harm, the nurse must take measures to ensure the client's safety. One way to do so is to provide and maintain a safe, secure environment for the client. This may require a change in the way a client's surroundings and living space are usually viewed. For example, a pencil or pen could be used as a dangerous weapon; an empty soda can could be used to deeply cut the wrists or to seriously injure someone else; and the glass from a bottle of make-up could cause great harm. These and all other potentially dangerous items must be removed from the client's immediate area.

well as any new orders or changes in orders must also be documented in the client's record (Eskreis, 1998).

Medical–Surgical Management

Medical

The client who is severely agitated, aggressive, actively suicidal, and/or homicidal and who is exhibiting or threatening violent acts may need to be restrained or placed in seclusion in order to be safely contained. The physical holding of someone or use of mechanical restraints severely restricts movement and can constitute a violation of the client's rights unless sufficient clinical justification exists. Thus, all of the client's comments and behaviors plus any nursing interventions must be documented in the client record per agency policy. This documentation provides the necessary justification for the use of restraints or seclusion. In addition, the physician must write a specific, time-limited order that spells out the reason restraints or seclusion was indicated for use with the client.

Physical Restraints Physical restraints, usually leather straps, are used to immobilize a person who is clearly dangerous to self or others and who poses sufficient risk of harm. Physical restraints may be applied only under the direction and supervision of a registered nurse (RN) and must comply with state laws regarding their use. In almost all cases, there must be a physician's order to apply the restraints, and there must be clearly documented evidence that the restraints were needed. Some of the observable behaviors indicating that restraints are necessary include increased motor activity, verbal and/or physical threats, overresponsiveness to stimuli, and actual physical assault (Frisch & Frisch, 1998).

Seclusion Seclusion is the process of confining a client to a single room. The room may be locked or

PROFESSIONAL TIP

Level of Observation

The frequency of client observation is determined by the degree of suicide risk and is written as a specific order from the physician. Observations of the client are documented. Some clients must be checked a minimum of once every 15 minutes. Other clients may require more frequent observation and monitoring. If the client is *actively* suicidal and/or homicidal and is indicating an imminent intent to harm self or others, a specific staff member will be assigned to that client at all times on a one-to-one basis.

PROFESSIONAL TIP

No-Suicide Contract

Obtaining a "No-Suicide Contract" from the client is one way to help reduce the risk of suicide attempts. There are several guidelines to follow in working through this process:

- Ask the client whether he is able to make a promise *to himself* that he will not do anything to harm himself. **Rationale**: It is important for the client to make the contract with himself, because if the contract is made with someone else, such as a nurse, and the client later becomes angry or upset with that person, he may then harm himself in order to "get back" at that person.
- If the client is unable to commit to the No-Suicide Contract for the rest of his life, work with him on establishing a time frame to which he can commit, for example, 1 week, 24 hours, 8 hours, or some other time frame. Always meet with the client at the end of the allotted time frame and review/renew the contract at that time. **Rationale**: The suicidal individual may feel overwhelmed at the thought of promising *never* to harm himself, but may be able to sincerely commit for a shorter length of time.
- Ask the client whether he is able to maintain the No-Suicide Contract *no matter what happens*. **Rationale:** Some clients will leave a way out of the contract. For example, the suicidal client may outwardly make a promise to not commit suicide but inwardly think "unless something really bad happens, like if my wife leaves me." If the wife then files for a divorce, the client may feel that he has "permission" to kill himself. Adding the *no matter what happens* clause blocks off this avenue of escape from the contract.
- Ask the client whether he can make a promise to himself that if thoughts of suicide return, he will talk to someone and let them know before taking any action. **Rationale**: If the client talks to someone regarding his thoughts of suicide *before* he attempts suicide, a successful intervention and suicide prevention are more likely.
- Assist the client in developing a detailed plan of action regarding those persons he will contact in the event that he again experiences suicidal thoughts. Include names and phone numbers of all significant and supportive individuals. **Rationale**: During a crisis, the suicidal individual is not able to think rationally and will behave and act in an impulsive manner. Having a well-developed plan of action increases the likelihood that the suicidal individual can follow these guidelines.
- At the bottom of the list put the name and phone number of the local suicide crisis hotline and/or local emergency number (911). **Rationale**: Including these numbers ensures that there will always be someone available for the suicidal client to talk to 24 hours a day, 7 days a week, 365 days a year.
- Assist the client in putting the No-Suicide Contract in writing and in his own words. Give the client the original and put a copy in the client's chart. **Rationale**: When the contract is in writing and the client has a copy, he will be more likely to follow through with his promise to not commit suicide.

---

unlocked, and it may or may not have furnishings. The purpose of seclusion is to provide security, to remove the client from a situation of escalating anger and violence, and to remove the client who is hypersensitive to environmental stimuli from the stimulation of a hospital unit. Seclusion, like the use of physical restraints, can be used only when all other avenues for control have been exhausted. The client must be told what is happening and why. He must not be left alone; a staff member should be assigned to observe the client, usually from the doorway. Seclusion is an enforced "time-out," where the client is removed from the situation only long enough to allow him to calm down, regain a sense of control, and then reenter the unit.

Therapy Psychotherapy is often indicated and initially may focus on personal and social conditions that bring about and/or perpetuate suicidal thoughts. Cognitive-behavioral therapy may be particularly useful, as may techniques to deal with frustration and anger. Substance use and abuse are often involved and may require separate outpatient or inpatient interventions.

Pharmacological

The severely agitated, aggressive, suicidal, and/or homicidal client who is violent or threatening violence may require a medication with strong anxiolytic (antianxiety) and/or sedative properties, such as one of the antianxiety agents or a sedative-hypnotic (refer back to Table 45-2). Additionally, the suicidal client who is depressed may be evaluated for treatment with one of the many available antidepressants such as fluoxetine hydrochloride (Prozac), sertraline hydrochloride (Zoloft), paroxetine hydrochloride (Paxil), fluvoxamine maleate (Luvox), mirtazapine (Remeron), or one of the many others (refer back to Tables 45-4, 45-5, 45-6, and 45-7).

Diet

Foods are not necessarily restricted for the client who is severely agitated, aggressive, actively suicidal, and/or homicidal; however, the food tray should be inspected for any potentially dangerous objects such as glassware or silverware. Even plasticware can be broken in such a way as to yield a very dangerous weapon for hurting self or others.

Activity

The activity level of the client who is severely agitated, aggressive, actively suicidal, and/or homicidal their may need to be restricted for a period of time in order to maintain the client's safety and the safety of others.

▶ NURSING PROCESS

▶ Assessment

▶ Subjective Data

The client who is severely agitated, aggressive, and/or homicidal may argue, yell, curse, and make numerous verbal threats in a loud voice. The suicidal client may indicate intentions verbally, nonverbally, or a combination of the two. The client contemplating suicide may verbalize his thoughts either directly or indirectly. A direct statement may be something as straightforward as "I am planning to kill myself." An indirect statement might be "I'm not going to be around here anymore" or "Everyone will be better off without me" (Gorman, Sultan, & Raines, 1996).

▶ Objective Data

The client who is severely agitated, aggressive, and/or homicidal may exhibit restlessness, pacing, and "poor impulse control"; may be physically intimidating; and may use or try to use a variety of available weapons such as books, furniture, or a coffee pot (Gorman et al., 1996). A nonverbal signal of possible intentions of suicide may be seen in the client who begins making arrangements for people and pets to be taken care of, putting personal affairs in order, and giving away personal possessions, especially treasured items.

Nursing diagnoses for the client who is severely agitated, aggressive, actively suicidal, and/or homicidal may include the following:

Nursing Diagnoses	Planning/Goals	Nursing Interventions
Violence, Risk for, Self-Directed, related to risk factors such as mental health, emotional status, or suicidal plan.	The client will not harm self.	Assess for the presence of suicidal thoughts and whether a specific plan is present (Badger, 1995).
		Evaluate the degree of risk associated with the client's verbalization of suicide intent.
		Contact the attending physician or psychiatrist and inform of the client's intentions and current condition (Isaacs, 1998).
		Assess and evaluate the client's surroundings and environment for any potentially dangerous items or objects that could be used for self-harm.
		Remove or secure any potentially harmful items after thoroughly evaluating the situation (Badger, 1995).
		Increase the level of observation so that the client is frequently monitored (Badger, 1995).
		Assist the client in developing a No-suicide Contract (Badger, 1995).
Violence, Risk for, Directed at Others, related to risk factors such as history of violence against others, suicidal behavior, impulsivity.	The client will not harm anyone.	Assess for the presence of homicidal ideations.
		If the client is verbalizing a plan to harm someone, immediately notify the proper authorities so they can alert this individual.

Evaluation Each goal must be evaluated to determine how it has been met by the client.

SAMPLE NURSING CARE PLAN

THE SUICIDAL CLIENT WITH MAJOR DEPRESSION

Alice is a 27-year-old female who was brought to the emergency department of a county hospital by ambulance following a serious suicide attempt via ingesting a bottle of insecticide. After being treated in the emergency room, she spent 2 days in the intensive care unit (ICU) and then was transferred to a locked

continued

adult inpatient psychiatric unit for evaluation and treatment. Alice reports she became suicidal following the recent ending of a 4 year relationship with her boyfriend and decided to take her life because she felt "completely hopeless," that "there was nothing left to live for," that "no one would miss her" if she were dead, that she "would never be loved," and that she "could never be happy again." Prior to the suicide attempt, Alice reports that she had not been eating, had only been sleeping 1 to 2 hours per night, and had been crying almost continuously throughout the day. Since admission to the psychiatric unit, Alice has been started on sertraline (Zoloft).

Nursing Diagnosis 1 *Violence, Risk for, Self-directed, related to recent loss, feelings of abandonment, and impulsive behavior as evidenced by suicide attempt of drinking bottle of insecticide, verbalizations that "there was nothing left to live for" and that "no one would miss her" if she were dead*

PLANNING/GOALS	NURSING INTERVENTIONS	RATIONALE	EVALUATION
Alice will verbalize that she is no longer at risk of harming herself.	Assist Alice in developing a No-suicide Contract. Obtain in writing if possible, make a copy for her chart, and give her the original.	A written No-suicide Contract may help deter self-destructive behavior in the future.	At the time of discharge from the adult inpatient psychiatric unit, Alice was no longer actively suicidal or intent upon harming herself. She still had occasional suicidal ideations; however, she did not feel compelled to act on them. She had made a promise to herself that she would never try to kill herself again no matter what happened, and that if those thoughts returned, she would find someone to talk to before she did anything. She also had developed a written list of friends and relatives she could call if she again experienced thoughts of suicide.
	Explore with Alice factors that contributed to her becoming suicidal.	Knowledge of those things that led to the current suicide attempt can be the first step in preventing another.	
	Encourage Alice to verbalize her feelings related to the recent break-up and to explore any unresolved past issues that this loss might have triggered.	Current feelings of loss and abandonment are often magnified and intensified by unresolved past situations and circumstances that were never effectively handled.	
	Explore with Alice her usual methods of coping with stressful situations and whether these have been effective for her.	Looking at one's behaviors and their effectiveness or ineffectiveness can lead to a better understanding of those behaviors that must be changed.	
	Assist Alice in identifying and then developing stress-management methods as alternatives to attempting suicide.	Identifying healthier behaviors is necessary before any changes can be made. This assists the client in recognizing alternate methods of managing stressful situations.	
	Assist Alice in developing a suicide-prevention plan and in identifying	Plans to prevent suicide must be developed ahead of time, because	

continued

supportive individuals and resources that she can turn to in the event that she begins to again have suicidal thoughts.

individuals contemplating suicide are impulsive and unable to problem solve or think clearly. They may, however, be able to follow through with a previously defined plan of action.

Teach Alice about possible side effects associated with sertraline (Zoloft), such as nausea and GI upset, and encourage her to have something to eat prior to taking this medication.

Medication education is an integral part of treatment.

Emphasize the importance of taking this medication as prescribed and not stopping the medication on her own, even if she starts to feel better and thinks that she no longer needs it.

Clients often stop taking prescribed medications when their symptoms disappear, because they think that the medications are no longer needed. However, if medications are discontinued prematurely, symptoms usually reappear and are often much more serious.

Encourage Alice to keep a journal to reflect on her thoughts and feelings.

Writing in a journal can be a safe and effective method of identifying, expressing, and releasing feelings and emotions.

Encourage Alice to keep follow-up appointments for medication to monitor progress.

Follow-up appointments for medication are recommended to evaluate effectiveness and to monitor for any side effects.

Assist Alice in setting up an appointment for outpatient counseling/therapy upon discharge per recommendation from the treatment team. Encourage Alice to keep counseling appointments.

Follow-up treatment with counseling and/or therapy is recommended after a suicide attempt in order to address the underlying issues and to prevent future attempts.

continued

Nursing Diagnosis 2 *Hopelessness related to feelings of loss about her life and future as evidenced by verbalizations of feeling: "completely hopeless," that she "would never be loved," and that she "could never be happy again"*

PLANNING/GOALS	NURSING INTERVENTIONS	RATIONALE	EVALUATION
Alice will be less hopeless as indicated by verbalizations of plans for her future.	Develop a therapeutic nurse–client relationship with Alice utilizing the components of trust, rapport, respect, genuineness, and empathy.	Implementing the components of trust, rapport, respect, genuineness, and empathy will foster the development of a therapeutic nurse–client relationship.	Alice continued to have fleeting thoughts of hopelessness as far as ever having another significant relationship or being in love again; however, she now was beginning to catch herself and could identify these thoughts as being irrational and negative in nature and not helpful to her in any way.
	Encourage Alice to become involved in activities on the unit, for example, interacting with staff and other clients and attending and participating in therapy groups and recreational activities.	Being involved in some type of activity helps distract the mind from a preoccupation with losses, overwhelming feelings of depression, and suicidal ideations.	
	Provide things for Alice to do when she is feeling down, for example, go for a walk with the staff, read a newspaper or book, or play a game.	Clients who are severely depressed and suicidal have tunnel vision and are unable to see any other options or choices available to them. It is important to somehow buy enough time to allow for something to shift for them—for them to see the situation as not so utterly and permanently hopeless or for them to begin to feel better and think differently once they have started responding to medication.	
	Provide a message of hope for the future, for example, "Things might look a little different tomorrow."		
	Assist Alice in identifying the irrational beliefs or thoughts that she is having, for example, when she says no one will *ever* love or want her again.	Cognitive theory states that it is the thoughts or messages that we tell ourselves in our heads that cause us to feel a certain way. Therefore, if we change the way we are thinking by replacing irrational thoughts with rational or healthier ones, we will change the way we feel (Ellis, 1975).	

THE CLIENT WHO IS PSYCHOTIC

Psychosis is a state wherein an individual loses the ability to recognize reality. A psychotic person may experience hallucinations, wherein he hears voices or sees images of persons or things that others cannot see or hear. A psychotic person is frequently unable to care for basic needs of safety, security, nutrition, and so on. Such an individual is hospitalized for their own safety and to initiate treatment (usually involving some form of medication) to bring the symptoms under control. A psychotic person may slip into and out of reality.

Psychosis can be a component of several different psychiatric illnesses. In addition to Panic Anxiety and Major Depressive Disorder, other psychiatric diagnoses, including Schizophrenia and Bipolar Disorder, may involve psychosis.

THE CLIENT WITH SCHIZOPHRENIA

The client with schizophrenia can be very difficult to understand and treat. One of the reasons for this is that the symptoms of schizophrenia can be confusing and frightening to caregivers. Clients with schizophrenia frequently have belief systems that have become distorted in some manner, so that they hold firmly to false ideas or delusions, even when presented with evidence to the contrary. When confronted with an opposing belief system, they may become even more entrenched in their mistaken views and begin to believe others are "against them," when, in fact, they are not. Unfortunately, this makes them even more paranoid and suspicious, adding further to their already distorted views of reality. As a result, these individuals are often struggling to determine the difference between that which is real and that which is unreal or delusional.

Hallucinations can occur in relation to any of the five senses (hearing, sight, touch, taste, and smell), but the most common types of hallucinations are auditory and visual. Individuals experiencing **auditory hallucinations** think they are hearing someone talk to them, when, in reality, no one is. The voice may be that of someone the individual recognizes, or the voice may be unknown to the person. If the voice or voices are comforting, the individual will be very resistant to "giving them up." Most of the time, however, the voices are derogatory in nature, telling the person that there is something wrong with him. The most serious type of hallucination is referred to as the **command hallucination**, which occurs when the voice or voices tell the individual to harm himself or someone else in some manner. For example, the voices may tell the individual

to jump off of a bridge or building, step in front of a moving motor vehicle, or take an overdose of medication. These hallucinations are extremely dangerous because the demands are so strong that the individual is very likely to act on them.

The individual experiencing a **visual hallucination** will perceive or see someone or something that is not actually there. Depending on the nature of the hallucination and whether the individual perceives it as threatening, the situation can be very frightening.

Medical–Surgical Management

Medical

At this time, there is unfortunately no cure for schizophrenia; however, it is possible for a number of these individuals to lead functional lives with minimally debilitating symptoms through psychosocial treatments.

The goals of psychosocial treatment interventions can be conceived in a number of different ways, but one useful approach has been to divide interventions into three categories: clinical and family support services, rehabilitative services, and humanitarian aid/public safety (Hargreaves & Shumway, 1989). The goal of clinical interventions is to reduce both positive and negative symptoms and to maximize functional outcome. Clinical support involves outpatient management and family/community services. Rehabilitation involves increasing clients' capacities, both for social interactions and for productive activity (including gainful employment, when feasible). Humanitarian interventions are those efforts that maximize an individual's independence and quality of life within the bounds of her mental disability. Public safety involves balancing personal liberty with the recognition that some social control may be needed to prevent harm, both to the individual and to society.

Electroconvulsive therapy (ECT) may be a consideration for the client in the acute phase of schizophrenia; however, ECT is contraindicated in cases of chronic schizophrenia, as it has not proven to be effective for this disorder (Endler & Persad, 1988).

Pharmacological

The most commonly prescribed classification of medications for the client experiencing schizophrenia is the antipsychotics (Tables 45-9 and 45-10). This group of medications is given to reduce the signs and symptoms of psychosis, with a long-term goal of the client eventually being symptom free. If this is not possible, the goal is to reduce symptoms to a manageable level.

Because a number of side effects are associated with the antipsychotics, client teaching is an important part of the nurse's role. In addition to common side effects, some antipsychotic medications also have the potential for causing adverse reactions such as

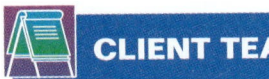

CLIENT TEACHING

Adverse Reactions to Antipsychotic Medications

- *Extra-pyramidal side effects:* a common adverse reaction of some antipsychotic medications (especially the older ones) involving muscle rigidity and involuntary muscle movements; reversible if the dose is lowered or an antiparkinson agent is administered
- *Tardive dyskinesia:* irreversible reaction to antipsychotics (usually associated with high doses over a long period of time) consisting of involuntary muscle and body movements
- *Neuroleptic malignant syndrome:* a rare and potentially fatal reaction to antipsychotic medications characterized by a very high fever, severe muscle stiffness, and changes in sensorium progressing to coma

extrapyramidal symptoms (EPS), tardive dyskinesia (TD), and neuroleptic-malignant-syndrome (NMS).

One of the most important factors in symptom management for schizophrenia is medication compliance. In most cases, individuals who are schizophrenic must

Table 45-9 ATYPICAL ANTIPSYCHOTICS

GENERIC NAME	TRADE NAME	POTENTIAL SIDE EFFECTS
clozapine	Clozaril	Agranulocytosis, constipation, dizziness, EPS, hypotension, increased salivation, leukopenia, NMS, sedation, seizures, tachycardia, weight gain
olanzapine	Zyprexa	Agitation, amblyopia, constipation, dizziness, dry mouth, headache, NMS, orthostatic hypotension, restlessness, rhinitis, sedation, seizures, tachycardia, TD, tremors, weakness, weight gain
quetiapine fumerate	Seroquel	Dizziness, EPS, NMS, seizures, TD, weight gain
risperidone	Risperdal	Aggressive behavior, constipation, cough, decreased libido, diarrhea, dizziness, dry mouth, dysmenorrhea/menorrhagia, EPS, headache, increased dreams, increased sleep duration, insomnia, itching/skin rash, nausea, NMS, pharyngitis, rhinitis, sedation, visual disturbances, weight gain

Compiled from Davis's Drug Guide for Nurses *(6th ed.), by J. H. Deglin and A. H. Vallerand, 1999, Philadelphia: F. A. Davis.*

CLIENT TEACHING

Atypical Antipsychotics

Be sure to instruct each client taking an atypical antipsychotic medication in the following:

- Do not drink alcohol while taking the medication.
- Do not take any other medications, prescription or OTC, unless prescribed by your physician.
- Do not stop taking the medication without authorization from your physician.
- Do not stop taking the medication abruptly.
- The ability to drive and/or operate heavy machinery may be impaired while taking the medication.
- Rise slowly from a lying position to prevent dizziness and a sudden drop in blood pressure.
- The medication is contraindicated during pregnancy and lactation. Reliable contraception should be utilized while taking the medication. Female clients should advise their physicians immediately if they suspect they are either pregnant or planning to become pregnant.
- Be aware of the potential side effects of the medications.
- Notify your physician immediately of unexplained fever, sore throat, bleeding, bruising, or petechiae.
- Wear sunscreen and protective clothing while outdoors, as olanzapine (Zyprexa) and risperidone (Risperdal) increase susceptibility to sunburn.
- Avoid temperature extremes if taking olanzapine (Zyprexa), quetiapine fumerate (Seroquel), or risperidone (Risperdal), as the body's ability to regulate internal temperature is affected by these medications.
- Utilize good oral hygiene in conjunction with sugarless candy or gum to minimize the discomforting side effect of dry mouth associated most frequently with clozapine (Clozaril) and olanzapine (Zyprexa).
- Beware of associated risks including EPS, NMS, and a high risk of agranulocytosis and seizures with clozapine (Clozaril); EPS, TD, and NMS with olanzapine (Zyprexa), quetiapine (Seroquel), and risperidone (Risperdal); and seizures with olanzapine (Zyprexa) and quetiapine fumerate (Seroquel).
- Treatment with clozapine (Clozaril) requires *weekly* white blood cell (WBC) monitoring to assess for onset of agranulocytosis. Medication is dispensed in 7-day increments to maintain policy compliance and prevent this potentially life-threatening occurrence.

Table 45-10 PHENOTHIAZINES (ANTIPSYCHOTICS)

GENERIC NAME	TRADE NAME	POTENTIAL SIDE EFFECTS
chlorpro-mazine	Thorazine	Agranulocytosis, blurred vision, constipation, dry eyes, dry mouth, hypotension, NMS, photosensitivity, sedation, TD
fluphenazine hydrochloride	Prolixin	Agranulocytosis, EPS, photosensitivity, TD
thioridazine hydrochloride	Mellaril	Agranulocytosis, blurred vision, constipation, dry eyes, dry mouth, hypotension, NMS, photosensitivity, sedation, TD

Compiled from Davis's Drug Guide for Nurses *(6th ed.), by J. H. Deglin and A. H. Vallerand, 1999, Philadelphia: F. A. Davis.*

take some type of antipsychotic medication for the remainder of their lives. Clients suffering from schizophrenia are often extremely resistant to taking their medications as prescribed and usually require multiple repeat hospitalizations for stabilization. Multiple reasons exist for noncompliance, one being the client's denial of the diagnosis or the illness itself or of the seriousness of the illness. As a result of denial, the individual with schizophrenia resists taking medication, because to the client, taking medication equates to acceptance of having a serious mental disorder. Clients may also become noncompliant after a period of time on medication; once they start to feel better, they think the medication is no longer needed and stop taking it. After a short time of being off the prescribed medication, however, most individuals with schizophrenia will experience a return or significant worsening of their previous symptoms.

Probably the most common reason for medication noncompliance, however, is the number of troublesome side effects and potentially dangerous adverse reactions historically associated with antipsychotic medications. Fortunately, a number of newer antipsychotic medications are now available that have fewer side effects and are much better tolerated. Even with the advent of these newer and more effective medications, however, many individuals are unable to benefit from them due to the high cost and the difficulties sometimes associated with accessing these medications.

Diet

Some of the antipsychotics such as clozapine (Clozaril), olanzapine (Zyprexa), quetiapine fumerate (Seroquel), and risperidone (Risperdal) can cause weight gain over time. For the individual who has schizophrenia and its multiple associated problems, weight gain can constitute yet one more stressor. Teaching for

CLIENT TEACHING

Phenothiazines

Be sure to instruct each client taking a phenothiazine medication in the following:

- Do not drink alcohol while on the medication.
- Do not take any other medications unless prescribed by your physician.
- Do not stop taking the medication abruptly.
- The ability to drive and/or operate heavy machinery may be impaired while taking the medication.
- Be aware of possible side effects of the medication.
- Increase fluid intake to minimize the side effects of dry mouth and constipation.
- Increase dietary fiber to minimize the side effect of constipation.
- Rise slowly from a lying position to prevent dizziness and a sudden drop in blood pressure.
- These medications are contraindicated during pregnancy and lactation. Female clients should advise their physicians immediately if they are either pregnant or planning to become pregnant.
- Wear sunscreen and protective clothing while outdoors, as the medication increases susceptibility to sunburn.
- Some of the side effects may diminish in intensity after an initial period of adjustment.
- The medication may increase your risk of developing EPS, TD, and NMS.

the client who is at risk for gaining weight must therefore emphasize the importance of being cognizant of and conservative with regard to caloric and fat intake,

CLIENT TEACHING

Schizophrenia

Family involvement is important for all clients, but it is especially critical for the client with schizophrenia. Because the client may be too ill or confused to be trusted to take medications reliably, it becomes the responsibility of family members to help ensure medication compliance. Most hospital readmissions for the client with schizophrenia are due to noncompliance with the prescribed medication regimen. If the family understands the important role psychotropic medications can play in preventing decompensation (a return of the psychiatric symptoms) and subsequent hospital readmission, the client has a much better chance of remaining stabilized.

avoiding a sedentary lifestyle, and increasing physical activity.

Activity

Clients with schizophrenia tend to be tired and lethargic, probably due to multiple factors including the disease process and, possibly, the sedative properties associated with some of the antipsychotics, especially some of the older ones such as chlorpromazine (Thorazine) and thioridazine (Mellaril).

▶ NURSING PROCESS

▶ Assessment

▶ Subjective Data

The client with schizophrenia may be very frightened, confused, and disorganized in thought process. The client may use a nonsensical combination of words that is meaningless to others (**word salad**), talk out loud even when no one is present, or respond to internal stimulation or hallucinations.

▶ Objective Data

The client with schizophrenia may be isolated, withdrawn, and experience great difficulty in any type

PROFESSIONAL TIP

Refraining from Making Judgments

Sometimes nurses stereotype clients and may make judgments based on their own values, cultural biases, and personal beliefs. Such behavior can adversely affect their work with clients. The nurse's words can have a strong impact on the client, either favorable or unfavorable, even without the nurse's being aware of it. Something as simple as changing the words we use may help the client and family feel less defensive and may open the door for more effective communication. One example of an often-used term that carries negative connotations is *noncompliance*. Ward-Collins (1998) encourages nurses to consider using another term such as *nonadherence*, which does not carry the same degree of negative connotations.

of social interaction or situation. The client may be very lethargic and not want to do much of anything except stay in bed and sleep. Thus, the client may require a great deal of assistance and encouragement to perform ADL and complete basic hygiene needs.

Nursing diagnoses for the client with schizophrenia may include the following:

Nursing Diagnoses	Planning/Goals	Nursing Interventions
▶ *Sensory/Perceptual Alterations, Visual and Auditory, related to altered sensory perception*	The client will experience a decrease in the intensity and frequency of symptoms.	Assess for the presence of hallucinations. Assist the client in beginning to exert some control over the hallucinations. Educate the client about ways to decrease the intensity and power of the hallucinations.
▶ *Knowledge Deficit, related to medication therapy*	Client will verbalize an understanding of the disorder and the ongoing need for medications.	Educate the client and family about the disorder of schizophrenia. Educate the client and family about the need for antipsychotic medications. Educate the client and family about the importance of continuing the prescribed medication regimen.

Evaluation Each goal must be evaluated to determine how it has been met by the client.

THE CLIENT WITH BIPOLAR DISORDER

Bipolar Disorder (previously known as manic–depressive disorder) is a psychiatric diagnosis characterized by wide fluctuations in **mood** (the way an individual reports feeling, e.g., depressed, elated, happy, sad) and **affect** (the objective or outward manifestation of the way an individual is feeling, e.g., avoids eye contact, smiles occasionally). In addition to having a

wide range of both affect and mood, the individual with bipolar disorder may experience fluctuations between depression and **mania** (extremely elevated mood with accompanying agitated behavior). The client with bipolar disorder may experience these fluctuations in mood and affect in varying degrees and over varying time frames. For example, an individual may experience changes in mood and affect every few years, at certain times of the year, every few months, every few weeks, or even every few days. The alterations in mood between depression and mania are often referred to as **cycling**. Individuals who suffer what is known as rapid cycling may experience multiple swings between depression and mania in the same day. There are also several degrees of both depression and mania that the individual can experience. As is the case with depression, an individual can experience mild, moderate, or severe mania. The degrees of mania range on a continuum from **hypomania** (a mild form of mania without significant impairment) to severe or delirious mania (Goodwin & Jamison, 1990).

An individual in the depressed phase of bipolar disorder will manifest the same signs and symptoms as an individual with depression. The client in the manic phase of bipolar disorder may be very irritable and agitated and can be intimidating toward others, both verbally and physically. The client exhibiting manic behavior is often hyperactive, unable to sit down or remain still, and may display a **euphoric** (being elated out of context to the situation) affect and mood. Once in the manic phase of illness, clients will often exhibit behaviors incongruent with their usual personalities. For example, the manic client may dress in a flamboyant and provocative manner; spend money and buy things in a very lavish fashion; and become sexually promiscuous and engage in risky behaviors that would otherwise be out of character. After a while, the client in the manic phase of bipolar disorder can experience a great deal of conflict in social, familial, and personal relationships. It often becomes the responsibility of a significant other or family member to seek professional assistance for the individual. This already difficult situation is compounded by the fact that the client in the manic phase of bipolar disorder is frequently in denial about the illness, does not perceive the erratic behavior as problematic, and enjoys the "high" created by the disorder. As a result, the individual often refuses any type of help, and the family may be required to seek involuntary hospitalization in order to obtain the much-needed treatment.

Medical–Surgical Management

Medical

The severely agitated client in the manic phase of bipolar disorder may need to be secluded and/or re-strained in order to protect against self-inflicted injury and/or the risk of injury to others.

Psychotherapy may be helpful to the client experiencing bipolar disorder, but it is not recommended as the only intervention. These clients typically require some type of medication management for the remainder of their lives in order to function adequately.

Pharmacological

The drug of choice for treatment of bipolar disorder is lithium carbonate (Lithonate) (Table 45-11). Lithium is a naturally occurring salt that has proven highly effective for many individuals in managing the severe mood swings associated with bipolar disorder. Lithium is referred to as a "mood stabilizer," meaning that it helps level or even out the wide mood swings associated with the disorder. However, some individuals

CLIENT TEACHING

Lithium

Be sure to instruct each client taking lithium in the following:

- Do not drink alcohol while taking this medication.
- Do not take any other medications, prescribed or OTC, unless authorized by your physician.
- Do not stop taking this medication without authorization from your physician.
- Female clients should utilize a reliable form of contraception while taking this medication. Immediately inform your physician if pregnancy is suspected.
- Drink 2,000 to 3,000 cc of fluid (9–10 glasses) per day.
- Maintain a consistent level of salt in the diet.
- The ability to drive or operate heavy machinery may be impaired while on this medication.
- Serum lithium level must be checked at scheduled intervals throughout therapy.
- Be aware of signs and symptoms of lithium toxicity.

Table 45-11 MOOD STABILIZER: ANTIMANIC			
GENERIC NAME	**TRADE NAME**	**POTENTIAL SIDE EFFECTS**	**SIGNS AND SYMPTOMS OF TOXICITY**
lithium carbonate	Eskalith, Lithane, Lithonate	Abdominal pain, acneiform eruption, anorexia, arrhythmia, bloating, diarrhea, dizziness, drowsiness, EKG changes, fatigue, folliculitis, GI upset, headache, hypothyroidism, impaired memory, irritability, leukocytosis, muscle weakness, nausea, polyuria, seizures, tinnitus, tremors	Ataxia, change in level of orientation, confusion, diarrhea, drowsiness, excessive urination, lack of coordination, muscle weakness, tremors, vomiting

Compiled from *Davis's Drug Guide for Nurses* (6th ed.), by J. H. Deglin and A. H. Vallerand, 1999, Philadelphia: F. A. Davis.

either cannot tolerate lithium therapy or become resistant to its therapeutic effectiveness after a period of time. Fortunately, there are some other medications that are often prescribed for clients who cannot take lithium. These include the anticonvulsants valproic acid (Depakene) and carbamazepine (Tegretol) and the anxiolytic/anticonvulsant clonazepam (Klonopin) (Table 45-12).

Lithium has a very narrow range of therapeutic effectiveness. The amount of lithium the individual has available and whether this level is appropriate is measured by a blood test called **serum lithium level**. As a rule of thumb, the acceptable therapeutic range for the serum lithium level is 0.5 to 1.5mEq/L; however, the value may vary slightly depending on the laboratory that is performing the test (Deglin & Vallerand, 1999). A lithium level that is too low will not produce any benefit, and one that is too high may be **toxic**, or poisonous. It is therefore critical that the serum lithium level be obtained every 5 days until the client is stabilized on the medication. Blood should then be

Table 45-12	MOOD STABILIZERS: ANTICONVULSANTS	
GENERIC NAME	**TRADE NAME**	**POTENTIAL SIDE EFFECTS**
carbamazepine	Tegretol	Aganulocytosis, aplastic anemia, ataxia, drowsiness, drug-induced hepatitis, thrombocytopenia
valproic acid	Depakene	Confusion, dizziness, indigestion, hepatotoxicity, leukopenia, nausea, thrombocytopenia, vomiting

Compiled from Davis's Drug Guide for Nurses *(6th ed.), by J. H. Deglin and A. H. Vallerand, 1999, Philadelphia: F. A. Davis.*

drawn at regular intervals, approximately every 12 to 16 weeks, for as long as the client is taking the medication (Bailey, 1998). Prior to initiating lithium therapy, a 24-hour urine creatinine clearance test is done to evaluate the functioning of the kidneys and their ability to adequately excrete the lithium.

Diet

Because lithium is a salt that is chemically similar to sodium chloride (table salt), lithium and sodium compete for absorption at receptor sites. This relationship is inversely proportional; thus, any changes in the body's sodium level will directly affect lithium level. Adequate fluid intake is very important for the client on lithium therapy. It is recommended that the client taking lithium consume a minimum of 2,000 to 3,000 cc of water per day. Due to the stimulating effects of caffeine, clients taking lithium should avoid any beverages containing caffeine.

Activity

The balance of sodium chloride to lithium can also be affected by the client's level of activity. An increase in activity, especially in hot and/or humid conditions when excessive perspiration is likely, can deplete the client's sodium level, thereby causing a drastic increase in lithium level and, potentially, lithium toxicity. A sudden increase in a client's activity level requires close monitoring and replacement of both fluid and electrolytes in order to prevent a sudden increase in the lithium level.

CLIENT TEACHING

Anticonvulsants

Be sure to instruct each client taking an anticonvulsant medication in the following:

- Do not drink alcohol while taking the medication.
- Do not take any other medications, prescribed or OTC, unless authorized by your physician.
- Take the medication exactly as prescribed.
- Do not stop taking the medication without authorization from your physician.
- Do not stop taking the medication abruptly.
- The medications is contraindicated during pregnancy and lactation. Female clients should advise their physicians immediately if they are either pregnant or planning to become pregnant.
- Carbamazepine (Tegretol) can impair the effectiveness of hormonal forms of contraception. Female clients should practice an alternate form of birth control while on this medication.
- The ability to drive or operate heavy machinery may be impaired while on the medication.
- Laboratory tests monitoring complete blood count (CBC), platelet count, bleeding time, and hepatic functioning must be performed periodically throughout therapy.
- Notify your physician immediately of unexplained fever, sore throat, bleeding, bruising, or petechiae.
- Serum level must be checked at scheduled intervals throughout therapy.

LIFE CYCLE CONSIDERATIONS

Creatinine Clearance

Because elders have reduced creatinine clearance, they are at a greater risk for developing toxicity while taking lithium (Andresen, 1998).

▶ NURSING PROCESS

▶ Assessment

▶ Subjective Data

The client with bipolar disorder may deny having a problem or may view the problem as residing in other people. The client may also be quite loud, flamboyant, and grandiose in verbalizations and manifest very quick and **pressured speech** (rapid, intense speech).

▶ Objective Data

The client may be sleeping very little or not at all and may not be eating or drinking, if in the manic phase. The client may at times be very irritable, agitated, quick to anger, and, possibly, violent. Clients with bipolar disorder often have extreme difficulty in interpersonal and social relationships, as they have no personal boundaries. They may also be very invasive and intrusive in their interactions with others, both verbally and physically.

Nursing diagnoses for the client with bipolar disorder may include the following:

Nursing Diagnoses	Planning/Goals	Nursing Interventions
▶ *Sleep Pattern Disturbance, related to sensory alterations*	The client will sleep 6 hours per night.	Provide a quiet, peaceful environment.
		Decrease external stimulation and environmental distractions.
		Teach client relaxation exercises.
▶ *Noncompliance (medication and treatment regimen) related to health beliefs*	The client will demonstrate increased compliance with medication and treatment.	Educate the client and family about the disease process and the progression of the illness over time.
		Educate the client and family about prescribed medication, indications for use, dosage, times, and any possible side effects or untoward reactions.
		Educate the client and family about the importance of taking the medication as prescribed.
		Teach the client to continue taking medication and to not miss doses *even if the condition improves dramatically.*

Evaluation Each goal must be evaluated to determine how it has been met by the client.

THE CLIENT REQUIRING SPECIAL CONSIDERATION

Several categories of psychiatric disorders require special attention and consideration on the part of the nurse. These include disorders commonly associated with childhood and adolescence and with individuals who have been violated in some manner, such as via neglect and/or abuse.

THE CLIENT WITH ATTENTION-DEFICIT/HYPERACTIVITY DISORDER

The *DSM-IV* identifies 18 diagnostic criteria for Attention-Deficit/Hyperactivity Disorder (ADHD) that fall under the categories of *inattention, hyperactivity,* and *impulsivity* (APA, 1994). There are three varieties of Attention-Deficit/Hyperactivity Disorder listed in the *DSM-IV:* Attention-Deficit/Hyperactivity Disorder, Pre-

dominantly Hyperactive-Impulsive Type; Attention-Deficit/Hyperactivity Disorder, Predominantly Inattentive Type; and Attention-Deficit/Hyperactivity Disorder, Combined Type. The child with ADHD may exhibit one or more of these behaviors in any combination (inattention, hyperactivity, and impulsivity). The problematic behaviors associated with these disorders vary in severity for each individual. Once thought to be a disorder only of childhood, it is now known that ADHD may continue well into adulthood. Individuals with ADHD are extremely sensitive to their environments and surroundings and respond immediately to any type of stimuli or distraction that most individuals would not even notice.

PREDOMINANTLY HYPERACTIVE-IMPULSIVE TYPE

As the name suggests, hyperactivity is considered to be a hallmark feature of Predominantly Hyperactive-

Impulsive Type ADHD, which is usually diagnosed in childhood when the symptoms first manifest. The pediatric client with ADHD may be referred for evaluation and treatment by parents or teachers because of impulsive and disruptive behavior in the classroom setting and/or at home. Research indicates that among the children with ADHD, the ratio of males to females ranges anywhere from 4 : 1 to 9 : 1 (APA, 1994). In many cases, there seems to be a familial or possible genetic link, as seen in health histories, which often reveal a parent or immediate family member as having had a similar problem as a child.

PREDOMINANTLY INATTENTIVE TYPE

In some children with ADHD predominantly inattentive type, the symptom of hyperactivity is not always present. This is the case in children who have problems primarily with attention span. The inattentive child cannot maintain attention on one task, does not appear to listen when spoken to, and is easily distracted and forgetful.

COMBINED TYPE

As the name suggests, children with ADHD of the combined type exhibit symptoms of hyperactivity, impulsivity, and inattention. The characteristics must typically be exhibited for a period of at least 6 months in order to qualify for the diagnosis.

Medical–Surgical Management

Medical

Counseling and therapy are often recommended to the client and family to assist in managing the child with this disorder. The parents will require assistance in developing an effective behavior-modification program, such as a token-economy system that rewards desired behaviors, to help manage some of the child's problematic behaviors (Glod, 1997).

Pharmacological

The central nervous system (CNS) stimulants, which include methylphenidate hydrochloride (Ritalin), pemoline (Cylert), dextroamphetamine (Dexedrine), and, most recently, a combination of both dextroamphetamine and amphetamine (Adderal), is the class of medications usually prescribed to treat ADHD (Glod, 1997) (Table 45-13). As a rule, these medications have the tendency to stimulate an individual and therefore increase activity level often to the point of hyperactivity. When one of the CNS stimulants is given to someone with ADHD, however, it has the opposite effect, or

PROFESSIONAL TIP

Token-Economy System

A token-economy system is a form of behavior modification used to shape a client's behavior over time. The client receives a "token" (poker chips work well) each time an appropriate or desired behavior is exhibited. In the classroom, the desired behavior might be working 15 minutes on a math assignment; at home, it might be picking up dirty clothes off the bedroom floor. Receiving the token is a form of positive reinforcement for the client and provides immediate gratification. At the end of a designated period of time, the client may "cash in" earned tokens for a prize (game, puzzle) or a special privilege (going to get an ice cream). The cashing in of tokens emphasizes the concept of delayed gratification, which in turn teaches patience.

paradoxical reaction. Thus, instead of making someone with ADHD more hyperactive, it actually helps calm him. Because most of the symptoms of the child with ADHD, such as hyperactivity and the inability to concentrate and remain on task, are manifested in the classroom, it is in this setting that any improvement will likely first be noted. When a child begins a new medication it is vitally important that the family communicate openly with the child's teacher to ensure close monitoring of the child's response to medication. The child with ADHD who has been hyperactive, unable to stay on task, or complete assignments before receiving medication may now be less disruptive in the classroom and better able to remain on task and complete assignments. In addition, the medication can be a useful adjunct to facilitate the child's ability to develop and strengthen internal mechanisms for improving behavior.

Teaching the client and family about the prescribed medication is very important, as there are some common side effects associated with the CNS stimulants, such as insomnia. To help decrease the risk of insomnia, these medications are usually given in the morning at breakfast, and if more is needed, another dose is given again at lunchtime. In some cases, a late-afternoon dose may be needed after school; however, this decision must be made very cautiously, because the later in the day that the dose is given, the greater the risk of insomnia that night for the child.

The client on CNS stimulants must be monitored for any vocal or motor tics, which might indicate the development of Tourette's syndrome. The CNS stimulant should be discontinued immediately if these symptoms are noted.

Table 45-13 CENTRAL NERVOUS SYSTEM STIMULANTS

GENERIC	TRADE NAME	POTENTIAL SIDE EFFECTS
dextroamphetamine	Dexedrine	Anorexia, headache, hyperactivity, hypertension, insomnia, palpitations, physical and psychological dependence, restlessness, tachycardia, tolerance, tremors, urticaria, weight loss
dextroamphetamine/amphetamine	Adderal	Anorexia, hyperactivity, insomnia, palpitations, physical and psychological dependence, restlessness, tachycardia, tremors
methylphenidate hydrochloride	Ritalin	Anemia, anorexia, hyperactivity, hypertension, insomnia, leukopenia, physical and psychological dependence, restlessness, skin rash, suppression of weight gain, tolerance, tremors
pemoline	Cylert	Anorexia, aplastic anemia, decreased growth, drug-induced hepatitis, insomnia, nausea, physical or psychological dependence, seizures, stomachache, tolerance, weight loss

Compiled from Davis's Drug Guide for Nurses *(6th ed.), by J. H. Deglin and A. H. Vallerand, 1999, Philadelphia: F. A. Davis;* Lippincott's Need-to-know Psychotropic Drug Facts, *by K. P. Bailey, 1998, Philadelphia: Lippincott; PDR Nurses Handbook, by G. Spratto and A. Woods, 1999, Albany, NY: Delmar Publishers; and "Attention Deficit Hyperactivity Disorder throughout the Lifespan: Diagnosis, Etiology, and Treatment," by C. A. Glod, 1997,* Journal of the American Psychiatric Nurses Association, 3(3), *89–92.*

Diet

One potential problem associated with the CNS stimulants is that of decreased appetite, which can become serious if the child begins losing weight as a side effect of the medication. In such an instance, the medication may need to be given immediately after a meal to decrease the chance of suppressing the appetite. The family can be educated on the need to adjust the timing and amount of food intake. The child may have to eat larger meals later in the day, when the effects of the medication have worn off, or consume a larger snack in the evening prior to bedtime.

The role and importance of diet in the management of ADHD continues to be highly controversial; however, some data supports the restriction of certain foods as an effective method of managing this disorder. Foods that contain sugar and caffeine are sometimes recommended to be excluded from the diet of the child with ADHD. The theory behind this recommendation is that sugar and caffeine tend to energize and increase any child's activity level, and in the case of some children with ADHD, this effect seems to be even more accentuated. Another controversial issue surrounding the significance of diet is that of food sensitivities and allergies. Food allergies sometimes manifest in symptoms such as irritability and hyperactivity, which may then be confused or misdiagnosed as ADHD.

Activity

The child with ADHD will usually respond best to a highly structured environment, which includes clear expectations and firm, consistent limits as well as appropriate consequences for unruly and disruptive behaviors. For example, a "time-out" may be used when the child must be temporarily removed from a setting or the environment.

 CLIENT TEACHING

CNS Stimulants

For each client taking a CNS-stimulant medication, instruct the client or, if the client is too young to understand or reliably carry out the instructions, the client's caregivers in the following:

- Take the medication only as prescribed.
- Do not take any other medications without physician approval.
- Be alert for decreased appetite and adjust meals and mealtimes accordingly.
- Do not take any doses after 5 P.M. as doing so will increase the risk of insomnia.
- Obtain periodic liver function tests if taking pemoline (Cylert).
- Obtain periodic CBC, platelet count, and differential if taking methylphenidate (Ritalin).
- Limit caffeine intake.

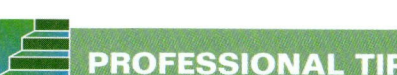 **PROFESSIONAL TIP**

CNS-Stimulant Abuse

Another consideration often overlooked in terms of the CNS stimulants is the risk for abuse due to the strong addictive potential of these medications. Not only is the client with ADHD at risk for abusing these medications, but sometimes the client "shares" prescribed medication with schoolmates and friends interested in drug experimentation. Another problem that may be encountered is abuse of the prescribed medication by a family member with a substance-abuse problem.

▶ NURSING PROCESS

▶ Assessment

▶ Subjective Data

The child or adolescent with ADHD frequently verbalizes feeling "bad" about being unable to control hyperactive and disruptive behaviors. After numerous negative encounters with teachers and the principal, the child's esteem begins to erode, and he may verbalize feeling like a failure, especially in the classroom. After only a single dose of medication, however, the child sometimes states a noticeable difference in the ability to remain centered and focused.

▶ Objective Data

Although usually described as being hyperactive, unable to concentrate, unable to focus, and unable to remain on task, children with ADHD may sometimes be able to concentrate and remain quite attentive and focused. This usually happens in situations that the child enjoys, and sometimes in situations that are new to the child. It can be quite frustrating for parents to bring in their child for an evaluation or screening, only to have the child not exhibit any of the usual problem-

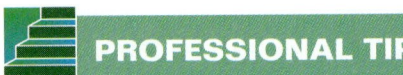

PROFESSIONAL TIP

Time-Outs

A time-out should be a consequence for an undesired behavior and should not be administered in a punitive manner. The child is asked to leave the current situation and go to a designated place, usually a specific chair or place in the room, for a brief period of time. If unable to leave in response to a verbal request, the child may need to be physically removed from the situation until calm enough to return. A rule of thumb is not to exceed 1 minute of time-out for each year of the child's age. For example, a maximum time-out for a 3-year-old child would be 3 minutes (although much less is usually indicated due to the child's inability to comprehend time), and a time-out for a 7-year-old child would never exceed 7 minutes.

atic behaviors. The knowledgeable practitioner or evaluator will be aware of what is happening and will obtain the necessary information from the parental report of the child's health history.

Nursing diagnoses for the child with ADHD may include the following:

Nursing Diagnoses	Planning/Goals	Nursing Interventions
▶ *Knowledge Deficit (medications and disease process), related to new diagnosis of disorder and treatment regimen*	The child and parents will verbalize an increased understanding of the disorder. The child and parents will verbalize an understanding about the role medications can play in treatment.	Educate the child and family about the disorder, including signs and symptoms. Educate the child and family about the medication, including indications for use, dosages, when to take the medication, and possible side effects. Educate the child and family about the benefits that can be expected with the particular medication. Emphasize the importance of taking the medication as prescribed.
▶ *Social Interaction, Impaired, related to unaccepted social behaviors*	The child will demonstrate an increase in appropriate peer interactions.	Explain to the child those behaviors that are expected. Observe the child in social situations with peers. Provide positive reinforcement for demonstration of appropriate behaviors. Immediately intervene when unacceptable behaviors are observed.

Evaluation Each goal must be evaluated to determine how it has been met by the client.

THE CLIENT EXPERIENCING NEGLECT AND/OR ABUSE

There are many types of **neglect** (a situation wherein a basic need of the client is not being provided) and **abuse** (an incident involving some type of violation to the client). Neglect can be quite evident, such as a lack of adequate food, clothing, or shelter, or less tangible, such as emotional neglect or an absence

of nurturing. Abuse can be physical, emotional, psychological, financial, or sexual in nature, or any combination of these. Abuse can also take the form of **domestic violence**, which is aggression and violence involving family members. Oftentimes, neglect and abuse go hand in hand.

A client experiencing neglect or abuse is usually dependent on another individual for the meeting of basic care and needs. In many neglectful or abusive situations, the clients are vulnerable individuals such as children, adolescents, or elders. Others who are neglected or abused include individuals with some type of illness or incapacitation. Neglect and abuse can take many shapes and forms, ranging anywhere from mild cases to situations so severe that death is the end result.

CHILD ABUSE AND NEGLECT

Parents and caregivers who physically discipline children believe that physical punishment is essential to making children responsible citizens. Most parents do not intentionally permanently injure their children. Some family violence experts believe that parents who hit their children are modeling that interpersonal violence is acceptable behavior. Spanking children may not be considered physical abuse by legal authorities, but whipping children with belts on their bare skin might legally be considered physical abuse. Psychological abuse, sexual abuse, and severe neglect can be as damaging to children as is physical abuse.

The following definitions of child abuse and neglect have been adopted from the Victims of Child Abuse Act of 1990.

- *Child abuse* is any physical or mental injury, sexual abuse, exploitation, negligent treatment, or maltreatment of a child under the age of 18 (or the age specified by the child protection law of the state in question) by a parent or parent substitute.
- *Negligent treatment* is the failure of a parent or parent substitute to provide, for reasons other than poverty, adequate food, clothing, shelter, or medical care such that the physical health of the child is seriously endangered.
- *Physical injury* includes, but is not limited to, lacerations, fractured bones, burns, internal injuries, severe bruising, or serious bodily harm.
- *Mental injury* is harm to a child's psychological or intellectual functioning. It may manifest as severe anxiety, depression, withdrawal, or outward aggressive behavior or a combination of these behaviors, which may be demonstrated by a change in behavior, emotional response, or cognition.
- *Sexual abuse* includes the employment, use, persuasion, inducement, enticement, or coercion of a child to engage in or assist another person to engage in sexually implicit conduct. It is the rape, molestation, prostitution, or other forms of sexual exploitation of children or incest with children.
- *Sexually explicit conduct* is actual or simulated sexual intercourse whether with persons of the same sex or of the opposite sex, bestiality, masturbation, lascivious exhibition of the genitals or pubic area of a person or animal, or sadistic or masochistic abuse.
- *Child molestation* is sexual involvement such as oral–genital contact, genital fondling and viewing, or masturbation.

LIFE CYCLE CONSIDERATIONS

Childhood Sexual Abuse

Children are frequently reluctant to tell anyone about sexual abuse and may keep the horrible secret for many years. Sexually abused children may not disclose the incident for a number of reasons "including fear, confusion, guilt, shame, and ignorance about the incident and who they could turn to for help" (Johnson & Cheffer, 1996). DiVitto (1998) states, "The victim of incest often experiences a secondary trauma if he or she is not believed or is blamed for the abuse by the person in whom the child has confided."

- *Sexual exploitation* is child pornography, sexually explicit reproduction of a child's image, or child prostitution (U.S. Code Annotated, Title 42, 1990, P.L. 104, pp. 4806–4807).
- *Incest* is sexual relations between children and blood relatives or surrogate family members.

All states, Washington, DC, Puerto Rico, and the Virgin Islands have statutes that mandate nurses who know or suspect child abuse to report it. The report is made to an agency designated by the state, usually the county welfare or social service's child protective unit. The laws provide that nurses who report child abuse be protected from civil and criminal liability unless they make a false report. Failure to report is a misdemeanor in many states. In an attempt to keep lines of communication open, nurses should ideally tell

PROFESSIONAL TIP

Child Abuse Reports

The report should carefully document the physical evidence of abuse and neglect without making judgments about the family. Child abuse reports should include the following:
- The name of the victim.
- Current location of the victim.
- Type of abuse you are reporting.
- Types and severity of injuries you observed.
- Parent or caregiver's account of the injuries.
- When possible, child's account of the injuries.
- The reasons you suspect the child is being abused or neglected.
- In the client's record, chart your observations and your report to the child protective agency.

From Psychiatric Mental Health Nursing, *by N. Frisch and L. Frisch, 1998, Albany, NY: Delmar Publishers.*

abusive parents that they are legally required to report the suspected child abuse. Nurses should not, however, put themselves at risk for injury if they think that informing families will lead to personal harm (Frisch & Frisch, 1998).

ELDER ABUSE AND NEGLECT

Elder abuse became nationally recognized in 1981 after the House Select Committee on Aging issued its landmark report *Elder Abuse: An Examination of a Hidden Problem*. The committee found that elder abuse was simply "alien to the American ideal." Because it is such a difficult concept to come to grips with, even abused elders are reluctant to admit their loved ones have abused them.

The committee defined the following types of elder abuse: physical, passive physical, financial, psychological, sexual, and violation of rights. There is no federal legislation to protect elders from abuse, neglect, or exploitation. Forty-eight states, including the District of Columbia, have laws that offer some form of protection for elders or dependent adults. Adult abuse and protection laws are based on the legal premise that society (represented by the state) has the authority to act in a parental capacity for persons who are unable to care for and protect themselves and thus prevent them from suffering from abuse, neglect, or exploitation by those responsible for their care or from self-abuse (Frisch & Frisch, 1998). The purposes of adult protection service laws are to facilitate the identification of functionally impaired elders who are being abused, neglected, or exploited by others; to encourage expeditious reporting; and to extend protective services while protecting the rights of the abused. In most states, the adult protective services agency (APS) is the principal public agency that is designated to receive and investigate allegations of elder abuse and neglect.

LIFE CYCLE CONSIDERATIONS

Abuse of Elders

Due to a loss of independence and a forced reliance on others, elders are vulnerable to being abused in a number of ways. Morris (1998) defines a vulnerable adult "as a person with a physical or mental condition—such as Alzheimer's disease or an infirmity related to aging—that substantially impairs his ability to care for himself." Laws have been developed to protect elders from abusive situations, and agencies such as APS have been established to facilitate this process.

In most jurisdictions, the county departments of social services maintain the APS unit (Thobaben, 1989).

DOMESTIC VIOLENCE

Domestic violence occurs in relationships where intentional or controlling behavior is perpetrated by persons with whom a survivor has had or currently has an intimate relationship. The syndrome may include actual or threatened physical injury, sexual assault, psychological abuse, economic control, and/or progressive isolation (Medical Education Group Learning Systems, 1995).

Domestic violence occurs in relationships where conflict is the continuous result of power inequality between partners. One of the partners is afraid of and harmed by the other. This should not be confused with domestic strife, which is present in most relationships where neither partner has more power or control than the other and, thus, neither is victim or abuser. Domestic strife can be caused or made worse by many things, such as financial hardship, sexual infidelity, alcohol or other substance use, work pressure, jealousy, and differences in expectations about the relationship (Women's Issues and Social Empowerment [W.I.S.E.], 1997).

As of March 1994, all but five states have laws that, to varying extents, require nurses to report cases of domestic violence. Most states have general laws that mandate health care providers to report incidents when injuries are caused by a weapon (gun, knife, or other deadly weapon). Each state's statute has its definitions of terms, such as what constitutes "violence," "weapon," or "grave" injury, and when health professionals are mandated to report (Hyman, Schillinger, & Lo, 1995). Mandatory reporting laws have relieved some battered clients of the onus of reporting their batterers. However, some battered women are reluctant to seek medical care because they are afraid to admit that their injuries have been caused by abuse. They are ashamed or fear their partners will retaliate against them. They are also reluctant to call the police because they do not believe it will help their situation or they fear retaliation from their partners after the police leave or the abusers are released from jail. When nurses are required to report abused women to law enforcement, they should inform clients of their legal obligations and try to ensure the survivor's safety.

RAPE

Rape is a legal term, not a medical entity. It is a crime of violence. Rapists use sexual violence to dominate and degrade their victims and to express their own anger. It is not an act of lust or an overzealous release of passion done to satisfy a sexual urge (Frisch & Frisch, 1998).

According to Aguilera (1997), there are three basic types of rape: (1) rape by a person known to the survivor, for example, father, former and current friends (date rape), neighbors, partner or separated partner, dissatisfied clients of prostitutes; (2) gang rape; and (3) stranger-to-stranger rape. The latter, which women fear the most, follows an identifiable pattern. Such rapists look for women who are vulnerable, even though they differ on defining who is vulnerable. They might attempt to rape elders, people who are developmentally, physically, or mentally challenged, or intoxicated people. They might look for environments that are easy to enter and relatively safe (e.g., women's bedrooms) and where they will not be interrupted. They often select their victims long before they approach them and repeat the same pattern of victim selection over and over again. All types of rape can be an emotionally terrorizing experience for the survivors.

Medical–Surgical Management

Medical

Planning care for survivors of neglect and abuse and their families will require input from the clients and a survey of their resources to ensure that the targeted care is in line with their expectations and commitments. Nursing interventions directed at primary prevention of interpersonal violence are those that reduce or control the causative factors associated with interpersonal violence and sexual assaults. By identifying families at high risk for abuse, nurses can help the family plan efforts to modify those risk factors.

Health Promotion

Primary prevention includes empowering survivors of abuse by helping them learn to care for and protect themselves from the imposition by others. For example, children can be taught in health care settings or schools those things to do if they are being abused. It also includes changing the family's perceptions of violence as an acceptable mode of conflict resolution (Clark, 1999).

Also included is providing anticipatory guidance. For example, by anticipating the challenges of toddlerhood, nurses can acknowledge that this can be a difficult period for parents and can provide practical advice about constructive discipline. They can teach college freshmen about date rape and to avoid vulnerable situations. They can encourage families with dependent elderly members to use respite care services

PROFESSIONAL TIP

Caring for the Abused Client

When questioning clients about the possibility of interpersonal violence or sexual assault, the nurse must quickly develop a rapport and create an environment that indicates that their personal experiences are acceptable topics to discuss. This allows them the opportunity to express their fears and concerns. This can be done by:

- Treating them with dignity and concern,
- Giving priority to them over nonemergency clients,
- Placing them in quiet and private areas,
- Not leaving them alone,
- Speaking quietly and in a nonjudgmental manner,
- Using active and empathic listening skills,
- Not acting shocked or surprised at the details of their experiences,
- Reassuring them that the abuse was not their fault,
- Explaining any delays in treatment,
- Asking permission to call family members, friends, or in the case of rape, rape crisis advocates, and
- Providing information about community resources.

PROFESSIONAL TIP

Interviewing the Survivor of Abuse or Violence

The type of questions will depend on the type of violence and whether survivors have told you they have been abused. If they have told you they have been abused, you must ask specific questions about the abuse. If they have not, you must ask more open-ended questions to allow them to disclose sensitive information. Generally speaking:

- Inform the client that it is necessary to ask some very personal questions;
- Use language appropriate for the age and developmental level of the survivor;
- Use conversational language or street language;
- Keep questions simple, nonthreatening, and direct;
- Pose questions in a manner that permits brief answers;
- Indicate sensitivity to and acceptance of the client's state of confusion;
- Avoid using leading statements that can distort the client's report;
- Do not criticize the client's family; and
- Do not promise not to report the abuse; indicate that you are required by law to report the abuse.

and day care programs. Such support and anticipatory guidance can enhance the family's and client's competence and diminish the likelihood of violence or abuse.

▶ NURSING PROCESS

▶ Assessment

▶ Subjective Data

There is no comprehensive assessment tool that offers conclusive evidence that neglect, abuse, or violence has occurred. Nurses must act like detectives when assessing clients, given that clients or their abusers will rarely admit to abuse or violence. The nurse must make direct observations of the client and family members. For example, does the child seem afraid of the caregiver? Does the caregiver hit the child? These observations are clues that more probing is necessary.

In order to properly assess survivors of abuse, nurses must know the symptoms that are commonly seen in interpersonal violence and sexual assaults and the common characteristics of the abusers. Many of the symptoms are subjective, so the nurse and the health care team must piece together the evidence to ascertain whether interpersonal violence has occurred or clients are at risk for violence. Psychological abuse is a particularly difficult area to assess, as emotional relationships are very culture bound, and words and emotions that may be harmful in one family are not necessarily so in another family.

▶ Objective Data

A more extensive examination is warranted when the history or behavioral symptoms indicate interpersonal abuse. Clients will need to have physical examinations to assess the extent of their injuries and to collect forensic evidence to prove who assaulted them. A traumagram, or body map (a drawing of the front and back of a nude human figure), is generally used to mark the location of all visible injuries. Each state has legally mandated procedures for collecting evidentiary material, and nurses must be sure that the legal "chain of evidence" pertaining to collection of forensic samples is unbroken. The medical record should document the injuries and nursing and medical treatment that may serve as legal evidence of the client's condition.

Nursing diagnoses for the client experiencing neglect or abuse may include the following:

Nursing Diagnoses	Planning/Goals	Nursing Interventions
▶ *Family Processes, Altered, related to neglect*	The client will not experience any further neglect.	Provide support for the client.
		Document the evidence of neglect with which the client presents via written observations, laboratory reports, and/or pictures, if indicated.
		Report the case of neglect to the proper authorities: police, child protective services (CPS), APS, and any others that might be indicated.
▶ *Fear related to abuse*	The client will verbalize being less fearful.	Reassure the client that the client is in a safe place and that you are there to help in any way that you can.
		Provide emotional support to the client in a nonjudgmental manner.
▶ *Injury, Risk for, related to abusive home life*	The client will not experience any further injury or abuse.	Address the client's safety needs and attempt to assess whether abuse is occurring.
		If you suspect that abuse is occurring or a child is being harmed in any way, notify your supervisor and contact the proper authorities (Ladebauche, 1997).

Evaluation Each goal must be evaluated to determine how it has been met by the client.

THE CLIENT WITH AN EATING DISORDER

Eating disorders include anorexia nervosa and bulimia nervosa. **Anorexia nervosa** is characterized by self-imposed starvation by restricting caloric intake and compulsive exercising. **Bulimia nervosa** is characterized by periods of binge eating of up to 10,000 calories at one time followed by self-induced vomiting and other forms of purging such as laxative and diuretic abuse. In bulimia nervosa, the client's weight is normal or above normal. In anorexia nervosa, body weight is low and keeps getting lower. Almost all clients with these disorders are female and below the age of thirty.

Complications can be serious and include cardiac abnormalities such as bradycardia, hypotension, arrhythmias, CHF, and cardiovascular collapse; oral and esophageal erosions and dental caries from vomiting;

renal abnormalities that affect the kidney's ability to filter urine; skin rashes from malnutrition; and bruising from vomiting.

Clients with anorexia nervosa tend to be high achievers, perfectionists, have a distorted body image in that they see themselves as fat, and are rigid and ritualistic.

Bulimia nervosa occurs more frequently than anorexia nervosa, with clients experiencing a fear of not being able to stop eating. Clients often experience guilt and depression after a binge.

Medical–Surgical Management

Diet

During severe cases, clients may be admitted for enforced feeding, including the placement of a feeding tube or TPN, IV fluid rehydration, and electrolyte replacement. Clients need to be monitored for refeeding complications such as pancreatitis and gastric dilation. Small quantities are given at first and very gradually the amount is increased.

Other Therapies

Treatment is primarily psychiatric, involving the client and family, and is typically done on an outpatient basis.

▶ NURSING PROCESS

▶ Assessment

▶ Subjective Data

Clients with both anorexia nervosa and bulimia nervosa may verbalize feelings of helplessness and being out of control, and may exhibit low self-esteem. They may also have overprotective parents. Clients with anorexia nervosa may also describe bad dreams and cold intolerance.

▶ Objective Data

Assessment of clients with anorexia nervosa may show low weight, usually lost over a short period of time, reluctance to eat with others, moving food around the plate without eating it, hypotension, heart irregularities, and altered thinking patterns.

Objective assessment of clients with bulimia nervosa may show normal weight, tooth erosions and dental caries, puffy face, callused knuckles, broken blood vessels in the eyes and face, reluctance to eat with others, and going to the bathroom immediately after eating.

Laboratory analysis will include a CBC, which may show low Hgb, Hct, and platelets; electrolytes, which may show low sodium, potassium, and chloride; an SMA-22 that shows low protein, phosphate, and magnesium; and elevated BUN.

Nursing diagnoses for a hospitalized client with anorexia nervosa or bulimia nervosa may include the following:

Nursing Diagnoses	Planning/Goals	Nursing Interventions
Nutrition, Altered, Less than Body Requirements, related to psychological restriction of food intake, excessive activity	The client will demonstrate increased consumption of nutrients as evidenced by weight gain daily and improved laboratory values.	Weigh daily. Monitor calorie intake. Monitor I & O every shift. Administer IV rehydration, electrolyte replacement, and TPN or tube feedings as ordered. Monitor behavior at and around meal time, such as going to the bathroom right after eating. Monitor exercise patterns.
Fluid Volume Deficit, High Risk for, related to inadequate intake of liquids, self-induced vomiting, laxative and diuretic use	The client's intake and output will be approximately equal by the fourth hospital day. The client's electrolytes will be within normal limits, by the third hospital day. The client's fluid intake will be at least 2000 mL per day.	Monitor I & O every shift and bowel movements for diarrhea (a sign of continued laxative abuse). Monitor laboratory reports for electrolyte levels as ordered. Administer IV fluid and electrolyte replacement as ordered.
Coping, Ineffective, Individual, related to maturational crisis and attempting to control environment	The client will verbalize feelings regarding disease process and hospitalization, by discharge. The client will identify current coping strategies, by discharge. The client will identify personal strengths, by discharge.	Provide opportunities for the client to express feelings regarding hospitalization. Encourage client to identify coping mechanisms and strengths. Give positive feedback regarding identified personal strengths.

Evaluation Each goal must be evaluated to determine how it has been met by the client.

CASE STUDY

Michael is a 7-year-old boy who was referred to the school nurse today by his physical education teacher, Mrs. Epstein. Michael regularly comes to school in soiled, torn clothes that do not fit. He is usually dirty and unkempt and often smells like he has not bathed for several days. In the school cafeteria, he frequently is seen asking his classmates for food from their trays. He also has been observed stuffing his pockets with food when he leaves the cafeteria. Michael is a bright student, but recently he has started having some problems in the classroom. His classroom difficulties consist primarily of restlessness, trouble concentrating and remaining on task, and preoccupation. Additionally, he has had multiple conflicts with his classmates and has been sent to the principle's office two times this year for aggressiveness. Today, Mrs. Epstein noticed multiple bruises and small burns on both of Michael's arms when he took off his jacket during a game of kickball. When the teacher took Michael aside and asked what had happened, Michael's only response was, "Nothing." Mrs. Epstein then explained to Michael that she wanted him to go to the nurse's office with her so that the nurse could examine him. Mrs. Epstein also told Michael that he was not in trouble and that she was concerned about him.

The following questions will guide your development of a nursing care plan for the case study.

1. What do you suspect is happening to Michael?

2. As a nurse, what must you do if you suspect child abuse?

3. List some signs and symptoms, in addition to Michael's, that a child who is being abused might exhibit.

4. List subjective and objective data that the nurse should obtain.

5. Write two individualized nursing diagnoses and goals for Michael.

SUMMARY

- The components of a therapeutic nurse–client relationship include trust, rapport, respect, genuineness, and empathy.
- An individual's anxiety level may range anywhere from mild to panic level.
- The nurse often encounters clients and/or family members who are angry, aggressive, homicidal, and/or suicidal in the midst of a crisis situation.
- The depressed individual must be evaluated for risk of suicide.
- The individual with schizophrenia may be out of touch with reality and influenced by delusions and/or hallucinations.
- Individuals with bipolar disorder may experience wide mood swings ranging from depression to mania.
- Neglect and abuse can occur among any age group.
- Anorexia nervosa and bulimia nervosa are psychological disorders affecting mostly women. Severe nutritional imbalances can occur leading to serious effects on the cardiovascular system.

Review Questions

1. The client who is experiencing severe or panic level anxiety should:

   a. be left alone to calm down.
   b. be taught new information.
   c. never be left alone.
   d. be given an antidepressant immediately.

2. Two of the newest antidepressants are:

   a. pemoline (Cylert) and methylphenidate (Ritalin).
   b. mirtazapine (Remeron) and venlafaxine (Effexor).
   c. quetiapine (Seroquel) and olanzapine (Zyprexa).
   d. alprazolam (Xanax) and lorazepam (Ativan).

3. Clients receiving MAOIs must avoid foods containing which of the following?

   a. Thiamine
   b. Tyramine
   c. Tryptophan
   d. Thorazine

4. A nurse who is aware of a client's plan to kill someone else should do which of the following?

   a. Nothing; it is not her responsibility.
   b. Contact the physician and alert the proper authorities.
   c. Discourage the client from following through with the plan.
   d. Continue preparing the client for discharge per orders in the chart.

5. The client who is contemplating suicide may demonstrate which of the following behaviors?

   a. Giving away prized personal possessions
   b. Buying new personal items
   c. Purchasing an expensive item
   d. Purchasing an inexpensive item

6. Schizophrenia is usually treated with which of the following classification of medications?

   a. Antidepressants
   b. Antipsychotics
   c. Mood stabilizers
   d. CNS stimulants

7. Signs and symptoms of schizophrenia include:

   a. hyperactivity and decreased concentration.
   b. crying spells and decreased appetite.
   c. compulsive rituals.
   d. hallucinations and/or delusions.

8. Which of the following is the drug of choice for treating bipolar disorder?

   a. Librium
   b. Valium
   c. Thorazine
   d. Lithium

9. A client with bipolar disorder may manifest which of the following symptoms?

   a. Mood fluctuations alternating between mania and depression
   b. An addiction to drugs and alcohol
   c. Overwhelming feelings of fear and dread
   d. An over-exaggeration of physical symptoms

10. The child with ADHD will probably be prescribed a medication from which of the following classifications?

   a. Antipsychotics
   b. Antianxiety medications
   c. Mood stabilizers
   d. CNS stimulants

11. The client experiencing abuse will:

   a. always tell the truth about what is happening.
   b. often lie about what is happening in order to protect the abuser.
   c. always contact the authorities.
   d. never withhold significant information from health care providers.

Critical Thinking Questions

1. Consider your feelings after treating a client believed to be suffering from domestic abuse. What was your reaction to this client? Were you able to respond appropriately? How would you have felt if the client refused your attempts to help remove her from the abusive situation?

2. What actions would you take if you felt a co-worker was suffering from depression?

⚡ WEB FLASH!

- What resources can you find on the Web to help clients or families cope with schizophrenia?
- Can you find more information on the uses of ECT by searching the Web using *electroconvulsive therapy* as a key word?
- What research related to new drug treatments and psychiatric disorders can you find by searching the Web?

CHAPTER 46

NURSING CARE OF THE CLIENT: SUBSTANCE ABUSE

MAKING THE CONNECTION

Refer to the following chapters to increase your understanding of substance abuse:

- **Chapter 6, Legal Responsibilities**
- **Chapter 7, Ethical Responsibilities**
- **Chapter 15, Wellness Concepts**
- **Chapter 25, Assessment**

- **Chapter 31, Nursing Care of the Client: Respiratory System**
- **Chapter 34, Nursing Care of the Client: Gastrointestinal System**
- **Chapter 55, Nursing Care of the Older Client**

LEARNING OBJECTIVES

Upon completion of this chapter, you should be able to:
- *Define key terms.*
- *Differentiate among dependence, abuse, and intoxication.*
- *Describe issues related to drug testing.*
- *Discuss substances frequently abused.*
- *Use assessment skills to identify possible substance abuse.*
- *Describe nursing interventions in working with substance abusers.*
- *Describe stages of alcoholism and the impact on the individual, family, and society.*
- *Discuss medications frequently used in the treatment of substance abuse.*
- *Describe an impaired nurse.*
- *Identify goals of programs for impaired nurses.*

INTRODUCTION

Substance use has taken place for many centuries. It is not a new problem for society. A **substance** is a drug, legal or illegal, that may cause physical or mental impairment. With the great increase in world population there are more people involved in substance abuse. Today's speed of travel and communication has facilitated the broad distribution of substances.

Many street drugs are "cut" (mixed) with substances that should not be consumed, such as talcum powder, rodent exterminating powder, or even strychnine. The

KEY TERMS

abuse	misuse
addiction	opisthotonos
behavioral tolerance	relapse
codependent	reverse tolerance
confabulation	substance
cross-tolerance	synthesiasis
dependence	teratogenic
detoxification	tolerance
hallucination	withdrawal
intoxication	
Johnsonian intervention	

purity (strength) of the drug is then not known and overdose easily occurs. Fatalities can occur from the substance with which the drug is cut.

In the United States, substance disorders affect males and females, all ethnic groups, and persons of all levels of education and income. From the newborn to the elderly, all ages can be affected.

Substance disorders may be classified as intoxication, abuse, or dependence (addiction); definitions are based on the criteria presented in the American Psychiatric Association's *Diagnostic and Statistical Manual of Mental Disorders,* fourth edition (*DSM-IV*). The reversible effect on the central nervous system (CNS) soon after the use of a substance is termed **intoxication**. **Abuse** is the misuse, excessive, or improper use of a substance, the abstinence of which does not cause withdrawal symptoms. **Dependence** (**addiction**) is reliance on a substance to such a degree that abstinence causes functional impairment, physical withdrawal symptoms, and/or a psychological craving for the substance. The person has no control over use of the substance and feels pleasure only when using the substance. Table 46-1 shows diagnostic criteria for abuse and dependence.

HISTORICAL PERSPECTIVES

Nearly 6,500 years ago, ancient Egyptians used opium for pain relief. Later they used it for recreation when they discovered it provided anxiety relief, a pleasurable experience, and an escape from reality. Drug problems began in the United States with the Civil War in 1861. Wounded soldiers were given their own supply of morphine. Its use was uncontrolled. Dependence-producing drugs such as cocaine, heroin, and morphine were given freely to clients by doctors. Patent medicines, many containing alcohol, cocaine, and heroin, were said to cure almost any ailment a person might have.

The Pure Food and Drug Act of 1906, requiring accurate labeling of drugs, was the first measure designed to control drugs in the United States. In 1914, The Harrison Act made the use of certain narcotics illegal. Physicians then became unwilling to give individuals these drugs and drug use actually increased as those persons already using drugs turned to illegal markets for a supply. In 1919 Congress passed the 19th Amendment to the Constitution declaring the making and selling of alcohol illegal. Prohibition lasted until 1933 when the 19th Amendment was finally repealed because it had not controlled drunkenness or alcoholism as it was intended.

Many medical, law enforcement, and legislative efforts in the 1930s slowed narcotic abuse and addiction. Then marijuana flooded the market. The Marijuana Tax Act of 1937 was intended to raise revenue, identify the persons involved in its use, and discourage the recreational use of marijuana. Marijuana was removed in 1941 from the official list of drugs United States physicians could prescribe. World War II disrupted supply routes of drugs from Asia and Europe, and large-scale drug use disappeared in the United States.

Table 46-1 DIAGNOSTIC CRITERIA FOR SUBSTANCE ABUSE AND DEPENDENCE

SUBSTANCE DEPENDENCE

A maladaptive pattern of substance use, leading to clinically significant impairment or distress, as manifested by three (or more) of the following, occurring at any time in the same 12-month period:

(1) tolerance, as defined by either of the following:

    (a) a need for markedly increased amounts of the substance to achieve intoxication or desired effect

    (b) markedly diminished effect with continued use of the same amount of the substance

(2) withdrawal, as manifested by either of the following:

    (a) the characteristic withdrawal syndrome for the substance (refer to Criteria A and B of the criteria sets for Withdrawal from the specific substances)

    (b) the same (or a closely related) substance is taken to relieve or avoid withdrawal symptoms

(3) the substance is often taken in larger amounts or over a longer period than was intended

(4) there is a persistent desire or unsuccessful efforts to cut down or control substance use

(5) a great deal of time is spent in activities necessary to obtain the substance (e.g., visiting multiple doctors or driving long distances), use the substance (e.g., chain-smoking), or recover from its effects

(6) important social, occupational, or recreational activities are given up or reduced because of substance use

(7) the substance use is continued despite knowledge of having a persistent or recurrent physical or psychological problem that is likely to have been caused or exacerbated by the substance (e.g., current cocaine use despite recognition of cocaine-induced depression, or continued drinking despite recognition that an ulcer was made worse by alcohol consumption)

SUBSTANCE ABUSE

A. A maladaptive pattern of substance use leading to clinically significant impairment or distress, as manifested by one (or more) of the following, occurring within a 12-month period:

    (1) recurrent substance use resulting in a failure to fulfill major role obligations at work, school, or home (e.g., repeated absences or poor work performance related to substance use; substance-related absences, suspensions, or expulsions from school; neglect of children or household)

    (2) recurrent substance use in situations in which it is physically hazardous (e.g., driving an automobile or operating a machine when impaired by substance use)

    (3) recurrent substance-related legal problems (e.g., arrests for substance-related disorderly conduct)

    (4) continued substance use despite having persistent or recurrent social or interpersonal problems caused, or exacerbated by the effects of the substance (e.g., arguments with spouse about consequences of intoxication, physical fights)

B. The symptoms have never met the criteria for Substance Dependence for this class of substance.

Reprinted with permission from the Diagnostic and Statistical Manual of Mental Disorders, Fourth Edition. *Copyright 1994 American Psychiatric Association.*

The 1960s saw drug use move into the mainstream of life in the United States. Drugs were used as a form of relaxation. The Comprehensive Drug Abuse Prevention and Control Act was passed in 1970; it is commonly referred to as the Controlled Substance Act. This act regulates the manufacture, distribution, and dispensing of controlled substances. To enforce the provisions of this act, the Drug Enforcement Administration (DEA) was organized.

There are five classifications or schedules of controlled substances. The categories are based on the drugs' potential to cause psychological and/or physical dependence, and also on their potential for abuse. Table 46-2 identifies and explains the five schedules.

In the 1980s, marijuana and other drug use declined, especially among high school students. Cocaine and its derivative, crack, were the new drugs of choice. The increased supply hooked many people into heavy drug use. The 1990s have seen an increase in the use of all substances.

FACTORS RELATED TO SUBSTANCE ABUSE

There are many factors that interact to influence a person's substance abuse. Many people who have stopped substance abuse **relapse** (return to a previous behavior or condition) because of these same factors.

Table 46-2	SCHEDULES OF CONTROLLED SUBSTANCES
Schedule I (C-I)	High abuse and dependence potential. No accepted medical use in the United States. Includes heroin, mescaline, LSD, marijuana, and other hallucinogens and certain opiates. Can be obtained legally for limited research programs.
Schedule II (C-II)	High abuse and dependence potential. Have currently accepted medical use. Includes narcotics, barbiturates, and amphetamines. Obtained only with physician's prescription, nonrefillable.
Schedule III (C-III)	Less abuse potential, moderate dependence likely. Includes nonbarbiturate sedatives and some narcotics in limited doses. Prescription refills good for 6 months. Fewer controls than for Schedule II.
Schedule IV (C-IV)	Even less abuse potential, limited dependence likely. Includes some sedatives and antianxiety agents and nonnarcotic analgesics.
Schedule V (C-V)	Limited abuse potential. Includes cough medicines containing codeine and antidiarrheals. May be sold over-the-counter in pharmacies to persons over 18 years old. A record is kept of the buyer's name.

These factors may be categorized as individual, family, lifestyle, environmental, and developmental.

Individual Factors

Genetic factors are being researched as a possible reason for a person's susceptibility to substance abuse. According to Santomier and Hogan (1991), research has produced some evidence to suggest the presence of an abnormal chromosome in addicted individuals. This does not guarantee addiction but may predispose the person to addiction.

Other research suggests that variations in the intensity of the flow of neurotransmitters may cause certain individuals to be more susceptible to addiction. The personality traits of sensation seeking and being impulsive may make it easier for the person to experiment with substances.

Family Patterns

Substance abuse, especially in the adolescent, seems to be related to family relationships. Close family relationships, with the parents involved in their children's activities, appear to discourage substance abuse. Families with positive relationships between parents and children generally have less use of illicit drugs. Parent-child interactions that show a lack of closeness, lack of involvement in the children's activities, lack of or inconsistent discipline, and low aspirations for the children's education contribute to the prediction of substance abuse by the children.

Families of adolescent substance abusers generally have negative communication patterns. That is, there is a lack of praise and a great deal of blaming and criticism. Often there are unreal expectations of the children by the parents, inconsistent or unclear behavioral limits, and a pattern of self-medication by family members.

Lifestyle

All dimensions of a person's life that influence how that person lives are termed lifestyle. First is the physical dimension which includes food, clothing, shelter, and health care. The second is the social dimension, which includes friends, organizations, and activities with others. Third is the intellectual/emotional dimension, including education, parental support of education, self-esteem, and how the individual is treated by others. The fourth dimension is spiritual and includes a belief in a "higher being," caring and compassion for others, and being in touch with the inner self. Substance use, abuse, or dependence may be the coping mechanism used by an individual who has problems in any dimension of lifestyle.

Environmental Factors

There are many environmental factors that may encourage or predispose an individual to substance abuse. The social environment in which persons find themselves, the groups, clubs, gangs, sororities, fraternities, and other organizations influence the acceptance or rejection of substance abuse. The stresses in a person's life, including accidents, disabilities, illnesses, stressful family relations, frequent job changes, divorce, death, or precarious financial conditions may be too much for that person to handle. The maladaptive coping of substance abuse offers temporary relief. Because the symptoms of the stressors are reduced, substance abuse is reinforced.

Advertising can influence people in subtle ways to become involved in substance use and abuse. Landau (1995) describes how use of Camel cigarettes by the 18 to 24-year-old age group soared when the character Joe Camel was introduced in advertising promotions in 1988. It was "cool" to be associated with Joe Camel. Other advertising connects caffeine, nicotine, or alcohol with success, sexuality, and power.

Social traditions, especially in the use of alcohol, may open the door for abuse in certain individuals. Some examples of these social traditions include having wine with meals, making toasts at weddings and other celebrations, serving "holiday cheer," and going to "happy hour." For some individuals, these situations may predispose them to alcohol abuse or dependence.

Peer activities, especially during adolescence, may result in substance abuse. Even adults often feel they must go along with certain activities, such as drinks after work or cocktail hour, to get ahead in their career.

Some occupations, like health care, seem to be more associated with substance problems than others. Physicians and nurses, particularly, have access to many substances of abuse.

Developmental Factors

Many individuals have not had good role models in their life. They have not learned to identify with others and do not understand that their behavior affects others. Not learning the skills and attitudes of problem solving leaves the individual unable to apply personal resources to situations, and escape seems the only answer. Substances provide that escape.

Learning the intrapersonal skills of self-discipline, self-control, and self-assessment helps the individual to cope with tension and stress. These skills also work to prevent dishonesty with self, inability to defer gratification, and low self-esteem. A lack of interpersonal skills results in dishonesty with others, resistance to feedback, and inability to share feelings and give or accept help. Not learning to take responsibility or adapt one's behavior to a situation results in irresponsibility, not accepting the consequences of behavior, and seeing oneself as a victim of circumstances. Individuals who do not view themselves as empowered may choose substance use as a means of gratification.

PREVENTION

Prevention of substance abuse must be a proactive process to empower people to constructively confront stressful situations in their lives in adaptive ways. There are three levels of prevention. Primary prevention focuses on preventing the initial use or preventing further uses that may lead to abuse or dependence. This is usually aimed at school-age children. Children need to hear the message that drugs are not good for them. Education about substances and their effects must also emphasize personal, social, and health risks. Children need role models to teach them how to cope with life without drugs, to resist social and peer pressure, and to make effective decisions.

Secondary prevention focuses on preventing ongoing use from becoming a situation of abuse or dependence. If abuse is already evident, the focus is to return the client to a state of abstinence or at least reduced use.

Tertiary prevention focuses on returning the client to a drug-free state. If this is not possible, the goal is then to prevent physical and psychosocial problems from getting worse.

DIAGNOSTIC TESTING

Clients who have a problem with substance abuse or dependence often have abnormal liver function tests and electrolyte levels. Diagnostic criteria for specific substance-related disorders can be found in DSM-IV.

Tests may be done with either a blood or urine specimen. A positive test indicates only that the person has been exposed to the substance. It does not indicate abuse, addiction, or intoxication (except alcohol). Positive screening tests should be confirmed by a more specific test using a different process. Drugs for which tests can be done include alcohol, benzodiazepines, barbiturates, cocaine, crack, amphetamines, opiates, synthetic narcotic analgesics, cannabis, and PCP.

Urine is usually the body fluid tested because it is easily obtained and tested. When obtaining a urine specimen for drug screening, the client should be observed so as to prevent adulteration of the specimen by the client, such as substituting another person's drug-free urine. A "chain of custody" is maintained by having each person who handles the specimen sign an attached paper until the specimen has been tested.

Detection of a substance depends on the amount used and the time since last used. Most substances are detectable for less than 7 days. Chronic marijuana use, however, may be detected for up to 30 days. Cocaine, barbiturates, amphetamines, and opiates are detectable for less than 2 days and alcohol less than 1 day. A false negative may result if the client's drug level falls below the threshold of sensitivity for the test.

Positive results for reasons other than substance abuse can occur. This is called a false positive. Poppy seeds may give a positive result for opiates for up to 60 hours after ingestion. Using a Vicks® Inhaler or over-the-counter diet aids may give a positive result for amphetamines. The client should be asked about the use of these items.

Breath specimens can be used to determine alcohol levels. Law enforcement officials do this with the breathalyzer tests. If hair is not cut, hair analysis can detect substance use for up to a year after the person has used a drug for only 2 or 3 days. Testing meconium (first stools) from a newborn can detect illicit drug use by the mother during pregnancy.

TREATMENT/RECOVERY

Treatment depends on many factors, including the amount and frequency of substance use, age, health, diet, and overall lifestyle of the individual. Infection from the use of unsterile needles and/or tissue or organ damage caused by the substance used, such as lung damage from smoking crack or marijuana or using inhalants, will also require treatment.

Recovery requires abstinence along with intrapersonal and interpersonal changes. Most individuals need professional treatment and participation in a self-help program. Daley, Moss, and Campbell (1993) describe four areas of recovery: physical recovery, psychological and behavioral recovery, social and family recovery, and spiritual recovery.

Physical recovery means eliminating the substance from the body. This is termed **detoxification**. If the client cannot stop using the substance or if withdrawal symptoms are present, admission to a detoxification unit is usually necessary. After detoxification, treatment must focus on restoring the client's physical health and dealing with the cravings for the substance now removed from the client's body. It helps if environmental cues such as drug paraphernalia and alcohol bottles or cans are removed.

Psychological and behavioral recovery becomes evident when the client no longer denies the problem and accepts the inability to consistently control the substance abuse. The client will have developed a desire for abstinence and accepted the need for long-term recovery and support. Emotional stability will be restored when the client learns to cope with uncomfortable emotional states without the use of the abused substance.

Social and family recovery occurs when the client no longer denies the impact on the family and makes amends to family members and significant others who have been negatively affected by the substance abuse. The client works to improve family relationships and develops a recovery support system. Also, the client learns to resist social pressures to use alcohol or other drugs and participates in healthy leisure-time activities. The client's family should also attend a program for recovery. If a client returns to a dysfunctional family, it may be difficult for the client to maintain recovery.

Spiritual recovery is attained when the client has resolved the feelings of guilt and shame and developed a meaning for life and a relationship with a higher power.

SUBSTANCE USE PATTERNS

Patterns of substance use have changed throughout the years. Coffee (caffeine) and cigarettes (nicotine) are legal in our society and widely used. While many people still drink coffee, more and more are using decaffeinated coffee. Cigarette use has decreased in the older population as the addictive nature and negative effects of nicotine have become more evident. However, cigarette use has increased in the adolescent population.

The substance of choice is alcohol. It is legal and easily obtained. Many high school seniors have been drunk and some are already regular drinkers. There are still more alcoholic men than women, but the number of identified women alcoholics is increasing.

Elderly persons are more commonly addicted to prescription medications, especially minor tranquilizers and sleeping pills. Alcohol may be used by the elderly to soothe feelings of isolation and loneliness. Depression and paranoia may be misidentified as senility rather than a problem with alcohol.

Moderate consumption of alcohol may have been influenced by Mothers Against Drunk Driving (MADD) and Students Against Drunk Driving (SADD). Laws that make bars and individuals liable if they let guests leave and drive while drunk, and famous people like Betty Ford and Liza Minelli sharing with the public their illness and recovery, are other influences.

Johnston, O'Malley, and Bachman (1998) report on the ongoing study of illicit drug use among 8th-, 10th-, and 12th-grade students, which shows a decline in use. This is the second year of decline for 8th graders and the first year of decline for 10th and 12th graders.

CNS DEPRESSANTS

Central nervous system depressants usually decrease the heart and respiratory rates as well as voluntary muscle responses. Substances in this category include alcohol, benzodiazepines, and cannabis.

ALCOHOL

Low doses of alcohol depress areas of the brain that are inhibitory, causing diminished self-control and

Table 46-3 ALCOHOL CONTENT IN SELECTED BEVERAGES		
BEVERAGE	**PERCENT ALCOHOL**	**EQUIVALENT AMOUNTS**
Beer	4	12 ounces
Wine cooler	4	12 ounces
Wine	14	4 ounces
Hard liquor	40	1½ ounces

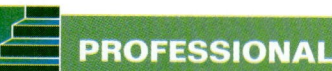

PROFESSIONAL TIP

Alcohol Use

According to the National Institute on Alcohol Abuse and Alcoholism (NIAAA) (1999b), 32% of all traffic crash fatalities were alcohol-related. The estimated cost of alcohol abuse for 1995 is $166.5 million (NIAAA, 1999c).

impaired judgment. Continued alcohol ingestion may cause unconsciousness and even death.

The active ingredient in alcoholic beverages is ethanol. Depending on the alcoholic beverage consumed, varying amounts of ethanol are ingested. It is metabolized at an average rate of 10 mL/hr. Table 46-3 shows the alcohol content in some beverages.

One ounce of alcohol provides 200 Kcal but no other nutrients. It is not converted to glycogen. The blood alcohol level depends on the size of the person, the amount ingested, and the time since ingestion. Most states have set the legal limit for blood alcohol while driving a motor vehicle at 100 mg/dL (0.1%), but some have reduced it to 0.08%.

Incidence

Several national surveys have found that approximately two-thirds of the population have more than an occasional drink. Men are likely to drink more frequently and in greater quantity than women. The vast majority of individuals with an alcohol problem are blue- or white-collar men and women. Some alcoholics drink little or nothing in public or with friends. They are "at home" or "hidden" alcoholics and are more likely to be women. It often takes a family quite awhile to realize that one of its members has an alcohol problem.

The individual with an alcohol problem often learns **behavioral tolerance**, a compensatory adjustment made by an individual under the influence of a particular substance. The person under the influence of alcohol learns how to compensate for the deterioration of motor performance and speech.

Signs and Symptoms

The ingestion of alcohol causes a feeling of euphoria, relaxation of skeletal muscles, changes in mental activity such as altered judgment, and reduced self-control. It has a diuretic effect that, in heavy drinkers, may cause increased loss of electrolytes, especially potassium, magnesium, and zinc. An increased level of alcohol depresses the cardiovascular and respiratory systems and produces a toxic effect on the intestinal mucosa, resulting in decreased absorption of thiamine,

folic acid, and vitamin B_{12}. Excess long-term consumption of alcohol often results in a severe lack of nutrient intake.

Psychosocial aspects include memory blackouts, secretive drinking, rationalization of drinking behavior, trouble with family and employer, loss of outside interests, neglect of food intake, impaired thinking, and moral deterioration. **Confabulation**, making up information to fill in memory gaps, is used by individuals abusing or depending on alcohol. Alcohol may be detected in the blood for 6 to 10 hours.

Potential for Addiction

The potential for addiction is high. Alcohol is not a scheduled or controlled drug.

Associated Problems/Disorders

Excessive and prolonged alcohol intake can affect numerous body systems.

Liver Deterioration

Chronic alcohol abuse causes three distinct diseases of the liver. They are fatty liver, an accumulation of triglycerides in the liver caused by obesity, excessive alcohol consumption, and certain drugs; alcoholic hepatitis, an acute toxic liver injury from excess alcohol consumption; and cirrhosis, a chronic degenerative liver disease that can be caused by alcohol consumption. Fatty liver is reversible, but alcoholic hepatitis and cirrhosis are not. Liver cells will not function once the scar tissue of cirrhosis develops. In 1995, 88.7% of deaths from cirrhosis of the liver were related to alcohol consumption (NIAAA, 1999a). Esophageal varices are associated with cirrhosis and could cause death if they bleed.

Gastrointestinal Disturbances

Alcohol damages the lining of the stomach and esophagus by irritating the mucosa and causing inflammation or ulcer formation. Aspirin with alcohol can result in greater irritation and bleeding in the gastrointestinal (GI) tract. Gastric pain, vomiting, and diarrhea are common in alcohol abuse and are often what brings the individual to the health care system.

Pancreatitis

An alcoholic has a higher risk of developing pancreatitis than an abstainer. Severe pancreatitis can result in death.

Wernicke's Encephalopathy

This inflammatory hemorrhagic and degenerative condition of the brain is caused by a thiamine deficiency. It is characterized by delirium, memory loss, unsteady gait, a sense of apprehension, and an altered level of consciousness. Thiamine intake improves the situation.

Korsakoff's Psychosis

Disorientation, amnesia, insomnia, hallucinations, and peripheral neuropathologies characterize this psychosis. Both thiamine and B_{12} deficiencies contribute to the degeneration of the brain and peripheral nervous system. Frequently, there is bilateral foot drop and pain over the long nerves. Thiamine and B_{12} intake may improve the situation.

Cardiovascular Disturbances

Moderate amounts of alcohol cause cutaneous vasodilation (flushed skin). This causes rapid heat loss, and the core temperature may drop to a dangerous level. Blood pressure decreases with intoxicating doses of alcohol. There may be irregularities in cardiac rhythm. Hematologic alterations such as bone marrow depression, anemia, leukopenia, or thrombocytopenia may also occur.

Fetal Alcohol Syndrome

Fetal alcohol syndrome is caused by the **teratogenic** (causing abnormal development of the embryo) effects of alcohol related to the amount of alcohol ingested and the stage of pregnancy when the alcohol is ingested. Even a small amount of alcohol can be detrimental and have lifelong consequences for the infant. For a diagnosis of FAS, the infant must meet certain criteria. Table 46-4 gives these criteria.

If only some of the FAS criteria are met, it is called fetal alcohol effects (FAE). The only treatment for FAS or FAE is prevention. Women who are pregnant or are trying to get pregnant should abstain from alcohol consumption.

Withdrawal

Withdrawal refers to the symptoms produced when a substance on which an individual has dependence is no longer used by that individual. Alcohol withdrawal syndrome (AWS) appears when the blood alcohol concentration of the alcoholic decreases. The onset of symptoms usually occurs 6 to 12 hours after drinking stops and may last up to 8 days. Chronologically, how long the drinking has occurred and the amount of alcohol consistently consumed are factors in the severity of the withdrawal symptoms. Figure 46-1 shows alcohol withdrawal patterns.

Alcohol withdrawal occurs in three stages:

- Stage 1 (minor withdrawal) includes restlessness, anxiety, sleeping problems, agitation, and tremors; other signs include low-grade fever, tachycardia, diaphoresis, and hypertension.
- Stage 2 (major withdrawal) includes stage 1 signs and symptoms plus visual and auditory hallucinations, whole-body tremors, pulse greater than 100, diastolic BP greater than 100, pronounced diaphoresis, and possibly vomiting.
- Stage 3 (delirium tremens) includes a temperature over 37.8°C (100°F); disorientation to time, place, and person; global confusion; and inability to recognize familiar objects or persons. This is a medical emergency with a mortality rate of 2% to 5% (National Institute on Drug Abuse [NIDA], 1997).

If alcohol abuse continues, symptoms of subsequent withdrawals are generally more severe. It is recommended that withdrawal be medically monitored to decrease the chance of fatality.

Table 46-4 INFANT CRITERIA FOR FETAL ALCOHOL SYNDROME

- Prenatal and/or postnatal growth retardation (weight, length, or head circumference below the 10th percentile)
- CNS involvement (signs of neurologic abnormality, developmental delay, or intellectual impairment)
- Craniofacial anomalies, at least two of the following (microcephaly or head circumference below 3rd percentile, microopthalmia or short palpebral fissure, poorly developed philtrum, thin upper lip, or flattening of maxillary area)

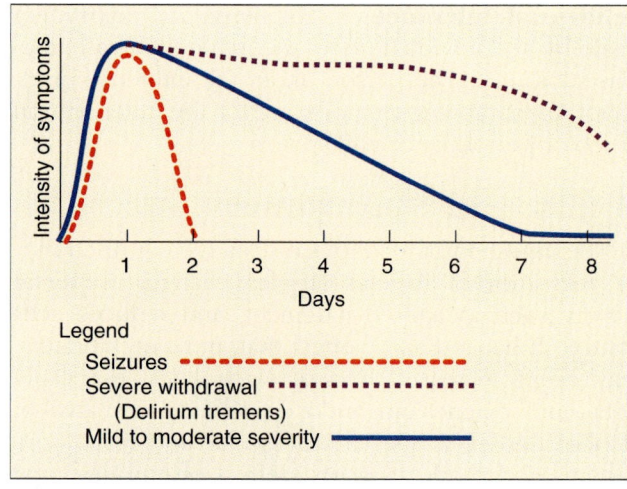

Figure 46-1 Alcohol Withdrawal Patterns

Treatment/Rehabilitation

Many treatment programs are based in hospital or residential treatment centers. These are generally called inpatient programs and last 30 days. Many insurance companies are encouraging clients to participate in lower-cost outpatient programs. Currently, there is no evidence that inpatient programs are more effective than outpatient programs.

Many outpatient programs have both day and evening sessions so clients can maintain their usual occupations. The programs usually consist of a 4-week intensive session with follow-up sessions for 6 to 24 months. The first part of either type of treatment program is detoxification.

Detoxification

The goal of detoxification (DETOX) is to halt or control the neuronal overactivity that occurs when the alcohol level is reduced or alcohol is no longer present in the client's body. This is done by substituting a pharmacologically similar drug and gradually reducing the dose given. The benzodiazepine drugs, chlordiazepoxide (Librium), diazepam (Valium), lorazepam (Ativan), and clorazepate dipotassium (Tranxene), are the most commonly used.

During DETOX, other problems such as malnutrition, vitamin deficiencies (B vitamins, especially thiamine), dehydration, and potassium and magnesium deficiencies must also be treated. A client with hypoglycemia should be given thiamine before administering dextrose to prevent Wernicke's encephalopathy. Ignoring these problems complicates the management of detoxification.

Psychologic Intervention

The classic psychologic intervention technique was originally described by Johnson (1973). Although several modifications have been published and used since then, the technique is still used and is known as **Johnsonian intervention**, which is a confrontational approach to a client with a substance problem that lessens the chance of denial and encourages treatment before the client "hits bottom." The client's significant others (spouse, teenage or older children, 1 or 2 close friends, possibly employer) meet with a professional addiction counselor. This group rehearses so that they may present a united front when confronting the client. They present specific examples of painful or embarrassing behaviors by the client while intoxicated that caused problems and concerns. It is difficult for the client to maintain denial in this situation. Then the group encourages the client to accept professional help. If the client refuses help, each individual of the group must plan to minimize codependent behavior in the future. This technique can also be used for substances other than alcohol. Examples of confrontations may be found in Johnson's books (1973, 1988). Codependency is discussed later in the chapter.

Education

The abuse of or dependence on alcohol is a maladaptive way to cope with life stressors. Learning basic life skills to improve personal competence and provide adaptive coping mechanisms helps the individual resist the use of alcohol.

One adaptive coping mechanism is exercise. Assist clients to become active in an exercise program and encourage them to participate. Exercise helps relieve feelings of stress and promotes feelings of well-being.

Teach clients about the Food Guide Pyramid for an adequate, balanced diet. Most alcoholics have, in the past, received the majority of their calories from alcohol. They must now learn how to maintain health by eating nutritious foods.

The interaction of alcohol with other drugs should also be taught. Some effects can be life-threatening. Table 46-5 shows the interaction of alcohol with some classifications of drugs.

Table 46-5 ALCOHOL INTERACTION WITH OTHER DRUGS

DRUG CLASSIFICATIONS WITH EXAMPLES	INTERACTION	DRUG CLASSIFICATIONS WITH EXAMPLES	INTERACTION
Narcotic analgesics • meperidine hydrochloride (Demerol) • proproxyphene HCl (Darvon) • hydromorphone HCl (Dilaudid)	• Loss of effective breathing (respiratory arrest) • Can be fatal	Antidepressants • imipramine HCl (Tofranil) • desipramine HCl (Pertofrane) • perphenazine and amitriptyline HCl (Triavil)	• Reduces CNS functioning • Chianti wine may cause hypertensive crisis
Nonnarcotic analgesics • aspirin (Bayer Aspirin)	• Stomach and intestinal bleeding	Antihistamines • Most cold remedies • pseudoephedrine HCl and triprolidine HCl (Actifed) • chlorpheniramine maleate and acetaminophen (Coricidin)	• Increased calming effect • Person becomes very drowsy • Driving is hazardous
Anticoagulants • warfarin sodium (Coumadin, Panwarfin) • dicumarol	• Increases drugs' ability to stop blood clotting • May cause life-threatening or fatal hemorrhage		

continued

Table 46-5 ALCOHOL INTERACTION WITH OTHER DRUGS (continued)

DRUG CLASSIFICATIONS WITH EXAMPLES	INTERACTION	DRUG CLASSIFICATIONS WITH EXAMPLES	INTERACTION
Antihypertensives • reserpine (Serpasil) • methyldopa (Aldomet)	• Orthostatic hypotension	Antipsychotics • thioridazine HCl (Mellaril) • chlorpromazine HCl (Thorazine)	• Added CNS depression and impairs voluntary movements • Causes respiratory depression • Can be fatal
Antimicrobials • metronidazole (Flagyl) • cefotetan disodium (Cefotan) • rifampin (Rifadin)	• Possible disulfiram-like reaction, nausea, cramps, vomiting, headache, flushing or hepatotoxicity	Sedative-hypnotics • glutethimide (Doriden) • pentobarbital (Nembutal)	• Reduces CNS functioning • Sometimes causes coma and respiratory arrest • Can be fatal
CNS stimulants • Most diet pills • dextroamphetamine sulfate (Dexedrine) • caffeine (No Doz) • methyphenidate HCl (Ritalin)	• May reverse depressant effect of alcohol and give a false sense of security	Antianxiety agents • diazepam (Valium) • chlordiazepoxide (Librium)	• Reduces CNS functioning • Decreased alertness and judgment • Can lead to household and driving accidents
Diuretics • chlorothiazide (Diuril) • furosemide (Lasix)	• May reduce blood pressure and cause dizziness		

Self-Help Groups

Alcoholics Anonymous (AA), begun in 1935, is the model for other self-help groups such as AL-ANON for adults, AL-ATEEN for teenage children, and AL-ATOT for younger children in the family of an alcoholic. The holistic approach of AA to the individual with alcohol problems is described in the Twelve Steps (Table 46-6).

Disulfiram

Disulfiram (Antabuse) may be given to some alcohol abusers as a deterrent to drinking. It inhibits the enzyme needed to metabolize alcohol. Drinking alcohol with disulfiram in the body causes flushing of the neck and face, blurred vision, nausea, vertigo, anxiety, palpitations, tachycardia, and hypotension. Clients must be instructed not to use cologne, mouthwash, aftershave, over-the-counter cold preparations, cough syrups, vitamin-mineral tonics, as well as candies, sauces, and foods made with alcohol. These items will cause the same reaction as if the person took a drink of alcohol.

Therapy should not be started until at least 12 hours after the last drink of alcohol. The effects of disulfiram with alcohol can occur for 6 to 12 days after taking the disulfiram. As with any drug, there are side effects such as drowsiness, fatigue, and impotence. Garlic-like breath occurs frequently and is sometimes used as an indicator of compliance in taking the disulfiram. Disulfiram is contraindicated in clients with cardiovascular disease, hypothyroidism, suicide ideation, and in clients receiving antihypertensives or monoamine oxidase inhibitors (MAOI).

Table 46-6 ALCOHOLICS ANONYMOUS

1. We admitted we were powerless over alcohol—that our lives had become unmanageable.
2. Came to believe that a Power greater than ourselves could restore us to sanity.
3. Made a decision to turn our will and our lives over to the care of God *as we understood Him*.
4. Made a searching and fearless moral inventory of ourselves.
5. Admitted to God, to ourselves and to another human being the exact nature of our wrongs.
6. Were entirely ready to have God remove all these defects of character.
7. Humbly asked Him to remove our shortcomings.
8. Made a list of all persons we had harmed, and became willing to make amends to them all.
9. Made direct amends to such people wherever possible, except when to do so would injure them or others.
10. Continued to take personal inventory and when we were wrong promptly admitted it.
11. Sought through prayer and meditation to improve our conscious contact with God, *as we understood Him*, praying only for knowledge of His will for us and the power to carry that out.
12. Having had a spiritual awakening as the result of these steps, we tried to carry this message to alcoholics, and to practice these principles in all our affairs.

The Twelve Steps are reprinted with permission of Alcoholics Anonymous World Services, Inc. Permission to reprint the Twelve Steps does not mean that A. A. has reviewed or approved the contents of this publication, nor that A. A. agrees with the views expressed herein. A. A. is a program of recovery from alcoholism only—use of the Twelve Steps in connection with programs and activities which are patterned after A. A., but which address other problems, or in any other non-A. A. context, does not imply otherwise.

BENZODIAZEPINES AND OTHER SEDATIVE-HYPNOTICS

With the introduction in 1961 of chlordiazepoxide (Librium), the benzodiazepines have replaced most of the short-acting barbiturates and other nonbarbiturate sedative-hypnotics that were in use prior to that time. Examples include diazepam (Valium), secobarbital (Seconal), and paraldehyde (Paral). Street names include roofies, tranks, ludes, barbs.

Incidence

Benzodiazepines are not commonly used as recreational drugs but are widely prescribed and are thus available for abuse. Statistics are not available because some clinicians are still denying that addiction to these drugs occurs. Withdrawal symptoms are subtle and delayed, and the symptoms are not always connected to the benzodiazepines.

Barbiturates and other sedative-hypnotics are more abused but less prescribed. These are available on the illegal market.

Signs and Symptoms

Benzodiazepines in low doses produce drowsiness or sedation. Larger doses produce sleep, but surgical anesthesia cannot be induced. Respirations are not depressed and there is little effect on the cardiovascular system unless extremely large doses are taken. Then a decrease in systolic blood pressure and an increase in heart rate may result. Side effects may include motor incoordination, ataxia, increased hostility or rage, confusion, metallic-like aftertaste, headache, and blurred vision. **Tolerance** (a decreased sensitivity to subsequent doses of the same substance; an increased dose of a substance is needed to produce the same desired effect) to other benzodiazepines and **cross-tolerance** (a decreased sensitivity to other substances in the same category) to other CNS depressants occur with chronic use.

Barbiturates depress all areas of the CNS, some selectively according to the dosage. They do not reduce pain. Respirations are depressed but not significantly when therapeutic doses are taken. When a barbiturate is given to a client in pain, excitement rather than sedation may occur. Side effects may include drowsiness, residual effects on motor skills, and especially in the elderly, excitement, irritability, or delirium. An overdose of barbiturates causes decreased respirations, rapid and weak pulse, cyanosis, coma, and sometimes respiratory paralysis. Tolerance results from chronic use or abuse. Benzodiazepines may be detected for 1 to 6 weeks.

Potential for Addiction

The potential for addiction is high for all of these substances. Benzodiazepines are schedule IV drugs; barbiturates may be either schedule II, III, or IV drugs; and methaqualone is a schedule I drug.

Withdrawal

Symptoms of withdrawal for benzodiazepines, which may not manifest for a week or more, include cramping, sweating, disorientation, confusion, tremors, depression, hallucinations, and paranoia. Barbiturate withdrawal symptoms include anxiety, weakness, anorexia, insomnia, tremors, delirium, and seizures that occur within 72 hours of the last use. Withdrawal reactions related to other sedative-hypnotics include nausea, headache, cramping, toxic psychosis, insomnia, and convulsions.

The withdrawal pattern is the same as for alcohol.

Treatment/Rehabilitation

Ideally, treatment for benzodiazepine abuse is a gradual reduction in the amount taken until the client is no longer taking any. A cross-tolerant drug such as phenobarbital is sometimes given to control symptoms and then its dosage is reduced. Hospital treatment is likely to be needed. Treatment for barbiturate and other sedative-hypnotics overdose or withdrawal is symptomatic.

Rehabilitation that focuses on teaching clients alternative methods of coping with the anxiety and stressors in their lives is necessary. Supportive individual psychotherapy or a self-help recovery group is almost always advisable. The goal is to assist the client to identify the consequences of the behavior and to understand the risks of relapse.

CANNABIS

Marijuana is the most common type of cannabis used. It is composed of dried leaves, stems, and flowers of the plant *Cannabis sativa* and can be smoked or added to food. Hash or hashish is a potent concentrate of the resin from the flowers. Hash oil is extremely concentrated, made by boiling hashish in a solvent and filtering out the solid matter. Street names include grass, pot, reefer, smoke, weed, and Mary Jane. "Blunts" are cigars emptied of tobacco and refilled with marijuana.

Incidence

Use in the United States began in the early 1900s, peaked in the period 1978 to 1980, and has steadily decreased since. According to Johnston, O'Malley, and Buchman (1991 and 1998), the prevalence of marijuana use by high school seniors increased from 20% in the class of 1969 to 60.4% in the class of 1979 and fell to 50.2% in the class of 1987 and fell again to 40.7 percent in the class of 1990. Use increased between 1990 and 1997 but declined in 1998 to 49%.

Signs and Symptoms

Short-term effects of marijuana use include memory and learning problems; distorted perception; difficulty in thinking and problem solving; loss of coordination; and increased heart rate, anxiety, and panic attacks. Long-term use produces changes in the brain similar to those seen after long-term use of other major drugs of abuse (NIDA, 1999j). A **reverse tolerance** can develop whereby a smaller amount of marijuana will elicit the desired psychic effects. Marijuana may be detected for up to 5 weeks.

Potential for Addiction

The potential for psychologic addiction is moderate. More than 120,000 persons seek treatment each year for their primary marijuana addiction (NIDA, 1999j). Marijuana is a schedule I drug.

Associated Problems/Disorders

Critical skills related to attention, learning, and memory are impaired in heavy marijuana users even 24 hours after the last use. Also, persons below college age who use marijuana tend to be more accepting of deviant behavior, have more aggression and delinquent behavior, act more rebellious, and have poorer relationship with parents (NIDA, 1999j).

Withdrawal

Nausea, myalgia, restlessness, irritability, nervousness, insomnia, and depression may appear after ceasing marijuana use. Symptoms may not appear for up to 1 week after the last use.

Treatment/Rehabilitation

Treatment focuses on relapse prevention and the development of new coping mechanisms, ways of liv-

ing, and means of having fun without drugs. Weekly group therapy sessions to maintain a commitment to abstinence and enhance interpersonal skills are often used. Participation in a self-help group is encouraged.

CNS STIMULANTS

Drugs that stimulate the CNS include cocaine, amphetamines, caffeine, nicotine, and methylphenidate hydrochloride (Ritalin). They increase cortical alertness and electrical activity in the brain and spinal cord. There is tachycardia and an increase in blood pressure.

COCAINE

Cocaine is extracted from the leaves of the coca plant, *Erythroxylum coca*. It may be heated and the fumes inhaled. This is termed *free-basing*. As a white powder, cocaine may be snorted by inhaling it through the nose. It may also be heated to a liquid state and injected intravenously. Crack is a crystallized form of cocaine that is melted in a water pipe and smoked. Street names include coke, crack, flake, rocks, snow, "C," and blow.

Incidence

Cocaine abuse and dependence was the major illicit drug problem for the United States in the 1980s. The introduction of crack dramatically increased cocaine abuse among the poor. Crack is low cost and gives an intense "high." It is estimated that 3.6 million persons in the United States are chronic cocaine users (NIDA, 1999c).

Signs and Symptoms

The immediate reaction, less than 10 seconds, is an intense euphoria that lasts 10 to 15 minutes. This short response time leads people to binge on cocaine. That is, they repeatedly use cocaine trying to maintain the euphoria.

The heart rate increases, blood pressure goes up, pupils dilate, peripheral blood vessels constrict, and temperature increases. Normal pleasures are magnified, anxiety decreases, self-confidence increases, social inhibitions are reduced, communication is facilitated, and sexual feelings are enhanced. Other psychological effects are inability to concentrate, insomnia, reduced sense of humor, antisocial behavior, hallucinations, and compulsive behavior.

An overdose may occur with the first use because there is little quality control of drug strength in the street drug culture. A client with an overdose may have arrhythmias, tremors, convulsions, respiratory failure, cardiovascular collapse, and death. Cocaine may be detected for up to 4 days.

LIFE CYCLE CONSIDERATIONS

Marijuana Use

- Toddlers whose parents use marijuana have more anger and regressive behavior (thumb sucking, temper tantrums) than toddlers whose parents do not use marijuana.
- During pregnancy, marijuana use may interfere with maternal and thus fetal nutrition, rest, and immune system functioning.
- Smaller babies are born to mothers who use marijuana during pregnancy and smaller babies more often develop health problems.
- Marijuana use during the first month of lactation can impair the infant's motor development (NIDA, 1999j).

Potential for Addiction

The potential for addiction is high. Cocaine is a schedule II drug.

Associated Problems/Disorders

Many types of heart disease are linked to cocaine use, especially ventricular fibrillation, heart attack, and hypertension. When cocaine is snorted regularly, respiratory problems occur, including loss of sense of smell, nosebleeds, hoarseness, and respiratory failure.

When cocaine is taken with alcohol, the two drugs are converted in the body to cocaethylene, which is more toxic than either drug alone (NIDA, 1999c).

Withdrawal

The crash, a period of exhaustion, occurs in the client; there are symptoms of depression, anxiety, and a great need for sleep. The depression may be to the point of suicidal behavior. The client has no energy, shows little interest in the surroundings, and seems to have little ability to experience pleasure. These symptoms are the most intense during the first 3 days but continue for 1 to 4 months. An intense craving for cocaine is felt, including dreaming about cocaine. Then there is a period of less intense craving for cocaine called extinction, which may last months or even years. Withdrawal does not result in a medical emergency as seen with alcohol.

Treatment/Rehabilitation

Treatment is aimed at reducing the craving and managing the severe depression. Careful monitoring of the client is necessary to identify and prevent actions aimed at carrying out the idea of suicide. The intense craving for cocaine and strong denial that cocaine is addicting creates a problem in engaging an individual, with a history of cocaine usage, in treatment. Inpatient programs for some clients with cocaine dependence should therefore be recommended, while other clients can be effectively treated in outpatient programs.

Medications

Bromocriptine mesylate (Parlodel) in small doses seems to reduce the withdrawal symptoms. Amantadine hydrochloride (Symmetrel) also has some success in treating cocaine withdrawal. Desipramine hydrochloride (Pertofrane) seems to reduce the craving for cocaine.

Education

Individual or group therapy should focus on helping the client feel pleasure again, improve energy level, and reduce cocaine craving. Peer support groups and self-help groups, such as Cocaine Anonymous, may be very effective. Random and regular urine testing is an external support to promote abstinence.

AMPHETAMINES

Amphetamines (also called uppers, speed, bennies) include dextroamphetamine sulfate (Dexedrine), amphetamine sulfate (Amphetamine), and methamphetamine hydrochloride (Desoxyn). Medically they are used to treat attention deficit hyperactivity disorder (ADHD), narcolepsy, and obesity.

Incidence

Amphetamines have been abused since the early 1930s. World War II greatly increased use and abuse when military personnel used amphetamines to decrease fatigue and increase alertness. Today, abuse ranges from truck drivers and college students who want to ward off sleep and increase alertness to the heavy abuser who injects or smokes homemade methamphetamine, known as meth, chalk, ice, crystal, crank, and glass. An estimated 4.9 million people in the United States have tried methamphetamine at some time (NIDA, 1999k).

Signs and Symptoms

Besides suppressing fatigue and increasing alertness, amphetamines enhance psychomotor performance, induce a temporary state of well-being, and give an instantaneous euphoria. Like cocaine, after several days the person becomes exhausted and lapses into a long period of sleep and depression (crash). The action of amphetamines lasts much longer than that of cocaine and there is a greater potential for adverse reactions and severe toxicity.

High abuse doses may cause insomnia, tachycardia, headache, arrhythmias, hypertension followed by hypotension, nausea, vomiting, cramping, diarrhea, hyperreflexia, convulsions, and death. The psychologic effect is termed amphetamine psychosis and closely resembles paranoid schizophrenia. Symptoms include paranoid ideation, confusion, compulsive behaviors, and visual and auditory hallucinations. Tolerance does develop. Amphetamines may be detected for up to 2 days.

Potential for Addiction

The potential for addiction is high. Amphetamines are schedule II drugs.

Associated Problems/Disorders

Cardiovascular problems occur, including irregular and rapid heartbeat; hypertension; and irreversible, stroke-producing damage to small blood vessels in the brain (NIDA, 1999k). Injecting the drug may damage blood vessels and cause skin abscesses, and if injection equipment is shared, there is an increased risk of HIV/AIDS and hepatitis B and C transmission.

Withdrawal

There are no physical manifestations of withdrawal. Psychological changes include apathy, irritability, depression, disorientation, anxiety, paranoia, aggression, and an intense craving for the drug.

Treatment/Rehabilitation

Urinary acidifiers, such as ascorbic acid (vitamin C), increase the excretion of amphetamines. Diazepam (Valium) is given for sedation to ease the withdrawal crash. Bromocriptine mesylate (Parlodel) or levodopa (Dopar) may help decrease the craving. A quiet environment is also helpful.

Behavioral therapy is used to help the client recognize and accept the need to stop using amphetamines. Supportive individual or group therapy, and especially self-help groups, aids the client to stay abstinent and in treatment.

CAFFEINE

Caffeine is found in coffee, tea, cola beverages, cocoa, chocolate, and some nonprescription drugs.

Incidence

Caffeine is probably the best known and most frequently used and abused CNS stimulant.

Signs and Symptoms

Caffeine causes relaxation of smooth muscles in blood vessels and bronchi, diuresis, an increased gastric acid secretion, suppression of appetite, increased feeling of energy, and constriction of cerebral blood vessels. An increased level of caffeine intake causes jitteriness, restlessness, nervousness, excitement, flushed face, palpitations, and nausea.

Potential for Addiction

The potential for addiction is moderate. Caffeine is not a scheduled drug.

Withdrawal

Withdrawal produces headache, irritability, and tremulousness.

Treatment/Rehabilitation

A gradual reduction of caffeine intake can reduce or eliminate the withdrawal symptoms. The client can then drink decaffeinated coffee and tea and caffeine-free soft drinks. The intake of cocoa and chocolate should be greatly reduced or eliminated. Caffeine can be avoided by reading labels and not using nonprescription products that contain caffeine.

NICOTINE

Nicotine is found in tobacco in a 1% to 2% concentration. There is no therapeutic use for nicotine. Smoking and other uses of tobacco have been in and out of favor several times during the past 5 centuries. This century has seen the greatest degree of abuse. Reasons for this increase are related to the mass production of tobacco products, mass advertising campaigns, and the psychological dependence produced by the nicotine. Tobacco, even when used in moderation, will likely produce disease and death. Tobacco kills more than 430,000 U.S. citizens each year. That is more than alcohol, cocaine, heroin, homicide, suicide, car accidents, fire, and AIDS combined (NIDA, 1998b).

Incidence

About 29% of the population age 12 and over uses tobacco (NIDA, 1999b). In high school students, smoking increased from 27.5% in 1991 to 36.4% in 1997 (NIDA, 1998b).

Signs and Symptoms

Nicotine causes decreased skeletal muscle tone, decreased sensitivity of some receptor sites (pain, heat, taste buds), reduced appetite, vasoconstriction, decreased body temperature, and increased blood pressure. Tolerance develops so the daily intake must increase to continue the desired effect.

Potential for Addiction

The potential for addiction is high. Even first-time users can become dependent within weeks of their initial use. Nicotine is not a scheduled drug.

Associated Problems/Disorders

Other ingredients in the smoke (tar, carbon monoxide, and incompletely burned waste products) are largely responsible for the negative health consequences.

Respiratory

Chronic obstructive pulmonary disease is caused by the many changes tobacco use makes in the respiratory system. Smokers are more prone to developing pneumonia, and asthma is exacerbated by smoking. Chronic exposure to smoke inhalation gives children higher rates of otitis media and respiratory illnesses.

Cardiovascular

Ischemic heart disease is twice as likely to develop in a smoker than in a nonsmoker. Cerebrovascular accidents and peripheral vascular disease are strongly associated with smoking. Cessation of smoking, about 10 years, reduces the risks for these 3 vascular diseases to the nonsmoker's level. Nearly 20% of deaths due to heart disease are attributable to smoking (NIDA, 1998b).

Cancer

Many cancers—oral, pharyngeal, laryngeal, esophageal, lung, pancreatic, kidney, and bladder—are strongly associated with tobacco. Secondhand smoke causes lung cancer in nonsmoking adults. Cigarette smoking is linked to approximately 90% of all lung cancer cases (NIDA, 1998b). The Surgeon General's report in 1982 stated that cigarette smoking is the major single cause of cancer mortality in the United States.

Withdrawal

Short-term effects of nicotine withdrawal include nausea, diarrhea, headache, drowsiness, insomnia, irritability, and poor concentration. Increased appetite along with an intense craving for tobacco may persist for 6 months or longer.

Treatment/Rehabilitation

Nicotine replacement therapy by patch, nasal spray, inhaler, or gum helps individuals break the habit. It is important that the client not smoke while using the patch. Serious adverse effects may be experienced with a high serum nicotine level. It can be toxic. Later, a gradual withdrawal of the nicotine patch can be accomplished. The first nonnicotine prescription drug to treat nicotine addiction, bupropion (Zyban), was approved by the Food and Drug Administration in 1996.

The availability of these products has produced a 20% increase in successful quitting each year (NIDA, 1998b).

An exercise program will help with stress management and minimize possible weight gain. Relaxation techniques will also reduce stress. Support by family and significant others for the person quitting tobacco use may help the process. A lack of support may greatly increase the difficulty of quitting for the individual. The rate of relapse is highest in the first few weeks, and diminishes considerably after 3 months.

METHYLPHENIDATE HYDROCHLORIDE (RITALIN)

Currently, there is an increase in the use (misuse and overuse) of Ritalin that is becoming a growing problem. Ritalin is an accepted treatment for children with attention deficit hyperactivity disorder (ADHD). Although Ritalin is a CNS stimulant, there is a paradoxical calming effect on children with ADHD. Many children are being given Ritalin without thorough testing to eliminate other causes of attention deficit. These children have the potential for dependence. Ritalin is also used for narcolepsy. It can be detected for 1 to 2 days and is a schedule II drug.

HALLUCINOGENS

Hallucinogens refers to a group of naturally occurring and synthetic agents that produce essentially the same mind-altering effects.

Psilocybin and psilocin are naturally occurring organic compounds found in some mushrooms that grow in the United States and Mexico. These mushrooms have been used for centuries in southern Mexico, primarily in religious ceremonies. Fresh or dried mushrooms, sometimes mixed with food, are ingested orally.

Dimethyltryptamine (DMT) and diethyltryptamine (DET) are found in tropical plant leaves and seeds. For centuries they have been dried and powdered and

LIFE CYCLE CONSIDERATIONS

Smoking

- Menopause generally occurs earlier in women who smoke.
- The use of oral contraceptives and smoking predispose women to cardiovascular and cerebrovascular disease especially when over 30 years of age.
- Pregnant women who smoke have increased risk of stillborn, preterm, or low birth weight infants.
- Female children of women who smoked during pregnancy are more likely to smoke and persist in smoking.
- Secondhand smoke increases the risk of respiratory illnesses and otitis media in children, and sudden infant death (NIDA, 1999b).
- The older smoker is often less motivated to quit because of the feeling that "I've survived this long."

CULTURAL CONSIDERATIONS

Mescaline

Mescaline is the active ingredient in peyote cactus found growing in the southwestern United States and Mexico. It is the only legally used hallucinogen. Members of the Native American Church of the United States may use it for religious purposes. It is ingested orally. A cross-tolerance to LSD and psilocybin occurs.

used as snuff. They are not orally active. Sometimes the powder is added to tobacco or marijuana.

There are several amphetamine-like hallucinogens. Probably the two best known are 2,5 dimethyl-4-ethyl-amphetamine (DOM) and methylene-dioxyamphetamine (MDMA, ecstasy), which are chemically manufactured compounds. These are usually taken orally but may be injected intravenously or inhaled.

LYSERGIC ACID DIETHYLAMIDE

Lysergic acid diethylamide (LSD), a manufactured chemical compound, is perhaps the most widely known and used hallucinogen. In the past, LSD has been used as a legitimate medication and in research. In the 1960s when its abuse became so widespread, the manufacturer refused to supply it for research. It had already been discontinued as a useful medication. It is generally taken orally but can be injected intravenously.

Incidence

The use of hallucinogens declined throughout the 1980s. The early 1990s indicated that LSD was making a comeback. The 1990 and 1991 annual survey of high school seniors found that for the first time since 1976, more seniors had used LSD than cocaine in the previous 12 months. The 1998 survey showed a slight downward movement in LSD use (Johnston et al., 1998). Other names for LSD are acid and microdot.

Signs and Symptoms

The functioning of both the peripheral nervous system and the central nervous system is altered by LSD. Physical effects include hypertension, increased temperature, sweating, loss of appetite, dilated pupils, and dry mouth. Time and distance are distorted, rational judgment is impaired, and visual **hallucinations** (perceiving things that are not really there) and delusions along with **synthesiasis** (hearing colors and seeing sounds) occur. A state of either euphoria or depression is experienced. The depression with feelings of anxiety, panic, or suicidal tendencies is termed a "bad trip." Flashbacks occur suddenly days or years after LSD use. Their occurrence and frequency are unpredictable but seem to happen in times of high stress. LSD may be detected up to 8 hours.

Potential for Addiction

LSD is not considered an addictive drug, but it does produce tolerance. It is a schedule I drug.

Associated Problems/Disorders

Personality changes occur with LSD use and may happen after a single LSD experience. Acceptable social behaviors seem to diminish with use.

Withdrawal

There is no withdrawal seen.

Treatment/Rehabilitation

A person on a "bad trip" should be carefully watched to prevent self-injury. Reassurance, support, and "talking down" should be done in a quiet, pleasant manner. The person should be encouraged to sit up or walk. Closing the eyes intensifies the "bad trip." The person should be reminded that the drug is causing the effects, which will soon go away.

After cessation of chronic LSD use, long-term psychotherapy is usually required to determine what needs were fulfilled by the use of this drug. A 12-step program and family assistance are usually necessary to reinforce the decision to remain abstinent. If the client is upset by flashbacks or the fear of flashbacks, an anxiolytic drug such as diazepam (Valium) may be ordered.

PHENCYCLIDINE

Phencyclidine (PCP) was made for use as an anesthetic agent, but it produced such adverse reactions that it was withdrawn from clinical trials. However, it can easily be manufactured in an unsophisticated laboratory from simple materials. The degree of purity varies widely. It is often found as a contaminant in other street drugs. The anesthetic is used in veterinary medicine.

Incidence

PCP is primarily used by adolescents and young adults with the first use between the ages of 13 and 15 years. Approximately 3% of those between the ages of 12 and 17 years had used PCP in 1991. The use increased to approximately 4% in 1997 (NIDA, 1999l). Other names for PCP are angel dust, ozone, wack, and rocket fuel. Marijuana combined with PCP is called killer joints or crystal super grass.

Signs and Symptoms

There are usually four phases, with the symptoms dose related. Acute toxicity is characterized by visual disturbances, auditory hallucinations, combativeness, catatonia, convulsions, and coma, and lasts about 3 days. The toxic psychosis phase has visual and auditory hallucinations, agitation, paranoid delusions, and disturbed judgment, and lasts about 7 days. The third phase has psychotic episodes, including thought disorders, paranoid ideation, and affect disorders much like schizophrenia and lasts a month or more. Depression is the fourth phase that may end in suicide. The use of other street drugs may alleviate the depression. Behavior is highly unpredictable. Death can occur from respiratory depression. For 2 to 8 days PCP can be detected.

Potential for Addiction

Even chronic use does not produce physical dependence. Psychological dependence does develop as evidenced by a craving for PCP. It is a schedule I and II drug.

Associated Problems/Disorders

Seizures are a common occurrence with PCP. Hypertension and hyperthermia must be treated before they become a crisis situation. **Opisthotonos**, a complete arching of the body with only the head and feet on the bed, usually is relieved as the blood level of PCP decreases. Cardiac arrhythmias may need interventions by a cardiologist. Acute renal failure may result from the use of PCP. Strokes also have been reported.

Withdrawal

PCP is fat soluble and its effects are felt weeks after the last use as it is gradually released from the fatty tissue into the circulation.

Treatment/Rehabilitation

Treatment should begin in an inpatient setting because of the high risk of suicide. The goal is to keep the client from resuming drug use. Sedatives may be used and urinary acidifiers such as ascorbic acid may be given to increase excretion of PCP. Minimal confrontation should be used in a nonthreatening, nonstimulating, supportive environment. No effort should be made to "talk down" or calm the individual. Diazepam (Valium) may be ordered.

Vocational counseling and training may enhance self-esteem. Body awareness, yoga, and progressive relaxation help the client focus and improve attention span and concentration. Participation in a self-help group such as Narcotics Anonymous (NA) should be encouraged, though initial involvement is usually minimal.

OPIOIDS

Opioids is a term used to refer to naturally occurring opiates, semisynthetic opiates, synthetic opiates, and agonist-antagonists. Table 46-8 provides examples of these opioids. Heroin is the most abused and the most rapid acting of the opioids (NIDA, 1999g).

Incidence

Kleber (1994) described the 1990s as the decade of heroin. Cocaine addicts switched to heroin. Heroin was easily available, the purity was higher than in decades, and it could now be sniffed or smoked instead of injected (NIDA, 1999g). By 1998, the increase in heroin

Table 46-8 OPIOIDS	
TYPE	**EXAMPLE**
Natural Opiates	morphine sulfate codeine sulfate
Semisynthetic Opiates	heroin hydromorphone hydrochloride (Dilaudid) oxymorphone hydrochloride (Numorphan) oxycodone (in Percodan) hydrocodone (in Hycodan)
Synthetic Opiates	meperidine hydrochloride (Demerol) methadone hydrochloride (Dolophine) propoxyphene (Darvon)
Agonist-Antagonists	pentazocine (Talwin) nalbuphine hydrochloride (Nubain) butorphanol tartrate (Stadol)

use by high school students had stopped (Johnston et al., 1998). Other names for heroin are horse, smack, "H," skag, and junk.

Signs and Symptoms

All of these drugs affect the central nervous system, causing mental changes, euphoria, drowsiness, analgesia, constricted pupils, and depressed respirations. These changes become more pronounced as the dose is increased.

Opioids increase stomach tone, decrease intestinal peristalsis, and increase the tone of the anal sphincter. This all adds up to constipation. Prolonged drug use may result in a fecal impaction.

Peripheral blood vessels are dilated by opioids, and orthostatic hypotension frequently occurs. The work of the heart is not changed by opioids, so they are frequently used to treat the severe pain of a myocardial infarction.

Tolerance may develop to one or more of the effects of opioids but not to others. For example, morphine addicts will always have pinpoint pupils even when the euphoric effects are not experienced. Tolerance to one opioid usually means tolerance to other opioids as well. Withdrawal symptoms from one opioid can be suppressed by using another opioid.

Potential for Addiction

The potential for addiction is high. Heroin is a schedule I drug; methadone, schedule II; morphine, schedule II or III; and codeine and opium are schedule II, III, or IV.

Associated Problems/Disorders

Chronic heroin injection may cause scarred and collapsed veins, bacterial infections of the heart valves and blood vessels, abscesses, and liver or kidney disease. Pneumonia may result from the respiratory-depressing effect of heroin. Additives to street heroin may clog blood vessels or cause immune reactions, leading to arthritis or other rheumatologic conditions. Sharing injection equipment can lead to infections of hepatitis B and C, HIV, and other blood-borne viruses, which can then be passed on to sexual partners and children.

Withdrawal

Withdrawal symptoms are dependent on drug purity, dose, and route of administration. Withdrawal is characterized by a rebound excitability of those functions that had been depressed. Symptoms include stomach cramps, nausea, vomiting, diarrhea, diaphoresis, hypertension, aching of bones and muscles, lacrimation, rhinorrhea, cold flashes with goose bumps, yawning, mydriasis, anxiety, irritability, restlessness, and sometimes paranoia, violence, fear, or depersonalization.

Morphine withdrawal symptoms begin within 8 to 12 hours after the last dose, and the acute phase is over in about 10 to 14 days. Figure 46-2 illustrates the signs and symptoms of morphine withdrawal. This is the basic pattern of withdrawal for all opioids.

Codeine withdrawal symptoms may be a little less

LIFE CYCLE CONSIDERATIONS

Heroin Use
- During pregnancy, heroin use may cause a miscarriage or preterm birth.
- Infants of addicted mothers have a greater risk of sudden infant death syndrome (SIDS).

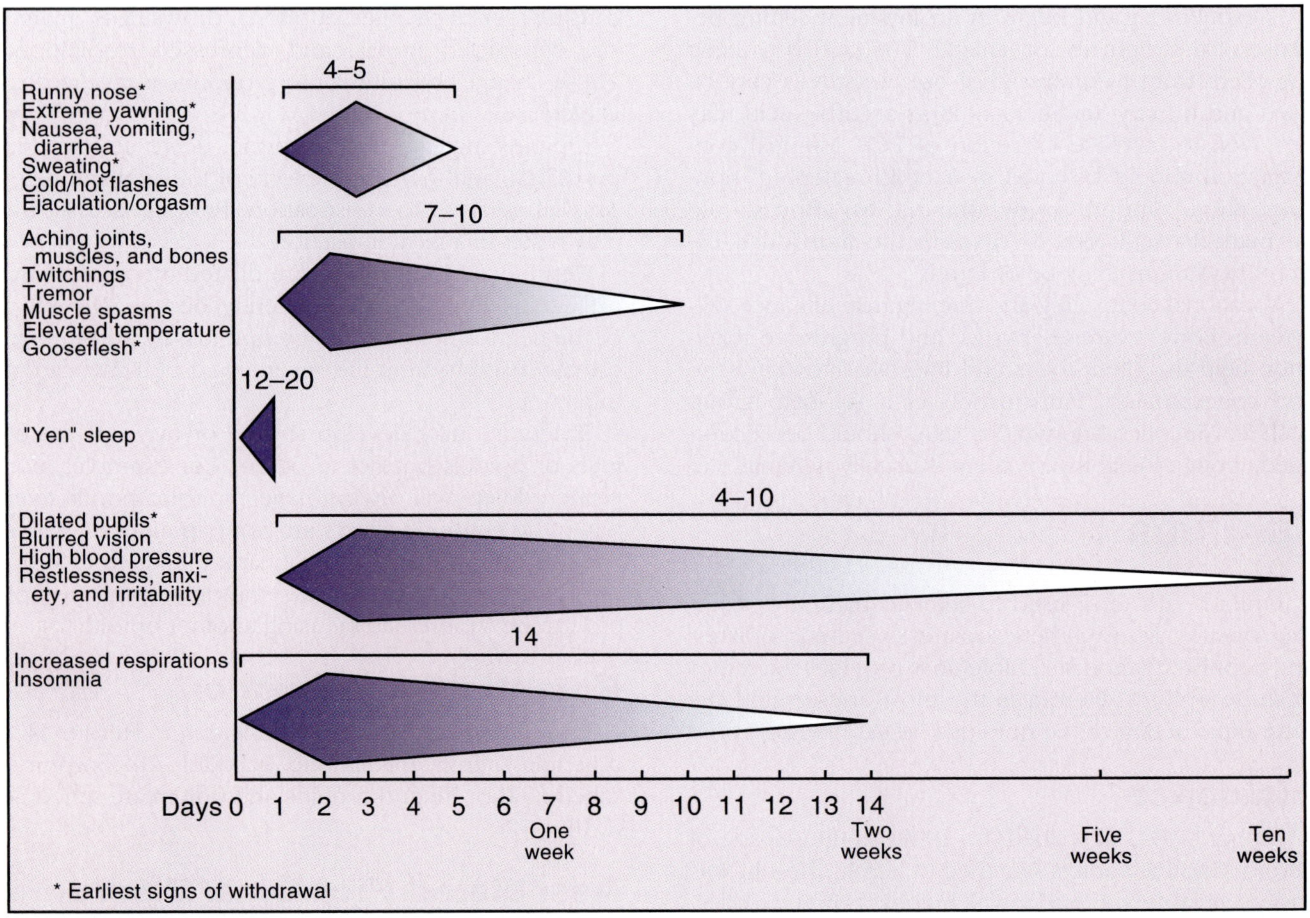

severe than those of morphine withdrawal. Dilaudid and heroin withdrawal may begin slightly earlier than morphine withdrawal. Meperidine (Demerol) withdrawal begins within 3 hours and peaks in 8 to 12 hours. Propoxyphene (Darvon) withdrawal is considerably milder.

Methadone withdrawal is slower to develop and lasts longer. Symptoms may not occur for 1 to 2 days, with acute symptoms lasting 2 to 3 weeks but not disappearing until 6 weeks after abstinence begins. Symptoms of fatigue, sluggishness, and irritability may last up to 6 months.

Withdrawal from the agonist-antagonists begins in 6 to 8 hours and is usually over in 8 days. The symptoms are the same as for morphine only in a milder form.

Figure 46-2 Duration of Morphine Withdrawal Signs and Symptoms

Treatment/Rehabilitation

Initial treatment is symptomatic and supportive of vital functions until the acute phase is over.

Detoxification

Several methods currently used for opioid detoxification are methadone, LAAM, and naltrexone.

Methadone Methadone is given and the dose adjusted to keep withdrawal symptoms under control. The daily dose is gradually reduced over a period of 3 to 6 months. Routine and random urine testing is usually done to ensure no other drug use.

Levo-alpha-acetyl-methadol Levo-alpha-acetyl-methadol (LAAM) is a synthetic opiate, like methadone, used to treat heroin addiction. It blocks the effects of heroin for up to 72 hours, so it need be taken only 3 times a week.

Naltrexone Naltrexone (ReVia) blocks the effects of morphine, heroin, and other opiates. Its effects last 1 to 3 days depending on the dose. The pleasurable effects of heroin are blocked, making it useful to treat highly motivated individuals. It is also used to prevent relapse in former opiate addicts.

Counseling/Self-Help Groups

Individual and/or group counseling must go hand in hand with the detoxification to help the client learn new methods of coping with life's stresses. Participation in Narcotics Anonymous (NA) helps the client maintain abstinence from drugs.

Behavioral Therapy

Contingency management therapy employs a voucher system. Clients earn "points" for having negative drug tests. These can be exchanged for items encouraging healthy living (NIDA, 1999g).

INHALANTS

Inhalants are inexpensive and easy to obtain. Examples are toluene (glues), gasoline, kerosene, isopropyl alcohol, lacquer thinner, acetone, benzene, naptha, carbon tetrachloride, fluorocarbons (aerosol propellants), correction fluid, and nitrous oxide. They are rapidly absorbed into the brain and stored in body fat.

Incidence

In 1997, 21% of 8th graders, 18.3% of 10th graders, and 16.1% of 12th graders reported using inhalants at least once (NIDA, 1999h). Inhalants are not scheduled drugs.

Signs and Symptoms

The desired effect of euphoria is followed by nausea, headache, and amnesia. Other effects of using inhalants include dizziness, unsteady gait, slurred speech, auditory and visual hallucinations, drowsiness, hypo-tension, heightened sexual response due to profound vasodilation, stupor, unconsciousness, and coma. Heavy use can lead to hypoxia, multiple organ damage, and death. Airway freezing and/or laryngospasm can be caused by nitrous oxide.

Behaviors that may indicate inhalant abuse include decreased school performance; loss of interest in extracurricular, family, and social activities; and the onset of legal problems.

Potential for Addiction

The potential for addiction is high for psychological dependence only.

Associated Problems/Disorders

Chronic pulmonary irritation and/or chemical pneumonitis may be caused by the use of inhalants. Toluene may cause renal tubular acidosis, hearing loss, and brain damage. Fluorocarbons sensitize the myocardium to catacholemines and may cause arrhythmias.

Withdrawal

There are no withdrawal symptoms.

Treatment/Rehabilitation

Initial treatment is to provide oxygen and respiratory support. Participation in a traditional chemical dependency program is often needed. An adolescent 12-step group is very helpful. Individual and family counseling are essential.

ANABOLIC STEROIDS

Anabolic steroids are synthetic derivatives of testosterone. They cause both androgenic (masculinizing) and anabolic (tissue building) effects. Most people use anabolic steroids for their anabolic effects. Medically, they are used in the treatment of some anemias and in some cancer therapies. The use of anabolic steroids is banned by the International Olympic Committee and the National Collegiate Athletic Association.

Incidence

Primary users are athletes seeking to improve their performance. Other people use anabolic steroids to improve their physical appearance. In 1997, 1.8% of 8th graders, 2% of 10th graders, and 2.4% of 12th graders had used anabolic steroids (NIDA, 1999m).

 LIFE CYCLE CONSIDERATIONS

Anabolic Steroid Use
In adolescents, anabolic steroid use can halt growth prematurely.

Signs and Symptoms

The commonly perceived effects of anabolic steroids are an increase in skeletal muscle mass, enhanced physical performance of the skeletal muscles, increased body weight, and improved athletic ability. However, there is no conclusive evidence that these perceived effects are medically accurate.

Potential for Addiction

The potential for addiction is moderate. Anabolic steroids are schedule III drugs.

Associated Problems/Disorders

Other effects found when anabolic steroids are used include hepatocellular damage, cholestasis, hepatoadenoma, hepatocarcinoma, acne, hirsutism, male-pattern baldness, a deepening of the voice, increased cholesterol level, increased blood pressure, decreased glucose tolerance, mood swings, aggressiveness, depression, psychosis, and hepatitis or HIV infection if needles are shared. In males, there is also testicular atrophy, oligospermia, impotence, prostatic hypertrophy, prostatic carcinoma, and gynecomastia. In females, there is also amenorrhea, clitoromegaly, uterine atrophy, breast atrophy, facial hair growth, and teratogenicity.

These effects seem to be reversible when the anabolic steroids are no longer taken, except for the male-pattern baldness, liver tumors, and gynecomastia in males and clitoral enlargement, virilization, and male-pattern baldness in females. The increased aggressiveness and euphoria are probably beneficial during athletic competitions but otherwise may cause severe social problems.

Withdrawal

Symptoms of withdrawal include lethargy, abdominal muscle cramps, constipation, headache, and depression.

Treatment/Rehabilitation

Treatment of withdrawal focuses on providing symptom relief for the client and counseling to build self-esteem and self-confidence in abilities without the use of anabolic steroids.

▶ NURSING PROCESS

Nursing care is an essential component of the multidisciplinary approach to substance abuse treatment.

▶ Assessment

The subjective and objective data given are related to substance abuse and dependence in general.

▶ Subjective Data

The client will often describe being very relaxed; feeling wonderful; or having a headache, fatigue, depression, sleep disturbance, suppression of appetite, dizziness, hallucinations, paranoia, anxiety, emotional lability, memory loss, heightened sexual desire (with early use), or loss of sexual desire (with continued use). Problems in various areas of life are common, such as frequent job changes; marital conflict, separation and/or divorce; work-related accidents, lateness, absenteeism; and legal problems, including arrest for driving while intoxicated. The client may describe having falls or fights and financial problems. Normal diet pattern and the presence of any disease conditions should be noted.

The client should be asked, "How often do you use drugs/alcohol? How much do you usually use? Have you ever used drugs/alcohol more than you use them now? When? Under what circumstances? What substance did you last use?" The information received from the client may not always be accurate. Validation with the family or significant other is helpful.

▶ Objective Data

Neglect of health and personal care is often evident. The client may have dental caries, bad breath, gingivitis, unkempt appearance, and be undernourished or malnourished. If substances have been inhaled, there may be irritation and bleeding of the nasal mucosa, destruction of the nasal mucosa and cartilaginous structures, or depression of respirations. If substances have been injected intravenously, there will be scarring of veins (needle marks, track marks), possibly skin infections, enlarged lymph nodes, and hematomas.

The client may appear older than the stated age and have chronic cough producing brown to black sputum, dilated or pinpoint pupils, tremors, slurred speech, lack of coordination, frequent episodes of sexually transmitted diseases, jaundice, or vomiting. There may be tachycardia, hypertension, ascites, or petechiae.

▶ Nursing Diagnoses

Nursing diagnoses for a client with substance abuse or dependence may include the following:

- *Nutrition, Altered, Less than Body Requirements*
- *Self-Care Deficit*
- *Injury, Risk for*
- *Sleep Pattern Disturbance*
- *Activity Intolerance*
- *Mobility, Impaired, Physical*
- *Sensory/Perceptual Alterations*
- *Communication, Verbal, Impaired*
- *Infection, Risk for*
- *Fluid Volume Excess or Deficit*
- *Thought Processes, Altered*
- *Coping, Individual, Ineffective*

- *Self-Esteem Disturbance*
- *Violence, Risk for, Directed at Others or Self-Directed*
- *Anxiety*
- *Social Interaction, Impaired*
- *Hopelessness*
- *Powerlessness*
- *Coping, Family, Ineffective, Compromised*

▶ Planning/Outcome Identification

There are several overall goals for the care of a client with a substance abuse problem. The client will do the following:

1. Abstain from using psychoactive substances
2. Adhere to the treatment plan
3. Make lifestyle changes to maintain abstinence
4. Engage in behaviors that foster good health

Other goals specific to nursing diagnoses must be formulated on an individual basis.

▶ Nursing Interventions

Nursing interventions include active listening, providing care in a nonjudgmental manner, teaching health promotion, and referral to self-help groups or individual counseling. Other nursing interventions must be specific for the goals and nursing diagnoses identified for the individual client. Examples might include the following:

1. Provide well-balanced diet. Monitor intake and lab tests results. Assess for GI bleeding.
2. Assist with personal hygiene. Encourage self-care.
3. Administer medications as ordered to decrease or prevent symptoms of withdrawal. Keep call light in client's reach. Keep side rails up.
4. Provide warm milk at bedtime. Plan with client a time for bed. Encourage use of relaxation techniques. Reassure client that insomnia will improve.
5. Encourage client to do active ROM exercises.
6. Assist client to turn in bed. Assist client to ambulate as able. Answer call light promptly.
7. Do not argue with a client having hallucinations. Remind client of day, time, and place.
8. Watch client's nonverbal communication.
9. Encourage good personal hygiene. Inspect skin for integrity.
10. Administer antibiotics as ordered. Monitor vital signs. Monitor I & O. Monitor lab tests results.
11. Administer vitamins as ordered. Provide cues as needed. Encourage adequate diet intake.
12. Assess coping patterns to identify strengths and weaknesses. Actively listen to client. Refer to appropriate community agencies.
13. Assist client to identify areas of low self-esteem. Encourage client participation in group therapy. Refer to individual counseling as needed.

LIFE CYCLE CONSIDERATIONS

Substance Misuse or Abuse

- The fetus is especially vulnerable to any substances used by the mother.
- Adolescents often progress from lighter to heavier illicit substance use leading to more serious multisubstance use.
- Indicators of adolescent substance abuse include a decline in academic performance, mood swings, personality changes, fatigue, drowsiness, and behaviors indicating depression.

In the elderly:
- **Misuse** (using a legal drug for something other than intended or exceeding the recommended dose of a drug) is more common than abuse or dependence.
- Substances that decrease respirations can increase the frequency of mental confusion.
- Decreased coordination from alcohol or other substances is associated with falling more often and fracturing the wrist, back, and hips.
- Chronic medical conditions can be made worse from even minimal use of alcohol or other drugs as these substances can change the effect of prescribed medications.
- Unrealistic expectations of retirement may lead to use of mood-altering substances to relieve depression and boredom.

14. Monitor client closely. Use restraints as ordered. Keep bed in low position and side rails up.
15. Introduce client to other recovering persons. Encourage client to participate in self-help group.
16. Provide spiritual support if asked.
17. Involve client in decision making when possible. Give positive reinforcement for abstinence.
18. Encourage family to participate in treatment program.

▶ Evaluation

Each goal must be evaluated to determine how it has been met by the client.

CODEPENDENCY

Codependency was first recognized by those working with families of alcoholics. It is a learned pattern of feeling and behaving, a problem with relationships. In healthy relationships, people share love, concern, and respect for each other. There is equal give-and-take. This is termed interdependence. In unhealthy relationships, people are often out of touch with their own needs and feelings. They may be unwilling or unable to take care of themselves and have little self-esteem. Only by fulfilling the expectations of others do they feel good about themselves. This is termed codependence. **Codependent** persons live based on what others think of them. They always try to meet the needs of others, demand love from others, and manipulate and control the lives of others.

Serious family problems like addictions, abuse, family secrets, or other major stresses cause confusion and put a family at risk. Codependent behavior thrives when fear, guilt, blame, and low self-esteem become evident. When family members do not relate to each other in positive ways or when their interactions do not provide a healthy environment, the family is called dysfunctional. Many children grow up in dysfunctional families and learn to be codependent.

Codependency tends to run in families. Parents cannot teach their children how to cope in healthy ways if they do not know how themselves. Without intervention or a conscious change by the individual, a pattern of codependent behavior will continue in other relationships.

Characteristics

Persons who are codependent have specific characteristics or traits. They have low self-esteem, never feel they are good enough, and often feel shame. Emotions are denied. They are out of touch with their own feelings and deny their own needs. Their smile is phony much of the time. Problems with communication become evident as they have trouble expressing their needs and feelings. Often they say the opposite to hide their true feelings. They expect others to read their mind. Relationship problems occur because they are afraid of being hurt or that others might learn of their secret feelings and reject them. They cannot risk loving and losing. Relationships are desired but walls are always put up.

Codependent persons live through others. They are people pleasers who would rather give than take. The approval of others means they are "OK." They think they can fix others. The feeling of powerlessness occurs because they give power to others by looking to them for approval. They go to extremes. For a while they will try very hard for approval and then they will not try at all or they will keep negative feelings inside with a smile on their face and then blow up over some little thing. Table 46-9 lists some characteristics of the codependent person.

Treatment

Professional help is usually necessary to change codependent behavior. The goal of treatment is to help the codependent person feel happy and good about himself or herself. Therapy sessions focus on identifying and reconnecting with the true self, dealing with feelings, learning how to communicate feelings,

learning to trust, setting boundaries for relationships, and taking charge of their own life.

THE IMPAIRED NURSE

Most states now have peer assistance programs to help nurses impaired by either alcohol or other substances. Substance abuse and dependence are greater problems among nurses than among the general public because nurses have access to many controlled substances. The impaired nurse often requests to give medications, makes medication errors, and "wastes" drugs frequently. This nurse may wear long sleeves and spend an extraordinary amount of time in the bathroom.

Peer assistance programs first appeared in 1980. They have been formed through the state nursing association or the state board of nursing, or through joint effort of both. The goals of the peer assistance programs are to assist the impaired nurse to receive treatment; protect the public from impaired nurses; help the recovering nurse reenter the nursing work force in a planned, safe manner; and monitor the nurse's recovery for a time. The state board of nursing may restrict access to controlled substances for the recovering nurse for some period of time.

Prior to the peer assistance programs, impaired nurses were generally just dismissed from employment. Then they would find employment at another health care agency where substance abuse or dependence would continue. This often went on for years.

As the name implies, peer assistance programs are staffed with nurses to help nurses. Many of the staff are volunteers who work in psychiatric nursing or substance abuse centers or who are themselves recovering from substance abuse. It is best not to cover up for a colleague with a substance abuse problem; rather, the nurse should report the situation to a supervisor who can arrange for the nurse to receive help. Some boards of nursing will discipline a nurse for failing to report a fellow nurse who is abusing drugs.

Table 46-9 CHARACTERISTICS OF THE CODEPENDENT PERSON	
Caretaking	"I always give to others. No one gives to me."
Obsession	"I can't stop worrying about ___ problems."
Denial	"I pretend I don't have problems."
Poor communication	"No one understands me."
Lack of trust	"I don't trust myself."
Anger	"I resent feeling controlled and manipulated."

From Mental Health Concepts *(4th ed.), by C. Waughfield, 1998, Albany, NY: Delmar Publishers. Copyright 1998 by Delmar Publishers. Adapted with permission.*

CASE STUDY

Joe, age 19, quit school 3 years ago. He has a part-time job at a fast-food place but has been tardy or absent quite often lately. Sometimes he is easy to get along with, and sometimes he is aggressive and difficult. His mother, with whom he lives, says he is a good boy and does not give her any trouble. Joe was brought to the emergency room by a friend after he passed out. His temperature is 99°F, respirations 10, and pupils are pinpoint. There are track marks on both arms.

The following questions will guide your development of a nursing care plan for the case study.

1. List signs and symptoms, other than Joe's, that a client may experience as a heroin addict.
2. List diagnostic tests that may be ordered.
3. List subjective and objective data the nurse should obtain.
4. Write three individualized nursing diagnoses and goals for Joe.
5. List resources within the medical center and local area that could assist Joe.
6. Describe the use of methadone in heroin addiction.
7. List teaching that Joe will need as a part of his rehabilitation.

SUMMARY

- Substance abuse and dependence have been problems for centuries.
- Factors related to substance abuse include individual, family patterns, lifestyle, environmental, and developmental factors.
- A false positive result on a drug screening test may be caused by ingestion of poppy seeds or use of a Vicks® inhaler.
- Detoxification is the first step in the treatment and rehabilitation of a substance abuser.
- Street drugs vary in strength and purity. Higher priced drugs are often mixed with cheaper or easier to obtain drugs.
- Neglect of health and personal care are often evident in substance abuse and dependence.
- Nurses have a higher incidence of substance abuse and dependence than the general public.
- Most states have peer assistance programs for impaired nurses.

Review Questions

1. Schedule II substances:
   a. can be sold as over-the-counter drugs.
   b. have high abuse and dependence potential.
   c. can have prescription refilled for 6 months.
   d. have no accepted medical use in the United States.

2. Substance use and abuse are:
   a. influenced by advertising.
   b. caused by a lack of education.
   c. rejected by all religious groups.
   d. caused by a chromosomal abnormality.

3. Prevention of substance abuse must be focused on:
   a. parents.
   b. children.
   c. teenagers.
   d. young adults.

4. Drug screening tests:
   a. are very accurate.
   b. indicate the level of abuse.
   c. indicate exposure to a substance.
   d. can test for all substances of abuse.

5. The substance most often chosen for abuse or dependence is:
   a. heroin.
   b. cocaine.
   c. alcohol.
   d. marijuana.

6. Alcoholics Anonymous is:
   a. the newest self-help group.
   b. a short-term temporary help group.
   c. a government agency to help those with an alcohol problem.
   d. a self-help group providing a holistic approach to abstinence.

7. Urinary acidifiers are used in the treatment of:
   a. opioids and LSD.
   b. amphetamines and PCP.
   c. alcohol and CNS stimulants.
   d. inhalants and benzodiazepines.

8. The use of inhalants:
   a. can be fatal.
   b. includes only glue and paints.
   c. has severe withdrawal symptoms.
   d. is a harmless activity of young male teenagers.

Critical Thinking Questions

1. What is your attitude toward substance abusers?

2. Should drug testing of all health care workers be required? How would you feel if requested to comply?

WEB FLASH!

- Search the Internet for information about the various illicit substances. What type of information do you find? Will it be helpful in caring for a client with a substance abuse problem?
- Visit the resources for this chapter on the Web. Do you find them on the Internet? What type of information or services do they provide?

Maternal/Child Health Nursing

CHAPTER 47

PRENATAL CARE

MAKING THE CONNECTION

Refer to the following chapters to increase your understanding of prenatal care:

- **Chapter 18, Basic Nutrition**
- **Chapter 35, Nursing Care of the Client: Reproductive System**

LEARNING OBJECTIVES

Upon completion of this chapter, you should be able to:
- *Define key terms.*
- *Discuss historical factors affecting pregnancy and childbirth.*
- *Describe fetal development from conception to birth.*
- *Identify the physical and psychological maternal changes during pregnancy.*
- *Describe the assessments to be performed at each prenatal visit.*
- *Discuss the nutritional needs of a woman during pregnancy.*
- *List the discomforts of pregnancy and one way a client might alleviate each.*
- *Use the nursing process to plan care for a pregnant client.*

INTRODUCTION

For centuries birth was part of family life and took place at home. Women learned about pregnancy and childbirth by asking female family members or friends and by being present when other women gave birth. In the United States in 1900 more than 90% of births were in the home.

In 1908 the American Red Cross and the Maternity Center Association offered the first formal programs for prenatal education. These early classes taught women about pregnancy, nutrition, and health care during pregnancy. By the 1950s the classes included preparation for birth. In 1960 the American Society for Psychoprophylaxis in Obstetrics (ASPO/Lamaze) and

KEY TERMS

abortion	linea nigra
age of viability	meconium
amenorrhea	multigravida
amnion	multipara
anticipatory guidance	nesting
ballottement	nulligravida
Braxton-Hicks contractions	nullipara
Chadwick's sign	para
chloasma	physiologic anemia of pregnancy
chorion	pica
coitus	placenta
colostrum	postterm
copulation	prenatal care
cotyledon	preterm
couvade	primigravida
ductus arteriosus	primipara
ductus venousus	pseudocyesis
fertilization	psychoprophylaxis
foramen ovale	quickening
fundus	striae gravidarum
funic souffle	supine hypotensive syndrome
Goodell's sign	teratogen
GP/TPAL	term
gravida	umbilical cord
Hegar's sign	uterine souffle
implantation	vernix caseosa
lanugo	Wharton's jelly
Leopold's maneuvers	zygote
let-down reflex	

the International Childbirth Education Association (ICEA) were founded. They both promote the idea that birth is a healthy process and that parents should have choices about the process.

In 1969, the Nurses Association of the American College of Obstetricians and Gynecologists (NAACOG) was formed with a goal of improving the health of women and newborn infants. The organization was renamed Association of Women's Health, Obstetric and Neonatal Nurses (AWHONN) in 1993. In conjunction with the American Nurses Association, AWHONN offers certification examinations for nurses engaged in obstetrical-gynecological nursing.

Today, many couples postpone pregnancy to obtain advanced education or establish careers; they may expect to participate in every aspect of the pregnancy, including decision making, and are much more informed than in the past of the educational offerings available. Today's nurse must have a firm understanding of the physical and psychological changes brought about by pregnancy, as well as the application of the nursing process in meeting the needs of the childbearing family.

PRECONCEPTION EDUCATION AND CARE

It has long been known that prenatal education and care identifies and reduces some problems in pregnancy and improves many outcomes. Yet, the United States continues to rank 21st in infant mortality rankings of industrialized nations in the world (Guyer et al., 1996). More and more, perinatal health experts are recognizing that a healthy pregnancy begins before conception.

Preconception education and care are focused on helping a couple prepare to conceive and identifying their reproductive risks prior to conception. The main goal is to protect the fetus during embryogenesis. Unhealthy habits can harm the fetus before the mother knows she is pregnant. Adopting a healthy lifestyle before pregnancy means eating a low-fat, high-fiber diet rich in vegetables and fruits; exercising at least 3 times a week; and getting to within 15 pounds of one's ideal weight. Another goal is to help the couple identify genetic factors that may affect a pregnancy. Several of the topics covered in preconcpetion visits are discussed following.

Immunizations and Disease Status

Immunization status should be confirmed and testing for infectious diseases such as syphilis, hepatitis, HIV, chlamydia, gonorrhea, human papilloma virus, and herpes simplex should be performed. These diseases can be treated to minimize adverse effects on the mother and fetus. Some states, such as New York, also test for group B streptococcus. Needed immunizations, especially rubella and hepatitis B, should be completed before a pregnancy is begun. Chronic diseases such as hypertension, cardiac disease, diabetes, epilepsy, thyroid dysfunction, asthma, renal disease, and phenylketonuria should be under control for the best outcome of pregnancy.

Medications

Known teratogens to be avoided are warfarin (Coumadin), gold salts, isotretinoin (Accutane), valproic acid (Depakene), lithium (Eskalith), diethylstilbestrol, DES (stilphostrol), live-virus vaccines, and folic acid antagonists (Cefalo & Moos, 1995). Taking any medication, either over-the-counter (OTC) or prescription, should first be discussed with the health care provider. It is best to have the system cleared of medications prior to conception, if possible.

Smoking, Alcohol, and Illicit Drugs

Smoking, alcohol, and illicit drugs all have negative effects on pregnancy. Smoking may cause spontaneous abortions and low-birth-weight infants. Fetal alcohol syndrome may be caused by excessive intake of alcohol, especially in the first trimester. Use of illicit drugs can lead to any number of fetal anomalies or disorders. Clients should be encouraged to discontinue use of these substances prior to and throughout pregnancy.

Genetic Risk Factors

A review of family history helps identify genetic risk factors. If any are identified, the couple is encouraged to have genetic counseling. Genetic services may be used preconceptually to determine the risk to a fetus of a particular disorder that has appeared in either parent's family, or by individuals believed to be at risk for a genetic disorder but who have no symptoms, and by individuals who have clinical findings indicative of a genetic disorder.

Male Contributions

A lower birth weight, mean deficit of 88 g, has been found in the infants of fathers who smoked and whose

CULTURAL CONSIDERATIONS

Childbearing

Caring for a pregnant client from another culture can be a very rewarding experience for the nurse who takes time to learn and who shows sensitivity and respect toward cultural differences. Journal articles may be found about the childbirth practices of other cultures, such as those by Hutchinson and Baqi-Aziz (1994) and Schneiderman (1996).

mothers did not (Martinez et al., 1994). Also, smoking affects spermatogenesis and sperm mobility. Male exposure to occupational chemicals has been associated with spontaneous abortion, stillbirth, preterm delivery, and small-for-gestational-age babies (Robaire & Hales, 1993). Since spermatogenesis is continuous so that a new supply of sperm are generated every 12 weeks, men can avoid smoking and exposure to occupational chemicals for the period of time when the couple is planning a pregnancy, and thus eliminate their effects.

PREGNANCY

Pregnancy refers to the condition of carrying an offspring within the body. It is a form of reproduction that unites the cells of two individuals to form a unique new individual who embodies characteristics of both parents.

Fertilization

Pregnancy typically begins as a result of **coitus** or **copulation**, which is the sexual act that delivers sperm to the cervix by ejaculation of an erect penis. Sperm entering the vagina by other means such as artificial insemination may also result in fertilization. **Fertilization** or conception occurs when a sperm and ovum unite. This union generally occurs in the distal third of the fallopian tube. The fertilized ovum is now called a **zygote**.

The gender of the zygote is determined at the time of fertilization. When the ovum and sperm each contribute an X chromosome, the result is a female. When the ovum contributes an X chromosome and the sperm a Y chromosome, the result is a male.

Cell division occurs as the zygote travels the fallopian tube to the uterus. It takes 3 to 4 days of cell division, or mitosis, for the zygote to become a morula, which resembles a mulberry. The morula entering the uterus is now called a blastocyst. The cells have differentiated into an inner mass of embryonic cells, which becomes the embryo; and an outer layer called the trophoblast, which is involved in implantation, hormone secretion, and membrane and placental formation (Figure 47-1).

Implantation

About 7 days after ovulation or 5 days after fertilization, the trophoblast burrows into the endometrium, usually in the upper part of the uterus. This process is called **implantation**, or embedding of the fertilized egg into the uterine lining. The trophoblast puts out villi, fingerlike projections, to anchor the blastocyst.

Multiple pregnancy occurs when more than one fetus develops at the same time. When twins result from two ova being fertilized by two sperm, the twins are fraternal or dizygotic. They are nonidentical and may be two males, two females, or one male and one female. There are two amnions, two chorions, and two placentas.

If one ovum is fertilized by one sperm and the inner cell mass of the blastocyst splits in two to form two embryos, the twins are identical or monozygotic. They may be two males or two females. There are two amnions, one chorion, and one placenta. The genetic makeup is identical in each fetus (Figure 47-2).

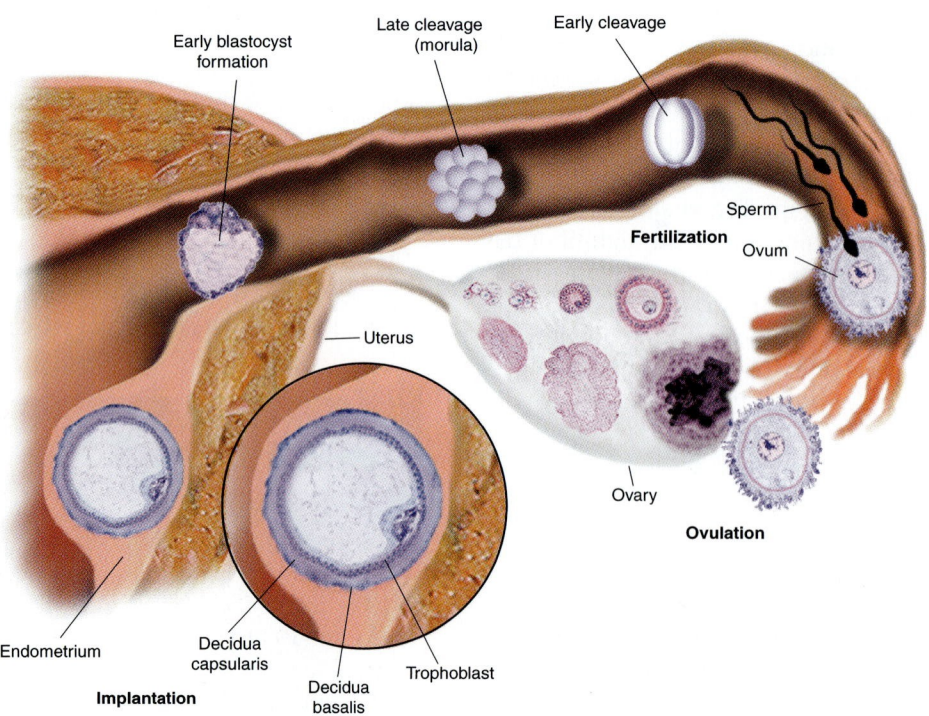

Figure 47-1 Ovulation, Fertilization, and Implantation

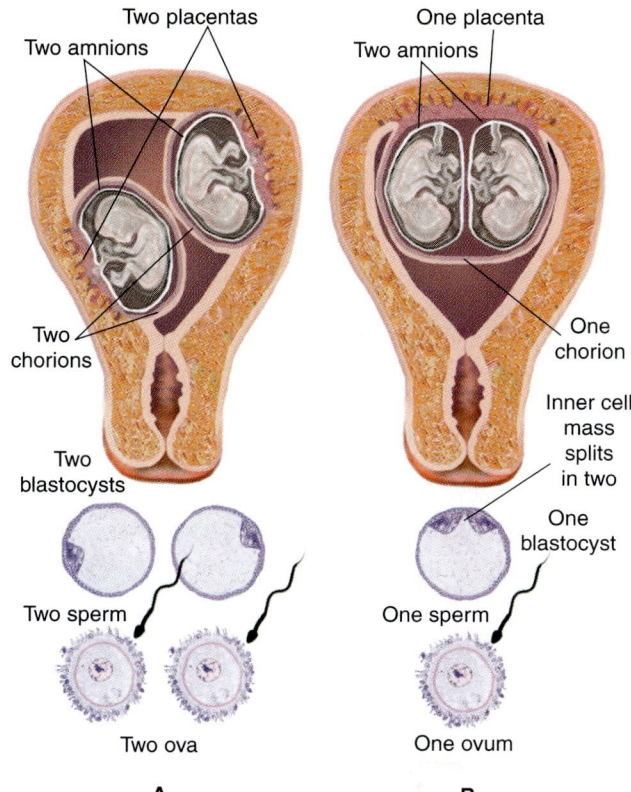

Figure 47-2 Formation of Twins: A. Fraternal (nonidentical); B. Identical

The outer fetal membrane is the **chorion**, formed from the trophoblast. The chorionic villi degenerate, except for those attached to the uterine wall, which become the placenta. The inner membrane, the **amnion**, originates in the blastocyst during the early stages of development. The amnion expands as the fetus grows until it slightly adheres to the chorion. These two fetal membranes form the amniotic sac or bag of water (BOW).

Amniotic Fluid

The amniotic fluid is formed by the secretions from the amniotic cells, lungs and skin of the fetus, and fetal urine. It is 98% water, but also has traces of glucose, proteins, urea, creatinine, **lanugo** (fine hair covering body of fetus), and **vernix caseosa** (white, creamy covering on the fetus's body). Amniotic fluid is slightly alkaline. Approximately every 3 hours the fluid is replaced. The amnionic cells and the fetus urinating and swallowing regulate the secretion and reabsorption of the fluid.

The amniotic fluid has several important functions in that it:

- Equalizes the pressure around the fetus.
- Cushions the fetus from injury.
- Provides a constant temperature and fluid for the fetus to swallow.
- Allows freedom of movement for the fetus.
- Prevents the membranes from sticking to the fetus.

The yolk sac develops as a second cavity in the blastocyst. It forms primitive red blood cells until the liver is able to take over the process in about 6 weeks. Gradually, the yolk sac is incorporated into the umbilical cord.

Placenta and Umbilical Cord

The chorionic villi at the base of the implanted fertilized ovum and the decidua basalis, the endometrium at the site of implantation, form the placenta. The **placenta** is a membranous vascular organ connecting the fetus to the mother, which produces hormones to sustain a pregnancy, supplies the fetus with oxygen and food, and transports waste products out of the fetal system. The development of the placenta, stimulated by progesterone secreted by the corpus luteum, begins about the third week following fertilization. The placenta is fully functional by the twelfth week.

There is a maternal side to the placenta and a fetal side. The maternal side is irregular and is divided into subdivisions called **cotyledons**. It resembles liver both in color and texture. The fetal side is covered by the amnion so it is smooth and shiny.

The chorionic villi contain blood vessels that join to form larger and larger vessels, eventually becoming the umbilical cord. The **umbilical cord**, a structure that connects the fetus to the placenta, has two arteries and one vein. It is surrounded and protected by a thick substance called **Wharton's jelly** and covered by the amnion. The two umbilical arteries carry deoxygenated blood from the fetus to the placenta where carbon dioxide and other waste products are eliminated. The one umbilical vein carries oxygenated blood to the fetus along with nutrients, hormones, antibodies, and whatever drugs or toxic substances the mother may have in her body. This is one instance in which arteries carry deoxygenated blood and a vein transports oxygenated blood. Generally, the cord is attached to the center of the placenta, but it can be attached any place on the placenta.

The circulatory systems of the mother and fetus are separate. Maternal blood enters the intervillous spaces of the placenta. Fetal blood is in the vessels of the chorionic villi. Thus the cells of the fetal blood vessels and the chorion keep maternal blood and fetal blood separate.

Functions of the Placenta

The placenta has three major functions: transport, endocrine, and metabolic. All are necessary to maintain the pregnancy and promote normal fetal growth and development. The placenta provides the respiratory and excretory functions for the fetus as well as providing nutrition to the fetus.

Transport There are several mechanisms by which the placenta transports substances.

- Substances may move by diffusion from an area of higher concentration to an area of lower concentration. Those transported by this mechanism are: oxygen, carbon dioxide, carbon monoxide, water, electrolytes, fat-soluble vitamins, anesthetic gases, and drugs.

- Facilitated diffusion uses a carrier system to move molecules more rapidly than simple diffusion. Some glucose and oxygen are transported by this method.
- Active transport allows molecules to move from an area of lower concentration to an area of higher concentration. Substances moved across the placenta by active transport are: amino acids, glucose, iron, calcium, iodine, and water-soluble vitamins.
- Pinocytosis transfers larger molecules such as albumin, globulins, antibodies, and viruses through cell membranes.
- Osmotic pressure and hydrostatic pressure move most of the water.

Very large molecules such as insulin, heparin, IgM, and blood cells do not move across the placenta unless there is a tear in the placenta.

Endocrine The placenta secretes five hormones that are essential to pregnancy: human chorionic gonadotropin (hCG), which is the basis for pregnancy tests; human placental lactogen (hPL); estrogen; progesterone; and relaxin.

The trophoblast secretes hCG during early pregnancy. The hCG prevents involution of the corpus luteum and stimulates it to continue producing progesterone and estrogen for 11 to 12 weeks. Eight to ten days after fertilization, hCG is present in maternal blood serum; a few days after the missed menstrual period, hcG is found in maternal urine. After eleven weeks, the placenta is producing enough estrogen and progesterone to maintain the pregnancy.

Human placental lactogen makes a sufficient supply of protein, glucose, and minerals available to the fetus by stimulating changes in maternal metabolism. Human placental lactogen is an insulin antagonist, thus decreasing maternal metabolism of glucose. It also ensures that the mother's body is prepared for lactation.

The placenta secretes primarily the estrogen estriol. Essential precursors from the fetal adrenal glands are used by the placenta for conversion to estriol. Estrogen stimulates development of uterine and breast tissues in the mother. It also increases vascularity and vasodilation in the villous capillaries.

After eleven weeks of pregnancy, the placenta takes over the production of progesterone from the corpus luteum. Progesterone, a smooth muscle relaxant, prevents uterine contractions by decreasing its contractility. It also maintains the endometrium.

Relaxin causes changes in collagen. The connective tissue of the symphysis pubis and sacroiliac joints are softened and become slightly flexible.

Metabolic The placenta produces fatty acids, glycogen, and cholesterol for fetal use and hormone production. The enzymes required for fetoplacental transfer are also produced by the placenta. It breaks down epinephrine and histamine and stores glycogen and iron.

FETAL DEVELOPMENT

Fetal development is divided into three stages. The preembryonic or germinal stage is the first 14 days after fertilization. The second stage, the embryonic stage, is from the beginning of the third week (day 15) through week eight. The fetal stage is from week nine until 38 to 40 weeks or full term.

Development occurs in a systematic manner from head to toe (cephalo-caudal), from proximal to distal (close to body–farthest from body), and from general to specific. This means that the head develops before the arms and the arms develop before the legs; the arms and legs develop before the fingers and toes; and the fetus moves its arms before grasping with the hands.

Fetal development is sometimes described in general terms of trimester. The first trimester is the first 12 weeks, second trimester weeks 13 through 27, and third trimester weeks 28 to 40.

Pregnancy generally lasts 10 lunar (28 days) months, 40 weeks, or 280 days. It is calculated from the first day of the mother's last menstrual period (LMP). Table 47-1 identifies stages of fetal development and gives the weight and length (crown-rump length, or C-R) or crown-heel (C-H) beginning in week four.

System Development

All systems in the fetus have begun forming by the eighth week. They grow, develop, and mature at different rates, and some do not mature until years after birth.

Cardiovascular System

With the primitive heart beginning to beat on the 21st day following conception, the cardiovascular system is the first to function in the embryo. Most congenital malformations of the heart and great vessels develop during the sixth to eighth weeks.

Fetal Circulation Fetal circulation has several unique features. Oxygenated blood comes from the placenta and enters the fetus, at the umbilicus, through the umbilical vein. It divides at the liver with a small branch going to the liver and the other branch, the **ductus venosus**, entering the inferior vena cava. The blood is now partially deoxygenated by the blood coming from the lower part of the fetus's body.

This blood enters the right atrium and moves through the **foramen ovale** (a flap opening in the atrial septum that allows only right to left movement of blood) to the left ventricle. A small portion of this blood passes into the right ventricle. The left ventricle pumps the blood out through the aorta.

Table 47-1 STAGES OF FETAL DEVELOPMENT

STAGE	FETAL DEVELOPMENT	STAGE	FETAL DEVELOPMENT
Preembryonic or Germinal Stage		**Second Trimester**	
Weeks 1 and 2	Rapid cell division and differentiation. Germinal layers form.	Week 16 Wt 200 g (7 oz) L 13.5 cm (5.5 in) (C–R) 15 cm (6 in) (C–H)	Meconium forms in bowels. Scalp hair appears. Frequent fetal movement. Skin thin, pink. Sensitive to light. 200 mL amniotic fluid. (Amniocentesis possible.)
Embryonic Stage			
Week 3	Primitive nervous system, eyes, ears, red blood cells present. Heart begins to beat day 21.		
Week 4 Wt 0.4 g L 4–6 mm (crown–rump, C–R)	Half the size of a pea. Brain differentiates. GI tract begins to form. Limb buds appear.	Week 20 Wt 435 g (15 oz) L 19 cm (7.5 in) (C–R) 25 cm (10 in) (C–H)	Myelination of spinal cord begins. Peristalsis begins. Lanugo covers body. Vernix caseosa covers body. Brown fat deposits begun. Sucks and swallows amniotic fluid. Heart beat heard with fetoscope. Hands can grasp. Regular schedule of sucking, kicking, and sleeping.
Week 5 L 6–8 mm (C–R)	Cranial nerves present. Muscles have innervation.		
Week 6 L 10–14 mm (C–R)	Fetal circulation established. Liver produces red blood cells. Central autonomic nervous system forms. Primitive kidneys form. Lung buds present. Cartilage forms. Primitive skeleton forms. Muscles differentiate.	Week 24 Wt 780 g (1 lb, 12 oz) L 23 cm (9 in) (C–R) 28 cm (11 in) (C–H)	Alveoli present in lungs, begin producing surfactant. Eyes completely formed. Eyelashes and eyebrows appear. Many reflexes appear. Chance of survival if born.
		Third Trimester	
Week 7 L 22–28 mm (C–R)	Eyelids form. Palate and tongue form. Stomach formed. Diaphragm formed. Arms, legs move.	Week 28 Wt 1200 g (2 lb, 10 oz) L 28 cm (11 in) (C–R) 35 cm (14 in) (C–H)	Subcutaneous fat deposits begun. Lanugo begins to disappear. Nails appear. Eyelids open and close. Testes begin to descend.
Week 8 Wt 2 g L 3 cm (1.5 in) (C–R)	Resembles human being. Eyes moved to face front. Heart development complete. Hands and feet well formed. Bone cells begin replacing cartilage. All body organs have begun forming.	Week 32 Wt 2,000 g (4 lb, 6.5 oz) L 31 cm (12 in) (C–R) 41 cm (16 in) (C–H)	More reflexes present. CNS directs rhythmic breathing movements. CNS partially controls body temperature. Begins storing iron, calcium, phosphorus. Ratio of the lung surfactants lecithin and sphingomyelin (L/S) is 1.2:2.
Fetal Stage			
Week 9	Finger and toe nails form. Eyelids fuse shut.		
Week 10 Wt 14 g (½ oz) L 5–6 cm (2 in) crown–heel (C–H)	Head growth slows. Islets of Langerhans differentiated. Bone marrow forms, RBCs produced. Bladder sac forms. Kidneys make urine.	Week 36 Wt 2,500– 2,750 g (5 lb, 8 oz) L 35 cm (14 in) (C–R) 48 cm (19 in) (C–H)	A few creases on soles of feet. Skin less wrinkled. Fingernails reach fingertips. Sleep-wake cycle fairly definite. Transfer of maternal antibodies.
Week 11	Tooth buds appear. Liver secretes bile. Urinary system functions. Insulin forms in pancreas.		
		Week 38	L/S ratio 2:1
Week 12 Wt 45 g (1.5 oz) L 9 cm (3.5 in) (C–R) 11.5 cm (4.5 in) (C–H)	Lungs take shape. Palate fuses. Heart beat heard with Doppler. Ossification established. Swallowing reflex present. External genitalia, male or female distinguished.	Week 40 Wt 3,000– 3,600 g (6 lb, 10 oz– 7 lb, 15 oz) L 50 cm (20 in) (C–H)	Lanugo only on shoulders and upper back. Creases cover sole. Vernix mainly in folds of skin. Ear cartilage firm. Less active, limited space. Ready to be born.

Blood entering the right atrium from the superior vena cava flows to the right ventricle. It is pumped out through the pulmonary arteries. Most of this blood goes into the aorta through the **ductus arteriosus**, a fetal vessel connecting the pulmonary trunk to the aorta. Normally this closes at birth. A small amount of blood goes to the lungs to nourish the lung tissue.

The aorta and its branches supply blood to the rest of the body. The two umbilical arteries branch from the internal iliac arteries and return blood to the placenta to be oxygenated. Figure 47-3 shows fetal circulation.

Hematologic Development The formation of blood goes along with cardiovascular development. About day 14, primitive blood cells are formed in the yolk sac. It is the fifth week of gestation before the fetal liver begins hematopoiesis.

Fetal hemoglobin (Hgb F), found only during gestation and the early neonatal period, has a great attraction for oxygen. This ensures an adequate oxygen supply. Blood type is genetically determined at conception.

Gastrointestinal System

During the fourth week of gestation, the gastrointestinal tract begins forming. The fetus begins swallowing amniotic fluid by the twentieth week, but there is no coordination of the swallow and suck reflexes until about 34 weeks.

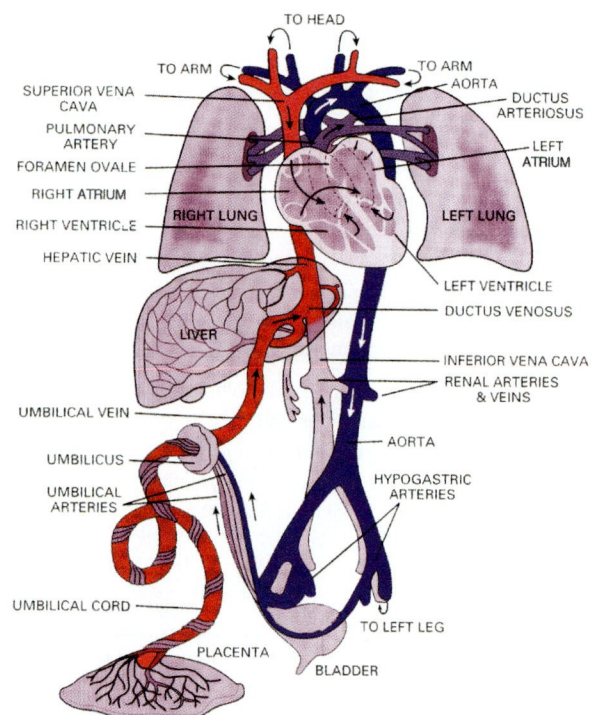

Figure 47-3 Fetal Circulation. Red shows arterial blood, dark purple shows venous blood, and light purple shows mixed arterial–venous blood.

Meconium (fecal material stored in the fetal intestines) begins to form about week 16. However, there should not be passage of meconium in utero. If the fetus encounters hypoxic stress, the anal sphincter may relax and meconium may be passed, causing meconium staining of the amniotic fluid.

Musculoskeletal System

Limb buds appear late in the fourth week and development is complete by the eighth week. Growth of the skeleton is determined by genetics and maternal supply of calcium and phosphorus. Cartilage is noted about 5 weeks and ossification begins about 12 weeks but is not completed until after puberty, when growth is complete.

By the end of the twelfth week, skeletal muscles begin involuntary movements. Skeletal muscle development depends on an adequate volume of amniotic fluid to allow plenty of fetal movement.

Genitourinary System

Kidneys begin forming at about 3 weeks and pass through several changes. Around 12 weeks they begin to produce a hypotonic urine. The placenta and the maternal kidneys are still responsible for fetal waste removal. All the nephrons are in the kidneys at birth.

The reproductive system develops at the same time as the urinary system. Testes can be seen in the abdomen by 7 weeks and begin descending to the scrotum about 30 weeks. The ovaries develop in the abdomen and stay in the pelvic cavity. All of the ova a female will ever have are in the ovaries at birth. Visual determination of fetal gender can be made through ultrasound by the end of week 12.

Integumentary System

The skin protects the underlying tissues. Vernix caseosa protects the skin, with the amount present decreasing as the pregnancy progresses. Creases form on the palms, fingers, and soles during week 11, with permanent designs formed by week 17. Skin color is genetically determined.

Lanugo appears during week 20 and slowly disappears; most is gone by birth. Tooth buds for the deciduous (baby) teeth appear during week 6 while tooth buds for permanent teeth do not appear until week 10. Second and third permanent molar tooth buds do not appear until after birth.

Mammary glands develop during the sixth week.

Respiratory System

Lung buds begin forming during week 6, with bronchi forming by week 16. Primitive lungs are formed by 23 weeks, but there are not enough alveoli for sufficient gas exchange. Surfactant production begins between weeks 20 and 24. Surfactant reduces the surface tension of the fluid lining the alveoli in the lungs, thus facilitating breathing. Surfactant production matures between weeks 35 and 37. After 23 weeks' gestation the lungs are capable of borderline support of extrauterine respiration. Therefore, the **age of viability**, or gestational age at which a fetus could live outside the uterus, is considered to be 24 weeks. Adequate lung functioning also depends on surfactant production and neurologic maturation.

Immunologic System

Between the twelfth and fifteenth weeks, immune capability begins developing. It functions very minimally since the fetus lives in a sterile environment. The fetus produces small amounts of the immunoglobins IgG, IgA, and IgE before 20 weeks. IgG provides the most immunity. Maternal IgG is actively transported across the placenta to provide passive immunity against many infectious diseases. Blood group antibodies are a type of IgG. They can move across the placenta by active transport and cause hemolytic disease of the newborn.

Factors Affecting Fetal Development

Many factors influence fetal development, especially during the first trimester. Even before the mother knows she is pregnant many factors are affecting embryonic development. One of the very first is the quality of the sperm and the ovum and the genetic code. **Teratogens** (any agent, such as radiation, drugs, viruses, or other microorganisms, capable of causing abnormal fetal development) exert the greatest influence on cells undergoing the most rapid growth. Each organ has a period when teratogenic agents or other insults can cause physical and functional defects.

A well-provided maternal environment is also important. Maternal malnutrition, acute and chronic diseases, drugs, alcohol, and smoking all can exert potentially harmful effects on the fetus before birth.

PHYSIOLOGICAL CHANGES OF PREGNANCY

Many physiological changes take place when a woman is pregnant. Every system of the mother's body undergoes some change during pregnancy.

Reproductive System

The most obvious physiological changes occur in the reproductive system.

Uterus

The most dramatic change occurs in the size of the uterus. Before pregnancy it is a small, pear-shaped, thick-walled, muscular organ weighing 60 g (2 oz). At the end of pregnancy it is a large, thin-walled organ

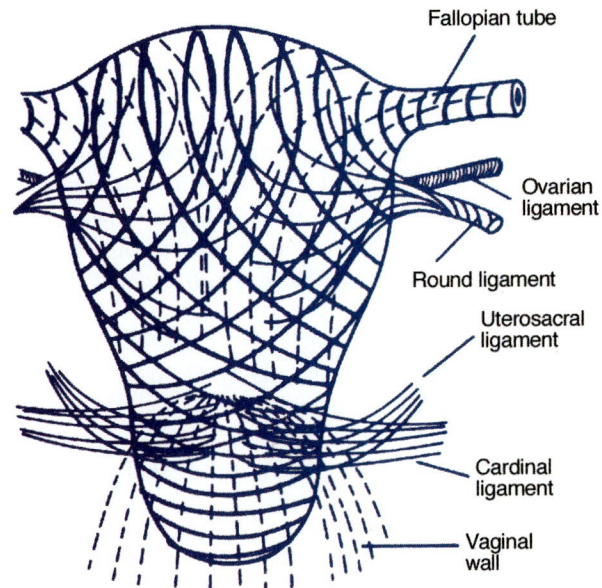

Figure 47-4 Muscle Layers of the Uterus

weighing 1,000 g (2 lb). Its capacity has increased from 10 mL to 5 L. The uterus enlarges mainly by hypertrophy of the muscle cells stimulated by estrogen and the growing fetus. There are three layers of smooth (involuntary) muscles in the uterus (Figure 47-4). The outer layer is made of longitudinal muscles. The muscle fibers of the middle layer are interlaced in a figure eight pattern. Circular fibers that form sphincters at the openings of the fallopian tubes and at the internal os of the cervix make up the inner layer of uterine muscle. This configuration of muscle layers allows the uterus to expand evenly in all directions during pregnancy. One-sixth of the mother's blood volume is in the vascular system of the uterus by the end of pregnancy.

Irregular, painless uterine contractions occur throughout pregnancy. About 16 weeks or later the mother may become aware of these **Braxton-Hicks contractions**. These painless contractions assist in uterine and placental circulation. A softening of the uterine isthmus about the sixth week of pregnancy, noted during a pelvic exam, is called **Hegar's sign**.

Cervix

The cervix increases in cell number by the influence of estrogen. It secretes a thick, sticky mucus that forms a plug in the cervix. This plug prevents microorganisms from entering through the vagina. During labor, as the cervix dilates, this mucus plug is expelled. **Goodell's sign** (softening of the cervix) and **Chadwick's sign** (a purplish-blue color of the cervix and vagina due to the increased vascularity) are both noted at about 8 weeks.

Ovaries

Follicles do not mature and ovulation does not occur during pregnancy. The corpus luteum produces progesterone and estrogen for about 12 weeks, at which time the placenta takes over the production.

Vagina

Estrogen causes a loosening of connective tissue and an increase in vaginal secretions. The acidic secretions prevent bacterial infections. The increased level of glycogen in cells may enhance growth of organisms such as *Trichomonas vaginalis* or *Candida albicans*.

Breasts

In addition to breast enlargement from hormonal influence, the nipples become more erect, the areolas darken, and Montgomery's tubercles enlarge. **Colostrum**, an antibody-rich yellow fluid, is secreted by the breasts during the last trimester and first 2–3 days after birth, and gradually changes to milk a few days after delivery.

Cardiovascular System

Blood flow increases to the uterus and kidneys where the workload is increased. The pulse increases by 10 to 15 beats/minute by the end of pregnancy. Cardiac output increases 30% to 50% early in pregnancy. Blood pressure decreases, is lowest during the second trimester, and increases gradually to near the prepregnant level during the third trimester. This occurs because of the progesterone's relaxing effect on the smooth muscles.

Stasis of blood in the lower extremities, caused by the enlarged uterus interfering with return blood flow, may lead to dependent edema and varicose veins of the legs, vulva, or rectum.

Supine hypotensive syndrome, also known as vena caval syndrome, occurs when the mother lies supine. The enlarged, heavy uterus presses on the inferior vena cava causing a reduced blood flow back to the right atrium (Figure 47-5). The mother experiences dizziness, clammy-pale skin, and a lowering of her blood pressure. The situation is relieved when the mother lies on her side.

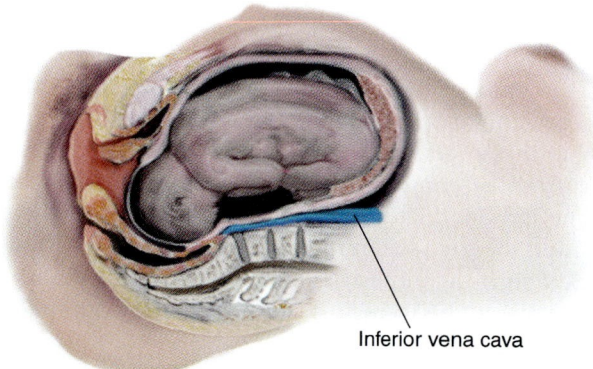

Inferior vena cava

Figure 47-5 Supine Hypotensive Syndrome. Enlarged uterus presses on vena cava when mother is supine. Side-lying position relieves pressure.

Maternal blood volume increases 30% to 50%, reaching its peak about 30 weeks. There is some increase in red blood cells, but most of the increase is plasma. This hemodilution is manifested by a lower hematocrit (34% to 40%) and is termed **physiologic anemia of pregnancy**.

The white blood cell count begins to increase by about 8 weeks and may reach 18,000/mm³ by the time of delivery. Platelets, fibrin, fibrinogen, and coagulation factors VII, IX, and X increase. This increase with possible venous stasis in late pregnancy increases the risk of venous thrombosis.

Respiratory System

Progesterone decreases airway resistance, allowing an increase in oxygen consumption. The enlarging uterus presses upward on the diaphragm. The rib cage flares and the chest circumference expands to keep the intrathoracic volume the same as when not pregnant. Estrogen causes edema and vascular congestion of the nasal mucosa.

Musculoskeletal System

The relaxation of the pelvic joints in preparation for delivery is caused by relaxin. As pregnancy progresses, the mother's center of gravity gradually changes because of the increased size and weight of the uterus anteriorly. To compensate, the mother increases the curve of the lumbosacral spine (lordosis), which frequently results in a low backache, and may cause the woman to have a waddling gait. Figure 47-6 illustrates this change throughout pregnancy.

Gastrointestinal System

Nausea and/or vomiting, known as "morning sickness," are common in early pregnancy but usually disappear by 12 weeks. The smooth muscle relaxation effect of progesterone results in delayed gastric emptying and decreased peristalsis. The enlarging uterus displaces the stomach and intestines. All these changes contribute to constipation. Relaxation of the cardiac sphincter may allow reflux of acidic gastric contents into the esophagus, giving the mother heartburn.

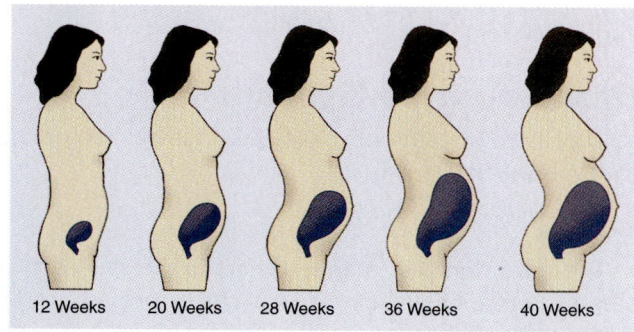

| 12 Weeks | 20 Weeks | 28 Weeks | 36 Weeks | 40 Weeks |

Figure 47-6 Increasing Lordosis throughout Pregnancy

Urinary System

Urinary frequency occurs in the first trimester as the enlarging uterus presses on the bladder and in the third trimester as the fetus settles into the pelvis and presses on the bladder. Progesterone causes the ureters to relax and dilate. Glomerular filtration rate (GFR) begins rising in the second trimester. Tubular reabsorption also increases.

Glycosuria (excretion of glucose in the urine) may develop if the kidneys are unable to reabsorb all the glucose filtered by the glomeruli. Any amount more than a trace of glucose in the urine should be investigated.

Integumentary System

Several skin pigment changes generally occur during pregnancy. The nipples, areola, vulva, and perineal area darken. **Linea nigra** is a pigmented line on the abdomen from umbilicus to symphysis pubis. **Chloasma**, also called "mask of pregnancy," is a darkening of the skin of the forehead and around the eyes. It is generally more pronounced in dark-haired women. **Striae gravidarum** or "stretch marks" are reddish streaks frequently found on the abdomen, thighs, buttocks, and breasts. They are the result of separation of the underlying connective tissue of the skin (Figure 47-7).

Endocrine System

The anterior pituitary hormone prolactin is responsible for initial milk production. The posterior pituitary hormone oxytocin causes uterine contractions and the ejection of milk from the breasts (**let-down reflex**) after delivery.

The placental hormones, especially hPL, are insulin antagonists so a greater insulin production is required. This puts an increased stress on the islets of Langerhans in the pancreas to put out more insulin. A woman with a marginally functioning pancreas may show signs of gestational diabetes.

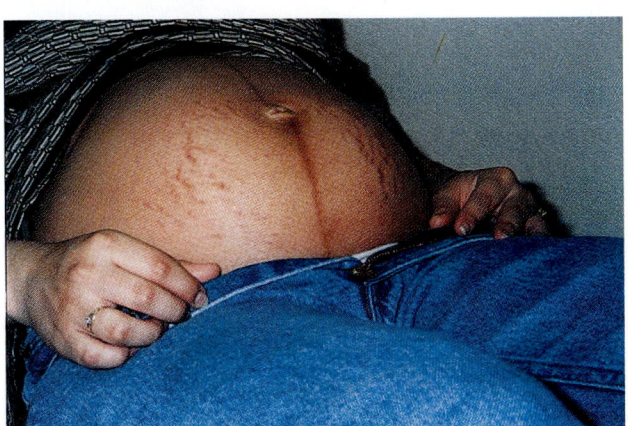

Figure 47-7 Linea Nigra and Striae Gravidarum (*From Health Assessment and Physical Examination, by M. E. Z. Estes, 1998. Albany, NY: Delmar Publishers.*)

A slight increase in the size of the thyroid often occurs as well as an increase in its capacity to bind thyroxine. This results in a higher level of serum protein bound iodine (PBI).

Metabolism

The metabolic rate of the mother increases during pregnancy as the demands of the growing fetus increase. The mother must meet her own and the fetus's nutritional needs.

SIGNS OF PREGNANCY

The many physiological changes that a woman experiences during pregnancy can be categorized as presumptive, probable, or positive signs of pregnancy.

Presumptive Signs

Changes that the woman experiences and reports are termed presumptive or subjective signs. They may be caused by other conditions, so are not diagnostic of pregnancy. Presumptive signs include:

- **Amenorrhea** (absence of menses), usually the first sign that a woman notices causing her to think she is pregnant.
- Nausea and vomiting, often referred to as "morning sickness" but can occur any time of the day. This sign usually disappears by 12 weeks of pregnancy.
- Breast changes, tenderness, or tingling.
- Urinary frequency, as the growing uterus presses against the bladder, giving the woman the sensation of needing to urinate.
- Excessive fatigue, often noted after the first missed menstrual period. It may last for several months.
- Abdominal enlargement usually noticed by the woman, generally after 12 weeks.
- **Quickening**, perception of fetal movement by the mother, usually between 16 and 20 weeks. It begins as a fluttering sensation and gradually gets stronger and more frequent.

A positive diagnosis of pregnancy is usually made before these last two signs are noted by the woman. However, there is a condition called **pseudocyesis** or false pregnancy, in which the woman believes so strongly that she is pregnant that she appears to have all the early presumptive signs of pregnancy.

Probable Signs

The examiner can identify these objective changes, but since they can be caused by conditions other than pregnancy they are not diagnostic of pregnancy.

Pelvic Signs

Goodell's sign (softening of the cervix), Hegar's sign (softening of the uterine isthmus), and Chadwick's sign (purplish discoloration of the vagina, cervix, and vulva) can be identified by the examiner during the first 12 weeks of pregnancy.

Uterine enlargement can be identified after the eighth week of pregnancy. The fundus is palpable just above the symphysis at 12 weeks and at the umbilicus at 20 weeks (Figure 47-8). If these uterine enlargement milestones are reached earlier, multiple pregnancy should be suspected.

Braxton-Hicks Contractions

After the 28th week, these painless contractions can be felt by the examiner and also by the client.

Uterine and Funic Souffle

When auscultating the abdomen over the uterus a soft blowing sound may be heard. The sound occurring at the same rate as the mother's pulse is called the **uterine souffle**. It is due to the blood pulsating through the uterus and placenta. The sound occurring at the same rate as the fetal heart rate is called the **funic souffle**. It is due to blood pulsating through the umbilical cord.

Increased Pigmentation

The nipples and areola darken. Linea nigra may appear on the abdomen, chloasma may mark the face, and striae gravidarum may be noticed on the breasts and abdomen.

Ballottement

During the fourth or fifth month, if the fetus is pushed upward through the vagina or abdomen, the floating fetus rebounds against the examiner's fingers; this is known as **ballottement** (Figure 47-9). This occurs only while the fetus is small in comparison to the amount of amniotic fluid.

Pregnancy Test

The basis for a pregnancy test is the presence of hCG in either the urine or blood of the woman. A test of the blood is positive 8 days after conception, and a test of the urine is positive 10 to 14 days after conception.

Positive Signs

A positive sign of pregnancy proves conclusively that the woman is pregnant. No other condition can cause these signs to appear. There are only three positive signs of pregnancy: hearing the fetal heartbeat, visualization of the fetus, and the examiner feeling fetal movement.

Hearing the Fetal Heartbeat

The fetal heartbeat can be detected by 8 weeks using the Doppler ultrasound method, but generally is heard at 10 to 12 weeks. A fetoscope can detect the fetal heartbeat by 18 to 20 weeks (Figure 47-10).

Visualization of the Fetus

An abdominal ultrasound examination can detect a pregnancy by the sixth week after the last menstrual period (LMP). An endovaginal ultrasound examination, using a vaginal probe, can detect a gestational sac 10 days after implantation.

Examiner Feeling Fetal Movement

Fetal movement felt by the examiner, not the mother, is a positive sign of pregnancy.

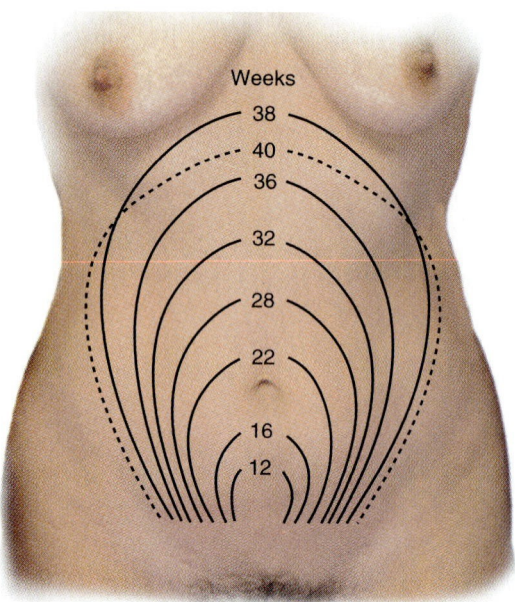

Figure 47-8 Fundal Height Milestones (*Adapted from Health Assessment and Physical Examination, by M. E. Z. Estes, 1998. Albany, NY: Delmar Publishers.*)

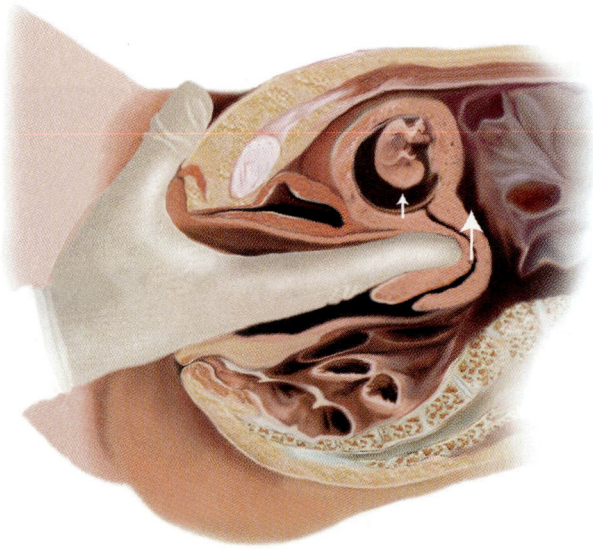

Figure 47-9 Ballottement

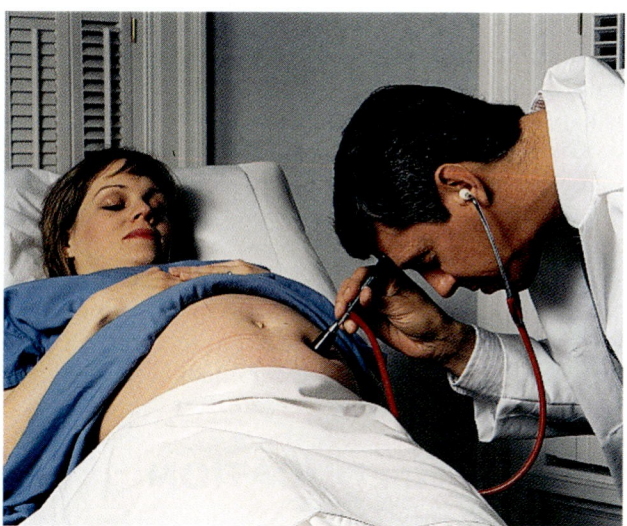

Figure 47-10 Fetoscope in Use

PSYCHOLOGICAL ADAPTATION TO PREGNANCY

Pregnancy is often viewed as a developmental stage having its own developmental tasks. Both the expectant mother and father deal with significant changes and major psychosocial adjustment.

Developmental Tasks

Four major developmental tasks have been identified for pregnancy. They are pregnancy validation, fetal embodiment, fetal distinction, and role transition. These developmental tasks are met in this order. The rate at which they are met will vary. According to Malnory (1996), completion of the developmental tasks is critical to positive parenting.

Pregnancy Validation

During the first trimester, the pregnant woman's task is to validate and accept the pregnancy. Until the woman meets this task, she cannot meet the rest of the developmental tasks. Even when pregnancy is planned, there are normal feelings of ambivalence and disbelief about the pregnancy. Many women become introspective or have mood swings due to hormone fluctuations.

Fetal Embodiment

Fetal embodiment occurs as the mother incorporates the growing fetus into her body image. The physical changes she is experiencing, especially the growing uterus, help her meet this task. She feels that the fetus is a part of her. Self-involvement, depression, or regressive behavior may be signs of difficulty in meeting this task.

Fetal Distinction

When fetal movement is felt, it becomes easier for the mother to think of the fetus as a separate being.

She may daydream about what the baby will be like and think about the kind of mother she wants to be.

Role Transition

The last trimester is a time of preparation. Many expectant parents attend childbirth classes to learn about and prepare for labor, delivery, infant care, and self-care. Preparing a nursery, buying baby clothes, and selecting a day care are all ways of preparing for the infant's arrival.

At the end of pregnancy, many mothers experience a surge of energy and see to it that the entire household is organized for the coming of the infant. This is called **nesting**. All these preparations assist the pregnant woman in the transition to her new role of mother.

Partners' Tasks

Fathers and other partners must meet the same developmental tasks as the expectant mother but in a more abstract way. Accepting the fact that *they* (as a couple) are pregnant and announcing it to family and friends meets the first task. The partner may also have ambivalent feelings about the pregnancy. By accepting the changes in the pregnant partner, both physical and psychological, the task of fetal embodiment is met. Fetal distinction is generally met when the partner hears the fetal heartbeat and feels the fetus moving. Role transition is met in virtually the same way as is done by the pregnant woman.

Factors Affecting Psychological Response

Factors that contribute to a woman's psychological response to her pregnancy include body image, financial situation, cultural expectations, emotional security, and support from significant others.

Body Image

The mother's body image, or perception of her own body, may change in several areas. The noticeable changes in body shape and the speed with which those changes occur may be very threatening to some

CULTURAL CONSIDERATIONS

Preparation for the Infant

A lack of preparation for the birth of the baby may indicate a problem in meeting the task of role transition. However, some cultures or families do not actually purchase any items for the baby until after birth because this practice is believed to bring bad luck. The nurse must be sensitive to cultural practices different from her own and not assume that the couple who has not established a nursery prior to the birth is not eagerly awaiting the new baby's arrival.

women. Some women feel "fat" and "ugly" when they are pregnant, and others feel "so good" and "beautiful" when they are pregnant.

The physical discomforts of pregnancy may cause the mother to feel a lack of control over her own body. For example, urinary frequency or urinary incontinence may increase negative feelings about the pregnancy.

Pregnant women often feel restricted in their physical activities. As long as there is no problem with the pregnancy, they should be encouraged to continue their regular activities, keeping in mind that moderation is the key.

Financial Situation

A poor financial situation may be the cause of anxiety about paying bills, buying needed items for infant care, or having enough and proper foods for good nutrition. Financial consideration may also be a significant concern for the expectant mother's partner.

Cultural Expectations

Cultural expectations of the family may cause conflicts for the pregnant woman and her partner if their ideas are different from their families' expectations. Conflicts may also occur if the cultural expectations of the mother are different from the cultural expectations of the father or partner.

Emotional Security

A pregnant woman's satisfaction with herself and her life situation will also have an impact on how she responds to being pregnant. If the woman is secure in her feelings about herself and her perceived abilities as a mother, the pregnancy is more likely to be enjoyable. A pregnancy that was planned or long anticipated will likely be received with joy and excitement, whereas an unexpected or unwanted pregnancy may be met with fear, dread, or uncertainty.

Support from Significant Others

It is important for the nurse and the expectant mother to also take into consideration the psychological responses of significant others, namely, the father/partner, siblings, and grandparents.

Fathers/Partners The expectant father or partner must shift thinking from being a person without children to a person with a child. He may feel left out, neglected, or resent the attention focused on the expectant mother.

Couvade is the development of physical symptoms by the expectant father such as fatigue, depression, headache, backache, and nausea. Longobucco and Freston (1989) found that men who show couvade have greater paternal role preparation.

Siblings A new baby may be seen by siblings as a threat to their relationship with the parents. Siblings should be included in the pregnancy and preparations for the new baby on an age-appropriate basis. Feeling the fetus kick or hearing the heartbeat are often help-

ful activities for siblings. Parents must be sure to maintain some special time just for the siblings. Many areas have classes for siblings to help them understand what is happening in their lives.

Grandparents Grandparents are usually the first ones told about the pregnancy. It is often difficult for grandparents to know how much to become involved in the process. Some grandparents feel they are not ready or are too young to become grandparents.

Practices of childbearing and child rearing often change greatly from one generation to another. Some areas have classes to provide information to grandparents about these changes.

PRENATAL EDUCATION AND CARE

Prenatal care (care of a woman during pregnancy, before labor) is credited with the reduction of perinatal mortality over the last 50 years. The earlier prenatal care is begun the better. This provides an opportunity for the health care provider to obtain baseline data on physical assessments and laboratory test results.

Anticipatory guidance (providing information, teaching, or guidance to a client in anticipation of an

CULTURAL CONSIDERATIONS

Beliefs Influencing Pregnancy

Some cultural practices may not always be observed by a client, but some general practices that have cultural influences include the following:

- Muslim women are to keep hair, body, arms to the wrist, and legs to the ankles covered at all times (Hutchinson & Baqi-Aziz, 1994).
- A Muslim woman may not be alone in the presence of a man other than her husband or a male relative, including during a physical examination (Hutchinson & Baqi-Aziz, 1994).
- Korean women defer to elders, especially the mother-in-law, for care decisions (Schneiderman, 1996).
- Korean women are very modest and often prefer to have their husbands leave the room during potentially embarrassing procedures (Schneiderman, 1996).
- Koreans do not like having their name written in red ink, as red ink is used for the deceased (Howard & Berbiglia, 1997).
- Guatemalan women believe that a pregnant woman and her unborn child are physically and spiritually weak and may be vulnerable to illnesses and evil forces (Callister & Vega, 1998).
- In Malawi, Africa, the father determines family size and the timing of the pregnancies (Gennaro et al., 1998).

expected event) is probably the most important aspect of prenatal care. It is based on the assessment of mother and fetus and knowledge of the normal process of pregnancy and possible complications.

Prenatal Care

The goals of prenatal care are:

- A healthy, prepared mother having minimal discomforts
- Identification of potential problems or complications as early as possible
- Safe delivery of a healthy infant
- A prepared father or partner who participates as much or as little as the couple desires
- Prepared siblings and grandparents

Initial Visit

A comfortable environment, open communication, and the nurse's attitude will help put the woman at ease during the initial prenatal visit. The first visit is often quite lengthy. A complete history is recorded to identify factors that may negatively affect the pregnancy and a physical examination is performed. If the woman did not seek preconception care, all of the topics covered in that section would then be discussed at the first prenatal visit. Important terms used in describing a pregnant client are provided in Table 47-2.

Initial History The history provides the health care provider with the client's past and present health. Figure 47-11 shows a sample health history summary.

Table 47-2 TERMS USED IN DESCRIBING A PREGNANT CLIENT

Abortion Loss of pregnancy before the age of viability (usually 24 weeks' gestation)

GP/TPAL Gravida, para/term, preterm, abortions, living

Examples: Mary Jo is G2 P1/T2 P0 A0 L2; second pregnancy, one delivery/two infants at term (twins), both living.

Susan is G4 P2/T1 P1 A1 L2; fourth pregnancy, two deliveries/one term infant, one preterm infant, one born before 24 weeks, two living children.

Gravida Pregnancy, regardless of duration, includes present pregnancy

Para Delivery (birth) after 24 weeks' gestation, whether infant born alive or dead or number of infants born

Preterm Delivery after 24 weeks' gestation but before 38 weeks (full term)

Term A pregnancy between 38 and 42 weeks' gestation

Nulligravida Never been pregnant

Primigravida Pregnant for first time

Multigravida Pregnant two or more times

Nullipara Never having delivered an infant after 24 weeks' gestation

Primipara Has delivered once after 24 weeks' gestation

Multipara Has delivered twice or more after 24 weeks' gestation

Postterm Delivery after 42 weeks' gestation

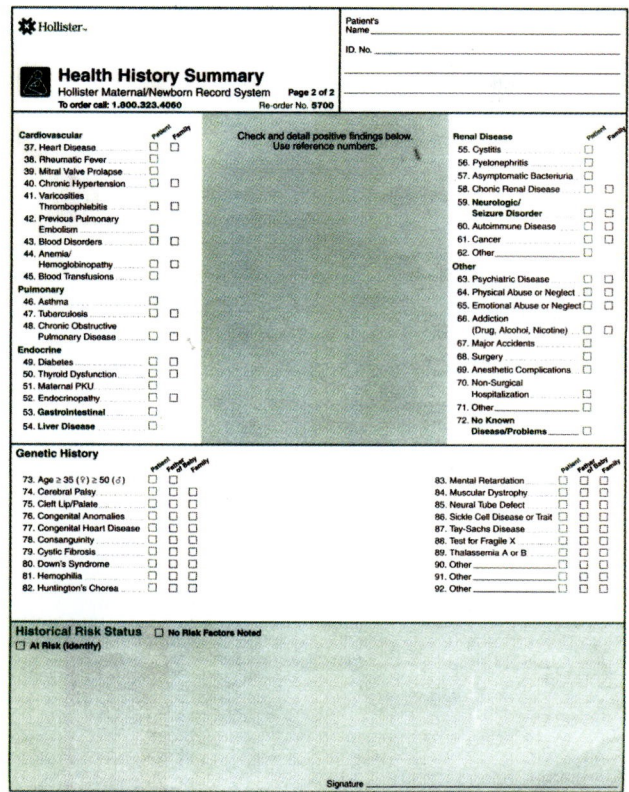

Figure 47-11 Representative Health History Forms (*Permission to use this copyright material has been granted by the owner, Hollister Incorporated.*)

Estimating Duration of Pregnancy Every family wants to know the "due date," the estimated date when the infant is to be born. The estimated date of birth (EDB) or estimated date of delivery (EDD) is 40 weeks from the first day of the woman's LMP. Many women do not keep track of their menstrual periods, or have irregular periods; but an EDB can be identified based on other factors such as uterine size, date of quickening, date when the fetal heartbeat is heard, and ultrasound fetal measurements.

Naegele's Rule Naegele's rule is the most common method of calculating the EDB. The rule is: take the date of the first day of the last menstrual period, subtract 3 months, and add 7 days. For instance, if the LMP was June 28, the calculation would be as follows:

Month	Day
6 (June)	28
− 3 months	+ 7 days
3 (March)	35

Since there are 31 days in March, the EDB moves forward to April 4.

Gestation Calculator A gestation calculator, in the shape of either a chart or a wheel, allows a quick EDB calculation. The wheel generally provides other information also, such as fetal weight and body length for each week (Figure 47-12).

Fundal Height Fundal height generally is indicative of gestational age through the second trimester (refer back to Figure 47-8). The **fundus** (top of the uterus) is measured in centimeters from the top of the pubic symphysis to the top of the uterine fundus (McDonald's method). This is fairly accurate between 18 and 30 weeks' gestation. The fundal height, for example, is generally 20 cm (at the umbilicus) at 20 weeks' gestation and 25 cm at 25 weeks' gestation in the average height woman. Evaluating the visit-to-visit fundal height measurements provides a general pattern of fetal growth. A sudden increase may indicate twins or hydramnios (excessive amount of amniotic fluid) while a smaller increase may indicate growth retardation (Figure 47-13).

Other Indicators Additional assessments that indicate the gestational week of pregnancy include: ultrasound, fetal heartbeat, and quickening.

- Ultrasound: Five to six weeks after the LMP an ultrasound can detect a gestational sac. It shows fetal heartbeat activity at 9 to 10 weeks' gestation. By 12 to 13 weeks the biparietal diameter (BPD), or distance between the parietal bones of the fetal skull, can be measured.

- Fetal Heartbeat: The fetal heartbeat is generally heard by 10 to 12 weeks with the Doppler device, but may be heard as early as 8 weeks' gestation. It is usually 18 to 20 weeks before the fetal heartbeat can be heard with a fetoscope.

- Quickening: Fetal movement is usually felt by the mother at about 20 weeks' gestation. Women may identify these movements as early as 16 weeks or as late as 22 weeks. Typically, the woman will detect this movement earlier with a second pregnancy than with a first.

Physical Examination The physical examination begins with measuring the client's height and weight and vital signs. A head-to-toe examination is performed by the health care provider. Special attention is given to the assessment of the heart, lungs, pelvis, breasts, and nipples. Figure 47-14 shows an initial pregnancy profile form, and Figure 47-15 shows a prenatal flow record.

The pelvic examination is performed last. The external genitalia are examined for scars, lesions, or infection. A Pap smear for cervical cancer and a specimen of cervical mucous for gonorrhea are usually obtained. A bimanual examination is performed to determine uterine changes (Figure 47-16) and pelvic

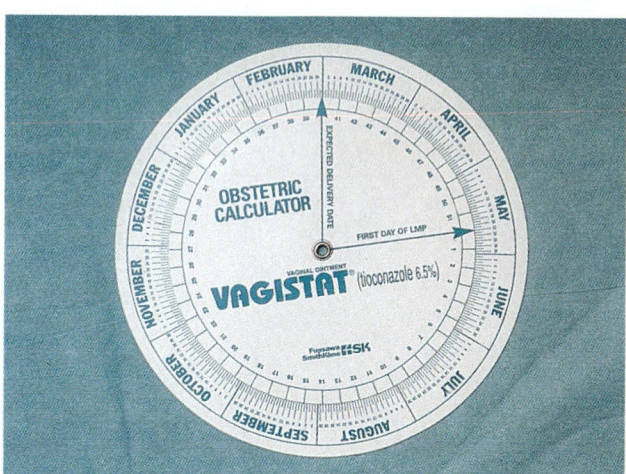

Figure 47-12 Gestation Calculation Wheel. Place arrow labeled *last menses began* on date of LMP. Read date at arrow labeled *40*.

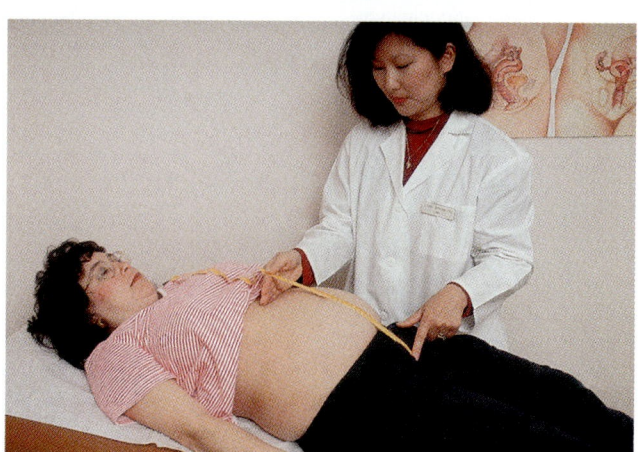

Figure 47-13 Measuring Fundal Height

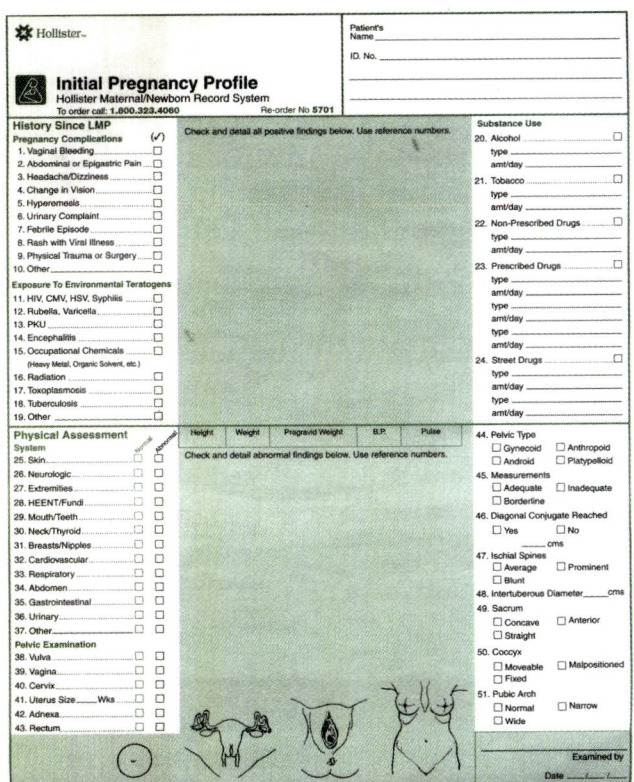

Figure 47-14 Representative Initial Pregnancy Profile *(Permission to use this copyright material has been granted by the owner, Hollister Incorporated.)*

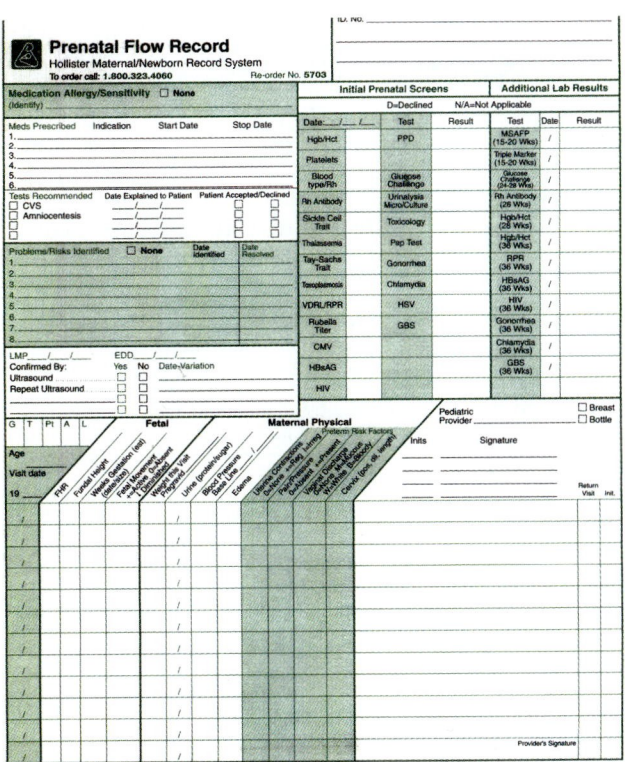

Figure 47-15 Representative Prenatal Flow Record *(Permission to use this copyright material has been granted by the owner, Hollister Incorporated.)*

size to estimate adequacy of the pelvic opening for delivery.

Pelvic size is estimated by the examiner during the manual examination. The diagonal conjugate (distance from the lower border of the pubic symphysis to the

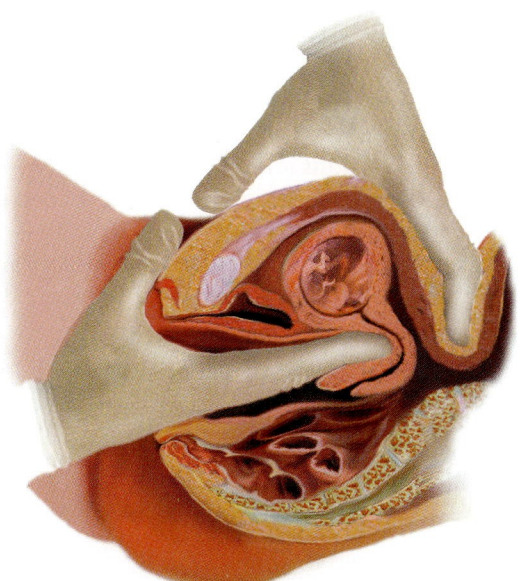

Figure 47-16 Bimanual Examination to Determine Uterine Changes *(From Health Assessment and Physical Examination, by M. E. Z. Estes, 1998. Albany, NY: Delmar Publishers.)*

sacral promontory) is an estimate of the pelvic inlet. It is generally 11.5 cm. The anteroposterior diameter (9.5 to 11.5 cm), measured from the lower border of the pubic symphysis to the tip of the sacrum, is an estimate of the pelvic outlet.

Screening Tests

During the first visit, screening tests are performed to determine the mother's health and to have baseline data with which to compare subsequent test results. The tests may vary for a specific client but generally include those listed in Table 47-3.

Return Visits

Return visits for an uncomplicated pregnancy generally are:

- Every 4 weeks for the first 28 weeks
- Every 2 weeks during weeks 29 to 36
- Every week, after 36 weeks, until birth of infant

Subjective Data The following subjective data should be collected at each return visit:

- How the client is feeling
- Any discomforts, concerns, or questions the client may have
- Any body changes noticed by the client
- How developmental tasks are being met

Table 47-3 SCREENING TESTS IN PREGNANCY

TEST	RESULTS
Complete Blood Count	
RBC	3.75 million/mm³ due to hemodilution.
WBC	Rises to 18,000/mm³ by late pregnancy. Mostly an increase in neutrophils.
Hemoglobin (Hgb)	May decrease to 11.5g/dL later in pregnancy due to hemodilution. Repeat at 28 and 36 weeks.
Hematocrit (Hct)	33% lowest acceptable, due to hemodilution.
Blood Type	A, B, AB, or O
Rh factor	Positive or negative. If negative, do indirect Coomb's test. Check father's Rh.
Coomb's Test	Should remain negative. Retest Rh negative woman at 28 weeks.
Rubella Titer (HAI)	> 1:10 indicates immunity. < 1:10, immunize after birth of infant.
Blood Glucose	Should be 60–110 mg/dL. Retest at 24 and 32 weeks.
VDRL or RPR (Syphilis)	Should be negative.
Cervical/Vaginal Culture	Should be negative.
Gonorrhea	
Chlamydia	
Group B Streptococcus	
Hepatitis B Surface Antigen (HB₅Ag)	Positive indicates either active hepatitis or carrier state.
Antibody Titer HB₅Ag	Positive indicates immunity to hepatitis.
HIV (many states mandate that it be offered)	Should be negative.
Tuberculosis	Should be negative.
Skin tests: Mantoux or Tine	If positive, do chest x-ray.
Urinalysis	
Color, specific Gravity, pH, ketones, albumin, glucose	Same as nonpregnant. Repeat at 28 weeks. Trace of glycosuria may occur in pregnancy.
Alpha-fetoprotein (AFP)	Check with laboratory for normal range for each week of gestation. If elevated, may have neural tube defects. If decreased, may have Down syndrome.

PROFESSIONAL TIP

Prenatal Diagnostic Tests

"AFP testing is accepted as the standard of care and must be offered to pregnant women between the 16th and 20th weeks of pregnancy. . . . [H]ealth care providers need to keep a record of patients' refusal of any diagnostic tests offered to them" (Rhodes, 1995).

At an early return visit, the mother's expectations for childbirth should be discussed. Closer to the EDB, preparations for the baby should also be covered.

Objective Data On each return visit, the following objective data should be collected and compared to data collected on previous visits and to prepregnant data, if known.

Blood Pressure Any increase of 30 mm Hg systolic or 15 mm Hg diastolic from one visit to the next should be reported to the health care provider. If there is no previous BP to compare to, a blood pressure of 140/90 should be reported.

Weight Total weight gain should be approximately 25 to 35 pounds, distributed as follows:

- Weeks 1 to 12:   3 to 4 pounds
- Weeks 13 to 40:   1 pound/week

Uterine Size The fundal height in centimeters is indicative of the weeks of gestation between 18 and 30 weeks.

Edema A small amount of dependent edema is often present in the last few weeks of pregnancy. Edema of the hands and face should be reported to the health care provider. Sometimes it is difficult to detect small amounts of edema in the hands, so the nurse should ask the client if her rings are tighter or if she has had to remove her rings.

Fetal Position Assessment of fetal position is performed using **Leopold's maneuvers**, a series of specific palpations of the pregnant uterus to determine fetal position and presentation. The client is placed in the supine position with knees bent, and the examiner stands at the client's right side facing her head.

- First, the examiner palpates to determine which fetal part is in the fundus. Generally, it is the breech (buttocks).
- Second, the examiner moves hands to the sides of the uterus and determines on which side of the mother the fetal back is located.
- Third, the examiner's right hand is placed above the symphysis pubis to note whether the head or breech is near the pubic symphysis (this should correlate with the first maneuver).
- Fourth, the examiner changes position to face the client's feet, and palpates the sides of the abdomen

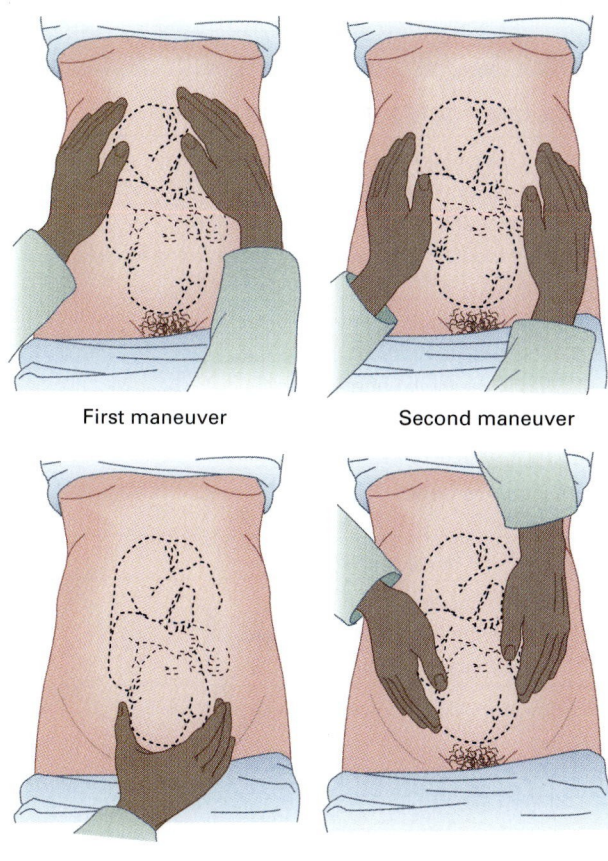

First maneuver   Second maneuver

Third maneuver   Fourth maneuver

Figure 47-17 Leopold's Maneuvers (*From* Health Assessment and Physical Examination, *by M. E. Z. Estes, 1998. Albany, NY: Delmar Publishers.*)

to determine on which side the cephalic prominence presents (Figure 47-17).

Fetal Heartbeat After Leopold's maneuvers have determined fetal position, the fetal heartbeat should be assessed over the location of the fetal back. The rate should be 120 to 160 beats/minute. The rate is recorded, indicating the abdominal quadrant in which the heartbeat was noted.

Laboratory Tests At each visit a urine sample is tested with a dipstick for protein, glucose, and ketones. If the results are positive for any of these three, the health care provider must be notified.

Anticipatory Guidance

Many of the nursing interventions during pregnancy are anticipatory guidance (teaching). The order in which topics are covered and the time frame when topics are covered may vary from client to client, depending on when prenatal care was begun and if there are any complications.

Environmental Hazards

Any chemicals, metals, anesthetic agents, antineoplastic and viral drugs and x-ray examinations should be avoided. Excessive heat from saunas, hot tubs, or exercise in hot humid weather should be avoided to prevent maternal hyperthermia (core temperature above 38.9°C/102°F). This has been associated with neural tube defects. Rogers and Davis (1995) report that the time needed to reach this core temperature is 15 minutes in a 39°C (102.2°F) tub and 10 minutes in a 41.1° C (106°F) tub.

Discomforts of Pregnancy

The physiological changes in pregnancy often cause discomforts to the woman. Table 47-4 identifies the common discomforts of pregnancy, possible causes, and interventions the client can try to alleviate or reduce the discomfort.

Warning Signs

The client should be taught to immediately report to the health care provider the warning signs listed in Table 47-5. They may indicate complications of pregnancy. Generally, the sooner interventions are begun the better the outcome.

Nutrition

There is very little change needed in the diet of a pregnant woman if she is already following the food guide pyramid. A woman eating a balanced, adequate diet needs to add only 300 kcalories a day to her diet when pregnant and 500 kcalories a day when breastfeeding. The addition of two milk servings and one meat serving will meet the 300 kcalorie increase as well as the increased need for calcium and protein.

Many health care providers have their pregnant clients take a multivitamin with calcium and iron to ensure an adequate intake of these essential nutrients. Folic acid in the multivitamin prevents neural tube defects, calcium is needed for bone and teeth, and iron is needed to prevent anemia in mother and fetus. Based on a nutritional assessment, suggestions can be made to the client for a more adequate dietary intake, taking into account personal and cultural preferences.

Some pregnant women eat substances that are not considered edible and have no nutritive value. This is called **pica**. Substances generally eaten in the United States are laundry starch, dirt, clay, and freezer frost. Eating laundry starch interferes with absorption of nutrients. Clay, dirt, and laundry starch contribute to constipation and possible fecal impaction.

 CLIENT TEACHING

Pregnancy and Fluid Intake

A pregnant woman should drink at least 8 to 10 (8-oz) glasses of fluids each day. At least 4 to 6 glasses should be water.

Table 47-4 DISCOMFORTS OF PREGNANCY

DISCOMFORT	CAUSE	CLIENT INTERVENTIONS
Nausea/vomiting	Elevated hCG level. Decreased gastric emptying time due to progesterone. Ambivalence about pregnancy. Fatigue.	Limit fluid intake at meals and upon waking. Eat crackers or toast upon waking. Eat small amounts more frequently. Avoid fried, spicy, odorous, or gas-forming foods.
Heartburn	Gastric reflux—cardiac sphincter relaxed due to progesterone.	Avoid overeating. Eat small, frequent meals. Avoid greasy foods. Sit up 30 minutes after eating. Take antacid only with health care provider's approval.
Urinary frequency	Pressure of uterus on bladder (early and late in pregnancy). Urinary tract infection	Empty bladder when urge is felt. *Do not* restrict fluid intake.
Breast tenderness	Effect of estrogen and progesterone.	Wear well-fitting, supportive bra.
Flatulence	Relaxation of GI tract due to progesterone.	Eat small meals. Omit gas-forming foods from diet. Have regular elimination.
Constipation	Bowel sluggishness due to progesterone. Pressure of uterus on bowel. Decreased activity and fluid intake. Inadequate fiber in diet. Iron supplement.	Have regular schedule for bowel movement. Increase activity and fluid intake. Increase fiber in diet (raisins, prunes, fresh fruits and vegetables).
Hemorrhoids	Constipation. Straining to have bowel movement. Pressure of gravid (pregnant) uterus on veins. Prolonged standing.	Prevent constipation (see above). Apply ice packs. Use topical anesthetic ointments. Take sitz bath. Gently push hemorrhoids back into rectum.
Ankle edema	Prolonged standing or sitting. Sodium and water retention from hormonal influence. Increased capillary permeability.	Dorsiflex feet when prolonged standing or sitting necessary. Elevate legs when sitting or resting. Increase number of rest periods.
Vericose veins (legs)	Increased blood volume. Congenital predisposition to weak vascular walls. Relaxation of vessel walls due to progesterone. Inactivity. Poor muscle tone. Prolonged standing. Obesity.	Rest with feet and legs elevated. Avoid crossing legs, standing still, garters and restrictive clothing. Wear support hose.
Backache	Relaxation of joints due to estrogen and relaxin. Exaggerated lordosis from change in center of gravity. Wearing high-heeled shoes. Excessive weight. Fatigue. Poor body mechanics.	Get adequate rest. Use proper posture. Use proper body mechanics. Wear low-heeled shoes.
Dyspnea	Supine hypotensive syndrome. Decreased lung capacity from pressure of uterus on diaphragm.	Lie on either side. Sleep in semi-Fowler's position.
Leg cramps	Calcium/phosphorus imbalance. Pointing toes. Fatigue or muscle strain. Pressure of gravid uterus impairs circulation to legs.	Evaluate diet for adequate calcium intake. Pull toes up toward knees. Rest with legs elevated.

continued

Table 47-4 DISCOMFORTS OF PREGNANCY *continued*

DISCOMFORT	CAUSE	CLIENT INTERVENTIONS
Dizziness and fainting	Supine hypotensive syndrome. Sudden change of position. Standing for long period in warm area. Hyperventilation. Hypoglycemia. Anemia.	Lie on either side, not on back. Arise slowly. Avoid standing in warm area. Practice slow, deep respirations. Drink orange juice for fast-acting sugar.
Bleeding gums, nasal stuffiness, and epistaxis	Increased estrogen level. Increased blood volume. Lack of vitamin C.	Avoid use of decongestants. Keep nasal passages lubricated. Drink orange juice. Have dental checkup.
Vaginal discharge	Increased estrogen causes more cervical mucous.	Practice good personal hygiene. Avoid douching.
Itchy skin	Tissue stretching. Soap use. Dehydration.	Use lotion on skin. Change soap, rinse well. Drink more fluids.
Mood swings	Hormonal changes. Inadequate rest. Inadequate diet. Ambivalence about pregnancy.	Get more rest. Eat balanced diet. Express fears, feelings, and concerns.

Table 47-5 WARNING SIGNS DURING PREGNANCY

WARNING SIGN	POSSIBLE CAUSE
Vaginal bleeding (any), "bloody show"	Abortion (miscarriage), placenta previa, placenta abruptio, lesions of cervix or vagina
Sudden gush of fluid from vagina	Rupture of membranes
Persistent vomiting	Hyperemesis gravidarum, infection
Severe, continuous headache	Hypertension, preeclampsia
Swelling of face, hands, legs, feet when arising in morning	Preeclampsia
Visual disturbances: blurring, double vision, flashes of light, spots before eyes	Hypertension, preeclampsia
Dizziness	Hypertension, preeclampsia
Fever over 100°F (37.8°C) and chills	Infection
Pain in abdomen or cramping	Ectopic pregnancy, abortion (miscarriage), placenta abruptio, labor
Epigastric pain	Preeclampsia
Irritating vaginal discharge	Vaginal infection
Dysuria	Urinary tract infection
Oliguria	Dehydration, renal impairment
Noticeable reduction or absence of fetal movement	Fetal distress, fetal death

Factors that place a woman at risk for nutritional inadequacy during pregnancy include:

- Adolescence, due to demands for own growth and pregnancy; and possible poor dietary habits
- Inadequate nutritional intake
- Pica
- Smoking, alcohol use, or drug addiction
- Short interval between pregnancies—no time to replenish nutrient stores
- Medical conditions such as diabetes or kidney problems
- Depression

Self-Care

Physical care during pregnancy generally involves minor adjustments in or moderation of normal habits.

Breast Care

Proper support of the breasts is important during pregnancy whether the woman is planning to breast-feed or bottle-feed her baby. A properly fitted maternity or nursing bra promotes comfort, retains breast shape, and prevents back strain if breasts are very large.

Cleanliness of the breasts is very important. Washing with water is sufficient as soap removes the natural lubricant provided by Montgomery's tuburcles, causing drying and possible cracking of the nipples. If leakage is experienced, a nursing pad can be worn inside the bra, and the pregnant woman encouraged to rub the fluid into the nipple to lubricate the skin. Air-drying the nipples after leaking will also promote breast health.

Personal Hygiene

Daily bathing is important since the pregnant woman generally has increased perspiration and vaginal mucous. Either a tub bath or shower may be taken, depending on the woman's preference and facilities available. Later in pregnancy, a tub bath may require that the mother have help in getting out of the tub. Douching should not be done as it changes the pH of the vagina and alters the normal flora.

Activity/Rest

The pregnant woman should have some type of regular physical activity. Walking, swimming, and cycling are perhaps the best activities for most women. A woman who routinely participates in strenuous activity before pregnancy can usually continue in that activity as long as there are no complications of the pregnancy. Fatigue should be avoided. Pregnant clients should exercise for no longer than 15 minutes at a

---

 CLIENT TEACHING

Exercises for Pregnancy

Specific exercises can be taught to clients to help strengthen muscle tone in preparation for birth.

- The pelvic tilt reduces back strain and strengthens the abdominal muscles. Figure 47-18 illustrates how to perform the pelvic tilt in both a standing and kneeling position. Exhale, roll the hips and buttocks forward, hold for a count of five, then inhale and relax.
- Abdominal muscle tightening with every breath increases abdominal muscle tone. This can be done anywhere in any position. While slowly taking in a deep breath, expand the abdomen. Then exhale slowly while pulling the abdomen in until

the muscles are completely contracted. Relax a few seconds and repeat the exercise.

- Kegel's exercises strengthen and tighten the perineal muscles. Tighten these muscles and pull them up toward the vagina as if trying to stop urination midstream. This exercise also can be done anytime, anyplace.
- The tailor sit (cross-legged sit) stretches the inner thigh muscles; adding arm reaches stretches the sides and upper body and helps relieve upper backache. Sit cross-legged and stretch one arm high over head, then release and exhale and repeat on other side. Figure 47-19 illustrates the tailor sit and arm reaches.

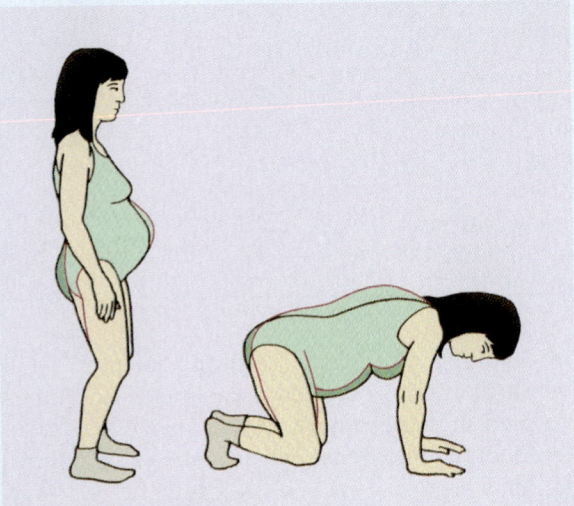

Figure 47-18 Pelvic Tilt

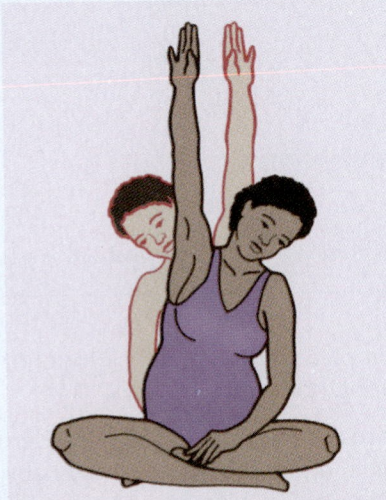

Figure 47-19 Tailor Sit and Arm Reaches

time, keeping the maternal heart rate to 140 beats/minute or less. They should avoid hyperthermia and drink plenty of fluids before and after exercise to prevent dehydration.

Adequate rest is important for the pregnant woman, as it is for everyone, for physical and mental health. Especially during the first and last trimester, she needs more sleep. It may be a challenge to find rest time during the day, especially for women who work outside the home or have small children.

Clothing

Clothing is an important aspect of a woman's self-image. This is especially true during pregnancy when the physical changes may have a negative impact on her self-image. The clothes should be attractive, yet loose and nonconstricting. Maternity clothes are often shared among friends since they are worn for a relatively short time and can be expensive. The pregnant woman should avoid wearing knee-high or thigh-high stockings or garters as they can interfere with circulation in the legs.

Low-heeled shoes are usually suggested. However, if the woman does not have a problem with backache and can maintain her balance, there is no medical reason for not wearing high-heeled shoes. Edema in the feet toward the end of pregnancy may require switching to a larger size shoe.

Employment

How long to work when pregnant depends on the type of work done by the woman and how the pregnancy is progressing. The major factors to consider are whether there are teratogenic hazards in the work environment, if the woman will be subject to physical strain or overfatigue, and if there are obstetrical or medical complications of the pregnancy. Rest periods should be available during the workday.

Travel

Unless there are obstetrical or medical complications, travel need not be restricted. When traveling by car, the pregnant client should be encouraged to stop every 2 hours and walk around for 10 minutes or so. It is imperative always to wear the seat belt, both lap and shoulder, and to keep the lap belt snug below the abdomen. Possible bladder trauma, in case of an accident, can be decreased by keeping the bladder empty. Travel by air should be considered for long trips. Clients should be aware that many airlines and cruise ships will not accept passengers past a certain week of pregnancy.

Dental Care

Regular oral hygiene should continue during pregnancy. Dental care can be performed during pregnancy. The woman should inform her dentist that she is pregnant. If possible, x-rays should be delayed until after the infant is born. If x-rays must be done, a lead apron must be used.

Sexual Activity

There is no reason to limit sexual activity in a healthy pregnancy. Only when there is bleeding or the membranes have ruptured is sexual intercourse contraindicated. As always, barrier protection should be used to prevent sexually transmitted diseases.

The expectant woman's sexual desire may decrease during the first trimester because of fatigue, nausea/vomiting, and breast tenderness. Often during the second trimester, when the discomforts have lessened, she has greater sexual satisfaction than when not pregnant. By the third trimester, the discomforts of fatigue, dyspnea, urinary frequency, and painful pelvic ligaments may decrease her sexual desire.

After the fourth month, the woman should not lie flat on her back during intercourse because of supine hypotensive syndrome. A pillow can be placed under her right hip to displace the uterus or an alternate position used.

Men may find a change in their desire too. This may be related to their feelings about their partner's changing appearance, concern about hurting her or the fetus, and having sexual intercourse with a pregnant woman.

CHILDBIRTH EDUCATION

Many health care providers recommend that their clients attend a prepared childbirth class. When a woman understands what is happening in her body, she has less fear and is less tense. She will then be more relaxed during labor and will be able to help more effectively during the birth process.

Several persons have gained recognition for developing childbirth education programs. The three most commonly known are Dick-Read, Bradley, and Lamaze. The most popular is the Lamaze method, or more accurately, some adaptation of the Lamaze method.

Dick-Read

In the 1930s, Dr. Grantly Dick-Read proposed the fear-tension-pain syndrome. That is, the woman during childbirth experiences fear because she does not understand what is happening in her body. This causes tension which causes the woman to perceive pain more intensely. Classes based on this method include the physiology of childbirth, exercises for the abdomen and perineal muscles, and relaxation techniques. Classes also focus on teaching the woman to visualize what is happening inside her body, and to use abdominal breathing, not chest breathing.

Bradley

Dr. Robert Bradley stressed that labor is a normal process and focused on environmental variables. He felt that husband or partner support is most important.

During early labor, diversionary activities are encouraged. When not walking, the tailor sit or Sims position are encouraged. During a contraction, the woman is to close her eyes and relax with slow, deep abdominal breathing. The husband/partner is to be supportive, touch the laboring woman, and put a hand on her abdomen during a contraction.

Lamaze

Dr. Fernand Lamaze introduced the childbirth preparation method called **psychoprophylaxis** (mental and physical preparation for childbirth). It combines controlled muscle relaxation and breathing techniques. The pregnant woman is taught to contract a specific group of muscles and relax the rest of her body. This conditions her to relax when the uterus contracts.

Abdominal effleurage, light stroking of the abdomen, is used to relieve mild pain but not intense pain. Back pain can be relieved by pressure on the sacrum.

NURSING PROCESS

The nurse's role centers on helping the client maintain a healthy pregnancy and preparing the client for childbirth and delivery.

Assessment

The information presented in this chapter encompasses the possible subjective data and objective data that may be gathered about a specific client.

Nursing Diagnoses

Nursing diagnoses applicable to a pregnant client may include:

- *Activity Intolerance*
- *Anxiety*
- *Breathing Pattern, Ineffective*
- *Body Image Disturbance*
- *Constipation*
- *Fatigue*
- *Family Coping: Potential for Growth*
- *Fear*
- *Fluid Volume Deficit*
- *Fluid Volume Excess*
- *Health Maintenance, Altered*
- *Health Seeking Behaviors*
- *Individual Coping, Ineffective*
- *Injury, Risk for*
- *Knowledge Deficit* (specify)
- *Noncompliance* (specify)
- *Nutrition: Altered, Less Than Body Requirements*
- *Physical Mobility, Impaired*
- *Self-Care Deficit*
- *Sexual Dysfunction*
- *Sleep Pattern Disturbance*

Planning/Outcome Identification

At least one goal must be set with the client to meet the need of the client as identified by the nursing diagnoses.

Nursing Interventions

Nursing interventions must be individualized and specific for the client based on the assessment, nursing diagnoses, and goals. Nursing interventions for prenatal care are focused on teaching the client and providing anticipatory guidance.

Evaluation

Each goal must be evaluated to determine how it has been met by the client.

SAMPLE NURSING CARE PLAN

PRENATAL CARE

Penny, age 23, first pregnancy, states she has been nauseated and has not eaten for about 3 weeks, feels very tired all the time, takes a nap after work, and then has trouble sleeping because she has to go the bathroom frequently. Her LMP was six weeks ago, menstrual periods have always been regular every 28 days. She smokes 1 pack/day and drinks beer on the weekends. She does not like to cook so most meals are eaten out. She has lost 3 pounds in the last month.

Nursing Diagnosis 1 *Knowledge Deficit of Self-Care in Pregnancy, related to inexperience as evidenced by eating, drinking, and smoking habits*

continued

PLANNING/GOALS	NURSING INTERVENTIONS	RATIONALE	EVALUATION
Penny will competently care for herself during pregnancy.	Teach physiology of pregnancy, discomforts of pregnancy, things she can do to relieve the discomforts, self-care aspects, and fetal development. Gather more data about her work environment and psychosocial aspects of nutrition, smoking, and drinking.	Knowledge of pregnancy and fetal development gives Penny reason to take care of herself.	Penny states that she now understands the changes pregnancy makes in her body.

Nursing Diagnosis 2 *Nutrition, Altered, less than body requirements related to inadequate food intake as evidenced by nausea and weight loss*

PLANNING/GOALS	NURSING INTERVENTIONS	RATIONALE	EVALUATION
Penny will have sufficient nutritional intake during pregnancy.	Teach basic nutrition, food guide pyramid, and nutritional needs during pregnancy.	Understanding the nutritional needs in pregnancy will encourage changes in Penny's eating pattern.	Penny follows the food guide pyramid most of the time and is drinking 4 glasses of milk a day.

Nursing Diagnosis 3 *Injury, Risk for, related to teratogenic substances as evidenced by smoking and alcohol consumption*

PLANNING/GOALS	NURSING INTERVENTIONS	RATIONALE	EVALUATION
Penny will stop smoking and drinking alcohol.	Teach effects of smoking and alcohol on fetal development.	Knowledge of the effects of smoking and alcohol on fetal development will encourage Penny to abstain from both.	Penny has cut her smoking in half and only drinks one beer on the weekend.

CASE STUDY

Beth, age 30, and John, age 30, have been married 4 years. Beth's LMP was 12 weeks ago, but her menstrual periods have always been very irregular. She is tired all the time and nauseated every day, her clothes are very tight around her waist, and her abdomen is protruding.

The following questions will guide your development of a nursing care plan for the case study.

1. What other data would you collect about Beth?
2. What diagnostic tests would you anticipate the health care provider performing or ordering?
3. What anticipatory guidance would be appropriate for Beth?
4. When should Beth return for a checkup?

SUMMARY

- Ideally, planning for pregnancy should begin before conception.
- Fetal development proceeds in an orderly and predictable manner.
- Prenatal care involves all aspects of the couple's life.
- A complete history for a pregnant client includes her own medical and obstetrical history, family history, and the fetus's father's history.
- Nutrition increase for pregnancy is 300 kcalories/day. Two extra glasses of milk and one extra serving of meat will meet this need and supply the extra calcium and protein needed.
- Anticipatory guidance comprises the majority of nursing interventions when caring for a pregnant client.

Review Questions

1. Using Naegele's rule, when is a client expected to deliver if her LMP began on March 15?

    a. November 15
    b. November 23
    c. December 8
    d. December 22

2. A client pregnant for the first time is termed a:

    a. primipara.
    b. multipara.
    c. primigravida.
    d. multigravida.

3. Which of the following should the nurse recognize as the desired weight gain during pregnancy?

    a. 25 to 35 pounds
    b. 12 to 20 pounds
    c. 15 to 28 pounds
    d. 10 to 15 pounds

4. A prenatal client asks how the sex of her baby is determined. The nurse correctly explains that the sex is determined by a:

    a. gene in the ovum.
    b. gene in the sperm.
    c. chromosome in the ovum.
    d. chromosome in the sperm.

5. Which of the following should the nurse recognize as a positive sign of pregnancy?

    a. Ballottement
    b. Hearing fetal heartbeat
    c. A positive pregnancy test
    d. Increase in abdominal size

6. Which of the following lunches would the nurse encourage for a pregnant woman?

    a. Bologna sandwich, potato chips, cola
    b. Cold chicken, french fries, roll, milk

    c. Bowl of bean soup, crackers, glass of ice tea
    d. Cottage cheese, tossed salad and cracker, orange, water

7. The nurse is aware that which of the following statements made by a pregnant couple indicates a correct understanding of sexual activity during pregnancy?

    a. "There are no restrictions on sexual activity during an uncomplicated pregnancy."
    b. "Sexual activity should be avoided from the beginning of the second trimester."
    c. "Sexual activity on a limited basis is permitted until the last six weeks of pregnancy."
    d. "All sexual activity should be omitted during the time that the regular menstrual period would have occurred."

8. Which of the following hormones plays the most important role in preparing the uterus for pregnancy?

    a. Proscretin
    b. Progesterone
    c. Human growth hormone
    d. Follicle-stimulating hormone

9. The union of a sperm and an ovum is termed:

    a. gestation.
    b. reception.
    c. fertilization.
    d. ligamentation.

Critical Thinking Questions

1. How would you feel taking care of a pregnant drug addict?

2. What approach would you use when providing anticipatory guidance to a pregnant alcoholic?

3. How would the cultural considerations given in the chapter affect your nursing care of clients with those beliefs?

 WEB FLASH!

- Search the Internet for information about pregnancy, prenatal care, prenatal education, Lamaze and psychoprophylaxis. What information is available?
- Is the information on the Web for health care professionals or the general public?

COMPLICATIONS OF PREGNANCY

MAKING THE CONNECTION

Refer to the following chapters to increase your understanding of the complications of pregnancy:

- **Chapter 17, Loss, Grief, and Death**
- **Chapter 32, Nursing Care of the Client: Cardiovascular System**
- **Chapter 33, Nursing Care of the Client: Blood and Lymph Systems**
- **Chapter 36, Nursing Care of the Client: Sexually Transmitted Diseases**
- **Chapter 37, Nursing Care of the Client: Endocrine System**
- **Chapter 46, Nursing Care of the Client: Substance Abuse**

- **Chapter 47, Prenatal Care**
- **Chapter 49, The Birth Process**
- **Procedures:** B1, Handwashing; B2, Use of Protective Equipment; B6, Assessing Blood Pressure; B29, Measuring Intake and Output; I1, Surgical Asepsis: Preparing and Maintaining a Sterile Field; I2, Performing Open Gloving and Removal of Soiled Gloves; I4, Performing Urinary Catheterization: Female Client

LEARNING OBJECTIVES

Upon completion of this chapter, you should be able to:
- *Define key terms.*
- *Discuss therapy for a client with hyperemesis gravidarum.*
- *Compare and contrast the etiology, medical–surgical management, and nursing care for the bleeding situations in pregnancy.*
- *Describe the development, medical–surgical management, and nursing care of a client with pregnancy-induced hypertension.*
- *Describe the nursing care for a client with a chronic medical problem: diabetes, hypertension, heart disease, maternal PKU.*
- *Discuss the effects of infection on a pregnant woman and her fetus and ways of preventing the infections.*
- *Compare and contrast the etiology, medical–surgical management, nursing care, and effect on the fetus of Rh incompatibility and ABO incompatibility.*

- *Describe the effects of multiple pregnancies on the mother, fetuses, and family.*
- *Describe the effects of addiction on the mother and fetus.*
- *Summarize the needs of a woman in preterm labor.*

KEY TERMS

abortion	hyperemesis gravidarum
abruptio placenta	incompetent cervix
amniocentesis	kernicterus
early deceleration	late deceleration
eclampsia	macrosomia
ectopic pregnancy	miscarriage
euglycemia	placenta previa
fetal biophysical profile	preeclampsia
	surfactant
HELLP syndrome	tocolysis
hydatidiform mole	variable deceleration
hydramnios	

INTRODUCTION

It is truly impressive that most pregnancies have no complications. For those clients who do have complications, it can be a very frightening and guilt-ridden situation. Regular prenatal care is the best way to identify clients who have high-risk factors. These clients can then be assessed and monitored more closely, and signs and symptoms of complications detected as early as possible. Medical–surgical management and effective nursing care can then be implemented. Many of the causes of high-risk pregnancies are given in Table 48-1.

This chapter covers the common complications of pregnancy including etiology, medical–surgical management, and the nursing process.

ASSESSMENT OF FETAL WELL-BEING

When complications arise in a pregnancy, more intense and specific assessments of the fetus are required. The fetal assessments described in Chapter 47 are also to be used. High-frequency, inaudible sound waves are directed toward the uterus. The sound waves reflected back are converted into a visual image (Figure 48-1).

Ultrasound

Ultrasound allows visualization of the uterine contents.

Ultrasound provides the following information.

First Trimester
- Early positive diagnosis of pregnancy about 5 or 6 weeks after LMP
- Identification of more than one fetus
- Observation of cardiac activity at 21 days and respiratory movements about 11th week of gestation
- Diagnosis of an ectopic pregnancy

Second and Third Trimester
- Measurement of biparietal diameter, femur length, overall length (crown-heel and crown-rump), ges-

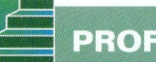

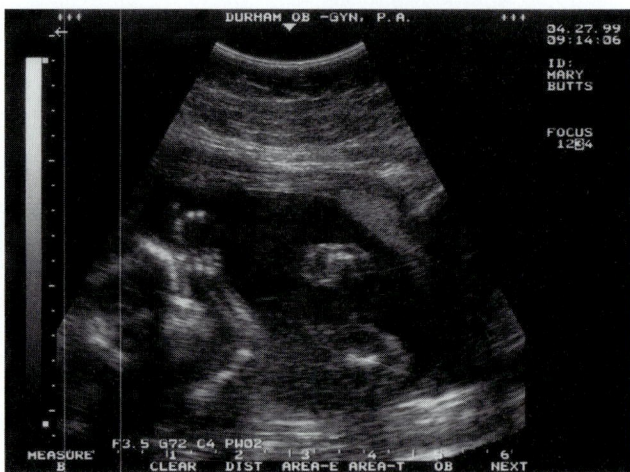

Figure 48-1 Ultrasound provides a visual image of uterine contents.

tational age, and intrauterine growth retardation (IUGR)
- Detection of some fetal anomalies, especially anencephaly and hydrocephalus
- Detection of hydramnios (excessive amniotic fluid, or polyhydramnios) or oligohydramnios (deficiency of amniotic fluid), either of which is frequently associated with fetal anomalies
- Identification of amniotic fluid pockets; a vertical pocket of 2 cm is associated with normal fetal status
- Location of the placenta, which is necessary prior to an amniocentesis and to determine placenta previa
- Determination of fetal position and presentation
- Detection of fetal death; fetal heart beating is not visualized, and the bones in the fetal head separate

Table 48-1 CAUSES OF HIGH-RISK PREGNANCY

GENERAL	OBSTETRICAL	MEDICAL	OTHER
Age (under 15 or over 35 years)	Previous problems	Chronic diseases	Smoking
Unmarried	Abortion	Diabetes	Drug abuse
Low socioeconomic group, little education	Excessive size of infant	Hypertension	Alcohol abuse
Prenatal care begun 27 weeks or later	Cesarean birth	Sickle cell anemia	Nutritional deficit
	Postterm birth	Thyroid disease	
	Incompetent cervix	Sexually transmitted disease	
	Abnormal fetal presentation	Cervical neoplasia	
	Rh negative and sensitized	Urinary tract infection	
	Preeclampsia	Neurological problem	
	Multiple pregnancy	Psychiatric problem	

Transabdominal Ultrasound

The mother is asked to have a full bladder when the ultrasound is performed. This allows the other structures to be assessed in relation to the bladder. The transducer is moved slowly over the abdomen while the client lies on her back. This position may cause shortness of breath. The procedure takes about 20 to 30 minutes.

Endovaginal Ultrasound

A probe is inserted into the vagina, putting it close to the structures being imaged. This produces a clearer image. The client is in the lithotomy position and has an empty bladder.

Nonstress Test

A nonstress test (NST) requires an electronic fetal monitor to record fetal movement and fetal heart rate (FHR) accelerations (short-term increases in fetal heart rate caused by fetal movement). Specific equipment may vary. The mother reclines in a chair or in bed in semi-Fowler's or side-lying position. This noninvasive test is used once or twice a week after 30 weeks' gestation in high-risk clients (Figure 48-2).

The test is reactive if there are two accelerations of 15 beats/minute, lasting 15 seconds in a 20-minute period. This indicates that the fetus has adequate oxygenation and an intact central nervous system.

The test is nonreactive if the criteria for reactive are not met. This may indicate that the fetus is asleep or is having problems.

An unsatisfactory test is identified if there is inadequate fetal activity or the data cannot be interpreted. If decelerations of the FHR are noted, the health care provider should be notified.

Fetal Acoustic Stimulation Test and Vibroacoustic Stimulation Test

The fetal acoustic stimulation test (FAST) and vibroacoustic stimulation test (VST) are used in conjunction with the NST. A small battery-operated device is placed on the mother's abdomen over the fetal head. A low-frequency vibration and a buzzing sound are emitted from the device to stimulate the fetus who had a nonreactive NST. The sounds emitted last no more than 3 seconds and are repeated every minute if no accelerations occur.

Two FHR accelerations of 15 beats/minute, lasting 15 seconds, in a 10-minute period are considered to be a reactive test. Some institutions use the FAST and VST instead of an NST.

Fetal Biophysical Profile

The **fetal biophysical profile** (FBPP) assesses five biophysical variables: fetal breathing movement, fetal movements of body or limbs, fetal tone (extension/flexion of extremities), amniotic fluid volume, and reactive NST (Table 48-2). The first four are assessed by ultrasound. A score of 8 or more shows probable fetal well-being.

Fetal Movements

From the time of quickening (16 to 20 weeks), fetal movement is reassuring to the mother. Counting fetal

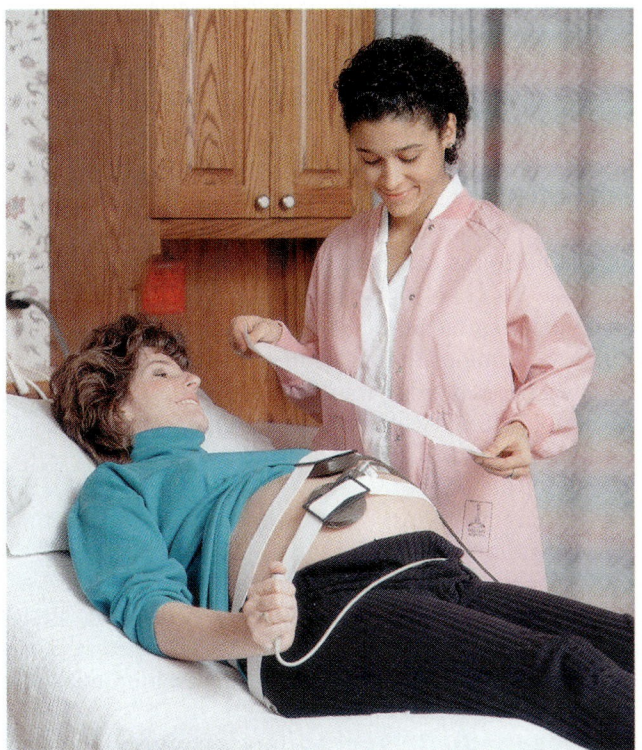

Figure 48-2 Nonstress Test (NST) to Assess Fetal Well-being

Table 48-2 BIOPHYSICAL PROFILE		
	SCORE 2	**SCORE 0**
Fetal Breathing	One or more episodes lasting 30 seconds in 30 minutes.	Not present or not lasting 30 seconds.
Fetal Movement	Three or more body/limb movements in 30 minutes.	Two or fewer body/limb movements in 30 minutes.
Fetal Tone	One or more episodes of active flexion/extension.	Slow extension with return to partial flexion, or movement absent.
Fluid Assessment	One or more pockets of amniotic fluid 1 cm in two perpendicular planes.	No pocket, or no pocket 1 cm in two perpendicular planes.
Fetal Reaction	Reactive NST.	Nonreactive NST.

movement daily provides evidence that the fetus is not having difficulty.

One method is to count fetal movements for 10 minutes three times a day. Another, which is the Cardiff method, requires the mother to count fetal movements at the same time each day until 10 movements are felt. The start and stop times are recorded.

The health care provider should be contacted if there are:

- fewer that 10 movements in 12 hours.
- no movements for 8 hours.
- sudden violent movements followed by reduced movements.

Biochemical Assessments

Three tests include maternal serum alpha-fetoprotein, estriol, and human placental lactogen.

Maternal Serum Alpha-Fetoprotein

Maternal serum alpha-fetoprotein (MSAFP) identifies some birth defects and chromasomal anomalies during the antepartum period. AFP is found in maternal serum about 7 weeks' gestation and rises steadily until the last trimester. All women should have the test between 16 and 18 weeks' gestation. Since there is a normal range for each week of pregnancy, a correct gestational age is important to the interpretation of the test.

If the MSAFP level is high, it may indicate a fetal open neural tube defect, multiple gestation, Rh isoimmunization, maternal diabetes mellitus, or fetal distress and death. If the MSAFP level is low, the fetus may have Down's syndrome or there may be a maternal hypertensive state.

Estriol

Maternal estriol level indicates fetoplacental function. Essential precursors from the fetal adrenal glands are converted by the placenta to estriol. The level in maternal serum and urine usually increases throughout pregnancy, so there must be a series of tests throughout pregnancy. The gradual increase in the maternal estriol level indicates that the fetal adrenal glands and the placenta are functioning normally.

Human Placental Lactogen

Human placental lactogen (hPL) increases throughout pregnancy correlating with increased fetal weight.

Amniocentesis

Amniocentesis is a procedure in which a needle is inserted through the abdomen into the amniotic sac. Amniotic fluid is withdrawn and sent to the laboratory for testing. At 14 to 16 weeks' gestation, an amniocentesis may be performed for diagnosis of genetic diseases or birth defects if the mother is over 35 or either parent has a family history of genetic disease (Figure 48-3).

Later in pregnancy, amniocentesis is most often

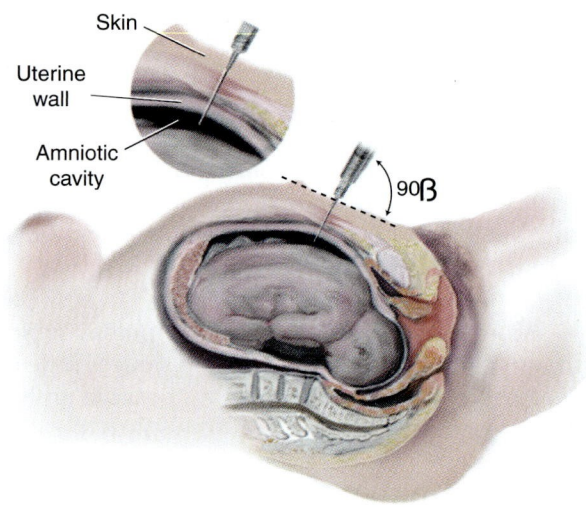

Figure 48-3 In amniocentesis, a small amount of amniotic fluid is withdrawn for study.

used to determine fetal lung maturity. In a problem pregnancy when preterm delivery of the fetus is a possibility, the physician will often try to maintain the pregnancy until the lungs are mature.

The nurse assists the physician performing the amniocentesis and provides emotional support to the client.

Safety: Amniocentesis

- Wash hands.
- Wear goggles or face mask, splash apron, and disposable gloves.
- Label specimen clearly so laboratory personnel can use appropriate precautions.
- Wash hands after removal of gloves.

Tests on Amniotic Fluid

Both the fluid and the cells in the amniotic fluid are used for testing. The fluid should be clear, colorless, and may have flecks of vernix caseosa floating in it.

Lecithin/Sphingomyelin Ratio **Surfactant** is phospholipids in the lungs that lower surface tension and stabilize the alveoli so they do not collapse on exhalation. The ratio of two phospholipids that are components of surfactant, lecithin and sphingomyelin (L/S ratio), determines the maturity of the lungs.

Early in pregnancy the lecithin level is low and the sphingomyelin level is high. About 32 weeks' gestation, this relationship begins to change. By 35 weeks' gestation the lecithin level is twice as high as the level of sphingomyelin. An L/S ratio of 2:1 is considered indicative of lung maturity.

Some conditions may accelerate lung maturation, such as severe pregnancy-induced hypertension (PIH), chronic maternal hypertension, or prolonged rupture of membranes. Diabetes and Rh isoimmunization seem to delay fetal lung maturity.

Phosphatidylglycerol Another phospholipid in surfactant, phosphatidylglycerol (PG), appears in the amniotic fluid when the lungs are mature, about 35 weeks' gestation.

Bilirubin In clients with Rh incompatibility, there is bilirubin in the amniotic fluid. The level of bilirubin corresponds to the degree of fetal anemia.

Sex Determination The sex of the fetus can be accurately determined by cell studies. This is important in sex-linked genetic abnormalities.

Chorionic Villi Sampling

In chorionic villi sampling (CVS), samples of chorionic villi from the developing placenta are obtained to assess for the same genetic disorders as in amniocentesis. CVS is performed between 8 and 10 weeks' gestation. Either a vaginal or abdominal approach may be used (Figure 48-4).

Contraction Stress Test

A contraction stress test (CST) evaluates the respiratory function of the placenta. During a uterine contraction, blood flow to the intervillous spaces is momentarily reduced, thus decreasing oxygen available to the fetus. A healthy fetus tolerates this well. Fetal hypoxia, myocardial depression, and a decrease in fetal heart rate (FHR) occur if the placenta's reserve is not sufficient.

This test is used with clients who have heart disease, hypertension, pregnancy-induced hypertension (PIH), sickle cell anemia, previous stillbirths, Rh sensitization, or a nonreactive NST. It is most often performed on the client with diabetes (chronic or gestational).

The vascular changes that take place in diabetes will also affect the placenta. Vascular changes in the placenta cause placental insufficiency so the fetus will not tolerate a CST well. Contraindications for use of this test are: placenta previa, abruptio placenta, prema-

ture rupture of membranes, a history of preterm labor, or previous cesarean birth.

The uterine contractions are induced by either intravenous oxytocin or breast self-stimulation. An electronic fetal monitor provides continuous information of the FHR and uterine contractions. A 15-minute baseline recording on the fetal monitor is obtained before contractions are stimulated. Intravenous oxytocin is given piggy-back to another IV so it can be stopped when necessary. When three uterine contractions lasting 40 to 60 seconds occur in 10 minutes, the oxytocin is stopped. If three late decelerations occur, the oxytocin is stopped.

For nipple stimulation, warm washcloths are applied to the breasts and/or one nipple is manually rolled by the client. When three uterine contractions lasting 40 to 60 seconds occur in 10 minutes, the stimulation is discontinued. If a decrease in FHR occurs with a contraction, the nipple stimulation is stopped.

A negative CST with no late decelerations is the desired result. The fetus is able to tolerate the hypoxia of uterine contractions. A positive CST with late decelerations that occur with more than half of the contractions is not the desired result.

Electronic Fetal Monitoring

Electronic fetal monitoring (EFM) provides a visual record of the FHR in relation to the uterine contractions. It allows early detection of fetal distress and abnormal uterine activity. High-risk clients and clients with a problem in their pregnancy are candidates for EFM. Some birthing places routinely have all clients on EFM.

External (Indirect) Monitoring

A tocodynamometer (for uterine activity) is placed on the mother's abdomen near the fundus. A strap around the mother holds it securely in place. A Doppler transducer (ultrasonic device) is placed on the mother's abdomen and moved around until the fetal heart is heard the best. A strap around the mother holds it in place also (Figure 48-5A). Sounds waves are bounced off the fetal heart and picked up and displayed by the monitor.

Internal (Direct) Monitoring

This is a more reliable method then external monitoring. An ECG electrode to directly monitor FHR is attached to the fetal presenting part (head) (Figure 48-5B). For this to be initiated, the membranes must be ruptured, the cervix must be dilated at least 2 cm, the presenting part must be down against the cervix, and the presenting part must be known. Only a person specially trained for this procedure should perform it.

Either the external tocodynamometer or an intrauterine catheter may be used to assess uterine contractions. A thin, flexible polyethylene catheter filled

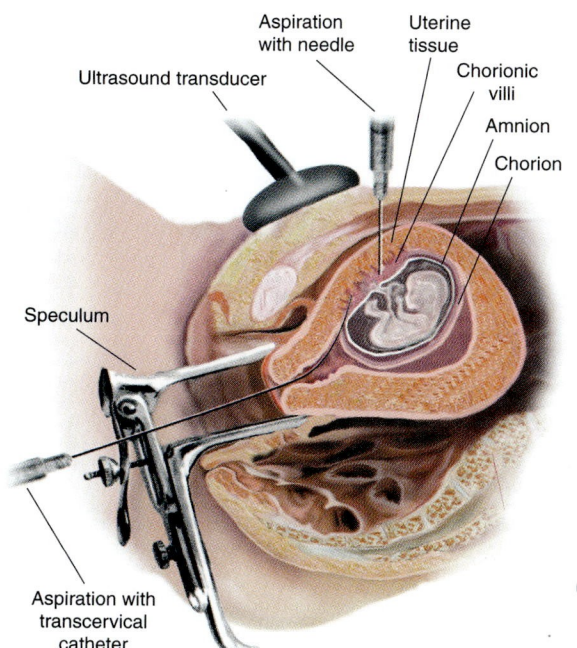

Ultrasound transducer
Aspiration with needle
Uterine tissue
Chorionic villi
Amnion
Chorion
Speculum
Aspiration with transcervical catheter

Figure 48-4 Chorionic Villi Sampling (performed between 8 and 10 weeks gestation)

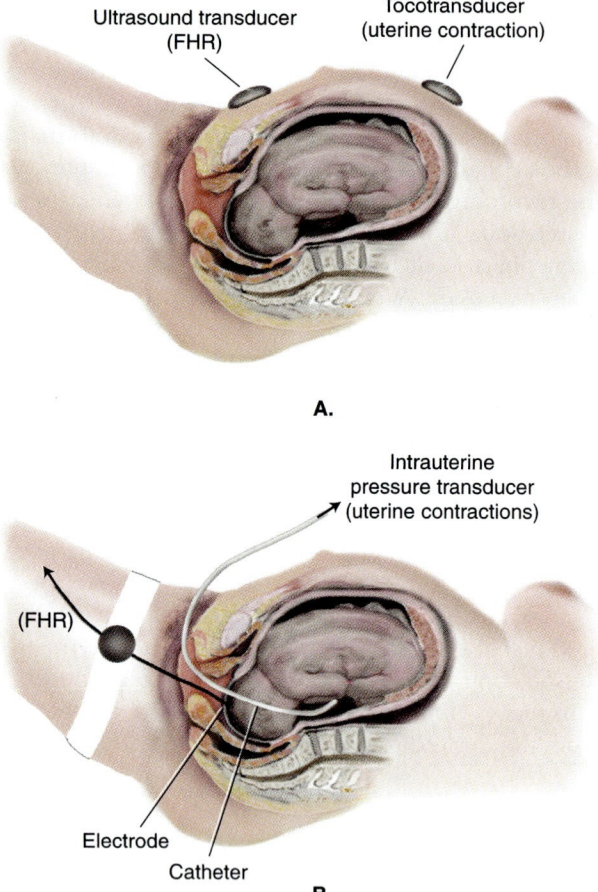

Ultrasound transducer (FHR)

Tocotransducer (uterine contraction)

A.

Intrauterine pressure transducer (uterine contractions)

(FHR)

Electrode

Catheter

B.

Figure 48-5 Fetal Monitoring: A. External (indirect). The top transducer picks up the uterine contraction and the lower transducer picks up the fetal heart and transmits the signal as an electrical impulse to the monitor where they are recorded; B. Internal (direct). The ECG electrode on the fetus's scalp picks up the fetal heart rate and the intrauterine catheter picks up uterine contractions.

with sterile, distilled water is inserted into the amniotic fluid in the uterus. The increased pressure on the fluid during a contraction is translated into an electrical signal. This provides reliable information about the contractions. Sterile technique is used when inserting both the scalp electrode and the catheter.

Interpretations

New definitions have been recommended by the National Institute of Child Health and Human Development Research Planning Workshop. These are being tested and so may be found in practice in specific institutions.

The interpretations currently in use will be presented here.

Baseline Rate Baseline rate is the average FHR during a 10-minute period. The normal rate is 120 to 160 beats/minute. A rate above 160 beats/minute is tachycardia, and a rate below 120 beats/minute is bradycardia.

Baseline Variability Short-term variability is the beat-to-beat change in FHR. Long-term variability is the waviness (called cycles) that occurs 3 to 5 times a minute.

Accelerations Accelerations are short-term increases in FHR usually caused by fetal movement. This is the basis for the NST.

Early Deceleration **Early decelerations** are reductions in fetal heart rate that begin early with the contraction and typically mirror the contraction. Head compression during contractions causes a decrease in cerebral blood flow which shows as early deceleration. No intervention is required (Figure 48-6).

PROFESSIONAL TIP

Electronic Fetal Monitoring

The National Institute of Child Health and Human Development Research Planning Workshop recommended new definitions for the interpretation of electronic fetal monitoring (Harvey, 1997; NICHD, 1997). There will be research and refinement of the definitions, over time. Some institutions may implement the new definitions and some may wait until the tested results are published before implementing them. Communication of which definitions are being used is most important.

The new definitions are as follows:

- *Baseline rate:* The rate is measured over 10 minutes and is typically between 110 and 160 beats/minute in a term fetus.
- *Baseline variability:* Classified into one of four categories: absent, minimal, moderate, and marked; defined by the amplitude of the FHR. No distinction is made between short- and long-term variability. A picture will be used for a visual reference.
- *Accelerations:* A change in FHR that is a "visually apparent abrupt increase" (onset of acceleration to peak less than 30 seconds) by at least 15 beats/minute, lasting at least 15 seconds.
- *Decelerations:* Will still be classified as early, late, or variable, but the biologic and clinical significance of the pattern may no longer be assumed from the descriptive definition (Harvey, 1997).
- *Early deceleration:* Gradual onset, occur early, mirror image of contraction.
- *Late deceleration:* Gradual onset, delayed in onset, nadir (the lowest point), and recovery in relation to contraction. (When a timing discrepancy exists and early or late is in question, the nadir of the deceleration and peak of the contraction will differentiate early and late.)
- *Variable deceleration:* All abrupt onset decelerations reaching nadir within 30 seconds.

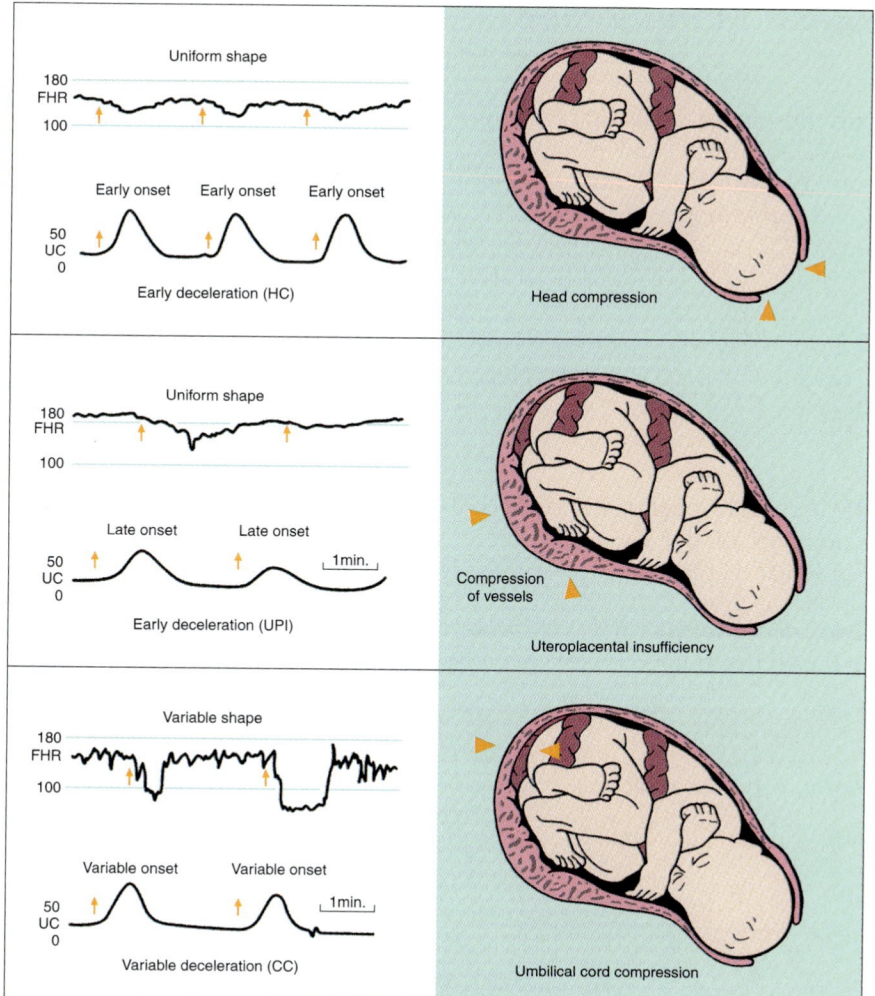

Figure 48-6 Fetal Heart Rate Patterns from Continuous Electronic Fetal Monitoring (*Adapted from* Basic Maternal Newborn Nursing, *by B. Anderson & P. Shapiro, 1994. Albany, NY: Delmar Publishers.*)

Late Deceleration **Late decelerations** are reductions in fetal heart rate that begin at the peak of the contraction and increase to the baseline level after the contraction has ceased. They are due to uteroplacental insufficiency. Oxygen administered to the mother may be started. Late decelerations should be reported to the health care provider (Figure 48-6).

Variable Deceleration **Variable decelerations** are reductions in fetal heart rate that have no relationship to contractions of the uterus. They occur when compression of the umbilical cord reduces blood flow between fetus and placenta. A change in the mother's position may take pressure off the cord. These should also be reported immediately (Figure 48-6).

HYPEREMESIS GRAVIDARUM

Hyperemesis gravidarum is excessive vomiting during pregnancy. The cause is unknown but may be related to an increased estrogen level, gonadotropin production, or trophoblastic activity. Psychological factors may also be involved. The vomiting progresses to the point that the woman vomits everything swallowed. It does not subside at about 12 weeks' gestation as does "morning sickness."

Dehydration leads to fluid and electrolyte imbalance and alkalosis from the loss of hydrochloric acid. As the situation becomes worse, the client experiences tachycardia and may have hypovolemia, hypotension, an increase in hematocrit and blood urea nitrogen (BUN), and a decrease in urine output.

The starvation situation causes protein and vitamin deficiencies. Cardiac functioning may be disrupted by severe potassium loss. Untreated, the client may experience metabolic changes or death. Embryonic or fetal death may occur.

The treatment goals are to control vomiting, correct dehydration, restore electrolyte balance, and maintain adequate nutrition.

Medical–Surgical Management

Medical

The client is usually hospitalized and intravenous fluids containing glucose, vitamins, and electrolytes are started immediately. IV therapy is continued until all vomiting has stopped for 48 hours. Psychotherapy may be recommended.

Pharmacological

A sedative may be given. However, medications are kept to a minimum because of potential teratogenic (harmful) effects to the fetus.

Diet

The client is kept NPO until all vomiting has stopped for 48 hours. Small amounts of dry foods are then tried. Progression to a regular diet is done slowly.

Activity

Bed rest is usually maintained until the condition begins to improve. Visitors may be restricted for a few days to allow the client to rest.

▶ NURSING PROCESS

▶ Assessment

▶ Subjective Data

Especially important is the client's emotional state and her feelings about the pregnancy, the fetus, and her mate. The nurse should ask what triggers her nausea and vomiting.

▶ Objective Data

These include the amount and character of all emesis, intake and output, and fetal heart rate. Signs of jaundice and vaginal bleeding should be noted.

Nursing diagnoses for a client with hyperemesis gravidarum may include the following:

Nursing Diagnoses	Planning/Goals	Nursing Interventions
▶ *Nutrition, Altered, Less Than Body Requirements, related to persistent vomiting*	The client will cease vomiting.	Maintain relaxed, quiet environment. Monitor amount and character of all emesis. Maintain accurate I & O record. Ensure good oral hygiene after each vomiting episode. When vomiting stops, provide bland foods and oral fluids as ordered. Maintain cheerful, optimistic attitude.
▶ *Fluid Volume Deficit, related to decreased fluid intake and excessive fluid loss*	The client will have fluid balance.	Administer IV fluids as ordered. Monitor laboratory reports for electrolyte levels. Assess skin turgor and mucous membranes. Provide small amounts of oral fluids when tolerated. Maintain accurate I & O record.
▶ *Fear, related to fetal well-being*	The client will discuss fears with health caregivers.	Provide opportunities for client to express fears. Show acceptance of client's perceptions. Assist client to identify personal strengths. Listen to what the client says. Help client identify sources of support.

Evaluation Each goal must be evaluated to determine how it has been met by the client.

BLEEDING

Bleeding disorders include abortion, ectopic pregnancy, hydatidiform mole, placenta previa, abruptio placenta, and disseminated intravascular coagulation.

ABORTION

Abortion is the spontaneous (natural) or induced (purposeful) termination of a pregnancy before viability of the fetus. A fetus is considered viable at 24 weeks' gestation. With medical intervention, a fetus between 20 and 24 weeks' gestation may survive. Some states have defined viability as 20 to 24 weeks' gestation and a weight of 500 g.

A spontaneous abortion is often called a **miscarriage**. Spontaneous abortions may be related to chromosomal abnormalities, faulty implantation, teratogenic substances, placental abnormalities, incompetent cervix, chronic maternal diseases, maternal infections, and endocrine imbalances. Clinically, spontaneous abortions are classified as:

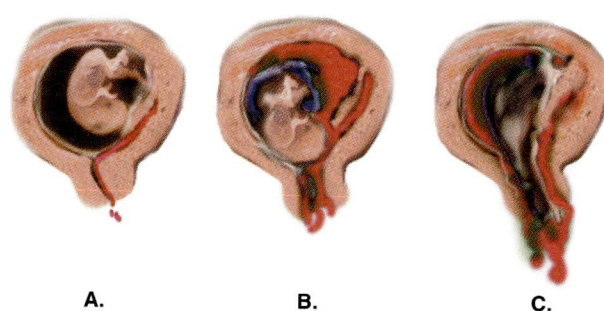

A. **B.** **C.**

Figure 48-7 Types of Spontaneous Abortions: A. Threatened; B. Inevitable; C. Incomplete

- Threatened: Unexplained bleeding and cramping. The cervix is closed and membranes are intact (Figure 48-7A).
- Inevitable: Increased bleeding and cramping. The cervix begins to dilate and the membranes may rupture (Figure 48-7B).
- Incomplete: Some of the products of conception are expelled. Most often the placenta is not expelled. Bleeding is heavy and cramping severe (Figure 48-7C).
- Complete: All products of conception are expelled.
- Missed: Embryo or fetus dies but is retained. The cervix is closed. If the fetus is not expelled within 6 weeks, disseminated intravascular coagulation (DIC) may develop.
- Habitual: Any of the above occurring in 3 consecutive pregnancies. Most commonly, the cervix begins to dilate in the second trimester. This is called an **incompetent cervix**.

Medical–Surgical Management

Medical

For threatened abortion, the client is usually told to limit activities for 24 to 48 hours. If the bleeding is going to stop, it will usually do so in 48 hours. If the bleeding stops, it is suggested that the client avoid stress, fatigue, strenuous activity, and sexual intercourse. Having one or two rest periods during the day

PROFESSIONAL TIP

Spontaneous Abortion

The client who has a miscarriage may experience a wide spectrum of emotions, from shock, disbelief, and guilt to anger and despair. She may have difficulty managing these feelings as well as responding to the reactions of partner, family, and friends. The nurse can assist by answering the woman's questions, allowing her to express her emotions, and respecting her need to grieve.

is also recommended until the pregnancy seems to be progressing normally.

Surgical

A client with an inevitable or incomplete abortion generally is hospitalized to remove the products of conception from the uterus. A dilatation and curettage (D & C) or suction evacuation is performed. Depending on the amount of blood loss, the client may be given blood transfusions.

When the products of conception, in a missed abortion, are not expelled in 4 to 6 weeks, the client is hospitalized. For a 12 weeks' gestation or less, a D & C is performed. If more than 12 weeks' gestation, induction of labor with oxytocin may be used.

When habitual abortions are caused by an incompetent cervix, it can be treated surgically by cerclage (Shirodkar procedure, Figure 48-8). Suture material is placed in the cervix in a purse-string fashion at the level of the internal os. This is done about 16 weeks' gestation. The suture can be left in for future pregnancies and a cesarean birth planned, or the suture may be removed at term and a vaginal birth allowed. If the mother goes into labor or the membranes rupture, she must call her health care provider and go to the hospital immediately.

▶ NURSING PROCESS

▶ Assessment

▶ Subjective Data

The client may describe abdominal cramping and vaginal bleeding, and may have feelings of fear and guilt.

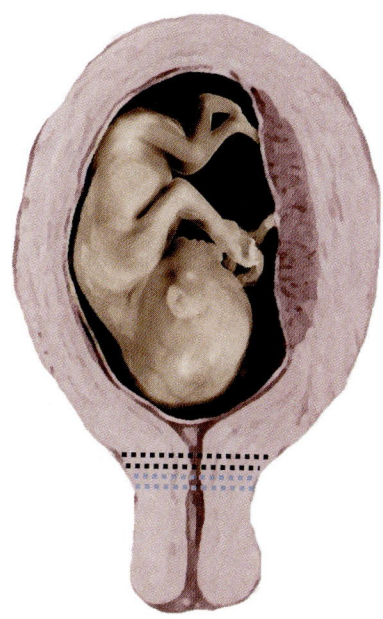

Figure 48-8 Shirodkar Procedure: Purse-String Suturing for an Incompetent Cervix

▶ Objective Data

Amount of bleeding and presence of clots should be noted. Any tissue expelled should also be noted and documented. Vital signs may indicate excessive blood loss (hypovolemia).

Nursing diagnoses for a client having an abortion may include the following:

Nursing Diagnoses	Planning/Goals	Nursing Interventions
▶ *Self-esteem, Disturbance of, related to feelings of guilt for doing something to cause abortion*	The client will maintain usual level of self-esteem.	Provide information about causes of a spontaneous abortion. Assist client to identify personal strengths. Actively listen to the client.
▶ *Pain, related to contractions (cramping) of uterine muscle*	The client will describe having less pain.	Administer analgesic as ordered. Monitor effect of analgesic.
▶ *Fear, related to potential loss of pregnancy*	The client will discuss fear with family.	Provide opportunities for the client to express fears. Help client identify sources of support. Show acceptance of client's perceptions.

Evaluation Each goal must be evaluated to determine how it has been met by the client.

SAMPLE NURSING CARE PLAN

THE CLIENT HAVING AN ABORTION

Pat, age 25, G4, P3, T2, P1, A0, L3, is admitted to the hospital with some bleeding and cramping. She states, "I'm scared, I don't understand what's happening." Vital signs are BP 108/66, T 98.6, P 86, R 24. Her skin is cool. At her first prenatal visit 3 weeks ago, the fetus was 12 weeks' gestation. Crying, she says, "I don't know what I did to cause this to happen."

Two hours later, Pat's cramping is severe and the bleeding heavy, bright red. Vital signs are BP 88/60, P 100, and R 28. Her skin is cold and clammy.

Nursing Diagnosis 1 *Fluid Volume Deficit, Active Loss, related to heavy bleeding as evidenced by hypotension and decreased pulse pressure*

PLANNING/GOALS	NURSING INTERVENTIONS	RATIONALE	EVALUATION
Pat will have vital signs return to baseline values.	Administer IV fluids and/or blood as ordered.	Replaces fluid volume lost by bleeding.	After a D & C, Pat's vital signs returned to baseline values.
	Monitor Pat's vital signs every 15 minutes or less.	Clinical indicators of fluid volume.	
	Save all vaginal pads and clots or tissue passed for physician to see.	Allows physician to estimate blood loss and identify any tissue passed.	
	Administer analgesic as ordered.	Relieving pain will make Pat more comfortable.	
	Prepare Pat for surgery as ordered.	Most likely, a D & C will be performed.	*continued*

Nursing Diagnosis 2 *Anxiety, Moderate, related to changes in her pregnancy as evidenced by statement "I'm scared, I don't understand what's happening."*

PLANNING/GOALS	NURSING INTERVENTIONS	RATIONALE	EVALUATION
Pat will verbalize her feelings about bleeding and cramping while pregnant.	Speak slowly and calmly to Pat.	Voice will convey calmness and sense of security.	Pat shared feelings of fear and guilt about the bleeding and cramping.
	Evaluate Pat's understanding of what is happening and possible treatment options.	Provides information for educational needs.	
	Involve spouse/significant other in discussion.	Gives family information and a feeling of control.	
	Be direct and focus on the specific topic.	Anxiety decreases ability to concentrate.	
	Help Pat identify coping methods used in the past.	Important to know how Pat has coped in the past.	

Nursing Diagnosis 3 *Grieving, Anticipatory, related to probable loss of pregnancy as evidenced by crying and statement "I don't know what I did to cause this to happen"*

PLANNING/GOALS	NURSING INTERVENTIONS	RATIONALE	EVALUATION
Pat will verbalize what losing a pregnancy means to her.	Allow Pat to express her feelings.	Expression of feelings releases energy and is calming.	Pat is having trouble talking about losing the pregnancy.
	Assess Pat's coping skills.	Coping skills may need to be reinforced or adapted.	
	Assist Pat to identify personal resources and strengths.	Promotes integrity of self.	
	Provide privacy for Pat and her family.	Allows them a chance to discuss the situation and make plans.	

ECTOPIC PREGNANCY

An **ectopic pregnancy** occurs when a fertilized ovum implants outside the uterine cavity. The most common site is in the fallopian tube. This generally happens when the fertilized ovum is unable to move through the tube. Figure 48-9 illustrates other possible sites of implantation in an ectopic pregnancy.

More than 70,000 ectopic pregnancies occur annually in the United States. Risk factors include pelvic inflammatory disease, in utero exposure to diethylstilbestrol, sexually transmitted diseases, pharmacologic treatment of infertility, and endometriosis (Minnick-Smith & Cook, 1997).

The pregnancy appears normal at first with the usual signs and symptoms including the presence of hCG in the blood and urine. Symptoms of ectopic

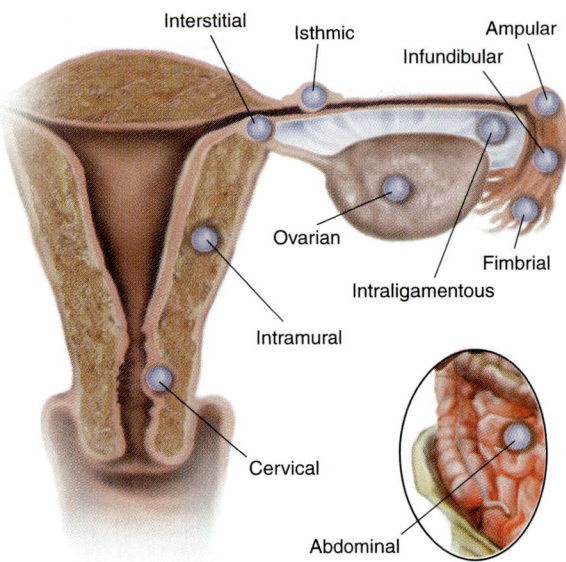

Figure 48-9 Possible Sites of Implantation in Ectopic Pregnancy

pregnancy begin gradually about 3 to 5 weeks after the first missed menstrual period. Pain is noted as the fallopian tube stretches with the growing embryo. The tube finally ruptures (a severe pain occurs) and bleeds into the peritoneal cavity. Some vaginal bleeding may be apparent. The client may rapidly show signs of hypovolemic shock. The signs of shock are out of proportion to the apparent blood loss. Ectopic pregnancy is a significant cause of maternal morbidity and mortality, and is nearly always fatal to the embryo.

Medical–Surgical Management

Medical

The menstrual history is reviewed and a pelvic examination performed to identify abnormal pelvic masses and tenderness. Severe pain occurs when the cervix is moved. A transvaginal ultrasound is also done. Serial testing of hCG shows a slower increase than in a normal pregnancy, in which the hCG level doubles every 48 to 72 hours. A serum progesterone level of 25 ng/mL strongly suggests a normal pregnancy, while a level of 5 ng/mL or less indicates a nonviable pregnancy. A level between 5 ng/mL and 25 ng/mL is uncertain, and a transvaginal ultrasound is needed.

Surgical

Rapid surgical treatment is generally necessary to remove the products of conception and to control bleeding. Laparotomy is seldom used now unless the client has orthostatic hypotension, tachycardia, or a falling hematocrit. Laparoscopic salpingostomy or salpingectomy are preferred. The procedure of choice is salpingostomy when future fertility is desired (Minnick-

Smith & Cook, 1997). If the fallopian tube is badly damaged, a salpingectomy is performed. The ovary is left in place if not damaged. Blood transfusions are often required.

Pharmacological

Methotrexate (Mexate, Folex) may be given to resolve an ectopic pregnancy.

Diet

If the client has surgery, she will be NPO prior to and after surgery.

Activity

The client is usually on bed rest until the situation is resolved.

▶ NURSING PROCESS

▶ Assessment

▶ Subjective Data

The client describes amenorrhea, nausea, breast tenderness, and a dull ache on one side that has increasingly become more severe. When the tube ruptures, the client will describe a single excruciating pain in the abdomen and may also have referred shoulder pain.

▶ Objective Data

Some vaginal bleeding may be apparent. Laboratory reports may show a low hemoglobin and hematocrit, a rising leukocyte level, and a slowly rising hCG level. The RBC count is low and sedimentation rate elevated. The abdomen may be rigid and tender. Vital signs may indicate hypovolemic shock.

Nursing diagnoses for a client with an ectopic pregnancy may include the following:

Nursing Diagnoses	Planning/Goals	Nursing Interventions
▶ *Grieving, Anticipatory, related to the loss of the pregnancy*	The client will understand that grieving may last several months.	Encourage client and family to talk about their feelings. Allow them privacy to grieve. Listen actively to concerns about this and future pregnancies. Provide information about causes of ectopic pregnancy. Refer to other professionals for help as needed.
▶ *Tissue Integrity, Impaired, related to the rupture of a fallopian tube*	The client will regain tissue integrity of the fallopian tube or it will be removed.	Prepare client for surgery as ordered. Begin preoperative teaching.
▶ *Pain, related to tubal rupture and blood in the abdomen*	The client will express less pain.	Administer analgesic as ordered and evaluate its effectiveness. Provide information about cause of pain.

Evaluation Each goal must be evaluated to determine how it has been met by the client.

HYDATIDIFORM MOLE

Hydatidiform mole (trophoblastic disease) is an abnormality of the placenta. The chorionic villi become fluid-filled, grapelike clusters; the trophoblastic tissue proliferates; and there is no viable embryo. In effect, the fertilized ovum dies and the chorion develops into vesicles. There is a possibility of developing choriocarcinoma.

The complete mole has only paternal genetic material. There is no embryonic tissue, only the fluid-filled cystic villi. A large amount of hCG is produced because the chorionic villi are proliferating. The classic signs are bleeding (usually brownish but may be red), uterine enlargement greater than would be expected for the gestation, and no fetal heart tones (FHT) heard (Figure 48-10). If any of the grapelike clusters are passed, it is diagnostic.

The partial mole has only focal areas of the fluid-filled cystic villi; some chorionic villi are formed normally. There is a fetus with multiple chromosomal anomalies and little chance for survival. A partial mole may not be recognized until the products of conception are examined after a spontaneous abortion.

The client may experience hyperemesis gravidarum because of the higher serum hCG level. If symptoms of pregnancy-induced hypertension appear before 24 weeks' gestation, a molar pregnancy is very probable. The primary diagnostic tool is ultrasound.

Medical–Surgical Management

Medical

After surgery to remove the mole, the client must be followed for 1 to 2 years. The care includes: chest x-rays to detect metastases, physical examinations with a pelvic examination, and regular (usually weekly) laboratory measurement of hCG level. The client is advised not to become pregnant during the follow-up time.

Surgical

The desire of the client for future fertility influences the surgical procedure to be used to empty the uterus. A D & C may be performed, but it is difficult to make certain that no fragment of the molar pregnancy is left in the uterus. A hysterotomy, cutting the uterus open (like cesarean birth), allows visual determination that the uterus is completely emptied. If the client is older and no future fertility is desired or there is excessive bleeding, a hysterectomy if performed.

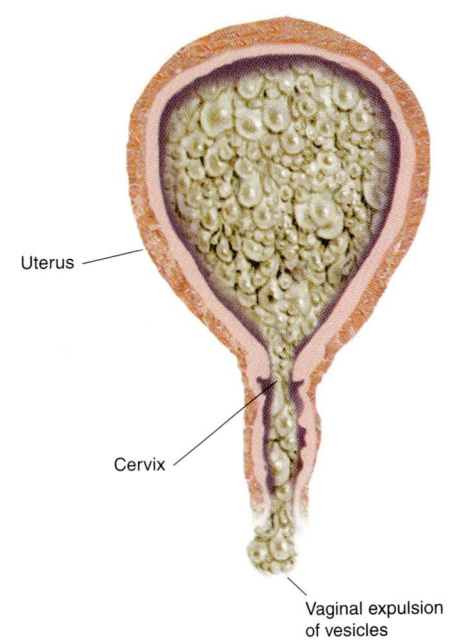

Uterus

Cervix

Vaginal expulsion of vesicles

Figure 48-10 Hydatidiform Mole

Pharmacological

If the hCG level remains high or rises after the uterus is evacuated, methotrexate (Mexate, Folex) is given. Oxytocin is given to keep the uterus contracted to control bleeding. Typed and cross-matched blood must be available.

CLIENT TEACHING

Methotrexate

• There is a risk of photosensitivity when taking methotrexate (Mexate, Folex) to reduce hCG levels following treatment for hydatidiform mole.

• Clients should avoid sun exposure while taking this medication.

Activity

Bed rest is maintained until after surgery, then ambulation is progressively increased.

▶ NURSING PROCESS

▶ Assessment

▶ Subjective Data

The client may describe severe nausea and vomiting and may be having some brownish vaginal discharge.

▶ Objective Data

There is vaginal bleeding, usually brownish but may be bright red. Uterine enlargement is greater than expected for gestational age. Ultrasound reveals a characteristic molar pattern. The client may have symptoms of pregnancy-induced hypertension (BP 140/90 or an increase of 30/15, proteinuria, and edema measured by sudden weight gain).

Nursing diagnoses for a client with hydatidiform mole may include the following:

Nursing Diagnoses	Planning/Goals	Nursing Interventions
▶ *Fear, related to the possible development of choriocarcinoma*	The client will discuss fears with health care provider or other professional.	Provide opportunities for client to express fears. Help client identify sources of support. Refer to other professionals as needed.
▶ *Knowledge Deficit, related to lack of understanding for regular monitoring of hCG level and delaying pregnancy*	The client will discuss reasons for regular monitoring of hCG level and why pregnancy should be delayed.	Present information as to how hCG level indicates whether choriocarcinoma is developing. Provide reasons for delaying another pregnancy. Allow client to express feelings about regular laboratory testing of blood.

Evaluation Each goal must be evaluated to determine how it has been met by the client.

PLACENTA PREVIA

Placenta previa occurs when implantation is in the lower uterine segment with the placenta lying over or very near the internal cervical os (Figure 48-11). The cause is unknown, but predisposing factors may be multiparity, uterine scarring from D & C or cesarean birth, or uterine infections.

The classic symptom is *painless bleeding* in the last half of pregnancy. There may be occasional bright red spotting or intermittent gushes of blood. Rarely is bleeding continuous. The uterus is relaxed and not tender. Bleeding is unrelated to maternal activity. Placenta previa is classified in three ways:

• Low-lying or Marginal: Placenta is near the internal cervical os but does not cover any part of opening.

• Partial: Placenta covers part of internal cervical os opening.

• Complete or Total: Placenta completely covers internal cervical os opening.

Toward the last part of pregnancy, the cervix effaces (thins). This movement of the cervix pulls away

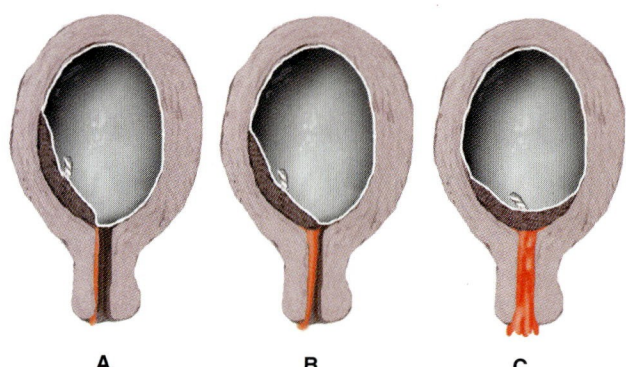

Figure 48-11 Placenta Previa: A. Low implantation (marginal); B. Partial placenta previa; C. Total placenta previa

from the placenta, and the exposed placental sinuses begin to bleed. The earlier this happens the more serious the situation.

Effects on the Fetus/Neonate

The gestational age of the fetus and the amount of bleeding determine the effects on the fetus/neonate. During profuse bleeding the fetus may suffer from hypoxia. After delivery, the neonate should be checked to see if the bleeding resulted in anemia.

Medical–Surgical Management

Medical

The goal is to maintain the pregnancy until the fetus is mature enough to survive outside the uterus. Fetal maturity is assessed by checking the lecithin/sphingomyelin ratio for lung maturity. The mother is usually hospitalized. Hemoglobin and hematocrit (H & H) is usually determined every 12 hours. The laboratory will type and cross-match, and 2 units of blood will be kept on call in the event of severe blood loss.

Diagnosis is made with an ultrasound. Once the diagnosis is made, no vaginal examinations are performed because of the risk of causing more bleeding by disturbing the placenta. If an ultrasound is unavailable, vaginal bleeding profuse, and the pregnancy near term, the health care provider may examine the client vaginally. This is done in the delivery room with a setup for vaginal delivery and a setup for a cesarean delivery.

Surgical

If the maternal situation becomes worse or there is fetal distress, a cesarean birth is immediately begun.

Pharmacological

In an attempt to accelerate fetal lung maturity, a drug such as betamethasone (Celestone) may be given to the mother.

Activity

The client is on bed rest with bathroom privileges as long as no bleeding occurs. If bleeding begins, the client is on complete bed rest.

▶ NURSING PROCESS

▶ Assessment

▶ Subjective Data

The client describes painless bleeding.

▶ Objective Data

Vaginal bleeding may range from spotting to profuse bleeding. The uterus remains soft and relaxes fully between contractions if labor begins. FHR generally remains stable unless bleeding is profuse and maternal shock occurs.

Nursing diagnoses for a client with placenta previa may include the following:

Nursing Diagnoses	Planning/Goals	Nursing Interventions
▶ *Fluid Volume Deficit, related to blood loss*	The client will maintain perfusion to placenta and vital organs.	Observe, report, and record blood loss (count and/or weigh pads). Monitor client's vital signs. Monitor I & O. Inspect skin for pallor, cyanosis, clamminess, and coldness. Evaluate state of consciousness. Monitor FHR. Monitor laboratory reports.
▶ *Fetal Gas Exchange, Impaired, High Risk for, related to decreased maternal blood volume and hypotension*	FHR will remain within normal limits.	Monitor FHR, baseline variability, and decelerations. Observe amniotic fluid for meconium.

Evaluation Each goal must be evaluated to determine how it has been met by the client.

ABRUPTIO PLACENTA

The premature separation from the wall of the uterus of a normally implanted placenta is called **abruptio placenta**. It occurs spontaneously after the 20th week of gestation in one out of 75 to 90 pregnancies (Bougere, 1998). The cause is unknown. Contributing factors may include: maternal hypertension, multiple pregnancy, smoking, use of alcohol, or use of cocaine. Generally, it occurs late in pregnancy or during labor. There are three types of abruptio placenta (Figure 48-12).

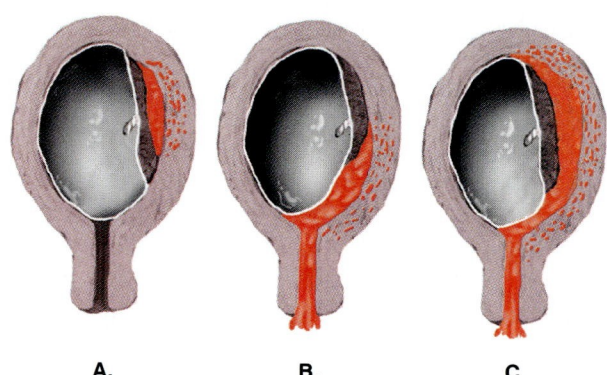

A.   **B.**   **C.**

Figure 48-12 Abruptio Placenta: A. Central abruption, concealed hemorrhage; B. Marginal abruption, external hemorrhage; C. Complete abruption, external hemorrhage (could also be concealed)

- Central: Center of the placenta separates with blood trapped between placenta and uterine wall; there is no apparent bleeding.
- Marginal: Edge of placenta separates and bright red bleeding is apparent vaginally.
- Complete: Entire placenta separates with profuse bleeding apparent vaginally.

A central abruption may progress to a complete abruption. In central and complete, blood invades the uterine muscle (bruising called *Couvelaire uterus*) causing a rigid, painful abdomen. After delivery the uterus contracts poorly and the client may require a hysterectomy to control the bleeding. The damage to the uterine muscle and the retroplacental clotting can cause a large release of thromboplastin. This can trigger the development of disseminated intravascular coagulation (DIC). Maternal mortality is relatively low. Problems after the delivery depend on the severity of the bleeding. Table 48-3 compares placenta previa and the various types of abruptio placenta.

Effects on the Fetus/Neonate

Perinatal mortality is about one-third of the cases of abruptio placenta. The outcome depends on fetal maturity and severity of the abruption. Preterm labor, hypoxia, and anemia are the most serious complications. Irreversible brain damage or fetal death may occur if hypoxia is not reversed quickly.

Medical–Surgical Management

Medical

Intravenous fluids, generally lactated Ringer's solution, are given to prevent or reverse hypovolemia. Laboratory tests to evaluate client's status and the clotting mechanism are ordered: H & H, platelet count, fibrinogen level, fibrin split products, thrombin time, prothrombin time, partial thromboplastin time, and bleeding time. Also, a type and cross-match for 3 to 4 units of blood or packed cells is requested (Bougere, 1998). If the mother is Rh negative, she is checked for Rh sensitization. An indwelling urinary catheter is inserted.

If separation is small and the pregnancy near term, induction of labor and vaginal delivery may be possible. If labor is not progressing in 8 hours, a cesarean birth is performed. If separation is moderate or severe, a cesarean birth is performed as soon as possible.

Surgical

Cesarean delivery is performed in many cases to prevent fetal demise. A hysterectomy may be required to control hemorrhage.

Pharmacological

RhoGAM is given to the nonsensitized Rh negative mother. Cryoprecipitate or plasma is given to treat hypofibrinogenemia. Analgesics are given as ordered.

Diet

No special diet or restrictions are required, though the client will be NPO if surgery is necessary.

Activity

The client will remain on bed rest until the situation is resolved.

▶ NURSING PROCESS

▶ Assessment

▶ Subjective Data

The client may describe moderate to severe pain in the abdomen. Fetal movement may become hyperactive and then may cease.

Table 48-3 COMPARISON OF PLACENTA PREVIA AND ABRUPTIO PLACENTA

CONDITION	BLEEDING	ABDOMEN	PAIN	BP
Placenta Previa	Bright red	No rigidity	None	Depends on amount of bleeding
Abruptio Placenta				
Central	None	Rigid	Acute	Decreased
Marginal	Dark red	No rigidity	Uterine tenderness	Decreased
Complete	Profuse	Rigid	Acute	Shock

▶ Objective Data

Vaginal bleeding is assessed. External fetal monitor will show uteroplacental insufficiency, baseline changes, and reduced variability. The contraction pattern will change and the resting tone will increase. Vital signs show indications of shock.

Nursing diagnoses for a client with abruptio placenta may include the following:

Nursing Diagnoses	Planning/Goals	Nursing Interventions
▶ Gas Exchange, Impaired, Fetal, related to altered uteroplacenta oxygen transfer due to placental separation	The fetus will not have hypoxia.	Watch external fetal monitor for decelerations, decreased baseline variability, and FHR. Provide nasal oxygen to mother. Have mother lie on left side.
▶ Grieving, Anticipatory, related to possible loss of pregnancy	The client will be able to verbalize feelings about possible loss of pregnancy.	Encourage client and family to talk about their feelings. Allow them some privacy to grieve. Contact minister, priest, or rabbi as requested by the client.
▶ Pain, related to retroplacental bleeding and possibly contractions	The client will verbalize an understanding of the cause of the pain.	Provide simple explanation for cause of pain. Encourage client to relax. Verbally tell client what and how to relax.
▶ Fluid Volume Deficit, related to blood loss	The client will regain fluid balance.	Monitor vital signs. Administer IV fluids as ordered. Accurately monitor I & O. Assess client for cold, clammy, cyanotic skin. Evaluate client's state of consciousness.

Evaluation Each goal must be evaluated to determine how it has been met by the client.

DISSEMINATED INTRAVASCULAR COAGULATION

Disseminated intravascular coagulation (DIC) is an overstimulation of the normal clotting process. Rapid, massive fibrin formation causes small thrombi to form throughout the circulatory system. This depletes the clotting factors and platelets. Generalized bleeding may then occur, leading to anemia or ischemia to vital organs because of the clots in the blood vessels.

DIC occurs as a complication of a primary problem. It is not only a complication of obstetrical situations, but also of many medical–surgical situations such as neoplasms, blood transfusion reaction, traumas, and infections. Men can also experience DIC. Obstetrical problems that may precipitate DIC include: abruptio placenta, placenta previa, hydatidiform mole, PIH, retained products of conception, amniotic fluid embolism, and infections.

Effects on the Fetus/Neonate

The primary problem may require immediate delivery of the fetus, even if preterm. The fetus may experience hypoxia to varying degrees. Fetal death can occur.

Medical–Surgical Management

Medical

Symptom onset is sudden with the client complaining of dyspnea or chest pain and becoming very restless and cyanotic and spitting frothy, blood-tinged mucous.

The underlying cause must be identified and corrected. If the fetus is not yet born, delivery should be facilitated. Diagnostic tests that may be used are: hemoglobin, hematocrit, fibrinogen level, platelet count, prothrombin time, and partial thromboplastin time.

Pharmacological

Intravenous administration of blood, fibrinogen, or cryoprecipitate is begun. Heparin given by continuous infusion pump inhibits thrombin activity and thus prevents formation of microemboli. There is no effect on already existing clots.

Oxygen therapy is often begun.

▶ NURSING PROCESS

▶ Assessment

▶ Subjective Data

The client may describe dyspnea or chest pain.

▶ Objective Data

The client may be extremely restless or cyanotic, and be expectorating blood-tinged frothy mucous.

Bleeding gums, epistaxis (nose bleed), petechiae under the blood pressure cuff around the client's arm, or bleeding from injection sites may also be present.

Nursing diagnoses for a pregnant client with DIC may include the following:

Nursing Diagnoses	Planning/Goals	Nursing Interventions
▶ *Anxiety, Moderate to Severe, related to the sudden change in health status*	The client will express understanding of what is happening to her and will feel less anxious.	Maintain a calm, positive manner. Explain to client what is happening, procedures, and treatment to be implemented. Remain with client. Allow client to express her anxiety. Answer client's questions.
▶ *Gas Exchange, Impaired, High Risk for, related to reduced oxygen-carrying capacity and ischemia of lung tissue*	The client will maintain adequate gas exchange to prevent tissue death.	Administer IV fluids, blood, or other substance to help restore a normal clotting mechanism. Administer heparin as ordered. Provide oxygen as ordered. Monitor lung sounds and respiratory rate. If fetus not yet delivered, monitor continuously with electronic fetal monitor.

Evaluation Each goal must be evaluated to determine how it has been met by the client.

PREGNANCY-INDUCED HYPERTENSION

Pregnancy-induced hypertension (PIH), the most common hypertensive disorder in pregnancy, appears after 20 weeks' gestation. The classic symptoms are hypertension, edema, and proteinuria. It is seen most often in primigravidas, especially those under 20 or over 35 years of age, who are in the lower socioeconomic group and have poor nutritional status. Diabetes, multiple pregnancy, or a family history of PIH also increase a client's risk.

Peripheral arteriole vasoconstriction and vasospasm lead to increased blood pressure and decreased perfusion of the uterus and placenta. Renal blood flow is lowered, renal glomerular filtration rate is lowered, and proteinuria results. Cerebral edema causes headaches and visual disturbances, Deep tendon reflexes become hyperactive. The liver enlarges, putting pressure on the liver capsule which causes epigastric pain. The condition may progress to **eclampsia**, or convulsions.

Despite decades of research, the cause remains unknown. It was previously called *toxemia* because it was thought that a toxin was produced in a pregnant woman's body. This term is no longer used. The only cure is delivery of the baby. PIH is a progressive condition developing from mild to severe **preeclampsia** to eclampsia and HELLP syndrome.

Effects on the Fetus/Neonate

Abruptio placenta and placental infarction may occur. Intrauterine growth retardation (IUGR) may occur as well as acute hypoxia and intrauterine death. A preterm infant may be born either because of spontaneous labor or obstetrical intervention.

Mild Preeclampsia

In mild preeclampsia the blood pressure increases 30 mm Hg systolic *or* 15 mm Hg diastolic over the client's baseline blood pressure on two occasions at least 6 hours apart, or a BP of 140/90 is noted. For example, a client with a baseline BP of 92/64 would be considered hypertensive at 122/80. Thus it is very important to have a baseline BP early in pregnancy.

Edema may be noted in the face and hands. It is objectively defined as weight gain of more than 1 pound a week.

Urine may show 1+ or 2+ albumin on a dipstick or 300 mg/L in 24 hours. Proteinuria is usually the last of the three classic symptoms to appear.

Severe Preeclampsia

Blood pressure increases to 160/110 or higher on two occasions 6 hours apart in severe preeclampsia. Generalized edema is easily noted in the face, hands, sacral area, lower extremities, and abdomen. Weight gain may be 2 pounds in a few days to a week.

Urinary albumin is 3+ or 4+ on dipstick. Urine output may drop to less than 500 mL/24 hours. Hematocrit, uric acid, and serum creatinine levels are elevated. The client may exhibit other symptoms such as: continuous headache, blurred vision, scotomata (spots before the eyes), nausea, vomiting, irritability, hyperreflexia, cerebral disturbances, pulmonary edema, dyspnea, cyanosis, and epigastric pain. Epigastric pain is often the last symptom identified before the client moves into eclampsia.

Eclampsia

The grand mal seizure experienced by the client has a tonic phase (pronounced muscular contractions) and a clonic phase (alternate contraction and relaxation of muscles). Then the client slips into a coma lasting from minutes to hours. With no treatment, the seizure/coma sequence may be repeated one or more times and death may follow.

Seizure activity may trigger uterine contractions, but the client in a coma is unaware of them and unable to let anyone know.

HELLP Syndrome

HELLP syndrome is PIH with liver damage. It is characterized by **h**emolysis, **e**levated **l**iver enzymes, and **l**ow **p**latelet count.

- Hemolysis is caused when intra-arterial lesions develop due to vasospasm, causing platelets to aggregate and a fibrin network to be formed. The RBCs are forced through the fibrin network and lysed, resulting in a large drop in hematocrit.
- Elevated liver enzymes (AST and ALT) may be due to microemboli in the vessels of the liver, causing ischemia.
- Low platelet count (must be less than 100,000/mm^3) results when the platelets are entrapped at the intra-arterial lesions.

The result of this syndrome is ischemia and tissue damage. The client may also show signs of hypoglycemia. A blood sugar less than 40 mg/dL is often associated with maternal mortality.

Medical–Surgical Management

Medical

The goals of treatment are to lower blood pressure, prevent convulsions, and deliver a healthy baby.

A client with mild preeclampsia may be allowed to stay home but is advised to stay in bed, lying on either side. This increases renal and placental blood flow. The client generally feels well, so education is very important to improve compliance with the plan of care.

Laboratory tests may include: hematocrit, platelet count, electrolytes, liver function (AST and ALT), es-

CLIENT TEACHING

Home Management of Mild Preeclampsia

- Bed rest is essential.
- Lie on either side but not on the back.
- Reduce anxiety.
- Take medications as prescribed.
- Eat a high-protein, moderate-sodium diet.
- Keep all prenatal appointments (may be 2/week).
- Report immediately: headache, visual disturbances, edema of face or hands, severe nausea and vomiting, and epigastric pain.

triol level, 24-hour urine for protein and creatinine, and serum creatinine.

Surgical

When the mother's condition continues to deteriorate or the environment within the uterus becomes harmful to fetal well-being, a cesarean birth may be necessary.

Pharmacological

Magnesium sulfate (MgSO$_4$) is a CNS depressant that decreases the possibility of convulsions. It also relaxes smooth muscles and may decrease blood pressure to some degree. MgSO$_4$ is usually given intravenously for greater accuracy of dosage, but may be given intramuscularly by Z-track. It is excreted by the kidneys and may reach a toxic level if the client has impaired renal function. An indwelling catheter is generally inserted to accurately measure output.

Calcium gluconate, the antidote for MgSO$_4$, must be kept in a syringe at the bedside ready to be given should signs of magnesium toxicity be noted. MgSO$_4$ is usually given for 24 to 48 hours after delivery to ensure that convulsions do not occur.

An antihypertensive drug may be given. Hydralazine (Apresoline) is the drug of choice except for

PROFESSIONAL TIP

Magnesium Sulfate Administration

- Respirations must be at least 12 to 14/minute.
- Deep tendon reflexes must be kept at normal response.
- Urine output must be at least 30 cc/hr.
- Serum magnesium level must be monitored (therapeutic level 4.0 to 8.0 mEq/dL).

clients with cardiac dysfunctions. They are given labetalol hydrochloride (Normodyne, Trandate).

A sedative such as phenobarbital or diazepam (Valium) may be given to help the client rest quietly.

Oxytocin may be given to induce labor. It may be given along with magnesium sulfate.

Diet

A well-balanced, high-protein, moderate-sodium diet should be provided. Excessively salty foods should not be eaten, but sodium restriction is no longer recommended. If the client is nauseated or there are signs of impending convulsions, the diet is withheld.

Activity

Bed rest, lying preferably on the left side but not on the back, must be complete.

▶ NURSING PROCESS

▶ Assessment

▶ Subjective Data

The client should be asked about headache, visual disturbances, epigastric pain, swelling of hands and face, nausea, and dyspnea.

▶ Objective Data

Vital signs and weight must be checked and compared to previous figures, and urine checked for protein. Edema may be found in the face, hands, sacral area, lower extremities, or abdomen. Laboratory reports of electrolytes, platelet count, liver enzymes, and hematocrit should be checked, and I & O monitored.

Nursing diagnoses for a client with PIH may include the following:

Nursing Diagnoses	Planning/Goals	Nursing Interventions
▶ *Family Processes, Altered, related to illness and bed rest or hospitalization of mother*	The family will work together to maintain family functioning.	Involve client and family in decisions when possible. Encourage client and family to verbalize feelings about situation. Encourage family to visit client as client's condition allows. Assist client and family to plan how to deal with situation. Help client and family identify sources of support.
▶ *Knowledge Deficit, related to lack of information about PIH, its treatment, and implications for mother and baby*	The client will verbalize an understanding of PIH, its treatment, and implications for herself and her baby.	Discuss PIH and implications with client. Explain the purpose and importance of each aspect of the plan of care. Encourage client to express feelings about her situation.
▶ *Fluid Volume Deficit, related to shift in fluids from intravascular to interstitial*	The client will maintain intravascular fluid volume.	Assess BP every 1 to 4 hours. Weigh daily. Maintain client on bed rest, lying on side, especially the left side. Assess for edema. Accurately record I & O. Test urine for protein as ordered. Monitor laboratory test results.

Evaluation Each goal must be evaluated to determine how it has been met by the client.

CHRONIC MEDICAL PROBLEMS

Conditions in this group include diabetes mellitus, chronic hypertension, heart disease, and maternal phenylketonuria.

DIABETES MELLITUS

Diabetic clients who wish to become pregnant should have their diabetes well under control before conception.

Gestational diabetes mellitus (GDM) is an abnormal glucose metabolism that appears only during pregnancy. Many women with GDM will have diabetes later in life. Whether the mother has chronic diabetes or GDM, the effects during pregnancy are the same.

Pregnancy and Carbohydrate Metabolism

Insulin production is increased in early pregnancy due to the stimulation of the mother's pancreas by the increased levels of estrogen, progesterone, and other hormones. The tissue response to insulin is also increased along with increased storage of glycogen in the liver and muscles. An increased resistance to insulin develops in the last half of pregnancy due to hPL (an insulin antagonist), prolactin, and elevated levels of cortisol and placental enzymes called insulinases, which destroy insulin. This diabetogenic effect of pregnancy occurs after about 20 weeks' gestation. The result is a catabolic state after a meal is absorbed and also during the night. Fat, at this time, is more readily metabolized, and ketones may be found in the mother's urine. Glucose from the mother provides the growing fetus with energy, thus putting stress on the balance of glucose production and utilization. Diabetes already present is more difficult to control. In a case where the pancreas has little insulin reserve, gestational diabetes occurs.

Effects of Pregnancy on Diabetes

The insulin requirements change throughout pregnancy. The need for insulin may decrease during the first trimester. The risk of hypoglycemia or hyperinsulinemia are increased if nausea and vomiting are present. Placental maturation and the increasing production of hPL cause the insulin requirements to rise during the second trimester, and they may even be 4 times higher by the end of pregnancy. After the placenta is passed, removing the source of hPL, there is generally an immediate decrease in the amount of insulin required.

There is a physiological decrease in the renal threshold for glucose. The risk of ketoacidosis is greater during pregnancy, as is an acceleration of vascular disease.

Effects of Diabetes on Pregnancy

Pregnancy in a diabetic client has a higher risk of complications than for a nondiabetic client. If vascular changes already exist, the chance for PIH is greater.

Hydramnios, an excessive amount of amniotic fluid, may occur. This may lead to preterm labor or premature rupture of the membranes.

Hyperglycemia can result in ketoacidosis caused by increased fat metabolism. Often, ketoacidosis develops slowly, but can result in maternal and fetal death if untreated. Maternal complications are directly related to the degree of blood glucose control.

Effects on the Fetus/Neonate

Macrosomia, excessive fetal growth, results from maternal hyperglycemia. The hyperglycemia stimulates fetal insulin production to utilize the available glucose. After birth, there is no more maternal glucose, but the fetal pancreas continues to produce a high level of insulin. In 2 to 4 hours the neonate is hypo-

glycemic. Fetal insulin production gradually decreases to an appropriate level.

Intrauterine growth retardation (IUGR) may result when the mother has vascular changes. Vascular changes also occur in the placenta. This decreases perfusion of the placenta and the fetus does not receive adequate amounts of nutrients.

A high fetal insulin level inhibits the production of surfactant in the lungs, making the possibility of respiratory distress syndrome very high. The decreased ability of maternal glycosylated hemoglobin (hemoglobin with glucose attached) to release oxygen causes the fetus to have polycythemia (excessive number of red blood cells). The polycythemia is a direct cause of hyperbilirubinemia since the immature liver is unable to metabolize the increased amount of bilirubin.

Congenital anomalies are several times higher in diabetic pregnancies and may be due to hyperglycemia in early pregnancy. Many anomalies involve the heart, central nervous system, and skeletal system.

Medical–Surgical Management

Medical

The goals of care are to maintain **euglycemia** (normal blood glucose level) between 70 mg/dL and 120 mg/dL, and to have a healthy mother and baby. The client is usually followed by both her endocrinologist and obstetrician.

Clients are taught to monitor their blood glucose level and give themselves insulin according to a sliding scale. For clients with GDM, this may be very difficult since diabetes is new to them.

Fetal status is evaluated throughout the pregnancy. AFP screening is performed because diabetic pregnancies have an increased risk of fetal neural tube defects. Gestational age is established by ultrasound about 18 weeks' gestation and repeated every 4 to 6 weeks to monitor fetal growth and assess for congenital abnormalities. The mother monitors fetal activity daily beginning about 28 weeks' gestation. An NST is often scheduled weekly beginning also about 28 weeks. A CST may be performed about 32 weeks, and may be scheduled weekly until a positive result occurs, indicating that the fetus is having trouble handling the contractions.

Many clients with diabetes are hospitalized several times during the pregnancy. The timing of birth is based mainly on fetal well-being but should never be past 40 weeks' gestation. The L/S ratio and presence of Pg in the amniotic fluid is usually checked about 38 weeks or earlier if an NST is nonreactive.

Surgical

If fetal well-being is deteriorating, a cesarean birth is often performed.

Pharmacological

Humalin is generally used, as it is unlikely to cause an allergic reaction. Insulin is given, most commonly, by multiple injections. This may be scheduled twice a day or 4 to 6 times a day after a blood glucose check. Oral hypoglycemics should be discontinued, with the physician's knowledge, when the client plans to become pregnant, or immediately when she becomes pregnant.

Diet

Pregnant women should increase their caloric intake about 300 kcal/day (35 to 40 kcal/Kg/day of ideal weight is recommended). Total kilocalories for the day should be divided among three meals and three snacks. The bedtime snack, eaten as late as possible, should have complex carbohydrates and protein to prevent hypoglycemia during the night. There should be no more than 10 hours between the bedtime snack and breakfast. A dietician should assist the pregnant diabetic client with meal plans based on food preferences, lifestyle, and culture.

Activity

Activity should be maintained throughout pregnancy unless contraindicated by complications. Activity level is taken into account when the diet and insulin prescribed are determined.

▶ NURSING PROCESS

▶ Assessment

▶ Subjective Data

Questions should be asked regarding a family history of diabetes, congenital abnormalities, neonatal deaths, or unexplained stillbirths. At each prenatal visit, questions should be asked about diet, activity, and medication compliance. After 28 weeks, maternal evaluation of fetal activity should be determined.

▶ Objective Data

The nurse should check urine for sugar, and also measure vital signs and weight. NST results and results of laboratory tests must be evaluated. Signs of infection should be noted.

Nursing diagnoses for a client with diabetes during pregnancy may include the following:

Nursing Diagnoses	Planning/Goals	Nursing Interventions
▶ *Knowledge Deficit, related to disease process of diabetes, control of diabetes, and implications for pregnancy*	The client will verbalize an understanding of the disease process of diabetes, control of diabetes, and implications for the pregnancy.	Present to or review with the client the pathophysiology of diabetes. Clarify client misconceptions. Teach how to monitor blood glucose level, the desired range, and importance of good control. Teach self-administration of insulin (if applicable) to client and significant other. Review effects of diabetes on client and fetus. Teach danger signs and whom to notify. Refer to diabetic support group in the community.
▶ *Injury, Risk for, Fetus, related to decreased uteroplacental functioning*	The client will verbalize an understanding of the various antepartal tests and what to expect during the procedures.	Teach client the possible effects of poor uteroplacental functioning. Explain purpose of periodic ultrasound, fetal activity record, weekly NST, amniocenteses for L/S ratio and Pg level, and biophysical profile.
▶ *Noncompliance, related to need for close monitoring and extra prenatal visits*	The client will perform blood glucose testing on schedule and attend all scheduled prenatal visits.	Review the importance of maintaining euglycemia. Assist client in making a chart on which to record results of blood glucose testing. Review importance of attending all scheduled prenatal visits. Work to schedule prenatal visits when most convenient for the client.

Evaluation Each goal must be evaluated to determine how it has been met by the client.

CHRONIC HYPERTENSION

A BP 140/90 or higher before pregnancy or before the 20th week of gestation that lasts longer than 6 weeks after delivery is termed chronic hypertension. A diastolic pressure of more than 80 mm Hg in the second trimester may indicate chronic hypertension.

A client with untreated or poorly controlled hypertension may show signs of hypertensive vascular disease such as arteriosclerosis and retinal hemorrhage.

Renal disease may be present. The placenta may have infarcts, and placenta abruptio may occur.

Effects on the Fetus/Neonate

A placenta with infarcts has reduced perfusion. This may cause IUGR and fetal hypoxia.

PIH Superimposed on Chronic Hypertension

Clients who have moderate to severe chronic hypertension are most at risk to develop PIH. In these women PIH develops rapidly and moves to a crisis state faster than in women without chronic hypertension. More stillbirths, abruptio placenta, and severe renal failure are found in clients with chronic hypertension. Any of the classic signs indicate PIH. These clients are hospitalized for medical management and nursing care.

Medical–Surgical Management

Medical

The goals of care are to prevent development of preeclampsia and to ensure a healthy fetus. Prenatal visits are generally scheduled every 2 weeks. An ultrasound is performed early to establish, or verify, the EDB. Around 22 and 32 weeks' gestation, an ultrasound checks for IUGR. If renal disease is suspected, creatinine clearance is determined early and repeated every 2 months.

Pharmacological

Antihypertensive medication, such as methyldopa (Aldomet), is continued throughout the pregnancy.

Diet

A well-balanced diet providing 1.5 g/Kg/day of protein is recommended. Salt intake should remain as it was before pregnancy.

Activity

Daily rest periods, with the client preferably lying on her left side (never on the back), are important to maintain adequate perfusion to the placenta and relieve dependent edema.

◗ NURSING PROCESS

◗ Assessment

◗ Subjective Data

Most clients have no symptoms of hypertension unless it becomes severe. Then headaches or visual disturbances may occur.

◗ Objective Data

Blood pressure will be 140/90 or higher.

Nursing diagnoses for a pregnant client with chronic hypertension may include the following:

Nursing Diagnoses	Planning/Goals	Nursing Interventions
◗ *Injury, High Risk for, Fetus, related to placental infarcts and poor placental perfusion*	The client will verbalize an understanding of possible placental changes leading to fetal injury and interventions to prevent this.	Teach client the possible placental changes related to hypertension. Assist client to plan for rest periods throughout the day. Administer antihypertensive medications as ordered.
◗ *Knowledge Deficit related to disease process and effects on pregnancy*	The client will verbalize an understanding of the disease process and effects on pregnancy.	Provide the client with information about the disease process and how pregnancy may be affected. Allow opportunity for client to ask questions.

Evaluation Each goal must be evaluated to determine how it has been met by the client.

HEART DISEASE

The normal physiological increase in blood volume that peaks about 28 to 32 weeks' gestation, and the increased cardiac output and heart rate, may cause problems in the client with heart disease. The heart compensates at first by tachycardia, and ventricular dilation and hypertrophy. When these mechanisms fail, the heart is no longer able to compensate and congestive heart failure occurs.

The results of having had rheumatic fever often restrict cardiac output and cause pulmonary congestion. The effects of congenital heart disease on pregnancy depend on the specific defect. Hypertension may cause cardiac insufficiency.

Effects on the Fetus/Neonate

IUGR and hypoxia may occur.

Medical–Surgical Management

Medical

Many clients are cared for by both their cardiologist and obstetrician. Early diagnosis and ongoing management is assessed by the use of chest x-rays, auscultation of heart sounds, ECG, echocardiogram, and sometimes cardiac catheterization. Prenatal care appointments may be increased to 2 or 3 a week between 28 and 32 weeks' gestation, when blood volume is highest. Sometimes hospitalization is necessary.

Pharmacological

Antibiotics are often used as a prophylaxis for all pregnant women with heart disease. Heparin may be used if coagulation problems develop, as heparin does not cross the placenta. Thiazide diuretics and furosemide (Lasix) may be used for congestive heart failure.

Diet

The diet should be high in iron and protein but low in sodium. Adequate kilocalories for normal weight gain should be provided.

Activity

Physical activity may be restricted depending on the client's symptoms. Eight to 10 hours of sleep and frequent rest periods throughout the day are important. The side-lying position is best to prevent compression of the inferior vena cava.

▶ NURSING PROCESS

▶ Assessment

▶ Subjective Data

Questions should be asked about activity level, amount of rest, increasing fatigue with activity, dyspnea, palpitations, cough, and anxiety. The nurse should also inquire about the availability of household help and the support system, to ascertain the client's ability to rest and relax.

▶ Objective Data

These data should include weight gain (fluid retention), edema, vital signs, signs of infection, anemia, heart murmurs, or crackles heard when the lungs are auscultated.

Nursing diagnoses for a pregnant client with heart disease may include the following:

Nursing Diagnoses	Planning/Goals	Nursing Interventions
▶ *Gas Exchange, Impaired, High Risk for, related to pulmonary edema*	The client will maintain adequate gas exchange.	Monitor and accurately record I & O. Assess vital signs frequently. Administer medications as ordered.
▶ *Activity Intolerance related to generalized decreased perfusion*	The client will be able to tolerate some activity.	Assess activity tolerance frequently. Promote activity level established by the physician. Discuss activity limitations and the need for sleep and rest periods.
▶ *Fear related to effects of maternal cardiac condition on fetal well-being*	The client will express her fears about fetal well-being.	Provide information on how fetal well-being may be affected by maternal cardiac condition. Listen to the client express her fears about fetal well-being.

Evaluation Each goal must be evaluated to determine how it has been met by the client.

MATERNAL PHENYLKETONURIA

Phenylketonuria (PKU) is an inborn error of metabolism in which there is a deficiency of the enzyme necessary to metabolize the amino acid phenylalanine. It is genetically inherited by a recessive gene. The accumulation of this amino acid and its metabolites leads to irreversible brain damage.

Since 1967 all newborns in the United States have had a screening blood test for PKU. The infants diagnosed with PKU were put on a phenylalanine-free diet. For years it was thought that the child treated with a phenylalanine-free diet outgrew the problem by about age 9. It is now known that the modified diet should be continued. When a woman with PKU keeps her phenylalanine level less than 2.0 mg/dL while pregnant, the outcome of pregnancy is better (Acosta & Wright, 1992).

Effects on the Fetus/Neonate

A poorly regulated maternal phenylalanine level causes an increase in the incidence of IUGR, mental retardation, microcephaly, and heart defects.

Medical–Surgical Management

Medical

The mother's blood phenylalanine level should be checked every 2 to 4 weeks during the first half of pregnancy. It may be checked every week in the last half of pregnancy. Iron and zinc levels are also checked.

Diet

A very expensive modified protein supplement can be used before and during pregnancy. Fruits, vegetables, fats, and some low-protein cereals make up the rest of the diet.

INFECTIONS

Any infection is a risk factor during pregnancy and should be diagnosed and treated promptly. Untreated infections may cause abortion, congenital anomalies, fetal infections, IUGR, preterm labor, mental retardation, or death.

TORCH GROUP

The TORCH group of infections include **to**xoplasmosis, **r**ubella, **c**ytomegalovirus, and **h**erpesvirus type 2.

TOXOPLASMOSIS

Toxoplasmosis is caused by the protozoan *Toxoplasma gondii*. This disease goes almost unnoticed by adults because the symptoms are mild, vague, and flu-like. The organism may be picked up by eating raw or partially cooked meat or from the feces of an infected cat. Maternal toxoplasmosis prior to pregnancy seems to offer protection against fetal infection.

Effects on the Fetus/Neonate

There is an increased incidence of abortion, preterm birth, stillbirth, and neonatal death if the mother contracts toxoplasmosis when she is pregnant. Damage to the fetus is generally more severe if the disease is acquired before 20 weeks' gestation. The neonate may have microcephaly, hydrocephaly, and convulsions. Many infants die soon after birth. Those who survive may be blind, deaf, or severely retarded.

Medical–Surgical Management

Medical

The goals are to identify the pregnant client at risk and treat the disease promptly when diagnosed. The incubation period is 10 days.

Pharmacological

The client may be treated with sulfadiazine (Microsulfon) or pyrimethamine (Daraprim).

Diet

No raw or partially cooked meats should be eaten. Fruits and vegetables should be washed before they are eaten.

Activity

Contact with a cat litter box should be avoided. Gloves should be worn when gardening. The cat's favorite place in the garden should be avoided.

▶ NURSING PROCESS

▶ Assessment

▶ Subjective Data

The nurse should ask about the presence of a cat in the home, and ask who cleans the litter box. The client may have no symptoms or may have malaise and/or myalgia.

▶ Objective Data

A rash may be evident as well as splenomegaly and enlarged cervical lymph nodes.

Nursing diagnoses for a pregnant client with toxoplasmosis may include the following:

Nursing Diagnoses	Planning/Goals	Nursing Interventions
▶ *Knowledge Deficit related to lack of knowledge about toxoplasmosis disease process*	The client will verbalize an understanding of toxoplasmosis disease process.	Provide information about toxoplasmosis, incubation period, how acquired, and ways to prevent it. Allow time for client to ask questions. Clarify client's misconceptions.
▶ *Grieving, Anticipatory, related to effects of toxoplasmosis on fetus/neonate*	The client will express feelings about possible effects on fetus/neonate.	Encourage client to discuss feelings about possible effects of toxoplasmosis on her fetus. Provide a private place for client and family to discuss the situation.

Evaluation Each goal must be evaluated to determine how it has been met by the client.

RUBELLA

Rubella, German measles, and three-day measles are all names for the same disease. After an incubation period of 14 to 21 days, a maculopapular rash appears and vanishes in 3 days. Rubella is highly contagious and is spread by airborne droplets.

Effects on the Fetus/Neonate

The earlier in pregnancy the infection occurs, the more severe the fetal effects. Congenital rubella syndrome occurs in many of the infections that occur before 8 weeks' gestation. It is characterized by cataracts, deafness, and patent ductus arteriosus. The infant may also have IUGR, mental retardation, and hyperbilirubinemia. Sometimes a petechial rash may be seen. These infants are infectious and may shed the virus for months.

Medical–Surgical Management

Medical

Prevention is the best cure. The prenatal laboratory screening includes the hemagglutination inhibition (HAI). A titer of 1:16 or higher signifies immunity, while a titer of less than 1:8 signifies a susceptibility to rubella. The client who is susceptible should avoid exposure to rubella while pregnant.

A pregnant woman who becomes infected with rubella during the first trimester may be counseled for a therapeutic abortion.

Pharmacological

All children should be immunized with the live attenuated vaccine by age 1. Susceptible pregnant women should be immunized very soon after delivery, and avoid becoming pregnant for 3 months following immunization to avoid the chance of infecting a fetus.

▶ NURSING PROCESS

▶ Assessment

▶ Subjective Data

There may be no symptoms or the client may describe muscle aches and joint pain.

▶ Objective Data

Temperature may be slightly elevated, and a maculopapular rash and lymphadenopathy may be present.

Nursing diagnoses for a pregnant client with rubella may include the following:

Nursing Diagnoses	Planning/Goals	Nursing Interventions
▶ *Health Maintenance, Altered, related to lack of knowledge about her need for rubella immunization before becoming pregnant*	The client will receive rubella vaccine soon after delivery.	Provide information about the implications of rubella when the HAI results are known. Provide information about rubella immunization. Answer client questions and clarify any misunderstandings.
▶ *Family Processes, Altered, related to the probability of fetal anomalies caused by maternal rubella*	The client and family will verbalize understanding of the probability of fetal anomalies and make a decision about continuing the pregnancy.	Discuss with client and family the probability and types of fetal anomalies that generally occur with maternal rubella. Provide a private place for client and family to discuss the situation. Answer questions and clarify misconceptions.

Evaluation Each goal must be evaluated to determine how it has been met by the client.

CYTOMEGALOVIRUS

Cytomegalovirus (CMV) is a member of the herpesvirus group. More than half of all adults have antibodies for CMV. CMV is found in saliva, breast milk, cervical mucous, urine, and semen. It spreads by close contact. It is asymptomatic in adults and children but can affect the fetus in utero or during delivery.

Effects on the Fetus/Neonate

The fetus may have extensive damage leading to fetal death. However, the fetus may survive with hydrocephaly, microcephaly, mental retardation, cerebral palsy, or with no noticeable damage.

An infected newborn is usually small for gestational age (SGA). Mental retardation, auditory deficits, or learning disabilities may not be noticed right away.

Medical–Surgical Management

Medical

Diagnosis is made when CMV is found in the maternal urine and an elevated IgM level with CMV antibodies identified.

There is no treatment for the mother or neonate.

HERPES GENITALIS (HERPES SIMPLEX VIRUS TYPE 2)

Herpes simplex virus type 2 (HSV-2) causes painful, vesicular genital lesions. The lesions appear within a few hours to 20 days after exposure. The primary episode is the most severe. Women who have their first infection close to the time of delivery have a greater chance of neonatal infection. After the membranes rupture, the virus ascends from active lesions to the fetus, or the fetus comes in contact with the lesions during a vaginal delivery. HSV-2 is not found in breast milk, so the mother may breast-feed.

Effects on the Fetus/Neonate

When there is an active HSV-2 infection in the first trimester, about one-half will end in spontaneous abortion or stillbirth. Most infected infants have no symptoms at birth. Symptoms of poor feeding, jaundice, and seizures develop after a 2- to 12-day incubation period. Many of these infants will also have the vesicular lesions.

Medical–Surgical Management

Medical

Diagnosis is made by culturing active lesions. Treatment is mainly to relieve pain. When no lesions are visible at the time of delivery, a vaginal birth is acceptable. Pregnancy is one of many causes of recurrence. There is no known cure.

Surgical

When active lesions are visible at the time of delivery, a cesarean birth is best to prevent fetal contact with the lesions (virus).

Pharmacological

Acyclovir (Zovirax) reduces healing time and the time the lesions contain the live virus. So far, studies have not shown an increased risk of birth defects for infants born to clients given Zovirax during pregnancy (*Nursing98 Drug Handbook,* 1998).

Cleansing with povidone-iodine (Betadine) may help prevent a secondary infection. Burrow's solution may relieve discomfort.

▶ NURSING PROCESS

▶ Assessment

▶ Subjective Data

The nurse should ask whether the client or her partner have ever had a herpes infection. Client may describe pain and discomfort from the lesions if she has a herpes infection.

▶ Objective Data

Lesions may be seen when infection is active. A cervical culture may indicate presence or absence of the virus.

Nursing diagnoses for the pregnant client with HSV-2 infection may include the following:

Nursing Diagnoses	Planning/Goals	Nursing Interventions
▶ *Pain related to local, open vulvar lesions*	The client will describe a decrease in pain after treatment is begun.	Administer medications as ordered. Suggest a sitz bath several times a day followed by air-drying of the vulva. Suggest wearing cotton underwear.
▶ *Sexuality Patterns, Altered, High Risk for, related to unwillingness to engage in sexual intercourse*	The client will maintain sexuality patterns.	Provide client with information about disease process, and the method of transmission. Refer client to community resources. Encourage client to engage in forms of sexual expression that do not involve genital contact.
▶ *Individual Coping, Ineffective, related to depression about risk to fetus if herpes lesions are present at birth*	The client will verbalize an understanding about how decision is made regarding the type of delivery when herpes lesions are present.	Provide client with information about the factors relative to type of delivery performed. Encourage client to have appropriate cultures run as recommended by her health care provider. Encourage client to report any changes that may indicate a recurrence of lesions.

Evaluation Each goal must be evaluated to determine how it has been met by the client.

HIV/AIDS

Weight gain or even maintenance of weight during pregnancy is a challenge for an HIV-infected client. Counseling should be provided regarding optimum nutrition, exercise, rest, and sleep.

Pregnancy is considered to be a somewhat immunosuppressive state, and may theoretically speed up the process of going from being HIV positive to an AIDS diagnosis.

Effects on the Fetus/Neonate

HIV may be transmitted to the fetus through the placenta, at the time of birth when exposed to maternal blood and vaginal secretions, or through breast milk. Infants often have a positive antibody titer for as long as 15 months after birth due to the transfer of maternal antibodies. Those infants who are not infected with HIV will seroconvert to a negative antibody titer.

Medical–Surgical Management

Medical

There is no cure for HIV or AIDS. Routine prenatal testing should be expanded to include a CD 4 lympho-cyte count and serologic testing for changes indicating that AIDS is progressing. NST and ultrasound are performed at 32 weeks' gestation. NST is continued weekly to monitor fetal status, and ultrasound is performed every few weeks depending on what is seen.

Diet

Nutritional counseling and support regarding food handling, food preparation, and diet choices is often necessary.

▶ NURSING PROCESS

▶ Assessment

▶ Subjective Data

The client may be asymptomatic or may describe having fatigue, malaise, loss of appetite, or diarrhea.

▶ Objective Data

Signs of anemia, cell-mediated immunodeficiency, progressive weight loss, lymphadenopathy, and neurologic dysfunction may be present. Purplish lesions may also be noted during assessment.

Nursing diagnoses for a pregnant client who has HIV/AIDS may include the following:

Nursing Diagnoses	Planning/Goals	Nursing Interventions
▶ *Infection, High Risk for, related to altered immune status*	The client will not develop infections during pregnancy.	Use Standard Precautions at all times. Monitor client for signs of infection (fever, cough, sore throat). Teach client to report changes that may indicate infection.
▶ *Fear, related to outcome of pregnancy and disease*	The client will verbalize fears about her pregnancy and HIV/AIDS.	Discuss HIV/AIDS disease process and how it can affect pregnancy. Provide opportunities for client to ask questions and clarify misconceptions. Assess client's support system. Refer client to community resources.
▶ *Nutrition, Altered, Less Than Body Requirements, related to lack of appetite*	The client will maintain weight or gain weight.	Monitor client's weight. Obtain 24-hour diet recall from client. Provide information about nutritional needs. Assist client in planning a high-protein, high-calorie diet.

Evaluation Each goal must be evaluated to determine how it has been met by the client.

OTHER INFECTIONS

Maternal infections may result in spontaneous abortion, a preterm infant, or an infected infant. Table 48-4 provides a summary of other infections affecting pregnancy. Most of these are covered in detail in Chapter 35 and Chapter 36.

HEMOLYTIC DISEASES

There are two types of hemolytic diseases: Rh incompatibility and ABO incompatibility. Rh incompatibility can be very devastating to the fetus, but it can be prevented. ABO incompatibility is naturally occurring and much less severe, but cannot be prevented.

Table 48-4 SELECTED INFECTIONS AND PREGNANCY

INFECTION	TREATMENT	MATERNAL EFFECTS	FETAL EFFECTS
Sexually Transmitted			
Syphilis	penicillin G benzathin (Bicillin L-A) or doxycycline (Vibramycin). Sexual partner should also be treated.	Chancre, slight fever, malaise. Progresses through secondary and tertiary stages if untreated.	Spontaneous abortion, stillbirth, congenital syphilis, sniffling, peeling of soles and palms.
Gonorrhea	ceftriaxone (Rocephin) plus erythromycin (Erythrocin Lactobionate). Partners must be treated.	Often no symptoms. May have purulent vaginal discharge, dysuria, or urinary frequency.	Ophthalmia neonatorum.
Chlamydia	erythromycin ethyl succinate (ABO-Erythro-ES).	Often no symptoms. May have purulent or thin vaginal discharge, burning on urination, preterm labor.	Conjunctivitis, chlamydial pneumonia, fetal death.
Condylomata acuminata (venereal warts)	Cryosurgery, laser surgery, electrocautery, or trichloro-acetic acid.	Soft, grayish, raised lesions.	Laryngeal papillomatosis if infection is present at birth.
Hepatitis B (HBV)	Supportive. Vaccine available.	Often no symptoms.	Most become carriers.
Vaginal Infections			
Monilia	miconazole (Monistat), clotrimazole (Gyne-Lotrimin).	Thick, white, cheesy discharge. Itching, dysuria.	Thrush.
Trichomoniasis	clotrimazole (Gyne-Lotrimin) in early pregnancy, metronida-zole (Flagyl).	Foamy, green-gray discharge, prutitis.	
Urinary Tract Infection			
Cystitis	Oral sulfonamides in early pregnancy, nitrofurantoin (Furadantin) in late pregnancy.	Dysuria, urgency, low-grade fever. If not treated, may result in acute pyelonephritis.	Hyperbilirubinemia if sulfonamides taken in last few weeks of pregnancy.

RH INCOMPATIBILITY

Rh incompatibility can happen only when the mother is Rh negative and the fetus is Rh positive. That is, the mother does not have the Rh factor and the fetus does have the Rh factor. In this case, the father must be Rh positive for the fetus to be Rh positive. If the father is Rh negative, there is no problem because the fetus will also be Rh negative.

The placenta keeps the mother's blood and the fetus's blood separated. In cases of ectopic pregnancy, abortion, infection of the placenta, abruptio placenta, birth, or at the time of placental separation, small tears may occur in the placenta and fetal blood may enter maternal circulation. The mother is then sensitized by the fetal Rh positive blood. She may also be sensitized by having a transfusion of Rh positive blood, even the smallest amount.

Fetal (Rh positive) blood in maternal (Rh negative) circulation stimulates maternal production of Rh antibodies. The Rh antibodies, like many other antibodies, pass through the placenta and destroy fetal red blood cells (Figure 48-13). Since this usually occurs at the time of birth, the first infant is usually not affected.

Effects on the Fetus/Neonate

If a tear occurred and there was no treatment, the next Rh positive fetus will have red blood cells destroyed by the maternal Rh antibodies. This causes anemia which in turn causes fetal edema (hydrops fetalis).

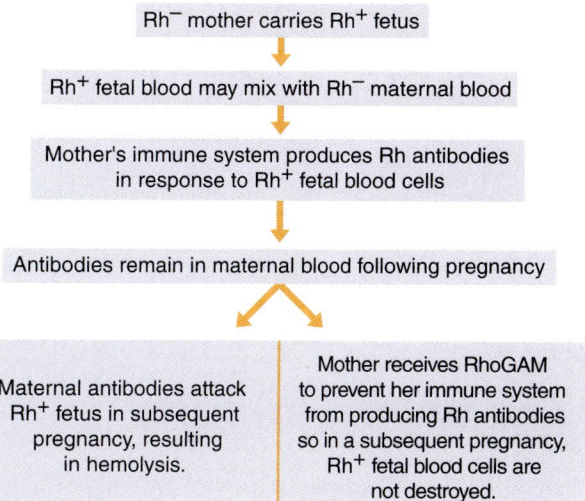

Figure 48-13 Rh Sensitization and Prevention

The next step is congestive heart failure and severe jaundice. Severe jaundice can cause neurologic damage called **kernicterus**. This entire syndrome, the most severe of the two hemolytic diseases of the newborn, is called erythroblastosis fetalis.

Medical–Surgical Management

Medical

One of the screening tests performed at the first prenatal visit determines the mother's Rh factor. When the mother is found to be Rh negative and the father is Rh positive or unknown, additional tests are run. An indirect Coombs' test detects Rh antibodies in maternal serum. The Rh antibody titer monitors what is happening when an Rh negative woman is carrying an Rh positive fetus. A rising titer may indicate the need for immediate intervention.

Ultrasound is performed about 15 weeks to determine gestational age. It is repeated several times throughout the pregnancy to measure fetal growth and assess fetal heart size and for hydramnios.

Amniocentesis may also be performed several times to determine the bilirubin (product of red blood cell breakdown) level and lung maturity. A fetal intrauterine blood transfusion may be indicated to maintain the fetus in the uterus until the lungs are more mature. The fetus is given Rh negative erythrocytes to replace those destroyed by the Rh positive antibodies. The erythrocytes are put into the peritoneal cavity where they are absorbed. Rh positive antibodies will not harm the Rh negative blood given to the fetus.

Pharmacological

Rh immune globulin (RhoGAM) is given to an Rh negative mother who is not sensitized (has a negative indirect Coombs' and antibody titer) and whose Rh positive infant has no antibodies on the infant's RBCs (negative direct Coombs'). RhoGAM must be administered within 72 hours of the infant's birth. It prevents the mother's body from making the Rh antibodies by providing temporary passive immunity.

It is recommended that RhoGAM be given at 28 weeks' gestation and after the delivery. RhoGAM is also given to an Rh negative woman after an abortion (spontaneous or induced), an ectopic pregnancy, and amniocentesis. It is never given to an Rh positive woman.

ABO INCOMPATIBILITY

In ABO incompatibility, the way in which a tear in the placenta may occur and fetal and maternal blood mix is the same as for Rh incompatibility. In this situation the problem occurs when maternal blood enters fetal circulation. Possible combinations for ABO in-

Table 48-5 POSSIBLE COMBINATIONS FOR ABO INCOMPATIBILITY

MOTHER	FETUS
A	B
B	A
O	A, B, AB

compatibility are given in Table 48-5. The most common type of ABO incompatibility occurs when the mother is type O and the fetus is either type A, B, or AB. The mother's plasma naturally contains anti-A and anti-B antibodies. These antibodies have a weaker hemolytic effect than Rh antibodies and they only affect mature RBCs. The number of antibodies is limited to the amount of maternal blood that entered fetal circulation. There is not a continuous supply of antibodies. Since ABO incompatibility is naturally occurring, it may affect the fetus of the first pregnancy. The affected newborn will have a positive direct Coombs' and will become jaundiced in the first 3 days of life.

MULTIPLE PREGNANCY

Fundal height greater than expected for the weeks of gestation is often the first clue of a multiple pregnancy. An ultrasound will verify 2 or more fetuses. Two or more heartbeats that differ by 10 beats/minute will be heard. The alpha fetoprotein level may be elevated. The first trimester proceeds much the same as with a single fetus except that maternal blood volume has a greater increase. Some women have more severe nausea and vomiting as well as shortness of breath on exertion, dyspnea, and backache.

As the uterus grows, there is greater pressure on and displacement of the internal organs. Pressure on the ureters favors urinary stasis and possible infection. Digestive problems and constipation may be more disturbing, dependent edema more marked, and varicose veins more prominent. PIH is more frequent than with a single fetus.

Effects on the Fetus/Neonate

Each fetus may have a decreased intrauterine growth rate (low birth weight). There is a greater risk of fetal anomalies, abnormal presentations, and preterm birth. Perinatal mortality is much greater for twins than for a single fetus.

Medical–Surgical Management

Medical

The goals are to promote normal fetal development for all fetuses and to prevent delivery of preterm infants. Prenatal visits are more frequent, and serial ultrasounds assess the growth of each fetus. NST and FBPP testing usually begin about 30 weeks' gestation and are repeated every 3 to 7 days until delivery.

Surgical

The method of birth may not be determined until the mother is in labor. Depending on complications that may occur, a cesarean birth may be required.

Pharmacological

A prenatal vitamin/mineral preparation is doubly important with a multiple pregnancy. An extra calcium supplement and folic acid may be required.

Diet

A well-balanced diet of 4,000 kcal with 135 g of protein is recommended. A weight gain of 40 to 50 pounds is acceptable with 15 to 20 pounds being gained by 20 weeks' gestation.

Activity

Frequent rest periods should be planned during the day. Resting in the side-lying position increases uteroplacental blood flow. The legs and feet should be elevated to reduce edema. Good posture should be maintained and good body mechanics used when lifting or moving objects.

SUBSTANCE ABUSE

Drugs commonly abused include: alcohol, cocaine, crack, marijuana, and heroin. The use of any of these substances is a threat to pregnancy. Substance abusers may not seek prenatal care, or they seek prenatal care very late in pregnancy. Most substance abusers do not voluntarily admit their addiction. These mothers may have an increased rate of PIH, abruptio placenta, poor nutrition, and sexually transmitted diseases. They often use available money for the drug habit instead of food.

Effects on the Fetus/Neonate

Alcohol may result in fetal alcohol syndrome, which manifests as both physical and mental abnormalities. Cocaine/crack increases the risk for IUGR, short body length, small head circumference, preterm birth, irritability, and low Apgar scores (an assessment of infant at 1 and 5 minutes after birth). Marijuana causes fine tremors and irritability. Heroin increases the risk for IUGR, hypoxia, preterm birth, irritability, and meconium aspiration. Irritability and poor consolability may interfere with maternal-infant bonding and attachment and increase the risk of infant abuse and neglect.

Medical–Surgical Management

Medical

When a client is known or discovered to be a substance abuser, a multidisciplinary approach is best to manage the medical, legal, and socioeconomic considerations, and provide a safe labor and delivery. The client may require hospitalization for detoxification. "Cold turkey" withdrawal is not recommended during pregnancy because of possible fetal risks. Urine screening is performed regularly.

▶ NURSING PROCESS

▶ Assessment

▶ Subjective Data

The client should be asked questions about the use of caffeine, tobacco, and over-the-counter drugs, and then about alcohol use and drug use. The client may have altered perceptions, so validation through other sources, if possible, is desirable.

▶ Objective Data

The client should be assessed for irritability, psychomotor problems, poor nutrition, and possible infections.

Nursing diagnoses for a pregnant client who is a substance abuser may include the following:

Nursing Diagnoses	Planning/Goals	Nursing Interventions
▶ *Nutrition Altered, Less than Body Requirements related to inadequate intake of food*	The client will gain appropriate weight during pregnancy.	Refer client to WIC (women, infant, and children) nutrition program. Monitor weight gain. Collect 24-hour diet recall from client. Explain foods client should include and why. Assist the client to plan meals.
▶ *Knowledge Deficit related to not understanding how substance abuse affects the fetus*	The client will verbalize how substance abuse can affect the fetus.	Explain how substance abuse affects the fetus. Allow time for client questions and for clarification of misconceptions.

continued

Nursing Diagnoses	Planning/Goals	Nursing Interventions
▶ *Infection, High Risk for, related to use of dirty needles and syringes*	The client will not have an infection from dirty needles and syringes.	Explain how client may pick up an infection from dirty needles and syringes.
		Refer client to community resources where clean syringes and needles may be available.
		Refer client to drug counseling program.

Evaluation Each goal must be evaluated to determine how it has been met by the client.

PRETERM LABOR

Preterm labor is labor that begins after viability but before 38 weeks' gestation. The causes of preterm labor may be maternal, fetal, or placental. Maternal factors that may cause preterm labor include: PIH, diabetes, heart or renal disease, an incompetent cervix, premature rupture of membranes, and maternal infection. Fetal factors include: fetal infection, multiple pregnancy, and hydramnios. Placental factors are placenta previa and abruptio placenta.

Effects on the Fetus/Neonate

Preterm labor may produce a neonate not able to cope well with extrauterine life.

Medical–Surgical Management

Medical

Preterm labor is confirmed by documented uterine contractions, ruptured membranes, and cervical dilation and effacement. No attempt is made to stop labor if any of the following conditions exist: the cervix dilated 4 cm or more, severe PIH, prolonged rupture of membranes, hemorrhage, abruptio placenta, fetal complications, or fetal death.

Pharmacological

The process of stopping labor with medications is called **tocolysis**. The drugs used in an attempt to stop preterm labor are called *tocolytics*.

Ritodrine hydrochloride (Yutopar) is a beta andrenergic agonist that inhibits contractility of the uterus. Maternal pulse, BP, lung sounds, and fetal heart rate must be closely monitored.

Turbutaline sulfate (Brethine) is also a beta-andrenergic agonist that relaxes the uterine muscle. It is being used more frequently even though the FDA has not approved it for tocolysis.

Magnesium sulfate ($MgSO_4$) has fewer side effects than the beta-andrenergic agonists and is being used more in preterm labor. A loading dose is given and then continued at the lowest rate necessary to maintain a noncontracting uterus (Mandeville & Troiano, 1998). Tocolysis is usually maintained with a maternal serum level of 5 to 8 mg/dL.

▶ NURSING PROCESS

▶ Assessment

▶ Subjective Data

Client may describe having contractions or that "my water broke." The client may also express concern about what is happening.

▶ Objective Data

Contractions may be documented, cervix dilating and effacing, or membranes ruptured. The client may experience tension, restlessness, or vital sign changes.

Nursing diagnoses for a client in preterm labor may include the following:

Nursing Diagnoses	Planning/Goals	Nursing Interventions
▶ *Anxiety, Moderate, related to perception of what is happening and not having time to prepare for labor*	The client will express less anxiety about being in preterm labor.	Explain what is happening to client and all tests and procedures before beginning them.
		Spend time with client so she can express her anxieties and ask questions.
		Keep client informed about how the preterm labor is responding to treatment.
▶ *Knowledge Deficit, related to lack of information about preterm labor causes, determination, and treatment*	The client will verbalize an understanding about preterm labor and treatments.	Explain what preterm labor is, possible/probable causes, and treatment.
		Allow client time to ask questions.
		Clarify any misunderstandings.

continued

Nursing Diagnoses	Planning/Goals	Nursing Interventions
▶ *Fear, related to risk for fetus*	The client will express her fears for fetal welfare.	Encourage client to express fears related to fetal well-being. Keep client informed about fetal status. Encourage family to spend time with client.

Evaluation Each goal must be evaluated to determine how it has been met by the client.

CASE STUDY

Part A: *Mary Jo, age 32, is G 3, P 2, T 1, P 1, A 0, L 2. The children are ages 1½ and 3. Bob, her husband, works 8 to 5. She is 32 weeks' gestation. Her BP has been 104/68 at her prenatal visits. Today her BP is 136/84. She has gained 6½ pounds in the 4 weeks since her last visit. There is edema in both feet.*

Part B: *Two weeks later, Mary Jo's BP is 140/90 and she has gained 4 more pounds. She states that she had to take her rings off because they were too tight. The physician admits her to the hospital with orders for bed rest in side-lying position, MgSO₄ IV drip, and a high-protein diet.*

Part C: *The electronic fetal monitor shows a sustained increase in the baseline fetal heart rate. Mary Jo's deep tendon reflexes are very reactive.*

The following questions will guide your development of a nursing care plan for the case study.

Part A:

1. What other assessments should be made?
2. What advice would you anticipate the physician giving Mary Jo?
3. How can you assist Mary Jo to implement the physician's advice?

Part B:

4. What are the goals for Mary Jo's care?
5. What nursing assessments must now be obtained?
6. What diagnostic tests might be ordered?

Part C:

7. Identify three nursing diagnoses and goals for Mary Jo.
8. Identify nursing interventions for each nursing diagnosis.

SUMMARY

- High-risk factors can often be identified early in prenatal care.
- Continuing prenatal care allows for signs of complications to be identified as early as possible.
- Many procedures and tests are available to assess fetal well-being.
- When bleeding occurs in pregnancy, mothers often feel guilty that they may have done something to cause the bleeding.
- Mothers with chronic medical conditions are often cared for by both the medical physician and the obstetrician during pregnancy.
- Complications of pregnancy add to the emotional and financial stress for the client and family.

Review Questions

1. Judy is a 16-year-old primigravida at 38 weeks whose membranes ruptured spontaneously. Her chart indicates that she was seen by a physician for the first time 2 weeks ago. She is having contractions 10 to 12 minutes apart. Which of the following assessment findings would be indicative of a high-risk pregnancy?

   a. Lack of prenatal care and age
   b. She is not considered high risk
   c. The membranes rupturing spontaneously
   d. The contractions being 10 to 12 minutes apart

2. The maturity of which organ is based on the ratio of lecithin to sphingomyelin?

   a. Placenta
   b. Fetal lungs
   c. Acini glands
   d. Fetal kidneys

3. In planning the care of a client with DIC, the nurse would include which of the following?

   a. Giving coagulants
   b. Turning every 2 hours
   c. Watching for signs of bleeding
   d. Massaging the fundus frequently

4. The nurse appropriately documented that client teaching for a client with PIH included which of the following?

   a. The date of her next visit
   b. The importance of pushing fluids throughout the day
   c. Review of the basic food groups and recommended daily allowances
   d. The importance of resting on her side in a quiet, stress-free environment

5. A pregnant client is receiving magnesium sulfate. The nurse observes that the client's respirations are 8 and her patellar reflexes have decreased. The nurse should recognize that these observations should be:

   a. considered to be the desired result.
   b. recorded and monitored to see if they continue.
   c. brought to the attention of the charge nurse immediately.
   d. considered as an indication that a higher dose of medication is needed.

6. The diabetic woman who becomes pregnant experiences complications in terms of her own control and in terms of fetal welfare. What accounts for both areas of difficulty?

   a. Uterus
   b. Pancreas
   c. Placenta
   d. Vascular system

7. After delivery of the diabetic mother, the baby is usually placed in the neonatal intensive care unit for close observation because the nursing assessment is most likely to reveal which of the following complications?

   a. Anemia
   b. Rh problems

   c. Hypoglycemia
   d. Hyperglycemia

8. What is the primary purpose of an oxytocin stress test for the diabetic mother?

   a. Detect genetic defects in the fetus
   b. Estimate the size of the fetal skull
   c. Find the area of placental attachment in the uterus
   d. Determine how well the fetus will tolerate the stress of labor

9. Pregnant women should avoid eating raw or improperly cooked meat and having contact with feces of animals, especially cats, to prevent which complication?

   a. Rubella
   b. Candidiasis
   c. Toxoplasmosis
   d. Cytomegalovirus

10. A pregnant woman's blood is found to be Rh negative. Which of the following must be true for Rh incompatibility to be possible?

    a. Father's blood is found to be Rh positive.
    b. Father's blood is found to be Rh negative.
    c. Mother does not develop a secondary anemia during pregnancy.
    d. Mother has at least 2 blood transfusions during pregnancy.

Critical Thinking Questions

1. What would you do if you knew a client was a substance abuser but would not tell anyone at the prenatal clinic?

2. What would you do if a client with severe PIH who was on bed rest told you she just could not stay in bed and was getting up when no one was around?

 WEB FLASH!

- Search the Internet for information about the various conditions covered in this chapter. Are all of the sites accessible to you? Is the information for the general public or professionals?

THE BIRTH PROCESS

MAKING THE CONNECTION

Refer to the following chapters to increase your understanding of the birth process:

- **Chapter 25, Assessment**
- **Chapter 26, Pain Management**
- **Chapter 28, Anesthesia**
- **Chapter 47, Prenatal Care**
- **Chapter 48, Complications of Pregnancy**

LEARNING OBJECTIVES

Upon completion of this chapter, you should be able to:
- *Define key terms.*
- *Differentiate between true labor and false labor.*
- *Discuss signs of impending labor.*
- *Describe possible causes of labor.*
- *Identify the variables that affect the progress of labor.*
- *Describe the four stages of labor.*
- *Describe the mechanisms of labor.*
- *Discuss the maternal systemic responses to labor.*
- *Identify nursing actions necessary when admitting a woman to the labor unit.*
- *Discuss the specific assessments used when caring for a woman in labor: fetopelvic relationships, fetal assessment, contractions, Leopold's maneuvers, vaginal examination.*
- *Describe the most common complications of labor—dystocia and fetal distress.*
- *Identify possible medical-surgical interventions for labor: cesarean birth, induction and augmentation of labor, amniotomy, episiotomy, forceps, vacuum extractor, and analgesia/anesthesia.*
- *Discuss possible nursing diagnoses and nursing interventions for a client during labor and delivery.*
- *Appropriately care for a client during labor and delivery.*

KEY TERMS

acme	forceps
amniotomy	frequency
augmentation of labor	fundus
bloody show	increment
Braxton Hicks contractions	induction of labor
	intensity
cephalopelvic disproportion	interval
	lightening
cervical dilatation	macrosomia
cesarean birth	mechanism of labor
crowning	
decrement	molding
duration	nuchal cord
dysfunctional labor	precipitate birth
dystocia	precipitate labor
effacement	presenting part
engagement	preterm birth
episiotomy	preterm labor
external version	prolapsed cord
false labor	pudendal block
Ferguson's reflex	restitution
fetal attitude	station
fetal lie	suture
fetal position	tocolytic agent
fetal presentation	uterine retraction
fontanelle	

INTRODUCTION

The past decade has brought great changes in birthing practices. For hospital births, the concept of labor, delivery, recovery, postpartum (LDRP) rooms has given the expecting couple a more homelike environment and the mother is not moved from the labor room to the delivery room, to the recovery room, to the postpartum room during the birthing process (Figure 49-1). Family and friends, even the baby's siblings, may be present in the LDRP room during the birth process.

Community birthing centers and other settings offer alternatives for the laboring couple. Many clients attend childbirth classes and have in mind a birthing plan or expectations of what they anticipate the birthing process will be like.

This chapter outlines the birth process, from the onset of labor through the birth of the infant.

ONSET OF LABOR

For 38 to 40 weeks the pregnancy has been advancing and the fetus developing. Now, as the fetus reaches maturity, the birth process begins. Researchers are still trying to determine exactly what causes the onset of labor. However, there are two theories relative to why labor begins.

Theories Regarding Onset of Labor

The mechanical theory is based on the principle that as a hollow organ in the body becomes filled and distended, the organ tends to empty itself. Examples of this phenomenon are the bladder and sigmoid colon. This mechanism alone is not enough to fully explain

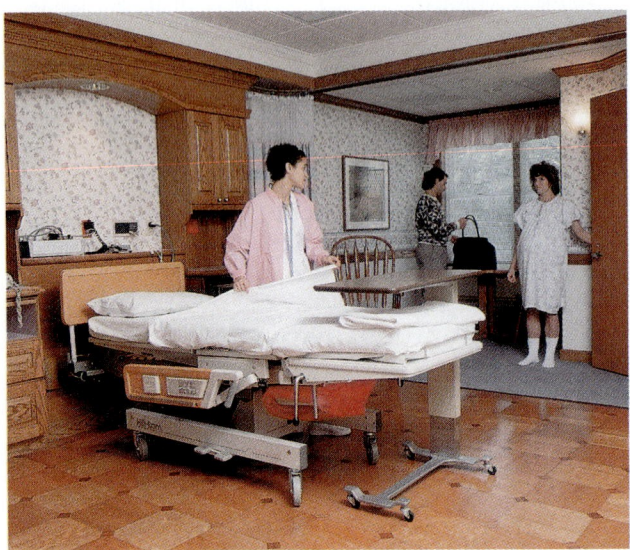

Figure 49-1 The LDRP concept allows the laboring couple to remain in the same room throughout the birth experience.

the onset of labor since a woman can have a full-term 6½ lb baby with one pregnancy and full-term twins each weighing 5½ lb with the next pregnancy.

The hormonal theory of the onset of labor relates to the changes in maternal progesterone and estrogen levels, the maternal production of oxytocin and prostaglandin, and the increase in fetal production of cortisol. There seems to be a highly integrated relationship among these hormones.

As the pregnancy nears its end, the placental production of progesterone decreases, thus decreasing the relaxing effect of progesterone on the uterus. The estrogen level rises, causing an increased sensitivity of the myometrium to oxytocin. Oxytocin, now produced by the mother's posterior pituitary gland, stimulates the uterus to contract. As the pregnancy nears 40 weeks of gestation, the uterus becomes more sensitive to oxytocin. Fetal cortisol production increases as the pregnancy nears term. It is believed to decrease the placental production of progesterone and stimulate the precursors of prostaglandin.

Signs of Impending Labor

There are several signs that indicate labor will soon begin. The signs are lightening, Braxton Hicks contractions, cervical softening, bloody show, rupture of membranes, and a sudden burst of energy.

Lightening

Lightening is the descent of the fetus into the pelvis. This may occur as early as 2 weeks before labor begins in the primigravida client but may not occur until a multigravida client is already in labor. The downward movement of the fetus and thus the uterus makes the upper part of the abdomen flatter. This relieves pressure on the diaphragm, allowing the mother to breathe easier, but she may experience:

- Leg cramps from pressure now on pelvic nerves,
- Urinary frequency from pressure now on the bladder, and
- Increased venous stasis from pressure now on the veins, resulting in edema of the lower extremities.

Braxton Hicks Contractions

Braxton Hicks contractions are irregular, intermittent contractions felt by the pregnant woman toward the end of pregnancy. The tightening sensation in the abdomen may become fairly regular and uncomfortable. The woman may go to the care provider's office or the hospital thinking she is in labor. If the cervix is not dilated and then the contractions stop, this is called **false labor**. Table 49-1 compares false labor and true labor.

Cervical Changes

At about 34 weeks of gestation, because of the changing ratio of estrogen to progesterone and the

Table 49-1	COMPARISON OF FALSE LABOR AND TRUE LABOR
FALSE LABOR	**TRUE LABOR**
Contractions often irregular but may be regular for a short time (1 to 2 hours).	Contractions occur at regular intervals.
Interval between contractions stays the same.	Interval between contractions gradually shortens.
Contraction intensity and duration remain the same.	Contractions increase in intensity and duration.
Contractions frequently stop when the client ambulates or changes position.	Contractions continue and often become stronger when the client ambulates.
Contractions eventually cease with controlled breathing or other relaxation techniques.	Contractions are usually not stopped with controlled breathing, other relaxation techniques, or sedation.
Cervix may soften but does not efface or dilate.	Cervix softens, effaces, and dilates.

production of prostaglandin, the cervix begins to "mature" or "ripen." That is, the cervix becomes softer and more spongy. **Effacement**, thinning of the cervix, may begin, especially when the woman is a primigravida. These cervical changes increase during labor to allow delivery of the fetus.

Bloody Show

Bloody show consists of cervical secretion, blood-tinged mucus, and the mucous plug that blocked the cervix during pregnancy. Labor often begins within 24 to 48 hours after the bloody show is noticed. However, a vaginal examination that includes cervical manipulation may result in a blood-tinged discharge. This may be confused with bloody show.

Rupture of Membranes

Rupture of membranes (ROM) usually occurs after labor has begun. However, in about 12% of women, the amniotic membranes rupture before the onset of labor (Ladewig, London, & Olds, 1998). When this occurs, the pregnant woman should notify her certified nurse midwife (CNM)/physician and proceed to the birthing facility. If **engagement** (when the widest diameter of the fetal presenting part [head] enters the inlet to the true pelvis) has not yet occurred, there exists the danger that the umbilical cord will wash out with the amniotic fluid (prolapsed cord).

If labor does not begin spontaneously within 12 to 24 hours after the membranes rupture and the pregnancy is near term, labor is often induced to avoid infection.

It is sometimes difficult for the woman to determine whether the membranes have ruptured or whether urine has escaped from her bladder. A simple test with nitrazine paper is helpful. When moistened in the discharge, the nitrazine paper will turn blue (react) if the discharge is amniotic fluid; the paper will usually not react if the membranes are still intact.

Sudden Burst of Energy

A few days before labor begins, some women will have a sudden burst of energy. The reason for this is unknown. The prospective mother should be careful not to tire herself. She will need the energy when labor begins.

MATERNAL SYSTEMIC RESPONSES TO LABOR

Knowing how the various systems of the mother's body respond to labor is important when making assessments and performing nursing interventions.

Cardiovascular System

Cardiac output increases because 400 mL of blood is squeezed from the uterus into maternal circulation with each contraction (Lowdermilk, Perry, & Bobak, 1999). The client's blood pressure increases during the first and second stages of labor due to the contractions. Blood pressure is highest during a contraction, so blood pressure should be taken *between* contractions. Anxiety and pain may also make the blood pressure increase. About 10% to 15% of women in labor will experience supine hypotensive syndrome, or decreased blood pressure when in a supine position (Burroughs, 1997).

Respiratory System

Oxygen consumption during labor is equal to that of moderate to strenuous exercise. As long as the respiratory center is not depressed by medication, the increased respiratory rate continues with oxygen consumption almost double the normal amount. If the mother develops hypoxia or acidosis, the fetus may be compromised. Hyperventilation may decrease the level of carbon dioxide in the mother's blood.

Renal System

When engagement occurs, the bladder, now an abdominal organ, is pushed forward and upward. A distended bladder may impede fetal descent. Pressure from the presenting part, especially during a contraction, may cause edema of the tissues because of impaired blood and lymph drainage. Urinary flow is decreased, especially when the woman is supine, because the uterus compresses the ureters. Often there is a lessened urge to void, so the client must be encouraged to do so.

Gastrointestinal System

During labor, peristalsis and absorption decrease. Gastric emptying time is prolonged and gastric contents increase in acidity (Blackburn & Loper, 1992). The staff in many hospitals do not allow the client in labor to eat solid food because there is always a possibility of an obstetrical emergency requiring surgery. Eating solid food would increase the risk of aspirating vomitus. The absorption of liquid is unchanged during labor. The lips and mouth become dry as a result of mouth breathing.

Fluid and Electrolyte Balance

Because of the muscular activity of labor, the mother's body temperature increases and she perspires profusely. The normal increase in respiratory rate and the tendency of women in labor to hyperventilate both cause an increase in fluid loss. The hyperventilation also affects electrolyte balance. To prevent dehydration, the staff in many hospitals routinely have intravenous fluids running on all clients in labor.

Immune System

The white blood count (WBC) increases, sometimes up to 25,000/mm³, during labor and stays elevated during the early postpartum period. The natural increase makes it difficult to identify any infectious process the woman may have.

Integumentary System

The vagina and perineum have a great ability to stretch. The degree of stretching varies with each client. However, there may still be minute tears in the vagina and/or perineum after the birth of the baby.

Musculoskeletal System

The marked increase in muscle activity during labor is accompanied by increased body temperature, di-

CULTURAL CONSIDERATIONS

Regarding Childbirth

- In Malawi, Africa, women are advised not to stand in doorways or peep through windows because this will cause the fetus to be stuck in the pelvis (Gennaro et al., 1998).
- Muslim laws of modesty require that women's hair, arms to the wrist, and legs to the ankles be covered at all times. The women may not be alone with a man other than their husband or a blood relative (Hutchinson & Baqi-Aziz, 1994).
- Southeast Asian women must lie on their side with a pillow under the head during labor (Mattson, 1995).

CULTURAL CONSIDERATIONS

Pain in Childbearing Women

- Chinese believe they will dishonor themselves and their family by any wild or loud response to pain (Weber, 1996).
- Mayan women overcome with fatigue and pain may be scolded or physically restrained (Weber, 1996).
- South and Central American cultures believe that the more intense the pain the stronger the love for the infant (Scott-Ramos, 1995).
- Muslim women either freely vocalize their pain and pray to Allah or stoically endure the pain. Some believe that the husband will be more concerned for them after delivery if the suffering was loud and obvious (Ahmed, 1994; Hutchinson & Baqi-Aziz, 1994).
- Korean women may stoically endure pain during labor because sanskin (goddess of three spirits) dislikes screaming (Howard & Berbiglia, 1997).
- In Malawi, Africa, women are considered a disgrace to the family and cultural group if they cry during labor (Gennaro, Kamwendo, Mbweza, & Kershbaumer, 1998).
- Guatemalan women may vocalize their pain by moaning rhythmically while rubbing their thighs and abdomen (Callister & Vega, 1998).

aphoresis, fatigue, and some proteinuria (1+) (Lowdermilk et al., 1999). The relaxation of pelvic joints, due to the influence of relaxin, may result in backache. Leg cramps also may be experienced.

Neurological System

The client may be euphoric at the beginning of labor. This often changes to seriousness and then to amnesia between contractions during the second stage of labor. Endogenous endorphins (a morphinelike chemical produced naturally by the body) increase the client's pain threshold and have a sedative effect. Pressure on the perineum, by the fetus descending through the birth canal, causes physiologic anesthesia in the perineal tissues.

Pain

The discomfort and pain of labor and birth are individual, subjective, very personal, and have a wide range of expression (Lowe, 1996). Visceral pain usually predominates the first stage of labor, with the stimuli originating in the uterus, cervix, adnexa, and pelvic ligaments. With fetal descent increasing during the late first stage and beginning second stage of labor, the traction and distention on the pelvic structures around the vagina are the primary stimuli for pain. The distention of the perineum is the stimulus for pain during the remainder of the second stage of labor and is transmitted primarily by the pudendal nerves. Figure 49-2 illustrates the intensity and distribution of discomfort during various stages of labor. Stages of labor are discussed later in this chapter.

The softness of pelvic tissues in parous women (women who have delivered at least one child) seems to cause less nociceptive stimuli than in nulliparous women (women who have never delivered a child) during the first stage of labor. However, during the second stage of labor, parous women have increased nociceptive stimuli because of the speed and intensity of fetal descent (Lowe, 1996). As with pain from any other cause, individuals respond in ways that are acceptable in their culture. Health care providers must be sensitive to the fact that expression of pain is rooted in cultural heritage.

VARIABLES AFFECTING LABOR

There are four major variables that affect labor. They are known as the 4 Ps: passage, passenger, pow-

ers, and psyche (Burroughs, 1997; Gorrie, McKinney, & Murray, 1998).

Passage

The passage consists of the bony pelvis, uterus, cervix, vagina, and perineum.

Pelvis

The size and shape of the true pelvis must be adequate for the fetal head to pass through for a vaginal birth. The CNM/physician can use several methods to determine the adequacy of the true pelvis such as:

- Palpation—Internally the bony prominences can be felt; externally the distance between the ischial tuberosities can be measured and then the distance between the ischial spines estimated.
- Ultrasound—An ultrasound is used to estimate pelvic adequacy as well as fetal growth, multiple pregnancy, placenta location, and fetal presentation.
- Pelvimetry—X-ray of the pelvis is seldom performed during pregnancy because of the radiation involved.

Uterus

The upper part of the uterus (fundus) becomes thicker with contractions and the lower section becomes thinner, forming a tube.

Cervix

The uterine contractions put pressure on the fetus, which in turn puts pressure on the cervix, causing the cervix to efface and dilate.

Vagina

The vagina sustains many changes throughout pregnancy. Various hormones cause an increase in vascularity, loosening of connective tissue, and hypertrophy of the smooth muscle cells. These changes allow the vagina to stretch enough for the fetus to pass through.

Perineum

The pressure of the fetus on the perineum causes stretching and thinning of the perineum.

Passenger

The size of the fetus as well as the fetal attitude, fetal lie, fetal presentation, and fetal position affects how easily the fetus can advance through the passage.

Size

The largest part of the fetal body is usually the head. Because the bones of the fetal skull are not fused, the bones can move, sometimes even overlap, as the fetus moves through the mother's bony pelvis. The shaping of the fetal head to adapt to the mother's pelvis during labor is called **molding**.

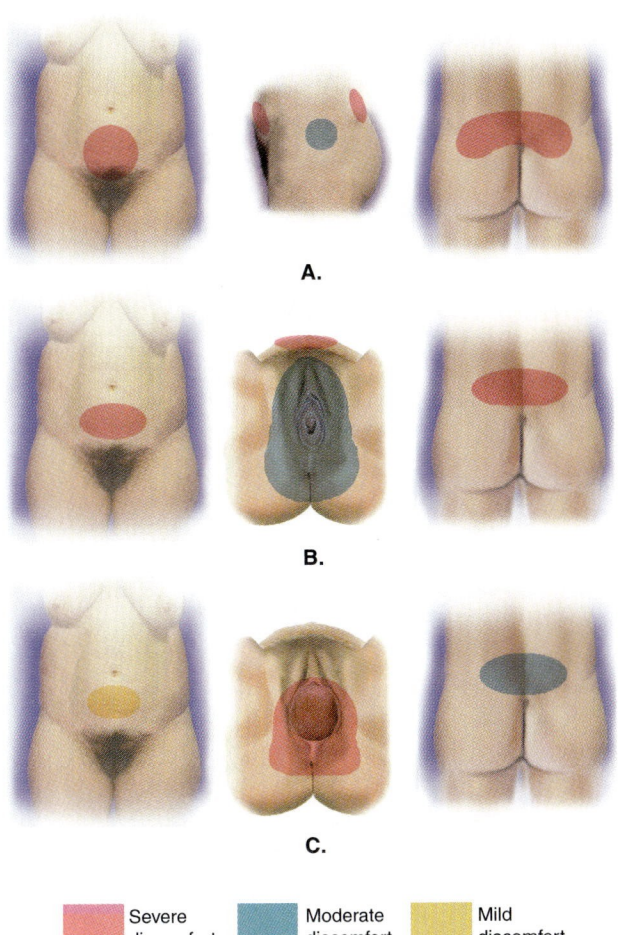

A.

B.

C.

| Severe discomfort | Moderate discomfort | Mild discomfort |

Figure 49-2 Intensity and Distribution of Discomfort during Various Stages of Labor: A. First stage; B. Early second stage; C. Late second stage and birth

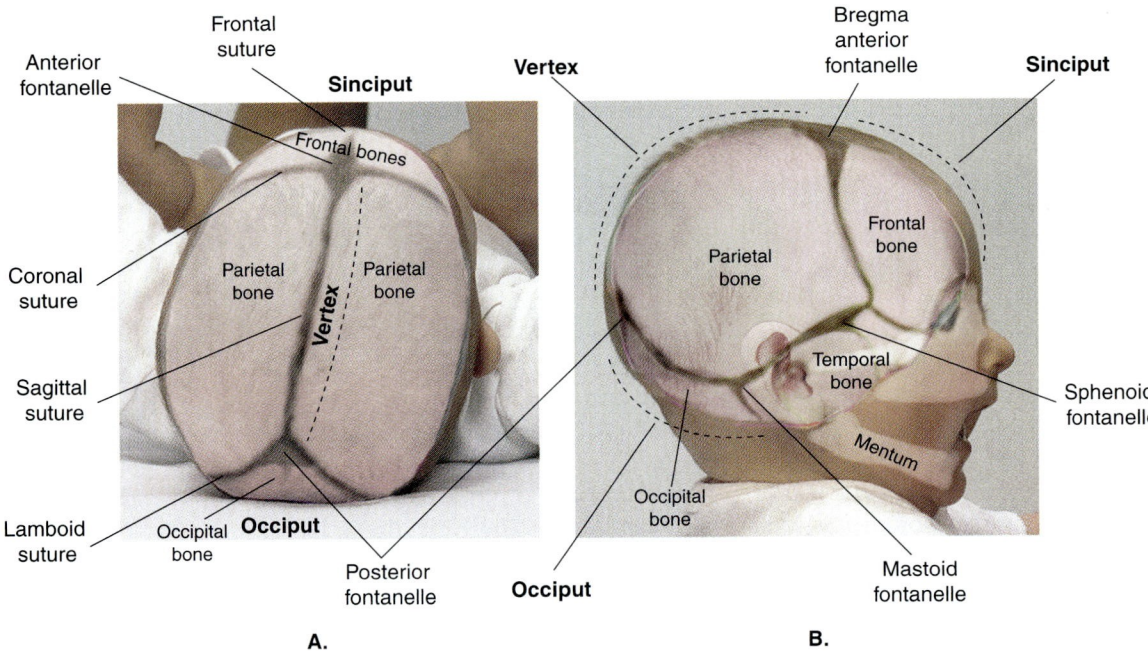

Figure 49-3 Fetal Skull—Sutures and Fontanelles: A. Superior view; B. Lateral view

The major bones of the skull are two frontal bones, two temporal bones, two parietal bones, and the occiput. The bones are joined by thin, fibrous, membrane-covered spaces called **sutures**. Where the sutures meet, there are larger membranous areas called **fontanelles** (Figure 49-3). The largest is the diamond shaped anterior fontanelle. The posterior fontanelle is triangular and smaller. The care providers can palpate the two fontanelles and the suture connecting them through the cervix and determine fetal position.

Fetal Attitude

Fetal attitude is the relationship of fetal body parts to one another. The ideal attitude of the fetus at term is flexion, with the head flexed onto the chest, the arms flexed over the chest, and the hips and knees flexed on the abdomen. If any part of the fetus is extended, especially the head or the legs, labor is usually more difficult. The attitude is then called extension.

Fetal Lie

The relationship of the cephalocaudal (head to foot) axis of the fetus to the cephalocaudal axis of the mother is called the **fetal lie**. When the fetal cephalocaudal axis is parallel to the mother's, it is called a longitudinal lie. At term, the fetus has a longitudinal lie in 99% of pregnancies (Dickason, Silverman, & Schult, 1997). When the fetal cephalocaudal axis is at a right angle to the mother's, it is called a transverse lie (Figure 49-4).

Fetal Presentation

Fetal presentation is determined by the fetal lie and the part of the fetus that enters the pelvis first. The part of the fetus in contact with the cervix is called the

presenting part. The most common type of presentation is cephalic (head), in 95% of deliveries, with breech (buttocks) being 4%, and shoulder 1% of deliveries (Burroughs, 1997) (Figure 49-5).

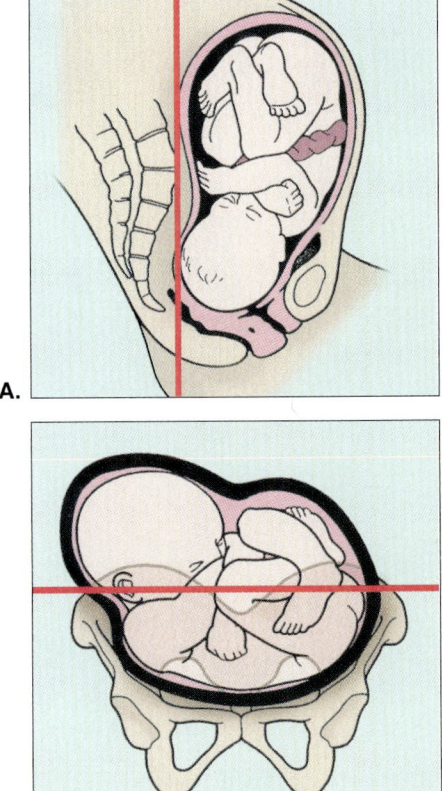

Figure 49-4 Fetal Attitude and Fetal Lie: A. Fetal attitude flexion, fetal lie longitudinal; B. Fetal attitude flexion, fetal lie transverse

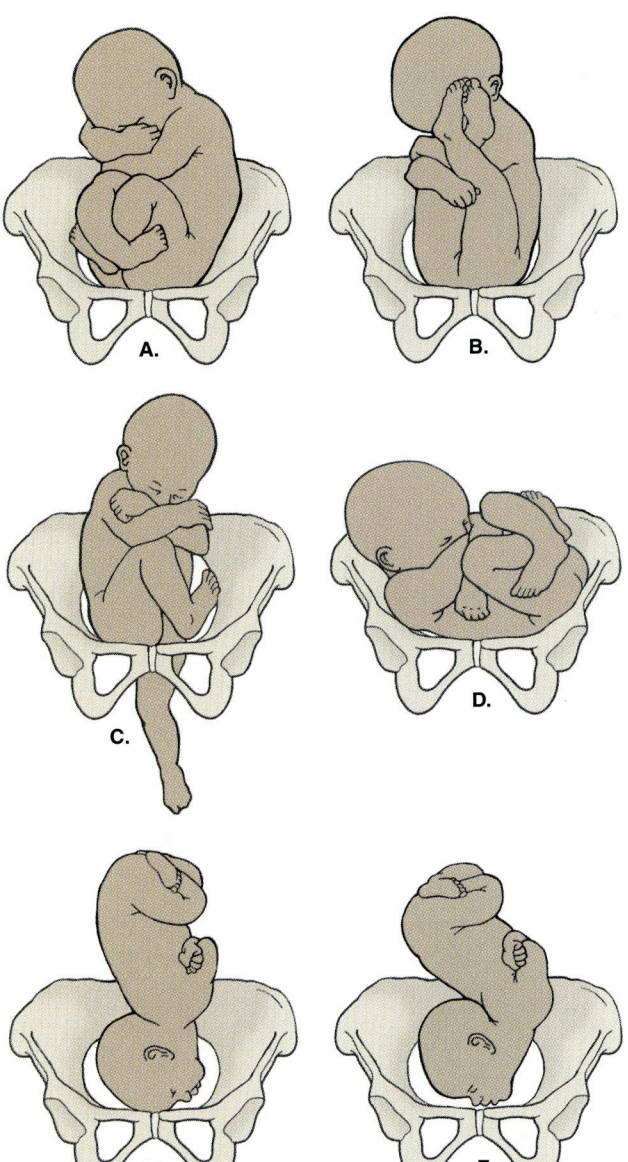

Figure 49-5 Fetal Presentation: A. Complete breech; B. Frank breech; C. Footling breech; D. Shoulder; E. Brow; F. Face

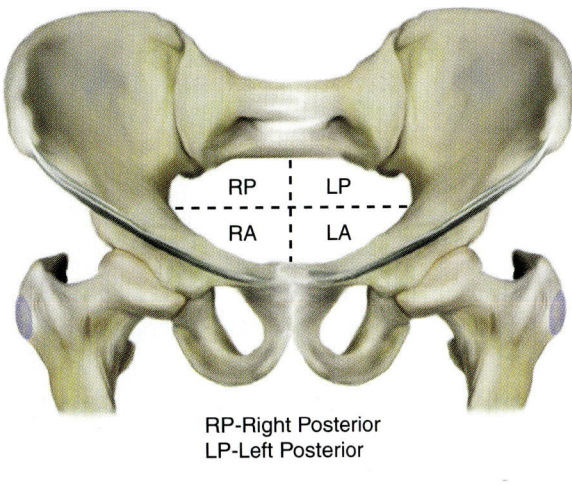

RP-Right Posterior
LP-Left Posterior

RA-Right Anterior
LA-Left Anterior

Figure 49-6 Pelvic Quadrants

- Footling breech: The hips and knees are extended with the foot as the presenting part (may be single footling or double footling).

Shoulder Presentation A shoulder presentation occurs in a transverse lie. The presenting part is usually the shoulder but may be the arm, back, abdomen, or side.

Fetal Position

Fetal position refers to the relationship of the identified landmark on the presenting part to the four quadrants of the mother's pelvis (Figure 49-6). The identified landmarks on various presenting parts are shown in Table 49-2.

The brow presentation does not have an identified landmark. The brow usually changes either to a vertex or face presentation. Because the shoulder presentation cannot be delivered vaginally, a landmark to designate position is of no value.

There are six possible positions for each presenting part as follows:

- Right occiput anterior (ROA) mentum (RMA) sacrum (RSA)
- Right occiput transverse (ROT) mentum (RMT) sacrum (RST)

Cephalic Presentation Cephalic presentations may be further differentiated by the part of the head entering the pelvis first. They may be:

- Vertex—with the occiput as the presenting part,
- Brow—with the sinciput as the presenting part, or
- Face—with the face as the presenting part.

Breech Presentations Breech presentations are differentiated by the attitude of the fetus's legs. The various breech presentations are as follows:

- Complete breech: Hips and knees are flexed on the abdomen in an attitude of flexion, with the buttocks as the presenting part.
- Frank breech: The hips are flexed, but the knees are extended with the buttocks as the presenting part.

Table 49-2	IDENTIFIED LANDMARKS ON VARIOUS PRESENTING PARTS
PRESENTING PART	**IDENTIFIED LANDMARK**
Vertex	Occiput (O)
Face	Mentum (M)
Breech (all)	Sacrum (S)

- Right occiput posterior (ROP) mentum (RMP) sacrum (RSP)
- Left occiput anterior (LOA) mentum (LMA) sacrum (LSA)
- Left occiput transverse (LOT) mentum (LMT) sacrum (LST)
- Left occiput posterior (LOP) mentum (LMP) sacrum (LSP)

Figure 49-7 illustrates the six positions of a vertex presentation. The same six positions apply to the face and breech presentations. The most common position is LOA, which is considered to be the most favorable for the welfare of both mother and baby.

Powers

The primary power during labor is the involuntary contractions of the uterus, which cause cervical effacement and dilatation during the first stage of labor. The secondary power is the voluntary use of the abdominal muscles by the mother to push during the second stage of labor.

Uterine Contractions

The smooth muscle of the uterus has the ability to contract and relax in a rhythmic manner. The relaxation period between contractions allows the muscles and the mother to rest. Uterine relaxation also restores uteroplacental circulation, which is important to fetal oxygenation and effective circulation in the uterus. Contractions begin in the **fundus**, top of the uterus, and spread over the uterus in about 15 seconds (Burroughs, 1997).

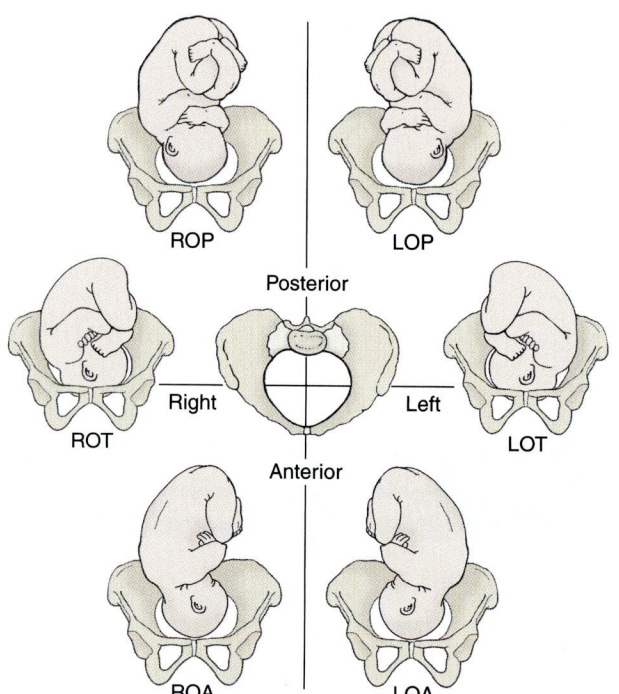

Figure 49-7 Various Positions of a Vertex Presentation

PROFESSIONAL TIP

Fetal Positions
- The right or left and anterior, posterior, or transverse always refer to the mother's pelvis.
- The middle word or letter refers to the identified landmark on the fetus, either occiput, mentum, or sacrum.

The muscle fibers of the uterus have the unique property of remaining permanently shortened to a small degree after each contraction. This is called **uterine retraction**. The shortening of the muscle fibers results in a gradual decrease in the uterine cavity size and a thickening of the muscle in the fundus. As the muscle fibers in the fundus retract, the lower uterine segment is pulled up. These two actions efface and dilate the cervix (Figure 49-8).

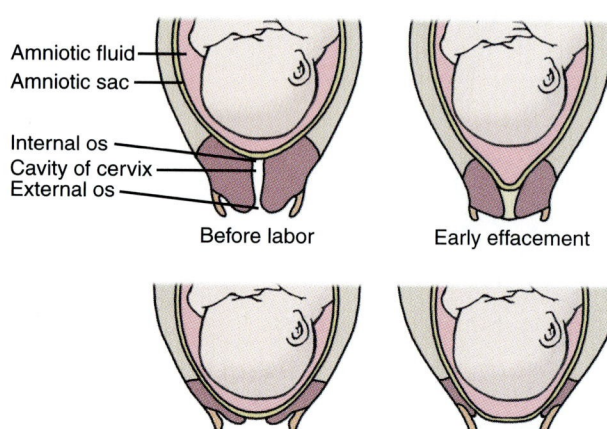

A. Primigravida

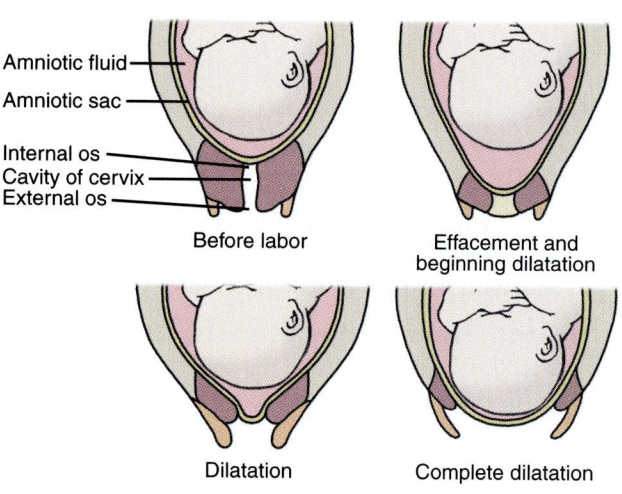

B. Multigravida

Figure 49-8 Effacement and Dilatation: A. Primigravida; B. Multigravida

Each contraction has three phases:

1. **Increment**: increasing intensity of a contraction (the longest phase)
2. **Acme**: peak of a contraction
3. **Decrement**: decreasing intensity of a contraction

Contractions are described in terms of frequency, duration, and intensity. **Frequency** is the time from the beginning of one contraction to the beginning of the next contraction. It includes one contraction and one resting period between contractions (**interval**). **Duration** is the length of one contraction, from the beginning of the increment to the conclusion of the decrement. **Intensity** is the strength of the contraction at the acme. Figure 49-9 illustrates these aspects of a contraction.

The duration of a contraction should not be longer than 90 seconds nor should the interval be less than 60 seconds. The uterus should completely relax between contractions. Contractions lasting longer than 90 seconds reduce uterine and placental circulation because of the prolonged compression of the blood vessels. This in turn compromises the fetus.

Contractions are affected by the mother's position. When the mother lies on her back the contractions are often more frequent but have less intensity. When she lies on her side, the contractions are usually less frequent but have greater intensity. Thus, a side-lying position improves progress in labor. Lying on the side also prevents supine hypotension syndrome in the mother and improves oxygenation of the uterus, placenta, and fetus because the heavy uterus is not compressing the inferior vena cava.

Mother's Pushing

Once the cervix has dilated completely, it is time for the fetus to navigate through the remaining mechanisms of labor. The accepted procedure has been for the mother to take a deep breath at the beginning of a contraction, hold her breath, and voluntarily push in a Valsalva-type bearing down throughout a contraction. This pushing technique is directed by the nurses and/or the CNM/physician.

The spontaneous onset of the urge to bear down is triggered when the presenting part reaches the pelvic floor where stretch receptors in the posterior vagina cause the release of oxytocin, which spontaneously increases the pushing sensation (Cosner & deJong, 1993). This spontaneous, involuntary urge to bear down is known as **Ferguson's reflex**.

Psyche

Psyche refers to the mother's attitude toward labor and her preparation for labor. The mother's attitude toward labor is shaped by her experiences and expectations. Culture shapes values about and responses to childbirth. It provides the mother with ideas about

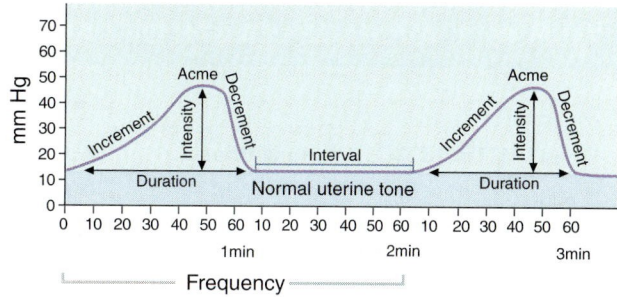

Figure 49-9 Aspects of a Contraction (frequency 2 minutes, duration 60 seconds, intensity moderate)

how to behave during labor and how to interact with her baby.

Anxiety or fear causes the mother's body to secrete catecholamines, which can suppress uterine contractions and restrict placental blood flow. Relaxation increases the progress of labor. Childbirth preparation classes enhance the mother's ability to work with her body rather than working against it. When a woman has realistic expectations about childbirth, she is more likely to have a positive experience.

STAGES OF LABOR

For many years, labor was divided into three stages. In each of these three stages, specific events can be identified. A fourth stage has been acknowledged as being critical to the birth process, the recovery period after the birth of the baby. This chapter discusses four stages of labor. Table 49-3 presents an overview of the average duration of the first two stages. Stages 1 and 2 vary in the average length for primigravida clients and multigravida clients. Stages 3 and 4 are approximately the same length for all clients and are not included in this table.

First Stage: Dilatation and Effacement

The first stage of labor begins with the onset of regular contractions and ends when **cervical dilatation**, the enlargement of the cervical opening (os), is complete (10 cm). This is usually the longest stage of labor and is divided into three phases: latent, active, and transition.

Latent Phase

The latent phase of the first stage of labor ends when the cervix is dilated 4 cm. Contractions occur every 10 to 20 minutes at first and become more frequent, every 5 to 7 minutes. The duration of the contractions begin at 15 to 20 seconds and progress to 30 to 40 seconds. The contraction intensity begins as mild and gradually becomes moderate.

The client is usually alert and often talkative. She is

Table 49-3 AVERAGE LENGTH OF LABOR STAGES 1 AND 2

CHARACTERISTIC	FIRST STAGE			SECOND STAGE
	Latent Phase	Active Phase	Transition Phase	
Primigravida	8 to 10 hours	6 hours	2 hours	1 hour
Multigravida	5 hours	4 hours	1 hour	15 minutes
Cervical dilatation	0 to 4 cm	4 to 8 cm	8 to 10 cm	
Contractions				
Frequency	10 to 20 progressing to 5 to 7 minutes	3 to 5 minutes	2 to 3 minutes	2 to 3 minutes
Duration	15 to 20 progressing to 30 to 40 seconds	40 to 60 seconds	60 to 90 seconds	60 to 90 seconds
Intensity	Mild progressing to moderate	Moderate progressing to strong	Strong	Strong

often relieved that labor has begun, yet anxious about what is ahead for her. This is a good time to review the client's preparations for labor and expectations of how labor and delivery will be handled (e.g., medications, persons present). Any needed teaching, especially breathing techniques, should be undertaken at this time. If the membranes have not ruptured, many women prefer to walk during this time.

Active Phase

The active phase of the first stage of labor begins when the cervix is dilated 4 cm and ends when the cervix is dilated 8 cm. Contractions occur every 3 to 5 minutes with a duration of 40 to 60 seconds. They are of moderate intensity, progressing to strong. Clients perceive varying degrees of discomfort. The client now focuses more on the breathing techniques during contractions and is less talkative.

Transition Phase

The transition phase of the first stage of labor begins when the cervix is dilated 8 cm and ends when the cervix is dilated 10 cm. Contractions occur every 2 to 3 minutes with a duration of 60 to 90 seconds. There is little rest for the client between contractions. The intensity of the contractions is strong. The client usually needs to be reminded to focus, relax, and breathe with each contraction. She is very aware of the increasing intensity of the contractions, may become very restless, and may fear being left alone. Requests for medication often accompany statements like "I can't take it any more." Following are characteristics of the transition phase:

- Restlessness
- Hyperventilation
- Bewilderment and sometimes anger
- Difficulty following directions
- Focus on self
- Irritability

- Statements like "Don't touch me"
- Nausea, occasionally vomiting
- Very warm feeling
- Perspiration on upper lip
- Increasing rectal pressure

 Safety: Use of Stirrups during Birth

Clients who are delivering in a modified lithotomy position may have their feet placed in stirrups to open the pelvis and facilitate access to the perineum.

- Stirrup height and lower leg length must be adjusted for each client.
- Both legs must be raised into the stirrups at the same time to prevent strain on the pelvic ligaments.

Second Stage: Birth of Baby

The second stage of labor begins when cervical dilatation is complete and ends with the birth of the baby. Contractions continue at a frequency of 2 to 3 minutes, duration of 60 to 90 seconds, and strong intensity. Now that the cervix is completely dilated, the mother can actively assist in the descent of the fetus by contracting the abdominal muscles and bearing down with each contraction. This active participation in the process often gives her a sense of control.

 CLIENT TEACHING

Effective Pushing in Upright or Squatting Position

The mother can push more effectively if she:
- Flexes chin on her chest and bends over her uterus,
- With elbows *bent,* pulls on her flexed knees, and
- Exhales and vocalizes when pushing.

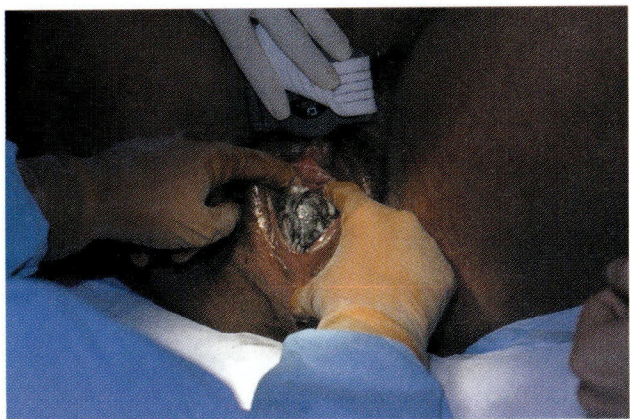

Figure 49-10 Crowning

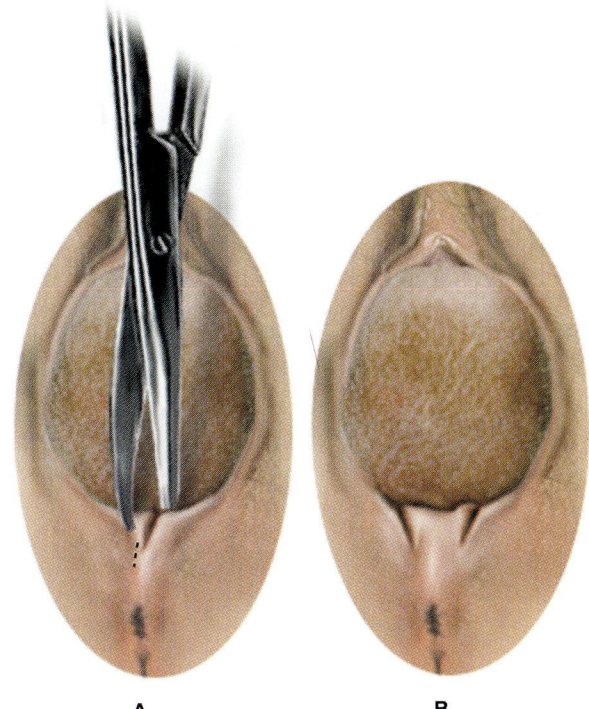

A.   **B.**

Figure 49-11 Episiotomy: A. Midline; B. Right or left medio-lateral

As the fetal head descends, it puts pressure on the pelvic nerves and the mother has a greater desire to push. Pressure from the fetal head makes the perineum bulge, then flatten and move anteriorly. With each contraction the labia begin to separate and the baby's head is seen, but the head recedes between contractions. When the largest diameter of the fetal head is past the vulva (head can be seen between contractions), **crowning** has occurred and the birth is imminent (Figure 49-10). It is at this time that an **episiotomy**, an incision in the perineum to facilitate passage of the baby, may be performed (Figure 49-11). A few more contractions will push the head out, and a few more will deliver the body.

As the fetus moves through the pelvis and birth canal, several changes in position must occur. This series of movements is collectively called the **mechanisms of labor** or cardinal movements.

Mechanisms of Labor

The mechanisms of labor are engagement, descent, flexion, internal rotation, extension, external rotation, and expulsion (Figure 49-12). The first three generally occur during the first stage of labor.

Engagement As explained earlier, engagement occurs when the presenting part of the fetus (usually head) fully enters the true pelvis. It generally happens before labor begins in primigravidas and after labor begins in multigravidas.

Descent Descent begins with engagement and continues with each contraction throughout the labor process.

Flexion The fetal head is bent forward as it meets resistance during descent, causing the chin to rest on the sternum. This allows the narrowest part of the head to enter the pelvic outlet.

Internal Rotation Internal rotation takes place mainly during the second stage of labor. The head rotates so the occiput is next to the symphysis pubis.

Extension As the fetal head continues to descend, the occiput pivots under the symphysis pubis and the

fetal head becomes unflexed (extended) and pushes upward out of the vagina. The head is actually born at this time.

Restitution and External Rotation Once the head has emerged, it rotates back to be in normal alignment with the shoulders. This is called **restitution**. Fetal position in the uterus can be identified by observing this turning of the head. The shoulders now rotate to be in an anteroposterior position under the symphysis pubis.

Expulsion The health care provider assisting with the birth applies gentle downward pressure on the baby's head to allow the anterior shoulder to emerge. Then the baby's head is gently raised so the posterior shoulder can be delivered. The rest of the baby's body then just slides out. This is called expulsion (Figure 49-13).

Third Stage: Delivery of Placenta

The third stage of labor begins with the birth of the baby and ends with the delivery of the placenta. This should occur in 30 minutes or less. After the baby is born, the uterus continues contracting, decreasing its capacity and thereby reducing the surface area of placental attachment. The reduced surface area causes the placenta to separate from the uterine wall. As it separates, bleeding occurs, causing the formation of a retroplacental (behind the placenta) hematoma. This hematoma facilitates the separation process. The membranes are peeled from the uterine wall as the placenta slides into the vagina.

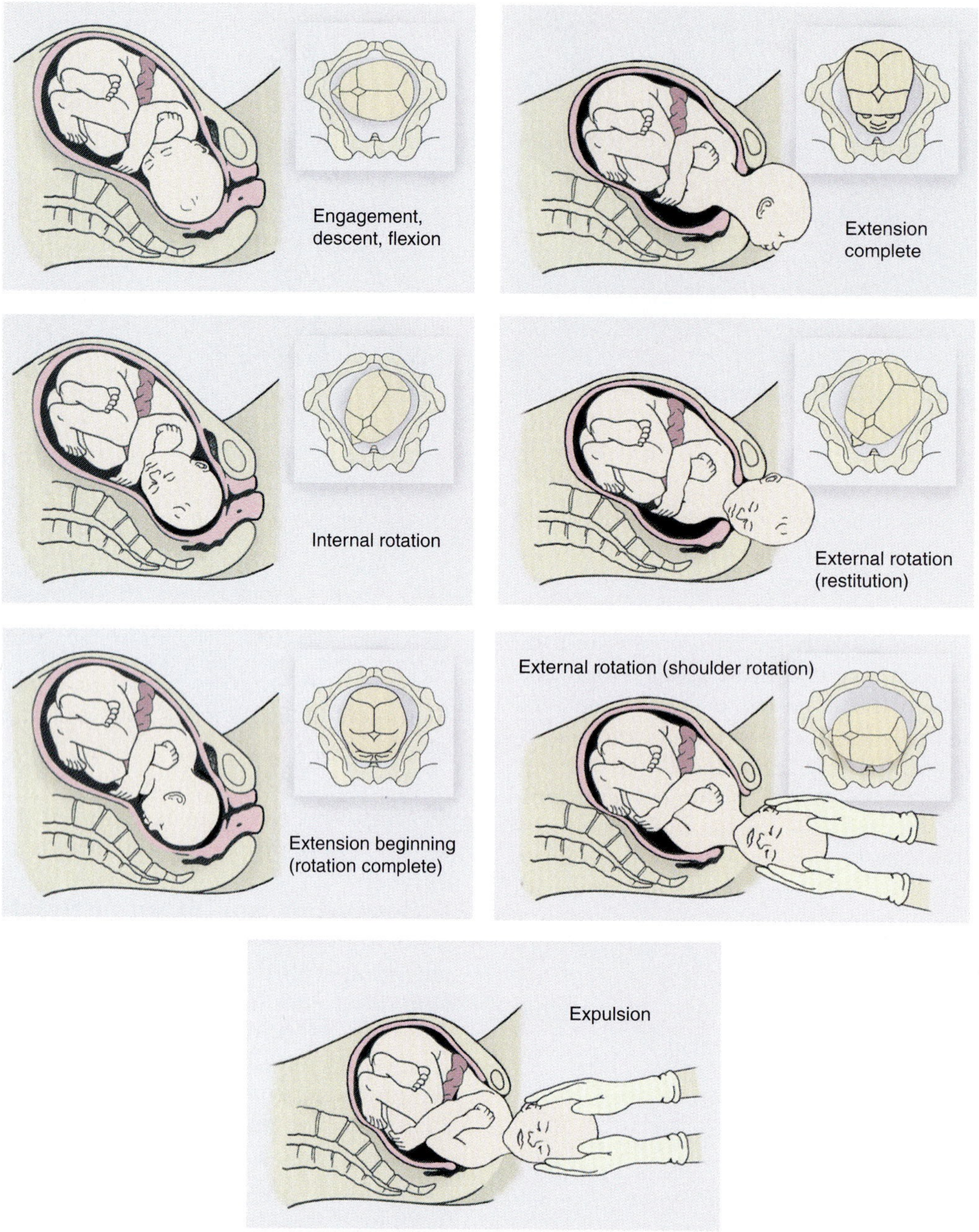

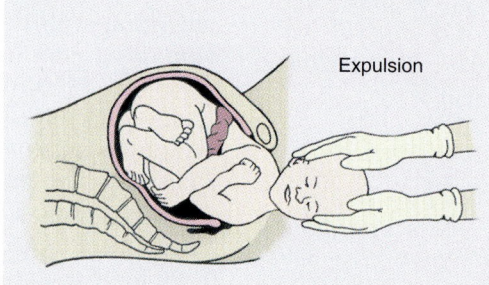

Figure 49-12 Mechanisms of Labor

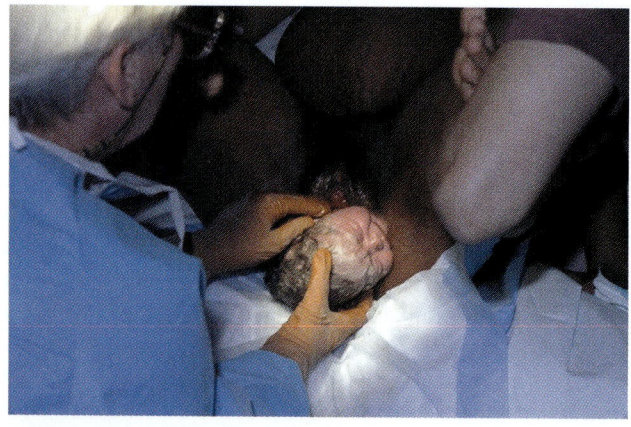

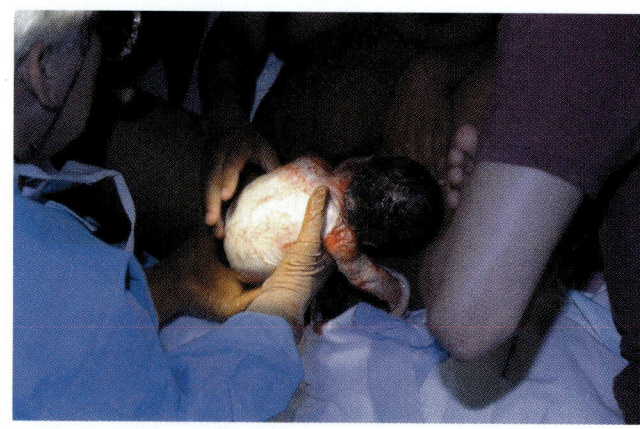

Figure 49-13 Birth of an Infant

Signs that the placenta has separated should be observed about 5 to 10 minutes after the birth of the baby. These signs are:

- Globular shape of the uterus,
- Gush of blood from the vagina, and
- More of the cord protrudes from the vagina (is visible).

When these signs of placental separation have appeared, the client is asked to push one last time to deliver the placenta.

The birthing facility disposes of the placenta after the delivery. Occasionally, a client may request to have the placenta to uphold cultural expectations.

Fourth Stage: Recovery

The fourth stage of labor is the first 2 hours after the birth of the baby when the mother's body begins its physiological readjustments. Blood loss is usually between 250 mL and 500 mL. There is a moderate decrease in the systolic and diastolic blood pressure and an increase in pulse rate. The uterus should remain contracted to control bleeding and be positioned in the midline of the abdomen about midway between the symphysis and the umbilicus.

The new mother may be very hungry and thirsty. A shaking chill may be experienced in response to the ending of the physical work of labor. The bladder may be hypotonic due either to trauma during the second stage of labor and/or to decreased sensation from anesthesia. This may result in urinary retention.

ADMISSION OF CLIENT IN LABOR

Admission of a client in labor may be different for each person. Although there are standard nursing assessments and interventions for a woman in labor, each client must be cared for individually based on her particular situation. The priorities of establishing a nurse/client relationship and assessing the condition of mother and fetus may be undertaken in a sequential order or may need to be performed simultaneously.

It is important to determine which stage of labor the mother may be in at the time of admission. A few specific questions might include the following:

- When did your labor begin?
- How frequent are the contractions and how long do they last?
- Have the membranes ruptured? (Has your water broken?)
- How many pregnancies is this for you? How long were your other labors (if this is not the first pregnancy)?

Depending on the answers to these questions, a determination is made about how to proceed with the admission. When a woman is admitted in early labor, time can be taken to establish the nurse/client relationship by:

- Making the woman and her partner or family feel welcome,
- Determining their expectations about the birth (did they attend childbirth classes?), and
- Identifying cultural values and preferences related to the birth process.

Initial Assessment

After the nurse/client relationship has been established on admission, more specific assessments are made. Figure 49-14 shows a sample obstetric admitting record. A copy of the prenatal record is generally sent to the birthing facility and is added to the client's record

Obstetric Admitting Record
Hollister Maternal/Newborn Record System   Page 1 of 2
To order call: 1.800.323.4060   Re-order No. 5710

Basic Admission Data   Date ___/___/___ Time ___
☐ Ambulatory   ☐ Stretcher   ☐ Oriented to Unit
☐ Wheelchair   ☐ Transfer From ___   ☐ Safety/Security

G ___ T ___ P ___ Ab ___ L ___ / M P ___   Wks ___
☐ By Fetal Assessment ___/___/___

Race/Ethnicity ___   Age ___
Advance Directives ☐ None   ☐ Living Will
☐ Medical Power of Attorney
Organ Donor ☐ Yes ☐ No
Last Oral Intake
Fluids ___/___/___ Time ___
Solids ___/___/___ Time ___
Medications
Type/Dose   Last Taken   With Patient   Disposition

MD/CNM ___ Tel No ___ Support Person/Relationship ___ Tel No ___

Patient Triage Data   ☐ See Triage Record
Contractions   ☐ None   ☐ Palpation   ☐ Tocotransducer
Frequency ___   Duration ___   Intensity ___
Began on ___/___/___ Time ___
Membranes   ☐ Intact   ☐ Bulging
☐ Ruptured (Date ___/___/___ Time ___)
☐ Nitrazine test ☐ pos ☐ neg   ☐ Sterile Speculum Exam
☐ Fern test ☐ pos ☐ neg   (findings ___)

Physical Assessment
Height ___ Wt Pregrav/Grav ___ Temp ___ Pulse ___ Resp ___ BP ___
Detail Abnormal Findings
System (Normal/Abnormal)
HEENT
Neurologic
Skin
Breasts
Extremities
Cardiovascular
Respiratory
Abdomen
Gastrointestinal
Urinary
Genitalia
Initial Problems Identified ☐ None   Plan
1.
2.
3.

Allergies/Sensitivities ☐ None
☐ Medication ___
☐ Other ___

Reasons for Admission
☐ Onset of Labor
☐ Induction of Labor
☐ Spontaneous Abortion
☐ Cesarean Section
☐ Primary ☐ Repeat (reason for primary ___)
☐ Tubal Ligation
☐ Vaginal Bleeding
☐ ROM ☐ Premature ☐ Prolonged
☐ Preterm Labor
Detail Reasons for Admission ___

Observation Evaluation
☐ Fetal Status
☐ Ultrasound
☐ Amniocentesis
☐ NST ☐ CST
☐ Medical Complications
☐ Obstetric Complications

Personal Effects   Disposition
Item | With Patient | With Support Person | Other (Describe)

Fluid   ☐ Clear   ☐ Bloody   ☐ Meconium Stained
☐ Foul Odor ☐ No Foul Odor ☐ None Observed
Vaginal Bleeding ☐ None ☐ Normal Show
☐ Bleeding (Describe ___)
Cervical Exam By ___
Station ___ Effacement ___ Dilatation ___ cms
Presentation ☐ Vertex   ☐ Transverse Lie
☐ Face/Brow   ☐ Compound
☐ Breech (type ___)   ☐ Unknown

Fetal Evaluation Data   Multiple Gestation ☐ No ☐ Yes
Fundal Height ___ cms   Presentation   Position
Fetal Weight (est.) ___   1.
FHR ___   2.
☐ Fetoscope ☐ Fetal Monitor   3.
☐ Doppler ☐ Other ___

Specimens Obtained (Check all that apply)
Urine Test | Time | Results || Blood Test | Time | Results
☐ Urinalysis || ☐ Hgb
☐ C + S || ☐ Hct
☐ Glucose || ☐ VDRL/RPR
☐ Albumin || ☐ Type/Screen
☐ Ketones ||
☐ pH || Cervical Culture
☐ Blood || ☐ GBS
☐ Toxicology ||

Admitting Signature ___ Date/Time ___ Examiner Signature ___ Date/Time ___

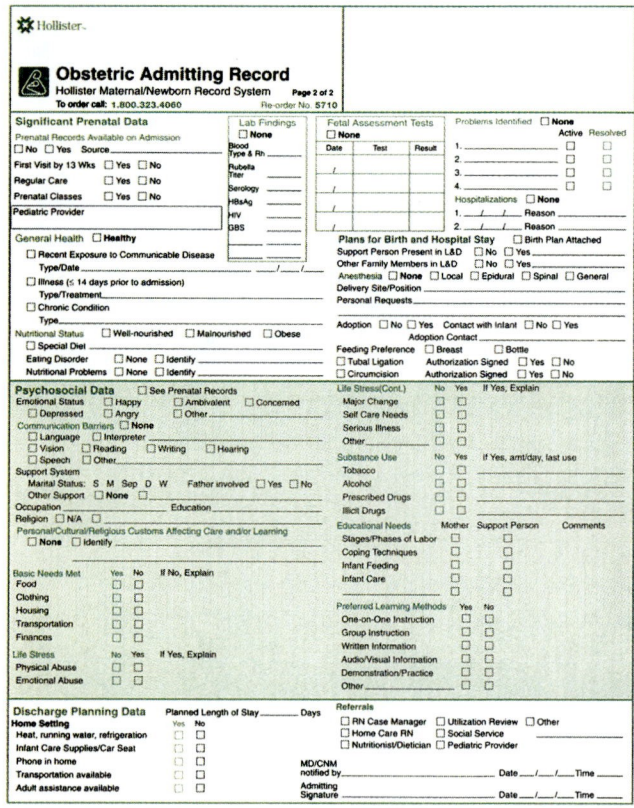

Obstetric Admitting Record
Hollister Maternal/Newborn Record System   Page 2 of 2
To order call: 1.800.323.4060   Re-order No. 5710

Significant Prenatal Data
Prenatal Records Available on Admission
☐ No ☐ Yes Source ___
First Visit by 13 Wks ☐ Yes ☐ No
Regular Care ☐ Yes ☐ No
Prenatal Classes ☐ Yes ☐ No
Pediatric Provider ___

General Health ☐ Healthy
☐ Recent Exposure to Communicable Disease
Type/Date ___
☐ Illness (≤ 14 days prior to admission)
Type/Treatment ___
☐ Chronic Condition
Type ___
Nutritional Status ☐ Well-nourished ☐ Malnourished ☐ Obese
☐ Special Diet
Eating Disorder ☐ None ☐ Identify ___
Nutritional Problems ☐ None ☐ Identify ___

Psychosocial Data ☐ See Prenatal Records
Emotional Status ☐ Happy ☐ Ambivalent ☐ Concerned
☐ Depressed ☐ Angry ☐ Other ___
Communication Barriers ☐ None
☐ Language ☐ Interpreter
☐ Vision ☐ Reading ☐ Writing ☐ Hearing
☐ Speech ☐ Other ___
Support System
Marital Status: S M Sep D W   Father involved ☐ Yes ☐ No
Other Support ☐ None ☐ ___
Occupation ___ Education ___
Religion ☐ N/A ☐ ___
Personal/Cultural/Religious Customs Affecting Care and/or Learning
☐ None ☐ Identify ___

Basic Needs Met   Yes No   If No, Explain
Food
Clothing
Housing
Transportation
Finances
Life Stress   No Yes   If Yes, Explain
Physical Abuse
Emotional Abuse

Discharge Planning Data   Planned Length of Stay ___ Days
Home Setting   Yes No
Heat, running water, refrigeration
Infant Care Supplies/Car Seat
Phone in home
Transportation available
Adult assistance available

Lab Findings
☐ None
Blood Type & Rh ___
Rubella Titer ___
Serology ___
HBsAg ___
HIV ___
GBS ___

Fetal Assessment Tests
☐ None
Date | Test | Result

Problems Identified ☐ None   Active Resolved
1.
2.
3.

Hospitalizations ☐ None
1. ___ Reason ___
2. ___ Reason ___

Plans for Birth and Hospital Stay
Support Person Present in L&D ☐ Yes ☐ No ___ ☐ Birth Plan Attached
Other Family Members in L&D ☐ No ☐ Yes ___
Anesthesia ☐ None ☐ Local ☐ Epidural ☐ Spinal ☐ General
Delivery Site/Position ___
Personal Requests ___
Adoption ☐ No ☐ Yes   Contact with Infant ☐ No ☐ Yes
Adoption Contact ___
Feeding Preference ☐ Breast ☐ Bottle
☐ Tubal Ligation   Authorization Signed ☐ Yes ☐ No
☐ Circumcision   Authorization Signed ☐ Yes ☐ No

Life Stress(Cont.)   No Yes   If Yes, Explain
Major Change
Self Care Needs
Serious Illness
Other ___
Substance Use   No Yes   If Yes, amt/day, last use
Tobacco
Alcohol
Prescribed Drugs
Illicit Drugs
Educational Needs   Mother Support Person   Comments
Stages/Phases of Labor
Coping Techniques
Infant Feeding
Infant Care
Preferred Learning Methods   Yes No
One-on-One Instruction
Group Instruction
Written Information
Audio/Visual Information
Demonstration/Practice
Other ___

Referrals
☐ RN Case Manager ☐ Utilization Review ☐ Other ___
☐ Home Care RN ☐ Social Service ___
☐ Nutritionist/Dietician ☐ Pediatric Provider
MD/CNM notified by ___ Date ___/___/___ Time ___
Admitting Signature ___ Date ___/___/___ Time ___

Figure 49-14 Representative Obstetric Admitting Record *(Permission to use this copyright material has been granted by the owner, Hollister Incorporated.)*

when she is admitted. Information can be obtained from the prenatal record. Clients who have not received prenatal care will need a more extensive assessment.

A physical examination is performed, including the following:

- Vital signs
- Auscultation of heart and lungs
- Leopold's maneuvers (described in Chapter 47) to determine fetal lie and presentation
- Fetal heart rate (FHR) (described in Chapter 47), continuous electronic fetal monitoring may be used during the birthing process (described in Chapter 48)
- Contractions for frequency, duration, and intensity
- Nitrazine test if mother is not sure whether the membranes have ruptured
- Vaginal examination (Figure 49-15) to determine cervical effacement and dilatation, fetal position, and station; usually done by the registered nurse (RN) or CNM/physician
- Inspection for signs of edema of face, hands, legs, and sacrum

The FHR may be heard in various places on the mother's abdomen depending on the position of the fetus (Figure 49-16).

Station is the relationship of the fetal presenting part to the ischial spines. It is measured in centimeters above (−) or below (+) the ischial spines (Figure 49-17).

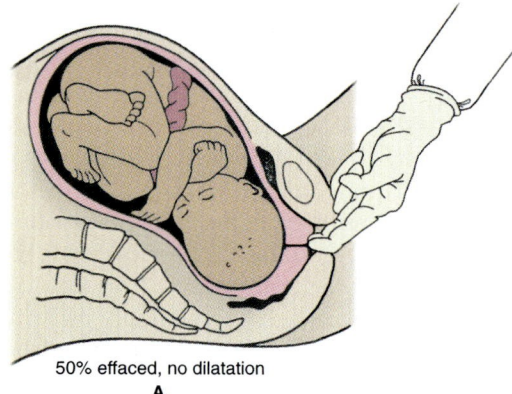

50% effaced, no dilatation
A.

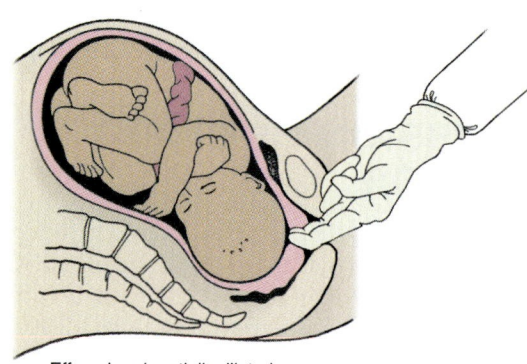

Effaced and partially dilated
B.

Figure 49-15 Vaginal Examination: A. 50% effaced, no dilatation; B. 100% effaced, partly dilated

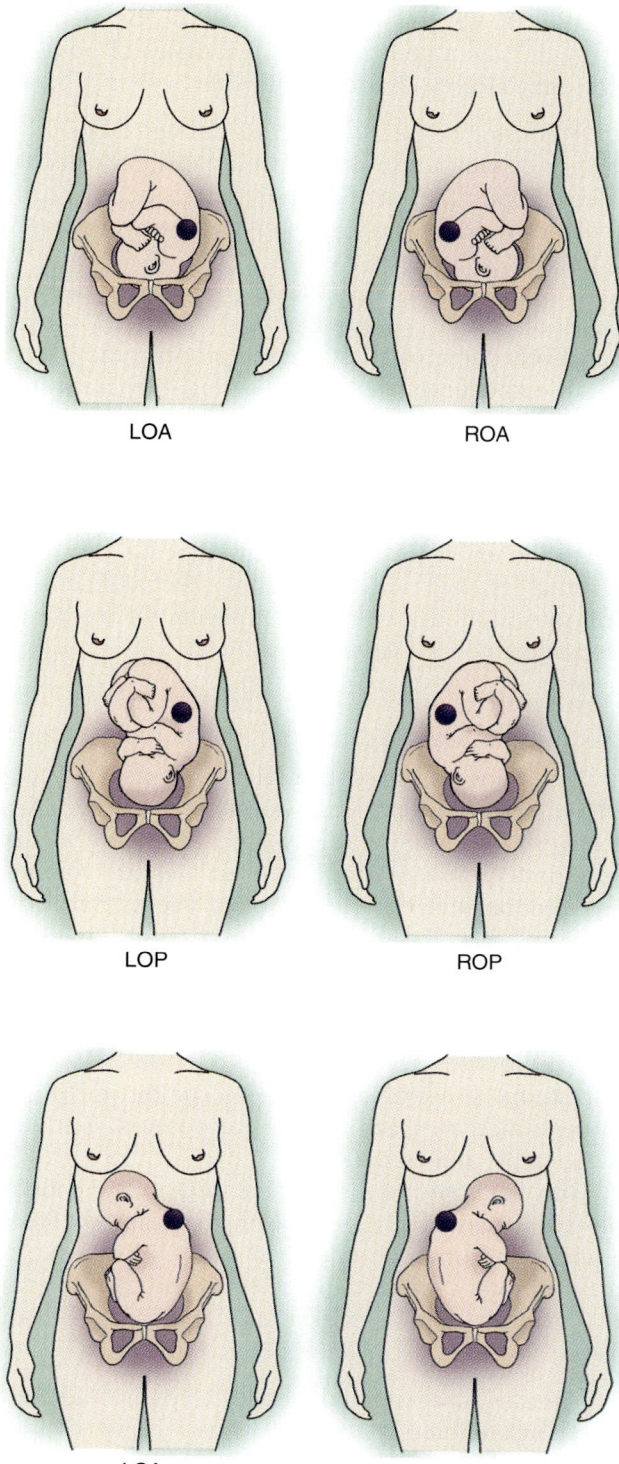

LOA   ROA

LOP   ROP

LSA   RSA

Figure 49-16 Based on Leopold's maneuvers, FHR will best be heard in the marked areas for the various positions.

Contractions are assessed by placing the fingers of one hand on the fundus of the uterus, and using light pressure to keep the fingers still. Contractions begin in the fundus and spread down the uterus. The person assessing the contractions can feel the tightening of the uterus before the mother is aware of it.

At least three contractions in a row should be as-

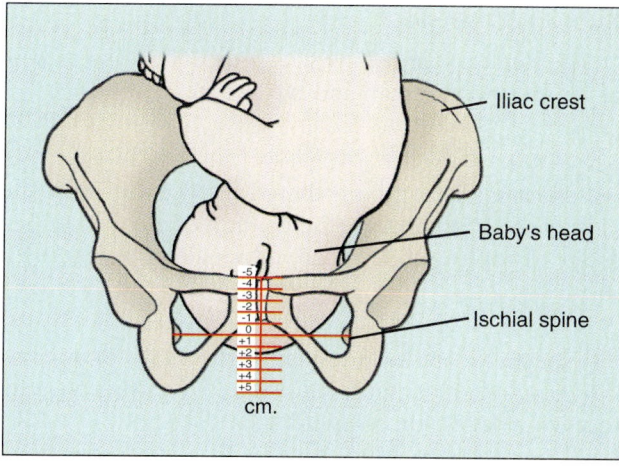

Iliac crest

Baby's head

Ischial spine

cm.

Figure 49-17 Station. Relationship of the fetal presenting part to the ischial spines. The station illustrated is +2.

sessed. The time each contraction begins and ends and the time lapse between contractions should be noted. The intensity can be estimated by how easily the uterus can be indented during a contraction.

- Mild contraction: uterus is easily indented with the fingertips; feels like the tip of the nose
- Moderate contraction: uterus is more difficult to indent with the fingertips; feels similar to the chin
- Strong contraction: uterus unable to be indented with the fingertips; feels like the forehead

 Infection Control: Standard Precautions

- Disposable gloves should be worn any time hands might come in contact with amniotic fluid, blood, bloody show, urine, or feces.
- Wear a splash apron and eye covering (goggles or face mask) when the splashing of body fluids is possible.
- Wash hands before putting on gloves and immediately after removing them.

NURSING PROCESS

The nurse is an important member of the team that helps the mother to successfully progress through the birth experience.

 PROFESSIONAL TIP

Station

- It is often a challenge to remember the notations of station.
- Remember, plus (+) is what is desired; the presenting part is below the level of the ischial spines. Minus (−) means the presenting part is not yet to the level of the ischial spines.

Assessment

The nurse's role begins with a thorough assessment of the laboring woman and her progress.

Subjective Data

Subjective data to be gathered throughout labor and birth of the infant include the comfort of the mother, her ability to cope, and her desire to urinate or defecate.

Objective Data

Objective data include vital signs; FHR; frequency, duration, interval, and intensity of contractions; fetopelvic relationships, including fetal attitude, fetal lie, fetal presentation, and station; condition of membranes; maternal behavior, including tone of voice and facial expressions; and maternal verbalizations. Table 49-4 provides suggested time frames for selected assessments.

Nursing Diagnoses

Many different nursing diagnoses may be appropriate for a client during labor and the birthing process. Selected nursing diagnoses appropriate for the first three stages of labor are listed.

- *Communication, Verbal, Impaired*
- *Pain*
- *Fatigue*
- *Anxiety*
- *Fear*
- *Knowledge Deficit*
- *Infection, Risk for*
- *Fluid Volume, Deficit, Risk for*
- *Urinary Elimination, Altered*
- *Gas Exchange, Impaired (fetal)*
- *Tissue Perfusion, Altered (maternal)*
- *Physical Mobility, Impaired*
- *Coping, Individual, Ineffective*
- *Injury, Risk for*
- *Social Isolation*
- *Family Processes, Altered*

Planning/Outcome Identification

Based on the client's expectations of labor and the birthing process and the assessments performed by the facility staff, the planning and goals can be mutually set by the client and the nurse. Examples of possible goals may include that the client will:

- Demonstrate expected progress through labor,
- Express satisfaction with the assistance provided by her support person and facility staff,
- Maintain adequate hydration with oral and/or IV intake,
- Void at least every 2 hours to prevent bladder distention,
- Actively participate in the labor process, and
- Not experience any injury during the labor and birthing process.

Nursing Interventions

Nursing interventions focus on continuing assessment of labor progress and fetal well-being, providing maternal physical care, assisting the client and her support person, and providing or assisting with pharmacologic comfort measures.

Continuing Assessment of Labor and Fetal Well-Being

Continuing assessment of labor progress and fetal well-being is performed as previously discussed. Any changes outside the normally expected changes must be reported immediately. Some facilities use continuous electronic fetal monitoring on all clients. However, the nurse should still personally assess and time contractions and listen to the FHR at regular intervals. Figure 49-18 presents a sample labor in progress record.

Providing Maternal Physical Care

Maternal physical care includes comfort measures, hygiene measures, ambulation and position, food and fluid intake, and elimination.

Comfort Measures There are many comfort measures that can be used with the client in labor. Some may work with one client and not the next, or may work for a while with one client and then she will not want that comfort measure used any more. Comfort measures to try include the following:

- Offering the client fluids and ice chips as ordered or per institutional policy
- Providing oral care

Table 49-4 **SUGGESTED TIME FRAMES FOR SELECTED ASSESSMENTS**				
ASSESSMENT	**LATENT PHASE**	**ACTIVE PHASE**	**TRANSITION PHASE**	**SECOND STAGE**
BP, P, R	q 1 h	q 1 h	q 30 min	q 5 min
Temperature	q 4 h	q 4 h	q 4 h	
(if ROM)	q 2 h	q 2 h	q 2 h	
FHR	q 1 h	q 30 min	q 15 min	q 5 min
Contractions	q 1 h	q 30 min	q 15 min	continuously

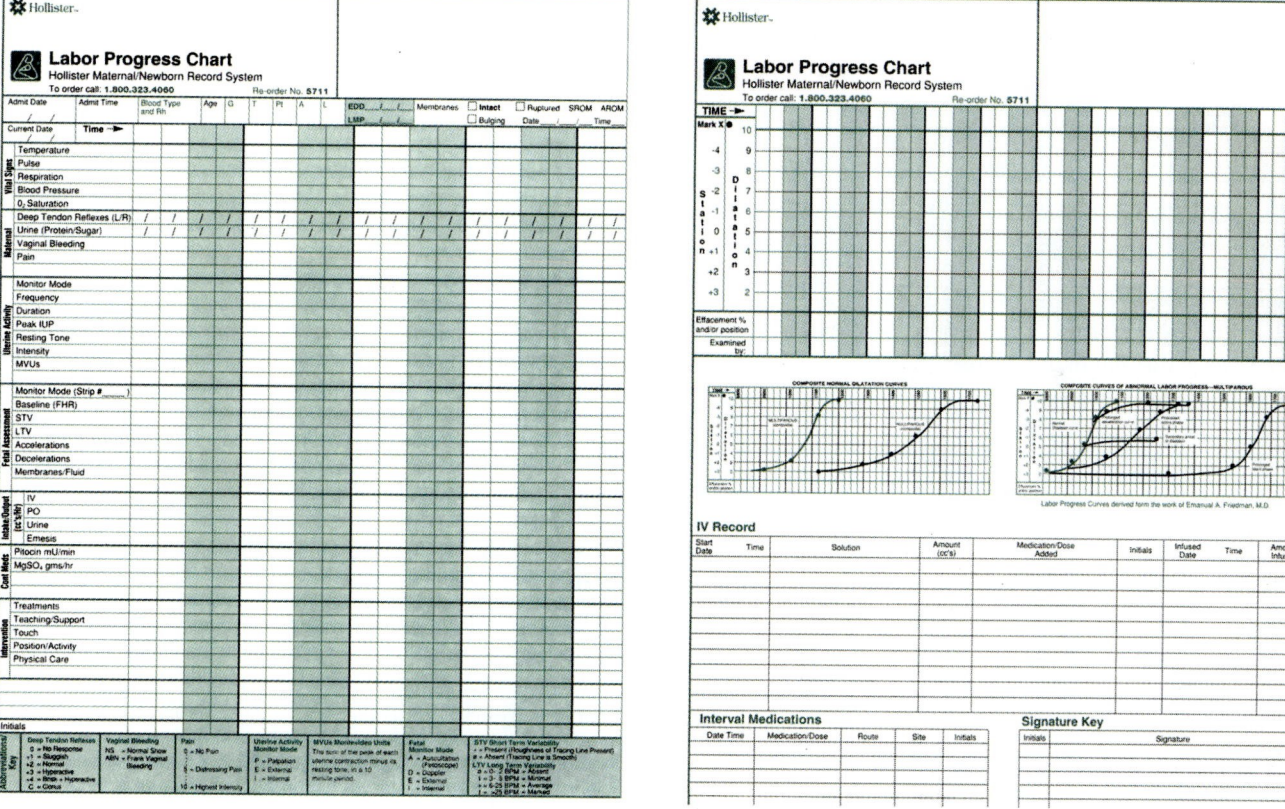

Figure 49-18 Representative Labor Progress Record (*Permission to use this copyright material has been granted by the owner, Hollister Incorporated.*)

- Assisting the client with frequent position changes, encouraging side-lying or upright positions
- Encouraging voluntary relaxation of specific muscle groups and the use of effleurage
- Suggesting the use of a cold washcloth on the forehead or nape of the neck
- Providing encouragement and praise
- Keeping the client informed of progress
- Checking the client's bladder and encouraging urination every 2 hours
- Giving back rub or applying counterpressure to sacrococcygeal area
- Assisting the client in walking and using a shower or Jacuzzi
- Offering the client analgesics as ordered

Hygiene Measures If showers or Jacuzzis are available and are not contraindicated for the client, their use should be offered to the client. The discomfort of labor is often reduced by these measures. Bed linens should be kept clean and dry. Linen savers should be changed frequently.

Ambulation and Position Ambulation may increase uterine activity, provide distraction from the discomforts of labor, and enhance maternal control of the situation. The client should be encouraged to walk only if the membranes are still intact, the presenting part is engaged after ROM, and if she has not had pain medication.

The side-lying position promotes utero-placental blood flow (and thus fetal oxygenation) and renal blood flow. If the client wants to lie on her back, a pillow can be placed under one hip to keep the uterus from compressing the aorta and vena cava. Both the squatting position and the hands-and-knees position seem to facilitate an occiput posterior fetal position to rotate to an anterior position.

Food and Fluid Intake Clear liquids and ice chips are usually all that is offered to clients in labor. Because regional anesthesia has almost replaced general anesthesia in childbirth, the risk of aspiration is also almost eliminated and the practice of giving clear liquids only is being challenged (Lowdermilk et al., 1999).

In some facilities, IV fluids are started on every client. It is very important to keep an accurate I & O when IV fluids are running because of the danger of hypervolemia.

Elimination The client should be encouraged to void every 2 hours. A distended bladder may impede descent of the presenting part, cause undue discomfort to the client, and lead to bladder atony after the birth.

If allowed, getting up to go to the bathroom may be the easiest for the client. Sitting on a bedpan at the edge of the bed with feet on a chair may be the next best option.

Catheterization may be required if the client cannot void and the bladder is distended. The vulva and perineum must be thoroughly cleaned to remove any amniotic fluid and bloody show before catheterization. If the catheter cannot be inserted, the presenting part is probably compressing the urethra; the procedure must be discontinued and the RN or CNM/physician notified.

Because of the decrease in intestinal motility, most women do not have a bowel movement during labor. However the pushing and birth of the infant during the second stage of labor may cause some stool to be expelled from the rectum. This should be cleaned immediately and the client reassured that this is a normal and expected occurrence.

Assisting Client and Support Person

The support person many times is the father, but it may be another woman or man. The person the mother has chosen to be the support person should be treated with the same respect as the mother, regardless of the relationship to the mother or the fetus.

The client who has participated in childbirth preparation classes with a support person already has some skills and a plan for coping with labor and birth. The nurse should determine what that plan is and assist, as needed, in carrying out that plan.

The client and support person who have not attended childbirth preparation classes should be taught the various techniques of coping with labor during the latent phase of labor. The nurse may actually provide more of the supportive care in this situation.

Breathing Techniques Three different breathing patterns are used. The first pattern is used until it is no longer effective, then the next pattern is used. Each breathing pattern begins and ends with a deep cleansing breath, with inhalation through the nose and exhalation through pursed lips, moving only the chest. The breathing techniques:

- Provide adequate oxygenation of mother and fetus,
- Provide a focus of attention,
- Decrease pain and anxiety, and
- Increase mental and physical relaxation.

These breathing patterns are used only during a uterine contraction. Between contractions, breathing returns to the woman's regular breathing pattern.

Slow, Deep Chest Breathing For this pattern, the client takes a cleansing breath, then inhales through the nose and exhales through pursed lips, 6 to 9 breaths per minute. At the end of the contraction, she takes another cleansing breath. It takes concentration to breathe this slowly.

Shallow Breathing A cleansing breath is taken first. The client inhales and exhales through the mouth about 4 times every 5 seconds. This may be increased to 2 breaths per second, usually at the peak of a contraction.

Pant-Blow Breathing The pant-blow breathing is generally used when the contractions become very intense. This pattern is very similar to the shallow breathing except that every three or four breaths a forceful exhalation (blow) is made through pursed lips. A cleansing breath is taken at the beginning and end of the contraction. It takes great concentration to maintain this pattern during a contraction.

All clients should be kept informed of their progress in labor. Positive feedback to the client and support person regarding how they are coping with the labor process is also important.

If siblings are to be present for labor and the birth, another person should be there to watch over the children and provide them with explanations, diversions, and comfort as needed. Neither the support person nor the nurses should be responsible for the children. Their focus should be on the client.

Providing Pharmacologic Comfort Measures

The nonpharmacologic comfort measures may be all that is needed for some women in labor. For other women, the increasing discomfort interferes with their ability to relax, use the breathing techniques appropriately, and maintain a sense of control. Pharmacologic comfort measures include systemic medications, regional blocks, and general anesthesia.

Systemic Medications Systemic medications should be administered only if:

- The client is willing to receive them and her vital signs are stable,
- The fetus is at term, exhibits normal movement, has a FHR between 120 and 160 with no late or variable decelerations, and does not exhibit meconium staining of the amniotic fluid, and
- Contractions are well established with the cervix dilated at least 4 to 5 cm in a nullipara or 3 to 4 cm in a multipara, the presenting part is engaged, and no complications are identified.

Effect on the fetus depends on the dosage given, timing and route of administration, and the pharmacokinetics of the drug. The intravenous (IV) route is gen-

PROFESSIONAL TIP

Pain Relief Medications

Before receiving a medication, the client should understand the following:
- Type of medication
- Route of administration
- Expected effects of the medication
- Possible side effects of the medication
- Implications for the fetus/neonate
- Safety measures to be followed (e.g., stay in bed, have side rails up)

Table 49-5 PAIN MANAGEMENT DRUGS COMMONLY USED DURING LABOR

DRUG	ROUTE	ONSET	PEAK EFFECT	LASTING
Narcotic Analgesics				
meperidine	IV	30 sec	5 to 10 min	2 to 4 hr
(Demerol)	IM	10 to 15 min	40 to 50 min	2 to 4 hr
fentanyl citrate	IV	1 to 2 min	3 to 5 min	½ to 1 hr
(Sublimaze)	IM	7 to 10 min	20 to 30 min	1 to 2 hr
Narcotic Agonist-Antagonists				
nalbuphine hydrochloride	IV	2 to 3 min	30 min	3 to 4 hr
(Nubain)	IM	15 min	60 min	3 to 6 hr
butorphanol tartrate	IV	2 to 3 min	½ to 1 hr	2 to 4 hr
(Stadol)	IM	10 to 30 min	½ to 1 hr	3 to 4 hr
pentazocine lactate	IV	2 to 3 min	15 to 30 min	2 to 3 hr
(Talwin)	IM	15 to 20 min	30 to 60 min	2 to 3 hr
Narcotic Antagonist				
naloxone	IV	1 to 2 min	unknown	depends on dose
(Narcan)	IM	2 to 5 min	unknown	longer than IV
Analgesic Potentiators				
promethazine hydrochloride	IV	3 to 5 min	unknown	12 hr
(Phenergan)	IM	20 min	unknown	12 hr
hydroxyzine hydrochloride Z-track (Atarax, Vistaril)	IM only	unknown	unknown	4 to 6 hr

erally preferred over the intramuscular (IM) route because the drug's effect is faster and more reliable. Table 49-5 lists drugs commonly used for pain management during labor.

Regional Blocks There are several types of regional blocks that may be used during labor and/or birth, including epidural block, intrathecal block, local infiltration, and pudendal block.

Epidural Block An epidural block may be used for pain control during labor and birth. It may be a continuous or intermittent infusion of a local anesthetic drug through a catheter placed in the epidural space. A very small dose of morphine (Duramorph), fentanyl (Sublimaze), or sufentanyl (Sufenta) may be added to the local anesthetic drug for faster and longer-lasting relief of pain. Advantages are good pain control, yet the client can participate in the birth process and interact with her infant and support person. Disadvantages may include maternal hypotension, bladder distention,

epidural catheter migration, nausea and vomiting, pruritis, and delayed respiratory depression.

Intrathecal Block Intrathecal injection of an opioid analgesic such as fentanyl (Sublimaze), sufentanyl (Sufenta), or morphine (Duramorph) is a pain management option for labor that is gaining acceptance (Gorrie et al., 1998). A much smaller dose than is given systemically is injected into the subarachnoid space. Advantages are rapid onset yet no sedation, no hypotensive effect, and no motor block so the client may walk during labor. Disadvantages may include the short duration of action so that the client may require another injection and the inadequate relief of pain in late labor and during birth so that another pain relief measure is required.

Local Infiltration Local infiltration anesthesia of the perineum is achieved by injecting a local anesthetic into the perineum. This is used just before the time of

PROFESSIONAL TIP

Meperidine (Demerol) Use in Labor

When meperidine (Demerol) is given IM during labor, the birth of the infant should ideally occur in less than 1 hour after administration or more than 4 hours after administration (time of peak affect) to minimize respiratory depression of the neonate.

PROFESSIONAL TIP

Narcotic Agonist-Antagonists and Narcotic Antagonists Administration

The drugs nalbuphine hydrochloride (Nubain), butorphanol tartrate (Stadol), pentazocine lactate (Talwin), and naloxsone (Narcan) should not be given to substance-dependent clients because these drugs may precipitate withdrawal symptoms.

birth in preparation for performing an episiotomy, suturing a laceration, or when a pudendal block cannot be performed. Local anesthetics such as procaine hydrochloride (Novocain), chloroprocaine hydrochloride (Nesacaine), and tetracaine hydrochloride (Pontocaine), which metabolize rapidly, and bupivacaine hydrochloride (Marcaine), lidocaine hydrochloride (Xylocaine), mepivacaine hydrochloride (Carbocaine), which are more powerful and longer-acting, are often used. Advantages are that the procedure is technically uncomplicated and practically free of complications. A disadvantage is that a large amount of local anesthetic may be required.

Pudendal Block A **pudendal block** is the injection of a local anesthetic into the pudendal nerve to provide perineal, external genitalia, and lower vaginal anesthesia (Figure 49-19). The pudendal block may be performed during the transition phase of the first stage or the second stage of labor. The advantage is that there are no changes in maternal vital signs or the FHR. Disadvantages may include rectal puncture, sciatic nerve block, or a hematoma.

General Anesthesia Because general anesthesia involves loss of consciousness, it is rarely used in vaginal births. It may, however, be used for cesarean births, especially in emergency situations. The greatest danger is fetal depression because most general anesthetics reach the fetus in about 2 minutes.

RISKS OF LABOR AND BIRTH

Most labors and births proceed as expected. However, there are complications that may be anticipated and some that happen unexpectedly. The most common risks—preterm labor and birth, premature rupture of membranes, dystocia, abnormal duration of labor, and prolapsed cord—are discussed.

Preterm Labor and Birth

Preterm labor is the onset of regular contractions of the uterus that cause cervical changes between 20 and 37 weeks of gestation. **Preterm birth** is a birth

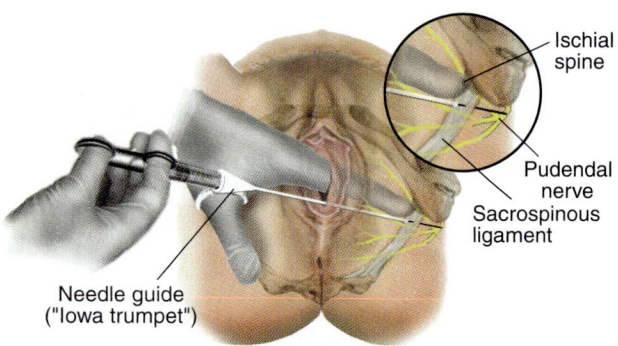

Figure 49-19 Pudendal block provides anesthesia to the perineum, external genitalia, and lower vagina.

Labels in figure:
Ischial spine
Pudendal nerve
Sacrospinous ligament
Needle guide ("Iowa trumpet")

LIFE CYCLE CONSIDERATIONS

Risks of Labor and Birth

- Adolescents (under age 15) have a greater risk of preterm labor, prolonged labor, and dystocia related to the small size of the pelvis because they have not yet reached bone growth maturity, which results in cephalopelvic disproportion (CPD).
- Mature women (over age 35) have a greater risk of preterm labor, longer labor, cesarean birth, and dystocia related to fetal anamolies.

(Lowdermilk et al., 1999)

that takes place before the end of the 37th week of gestation. Only about half of the time can a precipitating cause be identified. The single most important factor predisposing to preterm labor and birth is having already had a preterm birth. Other factors often associated with preterm labor and birth include premature rupture of the membranes (PROM), multiple gestation, bacterial vaginosis, intraamniotic infection, bleeding, and uterine/cervical abnormalities (Simpson, 1997).

Most women in preterm labor are admitted to the hospital for further evaluation. A urine specimen is examined for evidence of a urinary tract infection. Cervical or vaginal secretions are obtained during a sterile speculum examination to culture for *Chlamydia trachomatis,* group B streptococcus, or gonococcus infections.

If contractions are continuing and cervical changes are occurring, tocolytic agents may be prescribed. **Tocolytic agents** are medications that inhibit contrac-

HOME HEALTH CARE

Preterm Labor

- Follow instructions regarding activity limitation.
- Monitor uterine contractions 2 to 3 times a day for 30 minutes to 1 hour.
- Count fetal movements as instructed.
- Practice relaxation techniques.
- Drink 8 to 10 (8 oz) glasses of fluids each day.
- Empty bladder frequently.
- Avoid smoking, alcohol, and nontherapeutic drugs.
- Limit caffeine intake (colas, coffee, tea, chocolate).
- Avoid activities that can stimulate labor (e.g., nipple stimulation, any sexual activity that causes orgasm).
- Take medications as prescribed.
- Keep appointments with CNM/physician.

tions. The most commonly used are ritodrine (Yutopar), terbutaline (Brethine), and magnesium sulfate. A corticosteroid may also be given to accelerate fetal lung maturation. There is greater fetal benefit if at least 24 hours elapse between the first dose and the birth.

If contractions subside and cervical dilatation and effacement remain the same, the client may be discharged with instructions to limit activities and medication to prevent labor.

Premature Rupture of Membranes

When the membranes rupture before labor begins, it is called premature rupture of membranes (PROM). This is the most common cause of preterm labor and occurs in 2% to 18% of pregnancies (Varney, 1997). Contractions usually begin within 24 hours when the client is at term. In pregnancies of 28 to 34 weeks' gestation, labor may not start for a week or more.

In most cases of PROM, the cause is unknown. Besides preterm labor and birth, PROM can result in prolapse of the cord and intrauterine infection. A positive identification of amniotic fluid is made by observation of amniotic fluid escape from the cervix during a sterile speculum examination, a positive nitrazine test, or the presence of ferning when the fluid is viewed under a microscope (Gilbert & Harmon, 1998). The client may be hospitalized until after the birth of the infant, or if there are no signs of infections or fetal distress, she may be sent home. If hospitalized, continuing assessments include maternal vital signs; FHR; fetal movements; vaginal discharge for odor, color, and amount; and palpation of the uterus for tenderness.

Dystocia

Dystocia is a long, difficult, or abnormal labor caused by any of the four major variables (4 Ps) that affect labor. The following may be causes:

- Dysfunctional labor: ineffective contractions or maternal pushing efforts (powers)
- Pelvic structure variations (passage)
- Fetal variations: anomalies, abnormal presentation or position, very large size, or number of fetuses (passenger)
- Mother's responses: related to preparation for childbirth, past experiences, culture, and support persons (psyche)

Dysfunctional Labor

Dysfunctional labor is a labor with problems of the contractions or with maternal bearing-down efforts. The contractions may be hypertonic or hypotonic.

Hypertonic Uterine Contractions Hypertonic uterine contractions, usually occurring in the latent phase of labor, are very frequent and uncoordinated

HOME HEALTH CARE

Premature Rupture of Membranes

- Stay in bed, lying on either side, except to go to the bathroom (or as instructed).
- Take temperature every 4 hours when awake.
- Count fetal movements daily (report if less than 4 in 1 hour or an abnormal increase).
- Be aware of uterine contractions; if frequency is less than 10 minutes, notify CNM/physician.
- Use good perineal hygiene (e.g., wipe from front to back).
- Report any foul-smelling vaginal discharge or uterine tenderness.
- Take showers or sponge baths, not a tub bath.
- Avoid breast stimulation, sexual stimulation, and sexual intercourse.

and have an increased resting tone. The mother has discomfort out of proportion to the intensity of the contractions, which do not dilate or efface the cervix. The excessive pain results from anoxia of the uterine muscle cells. A prolonged latent phase is generally the result.

The client may become fatigued and dehydrated and may express fear that she is losing control with the lack of progress. The fetus may experience distress because the hypertonic contractions and increased resting tone of the uterus interfere with uteroplacental blood flow. The increased and prolonged pressure on the fetal head may cause excessive molding, caput succedaneum, or cephalhematoma (discussed in Chapter 51).

Bed rest and analgesics such as morphine sulfate or meperidine hydrochloride (Demerol) are given to relieve pain, promote relaxation, and induce sleep. When the client awakens, uterine contractions are often normal and labor proceeds.

Hypotonic Uterine Contractions Hypotonic uterine contractions, also called uterine inertia, usually occur in the active phase of labor. After normal progress through the latent phase of labor, the contractions become weak and inefficient in the active phase and may even cease. Common causes are cephalopelvic disproportion (CPD) (discussed later), malposition of the fetus, an overstretched uterus from multiple fetuses, a fetus of very large body size, hydramnios, or grand-multiparity (having delivered more than six infants).

The risks for the mother include intrauterine infection, especially if the membranes are ruptured and labor is prolonged; postpartum hemorrhage due to inefficient uterine contractions after birth; exhaustion; and decreased coping ability. The fetus may experience distress because of the length of labor and sepsis from maternal pathogens ascending the birth canal.

An ultrasound is usually performed to rule out CPD. If all factors are normal, one or more measures for augmentation of (increasing) labor are instituted, including ambulation, enema, amniotomy, nipple stimulation, and oxytocin infusion (discussed later) (Varney, 1997).

Amniotomy An **amniotomy**, artificial rupture of membranes (AROM), is performed by the CNM/physician. Several linen savers and a folded bath towel are placed under the client to absorb the amniotic fluid. A disposable plastic hook is generally used (Figure 49-20). A vaginal examination is performed to determine dilatation, effacement, presenting part, and station, and FHR is assessed to determine that the fetus is doing well. If the presenting part is not engaged or if the presentation is not cephalic, the risk of a prolapsed cord is high and the amniotomy is generally not performed.

After an amniotomy, the FHR must be assessed for 1 full minute. A monitor pattern that is nonreassuring or has any significant changes must be promptly reported to the CNM/physician. If the cord is compressed, the FHR is usually less than 100 beats/minute becoming even less during contractions. Amniotic fluid odor, color, and quantity are documented. The fluid should be clear (sometimes flecks of vernix are present) with a mild odor. Greenish meconium-stained fluid may indicate placental insufficiency. Foul-smelling fluid or fluid with a strong odor with a cloudy appearance or yellow color often indicates chorioamnionitis. Maternal temperature should be taken every 2 hours after ROM and any elevation above 38°C (100.4°F) reported to the CNM/physician.

Maternal Bearing-Down Efforts Analgesia and/or anesthesia may block Ferguson's reflex and thus decrease the effectiveness of maternal bearing down. Lack of sleep, a long labor, inadequate hydration, and maternal position may also have an adverse effect on the mother's bearing-down efforts.

Pelvic Structure Variations

A woman with a small or abnormally shaped pelvis may experience a long and difficult labor. Only about 50% of women have the pelvic shape (gynecoid) most conducive to labor, fetal descent, and birth (Gorrie et al., 1998).

A distended bladder reduces the space available in the pelvis and is an obstruction to fetal descent. This greatly increases the client's discomfort. Other, less common obstructions are uterine fibroids or pelvic cysts.

Fetal Variations

Variations of the fetus that may cause dystocia include the following:

- Anomalies
- Abnormal presentation or position
- Size
- Number of fetuses

Anomalies Fetal anomalies such as hydrocephalus may prevent descent of the fetus. Anomalies are often discovered by an ultrasound during pregnancy. If a vaginal birth is not advisable or not possible, a cesarean birth is scheduled.

Abnormal Presentation or Position A cephalic presentation other than vertex makes a larger diameter of the fetal head move through the birth canal. Labor generally takes longer and is more difficult.

In a breech presentation, cervical effacement and dilatation are often slower because the buttocks are softer than the head and do not put firm pressure on the cervix to aid in dilatation. Following are risks to the fetus born in a breech presentation:

- Cord compression
- Aspiration of fluids in the vagina
- Head becoming stuck

External version (manipulation of the fetus through the mother's abdomen to a presentation facilitating birth) may be tried to change the presentation to cephalic.

It is not always possible to change the presentation of the fetus. Figure 49-21 illustrates the birth of a fetus in a complete breech presentation.

A position of occiput posterior or occiput transverse can contribute to dysfunctional labor. Labor is generally longer and causes more discomfort because the head has farther to rotate during internal rotation. Many women describe severe back pain and have leg pain on the side where the head is positioned. A change in the mother's position may promote rotation of the fetal head. When the mother's abdomen is de-

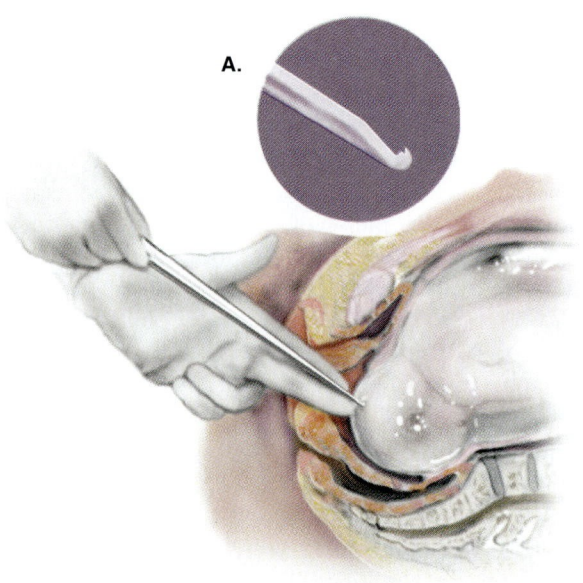

A.

B.

Figure 49-20 A. Disposable plastic hook to rupture membranes; B. Technique for rupturing membranes

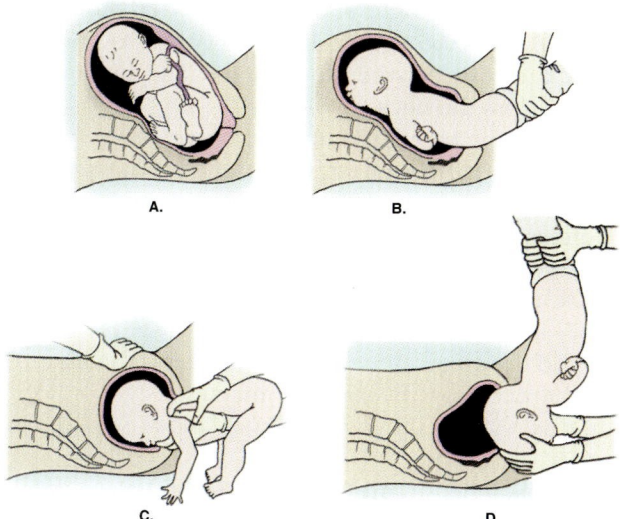

Figure 49-21 Birth of Fetus in Complete Breech Presentation: A. Descent and internal rotation; B. Extension of fetal back under symphysis (towel on legs used for traction); C. CNM/physician maintains head flexion by putting pressure on lower face with fingers of left hand (suprapubic pressure is applied by assistant to keep fetal head flexed); D. Assistant holds fetal legs with towel while CNM/physician assists the face and head over the perineum.

pendent to her spine, as in the hands-and-knees position, fetal rotation is encouraged (Figure 49-22).

Size An infant weighing more than 4,000 g (8.8 lb) is said to be **macrosomic**—having a very large body size. This may cause problems for a vaginal birth. As long as the mother's pelvis is of a size and shape to accommodate an infant this size, there is no problem. When the fetal head will not fit through the mother's pelvis, it is called **cephalopelvic disproportion** (CPD). The cause can be either fetal or maternal. The fetal head may be abnormally large and the mother's pelvis of normal size and shape, or the fetal head may be of average size and the mother's pelvis small or abnormally shaped. Whatever the cause, a cesarean birth is required.

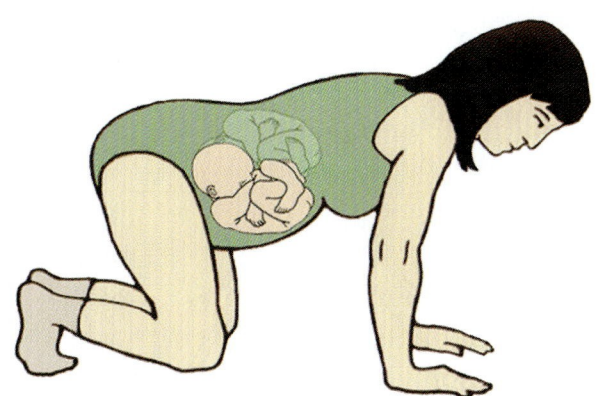

Figure 49-22 Fetus tends to rotate from occiput posterior to occiput anterior when mother is in a hands-and-knees position.

Number of Fetuses When more than one fetus is present, the uterus is overdistended. One or more of the fetuses may be in a presentation less desirable than vertex. Twins often have a cesarean birth, and when there are three or more fetuses, birth is almost always cesarean (Gorrie et al., 1998).

Mother's Responses

The mother's perception of labor is more important than her actual experience in labor. Tales from family and friends, a bad experience with a previous labor, and cultural expectations can add to the stress of labor. Excessive or prolonged stress experienced by the woman in labor may interfere with the progress of labor in several ways:

- Secretion of catecholamines (epinephrine and norepinephrine) by the adrenal glands in response to stress inhibits uterine contractions and decreases blood supply to the uterus and placenta while increasing blood supply to the skeletal muscles.
- Tense abdominal and pelvic muscles make contractions less effective.
- Contractions working against tense abdominal muscles increase pain, which adds stress to the situation and makes the mother more anxious.

The nurse can help allay the client's fears by offering encouragement, answering her questions honestly, and offering tips on how to make labor more successful. For instance, the nurse might suggest a change of position to a squatting bar to aid in fetal descent, or may offer a mirror so the mother can see the baby crown and be encouraged by her progress.

Abnormal Duration of Labor

Labor may be prolonged or abnormally short (precipitate).

Prolonged Labor

Many of the conditions previously discussed, such as hypotonic uterine contractions, CPD, abnormal fetal presentations or positions, or early use of analgesics may cause prolonged labor. Labor progress in either the first or second stage may be prolonged or arrested (stopped). The plotting of cervical dilatation on a labor graph, as found in Figure 49-18, helps in identifying these situations. Once the cause of the prolonged labor is identified, the CNM/physician can take steps to remedy the situation. A possible course of action might be induction of labor, a forceps- or vacuum-assisted birth, or cesarean birth (all discussed later).

When the active phase of the first stage of labor lasts more than 15 hours, the risk of fetal death increases sharply (Lowdermilk et al., 1999). With prolonged labor, maternal morbidity and mortality may result from infection, uterine rupture, serious dehydration, and postpartum hemorrhage.

Precipitate Labor/Precipitate Birth

A labor lasting less than 3 hours from the onset of contractions to the birth of the infant is considered a **precipitate labor**. Although a precipitate labor may end with a precipitate birth, they are not the same. Possible maternal complications during a precipitate labor include a loss of coping ability; an increased risk of uterine rupture; lacerations of the cervix, vagina, and perineum; and postpartum hemorrhage. Possible fetal complications include hypoxia, distress, and cerebral trauma.

A **precipitate birth** is a birth occurring suddenly and unexpectedly without a CNM/physician present to assist. When a client says "the baby's coming" or words to that effect, the health care provider should always look to see whether she is correct. Most of the time a large part of the fetal head is visible, if not already crowning. In this situation the nurse should do the following:

- Stay with the mother.
- Call for assistance or send support person to get assistance. Other staff members can notify the CNM/physician.
- Remain calm and reassure mother.
- Open emergency birth pack.
- If time permits, scrub hands, put on sterile gloves, and place sterile drape under mother's buttocks.
- As the head crowns, instruct mother to pant.
- If membranes are still intact, tear the sac, allowing amniotic fluid to flow out.
- Apply gentle pressure to the fetal head with one hand to prevent it from popping out. *Do not hold the head back with force enough to prevent it from being born.*
- With the mother still panting, check at the back of the fetal head for the umbilical cord. If there is a **nuchal cord** (umbilical cord around the neck) and

it is loose enough, slip the cord over the baby's head. If it is too tight, place two clamps on the cord, cut the cord between the clamps, and unwind the cord from the neck.

- Suction the baby's mouth, throat, and nose.
- With one hand on each side of the head, push gently downward until the anterior shoulder comes under the symphysis. Then gently raise the baby's head so the posterior shoulder is born.
- Ask the mother to push gently to assist in the birth of the rest of the infant's body.
- Hold the infant at the level of the uterus, being careful not to drop the slippery infant.
- Again, suction the mouth, throat, and nose of the infant.
- Dry the infant to prevent heat loss and place the infant on the mother's abdomen. Cover with a dry blanket.
- Document on the birth record the fetal position, nuchal cord, time of birth, Apgar scores (addressed later in this chapter) at 1 and 5 minutes after birth, gender, time and method of placental expulsion, and mother's condition.

Prolapsed Cord

When the umbilical cord lies below the presenting part of the fetus, it is termed a **prolapsed cord**. Prolapse of the cord may occur anytime and may be hidden (occult, not visible) or visible (Figure 49-23). It most commonly occurs with ROM, either spontaneous rupture of membranes (SROM) or AROM, as the cord washes down with the amniotic fluid. This happens in 1 out of 400 births (Lowdermilk et al., 1999).

A cord below the presenting part is compressed between the fetus and the mother's pelvis, resulting in decreased blood flow to the fetus. The fetus will have bradycardia with variable decelerations during uterine

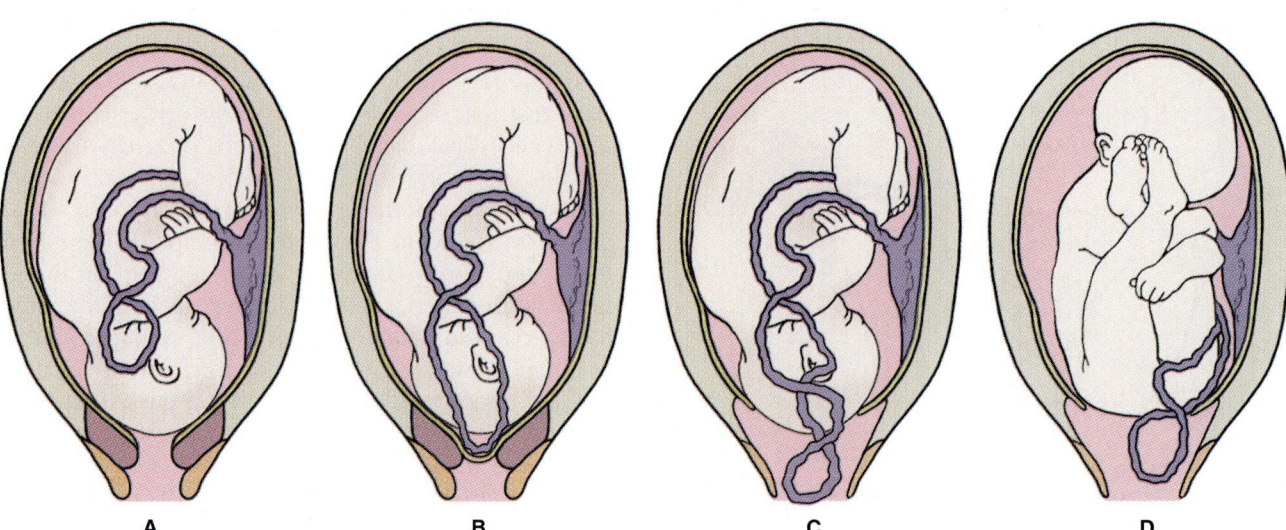

A.   B.   C.   D.

Figure 49-23 Prolapsed Cord: A. Hidden (occult, not visible); B. Prolapse with membranes still intact; C. Cord may be seen in vagina; D. Breech with prolapsed cord

contractions. Contributing factors include a long cord (greater than 100 cm or 40 in), unengaged presenting part, breech presentation, or transverse lie.

When a prolapsed cord is identified, pressure on the cord must be relieved immediately. The provider must call for assistance, don a sterile glove, insert 2 fingers into the vagina, and put pressure on the presenting part to relieve the compression of the cord. The client can then be assisted into a modified Sims' position with her hips up on pillows, the knee-chest position, or place the bed in Trendelenburg position. In these positions, gravity keeps the pressure of the presenting part off the cord (Figure 49-24). Occasionally, a vaginal birth may be possible, but generally a cesarean birth is preferred.

INDUCTION/AUGMENTATION OF LABOR

Induction of labor and augmentation of labor both relate to the stimulation of uterine contractions, but at different times in the labor process.

Induction of Labor

Induction of labor is the stimulation of uterine contractions *before* they begin spontaneously for the purpose of birthing an infant. Both chemical and mechanical methods can be used to induce labor. The most common methods used in the United States are intravenous oxytocin and amniotomy. Induction of labor may be considered in situations of preexisting

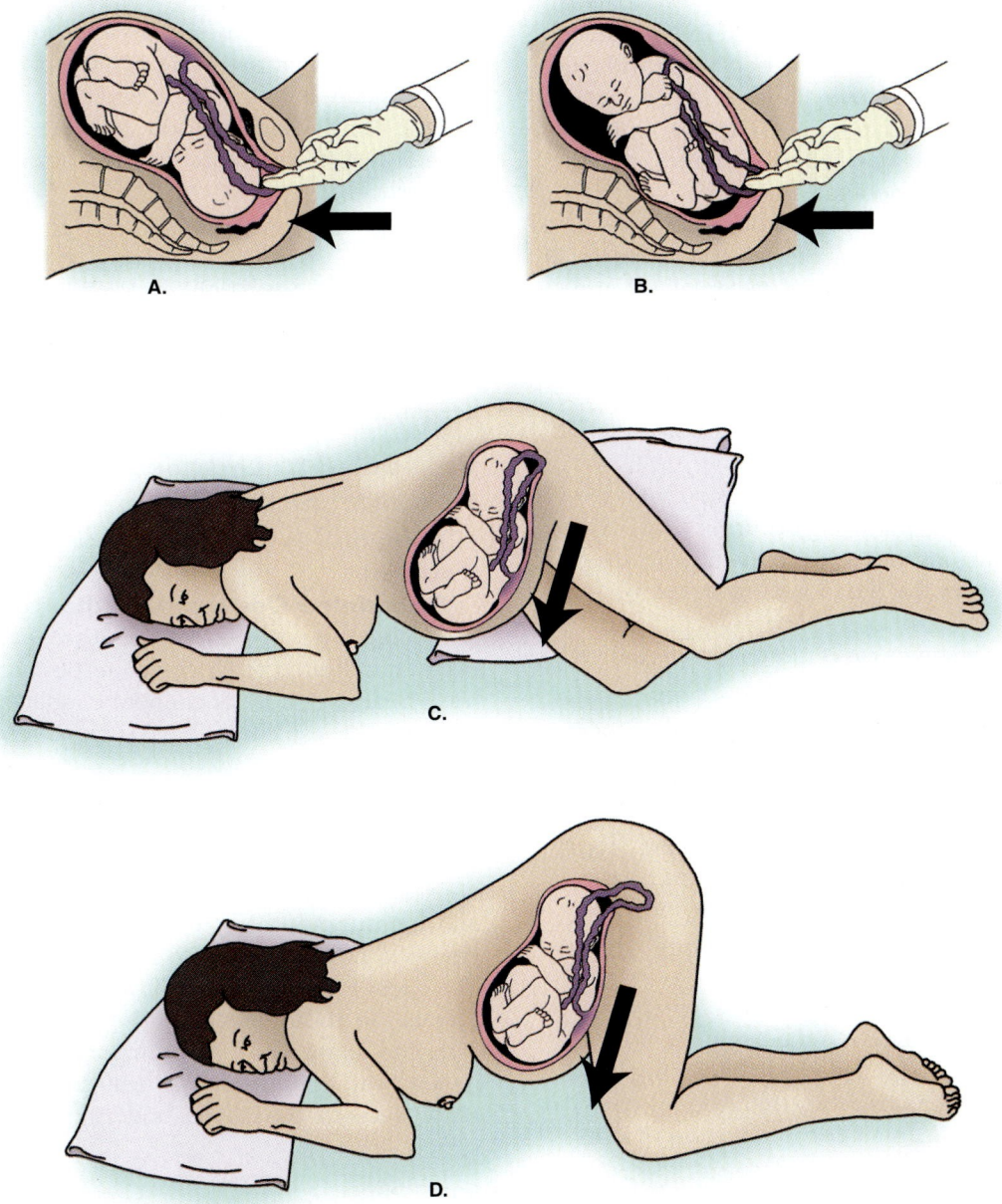

Figure 49-24 Examiner's fingers relieve pressure on prolapsed cord in (A) vertex presentation and (B) breech presentation; Gravity relieves pressure on prolapsed cord with mother in (C) modified Sims' position and (D) knee-chest position

maternal disease, PIH, PROM, postterm gestation, or fetal demise. Fetal maturity, especially lung maturity, must also be considered. Contraindications to induction are the same as those to spontaneous labor and vaginal birth (e.g., hydrocephaly, transverse lie).

If the cervix is "ripe" (soft), the probability of induction success is greater. If the cervix is not "ripe," prostaglandins are often used first to "ripen" the cervix. Dinoprostone (Prepidil) is often used, and the next day oxytocin infusion is begun. Frequently, oxytocin infusion and amniotomy are both used.

Oxytocin Infusion

A primary IV infusion of 1,000 mL of an electrolyte solution (e.g., lactated Ringer's) is started. A secondary infusion of 1,000 mL of the same solution is prepared with 10 units of oxytocin (Pitocin). The secondary infusion (with the oxytocin) is regulated by an infusion pump. The rate is very slow at the beginning with very small increases at regular intervals according to agency protocol or CNM/physician orders. The goal is to have contractions with a frequency 2 to 3 minutes, duration 40 to 60 seconds, and moderate intensity.

A fetal monitor is used to provide continuous data about FHR and contractions. Before each increase of the infusion rate, assessments of maternal BP and P, FHR (bradycardia or decelerations), and contractions should be made and documented. An intake and output record is maintained throughout the induction process.

Safety: Oxytocin Infusion
Discontinue the secondary infusion with the oxytocin if the following occur:
- Contractions are more frequent than every 2 minutes or the duration is more than 90 seconds
- Uterus resting tone is more than 20 mm Hg
- Fetal monitor shows:
  repeated late decelerations
  prolonged decelerations
  no variability
And then:
- Keep mother in side-lying position.
- Increase rate of primary IV fluid.
- Administer oxygen by face mask.
- Notify CNM/physician.

Augmentation of Labor

Augmentation of labor is the stimulation of uterine contractions *after* spontaneously beginning but the progress of labor is unsatisfactory. Intravenous oxytocin is used in the same manner as for induction of labor.

OBSTETRIC PROCEDURES

Sometimes a special obstetric procedure is needed to assist with the birth of an infant. These procedures

are cesarean birth, forceps-assisted birth, and vacuum-assisted birth.

Cesarean Birth

Cesarean birth is the birth of an infant through an incision in the abdomen and uterus. Indications for cesarean birth include placenta previa, placenta abruptio, CPD, prolapsed cord, breech presentation, active genital herpes, dystocia, pregnancy-induced hypertension, hydrocephaly, multifetal pregnancy, and repeat cesarean birth.

Incisions

The skin incision and uterine incision are not necessarily the same. The skin incision may either be transverse (Pfannenstiel) or vertical. The uterine incision may be vertical in either the upper uterus (classic) or lower uterine segment or transverse in the lower uterine segment (Figure 49-25). Which incisions are used are determined by the client and physician depending on the time factor, reason for the cesarean birth, client's desire for future pregnancies, and physician preference.

Anesthesia

Regional block, epidural, or spinal anesthesia are the most popular because the mother is awake and aware of the birth of her infant. When time is of the essence or when an epidural or spinal cannot be used, general anesthetic is used.

Scheduled or Unscheduled Cesarean Birth

A cesarean birth may either be scheduled or unscheduled.

Scheduled Cesarean Birth A cesarean birth is scheduled if it is to be a repeat cesarean birth, if labor is contraindicated (e.g., complete placenta previa, hydrocephaly), or if labor cannot be induced and birth is necessary. These clients have some time to prepare for the cesarean birth.

Unscheduled Cesarean Birth Unscheduled cesarean births are usually the result of some difficulty in the labor process. Besides concern about the situation causing the need for a cesarean birth, the client and her support person often experience a sense of failure at not being able to have the baby "normally." The client is generally tired from the labor process and forgets or misunderstands any explanations given. After the infant's birth, it is important for the client to review with the nurse the events prior to the cesarean birth to ensure the client's understanding of what happened.

Preoperative procedures must be performed quickly. Generally a Foley catheter is inserted to keep the bladder empty; an abdominal-mons surgical shave prep is completed; intravenous fluids are started (if not already running); blood and urine tests are ordered; and,

Skin incision   **Uterine incision**

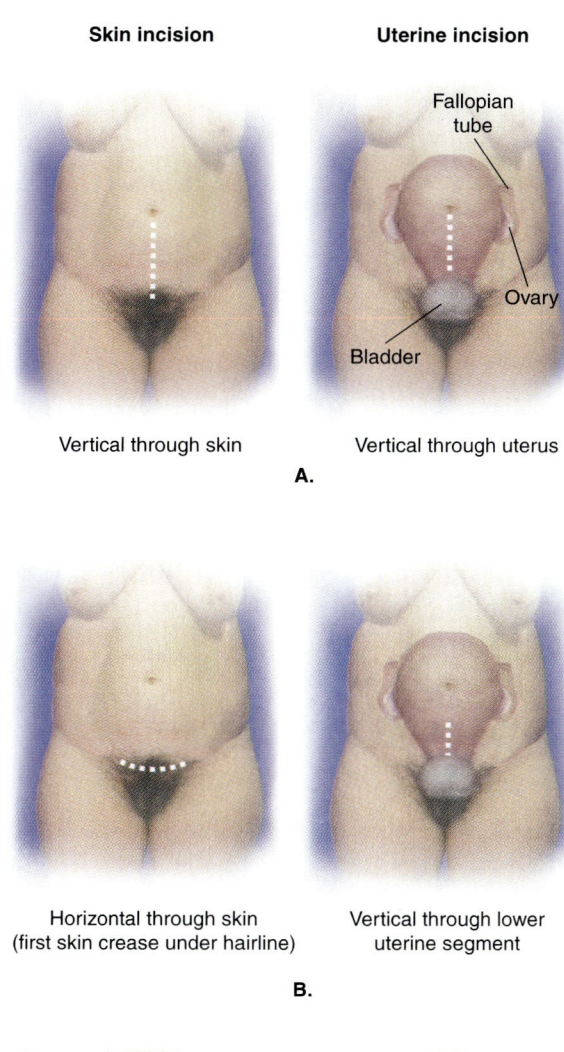

Vertical through skin   Vertical through uterus

A.

Horizontal through skin   Vertical through lower
(first skin crease under hairline)   uterine segment

B.

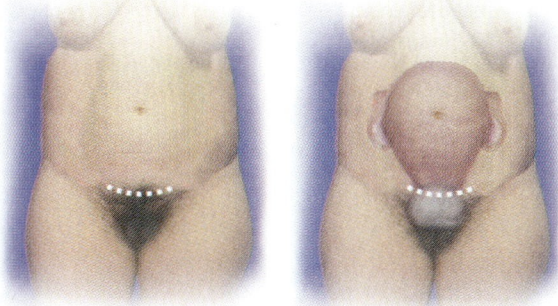

Horizontal through skin   Horizontal through lower
(first skin crease under hairline)   uterine segment

C.

Figure 49-25 Cesarean Birth: Skin and Uterine Incisions:
A. Classic, vertical skin incision with high uterine incision; seldom used except in emergency situation; B. Horizontal skin incision with low vertical uterine incision; C. Horizontal skin incision with horizontal uterine incision

if time is available, preoperative teaching may be instituted. The support person is encouraged to remain with the mother even in surgery to provide emotional support.

When the mother is awake during the cesarean birth, she is involved in seeing and holding her infant

just as in a vaginal birth, unless infant resuscitation is required. A pediatrician is usually present to care for the infant. It is extremely important to keep the mother informed about what is happening.

Vaginal Birth after Cesarean

When the reason for the initial cesarean birth is a nonrecurring situation such as placenta previa, prolapsed cord, or breech presentation, the client may be able to have a vaginal birth with the next pregnancy. If a low transverse uterine incision was made for the cesarean birth, a trial of labor is often recommended. If a classic uterine incision was made in the uterus, a trial of labor is contraindicated because the possibility of uterine rupture is very great. The possibility of a vaginal birth after cesarean (VBAC) is discussed throughout the pregnancy with the obstetrician.

Forceps-Assisted Birth

Forceps are metal instruments used on the fetal head to provide traction or to provide a method of rotating the fetal head to an occiput-anterior position. There are several types of forceps. Some forceps have fenestrated (open) blades and some solid blades, but they all have a locking mechanism that prevents the blades from compressing the fetal skull (Figure 49-26).

Forceps may be applied as:

- *Outlet forceps*—when head is crowning (Figure 49-27)
- *Low forceps*—when head is at +2 station or lower but not yet crowning
- *Midforceps*—when head is engaged but above +2 station

Indications

Any situation that threatens the mother or fetus that can be relieved by a vaginal birth is an indication for

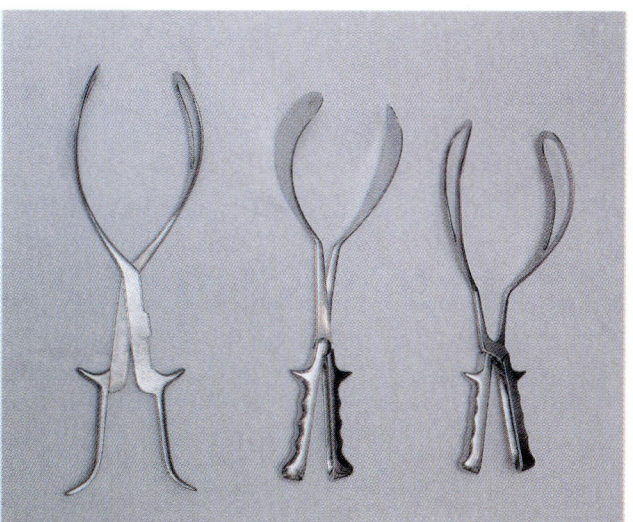

Figure 49-26 Types of Forceps

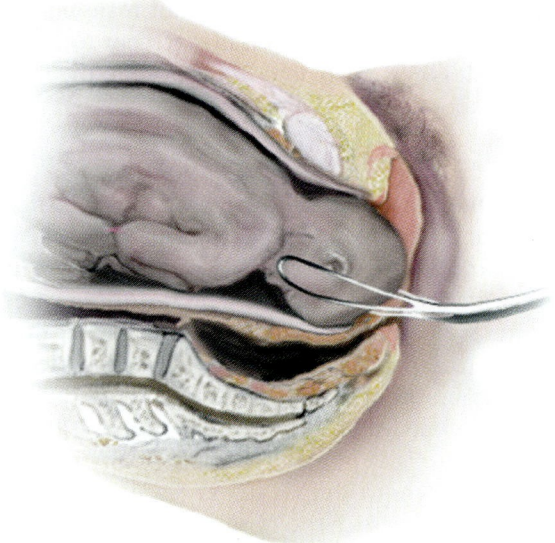

Figure 49-27 Outlet Forceps. Traction is applied downward and outward during contractions.

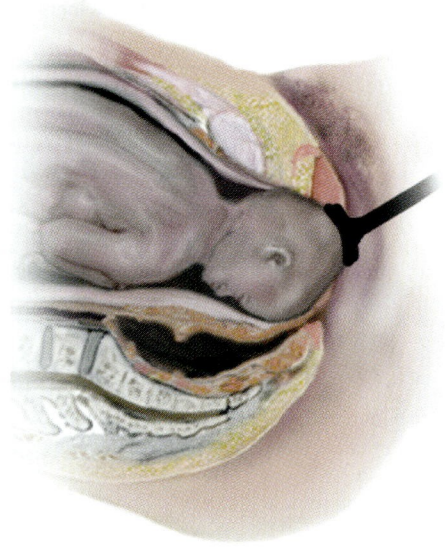

Figure 49-28 Vacuum-Assisted Birth

forceps use. Examples are an exhausted mother or one who has heart disease and a fetus in distress, in arrested rotation, or breech position (aftercoming head).

Application of Forceps

Before forceps are applied, the cervix must be completely dilated, membranes must be ruptured, and position and station of the fetal head must be known. The FHR must be checked, reported, and recorded *before* forceps are applied and again *after* forceps are applied to make sure the cord is not being compressed by the forceps. It may help the mother to understand about the forceps if it is explained that the forceps blades fit around the baby's head like two teaspoons fit around an egg (Lowdermilk et al., 1999). Traction is applied to the forceps only during contractions. Rotation is performed between contractions.

After the birth of the infant, the mother must be assessed for vaginal and cervical lacerations, hematoma, and bruising. The newborn infant may have facial bruising or edema.

Vacuum-Assisted Birth

A cup connected to suction is placed over the occiput on the fetal head. After the suction (negative pressure) is attained, traction downward and outward is applied during contractions (Figure 49-28). Indications are the same as for forceps-assisted birth.

Maternal risks include vaginal and rectal lacerations. Fetal risks include cephalhematoma, brachial plexus palsy, retinal and intracranial hemorrhage, and hyperbilirubinemia (O'Brian & Cefalo, 1996).

IMMEDIATE INFANT/ MOTHER CARE

During the first 20 to 30 minutes after the infant's birth, specific care is given to the infant and the mother.

 Infection Control: Standard Precautions
Disposable gloves should be worn when:
- Caring for the newborn until after the infant has received the initial bath,
- Assessing the amount of lochia and the perineum, and
- Cleansing the perineum.

Care of the Infant

Following are the immediate needs of the newborn infant:

- A—airway
- B—breathing
- C—circulation
- W—warmth

Identification of the infant is the top priority after the immediate needs are met.

Airway

The CNM/physician suctions secretions from the mouth and nose of the infant at the time of birth. Shortly thereafter, the infant takes the first breath and may begin to cry. The mouth and nose of the infant are suctioned by the nurse as needed to maintain an open airway. The bulb syringe must be compressed before inserting into mouth or nose of infant.

Breathing/Circulation

The infant's cardiopulmonary adaptation to extrauterine life is assessed by using the Apgar score (Table 49-6).

Each of the five items are assessed at 1 and 5 minutes after birth, providing a quick evaluation of how the heart and lungs are adapting. The five items to be assessed are arranged in priority from most important (heart rate) to least important (color). The infant is given a score, from 0 to 2, for each item. The five scores are then totaled.

When the Apgar score is 8 or higher, no special interventions are required. When the Apgar score is between 4 and 8, gentle rubbing of the infant's back for stimulation and administration of oxygen will usually result in an increase in the Apgar score at 5 minutes. It must be determined whether and when the mother received a narcotic for pain management during labor. Naloxone (Narcan) may be administered if the mother received a narcotic during labor.

When the Apgar score is between 0 and 4, the infant requires resuscitation. The infant must be kept on one side with the head flat or slightly elevated, as a head down position makes it more difficult to breathe because the intestines put pressure on the diaphragm.

Warmth

The infant must be dried to prevent heat loss by evaporation. A prewarmed radiant warmer is used while giving initial care. Skin-to-skin contact with a parent can also be used to provide warmth. A stockinette cap on the infant's *dry head* also helps prevent heat loss.

Identification

A set of four identification bands, two long and two short, imprinted with the same number are used. The mother's name, sex of infant, time of birth, and CNM/physician's name are written on each band. The two small bands are put on the infant (both ankles or a wrist and an ankle). The bands must fit the infant snugly but not too tightly (Figure 49-29).

Table 49-6 APGAR SCORE			
ITEM ASSESSED	**SCORE**		
	0	**1**	**2**
Heart rate	Absent	Slow (< 100)	Over 100
Respiratory rate	Absent	Slow, weak cry	Good cry
Muscle tone	Flaccid	Some flexion of extremities	Well flexed
Reflex irritability	No response	Grimace	Cry
Color	Blue, pale	Body pink, extremities blue	Completely pink (light skinned); absence of cyanosis (dark skinned)

A long band is applied to the mother's wrist. The other long band is usually applied to the father's wrist or other person serving as primary support. In multiple births, the mother and father have a band for each infant.

Most hospitals also footprint the newborn infant and either fingerprint or thumbprint the mother. The soles of the infant's feet must be dried and any vernix caseosa removed before footprinting.

Care of the Mother

If an oxytocic medication is to be given when the placenta is delivered, the blood pressure is taken both before and after the medication is administered. Maternal blood pressure is monitored every 5 to 15 minutes. The oxytocic medication may increase the BP. Excessive blood loss will cause the BP to fall.

The fundus of the uterus is palpated for firmness. It should be firm, about the size of a grapefruit, in the midline, below the umbilicus. The proper method of palpating the uterus is illustrated in Figure 49-30.

After the CNM/physician has completed repairing

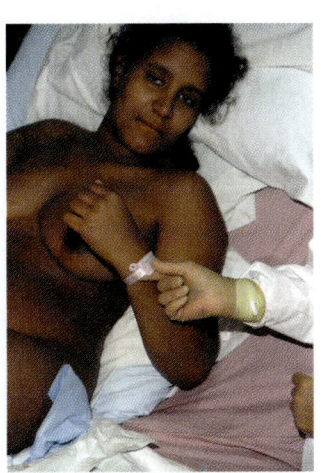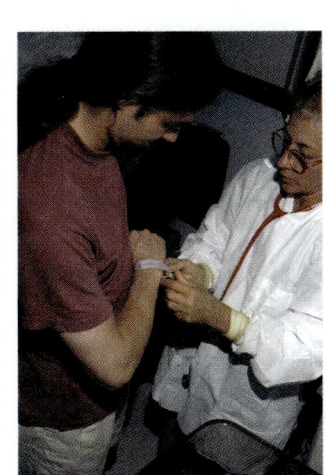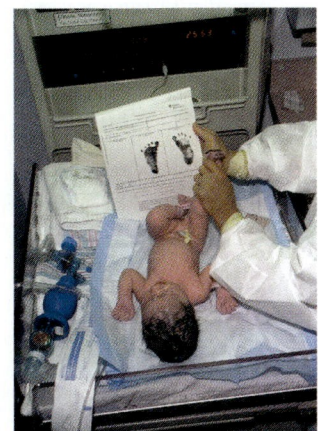

Figure 49-29 Matching identification bands are placed on infant, mother, and partner; infant is footprinted.

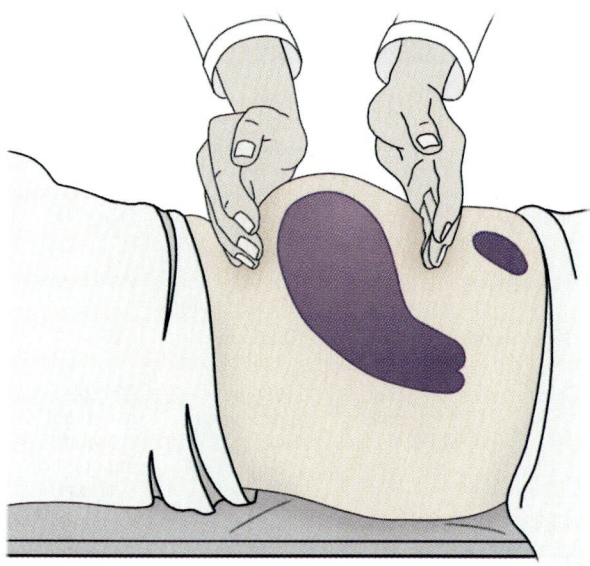

Figure 49-30 Palpation of Uterus after Delivery of Placenta

the episiotomy (if one was made) and/or any lacerations, the perineum is washed with warm sterile water and dried with a sterile towel. Maternity vaginal pads are then applied.

 Safety: Removing Legs from Stirrups
If legs were in stirrups during the birth:
- Two persons are needed to remove them,
- Each person places one hand under the knee and one under the heel (the mother generally has little control over leg movement),
- At the same time, both legs are lowered to the bed, and
- If the legs are numb, they may be bicycled to aid circulation return.

The mother may remain in the same bed (LDRP) or be moved to a recovery room bed. If the client is cold and begins to shiver, she should be covered with a warmed blanket, and a second blanket placed over it.

Mother, infant, and father or other support person are allowed time together to further the bonding and attachment process.

SAMPLE NURSING CARE PLAN

THE CLIENT IN LABOR

Anna Llanas, a 23-year-old gravida 1, para 0, is admitted in early labor. Her cervix is dilated 3 cm and is completely effaced. The fetus is at station 0. Contractions are every 5 minutes, duration 50 seconds, and of mild intensity. Her husband, Joe, is with her. They attended only the first 2 of the 6 childbirth preparation classes due to Joe's work schedule. Anna is tightly holding Joe's hand. Her voice is quivering as she says, "My water just broke. I'm scared. I don't know if I can do this. I've never done this before."

Nursing Diagnosis 1 *Anxiety related to the situational crisis of labor and the birthing process as evidenced by gravida 1, para 0, attended only first 2 childbirth classes, voice quivering, statement that she is scared and doesn't know if she can do this*

PLANNING/GOALS	NURSING INTERVENTIONS	RATIONALE	EVALUATION
Anna will express less anxiety within an hour.	Maintain calm and confident manner.	Provides verbal and nonverbal message that labor is a normal process.	Anna says she feels a little better and is now gently holding Joe's hand.
	Orient Anna and Joe to birthing room and explain admission procedure.	Allays feelings of anxiety regarding unfamiliar environment.	
	Determine Anna's and Joe's knowledge and expectation of labor.	Establishes a baseline for intervention and enhances their sense of control.	

continued

	Discuss the expected progress of labor and what will happen during the process.	Lessens anxiety associated with the unknown.	
	Involve Anna and Joe in decisions about care and share information on progress of labor.	Increases their sense of control.	
	Involve Joe in the care of Anna.	Strengthens Anna's ability to cope.	

Nursing Diagnosis 2 *Infection, Risk for, related to rupture of membranes as evidenced by statement "My water just broke."*

PLANNING/GOALS	NURSING INTERVENTIONS	RATIONALE	EVALUATION
Anna will show no evidence of infection.	Assess amniotic fluid's color, odor, amount, and presence of meconium.	May indicate intrauterine infection or fetal distress.	There are no signs of intrauterine infection or fetal distress.
	Monitor maternal vital signs and the FHR.	Evaluates for signs of infection and fetal distress.	
	Maintain Standard Precautions by following good handwashing technique, wearing gloves when providing perineal care to Anna, and using aseptic technique when indicated.	Prevents spread of microorganisms.	

Anna's vital signs are normal: T 98.6°F, P 84, R 20, and BP 114/70. FHR is 138. Anna reports back pain. Contractions are now every 3 to 4 minutes, duration 60 seconds, and of moderate intensity. The cervix is dilated 5 cm with station +1.

Nursing Diagnosis 3 *Pain related to increasing frequency, duration, and intensity as evidenced by contraction assessment*

PLANNING/GOALS	NURSING INTERVENTIONS	RATIONALE	EVALUATION
Anna will be able to cope with the discomfort.	Encourage Anna to change position frequently (every 30 minutes), using such positions as leaning forward when sitting or standing, side-lying, and hands and knees.	Shifts weight of fetus away from the back, relieving back pain; relieves strain and constant pressure; and helps fetus descend through pelvis.	Anna is able to handle the discomfort with Joe's help with focused breathing and by applying counterpressure to her back.

continued

	Instruct Anna and Joe to use focused breathing, effleurage, massage, sacral pressure, and conscious relaxation.	Increases relaxation and counteracts some of the discomfort.	
	Offer the use of shower or Jacuzzi.	Increases ability to relax. Heat interferes with transmission of pain impulses.	
	Palpate for distended bladder and encourage regular voiding (at least every 2 hours).	Prevents discomfort and the impediment of fetal descent.	
	Share with Anna and Joe about the progress in labor.	Increases willingness to continue when Anna knows efforts are having desired results.	
	Provide comfort measures such as oral care; ice chips; and cool, damp cloth to head or neck, and change damp gown and bed linens.	Relieves discomforts of dry mouth, diaphoresis, and leaking amniotic fluid.	
	Inform Anna about the pharmacologic pain relief measures available to her.	Gives Anna a sense of control when she can choose when to use medication for pain.	

Nursing Diagnosis 4 *Urinary Elimination, Altered, Risk for, related to sensory impairment as evidenced by progress of labor, station +1*

PLANNING/GOALS	NURSING INTERVENTIONS	RATIONALE	EVALUATION
Anna's bladder will not exhibit signs of distention.	Palpate Anna's bladder at least every 2 hours.	Identifies a full bladder when Anna is unable to feel the urge to void.	Anna voids every 2 hours.
	Encourage frequent voiding; catheterize if necessary.	Avoids bladder distention that may impede descent of fetus and result in trauma to bladder.	

Anna's cervix is now 8 cm dilated, station is +2. Contractions are every 2 to 3 minutes, duration 70 seconds, and strong intensity. She is very uncomfortable, requests the pain medication, and says, "I can't take it anymore." Joe is concerned and asks, "Is she alright?" FHR and maternal vital signs remain close to the admission assessment. Anna is given meperidine (Demerol) 50 mg IV. She is now resting well between contractions. In 30 minutes Anna's cervix is completely dilated, station is +3. She pushes spontaneously several times during each contraction. When she pushes her back stiffens, her arms push on the bed, and she holds her breath. Anna prefers a semi Fowler's position.

continued

Nursing Diagnosis 5 *Knowledge Deficit, Effective Pushing Technique related to lack of exposure to information since only attended first 2 classes as evidenced by posture during pushing and breath holding*

PLANNING/GOALS	NURSING INTERVENTIONS	RATIONALE	EVALUATION
Anna will push more effectively after instructions until birth of infant.	Teach Anna techniques to push more effectively.	Makes pushing more effective	In 30 minutes Anna and Joe have a 6 lb 10 oz (3,005 g) baby girl. The baby's Apgar scores are 8 at 1 minute and 9 at 5 minutes.
	During each contraction, Anna should do the following:		
	• Sit upright or squat	• Takes advantage of gravity; squatting slightly enlarges the pelvic outlet	
	• Flex chin on chest and curl over uterus	• Directs force of push into pelvis	
	• *With elbows bent,* pull on her flexed knees	• Provides more force to push	
	• Exhale and vocalize when she pushes	• Prevents Valsalva maneuver, which causes a decrease in placenta blood flow and thus oxygenation to the fetus	
	Observe Anna's perineum for crowning.	Keeps everyone informed of progress.	
	Allow Anna to rest between contractions (no unnecessary talking).	Allows Anna to gain strength for next contraction.	

CASE STUDY

Peggy Kazmierski, a 30-year-old gravida 4, para 3, has been in labor 3 hours. Her cervix is 7 cm dilated, station is −1. The fetus is in a vertex presentation, LOA position. When the membranes rupture during a strong contraction, the umbilical cord prolapses from the vagina, and the head is making the perineum bulge. Peggy begins to cry and asks, "What is happening? I feel something hanging out of me."

The following questions will guide your development of a nursing care plan for the case study.

1. What are the first actions the nurse should take?
2. What assessments should be made?
3. Identify two nursing diagnoses and goals for Peggy.
4. Identify appropriate nursing interventions for the diagnoses.

SUMMARY

- There are two theories relative to why labor begins: the mechanical theory and the hormonal theory.
- Signs of impending labor are lightening, Braxton Hicks contractions, cervical softening, bloody show, and rupture of membranes, and a sudden burst of energy.
- The four major variables that affect labor are known as the 4 Ps: passage, passenger, powers, and psyche.
- Labor is divided into four stages, which include first stage (dilatation and effacement), second stage (birth of baby), third stage (delivery of placenta), and fourth stage (recovery).
- The mechanisms of labor describe how the fetus moves through the maternal pelvis and birth canal.
- There are many cultural aspects of labor and birth for the nurse to consider when caring for a client from another culture.
- Standard Precautions must be kept in mind when caring for a client during labor and birth because of the many opportunities for contact with body fluids and blood.
- Contractions are assessed for frequency, duration, interval, and intensity.
- Pain management is an important nursing intervention with both nonpharmacological and pharmacological measures.
- The most common risks of labor and birth are preterm labor and birth, premature rupture of membranes, dystocia, abnormal duration of labor, and prolapsed cord.
- Obstetric procedures that may be required to assist with the birth of an infant are cesarean birth, forceps-assisted birth, and vacuum-assisted birth.

Review Questions

1. Fetal lie is:

   a. how deep the fetus's head had dropped into the pelvis.
   b. how long it takes for the fetus to move down the birth canal.
   c. the fetus's head being on the right or left side of the mother.
   d. the relation of the long axis of the fetus to that of the mother.

2. Which of the following measures should the nurse take when supporting a prepared couple during labor?

   a. Verbally encouraging them
   b. Staying with them all the time
   c. Taking FHR after each contraction
   d. Leaving them alone to do "their own thing"

3. It is important for the nurse caring for a client in labor to make sure the bladder is kept empty because a full bladder may:

   a. cause glucosuria.
   b. cause proteinuria.
   c. impede the progress of labor.
   d. make the mother's back ache more.

4. Following rupture of membranes, what is the most appropriate next action for the nurse to take?

   a. Listen to the FHR.
   b. Remove the wet linen.
   c. Time the contractions.
   d. Report the color and odor of the fluid.

5. A client is admitted for induction of labor with an oxytocic drug. She is 2 weeks past her EDB. Which of the following findings, if present, would it be essential to report to the CNM/physician before the oxytocic infusion is started?

   a. Low backache
   b. Regular contractions of 60 seconds' duration
   c. Irregular contractions of 20 seconds' duration
   d. A rise in blood pressure from 122/80 to 130/84

6. A client has an intravenous infusion running, to which oxytocin (Pitocin) has been added. Which of the following conditions would warrant immediate discontinuation of the intravenous infusion of Pitocin?

   a. Increase in bloody show
   b. Rupture of the membranes
   c. A contraction of 90 seconds' duration
   d. A fetal heart rate of 120 during a contraction

7. When monitoring the FHR during IV Pitocin induction, which of the following should be reported to the RN or CNM/physician?

   a. FHR consistently between 120 and 160
   b. Slowing of FHR to 118 during a contraction
   c. FHR of 172 during three consecutive contractions
   d. Increase in FHR from 132 to 140 during most contractions

8. The client in labor is encouraged to position herself on her side or with the head of the bed elevated to:

   a. prevent maternal hypotension.
   b. prevent maternal hypertension.
   c. reduce chance of nausea and backache.
   d. reduce the discomfort of the contractions.

9. Which of the following nursing observations would indicate the client was in the transitional phase of labor?

   a. Drowsiness, slow pulse, decrease in contractions

   b. Irritability, nausea/vomiting, perspiration on upper lip

   c. More frequent hypertonic contractions, severe pain, hypertension

   d. Contractions become intermittent with a longer relaxation phase, quietness

10. A client is having a precipitate birth. The most appropriate nursing action is to:

    a. stay with her and call for help.

    b. quickly move her to the delivery room.

    c. carefully monitor the FHR and contractions.

    d. assist her to change her position and breathe deeply.

Critical Thinking Questions

1. A client gravida 1, para 0 in labor is 7 cm dilated, station +1, and says that she wants to push. Her grandmother told her that she would have to push hard to have a baby so the client wants to push and get it over with. How should the nurse respond?

2. How does the care of the client change as she moves through the phases and stages of labor?

 WEB FLASH!

- Search the Web for organizations providing information about the labor and birth process. What type of information is available?
- Look on the Internet for alternative/complementary approaches to labor and delivery. What techniques can you find?

MAKING THE CONNECTION

Refer to the following chapters to increase your understanding of postpartum care:

- **Chapter 35, Nursing Care of the Client: Reproductive System**
- **Chapter 47, Prenatal Care**
- **Chapter 49, The Birth Process**

LEARNING OBJECTIVES

Upon completion of this chapter, you should be able to:
- *Define key terms.*
- *Describe the various aspects of family adaptation.*
- *Discuss the mother's physiologic changes after the birth of her baby.*
- *Describe the expected and unexpected emotional/behavioral changes in the new mother.*
- *Demonstrate the postpartum assessments for every new mother and the additional assessments for a mother who has had a cesarean birth.*
- *Discuss the possible postpartum complications of hemorrhage and puerperal infection, including endometritis, mastitis, and thrombophlebitis.*
- *Explain the advantages and disadvantages of the various methods of family planning.*
- *Plan and provide the care of a woman who has had a baby.*

KEY TERMS

afterpains
attachment
bonding
claiming process
colostrum
disseminated intra-
 vascular coagulation
dyspareunia
engorgement
engrossment
entrainment
involution
let-down reflex
lochia
mastitis
metritis

neonate
oophoritis
postpartum blues
postpartum
 depression
postpartum
 hemorrhage
postpartum
 psychosis
puerperal (postpar-
 tum) infection
puerperium
salpingitis
subinvolution
thrombophlebitis

INTRODUCTION

Postpartum period, or **puerperium**, is the term for the first 6 weeks after the birth of an infant. During this time the mother and family will experience many changes, including changes in the structure and function of a family. The mother and, if she has one, her partner begin to establish a relationship with their newborn infant and adjust their lives to include the newborn. The mother and partner must also redefine their own relationship. If there are siblings, they must adjust to their new place in the family structure and the newborn's claim on the time and love of the parents.

Many factors influence family adaptation, including previous experience with a newborn and the convenience of a support system. Previously, postpartum care was focused on the mother and newborn, but now the father or partner, siblings, and sometimes grandparents are included. This chapter explores the events of the postpartum period, including the various ways a family adapts to the newborn; the physiologic and psychosocial changes the mother experiences; preparation for discharge; health promotion; post-cesarean section care; and possible postpartum complications.

FAMILY ADAPTATION

Family roles and relationships must be reorganized with the birth of a baby. Bonding and attachment are the terms used to describe this process of becoming acquainted with the **neonate** (a newborn from birth to 28 days of life). The terms *bonding* and *attachment* are often used interchangeably, although they do have different meanings.

Bonding refers to a rapid process of attachment, parent to child only, taking place during the *sensitive period*, the first 30 to 60 minutes after the birth. The bonding is enhanced when parent and infant touch and interact with each other (Figure 50-1). Immediately after birth, the neonate generally is in a quiet, alert state and is ready for bonding and closeness.

Attachment, a long-term process that begins during pregnancy and intensifies during the postpartum period, establishes an enduring bond between parent and child and develops through reciprocal (parent to child and child to parent) behaviors. Becoming acquainted with the neonate is an important part of attachment. Touching, exploring, talking to, and using eye contact are all methods used to become acquainted.

The family identifies the infant's "likeness" to and the infant's "differences" from family members, and then the infant's unique qualities. This is often referred to as the **claiming process**.

Mother's Adaptation to Neonate

A mother's touch changes as she moves through a discovery phase with her infant. The mother usually begins by using her fingertips to explore her infant's face, fingers, and toes. This is called *finger-tipping*. The mother may then change to using her palm to stroke her infant's back, chest, arms, and legs. The

mother uses her arms to enfold and bring her infant close to her body (Figure 50-2). She may smooth her infant's hair and rub her cheek on the infant's cheek or head. A parent's intense interest and preoccupation in the newborn is termed **engrossment**.

Most mothers speak in a high-pitched voice spontaneously to their infants, seeming to know intuitively that infants respond to higher-pitched voices. Soon after birth, infants can distinguish their mother's voice from others.

Father/Partner's Adaptation to Neonate

A father or partner may also exhibit engrossment and display an intense interest in how the baby looks and responds (Figure 50-3). The father also has a desire to touch and hold his baby.

Research has shown that, for fathers and partners, variables other than being an active participant in the birth process are important in developing attachment to the newborn. They include the father or partner's relationship with his own parents, relationship with the infant's mother, and previous experience with children.

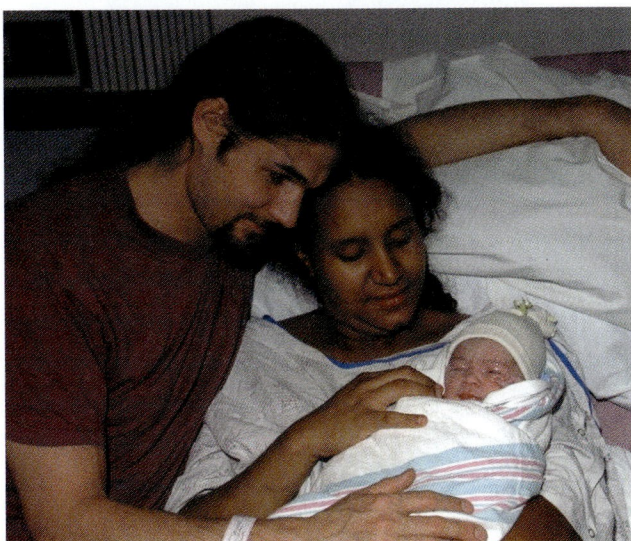

Figure 50-1 Bonding between Parents and Infant after the Birth

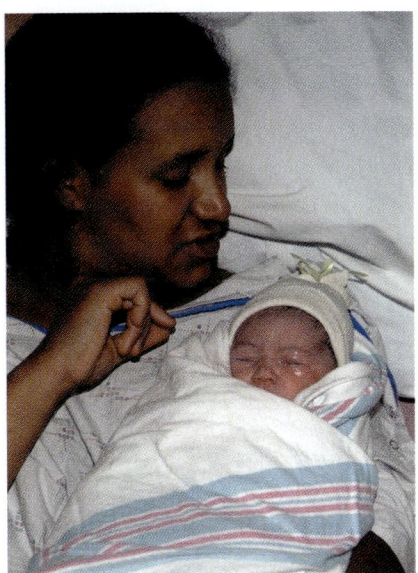

Figure 50-2 Mother Enfolding and Cuddling her Infant

LIFE CYCLE CONSIDERATIONS

Neonates' Reciprocal Behaviors

Neonates have the ability to:

• Make eye contact and move eyes to follow parent's face,
• Engage in intense, prolonged mutual gazing,
• Grasp parent's finger and hold on, and
• Move in rhythm to the parent's voice. This is called **entrainment**.

Most fathers want to be involved, but many lack confidence in caring for an infant. Tiller (1995) suggests that information about child care be presented, or reviewed if the father attended prenatal classes, after the infant is born. At this time the father is eager to learn because the information is now relevant.

Siblings' Adaptation to Neonate

The response of a sibling to the birth of a new sister or brother depends on age and developmental level of the older sibling. The adaptation is probably most difficult for toddlers, who often view the new baby as competition, someone who takes the parent's time and love. Negative behavioral changes may occur in the toddler, such as a return to thumb sucking or bed wetting; sleep problems; or hostility toward the mother, especially when she is caring for the new baby. Positive behavioral changes may be increased independence and taking an interest in the care of the newborn.

Parents' attitudes toward the newborn and their preparation of the siblings for the new arrival guide the older children's reactions. Parents can include each

child in the care of the baby according to their capabilities. For example, toddlers may be able to bring a clean diaper to the parent; preschoolers may help prepare for the baby's bath; and older children may hold, carry, or feed the baby (Figure 50-4).

Grandparents' Adaptation to Neonate

Grandparents go through a transition to grandparenthood just as parents go through a transition to parenthood. Practices and attitudes about childbirth and child rearing change from one generation to another as do the roles of men and women. The extent to which grandparents understand and accept the current practices and attitudes affects their relationship with their children and how supportive they may be (Figure 50-5).

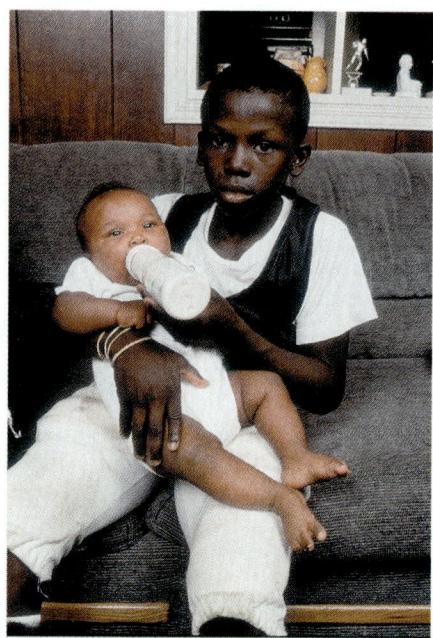

Figure 50-4 Older sibling can hold or help feed the baby.

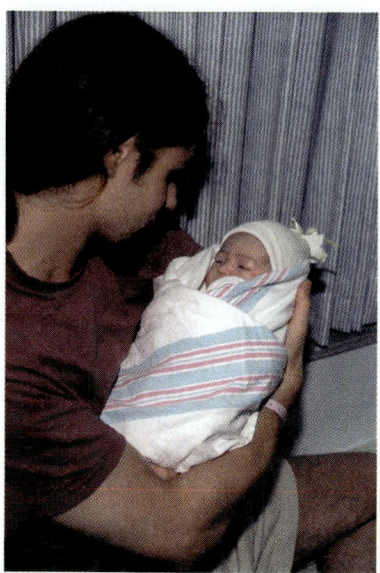

Figure 50-3 Father Displaying Engrossment

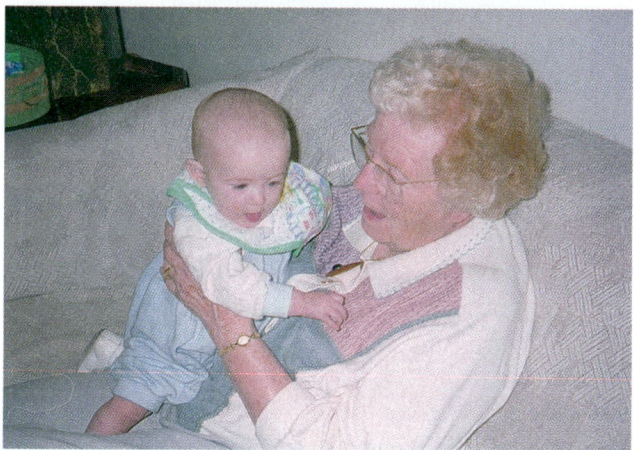

Figure 50-5 Grandparent Enjoying Grandchild

MATERNAL PHYSIOLOGIC CHANGES

Many of the physiologic changes postpartum (following birth) are a reversal of the changes in the various body systems that occurred during pregnancy. The initiation of lactation and reestablishment of normal menstrual cycles also occur.

Reproductive System

Changes occur in the uterus, cervix, vagina, and perineum.

Uterus

Involution is the return of the reproductive organs, especially the uterus, to their prepregnancy size and condition. There are three processes involved in involution:

- Muscle fiber contraction: With the uterus now empty, the uterus firmly contracts to control bleeding from the area of placental attachment; the muscle fibers gradually regain their former size and shape.
- Catabolism: The enlarged muscle cells of the uterus experience catabolic changes in protein cytoplasm that reduce the size of each cell. Catabolic products are excreted as nitrogenous wastes in the urine.
- Regeneration: The endometrium is regenerated within 2 to 3 weeks, except for the placental site, which is healed and regenerated by approximately 6 weeks.

Uterine Fundal Descent Following the birth, the uterus is about the size of a grapefruit with the fundus about halfway between the umbilicus and symphysis pubis. The fundus rises to the umbilicus in a few hours and stays there about 24 hours. Then the fundus descends about 1 cm, 1 finger breadth, each day for about 10 days when it is once again in the pelvis and unable to be palpated abdominally. A full bladder will push the uterus upward.

The contracting uterus may be a source of discomfort for some women after the infant's birth, especially for multiparas and those who are breastfeeding. Breastfeeding stimulates the release of oxytocin from the posterior pituitary, which stimulates strong uterine contractions as well as the "let down" reflex. These contractions are known as **afterpains**.

Lochia **Lochia** is the uterine/vaginal discharge after childbirth. It is initially bright red, then changes to a pink or pinkish brown, and then to a yellowish white. The odor of lochia is like a normal menstrual flow. A foul odor is indicative of infection.

For the first 3 days, the lochia is mostly blood with small pieces of decidua and mucus. This is called *lochia rubra*. About the fourth day the amount decreases and the color changes to a pink or pinkish brown called *lochia serosa*. It is mostly a serous exudate with cervical mucus, erythrocytes, and leukocytes. After the 10th day, the erythrocyte level decreases and the discharge becomes yellowish white, *lochia alba*. Now the lochia consists of leukocytes, epithelial cells, decidua, mucus, serum, and bacteria. This discharge may last for 6 weeks or more (Visness, Kennedy, & Ramos, 1997).

Cervix

Within 18 hours after birth, the cervix has become firm, has shortened, and has regained its shape (Lowdermilk, Perry, & Bobak, 1999). By the end of 2 weeks the cervical os is closed, but after delivery the opening is more like a slit than a circle.

Vagina and Perineum

The vagina was greatly stretched during labor. It takes 6 weeks for the vagina to complete involution and regain the contour it had prior to pregnancy. It never does regain the size it had prior to pregnancy. The vaginal mucosa is atrophic in lactating women, at least until menstruation returns. The reduced level of estrogen causes a decrease in vaginal lubrication, which may cause **dyspareunia**, or coital discomfort.

The stretching and thinning of the perineum during labor may cause edema and bruising of the perineum after the birth. Many women have an episiotomy (surgical incision of the perineum) before the infant's birth. Lacerations of the perineum also may occur. Both lacerations and episiotomies are classified according to the tissues involved and will take time to heal:

First degree: skin and mucous membrane

Second degree: skin, mucous membrane, and muscle

Third degree: skin, mucous membrane, muscle, and rectal sphincter

Fourth degree: skin, mucous membrane, muscle, rectal sphincter, and rectal mucosa

Even when the episiotomy or laceration is small, it can cause a great deal of discomfort because the muscles of the perineum are used when sitting, stooping, bending, squatting, walking, and defecating.

Endocrine System

After the expulsion of the placenta, the levels of the placental hormones estrogen, progesterone, human placental lactogen (hPL), human chorionic gonadotropin (hCG), and relaxin rapidly decline. The decrease in hPL, estrogen, and cortisol causes a reversal of the diabetogenic effect of pregnancy. This rapid change necessitates frequent assessment of the diabetic mother's blood glucose level.

Lactation

The rapid decline of the estrogen and progesterone levels allows the prolactin to initiate milk production within 2 to 3 days after the infant's birth. Oxytocin, a posterior pituitary hormone, causes the milk to be expressed from the alveoli into the lactiferous ducts. This is called "let down." The **let-down reflex** is a neurohormonal reflex; that is, either neuro (the mind) or the hormone (oxytocin) may initiate "let down." A breastfeeding mother hearing a baby cry or thinking about feeding her infant often stimulates the let-down reflex and milk will drip from the nipples (neuro). The release of oxytocin in response to the infant's sucking also stimulates the let-down reflex (hormonal). Many women describe a tingling/burning feeling in the breasts when the milk is "let down."

Menstrual Cycle

There is a great difference when ovulation and menstruation are reestablished based on whether the mother is breastfeeding or not breastfeeding. The level of follicle-stimulating hormone (FSH) is the same in both breastfeeding and nonbreastfeeding mothers. It is believed that the increased level of prolactin in breastfeeding mothers causes the ovaries to not respond to the FSH and ovulation does not occur (Bowes, 1996). The prolactin level remains high in breastfeeding women for approximately 6 weeks. The prolactin level is influenced by three factors: frequency and duration of feedings, supplemental feedings, and possibly the strength of the infant's sucking (Lowdermilk et al., 1999). In nonbreastfeeding mothers, the prolactin level returns to the prepregnant level within 2 weeks.

Ovulation in nonbreastfeeding mothers takes place as early as 27 days after the birth and usually has resumed by 2 months (Bowes, 1996). Most nonbreastfeeding mothers resume menstruating within 3 months after the birth.

The average time for ovulation to take place in breastfeeding mothers is approximately 190 days (Bowes, 1996). The return of ovulation and menstruation in breastfeeding mothers is determined, to a large measure, by the breastfeeding pattern. Approximately 25% of breastfeeding mothers ovulate before their menstrual periods return (Zlatnik, 1999). This underscores the fact that breastfeeding is not a reliable form of birth control.

Breasts

During the last few weeks of pregnancy, the breasts begin to fill with a fluid called colostrum. **Colostrum** is a yellowish fluid rich in antibodies and high in protein. As milk production begins, 2 to 3 days after birth, the breasts feel firm, warm, and may be tender. This lasts about 48 hours. By day 3 or 4 after the birth, **engorgement** may occur; the breasts become quite distended (swollen), tender, and warm. This is caused mainly by vasocongestion, especially of the veins and lymphatics.

The changes in the breasts after the birth of a baby are partly determined by whether the mother is breastfeeding or not. For the nursing mother, frequent breastfeeding sessions will encourage milk production and sustain lactation.

If the mother does not intend to breastfeed, although milk is present it should not be expressed because this causes more milk to be produced. Engorgement spontaneously disappears and discomfort decreases in 24 to 48 hours if the breasts are not emptied of milk. If breastfeeding is never begun or is stopped, lactation ceases within a week.

Gastrointestinal System

Most new mothers are hungry and thirsty after giving birth because of the energy expended during labor. Following recovery from any analgesia or anesthesia the mother may have received, she may request extra food.

Mothers may encounter difficulty in having a bowel movement after giving birth. There are several reasons, including:

- Peristalsis has been decreased due to the effects of the increased progesterone level during pregnancy; this may take several days to become normal again,
- Prelabor diarrhea,
- Lack of food during labor,
- Dehydration,
- Perineal trauma, episiotomy repair, or hemorrhoids, and
- Mother's anticipation of discomfort.

Cardiovascular System

The increase in blood volume during pregnancy allows a significant loss of blood without any ill effects to the mother. In a vaginal birth, blood loss averages 500 mL, while a cesarean birth averages a 1,000 mL blood loss.

Vital Signs

The new mother's temperature may rise to 100.4°F (38°C) during the first 24 hours because of dehydration during labor and the trauma of delivery. After 24 hours, the temperature should be normal, though may rise again when milk production begins.

The pulse, which increased during pregnancy, re-

CULTURAL CONSIDERATIONS

Breastfeeding

- Some Hispanic, Southeast Asian, Vietnamese, Cambodian, and Laotian women may choose not to breastfeed until the milk comes in (Mattson, 1995).
- Many women will breastfeed until the child is 2 years old, based on cultural practices and expectations (Hutchinson & Baqi-Aziz, 1994).

mains elevated or may even rise for up to 24 to 48 hours, but should not exceed 100 beats per minute. Periods of bradycardia may also be experienced. The pulse returns to the prepregnant rate in approximately 8 weeks (Bowes, 1996).

The diaphragm descends when the uterus is emptied, making respirations much easier. In 6 to 8 weeks respiratory function will return to the prepregnant rate. The blood pressure may have a small increase in both the systolic and diastolic aspects that lasts about 4 days (Bowes, 1996). The rapid decrease in intra-abdominal pressure after birth results in visceral blood vessel dilation, which may cause orthostatic hypotension.

Cardiac Output

Cardiac output, which increased during pregnancy, may increase even higher for up to 60 minutes following delivery. This increase occurs following both vaginal and cesarean births (Bowes, 1996). Cardiac output remains elevated for at least 48 hours, and then rapidly decreases in the first 2 weeks postpartum. The return of cardiac output to the prepregnancy level takes about 24 weeks (Simpson and Creehan, 1996).

Blood Volume

The changes in blood volume are rapid and dramatic. There are three physiologic changes that protect from excessive blood loss:

CULTURAL CONSIDERATIONS

Foods in the Postpartum Period

A nurse must be sensitive to the fact that a new mother's food choices and preferences may have cultural or ethnic foundations. For instance:

- Korean women may wish to eat seaweed soup and steamed rice, as they are believed to cleanse the body of lochia and increase the production of breast milk (Howard & Berbiglia, 1997; Schneiderman, 1996).
- Muslim women may request a vegetarian or kosher diet following childbirth (Hutchinson & Baqi-Aziz, 1994).

- Loss of the uteroplacental circulation (when the placenta is expelled) reduces the maternal vascular bed by 10% to 15%.
- Stimulus for vasodilation is removed with the loss of placental endocrine function.
- Movement of extravascular water, stored during pregnancy, into the blood vessels increases blood volume.

The excess plasma volume is eliminated from the body by both diuresis and diaphoresis. Diuresis (excessive urine excretion) results from a decrease in aldosterone, which was increased during pregnancy. It is not uncommon for a new mother to have a urinary output of 3,000 mL per day for 2 to 3 days (Gorrie, McKinney, & Murray, 1998). Diaphoresis (profuse perspiration), while not clinically significant relative to fluid elimination, may be uncomfortable for the mother, especially if she is not expecting it to occur. It often occurs at night for 2 to 3 nights following delivery.

Blood Values

The white blood cell count, which increased slightly during pregnancy (to 12,000/mm^3), now increases to 20,000 or even 30,000/mm^3 during the first 10 to 12 days after the infant's birth (Cunningham, MacDonald, Grant, Leveno, Gilstrap, and Hankins, 1997). The neutrophil level increases the most for protection against invading organisms.

The large loss of plasma volume during the first 3 days after the birth results in a rise in both the hemoglobin and hematocrit levels by the seventh day, unless excessive blood loss has occurred.

Coagulation

The increased levels of clotting factors and fibrinogen during pregnancy remain elevated for a few days as protection against postpartum hemorrhage. Thus, there is an increased risk for thrombus (clot) formation. Mothers having varicose veins, a cesarean birth, or a history of thrombophlebitis are at greater risk for thrombus formation.

Varicosities

Varices of the legs, anus (hemorrhoids), and vulvar area empty rapidly immediately after the birth.

Urinary System

Physical changes take place in the structures of the urinary system; there are also chemical changes in the urine.

Physical Changes

The hypotonia of the bladder and dilation of the ureters during pregnancy take approximately 2 to 8 weeks to return to the prepregnant state (Cunningham et al., 1997). Also, the bladder, urethra, and tissue around the urinary meatus may have been traumatized and become edematous during labor and birth, which may result in difficulty in urination.

The mother may have a problem with overdistention and incomplete emptying of the bladder and residual retention of urine because the diuresis causes the bladder to fill quickly. Those mothers who received a regional anesthesia are especially at risk for bladder distention and difficulty voiding until the anesthesia wears off.

Postpartum hemorrhage and urinary tract infection are two complications related to urinary retention and bladder overdistention. Urinary stasis provides the bacteria with enough time to multiply and cause an infection. A full bladder displaces the uterus up and to the side, resulting in uterine atony (inability of the uterus to contract). This is the primary cause of excessive bleeding. Adequate emptying of the bladder helps the bladder regain its tone in 5 to 7 days after the birth (Lowdermilk et al., 1999).

Chemical Changes

The catabolic processes of uterine involution cause a mild proteinuria for 1 to 2 days in approximately 50% of new mothers (Simpson & Creehan, 1996). Ketonuria and elevated blood urea nitrogen (BUN) may also be present.

Musculoskeletal System

The musculoskeletal changes that occur during pregnancy are reversed during the postpartum period.

Joints, Ligaments, and Cartilage

As the level of the hormone relaxin decreases, the ligaments and cartilage, especially of the pelvis, begin to revert to their prepregnant positions. Hip or joint pain may be noticed as these changes take place. Joints, cartilage, and ligaments are stabilized by 6 to 8 weeks after the birth.

All joints return to their normal prepregnant state except those in the feet. The new mother may discover a permanent increase in her shoe size (Lowdermilk et al., 1999).

Abdominal Muscles

Many new mothers, when they stand up, are dismayed when the abdominal muscles protrude, giving a still-pregnant appearance. It usually takes 6 weeks for the abdominal muscles to return almost to their prepregnant state (Lowdermilk et al., 1999). Previous muscle tone, proper exercise, and the amount of adipose tissue all influence the return of muscle tone.

Integumentary System

The level of melanocyte-stimulating hormone (MSH) declines rapidly after the birth and the areas of hyperpigmentation begin to lighten in color. In some women, however, the linea nigra and the darkened nipple areola may remain dark. Most of the skin's elasticity returns, but some striae may still be visible as small or large silver streaks on the breasts, abdomen, buttocks, or thighs.

Spider angiomas (nevi) and palmar erythema usually fade with the decrease in the estrogen level. In some women, however, they do stay.

Any fine hair appearing during pregnancy usually disappears. However, any coarse or bristly hair appearing during pregnancy may remain.

Neurologic System

Any pregnancy-induced neurologic discomforts usually lessen after birth (Lowdermilk et al., 1999). However, fatigue, afterpains, muscle aches, episiotomy or abdominal incision pain, and breast engorgement all may give rise to maternal discomfort. If the mother received an analgesic or anesthesia, she may experience a temporary loss of feeling in her legs and dizziness.

The mother who has a headache must be carefully assessed. If the mother had a regional anesthesia (epidural or spinal), the headache may be caused by a leakage of cerebrospinal fluid into the extradural space during needle placement; this is known as a spinal headache. This headache is generally more severe when the mother sits or stands and is relieved when she lies down. If the mother has blurred vision, photophobia, and abdominal pain with a headache, it may indicate that she is developing pregnancy-induced hypertension (PIH), or if she had PIH during pregnancy, that it is getting worse.

Weight Loss

Immediate weight loss is the sum of the infant's weight, placenta, amniotic fluid, and blood loss. Typically, this is approximately 13 lbs. During the first 2 weeks postpartum, an additional 8 to 9 lbs is lost as the result of diuresis, diaphoresis, and the involution of the reproductive organs. It takes most mothers approximately 6 months to return to their prepregnant weight, and some may take an entire year. The energy required for breastfeeding may assist in the weight loss process.

MATERNAL PSYCHOSOCIAL CHANGES

There are both expected and unexpected emotional/behavioral changes that may be encountered. The effects of early discharge must also be considered.

Expected Changes

Expected emotional/behavioral changes include those restorative/adaptive phases described by Reva Rubin, postpartum "blues," and those related to a cesarean birth.

Rubin's Restorative/Adaptive Phases

Rubin (1961) described three phases of maternal restoration/adaptation. These phases are called *taking-in, taking-hold, and letting-go.*

Taking-In Phase This phase is focused mainly on the mother's need for food, fluid, and sleep. The mother's behavior is passive as she takes in the physical care and attention from others. She depends on others to meet her needs. Rubin (1961) described this as the phase of nurturing and protective care lasting 2 to 3 days. Studies by Ament (1990) and Wrasper (1996) confirmed the behavior described by Rubin but noted that the behavior was present only during the first 24 hours after birth.

Integration of the labor and birth experience into reality is the major task of the mother at this time. It is important for her to discuss the details of the labor and birth, especially with the nurse(s) who cared for her. She is thus able to clarify details about her experience that she may not remember because of the effects of medication or the natural sleep and amnesia between contractions, especially in the second stage of labor. By describing to family and friends the birth experience, the mother realizes that the pregnancy is past and the infant is now a separate individual.

The father or partner may also experience a taking-in phase as he is congratulated on the birth of the infant. Family members often treat him in a special way.

Taking-Hold Phase In the taking-hold phase, the mother becomes more independent as she takes an interest in and responsibility for her own physical care. Her focus shifts to the care of her infant. She welcomes opportunities to learn about the behavior of infants and to practice caring for her infant. Martell (1996) and Wrasper (1996) believe that childbirth preparation classes, pain management practices, early newborn contact, rooming-in, and early discharge enhance taking-hold behaviors. Because most mothers are discharged during this phase, which lasts approximately 10 days,

HOME HEALTH CARE

Coping with Taking-Hold Phase
- Acknowledge parents' anxiety about caretaking abilities.
- Provide information about infant behaviors.
- Allow parents to provide infant care (nurse should not take over) even if performed awkwardly.
- Praise parents' caregiving efforts.
- Provide parents with a contact and phone number in the event they have questions.

continued coping with the physical and emotional/behavioral changes at home is required.

The father or partner's interest in infant behaviors and care is similar to the mother's in the taking-hold phase. He may also be anxious but is usually willing to learn.

Letting-Go Phase If this is a first baby, the mother and father/partner must give up the role and carefree lifestyle of being only a couple. They are now a couple with a child.

The expected birth experience may not have been realized. For example, a planned vaginal birth with no anesthesia may have changed to a cesarean birth and/or use of regional anesthesia. The parents must let go of the planned experience and accept what really happened.

For some mothers and/or fathers, the newborn infant does not fit the expected baby they dreamed of and talked about during pregnancy. They may be disappointed in the gender, size, or other characteristics of the infant. Now they must let go of their expectations and accept the reality of their infant.

The mother and father let go of their role of "expecting" and move forward as a unit with a new member. They establish a lifestyle that includes the child and their role as parents. Time must be made for sharing adult activities and interests.

Postpartum Blues

Postpartum blues or "baby blues" is a mild, transient condition of emotional lability and crying for no apparent reason that affects up to 80% of women who have just given birth and lasts about 2 weeks (Albright, 1993). Other symptoms include fatigue, anxiety, restlessness, let-down feeling, headache, and sadness. The etiology is unknown. This is a self-limiting situation that begins about 3 days, peaks about 5 days, and disappears approximately 10 days after birth.

Cesarean Birth

When a cesarean birth is an emergency (unplanned), the taking-in phase may last longer because these mothers also need to accept and understand the events that made the cesarean birth necessary. It is important for the nurse to understand that these mothers are surgical clients requiring immediate physical care to restore or maintain physiologic health. When pain, bleeding, and incision care are under control, the nurse can help the mother understand the birth and incorporate the experience into her reality.

Some mothers may have feelings of frustration, anger, low self-esteem, or disappointment that they could not have their baby the "normal way" (vaginal birth). At the same time they are relieved, happy, and filled with gratitude that the infant had a safe birth and is healthy. It may be a time of many, often opposing, emotions.

Unexpected Changes

Unexpected emotional/behavioral changes include postpartum depression, postpartum psychosis, and reaction to an infant with problems.

Postpartum Depression

Postpartum depression (PPD) is similar to postpartum blues but is more serious, intense, and persistent. Approximately 12% of new mothers experience a syndrome more severe than postpartum blues (Albright, 1993; Green & Adams, 1993; Lowdermilk et al., 1999). PPD may be mild, moderate, or severe with symptoms becoming more numerous and intense as the severity increases.

The mother with mild PPD cares lovingly for her infant but is unable to feel the love. She may express feelings of irritability, guilt, shame, unworthiness, and a sense of loss of self. Symptoms persist past the first few weeks after the infant's birth.

Moderate PPD is characterized by spontaneous crying, insomnia or hypersomnia, fatigue, decreased concentration, and sometimes food cravings.

With severe PPD the irritability of the mother may explode into violent outbursts or uncontrollable crying often directed toward significant others. She often will not discuss her symptoms or negative feelings toward the infant, which may include disinterest, annoyance with care demands, or even thoughts of harming the infant.

Psychotherapy and pharmacological interventions are generally required. Sometimes, hospitalization is necessary.

Postpartum Psychosis

Postpartum psychosis is more severe than PPD and is characterized by delusions and thoughts of self-harm or infant harm. This condition is rare, occurring in 0.1% to 0.2% of births (Kaplan, Sadock, & Grebb, 1998). Symptoms usually begin within 2 to 3 weeks after the birth. The symptoms include fatigue, restlessness, insomnia, crying, labile emotions, inability to move, irrational statements, incoherence, confusion, and obsessive concerns about the infant's health. Approximately 50% have delusions and 25% have hallucinations (Lowdermilk et al., 1999).

Postpartum psychosis is a psychiatric emergency. Kaplan et al. (1998) report on a study in which 5% of clients with postpartum psychosis committed suicide and 4% committed infanticide. The mother is usually hospitalized and provided both pharmacological support and psychotherapy.

Infant with a Problem

It may be difficult for the mother and/or father to bond with and attach to an infant born preterm or with physical or functional anomalies (Figure 50-6). The parents may have feelings of guilt that they, somehow,

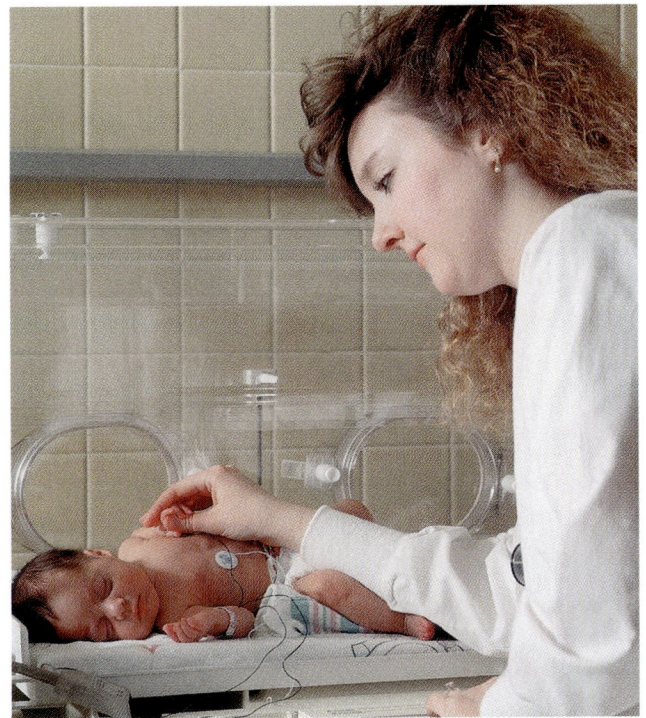

Figure 50-6 Parents of an infant who requires special medical care should be encouraged to spend as much time with their child as possible.

caused the infant's problem. Either or both of the parents may not be able to accept an infant who does not look like a normal, healthy infant. When one parent's reaction to the infant with a problem is opposite that of the other's, there may be a terrific strain on their relationship.

DISCHARGE

In an effort to reduce health care costs and meet consumer demand for a more family-centered experience with less medical intervention, the short hospital stay came into existence (Wilkerson, 1996). In the 1950s, most new mothers remained in the hospital 5 days for a vaginal birth and 7 days for a cesarean birth. The stays were gradually reduced to 3 days for a vaginal birth and 5 days for a cesarean birth. For several years in the early 1990s, third-party payers (health plans and insurance companies) mandated discharge within 24 hours for a vaginal birth and 72 hours or less for a cesarean birth.

Health care professionals became concerned about client (mother and infant) safety because many problems do not show up in the first 24 hours after birth. The time for assessing bonding/attachment and parenting behaviors was almost eliminated. Parents were barely acquainted with their infant and client teaching about newborn care, and identifying health problems such as dehydration, jaundice, and breastfeeding difficulties had to be rushed (Havens & Hannan, 1996).

The federal government passed the Newborns' and Mothers' Health Protection Act of 1995, which requires all health plans to allow a stay of 48 hours following vaginal birth and 96 hours following a cesarean birth (Ferguson & Engelhard, 1996).

Follow-up home care is being utilized in many areas. This may be a telephone call or two to see how the mother and infant are doing, or it may include actual home visits.

▶ NURSING PROCESS

▶ Assessment

Assessments specific to the first few days postpartum include BUBBLE (breasts, uterus, bladder, bowel, lochia, and episiotomy), vital signs, lower extremities and Homans' sign, bonding/attachment, parenting, activity, comfort, and self-care. These assessments are usually performed, at least once a shift, until the mother is discharged. A sample initial postpartum profile sheet is shown in Figure 50-7.

 Infection Control: Standard Precautions in Postpartum Care

Gloves should be worn when:
- Assessing the breasts if there is leakage of colostrum or milk,
- Handling used breast pads,
- Assessing lochia and the perineum,
- Changing peripads or chux, and
- Handling anything on which there is lochia (bed linen, towels, washcloth, clothing, peripads, chux).

▶ Subjective Data

The nurse should ask the mother whether the milk has come in or whether there is any breast discomfort; whether the bladder feels empty after urination; whether the mother is able to pass gas rectally or has the urge to have a bowel movement; whether any clots are passed vaginally and when the peripad was last changed; whether there is dizziness when getting up; whether contractions are felt during breastfeeding; or whether there is discomfort or pain especially in the perineal area.

 CLIENT TEACHING

Breast Assessment
- Explain the characteristics of the breast and what to expect depending on whether the mother is breastfeeding or not.
- Describe how to recognize problems such as mastitis and nipple fissures or cracks.

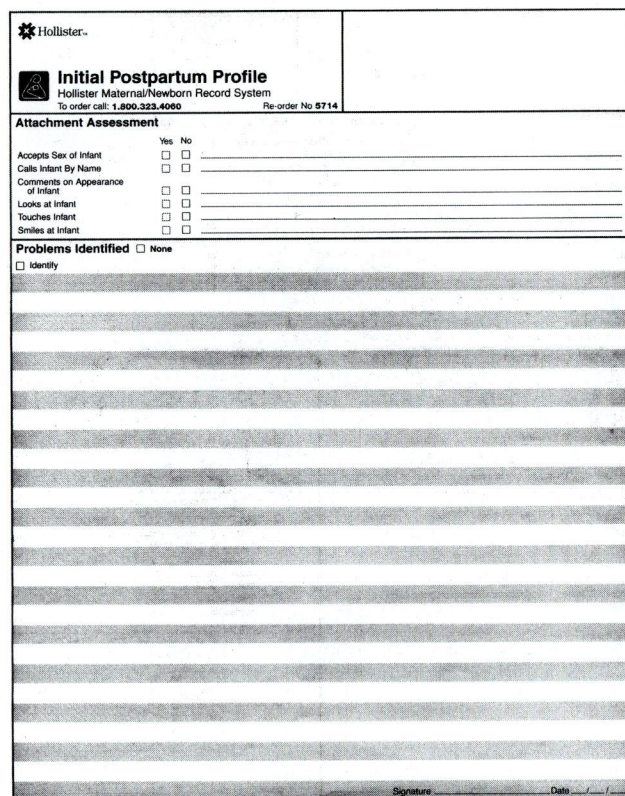

Figure 50-7 Representative Initial Postpartum Profile *(Permission to use this copyright material has been granted by the owner, Hollister Incorporated.)*

▶ Objective Data

Breasts

The nurse should note the size and shape of the breasts, and any abnormalities or reddened areas. The breasts should be gently palpated for softness, firmness, engorgement, warmth, or tenderness. The nipples must be checked for cracks, fissures, soreness, and inversion.

Uterus

The abdomen is palpated to find the top (fundus) of the uterus by pressing in and down with the side of one hand, and placing the other hand above the symphysis to support the uterus. The size, consistency, and placement (midline or off to one side) of the uterus is noted. It should be the size of a grapefruit, firm (not boggy), and in the midline. Each day it should descend approximately 1 cm (1 finger breadth). Fundal descent is documented in relation to the umbilicus (Figure 50-8).

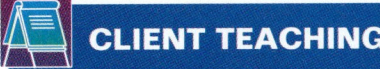

CLIENT TEACHING

Assessing the Fundus

• Explain why it is important for the uterus to be firmly contracted.
• Demonstrate how to palpate the uterine fundus.
• Demonstrate the way to gently massage the fundus.

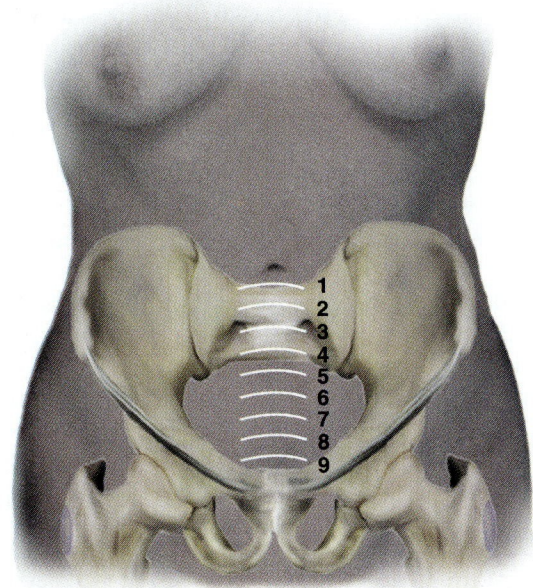

Figure 50-8 Uterine Involution. Uterine fundal descent is approximately 1 cm/day.

CLIENT TEACHING

Bladder and Bowel Elimination

Encourage the new mother to:

- Drink plenty of fluids,
- Ambulate frequently and use the bathroom, not a bedpan,
- Eat a well-balanced diet with increased fiber and fluids, and
- Promptly answer nature's call to urinate or defecate.

Bladder

When the abdomen is palpated for the uterine fundus, the bladder can also be palpated for distention. A full, distended bladder is very often the cause for the fundus to be higher than it should be and to be positioned off to one side (not in the midline) (Figure 50-9). An intake and output (I&O) record is kept during the first 24 hours, at least, to assist in identifying urine retention.

Bowels

The nurse should inspect the abdomen for distention and auscultate for the presence of bowel sounds. The client's labor record should be reviewed to check whether she received an enema. The anus can be inspected when the episiotomy is checked.

CLIENT TEACHING

Lochia Assessment

- Describe the expected changes in the color and amount of lochia.
- Advise the mother that if the lochia changes from serosa back to rubra, she is either doing too much heavy work or the uterus is not firmly contracted. The mother should check fundal firmness and rest for a while.
- Instruct mother to notify her CNM/physician if clots are passed or if the lochia has an unusual or unpleasant odor.

Lochia

The mother should be asked to lie on her back with knees flexed so the peripad can be lowered in the front. Lochia is assessed for color, amount, odor, and presence of clots. The mother is then asked to turn to her side to see whether any lochia has pooled under her buttocks.

Amount It is difficult to estimate the amount of lochia on a perineal pad. Luegenbiehl, Brophy, Artigue, Phillips, and Flack (1990) identified a method to estimate the amount of lochia discharged in 1 hour (Figure 50-10).

The mother who has had a cesarean birth will have less lochia after the first 24 hours than a mother who

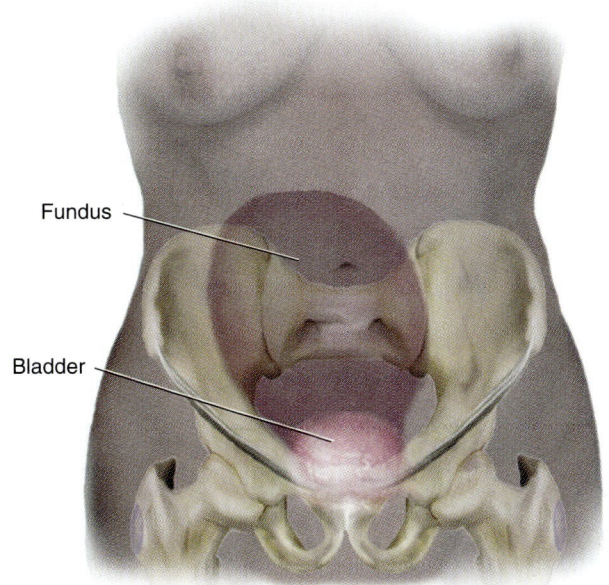

Figure 50-9 A full bladder displaces the uterus and prevents its contraction.

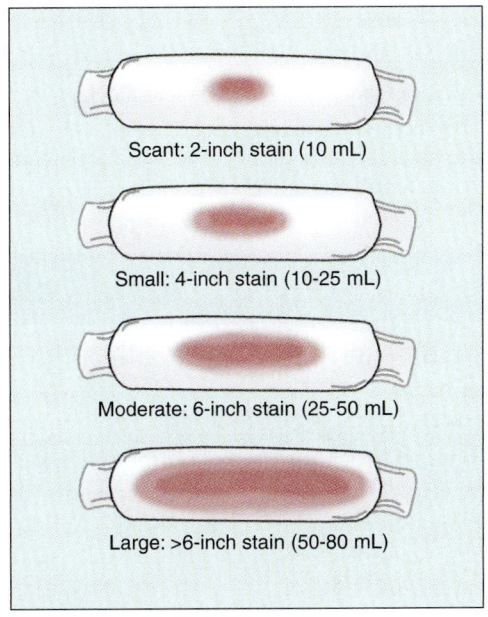

Scant: 2-inch stain (10 mL)

Small: 4-inch stain (10-25 mL)

Moderate: 6-inch stain (25-50 mL)

Large: >6-inch stain (50-80 mL)

Figure 50-10 Method for Assessing the Volume of Lochia from the Stain Size on a Peripad

had a vaginal birth. The lochia usually changes from rubra to serosa sooner also. This is because the inside of the uterus is wiped with sponges during a cesarean birth, removing some of the endometrium.

Odor Lochia has a nonoffensive odor. If the lochia has a foul odor, an infection is present and the CNM/physician must be notified at once.

Presence of Clots A few small clots, which occur when blood pools in the vagina, are normal. Passing many or large clots is not normal and requires further investigation.

Episiotomy

The episiotomy is assessed with the mother in Sims' position (Figure 50-11). This can be done when the mother is on her side for lochia assessment. With a gloved hand, the nurse very gently raises the upper buttock just enough to see the episiotomy. Changes in the episiotomy should be noted, such as the following:

- Redness—inflammation
- Ecchymosis—bruising
- Edema—swelling
- Discharge—from incision
- Approximation of suture line

With the client in the same position, the nurse should gently touch the external labia and note

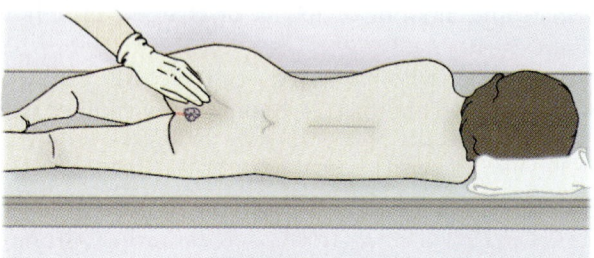

Figure 50-11 The episiotomy is assessed with the mother in Sims' position. The upper buttock is raised very gently, just enough to see the episiotomy. The anal area can be assessed for hemorrhoids at the same time.

CLIENT TEACHING

Techniques to Decrease Episiotomy Discomfort

Instruct mother to:
- Tighten her buttocks and perineum before sitting to prevent pulling on the episiotomy and perineal area, and to release the tightening after being seated.
- Rest several times a day with feet elevated.
- Practice the Kegel exercise many times a day to increase circulation to perineal area and to strengthen the perineal muscles.

whether this causes pain. The labia should also be inspected for ecchymosis and edema. The anus can be inspected for hemorrhoids.

Vital Signs

Vital sign assessment should be made every 15 minutes for the first 1 to 2 hours after birth. If no problems are identified, vital signs may then be checked every 8 hours.

Temperature Temperature may increase to 100.4°F (38°C) during the first 24 hours. After the first 24 hours, a temperature over 100.4°F suggests an infection.

Pulse After the first hour following the birth, the mother's pulse rate may decrease to 50 to 70 beats/minute for 6 to 8 days. An elevated pulse may indicate excessive blood loss, infection, anxiety, or pain.

Blood Pressure Blood pressure should remain consistent with the baseline during pregnancy. An increase suggests PIH, while a decrease may indicate excessive bleeding.

Lower Extremities and Homans' Sign

The nurse should examine the mother's legs for signs of thrombophlebitis such as redness, heat, edema, and tenderness. The pedal pulses should be palpated. The assessment for Homans' sign must also be performed.

To assess for Homans' sign, the nurse supports the client's leg under the knee while sharply dorsiflexing the foot (Figure 50-12). Homans' sign is positive if the client experiences calf discomfort when the foot is dorsiflexed and negative if the client does not experience discomfort in the calf. When Homans' sign is positive, it must be reported at once to the CNM/physician because it may indicate thrombophlebitis.

Bonding/Attachment

The interaction of mother with her infant are assessed for the expected behaviors of bonding and beginning attachment. The manner in which the mother

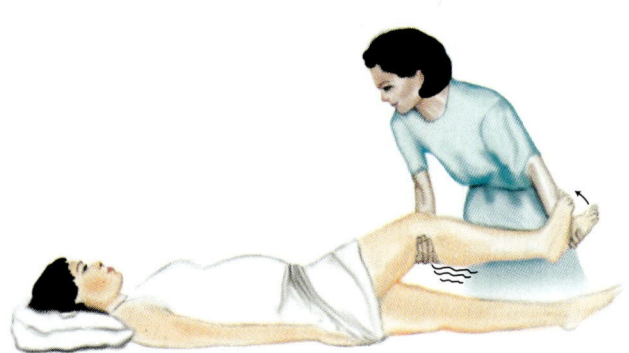

Figure 50-12 Homans' Sign Assessment. Discomfort experienced in the calf when foot is sharply dorsiflexed is considered positive and may indicate thrombophlebitis.

CULTURAL CONSIDERATIONS

Rest

Expectations of maternal activity during the postpartum period may be influenced by cultural norms. For example:

- Korean women rest an average of 21 days following birth (Howard & Berbiglia, 1997).
- Southeast Asian, Vietnamese, Cambodian, and Laotion women stay in bed without a pillow and keep warm for 2 days (Mattson, 1995).

quently walking around. Many complications such as thromboses, emboli, and hypostatic pneumonia occur when the mother is in bed for extended periods of time.

Rest is just as important as activity. The mother expended a great deal of energy during labor and birth. Care should be planned so the mother has some uninterrupted periods of rest.

Safety: First Ambulation

The first time a new mother gets out of bed, the nurse should be at her side and ready to assist in case the mother becomes light-headed, weak, or dizzy.

Comfort

Comfort is essential to rest. Many new mothers never say anything about discomforts because they are so excited and pleased with their new infant. The nurse must be alert to any behavioral signs of discomfort. Most discomfort is related to perineal pain or afterpains.

Self-Care

Assessment of self-care includes the mother's knowledge of how to care for herself and also whether she actually performs the care. Self-care includes showering, perineal care, checking the fundus, breast care, and rest. The nurse can support the client's recovery by encouraging her to bathe, toilet, and feed herself independently.

holds, examines, and speaks to the infant is important. For instance, the mother who cradles her infant, gazes at her infant's face, and speaks in a pleasant manner to the infant is exhibiting signs of bonding and attachment.

Parenting

The skill with which the mother cares for her infant is also assessed. For example, the nurse may wish to observe feeding, diapering, bathing, and consoling skills to determine whether additional teaching is required.

Activity

The nurse must determine that the mother is ambulating, that is, getting up to go to the bathroom and fre-

Nursing diagnoses for a postpartum mother may include the following:

Nursing Diagnoses	Planning/Goals	Nursing Interventions
▶ *Urinary Elimination, Altered, related to sensory motor impairment from bladder trauma during labor and birth*	The mother will have appropriate urinary elimination (no bladder distention).	Monitor intake for adequate amount. Assess for bladder distention every 2 to 4 hours. Assist client to bathroom for elimination. Pour warm water over vulvar area or run water in the sink to stimulate urination. Catheterize, if necessary, as ordered.
▶ *Infection, Risk for, related to episiotomy*	The mother will have no signs of infection.	Assess episiotomy for redness and swelling. Teach mother pericare: wash hands, remove peripad from front to back, pour warm water over perineum, pat dry from front to back, apply clean peripad front first then toward the back, wash hands. Advise client to change peripad every 2 to 4 hours and every time she goes to the bathroom.
▶ *Pain, related to episiotomy, engorged breasts, or involution of the uterus*	The mother will state that discomfort has decreased.	*Episiotomy* Assess perineum for edema. Apply ice pack for 20 minutes; remove for at least 10 minutes before reapplying. Assist mother with Sitz bath as ordered, and watch for dizziness, floating feeling, or difficulty hearing (signs of possible fainting).

continued

Nursing Diagnoses	Planning/Goals	Nursing Interventions
		Apply Dermoplast spray or Americain spray (topical anesthetics) to perineum after a sitz bath or pericare, as ordered.
		Emphasize the need to wash hands before and after any care of the episiotomy.
		Teach mother to squeeze buttocks together before sitting, release after sitting.
		Encourage mother to practice Kegel exercise 4 or 5 times a day.
		Administer analgesic as ordered.
		Engorged Breasts (not breastfeeding)
		Encourage mother to wear a well-fitting supportive bra, removing it only for showers, to suppress lactation.
		Provide ice pack to axillary area and side of breast for 20 minutes 4 times a day to suppress lactation.
		Advise mother to avoid any stimulation to breast; stand with back to shower so warm water does not hit breasts.
		Administer analgesic as ordered.
		Engorged Breasts (breastfeeding)
		Encourage the mother to feed her infant approximately every 2 hours; empty (until soft) one breast; then feed from second breast or pump to soften.
		Administer antiinflammatory pain medication as ordered.
		Apply ice pack between feedings for 15 minutes on and 45 minutes off as ordered.
		Involution of Uterus (afterpains)
		Assess fundus for firmness and position.
		Determine when mother has pain.
		Explain, if mother is breastfeeding, that the oxytocin released in response to breastfeeding causes the uterus to contract. The discomfort lasts only a few minutes at the beginning of each breastfeeding session for the first 4 to 6 days.
		Administer analgesic as ordered.

Evaluation Each goal must be evaluated to determine how it has been met by the client.

HEALTH PROMOTION

The mother's record must be checked to determine the mother's need for Rh immune globulin (RhoGAM) and rubella immunization. When required, these two items protect the fetuses of future pregnancies.

PROFESSIONAL TIP

Rh Immune Globulin (RhoGAM) Administration

RhoGAM is administered intramuscularly to Rh-negative, antibody negative (Coombs' negative) mothers who gave birth to an Rh-positive infant. It is never given to the infant.

Rh Immune Globulin

Rh immune globulin (RhoGAM) is given within 72 hours after birth to prevent sensitization of Rh-negative mothers who gave birth to Rh-positive infants. The RhoGAM promotes lysis of fetal Rh-positive red blood cells before the mother's body is able to form antibodies against them.

Rubella Immunization

It is recommended that all women who have not had rubella or who have a 1:8 rubella titer be given rubella vaccine in the immediate postpartum period. This will prevent fetal anomalies in future pregnancies if the mother is exposed to rubella. Breastfeeding is not a contraindication to receiving the immunization. Because the vaccine may be teratogenic, pregnancy must be avoided for 2 to 3 months.

SAMPLE NURSING CARE PLAN

THE POSTPARTUM CLIENT

Sophia and Jack Viernot have just participated in the birth of their first child, a daughter, weighing 6 lbs, 8 oz and measuring 21 inches long. A small episiotomy was made. Jack has "always wanted a son" and is "disappointed about having a daughter." He looks at the infant but does not touch her or speak to her.

Sophia is exhausted from the labor and birth, says she is too tired to hold the baby, and wants only to sleep. Her vital signs are within normal range, and the uterus tends to relax. Within 1½ hours, she has saturated three peripads. A bulge is noted above the symphysis. Sophia is unable to urinate at this time.

Nursing Diagnosis 1 *Fluid Volume Deficit, Risk for, related to early postpartum hemorrhage as evidenced by saturating three peripads in 1½ hours*

PLANNING/GOALS	NURSING INTERVENTIONS	RATIONALE	EVALUATION
Sophia's fluid volume will be maintained by reducing the amount of lochia discharge.	Palpate and monitor fundal height, location, and consistency.	Determines status of uterus (firm or boggy) and height and location relative to umbilicus.	Sophia's fluid volume is maintained when voiding allows the uterus to contract and the amount of lochia to decrease.
	For boggy uterus, gently massage and assess muscle tone.	Promotes uterine contraction and increases uterine tone.	
	Monitor lochia (amount and color), time peripad changed, and degree of peripad saturation.	Evaluates the amount of lochia.	
	Assess for bladder fullness and encourage voiding.	A full bladder interferes with contracting of the uterus.	
	Monitor intake and output.	Identifies potential need to urinate.	
	Monitor vital signs, skin temperature, and color.	Detects signs of shock.	
	Administer oxytocic agent as ordered.	Promotes uterine contraction.	
	Explain involution process to Sophia and teach her to check and gently massage her uterus.	Involves Sophia in self-care.	

Nursing Diagnosis 2 *Altered Parenting, Risk for, related to not gender desired as evidenced by Jack expressing a desire for a son, showing seeming disappointment with a daughter, not touching or speaking to the infant, and Sophia saying she is too tired to hold the baby*

continued

PLANNING/GOALS	NURSING INTERVENTIONS	RATIONALE	EVALUATION
Sophia and Jack will demonstrate bonding and attachment behaviors with their daughter.	Assist Sophia in holding her daughter.	Emphasizes holding infant as important.	Sophia follows nurse's example and strokes the infant's head and face with her fingertips and talks to her. Jack touches the infant's fingers but does not watch her intently or for longer than a few seconds.
	Point out unique characteristics about the infant (e.g., dimple in right cheek, long fingers).	Helps Sophia and Jack get acquainted with their daughter.	
	Ask Sophia and Jack who the infant looks like.	Assists Sophia and Jack in identifying family characteristics.	
	Model bonding and attachment behaviors for Sophia and Jack such as talking to infant, finger-tipping, and examining infant.	Shows Sophia and Jack how to interact with their daughter.	
	Describe infant's behavior and explain that the infant can see and hear her parents.	Enables Sophia and Jack to understand their infant and her abilities.	

Nursing Diagnosis 3 *Urinary Elimination, Altered, related to sensory motor impairment as evidenced by inability to urinate and bulge noted above the symphysis*

PLANNING/GOALS	NURSING INTERVENTIONS	RATIONALE	EVALUATION
Sophia will have regular urinary elimination with no bladder distention.	Palpate bulge above symphysis while asking Sophia whether bladder feels full.	Confirms that bulge is a full bladder.	Sophia empties her bladder when assisted to the bathroom.
	Assist Sophia to the bathroom or onto bedpan if she is unable to ambulate.	Allows Sophia to empty her bladder.	
	Run water in sink, place Sophia's hands in warm water, or pour water over her perineum.	Stimulates urination.	
	Administer analgesic as ordered if Sophia has vulvar/perineal discomfort and is afraid to void.	Relieves discomfort; may help Sophia relax and void.	
	Catheterize if necessary, as ordered.	Empties bladder, allowing uterus to contract and promoting comfort.	

continued

Nursing Diagnosis 4 *Infection, Risk for, related to inadequate primary defenses as evidenced by episiotomy and low pH of lochia*

PLANNING/GOALS	NURSING INTERVENTIONS	RATIONALE	EVALUATION
Sophia will have no evidence of infection.	Follow Standard Precautions, especially good handwashing before and after providing care, and wear gloves when contact with lochia or urine is possible.	Prevents spread of infection.	Sophia has no signs of infection.
	Use strict aseptic technique when inserting a catheter or starting an intravenous infusion.	Reduces the risk of a nosocomial infection.	
	Monitor vital signs.	If elevated, may indicate an infection.	
	Monitor for loss of appetite, malaise, and chills.	May indicate infection.	
	Assess episiotomy for redness, edema, drainage, and pain; and lochia for a foul odor.	Indicates infection.	
	Teach Sophia proper perineal care.	Keeps perineum clean and prevents contamination of episiotomy by anal organisms.	

CESAREAN BIRTH

All of the assessments just discussed are also performed on a mother who has had a cesarean birth. In addition, postoperative assessments are performed, including incision, respirations and breath sounds, abdomen and bowel sounds, fluid intake, urine output, and the degree of pain.

Incision

The dressing is inspected for intactness and any bleeding or discharge. After the dressing is removed, the incision is assessed for signs of infection such as redness, heat, pain, or edema and the suture line for approximation.

Respirations and Breath Sounds

If the mother received narcotics either epidurally or with patient-controlled analgesia (PCA), her respirations must be assessed frequently because narcotics depress the respiratory center. Respiratory rate and depth are assessed every 15 minutes for the first hour, every 30 minutes for the next 4 to 5 hours, and every hour for the remainder of the first 24 hours. Some institutions may use an apnea monitor. Breath sounds are auscultated at each respiratory check to identify whether secretions are beginning to pool in the bronchioles. The client's efforts of turning (changing position), coughing, deep breathing, and use of the incentive spirometer must also be assessed.

Abdomen and Bowel Sounds

In addition to the incision, the abdomen is assessed for softness or distention. Bowel sounds are auscultated until peristalsis is noted in all four quadrants. The mother should be asked whether she has been able to pass any flatus (gas) rectally.

Fluid Intake

The flow rate of intravenous fluids as well as the site must be frequently assessed. The amount of intravenous fluid and any oral fluid intake are recorded.

Urine Output

A Foley catheter is generally inserted into the bladder before the cesarean birth. The amount of urine output as well as the clarity and color are assessed and recorded.

Pain

Most new mothers who have a vaginal birth are eager to interact with their newborn infant. This is no different following a cesarean birth; however, these mothers will need to be taught how to hold and carry the infant in a way that will not disturb or irritate the incision. The mothers may not want pain medication because they want to stay awake with and enjoy their infants.

Breastfeeding mothers who have had a cesarean birth may also not admit to having pain because they are concerned that pain medication will be present in the breast milk. Pain medication is generally required for 24 to 48 hours following a cesarean birth. These mothers can be taught to support the baby with a pillow so as to avoid incisional pain while nursing.

COMPLICATIONS

The most common complications of childbirth are postpartum hemorrhage, infection, thromboembolic conditions, and disseminated intravascular coagulation.

POSTPARTUM HEMORRHAGE

Postpartum hemorrhage is defined as a blood loss of more than 500 mL after the third stage of labor or 1,000 mL after a cesarean birth. The hemorrhage is identified as either early, within the first 24 hours, or late, generally occurring 1 to 2 weeks after the birth, but may occur up to 6 weeks after the birth.

EARLY POSTPARTUM HEMORRHAGE

Early postpartum hemorrhage has several possible causes: uterine atony, retained placental fragments, lacerations of the birth canal, and hematomas. Predisposing factors for postpartum hemorrhage include the following:

- Overdistention of the uterus (large infant, multiple gestation, or hydramnios)
- Grandmultiparity (more than 5)
- Precipitate labor or birth
- Prolonged labor
- Use of forceps or vacuum extractor
- Use of tocolytic drugs
- Use of oxytocin to augment or induce labor,

- Cesarean birth
- Manual removal of the placenta
- Clotting disorders

Uterine Atony

Uterine atony is a lack of muscle tone in the uterus. The uterus feels soft and boggy. Hemorrhage from uterine atony is usually a steady flow. Blood pressure and pulse changes may not occur until the blood loss is severe because during pregnancy there is an increase in blood volume.

Retained Placental Fragments

Occasionally, small pieces of the placenta may not be expelled. These pieces prevent the uterus from contracting effectively, and bleeding continues.

Lacerations of the Birth Canal

Factors predisposing a woman to lacerations of the birth canal include the following:

- Nulliparity
- Forceps-assisted or vacuum cup-assisted birth
- Precipitous birth
- Macrosomia
- Epidural anesthesia

Lacerations may occur in the perineum, vagina, cervix, or around the urethral meatus. Most lacerations are identified and repaired by the CNM/physician immediately following the birth. Occasionally, a laceration is overlooked and bright red bleeding persists when the uterus is firmly contracted.

Hematoma

A hematoma forms when there is bleeding into the tissues; there is no external laceration. Spontaneous or forceps-assisted births may result in hematoma formation. The most common sites are the vulva, vagina, and retroperitoneal area (Figure 50-13). A hematoma is a bluish-purple mass that produces deep, severe, unrelenting pain and a feeling of great pressure. When the uterus is firmly contracted, the amount of lochia is within normal limits, and the mother has a falling blood pressure or tachycardia and persistently describes severe pain, a hematoma should be suspected.

LATE POSTPARTUM HEMORRHAGE

A late postpartum hemorrhage usually occurs 1 to 2 weeks after the birth because of **subinvolution** (incomplete return of the uterus to its prepregnant size and consistency) or retained placental fragments. Clots may form around the retained placental fragments immediately postpartum, thus keeping lochia within

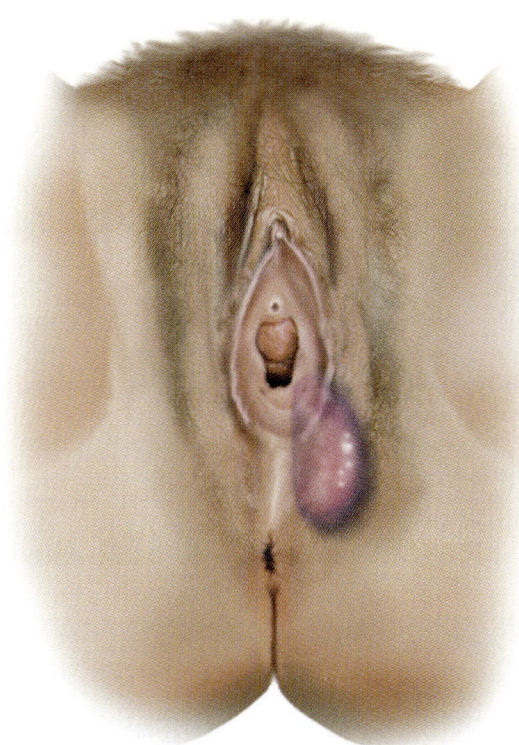

Figure 50-13 Hematoma of the Vulva

normal limits. Several days later, when the clots slough, excessive bleeding occurs. There is usually no warning of a late postpartum hemorrhage.

Medical–Surgical Management

Medical

The CNM/physician carefully palpates the uterus to make sure it is contracting after the birth. A thorough examination of the birth canal for lacerations or hematomas is also undertaken. A sonogram may be used to determine the presence of retained placental fragments.

Surgical

Cunningham et al. (1997) report that curettage, formerly the usual treatment, is now believed to cause more bleeding because of the trauma to the placental site. It now is performed when other methods have failed to control the bleeding.

Surgical evacuation of a large hematoma or one increasing in size may be necessary to attain hemostasis. The bleeding vessel is identified and ligated (tied).

Pharmacological

Oxytocin (Pitocin), methylergonovine maleate (Methergine), or prostaglandins may be given to contract the uterus. The strong contractions produced by these medications often loosen the retained placental fragments, which are then discharged with the lochia. Antibiotics are often used prophylactically to prevent infection. Blood transfusion or replacement of coagulation factors may be necessary depending on the amount of blood lost.

Activity

The mother is usually kept in bed until the bleeding is under control.

▶ NURSING PROCESS

▶ Assessment

▶ Subjective Data

The mother may either describe feeling like a lot of blood is coming from her vagina, or a severe pain in the vulvar or perineal area.

▶ Objective Data

The fundus is palpated for size, consistency, and position. The nurse should check how long the peripad has been in place, how much lochia is present, and whether the bladder is distended. Vital signs will probably be within the normal range.

Nursing diagnoses for a client with a postpartum hemorrhage may include the following:

Nursing Diagnoses	Planning/Goals	Nursing Interventions
▶ *Fluid Volume Deficit related to blood loss from uterine atony, lacerations, retained placental fragments, or hematoma*	The client will maintain adequate fluid volume.	Assess vital signs.
		Assess fundal height, firmness, and location as per agency protocol. If client has predisposing factors for postpartum hemorrhage, assess more frequently.
		Assess lochia amount and color and relate to firmness of fundus. Notify CNM/physician about excessive bleeding.
		Assess bladder for distention.
		Maintain mother on bed rest.
		Call for assistance; one nurse to monitor vital signs while a second nurse monitors fundus and lochia.

continued

Nursing Diagnoses	Planning/Goals	Nursing Interventions
		Save all peripads, linen, and linen savers for more accurate estimate of blood loss.
		Document all assessments, interventions, and each time CNM/physician is notified.
		Administer medications as ordered.
▶ *Pain related to tissue damage from hematoma formation*	The client will describe having less pain.	Apply ice pack to hematoma.
		Continue assessment of hematoma size.
		Assess client's pain using 0 to 10 pain scale (0 = no pain, 10 = most pain).
		Notify CNM/physician of hematoma and pain assessment.
		Administer medications as ordered.
		Document all assessments, interventions, and each time CNM/physician is notified.

Evaluation Each goal must be evaluated to determine how it has been met by the client.

INFECTIONS

Puerperal (postpartum) infection is an infection following childbirth occurring between the birth and 6 weeks postpartum. It is defined as a temperature of 38°C (100.4°F) or more on 2 consecutive days during the first 10 days after the birth, not counting the first 24 hours (Hamadeh, Dedmon, & Mozley, 1995).

Because all parts of the reproductive tract are connected to each other, it is easy for organisms to move from the vagina through the cervix, to the uterus, through the fallopian tubes, and out to the ovaries and peritoneal cavity. The increased blood supply to the reproductive tract during pregnancy provides more avenues for invading bacteria to be spread throughout the body with the possibility of causing a life-threatening septicemia.

Amniotic fluid and lochia are alkaline, so during labor and in the postpartum period the normal acidity of the vagina is reduced, which encourages bacterial growth.

It is seldom necessary to keep the baby separated from the mother during maternal infection, as they generally share the same organisms. Someone should be available to care for the infant because the mother is usually tired and does not have the energy to fully care for her infant.

Common postpartum infections are wound infection, metritis, mastitis, and urinary tract infection. Predisposing factors for puerperal infection are listed in Table 50-1.

WOUND INFECTION

The break in the skin from lacerations, episiotomies, and surgical incisions from cesarean birth provides an easy portal of entry for bacteria. Localized signs of infection (redness, warmth, edema, and tenderness)

Table 50-1 PREDISPOSING FACTORS FOR POSTPARTUM INFECTION

PREDISPOSING FACTORS	DESCRIPTION/ EXPLANATION
Antepartum	
Medical conditions • Diabetes • Alcoholism • Drug abuse • Anemia • Poor nutrition/malnutrition • Immunosuppression	Ability to defend against any infection is decreased.
History of previous infections	Possibly more vulnerable to infections
Intrapartum	
Prolonged rupture of membranes	Provides direct access to interior of uterus
Chorioamnionitis	Organisms already in uterus
Prolonged labor	More time for bacteria to multiply
Excessive number of vaginal examinations	Increases opportunity for organisms from outside source or vagina to be introduced into the uterus
Internal fetal monitoring	Provides opportunity for introduction of organisms
Bladder catheterization	Possible introduction of organisms into bladder
Episiotomy, lacerations, and cesarean birth	Provide portals of entry for organisms
Postpartum	
Retained placental fragments	Good medium for bacterial growth
Hematoma	Makes tissues more susceptible
Hemorrhage	Infection-fighting components of blood are lost

are assessed at the skin break, which, if untreated, will develop into generalized signs of infection, including an elevated temperature and malaise. Wound edges may separate and drainage may be evident.

METRITIS

Metritis, inflammation of the uterus, includes both endometritis (inflammation of the inside of the uterus, or endometrium) and parametritis (inflammation of the outside of the uterus, or parametrium, including the connective tissue of the broad ligaments). The usual causes are the organisms that normally inhabit the vagina and cervix. This infection easily spreads through the fallopian tubes (**salpingitis**) to the ovaries (**oophoritis**).

MASTITIS

Mastitis is inflammation of the breast, generally during breastfeeding. The usual cause is *Staphylococcus aureus* but may also be *Candida albicans*. Symptoms appear between 2 and 4 weeks after birth. There is usually a crack or fissure in the nipple for the portal of entry. Nipple soreness may result in shorter breastfeeding times, allowing milk stasis, which is a good medium for bacterial growth.

URINARY TRACT INFECTION

Approximately 2% to 4% of new mothers will have a urinary tract infection (UTI) (Gorrie et al., 1998). Trauma to the bladder and urethra during labor and birth, urinary stasis after the birth, and catheterization all contribute to the development of a UTI.

Medical–Surgical Management

Medical

The goal of treatment is to confine the infection and prevent it from spreading systemically.

A culture of drainage from a wound, the uterine cavity, or urine is performed to identify the causative agent of the infection. Breastfeeding should continue during an infection unless the antibiotic used is contraindicated during lactation. Even with mastitis, breastfeeding should continue; emptying the breast at regular intervals is beneficial. If an abscess forms and ruptures into the breast ducts, the breast should be pumped and the milk discarded. Breastfeeding should continue with the unaffected breast.

Surgical

Some sutures may be removed from the episiotomy, laceration repair, or abdominal incision to allow for drainage. If an abscess forms in mastitis, it may require an incision to allow drainage.

Pharmacological

As soon as a culture is taken, a broad-spectrum antibiotic is usually administered pending the results of the culture.

- *Wound infection:* Iodoform gauze may be placed in the open incision. An analgesic may be necessary.
- *Metritis:* Intravenous administration of antibiotics may be required initially. An antipyretic is given to reduce fever, and methylergonovine maleate (Methergine) is given to increase lochia drainage and promote involution.
- *Mastitis:* Early antibiotic therapy usually prevents abscess formation. An analgesic may be necessary.

Diet

A diet high in protein and vitamin C is needed for wound healing. Fluid intake should be increased to 3,000 mL/day for mothers with a urinary tract infection. Maintaining the increased fluid intake necessary for breastfeeding is essential even when the mother has mastitis.

Activity

Extra rest periods are necessary for all new mothers with an infection. This is especially important for mothers with metritis and mastitis, who should ambulate only enough for their own self-care initially. While in bed, the mother with metritis should be in Fowler's position to aid in lochial drainage from the uterus.

Health Promotion

Strict aseptic technique during labor and birth as well as frequent handwashing by those providing care to the mother are major factors in preventing postpartum infections.

◗ NURSING PROCESS

◗ Assessment

◗ Subjective Data

The mother may describe nausea, fatigue, malaise, pelvic pain or heaviness, leg tenderness, or breast tenderness.

◗ Objective Data

The objective data may include fever; chills; foul-smelling lochia; redness, edema, drainage, or wound separation; dysuria, frequency, or urgency; cracked nipple; and redness and edema of the breast.

Nursing diagnoses for a client with a postpartum infection may include the following:

Nursing Diagnoses	Planning/Goals	Nursing Interventions
▶ *Knowledge Deficit related to lack of exposure to information about the etiology, management, or prevention of puerperal infections*	The client will follow the management plan for her infection.	Teach client how changes after birth predispose to infection. Explain the specific management for client's infection. Answer client's questions.
▶ *Pain related to wound infection, metritis, mastitis, or urinary tract infection*	The client will describe less discomfort.	Administer analgesics and antibiotics as ordered. Continue assessing degree of pain using 0 to 10 pain scale (0 = no pain, 10 = worst pain).
▶ *Family Processes, Altered, related to shift in health status of family member (mother)*	The family will make adjustments for the mother's infection.	Assist family in understanding mother's limitations. Help family identify resources, people that can help out, until the mother is well.

Evaluation Each goal must be evaluated to determine how it has been met by the client.

THROMBOEMBOLIC CONDITIONS

Thrombophlebitis refers to the formation of a clot in an inflamed vein. Superficial thrombophlebitis is more common when the mother had preexisting varicose veins. Deep vein thrombosis (DVT) may or may not be related to vein inflammation and is seen more in women with a history of thromboses. Pulmonary embolism may be a complication of DVT. Septic pelvic thrombophlebitis is more commonly found in a mother with metritis as the inflammation spreads to the pelvic veins.

The incidence of thromboembolic conditions has decreased over the past 20 years since early ambulation has become a standard practice after childbirth (Lowdermilk et al., 1999). Venous stasis and hypercoagulation, which are present during pregnancy, are the major causes. Other risk factors include maternal age over 35, cesarean birth, prolonged time in stirrups during second stage of labor, obesity, smoking, and a history of varicosities or venous thromboses.

Medical–Surgical Management

Medical

Thrombophlebitis is usually managed with rest, elevation of the affected leg, and local application of heat. Elastic stockings are fitted for use when the mother is able to ambulate. Doppler ultrasound is an accurate diagnostic test for DVT. The mother who is receiving a broad-spectrum antibiotic for metritis and whose symptoms are not diminishing should be suspected of having septic pelvic thrombophlebitis.

Pharmacological

An analgesic is given to relieve discomfort. Antibiotics are often given if the mother has a fever. DVT and septic pelvic thrombophlebitis are usually treated with intravenous heparin for 5 to 7 days. During this time, warfarin sodium (Coumadin) is begun and is usually continued for several months.

Activity

Bed rest is required for all thromboembolic conditions. When the mother is allowed to ambulate, she must wear elastic stockings. In thrombophlebitis and DVT, the affected leg is elevated until symptoms decrease.

Health Promotion

The client should be instructed to avoid prolonged standing or sitting. Legs are not to be crossed when sitting. Walking increases venous return and is therefore encouraged. Stirrups should be padded and properly adjusted for correct support and to prevent pressure on the legs.

▶ NURSING PROCESS

▶ Assessment

▶ Subjective Data

The mother may describe discomfort or pain in the leg affected with superficial thrombophlebitis or DVT, and a fullness/heaviness or pain in the pelvis if septic pelvic thrombosis occurs.

▶ Objective Data

Signs of superficial thrombophlebitis include redness, warmth, and swelling where the vein is inflamed. Deep vein thrombosis may manifest as edema and calf pain. A positive Homans' sign may be present, but may also be caused by a strained muscle or improper use of stirrups during the birth. The classic sign of septic pelvic thrombophlebitis is fever of unknown origin. When it is untreated, tachycardia, ileus, and an elevated white count develop.

A nursing diagnosis for clients with thromboembolic conditions may be:

Nursing Diagnosis	Planning/Goals	Nursing Interventions
▶ *Tissue Perfusion, Altered (peripheral), related to mechanical reduction of venous blood flow*	The client will maintain adequate tissue perfusion.	Ensure affected leg is properly elevated.
		Apply heat to affected leg, as ordered.
		Measure client for antiembolic stockings and teach proper application when able to ambulate.
		Encourage fluid intake to prevent dehydration.
		Administer analgesics, antibiotics, heparin, and Coumadin as ordered.
		Assess for signs of pulmonary embolism (chest pain and dyspnea) and evidence of bleeding (i.e., petechiae, bruising, nosebleed, hematoma) related to heparin therapy.
		Emphasize importance of having prothrombin time checked while taking warfarin sodium (Coumadin).
		Keep protamine sulfate, the heparin antagonist, readily available.

Evaluation Each goal must be evaluated to determine how it has been met by the client.

DISSEMINATED INTRAVASCULAR COAGULATION

Disseminated intravascular coagulation (DIC) is an abnormal stimulation of the clotting mechanism, which consumes clotting factors, causing small clots throughout the vascular system and widespread bleeding internally, externally, or both. This results in platelet and clotting factor depletion. DIC may result from a missed abortion, abruptio placenta, amniotic fluid embolism, severe preeclampsia, hemorrhage, and a dead fetus. It is a complication of a preexisting problem.

Correction of the underlying cause is the main aspect of medical management. Blood replacement products including whole blood, packed red cells, or cryoprecipitate may be administered. Nursing care includes continued assessment for signs of bleeding and of complications from the blood products. Intake and output is recorded; urinary output must be maintained at more than 30 mL/hour.

CASE STUDY

Jeff and Meli Lahoti had their third child, a second son, yesterday. The baby weighed 8 lbs, 10 oz, the largest of their three children. The labor lasted 5 hours. An episiotomy was performed this time but had not been for the previous births.

Meli is having problems walking to the bathroom and says she feels faint and dizzy when she stands up. She talks constantly about the pain from the episiotomy. A bruised, edematous area is noted beside the episiotomy. Analgesics provide little relief. Plans were to breastfeed this infant as she had the first two. Today she does not want to feed the baby because she "hurts too much."

continued

CASE STUDY *continued*

The following questions will guide your development of a nursing care plan for this case study.

1. What assessments should be made?
2. Identify three nursing diagnoses for Meli.
3. Identify planning/goals for Meli.
4. List nursing interventions to help Meli meet the goals.
5. How can the effectiveness of this plan be evaluated?

SUMMARY

- The first 6 weeks after the birth of an infant is called the puerperium or postpartum period.
- Mothers, fathers, siblings, and grandparents all make special adaptations for the neonate.
- During the postpartum period, most of the physiologic changes of pregnancy are reversed and the mother's body returns to its prepregnant state.
- Immediate weight loss of the mother is 13 lbs with an additional 8 to 9 lb loss during the first 2 weeks postpartum.
- Rubin describes three phases of maternal restoration/adaptation—taking in, taking hold, and letting go.
- Unexpected emotional/behavioral changes include postpartum depression, postpartum psychosis, and reaction to an infant with problems.
- Specific assessments for the first few days postpartum include BUBBLE (breasts, uterus, bladder, bowel, lochia, and episiotomy), vital signs, Homans' sign, bonding/attachment, parenting, activity, comfort, and self-care.

Review Questions

1. When checking the height of the uterine fundus on the second postpartum day, the nurse should expect to find the fundus:

   a. at the umbilicus.
   b. at the ischial spines.
   c. 2 finger widths above the umbilicus.
   d. 2 finger widths below the umbilicus.

2. The nurse observes passive and dependent behaviors displayed by a postpartum client. According to Reva Rubin, the client is in the:

   a. taking-in phase.
   b. letting-go phase.
   c. taking-hold phase.
   d. transitional phase.

3. A client has excessive vaginal bleeding after delivery. The assessment reveals a soft, boggy uterus located above the level of the umbilicus and displaced to the right side. The first action of the nurse should be to:

   a. notify the CNM/physician.
   b. massage the fundus and take vital signs.
   c. initiate measures that encourage voiding.
   d. put the client flat, take vital signs, and notify the CNM/physician.

4. Six hours postpartum, a client is placed on the bedpan to void. After trying for a period of time, she states that she is unable to void. Her bladder is distended. Which of these measures would it be best for the nurse to use to help the client void?

   a. Pour warm water over the client's vulva.
   b. Encourage the client to drink more fluids.
   c. Apply gentle manual pressure to the client's bladder.
   d. Explain to the client that she will have to be catheterized if she does not void.

5. A new mother tells the nurse that she is afraid of her baby and that she doubts she will be able to love the baby. The most appropriate action for the nurse would be to:

   a. tell the client she will learn fast.
   b. tell the client what a beautiful baby she has.
   c. encourage the client to talk about her feelings.
   d. have a psychiatrist visit the client immediately.

6. When massaging the fundus, the most appropriate nursing action is to:

   a. put firm pressure on the fundus in a downward direction.
   b. vigorously rub the low abdomen while simultaneously exerting downward pressure.

c. rub the low abdomen vigorously and continuously for at least 10 minutes each time.

d. place one hand over the fundus and the other just above the pubic bone and gently massage the fundus in a circular motion.

7. A client has excessive vaginal bleeding following the birth. The nurse should suspect a cervical or vaginal tear if client assessment reveals:

a. acute pelvic pain.

b. a hard, contracted uterus.

c. an elevation of blood pressure.

d. pieces of the placenta still attached to the uterine wall.

8. The postpartum client usually experiences diuresis:

a. immediately after the birth.

b. the first few days after the birth.

c. after the client has had sufficient oral intake.

d. when the infant has been breastfeeding for 10 minutes.

9. A client wants to know when she can begin breastfeeding and is anxious for her milk to start. The best response of the nurse would be:

a. "Ask your CNM/physician."

b. "Your baby will be brought to you at the next feeding time. Your milk will start right after that."

c. "We encourage you to breastfeed as soon as you wish. Your milk will probably 'come in' in about 3 days."

d. "The baby can breastfeed anytime after birth. After your colostrum is gone (3 to 4 days), your milk will come in (5 to 6 days)."

10. Which of the following actions will help suppress lactation?

a. Breast pumping

b. Restriction of oral fluids

c. Wearing a firm, supportive bra and applying ice packs

d. Application of warm, moist compresses to the breasts

Critical Thinking Questions

1. A client with a well-contracted uterus is having a very heavy lochia discharge. Why might this be happening? What care should be given to this client?

2. Identify the rationale for each nursing intervention given for the possible nursing diagnoses in this chapter.

WEB FLASH!

- Search the Web for information about postpartum depression and postpartum psychosis. Would this information be appropriate for or helpful to clients? What organizations are available to help clients?
- What information is available on the Internet about the various complications that can affect a client during the postpartum period?

CHAPTER 51

NEWBORN CARE

MAKING THE CONNECTION

Refer to the following chapters to increase your understanding of newborn care:

- **Chapter 14, The Life Cycle**
- **Chapter 48, Complications of Pregnancy**
- **Chapter 49, The Birth Process**
- **Chapter 50, Postpartum Care**
- **Chapter 52, Basics of Pediatric Care**
- **Chapter 53, Infants with Special Needs: Birth to 12 Months**

- **Procedures:** B1, Handwashing; B2, Use of Protective Equipment; B3, Measuring Body Temperature; B4, Assessing Pulse Rate; B5, Assessing Respirations; B37, Performing Cardiopulmonary Resuscitation (Infant); I14, Administering an Intramuscular Injection; I21, Administering Oxygen; I26, Skin Puncture

LEARNING OBJECTIVES

Upon completion of this chapter, you should be able to:
- *Define key terms.*
- *Describe the immediate needs of the newborn.*
- *Discuss what initiates breathing in the newborn.*
- *Describe the newborn's methods of heat production and heat retention.*
- *Identify the four ways heat is lost and nursing interventions to prevent heat loss.*
- *Describe the immediate care of the newborn.*
- *Discuss the Apgar score and how it is used.*
- *Describe the physical characteristics of the newborn.*
- *Identify the common variations in the newborn.*
- *Elicit the newborn's reflexes.*
- *Determine the gestational age of a newborn.*
- *Discuss the newborn's nutritional needs and how they can be met by breastfeeding and bottle feeding.*
- *Identify common problems the newborn may encounter and nursing interventions for each.*
- *Plan the care and then care for a newborn.*

INTRODUCTION

At the time of birth, the newborn must quickly make changes in the respiratory system to allow gas exchange to take place in the lungs and also make changes in the circulatory system to support the change

KEY TERMS

acrocyanosis
appropriate for
   gestational age
caput succedaneum
cephalhematoma
circumcision
cold stress
conduction
convection
cryptorchidism
Down syndrome
Epstein's pearls
erythema toxicum
   neonatorum
evaporation
foremilk
hallux varus
hindmilk
hydrocele
hyperbilirubinemia
hypospadias
kernicterus
lanugo
large for gestational age
meconium
meningocele
milia

molding
mongolian spots
myelomeningocele
neonatal transition
neutral thermal
   environment
nevus flammeus
nevus vascularis
nonshivering
   thermogenesis
ophthalmia
   neonatorum
phimosis
pseudomenstruation
radiation
small for gestational
   age
spina bifida occulta
syndactyly
talipes equinovarus
   (clubfoot)
telangiectactic nevi
thermogenesis
thermoregulation
vernix caseosa
witch's milk

to respiratory gas exchange. These profound, vital changes are critical to maintaining extrauterine life. The first few hours after birth wherein the newborn makes these changes and stabilizes respiratory and circulatory functions is called the **neonatal transition** period. Other body systems also make changes in their functioning over a longer period of time, though they are not crucial to the immediate survival of the infant.

Nurses are instrumental in assisting the newborn and mother through the neonatal transition period.

IMMEDIATE NEEDS OF THE NEWBORN

The immediate needs of the newborn are airway, breathing, circulation, and warmth.

Airway

A clear airway is necessary for adequate gas exchange.

Breathing

In utero, the fetus relied on the placenta and the mother's respirations for gas exchange. However, fetal breathing movements, from approximately 11 weeks' gestation, help develop the chest wall muscles and the diaphragm (Ladewig, London, & Olds, 1998). By approximately 35 weeks' gestation, the surfactant produced by the alveoli is sufficient in amount (L/S ratio 2:1) to allow the alveoli to remain partially expanded when the newborn begins to breathe at birth.

For the lungs to function, two changes must happen:

- Pulmonary ventilation must be established with lung expansion at the first breath.
- Pulmonary circulation must greatly increase.

The initiation of breathing is influenced by four factors—physical, chemical, thermal, and sensory—which work together.

Physical Factors

The physical (sometimes called mechanical) factors include the compression of the fetal chest as it moves through the birth canal, which squeezes fluid from the lungs and increases intrathoracic pressure; and the chest wall recoil, which occurs as the newborn's trunk emerges. The chest recoil creates negative intrathoracic pressure, which causes a small amount of air to replace the fluid that was squeezed out of the lungs and some of the lung fluid to move across the alveolar membranes into the interstitial tissue of the lungs. Each breath allows more air into the alveoli and more fluid moves into the interstitial tissue. Because the protein concentration is higher in the capillaries, the interstitial fluid is drawn into them. All the alveolar fluid is absorbed within the first day after birth.

Chemical Factors

When the cord is clamped, placental gas exchange ceases, causing an increase in $PaCO_2$ and a decrease in PaO_2 and pH (a transitory asphyxia). These changes stimulate the carotid and aortic chemoreceptors, which send impulses to the respiratory center in the medulla, which in turn stimulates respirations. A brief period of asphyxia stimulates respirations whereas prolonged asphyxia is a central nervous system (CNS) respiratory depressant.

Thermal Factors

The change in temperature from the intrauterine environment to the extrauterine environment, a decrease of more than 20°F, is also a stimulus to breathing. The colder temperature stimulates the skin nerve endings and the newborn breaths as a response. Cold stress and respiratory depression result from excessive cooling of the newborn.

Sensory Factors

The comfortable, relatively quiet uterine environment is left behind for an environment full of sensory stimuli. The auditory and visual stimuli associated with birth, along with the tactile stimulation of being handled, assist in the initiation of respirations.

Circulation

Several circulatory changes are necessary for the successful change from fetal circulation to neonatal circulation. These changes involve the pulmonary blood vessels, ductus arteriosus, foramen ovale, and ductus venosus.

Pulmonary Blood Vessels

The dilation of these blood vessels begins with the first breath taken by the newborn. This results in lower pulmonary resistance, which allows the blood to freely circulate through the lungs to be oxygenated.

Ductus Arteriosus

Within minutes after birth, the ductus arteriosus has a reversal of blood flow caused by the increased pressure in the aorta and the increase of oxygen in the blood. This results in more blood flowing through the pulmonary arteries for oxygenation. Closure of the ductus arteriosus is complete within 24 hours and is permanent in 3 to 4 weeks.

Foramen Ovale

The foramen ovale also closes within minutes after birth because of the higher pressure in the left atrium than in the right atrium. The increased blood flow in the lungs decreases pressure in the right atrium and the return of blood from the lungs increases the pressure in the left atrium. Closure of the foramen ovale is permanent in approximately 3 months.

Ductus Venosus

When the cord is clamped, the blood ceases flowing through the umbilical vein to the ductus venosus and into the inferior vena cava. Blood now flows through the liver and is filtered as in adult circulation.

Warmth

At birth the newborn must begin **thermoregulation**, maintenance of body temperature. Three factors are instrumental in thermoregulation: heat production, heat retention, and heat loss.

Heat Production

The newborn produces heat (**thermogenesis**) through general metabolism, muscular activity, and nonshivering thermogenesis (unique to the newborn). Newborns rarely shiver as adults do to increase heat production. Shivering seen in a newborn indicates that the metabolic rate has already doubled (Ladewig et al., 1998).

When the infant is in a cool environment and requires more heat, the metabolic rate increases, producing more heat. The newborn may cry and have muscular activity when cold, but there is no voluntary control of muscular activity.

If the infant's temperature is not adequately raised through increased metabolism, **nonshivering thermogenesis**, the metabolism of brown fat, begins. Brown fat is a special fat found only in newborns. It appears at about 26 to 30 weeks of gestation and increases until 2 to 5 weeks of age (unless depleted by cold stress). The fat is highly vascularized, which gives it the brown color. The brown fat is located at the back of the neck, between the scapula, around the kidneys and adrenals, in the axilla, and around the heart and abdominal aorta (Figure 51-1). Once the brown fat has been metabolized, the infant no longer has this method of heat production available.

Heat Retention

Newborns retain heat by staying in a flexed position. This reduces the area of skin exposed to the environmental temperature, thus decreasing heat loss. They also use the mechanism of peripheral vasoconstriction to retain heat.

Heat Loss

The newborn has thin skin with blood vessels close to the surface and little subcutaneous fat to prevent heat loss. Heat moves from the warm internal areas to the cooler skin surface and then to the surrounding environment. Excessive heat loss is called **cold stress**. An increase in metabolism leads to a significant increase in the need for oxygen. When oxygen is used for metabolism (heat production), the infant may experience hypoxia. There may not be enough oxygen for the metabolic rate to increase, and the newborn will not be able to maintain body temperature. Prolonged cold stress causes respiratory difficulties and a decrease in surfactant production. Less surfactant hinders lung expansion, which in turn leads to more respiratory distress. Decreased blood oxygen may cause vasoconstriction of the pulmonary vessels with a return to fetal circulation patterns, which further increases respiratory distress.

The glucose necessary for increased metabolism is made available when glycogen stores are converted to glucose. If the glycogen is depleted, hypoglycemia results.

Brown fat metabolism results in the release of fatty acids. Continuous brown fat metabolism, when the newborn is in a cold stress situation for a considerable time, results in metabolic acidosis, which can be life-threatening. Excess fatty acids in the blood interfere with bilirubin transportation to the liver, which increases the risk of jaundice.

There are four methods by which the newborn loses heat: conduction, convection, evaporation, and radiation.

Conduction Conduction is the loss of heat by direct contact with a cooler object. When a newborn is

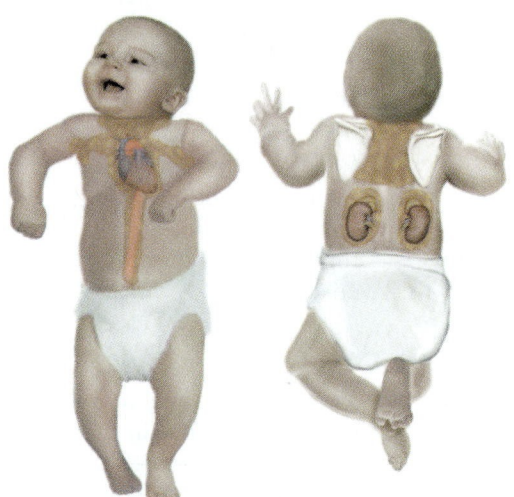

Figure 51-1 Brown Fat Distribution in the Newborn

PROFESSIONAL TIP

Effects of Cold Stress
- Oxygen need increased
- Respiratory distress
- Surfactant production decreased
- Hypoglycemia
- Metabolic acidosis
- Jaundice

touched by cold hands or a cold stethoscope or is placed on a cold surface such as a scale, heat is lost. Heat loss can be prevented by warming objects touching the newborn. If a newborn is wrapped in a warmed blanket or placed against the mother's warm skin, heat will be lost by the blanket or mother's skin to the cooler newborn and the newborn is warmed.

Convection **Convection** is the loss of heat by the movement of air. When air moves (air currents), heat is transferred to the air. Air currents from an open door or window, air conditioning, or from people moving around increase heat loss. A radiant warmer is often used for the newborn immediately after birth to prevent heat loss by convection (Figure 51-2). Heat loss, in the newborn, can be prevented by wrapping the infant in a blanket and placing a stocking cap on the head and by keeping the newborn out of any drafts.

Evaporation **Evaporation** is the loss of heat when water is changed to a vapor. When a wet body dries, heat is lost, such as a newborn wet with amniotic fluid or during a bath. The insensible water loss from the skin and respiratory tract also results in heat loss. Heat loss can be prevented by immediately drying the newborn at birth and after receiving a bath, and by changing wet clothing and diapers promptly.

Radiation **Radiation** is the loss of heat by transfer to cooler objects nearby, but not through direct contact. An infant placed near a cold window loses heat by radiation to the sides of the crib and the window. If the walls of an incubator are cold, the infant loses heat. Heat loss can be prevented by keeping cribs and incubators away from cold windows.

IMMEDIATE CARE OF THE NEWBORN

The immediate care of the newborn includes obtaining the Apgar score, resuscitation (if needed), providing a neutral thermal environment, proper identification of the infant, parent/infant bonding, and prophylactic care.

PROFESSIONAL TIP

Newborns and Standard Precautions
Penny-MacGillivray (1996) explains that blood and amniotic fluid, once believed to be sterile, are now considered contaminated with blood-borne pathogens. All newborns are now also considered contaminated until the first bath has removed all blood and amniotic fluid from the infant's body. The nurse performing the assessment and giving the first bath *must wear gloves.*

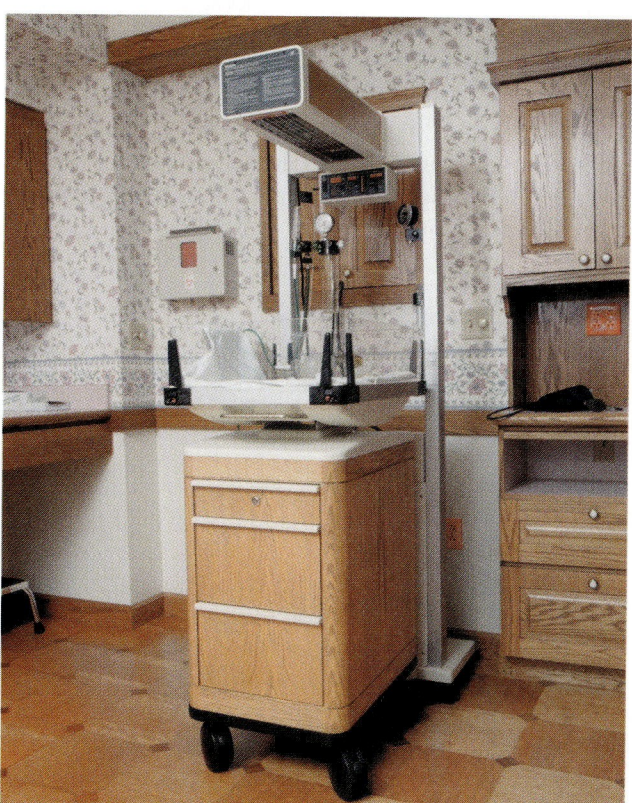

Figure 51-2 A radiant warmer keeps the air around the newborn warm, preventing heat loss by convection.

Apgar Score

The Apgar score, which assesses the infant's cardiopulmonary adaptations to extrauterine life, was discussed in Chapter 49, Birth Process.

Resuscitation

Resuscitation is begun if no respirations are initiated by the infant. The licensed practical/vocational nurse (LP/VN) may be asked to use a bulb syringe to suction mucus from the infant's oropharynx, gently rub the infant's back for stimulation, or provide oxygen. More intense resuscitation would typically be performed by a registered nurse (RN) or physician.

Neutral Thermal Environment

A **neutral thermal environment** is an environment in which the newborn can maintain internal body temperature with minimal oxygen consumption and metabolism. In this environment the newborn's body does not have to focus on temperature maintenance but can focus on growth and development.

Identification

Proper identification of the newborn is vital. The identification bands must be checked and compared to the mother's band each time the baby is brought into the mother's room. The process of applying the identification bands is discussed in Chapter 49, Birth Process.

Parent/Infant Bonding

Interaction between the parents and infant should be promoted as soon as the infant is stable. The nurse may need to assist the parents in holding their baby or to give them permission to examine the infant.

Prophylactic Care

Prophylactic care includes the administration of vitamin K and hepatitis B vaccine, instillation of an antibiotic ophthalmic ointment, and umbilical cord care.

Vitamin K

At birth, newborns lack vitamin K, which is necessary for the clotting process. Vitamin K is synthesized in the intestine and requires food and normal intestinal flora for the process. Because the intestines are sterile at birth, no vitamin K can be produced for several days. An intramuscular (IM) injection of vitamin K, phytonadione (aquaMEPHYTON) is generally given within the first hour after birth to prevent hemorrhagic disorders. A normal newborn is able to produce vitamin K by the eighth day (Lowdermilk, Perry, & Bobak, 1999).

Hepatitis B Vaccination

The Centers for Disease Control and Prevention (CDC) along with the Advisory Committee on Immunization Practices (ACIP), the American Academy of Pediatrics (AAP), and the American Academy of Family Physicians (AAFP) recommend that newborns be given the first dose of hepatitis B (Hep B) vaccine within 12 hours of birth (see Appendix A). Infants whose mothers have hepatitis B should also receive hepatitis B immune globulin (HBIG) at the same time, but at a different site than the vaccine. The HBIG provides passive immunity until the newborn develops antibodies. In many agencies, the parents must give written permission for the infant to receive the hepatitis B vaccine.

Eye Prophylaxis

In the United States it is mandatory that a prophylactic agent be instilled in the eyes of all neonates to prevent **ophthalmia neonatorum**. This is an inflammation of the newborn's eyes that results from passing through the birth canal when a gonorrheal or chlamydial infection is present. The medication used for prophylaxis varies with agency protocol but is generally erythromycin (Ilotycin Ophthalmic Ointment) or tetracycline (Achromycin Ophthalmic Ointment) (Lowdermilk et al., 1999). Silver nitrate 1% is now seldom used because it protects only against gonorrheal infection and not chlamydial infection. To promote parent/infant eye contact, bonding, and attachment, some agencies delay the eye prophylaxis for an hour or so.

Umbilical Cord Care

Umbilical cord care is the same as for any surgical wound (Krebs, 1998). The cord and the skin at its base are assessed for redness, edema, and purulent drainage each time the diaper is changed. The cord and skin are cleaned as per agency protocol (i.e., triple blue dye, alcohol, or erythromycin solution). The prevention of or early identification of any hemorrhage or infection is the goal of care.

Safety: Cord Hemorrhage
- When bleeding from the cord is noted, check the clamp and apply a second clamp on the body side of the first one.
- If the bleeding does not immediately stop, notify the health care provider.

PHYSICAL CHARACTERISTICS OF THE NEWBORN

The newborn infant is not just a miniature adult. Identification of the physical characteristics and common variations of the newborn found in the infant are documented. This provides a basis for nursing diagnoses and care. Agencies generally have a form to follow such as the one shown in Figure 51-3. This form incorporates data about the mother, the delivery, Apgar score, and gestational age along with the physical assessment of the infant.

Weight and Length

Most full-term newborns weigh between 2,500 g and 4,000 g or approximately 5 lb, 8 oz to 8 lb, 13 oz. Newborns lose 5% to 10% of their body weight in the first 3 to 4 days. This is a result of small fluid intake, volume of **meconium** (first bowel movements of newborn, black and tarry) (Figure 51-4), and urination. Birth weight is generally regained by 10 days of age.

Their head to heel length is 48 cm to 53 cm (approximately 19 in. to 21 in.), and crown to rump length is 31 cm to 35 cm (approximately 12 in. to 14 in.) or approximately equal to the head circumference.

Vital Signs

The axillary temperature should be between 36.5°C and 37.2°C (97.6°F and 98.9°F). A continuous skin probe is best for small newborns or those in a radiant warmer. Normal skin temperature is 36°C to 36.5°C (96.8°F to 97.6°F). Crying may slightly increase temperature.

The apical heart rate is 120 to 140 beats/minute. When the newborn is sleeping, the heart rate decreases, and when crying, the heart rate increases.

Respirations are 30 to 60 breaths/minute. As with the heart rate, sleep decreases respirations and crying increases respirations.

Initial Newborn Profile

❋ Hollister.

Initial Newborn Profile
Hollister Maternal/Newborn Record System
To order call: 1.800.323.4060   Re-order No. 5720

Admit Data Date____/____ Date_____	Newborn Data	☐ male ☐ Breast ☐ Female ☐ Bottle	Maternal Data	G	T	Pt	A	L

Admit Data Date____/____ Date_____
ID/Band No. _____ Name _____
Admitted By _____
Medications ☐ None ☐ See Delivery Data
Date   Time Medication   Dose   Route Inits
         Eye Prophylaxis   Site
_____ Erythromycin _____
_____ _____ Vitamin K _____

Newborn Data
Birthdate ____/____/____
                          Time _____
Place of Birth ☐ Hospital _____
☐ Vertex ☐ Breech ☐ Vaginal ☐ Cesarean
Delivered by _____
Apgar __1min __5min __10min
Cord Blood pH ___ Type/Rh ___ Coombs ___
Intrapartum Problems Identified ☐ None
1.
2.
3.

Maternal Data
Name_____   Age_____
Record No._____ Room No._____
Blood Type/Rh _____ Antibody + -
Screens   Neg Pos   Comments
STD   ☐   ☐
Urine Tox   ☐   ☐
Hepatitis B   ☐   ☐

Measurements/Gestational Age Assessment
See
Delivery
Data
☐ Weight ____lbs ____gms Gest Age by Dates ____ Wks
                          Gest Age by Exam ____ Wks
☐ Length ____cms ____ins   ☐ Preterm
☐ Head Circ ____cms ____ins ☐ Term
☐ Chest Circ ____cms ____ins ☐ Postterm
☐ Abd Circ ____cms ____ins   ☐ SGA ☐ AGA ☐ LGA

Physical Assessment
Date __/__/__   Time_____ Age _____ hrs
Temp_____ Pulse Rate/Rhythm_____ Resp_____ BP ___ ☐ Not done
Head/Neck   Detail Abnormal Findings
1. Fontanels   Level Bulging Depressed
   Anterior
   Posterior
2. Sutures ☐ Open ☐ Closed ☐ Overriding
3. Variations ☐ None ☐ Molding ☐ Caput ☐ Cephalhematoma
4. Lacerations ☐ No ☐ Yes
                                Normal Abnormal
5. Face ....   ☐   ☐
6. Eyes ....   ☐   ☐
7. Ears ....   ☐   ☐
8. Nose ....   ☐   ☐
9. Mouth ....   ☐   ☐
10. Neck ....   ☐   ☐
Chest
11. Breath sounds.. ☐   ☐
12. Thorax ....   ☐   ☐
13. Clavicles ....   ☐   ☐
Cardiovascular
14. Heart sounds... ☐   ☐
15. Pulses .... ☐   ☐
Abdomen
16. Structure ......   ☐   ☐
17. Bowel sounds.. ☐   ☐
18. Cord ....   ☐   ☐
19. Liver ....   ☐   ☐
20. Spleen ....   ☐   ☐
21. Kidneys ....   ☐   ☐
Genitalia
22. Female .... ☐   ☐
23. Male ....   ☐   ☐

Musculoskeletal   Normal Abnormal   Detail Abnormal Findings
24. Tone ....   ☐   ☐
25. Extremities ...... ☐   ☐
26. Hips ....   ☐   ☐
27. Spine ....   ☐   ☐
Neurologic
28. Reflexes ....   ☐   ☐
29. Cry ....   ☐   ☐
Skin
30. Condition ☐ Smooth ☐ Dry ☐ Peeling ☐ Vernix ☐ Mec Stain
31. Color ☐ Pink ☐ Ruddy ☐ Pale ☐ Mottled ☐ Cyanotic
          ☐ Jaundice (time noted ___)
32. Variations (i.e. rash, lesion, birthmark)
Elimination
33. Bowel Anus Patent ☐ Yes ☐ No _____
                    First Meconium (date, time)_____
34. Urine First Void (date, time)_____

Problems identified ☐ None
1.
2.
3.
Comments/Plan

Newborn Risk Indicators

Observable at birth	Within 24 hrs. postpartum
☐ **No risk factors noted**	☐ **No risk factors noted**
☐ Abnormal presentation	☐ Abdominal presentation
☐ Multiple birth	☐ Vomiting
☐ Low birth rate	☐ Failure to pass meconium (if skin not stained)
☐ Resuscitation at birth	
☐ 1 min. Apgar <5	☐ Melena
☐ 5 min. Apgar <7	☐ Apneic episodes (>20 seconds)
☐ Placental Abnormalities	☐ Tachypnea (transient)
☐ Two cord vessels	☐ See-saw breathing
☐ Difficult catheterization	☐ Cyanosis
☐ > 20 ml. of gastric aspirate	☐ Petechiae/Ecchymoses
☐ Small mandible with cleft palate	☐ Jaundice
☐ Grunting	☐ Pallor
☐ Deep retractions	☐ Plethora
☐ Imperforate anus	☐ Fever
☐ Pallor	☐ Hypothermia
☐ Jaundice	☐ Arrhythmias
☐ Plethora	☐ Murmur
☐ Convulsions	☐ Lethargy
☐ Decreased tone	☐ Tremors (jitters)
☐ Congenial malformations	☐ Convulsions
☐ _____	☐ _____
☐ _____	☐ _____
☐ _____	☐ _____

Signature _____

Figure 51-3 Initial Newborn Profile with Newborn Risk Indicators (*Permission to use this copyright material has been granted by the owner, Hollister Incorporated.*)

Blood pressure ranges between 60 and 80 mm Hg systolic and 40 and 45 mm Hg diastolic. By 10 days of age, it is 100/50 mm Hg. Activity and crying will increase the newborn's blood pressure.

General Appearance

Full-term newborns have a flexed posture. The head is flexed, the arms are flexed on the chest, and the legs are flexed on the abdomen.

Skin

At birth the skin is red, puffy, and smooth. Some **vernix caseosa** (a white, creamy substance) may thinly cover the skin, with large amounts found in body creases. **Lanugo** (fine, downy hair) may still be seen on the forehead and shoulders, or it may all have

disappeared. **Acrocyanosis**, blue coloring of the hands and feet, is generally present for several hours until the cardiopulmonary changes have stabilized and fully oxygenated blood has reached the hands and feet. Edema may be present around the eyes, face, dorsa of hands, legs, feet, and labia or scrotum.

Head

The head circumference, measured over the most prominent part of the occiput and just above the eyebrows, is between 33 cm and 35 cm (approximately 13 in. to 14 in.). There are two fontanelles, one anterior and one posterior. The anterior fontanelle is largest, diamond shaped, and closes by 18 months of age. The posterior fontanelle is triangular in shape and closes about 2 months after birth. The fontanelles should be firm and flat but may bulge when the infant cries or coughs.

Eyes

Eye color varies, being either slate gray, blue, or brown. Permanent eye color is usually established by 3 months of age. The eyelids are usually edematous, and there are no tears.

Ears

The ears are soft, pliable, and recoil swiftly when bent and released. Ear placement should be so the top

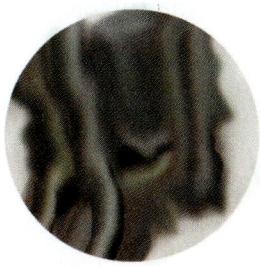

Figure 51-4 Meconium Stool

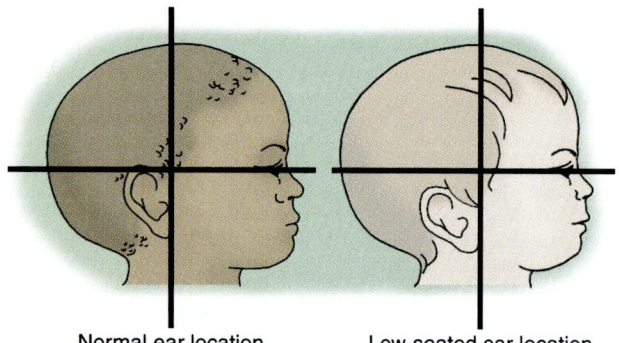

Normal ear location   Low-seated ear location

Figure 51-5 Ear Placement. Top of ear should be in line with outer canthus of the eye.

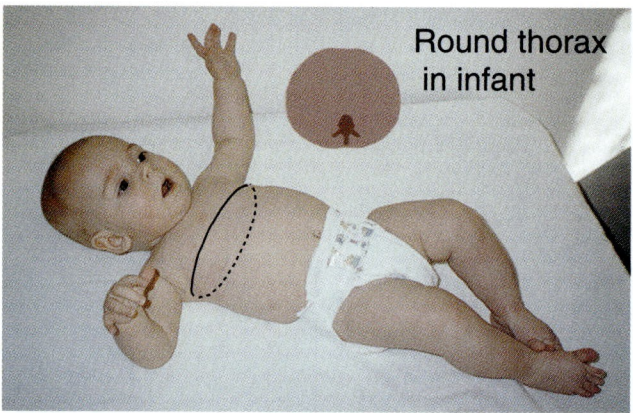

Round thorax in infant

Figure 51-6 Newborn chest is round, having the same diameter front to back and side to side.

of the ear is in line with the outer canthus of the eye (Figure 51-5).

Neck

The neck is short, thick, and usually has several skin folds.

Chest

Chest circumference is 30.5 cm to 33 cm (approximately 12 in. to 13 in.). It is measured directly over the nipple line and lower edge of the scapulas. The chest circumference is 2 cm to 3 cm smaller than the head circumference. The diameters front to back and side to side are equal (Figure 51-6).

Safety: Disposable Paper Tape Measure
When a measurement has been completed, either roll the infant off the paper tape measure or lift the newborn and remove the paper tape measure. Never pull the tape measure out from under the newborn; a paper cut on the newborn's body may result.

Abdomen

The abdomen is cylindrical in shape. The bluish-white umbilical cord protrudes from the center.

Genitalia

The labia are usually edematous with vernix caseosa between the labia.

If the testes are descended, the scrotum is large, pendulous, and edematous; if the testes are not descended, the scrotum is small. In either case the scrotum is covered with rugae. The newborn with dark skin has a deeply pigmented scrotum. The newborn should urinate within 24 hours.

Back

The spine should be intact with no openings, masses, or prominent curves.

Extremities

The extremities are usually flexed, have a full range of motion, and are symmetrical. Ten fingers and ten toes should be present with creases visible on the anterior two-thirds of the sole of the foot.

COMMON VARIATIONS IN THE NEWBORN

There are many variations seen in the newborn that are perfectly normal and cause no trouble. Any one newborn may have some of these variations but not all. Most of these variations disappear in a few days or weeks, a few in several years.

Skin

There are several colorations or skin eruptions that may be present, including jaundice, ecchymoses, milia, erythema toxicum neonatorum, telangiectactic nevi, nevus flammeus, nevus vascularis, and mongolian spots.

Jaundice

Jaundice occurring *after* the first 24 hours of life is related to the normal destruction of the excess red blood cells (RBCs) in the newborn. With direct oxygenation of the blood in the newborn's lungs, the extra RBCs of the fetus are no longer needed. The infant's immature liver is often unable to conjugate all the bilirubin released by the destroyed RBCs, and this is evident as jaundice. The jaundice usually peaks at 72 hours then disappears in a couple of weeks. Jaundice appearing *within* the first 24 hours of life is discussed later in this chapter.

Ecchymosis

Areas of ecchymosis (bruising) may be evident following a difficult delivery. Petechiae may also be present.

CLIENT TEACHING

Milia

Milia are not whiteheads and should never be squeezed.

Milia

Milia are white, pin head-size, distended sebaceous glands on the cheeks, nose, chin, and occasionally on the trunk. After a few weeks of bathing, they usually disappear.

Erythema Toxicum Neonatorum

Erythema toxicum neonatorum is a pink rash with firm, yellow-white papules or pustules found on the chest, abdomen, back, and buttocks of some newborns. This may appear 24 to 48 hours after birth and disappear in a few days without any treatment.

Telangiectactic Nevi

Telangiectactic nevi ("stork-bites") are birthmarks of dilated capillaries that blanch with pressure. They may appear on the eyelids, nose, occipital area, or nape of the neck and fade between 1 and 2 years of age.

Nevus Flammeus

Nevus flammeus (port-wine stain) is a large reddish-purple birthmark usually found on the face or neck that does not blanch with pressure. It is not raised above the skin. This does not spontaneously disappear but may be lightened with special laser treatments.

Nevus Vascularis

Nevus vascularis (strawberry mark) is a birthmark of enlarged superficial blood vessels. They are elevated, red in color, and of variable size and shape. They are most often found on the head, face, neck, and arms. By school age, they have generally disappeared.

Mongolian Spots

Mongolian spots are deep blue areas of coloration, usually in the sacral region, at birth. They are seen mainly in infants of African, Asian, American Indian, Hispanic, and Southern European descent.

PROFESSIONAL TIP

Mongolian Spots

Carefully document the presence of mongolian spots on the newborn's record. This may prevent charges of child abuse being filed later against the parents or caregivers.

Head

Three common variations in newborns involve the head: molding, caput succedaneum, and cephalhematoma.

Molding

Molding is the shaping of the fetal head to adapt to the mother's pelvis during labor. In 2 to 3 days the cranial bones typically return to their proper placement (Figure 51-7).

Caput Succedaneum

Caput succedaneum, edema of the newborn's scalp that is present at birth, may cross suture lines and is caused by head compression against the cervix (Figure 51-8A). The edema disappears in 2 to 3 days. No treatment is needed.

Cephalhematoma

Cephalhematoma is a collection of blood between the periosteum and the skull of a newborn. It appears several hours to a day after birth, does not cross suture lines, and is caused by the rupturing of the periosteal bridging veins due to friction and pressure during labor and delivery (Figure 51-8B). It is usually the largest on the second or third day and spontaneously resorbs in 3 to 6 weeks. Table 51-1 compares caput succedaneum and cephalhematoma.

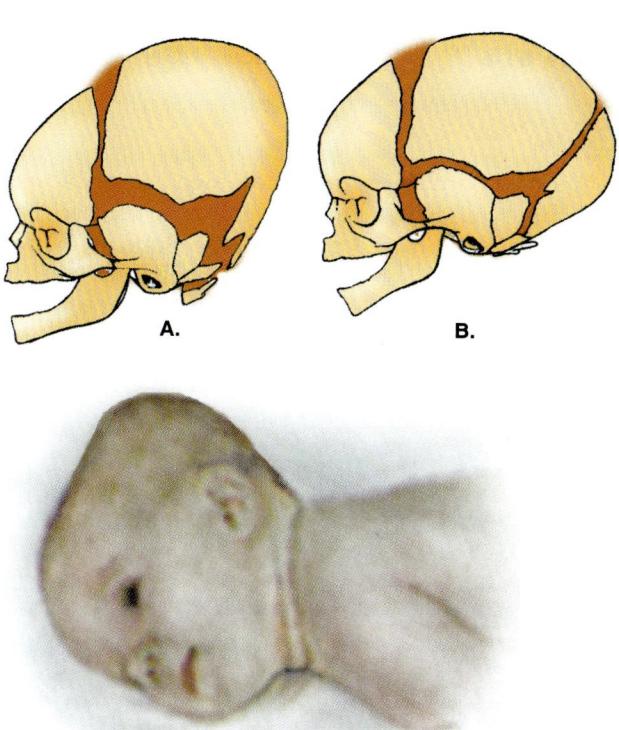

Figure 51-7 Molding: A. Movement of cranial bones during labor; B. Cranial bones return to their proper placement in 2 to 3 days; C. Infant exhibiting molding.

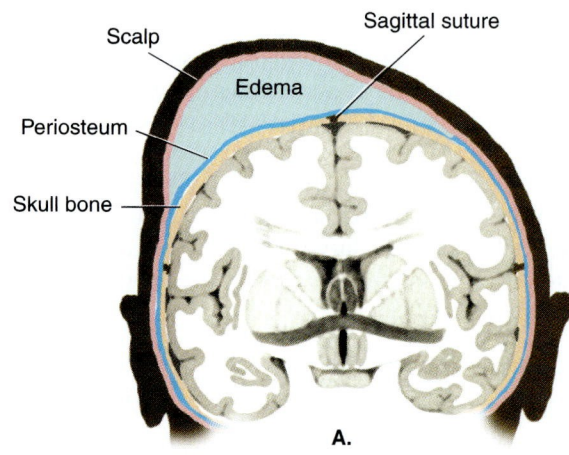

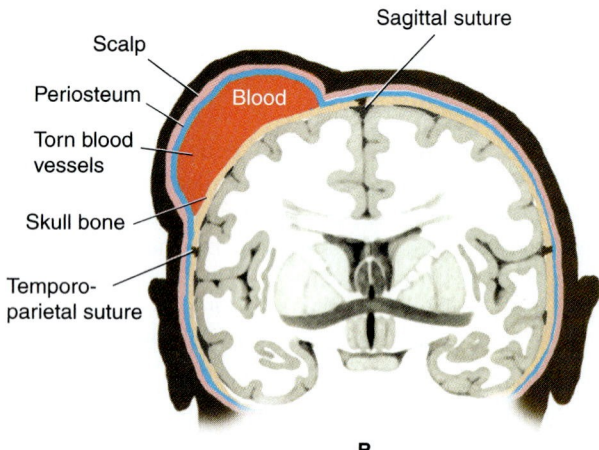

Figure 51-8 A. Caput Succedaneum; B. Cephalhematoma

Eyes

The newborn's eyes may show signs of strabismus, which is caused by poor neuromuscular control. This usually disappears in 3 to 4 months. Subconjunctival hemorrhages are present in approximately 10% of newborns (Ladewig et al., 1998). Change in vascular tension or ocular pressure during birth causes these hemorrhages. They last for a few weeks and do not impair vision.

Ears

The ears may be of irregular shape and size. The pinna may be flat against the head.

Mouth

Precocious teeth may be present at birth in the center of the lower gum. If loose, they should be removed to prevent aspiration. **Epstein's pearls**, small, whitish-yellow epithelial cysts, are found on the hard palate. They disappear within a few weeks.

Chest

Many newborns, both male and female, have engorged breasts as a result of maternal hormones. This occurs by the third day and may last 2 weeks. The nipples may secrete a whitish fluid, often called "**witch's milk**."

Genitalia

There several variations in the female and male genitalia.

Female

Pseudomenstruation, a blood-tinged mucous discharge from the vagina, may be evident in the first week after birth. It is caused by the withdrawal of maternal hormones. A vaginal tag or hymenal tag may be present but will disappear in a few weeks.

Male

Hypospadias, placement of the urinary meatus on the underside of the penis, may be present. **Phimosis**, when the opening in the foreskin is so small that it cannot be pulled back over the glans, may interfere with urination. **Cryptorchidism**, failure of one or both testes to descend, may be evident. **Hydrocele**, fluid around the testes in the scrotum, usually disappears without any treatment.

Extremities

There may be partial **syndactyly** (fusion of two or more fingers or toes) of the second and third toes. **Hallux varus**, placement of the great toe farther from other toes, may be present.

REFLEXES

Many of the newborn's movements are reflexive in nature. Some reflexes, like sneezing, coughing,

Table 51-1 COMPARISON OF CAPUT SUCCEDANEUM AND CEPHALHEMATOMA		
CHARACTERISTIC	**CAPUT SUCCEDANEUM**	**CEPHALHEMATOMA**
Fluid	Edema	Blood
Layer involved	Scalp	Between periosteum and skull
Relationship to suture lines	May cross suture lines	Does not cross suture lines
Appears	Present at birth	First or second day
Disappears	2 to 3 days	3 to 6 weeks

swallowing, blinking, yawning, and hiccupping are present throughout life. Others disappear at various times throughout the first 2 years of life; these are discussed next. These neonatal reflexes must be lost before motor development can proceed (Estes, 1998). The presence of the reflexes indicates neurological integrity.

Rooting Reflex

The rooting reflex is elicited by stroking the skin at one corner of the infant's mouth. The infant will turn the head toward the side stroked (Figure 51-9). This reflex is present up until 3 or 4 months of age. Absence of the reflex during this time frame may indicate a frontal lobe lesion.

Sucking Reflex

Touching the newborn's lips elicits the sucking reflex (Figure 51-10). This reflex occurs until approximately 10 months of age. Preterm infants or an infant who is breastfed by a mother taking barbiturates will not exhibit the sucking reflex because of CNS depression.

Extrusion Reflex

When the tip of the tongue is touched or depressed, the infant will force the tongue outward. This reflex disappears at approximately 4 months of age. Feeding an infant food with a spoon before 4 months of age is difficult because of the extrusion reflex.

Palmar Grasp Reflex

When a finger is placed across the palm, the infant's fingers flex and grasp the examiner's finger (Figure 51-11). If the palmar grasp reflex is present after 4 months of age, frontal lobe lesions are suspected.

Plantar Grasp Reflex

When the infant's leg is held in one hand, and the plantar surface of the foot is touched below the toes with the other hand, the infant's toes will curl downward (Figure 51-12). This reflex lasts until 8 months of age. If the plantar grasp reflex is absent on one foot, an obstructive lesion is suspected. Absence of the reflex in both feet is seen with neurological alterations such as cerebral palsy.

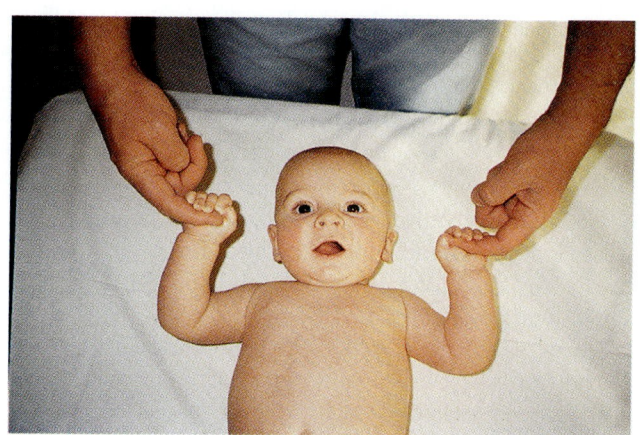

Figure 51-11 Palmar Grasp Reflex

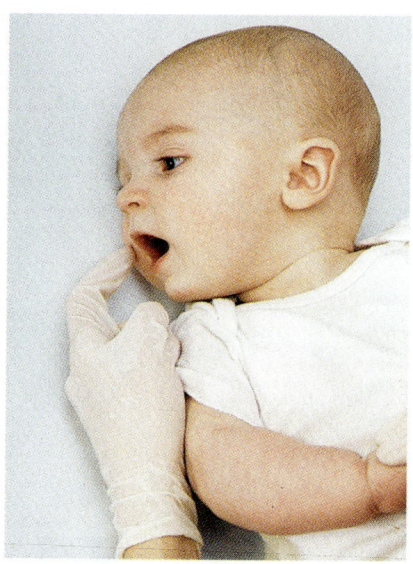

Figure 51-9 Rooting Reflex

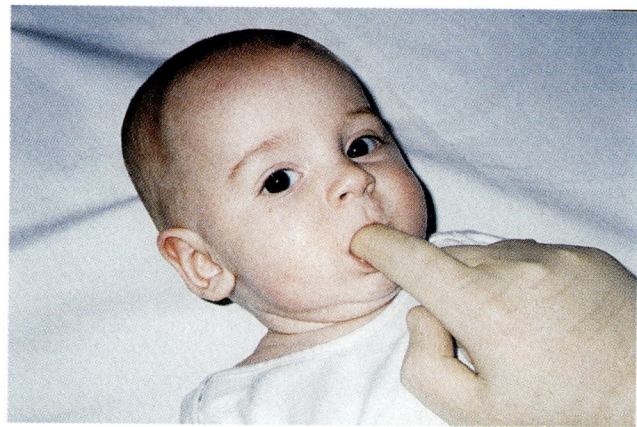

Figure 51-10 Sucking Reflex

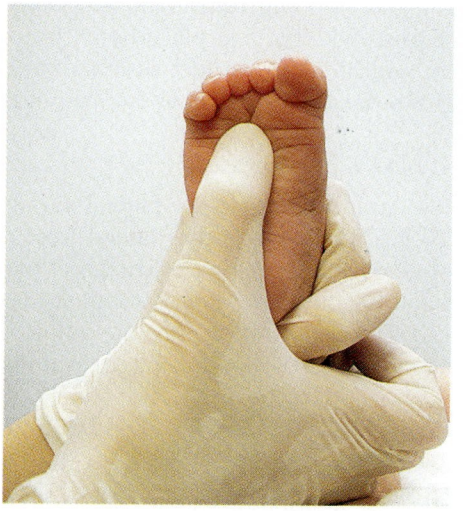

Figure 51-12 Plantar Grasp Reflex

Tonic Neck Reflex

The tonic neck reflex is sometimes referred to as the "fencing" reflex because of the position assumed by the infant. This reflex is elicited by placing the infant supine and rotating the head to one side. The arm and leg on the side to which the jaw is turned will extend and the opposite arm and leg will flex (Figure 51-13). Sometimes, this reflex may not be displayed until 6 to 8 weeks of age. If it is still seen after 6 months of age, cerebral damage is suspected.

Moro Reflex

The Moro reflex is sometimes called the startle reflex. It is elicited either by holding the newborn in a semisitting position and then allowing the head to fall backward to an angle of 30°, or having the infant lying on a flat surface and then hitting the surface to startle the infant. The response by the infant less than 4 months of age is to quickly extend and abduct the arms with the fingers fanning out. The thumb and forefinger form a "C" followed by adduction of the arms in an embracing motion. A slight tremor may be noted. The legs may also extend and then flex (Figure 51-14). The Moro reflex is present at birth and disappears between 4 and 6 months of age. Possible brain damage is indicated if the response persists after 6 months of age. An asymmetrical response may be caused by an injury to the clavicle, humerus, or brachial plexus.

Gallant Reflex

The Gallant reflex is elicited with the infant lying prone with the hands under the abdomen. The infant's skin is stroked along one side of the spine; the infant's shoulders and pelvis turn toward the stimulated side (Figure 51-15). A spinal cord lesion is suspected if there is no response from an infant under 2 months of age. This reflex is present from birth to age 2 months.

Stepping Reflex

To elicit the stepping reflex, the newborn is held under the arms with the feet placed on a firm surface. The infant will lift alternate feet as if walking (Figure 51-16). This reflex disappears at about 3 months of age.

Babinski's Reflex

To elicit Babinski's reflex, the plantar surface of the infant's foot is stroked from the lateral heel area upward and across under the toes. The great toe should dorsiflex and the other toes fan out (Figure 51-17). The presence of Babinski's reflex after the infant has mastered walking (12 to 18 months of age) is abnormal.

Crossed Extension Reflex

The crossed extension reflex is elicited with the infant supine by holding one leg extended with the knee pressed down and stimulating the bottom of that foot.

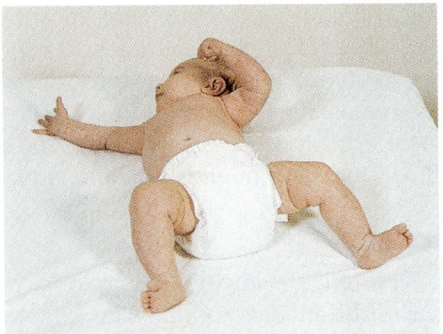
Figure 51-13 Tonic Neck Reflex

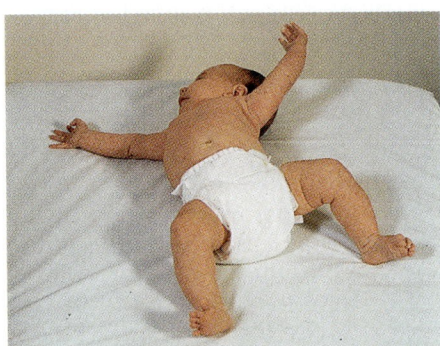
Figure 51-14 Moro (Startle) Reflex

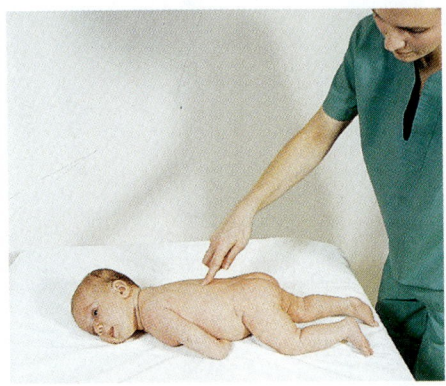
Figure 51-15 Gallant Reflex

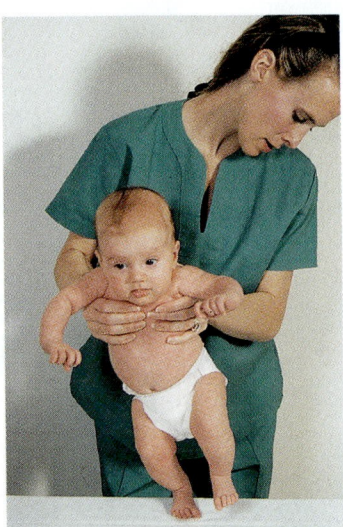
Figure 51-16 Stepping Reflex

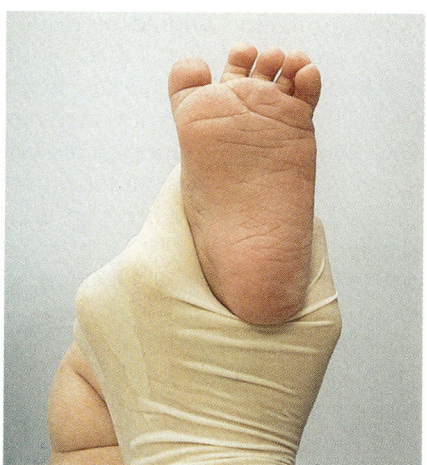

Figure 51-17 Babinski's Reflex

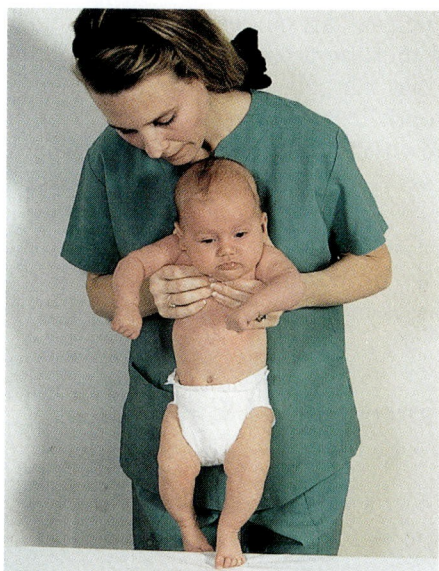

Figure 51-18 Placing Reflex

LIFE CYCLE CONSIDERATIONS

Babinski's Reflex

The expected response from an infant is opposite that of an older child or adult.

- The expected response from an infant (until walking is mastered) is dorsiflexion of the great toe and fanning of the other toes. This is a positive (normal) response.
- The expected response from a child who has mastered walking and for an adult is flexion of the great toe and other toes. This is a negative (normal) response.
- If an infant has a negative Babinski response or an older person has a positive Babinski response, a neurologic evaluation is required.

periods of reactivity. Following that, the infant will exhibit various behavioral states, divided into sleeping and waking phases.

Periods of Reactivity

There are two periods of reactivity that occur during the first few hours of life, separated by a period of sleep.

First Period of Reactivity

During the first period of reactivity, the first 30 minutes after birth, the newborn is awake, alert, and active. It is a prime time for parent/infant interaction. The newborn may act hungry, with a strong sucking reflex evident. If the mother plans to breastfeed, this is the ideal time for her to begin. During this period, the newborn's heart rate and respirations are rapid, and bowel sounds are seldom heard.

Sleep Period

The newborn enters a sleep period that usually lasts from 2 to 4 hours. This is a time of deep sleep, from which it is difficult to awaken the newborn. The heart and respiratory rates return to baseline and bowel sounds become audible.

Second Period of Reactivity

The second period of reactivity lasts from 4 to 6 hours. The newborn is once again awake and alert.

The other leg should flex, adduct, and then extend as if trying to push away the stimulus. This reflex should be present during the first 4 weeks of life.

Placing Reflex

To elicit the placing reflex, the infant is held under the arms from behind then brought to a standing position, touching the dorsum of one foot on the edge of the table. The tested leg will flex and lift onto the table (Figure 51-18). It is abnormal for there to be no response. An infant born in a breech presentation or one with paralysis or cerebral cortex difficulties may not respond to this stimulus.

BEHAVIORAL CHARACTERISTICS

During the first 6 to 10 hours after birth, the infant has a fairly predictable pattern of behavior called the

PROFESSIONAL TIP

Stepping Reflex and Placing Reflex

While fairly similar, the stepping and placing reflexes are two different reflexes and should not be tested at the same time.

Physiologic responses vary. The heart and respiratory rates increase, yet there may be periods of apnea, which may cause the heart rate to decrease. During these fluctuations, the newborn may become mottled or slightly cyanotic.

The newborn may gag, spit up, or choke as gastric and respiratory mucus increases. Close observation is a must during this period of activity so that appropriate interventions may be taken to maintain a clear airway for the infant.

The first meconium stool is often passed as the gastrointestinal tract becomes more active. The first voiding may now occur. The newborn may begin rooting, sucking, and swallowing, indicating a readiness for feeding.

Behavioral States

Brazelton (1984) identified that newborns have different states of being. He categorized them as sleep states and alert states.

Sleep States

Two sleep states have been identified for the newborn: quiet sleep and active sleep. At term, a newborn changes from one sleep state to the other approximately every 45 to 50 minutes during sleep. Of the total amount of sleep, 45% to 50% is active sleep, 35% to 45% is quiet sleep, and 10% is shifting between the two sleep states (Ladewig et al., 1998).

Quiet Sleep State In quiet sleep, the eyes are closed and there are no eye movements. Respirations are regular, quiet, and slower than in any other state. The heart rate is 100 to 120 beats/minute. There are startles or jerky movements at regular intervals. Stimuli in the environment are not likely to cause a change in the newborn's state.

Active Sleep State During active sleep, respirations are rapid and irregular and sucking movements may be observed. The infant stretches, moves extremities, makes faces, and may fuss briefly. Rapid eye movements (REM) occur. Environmental stimuli may startle the infant, who may then go back to sleep or awaken.

Alert States

There are four alert states: drowsy, quiet alert, active alert, and crying.

Drowsy State The transition between sleep and awake is called the drowsy state. The eyes open and then slowly close, as if unable to stay open. When open, the eyes appear glazed and unfocused. From this state the infant may go back to sleep or awaken.

Quiet Alert State In the quiet alert state, the infant focuses on people or objects, responds with intense gazing, and seems very interested in the immediate environment. Body movements are minimal. When the infant is in the quiet alert state, it is a good time to

enhance bonding. Parents should be made aware of this so they can take advantage of this opportunity.

Active Alert State The infant is often fussy and restless in the active alert state, with more rapid and irregular respirations. The awareness of discomfort from hunger or cold is more intense. Motor activity is quite frequent. The infant is less focused on visual stimuli than in the quiet alert state.

Crying State Crying is generally accompanied by jerky motor activity. Crying serves as a distraction from disturbing stimuli, allows a discharge of energy, and is a method of communication to elicit appropriate responses from parents or caregivers.

GESTATIONAL AGE

According to Alexander and Allen (1996), gestational age must be determined in the first 4 hours after birth so that age-related problems can be identified and appropriate care initiated.

The New Ballard Score is the most commonly used tool (Figure 51-19). It has two elements: external physical characteristics and neuromuscular maturity. If the findings of neuromuscular maturity are not in line with the findings of the external physical characteristics, a second assessment should be performed within 24 hours.

Assessment of External Physical Characteristics

The nurse should begin with resting posture, then skin, lanugo, plantar creases, breast, eye/ear, and then genitals.

Resting Posture

Although resting posture is a characteristic of neuromuscular maturity, it should be assessed first. The posture the newborn assumes when lying undisturbed is to be assessed. The very preterm infant has no flexion of the extremities, while the full-term infant is fully flexed.

Skin

The skin of a preterm infant is very transparent and thin. As gestation progresses, the veins disappear from view as subcutaneous fat is deposited. Vernix caseosa disappears near term but may remain in the creases. There may be some cracking and peeling of the skin, especially around the ankles and feet. As the skin loses moisture after birth, peeling is more apparent.

Lanugo

Lanugo is most abundant between 28 and 30 weeks' gestation. It disappears as the gestational age increases, first disappearing from the face, then the extremities

NEWBORN MATURITY RATING & CLASSIFICATION

ESTIMATION OF GESTATIONAL AGE BY MATURITY RATING

SYMBOLS: X - 1ST EXAM   O - 2ND EXAM

Gestation by Dates _____ wks

Birth Date _____ Hour _____ am/pm

APGAR _____ 1 min _____ 5 min

NEUROMUSCULAR MATURITY

	-1	0	1	2	3	4	5
Posture							
Square Window (wrist)	>90°	90°	60°	45°	30°	0°	
Arm Recoil		180°	140°-180°	110°-140°	90°-110°	<90°	
Popliteal Angle	180°	160°	140°	120°	100°	90°	<90°
Scarf Sign							
Heel to Ear							

MATURITY RATING

score	weeks
-10	20
-5	22
0	24
5	26
10	28
15	30
20	32
25	34
30	36
35	38
40	40
45	42
50	44

PHYSICAL MATURITY

Skin	sticky friable transparent	gelatinous red, translucent	smooth pink, visible veins	superficial peeling and or rash few veins	cracking pale areas rare veins	parchment deep cracking no vessels	leathery cracked wrinkled	
Lanugo	none	sparse	abundant	thinning	bald areas	mostly bald		
Plantar Surface	heel-toe 40 - 50mm: -1 <40 min: -2	>50mm no crease	faint red marks	anterior transverse crease only	creases ant. 2/3	creases over entire sole		
Breast	imperceptible	barely perceptible	flat areola no bud	stippled areola 1-2mm bud	raised areola 3-4mm bud	full areola 5-10mm bud		
Eye/Ear	lids fused loosely: -1 tightly: -2	lids open pinna flat stays folded	sl. curved pinna; soft slow recoil	well curved pinna; soft but ready recoil	formed and firm instant recoil	thick cartilage ear stiff		
Genitals Male	scrotum flat, smooth	scrotum empty faint rugae	testes in upper canal rare rugae	testes descending few rugae	testes down good rugae	testes pendulous deep rugae		
Genitals Female	clitoris prominent labia flat	prominent clitoris small labia minora	prominent clitoris enlarging minora	majora & minora equally prominent	majora large minora small	majora cover clitoris and minors		

SCORING SECTION

	1st Exam=X	2nd Exam=O
Estimating Gest Age by Maturity Rating	Weeks	Weeks
Time of Exam	Date _____ Hour _____ am pm	Date _____ Hour _____ am pm
Age at Exam	Hours	Hours
Signature of Examiner	M.D.	M.D.

Figure 51-19 New Ballard Score (*Courtesy of Bristol Myers Squibb*)

and trunk. A small amount may remain on the shoulders, ears, and sides of the forehead at full term.

Plantar Creases

During the first 12 hours of life the plantar creases are reliable signs of gestational age. Sole creases develop from the top (under toes) beginning about 32 weeks of gestation. The creases cover two-thirds of the sole by 37 weeks and cover the sole at 40 weeks' gestation.

Breast

The size of the breast bud tissue is measured by placing the forefinger and middle finger on each side of the breast tissue and measuring between the fingers. At term, the breast bud tissue should be 1 cm. This should be performed gently to prevent tissue damage.

Eye/Ear

The eyelids are fused until 26 to 28 weeks of gestation. The upper pinna begins to curve over at about 33 to 34 weeks of gestation. The curving over continues until it is complete at 39 to 40 weeks of gestation.

The infant at less than 32 weeks of gestation has almost no ear cartilage. When folded, the ear remains folded. By 36 weeks there is enough cartilage for the ear to slowly return to its original state when folded. The ear of a full-term infant springs back quickly when folded.

Male Genitals

The male genitals are evaluated for descent of the testes, presence of rugae on the scrotum, and scrotal size. The testes are formed in the abdomen, move into the inguinal canal at 30 weeks of gestation, then into

CULTURAL CONSIDERATIONS

Lanugo

There may be more lanugo on infants with dark skin coloring than on fair-skinned infants with light-colored hair.

PROFESSIONAL TIP

Ears

When caring for an infant of 32 weeks' gestation or less, be sure the infant's ears are flat to the head and not bent over. Lying on a bent ear can impair circulation to the ear.

the upper scrotum by 37 weeks of gestation, and are fully descended by full term. Before 36 weeks, there are few rugae on the scrotum. By 38 weeks, rugae have formed on the anterior part of the scrotum and cover the scrotum by 40 weeks of gestation. The scrotum is large and pendulous by 40 weeks.

Female Genitals

Deposits of subcutaneous fat related to nutritional status as well as gestational age determine the appearance of the female genitals. The clitoris and labia minora seem large in comparison to the labia majora, which are small and widely separated at 30 to 32 weeks of gestation. By 36 to 38 weeks of gestation, the clitoris is mostly covered by the labia majora. By 40 weeks of gestation, the labia majora covers the labia minora and clitoris.

Neuromuscular Maturity

The five remaining neuromuscular characteristics to be evaluated are square window, arm recoil, popliteal angle, scarf sign, and heel to ear.

Square Window

The square window sign is elicited by bending the wrist so the palm is as flat against the arm as possible. If the angle between the palm and arm is 90° and looks like a square window, the gestational age is 32 weeks or less and receives a score of 0. If the angle is greater than 90°, the score is −1. The angle becomes smaller the more mature the infant is, until the palm can fold flat against the arm in a full-term newborn.

Arm Recoil

The infant's arms are held with the elbows fully flexed for 5 seconds. Then the arms are pulled straight down at the infant's sides and quickly released. The elbows of a full-term newborn, when released, rapidly recoil and have an angle less than 90°. That infant is given a score of 4. Very preterm infants may not move their arms (no recoil) and receive a score of 0.

Popliteal Angle

The popliteal angle is measured when the thigh is flexed on the abdomen, the hips remain flat on the table, and the lower leg is straightened just until met by resistance. Then the angle behind the knee is scored. When the leg can be fully extended, a score of −1 is given, but if the popliteal angle is less than 90°, a score of 5 is given.

Scarf Sign

The newborn's arm is drawn across the body toward the opposite shoulder until resistance is felt. The shoulder of the arm being tested should remain on the table. The relation of the elbow to the infant's midline is noted for scoring. If the elbow does not reach near the midline, it is a score of 4. When the elbow goes across and beyond the infant's body, a score of −1 is given.

Heel to Ear

With the hips remaining on the surface of the table, the newborn's foot is moved toward the ear on the same side. When resistance is felt, foot position relative to the ear and the degree of knee extension is noted. The preterm infant's leg will remain straight and the foot will be near the ear. The more mature the infant the more resistance will be felt and more flexion will be noted.

Gestational Age Relationship to Intrauterine Growth

There is a normal range of birth weight for each week of gestation as well as for length, head circumference, and intrauterine weight-length ratio (Figure 51-20). Birth weight is classified as follows:

- **Large for gestational age** (LGA): Infant's weight falls above the 90th percentile for gestational age.
- **Appropriate for gestational age** (AGA): Infant's weight falls between the 90th and 10th percentile for gestational age.
- **Small for gestational age** (SGA): Infant's weight falls below the 10th percentile for gestational age.

The correlation of the infant's measurements for length and head circumference also documents the infant's level of maturity and appropriate classification of LGA, AGA, or SGA.

All of these determinations assist caregivers to expect possible physiologic complications, and together with the results of a physical assessment are the basis for preparing an appropriate care plan for the infant.

FIRST BATH AND CORD CARE

The infant's first bath, and the type of bath for the next 10 days to 2 weeks, is a sponge bath. Newborns are not generally given a tub bath until after the cord has fallen off and healing is complete. Placing the infant under a radiant warmer during a sponge bath helps prevent heat loss.

Begin by wiping each eye with either a separate cotton ball or a separate place on a washcloth. The eyes are wiped from the inner to outer canthus. The entire face is washed. All of the creases of the ears are cleaned with a corner of a washcloth; a cotton-tipped applicator should *never* be used in the ears.

Soap or a cleansing agent is used on the rest of the body according to agency protocol. Creases must have special attention to be sure that all traces of blood and the majority of vernix caseosa are removed. When completely washed and rinsed, the infant is dried and wrapped in a dry, warm blanket.

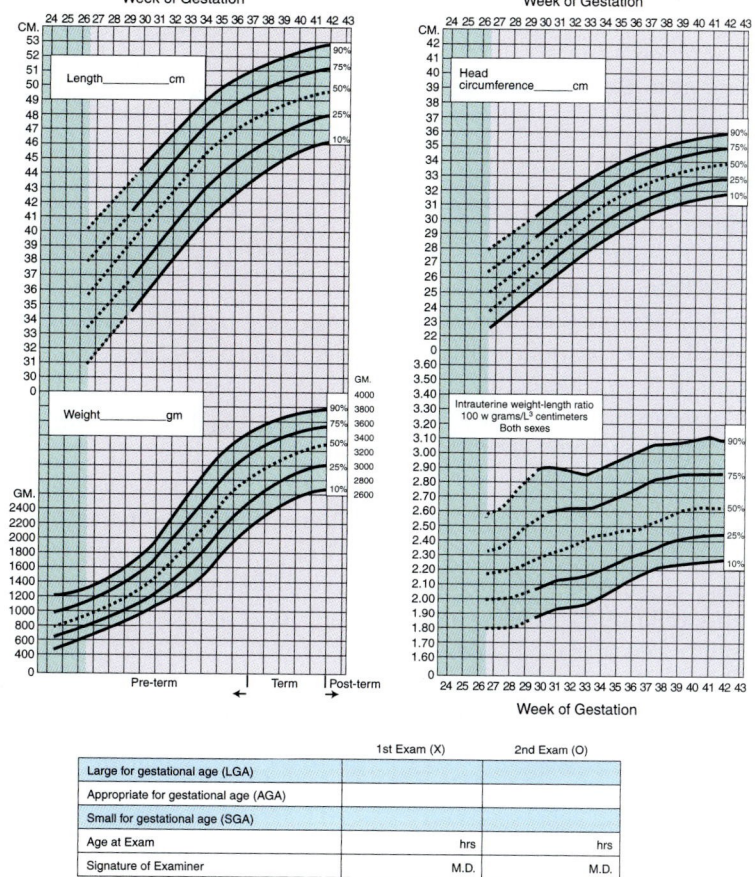

Figure 51-20 Intrauterine Growth Grids *(Courtesy of Mead Johnson Nutritionals.)*

The hair is washed last to prevent heat loss from a wet head during the bath. Using gauze squares and the approved soap, the head should be firmly scrubbed to remove all blood and body fluids. Infants with a large amount of hair may require the use of a comb to remove all traces of substances in the hair. A second washing and rinsing of the head may be necessary. The head must be well dried when finished.

The infant may remain in the radiant warmer on dry linens or may be dressed, wrapped in a blanket with a hat on the head, and placed in a regular crib and covered with another blanket. Within 30 minutes to 1 hour, the infant's temperature should be checked.

CULTURAL CONSIDERATIONS

Umbilical Cord

In Malawi, Africa, infants are kept indoors and are not named until the umbilical cord falls off, typically within the first 2 weeks (Gennaro, Kamwendo, Mbweza, & Kershbaumer, 1998).

CULTURAL CONSIDERATIONS

Infant Care

Nurses must be aware of different cultural practices in order to provide sensitive care. A few examples include:

- Korean tradition is to consider a newborn 1 year old at the time of birth.
- Korean parents will often tightly wrap a newborn in a blanket to prevent possible harm from the wind (Howard & Berbiglia, 1997).
- Japanese parents often choose to immerse the infant for a bath before the cord is healed (Sharts-Hopko, 1995).
- Muslim fathers traditionally call praise to Allah in the newborn's right ear prior to cleansing the infant.
- Most infants of Muslim parents are not named until they are 7 days old (Hutchinson & Baqi-Aziz, 1994).
- Babies of Southeast Asian parents are kept swaddled for the first few days (Mattson, 1995).

Following the first bath, a bacteriostatic agent is applied to the cord stump and clamp according to agency protocol.

The cord should be cleaned, at least daily, with alcohol. The diaper should be folded under to allow the cord to dry and prevent urine from getting on the cord.

CIRCUMCISION

Circumcision is the surgical removal of the prepuce (foreskin), which covers the glans penis. In 1989, the American Academy of Pediatrics took the position that "newborn circumcision has potential medical benefits and advantages as well as disadvantages and risks" (AAP, 1989). Circumcision is considered an elective procedure for which parents must give written consent. Only full-term, healthy newborns should be circumcised.

Procedure

The infant is placed on a circumcision board just before the procedure begins (Figure 51-21). Because infants prefer a flexed position, being placed on a circumcision board is frustrating to the newborn. Crying often begins at this point, before the procedure is started.

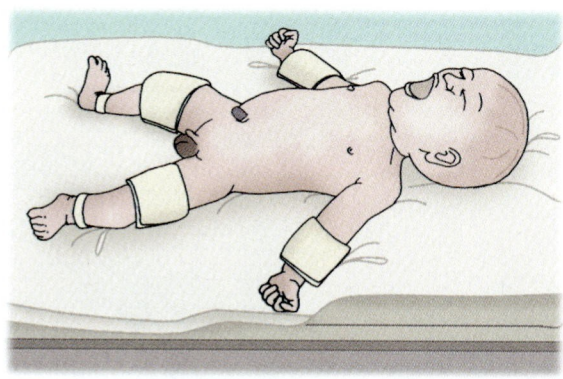

Figure 51-21 Circumcision Board. Infant is restrained just before the procedure begins.

Traditionally, no anesthesia was used and still is seldom used. Some physicians may now use a lidocaine injection or a topical anesthetic cream. The physician then makes a slit in the prepuce and then uses either a Gomco (Yellen) clamp (Figure 51-22) or Plastibell (Figure 51-23) to control bleeding when the prepuce is cut off. After a circumcision with the Gomco clamp, A+D ointment or petroleum jelly is put on the penis to prevent the diaper from sticking to the site. At each diaper change, new ointment is applied for at least 24 to 48 hours.

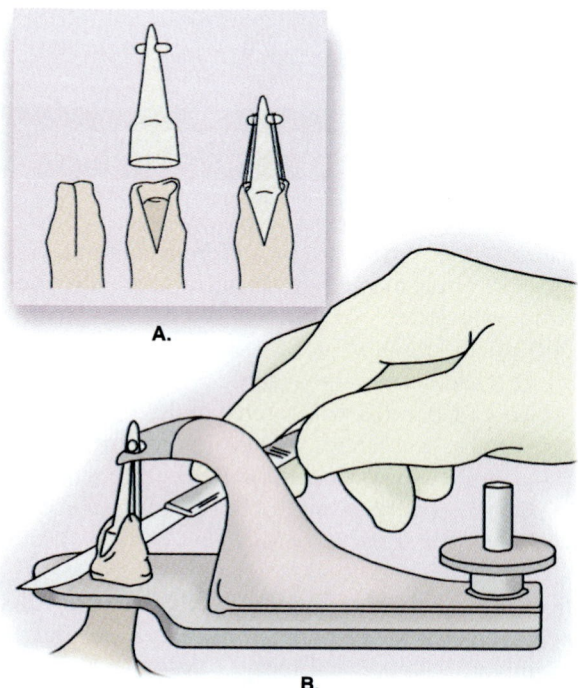

Figure 51-22 Gomco (Yellen) Clamp Used for Circumcision: A. After slit is made in prepuce, the cone is placed over the glans and the prepuce is pulled up around the cone; B. The cone is placed in the clamp, which is tightened to obliterate the blood vessels. This prevents bleeding. The prepuce is cut away and the clamp is removed in 3 to 5 minutes.

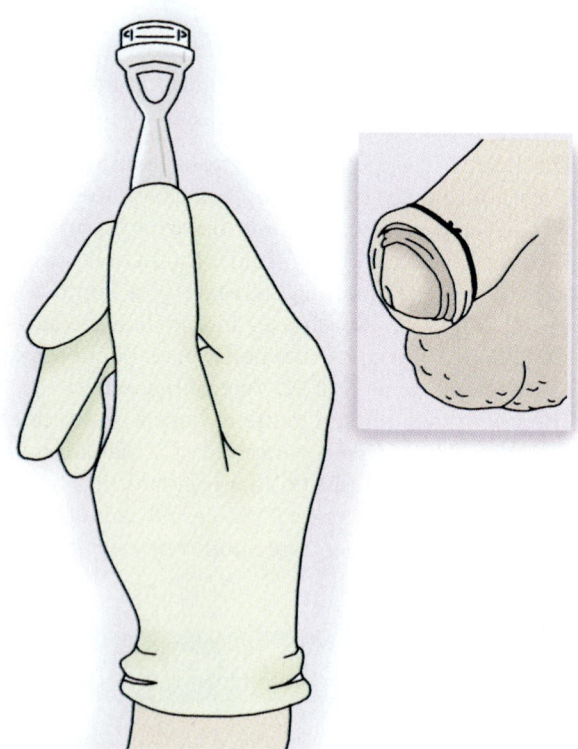

Figure 51-23 Plastibell Used for Circumcision. The plastibell is placed over the glans after a slit is made in the prepuce. A suture is tied around the ring. This prevents bleeding when the prepuce is cut away. The handle is removed, leaving the ring to fall off in 5 to 8 days after healing.

PROFESSIONAL TIP

Reasons for and against Circumcision

For
- Religious rite
- Easier to keep clean
- So child looks like circumcised father
- Prevent need for procedure later in life
- May reduce urinary tract infections

Against
- Procedure is painful
- Believe sexual pleasure is decreased later
- Possibility of hemorrhage or infection
- Removes natural protection of glans

Nursing Responsibilities

The nurse ensures that the circumcision permit has been signed by a parent. Equipment and supplies are set up, and the infant is placed on the circumcision board with diaper removed. Most infants are not fed for 2 to 4 hours before the procedure to prevent regurgitation.

Safety: Circumcision Procedure
Keep a bulb syringe nearby in case the infant requires suctioning.

During the procedure, the nurse should comfort the infant by talking to the infant, playing a tape of soft music or intrauterine sounds, or lightly stroking the infant. After the procedure the infant should be held to provide comfort. Care following a circumcision includes checking hourly for 12 hours to see if any bleeding is occurring and that the infant is voiding.

If the infant goes home within the first 12 hours after circumcision, bleeding must be minimal and the infant must have voided. The nurse must ensure that

CULTURAL CONSIDERATIONS

Circumcision
- Jewish parents have a special religious ceremony on the eighth day after birth when the infant is circumcised and named.
- Muslim parents practice circumcision as a religious rite.
- In the United States, circumcision is generally culturally accepted.
- In European countries, circumcision is performed infrequently.

HOME HEALTH CARE

Circumcision
- Wash hands before touching penis.
- Continue checking circumcision hourly until 12 hours after procedure.
- If bleeding, apply gentle pressure with sterile 4 × 4 gauze. If bleeding does not stop, call physician.
- Check that infant has a wet diaper 6 to 10 times in 24 hours.
- Change diaper frequently. Use warm water to gently clean penis and reapply A+D ointment or petroleum jelly after each change, except when Plastibell is used.
- Check for redness, swelling, or discharge, which are signs of infection.
- Provide comfort by holding and talking soothingly to infant.

the parents know how to care for the circumcision and that they have the physician's telephone number.

NUTRITION

Feeding the newborn is an important aspect of parenting. Nurses assisting in the choice of a feeding method must have knowledge of the newborn's nutritional needs. The American Academy of Pediatrics recommends breast milk for at least 12 months (AAP, 1997).

Nutritional Needs of Newborn

The full-term newborn needs a sufficient intake of calories to meet energy and growth requirements. There should be adequate carbohydrates and fats for energy so that proteins can be used for growth. A newborn requires 110 to 120 kcal/kg (50 to 55 kcal/lb) each day to meet these needs.

This equates to approximately 20 oz of breast milk or formula each day. Newborns lose weight the first few days of life partly because their intake of calories is less than their requirement. One reason is that the newborn's stomach capacity is only 20 mL (30 mL = 1 oz). This capacity increases rapidly so that by 7 days of age the infant may consume 2 to 3 oz at each feeding. The infant regains birth weight by age 10 days.

Breast Milk and Infant Formula Composition

The compositions of breast milk and infant formula are different.

Breast Milk

Breast milk is biologically designed to meet the needs of human infants. Its composition changes to meet the changing nutritional and immunologic needs of the infant. Breast milk is easily digested.

The colostrum (first few days) is rich in immunoglobulins to protect the newborn's gastrointestinal tract from infection. Colostrum helps establish normal intestinal flora and has a laxative effect that assists in the passage of meconium.

In 2 weeks, mature milk is being produced. It contains sufficient nutrients to meet the infant's needs and has 20 kcal/oz. Breast stimulation and removal of milk from the breast stimulates the secretion of prolactin by the anterior pituitary of the mother. Prolactin increases milk production. As the demand becomes greater (infant feeding longer and more frequently), the milk supply increases.

The mother's diet makes little difference in the proportions of carbohydrates, protein, and most minerals in her breast milk, but fat content and the amount of vitamins are affected. The breastfeeding mother must eat a well-balanced diet to provide the most nutritious milk for her infant and to maintain her own health and energy level. An extra 500 calories a day is needed to support breastfeeding.

Infant Formula

There are many infant formulas that are modified to match the components in breast milk as nearly as possible. Most formulas are modified cow's milk. Protein is reduced, saturated fat is removed and replaced with vegetable fats, and vitamins and some minerals are added. Soy formulas are used for infants with allergies or who do not tolerate cow's milk-based formula. Nutramigen is a protein hydrolysate formula made from cow's milk but treated to be hypoallergenic.

Special formulas are made to meet special needs of some infants. Preterm infants need more calories but less quantity; these formulas provide 24 kcal/oz. Other formulas are modified to be low in the amino acid phenylalanine for infants with phenylketonuria (PKU), who cannot digest phenylalanine.

Feeding Method

Nutrition is provided for the newborn either through breastfeeding or bottle feeding. Whichever the parents choose, nurses must support and assist the parents to make the experience meaningful. Some of the advantages and disadvantages of breastfeeding and bottle feeding are identified in Table 51-2

Other factors besides the advantages and disadvantages of breastfeeding and bottle feeding enter into the decision of how to feed the newborn. These factors include support offered by the infant's father; support by other family members; the need to work outside the home by the mother; and age, educational level, and income level of the parents.

When the mother is breastfeeding (8 to 12 times a day at first) she is focused on the infant. Various tasks

---

Table 51-2 BREASTFEEDING/BOTTLE FEEDING, ADVANTAGES AND DISADVANTAGES

	BREASTFEEDING	BOTTLE FEEDING
Advantages	Nonallergenic Meets infant's specific nutritional needs Immunologic properties help prevent infections Easily digested Constipation unlikely (Figure 51-24A) Overfeeding less likely Convenient, always available No formula or bottles to buy No formula and bottles to prepare Oxytocin release helps involution Mother more likely to eat well-balanced diet May help with mother's weight loss Enhances mother/infant attachment through skin-to-skin contact	Father or others may feed infant day or night Feed less frequently (3 to 4 hours) Amount of milk taken at each feeding known
Disadvantages	Feed more frequently (2 to 3 hours) More frequent diaper changes Amount of milk taken at each feeding unknown Medications taken by mother present in milk Discomfort of some mothers to nurse in public Expense of pumping and storing milk for periods when mother is unavailable (such as work hours)	Expense of formula, bottles Washing bottles Fixing and refrigerating formula Carrying bottles on outings May cause constipation (Figure 51-24B)

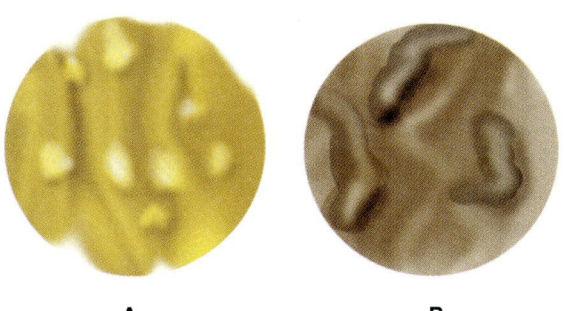

A. **B.**

Figure 51-24 A. Stool of breastfed infant; B. Stool of bottle-fed infant

around the home may need to be left undone or the father will need to do them. Support from other family members may be based on how other family members have chosen to feed their infants.

Breastfeeding

Many factors influence breastfeeding, including positions for feeding, latching on, and length of feeding.

Positions for Feeding

The infant should be held with the head slightly higher than the rest of the body. The cradle hold, with the infant's head in the bend of the mother's elbow and the arm supporting the infant's body, is probably the most common. It can be used whether breastfeeding or bottle feeding. Other positions that are particularly adaptable to breastfeeding are the football hold, side-lying position, and across the lap position (Figure 51-25). The mother's free hand should be in a "C" position, supporting the underside of her breast with the fingers.

Latching On

The mother should use the infant's rooting reflex to allow proper positioning of the nipple in the infant's mouth. Brushing the nipple against the infant's lower lip will cause the infant to open the mouth. When the mouth is wide open and the tongue is down, the mother quickly brings the infant closer to the breast so the infant can latch on to the nipple and areola. When properly positioned, the tongue is on top of the lower gum and under the breast, with the lips flared outward. When the infant is properly latched on, the suction is strong. To remove the infant from the breast, the mother should insert a finger into the corner of the infant's mouth between the gums to break the suction and quickly remove the breast. The nipple should never be simply pulled out from the infant's mouth because this will cause the mother pain and may also result in tissue damage to the nipple.

CLIENT TEACHING

Timing of Feedings

Feedings should be given when the infant is hungry (demand feeding) rather than on a fixed schedule. The infant is ready to eat when wide awake, sucking on hands, rooting, and slightly fussy.

Length of Feeding

Feeding length varies with each mother/infant unit. However, the feeding should be long enough to remove all the **foremilk**, the watery first milk from the breast, which is high in lactose, like skim milk, and is effective in quenching thirst. This allows the infant to receive the **hindmilk**, which is higher in fat content, leads to weight gain, and is more satisfying.

The average time for a feeding session is approximately 30 minutes. It is more important to know when the infant is finished feeding than to go by the clock. When an infant is satisfied, the sucking and swallowing will be much slower and the breast will be soft. The infant may fall asleep and release the nipple.

The first breast should be emptied (very soft) before moving the infant to the other breast. At the next feeding, the breast used last at the previous feeding should be used first. This ensures that each breast is emptied at least at every other feeding. As the infant grows and requires more milk, both breasts may be emptied at each feeding.

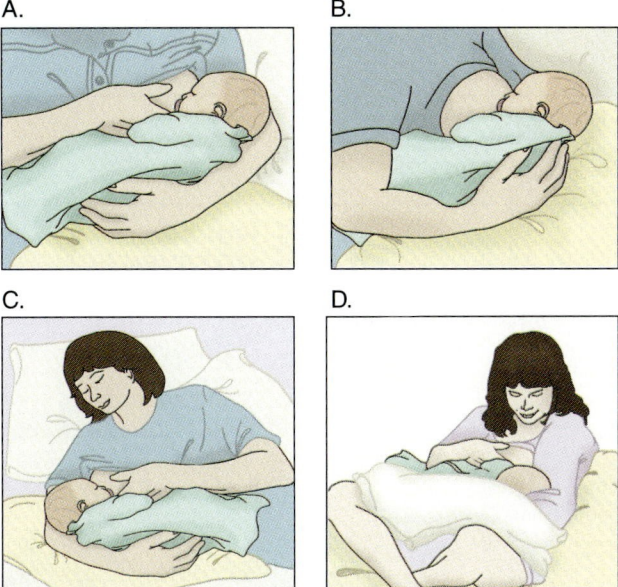

A.   B.

C.   D.

Figure 51-25 Positions for Feeding Infant: A. Cradling, used for breast and bottle feeding; B. Football hold; C. Lying down; D. Across lap

Bottle Feeding

Factors related to bottle feeding include bottles, formula preparation, and amount of feeding.

Bottles

Babies will generally feed well from any bottle and nipple, though many babies will eventually develop a preference and may refuse a new type of nipple. Whatever choice the parents make will be fine. Washing the bottles and nipples with a bottle and nipple brush in warm soapy water is necessary for thorough cleaning. Rinsing thoroughly will remove all traces of soap. Only if there is a question regarding the safety of the water supply (e.g., well water on a farm or ranch) is boiling of the bottles and nipples necessary.

Formula Preparation

Formulas are available in three forms: ready to feed, concentrated, and powdered. The latter two require addition of water. The choice of formula is generally left up to the parents. There is a great difference in price, so the choice may be made based on finances. Mixing of formula must be accurate to provide the 20 kcal/oz.

Amount of Feeding

Most newborns begin by drinking 7.5 mL to 15 mL (¼ to ½ oz) at a feeding but gradually increase to approximately 90 mL to 120 mL (3 to 4 oz) at each feeding in 2 weeks. The infant's appetite will generally increase during growth spurts at 2 weeks, 6 to 9 weeks, and 3 to 6 months, so the amount of formula should be increased by 30 mL (1 oz) in each bottle to meet this need.

Burping

All infants require burping, whether breastfed or bottle fed. Burping is needed to expel the air swallowed when the infant sucks. Some infants swallow more air than others and require more frequent burping.

To facilitate burping, the infant can be held upright on the feeder's shoulder, in a sitting position on the feeder's lap with the head and chest supported with one hand, or prone across the feeder's lap. The other hand is used to gently pat or rub the infant's back.

Burping should be done generally about halfway through the feeding for bottle feeding and when changing breasts for breastfeeding. Parents soon learn the infant's cues regarding the need to be burped.

SAMPLE NURSING CARE PLAN

NEWBORN INFANT

Selena Sauve, born at 36 weeks gestation, weighs 6 pounds 3 ounces and is 19 inches long. Her Apgar score was 8 at 1 minute and 9 at 5 minutes. Axillary temperature is 96.5°F (35.8°C), respirations 56, and apical pulse 148. The parents are very excited about Selena, their first child. Selena is very sleepy and is not breastfeeding well.

Nursing Diagnosis 1 *Thermoregulation, Ineffective, related to immaturity as evidenced by birth at 36 weeks gestation*

PLANNING/GOALS	NURSING INTERVENTIONS	RATIONALE	EVALUATION
Selena's temperature will be between 97.5°F (36.4°C) and 98.9°F (37.2°C).	Keep Selena adequately clothed and covered.	Maintains her temperature.	Selena's temperature is 97.8°F.
	Maintain ambient room temperature between 77.2°F (25.1°C) and 78.1°F (25.6°C).	Is optimum environmental temperature.	
	Keep Selena away from air conditioning vents, drafts, and fans.	Prevents heat loss by convection.	
	Use warm water when bathing Selena, wrap her in a towel, and dry	Prevents heat loss by evaporation.	

continued

her quickly. Wash her head after she is dried and dressed. Dry her head thoroughly and put a cap on her head.

Cover scales and examination area before Selena is laid down.	Prevents heat loss by conduction.	
Keep Selena's crib away from outside windows.	Prevents heat loss by radiation.	
Teach Selena's parents how to maintain a neutral thermal environment for Selena.	Prevents Selena from using her brown fat too fast.	

Nursing Diagnosis 2 *Infection, Risk for, related to risk factor of inadequate primary defenses as evidenced by cut umbilical cord and immature immune system*

PLANNING/GOAL	NURSING INTERVENTIONS	RATIONALE	EVALUATION
Selena will have no signs of infection of the eyes, diaper area, or umbilical cord.	Use good handwashing technique (caregivers and parents) before and after caring for Selena.	Prevents spread of infection.	Selena shows no signs of infection.
	Provide prescribed eye prophylaxis and keep eyes clean.	Prevents infection.	
	Keep diaper area clean and dry.	Prevents skin irritation and infection.	
	Place diaper below the umbilical cord.	Allows cord to dry and heal.	
	Provide prescribed cord prophylaxis and clean umbilical cord daily with alcohol.	Prevents infection and removes exudate.	

Nursing Diagnosis 3 *Nutrition, Altered, Less than Body Requirement related to limited nutritional intake as evidenced by being very sleepy and not breastfeeding very well*

PLANNING/GOAL	NURSING INTERVENTIONS	RATIONALE	EVALUATION
Selena will lose only 5 to 10 ounces of weight during the first 3 days.	Assist mother in breastfeeding Selena.	Provides support for first time breastfeeding.	Selena lost 7 ounces during the first 3 days.
	Demonstrate use of rooting reflex to ensure proper latch on.	Uses natural response of infant for proper position of mouth and tongue.	

continued

Explain that Selena will suck in spurts.	Assists mother in knowing that Selena has not finished breastfeeding when she rests.
Explain that the breast has foremilk and hindmilk (needed for growth), so breasts must be emptied.	Ensures that mother will allow Selena to empty one breast before changing to the other breast.

PROBLEMS OF THE NEWBORN

Problems of the newborn identified either at birth or before discharge include hyperbilirubinemia, respiratory distress, cleft lip/palate, hydrocephalus, spina bifida, Down syndrome, and talipes equinovarus. Newborn problems may also occur when the mother is diabetic, HIV positive, or a substance abuser. Phenylketonuria must be tested for as soon as possible so treatment can begin immediately.

HYPERBILIRUBINEMIA

Hyperbilirubinemia, an excess of bilirubin in the blood, may be related to physiologic jaundice or pathologic jaundice. Physiologic jaundice does not appear until after 24 hours of age and is more commonly seen after the infant has gone home. It is discussed in Chapter 53.

Pathologic jaundice appears in the first 24 hours and may lead to **kernicterus** (deposits of bilirubin causing yellow staining in the brain, especially the basal ganglia, cerebellum, and hippocampus). The exact level of total bilirubin when kernicterus occurs is not known but may occur at 20 mg/dL in full-term infants and at a lower level in preterm neonates.

The most common cause is Rh incompatibility.

Medical–Surgical Management

Medical

Phototherapy is the most common treatment for jaundice. The "bili" lights are special flourescent lamps (in the blue-light spectrum) placed over the infant. Only a diaper and an eye covering are on the infant to expose the most skin surface to the light. A fiber-optic phototherapy blanket and the BiliBed® with the Bilicombi™ blanket (Figure 51-26) have been designed to provide phototherapy without the eyes needing to be covered. Because the infant is covered, thermal regulation is no longer a problem, and interaction with the parents can take place. The infant may experience frequent, green, loose stools as the bilirubin is excreted.

Surgical

If the bilirubin level cannot be reduced quickly or maintained below 12 mg/dL with phototherapy treatment, exchange transfusion is necessary. Blood type O, Rh negative blood is used. During this procedure 5 mL to 10 mL of blood are removed from the infant and replaced with a like amount of donor blood. This is a very slow process. Complications of hypervolemia, hypovolemia, infection, cardiac arrhythmias, and air embolism may occur.

This procedure is seldom necessary today because of the widespread use of RhoGAM to prevent Rh incompatibility.

Diet

Fluid intake is increased to assist in elimination of the bilirubin through the urine.

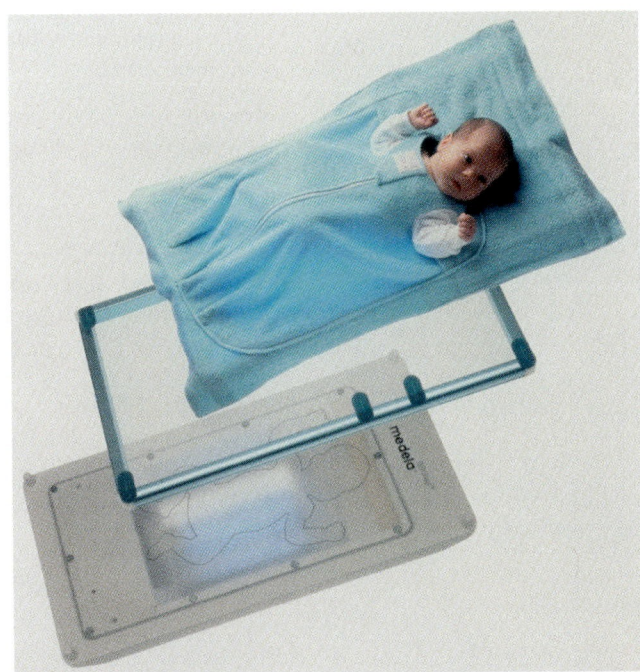

Figure 51-26 BiliBed® with Bilicombi™ Blanket © *1999 Medela, Inc. (Photo courtesy of Medela, Inc.)*

▶ NURSING PROCESS

▶ Assessment

▶ Subjective Data
None

▶ Objective Data
Prenatal and perinatal records are reviewed to identify factors predisposing to jaundice. Jaundice in light-skinned infants is assessed by blanching the skin (pressing firmly with the thumb) over a bony prominence such as the forehead, nose, or sternum. When the thumb is removed, the area has a yellowish appearance before normal color returns if jaundice is present. In darker-skinned infants, the infant's oral mucosa, posterior aspect of the hard palate, or conjunctival sacs will have a yellow coloring when jaundice is present.

Nursing diagnoses for an infant with hyperbilirubinemia may include the following:

Nursing Diagnoses	Planning/Goals	Nursing Interventions
▶ *Fluid Volume Deficit, Risk for, related to increased insensible water loss and frequent loose stools secondary to phototherapy*	The infant's intake will be at least 100 to 150 mL/kg/day.	Encourage adequate feedings of infant by mother. Provide extra water intake.
▶ *Skin Integrity Impaired, Risk for, related to frequent loose stools secondary to phototherapy*	The infant's diaper area will maintain skin integrity.	Check diaper frequently and change as soon as soiled. Apply A+D ointment or petroleum jelly to diaper area after cleansing.

Evaluation Each goal must be evaluated to determine how it has been met by the client.

RESPIRATORY DISTRESS

Two types of respiratory distress may occur in a newborn: respiratory distress syndrome (RDS) and transient tachypnea of the newborn (TTN).

Respiratory distress syndrome is associated with preterm infants and surfactant deficiency. Verma (1995) describes respiratory distress syndrome as due to alterations in surfactant quantity, composition, function, or production. These infants have hypoxia, respiratory acidosis, and metabolic acidosis.

Transient tachypnea of the newborn is found mainly in AGA and near-term infants (Ladewig et al., 1998). Either intrauterine or intrapartum asphyxia has been experienced by these infants. This results in the newborn's failure to clear the airway of lung fluid and mucus or aspiration of amniotic fluid. No respiratory difficulties are experienced at birth, but shortly after birth the newborn may have flaring of the nares and expiratory grunting. By 6 hours of age, tachypnea is noted, with respirations as high as 100 to 140 breaths/minute.

Medical–Surgical Management

Medical

The goal is to determine which type of respiratory distress is affecting the newborn and begin treatment. For RDS the goals of treatment are maintenance of adequate oxygenation and ventilation and correction of the respiratory and metabolic acidosis. Mild RDS is often treated only with increased, humidified oxygen concentration. Infants with moderate RDS may require continuous positive airway pressure (CPAP). Mechanical ventilation is required for severe RDS. The oxygen needs of infants with RDS increase over the first 48 hours.

Infants with TTN generally require ambient oxygen of 30% to 50% initially. This need for increased oxygen generally decreases over the first 48 hours. Treatment is usually required only for 4 days.

▶ NURSING PROCESS

▶ Assessment

▶ Subjective Data
None

▶ Objective Data
There will be cyanosis pallor or mottling of the skin, tachypnea, grunting respirations, retractions, and nasal flaring. To rate the infant's respiratory effort, the Silverman-Anderson index is often used (Figure 51-27). The heart rate is generally within normal limits.

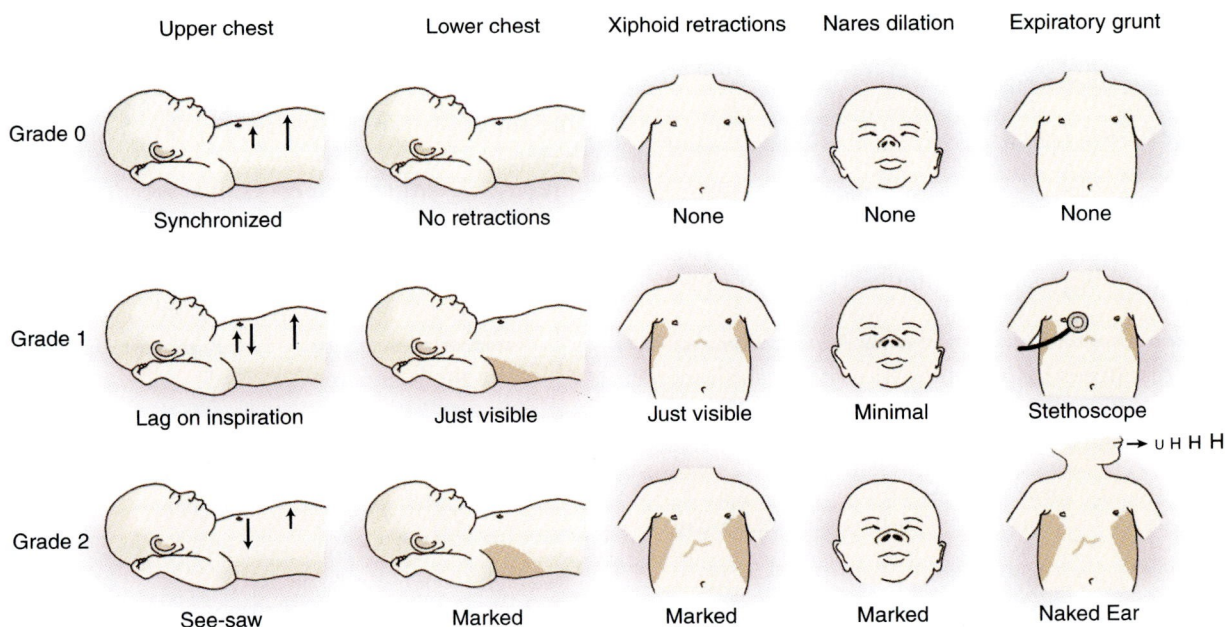

Figure 51-27 Silverman-Anderson Index

Nursing diagnoses for an infant with respiratory distress may include the following:

Nursing Diagnoses	Planning/Goals	Nursing Interventions
▶ *Gas Exchange, Impaired, related to ventilation perfusion imbalance*	The infant will have increased gas exchange as indicated by pulse oximetry.	Monitor pulse oximetry, respirations at least hourly. Provide oxygen as ordered. Monitor oxygen concentration.
▶ *Infection, Risk for, related to invasive procedures*	The infant will have no signs of infection.	Maintain strict aseptic technique in the care of the infant.

Evaluation Each goal must be evaluated to determine how it has been met by the client.

CLEFT LIP/PALATE

The immediate concern with cleft lip/palate (Figure 51-28) is the problem of feeding the infant. The size of the cleft and whether the palate is also involved determine the difficulty of feeding. Special nipples and feeding devices are available. The infant should be held in an upright sitting position when feeding. Frequent burping is necessary because these infants swallow more air than usual. When sleeping, the infant should be kept in a side-lying position.

Parents of an infant with any congenital anomaly need support, as they may need to grieve over the loss of a normal infant. The nurse must role model interacting with the infant. Complete coverage is found in Chapter 53.

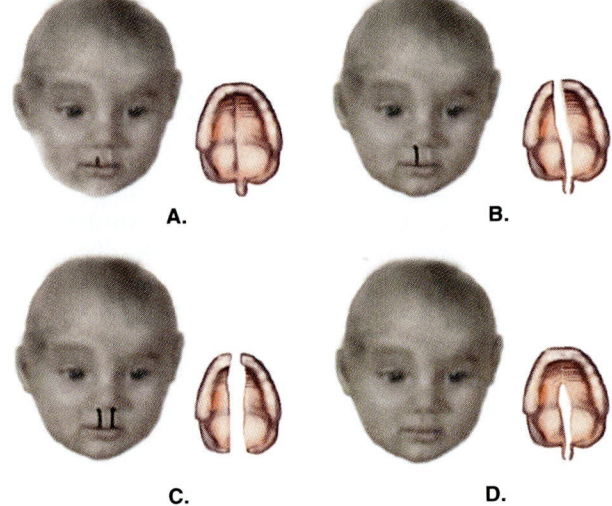

Figure 51-28 Types of Cleft Lip/Palate: A. Small notch in lip, palate normal; B. Cleft lip and cleft palate; C. Bilateral cleft lip and cleft palate; D. Lip normal, cleft palate

HYDROCEPHALUS

Hydrocephalus, excess cerebrospinal fluid in the cerebral ventricles, causes the infant's head to be enlarged. Head circumference is measured daily, fontanels checked to see whether they are flat or bulging, and the infant's position changed frequently. The infant usually cannot move the head. Complete coverage is found in Chapter 53.

SPINA BIFIDA

There are three types of spina bifida (neural tube defects): spina bifida occulta, meningocele, and myelomeningocele (Figure 51-29). **Spina bifida occulta** is a failure of the vertebral arch to close. There is a dimple on the back, which may have a tuft of hair in it. No care is required.

A **meningocele** is a saclike protrusion along the vertebral column filled with cerebrospinal fluid and meninges. Surgery is required to repair the defect, but there are no long-term effects.

A **myelomeningocele** is a saclike protrusion along the vertebral column filled with spinal fluid, meninges, nerve roots, and spinal cord. Because of the nerve root and spinal cord involvement, there will be paralysis at some level after surgical repair.

The saclike protrusions must be kept covered with sterile saline dressings, and the infant handled carefully when changing position from side to side. The sac must be kept free from contamination by urine and stool. Head circumference is measured and fontanels checked for bulging on each shift because hydrocephalus often develops. Complete coverage of myelomeningocele is found in Chapter 53.

DOWN SYNDROME

Down syndrome is caused by a chromosomal abnormality, also called trisomy 21. Routine care is provided in the newborn period. Complete coverage is found in Chapter 53.

TALIPES EQUINOVARUS

Talipes equinovarus, also called clubfoot, is a congenital deformity in which the foot and ankle are twisted inward and cannot be moved to a midline position (Figure 51-30). The foot or feet of some infants appear to turn inward, but if they can be moved to the midline the cause is intrauterine position. Range-of-motion exercises will often correct this.

Infants with true clubfoot may have a cast on before going home. Complete coverage is found in Chapter 53.

INFANT OF A DIABETIC MOTHER

The infant of a diabetic mother (IDM) requires close observation the first few hours to several days after birth. If the mother has vascular complications with the diabetes, the infant is generally SGA. If the mother has gestational diabetes or diabetes without vascular changes, the infant is generally LGA, especially if the diabetes has not been well-controlled. The large size is the result of fat deposits and increased size of all organs except the brain. The IDM has less total body water, especially in the extracellular spaces. Following are complications seen most often in the IDM:

- Hypoglycemia: The loss of maternal glucose at birth and the high level of insulin produced by the infant decrease the infant's blood glucose within hours after birth. It takes a period of time for insulin production to be reduced in the newborn.
- Respiratory distress: Insulin is antagonistic to the cortisol-induced stimulation of lecithin (phospholipid necessary for lung maturation) synthesis. This

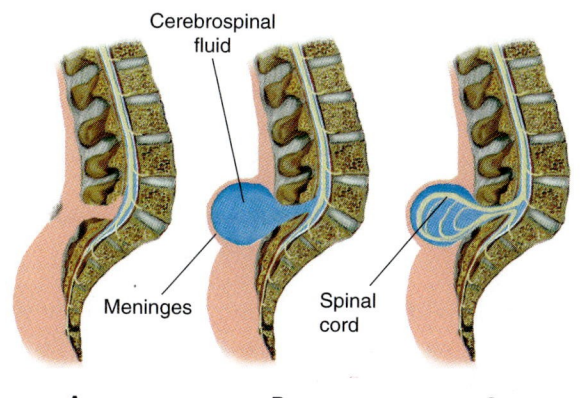

Figure 51-29 Types of Spina Bifida: A. Spina bifida occulta; B. Meningocele; C. Myelomeningocele

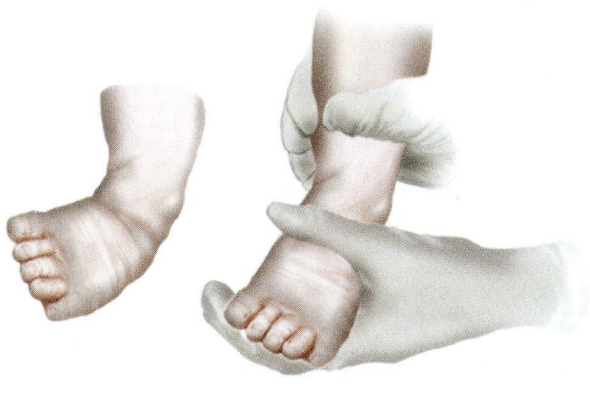

Figure 51-30 A. Talipes equinovarus (clubfoot); B. Foot moves to midline; positional, not clubfoot

results in less mature lungs than would be expected for the gestational age. This does not seem to be a problem if the mother has vascular complications with her diabetes.

- Hyperbilirubinemia: Hepatic immaturity and a decreased extracellular fluid volume, which increases hematocrit, may be the cause of the hyperbilirubinemia seen 48 to 72 hours after birth (Ladewig et al., 1998). Any bruises from a difficult delivery may also be a cause.
- Birth trauma: The large size of many IDMs predisposes them to trauma during labor and delivery.
- Congenital birth defects: Birth defects may include patent ductus arteriosus, ventricular septal defect, transposition of the great vessels, small left colon syndrome, and sacral agenesis (Tyrala, 1996).

Medical–Surgical Management

Medical

Blood glucose monitoring is performed hourly during the first 4 to 6 hours of life and then every 4 hours for 24 hours, or per agency protocol. Blood is generally obtained by heel stick (Figure 51-31)

Pharmacological

An intravenous infusion of glucose may be necessary if early feeding does not keep the blood glucose at 45 mg/dL or above.

Diet

A feeding of 5% glucose water may be given soon after birth, followed in 1 hour by a breast or formula feeding, which is continued on a regular basis.

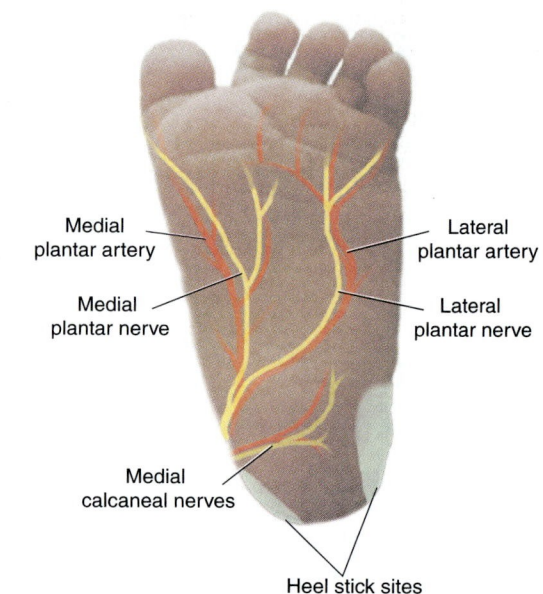

Figure 51-31 Shaded areas are heel stick sites.

▶ NURSING PROCESS

▶ Assessment

▶ Subjective Data
None

▶ Objective Data
Blood glucose screening of less than 45 mg/dL should be verified by laboratory analysis. The infant may show signs of jitteriness or tremors. Diaphoresis, though uncommon for a newborn, may occur with hypoglycemia. Poor muscle tone, low temperature, and rapid respirations may also be noted.

Nursing diagnoses for an infant with hypoglycemia may include the following:

Nursing Diagnoses	Planning/Goals	Nursing Interventions
▶ *Nutrition, Altered, Less Than Body Requirements related to increased glucose use secondary to being IDM*	The infant will maintain an adequate glucose level.	Ensure timely infant feedings. Monitor blood glucose level according to protocol. Prevent cold stress and identify other stressors (hypoxia, sepsis, RDS) that increase glucose use.
▶ *Pain related to physical injury of heel sticks for glucose monitoring*	The infant will decrease crying after each heel stick.	Properly perform heel stick to avoid nerves and arteries. Hold and comfort infant after heel stick procedure.

Evaluation Each goal must be evaluated to determine how it has been met by the client.

INFANT OF AN HIV POSITIVE MOTHER

The transmission rate of HIV infection from mother to infant is 28% to 35% (Merenstein, Adams, & Weisman, 1998). This transmission may occur through the placenta at various gestational ages, through maternal blood and secretions during labor and birth, and through breast milk after the birth (Fanaroff & Martin, 1997).

Every infant born to an HIV seropositive mother will have HIV antibodies that have crossed the placenta from the mother. By 8 to 15 months of age, uninfected infants have lost the maternal antibodies; but the infected infants have begun to develop their own antibodies and remain HIV seropositive (Fanaroff & Martin, 1997).

At birth the HIV infected infant typically has no symptoms. The appearance of an opportunistic disease between 3 and 6 months of age may alert caregivers to the presence of HIV infection. Lymphoid interstitial pneumonitis is considered a criterion for diagnosis (Fanaroff & Martin, 1997). As a basis for care, all infants of HIV positive mothers must be presumed to be HIV positive.

Breastfeeding is not recommended.

INFANT OF A SUBSTANCE-ABUSING MOTHER

The infant of a substance-abusing mother (ISAM) is a substance abuser at birth. When the umbilical cord is cut at birth, the newborn experiences withdrawal. The severity of withdrawal symptoms depends on the substance(s) abused by the mother and the time and amount of the last dose. The symptoms may occur within the first 24 to 48 hours after birth or not until 4 or 5 days of age. Alcohol withdrawal symptoms often appear within 6 to 12 hours after birth or at least within the first 3 days. Infant alcohol dependence is physiologic. It may be very difficult for the substance-abusing mother to care for her infant initially and/or long term.

Complications commonly found in an ISAM include withdrawal, respiratory distress, jaundice, behavior problems, congenital anomalies, and growth retardation. Infants of alcohol dependent mothers may also have fetal alcohol syndrome (FAS).

Medical–Surgical Management

Medical

Treatment is focused on the management of the previously mentioned complications that may be present. Approximately 50% of these infants experience withdrawal symptoms severe enough to require treatment.

PROFESSIONAL TIP

Narcotic Antagonists

The use of naloxone (Narcan) is contraindicated for infants born to narcotic abusers. It may cause severe signs and symptoms of narcotic withdrawal, especially seizures.

Pharmacological

Phenobarbital or tincture of opium may be used to control drug withdrawal symptoms. Phenobarbital or diazepam (Valium) may be used to control seizures in the alcohol-dependent infant.

Diet

Formula supplying 24 kcal/oz is recommended for the infant who experiences vomiting and diarrhea or who is excessively active.

▶ NURSING PROCESS

▶ Assessment

▶ Subjective Data
None

▶ Objective Data

The drug-dependent infant may experience hyperactivity, persistent high-pitched shrill cry, tremors, seizures, tachypnea, fever, disorganized sucking and swallowing, vomiting, diarrhea, stuffy nose, yawning, sneezing, and sweating. The alcohol-dependent infant may or may not have FAS, which includes mental retardation, hyperactivity, growth deficiency, distinctive facial abnormalities, and other congenital anomalies. This infant may also experience tremors, seizures, inconsolable crying, abdominal distention, great activity, and exaggerated rooting and sucking.

Nursing diagnoses for an infant experiencing withdrawal may include the following:

Nursing Diagnoses	Planning/Goals	Nursing Interventions
▶ *Nutrition Altered, Less Than Body Requirements, related to disorganized sucking and swallowing, vomiting, diarrhea, and hyperactivity*	The infant will not lose excessive weight (more than 10% of birth weight).	Monitor infant's temperature so environment can be adjusted to maintain normal infant temperature. Provide small frequent feedings. Administer medications as ordered. Position infant on the side to avoid possible aspiration. Maintain strict intake and output. Weigh infant every 8 hours. Monitor for signs of dehydration (sunken fontanel, dry mucous membranes, poor skin turgor, weight loss).
▶ *Injury, Risk for, related to effects of substance withdrawal (seizures, hyperactivity)*	The infant will not exhibit signs of seizures.	Administer medications as ordered. Decrease environmental activity. Plan care to necessitate minimum stimulation.

continued

Nursing Diagnoses	Planning/Goals	Nursing Interventions
		Wrap infant snugly.
		Monitor activity level.
▶ *Parenting, Altered, Risk for, related to substance abuse and difficult temperament of the infant*	The parent will show signs of bonding/attachment and an interest in infant care.	Explain effects of maternal substance abuse on infant and the process of withdrawal.
		Role model interacting with the infant.
		Encourage mother to interact with her infant.
		Explain and demonstrate infant care procedures, especially how to avoid excess stimulation of the infant.
		Make referrals to social agencies and infant development programs.

Evaluation Each goal must be evaluated to determine how it has been met by the client.

PHENYLKETONURIA

Most states require neonatal screening for the genetic disease phenylketonuria (PKU). It is an inborn error of metabolism in which the infant has a deficiency of the enzyme required to digest the amino acid phenylalanine. The infant must ingest an ample amount of phenylalanine, found in both breast milk and regular infant formulas, for the PKU test to be reliable. The test is performed at least 24 hours after the initial breast or formula feeding.

An infant with PKU must be put on a diet low in phenylalanine, preferably by 1 month of age. There are infant formulas available that are very low in phenylalanine. Without screening and diet modification, severe mental retardation results. Even with neonatal PKU screening, many affected children have some intellectual impairment (Lowdermilk et al., 1999).

PROFESSIONAL TIP

PKU

The time of the first breast or formula feeding is to be documented so at least 24 hours passes before the heel stick for the PKU test is performed.

CULTURAL CONSIDERATIONS

Phenylketonuria

The highest incidence of PKU is found in the white populations of Northern Europe and the United States; it is less common in populations of African, Chinese, and Japanese descent (AAP, 1996).

CASE STUDY

Baby boy Hren, a full-term newborn, is 36 hours old. He has type B, Rh positive blood and his mother type O, Rh positive blood. There is a small cephalhematoma on the right parietal bone. Routine assessment identified the appearance of jaundice when the skin was blanched on his forehead. His bilirubin level was 2 mg/dL on the cord blood and 4 mg/dL at 24 hours of age.

The following questions will guide your development of a nursing care plan for the case study.

1. What factors may be causing the jaundice?
2. What orders would you anticipate the physician would write?
3. What are the critical levels of bilirubin?
4. Phototherapy is begun using "bili" lights. What assessments and precautions must be taken when these lights are used?
5. Identify two possible nursing diagnoses and a goal for each for baby boy Hren.
6. Describe nursing interventions for meeting the goals.
7. How can the goals be evaluated?

SUMMARY

- The immediate needs of the newborn are airway, breathing, circulation, and warmth.
- The initiation of breathing is related to physical, chemical, thermal, and sensory factors.
- Circulatory changes include the closing of the three fetal structures: the ductus arteriosus, foramen ovale, and the ductus venosus.
- Nonshivering thermogenesis, metabolism of brown fat, is the newborn's unique method of heat production.
- Infants lose heat through conduction, convection, evaporation, and radiation.
- The immediate care of the newborn includes obtaining the Apgar score, resuscitation (if required), providing a neutral thermal environment, identification, parent/infant bonding, and prophylactic care.
- Common variations of the newborn must be carefully documented, especially mongolian spots, to possibly prevent parents from being charged with child abuse.
- Neurologic integrity can be assessed through the many reflexes of the newborn. Most of these reflexes disappear during the first 2 years of life.
- Six states of being have been identified for the newborn: quiet sleep, active sleep, drowsy, quiet alert, active alert, and crying.
- Gestational age can be determined by assessing 6 physical characteristics and 6 neuromuscular maturity characteristics.
- Infants are considered contaminated with blood-borne pathogens until after the first bath.
- Problems of the newborn include hyperbilirubinemia, respiratory distress, cleft lip/palate, hydrocephalus, spina bifida, Down syndrome, talipes equinovarus, and phenylketonuria.
- Infants need special care when the mother is a diabetic, HIV positive, or a substance abuser.

Review Questions

1. The nurse is aware that survival of a newborn infant depends primarily upon:

   a. the infant's regulation of body temperature.
   b. prompt expansion of the lungs and the establishment of gaseous exchange.
   c. the infant's energy provided from materials obtained from the environment.
   d. the rise in the infant's arterial oxygen tension and a rapid fall in carbon dioxide tension.

2. When assisting the establishment of respirations in a newborn, which of these actions should the nurse do first?

   a. Tie the cord.
   b. Provide continuous oxygen.
   c. Use a resuscitation machine.
   d. Remove mucus from the nose, mouth, and throat.

3. The nurse dries a newborn infant as soon after birth as possible, primarily to help:

   a. stimulate the infant's circulatory system.
   b. avoid excess heat loss from the infant's body.
   c. remove organisms from the infant's skin acquired during birth.
   d. remove the amniotic fluid so the infant is not so slippery.

4. The mother touches her infant's cheek gently with her finger and exclaims, "Look! He turns his head toward my finger." The nurse explains that this response to a touch on the cheek is called the:

   a. grasp reflex.
   b. sucking reflex.
   c. rooting reflex.
   d. startle reflex.

5. A new mother asks the nurse about the bluish area on the infant's buttocks. The nurse's response is based on knowledge that this discoloration:

   a. is called mongolian spots.
   b. may need to be removed surgically.
   c. is a birthmark that the infant will have for life.
   d. should be checked about twice a year for precancerous cells.

6. A new mother feels the soft spot on her baby's head and asks when it will close. The nurse responds that the anterior fontanelle normally is closed by the time the infant reaches the age of:

   a. 3 months.
   b. 6 months.
   c. 12 months.
   d. 18 months.

7. The nurse understands that vitamin K is administered shortly after birth primarily to help:

   a. peristaltic movements.
   b. stimulate respirations.
   c. improve blood coagulation.
   d. increase calcium absorption.

8. Following a circumcision, the newborn should be observed for complications. The most likely complication is:

   a. bleeding.
   b. retention of urine.
   c. blood in the urine.
   d. hematoma of the scrotum.

9. Blood between the periosteum and the skull bone of the newborn is called:

   a. melanoma.
   b. hemangioma.
   c. cephalhematoma.
   d. caput succedaneum.

10. The nurse is aware that the most generally accepted theory of the cause of physiologic jaundice is that it results from:

    a. dehydration fever.
    b. congenital obliteration of the bile ducts.
    c. rapid destruction of excess red blood cells.
    d. antibodies caused by the Rh negative factor in the maternal blood.

Critical Thinking Questions

1. Mrs. Salinas is trying to breastfeed her second child. She gave up in 3 weeks with her first child because of cracked, sore nipples. What factors may affect her success or failure? What nursing interventions should be planned and started?

2. Your personal opinion is that newborn circumcision should not be performed on a routine basis. You are assigned to assist with a routine circumcision. How will you handle this situation?

 WEB FLASH!

- Check the Internet for the most recent immunization schedule for children. Are there any changes from the previous year?
- What resources are available on the Internet for parents with new infants?

BASICS OF PEDIATRIC CARE

MAKING THE CONNECTION

Refer to the following chapters to increase your understanding of pediatric care:

- **Chapter 7, Ethical Responsibilities**
- **Chapter 12, Cultural Diversity and Nursing**
- **Chapter 14, The Life Cycle**
- **Chapter 15, Wellness Concepts**
- **Chapter 17, Loss, Grief, and Death**
- **Chapter 24, Medication Administration**
- **Chapter 26, Pain Management**
- **Chapter 28, Anesthesia**
- **Chapter 29, Nursing Care of the Surgical Client**

LEARNING OBJECTIVES

Upon completion of this chapter, you should be able to:

- *Define key terms.*
- *Discuss the role of the nurse in preparing a child and family for hospitalization.*
- *Explain the role of the nurse in admission and discharge of the pediatric client.*
- *Prepare children at different developmental stages for procedures.*
- *Discuss various methods for assessing basic needs and planning daily care.*
- *Safely perform supportive pediatric procedures.*
- *Identify the child's concept of death at various developmental stages.*
- *Describe common responses (child, family, siblings, nurses) to a dying child.*
- *Discuss sources of support for the dying child.*

KEY TERMS

assent
child life specialist
emancipated minor
family-centered care
rooming-in

INTRODUCTION

Nursing care of children centers on promoting, maintaining, and restoring the health of the child and family. While families are very important to all clients in the health care area, parents are essential to the care and nurturing of the young child. For this reason, when providing care to children, inclusion of the family is essential. Family-centered care recognizes the family as the constant in a child's life. **Family-centered care** is defined as: incorporating into policy and practice the recognition that the family is the constant in a child's life while the service systems and support personnel within those systems change (Shelton & Stepanek, 1994). An additional factor that impacts the health care of children is their rapidly evolving growth and development.

Children differ from adults in their physical, emotional, and cognitive responses. Physical, emotional, and cognitive immaturity will affect the child's response to comprehension of and reaction to illness or injury. For that reason a child's developmental level must always be assessed and care plans based on that level. Nursing care of children covers the neonatal period (birth to 28 days), infancy (1 month to 1 year), toddlerhood (12 months to 3 years), preschool age (3 to 6 years), school age (6 to 10 years), preadolescence (10 to 12 years), and adolescence (13 to 20 years). For more detailed information on physical, emotional, cognitive, and moral development, refer to Chapter 14 in this book.

Trends in health care, such as shorter hospital stays, provision of care in the home, outpatient surgery, and managed care, have changed the settings in which children and their families receive care. These settings include the home, school-based and outpatient clinics, 24-hour observation and outpatient surgery areas, emergency rooms, rehabilitative care, hospitals, and intensive care units. Nurses must be able to rapidly assess, plan, implement, and evaluate care in these diverse settings.

Although any illness of a child is a major stressor for a family, it can also result in a positive experience. Nurses can maximize the client/family/nurse contact by fostering parent-child relationships, providing educational opportunities, promoting self-mastery, and providing socialization.

This chapter discusses preparing the child and family for hospitalization, pediatric procedures, and the dying child.

PREPARING THE CHILD AND FAMILY FOR HOSPITALIZATION

Foremost in the preparation of children for hospitalization on any unit is preparing the family. If the family has sound information about the child's illness, confidence in their medical recommendations, and the support of understanding nurses, then they are more likely to be able to assist in preparing the child for the hospital experience. Hospitalization may be planned or unexpected. When the hospitalization is planned, parents and child have time to prepare for the event. Many hospitals and agencies concerned with the care of the young child provide age-appropriate materials to assist parents and children to prepare for the experience of hospitalization. These materials include tours of the hospital with dress-up in surgical attire and playing with equipment, photographs and videotapes, health fairs to explain procedures, and books and films to explain in age-appropriate terms what to expect. Adolescents need different approaches in preparation for hospitalization; they not only learn from written materials, models, and films but also benefit from peers who have experienced the same procedures. Allowing them to ask questions of health care workers without their parents being present is also beneficial.

When hospitalization is unexpected, it is of utmost importance that children be given opportunities to explore their new surroundings and encouraged to view hospitalization as an adventure that they can handle. All children and their families need to be treated with respect. They need to know that the nurse will listen attentively, in an open-minded, nonjudgmental way.

Many hospitals have **child life specialists**, who are health care professionals with extensive knowledge of

CLIENT TEACHING

Sample Teaching Materials for Children Requiring Hospitalization

Videotapes

- *Special Kids, Special Dads: Fathers of Children with Disabilities* (James May, Video), Association for the Care of Children's Health.
- *Super Asthma Kids: We Take Control* (Through Our Eyes Productions, Video), Association for the Care of Children's Health.

Books

- *Becky's Story.* Baznick, Donna. Association for the Care of Children's Health.
- *Curious George Goes to the Hospital.* Rey, M., & Rey, H. A. Houghton Mifflin Company.
- *Doctors and Nurses: What Do They Do?* Green, C. Harper & Row Junior Books.
- *The Moon Balloon.* Drescher, J. Association for the Care of Children's Health.
- *Fuzzy and Frankie.* Murray, S. Association for the Care of Children's Health.

Booklets

- *Pain, Pain, Go Away: Helping Children with Pain* (Pat McGrath, G. Allen Finley, & Judith Ritchie, 1993), Association for the Care of Children's Health.
- *Preparing Your Child for the Hospital—A Checklist,* Association for the Care of Children's Health.

psychology and early childhood development, trained to prepare the child and family for hospitalization, surgery, and procedures. Their goals include maintaining normalcy, minimizing psychological trauma, and promoting optimal development of the child and family. A collaborative effort between the nurse, the child life specialist, and other health care providers helps ensure the best possible hospital experience for the child and family.

Many hospitals provide various educational programs such as open house for well children and preadmission orientation. These programs are designed to orient the child and family to the environment and procedures and may incorporate such learning activities as audiovisuals, art, puppets, tours, and role-play.

The preparation of the child and family should be guided by consideration of the child's developmental level. Parents of infants and toddlers must be reassured of their important role as primary care providers, even during hospitalization (Figure 52-1). Parents must be encouraged to make the necessary arrangements that will allow them to room-in with the hospitalized child. **Rooming-in** is the practice of staying with a

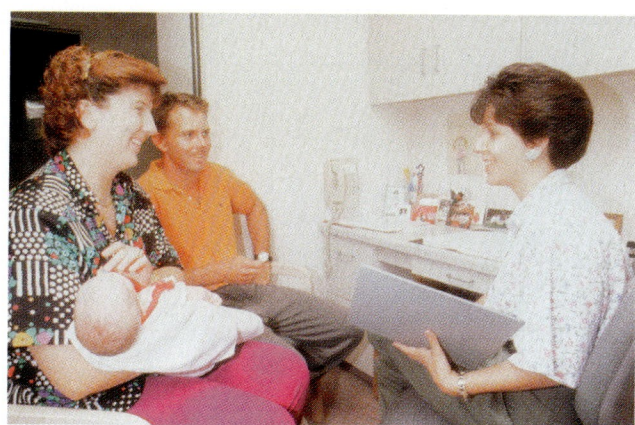

Figure 52-1 The nurse helps prepare the parents for a child's hospitalization.

hospitalized client (child) 24 hours a day to provide care and comfort to that child. It may also be the method of choice when parents need to learn and practice specialized treatments that they will be performing at home for the child.

Admission

In the past the majority of care provided to ill children was in the hospital setting. The current trend is to utilize community-based areas such as clinics, freestanding surgical units, schools, and the home. Children admitted to the hospital are more acutely ill yet the time spent in the agency is shorter. The nurse's role in the care of children is changing and expanding. In planning care for children, prevention will be a key component as well as teaching for the child and family. The nurse is frequently the first person who sees the child and family when they enter the health care system. The nurse's ability to assess the child and family for physical, psychosocial, cultural, spiritual, and growth and developmental factors will set the stage for the plan of care.

The plan of care begins with the admission to the health care facility. The completion of admission information includes: previous data regarding the child and family as well as information regarding peers and play patterns, eating patterns, sleeping patterns, school history, normal activity patterns, fears, habits, primary language spoken, language development and level of understanding, usual reaction to pain, special routines, and perception of parents regarding prior or present hospitalizations. In addition, an assessment of basic needs and daily care planning information will be obtained. Most agencies have policies and procedures for admission. Many institutions have a form for parents to complete regarding the child's routines, prior illnesses, current medications, and specific adaptations needed for the child and family. This form is usually signed by the parent and kept in the medical record. Although

the agency may have a set policy for admission, the routine may need to be altered based on the needs of the child and family. For example, a fearful child in pain may need to have pain medication and support prior to being interviewed. The nurse always focuses on the needs of the client and family in order to support and assist in mobilizing coping mechanisms rather than data gathering.

The initial assessment determines the need for immediate care. After the family and child are made comfortable or stabilized, a more thorough physical assessment and health history may be obtained. The standard data collected are: history of the client, allergies, nutritional intake, sleep, elimination, psychosocial information, spiritual and cultural factors, and the initial physical assessment. Data collected at the time of admission are used to identify nursing diagnoses and to establish a plan of care; these are placed in the child's chart. Figure 52-2 shows an example of a pediatric admission form.

Many agencies have standardized care plans based on the most common problems identified by the assessment. These care plans are also placed on the chart and are the basis of care. In addition to standardized care plans, many agencies are developing clinical paths or care paths for specific disease states. These tools assist the nurse in giving care based on protocols that result in more rapid recovery, prevention of complications, reduction of length of stay, and cost-containing care for the client and family.

Protection/Safety

Situations may arise during hospitalization that may jeopardize the safety and well-being of the child. Nurses must be ever mindful of who has custody of the child and screen visitors if there are threats to the child's safety. Issues of custody, disputes among family members, and kidnapping of children are no longer remote problems for hospital personnel. Security measures have been put in place in most pediatric units with visible identification of parents, approved visitors, and personnel. Many units utilize electronic surveillance for visitors and monitoring devices for the hospitalized children.

Informed consent of the legal guardian is obtained at the time of admission for general treatment including procedures such as IV insertions, specimen collection, and medication and oxygen administration. Separate informed consents of the legal guardian must be obtained for procedures such as lumbar punctures, chest tube insertion, and bone marrow aspirations. Federal guidelines state that children over 7 years of age have the right to give **assent** (the child's voluntary agreement to participate in a research project or to accept treatment) for treatment and research procedures. In most states, clients over 18 years of age can legally give informed consent. In addition, most states allow

ADMISSION FORM PART 1 OF 2
PARENT / PATIENT INFORMATION

Dear Parent,
We want to work with you to individually plan the care which your child will receive. You can help us by completing this form. The information will help us learn about your child's illness or condition and about his/her general health. If you have any questions or if you do not want to answer any or all of the questions, please return the form to the nurse. Your nurse will review your answers and together we will develop a plan for your child's care.
Thank you for your cooperation.

The DCH Nursing Staff

GENERAL INFORMATION

Primary language _____ Interpreter _____
Where will you be staying during your child's hospitalization? _____
Whom should we call in case of emergency. NAME: _____ RELATIONSHIP: _____
in case you are not available: _____ Phone, days _____ Phone, nights _____
What do you expect to happen during this hospitalization? _____
What childhood disease has your child had? ☐ measles; ☐ chicken pox, ☐ mumps; ☐ rubella;
Has your child been exposed to any of these within the past two weeks? ☐ Yes ☐ No
Do you have child's immunization card? ☐ Yes ☐ No
Are your child's immunizations current? ☐ Yes ☐ No   Check those which your child has had.
DPT ☐ 2 mo. ☐ 4 mo. ☐ 6 mo. ☐ 15 mo. ☐ 4-6 yrs.   OPV ☐ 2 mo. ☐ 4 mo. ☐ 15-18 mo. ☐ 4-6 yrs
HIB ☐ 2 mo. ☐ 4 mo. ☐ 6 mo. ☐ 12-15 mo.   MMR ☐ 15 mo. ☐ 11-12 yrs
Td ☐ 14-16 yrs.   Hepatitis ☐ Birth ☐ 1-2 mo. ☐ 6-18 mo.
What is your child's grade in school? _____   TB Skin Test _____ Boosters _____
Previous hospitalization _____
(Patient only) Do you...smoke? ☐ No ☐ Yes _____ packs/day   use alcohol? ☐ No ☐ Yes...
Where? _____ Why? _____

DISCHARGE PLANNING INFORMATION

Parent/Guardian: present ☐ Not available ☐ Telephone interview ☐
Have you been receiving help from any agencies? ☐ Yes ☐ No
☐ Home Health ☐ Visiting Nurse ☐ WIC ☐ AFDC ☐ CIDCS ☐ Early Childhood Intervention
If you need help with your child at home, who can assist you? _____
Does your child require any special equipment or supplies in his/her daily home care? ☐ Yes ☐ No
(apnea monitor, oxygen, suction, etc...)
What information do you need regarding your child's illness and/or hospitalization? _____

IF YOU NEED HELP ARRANGING FOR POSTHOSPITAL SERVICES INFORM YOUR PHYSICIAN OR NURSE THAT YOU WOULD LIKE TO TALK TO A PROFESSIONAL STAFF MEMBER WHO HANDLES DISCHARGE PLANNING.

MEDICATION HISTORY

In this section, please list for each medication your child takes, the dose, how often taken, the time of the last dose, and you/your child's understanding of the reason the drug has been prescribed. If there are problems taking the drug, please describe those also. While your child is in the hospital, ALL medications will be provided. If you have brought medications with you, please do not leave them. Please take them home. Thank you.

Medication	Dose	Frequency	Last Taken	Purpose/Problems Taking

Allergies: Not Known ☐ Medications _____ Foods _____ Other: _____

DRISCOLL CHILDREN'S HOSPITAL
CHILDREN'S MEDICAL CENTER OF SOUTH TEXAS

ADMISSION ASSESSMENT

For the following questions, please check your answer – yes or no – and use the space provided to describe or provide more information.

NUTRITIONAL METABOLIC

YES NO
☐   ☐ Use a pacifier, bottle, cup, special nipple, feeding tube? _____
☐   ☐ Type of diet? _____
☐   ☐ Take formula? Type _____ Amount? _____ How often? _____
☐   ☐ Has your child had any recent weight change? Loss _____ Gain _____
☐   ☐ Any changes in appetite or thirst? _____
☐   ☐ When did child last eat or drink? _____

ELIMINATION

☐   ☐ Is child potty trained? Special words _____
☐   ☐ Diapers? Type _____ Size _____
☐   ☐ Has your child experienced any changes or difficulties with urination? _____
☐   ☐ Does your child have a history of bed wetting? _____
☐   ☐ Does your child often have diarrhea or constipation? _____
☐   ☐ Are laxatives or other aids used for regularity? _____

ACTIVITY EXERCISE

☐   ☐ Does your child have preferred play activities? _____
☐   ☐ Does your child tire easily with play? _____
☐   ☐ Does your child have appliances or need assistance for walking or mobility? (walker, wheelchair) _____
Briefly describe your child's usual daily routine: _____

COGNITIVE-PERCEPTUAL

YES NO
☐   ☐ Does your child have any difficulty hearing? Use a hearing aid? Type: _____
☐   ☐ Does your child have any difficulty seeing? When were the eyes last checked? _____ Wear glasses? _____
☐   ☐ Does your child sometimes have difficulty learning? _____
What is the easiest way for him/her to learn? (books, film watching, demonstrations) _____
What do you do special to comfort your child when having pain/discomfort? _____

COPING-STRESS

☐   ☐ Are there any recent changes in family life that may affect this hospitalization? _____
☐   ☐ How have your child/you and your family responded to these changes? _____
☐   ☐ Are there other children in family? _____ Ages _____
☐   ☐ Do you have family or friends in the Corpus Christi area? _____
Whom do you define as your family or support system? _____
☐   ☐ Being in the hospital is stressful for many people. Is there anything we can do to make it easier for you or for your child? _____

ORIENTED TO
☐ Phone; ☐ Bed; ☐ Call light/intercom; ☐ Parent bed/regulations (Recliners up by 8 a.m.) ☐ Patient Rights & Responsibilities
☐ Playroom; ☐ Mealtimes; ☐ Smoking policy; ☐ IV, VS routine, a.m. wts ☐ Visitation Limits/hrs. ☐ Intake & Output Monitored
☐ Care of valuables; ☐ Side rails; ☐ TV; ☐ Isolation; ☐ ID Band ☐ Car seat for discharge ☐ Save diapers
☐ Bear Questionaires ☐ No electrical appliances
Oriented by: _____

Parent Signature: _____ Date: _____ Time: _____

Figure 52-2 Pediatric Admission Form *(Courtesy Driscoll Children's Hospital.)*

ADMISSION FORM PART 2 OF 2

TO BE COMPLETED BY ADMITTING NURSE.   Attn. Physician/Time Notified _____ by _____

Arrival to RM _____ Date _____ Time _____ Resident _____ by _____

Brief History _____

GENERAL APPEARANCE: _____

_____

NEUROLOGICAL: Responds to: ☐ Verbal ☐ Pain ☐ Nonresponsive

Gait: ☐ N/A ☐ Walks ☐ Unable to stand ☐ Uncoordinated   LOC: ☐ Lethargic ☐ Semi-Comatose ☐ Comatose ☐ Alert

Movement: ☐ Coordinated ☐ Voluntary ☐ Involuntary; Speech _____ Head Circ _____

Anterior Fontanel _____

Seizures _____   Pupil   1 2 3 4 5 6 7 8

Developmental level: _____   Scale: · • ● ● ● ● ● ●
                                           (mm)

CARDIO VASCULAR: HR _____

Apical pulse: rhythm _____ Peripheral pulses: RA _____ RL _____ LA _____ LL _____ BP _____

Clubbing: _____ Nailbed Color _____ Capillary Refill _____

Comments: _____

RESPIRATORY: Temp. _____

Breath Sounds: ☐ Clear ☐ Crackles ☐ Wheezing ☐ Coarse ☐ Diminished _____ RR _____

Retractions: ☐ None ☐ Substernal ☐ Intercostal ☐ Subcostal _____ Chest Circ _____

Effort: ☐ Shallow ☐ Deep ☐ Labored ☐ Unlabored; Cough _____ Sputum _____

Chest Symmetry _____ Comments: _____

GASTRO-INTESTINAL:

Abdomen: ☐ Soft ☐ Tender ☐ Nontender ☐ Rigid ☐ Distended; Last B.M. _____ Wt _____

Bowel Sounds: ☐ Active ☐ Hyperactive ☐ Hypoactive; Appetite _____ Ht _____

Tubes: ☐ OG ☐ NG ☐ GT ☐ JT _____ Abd girth _____

Comments: _____

GYNECOLOGICAL: ☐ No abnormalities reported ☐ Sexually active; LMP _____

Discharge _____ Lesions _____ Comments: _____

GENITOURINARY: Urine color _____ Amt. _____ Odor _____ Discharge _____

Incontinent _____ Last void _____

Comments: _____

MUSCULO-SKELETAL:

☐ Moves all extremities ☐ Limited ROM; Swelling _____

Contractures _____ Edema _____ Prosthetic devices _____

Comments: _____

INTEGUMENTARY: (on figure in box, note location of any items with the appropriate letter and check the box by the letter)

☐ Skin intact ☐ Warm ☐ Cool ☐ Cold ☐ Moist ☐ Dry; Color: ☐ Pale ☐ Pink ☐ Jaundiced ☐ Cyanotic ☐ Mottled

Turgor _____ Masses/Size _____ IV site, condition, fluids _____

Wounds/Dressings _____

Comments: _____

☐ B - Bruise
☐ D - Decubitus
☐ L - Laceration
☐ R - Rash
☐ S - Scar

Nursing Process/Plan of care inititated _____ Nurse initials _____

Allergies: Not Known _____ Medications _____

Foods _____ Environmental _____

R.N. _____ Date/Time _____

Figure 52-2 *continued*

some exceptions for parental consent in cases involving emancipated minors. An **emancipated minor** is a child who has the legal competency of an adult because of circumstances involving marriage, divorce, parenting a child, living independently without parents, or enlistment in the armed services.

Choking and falls are also areas of concern with hospitalized children. To avoid choking, the environment must be free of objects that could be placed in the mouth and possibly occlude the airway (e.g., broken

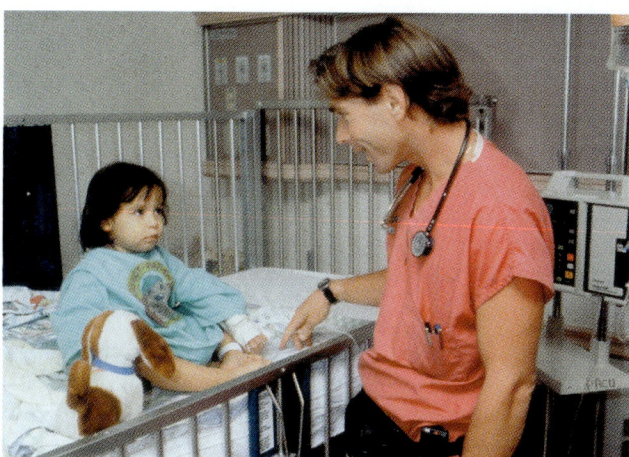

Figure 52-3 All hospitalized children will have an ID band, which will be placed on either the wrist or ankle.

PROFESSIONAL TIP

ID Bands

It is very important for all clients to have a hospital identification (ID) band on at all times (Figure 52-3). It is equally important that all health care providers check the band for proper client identification prior to performing any procedure. Any child not having an ID band needs to have the band replaced prior to treatments.

balloons, syringe caps, toys, food). An adult should always be present when a young child is eating. Other safety concerns in the hospital setting include machinery (e.g., IV pumps and equipment, needles). Doors to treatment rooms, staircases, supply closets, and rooms containing extra equipment need to be equipped with locks preventing access by children.

Side rails on cribs must be up at all times. If a toddler is able to climb over the rails, a safety cover may need to be placed over the crib, or a regular bed may be used. The nurse should never turn his or her back to a child or reach for materials when the side rail is down if the child is not properly secured.

The Child Undergoing Surgery

The child and family experience with surgery may be an elective procedure, planned in advance, or the result of an emergency with little time for planning. When possible, preadmission visits are an excellent way to prepare the child and family for surgery. Sessions should be scheduled within the week prior to admission. Table 52-1 contains suggestions for hospital preparation and surgery that are appropriate for planned procedures. As with any preparation, a multidisciplinary approach that includes parents, nursing staff, child life specialists, medical staff, and other involved professionals is best.

Preparation for surgery should include both psychosocial and physical preparation. The purpose of preoperative preparation is to reduce fear and anxiety associated with the surgical procedure and the surrounding environment. Play can facilitate preparation for hospitalization. Visits to units prior to the experience can familiarize the child and family with sights, sounds, smells, and equipment. Anatomically correct dolls and puppets, drawings, and models can be used to teach the child and family about the procedures. Through play, the child can experience the use of equipment to take vital signs and become familiar with other health care interventions.

Children need to be reassured that they will be transported to the operating room accompanied by parents and that their parents will be there when they wake up. Parents must be informed of the expected length of the surgery and be kept informed of the child's status throughout the procedure. It helps the child and parents if one nurse is designated to be the contact prior to, during, and after surgery.

Many hospitals and surgical units allow and encourage parents to be present during anesthesia induction. The presence of parents and familiar objects such as blankets and toys in the presurgical area decreases anxiety in the child as well as the parents. Decreased anxiety lessens the need for premedication for the child. Some common induction techniques for young children include concealing the breathing circuit in a play phone, behind a pacifier, or within a stuffed ani-

---

Table 52-1 NURSING RESPONSIBILITIES TO THE CHILD UNDERGOING SURGERY

PREPARATION FOR SURGERY	AGE CONSIDERATIONS
Psychological Explain surgery. Prepare for separation from family. Conduct preadmission visit.	*Infant:* Allow infant to remain on caregiver's lap as long as possible. *Toddler:* Use dolls, puppets, play hospital. *Preschooler:* Use books, videos, art. Assure toddlers and preschoolers that the surgery is not their fault and is not a punishment. *School-age Child:* Offer brief explanations with supporting visuals.
Physical Discontinue food and drink after specified time. Monitor fluid level (child has less fluid within body and can become dehydrated quickly). Perform specific preparation for procedure. Ensure that consent form is signed by guardian. Administer preoperative medication.	*Infant:* Explain to caregivers only. *Toddler:* Explain 3 days in advance. *Preschooler:* Prepare formally no more than 1 week in advance. *School-age Child:* Videos and tours.
Postoperative Care Make preparations for return of child. Obtain vital signs. Assess pain level. Inspect operative site. Check dressings for bleeding or other drainage. Check bowel and bladder function. Observe for signs of shock, dehydration, infection.	*Infant:* Maintain body warmth. Monitor intake and output. *Toddler and Preschooler:* Give favorite animal or try to provide comfort. *School-age Child:* Ask about comfort and preferred distraction activities. *All children:* Presence of parents on return to postop area and in child's room is important. Know the manifestations of pain and medicate as needed.

mal, and providing a choice of flavored gases (e.g., watermelon, grape, chocolate, etc.) (Zuckerberg, 1994).

During the postoperative period, the child will be monitored for bleeding, pain level, and pulmonary and circulatory status. When the child awakens, it is important that the parents be present to calm and comfort the child. Comfort objects from home such as favorite toys may assist the child in feeling at ease. Pain medication should be used as necessary. Most health care facilities have instructions to follow for general and specific surgical procedures.

The child may be discharged home or admitted to an inpatient unit for further care. Since children recuperate more quickly in a familiar environment, they are discharged as soon as is safely possible following surgery. Discharge planning should be initiated at admission. The ability of the parents to provide adequate care at home determines the extent of education provided prior to discharge and the need for involvement of a home health agency after discharge.

Discharge/Discharge Planning

Nurses play an important role in preparing the child and family for discharge and home care. A multidisciplinary approach should be used that includes the social service department, home care agencies, rehabilitation therapists, and the family to plan for equipment, procedures, and other home care needs. Discharge plans should begin with the admission of the child. Many agencies have a discharge planning nurse who coordinates the plans for home care. It is important for the nurse working with the client and family to take part in the planning and communicate frequently with the discharge nurse regarding information about the client and family.

Assessment of the family's ability to manage the child's care and the ability of the home environment to support the care needed by the child is important. Early planning provides the health care providers and family time to investigate financial support by agencies such as Medicaid and private insurance. If the child is school-aged, the school district should be involved in order to plan for continued education. This may require special assessment by the school system and a plan of educational care developed to include home tutors, specialized services such as speech therapists and occupational therapists, and/or transportation to school with specialized medical care to be delivered at the school.

Parents may need to learn special or rehabilitative procedures for the child's care. The parents are taught special procedures to be done at home. The nurse demonstrates, explains, and observes as the parents assume the care they will be responsible for at home. The education provided and the parents' ability to perform care are discussed with the public health nurse, home health nurse, or individual who will be managing the home care program. Parents will be assisted in exploring options for relief from the child's care, such as respite care, relatives, church groups, or lists of caregivers with ability to give specialized care.

The family is the most important advocate and spokesperson for the child. When a child needs long-term care, the family will need the services of many agencies and numerous health care personnel. To coordinate health care and to prevent gaps and overlaps, one person needs to be identified as a case manager. The parent may decide to act as the child's case manager with support and education from discharge planners.

PEDIATRIC PROCEDURES

In preparing the child and family for procedures performed either at home or in an agency, it is important to take into consideration the child's growth and development, cognitive abilities, and physical and psychosocial factors. It is important that procedures be conducted effectively and efficiently with the least amount of discomfort to the client and family. The following procedures are common to the care of children. While they are similar to procedures performed on adults, they also may differ in several ways. Nurses must be knowledgeable about variations in preparation, equipment, positioning, and specific steps when performing procedures on children.

Physical Assessment

Physical assessments for the child are similar to those for the adult with a few differences. Measurements of physical size are significant in evaluating a child's health status. Deviation from the established norms may indicate a significant health problem.

Growth Measurements

Growth measurements for children are recorded at each well-child visit as well as visits for disease episodes. Measurements must be taken correctly and accurately. Values for growth parameters are placed on percentile charts and evaluated with those of the general population. In general, percentiles from 5% to 95% are considered within normal ranges. All growth evaluations

HOME HEALTH CARE

Tips for Discharge
- Assess needs and resources.
- Plan for comprehensive care.
- Provide clear, concise written instructions.
- Link client with service provider.
- Coordinate services.
- Advocate for appropriate services.

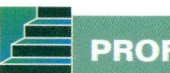

PROFESSIONAL TIP

General Instructions for All Pediatric Procedures

Preprocedure

Check physician's orders.

Review procedure in agency procedure manual.

Gather equipment and assistance if necessary.

Introduce yourself and assistants to child and parents.

Identify child by name band or approved identification method.

Give instructions and explanation to the child and parent and ask if there are any questions.

If parent is going to hold child, demonstrate exactly what you want done. Make sure the parent feels secure about assisting with the procedure. Make sure you know the agency policy regarding parents assisting with procedures by holding the child.

Wash your hands.

Don protective clothing if necessary.

During the Procedure

Maintain privacy.

Tell the child exactly what is expected of him or her, never threaten or tell a child you will have to "hold him/her down."

Have someone assist you if necessary and if it will facilitate the procedure being completed more quickly.

Maintain a conversation with parent and child, explaining what you are doing, in a calm soothing voice.

Keep the child and parent informed of the procedure's progress.

Tell the child when the procedure is nearly complete.

Support of Child and Family

Offer ways of coping with pain or discomfort (imagery, music). Give permission to cry.

Use developmentally appropriate words.

Give child as much choice over the procedure as possible.

---

take into consideration a child's genetic predisposition. As well as genetic concerns, ethnic and socioeconomic background may influence growth norms. It is unknown whether the differences within the ethnic and socioeconomic backgrounds are from the cultural norms or the result of nutritional differences.

The growth charts most commonly used in the United States are those from the National Center for Health Statistics (NCHS) and are available for boys and girls of different ages. There are growth charts available for children 2 to 3 based on whether their height is measured in a lying or standing position. Lying position is referred to as recumbent, and height while standing is referred to as stature. Most children under age 2 are measured in a recumbent position, and children over 2 are measured in a standing position.

Children Under Two Years of Age Growth measurements for children under 2 differ in the procedure and types of measurements taken. Typical mea-

surements taken for the child under 2 are: length; weight; and head, chest, and abdominal circumferences.

Length Measurement of length is taken with the child in a supine position. The method for children under 2 is as follows:

1. Use a paper sheet to lay the infant in a recumbent (lying down) position. Extend the infant's body.
2. Ensure that the infant's head is in midline and legs are extended. Gently grasp knees and push toward table to fully extend legs (Figure 52-4).
3. Place a mark on the paper at the crown of the infant's head.
4. Extend the leg and place a mark on the paper at the base of the heel (toes pointing upward).

PROFESSIONAL TIP

Growth

Growth is a continuous and uneven process, and the most important point for monitoring the growth of children is comparison over time.

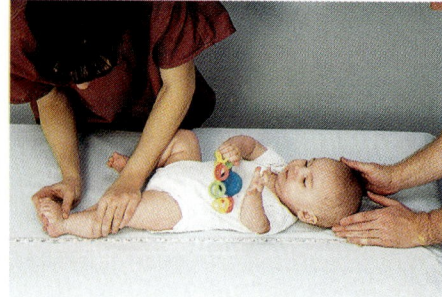

Figure 52-4 Measuring Recumbent Length in an Infant

5. If a measuring board is used, place the infant's head against the board and extend the legs, placing the heels of the feet on the footboard.
6. Measure the distance between the two marks or on the measuring board.
7. Record the length.

Weight Infants are weighed on a platform scale. They may be placed in either a sitting or supine position, depending on their ability to sit unsupported. Prior to weighing the infant the nurse must make sure the scale is cleaned, a paper cover is placed on the scale, and the room is warm. The scale should always be balanced prior to weighing the infant. The method for weighing is as follows:

1. Place the nude child on the scale, making sure never to turn your back to the child on the scale. Hold your hand over the infant but do not touch the infant while obtaining the weight (Figure 52-5).
2. Measure to the nearest 10 grams or 2 ounces and record the weight.

Head Circumference During the first year or two of life, head circumference is measured as an important indication of brain growth. The method for obtaining head circumference is as follows:

1. Measure the head at its greatest circumference.
2. Wrap a measuring tape around the infant's head, placing it above the brows, the pinna of the ears, and around the occipital prominence. Make sure the tape is flat against the skin.
3. Record the circumference.

Chest Circumference The chest circumference is often measured during the first year of life as an indicator of adequate growth. During the first year, head circumference is greater than chest circumference;

after age 1, chest circumference exceeds head circumference. The method for obtaining chest circumference is as follows:

1. Measure the chest at its greatest circumference.
2. Wrap a measuring tape around the infant's chest, placing it under the axilla and over the nipple line (Figure 52-6).
3. Measure between inspiration and expiration.
4. Record the circumference.

 Safety: Paper Tape Measures
Use care when placing paper tape measures. Place under the infant and wrap around carefully. Do not slide the tape around on infant as this may result in paper cuts on the baby.

Abdominal Circumference The abdominal circumference is obtained on very young or preterm infants to detect abdominal distention. The method for measuring abdominal circumference is as follows:

1. Measure the abdomen at its point of greatest girth.
2. Place a paper tape around the infant's abdomen at the umbilicus.
3. Record the circumference.

Children Over Two Years of Age Typical measurements taken on children over 2 years of age include height and weight.

Height After the age of 2 or 3, height is measured with the child standing upright. The child's shoes

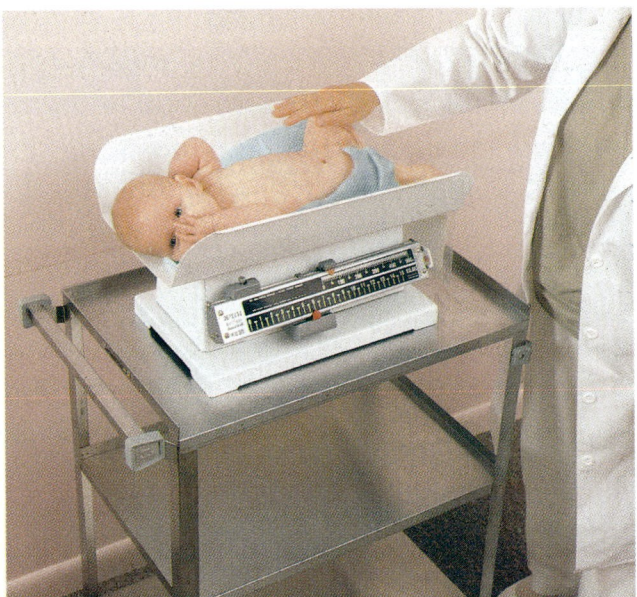

Figure 52-5 Measuring Weight in an Infant

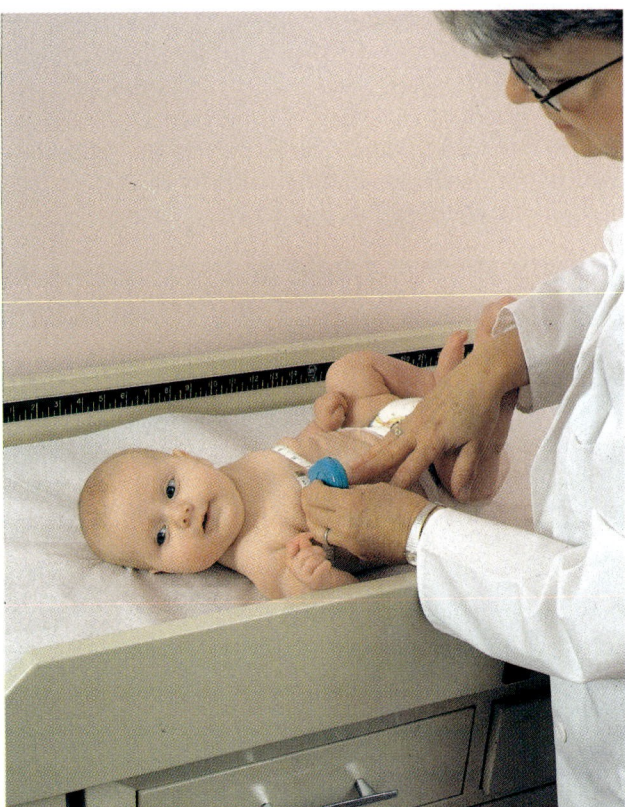

Figure 52-6 Measuring Chest Circumference in an Infant

should be removed before the measurement is taken, and the child should stand upright, with the back to the wall or scale. The child should be asked to stand very straight with head in midline and shoulders, buttocks, and heels touching the wall or the attachment to a balance scale. The method for measuring height is as follows:

1. On the balance scale, lower the ruler device until it touches the top of the child's head (Figure 52-7). Take the measurement.
2. If measuring the child against a wall, place a flat edge such as a ruler on top of the child's head. Make a mark on the wall; measure from the floor to the mark.
3. Record the height.

Weight After a child can stand and balance well, weight is taken on a standing scale. Standing scales are digital or balance. Shoes should be removed for all children. Toddlers are weighed in their underclothes, older children are weighed in street clothes with heavy jackets removed. The method for weighing is as follows:

1. Keep the room warm and ensure privacy.
2. Balance the scale prior to the child stepping on it.
3. Place child in center of scale and, with a balance scale, move the weights until the scale is balanced.
4. On digital scale, have child stand in center of scale and take reading.
5. Measure to the nearest 100 grams or ¼ pound and record the weight.

Vital Signs

Assessment of vital signs (temperature, pulse, respiratory rate, and blood pressure) is an important method for measuring and monitoring vital body functioning. In children, vital signs may change quickly

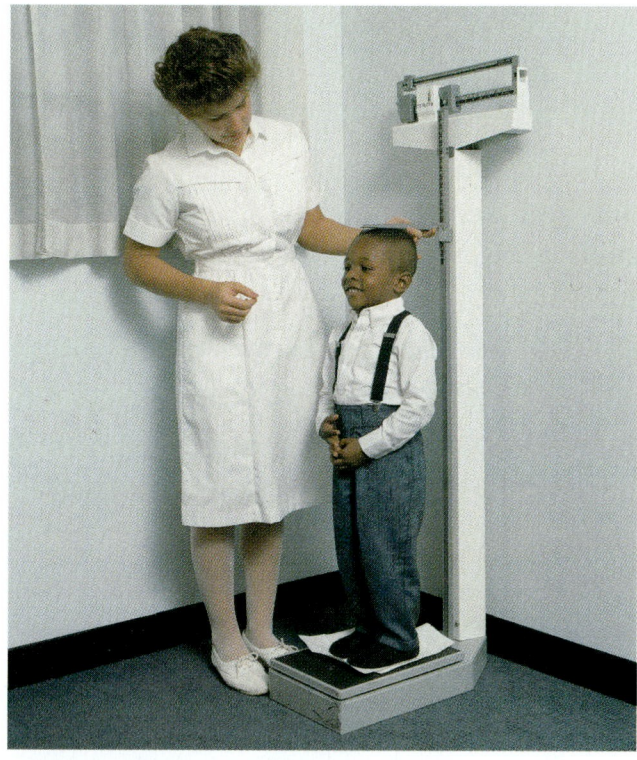

Figure 52-7 Measuring Height in Child

and will provide the basis for decisions regarding care. Table 52-2 describes normal vital signs by age.

Body Temperature Temperature assessment is a simple, objective, inexpensive, and reliable indicator of illness and is part of the pediatric assessment. Currently there are four types of thermometers utilized in pediatric agencies: glass, electronic, digital, and tympanic membrane. The electronic and tympanic membrane thermometers are the most common types utilized in acute care agencies. Another type of thermometer known as a thermograph (plastic strips or dots) is used

Table 52-2 NORMAL VITAL SIGNS BY AGE				
AGE	**TEMPERATURE**	**PULSE RATE**	**RESPIRATORY RATE**	**BLOOD PRESSURE**
Newborn	98.8–99°F	100–160	30–60	Systolic: 46–92 Diastolic: 38–71
6 months–1 year	97.5–98.6°F	90–130	24–40	Systolic: 72–106 Diastolic: 40–66
3 years	97.5–98.6°F	80–125	20–30	Systolic: 72–110 Diastolic: 40–73
6 years	97.5–98.6°F	70–110	16–22	Systolic: 46–92 Diastolic: 38–71
10–14 years	97.5–98.6°F	60–110	16–20	Systolic: 83–121 Diastolic: 45–79
14–19 years	97.5–98.6°F	55–90	15–90	Systolic: 93–131 Diastolic: 49–85

for screening only. Each agency will have guidelines to follow in taking temperatures.

Four routes are utilized for obtaining temperatures; axillary, oral, rectal, and tympanic. Axillary temperatures are usually taken on newborns, preterm infants, and infants and children under 3 years of age. The thermometer is placed in the axilla and the child's arm pressed close to the body for a minimum of 5 minutes if it is a mercury device or until the electronic thermometer registers.

An oral temperature may be taken in most children 6 years of age or older, including adolescents; the procedure is the same as for adults.

Because of the risk of rectal perforation, discomfort of the child and parent, concerns regarding sexual abuse, and difficulty comforting the child (Kai, 1993), rectal temperatures are taken when no other route is available. The child is positioned supine, prone, or side-lying, and a well-lubricated thermometer is inserted no more than a maximum of 2.5 cm for 3 to 5 minutes. Rectal temperatures are contraindicated on preterm infants, immunosuppressed children, and children with rectal surgery or gastrointestional disorders (i.e., diarrhea and any bleeding disorder). See Figure 52-8.

Tympanic temperature measurement is used in home care and inpatient settings. Measurements using these thermometers are more quickly and easily obtained. The procedure appears to be less upsetting to children and is easy to learn by parents for home care. Tympanic temperatures and rectal temperatures ap-

pear to strongly correlate. Technique is very important in using the tympanic thermometer. Position of the thermometer enhances the accuracy of the reading. The ear canal must be straightened as when using an otoscope. With the ear tugged correctly and the probe tip pointing at the midpoint between the eyebrow and the sideburn on the opposite side of the face, more accurate temperature readings are obtained. Size of the probe also influences temperature. Using appropriately sized ear probes for children increases the accuracy of the reading.

The method for taking a temperature is as follows:

1. Prepare the child and family for the procedure and assure them that little discomfort will arise from the procedure.
2. Select the appropriate method for obtaining the temperature measurement based on the child's age and condition.
3. Provide an explanation of the procedure to the child and family.
4. Assist the child into a position of comfort. The child may remain on the parent's lap if preferred.
5. Wash hands.
6. Don gloves and use Standard Precautions.
7. Obtain the child's temperature using method chosen.
8. Offer praise to the child for cooperating.
9. Document and report core temperatures of less than 36°C (96.8°F) or greater than 38.5°C (101.4°F) or specified parameters for individual child.
10. Reassess the child's temperature every one-half to 1 hour, or per instructions.
11. Document method of temperature assessment, measurement obtained, and any resulting action.

Safety: Thermometers

Regardless of the device utilized for temperature taking, *do not* lay it down in the child's bed for safety and for infection control reasons.

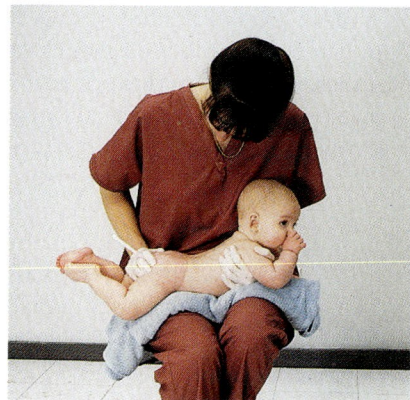

Figure 52-8 Taking a Rectal Temperature

PROFESSIONAL TIP

Measuring Temperature

Regardless of the type of thermometer used, the child's temperature should be measured at the same site and with the same type of device to maintain consistency and allow for reliable comparison and tracking of temperatures over time.

CLIENT TEACHING

Temperature Measurement

Most parents will need to learn to take their child's temperature at home. Demonstrate how it is done and then observe the parent in performing. Make sure the parent is comfortable with the procedure and is able to read the thermometer accurately. Digital thermometers are easy to read because the temperature is displayed on a small screen on the thermometer; they may be used to take oral, axillary, and rectal temperatures.

CLIENT TEACHING

Measuring Pulse Rate

Parents having children taking medication, such as digoxin, may need to learn to take a pulse rate on their child prior to administering the drug. For these parents it is important that the nurse demonstrate the method of taking the pulse and observe the parents as they take the pulse on their child. The parents need to know the acceptable pulse range for their child as well as the method of obtaining the pulse.

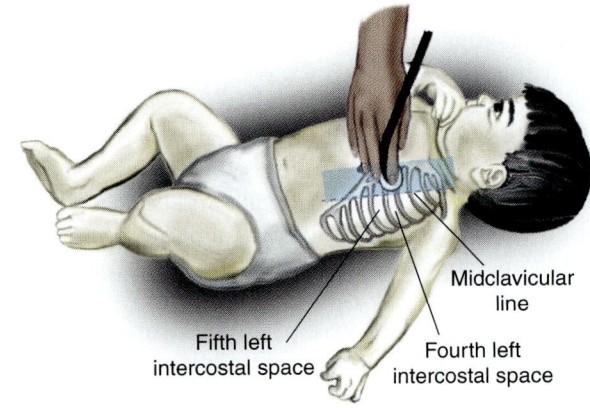

Figure 52-9 Apical Pulse Position for Infant and Child

Heart Rate or Pulse For children under the age of 2 and those having irregular heart rhythms or congenital heart disease, apical pulse is the preferred site. Radial pulse is taken for children above 3 years of age unless contraindicated. The method for taking a heart rate/pulse is as follows:

1. To count the pulse rate, place the stethoscope on the anterior chest at the fifth intercostal space in a midclavicular position (Figure 52-9).
2. Count the rate for 1 full minute.
3. Note whether the rhythm is regular or irregular.
4. Note whether the pulse is normal, bounding, or thready.
5. Compare the distal and proximal pulses for strength.
6. Pulse rates may be checked at sites other than the apex of the heart, for example, the carotid, brachial, radial, femoral, and dorsal pedis sites.
7. Record rate, quality, and rhythm.

Respiratory Rate The rate, depth, and ease of respiration are observed in the child. Respiratory rate will vary by age of the child. Since respiratory rate is irregular, it needs to be counted for 1 full minute. It is best if the child is unaware that respirations are being counted. The method for obtaining a respiratory rate is as follows:

1. Children's respirations are diaphragmatic, so observe abdominal movement to count respirations.
2. Count respirations prior to obtaining temperature or pulse rates (expect abdominal respirations to be irregular).
3. Count for 1 full minute.
4. Record rate, quality, and rhythm.

Blood Pressure Blood pressure measurement for the child is basically the same as for an adult. The size of the cuff is determined by the size of the child's arm or leg. Generally, the bladder of the cuff is two-thirds of the width of the limb in which the BP is being measured. If the bladder is too small, the pressure will be falsely high; if it is too large, the pressure will be falsely low. Blood pressure may be taken on the upper or lower extremities. General instructions for BP measurement are as follows:

Electronic Monitoring:
1. Place the cuff around the desired extremity.
2. Activate the equipment according to the manufacturer's recommendations.
3. Stabilize limb during inflation and deflation, because movement sometimes interferes with the device's ability to measure the blood pressure accurately.
4. For some devices the first reading is a priming reading and the second reading is considered the true blood pressure reading. Refer to manual.
5. Record the reading.

Manual Cuff:
1. Position limb at level of heart.
2. Rapidly inflate cuff to about 20 mm Hg above point at which radial pulse disappears.
3. Release cuff pressure at a rate of about 2 to 3 mm Hg per second during auscultation of artery.
4. Record systolic value as onset of a clear tapping sound.
5. Record diastolic pressure as disappearance of all sounds. Record systolic, diastolic pressures, limb used, position, cuff size, and method.

Developmental Assessment

Developmental assessment for the growing child is an important measure. A tool that is frequently used for the child under 6 years of age is the Denver II (DDST). The test is composed of four sections: personal-social, fine motor-adaptive, language, and gross motor. Of the 125 items on the test, responses can be obtained by observing the child, asking the parent, and having the child perform a task.

Informing the parent that the DDST is not an I.Q. (intelligence quotient) test but a helpful measure of the child's growth and development begins the test. The parent and child are made comfortable in the testing environment. Age-appropriate communication and approaches are directed toward the child (e.g., very young children may prefer to sit in parent's lap). The child is then evaluated on a series of tasks, and rated on each with a "P" for pass, "F" for refuse, and "NO" for no opportunity. A caution is given when the child fails to perform an item that has been achieved by 75% to 90% of children of the same age. A delay indicates the child's inability to perform a task that would be expected to be mastered by children in the developmental stage just prior to the child's current developmental stage. A suspect test is one with one or more delays and/or two or more cautions.

Current illness, lack of sleep, anxiety, chronic disability, or sensory deficits can affect a child's performance. If these factors can explain a child's failure to successfully complete the DDST, then the test may be readministered in 1 month, providing resolution of the problem has occurred. If a developmental delay exists, early detection can lead to intervention and possible resolution.

Child Safety Devices

Restraints are used for many reasons with pediatric clients. For the most part restraints are used to protect and prevent injury to the child. Restraints are regulated by the Omnibus Budget Reconciliation Act (OBRA), which states that restraints should be used only as a last resort for the protection of clients and others. The legislation further indicates that restraints may not be used for the convenience of the staff. Therefore, all possible alternatives should be considered prior to restraining the child. Some alternatives may be utilizing a person to sit with the child, using diversion with the child, and some behavior modification techniques. Physical restraints include safety vests, mittens, and ankle, elbow, and wrist restraints. The use of a restraint may require a physician's order stating why the restraint is needed and how long it will be left in place.

Prior to placing the restraint, check the extremity or area that will be restrained for any breaks in the skin, impaired circulation, and neurological deficits. Any orthopedic problem should also be noted. If these conditions exist, the physician should be notified prior to putting the restraint in place. General instructions for use of all restraints follow:

1. Explain to the child and family members why his/her body part will be restrained, where the restraint will be placed, what movement it will prevent, and how long it will be in place.
2. Puppets, dolls, or stories may be used assist the child in understanding.
3. Always check the restraint 15 minutes after applying and at least every hour thereafter, or more often if the child is very active.
4. Check the restrained extremity for temperature, pulses, and capillary refill.
5. Remove the restraints every 2 hours to allow for range of motion and repositioning.
6. Restrain as little and as loosely as possible to maintain safety while allowing enough freedom so that the child can touch some part of the body.
7. Provide age-appropriate stimulation for the child while he/she is restrained.
8. Documentation will include:
   a. behavior that led to applying restraints;
   b. attempts to calm client prior to restraining and client's response;
   c. explanation to parent regarding restraint use;
   d. circulatory and neuromuscular checks while restrained; and
   e. removal of the restraints, range of motion, and position changes every 2 hours.

See Table 52-3 for a summary of the types of mechanical restraints used with children.

Specimen Collection

Specimens are collected from children the same as adults with a few modifications. Children require more specific explanations and directions in an age-appropriate format. Any sensation that may be felt should be explained. Regardless of the type of specimen collected, Standard Precautions must be used.

Urine

A urine sample is obtained to assess for infection and to determine levels of blood, protein, glucose, acetone,

Table 52-3 MECHANICAL RESTRAINTS USED WITH CHILDREN		
TYPE OF RESTRAINT	**DESCRIPTION**	**USES**
Elbow restraint	Heavy fabric with compartments in which tongue blades are inserted; may also be heavy cardboard cylinders	Used to keep arms extended and away from target site; often used in head or neck surgery, and scalp vein infusion
Mummy restraint	Tightly wrapped blanket or sheet	Used for short procedures, usually on infant, to minimize movement
Jacket restraint	Jacket with ties that may be attached to bed	Used to keep child in bed after surgery
Crib top bubble restraint	Large plastic bubble attached to top of crib	Used for older infant and toddler to prevent falling and climbing out of bed

bilirubin, drugs, hormones, metals, and electrolytes excreted by the kidneys. Urine can also be assessed for concentration/specific gravity, pH, and other substances.

A collection bag is used to obtain a clean catch urine sample from an infant. Older children, after being given clear instructions, are usually capable of collecting their own urine.

The method of obtaining a urine sample for the infant is as follows:

1. Remove the diaper and clean the skin around the meatus; allow to dry thoroughly.
2. Attach the bag with the adhesive tabs, for girls, around the labia, and for boys, around the scrotum (Figure 52-10).
3. Make sure the seal is tight to prevent leakage.
4. Check the bag frequently for urine.
5. To remove the bag, pull away gently from the skin using moistened cotton balls to assist in releasing the adhesive.
6. Pour into container and cap tightly.
7. Send to lab immediately.
8. Document color, amount, clarity, and lab tests requested.

A clean catch sample for a male older child is collected in the following manner:

1. Instruct the older child to clean the head of his penis (after retracting the foreskin, if not circumcised) 3 times, each time using a different towelette, moving from the urethral meatus outward.
2. Have the child urinate a small amount into the toilet, stop the flow, then urinate into the sterile container.
3. Proceed as above.

A clean catch sample for a female older child is collected in the following manner:

1. Instruct the child to sit back on the toilet as far as possible with her legs apart. Have her spread her labia with her fingers and wipe each side with a separate towelette using a front-to-back stroke. Tell the child to use a third wipe to clean the meatus, repeating the front-to-back motion.
2. Have the child urinate a small amount into the toilet, stop the flow, then urinate into the sterile container.
3. Proceed as above.

Stool

Stool specimens are used in pediatric clients to check for the presence of fat, blood, bacteria, parasites, or reducing substances. If the stool specimen is needed from an infant or incontinent child, it can be scraped from the diaper and placed in the appropriate container. If the child is potty-trained, a bedpan or container may be used to collect the specimen. The

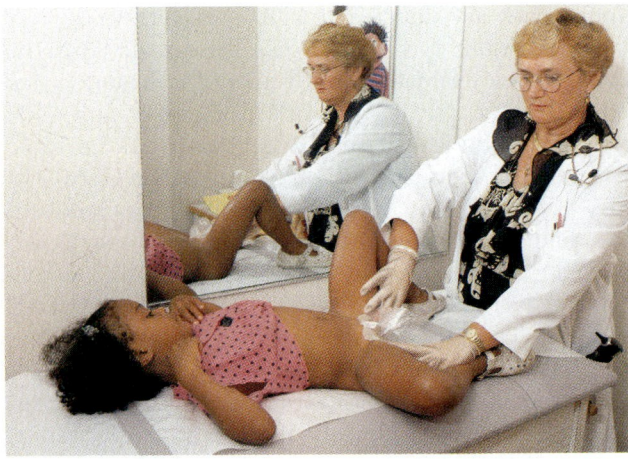

Figure 52-10 Applying a Urine Collection Bag to a Child

time the specimen is obtained, as well as color, consistency, any odor, and disposition all must be recorded.

Blood

Blood specimens are obtained from children by accessing veins of the hand or antecubital space, heelsticks, and femoral and jugular venipunctures. Collection of blood is very distressing to young children because of their lack of discrete body boundaries and the pain involved. The use of EMLA, a topical anesthetic cream, can reduce the discomfort of the needle penetrating the skin. EMLA contains lidocaine-prilocaine 5% and can be used to decrease pain associated with selected procedures: venipuncture, lumbar puncture, suture removal, immunizations, bone marrow aspiration, and removal of foreign bodies. EMLA is not ap-

PROFESSIONAL TIP

Urine Specimen in Non-Toilet-Trained Child

- If collecting urine and blood specimens, place a urine bag on prior to drawing blood. Most stressful procedures will precipitate urination.
- Stroking the abdomen with an alcohol prep and fanning it dry will frequently cause urination (Ellis, 1989).
- Urine for most tests except culture and sensitivity may be obtained from the diaper. Using gloves, remove the diaper, tear out the wettest portion of the diaper, place in a syringe with plunger removed, insert plunger, and squeeze the urine out of the diaper.
- Prior to placing a paper diaper on an infant or incontinent child, cut a vertical slit in the front of the diaper. Place a urine bag, and then the diaper on the child, then gently pull the urine bag through the slit. This allows visualization of urination (Ashwill & Droske, 1997).

proved for infants because of lack of testing and is not placed on skin that is broken. The cream is applied to the site liberally with an occlusive dressing and left in place 60 minutes prior to the procedure. The duration of the anesthesia is at least 2 and not more than 5 hours. Permission to use EMLA varies by institution; some may require a physician's order, and others allow the nurse to use it without an order. Children still may fear the needle stick; however, when the stick is not painful they are more content. Venipunctures that are the same as those in adults are not covered in this section.

Jugular Venipuncture Jugular and femoral venipunctures are performed by a physician, with the nurse assisting and monitoring the child. The blood specimen is obtained from the large superficial external jugular vein. The nurse assists the physician by doing the following:

1. Place child in mummy restraint (possibly just hold child's arms).
2. Position child with head and shoulders extended over the edge of a table or small pillow with neck area hyperextended (Figure 52-11).
3. Take care that circulation and breathing during the procedure are not impaired.
4. Make sure that the nose and mouth are not covered by the restrainer's hand.
5. Document in the chart the amount of blood drawn, the site, condition of the site, and the type of dressing applied.

Femoral Venipuncture The nurse assists the physician by doing the following:

1. Place child in modified mummy restraint with legs exposed.
2. Position child's legs in a froglike position to provide extensive exposure of the groin area (Figure 52-12).
3. Restrain legs in frog position with hands while controlling the child's arm and body movements with downward and inward pressure of forearms.

4. Cover genitalia to avoid contamination if the child urinates.
5. Document in chart amount of blood drawn, site, condition of the site, and type of dressing applied.

Lumbar Puncture Lumbar puncture (spinal tap) requires the infant or child to be held perfectly still. It is desirable to have an experienced staff member hold the child for the procedure. Lumbar puncture is performed as follows:

1. Place infant in sitting or side-lying position (neonates) with modified head extension to decrease respiratory distress during procedure.
2. Immobilize arms and legs with nurse's hands.
3. Observe child for difficulty in breathing.
4. Place child on side with back close to or extended over the edge of examining table, head flexed, and knees drawn up toward the chest.
5. Reach over the top of the child and place one arm behind child's neck and the other behind the knees (Figure 52-13).

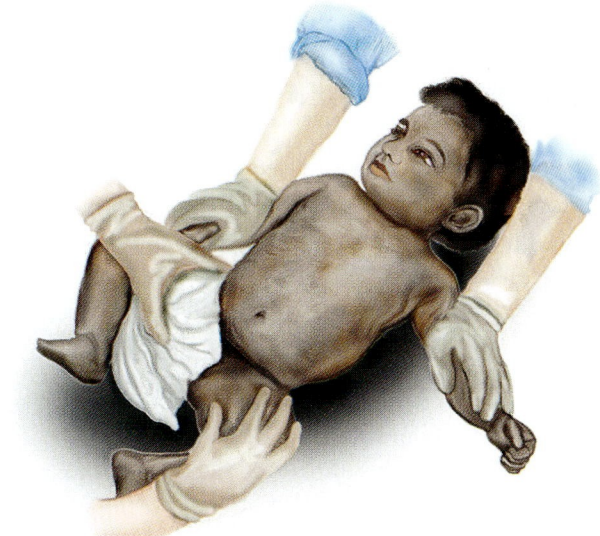

Figure 52-12 Positioning for Femoral Venipuncture

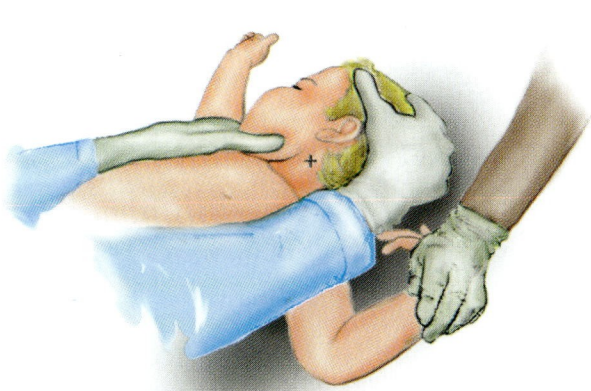

Figure 52-11 Positioning for Jugular Venipuncture

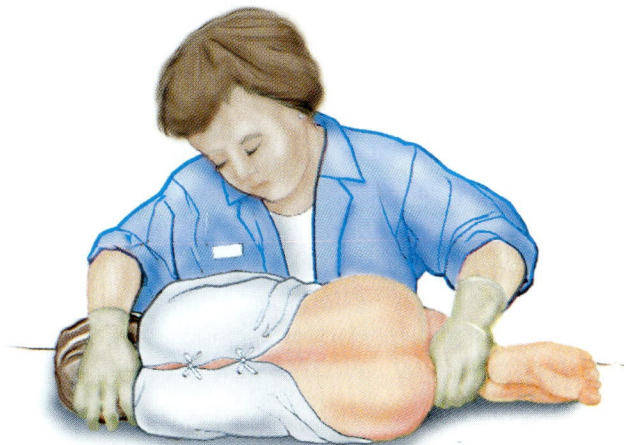

Figure 52-13 Positioning for Lumbar Puncture

6. Stabilize this position by clasping own hands in front of the child's abdomen.

7. Observe carefully for compromise in circulatory or respiratory systems. The restrainer's body should not cover the nose and mouth of the child.

8. Document number of attempts to obtain spinal fluid, number of cc's to lab, lab tests requested, color and consistency of spinal fluid, and response of child to procedure.

Intake and Output

Most children in acute care agencies will be on intake and output. Intake and output is critical for children with the following conditions:

- Anyone receiving IV fluids or TPN
- Major surgery
- Prematurity
- Renal disease or dysfunction
- Congestive heart failure
- Heart disease or anomalies
- Endocrine disorders
- Gastrointestinal disorders
- Shock
- Burns
- Medications such as digoxin, lasix, or corticosteriods
- Neurological conditions

To measure output for infants, the nurse should:

1. Weigh the diaper prior to placing it on the infant and then again when wet. For each mg the diaper weighs, record 1 cc of urine. Caution: For those diapers that protect against wetness, the accuracy may be distorted because of the absorbent material embedded in the diaper.

2. A urine bag with adhesive may be placed on the child and the urine collected measured in this way. This is not usually done because of the irritation of the adhesive over time.

For toddlers and older children, the nurse should measure urine and stool output in a bedpan or other container. All intake is measured and recorded on the intake and output sheet. If parents are present, they need to be instructed to measure and record fluids taken in and those eliminated. All fluids from IVs and other sources must be recorded. Drainage from stomas, colostomies, fistulas, and emesis should be measured and recorded.

Administration of Medications

Administration of medications to infants and children presents a number of adaptations. The medication dosage is determined by the physician; however, the nurse must observe the five rights of medication administration. All procedures or treatments to the child and parents are explained based on the child's

LIFE CYCLE CONSIDERATIONS

Medication Administration in Children

Suggestions to facilitate successful medication administration in infants and children:

- Be honest with the child.
- Allow the child choices when possible.
- Provide distraction when appropriate.
- Praise the child for doing his/her best.
- Expect success; use a positive approach.
- Allow the child opportunity to express feelings.
- Involve the child in order to gain cooperation.
- Provide a developmentally appropriate explanation.
- Do not use basic foods such as milk to disguise medication.
- Spend some time with the child after administering the medication.

developmental stage and the level of understanding of both parties. All questions posed by the parents and child must be answered prior to giving the medication.

Approaches to Pediatric Clients

Children's reactions to medication administration are affected by developmental characteristics such as physical skills and cognitive understanding, environmental influences, past experiences, cultural influences, parental responses, current relationship with the nurse, and perception of the present situation.

Calculating Dosages for Children

Standardized doses of medication for children do not exist. The most common method of determining medication amounts is based on the child's weight. This is a more reliable method of determining the medication amount because it allows for a more precise dose based on weight (see example in Professional Tip box). Medication doses also may be calculated by body surface area (BSA mg/m^2). The formula to calculate dosage using surface area is:

$$\text{Approximate dose} = \frac{\text{BSA of child (m}^2\text{)}}{1.7} \times \text{Adult dose}$$

PROFESSIONAL TIP

Dosage Calculations for Children

The recommended dose of Ampicillin is 50–100 mg/kg/day in equally divided doses every 6 hours. For a child weighing 5 kilograms, the dose would be 250–500 mg divided by 4, or 63–125 mg q6h.

Oral Medications

The oral route of medication is the preferred method of administering medication to a child. Oral medications may come in liquids, pills, tablets, and caplets. Pediatric medications are frequently in a liquid suspension that tastes "good" and is colorful. Many medications will have an unpleasant after-taste. Nurses become aware of medications that are bitter or unpleasant, and there are methods to decrease the unpleasant taste such as numbing the tongue prior to administration by giving a flavored ice popsicle or small ice cube. The method for administering oral medication to a child is as follows:

1. Select appropriate vehicle; for example, calibrated cup, syringe, dropper, measuring spoon, nipple.
2. Prepare medication.
3. Measure into appropriate vehicle.
4. Avoid mixing medications with essential food items such as milk, formula, etc. (The child may later refuse the essential food item because of the association with medication.)
5. Administer the medication, employing safety precautions in identification and administration.

Specific instructions for administering oral medications to infants are as follows:

1. Hold infant in semi-reclining position.
2. Place syringe, measuring spoon, or dropper with medication in mouth well back on the tongue or to the side of the tongue.
3. Administer slowly and wait for the child to swallow to reduce likelihood of choking or aspiration.
4. Allow infant to suck medication placed in nipple.

Specific instructions for administering oral medications to the older infant or toddler are as follows:

1. Explain in developmentally appropriate terms what you are going to do.
2. Allow the child to sit on your lap or the parent's lap in a sitting or modified supine position.
3. Use mild or partial restraint.
4. Administer the medication slowly with a syringe or small medicine cup.
5. Never force actively resistive children because of the danger of aspiration; postpone 20 to 30 minutes and offer medication again.

Specific instructions for administering oral medications to a preschool child are as follows:

1. Use a straightforward approach.
2. For a reluctant child, use the following:
   • Simple persuasion (e.g., "When you take your medicine, we can go to the playroom.").
   • Reinforcement, such as stickers or other rewards for compliance.

PROFESSIONAL TIP

Resistant Child

If the nurse holds the small child on his/her lap with the child's right arm behind the nurse, and the left hand firmly grasped by the nurse's hand, the medication can be slowly poured into the mouth of a resisting child (Figure 52-14).

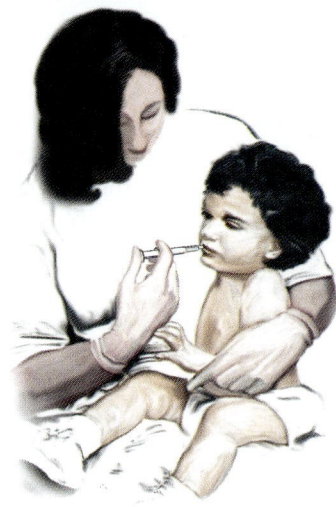

Figure 52-14 Administering Oral Medication to a Child

Intramuscular Injections

Intramuscular injections are used widely for pediatric clients. Medications given by the intramuscular route include immunizations, antibiotics, and other drugs. Children have reported that injections are one of the most stressful and painful experiences of health care (Eland & Anderson, 1977; Gedaly-Duff & Burns, 1992). The task for nurses is to support the child while administering the medication quickly, in a safe manner, and with the least amount of pain and stress to the child.

Otic Medications

Otic medication is used frequently in children who have ear infections. Because of pain associated with cold coming in contact with the tympanic membrane, all otic medications should be warmed to room temperature prior to administering. The child should receive an age-appropriate explanation regarding what will be felt and heard (e.g., "It may feel like a moth in your ear.") and what can be done to help. Assistance in restraining a young child may be needed.

The nurse should position the child on the side with the affected ear up, and clean any discharge with a clean gauze pad. The nurse will brace the administering hand above the ear on the head. To instill the solution for an infant, the pinna of the ear should be pulled back and down; for an older child, the pinna is pulled back and up. After instillation, the tragus of the ear is massaged to ensure the drops reach the tympanic membrane. Cotton may be loosely packed into the ear canal, if ordered.

Intravenous Medications

Children in acute care settings frequently receive intravenous (IV) medications. Children who have poor absorption as a result of dehydration, malabsorption syndromes, shock, and those in need of a high concentration of the drug quickly would receive IV fluids and medication. Children needing continuous pain relief benefit from IV medication administration. Advantages of IV medications are the immediate effect and the ability to control blood levels of the drugs used. Disadvantages are the same: side effects occur very quickly, and the drug may be very corrosive to the veins. Once the drug is administered into the bloodstream, further control is limited.

All drugs given by IV route require a specified minimum dilution and specific rate of flow. It is difficult to control the IV flow rate in children by gravity. Children are at risk for fluid overload when IV rates are not controlled. It is for this reason that all children receiving IV fluids or medications should receive those fluids through a volumetric infusion pump. IV medication may be delivered as a continuous infusion or intermittently. Syringe pumps are used in many agencies to deliver small amounts of medication.

Nursing care of the client receiving IV fluids and/or medication includes site assessment every hour for signs and symptoms of infiltration. Site assessment must include color of the site, tension of the skin, and skin temperature. When administering IV fluids and medications to the pediatric client, the nurse needs to know:

- Type of fluid
- Compatibility of medication and IV solutions
- Recommended dilution of the drug
- Recommended time frame for administration
- Amount of flush needed
- Any precautions to observe prior to administration; e.g., for aminophylline (Aminophyllin), take apical pulse prior to administering
- Side effects of the drug

THE DYING CHILD

Care of the dying child presents one of the greatest challenges to nurses. It involves sensitive, gentle physical care and comfort measures for the child as well as continuing emotional support for the family and caregivers.

Child

Children's understanding of death parallels their cognitive and psychosocial development. Preverbal infants and toddlers have no clear concept of death. Children between the ages of 3 and 5 may view death as a kind of sleep that is interchangeable with life. Due to their concrete thinking, school-age children begin developing the concept of death as final. Adolescents have a maturing understanding of death. In addition to their developmental level, children are greatly influenced by their life experiences and the attitudes of those around them.

Children can sense when they are seriously ill. They may realize they are dying because of the effects of disease and treatments on their body. The child usually experiences fear of death, of dying alone, and of pain. Nursing interventions include promoting socialization with family and peers, providing avenues for self-expression (i.e., drawings, fantasy play, storytelling), dealing directly with the child's questions, and allowing the death to occur in peace and with dignity.

Parents

When death is expected, the family begins a mourning process called anticipatory grieving. Manifestations of this process include denial, anger, and depression. It is important for the nurse to acknowledge the parents' feelings, encourage expression, and guide them through the gradual process to reorganization. Spouses may need additional support when they are at different levels of grieving to prevent a sense of loneliness and isolation.

It is important for nurses to explore options with the family concerning the child's care. The child and family have a right to request termination of treatment and to determine the care setting.

Parents who are caring for their dying child usually fear what the death will be like, not being present at the death, and pain the child will experience. The family needs to be encouraged to talk to the child about dying. Families need help to focus on the time that remains with the child. Openness and honesty will allow the health care providers and the family to provide effective care, to avoid misunderstandings, to see that the child and the family resolve problems, and to share their love.

Siblings

Like their parents, siblings may experience anticipatory grief in the form of anger, denial, or fear. They may resent the attention given the dying child. Siblings may fear that they caused their brother or sister to become ill or that the same thing will happen to them. They may need help in adapting to their parents' distraction, grief, and increased protectiveness.

The nurse can encourage parents to include siblings

in the care of the dying child, in discussions about dying, and in the funeral. Like the dying child and the grieving parents, siblings need acknowledgment of their feelings and opportunities for expression.

Nurse

Caring for the dying is usually a team effort, but often the nurse is the coordinator of the care. Working effectively with dying children and their families requires confidence, empathy, and competence in addition to attention to managing personal stress. Nurses who are comfortable with their own mortality can help make the remainder of the child's life more meaningful and the family's mourning experience more healing.

Nurses experience reactions to caring for dying children including denial, anger, depression, guilt, and ambivalent feelings. Nurses may even cry in the presence of the child and the family. A grieving father wrote of a nurse caring for his son who had just died, "We were grateful for her kindness and her tears" (Brown, 1992). Learning to care for the dying involves talking with other professionals, sharing concerns, comforting each other in stressful times, maintaining good general health, using distancing techniques, and focusing on the positive aspects of the caregiver role.

Sources of Support

Hospice care may be an option for the dying child. Hospice services provide palliative care for the dying to live life to the fullest without pain, with choices of dignity, and with family support including follow-up care postdeath. Self-help groups such as Compassionate Friends, an international organization for bereaved parents and siblings, are available in many communities.

CASE STUDY

Tillie, a 5-year-old with an inoperable abdominal tumor, lives with her parents and a 7-year-old sister, Tammie. The decision has been made to discontinue chemotherapy. Tillie has been involved in decisions about her care throughout her illness. When asked about her condition, she states, "I'm very sick and I'm not getting better." Tillie spends much of her time curled in a fetal position with her favorite toy, a tattered rag doll named Dolly. Tillie refuses physical exams and pills and gets little sleep due to her pain.

The following questions will guide your development of a nursing care plan for the case study.

1. List subjective and objective data a nurse would want to know about Tillie and her family.
2. List three nursing diagnoses and goals for Tillie.
3. What would you expect a 5-year-old to understand about death?
4. What nursing interventions will be required for Tillie and her family?
5. List three successful outcomes for Tillie and her family.

SUMMARY

- Even though hospitalization places great stress on children and their families, it can be a positive growth experience for the child.
- Teaching children and their families what to expect and explaining what is going to happen before, during, and after procedures helps reduce anxiety.
- Children's developmental stage and cognitive ability influence the preparation for treatments and procedures.
- Children must be protected from hazards that can cause harm to them.
- The child's stage of development, cognitive ability, and life experiences contribute to the child's understanding of death.

Review Questions

1. The major stressor of hospitalization for infants and young children is:
   a. pain.
   b. bodily injury.
   c. loss of control.
   d. separation anxiety.

2. Because of their stage of development, preschoolers may view hospitalization as:
   a. abuse.
   b. rejection.
   c. punishment.
   d. abandonment.

3. Prior to drawing blood on a 9-year-old, the nurse tells the child:

   a. a Band-Aid will not be necessary.
   b. the procedure will not be painful.
   c. not to worry about the tight tourniquet.
   d. the body will produce more blood to replace what is being taken.

4. An appropriate method for administering oral medication to a small child is to mix it with:

   a. milk.
   b. food from the child's plate.
   c. a large amount of water.
   d. sweet-tasting food or syrup.

Critical Thinking Questions

1. Prepare a preoperative plan for a 3-year-old Hispanic male undergoing surgery for an inguinal hernia. Include developmental, cultural, and physiological considerations for the child and his family.

2. A child has received multiple IM injections and has a real fear of the "needle." Parents threaten the child that if he does not follow what they say, the nurse will come and give him a "needle." How would you approach the parents? What interventions would assist the child to lessen his fear and regain control?

WEB FLASH!

- Search the Web for support groups for children with specific health conditions such as asthma or cancer. What do you find? Are resources available for families, parents, and siblings?
- Can you locate a hospice network on the Internet devoted to children? Is there a local chapter in your town?

INFANTS WITH SPECIAL NEEDS: BIRTH TO 12 MONTHS

MAKING THE CONNECTION

Refer to the following chapters to increase your understanding of infants with special needs:

- **Chapter 12, Cultural Diversity and Nursing**
- **Chapter 14, The Life Cycle**
- **Chapter 17, Loss, Grief, and Death**
- **Chapter 23, Fluid, Electrolyte, and Acid–Base Balance**
- **Chapter 25, Assessment**
- **Chapter 26, Pain Management**
- **Chapter 28, Anesthesia**
- **Chapter 29, Nursing Care of the Surgical Client**
- **Chapter 31, Nursing Care of the Client: Respiratory System**
- **Chapter 32, Nursing Care of the Client: Cardiovascular System**
- **Chapter 33, Nursing Care of the Client: Blood and Lymph Systems**
- **Chapter 34, Nursing Care of the Client: Gastrointestinal System**
- **Chapter 38, Nursing Care of the Client: Musculoskeletal System**
- **Chapter 39, Nursing Care of the Client: Immune System**
- **Chapter 40, Nursing Care of the Client: Integumentary System**
- **Chapter 41, Nursing Care of the Client: Nervous System**
- **Chapter 42, Nursing Care of the Client: Urinary System**
- **Chapter 43, Nursing Care of the Client: Sensory System**
- **Chapter 52, Basics of Pediatric Care**

LEARNING OBJECTIVES

Upon completion of this chapter, you should be able to:
- *Define key terms.*
- *Differentiate the most common respiratory conditions affecting infants.*
- *Describe nursing care for infants with circulatory conditions.*
- *Discuss nursing considerations for infants with digestive conditions.*
- *Explain the evaluative techniques used for infants suspected of having musculoskeletal alterations.*
- *Differentiate among the skin disorders most commonly seen in infants.*
- *Explain the causes and effects of nervous system disorders seen in infants.*

KEY TERMS

abduction
antipyretic
atresia
child abuse
circumoral cyanosis
colic
dislocation
dysplasia
erythematous
hypotonia
intussusception
jaundice
kernicterus
lecithin
meconium ileus
meningitis
milia
mongolian spots
myelomeningocele
myringotomy
projectile vomiting
pruritus
stridor

- *Describe nursing care for infants with genitourinary conditions.*
- *Outline teaching strategies for parents of infants with visual and hearing impairments and cognitive disorders.*
- *Implement nursing interventions for infants who have been abused.*
- *Describe teaching guidelines for families of infants who have unsafe environments.*

INTRODUCTION

The immaturity of all body systems leaves infants vulnerable to numerous illnesses and disorders. Most health problems during infancy are due to respiratory and gastrointestinal infections or congenital anomalies. Although infants can become ill rapidly, they usually recover quickly. This chapter describes common conditions and illnesses affecting all systems of the infant; typical medical and surgical management; and nursing care of infants.

RESPIRATORY SYSTEM

In the normal infant, breathing is quiet and shallow with variations in rate and rhythm. Respiratory movement is primarily abdominal. Respirations should be counted for 1 full minute while watching the rise and fall of the abdomen. The normal rate ranges from 30 to 50 breaths per minute. A persistent rate above 60 breaths per minute is an important sign of respiratory distress.

The child's respiratory tract is constantly changing and growing during the first 12 years of life. Differences between the respiratory tract of the adult and the infant contribute to the greater potential for obstruction, aspiration, infection, and airway resistance in the child (Table 53-1). In the infant, the most common respiratory disorders include otitis media, laryngotracheobronchitis, pneumonia, respiratory distress syndrome, cystic fibrosis, and sudden infant death syndrome.

OTITIS MEDIA

Otitis media is an inflammation of the middle ear. The eustachian tubes, which allow for drainage from the middle ear to the nasopharynx, are shorter, wider, and more horizontal in infants than in adults (Figure 53-1). As a result, drainage is frequently impaired, resulting in retention of secretions and air in the middle ear. This positioning also facilitates the movement of bacteria up the eustachian tube from the pharynx into the middle ear. An upper respiratory infection often

Table 53-1 RESPIRATORY TRACT DIFFERENCES BETWEEN INFANTS AND ADULTS

DIFFERENCES IN CHILDREN	SIGNIFICANCE
Small nares, oral cavity, and nasopharynx; large tongue	Increases risk for obstruction
Obligatory nose breathers (< 6 months) due to immature neurological function	Increases risk for obstruction
Rapid growth of lymph tissue	Increases risk for obstruction with infection
Larynx and glottis high in neck	Increases risk for aspiration
Large amount of soft tissues and loose, poorly anchored mucous membranes; long floppy epiglottis	Increases risk for obstruction with infection
Fewer functional airway muscles	Increases risk for aspiration
Immature cartilages that may collapse when neck is flexed	Increases risk for obstruction
Short neck resulting in structures being closer together	Increases risk for infection
Short, narrow airway	Increases risk for obstruction and aspiration; increases airway resistance/respiratory effort
Bifurcation of trachea at the third thoracic space	Increases risk for infection and aspiration
Immature intercostal muscles and cartilaginous ribs; primarily diaphragmatic breathers	Increases respiratory effort
Eustachian tube shorter, wider, and straighter	Increases risk for infection

precedes the development of otitis media in infants. *Haemophilus influenzae* is a common causative agent of otitis media in infants.

Infants with otitis media may be irritable, pull at the infected ear, or have diarrhea, vomiting, fever, and hearing loss. Upon inspection, the ear drum will be red, bulging, and nonmobile. Prolonged otitis media may result in sensorineural and/or conductive hearing loss, which is further discussed in the hearing impairment section of this chapter.

Medical–Surgical Management

Medical

Medical treatment focuses on elimination of the infection and follow-up evaluation to determine the extent of hearing loss, if any.

Surgical

If infections recur, **myringotomy** (surgical incision of the eardrum) may be performed and tympanoplasty tubes inserted to drain the fluid from the middle ear.

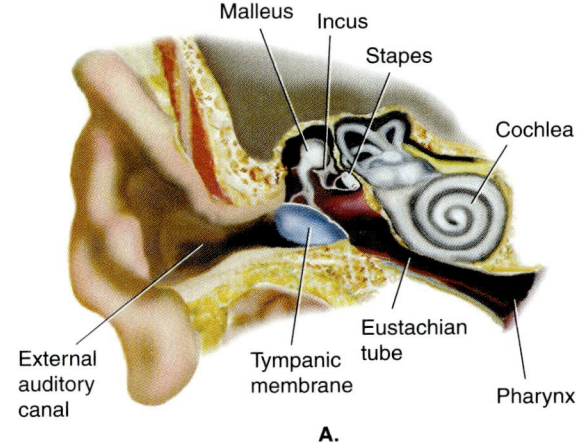

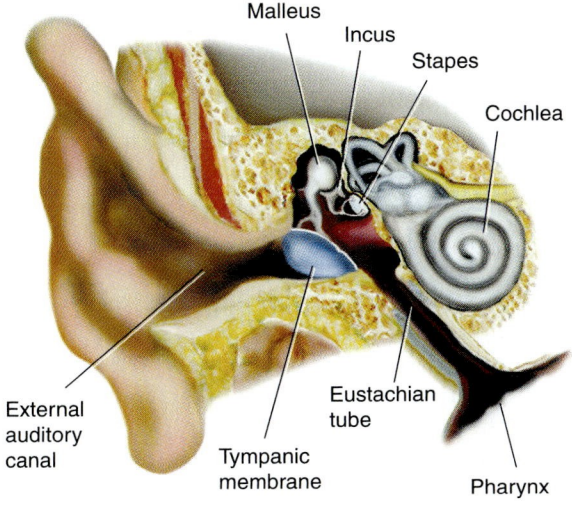

Figure 53-1 Eustachian Tubes: A. Infant; B. Adult

Pharmacological

Treatment usually includes antibiotics, **antipyretics** (drug used to reduce an abnormally high temperature), and analgesics. Considerations when deciding which antibiotic to administer include compliance of parents in giving the medication, the child's willingness to take oral medications, and the pain involved with injections. Studies have indicated that a single intramuscular dose of ceftriaxone (Rocephin) eliminates symptoms as effectively as does 10 days administration of oral amoxicillin (Green & Rothrock, 1993) or trimethoprim-sulfamethoxazole (Bactrim, Septra) (Barnett et al., 1997).

Nursing Management

The primary nursing concerns are relieving fever and pain and teaching the parents about signs and symptoms, management, and prevention of otitis media. Acetaminophen (Tylenol) or ibuprofen (Motrin) may be used to reduce fever. In addition to analgesic ad-

PROFESSIONAL TIP

Rocephin

Strategies to minimize the pain associated with the injection of ceftriaxone (Rocephin) include the use of lidocaine 1% as the diluent and the application of EMLA cream on the site prior to injection.

ministration, pain may be minimized by applying a heating pad on the low setting or an ice pack compress to the affected ear. Lying on the affected side will facilitate drainage, if the eardrum has ruptured or myringotomy has been performed. Providing liquids and soft foods may minimize pain due to chewing.

Parents must be taught to have the infant examined at the first sign of a possible ear infection. Early possible signs of infection include hearing difficulties, pulling or rubbing of the ears, and irritability.

If antibiotics are prescribed, it is imperative that the child be given all of the medication. Failure to adhere to prescribed treatment may lead to the need for additional antibiotics; hearing loss; and potential speech and language problems.

Prevention of otitis media involves ensuring proper positioning during feeding. Infants who are bottle-fed should be held with the head slightly elevated to prevent formula from draining into the middle ear through the wide eustachian tube. Studies have suggested that breastfed infants have fewer episodes of otitis media than do bottle-fed infants because of the semivertical positioning and the protection provided by immunoglobulin A contained in the breast milk (Duncan et al., 1993; Tully, Bar-Haim, & Bradley, 1995).

Providing a smoke-free environment is another important element of prevention. Parents must be aware of the relationship between environmental tobacco smoke and otitis media in young children. Passive smoking has been associated with an increase in blocked eustachian tubes, which can lead to nasopharyngeal congestion and upper respiratory infections (Kitchens, 1995).

LARYNGOTRACHEOBRONCHITIS

Laryngotracheobronchitis (LTB), the most common type of croup, is a viral illness that causes swelling (narrowing) of the upper airway (Figure 53-2).

Initial symptoms include inspiratory **stridor** (a high-pitched, harsh sound), a "barking" cough, and hoarseness. The child may have a persistent, low-grade fever and a history of profuse nasal drainage with increased respiratory effort for several days.

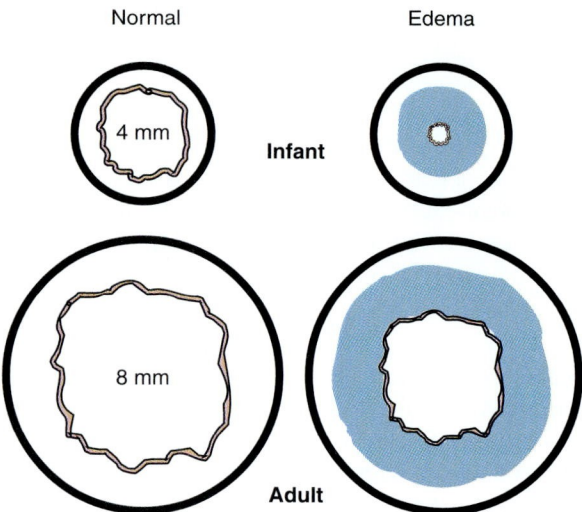

Figure 53-2 Effect of Edema on Airway Resistance in the Infant versus the Adult: Whereas 1 mm of circumferential edema (on right) can cause a 75% decrease in the cross-sectional area of an infant's airway, it causes only a 44% decrease in the adult's.

Medical–Surgical Management

Medical

Treatment is focused on maintaining a patent airway and improving respiratory effort by creating a highly humid, cool-mist environment.

Pharmacological

Use of medications such as bronchodialators, corticosteroids, and sedatives is controversial because of potential side effects. In severe cases caused by respiratory syncytial virus (RSV), ribavirin (Virazole), an aerosoled antiviral agent, may be used.

Nursing Management

Children with mild croup (no stridor at rest, mild retractions, no cyanosis, and restlessness only when disturbed) are managed at home. Parents are taught to monitor for signs of respiratory distress and ways to maintain high humidity and hydration.

Care for the hospitalized infant includes a mist hood or tent with oxygen and, if the child is refusing oral fluids or respirations are greater than 60 breaths per

PROFESSIONAL TIP

Throat Procedures

Procedures involving the throat (i.e., cultures and visual inspection) can cause laryngospasm and airway obstruction and should therefore be avoided when children present with symptoms such as inspiratory stridor, a barking cough, or hoarseness.

HOME HEALTH CARE

Managing LTB at Home

- Observe for early signs of respiratory distress, such as stridor at rest; lower rib retractions; difficulty swallowing; absence of cough; agitation; respiration > 50; flaring nares
- Maintain high humidity with cool-air vaporizer, 10 to 15 minutes in the bathroom with steam from a hot shower, cool air through a window
- Hydrate with cool, noncarbonated, nonacidic beverages of choice; ice pops; jello; small pieces of ice
- Provide rest by holding, rocking, soothing, and staying calm

minute, intravenous (IV) therapy. Infants may be held with the mist blowing in the face, if being in the tent causes distress. Parents should remain with the child and provide routine care throughout hospitalization in an effort to keep the infant calm, quiet, and in the tent. The presence of favorite toys and items from home can be also be comforting to the infant. It is important to keep linens and clothes dry and the child in a comfortable position (usually semireclined in an infant seat placed under the tent). If oxygen is administered, the concentration delivered is regulated to maintain arterial saturation above 95% (according to pulse oximetry).

As with home care, monitoring for early signs of impending airway obstruction is paramount. Intubation equipment should be readily available at all times.

PNEUMONIA

An inflammation of the bronchioles and alveolar spaces of the lungs, pneumonia is most commonly caused by RSV in infants. Pneumonia is often preceded by an upper respiratory infection. Viral infections render the infant more susceptible to secondary bacterial invasion. Pneumococcal pneumonia is the most common form of bacterial pneumonia found in infants.

Onset is usually abrupt, with rapidly increasing fever, flaring nostrils, **circumoral cyanosis** (bluish discoloration surrounding the mouth), chest retractions, pulse rate of 140 to 180 beats per minute, respiratory rate of 60 to 80 breaths per minute, and nonproductive cough. Chest x-rays and secretion cultures are used to confirm the diagnosis.

Medical–Surgical Management

Medical

Treatment involves oxygen and cool mist administration, chest physiotherapy, postural drainage, hydration, family support, antipyretics, antitussives, and antibiotics (if causative agent is bacterial).

Nursing Management

Nursing care focuses on monitoring respiratory status, hydrating, preventing further infection, and promoting safety. Monitoring for dehydration is accomplished by accurate intake and output (I & O) measurement and assessment of skin turgor and anterior fontanel. A bulb syringe should be used to suction the nose and nasopharynx as needed and prior to feeding. Saline nose drops may aid in clearing passages. The infant's position should be changed frequently to prevent both stasis of secretions in the lungs and secretion drainage into the eustachian tubes. Parents must be encouraged to be active participants in their infant's routine daily care.

RESPIRATORY DISTRESS SYNDROME

Preterm infants often have respiratory distress syndrome (RDS) because the lungs are deficient in surfactant, a soapy substance that reduces surface tension inside the air sacs. The lungs collapse after each breath, greatly reducing the infant's supply of oxygen. This, in turn, damages the lung cells, contributing to the formation of hyaline membrane. This membrane blocks gas exchange in the alveoli.

Clinical manifestations include tachypnea (70 to 120 breaths per minute in children), retractions, grunting, crackles, pallor, cyanosis, slow capillary refill, hypothermia, peripheral edema, flaccid muscle tone, gastrointestinal (GI) shutdown, jaundice, and acidosis. Chest radiographs confirm the diagnosis.

The first 96 hours are critical to the recovery of infants with RDS. Complications of RDS include complications of oxygen administration; intraventricular hemorrhage; bronchopulmonary dysplasia (BPD); and necrotizing enterocolitis.

Medical–Surgical Management

Medical

Treatment includes administration of surfactant through the endotracheal tube immediately at or soon after birth. In addition, continuous positive airway pressure (CPAP) helps keep the lungs partially expanded until they begin producing surfactant (approximately 5 days).

Health Promotion

Attempts may be made to prevent the occurrence of RDS. Surfactant may be administered to at-risk infants prior to the development of RDS. If preterm delivery is expected, **lecithin**, the major component of surfac-

tant, may be measured to determine lung maturity. If insufficient lecithin is present, the mother may be given a glucocorticosteroid that crosses the placenta and causes the infant's lungs to produce surfactant within 72 hours.

Nursing Management

Nursing care includes close monitoring, eliminating unnecessary physical stimulation and metabolic demands, and establishing a positive relationship with the parents. The infant will be placed in a warmer and be under an oxygen hood or mechanically ventilated.

CYSTIC FIBROSIS

Cystic fibrosis (CF), a major dysfunction of all exocrine glands, primarily affects the lungs, the pancreas, the liver, and the reproductive organs. Characteristics of this disease include increased viscosity of mucous gland secretions, elevated sweat electrolytes, increased organic and enzymatic constituents of saliva, and abnormalities in autonomic nervous system function. This disease is transmitted as an autosomal recessive trait, meaning that both parents must be carriers (Table 53-2). Therefore, it is common that infants with CF also have siblings with CF.

Most children show evidence of the disease by 1 year of age. The earliest manifestation of CF is **meconium ileus** (impacted feces in the newborn, causing bowel obstruction). **Intussusception** (telescoping of the bowel) may be another sign of the disorder. Rectal prolapse is a common problem resulting from difficulty passing the sticky, thick stools. These GI problems result from the lack of pancreatic enzymes. Most children have difficulty maintaining and gaining weight, despite a voracious appetite. Pulmonary complications, such as chronic moist, productive cough and frequent infections, are present in most children with CF. Many children develop barrel chests and clubbed fingers due to the chronic lack of oxygen. With few exceptions, males are sterile (White, Munro, & Pickler, 1995).

Parents frequently report that their infants taste like salt when they kiss them. This common manifestation

Table 53-2 **AUTOSOMAL RECESSIVE INHERITANCE**			
		Mother (Carrier: Has Trait)	
	Gametes	A	a
Father (Carrier: Has Trait)	A	**AA** (no disease/trait)	**Aa** (has trait)
	a	**Aa** (has trait)	**aa** (has disease)

is due to the elevated sweat electrolytes. Diagnosis is confirmed with the sweat chloride test.

Although CF is a life-threatening illness, families must be encouraged to focus on positive outcomes. The life expectancy continues to rise, and the search for improved treatments continues (Fiel, 1995; Knowles, Olivier, Hohneker, Robinson, Bennett, & Boucher, 1995; Shak, 1995).

Medical–Surgical Management

Medical

Treatment focuses on managing pulmonary complications, ensuring adequate nutrition, and assisting the child and family in adapting to a chronic disorder. Chest physiotherapy (CPT, postural drainage) is usually performed 1 to 3 times per day to maintain patent airways.

Pharmacological

Aerosol treatments, and antibiotic therapy may be used as indicated. Commercially prepared pancreatic enzymes are given with meals and snacks to aid digestion and absorption of fats and proteins.

CPX (a chemical derivative of existing lead compounds) is a new protein repair therapy that may interact directly with the cystic fibrosis transmembrane regulator (CFTR) protein, the product of the CF gene. It appears to repair the faulty protein, thereby curing the basic CF defect. Clinical studies of this new drug began in August of 1998. Researchers are evaluating the safety and pharmacodynamics of oral doses of CPX in as many as 50 adults with CF at multiple sites (Cystic Fibrosis Foundation, 1998).

Diet

Well-balanced, high-caloric diets should be maintained because children with CF often absorb only 50% of ingested foods.

▶ NURSING PROCESS

▶ Assessment

▶ Subjective Data

The nurse should assess the child and parents for indications of anxiety and fear. The family can be interviewed about activities or events leading up to the crisis, effects of illness on day-to-day functioning, previous hospitalizations, and knowledge about the condition.

▶ Objective Data

Physical assessment focuses on respiratory status, growth and development, hydration, and nutrition. The nurse observes for adventitious lung sounds, cough, finger clubbing, barrel chest, frequency and nature of stools, abdominal distention, weight loss, fatigue, and pallor. In addition, height and weight should be routinely plotted on a growth chart, and developmental level should be assessed using the Denver II.

Nursing diagnoses for the infant with CF may include the following:

Nursing Diagnosis	Planning/Goals	Nursing Interventions
▶ *Airway Clearance, Ineffective, related to thick, tenacious secretions*	The client will maintain a clear airway.	Initiate aerosol therapy, CPT, and breathing exercises as prescribed; schedule at least 1 hour before or after meals. Administer oxygen as prescribed and monitor closely for level of consciousness. Calculate and maintain required fluid intake. Observe for signs of infection. Assess respiratory status frequently. Administer antibiotics as prescribed.
▶ *Growth and Development, Altered, related to inability to digest nutrients and possible loss of appetite*	The client will exhibit signs of adequate growth and development.	Ensure high-caloric intake. Administer prescribed pancreatic enzymes with meals and snacks. Offer small, frequent feedings if appetite poor. Monitor weight and height (plot on growth chart). Assess developmental level (i.e., with the Denver II). Encourage physical activity limited only by the child's endurance.
▶ *Fear (family) related to long term care and prognosis*	The family will verbalize knowledge of disease and demonstrate proper techniques for care.	Teach the family the importance of carrying out prescribed therapeutic plan. Teach the family skills for carrying out prescribed therapeutic plan.

continued

Nursing Diagnosis	Planning/Goals	Nursing Interventions
	The family will verbalize lessened fears and anxiety.	Provide numbers for CF Foundation and community resources.
	The family will utilize available support systems and community resources.	Encourage expression of feelings and concerns.
		Refer the family for genetic counseling.

Evaluation Each goal must be evaluated to determine how it has been met by the client.

SUDDEN INFANT DEATH SYNDROME

Sudden infant death syndrome (SIDS), commonly called "crib death," is the sudden unexpected death of an apparently healthy infant in whom the postmortem fails to reveal an adequate cause. It is the leading cause of death in infants over 1 month of age, with 90% of deaths occurring by 6 months of age (The American SIDS Institute, 1999). Although numerous theories have been proposed regarding the cause of SIDS (including airway obstruction, abnormal cardiorespiratory control, and hyperactive airway reflexes), no single cause has been identified.

Typically, the child is found huddled in the corner of a disheveled bed, with blankets over the head. Frothy, blood-tinged fluid fills the mouth and nose, and the infant may be lying face down in the secretions. The diaper is wet and full of stool. The hands may be clenched.

Nursing Management

Nursing care involves empathic support of the family. Parents should be asked only factual questions, with no suggestion of responsibility. It is vital to reassure them that death caused by SIDS is not predictable or preventable. The family needs to know that an autopsy must be performed to confirm the diagnosis of SIDS. They should be encouraged to hold their child and say "good-bye." If the mother was breastfeeding, she needs information about abrupt discontinuation of lactation. Referrals should be made to the SIDS Foundation. The nurse should find someone to accompany the family to their home, if possible.

Ideally, the family will receive a visit from a competent, qualified professional as soon after the death as possible. Areas needing to be discussed include expression of feelings, coping mechanisms, siblings' reactions, and birth of a subsequent child.

CARDIOVASCULAR SYSTEM

Indications that the heart is functioning normally include warm skin, pink mucous membranes, easily palpated pulses, symmetrical chest, normal growth and development, and high activity tolerance. Upon auscultation of a healthy heart at the point of maximum intensity (PMI), two sounds (S1 ["lub"] and S2 ["dub"]) are heard. Heart sounds should be clear and distinct, regular and even. The rate should be the same as the radial pulse. In many children, a *sinus arrhythmia,* wherein the heart rate increases on inspiration and decreases on expiration, is considered normal.

During fetal life, the lungs are inactive and require only a small amount of blood to nourish their tissues. Blood is circulated through the umbilical arteries to the placenta, where waste products and carbon dioxide are exchanged for oxygen and nutrients. The blood is then returned to the fetus through the umbilical vein.

At birth, the umbilical cord is cut, and the infant's own independent system is established. The ductus arteriosus, the foramen ovale, and the ductus venosus are no longer needed. They normally close and atrophy during the first several weeks after birth. Figure 53-3 illustrates the circulatory patterns of the healthy prenatal and postnatal heart.

Congenital cardiac defects, called congenital heart disease, range from mild to severe. They may be detected immediately at birth or may not be detected for several months.

CONGENITAL HEART DISEASE

Congenital heart disease is among the leading causes of death during the first year of life (Anderson, Kochanek, & Murphy, 1997). Errors in formation of the heart or great vessels can occur prenatally, and persistence of fetal circulation can occur postnatally. Heart defects are best categorized according to blood flow patterns: (1) increased pulmonary blood flow, (2) decreased pulmonary blood flow, (3) obstructed blood

PROFESSIONAL TIP

SIDS

Health care providers may benefit from a debriefing session with the hospital chaplin or a counselor following an encounter with the family of a SIDS victim.

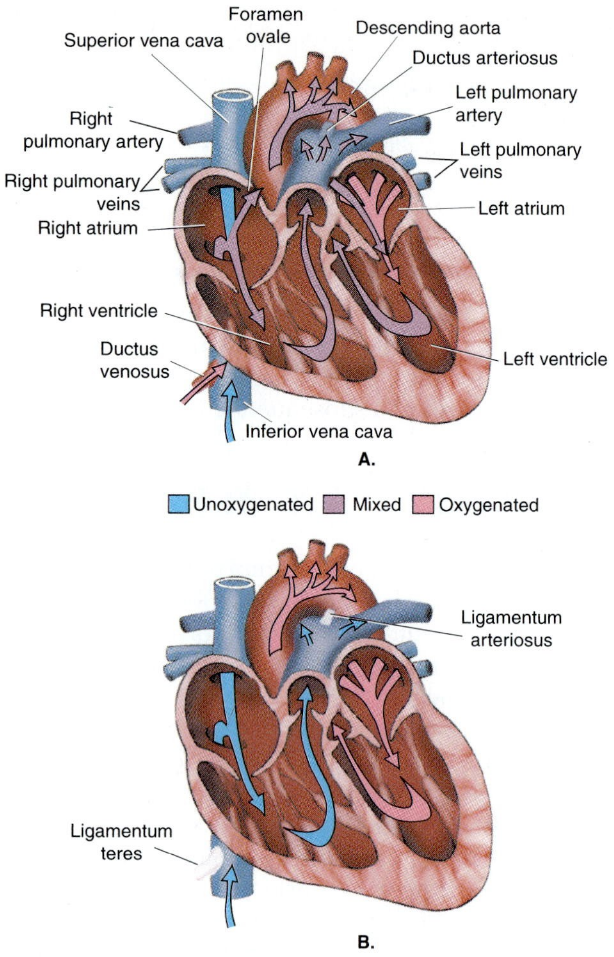

A.

☐ Unoxygenated ☐ Mixed ☐ Oxygenated

B.

Figure 53-3 Circulation of the Heart: A. Prenatal; B. Postnatal.

flow out of the heart, (4) mixed blood flow. Four of the most common heart defects in infants are listed in Table 53-3.

Rubella in the mother during the first trimester of pregnancy is a common cause of heart defects in infants. Other possible maternal causes include alcoholism, irradiation, ingestion of drugs, diabetes, malnutrition, and being over 40 years old (Hoffman, 1990). Heredity is also a contributing factor.

Infants with severe heart defects may be born with obvious distress due to hypoxia. Those with less serious defects may compensate and appear to be healthy at birth. Heart murmurs and delayed growth and development observed later may call attention to problems. Infants with severe defects will often manifest signs and symptoms of CHF, such as fatigability; orthopnea; failure to thrive; pale, mottled, or cyanotic skin; hoarse or weak cry; tachycardia; and signs of respiratory distress, such as rate over 60, costal retractions, orthopnea, wheezing and coughing.

Medical–Surgical Management

Surgical

Surgical intervention to repair a defect may be postponed until the child develops CHF. Generally, the older the infant, the better the surgical outcome. Refer to Table 53-3 for treatments of common heart defects.

Pharmacological

Digoxin (Lanoxin) is the drug most often used to improve the heart's contractility and increase its

Table 53-3 COMMON HEART DEFECTS IN INFANTS

	VENTRICULAR SEPTAL DEFECT (VSD)	**ATRIAL SEPTAL DEFECT (ASD)**	**PATENT DUCTUS ARTERIOSIS (PDA)**	**TETRALOGY OF FALLOT (TOF)**
Description	Opening between ventricles	Opening between atria; incompetent foramen ovale	Failure of fetal ductus arteriosus to close postnatally	Four defects: (VSD), pulmonic stenosis, overriding aorta, and right ventricular hypertrophy
Blood Flow Pattern	↑ Pulmonary flow, left-to-right shunting	↑Pulmonary flow; left-to-right shunting	↑ Pulmonary flow, left-to-right shunting	↓ Pulmonary flow; right-to-left shunting
Manifestations	↑ Respiratory infections; normal growth and development; congestive heart failure (CHF), if defect large	Usually asymptomatic, possible dysrhythmias, CHF if defect large	Usually asymptomatic, CHF possible, machinery-like murmur	Hypoxia, murmur, delayed growth and development
Treatment	Surgical correction by 2 years of age; prognosis dependent on extent of defect	Surgical correction by 6 years of age; excellent prognosis	Possibly indomethacin (Indocin) administration to premature babies; surgical correction by 2 years; excellent prognosis	Surgical correction by 1 year of age

output. Furosemide (Lasix) is the most commonly used diuretic. Because most diuretics cause potassium loss, serum potassium level is monitored, and potassium supplements may be ordered. Oxygen therapy and fluid management are also part of the treatment plan.

Diet

When infants experience significant dyspnea while feeding, special feeding techniques are needed, such as providing small, frequent feedings and softer nipples. Some infants need higher caloric formulas and diets to meet nutritional needs. Gavage feedings may be required if the infant becomes fatigued before taking an adequate amount of formula.

▶ NURSING PROCESS

▶ Assessment

▶ Subjective Data

The nurse should take a history of the child's previous hospitalizations and assess the family's knowledge about the condition. The family's anxiety level, coping strategies, and economic status should also be noted.

▶ Objective Data

The child's behavioral patterns, cardiac and respiratory function, fluid status, and growth and development should all be assessed. The nurse should obtain a detailed history of onset of symptoms and a typical day's activity schedule.

Nursing diagnoses for the infant with a heart defect may include the following:

Nursing Diagnosis	Planning/Goals	Nursing Interventions
▶ *Cardiac Output, Decreased, related to structural defect*	The client will demonstrate sufficient cardiac output to meet metabolic demands.	Administer digoxin as prescribed. Monitor vital signs (including apical pulse for 1 minute), potassium levels, urine output, cardiac rhythm, activity tolerance. Assess for signs of digoxin toxicity (vomiting, anorexia, dysrhythmias, bradycardia [pulse rate < 90 to 110]), peripheral perfusion. Provide periods of rest each hour.
▶ *Breathing Pattern, Ineffective, related to pulmonary congestion*	The client will breathe effortlessly at rest.	Keep the client in semi-Fowler's position (i.e., use infant seat). Administer humidified oxygen as prescribed. Assess respiratory rate and effort, color, and oxygen saturation. Employ comfort measures (i.e., holding, rocking, presence of parents). Respond quickly to crying.
▶ *Fluid Volume Excess related to fluid accumulation*	The client will experience decreased edema.	Administer diuretics as prescribed. Measure I & O. Weigh daily (same time and scale). Assess skin for edema, breakdown. Turn every 2 hours and elevate edematous extremities. Monitor electrolytes.
▶ *Nutrition, Altered, Less than Body Requirements, related to fatigue and dyspnea*	The client will demonstrate normal weight gain for age.	Give small, frequent, high-caloric feedings. Use soft nipple with large hole. Implement gavage feeding, if the infant tires before taking prescribed amount of formula. Make feeding time as stress free as possible. Hold the infant when bottle-feeding (preferably by primary caregiver).
▶ *Growth and Development, Altered, related to low energy level*	The client will meet developmental milestones for age.	Encourage age-appropriate activities, stimulation, and socialization. Allow the child to set own pace
▶ *Family Processes, Altered, related to child with life threatening illness/condition*	The family will receive needed support.	Teach the family as needed about medication administration, signs and symptoms of CHF and when to report, feeding techniques, and appropriate activities for the child. Refer the family to appropriate community resources.

Evaluation Each goal should be evaluated to determine how it has been met by the client.

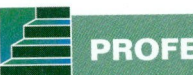

Stress at Feeding Time

Ways to decrease stress at feeding time include the following:

- Decrease the noise level.
- Hold the infant while sitting in rocker.
- Assess the infant's readiness to eat. (Infant is calm, demonstrates rooting, latches onto nipple eagerly, opens mouth voluntarily, looks at caregiver.)

BLOOD AND LYMPH SYSTEMS

The hematologic system regulates, directly or indirectly, the functions of all body tissues and organs. Some of the most common disorders occurring in infants include hyperbilirubinemia, iron-deficiency anemia, and sickle-cell anemia (SCA).

HYPERBILIRUBINEMIA

Hyperbilirubinemia, often referred to as jaundice, is a common occurrence in neonates. **Jaundice** refers to a yellow discoloration of the skin, sclera, mucous membranes, and body fluids due to excess bilirubin and deposition of bile pigments. Physiologically, hemoglobin is broken down by the liver into iron, protein, and bilirubin. The bilirubin binds to albumin and is transported to the liver, where it is conjugated. Conjugated bilirubin is then eliminated through the intestines. Neonates have an intestinal enzyme that can convert the conjugated bilirubin back to unconjugated bilirubin, which can be reabsorbed into the bloodstream. This process can contribute significantly to the amount of bilirubin that the immature liver must break down. As the bilirubin level rises, some of the excess bilirubin is deposited in body tissues, resulting in a temporary yellow discoloration of the skin and sclera. A high level of bilirubin can penetrate and damage brain cells, causing severe neural symptoms (**kernicterus**). Hyperbilirubinemia develops during the first few days of life in 45% to 60% of term infants and in as many as 80% of preterm infants.

Medical–Surgical Management

Medical

The main objective of treatment is to reduce the amount of unconjugated bilirubin and aid in the conversion of bilirubin to a form that can be excreted by the body (urobilinogen). Full-term infants with jaundice may benefit from early and frequent breastfeeding (every 2 hours). Otherwise, treatment usually begins with a phototherapy light, called a bililight, or a fiberoptic blanket. This light causes a chemical reaction in the skin and converts unconjugated bilirubin to a form that can be excreted by the body (lumirubin). Therapy is usually continual, with short breaks for feeding and holding. Phototherapy may be done at home, because it is less expensive than treatment in the hospital and the family will not have to be separated from their newborn.

Pharmacological

If the bilirubin level responds slowly to phototherapy, phenobarbital is sometimes given to enhance both the liver enzyme action and bilirubin excretion. Breastfeeding may have to be stopped for 24 to 48 hours if the level does not decrease with phototherapy. Ironically, breastfeeding and breast milk may cause hyperbilirubinemia as well as prevent it.

▶ NURSING PROCESS

▶ Assessment

▶ Subjective Data

Perinatal risk factors such as familial history of hyperbilirubinemia and induced delivery should be assessed.

▶ Objective Data

The nurse can assess for jaundice by applying light pressure to the skin over either the tip of nose or the sternum in natural day light. For dark-skinned infants, the sclera, conjunctiva, and oral mucosa are observed for a yellow color. Bruising, petechiae, and pallor are also suggestive of hyperbilirubenemia.

Nursing diagnoses for the infant with hyperbilirubinemia may include the following:

Nursing Diagnosis	Planning/Goals	Nursing Interventions
▶ *Fluid Volume, Risk for Deficit, related to insensible losses*	The client will maintain fluid balance.	Assess skin for signs of dehydration. Calculate needed fluid intake to compensate for losses. Monitor I & O.

continued

Nursing Diagnosis	Planning/Goals	Nursing Interventions
▶ *Skin Integrity, Impaired, Risk for, related to use of phototherapy and diarrhea*	The client's skin will remain intact.	Assess skin for breakdown. Monitor temperature every 2 to 4 hours. Keep skin clean and dry. Do not apply any oils or lotions.
▶ *Family Processes, Altered, related to situational crisis*	The family will receive needed support.	Encourage bonding by removing eye shields and allowing the parents to hold/feed the infant. Teach the importance of eye shields under light. Support the breastfeeding mother. Encourage pumping the breasts, if feeding must be stopped temporarily. Keep the parents informed.

Evaluation Each goal must be evaluated to determine how it has been met by the client.

IRON-DEFICIENCY ANEMIA

The incidence of iron-deficiency anemia is usually related to the infant's consuming large amounts of milk and foods that do not contain supplemental iron. These babies are often overweight due to excessive intake of cow's milk, which is a poor source of iron. In addition, cow's milk can cause loss of blood in the stool.

Because full-term infants have iron stores from fetal circulation that usually last for 5 to 6 months, iron-deficiency anemia usually surfaces between 9 and 24 months of age. Clinical manifestations may include extreme pallor (porcelain-like in fair-skinned infants), tachycardia, lethargy, irritability, and below-normal hemoglobin, hematocrit, and iron levels.

Medical–Surgical Management

Pharmacological

Iron therapy is usually prescribed and continued for 3 months after hemoglobin and hematocrit levels return to normal. An increase in hemoglobin level can be expected within 4 to 30 days. Ascorbic acid may also be prescribed in an attempt to facilitate iron absorption. Intramuscular (IM) or IV injections may be necessary if levels do not improve after 1 month of oral iron. Transfusions are indicated only for the most severe cases.

Diet

Long-term therapy is directed at increasing the dietary intake of iron and continuing the use of iron-fortified formula until 12 months of age.

Nursing Management

Primary nursing interventions include preventing anemia through educating the family, including the administration of iron. It is important to explore any mis-

PROFESSIONAL TIP

WIC
The federal supplemental food program called Women, Infants, and Children (WIC) is an excellent resource for nutritious food for low-income families with pregnant, postpartum, or lactating women and children up to 5 years of age. In addition to food, this program provides nutritional education and screening.

conceptions parents may have, such as "milk is a perfect food" and "excessive weight gain equates to a healthy child and good mothering."

Foods rich in iron, such as liver, dried beans, iron-fortified cereals, apricots, prunes, egg yolks, and dark-green, leafy vegetables, should be encouraged. Infants should remain on iron-fortified formulas until 12 months of age.

Caregivers should be instructed in the proper administration of oral iron. When administering IM preparations, no more than 1 mL should be given deep into

CLIENT TEACHING

Administration of Iron to Infants
When instructing caregivers in the administration of iron to infants, teach to:
- Administer with citrus fruit or juice in order to increase its absorption.
- Administer through a straw or medicine dropper placed at the back of the mouth, to decrease staining of the teeth.
- Brush or wipe the infant's teeth after administration.
- Expect dark, black stools.

the muscle using the Z-track method to prevent staining of tissues and to minimize irritation.

SICKLE-CELL ANEMIA

Sickle-cell anemia is a genetic disorder characterized by the production of abnormal hemoglobin and resulting in the red blood cells' (RBCs') taking on a "sickle" shape (Figure 53-4). Due to the presence of fetal hemoglobin, clinical symptoms usually do not appear until 6 months of age. Episodes of sickling may be triggered by infection, dehydration, hypoxia, trauma, or general physical or emotional stress resulting in impaired circulation and increased RBC destruction.

The most common symptoms of SCA include abdominal pain (due to sludging in the spleen and leading to its enlargement), fever, severe leg pain and hot, swollen joints. In addition, growth retardation, chronic anemia, and increased susceptibility to infection may be experienced. This disease occurs primarily among African Americans and is transmitted as an autosomal recessive trait wherein both parents are carriers (refer back to Table 53-2).

Medical–Surgical Management

Medical

Between episodes, the goal is to prevent crises with adequate hydration (1,500 to 3,000 mL/day). During crises, treatment may include bed rest, oxygen, analgesics (morphine), and fluids.

Pharmacological

Children with this disease must be immunized with pneumococcal, meningococcal, and hepatitis B vaccines due to increased susceptibility to infection and the likelihood of transfusion therapy. Prophylactic oral penicillin is often prescribed twice a day.

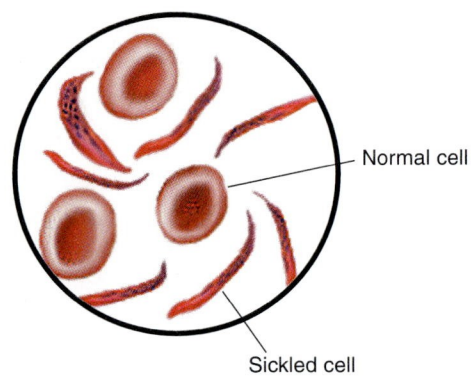

Figure 53-4 Sickling Cells

Health Promotion

High altitudes, poorly pressurized airplanes, and exposure to cold temperatures must be avoided. Maintaining hydration is of paramount importance. Neonatal screening, early intervention, prophylactic antibiotics, and parent education have allowed children with SCA to live into adulthood.

▶ NURSING PROCESS

▶ Assessment

▶ Subjective Data

The family should be interviewed about activities or events leading up to the crisis, a history of child's health, and previous episodes. The nurse should evaluate the family's level of knowledge about the condition.

▶ Objective Data

The nurse must assess all areas and systems that can be affected by circulatory obstruction, such as vital signs, vision, hearing, growth and development, and the respiratory, GI, renal, neurological, and musculoskeletal systems.

Nursing diagnoses for the infant with sickle cell anemia may include the following:

Nursing Diagnosis	Planning/Goals	Nursing Interventions
▶ *Tissue Perfusion, Altered, related to vaso-occlusion and anemia*	The client will maintain oxygen saturation levels at 95% or greater.	Administer oxygen as prescribed. Monitor oxygen saturation, capillary refill, and respiratory status. Maintain the client in a position of comfort (semi- to high-Fowler's). Administer packed RBCs as prescribed.
▶ *Pain related to vaso-occlusion and tissue ischemia*	The client will be pain free.	Apply heat to affected area; avoid cold compresses. Administer analgesics as prescribed (preferably morphine) and assess effectiveness by assessing behavior and vital signs. Reassure the family that opioids are appropriate, high doses may be needed, and addiction is rare. Position the client carefully and handle gently.

continued

Nursing Diagnosis	Planning/Goals	Nursing Interventions
▶ *Infection, Risk for, related to splenic malfunction*	The client will be infection free.	Provide one to one and one-half daily fluid requirement as determined by body weight.
		Provide daily food requirements as determined by body weight and length.
		Administer antibiotics as prescribed.
		Ensure that the infant avoids contact with known sources of infection.
		Ensure that immunizations are up-to-date.
▶ *Knowledge Deficit (family) related to cause and treatment of disease*	The family will verbalize an understanding of the risk factors and ways to minimize them.	Teach need for one to one and one-half times daily fluid requirement.
		Teach importance of handwashing and avoiding known sources of infection.
		Reinforce importance of up-to-date immunizations for the infant.
		Teach to shield the infant from overexertion, emotional stress, and low-oxygen environments.
		Teach early intervention for any sign of infection (e.g., temperature of 101.5°F or greater) or dehydration (weight loss, dry skin and mucous membranes, sunken fontanel).
		Teach medication administration as ordered.
▶ *Family Processes, Altered, related to child with chronic condition*	The family will adjust to lifelong, potentially fatal hereditary disease.	Explain procedures and planned treatments.
		Allow the family to provide care in the hospital.
		Provide information about appropriate developmental activities.
		Encourage the family to talk about feelings and concerns.
		Stress positive outcomes (i.e., that most of the time, children are asymptomatic and can participate in appropriate activities without restrictions).
		Provide information regarding transmission of the condition; refer for genetic counseling.
		Provide numbers for American Sickle Cell Anemia Association and available support groups.

Evaluation Each goal must be evaluated to determine how it has been met by the client.

GASTROINTESTINAL SYSTEM

Infants have minimal saliva, no voluntary control of swallowing, a small stomach, rapid intestinal motility, a relaxed cardiac sphincter, deficiency of enzymes in the duodenum, and immature liver function. This accounts for the numerous GI problems that occur during the first 12 months of life, such as vomiting, diarrhea, **colic** (sudden, recurrent bouts of abdominal pain), and failure to thrive. In addition, because the immune system is also immature, the infant is highly susceptible to infection. Congenital defects resulting in **atresia** (absence or closure of a body orifice), malposition, nonclosure, or other abnormalities can occur in any area of the GI tract. Any GI problem, whether a lack of nutrients, an infection, or a congenital disorder, can quickly affect other parts of the body and ultimately affect general health and growth and development. The GI disorders discussed following include thrush, acute gastroenteritis, colic, failure to thrive, cleft lip/palate, esophageal atresia with tracheoesophageal fistula, pyloric stenosis, Hirschsprung's disease, gastroesophageal reflux, and intussusception.

THRUSH

Thrush (moniliasis, candidiasis) is an oral fungal infection that is transmitted from the vaginal canal of an infected mother to the newborn. Other contributing factors include poor handwashing by care providers, inadequate washing of bottles and nipples, and antibiotic therapy. Thrush is characterized by painless, white patches that look like curdled milk on the oral mucosa (Figure 53-5).

Medical–Surgical Management

Pharmacological

Topical nystatin (Mycostatin) is the most commonly used treatment for thrush. It is applied to the oral mucosa four times per day with an applicator or a gloved

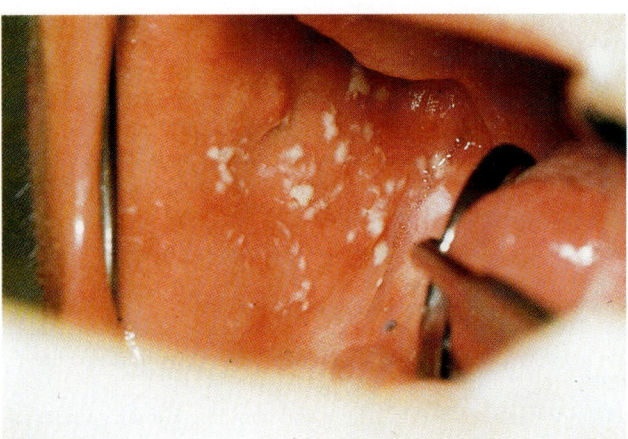

Figure 53-5 Thrush *(Courtesy of Dr. Joseph Konzelman, School of Dentistry, Medical College of Georgia)*

finger and then swallowed. The mouth should be rinsed prior to medicating. In addition, if infants are breastfed, the medication should be applied to the breasts.

Nursing Management

Caregivers are taught proper handwashing and hygiene. The boiling of bottles and nipples for 20 minutes will kill spores.

ACUTE GASTROENTERITIS

Acute gastroenteritis (AGE) is an inflammation of the stomach and intestines that may be accompanied by diarrhea and vomiting. This common condition may be caused by malnutrition, lactose intolerance, chronic conditions, or infections (commonly rotaviruses).

The infant with AGE will have an increased number of green, liquid stools tinged with mucous or blood. In addition, symptoms of fluid and electrolyte imbalance; cramping; extreme irritability; and vomiting may be exhibited. Depending on age and nutritional status and on the severity and duration of the diarrhea, the infant may become severely dehydrated and gravely ill.

Medical–Surgical Management

Medical

Regaining and maintaining fluid balance is paramount. Oral rehydrating fluids such as Pedialyte and Lytren may be used for mild dehydration. For severe dehydration, IV solutions are needed to replace fluids and electrolytes. Antibiotics may be prescribed if bacterial infection is indicated from stool cultures.

Diet

Once rehydration is attained, the usual diet is continued. Research has indicated that early reintroduction of normal nutrients is desirable, and delayed introduction of food may be harmful in terms of nutritional status and duration of illness. Breastfed infants should continue on supplemental oral rehydrating solutions throughout the illness. If formula or nonhuman milk feedings are not tolerated, lactose-free formulas may be suggested.

▶ NURSING PROCESS

▶ Assessment

▶ Subjective Data

Caregivers should be questioned regarding probable etiologic agents such as introduction of new food; exposure to infectious agents; travel to an area where the infectious agent is endemic; contact with foods that might be contaminated; crowded, dirty living conditions; and contact with pets that are known to be sources of enteric infections, such as pet turtles. Allergy, drug, health, and diet histories should also be obtained.

▶ Objective Data

Assessing for dehydration is paramount for infants with AGE (Table 53-4). In addition, the diaper area should be assessed for skin breakdown resulting from repeated contact with diarrheal stools.

Table 53-4 ASSESSING DEHYDRATION

SIGNS AND SYMPTOMS	MILD	MODERATE	SEVERE
Weight loss	< 5%	6–10%	> 10%
Skin turgor	Taut	Tenting	Tenting
Skin color	Pale	Grey	Mottled
Mucous membranes	Slightly dry, pale	Very dry, grey	Parched
Urine output	Decreased	Absent	Absent
Blood pressure	Normal	Normal	Decreased
Pulse	Normal or increased	Increased	Increased/thready
Fontanel	Flat	Depressed	Sunken

Nursing diagnoses for the infant with AGE may include the following:

Nursing Diagnosis	Planning/Goals	Nursing Interventions
▶ *Fluid Volume Deficit related to excessive GI losses*	The client will be adequately hydrated (specify).	Monitor I & O and notify physician if output < 1 mL/kg/h.
		Assess weight daily and compare with previous weights.
		Assess for degree of hydration.
		Monitor electrolyte levels.
		Administer fluids and electrolytes as prescribed.
		Encourage clear liquids and oral rehydrating solutions (Pedialyte, Lytren) in small doses every 30 minutes until rehydrated; after rehydration, alternate with water, breast milk, or half-strength formula, as needed.
▶ *Infection, Risk for, related to GI infection*	The client and family will be infection free.	Teach proper handwashing and diaper hygiene to care providers.
		Wear gloves when handling diapers.
▶ *Skin Integrity, Impaired, Risk for, related to frequent contact with diarrheal stools*	The client's skin will remain intact.	Change diapers every 2 hours, as needed.
		Cleanse skin with mild soap (Dove) and water.
		Apply barrier (A&D Ointment).
		Teach the family proper techniques.

Evaluation Each goal must be evaluated to determine how it has been met by the client.

PROFESSIONAL TIP

Potassium Administration

Urine output must be established before potassium can be administered.

Infection Control: Diaper Hygiene
- Change diapers as soon as they are soiled
- Wear gloves when changing diapers
- Fold the used diaper with soiled area to the inside and immediately place the diaper in a covered receptacle
- Cleanse the skin and dispose of wipes along with the diaper
- Remove gloves after disposal of wipes
- Rediaper
- Wash hands immediately after rediapering is complete
- Store soiled clothing, cloth diapers, and washcloths in a covered receptacle
- Cleanse surface of changing area

COLIC

Colic is a sudden, periodic attack of abdominal pain and cramping that is manifested by severe crying for several hours and by the drawing of the legs up to the abdomen. It usually occurs between birth and 3 months of age and at approximately the same time each day (late afternoon, early evening hours). During these episodes, the infant is generally inconsolable, which may interfere with parent–child attachment and family relations.

The child is usually eager to eat and is growing appropriately. There is no known cause of colic, however, speculation points to overfeeding, overly rapid feeding, improper burping, the swallowing of large amounts of air, and emotional stress between parent and child (Wong, Hockenberry-Eaton, Winkelstein, Wilson, Ahmann, & DiVito-Thomas, 1999).

Medical–Surgical Management

Medical

Sensitivity to formula; food allergies; peritoneal infection; and intestinal obstruction must be ruled out as specific causes of the distress. If sensitivity to formula is suspected, another brand of formula may be substituted. In the case of breastfeeding mothers, dairy products such as milk, ice cream, butter, yogurt, cheese, puddings, and creamed soups should be avoided for several days in an attempt to relieve the infant's symptoms.

CLIENT TEACHING

Calcium and Breast Milk

If the breastfeeding mother maintains a milk-free diet for more than several days, she must take calcium supplements in order to maintain the calcium content of the breast milk.

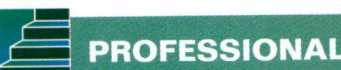

PROFESSIONAL TIP

Assessing Colic

Questions to consider when assessing the family with a colicky infant include the following:

- Which family members are usually present during the attacks?
- What is the caregiver doing prior to the episodes?
- What measures have been used to relieve the crying?

Pharmacological

Sedatives, antispasmodics, antihistamines, and antiflatulents are sometimes recommended in an attempt to relieve symptoms. Hydroxyzine hydrochloride (Atarax) and phenobarbital are most commonly used.

Nursing Management

Assessing circumstances surrounding the colicky event, exploring techniques to relieve symptoms, and supporting parents during the colicky period are the primary nursing goals. The nurse should observe the feeding technique in order to assess the parent's sensitivity and response to the infant's cues distress and and to evaluate the clarity of the infant's cues and the infant's responsiveness to the parent.

Parents should be reassured that colic usually resolves by 3 months of age and does not indicate poor or inadequate parenting. Further, they should be en-

CLIENT TEACHING

Suggestions for Alleviating Colic

- Provide rhythmic movement, such as rocking, swinging, and riding in the car
- Alternate positions, such as placing the infant face down across the lap
- Reduce environmental stimuli, especially during feedings
- Provide a variety of tactile stimulation, such as rubbing the head or abdomen or placing prone on a warm heating pad
- Provide small, frequent feedings
- Burp during and after feedings
- Respond immediately to crying

couraged to talk about their feelings toward the infant and any insecurities they may feel.

FAILURE TO THRIVE

Failure to thrive (FTT) is the label applied to infants who fail to gain weight and who show signs of delayed development. There are two categories of FTT: organic, which is caused by a physical defect or condition; and nonorganic, which is the result of psychosocial factors such as an impaired parent–child relationship. Manifestations of FTT include sustained growth failure (below the 5th percentile on the standardized growth chart), developmental delays in all areas, and poor feeding and sleeping patterns.

Medical–Surgical Management

Medical

If FTT is the result of a physical defect or condition, the condition is treated. Regardless of the cause, the primary goals are to provide adequate nutrition, promote growth and development, and assist parents in developing the skills needed to nurture their infant.

Health Promotion

In most cases of nonorganic FTT, a multidisciplinary health care team is needed to deal with the physical, psychosocial, mental, and emotional problems that may be occurring in the family. If the entire family is to become healthy, each member must be helped to change.

▶ NURSING PROCESS

▶ Assessment

▶ Subjective Data

The focus should be the infant's routine, respiratory status, and diet history. It is important to assess the family for depression, substance abuse, mental retardation, and psychosis as well as socioeconomic level, education, social isolation, stress factors, and support systems.

▶ Objective Data

The physical assessment should focus on signs of malnutrition (skin, hair, nails, mucous membranes, energy level, developmental milestones) and on parent–infant interactions (parent's cues, infant's cues, and synchrony).

Nursing diagnoses for the infant with FTT may include the following:

Nursing Diagnosis	Planning/Goals	Nursing Interventions
▶ Nutrition, Altered, Less than Body Requirements, related to insufficient intake of calories and/or impaired parent/child interaction	The client will demonstrate growth curve above the 5th percentile.	Provide consistent nursing staff around the clock. Feed the infant on demand and increase intake as tolerated. Develop a structured routine. Monitor I & O. Weigh daily. Encourage parental involvement in care, demonstrate and model appropriate care techniques, praise positive attempts at care, and provide for rooming-in. Use a variety of methods to teach child care to the parents.
▶ Development, Risk for Altered, related to inadequate stimulation	The client will attain age-appropriate developmental milestones.	Begin a program of play that stimulates interest and responsiveness. Teach the parents ways to play and interact with the infant. Teach parents to cuddle the infant.

Evaluation Each goal must be evaluated to determine how it has been met by the client.

CLEFT LIP/PALATE

The most common facial malformations are cleft lip and cleft palate. They may occur separately or together. Failure of the palates and/or lip to fuse is evident at birth. The defect may occur unilaterally on either side or bilaterally and with varying degrees of severity. The cause is unclear, but some genetic component seems likely.

Clinical manifestations include nasal, lip, and palate distortions. The child born with a cleft palate and intact lip does not manifest the external disfigurement so potentially distressing to parents, but the physical problems are more serious. The infants with a cleft palate is at risk for aspiration, feeding difficulties, and respiratory infections (Figures 53-6 and 53-7).

Medical–Surgical Management

Medical

Care is directed toward closing the defects, maintaining adequate nutrition, preventing complications, and fostering normal growth and development of the child. Total care may involve many specialists, including pediatricians, nurses, plastic surgeons, orthodontists, prosthodontists, otolaryngologists, speech therapists, and psychiatrists. The extent of multidisciplinary care depends on the severity of the defect. Infants with cleft lip and palate are prone to recurrent otitis media, which will likely be treated with antibiotics.

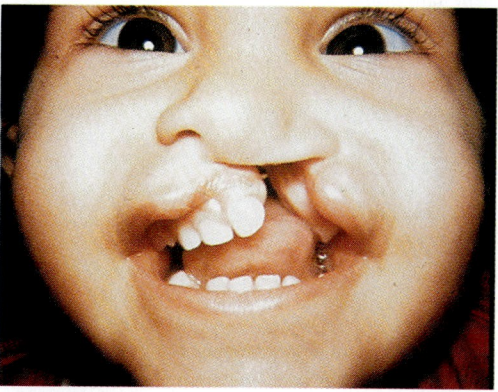

Figure 53-6 Older Child with Unrepaired Cleft Lip (Courtesy of Dr. Joseph Konzelman, School of Dentistry, Medical College of Georgia)

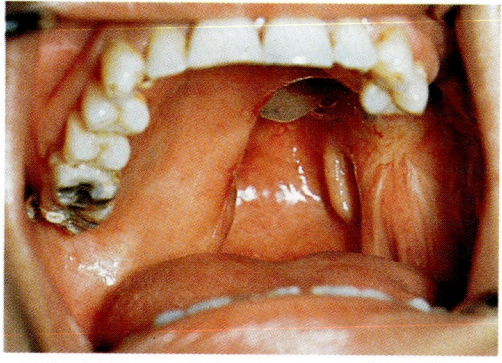

Figure 53-7 Older Child with Unrepaired Cleft Palate (Courtesy of Dr. Joseph Konzelman, School of Dentistry, Medical College of Georgia)

Surgical

Closure of the lip precedes that of the palate, usually at 6 to 12 weeks of age. The palate is usually closed surgically at 12 to 18 months of age to facilitate speech development.

Health Promotion

Maternal use of multivitamin supplements containing folic acid around the time of conception has been reported to reduce the risk of cleft malformations by up to 50% (Shaw, Lamamer, Wassernman, O'Malley, and Tolarova, 1995).

▶ NURSING PROCESS

▶ Assessment

▶ Subjective Data

The emotional impact of the birth of an infant with a facial deformity is assessed at birth. The family's acceptance of the child is assessed periodically, at various appointments and hospital admissions.

▶ Objective Data

Cleft lip and palate are observable at birth. A cleft palate is palpable with the finger, and the degree of involvement should be documented. Ability to suck, swallow, breathe, and handle secretions must be evaluated.

Nursing diagnoses for the infant with cleft lip or palate may include the following:

Nursing Diagnoses	Planning/Goals	Nursing Interventions
▶ *Coping, Family, Ineffective, related to birth of infant with visible and/or structural defect*	The family will bond with the infant.	Encourage the parents to hold the infant.
		Point out positive attributes of the infant (e.g., hair, eyes, alertness); convey attitude of acceptance of the infant and family.
		Explain expected outcomes of surgical repair; show pictures of repaired children.
		Allow expression of feelings.
		Assess the parents' knowledge, degree of anxiety, level of discomfort, interpersonal relationships.
		Explore reactions of extended family.
		Encourage the parents to participate in care of the infant.
		Provide information.
		Refer to parental support groups and to other families in similar situations.
▶ *Nutrition, Altered, Less than Body Requirements, related to infant's inability to form an adequate seal when sucking on the nipple*	The infant will maintain a growth curve above the 5th percentile.	Provide 100 to 150 cal/kg/d and 100 to 130 mL/kg/d.
		Assess output daily.
		Weigh daily.
		Observe for respiratory impairment (i.e., for adventitious breath sounds, increased respiratory rate).
		Facilitate breastfeeding; refer for ongoing support (i.e., to La Leche League).
		Position the infant in an upright or semi-sitting position for feeding.
		Use effective assistive devices (i.e., longer, softer nipples; feeders).
		Feed small amounts slowly, allowing ample time for sucking and swallowing; burp after 15 to 30 mL.
		Initiate nasogastric feeding if infant is unable to ingest sufficient calories by mouth.
▶ *Tissue Integrity, Impaired, related to surgical correction of cleft*	The client's tissue will heal with minimal scarring.	Position the infant on side or back.
		Use elbow restraints for 7 to 10 days as needed and teach proper application to parents.
		Medicate for pain around-the-clock for at least 24 hours postoperatively.
		Provide developmentally appropriate activities (e.g., music, mobiles, holding) to distract the infant's attention from the incision site.
		Do not use pacifiers, spoons, or straws for 7 to 10 days postoperatively.
		Progress to a soft diet appropriate to age and as ordered and tolerated within 48 hours.

continued

Nursing Diagnoses	Planning/Goals	Nursing Interventions
▶ *Infection, Risk for, related to surgical procedure and accumulation of formula and secretions in oral cavity*	The client's surgical site will be free of infection.	Assess vital signs and oral cavity every 2 hours. Cleanse suture line with normal saline or sterile water, as ordered. Give 5 to 15 mL water after each feeding to cleanse the mouth. Apply antibiotic cream as ordered. Ensure handwashing by all care providers. Include parents in care and prepare for home care.

Evaluation Each goal must be evaluated to determine how it has been met by the client.

ESOPHAGEAL ATRESIA WITH TRACHEOESOPHAGEAL FISTULA

Esophageal atresia and tracheoesophageal fistula are rare malformations that may occur alone or in combination and represent a failure of the esophagus to develop as a continuous passage (atresia) to the stomach and/or an unnatural connection between the esophagus and the trachea (fistula) (Figure 53-8). The cause is unknown.

Manifestations include excessive salivation, drooling, coughing, choking when feeding and cyanosis. A history of polyhydramnios (excessive production of amniotic fluid) during the prenatal period is common.

Medical–Surgical Management

Medical

The primary goal is prevention and treatment of aspiration pneumonia. The infant will be designated NPO and administered IV fluids. Removal of secretions from the mouth and esophagus requires frequent or continuous suctioning through an nasogastric tube (NGT). Antibiotics will be prescribed for any developing pneumonia.

Surgical

These defects represent a critical neonatal surgical emergency. Surgical correction may be accomplished in several stages depending on the size and condition of the infant and the extent of the defect. If closure of the gap requires staged repair, a gastrostomy tube will be placed for feeding. The prognosis is usually good with surgery.

Nursing Management

Nursing responsibility for detection of this malformation begins immediately after birth. The newborn is assessed for color, amount of saliva, ability to swallow, respiratory distress, and abdominal distention. A maternal history of polyhydramnios necessitates assessment for the defect with insertion of an NGT. No feedings should be initiated until the infant has been assessed. When the defect is diagnosed, the nurse prepares the infant and the family for immediate surgery. Postoperative care is the same as that provided to any high-risk newborn.

PYLORIC STENOSIS

Pyloric stenosis is a common disorder that occurs when the circular muscle surrounding the pylorus hypertrophies and blocks gastric emptying (Figure 53-9). It is rarely diagnosed before the third week of life. Manifestations include **projectile vomiting** (ejection of stomach contents up to 3 feet), ravenous hunger, hyperactive bowel sounds, irritability, FTT, decreased number and volume of stools, an olive-shaped mass in the right upper quadrant, and visible peristaltic waves.

Medical–Surgical Management

Medical

Diagnosis is usually made before malnutrition, dehydration, and alkalosis are severe. It is unusual for the infant to require IV fluid therapy prior to surgery.

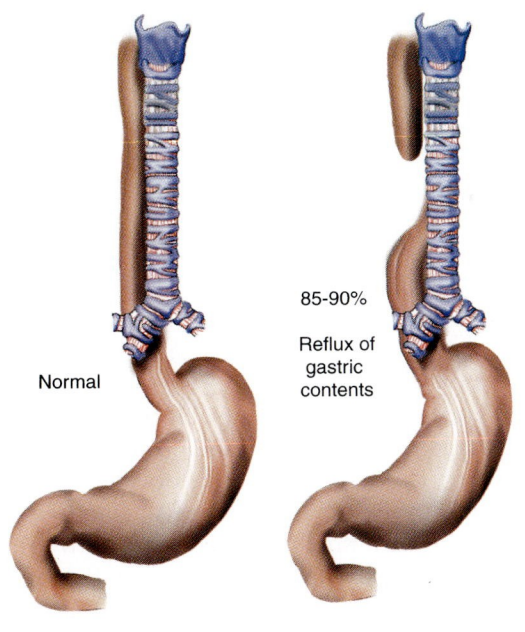

Normal

85-90%

Reflux of gastric contents

A.   B.

Figure 53-8 Esophagus: A. Normal; B. Atresia/Fistula

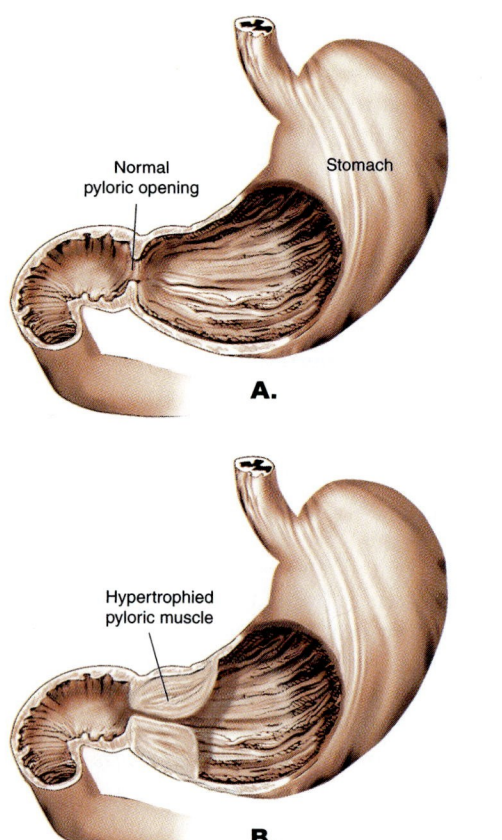

Figure 53-9 Stomach: A. Normal opening; B. Pyloric stenosis

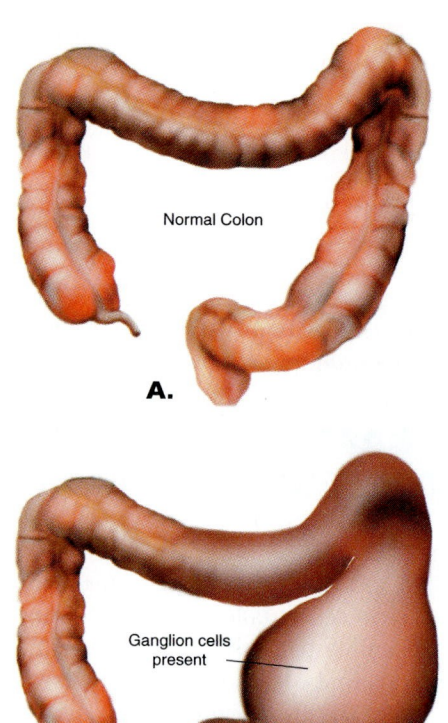

Figure 53-10 Colon: A. Normal; B. Hirschsprung disease/Megacolon

Surgical

The defect usually is discovered early and repaired immediately. Most infants recover rapidly and completely with surgery.

Nursing Management

Recognizing the signs and symptoms early is paramount. Pre- and postoperative care are the same as for any GI surgical client. Infants are allowed to resume feedings 4 to 6 hours postoperatively and may be discharged within 72 hours.

HIRSCHSPRUNG'S DISEASE/ MEGACOLON

Hirschsprung's disease is a congenital anomaly manifested as a partial or complete mechanical obstruction resulting from inadequate motility of part of the colon. There is an absence of parasympathetic ganglion cells and, thus, of peristalsis within the muscular wall of the distal colon and the rectum. As a result, the affected portion of the bowel narrows, and the portion directly above the affected area becomes greatly dilated and fills with feces and gas (Figure 53-10). Failure of the newborn to have a stool during the first 24 hours may be indicative of this defect.

Older infants may have constipation or ribbonlike stools and an enlarged, distended abdomen.

Medical–Surgical Management

Medical

For the child with a mild defect, management may involve dietary modification, stool softeners, and isotonic irrigations until the child is toilet trained. Most infants with Hirschsprung's require surgical intervention.

Surgical

Surgical intervention involves removal of the aganglionic bowel and creation of a temporary colostomy. Resection and colostomy closure are performed after the child reaches 10 kilograms.

Nursing Management

The nurse assesses the newborn for passage of stool during the first 24 hours and observes for signs of constipation and for malformed stools throughout infancy. All infants with Hirschsprung's must be assessed for weight gain, nutritional intake, and bowel habits. Parents are taught both to ensure regular bowel habits with daily saline irrigations and a balanced diet and to observe for signs of fluid and electrolyte imbalances, such as dry mucous membranes and increased thirst.

Postoperative care may include reduction of anxiety and preparation for home care of the colostomy.

GASTROESOPHAGEAL REFLUX

Gastroesophageal reflux (GER) is the return of abdominal contents into the esophagus due to an immature sphincter. Manifestations such as hunger, irritability, FTT, vomiting, and frequent upper respiratory infections usually occur during the first 6 weeks of life.

The majority of infants have mild reflux and generally improve without surgical intervention by 1 year of age. Severe cases of GER that do not respond to therapy can result in esophageal strictures, respiratory distress, and FTT.

Medical–Surgical Management

Medical

Gastroesophageal reflux often resolves with dietary modifications, medication, and positioning. Small, frequent feedings and frequent burping are measures for minimizing reflux. Thickening formula with cereal (1 to 3 teaspoons of cereal for each ounce of formula) may be recommended if FTT persists.

Placing the infant prone and with the head elevated 30 degrees (Figure 53-11) is generally thought to be the most effective positioning for reducing the frequency of reflux. Positioning in an infant seat may cause increased intra-abdominal pressure and is not recommended.

Surgical

Severe cases of GER that do not respond to medical interventions may be treated with a surgical procedure called fundoplication, which involves loosely wrapping the gastric fundus around the lower esophagus.

Pharmacological

Medications such as cimetidine (Tagamet), ranitidine (Zantac), or famotidine (Pepcid) may be effective in reducing gastric acid content.

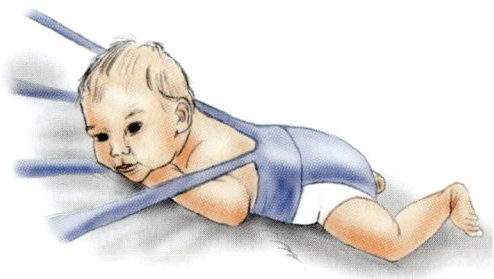

Figure 53-11 Thirty-Degree Elevated Prone Position to Counter Gastroesophageal Reflux

Nursing Management

Nursing care is directed at recognizing signs and symptoms of GER and educating parents regarding home care, including feeding, positioning, and medications. Pre- and postoperative care will be needed if the defect is surgically repaired.

INTUSSUSCEPTION

Intussusception is a disorder characterized by the telescoping of one portion of the bowel (usually the ileum) into a distal portion (usually the ascending colon). A previously healthy infant who develops intussusception will suddenly become pale, cry out sharply, and draw up the legs in a severe colicky spasm of pain. Such episodes last for several minutes and recur within 20 minutes. Vomiting and passage of "currant-jelly stools" (containing bloody mucous) also occur. Symptoms of shock, such as increased heart rate and changes in level of consciousness, appear quickly. If the intussusception is detected and reduced within 24 hours, morbidity is minimal. However, 5% to 10% of infants with intussusception die of complications such as perforation, peritonitis, and sepsis (Behrman, Kliegman, & Arvin, 1996).

Medical–Surgical Management

Medical

Initial treatment involves hydrostatic reduction with barium or air enema at the time of diagnosis, with a success rate of 70% to 85% (Behrman, Kleigman, & Arvin, 1996).

Surgical

If hydrostatic reduction fails or bowel damage is visualized during x-ray, surgical repair is done immediately. Surgery may consist of manual reduction of the telescoping, resection and anastamosis, or, possibly, colostomy, if the intestine is gangrenous.

Nursing Management

Early recognition of signs and symptoms of intussusception (i.e., abrupt onset of colicky pain and vomiting with currant-jelly stools) is most important. Nurses can help parents visualize telescoping by pressing the finger of an inflated rubber glove into the glove; pressing on the glove will then demonstrate hydrostatic reduction as the finger is pushed back to its normal position.

SAMPLE NURSING CARE PLAN

THE INFANT CLIENT WITH ABDOMINAL SURGERY

Eight-month-old Nathan was brought to the emergency room by his mother and father, who stated that he was perfectly fine until approximately 4 hours ago when he refused to eat lunch or take his bottle. He wanted to be held and became increasingly irritable. He began alternating between inconsolable crying and being quiet and limp. Physical examination revealed a palpable abdominal mass and passage of currant-jelly stool. Barium enema confirmed the diagnosis of intussusception, but attempts to reduce the blockage were unsuccessful. Nathan was admitted and prepared for surgery. Nathan weighs 8.8 kg and is maintaining a normal growth curve at the 50th percentile. He has attained all appropriate developmental milestones. This is Nathan's first illness and hospitalization. His mother begins to cry when she learns of the impending surgery and says, "What did I do wrong?" When the surgery is over, the doctor reports that Nathan has a temporary colostomy that will be closed in a few months. Nathan returns from surgery with an NGT and a urinary catheter in place and with dextrose 5% with normal saline being administered by IV at 40 cc per hour.

Nursing Diagnosis 1 *Injury, Risk for, related to physical risk factors as evidenced by surgical procedure, loss of fluids, altered nutrition, and chemical risk factor of anesthesia*

PLANNING/GOALS	NURSING INTERVENTIONS	RATIONALE	EVALUATION
Nathan will be free of injury, infection, and complications.	Assess vital signs, skin, hydration, and respiratory status every 4 hours.	Facilitates early detection of signs of complications.	Surgical site is infection free and show signs of healing.
	Administer antibiotics as prescribed.	Prevents infection.	
Nathan will demonstrate required fluid I & O.	Provide mouth care at least every 4 hours.	Mucous membranes become dry when clients are NPO.	Mucous membranes are moist.
	Maintain NPO and monitor IV as prescribed, and record I & O.	An empty stomach prevents aspiration, and fluids maintain hydration.	Fluid requirements are maintained.
	Assess bowel sounds every 2 hours.	Active bowel sounds are an indication of ability to tolerate food.	
Nathan will maintain growth curve at 50th percentile.	When diet is ordered, offer small sips of water and advance as tolerated.	Small, frequent feedings decrease vomiting.	Client loses less than 5% of admission weight.

Nursing Diagnosis 2 *Pain related to physical injury as evidenced by surgical procedure*

PLANNING/GOALS	NURSING INTERVENTIONS	RATIONALE	EVALUATION
Nathan will be pain free.	Administer pain medications every 3 to 4 hours as prescribed and around-the-clock.	If child is able to sleep and rest, recovery is faster.	Child sleeps quietly and shows no signs of restlessness.

continued

Position for comfort; allow caregivers to hold and comfort.

Lubricate nostrils, if NGT present.

Perform procedures such as dressing changes and respiratory therapy after analgesia.

Nursing Diagnosis 3 *Anxiety (parental) related to hospitalization, colostomy, and home care as evidenced by parental reaction and questioning*

PLANNING/GOALS	NURSING INTERVENTIONS	RATIONALE	EVALUATION
Nathan's parents will understand etiology, pathology, and treatment of illness.	Encourage expression of feelings.	It is important to maintain positive family interaction during hospitalization.	Family care providers demonstrate skill and knowledge in caring for their child's needs.
	Explain procedures, keep informed of progress, and answer questions.	Facilitates development of rapport with the family.	
Nathan's parents will provide comfort to their child.	Encourage parental presence and give positive re-enforcement to client and family for cooperation and participation in care.	Active participation facilitates coping and decreases anxiety.	
Nathan's parents will demonstrate proper techniques for home care procedures.	Teach parents to provide colostomy care, dressing changes, fluids, nutrition, and growth-fostering activities.	Provides parents with skills required to care for Nathan at home.	Parents verbalize decreased anxiety and return demonstrations of colostomy care and dressing changes.
	Refer to appropriate community resources.	Support personnel at home will decrease parents' anxiety and ensure that proper care is provided.	

MUSCULOSKELETAL SYSTEM

The musculoskeletal system provides protection to vital organs, supports weight, stores minerals, and supplies RBCs. Disorders may be congenital or acquired and require short- or long-term care. Most alterations of the arms and legs are mild variations of normal posturing, but some are severe anomalies. The two most common congenital skeletal defects are clubfoot and dislocated hip.

CONGENITAL TALIPES EQUINOVARUS (CLUB FOOT)

The equinovarus foot has a clublike appearance with the entire foot inverted, the heel drawn up, and the forefoot adducted (Figure 53-12). It can occur as a single anomaly or in connection with other defects such as **myelomeningocele** (a saclike protrusion situated along the vertebral column and filled with spinal fluid, meninges, nerve roots, and spinal cord). Club foot is

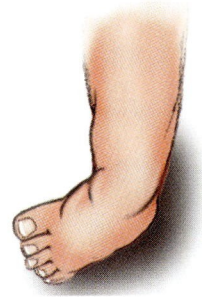

Figure 53-12 Club Foot

apparent at birth and may be bilateral or unilateral. The degree of malformation and likelihood for complete correction varies. Even with correction, recurrence is common.

Medical–Surgical Management

Medical

Correction is usually started during the neonatal period with manipulation and casting of the foot. The long leg cast is changed every few days for the first few weeks and then every week or two for several months. Correction is confirmed by x-ray. Following casting, a splint with shoes attached is used for several months to maintain correction.

Surgical

Children who do not respond to nonsurgical treatment within 3 to 6 months need surgical correction. Following surgery, a cast is applied with the knee in a flexed position. After 6 to 12 weeks, casting is discontinued, and corrective shoes or bracing may be prescribed. Even with aggressive therapy, the foot is seldom entirely normal, and atrophy of the calf is common.

 CLIENT TEACHING

Cast Care
Instruct parents in the following regarding cast care:
- Casts must be changed as prescribed to maintain growth and comfort.
- Wet casts should be handled with the palms (to prevent indentations).
- Hair dryers should not be used to facilitate drying of the cast.
- Plaster of paris casts should dry within 10 to 72 hours, depending on the size.
- Dry casts should be felt for "hot spots" and observed for visible stains due to drainage, which may indicate skin breakdown.
- Signs of swelling should be noted and reported immediately.
- Toes should be warm, pink, and moving.

Nursing Management

Initially, the nurse must assess and explore the parents' feelings about their less-than-perfect newborn and the family's knowledge about the defect, treatment, and need for long-term care. Nursing responsibilities include teaching the parents cast care, monitoring for complications, encouraging compliance with long-term follow-up, and facilitating normal development.

DEVELOPMENTAL DYSPLASIA OF THE HIP

Developmental **dysplasia** (abnormal development) of the hip (DDH) refers to a variety of conditions wherein the femoral head and the acetabulum are improperly aligned. These conditions include **dislocation** (displacement of the bone from its normal position in a joint), subluxation (partial dislocation), and acetabular dysplasia. These conditions can be congenital, but in some children, they develop after birth.

Manifestations include limited **abduction** (lateral movement away from body) of the affected hip, asymmetry of the gluteal and thigh fat folds, and telescoping or pistoning of the thigh. The walking infant may manifest minimal to pronounced variations in gait, with lurching toward the affected side. The longer the disorder goes untreated, the more pronounced the clinical manifestations become and the worse the prognosis.

Medical–Surgical Management

Early screening, detection, and treatment enable the majority of affected children to attain normal hip function.

Medical

For young infants, the Pavlik harness is used to maintain flexion, abduction, and external rotation (Figure 53-13). This harness is highly effective when used

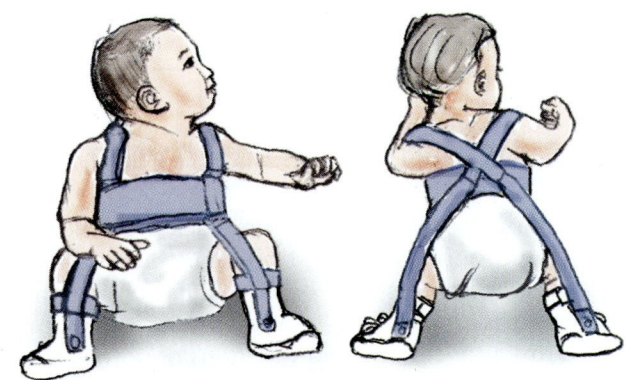

Figure 53-13 A Pavlik harness is used to treat an infant with developmental dysplasia of the hip.

as prescribed. A hip spica cast may be necessary when the harness is ineffective. Older infants may require traction for weeks, either at home or in the hospital.

Surgical

The older infant may require closed reduction under anesthesia and/or open reduction followed by a hip spica cast.

▶ NURSING PROCESS

▶ Assessment

▶ Subjective Data

The nurse is alerted to the possibility of DDH when the infant has a history of being delivered by cesarean section or frank breech, is large for gestational age, or is a twin.

▶ Objective Data

During the newborn assessment and routine nurturing activities, the infant is inspected for limited abduction of the hip, a wide perineum, and unequal gluteal folds (Figure 53-14). The walking infant is assessed for a limp or an unusual gait.

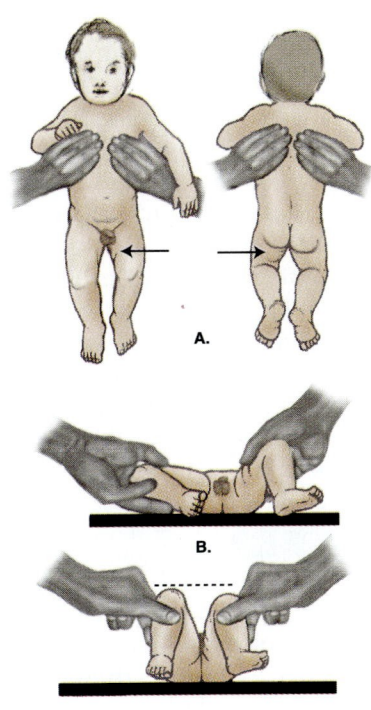

Figure 53-14 Assessing for DDH. A. Thighs and gluteal folds will show asymmetry. B. Flexion will show limited hip abduction. C. Knee height will show uneven level due to shortened femur.

Nursing diagnoses for the infant with DDH may include the following:

Nursing Diagnoses	Planning/Goals	Nursing Interventions
▶ *Anxiety (parental) related to having a less-than-perfect child and to the need to provide complex long-term care*	The parents will verbalize feelings about their child and the condition. The parents will carry out prescribed therapy and provide daily care with confidence.	Explore the parents' feelings about their less-than-perfect newborn and their knowledge about the defect, treatment, and need for long-term care. Teach the parents about harness use (i.e., the hips should be flexed without being tight, the harness should be worn 23 hours per day). Explore options for the safe transport of the infant (i.e., use of a special car seat, adaptation of stroller).
▶ *Skin Integrity Impaired, Risk for, related to devices*	The client's skin will remain intact.	Teach the parents to assess the infant's skin for irritation and to change the infant's position every 2 to 4 hours. Teach the parents ways of protecting the infant's skin from the brace (e.g., using a shirt that snaps at the crotch, long socks under the harness). Teach the parents to change diapers without removing the harness. Teach the parents to bathe the infant daily during the 1 hour that the harness is off.
▶ *Growth and Development, Risk for Altered, related to immobility and difficulty in positioning*	The client will attain milestones appropriate for age and limitations.	Teach the parents to provide activities that stimulate the infant's upper extremities and all five senses (e.g., blocks, musical toys, balls, bright mobiles) and to interact with the infant. Teach the parents methods of holding, nursing, feeding, and cuddling the infant when the harness is in use. Instruct the parents to include the infant in family activities and outings.

Evaluation Each goal must be evaluated to determine how it has been met by the client.

INTEGUMENTARY SYSTEM

Normally, infants have soft, smooth, dry, cool, taut, elastic skin. Color is evenly distributed but may display variations such as freckles, **mongolian spots** (large patches of bluish skin on the buttocks of dark-skinned infants), small hemangiomas called "stork bites" (on eyelids or back of the neck), and **milia** (pearly white cysts on the face). Most of these blemishes disappear within months and require no treatment.

The infant's skin is immature and, thus, susceptible to disorders. The most frequently seen skin disorders include milia rubra, diaper dermatitis, seborrheic dermatitis, and atopic dermatitis.

MILIA RUBRA

Milia rubra, also known as prickly heat, is most noticeable on the folds of the skin, chest, and neck. This rash appears as pinhead-sized **erythematous** (reddishness of the skin) papules. It commonly occurs when infants are febrile or overdressed in summer heat. Infants may be irritable because of itching.

Nursing Management

Treatment is primarily preventive. Caregivers should be taught to avoid bundling infants in hot weather. Tepid baths may help alleviate itching.

DIAPER DERMATITIS

Diaper dermatitis, also called diaper rash, is characterized by erythema (redness), edema, vesicles, papules, and scaling on the perineum, genitals, buttocks, and skin folds. It is caused by repetitive exposure to an irritant such as urine, feces, soap, detergent, ointment, friction, or infection resulting from bacteria or yeast (*Candida albicans*) (Figure 53-15). The incidence is generally reported to be greater among bottle-fed than among breastfed infants (Wong, et al., 1999).

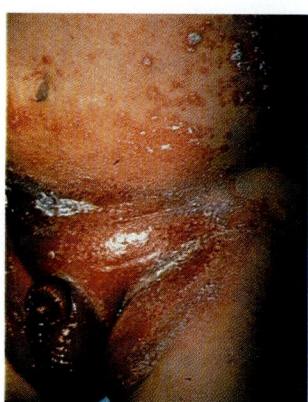

Figure 53-15 Candidiasis (*Courtesy of the Centers for Disease Control and Prevention [CDC]*)

Nursing Management

In order to prevent diaper rash, care providers must change diapers frequently and keep the infant's skin clean and dry. Use of disposable diapers and exposure of healthy skin to air, not heat, will help keep the skin dry. Ointments such as zinc oxide or petrolatum may be used to protect inflamed skin. Nystatin (Mycostatin) ointment or cream may be applied to treat Candida.

SEBORRHEIC DERMATITIS

Seborrheic dermatitis, also called cradle cap, is characterized by yellowish, scaly, or crusted patches on the scalp of infants up to 3 months of age (Figure 53-16) It typically results from excessive sebaceous gland activity.

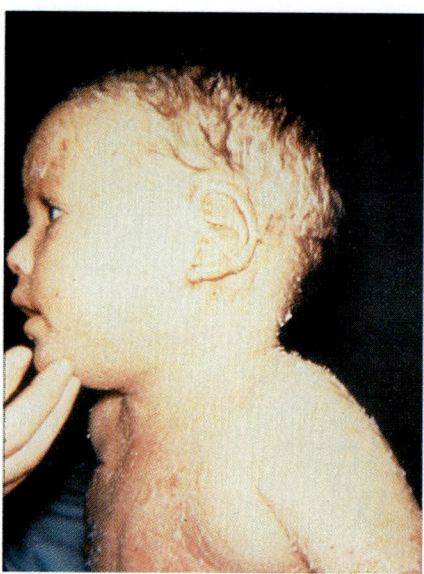

Figure 53-16 Seborrheic Dermatitis (*Courtesy of the Centers for Disease Control and Prevention [CDC]*)

LIFE CYCLE CONSIDERATIONS

Dressing Infants

Caregivers should be advised to dress infants as they themselves are dressed, being careful not to overdress the infant.

Nursing Management

Caregivers should be taught that cradle cap is not due to poor hygiene but, rather, to increased sebum production by the scalp. It will eventually disappear, although children with dry skin may continue to have flakes on the scalp. A mild shampoo or mineral oil may be left on the scalp for a few minutes to help soften and loosen the crust. The hair can then be rinsed and combed with a fine-tooth comb to loosen and remove the crust. In most cases, no further treatment is needed. The crusting can usually be prevented by washing the infant's head with a washcloth and using a fine-toothed comb.

ATOPIC DERMATITIS

Atopic dermatitis, also called eczema, is a chronic, superficial inflammatory skin disorder characterized by intense **pruritus** (severe itching). It is considered to be at least in part an allergic reaction to irritants (wool, nylon, plastics, detergents, perspiration, cosmetics, and perfumed lotions and soaps) and allergens (dust, pollens, and foods). A strong family history of eczema, asthma, food allergies, or allergic rhinitis usually predisposes a child to eczema. The disorder is uncommon among breastfed infants before other foods are added to the diet (Saarinen & Kajosaari, 1995).

Papules and vesicles usually begin forming on the cheeks and spread to the arms and legs and then to the trunk. Exudate and crust are often present.

Infantile eczema usually resolves by the age of 3 years. However, infants who have eczema tend to develop hay fever or asthma later in life.

Medical–Surgical Management

Medical

Treatment is aimed at relieving pruritus, hydrating skin, reducing inflammation, and preventing secondary infections. Baths and compresses may provide temporary relief.

Pharmacological

A variety of lotions, oral antihistamines, topical corticosteroids, and antibiotics may be prescribed.

Diet

A diet including a milk substitute such as soy formula, a vitamin supplement, and foods known to be hypoallergenic may be instituted to rule out offending foods. If the child's skin improves, foods are added back into the diet one at a time at intervals of approximately 1 week. The effects are then noted and any allergenic foods eliminated from the child's diet.

PROFESSIONAL TIP

Controlling Allergens

When teaching caregivers about the need to decrease allergens in the child's environment, the nurse should stress the following:

- "Smoking outside," rather than "not smoking"
- "Keeping pets outside," rather than "getting rid of pets"
- "Removing as much dust as possible from the child's room," rather than "removing as much dust as possible from the entire house"

Providing alternatives to the ideal situation may empower caregivers to set more realistic goals for improving their child's environment.

Health Promotion

Guidelines for preventing eczema include practicing breastfeeding; prohibiting cow's milk, eggs, fish, corn, citrus, peanuts, nuts, and chocolate for the first 12 months of life; and delaying introduction of solid foods until 6 months of age. Environmental control of dust, mold, animals, and cigarette smoke is also recommended.

Nursing Management

The major nursing goals are to soothe and relieve pruritus, maintain skin integrity, provide adequate nutrition and fluids, offer sensory stimulation, and teach the family about the condition. Caregivers may feel apprehensive or repulsed by their infant's appearance. They need to be encouraged to express their feelings but be assured that eczema, while potentially distressing, is a temporary condition.

NERVOUS SYSTEM

By the fourth week of gestation, the neural tube has closed, and the brain and the spinal cord have begun to form. By the second month of gestation, the brain is the most prominent part of the body. It grows rapidly and continues to grow through the fifth year of life. As myelinization of the peripheral nerves progresses, so do the child's coordination and fine motor abilities. The primitive reflexes (Moro, grasp, and rooting) disappear by 12 months of age. Alterations discussed following are spina bifida, hydrocephalus, febrile convulsions, **meningitis** (inflammation of the meninges), and cerebral palsy.

SPINA BIFIDA

Spina bifida is a neural tube defect wherein incomplete closure of the vertebrae and neural tube results in an opening through which meninges and spinal cord may protrude. Although the cause remains undetermined, genetic predisposition, maternal folic acid deficiency during pregnancy, and environmental factors such as pollution may be implicated. The severity of the defect can vary, with manifestations ranging from a dimple or small tuft of hair (which may be overlooked at birth) to a large, saclike protrusion anywhere along the lumbar or sacral area (Figure 53-17). The most severe form is myelomeningocele. The degree of neurological impairment depends on the location of the defect on the spinal cord and the size of the defect. The child may be asymptomatic or display neurological impairments varying from mild sensory loss to complete paralysis below the lesion. Associated defects may include hydrocephalus (present in 90% of clients) and genitourinary and orthopedic defects. Although these children often require lifelong therapy and care, many ultimately go on to live independently and become productive adults.

Medical–Surgical Management

Medical

Specialists such as neurologists, neurosurgeons, orthopedic specialists, pediatricians, urologists, and physical therapists may be needed to provide surgical repair and follow-up treatment.

Surgical

Surgery is required to close the defect but may not be performed immediately after birth. Waiting several days gives the family time to adjust to the initial shock and become involved in the decision-making process.

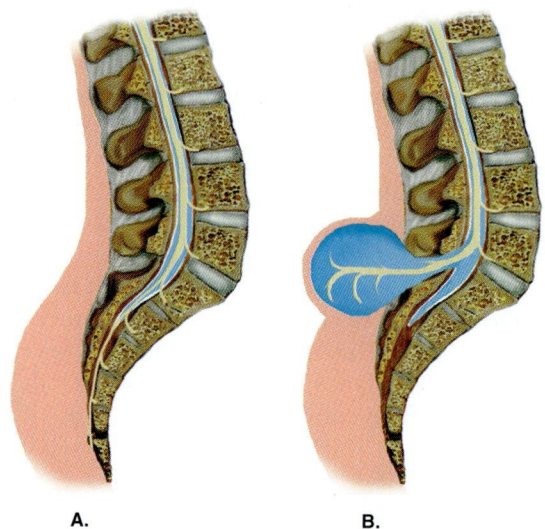

Figure 53-17 Spinal Cord: A. Normal closure; B. Myelomeningocele

Immediate closure reduces the risk of infection and allows for easier handling of the infant, which, in turn, facilitates earlier bonding.

▶ NURSING PROCESS

▶ Assessment

▶ Subjective Data

The parents' feelings about their less-than-perfect newborn and their knowledge about the defect, the treatment, and the need for long-term care must be assessed.

▶ Objective Data

At birth, the intactness of the membranous sac is assessed. Neurological impairment must be assessed by noting movement of the extremities; reflexes; anal reflex; urinary output; vital signs; fontanels; and head circumference.

Nursing diagnoses for the infant with spina bifida may include the following:

Nursing Diagnoses	Planning/Goals	Nursing Interventions
▶ *Anxiety (parental), related to having a less-than-perfect child and to the need to provide complex long-term care*	The parents will verbalize their feelings about the child and condition.	Explore the parents' feelings about their less-than-perfect newborn and their knowledge about the defect, the treatment, and the need for long-term care.
		Teach the parents ways to elicit sucking and to feed and cuddle the infant.
	The parents will carry out prescribed therapy and provide daily care with confidence.	Teach the parents to assess for signs of constipation, such as abdominal distention, vomiting, and poor feeding.
		Teach the parents to recognize signs of increased intracranial pressure, such as irritability, restlessness, and vomiting.
		Explore options for mobility, such as splints, a walker, or a wheelchair.
		Refer the family to the Spina Bifida Association and to local resources and support groups.

continued

Nursing Diagnoses	Planning/Goals	Nursing Interventions
▶ *Infection, Risk for, related to vulnerability of the sac, the surgical procedure, and the lack of bowel and bladder control*	The client will be infection free.	***Preoperative:*** Monitor the infant's vital signs, neurological status, and behavior. Administer prophylactic antibiotics, as ordered. Keep the sac covered with a moist, warm, sterile dressing and change every 2 hours. Maintain the infant in the prone position. Protect the sac from fecal contamination. ***Postoperative:*** Provide prescribed wound care. Instruct the parents in the use of intermittent, clean catheterization to keep bladder empty.
▶ *Growth and Development, Risk for Altered, related to immobility*	The client will attain milestones appropriate for age and limitations.	Teach the parents to provide activities that stimulate the infant's upper extremities and all five senses and to interact with the infant. Instruct the parents to include the infant in family activities and outings. Explore options for education and vocational training as the child grows older.

Evaluation Each goal must be evaluated to determine how it has been met by the client.

HYDROCEPHALUS

In hydrocephalus, the balance between the rate of cerebrospinal fluid (CSF) formation and absorption is disturbed. This disturbance may result from an obstruction in the circulation of CSF or from defective absorption. Hydrocephalus may be recognized at birth or weeks or months later. The condition may be congenital or occur as the result of a neoplasm, a head injury, or an infection.

Manifestations include an excessively large head at birth or rapid head growth along with widening cranial sutures. As pressure increases, the anterior fontanel becomes tense and bulges, and the eyes appear to be pushed downward, with the sclera visible above the iris ("sunset eyes"). Because of the increase in intracranial pressure, the infant may display irritability, restlessness, a high-pitched cry, vomiting, seizure, and change in level of consciousness.

Medical–Surgical Management

Surgical

Surgical intervention is the only effective means of relieving brain pressure and preventing further damage to the brain tissue. Surgery involves removing the obstruction or inserting a shunting device that bypasses the point of obstruction and drains the excess CSF into a body cavity, usually the peritoneum.

Nursing Management

Nursing assessment and care is similar to that for any infant with a neurological defect. Vital signs, head circumference, and neurological signs are monitored. Preventing infections, providing loving care to the child and support to the family, and increasing the family's knowledge about the condition are paramount. Realistic growth and development goals should be set. Many infants with hydrocephalus are able to ultimately live independently and become productive adults despite associated neurological disabilities.

FEBRILE CONVULSIONS

A convulsion or seizure involves involuntary muscle contraction and relaxation. Seizures may be a symptom of a wide variety of disorders. In infants and children, febrile seizures usually accompany such infections as otitis media, upper respiratory infections, and meningitis. Clinical manifestations include sudden occurrence, body stiffening, and loss of consciousness followed by quick, jerking movements of the arms, legs, and facial muscles. Breathing may be irregular, and swallowing ability may be absent.

Febrile seizures usually occur early in the course of a high fever. Usually, only one seizure occurs, and it will last less than 3 minutes. Febrile seizures carry little risk of neurological damage.

Medical–Surgical Management

Pharmacological

Most febrile seizures stop before the infant can be taken for medical attention. If the seizure continues, diazepam (Valium) is the drug of choice. Antipyretics such as acetaminophen (Tylenol) or ibuprophen (Motrin) may be used to reduce the infant's fever.

Nursing Management

Nursing care focuses on teaching parents about febrile seizures and treating a fever. Parents are naturally extremely anxious when their child has experienced a seizure, especially the first time. The nurse should reassure the parents that febrile seizures are not life threatening, do not cause neurological damage, are common in children under 5 years of age who are experiencing infection, usually do not recur, and usually last less than 3 minutes.

MENINGITIS

The most common infection of the central nervous system (CNS) in infants is meningitis. The three main types of causative organisms are bacterial, tubercular, and viral. Meningitis may also occur as the result of complications of neurosurgery, trauma, systemic infection, or sinus or ear infection. Bacterial meningitis is the most common and serves as the focus of this discussion.

Clinical manifestations may occur suddenly or gradually and include neurological symptoms such as a high-pitched cry, fever, seizures, irritability, as well as vomiting, a bulging anterior fontanel, and poor feeding. Early diagnosis and treatment are essential for uncomplicated recovery.

Medical–Surgical Management

Medical

Meningitis is a medical emergency. A spinal tap (lumbar puncture) is performed promptly whenever symptoms are present and prior to the administration of antibiotics. The causative organism usually can be ascertained from stained smears of the spinal fluid. Appropriate IV antibiotics are prescribed for bacterial

CLIENT TEACHING

Tips for Treating a Fever

Teach parents to care for their febrile infant by:

- Administering acetaminophen or ibuprophen, but *never* aspirin;
- Providing more clothing if the child is too cold and less clothing if the child is too warm, to prevent shivering;
- Applying cool, moist compresses to the forehead 1 hour after administering an antipyretic; and
- Encouraging fluid intake (e.g., water, juice, ice, popsicles).

meningitis. The infant is isolated from other clients for at least 24 hours.

Health Promotion

Current immunizations schedules include the *Haemophilus influenzae* type b conjugate vaccine (HbCV). The incidence of *H. influenza* type B (Hib) has greatly decreased since the advent of this immunization.

Nursing Management

After assisting with the spinal tap and starting the IV, the nurse should complete the history and physical. It is important to note any food and fluid intake, nausea, vomiting, or loss of appetite, as well as recent immunizations, illnesses, surgery, and injuries and previous lumbar puncture.

The physical examination must include a complete neurological assessment and an evaluation of head circumference. The fontanels are examined for bulging.

Nursing care includes maintaining isolation for at least 24 hours, administering antibiotics, monitoring neurological status every 4 hours, maintaining fluid balance, establishing trust with the parents and infant, teaching the parents about the disease and ways to care for their infant, and referring close contacts for possible prophylactic treatment.

CEREBRAL PALSY

Cerebral palsy (CP) is a nonprogressive motor disorder resulting from damage to the motor centers of the brain. This damage can occur during the prenatal, perinatal, or postnatal period.

Manifestations of CP vary in severity and may include delayed gross motor development (e.g., persistent head lag), alterations in muscle tone (e.g., body stiffness), abnormal motor performance (e.g., uncoordinated or involuntary movements), and reflex abnormalities (e.g., persistent tonic neck). In addition, the child may experience seizures, impaired vision and hearing, difficulty swallowing and speaking, and subnormal learning and reasoning. Less-severe cases of CP may not be diagnosed until 2 years of age.

Medical–Surgical Management

Medical

A multidisciplinary team including the family, pediatricians, neurologists, surgeons, nurses, nutritionists, therapists, social workers, and special education teachers is necessary to assist the child in developing maximum potential.

Surgical

Surgical intervention such as lengthening the Achilles' tendon and releasing the hamstrings may be necessary to improve ambulation.

▶ NURSING PROCESS

▶ Assessment

▶ Subjective Data

A history of conditions such as maternal diabetes, ABO or Rh incompatibilities, rubella in the first trimester, prematurity, prolonged labor, and postnatal infections or trauma may predispose an infant to brain damage and CP.

▶ Objective Data

The infant who feeds poorly and is rigid, tense, or hypotonic warrants further observation. Assessing for developmental delays with an instrument such as the Denver II is of utmost importance.

Nursing diagnoses for the infant with CP may include the following:

Nursing Diagnoses	Planning/Goals	Nursing Interventions
▶ *Nutrition, Altered, Less than Body Requirements, related to difficulty chewing and swallowing and to increased muscle activity*	The client will maintain a normal growth curve above the 5th percentile on the growth chart.	Encourage active swallowing by maintenance of a flexed sitting position, with the arms brought forward. Provide jaw stabilization from the front or side of the face. Provide a flexible feeding schedule with frequent, small feedings. Encourage use of adaptive utensils and foods to stimulate self-care (e.g., finger foods, foods that stick to utensils, spoon with padded handle). Refer to a nutritionist and an occupational therapist, as needed.
▶ *Growth and Development, Altered, related to neuromuscular impairment*	The client will achieve maximum potential.	Teach the parents to stimulate the infant and to interact on the infant's functional level. Encourage early intervention and participation in infant-stimulation programs.
▶ *Mobility, Impaired, Physical, related to spasticity and muscle weakness*	The client will attain mobility via assistive devices.	Refer to a physical therapist, as needed. Evaluate the need for special equipment. Ensure adequate rest. Perform prescribed range-of-motion and stretching exercises. Provide preoperative and postoperative care for the infant who requires corrective surgery. Select toys and activities that improve motor activity (e.g., place a desired toy such that the child must reach).
▶ *Communication, Verbal, Impaired, related to neuromuscular impairment and difficulty with articulation*	The client will develop methods of communication.	Refer to a speech therapist, as needed. Encourage the use of flash cards, articles, pictures, talking boards, a computer with a voice synthesizer. Encourage jaw-stabilization methods (as with feeding) to facilitate speech.

Evaluation Each goal must be evaluated to determine how it has been met by the client.

GENITOURINARY SYSTEM

During infancy, the kidneys are less able to concentrate urine, and output per kilogram of body weight is higher than that of an adult. Bladder capacity increases with age, from 20 to 50 mL at birth to 700 mL in adulthood, and the infant's urethra is shorter than the adult's. In addition, infants lack bladder control due to insufficient nerve development.

Most external defects of the genitourinary (GU) tract are not life threatening in the physical sense, but may present social problems with lifelong implications for the child and family. More severe disorders such as exstrophy of the bladder and ambiguous genitalia lead to concerns about penis size, appearance of the genitalia, altered elimination, potential ability to procreate, and rejection by peers. These children and their families need emotional support in order to adjust to these permanent alterations. Hypospadias, hydrocele, cryptorchidism, vesicoureteral reflux, and Wilm's tumor are the most common types of urinary alterations.

HYPOSPADIAS

Hypospadias is a condition wherein the urethral opening is on the ventral (under) surface of the penis (Figure 53-18). It is often associated with undescended testes and inguinal hernia and is visible on inspection at birth.

Medical–Surgical Management

Surgical

Hypospadias is surgically corrected during the first year of life. The infant is not circumcised at birth, because the foreskin may be used to correct the defect.

Nursing Management

Nursing care focuses on preparing parents for the surgical procedure and for postoperative and home care. Parents must be assured that normal urination will be restored and that sexual function will not be impeded. In addition, they must be told that the penis may never appear perfectly normal, even after the surgery. The infant may go home with a catheter in place until healing is complete. Parents must demonstrate catheter care prior to discharge.

HYDROCELE

Hydrocele is the result of the processus vaginalis failing to close, which allows fluid to enter the scrotum. The scrotum contains a palpable, round, nontender mass. This defect is often associated with inguinal hernia.

Medical–Surgical Management

Medical

Most hydroceles will close by 1 year of age without intervention.

Surgical

If spontaneous closure does not occur by 1 year of age, surgical intervention may be done on an outpatient basis.

Nursing Management

Preoperative preparation and postoperative care are the focus of the nurse. Postoperative care focuses on pain management, infection control, and activity restriction. Parents must be alerted to the potential for temporary swelling and discoloration of the scrotum.

CRYPTORCHIDISM

Cryptorchidism is a condition wherein one or both testes do not descend into the scrotal sac. One or both

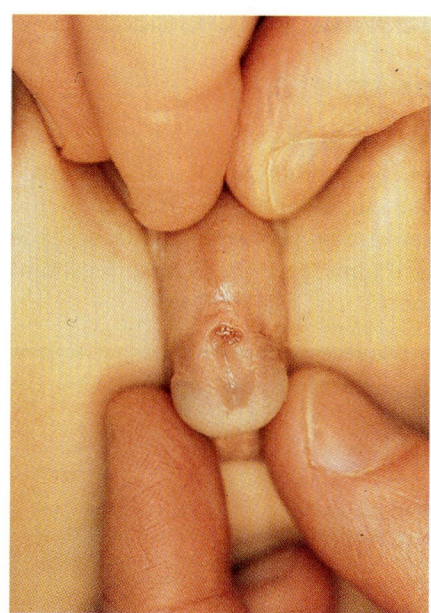

Figure 53-18 Hypospadias *(Courtesy of Dr. James Mandell, Chief Surgeon, Urology, Albany Medical College, Albany, NY)*

sides of the scrotum appear to be smaller than normal. When palpated, the scrotal sac is empty. This defect is often associated with inguinal hernia.

Medical–Surgical Management

Medical

The testes usually descend spontaneously by 1 year of age. If the testes have not descended after 1 year, hormone therapy may be prescribed.

 HOME HEALTH CARE

Infant with External GU Defect Repair

Pain Management
- Medicate for pain as prescribed for 24 to 48 hours postoperatively
- Protect the site by double diapering

Infection Control
- Handwash before and after diapering
- Carefully and thoroughly cleanse any area soiled with stool or urine
- Watch for signs of infection, such as fever, irritability, drainage, and redness
- Increase fluid intake

Activity Restriction
- Do not allow the infant to play on riding toys
- Do not allow the infant to straddle the caregiver's hip when being carried

Surgical

Surgical correction, if required, is performed by 3 years of age to prevent sterility.

Nursing Management

Preoperative preparation and postoperative care are the primary nursing concerns. Postoperative care focuses on pain management, infection control, and activity restriction.

VESICOURETERAL REFLUX

Vesicoureteral reflux refers to the backflow of urine from the bladder into the ureters and, possibly, the kidneys. Reflux can result from abnormal insertion of the ureters into the bladder or from a urinary tract infection (UTI). The primary manifestation of vesicoureteral reflux is recurrent UTIs. Specific clues of a UTI in the infant include poor feeding; vomiting; and failure to gain weight. A UTI is confirmed by detection of bacteria in the urine. Early diagnosis with radiological studies is important to prevent renal injury.

Medical–Surgical Management

Medical

The primary concern is preventing UTIs. Low-dose prophylactic antibiotic therapy is prescribed until the reflux is resolved. In addition, urine cultures, cystograms, and blood studies are necessary to monitor for UTI and kidney function. Less-severe refluxes will resolve spontaneously.

Surgical

Surgical reimplantation of the ureter(s) into the bladder may be necessary if UTIs persist.

Nursing Management

Nursing care includes treatment and prevention of UTIs (see Chapter 42). Parents must understand that medical treatment may be needed for years and that compliance as well as follow-up is important. If surgery is required, pre- and postoperative care will be needed.

WILMS' TUMOR

Wilms' tumor (nephroblastoma) is found in the kidney region and is one of the most common early childhood cancers. The tumor arises from bits of embryonic tissue remaining after birth. The etiology is unknown, but Wilm's tumor is associated with other anomalies such as GU defects, microcephaly, and mental retardation. The most common manifestations are an abdominal mass located to one side of the midline, abdominal pain, malaise, anemia, and fever.

Medical–Surgical Management

Surgical

Surgical removal of the involved kidney and lymph node is the treatment of choice. Chemotherapy and radiation may be used pre- and postoperatively, depending on the stage and size of the tumor.

Nursing Management

If a mass is felt in a child's abdomen, palpation should be stopped immediately, as it is possible to dislodge cells and spread the tumor. Nursing management focuses on pre- and postoperative care, chemotherapy administration, and family support.

COGNITIVE AND SENSORY SYSTEMS

Cognitive and sensory impairments result in a variety of lifelong challenges for infants and their families. Nursing care focuses on assessment of the degree of impairment and on appropriate interventions for individual and family adaptation. Some of the most common cognitive and sensory impairments occurring in infants include Down syndrome and visual and hearing impairments.

DOWN SYNDROME

Down Syndrome is a chromosomal anomaly resulting in moderate to severe mental retardation. There is evidence that supports trisomy 21 (an extra chromosome); translocation of chromosomes 15, 21, and 22; and advanced parental age as possible causes of Down syndrome.

Manifestations include a variety of facial and body abnormalities and intellectual, language, and social alterations. Typically, the child with Down syndrome has upward- and outward-slanted (almond-shaped) eyes; a depressed nasal bridge; a protruding tongue; small, short, low-set ears; a short, broad neck; transverse palmar crease; broad, short hands with stubby fingers; a protruding abdomen; **hypotonia** (lax muscle tone); and a blunted affect. Numerous medical conditions

PROFESSIONAL TIP

Wilm's Tumor

If a client has a Wilm's tumor, a sign stating, "Do not palpate the abdomen" should be posted at the head of the bed.

Feeding the Infant with Down Syndrome
- The tongue thrust represents a physiologic response rather than a refusal to eat
- Use a long, straight-handled spoon to place food to the back and side of the mouth
- Refeed food that is thrust out of the mouth
- Increase fluids and fiber to prevent constipation
- Monitor height and weight by plotting on a growth chart each month

may be associated with Down syndrome, including cardiac anomalies, GI defects, endocrine disorders, and leukemia.

Medical–Surgical Management

Medical

A multidisciplinary team of health care providers may be needed to assist the child with Down syndrome to reach personal maximum potential. During the first year, the focus is on monitoring for GI and cardiac disorders. Between the second and fourth years, medical emphasis is on sleep and behavioral difficulties, thyroid screening, and visual and dental assessment. Frequent infections are a common problem.

Surgical

Surgery may be required for correction of associated cardiac and GI anomalies.

Health Promotion

Prenatal diagnosis of Down syndrome is possible through genetic testing, alpha-fetoprotein (AFP) level, or amniotic fluid samples. As a result of increased prenatal diagnosis, approximately 40% of fetuses with Down syndrome in women over 35 years of age are now electively terminated (Ashwill & Droske, 1997). Therefore, the number of children born with Down syndrome is decreasing.

▶ NURSING PROCESS
▶ Assessment
▶ Subjective Data

At birth, it is especially important to elicit the family's health history, the results of amniocentesis (if done), and parental ages. As the infant grows, a thorough assessment is essential to evaluate interaction between the child and family, the family's coping abilities, and the degree to which the child is thriving.

▶ Objective Data

During the initial physical examination at birth, the nurse assesses for the unique features that indicate Down syndrome. As the child grows, assessment of developmental milestones will indicate delays in all areas (language, social, and motor).

Nursing diagnoses for the infant with Down syndrome may include the following:

Nursing Diagnoses	Planning/Goals	Nursing Interventions
▶ Social Isolation, related to fear of and embarrassment about the child's behavior or appearance	The family will achieve optimal socialization.	Assist in identifying positive features and behaviors in the infant.
		Emphasize that the infant needs play, discipline, and social interaction, as does any infant.
		Encourage the family to teach the child socially acceptable behaviors (e.g., manners and appropriate touch).
		Encourage the family to express feelings and concerns.
		Refer the family to support groups.
▶ Growth and Development, Altered, related to poor sucking abilities and anomalies	The client will maintain a normal growth curve above the 5th percentile.	Explore options for ensuring optimal fluid and calorie intake (e.g., adaptive utensils).
		Encourage self-feeding, when age appropriate.
		Maintain routine.
		Refer to dietitian, as needed.

Evaluation Each goal must be evaluated to determine how it has been met by the client.

VISUAL IMPAIRMENT

The eye is not fully developed until approximately 10 to 12 years of age. Visual acuity normally increases from a range of 20/50 to 20/80 at birth to a range of 20/20 to 20/30 by age 5 years.

Visual impairments are classified as follows: sighted with eye problems, partially sighted (20/70 to 20/200), and legally blind (20/200 or less). Refractory errors are the most common type of childhood visual disorders.

Strabismus (crossed eye) is due to lack of coordination of the extraocular muscles. When both eyes are unable to focus simultaneously, the brain suppresses the image from the deviating eye to prevent double vision (diplopia). Amblyopia (blindness from disuse) can develop if strabismus is not treated early. If untreated amblyopia occurs in a child younger than 4 years of age, permanent loss of vision in the deviated eye may result.

Manifestations of visual impairment may include failure to follow an object or to react to bright light, excessive rubbing of the eyes, squinting, tilting of the head, and crossed eyes (after 6 months of age). Visual impairments may be caused by perinatal and postnatal infections; conditions such as sickle-cell disease, juvenile rheumatoid arthritis, glaucoma, cataracts and retinoblastoma; and injuries.

Medical–Surgical Management

Medical

Most visual disorders are treated with corrective lenses. Strabismus may require patching of the stronger eye to increase visual stimulation of the weaker eye. The earlier the treatment, the better the chances of normal development and function and adequate vision.

Surgical

Surgical intervention is required for glaucoma, cataracts, and, sometimes, strabismus.

Nursing Management

Early detection and referral are crucial in preventing childhood visual impairment. At birth, the nurse assesses response to visual stimuli, ability to fixate and follow an object to midline, and ability to make eye contact. At 3 months of age, the infant is assessed for ability to follow moving objects. Crossed eyes after 6 months of age warrants further evaluation. Referrals are made to available associations and support groups as needed (see the Resources listed at the end of this book).

Preoperative and postoperative care are provided when surgical intervention is required. It is most important that the nurse educate the parents about the condition, the prescribed treatment, home care, and follow-up.

HEARING IMPAIRMENT

At birth, the ear is completely developed. Hearing impairments range from mild to profound and include deaf as well as hard of hearing. Hearing loss is divided into four categories. Conductive (middle-ear hearing loss) is the most common type of hearing impairment and results from interference of transmission of sound to the middle ear. It is usually caused by otitis media. Sensorineural hearing loss (nerve deafness) involves damage to the inner-ear structures and/or auditory nerves. Mixed hearing loss is a combination of conductive and sensorineural loss. It is usually caused by recurrent otitis media. Central hearing loss results from damage to the conduction system between the brain stem and the cerebral cortex.

Infants at risk for hearing loss include those with prenatal, perinatal, and postnatal conditions including a family history of hearing impairments; malformations; low birth weight; asphyxia; infection; CP; Down syndrome; or a history of being administered ototoxic drugs.

Manifestations of hearing impairment in the infant include failure to startle or awaken to a loud sound, to turn the head to sound by 4 months of age, and to babble by 3 months of age. As the child with a hearing impairment matures, language skills are affected, and the child may be perceived as having cognitive as well as behavioral problems.

Medical–Surgical Management

Medical

Treatment depends on the cause and type of loss. Antibiotics are prescribed for otitis media, which is the most common cause of conduction loss. Sensorineural loss is usually irreversible. Hearing aids or cochlear implants may be recommended.

Surgical

Insertion of tympanostomy tubes for chronic otitis media is controversial.

Nursing Management

Detection and prevention are the most important goals for the nurse. All children should be assessed for hearing acuity at birth, at well-child visits, and whenever there is a complaint specific to the ears. Developmental assessments will reveal language delays in infants and children with hearing impairments. When delays are noted, the child is referred for further evaluation.

CHILD ABUSE

Child abuse is any intentional act of physical neglect or physical, emotional, or sexual abuse committed by a person responsible for the care of a child. Child abuse can be detected at any age, even in utero. However, adolescents experience the greatest incidence of abuse.

PHYSICAL NEGLECT

Physical neglect is failure to provide the adequate hygiene, health care, nutrition, love, nurturing, and supervision required for an infant's normal growth and development. Clinical manifestations of physical neglect in the infant may include inadequate weight gain, dental caries, poor hygiene, and lack of immunizations.

PHYSICAL ABUSE

Physical punishment that leaves marks, causes injury, or threatens the child's physical or emotional well-being is considered physical abuse. Typical clinical manifestations of physical abuse include bruises on the abdomen, buttocks, genitalia, thighs, and mouth; bruises with distinctive outlines indicative of such things as hangers, belt buckles, hands, teeth, and sticks; bone fractures at various stages of healing; spiral fractures; cerebral edema or hemorrhage; and burns (e.g., from immersion of feet in hot water or from cigarettes). The child may appear sad and forlorn or may actively seek to please.

Predisposing factors to physical abuse include characteristics of the parent, child, and environment. Parents who abuse their children may have been severely punished as children, have difficulty controlling aggressive impulses, be socially isolated, and have few supportive relationships. Children at greatest risk for abuse are those who are premature, illegitimate, unwanted, brain damaged, hyperactive, physically disabled, or "difficult" (Ashwill & Droske, 1997; Wong, et. al., 1999). A stressful environment due to divorce, poverty, unemployment, poor housing, frequent relocation, and drug addiction may contribute to physical abuse. However, abuse occurs at all educational, social, and economic levels.

A more unusual type of abuse is Munchausen syndrome, wherein one person either fabricates or induces illness in another to get attention. Usually, the mother has the syndrome and inflicts injury on her child.

EMOTIONAL ABUSE

Emotional abuse includes acts or omissions by the caregiver that could cause serious behavioral, cognitive, emotional, or mental disorders. Emotional abuse may involve shaming, ridiculing, embarrassing, or insulting the child, and destruction of the child's personal property. Clinical manifestations in the emotionally abused child may include developmental delays, failure to thrive, disruptive behavior, extreme behavior (withdrawal, aggression), and unusual fearfulness, obsessions, and suicide attempts.

SEXUAL ABUSE

Sexual abuse is the exploitation of a child for the sexual gratification of an adult. Common forms of sexual abuse are oral–genital contact, fondling and caressing of the genitals, intercourse (vaginal or anal), rape, sodomy, and prostitution. Possible clinical manifestations in the infant include vaginal discharge; blood-stained diapers; genital redness, pain, itching, or bruising; lax rectal tone; difficulty sitting; and UTIs

Medical–Surgical Management

Medical

Diagnosis of abuse is based on a careful history and thorough physical examination. Injuries are treated as needed. All health care providers are legally required to report any suspected child abuse to the local child protective agency.

▶ NURSING PROCESS

▶ Assessment

▶ Subjective Data

The nurse obtains information about parental concerns; a general family history; and a specific child history. Beginning with nonthreatening topics allows the nurse to demonstrate concern before asking about suspected abuse. Details about the way the injuries occurred should be documented verbatim and using quotation marks.

▶ Objective Data

Physical assessment and documentation must be thorough. Figure diagrams should be used to document skin injuries. Inconsistencies between what reportedly happened and the extent of injuries constitute a strong indicator of child abuse.

Nursing diagnoses for the abused child may include the following:

Nursing Diagnoses	Planning/Goals	Nursing Interventions
▶ *Injury, Risk for, related to family history of abuse/ neglect*	The client will be free from abuse/neglect.	Use a nonthreatening, nonjudgmental manner when interacting with the parents.
		Assess and document the child's history and physical examination results, family history, parent–child interactions, the child's response to surroundings and strangers, and the child's developmental level.

continued

Nursing Diagnoses	Planning/Goals	Nursing Interventions
		Report all cases of suspected child abuse.
		Assist in removing the child from the unsafe environment.
		Refer the family to social services, as needed.
▶ *Parenting, Altered, related to lack of knowledge*	The family will respond to the child's needs appropriately.	Assess the family's strengths, weaknesses, coping mechanisms, and support systems.
		Assess the parents' expectations of the child; choice and use of comfort measures; responses to the child; and general knowledge about the child.
		Discuss the parenting that the parents received as children.
		Provide information regarding normal growth and development, nutrition, well-child care, and nurturing.
		Role-model when interacting with the child.
		Encourage the parents to participate in the child's care.
		Reinforce positive behaviors on the part of the parents.
		Assist the family in identifying stressors and options for decreasing stress.
		Refer the parents to a support group such as Parents Anonymous.

Evaluation Each goal must be evaluated to determine how it has been met by the client.

ENVIRONMENTAL SAFETY

As infants develop and become mobile explorers, environmental safety becomes a major concern for all caregivers. An important role of the nurse is to educate caregivers regarding maintaining a safe environment and administering appropriate aid in the event of an accident. Common environmental safety hazards include poisoning, trauma, suffocation, and drowning.

POISONING

Poisonous substances can be found everywhere. Commonly ingested substances include cosmetics and other personal care products, medicines, cleaning products, plants, gasoline, toys, lead-based paint, and other miscellaneous foreign substances.

Medical–Surgical Management

Medical

The poison control center should be called initially and immediately to ascertain whether the child should be treated at home or taken to a treatment center. When the exact substance and amount are unknown, the child should be taken to a treatment center, where complications can be anticipated and life support provided, if needed.

Vomiting is usually initiated immediately to the conscious child, unless the ingested substance is corrosive or highly irritating. Corrosives and irritants can cause further damage to mucous membranes of the esophagus and pharynx if vomited.

When emesis is contraindicated, gastric lavage is used to evacuate the stomach contents. In addition, activated charcoal may be administered to prevent further absorption of the poison.

Pharmacological

The drug of choice for inducing vomiting is ipecac syrup. Children 6 to 12 months of age should be given 10 mL orally followed by approximately 8 oz of a fluid of choice. Results should occur within 30 minutes (Eisenhauer, Nichols, Spencer, & Bergan, 1998).

Activated charcoal may be administered orally or through an orogastric tube to further absorb the poison and remove it from the body. Because activated charcoal inactivates ipecac syrup, it is best administered after emesis. Activated charcoal may be mixed with a cathartic such as magnesium sulfate (Epsom salts). An antiemetic is sometimes needed.

Magnesium sulfate may be prescribed to promote rapid elimination, thereby decreasing absorption of the poison. Mixing magnesium sulfate with a sweet liquid may enhance its palatability. Results should occur within 2 to 4 hours.

Nursing Management

The nurse focuses on poison prevention as well as on care of the poisoned child. Through printed materials such as checklists for poison proofing a home and illustrated first-aid guidelines, nurses should educate the public about ways to decrease the incidence of poisonings. Consciousness-raising efforts should be included in each plan of care. Parents must be reminded of the importance of keeping the phone number of the poison control center on the phone and having ipecac syrup and magnesium sulfate on hand at all times.

When confronted with a poisoning incident, the nurse focuses on maintaining vital functions, preventing continued absorption of the poison, preventing complications related to the poisoning and treatment, reducing fear, and educating the caregiver about poison prevention. Once the child's condition is stabilized, exposure to the poison must be terminated. Substances should be removed from the mouth first manually and then by a sip of water; from the eye with a continuous flush of normal saline; and from the skin by removing contaminated clothing and washing the skin with soap and water.

Once exposure is terminated, the substance should be identified and the poison control center consulted. Procedures to induce vomiting and prevent absorption are initiated as directed by the poison control center.

TRAUMA

Falls and motor vehicle injuries are the most common causes of trauma in infants. Medical–surgical management is dictated by the location and extent of the injury.

Nursing Management

Preventing trauma or injuries is of utmost importance. Parents must stay aware of their infant's abilities as the infant grows and develops and be prepared to

CLIENT TEACHING

Poison Prevention

Advise caregivers of the following poison prevention measures:

- Keep all medicines and household cleaners in original containers with childproof caps and out of reach of children
- Do not treat medicine like candy *or* candy like medicine
- Read labels carefully before using medicines and household cleaners
- Attach the poison control center's phone number to the phone
- Keep ipecac syrup and magnesium sulfate on hand at all times (even on trips)
- Prevent children from chewing or ingesting plants
- Be aware of those things at a child's eye level by crawling around the house on hands and knees
- Mop floors and woodwork with a wet mop at least once a week (especially if the house was built prior to 1960)

provide a safe environment. Everytime a nurse encounters a parent, developmentally appropriate safety information and reminders should be provided. In addition, car seat safety must be stressed.

SUFFOCATION/DROWNING

Suffocation occurs when air exchange is hindered by covering the mouth or nose, applying pressure to the throat and chest, or excluding air (e.g., via refrigerator entrapment).

CLIENT TEACHING

Tips for Maintaining a Safe Environment throughout Infancy

At 4 months, infants begin to roll and become very active:

- Keep crib side rails all the way up
- Do not leave the infant unattended on raised areas like beds, sofas, changing tables; instead, place on the floor or in a playpen
- Use walkers away from the stairs
- Never leave the infant unattended in the tub
- Place car seat in the center of the back seat and facing backward until the infant is 20 pounds or 12 months old. *Always use a car seat.*

At 6 months, infants begin to crawl, reach, and put things in their mouths:

- Keep the floor swept and be alert for small objects that may be put in the mouth.
- Put gates at the tops and bottoms of stairways
- Keep bathroom doors closed
- Dress the infant in clothing that allows freedom of movement
- Do not leave the infant unattended in high chair
- Keep cords and plastic bags out of the infant's reach

At 8 months, infants begin to pull up and walk around furniture:

- Ensure that furniture both inside and outside the house is sturdy enough for the infant to pull self to standing
- Eliminate containers of water inside and outside the house
- Avoid dressing the infant in socks without shoes

At 10 to 12 months, infants may begin to walk:

- Keep exterior doors secure
- Secure gates around swimming pools
- Keep appliance doors closed at all times
- Place the infant over 20 pounds in a front-facing car seat

Drowning can occur in only inches of water. Drowning is a great concern when an infant is in the tub.

Nursing Management

Educating parents and care providers is of utmost importance. Safe cribs have no more than 2⅜ inch space between the slats, and the crib mattress fits snugly against the slats. The crib is placed out of reach of windows and other furniture that may have cords or strings that could entrap or strangle a child. Other objects that may contribute to suffocation are electrical cords, toys with strings, plastic bags, pieces of balloons, crib mobiles, pieces of hard food, and restraining straps.

Drowning may occur in toilets, buckets of water, tubs, and pools. Nurses should remind caregivers that an infant or young child will not roll from the back to the stomach when the child's face is covered with water and that infants are top heavy and do not have the strength to pull themselves out of a bucket should they fall in head first.

CASE STUDY

Janie is a 10-month-old female who was brought to the clinic by her grandmother. The grandmother reports that Janie is irritable, refuses to eat, and does not want to be rocked or cuddled. Janie's temperature is 102°F. She had been treated for an upper respiratory infection 10 days ago. A spinal tap indicates that Janie has meningitis. An IV is started, and antibiotics are administered.

The following questions will guide your development of a nursing care plan for the case study.

1. List subjective and objective data a nurse should obtain about Janie.
2. List three nursing diagnoses and goals for Janie.
3. List three successful outcomes for Janie.
4. How can the spread of this infection be prevented?
5. What must be included in discharge planning if Janie's recovery is uneventful?

SUMMARY

- The most common skin disorders of infancy are diaper rash, eczema, and cradle cap.
- The immaturity of the respiratory system creates hazards for the healthy infant and places the compromised infant at even greater risk of infection.
- Sudden infant death syndrome is the leading cause of death among infants.
- Signs of congenital heart disease in the infant include poor weight gain, poor feeding habits, fatigue, and respiratory infections.
- Iron-deficiency anemia can be prevented largely by teaching parents the importance of providing iron-fortified formula to infants until the age of 12 months.
- Possible signs of GI obstruction in the infant include abdominal pain, nausea and vomiting, abdominal distention, and decreased stool output.
- Treatment of colic may involve a change in feeding practices, correction of a stressful environment, and support of the parents.
- The most common defects of the GU tract include cryptorchidism, hydrocele, and hypospadias.
- The nursing goals when caring for infants with musculoskeletal impairments focus on preventing both skin breakdown and developmental delays.
- Infants become feverish quickly and must be observed for febrile seizures and protected from injury.
- Routine immunization of infants against *H. Influenzae* type B infection has reduced the incidence of bacterial meningitis.
- Developmental assessment will reveal language and social delays in infants with hearing and visual impairments.
- Inconsistencies between what reportedly happened and the extent of injuries constitute a strong indicator of child abuse.

Review Questions

1. An appropriate nursing intervention when caring for an infant with an upper respiratory infection and elevated temperature is to:
   a. give tepid water baths to reduce fever.
   b. encourage food intake to maintain caloric needs.

c. dress the infant in heavy clothing to prevent chilling.

d. give frequent, small amounts of favorite fluids to prevent dehydration.

2. An early clinical manifestation of CF is:

a. meconium ileus.

b. foul-smelling, frothy, greasy stools.

c. a history of poor intestinal absorption.

d. recurrent pneumonia and lung infections.

3. A 2-month-old breastfed infant with acute diarrhea is successfully rehydrated with oral solutions. The mother will now be instructed to:

a. continue breastfeeding.

b. stop breastfeeding until the breast milk can be cultured.

c. stop breastfeeding until diarrhea is absent for 24 hours.

d. express breast milk and dilute with sterile water before feeding.

4. During the first few days following surgical repair of an infant's cleft lip, the nurse will instruct the mother to:

a. provide crib toys for distraction.

b. remove restraints periodically to cuddle the infant.

c. keep the infant heavily sedated to prevent suture strain.

d. leave the infant in the crib at all times to prevent suture strain.

5. A new mother asks the nurse, "How can diaper rash be prevented?" The nurse's best response is:

a. "Wash the area with soap and water after every diaper change."

b. "Wash the area with mild soap and water and dry thoroughly after stools."

c. "Wash the area with soap before applying a thin layer of oil after stools."

d. "Wipe the buttocks with oil and apply powder to creases after every diaper change."

6. When caring for an infant with eczema, the priority nursing intervention is:

a. relieving pruritus.

b. keeping lesions dry.

c. keeping the infant content.

d. maintaining adequate nutrition.

7. A clinical manifestation of increased intracranial pressure in infants is:

a. irritability.

b. diarrhea.

c. photophobia.

d. flat anterior fontanel.

8. After an infant's myelomeningocele has been repaired, the major long-term threat to life will be:

a. renal disease.

b. heart disease.

c. endocrine problems.

d. reparative problems.

Critical Thinking Questions

1. What would you say to a parent who refused to have a child immunized?

2. What can nurses do to decrease the incidence of alterations in sensory function among children?

 WEB FLASH!

- Find the Web site for updated immunization practices.
- Search under some of the disorders covered in this chapter, such as cystic fibrosis and Down syndrome. Are there Web sites offering information specific to infants? Families? Nurses?
- What resources (books, video, chat rooms) can you locate on the Web that are devoted to families caring for infants with specific disorders?

COMMON PROBLEMS: 1–18 YEARS

LEARNING OBJECTIVES

Upon completion of this chapter, you should be able to:
- *Define key terms.*
- *Discuss the common disorders of the integumentary system in children.*
- *Differentiate the pathophysiology, common diagnostic tests, treatment, and nursing care for skin conditions in children as compared to adults.*
- *Differentiate the etiology, medical–surgical management, and nursing care for respiratory conditions in children as compared to adults.*
- *Describe the causes, assessment, and management of rheumatic fever in children.*
- *Differentiate the pathophysiology, common diagnostic tests, treatment, and nursing care for digestive conditions in children as compared to adults.*
- *Differentiate the etiology, medical–surgical management, and nursing care for genitourinary conditions in children as compared to adults.*
- *Discuss communicable and infectious diseases of childhood, including their causative agents, transmission, incubation periods, contagious periods, prevention, signs and symptoms, treatment, and nursing care.*
- *Differentiate the etiology, medical–surgical management, and nursing care for orthopedic conditions in children as compared to adults.*
- *Briefly describe behavioral problems in children, including symptoms, treatment, and nursing care.*
- *Plan care for a child with any of the common pediatric disorders.*

INTRODUCTION

Pediatric nursing focuses on protecting children from illness and injury as well as assisting them to attain optimal levels of functioning, regardless of health status. In addition, the pediatric nurse must understand the phases of a child's growth and development (refer to Chapter 14) and be sensitive to the importance of family interactions. This chapter focuses on common childhood conditions and illnesses affecting all systems of the body; the typical medical and surgical management for these conditions; and nursing management of the child and family.

RESPIRATORY SYSTEM

Disorders of the respiratory system that occur most often in children include upper-respiratory infections, allergic rhinitis, tonsillitis, asthma, and foreign-body aspiration.

UPPER-RESPIRATORY INFECTIONS

Common upper-respiratory infections include naso-pharyngitis (the common cold), pharyngitis, and in-fluenza. Nasopharyngitis is usually credited with being the most common childhood respiratory illness. These disorders are generally responsive to supportive thera-pies, and symptoms typically improve within 3 days. Clinical manifestations, etiology, and management of these common upper-respiratory disorders are pre-sented in Table 54-1.

Nursing Management

Maintaining fluid intake, providing comfort mea-sures, and preventing spread of infection are the main goals of care for the child with an upper-respiratory in-fection. The child should not be forced to eat if ap-petite is decreased. An appropriate diet may include cool, bland fluids and soft foods such as gelatin, soup, mashed potatoes, puddings, hot cereals, and ice pops. Parents should be taught to observe for urinary output and for moist mucous membranes as signs of adequate hydration.

Comfort measures may include warm salt-water gar-gles (¼ tsp salt per 8 oz glass of water) and warm or cool compresses applied to the throat. Nasal decon-gestion may be relieved with normal saline drops be-fore feedings and at bedtime. A cool-mist humidifier at the bedside may also relieve symptoms.

It is important that parents know how both to take a child's temperature and to safely administer nonsalicy-late antipyretics, such as acetaminophen (Tylenol). Salicylates, such as aspirin, are not used because of the associated risk of Reye's syndrome.

Parents and children should be taught methods for preventing the spread of infection, such as conscien-tious handwashing, proper disposal of tissues, and covering of the nose and mouth when coughing and sneezing. It is also important to avoid contact with in-fectious persons. Preventing the spread of infection is especially challenging in school and crowded living

Table 54-1 DISTINGUISHING CHARACTERISTICS OF COMMON URIs

	NASOPHARYNGITIS	PHARYNGITIS	INFLUENZA
Manifestations	**Rhinorrhea** (watery nasal discharge), conges-tion, sneezing, fever, cough, sore throat, muscular aches, and, possibly, enlarged lymph nodes	Sore throat, erythema and inflamma-tion of the pharynx and tonsils, fever, enlarged, tender cervical lymph nodes *Viral:* gradual onset, hoarseness, cough, rhinitis, malaise *Bacterial:* abdominal pain, vomiting, headache	Chills, fever, flushed face, myalgia (pain in muscles), cough, rhinitis, headache, sore throat, photophobia, conjunctivitis
Etiology	Viral	Viral (80%) or bacterial (20%)	Influenza virus
Incidence	Typically 6 to 9 colds per year, most commonly in the fall and spring	Most common among 4 to 7-year-olds	Highest among school-age children
Management	Rest, fluids, nonsalicylate antipyretics, oral decon-gestants, sterile saline nose drops	Rest; fluids; nonsalicylate antipyretics or ibuprophen; warm salt-water gar-gles; cool, bland liquids; antibiotics for streptococcal infections	Rest, fluids, nonsalicylate antipyretics

CLIENT TEACHING

Administering Normal Saline Drops
1. Instill two drops
2. Wait 5 minutes
3. Instill two more drops
4. Drops should not be used for more than 3 days.

PROFESSIONAL TIP

Throat Culture
The only reliable means of determining whether pharyngitis is viral or bacterial is with a throat culture. The nurse is most often the person who performs a throat smear for culture, which requires a physician's order. The applicator is swabbed across the tonsils, the posterior edge of the soft palate, and the uvula.

environments. Children in day care centers suffer a higher rate of infection than do children who spend their days in the home.

Untreated streptococcal infections may lead to complications such as rheumatic fever, meningitis, and glomerulonephritis. Parents of children with pharyngitis due to streptococcal infection ("strep throat") must understand the importance of completing the course of prescribed antibiotics.

ALLERGIC RHINITIS

Allergic rhinitis ("hay fever") is an inflammatory disorder of the nasal mucosa. Most often, it is a seasonal, recurrent response to allergens such as animal dander, house dust, pollens, and molds. Manifestations include rhinorrhea, postnasal drip, sneezing, allergic conjunctivitis, sniffing, itchy nose and palate, dark circles under the eyes, and the "allergic salute" (transverse nasal crease that results from repeatedly pushing nose upward and backward to relieve itching).

Medical–Surgical Management

Pharmacological

Antihistamines, decongestants, and bronchodilators may be given to relieve symptoms of congestion and difficulty with breathing. Topical intranasal corticosteroids are quite effective in children who do not respond to antihistamines and decongestants. Systemic corticosteroids may be used in extreme cases. Immunotherapy or desensitization to allergens may be initiated if antihistamines and decongestants are not effective in relieving symptoms or are needed chronically. Desensitization is performed for those allergens that produce a positive reaction on skin testing. The allergist sets up a schedule for injections in gradually increasing doses until a maintenance dose is reached. Desensitization is considered to be a safe procedure with considerable benefit for some children. Severe reactions are uncommon. During immunotherapy, children must be observed for signs of anaphylaxis for 30 minutes after each injection.

Health Promotion

The treatment of choice is to eliminate the allergen from the child's environment. Recommendations for limiting the child's exposure to allergens include avoiding wool and down; using dust proof covers on bedding; removing carpets, draperies, and blinds from the child's room, if not the whole house; keeping humidity lower than 50%; keeping pets outside; and using air filters.

Nursing Management

Nursing care focuses on therapeutic management of the disease. After identification of the allergens, the family may need assistance with allergy proofing the home and administering medications.

Drowsiness, dry mouth, and excitability are side effects of some antihistamines. Combining an antihistamine and decongestant may prevent drowsiness.

TONSILLITIS

Tonsillitis, a common illness among children, is an inflammation of the tonsils (two masses of lymphoid tissue located at the back of the mouth), resulting from pharyngitis. Tonsils filter and protect the respiratory and alimentary tracts from infection. They normally enlarge progressively between 2 and 10 years of age and reduce during preadolescence. If the tonsils become enlarged from infection, they can interfere with breathing and swallowing and cause partial deafness. Clinical manifestations of tonsillitis include sore throat; enlarged, bright-red tonsils; mouth breathing; halitosis; nasal speech; and snoring.

Medical–Surgical Management

Surgical

Tonsillectomy may be warranted in cases of abscesses, upper airway obstruction, and obstructive sleep apnea. Adenoidectomy (removal of lymphoid tissue in the nasal pharynx) is performed in cases of recurrent otitis media with eustachian tube obstruction or for persistent nasal or airway obstruction. If tonsillectomy can be postponed until 4 or 5 years of age, the apparent need often will have disappeared.

Pharmacological

Medical treatment includes analgesics for pain, antipyretics for fever, and antibiotics for streptococcal infections.

▶ NURSING PROCESS

▶ Assessment

▶ Subjective Data

The nurse must be sensitive to the child's and family's level of anxiety and offer opportunities for expression of concerns. The use of puppets, dolls, and other materials may be an effective way to allow the child to act out the pending surgical experience and to express concerns and fears.

▶ Objective Data

Presurgical assessments such as complete blood count (CBC), clotting time and urinalysis are usually done on an outpatient basis.

Upon admission on the day of surgery, vital signs and laboratory results are reviewed for abnormalities, and the child is assessed for signs of infection (fever, elevated white blood count [WBC], and redness and exudate of the throat). In addition, the child's mouth is observed for loose teeth that could be aspirated during anesthesia.

Postoperatively, assessment focuses on monitoring vital signs and observing for hemorrhage, ability to swallow, and dehydration. The most obvious signs of bleeding from the surgical site are restlessness or anxiety, frequent swallowing, and rapid pulse. Each time vital signs are taken, a flashlight should be used to observe the pharynx for bleeding.

Nursing diagnoses for the child following a tonsillectomy may include the following:

Nursing Diagnoses	Planning/Goals	Nursing Interventions
▶ *Aspiration, Risk for, related to unswallowed saliva and postoperative bleeding*	The client's airway will remain patent.	Maintain the child in a prone or side-lying position. Monitor vital signs every 15 minutes for 1 hour and hourly for the next 4 hours. Ensure availability of suction equipment. Do not give oral fluids until the child is completely awake. Avoid hot liquids, irritating foods, and use of straws. Instruct the child to avoid coughing and clearing the throat; encourage the child to expectorate secretions into a tissue.
▶ *Fluid Volume, Risk for Deficit, related to blood loss and decreased oral intake*	The client will maintain appropriate fluid intake and demonstrate minimal fluid loss.	Observe for signs of blood loss, such as frequent swallowing, elevated pulse and respirations, pallor, restlessness and anxiety; report to physician immediately. Maintain intravenous (IV) fluids until the child is taking oral fluids. Encourage intake of cold or cool liquids such as ice pops (no red), noncitric juices, gelatin (no red), and ice chips; introduce milk products only after clear liquids are tolerated. Record hourly intake and output (I & O).
▶ *Pain related to surgical procedure*	The client will have pain relief (< 3 on a scale of 1 to 10).	Provide nonaspirin analgesic every 4 hours for at least the first 24 hours postoperative. Use age-appropriate pain assessment tools. Encourage the parents to stay at the child's bedside to provide reassurance and comfort.
▶ *Knowledge Deficit (family) related to discharge care*	The caregivers will verbalize an understanding of discharge care.	Instruct the caregivers to: • Watch for signs of hemorrhage especially between the fifth and tenth postoperative days. • Watch for signs of infection (persistent earache, temperature over 102°F). • Call physician if bleeding or signs of infection occurs. • Encourage liquids and soft foods as tolerated for 10 days. • Avoid rough, scratchy foods for 3 weeks. • Maintain pain control with nonaspirin analgesics every 4 hours as needed during first week. • Restrict the child's activity for 10 days (i.e., no school or vigorous exercise). • Expect the throat to be white in appearance and the mouth odor to be bad for the first week. • Bring child for follow-up visit in 1–2 weeks.

Evaluation Each goal must be evaluated to determine how it has been met by the client.

ASTHMA

Asthma, a reactive airway disease (RAD), is defined as narrowing or obstruction of the airway triggered by stimuli (such as cold air, smoke, viral infection, exercise, stress, drugs, or allergens) and inflammation that leads to mucosal edema and mucus hypersecretion. Asthma is the leading cause of school absenteeism and the most common admitting diagnosis in children's hospitals (Behrman, Kliegman, & Arvin, 1996). Clinical manifestations of asthmatic attacks or episodes include a dry, hacking cough; wheezing; and difficulty breathing. The child may need to sit up to breathe. Attacks may last for hours or days. Thick, tenacious mucus may be expectorated after a coughing episode. In children with repeated acute exacerbations, barrel chest and the use of accessory muscles of respiration are common findings. Chronic asthmatics are usually small according to the standard growth charts. In some cases, episodes no longer occur after puberty, and growth usually catches up in adolescence. There is evidence suggesting that RAD is hereditary (Behrman, Kliegman, & Arvin, 1996). A definitive diagnosis of asthma can be made when the airway obstruction (indicated by pulmonary function tests) is reversed with bronchodilators.

Medical–Surgical Management

Medical

Medical treatment is aimed at preventing airway damage resulting from repeated and severe episodes of asthma. Care is focused on early recognition and treatment of episodes, identification and elimination of allergens, and education of the child and family. Allergy proofing the home along with skin testing followed by desensitization are methods used to control allergens (Refer to the section on Allergic Rhinitis).

Families are educated about the disease, including ways to prevent attacks; early signs of episodes; drug therapy; appropriate exercise; and chest physiotherapy (CPT), if needed. Early symptoms include increasing cough at night, in the early morning, or in conjunction with activity; respiratory retractions; and wheezing. Using a peak flowmeter is an objective way to measure airway obstruction: families must learn how both to use this device and to record the results.

Pharmacological

A combination of bronchodilators and anti-inflammatory agents is used to treat asthma. The most commonly prescribed bronchodilators are albuterol

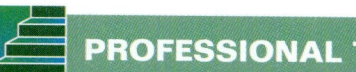

PROFESSIONAL TIP

Theophylline

The margin of safety is narrow with theophylline. Early adverse effects include irritability, restlessness, insomnia, headache, vomiting, and diarrhea.

(Ventolin), metaproterenol sulfate (Alupent), and terbutaline (Brethine). These drugs cause relaxation of bronchial smooth muscle and inhibit the release of mediators from mast cells. Small doses by inhalation are the most effective mode of administration. Bronchodilators may be taken together by inhalation and be given parenterally for additional effect. Repetitive use may mask increasing airway inflammation and hyper-responsiveness. Correct use of metered-dose inhaler (MDI) is important for maintaining control of asthma symptoms.

Theophylline is the oldest effective bronchodilator. It requires continuous oral or IV administration and is most therapeutic when the serum level measures 10–20 μg/mL.

Anti-inflammatory drugs of choice include cromolyn sodium (Crolom) and corticosteroids such as prednisone (Deltasone). Cromolyn is an antiasthmatic, mast cell stabilizer that prevents asthma symptoms by blocking the release of mast cell mediators. Once symptoms start, however, cromolyn is ineffective. Adverse effects associated with cromolyn are airway irritation with mild cough and a bad taste. Corticosteroids effectively reduce mucosal edema and potentiate the effect of bronchodilators. Steroids may be given in inhaled form to reduce the oral dose required and to decrease systemic effects that accompany oral administration. Long-term use of oral steroids is reserved for chronic asthma that has not responded to other drugs. Adverse side effects of long-term oral therapy include Cushing's syndrome, growth suppression, osteoporosis, glaucoma, cataracts, peptic ulcer, hyperglycemia, and decreased resistance to infection (Eisenhauer et al., 1998).

Activity

Children with asthma should not be automatically restricted from physical activity. With adequate treatment, a child with asthma can participate in most physical activities. Sports that do not require sustained exertion, such as gymnastics, baseball, and weight lifting, are well tolerated. Swimming is frequently recommended as an ideal sport because the air is humidified, and breathing increases end expiratory pressure.

SAMPLE NURSING CARE PLAN

THE CHILD WITH ASTHMA

Mikala, a 5-year-old girl, was admitted to the emergency room (ER) with severe coughing, fever, and difficulty breathing. Crackles and wheezing were evident in all fields upon auscultation. Vital signs were temperature 102°F; pulse, 160; and respirations, 40. Pulse oximetry was 90%. Her parents had given her Tylenol for what they thought was a "cold." When her condition worsened during the night, they brought her to the ER. Mikala has no history of asthma but has eczema. She has just started kindergarten. Her parents are extremely distraught and are asking many questions. Mikala cries every time anyone enters the room.

Nursing Diagnosis 1: *Airway Clearance, Ineffective, related to secretions in the bronchi and exudate in the alveoli as evidenced by difficulty breathing, crackles, and wheezing*

PLANNING/GOALS	NURSING INTERVENTIONS	RATIONALE	EVALUATION
Mikala will have effective airway clearance.	Monitor vital signs, auscultate breath sounds, assess respiratory effort and rate, and assess skin color every 15 to 30 minutes.	Subtle changes may serve as an early warning of increased airway obstruction.	Mikala's airway is clear.
	Monitor arterial blood gases (ABGs), pulse oximetry, and pulmonary function tests results.		
	Administer oxygen at the ordered flow rate (if chronic asthmatic, not to exceed 2 L/min).	Decreases hypoxia. Administration of oxygen to a child with chronic carbon dioxide retention may cause respiratory depression.	
	Position the client upright or for comfort.	Enhances lung expansion.	
	Ensure availability of suction equipment and tracheostomy tray.	Condition can deteriorate rapidly.	
	Provide at least 1,600 cc fluids (IV/p.o.)/24 hours.	Liquefies secretions and replaces insensible fluid losses.	
	Initiate nothing-by-mouth (NPO) status during periods of severe respiratory distress.	Oral fluid intake during periods of distress can cause aspiration.	
	Administer ordered medications and assess for therapeutic effect.	Bronchodilators and steroids open airways and decrease edema.	

continued

		Theophylline level of > 30 can cause serious complication.	
Assess breath sounds before and after CPT.		CPT, coughing, and deep breathing help loosen/eliminate secretions.	
Encourage client to cough and deep breathe by blowing bubbles through a wand.			

Nursing Diagnosis 2: *Anxiety related to threat to or change in health status as evidenced by respiratory distress and hospitalization*

PLANNING/GOALS	NURSING INTERVENTIONS	RATIONALE	EVALUATION
Mikala and her parents will be relaxed.	Maintain a calm, quiet environment and a reassuring manner.	Decreases oxygen demand and the work of breathing.	Mikala cooperates with the staff.
	Play with the child.	Build rapport and trust.	The parents participate in Mikala's care.
	Keep the parents informed of procedures, treatments, and condition of their child.	Builds rapport and trust. Calming the parents can help calm child.	

Nursing Diagnosis 3: *Knowledge Deficit related to lack of exposure as evidenced by many questions*

PLANNING/GOALS	NURSING INTERVENTIONS	RATIONALE	EVALUATION
Mikala's parents will verbalize accurate knowledge about asthma.	Teach the family about the disease, its triggers, and prescribed medications and treatment	Understanding increases compliance with treatment.	Mikala's parents verbalize accurate knowledge about the disease and its treatment.
	Assess the family's knowledge about triggers, precipitating factors (such as colds), and allergen control.	Triggers may have been assessed, given that the child has eczema. Knowledge of allergen control may decrease the likelihood of future episodes.	Mikala resumes normal activities.
	Teach the importance of taking medications as prescribed.	Maintains therapeutic levels.	
	Teach the importance of exercise and ways to choose appropriate activities based on the child's condition.	Promotes pulmonary and cardiovascular health, enhances self-esteem, and offers peer interaction.	

FOREIGN-BODY ASPIRATION

Foreign-body aspiration is the inhalation of any object into the respiratory tract. Commonly aspirated items among children include nuts, grapes, popcorn, hard candy, dried beans, bones, coins, parts of toys, screws, and balloons. Aspiration may occur at any age but is most common between the ages of 6 months and 4 years. Clinical manifestations may include spasmodic coughing, respiratory distress, or gagging in the absence of fever or other symptoms of illness.

Medical–Surgical Management

Medical

Removal of foreign bodies from the respiratory tract is done by direct laryngoscopy or bronchoscopy. After the procedure, the child should remain hospitalized for observation of laryngeal edema and respiratory distress. Cool mist is provided and antibiotic therapy ordered if appropriate.

Health Promotion

It is important that parents and child care providers remain watchful as the child gains increased locomotor and manipulative skills and becomes more curious about the environment.

Nursing Management

After the object has been removed, the main focus of care is prevention. The nurse must assess the parents' knowledge of safety in relation to the child's developmental level. Parents are encouraged to keep cylindric, spheric, and pliable objects smaller than 1¼ inches out of children's reach. In addition, children must be supervised when eating, and food must be cut into small, irregular pieces.

CARDIOVASCULAR SYSTEM

A major threat to the child's cardiovascular system is rheumatic fever, which may lead to permanent heart damage and disability.

RHEUMATIC FEVER

Rheumatic fever is a chronic childhood disease affecting the heart, joints, lungs, and brain. It results from an autoimmune response to untreated group A beta-hemolytic streptococcal infections. Clinical manifestations are classified as minor and major. Minor clinical manifestations include fever, listlessness, anorexia, pallor, weight loss, and vague muscle, joint, or abdominal pain. Major clinical manifestations include polyarthritis, chorea (spasmodic twitchings), carditis, erythema marginatum (red skin lesions), and subcutaneous nodules. An elevated antistreptolysin-O (ASO) titer (indicative of recent streptococcal infection) is common among children with rheumatic fever.

Medical–Surgical Management

Medical

Diagnosis is made by evaluating presenting signs and symptoms and laboratory test results. A throat culture determines whether the infection is active. Erythrocyte sedimentation rate (ESR), C-reactive protein, and leukocyte counts are elevated in the presence of inflammatory processes. Chest x-ray, electrocardiogram, and echocardiogram may demonstrate evidence of carditis.

The goals of medical management are to treat any existing strep infection, prevent recurrences and heart damage, and alleviate pain and fever. Bed rest is prescribed for the child with carditis until ESR and heart rate are within normal limits.

Pharmacological

Penicillin, salicylates, and corticosteroids are used to treat rheumatic fever. Long-term administration (as long as 5 years) of penicillin helps prevent the recurrence of rheumatic heart disease. Salicylates relieve pain, reduce inflammation of polyarthritis, and reduce fever. Corticosteroids are used in the presence of carditis. Residual heart disease (congestive heart failure) is treated as needed with digitalis and diuretics. Anticonvulsants may be prescribed to alleviate severe chorea.

Diet

A low-sodium diet may be prescribed in the presence of congestive heart failure.

Activity

Bed rest is essential to reduce the workload of the heart. The length of bed rest can range from weeks to months depending on the cardiac status.

Health Promotion

Continual health supervision for children is the key to prevention of rheumatic fever and resulting heart disease. It is important that children with upper respiratory infections be evaluated for group A *beta-hemolytic streptococcus* and treated with penicillin as prescribed.

▶ NURSING PROCESS

▶ Assessment

▶ Subjective Data

Initially, the nurse determines whether any family members have had a sore throat or unexplained fever within the past 2 months. The nurse should find out when symptoms began; what, if any, treatment was obtained; and if an antibiotic was prescribed, whether it was taken as directed.

▶ Objective Data

The child is monitored for cardiac complications such as abnormal vital signs, shortness of breath, edema, and precordial pain. Joints are assessed for tenderness, small lumps, and rapid, purposeless movements. Age-appropriate tools should be used to assess pain.

Nursing diagnoses for the child with rheumatic fever may include the following:

Nursing Diagnoses	Planning/Goals	Nursing Interventions
▶ *Pain related to inflamed joints*	The client will be comfortable.	Alternate applying heat and cold to affected joints. Handle joints gently. Reposition the child every 2 hours. Provide distraction such as guided imagery and relaxation.
▶ *Activity Intolerance related to shortness of breath and pain*	The client will tolerate restricted activities.	Limit activites to bed and chair, with bathroom privileges, and meals at the table. Include rest periods alternated with activities such as board games, computer use, movies, puzzles, books, art, and crafts.
▶ *Injury, Risk for, related to weakness and chorea*	Child will be injury free.	If the child is experiencing chorea, the mattress may need to be placed on the floor and the child may require assistance going up and down stairs. Seizure precaution should be taken. Nurses must teach the importance of evaluating children with upper respiratory infections for streptococcus, and treating with penicillin.
▶ *Knowledge Deficit related to medication administration*	The client and family understand the importance of antibiotic therapy in preventing recurrence of the disease and further heart damage.	Stress the importance of taking penicillin as prescribed even if symptoms disappear.

Evaluation Each goal must be evaluated to determine how it has been met by the client.

BLOOD AND LYMPH SYSTEMS

Leukemia, idiopathic thrombocytopenic purpura, and hemophilia are blood disorders that commonly occur during childhood.

LEUKEMIA

Leukemia is the uncontrolled production of lymphocytes (immature white blood cells). It is the most common childhood cancer. The most common form of leukemia is acute lymphocytic leukemia (ALL). The prognosis has been improving dramatically thanks to vigorous therapy. However, there is concern related to adverse effects of the therapy. Clinical manifestations, the results of neutropenia and decreased red blood cells (RBCs) and platelets, include pallor, weakness, fever, excessive bruising, petechiae, purpura, bone or joint pain, and abdominal pain.

Medical–Surgical Management

Medical

In addition to the client's history, symptoms, and laboratory studies, bone marrow aspiration is done to confirm the diagnosis of leukemia. The goals of medical intervention are to eradicate the leukemic cells via chemotherapy and to provide supportive care during treatment.

Surgical

Bone marrow transplant may be recommended after the second remission.

Pharmacological

A combination of drugs is administered through a subclavian catheter and/or intrathecally to bring about remission. Treatment may last 2 to 3 years. After 30 days of initial treatment, remission can be verified via bone marrow aspiration and lumbar puncture. If remission occurs, the prognosis is good. For the child who suffers a relapse, different drugs are used in an attempt to reinduce a remission. Relapses decrease the probability of survival.

Nursing Management

The emotional states of the child and the family members must be assessed and needs identified so that a plan can be made to assist them in working through and resolving their feelings and fears. The nurse must explore how the child and family are coping with the illness as well as the treatment.

IDIOPATHIC THROMBO-CYTOPENIC PURPURA

Idiopathic thrombocytopenic purpura (ITP) is a blood disorder associated with a deficit of platelets in the circulatory system. An autoimmune disorder often preceded by a viral infection, ITP may be acute and self-limiting or be chronic and require therapy. The peak age of occurrence is 2 to 4 years. Manifestations include bruising and petechiae.

Medical–Surgical Management

Medical

Diagnostic evaluation involves gathering a history of viral illness, information about any medications, and a CBC. The CBC will be normal except for a low platelet level. If the history and CBC suggest ITP, bone marrow aspiration may be done to rule out oncological disorders. Most cases are self-limiting, with the platelet count returning to normal within 6 months without therapy. Platelet transfusions may be necessary for the child with chronic ITP if active uncontrolled bleeding occurs.

PROFESSIONAL TIP

Life-threatening Illness

The following questions can be used in assessing the feelings and fears associated with the diagnosis of life-threatening illness:

- Has the child and/or family been associated with hospitals, nurses, and doctors in the past? If yes, what were the positive and negative aspects of the experience?
- Does the family know anyone diagnosed with a life-threatening illness? If yes, what happened to that person?
- Are there concerns about the child's future? The family's future?

Surgical

When drugs no longer control the thrombocytopenia in a child with chronic ITP, a splenectomy may be indicated. Splenectomy is usually not performed before 5 years of age due to the immaturity of the child's immune system.

Pharmacological

Steroids and immune globulin are given to block the autoimmune destruction of platelets.

▶ NURSING PROCESS

▶ Assessment

▶ Subjective Data

Parents may bring their child to the doctor because of a "red rash" or bruising. The child's activity level may be reported to be normal.

▶ Objective Data

The nurse observes for further bleeding (e.g., epistaxis, hematuria, blood in stools), and level of consciousness.

Nursing diagnoses for the child with ITP may include the following:

Nursing Diagnoses	Planning/Goals	Nursing Interventions
▶ *Injury, Risk for, related to low platelet count*	The client will be free of injury.	Have the child curtail physical activities and sports until platelets return to normal.
		Encourage the use of a soft-bristled toothbrush to minimize gum bleeding.
		Observe for signs of bleeding.
		Flush the catheter with saline to confirm proper placement of an IV line.

continued

Nursing Diagnoses	Planning/Goals	Nursing Interventions
▶ *Knowledge Deficit (family) related to disorder and treatment*	The family will verbalize an understanding of the disorder and treatment.	Teach the family that ITP should subside within 6 months. Teach the family side effects of steroids, such as edema, insomnia, mood changes, poor healing, peptic ulcers, and growth retardation. Establish a safe, age-appropriate home environment (e.g., pad table corners, crib rails, and knees and elbows to decrease injury). Instruct parents to use nonaspirin analgesics and antipyretics. Evaluate the child's platelet count weekly.
▶ *Infection, Risk for, related to chronic use of steroids and/or splenectomy*	The client will be free of infection.	Teach the family the signs and symptoms of infection. Administer pneumococcus vaccine and/or daily antibiotics, if the child has a splenectomy.

Evaluation Each goal must be evaluated to determine how it has been met by the client.

HEMOPHILIA

Neonatal bleeding from the umbilical cord or circumcision site may be an early manifestations of severe hemophilia. Mild hemophilia may not be detected until the toddler becomes mobile, and unusual bruising and bleeding occur from small injuries.

Nursing interventions center on prevention and teaching. Regular physical exercise strenghtens muscles and joints and may decrease the number of bleeding episodes. Adolescents who have seroconverted to human-immunodeficiency-virus–(HIV-)positive status must be especially knowledgeable about safe sexual behavior (see Chapter 36, Nursing Care of the Client: Sexually Transmitted Diseases).

GASTROINTESTINAL SYSTEM

Gastrointestinal (GI) disorders in children interfere with nutrition and fluid and electrolyte balance and have the potential for impairing growth. Common GI disorders of childhood include constipation and parasitic infections.

CONSTIPATION

Constipation is the infrequent or difficult passage of hard, dry stools. It is most common during the toddler and preschool years because of the child's (and parents') efforts at toilet training. School-age children may experience constipation as a result of busy schedules, hesitation to use unfamiliar bathrooms, and limited bathroom privileges. Other potential causes of constipation include lack of fresh fruit and vegetables and grains in the diet, dehydration, lack of exercise, emotional stress, certain drugs, pain from passage of hard stool, excessive milk intake, and a variety of GI tract and systemic disorders and spinal lesions.

Chronic constipation causes an enlarged rectum, which impairs sphincter control, resulting in **encopresis** (the passage of watery colonic contents around a hard fecal mass). Predisposing factors for encopresis include inadequate or inconsistent toilet training or psychological stress such as that related to starting school or the birth of a sibling. Clinical manifestations of constipation include abdominal pain and cramping without distention; palpable, movable fecal mass and a large amount of stool inside rectum; diarrhea; malaise; anorexia; and headache.

Medical–Surgical Management

Medical

Abdominal x-rays may reveal a rectum enlarged with stool and gas. The impaction is removed with enemas.

 CLIENT TEACHING

Guidelines for Preventing Constipation in Children

For toddlers and preschool children:
- Increase cereal, fruit, vegetable, and fluid intake
- Encourage sitting on the toilet for 5 to 10 minutes after breakfast and after dinner

For school-age children:
- Allow 1 hour to finish breakfast prior to leaving for school to allow sufficient time for bathroom use
- Encourage children to take responsibility for including cereals, fruits, vegetables, and fluids in their diets
- Encourage children to exercise daily
- Decrease the anxiety of children by taking time each day to communicate about their days, activities, concerns, and fears.

Pharmacological

Stool softeners or laxatives may be prescribed in an effort to retrain the rectum after the impaction has been removed. Mineral oil may be prescribed to decrease the pain of defecation.

Diet

Increasing water and fiber intake and limiting milk intake will often decrease constipation and promote defecation.

Health Promotion

Counseling may be part of the treatment plan, if there is no evidence of physiologic disorders. Establishing and maintaining regular toileting habits, drinking fluids, eating a high-fiber diet, and participating in regular exercise will also help prevent constipation.

Nursing Management

Nursing care focuses on teaching parents about normal bowel patterns in children and the importance of diet and exercise in maintaining those patterns. Assessing the child's diet history and eliciting a description of bowel patterns may provide clues to the cause of constipation. Dietary changes may be all that is required to resolve constipation.

Requiring the child to sit on the toilet for 10 minutes approximately 30 minutes after meals will encourage regular bowel habits. Parents must be cautioned about the overuse of laxatives, stool softeners, and enemas. Use of mineral oil may cause soiling due to leakage, which should not be mistaken for encopresis.

INTESTINAL PARASITIC INFECTIONS

Common parasitic infections include giardiasis (a protozoan) and helminths (i.e., pinworms, roundworms, hookworms). Children are more commonly infected than adults because they frequently put their hands in their mouths. Temperate climates, crowded conditions (i.e., day care centers, schools), untreated water, and poor hygiene practices may contribute to outbreaks of parasitic infections. Appearance, mode of transmission, and clinical manifestations vary, depending on the parasite (Table 54-2).

Medical–Surgical Management

Medical

Identification of a parasitic infection is done with fecal smear or a microscopic examination. Pinworms may be diagnosed by using cellophane tape to capture eggs from around the anus and then examining them under a microscope.

PROFESSIONAL TIP

Quinacrine Hydrochloride (Atabrine HCl)
To disguise the bitter taste of quinacrine tablets, pulverize and mix with jam or honey.

Table 54-2 COMMON INTESTINAL PARASITES

	APPEARANCE	MODE OF TRANSMISSION	CLINICAL MANIFESTATIONS
Giardiasis	Microscopic	Ingested cysts Person to person Untreated water Contaminated food Animals Soil Feces	Diarrhea Weight loss Abdominal cramping
Pinworm	White, threadlike worm	Person to person Ingested or inhaled eggs	Itching around the anus Irritability Distractibility
Roundworm	Pink worm, 9 to 12 inches in length	Eggs passed from hand to mouth (may migrate to liver and lungs)	Abdominal pain, distention, or obstruction Vomiting Jaundice Pneumonitis
Hookworm	Microscopic	Skin penetration by contact with contaminated soil (may migrate to lungs)	Dermatitis Anemia Pneumonitis Malnutrition

CLIENT TEACHING

Preventing Parasitic Infestations

- Care providers should wash hands thoroughly after changing diapers.
- Soiled diapers should be disposed of in trash receptacles.
- Children should be taught to wash their hands and fingernails after using the toilet and before eating.
- Bedding and undergarments should be washed in hot water.
- Cleaning agents containing bleach should be used regularly in bathrooms.
- All raw fruits and vegetables should be washed prior to eating.
- Sandboxes should be covered when not in use.
- Swimming pools that allow diapered children should be avoided.
- Shoes should be worn outside.

Pharmacological

Helminths are treated with oral anthelmintic medications such as pyrantel pamoate (Antiminth) or mebendazole (Vermox). Medication should be repeated 2 to 3 weeks later to eliminate any parasites that may hatch after the initial treatment. All family members should also be treated.

Metronidazole (Flagyl) or quinacrine hydrochloride (Atabrine HCl) are effective in treating giardiasis. Child care providers should be alerted to the possibility of a yellow discoloration to the skin for the child on quinacrine hydrochloride (Atabrine HCl).

HOME HEALTH CARE

Instructions for the Tape Test for Pinworms

Perform the test early in the morning, before the child awakens,

1. Wind the tape around the end of a tongue blade, sticky side out.
2. Spread the child's buttocks and press the tape against the anus, rolling the blade from side to side.
3. Place the tongue blade in a glass jar or plastic bag.
4. Take to the lab for microscopic examination. If a glass slide is available, remove the tape from the tongue blade and place it smoothly on the slide, sticky side down.

Diet

A well-balanced diet with additional protein and iron may be prescribed for the child with hookworms. These nutrients may be depleted due to blood loss and malnutrition.

Health Promotion

Attention to meticulous sanitary practices is essential.

Nursing Management

Nursing care includes assisting with collection of specimens, treatment of infections, and prevention of reinfection. Stool specimens can be collected from diapers, potty chairs, or a toilet covered with clear plastic wrap. A tongue blade can be used to place the specimen into the designated and properly labeled container. Parents may also need detailed instructions for performing the tape test (see the accompanying Home Health Care box). The nurse also provides education regarding the course of treatment and home care.

ENDOCRINE SYSTEM

A common endocrine disorder in children is type 1, formerly called insulin-dependent diabetes. The management of diabetes in children presents some unique challenges due to their physical immaturity and dependence on family for care. Stabilizing insulin needs during puberty requires vigilant monitoring of the glucose level and regulating diet, insulin, and exercise. The lifestyle of the entire family must change in order to effectively treat the child with diabetes. Family members should be familiar with and adhere to the prescribed regimen. Most school-age children are ready and able to learn to give their own injections and should be encouraged to do so.

For medical–surgical management and nursing management of the client with endocrine disorders, see Chapter 37, Nursing Care of the Client: Endocrine System.

MUSCULOSKELETAL SYSTEM

Common musculoskeletal disorders in children include scoliosis, Legg-Calvé-Perthes disease, muscular dystrophy, juvenile arthritis, and fractures.

SCOLIOSIS

Scoliosis, the most common spinal deformity in children, involves lateral curvature greater than 20 degrees, spinal rotation, rib asymmetry, and thoracic hypokyphosis (Figure 54-1). It occurs most frequently in

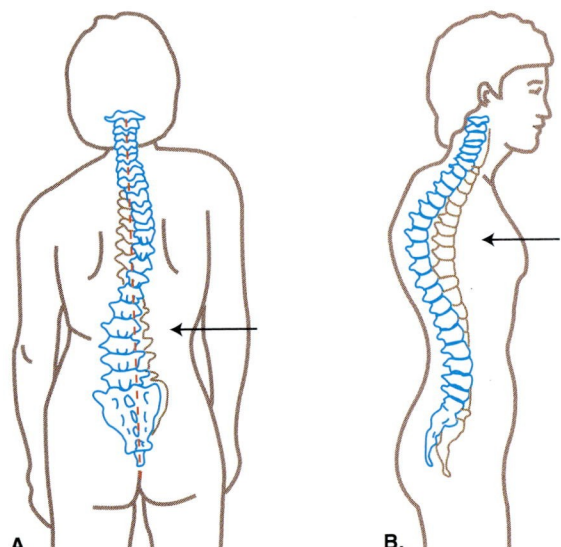

Figure 54-1 A. Scoliosis; B. Kyphosis

prepubescent girls and is usually not caused by any other injury or disease.

Clinical manifestations include visible curve of the spine, posterior rib hump when bending forward, asymmetrical rib cage, and uneven shoulder or pelvic heights. Parents may notice that the child's clothes do not fit properly (e.g., uneven hems).

Medical–Surgical Management

Medical

The goal of medical treatment is to stop the curvature of the spine. Early detection and treatment of scoliosis are essential to successful management. The treatment regimen depends on the degree and progression of the curvature and the reaction of the child and family. Children with mild curvatures may simply be monitored throughout the growth cycle. Electrical stimulation, bracing, and exercise may be prescribed for children with mild to moderate curvatures.

Surgical

Surgical intervention may be required for children with curvatures greater than 40 degrees. The goal of surgery is to correct the curvature of the spine with internal fixation and instrumentation.

▶ NURSING PROCESS

▶ Assessment

▶ Subjective Data

Initially, the child may complain of a sore back, improperly fitting clothing, or a slight limp. When being treated with a brace, the child is assessed for problems related to self-esteem and body image. In addition, the child and parents are asked to report on the degree of compliance with the prescribed regimen. If the child requires surgery, feeling and fears of the child and the family must be assessed.

▶ Objective Data

Screening for scoliosis is an important role of the nurse. Children 10 years of age and older are assessed. With clothes removed, the back is observed for uneven shoulders and hips, prominent shoulder blade on one side, and curved spine. While bending at the waist and touching the toes, the child's back is assessed for a rib hump and curved spine (Figure 54-2).

When the brace is in place, it is important to continue monitoring the degree of the curvature and to assess the skin at pressure points for irritation. Progression of the curve may be indicative of either noncompliance with the prescribed treatment or the need for more aggressive therapy.

Postoperatively, the child is assessed for neurological status, pain, fluid balance, bleeding, and bowel and bladder function. Mobility and nutrition are quickly resumed if there are no complications.

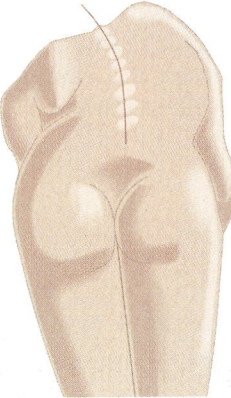

Figure 54-2 Scoliosis screening reveals a rib hump and curved spine.

Nursing diagnoses for the child with scoliosis may include the following:

Nursing Diagnoses	Planning/Goals	Nursing Interventions
▶ *Knowledge Deficit (family and child) related to lack of information about scoliosis, including treatment and surgery*	The client and family will verbalize an understanding of and comply with the medical regimen.	Identify the client's and family's knowledge level and areas of concern. Inform the child and family that the brace must be worn for 16 to 23 hours/day for years.

continued

Nursing Diagnoses	Planning/Goals	Nursing Interventions
		Inform the child and family that use of brace may eliminate need for surgery.
		If surgery is necessary, prepare the child and family for the need to log roll the child and the need for the child to cough and have them demonstrate preoperatively.
▸ *Body Image Disturbance related to deformity, bracing, and surgical scar*	The client will talk about feelings. The client will demonstrate self-confidence.	Involve the child in the plan of care. Provide the child with opportunities to ventilate feelings about being different. Encourage the child to talk about experiences with friends. Help the child select clothing that is stylish yet loose enough to fit over the brace. Help the child focus on positive body features (e.g., hair, complexion). Help the child select activities that will enhance abilities. Provide the child with privacy during hospitalization.
▸ *Skin Integrity, Impaired, Risk for, related to wearing of a brace*	The client's skin will remain intact.	Have the child wear a knit cotton shirt under the brace. Place a protective pad over bony prominences. Report reddened areas so that the brace can be adjusted.
▸ *Mobility, Impaired, related to restricted movement (brace/surgery)*	The client will adjust to restricted movement.	Perform exercises as prescribed. Instruct the child in how to move with the brace (i.e., climb stairs, get in and out of a vehicle, chair, desk, and bed).
▸ *Injury, Risk for, related to neurovascular deficit secondary to instrumentation*	The client will regain all body functions postoperatively.	Assess all extremities for color, capillary refill, warmth, sensation, and motion. Monitor signs of bowel distention and urinary retention. Maintain body alignment by log rolling every 2 hours and rolling from a side-lying position to a sitting position. Assist with early ambulation postoperatively.
▸ *Pain related to operative procedure*	The client will experience pain reduction to an acceptable level.	Assess pain level postoperatively, using pain scale. Provide prescribed analgesics around the clock for the first 24 to 48 hours. Explore alternate means of relieving pain (e.g., dim lights, music). Assess and document the child's response to relief measures.
▸ *Knowledge Deficit (family and child) related to home care*	The client and family will successfully manage postoperative treatment at home.	Teach proper wound care. Discuss the importance of a well-balanced diet in maintaining healthy bones. Discuss activity restrictions (e.g., lifting no more than 10 pounds) and the length of time they will be in place. Have the child demonstrate moving without twisting or bending at the waist. Emphasize the importance of keeping follow-up appointments.

Evaluation Each goal must be evaluated to determine how it has been met by the client.

LEGG-CALVÉ-PERTHES DISEASE

Legg-Calvé-Perthes disease is necrosis of the head of the femur. The disease occurs most commonly in Caucasian boys between the ages of 4 and 8 years. The cause is unknown. Clinical manifestations include hip and knee soreness or stiffness, painful limp, and quadricep muscle atrophy.

Medical–Surgical Management

Medical

Diagnosis is made by x-ray. The goal of treatment is to maintain the shape of the femoral head and reduce the risk of permanent stiffness and degenerative arthritis. Methods used to accomplish this goal include traction, bracing, and surgery.

Initially, the child is hospitalized for non–weight-bearing range-of-motion exercises and bed rest. If there is no improvement within 10 days, alternate methods of treatment are usually begun.

Nonsurgical intervention may involve traction followed by the use of a non–weight-bearing abduction brace to position the femoral head in the acetabulum. Exercises are needed to maintain muscle integrity during the time period that the child is required to wear the brace, for as long as 1 to 3 years.

Surgical

Surgical intervention is often the treatment of choice because it reduces treatment time and eliminates compliance problems. The child is usually able to resume normal activities in 3 to 4 months.

Nursing Management

Maintaining mobility and educating the child and family are the primary nursing goals. The family and child are encouraged to adhere to treatment plans and keep follow-up visits. Proper application of the abduction brace must be demonstrated. In addition, skin assessments must be performed daily. The child must be encouraged to maintain muscle integrity via prescribed exercises. Involvement in activities such as horseback riding and swimming may be permitted.

DUCHENNE MUSCULAR DYSTROPHY

Duchenne muscular dystrophy is an x-linked, recessive, hereditary, progressive, degenerative disease of the muscles. The disease occurs almost exclusively among males and is carried by females. Clinical manifestations include delayed motor development, difficulty standing or walking, progressive muscle weakness, increasing abnormalities in gait and posture, lordosis, pelvic waddling, frequent falling, **Gowers' sign** (walking the hands up legs to move from a sitting to a stand-

ing position), and a flat affect and smile. The disease continues into adolescence and young adulthood, when the client usually succumbs to respiratory failure. Children with Duchenne muscular dystrophy rarely live beyond 20 years of age. Complications include obesity, contractures, respiratory infections, and cardiac failure. Diagnosis is confirmed by serum enzyme assay, muscle biopsy, and electromyography .

Medical–Surgical Management

Medical

Initially, therapeutic management is aimed at maintaining ambulation and independence for as long as possible with bracing and physical therapy. Later, therapy is directed at maximizing sitting capabilities, respiratory function, and self-care. Genetic counseling is recommended for parents, female siblings, and maternal aunts and their female offspring.

Surgical

Contractures may be released surgically in order to keep the child as mobile as possible.

▶ NURSING PROCESS

▶ Assessment

▶ Subjective Data

When there is family history of muscular dystrophy, the child should be monitored carefully. Assessing both the family's ability to cope with a chronic, debilitating illness and the support systems available to the family is also important.

▶ Objective Data

The child is routinely monitored for mobility, self-care abilities, weight gain, and infections.

Nursing diagnoses for the child with Duchenne muscular dystrophy may include the following:

Nursing Diagnoses	Planning/Goals	Nursing Interventions
▶ *Mobility, Impaired, Physical, related to progressive muscle wasting and contractures*	The client will remain physically active.	Reinforce physical therapy exercise regimen.
		Encourage activity (e.g., school attendance, swimming).
		Encourage the use of adaptive equipment as needed (e.g., a back brace).
▶ *Self-Care Deficit related to progressive weakness*	The client will be able to perform activities of daily living (ADL) as long as possible.	Instruct the family in ways to adapt the home as needed (e.g., grab bars, overhead sling, raised toilet, wheelchair access).
		Focus on those things the child can do to prevent frustration.
		Maintain the child's independence as long as possible (e.g., via an electric wheelchair and portable phone).

continued

Nursing Diagnoses	Planning/Goals	Nursing Interventions
▶ *Coping, Family, Ineffective, related to increased demands of care, financial burdens, and needs of other children*	The family will cope effectively with the disease process.	Refer the family to resource and support groups. Assist the family in anticipating needs and coordinating services. Encourage involvement of extended family and friends. Encourage the family to express feelings.

Evaluation Each goal must be evaluated to determine how it has been met by the client.

JUVENILE ARTHRITIS

Juvenile arthritis (JA) is a systemic, multisystem disorder that affects the body's connective tissue; it is also known as an autoimmune inflammatory disease. There are many different forms of the disease, including juvenile rheumatoid arthritis.

Clinical manifestations include joint swelling accompanied by limited range of motion; pain; tenderness; and inflammation lasting longer than 6 weeks. Complications include blindness and disability. Prognosis is generally good with early detection and treatment.

Medical–Surgical Management

Medical

The goal of treatment is to maintain mobility and preserve joint function. The therapeutic regimen includes drugs, physical therapy, and/or surgery.

Surgical

Depending on the severity of the disease, surgery may be necessary to release contractures, correct leg length discrepancies, and replace joints.

Pharmacological

Drug therapy includes aspirin, nonsteroidal anti-inflammatory drugs such as ibuprofen (Motrin) and naproxen (Naprosyn), slower acting antirheumatic drugs such as gold sodium thiomalate (Myochrysine), and D-penicillamine (Cuprimine). Cytotoxic drugs may be used for severe disease that does not respond to other drugs. Corticosteroids may be used sparingly when the disease is life threatening.

HOME HEALTH CARE

Juvenile Arthritis

Home treatment for juvenile rheumatoid arthritis may include the following:
- Exercise, such as swimming and bicycling, to maximize muscle strength and range of motion
- Splints, positioning, and application of heat and cold to provide comfort during painful episodes

Nursing Management

Refer to Chapter 39: Nursing Care of the Client: Immune System.

FRACTURES

Fractures in children tend to be less complicated and heal more quickly than do those in adults. The bones most commonly fractured in children include the clavicle, femur, tibia, humerus, wrist, and fingers. Fractures in the area of the epiphyseal plate (growth plate) can cause permanent damage and severely impair growth. Greenstick fractures are common among young children due to incomplete ossification. Evidence of old fractures in a young child is suggestive of possible child abuse, whereas fractures in infants may indicate osteogenesis imperfecta (brittle bone disease).

Treatment usually involves realignment and immobilization using traction or closed manipulation and casting.

Refer to Chapter 38, Nursing Care of the Client: Musculoskeletal System for medical management and the nursing process.

IMMUNE SYSTEM

Infectious or communicable diseases are not life threatening to most children. However, children with immature or compromised immune systems are at greater risk of developing severe and even fatal complications as the result of communicable diseases.

COMMUNICABLE DISEASES

A communicable disease is an illness that is directly or indirectly transmitted from one person to another. Infants and young children are more susceptible to infectious diseases because their immune systems are not fully developed until 6 years of age, and their hygiene habits (e.g., covering the mouth when coughing) are lacking. Selected communicable diseases, along with causal agent, transmission mode, communicable period, incubation period, clinical manifestations, potential complications, treatment and immunity conferment are listed in Table 54-3.

Table 54-3 SELECT COMMON COMMUNICABLE DISEASES

DISEASE (CAUSAL AGENT)	TRANSMISSION MODE AND COMMUNICABLE PERIOD	INCUBATION PERIOD	CLINICAL MANIFESTATIONS AND POTENTIAL COMPLICATIONS	TREATMENT AND IMMUNITY CONFERMENT
Chicken pox (varicella-zoster virus, Figure 54-3)	*Transmission mode:* direct contact, respiratory droplet, airborne particles *Communicable period:* 1 day before lesions appear until all lesions crust over	10 to 21 days	*Clinical manifestations:* Fever, malaise, irritability, and a rash that begins as macules and progresses to fluid-filled papules to crusted lesions *Potential complications:* Reye's syndrome, skin infections, encephalitis	*Treatment:* antihistamines, baths, and lotions for itching *Immunity conferment:* Natural or with vaccine; may reactivate in adults as herpes zoster
Diphtheria (*Corynebacterium diphtheriae*)	*Transmission mode:* direct contact, contact with contaminated articles, or consumption of unpasteurized milk *Communicable period:* 2 to 4 weeks in presence of antibiotic treatment, months without treatment	2 to 5 days	*Clinical manifestations:* Fever, cough, pharyngitis, anorexia, membranous lesion on tonsils, pharynx, or larynx *Potential complications:* neuritis, carditis, congestive heart failure, respiratory failure	*Treatment:* Isolation, antitoxin, antibiotics, and analgesics *Immunity conferment:* diphtheria, tetanus, and acellular pertussis (DTaP) vaccine; passive immunity conferred by maternal antibodies
Erythema infectiosum, or Fifth disease (Parvovirus B19, Figure 54-4)	*Transmission mode:* Contact with respiratory secretions and blood *Communicable period:* unknown	4 to 20 days	*Clinical manifestations:* Fiery-red cheeks ("slapped face" appearance); erythematous, maculopapular, lacy rash on trunk then limbs *Potential complications:* none	*Treatment:* Supportive *Immunity conferment:* no vaccine
Hepatitis B, or serum hepatitis (hepatitis B virus [HBV])	*Transmission mode:* blood, secretions, prenatally, perinatally, sexual contact *Communicable period:* Throughout clinical course	50 to 180 days	*Transmission mode:* mild flulike symptoms, jaundice in adolescents *Potential complications:* Liver failure	*Treatment:* supportive care *Immunity conferment:* hepatitis B vaccine (Hep B)
Measles, or rubella (measles virus, Figure 54-5)	*Transmission mode:* direct or indirect contact with respiratory droplets *Communicable period:* 4 days before to 5 days after appearance of rash	10 to 21 days	*Clinical manifestations:* fever, runny nose, cough, enlarged lymph nodes, Koplik's spots (small, red spots with blue-white centers on oral mucosa, Figure 54-6), photophobia, maculopapular rash from hairline over entire body *Potential complications:* otitis media, pneumonia, encephalitis, airway obstruction	*Treatment:* supportive care *Immunity conferment:* measles, mumps, rubella (MMR) vaccine *Active:* from infection with causative agent
Mononucleosis (Epstein-Barr virus)	*Transmission mode:* direct contact with saliva; blood transfusions; most common in adolescents and young adults *Communicable period:* Unknown	30 to 50 days	*Clinical manifestations:* fever, pharyngitis, fatigue, sore throat, enlarged lymph nodes *Potential complications:* splenic rupture, hepatitis, meningitis, encephalitis, Guillain-Barré syndrome	*Treatment:* supportive care, antipyretics, analgesics *Immunity conferment:* no vaccine

continued

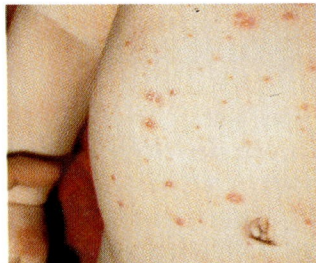

Figure 54-3 Varicella (*Courtesy of Robert A. Silverman, MD, Clinical Associate Professor, Department of Pediatrics, Georgetown University*)

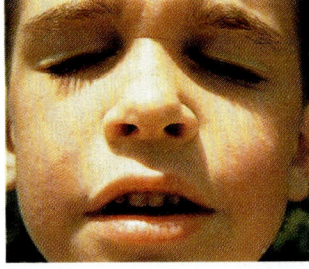

Figure 54-4 "Slapped Face" in Erythema Infectiousum (Fifth Disease) (*Courtesy of the Centers for Disease Control and Prevention [CDC]*)

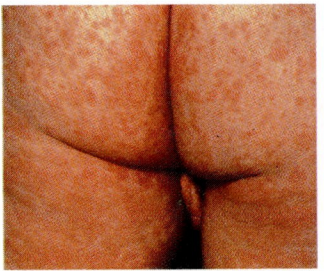

Figure 54-5 Rubeola/Measles (*Courtesy of the Centers for Disease Control and Prevention [CDC]*)

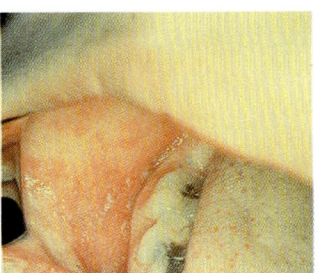

Figure 54-6 Koplik's Spots in Rubeola (*Courtesy of the Centers for Disease Control and Prevention [CDC]*)

Table 54-3 SELECT COMMON COMMUNICABLE DISEASES *continued*

DISEASE (CAUSAL AGENT)	TRANSMISSION MODE AND COMMUNICABLE PERIOD	INCUBATION PERIOD	CLINICAL MANIFESTATIONS AND POTENTIAL COMPLICATIONS	TREATMENT AND IMMUNITY CONFERMENT
Mumps, or parotitis (paramyxovirus)	*Transmission mode:* direct or indirect contact with saliva *Communicable period:* 7 days before swelling until 2 to 3 days after swelling subsides	14 to 21 days	*Clinical manifestations:* fever; headache; malaise; anorexia; "earache" aggravated by chewing; enlarged parotid gland (Figure 54-7) *Potential complications:* orchitis, meningoencephalitis, hearing loss	*Treatment:* supportive care, antipyretics, analgesics *Immunity conferment:* MMR vaccine; natural; passive: mumps immune globulin
Pertussis, or whooping cough (*Bordetella pertussis*)	*Transmission mode:* direct contact or respiratory droplets *Communicable period:* 1 week after exposure until 4 to 6 weeks	5 to 21 days	*Clinical manifestations:* upper respiratory symptoms progressing to severe paroxysmal cough with inspiratory whoop *Potential complications:* pneumonia, otitis media, hemorrhage, convulsions	*Treatment:* antibiotics, supportive care with high humidity *Immunity conferment:* DTaP vaccine; active: from infection with causative agent
Poliomyelitis, or infantile paralysis (poliovirus types I, II, III)	*Transmission mode:* fecal–oral, respiratory droplets *Communicable period:* unknown prior to symptoms, 1 week after symptoms for respiratory contact, up to 6 weeks for fecal contact	5 to 14 days	*Clinical manifestations:* fever, headache, abdominal pain, stiff neck, pain and tenderness in lower extremities, paralysis *Potential complications:* permanent paralysis, respiratory arrest	*Treatment:* supportive, rehabilitative care *Immunity conferment:* poliovirus vaccine (inactivated [IPV] or live oral [OPV]); active: immunity against a specific strain conferred by disease
Roseola, or exanthema subitum (herpesvirus type 6, Figure 54-8)	*Transmission mode:* unknown; appears between 6 months and 2 years of age *Communicable period:* unknown	Unknown	*Clinical manifestations:* rose-pink, nonpruritic maculopapules on trunk then face, neck, and limbs that fade on pressure *Potential complications:* febrile seizures	*Treatment:* antipyretics, supportive care *Immunity conferment:* no vaccine
Rubella, or German measles, 3-day measles (Rubella virus, Figure 54-9)	*Transmission mode:* airborne, direct contact with droplets, transplacental *Communicable period:* 10 days before symptoms and 15 days after rash appears	14 to 21 days	*Clinical manifestations:* fever, headache, malaise, runny nose, anorexia, maculopapular rash progressing from head to extremities *Potential complications:* risks for unborn fetus of infected mother: spontaneous abortion, stillbirth, ear, eye, and cardiac anomalies	*Treatment:* supportive care *Immunity conferment:* MMR vaccine

continued

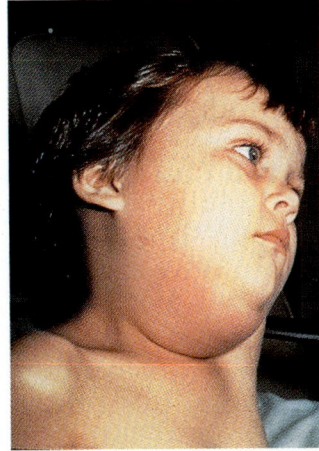

Figure 54-7 Mumps *(Courtesy of the Centers for Disease Control and Prevention [CDC])*

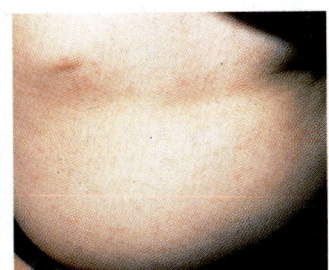

Figure 54-8 Roseola *(Courtesy of Robert A. Silverman, M.D., Clinical Associate Professor, Department of Pediatrics, Georgetown University)*

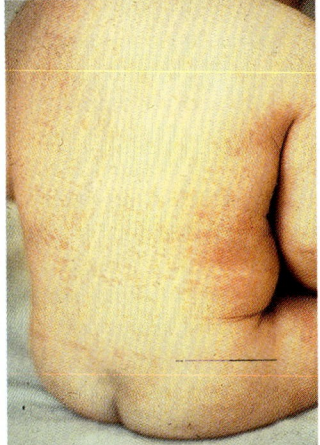

Figure 54-9 Rubella *(Courtesy of the Centers for Disease Control and Prevention [CDC])*

Table 54-3 SELECT COMMON COMMUNICABLE DISEASES *continued*

DISEASE (CAUSAL AGENT)	TRANSMISSION MODE AND COMMUNICABLE PERIOD	INCUBATION PERIOD	CLINICAL MANIFESTATIONS AND POTENTIAL COMPLICATIONS	TREATMENT AND IMMUNITY CONFERMENT
Scarlet fever, or scarlatina (group A beta-hemolytic streptococci, Figure 54-10)	*Transmission mode:* airborne respiratory droplets and contaminated articles *Communicable period:* from onset of symptoms until 24 hours after antibiotic therapy is initiated	1 to 7 days	*Clinical manifestations:* fever, headache, "strawberry tongue," abdominal pain, sore throat, skin on hands and feet peels in sheets after first week *Potential complications:* glomerulonephritis, rheumatic fever	*Treatment:* penicillin, antipyretics, analgesics *Immunity conferment:* no immunity
Tetanus, or lockjaw (*Clostridium tetani*)	*Transmission mode:* direct contact of skin wound with contaminated soil or implements *Communicable period:* not communicable	3 to 21 days	*Clinical manifestations:* stiffness of neck and jaw, difficulty breathing *Potential complications:* laryngospasm, death	*Treatment:* supportive care *Immunity conferment:* DTaP vaccine: passive: from tetanus antitoxin or immune globulin (TIG)

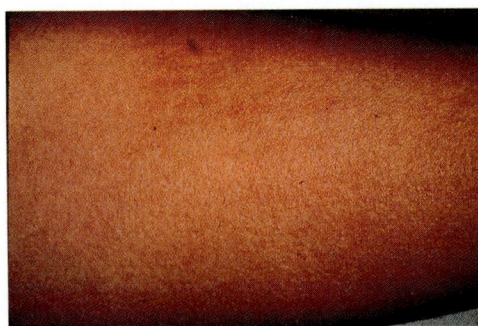

Figure 54-10 Scarlet Fever *(Courtesy of the Centers for Disease Control and Prevention [CDC])*

Nursing Management

Immunization is critical to the health of children. One of the goals of the United States government is to immunize 90% of children aged 2 years by the year 2000 (U.S. Department of Health and Human Services, 1990). Nurses and health care providers must be familiar with immunization schedules and the various frequent revisions to these schedules. The Advisory Committee on Immunization Practices (ACIP) of the United States Public Health Service Centers for Disease Control (CDC) and the American Academy of Pediatrics (AAP) Committee on Infectious Diseases are responsible for recommendations regarding vaccinations. Changes in recommendations are published in the *Morbidity and Mortality Weekly Report* for the ACIP and in *Pediatrics* for the AAP.

Nurses must be able to recognize barriers to immunizations and be prepared to educate families about vaccine safety, administration, precautions, and contraindications. Barriers to immunization include long waiting lines, appointment-only systems, inaccessible clinic sites, and inability to speak English. Every opportunity must be taken to immunize children whenever they enter any health care facility.

Federal law requires health care providers to provide general information about immunizations prior to administration. This general information includes nature, prevalence, and risks of the disease; type of immunization product to be used; the expected benefits and the risk of side effects of the vaccine; and the need for accurate immunization records. If possible, this lengthy information should be provided prior to the immunization appointment so that families have time to read and understand the information and to ask questions. Otherwise, the health care provider must inform parents at the time of administration. Informed consent of the parent(s) should be documented.

Nurses must also be knowledgeable about the safe administration of immunizations. This includes proper storage, reconstitution, sequence (see Appendix A), injection site, and technique.

The nurse is responsible for documenting on the child's immunization record the type of vaccine, the date of administration, the manufacturer and lot number, the expiration date, and the administration site. Parents are encouraged to keep and provide immunization records at every health care visit.

INTEGUMENTARY SYSTEM

Because they are visible and often disfiguring, skin disorders can prove emotionally and psychologically stressful for the child and family. It is important that the pediatric nurse teach families and children strategies to maintain healthy skin. Skin disorders may be caused by infections (bacterial, fungal, viral), infestations (pediculosis, scabies), insects, substances (contact dermatitis), acne, and injuries such as burns.

BACTERIAL INFECTIONS

Bacterial infections of the skin are usually caused by staphylococci or streptococci. The two most common skin disorders of childhood resulting from bacterial infections are impetigo and cellulitis.

IMPETIGO

Impetigo, the most common skin infection of childhood, often begins in an area of broken skin, such as that caused by an insect bite or eczema. The face, mouth, hands, neck, and extremities are the most common sites.

Clinical manifestations include primary lesions (macules that change rapidly to form small, thin-walled vesicles with an erythematous halo), secondary lesions (ruptured vesicles covered by a honey-colored crust over an ulcerated base), pruritus, burning, and lymph node enlargement (Figure 54-11). Lesions usually resolve within 2 weeks. Because impetigo is commonly caused by streptococci, rheumatic fever or glomerulonephritis are possible complications.

Medical–Surgical Management

Pharmacological

A topical bactericidal ointment such as polymyxin B sulfate-neomycin (Neosporin) is applied for 5 to 7 days. Children with multiple lesions may require oral antibiotics such as erythromycin (AK-Mycin). In extreme and extended situations, parenteral antibiotics may be required.

Nursing Management

The primary nursing goals are to prevent the spread of infection and promote healing. The child with impetigo is treated at home and should not return to school for 2 days after antibiotics are initiated. The nurse must emphasize the importance of taking antibiotics as prescribed.

Caregivers must be encouraged to employ preventive hygiene practices such as sleeping alone, bathing

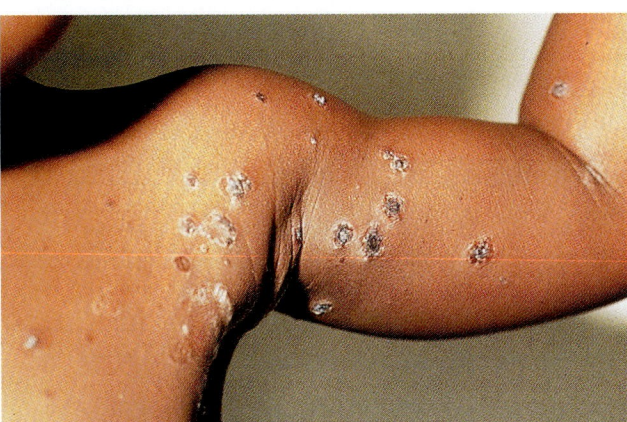

Figure 54-11 Impetigo *(Courtesy of Robert A. Silverman, M.D., Clinical Associate Professor, Department of Pediatrics, Georgetown University)*

HOME HEALTH CARE

Preventing Children from Scratching Lesions

To prevent children from scratching lesions:

- Cut the fingernails short;
- Give cool baths;
- Cover the lesions with clothing, when possible;
- At nighttime, cover the hands with socks or gloves;
- During the day, encourage activities that require use of the hands; and administer antihistamines or sedatives as needed to control itching;
- Keep the child cool.

daily with antibacterial soap, using a separate towel, washing hands properly, and using separate eating utensils. The lesions should be washed gently 3 times per day with a warm, soapy washcloth. Soaked crusts should be removed and topical bactericidal ointment applied. A small amount of bleeding after crust removal is common. The lesions are left uncovered. Children must learn to keep their fingers away from the lesions.

CELLULITIS

Cellulitis is a bacterial infection of the skin and subcutaneous tissue. The condition usually affects the face (buccal and periorbital regions) or lower extremities. Children with cellulitis have a history of trauma, impetigo, upper respiratory infections, sinusitis, otitis media, or tooth abscess. Common causative organisms are staphylococci and streptococci. Clinical manifestations include rapid onset of red or lilac color; tender, hot, edematous skin; and enlarged lymph nodes. Possible complications of cellulitis include septic arthritis, osteomyelitis, meningitis, brain abscess, or blindness.

Medical–Surgical Management

Medical

Cellulitis of the extremities is usually treated at home with oral antibiotics and warm compresses. Cellulitis involving the joints or face is extremely serious, requiring hospitalization and IV antibiotics.

Surgical

Incision and drainage of the affected area may be necessary if the condition does not improve with treatment.

Nursing Management

The affected extremity should be elevated and immobilized. Warm, moist soaks applied every 4 hours increase circulation to the affected area, relieve pain, and promote healing. Parents must be informed that failure to administer the entire course of antibiotics as ordered may result in a more serious infection.

FUNGAL INFECTIONS

Fungal infections are named using the term *tinea* (ringworm) followed by the Latin word for the affected part of the body (Table 54-4).

Nursing Management

Adequate teaching is essential for successful treatment of tinea. Lotion and cream should be applied to the entire lesion and extending to approximately 1 inch beyond the lesion. Oral medication must be taken for the full course of treatment, even if symptoms disappear. Proper hygiene is essential.

VIRAL INFECTIONS

Viral skin infections can produce lesions such as rashes, macules, papules, vesicles, urticaria (hives), and warts. Common communicable diseases of childhood that produce rashes and are preventable through immunizations include rubeola, rubella, and varicella (refer back to Table 54-3). Herpes simplex virus type 1 is a common, contagious skin infection for which there is no cure or prevention.

HERPES SIMPLEX VIRUS TYPE 1

Herpes simplex virus type 1 (HSV-1) is an often recurrent infection of the mouth ("cold sore," "fever blister"), throat, eyes, or fingers (Figure 54-12). After initial infection, the virus remains dormant within nerve cells and can be reactivated by fever, stress, trauma, sun exposure, menstruation, or immunosuppression. Children suffering from burns, eczema, diaper rash, or immunosuppression are particularly susceptible to HSV-1. Clinical manifestations include clusters of fluid-filled vesicles; ulcerations; swelling; inflammation; pruritus; and severe pain. Lesions usually dry and crust within 7 to 10 days.

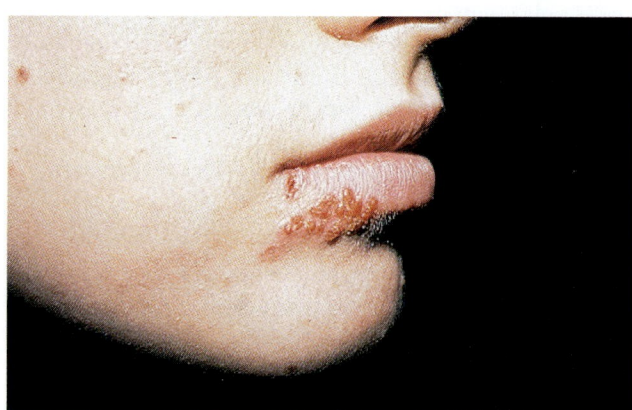

Figure 54-12 Herpes Simplex Virus Type I *(Courtesy of Robert A. Silverman, M.D., Clinical Associate Professor, Department of Pediatrics, Georgetown University)*

Table 54-4 COMMON FUNGAL INFECTIONS

INFECTION (SITES)	CLINICAL MANIFESTATIONS	AFFECTED POPULATION	TREATMENT AND PREVENTION
Tinea capitis (scalp)	Erythema, pruritus, scaly scalp with round patches of alopecia	2- to 10-year-old children	*Treatment:* oral griseofulvin (Fulvicin P/G, Grifulvin V) *Prevention:* Avoid sharing combs, barber scissors, hats, and towels; avoid direct contact with infected scalp
Tinea corporis (trunk, face, extremities)	Ringlike, scaly plaques measuring ½ to 1 inch and having pale centers and red margins	Young boys living in hot, humid climates	*Treatment:* antifungal cream applied three times per day until lesions have been gone for 1 week (usually 2 to 4 weeks). *Prevention:* treat infected pets
Tinea pedis (feet, toes; "athletes foot")	Fissures, red scaly lesions	Adolescents and adults	*Treatment:* daily washing and application of antifungal cream for up to 6 weeks. *Prevention:* avoid contaminated floors, sidewalks, and showers; nylon socks; plastic shoes; closed shoes
Tinea cruris (inner thighs, inguinal area; "jock itch")	Scaly lesions, erythema, pruritus, possible papules or vesicles	Most commonly, athletes and obese individuals	*Treatment:* oral griseofulvin (Fulvicin P/G, Grifulvin V), sitz baths to soothe *Prevention:* wear loose-fitting undergarments to promote dryness

Medical–Surgical Management

Medical

Given that there is no cure for HSV-1, treatment is directed toward relieving symptoms. Usually, children are managed at home by ensuring adequate hydration, pain management, and secondary-infection prevention.

Pharmacological

Antibiotic ointment may be used to treat secondary infections. Acetaminophen (with or without codeine) and topical and mouthrinse anesthetics may be prescribed for pain relief.

Nursing Management

Monitoring for dehydration due to painful swallowing and for prevention of secondary infection is the focus of nursing care. Offering frozen ice pops, jello, noncitrus juices, milk, and flat sodas helps ensure adequate fluid intake despite painful swallowing. Small, frequent feedings of bland, soft foods should be encouraged. Parents must be reassured that fluids are more important than solid food for the first few days.

The hospitalized child is placed in contact isolation or under drainage and secretion precautions. The child is considered contagious until lesions have fallen off or mucous membrane ulcerations have healed.

HOME HEALTH CARE

Caring for the Child with HSV-1
- Wear gloves when suctioning or providing oral care and when handling soiled linens and clothing
- Practice proper handwashing (remembering to wash hands after removing gloves)
- Wash all eating utensils and towels in hot, soapy water
- Do not eat after the child
- Prevent the child from putting the fingers in the mouth (using elbow restraints on infants, if needed)
- Use a protective cover such as a sheet when holding and cuddling the child
- Provide oral fluids that do not irritate the mucous membrane, such as noncitrus juices, flat sodas, milk, and ice pops
- Provide at least 100 mL (approximately ½ cup)/kg/day for a child under 20 kg
- Watch for signs of dehydration, such as dry skin and mucous membranes and decreased urine output (< 3 to 4 times/day)
- Administer medications as prescribed

INFESTATIONS

Infestations are one of the major health problems in schools. Common infestations are pediculosis and scabies.

PEDICULOSIS

Pediculosis (lice) is an infestation that most typically affects the head, body, or pubic area. Pediculosis of the head (head lice) is the most common infestation seen in children. Lice attach their eggs (nits) to hair shafts close to the scalp. The nits then hatch in approximately 1 week. Clinical manifestations of head lice infestation include "dandruff" (nits) that is not easily removed, severe itching of the scalp, and "bugs" in the hair (usually behind the ears and at the back of the head) (Figure 54-13). Signs and symptoms of body lice infestation include intense pruritus and papular, rose-colored dermatitis in areas under tight-fitting clothing.

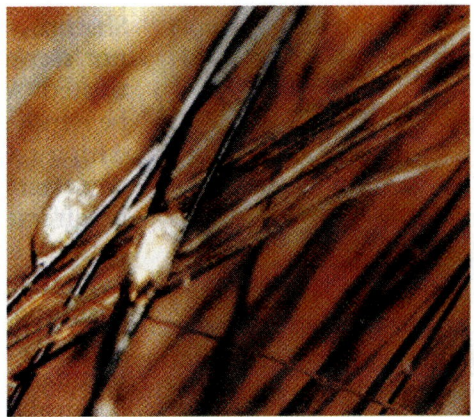

Figure 54-13 Nits *(Courtesy of Hogil Pharmaceutical Corporation)*

PROFESSIONAL TIP

Checking for Lice

Because lice do not transmit from hair to hands, the use of gloves during head checks is neither necessary nor cost effective.

PROFESSIONAL TIP

Manual Removal of Lice

The National Pediculosis Association advocates early detection and manual removal of nits and lice to prevent the unnecessary use of chemicals such as lindane.

HOME HEALTH CARE

Guidelines for Managing Infestations

- Wash bedding, clothing, and stuffed animals in hot water and dry in a hot dryer
- Vacuum carpets, upholstered seats (in the car and house), and mattresses and discard used vaccuum bags
- Dry clean or seal in plastic for 2 weeks any nonwashable items such as hats.
- Soak hair-care products in a scabicide or pediculicide for at least 1 hour.

Lice are easily passed from child to child in close-contact situations (the home, day care centers, and schools) via the sharing of headgear, hair-care products, pillows, blankets, and towels.

Medical–Surgical Management

Pharmacological

Several antilice products are available (Table 54-5).

Nursing Management

Nursing care for children with pediculosis focuses on screening and education. Parents and teachers are encouraged to incorporate checking for lice into routine daily hygiene. Early detection facilitates immediate removal. There is no need to cut long hair or to shave the child's head; which only draws more attention to the fact that the child is infested.

Children should be taught that anyone can get lice and that taunting a child who has lice may hurt the child's feelings. Because lice are transmitted from person to person, children should be cautioned about using hair-care products and hats that do not belong to them.

SCABIES

Scabies results from the impregnated "itch mite" burrowing into the epidermis to lay her eggs. Clinical manifestations include intense pruritus and rash (papules, vesicles, and nodules) found most often on the wrists, finger webs, elbows, axillae, feet, ankles, head, neck, abdomen, waist, groin, and buttocks (Figure 54-14). Secondary infections often occur as a result of scratching of the lesions.

Medical–Surgical Management

Pharmacological

Lindane (Kwell, Scabene) lotion (refer back to Table 54-5) is recommended for children and family members over 2 years of age. Crotamiton (Eurax) lotion is used for children under 2 years of age, because it is considered less toxic than lindane. An oral antihistamine such as diphenhydramine hydrochloride (Benadryl) or hydroxyzine (Atarax) may be prescribed to relieve pruritus.

Nursing Management

Nursing management for the child with scabies focuses on promoting healing, preventing secondary infections, and preventing further transmission of the condition. All persons having direct contact with the child, including care providers and those living in the child's house, should be treated. Itching and rash may endure for 2 to 3 weeks.

BITES/STINGS

Animals (usually dogs), spiders, ticks, and insects (e.g., mosquitoes, fleas) account for the many bites

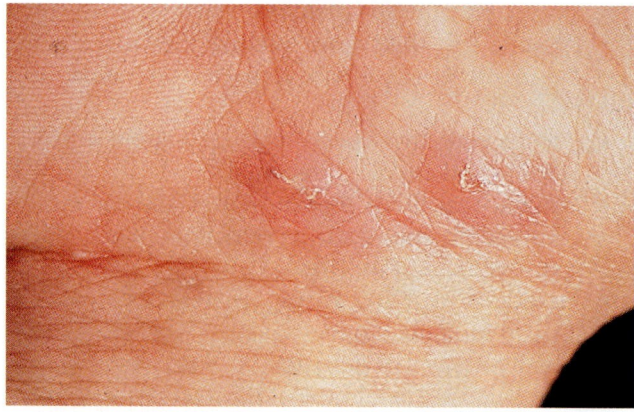

Figure 54-14 Scabies *(Courtesy of Robert A. Silverman, M.D., Clinical Associate Professor, Department of Pediatrics, Georgetown University)*

Table 54-5	ANTILICE PRODUCTS	
PRODUCT	**TREATMENT**	**EFFECT**
lindane (Kwell, Scabene)	Apply to hair, leave on for 4 to 5 minutes, and rinse out of hair with water; reapply in 1 week to kill hatched nits	Kills lice but does *not* effectively kill nits; may be re-absorbed through the skin and cause neurotoxicity
permethrin (Nix)	Apply to shampooed hair, leave on for 10 minutes, and rinse out of hair with water: do not re-shampoo for 24 hours	Safely kills lice and nits with one application
pyrethrins (TripleX, RID)	Apply to hair as directed; repeat treatment in 1 to 2 weeks, if live nits are present	Safely kills lice and nits; product of choice for those under 2 years of age and for pregnant adolescents

and stings suffered by children. Bites and stings generally cause mild discomfort and are simple to treat. However, in some cases, life-threatening situations result.

ANIMAL BITES

Animal bites may result from domestic or wild animals, but are most commonly caused by a familiar dog. Children less than 4 years of age are bitten most frequently, because of their height and the associated tendency to be near the dog's face. Dog bites usually occur on the face or extremities and can result in crushing and puncture wounds and lacerations.

Medical–Surgical Management

Medical

The primary medical concerns for the child who has suffered an animal bite are infections from rabies and tetanus and scarring, especially on the face. Generally, after the wound and surrounding area are thoroughly washed with mild soap and water, a clean dressing is applied.

Pharmacological

If the animal is unvaccinated for rabies, the child will be given a series of immunizations to prevent rabies. Antibiotics may be indicated if the wounds are deep. Tetanus toxoid may be administered, depending on the child's immunization history and the severity of the wound.

Nursing Management

Nursing care focuses on prevention and wound care. It is important for children to learn "animal safety rules" in order to prevent bites.

Parents and children should be taught to cleanse wounds properly and observe for signs of infection.

CLIENT TEACHING

Animal Safety Rules
- Stay away from strange or wild animals such as raccoons, skunks, bats, and squirrels
- Stay away from a dog's face
- Pet animals by rubbing, stroking, scratching, and patting; never hit, bite, or pinch
- Allow unfamiliar animals to smell you before attempting to touch them
- Ask the permission of the owner before petting an animal
- Never approach an animal while it is eating, sleeping, injured, or tending to its babies

Also parents should be encouraged to keep their child's immunizations up to date. If rabies immunizations are required, parents must understand the importance of returning for the injections on the appropriate days. Animal bites should be reported to the community animal control agency.

SPIDER BITES

Bites from black widow and brown recluse spiders demand medical attention. Characteristically, these spiders are nonagressive, avoid light, and bite only in self-defense. Although both spiders inject toxic venom when they bite, the initial bite itself may go unnoticed. Within a few hours after the bite, however, manifestations such as swollen, painful erythema, and systemic reactions surface. Black widow venom is neurotoxic and may cause dizziness, weakness, abdominal pain, paralysis, seizures, and, possibly, death due to shock and renal failure. Brown recluse venom is necrotoxic, with the bite progressing to a necrotic ulcer within 1 to 2 weeks. Systemic reactions may include fever, nausea and vomiting, and joint pain. The recluse bite is not fatal, but the ulcer may take months to heal.

Medical–Surgical Management

Medical

The child with a black widow spider bite will be hospitalized for supportive care until neurological symptoms subside and renal function is confirmed. The child with a brown recluse bite will require wound care and pain management but will usually not require hospitalization.

Surgical

Skin grafting may be required for large ulcers resulting from the brown recluse spider bite.

Pharmacological

Antivenin (Lactrodectus mactans) is administered to the child with a black widow spider bite, if the child has no allergy to horse serum. In addition, analgesics, muscle relaxants, and tetanus prophylaxis may be required.

There is no antivenin for the brown recluse spider bite. Antibiotics, corticosteroids, analgesics, and tetanus prophylaxis may be prescribed for the time period during which the wound is healing.

Nursing Management

Nursing management focuses on wound care, proper administration of medications, and prevention. Parents and children should be taught to be cautious in areas where spiders are likely to live, such as woodpiles and closets.

Guidelines for Preventing Tick Bites
- When walking in fields or woods, wear long-sleeved shirts, tuck long pants into socks, and use insect repellent. Wearing light colors facilitates finding ticks.
- When returning from a tick-infested area, look for ticks and remove ticks as soon as possible.
- Bathe dogs with a shampoo containing permethrin.

TICK BITES

Ticks live in fields and woods. They feed on the blood of mammals (e.g., humans, dogs, livestock, and deer) by embedding their heads into the skin. Tick bites cause pruritic nodules at the site of attachment and, rarely, systemic reactions such as fever, rash, and paralysis. Lyme disease and Rocky Mountain spotted fever are caused by organisms that are transmitted by ticks.

Nursing Management

Preventing tick bites and removing embedded ticks are the primary focus. Ticks are removed by applying vaseline or nail polish for 30 minutes to suffocate the tick. The tick's body is then grasped with tweezers and pulled straight up in an attempt to remove the embedded head along with the body. Any remaining part of the head should be removed using a sterile needle. Hands should then be thoroughly washed.

INSECT BITES

Insects such as mosquitoes, flies, fleas, and gnats inject foreign proteins when they penetrate the skin to suck blood. Insect bites usually result in itching, erythema, and small wheal. The severity of the reaction depends on the degree of the child's hypersensitivity.

Medical–Surgical Management

Medical

Medical management focuses on alleviating itching and preventing infection. Baths and cool compresses may relieve itching and prevent scratching, which can lead to bacterial infections.

Pharmacological

Antipruritics and antihistamines may be prescribed to control severe itching and facilitate sleep.

Nursing Management

Nursing management focuses on preventing bites, alleviating itching, and preventing infection. Mattresses, carpets, furniture, and pets may require treatment with insecticides.

CONTACT DERMATITIS

Contact dermatitis is an inflammatory reaction of the skin to allergens, such as rubber, dyes, nickel, or poison ivy, or to irritants, such as soaps, wool, urine, or stool. Manifestations of allergic contact dermatitis include tiny, itching, weeping blisters over an area of skin (Figure 54-15). Manifestations of irritant contact dermatitis include localized, dry, inflamed, pruritic skin.

Medical–Surgical Management

Medical

Treatment involves discontinuing exposure to the offending agent, washing the skin thoroughly, and applying cool compresses.

Pharmacological

Steroid cream (1%) may be applied in a thin layer several times per day after the application of cool compresses. Oral steroids may be prescribed for severe cases.

Nursing Management

Nursing care is aimed at relieving itching, preventing infection, and identifying and removing offensive substances. In addition to cool compresses, oral antihistamines, antipruritic lotions, and tepid Aveeno baths may relieve itching. Overheating should be avoided. Children should be taught to recognize and avoid poison ivy, oak, and sumac.

ACNE

Acne, one of the most common health problems of adolescence, is a noninfectious, inflammatory disease

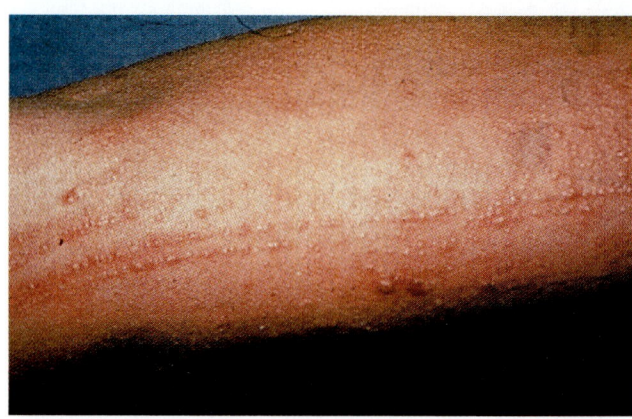

Figure 54-15 Contact Dermatitis *(Courtesy of the Centers for Disease Control and Prevention [CDC])*

of the skin involving the sebaceous glands and hair follicles (Figure 54-16). Pathophysiologic factors having the greatest influence on acne development are overproduction of sebum; formation of **comedones**, or whiteheads and blackheads (Figure 54-17); and proliferation of *Propionibacterium acnes* bacteria in the hair follicles (Hurwitz, 1995).

Manifestations include comedones, papules, pustules, and nodules on the face, neck, back, shoulders, and upper chest. Factors related to the development of acne include elevated hormone levels (especially androgens); predisposition; emotional stress; hot, humid environments; the premenstrual period, in females; and the growth of anaerobic bacteria. The visual lesions of acne, although usually temporary, may be extremely distressing to the adolescent, who is typically very concerned about appearance.

Medical–Surgical Management

Pharmacological

Treatment is individualized, depending on the severity and types of lesions. The goal is to decrease sebum production and prevent infection with *P. acnes*. Topical agents benzoyl peroxide (Clearasil, Benoxyl) and tretinoin (Retin-A) are available as cleansers, lotions, creams, sticks, pads, gels, and bars and may be effective for mild cases. Other topical keratolytic agents containing sulfur, resorcinol, or salicylic acid may be prescribed for drying and peeling effects. Topical or oral antibiotics, such as erythromycin and tetracycline preparations, may be administered for infections.

CLIENT TEACHING

Isotretinoin (Accutane)

It is important that adolescent females on isotretinoin, who are sexually active, use contraceptives 1 month before treatment is started; during treatment; and 1 month after discontinuation of treatment. In addition, clients tacking isotretinoin should not donate blood during this period of time.

Isotretinoin (Accutane) may be used for nodulocystic acne. Side effects of isotretinoin include dry lips and skin, eye irritation, temporary worsening of acne, **epistaxis** (nosebleed), bleeding and inflammation of the gums, itching, photosensitivity, and joint and muscle pain. In addition, isotretinoin may cause central nervous system, heart, thymus, and craniofacial abnormalities in the fetus.

If isotretinoin is to be prescribed, preganancy tests are done 2 weeks prior to initiating, every month during, and 1 month after discontinuing the treatment. All women of childbearing potential are placed on contraception during treatment.

Nursing Management

A healthy lifestyle, including adequate rest, exercise, and diet, promotes healing of lesions. The nurse must be especially sensitive to the adolescent's feelings about the condition, no matter how mild the case may seem.

The adolescent and family must be educated about acne and the prescribed treatment. Adolescents should take responsibility for implementing the prescribed care.

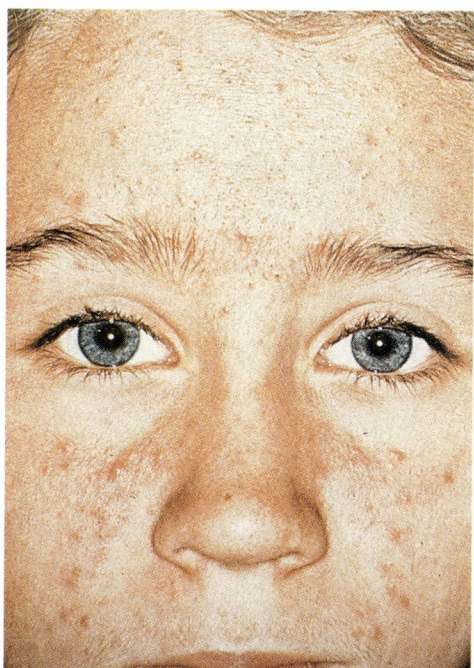

Figure 54-16 Acne (*From* Acne Vulgaris, *by G. Plewig and A. B. Kligmann (Eds.). 1975 Berlin/Heideberg, Germany: Springer-Verlag. Used with permission.*)

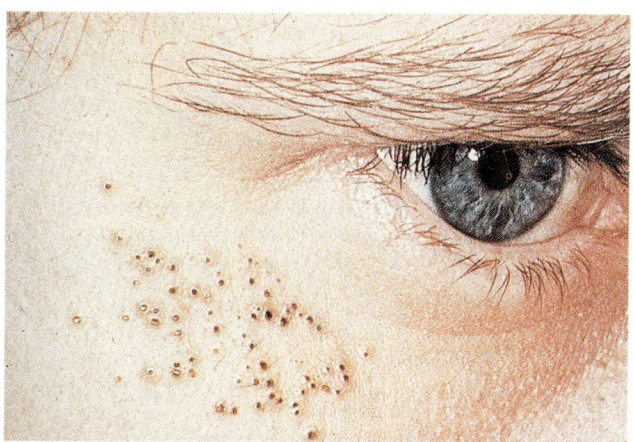

Figure 54-17 Open Comedones (*From* Acne Vulgaris, *by G. Plewig and A. B. Kligmann (Eds.), 1975 Berlin/Heideberg, Germany: Springer-Verlag. Used with permission.*)

BURNS

Burns are the second leading cause of injury deaths among children between 1 and 14 years of age (Ashwill & Droske, 1997). Carelessness of adults, the children's curiosity and increasing mobility, and caretakers' failure to adequately supervise children all contribute to the high incidence of burns among children. In addition, burns are a common form of child abuse (Herrin & Antoon, 1996). Thermal burns (e.g., from scalding liquids, house fires) are most common, followed by chemical (e.g., from touching or ingesting caustic agents) and electrical (e.g., from wires, curling irons, ovens), respectively.

The major manifestations of burns include severe wounds, pain, fluid and nutritional deficits, respiratory complications, and secondary infections. All systems of the burned child are at risk for complications.

Medical–Surgical Management

Medical

The severity of the burn injury is assessed on the basis of the percentage of surface burned and the depth of the wound. The standard "rule of nines" used with adults yields an inaccurate estimate of distribution of burns in children because of the differences in body proportion between children and adults. Adaptations of the Lund and Browder (1944) chart for determining percentage of body surface area in pediatric burn injuries are frequently used (Figure 54-18).

The involvement of specific body parts or certain specific burn distributions increase burn severity, regardless of body surface area affected. Burns to the face, hands, feet, perineal area, or anterior chest, and circumferential burns of the thorax or extremity are treated as major because of the potential for functional impairment. Regardless of the amount of tissue destroyed, if smoke inhalation is suspected, there is risk for airway obstruction.

Pharmacological

Tetanus antitoxin or toxoid should be ordered according to the child's immunization status. Intravenous morphine sulfate is the drug of choice for pain control. Analgesics must be administered 20 to 30 minutes prior to dressing changes and debridement to provide the most relief possible. Itching may persist for months and may be relieved with medication.

Health Promotion

Prevention of scarring and contractures is essential for optimal cosmetic and functional recovery. Pressure dressings and suits may need to be worn for more than 1 year to minimize scarring. Physical therapy, initiated

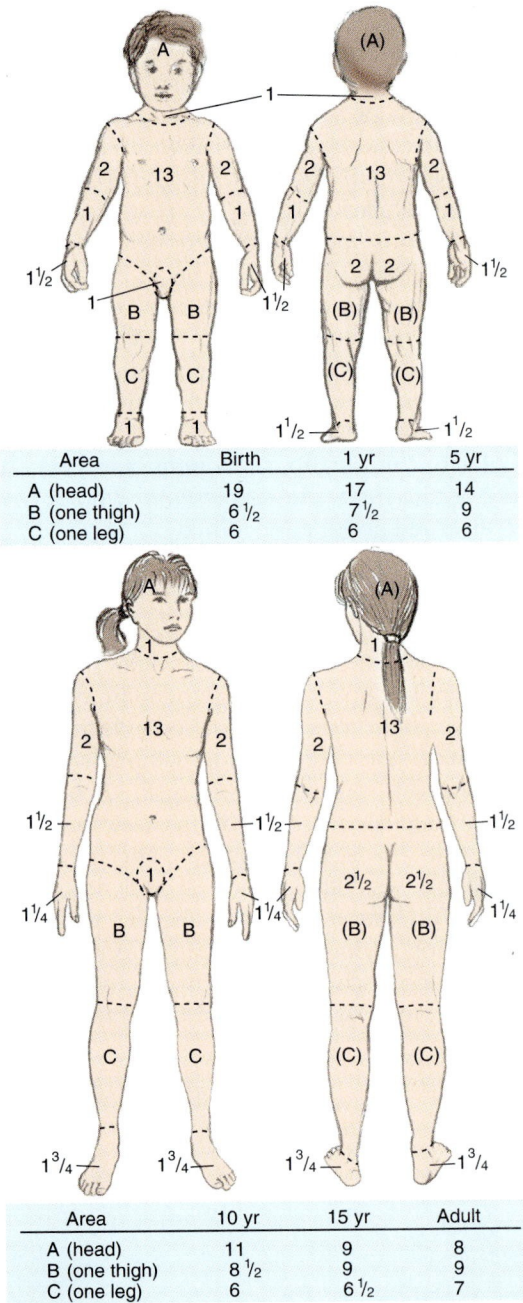

Area	Birth	1 yr	5 yr
A (head)	19	17	14
B (one thigh)	6 1/2	7 1/2	9
C (one leg)	6	6	6

Area	10 yr	15 yr	Adult
A (head)	11	9	8
B (one thigh)	8 1/2	9	9
C (one leg)	6	6 1/2	7

Figure 54-18 Estimation of Distribution of Burns (*From Whaley and Wong's Nursing Care of Infants and Children (6th ed.), D. Wong, M. Hockenberry-Eaton, M. Winkelstein, D. Wilson, E. Ahmann, and P. DiVito-Thomas, 1999, St. Louis, MO: Mosby. Copyright 1999 by Mosby. Adapted with permission.*)

at the time of admission and continued until the scars mature, prevents flexion contractures. These treatments add to the child's discomfort.

Nursing Management

Refer to Chapter 40, Nursing Care of the Client: Integumentary System, for information on nursing management of the client who has been burned.

URINARY SYSTEM

Acute poststreptococcal glomerulonephritis, nephrotic syndrome, and enuresis are discussed following.

ACUTE POSTSTREPTOCOCCAL GLOMERULONEPHRITIS

Glomerulonephritis is an inflammation of the glomeruli of the kidneys. Acute poststreptococcal glomerulonephritis (APSGN) occurs as an immune reaction to streptococcal infection of the throat or skin.

Clinical manifestations of hematuria and periorbital edema usually appear 1 to 3 weeks after a streptococcal infection. Other possible manifestations include decreased urine output, hypertension, fever, and fatigue. The prognosis is excellent.

Medical–Surgical Management

Medical

The diagnosis of APSGN can be made based on history, presenting symptoms, and laboratory results. There is no treatment for APSGN. Medical management focuses on presenting signs and symptoms and the degree of renal dysfunction. Laboratory values usually return to normal within 6 to 12 weeks.

Pharmacological

Hypertension may be treated by limiting sodium and water intake or by administering diuretics or antihypertensives.

Nursing Management

Refer to Chapter 42, Nursing Care of the Client: Urinary System, for information on nursing management of the client with APSGN.

NEPHROTIC SYNDROME

Nephrotic syndrome refers to kidney disorders characterized by proteinuria, hypoalbuminemia, and edema. The most common childhood nephrotic disorder, minimal change nephrotic syndrome (MCNS), results from minimal alterations of the glomerulus. The cause of the alteration is unknown.

Clinical manifestations include pitting edema (periorbital and dependent), anorexia, fatigue, abdominal pain, increased weight, and normal blood pressure. Potential complications include respiratory compromise and peritonitis. Although the child may experience remissions and exacerbations for months, the prognosis in most cases is good.

Medical–Surgical Management

Medical

Diagnosis is made based on clinical presentation, age of the child, massive proteinuria (50 mg/kg/day), and hypoalbuminemia (below 27g/L) (Kelsch & Sedman, 1993).

Surgical

A kidney biopsy may be done if a lesion other than MCNS is suspected or the child does not respond as expected to pharmacological treatments.

Pharmacological

The use of corticosteroids such as prednisone (Cortan) induces remission in most cases. Corticosteroid therapy usually produces diuresis within 7 to 14 days. After diuresis occurs, prednisone is continued every other day for 3 days per week. Urine is tested daily for protein until protein has been absent from the urine for up to 7 days. The drug dosage is then gradually decreased and discontinued over a 4-week period. Repeat corticosteroid therapy is administered to children who have relapses after drug therapy is discontinued.

Alkylating agents such as cyclophosphamide (Cytoxan) may be used to reduce symptoms and prevent further relapses in children who do not respond adequately to repeated corticosteroid therapy. The risks and benefits of this therapy must be carefully considered.

When the child is in remission, administration of vaccines for pneumococci and flu should be considered, because an exacerbation of nephrotic syndrome can occur following an infection.

Diet

A general "no-added-salt" diet is recommended. Appealing, small, frequent meals should be offered to the child, who typically has a poor appetite.

▶ NURSING PROCESS

▶ Assessment

▶ Subjective Data
The family should be questioned about symptom onset, appetite, urine output, irritability, and signs of fatigue.

▶ Objective Data
Areas of assessment include daily weight, abdominal girth, and vital signs. Skin is assessed for pallor, irritation, breakdown, and edema.

Nursing diagnoses for the child with MCNS may include the following:

Nursing Diagnoses	Planning/Goals	Nursing Interventions
▶ *Fluid Volume Excess related to compromised regulatory mechanism*	The client will maintain fluid balance.	Monitor I & O hourly; report urinary output of < 2 mL/kg/hr. Weigh daily. Measure abdominal girth daily at the level of the umbilicus. Test urine albumin daily with reagent strips.
▶ *Skin Integrity, Impaired, Risk for, related to altered circulation*	The client's skin will remain intact.	Inspection the child's skin for breakdown. Turn and reposition the child every 2 hours. Keep the child's skin clean and dry. Use a protective mattress (e.g., eggcrate).
▶ *Infection, Risk for, related to immunosuppression*	The client will remain infection free.	Screen visitors for signs of infection. Practice proper handwashing technique. Monitor the child for signs of infection, such as sore throat, cough, fever, abdominal pain. Monitor laboratory values daily.
▶ *Knowledge Deficit (family) related to treatment regimen*	The family will follow through with the prescribed treatment.	Educate the family about the disease process. Instruct the family to test urine for albumin, assess for edema and infection, and administer drugs. Instruct the family to allow a return to ADL once the child is free of edema.

Evaluation Each goal must be evaluated to determine how it has been met by the client.

ENURESIS

Enuresis is involuntary urination beyond the age when control of urination commonly is acquired. It is not unusual for nocturnal enuresis, or bedwetting, to occur until 8 years of age, due to small bladder capacity and delayed maturation of the neuromuscular system. Most children will outgrow bedwetting without therapeutic intervention.

When enuresis continues to occur beyond the eighth year or reoccurs in a child who has been dry both day and night for a prolonged period, there may be cause for concern. Possible causes of reoccurring enuresis include urinary tract infections, minor abnormalities of the urinary tract, pinworm infestation, constipation, diabetes, sickle-cell anemia, sexual abuse, stress, and sleep disorders.

Medical–Surgical Management

Medical

Urinalysis and urine culture are done to rule out infection. Other diagnostic studies are performed to rule out all possible causes. Common treatment approaches for enuresis without a physiologic cause include fluid restriction, bladder stretching exercises, behavioral conditioning (e.g., enuresis alarm), and reward systems.

Pharmacological

An anticholinergic such as oxybutynin chloride (Ditropan) may reduce uninhibited bladder contractions. Vasopressins such as desmopressin acetate (DDAVP) nasal spray may reduce nighttime urine output. Antidepressants such as imipramine hydrochloride (Tofranil) may be prescribed.

Other Therapies

If emotional factors are precipitating enuresis, psychosocial support may be an essential part of care. A multidisciplinary team approach is most effective.

PROFESSIONAL TIP

Enuresis

It is most important to provide the family and the child with opportunities to ventilate feelings. The family and the child must be active and willing participants in any plan of care that is implemented. Parents must be told that reprimanding the child will not improve the outcome.

PSYCHOSOCIAL DISORDERS

Psychosocial disorders are responses to stressors. Factors influencing an individual's response to stressors include temperment, developmental level, nature and duration of the stressors, past experiences, and coping and adaptive abilities of the family. Possible manifestations in children include depression, anxiety, encopresis, enuresis, passive–agressive behavior, and learning problems (Ashwill & Droske, 1997). Some of the psychosocial disorders of childhood include obesity, anorexia nervosa and bulimia nervosa, autism, attention deficit hyperactivity disorder, and suicide.

OBESITY

Obesity is the excessive accumulation of fat resulting in an increase in body weight to 20% or more above ideal weight. Obesity can be a precursor of cardiovascular disease, hypertension, and diabetes. Factors contributing to obesity include an overconsumption of food; a sedentary lifestyle; a lack of parental knowledge regarding nutrition and food preparation; unstructured meals; genetic predisposition; and peer pressure.

The obese child may overeat to compensate for lack of parental love and to relieve stress. As a result of obesity, the child may have low self-esteem, poor body image, difficulty in relationships, and recurring bouts of anxiety and depression.

Medical–Surgical Management

Medical

Obesity is difficult to treat. Positive outcomes are more likely when the child has a support system, understands the importance of weight reduction, and is actively involved in the plan of care.

Diet

Meals and snacks should consist of small servings of nutritional foods. The family and child should be taught ways to select and prepare foods. Favorite foods should be incorporated into the menu whenever possible.

Activity

Physical exercise must be incorporated into the child's daily routine.

Nursing Management

Nursing care focuses on meeting nutritional needs, managing related problems, and promoting self-esteem. Weight, exercise, and nutritional intake should be assessed at predetermined intervals. Positive feedback

CLIENT TEACHING

Caring for the Child Who Is Obese
Share the following ideas with caregivers of obese children.

Nutrition
- Keep a food diary for 1 week; include time, place, type, and amount of food eaten, and the reasons for eating
- Set a reasonable weight-loss or weight-maintenance goal
- Establish and maintain regular mealtimes
- Serve meals at the table only, preferably with the family
- Serve meals on a small plate in an effort to decrease quantity of food consumed
- Encourage the child to eat slowly
- Keep low-calorie snacks on hand.

Exercise
- Get the child involved in regular outside activities.
- Walk instead of ride whenever possible.

Self-Esteem
- Weigh the child only one time per week
- Focus on the child's positive assets
- Provide positive feedback for positive behavior

Support
- Establish a group or buddy system
- Participate in a support group

should be provided for accomplishments, no matter how small. Goals should be discussed and revised as needed.

Support groups such as Weight Watchers and Overeaters Anonymous may be helpful. In addition, support groups may be available through schools, summer camps, or children's hospitals. A team approach utilizing a psychiatrist or psychologist, a nutritionist, and a nurse may be appropriate.

ANOREXIA NERVOSA AND BULIMIA NERVOSA

Anorexia nervosa and bulimia nervosa are two of the most common eating disorders among children. Anorexia nervosa is self-inflicted starvation; bulimia nervosa is binge-eating followed by purging. These disorders usually begin in middle to late adolescence and can last indefinitely, depending on response to treatment. The incidence is highest among white girls in the higher socioecomonic classes (Wong, et al.,

1999). Possible causes of these disorders include sensitivity to social pressure for thinness; distorted body image; and longstanding dysfunctional family patterns.

Clinical manifestations include body weight 15% below that expected for age and height, intense fear of gaining weight, dry skin, brittle nails, downy hair on the back and extremities, amenorrhea, constipation, hypothermia, bradycardia, low blood pressure, fluid and electrolyte imbalances, and anemia. Depression, crying spells, feelings of isolation and loneliness, and suicidal thoughts and feelings are common. Clues to frequent vomiting include dental caries and erosion and throat irritation. Callouses or abrasions may be noted on the back of the hands, from frequent contact with the teeth while inducing vomiting.

Medical–Surgical Management

Medical

The goal of medical treatment is to correct malnutrition and resulting complications. A weight gain of 0.1 to 0.2 kg/d is emphasized until the desired weight is attained. Enteral feedings or total parenteral nutrition (TPN) may be necessary to replace lost fluids, protein, and nutrients.

Pharmacological

Antidepressants such as imipramine hydrochloride (Tofranil) or desipramine hydrochloride (Norpramin) may be prescribed.

Other Therapies

Individual and family therapy are used to address dysfunctional family patterns and assist the adolescent in identifying and dealing with self-esteem and body image issues. Treatment is typically long-term.

Nursing Management

Refer to Chapter 45, Nursing Care of the Client: Mental Illness, for possible nursing diagnoses for the client with anorexia or bulimia nervosa and to the Resources listing at the end of this book.

AUTISM

Autism is a complex disorder of brain function involving abnormal emotional, social, and linguistic development. The cause of autism is unknown. However, research suggests it may result from a disturbance in language comprehension, a biochemical problem involving neurotransmitters, or abnormalities in the central nervous system.

Possible clinical manifestations include lack of eye contact, aversion to touch, delayed language development, blank expression, lack of response to verbal stimulation, repetitive behaviors, bizarre body movements, and self-destructive behaviors. Manifestations may vary from mild to severe. The prognosis depends on early detection and the child's response to treatment.

Medical–Surgical Management

Medical

Diagnosis is based on the presence of specific criteria as listed in the *Diagnostic and Statistical Manual of Mental Disorders,* fourth edition (DSM-IV) (American Psychiatric Association, 1994). In addition, a complete physical and neurological examination is necessary to rule out other disorders such as lead poisoning, phenylketonuria, congenital rubella, and measles encephalitis.

Treatment is provided by a multidisciplanary team and focuses on promoting normal development, social interaction, and learning. Behavior-modification techniques are used to reward desirable behaviors and foster positive coping skills.

Nursing Management

Nursing care focuses on early detection, decreasing environmental stimuli, providing supportive care, maintaining a safe environment, and giving parents anticipatory guidance. Assessment must include monitoring growth and development, especially language and social skills. When caring for a child with autism, it is important to ascertain the child's routines, rituals, and likes and dislikes. Because autistic children do not do well in unfamiliar environments, it is important that they be surrounded by familiar objects. The child may need assistance with self-care. Schedules and care providers should be kept as consistent as possible. Close supervision is usually required at all times.

Parents need a great deal of support to cope with the challenges of having an autistic child. Children should be assisted to reach their maximum potential

CLIENT TEACHING

Modifying Behavior in the Child Who Is Autistic

- Emphasize the child's positive skills
- Provide immediate feedback for appropriate behavior
- Continue social interactions even when the child is unresponsive
- Provide tactile stimulation such as tickling, holding, cuddling, and shaking hands
- Teach the child to embrace, kiss, and shake hands
- Speak in short sentences
- Use a firm but caring approach
- Maintain daily routines

through enrollment in special education programs and participation in behavior modification. Some children may achieve independence by adulthood. Parents should be informed about local support groups and referred to the Autism Society of America for current information.

ATTENTION DEFICIT HYPERACTIVITY DISORDER

Attention deficit hyperactivity disorder (ADHD) is a developmental disorder characterized by developmentally inappropriate degrees of inattention, overactivity, and impulsivity. The child is usually diagnosed between the ages of 3 and 6 years. Possible clinical manifestations include poor impulse control, distractibility, fidgeting with hands, squirming in seat, excessive talking, and difficulty following instructions.

Medical–Surgical Management

Medical

Diagnosis may be made based on diagnostic criteria in the DSM-IV (American Psychiatric Association, 1994) as well as a complete multidisciplinary evaluation. Treatment focuses on decreasing distractions, modifying behavior (e.g., setting limits, ensuring consistency, praising accomplishments), and/or initiating pharmacological therapy.

Pharmacological

The most commonly prescribed medications include methylphenidate (Ritalin), pemoline (Cylert), and dextroamphetamine (Dexedrine). These drugs stimulate the area of the child's brain that facilitates concentration. Potential side effects include loss of appetite resulting in delayed growth.

CLIENT TEACHING

Caring for the Child with ADHD
- Praise positive behaviors and set limits
- Administer medication as prescribed and with meals
- Give clear, simple instructions and provide frequent reminders to follow instructions
- Reduce stimuli in the child's environment, for example, turning off the TV when the child is to do homework
- Allow for a shortened attention span by providing short teaching sessions and activities that allow for mobility
- Consult with trained professional for behavior-modification therapy

Nursing Management

Nursing care focuses on improving the child's social interaction and educating the family and teachers.

SUICIDE

Suicide is the third leading cause of death among adolescents. Boys complete suicide four times more often than do girls, but girls attempt suicide five times more often than do boys. Males tend to use lethal methods such as guns, hanging, and jumping from high elevations, whereas girls more often overdose or cut the wrists. Adolescents who have attempted suicide once are at greatest risk for attempting again. Attempted suicide rarely occurs without warning (Centers for Disease Control and Prevention, 1997a).

Clinical manifestations in the suicidal adolescent may include depression, boredom, restlessness, concentration problems, irritability, lethargy, and intentional misbehavior. Children at high risk for committing suicide may be experiencing depression; pregnancy; failure in school; drug use; death of a friend or parent; problems with a relationship; sexual abuse; chronic illness; or a broken home.

Medical–Surgical Management

Medical

The child thought to be at high risk for suicide is usually admitted to a psychiatric unit for care. Treatment may include individual, group, and/or family therapy. Negotiating a "No-Suicide" contract is one method that may be used with a suicidal child. In this written and signed contract, the child agrees not to attempt suicide for a negotiated period of time (e.g., weeks, days, minutes). If at any time the child feels unable to keep the contract, the child agrees to contact help. Children with severe self-abusive behavior may need to be physically or chemically restrained.

Pharmacological

Drugs that may be used for chemical restraint include diphenhydramine hydrochloride (Benadryl), thioridazine hydrochloride (Mellaril), chlorpromazine (Thorazine), and lorazepam (Ativan). The suicidal child may also require antidepressant and/or antipsychotic medications.

▶ NURSING PROCESS

▶ Assessment

▶ Subjective Data

The nurse assesses the suicidal child for behaviors; attitudes; risk factors; lethality of the proposed method of suicide; coping mechanisms; and support systems.

▶ Objective Data

The nurse observes the child for signs of physical and sexual abuse, self-destructive behaviors, and sudden changes in behavior.

Nursing diagnoses for the child who is suicidal may include the following:

Nursing Diagnoses	Planning/Goals	Nursing Interventions
▶ *Violence, Risk for, Self-directed, related to desire to ease emotional pain, solicit attention of others, or avoid responsibility*	The client will be less likely to repeat the suicide attempt.	Use a nonjudgmental, empathic approach and a voice and demeanor that are clear, direct, and supportive to discuss feelings and the suicidal event.
		Remove potentially harmful objects from the environment (e.g., belts, scarves, shoestrings, matches, lighters).
		Monitor the high-risk child at all times, even during bathroom use and sleep.
		Administer prescribed medications.
		Suggest alternate activities for those times when impulsive behavior occurs.
		Restrain the child (as ordered) as an act of care, not punishment.
▶ *Family Processes, Altered, related to relational disturbance or abuse/neglect*	The client will feel safe and receive support from others to meet needs.	Encourage individual and group therapy for the entire family to explore personal issues and the need for social support.
		Assist the parents to regain the ability to assist their child and manage the home environment.
		Foster parent–child interaction.
		Teach the family to monitor the child for sudden changes in behavior.
		Teach the family and child about medication administration.
		Encourage the family to keep follow-up appointments.

Evaluation Each goal must be evaluated to determine how it has been met by the client.

CASE STUDY

Jaime is a 14-year-old male. He was diagnosed with DMD at 5 years of age. His older brother also had DMD and died 2 years ago at the age of 16. Jaime lives with his parents and 10-year-old sister, Liza. Associated problems include confinement to a wheelchair; contractures of the hips, knees, and ankles; scoliosis requiring a brace; frequent respiratory infections; and obesity. Jaime attends the ninth grade, is a member of the chess club, and enjoys the youth group at his church.

The following questions will guide your development of a nursing care plan for the case study.

1. List the characteristic progression of DMD.
2. Cite three nursing diagnoses and goals for Jaime.
3. Identify interventions to help Jaime and his family address the nursing diagnoses identified in question 2.
4. How might genetic counseling benefit this family?
5. Identify resources available to help Jaime and his family cope with DMD.

SUMMARY

- The most common skin disorders among toddlers and preschoolers are impetigo and dog bites.
- The most common skin disorders among school-age children are pediculosis and scabies.
- The most common skin disorder among adolescents is acne.
- Common respiratory tract infections of childhood include nasopharyngitis, pharyngitis, and influenza.
- Asthma is the leading cause of chronic illness among children.
- Treatment of asthma involves allergen control, drug therapy, controlled exercise, physical therapy, and desensitization.
- Prevention or treatment of group A streptococcal infection in turn prevents rheumatic fever.
- Nursing care of the child with leukemia focuses on preparing the child and family for diagnostic and therapeutic procedures, preventing complications of myelosuppression, managing problems of drug toxicity, and providing emotional support.
- Parents of a child with ITP must be able to detect signs of bleeding and know ways to prevent injuries.
- Constipation can be prevented by establishing and maintaining regular toileting habits, drinking fluids, eating a diet high in fiber, and participating in regular exercise.
- Children are more commonly infected with intestinal parasites than are adults because they put their fingers in their mouths more often.
- Obesity can be a precursor to cardiovascular disease, hypertension, and diabetes.
- Acute poststreptococcal glomerulonephritis occurs as an immune reaction to streptococcal infection of the throat or skin.
- Goals for the child with nephrotic syndrome include fluid balance, intact skin, freedom from infection, and compliance with urine testing and drug therapy.
- Goals for children with structural anomolies, such as scoliosis or Legg-Calve-Perthes disease, and injuries may include preventing skin breakdown (due to casts and braces) and keeping follow-up appointments.
- Nursing care for the child with DMD focuses on maintaining physical activity, promoting respiratory function, managing weight, and encouraging age-appropriate social activities.
- Nursing care for the child with juvenile rheumatoid arthritis focuses on preventing injury, controlling pain, enhancing mobility, and encouraging age-appropriate activities.
- Nursing goals for the autistic child may include decreasing environmental stimuli, providing supportive care, maintaining a safe environment, and giving parents anticipatory guidance.

- Treatment for the child with ADHD focuses on decreasing distractions, modifying behavior, and initiating drug therapy.
- Suicide is the third leading cause of death among adolescents.
- Child abuse can be classified as physical abuse, physical neglect, emotional abuse, or sexual abuse.

Review Questions

1. Determining the causative agent and administering the proper treatment for skin and throat infections may prevent further complications such as:
   a. leukemia.
   b. mononucleosis.
   c. idiopathic thrombocytopenia purpura.
   d. acute post-streptococcal glomerulonephritis.

2. The safest option for treating pediculosis is to:
   a. detect early and spray with insecticides.
   b. wash with regular shampoo.
   c. wash with treated shampoo.
   d. detect early and remove manually.

3. The best way to prevent allergic rhinitis and asthma is to:
   a. force fluids.
   b. take antibiotics.
   c. control allergens.
   d. take antihistamines.

4. Children with leukemia are at high risk for infection because of:
   a. decreased lymphocytes
   b. increased red blood cells
   c. decreased platelets
   d. decreased neutrophils

5. Intestinal parasitic infections are more prevalent among children than among adults because:
   a. children are not toilet trained.
   b. adults maintain better hygiene.
   c. adults eat more nutritious meals.
   d. children put their hands in their mouths more often.

6. Nursing diagnoses for the child with nephrotic syndrome may include:
   a. *Fluid Volume Excess related to fluid retention.*
   b. *Pain related to operative procedure.*
   c. *Mobility, Impaired, Physical, related to use of a brace.*
   d. *Body Image Disturbance related to loss of hair.*

7. A clinical manifestation of scoliosis is:

    a. lateral curvature of the spine.
    b. necrosis of the femoral head.
    c. quadricep muscle atrophy.
    d. Gower's sign.

8. Treatment for the child with ADHD includes:

    a. decreasing distractions.
    b. placing in special education class.
    c. prescribing sedatives.
    d. eating a special diet.

Critical Thinking Questions

1. What is the most important data to gather when assessing a child for fluid volume deficit?

2. What would you say to a parent who smokes around a child who has asthma?

WEB FLASH!

- Search the Web for current legal/ethical issues related to pediatric health care.
- What Internet resources can you find directed toward parents on the subject of communicable diseases? Are prevention guidelines included? What hotline numbers can you locate?

Chapter 55
Nursing Care of the Older Client

55

NURSING CARE OF THE OLDER CLIENT

MAKING THE CONNECTION

Refer to the following chapters to increase your understanding of the older adult:

- **Chapter 8, Communication**
- **Chapter 23, Fluid, Electrolyte, and Acid–Base Balance**
- **Chapter 29, Nursing Care of the Surgical Client**
- **Chapter 31, Nursing Care of the Client: Respiratory System**
- **Chapter 32, Nursing Care of the Client: Cardiovascular System**
- **Chapter 34, Nursing Care of the Client: Gastrointestinal System**
- **Chapter 35, Nursing Care of the Client: Reproductive System**
- **Chapter 37, Nursing Care of the Client: Endocrine System**

- **Chapter 38, Nursing Care of the Client: Musculoskeletal System**
- **Chapter 40, Nursing Care of the Client: Integumentary System**
- **Chapter 41, Nursing Care of the Client: Nervous System**
- **Chapter 42, Nursing Care of the Client: Urinary System**
- **Chapter 43, Nursing Care of the Client: Sensory System**
- **Chapter 45, Nursing Care of the Client: Mental Illness**
- **Chapter 46, Nursing Care of the Client: Substance Abuse**

LEARNING OBJECTIVES

Upon completion of this chapter, you should be able to:
- *Define key terms.*
- *Describe stereotypes associated with older adults.*
- *Discuss the biological and psychosocial theories of aging.*
- *Cite the normal physiologic changes that occur with aging.*
- *List the normal functional changes that occur with aging.*
- *Describe key factors of optimal health maintenance in the aging adult.*
- *Identify funding and policy changes that have influenced elder care.*
- *Identify common disorders related to aging.*
- *Detail nursing interventions for each disorder.*
- *Discuss areas wherein the nurse can advocate for older adults on the individual, community, state, and national levels.*

KEY TERMS

activities of daily living	gerontology
Balanced Budget Act	Health Care Financ-
delirium	ing Administration
dementia	Omnibus Budget
gerontological nursing	Reconciliation Act
gerontologist	polypharmacy

INTRODUCTION

Gerontology is the study of the effects of normal aging and age-related diseases on human beings. It is a general term used by all health care and social services disciplines. Aging (senescence) is a complex phenomenon that occurs on the continuum of human life, beginning with birth and continuing throughout the lifespan, and on into the end stages of life and death.

The phrase *older adult* is very subjective and has historically meant persons who are 65 years of age and older. However, there is a great deal of debate among **gerontologists** (gerontological specialists in advanced practice nursing, geriatric psychiatry, medicine, and social services) as to whether this specific age delineation should continue to be used as we enter the 21st century. The practice of using 65 years of age as a dividing line for social welfare benefits began in the 1880s when Otto von Bismark randomly selected that age for benefits in Germany. It should be noted that there was no standardized clinical basis for establishing this age as the dividing line between young and old. Longer average life-expectancy rates (75.6 years for both genders, 72.1 years for men, and 79.0 years for women [U.S. Senate Special Committee on Aging, 1990]) along with a decline in the average number of children per family since the late 1960s have changed U.S. demographics. As a result, there is a great need to support and strengthen independence among older adults, and to value and utilize their life experiences in the areas of career, family, and community.

Retirement age is now less consistently determined by a mandatory age limit. Rather, retirement frequently is offered when the employee meets a formula of combined age and years of service. Since the 1990s, benefit penalties have been imposed on Social Security beneficiaries who are 65 to 70 years of age and who continue to earn incomes over a minimum amount. This action has had the social impact of encouraging either full or partial retirement by 65 years of age and limiting the income of those elders (especially older women) who do not have retirement plans. The original goal was to provide assistance to those individuals who were most needy. However, this practice may also inadvertently be penalizing those elders who financially need to work and at the same time be sending a message to industry and society that the expertise of those individuals who are 65 to 70 years of age is not needed or valued. Along with the challenges of financing access to basic health care, that will bring older adults and their caregivers; policymakers; and gerontologists to the table as future social and health policies for America's elderly are developed.

Currently, the clinical delineation of an older adult is still someone who is 65 years of age or older; older-old adults are defined as those individuals 85 years of age or older. In 1900, there were a total of 3.1 million individuals over the age of 65 in the United States (Dychtwald & Flower, 1989); by 1994, there were 33.2 million, 3.5 million of whom were over the age of 85 years (Campion, 1994). It is projected that by the year 2030, the number of older individuals in the United States will reach 70.2 million (Figure 55-1). The most rapid increase is expected to occur in the years 2010–2030, when the "baby-boomers" reach age 65.

The aging of the United States and the world is a phenomenon that will impact all areas of society. The age range of 65 to 100+ years potentially comprises three generations: parents, grandparents, and great-grandparents. No other age group has the potential for as much diversity in both strengths and needs, both psychosocial and physical.

The future will also place demands on those who were born from the late 1950s to the late 1960s. Many in this age group chose to focus first on career, delaying marriage and childrearing until in their thirties. They have thus been labeled "the sandwich generation" to denote the challenges they will face in meeting social and financial responsibilities later in life as they work to provide for children entering college and for aging parents and, sometimes, grandparents and, in a few instances, great-grandparents.

This chapter presents an overview of influences on the older client, including the social impacts of aging. Also examined are theories of aging; myths and realities of aging; health promotion and aging; physiologic and functional changes that normally occur with aging; and some common disorders of aging along with nursing interventions to assist clients to achieve optimal outcomes related to those disorders.

As caregivers for older adults, nurses and other members of the client's health care team must also understand the budgetary and policy decisions that can affect the care they will provide to their clients. Thus, this chapter concludes with a short discussion on health care financing for elder care in the 21st century.

GERONTOLOGICAL NURSING

The acceptance of **gerontological nursing** as a separate nursing specialty that addresses and advocates for the special care needs of older adults has not been realized without a struggle. In 1961, gerontological nursing attained national recognition with the creation

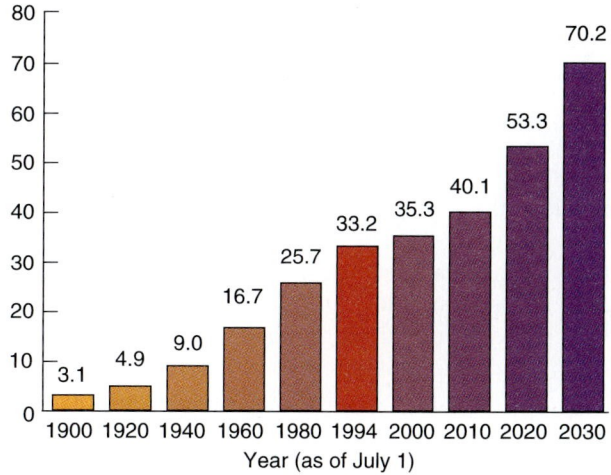

Number of persons 65+: 1900 to 2030

Figure 55-1 Number of Persons over Age 65: 1900–2030 (*From* A Profile of Older Americans, *by The Administration on Aging and the AARP, 1995*)

of its own division of nursing within the American Nurses Association (ANA). Nurses in the United States who were aware of the trends toward an aging population realized the importance of taking such a step. The charter members of the Division of Gerontological Nursing deserve a great deal of credit for their vision and commitment to developing gerontology education and recognizing the special nursing care needs of older adults. The major topics addressed in the overview of the expanding scope of practice for gerontological nursing included (Bahr, 1994):

- The historical evolution of gerontological nursing practice based on population statistics;
- The way that ageism in U.S. society has affected the profession of nursing, the health care delivery system, and the care of older adults;
- Nursing education and care of older adults with a perspective derived from studies of the attitudes and interests of nursing personnel and nursing students;
- The delineation of various aspects of nursing care of older adults, including clinical practice based on the ANA Standards of Nursing Practice; select theories of nursing applied to the care of older adults; and the expanding scope of gerontological nursing, in general, and the roles of clinical nurse specialists and geriatric nurse practitioners, in particular; and
- Trends in gerontological nursing and long-term care.

The battle continues against the stereotyping of older adults, both in the health professions and in the community at large. There are many stereotypes or preconceived notions associated with aging and being old. Stereotypes are usually generated in an attempt to categorize people or to set standards that can be applied to large groups of people. They are often based on an individual's experience with persons in that group. Stereotypes may be true of some individuals, but not of a collective group.

Health professionals, in particular, must be diligent in avoiding age prejudice, as believing stereotypes can influence interactions between older adults and caregivers. The caregiver may treat the older adult as a child in an old body. This approach is demeaning to elders and strips individuals of their self-esteem and dignity. Clients with cognitive or expressive deficits cannot always process questions or comments quickly or follow through with responses. Nurses and caregivers must never make the mistake of believing that clients do not understand verbal and, especially, nonverbal messages. Elders are a diverse group; they deserve respect and, through their memories and life examples, can teach a great deal to younger persons about life and survival and coping skills. Learning from clients and their families and assisting clients to find activities that enhance the quality of life (regardless of state of health) make caring for older adults a rewarding and satisfying experience.

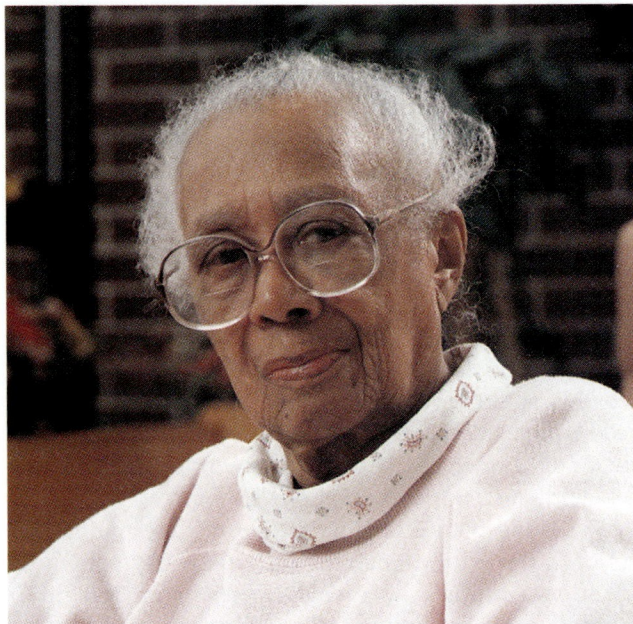

Figure 55-2 The aging process is a normal and natural part of growth and development.

Aging is universal, progressive, and irreversible and eventually leads to death. The aging process itself, however, is very individualized and is independent of chronological age. The way whereby an individual ages is influenced by genetics; lifestyle; availability and quality of health services; cultural beliefs; and socioeconomic status. Certain physiologic changes are expected with aging (Figure 55-2), although there exists considerable variation in the time of onset, rate, and degree of these changes. In order to render effective and compassionate care to elderly clients, nurses working in gerontology must be familiar with the normal processes as well as the common disorders of aging.

THEORIES OF AGING

At this time, no single theory of aging has been universally accepted by practitioners in gerontology. Aging is a complex issue that must take into account the psychosocial, cultural, and experiential aspects of living. Several biological theories of aging have been proposed to explain the physiologic and functional changes that are observed in older adults. Psychosocial theories of aging strive to explain the behaviors and social interactions of older adults. These theories are summarized in Table 55-1. It should be noted, however, that each generation is unique and that biological and psychosocial theories of aging are thus unlikely to be universal. Also, as more knowledge is garnered from scientific studies (e.g., the study of the impact on cells of auto-oxidization by free radicals and the study of dietary chemical exposure) and gene sequencing efforts (e.g., the human genome project), it is likely that the biological theories of aging will change as well.

Table 55-1 THEORIES OF AGING

BIOLOGICAL THEORIES

Title	Major Premise
Somatic mutation theory	Radiation or miscoding of enzymes causes changes in the DNA. Changes associated with aging are the result of decreased function and efficiency of the cells and organs.
Programmed aging theory	The life span is programmed within the cells. This genetic clock determines the speed at which the person ages and eventually dies.
Cross-linkage, or collagen, theory	Collagen is the principal component of connective tissue and is also found in the skin, bones, muscles, lungs, and heart. Chemical reactions between collagen and cross-linking molecules cause loss of flexibility, resulting in diminished functional mobility.
Immunity theory	The thymus becomes smaller with age. The ability to produce T-cell differentiation decreases. This impairs immunologic functions and results in increased incidence of infections, neoplasms, and autoimmune disorders.
Stress theory	Stress throughout the lifetime causes structural and chemical changes in the body. These changes eventually cause irreversible tissue damage.

PSYCHOSOCIAL THEORIES

Title	Major Premise
Activity theory	Roles and responsibilities change throughout the lifetime. Life satisfaction depends on maintaining an involvement with life by developing new interests, hobbies, roles, and relationships.
Disengagement theory	There is decreased interaction between the older person and others in his social system. The disengagement is inevitable, mutual, and acceptable to both the individual and society.
Continuity theory	Successful methods used throughout life for adjusting and adapting to life events are repeated. Characteristic traits, habits, values, associations, and goals remain stable throughout the lifetime, regardless of life changes.

MYTHS AND REALITIES OF AGING

Myths are fictitious ideas. Myths about elders are abundant and do not reflect the reality of the aging population. Following are some common myths associated with aging, based (in part) on data from the United States Bureau of Census and *A Profile of Older Americans* developed by the American Association of Retired Persons (AARP) in 1995.

Myth: Senility is an expected result of aging.

Reality: Senility is an outdated term once used to refer to any form of dementia that occurred in older

CULTURAL CONSIDERATIONS

Aging

At the same time that diversity continues to broaden in the United States, it remains important to understand the individual needs of clients. As with all clients, it is important to assess the older client's religious beliefs, traditions, and culture and to evaluate the ways that these may influence the client's health beliefs and health practices. Not only can caregivers make the mistake of not fully assessing the client's beliefs about health in elders, they can also be misled themselves by myths about aging that exist in U.S. society.

people. Dementia is a result of disease, can affect adults of all ages, and is not a natural consequence of aging. Although some slight declines are noted in short-term memory from the age of 40 on, most people adjust through the use of memory aids such as lists and calendars. Long-term memory can actually become clearer with age. Even for a client with dementia, long-term memory can remain somewhat intact long into the disease process. Thus, nurses and caregivers find that interventions such as reminiscence, memory photo books, and activities that draw on the client's long-practiced skills provide positive client outcomes (Figure 55-3).

Myth: Incontinence is an expected result of aging.

Reality: Incontinence is not an expected outcome of aging and, in most cases, can be reversed through assessment and treatment. The challenge is that many people are embarrassed to discuss this problem with family or primary providers. Also, in long-term care settings, both the belief in this myth and the historically low staffing levels have served to dissuade clinical efforts at providing the needed nursing interventions (prompted voiding; consistent,

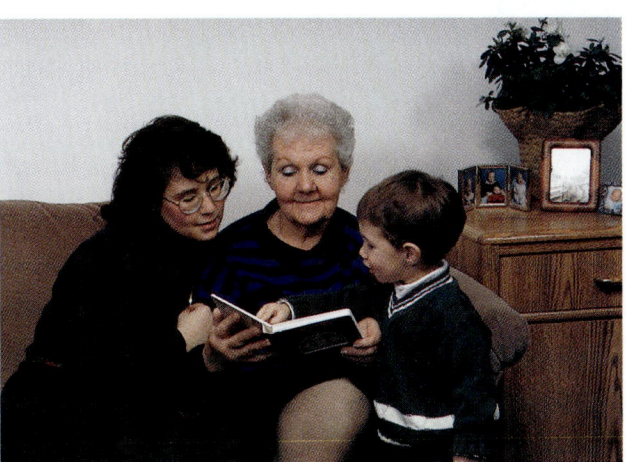

Figure 55-3 Sharing memories and photographs with younger family members is valuable for all generations.

nonhurried, timed voiding) to reverse urinary incontinence. In settings where care is provided to older adults, lack of funding, lack of policy support and education, and inconsistent enforcement of adequate staffing levels have often had a negative impact on client health outcomes. By developing urinary incontinence treatment programs, care facilities could improve clinical outcomes for clients and also reduce health care costs. A highly conservative estimate of the current direct costs of urinary incontinence in nursing homes is $3.3 billion (Hu, 1990), based on 1987 dollars.

Myth: Older adults are no longer interested in sexuality or sexual activity.

Reality: Sexuality is a lifelong need. Elders can be and are sexually active, regardless of age. Although sexual function may be affected by changes in the reproductive systems, persons of both genders are capable of orgasm into old age. Despite interest and desire, physiologic or psychological problems and medication side effects may present barriers to intercourse. In such situations, sexuality without coitus can provide elders with love and intimacy. It is important to remember that human beings are social beings. Just as small babies can fail to thrive without human touch (hugs, nurturing, companionship, valuing of the individual), so can older adults fail to thrive without these same human interactions and support (Figure 55-4).

The medication sildenafil citrate (Viagra) has proven beneficial to many older couples as they work to meet their sexual health needs. The debate over the acceptance and funding of this medication for erectile dysfunction sheds light on just how far U.S. society still has to go in debunking this myth and replacing it with the truth that normal human sexuality needs continue throughout the life span.

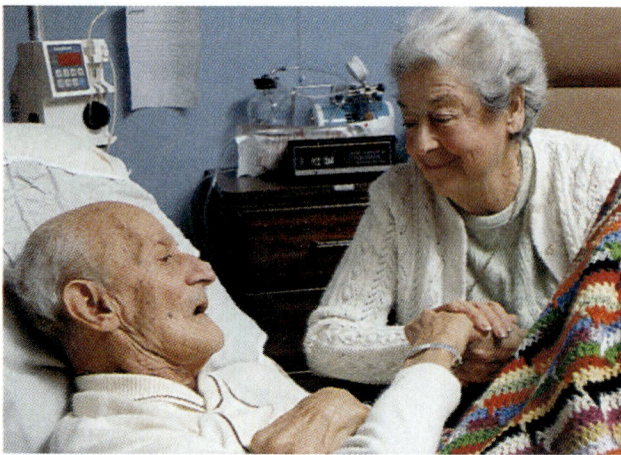

Figure 55-4 Individuals of all ages benefit from intimacy and companionship.

Myth: Most people spend the last years of their lives in nursing homes.

Reality: Projections are that from 10% to 40% of elderly in the U.S. will spend some time in extended care facilities, depending on the report and the age group discussed. For many, that stay will involve rehabilitation following surgery, a fracture, or stroke before returning home after a short hospital stay. The late 1990s have seen a growing interest in the use of alternative care options for elders (retirement communities, assisted living centers, group homes, respite care, and partial hospitalization/adult day programs). However, the majority of older adults continue to live in communities with varying levels of assistive services or support as they age. The projected trends in long-term care needs are for continued use of alternate settings that will support interventions to meet residents' physical, psychosocial, cultural, spiritual, cognitive, and mental health needs.

Traditionally, elders in long-term care facilities have been taken from home environments where they have likely experienced the highest level of independence they have had in their lifetimes (to choose when to get up, eat, go to bed, and the like), and have been placed in settings where very few, if any, choices, including care decisions, are made based on their preferences. Gerontological nurses have an ongoing responsibility to help recreate the way care is provided to elderly clients and to advocate for individual choices for older clients in long-term care facilities in the 21st century. Nurse leaders must learn to think in new ways about long-practiced trends in elder care in the United States and to work with older clients and their families to envision and create better trends.

Myth: All elderly persons are financially impoverished.

Reality: Income range varies among those over 65 years of age, just as it does among those in younger groups. However, the high costs of medications does disproportionately affect those over age 65, who are more likely to have one or more chronic conditions that require management with medication. In the past, lack of reimbursement for preventive assessment, treatments, and medications led many elders to go without medications or to delay care until they were too ill to wait any longer. This resulted in increased use of acute care services in hospitals.

In 1992, families headed by persons over 65 years of age had a median income of $25,315, despite the fact that the median net worth of older households (assets over expenses) is $73,500. The challenge for most elders below the median (especially older women, who often have lower retirement incomes) is that most of their assets are tied up in the family home or in other nonliquid holdings. Thus, when an acute illness strikes, there is little financial reserve to help cover costs.

HEALTH AND AGING

Like all age groups, elders can do much to adopt a healthy lifestyle that will enhance their remaining years.

Activities of Daily Living

Being well groomed enhances the self-esteem of all older adults. Adaptive devices and techniques are available for those who need assistance with the **activities of daily living** (ADL), basic care activities that include mobility, bathing, hygiene, grooming, dressing, eating, and toileting.

Mobility

Many assistive devices are available to help the older client maintain mobility and independence. Handrails can decrease the risk of falls while the person is walking (Figure 55-5); they are also useful in the tub and, when used in conjunction with a plastic riser, can help the older adult get on and off the toilet safely.

Bathing

Skin dryness increases with aging; thus, it may be preferable for older adults to bathe or shower only two to three times per week and to take sponge baths in between. A gentle soap should be used sparingly for the bath, after which a moisturizing lotion should be applied. The individual or caregiver should be instructed to inspect the skin during bathing for any indication of skin breakdown, lumps, or changes in moles.

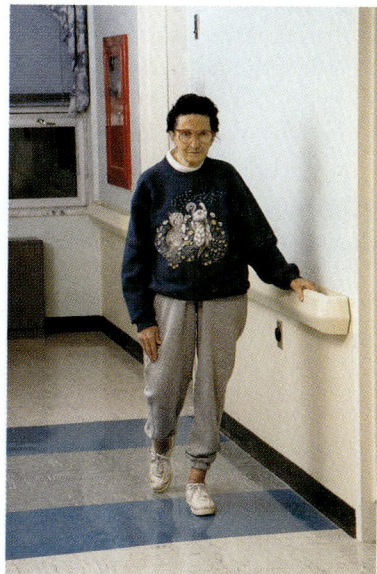

Figure 55-5 Handrails allow clients more independence when ambulating.

With aging oil secretion decreases in the scalp, and hair can thus become dry. Shampooing one or two times per week is usually adequate for most elders, and a simplified hairstyle may be helpful to those with limited mobility in the arms. The use of mild shampoos and conditioners can also enhance hair texture.

Hygiene

Fingernails may become more brittle with aging. Keeping the client's fingernails clean and short can prevent accidental injury or scratches to fragile older skin. Impaired circulation is common among older adults, and special attention should thus be given to care of the feet and lower extremities. Because toenails frequently become thick and tougher with aging, soaking the feet prior to trimming the toenails may ease the task. For clients with circulation or skin integrity problems of the feet and toes or for clients with diabetes, a referral to a podiatrist should be made for nail trimming. During bathing, the client's feet should be monitored for discomfort; inflammation; broken skin; color changes such as redness, pallor, or cyanosis (blue or purple discoloration resulting from lack of circulation); heat or coldness; cracking between toes; and corns or calluses.

The need for adequate oral care does not diminish with aging. Dental problems can result in poor eating habits and inadequate nutrition. Inadequate brushing and dental check-ups can lead to gingivitis (bleeding and edematous gums), which, if left untreated, can progress to periodontal disease that can destroy connective tissue, alveolar bone, and periodontal ligaments. The nurse must therefore monitor clients for proper oral care. For those clients with dentures, the nurse must inspect the dentures for cleanliness and proper fit. Clients with dentures must brush the dentures and the gums regularly with a soft brush and a mild cleanser. It is helpful to label dentures with the client's name to facilitate identification of the dentures in the event that the client is admitted to a hospital or an assistive care setting.

Grooming

Good grooming is important in promoting the older client's self-esteem and confidence. Keeping the hair neat and tidy, choosing attractive clothing and jewelry, and making decisions about makeup and other personal care practices will all contribute to the older client's sense of well-being and independence (Figure 55-6).

Male clients may feel much better with a clean shaven face. Infection-control principles demand that each razor (either electric or blade) be used for only one individual, and that that razor be marked with the client's name. Women may also require attention to facial hair, as estrogen levels decrease after menopause. It is not uncommon for older women to notice hairs on

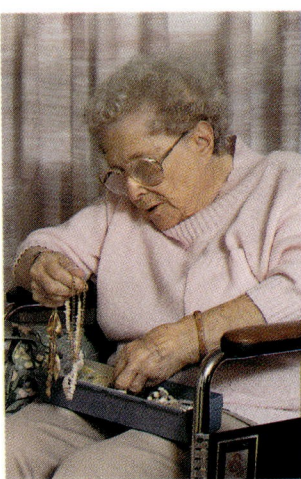 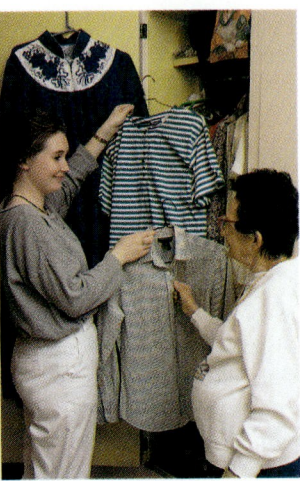

Figure 55-6 Good grooming for the older client includes choosing personal items such as jewelry and clothing.

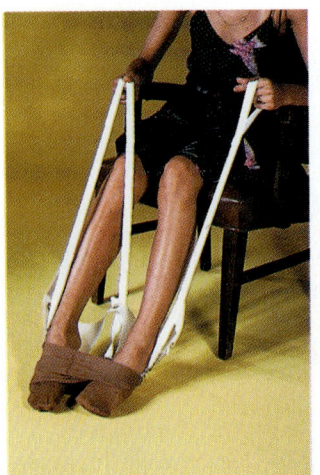 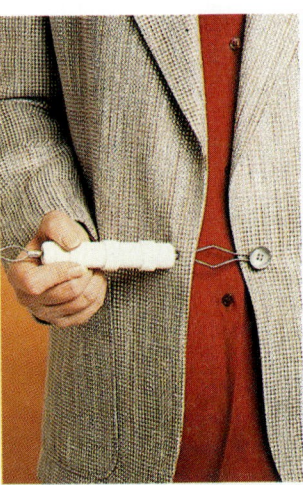

Figure 55-7 Assistive devices such as these for pantyhose and buttons are available to help clients dress independently. *(Courtesy of Maddak Inc.)*

the chin or upper lip that were not there in younger days. Also, both men and women are likely to notice graying and diminished hair on legs, underarms, and pubic areas as they age.

Dressing

Dressing may be difficult for clients who have restricted joint movement, paralysis, or limited endurance due to health problems. Many choices are available to ease dressing, such as elastic waists, velcro fasteners, and assistive reaching and dressing devices (Figure 55-7).

Eating

Many older adults are able to maintain the ability to self-feed, thereby promoting independence and self-esteem. Neurological and musculoskeletal alterations may, however, affect ability to self-feed. Dysphagia, or difficulty swallowing, may place the older client at increased risk of choking, and diminished taste sensation may affect the desire to eat.

Toileting

Toileting habits also change with aging. Bowel elimination problems can often be prevented as clients age by:

- Ensuring adequate fiber intake,
- Ensuring adequate fluid intake,
- Ensuring regular daily exercise, and
- Developing regular elimination habits.

For the client in the hospital or a long-term care facility, it is helpful to:

- Maintain previously effective habits such as reading on the toilet or drinking warm liquids upon arising, and
- Assist the client to the toilet approximately 30 minutes after eating, to take advantage of the gastrocolic reflex.

As a result of the physical changes that occur with aging, increased frequency of urination may be noted in elders of both genders. It is not uncommon for older adults to self-limit fluid intake due to a fear of incontinence. This habit is unhealthy and should thus be discouraged. Cases of incontinence should be assessed to determine the cause and type, so that appropriate interventions and treatment can be implemented. Timing the use of prescribed diuretics in the morning rather than the evening can prevent the increased need for urination at night, which is especially helpful to older clients who are being treated for congestive heart failure (CHF).

Exercise

What was once accepted as the normal deterioration of old age is now considered the result of disuse through sitting and bed rest. Research indicates that high-intensity, progressive resistance training can improve muscle strength and muscle size in frail elderly clients. Walking and all other maneuvers required for ADL are also beneficial. Exercise programs should be

PROFESSIONAL TIP

Bowel Patterns in Elderly Clients

It is extremely important that caregivers of older adults monitor bowel patterns. Long periods of constipation (> than 2 to 3 days) should alert caregivers to the need for interventions to minimize the likelihood of bowel impaction, which can ultimately be life threatening if left untreated. Evacuation aids such as laxatives, lubricants, stool softeners, and enemas all have side-effects and should thus be avoided if at all possible. Dietary changes or an exercise regimen should be introduced first.

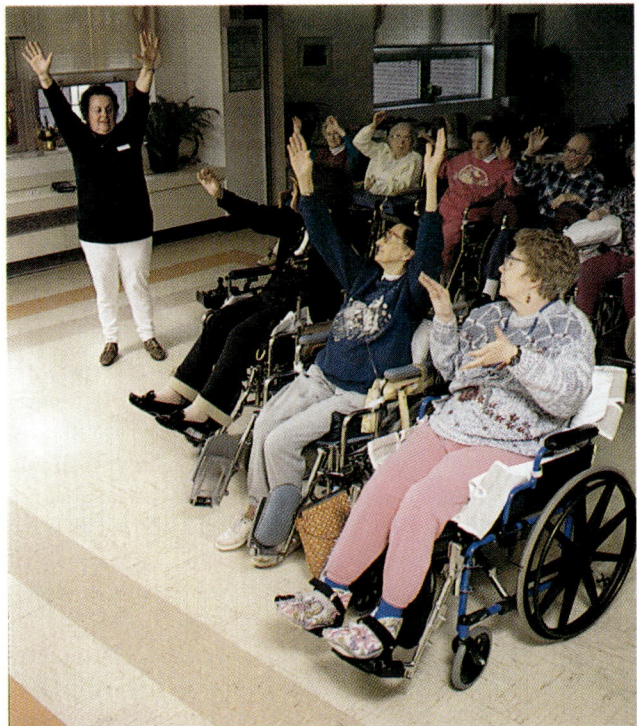

Figure 55-8 Exercise is important to all clients and should be tailored to interests and ability levels.

individually planned and should take into consideration the older person's:

- General health status (Figure 55-8),
- Physiologic disorders (if present),
- Preference for solidarity or group activity,
- Physical environment, and
- Financial status.

Nutrition

For many older adults, cultural heritage, religious rites, ethnic practices, and family traditions are linked to food. The physiologic, psychological, sociological, and economic changes of aging may compromise nutritional status. Elders must follow a balanced diet, often with lowered intakes of sugar, caffeine, and sodium. There are no universally accepted dietary guidelines specific to older adults. A dietitian can determine the needed food intake for a specific individual by taking into account the individual's height, ideal weight, activity level, and disease processes.

The National Institutes of Health (NIH) recommends 1,000 mg of calcium per day for both men and women over the age of 25. Postmenopausal women 50 to 65 years of age who are not receiving estrogen therapy have been reported to need 1,500 mg of calcium per day (Yen, 1995). It is important to note that calcium supplements should also contain vitamin D to provide for optimal metabolism by the body. The need for additional supplements depends on the older individual's nutritional status and ability to maintain an ad-

equate diet. Growing discussion supports the needs for adequate protein intake, to maintain both skin integrity and bone density; moderate carbohydrates intake due to the metabolism of carbohydrates to sugars; and, whenever possible, the acquisition of needed calcium from dietary intake of unprocessed natural cheeses (Peskin, 1999).

It is important that nurses be knowledgeable about community services designed to help older clients meet their nutritional needs. Such services include grocery transportation and delivery services, homebound meals (e.g., Meals on Wheels), group meals at senior food sites, and the Food Stamp program. Nurses and caregivers should also realize that socialization and companionship are necessary components of adequate dietary intake, and should thus ensure that these areas are addressed as part of any food-assistance intervention.

Psychosocial Considerations

Older adults, like all individuals, have psychosocial and cognitive needs for lifelong learning. Many colleges have developed education program options for elder students (often at no tuition), and employers are beginning to recruit older workers for part-time positions (recognizing their historically good work ethic and experience). Many elders continue to volunteer countless hours each year, offering to help meet the social service needs of their communities. These efforts can result in feelings of productivity and self-worth for the older adult. Mental activity and emotional involvement are as necessary to the overall well-being as is physical activity. Older clients can benefit from building on their long-practiced skills to develop interesting and stimulating activities or hobbies. Such activities may be of an individual or group nature. Socialization with people of all age groups can help not only the older participants, but also the young and middle-age participants, by illustrating that aging is not a disease but, rather, a rich and natural part of the life process.

Strengths

Older adults generally have suffered many losses over the years. Some losses are slight and require only minor adaptation, whereas others may significantly affect the person. Physiologic changes or disease processes may result in losses, causing impairments in:

- Communication,
- Vision and learning,
- Mobility,
- Cognition, or
- Psychosocial skills.

If the impairment is severe, the individual could lose some degree of independence, and adaptations may be required. Furthermore, losses can cascade for the older client, as one loss contributes to another. For example, if an elderly person with diabetes were to lose her driver's license due to impaired vision related to diabetic retinopathy, socialization might be restricted, which in turn might increase her feelings of loneliness and diminished self-esteem. If, however, her spouse provides caregiving and transportation, these adaptations might allow her to remain active socially while still living in her home. If her spouse later dies, and her health continues to decline, a move to an assisted living facility may become necessary, if other community adaptations are unavailable. She would then be faced with adapting to the loss of both her home and her spouse.

Health care professionals should remember that persons who have lived for many years are survivors and can adapt to life changes better if they are allowed to utilize their existing strengths. They are often much stronger and more ingenious and enterprising than they are given credit for. The strengths of each individual (including past coping skills) must be identified and utilized when planning care and assisting the older client to find new ways to adapt and maintain optimal independence in a new setting.

Health Promotion and Disease Prevention

Older adults must be alerted to means of preventing disease and reducing risks. Being knowledgeable about self-care and participating in screening tests are important components of health maintenance. For older men, annual prostate examinations and a regular prostate specific antigen (PSA) level lab test, which can detect prostate cancer in the early stages, are recommended every 1 to 2 years. For older women, annual mammograms and Pap smears, and monthly breast self-examinations represent means of detecting breast and gynecological cancers in the early stages. Nurses can teach their clients habits for healthy living and inform them of signs and symptoms that require medical investigation. Older clients who have been exposed to environmental chemicals, tobacco, or extensive alcohol use over many years often experience serious health consequences as they reach older age. Older clients of any age can benefit from healthy lifestyles and from disease-prevention interventions such as being inoculated yearly against influenza and

PROFESSIONAL TIP

Identifying Strengths of Older Adults as Part of Assessment

Assessment should include the identification of strengths as well as problems. Strengths are utilized to achieve or maintain optimal physical, mental, and emotional function. All of the following can be considered strengths:

- Cognitive health
- Freedom from or successful adaptation to deficits or impairments
- A history of healthy lifestyle with regard to diet, sleep, stress management, exercise, and chemical abuse (none)
- Adequate functional ability to carry out ADL
- Freedom from incapacitating physical discomfort and pain
- A physically safe living environment
- Feelings of security in present environment
- Realistic knowledge about capabilities
- Pattern of avoiding dangerous situations and unnecessary risks
- Compliance with health care regimen
- Capability with regard to managing own environment
- An intact support system
- Satisfying relationships with others
- Opportunities for sexual expression
- Access to transportation
- Adequate functional mobility
- Successful adaptation to life changes and crises
- History of relinquishing roles as phases of life require and replacing them with satisfying new roles
- A pattern of successful mourning for losses

- Participation in groups: religious, community, hobbies
- Membership in family whose members respect each other and are willing to give and receive help when necessary
- Successful problem-solving skills
- Willingness to seek information to improve situation
- Evidence of initiative and self-confidence in abilities and judgment
- Participation in self-care by making decisions and accepting responsibility for decisions
- A well-defined value system
- Acceptance of that which cannot be changed
- Successful use of assertive skills
- Strong spiritual beliefs and ability to find comfort and strength in spiritual and religious practices
- Enthusiastic appreciation for aging, with demonstrative embrace of the positive aspects and adaptation to the negative aspects
- Participation in healthy reminiscing; evidence of few regrets about life past
- Joyful appreciation for nature, art, music, hobbies, and activities
- A well-developed sense of humor

every 6 years against pneumonia; assessment of tuberculosis (TB) status; and adequate safe food and clean water intake.

In many cases, by the time a person reaches 65 to 70 years of age, that person has been prescribed medication to address at least one ongoing (chronic) medical problem (e.g., hypertension, heart disease, diabetes, allergies, gastrointestinal disorders). The challenge many elders face is that side effects from one medication are often treated with another prescription medication. If the client then goes to different doctors, these doctors may prescribe even more medications to address the same or other health concerns. This is called **polypharmacy**, or the problem of clients taking numerous prescription and over-the-counter medications for the same or various disease processes, with unknown consequences from the resulting combinations of chemical compounds and cumulative side effects. In many settings, primary care providers, nurses, clinical pharmacists, and social workers collaborate on interdisciplinary teams to assist the older client and the family to oversee the client's medication management, as well as other health needs.

Among the biggest challenges facing older clients are shorter hospitalization stays and reduced time with physicians in the physician's offices. There is less time to ensure that the follow-up services the client will need are understood and in place and less time to educate client and family about medication regimens, including timing and possible interactions with other prescription and over-the-counter drugs or herbal remedies that the client may also be taking. The nurse, as part of the interdisciplinary team, plays a vital role as client advocate when ensuring that older clients have the teaching, services, and follow-up care they need.

PHYSIOLOGIC CHANGES ASSOCIATED WITH AGING

Although the aging process brings with it many physiologic changes, it should be remembered that aging and disease are not synonymous. Whereas the physiologic changes of aging described following are normal for most people, the medical disorders described are not considered normal.

Respiratory System

See Chapter 31 for an anatomy and physiology review of the respiratory system. The following respiratory changes result from the aging process:

- The muscles of respiration become less flexible, causing decreased vital capacity of the lungs.
- Decrease in functional capacity results in dyspnea on exertion or stress; usual activity does not affect breathing.

- Effectiveness of the cough mechanism lessens, increasing the risk of lung infection.
- The alveoli thicken and decrease in number and size, causing less effective gas exchange and, in individuals who also have chronic lung disease, intensifying respiratory deficits.
- Structural changes in the skeleton, such as kyphosis (seen in clients with osteoporosis as an often asymetrical convex curve of the spine, can decrease diaphragmatic expansion. Kyphosis in older clients can lead to a need for small, more frequent meals to balance nutritional requirements and respiratory function due to the restriction of adequate space for expansion and contraction of the diaphragm. It can also create skin integrity risks, as the bony prominences of the client's back press against the backs of chairs.

Common respiratory disorders related to aging include the following:

- Respiratory tract infection (RTI)
- Chronic obstructive pulmonary disease (COPD)
- Pulmonary tuberculosis (TB)

Nursing Interventions: Respiratory Tract Infections

1. Advise discussing the pneumovaccine with the primary care provider.
2. Advise obtaining annual influenza vaccine.
3. Assist the client to assume a position of comfort and assist with medications and respiratory treatments, as ordered.
4. Avoid distention of bowel, bladder, or stomach, any of which can increase breathing discomfort.
5. Allow adequate time for nursing care.

LIFE CYCLE CONSIDERATIONS

TB in the Elderly Client

Elders can be vulnerable to TB because of:

- An ineffective cough reflex and the resulting inability to clear the lungs.
- An altered immune system and a reduced response to extrinsic antigens. Not only are elders at increased risk of infection via a new contagion, but older clients who contracted TB years ago and have been in remission since can experience reexacerbation. The risk of reexacerbation increases in cases where the initial infection was remote and healed (encapsulated) such that the immune system's memory of the T cells has been lost. Facilities where health care is provided to older clients and to immune compromised clients thus must regularly assess the TB status of both their clients and their employees.

6. Administer humidified oxygen therapy, as prescribed.
7. Administer analgesics and antipyretics, as prescribed.
8. Assess for signs of dehydration and ensure that fluids are accessible to the client, unless contraindicated.
9. Review diagnostic data and monitor lung sounds and intake and output every 8 hours or as needed given changes in the client's condition. Weigh the client daily, assessing for fluid retention.
10. Monitor for any signs of respiratory distress (cyanosis of lips, mucous membranes, or nailbeds) and obtain pulse-oximetry readings, as needed.

Nursing Interventions: Chronic Obstructive Pulmonary Disease

1. Assist the client to a position of comfort.
2. Teach the client to use pursed-lip breathing to avoid hyperventilation when short of breath.
3. Teach the client diaphragmatic breathing for use when active.
4. Teach proper use of inhalers. Steroid inhalers should be used first, with a full 60-second wait between puffs; after waiting 3 minutes, any bronchodilator inhalers that are prescribed should then be used, also with a 60 second wait between puffs.
5. Teach the client to cough and clear the airway.
6. Adminster chest physiotherapy (e.g., percussion, postural drainage), if prescribed.
7. Establish a schedule for ambulation, gradually increasing the distance ambulated.
8. Assist with active assistive range of motion exercises.
9. Monitor for signs and symptoms of infections (e.g., fever, blood-tinged or thick, greenish colored sputum, and diminished lung sounds) and immediately report same to the registered nurse and the primary care provider.

PROFESSIONAL TIP

COPD

Remember that in the client with COPD, breathing may not be triggered by a higher level of carbon dioxide as it would in clients without COPD, because the client with COPD always has a consistently high CO_2 level. The breathing impulse is instead triggered by a low level of oxygen. Increasing the oxygen level by more than 1 to 2 L/h in the client with COPD can shut shut down the trigger to breathe, and can drive the client into respiratory failure.

10. Monitor breathing and pulse rate and administer oxygen, if necessary, during periods of increased activity.
11. Suggest smoking cessation programs, if the client is a smoker.

Safety: Oxygen and Smoking
Ensure that no smoking is allowed around clients on oxygen therapy.

Nursing Interventions: Pulmonary Tuberculosis

1. Monitor clients for TB status and for symptoms including fever, night sweats, weight loss, and cough producing blood-tinged sputum.
2. Inform the client, family, and caregivers of the need for adequate isolation techniques.

Infection Control: TB
Remember that TB is spread through droplets when a client sneezes or coughs (direct and indirect contact). Consult the infection-control nurse on the client's interdisciplinary team and work to protect the client and others from transmission of *Mycrobacterium tuberculosis* and other infections.

3. Evaluate the client's risk for infection with the human immunodeficiency virus (HIV) and related pneumocystic pneumonia.
4. Monitor that the client's psychosocial needs are being adequately met while the disease is being pharmacologically addressed with medications like isoniazid (Laniazid). Tell the client and family that the entire course of medication must be completed.
5. Monitor the client's nutrition intake and provide supplements as necessary to maintain adequate body weight.
6. Provide for rest periods throughout the day. Encourage the older client with TB to monitor activity level and length of visits by family so as not to become overtired.

Cardiovascular System

See Chapter 32 for an anatomy and physiology review of the cardiovascular system. The following cardiovascular changes result from the aging process:

- Cardiac output and recovery time decline. The heart requires more time to return to a normal rate after a rate increase in response to activity.
- The heart rate slows.
- Blood flow to all organs decreases. The brain and coronary arteries continue to receive a larger volume than do other organs.
- Arterial elasticity decreases, causing increased peripheral resistance and, in turn, a rise in systolic

blood pressure and a slight rise in diastolic blood pressure.

- Veins dilate, and superficial vessels become more prominent.

Common cardiovascular disorders related to aging include the following:

- Peripheral vascular disease (PVD)
- Hypertension
- Chronic CHF

Nursing Interventions: Peripheral Vascular Disease

1. Assess the lower extremeties, including the peripheral pulses, for signs of arterial or venous insufficiency.
2. Evaluate lifestyle factors that may aggravate or advance atherosclerosis, such as a high-carbohydrate, high-fat diet and little exercise.
3. Teach the client about the disease, including treatment, medication actions and side effects, and signs of thrombosis.
4. Educate the client and caregivers about the care and inspection of the lower extremeties.
5. Provide instructions on interventions specific to the client's type of PVD (arterial or venous).

Nursing Interventions: Hypertension

1. Evaluate food intake patterns, especially of cholesterol, fats, sodium, and carbohydrates. Make recommendations based on findings.
2. Evaluate for fluid retention.
3. Recommend a smoking cessation program, if necessary.
4. Advise the client to avoid alcohol use.
5. Recommend and facilitate a consistent and appropriate exercise program.
6. Discuss the relationship of stress to hypertension and provide resources from which the client can learn relaxation techniques.
7. Provide information on medications and the importance of taking daily blood pressure medications as prescribed, regardless of health status on any given day.
8. Arrange for and encourage regular blood pressure checks and teach the client or significant others proper use of blood pressure equipment, if applicable.

Nursing Interventions: Chronic Congestive Heart Failure

1. Frequently monitor serum digitalis level and monitor for any signs of digoxin toxicity, for which older clients are at increased risk due to the decreased rate of renal clearance of the drug. Withhold the digoxin and immediately contact the registered nurse and the physician if abnormal

 **CLIENT TEACHING**

Digoxin Toxicity

Possible signs and symptoms of digoxin toxicity include the following:

- Disturbances in cardiac rhythms
- Fatigue
- Listlessness
- Anorexia
- Nausea
- Visual disturbances (halos around lights)
- Shaking
- Unsteady gait
- Confusion

serum level or signs and symptoms of toxicity are present.
2. Take the apical pulse for a full 1 minute before administering digoxin. Withhold the medication if the apical pulse is below 60, and consult the registered nurse and the physician if this or any other significant changes in vital signs are noted.
3. Monitor the client's blood pressure and lung sounds.
4. Monitor electrolyte levels, blood urea nitrogen (BUN), and creatinine level to observe system changes including decreased kidney efficiency.
5. Monitor for signs of fluid retention such as intake and output (output too small), weight gain, shortness of breath, or coughing.
6. Encourage alternating periods of activity with periods of rest.
7. Encourage the client to maintain a level of exercise/physical activity appropriate to physical condition.
8. Teach the client and family about the safe use of the prescribed medications.
9. For clients on diuretics, which deplete potassium, monitor fluid intake and level of potassium, ensuring adequacy of each. Encourage administration of diuretics early in the day, unless contraindicated, to prevent increased urination at night.

Gastrointestinal System

See Chapter 34 for an anatomy and physiology review of the gastrointestinal system. The following gastrointestinal changes result from the aging process:

- Tooth enamel thins.
- Periodontal disease rate increases.
- Taste buds decrease in number, and saliva production diminishes.
- Effectiveness of the gag reflex lessens, resulting in an increased risk of choking.

- Esophageal peristalsis slows, and the effectiveness of the esophageal sphincter lessens, causing delayed entry of food into the stomach and increasing the risk of aspiration.
- Hiatal hernia may occur.
- Gastric emptying slows. Food remains in the stomach longer, decreasing the capacity of the stomach.
- Peristalsis and nerve sensation of the large intestine decreases, contributing to constipation.
- The incidence of diverticulosis increases with age.
- Liver size decreases after age 70.
- Liver enzymes decrease, slowing drug metabolism and the detoxification process.
- Emptying of the gallbladder lessens in efficiency, resulting in thickened bile, increased cholesterol content, and increased incidence of gallstones.

PROFESSIONAL TIP

Determining Alterations in Nutrition

- Height and weight: Record actual body weight, usual body weight, and ideal body weight. If usual weight has varied significantly from the ideal for several years, the use of height/weight tables may be meaningless. Compare actual body weight to usual body weight to determine present status.
- Review laboratory values: hematocrit, hemoglobin, total iron-binding capacity, total protein, BUN.
- Determine whether client is on a weight-loss diet.
- Determine whether client was edematous when initially weighed and has lost weight with treatment.
- Evaluate cognitive status. Cognitively impaired clients may be unaware of hunger or be unable to attend to the task of eating.
- In clients with central nervous system damage, evaluate the presence of sensory–perceptual deficits that interfere with eating.
- Evaluate ability to pick up utensils and glasses and to get items from table to mouth.
- Evaluate dental/oral status: status of teeth/dentures, gums, presence of oral dryness (xerostomia).
- Determine presence of impaired swallowing.
- Determine whether client has distaste for certain food groups.
- Assess knowledge in regard to nutrition and food purchase and preparation.
- Determine whether client is taking medications that interfere with taste or food absorption.
- Determine whether financial status interferes with food purchasing.
- Evaluate for history of compulsive eating.

Common gastrointestinal disorders related to aging include the following:

- Over-/undernutrition
- Constipation
- Dehydration
- Dental disorders

Nursing Interventions: Over-/Undernutrition

1. Assess nutritional status.
2. Provide nutritional instruction based on assessment findings.
3. Advise on community nutrition programs (e.g., Meals-on-Wheels, senior center food sites, food pantries, and Food Stamp program).

Nursing Interventions: Constipation

1. Assess food and fluid intake.
2. Make recommendations based on assessment findings (e.g., increase fiber intake, increase fluid intake).

HOME HEALTH CARE

Nutritional Status

Evaluate the following when assessing a client's nutritional status in the home:

- Ability to shop for and prepare meals (Figure 55-9)
- Mealtime environment, for unpleasant odors, noises, and visual stimuli
- Table setting, for appealing table cover, centerpiece, colorful dishes
- Appropriateness of food storage system (cabinets, refrigerator, freezer)

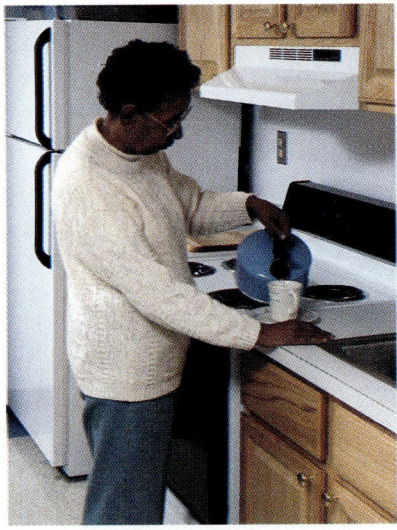

Figure 55-9 Cooking and preparing foods in the home are important skills to maintaining a nutritionally healthy lifestyle.

3. Discuss the relationship of exercise to bowel activity.
4. Discuss the importance of routine for regular bowel elimination.
5. Advise avoiding the overuse of laxatives.
6. Monitor adequate bowel elimination and provide interventions (e.g., prune juice, senna bars, milk of magnesia, as ordered) to assist the client in returning to a normal bowel elimination routine.

Nursing Interventions: Dehydration

1. Identify the reason for dehydration (i.e., inadequate fluid intake or excessive fluid output).
2. Identify the reason and corresponding interventions for inadequate fluid intake:
   - Fluids are inaccessible due to the client's physical limitations: offer fluids on a regular basis throughout the day.
   - The client dislikes water or other available fluids: identify fluid choices.
   - The client restricts fluids due to a fear of incontinence: explain the relationship of decreased fluid intake to bladder infections and arrange for assistance, as needed, for toileting.
3. Identify the reasons for any excessive fluid output and treat accordingly.

Nursing Interventions: Dental Disorders

1. Teach the oral hygiene procedures of brushing and flossing and facilitate and encourage brushing of the teeth and gums and flossing of the teeth, as tolerated.
2. Inspect the mouth regularly for signs of dental disorders.
3. Advise regular dental checkups.

Reproductive System: Female

See Chapter 35 for an anatomy and physiology review of the female reproductive system. The following reproductive changes result from the aging process:

- Estrogen production decreases with the onset of menopause.
- Ovaries, uterus, and cervix decrease in size.
- The vagina shortens, narrows, and becomes less elastic, and the vaginal lining thins. Secretions decrease and become more alkaline, resulting in increased incidence of atrophic vaginitis. These changes may result in discomfort during coitus, which can often be rectified with the use of a water-based lubricant. As at any age, protected intercourse (safe sex) through the use of a latex condom should be advised with new partners.
- Supporting musculature of the reproductive organs weakens, increasing the risk of uterine prolapse.
- Breast tissue diminishes, and nipple erection lessens during sexual arousal.

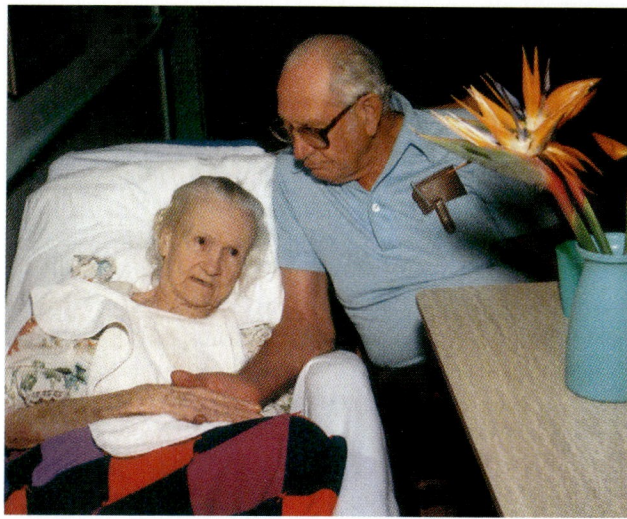

Figure 55-10 Sexuality and companionship remain important throughout the life span.

- Libido and the need for intimacy and companionship in older women remain unchanged (Figure 55-10).

Common female reproductive system disorders related to aging include the following:

- Breast cancer (the risk of which increases with age)
- Altered sexuality patterns related to physiologic changes, medications, changes in body image, or psychosocial changes such as the loss of significant other or a move to a setting that provides some level of assistive care (i.e., group home, assisted living center, or care facility)

Nursing Interventions: Female Reproductive System Disorders

1. Teach and encourage monthly breast self-exams and yearly mammograms for early detection and treatment of disorders.
2. Establish rapport and encourage the client to verbalize feelings and concerns related to sexuality, body image, and self-esteem.
3. Complete a sexual history and recommend interventions based on findings. Support the client's needs for companionship and intimacy throughout the life span.
4. Recommend that a bone density scan be discussed with the client's primary care provider to allow for early detection and treatment of osteoporosis.
5. Encourage annual gynecological examinations with the client's primary care provider.

Reproductive System: Male

See Chapter 35 for an anatomy and physiology review of the male reproductive system. The following reproductive changes result from the aging process:

- Testosterone production decreases, resulting in decreased size of the testicles.
- Sperm count and viscosity of seminal fluid decrease.
- Although more time is required to obtain erection, the older man often finds that he and his partner can enjoy longer periods of lovemaking (greater control) prior to ejaculation. As at any age, protected intercourse (safe sex) through the use of a latex condom should be advised with new partners.
- The prostate gland may enlarge.
- Impotency may occur. Medications and other medical interventions have been successful in reversing impotency problems in many older males. A thorough evaluation by the primary care provider and a urologist can provide clients with available options given health status and current medication regimen.
- Libido and the need for intimacy and companionship remain unchanged in older males.

Common male reproductive disorders related to aging include the following:

- Altered sexuality patterns related to physiologic changes, medications, changes in body image, or psychosocial changes such as the loss of significant other or a move to a setting that provides some level of assistive care (i.e., group home, assisted living center, or care facility)
- Benign prostatic hypertophy (BPH)

Nursing Interventions: Male Reproductive System Disorders

1. Establish rapport and encourage the client to verbalize feelings and concerns related to sexuality, body image, and self-esteem.
2. Complete a sexual history and recommend interventions based on findings. Support the client's needs for companionship and intimacy throughout the life span.
3. Provide client and family education regarding the signs and symptoms of prostate disorders (e.g., difficulty in starting the urine stream, a smaller urine stream, frequent urination, frequent nighttime awakening for the purpose of urinating, or, in severe cases, the failure or inability to urinate).
4. Teach and encourage monthly testicular self-exam and yearly digital rectal examinations of the prostate gland by a primary care provider. The benefits of a PSA lab test performed every 1 to 2 years to facilitate early detection and treatment of prostate cancer are currently under research and debate.

Endocrine System

See Chapter 37 for an anatomy and physiology review of the endocrine system. The following endocrine changes result from the aging process:

- Alterations occur in both the reception and the production of hormones.
- Release of insulin by the beta cells of the pancreas slows, causing an increase in blood sugar.
- Thyroid changes may lower the basal metabolic rate.

The most common endocrine disorder related to aging is diabetes mellitus, type 2.

Nursing Interventions: Diabetes Mellitus Type 2

1. Arrange for a consultation with a dietitian to assess nutritional status and to provide food-management instruction.
2. Teach the client, family members, or caregivers (as appropriate) the procedure for blood glucose monitoring specific to the equipment the client will be using.
3. Develop a personal exercise program with the client based on the client's physical condition, mental status, resources, and interests.
4. Provide information on prescribed oral hypoglycemic medications.
5. Teach the causes, signs, and treatment of hypoglycemia and hyperglycemia.
6. Advise on self-care and on careful monitoring of the extremities and of sores on the skin, to minimize threats to skin integrity.
7. Encourage the client to wear shoes and to have nails trimmed by a podiatrist, if unable to safely perform self-care.

Musculoskeletal System

See Chapter 38 for an anatomy and physiology review of the musculoskeletal system. The following musculoskeletal changes result from the aging process:

- Muscle mass and elasticity diminish, resulting in decreased strength, endurance, coordination, and increased reaction time.
- Bone demineralization occurs, causing skeletal instability and shrinkage of intervertebral disks. The flexibility of the spine lessens, and spinal curvature often occurs.
- Joints undergo degenerative changes, resulting in pain, stiffness, and loss of range of motion.

Common musculoskeletal system disorders related to aging include the following:

- Osteoporosis
- Degenerative arthritis
- Fractured hip

Nursing Interventions: Osteoporosis

1. Make dietary recommendations to ensure adequate intake of calcium, protein, and vitamin D.

2. Recommend a smoking cessation program, if necessary.

3. Advise the client to avoid alcohol.

4. Encourage the client to take a calcium supplement in conjunction with vitamin D, as ordered by the client's primary care provider.

5. Recommend consultation with the primary care provider regarding either estrogen replacement therapy (ERT) options for females, or the use of medications like alendronate sodium (Fosamax) to address bone density loss associated with osteoporosis.

6. Teach the client, family, and caregivers about measures to reduce the risk of falling and sustaining fractures.

7. Recommend evaluation (via x-ray) for the presence of stress, or compression, fractures of the spine in cases of severe back pain that occurs with or without a fall. In clients with osteoporosis, these fractures can occur more easily because the vertebrae are compacted by shrinkage of the intervertebral spaces as a consequence of aging.

8. Provide adequate pain control for back pain or other musculoskeletal discomfort.

9. Monitor for adequate dietary intake of calories and fluids and for effective elimination patterns.

10. Teach, encourage, and assist clients to establish exercise programs appropriate to their capabilities. Especially promote exercise programs that include walking or other weight-bearing activities, as tolerated (Figure 55-11).

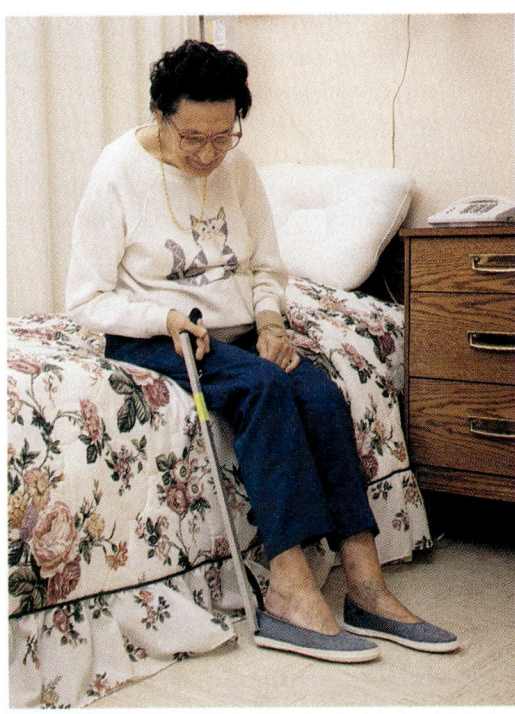

Figure 55-11 This elderly client is able to ambulate and remain active with the help of an assistive device.

Nursing Interventions: Degenerative Arthritis

1. Suggest a schedule for alternating periods of activity and rest.

2. Advise a weight reduction plan, if necessary, to eliminate extra strain on affected joints.

3. Teach, assist, and encourage the client to establish an exercise program that emphasizes gentle stretching and movement of all joints. For those clients who are more independent, exercise programs in warm water can have positive outcomes.

4. Provide adequate pain control. Teach clients and caregivers to monitor for gastrointestinal distress related to arthritis medications such as nonsteroidal anti-inflammatory drugs (NSAIDs) and to be aware that enteric coated medications cannot be crushed, as they are designed to protect the stomach by dissolving in the duodenum.

5. Encourage the client to seek ongoing evaluation by the physician, as new arthritis medications such as celecoxib (Celebrex) are continually being developed and trialed.

Nursing Interventions: Fractured Hip

NOTE: Nursing interventions may vary depending on whether the older client has an open reduction/internal fixation fracture (ORIF) or total hip arthoplasty (THA).

1. Maintain postoperative positioning as appropriate to the client's form of treatment.

2. Provide adequate pain control prior to physical therapy and on an ongoing basis through the recovery process.

3. Prevent complications, including skin breakdown, RTIs, infections at the surgical site, and dislocation of the prosthesis or internal fixation device.

4. Facilitate and monitor with the registered nurse the client's consistent use of antiembolism stockings as ordered and the administration of anticoagulant medications and the related monitoring of lab values, to decrease the risk of pulmonary embolism (which can be a significant risk to older clients after hip fracture and/or hip replacement).

5. Teach the client about fall prevention. Evaluate the client's environment (home, room, bathroom) for safety with regard to mobility and make recommendations for rectifying any threats to safety.

Integumentary System

See Chapter 40 for an anatomy and physiology review of the integumentary system. The following integumentary changes result from the normal aging process:

• Subcutaneous tissue and elastin fibers diminish, causing the skin to become thinner and less elastic.

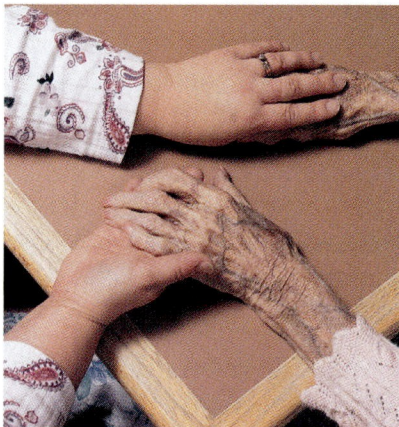

Figure 55-12 Hyperpigmentation is a normal result of the aging process.

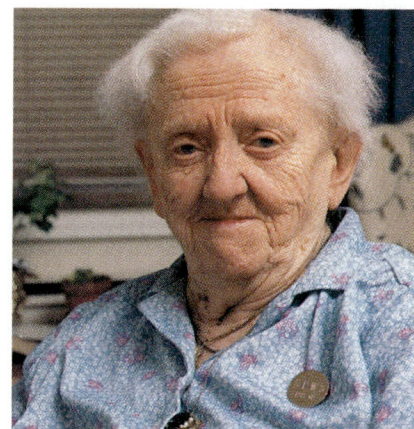

Figure 55-13 Gray hair results from a reduction in melanin production.

- Ability of melanocytes to produce even pigmentation diminishes, resulting in hyperpigmentation or liver spots, typically on the hands and wrists (Figure 55-12).
- Eccrine, apocrine, and sebaceous glands decrease in size, number, and function, resulting in diminished secretions and moisturization and, thus, pruritis.
- Body temperature regulation diminishes due to decreased perspiration and, many times, decreased circulation.
- Capillary blood flow decreases, resulting in slower wound healing.
- Blood flow decreases, especially to lower extremities.
- Vascular fragility causes senile purpura.
- Cutaneous sensitivity to pressure and temperature diminishes.
- Melanin production decreases, causing gray-white hair (Figure 55-13).
- Scalp, pubic, and axillary hair thin, and women display increased facial hair on the upper lip and chin.
- Nail growth slows, nails become more brittle, and longitudinal nail ridges form.

Common integumentary disorders related to aging include the following:

- Pressure ulcers (alteration in skin integrity)
- Herpes zoster (shingles)
- Skin cancer (included because the risk of skin cancer increases with age)

Nursing Interventions: Alteration in Skin Integrity

1. Perform a pressure ulcer risk assessment upon the client's admission to the health care setting (Figure 55-14).
2. Implement pressure ulcer prevention protocol for clients at risk for pressure ulcer formation. It is important to consider and document pressure relieving interventions for all surfaces that the client will sit or lay on during the course of the day (Table 55-2).
3. Encourage adequate intake of protein and fluids to help ensure good skin integrity.

Infection Control: Skin Integrity
It is the nurse's responsibility to educate caregivers (including other staff members, as necessary) about the need to thoroughly wash and dry the client's perineal area, and to keep linens and clothing clean and dry, especially when incontinence is a problem. Such education may also include instruction on maintaining client privacy; properly retracting, cleansing, and repositioning the foreskin of an uncircumcised older male client; and proper cleansing of the skin folds of an older female client's perineal area. Clients and caregivers should also be instructed to cleanse front to back only and to not rinse and reuse washcloths again or use them on other body areas. These simple hygiene and infection-control guidelines can help maintain the client's skin integrity and can also prevent unnecessary infections.

Nursing Interventions: Herpes Zoster
1. Treat the pain.
2. Treat the ulcer with medications (e.g., acyclovir [Zovirax] topical cream), as ordered, to reduce the length of time of the outbreak.
3. Develop a plan to ensure continuity in meeting the client's psychosocial needs, and allow the client time to share concerns.

Infection Control: Herpes Zoster
Prevent cross-infection from drainage from the vesicular eruptions by practicing proper hand-washing and implementing appropriate isolation procedures, especially if the client is in the hospital or another health care facility.

Date of assessment: _____   Nurse: _____

Pressure ulcer present on admission: No ____ Yes ____ Stage ____

A score of 11 or more places a client at risk for pressure ulcer formation. Preventive protocol should be established.

Activity		Total	Level of Consciousness		Total
Ambulant without assistance	0		Alert	0	
Ambulant with assistance	2		Slow verbal response	1	
Chairfast	4		Responds to verbal or painful stimuli	2	
Bedfast	6	_____	Absence of response to stimuli	3	_____
Mobility—Range of Motion			**Nutritional Status**		
Full range of motion	0		Good (eats 75% or more of required intake)	0	
Moves with minimal assistance	2		Fair (eats less than 75% of required intake)	1	
Moves with moderate assistance	4		Poor (minimal intake, consistent weight loss)	2	
Immobile	6	_____	Unable/refuses to eat/drink, emaciated	3	_____
Skin Condition			**Incontinence—Bladder**		
Hydrated and intact	0		None	0	
Rashes or abrasions	2		Occasional (fewer than 2/24 hours)	1	
Decreased turgor, dry	4		Usually (more than 2/24 hours)	2	
Edema, erythema, pressure ulcers	6	_____	Total (no control)	3	_____
Predisposing Disease Process			**Incontinence—Bowel**		
No involvement	0		None	0	
Chronic, stable	1		Occasional (formed stool)	1	
Acute or chronic, unstable	2		Usually (semi-formed stool)	2	
Terminal	3	_____	Total (no control, loose stool)	3	_____

Figure 55-14 Pressure Ulcer Risk Assessment

Table 55-2 PROTOCOL FOR CLIENTS AT RISK FOR PRESSURE ULCERS

OBJECTIVE	INTERVENTIONS	OBJECTIVE	INTERVENTIONS
Relieve pressure	• Establish positioning schedule. • Place pressure relieving mattress on bed, cushions on chair. • Teach client wheelchair exercises. • Stand and/or ambulate client in chair frequently. • Use wheelchair for transporting only. • Allow client to sit on bedpan, commode, or toilet for only brief periods. • Check areas of pressure under casts, braces, splints, slings, prostheses.	Prevent spasticity and contractures	• Avoid quick, rough movements. • Do range of motion exercises at least twice daily. • Assess for synergy patterns when positioning. • Administer oral antispasmodics if ordered.
Relieve friction and shearing	• Use turning sheet for positioning in bed and chair. • Keep head of bed lower than 30 degrees unless contraindicated. • Use supportive devices to prevent sliding in chairs. • Use appropriate transfer techniques. • Do not use powder on skin. • Place bed cradle under top covers.	Maintain hydration/ nutritional status	• Assess nutritional status. • Investigate causes of anorexia. • Correct underlying nutritional deficits. • Encourage additional fluids, unless contraindicated. • Give high protein supplement, if necessary. • Monitor weight weekly.
Prevent moisture/ maceration	• Implement scheduled toileting or bladder retraining program. • Use absorbent incontinent briefs or pads. • Check incontinent clients frequently. Wash and rinse thoroughly. Apply moisture barrier. • Avoid use of plastic/rubber sheets, protectors.		Continue with routine skin care. Do skin checks with each position change.

Nursing Interventions: Skin Cancer

1. Teach clients and caregivers both cancer prevention methods and skin self-examination to detect lesions early. Early detection and treatment of skin cancers are essential to optimal client outcomes.
2. Provide information in both verbal and written form and in collaboration with the client's multidisciplinary team, regarding treatment (surgery, chemotherapy, radiation, and other options).
3. Monitor for signs of infection at the lesion site.
4. Ensure that the client's psychological, psychosocial, spiritual, and dietary needs are also addressed.

Nervous System

See Chapter 41 for an anatomy and physiology review of the nervous system. The following neurological changes result from the aging process:

- Neurons in the brain decrease in number, resulting in decreased production of neurotransmitters and, thus, reduced synaptic transmission.
- Cerebral blood flow and oxygen utilization decrease.
- Time required to carry out motor and sensory tasks requiring speed, coordination, balance, and fine-motor hand movements increases.
- Short-term memory may somewhat diminish without much change in long-term memory.
- Night sleep disturbances occur due to more frequent and longer wakeful periods.
- Deep-tendon reflexes decrease, although reflexes at the knees remain fairly intact.

Many disorders that affect the neurological system are not unique to elders. However, the risk of acquiring one of these disorders increases with age. One of the most common diagnoses among elders in long-term care facilities is dementia, particularly one form of dementia called Alzheimer's disease (AD). **Dementia** is an organic brain pathology characterized by losses in intellectual functioning. The clinical manifestations associated with dementia are never considered normal aging changes.

It is important for care providers to assess the length of onset of confusion or cognitive changes in the client. Generally, dementia describes declines that have a slow onset of greater than 6 months, whereas **delirium** (or acute confusion) describes cognitive changes

that have a shorter onset of 6 months or less. Acute confusion can occur independently or as an exacerbation of a current dementia-related disorder in the client. Acute confusion can result from many stresses such as infections, medication side effects, drug interactions, metabolic imbalances, dehydration, or injuries from falls (e.g., subdural hematomas). Elimination of the causative factor can often turn the acute confusion around in a relatively short period of time to the pre-exacerbation level of functioning, unless further pathology to the brain has occurred.

Nursing Interventions: Alzheimer's Disease

1. Before diagnosis, encourage a medical and psychological diagnostic workup including a mental status examination.
2. Facilitate orientation in the early stages of the disease with calendars, lists, and consistent schedules.
3. Arrange an environment that is therapeutic, consistent, calm, and safe and that alternates rest with activities that require the use of long-practiced skills.
4. Encourage and facilitate access for the client and family to support groups where they can independently share their feelings and concerns and have questions addressed.
5. When assistance is needed with ADL, implement consistent routines with consistent caregivers but allow for delay of care if needed due to client stress or irritability. Encourage independence of the client while assisting with ADL (e.g., offer a warm washcloth for client to wash the face and assist with those ADL that the client cannot complete without assistance).

LIFE CYCLE CONSIDERATIONS

Mental Health in the Elderly

Mood disorders including depression, bipolar disorder, anxiety disorders, late onset psychosis, sleep disorders, substance abuse, schizophrenia (chronic and late onset), and other psychiatric diseases certainly occur among older clients and often go unaddressed or are ineffectively treated. Appropriate assessment, treatment, and clinical management of these clients require effective interdisciplinary teams comprising a geriatric psychiatrist; a neurologist; a clinical nurse specialist specializing in gerontology and mental health; a licensed social worker; a clinical pharmacist; other multidisciplinary team members (including direct care nurses and staff and activity therapists); and the client's family and, whenever possible, the client.

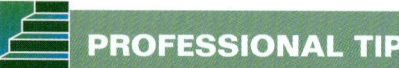

PROFESSIONAL TIP

Nervous System in the Elderly Client

In the absence of pathology, intellect and capacity for learning remain unchanged with aging.

6. Monitor general health status. Treat any underlying medical problems. Provide adequate pain control, as needed, and monitor for lack of sleep to minimize the risk of violent behavior (Andersen, 1999). Observe for the client's better times of the day, and plan activities or interventions accordingly.

7. Build a trusting relationship with the client. Use clear, simple directions and treat clients with respect and as individuals, building on their strengths and their unique interests and histories. Doing so demonstrates appreciation for the individual and can help build the client's self-esteem.

8. Be aware that as much is communicated to the AD client through the caregiver's nonverbal behavior and tone and volume of voice as is communicated through actual words. A calm attitude allows the client time to process and retrieve information when spoken to or asked a question.

9. Support the client's mobility within a safe environment, recognizing that as the disease progresses, baseline wandering often increases as a coping skill, whereas verbal communication often decreases (Fetters, 1994). Bean bag chairs, low mattresses, bed and chair alarms, positional (anti-sliding) wedges for chairs, merry walkers that support independent mobility, and assisted-ambulation programs to build leg strength are all therapeutic interventions for AD clients as the disease progresses and represent preferable alternatives to the use of restraints.

10. Monitor for changes in baseline behaviors and for intensity of wandering (both pacing or lethargy), as either often indicates underlying infections, metabolic imbalances, or stress. Encourage clients to alternate periods of activity and rest.

Nursing Interventions: Depression

1. Assess for signs of a physical basis for any fatigue (e.g., infection, pain, altered nutritional status, or shortness of breath upon exertion).

2. Administer treatment for underlying physiologic problems, if applicable.

3. If symptoms persist, encourage the client to have a medical diagnostic workup with a geriatric psychiatrist, if such a workup has not yet been done.

4. Monitor for verbal or nonverbal signs of suicidal thoughts/intent. Determine whether the client has a plan.

5. Provide one-on-one supervision of the client as needed and assure the client that the caregiver will keep him safe. If appropriate for the client, seek an agreement that he will not try to harm himself.

6. Administer antidepressant medication as ordered. Provide client and family education regarding

medication, including length of time before therapeutic results should occur, and potential side effects. Report immediately to the registered nurse and primary care provider any extrapyramidal side effects (e.g., tremors, drooling, pin rolling of the fingers, shuffling gait) that are observed.

7. If the client is not assessed as being at risk for suicide but is isolating in his room, establish small goals with the client (e.g., coming out of the room and sitting safely in the hallway with the nurse for 5 minutes two times per day and for meals). Advance to more challenging goals as the client demonstrates increased tolerance for social interaction.

8. Facilitate the client's reintegration into a healthy support system and provide small community group time for the client to share his views.

Nursing Interventions: Transient Ischemic Attack

1. Assess for risk factors for stroke and for the existence of any previous carotid vascular tests for potential blockage (stenosis).

2. Provide client and family education explaining the relationship between risk factors and TIA and stroke.

3. Provide teaching to assist in reducing risk factors.

4. Monitor orthostatic blood pressure and encourage clients to change positions slowly to decrease the risk of falling.

Urinary System

See Chapter 42 for an anatomy and physiology review of the urinary system. The following urinary changes result from the aging process:

- Nephrons in the kidneys decrease in number and function, resulting in decreased filtration and gradual decrease in excretory and reabsorbtive functions of the renal tubules.
- Glomerular filtration rate decreases, resulting in decreased renal clearance of drugs.
- Blood urea nitrogen increases. The creatinine clearance test is a better indicator than is BUN of renal function in elders.
- Sodium-conserving ability diminishes.
- Bladder capacity decreases, causing increased frequency of urination, including nocturia.
- Renal function increases when the older client lies down, sometimes causing a need to void shortly after going to bed.
- Bladder and perineal muscles weaken, resulting in the inability to empty the bladder and predisposing the elderly client to cystitis.
- Incidence of stress incontinence increases in older females.
- The prostate may enlarge in older males, causing urinary frequency or dribbling.

Common urinary disorders related to aging include the following:

- Incontinence
- Urinary tract infections (UTIs)

Nursing Interventions: Incontinence

1. Complete an assessment for bladder management (Figure 55-15).
2. Identify the type of incontinence present (Table 55-3).
3. Implement an appropriate bladder management program (Table 55-4).
4. Frequently monitor for skin impairment.
5. Offer absorbent incontinent pads or briefs that draw the moisture away from the skin.
6. Teach all caregivers, the client, and the family the importance both of adequate cleansing of the genital area (proper retraction and cleansing of the foreskin in the older uncircumcised male and proper cleansing of the skin folds of the older female), legs, and back and of the use of clean linens, to ensure that the client's skin is kept clean and dry. Apply a moisture barrier cream as needed to prevent skin maceration from excessive exposure to moisture.
7. Teach and employ effective infection-control techniques (e.g., wipe and clean [from front to back only] after toileting and when bathing).
8. Encourage referral to discuss medical options (in addition to nursing interventions) for treatment of incontinence.
9. Allow the client to voice concerns over incontinence and assist to overcome any adverse effects on psychosocial functioning.

Table 55-3 TYPES OF URINARY INCONTINENCE

TYPE	CHARACTERISTICS
Functional	Bladder emptying is unpredictable but complete. Incontinence is related to impairment of cognitive, physical, or psychological functioning or to environmental barriers.
Urge	Incontinence occurs immediately after the sensation to void is perceived.
Reflex	Incontinence is related to neurogenic bladder and central nervous system or spinal cord injury. Bladder fills, and uninhibited bladder contractions cause loss of urine.
Stress	Increased abdominal pressure is higher than urethral resistance. Stress associated with coughing or laughing causes incontinence.
Total	Unpredictable, unvoluntary, continuous loss of urine.

Nursing Interventions: Urinary Tract Infections

NOTE: Elderly persons frequently do not present with the usual signs and symptoms of UTIs. Falling or signs of acute confusion (more than usual) may often be the major clinical manifestations.

1. Monitor fluid intake and output. Increase intake unless contraindicated. Offer cranberry juice frequently, per ordered diet.

To be completed and reviewed every 90 days or as frequently as needed based on outcome and response.

CLIENT_____ Adm No. _____ Date_____ Diagnoses_____ Birthdate_____

Bladder function: History of infection or other urinary problem._____ Urinalysis: Date_____

Protein____ Glucose__ Ketones__ RBC__ WBC__ Bacteria__ Crystals__ Sp.Gr.__ Culture: Date_____ Result_____

Treatment_____

BUN____ Ser.Creatinine____ Tot.Pro.____ FBS____ To be completed after 2-week assessment period

Frequency of voiding_____ Average amount_____ Is client aware of need to void?_____ Urgency?_____ Dribbling?_____

Incontinence preceded by laughing, sneezing_____

Medications affecting bladder function/continence_____

Mental status: Short-term memory_____ Orientation_____ Able to express self_____

    Able to follow directions_____ Reaction to incontinence_____

Hydration baseline: Daily average fluid intake: Days_____ Eve._____ Night_____

Mobility/self-care skills: Ambulatory/self_____ Cane_____ Walker_____ Requires assist of one or two_____

    Weight-bearing_____ Propels self by w/c_____ Transfers self_____ Requires assistance_____

    Can manage clothing_____ Cleanses self after toileting_____ Washes hands_____

Figure 55-15 Assessment for Bladder Management

Table 55-4 BLADDER MANAGEMENT TECHNIQUES

PROGRAM	DESCRIPTION
Kegel exercises	Used for stress incontinence in cognitively alert persons. Exercises strengthen pelvic floor musculature.
Scheduled toileting	Client is on a fixed schedule of toileting—usually every 2 hours. Technique can be used to facilitate voiding and emptying of the bladder.
Habit training	Client is toileted according to individual pattern of voiding. Several days must be spent assessing pattern.
Bladder retraining	Restores normal pattern of voiding/continence. Requires accurate assessment before establishing schedule with progressive shortening or lengthening of toileting intervals. Client must be cognitively alert.
Prompted voiding	Client is prompted to toilet at regular intervals and is given social reinforcement for appropriate toileting behavior.

2. Teach and encourage client to empty the bladder every 3 to 4 hours.
3. Encourage the client to take all medication as prescribed.
4. Use proper infection-control techniques to minimize the risk of infection, including maintaining sterile technique for any urinary catheterization procedure (for urinalysis, assessment for bladder retention, or insertion of indwelling catheter), to prevent unnecessary introduction of bacteria into the bladder.
5. Teach female clients to wipe from front to back only; cleanse thoroughly after bowel movements; avoid bubble baths, colored toilet paper, douches, and vaginal sprays; and wear underwear made from cotton rather than synthetic fibers.
6. Teach the client and caregivers that hematuria (blood in the urine) and fever indicate the need for immediate assessment and intervention, as these signs and symptoms can signify a potentially serious infection or condition. Any signs and symptoms of bladder infection should be immediately reported to the registered nurse and the physician.

Sensory Changes

See Chapter 43 for an anatomy and physiology review of the sensory system. The following sensory changes result from the aging process:

Vision

- With aging, the lens becomes less pliable and less able to increase its curvature in order to focus on near objects, causing presbyopia (trouble seeing objects up close) and decreased accomodation. The lens also yellows, causing distorted color perceptions, with greens and blues washing out and warm colors such as reds and oranges becoming more distinct. The incidence of cataracts also increases.
- Accommodation of pupil size decreases, resulting in both decreased adjustment to changes in lighting and decreased ability to tolerate glare. For instance, high-gloss tile floors in hallways can appear like hills and valleys to older clients, especially those with perceptual deficits; this may increase anxiety and safety risks.
- Vitreous humor changes in consistency, causing blurred vision. Changes in the anterior chamber may increase the pressure of the aqueous humor, resulting in glaucoma.
- Lacrimal glands secrete less fluids, causing dryness and itching. Entropion or ectropion (turning of the eyelids inward or outward) occasionally occurs in older clients. These conditions can not only impact vision, but can increase the risk of infection due to dryness and ineffective blinking. In these conditions, obtaining an order for artificial tears, lacrilube, and eye drop treatments for dryness or infection may be necessary.

Infection Control: Eye Care

To decrease infection risks, remind all caregivers to wash from the center outward when washing clients' eyes.

Common vision disorders related to aging include the following:

- Presbyopia
- Cataract
- Glaucoma
- Age-related macular degeneration

Nursing Interventions: Visual Impairment

1. Teach visually impaired clients adaptive techniques for ADL, such as extra lighting.
2. Advise regular examination by an ophthalmologist.
3. Provide preoperative and postoperative care and teaching to clients undergoing cataract surgery, including lifting and bending restrictions as well as measures to prevent infection.
4. Teach proper eye drop administration techniques to all clients who are prescribed eye drops, including holding the drop in the eye with the lid closed for 30 seconds after administration.
5. Ensure that older clients have their glasses on when needed to decrease perceptual and spatial deficits.

Hearing

- As aging occurs, the pinna becomes less flexible, the hair cells in the inner ear stiffen and atrophy, and cerumen (earwax) increases.

- The number of neurons in the cochlea decrease, and the blood supply lessens, causing the cochlea and the ossicles to degenerate.
- Presbycusis, the impairment of hearing in older adults, is often accompanied by a loss of tone discrimination. High-frequency tones are lost first; thus, keeping the voice low and calm and decreasing any background noise can improve the client's comprehension of the caregiver's message.

Nursing Interventions: Hearing Impairment

1. Assess for ear pain; drainage; inflammation; abnormalities; surgeries; perforations; or impacted cerumen.
2. Evaluate medication regimen and assess for ototoxicity, if medication history reveals such a risk.
3. Advise hearing testing by an audiologist, if the previous assessments are negative.
4. Monitor the care and use of a hearing aid by the older client with unilateral or bilateral aids (Figure 55-16). Provide teaching and assistance as needed for cleaning the hearing aid(s) and replacing batteries.
5. Instruct caregivers and family about the communication and socialization needs of the client. For some older clients, either the use of a small erasable board to augment verbal questions or

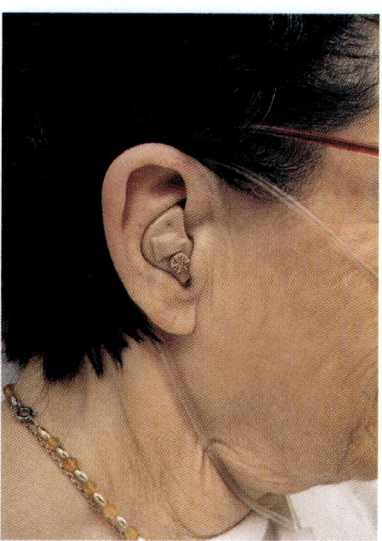

Figure 55-16 Hearing aids help compensate for hearing loss that results from aging.

communication with written text represents a therapeutic intervention for hearing impairment. If writing dexterity or ability is also impaired, a story board that has pictures indicating the client's needs (e.g., bathroom, food, rest) can assist the client to independently communicate needs to caregivers.

SAMPLE NURSING CARE PLAN

THE CLIENT WITH ALZHEIMER'S DISEASE (AD)

Mrs. Jane Rodriguez, 64 years old, was admitted to the Alzheimer's unit of a long-term care facility. Last month, Mrs. Rodriguez was visiting her daughter in another state and wandered away from the daughter's home. Mrs. Rodriguez was found 60 miles away, unharmed but completely disoriented and agitated. Mrs. Rodriguez had worked as a nursing assistant before she retired. She is a widow and has two children in the same community where the nursing home is located, in addition to the daughter who she was visting in another state. Unless reminded, Mrs. Rodriguez does not shower or change clothes. She awakens at least once each night and asks for breakfast.

Nursing Diagnosis 1 *Thought Processes, Altered, related to progressive dementia as evidenced by disorientation to time and place, loss of short-term memory, inability to concentrate, and periods of agitation*

PLANNING/GOALS	NURSING INTERVENTIONS	RATIONALE	EVALUATION
Mrs. Rodriguez will remain calm and will not experience agitation and anxiety as a result of her disorientation and memory loss.	Provide Mrs. Rodriguez with clues for orientation: "Good morning, Mrs. Rodriguez. My name is Jean, and I will help you today." Avoid	People in the early stages of Alzheimer's disease may become agitated because their world is always unfamiliar to them. The	Mrs. Rodriguez remained calm and showed no signs of agitation or anxiety.

continued

putting her on the spot by asking questions she may not answer, such as "Do you know what day this is?"

Place a large sign on Mrs. Rodriguez's door with her name printed in large letters to help her find her room.

Have family bring in snapshots and photos to stimulate reminiscence.

Avoid changing Mrs. Rodriguez's room. Put items back in the same place all the time.

Consult with activities staff in planning self-expressive, non-fail activities that require little concentration (e.g., painting with nontoxic paints, modeling with nontoxic clay).

If Mrs. Rodriguez is resistant to care, provide clear, simple, nonthreatening instructions and delay care as needed until she is calmer.

issue is not whether individuals with a dementia are oriented, but whether they can cope with their environment.

Short-term memory loss makes it impossible for Mrs. Rodriguez to remember where her room is or where the bathroom is. If she still recognizes her name, posting it on the door will help her find her way.

Reminiscing can be a satisfying activity. It is especially helpful if the photos are from an earlier, happier time such as when her children were young. Long-term memory may still be intact, allowing her to recall these happier times.

Consistency in the environment (as well as in routine and staff) reduces frustration.

Appropriate activities prevent boredom, which can lead to irritation. It is important to plan nonstressful, noncompetitive, failure-proof activities in order to prevent frustration.

Persons with cognitive deficits often vary between combativeness and cooperation. Often, delaying care for even 10 to 15 minutes when resistance is encountered improves client outcomes. Also, exploring and understanding the antecedents to a client's combative behavior allows caregivers to intervene early and to change the environment or the approach to better ensure positive client outcomes (Andersen, 1999).

continued

Nursing Diagnosis 2 *Injury, Risk for, related to risk factors of mode of transportation and cognitive and affective factors as evidenced by wandering behavior, impaired judgment, and disorientation*

PLANNING/GOALS	NURSING INTERVENTIONS	RATIONALE	EVALUATION
Mrs. Rodriguez will remain free of injury while retaining as much independence and freedom as possible.	Lock up tools, medicines, and chemicals. Keep only nonpoisonous plants on the unit. Arrange furniture so that walkways are open. Pad sharp corners of tables and chests. Cover electrical outlets and hot radiators. Place electrical cords and telephone wires out of reach.	Persons with Alzheimer's disease do not recognize unsafe acts or conditions due to loss of impulse control and loss of judgment. They do not comprehend cause and effect.	Mrs. Rodriguez has experienced no injury.
	Provide assurance during fire drills.	Unusual activity of any sort increases agitation, especially when noise level is increased.	

Nursing Diagnosis 3 *Self-Care Deficit related to perceptual or cognitive impairment (memory loss and sensory–perceptual deficits) as evidenced by needing a reminder to shower and change clothes*

PLANNING/GOALS	NURSING INTERVENTIONS	RATIONALE	EVALUATION
Mrs. Rodriguez will complete ADL with minimal assistance now and with increasing assistance as the disease progresses.	Use verbal cues and hand-over-hand assistance with ADL. Instruct staff to avoid doing tasks that Mrs. Rodriguez can do by herself. Watch for signs of frustration and irritation and intervene when appropriate.	Using these simple techniques can minimize the need for assistance, thereby increasing feelings of self-esteem.	Mrs. Rodriguez participates in ADL.
	Ask family to bring in clothing that is easy to manipulate. Set clothing out in the order it is to be put on.	Dressing is one of the more difficult tasks to accomplish. Appropriate clothing can simplify the activity.	
	Consider tub baths rather than showers. Provide privacy, check the temperature of the bathroom, and do not leave the client alone.	Showers are frequently threatening or confusing to persons with Alzheimer's disease. Tub baths are also more relaxing.	

continued

Nursing Diagnosis 4 *Sleep Pattern Disturbance related to disorientation as evidenced by wakefulness at night*

PLANNING/GOALS	NURSING INTERVENTIONS	RATIONALE	EVALUATION
Mrs. Rodriguez will experience fewer periods of wakefulness during the night. If she awakens, she will remain calm and free of agitation.	Avoid stimulating activities prior to bedtime. Establish a consistent bedtime routine. Take Mrs. Rodriguez to the bathroom and allow sufficient time for complete bladder emptying.	Overstimulation prior to bedtime may increase anxiety, preventing sleep. Having the client participate in relaxation activities and repeating the client's long-practiced bedtime routine prior to bed may also be helpful.	Mrs. Rodriguez sleeps through the night several times a week.
	Help Mrs. Rodriguez with a sponge bath and with oral care; give her a back rub using warm lotion and slow, smooth strokes.	These activities are relaxing.	
	Provide a light snack of a warm, noncaffeinated beverage and a plain, easily digested cracker, cookie, or a piece of toast. Be patient and do not rush her.	Hunger or overeating can interfere with sleep.	
	Question family concerning previous bedtime routines and sleeping habits.	Individuals may have used specific sleep routines throughout their lifetimes, such as sleeping with a night light, having a window open, playing a radio, or wearing socks to bed.	
	Repeat bedtime routine when Mrs. Rodriguez awakens during night.	Mrs. Rodriguez will think it is time to go to bed.	
	Encourage a short nap early in the afternoon.	Sleep pattern disturbances may result from overfatigue.	
	Avoid the use of sleeping medications.	Sleeping medications are seldom effective and may increase confusion, disorientation, and restlessness.	

FINANCING ELDER CARE IN THE 21ST CENTURY

Since the 1960s, the U.S. Congress has developed and implemented a series of national entitlement programs to help ensure adequate income, housing, and access to medical care for older Americans. As the number of older clients (those over age 65, particularly those over age 85) continues to rise, caregivers and advocates for elder care should strive to understand the budgetary policies that have influenced and continue to influence the U.S. health care delivery system.

Medicare

Medicare (Title XVIII) is a nationwide health insurance program for Americans who are 65 years of age or older, for persons who are eligible for Social Security disability payments for longer than 2 years, and for certain workers and dependents who need kidney transplants or dialysis. The **Health Care Financing Administration** (HCFA) is the federal agency in charge of administering the Medicare program. The program was enacted as part of the Social Security Act of 1965 and became effective on June 1, 1966. It consists of two separate but coordinated programs: hospital insurance (called part A) and medical insurance (called part B), which covers physician's services, outpatient services, some medical supplies, and some skilled nursing and home health services. Medicare provides basic protection for the cost of health care but does not cover all expenses (U.S. Department of Health and Human Services, Social Security Administration, 1991). Among the expenses *not* covered by Medicare for older Americans are those associated with the following:

- Home health care that does not require skilled personnel (e.g., as of February 1998, expenses for a home health visit [skilled] for the purpose of obtaining a blood sample are not covered).
- Nursing home care (except for skilled care for a limited time)
- Some routine medical checkups and related tests
- Prescription drugs
- Eye and hearing tests and eyeglasses and hearing aids
- Routine dental care and checkups

In the late 1990s, many insurance policies were available to supplement at varying levels the benefits paid by Medicare. This led many older clients to "stack" insurance policies, or to buy numerous overlapping policies for fear of being underinsured. The insurance industry and Congress worked together to outlaw stacking of Medicare supplement policies.

Although there has been some improvement in insurance coverage for preventive screening tests such as mammograms, the lack of reimbursement for prescription drugs continues to significantly burden older Americans, many of whom must choose between costly medications and food.

Medicaid

The Medicaid program was also enacted as part of the Social Security Act of 1966 and is often referred to as Title XIX. This program, which is federally aided and state operated and administered, provides medical benefits to certain indigent, or low-income, Americans. Nursing home bills represent a staggering burden for many older Americans who require nursing care. In 1995, nursing home bills averaged $22,000 per person per year, and projections showed that two-thirds of elders who lived alone would run out of savings after 13 weeks in a nursing home (Gallo, Reichel, & Andersen, 1995). Medicaid takes into account government-determined poverty levels when providing benefits, with coverage being extended to persons who are at certain percentages of the poverty level (e.g., 200% of poverty level, 150% of poverty level, and 100% of poverty level). Long-term care facilities serve both private-pay clients (those whose expenses are paid by themselves, their families, or their long-term care insurance policies) and Title XIX- (Medicaid-) funded clients. Medicaid coverage for long-term care is not available until a person's assets have been depleted to a certain set level. Elder care advocates continue in their efforts to protect the assets of the spouse who is able to stay in the family home after the other spouse must be placed in a nursing home.

To some in the United States, the debate over Social Security, Medicare, and Medicaid financing is viewed as someone else's priority. However, the moral responsibility for providing access to quality services and care for our country's elderly is shared by all Americans. Elder care services should be developed to promote independence yet should provide assistance when needed.

Omnibus Budget Reconciliation Act

The **Omnibus Budget Reconciliation Act** (OBRA), first enacted in 1987 and reenacted in 1990, sought to ensure quality services for older Americans. The act included guidelines for services that were required to be made available to seniors, and promoted the rights of seniors. However, as was the case with all health care costs, elder care costs continued to rise in the United States, and discussions and proposed legislation for financial reforms intensified.

Balanced Budget Act of 1997

Among the most significant influences on the financing of elder care in the past decade is the **Balanced Budget Act** (BBA) of 1997. The BBA replaced cost-based reimbursement for care provided in skilled nursing facilities (SNFs) with a prospective payment system (PPS) based on client assessment within a resource utilization group system (RUGS). Reimbursement for home health services also shifted to a PPS.

The BBA also states that discharge from hospitals to SNFs or home care for 10 common but as yet unpublished diagnosis-related groups (DRGs) is to be considered as a transfer for payment purposes. Medicare's goal was to make a single blended payment that combined the traditional hospital DRG payment and the payment for postacute care services to be shared by the providers.

The intended implications for practice included reduced reimbursement to some SNFs, fewer discharges from hospitals to independent facilities for subacute care or home care, and, thus, encouraged the creation of integrated delivery systems and managed care. In reality, however, it has become more difficult to find placement in SNFs for clients with complex needs, because the new reimbursement system simply does not fund all their health care needs.

These reimbursement and regulatory changes surely represent only the beginning of such efforts to balance resources and need as the U.S. population continues to age. Certainly, significant work lies ahead for advocates of quality elder care in the United States and the world in the 21st century. Nurses will play a vital role in the ensuing debates, for they will see firsthand the positive and negative outcomes of their clients.

CASE STUDY

Mr. Jack Baroni, a 72-year-old male, was admitted to the skilled care facility for rehabilitation following an open reduction, internal fixation of the right hip. Mr. Baroni had fallen while going up the stairs of his home, suffering an intertrochanteric, comminuted fracture of the right femur. He has no recollection of what caused him to fall. He is married and, until his surgery, was working part time as a school-crossing guard. While in the hospital, Mr. Baroni exhibited mental status changes including disorientation and confusion. His wife reports that he never had this problem prior to the surgery. He is continent of bowel and bladder. Mr. Baroni was in relatively good health until the fall. He and his wife agree that he should return home after rehabilitation is complete.

The following questions will guide your development of a nursing care plan for the case study.

1. Identify specific admission assessments that would be required for Mr. Baroni because of his age and condition.
2. Identify complications for which Mr. Baroni is at risk.
3. List interventions to prevent each complication.
4. Cite possible reasons for Mr. Baroni's fall.
5. Describe methods for assessing Mr. Baroni's mental status.
6. Describe possible reasons for his altered mental status.
7. Write three individualized nursing diagnoses and goals for Mr. Baroni.
8. List nursing actions related to altered mental status.
9. List four successful outcomes for Mr. Baroni.
10. Develop a teaching plan for Mr. Baroni.
11. List the community resources Mr. Baroni may need after discharge.

SUMMARY

- The elderly population is rapidly growing.
- Although many stereotypes and myths are associated with aging, elders are in fact very diverse in their characteristics.

- Health maintenance is as important for older adults as it is for younger persons. A healthy lifestyle can enhance the quality of life.
- Many changes are associated with aging. The disorders commonly seen among elders are often the results of pathology and are thus not considered a

normal part of aging. However, the risk of acquiring these disorders increases with age.

- Nurses knowledgeable about aging can plan interventions that will prevent complications for which elders are at risk.
- Nurses have a responsibility to advocate for their older clients. Nurses should be active legislatively and should work collaboratively to develop elder-care services that are affordable, provide equal access for all older Americans, and promote optimal wellness and independence.

Review Questions

1. Which of the following is a true statement?

   a. All people eventually become senile if they live long enough.
   b. People lose interest in sex as they age.
   c. Most elders are financially impoverished.
   d. Incontinence is not an expected or normal change of aging.

2. The programmed aging theory states that:

   a. stress causes structural and chemical changes in the body, which, in turn, cause aging.
   b. a genetic clock determines the speed at which people age.
   c. changes in collagen are the cause of aging.
   d. the decreasing ability to produce T-cell differentiation causes aging.

3. The elderly individual can reduce the potential for acquiring RTIs by:

   a. obtaining an influenza vaccine each year.
   b. staying inside throughout the winter months.
   c. avoiding exercise.
   d. limiting fluid intake.

4. Research indicates that:

   a. weight-bearing exercise is not recommended for elders.
   b. high-intensity resistance training can improve muscle strength in elders.
   c. muscle deterioration in elders is to be expected.
   d. walking is the only healthy exercise for elders.

5. Integumentary changes associated with aging include:

   a. increased glandular secretions.
   b. increased capillary blood flow.
   c. increased melanin production.
   d. increased vascular fragility.

Critical Thinking Questions

1. What services are essential in a quality elder-care program?

2. How can you advocate as a nurse for your older clients?

3. If you were going to author an Older American client's bill of rights, what things would you include?

4. What myths or stereotypes have you observed that affect the elderly?

 ## WEB FLASH!

- Search federal sites for some of the legislation and policies that are discussed in this chapter and affect elder care (e.g., OBRA and BBA).
- What clinical guidelines are available on the Internet from the government or other sources for the care of elderly clients (e.g., for urinary incontinence or pain treatment)?

Health Care in the Community

REHABILITATION, HOME HEALTH, LONG-TERM CARE, AND HOSPICE

MAKING THE CONNECTION

Refer to the following chapters to increase your understanding of rehabilitation, home health, long-term care, and hospice:

- **Chapter 6, Legal Responsibilities**
- **Chapter 7, Ethical Responsibilities**
- **Chapter 12, Cultural Diversity and Nursing**
- **Chapter 17, Loss, Grief, and Death**

- **Chapter 25, Assessment**
- **Chapter 26, Pain Management**
- **Chapter 55, Nursing Care of the Older Client**

LEARNING OBJECTIVES

Upon completion of this chapter, you should be able to:
- *Define key terms.*
- *List three reasons why there has been a significant change in the growth of nonacute care services.*
- *Discuss the legal/ethical implications of:*
  1. *Limiting aggressive health care services (such as rehabilitation or intensive care) for the elderly as a cost saving measure for the preservation of Medicare funds.*
  2. *Determining nurses' responsibility for accepting decisions made by individuals with questionable mental competency.*
- *Describe the differences between Medicaid and Medicare.*
- *Distinguish among licensure, certification, and accreditation.*
- *Describe the role of the LP/VN as a member of the interdisciplinary health care team in various health care settings.*
- *Discuss the types of clients that would benefit from participation in a rehabilitation program.*
- *Identify the responsibilities of the LP/VN in rehabilitation nursing, nursing in long-term care, in-home care, and hospice.*
- *List the various types of long-term care services.*

KEY TERMS

accreditation	Medicaid
adult day care	Medicare
assisted living	Medigap insurance
certification	rehabilitation
hospice	respite care
licensure	subacute care
long-term care facility	synergy

INTRODUCTION

There has been a strong emergence in the past decade of nonacute health care services. The growth of these services is a reflection of several changes occurring in the United States:

- The Tax Equity and Fiscal Responsibility Act of 1983 initiated the Medicare Prospective Payment system and the diagnosis-related group (DRG) system. This has resulted in the discharge of clients from acute-care hospitals much earlier. Clients, particularly elderly individuals, often require continuing care.
- Lives are being saved that would have been lost a few years ago. Ongoing health care services are often necessary for these individuals.

- The number of Americans over the age of 65 has tripled in this century. The risk of acquiring a chronic disease increases as individuals age, requiring health care throughout life.
- The cost of acute care has reached critical proportions. Case management is an attempt to contain costs by assisting people in defining their service needs, locating and arranging services, and coordinating the services of multiple providers. The cost of health care can be managed by controlling client access to services (General Accounting Office, 1994).

These changes have resulted in a vast increase in rehabilitation, home health, long-term care, and hospice services. There is an intermingling of services and settings under each of these categories of care. Rehabilitative services for example, may be provided in an acute-care setting, in a rehabilitation hospital, in a long-term care facility, or in the client's home. Home care may provide the same services that would be available in a subacute care nursing facility. Long-term care refers to both home and community-based services. Hospice care may be provided in the home or institution. While many of the clients requiring these services are elderly, there are an increasing number of services specializing in pediatric care.

LEGAL AND ETHICAL RESPONSIBILITIES

The legal basis for the provision of care in long-term care facilities is found in the Omnibus Budget Reconciliation Act (OBRA) of 1987. This act was legislated after a lengthy study of the care delivery in long-term facilities throughout the country. The major components of the act concern the issues of nursing assistant training, the regulation of the use of physical and chemical restraints, the Minimum Data Set (MDS 2) as an assessment tool, and the legal foundation for residents' rights. Many of the regulations found in OBRA also apply to home health nursing agencies.

The rights of the health care consumer are regulated for both long-term care and home health care. Before receiving services from either, the consumer must be given a copy of these rights and indicate an understanding of their content (Tables 56-1 and 56-2). In addition to OBRA, there are many other regulatory acts

Table 56-1 RESIDENT'S RIGHTS

This is an abbreviated version of the Resident's Rights as set forth in the Omnibus Budget Reconciliation Act. This document must be given to all residents and/or their families prior to admission to any long-term care facility.

1. **The resident has the right to free choice, including the right to:**
   - choose an attending physician
   - full advance information about changes in care or treatment
   - participate in the assessment and care planning process
   - self-administration of medications
   - consent to participate in experimental research
2. **The resident has the right to freedom from abuse and restraints, including freedom from:**
   - physical, sexual, mental abuse
   - corporal punishment and involuntary seclusion
   - physical and chemical restraints
3. **The resident has the right to privacy including privacy for:**
   - treatment and nursing care
   - receiving/sending mail
   - telephone calls
   - visitors
4. **The resident has the right to confidentiality of personal and clinical records.**
5. **The resident has the right to accommodation of needs including:**
   - choices about life
   - receiving assistance in maintaining independence
6. **The resident has the right to voice grievances.**
7. **The resident has the right to organize and participate in family and resident groups.**

8. **The resident has the right to participate in social, religious, and community activities including the right to:**
   - vote
   - keep religious items in the room
   - attend religious services
9. **The resident has the right to examine survey results and correction plans.**
10. **The resident has the right to manage personal funds.**
11. **The resident has the right to information about eligibility for Medicare/Medicaid funds.**
12. **The resident has the right to file complaints about abuse, neglect, or misappropriation of property.**
13. **The resident has the right to information about advocacy groups.**
14. **The resident has the right to immediate and unlimited access to family or relatives.**
15. **The resident has the right to share a room with the spouse if they are both residents in the same facility.**
16. **The resident has the right to perform or not perform work for the facility if it is medically appropriate for the resident to work.**
17. **The resident has the right to remain in the facility except in certain circumstances.**
18. **The resident has the right to personal possessions.**
19. **The resident has the right to notification of change in condition.**

(As determined by Omnibus Budget Reconciliation Act [OBRA] of 1987)

Table 56-2 CLIENT'S RIGHTS IN HOME CARE

Clients receiving home health care services or their families possess basic rights and responsibilities. These include:

The right to:

1. be treated with dignity, consideration, and respect.
2. have their property treated with respect.
3. receive a timely response from the agency to requests for service.
4. be fully informed on admission of the care and treatment that will be provided, how much it will cost, and how payment will be handled.
5. know in advance if they will be responsible for any payment.
6. be informed in advance of any changes in care.
7. receive care from professionally trained personnel, to know their names and responsibilities.
8. participate in planning care.
9. refuse treatment and to be told the consequences of this action.
10. expect confidentiality of all information.
11. be informed of anticipated termination of service.
12. be referred elsewhere if denied services solely based on ability to pay.
13. know how to make a complaint or recommend a change in agency policies and services.

The responsibility to:

1. remain under a doctor's care while receiving services.
2. provide the agency with a complete health history.
3. provide the agency all requested insurance and financial information.
4. sign the required consents and releases for insurance billing.
5. participate in care by asking questions, expressing concerns, stating whether information is not understood.
6. provide a safe home environment in which care is given.
7. cooperate with the doctor, the staff, and other caregivers.
8. accept responsibility for any refusal of treatment.
9. abide by agency policies that restrict duties the staff may perform.
10. advise agency administration of any dissatisfaction or problems with care.

that affect the delivery of care in the settings described in this chapter. These include the Self-Determination Act of 1990, which is a federal regulation, and legislation related to the reporting of client abuse (state regulations).

There is a fine line between what is a legal issue and what is an ethical issue. It is beyond the scope of this chapter to provide answers to the questions arising from such problems. However, these situations are examples of common legal and ethical issues.

1. An 80-year-old client in the third stage of Alzheimer's disease falls and fractures his hip. Should this client be transferred to a rehabilitation hospital for intensive rehabilitation? If not, what are the alternatives?

2. The staff of a long-term care facility suspects that a client was abused by her son before admission to the facility. The son wishes to take the mother home, and the mother is in agreement with this plan. The discharge planner learns that the local social services agency had investigated the client's living situation for abuse prior to the mother's admission. The case worker also suspects abuse but could find nothing objective upon which to build a case. Do the nursing staff and social workers of the facility have a legal or ethical obligation to attempt intervention? If so, what actions should be taken?

3. J.B. is a young adult (23 years old) receiving rehabilitation after suffering a traumatic brain injury due to a motorcycle accident. He wishes to make decisions concerning his care and treatment. His mental competency is questionable. However, this has not been legally established, and his parents make decisions often in opposition to J.B.'s preferences. What are the legal and ethical responsibilities of the nurse in accepting the decisions of relatives versus client?

4. Mr. A. and Mrs. C. are both residents of a long-term care facility. Mr. A. is married and Mrs. C. is a widow. The two have developed an intimate relationship that appears to be mutually satisfying to them both. Both residents are mentally competent and consenting adults. Mrs. A. is troubled by this and expects the staff to intervene. Does the staff have the right to intervene? If so, does this conflict with the residents' rights?

SOURCES OF REIMBURSEMENT

Medicare and Medicaid have long been traditional sources of reimbursement for nonacute care. All health care providers must be certified by both Medicare and Medicaid to receive payment for services rendered. While virtually all hospitals are certified by both Medicare and Medicaid, many long-term care providers, including home health care and skilled care facilities, are not. Clients, families, and hospital discharge planners need to be aware of this when planning continuing care.

Medicare

In 1965, **Medicare** (Title XVIII) was signed into law as an amendment to the Social Security Act and is the major source of payment for acute care services for persons over 65 years old and for permanently disabled individuals who receive Social Security disability benefits. Medicare is administered by the federal government through the Health Care Finance Administration (HCFA). Medicare Part A covers inpatient hospital care, home health care, and hospice care. Payment may be made for care in a skilled nursing facility. However, there are many restrictions, and criteria for coverage frequently change. Medicare Part B covers partial costs for physician services, outpatient hospital and rehabilitation care, and certain services and supplies not covered by Part A.

Medicare pays for limited skilled care and rehabilitation services in certified long-term care facilities if the client and the services provided meet specific criteria. Certified home health care agencies may be reimbursed for intermittent visits if the client requires skilled health care by a registered nurse.

Medicaid

Medicaid (Title XIX) pays for health services for the aged poor, the disabled, and low-income families with dependent children (Abrams, Beers, & Berkow, 1995). The program is financed by federal and state funds and is administered at the state level. Thus, services provided vary from state to state. Medicaid is currently the primary health financing program for low-income families and disabled individuals. It is a means-tested program, providing funds only when all other financial resources have been exhausted (Buckwalter, 1995). Services covered include inpatient and outpatient hospital care, diagnostic services, physician services, skilled nursing care, and home health services. Medicaid finances health care for 32 million persons at a total annual cost of $125 billion, of which $31 billion is spent on the elderly. Of this amount, 73% provides long-term care services for 1.4 million elderly persons. Medicaid is the principal source of financial assistance for long-term care. Medicaid pays for skilled home health care in all states, and 29 states also cover the optional benefit of personal care in the home. In 1993, 300,000 persons received home health and personal care services at a cost of $2.8 billion to Medicaid (Buckwalter, 1995).

Private Insurance

Sixty-six percent of beneficiaries of Medicare purchase **Medigap insurance** to pay for costs not covered by Medicare. These policies are purchased from private insurance companies. Medigap insurance has been restricted by Congress to a basic plan with nine

possible expansions (Abrams, et al., 1995). Only 0.2% of all long-term care costs are covered by insurance (Fisher, 1995). About 50% of costs are paid by the clients and their families, about 3% by Medicare, and the remainder by Medicaid (Abrams, et al., 1995). Long-term care insurance is a relatively new concept and the benefits vary greatly depending on the insurance company.

LICENSURE, CERTIFICATION, AND ACCREDITATION

There are a number of processes that have been designed to assure the health care consumer that the facility, agency, or service meets minimal standards of care. **Licensure** is a mandatory system of granting licenses according to specified standards and is regulated by each state. **Certification** is a voluntary process that establishes and evaluates standards of care but is required for any provider who seeks reimbursement from government funds. Because government funding is regulated by the federal government, certification standards are generated by the federal government. **Accreditation** is an additional confirmation of quality and generally indicates that the provider has gone above the minimum standards in the delivery of care and service.

Licensure

All health care facilities must be licensed. Each state has a designated agency (often the Department of Public Health) that is responsible for licensing health care facilities. A team of surveyors visits each facility annually to determine whether the facility is in compliance with the rules and regulations of the state. Noncompliance in any area results in severe sanctions and financial penalties to the institution. The facility is given a limited amount of time to correct any deficiencies. In cases where residents' lives or well-being are threatened, the facility may lose its license to operate.

Certification

Certification is required for any facility that chooses to be reimbursed by government funds, Medicare, and Medicaid. There are standards that must be met for certification to be granted. HCFA contracts with the state agencies to perform this function. In some states the long-term care survey for licensure and certification is done concurrently. Because there are two regulatory agencies (state and federal), the states have adopted the federal regulations and in some cases have exceeded federal regulations. Certification may not be granted if the facility is not in compliance with regulations. This means the facility will not receive any reimbursement from Medicare or Medicaid funds.

Accreditation

Seeking accreditation is voluntary (not required by law). Accrediting organizations issue standards whereas state/federal licensure and certification agencies issue rules and regulations. The Joint Commission on Accreditation of Healthcare Organizations (JCAHO) has long been accrediting hospitals and skilled nursing facilities. The Commission on Accreditation of Rehabilitation Facilities (CARF) has been accrediting comprehensive inpatient rehabilitation programs since 1966. Facilities like a subacute care unit specializing in rehabilitation may seek accreditation from both commissions (Bailis, 1995).

REHABILITATION

Rehabilitation is a process designed to help individuals reach their optimal level of physical, mental, and psychosocial functioning. This goal is accomplished by preventing complications, modifying the effects of the disability, and increasing independence. By so doing, the individual's self-esteem is maximized, thus increasing quality of life (Habel, 1993). Rehabilitation is concerned with increasing the client's ability to complete the basic activities of daily living (ADL) and the instrumental activities of daily living (IADL). ADL include grooming and hygiene, eating, dressing, toileting, and mobility. The IADL include higher-level tasks such as household and money management, using the telephone, and driving a car. For persons who have limited potential for regaining total independence, the goal is to teach the client to manage his or her own care. For every dollar spent on rehabilitation, 30 dollars are saved (Huey, 1995).

The Interdisciplinary Health Care Team

The interdisciplinary health care team (IHCT) is an essential component to any rehabilitation process. The client and family are the focus of the team and are encouraged to participate in the planning of care. The degree to which the family participates is determined by the client. The professional members of the team are selected based on the needs of the client. Physical and occupational therapists, a speech/language pathologist, recreational therapists, rehabilitation nurses, the physician, social workers, dietitians, and mental health professionals are usually required to provide services (Figure 56-1).

Each discipline completes an assessment and pools

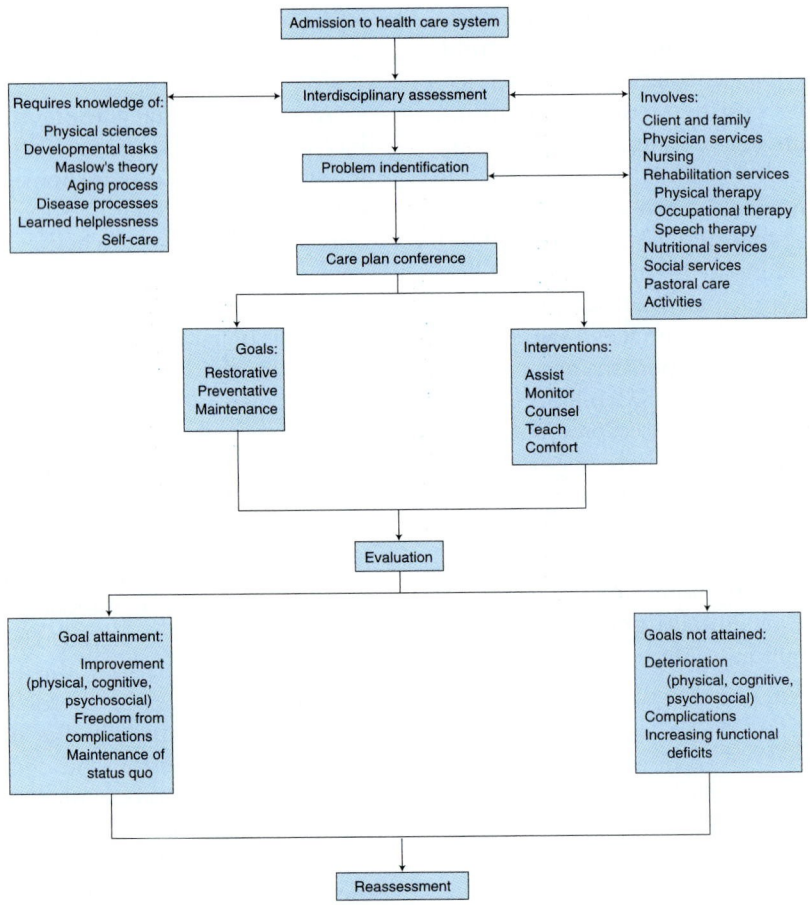

Figure 56-1 The Interdisciplinary Health Care Team Process

this information at the care planning conference so that a consensus among members (including the client and family) can be reached. The team process avoids both duplication of services and fragmented care. A holistic approach is utilized so that the client's physical, mental, and psychosocial needs will be identified (Wenckus, 1995).

Role of the LP/VN

Rehabilitation nursing is a specialty practice and requires specialized knowledge, skills, and attitudes. A sound knowledge base in the anatomy and physiology of the neurological, musculoskeletal, gastrointestinal, and urological systems is a prerequisite. The nurse must have excellent clinical skills in the areas of therapeutic positioning, range of joint motion exercises, transfers, ambulation, and activities of daily living. The nurse is responsible for planning measures to prevent complications such as impaired skin integrity and contractures and to implement interventions for dysphagia, incontinence, and other identified problems.

The nurse is a member of the interdisciplinary team and as such may function as caregiver, counselor, coordinator of care, and client advocate (Habel, 1993). The nurse needs an understanding of the roles and responsibilities of each discipline and how the nurse interrelates with each discipline. There is a steady demand for rehabilitation nurses in all settings.

Functional Assessment and Evaluation for Rehabilitation

Clients who need rehabilitation are screened before admission to a program. Assessments are completed by health care professionals whose services may be required by the client (Figure 56-2). The purpose of screening is to select the best setting for services. Criteria for admission to a program usually require that the client be:

- Medically stable
- Able to learn
- Able to sit supported for at least 1 hour a day and to actively participate in the program

Interdisciplinary programs may stipulate that the client has disabilities in 2 or more areas of function:

- Mobility
- Performance of ADL
- Bowel and bladder control
- Cognition
- Emotional function
- Pain management
- Swallowing
- Communication

There are a number of standardized assessment instruments that are designed to evaluate motor function, cognition, speech and language, mobility, and

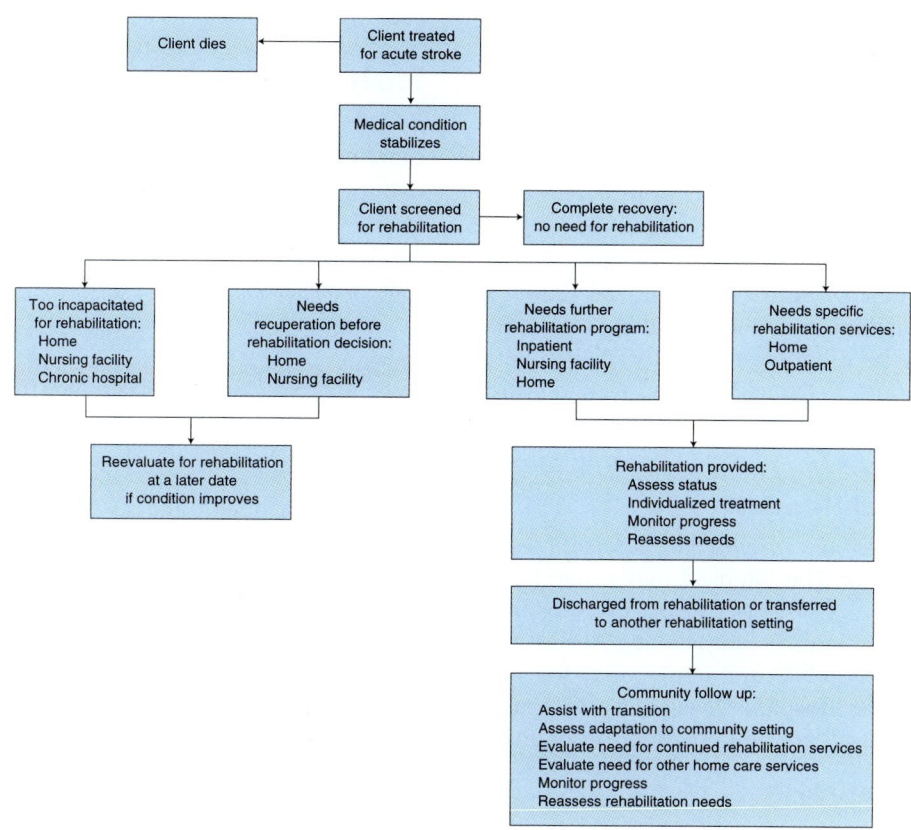

Figure 56-2 Assessing Potential—Stroke Rehabilitation

the client's performance of activities of daily living. There are additional tools that identify the client's risk for pressure ulcer formation, and potential for bowel and bladder management for incontinence. Refer to the AHCPR publication *Post-Stroke Rehabilitation, Clinical Guideline Number 16,* for a complete description of assessment instruments (Gresham, et al., 1995).

Rehabilitation Settings

Rehabilitation can be conducted in a variety of settings. Rehabilitation begins during the acute stage of illness when the client's medical condition stabilizes. Continuing rehabilitative services are often needed after discharge from acute care, necessitating transfer to a hospital inpatient program, a skilled nursing facility, an outpatient rehabilitation program, or a home rehabilitation program. Decisions about entry into a rehabilitation program should reflect a consensus among the client, family or significant others, physician, and the rehabilitation program.

Hospital Inpatient Program

Hospitals may have a separate rehabilitation unit, or services may be available in a freestanding hospital specializing in the delivery of rehabilitation services. In either case, the hospitals are staffed by a full range of rehabilitation professionals. Registered nurses and a physician skilled in rehabilitation (physiatrist) are available 24 hours a day. Hospital programs are generally more intense and comprehensive than programs in other settings, requiring greater physical and mental effort from the client.

Skilled Nursing Facility

Skilled nursing facilities often offer rehabilitation services. The facility may be hospital based or community based. The programs are similar to those offered in hospital settings with a full range of services and health care professionals. Physician coverage varies, but professional nursing care is rendered 24 hours a day. The program is usually less intense than a hospital program; this may be a benefit to elderly clients with limited energy resources. Families should research the services available because they differ greatly from one facility to the next.

Outpatient Rehabilitation

Outpatient services are offered by hospital-based rehabilitation programs. The intensity may range from occasional visits to 3 or 4 visits per week. Day hospital programs are another form of outpatient services but require the client to spend several hours a day for 3 to 5 days a week at the hospital. Availability of transportation is a prerequisite for all outpatient programs.

Home Rehabilitation

Some home health agencies provide a full scope of services, including nursing, all therapies, and social services. Service is usually provided on an intermittent basis for medically stable clients. The accessibility of services varies greatly depending on the availability of therapists in the area.

HOME HEALTH CARE

Home care encompasses a number of services delivered to persons in their homes and is the fastest growing segment of health care delivery. The total number of home health care agencies increased by 26% between 1989 and 1994 (Millea, 1995). Clients are receiving intravenous therapy, ventilator care, parenteral nutrition, and chemotherapy at home. Many agencies have nurse specialists on staff for complicated cases involving care required for wounds, intravenous therapy, diabetes, and cardiac or respiratory problems.

Medicare certified agencies provide intermittent care to persons meeting the criteria for care. A registered nurse may call on the client a specified number of times each week to assess the client's condition, supervise the work of LP/VNs and other nonlicensed staff, and deliver skilled nursing care. Nursing assistants are assigned to give personal care; check vital signs; and do positioning, transfers, and passive range-of-motion exercises. In addition to nursing staff, the agency may provide therapists and social workers to serve their clients, also on an intermittent basis. These services are time-limited by Medicare and are not reimbursable if the client is not deemed to require skilled care.

Role of the LP/VN

Although the role of the LP/VN in home care is expanding, current (1994) statistics indicate that LP/VNs make up the smallest number of home health care professionals. There were 254,643 registered nurses, 34,757 LP/VNs, 171,346 home health care assistants, and 48,460 physical therapists working in home care

HOME HEALTH CARE

Services

The home health agency may provide or arrange with other vendors for services needed by the client. This may include Meals-on-Wheels, homemaker services for light housekeeping tasks, companion services, transportation for outpatient care, intravenous therapy, pain management, and parenteral nutrition. The home health nurse needs to be aware of the availability of respite care because family members may need a break from the rigors of caregiving and may need encouragement from the nurse to do so.

(Millea, 1995). The responsibilities of the LP/VN vary among agencies. All nurses working in home care must have excellent assessment skills and a keen ability to identify actual and potential problems. Working with the family may be a greater challenge than meeting the needs of the client. Teaching the client and family is a major responsibility for the home health nurse. The educated client can assume more control. The client with a chronic health problem will have ongoing needs after the home health care is discontinued. Clients and their family caregivers must know the following:

The disease process
- Complications that may occur
- How to prevent the complications
- Signs and symptoms of the complications
- How to reduce risk factors such as dietary adaptations and exercise programs

Medications
- Actions of medications
- Special administration guidelines such as timing related to meals
- Side effects

Special skills
- Drawing up and administering insulin or other injectables
- Using a blood glucose monitor
- Changing dressings
- Monitoring vital signs
- Using special client care equipment, adaptive devices, and assistive devices

Documentation and communication
- How to keep records for nurse or physician visit; for example, blood glucose, blood pressure, and weight
- Communication with health care providers
- How and when to contact the home health nurse
- How and when to contact the physician
- How and when to contact emergency services

LONG-TERM CARE

Long-term care refers to a spectrum of services provided to individuals who have an ongoing need for health care. Long-term care has traditionally meant a community-based nursing home licensed for skilled or intermediate care. While there is a great demand for this type of care, there is also a market for other levels of health care. It is estimated that by the year 2030, more than 8 million seniors will be residing in nursing homes (American Health Care Association [AHCA], 1998). Currently 1.5 million persons live in 17,000 nursing homes. Of the residents, 90% are over age 65, but 24% are over age 85 (AHCA, 1998).

The increasing population of elderly persons has resulted in tremendous changes in health care delivery.

Housing options are often a component of the package of services available. The least restrictive level of care that is appropriate for the client's needs will generally be the most cost effective.

Long-Term Care Facilities

A **long-term care facility** may be licensed for either intermediate care or skilled nursing care. Long-term care facilities provide services to individuals who are not acutely ill, have continuing health care needs, and cannot function independently at home. Intermediate care facilities (ICF) are not certified for reimbursement from Medicare but may be certified for Medicaid funding. Skilled nursing facilities (SNF) are eligible for certification by both Medicare and Medicaid, but not all facilities choose to become certified. These facilities were formerly called nursing homes, rest homes, or convalescent centers. The term *extended care facility* (ECF) refers to any facility that renders care for a long period of time. It has no concrete definition and could refer to either an intermediate or skilled nursing facility. Facilities in every state that receive any government funds from any source are required by law to be in compliance with the OBRA regulations. It is estimated that 2 out of 5 persons in the United States will need long-term care sometime in their lives (AHCA, 1998).

Facilities of today bear little resemblance to those of the 1970s and 1980s. A restorative philosophy of care provides direction for the interdisciplinary team. Emphasis is placed on assisting the client (usually called resident) to attain and maintain the highest level of physical, mental, and psychosocial function. A holistic approach is utilized and families are important members of the care team.

A large number of facilities have special units devoted to the care of residents with specific problems. These units may care for persons with Alzheimer's disease, diabetes, respiratory disorders, wounds, and so on.

Subacute Care

Subacute care is a relatively new concept designed to provide services for clients who are out of the acute stage of their illnesses but who still require skilled nursing, monitoring, and ongoing treatments. The clients are not critically ill but do have complex medical needs. Subacute care is intended to fill the gap between the acute care hospital and the traditional long-term care facility (Glosner, 1995).

Subacute care facilities are usually housed in a section of a freestanding long-term care facility. The nurses may have a critical care background or are given additional training to equip them with the skills needed to provide care. Services may include intensive rehabilitation therapies, wound and pain management, care for clients with acquired immunodeficiency syndrome

(AIDS), oncology care, postsurgical services, intravenous therapy, nutritional support, peritoneal dialysis, ventilator care, and cardiac monitoring. Many subacute care units specialize in 1 or 2 of these areas. Clients stay from 20 to 30 days. Efficient discharge planning and client teaching are essential components to the plan of care.

Continuing Care Retirement Communities

Continuing Care Retirement Communities (CCRC) are designed to provide continuing levels of care as the individual's health care needs change. These levels include:

- Independent living in apartments located on the campus—housekeeping services and meals are provided
- **Assisted living**—a combination of housing and services for persons who need help with the activities of daily living
- Health care—either short-term for persons recovering from a temporary disorder or permanent for long-term illnesses such as Alzheimer's disease. The health care facility of the CCRC may be licensed as either skilled or intermediate

CCRCs usually charge a fee upon entry to the system and a monthly fee thereafter. The client must give proof of adequate financial resources in order to be accepted into the system. In exchange, individuals have the security of knowing that they will receive care for the remainder of their lives. Most CCRCs stipulate that persons must enter the system when they are able to live independently in the apartments. The health care facility of the CCRC may be certified for Medicaid if clients exhaust their financial resources. The health care facility may be certified for Medicare for clients who are qualified to receive such services. Neither Medicare nor Medicaid will pay for the independent living or assisted living sections of a CCRC.

Assisted Living

Assisted living combines housing and services for persons who require assistance with activities of daily living. Nursing care is not provided. These are persons who cannot live alone but who do not need 24-hour care. It is a less restrictive environment than a long-term care facility and maintains the individual's independence and freedom of choice. This level of care may be offered in a freestanding facility or as a section of a long-term care facility or CCRC as previously described. A monthly fee is charged and covers rent, utilities, housekeeping services, meals, transportation, health promotion, exercise programs, and assistance with ADL (Assisted Living Federation of America [ALFA], 1999).

There are an estimated 30,000 assisted living residences in the United States with more than 1 million residents (ALFA, 1999). The typical resident is a female (single or widowed) 83 years old or older (ALFA, 1999). Assisted living residences are licensed by the state. Costs range from $1,000 to $3,000 per month and are mainly paid from personal funds (AHCA, 1998).

Adult Day Care

Adult day care centers may be located in a separate unit of a long-term care facility, in a private home, or be freestanding. They provide a variety of services in a protective setting for adults who are unable to stay alone but who do not need 24-hour care. The centers are generally open from 7:00 A.M. to 6:00 P.M. 5 days a week and serve 2 or 3 meals a day. A daily or hourly fee is charged with an additional charge for meals. Services may be limited to socialization or may be comprehensive offering modest rehabilitation services and nursing care. Adult day care is often utilized by working persons who have a spouse or parent living with them who cannot be left alone. Fifty percent of clients in day care have some degree of cognitive impairment (Meng, 1995).

Respite Care

Respite care may be offered by adult day care centers, long-term care facilities, or in private homes. It is intended to provide a break to caregivers and may be utilized a few hours a week, for an occasional weekend, or for longer vacations. Planned activities, meals, and supervision are included in respite care services.

Foster Care

Some states are investigating the use of foster homes for individuals who cannot live independently but who do not require the services of a health care facility. A person with Alzheimer's disease who is mobile but who is unable to stay alone because of cognitive impairment would be a candidate for foster care. The legal structure is similar to the foster home concept for children.

Role of the LP/VN

There are probably more career opportunities available for the LP/VN in long-term care facilities than in the other types of health care described in this chapter. In a small facility the LP/VN might act as supervisor during the night or evening shifts. In larger facilities the LP/VN might be in charge of one unit with a registered nurse as a house supervisor. The nurse needs sharp assessment skills and a sound ability to make nursing judgments based on assessment findings. The LP/VN may also be expected to supervise and coordinate the work of nursing assistants. The nurse may wish to seek additional course work to acquire supervisory skills. LP/VNs may take the Certification Examination for Practical and Vocational Nurses in Long-Term Care (CEPN-LTC™) given by the National Council of State Boards of Nursing (NCSBN). Those who pass the examination are certified in long-term care and may use the initials "CLTC" to signify their certification.

HOSPICE

Hospice is humane, compassionate care provided to clients who can no longer benefit from curative treatment and have 6 months or less to live. The special care is designed to provide sensitivity and support, allowing clients to carry on an alert, pain-free life with other symptoms managed so the last days are spent with dignity and quality of life at home or in a home-like setting. This is sometimes referred to as palliative care.

The first hospice in the United States began in 1974. Today, there are more than 3,000 programs that are estimated to serve 450,000 terminally ill clients and their families each year (National Hospice Organization [NHO], 1999).

The primary physician must refer the client to hospice. Care and support are provided to both client and family by a team consisting of the physician, nurses, counselors, therapists, social worker, aides, and volunteers. The team regards dying as a normal process and does nothing to hasten or postpone death. Relief of

PROFESSIONAL TIP

Hospice Settings

Hospice care may be implemented in a variety of settings: the client's home, a special area of hospitals or nursing homes, or freestanding inpatient facilities. Most clients receive care at home. In 1995, 77% of hospice clients died in their home, 19% died in an institutional facility, and 4% died in other settings (NHO, 1999).

pain and other distressing symptoms is provided. The client is supported to live as actively as possible until death. The family is supported to help them cope during the client's illness and in their bereavement after the client's death.

Benefits for hospice are included in most private health care insurance, health maintenance organizations (HMOs), and managed care; Medicare; and in 43 states plus the District of Columbia by Medicaid. For hospice care in 1995, Medicare paid for 65.3% of the clients; private insurance, 12%; Medicaid, 7.8%; indigent (nonreimbursed) care, 4.2%; and other, 10.7% (NHO, 1999). As of 1999, 44 states had licensure laws for hospice programs. Some programs are certified voluntarily by Medicare and accredited by the JCAHO or Community Health Accreditation Program (CHAP) (NHO, 1999).

SAMPLE NURSING CARE PLAN

THE CLIENT REQUIRING REHABILITATIVE CARE

Mr. Jason, 65 years old, was admitted to a skilled nursing facility following hospitalization for a right cerebral hemisphere stroke. He is unable to purposefully change position without assistance. His gag reflex is weakened, swallowing is delayed, and there is coughing after swallowing. Mr. Jason has smoked for 50 years and is still doing so. Rehabilitation was initiated in the hospital. A feeding tube was put in place with the goal to assist Mr. Jason to regain his swallowing ability so the tube can be removed. Mr. Jason frequently expresses his discouragement with his dependency on the staff. He is married and lives in the community with his wife. Mr. Jason had been retired for 1 year before the stroke. Mrs. Jason works full time. Two adult children live in other states. Mrs. Jason hopes that her husband will regain adequate mobility skills so that she can eventually take him home.

Nursing Diagnosis 1 *Mobility, Impaired, Physical, related to left hemiplegia and sensory/perceptual impairments as evidenced by inability to purposefully change position of body without assistance*

PLANNING/GOALS	NURSING INTERVENTIONS	RATIONALE	EVALUATION
Mr. Jason will maintain current level of range of motion in all joints.	Change position at least every 2 hours; place affected extremities out of synergy.	Prevent contracture formation and pressure ulcers. Hemiplegic limbs are flaccid immediately	Range of joint motion is preserved. Complications related to immobility are *continued*

after stroke and then become spastic. **Synergy** patterns (abnormal patterns of movement that result from an overactive stretch reflex due to CNS damage) may develop in response to spasticity, causing contractures. Positioning out of synergy avoids contracture formation.

prevented. Progress in mobilization is achieved; movement in bed, transfers with 1 to 2 assists, transfer independently, and ambulation are noted.

Mr. Jason will remain free of contractures.

Do passive range-of-motion exercises twice a day on affected extremities. Assist with active range-of-motion exercises on unaffected extremities. Teach to do self-range-of-motion exercises when condition permits.

Range-of-motion exercises maintain joint mobility and prevent contracture formation. Active and self range-of-motion exercises will also increase strength and endurance.

Mr. Jason will begin program of progressive mobilization.

Teach Mr. Jason to move in bed:

– Client begins in supine position with the knees bent and feet flat in bed.

– Instruct client to raise the hips by pressing his heels down.

– Stabilize the affected limb by exerting pressure downward through the thigh just above the knee while assisting the client to lift the pelvis clear of the bed (Galarneau, 1993).

Increases the client's bed mobility. The recovery of a client with a stroke is dependent on the cooperative efforts of several interdisciplinary team members.

Consult with physical therapist about program for progressive mobilization.

The physical therapist is an expert in mobility.

Nursing Diagnosis 2 *Swallowing, Impaired, related to neuromuscular impairment as evidenced by weakened gag reflex, delayed swallowing, and coughing after swallowing*

PLANNING/GOALS	**NURSING INTERVENTIONS**	**RATIONALE**	**EVALUATION**
Mr. Jason will swallow without aspirating.	Consult with speech/language pathologist in regard to	A video-recorded fluoroscopy is used to make a definitive diag-	There are no signs of aspiration.

continued

video-recorded fluoroscopy for swallowing evaluation.

nosis of impaired swallowing. The results of the evaluation provide a basis for interventions suggested by the speech/language pathologist.

Serve semisolid foods of medium consistency. Use a commercial thickener for liquids. Avoid milk, citrus juices, and water.

These foods require less manipulation in the mouth and allow the client to concentrate on swallowing rather than chewing. Liquids are more manageable when thickened. Water provides minimal sensory stimulation, making it difficult for the client to manage water. Milk and citrus juices stimulate production of saliva.

Allow rest period before eating. Position client at 60°–90° angle before, during, and for 1 hour after eating.

Fatigue increases risk of aspiration.

Maintain head in midline with neck slightly flexed.

This position facilitates the passage of food through the pharynx.

Face the client, avoid haste.

Facing the client allows feeder to evaluate the eating process. If the feeder appears hurried, the client may try to eat faster.

Minimize distractions, keep conversation minimal.

The client's attention must focus only on eating.

Allow Mr. Jason to see and smell food. Give verbal descriptions. Use regular metal teaspoon, give one-half teaspoon at a time.

Sensory cues promote awareness of eating.

Place food on unaffected side of mouth. Teach to hold food in mouth, think about swallowing, and then swallow twice.

Buccal pocketing of food in the cheek on the affected side is common after a stroke.

continued

Nursing Diagnosis 3 *Self-Esteem, Situational Low, related to changes in functional abilities as evidenced by verbal expression of discouragement*

PLANNING/GOALS	NURSING INTERVENTIONS	RATIONALE	EVALUATION
Mr. Jason will verbalize acceptance of self, situation, and lifestyle changes.	Assess for signs of severe or prolonged grieving.	The client needs to grieve the loss of his former self. Prolonged grieving may indicate need for counseling.	Mr. Jason is progressing through all rehabilitation therapies and presents no signs of prolonged grieving.
	Assess client's interactions with significant others.	Other people may be reinforcing the concepts of helplessness and invalidism.	
	Listen in nonjudgmental fashion to comments about situation.	Each person responds differently to a crisis. Being nonjudgmental builds trust and encourages verbalization of thoughts.	

CASE STUDY

Mrs. Emma James, 72 years old, was admitted to Community Hospital for a left below knee amputation. Mrs. James has been an insulin dependent diabetic for 35 years. The amputation follows a long and unsuccessful period of treatment for venous stasis ulcers. Mrs. James was transferred from the hospital to a rehabilitation hospital on her fourth postoperative day. After 2 weeks at the rehabilitation hospital, she was transferred to a skilled care facility near her home for additional rehabilitation and regulation of the diabetes. She is now ready to be discharged to her home. Mrs. James has a prosthesis and is able to ambulate with a walker. She can perform her ADL with minimal assistance. She was on a sliding scale and blood glucose monitoring 4 times a day while in the long-term care facility. Her physician has now placed her on insulin twice a day with daily blood glucose checks. Her vision is somewhat impaired due to the diabetes. Mrs. James lives alone in a one-story home in a safe residential area. The discharge planner at the skilled care facility has arranged continuing care for Mrs. James through a local home health agency.

The following questions will guide your development of a nursing care plan for the case study.

1. Identify the assessment factors that are most important in planning Mrs. James's care.
2. List the nursing diagnoses that would be applicable to Mrs. James's assessment.
3. Describe the complications for which Mrs. James is at risk.
4. Describe nursing interventions for preventing the complications.
5. What specific actions would you take to prevent a recurrence of venous stasis ulcers?
6. What additional community services does Mrs. James need?
7. What nursing services (frequency of nurse visits, services from a nursing assistant, other home health services) would you plan to meet her needs? Which services would each person provide?
8. Describe the outcomes you would expect for Mrs. James.

SUMMARY

- There has been a significant increase in the growth of nonacute care settings.
- Medicaid (state and federal funds) and Medicare (federal funds) are major sources of health care payment, especially for the elderly and permanently disabled. The availability of these resources in the future is in jeopardy. Alternative funding sources are being explored by state and federal governments.
- Rehabilitation can be provided in a variety of settings.
- There is a need for the services and skills of the LP/VN in all of these health care services. Experience and additional education may be required for employment in special care settings.

Review Questions

1. One reason for the growth in nonacute care health services is:

   a. the diminishing supply of physicians.
   b. an increase in the number of hospitals in the country.
   c. the cost of acute care.
   d. the increase in Medicare reimbursement.

2. Medicare is a reimbursement system for health care providers that:

   a. is based upon the client's personal financial resources.
   b. is available to persons 65 years of age and over or who have been disabled for 2 or more years.
   c. pays the full cost of all medical care.
   d. is managed by each state.

3. Subacute care is most often provided:

   a. in a step-down unit of the hospital.
   b. in a special care unit of a skilled care facility.
   c. for clients who are terminally ill.
   d. for clients who require life support.

4. Which of the following clients would be most likely to benefit from rehabilitation services?

   a. Mr. J, 64 years old, had a stroke, is responsive and stable.
   b. Mrs. B, 89 years old, has Alzheimer's disease in the fourth stage.
   c. Miss Z, 26 years old, is recovering from pneumonia.
   d. Mr. K, 56 years old, has terminal cancer of the lung.

5. Which of the following is a legal requirement for health care facilities that is controlled by each state?

   a. Accreditation
   b. Certification
   c. Licensure
   d. Provision of free care

6. As a member of the interdisciplinary health care team, the LP/VN must be able to:

   a. participate in the planning of client care.
   b. plan the appropriate diet for clients.
   c. teach the new amputee how to walk with a prosthesis.
   d. provide alternative methods of communication for the client with recent stroke.

7. In the home health care setting, it is essential that the LP/VN possess skills in:

   a. advanced intravenous therapy.
   b. respiratory therapy treatments.
   c. physical assessment.
   d. planning and providing speech therapy.

8. In a long-term care facility, the LP/VN may serve as the:

   a. charge nurse of a unit.
   b. director of nursing.
   c. clinical nurse specialist.
   d. social worker.

Critical Thinking Question

1. What are the pros and cons related to working for a home health agency or a long-term care facility?

WEB FLASH!

Search the Internet for the various types of health care discussed in this chapter. What information is available? Is it focused for consumer or provider?

UNIT
15
Leadership/Work Transition

Chapter 57
Leadership/Work Transition

LEADERSHIP/ WORK TRANSITION

MAKING THE CONNECTION

Refer to the following chapters to increase your understanding of leadership/work transition:

- **Chapter 5, The Health Care Delivery System**
- **Chapter 6, Legal Responsibilities**
- **Chapter 8, Communication**
- **Chapter 10, Documentation**

LEARNING OBJECTIVES

Upon completion of this chapter, you should be able to:

- *Define key terms.*
- *Outline the skills needed for effective management.*
- *Summarize the five rights of delegation.*
- *Explain factors that must be assessed in establishing priorities of care.*
- *Compare and contrast the roles of the registered nurse, licensed practical/vocational nurse, and unlicensed assistive personnel.*
- *Describe the content and format of résumés.*
- *Outline actions to take prior to a job interview.*

KEY TERMS

accountability	laissez-faire
assignment	leadership
autocratic	management
competency	policy
delegation	procedure
democratic	résumé
job description	

INTRODUCTION

By now you may have mastered the nursing process and demonstrated competency in many of the technical skills you will be required to perform on a daily basis. There are still other skills you will need in order to become competent in practice, however. These are the leadership skills that will allow you to manage yourself and others, delegate and prioritize

tasks, and resolve conflicts and problems that may arise in the workplace. As a new graduate, you will not be expected to have yet mastered these skills; rather, they will develop as you progress in your career.

This chapter introduces these leadership skills as well as provides insight into the working environment. It explores the general organizational structure of the health care setting, defines nurses' roles within the health care system, and explores career options. The chapter walks you through the period from graduation to your first day on the job. Included are discussions of the examination process for licensure, preparations for a job search and interview, and continuing education.

LEADERSHIP

Leadership is the ability to direct or motivate others to achieve goals. Many personal qualities are associated with leaders, such as self-direction, flexibility, and assertiveness. Leaders are considered critical thinkers, responsible decision makers, and role models. Often, leaders are considered to possess a vision that directs a group and elicits the group's best efforts (Figure 57-1). Nursing leaders critically examine the way nursing care is delivered and use their power to effect change.

Leadership Styles

Several leadership styles are recognized. The style varies with the personality of the leader. Most often, a leader exhibits some characteristics of each style of leadership, though one style will typically be more dominant. Not all leadership styles are effective in all situations. Three recognized styles of leadership are autocratic, democratic, and laissez-faire.

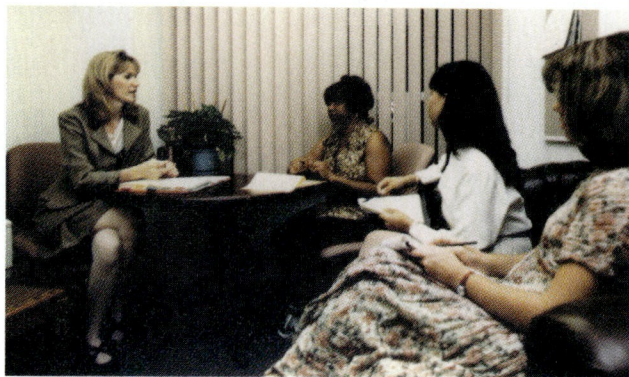

Figure 57-1 Leaders are often effective in unifying and directing groups.

Autocratic

Autocratic leadership is task-oriented and is based on the premise that the leader knows best. This leader is often viewed as controlling and inhibiting of the creativity and autonomy of workers. The leader problem solves and makes decisions without consulting the parties involved. All information is directed downward from leader to workers. The leader exercises responsibility for ensuring the work is done by issuing commands or orders to direct the work force. This leadership form is especially effective in crisis situations or situations requiring a quick response, or when leading a group with limited knowledge. When workers have a certain degree of knowledge, and teamwork is important, this style of leadership is not effective.

Democratic

The underlying belief of the **democratic** style of leadership is that every member of the team should have input (Figure 57-2). Although democratic leadership can be time consuming, the benefit is seen in increased cooperation and teamwork. Individual workers are encouraged to participate in decision making and to express their viewpoints. The leader acts more as a resource person and facilitator. This approach is less ef-

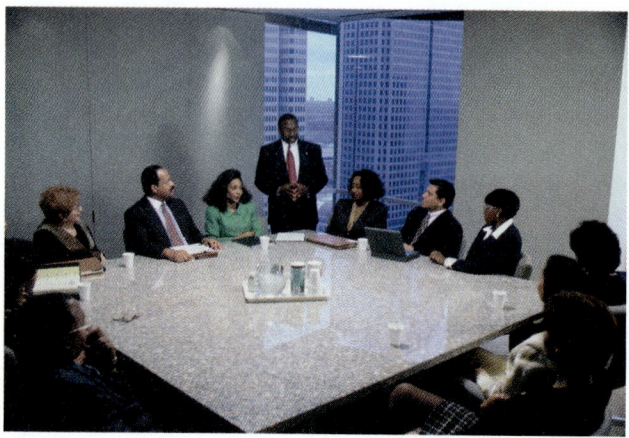

Figure 57-2 A democratic leader asks for input from the team during a brainstorming session. *(Courtesy of Photodisc)*

fective when there is conflict within the group or when time is short.

Laissez-Faire

The **laissez-faire** leadership style is a passive, nondirect approach that gives leadership responsibilities to the group rather than to one person. This style promotes optimal autonomy and creativity in group members. Task achievement is more difficult under this leadership form, so it is not a style of leadership used frequently in health care. The leader is almost unidentifiable, relying on the group's strengths and initiative to accomplish tasks.

Leadership Skills

Many theories of leadership cite several skills needed for effective leadership. These skills include communication, problem solving, self-evaluation, and management.

Communication

Strong communication skills foster trusting relationships with peers, subordinates, superiors, and clients, thus facilitating the leader's ability to motivate others. Additionally, leaders must be able to convey ideas and information clearly, concisely, and persuasively for the leader to effectively implement changes in the delivery of nursing care.

Problem Solving

Problem solving skills incorporate the ability to analyze all aspects of a problem, explore options, find solutions, and implement changes. Problem solving is a careful, deliberate process. Leaders seek information, consult experts, and use available resources to address problematic situations and enhance care.

Self-Evaluation

The self-evaluation skills necessary for effective leadership involve an honest assessment of personal strengths and weaknesses. Following such an assessment, efforts are made to enhance personal growth and development. An unwillingness to critically examine oneself hampers the leader's ability to critically examine, problem solve, and effect change in the workplace.

Management

Management skills involve the accomplishment of tasks either by doing them oneself or directing others to do them. Licensed practical/vocational nurses (LP/VNs) are in positions that require them to manage people and resources used to delivery quality client care.

MANAGEMENT

Management and leadership are closely related concepts. **Management** is the accomplishment of tasks through the effective use of people and resources. Management involves the practical, "nuts and bolts" of getting the job done with the available resources.

Every nurse is a manager. Managing the needs of a group of clients or managing the activities of a group of nursing assistants requires the same skills. Practice and education can help develop the management skills and, potentially, the leadership skills of every nurse.

As managers, LP/VNs are expected to plan, organize, supervise, and monitor the care that is provided to a group of clients. The actual care may be accomplished by the nurse or by others, typically certified nurse assistants (CNAs) or some other type of unlicensed assistive personnel (UAP). Each aspect of management encompasses several components.

- *Planning:* identifying tasks to be accomplished, determining available resources, assessing skill level of workers, identifying problems, and setting priorities
- *Organizing:* making client assignments, ensuring availability of resources, sharing pertinent information, and determining time tables (e.g., of breaks, lunch, completion of certain tasks)
- *Supervising:* directing care provided by others, investigating problems, communicating information, reallocating people and resources as needed, and educating staff as needed
- *Monitoring:* determining whether tasks have been accomplished, assessing need for further action, and ensuring that appropriate documentation is completed

TASK ASSIGNMENT

An array of activities is involved in caring for clients, and all personnel have specific tasks they can facilitate. The ability of a specific staff member to perform a specific task is based on level of education and experience. However, overlap exists, and determining who can legally do what is often confusing.

Tasks of the LP/VN

Registered nurses (RNs) and LP/VNs are individually licensed. Although some overlap exists in the scopes of practice of the LP/VN and the RN, there are also some significant differences. Licensed practical/vocational nurses are dependent practitioners, meaning that an RN, doctor, dentist, or some other health care provider must supervise them. Most often the supervisor is an RN.

In addition to a scope of practice, LP/VNs and RNs have given scopes of competence. Within the scope of practice, there are tasks and responsibilities the individual may or may not be competent to implement. For example, it is within the scope of practice for the LP/VN to perform phlebotomy, but this task does not fall within the scope of competence of every LP/VN.

LP/VN Services

Any time nursing services are provided by an LP/VN, the supervising RN must be on the premises or immediately available by telephone. Being available by an answering machine or service does not fall within the definition of "immediately available." The amount of supervision is a function of the setting. In home health care or long-term care settings, it is common practice for the supervising RN to be available by telephone rather than on the premises.

The scope of competence expands as new skills are acquired, but all skills must fall within the scope of practice.

Licensed practical/vocational nurses are qualified to care for clients with common illnesses and to provide basic and preventive nursing procedures. Licensed practical/vocational nurses can participate in data collection, planning, implementation, and evaluation of nursing care in all settings. In most states, some specific activities are considered beyond the scope of practice of the LP/VN. These activities, with some variances by state, include the following:

- Client assessments (can collect data but not perform physical assessments)
- Independent development of the nursing care plan
- Triage, case management, or mental health counseling
- Intravenous chemotherapy
- Administration of blood and blood products
- Administration of initial doses of any intravenous medication
- Any procedures involving central lines

Tasks of the UAP

Nursing UAP do not have a scope of practice. A task that falls within the protected scope of practice of any licensed profession (including registered nursing and licensed practical/vocational nursing) *cannot* be performed by a UAP. These personnel can perform only those health-related activities for which they have been determined competent to perform. These activities include the following:

- Activities of daily living (feeding, grooming, toileting, ambulating, dressing)
- Vital signs (Figure 57-3)
- Venipuncture
- Glucometer use
- Mouth care and oral suctioning
- Care of hair, skin, and nails

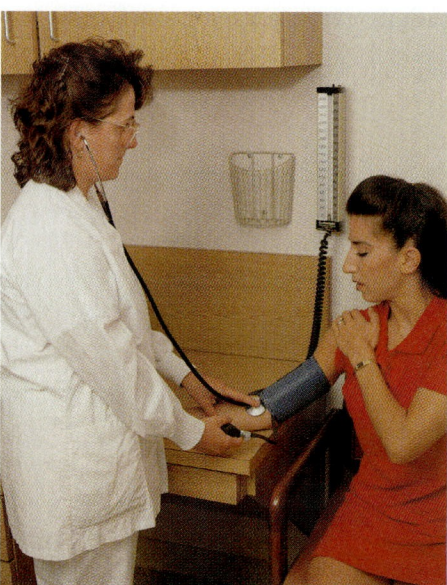

Figure 57-3 Unlicensed assistive personnel (UAP) can assist in many tasks, including measuring vital signs.

- Electrocardiogram measurements
- Applying clean dressings without assessment
- Non-nursing functions (clerical work, transport, cleaning)

DUTY DELEGATION

Delegation is the process of transferring to a competent individual the authority to perform a select task in a select situation. State provisions for the delegation of nursing tasks vary. Some states allow for the delegation of nursing tasks by an RN to both LP/VNs and UAP. In some states, LP/VNs may delegate certain nursing tasks to other LP/VNs or to UAP. Other states restrict delegation to licensed personnel only.

The licensed nurse retains accountability for the delegation. **Accountability** is defined as responsibility for actions and inactions performed by oneself or others. **Assignment**, another term frequently used to describe the transfer of activities from one person to another, involves the downward or lateral transfer of both responsibility and accountability for an activity.

At least one state differentiates between delegating nursing tasks to licensed nurses and assigning tasks to UAP. In New York, a nurse is not legally responsible for the process or outcome of care delegated to another licensed nurse. The nurse does remain responsible for tasks assigned to UAP, however. As an LP/VN, you are responsible for the decisions you make to delegate or assign tasks. Your knowledge of the client, activity, and worker will help you make sound decisions.

In most settings, RNs decide which nursing activities can be delegated or assigned to other licensed nurses (RNs or LP/VNs) and to UAP. Registered nurses and LP/VNs must consider five factors when making the decision to delegate or assign duties:

- *The potential for harm.* Certain nursing activities carry a risk for harming the client. Generally, the more invasive a procedure, the greater the potential for harm. Additionally, some activities carry a greater risk for certain kinds of clients (e.g., cutting the toenails of a diabetic). The greater the potential for harm, the greater the need for a licensed nurse to perform the activity.
- *The complexity of the task.* The cognitive skills and psychomotor skills needed for different nursing tasks vary considerably. As the skills increase in complexity, the level of education and competence becomes more critical. Some activities require a level of nursing assessment and judgment that can be provided only by a licensed professional.
- *The required problem solving and innovation.* As care is delivered, problems may develop. A successful outcome for the client may depend on a complex analysis of the problem and an individualized problem-solving approach. Alternatively, a simple activity may require special adaptation because of the client's condition. As problem solving increases in complexity and the need for innovation grows, so does the likelihood that a licensed nurse should provide the care.
- *The unpredictability of the outcome.* A client's response to an activity may be very predictable. If the client is unstable or the activity is new for the client, however, client response may be unpredictable and unknown. As unpredictability increases, so does the need for a licensed nurse.
- *The required coordination and consistency of the client's care.* Effective planning, coordination, and evaluation of client care requires the nurse to have direct client contact. The more stable the client and the more common the medical diagnosis, the more the care that can generally be delegated to support personnel. The need for a licensed nurse increases as the required coordination needed to delivery quality care increases.

The five rights of delegation provide further direction in making appropriate decisions about delegation. They are as follows:

- *Right Task:* The nurse must determine whether the task is delegable for a specific client.
- *Right Circumstance:* Factors to consider include the client setting, availability of resources, client's condition, and other factors.
- *Right Person:* The nurse must ask the question, "Is the right person delegating the right task to the right person to be performed on the right client?"
- *Right Direction/Communication:* A clear, concise description of the task should be conveyed, including all expectations for accomplishing the task.
- *Right Supervision:* Appropriate monitoring, implementation, evaluation, and feedback must be provided.

Registered nurses are frequently responsible for delegating care and assigning clients to the other nursing staff. In some settings, however, LP/VNs make these decisions. Licensed practical/vocational nurses should use the same guidelines to make decisions regarding delegating an activity to another LP/VN or assigning the task to UAP.

CARE PRIORITIZATION

Establishing priorities requires an understanding of the importance of different problems to the nurse, the client, the family, and other health care providers. For example, a client may be impatient to bathe because family is scheduled to visit. The nurse, however, does not want to remove the client's dressing for a bath until the physician has been able to examine the wound. Providing quality care while balancing such competing demands and ensuring completion of all tasks can be challenging.

Information obtained during the change-of-shift report is needed to appropriately establish priorities. This information can be useful in creating a worksheet identifying a list of tasks and target times for accomplishing these tasks. The time allotted for activities varies based on the condition of the client, the availability of support personnel, the availability of supplies, and a number of other factors. The effective use of time is important whether caring for one client, caring for a group of clients, or supervising the activities of others providing care.

While it is useful to get an overview of the day's activities, the clinical setting can change quickly and frequently. This is especially true in acute care settings. The nurse must be flexible and continually evaluate and reorder the priorities of care.

Given the same assignment, nurses will not necessarily establish the priorities of care in exactly the same way. If working closely with an RN, you should determine the priorities as she views them. When supervising UAP, you must be clear about your priorities and expectations. Among the factors that can be examined when establishing priorities are the following:

- *Safety:* You should ascertain whether a safety situation must be addressed immediately. A client experiencing a cardiac arrest, a fall, an insulin reaction, and other situations presenting an imminent threat must be tended to first.
- *Timing:* Medications, tests, and vital signs are frequently ordered at specific times. Often, there is very little flexibility in shifting the times. In hospitals, medications, for example, must be given within a specified time frame, usually ½ hour before or after the established time.
- *Interdependence of events:* You must ascertain whether some activity must occur before another

activity can take place. For example, a fasting blood sugar must be completed before the client receives either insulin or food; blood to ascertain the peak level of gentamyacin is drawn a specified time after the medication is given.

- *Client requests:* Quality care depends on meeting client needs. Some events—showers, bed changings, enema administration, and so on—can be scheduled after consulting with the client regarding personal preferences.
- *Availability of help:* If two people are needed to turn a client, ambulate a client, or provide other care, coordination of the health care team is essential for effective utilization of time. Ascertain which activities require assistance, then consult with coworkers about their availability.
- *Client's status:* Clients vary in the extent to which they can participate in their care. This factor influences the order of executing tasks and the length of time a task takes. A semi-independent client can be performing a task (e.g., bathing) with minimal assistance while the nurse attends to some other need.
- *Availability of resources:* If six clients are supposed to get out of bed and sit in chairs, and only two chairs are available, the clients clearly cannot get out of bed at the same time. Geri-chairs, wheelchairs, and other equipment are sometimes limited. Additionally, tasks may need to be delayed because supplies must be obtained from central supply.

Effectively organizing and establishing priorities with regard to care takes practice. Obtaining answers to certain questions when looking back at the day's events can help you hone this skill: Did you lack information that would have helped you prioritize more effectively? Did you fail to or inaccurately consider the client's status, the availability of help, or other factors? Did you establish priorities and set a schedule without getting client input? Did you fail to coordinate with coworkers? You must learn from experience. Both client and nurse feel the positive benefits of a day that flowed smoothly.

WORKPLACE TRANSITION

A successful employment experience depends on more than nursing knowledge and technical competence. Success requires competence in the particular job position. Success also depends on the nurse's integration into the health care team and the nurse's understanding of the overall health care organization.

The Nursing Team

Within the nursing staff are different team members. Nursing staff includes nursing UAP, CNAs, LP/VNs, RNs, and nurse practitioners (NPs). The roles, levels of education, skills, levels of independence, and lengths

Workplace Hierarchy

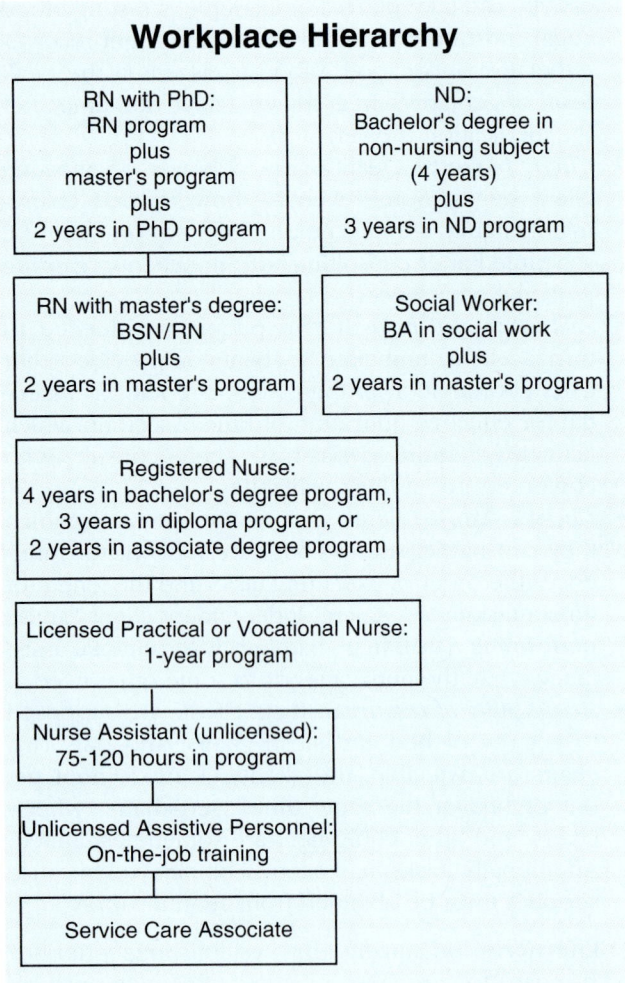

Figure 57-4 Workplace Hierarchy

of education vary considerably (Figure 57-4). Familiarizing yourself with the roles of other nursing staff will help ensure that your practice conforms to the scope of practice as outlined by law.

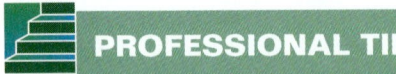

PROFESSIONAL TIP

Hierarchy

As defined in the Nursing Practice Acts, or in the state nursing board's rules and regulations, an LP/VN works under the direction of an RN, physician, or dentist. These are the professionals who will directly supervise your work. In some states, the language of the law indicates that "other health care providers" can supervise you. The question is, Who are the other health care providers? In your state, must you follow orders written by a physician's assistant? A nurse practitioner? A physical therapist? The answers vary by state. It is critical that you know who can direct your nursing activities.

Nursing UAP can have a number of different titles including UAP, patient care technician, clinical technician, and nursing assistant. These persons provide hands-on care to clients in addition to performing other duties. None of these personnel has a license to practice. Rather, training is provided by the employer and may last from 2 to 10 weeks. The tasks they are expected to perform are designated by the employer and typically include things such as phlebotomy, electrocardiogram measurement, intake and output reading, bed making, and assisting clients with activities of daily living.

A CNA is also unlicensed. In contrast to other UAP, however, the curriculum and length of training to become a CNA are prescribed. As a part of health care reforms in the long-term care setting, the primary employment setting of CNAs, a set curriculum of 100 hours duration must be completed to be certified.

Licensed practical/vocational nurses work very closely with registered nurses. The LP/VN attends a 1-year program and must pass the National Council Licensure Examination for Practical Nurses (NCLEX-PN). The RN is educated in a 3-year hospital-diploma program, a 2-year college associate-degree program, or a 4-year college baccalaureate program and must pass the National Council Licensure Examination for Registered Nurses (NCLEX-RN).

An NP is an RN who has obtained additional education (usually a master's degree) and is certified by the state. The role of the NP typically includes diagnosis and treatment of commonly occurring medical conditions. Outpatient clinics frequently employ NPs. Increasingly, they are also found working in hospitals, long-term care facilities, and rehabilitation centers.

Job Expectations and Responsibilities

Employees are hired to work at a specific site, for example, the fifth floor of the hospital or the internal medicine clinic at the outpatient health facility. The employer's expectations are summarized in job descriptions and in the policy and procedure manual. Although reading these papers is often viewed as bor-

PROFESSIONAL TIP

Unlicensed Personnel

Much controversy surrounds the role of UAP. Concerns have been raised that unlicensed personnel are functioning as de facto licensed nurses in violation of Nursing Practice Acts. Further, serious questions exist about the cost savings and quality of care in light of increased reliance on UAP and a corresponding reduction in licensed nurses. Understanding the role and limitations of UAP is critical.

ing and a waste of time, successful employment depends on understanding job expectations and the employer's policies.

Job Descriptions

A **job description** is a written outline of job responsibilities. Job responsibilities vary from employer to employer. For example, in long-term care facilities, LP/VNs are not routinely expected to bathe clients, as this task is performed by CNAs. In a hospital setting, however, job responsibilities of an LP/VN may include bathing clients. All the job expectations should fall within the scope of practice of the LP/VN.

In addition to summarizing job responsibilities, a job description frequently outlines requirements for the position (e.g., LP/VN, experience preferred), supervisor's title, supervisory responsibilities, and frequency and/or method of evaluation. A job description may also include a list of **competencies**, the specific skills or tasks (e.g., blood glucose monitoring) needed for a particular position. Employers are expected to assess competencies at the time of employment and periodically thereafter, usually annually.

A clear understanding of one's own job description is critical to the safe, effective practice of nursing in the specific employment setting. Failure to meet the job responsibilities as outlined in the job description can result in termination of employment. Familiarity with the job descriptions of supervisors and of persons who you may supervise is also very helpful in ensuring that you have a clear understanding of your role and those things you can expect of others.

Policies and Procedures

The employer's policies and procedures manual is also a very important reference document.

An employer's **policies** are written descriptions of the employer's expectations for handling various situations. Policies often are applicable to everyone working in the facility, rather than being nursing specific. Policies addressing confidentiality, dissemination of client information, handling of suspected cases of abuse, management of client valuables, and so on are common. A review of the policies and procedures manual is often required at the start of employment. A periodic self-initiated review of the manual is useful in ensuring that work performance meets the employer's expectations.

Procedures are step-by-step instructions describing the processes for performing various nursing tasks. Although these nursing procedures will likely already be familiar to you, it is important that you perform tasks as directed by your employer. There are usually several correct, safe methods for performing a procedure; the way you were taught in school may vary from your employer's procedure. This may require altering the way you perform certain procedures

Organizational Chart

An organizational chart is a visual representation of the relationships of one department to another within the facility and/or the relationship of the facility to other facilities in a health care network. Frequently included in the organizational chart are the names and/or titles of department leaders and the lines of authority. This information provides an understanding of the way your department fits into the larger organization.

All employees within a health care facility are part of a large organization. Every organization has a unique organizational culture of commonly held values, beliefs, and expectations directing the work force in the provision of services. For example, the organizational culture of a for-profit freestanding kidney dialysis center will be different from that of a free health clinic. Insights into the organizational culture of any health care facility can be garnered from the organization statement summarizing the facility's mission, vision, values, and goals. Although such statements often seem theoretical and far removed from job responsibilities, they do guide the organization in its provision of services.

FROM STUDENT TO EMPLOYEE

You have completed the licensed practical/vocational nursing educational program (Figure 57-5). Through formal education and clinical supervision, you have studied and learned the skills necessary to become competent in providing client care. Now you are ready to graduate and begin your career as a nurse.

Your first task as a graduate practical nurse is to take and pass the NCLEX-PN examination and obtain your nursing license. After you have obtained your license, you can begin the search for a job. The effort required in the period of time between the job search

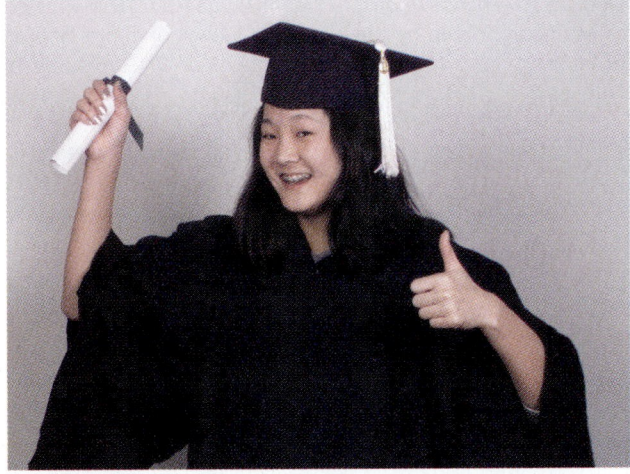

Figure 57-5 Congratulations! You have successfully completed your program.

and employment can be considered a job in and of it-self. There are many tasks to complete and skills to master to land your first job as an LP/VN.

STATE BOARD EXAMINATION AND LICENSURE

In some states, you can begin work as a graduate LP/VN. A graduate LP/VN has completed the educational requirements and either is waiting to take the NCLEX-PN or to receive test results and a license. Check with your state board of nursing to learn both the requirements for a temporary license to practice nursing as a graduate LP/VN and any restrictions put on your practice while working under this status. Figure 57-6 shows the states that allow graduates to apply for temporary permits. For most students, however, the time after graduation is used to prepare for the state board exams.

The NCLEX-PN

The examination that all practical nurses must pass in order to be licensed is the NCLEX-PN. The NCLEX tests the skills and knowledge required for entry-level practice. The state boards use the results of this examination to determine whether a license will be issued to the graduate. Figure 57-7 lists the steps each graduate must follow in order to take the examination. The NCLEX tests knowledge of client needs such as physiologic and psychological needs, safety, and health promotion, as well as the nursing process, including data collection, planning, and implementation. The test is administered via a computer using a method called computerized adaptive testing (CAT), wherein the computer selects the test questions as you take the examination. You must answer all of the questions as they are presented to you, and you may not skip questions. All of the questions are multiple choice in format. All LP/VN candidates answer a minimum of 85 questions and a maximum of 205 questions during the maximum 5-hour testing period (National Council State Boards of Nursing, 1997a). The results are mailed to the candidate by the state board 1 month or less after the examination. Candidates may retake the examination, however, the National Council requires a wait of at least 91 days between testings. Your state board may have other policies related to retaking the exam.

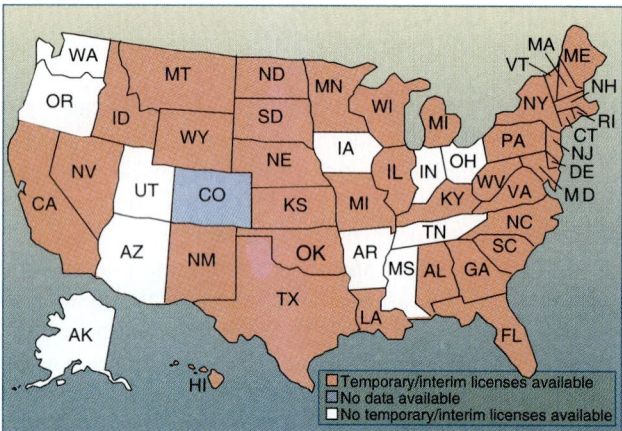

Figure 57-6 States Where You Can Apply for a Temporary License To Practice upon Graduation (*Data from* 1996 Profiles of Member Boards by the National Council of State Boards of Nursing, Inc., *1997, National Council of State Boards of Nursing.*)

PROFESSIONAL TIP

Temporary Permits

Although it is possible to work during the interim period between NCLEX-PN testing and licensure, most employers will postpone hiring until after you have received your permanent nursing license. Therefore, do not be discouraged if you are unable to obtain employment as a graduate LP/VN during this period.

1. Apply to the board of nursing for a license, following instructions from that board.

2. Candidate gets an *NCLEX® Examination Candidate Bulletin* from the board of nursing.

3. Candidate submits a registration form to The Chauncey Group (the National Council's contracted testing service) or registers by phone. The Chauncey Group will acknowledge the candidate's registration my mail.

Note: Candidates seeking licensure from Illinois and Massachusetts do not register directly with The Chauncey Group. Follow registration instructions provided by those boards of nursing.

4. The board of nursing will communicate the candidate's eligibility to test to The Chauncey Group.

5. The Chauncey Group will send the candidate an Authorization To Test (ATT) with a booklet called *Scheduling and Taking your NCLEX® Examination* and a list of test centers.

6. The candidate will call a Sylvan test center and schedule an appointment to test.

7. On the appointed day, the candidate will take the test at a Sylvan Technology Center.

8. Sylvan transmits the test results to The Chauncey Group. After verifying the accuracy of the results, The Chauncey Group transmits them to the designated board of nursing.

9. The board of nursing sends results to the candidate.

Figure 57-7 NCLEX Examination Testing Process (*Reprinted courtesy of the National Council of State Boards of Nursing, Inc.*)

Your License

After you have successfully passed the NCLEX, you will be issued your nursing license from your state board. It is your responsibility to maintain your license according to your state's standards and inform your state board of any changes in name, address, and employment. Once licensed, you are ready to practice.

EMPLOYMENT OPPORTUNITIES

A wide variety of employment opportunities exist for the LP/VN. These range from employment in the traditional settings of hospital and nursing home to that in less traditional settings such as correctional facilities and hospice care. In 1996, 32% of LP/VNs worked in hospitals, 27% worked in nursing homes, and 13% worked in doctor's offices and clinics (Bureau of Labor Statistics, 1998). Although the majority of LP/VNs are still employed in traditional settings, increasing opportunities are arising in the nontraditional settings because of changes in health care delivery. An overview of the various employment settings for the LP/VN follows. As a graduate, it is your task to determine the setting that constitutes the best fit for you.

Hospitals

Although the majority of LP/VNs are still working in the hospital setting, it is projected that the number of jobs for LP/VNs in hospitals will decline through the year 2006 (Bureau of Labor Statistics, 1998). Therefore, LP/VNs seeking to enter this setting will meet more competition than in the past. Employment opportunities outside of the client care unit, such as in hospital-based clinics, outpatient care units, and hospital-based long-term care units, are where most LP/VNs will typically find work in the hospital setting.

Long-Term Care Facilities/ Rehabilitation Centers

Employment for LP/VNs in long-term care and rehabilitation settings is projected to grow faster than average through the year 2006 (Bureau of Labor Statistics, 1998). Long-term care will offer the greatest number of new jobs for LP/VNs, due to the growing elderly population. Nurses in this setting will also provide care to clients who have been released by the hospital but who are not yet well enough to go home and who need additional rehabilitative services (Figure 57-8).

Community Health Agencies

In the community health setting, care is provided to clients through established health care programs. These programs are generally funded by local, state, or federal government or by voluntary agencies. Nurses in this setting will generally work in a community clinic or will travel to clients' homes to provide care and education.

Private Duty

Private duty nurses are self-employed, meaning the nurse is hired and paid directly by the client. The nurse works under the direction of a physician but must rely on knowledge and judgment to provide care. Private duty nurses are responsible for handling all matters of licensing and finances on their own.

Home Care Agencies

In the home care setting, care is provided to clients in their own homes. The nurse is generally employed by an agency but will work in the home of an assigned client. This area of nursing is rapidly expanding, due to both a consumer demand for home care and the lowered costs of caring for an individual in the home (Figure 57-9).

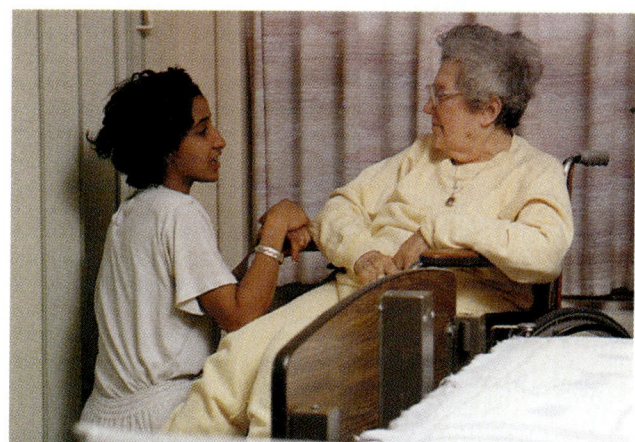

Figure 57-8 Care of elders in long-term care facilities is a growing career opportunity for the LP/VN.

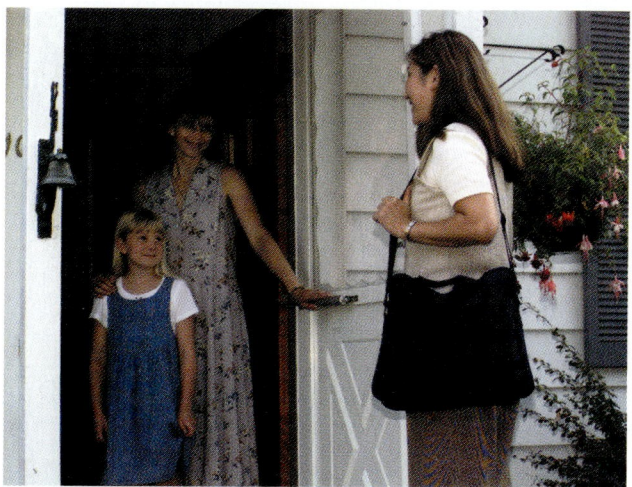

Figure 57-9 Nurses working in home health care agencies must be able to travel to the client's home to provide care.

Hospice

Hospice nursing care consists of providing comfort to dying clients and their families. The role of the nurse is to alleviate pain and other symptoms but not to provide curative care. The clients in the hospice setting are terminally ill and typically have fewer than 6 months to live. Hospice services are most often rendered in the home, but services can also be offered in other settings.

Occupational Health

Occupational health nursing serves to provide safe working environments in industrial workplaces. Occupational health nurses work within industries and corporations and collaborate with corporate administration to provide health education and promotion to employees in the workplace.

Correctional Facilities

Correctional nursing is the branch of nursing that provides care within prisons, youth detention centers, and probation divisions. Care provided ranges from ambulatory care to emergent care to comprehensive health care.

School

School nursing focuses on providing care to the school-age child. The school nurse serves to promote wellness and identify or prevent problems. Both public and private schools offer opportunities for school nursing.

Parish

Parish nurses provide health care education and support to a congregation. The care is designed to meet the common needs and beliefs of a specified group of people.

Insurance Companies

Nurses working in the insurance setting are often responsible for coding treatments, providing physical examinations for insurance policies, and reviewing medical records.

PREPARING FOR THE JOB HUNT

Job hunting for many people is synonymous with scanning the Sunday want ads. This is not necessarily a bad place to identify potential employers; after all, given that the employer is advertising, they probably are hiring. The problem with relying solely on this approach is it limits you to the jobs that are available rather than the job you want. Many job openings do not get advertised in the newspaper. Job vacancies exist well before they get advertised. Remember, using this method, you are in competition with all the other job seekers who are relying on want ads to identify employment options.

Other options exist for identifying potential employers. The telephone directory is a great place to identify health care facilities in your area. You are likely to find far more health care facilities in your local area than you ever imagined. All these facilities represent potential employers. Job counselors disagree on the usefulness of telephoning the employers to determine whether job vacancies exist: Some claim that a telephone call is a quick method of determining vacancies, whereas others believe a face-to-face visit to the facility yields better results.

A job club, perhaps formed with your nursing school classmates, is often an effective method of sharing information about employers, vacancies, job requirements, and the like. Additionally, a job club can be a morale booster, if landing that job is somewhat elusive. Your colleagues in the club may also offer insights into those areas of nursing to which they believe you are most suited.

After you have identified potential employers, be persistent in your job hunt. Most importantly, go after that job that looks interesting to you regardless of whether they have a known vacancy. But don't stop there. Apply at many different organizations. Apply not just at different facilities, but at many facilities. Concentrate on small employers. Every health care job seeker has heard about the local large medical center. However, right around the corner from your home may be the less well-known school for developmentally disadvantaged children and waiting there may be your ideal job!

Potential employers can be identified in several other ways. Nursing journals typically advertise positions. Sometimes, your instructors know of positions. The state or local employment office may offer assistance. Professional job placement services are also available. Increasingly, the Internet advertises job openings along with job-hunting information and tips. A little initiative in accessing such resources can prove an immeasurable help in finding the job you want, rather than just any job.

You graduated, passed the NCLEX, and were issued a license to practice; now it is time to begin seeking employment. The job search requires up-front preparation on your part to organize and pinpoint the areas where you would like to concentrate your efforts. After graduation, you must take the following steps to secure a job:

1. Identify your objective
2. Prepare a résumé
3. Prepare a cover letter
4. Prepare a list of references
5. Prepare a telephone call script

6. Complete a job application
7. Prepare for the interview
8. Prepare a thank you note

Completing these steps will obtain you the face-to-face meeting (the interview) that will ultimately result in an offer of employment.

Identify Your Objective

A common mistake among job hunters is identifying potential employers as a first step. Most employment counselors advise beginning the job search with *you*. Identify your job target or objective first. If you cannot envision yourself as a medication nurse in a long-term care facility (a very common position for LP/VNs), there is very little reason to apply for such employment in that setting.

Identifying your objective accomplishes two important things. First, once you know your objective, you will know where to focus your efforts in identifying potential employers. Second, you will have a reference point for choosing those things to say about yourself on a résumé or during a job interview. You will be prepared to tell prospective employers precisely the ways that you can be of benefit to them.

If you are having difficulty pinpointing your objective, think back to other jobs or volunteer projects in which you have been involved. What skills did you use? What did you like about the job or project? Make a list of your strongest four to six skills: These are the skills you want to use in your new job and that will be valuable in identifying your objective. Ascertain which jobs call for those skills. The skills needed for a particular job can be identified in a number of ways, including the following:

• Talking to people in nursing positions and asking them what they like and do not like about their jobs. During clinical in nursing school, you may have already talked to nurses and have more information than you realize.
• Reading the job descriptions in the classified ads.
• Calling places that employ LP/VNs and asking them to send you a job description.

Once you have matched your skills to the skills required in a particular job, you have effectively identified your job objective.

Prepare a Résumé

The **résumé** is a job-hunting tool that summarizes your employment qualifications. The content of the résumé should be factual, accurate, and honest. The focus should be on verifiable skills or accomplishments that suggest to the employer those things you can do for them should they hire you. The résumé may be targeted toward a specific job, a specific career field (e.g., licensed practical/vocational nursing), or a specific person. Some employers want a résumé, others rely on job applications, and still others ask for both a résumé and a job application.

Regardless of the format selected, the résumé will include the following information:

• Name, address, phone number, and e-mail, if you have an account
• Objective
• Educational experience including names of schools, dates of attendance, and course of study
• Employment history including employers' names and addresses, dates of employment, and descriptions of work experience.

In the course of developing your résumé, make a list of all your past jobs and then decide which jobs you want to include on the résumé. If you have very little work experience, list all jobs on the résumé. Definitely include jobs that show experience related to your job objective. Include unpaid or volunteer work, if it highlights skills and experience needed for the job you are seeking.

Having significant gaps in your employment history may give the impression that you are an unstable worker. Employment gaps can be explained in a number of ways. If the gap resulted because you were in school, include that information. If you did significant volunteer work during that period, describe those activities. Being a full-time parent or a full-time caregiver to a family member is a respectable activity that sufficiently explains gaps in paid employment.

Similarly, make a list of your training and education. You certainly want to include training and education you have completed. If you have an academic degree, include the college, your major, the degree granted, and the date the degree was awarded.

If you have completed only a portion of training, list the courses that are directly related to your objective. The same applies to college courses you may have taken. It is usually not necessary to mention a high school diploma, unless the position you seek calls for one or you have no other higher education.

The next step in creating a résumé is to select a format. The three most common résumé formats are chronological, functional, and combination. Each format contains the same basic information about you, but organized in different ways. Your background and job objective will determine the format you use.

The chronological format highlights your jobs (Figure 57-10). It arranges your work experience in order by dates of the jobs you have had. The most recent job is usually listed first. The functional format is organized around your work experience and the skills involved. For example, you may have experience in providing respite care for your aunt, who has sole responsibility for her invalid mother. Additionally, you may have done volunteer work providing respite care

Anita Jones, LPN
1234 Pleasant Street
Chicago, Illinois 60000
Telephone: (123) 456-7890

OBJECTIVE: Position as an LPN in long-term care setting

LICENSE NUMBER: State of Illinois #_____

**PROFESSIONAL
EXPERIENCE:**

**1992–present   General Hospital and Medical Center
Chicago, Illinois**

Position: LPN, medication nurse
Provide direct care as a team member on a 36 bed unit.
Distribute and maintain medications. Work in cooperation
with nonlicensed team members. Manage nursing outcomes
using assistive personnel. Received three letters of
commendation for patient care delivery.

1987–1992   City Teaching Medical Center
Chicago, Illinois

Position: LPN, general medical unit
Provided direct patient care on a 25-bed medical unit. Gained
experience caring for geriatric patients. Helped develop unit
procedures for shift rotation. Participated in an average of
12 hours of continuing-education contact hours per year.

EDUCATION: Chicago State University, Chicago, Illinois
Completed 24 credit hours of course work in BSN prerequisites,
focus on physiology and psychology

Highland Community College, Freeport, Illinois
Licensed Practical Nurse, 1987
Class representative to faculty council

**RELATED
EXPERIENCE:**   Lectured 25 preschool students on keeping healthy, repeated
program four times

AFFILIATIONS: Member, NFLPN

REFERENCES: Available upon request

Figure 57-10 Sample Chronological Résumé

for a local hospice, or you may have provided frequent care to your nephew with Down syndrome. These activities could all be listed under one heading that captures the skill of respite care. The résumé style that combines both the chronological and functional format is referred to as the combination format.

Numerous references are available to help you write a résumé. Tips on effective action words, examples of complete résumés, layout options, and other advice on résumé writing can help you create a high-quality résumé. Ask a friend, a teacher, a coworker, a classmate or someone else to give you feedback on your résumé. Even after you have revised your résumé 10 times, you will be amazed at the degree to which you can still refine it.

The appearance of your résumé is as important as the content. After all, your résumé may provide the employer with their first impression of you. The résumé should be concise enough to fit on one page and must be typed in a neat, readable typeface (e.g., Times Roman). Your final résumé must be absolutely free of typographical or grammatical errors, erasures, grease smudges and fingerprints. Good-quality résumé paper should be used: In health care, white paper is preferred, although ivory can also be used. Avoid using pastel papers and fancy script typefaces. Additionally, avoid logos of any kind. You want to convey compe-

tence through a résumé that is professional looking and easy to read.

Prepare a Cover Letter

You should prepare a cover letter to attach to your résumé when applying for a specific position. The letter should be one page in length, refer to the position you are applying for, explain the way you found out about the position, and briefly describe one of your skills that is pertinent to the position. You should also establish a time frame for contacting the prospective employer to follow up on your résumé. Be sure that you do follow up with a call to track the progress of your application. The letter should follow the standard format of a business letter, contain no grammatical or spelling errors, and be on the same quality paper as your résumé. Always use the full name and title of the person to whom you are sending the letter and résumé. You should not use a stock cover letter for all of the positions for which you are applying. The cover letter should always be individualized to the position and the company to which you are applying. Figure 57-11 shows a sample cover letter.

Prepare a List of References

References are people, such as colleagues, instructors, or employers, who can verify and support your professional and educational background claims.

1234 Pleasant Street
Chicago, IL 60000
September 12, 2000

Thomas DiNapoli
Human Resources Manager
St. Anne's Medical Center
P.O. Box 3476
Pittsburgh, PA 15230

Dear Mr. DiNapoli:

I am applying for the position of full-time medication nurse that you advertised in the September 11 *Pittsburgh Press and Post Gazette*. My resume is enclosed.

In the last year I worked with my health care team to establish new procedures and protocols for medication rounds. The procedures have been successfully implemented and I can bring these innovative ideas to your facility.

I would be happy to come in for an interview. I can be reached at (123) 456-7890 and will call you on September 19 to answer any questions you may have.

Sincerely,

Anita Jones, LPN

Enclosure

Figure 57-11 Sample Cover Letter

Through the use of references, prospective employers attempt to verify information you have provided on a job application or your résumé. Employers also use references to gather more information about you. Do not provide references unless the prospective employer requests them. If you must supply references, be sure they are typed and include all pertinent information (name, title, employer, address, and telephone number).

Given the likelihood that a potential employer will ask for references, it is a good idea to always be prepared to provide them. Contact the people you intend to list as references and ask whether they are willing to be references for you. Remember, however, that the willingness of a person to serve as a reference does not guarantee that the information provided will be positive; therefore, ask any prospective references how they may respond to questions that you anticipate from a prospective employer. For example, if the employer asks your nursing school instructor something about your record of tardiness, will the instructor focus on the three times you were late for clinical, or will the instructor comment favorably that you are prompt and efficient in completing your responsibilities?

Choose references who are prepared to comment on the skills you possess and need for the job in question. Provide all references with information about the position for which you applied and the job expectations. This information allows your references to tailor their comments to the demands of the prospective job.

Prepare a Telephone Call Script

A telephone call script outlines the information you want to learn and/or share with prospective employers. Preplanning the telephone call helps you organize the call, ensures that crucial information is learned or given, and generally helps you sound efficient and competent. Consider having several scripts. One script may address a request for information such as job descriptions and vacancies; another may be an introduction about you and an inquiry about the application process; and yet another may focus on the status of your application after you have had an interview. The key is to prepare for any contact with a potential employer, whether it be by phone or in person.

Complete a Job Application

Many employers will simply ask you to complete a job application. The job application should be completed totally and neatly. Most employers balk at job applications that say "see attached résumé" rather than provide the information as requested. Preparation is key. Come with the information you may need to complete an application. Such information typically includes a list of past employers, including addresses, telephone numbers, supervisors' names, and dates of employment. Information about schools you have at-

tended is also generally asked for on a job application. If you are nervous about completing an application "cold," ask the employer to send you a form. Practice completing it at home, so that you are certain you have all the information requested; then the practice application in the trash, and visit the employer to complete the form in person. Figure 57-12 shows a sample job application.

Prepare for the Interview

The interview is a crucial part of the job-search process. An interview is best thought of as an opportunity for you and the interviewer to exchange information. Your task is to convey pertinent information about your skills, abilities, education, and experience. The interviewer's task is to relay information about the particular job and the employer and to evaluate your qualifications. If both parties have fulfilled their responsibilities, appropriate decisions follow. The interviewer decides whether you are the most desirable candidate for the job—and you decide whether you want the job

Application for Employment
(pre-employment questionnaire) (an equal opportunity employer)

Personal Information   Date   September 20, 1999

Name   Anita Jones   Social security number   351-44-5751

Present address   1234 Pleasant Street   Chicago   IL   60000

Permanent address   same

Phone No.   (123) 456-7890   Are you 18 years or older?   yes   no

Are you either a U.S. citizen or an alien authorized to work in the United States?   yes   no

Employment Desired
Position   medication nurse   Date you can start   October 15   Salary desired   open

Are you employed now?   Yes   If so may we inquire of your present employer?   Yes

Ever applied to this company before?   No   where? _____ when? _____

Referred by   Ken Jenkins

Education	Name and location of school attended graduate?	No. of years	Did you	Subjects studied
Grammar school	Cambden Elementary School District #95	8	yes	general curriculum
High school	Cambden High School	4	yes	vocational curriculum, nursing
College	Highland Community College	1	yes	LPN
Trade, business or correspondence school				

Former Employers (list below the last three employers, starting with the last one first)

Date, month and year	Name and address of employer	Salary	Position	Reason for leaving
from June 1992 to present	General Hospital and Medical Center	6.85 hr.	medication nurse	currently employed
from June 1987 to May 1992	City Teaching Medical Center	4.30 hr.	nurse	part-time only

Which of these jobs did you like best?   City Teaching Medical Center
What did you like most about this job?   geriatrics

References: give the names of the three persons not related to you, whom you have known at least one year

Name			
Denise Thompson			1.5
Phylis Hunter			2.0
Frank Hopkins	Highland Community College - Freeport, IL	nursing instructor	1.0

Figure 57-12 Sample Job Application

Preparation is the key to a successful interview. Well before the actual interview, the stage for a meeting is set. You have determined your objective, identified a potential employer, and filled out a job application or provided a resumé. The prospective employer has screened your information and selected you for an interview. But you still have work to do before the actual interview.

Research the Employer

Part of preparing for an interview involves researching the employer. You want to learn everything you can about the employer. Showing such initiative gives the interviewer the impression that you have a sincere interest in employment with the organization. Information you learn may also help you develop questions to ask the employer or anticipate questions that the employer may ask you.

Anticipate Questions

Try to anticipate questions the employer may ask you. For example, if after investigating an outpatient clinic, you learn that electrocardiogram and phlebotomy are performed on site, you can be fairly certain that the employer will ask whether you have performed these skills. Typical questions asked by an employer focus on strengths and weaknesses, interest in the position, past experience, future plans, and potential contributions to the open position.

As a general rule, law forbids the employer to ask personal questions. For instance, questions about child care arrangements, plans to have a family, height, weight, and religion are not allowed. With severe limitations, the employer can ask about age (e.g., "Are you over 18 or under 70?") and disabilities or illnesses (e.g., "Is there anything that would interfere with your performance of the job?").

Be Prepared

Anticipate questions and plan your responses. Examine your resumé again. Reflect on your goals. Assess your skills and knowledge. Decide the information you want to convey to the interviewer. Develop complete but concise answers to anticipated questions. Employers have a limited amount of time for interviews and want you to get to the point as quickly as possible.

Bring your resumé and references, even if you have provided these to the potential employer at a prior time. You want to be certain the interviewer has information about you at hand as you talk.

Be prompt for the interview. An overly early arrival will tend to increase your nervousness; and a late arrival is simply unacceptable. Plan your route to the facility ahead of time. Anticipate traffic delays or parking problems. Allow time to compose yourself before the interview.

During the actual interview you want to make a positive impression. Your physical appearance is probably the first thing the interviewer will notice. Dress conservatively, neatly, and clean. You want to project confidence and competence. Excessive jewelry or make-up, trendy body piercing or hairstyle, casual attire, and overdressing tend to detract from the image you want to present.

Attempt to strike a balance between a friendly but not too familiar, professional but not too aloof demeanor. Greet the interviewer by shaking hands, and wait for the interviewer to offer you a seat. Do not smoke or chew gum. Answer questions directly and honestly, but do not ramble on or offer extraneous information (Figure 57-13).

A common tendency is to view the interview as a one-sided interaction—as the employer's opportunity to scrutinize prospective employees. The interviewer's task is to confirm the information you have provided on your job application or resumé. In addition to gathering more detailed information about you, the interviewer is interested in the way you handle yourself and whether you are a good match for the job and the employer. After a screening and selection process, the employer offers employment to the most desirable candidate. But remember, securing employment is a two-sided process: You also are interviewing the interviewer to gather information about the employer, to ascertain whether the job opportunity is the right fit for you.

Any offer of employment you receive can be accepted or rejected. You should already have obtained information about the employer that was enticing enough to cause you to apply for employment. The interview is, however, your opportunity to gather more information about the employer. This information serves as the basis for determining whether you really

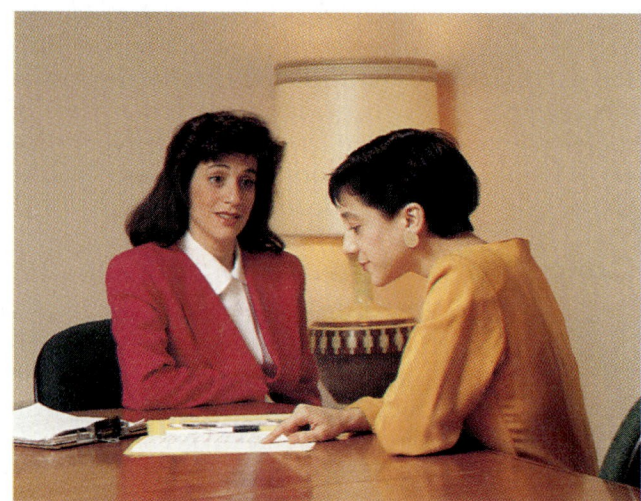

Figure 57-13 Be prepared for the interview; know those things you want to learn and those things you want to share with the interviewer.

want the job. Go to the interview with a written list of questions you have for the employer.

Your questions can address a number of topics including orientation, organization of the nursing staff, working conditions, and educational opportunities. For example, How long is the orientation? How often is overtime or floating required? On which unit will I be assigned to work? What are the five most common diagnoses on that unit? What is the ratio of RNs to LP/VNs to UAP? What is the schedule of a normal work week? The list of potential questions is endless.

The advice is often given not to ask about salary and benefits during the first interview. At some point, however, this information becomes crucial to your decision making. If the interviewer does not volunteer information about salary and benefits, at the very least wait until the end of the interview to discuss these matters. Employers want to know you are interested in work, because while everyone is interested in pay, not everyone is interested in the actual position available. Thus, you may want to consider waiting to learn about salary and benefits until a job offer has been made.

At the end of the interview, you may be offered employment. If you are confident that you want the position, accept the offer. If you have any hesitation, however, inform the employer that you will respond in a day or two. Do not turn the offer down at the interview. Go home, review the information you have available, discuss the offer with relevant people, and then notify the employer. Whether you decide to accept or decline the offer of employment, definitely respond to the employer's offer. Even in declining an employment offer, you want to leave a positive impression. You never know when you may encounter that recruiter in the future.

At the end of the interview, shake hands with the interviewer and offer thanks for the interviewer's time and consideration. If you believe you want the job, say so. Statements such as "After our discussion, I am very interested in working here" or "I really want to work with your client population and want the job" indicate your strong interest to the prospective employer.

Prepare a Thank You Note

The thank you note is critical to a successful job search. Always follow up an interview with a thank you note. Some employment counselors suggest you send a thank you note to everyone involved in the interview process. These people may include the person who suggested the employer, the receptionist and, certainly, the person who conducted the interview.

A thank you note can be handwritten or typed. The key is to send it the same day as the interview. The thank you note should be personal: say something about the way the person treated you, the highlights of the interview, or something you forgot to mention dur-

1234 Pleasant Street
Chicago, IL 60000
September 26, 2000

Thomas DiNapoli
Human Resources Manager
St. Anne's Medical Center
P.O. Box 3476
Pittsburgh, PA 15230

Dear Mr. DiNapoli:

Thank you for taking the time to speak with me yesterday about the position of medication nurse at St. Anne's Medical Center. I was very impressed with your company, and the job sounds wonderful. I'm more than ever convinced that my experience can benefit your company.

I appreciated the opportunity to meet you and learn about St. Anne's.

Sincerely,

Anita Jones, LPN

Figure 57-14 Sample Thank You Note

ing the interview. If the interview confirmed your interest in employment, say so. Even if you decide that the employment setting is not for you, write a thank you anyway. Your career interests may change at some point. Further, employers talk to each other; therefore, you want to leave a good impression any place you seek employment. Figure 57-14 shows a sample thank you note.

A FINAL WORD ABOUT EMPLOYMENT

As a new graduate, financial pressures or a seemingly limited pool of available jobs may influence your job search. You also may be considerably swayed by the advice that you should "get a year of experience in general medical–surgical nursing" before moving on to the job you really want. Financial pressures and the job market may indeed pose some limitations. Further, a year of medical–surgical experience is helpful. But resist taking a job for just these reasons.

As an occupation, licensed practical/vocational nursing offers much variety with regard to employment setting, client age, type of work, number of hours available to work, availability of days and shifts, amount of supervision, and a host of other factors. Such variety will become evident as you investigate available employment options.

A poor fit between the job and your interests, needs, or abilities is a setup for failure. As a newly employed LP/VN, you want to establish an employment record of success and increasing growth in your skills and knowledge. You want to build on your newfound confidence and competence. A thorough and honest evaluation of your strengths and weaknesses, a clearly identified objective, and a careful review of employment options will help ensure satisfying and rewarding employment.

SUMMARY

- Leadership styles are typically classified as autocratic, democratic, or laissez-faire.
- Skills necessary for effective leadership include communication, problem solving, self-evaluation, and management.
- Being a good manager means knowing how and when to assign tasks, delegate duties, prioritize care, and resolve conflict.
- In most instances, the RN will be in charge of delegating tasks to the LP/VN. The decision to delegate a task should be based on the potential for harm, the complexity of the task, the problem solving required, the unpredictability of the outcome, and the required coordination of care.
- The five rights of delegation include the right task, the right circumstance, the right person, the right direction, and the right supervision.
- Factors to assess when establishing priorities of care include safety, timing of tests and other tasks, interdependency of events, client requests, availability of help, client status, and availability of resources.
- The steps involved in securing a job include identifying your objective, preparing a résumé, preparing a cover letter, preparing a list of references, preparing a telephone call script, completing a job application, preparing for the interview, and preparing a thank you note.

Review Questions

1. The following information should be included on a résumé:

    a. name, address, telephone number, job objective.

    b. information about prior employment, name, family information.

    c. job objective, references, prior education and experiences.

    d. name, address, job objective, availability for interview.

2. Pauline, an LP/VN, is the evening-shift charge nurse on 3B, a 40-bed unit in a long-term care

facility. Christine is a CNA from another floor sent to work on 3B for the evening. She asks Pauline when she and the other three CNAs should take their lunch break. Pauline tells her to "work it out between themselves." Pauline is using a style of leadership called:

    a. participatory leadership.

    b. democratic leadership.

    c. autocratic leadership.

    d. laissez-faire leadership.

3. The five rights of delegation include the right

    a. task, time, circumstance, and supervision.

    b. supervision, task, person, and direction.

    c. person, task, time, and direction.

    d. time, task, person, and supervision.

Critical Thinking Questions

1. After a lengthy job search, Alicia secures employment at a long-term care facility. The facility residents are all retired nuns. Alicia enjoys geriatrics, management seemed fair and reasonable, the environment is clean and attractive, and financial benefits are competitive. However, Alicia finds the nuns to be demanding and unappreciative. Additionally, the religious underpinnings of the facility influence her work more than she anticipated. After 2 months, she now dreads going to work. What should she do?

2. Nancy works in a long-term care facility as the evening-shift charge nurse on 4 West. As part of her duties, she makes the client assignments to the CNAs. She also monitors their work and intervenes where necessary to ensure that clients receive safe and appropriate care. Lately, Nancy observes that Martha, a CNA, is not completing all her assigned responsibilities. How should Nancy address this problem?

WEB FLASH!

- Search the Web under broad categories such as *leadership, management, delegation,* and *employment.* What kind of sites do you locate?
- How is your search enhanced when you add qualifiers to narrow the search, such as *nursing, LPN, LVN,* or *UAP?*

Atlas of Nursing Procedures

BASIC PROCEDURES

Procedure B1   Handwashing

Equipment

- Soap
- Sink
- Paper or cloth towels
- Running water

Action	Rationale
1. Remove jewelry. Wristwatch may be pushed up above the wrist (midforearm). Push sleeves of uniform or shirt up above the wrist at midforearm level.	1. Provides access to skin surfaces for cleaning. Facilitates cleaning of fingers, hands, and forearms.
2. Assess hands for hangnails, cuts or breaks in the skin, and areas that are heavily soiled (follow agency policy regarding nail polish and artificial nails)	2. Intact skin acts as a barrier to microorganisms. Breaks in skin integrity facilitate development of infection and should receive extra attention during cleaning.
3. Turn on the water. Adjust the flow and temperature. Temperature of the water should be warm.	3. Running water removes microorganisms. Warm water removes less of the natural skin oils.
4. Wet hands and lower forearms thoroughly by holding under running water. Keep hands and forearms in the down position with elbows straight. Avoid splashing water and touching the sides of the sink.	4. Water should flow from the least contaminated to the most contaminated areas of the skin. Hands are considered more contaminated than arms. Splashing of water facilitates transfer of microorganisms. Touching of any surface during cleaning contaminates the skin.
5. Apply about 5 mL (1 teaspoon) of liquid soap. Lather thoroughly.	5. Lather facilitates removal of microorganisms. Liquid soap harbors less bacteria than bar soap.
6. Thoroughly rub hands together for about 10 to 15 seconds. Interlace fingers and thumbs and move back and forth to wash between digits (Figure B1-1). Rub palms and back of hands with circular motion. Special attention should be provided to areas such as the knuckles and fingernails, which are known to harbor organisms (Figure B1-2).	6. Friction mechanically removes microorganisms from the skin surface. Friction loosens dirt from soiled areas.

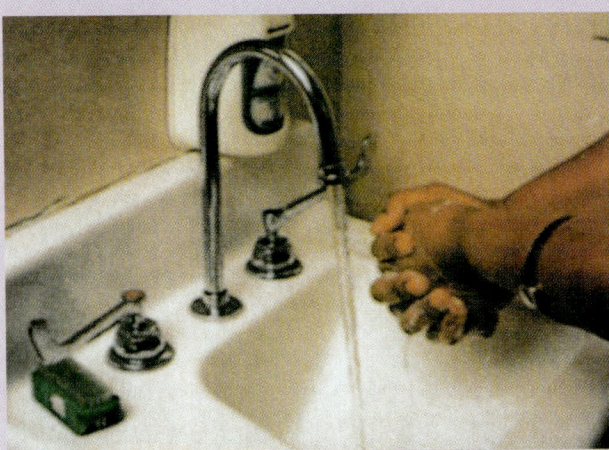

Figure B1-1 Interlace fingers to wash between the digits.

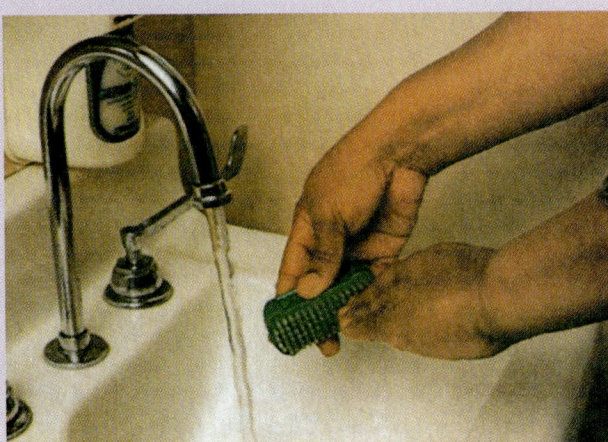

Figure B1-2 Provide special attention to washing knuckles and fingernails (brush may or may not be available).

continued

Action	Rationale
7. Rinse with hands in the down position, elbows straight. Rinse in the direction of forearm to wrist to fingers.	7. Flow of water rinses away dirt and micro-organisms.
8. Blot hands and forearms to dry thoroughly. Dry in the direction of fingers to wrist and forearms. Discard the paper towels in the proper receptacle.	8. Blotting reduces chapping of skin. Drying from cleanest (hand) to least clean area (forearms) prevents transfer of microorganisms to cleanest area.
9. Turn off the water faucet with a clean, dry paper towel (Figure B1-3).	9. Prevents contamination of clean hands by a less clean faucet.

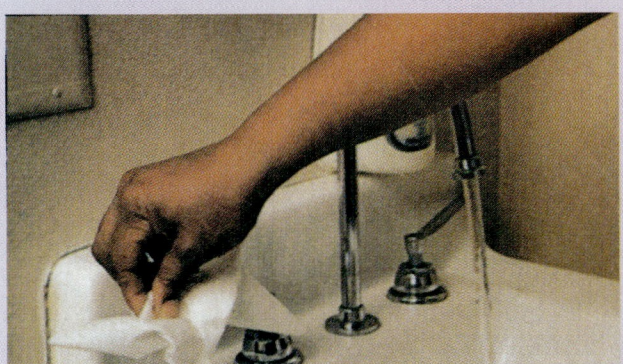

Figure B1-3 Turn off faucet with a clean, dry paper towel.

Procedure B2 — Use of Protective Equipment

Equipment

- Gloves
- Mask and goggles or face shield
- Gown

Action	Rationale
• *Wash your hands before applying any personal protective equipment (PPE)* •	

Applying Gloves (*Note:* If wearing full PPE, gloves are put on last.)

Action	Rationale
1. Wash hands.	1. Reduces spread of microorganisms.
2. Remove clean gloves from box.	2. Gloves are for one-time use.
3. Put hands into gloves, adjusting fingers for proper fit.	3. Proper fit is important for client care.

Applying Mask

Action	Rationale
4. Adjust mask over nose and mouth.	4. Ensures proper fit.
5. Tie top strings behind head first, then bottom strings. Or slip elastic over back of head.	5. Keeps mask from falling off.
6. Bend metal nosepiece over bridge of nose.	6. Provides better fit.
7. Replace mask if it becomes significantly damp with exhaled moisture.	7. Moisture can reduce the efficacy of some masks.

continued

Action	**Rationale**

Applying Protective Eyewear (*Note:* If mask is needed due to potential for splashing, goggles are also needed.)

8. Apply mask first, then apply the goggles or face shield. If eyeglasses are worn, eye protection is still required over eyeglasses to protect sides of eyes.

8. Protects eyes from splashing of body fluids.

Applying Gown (*Note:* If applying complete set of PPE, mask is applied before gown. Gloves are applied after gown.)

9. Hold the clean gown by the neck in front of you, letting it unfold. Do not let it touch the floor.

9. Reduces risk of contamination.

10. Place your arms in the sleeves and slide the gown up to your shoulders (Figure B2-1).

10. Reduces handling of front of gown.

11. Slip your hands inside the neck and grasp the ties. Tie them at the neck (Figure B2-2).

11. Secures gown.

12. Cover your uniform at the back with the gown and tie the ties at the waist. The gown must completely cover your clothing (Figure B2-3).

12. Reduces risk of contamination of nurse.

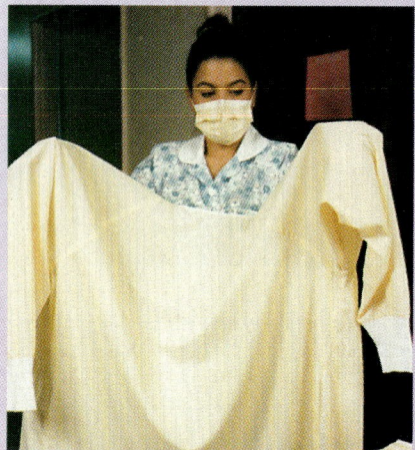 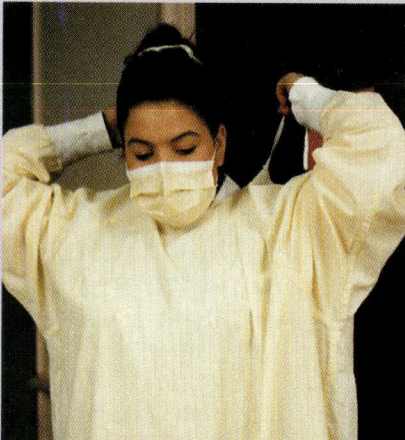 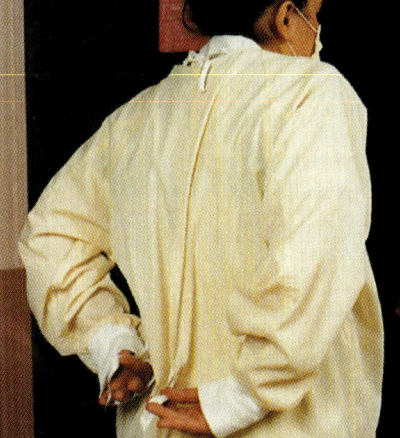

Figure B2-1 Place your arms in the sleeves and slide the gown up to your shoulders.

Figure B2-2 Slip fingers inside the neckband and tie gown.

Figure B2-3 Reach behind, overlap the edges of the gown so the uniform is completely covered, and tie the waist ties.

Removing Protective Clothing

Remove PPE in the following order:

- Untie front waist tie of the gown.
- Remove gloves.
- Wash your hands.
- Untie the neck tie of the gown and remove the gown.
- Wash your hands.
- Remove protective eyewear (if worn).
- Remove mask.
- Wash your hands.

See detailed procedure, which follows.

continued

Action	**Rationale**

Removing Gloves (Loosen waist tie on gown before removing gloves.)

13. Grasp the outside of the glove of the non-dominant hand (Figure B2-4).	13. Reduces risk of contaminating hands.
14. Pull the glove down, turning glove inside out with fingers inside while pulling it off the hand (Figure B2-5).	14. Reduces risk of contaminating hands.
15. Place this glove in the palm of the gloved hand.	15. Reduces risk of contaminating hands.
16. Using ungloved hand, reach under remaining glove, and pull glove off from underneath, turning glove inside out, and capturing other glove within (Figure B2-6).	16. Reduces risk of contaminating hands.
17. Discard gloves according to agency policy.	17. Reduces transmission of microorganisms.
18. Wash hands.	18. Reduces risk of transmitting microorganisms.

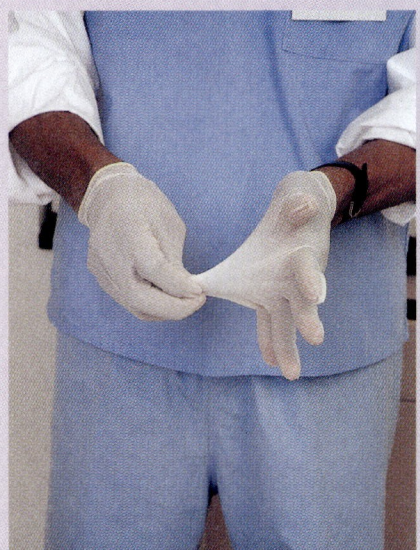

Figure B2-4 With fingers of one hand, grasp glove of other hand.

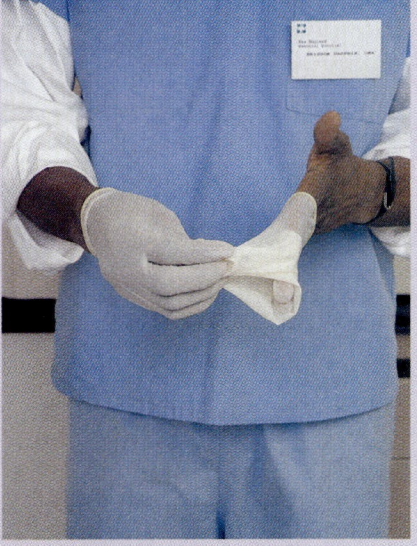

Figure B2-5 Pull the glove down over the hand and the fingers and remove it. The glove is inside out with the contaminated side inside.

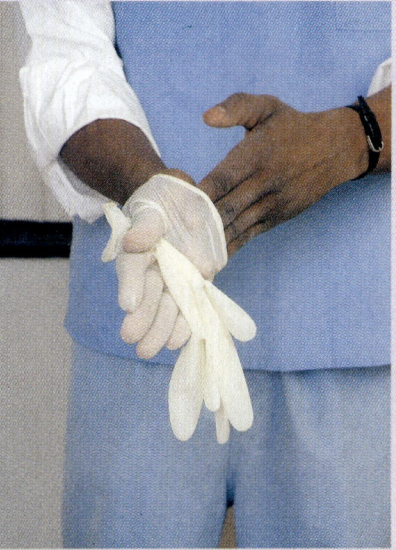

Figure B2-6 Hold the glove just removed in the gloved hand. Insert fingers of the ungloved hand inside the cuff of the other glove.

Removing Gown (*Note:* Waist tie should be loosened before gloves are removed.)

19. Untie neck ties of gown. Loosen gown at shoulders by touching only the inside of the gown (Figure B2-7).	19. Reduces risk of contaminating clothing.
20. Grasp the neck ties and pull the gown down and off, turning inside out.	20. Reduces risk of contaminating clothing.
21. Roll the gown away from your body (Figure B2-8). Discard according to agency policy. Wash your hands.	21. Reduces transmission of microorganisms.

continued

Action	**Rationale**

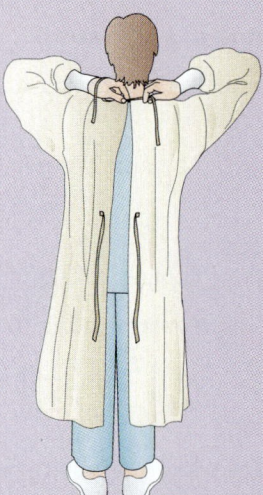

Figure B2-7 Untie neck ties of gown.

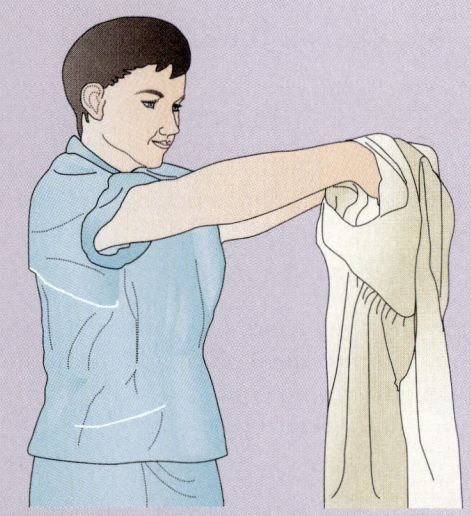

Figure B2-8 Pull the gown down off the arms, being careful that the hands do not touch the outside of the gown. Hold the gown away from your uniform and roll it up with the contaminated side inside. If gown is disposable, place it in the receptacle for contaminated trash. If gown is not disposable, place it in laundry hamper for contaminated linens.

Removing Protective Eyewear

22. Lift protective goggles or face shield away from face. Follow agency policy regarding disposal.

22. In some cases, clean goggles are re-used.

Removing Mask

23. Untie the upper tie first, then the lower tie, or pull the elastic from around the back of the head. Remove the mask by touching only the ties. (*Note:* Never wear a mask around the neck with the lower ties tied around the neck and the upper ties hanging down.)

23. Reduces risk of contaminating clothing.

Procedure B3   Measuring Body Temperature

Equipment

- Thermometer; glass (client's bedside); electronic and disposable protective sheath; disposable (chemical); tympanic
- Lubricant (rectal, glass thermometer)
- Two pairs of nonsterile gloves
- Tissues

Action	**Rationale**

• Wash your hands • Check the client's identification band •
• Explain the procedure to the client prior to beginning •

1. Review medical record for baseline data and factors that influence vital signs.

1. Establishes parameters for client's normal measurements, provides direction in device selection, and determines site to use for measurement. Vital signs are measured in the order of T-P-R and BP, usually without interruptions,

continued

Action	Rationale
	so as to provide the nurse with an objective clinical database to direct decision making.
2. Explain to the client that vital signs will be assessed. Encourage client to remain still and refrain from drinking, eating, or smoking.	**2.** Encourages participation, allays anxiety, and ensures accurate measurements. Cold or hot liquids or food and smoking alter circulation and body temperature.
3. Assess client's toileting needs and proceed as appropriate.	**3.** Prevents interruptions during measurements, communicates caring, and promotes client comfort.
4. Gather equipment indicated.	**4.** Facilitates organized assessment and measurement.
5. Provide for privacy.	**5.** Decreases embarrassment.
6. Wash hands and don gloves.	**6.** Hands are washed before and after every contact with a client. Gloves are worn to avoid contact with all bodily secretions and to reduce transmission of microorganisms.
7. Position the client in a sitting or lying position with the head of the bed elevated 45° to 60° for measurement of all vital signs except those designated otherwise.	**7.** Promotes comfort and site access for all measurements. Activity and movement can elevate heart and respiratory rates.
8. *Oral Temperature: Glass Thermometer*	
a. Select correct color tip of thermometer from client's bedside container.	**a.** Identifies correct device; a blue color tip usually denotes an oral thermometer.
b. Remove thermometer from storage container and cleanse under cool water.	**b.** Cleansing removes disinfectant that can cause irritation to oral mucosa. Cool water prevents expansion of the mercury.
c. Wipe thermometer dry with a tissue from bulb's end toward fingertips.	**c.** Wipe from area of least contamination to most contaminated area.
d. Read thermometer by locating mercury level. It should read 35.5°C (96°F).	**d.** Thermometer must be below normal body temperature to ensure an accurate reading.
e. If thermometer is not below a normal body temperature reading, grasp thermometer with thumb and forefinger and shake vigorously by snapping the wrist in a downward motion to move mercury to a level below normal.	**e.** Shaking briskly lowers level of mercury in the column. Because glass thermometers break easily, make sure that nothing in the environment comes in contact with the thermometer when shaking it.
f. Place thermometer in client's mouth under the tongue and along the gumline to the posterior sublingual pocket. Instruct client to hold lips closed.	**f.** Ensures contact with large blood vessels under the tongue. Prevents environmental air from coming in contact with the bulb.
g. Leave in place as specified by agency policy, usually 3–5 minutes.	**g.** Thermometer must stay in place long enough to ensure an accurate reading.
h. Remove thermometer and wipe with a tissue away from fingers toward the bulb's end.	**h.** Mucus on thermometer may interfere with disinfectant solution's effectiveness. Wipe from area of least contamination to most contaminated area.

continued

Action	Rationale
i. Read at eye level and rotate slowly until mercury level is visualized.	**i.** Ensures an accurate reading.
j. Shake thermometer down, and cleanse glass thermometer with soapy water, rinse under cold water, and return to storage container.	**j.** Mechanical cleansing removes secretions that promote growth of microorganisms. Hot water may cause coagulation of secretions and cause expansion of mercury in thermometer.
k. Inform client of temperature reading.	**k.** Promotes client's participation in care.
l. Remove and dispose of gloves in receptacle. Wash hands.	**l.** Reduces transmission of microorganisms.
m. Record reading and indicate site as "OT."	**m.** Accurate documentation by site allows for comparison of data.

9. *Oral Temperature: Electronic Thermometer*

Action	Rationale
a. Place disposable protective sheath over probe.	**a.** Prevents transmission of microorganisms.
b. Grasp top of the probe's stem. Avoid placing pressure on the ejection button.	**b.** Pressure on the ejection button releases the sheath from the probe.
c. Place tip of thermometer under the client's tongue and along the gumline to the posterior sublingual pocket lateral to center of lower jaw (Figure B3-1).	**c.** Sublingual pocket contains superficial blood vessels.

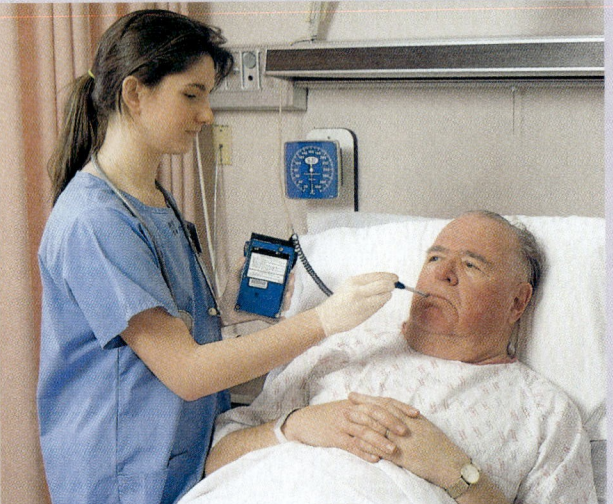

Figure B3-1 Place the tip of thermometer under client's tongue in posterior sublingual pocket lateral to center of lower jaw.

Action	Rationale
d. Instruct client to keep the mouth closed around thermometer.	**d.** Maintains thermometer in proper place and decreases amount of time for an accurate reading.
e. Thermometer will signal (beep) when a constant temperature registers.	**e.** Signal indicates temperature reading.
f. Read measurement on digital display of electronic thermometer. Push ejection button to discard disposable sheath into receptacle and return probe to storage well.	**f.** Reduces transmission of microorganisms. Ensures that the electronic system is ready for next use.

continued

Action	Rationale
g. Inform client of temperature reading.	**g.** Promotes client's participation in care.
h. Remove gloves and wash hands.	**h.** Reduces transmission of microorganisms.
i. Record reading and indicate site "OT."	**i.** Accurate documentation by site allows for comparison of data.
j. Return electronic thermometer unit to charging base plugged into electrical outlet.	**j.** Ensures thermometer is ready for next use.

10. *Rectal Temperature*

a. Place client in the Sims' position with upper knee flexed. Adjust sheet to expose only anal area.	**a.** Proper positioning ensures visualization of anus. Flexing knee relaxes muscles for ease of insertion.
b. Place tissues in easy reach. Don gloves.	**b.** Tissue is needed to wipe anus after device is removed.
c. Prepare the thermometer (refer to steps 8b, c, d, and e).	
d. Lubricate tip of rectal thermometer or probe (a rectal thermometer usually has a red cap).	**d.** Promotes ease of insertion of thermometer or probe.
e. With dominant hand, grasp thermometer. With nondominant hand, separate buttocks to expose anus.	**e.** Aids in visualization of anus.
f. Instruct client to take a deep breath. Insert thermometer or probe gently into anus: infant, 1.2 cm (0.5 in.); adult, 3.5 cm (1.5 in.) (Figure B3-2). If resistance is felt, do not force insertion.	**f.** Relaxes anal sphincter. Gentle insertion decreases discomfort to client and prevents trauma to mucous membranes.

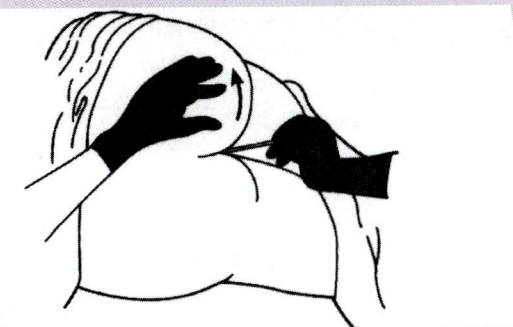

Figure B3-2 Insert probe or rectal thermometer into anus.

g. Length of time (refer to step 8g) or signal heard.	
h. Wipe secretions off glass thermometer with a tissue. Dispose of tissue in a receptacle.	**h.** Removes secretions and fecal material for visualization of mercury level. Prevents transmission of microorganisms.
i. Read measurement and inform client of temperature reading.	**i.** Encourages client participation.
j. While holding glass thermometer in one hand, use other hand to wipe anal area with tissue to remove lubricant or feces and dispose of soiled tissue. Cover client.	**j.** Prevents contamination of clean objects with soiled thermometer, decreases skin irritation, and promotes client comfort. Prevents embarrassment.

continued

Action	**Rationale**

k. Cleanse thermometer (refer to step 8j).

l. Remove and dispose of gloves in receptacle.

l. Decreases transmission of microorganisms.

m. Record reading and indicate site as "RT."

m. Accurate documentation by site allows for comparison of data.

11. *Axillary Temperature*

a. Remove client's arm and shoulder from one sleeve of gown. Avoid exposing chest.

a. Exposes axillary area.

b. Make sure axillary skin is dry; if necessary, pat dry.

b. Removes moisture and prevents a false low reading.

c. Prepare thermometer (refer to steps 8b, c, d, and e).

c. See Rationales 8b, c, d, and e.

d. Place thermometer or probe into center of axilla (Figure B3-3A). Fold client's upper arm straight down and place arm across client's chest (Figure B3-3B)

d. Puts device in contact with axillary blood supply. Maintains the device in proper position.

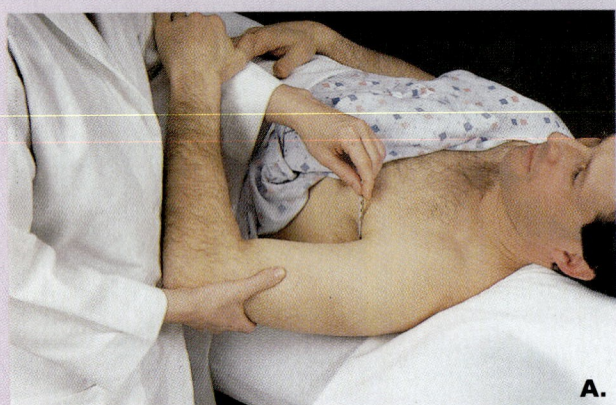 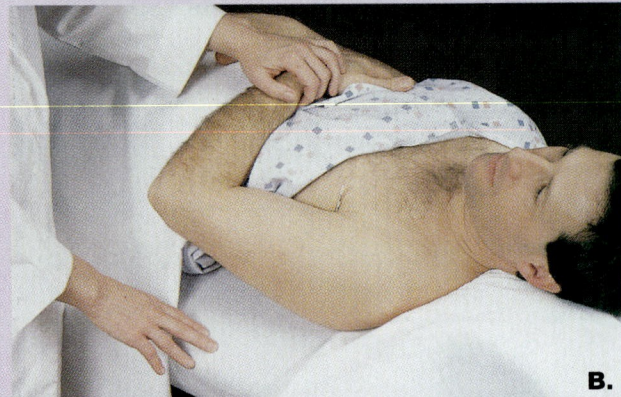

Figure B3-3 A. Insert thermometer into center of axilla. B. Place client's arm across chest.

e. Leave glass thermometer in place as specified by agency policy (usually 6–8 minutes). Leave an electronic thermometer in place until signal is heard.

e. Device must stay in place long enough to ensure an accurate reading. Signal indicates temperature reading.

f. Remove and read thermometer.

g. Inform client of temperature reading.

g. Encourages client participation.

h. Cleanse glass thermometer (refer to steps 8h and 8j) and return to storage container.

h. Prevents transmission of microorganisms and breakage of glass thermometer.

i. Assist client with replacing gown.

i. Promotes comfort.

j. Record reading and indicate site as "AT."

j. Promotes accurate documentation for data comparison.

12. *Disposable (Chemical Strip) Thermometer*

a. Apply tape to appropriate skin area, usually forehead.

a. Tape must be in direct contact with the client's skin.

continued

Action	Rationale
b. Observe tape for color changes.	**b.** Color reflects temperature reading (refer to the manufacturer's instructions).
c. Record reading and indicate method.	**c.** Promotes accurate documentation for data comparison.
13. *Tympanic Temperature: Infrared Thermometer*	
a. Position client in Sims' position.	**a.** Promotes access to ear.
b. Remove probe from container and attach probe cover to tympanic thermometer unit.	**b.** Prevents contamination.
c. Turn client's head to one side. For an adult, pull pinna upward and back; for a child, pull down and back. Gently insert probe with firm pressure into ear canal.	**c.** Provides access to ear canal. Gentle insertion prevents trauma to external canal. Firm pressure is needed to ensure probe contact against tympanic membrane.
d. Remove probe after the reading is displayed on digital unit (usually 2 seconds).	**d.** Reading is displayed within seconds.
e. Remove probe cover and replace in storage container.	**e.** Prevents damage to the reusable probe.
f. Return tympanic thermometer to storage unit.	**f.** Recharges batteries of unit.
g. Record reading and indicate site as "ET."	**g.** Promotes accurate documentation for data comparison.

Procedure B4 — Assessing Pulse Rate

Equipment

- Watch with a second hand
- Alcohol swab
- Stethoscope

Action	Rationale
• *Wash your hands* • *Check the client's identification band* • *Explain the procedure to the client prior to beginning* •	
1. *Radial Pulse*	
a. Inform client of the site(s) at which you will measure pulse.	**a.** Encourages participation and allays anxiety.
b. Flex client's elbow and place lower part of arm across chest.	**b.** Maintains wrist in full extension and exposes artery for palpation. Placing client's hand over chest will facilitate later respiratory assessment without undue attention to your action. (It is difficult for any person to maintain a normal breathing pattern when someone is observing and measuring.)
c. Place your index and middle finger on inner aspect of client's wrist over the radial artery and apply light but firm pressure until pulse is palpated (Figure B4-1).	**c.** Fingertips are sensitive, facilitating palpation of pulse. The nurse may feel own pulse if palpating with thumb. Applying light pressure prevents occlusion of blood flow and pulsation.

continued

Action	Rationale

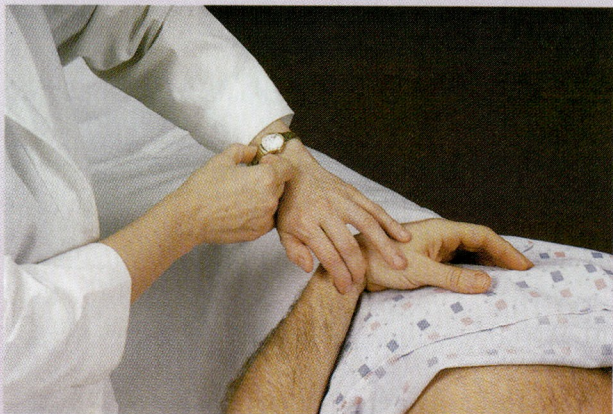

Figure B4-1 Place index and middle finger on inner aspect of client's wrist over the radial artery.

d. Identify pulse rhythm.

e. Determine pulse volume.

f. Count pulse rate by using second hand on a watch:

- For a regular rhythm, count number of beats for 30 seconds and multiply by 2.

- For an irregular rhythm, count number of beats for a full minute, noting number of irregular beats.

2. *Apical Pulse*

a. Raise client's gown to expose sternum and left side of chest.

b. Cleanse earpiece and diaphragm of stethoscope with an alcohol swab.

c. Put stethoscope around your neck.

d. Apex of heart:

- With client lying on left side (optional), locate suprasternal notch.

- Palpate second intercostal space to left of sternum.

- Place index finger in intercostal space, counting downward until fifth intercostal space is located.

- Move index finger along the fifth inter-costal space, left of the midclavicular line to palpate the point of maximal impulse (PMI) (Figure B4-2).

d. Palpate pulse until rhythm is determined. Describe as regular or irregular.

e. Quality of pulse strength is an indication of stroke volume. Describe as normal, weak, strong, or bounding.

f. An irregular rhythm requires a full minute of assessment to count an accurate rate.

a. Allows access to client's chest for proper placement of stethoscope.

b. Decreases transmission of microorganisms from one practitioner to another (earpiece) and from one client to another (diaphragm).

- Identification of landmarks facilitates correct placement of the stethoscope at the fifth intercostal space in order to hear point of maximal impulse.

continued

Action	Rationale

- Keep index finger of nondominant hand on the PMI.

• Ensures correct placement of stethoscope.

e. Inform client that you are going to listen to his heart. Instruct client to remain silent.

e. Elicits client support. Stethoscope amplifies noise.

f. With dominant hand, put earpiece of the stethoscope in your ears and grasp diaphragm of the stethoscope in palm of your hand for 5 to 10 seconds.

f. Dominant hand facilitates psychomotor dexterity for placement of earpiece with one hand. Heat warms metal or plastic diaphragm and prevents startling client.

g. Place diaphragm of stethoscope over the PMI and auscultate for sounds S_1 and S_2 to hear lub-dub sound (Figure B4-3).

g. Movement of blood through the heart valves creates S_1 and S_2 sounds. Listen for a regular rhythm (heartbeats are evenly spaced) before counting.

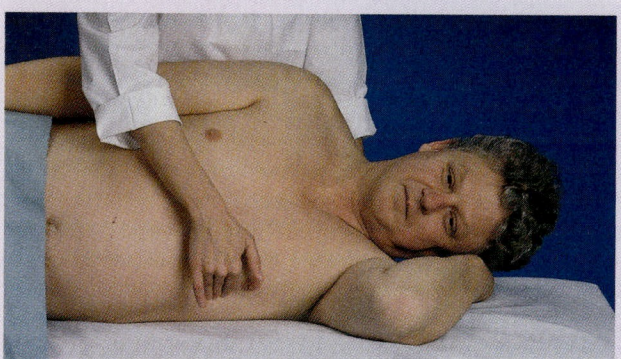

Figure B4-2 Palpating the Apical Pulse

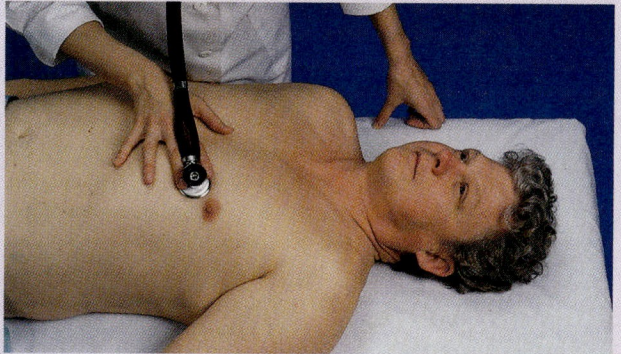

Figure B4-3 Place diaphragm of stethoscope over the PMI to auscultate for sounds. (Supine is alternative position.)

h. Note regularity of rhythm.

h. Establishment of a rhythm pattern determines length of time to count the heartbeats to ensure accurate measurement.

i. Start to count while looking at second hand of watch. Count lub-dub sound as one beat:

i. Ensures sufficient time to count irregular beats.

- For a regular rhythm, count rate for 30 seconds and multiply by 2.

- For an irregular rhythm, count rate for a full minute, noting number of irregular beats.

3. *Pedal (dorsalis pedis) Pulse*

a. Explain to the client that you need to check the circulation in the feet.

a. Encourages client participation and allays anxiety.

b. Position leg flat on the bed with foot in neutral position, or place foot flat on bed.

b. Provides access to artery.

c. Palpate the upper surface (dorsum) of the foot on an imaginary line drawn from the middle of the ankle to a space between the first and second toes.

c. Identifies the location of the artery.

d. Identify pulse rhythm.

d. Palpate pulse until rhythm is determined. Describe as regular or irregular.

continued

Action	Rationale
e. Determine pulse volume.	e. Quality of pulse is an indication of peripheral perfusion. Describe as normal, weak, strong, or bounding.
f. Share your findings with client.	f. Supports client participation in care.
g. Record by site the rate, rhythm, and, if applicable, number of irregular beats.	g. Recording rate and characteristics at bedside ensures accurate documentation.
h. Transfer information to client's record.	h. Facilitates communication among members of the health care team.

Procedure B5 — Assessing Respirations

Equipment

- Watch with a second hand

Action	Rationale
• Wash your hands • Check the client's identification band prior to beginning •	
1. Before replacing client's gown from auscultating heart sounds, assess respirations.	1. Facilitates observation of chest wall and abdominal movements.
2. Place your hand over client's wrist and observe one complete respiratory cycle.	2. Hand rises and falls with inspiration and expiration.
3. Start to count with first inspiration while looking at second hand sweep of watch.	3. Respiratory rate is one complete cycle (inspiration and expiration).
• Infants and children: count a full minute.	• Infants and children usually have an irregular rate.
• Adults: count for 30 seconds and multiply by 2. If an irregular rate or rhythm is present, count for a full minute.	• Respiratory rate reflects number of breaths per minute.
4. Observe depth of respirations by degree of chest wall movement and rhythm of cycle (regular or interrupted).	4. Reveals volume of air movement into and out of the lungs. Describe as shallow, normal, or deep.
5. Replace client's gown.	5. Prevents embarrassment and chilling.
6. Record rate and character of respirations.	6. Record rate and characteristics at bedside to ensure accurate documentation.

Procedure B6 — Assessing Blood Pressure

Equipment

- Alcohol swabs
- Stethoscope
- Sphygmomanometer with proper size cuff

continued

Action	**Rationale**

• Wash your hands • Check the client's identification band •
• Explain the procedure to the client prior to beginning •

Action	**Rationale**
1. Determine which extremity is most appropriate for reading. *Do not* take a pressure reading on an injured or painful extremity or one in which an intravenous line is running. Do not take blood pressure on the operative side of a woman after a mastectomy, or in the arm in which a dialysis shunt is present.	1. Cuff inflation can temporarily interrupt blood flow and compromise circulation in an extremity already impaired or a vein receiving intravenous fluids. Avoids vascular compromise.
2. Select a cuff size that completely encircles upper arm.	2. Provides equalization of pressure on the artery to ensure accurate measurement.
3. Move clothing away from upper aspect of arm.	3. Ensures accurate measurement.
4. Position arm at heart level, extend elbow with palm turned upward.	4. Blood pressure increases when arm is below level of heart and decreases when arm is above level of heart.
5. Make sure bladder cuff is fully deflated and pump valve moves freely.	5. Equipment must function properly to obtain an accurate reading.
6. Locate brachial artery in the antecubital space.	6. Designates placement of stethoscope.
7. Apply cuff snugly and smoothly over upper arm, 2.5 cm (1 in.) above antecubital space with center of bladder over brachial artery (Figure B6-1).	7. Ensures even pressure distribution over brachial artery. Prevents tubing from being constricted and allows visualization of aneroid manometer dial.
8. Connect bladder tubing to manometer tubing. If using a portable mercury-filled manometer, position vertically at eye level.	8. Maintains closed system; supports accurate reading of mercury level in manometer.
9. Palpate brachial artery (Figure B6-2). Turn valve clockwise to close and compress bulb to inflate cuff to 30 mm Hg above point where palpated pulse disappears, then slowly release valve (deflating cuff), noting reading when pulse is felt again.	9. Inflates the cuff's bladder with pressure and temporarily impairs flow of blood through artery. Provides an estimate of maximum pressure required to measure systolic pressure.

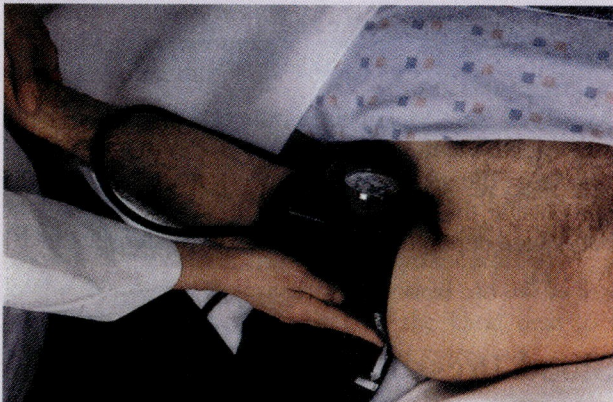

Figure B6-1 Wrap the blood pressure cuff on arm 1 inch above client's brachial pulsation, with bladder centered over brachial artery.

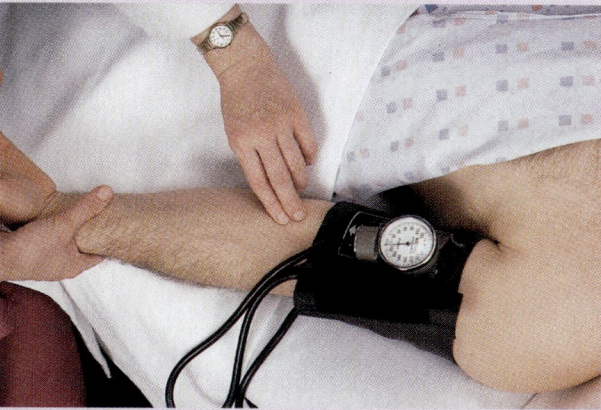

Figure B6-2 Palpate the brachial artery with fingertips below the pressure cuff.

continued

Action	**Rationale**
10. Insert earpiece of stethoscope into ears with a forward tilt, ensuring diaphragm hangs freely.	10. Enhances sound transmission from bell or diaphragm to ears.
11. Relocate brachial pulse with your nondominant hand and place bell or diaphragm directly over pulse. Bell or diaphragm should be in direct contact with skin and should not touch cuff (Figure B6-3).	11. Sound heard best directly over artery; decreases muffled sounds that cause inaccurate reading. Bell is more sensitive to low-frequency sound that occurs with pressure release.

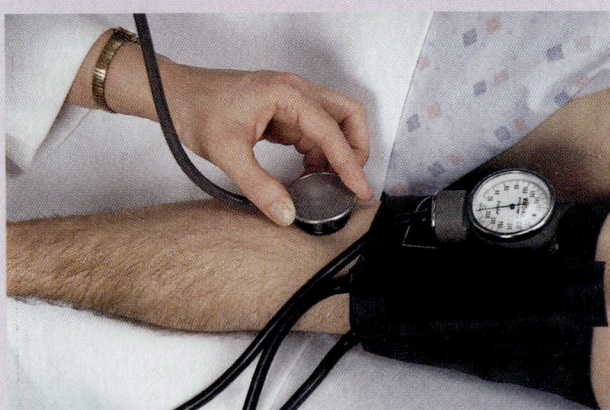

Figure B6-3 Bell Placed over Brachial Artery below Blood Pressure Cuff

Action	**Rationale**
12. With dominant hand, turn valve clockwise to close. Compress pump to inflate cuff until manometer registers 30 mm Hg above diminished pulse point identified in step 9.	12. Prevents air leak during inflation. Ensures the cuff is inflated to a pressure greater than the client's systolic pressure.
13. Slowly turn valve counterclockwise so that mercury falls at a rate of 2–3 mm Hg per second. Listen for five phases of Korotkoff's sounds while noting manometer reading:	13. Maintains constant release of pressure to ensure hearing first systolic sound. Identify manometer readings for each of the five phases.
• A faint, clear tapping sound appears and increases in intensity (phase I).	• Identify two consecutive tapping sounds to confirm systolic reading (phase I is systolic).
• Swishing sound (phase II).	
• Intense sound (phase III).	
• Abrupt, distinctive muffled sounds (phase IV).	
• Sound disappears (phase V).	• Phase V is the best index of diastolic blood pressure.
14. Deflate cuff rapidly and completely.	14. Prevents arterial occlusion and client discomfort from numbness or tingling.
15. Remove cuff or wait 2 minutes before taking a second reading.	15. Releases trapped blood in the vessels.
16. Inform client of reading.	16. Promotes client participation in care.
17. Record reading.	17. Ensures accuracy.
18. Lower bed, raise side rails, place call light within easy reach.	18. Promotes client safety.
19. Put all equipment in proper place.	19. Fosters maintenance of equipment.

continued

Action	Rationale
20. Wash hands.	**20.** Prevents transmission of microorganisms.
21. Document measurements in client's medical record on appropriate form, usually vital signs flow sheet.	**21.** Vital sign measurements are usually charted on the graphic section of the vital signs form.
22. Compare data with client's baseline and normal range for age group.	**22.** Provides for comparative data analysis.
23. If any measurements are abnormal, measure again and report abnormal findings to instructor or charge nurse.	**23.** Reporting abnormal measurements alerts staff to possible problems requiring intervention.

Procedure B7 — Weighing Client, Mobile and Immobile

Equipment

- Scale: standing electronic or balance scale (Figure B7-1); or sling scale (Figure B7-2)
- Plastic cover for sling scale
- Recommended disinfectant
- 1–3 other staff members to assist when using sling scale
- Gloves (when applicable)

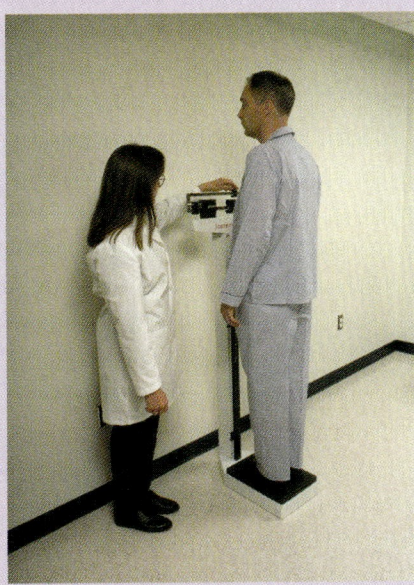

Figure B7-1 The standing balance scale is used to weigh ambulatory clients.

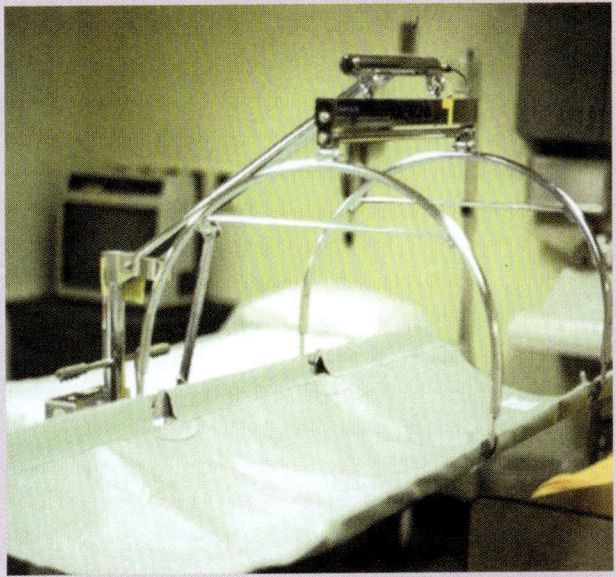

Figure B7-2 The sling scale is used to weigh clients in bed.

Action	Rationale

• Wash your hands • Check the client's identification band •
• Explain the procedure to the client prior to beginning •

Standing Scale

Action	Rationale
1. Place scale near client.	**1.** Reduces risk of fall or injury.
2. Turn on scale (if required) and calibrate to zero.	**2.** Ensures accurate reading.

continued

Action	**Rationale**
3. Ask client to step up on the scale and stand still (Figure B7-3).	**3.** Obtains weight.

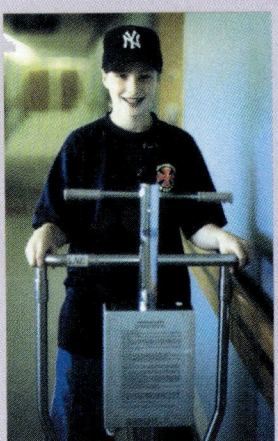

Figure B7-3 Have client stand straight and still while on the standing scale so accurate measurements of weight and height can be obtained.

Action	**Rationale**
Electronic scale: Read weight after digital numbers have stopped fluctuating.	Reading is not accurate when the numbers are still fluctuating.
Balance scale: Slide the scale's weight indicators on the blance beam until the balance rests in the middle. Add the two numbers to read the client's weight.	Weights on scale must be balanced to obtain accurate reading.
4. Ask client to step down and assist client back to the bed or chair, if necessary.	**4.** Reduces risk of injury if client needs assistance.
5. Wipe scale with appropriate disinfectant.	**5.** Reduces risk of spread of infection.
6. Wash hands.	**6.** Reduces transmission of microorganisms.

Sling Scale

Action	**Rationale**
7. Wash hands and put on gloves.	**7.** Reduces risk of nosocomial infection.
8. Introduce yourself to client and explain what you would like him to do.	**8.** Builds rapport; involves client in his care.
9. Place plastic covering on sling if available (can usually be ordered in bulk from the manufacturer).	**9.** Reduces risk of spreading infection between clients.
10. Remove pillows. Turn client to one side and place half of sling on bed next to client with remaining half rolled up against client's back (Figure B7-4).	**10.** Most accurate weight will be obtained by leaving no other bedding between client and sling.
11. Turn client to other side, and unroll rest of sling so it lies flat beneath client.	**11.** Turning in this manner maximizes client comfort.
12. Roll the scale over the bed so that the legs of the scale are underneath the bed (Figure B7-5). Open and lock the legs of the scale.	**12.** Ensures equipment is being used safely to reduce risk of injury.
13. Turn on scale and calibrate to zero.	**13.** Ensures accurate reading.

continued

Action	Rationale

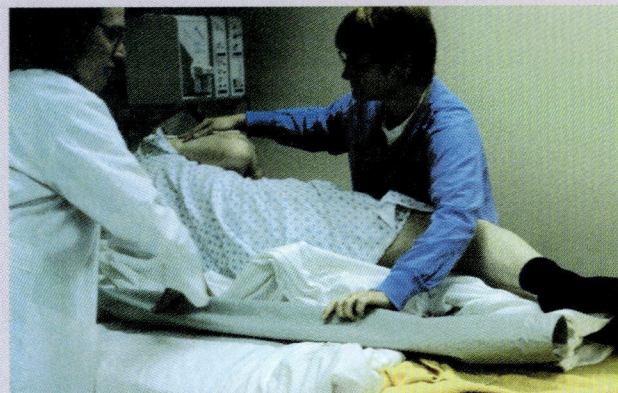

Figure B7-4 Turn client on one side and place sling on the bed.

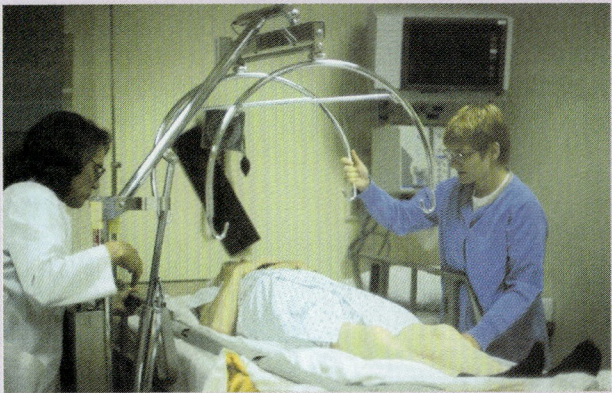

Figure B7-5 After unrolling the rest of the sling under the client, move the scale into position over the bed.

14. Lower arms of the scale and slip hooks through holes in sling (Figure B7-6).

14. Attaches sling to scale to obtain weight.

15. Pump scale until sling is completely off the bed (Figure B7-7).

15. Ensures accurate weight.

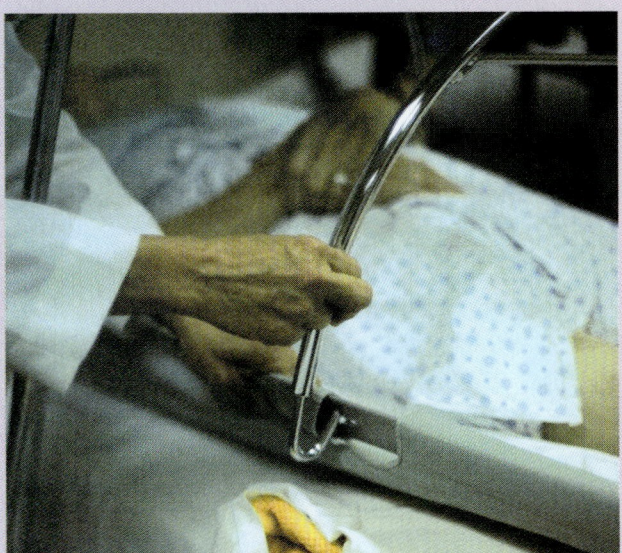

Figure B7-6 Attach the hooks through the holes in the sling.

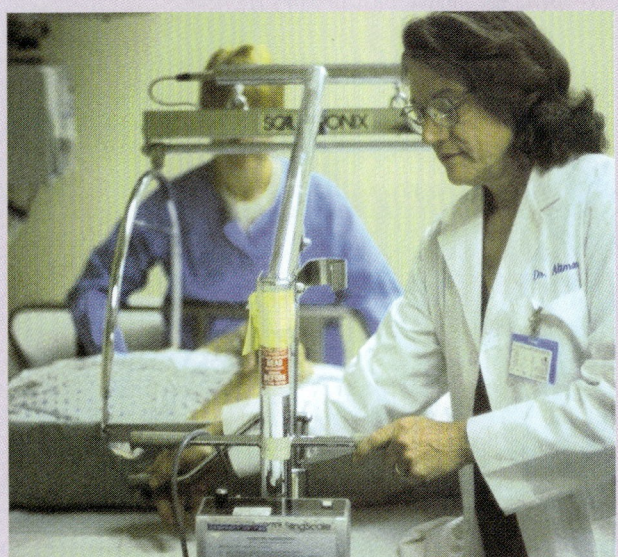

Figure B7-7 Pump the scale until the sling lifts completely off the bed.

16. Remind client to remain still. Read weight after digital numbers have stopped fluctuating (Figure B7-8).

16. Reading is not accurate when the numbers are still fluctuating.

17. Lower client back to bed and remove arms of scale from sling (Figure B7-9).

17. Prepare for removal of sling.

18. Unlock legs, return to their original position, and remove scale from bed.

18. Remove equipment to allow staff to remove sling from beneath client.

19. Turn client from side to side to remove sling from underneath client.

19. Remove sling.

20. Realign client with pillows and covers.

20. Ensures comfort and privacy.

continued

Action	Rationale

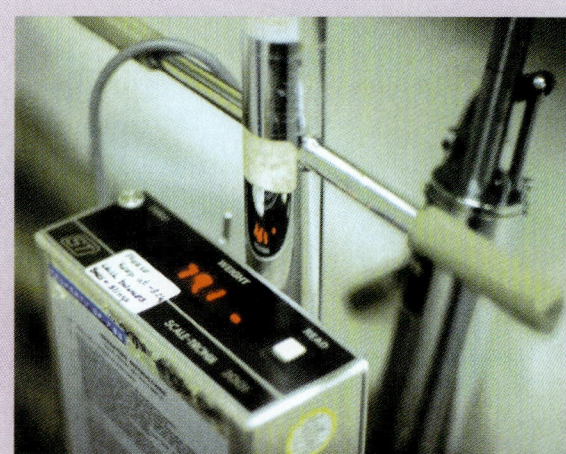

Figure B7-8 Read the weight after the numbers have stopped fluctuating.

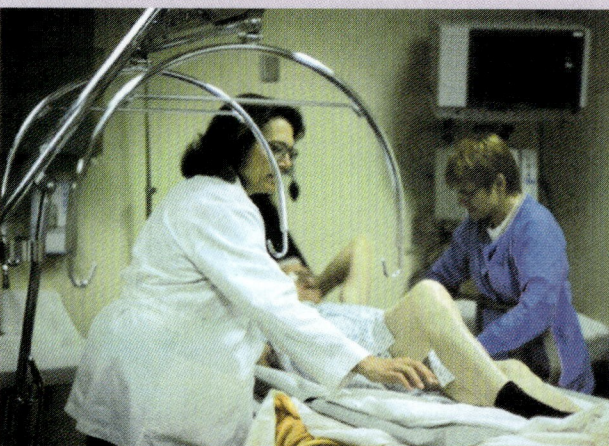

Figure B7-9 Lower the client back to the bed and prepare to remove the sling.

21. Remove plastic covering from sling and discard per hospital policy.

21. Reduces risk of spread of infection.

22. Remove gloves and wash hands.

22. Reduces transmission of microorganisms.

Procedure B8   Practicing Proper Body Mechanics

Equipment

- None required

Action	Rationale

1. Get a firm footing by keeping your feet apart.

1. Develops and maintains a stable base.

2. Bend at the knees; avoid bending at the waist. Hold the load close to your body (Figure B8-1).

2. Provides greater leverage for lifting.

3. Lift with the leg muscles.

3. Uses the strongest muscles, thereby reducing risk of injury.

4. Tighten abdominal muscles to lift.

4. Provides greater support to the back.

5. Turn by pivoting your feet, not your trunk, while lifting (Figure B8-2).

5. Maintains proper body alignment.

6. If the load is heavy, get help or use a mechanical lift.

6. Avoids strain and possible injury.

7. Push, do not pull.

7. Prevents back injury.

8. Use wheeled objects (e.g., a wheelchair).

8. Eases mobility.

9. Perform health-promoting activities.

9. Exercising, maintaining normal weight for height, pacing activities, and relaxing promote good body conditioning.

continued

Action	Rationale

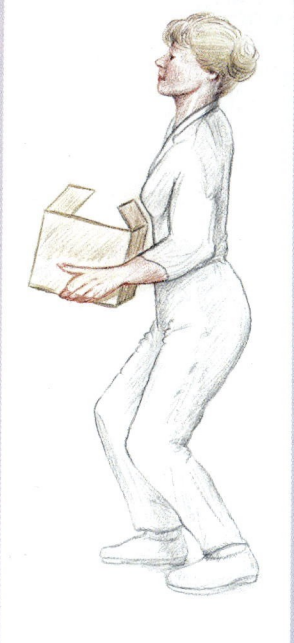

Figure B8-1 Bend knees to lift.

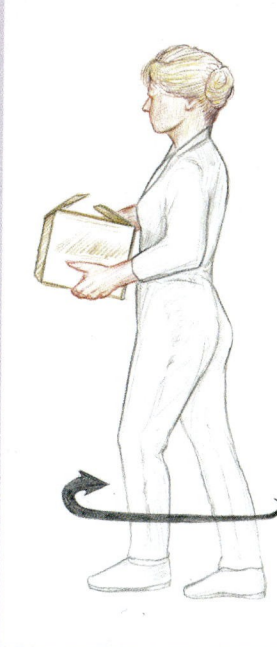

Figure B8-2 Pivot with feet.

Procedure B9   Performing Passive Range-of-Motion Exercises

Equipment

- Bed with side rails

Action	Rationale

• *Wash your hands* • *Check the client's identification band prior to beginning* •

Action	Rationale
1. Explain to the client the purposes of range-of-motion (ROM) exercises.	1. Reduces client anxiety and increases cooperation.
2. Elevate the bed.	2. Decrease nurse's muscle strain and promotes proper body mechanics.
3. Assist client to supine position in a warm, comfortable environment.	3. Promotes client's comfort level.
4. Start at head of client and perform ROM exercises down each side of the body.	4. Provides a systematic method to ensure that all body parts are exercised.
5. Repeat each range-of-motion exercise 5 times in a slow, firm manner.	
6. Cradle client's head with palms of hand while holding the extremities by the long bone areas.	6. Provides support to each body part, thus reducing strain on muscles and joints.
Head: Rotation—Turn the head from side to side. Flexion and extension—Tilt the head toward the chest and then tilt slightly upward (Figure B9-1). Lateral flexion—Tilt the head on each side so as to almost touch the ear to the shoulder.	

continued

Action	**Rationale**

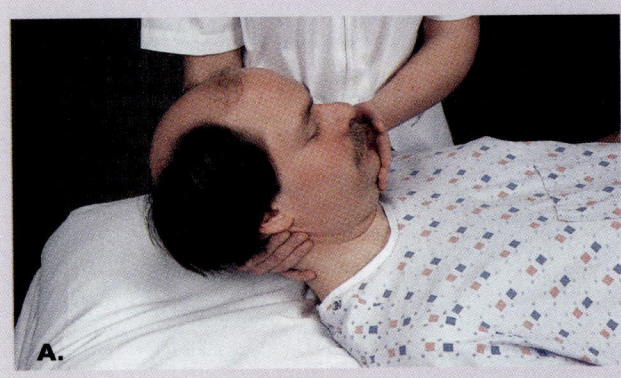 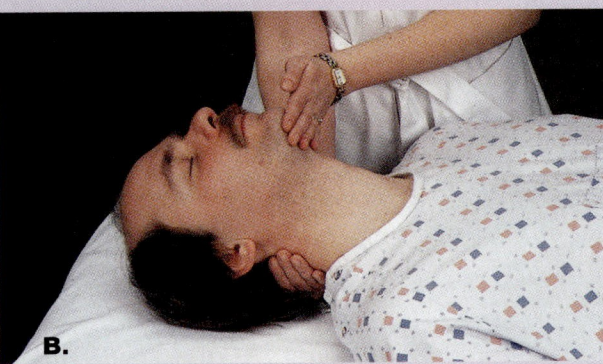

Figure B9-1 Passive ROM Exercises of Head. A. Flexion of neck; B. Extension of neck

Neck: Rotation—Place the client in a sitting position and rotate the neck in a semicircle while supporting the head.

Trunk: Flexion and extension—Bend the trunk forward, straighten the trunk, then extend slightly backward. Rotation—Turn the shoulders forward and return to normal position. Lateral flexion—Tip trunk to left side, straighten trunk, tip to right side.

Have the client resume a supine position.

Arm: Flexion and extension—Extend the arm in a straight position upward toward the head, then downward along the side. Adduction and abduction—Extend the arm in a straight position toward the midline (adduction) and away from the midline (abduction).

Shoulder: Internal and external rotation—Bend the elbow at a 90° angle with the upper arm parallel to the shoulder; rotate the shoulder by moving the lower arm upward and downward.

Elbow: Flexion and extension—Supporting the arm, flex and extend the elbow (Figure B9-2). Pronation and supination—Flex elbow, move the hand in palm-up and palm-down position.

Wrist: Flexion and extension—Supporting the wrist, flex and extend the wrist. Adduction and

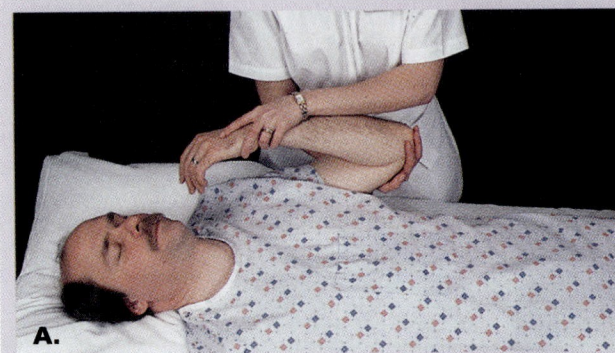 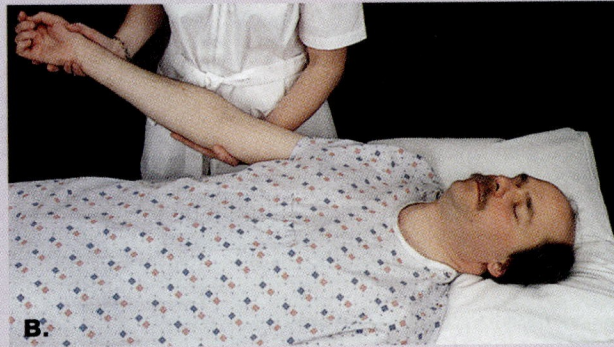

Figure B9-2 Passive ROM Exercises of Elbow. A. Flexion of elbow; B. Extension of elbow

continued

Action	Rationale

abduction—Supporting the lower arm, turn wrist right to left, left to right, then rotate the wrist in a circular motion.

Hand: Flexion and extension—Supporting the wrist, flex and extend the fingers. Adduction and abduction—Supporting the wrist, spread fingers apart and then bring them close together. Opposition—Supporting the wrist, touch each finger with the tip of the thumb.

Thumb: Rotation—Supporting the wrist, rotate the thumb in a circular manner.

Hip and Leg: Flexion and extension—Supporting the lower leg, flex the leg toward the chest and then extend the leg (Figure B9-3). Internal and external rotation—Supporting the lower leg, angle the foot inward and outward.

Knee: Flexion and extension—Supporting the lower leg, flex and extend the knee.

Ankle: Flexion and extension—Supporting the lower leg, flex and extend the ankle.

Foot: Adduction and abduction—Supporting the ankle, spread the toes apart and then bring them close together. Flexion and extension—Supporting the ankle, extend the toes upward and then flex the toes downward.

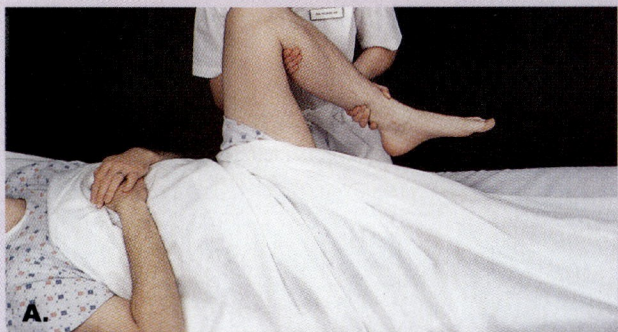 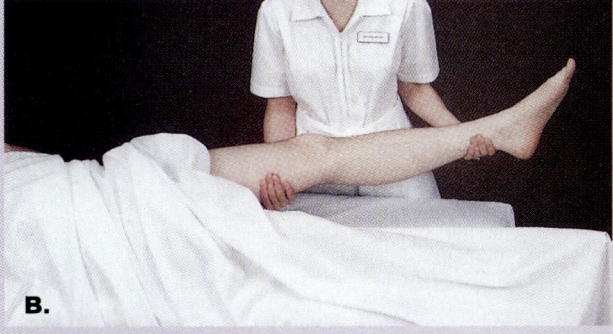

Figure B9-3 Passive ROM Exercises of Hip and Knee. A. Flexion of hip and knee; B. Extension of hip and knee

Procedure B10   Assisting a Client with Ambulation

Equipment

• None required

Action	Rationale

• Wash your hands • Check the client's identification band •
• Explain the procedure to the client prior to beginning •

1. Inform client of the purposes and distance of the walking exercise.	1. Reduces client anxiety and increases cooperation.

continued

Action	**Rationale**
2. Elevate the head of the bed and wait several minutes.	2. Prevents orthostatic hypotension.
3. Lower the bed height.	3. Reduces distance client has to step down, thus decreasing risk of injury.
4. With one arm under the client's back and one arm under the client's upper legs, move the client into the dangling position (Figure B10-1).	4. Provides client support and reduces risk of fall.

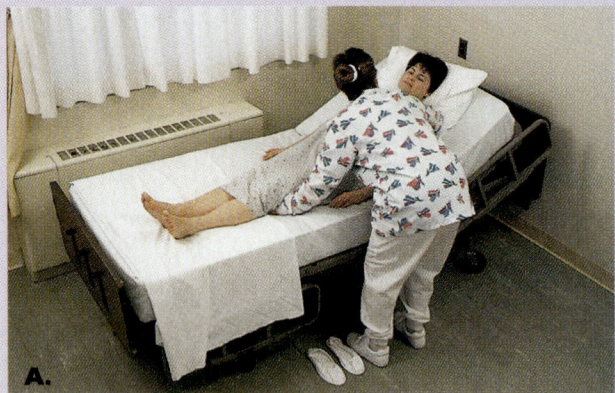 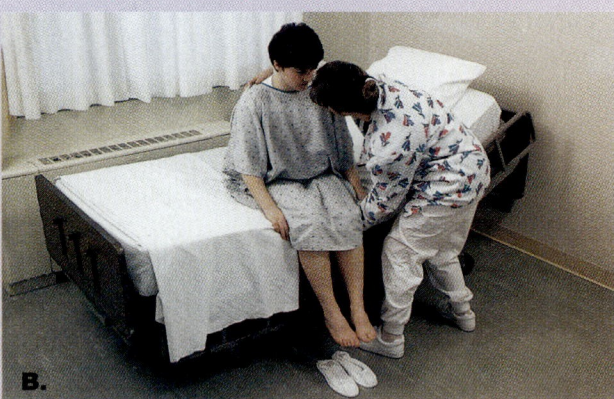

Figure B10-1 Assist the client from a supine to a seated position. A. Place one arm under the client's back and one arm under the client's legs. B. Help the client move into the dangling position.

5. Encourage client to dangle at side of bed for several minutes.	5. Prevents orthostatic hypotension. Allows for assessing tolerance for the sitting position.
6. Stand in front of client with your knees touching client's knees.	6. Prevents client from sliding forward if dizziness or faintness occurs.
7. Place arms under client's axillae (Figure B10-2).	7. Supports client's trunk.

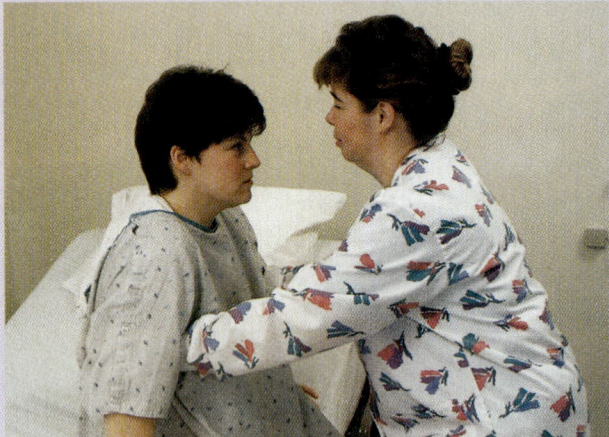

Figure B10-2 Assist client to a standing position by supporting the client's trunk with your arms under the client's axillae.

8. Assist client to a standing position, allowing client time to balance.	8. Reduces risk of fall.
9. Help client ambulate desired distance or distance of tolerance by placing your hand under the client's forearm and ambulating close to the client (Figure B10-3).	9. Provides assistance in achieving ambulatory goals.

continued

Action	Rationale

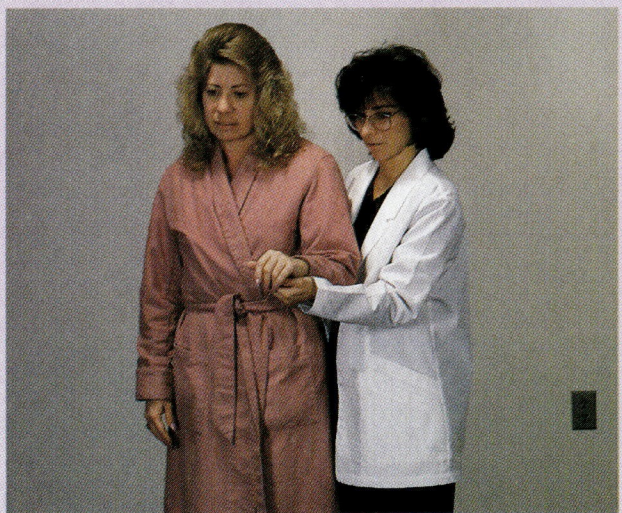

Figure B10-3 Assisting a Client with Ambulation

Action	Rationale
10. At the end of ambulation, assist the client back to bed or to chair beside bed.	10. Allows client to rest.
11. Document client's progress with ambulation.	11. Facilitates communication with members of the health care team.

Procedure B11 Positioning a Client in Bed

Equipment

- Hospital bed with side rails
- Pillows or foam wedges
- Foot board
- Turn sheet or draw sheet
- Hand cones
- High-top tennis shoes

Action	Rationale
• *Wash your hands* • *Check the client's identification band prior to beginning* •	
1. Inform client of reason for the move and how to assist (if able).	1. Reduces anxiety; helps increase comprehension and cooperation; promotes client autonomy.
2. Elevate bed to highest position.	2. Avoids strain on nurse's back muscles; promotes proper body mechanics.
3. Using two nurses, place turn (or draw) sheet under client's back and head.	3. Decreases shearing, which can precede formation of pressure ulcers.
Fowler's Position	
4. Place bed in a 15° to 30° angle for low-Fowler's position, 45° to 60° angle for Fowler's position, or 70° to 90° angle for high-Fowler's position.	4. The height of the head of the bed is determined by physician's order, client preference, client tolerance, or client's activity (e.g., eating).
5. If desired, place pillows at small of back, under ankles, under the arms, and under head of client.	5. Promotes client comfort. Pillows under ankles elevate heels to help prevent pressure ulcer formation. Pillows under the arms can assist with lung expansion.

continued

Action	Rationale
6. Slightly elevate the gatch of the lower portion of the bed.	6. Assists in maintaining correct client positioning.
7. Assess client for comfort.	7. Comfort is subjective.
8. Lower height of bed and elevate side rails.	8. Promotes client safety.

Supine Position

Action	Rationale
9. Follow steps 1–3.	
10. Place bed in a flat position.	
11. Place pillows at small of back, under head, and under ankles.	11. Adds to client comfort; relieves pressure on heels.
12. Assess client's comfort level.	12. Comfort is subjective.
13. Lower height of bed and elevate side rails.	13. Promotes client safety.

Side-Lying Position

Action	Rationale
14. Follow steps 1–3.	
15. Place client on side by logrolling (Procedure B15).	15. Places client on side for the proper positioning; reduces flexion of neck and spine.
16. Place a small pillow under client's head. Place pillow or foam wedges behind client's back. Place a pillow between client's legs. Put a pillow tucked by the client's abdomen.	16. Pillows at back and abdomen help maintain side-lying position. Small pillow under head is for comfort. Pillow between legs is for back alignment, comfort, and pressure relief. Pillow at abdomen supports upper arm, thus protecting the upper arm–shoulder joint positioning.
17. Run your hand under the client's dependent shoulder and move the shoulder slightly forward.	17. Removes pressure on upper arm-shoulder joint, promoting comfort.
18. Assess the client for comfort.	18. Comfort is subjective.
19. Lower the bed and elevate the side rails.	19. Promotes client safety.

Prone Position

Action	Rationale
20. Follow steps 1–3.	
21. Assist the client to lie on abdomen.	21. Prepares client to assume prone position.
22. Place a small pillow under client's head; head should be turned to side. The client's arms can be extended near side or flexed toward head. Place a small pillow under chest for female client and for client with a barrel chest.	22. Pillows at head and chest are for comfort. The arms are positioned according to client preference and flexibility. Pillow under chest protects breasts and promotes comfort.
23. Place a small pillow under ankles or have toes placed in space between foot of bed and the mattress.	23. Relieves pressure on toes.
24. Assess client for comfort.	24. Comfort is subjective.
25. Lower the bed and elevate the side rails.	25. Promotes client safety.

General Guidelines for Client Positioning

Action	Rationale
26. Use a hand cone for positioning the hand if needed. Place the cone in hand, with the wider portion near the little finger and the narrow portion nearer the index finger.	26. Helps prevent hand flexion contractures.

continued

Action	**Rationale**
27. Assess the client's skin frequently (at least every 2 hours) for pressure marks.	**27.** Immobile clients are prone to tissue ischemia with subsequent development of pressure ulcers.
28. Turn client frequently; every 2 hours or less.	**28.** Promotes blood circulation and prevents skin breakdown.
29. Use a footboard or high-top tennis shoes for clients in Fowler's and supine position if indicated.	**29.** Assists in prevention of foot drop.
30. Prepare a turn schedule for each client and place on chart at head of client's bed.	**30.** Stresses to all nursing personnel the importance of turning client frequently.
31. For all clients, be sure call bell is within reach.	**31.** Promotes safety; allows communication.

Procedure B12   Moving a Client in Bed

Equipment

- Hospital bed with side rails
- Turn sheet or draw sheet

Action	**Rationale**
• Wash your hands • Check the client's identification band prior to beginning •	
1. Inform client of reason for the move and how to assist (if able).	**1.** Reduces anxiety; helps increase comprehension and cooperation; promotes client autonomy.
2. Elevate bed to high position. Lower head of bed.	**2.** Lessens strain on nurse's back muscles; promotes proper body mechanics.
3. With two nurses, place turn/draw sheet under client's back and head (if not already present).	**3.** Reduces shearing force which can precipitate pressure sores.
4. Nurses stand on each side of client. Position client with knees flexed to push with feet if able to assist with move (Figure B12-1).	**4.** Client assistance lessens strain on nurse's back muscles; promotes client autonomy.
5. Have client use a bed trapeze, if available.	**5.** Lessens shearing force; decreases strain on both client and nurses.

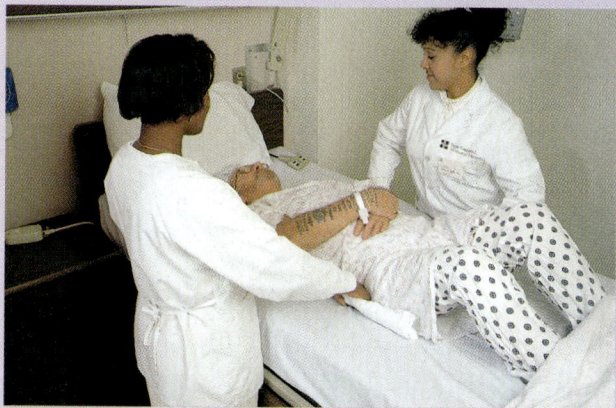

Figure B12-1 Moving Client in Bed: Client Positioned with Knees Flexed

continued

Action	Rationale
6. The lead nurse will give the signal to move. The nurses will lift up on the turn/draw sheet. The move is coordinated to transfer the client up toward the head of the bed.	6. Lessens strain on client and nurses. Reduces shearing force.
7. Position in bed can be maintained using bed gatch, if tolerated by client.	7. Elevated bed gatch maintains position by preventing client from sliding downward.
8. Elevate head of bed, if tolerated by client.	8. Promotes comfort; facilitates eating and drinking; facilitates communication.
9. Assess client for comfort.	9. Comfort is subjective.
10. Lower bed and elevate side rails.	10. Promotes client safety.

Procedure B13   Transferring a Client from Bed to Wheelchair

Equipment

- Bed   • Wheelchair

Action	Rationale
• *Wash your hands* • *Check the client's identification band prior to beginning* •	
1. Inform client about desired purpose and destination.	1. Reduces client anxiety and increases cooperation.
2. Assess client for ability to assist with the transfer and for presence of cognitive or sensory deficits.	2. Promotes safety.
3. Lower the height of the bed.	3. Reduces distance client has to step down, thus decreasing risk of injury.
4. Allow client to dangle for a few minutes.	4. Allows time to assess client's response to sitting; reduces possibility of orthostatic hypotension.
5. Bring wheelchair close to the side of the bed, toward the foot of the bed.	5. Minimizes transfer distance.
6. Lock wheelchair brakes and elevate the foot pedals.	6. Provides stability.
7. Assist client to side of bed until feet touch the floor.	7. Provides guidance and helps client maintain balance.
8. Assist the client to a standing position and provide support.	8. Helps client stand safely and gives time to assess status.
9. Pivot client so client's back is toward the wheelchair (Figure B13-1).	9. Moves client into proper position to be seated.
10. Place client's hands on the arm supports of the wheelchair.	10. Allows client to gain balance and judge distance to seat.
11. Bend at the knees, easing the client into a sitting position (Figure B13-2).	11. Increases stability and minimizes strain on back.

continued

Action	Rationale

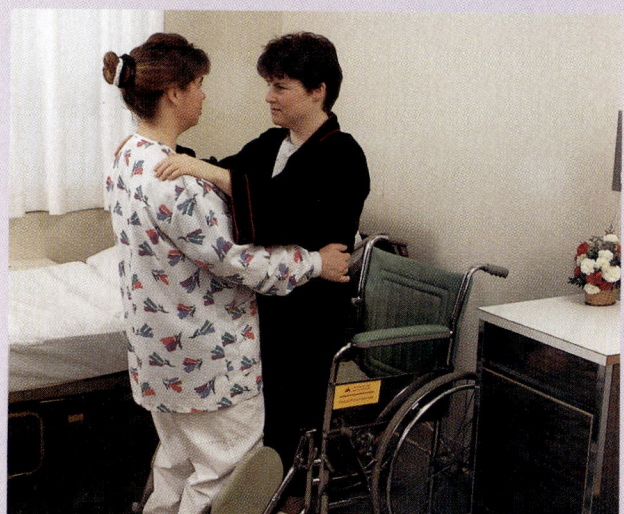

Figure B13-1 Pivot client so back is toward wheelchair.

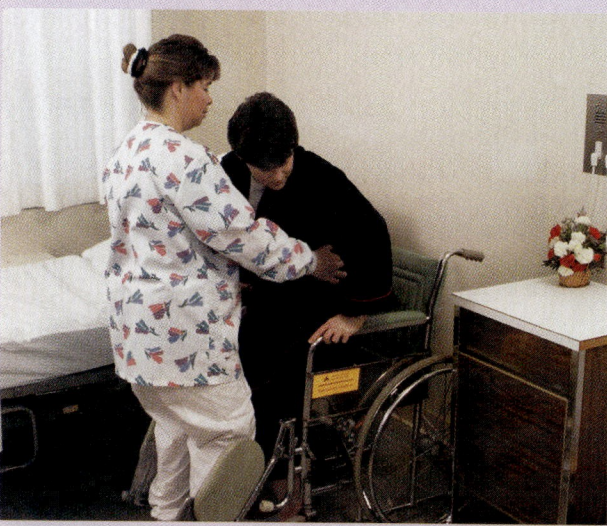

Figure B13-2 Ease client into wheelchair.

12. Assist client to maintain proper posture.

12. Broadest, and therefore safest, base of support is with client seated as far back on the seat as possible.

13. Secure the safety belt, place client's feet on feet pedals, and release brakes.

13. Ensures client safety; prepares client for movement.

Procedure B14 — Transferring a Client from Bed to Stretcher with Minimum Assistance/Maximum Assistance

Equipment

- Bed
- Pillows

- Stretcher
- Lift Sheet

Action	Rationale

• Wash your hands • Check the client's identification band •

1. Inform client about desired purpose and destination.

1. Reduces client anxiety and increases cooperation.

2. Raise the height of bed and lock brakes.

2. Reduces distance nurse must bend, thus preventing back strain; prevents bed from moving.

Minimum Assistance

3. Instruct client to move to side of bed close to stretcher. Lower side rails of bed and stretcher.

3. Decreases risk of client falling.

4. Stand at outer side of stretcher and push it toward bed. Lock stretcher brakes.

4. Diminishes the gap between bed and stretcher; secures the stretcher position.

5. Instruct client to move onto stretcher with assistance as needed.

5. Promotes client independence.

6. Cover client with sheet or bath blanket. Release brakes of stretcher.

6. Promotes comfort; protects privacy.

continued

Action	**Rationale**
7. Elevate side rails on stretcher and secure safety belts about client.	**7.** Prevents falls.
8. Stand at head of stretcher to guide it when pushing.	**8.** Pushing, not pulling, ensures proper body mechanics.

Maximum Assistance

Action	**Rationale**
9. Assess amount of assistance required for transfer. Usually two to four staff members are required for the maximum assisted transfer.	**9.** Promotes client independence; assures that enough staff are present before beginning transfer.
10. Lock wheels of bed and stretcher (Figure B14-1).	**10.** Prevents falls.

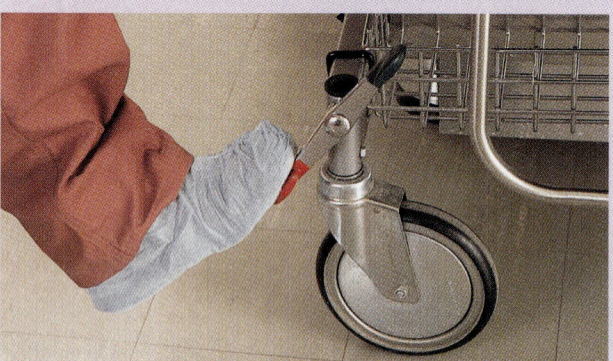

Figure B14-1 Lock wheels on the stretcher.

Action	**Rationale**
11. Have one nurse stand close to client's head.	**11.** Supports client's head during the move.
12. Logroll the client (see Procedure B15) and place a lift sheet under the client's back, trunk, and upper legs. The lift sheet can extend under the head if client lacks head control abilities.	**12.** Prevents flexion and rotation of client's hips and spine; maintains correct body alignment.
13. If urinary drainage bag is present, empty it and move it to side of bed closest to stretcher.	**13.** Prevents risk of urinary infection.
14. Move client to edge of bed near stretcher.	**14.** Prevents dragging, which causes shearing force.
15. Nurse on nonstretcher side of the bed rolls the lift sheet toward the client's side (Figure B14-2).	**15.** Provides the nurse with stronger gripping surface; provides maximum control of client movement; promotes good body mechanics for nurse.

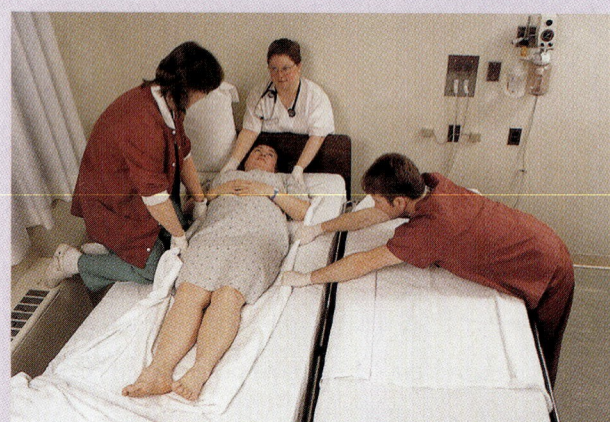

Figure B14-2 Transferring Client with Maximum Assistance; Grasping Lift Sheet

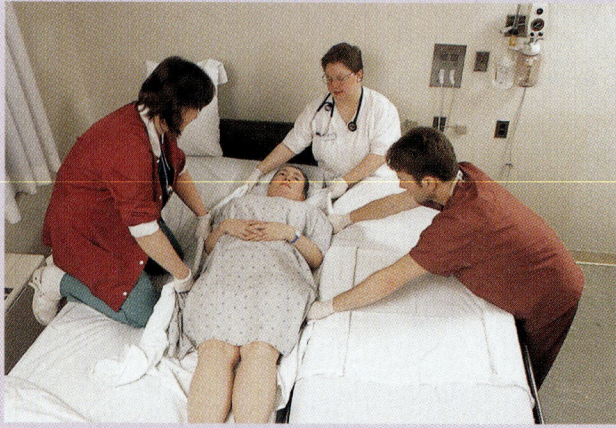

Figure B14-3 Transferring Client with Maximum Assistance; Moving Client from Bed to the Stretcher

continued

Action	Rationale
16. Place pillow overlapping the bed and stretcher.	**16.** Protects head from injury.
17. One nurse acts as team leader. Client is moved on count of three from team leader. One nurse is on each side of client, one nurse controls client's head. Client is lifted with lift sheet and moved from bed to stretcher by team (Figure B14-3). If client is heavy or difficult to move, it may require several small moves to get client from bed fully onto stretcher.	**17.** Promotes proper body mechanics and client safety.
18. Secure safety belts and elevate side rails of stretcher.	**18.** Prevents falls.
19. If IV is present, move it from bed IV pole to stretcher IV pole after client transfer.	**19.** Prevents tubing from being pulled and IV from being dislodged.
20. Empty all drainage bags (e.g., T-tube, Hemovac, Jackson-Pratt). Secure drainage system to client's gown prior to transfer.	**20.** Decreases possibility of spills; prevents dislodging of tubes.
21. Document where the client is going on the stretcher and client's response to move.	**21.** Provides record of client's whereabouts in building.

Procedure B15 Logrolling a Client with a Turn Sheet

Equipment

- Hospital bed with side rails
- Pillows
- Turn sheet or draw sheet
- Gloves (if chance of exposure to body fluids)

Action	Rationale

• *Wash your hands* • *Check the client's identification band prior to beginning* • *Wear gloves if indicated* •

Action	Rationale
1. Inform client of reason for the move and how to assist (if able).	**1.** Reduces anxiety; helps increase comprehension and cooperation; promotes client autonomy.
2. Elevate hospital bed to high position.	**2.** Avoids strain on nurse's back muscles; promotes proper body mechanics.
3. Using one or more staff members; place a turn/draw sheet under the client's back, buttocks, and head (if not already present).	**3.** Reduces shearing force, which can precipitate pressure ulcer formation.
4. The lead person tells the client and other personnel the direction of the move.	**4.** Cooperation and coordination place less strain on client and personnel.
5. One person stands on each side of the bed. The lead nurse gives the signal for the move. The staff member on the side of the bed in the direction of the move holds the turn/draw sheet to guide the move. The second staff member applies gentle pressure on client's back toward the direction of the move, assisting client to roll (Figure B15-1).	**5.** Two persons give more support to client than one person could and are better able to maintain proper alignment of client's spine and neck.

continued

Action	**Rationale**

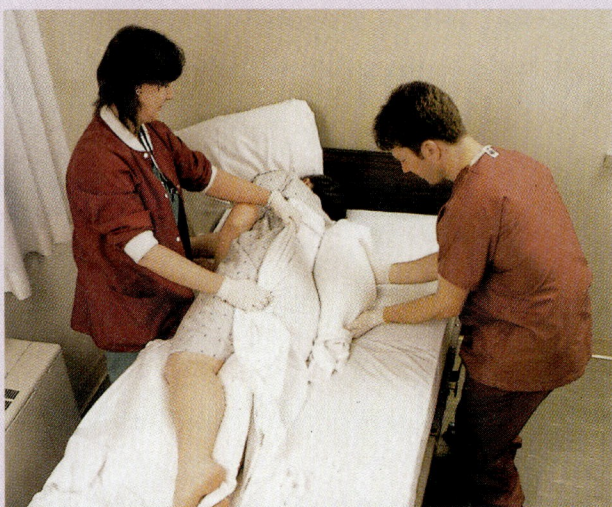

Figure B15-1 Logrolling: Two-Person Move

Action	**Rationale**
6. Tuck pillows at client's back and abdomen.	6. Maintains side-lying position.
7. Assess the client for comfort and proper alignment.	7. Comfort is subjective.
8. Elevate side rails and lower the bed height.	8. Promotes client safety.
9. This procedure can be reversed to reposition clients on their backs or opposite side.	9. Repositioning can prevent development of pressure sores.

Procedure B16   Bedmaking: Unoccupied Bed

Equipment

- Bottom sheet (fitted, if available)
- Draw sheet (regular top sheet may be used)
- Mattress pad (if available)
- Linen bag hamper outside the room
- Top sheet
- Pillowcase (each pillow on the bed)
- Antiseptic solution, washcloth, and towel
- Nonsterile gloves

Action	**Rationale**
Unoccupied Bed	
1. Wash hands.	1. Reduces transmission of microorganisms.
2. Place hamper by client's door if linen bags are not available. Explain procedure to client. Assess condition of blanket and/or bedspread.	2. Provides for proper disposal of soiled linens. Encourages client cooperation. Allows for organization of supplies.
3. Gather linen and gloves. Place linen on a clean, dry surface in reverse order of usage at the client's bedside (pillowcases, top sheet, draw sheet, bottom sheet).	3. Provides easy access to items.
4. Inquire about the client's toileting needs and attend as necessary.	4. Provides for client comfort and prevents interruptions during bedmaking.

continued

Action	Rationale
5. Assist client to a safe, comfortable chair.	**5.** Increases client's comfort and decreases risk for falls.
6. Don gloves.	**6.** Decreases risk of infection from soiled, contaminated linens.
7. Position bed: flat, side rails down, adjust height to waist level.	**7.** Promotes good body mechanics and decreases back strain.
8. Remove and fold blanket and/or bedspread. If clean and reusable, place on clean work area.	**8.** Keeps reusable bed linens clean.
9. Remove soiled pillowcases by grasping the closed end with one hand and slipping the pillow out with the other. Place soiled cases on top of soiled sheet and put pillows on clean work area.	**9.** Allows easy removal of the pillowcases without contamination of uniform by soiled linens and keep pillows clean.
10. Remove soiled linens: Start on the side of the bed closest to you; free the bottom sheet by lifting the mattress and rolling soiled linens to the middle of the bed. Go to the other side of the bed, repeat action.	**10.** Prevents tearing and fanning of linens. Linens are folded from cleanest area to most soiled to prevent contamination.
11. Fold soiled linens: head of bed to middle, foot of bed to middle. Place in linen bag or hamper, keeping soiled linens away from uniform.	**11.** Fanning linens increases number of microorganisms in air. Folding linens decreases the risk of transmission of infection to others.
12. Check mattress and pad, if used. If the pad is soiled, replace. If the mattress is soiled, clean with an antiseptic solution and dry thoroughly.	**12.** Reduces transmission of microorganisms.
13. Remove gloves, wash hands.	**13.** Reduces transmission of microorganisms to clean linens.
14. Open clean bottom sheet lengthwise onto the bed with the seamed side of the sheet toward the mattress. Unfold half of the sheet's width to center crease and smooth the sheet flat (refer to action 15 for placing sheet onto mattress).	**14.** Facilitates making bed in an organized, time-saving manner by not having to go from one side of the bed to the other.
15. Proceed with placing bottom sheet onto the mattress:	
a. Fitted sheet	
• Position yourself diagonally toward the head of the bed.	• Prevents back strain. Placement of seamed side toward mattress prevents irritation to the client's skin. Proper placement of linens ensures adequate sheeting for all sides of the bed.
• Start at the head with seamed side of the fitted sheet toward the mattress.	
• Lift the mattress corner with your hand closest to the bed; with your other hand, pull and tuck the fitted sheet over the mattress corner; secure at the head and sides.	
• Repeat action at foot of bed.	
b. Flat regular sheet	
• Lay the bottom edge of the sheet on the top of the mattress even with the foot of the bed.	• Ensures proper placement of the sheet so that it can be tightly secured at the top and on both sides of the bed.

continued

Action	Rationale
• Allow the sheet to hang 10 inches (25 cm) over the mattress on the side and at the top of the bed.	
• Position yourself diagonally toward the head of the bed. Lift the top of the mattress corner with the hand closest to the bed and smoothly tuck the sheet under the mattress (Figure B16-1).	• Prevents straining of back muscles; decreases the chance that the sheet will pull out from under the mattress.

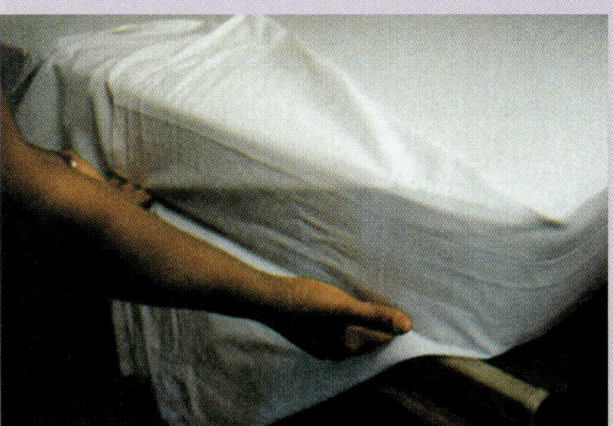

Figure B16-1 Tuck the sheet under the mattress corner.

Action	Rationale
16. Miter the corner at the head of the bed.	16. Secures sheet tightly to the mattress; with the triangular fold providing a smooth tuck to keep the linen in place.
a. Face the side of bed and lift and lay the top edge of the sheet onto the bed to form a triangular fold (Figure B16-2A).	
b. Tuck lower edge of sheet (hanging free at side of mattress) under mattress.	
c. Grasp the triangular fold, bring it down over the side of the mattress and tuck the sheet smoothly under the mattress (Figure B16-2B). Straighten the free hanging sheet on mattress side.	

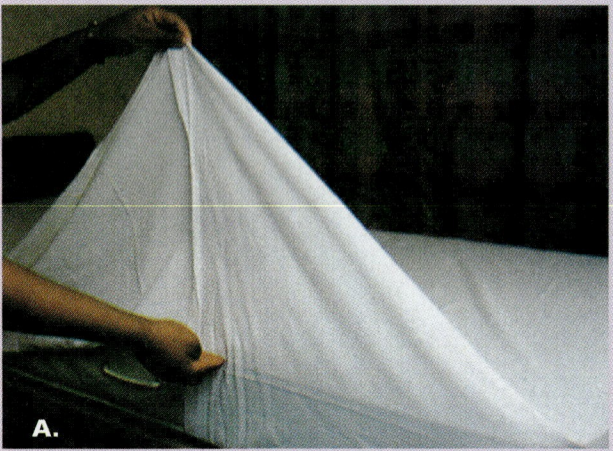 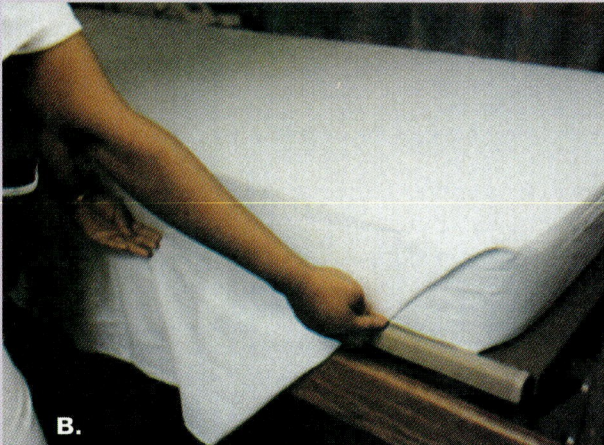

Figure B16-2 A. Lay the top edge of the sheet onto the bed to form a triangular fold. B. Bring the triangular fold down over the side of the mattress and tuck the sheet under the mattress.

continued

Action	Rationale
17. Place draw sheet onto top of bottom sheet and unfold to middle crease. Both sheets should hang 10 inches (25 cm) over the side of the mattress.	**17.** Provides a sheet to lift and move the client in bed without having to use the bottom sheet and remake the bed. Helps to keep bottom sheet clean.
18. Face the side of the bed, palms of hands down. Tuck both the bottom and draw sheets under the mattress. Ensure that the bottom sheet is tucked smoothly under the mattress all the way to the foot of the bed.	**18.** Keeps sheets taut, in place, and wrinkle-free, decreasing the risk of skin irritation.
19. Go to the other side of the bed, unfold the bottom sheet, repeating actions 14 to 16.	**19.** Unfolding decreases air current, which can spread microorganisms.
20. Unfold the draw sheet and grasp the free hanging sides of both the bottom and draw sheets. Pull toward you, keeping your back straight, and with a firm grasp (sheets taut) tuck both sheets under the mattress. Use your arms and open palms to extend the linen under the mattress.	**20.** Uses your body's weight in pulling the sheet taut and prevents strain on your back muscles.
21. Place the top sheet on top of bed and unfold lengthwise, placing the center crease (width) of the sheet in the middle of the bed. Place the top edge of the sheet (seam up) even with the top of the mattress at the head of the bed. Pull the remaining length toward the bottom of the bed.	**21.** Making one side of the bed at a time saves time and movement. Seam will be folded down to prevent contact with the client's skin, which can result in irritation.
22. Unfold and apply the blanket or spread; repeat action 21.	**22.** Provides warmth.
23. Miter the bottom corners as described in action 16.	**23.** Secures linen at the foot of the bed.
24. Face the head of the bed and fold the top sheet and blanket over 6 inches (15 cm). Fan-fold the sheet and blanket (from the head to the middle of the bed).	**24.** Allows the client to get under the covers easily.
25. Apply clean pillowcase on each pillow. With one hand, grasp the closed end of the pillowcase. Gather case and turn it inside out over hand. With same hand, grasp the middle of one end of the pillow. With the other hand, pull the case over the length of the pillow. The corners of the pillow should fit snugly into the corners of the case.	**25.** Keeps clean pillowcase away from your uniform.
26. Return the bed to the lowest position and elevate the head of the bed 30 to 45 degrees. Put side rails up on side, farthest from client.	**26.** Allows the client easy access to the bed. Provides for client safety.
27. Inquire about toileting needs of the client; assist as necessary.	**27.** Saves client energy and provides time to care for the client's needs.
28. Assist the client back into the bed and pull up the side rails; place call light in reach; take vital signs.	**28.** Promotes client safety and a means to call for assistance. Sitting up in a chair and movement may cause changes in the client's vital signs.
29. Document your actions and the client's response during the procedure and to being up in a chair.	**29.** Documents completion of procedure and assessment findings of client's tolerance.

continued

Action	Rationale

Surgical Bed

30. Follow steps 1-22 Bedmaking: Unoccupied Bed

30. See Rationales 1–22.

31. Face the head of the bed and fold the top sheet and blanket over 6 inches (15 cm). Face the foot of the bed and fold the top sheet and blanket up so the fold is even with the bottom of the mattress. Standing on the side of the bed where the client will be transferred from the stretcher, face the bed and bring the bottom corner and top corner to the center of the bed, forming a triangle. Fan-fold the top sheet and the blanket to the side of the bed opposite where the stretcher will be placed.

31. Allows easy transfer of client from stretcher into bed without linens getting in the way.

32. Apply clean pillowcase as in step 25, but do not put pillow on the bed.

32. Keeps bed free of obstacles for easy transfer of client; pillow may be contraindicated for client.

33. Maintain bed in high position with head flat.

33. Places bed in proper position to move client from stretcher to bed.

34. Move furniture out of the way to clear a path from doorway to bed.

34. Allows stretcher to be easily brought to bedside.

35. Have the following items available: tissues, emesis basin, blood pressure cuff and stethoscope, IV pole, I&O sheet, and any other equipment specific to client's needs.

35. Ensures supplies and equipment are easily accessible.

36. When client returns, assist with transfer from stretcher to bed (Procedure B14). Pull top sheet and blanket over client. Tuck in top sheet and blanket, leaving room for client's feet.

36. Provides warmth, secures linens, and allows space for feet.

37. Adjust head of bed according to client preference or postoperative orders. When immediate post-operative care is completed, raise side rails, place bed in low position, and put call bell within client's reach.

37. Provides for client safety.

38. Wash hands.

38. Prevents transmission of microorganisms.

39. Document your actions and the client's response.

39. Facilitates communication among members of the health care team.

Procedure B17 — Bedmaking: Occupied Bed

Equipment

- Linen hamper
- Pillowcase
- Bath blanket

- Top sheet, draw sheet, bottom sheet
- Blanket
- Gloves if risk of exposure to body fluids

Action	Rationale

1. Apply gloves if indicated.

1. Promotes asepsis.

2. Explain procedure to client.

2. Promotes client cooperation.

continued

Action	Rationale

3. Remove top sheet and blanket. Loosen bottom sheet at foot and sides of bed. Lower side rail on side of nurse. Client should be covered with a bath blanket.

3. Facilitates easy removal of linen. Lowering only side rail close to nurse reduces client's risk of falls. Bath blanket prevents exposure and chills.

4. Position client on side, facing away from you. Reposition pillow under head.

4. Provides space to place clean linen.

5. Fan-fold or roll bottom linens close to client toward the center of the bed (Figure B17-1).

5. Maintains soiled linen together. Promotes comfort when client later rolls to other side.

6. Place clean bottom linens with the center fold nearest the client. Fan-fold or roll clean bottom linens nearest client and tuck under soiled linen (Figure B17-2). Maintain an adequate amount of sheet at head for tucking. Sheet should be even with the bottom edge of mattress.

6. Provides for maximum fit of sheets and decreases chance of wrinkles.

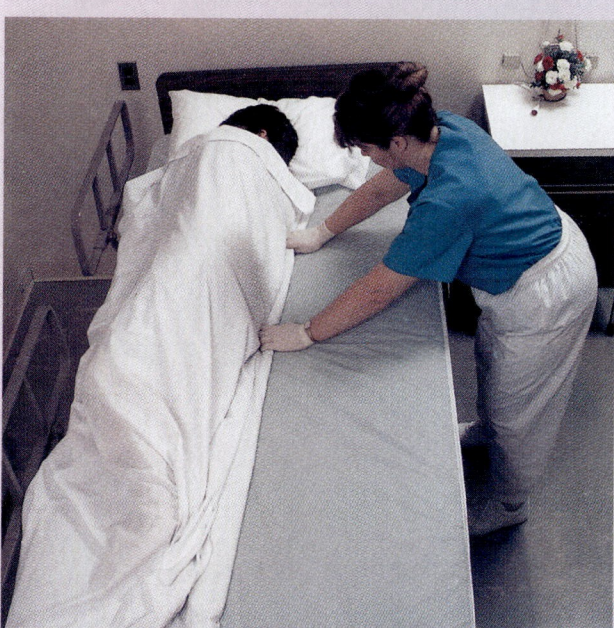

Figure B17-1 Fan-fold or roll the bottom linens close to the client toward the center of the bed.

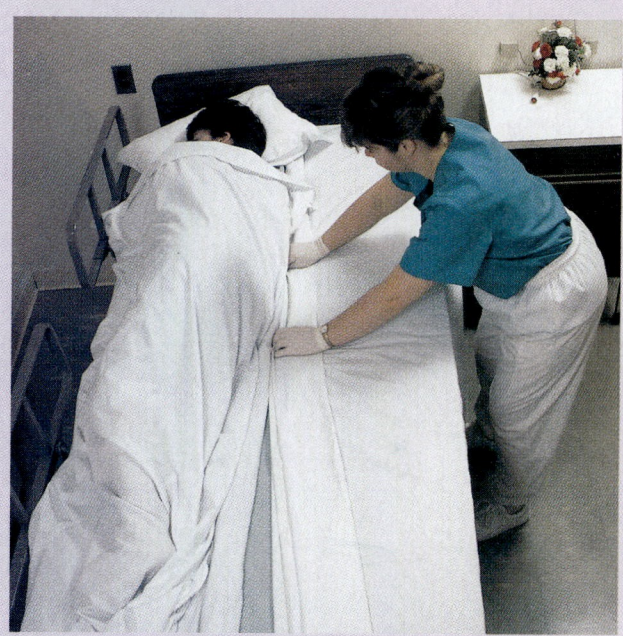

Figure B17-2 Fan-fold the clean bottom linens nearest the client and tuck under the soiled linens.

7. Miter bottom sheet at head of bed. To miter, lift mattress and tuck sheet over the edge of the mattress, lift edge of sheet that is hanging to form a triangle and lay upper part of sheet back onto bed; tuck the lower hanging section under the mattress. Tuck the sides of the sheet under the mattress.

7. Holds linens firmly in place.

8. Fold draw sheet in half. Identify the center of the draw sheet and place close to the client. Fan-fold or roll draw sheet closest to client and tuck under soiled linen; refer to Figure B17-3. Smooth linen. Tuck draw sheet under mattress, working from the center to the edges. Draw sheet should be positioned under the lower back and buttocks.

8. Draw sheet facilitates moving and lifting clients while in bed.

9. Log roll client over onto side facing you. Raise side rail.

9. Positions client off soiled linen. Protects client from falling.

continued

Action	Rationale
10. Move to other side of bed. Remove soiled linens by rolling into a bundle and place in linen hamper without touching uniform.	10. Prevents cross-contamination.
11. Unfold/unroll bottom sheet, then draw sheet. Look for objects left in the bed. Grasp each sheet with knuckles up and over the sheet and pull tightly while leaning back with your body weight (Figure B17-4). Client may be positioned supine or side-lying.	11. Tight sheets keep linens wrinkle-free and decrease risk of skin irritation. Leaning back uses body weight for good body mechanics.

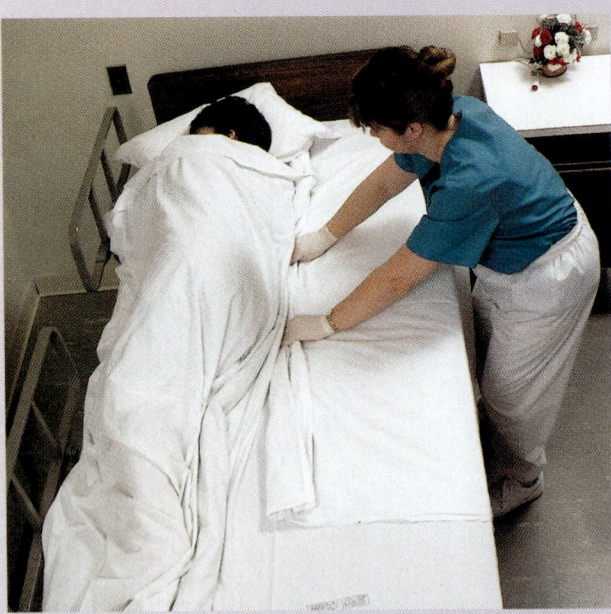

Figure B17-3 Fan-fold the draw sheet close to the client and tucking under the soiled linen.

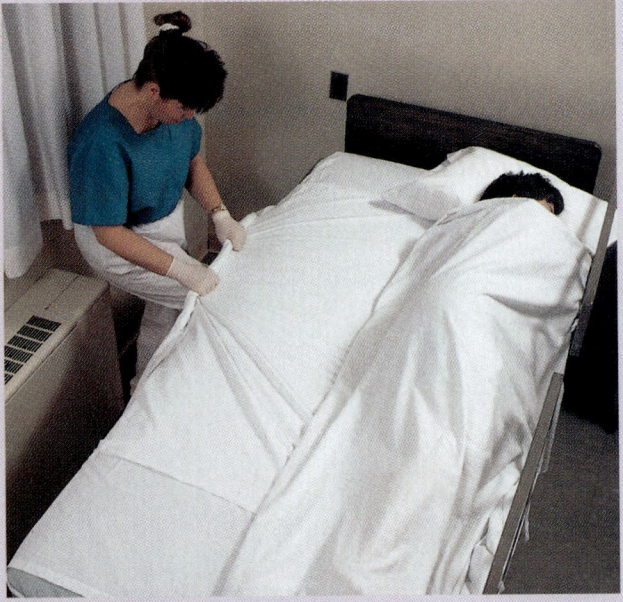

Figure B17-4 Grasp the bottom and draw sheets and pull tightly.

Action	Rationale
12. Place top sheet over client with center of sheet in middle of bed. Unfold top of sheet over client. Remove bath blanket left on client to prevent exposure during bedmaking. Place top blanket over client, as you did with the top sheet.	12. Provides client with top sheet and blanket to prevent chilling.
13. Raise foot of mattress and tuck the corner of the top sheet and blanket under. Miter the corner. Repeat with other side of mattress.	13. Secures top sheet and blanket in place.
14. Grasp top sheet and blanket over client's toes and pull upward, then make a small fan-fold in the sheet.	14. Permits client to move feet under the sheets. Provides room under the tight top sheet and blanket.
15. Remove soiled pillowcase. Grasp center of clean pillowcase and invert pillowcase over hand/arm. Maintain grasp of pillowcase while grasping center of pillow. Use other hand to pull pillowcase down over pillow. Place pillow under client's head. While changing pillowcase, client can be instructed to rest head on bed, or place a blanket under client's head.	15. Provides clean pillowcase without shaking pillow or pillowcases. Promotes comfort.
16. Document procedure used to change linen and client's condition during the procedure.	16. Provides documentation of nursing care and assessment of client's status.

Procedure B18   Adult Bath

Equipment

- Bath towels
- Bath blanket
- Soap
- Lotion
- Powder
- Clean linen

- Washcloths
- Washbasin
- Soap dish
- Deodorant
- Clean gown
- Disposable gloves

Action	Rationale
• Check the client's identification band prior to beginning •	
1. Assess client's preferences about bathing.	1. Provides client opportunity to participate in care.
2. Explain procedure to client.	2. Enhances cooperation.
3. Prepare environment. Close doors and windows, adjust temperature, provide time for elimination needs, and provide privacy.	3. Protects from chills during bath and increases sense of privacy.
4. Wash hands. Apply gloves. Gloves should be changed when emptying water basin.	4. Reduces potential for transmission of pathogens.
5. Lower side rail on the side close to you. Position client in a comfortable position close to the side near you.	5. Prevents unnecessary reaching. Facilitates use of good body mechanics.
6. If bath blankets are available, place bath blanket over top sheet. Remove top sheet from under bath blanket (Figure B18-1). Remove client's gown. Bath blanket should be folded to expose only the area being cleaned at that time. (Top sheets may also be used for bath blankets.)	6. Prevents exposure of client. Promotes privacy; protects from chills.

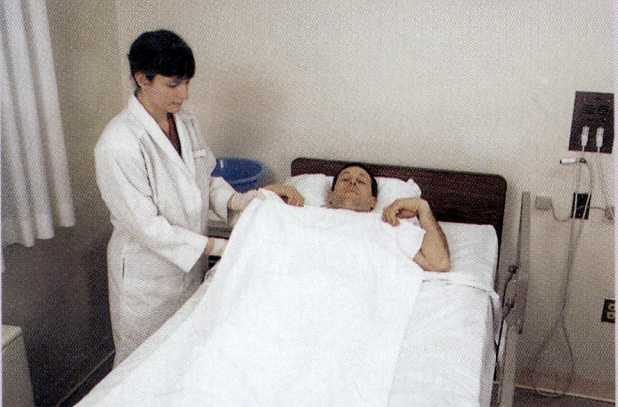

Figure B18-1 Place a bath blanket over the top sheet and remove the sheet from under the blanket.

7. Fill washbasin two-thirds full. Permit client to test temperature of water with his or her hand. Water should be changed when a soapy film develops or water becomes soiled.	7. Prevents accidental burns or chills.

continued

Action	Rationale
8. Make a bath mitten with the washcloth. To make a mitten: grasp the edge of the washcloth with the thumb; fold a third over the palm of the hand; wrap remainder of cloth around hand and across palm, grasping the second edge under the thumb; fold the extended end of the washcloth onto the palm and tuck under the palmar surface of the cloth.	8. Prevents ends of washcloth from dragging across skin. Promotes friction during bath.
9. Wash the face. Ask the client about preference for using soap on the face. Use a separate corner of the washcloth for each eye, wiping from inner to outer canthus (Figure B18-2). Wash neck and ears. Rinse and pat dry. Male clients may want to shave at this time. Provide assistance with shaving as needed.	9. Some clients may not use soap on their face. Using separate corners of washcloth reduces risk of transmitting microorganisms. Patting dry reduces skin irritation and drying.
10. Wash arms, forearms, and hands. Wash forearms and arms using long, firm strokes in the direction of distal to proximal (wrist to upper arm; Figure 18-3). Arm may need to be supported while being washed. Wash axilla. Rinse and pat dry. Apply deodorant or powder if desired. Immerse client's hand into basin of water. Allow hand to soak about 3 to 5 minutes. Wash hands, interdigit area, fingers, and fingernails. Rinse and pat dry.	10. Long strokes promote circulation. Soaking hands softens nails and loosens soil from skin and nails. Strokes directed distal to proximal promote venous return. Powder removes excess moisture.

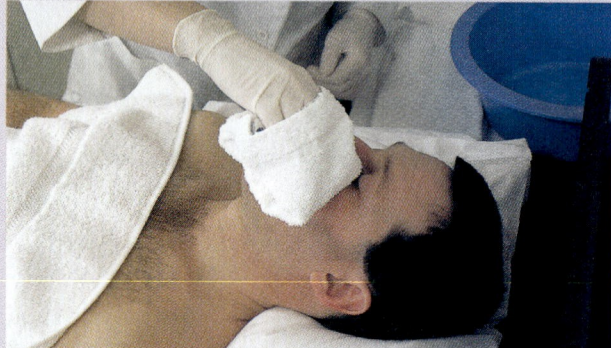

Figure B18-2 Clean the eye with the corner of the washcloth, wiping from the inner to the outer canthus.

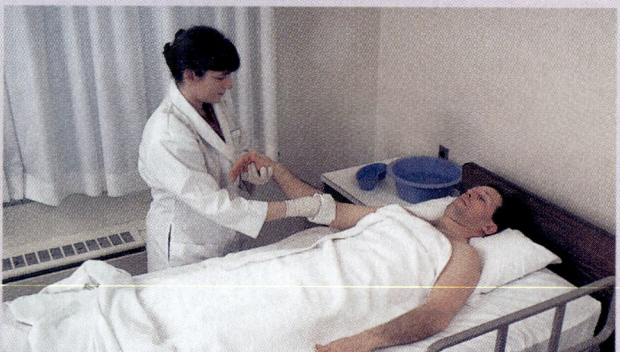

Figure B18-3 Wash forearms and arms in the direction of the wrist to upper arm.

Action	Rationale
11. Wash chest and abdomen. Fold bath blanket down to umbilicus. Wash chest using long, firm strokes. Wash skinfold under the female client's breast by lifting each breast. Rinse and pat dry. Fold bath blanket down to suprapubic area. Use another towel to cover chest area. Wash abdomen using long, firm strokes. Rinse and pat dry. Replace bath blanket over chest and abdomen. Cover chest or abdomen area in between washing, rinsing, and drying to prevent chilling.	11. Promotes privacy and prevents chills. Long strokes promote circulation. Perspiration and soil collect within skin folds.
12. Wash legs and feet. Expose leg farthest from you by folding bath blanket to midline. Bend the leg at the knee. Grasp the heel, elevate the leg from the bed and cover bed with bath towel. Place	12. Supports joint to prevent strain and fatigue. Soaking foot loosens dirt, softens nails, and promotes comfort.

continued

Action	**Rationale**
washbasin on towel. Place client's foot into washbasin. Allow foot to soak while washing the leg with long, firm strokes in the direction of distal to proximal (ankle to thigh; Figure B18-4). Rinse and pat dry. Clean soles, interdigits, and toes. Rinse and pat dry. Perform same procedure with the other leg and foot.	

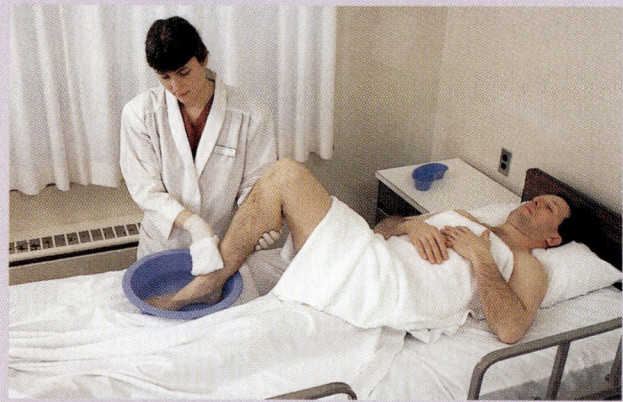

Figure B18-4 Wash the leg and foot in the direction of ankle to thigh.

Action	**Rationale**
13. Wash back. Assist client into prone or side-lying position facing away from you. Wash the back and buttocks using long, firm strokes. Rinse and pat dry. Give back rub and apply lotion.	**13.** Exposes back and buttocks for washing. Back rub promotes relaxation and circulation.
14. Perineal care: Assist client to supine position. Perform perineal care (see Procedure B19).	**14.** Removes genital secretions and oil.
15. Apply lotion and powder as desired. Apply clean gown.	**15.** Lotion lubricates skin. Powder absorbs excess perspiration.
16. Document skin assessment, type of bath given, and client outcomes and responses.	**16.** Provides evidence of nursing care.

Procedure B19   Perineal Care

Equipment

- Bath basin
- Soap
- Two or three washcloths
- Dry bath towel
- Bath blanket

- Waterproof pads
- Toilet tissue
- Lotion or ointment
- Disposable gloves

Action	**Rationale**
• *Check the client's identification band prior to beginning* •	
1. Explain procedure and purpose to client. Obtain permission. Close door and pull curtain around bed.	**1.** Promotes cooperation. Provides privacy.
2. Wash hands and apply gloves.	**2.** Reduces transmission of pathogens.

continued

Action	Rationale
3. Place waterproof pad under client's buttocks. Client may be placed on a bedpan for perineal care. Females usually assume the dorsal recumbent position. Males may assume the dorsal recumbent or supine position with knees and hips flexed.	**3.** Waterproof pad prevents wetting of linen. Dorsal recumbent position provides maximal visualization of genital area.
4. Expose perineal area. Fold client's gown up above the genital area. Place a bath blanket over the client using a "diamond" draping technique. Corners of bath blanket should point toward the head, sides of body, and between the client's legs. Fold top linen down to the end of the bed. Tuck side corners of bath blanket around client's legs. Lift corner between client's legs to expose perineal area (Figure B19-1).	**4.** Draping promotes a sense of privacy and decreases exposure.

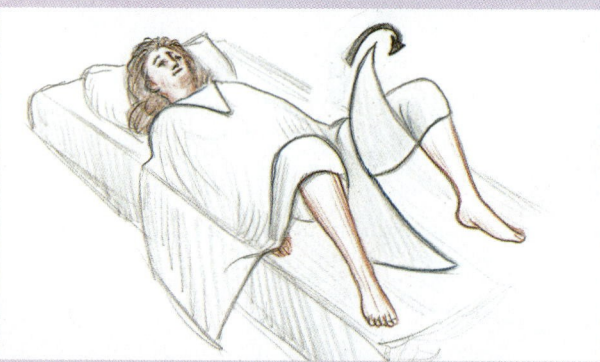

Figure B19-1 Drape the client for perineal care.

Action	Rationale
5. Moisten and lather washcloths. Female: Clean perineal area in the downward direction (from pubic area to rectum). Clean and dry upper thighs. Use separate quarters of the washcloth for each cleaning stroke. Discard soiled washcloths as necessary. Clean the labia majora. Separate the labia majora to clean between the labia majora and labia minora. With the labia separated, clean the clitoris, urethral meatus, and vaginal orifice (Figure B19-2). Rinse the area well with warm water. Pat perineal area dry. Apply lotion to upper thighs. Male: Gently raise penis. May place a bath blanket under the penis. If the client develops an erection, delay perineal care. Gently grasp the shaft of the penis. If the client is uncircumcised, retract the foreskin. Use a circular motion to clean the meatus of the penis and glans in an outward direction (Figure B19-3). Replace the foreskin after cleansing the glans. Clean the shaft of the penis. Rinse penis. Pat glans and shaft of penis dry. Clean and dry scrotum. Scrotum may need to be lifted during cleaning. Discard soiled washcloths as necessary.	**5.** Cleaning in the direction of the pubic area to rectum reduces risk of transmitting fecal material to the urinary tract. Using clean area of washcloth for each stroke reduces risk of transmitting organisms. Cleaning between the labia removes accumulated smegma. Gentle handling reduces chance of an erection. Smegma accumulates around the foreskin. Replacing of foreskin prevents phimosis. Cleaning moves from area of least to most soiled.

continued

Action	Rationale

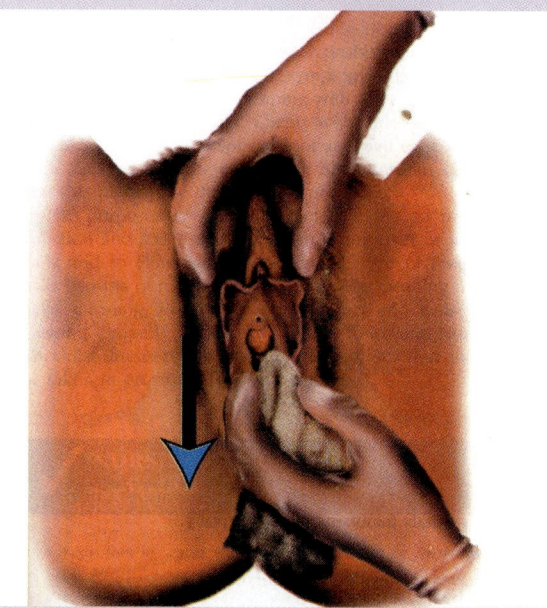

Figure B19-2 Clean the female perineal area.

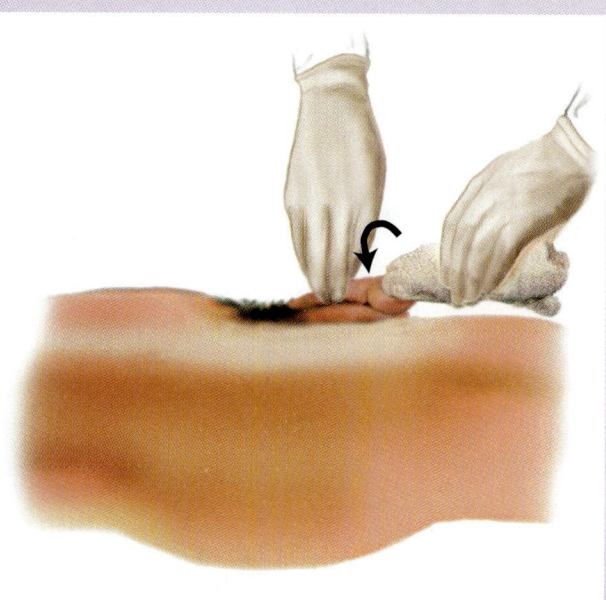

Figure B19-3 Clean the male perineal area.

6. Perform anal care. First remove any fecal material with toilet tissue. Clean perineal area by wiping from genitals to anus with one stroke. Discard soiled washcloths as necessary. Clean anus in circular motion. Rinse anal area. Pat dry.

6. Cleaning fecal material with toilet tissue removes the bulk of soil prior to washing. Cleaning from genitals to anus reduces chances of transmitting fecal microorganisms to urinary tract. Patting dry reduces skin irritation.

7. Remove gloves. Wash hands. Remove bath blanket. Place gown down over genitals. Place top linen on client.

7. Reduces transmission of microorganisms. Covering genitals maintains client's privacy.

8. Document procedure performed, client's response, and assessment findings.

8. Provides evidence of nursing care.

Procedure B20   Catheter Care

Equipment

- Clean gloves
- Waterproof pad to protect linens
- Wash cloths, soap, and water

Action	Rationale

• Wash your hands • Check the client's identification band •
• Explain the procedure to the client before beginning •

1. Provide privacy.

1. Protects client dignity.

2. Put on clean gloves.

2. Reduces transmission of microorganisms.

3. Place client in supine position and expose perineal area and catheter.

3. Allows for visualization of field. If unable to visualize the perineal area with the client supine, try placing the client in a side-lying position.

4. Place waterproof pad on bed.

4. Protects linens.

continued

Action	**Rationale**
5. Cleanse periurethral area with soap and water (Figure B20-1). Cleanse meatus in circular motion from the most inner surface to the outside.	5. Soap has antibacterial qualities adequate to clean the area and will usually not irritate the skin or mucous membranes. Moving from the cleanest area out decreases risk of recontamination.

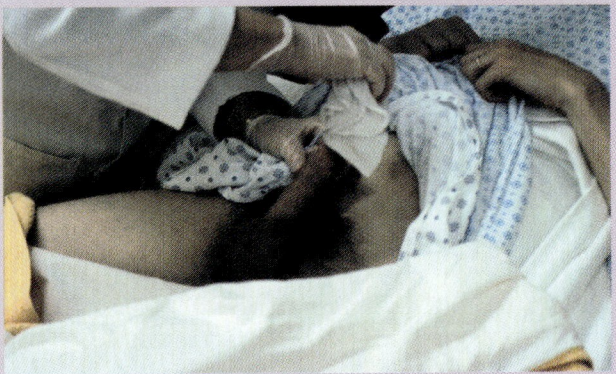

Figure B20-1 Using a washcloth, cleanse the penis and perineal area with soap and warm water.

6. With clean washcloth, cleanse catheter from meatus to end of catheter, taking care not to pull on catheter.	6. Decreases risk of contamination.
7. Be sure to repeat catheter care anytime the periurethral area becomes soiled with stool or other drainage.	7. Reduces risk of infection.
8. Place linen in proper receptacle for laundry or disposal.	8. Reduces transmission of infection to other clients.
9. Remove gloves and wash hands.	9. Reduces transmission of microorganisms.
10. Document care given.	10. Communicates to other caregivers what care was given.

Procedure B21   Oral Hygiene

Equipment

Brushing and Flossing
- Toothbrush
- Toothpaste
- Emesis basin
- Towel
- Cup of water
- Nonsterile gloves
- Dental floss
- Dental-floss holder
- Mirror
- Lip moisturizer

Denture Care
- Denture brush
- Denture cleaner
- Emesis basin
- Towel
- Cup of water
- Nonsterile gloves
- Tissue
- Denture cup

Special Care Items for Clients with Impaired Physical Mobility or Who Are Unconscious (comatose)
- Soft toothbrush or toothette
- Tongue blade

continued

Equipment *continued*

- 3 × 3 gauze sponges
- Cotton-tip applicators
- Prescribed solution and/or milk of magnesia

- Plastic Asepto syringe
- Suction machine and catheter

Action	Rationale

• Check the client's identification band • Explain the procedure to the client prior to beginning •

Self-Care Client

Flossing and Brushing

Action	Rationale
1. Assemble articles for flossing and brushing.	1. Promotes efficiency.
2. Provide privacy.	2. Relaxes the client.
3. Place client in a high-Fowler's position.	3. Decreases risk of aspiration.
4. Wash hands and don gloves.	4. Reduces microorganism transfer and exposure to body fluids.
5. Arrange articles within client's reach.	5. Facilitates self-care.
6. Assist client with flossing and brushing as necessary. Position mirror and emesis basin near client for use during activity.	6. Flossing and brushing decrease microorganism growth in mouth. Use of mirror permits cleaning back and sides of teeth.
7. Assist client with rinsing mouth.	7. Removes toothpaste and oral secretions.
8. Reposition client, raise side rails, and place call button within reach.	8. Promotes comfort, safety, and communication.
9. Rinse, dry, and return articles to proper place.	9. Promotes a clean environment.
10. Remove gloves, wash hands, and document care.	10. Prevents the transmission of microorganisms and documents nursing care.

Denture Care

Action	Rationale
11. Assemble articles for denture cleaning.	11. Promotes efficiency.
12. Provide privacy.	12. Relaxes the client.
13. Assist client to a high-Fowler's position.	13. Facilitates removal of dentures.
14. Wash hands and don gloves.	14. Reduces microorganism transfer and exposure to body fluids.
15. Assist client with denture removal:	15. Breaks seal created with dentures without causing pressure and injury to oral membranes.
a. Top denture:	
• With tissue, grasp the denture with thumb and forefinger and pull downward.	• Prevents breaking of dentures.
• Place in denture cup.	
b. Bottom denture:	
• Place thumbs on the gums and release the denture. Grasp denture with thumb and forefingers and pull upward.	
• Place in denture cup.	

continued

Action	**Rationale**
16. Apply toothpaste to brush and brush dentures either with cool water in the emesis basin or under running water in the sink.	**16.** Facilitates removal of microorganisms.
17. Rinse thoroughly.	**17.** Removes toothpaste.
18. Assist client with rinsing mouth and replacing dentures.	**18.** Freshens mouth and facilitates intake of solid food.
19. Reposition client, with side rails up and call button within reach.	**19.** Promotes comfort, safety, and communication.
20. Rinse, dry, and return articles to proper place.	**20.** Maintains a clean environment.
21. Remove gloves, wash hands, and document care.	**21.** Prevents the transmission of microorganisms and documents nursing care.

Full-Care Client

Brushing and Flossing

Action	**Rationale**
22. Assemble articles for flossing and brushing.	**22.** Promotes efficiency.
23. Provide privacy.	**23.** Relaxes client.
24. Wash hands and don gloves.	**24.** Reduces microorganism transfer and exposure to body fluids.
25. Position client as condition allows: high-Fowler's, semi-Fowler's, or lateral position with head turned toward side.	**25.** Decreases risk of aspiration.
26. Place towel across client's chest or under face and mouth if head is turned to one side.	**26.** Catches secretions.
27. Moisten toothbrush, apply small amount of toothpaste, and brush teeth and gums.	**27.** Moistens mouth and facilitates plaque removal.
28. Grasp the dental floss in both hands or use a floss holder and floss between all teeth, holding floss against tooth while moving floss up and down sides of teeth (Figure B21-1).	**28.** Removes plaque and prevents gum disease.
29. Assist the client in rinsing mouth.	**29.** Removes toothpaste and oral secretions.
30. Reapply toothpaste and brush the teeth and gums using friction in a vertical or circular motion. On inner and outer surfaces of teeth, hold brush at 45 degree angle against teeth and brush from sulcus to crowns of teeth. On biting surfaces, move brush back and forth in short strokes. All surfaces of teeth should be brushed from every angle (Figure B21-2).	**30.** Permits cleaning of back and sides of teeth and decreases microorganism growth in mouth.
31. Assist the client in rinsing and drying mouth.	**31.** Removes toothpaste and oral secretions.
32. Apply lip moisturizer, if appropriate.	**32.** Maintains skin integrity of lips.
33. Reposition client, raise side rails, and place call button within reach.	**33.** Promotes comfort, safety, and communication.
34. Rinse, dry, and return articles to proper place.	**34.** Provides an orderly environment.
35. Remove gloves, wash hands, and document care.	**35.** Prevents transmission of microorganisms and documents nursing care.

continued

Action	**Rationale**

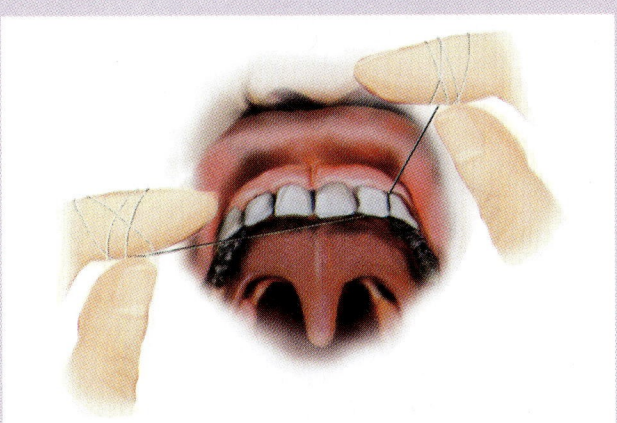

Figure B21-1 Floss teeth.

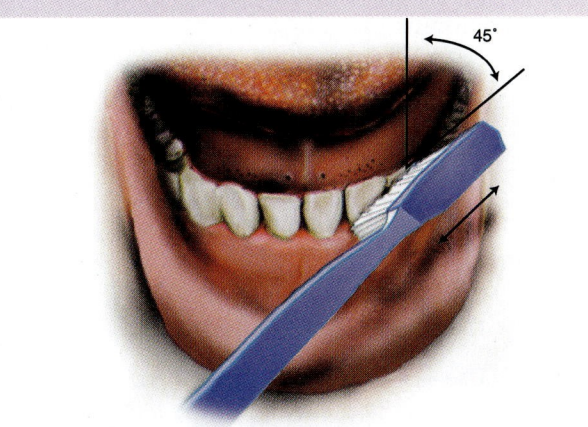

Figure B21-2 Brush teeth.

Clients at Risk for or with an Alteration of the Oral Cavity

Follow actions 22 through 24.

36. Bleeding:	**36.**
a. Assess oral cavity with a padded tongue blade and flashlight for signs of bleeding.	**a.** Determines if bleeding is present, amount, and specific areas.
b. Proceed with the actions for oral care for a full-care client, except:	
• Do not floss.	
• Use a soft toothbrush, toothette, or a tongue blade padded with 3 × 3 gauze sponges to gently swab teeth and gums.	• Decreases risk of bleeding.
• Dispose of padded tongue blade into a bio-hazard bag according to agency policy.	• Promotes proper disposal of contaminated waste.
• Rinse with tepid water.	• Cleanses mouth.
37. Infection:	**37.**
a. Assess oral cavity with a tongue blade and flashlight for signs of infection.	**a.** Determines appearance, integrity, and general condition of oral cavity.
b. Culture lesions as ordered.	**b.** Identifies growth of specific microorganisms.
c. Proceed with the actions for oral care for a full-care client except:	
• Do not floss.	• Prevents irritation, pain, and bleeding.
• Use prescribed antiseptic solution.	• Antiseptic solutions decrease growth of microorganisms.
• Use a tongue blade padded with 3 × 3 gauze sponges to gently swab the teeth and gums.	
• Dispose of padded tongue blade into a bio-hazard bag according to institutional policy.	• Promotes proper disposal of contaminated materials.
• Rinse mouth with tepid water.	• Cleanses mouth.

continued

Action	Rationale

38. Ulcerations:
 	
   a. Assess oral cavity with a tongue blade and flashlight for signs of ulcerations.
 	
   b. Culture lesions as ordered.
 	
   c. Proceed with actions for oral care for a full-care client except:
 	
     • Do not floss.
 	
     • Use prescribed antiseptic solution.
 	
     • Use a tongue blade padded with 3 × 3 gauze sponges to gently swab the teeth and gums.
 	
     • Dispose of padded tongue blade into a biohazard bag according to institutional policy.
 	
     • Rinse mouth with tepid water.
 	
     • Apply solution or paste as prescribed with cotton-tip applicators.
	38. Same as for action 37.
	
	• Provides a coating that promotes healing of the tissue.

Unconscious (Comatose) Client

Action	Rationale
39. Follow actions 22 to 24 for full-care client.	**39.** Same as for actions 22 to 24 for full-care client.
40. Explain the procedure to the client.	**40.** Demonstrates respect for the client.
41. Place the client in a lateral position, head turned toward the side.	**41.** Prevents aspiration.
42. Use a floss holder and floss between all teeth.	**42.** Prevents aspiration.
43. Moisten toothbrush, apply small amount of toothpaste, and brush the teeth and gums as described in action 30.	**43.** See rationale 30.
44. After flossing and brushing, rinse mouth with an Asepto syringe and perform oral suction (see Procedure I22 for a description of oropharyngeal/nasopharyngeal suctioning).	**44.** Promotes cleansing and removal of secretions and prevents aspiration.
45. Dry the client's mouth.	**45.** Prevents skin irritation.
46. Apply lip moisturizer.	**46.** Maintains skin integrity of lips.
47. Leave the client in a lateral position with head turned toward side for 30 to 60 minutes after oral hygiene care. Remove the towel from under the client's mouth and face.	**47.** Prevents pooling of secretions and aspiration.
48. Dispose of any contaminated items in a biohazard bag and clean, dry, and return all articles to the appropriate place.	**48.** Promotes proper disposal of contaminated materials.
49. Remove gloves, wash hands, and document care.	**49.** Prevents the transmission of microorganisms and documents nursing care.
50. Document type of oral care given and client's response.	**50.** Provides record of care given.

Procedure B22 Eye Care: Artificial Eye and Contact Lens Removal

Equipment

Artificial Eye
- Storage container
- Mild soap
- 3 × 3 gauze sponges
- Cotton balls
- Towel
- Emesis basins
- Eye irrigation syringe (optional)
- Running water
- Nonsterile gloves
- Biohazard bag
- Saline solution

Contact Lenses
- Lens container
- Soaking solution (type used by client)
- Towel
- Suction cup (optional)
- Scotch tape (optional)
- Nonsterile gloves

Action	Rationale
• Wash your hands • Check the client's identification band • *• Explain the procedure to the client prior to beginning •*	

Artificial Eye Removal

Action	Rationale
1. Inquire about client's care regimen and gather equipment accordingly.	1. Promotes continuity of care.
2. Provide privacy.	2. Relaxes the client.
3. Wash hands; don gloves.	3. Prevents transmission of microorganisms.
4. Place client in a semi-Fowler's position.	4. Facilitates procedure and client participation.
5. Place the cotton balls in emesis basin and half fill with warm tap water.	5. Dry cotton balls could cause irritation.
6. Place 3 × 3 gauze sponges in bottom of second emesis basin, and half-fill with mild soap and tepid water.	6. Gauze serves as padding to prevent breakage of the prosthesis.
7. Grasp and squeeze excess water from a cotton ball. Cleanse the eyelid with the moistened cotton ball, starting at the inner canthus and moving outward toward the outer canthus. After each use, dispose of cotton ball in biohazard bag. Repeat procedure until eyelid is clean (without dried secretions).	7. Eliminating the excess water prevents water from running down the client's face. Cleansing the eyelid prevents contamination of the lacrimal system (inner canthus area). Disposal of cotton balls prevents transmission of microorganisms to other health care workers.
8. Remove the artificial eye:	8. Promotes removal of artificial eye. Cupping prevents dropping and possible breaking of the eye. Applying pressure will help the prosthesis to slip out.
a. Using dominant hand, raise the client's upper eyelid with index finger and depress the lower eyelid with thumb (Figure B22-1).	
b. Cup nondominant hand under the client's lower eyelid.	
c. Apply slight pressure with index finger between the brow and the artificial eye and remove it.	

continued

Action	**Rationale**

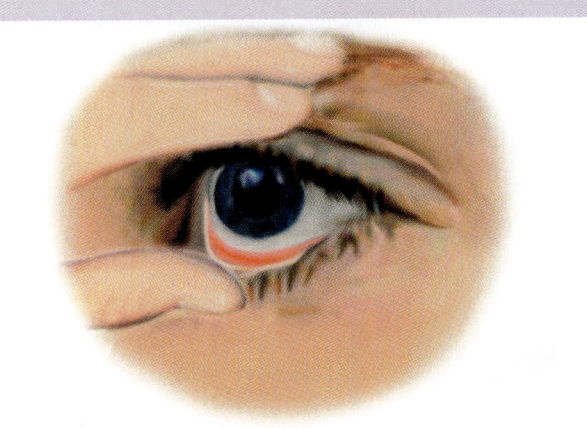

Figure B22-1 Removal of an Artificial Eye

9. Place the artificial eye in the emesis basin that has soap and water.

9. Prevents secretions from adhering to the prosthesis.

10. Grasp a moistened cotton ball and cleanse around the edge of the eye socket. Dispose of the soiled cotton ball into biohazard bag. Keep the prosthesis in the soap-and-water solution.

10. Cleanses the eye socket. Disposal of cotton ball prevents transmission of microorganisms to other health care workers. Keeping eye in solution during cleaning decreases risk of damage.

11. Inspect the eye socket for any signs of irritation, drainage, or crusting.

11. Indicates an infection.

Note: If the client's usual care regimen or physician order requires irrigation of the socket, proceed with step 12; otherwise, go to step 13.

12. Eye socket irrigation:

12.

a. Lower the head of the bed and place the client in a supine position. Place protector pad on bed; turn head toward socket side and slightly extend neck.

a. Cleanses the eye socket and removes secretions. Positioning of client facilitates ease in performing the procedure and client comfort.

b. Fill the irrigation syringe with the prescribed amount and type of irrigating solution (warm tap water or normal saline).

b. Assures compliance with client's regimen or prescribed orders.

c. With nondominant hand, separate the eyelids with your forefinger and thumb, resting fingers on the brow and cheekbone.

c. Keeps the eyelid open and the socket visible.

d. Hold the irrigating syringe in dominant hand several inches above the inner canthus; with thumb, gently apply pressure on the plunger, directing the flow of solution from the inner canthus along the conjunctival sac.

d. Prevents injury to the client.

e. Irrigate until the prescribed amount of solution has been used.

f. Wipe the eyelids with a moistened cotton ball after irrigating. Dispose of soiled cotton ball in biohazard bag.

continued

Action	Rationale
g. Pat the skin dry with the towel.	
h. Return the client to a semi-Fowler's position.	
i. Remove gloves, wash hands, and don clean gloves.	**i.** Prevents transmission of microorganisms to prosthesis.
13. Rub the artificial eye between index finger and thumb in the basin of warm soapy water.	**13.** Creates cleaning with friction and prevents breakage of the prosthesis.
14. Rinse the prosthesis under running water or place in the clean basin of tepid water. Do not dry the prosthesis. *Note:* Either reinsert the prosthesis (step 15) or store in a container (step 16).	**14.** Removes soap and secretions. Keeping the artificial eye wet prevents irritation from lint or other particles that might adhere to it and facilitates reinsertion.
15. Reinsert the prosthesis:	**15.** Facilitates reinsertion of the prosthesis without discomfort to the client.
a. With the thumb of the nondominant hand, raise and hold the upper eyelid open.	
b. With the dominant hand, grasp the artificial eye so that the indented part is facing toward the client's nose and slide it under the upper eyelid as far as possible.	
c. Depress the lower lid.	**c.** Allows the prosthesis to slide into place.
d. Pull the lower lid forward to cover the edge of the prosthesis.	
16. Place the cleaned artificial eye in a labeled container with saline or tap water solution.	**16.** Protects the prosthesis from scratches and keeps it clean.
17. Grasp a moistened cotton ball and squeeze out excessive moisture. Wipe the eyelid from the inner to the outer canthus. Dispose of the soiled cotton ball in a biohazard bag.	**17.** Squeezing the cotton ball removes moisture. Cleansing the eyelid prevents contamination of lacrimal system. Disposal of cotton ball prevents the transmission of microorganisms to other health care workers.
18. Clean, dry, and replace equipment.	**18.** Promotes a clean environment.
19. Reposition the client, raise side rails, and place call light in reach.	**19.** Promotes client's comfort, safety, and communication.
20. Dispose of biohazard bag according to agency policy.	**20.** Prevents the transmission of microorganisms to other health care workers.
21. Remove gloves and wash hands.	**21.** Same as step 20.
22. Document procedure, client's response and participation, and client teaching and level of understanding.	**22.** Demonstrates that the procedure was done and the level of client participation and learning.

Contact Lens Removal

Action	Rationale
23. Assemble equipment for lens removal.	**23.** Promotes efficiency.
24. Assess level of assistance needed, provide privacy, and explain the procedure to the client.	**24.** Level of assistance determines level of intervention. Privacy reduces anxiety. Explanation of procedure promotes cooperation.
25. Wash hands and don gloves.	**25.** Reduces transfer of microorganisms.

continued

Action	Rationale
26. Assist the client to a semi-Fowler's position.	**26.** Facilitates removal of lens.
27. Drape a clean towel over the client's chest.	**27.** Provides a clean surface and facilitates the location of a lens if it falls during removal.
28. Prepare the lens storage case with the pre-scribed solution. If storage case is not available, put each lens in a separate sterile specimen cup with saline. Label right and left.	**28.** Hard lenses can be stored dry or in a special soaking solution. Soft lenses are stored in sterile normal saline *without* a preservative.
29. Instruct the client to look straight ahead. Assess the location of the lens. If it is not on the cornea, either you or the client should gently move the lens toward the cornea with pad of index finger.	**29.** Client's position promotes easy removal of lens. Positioning lens on the cornea aids removal. Use of the finger pad of the index finger prevents damage to cornea and lens.
30. Remove the lens.	**30.** Cupping the hand under eye helps to catch the lens and prevent breakage. Pulling corner of the eye tightens eyelid against eyeball. Pressure on upper edge of lens causes lens to tip forward.
a. Hard lens:	
• Cup nondominant hand under the eye.	
• Gently place index finger on the outside cor-ner of the eye and pull toward the temple and ask client to blink (Figure B22-2).	
b. Soft lens:	
• With nondominant hand, separate the eyelid with your thumb and middle finger.	• Separating the eyelid exposes the lower edge of lens.
• With the index finger of the dominant hand gently placed on the lower edge of the lens, slide the lens downward onto the sclera and gently squeeze the lens.	• Positions lens for easy grasping with the pad of the index finger, which prevents injury to the cornea and lens. Squeezing the lens allows air to enter and release the suction.
• Release the top eyelid (continue holding the lower lid down) and remove the lens with your index finger and thumb (Figure B22-3).	

Figure B22-2 Removal of a Hard Contact Lens

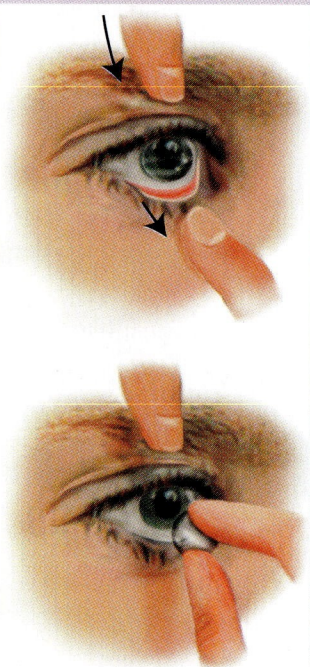

Figure B22-3 Removal of a Soft Contact Lens

continued

Action	Rationale
Note: If step 30 is unsuccessful, secure a suction cup to remove the contact lens. If you are unable to remove the lens, notify the physician.	Suction cup is used to remove a lens from an unconscious or dependent client.
31. Store the lens in the correct compartment of the case ("right" or "left"). Label with the client's name.	**31.** Storage prevents damage to the lenses and ensures that each lens will be reinserted into the correct eye.
32. Remove the other lens by repeating steps 30 and 31.	**32.** Refer to steps 30 and 31.
33. Assess eyes for irritation or redness.	**33.** Signs of corneal irritation.
34. Store the lens case in a safe place.	**34.** Prevents damage or loss.
35. Dispose of soiled articles; clean and return reusable articles to proper location.	**35.** Reduces transmission of infection.
36. Reposition the client, raise side rails, and place call light in reach. *Be aware that client may have trouble seeing if eyeglasses are not available.*	**36.** Promotes client comfort, safety, and communication.
37. Remove gloves and wash hands.	**37.** Prevents transmission of infection.
38. Document procedure, client's response and assessment findings, and the storage place of the lenses.	**38.** Documents the removal of lenses, condition of the cornea, and where the lenses are stored.

Procedure B23   Giving a Back Rub

Equipment

- Quiet environment, free of interruptions, with a comfortable room temperature
- Bath blanket
- Lotion, baby powder, or massage oil
- Comfortable bed or massage table that allows a client to lie in a side-lying or prone position
- Bath towel to absorb excess moisture, oils
- Gloves if necessary

Action	Rationale
• Check the client's identification band • Explain the procedure to the client prior to beginning •	
1. Wash your hands and don gloves if necessary.	1. Reduces the transmission of microorganisms.
2. Help client to a prone or side-lying position (Figure B23-1).	2. Exposes back and shoulder area.

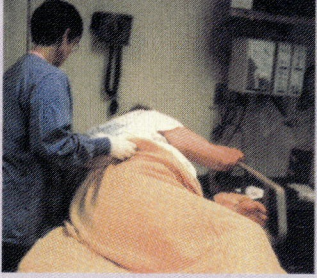

Figure B23-1 Position client in a prone or side-lying position.

continued

Action	**Rationale**
3. Drape the bath blanket, and undo the client's gown exposing the back, shoulder, and sacral area, keeping the remainder of the body covered (Figure B23-2).	**3.** Prevents chilling and excess exposure.
4. Pour a small amount of lotion in your hand and warm between your palms for a few moments. The lotion bottle can also be submerged in a bowl of warm water for a few minutes to warm the lotion. Baby powder may be substituted for oils or lotions (Figure B23-3).	**4.** Prevents cold lotion being applied to the body. Some clients may be sensitive to oils or lotions.

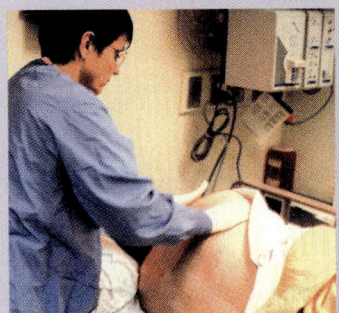

Figure B23-2 Expose the back, shoulder, and sacral area.

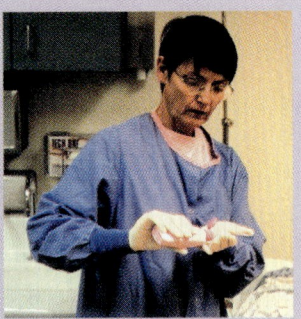

Figure B23-3 Pour lotion on your hand and warm between your palms.

5. Begin in the sacral area with smooth, circular strokes, moving upward toward the shoulders. Gradually lengthen the strokes (effleurage) to the upper back, scapulae, and upper arms. Apply firm, continuous pressure without breaking contact with the client (Figure B23-4).	**5.** Applying firm, continuous pressure increases circulation and relaxation.
6. Assess client's back as you are massaging for areas of redness and signs of decreased circulation.	**6.** Monitors for signs of early skin breakdown.
7. Provide a firm, kneading massage (petrissage) to areas of increased tension if desired, in areas such as the shoulders and gluteal muscles.	**7.** Firm, kneading strokes can decrease muscle tension, reducing pain and increasing relaxation.
8. Complete the massage with long, very light brush strokes, using the tips of the fingers.	**8.** A very relaxing stroke; signals end of the massage.

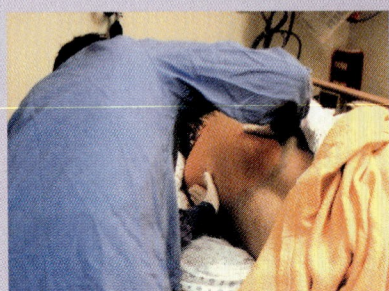

Figure B23-4 Apply firm continuous pressure without breaking contact between your hands and the client's skin.

continued

Action	Rationale
9. Gently pat or wipe excess lubricant off of the client and cover the client.	9. Prevents soiling of the bed with excess lotions and keeps the client warm.
10. Wash hands.	10. Reduces the transmission of microorganisms.
11. Document back rub, client's response to back rub, and any unusual findings.	11. Provides record of care and client's response.

Procedure B24 — Shaving a Client

Equipment

- Electric or disposable razor
- Warm water
- Washbasin
- Mirror
- Gloves
- Shaving cream or soap
- Washcloth and bath towel
- After-shave lotion (if the client has no skin irritation and prefers lotion)
- Sharp scissors and comb (if mustache care required)

Action	Rationale
• Check client's identification band • Explain the procedure to the client prior to beginning •	
1. Wash hands and apply gloves	1. Reduces the transmission of microorganisms.
2. Assist the client to a comfortable position. If the client can shave himself, set up the equipment and supplies, including warm water, and watch the client for safety. Adjust lighting as needed. Follow agency policy.	2. Facilitates comfort and ease of shaving. Encourages autonomy. Facilitates proper body mechanics and prevents injury to client.
3. Place a towel over the client's chest and shoulder.	3. Protects the client and gown from soil.
4. Fill a washbasin with water at approximately 44°C (110°F). Have client check temperature for comfort.	4. Warm water helps to soften the skin and beard; relaxes client.
5. Place the washcloth in the basin and wring out thoroughly. Apply the cloth over the client's entire face.	5. Same rationale as action 4.
6. Apply shaving cream.	6. Helps soften the whiskers.
7. Take the razor in the dominant hand and hold it at a 45° angle to the client's skin. Start shaving across one side of the client's face. Use the non-dominant hand to gently pull the skin taut while shaving. Use short, firm strokes in the direction of hair growth. Use short, downward strokes over the upper lip area (Figure B24-1).	7. Prevents razor cuts and discomfort during shaving.
8. Rinse the razor in water as cream accumulates.	8. Keeps the cutting edge of the razor clean.
9. Check the face to see if all facial hair is removed.	9. Ensures a neat appearance.
10. After all facial hair is removed, rinse the client's face thoroughly with a moistened washcloth.	10. Promotes comfort and cleanliness.

continued

Action	**Rationale**

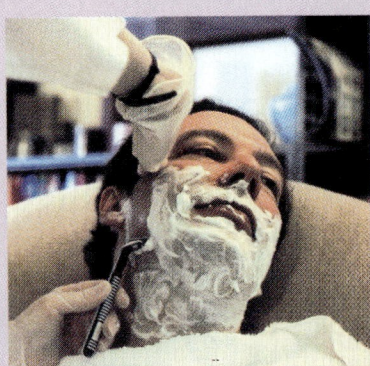

Figure B24-1 Shave with short, firm strokes in the direction the hair grows.

11. Pat client's face dry and apply after-shave lotion if desired.	**11.** Promotes skin integrity; stimulates and lubricates the skin.
12. Assist the client to a comfortable position and allow him to inspect the results of your shave with a mirror.	**12.** Facilitates comfort and a sense of control.
13. Dispose of equipment in proper receptacle.	**13.** Equipment should not be shared between clients in accordance with Universal Precautions since disruption of skin and bleeding may occur. The client may, however, keep his own razor. Clean and store it at the bedside.
14. Wash hands.	**14.** Reduces the transmission of microorganisms.
15. Document shaving client, any problems encountered, and client's response.	**15.** Provides record of client's care.

Procedure B25 — Applying Antiembolism Stockings

Equipment

- Antiembolism stockings and package directions
- Tape measure
- Powder or cornstarch (if client is not allergic)

Action	**Rationale**

• Wash your hands • Check the client's identification band • Explain procedure to client prior to beginning •

1. Review the orders, including the reason for the stockings and the type of stockings ordered (e.g., knee or thigh high).	**1.** Ensures accuracy; facilitates compliance.
2. With the client in a supine position in bed, measure the client's leg for the correct size:	**2.** Supine position encourages venous return and decreases swelling, thereby allowing accurate measurement for size of stockings.
• Thigh-high stockings: from Achilles tendon to the gluteal fold, circumference of the midthigh.	

continued

Action	Rationale
• Below the knee stockings: from the Achilles tendon to the popliteal fold, circumference of the midcalf.	
3. Compare the obtained measurements with the package insert to ascertain proper size.	3. Correct size is essential for stockings to apply the appropriate pressure for adequate venous return without compromise to circulation.
4. Evenly apply talc or cornstarch to the client's legs and feet if client is not allergic.	4. Allows for smoother appliance of stockings. Powders also absorb moisture.
5. Apply stockings. The best time to apply stockings is early in the morning, before the client gets out of bed, or immediately after surgery. Keep client in supine position until stockings are applied.	5. Feet are less swollen in the morning because the feet have been in a nondependent position during the night.
6. Open the package and turn stockings inside out. Place hands deep enough inside the stockings to grasp the stocking toe.	6. Because stockings contain strong elastic, application can be difficult if not initiated from the bottom up and if stockings are not turned inside out. Wrinkles in stockings can also occur if a systematic approach is not used for application.
7. Hold onto the client's toes with the same hand, invert the stocking with the other hand and pull it over the hand that is holding the client's toes. Remove the hand from the inside of the stocking.	7. See Rationale 6.
8. Hold each side of the stocking and pull the inverted stocking over the client's toes.	8. See Rationale 6.
9. Continuing to hold each side of the stocking, firmly pull the stocking from the client's toes to the heel in one motion. Pull the stockings up by using the thumbs to guide the stockings upward over the ankles and up the client's legs (Figures B25-1 and B25-2).	9. See Rationale 6.
10. Repeat with the other leg.	10. See Rationale 6.

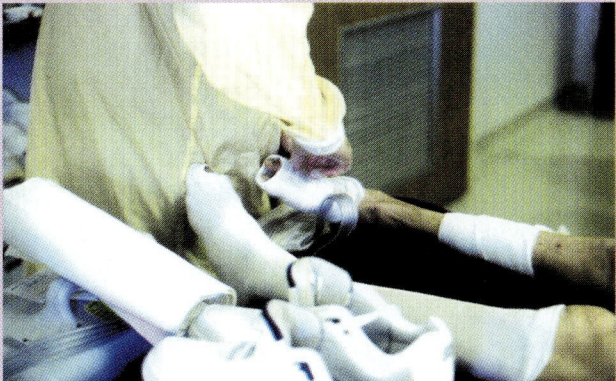

Figure B25-1 Place the stocking over the client's toes and foot.

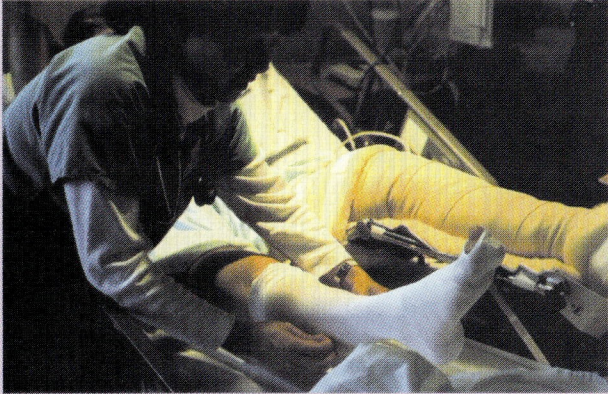

Figure B25-2 Pull the stocking smoothly and evenly up the client's leg.

continued

Action	Rationale
11. Remove any wrinkles in the stockings and smooth over (Figure B25-3).	**11.** Wrinkles can create skin breakdown and constrict the circulation.

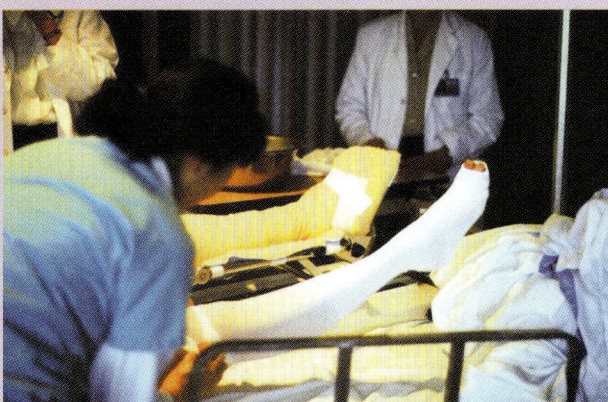

Figure B25-3 Smooth out any wrinkles and make sure the toes are comfortable.

Action	Rationale
12. Wash hands.	**12.** Reduces transmission of microorganisms.
13. Document application of antiembolism stockings.	**13.** Provides record of client care.

Procedure B26 — Positioning and Removing a Bedpan

Equipment

- Bedpan (regular or fracture)
- Disposable gloves
- Bedpan cover
- Toilet paper
- Washcloth and towel, soap

Action	Rationale
Positioning a Bedpan	
1. Close curtain or door.	**1.** Provides for privacy.
2. Wash hands, apply gloves.	**2.** Prevents transmission of microorganisms.
3. Lower head of bed so client is in supine position.	**3.** The supine position will increase ability of client to move to side-lying position.
4. Warm bedpan under warm water if needed, powder if necessary.	**4.** For comfort, prevents bedpan from sticking to the skin.
5. If client is able to lift buttocks, place bedpan under buttocks, with lower end near the lower back region (Figure B26-1).	**5.** Ensures proper placement of the bedpan before client rolls on top of bedpan.
6. If client is unable to lift buttocks, assist client to side-lying position using side rail.	**6.** Provides for best position for proper placement of bedpan.
7. While holding the bedpan against the client's buttocks with one hand, help the client to roll onto her back (Figure B26-2).	**7.** Prevents dislocation or misalignment of bedpan.
8. Check placement of bedpan by looking between client's legs.	**8.** May prevent spillage due to misalignment of bedpan.

continued

Action	**Rationale**

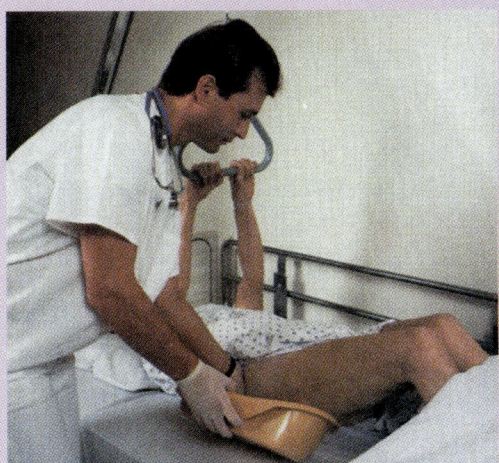

Figure B26-1 Slip the bedpan under the client's buttocks while client lifts herself with the trapeze.

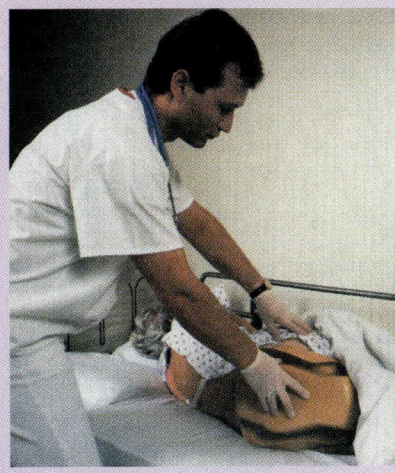

Figure B26-2 Place the bedpan against the client's buttocks and assist client to roll back.

9. If indicated, elevate head of bed to 45° angle.

9. Check physician order; bed remains flat if client has a spinal cord injury or spinal surgery. Elevating the head of bed creates a more normal elimination position.

10. Place call light within reach of client; place side rails in upright position and allow for privacy.

10. Privacy allows for a more comfortable elimination environment; elevated side rails provide for safety.

Removing a Bedpan

11. Wash hands, don gloves.

11. Prevents transmission of microorganisms.

12. Lower head of bed to supine position.

12. Increases client's ability to move to side-lying position.

13. While holding bedpan flat on bed with one hand, roll client to side. Or, if client is strong enough, have her lift buttocks.

13. Prevents possible spillage of bedpan contents.

14. Assist with cleaning or wiping if needed; always wipe from front to back.

14. Client may not be able to clean herself; wiping from front to back decreases chances of cross-contamination from anus to urethra.

15. Empty bedpan, clean it, and store it in proper place; if bedpan is to be emptied outside client's room, cover it during transport.

15. Promotes privacy and decreases the chance of spilling contents.

16. Remove gloves and wash hands.

16. Prevents transmission of microorganisms.

17. Allow client to wash hands.

17. Provides for physical hygiene and comfort.

18. Place call light within reach; recheck that side rails are in the upright position.

18. Ensures client safety and comfort.

19. If client is on I&O, record amount of urine voided.

19. Maintains accurate I&O record.

Procedure B27   Applying a Condom Catheter

Equipment

- Condom catheter
- Collection bag
- Supplies for cleansing skin
- Connecting tubing
- Disposable gloves

Action	Rationale

• Check the client's identification band • Explain the procedure to the client prior to beginning •

Action	Rationale
1. Wash hands and apply gloves.	1. Reduces risk of contamination.
2. Select an appropriate condom catheter.	2. The condom catheter must be sized correctly (refer to manufacturer's recommendations), contain a distal tip that resists twisting and occlusion, and contain an adhesive that prevents leakage. Latex condom catheters are avoided in men who are allergic to latex and in boys with myelodysplasia.
3. Cleanse the penile shaft.	3. Reduces surface dirt and pathogens.
4. Inspect the penile shaft for excessive hair.	4. Excessive penile hair is clipped to provide a watertight seal when the condom is applied.
5. Inspect the penis for altered skin integrity.	5. Small lesions may be protected by the use of a skin sealant; significant erosions or rashes require consultation with the enterostomal nurse specialist or a dermatologist before proceeding.
6. Stretch the shaft of the penis and unroll the condom to the base of the penis (Figure B27-1). Follow product directions for the application of the sealant (Figure B27-2). A securing strap may or may not be required, depending on the device.	6. The condom is applied over the entire penile shaft to maximize a watertight seal; the adhesive may be built into the wall of the condom, or a dual-sided sealant strip may be used to prevent leakage.

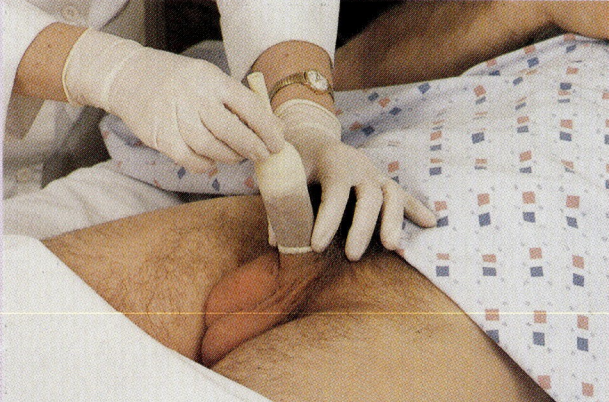

Figure B27-1 Unroll condom catheter to the base of the penis.

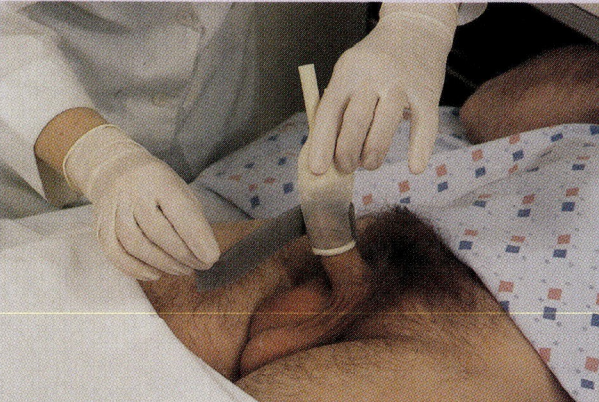

Figure B27-2 Secure the condom catheter with a strap (optional).

Action	Rationale
7. Attach the condom to the drainage apparatus; either a leg bag or bedside drainage bag.	7. Ensures adequate urine containment.
8. Remove gloves and wash hands.	8. Reduces the risks of contamination.

continued

Action	Rationale
9. Remove and reapply the condom catheter every 24 to 48 hours, or whenever leakage occurs.	9. Regular reapplication allows routine inspection of the penile skin and avoids bacterial overgrowth and altered skin integrity under the condom.
10. Document application of condom catheter, any problems encountered, and client's response.	10. Provides record of client care and client status.

Procedure B28 (Part 1)   Administering an Enema—Large/Small (Mini)

Equipment

- Enema bag (disposable comes with rectal tip catheter; reusable may need to have rectal tip catheter checked for damage and rectal tip may need to be replaced)
- Towel and washcloth
- Solution per physician's order
- Water-soluble lubricant
- Clean gloves
- Bedpan, commode, or toilet

Action	Rationale
• *Wash your hands* • *Check the client's identification band* • • *Explain the procedure to the client prior to beginning* •	
1. Introduce yourself and explain procedure; close door or curtain.	1. Client may be more relaxed if prepared for procedure, told what to expect, and provided with privacy.
2. Prepare the solution; assure temperature is between 99° and 102°F by using a thermometer or placing a few drops on your wrist.	2. Avoids harming the intestinal mucosa.
3. Wash hands and don gloves.	3. Protects from contamination.
4. Assist client to left side-lying position, with right knee bent.	4. Lying flat on left side allows fluid to flow through to colon with contour of bowel.
5. Place bedpan, commode, robe and slippers within easy reach.	5. Urgent evacuation of bowels or inability to retain fluid may occur.
6. Hang bag of enema solution 12 to 18 inches above anus.	6. This height allows for steady flow of fluid into the client by gravity; a bag placed at a height greater than 18 inches allows for too rapid an infusion rate and could result in cramping or discomfort for the client.
7. Lubricate 4 to 5 inches of catheter tip.	7. Eases catheter tip insertion.
8. Separate buttocks, insert catheter tip into anal opening, slowly advance catheter approximately 4 inches.	8. Further catheter advancement could cause damage to bowel.
9. Slowly infuse solution via gravity flow; bag height may be increased but should not exceed 18 inches above anal opening (Figure B28-1).	9. Rapid infusion caused by bag height over 18 inches may cause cramping and discomfort. Bowel perforation is also a risk.
10. If client complains of increased pain or cramping, or if fluid is not being retained, stop procedure, wait a few minutes, then restart.	10. Discomfort may cause poor retention of fluid.

continued

Action	**Rationale**

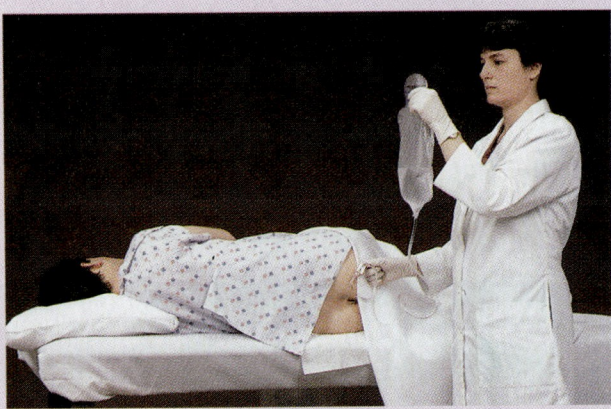

Figure B28-1 Raise the height of the enema container to allow infusion of the solution.

11. Clamp tubing when fluid finishes infusing; remove catheter tip.	11. Stops flow of fluid.
12. Assist client to bedpan, commode, or toilet; refer to Procedure B26 for positioning and removing bedpan.	12. If bedpan is used, place client in sitting position. Clients should be instructed to retain fluid for as long as possible.
13. Discard equipment in proper place. If equipment is reusable, properly clean and store it.	13. Prevents spread of microorganisms.
14. Remove gloves and wash hands.	14. Reduces spread of microorganisms.
15. Instruct client to call for assistance when finished eliminating, or if untoward feeling occurs, such as lightheadedness or dizziness.	15. Provides assistance and avoids potential harm to client.
16. Assist client with washing if needed.	16. Promotes client comfort.
17. Document solution given, client's reaction to procedure, and results obtained.	17. Provides information about procedure, client's reaction, and results obtained.

Procedure B28 (Part 2)   Administering an Enema (Small/Mini)

Equipment

- Enema—small and mini-enemas come premixed
- Disposable gloves
- Washcloth and towel
- Lubricant
- Bedpan, commode, toilet

Action	**Rationale**

• Wash your hands • Check the client's identification band •
• Explain the procedure to the client prior to beginning •

1. Introduce yourself, explain procedure, close door or curtain.	1. Client may be more relaxed with privacy and knowing what to expect.
2. Place commode next to bed; have robe and slippers available.	2. If client is able to use commode, easy access is necessary due to urgency after enema administration.

continued

Action	Rationale
3. Have bedpan easily available.	**3.** Bedpan is ready if client is unable to retain fluid.
4. Wash hands and don gloves.	**4.** Prevents cross-contamination of bacteria.
5. Lower head of bed to flat position.	**5.** Easier for client to roll to left side.
6. Assist client to roll to left side-lying position with right knee slightly bent.	**6.** Lying on left side helps solution flow with the contour of the bowel.
7. Remove catheter tip guard; gently squeeze bottle until fluid drips (for mini-enemas, tip needs to be punctured with needle or pin).	**7.** Most prepared enemas have perforated tips; a gentle squeeze will ensure this.
8. Lubricate catheter tip.	**8.** Most premixed solutions are prelubricated; however, additional lubrication may be needed.
9. Separate buttocks and insert enema tip into anal opening; gently squeeze contents into rectum.	**9.** Gentle insertion and infusion lessens risk of undue discomfort and damage to colon.
10. Remove tip and assist to bedpan, commode, or toilet. Ask client to retain fluid for as long as possible, at least 30 minutes.	**10.** Assistance ensures safe transfer for client. Better results occur when enema is retained for a longer period of time.
11. Dispose of contaminated material in proper receptacles.	**11.** Prevents contamination.
12. Remove gloves and wash hands.	**12.** Reduces risk of contamination.
13. Assist client with cleaning if needed.	**13.** Illness or fatigue may cause some clients to require assistance for cleaning.
14. Document solution given, client's reaction to procedure, and results obtained.	**14.** Provides information about procedure, client's reaction, and results obtained.

Procedure B29 — Measuring Intake and Output

Equipment

- I&O form at bedside
- Glass or cup
- Graduated container for output
- I&O graphic record in chart
- Bedpan, urinal, or bedside commode
- Nonsterile gloves

Action	Rationale
• Check client's identification band prior to beginning •	
1. Wash hands.	**1.** Reduces potential for transmission of pathogens.
2. Explain purpose of keeping I&O record to client. Explain that: • All fluids taken orally must be recorded. • Form for recording must be used. • Client must void into bedpan, urinal, or "hat" in toilet for collecting urine; not into toilet. • Toilet tissue should be disposed of in plastic-lined container, not in bedpan.	**2.** Elicits client support.

continued

Action	Rationale
Intake	
3. Measure all oral fluids in accord with agency policy: e.g., cup = 150 mL, glass = 240 mL.	**3.** Provides for consistency of measurement.
4. Record time and amount of all fluid intake in the designated space on bedside form (oral, tube feedings, IV fluids).	**4.** Documents fluids.
5. Transfer 8-hour total fluid intake from bedside I&O record to graphic sheet or 24-hour I&O record on client's chart, according to agency policy.	**5.** Provides for data analysis of client's fluid status.
6. Record all forms of intake, except blood and blood products, in the appropriate column of the 24-hour record.	**6.** Documents intake by type and amount.
7. Complete 24-hour intake record by adding the three 8-hour totals.	**7.** Provides consistent data for analysis of client's fluid status over a 24-hour period.
Output	
8. Don nonsterile gloves.	**8.** Reduces potential for transmission of pathogens.
9. Empty urinal, bedpan, commode "hat," or Foley drainage bag into graduated container and measure. Dispose of urine in toilet or hopper room, according to agency policy.	**9.** Provides accurate measurement of urine.
10. Remove gloves and wash hands.	**10.** Prevents cross-contamination.
11. Record time and amount of output (urine, drainage from nasogastric tube, drainage tube) on bedside I&O record.	**11.** Documents output.
12. Transfer 8-hour output totals to graphic sheet or 24-hour I&O record on the client's chart, according to agency policy.	**12.** Provides for data analysis of client's fluid status.
13. Complete 24-hour output record by totaling the three 8-hour totals.	**13.** Provides consistent data for analysis of client's fluid status over a 24-hour period.

Procedure B30   Urine Collection—Closed Drainage System

Equipment

- Rubber band or catheter clamp
- Tape and sign
- Examination gloves
- Sterile specimen container and label
- Sterile packages of 70% isopropanol (anti-infective) or povidone-iodine (antiseptic)
- Sterile 10-mL syringe with 23- or 25-gauge needle

Action	Rationale
• *Wash your hands* • *Check the client's identification band* • • *Explain the procedure to the client prior to beginning* •	
1. Gather equipment.	**1.** Promotes efficiency.
2. Manipulate the drainage tubing so that the urine in the tubing goes into the bag.	**2.** Facilitates urine to flow into the drainage bag; provides a fresh urine sample.

continued

Action	Rationale
3. Clamp the drainage tubing below the aspiration port; leave clamped 30 to 60 minutes.	3. Traps fresh urine in the tubing above the level of the aspiration port.
4. Tape a sign over the client's bed indicating that the Foley catheter's drainage tubing is temporarily clamped for a specimen.	4. Communicates to other personnel that the drainage tube is clamped.
5. Wash hands, don gloves.	5. Decreases transmission of microorganisms.
6. Provide for privacy.	6. Decreases embarrassment.
7. Cleanse the aspiration port with an anti-infective or antiseptic solution; let dry.	7. Inhibits growth and reproduction of microorganisms; povidone-iodine must dry to be effective antiseptic.
8. Remove all air from the needle and syringe.	8. Allow for withdrawal of the correct amount of urine.
9. Insert needle into aspiration port at a 45° angle, aspirate 10 mL from port, remove needle.	9. Prevents accidental puncture of the catheter wall on distant side of port; provides sufficient urine for analysis.
10. Transfer urine into sterile labeled container, secure lid on container, and place container in a biohazard bag.	10. Prevents contamination of sterile specimen, ensures client accuracy, prevents spillage.
11. Place needle and syringe unit into sharps container; *never recap a contaminated needle.*	11. Prevents accidental needle sticks.
12. Remove the notice from above the bed after removing clamp from tubing.	12. Clamp is no longer in place.
13. Remove and dispose of gloves, wash hands.	13. Decreases transmission of microorganisms.
14. Transport specimen to laboratory.	14. Prevents growth of bacteria or changes in the urine's analysis.
15. Document collection of urine specimen.	15. Provides information on collection of urine specimen.

Procedure B31 Urine Collection—Clean Catch, Female/Male

Equipment

- Examination gloves
- Sterile collection container and lid, label
- Sterile midstream kit
- 3 antiseptic towelettes or 3 cotton balls saturated with an antiseptic solution

Action	Rationale
• *Wash your hands* • *Check the client's identification band* • *Explain the procedure to the client prior to beginning*	
1. Gather equipment.	1. Promotes efficiency.
2. Don gloves, or ask the client to wash his or her hands.	2. Decreases transmission of microorganisms.
3. Provide for privacy.	3. Decreases embarrassment.

continued

Action	**Rationale**
4. *Instruct the female client to:*	4.
• Sit with legs separated on the toilet.	• Comfortable position, provides access to cleansing the labia.
• Open the sterile container, placing the lid up on a firm surface in easy reach.	• Prevents the inside of the container's lid from touching a soiled surface; prevents contamination of the specimen.
• Use the thumb and forefinger to separate the labia.	• Provides access for cleansing the labia.
• With the labia separated, using a downward stroke, cleanse one side of the labia with the towelette, discard the towelette, repeat procedure on the other side with the second towelette, repeat the procedure down the center with the third towelette, make sure the labia stay separated throughout the procedure (Figure B31-1).	• Prevents contamination of clean area.

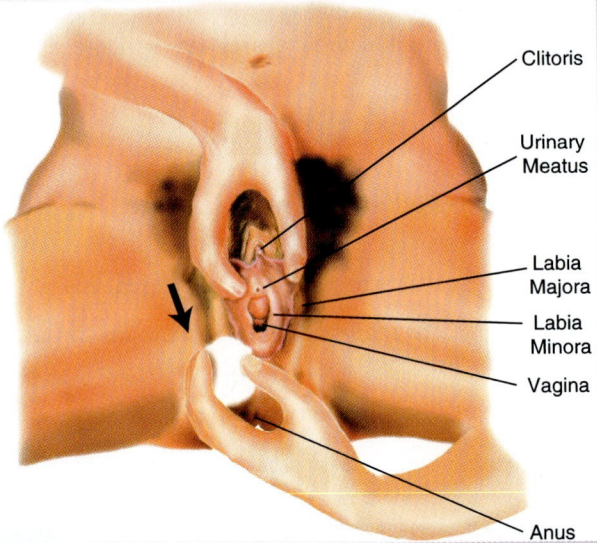

Clitoris

Urinary Meatus

Labia Majora

Labia Minora

Vagina

Anus

Figure B31-1 Client Cleansing Labia

• Begin to urinate into the toilet, place the collection cup under the stream of urine after a good flow of urine has been started. Fill the container half-way with urine.	• Initial flow of urine *is not* collected, can contain bacteria.
Instruct the male client to:	
• Stand in front of the toilet.	• Ensures position of comfort.
• Open the sterile container, placing the lid up on a firm surface in easy reach.	• Prevents the inside of the container's lid from touching a soiled surface; prevents contamination of the specimen.
• Retract foreskin, if necessary.	• Provides access for cleaning penis tip.
• Use a towelette to wipe the tip of the penis in a circular fashion. Repeat with the other two towelettes.	• Prevents contamination of clean area.

continued

Action	Rationale
• Begin to urinate into the toilet. Place the collection cup in the stream of urine, filling the cup approximately half-full.	• Initial flow of urine is not collected, because it can contain bacteria.
5. Place sterile lid back onto the container, close tightly, label, place in a biohazard bag, and transport to laboratory.	5. Prevents contamination of sterile specimen, prevents spillage, ensures accuracy of client.
6. Remove and dispose of gloves; wash hands.	6. Decreases transmission of microorganisms.
7. Document clean catch urine specimen collected.	7. Informs that clean catch urine specimen has been collected.

Procedure B32 — Collecting Nose, Throat, and Sputum Specimens

Equipment

- Two sterile swabs in sterile culture tubes
- Penlight
- Clean, disposable gloves
- Emesis basin or clean container
- Tongue blades
- Facial tissues
- Nasal speculum (optional)
- Sterile specimen cup or sputum specimen container

Action	Rationale
• Check the client's identification band • Explain the procedure to the client prior to beginning •	
1. Wash hands and put on clean gloves.	1. Reduces transmission of microorganisms.
2. Ask client to sit erect in bed or on chair facing nurse.	2. Provides easy access to nose or throat.
3. Prepare sterile swab for use by loosening top from container.	3. Prevents contamination of swab.

Collecting Throat Culture

Action	Rationale
4. Ask client to tilt head backward, open mouth, and say "ah."	4. Promotes visualization of pharynx, relaxes throat muscles, minimizes gag reflex.
5. Depress anterior one third of tongue with tongue blade for better visualization (Figure B32-1).	5. Promotes visualization of pharynx, but may induce gag reflex.
6. Insert swab without touching cheek, lips, teeth, or tongue.	6. Prevents contamination of the specimen with oral flora.

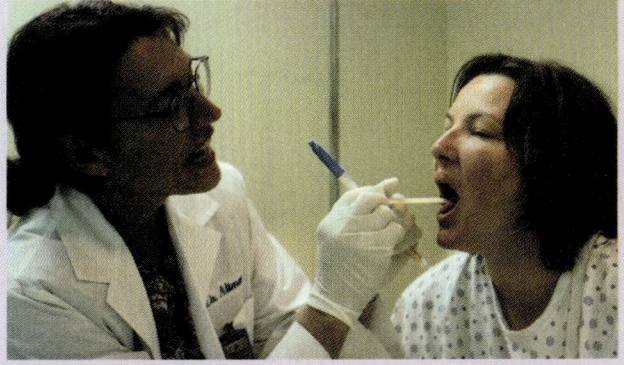

Figure B32-1 Depress the tongue with tongue blade.

continued

Action	Rationale

7. Swab tonsillar area from side to side in a quick, gentle motion (Figure B32-2).

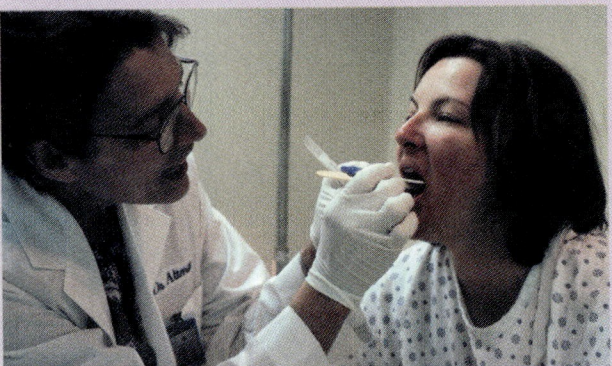

Figure B32-2 Swab the sample area using a quick gentle motion.

8. Withdraw swab without touching adjacent structures and place swab in culture tube. Crush ampule at bottom of tube and push swab into liquid medium.

9. Secure top to culture tube and label with client's name, according to agency policy.

10. Discard tongue depressor, place culture tube in biohazard bag, remove gloves and discard. Wash hands.

11. Send specimen to laboratory.

12. Document specimen collection.

Collecting Nose Culture

13. Instruct client to blow nose; check nostrils for patency with penlight.

14. Ask client to occlude one nostril, then the other, and exhale.

15. Ask client to tilt head back.

16. Insert swab into nostril until it reaches the inflamed mucosa and rotate the swab.

17. Withdraw the swab without touching adjacent structures and place swab in culture tube. Crush ampule at bottom of tube and push swab into liquid medium.

18. Secure top to culture tube and label with client's name.

19. Remove gloves and discard. Wash hands.

20. Send specimen to laboratory.

21. Document specimen collection.

---

7. Ensures collection of microorganisms.

8. Prevents contamination from outside microorganisms and erroneous culture results. Retains microorganisms in the culture tube and ensures the life of bacteria for testing.

9. Prevents identification mistakes, promotes accurate diagnosis for client.

10. Reduces transmission of microorganisms.

11. Provides most accurate results.

12. Provides record of physician's order being performed.

13. Clears nasal passages of mucus containing resident bacteria.

14. Determines the optimal nasal passage from which to obtain the specimen.

15. Promotes visualization of the sinuses.

16. Ensures the swab will be covered with the appropriate exudate.

17. Prevents contamination from normal nasal flora and erroneous culture results.

18. Prevents identification mistakes, promotes accurate diagnosis for client.

19. Reduces transmission of microorganisms.

20. Provides most accurate results.

21. Provides record of physician's order being performed.

continued

Action	Rationale

Collecting a Sputum Culture

22. Explain to the client that the specimen must be sputum coughed up from the lungs. Saliva is not diagnostic.

22. Promotes client cooperation.

23. Have a sterile specimen cup ready for the sample and some tissues at hand.

23. The specimen must be collected in a sterile cup to prevent contamination.

24. Have the client take several deep breaths and then cough deeply.

24. This helps to loosen secretions so the client will be able to provide a specimen.

25. Have client expectorate the sputum into the sterile cup without touching the inside of the cup.

25. Prevents contamination of the specimen.

26. Place the lid on the specimen container without touching the inside of the lid or the container.

26. Prevents contamination of the specimen.

27. Provide the client with tissues and make him comfortable.

27. Promotes client comfort.

28. Wash hands.

28. Reduces transmission of microorganisms.

29. Label specimen with client's name.

29. Promotes correct diagnosis for client.

30. Send specimen to laboratory.

30. Provides most accurate results.

31. Document sputum collection.

31. Provides record of physician's order being performed.

Procedure B33   Gathering a Stool Specimen

Equipment

- Clean or sterile bedpan, commode or "hat" for toilet
- Specimen card for occult blood testing, or sterile specimen cup, culture swab, or other special collection device according to test being done and agency policy, and proper identification for specimen

- Gloves
- Two tongue blades
- Paper towel

Action	Rationale

• Wash your hands • Check the client's identification band •

1. Explain that a stool specimen is needed, why it is needed, and how the client can assist.

1. Informs the client and promotes cooperation.

2. Depending on agency policy, assist client as needed to bedside commode or toilet. Have client void before moving bowels. Then, prepare for specimen collection. If client is not ambulatory, use a bedpan.

2. Allows client privacy and the ability to move his bowels in a more normal physiological position.

3. Instruct the client not to contaminate the specimen with urine, vaginal discharge, or toilet paper, if possible.

3. Minimizes risk of skewed laboratory results.

4. Ask the client to notify you as soon as the specimen is available.

4. Reduces the risk of contamination of specimen, allows the nurse to collect a fresh specimen, and reduces embarrassment to client.

continued

Action	Rationale
5. Assist the client with hygiene, help the client back to bed (as required) and ensure his or her comfort before turning attention to specimen.	5. Promotes client cleanliness and dignity.
6. Don gloves, wear gown if client is on isolation or at risk for infectious stool such as vancomycin-resistant enterococcus (VRE).	6. Reduces the risk of transmission of micro-organisms.
7. Assess the stool for color, consistency, and odor, and presence or absence of visible blood or mucus.	7. Facilitates comprehensive client assessment.
8. Using one or two tongue blades (depending on how much specimen is needed and for which test), transfer a representative sample of stool to the specimen card or container, taking care not to contaminate the outside of the container (or the inside of a sterile specimen cup). If using a culture swab, swab in a representative area of stool, particularly if any purulent material is visible. Check with laboratory regarding the volume of stool needed for a particular test.	8. Provides a high-quality sample for optimal results.
9. Close the card, place the lid on the container, or place the swab in the culture tube (according to agency policy) as soon as specimen is collected.	9. Reduces the risk of spread of microorganisms and reduces odor.
10. Place the specimen container in biohazard bag for transport to lab after proper labeling is done according to agency policy. Be careful not to contaminate outside of bag. Provide requisition for test according to agency policy.	10. Properly identifies specimen to client; makes transport of specimen to lab more aesthetic for personnel. Provides client privacy. Reduces spread of microorganisms.
11. Dispose of rest of stool according to agency policy.	11. Reduces spread of microorganisms.
12. Remove gloves and wash hands thoroughly.	12. Reduces spread of microorganisms.
13. Send specimen to laboratory immediately.	13. Maximizes quality of specimen for testing.
14. Document assessment of stool and time of specimen collection and that specimen was sent to laboratory.	14. Facilitates communication among members of the health care team.

Procedure B34 — Applying Abdominal, T-, Breast, and Scultetus Binders

Equipment

- Correct binder for intended purpose
- Safety pins or fasteners

Action	Rationale

• Wash your hands • Check the client's identification band •
• Explain the procedure to the client prior to beginning •

Abdominal Binders

1. Choose binder. If a stretch net binder is being used, select the correct circumference, and cut length to fit.	1. The correct size will make the binder most effective.

continued

Action	Rationale
2. Help the client into the proper position to place the binder.	**2.** Applying binders can be awkward if the client is not positioned correctly.

2. Help the client into the proper position to place the binder.

- For abdominal binders, the client should lie supine, and lift the hips, or position the client on one side, and roll the client onto the binder (Figure B34-1). For stretch net binders, slide the net over the head and neck, or slide the net up from the feet, depending on which is easier for the client.

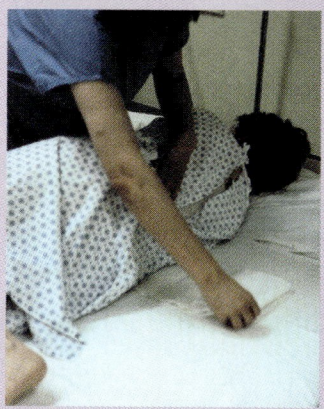

Figure B34-1 Place the binder under the client.

3. Wrap the abdominal binder snugly around client's waist, starting from the lower abdomen and working upward (Figures B34-2 and B34-3).

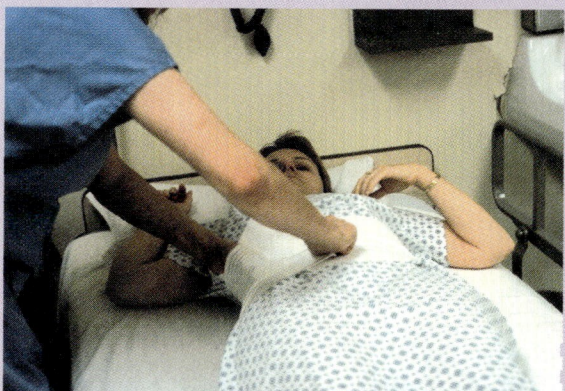

Figure B34-2 Wrap the binder snugly around the waist.

- Stretch net binders should be adjusted to cover the dressings they will be holding in place.

4. Secure binders with fasteners. If the binder does not have Velcro fasteners, secure with safety pins. Stretch net binders cling and stretch over the body part and do not need additional fastening. Check for snug fit.

2. Applying binders can be awkward if the client is not positioned correctly.

3. Correct application allows the client to get the most benefit from the binder.

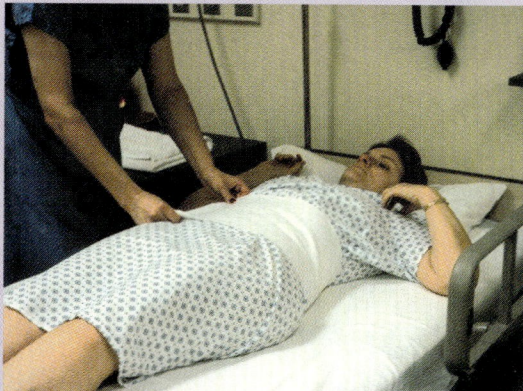

Figure B34-3 Secure the lower abdomen first and work upward.

4. Fasteners will keep binder in place. Be sure that all fasteners are closed securely to prevent possible client injury.

continued

Action	**Rationale**
5. Adjust if necessary. Be sure that binders are not restricting breathing or circulation (Figure B34-4). Be sure that sterile dressings are in place between the binder and any wound (Figure B34-5).	5. Binders that are too tight may make breathing difficult, and may contribute to skin irritation or breakdown. Binders are generally not sterile, so sterile dressings must be in place over the wound.

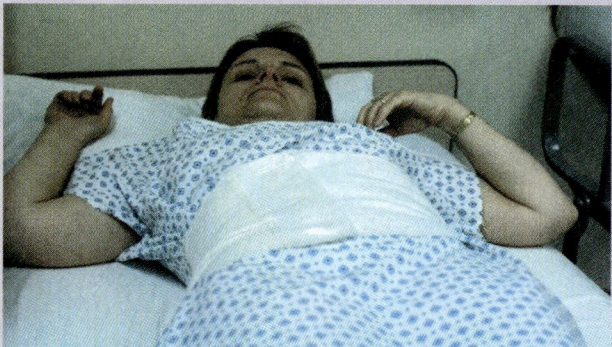

Figure B34-4 Assess the client to be sure the binder does not restrict breathing or circulation.

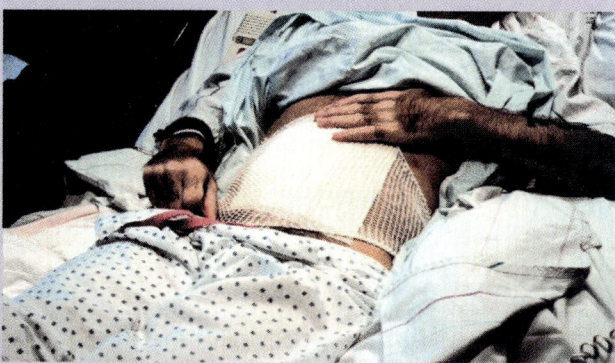

Figure B34-5 If a stretch net binder is used to cover a wound, make sure a sterile dressing is in place between the binder and the wound.

6. Wash hands.	6. Reduces transmission of microorganisms.

T-binder

7. Select the appropriate size binder; choose a single-tail for a female, and a double-tail for a male (Figure B34-6). (A double-tailed binder may be used for a female with a very large dressing.)	7. Proper sizing will keep binder and dressing in place.

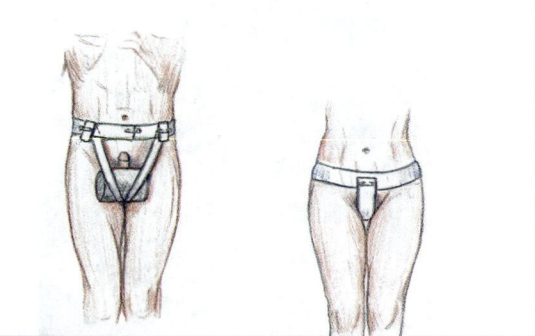

Figure B34-6

8. Place the binder smoothly under the client with the waistband at the waist, and the tail(s) running down the center of the back.	8. Facilitates application.
9. Wrap the waistband around the waist and secure it. Bring the tails up between the legs. For a male, each tail should be placed on either side of the testicles. Secure the tails to the waistband.	9. Secures dressings and promotes client comfort.
10. Wash hands.	10. Reduces transmission of microorganisms.

continued

Action	**Rationale**

Breast Binder

11. Assist the client to a sitting position.

11. Sitting will allow ease in placement of the binder. If not possible, turn client side-to-side while applying binder.

12. Apply binder, adjusting for a snug fit. Place padding under large breasts, if needed.

12. The tightness of the binder will be instrumental in adequate lactation suppression.

13. Adjust if necessary. Be sure that breast binder is not restricting breathing or causing skin irritation.

13. Breast binders that are too tight may make breathing difficult and/or may contribute to skin irritation or breakdown.

14. Use of adjunctive treatments (e.g., ice packs, analgesics) for additional comfort, if needed.

14. If breasts are engorged, adjunctive treatment may be required to increase client's level of comfort.

15. Wash hands.

15. Reduces transmission of microorganisms.

Scultetus Binder

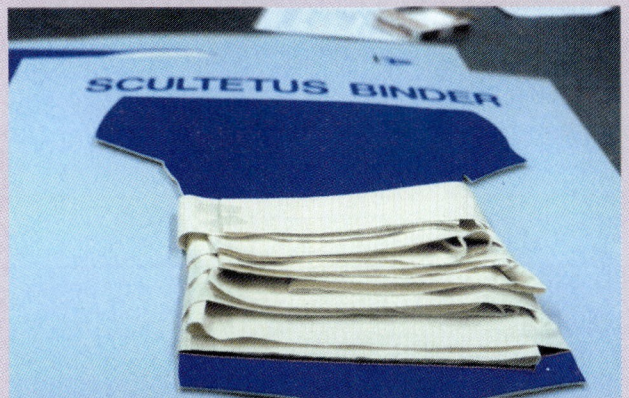

Figure B34-7 Scultetus binder

16. Place the scultetus binder (Figure B34-7) underneath the client, with the upper border no higher than the waist.

16. If the binder is too high, it will interfere with breathing.

17. Bring the tails across the center of the abdomen, one at a time, alternating sides, starting at the bottom. (For a postpartum client, work from the top down.) Each tail should overlap the next lower one by about half the width of tail for maximal support.

17. Supports the abdomen, and if needed, secures dressings.

18. Secure the last tail with a safety pin or other securing means, depending on the type of scultetus binder used.

18. Keeps the binder in place.

19. Wash hands.

19. Reduces transmission of microorganisms.

20. Document type of binder applied and client's reaction.

20. Informs health care providers of care given.

Procedure B35   Application of Restraints

Equipment

- Restraint

Action	Rationale

• Wash your hands • Check the client's identification band •

1. Explain rationale for application of restraint. Repeatedly reinforce rationale.

2. Select the proper type of restraint.

3. Assess skin for irritation.

4. Apply restraint to client assuring some movement of body part. One to two fingers should slide between restraint and client's skin. Tie straps securely with clove hitch knot. To make a clove hitch: make a figure-eight; pick up the loops; put the limb through the loops and secure (Figure B35-1). Pad bony prominences.

1. Explanations facilitate cooperation.

2. Least restrictive restraint that does not interfere with client's health status but provides safety should be selected.

3. Provides baseline skin assessment.

4. Maintains adequate circulation and mobility. Prevents skin breakdown.

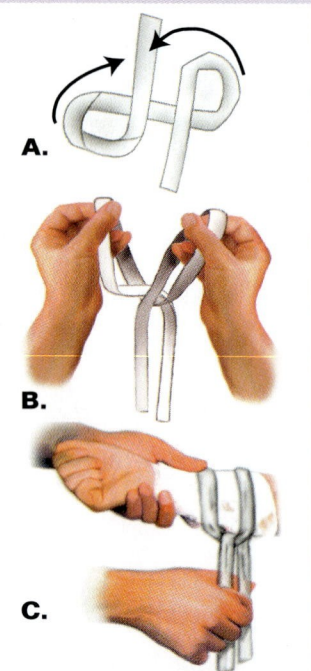

Figure B35-1 Making a Clove Hitch Knot: A. Make a figure-eight; B. Pick up the loops; C. Put the limb through the loops and secure.

5. Secure restraint to the bed frame; *do not* tie the straps to the side rail. Use a bow or slip knot that can be readily released in an emergency.

6. Assess restraints and skin integrity every 30 minutes. Release restraints at least every 2 hours.

5. Prevents accidental injury to client from moving side rails and decreases client's ability to untie restraints.

6. Permits muscle exercise. Promotes circulation.

continued

Action	Rationale
7. Continually assess the need for restraints (at least every 8 hours).	7. Assists in evaluating client's progress and response to restraints.
8. Document application and all assessments according to agency policy.	8. Many regulations govern restraint use.

Procedure B36 Clearing an Obstructed Airway

Equipment

- None required

Action	Rationale
1. Recognize the signs of airway obstruction. In the conscious person, airway obstruction is signaled by the inability to cough, speak, or breathe and often occurs during eating. In the unconscious person, note the absence of respiratory movements and the absence of air movement. A partial obstruction, indicated by high-pitched noises while breathing, a weak ineffective cough, and cyanosis, should be treated as a complete obstruction.	1. Allows you to react quickly and effectively. If the person with a partial airway obstruction has an effective cough, you must observe closely for exacerbation. Prompt intervention is necessary if the person is unable to dislodge the obstruction.
2. If the victim is conscious, ask, "Are you choking?" Announce that you can help. Position yourself behind the victim and wrap your arms around the victim's waist.	2. A person who cannot breathe is likely to panic; announcing your intentions will elicit cooperation.
3. Make a fist with one hand. Place the thumb side of the fist against the victim's abdomen just above the umbilicus and well below the xyphoid process. Grasp the fist with the other hand (Figure B36-1).	3. This position allows for rapid compressions of the diaphragm. Avoiding the xyphoid process (lower-most point of the sternum) reduces the risk of internal injury.

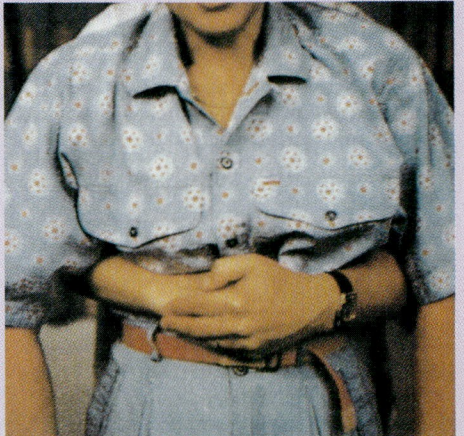

Figure B36-1 Placement of Fist into Abdomen

4. Press the fist into the victim's abdomen with quick, upward thrusts. Repeat thrusts until the object is expelled or the victim becomes unconscious.	4. The thrusts should be of sufficient force to produce an artificial cough.

continued

Action	Rationale
5. If the victim becomes unconscious, lower him to the floor and call for help by activating the Emergency Medical System (EMS) if outside the hospital or the internal emergency call system if inside the hospital.	**5.** At this point Advanced Life Support equipment and personnel should be mobilized.
6. Place the victim in a supine position. Perform a tongue-jaw lift, followed by a finger-sweep.	**6.** Potentially opens the airway and removes foreign body.
7. Open airway and try to ventilate; if still obstructed, reposition head and try to ventilate again.	**7.** Airway must be open for rescue breathing.
8. Kneel astride the victim with your body over the lower trunk or upper legs.	**8.** This position allows you to apply abdominal thrusts to the unconscious victim.
9. Place the heel of one hand on the victim's abdomen just above the umbilicus but well below the xyphoid process. Place the second hand on top of the first (Figure B36-2).	**9.** This position allows for rapid compressions of the diaphragm. Avoiding the xyphoid process (lower-most point of the sternum) reduces the risk of internal injury. *Note:* If the rescuer is too short to reach around the victim from behind, this position may also be used for the conscious victim.

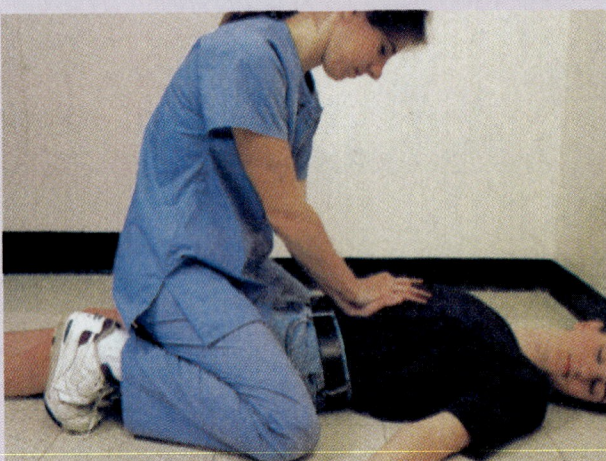

Figure B36-2 Placement of Hands on Abdomen for Unconscious Client

Action	Rationale
10. Press into the abdomen with quick, upward thrusts.	**10.** The thrusts should be of sufficient force to produce an artificial cough.
11. If the victim is in the late stages of pregnancy or is markedly obese, the hand position may be changed. In this case, place the fist over the midportion of the sternum, avoiding the xyphoid process.	**11.** A very large abdomen will make effective abdominal thrusts impossible.
12. After five abdominal thrusts in the unconscious victim, open the mouth and sweep with the index finger.	**12.** Abdominal thrusts may have raised the foreign body up to a level where it can be removed manually.
13. Open the airway using the head tilt–chin lift method (see Procedure B37) and attempt to ventilate. If successful, proceed with cardiopulmonary resuscitation sequence. If unsuccessful, repeat steps 8 through 12 in sequence until successful.	**13.** Until the obstruction is removed, no other resuscitation efforts will be successful.

continued

Action	**Rationale**
14. Document procedure, client's response, and outcome.	**14.** Communicates care given to health care team.

Procedure B37   Performing Cardiopulmonary Resuscitation

Equipment

- Backboard (optional)
- Personal protective equipment
- Resuscitation mask or face shield

Action	**Rationale**
1. Determine responsiveness of the victim by tapping or gently shaking and shouting, "Are you OK?"	**1.** Quickly determines whether an emergency exists. *Note:* If the victim has sustained an injury to the head or neck, to avoid furthering a spinal cord injury, move the victim only if absolutely necessary.
2. If the victim is unresponsive, call out for help and activate the EMS if outside the hospital, or the internal emergency paging system if inside the hospital.	**2.** Rapid initiation of advanced life support techniques, particularly defibrillation, is associated with increased success of resuscitation.
3. Position the victim for CPR by placing supine on a firm surface. If in a bed, roll the victim onto his or her side and place firm backboard under the torso, then roll back into a supine position. (Do not waste time searching for backboard if not readily available.)	**3.** Facilitates airway opening and chest compressions, and the firm surface increases the effectiveness of chest compressions.
4. Open the victim's airway using the head tilt–chin lift method (Figure B37-1) or the jaw thrust. Once the airway is open, place your cheek very close to the victim's mouth; look, listen, and feel for breathing.	**4.** Removal of the tongue from the posterior oropharynx may restore breathing in the unconscious adult victim. *Note:* If this maneuver restores breathing, place the victim in a side-lying position or continue to hold the airway open and monitor breathing until help arrives.

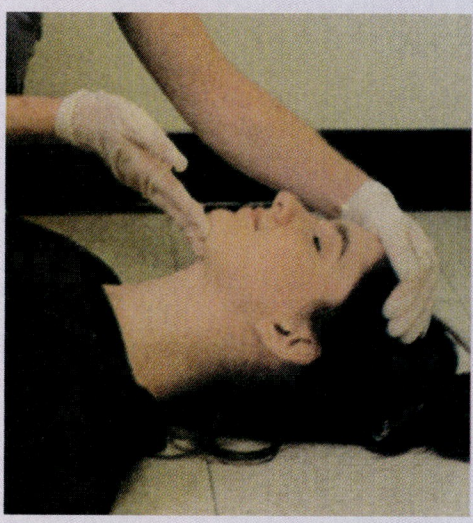

Figure B37-1 Open airway by head tilt–chin lift.

continued

Action	**Rationale**
5. If neck injury is present or suspected, open the airway by placing the fingertips of both hands under the angle of the victim's jaw and pulling the jaw forward.	**5.** Minimizes neck movement but is more difficult to perform.
6. If the victim is not breathing, position your mouth over the victim's mouth, forming an airtight seal. If a resuscitation mask or face shield is available, position it over the victim's mouth according to the product directions.	**6.** A mask or shield can be used to reduce the exposure of the rescuer to the oral secretions, blood, vomitus of the victim.
7. Give two slow, full breaths. Watch the chest rise as the breath is given, and allow for exhalation after the breath is given.	**7.** Slow breath delivery improves the distribution of air in the victim's lungs and decreases the risk that air will enter the stomach. Watching the chest rising verifies successful delivery of breaths.
8. Locate the carotid artery in the victim's neck (in the groove between the larynx and the large muscle of the neck). Palpate for at least 5 seconds to determine whether a pulse is present. If a pulse is present, continue to deliver breaths at a rate of 12 per minute, or a breath every 5 seconds.	**8.** Too-rapid pulse assessment may cause the rescuer to miss a slow or weak pulse. If a pulse is present, chest compression should not be performed.
9. If no pulse is present, begin chest compressions: Position yourself over the victim with your shoulders directly over the victim's chest (Figure B37-2). Place the heel of one hand over the lower half of the sternum, avoiding the xyphoid process. Place the second hand directly on top of the first, keeping the fingers up and off of the chest wall. Lock your elbows.	**9.** Correct hand position maximizes the effectiveness of compressions while minimizing the risk of injuries such as fractured ribs, pneumothorax, and lacerations of internal structures. Correct hand position may be achieved by running the middle finger along the bottom rib toward the sternum until the xyphoid process is felt. Place the opposite hand on the sternum two finger widths above this point.

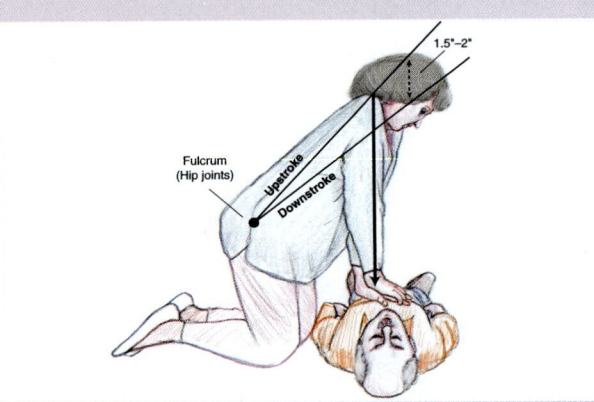

Figure B37-2 Proper Position of Rescuer

10. Compress the sternum 1½ to 2 inches, then release fully while maintaining correct hand position. Repeat the compression and release sequence 15 times at a rate equivalent to 80 to 100 compressions per minute.	**10.** Compression of the sternum forces blood to be ejected from the heart, mimicking normal ventricular systole. Release of the pressure moves blood into the heart, mimicking diastole.
11. After 15 chest compressions, return to the victim's head and open the airway as in step 4. Deliver two slow, full breaths as in steps 6 and 7. Repeat the sequence of 15 compressions to two breaths until help arrives or pulse and breathing are restored.	**11.** Repeated cycles of breaths and compressions are necessary to deliver oxygenated blood to the vital organs.

continued

Action	Rationale
12. Reassess for the return of breathing and pulse every few minutes; then resume CPR.	**12.** In rare instances, breathing and circulation may be restored with CPR. In most circumstances, CPR sustains minimal tissue oxygenation until Advanced Life Support measures are available.

Procedure B38 — Admitting a Client

Equipment

- Client education materials
- ID bracelet and bed tag
- Other equipment as dictated by client condition
- Valuables envelope
- Admission kit: wash basin, emesis basin, pitcher, and so on

Action	Rationale
• Wash your hands •	
1. Welcome client to unit. Introduce yourself by name and title. Ask client to state his name.	**1.** Verifies identification.
2. Orient client to room and nursing unit. Describe items such as nurse call bell system, location of bathroom, place for clothing, bed controls, television, telephone, visiting hours, meal times, Standard Precautions, and review items in client education materials such as client rights and other written information about the facility.	**2.** Reduces client anxiety; allows fuller participation in care.
3. Provide privacy for client to change into pajamas or hospital gown, if not already done.	**3.** Respects client privacy.
4. Show client ID bracelet to double-check proper identification. Attach bracelet to wrist. (This may have been done in Admitting Department.) Review drug allergies and attach allergy bracelet to same wrist, according to agency policy.	**4.** Confirms client identification; promotes client safety.
5. Document and store client's belongings and valuables according to agency policy.	**5.** Reduces the risk of loss.
6. Begin nursing assessment, according to agency policy.	**6.** Starts development of client database.
7. Perform any other actions, as directed by agency policy.	**7.** Different facilities have different needs, regulations, and guidelines for client admission.

Procedure B39 — Transferring a Client

Equipment

- Client medical record (if not electronic)
- Client's medications (if applicable)
- Client's imprinting plate
- Client's belongings
- Old records (if applicable)
- Stretcher or wheelchair

continued

Action	Rationale

• Wash your hands • Check the client's identification band •

Action	Rationale
1. Check to see if order is needed to initiate transfer according to agency policy.	1. Policies differ among facilities.
2. Call nursing unit of new location to see if bed is ready and to give report.	2. Provides continuity of care.
3. Explain the transfer to the client (and family, if appropriate). Answer any questions. Allay anxieties about moving.	3. Keeps client informed and promotes cooperation.
4. Review the valuables and belongings checklist completed on admission. Compare with belongings.	4. Ensures all of client's belongings are transferred with the client. Prevents loss.
5. Gather records and any other equipment that will be transferred with the client, according to agency policy, such as eye drops, other medications, IV pump, respiratory therapy equipment, and so on.	5. Helps make transfer more efficient and reduces multiple trips to new area.
6. Transfer client by appropriate vehicle (wheelchair, stretcher). Accompany client to new unit. Transfer care to another staff member in person. Ensure that call bell is within reach or staff member is in room before leaving client.	6. Enhances continuity of care. Promotes safety.
7. Document time of transfer and any other information required by agency policy.	7. Promotes communication among members of the health care team.
8. Upon return to unit, notify appropriate personnel according to agency policy that client has left the unit. Arrange for personnel to clean the bed and surroundings the client has left.	8. Prepares bed for new admission. Reduces transfer of microorganisms.

Procedure B40   Discharging a Client

Equipment

- Any required agency paperwork
- For discharge to home: prescriptions, client instructions

Action	Rationale

• Wash your hands • Check the client's identification band •

Action	Rationale
1. Check for order for discharge.	1. Most agency policies require order for discharge.

Discharge to Another Facility

Action	Rationale
2. Complete intra-agency transfer form, according to policy. Be sure to note last time of medication doses. Complete nursing discharge summary. Prepare transfer paperwork, according to policy.	2. Facilitates continuity of care. Promotes client safety.
3. Explain discharge to client, and family, if appropriate.	3. Includes client in care. Promotes cooperation.

continued

Action	Rationale
4. Notify receiving agency of impending transfer. Provide report, confirm ability to receive client.	4. Facilitates continuity of care. Ensures that new facility will accept client before client leaves current facility.
5. Arrange for transportation to new facility. Call transportation company according to agency policy.	5. Reduces waiting time; facilitates continuity of care.
6. Review the valuables and belongings checklist completed on admission. Compare with belongings.	6. Ensures all of client's belongings are transferred with the client. Prevents loss.
7. When personnel from transportation company arrive, assist client transfer to stretcher or wheelchair. Provide transportation personnel with required information, such as client's DNR status, for transfer. See that client's belongings accompany client, along with any required paperwork or equipment.	7. Provides continuity of care.

Discharge to Home

Action	Rationale
8. Discuss discharge with client, and family, if appropriate. Confirm that discharge teaching has been done. Ask client if there are any questions about self-care at home. If so, follow up with appropriate personnel (typically, RN).	8. Promotes client cooperation. Allays anxiety.
9. LP/VN or RN (according to agency policy) reviews with client: prescriptions to be filled, including telling client when next dose is due based on medications administered in the facility; food and drug interactions and any other essential medication information; care of incision or dressings, if indicated; dietary restrictions or other pertinent information; and when client should make appointment for follow-up with private physician.	9. Promotes continuity of care.
10. Have client/family provide return demonstration of skills required for self-care at home.	10. Demonstrates that learning has occurred.
11. Check that transportation to home is available. Check client room area for any personal belongings.	11. Reduces waiting time.
12. Complete any paperwork with client, as required by agency policy.	12. Meets regulatory requirements.
13. Escort client to transportation vehicle.	13. Promotes client safety.

For Any Discharge

Action	Rationale
14. Document time of discharge and any other information required by agency policy.	14. Promotes communication among members of the health care team.
15. Notify appropriate personnel according to agency policy that client has left the unit. Arrange for personnel to clean the bed and surroundings the client has left.	15. Prepares bed for new admission. Reduces transfer of microorganisms.

Procedure 11

Surgical Asepsis: Preparing and Maintaining a Sterile Field

Equipment

- Antimicrobial soap for handwashing
- Sterile materials (antiseptic solution, bowl, dressing, instruments)
- Additional sterile supplies (culture swab, gauze, or dressings to complement the type of procedure to be performed)
- Sterile drape (may be contained in dressing tray)
- Sterile solution
- Package of proper-sized sterile gloves
- Container for disposal of waste materials (follow agency policy), colored bag that designates infectious waste products

Action	Rationale
• *Wash your hands* • *Check the client's identification band* • *Explain the procedure to the client prior to beginning*	
1. Gather equipment for the type of procedure: a. Select only clean, dry packages marked sterile, and read listing of contents. b. Check the package for integrity and expiration date.	1. Prevents break in technique during procedure. If the package is moist or outdated, it is considered contaminated and cannot be used.
2. Select a clean area in the client's environment to establish the sterile field.	2. Promotes access to the sterile field during the procedure.
3. Explain procedure to the client; provide specific instructions if client assistance is required during the procedure.	3. Gains client's understanding and cooperation during the procedure.
4. Inquire about and attend to the client's toileting needs.	4. Prevents break in technique during the procedure.
5. Hospital environment: If the procedure is to be performed at the client's bedside, the client should be in a private room or moved to a clean treatment room if available.	5. Minimizes microorganisms in the environment.
6. Home environment: Secure privacy and remove pets from the room.	6. Puts the client at ease and promotes a clean environment.
7. Position client and attend to comfort measures; the client's position should provide the nurse easy access to the area and facilitate good body mechanics during the procedure.	7. Helps the client relax and prevents movement during the procedure; prevents reaching, decreasing the risk of contamination and back strain.
8. Wash hands; refer to Procedure B1.	8. Prevents transmission of infection.
9. Place sterile package (drape or tray) in the center of the clean, dry work area.	9. Prevents reaching over exposed sterile items when wrapper is removed.

Drape

Action	Rationale
10. Open the wrapper, pulling away from the body first.	10. Prevents contamination.
11. Grasp the folded top edge of drape with fingertips of one hand.	11. Edges are considered unsterile.
12. Remove the drape by lifting up and away from all objects while it unfolds; discard the outer wrapper with other hand.	12. If the drape touches an unsterile object, it is contaminated and must be discarded.

continued

Action	Rationale
13. With free hand, grasp the other drape corner, keeping it away from all objects.	**13.** Avoids contamination.
14. Lay the drape on the surface, with the drape bottom first touching the surface farthest from you; step back and allow the drape to cover the surface.	**14.** Prevents you from reaching over the sterile field; stepping back decreases risk that drape will touch your uniform.

Tray

Action	Rationale
15. Remove outer wrapping and place the tray on the work surface so that the top flap of the sterile wrapper opens away from you.	**15.** Prevents reaching over the sterile items.
16. Reach around the tray, not over it. With thumb and index fingertips grasping the wrapper's top flap, gently pull up, then down to open over the surface.	**16.** Only the edges of the field can be contaminated, pulling up frees the top folded flap.
17. Repeat the same steps to open the side flaps.	**17.** Keeps the arm from reaching over the sterile field.
18. Grasp the corner of the bottom flap with fingertips, step back, and pull flap down (Figure I1-1).	**18.** Creates a sterile work surface.

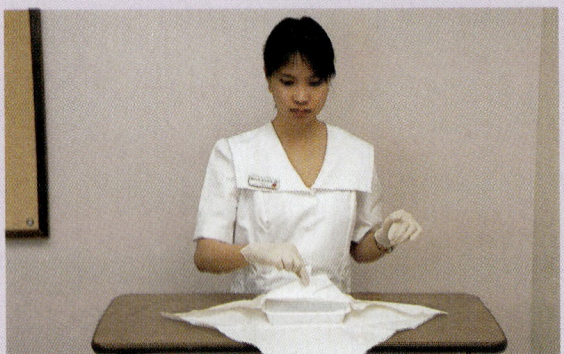

Figure I1-1 Grasp the corner of the bottom flap with fingertips, step back, and pull flap down (gloves not required for this procedure).

Adding Additional Sterile Items to Sterile Field

Action	Rationale
19. While facing the sterile field, step back, remove the outer wrapper, and grasp the item in your non-dominant hand so that the top flap will open away from you.	**19.** Keeps your dominant hand free; item remains sterile.
20. With your dominant hand, open the flaps as previously described.	**20.** Prevents reaching over the sterile item.
21. With your dominant hand, pull the wrapper back and away from the sterile field (toward your non-dominant arm holding the item) and place the item onto the field.	**21.** Prevents the wrapper from touching the sterile field.
22. When adding additional gauze or dressings to the sterile field, open the package as directed, grasp the top flaps of the wrapper and pull downward as shown in Figure I1-2, then drop the contents onto the center of the field as shown in Figure I1-3.	**22.** Prevents contamination of item and sterile field.

continued

Action	**Rationale**

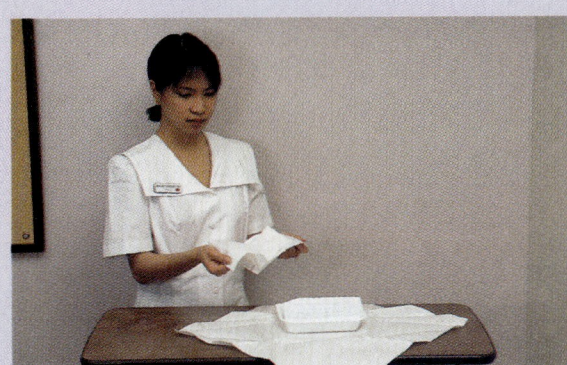

Figure I1-2 Grasp the flaps of the wrapped supply and pull downward.

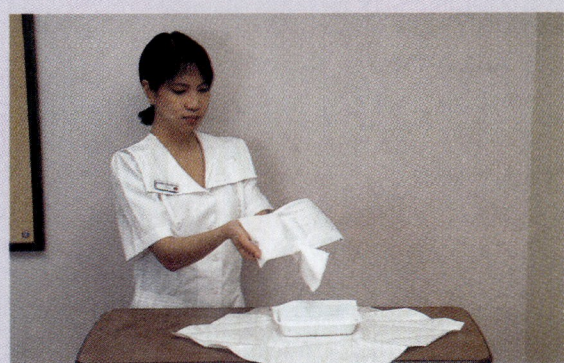

Figure I1-3 Add contents to the sterile field by holding the package 6 inches (15 cm) above the field and allowing the contents to drop onto the field.

Adding Solutions to Sterile Field

23. Read the labels and strengths of all solutions three times prior to pouring.

24. Remove the lid from the bottle of solution and invert the lid onto a clean surface.

25. Hold the bottle, label facing ceiling, 4 to 6 inches (10 to 15 cm) over the container on the sterile field; slowly pour the solution into the container to avoid splashing. Pour from the side of the sterile field. Do not reach over it.

26. Replace the lid on the container, label the container with the date and time, and initial the container.

Using Sterile Gloves

27. Wash hands and perform open gloving (see Procedure I2).

28. Continue with procedure, keeping gloved hands above waist level at all times, touching only items on the sterile field.

29. If using a solution to cleanse a site, use the sterile forceps to prevent contamination of gloves; dispose of forceps after use or process instruments according to agency policy.

30. Postprocedure, dispose of all contaminated items in colored plastic bag.

31. Remove gloves as shown in Procedure I2.

---

23. Ensures proper solution and strength.

24. Inverting the lid prevents contamination of the inner surface.

25. Prevents the label from getting wet. If the solution splashes onto the label, the field is contaminated because moisture conducts microorganisms from the nonsterile surface. Prevents contamination. If the solution splashes out of the container and the drape becomes wet, the field is contaminated.

26. Sterility of the solution will be lost if exposed to air for an extended period of time.

27. Prevents transmission of infection.

28. Decreases chance of contamination.

29. Prevents field contamination.

30. Decreases risk of transmission of infection to all health care workers.

31. Minimizes your risk of contact with infectious wastes on the gloves.

continued

Action	Rationale
32. Reposition the client.	**32.** Promotes client comfort.
33. Clean the environment; wash hands.	**33.** Prevents transmission of infection.
34. In the client's medical record, document the procedure, findings (i.e., description of infected area), and the response of the client.	**34.** Demonstrates compliance with sterile procedure and the effectiveness of therapy.

Procedure 12 — Performing Open Gloving and Removal of Soiled Gloves

Equipment

- Package of proper-sized sterile gloves

Action	Rationale
1. Wash hands (see Procedure B1).	**1.** Prevents transmission of infection.
2. Read the manufacturer's instructions on the package of sterile gloves; proceed as directed in removing the outer wrapper from the package, placing the inner wrapper onto a clean, dry surface.	**2.** Manufacturers package gloves differently; the instructions will tell you how to open properly to avoid contamination of the inner wrapper. Any moisture on the surface will contaminate the gloves.
3. Identify right- and left-hand gloves; glove dominant hand first.	**3.** Dominant hand should facilitate motor dexterity during gloving.
4. Grasp the 2-inch- (5-cm-) wide cuff with the thumb and first two fingers of the nondominant hand, touching only the inside of the cuff.	**4.** Maintains sterility of the outer surfaces of the sterile glove.
5. Gently pull the glove over the dominant hand, making sure the thumb and fingers fit into the proper spaces of the glove (Figure 12-1).	**5.** Prevents tearing the glove material; guiding the fingers into proper places facilitates gloving.

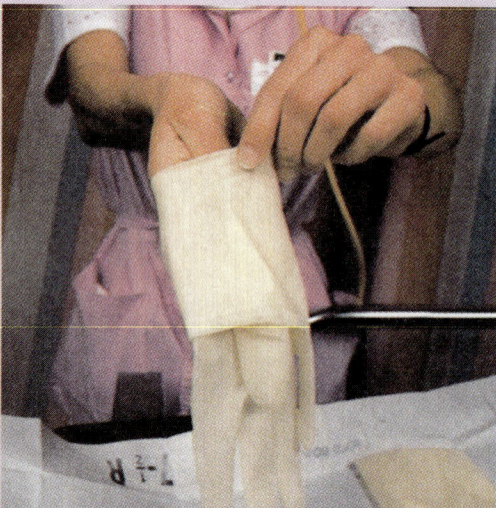

Figure 12-1 Pull the glove over the dominant hand.

6. With the gloved dominant hand, slip your fingers under the cuff of the other glove, gloved thumb	**6.** Cuff protects gloved fingers, maintaining sterility.

continued

Action	Rationale
abducted, making sure it does not touch any part of your nondominant ungloved hand.	
7. Gently slip the glove onto your nondominant hand, holding the thumb of the fully gloved hand apart from the other fingers and making sure the fingers slip into the proper spaces.	7. Contact is made with two sterile gloves; this reduces the risk of contamination from touching the arm.
8. With gloved hands, interlock fingers to fit the gloves onto each finger. When the gloves are soiled, remove by turning inside out as follows:	8. Promotes proper fit over the fingers.
9. Slip gloved fingers of the dominant hand under the cuff of the opposite hand or grasp the outer part of the glove at the wrist if there is no cuff (Figure I2-2).	9. Contact is made with two sterile gloves.

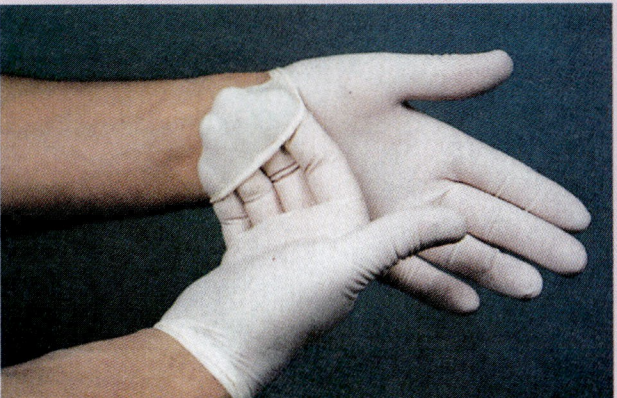

Figure I2-2 Insert gloved fingers under the cuff of the other glove.

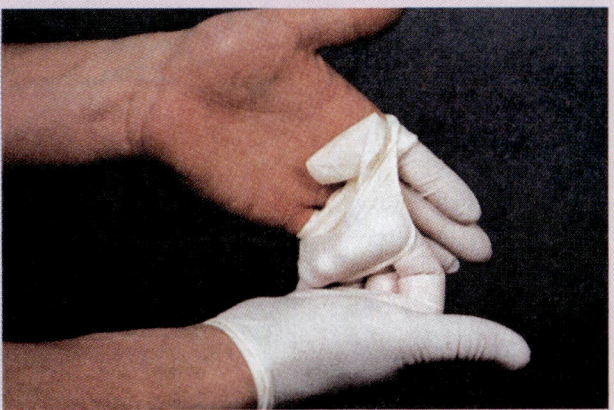

Figure I2-3 Pull the glove down to the fingers and off, turning the glove inside out.

Action	Rationale
10. Pull the glove down to the fingers and off, turning the glove inside out (Figure I2-3). Hold this glove in gloved hand.	10. Keeps the contaminated surface covered.
11. Slide two fingers of the bare hand between the wrist and the remaining glove. Slide this glove off, turning it inside out as it is removed, covering first glove removed.	11. Keeps the contaminated surface covered.
12. Dispose of soiled gloves according to institutional policy and wash hands.	12. Prevents the transfer of microorganisms.

Procedure I3 — Performing Urinary Catheterization: Male Client

Equipment

- Indwelling catheter with drainage system
- Adequate lighting source
- Blanket or drape
- Warm water
- Forceps
- Sterile catheterization kit
- Disposable gloves
- Soap and washcloth
- Towel
- Tape to secure catheter

continued

Action	**Rationale**

1. Provide for privacy.	1. Promotes cooperation and client dignity.
2. Set the bed to a comfortable height to work, and raise the side rail on the side opposite you.	2. Promotes proper body mechanics and assures client safety.
3. Assist the client to a supine position with legs slightly spread.	3. Relaxes muscles to facilitate insertion of the catheter.
4. Drape the client's abdomen and thighs, and place the penis over the thighs.	4. Promotes client comfort and warmth.
5. Ensure adequate lighting of the penis.	5. Facilitates proper execution of technique.
6. Wash hands, don disposable gloves, and wash perineal area.	6. Reduces transfer of microorganisms.
7. Remove gloves and wash hands. Choose correct catheter (Figure I3-1).	7. Reduces transfer of microorganisms.
8. Prepare a sterile field, apply sterile gloves, and connect the catheter and drainage system (if necessary).	8. The catheter and drainage system may be pre-connected; otherwise it is connected before catheterization to avoid exposing the client to ascending infection from an open-ended catheter.
9. Gently retract the foreskin (if present) and, using forceps, cleanse the glans penis with a povidone-iodine solution or other antimicrobial cleanser (Figure I3-2).	9. Removes dirt and minimizes the risk of urinary tract infection by removing surface pathogens.

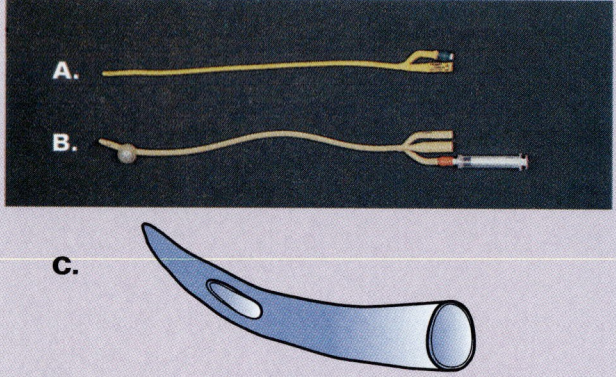

Figure I3-1 Types of Catheters: A. Foley Catheter; B. Three-Way Foley Catheter with Balloon Inflated; C. Coudé Catheter

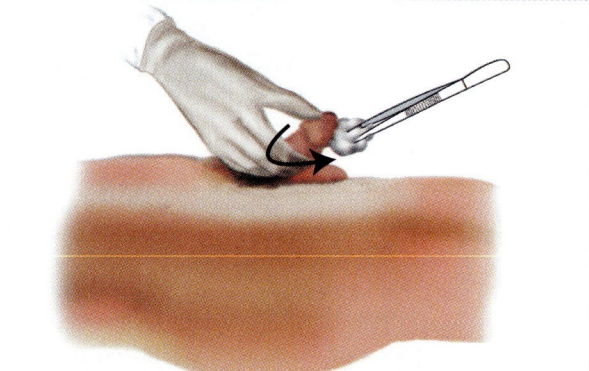

Figure I3-2 Cleanse the glans penis with a cotton ball held with forceps.

10. Inject 10 mL water-soluble lubricant (use a 2% xylocaine lubricant whenever feasible) into the urethra *before* catheter insertion; generously coat the distal portion of the catheter with water-soluble, sterile lubricant.	10. Avoids urethral trauma and discomfort during catheter insertion and facilitates insertion.
11. Hold the penis perpendicular to the body and pull up gently.	11. Facilitates catheter insertion by straightening urethra.
12. Steadily insert the catheter about 8 inches, until urine is noted. Continue inserting until the hub of the catheter (bifurcation between drainage port and retention balloon arm) is met.	12. Ensures adequate catheter insertion before retention balloon is inflated.

continued

Action	Rationale
13. Inflate the retention balloon using manufacturer's recommendations or according to physician orders.	**13.** Ensures retention of the balloon; up to twice the recommended volume of fluid may be inserted safely into the retention balloon if needed.
14. Instruct the client to immediately report discomfort or pressure during balloon inflation; if pain occurs, discontinue the procedure, deflate the balloon, and insert the catheter farther into the bladder.	**14.** Pain or pressure indicates inflation of the balloon in the urethra; further insertion will prevent misplacement and further pain or bleeding.
15. Gently pull the catheter until the retention balloon is snuggled against the bladder neck (resistance will be met) (Figure I3-3).	**15.** Maximizes continuous bladder drainage.

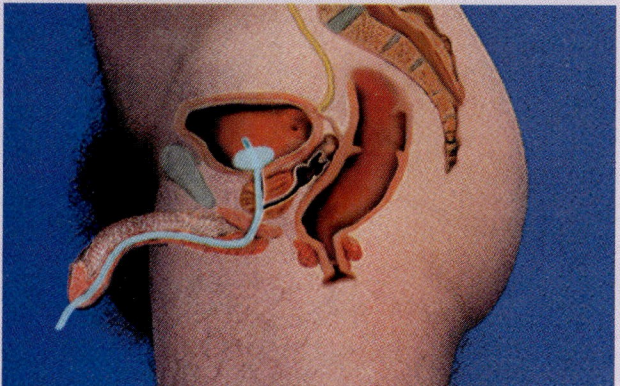

Figure I3-3 Correct Catheter Placement: Male Client

Action	Rationale
16. Secure the catheter to the abdomen or thigh.	**16.** Prevents excessive traction from the balloon rubbing against the bladder neck, inadvertent catheter removal, or urethral erosion.
17. Place the drainage bag below the level of the bladder.	**17.** Maximizes continuous drainage of urine from the bladder (drainage is prevented when the drainage bag is placed above the abdomen).
18. Remove gloves, dispose of equipment, and wash hands.	**18.** Prevents transfer of microorganisms.
19. Help client adjust position.	**19.** Promotes client comfort.
20. Document that catheterization was performed and amount of fluid in retention balloon.	**20.** Informs that catheter is in place; knowing amount of fluid assists when removing catheter.
21. Assess and document the amount, color, odor, and quality of urine.	**21.** Monitors urinary status.

Procedure I4 — Performing Urinary Catheterization: Female Client

Equipment

- See Procedure I3

continued

Action	**Rationale**

• Wash your hands • Check the client's identification band •
• Explain the procedure to the client prior to beginning •

1. See Procedure I3, steps 1 and 2.

2. Assist the client to a supine position with legs spread and feet together or to a side-lying position with upper leg flexed.

2. Facilitates visualization of area and promotes client comfort.

3. Drape client's abdomen and thighs.

3. Promotes client comfort and warmth.

4. Ensure adequate lighting of the perineum.

4. Facilitates proper execution of technique.

5. Refer to Procedure I3, steps 6, 7, and 8.

6. Generously coat the distal portion of the catheter with water-soluble, sterile lubricant.

6. Avoids urethral trauma and discomfort during catheter insertion.

7. Separate the labia and, using forceps, cleanse the periurethral mucosa with a povidone-iodine or other antimicrobial cleanser (Figure I4-1). Note that the gloved hand on the labia is no longer sterile.

7. Removes dirt and minimizes the risk of urinary tract infection by removing surface pathogens.

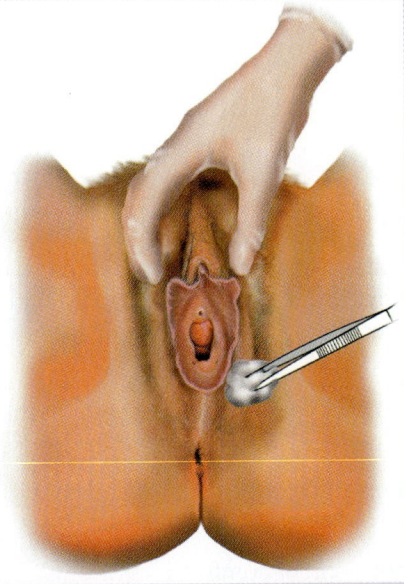

Figure I4-1 Cleanse the periurethral mucosa with a cotton ball held with forceps.

8. With your sterile, gloved hand, gently insert the catheter into meatus until urine is seen in the catheter tubing. Continue inserting for 1 to 3 additional inches.

8. Ensures adequate catheter insertion before retention balloon is inflated.

9. Inflate the retention balloon using manufacturer's recommendations or according to physician orders.

9. Ensures retention of the balloon; up to twice the recommended volume of fluid may be inserted safely into the retention balloon if needed.

10. Instruct the client to immediately report discomfort or pressure during balloon inflation; if pain occurs, discontinue the procedure, deflate the balloon, and insert the catheter further into the bladder.

10. Pain or pressure indicates inflation of the balloon in the urethra; further insertion will prevent misplacement and further pain or bleeding.

continued

Action	**Rationale**
11. Gently pull the catheter until the retention balloon is snuggled against the bladder neck (resistance will be met) (Figure 14-2).	**11.** Maximizes continuous bladder drainage.

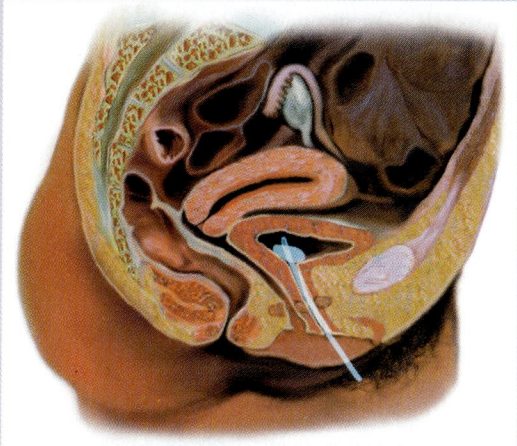

Figure 14-2 Correct Catheter Placement: Female Client

Action	**Rationale**
12. Secure the catheter to the abdomen or thigh.	**12.** Prevents excessive traction from the balloon rubbing against the bladder neck, inadvertent catheter removal, or urethral erosion.
13. Place the drainage bag below the level of the bladder.	**13.** Maximizes continuous drainage of urine from the bladder (drainage is prevented when the drainage bag is placed above the abdomen).
14. See Procedure 13, steps 18–21.	

Procedure 15   Irrigating an Open Catheter

Equipment

- Catheter tip irrigation syringe
- Sterile gloves
- Sterile basin

- Sterile solution in amount ordered by physician
- Sterile drape
- 5–10 alcohol wipes

Action	**Rationale**
• Wash your hands • Check the client's identification band • *• Explain the procedure to the client prior to beginning •*	
1. Open sterile drape and form a sterile field.	**1.** Promotes sterile environment.
2. Using sterile technique, open and place basin on sterile field.	**2.** Decreases the chances of bacteria being introduced into the bladder.
3. Pour solution into sterile basin. Solution should be no warmer than 99° to 102°F.	**3.** Maintains sterility of the solution.
4. Open syringe, remove tip and fill with solution, then place at opposite end of sterile field away from basin and solution.	**4.** Maintains sterile environment.
5. Open alcohol wipes exposing only half a wipe.	**5.** Facilitates handling of wipe.

continued

Action	**Rationale**
6. Don sterile gloves.	6. Prevents or inhibits contamination.
7. Clean junction between catheter and drainage tube with alcohol wipes.	7. Prevents contamination when juncture is disconnected.
8. Simultaneously twist and pull catheter and drainage tube apart.	8. Makes disconnection easy.
9. Hold both drainage tube and catheter in nondominant hand; with dominant hand take catheter tip syringe and place into catheter opening. Depending on the amount, syringe may need to be refilled and procedure repeated.	9. Holding both drainage and catheter tubing decreases the chances of falling and cross-contamination.
10. Slowly squeeze solution into the catheter using plunger.	10. Rapid infusion may cause bladder spasms.
11. Clean both tips with alcohol and reconnect.	11. Avoids reintroducing bacteria into catheter system.
12. Drain solution via gravity.	12. Pulling back solution through syringe may cause damage to bladder.
13. Clean work area and dispose of contaminated supplies properly.	13. Maintains safe, clean work environment.
14. Remove gloves and wash hands.	14. Prevents spread of bacteria.
15. Document amount of solution given; amount, color, and clarity of return; and client's response.	15. Provides record of procedure and client's status.

Procedure 16   Irrigating a Closed Catheter

Equipment

- Three-way indwelling catheter
- Sturdy IV pole
- Gloves
- Irrigation solution
- Large drainage bag
- Wipes

Action	**Rationale**

• *Wash your hands* • *Check the client's identification band* •
• *Explain the procedure to the client prior to beginning* •

Action	**Rationale**
1. Obtain irrigation solution from pharmacy as prescribed by the physician.	1. Irrigation solutions are selected for their antimicrobial properties or to remove clots and debris; a hypotonic or hypertonic solution may be absorbed through resected tissue, causing fluid and electrolyte imbalances.
2. Hang solution (1–3 L) from a sturdy IV pole (depending on anticipated rate of irrigation) using one-, two-, or three-port irrigation tubing. Flush tubing to remove air.	2. Relatively rapid irrigation may be used to remove debris or clots from the bladder; slower irrigations are used to treat local infection.
3. Connect the irrigation infusion tubing to the third irrigation port of the three-way catheter; refer to	3. Ensures proper irrigation and simultaneous drainage from the bladder.

continued

Action	Rationale

Action

the product for instructions and identification of the irrigation port (Figure 16-1). Use sterile technique.

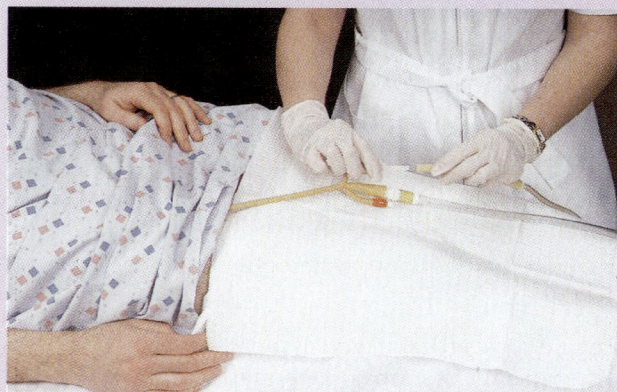

Figure 16-1 Connect the irrigation tubing to the irrigation port of the catheter.

4. Consult the physician concerning the rate of irrigation; *never* slow the irrigation rate because "pink urine" has been observed unless directed by the physician or urologic nurse specialist.

5. Regularly check the drainage container; empty the bag when filled two-thirds or more.

6. Document catheter irrigation; solution and amount used; amount, color, and clarity of return; and client's response.

Rationale

4. Clotting and catheter obstruction following transurethral resection of the prostate or transurethral sphincterotomy frequently occur because the nurse has prematurely slowed the irrigation; a pink solution is expected when an adequate irrigation is being performed; this finding does not mean that all bleeding has stopped.

5. Filling of the drainage bag occurs rapidly and can obstruct the irrigation.

6. Provides record of procedure and client's status.

Procedure 17   Changing a Colostomy Pouch

Equipment

- Appropriate pouch
- Skin barrier (Figure 17-1)
- Pouch clip or rubber band
- Skin paste
- Disposable gloves
- Soap and washcloth
- Warm water

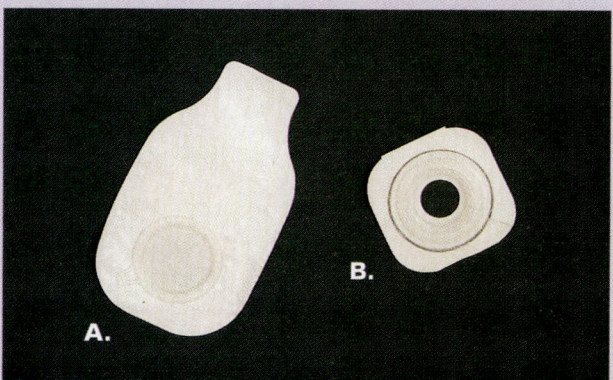

Figure 17-1 Equipment for Application of a Colostomy Pouch: A. Colostomy Pouch; B. Skin Barrier

continued

Action	**Rationale**

• Wash your hands • Check the client's identification band •
• Explain the procedure to the client prior to beginning •

Action	**Rationale**
1. Provide for privacy. Include caregivers in instruction if indicated.	1. Promotes cooperation and boosts caregiver confidence in ability to perform procedure.
2. Assist client to a standing (preferable) or sitting position.	2. Facilitates application of pouch by reducing wrinkles.
3. Don gloves.	3. Reduces risk of contamination.
4. Remove the soiled pouch by gently pressing on the skin while pulling the pouch.	4. Avoids trauma to the peristomal skin.
5. Discard the disposable pouch in a plastic bag after removing the clip used to seal the pouch.	5. Minimizes odor associated with the pouch change.
6. Cleanse the skin with soap and warm water. Rinse and dry thoroughly. (Soap may be omitted if the skin is irritated.)	6. Removes fecal material and pathogens and prepares the skin for pouch reapplication.
7. Inspect the peristomal skin for redness, altered skin integrity, or rashes; consult the enterostomal nurse if lesions of the peristomal skin are observed. Tissue or a gauze pad may be placed over stoma to absorb seepage during procedure.	7. Peristomal skin conditions cause morbidity and problems with pouch application unless managed promptly.
8. Remove excessive hair with a safety razor or electric razor as needed.	8. Excessive hair is removed to promote the seal between pouch adhesive and peristomal skin.
9. Inspect the pouch opening and ensure that it fits the stoma; use a pouch pattern to customize the fit if indicated (Figure 17-2).	9. Ensures appropriate-sized pouch and protects the peristomal skin.
10. Apply a skin sealant or skin paste if indicated; apply skin barrier (Figure 17-3).	10. Promotes an effective seal and protects the peristomal skin.
11. Gently apply the pouch and press into place (Figure 17-4). Seal the bottom of the pouch with the clip or a rubber band after air is expelled from the pouch.	11. Prevents leakage of effluent from the pouch.
12. Remove gloves and discard; wash hands.	12. Reduces risk of transfer of microorganisms.
13. Document type and size of pouch; condition of stoma (drainage amount and odor; surrounding skin); and client response.	13. Provides record of client status and condition of stoma.

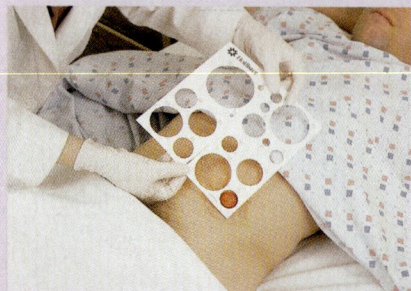

Figure 17-2 Measure the stoma for the colostomy pouch.

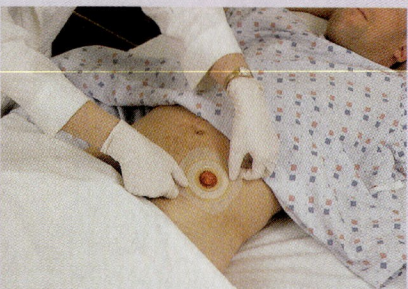

Figure 17-3 Apply the skin barrier to the stoma.

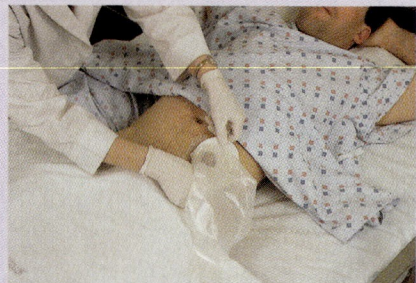

Figure 17-4 Press the pouch into place.

Procedure 18   Application of Heat and Cold

Equipment

- Heat-producing device with cover
- OR cold-producing device with cover

Action	Rationale
• Wash your hands • Check the client's identification band • *• Explain the procedure to the client prior to beginning •*	
1. Check the order for heat or cold therapy.	1. Ensures correct therapy is used.
2. Prepare the equipment according to manufacturer's instructions before preparing client if it will take time for equipment to become warm or cold.	2. Minimizes exposure time for client.
3. Position the client so that the body part requiring the heat or cold application can be exposed. Expose the body part while covering the rest of the client.	3. Respects client's dignity.
4. Review the circulatory status of the area to be treated and other client factors that can affect tolerance of heat or cold therapy, such as sensory defects. Carefully assess the area to be treated so that changes in appearance can be detected quickly. If open areas of skin exist, check with RN or physician before applying therapy directly to skin. Skin should be clean and dry before applying heat or cold therapy.	4. Promotes client safety by reducing the risk of complications.
5. Apply the heat or cold device on the client after applying cover over the device, according to manufacturer's instructions. (Use waterproof pads to protect linens, if indicated.)	5. Cover protects skin and reduces transfer of microorganisms.
6. Regularly assess the client for any complaints of discomfort, such as pain or burning. The frequency of assessment will depend on the client's underlying condition and experience with heat or cold therapy. If client has any complaints, remove heat or cold therapy immediately and reassess. Be sure the call bell is in reach.	6. Regular assessments will detect problems quickly and prevent injury.
7. Remove the heat or cold after 20 to 30 minutes, or according to physician order or agency policy.	7. Removes heat or cold before rebound phenomenon begins. (With heat application, vasoconstriction occurs to cool the area; with cold application, vasodilation occurs to warm the area.)
8. After removal, record client response to therapy, duration, and type of heat or cold therapy applied.	8. Facilitates communication among members of the health care team.

Procedure 19 — Administering an Oral, Sublingual, or Buccal Medication

Equipment

- Medication administration record (MAR)
- Medication cart or tray
- Glass of water or juice
- Medication cup
- Medication properly labeled
- Straw (if indicated)

Action	Rationale
Oral Medication	
1. Assess the client for potential problems, e.g., absence of a gag reflex.	1. Decreases the risk of aspiration.
2. Check the MAR against the physician's written orders.	2. Ensures accuracy in the administration of the medication.
3. Check for drug allergies.	3. Decreases risk of allergic reactions such as hives, urticaria, or anaphylactic shock.
4. Wash your hands.	4. Decreases transmission of microorganisms.
5. Prepare the medications for *one client at a time*.	5. Ensures that the right client receives the right medications.
• Select the correct medication and double check against MAR.	• Increases accuracy.
• Calculate the medication dose, if necessary.	• Determines the correct amount of medication to be given.
• Avoid touching the drug while pouring into cup. If unit dose is available leave drug in the wrapper until at the bedside.	• Decreases possibility of contaminating the medication and helps ensure accuracy.
• Prepare liquids by placing the label side of the medicine bottle against the palm of your hand and pouring the liquid at eye level (Figure 19-1).	• Prevents soiling and maintains legibility of the label. Ensures accurate measurement.
• Recheck prepared medications with MAR.	• Ensures right dose, route, and time.
• Check MAR to make sure all medications to be administered have been prepared.	• Promotes efficiency and decreases risk of error.
• Place medications on the tray or medication cart.	• Prevents spillage.

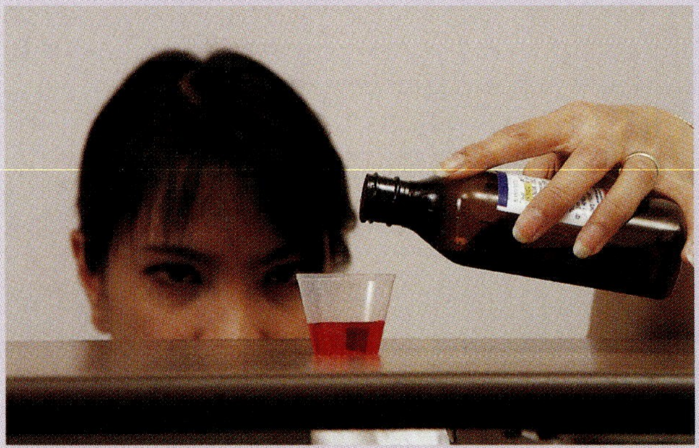

Figure 19-1 Measure oral medications at eye level to ensure accurate measurement.

continued

Action	Rationale
6. Check client's armband before administering the medications.	**6.** Ensures right client.
7. Identify the drug for the client and its therapeutic purpose.	**7.** Encourages client cooperation and increases client awareness of what to expect from the medication.
8. Assist client to a sitting position.	**8.** Prevents aspiration and promotes swallowing of the medication.
9. Offer liquids before and during ingestion of drug.	**9.** Facilitates downward movement of the medication in digestive system.
10. Remain with the client until all medications have been swallowed.	**10.** Ensures that all medications have been taken.
11. Wash your hands.	**11.** Decreases the transmission of microorganisms.

Sublingual Medication

Note: When administering more than one medication, administer the sublingual medication last.

Action	Rationale
12. Follow actions 2–4, 5 (except bullet 4), and 6 and 7.	**12.** See Rationales for actions 2–4, 5, and 6 and 7.
13. Don gloves.	**13.** Protects the nurse from spread of micro-organisms.
14. Explain to the client that this medicine is to dissolve under the tongue; it is not to be swallowed. Instruct client to allow tablet to dissolve completely and not to chew the tablet or drink water for an hour.	**14.** Promotes cooperation; enhances proper drug delivery.
15. Remove tablet from unit dose wrapper (if present), place tablet under client's tongue. (*Note:* If medication is nitroglycerin, have client wet the tablet with saliva before sliding it under the tongue, to speed absorption.)	**15.** Facilitates drug delivery.
16. Remove gloves and wash hands.	**16.** Decreases transmission of microorganisms.
17. After administering sublingual medication, check to be sure client did not swallow medication.	**17.** Swallowing interferes with drug absorption.

Buccal Medication

Note: When administering more than one medication, administer the buccal medication last.

Action	Rationale
18. Follow actions 12 and 13 for sublingual.	**18.** See Rationales 12 and 13.
19. Explain to client that this medicine is to dissolve between the cheek and gum; it is not to be swallowed. Instruct client to allow tablet to dissolve completely and not to chew or swallow the tablet or drink water while the tablet is in the mouth.	**19.** Promotes cooperation; enhances proper drug delivery; avoids risk of swallowing tablet.
20. Remove tablet from unit dose wrapper (if present); place tablet between client's cheek and gum.	**20.** Facilitates drug delivery.
21. Remove gloves and wash hands.	**21.** Decreases transmission of microorganisms.

continued

Action	Rationale
22. After administering buccal medication, check to be sure client did not swallow medication.	**22.** Swallowing interferes with drug absorption.
23. Record the administered medications on the MAR.	**23.** Provides documentation of medication administration.
24. Observe the client for side effects or adverse reactions.	**24.** Provides identification of potential problems related to the medications administered.

Procedure I10 — Withdrawing Medication from an Ampule

Equipment

- Medication administration record (MAR)
- Sterile syringe and needle
- Extra needle of proper gauge and length in accord with site
- Ampule of prescribed medication
- Sterile gauze or alcohol wipe
- Filter needle (check agency policy)

Action	Rationale
1. Wash your hands.	**1.** Decreases transmission of microorganisms.
2. Hold the ampule and quickly and lightly tap the top chamber until all fluid flows into the bottom chamber. Alternatively, hold the top chamber between the thumb and fingers, and make a large circle with the outstretched arm.	**2.** Moves the fluid trapped above the neck of the ampule to the lower chamber of the ampule. Centrifugal force will pull the fluid into the bottom chamber.
3. Place a sterile gauze or alcohol wipe around the neck of the ampule (Figure I10-1).	**3.** Contains the glass fragments and shields the nurse's fingers from the broken ampule.

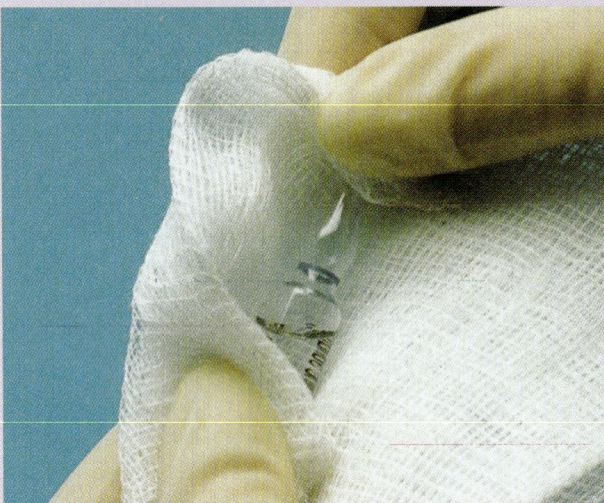

Figure I10-1 Snap open the ampule while holding a wipe or gauze around the neck of the ampule, to protect against glass fragments. (Gloves are optional.)

Action	Rationale
4. Firmly grasp the ampule and quickly snap the top off away from your body. Place the ampule on a flat surface.	**4.** Directs shattered glass fragments away from the nurse's face and fingers. Prevents spillage of medication.

continued

Action	**Rationale**
5. Withdraw the medication from the ampule, maintaining sterile technique.	5. Prevents the transmission of microorganisms.
• Check connection of needle to syringe by turning barrel to right while holding needle guard. *Note:* Some agencies require the use of a filter needle to withdraw medication from an ampule. Follow agency policy.	• Ensures an airtight system.
• Remove needle guard and hold syringe in dominant hand.	• Promotes dexterity.
• With nondominant hand grasp ampule and turn upside down, or hold ampule as shown.	• Provides access to medication.
• Insert the needle into the center of the ampule; do not allow the needle tip or shaft to touch the rim of the ampule.	• Prevents contamination of needle tip or shaft.
• Keep needle tip below level of meniscus (Figure I10-2).	• Prevents air from entering syringe and fluid from leaking out while the ampule is inverted.

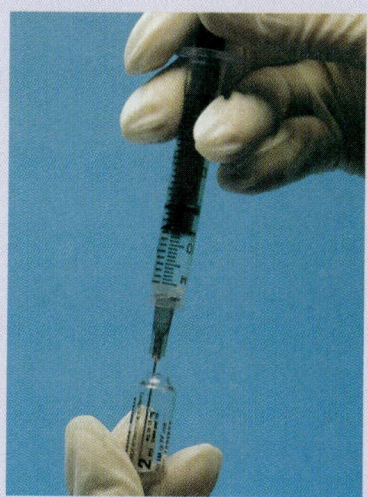

Figure I10-2 Hold the needle point below the level of fluid so the fluid does not leak out. (Gloves are optional.)

Action	**Rationale**
• Aspirate the medication by gently pulling on the plunger.	• Allows medication to enter the syringe.
• If air bubbles are aspirated, remove the needle from the ampule. Hold syringe with needle pointing up and tap sides of the syringe. Draw back slightly on plunger, and gently push the plunger upward to eject air. Reinsert the needle in the middle of the ampule and continue to withdraw the medication.	• Prevents loss of medication from the ampule caused from air pressure. Moves air bubbles above the fluid level in the syringe. Pulls medication from needle so only air is ejected from the syringe.
6. Remove excess air from the syringe and check the dosage of medication in the syringe. Recap with one-handed technique.	6. Allows for accurate measurement of medication dose; reduces risk of needle stick injury.
7. Change needle and properly discard used needle. Secure needle to syringe by turning the barrel to the right while holding the needle guard.	7. Changing needle reduces the risk that the drug will cause irritation to subcutaneous tissue.

Procedure 111   Withdrawing Medication from a Vial

Equipment

- Medication administration record (MAR)
- Sterile syringe and needle
- Alcohol wipe
- Vial of medication
- Sterile needle

Action	**Rationale**
1. Wash your hands. Gloves are optional.	1. Reduces transmission of microorganisms.
2. Prepare the vial.	2. Provides access to vial. Removes surface contamination. (*Note:* Manufacturer does not ensure sterility of rubber top.)
• Mix solution, if needed, by rotating vial between the palms. Do not shake.	
• Open the alcohol wipe.	
• New vial: remove cap from vial of medicine and cleanse the rubber top of the vial.	
• Used vial: cleanse the rubber top of the vial.	
3. Prepare syringe:	3. Ensures a closed system.
• Grasp needle and turn barrel of syringe to the right.	
• Remove the needle cap and pull back on plunger to fill syringe with an amount of air equal to amount of solution to be withdrawn from the vial.	• Displaces the solution with air to prevent the formation of a vacuum in the sealed vial.
4. Insert the needle into the center of the upright vial and, while keeping needle above the fluid level, inject air into the vial.	4. Creates positive pressure inside vial to allow accurate withdrawal of medicine. Avoids creating bubbles.
5. Invert vial; keep the vial at eye level and the needle's bevel below the fluid level, and remove the exact amount of medicine while touching only the syringe barrel and plunger tip (Figure I11-1).	5. Prevents contamination of the plunger, barrel, and medicine.

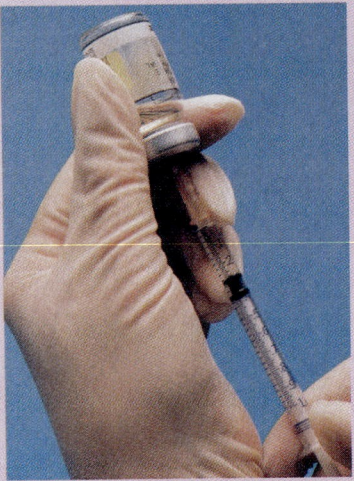

Figure I11-1 Invert the vial and keep the needle below the fluid level.

continued

Action	**Rationale**
6. Expel air from the syringe while needle remains within the inverted vial after tapping the side of the syringe with your finger.	6. Removes air bubbles created by the dead space in the needle's hub; allows for accurate measurement of the solution.
7. Check the amount of medicine in the syringe.	7. Ensures accurate dose.
8. Turn vial upright and remove the needle.	8. Prevents the leakage of solution from the vial.
9. Replace the needle cap using one-handed technique. Open the sterile package of the new needle. Remove used needle and dispose in the sharps container.	9. Prevents needle stick.
10. Attach the new needle to the syringe by turning the barrel to the right while holding the needle guard.	10. Provides a sharp needle for injection to decrease the client's discomfort.
11. Compare the medication in the syringe with the prescribed dosage in the MAR.	11. Complies with safety standards for ensuring the correct dosage.

Procedure I12 — Administering an Intradermal Injection

Equipment

- Medication administration record (MAR)
- Sterile tuberculin syringe and short bevel, 25 to 27 gauge, ⅜- to ½-inch needle
- Medication
- Alcohol swab and sterile 2 × 2 gauze pad
- Disposable gloves

Action	**Rationale**
• Check the client's identification band • Explain the procedure to the client prior to beginning •	
1. Check with the client and the chart for any known allergies.	1. Prevents the occurrence of hypersensitivity reactions such as hives or anaphylactic shock.
2. Check the MAR against the physician's written orders.	2. Ensures accuracy in administration of the correct medication.
3. Wash hands.	3. Reduces transmission of microorganisms.
4. Follow the five rights.	4. Promotes client safety.
5. Prepare the medication from an ampule or vial; refer to Procedure I10 or I11 as appropriate. Take the medication to the client's room and place on a clean surface.	
6. Place the client in a comfortable position; provide for privacy.	6. Promotes comfort. Promotes absorption of the medication. Decreases anxiety.
7. Wash hands and don nonsterile gloves.	7. Decreases contact with blood and body fluids.
8. Select and clean the site. • Assess the client's skin for bruises, redness, or broken tissue. • Select an appropriate site using appropriate anatomic landmarks.	8. Promotes absorption of the drug; reduces trauma to the body's tissue.

continued

Action	Rationale
• Cleanse the site with an alcohol wipe using a firm circular motion; cleanse from inside to outside; allow alcohol to dry.	• Aids in the removal of microorganisms on the skin.
9. Prepare the syringe for injection.	9. Ensures correct dosage of medication in the syringe.
• Remove the needle guard.	
• Express any air bubbles from the syringe.	
• Check the amount of solution in the syringe.	
10. Inject the medication.	10.
• Hold the syringe in dominant hand.	
• With nondominant hand, grasp the client's dorsal forearm and gently pull the skin taut on ventral forearm.	• Spreads the skin taut to facilitate needle insertion.
• Insert the needle at a 10° to 15° angle with the bevel facing upward until resistance is felt, and advance the needle approximately 3 mm below the skin surface; the needle's tip should be visible under the skin (Figure I12-1).	• Ensures that medication is injected into the intradermal tissue; initial resistance indicates the needle's tip is going through epidermis.

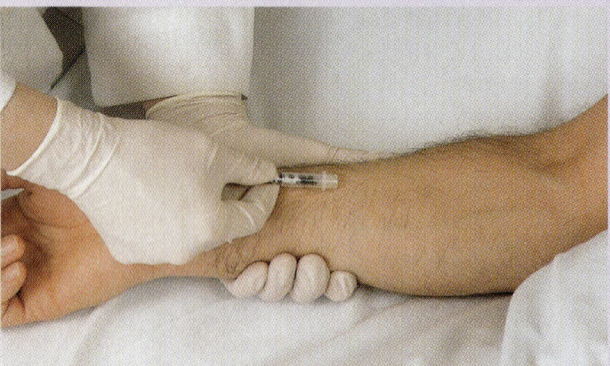

Figure I12-1 Spread the skin taut for an intradermal injection.

Action	Rationale
• Administer the medication slowly; observe the development of a bleb (small wheal that resembles a mosquito bite).	• Indicates that the medication was injected into the dermis.
• Withdraw the needle.	
• Pat area gently with a dry 2 × 2 sterile gauze pad.	
• Do not massage the area following the removal of the needle.	• Prevents spreading the medication beyond the point of injection.
11. Discard the needle and syringe in a sharps container. *Do not* recap needle.	11. Prevents needle sticks.
12. Remove gloves, dispose in appropriate receptacle, and wash hands.	12. Reduces the spread of microorganisms.
13. Observe for signs of an allergic reaction.	13. Ensures client safety.

continued

Action	Rationale
14. Draw a circle around the perimeter of the bleb with a ball point pen.	**14.** Allows for easy recognition and observation of the injection site.
15. Document medication, route, site, and time of injection on the MAR.	**15.** Provides a written description of the injection site and states the time the medication was administered.

Procedure I13   Administering a Subcutaneous Injection

Equipment

- Medication administration record (MAR)
- Sterile 3-mL syringe and ⅝-inch needle
- 2 alcohol swabs

- Medication as prescribed
- Disposable gloves

Action	Rationale
• *Check the client's identification band* • *Explain the procedure to the client prior to beginning* •	
1. Check with client and the chart for any known allergies.	**1.** Prevents the occurrence of hypersensitivity reactions such as hives or anaphylactic shock.
2. Check the MAR against the physician's written order.	**2.** Ensures accuracy of administration of the correct medication.
3. Wash your hands.	**3.** Reduces transmission of microorganisms.
4. Follow the five rights.	**4.** Promotes client safety.
5. Prepare the medication from an ampule or vial; refer to Procedure I10 or I11 as appropriate. Take medication to the client's room and place on a clean surface.	
6. Place the client in a comfortable position; provide for privacy.	**6.** Promotes relaxation of the muscles, decreasing discomfort from the injection.
7. Don nonsterile gloves.	**7.** Decreases contact with blood and body fluids.
8. Select and clean the site.	**8.** Promotes absorption of drug when injected into healthy tissue.
• Assess the client's skin for bruises, redness, hard tissue, or broken skin.	
• Cleanse the site with an alcohol swab; cleanse from inside outward.	• Removes the surface microorganisms.
9. Prepare for the injection.	**9.**
• Remove the needle guard and express any air bubbles from the syringe; check the dosage in the syringe.	• Prevents the injection of air into the subcutaneous tissue.
• With dominant hand, hold the syringe like a dart between your thumb and forefingers.	• Decreases risk for accidental contamination of the needle.
• Pinch the subcutaneous tissue between the thumb and forefinger with the nondominant hand. If the client has substantial subcutaneous tissue, spread the tissue taut.	• Ensures insertion of the needle into the subcutaneous tissue.

continued

Action	Rationale
10. Administer the injection.	**10.** Decreases the client's anxiety and the amount of discomfort.
• Insert the needle quickly at a 45° to 90° angle.	
• Release the subcutaneous tissue and grasp the barrel of the syringe with nondominant hand.	
• With dominant hand, aspirate by pulling back on the plunger gently, except when administering a heparin injection.	
• If blood appears, remove needle and discard in a sharps container.	• Indicates needle has entered a blood vessel.
• Inject medication slowly if there is no blood present.	• Prevents the injection of medication into the blood, which causes a faster absorption rate that may be dangerous to the client.
• Remove the needle quickly and lightly massage area with alcohol swab; do not massage the injection site after the administration of heparin.	• Promotes dispersement of medication in the tissues and facilitates absorption.
• Do not recap the needle; discard the needle and syringe in a sharps container.	• Prevents needle sticks.
11. Position client for comfort.	
12. Remove gloves and wash hands.	**12.** Reduces the spread of microorganisms.
13. Record on the MAR the medication, route, site, and time of injection.	**13.** Provides documentation that the medication was administered.
14. Observe the client for any side or adverse effects and assess the effectiveness of the medication at the appropriate time.	**14.** Alerts the nurse to hypersensitivity reactions; the peak plasma level is dependent on the drug's half-life.

Procedure 114   Administering an Intramuscular Injection

Equipment

- Medication administration record (MAR)
- Sterile 3-ml syringe and long bevel, 20 to 22 gauge, 1- to 2-inch needle (average-sized, adult client receiving a drug in an aqueous solution)
- Medication as prescribed
- Alcohol swab
- 2 × 2 gauze

Action	Rationale
• *Check the client's identification band* • *Explain the procedure to the client prior to beginning* •	
1. Check the MAR against the physician's written orders.	**1.** Ensures accuracy in medication administration.
2. Check with client and the chart for any known allergies.	**2.** Prevents the occurrence of hypersensitivity reactions.
3. Wash hands.	**3.** Reduces the spread of microorganisms.
4. Follow the five rights.	**4.** Promotes client safety.

continued

Action	Rationale
5. Prepare the medication from an ampule or vial; refer to Procedure I10 or I11 as appropriate.	**5.** Ensures that all of the medication is expelled from the needle's shaft.
• Add 0.1 to 0.2 mL of air to the syringe.	
• Take medication to the client's room and place on a clean surface.	
6. Place the client in an appropriate position to expose the site.	**6.** Provides access to the site, promotes relaxation of muscles, and decreases the discomfort from the injection.
• Deltoid: sitting position.	
• Ventrogluteal:	
– Side-lying: flex the knee; pivot the leg forward from the hip about 20° so it can rest on the bed.	
– Supine: flex the knee on the injection side.	
– Prone: point toes inward toward each other to internally rotate the femur.	
7. Don nonsterile gloves.	**7.** Decreases contact with blood and body fluids.
8. Select and clean the site.	**8.**
• Assess the client's skin for redness, scarring, breaks in the skin, and palpate for lumps or nodules.	• Avoids potential problems that may decrease the rate of the drug's absorption.
• Select site using the anatomic landmarks.	• Avoids tissue containing large nerves and blood vessels.
• Cleanse the area with an alcohol swab, cleanse from center outward using friction; wait 30 seconds to allow to dry.	• Removes the surface microorganisms and prevents the introduction of alcohol into subcutaneous tissue to avoid irritation.
9. Prepare for the injection.	
• Remove the needle cap by pulling it straight off, and expel any air bubbles from the syringe.	• Maintains the sterility of the needle; ensures the correct dosage in the syringe.
• Pull the skin down or to one side (Z-track technique) with nondominant hand.	• Decreases the risk of medication leaking into needle track and the subcutaneous tissue; reduces complications and discomfort.
10. Administer the injection.	**10.**
• Deltoid: quickly insert the needle with a dart-like motion at a 90° angle (Figure I14-1).	
• Ventrogluteal: quickly insert the needle using a dartlike motion and steady pressure at a 90° angle to the iliac crest in the middle of the V (Figure I14-2).	
• Z-track technique: With nondominant hand, pull the skin and subcutaneous tissue about 1 to 1.5 inches (2.5 to 3.5 cm) to one side of the injection site, out of alignment with the underlying muscle (Figure I14-3). (Do not use this technique in the deltoid; the dorsogluteal site in the buttocks is preferred.)	• Allows the medication to be "sealed" in the muscle after injection.

continued

Action	**Rationale**

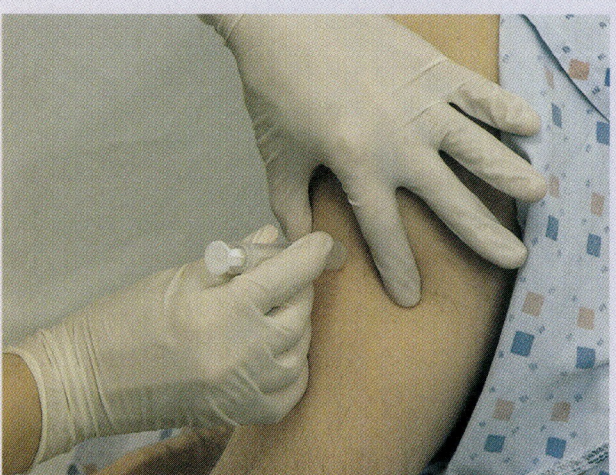

Figure 114-1 Administering Intramuscular Injection into the Deltoid Muscle

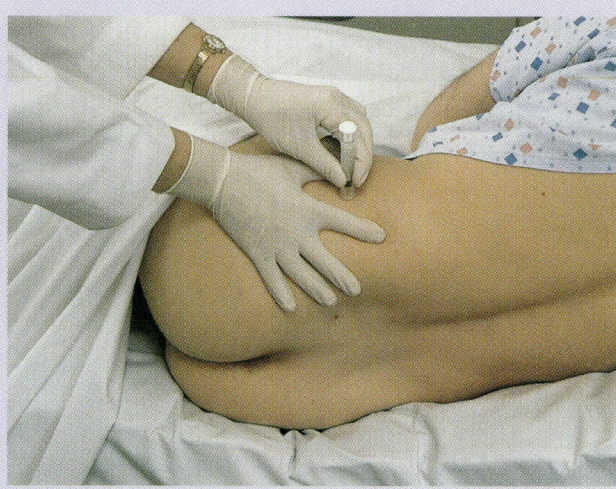

Figure 114-2 Administering Intramuscular Injection into the Ventrogluteal Site

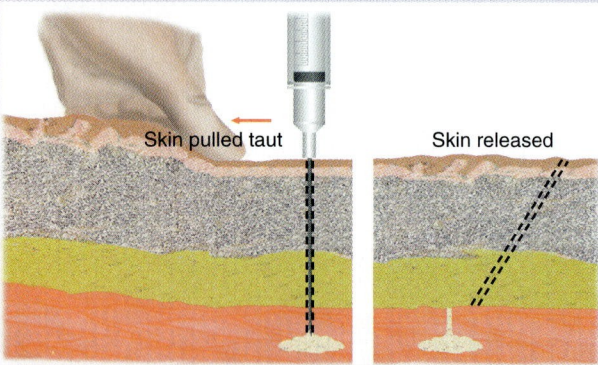

Skin pulled taut   Skin released

Figure 114-3 Administering Intramuscular Injection Using Z-Track Technique.

- While maintaining traction on the skin, insert the needle deeply. Aspirate with the same hand.

- Aspirate by pulling back on the plunger, and observe for blood.

- If blood appears, remove the needle and discard.

- If blood does not appear, inject the medication slowly, about 10 sec/mL.

- Wait 10 seconds after the medication has been injected, then smoothly withdraw the needle at the same angle of insertion.

- When finished with Z-track injection, maintain skin traction while removing the needle, then permit skin to return to normal position.

- Apply gentle pressure at the site with a dry, sterile 2 × 2 gauze; do not massage the injection site. Swab using gentle pressure.

- Allows medication to be injected 1 to 1.5 inches to the side of the skin entry site.

- Promotes comfort and allows time for the tissues to expand and begin absorbing the medication.

- Allows the medication to diffuse through the muscle.

- Releases pressure on tissues and seals medication in muscle.

- Decreases tissue irritation.

continued

Action	Rationale
• Discard the needle and syringe in a sharps container; do not recap the needle.	• Prevents needle sticks.
11. Position client for comfort; encourage client receiving ventrogluteal injections to perform leg exercises (flexion and extension).	11. Promotes the absorption of the medication.
12. Remove gloves, wash hands.	12. Prevents transmission of microorganisms.
13. Record on the MAR the medication, dosage, route, site, and time.	13. Provides documentation that the medication was administered.
14. Inspect the injection site within 2 to 4 hours and evaluate the client's response to the medication.	14. Alerts the nurse to hypersensitivity reactions; the peak plasma level is dependent on the drug's half-life.

Procedure 115 — Administering an Eye Medication

Equipment

- Medication administration record (MAR)
- Tissue or cotton ball
- Eye medication
- Nonsterile gloves

Action	Rationale
• Wash your hands • Check the client's identification band • Explain the procedure to the client prior to beginning •	
1. Check with the client and the chart for any known allergies or medical conditions that would contraindicate use of the drug.	1. Prevents occurrence of adverse reactions.
2. Check the MAR against the physician's written order.	2. Ensures accuracy in administration of the correct medication.
3. Gather the necessary equipment.	3. Promotes efficiency.
4. Follow the five rights of drug administration.	4. Promotes safety.
5. Take the medication to the client's room and place on a clean surface.	5. Decreases risk of contamination of bottle cap.
6. Ask if the client wants to instill own medication.	6. Some clients are used to instilling their own eyedrops.
7. Don nonsterile gloves.	7. Decreases contact with bodily fluids.
8. Place client in a supine position with the head slightly tilted back.	8. Minimizes drainage of medication through the tear duct.

Instilling Eyedrops

Action	Rationale
9. Remove cap from eye bottle and place cap on its side.	9. Prevents contamination of the bottle cap.
10. Squeeze the prescribed amount of medication into the eyedropper. (In some cases, drops will be administered directly from the bottle.)	10. Ensures correct dose.
11. Place a tissue below the lower lid.	11. Absorbs the medication that flows from the eye.

continued

Action	Rationale
12. With dominant hand, hold eyedropper ½ to ¾ inch above the eyeball; rest hand on client's forehead to stabilize.	**12.** Reduces risk of dropper touching eye structure.
13. Place nondominant hand on cheekbone and expose lower conjunctival sac by pulling on cheek while applying slight pressure to the inner canthus.	**13.** Stabilizes hand and prevents systemic absorption of eye medication.
14. Instruct the client to look up and drop prescribed number of drops into center of conjunctival sac (Figure I15-1).	**14.** Reduces stimulation of the blink reflex; prevents injury to the cornea.

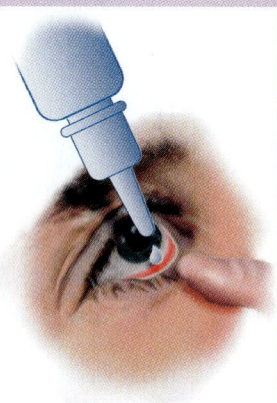

Figure I15-1 To administer an eye medication, gently press the lower lid down and have the client look upward while instilling drops into the lower conjunctival sac.

Action	Rationale
15. Instruct client to gently close and move eyes, but not to squeeze or rub them.	**15.** Distributes solution over conjunctival surface and anterior eyeball.
16. Recap container.	**16.** Prevents contamination.
17. Remove gloves, wash hands.	**17.** Reduces the transmission of microorganisms.
18. Record on the MAR the medication, dosage, route, site (which eye), and time administered.	**18.** Provides documentation that the medication was given.

Eye Ointment

Action	Rationale
19. Follow steps 1–9.	
20. Lower lid:	**20.**
• With nondominant hand, gently separate client's eyelids with thumb and finger, and grasp lower lid near margin immediately below the lashes; exert pressure downward over the bony prominence of the cheek.	• Provides access to the lower lid.
• Instruct the client to look up.	• Reduces stimulation of the blink reflex, and keeps cornea out of way of medication.
• Apply eye ointment along inside edge of the entire lower eyelid, from inner to outer canthus.	• Ensures drug is applied to entire lid.
21. Upper lid:	**21.**
• Instruct client to look down.	• Keeps cornea out of way of medication.

continued

Action	Rationale
• With nondominant hand, gently grasp client's lashes near center of upper lid with thumb and index finger, and draw lid up and away from eyeball.	
• Squeeze ointment along upper lid starting at inner canthus.	• Ensures medication applied to entire length of lid.
22. Follow steps 15–18.	

Medication Disk

Action	Rationale
23. Follow steps 1–8.	
24. Open sterile package and press dominant, gloved finger against the oval disk so that it lies lengthwise across fingertip. Remove from packet.	**24.** Promotes sticking of disk to fingertip.
25. Instruct the client to look up.	
26. With nondominant hand, gently pull the client's lower eyelid down and place the disk horizontally in the conjunctival sac.	**26.** Allows the disk to automatically adhere to the eye.
• Pull the lower eyelid out, up, and over the disk.	
• Instruct the client to blink several times.	
• If disk is still visible, repeat previous two steps.	
• Once the disk is in place, instruct the client to gently press his or her fingers against closed lid; do not rub eyes or move the disk across the cornea.	
• If the disk falls out, wash hands, don gloves, rinse the disk under cool water, and reinsert.	
27. If the disk is prescribed for both eyes (OU), repeat steps 24–26.	**27.** Ensures both eyes are treated at the same time.
28. Follow steps 17–18.	

Removing an Eye Medication Disk

Action	Rationale
29. Follow steps 4 and 6–8.	
30. Remove the disk.	**30.**
• With nondominant hand, evert the lower eyelid and identify the disk.	• Exposes the disk for removal.
• If the disk is located in the upper eye, instruct the client to close the eye, and place your finger on closed eyelid. Apply gentle, long, circular strokes; instruct client to open the eye. Disk should be located in corner of eye. With your fingertip, slide the disk to the lower lid, then proceed.	
• With dominant hand, use the forefinger to slide the disk onto the lid and out of the client's eye.	

continued

Action	Rationale
31. Remove gloves, wash hands.	**31.** Reduces transmission of microorganisms.
32. Record on the MAR the removal of the disk.	**32.** Provides documentation that the disk was removed.

Procedure 116 — Instilling an Ear Medication

Equipment

- Medication administration record (MAR)
- Sterile cotton balls, if ordered
- Ear medication
- Tissue

Action	Rationale
• Wash your hands • Check the client's identification band • *• Explain the procedure to the client prior to beginning •*	
1. Check with the client and chart for any known allergies.	**1.** Prevents the occurrence of hypersensitivity reactions.
2. Check the MAR against the physician's written orders.	**2.** Ensures accuracy in administration of the correct medication.
3. Follow the five rights of drug administration.	**3.** Promotes safety.
4. Don nonsterile gloves.	**4.** Reduces the transfer of microorganisms and decreases contact with bodily fluids.
5. Place the client in a side-lying position with the affected ear facing up.	**5.** Facilitates the administration of the medication.
6. Straighten the ear canal by pulling the pinna down and back for children or upward and outward for adults.	**6.** Opens the canal and facilitates introduction of medication.
7. Instill the drops into the ear canal by holding the dropper approximately ½ inch above the ear canal.	**7.** Prevents injury to the ear canal.
8. Ask the client to maintain the position for 2 to 3 minutes.	**8.** Allows for distribution of the medication.
9. Place a cotton ball on the outermost part of the canal, if ordered.	**9.** Prevents the medication from escaping when the client changes to a sitting or standing position.
10. Remove gloves and wash hands.	**10.** Reduces the transmission of microorganisms.
11. Document the drug, number of drops, time administered, and the ear medicated.	**11.** Documenting the actions of the nurse will reduce the number of medication errors.

Procedure 117 — Applying a Dry Sterile Dressing

Equipment

- Clean disposable gloves
- Moisture-proof bag
- Sterile gloves
- Bath blanket

continued

Equipment *continued*

- Sterile dressing set (if not available, gather the following):
  Sterile drape
  Gauze dressing and ABD pads (surgipads)
  Sterile container for cleansing solution
  Precut gauze if a drain is present
  Cotton-tip swabs

- Cleansing solution (per MD order or agency protocol)
- Adhesive remover
- Tape or Montgomery straps

Action	Rationale
• Check the client's identification band •	
1. Review medical and nursing orders for dressing change procedure and list of needed supplies.	1. A physician's order is needed to use a cleansing solution. Nursing orders will describe individualized client needs such as type and amount of dressing supplies needed.
2. Prepare the client. Assess the client's comfort level and medicate as needed for pain.	2. Dressing changes may cause the client pain.
3. Explain the procedure to the client.	3. Client cooperation is necessary to avoid contamination of the wound. Explanation decreases anxiety and increases cooperation.
4. Position the client. Using a bath blanket, drape the client so that only the wound is exposed.	4. Provides privacy and prevents chilling.
5. Place the moisture-proof bag within easy reach. Make a cuff on the bag by folding the top over.	5. Provides a receptacle for proper disposal of contaminated dressings.
6. Wash hands and don gloves. Remove the soiled dressing.	6. Prevents transmission of microorganisms.
a. If Montgomery straps or a binder was used, untie the tapes. If tape was used, gently remove tape by pulling up small sections at a time while holding down the skin in front of the tape (provides countertraction on the skin). If resistance is met, you may need to use adhesive remover (if skin is torn during tape removal, you have created another wound).	a. Careful removal of adhesive tapes prevents skin breakdown.
b. Carefully remove the outer protective dressing. Then remove the inner layers of gauze. If there is a drain present, use caution so it is not accidentally removed or dislodged.	b. Exposes the wound.
c. Place the soiled dressings in the moisture-proof bag.	c. Provides proper disposal and prevents contamination.
d. Remove and dispose of gloves in the moisture-proof bag.	
7. Assess the wound; note the odor and presence of any drainage	7. The wound needs to be assessed for signs of complications and healing.
8. Open sterile dressing tray or set up sterile supplies on sterile drape. Open cleansing solution (see Procedure I1).	8. Maintains sterile technique.

continued

Action	Rationale
9. Pour solution into sterile basin.	9. Keeps supplies sterile.
10. Wash hands and don sterile gloves.	10. Sterile gloves are needed if the wound is open and if drains are present to prevent introduction of microorganisms.
11. Clean the wound with the cleaning solution. Gauze may be held with the forceps or cotton swabs may be used. Be sure to cleanse from the area least contaminated to the area more contaminated, and use a new swab for each stroke. If a drain is present, cleanse this area last.	11. Always clean from the center of the wound to the outer area or top of incision to bottom to avoid contamination of the wound by pathogens present on surrounding skin surfaces.
12. If a drain is present, apply precut dressing around the drain. Apply a thick second layer of gauze over the drain.	12. To absorb exudate and isolate drainage from the wound.
13. Apply sterile dressing over wound. Cover with the ABD or surgipad.	13. Provides protection of the wound.
14. Secure the dressing with either tape or the ties from the Montgomery straps (Figure I17-1). Tapes should be placed at the edges of the dressing so that the edges cannot be lifted to expose the wound. Paper tape should be used on clients with thin fragile skin and clients who have sensitive skin.	14. Montgomery straps are used when a wound needs frequent dressing changes to prevent skin breakdown.

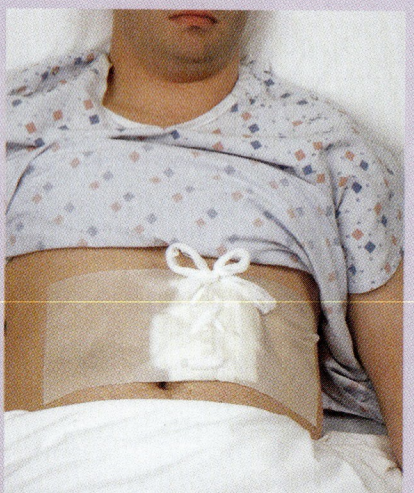

Figure I17-1 Montgomery Straps

Action	Rationale
15. Remove gloves, dispose, and wash hands.	15. Prevents transfer of pathogens.
16. Reassess client following dressing change to determine status and comfort level.	16. Determines effect of dressing change; alerts to any client needs.
17. Document all assessment findings and actions taken.	17. Records information for evaluation of progress of wound healing.

Procedure 118   Applying a Wet to Dry Dressing

Equipment

- Gather the equipment outlined in Procedure I17, plus:
- Sterile solution
- Fine mesh gauze
- Sterile forceps or sterile cotton swabs

Action	Rationale

• Wash your hands • Check the client's identification band •

1. Review medical and nursing orders for dressing change procedure and list of needed supplies.	1. A physician's order is needed to use a cleansing solution. Nursing orders will describe individualized client needs such as type and amount of dressing supplies needed.
2. Prepare the client. Assess the client's comfort level and medicate as needed for pain.	2. Dressing changes may cause the client pain.
3. Explain the procedure to the client.	3. Client cooperation is necessary to avoid contamination of the wound. Explanation increases cooperation by decreasing anxiety.
4. Position the client. Using a bath blanket, drape the client so that only the wound is exposed.	4. Provides privacy and prevents chilling.
5. Place the moisture-proof bag within easy reach. Make a cuff on the bag by folding the top over.	5. Provides a receptacle for proper disposal of contaminated dressings.
6. Remove the soiled dressing and assess the wound as outlined in Procedure I17, steps 6 and 7.	
7. Open sterile dressing tray. Using aseptic technique, place fine mesh gauze in sterile container. Pour enough cleansing solution into the container to soak gauze. Don sterile gloves.	7. Sterile technique is used to prevent introduction of pathogens into the wound.
8. Clean the wound as described in Procedure I17, step 11.	
9. Take one piece of fine mesh gauze and gently squeeze out the solution until the gauze is only slightly moist.	9. If the gauze is too moist, the wound bed can get too soupy, increasing the chance of bacterial growth.
10. Open the gauze and *gently* pack the gauze into the wound, using either forceps or the top of a cotton swab stick. Continue until all surfaces of the wound are in contact with gauze. *Do not* pack the wound too tightly and *do not* overlap wound edges with wet packing.	10. If the wound is packed too tightly, capillaries can be compressed. If the wet packing overlaps the wound edges, it can cause softening and breakdown of tissue.
11. Apply a layer of dry gauze over the wet gauze. Then cover with the ABD or surgipads.	11. Protects wound.
12. Secure the dressing with either tape or Montgomery straps and conclude the procedure (see Procedure I17, steps 14–17).	

Procedure 119 — Culturing a Wound

Equipment

- Disposable gloves
- Normal saline and irrigation tray
- Moisture-proof container or bag
- Sterile gloves and dressing supplies
- Culture tube and swab
- Sterile gauze

Action	Rationale
• Wash your hands • Check the client's identification band • *• Explain the procedure to the client prior to beginning •*	
1. Don disposable gloves and remove old dressing. Place old dressing in moisture-proof container, and remove and discard gloves. Wash hands again.	1. Prevents transmission of organisms.
2. Open the dressing supplies using sterile technique and don sterile gloves.	2. Maintains sterile environment.
3. Assess the wound's appearance; note quality, quantity, color, and odor of discharge.	3. Provides assessment of the amount and character of the wound's drainage prior to irrigation. Reddened areas and heavy drainage suggest infection.
4. Irrigate the wound with normal saline prior to culturing the wound if agency policy directs; do not irrigate with antiseptic.	4. Irrigation decreases the risk of culturing normal flora and other exudates such as protein; irrigating with an antiseptic prior to culturing may destroy the bacteria.
5. Using a sterile gauze pad, absorb the excess saline then discard the pad.	5. Removal of excess irrigant prevents maceration of tissue due to excess moisture.
6. Remove the culture swab from the culture tube and gently rotate the swab over the granulation tissue. Wipe only once with one swab. Avoid eschar and wound edges.	6. Decreases the chance of collecting superficial skin microorganisms.
7. Replace the swab into the culture tube, being careful not to touch the swab to the outside of the tube. Crush the ampule of medium in the bottom of the tube if present; recap the tube.	7. Avoids contamination with microorganisms. Releases the medium to surround the swab.
8. Wash hands and don sterile gloves. Dress the wound with sterile dressing (see Procedure 117).	8. Prevents contamination of the wound.
9. Label the specimen and arrange to transport the specimen to the laboratory.	9. Ensures proper handling of specimen.
10. Remove gloves and wash hands.	10. Prevents transmission of microorganisms.
11. Document all assessment findings and actions taken.	11. Records information for evaluation and promotes continuity of care.

Procedure 120

Irrigating a Wound

Equipment

- Sterile gloves
- Sterile irrigation kit (basin, piston irrigation or bulb syringe, solution container)
- Sterile dressing material to redress the wound after the irrigation procedure
- Disposable gloves
- Irrigation solution (per physician's order)
- Waterproof pad
- Moisture-proof container or bag
- Personal protective equipment (gown, gloves, goggles, mask (or face shield)

Action	Rationale
• Wash your hands • Check the client's identification band • *• Explain the procedure to the client prior to beginning •*	
1. Confirm the physician's order for wound irrigation, note the type and strength of the ordered irrigation solution.	1. Wound irrigation is a dependent nursing action.
2. Assess the client's pain level and medicate with analgesic 30 minutes before procedure if the medication is to be given po or IM.	2. Allows time for medication to be absorbed to increase the analgesic effect.
3. Place a waterproof pad on the bed. Assist the client onto the pad, then assist the client into a position that will allow the irrigant to flow through the wound and into the basin by gravity.	3. Positioning of the client and placement of a waterproof pad will decrease contamination of bed linen.
4. Don the disposable gloves; remove and discard the old dressing in moisture-proof container.	4. Prevents transmission of organisms.
5. Assess the wound's appearance and note quality, quantity, color, and odor of drainage.	5. Provides assessment of the status of the wound.
6. Remove and discard the disposable gloves, and wash hands.	6. Prevents transmission of organisms.
7. Don personal protective equipment except gloves.	7. Protects nurse from pathogens.
8. Prepare the sterile irrigation tray and dressing supplies. Pour the room-temperature irrigation solution into the solution container.	8. Aseptic technique is used to prevent introduction of microorganisms into the wound. Room-temperature solution reduces client discomfort.
9. Don sterile gloves.	9. Promotes sterile environment.
10. Position the sterile basin against the lower edge of the wound to "catch" the irrigant.	10. Decreases possibility of wound contamination.
11. Fill the piston or bulb syringe with irrigant and gently flush the wound. Refill the syringe and continue to flush the wound until the solution returns clear and no exudate is noted.	11. Gently irrigating the wound decreases trauma to granulation tissue.
12. Dry the edges of the wound by patting gently with gauze.	12. Drying the edges of the wound prevents maceration of tissues due to excess moisture.
13. Assess the wound's appearance and drainage.	13. Provides indication of change in wound status.
14. Apply a sterile dressing (see Procedure 117). Remove sterile gloves and wash hands.	14. Application of a sterile dressing protects the wound from microorganisms and trauma.
15. Document all assessment findings and actions taken.	15. Records information for evaluation.

Procedure 121   Administering Oxygen

Equipment

- Oxygen source (wall outlet or tank)
- Humidifier bottle, if used
- Nasal cannula and tubing

- Oxygen regulator or flowmeter
- Nipple adapter for flowmeter, if humidification is not used

Action	Rationale

• Check the client's identification band. •

1. Verify written order for oxygen therapy including method of delivery and flow rate.

2. Wash hands.

3. Explain procedure to client. Instruct the client and any other persons in the room to refrain from smoking or lighting matches while oxygen is in use. Check that all electrical equipment in use in the room has been inspected for electrical safety. Post appropriate signs in the room and on the door.

4. If using a wall outlet as oxygen source, plug flowmeter into outlet by pushing until it snaps into place. If a lock-release button is present, depress it as you insert the flowmeter.

   - If a tank is used as the oxygen source, the flowmeter should already be attached.

5. If humidification is used, remove the cover from the humidifier bottle to expose the adapter that connects the bottle to the flowmeter. Attach the bottle to the flowmeter by screwing the plastic nut on the adapter to the threaded outlet of the flowmeter.

6. If no humidification is used, attach the nipple adapter to the flowmeter by screwing it onto the threaded outlet of the flowmeter.

7. Attach oxygen tubing to the port on the humidifier bottle or the pointed end of the nipple adapter. Turn on oxygen flow by turning the thumbscrew (wall outlet) or knob (tank).

8. Adjust flow rate to the prescribed amount.

9. Gently position nasal prongs into client's nares, with curves of prongs pointing toward the floor of the nostrils (Figure 121-1).

---

1. Oxygen is a drug and its use must be ordered by a physician. Oxygen delivered by nasal cannula is prescribed in flow rates expressed as liters per minute (L/min).

2. Prevents transmission of pathogens.

3. Explanation reduces anxiety. Oxygen, while not itself flammable, makes fires burn more readily than they otherwise would, so strict fire safety must be observed. Faulty electrical equipment may produce sparks that could ignite materials nearby.

4. Wall outlets are sealed by heavy steel valves that prevent the escape of oxygen from the system. If you hear hissing from the valve, the flowmeter is not fully engaged.

   - Special tools are used to attach valves to oxygen tanks.

5. If long-term oxygen therapy is anticipated, flow is 6 L/min or higher, or drying of the respiratory mucosa and/or thick secretions are present, humidification of oxygen is indicated. Short-term and/or low-flow oxygen use, such as during a medical procedure, may not require humidification.

6. This adapter allows the oxygen tubing to be connected directly to the flowmeter.

7. Establishes proper functioning of equipment. If humidifier bottler is used, bubbling of oxygen through the bottle will be noted. In addition, verify flow by feeling for the flow of air from the cannula's nasal prongs.

8. As for any drug, correct dosing of oxygen is essential. Both insufficient and excessive amounts can be harmful to the client.

9. Directs the flow of oxygen into the nasal cavity, where it will mix with inspired room air.

continued

Action	Rationale
10. Loop the cannula tubing over the client's ears; adjust the fit of the tubing by sliding the adjuster upward to hold the cannula in place (Figure I21-2).	**10.** The fit of the cannula should be secure but not tight. A too-tight fit is uncomfortable, and may cause skin breakdown (especially above the ears).

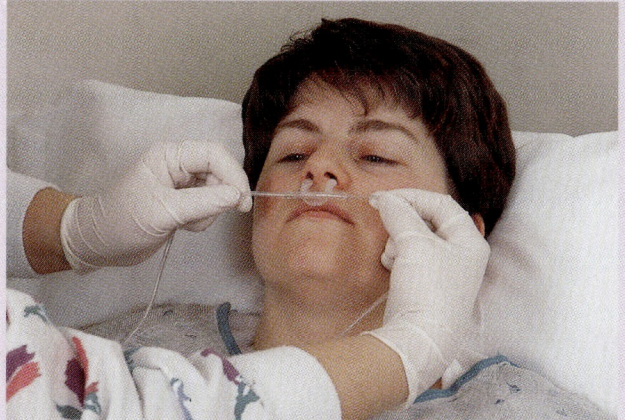

Figure I21-1 Insert cannula prong into nostrils (gloves are optional).

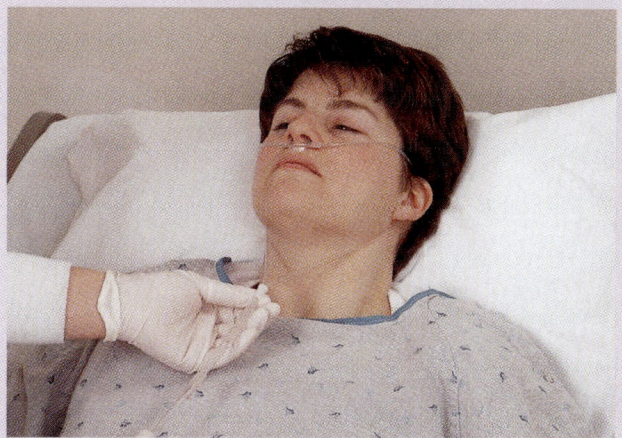

Figure I21-2 Adjust tubing.

11. Document the time oxygen is started, the liter flow, and the client's response.	**11.** Records information for evaluation and promotes continuity of care.
12. Assess the client's nares, face, and ears every 4 hours for signs of skin irritation or breakdown and document your findings. At the same time, inspect the nasal prongs for the presence of nasal secretions or crusts. If needed, wipe the prongs clean with a gauze pad or tissue.	**12.** Pressure from the tubing or cannula may cause skin breakdown. Accumulated secretions can impair the flow of oxygen.

Procedure I22 — Performing Nasopharyngeal and Oropharyngeal Suctioning

Equipment

- Suction source (wall suction regulator with collection bottle or portable suction machine)
- Sterile suction kit (contains suction catheter, sterile gloves, sterile solution container; may contain a small container of sterile normal saline)
- Sterile water-soluble lubricant
- Extension tubing connected to suction device
- Small bottle of sterile water or normal saline if not included in kit
- Personal protective equipment: gown, mask and goggles or face shield

Action	Rationale
• Check the client's identification band • Explain the procedure to the client prior to beginning •	
1. Assess the client's need for suctioning: inability to effectively clear the airway by coughing and expectorating; coarse bubbling or gurgling noises with respiration. Institutional policy will dictate which personnel are authorized to perform this procedure.	**1.** Suctioning is an uncomfortable and traumatic procedure and should be used only when needed.
2. Choose the most appropriate route (nasopharyngeal or oropharyngeal) for your client.	**2.** The oropharyngeal approach is easier but requires that the client cooperate; it may also

continued

Action	Rationale
If nasopharyngeal approach is considered, inspect the nares with a penlight to determine patency. Alternatively, you may assess patency by occluding each nare in turn with finger pressure while asking the client to breathe through the remaining nare.	produce gagging more readily. The nasopharyngeal route is more effective for reaching the posterior oropharynx but is contraindicated in clients with a deviated nasal septum, nasal polyps, or any tendency toward excessive bleeding (low platelet count, use of anticoagulants, recent history of epistaxis or nasal trauma).
3. Advise the client that suctioning may cause coughing or gagging but emphasize the importance of clearing the airway.	3. Promotes cooperation and reduces anxiety.
4. Wash your hands.	4. Reduces the transmission of pathogens.
5. Position the client in a high Fowler's or semi-Fowler's position.	5. Maximizes lung expansion and effective coughing.
6. If the client is unconscious or otherwise unable to protect his or her airway, place in a side-lying position.	6. Protects the client from aspiration in the event of vomiting.
7. Connect extension tubing to suction device if not already in place, and adjust suction control to between 110 and 120 mm Hg.	7. Excessive negative pressure can cause tissue trauma, whereas insufficient pressure will be ineffective.
8. Put on gown and mask and goggles or face shield.	8. Protects the nurse from splattering of body fluids.
9. Using sterile technique, open the suction kit. Consider the inside wrapper of the kit to be sterile, and spread the wrapper out carefully to create a small sterile field.	9. Produces an area in which to place sterile items without contaminating them.
10. Open a packet of sterile water-soluble lubricant and squeeze out the contents of the packet onto the sterile field.	10. Lubricant will be used to further lubricate the catheter tip if the nasopharyngeal route is used.
11. If sterile solution (water or saline) is not included in the kit, pour about 100 mL of solution into the sterile container provided in the kit.	11. This solution will be used to lubricate the catheter and to rinse the inside of the catheter to clear secretions.
12. If gloves are wrapped, carefully lift the wrapped gloves from the kit without touching the inside of the kit or the gloves themselves. Lay the wrapped gloves down next to the suction kit, and open the wrapper. Put on the gloves using sterile gloving technique (see Procedure I1).	12. The gloves should be kept sterile for handling the sterile suction catheter to avoid introducing pathogens into the client's airway.
13. If a cup of sterile solution is included in the suction kit, open it.	13. This solution will be used to lubricate the catheter and to rinse the inside of the catheter to clear secretions.
14. Designate one hand as *sterile* (able to touch only sterile items) and the other as *clean* (able to touch only unsterile items).	14. Usually, the dominant hand is the sterile hand, while the nondominant hand is clean. This prevents contamination of sterile supplies while allowing you to handle unsterile items.
15. *Using your sterile hand,* pick up the suction catheter. Grasp the plastic connector end between your thumb and forefinger and coil the tip around your remaining fingers.	15. Prevents accidental contamination of the catheter tip.

continued

Action	Rationale
16. Pick up the extension tubing *with your clean hand*. Connect the suction catheter to the extension tubing, taking care not to contaminate the catheter (Figure I22-1).	**16.** The extension tubing is not sterile.

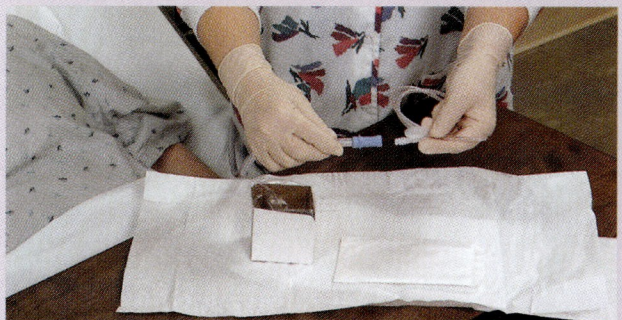

Figure I22-1 Attach catheter to tubing.

Action	Rationale
17. Position your clean hand with the thumb over the catheter's suction port.	**17.** Suction is activated by occluding this port with the thumb. Releasing the port deactivates the suction.
18. Dip the catheter tip into the sterile solution, and activate the suction. Observe as the solution is drawn into the catheter.	**18.** Tests the suction device as well as lubricates the interior of the catheter to enhance clearance of secretions.
19. For oropharyngeal suctioning, ask the client to open his or her mouth. Without activating the suction, gently insert the catheter and advance it until you reach the pool of secretions or until the client coughs. Do not poke catheter in oropharynx.	**19.** To minimize trauma, do not apply suction while the catheter is being advanced.
20. For nasopharyngeal suctioning, estimate the distance from the tip of the client's nose to the earlobe and grasp the catheter between your thumb and forefinger at a point equal to this distance from the catheter's tip.	**20.** Ensures placement of the catheter tip in the oropharynx and not in the trachea.
21. Dip the tip of the suction catheter into the water-soluble lubricant to coat catheter tip liberally.	**21.** Promotes the client's comfort and minimizes trauma to nasal mucosa.
22. Insert the catheter tip into the nare with the suction control port uncovered. Advance the catheter gently with a slight downward slant. Slight rotation of the catheter may be used to ease insertion (Figure I22-2). Advance the catheter to the point marked by your thumb and forefinger.	**22.** Guides the catheter toward the posterior oropharynx along the floor of the nasal cavity.
23. If resistance is met, *do not force the catheter*. Withdraw it and attempt insertion via the opposite nare.	**23.** Forceful insertion may cause tissue damage and bleeding.
24. Apply suction by occluding the suction control port with your thumb; at the same time, slowly rotate the catheter by rolling it between your thumb and fingers while slowly withdrawing it. Apply suction for no longer than 15 seconds at a time.	**24.** Prolonged suction applied to a single area of tissue can cause tissue damage.

continued

Action	**Rationale**

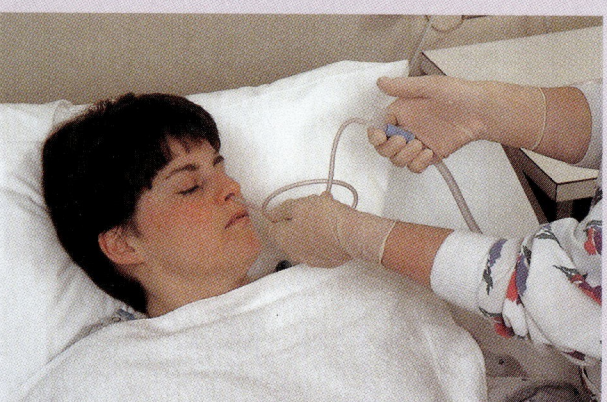

Figure 122-2 Insert catheter into nostril.

25. Repeat step 24 until secretions have been cleared, allowing brief rest periods between suctioning episodes.

26. Withdraw the catheter by looping it around your fingers as you pull it out.

27. Dip the catheter tip into the sterile solution and apply suction.

28. Disconnect the catheter from the extension tubing. Holding the coiled catheter in your gloved hand, remove the glove by pulling it over the catheter. Discard catheter and gloves in an appropriate container.

29. Discard remaining supplies in the appropriate container and wash your hands.

30. Provide the client with oral hygiene if indicated or desired.

31. Document the procedure, noting the amount, color, and odor of secretions and the client's response to the procedure.

25. Promotes complete clearance of the airway.

26. Allows you to maintain control over the catheter tip as it is withdrawn.

27. Clears the extension tubing of secretions that would promote bacterial growth and could block tubing.

28. Contains the catheter and secretions in the glove for disposal.

29. Prevents the transmission of pathogens.

30. Suctioning and coughing may produce an unpleasant taste.

31. Changes in the amount, color, or odor of pulmonary secretions may indicate infection.

Procedure 123   Performing Tracheostomy Care

Equipment

- Tracheostomy care kit (includes two sterile containers, sterile cotton-tip applicators, sterile pipe cleaner, sterile nylon brush, sterile 4 × 4 gauze pads, tweezers, sterile drapes, and tracheostomy ties)
- Two pairs of sterile gloves
- Plastic bag or biohazard container for disposal

- Sterile 0.9% sodium chloride solution
- Hydrogen peroxide solution
- Suction kit and suction equipment (see Procedure 124)
- Sterile precut 4 × 4 drain sponges
- Personal protective devices: gown, mask, and goggles or face shield

continued

Action	**Rationale**

• Check the client's identification band • Explain the procedure to the client prior to beginning •

1. Assist the client to a semi-Fowler's position. Remove pillows from behind the client's head.	**1.** Semi-Fowler's position allows comfortable access to the tracheostomy site, and removal of pillows reduces neck flexion.
2. Place plastic bag or disposal container within easy reach. Position in an area that does not require crossing over the sterile field or stoma to discard soiled items.	**2.** Prevents contamination of sterile field or stoma.
3. Place additional items on a clean overbed table or other easily accessible work space.	**3.** This space will be used to set up a sterile field for the tracheostomy care supplies.
4. Wash your hands.	**4.** Prevents the transmission of pathogens.
5. Loosen the caps on the bottles of sterile saline and hydrogen peroxide.	**5.** Permits easy opening of the bottles when ready.
6. Put on goggles, mask (or face shield) and gown.	**6.** Protects the nurse from splattering of body fluids (sputum).
7. Suction the client's tracheostomy tube (see Procedure I24); then remove the soiled tracheostomy dressing. Note the amount, color, and odor of any drainage around the stoma. Remove the gloves by pulling them over the discarded dressing, and discard the gloves and dressing.	**7.** Suctioning clears the airway of loose secretions. Inspection of the exudate reveals signs of possible peristomal infection. The old dressing and gloves used for suctioning are discarded to prevent reintroduction of pathogens. Removing the gloves over the old dressing permits containment of infectious exudate (if present).
8. Open the tracheostomy care kit, taking care to avoid touching the inside of the kit.	**8.** Prevents contamination of sterile items in the kit.
9. Using sterile gloving technique (Procedure I2), put on the gloves supplied in the tracheostomy care kit (if included) or a separate pair of sterile gloves.	**9.** Maintains sterility of the supplies in the kit.
10. Open the inner wrapper of the tracheostomy care kit to form a sterile field. Separate the two sterile containers and place them on the field. Lay the cotton applicators, pipe cleaners, nylon brush, and sterile 4 × 4 pads on the field. Place the sterile drape on the client's chest, with its upper edge as near to the tracheostomy tube as possible. Fold a tuck of the drape over your fingers as you position the drape.	**10.** Provides a sterile area in which to work. Prevents contamination of your sterile gloves.
11. Designate one hand as *sterile* (able to touch only sterile items) and the other as *clean* (able to touch only unsterile items).	**11.** Usually, the dominant hand is the sterile hand, while the nondominant hand is clean. This system prevents contamination of sterile supplies while allowing you to handle unsterile items.
12. *Using your clean hand,* open the bottles of sterile saline and peroxide, laying the caps outside of the sterile field. Pour about 100 mL of saline into one sterile container and about 100 mL of hydrogen peroxide into the other container. Set the bottles down outside of the sterile field. Remove oxygen tubing (if present), if the client can be without humidified oxygen for a short period of time.	**12.** These solutions will be used to clean the tracheostomy tube's inner cannula. Since the bottles and caps are unsterile, they should not be placed in the sterile field.

continued

Action	**Rationale**
13. *Using your sterile hand,* pick up a sterile cotton swab and saturate the tip with hydrogen peroxide. Swab the peristomal skin, including the area under the tracheostomy tube's faceplate. If you must touch the tracheostomy tube or the client, do so with your *clean* hand.	13. This action removes exudate and other material from the skin to maintain skin integrity.
14. *Using your clean hand,* gently loosen the inner cannula of the tracheostomy tube by twisting the outer ring counterclockwise; then withdraw the inner cannula in a smooth motion. Place the inner cannula into the basin of peroxide. *Note:* some tracheostomy tubes use disposable inner cannulae that would be replaced at this point in the procedure. If replacing a disposable inner cannula, skip to step 18.	14. Minimizes trauma to the client's tracheal tissues and reduces reflexive coughing. The hydrogen peroxide serves to dissolve crusted secretions.
15. *Using your sterile hand,* pick up the cannula. Using your clean hand, pick up the nylon brush and scrub to remove any visible crusts or secretions from inside and outside the cannula (Figure I23-1).	15. Any secretions retained on the inner cannula may be aspirated into the client's lungs, causing infection and possible airway obstruction. In some cases, the pipe cleaners may be needed to gain access to the inner surface of the cannula.

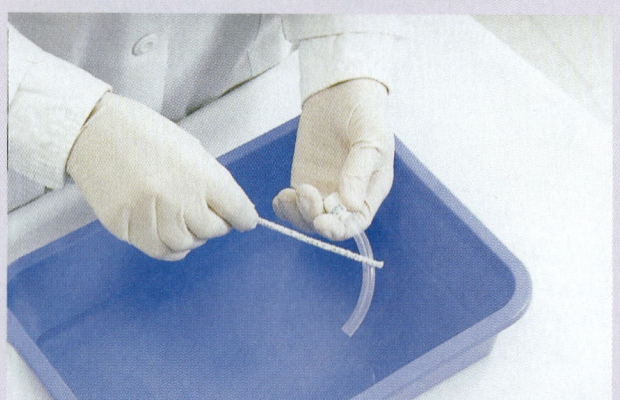

Figure I23-1 Clean lumen and inner cannula.

Action	**Rationale**
16. Place the cannula into the container of sterile saline. Agitate so that all surfaces are bathed in saline.	16. Rinses the peroxide off the cannula before it is returned to the client.
17. Inspect the inner cannula again to be sure it is clean; then remove excess saline from the lumen by tapping the cannula against a sterile surface.	17. Fluid trapped in the lumen of the cannula can be aspirated by the client.
18. Gently replace the inner cannula, following the curve of the tube. When fully inserted, lock the inner cannula in place by rotating the external ring clockwise until it clicks into place.	18. Minimizes tissue trauma and unintentional displacement.
19. Place a new precut sterile gauze dressing around the stoma, between the faceplate and the skin.	19. Protects the skin from irritation and breakdown due to friction with the faceplate and absorbs exudate if present. Using *precut* gauze dressings is important because cutting a regular 4 × 4 gauze will create loose fibers that may be inhaled by the client.

continued

Action	Rationale
20. Inspect the ties or strap securing the faceplate. If damp or soiled, carefully cut them (or loosen the Velcro™ to remove a strap). If cutting ties, be very careful not to cut the pilot balloon to the tracheostomy tube cuff. Remove the ties or strap and inspect the underlying skin for redness or breakdown.	**20.** Ties or straps that are wet contribute to skin breakdown and infection. *Note:* Tracheostomy ties should not be removed or changed for the first 24 hours after tracheostomy tube insertion to prevent dislodgement of the tube and bleeding from the stoma.
21. To replace ties (Figure I23-2), cut a length of twill tape about as long as the circumference of the client's neck. Fold over one end to 1 inch and cut a small (½ inch) slit into the folded end.	**21.** Creates a slit through which the end of the tie can be threaded and secured.

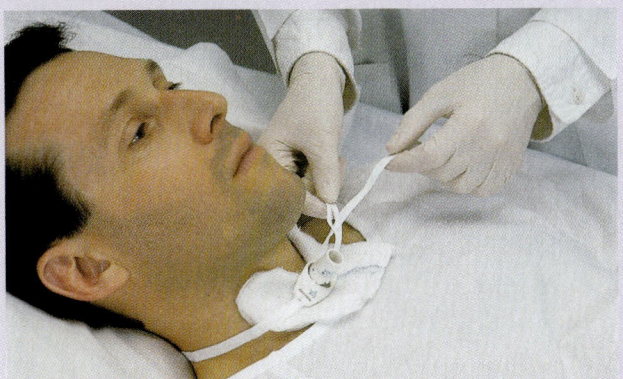

Figure I23-2 Change tracheostomy ties.

Action	Rationale
22. Thread the slit end of the tape through the eye of one side of the tracheostomy faceplate from the underside of the faceplate. Thread the end of the tie through the cut slit and secure it with a knot.	**22.** Creates a secure knot that can be easily cut when the tape needs to be removed and changed.
23. Slip the tape around the client's neck, keeping it smooth and flat against the skin.	**23.** Prevents excessive looseness or bunching of the tape.
24. Bring the loose end of the tape around to the other side of the faceplate. Ask the client to flex his or her neck and slip one of your fingers under the tape as you measure the desired tightness of the tie. (Do not move the head of a client with a neck injury.)	**24.** Flexion of the neck stimulates the increase in neck circumference that occurs with coughing. The tape should be secure but not tight. *Caution: Clients who have had neck surgery or injury should be monitored frequently for tightening of the tape due to neck swelling.*
25. Fold the end of the tape and cut a slit as in step 21, then tie the end as in step 22. Trim off excess tape from the end and knot the cut ends of the tape.	**25.** Prevents fraying of tape ends.
26. To replace a Velcro™ strap: Place new strap behind client's neck and thread ends through faceplate eyelets. Adjust tightness as above and secure Velcro™.	**26.** Velcro™ straps may be more comfortable for some clients and are easier to adjust for proper fit.
27. Reconnect the client to oxygen if necessary and reposition for comfort.	**27.** Restores supplemental oxygen and humidification to the client. *Note:* Some clients may not tolerate removal from supplemental oxygen during the entire tracheostomy care procedure. In this case, an assistant may be needed to intermittently replace and remove oxygen

continued

Action	Rationale
	throughout the procedure. Always work quickly, and continuously assess your client's response to the procedure.
28. Discard soiled items in the appropriate container. Remove and discard soiled gloves. Wash hands.	**28.** Prevents cross-contamination.
29. Document the procedure, noting the appearance of the stomal site and any exudate.	**29.** Increasing exudate or a change in its color or character may indicate infection.

Procedure 124   Performing Tracheostomy Suctioning

Equipment

- Suction source (wall suction regulator with collection bottle or portable suction machine)
- Sterile suction kit (contains suction catheter, sterile gloves, sterile solution container; may contain a small container of sterile normal saline)
- Extension tubing connected to suction device
- Small bottle of sterile water or normal saline if not included in kit
- Personal protective equipment: gown, mask and goggles or face shield

Action	Rationale
• Wash your hands • Check the client's identification band •	
1. Assess the client's need for suctioning: inability to effectively clear the airway by coughing and expectoration or coarse crackles auscultated over the upper airways.	**1.** Suctioning is an uncomfortable and traumatic procedure and should be used only when needed.
2. Explain the procedure to the client. Advise that suctioning may cause coughing; emphasize the importance of clearing the airway.	**2.** Promotes cooperation and reduces anxiety.
3. Position the client in a high Fowler's or semi-Fowler's position.	**3.** Maximizes lung expansion and effective coughing.
4. Connect extension tubing to suction device, if not already in place, and adjust suction control to between 80 and 100 mm Hg.	**4.** Excessive negative pressure can cause tissue trauma, hypoxemia, and atelectasis, whereas insufficient pressure will be ineffective.
5. Put on gown and mask and goggles or face shield.	**5.** Protects nurse from splattering body fluids.
6. Using sterile technique (see Procedure 122), open the suction kit. Consider the inside wrapper of the kit to be sterile, and spread the wrapper out carefully to create a small sterile field.	**6.** Produces an area in which to place sterile items without contaminating them.
7. If sterile solution (water or saline) is not included in the kit, pour about 100 mL of solution into the sterile container provided in the kit.	**7.** This solution will be used to lubricate the catheter and to rinse the inside of the catheter to clear secretions.
8. If gloves are wrapped, carefully lift the wrapped gloves from the kit without touching the inside of the kit or the gloves themselves. Lay the wrapped gloves down next to the suction kit, and open the wrapper. Put on the gloves using sterile gloving technique.	**8.** The gloves should be kept sterile for handling the sterile suction catheter thus avoiding introducing pathogens into the client's airway.

continued

Action	Rationale
9. If a cup of sterile solution is included in the suction kit, open it.	9. This solution will be used to lubricate the catheter and to rinse the inside of the catheter to clear secretions.
10. Designate one hand as *sterile* (able to touch only sterile items) and the other as *clean* (able to touch only nonsterile items).	10. Usually the dominant hand is the sterile hand while the nondominant hand is clean. This prevents contamination of sterile supplies while allowing you to handle unsterile items
11. *Using your sterile hand,* pick up the suction catheter. Grasp the plastic connector end between your thumb and forefinger and coil the tip around your remaining fingers.	11. Prevents accidental contamination of the catheter tip.
12. Pick up the extension tubing *with your clean hand.* Connect the suction catheter to the extension tubing, taking care not to contaminate the catheter.	12. The extension tubing is not sterile.
13. Instruct the client to take several slow, deep breaths.	13. Promotes optimal opening of airways and reduces suction-induced hypoxemia. *Note:* Clients should be preoxygenated by taking several deep breaths with supplemental oxygen set at 100% or by delivery of 100% oxygen via manual resuscitation bag. Always return oxygen flow to the prescribed rate after the suctioning procedure is completed.
14. Position your clean hand with the thumb over the catheter's suction port.	14. Suction is activated by occluding this port with the thumb. Releasing the port deactivates the suction.
15. Dip the catheter tip into the sterile solution, and activate the suction. Observe as the solution is drawn into the catheter.	15. Tests the suction device as well as lubricating the interior of the catheter to enhance clearance of secretions.
16. Using your clean hand, remove the oxygen delivery device from the tracheostomy tube and place it on a clean surface.	16. Permits access to the tracheostomy tube. Placing the oxygen device on a clean surface reduces contamination (the sterile glove wrapper may be used for this purpose).
17. Without occluding the suction control port, insert the catheter tip into the tracheostomy tube and advance it until the client coughs or resistance is met (Figure I24-1).	17. To minimize trauma, do not apply suction while the catheter is being advanced.

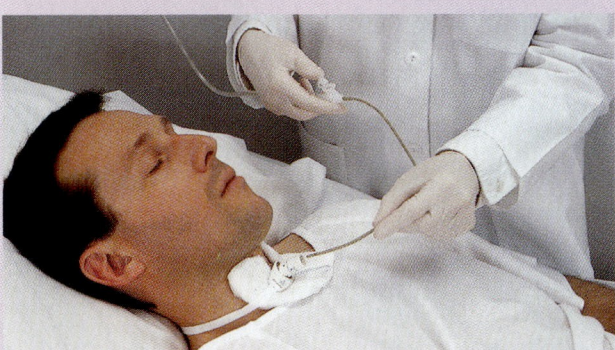

Figure I24-1 Suction tracheostomy.

continued

Action	Rationale
18. Withdraw the catheter slightly.	**18.** Do not want to apply suction when catheter tip is against the carina.
19. Apply suction by occluding the suction control port with your thumb; at the same time, slowly rotate the catheter by rolling it between your thumb and fingers while slowly withdrawing it. Apply suction for no longer than 15 seconds at a time.	**19.** Prolonged suction can cause tissue damage, atelectasis, and hypoxemia.
20. Repeat step 19 until all secretions have been cleared, allowing brief rest periods between suctioning episodes. Encourage client to breathe deeply between suctioning episodes. Provide oxygen between passes of the suction catheter.	**20.** Promotes complete clearance of the airway.
21. Withdraw the catheter and dip it into the cup of sterile saline, applying suction.	**21.** Cleans suction catheter of secretions.
22. Reapply oxygen delivery device.	**22.** Restores supplemental oxygen and humidification.
23. Ask the client to open his or her mouth. Insert the catheter and advance it along the oropharynx until resistance is felt. Apply suction and slowly withdraw the catheter.	**23.** *Note:* At this point the catheter is contaminated. If another suctioning pass into the tracheostomy is needed, a new sterile catheter must be used.
24. Dip the catheter tip into the sterile solution and apply suction.	**24.** Clears the extension tubing of secretions, which would promote bacterial growth.
25. Disconnect the catheter from the extension tubing. Holding the coiled catheter in your gloved hand, remove the glove by pulling it over the catheter. Discard catheter and gloves in an appropriate container.	**25.** Contains the catheter and secretions in the glove for disposal.
26. Discard remaining supplies in the appropriate container.	**26.** Follow institutional policy regarding the disposal of client care supplies.
27. Wash your hands.	**27.** Prevents the transmission of pathogens.
28. Provide the client with oral hygiene if indicated/desired.	**28.** Suctioning and coughing may produce an unpleasant taste.
29. Document the procedure, noting the amount, color, and odor of secretions and the client's response to the procedure.	**29.** Changes in the amount, color, or odor of pulmonary secretions may indicate infection.

Procedure 125 — Postoperative Exercise Instruction

Equipment

- Educational materials
- Tissue
- Disposable volume-oriented incentive spirometer or one with disposable mouthpiece
- Pillow
- Nonsterile gloves

continued

Action	Rationale
• Wash your hands • Check the client's identification band • *• Explain the procedure to the client prior to beginning •*	
1. Organize equipment.	**1.** Promotes efficiency.
2. Place client in a sitting position.	**2.** Promotes full chest expansion.
3. Demonstrate deep breathing exercise.	**3.** Shows the client how to breathe deeply.
4. Have the client return demonstrate deep breathing:	**4.** Fosters learning.
• Place one hand on abdomen (umbilical area) during inhalation.	• Exerts counterpressure during inhalation.
• Expand the abdomen and rib cage on inspiration.	• Promotes maximum chest expansion.
• Inhale slowly and evenly through your nose until you achieve maximum chest expansion.	• Maintains full expansion of the alveoli.
• Hold breath for 2 to 3 seconds.	• Increases the pressure, preventing immediate collapse of the alveoli.
• Slowly exhale through your mouth until maximum chest contraction has been achieved.	• Promotes maximum chest contraction.
• Repeat the exercise three or four times; allow client to rest.	• Enforces learning.
5. Demonstrate splinting and coughing.	**5.** Shows the client how to raise mucous secretions from the tracheobronchial tree.
6. Don gloves.	**6.** Reduces transmission of microorganisms.
7. Keep the client in a sitting position, head slightly flexed, shoulders relaxed and slightly forward, and feet supported on the floor.	**7.** Promotes full expansion of chest cage and use of accessory muscles to produce a deep, productive cough.
8. Have the client return demonstrate splinting and coughing:	**8.** Fosters learning.
• Have the client slowly raise head and sniff the air.	• Increases the amount of air and helps to aerate the base of the lungs.
• Have the client slowly bend forward and exhale slowly through pursed lips.	• Dries the tracheal mucosa as air flows over it; there is a slight increase in the carbon dioxide level, which stimulates deeper breathing.
• Repeat breathing two or three times.	• Loosens mucous plugs and moves secretions to the main bronchus.
• When the client is ready to cough, have client place a folded pillow against the abdomen (for abdominal incision) and grasp the pillow against the abdomen with clasped hands (Figure I25-1).	• Elevates the diaphragm and expels air in a more forceful cough; supports the abdominal muscles and reduces pain when coughing if the client has an abdominal incision.
• Have client take a deep breath and begin coughing immediately after inspiration is completed by bending forward slightly and producing a series of soft, staccato coughs.	• Removes secretions from the main bronchus.
• Have a tissue ready.	• Provides a tissue for sputum disposal.

continued

Action	**Rationale**

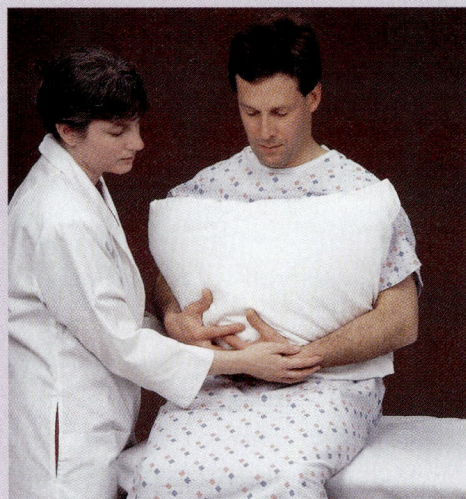

Figure I25-1 Splinting

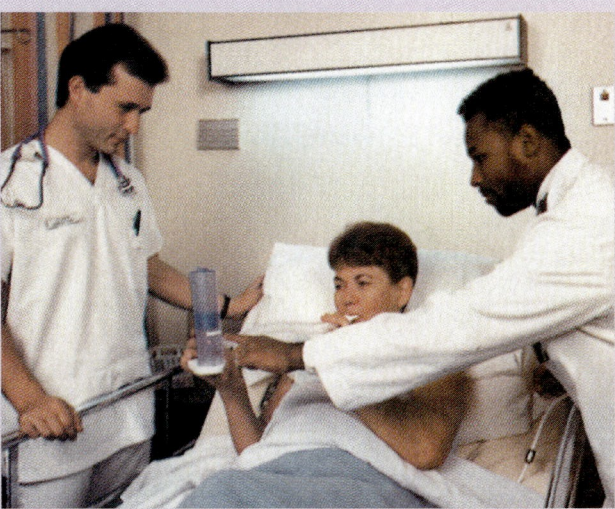

Figure I25-2 Incentive Spirometer

9. Instruct the client on the use of an incentive spirometer (Figure I25-2). Have the client:	**9.** Reinflates the alveoli and removes mucous secretions.
• Hold the incentive spirometer upright.	• Promotes proper functioning of the device.
• Take a normal breath and exhale, then seal lips tightly around the mouthpiece; take a slow, deep breath to elevate the balls in the plastic tube, hold the inspiration for at least 3 seconds.	• Allows for greater lung expansion; holding the inspiration increases the pressure, preventing immediate collapse of the alveoli.
• The client simultaneously receives feedback about the amount of inspired air volume on the calibrated plastic tube.	• Encourages the client to do respiratory exercises.
• Remove the mouthpiece, exhale normally.	• Allows normal expiration.
• Take several normal breaths.	• Provides client the opportunity to relax.
• Repeat the procedure four to five times.	• Encourages sustained maximal inspiration and loosens secretions.
• Tell client after surgery, incentive spirometer should be used for 10 to 12 breaths every hour, while awake.	
• Have the client cough after the incentive effort; repeat Step 8. Have a tissue ready.	• Facilitates removal of secretions.
• Have client clean mouthpiece under running water and place in clean container (disposable mouthpiece changed every 24 hours).	• Prevents transmission of microorganisms.
10. Explain leg and foot exercises (Figure I25-3).	**10.** Elicits client cooperation.

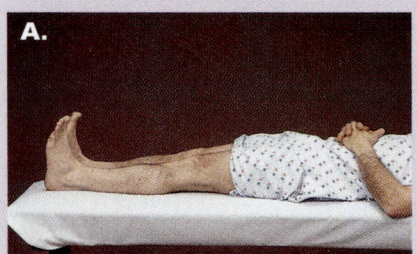 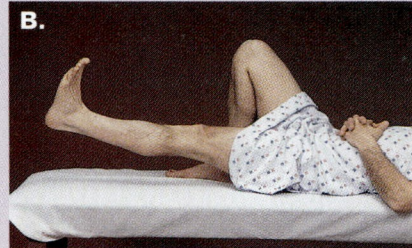 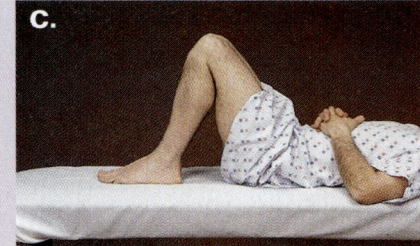

Figure I25-3 Leg Exercises

continued

Action	Rationale
11. Instruct client to return demonstrate in bed:	11. Fosters learning of how to improve venous blood return:
• Have the client, with heels on bed, push the toes of both feet toward the foot of the bed (plantar flexion) until the calf muscles tighten, then relax feet. Pull the toes toward the chin (dorsiflexion) until calf muscles tighten, then relax feet (Figure I25-3A).	• Causes contraction and relaxation of the calf muscles.
• With heels on bed, lift and circle each ankle, one at a time, first to the right and then to the left. Repeat three times and relax (Figure I25-3B).	• Causes contraction and relaxation of the quadriceps muscle.
• Flex and extend each knee alternately, sliding foot up along the bed and relax (Figure I25-3C).	• Causes contraction and relaxation of the quadriceps muscles.
12. Instruct clients with orthopedic surgery (e.g., hip surgery) how to use a trapeze bar.	12. Facilitates movement in bed without putting pressure on a leg or hip joint.

Procedure I26   Skin Puncture

Equipment

- Antiseptic—70% isopropanol or povidone-iodine
- Sterile 2 × 2 gauze
- Sterile lancet
- Hand towel or absorbent pad
- Collection tubes, strip for testing glucose, or other device for testing blood at bedside
- Nonsterile gloves

Action	Rationale
• *Wash your hands* • *Check the client's identification band* • • *Explain the procedure to the client prior to beginning* •	
1. Review client's medical record.	1. Verifies physician's order.
2. Prepare supplies:	2. Ensures efficiency.
• Open sterile packages.	
• Label specimen collection tubes (if used).	
• Place within easy reach.	
3. Don gloves.	3. Decreases the health care provider's exposure to blood-borne organisms.
4. Select site:	4. Avoids damage to nerve endings and calloused areas of the skin.
• Lateral aspect of the fingertips in adults/children.	
• Lateral aspect of the heel in infant.	
5. Place the hand or heel in a dependent position; apply warm compresses if fingers or heel are cool to touch.	5. Increases the blood supply to the puncture site.
6. Place hand towel or absorbent pad under the extremity.	6. Prevents soiling the bed linen.
7. Cleanse puncture site with an antiseptic and allow to dry; use 70% isopropanol if client is allergic to iodine.	7. Reduces skin surface bacteria (povidone-iodine must dry to be effective).

continued

Action	Rationale
8. With nondominant hand, apply light pressure by gently squeezing the area above/around the puncture site. Do not touch puncture site.	8. Increases blood supply to puncture site; maintains asepsis.
9. With the sterile lancet at a 90° angle to the skin, use a quick stab to puncture the skin (about 2 mm deep) (Figure 126-1).	9. Provides a blood sample with minimal discomfort to the client.

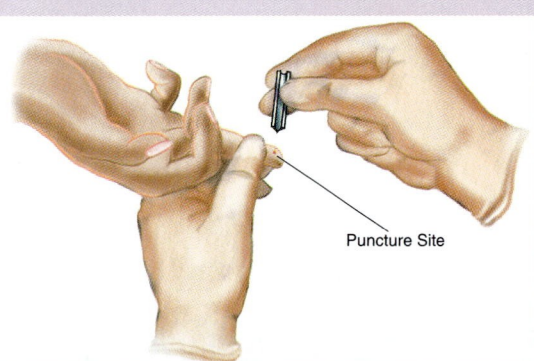

Puncture Site

Figure 126-1 Capillary Puncture of Fingertip

Action	Rationale
10. Wipe off the first drop of blood with a sterile 2 × 2 gauze; allow the blood to flow freely.	10. Pressure at the puncture site can cause hemolysis.
11. Collect the blood using tube, strip, or other device. Do not squeeze finger or heel.	11. Pericellular fluid may dilute blood and skew results.
12. Apply pressure to the puncture site with a sterile 2 × 2 gauze.	12. Controls bleeding.
13. Place contaminated articles into a sharps container.	13. Reduces risk for needle stick.
14. Remove gloves; wash hands.	14. Reduces transmission of microorganisms.
15. Position client for comfort with call light in reach.	15. Provides for comfort and communication.
16. Transport specimen to laboratory if indicated, or write results in the medical record.	

Procedure 127   Assisting a Client with Crutch Walking

- One pair of crutches
- Gait belt (optional)
- Measuring tape

Action	Rationale
1. Review client's medical record.	1. Verifies physician's order.
2. Inform client that you will be assisting with ambulation using crutches.	2. Reduces anxiety; helps increase comprehension and cooperation; promotes client autonomy.
3. Assess client for strength, mobility, range of motion, visual acuity, perceptual difficulties, and balance. *Note:* The nurse and physical therapist often collaborate on this assessment.	3. Helps determine the capabilities of client and amount of assistance required.

continued

Action	Rationale
4. Adjust crutches to fit the client. With the client supine, measure from the heel to the axilla. When client is standing, the crutch pad should fit 1.5 to 2 in. below the axilla (Figure I27-1). The hand grip should be adjusted to allow for the client to have elbows bent at 30° flexion.	**4.** Space between the crutch pad and the axilla prevents pressure on radial nerves. The elbow flexion allows for space between the crutch pad and axilla.

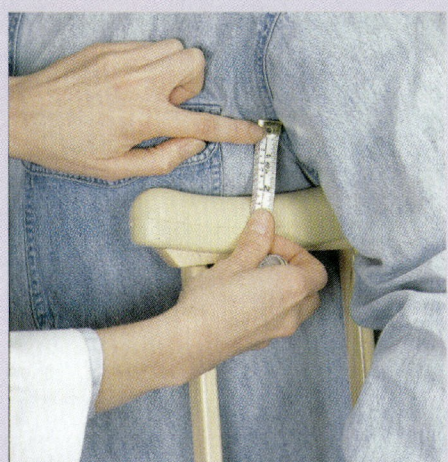

Figure I27-1 Adjusting Crutches to Fit Client

Action	Rationale
5. Lower the height of the bed.	**5.** Allows client to sit with feet on floor for stability.
6. Dangle the client at the side of bed for several minutes. Assess for vertigo.	**6.** Allows for stabilization of blood pressure, thus preventing orthostatic hypotension.
7. Instruct client on method to hold the crutches; that is, with elbows bent 30° and pad 1.5 to 2 in. below the axilla. Instruct client to position crutches lateral to and forward of feet. Demonstrate correct positioning. Tell client to place weight on hands, not axilla.	**7.** Increase client comprehension and cooperation. Pressure on axilla can cause nerve damage.
8. Apply the gait belt around the client's waist if balance and stability are unreliable.	**8.** Provides support; promotes client safety.
9. Assist the client to a standing position with crutches. Support as needed.	**9.** Standing for a few minutes will assist in preventing orthostatic hypotension.
10. Set realistic goals and opportunities for progressive ambulation using crutches.	**10.** Crutch walking takes up to 10 times the energy required for unassisted ambulation.
11. Consult with a physical therapist for clients learning to walk with crutches.	**11.** The physical therapist is the expert on the health care team for crutch-walking techniques.

Four-Point Gait

Action	Rationale
12. Position the crutches 4.5 to 6 in. to the side and in front of each foot. Move the right crutch forward 4 to 6 in. and move the left foot forward, even with the left crutch (Figure I27-2A). Move the left crutch forward 4 to 6 in. and move the right foot forward, even with the right crutch (Figure I27-2B). Repeat the four-point gait.	**12.** The four-point gait (used for partial or full weight bearing) provides greater stability. Weight bearing is on three points (two crutches and one foot or two feet and one crutch) at all times. The client must be able to bear weight with both legs.

continued

Action	**Rationale**

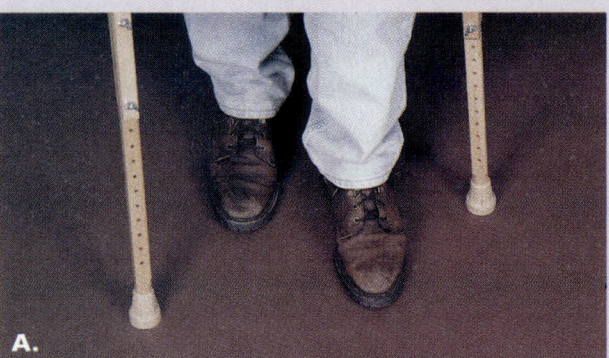 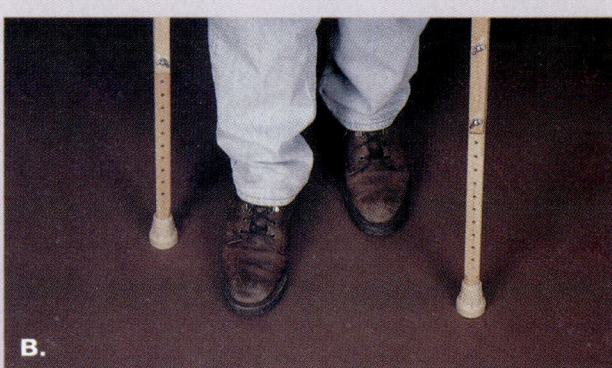

Figure I27-2 Four-Point Gait. A. Moving Right Crutch Forward and Left Foot Forward; B. Moving Left Crutch Forward and Right Foot Forward, Even with Right Crutch

Three-Point Gait

13. Advance both crutches and the weaker leg forward together 4 to 6 in. (Figure I27-3). Move the stronger leg forward, even with the crutches. Repeat the three-point gait.

Two-Point Gait

14. Move the left crutch and right leg forward 4 to 6 in. Move the right crutch and left leg forward 4 to 6 in. Repeat the two-point gait.

Swing-Through Gait

15. Move both crutches forward together 4 to 6 in. Move both legs forward together in a swinging motion, even with the crutches (Figure I27-4). Repeat the swing-through gait.

13. The three-point gait (used for partial or non-weight bearing) provides a strong base of support. This gait can be used if the client has a weak or non-weight-bearing leg.

14. The two-point gait (used for partial weight bearing) provides a strong base of support. The client must be able to bear weight on both legs. This gait is faster than the four-point gait.

15. The swing-through gait (used for people with severe weakness or paralysis of knees or hips) permits a faster pace. This gate requires greater balance and more strength.

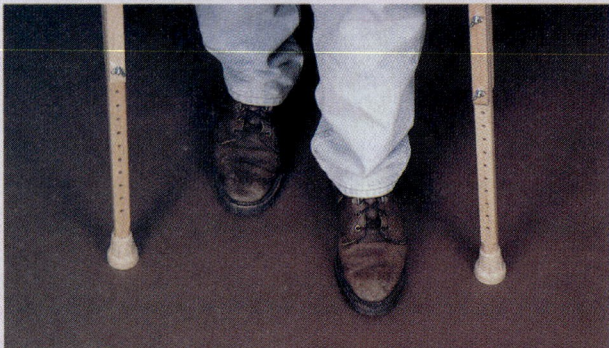

Figure I27-3 Crutch Walking: Three-Point Gait, Advancing Both Crutches and Weaker Leg Forward Together

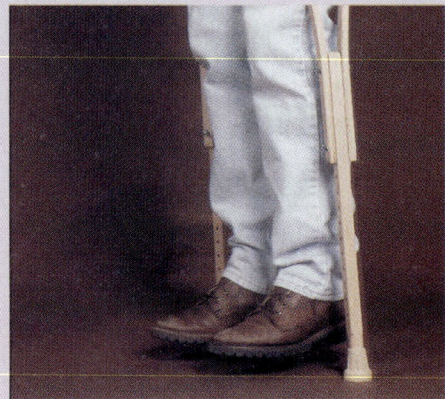

Figure I27-4 Crutch Walking: Swing-Through Gait

Procedure 128   Administering Enteral Tube Feedings

Equipment

- Asepto syringe or 20- to 50-mL syringe
- Clean towel
- Formula
- Water to follow feeding
- Emesis basin
- Disposable gavage bag and tubing
- Infusion pump for feeding tube
- Nonsterile gloves

Action	Rationale
• Wash your hands • Check the client's identification band • *• Explain the procedure to the client prior to beginning •*	
1. Review client's medical record.	1. Verifies physician's prescription for appropriate formula and amount.
2. Gather and assemble equipment. If using a bag, fill with prescribed amount of formula.	2. Promotes efficiency during procedure.
3. Place client on right side in high Fowler's position.	3. Reduces risk of pulmonary aspiration in event client vomits or regurgitates formula.
4. Don nonsterile gloves.	4. Reduces transmission of pathogens from gastric contents.
5. Provide for privacy.	5. Places client at ease.
6. Observe for abdominal distention; auscultate for bowel sounds.	6. Assesses for delayed gastric emptying; indicates presence of peristalsis and ability of GI tract to digest nutrients.
7. Check feeding tube: Insert syringe into adapter port, aspirate stomach contents, and determine amount of gastric residual.	7. Indicates whether gastric emptying is delayed.
• If residual is greater than 50 to 100 mL (or in accordance with agency protocol), hold feeding until residual diminishes.	• Reduces risk of regurgitation and pulmonary aspiration related to gastric distention.
• Instill aspirated contents back into feeding tube.	• Prevents electrolyte imbalance.
8. Administer tube feeding:	8. Provides nutrients as prescribed.

Intermittent—Bolus

• Pinch the tubing.	• Prevents air from entering tubing.
• Remove plunger from barrel of syringe and attach to adapter.	• Provides system to delivery feeding.
• Fill syringe with formula (Figure 128-1).	• Allows gravity to control flow rate, reducing risk of diarrhea from bolus feeding.

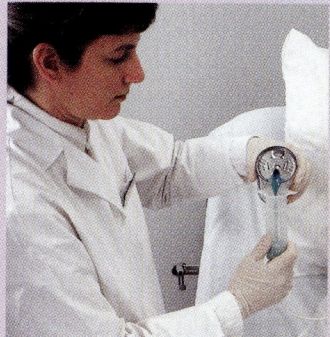

Figure 128-1 Adding Formula to Nasogastric Tube

continued

Action	Rationale
• Raise or lower syringe to control rate of feeding.	
• Allow formula to infuse slowly; continue adding formula to syringe until prescribed amount has been administered. Do not allow syringe to empty between fillings.	• Prevents air from entering stomach and reduces risk for gas accumulation.
• Flush tubing with 30 to 50 mL (or prescribed amount) of water.	• Maintains patency of feeding tube.

Intermittent—Gavage Feeding

Action	Rationale
• Hang bag on IV pole so that it is 18 inches above the client's head.	• Allows gravity to promote infusion of formula.
• Remove air from bag's tubing.	• Prevents air from entering stomach.
• Attach distal end of tubing to feeding tube adapter and adjust drip to infuse over prescribed time.	• Decreases risk of diarrhea.
• When bag empties of formula, add 30 to 60 mL (or prescribed amount) of water; after water is instilled, close clamp.	• Ensures that remaining formula in tubing is administered and maintains patency of tube; prevents air from entering the stomach.
• Wash reusable gavage bag with soap and hot water every 24 hours.	• Decreases risk of multiplication of microorganisms in bag and tubing.

Continuous Gavage

Action	Rationale
• Check tube placement at least every 4 hours or according to agency policy.	• Ensures that feeding tube remains in stomach.
• Check residual at least every 8 hours or according to agency policy.	• Indicates ability of GI tract to digest and absorb nutrients.
• If residual is greater than 1 to 2 times the hourly rate, hold feeding.	• Reduces risk of regurgitation and pulmonary aspiration related to gastric distention.
• Add prescribed amount of formula to bag for a 3- to 4-hour period; dilute with water if prescribed.	• Provides client with prescribed nutrients and prevents bacterial growth (formula is easily contaminated).
• Hang gavage bag on IV pole.	
• Prime tubing.	• Removes air from tubing.
• Thread tubing through feeding pump and attach distal end of tubing to feeding tube adapter; keep tubing straight between bag and pump.	• Provides for controlled flow rate; prevents loops in tubing.
• Adjust drip rate.	• Infuses formula over prescribed time.
• Monitor infusion rate and signs of respiratory distress or diarrhea.	• Prevents complications associated with continuous gavage.
• Flush tube with water every 4 hours as prescribed or following administration of medications.	• Maintains patency of tube.
• Replace disposable feeding bag at least every 24 hours, in accord with agency's protocol.	• Decreases risks of microorganisms.
• Turn client every 2 hours.	• Promotes digestion and reduces skin breakdown.

continued

Action	Rationale
• Provide oral hygiene every 2 to 4 hours.	• Provides comfort and maintains the integrity of buccal cavity.
9. Administer water as prescribed with and between feedings.	9. Ensures adequate hydration.
10. Clamp proximal end of feeding tube after formula has been administered.	10. Prevents air from entering the tube.
11. Remove gloves and wash hands.	11. Reduces risk of transmission of microorganisms.
12. Record total amount of formula and water administered on I&O form, and client's response to feeding.	12. Documents administration of feeding and achievement of expected outcome; e.g., client tolerates feeding and weight is maintained or increased.

continued

Atlas of Nursing Procedures

Procedure A1

Initiating Strict Isolation Precautions

Equipment

- Isolation sign
- Disposable gowns
- Gloves (nonsterile and sterile)
- Tape or bag ties
- Room with sink and running water
- Soap and paper towels
- Water pitcher, cups, and fresh water
- Other supplies relative to client's condition for example, dressings for wound care

- Goggles or face shield
- Disposable cups
- Disposable masks or face shield
- Impermeable bags (linen and trash)
- Disposable vital signs equipment (single-use thermometers, stethoscope, and sphygmomanometer), if available
- Linen
- Specimen containers and labels

Action	Rationale

• Wash your hands • Check the client's identification band • Explain the procedure to the client prior to beginning • Note: You must don barrier protection before checking the client's ID •

1. Review physician orders and agency protocols relative to the type of isolation precautions:

   a. Implement protocol related to the type of disinfectants needed to eliminate specific microorganisms.

   b. Alert housekeeping regarding the room number and type of isolation supplies needed in the room.

   c. Make sure the room has proper ventilation (the door will have to remain closed at all times) and that the bed and other electrical equipment are functioning properly.

2. Place appropriate isolation supplies outside the client's room and place isolation sign on the door.

3. Gather appropriate supplies to take in the room:

   a. Soap and paper towels

   b. Linen

   c. Impermeable bags

   d. Disposable vital signs equipment, if available

   e. Wound care supplies, if appropriate

4. Remove jewelry, lab coat, and other items not necessary for providing client care.

5. Wash hands and don disposable clothing:

   a. Apply mask by placing the top of the mask over the bridge of your nose (top part of mask has a lightweight metal strip) and pinch the metal strip to fit snugly against your skin.

1. Ensures compliance without unnecessary stress being placed on the client and family. Allows housekeeping to have the necessary supplies on their cleaning carts. Provides for client comfort and decreases the spread of microorganisms. Limits the number of personnel coming into the client's room and the client's exposure to microorganisms.

2. Ensures staff follows isolation protocol and alerts visitors to check with the nurses' station before entering the room.

3. Provides for organized care, handwashing, proper isolation, and client care materials. Decreases the spread of microorganisms and the number of times caregivers have to go into and out of the room.

4. Decreases the spread of resident and transient microorganisms.

5. Disposable garments act as a barrier protecting the nurses from contact with pathogens.

continued

Action	**Rationale**

b. Apply cap to cover hair and ears completely, if policy requires cap.

c. Apply gown to cover outer garments completely: Hold gown in front of body and place arms through sleeves (Figure A1-1A). Pull sleeves down to wrist. Tie gown securely at neck and waist (see Figure A1-1B, C).

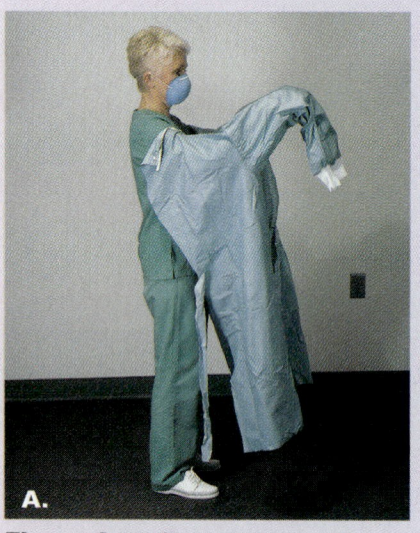 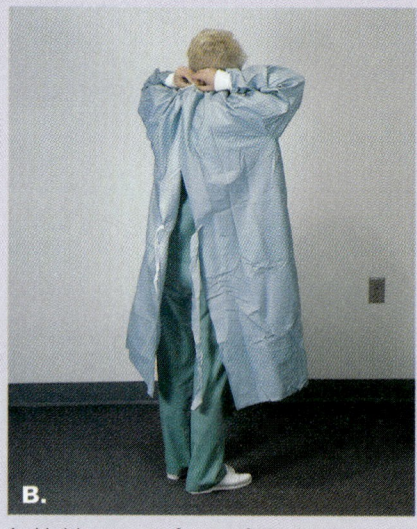 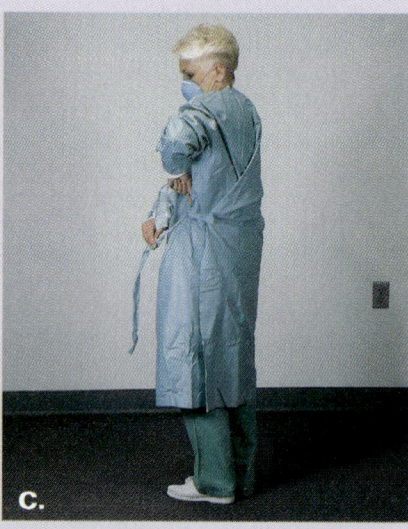

Figure A1-1 Donning disposable gown: A. Hold gown in front of the body and place arms through the sleeves. B. Fasten neck ties. C. Fasten waist ties.

d. Don nonsterile gloves and pull gloves to cover gown's cuff.

e. Don goggles.

e. Eyeglasses do not offer adequate protection.

6. Enter client's room with all gathered supplies; if client is to receive medications, bring them with you at this time. Arrange and store supplies and equipment.

6. Prevents trips into and out of client room and keeps supplies clean.

7. Assess client and family knowledge relative to client's diagnosed infection and isolation:

7. Client's and family's understanding of isolation procedures will increase their participation in care.

a. Reason isolation initiated

b. Type of isolation

c. Duration of isolation

d. How to apply barrier protection

8. Assess vital signs, administer medications if appropriate, and perform other functions of nursing care to meet the needs of the client. Record assessment data on a piece of paper, avoiding contact with any articles in the client's room.

8. Allows for data collection and the performance of client care measures.

9. Dispose of soiled articles in the impermeable bags, which should be labeled correctly according to contents. If soiled reusable equipment is removed from the room, label bag accordingly.

9. Impermeable bags prevent the leakage of contaminated materials, thereby preventing the spread of infection. Labeling is a warning to other personnel that the contents are infectious.

continued

Action	Rationale
10. Double bag soiled linen according to agency policy in an impermeable bag or in plastic linen bag.	10. Double bagging allows the washing of soiled linen without human contact. When linen is double bagged, the first bag is removed prior to washing and the second bag goes into the machine with the dirty linen and dissolves.
11. Replenish supplies before leaving the client's room by having another staff member bring the clean supplies and transfer at the door. Ask client if anything is needed (e.g., juice or personal care items).	11. Decreases the number of times staff members have to go in and out of the room and exposure to microorganisms.
12. Before leaving, let the client know when you will return and make sure call light is accessible.	12. Decreases a feeling of abandonment; provides client with a means of communication.
13. Exiting the isolation room: a. Untie gown at waist. b. Remove one glove by grasping the glove's cuff and pulling down so that the glove turns inside out (glove on glove) and dispose of it. With your ungloved hand, slip your fingers inside the cuff of the other glove, pull it off, inside out, and dispose of it. c. Grasp and release the ties of the mask, and dispose of it. d. Release neck ties of the gown and allow the gown to fall forward. Place fingers of dominant hand inside cuff of other hand and pull down over other hand (Figure A1-2A). With gown covered hand, pull gown over the dominant hand (Figure A1-2B). While gown is still on arm, fold outside of gown together, remove, and dispose of it (Figure A1-2C).	13. Gloves are removed inside out to avoid contact with skin. The gown is removed and folded with hands touching only the inside of the garment. Only the ties and the inside of the cap are touched with your hands. All articles are disposed of as soon as they are removed. c. If a client has a disease spread by airborne pathogens, you may remove the mask last.

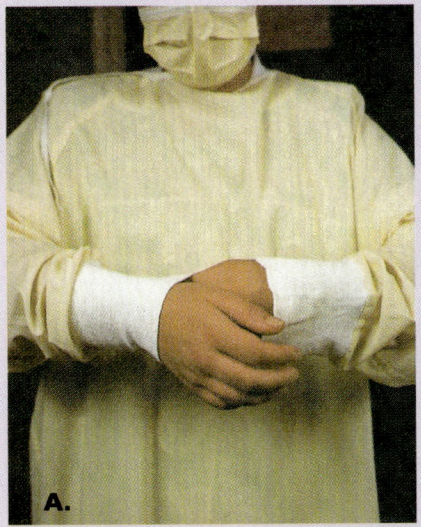
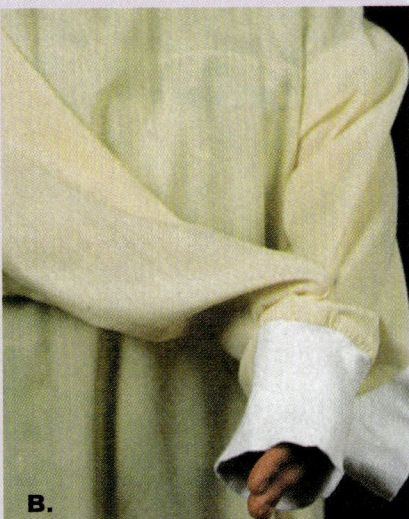
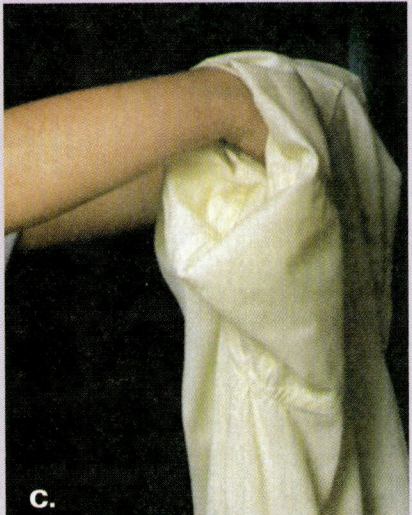

A. B. C.

Figure A1-2 Removing disposable gown: A. Place fingers of dominant hand inside the cuff of other hand and pull gown down over other hand. B. With the gown-covered hand, pull gown down over dominant hand. C. As the gown is removed, fold the outside of the gown together and dispose of it.

continued

Action	Rationale

e. Remove cap by slipping your finger under the cap and removing from the front to back and dispose of it.

14. Wash hands for 10 minutes. Don nonsterile gloves and remove bags from the client's room. Exit room and close door. Dispose of bags according to agency protocol. Remove gloves and wash hands.

14. Decreases likelihood of transmission of microorganisms.

Procedure A2 — Inserting a Nasogastric or Nasointestinal Tube for Suction and Enteral Feedings

Equipment

- Nonsterile gloves
- Cup of ice or water and straw
- Towel and tissues
- Flashlight or penlight
- Hypoallergenic tape, rubber band, safety pin
- 20-mL syringe or asepto syringe
- Disposable irrigation set (optional)
- Wall mount or portable suction equipment as available
- Stethoscope
- Personal protective equipment: gown, gloves, face shield (or goggles and mask)

- Ice chips in an emesis basin
- Water-soluble lubricant
- Tongue blade
- pH chemstrip
- Number 6, 8, 12 French tube for gastric suction (Levine, Salem, or Anderson) or a small-bore feeding tube, 8 or 12 French tube (Keofeed, Dubbhoff, Moss)
- Administration set with pump or controller for feeding tube

Action	Rationale

• Wash your hands • Explain the procedure to the client prior to beginning •
• Check the client's identification band •

1. Review client's medical record.

1. Confirms physician's prescription for inserting a nasogastric tube; history of nasal or sinus problems.

Nasogastric Tube Insertion

2. Gather equipment. Place rubber tubes only in basin of ice. Wash hands.

2. Promotes efficiency. Stiffens tube for easier insertion. Reduces transfer of microorganisms.

3. Provide for privacy.

3. Reduces anxiety.

4. Place client in Fowler's position, at least a 45° angle or higher, with a pillow behind client's shoulders. *Place comatose clients in semi-Fowler's position.*

4. Facilitates passage of the tube into the esophagus and swallowing.

5. Place towel over client's chest; put tissues in reach.

5. Prevents soiling of gown and bedding; lacrimation can occur during insertion through nasal passages.

6. Examine nostrils and assess as client breathes through each nostril.

6. Determines the most patent nostril to facilitate insertion.

continued

Action	Rationale
7. Measure length of tubing needed by using tube as a tape measure (gloves are optional at this step).	**7.** Approximates length of tube needed to reach stomach.

- Measure from end of client's nose to earlobe to xyphoid process of sternum (Figure A2-1).

- If tube is to go below stomach (nasoduodenal or nasojejunal), add an additional 15 to 20 cm.

- Place a small piece of tape on tube to mark length.

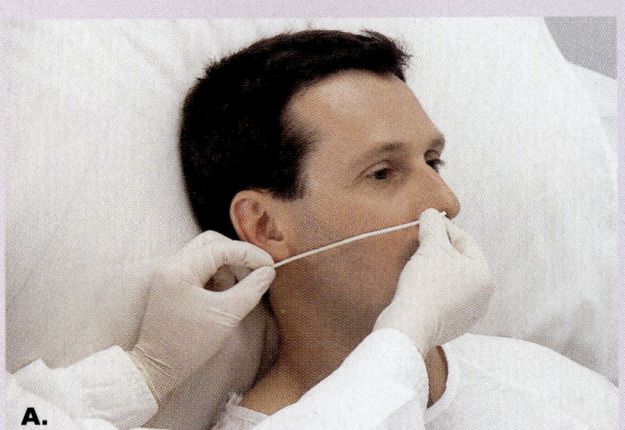 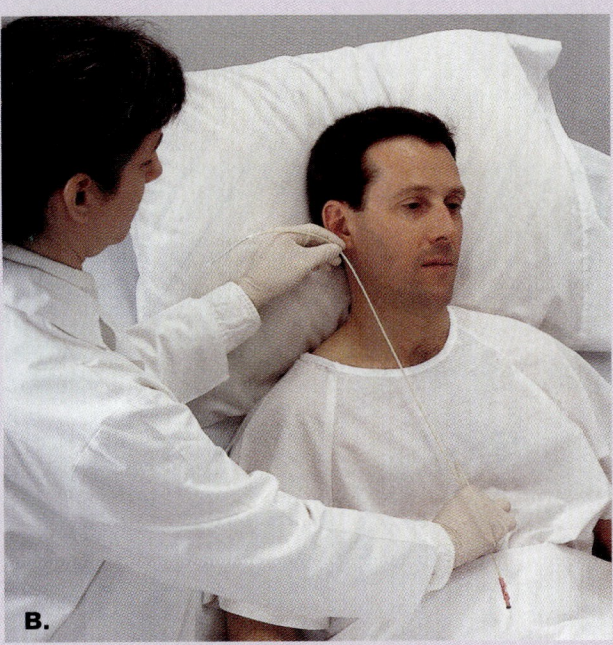

A.

B.

Figure A2-1 A. Measuring From End of Nose to Earlobe; B. Measuring From Earlobe to Xyphoid Process

Action	Rationale
8. Have client blow nose and encourage swallowing of water if level of consciousness and treatment plan permit.	**8.** Clears nasal passage without pushing microorganisms into inner ear; facilitates passage of tube.
9. Apply personal protective equipment.	**9.** Protects nurse from body fluids.
10. Lubricate first 6 to 8 inches of tube with water-soluble lubricant.	**10.** Facilitates passage into the nares.
11. Insert tube as follows (institutional policy will dictate which personnel are authorized to perform steps 11 to 13):	**11.** Promotes passage of tube with minimal trauma to mucosa.

- Gently pass tube into nostril to back of throat (client may gag); aim tube toward back of throat and down.

- When client feels tube in back of throat, use flashlight or penlight to locate tip of tube.

  - Ensures tip's placement.

- Instruct client to flex head toward chest.

  - Opens esophagus and assists in tube insertion after tube has passed through nasopharynx and reduces risk of tube entering trachea.

- Instruct client to swallow, offer ice chips or water, and advance tube as client swallows.

  - Assists in pushing tube past oropharynx.

- If resistance is met, rotate tube slowly with downward advancement toward client's closest ear; do not force tube.

  - Tube may be coiled or kinked or in the oropharynx or trachea.

continued

Action	Rationale
12. Withdraw tube immediately if changes occur in respiratory status.	**12.** Indicates placement of tube in the bronchus or lung.
13. Advance tube, giving client sips of water, until taped mark is reached.	**13.** Assists with tube insertion.
14. Check placement of tube:	**14.** Ensures proper placement in the stomach; pH below 3, tube is in stomach; a pH range of 6 to 7 indicates intestinal sites.

• Attach syringe to free end of tube and aspirate sample of gastric contents and measure with chemstrip pH (Figure A2-2).

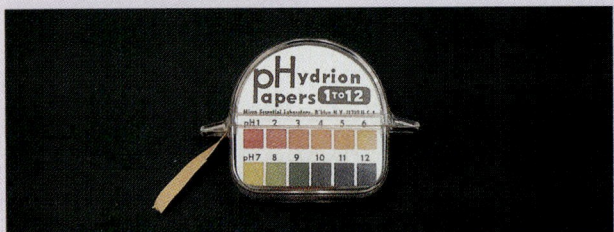

Figure A2-2 For Measuring pH of Aspirate

• Inject 10 mL of air into tube and listen, using a stethoscope, for simultaneous gurgling over epigastrum.

Action	Rationale
15. Leave syringe attached to free end of tube.	**15.** Prevents leakage of gastric contents.
16. If prescribed, obtain x-ray.	**16.** Confirms correct placement; if nasoduodenal or nasojejunal feedings are required, passage through pylorus may require several days.
17. Secure tube with tape as shown in Figure A2-3.	**17.** Prevents tube from becoming dislodged.

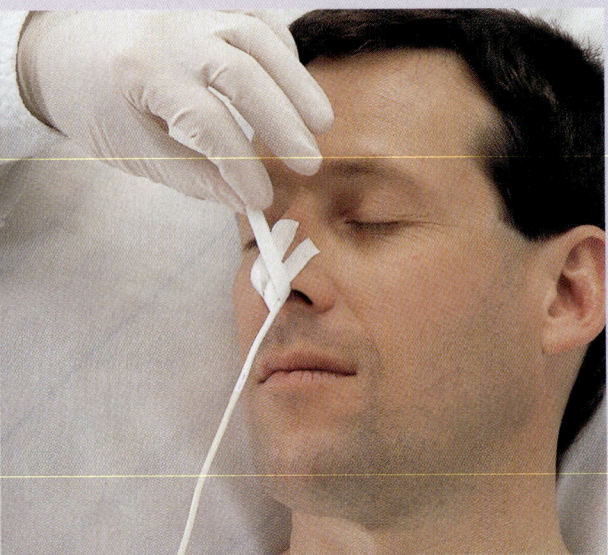

Figure A2-3 Securing Tube to the Client's Nose with Tape

• Split a 4-inch piece of tape to a length of 2 inches and secure tube with tape by placing the intact end of the tape over the bridge of the nose. Wrap split ends around the tube as it exits the nose.

• Prevents trauma to nasal mucosa by reducing pressure on nares.

continued

Action	Rationale
• Place a rubber band, using a slip knot, around the exposed tube (12–18 inches from nose toward chest); after x-ray, pin rubber band to client's gown.	• Allows client movement without causing friction on nares; metal devices are removed for x-rays to prevent artifacts.
18. Instruct client about movements that can dislodge the tube.	18. Reduces anxiety and teaches client how to prevent tugging on tube with head movement.
19. Gastric decompression:	19. Provides for decompression as prescribed by physician; intermittent or continuous suctioning is determined by type of tube inserted.
• Remove syringe from free end of tube and connect tube to suction tubing; set machine on type of suction and pressure as prescribed.	
• Levine tubes are connected to intermittent low pressure.	
• Salem sump or Anderson's tube may be connected to continuous low suction.	
• Observe nature and amount of gastric tube drainage.	• Provides information about patency of tube and gastric contents.
• Assess client for nausea, vomiting, and abdominal distention.	• Indicates effectiveness of intervention.
20. Provide oral hygiene and cleanse nares with a tissue.	20. Promotes comfort.
21. Remove personal protective equipment, dispose of in proper container, and wash hands.	21. Reduces transmission of microorganisms; protects other workers from coming into contact with objects contaminated with body fluids.
22. Position client for comfort, and place call light in easy reach.	22. Promotes comfort and safety.
23. Document:	23. Promotes continuity of care and shows implementation of intervention.
• The reason for the tube insertion.	
• The type of tube inserted.	
• The type (intermittent or continuous) of suctioning and pressure setting.	
• The nature and amount of aspirate and drainage.	
• The client's tolerance of the procedure.	
• The effectiveness of the intervention, such as nausea relieved.	

Insertion of a Small-Bore Feeding Tube

Action	Rationale
24. Follow steps 1 through 8 as stated earlier.	24. See steps 1 through 8.
25. Open adapter cap on tube, snap off end of water vial, and inject water into feeding tube adapter.	25. Activates Keolube lubricant in tube's lumen.
26. Close adapter cap.	26. Ensures a tight fit so water does not leak from adapter site.
27. Check that stylet does not protrude through holes in feeding tube; adjust as necessary.	27. Prevents mucosa trauma.

continued

Action	Rationale
28. Follow steps 9 through 13 as stated earlier.	**28.** See steps 9 through 13.
29. Check placement of tube: • Aspirate gastric contents with Luer-Lok syringe; see Figure A2-4.	**29.** Assures correct placement has been achieved; provides measurement of pH of secretions, as explained in step 14.

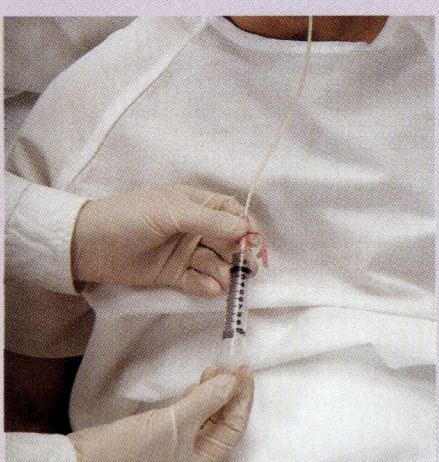

Figure A2-4 Aspirating Gastric Contents with Luer-Lok Syringe with Stylet in Place

Action	Rationale
• Measure pH of aspirate with chemstrip pH.	
30. Leave stylet in place until x-ray confirms placement in case tube needs to be advanced into the duodenum or jejunum.	**30.** Provides a safety measure.
31. Obtain x-ray. Remove stylet from feeding tube after x-ray, and plug open end of tube until feeding.	**31.** Confirms placement of tube prior to instilling formula; prevents gastric juices from seeping out of the tube.
32. Follow steps 20 through 23.	**32.** See steps 20 through 23.
33. Replace small-bore tube every 3 to 4 weeks.	**33.** Prevents obstruction and sepsis of small-bore tubes.

Procedure A3   Venipuncture

Equipment

- Sterile packages of 70% isopropanol (antiseptic) and povidone-iodine (topical antiinfectant)
- Sterile needle and syringe or vacutainer system (20- or 21-gauge needle for cubital vein puncture on an adult)
- Sterile 2 × 2 cotton gauze
- Tourniquet
- Nonsterile gloves
- Bandage or sterile adhesive bandage
- Collecting tubes

continued

Action	**Rationale**

• Wash your hands • Check the client's identification band •
• Explain the procedure to the client prior to beginning •

1. Place client in a sitting or supine position; lower side rail.

1. Promotes client comfort; provides access to the site.

2. Prepare supplies:

- Open sterile packages.

- Label specimen tubes with the client's data, according to agency policy.

2. Promotes efficiency; ensures accuracy of specimen collection regarding the client's identifying data, date and time of collection.

3. Position arm straight. If possible, place extremity in dependent position.

3. Provides access to vein. Increases venous dilation and visibility.

4. Apply the tourniquet 6 to 10 cm above the elbow. Tourniquet should only obstruct venous blood flow, not arterial. Check for a distal pulse.

4. Restricted arterial blood flow prevents venous filling.

5. Select a dilated vein (Figure A3-1). If a vein is not visible, instruct client to open and close a fist; or stroke extremity from proximal to distal, tap lightly over a vein, apply warmth.

5. Assists in veins filling with blood.

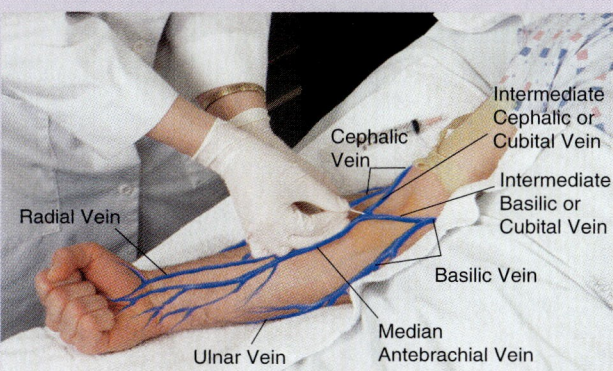

Figure A3-1 Nurse selects site for venipuncture and holds skin taut over site with needle held at 30° angle.

6. Palpate the vein for size and pliancy; be sure it is well seated.

6. Locates a well dilated vein; vein does not roll.

7. Release the tourniquet if it has been on for a lengthy period of time, or if the client is uncomfortable.

7. Prevents hemoconcentration.

8. Cleanse puncture site with isopropanol, let dry and cleanse with povidone-iodine, let dry or wipe with sterile gauze; do not touch site after cleansing. If the client is allergic to iodine, only use isopropanol and cleanse skin for 30 seconds (or according to agency policy).

8. Povidone-iodine reduces bacteria on the skin's surface; it must dry to be effective.

9. Place equipment in easy reach and position yourself to access the puncture site.

9. Promotes efficiency.

10. Reapply the tourniquet (time should not exceed 3 minutes).

10. Restricts blood flow, distends vein.

continued

Action	Rationale
11. Don gloves.	**11.** Decreases exposure to blood-borne organisms.
12. Perform venipuncture:	**12.**
• Remove cap from 20- or 21-gauge needle.	• Large-bore needle prevents hemolysis.
• With nondominant hand, stabilize the vein by holding the skin taut over the puncture site (apply downward tension on the forearm with your thumb).	• Prevents the vein from rolling when the needle is pushed against the outer wall of the vein.
• With dominant hand, hold the needle bevel facing upward at an approximately 10° to 30° angle to the arm (refer back to Figure A3-1).	• Provides for a downward movement toward vein.
• Puncture the skin into the straightest part of vein with a steady, moderately fast movement, (When the vein is entered you will feel a slight give and can see blood at the needle's hub.)	• Decreases risk of going through the vein, decreases discomfort.
• Apply moderate negative pressure by puncturing the vacuum tube or by gently retracting the syringe plunger. (When first performing a venipuncture, use a syringe. It takes greater dexterity to puncture the vacuum tube with a two-sided needle; if you apply too much pressure you will go through the vein.)	
13. Remove the tourniquet once blood is flowing into the tube or syringe; collect the specimen(s).	**13.** Prevents hemolysis.
14. Remove the needle and immediately apply pressure to site for 2 to 3 minutes or 5 to 10 minutes if client is taking anticoagulant medication. Keep the arm straight.	**14.** Decreases bleeding. Bending the arm can reopen the puncture site.
15. Have the client maintain pressure on the puncture site.	**15.** Facilitates clotting.
• *Note:* Green stoppers contain sodium heparin (anticoagulant); they must be mixed promptly after collection.	• Prevents coagulation of blood in test tube.
16. Apply a sterile bandage or adhesive bandage to puncture site.	**16.** Facilitates clotting.
17. If using a needle and syringe, transfer the blood into test tube under moderate pressure.	**17.** Prevents hemolysis.
18. Dispose the needle or needle-syringe into a sharps container.	**18.** Prevents needle stick.
19. Remove gloves; wash hands.	**19.** Decreases transmission of microorganisms.
20. Document venipuncture, amount of blood collected, and client's response.	**20.** Provides record of venipuncture and client's status.

Procedure A4   Preparing an Intravenous Solution

Equipment

- IV solution (bag or bottle)
- Extension set
- IV line filter
- Administration set (vented or nonvented)
- IV pole

Action	Rationale
1. Wash hands before preparing IV equipment.	1. Decreases the transmission of microorganisms.
2. Check the physician's order for the type and amount of solution.	2. Ensures the correct type and amount of fluid.
3. Check IV solution and equipment for expiration dates.	3. Ensures the sterility of the solution and item.
4. Select IV tubing in accord with agency policy.	4. Agency protocols reflect which items of equipment are to be used with specific IV solutions and to complement volume control devices.
5. Prepare IV solution label with client's name, date, time, additives, and your initials (according to agency policy).	5. Provides information to other health care workers relative to when the solution was hung and what additives are infusing in the solution.

Plastic Bag

6. Prepare the IV solution bag for administration:

- Remove outer wrapper around IV bag of solution.

- Inspect bag for tears or leaks by noting any moisture on the protective covering.

- Apply gentle pressure and observe for leakage.

- Examine solution for discoloration, cloudiness, or particulate matter by holding the bag against a dark and light background; if there is any evidence of contamination, do not use, and return bag to agency's dispensing department.

6. Ensures that solution is free of contamination; contaminated solutions are returned to central supply or pharmacy for manufacturer notification.

7. Remove administration set from the package and close the roller clamp on the IV tubing (Figure A4-1).

7. Prevents solution from escaping into the tubing until the drip chamber on the tubing has been primed.

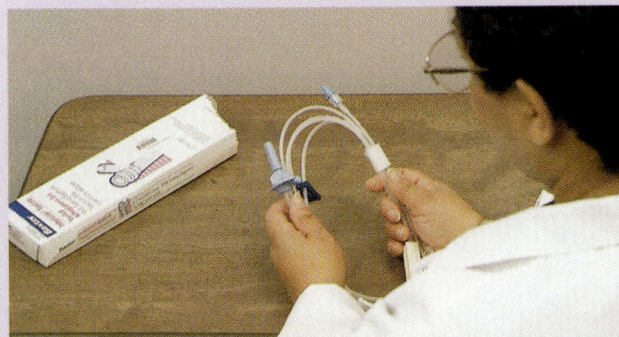

Figure A4-1 Remove tubing from the package, leaving the protective caps on both ends intact.

continued

Action	Rationale
8. Remove the protective cap from the nonvented IV tubing spike and maintain the sterility of the spike.	8. Prepares the sterile spike for insertion into the IV container; IV bags have a vented port.
9. Grasp the port of the IV bag with your nondominant hand. With your dominant hand, remove the plastic tab covering the port (Figure A4-2) and insert the full length of the spike into the bag's port (Figure A4-3).	9. Prevents contamination of both the port and the spike.

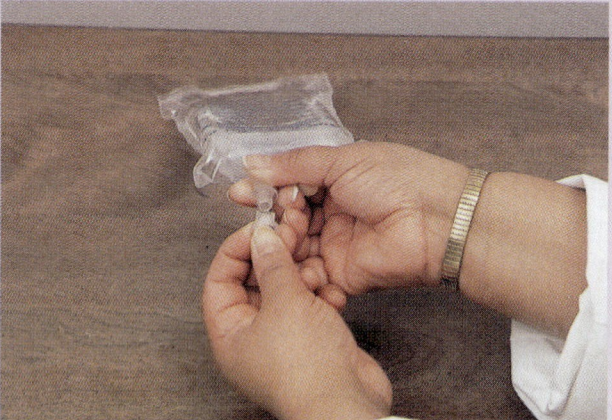

Figure A4-2 Open the IV plastic bag and pull down the plastic tab covering the port with one hand while pinching the port with the other hand.

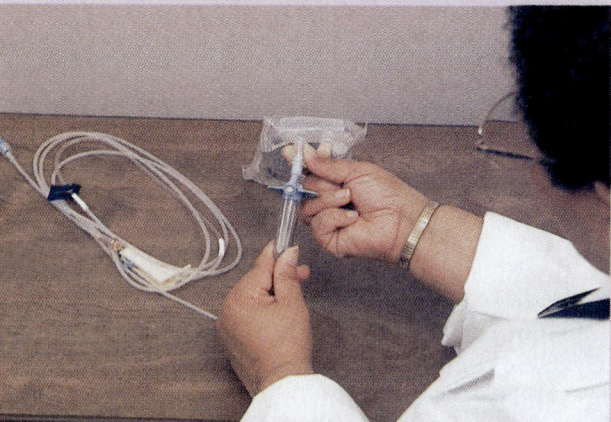

Figure A4-3 Remove the cap from the spike and spike the IV port.

Action	Rationale
10. Squeeze and quickly release pressure on the drip chamber of the IV tubing until the chamber is one-third to one-half full. Hang bag on IV pole.	10. Primes the chamber by displacing air with IV solution, allowing half of the chamber to remain free of solution.
11. Connect IV filter to tubing (if required).	11. Reduces the risk for bacteremia and the incidence of infusion phlebitis; tapping the filter as the solution runs through it eliminates any air bubbles trapped in the filter's membrane.
• Remove cap from filter.	
• Fit tubing's male adapter into filter's female connector, and twist to ensure tight connection.	
• Hold filter so connector joint is pointed down.	
• Hold tubing's end tip higher than the tubing's dependent loop to displace the air.	
• Open roller clamp on IV tubing to prime the tubing and filter (Figure A4-4).	
• Tap the filter as the IV solution runs through.	
• Close the roller clamp on the IV tubing.	
12. Replace the cap on the IV tubing's free end.	12. Maintains the sterility of the system.
13. Attach a Dial-a-Flo fluid regulator at the end of the IV tubing if fluids are to be administered with this device. With the cap off the end of the tubing, turn the Dial-a-Flo to the open position, open all the tubing regulator clamps, and clear the tubing of air; close the regulator clamp and replace the cap on the end of the tubing.	13. Controls the rate of infusion.

continued

Action	Rationale

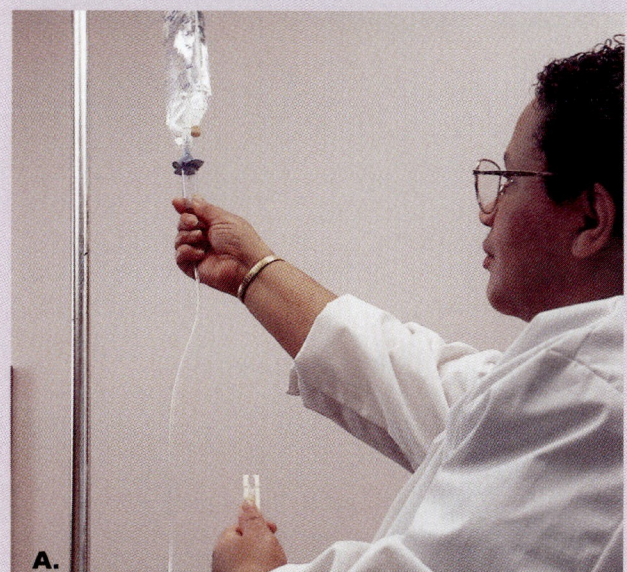
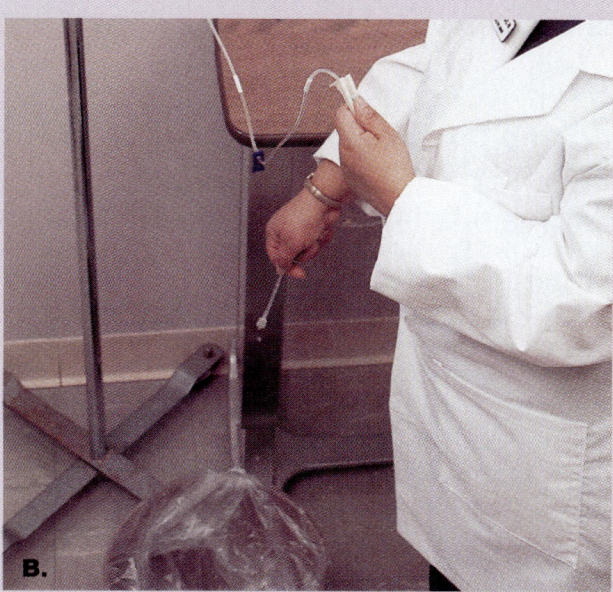

Figure A4-4 A. Prime the IV Tubing. B. Open the roller clamp on the tubing to allow the fluid to enter the tube and expel the air.

Action	Rationale
14. Tag tubing with date and time and your own initials (according to agency policy).	**14.** Indicates when tubing replacement is due (no more frequently than every 72 hours, in accord with agency protocol).
15. Explain to the client what you are doing before taking the IV equipment into the client's room.	**15.** Elicits client's cooperation.

Glass Bottle

Action	Rationale
16. Follow steps 1–5. • Vented tubing is used for glass bottles that are not vented.	

17. Prepare the IV solution for administration.
 	
  • Check bottle for cracks or leaks.
 	
  • Remove metal cap, metal disk, and rubber diaphragm from top of glass bottle, or remove protective additive cap if pharmacy has added medications to the IV bottle.
 	
  • Listen for the escape of air when the rubber diaphragm is removed.
	17. Ensures that solution is free of contamination; contaminated solutions are returned to central supply or pharmacy for manufacturer notification. Escape of air indicates the breaking of the vacuum inside the bottle, which will allow the fluid to flow into the tubing.

18. Close the roller clamp on the IV tubing.	**18.** Stops flow of fluid.
19. Remove the protective cap from the IV tubing spike and maintain the sterility of the spike.	**19.** Prevents contamination.
20. Place the glass bottle on a firm surface, and, using firm downward pressure, insert the spike through designated port on the bottle cap.	**20.** Pressure is required to puncture the rubber stopper in the neck of the IV bottle.
21. Invert IV bottle (if the bottle is vented, the fluid inside the vent tube will escape), and hang the bottle on an IV pole.	**21.** Allows gravity to displace the air in the IV tubing when the roller clamp is opened.
22. Continue steps 10–15.	

Procedure A5

Administering an IV Solution

Equipment

Adding Solution to a Continuous Infusion Line
• Prepared IV solution and medication

Adding a Solution to an Existing Heparin or PI Lock
• Prepared IV solution system with needleless locking cannula
• Alcohol or iodophor swab

• Needleless injection cap (if one is not in place)
• 2 prefilled syringes of 2 mL each of normal saline
• Nonsterile gloves

Action

Rationale

• Wash your hands • Check the client's identification band •
• Explain the procedure to the client prior to beginning •

Action	Rationale
1. Gather prepared equipment (solution labeled with the client's name, and time-taped for fluids to infuse per hour, according to agency policy.	1. Ensures correct fluids to be administered to the right client at the prescribed infusion rate.
2. Don gloves if you have to perform a veni-puncture or connect the tubing to an existing PI. *Gloves are not necessary if you are adding fluids to an existing infusion line.*	2. Decreases risk of transmission of micro-organisms.
3. Assess the puncture site.	3. Indicates signs of infiltration or infection.
• Observe for redness and puffiness.	
• Palpate for tenderness.	
4. Check patency of infusion site.	4. Verifies patency of IV system with venous access device in the client's vein.
• Verify that fluid is infusing.	
• If necessary, remove IV container from the pole and lower the container below the level of infusion site.	
• Observe for backflow of blood into the hub of the venous access device.	
• Replace container on IV pole.	

Adding Solution to a Continuous Infusion Line

Action	Rationale
5. Check the date on the tubing tag; if the tubing needs changing, refer to Procedure A4.	5. Indicates when tubing replacement is due.
6. Hang the new bag of fluids on the IV pole and remove the cover from the port.	6. Provides easy access to the fluids.
7. Remove the current infusion bag of fluids from the IV pole.	7. Makes it easier to remove tubing spike.
8. While maintaining aseptic technique, remove the tubing spike from the port of the infusing bag of fluids and reinsert the tubing spike into the port on the new bag of fluids; push the full length of the spike into the port.	8. Maintains the sterility of the IV system.
9. Set the infusion rate.	9. Produces correct drip rate.

continued

Action	**Rationale**

Manual Rate Regulation

- Open regulator clamp; close slowly while observing the drip chamber until the fluid is dripping at a slow, steady pace.

- Count the number of drops for a full minute; for example, if the drop factor of tubing is 10 drops/mL then the drop rate should be 21 drops/minute to infuse 1000 mL/8 hours (Figure A5-1).

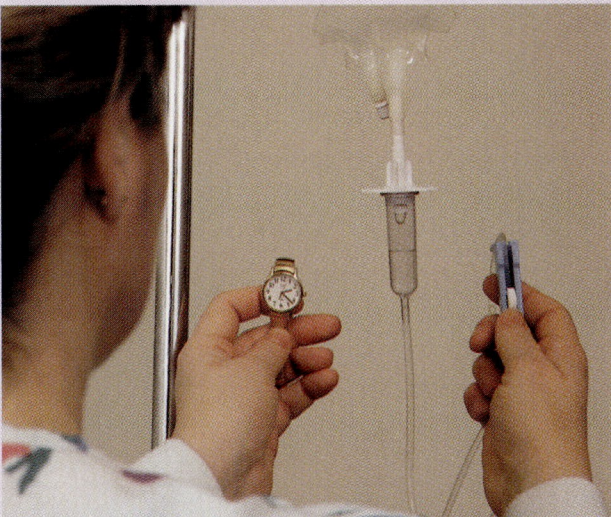

Figure A5-1 Manual Rate Regulation: Counting the Number of Drops for a One-Minute Interval

- Open the regulator clamp slowly to increase the drip flow rate; close the regulator clamp to decrease the drip rate to achieve 21 drops/minute.

- Recount the drop rate after 5 and 15 minutes.

- Proceed to steps 10–17.

Dial-a-Flo Regulation

- Turn Dial-a-Flo regulator until arrow is aligned with desired volume of fluid to infuse over 1 hour.

- Check drip rate for a full minute.

- Adjust height of IV pole if necessary.

- Recount drip rate after 5 minutes and again after 15 minutes.

- Proceed to steps 10–17.

Infusion Controller or Pump Regulation

- Insert tubing into infusion controller or pump in accord with manufacturer's instruction (Figure A5-2).

Rationale column:

- Determines patency of venous access device.

- Determines number of drops falling per minute.

- Controls drip rate with regular clamp.

- Detects changes in rate due to expansion and contraction of tubing.

- Regulates infusion of fluid at the desired rate.

- Verifies calculated drip rate with infusion rate.

- Facilitates flow by gravity.

- Detects changes in rate due to expansion and contraction of tubing.

- Ensures proper functioning of the device.

continued

Action	**Rationale**

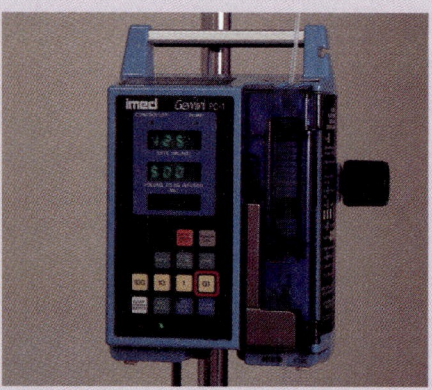

Figure A5-2 IV Tubing Threaded into an Infusion Pump with Controls Set

- Close door to controller or pump and open all tubing clamps and regulators.

- Set machine to regulate the volume to infuse per hour or drops per minute in accord with the type of machine. Also set the total volume to be infused.

- Push the *start* or *on* button.

- Proceed to steps 10–17.

Volume Control Chamber (Buretrol) Regulation

- Close regulators both above and below the chamber.

- If adding a new Buretrol, open regulator above the chamber and fill the chamber with 10 mL of fluid, close the top regulator, and slowly open the regulator below the chamber to remove air from the tubing. Close the bottom regulator (Figure A5-3).

- Allows controller or pump to regulate the infusion rate.

- Determines amount of fluid the device will deliver.

- Initiates the device's regulation of the fluid flow.

- Allows for precise release of fluids into the chamber.

- Facilitates priming the drip chamber and clearing the tubing below the chamber of air.

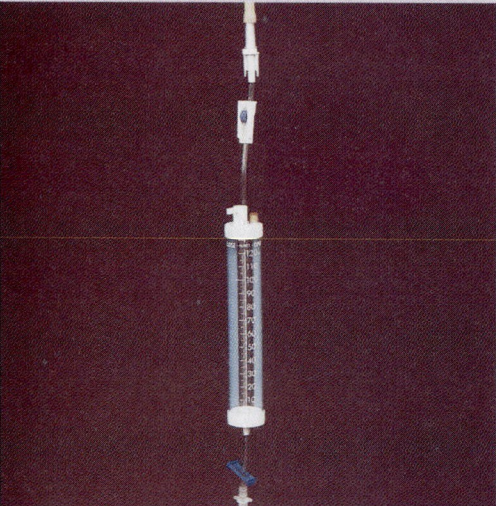

Figure A5-3 Volume Control Chamber

continued

Action	Rationale
• Open the top regulator and fill the chamber with the volume of fluid to infuse in 1 hour or 2 hours if the volume is small.	• Facilitates close monitoring of fluid volume.
• Close top regulator and ensure that air vent is open.	• Allows fluid to escape from the chamber.
• Open bottom regulator and regulate drops to calculated drip rate in accord with the drop factor.	• Determines volume to infuse over an hour.
• Count drip rate for a full minute.	• Verifies rate of infusion.
• Time-tape the chamber if a controller or pump is not used.	• Facilitates easy check of fluid infusion and shows when to add fluid to the chamber.
• Check chamber every 1 to 2 hours depending on the volume placed in the chamber.	• Maintains fluid infusion and prevents air from entering the chamber and tubing if all fluid is infused.
• Proceed with steps 10–17.	
10. On the time tape, write the time the fluids were initiated and your initials.	10. Facilitates easy check of fluid infusion progress as prescribed.
11. Monitor the volume delivered every 1 to 2 hours and compare with the time tape.	11. Ensures the actual volume being delivered.
12. If fluids are not infusing at the prescribed rate as indicated by time tape:	12. Ensures that prescribed amount of fluid is delivered.
• Check setting on controller or pump or Dial-a-Flo and adjust as indicated.	
• Increase height of IV pole.	• Allows gravity to facilitate the drip rate.
• Assess puncture site, reposition the venous access device, lower the IV fluid container below the puncture site and observe for a back-flow of blood. Replace container on pole.	• Ensures that venous access device is still in the vein.
13. Instruct client to limit movement of puncture site and to notify a nurse of any problems or discomfort.	13. Facilitates early detection of problems.
14. Apply an armboard as a last resort (Figure A5-4).	14. Immobilizes the extremity receiving the infusion.

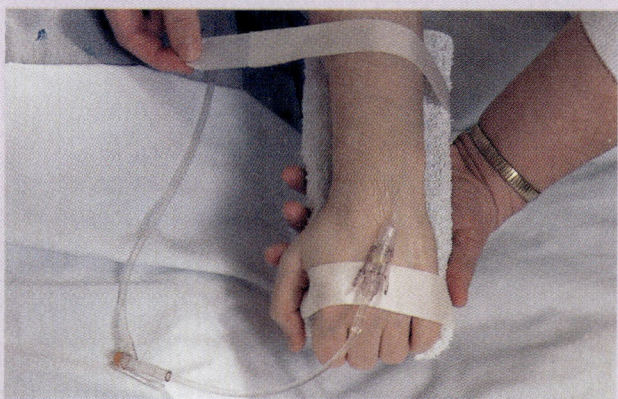

Figure A5-4 Positioning of Client with an IV Armboard

continued

Action	**Rationale**
15. Position the client for comfort and place the call light in easy reach.	**15.** Promotes client comfort and safety.
16. Wash hands and dispose of used supplies.	**16.** Decreases transmission of microorganisms.
17. Document on the client's medical record:	**17.** Provides a record of the nursing intervention and the client's response.
• Time of initiation of fluid infusion.	
• Type and volume of fluid infusing.	
• Infusion device used, if applicable.	
• Status of the venous access insertion site.	
• Problems encountered: for example, if venous access device is repositioned.	
• Client's tolerance to the fluid infusion.	
• Client teaching and learning.	

Adding a Secondary Line, Additive Bag (IV Piggyback)

Refer to Procedure A6.

Adding a Solution to an Existing Heparin or PI Lock

Action	**Rationale**
18. Follow steps 1–3.	
19. Hang IV solution on IV pole.	**19.** Provides easy access to system.
20. Don nonsterile gloves and cleanse needleless injection port with alcohol or iodophor swab. Allow to dry.	**20.** Reduces risk of transmission of microorganisms.
21. Insert saline syringe into port, slowly aspirate, and observe for blood; flush system and observe for swelling at puncture site.	**21.** Indicates a patent system and, with the presence of blood and lack of swelling, that the needle is probably in the vein.
22. Connect needleless locking cannula into injection port, open tubing clamp, and adjust rate as indicated in step 9.	**22.** Ensures administration of solution at the correct drip rate.
23. Dispose of equipment and gloves in proper receptacle and wash hands.	**23.** Reduces risk of transmission of pathogens.
24. When secondary bag and drip chamber are empty, don gloves, close the clamp, and disconnect the needleless locking cannula from the port's lock.	**24.** Indicates infusion of the solution.
25. Flush port with second saline syringe and place sterile needleless injection cap on the port.	**25.** Clears the line and reduces the risk of contaminating the port.
26. Dispose of equipment and gloves in proper receptacle and wash hands.	**26.** Reduces risk of transmission of pathogens.
27. Record fluid administration on MAR and client response in nurses' notes.	**27.** Documents nursing intervention and any client adverse reactions.

Procedure A6

Administering Medications by IV Piggyback to an Existing IV

Equipment

- Prepared and labeled medication solution bag
- Alcohol swab
- Secondary administration set
- Needle or needleless locking cannula if needleless system used.

Action	Rationale
• *Check the client's identification band* • *Explain the procedure to the client prior to beginning* •	
1. Gather prepared equipment (medication labeled with the client's name, and time tape for fluids to infuse per hour).	1. Ensures correct fluids to be administered to the right client at the infusion rate prescribed by the physician.
2. Wash hands. *Gloves are not necessary if you are adding fluids to an existing infusion line.*	2. Decreases risk of transmission of microorganisms.
3. Assess the puncture site.	3. Indicates signs of infiltration or infection.
• Observe for redness and puffiness.	
• Palpate for tenderness.	
4. Check patency of infusion site.	4. Verifies patency of IV system with venous access device in the client's vein.
• Observe fluid infusing.	
• If necessary, remove IV container from the pole and lower the container below the level of infusion site.	
• Observe for backflow of blood into the hub of the venous access device.	
• Replace container on IV pole.	
5. Secure medication bag and check physician's order and the MAR.	5. Ensures the correct client, medication, dosage, route, and frequency.
6. Check the client's chart for allergies and check the drug compatibility chart.	6. Ensures that the client is not allergic to the drug and that the prescribed drug is compatible with the primary IV solution.
7. Hang the secondary bag on IV pole.	7. Provides easy access for preparation.
8. Add the administration set to the secondary bag and prime the tubing.	8. Removes the air from the tubing.
9. Affix a needleless locking cannula to the end of tubing (Figure A6-1A).	9. Reduces risk of exposure to IV needles.
10. Cleanse needleless Y-site injection port of primary IV tubing closest to infusion site with an alcohol swab, allow to dry.	10. Reduces risk of transmission of microorganisms.
11. Insert needleless locking cannula of secondary bag set into Y-site injection port of primary set (Figure A6-1B).	11. Provides access for infusion and prevents dislodgement of needleless locking cannula.
12. Affix the extension hook to the primary bag on the IV pole so that the primary bag hangs below the level of the secondary bag.	12. Ceases flow of primary solution because of an increased hydrostatic pressure in secondary bag.

continued

Action	**Rationale**
13. Open clamp of secondary tubing and adjust drip rate to desired infusion rate.	**13.** Allows solution in the secondary bag to infuse at the prescribed drip rate.
• Slowly close the regular clamp while observing the drip chamber until the fluid is dripping at a slow, steady pace (Figure A6-1C).	

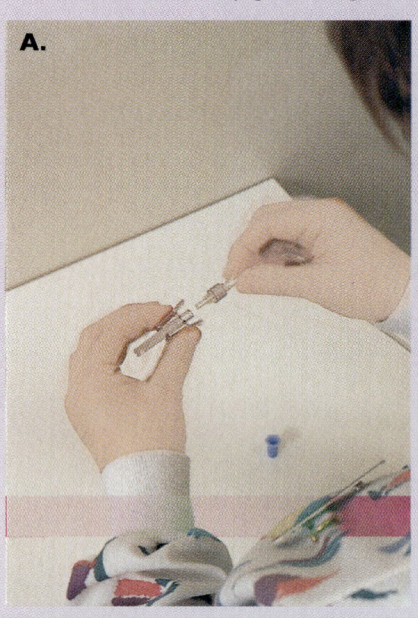 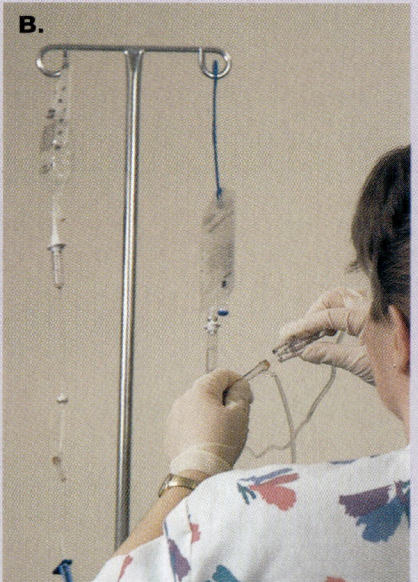 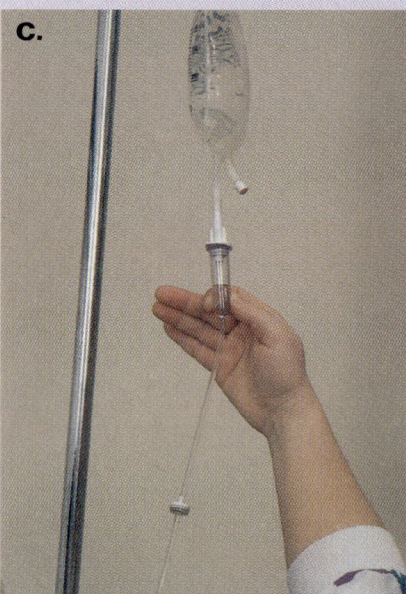

Figure A6-1 Administering Medications by IV Piggyback. A. Connect a needleless locking cannula to a secondary infusion line. B. Connect locking cannula to a Y-site injection port of primary infusion set. C. Monitor the infusion rate. (Gloves are not required for this procedure.)

• Count the drops for a full minute, e.g., if the drop factor of tubing is 10 drops/mL then the drop rate should be 10 drops/minute to infuse 50 mL in 50 minutes.	• Determines number of drops falling per minute.
• Recount the drop rate in 5 minutes.	• Detects changes in rate due to expansion and contraction of tubing.
14. Observe client for any signs of adverse reactions to the medication.	**14.** Provides for immediate intervention if client has an adverse reaction.
15. When secondary bag and drip chamber are empty, close the clamp on secondary system, readjust drip rate of primary solution as indicated, and remove the secondary system (or leave in place, according to agency policy).	**15.** Allows the primary solution to infuse at prescribed drip rate.
16. Record medication infusion on the MAR and note any client responses in the nurses' notes.	**16.** Documents the nursing intervention.

Procedure A7

Managing IV Therapy and Dressing Change

Equipment

Assessing and Changing IV Tubing
- Nonsterile gloves (use with contact with bodily fluids)

Troubleshooting an IV System
- Nonsterile gloves
- Sterile needle and 5-cc syringe with 2 mL normal saline or needleless system.

Changing a Gown
- Clean gown

Converting to an Intermittent Infusion Device
- Nonsterile gloves
- Protective pad
- Needleless injection cap

Changing a Peripheral IV Dressing
- Protective pad
- Tape (check for client allergy to tape)
- 70% isopropyl alcohol or povidone-iodine swab (check for client allergy to iodine)
- Antimicrobial ointment

Discontinuing an IV Line
- Sterile 2 × 2 gauze
- Tape or Band-Aid

- Administration sets (as determined by tubing to be replaced

- 70% isopropyl alcohol or povidone-iodine swab (check for client allergy to iodine)

- Sterile needle and 3-cc syringe with 2 mL of normal saline or needleless system

- Sterile IV dressing tray, sterile 2 × 2 gauze dressing, sterile adhesive, or transparent semipermeable membrane dressing and sterile gloves
- Receptacle for contaminated items

- Nonsterile gloves

Action	Rationale

• Wash your hands • Check the client's identification band •
• Explain the procedure to the client prior to beginning •

1. Gather equipment.

2. Place bed at comfortable working height and lower side rails as necessary.

Managing IV Site

3. Don gloves and assess IV site (according to agency protocol and CDC guidelines) at least every 8 hours for signs and symptoms of complications (phlebitis, infiltration, infection at site, allergic reaction).

4. Assess dressing.
   - Determine when dressing was applied by checking date and time written on dressing itself.

   - Observe dressing for moisture.

   - Observe that dressing is intact.

   - Gently palpate over the intact dressing.

1. Promotes efficiency.

2. Promotes proper body mechanics and provides access to area.

3. Decreases risk of contact with bloodborne pathogens; provides early detection of symptoms of complications and appropriate intervention.

4. Allows for assessment without disrupting in intact IV dressing.

   - Monitors medium for bacterial growth that would render sterile dressing contaminated.

   - Decreases risk of bacterial contamination to venipuncture site from nonadhering dressing.

   - Detects IV site swelling and edema around venipuncture site.

continued

Action	**Rationale**
• If client complains of tenderness or pain, remove dressing and inspect site.	• Detects early signs of phlebitis.
5. Change dressing immediately if it becomes wet, soiled, or loose.	**5.** Decreases risk of bacterial infection.
6. Observe patency of IV line and needle.	**6.** Ensures proper infusion rate; IV line and needle must be free of kinks, knots, and clots.
• Open roller clamp and observe for rapid flow of fluid into drip chamber; close roller clamp and set drip rate to prescribed flow rate.	• Denotes patency of IV line and prevents fluid overload.
• If fluid does not flow, remove IV container from pole, place below level of infusion site, and observe for blood return.	• Determines patency of needle or cannula and placement of the device in the vein; venous pressure should be greater than IV tubing pressure.
7. Peripheral cannulas are removed and changed to a new site every 48–72 hours.	**7.** Supports CDC recommendations for changing peripheral cannulas to a new site every 48–72 hours to decrease the risk of complications.
8. Change administration sets.	**8.** Promotes compliance with CDC guidelines to prevent infection.
• Use IV sets for blood or blood products only once.	
• Every 24 hours, change tubing for lipids if the solution is infusing continuously; use new tubing with each infusion if solution is infusing intermittently.	
• Every 24 hours, change IV tubing used for hyperalimentation.	
• Routine IV tubing should not be changed more frequently than every 72 hours.	

Troubleshooting an IV system

9. Overfilled drip chamber:	**9.** Maintains air in chamber to allow for flow-rate calculation.
• Close drip chamber.	
• Remove container from IV pole and turn it upside down.	
• Squeeze drip chamber until it is one-third to one-half full.	
10. Air in tubing:	**10.** Prevents infusion of air into the bloodstream.
• Observe fluid level in drip chamber.	
• Check tubing connections.	
• Disinfect injection port distal to air.	
• Insert sterile needle and syringe into injection port, and aspirate or use needleless system (if available).	
11. Blood is backing up IV tubing:	**11.** Prevents clot formation at the needle or cannula tip inside the vein.
• Check that IV container is above the level of the site and heart.	

continued

Action	Rationale
• Check security of tubing connections.	
• Check fluid level in tubing chamber and IV container.	
12. IV is positional:	**12.** Maintains bevel of needle or tip of cannula away from the inner lumen of the vein.
• Reposition hand or arm.	
13. Infusion controller or pump alarms:	**13.** Indicates flow problem. Follow agency policy.
• Check device for type of alarm.	
• Follow manufacturer's instructions for each alarm condition.	

Changing a Gown, Continuous IV Infusion in Hand or Arm

Action	Rationale
14. Untie back or side of gown.	**14.** Allows gown to slip freely from arms.
15. Remove gown's sleeve from arm and hand without IV.	**15.** Frees the gown for removal from the involved arm.
16. Adjust the tubing to extend over IV hand, then slip the sleeve down arm; avoid tugging on tubing.	**16.** Prevents pressure on the tubing, which could disturb the venipuncture site or dislodge the IV.
17. Place clean gown over client's chest and abdomen.	**17.** Prevents unnecessary exposure and maintains client warmth.
18. Remove IV container from pole and slip sleeve over container, keeping container above client's arm.	**18.** Prevents backflow of blood into tubing.
19. Place your hand up through distal end of clean gown sleeve and grasp container; pull container and tubing out through clean gown sleeve.	**19.** Maintains integrity of the IV system.
20. Hang container on pole and check flow rate.	**20.** Ensures that solution is infusing at prescribed rate.
21. Slip sleeve over client's IV arm and then on other arm; tie gown at back.	**21.** Maintains client's warmth and comfort.

Converting to an Intermittent Infusion Device

Action	Rationale
22. Perform steps 1 and 2.	
23. Check physician's order.	**23.** Verifies action to establish an intermittent infusion device.
24. Don clean gloves and close roller clamps on tubing.	**24.** Decreases risk of contact with bloodborne pathogens; prevents escape of solution from tubing.
25. Place protective pad under arm or hand with venipuncture site.	**25.** Prevents soiling of bed linen.
26. Open sterile package containing needleless injection cap and place in easy reach near venipuncture site.	**26.** Provides easy access.
27. With your nondominant hand, grasp hub of needle or cannula. With your dominant hand, disconnect IV tubing and attach needleless injection cap to hub.	**27.** Prevents dislodgement of needle or cannula.

continued

Action	**Rationale**
28. While stabilizing hub with nondominant hand, inject needleless injection cap port with 2 mL of normal saline.	**28.** Maintains patency of lock.
29. Discard old tubing and used supplies in receptacle.	**29.** Promotes a clean environment.

Changing a Peripheral IV Dressing

Action	**Rationale**
30. Perform steps 1 and 2.	
31. Place protective pad under IV site; don gloves.	**31.** Prevents soiling of bed linens; reduces risk of contact with bloodborne pathogens.
32. Remove transparent or gauze dressing in direction that client's hair grows; keep pressure over IV site and leave in place the tape that secures IV needle or cannula (Figure A7-1).	**32.** Decreases client's discomfort when removing tape; prevents dislodgement of needle or cannula.

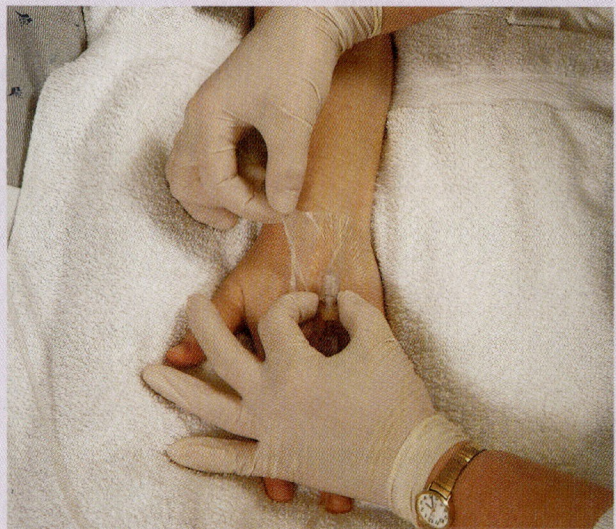

Figure A7-1 Removing Tape from a Peripheral IV. Remove tape with one hand while stabilizing the catheter's hub with the other hand.

Action	**Rationale**
33. Discard dressing and gloves in receptacle; wash hands.	**33.** Reduces risk for transmission of microorganisms.
34. Don gloves; inspect IV site for erythema, edema, infiltration.	**34.** Reduces risk of contact with bloodborne pathogens; denotes complications—for example, phlebitis, infiltration—that would necessitate changing IV site.
35. Cleanse IV site with alcohol or povidone-iodine. Using a circular motion, start at the puncture site and move outward peripherally; allow to dry (1 minute). Apply antimicrobial ointment over IV site, if dictated by agency protocol.	**35.** Reduces skin surface bacteria and prevents cross-contamination from skin bacteria near venipuncture site.
36. Replace tape:	**36.** Allows for stabilization of needle or catheter without tape's covering the insertion site, and eliminates positional flow of IV solution.

continued

Action	**Rationale**

Butterfly

- Place smallest pieces of tape across wings of butterfly.
- Place another piece of tape across middle to form an H; or
- Place small piece of tape under wings (Figure A7-2).

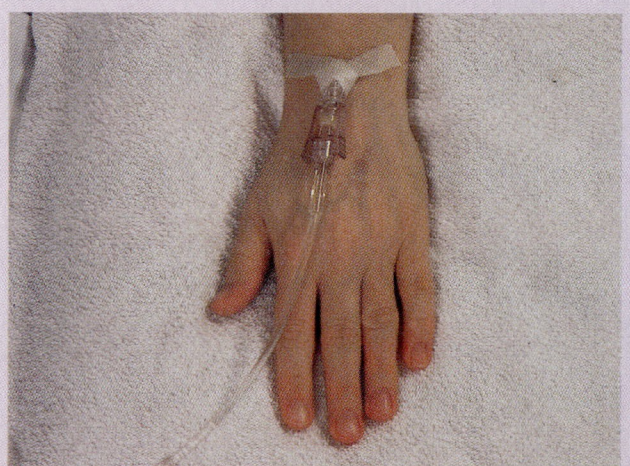

Figure A7-2 Retaping a Butterfly Needle via the Crisscross (V) Method

- Tape over to form a V.
- Place piece of tape across V.
- Avoid placing tape over insertion site.

Over-the-Needle Catheter (Angiocath)

- With tape edges sticking to your thumb and fingertip, slide small piece of tape under catheter hub with adhesive side up.
- Cross tape over hub to form a U (Figure A7-3).
- Place another small piece of tape across catheter hub.
- Avoid placing tape over insertion site.

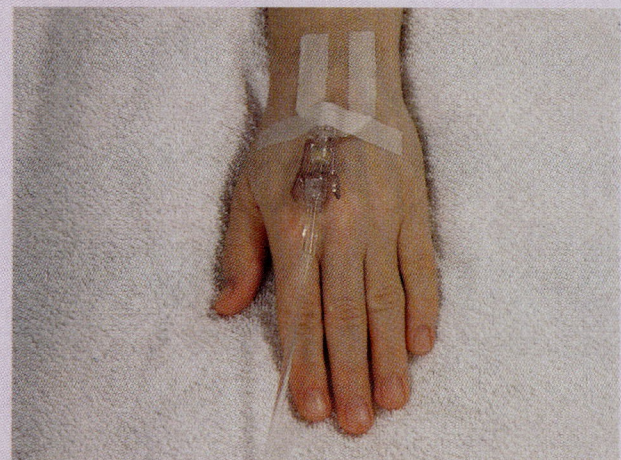

Figure A7-3 Retaping a Catheter via the U Method

37. Apply antimicrobial ointment over IV site if dictated by agency protocol.

38. Using aseptic technique, apply transparent or gauze dressing over IV insertion site; avoid wrinkling transparent dressing.

39. Place date, time, and your initials directly on dressing.

40. Discard soiled items and gloves in receptacle; wash hands.

41. Reassess patency of IV system, flow rate, and client's response to dressing change.

38. Provides protective barrier against bacteria.

39. Documents dressing change.

40. Reduces risk of transmission of microorganisms.

41. Validates patency of IV system and infusion of solution at prescribed flow rate.

continued

Action	Rationale
42. Record in nurses' notes: time and type of dressing change, nature of venipuncture site, patency, and IV flow rate.	**42.** Documents actions taken and condition of IV site and system.

Discontinuing an IV Line

Action	Rationale
43. Perform steps 1 and 2. Don nonsterile gloves.	
44. Assess if device is in place before discontinuing.	**44.** Allows for verification of complete removal of device.
45. Close roller clamp on IV tubing. If infusing, note amount of solution left in IV container.	**45.** Prevents spillage of solution when needle or catheter is removed; provides accurate amount of solution infused.
46. Stabilize needle or cannula with nondominant hand and remove tape in direction of hair growth.	**46.** Prevents unnecessary movement that could injure the vein; decreases discomfort when tape is removed.
47. Place sterile 2 × 2 gauze over puncture site and, while applying pressure, quickly and smoothly remove needle or catheter. Avoid pressing down on top of needle point while it is still in the vein.	**47.** Decreases bleeding and prevents injury to the vein.
48. Discard needle or catheter in receptacle.	**48.** Reduces risk of transmission of microorganisms.
49. Apply pressure over puncture site with sterile 2 × 2 gauze until bleeding stops. Apply tape firmly over the gauze; place gloves in receptacle and wash hands.	**49.** Promotes clot formation; keeps puncture site clean.
50. Inspect site for redness, swelling, or hematoma formation. Inspect removed cannula to assure it is intact.	**50.** Determines whether bleeding is occurring in the tissue.
51. Note whether there is any exudate on the catheter tip or at insertion site. Check site again in 15 to 30 minutes.	**51.** May indicate infection. Follow agency policy.
52. Record in nurses' notes time, amount of IV solution left in container when discontinued, and nature of puncture site.	**52.** Documents actions taken; promotes accurate intake recording and documents condition of puncture site.

References/Suggested Readings and Resources

Please note that because Internet resources are of a time-sensitive nature and URL addresses may change or be deleted, resource searches should also be conducted by association and/or topic.

CHAPTER 1
Holistic Care

REFERENCES/SUGGESTED READINGS

American Holistic Nurses' Association. (1994). AHNA Philosophy. *Journal of Holistic Nursing, 12*(3), 350–351.

Berggren-Thomas, P., & Griggs, M. (1995). Spirituality in aging: Spiritual need or spiritual journey? *Journal of Gerontological Nursing, 21*(3), 5–10.

Burkhardt, M. (1993). Characteristics of spirituality in the lives of women in rural Appalachian community. *Journal of Transcultural Nursing, 4*(2), 12–18.

Cerrato, P. (1998a). Understanding the mind/body link. *RN, 61*(1), 28–31.

Cerrato, P. (1998b). Spirituality and healing. *RN, 61*(2), 49–50.

Dossey, B. (1998). Holistic modalities & healing moments. *American Journal of Nursing (AJN), 98*(6), 44–47.

Dossey, B., & Dossey, L. (1998). Attending to holistic care. *AJN, 98*(8), 35–38.

Dossey, B., Keegan, L., Guzzetta, C., & Kolkmeier, L. (1995). *Holistic nursing: A handbook for practice* (2nd ed.). Gaithersburg, MD: Aspen.

Dyer, E. (1998, April 6). Faith & healing. *Corpus Christi Caller-Times.*

Hill, S., & Howlett, H. (1997). *Success in Practical Nursing: Personal and Vocational Issues.* (3rd ed.) Philadelphia: W. B. Saunders.

Hughs, C. (1997). Prayer and healing: A case study. *Journal of Holistic Nursing, 15*(3), 318.

Jerome, A. et al, (1992). Nurse self-awareness in therapeutic relationships. *Pediatric Nursing, 18*(2), 153–156.

Kahn, S., & Saulo, M. (1995). *Healing yourself.* Albany, NY: Delmar Publishers.

Kurzen, C. (1996). *Contemporary practical/vocational nursing* (3rd ed.). 3rd ed. Philadelphia: J. B. Lippincott.

Maslow, A. (1954). *Motivation and personality.* New York: Harper & Row.

Selye, H. (1956). *The stress of life.* New York: McGraw-Hill.

Taber's Cyclopedic Medical Dictionary. (1997). Philadelphia: F. A. Davis.

Waughfield, C. (1998). *Mental health concepts* (4th ed.). Albany, NY: Delmar Publishers.

Webster's New World College Dictionary (1997). Springfield, MS: Merriam-Webster.

World Health Organization. (1974). *Chronicle of WHO.* Geneva: The Organization Interim Commission.

Wright, K. (1998). Professional, ethical, and legal implications for spiritual care in nursing. *Image: Journal of Nursing Scholarship, 30*(1) 81–83.

RESOURCES

American Holistic Nurses' Association, P.O. Box 2130, Flagstaff, AZ, 86003-2130, 1-800-278-AHNA (1461), http://www.ahna.com e-mail: AHNA-flag@flaglink.com

Nurse Healers—Professional Associates International, Inc., 1211 Locust Street, Philadelphia, PA, 19107, 215-545-8079

Videos

- *Holistic Nursing* (1996), American Holistic Nurses' Association, 1-800-278-2462
- *At the Heart of Healing: Experiencing Holistic Nursing*, Kineholistic Foundation, 1-800-255-1914

CHAPTER 2
Critical Thinking

REFERENCES/SUGGESTED READINGS

Baker, C. R. (1996). Reflective learning: A teaching strategy for critical thinking. *Journal of Nursing Education, 35,* 19–22.

Bevis, E. O. (1993). All in all, it was a pretty good funeral. *Journal of Nursing Education, 32,* 101.

Birx, E. (1993). Critical thinking and theory-based practice. *Holistic Nursing Practice, 7* (3).

Bowers, B., & McCarthy, D. (1993). Developing analytic thinking skills in early undergraduate education. *Journal of Nursing Education, 32,* 107–113.

Brigham, C. (1993). Nursing education and critical thinking: Interplay of content and thinking. *Holistic Nursing Practice, 7* (3).

Brookfield, S. (1993). On impostership, cultural suicide and owners dangers: How nurses learn critical thinking. *Journal of Continuing Education in Nursing, 24* (5), 179–205.

Center for Critical Thinking. (1998, April 11). *A brief history of the idea of critical thinking.* [On-line]. Available: http://www.criticalthinking.org/University/univlibrary/cthistory.nclk

Duncan, G. (1996). An investigation of learning styles of practical and baccalaureate nursing students. *Journal of Nursing Education, 35,* 40–42.

Ennis, R. H. (1985). A logical basis for measuring critical thinking skills. *Educational Leadership, 43,* 44–48.

Heaslip, P. (1993, September). Intellectual standards: What are they? *Critical Connections* [Newsletter of the Critical Thinking Interest Group, University College of the Cariboo, Kamloops, B.C.]

Heaslip, P. (1994, November). Defining critical thinking. *Dialogue: A Critical Thinking Newsletter for Nurses, 3.*

Kurfiss, J. (1988). *Critical thinking: Theory, research, practice and possibilities.* Washington, DC: Association for the Study of Higher Education. (ASHE-ERIC Higher Education Report No. 2.)

Miller, M. A., & Malcolm, N. S. (1990). Critical thinking in the nursing curriculum. *Nursing & Health Care, 11,* 66–73.

Norris, S. P., & Ennis, R. H. (1989). *Evaluating critical thinking.* Pacific Grove, CA: Midwest Publication.

Paul, R. (1990). *Critical thinking: What every person needs to survive in a rapidly changing world.* Rohnert Park, CA: Center for Critical Thinking and Moral Critique, Sonoma State University.

Paul, R., & Willsen, J. (1993). *Critical thinking, from an ideal evolves an imperative.* Santa Rosa, CA: The Foundation for Critical Thinking.

Scriven, M., & Paul, R. (1996). *Defining critical thinking* [On-line]. (Center for Critical Thinking at Sonoma State University, Rohnert Park, CA). Available: http://www. criticalthinking.org/University/univclass/defining.nclk

Worrell, P. J. (1990). Metacognition: Implications for instruction in nursing education. *Journal of Nursing Education, 29*(4), 170–175.

RESOURCES

California Academic Press, 217 La Cruz Avenue, Millbrae, CA, 94030, 650-697-5628, www.calpress.com/, email: info@calpress.com

Center for Critical Thinking and Moral Critique, Sonoma State University, 1801 East Cotati Avenue CH65, Rohnert Park, CA, 94928-3609, 707-664-2940, 1-800-833-3645, www.criticalthinking.org

Foundation for Critical Thinking, P.O. Box 302, Wye Mills, MD, 21679, 410-364-5082

International Center for the Assessment of Higher Order Thinking, 707-664-4082, http://www.criticalthinking.org/icat.nclk

National Council for Excellence in Critical Thinking, 707-664-4275, www.criticalthinking.org/ncect.nclk

CHAPTER 3
Student Nurse Skills for Success

REFERENCES/SUGGESTED READINGS

Arnett, P. (1988). *How to Categorize Questions According to the "New" NCLEX-RN Test Plan*. SC: Arnett Development.

Brown, J., & Duguid P. (1996, July/August). Universities in the digital age, Change. *The Magazine of Higher Learning.*

Chenevert, M. (1995). *Mosby's tour guide to nursing school: A student's road survival kit* (3rd ed.). St. Louis, MO: Mosby.

The Center for New Discoveries in Learning Personal Learning Style Inventory/School Smart Kids. *Newsletter,* Vol. 1, No. 4 [on-line]. Available: http://www.howtolearn.com/ndil3.html

Chopra, D. (1997, May–June). How can I keep up? *Natural Health,* 208

Cohen, B., & Wood, D. (2000). *Memmler's the human body in health and disease* (9th ed.). Philadelphia: Lippincott.

Dale, E. (1954). *Audiovisual methods in teaching.* New York: Dryden Press.

DeLaune S., & Ladner, P. (1998). *Fundamentals of nursing: Standards & practice.* Albany, NY: Delmar Publishers.

DeWit, S. (1995). *Saunders student nurse planner.* Philadelphia: Saunders.

Dirkx, J. & Prenger, S. (1997). *A guide for planning and implementing instruction for adults—A theme-based approach.* San Francisco: Jossey-Bass.

Gylys, B., & Masters, R. (1998). *Medical terminology simplified, A programmed learning approach by body system.* (2nd ed.) Philadelphia: F.A. Davis.

Harrington, N., Smith N., & Spratt W. (1996). *LPN to RN transitions.* Philadelphia: Lippincott-Raven.

Highfield, M., & Wong, J. (1992, October). How to take multiple-choice tests. *Nursing92,* 22(10) 117–119.

Hoffman, K. (1997). *Effective college planning* (5th ed.). Orchard Park, NY: WNY Collegiate Consortium of Disability Advocates.

Holkeboer, R., and Walker, L. (1999). *Right from the start.* Belmont, CA: Wadsworth.

Lagerquist, S. (1996). *Little, Brown's nursing Q&A critical thinking exercises.* Boston: Little, Brown.

Lesar, T. S. (1998). Errors in the use of medication dosage equations. *Archives of Pediatric Adolescent Medicine, 152*(4), 340–344.

Matthews, K. H. (1997). Learning out of the box, Tuning in to your unique cluster of intelligences, *The Next Step Magazine,* 22–27.

Meltzer, M., & Marcus-Palau, S. (1997). *Learning strategies in nursing, Reading, studying and test taking* (2nd ed.). Philadelphia: Saunders.

Meltzer, M., & Palau, S. M. (1996a). *Acquiring critical thinking skills.* Philadelphia: Saunders.

Meltzer, M., & Palau, S. M. (1996b). *Learning strategies for allied health students.* Philadelphia: Saunders.

Mind tools: How your learning style affects your use of mnemonics [on-line]. Available: (1998) *http://www.mindtools. com/mnemlsty.html*

National Center for Learning Disabilities, Inc. Information About Learning Disabilities. (1999, January 24). Available: *www.ncld.org*

Nugent, P. M. & Vitale, B. A. (1997). *Test taking techniques for beginning nursing students* (2nd ed.). Philadelphia: F. A. Davis.

Ott, B., & Hardie, T. (1997). Readability of advanced directive documents. *Image: Journal of Nursing Scholarship, 29*(1), 53–57.

Phillips, A., & Sotiriou, P. (1996). *Steps to reading proficiency* (4th ed.). Belmont: Wadsworth.

Scheffer, B. (1996). *Critical thinking in nursing: An interactive approach* (2nd ed.). Philadelphia: Lippincott.

Sides, M. B., & Korchek, N. (1998). *Successful test-taking; Learning strategies for nurses* (3rd ed.). Philadelphia: Lippincott.

Woo, E. (1995, January 10). Teaching that goes beyond IQ. *Los Angeles Times.*

RESOURCES

The Center for New Discoveries in Learning, P.O. Box 1019, Windsor, CA, 95492, 707-837-8180

The Center for New Discoveries in Learning Personal Learning Style Inventory/School Smart Kids Newsletter Vol. 1, No. 4, http://www.howtolearn.com/ndil3. html

Choosing a College for Students with Learning Disabilities, http://www.ldresources.com/collegechoice.html

Closing the Gap, A Resource Directory, P.O. Box 68, 526 Main Street, Henderson, MN, 56044, 507-248-3294

Directory of Adaptive Technology: Trace Research and Development Center, 5-151 Waisman Center, 1500 Highland Avenue, University of Wisconsin, Madison, WI, 53705, 608-262-6966, http://trace.wisc.edu/CRERO/trace. html

Identifying Your Best Learning Styles, http://www.marin. cc.ca.us/~don/Study/13styles.html

The Institute for Learning Sciences, 1890 Maple Avenue, Evanston, IL, 60201, 847-491-3500

Mind Tools: The Old School House, Yapton, West Sussez, United Kingdom, BN18 ODU

Mind Tools: How Your Learning Style Affects Your Use of Mnemonics, http://www.mindtools.com/mnemlsty.html

The National Adult Literacy and Learning Disabilities Center (National ALLD), Academy for Educational Development, 1875 Connecticut Avenue, NW, Washington, DC, 20009-1202, 202-884-8185, 1-800/953-ALLD (953-2553), FAX: 202/884-8429, http://novel.nifl.gov/nalldtop.htm

National Center for Learning Disabilities, Inc., 381 Park Avenue South, Suite 1401, New York, NY, 10016, 212-545-7510, 1-888-575-7373, http://www.ncld.org/

CHAPTER 4
Nursing History, Education, and Organizations

REFERENCES/SUGGESTED READINGS

American Nurses Association. (1990). *Standards for nursing staff development.* Kansas City, MO: Author.

American Nurses Association. (1991). *American Nurses Association bylaws.* Washington, DC: Author.

American Nurses Association. (1998). *Mission statement* [On-line]. Available: http://www.nursingworld.org/about/mission.htm

Anglin, L. T. (1997). Historical perspectives: Influences of the past. In J. Zerwekh & J. C. Claborn (Eds.), *Nursing today: Transitions and trends* (2nd ed.). Philadelphia: Saunders.

Baker, C. M. (1994). School health: Policy issues. *Nursing & Health Care, 15*(4), 178–184.

Bell, P. (1993). "Making do" with the midwife: Arkansas' Mamie O. Hale in the 1940s. *Nursing History Review,* 155–169.

Boykin, A. B., & Schoenhofer, L. C. (1993). *Nursing as caring: A model for transforming practice* (#0-88737-601-1). New York: National League for Nursing.

Bullough, B., & Bullough, V. (Eds.). (1994). *Nursing issues for the nineties and beyond.* New York: Springer.

Bullough, V., & Bullough, B. (1993). Medieval nursing. *Nursing History Review,* 89–104.

Calhoun, J. (1993, March). The Nightingale pledge: A commitment that survives the passage of time. *Nursing & Health Care, 14*(3), 130–136.

Chinn, P. L. (1994). *Developing the discipline: Critical studies in nursing history and professional issues.* Gaithersburg, MD: Aspen.

Cushing, A. (1995, Summer). An historical note on the relationship between nursing and nursing history. *International History Nursing Journal, 1*(1), 57–60.

Dossey, B. (1995). Endnote: Florence Nightingale today. *Critical Care Nursing, 15*(4), 98.

Edelman, C. L., & Mandle, C. L. (1998). *Health promotion throughout the lifespan* (4th ed.). St. Louis: Mosby.

Estabrooks, C. A. (1995). Lavinia Lloyd Dock: The Henry Street years. *Nursing History Review, 3,* 143–172.

Hall-Long, B. A. (1995, February–March). Nursing's past, present, and future political experience. *Nursing and Health Care Perspective Community, 16*(1), 24–28.

Johnson, B. S. (1997). *Psychiatric–mental health nursing: Adaptation and growth* (4th ed.). Philadelphia: Lippincott.

Joint Commission on the Accreditation of Healthcare Organizations. (1996). *Accreditation standards and scoring guidelines for hospital-based mental health.* Oak Brook Terrace, IL: Author.

Macrae, J. (1995). Nightingale's spiritual philosophy and its significance for modern nursing. *Image: Journal of Nursing Scholarship, 27*(1), 8–10.

Maroun, V. M. (1994). An enduring collaborative model. *Nursing Outlook, 42*(3), 130–134.

Mason, D. J., & Leavitt, J. K. (1995). The revolution in health care: What's your readiness quotient? *American Journal of Nursing, 95*(6), 50–54.

National Association for Practical Nurse Education and Service, Inc. (1998). *History of NAPNES.* Silver Spring, MD: Author.

National Council of State Boards of Nursing, Inc. (1996). *Creating new national certification examination for LPN/VNs* [On-line]. Available: http://www.ncsbn.org/files/online/ar1996/creat/nc.html

National Council of State Boards of Nursing, Inc. (1998a). *National Council mission and purpose* [On-line]. Available: http://www.ncsbn.org/files/aboutnc.mission.asp

National Council of State Boards of Nursing, Inc. (1998b). *Overview: Programs and services of the National Council* [On-line]. Available: http://www.ncsbn.org/files/aboutnc/overview.asp

National Federation of Licensed Practical Nurses, (1998). *All about NFLPN* [On-line]. Available: http://www.nflpn.org/allaboutnflpn.htm

National League for Nursing. (1994a). Healing at home. *Nursing & Health Care,* 66–73.

National League for Nursing. (1994b). *Nursing data source 1994* (Vols. 1 & 2). New York: Author.

National League for Nursing. (1995). *Bylaws.* New York: Author.

National League for Nursing. (1998). Research Department, Communication. New York: Author.

National League for Nursing History. (1997). Adapted from *The Entry Dilemma* by Shirley H. Fondiller, National League for Nursing. Available: http:// www.nln.org/info-history.htm

Nightingale, F. (1969). *Nursing: What it is and what it is not.* New York: Dover Publications.

Ogren, K. (1994). The risk of not understanding nursing history. *Holistic Nursing Practice, 8*(2), 10.

Olsen, T. (1995). Recreating past separations and the employment pattern of nurses, 1900–1940. *Nursing Outlook, 43*(5), 210–214.

Secretary's Commission on Nursing. (1988). *Final report.* Washington, DC: Department of Health & Human Services.

Selanders, L. C. (1993). *Florence Nightingale: An environmental adaptation theory.* Newberry Park, CA: Sage.

Silverstein, N. G. (1994). Lillian Wald at Henry Street, 1893–1895. In P. L. Chinn (Ed.), *Developing the discipline: Critical studies in nursing history and professional issues.* Gaithersburg, MD: Aspen.

Strickland, O., & Fishman, D. (1994). *Nursing issues in the 1990s.* Albany, NY: Delmar Publishers.

Wall, B. (1993). Grace under pressure: The nursing sisters of the Holy Cross, 1861–1865. *Nursing History Review,* 71–88.

U.S. Department of Health and Human Services. (1996). *The registered nurse population.* Washington, DC: Author.

U.S. Department of Health and Human Services. (1995). *Healthy people 2000: Midcourse review & 1995 revisions.* Washington, DC: U.S. Government Printing Office.

RESOURCES

American Nurses Association (ANA), 600 Maryland Avenue SW, Suite 100 West, Washington, DC, 20024-2571, 202-651-7000, 1-800-274-4ANA (262), www.nursingworld.org

National Association of Practical Nurse Education and Service, Inc. (NAPNES), 1400 Spring Street, Suite 330, Silver Spring, MD, 20910, 301-588-2491

National Council of State Boards of Nursing, Inc. (NCSBN), 676 North St. Clair Street, Suite 550, Chicago, IL, 60611-2921, 312-787-6555, www.ncsbn.org

National Federation of Licensed Practical Nurses, Inc. (NFLPN), 1418 Aversboro Road, Garner, NC, 27529, 800-948-2511, www.nflpn.org

National League for Nursing (NLN), 61 Broadway, 33rd Floor, New York, NY, 10006, 212-363-5555, 1-800-669-1656, www.nln.org

CHAPTER 5
The Health Care Delivery System

REFERENCES/SUGGESTED READINGS

Aiken, L. H. (1995). Transformation of the nursing workforce. *Nursing Outlook, 43*(5), 201–209.

American Health Consultants. (1994). RNs fight PFC as hospitals struggle to cut costs—The battle is far from over. *Patient-Focused Care, 2*(11), 149–160.

American Nurses Association. (1991). *Nursing's agenda for health care reform.* Kansas City, MO: Author.

American Nurses Association. (1993a, September). *Consumers willing to see a nurse for routine "doctoring" according to Gallup poll* [news release]. Washington, DC: Author.

American Nurses Association. (1993b, September). *States with some form of nurse privileging.* Washington, DC: Author.

American Nurses Association. (1994). *Health care reform and America's nurses: Agenda for change.* Washington, DC: Author.

American Nurses Association. (1995). Managed care: Challenges and opportunities for nursing. *Nursing Facts* (Item PR-27). Washington, DC: Author.

American Nurses Association & American Association of Occupational Health Nurses. (1993). *Innovation at the work site: Delivery of nurse-managed primary health care services.* Washington, DC: American Nurses Association.

Baker, C. M. (1994). School health: Policy issues. *Nursing and Health Care, 15*(4),178–184.

Brown, S. A., & Grimes, D. E. (1993). *A meta-analysis of process of care, clinical outcomes, and cost effectiveness of nurses in primary care roles: Nurse practitioners and nurse–midwives* [executive summary]. Washington, DC: American Nurses Association.

Centers for Disease Control and Prevention (CDC). (1998). *Combating Complacency—HIV Prevention, Geneva '98. Trends.* Available: www.cdcnpin.org

Chamberlain, P., Chen, Y., Osuna, E., & Yamamoto, C. (1995). Innovative culture shock prescribed for health care. *Nursing Outlook, 43*(5), 232–234.

Deparle, N. (1998). *The state of the Children's Health Insurance Program.* Health Care Financing Administration. Available: www.hcfa.gov/init/testm918.htm

Feldstein, P. J. (1999). *Health care economics* (5th ed.). Albany, NY: Delmar Publishers.

Friedman, E. (1997). The uninsured: From dilemma to crisis. In P. Lee & C. Estes (Eds.), *The nation's health* (5th ed.). Boston: Jones & Bartlett.

Grace, H. K. (1997). Can medical costs be contained? In J. C. McCloskey, & H. K. Grace (Eds.), *Current issues in nursing* (5th ed.). St. Louis, MO: Mosby-Yearbook.

Grace, H. K., & Brock, R. M. (1997). Solving the health care dilemma: What will work? In J. C. McCloskey & H. K. Grace (Eds.), *Current issues in nursing* (5th ed.). St. Louis, MO: Mosby-Yearbook.

Harrison, B. S., Faircloth, J. W., & Yaryan, L. (1995). The impact of legislation on the role of the school nurse. *Nursing Outlook, 43*(2), 57–61.

Health Care Financing Administration (HCFA). (1998). *Medicare and Medicaid Expenses, 1997.* Available: www.hcfa.gov/pubforms/finance/97/ch2n1216.htm

Hicks, L. L., & Boles, K. E. (1997). Why health economics? In C. Harrington & C. L. Estes (Eds.), *Health policy and nursing: Crisis and reform in the U.S. health care delivery system* (2nd ed). Boston: Jones & Bartlett.

Hull, K. (1997). Hospital trends. In C. Harrington & C. L. Estes (Eds.), *Health policy and nursing: Crisis and reform in the U.S. health care delivery system* (2nd ed). Boston: Jones & Bartlett.

Igoe, J., & Giordano, B. (1992). *Expanding school health services to serve families in the 21st century.* Washington, DC: American Nurses Association.

Kellogg Foundation. (1994, June 24). *How people view their providers. Report of a survey.* Battle Creek, MI: Author.

Kelly, L., & Joel, L. (1995). *Dimensions of professional nursing* (7th ed.). New York: McGraw-Hill.

Kyle, S. M., & Coulter, J. S. (1995). The national immunization campaign: Implementation in a rural setting. *Nursing Outlook, 43*(2), 62–65.

Lee, P. R., Soffel, D., & Luft, H. (1997). Costs and coverage: Pressures towards health care reform. In P. Lee, C. Estes, & N. Ramsay (Eds.), *The nation's health* (5th ed.). Boston: Jones & Bartlett.

Levit, K. R., Lazenby, H. C., Cowan, C. A., & Letsch, S. W. (1997). National health expenditures. In C. Harrington & C. L. Estes (Eds.), *Health policy and nursing: Crisis and reform in the U.S. health care delivery system* (2nd ed). Boston: Jones & Bartlett.

Maraldo, P. J. (1997). Nursing's agenda for health care reform. In J. C. McCloskey & H. K. Grace (Eds.), *Current issues in nursing* (5th ed.). St. Louis, MO: Mosby-Yearbook.

McCloskey, J. C., & Grace, H. K. (Eds.). (1997). *Current issues in nursing* (5th ed.). St. Louis, MO: Mosby-Yearbook.

Miller, S. E. (1995). The role of the clinical nurse specialist in health care. *Journal of Home Health Care Practice, 7*(2), 62–72.

Moyer, M. E. (1997). A revised look at the number of uninsured Americans. In C. Harrington & C. L. Estes (Eds.), *Health policy and nursing: Crisis and reform in the U.S. health care delivery system* (2nd ed.). Boston: Jones & Bartlett.

O'Neil, E. H. (1993). *Health professions education for the future: Schools in service to the nation.* San Francisco: Pew Health Professions Commission.

Parris, N. M., & Hines, J. (1995). Payer and provider relationships: The key to reshaping health care delivery. *Nursing Administration Quarterly, 19*(3), 13–17.

Pearson, L. J. (1996). Annual update of how each state stands on legislative issues affecting advanced nursing practice. *Nurse Practitioner, 21*(1), 10–701.

Peck, S. P. (1997). Community nursing centers: Implications for health care reform. In J. C. McCloskey & H. K. Grace (Eds.), *Current issues in nursing* (5th ed.). St. Louis, MO: Mosby-Yearbook.

Pruitt, R. H., & Campbell, B. F. (1994). Educating for health care reform and the community. *Nursing and Health Care, 15*(6), 308–311.

Rosenberg, S. N., Allen, D. R., Handte, J. S., Jackson, T. C., Leto, L., Rodstein, B. M., Stratton, S. D., Westfall, G., & Yasser, R. (1995). Effect of utilization review in a fee-for-service health insurance plan. *New England Journal of Medicine, 333*(20), 1326–1330.

Rowe, J. W. (1996). Health care myths at the end of life. *Bulletin of the American College of Surgeons, 81*(6), 11–18.

Salmon, M. E. (1995). Public health policy: Creating a healthy future for the American public. *Family & Community Health, 18*(1), 1–11.

Schieber, G. J., Poullier, J. P., & Greenwald, L. M. (1997). U.S. health expenditure performance: An international comparison and data update. In C. Harrington & C. L. Estes (Eds.), *Health policy and nursing: Crisis and reform in the U.S. health care delivery system* (2nd ed.). Boston: Jones & Bartlett.

Sklar, C. J. (1995). The politics of health care reform. *Journal of Neuroscience Nursing, 27*(1), 4–10.

Society for Ambulatory Care Professionals. (1994). *Glossary of managed care terms: An issue briefing.* Chicago: American Hospital Association.

Stachenko, S. (1994). National opportunities for health promotion: The Canadian experience. *Health Promotion International, 9*(2), 105–110.

Stafford, M., & Appleyard, J. (1997). Clinical nurse and nurse practitioners. In J. C. McCloskey & H. K. Grace (Eds.), *Current issues in nursing* (5th ed.). St. Louis, MO: Mosby-Yearbook.

Tlusty, M. (1994). Higher mortality for women with PCP [brief item]. *Nursing and Health Care, 15*(4), 211.

Uphold, C. R., & Graham, M. V. (1993). Schools as centers for collaborative services for families: A vision for change. *Nursing Outlook, 41*(5), 204–211.

U.S. Department of Health & Human Services. (1993). *Medicare benefits booklet.* Washington, DC: U.S. Government Printing Office.

Vrabec, N. J. (1995). Implications of U.S. health care reform for the rural elderly. *Nursing Outlook, 43*(6), 260–265.

Washington Consulting Group. (1994, February). *Survey of certified nurse practitioners and clinical nurse specialists: December 1992, final report.* Rockville, MD: Division of Nursing.

Zerwekh, J., & Claborn, J. C. (1997). *Nursing today: Transitions and trends.* Philadelphia: Saunders.

RESOURCES

American Nurses Association (ANA), 600 Maryland Avenue SW, Suite 100 West, Washington, DC, 20024-2571, 1-800-274-4ANA (262), www.nursesworld.com

National Federation of Licensed Practical Nurses, Inc. (NFLPN), 1418 Aversboro Road, Garner, NC, 27529, 1-800-948-2511, www.nflpn.org

Society for Ambulatory Care Professionals, One North Franklin, 31st Floor, Chicago, IL, 60606, 312-422-3900, www.sacp-net.org

CHAPTER 6
Legal Responsibilities

REFERENCES/SUGGESTED READINGS

Beare, P., & Myers, J. (1998). *Principles and practices of adult health nursing* (3rd ed.). St. Louis, MO: Mosby-Year Book.

Becker, B., & Fendler, D. (1994). *Vocational and personal adjustments in practical nursing.* (7th ed.) St. Louis, MO: Mosby.

Bernzweig, E. (1995). *The nurse's liability for malpractice: A programmed course* (6th ed.). St. Louis, MO: Mosby.

Braun, J., & Lipson, S. (1993). *Toward a restraint-free environment.* Baltimore: Health Professions Press.

Calfee, B. (1995). Going before the board: How to prepare yourself. *Nursing95, 25*(3), 56–58.

Curtain, L. (1993). Informed consent: Cautious, calculated candor. *Nursing Management, 24*(4), 18, 20.

DeLaune, S., & Ladner, P. (1998). *Fundamentals of nursing: Standards & practice.* Albany, NY: Delmar Publishers.

Eggland, E. (1995). Charting smarter: Using new mechanisms to organize your paperwork. *Nursing95, 25*(9), 35–41.

Flight, M. (1998). *Law, liability, and ethics* (3rd ed.). Albany, NY: Delmar Publishers.

Green, A. (1995). Are you at risk for disciplinary action? *AJN, 95*(7), 36–42.

Hill, S., & Howlett, H. (1997). *Success in practical nursing: Personal and vocational issues* (3rd ed.). Philadelphia: W. B. Saunders

Hughes, T. (1994). Is your colleague chemically dependent? *AJN, 94*(9), 31–35.

Idemoto, B., Daly, B. et al. (1993). Implementing the patient self-determination act, *AJN, 93*(1), 20, 22–25.

Joint Commission on Accreditation of Healthcare Organizations (JCAHO). (1993). *Accreditation Manual for Hospitals.* Oakbrook Terrace, IL: Author.

Lippman, H. (1992, April). Addicted nurses: Tolerated, tormented, or treated. *RN, 36*–41.

Mandell, M. (1994). Not documented, not done. *Nursing94, 24*(8), 62–63.

Mayer, T. (1995, April). *Director of nurses' attitudes toward restraint usage in long-term care.* Master's Thesis, Indiana Wesleyan University.

Meyer, C. (1993). "End-of life" care: Patients, choices, nurses' challenges. *AJN, 93*(2), 40–47.

Mitchell, P., & Grippando, G. (1993). *Nursing perspectives and issues* (5th ed.). Albany: Delmar Publishers.

Monahan, F.D., Drake, T., & Neighbors, M. (1998). *Nursing care of adults* (2nd ed.). Philadelphia: W. B. Saunders.

Sandler, R. L. (1995). Restraining devices. *American Journal of Nursing, 95*(7), 34–35.

Skinner, K. (1993, December). The hazards of chemical dependency among nurses. *The Journal of Practical Nursing, 8*–11.

Taylor, C., Lillis, C., & LeMone, P. (1997). *Fundamentals of nursing: The art and science of nursing care* (3rd ed.). Philadelphia: J.B. Lippincott.

Walsh, S. M. (1995). Resuscitation decisions: Showing a family the way. *Nursing95, 25*(8), 50–51.

Zerwekh, J., & Claborn, J. C. (1997). *Nursing today: Transitions and trends.* Philadelphia: W. B. Saunders.

RESOURCES

Choice in Dying, Inc., 1035 30th Street NW, Washington, D.C., 20007, 202-338-9790, 1-800-989-9455, www.choices.org

Living Wills, Films for the Humanities and Sciences, P.O. Box 2053, Princeton, NJ, 08543-2053, 1-800-257-5126

Medcom, Inc., 6060 Phyllis Drive, Cypress, CA, 90630, 1-800-877-1443, www.medcomsolutions.com

The Verdict Is, Medical Electronic Educational Services, Inc., 930 Pitner Avenue, Evanston, IL, 60202, 1-800-323-9084

CHAPTER 7
Ethical Responsibilities

REFERENCES/SUGGESTED READINGS

American Hospital Association. (1992). *A patient's bill of rights.* Chicago: Author.

Aroskar, M. A. (1993). Ethical issues: Politics, power, and policy. In D. J. Mason, S. W. Talbott, & J. K. Leavitt (Eds.), *Policy and politics for nurses* (2nd ed.). Philadelphia: Saunders.

Aroskar, M. A. (1994). Politics and ethics in nursing: Implications for education. *Journal of Professional Nursing, 10*(3), 129.

Awong, L., & Miles, A. (1998a). When an adolescent wants to forgo therapy. *American Journal of Nursing, 98*(7), 67–68.

Awong, L., & Miles, A. (1998b). When the physician disregards the patient's expressed wishes. *American Journal of Nursing, 98*(2), 71.

Bandman, E. L., & Bandman, B. (1995). *Nursing ethics through the life span* (3rd ed.). Norwalk, CT: Appleton-Lange.

Beare, G., & Myers, J. (1998). *Adult health nursing* (2nd ed.) St. Louis, MO: Mosby-Year Book.

Callahan, J. (1994). The ethics of assisted suicide. *Health and Social Work, 19*(4), 237–243.

Curtin, L. (1993). Damage control and the whistleblower. *Nursing Management, 24*(5), 34–35.

Curtin, L. (1995). Nurses take a stand on assisted suicide. *Nursing Management, 26*(5), 71–76.

Davis, A. J., & Aroskar, M. A. (1997). *Ethical dilemmas and nursing practice* (4th ed.). Norwalk, CT: Appleton-Lange.

DeLaune, S., & Ladner, P. (1998). *Fundamentals of nursing: Standards of practice*. Albany, NY: Delmar Publishers.

Edge, R., & Groves, J.R. (1999). *The ethics of health care: A guide for clinical practice* (2nd ed.). Albany, NY: Delmar Publishers.

Gordon, M., Murphy, C., Candee, D., & Hiltunen, E. (1994). Clinical judgment: An integrated model. *Advances in Nursing Science, 16*(4), 55–70.

Haddad, A. (1995). Ethics in action. *RN, 58*(5), 21–23.

Haddad, A. (1998). Ethics in action. *RN, 61*(3), 21–24.

International Council of Nurses. (1973). *ICN code for nurses: Ethical concepts applied to nursing*. Geneva, Switzerland: Imprimeries Populaires.

Kristoff, B., Sellin, S., & Miller, M. (1994). Patients' rights and ethical dilemmas in home care: Incorporation of psychological concepts. *Home Healthcare Nurse, 12*(5), 45–50.

Mitchell, P., & Grippando, G. (1993). *Nursing perspectives and issues*. Albany, NY: Delmar Publishers.

National Federation of Practical Nurses, Inc. (NFLPN). (1996). *Nursing practice standards for the licensed practical/vocational nurse*. Garner, NC: Author.

Pappas, A. (1997). Ethical issues. In J. Zerwekh & J. Claborn (Eds.), *Nursing today: Transitions and trends*. Philadelphia: W.B. Saunders.

Pinch, W. J. (1990). Nursing ethics: Is covering up ever harmless? *Nursing Management, 21*(9), 60–62.

Raths, L., Harmin, M., & Simon, S. (1978). *Values and teaching* (2nd ed.). Columbus, OH: Merrill.

Rice, V. H., Beck, C., & Stevenson, J. S. (1997). Ethical issues relative to autonomy and personal control in independent and cognitively impaired elders. *Nursing Outlook, 45*(1), 25–34.

Salladay, S. (1995). Ethical problems. *Nursing95, 25*(2), 29–30.

Salladay, S. (1998). Ethical problems. *Nursing98, 28*(7), 30.

Schildmeier, D. (1997). Using public opinion to protect nursing practice. *American Journal of Nursing, 97*(3), 56–58.

Sumodi, V. (1995). Legalization of physician-assisted suicide: Point/counterpoint. *Nursing Forum 30*(1), 11–17.

Ustal, D. (1993). *Clinical ethics and values: Issues and insights*. East Greenwich, RI: Educational Resources in Health Care.

Wilson, D. M. (1996). Highlighting the role of policy in nursing practice through a comparison of "DNR" policy influences and "No CPR" decision influences. *Nursing Outlook, 44*(6), 272–279.

Zerwekh, J. V. (1997). Do dying patients really need IV fluids? *American Journal of Nursing, 97*(3), 26–30.

Zollo, M. B., & Derse, A. (1997). The abusive patient: Where do you draw the line? *American Journal of Nursing, 97*(2), 31–35.

RESOURCES

American Red Cross, Transplant Services, 2025 E Street N.W., Suite 108, Washington, D.C., 20006, 1-800-2-TISSUE (84-7783)

The Living Bank International, P.O. Box 6725, Houston, TX, 77265, 1-800-528-2971, www.livingbank.org

National Association for Practical Nurse Education and Service, Inc. (NAPNES), 1400 Spring Street, Suite 330, Silver Spring, MD, 20901, 301-588-2491

National Federation of Licensed Practical Nurses, Inc. (NFLPN), 1418 Aversboro Road, Garner, NC, 27529, 1-800-948-2511, www.nflpn.org

United Network of Organ Sharing (UNOS), 1100 Boulders Parkway, Suite 500, P.O. Box 13770, Richmond, VA, 23225-8770, 1-888-894-6361, 804-330-8541, www.unos.org

CHAPTER 8
Communication

REFERENCES/SUGGESTED READINGS

Bailey, D., & Bailey, D. (1997). *Therapeutic approaches to care of the mentally ill* (4th ed.). Philadelphia: F. A. Davis Company.

Barnsteiner, J. (1996). Newest online journal users: Clinicians. *Reflections, 22*(2), 21.

Barry, P. (1997). *Mental health and mental illness* (6th ed.). Philadelphia: J. B. Lippincott Company.

Brandt, M. (1995, March). Making the CPR vision a reality: Where should you start? *Journal of the American Health Information Management Association, 66*(3), 26–30.

Burtt, K. (1997, November/December). Nurses use telehealth to address rural health care needs, prevent hospitalizations. *The American Nurse, 21*.

Callanan, M., & Kelley, P. (1992). *Final gifts*. New York: Poseiden Press.

deWit, S. (1994). *Rambo's nursing skills for clinical practice*. Philadelphia: W. B. Saunders Company.

Dick, R., & Steen, E. (Eds.). (1991). *The computer-based patient record: An essential technology for health care*. Washington, DC: National Academy Press.

Earnest, V. (1993). *Clinical skills in nursing practice*. Philadelphia: J.B. Lippincott Company.

Frawley, K., & Asmonga, D. (1996, January). Update on the Medical Records Confidentiality Act. *Journal of the American Health Information Management Association, 67*(1), 12.

Frisch, N., & Frisch, L. (1998). *Psychiatric mental health nursing*. Albany, NY: Delmar Publishers.

Gay, K. (1993). *Getting your message across*. New York: Macmillan Publishing.

Goldsmith, J. (1996). Computers and nurses changing hospital care. *Reflections, 22*(2), 8–10.

Granade, P. (1997). The brave new world of telemedicine. *RN, 60*(7), 59–62.

Hall, E. (1959). *The silent language*. New York: Doubleday.

Jack, L. (1997). Effective communication. In J. Zerwekh, & J. Claborn (Eds.). *Nursing today: Transition and trends*, (2nd ed.). Philadelphia: W. B. Saunders Company.

Kübler-Ross, E. (1969). *On death and dying*. New York: MacMillan.

Kübler-Ross, E. (1975). *Death: The final stage of growth*. Englewood Cliffs, NJ: Prentice Hall.

Kübler-Ross, E. (1978). *To live until we say good-bye*. Englewood Cliffs, NJ: Prentice Hall.

Lorton, L., & Legler, J. (1996, April). A telemedicine trial. *Journal of the American Health Information Management Association, 67*(1), 40–42.

Medical Records Institute. (1994). Legality of electronic patient record systems. *Toward an electronic patient record, 2*(7).

Meranda, D. (1995, March). Administrative and security challenges with electronic patient record systems. *Journal of the American Health Information Management Association, 66*(3), 58–60.

Milliken, M. (1993). *Understanding human behavior.* Albany: Delmar Publishers Inc.

Pagano, M., & Ragan, S. (1992). *Communication skills for professional nurses.* Newbury Park, CA: Sage.

Ravitch, S. (1996). The Medical Records Confidentiality Act. *For The Record, 8*(9) 8–11.

Rhodes, A. (1995, November/December). The need for security with computerized records. *MCN, 20*(6), 299.

Roter, D., & Hall, J. (1993). *Doctors talking with patients/patients talking with doctors.* Westport, CT: Auburn House.

Ruben, B. (1992). *Communicating with patients.* Dubuque, IA: Kendall-Hunt.

Sherman, K. (1994). *Communication and image in nursing.* Albany, NY: Delmar Publishers Inc.

Smith, S. (1992). *Communications in nursing.* St. Louis: Mosby-Yearbook, Inc.

Tamparo, C., & Lindh, W. (1993). *Therapeutic communications for allied health professions.* Albany: Delmar Publishers Inc.

Telemedicine Research Center. (1997). *What is telemedicine?* Portland, OR: Author.

Waughfield, C. (1998). *Mental health concepts.* Albany, NY: Delmar Publishers.

RESOURCES

American Health Information Management Association, 919 North Michigan Avenue, Suite 1400, Chicago, IL, 60611-1683, 312-787-2672, www.ahima.org

CHAPTER 9
Nursing Process

REFERENCES/SUGGESTED READINGS

Alfaro-LeFevre, R. (1999). *Critical thinking in nursing: A practical approach.* (2nd ed.). Philadelphia: Saunders.

Alfaro-LeFevre, R. (1998). *Applying nursing process* (4th ed.). Philadelphia: Lippincott.

American Nurses Association. (1991). *Standards of nursing practice.* Kansas City, MO: Author.

Bevis, E. O. (1989). *Curriculum building in nursing: A process* (3rd ed., Publication No. 15–2277). New York: National League for Nursing.

Carpenito, L. J. (1995). *Nursing diagnosis: Application to clinical practice* (6th ed.). Philadelphia: Lippincott.

Clark, M. (1998). Implementation of nursing standardized languages NANDA, NIC, and NOC. *On-line Journal of Issues in Nursing,* [On-line] 2(2). Available: www.nursingworld.org

Edelman, C. L., & Mandle, C. L. (1998). *Health promotion throughout the lifespan* (4th ed.). St. Louis, MO: Mosby.

Fry, V. S. (1953). The creative approach to nursing. *American Journal of Nursing 53*(3), 301–302.

Gebbie, K. M., & Lavin, M. A. (1974). Classifying nursing diagnoses. *American Journal of Nursing 74,* 250–253.

Gordon, M. (1997)

Gordon, M. (1997). *Manual of nursing diagnoses 1997–1998 edition.* St. Louis, MO: Mosby.

Gordon, M. (1998, September 30). Nursing nomenclature and classification system development. *On-line Journal of Issues in Nursing,* [On-line] Available: www.nursingworld.org

Humphrey, C. J. (1998). *Home care nursing* (3rd ed.). Gaithersburg, MD: Aspen.

Iowa Interventions Project. (1993). The NIC taxonomy structure. *Image: Journal of Nursing Scholarship, 25*(3), 187–192.

Iowa Interventions Project. J. C. McCloskey & G. M. Bulechek (Eds.) (1996). *Nursing interventions classification (NIC)* (2nd ed.). St. Louis, MO: Mosby.

Iowa Outcomes Project. M. Johnson & M. Maas (Eds.) (1997). *Nursing Outcomes Classification (NOC).* St Louis, MO: Mosby.

Iyer, P. W., Taptich, B. J., & Bernocchi-Losey, D. (1994). *Nursing process and nursing diagnosis* (3rd ed.). Philadelphia: Saunders.

Johnson, D. (1959). A philosophy for nursing diagnosis. *Nursing Outlook, 7,* 198–200.

Johnson, M. (1998). Overview of the Nursing Outcomes Classification (NOC). *On-line Journal of Nursing Informatics* [On-line] 2(2). Available: http://cac.psu.edu/~dxm12/OJNI.htm

Johnson, M., & Maas, M. (1998). Implementing the nursing outcomes classification in a practice setting. *Outcomes Management for Nursing Practice, 2*(3), 99–104.

McCloskey, J. C. & Bulechek, G. M. (1998). Nursing interventions classification (NIC): Current status and new directions. *On-line Journal of Nursing Informatics, 2*(2). [On-line], available: http://gort.ucsd.edu/newjour/o/msg02267.html

McCloskey, J. C. & Maas, M. (1998). Interdisciplinary team: The nursing perspective is essential. *Nursing Outlook, 46*(4), 157–163.

National Federation of Licensed Practical Nurses (NFLPN). (1996). *Nursing practice standards for the licensed practical/vocational nurse.* Garner, NC: Author.

North American Nursing Diagnosis Association (NANDA) (1999). *Nursing diagnoses: Definitions & classifications 1999–2000.* Philadelphia: Author.

Nursing Interventions Classification. (1995). *The NIC Letter, 3*(1), 1–5.

Orlando, I. (1961). *The dynamic nurse–patient relationship.* New York: G. P. Putnam's Sons.

Orem, D. E. (1995). *Nursing: Concepts of practice* (5th ed.). St. Louis, MO: Mosby.

Paul, R. W. (1995). *Critical thinking: How to prepare students for a rapidly changing world.* Santa Rosa, CA: Foundation for Critical Thinking.

Wiedenbach, E. (1963). The helping art of nursing. *American Journal of Nursing, 63*(11), 54–57.

Wilkinson, J. M. (1996). *Nursing process in action: A critical thinking approach.* Redwood City, CA: Addison-Wesley Nursing.

Yoder Wise, P. S. (1998). *Leading and managing in nursing* (2nd ed.). St. Louis, MO: Mosby.

Yura, H., & Walsh, M. B. (1967). *The nursing process.* Washington, DC: The Catholic University of America Press.

RESOURCES

Center for Nursing Classification, College of Nursing, The University of Iowa, 407 Nursing Building, Iowa City, IA, 52242-1121, 319-335-7051, www.nursing.uiowa.edu

North American Nursing Diagnosis Association (NANDA), 1211 Locust Street, Philadelphia, PA, 19107, 215-545-8105, Fax: 215-545-8107

Nursing Diagnosis (journal), 1211 Locust Street, Philadelphia, PA, 19107, 800-242-6757

CHAPTER 10
Documentation

REFERENCES/SUGGESTED READINGS

American Health Consultants. (1995). Congress mandates study of PSDA effectiveness. *Medical Ethics Advisor, 11*(7), 95.

Burke, L. J., & Murphy, J. (1995). *Charting by exception applications*. Albany, NY: Delmar Publishers.

Colson, A. R., Bounds, J. A., Alt-White, A. C., & McDermott, S. (1995). Preparing for an ICU bedside computer. *Nursing Management, 26*(5), 48A–48B.

Estes, M. E. Z. (1998). *Health assessment & physical examination*. Albany, NY: Delmar Publishers.

Eggland, E. T., & Heinemann, D. S. (1994). *Nursing documentation: Charting, recording, and reporting*. Philadelphia: Lippincott.

Fiesta, J. (1991). If it wasn't charted, it was done! *Nursing Management, 22*(8), 17.

Grane, N. B. (1995). Documenting a "harmless" medication error. *Nursing95, 25*(4), 80.

Grobe, S. J. (1992). Nursing lexicon and taxonomy: Preliminary categorisation. In K.C. Lun et al. (Eds.), *Med-Info92: Proceedings of the 7th World Congress on Medical Information* (pp.) Amsterdam, Netherlands: Elsevier.

Grulke, C. C. (1995). Seven ways to help a student nurse. *American Journal of Nursing, 96* (60), 24L.

Hayes, B., Norris, J., Martin, K. S., & Androwich, I. (1994). Informatics issues for nursing's future. *Advances in Nursing Science, 16*(4), 71–81.

Iyer, P. W., & Camp, N. H. (1999). *Nursing documentation: A nursing process approach* (3rd ed.). St. Louis, MO: Mosby Yearbook.

Johnson, M., & Maas, M. (Eds.). (1997). *Nursing outcomes classfication (NOC)*. St. Louis, MO: Mosby.

Joint Commission on Accredation of Healthcare Organizations. (1998). *1998 Hospital accreditation standards*. Oakbrook Terrace, IL: Author.

Long, G. (1994). Measuring the benefits of bedside documentation systems. *Aspen's Advisor for Nurse Executives, 10*(3), 1–4.

McCloskey, J. C., & Bulechek, G. M. (1994). Standardizing the language for nursing treatments: An overview of the issues. *Nursing Outlook, 42*(2), 56–63.

McCloskey, J. C., & Bulechek, G. M. (1995). Validation and coding of the NIC taxonomy structure. *Image: Journal of Nursing Scholarship, 27*(1), 43–49.

McCloskey, J. C., & Bulechek, G. M. (1996). *Nursing interventions classification (NIC)* (2nd ed.). St. Louis, MO: Mosby.

National Library of Medicine. (1998). *Fact sheet, UMLS* [Online]. Available: www.nlm.nih.gov/pubs/factsheets/umls.html

North American Nursing Diagnosis Association. (1999). *NANDA Nursing diagnoses: Definitions and classification: 1999–2000*. St. Louis, MO: Author.

Nursing Interventions Classification (NIC). (1995). *The NIC letter, 3*(1), 4.

Ozbolt, J. G., Fruchtnight, J. N., & Hayden, J. R. (1994). Toward data standards for clinical nursing information. *Journal of the American Medical Informatics Association, 1*(2), 175–185.

Reiner, A. (Ed.). (1995). *Manual of patient care standards*. Gaithersburg, MD: Aspen.

Russell-Babin, K. (1994). Critical paths: From NASA to St. Peter's Medical Center. *Case Management Newsletter, 5*(1), 4–5.

Simmons, P. B., & Meadors, B. (1995). Eliminating friendly fire: Successful nursing documentation strategies. *Journal of Nursing Staff Development, 11*(2), 79–82.

Springhouse. (1999). *Mastering documentation* (2nd ed.). Springhouse, PA: Springhouse Corporation.

Steelman, V. M., Bulechek, G. M., & McCloskey, J. C. (1994). Toward a standardized language to describe perioperative nursing. *AORN Journal, 60*(5), 786–795.

Thompson, C. (1995, May). Writing better narrative notes. *Nursing95, 25*(5), 87.

Tucker, J. L. (1995). Interdisciplinary record improves documentation. *Patient Education Management, 2*(3), 45–47.

Voigt, L., Paice, J. A., & Pouliot, J. (1995). Standardized pain flowsheet: Impact on patient-reported pain experiences after cardiovascular surgery. *American Journal of Critical Care, 4*(4), 308–313.

Werley, H. H., & Lang, N. M. (1988). The consensually derived nursing minimum data set: Elements and definitions. In H. H. Werley & N. M. Lang (Eds.), *Identification of the nursing minimum data set* (pp. 402–411). New York: Springer.

Williams, S. (1990). *Decision making in critical care nursing*. Philadelphia: Decker.

RESOURCES

Center for Nursing Classification, NB 407, The University of Iowa, College of Nursing, Iowa City, IA, 52252-1121, www.nursing.uiowa.edu

North American Nursing Diagnosis Association (NANDA), 1211 Locust Street, Philadelphia, PA, 19107, 1-800-647-9002, www.nanda.org

CHAPTER 11
Client Teaching

REFERENCES/SUGGESTED READINGS

American Hospital Association. (1973). *A patient's bill of rights*. Chicago: Author.

Bandura, A. (1977). *Social learning theory*. Englewood Cliffs, NJ: Prentice Hall.

Barnes, L. (1997). Developing educational materials for patients. *MCN—The American Journal of Maternal/Child Nursing, 22*(1), 55.

Beare, P. G., & Myers, J. L. (1998). *Principles and practice of adult health nursing* (3rd ed). St. Louis, MO: Mosby.

Biddinger, L. A. (1993). Bruner's theory of instruction and preprocedural anxiety in the pediatric population. *Issues in Comprehensive Pediatric Nursing, 16,* 147–154.

Bloom, B. S. (1977). *Taxonomy of educational objectives: The classification of educational goals, handbook I: Cognitive domain*. New York: Longman.

Cirone, N. (1997). Patient education handbook. *Nursing97, 27*(8), 44–45.

Cordell, B., & Smith-Blair, N. (1994). Streamlined charting for patient education. *Nursing94, 24*(1), 57–59.

DeLaune, S. C. (1991). Altered patterns of degenerative origin. In J. L. Davies (Eds.), *Mental health and psychiatric nursing* (3rd ed), Boston: Jones and Bartlett.

Doak, C. C., Doak, L. G., & Root, J. H. (1995). *Teaching patients with low literacy skills* (2nd ed.). Philadelphia: J. B. Lippincott.

Duffy, B. (1997). Using creative teaching process with adult patients. *Home Healthcare Nurse, 15*(2), 102–108.

Edelman, C. L., & Mandle, C. L. (1998). *Health promotion throughout the lifespan* (4th ed.). St. Louis, MO: Mosby.

Freda, M. (1997). Don't give it away. *MCN—The American Journal of Maternal/Child Nursing, 22*(6), 330.

Joint Commission for Accreditation of Healthcare Organizations. (1998). *Accreditation manual.* Chicago: Author.

Jubeck, M. E. (1994). Teaching the elderly: A commonsense approach. *Nursing94, 24*(5), 70–71.

Katz, J. R. (1997). Bach to basics: Providing effective patient teaching. *American Journal of Nursing, 97*(5), 33–36.

Knowles, M. S., Holton, E. F., & Swanson, R. A. (1998). *The adult learner* (5th ed.). Houston: Gulf Publishing.

Messner, R. L. (1997). Patient teaching tips from the horse's mouth. *RN, 60*(8), 29–31.

Nightingale, C. (1992). Pointing to the way ahead: Health education for people with learning disabilities. *Professional Nurse, 7*(9), 612–613, 615.

Poroch, D. (1995) The effect of preparatory patient education on the anxiety and satisfaction of cancer patients receiving radiation therapy. *Cancer Nursing, 18*(3), 206–214

Redman, B. K. (1997). *The practice of patient education* (8th ed.). St. Louis, MO: Mosby Yearbook.

Seley, J. J. (1994). 10 strategies for successful patient teaching. *American Journal of Nursing, 94*(11), 63–65.

Weissman, M., & Jasovsky, D. (1998). Discharge teaching for today's times. *RN, 61*(6), 38–40.

CHAPTER 12
Cultural Diversity and Nursing

REFERENCES/SUGGESTED READINGS

Agre, P., & Spincola, L. (1996). Helping staff meet the needs of a culturally diverse patient population. *Nursing Forum, 23*(2), 347.

Andreola, N., Steerfel, L., & O'Sullivan, C. (1993). A different way: A look at alternative therapies. *Nursing Spectrum, 6*(18), 7–9.

Andrews, M., & Boyle, J. S. (1998). *Transcultural concepts in nursing care* (3rd ed.). Philadelphia: Lippincott.

Andrews, M. M. (1997). Cultural diversity and community health nursing. In J. M. Swanson & M. Nies (Eds.), *Community health nursing: Promoting the health of aggregates* (2nd ed., pp. 433–458). Philadephia: W. B. Saunders.

Andrews, M. M., & Bolin, L. (1997). The African American community. In J. M. Swanson & M. Nies (Eds.), *Community health nursing: Promoting the health of aggregates* (2nd ed., pp. 433–458). Philadephia: W. B. Saunders.

Andrews, M. M., & Hanson, P. (1998). Religion, culture, and nursing. In M. M. Andrews & J. Boyle (Eds.), *Transcultural concepts in nursing care* (3rd ed.). Philadelphia: Lippincott.

Boutell, K. A., & Bozett, R. W. (1990, July). Nurses' assessment of patient's spirituality: Continuing education implications. *Journal of Continuing Education in Nursing, 21,* 172–76.

Boyle, J. (1998). Culture and community. In M. M. Andrews & J. Boyle (Eds.), *Transcultural concepts in nursing care* (3rd ed.). Philadelphia: Lippincott.

Brewer, J. A., & Bonalumi, N. M. (1996). Cultural diversity in the emergency department: Health care beliefs and practices among the Pennsylvania Amish. *Journal of Emergency Nursing, 21*(6), 494–497.

Carpenito, L. J. (1997). *Nursing diagnosis: Applications in clinical practice* (7th ed.). Philadelphia: J. B. Lippincott.

Cassetta, R. (1993). Emphasizing cultural diversity to improve nursing education. *American Nurse, 25*(8), 6.

Chan, S. (1991). *Asian Americans: An interpretive history.* Boston: Twayne Publishers.

Charnes, L. S., & Moore, P. S. (1992). Meeting patient's spiritual needs: The Jewish perspective. *Holistic Nursing Practice, 6*(3), 64–72.

Clark, C. (1996). *Nursing in the community* (2nd ed.). Stamford, CT: Appleton and Lange.

Clark, M. (1999). *Nursing in the community* (3rd ed.). Stamford, CT: Appleton & Lange.

Davidhizar, R., Dowd, S., & Giger, J. (1998). Educating the culturally diverse health care student. *Nurse Educator, 23*(2), 38–42.

Degazon, C. (1996). Cultural diversity and community health nursing practice. In M. Stanhope & J. Lancaster (Eds.), *Community health nursing: Promoting health of aggregates, families, and individuals* (4th ed.). St. Louis, MO: Mosby-Yearbook.

Diaz-Gilbert, M. (1993). Caring for culturally diverse patients. *Nursing93, 23*(10), 44.

Doherty, W. (1992). Private lives, public values. *Psychology Today, 25*(3), 32–27.

Doswell, W., & Erlen, J. (1998). Multicultural issues and ethical concerns in the delivery of nursing care interventions. *Nursing Clinics of North America, 33*(2), 353–361.

Edelman, C., & Mandle, C. (1998). *Health promotion throughout the lifespan* (4th ed.). St. Louis, MO: Mosby.

Edmission, K. W. (1997). Psychosocial dimensions of medical–surgical nursing. In J. M. Black & E. Matassarin-Jacobs (Eds.), *Medical surgical nursing: Clinical management for continuity of care.* Philadelphia: Saunders.

Eliason, M. (1993). Ethics and transcultural nursing care. *Nursing Outlook, 41*(5), 225–228.

Eshleman, J. (1992, November). Death with dignity: Significance of religious beliefs and practices in Hinduism, Buddhism, and Islam. *Today's OR Nurse,* 19–20.

Fawcett, C. (1993). *Family psychiatric nursing.* St. Louis, MO: Mosby-Year Book.

Fish, S., & Shelley, J. (1988). *Spiritual care: The nurse's role.* (3rd ed.). Downers Grove, IL: Inter Varsity Press.

Galanti, G. (1991). *Caring for patients from different cultures.* Philadelphia: University of Pennsylvania Press.

Galanti, G. (1997). *Caring for patients from different cultures: Case studies from American hospitals* (2nd ed.). Philadephia: University of Pennsylvania Press.

Giger, J., & Davidhizar, R. (2000). *Transcultural Nursing: Assessment and intervention* (3rd ed.). St. Louis, MO: C. V. Mosby.

Green, J. (1992). Death with dignity: Jehovah's Witnesses. *Nursing Times, 88*(5), 36–37.

Grensing-Pophal, L. (1997). Dealing with diversity in the workplace. *Nursing97, 27*(9), 78.

Grossman, D. (1996). Cultural dimensions in home health nursing. *American Journal of Nursing, 96*(7), 33–36.

Grossman, D., & Taylor, R. (1995). Cultural diversity on the unit. *American Journal of Nursing, 95*(2).

Grudyknust, W. (1992). *Communicating with strangers: An approach to intercultural communication.* New York: McGraw-Hill.

Hoeman, S. (1996). Intraethnic diversity. *Home-Healthcare Nurse, 14*(7), 568.

Iverson, P. (1990). *The Navajos.* New York: Chelsea House Publishers.

Kelz, R. (1997). *Delmar's English–Spanish Pocket Dictionary for Health Professionals.* Albany, NY: Delmar Publishers.

Kirkpatrick, M., Brown, S., & Atkins, T. (1998). Using the internet to integrate cultural diversity and global awareness. *Nurse Educator, 23*(2), 15–17.

Lee, E. (Ed.). (1997). *Working with Asian Americans: A guide for clinicians.* San Francisco: Richman Area Multi-Services, Inc.

Leininger, M. (1994). *Transcultural nursing: Concepts, theories, and practices*. Columbus, OH: Greyden Press.

Lock, D. (1992). *Increasing multicultural understanding: A comprehensive model*. Newbury Park, CA: Sage.

Luckmann, J. (1999). *Transcultural communication in nursing*. Albany, NY: Delmar Publishers.

Malone, B. (1998). Diversity, divisiveness and divinity. *American Nurse, 30*(1), 5.

McManus, R. J. (1993). Medicine and ethics at the crossroad: A Roman Catholic perspective. *Rhode Island Medicine, 76*(2), 79–81.

Meleis, A. I. (1997). Immigrant transitions and health care: An action plan [News]. *Nursing Outlook, 45*(1), 42.

Morley, P., & Wallis, R. (Eds.). (1978). *Culture and curing: Anthropological perspectives on traditional medical beliefs and practices*. Pittsburgh, PA: University of Pittsburgh Press.

Roberson, M. (1993). Defining cultural and ethical differences to adapt to a Chinese patient population. *American Nurse, 25*(8), 6–10.

Robinson, A. (1994). Spirituality and risk: Toward an understanding. *Holistic Nursing Practice, 8*(2), 1–7.

Rourden, B., & Higgs, R. (1992, March). When your patient is a Hmong Refugee. *American Journal of Nursing, 92*, 52–55.

Sherman, K. (1994). *Communication and image in nursing*. Albany, NY: Delmar Publishers.

Singelenberg, R. (1990). The blood transfusion taboo of Jehovah's Witnesses: Origins, development and function of a controversial doctrine. *Social Science Medicine, 31*(4), 515–523.

Smith, L. (1998). Concept analysis: Cultural competence. *Journal of Cultural Diversity, 5*(1), 4–10.

Specter, R. (1995). *Cultural diversity health and illness* (4th ed.). Norwalk, CT: Appleton & Lange.

Spector, R. E. (1996). *Cultural diversity in health and illness*. (4th ed.). New York: Appleton-Century-Crofts.

Spradley, B. W., and Allender, J. A. (1996). *Community health nursing* (4th ed.). Philadelphia: J. B. Lippincott.

Stanhope, M., & Knollmueller, R. (1996). *Handbook of community health and home health nursing* (2nd ed.). St. Louis, MO: Mosby-Year Book.

Stanhope, M., & Lancaster, J. (1996). *Community Health Nursing* (4th ed.). St. Louis, MO: Mosby.

Sue, D. W., & Sue, D. (1990). *Counseling the culturally different: Theory and practice* (2nd ed.). New York: Wiley.

Talabere, L. (1996). Meeting the challenge of culture care in nursing: Diversity, sensitivity, competence, and congruence. *Journal of Cultural Diversity, 3*(2), 53–61.

U.S. Department of Commerce, Bureau of the Census. (1992). *Statistical abstract of the United States: 1992* (112th ed.). Washington, DC: U.S. Government Printing Office.

West, E. (1993). The cultural bridge model. *Nursing Outlook, 41*(5), 229–234.

RESOURCES

Cultural Diversity in Health Care (video), American Journal of Nursing, 345 Hudson Street, New York, NY, 10014

CHAPTER 13
Alternative/Complementary Therapies

REFERENCES/SUGGESTED READINGS

Achterberg, J., Dossey, B., & Kolkmeier, L. (1994). *Rituals of healing: Using imagery for health and wellness*. New York: Bantam Books.

Association of Psychophysiology and Biofeedback (AAPB). (1998). *What is biofeedback?* [On-line]. Available: www.aapb.org

Benson, H. (1975). *The relaxation response*. New York: William Morrow.

Borysenko, J., & Borysenko, M. (1994). *The power of the mind to heal*. Carson, CA: Hay House.

Brooke, P. (1998). Legal risks of alternative therapies. *RN, 61*(5), 53–58.

Brown, H., Cassileth, B. R., Lewis, J. P., & Renner, J. H. (1994, June 15). Alternative medicine—Or quackery? *Patient Care*, 80–98.

Budesheim, S., Neuberger, G., Kasal, S., Vogel-Smith, K., Hassanein, R., & DeViney, S. (1994). Determinants of exercise and aerobic fitness in outpatients with arthritis. *Nursing Research, 43*, 11–17.

Byrd, C., & Sherrill, J. (1995). The therapeutic effects of intercessory prayer. *Journal of Christian Nursing, 12*(1), 21–23.

Cerrato, P. (1998). Aromatherapy: Is it for real? *RN, 61*(6), 51–52.

Chiropractic Arts Center. (1998). *Common questions about chiropractic care*. [On-line] Available: www.chiroarts.com/page7.html

Chopra, D. (1993). *Ageless body, timeless mind*. New York: Harmony Books.

Coulter, A. H. (1995, November–December). The role of prayer in healing: Can it really help? *Alternative & Complementary Therapies*, 351–356.

Cousins, N. (1979). *Anatomy of an illness*. New York: Norton.

Cowens, D. (1996). *A gift for healing: How you can use therapeutic touch*. New York: Crown Trade Paperbacks.

DeLaune, S., & Ladner, P. (1998). *Fundamentals of Nursing: Standards & Practice*. Albany, NY: Delmar Publishers.

Dossey, B. M. (1995a). Using imagery to help your patient heal. *American Journal of Nursing, 95*(6), 41–46.

Dossey, B. M., (1995b). Imagery: Awakening the inner healer. In B. M. Dossey, L. Keegan, C. E. Guzzetta, & L. G. Kolkmeier (Eds.), *Holistic nursing: A handbook for practice* (2nd ed.). Gaithersburg, MD: Aspen.

Dossey, B. M. (1995c). The psychophysiology of bodymind healing. In B. M. Dossey, L. Keegan, C. E. Guzzetta, & L. G. Kolkmeier (Eds.), *Holistic nursing: A handbook for practice* (2nd ed.). Gaithersburg, MD: Aspen.

Dossey, B. M. (Ed.). (1997). *Core curriculum for holistic nursing*. Gaithersburg, MD: Aspen.

Dossey, B. M., & Guzzetta, C. E. (1995). Holistic nursing practice. In B. M. Dossey, L. Keegan, C. E. Guzzetta, & L. G. Kolkmeier (Eds.), *Holistic nursing: A handbook for practice* (2nd ed., pp. 5–24). Gaithersburg, MD: Aspen.

Dossey, L. (1995). *Healing words: The power of prayer and the practice of medicine*. San Francisco: Harper.

Dumoff, L. (1997). Expanding the OAM into a center for integral medicine and creating access to medical treatment: Two goals for the 105th congress. *Alternative & Complementary Therapies, 3*(1), 59.

Eisenberg, D. (1993). Medicine in a mind/body culture. In B. Moyers (Ed.), *Healing and the mind*. New York: Doubleday.

Eisenberg, D. M., Kessler, R. C., & Foster, C. (1993). Unconventional medicine in the United States: Prevalence, costs, and patterns of use. *New England Journal of Medicine, 328*(4), 246–252.

Feuerstein, G. (1998). *Yoga and yoga therapy* [On-line]. Available: http://members.aol.com/yogareserch/yogatherapy.htm

Fonnesbeck, B. Are you kidding? *Nursing98, 28*(3), 64.

Foster, S. (1995). Herbs for health. *The Herb Companion, 8*(1), 63–86.

Frisch, N. (1997). Changing of the guard. *Beginnings, 17*(1), 1, 11.

Frisch, N., & Frisch, L. (1998). *Psychiatric mental health nursing.* Albany, NY: Delmar Publishers.

Gagne, D., & Toye, R. C. (1994). Decreasing anxiety in psychiatric patients with therapeutic touch. *Archives of Psychiatric Nursing, 8*(3), 184–189.

Gates, R. (1997). Legal issues in alternative medicine. *Alternative Therapies in Clinical Practice, 4*(4), 143.

Guinness, A. (1993). *Family guide to natural medicine: How to stay healthy the natural way.* Pleasantville, NY: Reader's Digest.

Healing touch and energy therapy [On-line]. (1997). Available: www.altherapy.com/hlgtch.htm

Hover-Kramer, D. (1996). *Healing touch: A resource for health care professionals.* Albany, NY: Delmar Publishers.

Japsen, B. (1995, August 21). Cost-conscious providers take to holistic medicine. *Modern Healthcare,* 138–142.

Kahn, S., & Saulo, M. (1995). *Healing yourself: A nurse's guide to self-care and renewal.* Albany, NY: Delmar Publishers.

Keegan, L. (1994). *The nurse as healer.* Albany, NY: Delmar Publishers.

Keegan, L. (1995a). Nutrition, exercise, and movement. In B. M. Dossey, L. Keegan, C. E. Guzzetta, & L. G. Kolkmeier (Eds.), *Holistic nursing: A handbook for practice* (2nd ed., pp. 257–285). Gaithersburg, MD: Aspen.

Keegan, L. (1995b). Touch: Connecting with the healing power. In B. M. Dossey, L. Keegan, C. E. Guzzetta, & L. G. Kolkmeier (Eds.), *Holistic nursing: A handbook for practice* (2nd ed., pp. 539–567). Gaithersburg, MD: Aspen.

Keegan, L. (1998). Alternative & complementary therapies. *Nursing98, 28*(4), 50–53.

Keville, K., & Green, M. (1995). *Aromatherapy: A complete guide to healing arts.* Freedom, CA: Crossing Press.

Kolkmeier, L. G. (1995). Relaxation: Opening the door to change. In B. M. Dossey, L. Keegan, C. E. Guzzetta, & L. G. Kolkmeier (Eds.), *Holistic nursing: A handbook for practice* (2nd ed., pp. 573–608). Gaithersburg, MD: Aspen.

Krieger, D. (1993). *Accepting your power to heal: The personal practice of therapeutic touch.* Santa Fe, NM: Bear & Company Publishing.

Lanfranco, J. (1997). *Acupressure and shiatsu information* [On-line] Available: www.geocities.com/HotSprings/4416/acusci.html

Long, J. (1995). Down to earth: An ancient herb for a modern garden. *The Herb Companion, 8*(1), 22.

Mackey, R. B. (1995). Discover the healing power of therapeutic touch. *American Journal of Nursing, 95*(4), 27–33.

Marwick, C. (1995). Should physicians prescribe prayer for health? Spiritual aspects of well-being considered. *Journal of the American Medical Association, 273*(20), 1561–1562.

McGhee, P. (1996). *Health, healing, and the amuse system.* Dubuque, IA: Kendall/Hunt.

McGhee, P. (1998). Rx: Laughter. *RN, 69*(7), 50–53.

Meehan, T. C. (1993). Therapeutic touch and postoperative pain: A Rogerian research study. *Nursing Science Quarterly, 6*(2), 69–78.

Mentgen, J. (1995). The clinical practice of healing touch. In D. Hover-Kramer (Ed.), *Healing touch: A resource for health care professionals* (pp. 155–165). Albany, NY: Delmar Publishers.

Mills, E. M. (1994). The effect of low-intensity aerobic exercise on muscle strength, flexibility, and balance among sedentary elderly persons. *Nursing Research, 43,* 206–211.

Mornhinweg, G. C., & Voignier, R. R. (1995). Holistic nursing interventions. *Orthopaedic Nursing, 14*(4), 20–24.

Moyers, B. (1993). *Healing and the mind.* New York: Doubleday.

National Institutes of Health. (1998). *About the Office of Alternative Medicine* [On-line] Available: http://altmed.od.nih.gov/oam/about/general.shtml#budget

Nightingale, F. (1969). *Nursing: What it is and what it is not.* New York: Dover Publications.

Nurse Healers-Professional Associates, Inc. (1992). *Therapeutic touch: Teaching guidelines: Beginner's level Krieger/Kunz method.* New York: Author.

Olsen, M., & Sneed, N. (1995). Anxiety and therapeutic touch. *Issues in Mental Health Nursing, 16*(2), 97–108.

Pert, C. (1986). The wisdom of the receptors: Neuropeptides, the emotions, and bodymind. *Advances, 3,* 8–16.

Polunin, M., & Robbins, C. (1995). Eight healing herbs, 1995–1996. *Holistic Health Directory,* 30–34.

Quinn, J. (1993). Psychoimmunologic effects of therapeutic touch on practitioners and recently bereaved recipients: A pilot study. *Advances in Nursing Science, 15*(4), 13–26.

Rossi, E. L. (1993). *The psychobiology of mind body healing: New concepts of therapeutic hypnosis* (rev. ed.). New York: Norton.

Schar, D. (1995). *The backyard medicine chest: An herbal primer.* Washington, DC: Elliot & Clark.

Schroeder-Shecker, T. (1994). Music for the dying. *Journal of Holistic Nursing, 12*(1), 83–99.

Simons, S. (1997). Vegetables and fruits: Natural "Phyters" against disease. Paper presented at the Texas Agricultural Extension service conference.

Stedman, M. (1999). Alternatives: You'd better shop around. *Health, 13*(1), 60–66.

Stevenson, C. (1994). The psychophysiological effects of aromatherapy massage following cardiac surgery. *Complementary Therapies in Medicine, 2*(1), 27.

Swackhamer, A. N. (1995). It's time to broaden our practice. *American Journal of Nursing, 95*(1), 49–51.

Trevelyan, J. (1993). Aromatherapy. *Nursing Times, 89*(25), 38–40.

Vacca, V. (1998). Back to high touch. *RN, 69*(7), 88.

Walton, J. (1996). Spiritual relationships: A concept analysis. *Journal of Holistic Nursing, 14*(3), 237–250.

Weil, A. (1995a). *Natural health, natural medicine: A comprehensive manual for wellness and self-care* (rev ed.). New York: Houghton Mifflin.

Weil, A. (1995b). *Spontaneous healing: How to discover and enhance your body's natural ability to maintain and heal itself.* New York: Alfred A. Knopf.

Weiss, R. R., & James, W. D. (1997). Allergic contact dermatitis from aromatherapy. *American Journal of Contact Dermatology, 8*(4), 250.

Wetzel, W. (1993). Healing touch as nursing intervention. *Journal of Holistic Nursing, 11*(3), 277–285.

Wilkinson, S. (1995). Aromatherapy and massage in palliative care. *International Journal of Palliative Nursing, 1*(1), 21.

Wilson, D. F. (1995). Therapeutic touch: Foundations and current knowledge. *Alternative Health Practitioner, 1*(1), 55–63.

Zahourek, R. P., & Larkin, D. (1995). Hypnosis and therapeutic suggestion for managing pain and stress. *Alternative Health Practitioner, 1*(19), 43–55.

Zisselman, M. H., Rovner, B. W., Shmuely, Y., & Ferrie, P. (1996). A pet therapy intervention with geriatric psychiatry inpatients. *American Journal of Occupational Therapy, 50*(1), 47–51.

RESOURCES

The American Association of Therapeutic Humor, 222 South Meramec, Suite 303, St. Louis, MO, 63105, 314-863-6232, http://aath.org

American Holistic Nurses' Association, P.O. Box 2130, Flagstaff, AZ, 86003-2130, 1-800-278-AHNA (1461), www.ahna.org

Association for Applied Psychophysiology and Biofeedback, 10200 West 44th Avenue, Suite 304, Wheat Ridge, CO, 80033-2840, 1-800-477-8892, 303-422-8436, www.aapb.org

Colorado Center for Healing Touch, 198 Union Boulevard, Suite 204, Lakewood, CO, 80220, 303-989-0581, www.healingtouch.net

Holistic Alliance of Professional Practitioners Entrepreneurs Networkers, Inc. (HAPPEN), P.O. Box 90177, Gainesville, FL, 32607, 1-888-8HAPPEN (42-7736)

Journal of Nursing Jocularity, P.O. Box 40416, Mesa, AZ, 85274, 602-835-6165, www.jocularity.com, email: cardace@jocularity.com

The Laughter Remedy, 45 North Fullerton, Suite 402, Montclair, NJ, 07042, 973-783-8383

Office of Alternative Medicine, OAM Clearinghouse, P.O. Box 8218, Silver Spring, MD, 20907-8218, 1-888-644-6226, http://altmed.od.nih.gov/nccam

Yoga Research Center, P.O. Box 1386, Lower Lake, CA, 95457, 707-928-9898, http://members.aol.com/yogaresrch

CHAPTER 14
The Life Cycle

REFERENCES/SUGGESTED READINGS

American Academy of Pediatrics. (1994). *1994 red book: Report of the Committee on Infectious Diseases* (23rd ed.). Elk Grove, IL: Author.

American Academy of Pediatrics. (1998). Guidance for effective discipline. *Pediatrics, 101*(4), 723.

American Nurses Association. (1990). *Nursing's agenda for health care reform*. Washington, DC: Author.

Baker, C. M. (1994). School health: Policy issues. *Nursing & Health Care, 15*(4), 178–184.

Beare, P. G., & Myers, J. L. (1998). *Adult health nursing* (3rd ed.). St. Louis: Mosby-Yearbook.

Biddinger, L. E. (1993). Bruner's theory of instruction and preprocedural anxiety in the pediatric population. *Issues in Comprehensive Pediatric Nursing, 16*, 147–154.

Campbell, M., & Kreidler, M. (1994). Older adults' perceptions about wellness. *Journal of Holistic Nursing, 12*(4), 437–447.

Copenhaver, M. M. (1995). Better late than never: Of reminiscence and resolution. *Journal of Psychosocial Nursing, 33*(7), 18–22.

Davidson, D. A. (1995). Physical abuse of preschoolers: Identification and intervention. *American Journal of Occupational Therapy, 49*(3), 235–243.

de Anda, D., & Smith, M. A. (1993). Differences among adolescent, young adult, and adult callers of suicide help lines. *Social Work, 38*(4), 421–428.

Dombeck, M. B. (1995). Dream telling: A means of spiritual awareness. *Holistic Nursing Practice, 9*(2), 37–47.

Edelman, C. L., & Mandle, C. L. (1998). *Health promotion throughout the lifespan* (4th ed.). St. Louis: Mosby-Yearbook.

Eliopoulos, C. (1997). *Gerontological nursing* (4th ed.). Philadelphia: Lippincott.

Erikson, E. (1968). *Childhood and society*. New York: Norton.

Estes, M. E. Z. (1998). *Health assessment & physical examination*. Albany, NY: Delmar Publishers.

Firth, P. A., & Watanabe, S. J. (1996). *Women's health: Instant nursing assessment*. Albany, NY: Delmar Publishers.

Foley, D. (1995). *Women's encyclopedia of health & emotional healing*. Emmaus, PA: Rodale Press.

Fowler, J. W. (1995). *Stages of faith: The psychology of human development and the quest for meaning*. New York: Harper & Row.

Freud, S. (1961). *Civilization and its discontents*. New York: Norton.

Fuller, J., & Schaller-Ayers, J. (2000). *Health assessment: A nursing approach* (3rd ed.). Philadelphia: Lippincott.

Gilligan, C. (1982). *In a different voice: Psychologic theory and women's development*. Cambridge, MA: Harvard University Press.

Gilligan, C., & Attanucci, D. (1988). Two moral orientations: Gender differences and similarities. *Merrill-Palmer Quarterly, 34*(3), 332–333.

Guyton, A. C., & Hall, J. (1996). *Textbook of medical physiology* (9th ed.). Philadelphia: Saunders.

Hale, P. J. (1996). HIV, hepatitis, and sexually transmitted diseases. In M. Stanhope & J. Lancaster (Eds.), *Community health nursing: Promoting health of aggregates, families, and individuals* (4th ed.). St. Louis: Mosby-Yearbook.

Harkness, G. A., & Dincher, J. R. (1996). *Medical–surgical nursing: Total patient care* (9th ed.). St. Louis: Mosby-Yearbook.

Havighurst, R. J. (1972). *Developmental tasks and education*. New York: Longman.

Heriot, C. S. (1995). Developmental tasks and development in the later years of life. In M. Stanhope & P. Beare (Eds.), *Gerontological nursing*. Philadelphia: Davis.

Ineicher, B. (1995). Breastfeeding 2. Strategies to promote breastfeeding in inner cities. *Health Visit, 68*(2), 61–62.

Johnson, B. S. (1995). *Child, adolescent, and family psychiatric nursing*. Philadelphia: Lippincott.

Johnson, B. S. (1997). *Psychiatric–mental health nursing: Adaptation and growth* (4th ed.). Philadelphia: Lippincott.

Kahn, K. L., & Steeves, R. H. (1994). Witnesses to suffering: Nursing knowledge, voice, and vision. *Nursing Outlook, 42*(6), 260–264.

Kohlberg, L. (1977). *Recent research in moral development*. New York: Holt, Rinehart, & Winston.

Levin, J. D. (1995). *Introduction to alcoholism counseling: A bio-psycho-social approach* (2nd ed.). Washington, DC: Taylor & Francis.

Levinson, D. (1978). *The seasons of a man's life*. New York: Knopf.

Murray, R. B., & Zentner, J. P. (1997). *Health assessment & promotion strategies through the life span* (6th ed.). East Norwalk, CT: Appleton & Lange.

Nugent, E. (1995). Try to remember: Reminiscence as a nursing intervention. *Journal of Psychosocial Nursing, 33*(11), 7–11.

O'Neil, E. H. (1993). *Health professions education for the future: Schools in service to the nation*. San Francisco: Pew Health Professions Commission.

Orpinas, P. K. (1995). The co-morbidity of violence-related behaviors with health-risk behaviors in a population of high school students. *Journal of Adolescent Health, 16*(3), 216–225.

Piaget, J. (1963). *The origins of intelligence in children*. New York: Norton.

Piaget, J., & Inhelder, B. (1969). *The psychology of the child*. New York: Basic Books.

Randolph, N. (1998). *American nursing review of psychiatric and mental health nursing certification.* Springhouse, PA: Springhouse Corporation.

Roye, C. F. (1995). Breaking through to the adolescent patient. *AJN, 95*(12), 19–23.

Sapp, M., & Bliesmer, M. (1995). A health promotion/protection approach to meeting elders' healthcare needs through public policy and standards of care. In M. Stanley & P. Beare (Eds.), *Gerontological nursing.* Philadelphia: Davis.

Smith, A. (1986). *The body.* New York: Viking Penguin, Inc.

Sullivan, H. S. (1953). *Interpersonal theory of psychiatry.* New York: Norton.

U.S. Department of Health & Human Services, Public Health Service. (1990). *Healthy people 2000: National health promotion and disease prevention objectives* (DHHS Publication No. PHS 91-5012). Washington, DC: Author.

Wong, D. L., Hockenberry-Eaton, M., Wilson, D., Winkelstein, M. L., Ahmann, E., & DiVito-Thomas, P. (1999). *Whaley & Wong's nursing care of infants and children* (6th ed.). St. Louis, MO: Mosby-Yearbook.

RESOURCES

American Academy of Pediatrics, 141 Northwest Point Boulevard, Elk Grove Village, IL, 60007-1098, 847-228-5005, www.aap.org

American Association of Retired Persons, 601 E Street N.W., Washington, DC, 20049, 1-800-424-3410, www.aarp.com

American Foundation for Suicide Prevention, 120 Wall Street, 22nd floor, New York, NY, 10005, 1-888-333-2377, www.afsp.org

American Society on Aging, 833 Market Street, Suite 511, San Francisco, CA, 94103, 415-974-9600

Centers for Disease Control and Prevention (CDC), 1600 Clifton Road N.E., Atlanta, GA, 30333, 404-639-3311, www.cdc.gov

CHAPTER 15
Wellness Concepts

REFERENCES/SUGGESTED READINGS

Baughcum, A. (1998). Mom's beliefs may cause child obesity. *Archives of Pediatric and Adolescent Medicine, 152,* 1010–1014.

Browder, S. (1998). *Attention, women over 50* [On-line]. Available: www.seniornews.com/new-choices/article593.html

Brown, E. (1995, August). An inexpensive and painless alternative to colonoscopy? (coprocytobiology). *Medical Update, 19,* 1.

Carey, B. (1996, July/August). The slumber solution. *Health,* 70–75.

Centers for Disease Control and Prevention (CDC). (1998). Uninsured women miss mammograms. *Morbidity and Mortality Weekly Report, 47,* 825–829.

Chase, M. (1996, February 5). Simple handwashing gets new scrutiny for disease control. *The Wall Street Journal,* B1(E&W).

Dixon, B. (1995). *Good health for African Americans.* New York: Random House.

Don't overdo it: Alcohol paradox. (1996, February 5). *Industry Week, 245*(1), 19.

Eastman, P. (1996, January 17). Task force issues new screening guidelines. *Journal of the National Cancer Institute, 88*(3), 74.

Edlin, G., Golanty, E., & McCormack-Brown, K. (1997). *Essentials for Health and Wellness.* Boston: Jones and Bartlett.

Floyd, P., Mimms, S., & Yelding-Howard, C. (1995). *Personal health: A multicultural approach.* Englewood, CO: Morton Publishing Co.

Hafen, B., & Hoeger, W. (1997). *Wellness: Guidelines for a healthy lifestyle* (2nd ed.). Englewood, CO: Morton Publishing Co.

Health-club hygiene. (1995, November). *Industry Week, 244,* 31.

Hoeger, W., & Hoeger, S. (1995). *Lifetime physical fitness and wellness* (4th ed.). Englewood, CO: Morton Publishing.

Hoffman, E. (1995). *Our health, our lives.* New York: Pocket Books.

Ince, S. (1995, June). A bite of the apple. *Harvard Health Letter, 20,* 3.

Inlander, C., & Moran, C. (1994). *77 Ways to beat colds and flu.* New York: Walker Publishing.

Lee, I., & Paffenbarger, R. (1998). Exercise can cut stroke risk 50%. *Stroke, 29,* 2049–2054.

Liviton, R. (1995). *Brain builders.* West Nyack, NY: Parker Publishing.

Lowell, B. (1995). *Body signals.* New York: HarperCollins Publishers.

Malaty, H. (1998). Twin study: H pylori tied to hygiene. *American Journal of Epidemiology, 148,* 793–797.

Matthews, K. (1998). Suppressed anger hard on women's hearts. *Psychosomatic Medicine, 60,* 633–638.

Mayell, M. (1995). *52 Simple steps to natural health.* New York: Pocket Books.

Oman, D., & Reed, D. (1998). Religious elderly tend to live longer. *American Journal of Public Health, 88,* 1469–1475.

Osteoporosis, a silent disease, finds a louder voice. (1995, November–December). *Menopause News, 5,* 1.

Payne, W., & Hahn, D. (1995). *Understanding your health* (4th ed.). St. Louis, MO: Mosby-Year Book.

Quaid, K. (1993, September 30). Psychological and ethical considerations in screening for disease. *American Journal of Cardiology, 72,* 64D.

Quench strokes with every sip. (1995, October) *Prevention, 47,* 66.

Reed, D. (1998). Four factors predict "Healthy Aging." *American Journal of Public Health, 88,* 1463–1469.

Reichman, L., & Mangura, B. (1996, February). State-of-the-art tuberculosis prevention. *Chest, 109,* 301.

Robertson, J. (1996). *Peak-performance living.* New York: HarperCollins.

Seiger, L., Vanderpool, K., & Barnes, D. (1995). *Fitness and wellness strategies.* Dubuque, IA: Wm. C. Brown Communications.

Simon, H. (1992). *Staying well.* Boston: Houghton Mifflin Co.

Smith, C., & Maurer, F. (1995). *Community health nursing: Theory and practice.* Philadelphia: W. B. Saunders.

Smith, S., & Lancashire, J. (1995, November–December). Health promotion and disease prevention progress report. *Public Health Reports, 110,* 790.

Social stigma of colon and rectal problems thwarts life-saving cancer screenings. (1995, October). *Executive Health's Good Health Report, 32,* 1.

Sox, H. (1994, June 2). Preventive health services in adults. *New England Journal of Medicine, 330,* 1589.

U.S. Department of Agriculture, U.S. Department of Health & Human Services. (1995). *Home and Garden Bulletin No. 232* (4th ed.).

U.S. Department of Health & Human Services. (1990). *Healthy People 2000: National health promotion and disease prevention objectives.* (DHHS Publication No. [PHS] 91-50212). Washington, DC.

U.S. Department of Health & Human Services (USDHHS), Public Health Service. *Healthy people 2000: National health promotion and disease prevention objectives and first draft healthy people 2010: National health promotion and disease prevention objectives. [On-line] Available: http://web.health.gov/healthypeople*

U.S. Department of Health & Human Services (USDHHS), Public Health Service (PHS). (1998). 1997–1998 Progress Review [On-line]. Available: http://odphp.osophs.dhhs.gov/pubs/hp2000

Wash your hands (to help prevent colds). (1996, January). *Consumer Reports on Health, 2*(1).

Weil, A. (1995). *Natural health, natural medicine.* Boston: Houghton Mifflin.

Williams, R., & Williams, V. (1994). *Anger kills: Seventeen strategies for controlling the hostility that can harm your health.* New York: Random House.

RESOURCES

Aerobics and Fitness Association of America, 15250 Ventura Boulevard, Suite 200, Sherman Oaks, CA, 91403-3297, 1-800-446-2322, www.aerobics.com/

American Dietetic Association, 216 West Jackson Boulevard, Suite 800, Chicago, IL, 60606-6995, 1-800-366-1655, www.eatright.org

American Health Care Association, 1201 L Street, NW, Washington, DC, 20005, 202-342-4444, www.ahca.org

American Holistic Nurses' Association, P.O. Box 2130, Flagstaff, AZ, 86003-2130, 1-800-278-2462, www.ahna.org

Center for Science in the Public Interest, 1875 Connecticut Avenue, NW, Suite 300, Washington, DC, 20009-5728, 202-332-9110, www.cspinet.org

Centers for Disease Control and Prevention, *Morbidity and Mortality Weekly Report*, http://www.cdc.gov/cdc.html

Centers for Disease Control and Prevention, 1600 Clifton Road, NE, Atlanta, GA, 30333, 404-639-3311, www.cdc.gov

Consumer Product Safety Commission, Washington, DC, 20207, 1-800-638-2772, 1-800-638-8270 TDD, 1-800-492-8104 TTD in MD only

Dental Disease Prevention, Centers for Disease Control and Prevention (CDC), 1600 Clifton Road, NE, Atlanta, GA, 30333

Environmental Protection Agency (EPA), Public Information Center, 401 M Street, SW, Washington, DC, 20466, 1-800-424-9065, 202-260-2090, www.epa.gov

Food and Drug Administration, Office of Consumer Affairs, 5600 Fishers Lane, Rockville, MD, 20857, 1-888-463-6332, www.fda.gov

Food and Nutrition Information Center, National Agricultural Library Building, Room 304, 10301 Baltimore Avenue, Beltsville, MD, 20705-2351, 301-504-5719, www.nal.usda.gov/fnic/

Healthy People 2010, Office of Disease Prevention and Health Promotion, 738-6 Humphrey Building, 200 Independence Avenue SW, Washington, DC, 20201, 202-205-8583

Medic Alert Foundation International, P.O. Box 819008, Turlock, CA, 95381-1009, 1-800-344-3226, 209-668-3333, www.medicalert.org

National Cholesterol Education Program Information Center, 4733 Bethesda Avenue, Room 530, Bethesda, MD, 20814, 301-951-3260

National Council Against Health Fraud, Resource Center, 300 East Pink Hill Road, Independence, MO, 64057, 816-228-4595, www.ncahf.org

National Health Information Center, P.O. Box 1133, Washington, DC, 20013-1133, 1-800-336-4797, http://nhic-nt.health.org

National Highway Traffic Safety Administration, NES-11 HL, U.S. Department of Transportation, 400 7th Street, SW, Washington, DC, 20590, 202-366-9294, Auto Hotline: 1-800-424-9393, www.nhtsa.dot.gov

National Institute for Occupational Safety and Health, Clearinghouse for Occupational Safety and Health Information, Technical Information Branch, 4676 Columbia Parkway, Cincinnati, OH, 45226, 1-800-356-4674

The National Institute on Aging, P.O. Box 8057, Gaithersburg, MD 20898-8057, 1-800-222-2225, www.nih.gov/nia

National Institutes of Health, 9000 Rockville Pike, Bethesda, MD, 20892, 301-496-1776, www.nih.gov

National League for Nursing, 61 Broadway, New York, NY, 10006, 212-363-5555, 1-800-669-9656, Fax: 212-812-0393, www.nln.org

National Safety Council, 1121 Spring Lake Drive, Itasca, IL, 60143-3201, 630-285-1121, www.national-safety-council.ie

National Wellness Association/National Wellness Institute, 1300 College Court, P.O. Box 827, Stevens Point, WI, 54481-0827, 715-342-2961, www.wellnesswi.org

National Women's Health Network, 514 Tenth Street, NW, Washington, DC, 20004, 202-347-1140

U.S. Department of Agriculture, 14th & Independence Avenue, SW, Washington, DC, 20250, 1-800-535-4555, 202-720-2791, www.usda.gov

U.S. Department of Health and Human Services, Office of Disease Prevention and Health Promotion, 638-East Humphrey Building, 200 Independence Avenue, SW, Washington, DC, 20201, 202-690-6343, www.hhs.gov

World Health Organization, 525 23rd Street, NW, Washington, DC 20037, 202-974-3000, Headquarters Avenue Appia 20, 1211 Geneva 27, Switzerland, www.who.int

CHAPTER 16
Stress, Adaptation, and Anxiety

REFERENCES/SUGGESTED READINGS

Aguilera, D. C. (1998). *Crisis intervention: Theory and methodology* (8th ed.). St. Louis, MO: Mosby.

Alfaro-LeFevre, R. (1995). *Critical thinking in nursing: A practical approach.* Philadelphia: Saunders.

Badger, J. M. (1994). Calming the anxious patient. *American Journal of Nursing, 94*(5), 46–50.

Badger, J. M. (1995). Tips for managing stress on the job. *American Journal of Nursing, 95*(9), 31–33.

Beck, A. (1976). *Cognitive therapy and emotional disorders.* New York: International Universities Press.

Borman, J. S. (1993). Chief nurse executives balance of their work and personal lives. *Nursing Administration Quarterly, 18*(1), 30–39.

Bowman, A. M. (1993). Victim blaming in nursing. *Nursing Outlook, 41*(6), 268–273.

Bru, G., Carmody, S., Donohue-Sword, B., & Bookbinder, M. (1993). Parental visitation in the post-anesthesia care unit: A means to lessen anxiety. *Children's Health Care, 22*(3), 217–226.

Cullen, A. (1995). Burnout: Why do we blame the nurse? *American Journal of Nursing, 95*(11), 23–27.

DeLaune, S. C. (1993). Learned optimism. *Aspen's Advisor for the Nurse Executive, 8*(11), 8.

DeLaune, S. C. (1996). Applying the nursing process for clients with anxiety, somatoform, and dissociative disorders. In H. S. Wilson & C. R Kneisl (Eds.), *Psychiatric nursing* (5th ed., p. 368). Menlo Park, CA: Addison-Wesley.

Freud, S. (1959). Inhibitions, symptoms and anxiety. In J. Strachey (Trans.), *The standard edition of the complete psychological works of Sigmund Freud* (Vol. 20). London: The Hogarth Press.

Frisch, N., & Frisch, L. (1998). *Psychiatric mental health nursing.* Albany, NY: Delmar Publishers.

Gillies, D. A. (1994). *Nursing management: A systems approach* (3rd ed.). Philadelphia: Saunders.

Heinrich, K., & Killeen, M. E. (1993). The gentle art of nurturing yourself. *American Journal of Nursing, 93*(10), 41–44.

Holmes, T. H., & Rahe, R. (1967). The social readjustment rating scale. *Journal of Psychosomatic Research, 2,* 213–218.

Huebner, E., & Nelson, P. B. (1994, October). Managing change—The challenge of the '90s. *Caring,* 94–100.

Kahn, S., & Saulo, M. (1994). *Healing yourself: A nurse's guide to self-care and renewal.* Albany, NY: Delmar Publishers.

Keegan, L. (1995). Nutrition, exercise, and movement. In B. M. Dossey, L. Keegan, C. E. Guzzetta, & L. G. Kolkmeier (Eds.), *Holistic nursing: A handbook for practice* (2nd ed., pp. 257–288). Gaithersburg, MD: Aspen.

Kneisl, C. R., & Riley, E. (1996). Crisis intervention. In H. S. Wilson & C. R. Kneisl (Eds.), *Psychiatric nursing* (5th ed., pp. 711–731). Menlo Park, CA: Addison-Wesley.

Kobasa, S. C. (1979). Stressful life events, personality and health. An inquiry into hardiness. *Journal of Personality and Social Psychology, 37*(1), 1–11.

Kobasa, S. C., Maddi, S. R., & Kahn, S. (1982). Hardiness and health: A prospective study. *Journal of Personality and Social Psychology, 45*(4), 839–850.

Lauver, D. (1995). Optimism and coping with breast cancer symptoms. *Nursing Research, 44*(4), 202–207.

Lehman, L. (1993). Nursing interventions for anxiety, depression, and suspiciousness in the home care setting. *Home Healthcare Nurse, 11*(3), 35–40.

Lewin, K. (1951). *Field theory in social science.* New York: Harper.

Lippitt, R., Watson, J., & Westley, B. (1958). *The dynamics of planned change.* New York: Harcourt Brace.

Mandle, C. L., & Gruber-Wood, R. (1998). Health promotion and the individual. In C. L. Edelman & C. L. Mandle (Eds.), *Health promotion throughout the life-span* (4th ed.). St. Louis, MO: Mosby.

North American Nursing Diagnosis Association. (1999). *Nursing diagnoses: Definitions & classification.* 1999–2000. Philadelphia: Author.

Peplau, H. (1952). *Interpersonal relations in nursing.* New York: Putnam.

Poole, E. (1993). The effects of postanesthesia care unit visits on anxiety in surgical patients. *Journal of Post Anesthesia Nursing, 8*(6), 386–394.

Selye, H. (1974). *Stress without distress.* New York: New American Library.

Selye, H. (1976). *Stress in health and disease* (rev. ed.). Boston: Butterworths.

Stubblefield, C. (1995). Optimism: A determinant of health behavior. *Nursing Forum, 30*(1), 19–24.

Sullivan, H. S. (1953). *The interpersonal theory of psychiatry by H. S. Sullivan.* New York: Norton.

Talbott, S. W. (1993). Political analysis: Structure and process. In D. J. Mason, S. W. Talbott, & J. K. Leavitt (Eds.), *Policy and politics for nurses* (2nd ed., pp. 129–148). Philadelphia: Saunders.

Waughfield, C. (1998). *Mental health concepts* (4th ed.). Albany, NY: Delmar Publishers.

Woodhouse, D. K. (1993). The aspects of humor in dealing with stress. *Nursing Administration Quarterly, 18*(1), 80–89.

RESOURCES

American Holistic Nurses' Association, P.O. Box 2130, Flagstaff, AZ, 86003-2130, 800-278-AHNA (1461), 520-526-2196, www.ahna.org

Stress Reduction Clinic, University of Massachusetts Medical Center, 55 Lake Avenue North, Worcester, MA, 01655, 508-856-2656

CHAPTER 17
Loss, Grief, and Death

REFERENCES/SUGGESTED READINGS

American Nurses Association (ANA). (1992). Promotion of comfort and relief of pain in dying patients. In *Compendium of position statements on the nurse's role in end-of-life decisions.* Washington, DC: Author.

Andreas, L. (1998). Controlling pain: Keeping a dying patient comfortable. *Nursing98, 28*(1), 70.

Backer, B. A., Hannon, N. R., & Russell, N. A. (1994). *Death and dying: Understanding and care* (2nd ed.). Albany, NY: Delmar Publishers.

Barbus, A. J. (1975). The dying person's bill of rights. *American Journal of Nursing, 75*(1), 99.

Beckel, J. (1996). Resolving ethical dilemmas in long-term care. *Journal of Gerontological Nursing, 22*(1), 20–26.

Boon, T. (1998). Don't forget the hospice option. *RN, 61*(2), 30–33.

Bowlby, J. (1982). *Attachment and loss: Vol. 2. Separation anxiety and anger.* New York: Basic Books.

Bral, E. (1998). Caring for adults with chronic cancer pain. *American Journal of Nursing, 98*(4), 27–32.

Bridges, W. (1991). *Managing transitions: Making the most of change.* Reading, MA: Addison-Wesley.

Carpenito, L. J. (1997). *Handbook of nursing diagnosis* (7th ed.). Philadelphia: Lippincott.

Cerrudo, J. (1998). Letting go of Abuelo. *American Journal of Nursing, 98*(8), 53.

Corless, I., Germino, B., & Pittman, M. (Eds.). (1995). *A challenge for living: Death, dying, and bereavement.* Boston: Jones and Bartlett.

Czerwiec, M. (1996). When a loved one is dying: Families talk about nursing care. *American Journal of Nursing, 96*(5), 32–36.

deBlois, J. (1994, March). Changing the way we care for the dying. *Health Progress,* 48–52.

Doka, K., Rushton, C. H., & Thorstenson, T. A. (1994). HealthCare Ethics Forum '94: Caregiver distress: If it is so ethical, why does it feel so bad? *American Association Critical-Care Nurses Clinical Issues, 5*(3), 346–352.

Down, M. (1984). The hospice team. In S. H. Schraff (Ed.), *Hospice: The nursing perspective* (pp. 47–57). New York: National League for Nursing.

Durham, E., & Weiss, L. (1997). How patients die. *American Journal of Nursing, 97*(12), 41–46.

Edelman, C. L., & Mandle, C. L. (1998). *Health promotion throughout the lifespan* (4th ed.). St. Louis, MO: Mosby.

Engle, G. L. (1961). Is grief a disease? *Psychosomatic Medicine, 23,* 18–22.

Engle, G. L. (1964). Grief and grieving. *American Journal of Nursing, 64*(9), 93–98.

Estes, M. E. Z. (1998). *Health assessment & physical examination.* Albany, NY: Delmar Publishers.

Fauri, D. P., & Grimes, D. R. (1994). Bereavement services for families and peers of deceased residents of psychiatric institutions. *Social Work, 39*(2), 185–190.

Ferrell, B. (1998). End-of-life care. *Nursing98, 28*(9), 58.

Forbes, V. (1998). The dying game. *American Journal of Nursing, 98*(9), 50.

Haynor, P. (1998) Meeting the challenge of advance directives. *American Journal of Nursing, 98*(3), 27–32.

Kübler-Ross, E. (1969). *On death and dying.* New York: Macmillan.

Kübler-Ross, E. (1974). *Questions and answers on death and dying.* New York: Macmillan.

Kübler-Ross, E. (1997). *Meaning of our suffering.* Barrytown, NY: Barrytown, Ltd.

Lindemann, E. (1944). Symptomatology and management of acute grief. *American Journal of Psychiatry, 101,* 141–148.

MacGregor, P. (1994). Grief: The unrecognized parental response to mental illness in a child. *Social Work, 39*(2), 160–166.

McCaffery, M., & Pasero, C. (1999). *Pain: Clinical manual for nursing practice* (2nd ed.). St. Louis, MO: Mosby-Year Book.

McClain, M. E., & Shafer, S. M. (1996). Supporting families after sudden infant death. *Journal of Psychosocial Nursing and Mental Health Services, 34*(4), 30–34.

McGowan, D. (1998). The right to say goodbye. *RN, 61*(5), 84.

North American Nursing Diagnosis Association. (1999). *Nursing diagnoses: Definitions & classification. 1999–2000.* Philadelphia: Author.

Pasternak, R. E., Reynolds, C. F., Houck, P. R., Schlernitzauer, M., Buysse, D. J., Hoch, C. C., & Kupfer, D. J. (1994, April–June). Sleep in bereavement-related depression during and after pharmacotherapy with nortriptyline. *Journal of Geriatric Psychiatry and Neurology, 7,* 69–73.

Pritchett, K., & Lucas, P. (1997). Death and dying. In B. S. Johnson (Ed.), *Psychiatric–mental health nursing: Adaptation and growth* (4th ed., pp. 206–207). Philadelphia: Lippincott.

Pritchett, K., & Lucas, P. (1997). Grief and loss. In B. S. Johnson (Ed.), *Psychiatric–mental health nursing: Adaptation and growth* (4th ed., pp. 199–218). Philadelphia: Lippincott.

Reese, C. D. (1996). Please cry with me: Six ways to grieve. *Nursing96, 26*(8), 56.

Rhymes, J. (1993). Hospice care in the nursing home. *Nursing Home Medicine, 1*(6), 14–16, 22–24.

Roach, S. S., & Nieto, B. C. (1997). *Healing and the grief process.* Albany, NY: Delmar Publishers.

Smith-Stoner, M., & Frost, A. (1998). Coping with grief and loss: Bringing your shadow self into the light. *Nursing98, 28*(2), 49–50.

Taylor, M. (1995). Benefits of dehydration in terminally ill clients. *Geriatric Nursing, 16*(6), 271–272.

Taylor, P., & Ferszt, G. (1994). Letting go of a loved one. *Nursing94, 24*(1), 55–56.

Thompson, L. M. (1994). The future of death: Death in the hands of science. *Nursing Outlook, 42,* 175–180.

Ufema, J. (1995a). How to help dying clients feel "safe." *Nursing95, 25*(9), 59.

Ufema, J. (1995b). Insights on death and dying. *Nursing95, 25*(11,12), 19, 22–23.

Wong, M. M. (1996). *The 1996 national directory of bereavement support groups and services.* Forest Hills, NY: ADM Publishing.

Worden, J. W. (1991). *Grief counseling and grief therapy: A handbook for the mental health practitioner* (2nd ed.). New York: Springer.

RESOURCES

Association for Death Education & Counseling, 638 Prospect Ave., Hartford, CT, 06105, 860-586-7503

Choice in Dying, 475 Riverside Drive, New York, NY, 10115, 800-989-9455

Hospice Foundation of America, 777 17th Street, #401, Miami Beach, FL, 33139, 1-800-854-3402, www.hospicefoundation.org

The National Hospice Organization, 1901 North Moore St., Suite 901, Arlington, VA, 22209-1714, 703-243-5900, www.nho.org

CHAPTER 18
Basic Nutrition

REFERENCES/SUGGESTED READINGS

American Heart Association. (1999). *Non-AHA-Approved Diets.* [On-line] Available: www.deliciousdecisions.org/ff/tsd_nondiets_fad.html

Barrett, S. (1998). *Dietary reference intakes (DRIs): New guidelines for calcium and related nutrients.* [On-line] Available: http//www.quackwatch.com/03healthpromotion/dr01.html

Centers for Disease Control and Prevention. (1997). Update: Prevalence of overweight among children, adolescents, and adults—United States, 1988–1994. *MMWR, 46*(9), 199.

Cobb, M. (1997). Improving your patient's nutritional status. *Nursing97, 27*(6), 32hhr,32hh6.

Costello, M. (1996). Home health nutrition. *MedSurg Nursing, 5*(4), 229–238.

Couig, M. (1993). The New Food Label. *American Journal of Nursing, 93*(2), 68–71.

Craig, W. (1997). Phytochemicals: Guardians of our health. *Journal of the American Dietetic Association, 97*(10 Suppl. 2), S199–S204.

Dudek, S. (1997). *Nutrition handbook for nursing practice* (3rd ed.). Philadelphia: Lippincott.

Estes, M. E. Z. (1998). *Health assessment & physical examination.* Albany, NY: Delmar Publishers.

Frankel, E., Waterhouse, A., & Teissedra, P. (1995). Principal phenolic phytochemicals in selected California wine and their antioxidant activity in inhibiting oxidation of human low-density lipoproteins. *Journal of Agricultural & Food Chemistry, 43,* 890–894.

Gravely, M. (1993, Spring/Summer). Answering your questions on nutrition and nutrition labeling. *Food News for Consumers.* USDA, Food Safety and Inspection Service.

Institute of Medicine. (1997). *Dietary reference intakes for calcium, phosphorus, magnesium, vitamin D, and fluoride.* [On-line] Available: http//www2.nas.edu/whatsnew/276a.html

Institute of Medicine. (1998). *Dietary reference intakes: Thiamin, riboflavin, niacin, vitamin B_6, folate, vitamin B_{12} pantothenic acid, biotin, and choline.* [On-line] Available: http//www2.nas.edu/whatsnew/287e.html

Lee, R., & Nieman, D. (1993). *Nutritional assessment.* Madison, WI: Brown & Benchmark.

Loan, T., Magnuson, B., & Williams, S. (1998). Debunking six myths about enteral feeding. *Nursing98, 28*(8), 43–48.

McConnell, E. (1998). Administering parenteral nutrition. *Nursing98, 28*(7), 18.

National Academy of Sciences. (1989). *Recommended dietary allowances: 10th edition.* Washington, DC: National Academy Press.

Navder, K. (1993, Summer). Food and nutrition labeling: Past, present and future. *Journal of Home Economics,* 43–50.

O'Brien, B. (1993, Spring/Summer). Answering your questions on nutrition and nutrition labeling. *Food News for Consumers.* USDA, Food Safety and Inspection Service.

Oldways Preservation & Exchange Trust. (1997). *Vegetarian Diet Pyramid.* [On-line] Available: www.oldwayspt.org/html/p_veg.htm

Pace-Asciak, C., Hahn, S., Diamandis, P., Soleas, G., & Goldberg, D. (1995). The red wine phenolics trans-resveratrol and quercetin block human platelet aggregation and eicosanoid synthesis: Implications for protection against coronary heart disease. *Clinica Chimica Acta., 235,* 207–219.

Position of the American Dietetic Association: Phytochemicals and functional foods. (1995). *Journal of the American Dietetic Association, 95,* 493–498.

Sharpe, P., McGrath, L., McClean, E., Young, I., & Archbold, G. (1995). Effect of red wine consumption on lipoprotein (a) and other risk factors for atherosclerosis. *QJM, 88,* 101–108.

Simons, S. (1997). *Vegetables and fruits: Natural "Phyters" against disease.* Texas Agriculture Extension Service.

Staff. (1993, Jan/Feb). Food labeling . . . Finally. *Nutrition Action Healthletter, 20*(1), 5–6.

Stanfield, P. (1997). *Nutrition and diet therapy.* (3rd ed.). Boston: Jones and Bartlett.

Steinmetz, K., & Potter, J. (1996). Vegetables, fruit, and cancer prevention: A review. *Journal of the American Dietetic Association, 96,* 1027–1036.

Townsend, C. & Roth, R. (2000). *Nutrition & diet therapy.* (7th ed.). Albany, NY: Delmar Publishers.

USDA. (1990). *Nutrition and your health: Dietary guidelines for Americans* (3rd ed., Home and Garden Bulletin, No. 232). Washington, DC: United States Department of Agriculture and United States Department of Health and Human Services.

USDA. (1992). *Food guide pyramid* (Home and Garden Bulletin, No. 252). Washington, DC: United States Department of Agriculture, Human Nutrition Information Service.

USDA Human Nutrition Information Service and Food Marketing Institute. (1992). *The food guide pyramid . . . Beyond the basic 4.* Hyattsville, MD: United States Department of Agriculture.

Washington, H. (1998). The vitamin revolution. *Health, 12*(6), 104–110.

Williams, S. (1995). *Basic nutrition and diet therapy.* (10th ed.). St. Louis, MO: Mosby Year Book.

RESOURCES

American Dietetic Association, 216 West Jackson Blvd., Chicago, IL, 60606-6995, 312-899-0040, 1-800-877-1600, Fax: 312-899-1979, www.eatright.org, e-mail: webmaster@eatright.org

Food and Nutrition Board, Institute of Medicine, 2101 Constitution Avenue, N.W., Washington, DC, 20418, 202-334-2169

Food and Nutrition Information Center, USDA/National Agricultural Library, 10301 Baltimore Boulevard, Room 304, Beltsville, MD, 20705-2351, 301-504-5755, www.nal.usda.gov/fnic/

CHAPTER 19
Rest and Sleep

REFERENCES/SUGGESTED READINGS

American Psychiatric Association (APA). (1994). *DSM-IV.* Washington, DC: Author.

Brown, W. (1997). *What sleep disturbances do preschool children experience?* (From "Best Practices" series). [On-line]. Available: www.psychlink.com/resourc/consultn/article 28.html

Carter, A. (1997). *Restless legs syndrome (RLS)* [On-line], Clinical Reference Systems. Available: www.realage.com/Library/M_behavior.htm

Coleman, R. M. (1986) *Wide awake at 3:00 AM: By choice or by chance?* New York: Freeman.

Cooper, P. (1998). *Insomnia* [On-line], Clinical Reference Systems. Available: www.realage.com/Library/M_behavior.htm

Coren, S. (1996). *Sleep thieves: An eye-opening exploration into the science and mysteries of sleep.* New York: Free Press.

DeRoin, D. (1997). *Snoring.* [On-line] Clinical Reference Systems. Available: www.realage.com/Library/M_behavior.htm

Hogstel, M. O. (1994). *Nursing care of the older adult* (3rd ed.). Albany, NY: Delmar Publishers.

McCaffery, M., & Pasero. (1999). *Pain: Clinical manual for nursing practice* (2nd ed.). St. Louis, MO: Mosby.

McNeil, R. Padrick, K. & Wellman, J. (1986). "I didn't sleep a wink." *AJN, 86*(1), 26–27.

Moorcraft, W. (1993). *Sleep, dreaming & sleep disorders: An introduction* (2nd ed.). Lanham, MD: University Press of America.

Morgan, D. (1996). *Sleep secrets for shift workers & people with off-beat schedules.* Duluth, MN: Whole Person Associates.

National Sleep Foundation (NSF). (1998a). *ABCs of ZZZs* [On-line]. Available: www.sleepfoundation.org

National Sleep Foundation (NSF). (1998b). *The Nature of Sleep* [On-line]. Available: www.sleepfoundation.org

National Sleep Foundation (NSF). (1998c). *Sleep & Aging* [On-line]. Available: www.sleepfoundation.org

National Sleep Foundation (NSF). (1998d). *Sleep and the Traveler* [On-line]. Available: www.sleepfoundation.org

National Sleep Foundation (NSF). (1998e). *Why Target Sleep?* [On-line]. Available: www.sleepfoundation.org

North American Nursing Diagnosis Association. (1999). *Nursing diagnoses: Definitions and classification, 1999–2000.* Philadelphia: Author.

Pillow Firmness Key to Sleeping Well (1998). [On-line]. Available: www.thirdage.com

Simpson, C. (1996). *Coping with sleep disorders.* New York: Rosen Publishing Group.

Summerfield, C. (1998). *Napping: Men have the edge* [On-line]. Available: www.thirdage.com/health

RESOURCES

National Sleep Foundation, 729 Fifteenth Street, NW, Fourth Floor, Washington, DC, 20005, www.sleepfoundation.org, E-mail: natsleep@erols.com

CHAPTER 20
Safety/Hygiene

REFERENCES/SUGGESTED READINGS

Alexander, B. H., Rivara, F. P., & Wolf, M. E. (1992). The cost and frequency of hospitalization for fall-related injuries in older adults. *American Journal of Public Health, 82*(7), 1020–1023.

Bailey, S. L. (1992). Adolescents' multisubstance use patterns: The role of heavy alcohol and cigarette use. *American Journal of Public Health, 82*(9), 1220–1224.

Bouman, C. C. (1998). Functions of the immune system. In J. Myers & P. Beare, *Adult Health Nursing* (3rd ed.). St. Louis, MO: Mosby.

Carroll, P. (1998). Preventing nosocomial pneumonia. *RN, 61*(6), 44–47.

Easterling, M. (1990). Which of your clients is heading for a fall? *RN, 53*(1), 56–58.

Eriksson, J. H. (1994). *Oncologic nursing* (2nd ed.). Springhouse, PA: Springhouse Corporation.

Food and Drug Administration. (1995, August 23). *FDA safety alert: Entrapment hazards with hospital bed side rails* [On-line]. Available: http://www.fda.gov/cdrh/bedrails.html

Guyton, A. C., & Hall, J. (1996). *Textbook of medical physiology* (9th ed.). Philadelphia: Saunders.

Joint Commission on Accreditation of Healthcare Organizations. (1998). *Hospital accreditation standards*. Oakbrook Terrace, IL: Author.

Mion, L. C., Gregor, S., Buettner, M., Chwirchak, D., Lee, O., & Paras, W. (1989). Falls in the rehabilitation setting: Incidence and characteristics. *Rehabilitation Nursing, 14,* 17–22.

North American Nursing Diagnosis Association. (1999). *Nursing diagnoses: Definitions & classification 1999–2000.* Philadelphia: Author.

Richman, D. (1998). To restrain or not to restrain? *RN, 61*(7), 55–60.

Ruthazer, R., & Lipsitz, L. A. (1993). Antidepressants and falls among elderly people in long-term care. *American Journal of Public Health, 83,* 746–749.

Salladay, S. (1998). Severing the ties that bind. *Nursing98, 28*(5), 30.

Shaffer, S. (1997). Protective mechanisms. In S. Otto (Ed.), *Oncology nursing* (3rd ed.). St. Louis, MO: Mosby.

Stanhope, M., & Knollnueller, R. (1996). *Handbook of community and home health nursing: Tools for assessment, intervention, and education* (2nd ed.). St. Louis, MO: Mosby.

Stillwell, E. (1991). Nurses' education related to the use of restraints. *Journal of Gerontological Nursing, 17*(2), 23–25.

Sullivan-Marx, E. M. (1994). Delirium and physical restraint in the hospitalized elderly. *Image: The Journal of Nursing Scholarship, 26,* 295–300.

Walker, B. (1996). *Injury prevention in the elderly: Preventing falls.* Gaithersberg, MD: Aspen Publishers.

Walker, B. (1998). Preventing falls. *RN, 61*(5), 40–42.

Whedon, M., & Shedol, P. (1989). Prediction and prevention of patient falls. *Image: The Journal of Nursing Scholarship, 21*(2), 108–114.

RESOURCES

Consumer Product Safety Commission, Washington, DC, 20207, 1-800-638-2772

Environmental Protection Agency, Public Information Center, 401 M Street S.W., Washington, DC, 20460, 202-260-2090, www.epa.gov

Food and Drug Administration, Office of Consumer Affairs, 5600 Fishers Lane, Rockville, MD, 20857, 1-888-463-6332, www.fda.gov

Joint Commission on Accreditation of Healthcare Organizations (JCAHO), One Renaissance Boulevard, Oakbrook Terrace, IL, 60181, 630-792-5000, www.jcaho.org

National Institute for Occupational Health and Safety, Clearinghouse for Occupational Safety and Health Information, Technical Information Branch, 4676 Columbia Parkway, Cincinnati, OH, 45226, 1-800-356-4674

CHAPTER 21
Infection Control/Asepsis

REFERENCES/SUGGESTED READINGS

Association for Professionals in Infection Control and Epidemiology, Inc. (APIC). (1996). *Infection control tips on handwashing* [On-line]. Available: www.apic.org/html/cons/washtips/html

Beaumont, E. (1997). Technology scoreboard: Focus on infection control. *American Journal of Nursing, 97*(12), 51–54.

Benenson, A. S. (Ed.). (1995). *Control of communicable diseases in man* (16th ed.). Washington, DC: American Public Health Association.

Benner, J. (1998). Combating infection: Help from the web. *Nursing98, 28*(11), 71–72.

Berlinguer, G. (1992). The interchange of disease and health between the old and new worlds. *American Journal of Public Health, 82*(10), 1407–1414.

Black, J. M., & Matassarin-Jacobs, E. (1997). Medical–surgical nursing: Clinical management for continuity of care (5 ed.). Philadelphia: W.B. Saunders.

Bouman, C. C. (1998). Functions of the immune system. In J. Myers & P. Beare, *Adult health nursing* (3rd ed.). St. Louis, MO: Mosby.

Centers for Disease Control (CDC). (1991). *Recommendations for preventing transmission of human immunodeficiency virus, hepatitis B virus to patients during exposure—prone invasive procedures.* Washington, DC: U.S. Government Printing Office.

Centers for Disease Control. (1992). *Principles of epidemiology: Agent, host, environment* (2nd ed.). Atlanta, GA: Public Health Practice Program Office.

Combating Infection. (1997). Tackling disease transmission. *Nursing97, 27*(7), 65.

Compliance Control Center. (1998). *Hand-transmitted infection* [On-line]. Available: http:\\users.aol.com/comcontrol/cc12htm

DeLaune, S., & Ladner, P. (1998). *Fundamentals of nursing: Standards & practice.* Albany, NY: Delmar Publishing.

Department of Labor. (1991). Bloodborne pathogens rules and regulations. *Federal Register, 58,* 64175–64182.

Ellner, P. D., & Neu, H. C. (1992). *Understanding infectious disease.* St. Louis, MO: Mosby.

Finkelstein, L., & Mendelson, M., with Bailey, E. (1998). Exposure to bloodborne pathogens. *American Journal of Nursing, 98*(3), 67–68.

Guyton, A. C., & Hall, J. (1995). *Textbook of medical physiology* (9th ed.). Philadelphia: Saunders.

Hartstein, A. (1995). Control of methicillin-resistant *Staphylococcus aureus* in a hospital and an intensive care unit. *Infection Control and Hospital Epidemiology, 16*(7), 405–411.

Hegner, B., & Caldwell, E. (1999). *Nursing assistant: A nursing process approach* (8th ed.). Albany, NY: Delmar Publishers.

Hospital Infection Control Practices Advisory Committee (HICPAC). (1995). Recommendations for preventing the spread of vancomycin resistance. *Infection Control and Hospital Epidemiology, 16*(2), 105–113.

Ikeda, R., et al. (1995). Nosocomial tuberculosis: An outbreak of a strain resistant to seven drugs. *Infection Control and Hospital Epidemiology, 16*(3), 152–159.

Infection Control Update 1997. (1997). How to prevent IV catheter contamination. *Nursing97, 27*(6), 60.

National Center for Infectious Disease (NCID). (1997). *Sterilization or disinfection of medical devices: General principles* [On-line]. Available: www.cdc.gov/ncidod/diseases/hip/sterilgp.htm

Nicolle, L. E., & Garibaldi, R. A. (1995). Infection control in long-term-care facilities. *Infection Control and Hospital Epidemiology, 16,* 348–353.

North American Nursing Diagnosis Association (NANDA). (1999). *Nursing diagnoses: Definitions & classification 1999–2000.* Philadelphia: Author.

OSHA Regulations (1996). Bloodborne Pathogens 1910.1.3.(d)(4)(111)(A)(1) [On-line]. Available: http://www.osha.gov/oshstd_data/1910_1030html

Porche, D. J. (1991). Universal precautions. In R. L. Nichols, N. E. Hyslop, & J. G. Bartlett (Eds.), *Decision making in surgical sepsis*. Philadelphia: Decker.

Porche, D. J. (1998). Nursing management of adults with immune disorders. In J. Myers & P. Beare (Eds.), *Adult health nursing* (3rd ed.). St. Louis, MO: Mosby.

Pugliese, G. (1994). EPA begins testing hospital disinfectants as sterilant testing program nears completion. *Infection Control and Hospital Epidemiology, 16*(4), 248–250.

Pugliese, G. (1995). Nursing home fined $75,000 for isolating patient for 9 months. *Infection Control and Hospital Epidemiology, 16*(7), 418.

Satterfield, N. (1995). CDC publishes draft guidelines for isolation. Association for Professionals in Infection Control and Epidemiology, Inc. *Newsletter, 6*(1), 1–2.

Voss, A., & Widner, A.F. (1997). No time for handwashing!? Handwashing versus alcoholic rub: Can we afford 100% compliance? *Infection Control and Hospital Epidemiology, 18*(3), 205–208.

Weltman, A. C., Short, L. J., & Mendelson, M. H. (1995). Disposal-related sharps injuries at a New York City teaching hospital. *Infection Control and Hospital Epidemiology, 16*(5), 268–274.

RESOURCES

Association for Professionals in Infection Control and Epidemiology, Inc. (APIC), 1275 K Street, NW, Suite 1000, Washington, DC, 20005-4006, 202-789-1890, www.apic.org

Environmental Protection Agency (EPA), Disinfectant Hotline, 401 M Street, SW, Washington, DC, 20460-0003, 800-447-6349, Antimicrobial Program Branch, 703-305-7443

Hospital Infection Program (HIP), Office of the Director, HIP Mailstop A07, National Center for Infectious Diseases, Centers for Disease Control and Prevention, 1600 Clifton Rd., Atlanta, GA, 30333, www.cdc.gov/ncidod/hip/

National Foundation for Infectious Diseases, 4733 Bethesda Ave., Suite 750, Bethesda, MD, 20814, 301-656-0003, www.nfid.org

Society for Healthcare Epidemiology of America, 19 Mantua Road, Mt Royal, NJ, 08061, 609-423-0087

CHAPTER 22
Standard Precautions and Isolation

REFERENCES/SUGGESTED READINGS

Borton, D. (1996). Gloves on or off. *Nursing96, 26*(9), 46.

Borton, D. (1997). Isolation precautions: Clearing up the confusion. *Nursing97, 27*(1), 49.

Centers for Disease Control and Prevention (CDC). (1975). *Isolation techniques for use in hospitals* (2nd ed.), (HHS [CDC] Publication No. 80-8314). Washington, DC: U.S. Government Printing Office.

Centers for Disease Control and Prevention (CDC). (1985). Recommendations for preventing transmission of infection with human T-lymphotropic virus type III/lymphadenopathy-associated virus in the workplace. *Morbidity and Mortality Weekly Report (MMWR), 34*, 681–686, 691–695.

Centers for Disease Control and Prevention (CDC). (1987). Recommendations for prevention of HIV transmission in health-care settings. *MMWR, 36*(2S), 1S–18S.

Centers for Disease Control and Prevention (CDC). (1988). Update: Universal precautions for prevention of transmission of human immunodeficiency virus, hepatitis B virus, and other blood borne pathogens in health-care settings. *MMWR, 37*, 377–382, 387–388.

Centers for Disease Control and Prevention (CDC). (1996). Guideline for isolation precautions in hospitals. In *Guidelines for the prevention and control of nosocomial infections*. Atlanta, GA: Author.

Centers for Disease Control and Prevention (CDC)/ Hospital Infection Control Practices Advisory Committee (HICPAC). (1997a). *Part I: Evolution of isolation practices* [On-line]. Available: www.cdc.gov/ncidod/hip/isolat/isopart1.htm

Centers for Disease Control and Prevention (CDC)/ Hospital Infection Control Practices Advisory Committee (HICPAC). (1997b). *Part II. Recommendations for isolation precautions in hospitals* [On-line]. Available: www.cdc.gov/ncidod/hip/isolat/isopart2.htm

Centers for Disease Control and Prevention (CDC)/ Hospital Infection Control Practices Advisory Committee (HICPAC). (1997c). *Table I. Synopsis of types of precautions and patients requiring precautions* [On-line]. Available: www.cdc.gov/ncidod/hip/isolat/isotab_1.htm

Centers for Disease Control and Prevention (CDC)/ Hospital Infection Control Practices Advisory Committee (HICPAC). (1997d). *Table II. Clinical syndromes warranting additional emperic precautions to prevent transmission of epidemiologically important pathogens pending confirmation of diagnosis* [On-line]. Available: www.cdc.gov/ncidod/hip/isolat/isotab_2.htm

Centers for Disease Control and Prevention (CDC)/ Hospital Infection Control Practices Advisory Committee (HICPAC). (1997e). *Appendix A: Type and duration of precautions needed for selected infections and conditions* [On-line]. Available: www.cdc.gov/ncidod/hip/isolat/isoapp_a.htm

Department of Labor. (1991). Bloodborne pathogens rules and regulations. *Federal Register, 58*, 64175–64182.

Ellner, P. D., & Neu, H. C. (1992). *Understanding infectious disease*. St. Louis, MO: Mosby.

Gage, N. D., Landon, J. F., & Sider, M. T. (1959). *Communicable disease*. Philadelphia, PA: F. A. Davis.

Garner, J. S. (1984). Comments on CDC guideline for isolation precautions in hospitals, 1984. *American Journal of Infection Control, 12*, 163.

Garner, J. S., & Simmons, B. P. (1983). *CDC Guideline for Isolation Precautions in Hospitals* (HHS [CDC] Publication No. 83-8314). Atlanta, GA: U.S. Department of Health and Human Services, Public Health Service, Centers for Disease Control. *Infection Control* (1983) 4:245–325; and *American Journal of Infection Control* (1984) 12:103–163.

Haley, R. W., Garner, J. S. & Simmons, B. P. (1985). A new approach to the isolation of patients with infectious diseases: Alternative systems. *Journal of Hospital Infection, 6*, 128–138.

Haley, R. W., & Shachtman, R. H. (1980). The emergence of infection surveillance and control programs in U.S. hospitals: An assessment, 1976. *American Journal of Epidemiology, 111*, 574–591.

Hospital Infection Control Practices Advisory Committee (HICPAC). (1995). Recommendations for preventing the spread of Vancomycin resistance. *Infection Control and Hospital Epidemiology, 16*(2), 105–113.

Lynch, P., Jackson, M. M., Cummings, J., & Stamm, W. E. (1987). Rethinking the role of isolation practices in the prevention of nosocomial infections. *Annals of Internal Medicine, 107*, 243–246.

Lynch, T. (1949). *Communicable Disease Nursing*. St. Louis, MO: Mosby.

National Communicable Disease Center. (1970). *Isolation techniques for use in hospitals* (1st ed., PHS Publication No. 2054). Washington, DC: U.S. Government Printing Office.

North American Nursing Diagnosis Association. (1999). *Nursing diagnoses: Definitions & classification 1999–2000*. Philadelphia: Author.

Occupational Safety and Health Administration (OSHA). (1991). Occupational exposure to bloodborne pathogens: Final rule, 29CRF 1919;1030. *Federal Register, 56,* 64175.

Porche, D. J. (1991). Universal precautions. In R. L. Nichols, N. E. Hyslop, & J. G. Bartlett (Eds.), *Decision making in surgical sepsis*. Philadelphia: Decker.

Porche, D. J. (1998). Nursing management of adults with immune disorders. In P. Beare & J. Myers (Eds.), *Adult health nursing* (3rd ed.). St. Louis, MO: Mosby.

Satterfield, N. (1995). CDC publishes draft guidelines for isolation. *Association for Professionals in Infection Control and Epidemiology, Inc. Newsletter, 6*(1), 1–2.

Schaffner, W. (1980). Infection control: Old myths and new realities. *Infection Control, 1,* 330–334.

RESOURCES

Centers for Disease Control and Prevention, 1600 Clifton Road, Atlanta, GA, 30333, 404-639-3311, www.cdc.gov

CHAPTER 23
Fluid, Electrolyte, and Acid–Base Balance

REFERENCES/SUGGESTED READINGS

Bulechek, G., & McCloskey, J. (1992). *Nursing interventions: Essential nursing treatments* (2nd ed). Philadelphia: Saunders.

Burke, S. (1992). *Human anatomy & physiology in health and disease* (3rd ed.). Albany, NY: Delmar Publishers.

Clayton, K. (1997). Cancer-related hypercalcemia: How to spot it how to manage it. *American Journal of Nursing, 97*(5), 42–48.

DeLaune, S., & Ladner, P. (1998). *Fundamentals of nursing: Practice & standards*. Albany, NY: Delmar Publishers.

Estes, M. E. Z. (1998). *Health assessment & physical examination*. Albany, NY: Delmar Publishers.

Fong, E., Scott, A., Ferris, E., & Skelley, E. (1998). *Body structures and functions* (9th ed.). Albany, NY: Delmar Publishers.

Hartshorn, J., Lamborn, M., & Noll, M. (1997). *Introduction to critical care nursing* (2nd ed.). Philadelphia: Saunders.

Hogstel, M. (1994). *Nursing care of the older adult* (3rd ed.). Albany, NY: Delmar Publishers.

I.V. therapy: Update97. (1997). *Nursing97, 27*(11), 60–61.

Josephson, D. L. (1999). *Intravenous infusion therapy for nurses: Principles and practice*. Albany, NY: Delmar Publishers.

Kee, J., & Paulanka, B. (1999). *Fluids and electrolytes with clinical applications* (6th ed.). Albany, NY: Delmar Publishers.

Mader, S., & Templin, J. M. (1996). *Understanding human anatomy & physiology* (3rd ed.). Dubuque, IA: Wm. C. Brown Publishers.

Marieb, E. (1997). *Essentials of human anatomy & physiology* (5th ed.). Redwood City, CA: The Benjamin/Cummings Publishing Co.

Martini, F., & Welch, K. (1997). *Fundamentals of anatomy and physiology* (4th ed.). Englewood Cliffs, NJ: Prentice-Hall.

Masoorli, S. (1995). Know the pitfalls of I.V. therapy. *NSO Risk Advisor, 20*(2), 1,4.

McFarland, M., & Grant, M. (1994). *Nursing implications of laboratory tests* (3rd ed.). Albany, NY: Delmar Publishers.

Memmler, R., Cohen, B., & Wood, D. (1996). *The human body in health and disease* (8th ed.). Philadelphia: J. B. Lippincott.

Noe, D., & Rock, R. (1994). *Laboratory medicine*. Baltimore: Williams & Wilkins.

North American Nursing Diagnosis Association (NANDA). (1999). *Nursing diagnoses: Definitions & classification 1999–2000*. Philadelphia: Author.

Scanlon, V., & Sanders, T. (1995). *Essentials of anatomy and physiology* (2nd ed.). Philadelphia: F. A. Davis.

Tasota, F., & Wesmiller, S. (1998). Balancing act: Keeping blood pH in equilibrium. *Nursing98, 28*(12), 34–40.

Tate, P., Seeley, R., & Stephens, T. (1994). *Understanding the human body*. St. Louis, MO: Mosby-Year Book.

Thibodeau, G. (1996). *Structure & function of the body* (10th ed.). St. Louis, MO: Mosby-Year Book.

White, J., & Barnes, R. (1983). *Hands on biology, manual* (2nd ed.). Corpus Christi, TX: L P Enterprises.

White, V. (1997). Hyperkalemia. *American Journal of Nursing, 97*(6), 35.

RESOURCES

Intravenous Nurses Society, Fresh Pond Square, 10 Fawcett Street, Cambridge, MA, 02138, 617-441-3008, www.ins1.org

CHAPTER 24
Medication Administration

REFERENCES/SUGGESTED READINGS

American Hospital Formulary Service. (1996). *AHFS drug information 96*. Bethesda, MD: American Society of Hospital Pharmacists.

American Nurses Association. (1997, March/April). *American Nurse, 29*(2), 11.

Asbaghi, Z. (1995). Questions and answers about blood transfusions. *Nursing95, 25*(2), 32C–32G.

Behrman, R. E., Kliegman, R., & Arvin, A. M. (Eds.). (1996). *Nelson textbook of pediatrics* (15th ed.). Philadelphia: Saunders.

Beyea, S. C., & Nicoll, L. H. (1995). Administration of medication via intramuscular route: An integrative review of the literature and research-based protocol for the procedure. *Applied Nursing Research, 8*(1), 23–33.

Beyea, S. C., & Nicoll, L. H. (1996). Back to basics: Administering IM injections the right way. *American Journal of Nursing, 96*(1), 34–35.

Bulechek, G.M., & McCloskey, J.C. (2000). *Nursing interventions: Essential nursing treatments* (3rd ed.). Philadelphia: Saunders.

Daniels, J., & Smith, L. (1999). *Clinical calculations* (4th ed.). Albany, NY: Delmar Publishers.

Drug information for the health care professional (17th ed.). (1997). Rockville, MD: USP Convention.

Fitzpatrick, L., & Fitzpatrick, T. (1997). Blood transfusion: Keeping your patient safe. *Nursing97, 27*(8), 34–41

Goldy, D. (1998). Circulatory overload secondary to blood transfusion. *American Journal of Nursing, 98*(7), 33.

Hartshorn, J., Lamborn, M., & Noll, M. (1997). *Introduction to critical care nursing* (2nd ed.). Philadelphia: Saunders.

I.V. therapy: Update97. (1997). *Nursing97, 27*(11), 60–61.

Josephson, D. L. (1999). *Intravenous infusion therapy for nurses: Principles and practice*. Albany, NY: Delmar Publishers.

Kee, J., & Paulanka, B. (1999). *Fluids and electrolytes with clinical applications* (6th ed.). Albany, NY: Delmar Publishers.

Lehne, R. (1998). *Pharmacology for nursing care* (3rd ed.). Philadelphia: Saunders.

Masoorli, S. (1995). Know the pitfalls of I.V. therapy. *NSO Risk Advisor, 20*(2), 1, 4.

Matheny, N., Wehrle, M. A., Wiersema, L., & Clark, J. (1998). Testing feeding tube placement: Ascultation vs. pH method. *American Journal of Nursing, 98*(5), 37–42.

McConnell, E. (1998). Giving medications through an enteral feeding tube. *Nursing98, 28*(3), 6.

McConnell, E. (1999). Administering a Z-track IM injection. *Nursing99, 29*(1), 26.

North American Nursing Diagnosis Association. (1999). *Nursing diagnoses: Definitions & classification 1999–2000.* Philadelphia: NANDA.

Obenour, P. (1998). Administering an S.C. medication continuously. *Nursing98, 28*(6), 20.

Pickar, G. (1996). *Dosage calculation* (5th ed.). Albany, NY: Delmar Publishers.

Remington: The science and practice of pharmacology (19th ed.). (1995). Easton, PA: Mack Publishing.

Rice, J. (1998). *Medications & mathematics for the nurse* (8th ed.). Albany, NY: Delmar Publishers.

Saxton, D., & O'Neill, N. (1998). *Math and meds for nurses.* Albany, NY: Delmar Publishers.

Shannon, M., Wilson, B., & Stang, C. (1990). *Appleton & Lange's 1999 drug guide.* Norwalk, CT: Appleton & Lange.

Springhouse Corporation. (2000). *Nursing2000 drug handbook.* Springhouse, PA: Author.

Wilson, B., & Shannon, M. (1997). *Dosage calculations: A simplified approach* (3rd ed.). Norwalk, CT: Appleton & Lange.

Wise, M. (1997). Understanding needle-free access devices. *Nursing97, 27*(7), 32.

Spratto, G. & Woods, A. (2000). *PDR nurse's handbook 2000.* Albany, NY: Delmar Publishers.

Wolfrum, J. (1994). A follow-up evaluation to a needle-free IV system. *Nursing Management, 25*(12), 33–35.

RESOURCES

U.S. Pharmacopeia, 12601 Twinbrook Parkway, Rockville, MD, 20852, 800-822-8772, www.usp.gov

CHAPTER 25
Assessment

REFERENCES/SUGGESTED READINGS

American Heart Association (AHA). (1987). *Recommendations for human blood pressure determination.* (AHA Publication No. 701005). Dallas, TX: Author.

Andresen, G. (1998). Assessing the older patient. *RN, 61*(3), 46–55.

Bickley, L. S. (1999). *A guide to physical examination and history taking* (7th ed.). Phildelphia: J. B. Lippincott Company.

Bolander, V. B. (1994). *Basic nursing: A psychophysiologic approach* (3d ed.). Philadelphia: Springhouse.

Bosley, C. L. (1995). Assessing cardiac output: Don't stop at the heart. *Nursing95, 25*(9), 43–45.

Crow, S. (1997). Your guide to gloves. *Nursing97, 27*(3), 26–28.

DeLaune, S., & Ladner, P. (1998). *Fundamentals of nursing: Standards & practice.* Albany, NY: Delmar Publishers.

Estes, M. E. Z. (1998). *Health assessment & physical examination.* Albany, NY: Delmar Publishers.

Firth, P., & Watanabe, S. (1996). *Women's health.* Albany, NY: Delmar Publishers.

Fuller, J., & Schaller-Ayers, J. (1999). *Health assessment: A nursing approach.* Philadelphia: J. B. Lippincott Company.

Gallauresi, B. A. (1998). Pulse oximeters. *Nursing98, 28*(9), 31.

Hanson, C. (1996). *Delmar's instant nursing assessment: Gerontologic.* Albany, NY: Delmar Publishers.

Kirton, C. A. (1997). Assessing bowel sounds. *Nursing97, 27*(3), 64.

Murray, R. B., & Zentner, J. P. (1997). *Health assessment and promotion through the lifespan* (6th ed.). Norwalk: Appleton & Lange.

O'Hanlon-Nichols, T. (1999). Neurologic assessment. *American Journal of Nursing, 99*(6), 44–50.

O'Hanlon-Nichols, T. (1998). Basic assessment series: Musculoskeletal system. *AJN, 98*(6), 48–52.

O'Hanlon-Nichols, T. (1998). Basic assessment series: Gastrointestinal system. *AJN, 98*(4), 48–53.

O'Hanlon-Nichols, T. (1998). Basic assessment series: The adult pulmonary system. *AJN, 98*(2), 39–45.

O'Hanlon-Nichols, T. (1997). Basic assessment series: The adult cardiovascular system. *AJN, 97*(12), 34–40.

Owen, A. (1998). Respiratory assessment revisited. *Nursing98, 28*(4), 48–49.

Rice, K. L. (1998). Sounding out blood flow with a doppler device. *Nursing98, 28*(9), 56–57.

Taylor, C., Lillis, C., & LeMone, P. (1996). *Fundamentals of nursing: The art and science of nursing care* (3d ed.). Philadelphia: J. B. Lippincott Company.

Warner, P., Rowe, T., & Whipple, B. (1999). Shedding light on the sexual history. *AJN, 99*(6), 34–40.

Weber, J. (1997). *Health assessment in nursing.* Philadelphia: J. B. Lippincott Company.

CHAPTER 26
Pain Management

REFERENCES/SUGGESTED READINGS

Agency for Health Care Policy and Research. (1992). *Clinical practice guideline: Acute pain management: Operative or medical procedures and Trauma.* (AHCPR Publication No. 92–0032). Rockville, MD: U.S. Department of Health and Human Services.

Agency for Health Care Policy and Research. (1994). *Clinical practice guideline: Management of cancer pain.* (AHCPR Publication No. 94–0592). Rockville, MD: U.S. Department of Health and Human Services.

American Pain Society. (1992). *Principles of analgesic use in the treatment of acute and chronic cancer pain* (3d ed.). Skokie, IL: Author.

Beecher, H. K. (1956). Relationship of significance of wound to pain experienced. *JAMA, 161,* 1609–1613.

Berkowitz, C. (1997). Epidural pain control—Your job, too. *RN, 60*(8), 22–27.

Bonica, J. J. (Ed.). (1990). *The management of pain* (2d ed.). Philadelphia: Lea and Febiger.

Brand, P., & Yancey, P. (1993). *Pain: The gift nobody wants.* New York: HarperCollins.

Cleeland, C. S., Gonin, R., Hatfield, A. K., Edmonson, J. H., Blum, R. H., Stewart, J. A., & Pandya, K. J. (1994). Pain and its treatment in outpatients with metastatic cancer. *New England Journal of Medicine, 330,* 592–596.

Cousins, N. (1979). *Anatomy of an illness as perceived by the patient.* Toronto: Bantam.

Donovan, M., Dillon, P., & McGuire, L. (1987). Incidence and characteristics of pain in a sample of medical-surgical inpatients. *Pain, 30,* 69–78.

Dubner, R. (1991). Pain and hyperalgesia following tissue injury: New mechanisms and new treatments. *Pain, 44,* 213–214.

Faries, J. (1997a). Taking another route to pain relief. *Nursing97, 27*(6), 28.

Faries, J. (1997b). Assessing pediatric pain. *Nursing97, 27*(8), 18.

Faries, J. (1998a). Easing your patient's postoperative pain. *Nursing98, 28*(6), 58–60.

Faries, J. (1998b). Making a smooth switch from IV analgesia. *Nursing98, 28*(7), 26.

Gordin, P. C. (1990). Assessing and managing agitation in the critically ill infant. *American Journal of Maternal-Child Nursing Journal, 15,* 27–32.

Gordon, D., & Ward, S. (1995). Correcting patient misconceptions about pain. *American Journal of Nursing, 95*(7), 43–45.

Juarez, G. (1995). When culture clashes with pain control. *Nursing95, 25*(5), 90.

Kedziera, P. (1998). The two faces of pain. *RN, 61*(2), 45–46.

Liebeskind J., & Melzack, R. (1987). The International Pain Foundation: Meeting a need for education in pain management. *Pain, 30,* 1–2.

Markey, B. T., & Graham, M. (1997). Management of chronic pain with epidural steriods. *AORN Journal, 65*(4), 791.

McCaffery, M. (1979). *Nursing management of the patient with pain* (2d ed.). Philadelphia: J. B. Lippincott Company.

McCaffery, M., & Beebe, A. (1989). *Pain: Clinical manual for nursing practice.* St. Louis, MO: Mosby.

McCaffery, M., & Pasero, C. (1999). *Pain: Clinical manual* (2nd ed.). St. Louis, MO: Mosby.

McDevitt, M. J. (1995). A(TENS)tion! *Nursing95, 25*(12), 46–47.

McGuire, D. B., Yarbro, C. H., & Ferrell, B. R. (1995). *Cancer pain management* (2d ed.). Boston: Jones and Bartlett.

Melzack, R., & Wall, P. D. (1965). Pain mechanisms: A new theory. *Science, 150,* 971–979.

Merskey, J., & Bogduk, N. (Eds.). (1994). *Classification of chronic pain* (2d ed., pp. 209–214). Task Force on Taxonomy. Seattle, WA: IASP Press.

North American Nursing Diagnosis Association. (1999). *Nursing diagnoses: Definitions and classification, 1999–2000.* Philadelphia: Author.

Olsson, G., & Berde, C. (1993). Differences between nociceptive pain and neuropathic pain. In N. L. Schecter, C. B. Berde, & M. Yaster (Eds.), *Pain in infants, children, and adolescents* (p. 474). Baltimore: Williams & Wilkins.

Page, G. G., Ben-Eliyahu, S., Yirmiya, R., & Liebeskind, J. C. (1993). Morphine attenuates surgery-induced enhancement of metastatic colonization in rats. *Pain, 54*(1), 21–28.

Poulain, P., Langlade, A., & Goldberg, J. (1997). Cancer pain management in the home. *Pain Clinical Updates, 5*(1). Internet access www.halcyon.com/iasp/PCU97a.html.

Schecter, N. L., Berde, C. B., & Yaster, M. (Eds.). (1993). *Pain in infants, children, and adolescents.* Baltimore, MD: Williams & Wilkins.

Spratto, G., & Woods, A. (2000). *PDR® Nurse's Drug Handbook™.* Albany, NY: Delmar Publishers.

Stevens, B. (1994). Nursing management of pain in children. In C. L. Betz, M. M. Hunsberger, & S. Wright (Eds.), *Family-centered nursing care of children* (2nd ed.). Philadelphia: Saunders.

Strevy, S. (1998). Myths and facts about pain. *RN, 61*(2), 42–45.

Thomas, M., & Lundeberg, T. (1996). Does acupuncture work? *Pain Clinical Updates, 4*(3). Internet access www.halcyon.com/iasp/PCU96c.html.

Travell, J., & Rinzler, S. H. (1952). The myofascial genesis of pain. *Postgraduate Medicine, 11,* 425.

Travell, J. G., & Simons, D. G. (1983, 1992). *Travell & Simon's myofascial pain and dysfunction: The trigger point manual* (2d ed.), (Vols. 1 & 2). Baltimore: Williams & Wilkins.

Vasudevan, S. V. (1993). *Pain: A four letter word you can live with.* Milwaukee, WI: Montgomery Media.

Wong, D. L., Hockenberry-Eaton, M., Wilson, D., & Winkelstein, M. L. (1999). *Whaley & Wong's nursing care of infants and children* (6th ed.). St. Louis, MO: Mosby.

World Health Organization. (1986). *Cancer pain relief.* Geneva, Switzerland: Author.

World Health Organization. (1990). Cancer pain relief and palliative care. *Report of a WHO expert committee [World Health Organization Technical Report Series, 804].* Geneva, Switzerland: Author.

Yaster, M., Tobin, J. R., Fisher, Q. A., & Maxwell, L. G. (1994). Local anesthetics in the management of acute pain in children. *Journal of Pediatrics, 124*(2), 165–176.

RESOURCES

Agency for Health Care Policy and Research (AHCPR), Office of Health Care Information, Executive Office Center, Suite 501, 2101 East Jefferson St., Rockville, MD, 20852, www.ahcpr.gov

AHCPR Clearinghouse, P.O. Box 8547, Silver Spring, MD, 20907-8547, 800-358-9295, www.ahcpr.gov

- Clinical Practice Guideline for managing acute pain. Available in three formats: (1) The clinical practice guideline (Publication No. 92-0032); (2) Quick reference guides (Adults—No. 92-0019 and Pediatric—No. 92-0020); and (3) Pain Control after Surgery: A Patient's Guide (No. 92-0021)
- Clinical Practice Guideline for managing cancer pain. Available in three formats: (1) The clinical practice guideline (Publication No. 94-0592); (2) Quick reference guides (Adults—No. 94-0593 and Pediatric—No. 92-0594); and (3) Patient's Guide (No. 94-0595)

American Chronic Pain Association, c/o P. Cowan, P.O. Box 850, Rocklin, CA, 95677-0850, 916-632-0922, www.theacpa.org/

American Pain Society (APS), 4700 W. Lake Avenue, Glenview, IL, 60025, 375-4715, www.ampainsoc.org

American Society of Pain Management Nurses, 7794 Grow Drive, Pensacola, FL, 32514, 888-342-7766

International Association for the Study of Pain (IASP), 909 Forty-third Street N.E., Suite 306, Seattle, WA, 98105-6020, 206-547-6409, www.halcyon.com/iasp

National Chronic Pain Outreach Association, P.O. Box 274, Millboro, VA, 24460-0274

National Committee on Treatment of Intractable Pain, P.O. Box 9553, Friendship Station, Washington, DC, 20016-1553, 202-944-8140

National Headache Foundation, 428 W. St. James Place, 2nd Floor, Chicago, IL, 60614-2750, 800-843-2256, www.headaches.org

National Hospice Organization, 1901 North Moore Street, Suite 901, Arlington, VA, 22209-1714, 703-243-5900, 800-646-6460, www.nho.org

Journals

Chronic Pain Letter, Box 1303, Old Chelsea Station, New York, NY, 10011

The Clinical Journal of Pain, Lippincott Williams & Wilkins, 2275 Washington Square, Philadelphia, PA, 19106, 800-638-3030

The Journal of Pain and Symptom Management, Elsevier Publishing Co., Inc., Journal Fulfillment Department, P.O. Box 882, Madison Square Station, New York, NY, 10160-0200

Pain, International Association for the Study of Pain, 909 Forty-third Street N.E., Suite 306, Seattle, WA, 98105-6020, 206-547-6409

CHAPTER 27
Diagnostic Tests

REFERENCES/SUGGESTED READINGS

Baer, D., Baillie, A., & Naito, H. (1993). A guide to in-office testing. *Patient Care, 28*(3), 78–101.

Beattie, S. (1999). Cut the risks for cardiac cath patients. *RN, 62*(1), 50–54.

Dammel, T. (1997). Fecal occult-blood testing: Looking for hidden danger. *Nursing97, 27*(7), 44–45.

DeLaune, S., & Ladner, P. (1998). *Fundamentals of nursing: Standards & Practice.* Albany, NY: Delmar Publishers.

Gallauresi, B. (1998). Pulse oximeters. *Nursing98, 28*(9), 31.

Gibbar-Clements, T., Shirrell, D., & Free, C. (1997). PT and APTT: Seeing beyond the numbers. *Nursing97, 27*(7), 49–51.

Guyton, A. C. & Hall, J., (1996). *Textbook of medical physiology* (9th ed.). Philadelphia: Saunders.

Hill, J., & Newton, J. (1998). Contrast echo: Your role at the bedside. *RN, 61*(10), 32–35.

Hospital Nursing Section. (1995). Interpreting ECF waveform components. *Nursing95, 25*(6), 32C-32F.

Laxson, C., & Titler, M. (1994). Drawing coagulation studies from arterial lines: An integrated literature review. *American Journal of Critical Care, 3*(1), 16–23.

McFarland, M., & Grant, M. (1994). *Nursing implications of laboratory tests* (3rd ed.). Albany, NY: Delmar Publishers.

Montes, P. (1997). Managing outpatient cardiac catheterization. *American Journal of Nursing, 97*(8), 34–37.

National Center for Health Statistics. (1998). *Deaths/mortality* [On-line]. Available: www.cdc.gov/nchswww/fastats/deaths.htm

Noe, D., & Rock, R. (1994). *Laboratory medicine.* Baltimore: Williams & Wilkins.

Siconolfi, L. (1995). Clarifying the complexity of liver function test. *Nursing95, 25*(5), 39–44.

Somerson, S., Husted, C. & Sicilia, M. (1995). Insights into conscious sedation. *American Journal of Nursing, 95*(6), 26–33.

Thompson, M., & Coppens, N. (1994). The effects of guided imagery on anxiety levels and movement of clients undergoing magnetic resonance imaging. *Holistic Nurse Practice, 8*(2), 59–69.

Wolfe, S. (1997). The great mammogram debate. *RN, 60*(8), 41–44.

RESOURCES

National Library of Medicine, www.nlm.nih.gov (then click on "Search MEDLINE")

National Network of Libraries of Medicine (NN/LM) Regional Medical Libraries, 1-800-338-7657

CHAPTER 28
Anesthesia

REFERENCES/SUGGESTED READINGS

Abouleish, E., Rawal, N., & Rashad, M. N. (1991). The addition of 0.2 mg subarachnoid morphine to hyperbaric bupivacaine for cesarean delivery: A prospective study of 856 cases. *Regional Anesthesia, 16,* 137–140.

Ben-David, B., Vaida, S., Collins, G., Naum, M., & Gaitini, L. (1994). Transient paraplegia secondary to an epidural catheter. *Anesthesia & Analgesia, 79,* 598–600.

Berkowitz, C. (1997). Epidural pain control—Your job, too. *RN, 60*(8), 22–27.

Brockway, M. S., Noble, D. W., Sharwood-Smith, G.H., & Mc-Clure, J. H. (1990). Profound respiratory depression after extradural fentanyl. *British Journal of Anaesthesia, 64,* 243–245.

Bromage, P. R. (1993). Nerve injury and paralysis related to spinal and epidural anesthesia. *Regional Anesthesia, 18,* 481–484.

Camann, W. R., Murray, R. S., Mushlin, P. S., & Lambert, D. H. (1990). Effects of oral caffeine on postdural puncture headache: A double-blind, placebo-controlled trial. *Anesthesia & Analgesia, 70,* 181–184.

Carp, H., Singh, P. J., Vadhera, R., & Jayaram, A. (1994). Effects of the serotonin-receptor agonist sumatriptan on postdural puncture headache: Report of six cases. *Anesthesia & Analgesia, 79,* 180–182.

Cohen, D. E., Van Duker, B., Siegel, S., & Keon, T. P. (1993). Common peroneal nerve palsy associated with epidural analgesia. *Anesthesia & Analgesia, 76,* 429–431.

Dickman, C. A., Shedd, S. A., Spetzler, R. F., Shetter, A.G., & Sonntag, V. K. H. (1990). Spinal epidural hematoma associated with epidural anesthesia: Complications of systemic heparinization in patients receiving peripheral vascular thrombolytic therapy. *Anesthesiology, 72,* 947–950.

Horlocker, T. T., Wedel, D. J., & Offord, K. P. (1990). Does preoperative antiplatelet therapy increase the risk of hemorrhagic complications associated with regional anesthesia? *Anesthesia & Analgesia, 70,* 631–634.

Horlocker, T. T., Wedel, D. J., Schroeder, D. R., Rose, S. H., Elliott, B.A., McGregor, D. G., & Wong, G. Y. (1995). Preoperativeantiplatelet therapy does not increase the risk of spinal hematoma associated with regional anesthesia. *Anesthesia & Analgesia, 80,* 303–309.

Kilbride, J. M., Senagore, A. J., Mazier, W. P., Ferguson, C., & Ufkes, T. (1992). Epidural analgesia. *Gynecology and Obstetrics, 174,* 137–140.

Kroll, D. A., Caplan, R. A., Posner, K., Ward, R. J., & Cheney, F. W. (1990). Nerve injury associated with anesthesia. *Anesthesiology, 73,* 202–207.

Liu, S., Chiu, A. A., Carpenter, R. L., Mulroy, M. F., Allen, H. W., Neal, J. M., & Pollock, J. E. (1995). Fentanyl prolongs lidocaine spinal anesthesia without prolonging recovery. *Anesthesia & Analgesia, 80,* 730–734.

Naber, L., Jones, G., & Halm, M. (1994). Epidural analgesia: For effective pain control. *Critical Care Nurse, 14*(5), 69.

Onishchuk, J. L., & Carlsson, C. (1992). Epidural hematoma associated with epidural anesthesia: Complications of anticoagulant therapy. *Anesthesiology, 77,* 1221–1223.

Phillips, S., Hutchinson, S., & Davidson, T. (1993). Preoperative drinking does not affect gastric contents. *British Journal of Anaesthesia, 70,* 6–9.

Scott, J. C., & Stanski, D. R. (1987). Decreased fentanyl and alfentanil dose requirements with age: A simultaneous pharmacokinetic and pharmacodynamic evaluation. *Journal of Pharmacology and Experimental Therapeutics, 240,* 159–166.

Soreide, E., Holst-Larsen, H., Reite, K., Mikkelsen, H., Sorejde, J. A., & Steen, P. A. (1993). Effects of giving water 20–450 ml with oral diazepam premedication 1–2 h before operation. *British Journal of Anaesthesia, 71,* 503–506.

Yasuda, N., Lockhart, S. H., & Eger, E. I., II (1991). Kinetics of desflurane, isoflurane, and halothane in humans. *Anesthesiology, 74,* 489–498.

RESOURCES

American Association of Nurse Anesthetists, 222 South Prospect Avenue, Park Ridge, IL, 60068-4001, 847-692-7050, Fax 847-692-6068, www.aana.com

American Journal of Anesthesiology, 26 Main Street, Chatham, NJ, 07928-2402, 973-701-8900, www. amjanesthesiology.com

American Society of Anesthesiologists, 520 N. Northwest Highway, Park Ridge, IL, 60068-2573, 847-825-5586, Fax 847-825-1692, www.asahq.org

American Society of Peri Anesthesia Nurses, 6900 Grove Road, Thorofare, NJ, 08086, 609-845-5557, Fax 609-848-1881, www.aspan.org

American Society of Regional Anesthesia, PO Box 11086, Richmond, VA, 23230-1086, 804-282-0010, Fax 804-282-0090, www.asra.com

Anesthesia Patient Safety Foundation, Room 9562 E. B., 1400 Locust Street, Pittsburgh, PA, 15219-5166, e-mail info@apsf.org

Foundation for Anesthesia Education and Research, Charlton Building, Mayo Clinic, 200 First Street SW, Rochester, MN, 55905, 507-266-6866, Fax 507-284-0120, www.faer.org

Society for Education in Anesthesia, 1910 Byrd Avenue, Suite 100, PO Box 11086, Richmond, VA, 23230-1086, 804-282-5427, http://anesthesia.ccf.org:8080/sea

CHAPTER 29
Nursing Care of the Surgical Client

REFERENCES/SUGGESTED READINGS

Aldrete, J. (1995). The post-anesthesia recovery score revisited. *Journal of Clinical Anesthesiology, 7*(1), 89–91.

Association of Operating Room Nurses (1995a). *Standards and recommended practices.* Denver, CO: Author.

Association of Operating Room Nurses. (1995b) Surgical attire; recommended practices; biological monitors; sterile packages. *AORN Journal, 61*(5).

Atkinson, L., & Fortunato, N. (1996). *Berry & Kohn's operating room technique* (8th ed.). St. Louis, MO: Mosby-Year Book.

Beare, P. G., & Myers, J. L. (1998). *Adult health nursing* (3rd ed.). St. Louis, MO: Mosby-Year Book.

Black, J. M., & Matassarin-Jacobs, E. (1997). *Luckmann and Sorensen's medical–surgical nursing: A psychophysiologic approach* (5th ed.). Philadelphia: W.B. Saunders.

Bryant, R. A. (Ed.). (1992). *Acute and chronic wounds: Nursing management.* St. Louis, MO: Mosby-Year Book.

Burden, N. (1993). *Ambulatory surgical nursing.* Philadelphia: W. B. Saunders.

Cizzell, J. (1994). Back to basics: Test your wound assessment skills. *AJN, 94*(6), 34–35.

Erwin-Toth, P., & Hocevar, B. (1995). Wound care: Selecting the right dressing. *AJN, 95*(2), 46–51.

Fairchild, S. (1993). *Perioperative nursing: Principles and practice.* Boston: Jones and Bartlett.

Gilchrist, B. (1990). Washing and dressings after surgery. *Journal of the Wound Care Society, 86*(50), 71.

Goodman, K. (1995, September). Transitional diet. *Current topics in nutrition support.* Fort Wayne, IN: Lutheran Hospital of Indiana, Inc.

Goodman, K. (1995, October). Post-op or transitional feeding. *Current topics in nutrition support.* Fort Wayne, IN: Lutheran Hospital of Indiana, Inc.

Hogstel, M. (1994). *Nursing care of the older adult* (3rd ed). Albany, NY: Delmar Publishers.

Ignatavicius, D. D., Workman, M. L., & Mishler, M. A. (1999). *Medical–surgical Nursing Across the Health Care Continuum* (3rd ed.). Philadelphia: W. B. Saunders.

Lewis, S. M., Collier, I. C., & Heitkemper, M. M. (1996). *Medical–surgical nursing: Assessment and management of clinical problems* (4th ed.). St. Louis, MO: Mosby-Year Book.

Litwack, K. (1995). *Post anesthesia care nursing* (2nd ed.). St. Louis, MO: Mosby-Year Book.

Motta, G. (1993). How moisture retentive dressings promote healing. *Nursing 93, 23*(12), 26–33.

Phipps, W. J., Cassmeyer, V. L., Sands, J. K., & Lehman, M. K. (1999). *Medical–surgical nursing: Concepts and clinical practice* (6th ed.). St. Louis, MO: Mosby-Year Book.

Smeltzer, S. C., & Bare, B. G. (1996). *Brunner and Suddarth's textbook of medical–surgical nursing* (8th ed.). Philadelphia: Lippincott-Raven.

Talabiska, D. G. (1995). Malnutrition in the elderly. *Newlines in Multi-Vitamin Infusion, 4*(2), 1, 2, 6.

RESOURCES

American Board of Post Anesthesia Nursing Certification, 6900 Grove Road, Thorofare, NJ, 08086, 609-845-5557

Association of Operating Room Nurses (AORN), 2170 South Parker Road, Suite 300, Denver, CO, 80231, 303-755-6300

National Second Surgical Opinion Program, Administrative Office of Public Affairs, 330 Independence Avenue SW, Washington, DC, 20201, 1-800-638-6833, 202-245-6183

CHAPTER 30
Nursing Care of the Oncology Client

REFERENCES/SUGGESTED READINGS

Agency for Health Care Policy and Research. (1994). *Clinical practice guidelines: Management of cancer pain* (AHCPR Publication No. 94-0592). Rockville, MD: U.S. Department of Health & Human Services.

Alfaro-LeFevre, R., Blicharz, M., Flynn, A., & Boyer, M. (1992). *Drug Handbook: A nursing process approach.* Redwood, CA: Addison-Wesley.

American Cancer Society. (1998). Cancer facts and figures—1998. Atlanta, GA: Author.

American Pain Society. (1992). *Principles of analgesic use in the treatment of acute and chronic cancer pain* (3d ed.). Skokie, IL: Author.

Baird, S., Donehower, M., Stalsbroten, V., & Ades, T. (Eds.) (1997). *A cancer source book for nurses* (7th ed.). Atlanta, GA: American Cancer Society.

Belcher, A. (1992). *Cancer nursing.* St. Louis, MO: Mosby-Year Book.

Blackburn, G. (1998). Wasting away: Cancer cachexia. *Health News, 4*(4), 4. Waltham, MA: Massachusetts Medical Society.

Bral, E. (1998). Caring for adults with chronic cancer pain. *American Journal of Nursing, 4*(98), 27–32.

Carrol, D. (1993, September). Managing cancer pain. *Nursing Times, 89*(38), 69–70.

Chiramannil, A. (1998). Lung Cancer. *American Journal of Nursing, 4*(98), 46–47.

Erickson, J. (1994, November). Update on Hodgkin's Disease. *Nurse Practitioner,* 63–67.

Estes, M. E. Z. (1998). *Health assessment & physical examination.* Albany, NY: Delmar Publishers.

Frye, J. (1993). An overview on oncologic emergencies. *Highlights on Antineoplastic Drugs, 11*(1), 2–4.

Hansen, C. (1995, January). Colorectal cancer: A preventable disease. *Physician Assistant,* 15–26.

Held-Warmkessel, J. (1998). Chemotherapy complications: Helping your patient cope with adverse reactions. *Nursing98 4*(28), 41–45.

Kediziera, P. (1998). The two faces of pain. *RN, 61*(2), 45–46.

Kohr, J. (1995). Measuring your patient's pain. *RN, 58*(4), 39–40.

Lewis, S. & Collier, I. (1996). *Medical–surgical nursing: Assessment and management of clinical problems* (4th ed.). St. Louis, MO: Mosby-Year Book.

Lundquist, D., & Stewart, F. M. (1994, October). An update on non-Hodgkin's lymphomas. *Nurse Practitioner,* 41–54.

Mandel, J. S., Bond, J. H., et al. (1993). Reducing mortality from colorectal cancer by screening for fecal occult blood. *New England Journal of Medicine, 328*(19), 1365.

McCaffery, M., & Ferrell, B. (1994, July). How to use the new AHCPR cancer pain guidelines. *American Journal of Nursing,* 42–47.

McCarron, E. (1995, June). Supporting the families of cancer patients. *Nursing95,* 48–51.

Noonan, E. (1998, May 4). Drug combination found to eliminate cancer in mice. *Corpus Christi Caller Times.*

Ottery, F. (1994, March/April). Cancer cachexia prevention, early diagnosis and management. *Cancer Practice, 2*(2), 123–131.

Otto, S. (1997). *Oncology nursing* (3rd ed.). St. Louis, MO: Mosby-Year Book.

Phipps, W. J., Sands, Marek, J. F., (1999). *Medical-Surgical Nursing: Concepts and Clinical Practice* (6th ed.). St. Louis, MO: Mosby-Yearbook.

Porth, C. (1998). *Pathophysiology concepts of altered health states* (5th ed.), Philadelphia: J. B. Lippincott Company.

Researchers say new drug may boost effects of cancer radiation. (1998, May 12). *Corpus Christi Caller Times.*

Robuck, J., & Fleetwood, J. (1993). Nutritional support of the patient with cancer. *Capsules and Comments in Oncology Nursing, 1*(1), 20–30.

Scherer, J., & Timby, B. (1999). *Introductory medical–surgical nursing* (7th ed.). Philadelphia: J. B. Lippincott Company.

Schweid, L., & Werner-McCullough, M. (1994, September). Will you recognize these oncological crises? *RN,* 23–27.

Smeltzer, S., & Bare, B. (1996). *Brunner and Suddarth's textbook of medical–surgical nursing* (8th ed.). Philadelphia: J. B. Lippincott Company.

Tamoxifen for breast cancer prevention. (1998, December 15). *Healthnews, 4*(15).

Varricchio, C. (1994, July/August). Human and indirect cost of home care. *Nursing Outlook,* 151–157.

Weber, M. (1995, April). Clinical snapshot: Chemotherapy-induced nausea and vomiting. *American Journal of Nursing.*

White, L., & Spitz, M. (1994). Cancer risk and early detection assessment. *Capsules and Comments in Oncology Nursing, 2*(1), 2–3.

Wood, L., & Gullo, S. (1993). IV Vesicants: How to avoid extravasation. *American Journal of Nursing, 93*(4), 42–46.

Woodward, W., & Thobaben, M. (1994). Special home health care nursing challenges: Patients with cancer. *Home Health Care Nurse, 12*(3), 33–37.

RESOURCES

American Cancer Society (ACS), 1599 Clifton Road, NE, Atlanta, GA, 30329, 1-800-ACS-2345

National Alliance of Breast Cancer Organizations, 212-719-0154

National Coalition for Cancer Survivorship, 301-650-8868

Office of Cancer Communications, National Cancer Institute, Building 31, Room 10A24, Bethesda, MD, 20892, 1-800-4-CANCER, www.nci.nih.gov

Y-ME National Organization for Breast Cancer Information and Support, 1-800-221-2141

CHAPTER 31
Nursing Care of the Client: Respiratory System

REFERENCES/SUGGESTED READINGS

American Cancer Society (ACS). (1998). *Cancer facts and figures 1998.* Atlanta, GA: Author.

Avey, M. A. (1993). TB skin testing: How to do it right. *American Journal of Nursing, 93*(9), 42–44.

Borkgren, M. W., & Gronkiewicz. (1995). Update your asthma care: From hospital to home. *American Journal of Nursing, 95*(1), 26–34.

Boutotte, J. (1993, May). T.B.: The second time around and how you can help to control it. *Nursing93, 23*(5), 42–49.

Centers for Disease Control and Prevention (CDC). (1993). *TB facts for health care workers.* (No. 00-5655). Atlanta, GA: Author.

Centers for Disease Control and Prevention (CDC). (1994a). *Core curriculum on tuberculosis.* Atlanta, GA: U.S. Department of Health & Human Services.

Centers for Disease Control and Prevention (CDC). (1994b). *Questions and answers about TB* [On-line]. Available: www.cdc.gov/nchstp/faqs/qa.htm#intro_3

deWit, S. (1998). *Keane's essentials of medical–surgical nursing.* (4th ed.). Philadelphia. W. B. Saunders Company.

Grimes, D. E., & Grimes, R. M. (1995). Tuberculosis: What nurses need to know to control the epidemic. *Nursing Outlook, 43*(4), 164–173.

Jones, L., & Hannum, D. (1998). Playing it safe with a particulate respirator. *Nursing98, 28*(1), 50–51.

Loeb, S., et al. (Eds.). (1991). *Diagnostic test implications.* Springhouse, PA: Springhouse Corporation.

O'Hanlon-Nichols, T. (1998). Basic assessment series: The adult pulmonary system. *American Journal of Nursing, 98*(2), 39–45.

Owen, A. (1998). Respiratory assessment revisited. *Nursing98, 28*(4), 48–49.

Prentice, D., & Ahrens, T. (1994). Pulmonary complications of trauma. *Critical Care Nursing Quarterly, 17*(2), 24–33.

Ritchie, J. A., & Hagel, C. L. (1994). Asthma: A new look at helium therapy. *RN, 57*(9), 18–21.

Robertson, O. (1995, March). Penetrating chest trauma. *Nursing95, 25*(3), 33.

Shaw, T. (1995). The resurgence of tuberculosis: Current issues for nursing. *Nursing Times, 91*(40), 35–37.

Skelskey, C., & Leshem, O. (1997). Tuberculosis surveillance in long-term care. *American Journal of Nursing, 97*(10), 16BBBB–16DDDD.

Smith, R. N., Fallentine, J., & Kessel, S. (1995, February). Underwater chest drainage: Bringing the facts to the surface. *Nursing95, 25*(2), 60–67.

Steismeyer, J. (1993). A four step approach to pulmonary assessment. *American Journal of Nursing, 93*(8), 22–31.

Ulrich, S. A., Canale, S. W., & Wendall, S. A. (1997). *Medical–surgical nursing care planning guide* (4th ed.). Philadelphia: W. B. Saunders Company

Wallace, C. (1998). Emergency! Acute pulmonary edema. *RN, 61*(1), 37–40.

RESOURCES

American Cancer Society (ACS), 1599 Clifton Road, NE, Atlanta, GA, 30329, 1-800-ACS-2345, www.cancer.org

American Lung Association, 1740 Broadway, New York, NY, 10019, 212-315-8700

American Thoracic Society, 1740 Broadway, New York, NY, 10019-4374, 212-315-8808

Centers for Disease Control and Prevention (CDC), Division of Tuberculosis Elimination, 1600 Clifton Road, Mailstop E-10, Atlanta, GA, 30333, 404-639-8120

Cystic Fibrosis Foundation, 6931 Arlington Road, Bethesda, MD, 20814, 1-800-FIGHT-CF (344-4823), www.cff.org

International Association of Laryngectomies, 7440 North Shadeland Avenue, Suite 100, Indianapolis, IN, 46250, 317-570-4568, www.larynxlink.com/ial/ial/.htm, (Lost Chord and New Voice clubs are member clubs of this organization.)

CHAPTER 32
Nursing Care of the Client: Cardiovascular System

REFERENCES/SUGGESTED READINGS

American Heart Association. (1997). "Borderline" high systolic blood pressure raises risk of stroke, heart attack, and death [On-line]. Available: www.americanheart.org/Whats_News/AHA_News_Release/974510.html

American Heart Association. (1999a). Cardiovascular diseases [On-line]. Available: www.amhrt.org/statistics/03cardio.html

American Heart Association. (1999b). Cardiovascular disease statistics [On-line]. Available: www.amhrt.org/Heart_and_Stroke_A_Z_Guide/cvds.html

American Heart Association. (1999c). Coronary heart disease and angina pectoris [On-line]. Available: www.amhrt.org/Statistics/04crnry.html

American Heart Association. (1999d). High blood pressure [On-line]. Available: www.americanheart.org/statistics/06/hghbld.html

American Heart Association. (1999e). Rheumatic heart disease statistics [On-line]. Available: www.amhrt.org/Heart_and_Stroke_A_Z_Guide/hds.html

American Heart Association. (1999f). Risk factors and coronary heart disease [On-line]. Available: www.amhrt.org/Heart_and_Stroke_A_Z_Guide/cvds.html

American Heart Association. (1999g). Women, heart disease and stroke [On-line]. Available: www.amhrt.org/Heart_and_Stroke_A_Z_Guide/women.html

Arbour, R. (1994). Complete heart block. *Nursing94, 8, 33.*

Beare, P., & Myers, J. L. (1998). *Principles and practice of adult health nursing* (3d ed.). St. Louis, MO: Mosby-Year Book.

Beattie, S. (1993). CABG surgery: The second time around. *American Journal of Nursing, 8,* 42–45.

Beattie, S. (1999). Cut the risks for cardio cath patients. *RN, 62*(1), 50–54.

Bove, L. A. (1995). Now! Surgery for heart failure. *RN, 5,* 26–31.

Bright, L. D. (1995). Deep vein thrombosis. *American Journal of Nursing, 6,* 48–49.

Clinical update 95: Hypertension white-coat warning. (1995). *Nursing95, 6,* 54.

Coronary angiography: Heads up. (1994). *Nursing94, 12,* 32Q.

Cuddy, R. (1995). Hypertension: Keeping dangerous blood pressure down. *Nursing95, 8,* 34–43.

Goldman, H. (1994). Myocardial infarction—Diagnosis and treatment. *Nursing Times, 90*(16), 33–37.

Halm, M., & Penque, S. (1999). Heart disease in women. *American Journal of Nursing, 99*(4), 26–31.

Hasemeier, C. (1996). Permanent pacemaker: What you need to know to prepare a patient for this intervention. *American Journal of Nursing, 96*(2), 30–31.

Heart and stroke facts: 1996 Statistical supplement. (1996). American Heart Association.

Hickey, A. (1994). Catching deep vein thrombosis in time. *Nursing94, 10,* 34–42.

Hicks, S. L. (1994). Standing guard against silent ischemia and infarction. *Nursing94, 1,* 34–39.

Hiller, G. (1999). Atrial fibrillation. *Nursing99, 29*(2), 27–31.

Hole, Jr., J. W. (1993). *Human anatomy and physiology* (6th ed.). Dubuque, IA: Wm. C. Brown Publishers.

Janowski, M. J. (1996). Managing heart failure. *RN, 2,* 34–39.

Kudenchuk, P., Maynard, C., Martin, J., Wirkus, M., & Weaver, W. D. (1996). Comparison of presentation, treatment, and outcome of acute myocardial infarction in men versus women (the Myocardial Infarction Triage and Intervention Registry). *American Journal of Cardiology, 78,* 9–14.

Lazzara, D. (1999). Shocking facts about semiautomatic defibrillation. *Nursing99, 29*(4), 55–57.

Lewis, A. M. (1999). Cardiovascular emergency. *Nursing99, 29*(6), 49–51.

Lewis, S., & Collier, I. (1996). Medical–surgical nursing: Assessment and management of clinical problems (4th ed.). St. Louis, MO: Mosby–Year Book, Inc.

Linton, A., Matteson, M. A., & Maebius, N. K. (1995). *Introductory nursing care of adults.* Philadelphia: W. B. Saunders Company.

Mancini, M. E., & Kaye, W. (1999). AEDs: Changing the way you respond to cardiac arrest. *American Journal of Nursing, 99*(5), 26–30.

McDermott, B., & Deglin, J. (1994). *Understanding basic pharmacology: Practical approaches for effective application.* Philadelphia: F. A. Davis Company.

McKinney, B. (1999). Solving the puzzle of heart failure. *Nursing99, 29*(5), 33–39.

Megerman, J. (1995). Prophylaxis against venous thromboembolism after hip surgery. *JAMA, 273*(4), 287.

Merriam Webster Medical Dictionary. (1995). America on Line Reference Desk.

Monahan, F. D., Drake, T., & Neighbors, M. (1998). *Nursing care of adults* (2nd ed.). Philadelphia: W. B. Saunders Company.

Mosca, L., Manson, J. E., Sutherland, S. E., Langer, R. D., Manolio, T., & Barrett-Connor, E. (1997). Cardiovascular disease in women. American Heart Association [On-line]. Available: www.amhrt.org/Scientific/statements/1997/109701.html

Mosley, M., Oenning, V., & Melinik, G. (1999). Methemoglobinemia. *American Journal of Nursing, 99*(5), 47.

Olbrych, D. D. (1993). Interpreting C.P.K. and L.D.H. results. *Nursing93, 1,* 48–49.

Pagana, K. D., & Pagana, T. J. (1995). *Mosby's diagnostic and laboratory test reference.* St. Louis, MO: Mosby–Year Book, Inc.

Phipps, W. J., Cassemeyer, V. L., Sands, J. K., & Lehman, M. K. (1999). *Medical–surgical nursing: Concepts and clinical practice* (6th ed.). St. Louis, MO: Mosby–Year Book, Inc.

Raimer, F., & Thomas, M. (1995). Clot stoppers. *Nursing95, 3,* 34–43.

Research roundup. (1994). *Nursing94, 12,* 32Q.

Roger, V. L., Pellikka, P. A., Bell, M. R., Chow, C. W., Bailey, K. R., & Seward, J. B. (1997). Sex and test verification bias. Impact on the diagnostic value of exercise echocardiography. *Circulation, 95,* 405–410.

Ross, G. K., & DeJong, M. J. (1999). Pericardial tamponade. *American Journal of Nursing, 99*(2), 35.

Rowland, R. (Medical Correspondent). (1995, December 20). High blood pressure can lower men's cognitive skills. *Internet CNN Health Briefs.*

Sandler, R. L. (1994). Atrial fibrillation. *American Journal of Nursing, 12,* 26–27.

Sandler, R. L. (1995). Abdominal aortic aneurysm. *American Journal of Nursing, 1,* 38–39.

Scherer, J.C., & Timby, B. K. (1999). *Introductory medical–surgical nursing* (7th ed.). Philadelphia: J.B. Lippincott Company.

The Sixth Report of the Joint National Committee on Prevention, Detection, Evaluation, and Treatment of High Blood Pressure. (1997). NIH Publication 98-4080. Joint National Committee on Prevention, Detection, Evaluation, and Treatment of High Blood Pressure. Bethesda, MD: National Institutes of Health.

Sommers, M. (1994). *Concepts and activities: Medical–surgical nursing.* Springhouse, PA: Springhouse Corporation.

Spratto, G.R., & Woods, A.L. (2000). *PDR® Nurse's Drug Handbook™.* Albany, NY: Delmar Publishers.

Spratto, G. R., & Woods, A. L. (1997). *RN Magazine's NDR-95: Nurse's Drug Reference.* Albany, NY: Delmar Publishers.

Stephenson, J. (1992). The cold facts. *Harvard Health Letter, 17*(3), 1–4.

Strimike, C. L. (1995). Caring for a client with an intracoronary stent. *American Journal of Nursing, 1,* 40–46.

Swearingen, P. L. (1998). *Manual of medical–surgical nursing care: Nursing interventions and collaborative management* (4th ed.). St. Louis, MO: Mosby–Year Book, Inc.

Therapy in action: AICD patient handbook. (1995). Guidant Corporation Cardiac Pacemakers.

Whitaker, L., & Kelleher, A. (1994). Raynaud's syndrome: Diagnosis and treatment. *Journal of Vascular Nursing, 12*(1), 10–13.

Williams, N. (1994). Hand arm vibration syndrome. *Occupational Health, 3,* 89–90.

Woods, A. D. (1999). Managing hypertension. *Nursing99, 29*(3), 41–46.

RESOURCES

American Heart Association, National Center, 7272 Greenville Avenue, Dallas, TX, 75231-4596, 800-242-8721, http://www.amhrt.org

The Coronary Club, Inc., 9500 Euclid Avenue, Mail Code A42, Cleveland, OH, 44195, 216-444-3690

The Mended Hearts, Inc., 7272 Greenville Avenue, Dallas, TX, 75231, 214-706-1442, www.mendedhearts.org

National Cholesterol Education Program Information Center, P.O. Box 30105, Bethesda, MD, 20824-0105, 301-251-1222, 301-951-3260, www.nhlbi.nih.gov/nhlbi

National Heart, Lung, and Blood Institute Information Center, Public Health Service, P.O. Box 30105, Bethesda, MD, 20824, 301-251-1222, www.nhlbi.nih.gov

President's Council on Physical Fitness and Sports, Hubert Humphrey Building, Room 758H, 200 Independence Avenue S.W., Washington, DC, 20201, 202-690-9000, www.surgeongeneral.gov/ophs

CHAPTER 33
Nursing Care of the Client: Blood and Lymph Systems

REFERENCES/SUGGESTED READINGS

Anderson, K. N. (Ed.). (1994). *Mosby's medical nursing and allied health dictionary* (4th ed.). St. Louis, MO: Mosby-Year Book.

Beare, P., & Myers, J. L. (1998). *Principles and practice of adult health nursing* (3d ed.). St. Louis, MO: Mosby-Year Book.

Black, J. M., & Mastassarin-Jacobs, E. (1997). *Clinical Management for Continuity of Care* (5th ed.). Philadelphia: W. B. Saunders.

Campbell. K. (1995). Understanding acute and chronic myeloid leukaemia. *Nursing Times, 91*(47), 36–38.

Erickson, J. M. (1994). Update on Hodgkin's disease. *Nurse Practitioner, 19*(11), 63–68.

Fitzpatrick, L., & Fitzpatrick, T. (1997). Blood transfusion: Keeping your patient safe. *Nursing97, 27*(8), 34–41.

Gioia, K., Kleinert, D., & Hannon, M. (1999). What's wrong with this patient? *RN, 62*(2), 43–45.

Gorman, K. (1999). Sickle cell disease. *American Journal of Nursing, 99*(3), 38–43.

Hawley, K. (1996). Pernicious anemia. *American Journal of Nursing, 96*(11), 96.

Hutson, C. (1996). Emergency! Hemolytic transfusion reaction. *American Journal of Nursing, 96*(3), 47–48.

Interferon approved for chronic myelogenous leukemia. (1996). *RN, 59*(2), 78.

Leukemia Society of America. (1998a). Facts and statistics [On-line]. Available: www.leukemia.org/docs/leuk_rel/facts.html.

Leukemia Society of America. (1998b). Hodgkin's disease [On-line]. Available: www.leukemia.org/docs/leuk_rel/facts.html.

Leukemia Society of America. (1998c). Lymphoma [On-line]. Available: www.leukemia.org/docs/leuk_rel/facts.html.

Leukemia Society of America. (1998d). Myeloma [On-line]. Available: www.leukemia.org/docs/leuk_rel/facts.html.

Lewis, S., Collier, I., & Heitkemper, M. M. (1996). *Medical-surgical nursing* (4th ed.). St. Louis, MO: Mosby-Year Book.

Lundquist, D. M., & Stewart, F. M. (1994). An update on non–Hodgkin's lymphomas. *Nurse Practitioner, 19*(10), 41–54.

Matteson, M. A., McConnell, E. J., & Linton, A. D. (1997). *Gerontological Nursing* (2nd ed.). Philadelphia: W. B. Saunders.

McBrien, N. (1997). Clinical snapshot: Thrombocytopenic purpura. *American Journal of Nursing, 97*(2), 28–29.

Mitchell, R. (1999). Sickle cell anemia. *American Journal of Nursing, 99*(5), 36–37.

Monahan, F. D., Drake, T., & Neighbors, M. (1994) *Nursing care of adults.* Philadelphia: W. B. Saunders.

National Cancer Institute. (1992). *What you need to know about non-Hodgkin's Disease* (2nd ed.) (Brochure). Bethesda, MD: National Cancer Institute.

Pagana, K. D., & Pagana, T. J. (1999). *Mosby's diagnostic and laboratory test reference* (4th ed.). St. Louis, MO: Mosby-Year Book.

Phipps, W. J., Cassmeyer, V. L., Sands, J. K., & Lehman, M. K. (1999). *Medical-surgical nursing: Concepts and clinical practice* (6th ed.). St. Louis, MO: Mosby-Year Book.

Smeltzer, S. C., & Bare, B. G. (1996). *Brunner and Suddarth's textbook of medical-surgical nursing* (8th ed.). Philadelphia: Lippincott-Raven Publishers.

Spratto, G., & Woods, A. (2000). *PDR® Nurse's drug handbook™.* Albany, NY: Delmar Publishers.

Spraycar, M. (Ed.) (1995). *Stedman's medical dictionary* (26th ed.). Baltimore, MD: Williams and Wilkins.

Thibodeau, G. A., & Patton, K. T. (1995). *Anatomy and physiology* (3d ed.) St. Louis, MO: Mosby-Year Book.

Thomas, C. L. (Ed.). (1997). *Taber's cyclopedic medical dictionary* (18th ed.). Philadelphia: F. A. Davis.

Tranter, J. (1995). Making sense of blood transfusion. *Nursing Times, 910*(36), 34–36.

Warmkessel, J. H. (1997). Caring for patients with non-Hodgkin's lymphoma. *Nursing97, 27*(6), 48–49.

Wasilewski, A. (1995). *Roferon-A (Interferon Alfa-2a, Recombinant) Cleared for Marketing by FDA—First Interferon for Treatment for Chronic Myelogenous Leukemia.* Internet: OncoLink.

RESOURCES

American Cancer Society (ACS), 1599 Clifton Road, N.E., Altanta, GA, 30329, 800-ACS-2345, www.cancer.org

Aplastic Anemia Foundation, Inc., P.O. Box 613, Annapolis, MD, 21404, 800-247-2820, www.aplastic.org

BMT (Bone Marrow Transplant) Newsletter, 1985 Spruce Ave., Highland Park, IL, 60035, 708-831-1913, www.bmtnews.org

Cancer Information Service (CIS), 800-4-CANCER

Center for Sickle Cell Disease, 202-806-7930

Cooley's Anemia Foundation, 105 E. 22nd St., Room 911, New York, NY, 10010, 800-221-3571

Cure for Lymphoma Foundation, 215 Lexington Ave., New York, NY, 10016, 800-CFL-6848, www.cfl.org

The Leukemia Society of America, Inc. (LSA), 600 Third Ave., New York, NY, 10016, 800-955-4LSA, 212-573-8484, www.leukemia.org

National Association for Sickle Cell Disease, 4221 Wilshire Boulevard, Suite 360, Los Angeles, CA, 90010, 213-936-7205, 800-421-8453

National Heart, Lung, and Blood Institute, 9000 Rockville Pike, Bethesda, MD, 20892, 301-496-4236

The National Hemophilia Foundation, SOHO Building, Suite 406, 110 Greene St., New York, NY, 10012, 212-219-8180

National Marrow Donor Program, 3433 Broadway St. N.E., Minneapolis, MN, 55413, www.marrow.org

Office of Cancer Communications, National Cancer Institute, Building 31, Room 10A24, Bethesda, MD, 20892, 800-4-CANCER

Sickle Cell Disease Foundation of Greater New York, 1 West 125th St., Room 206, New York, NY, 10027

CHAPTER 34
Nursing Care of the Client: Gastrointestinal System

REFERENCES/SUGGESTED READINGS

Bradley, M., & Pupiales, M. (1997). Essential elements of ostomy care. *American Journal of Nursing, 97*(7), 38–45.

Butler, R. (1994, March). Managing the complications of cirrhosis. *American Journal of Nursing, 94*(3), 46–49.

Cameron, J. L. (1998). *Current surgical therapy* (6th ed.). St. Louis, MO: Mosby-Year Book.

Carpenito, L. J. (2000). *Nursing diagnosis: Application to clinical practice* (8th ed.). Philadelphia: J. B. Lippincott Company.

Giacchino, S., & Houdek, D. (1998). Ruptured varices! Act fast. *RN, 61*(5), 33–36.

International Working Party. (1995, February). Terminology of chronic hepatitis. *The American Journal of Gastroenterology, 90,* 181–189. Author.

Krupp, K., & Heximer, B. (1998). Going with the flow: How to prevent feeding tubes from clogging. *Nursing98, 28*(4), 54–55.

Lisant, P. & Talotta, D. (1994, May). An overview of viral hepatitis, A through E. *AORN Journal, 59,* 997–1005.

Martin, F. (1997). Ulcerative colitis. *American Journal of Nursing, 97*(8), 38–39.

McConnell, E. (1994, March). Loosening the grip of intestinal obstruction. *Nursing94, 24*(3), 34–41.

McConnell, E. (1998). Giving medications through an enteral feeding tube. *Nursing98, 28*(3), 66.

Meissner, J. (1994, July). Caring for patients with ulcerative colitis. *Nursing94, 24*(7), 54–55.

Metheny, N., Wehrle, M. A., Wiersema, L., & Clark, J. (1998). pH, color, and feeding tubes. *RN, 61*(1), 25–27.

Metheny, N., Wehrle, M. A., Wiersema, L., & Clark, J. (1998). Testing feeding tube placement: Ascultation vs. pH method. *American Journal of Nursing, 98*(5), 37–42.

Neergaard, L. (1996, February 24). Breath test detects bacteria causing ulcers. *Associated Press;* Daily Camera.

O'Hanlon-Nichols, T. (1998). Basic assessment series: Gastrointestinal system. *American Journal of Nursing, 98*(4), 48–53.

Spiro, C., Grant, E., & Gilley, M. (1994, March). Diverticular disease. *AORN Journal, 59,* 625–634.

Springhouse Corporation. (1999). *Illustrated guide to diagnostic tests.* Springhouse, PA: Author.

RESOURCES

American Liver Foundation, 75 Maiden Lane, Suite 603, New York, NY, 10038, 1-800-GO-LIVER (465-4837), http://liverFoundation.org/

National Digestive Diseases Clearinghouse, 2 Information Way, Bethesda, MD, 20892, 301-654-3810, www.niddk.nih.gov

National Foundation for Ileitis and Colitis, 386 Park Avenue South, New York, NY, 10016, 212-685-3440, www.ccfa.org

United Ostomy Association, 19772 McArthur Boulevard, Suite 200, Irvine, CA, 92612, www.uoa.org

CHAPTER 35
Nursing Care of the Client: Reproductive System

REFERENCES/SUGGESTED READINGS

American Cancer Society (ACS) (1998). *Cancer facts and figures—1998.* Atlanta: Author.

Angelucci, P. (1997). Benign prostatic hyperplasia. *Nursing97, 27*(11), 54–55.

Baird, S., Donehower, M., Stalsbroten, V., & Ades, T. (Eds.). (1997). *A cancer source book for nurses* (7th ed.). Atlanta: American Cancer Society.

Baron, R. H., & Walsh, A. (1995). Nine facts everyone should know about breast cancer. *American Journal of Nursing, 95*(7), 29–33.

Brenner, Z. R., & Krezner, M. E. (1995). Update on cryosurgical ablation for prostate cancer. *American Journal of Nursing, 95*(4), 44–48.

Chapman, K. (1994). When the prognosis isn't as good. *RN, 57*(7), 55–57.

Clowers, D. (1995). Personal communication. *Urodynamics, SCI-Urology.* Erectile Dysfunction Clinic Department of Veterans' Affairs: Seattle, WA.

Crandall, L. (1997). Menopause made easier. *RN, 60*(7), 46–50.

Cummings, J. M., Parra, R. O., & Boullier, J. A. (1995). Laser prostatectomy: Initial experience and urodynamic follow-up. *Urology, 45*(3), 414–19.

Dest, V. M., & Fisher, S. M. (1994). Breast cancer, dreaded diagnosis, complicated care. *RN, 57*(6), 48–58.

Donaldson, K. E., Briggs, J., & McMaster, D. (1994). RU-486: An alternative to surgical abortion. *JOGNN, 23*(7), 555–9.

Estes, M. E. Z. (1998). *Health assessment & physical examination.* Albany, NY: Delmar Thomson Learning.

Fowler, G. C., Hassalquist, M. B., & Zacur, H. A. (1994). Menstrual irregularities: A focused evaluation. *Patient Care, 28*(7), 155–60, 163–64.

Fox, S. M., & Haney, L. G. (1994). Taxol: New hope for cancer patients. *RN, 57*(11), 33–36.

Gerber, G. S. (1995). Lasers in the treatment of benign prostatic hyperplasia. *Urology, 45*(3), 193–98.

Gordon, S., Brenden, J., Wyble, J., & Ivey, C. (1997). When the Dx is penile cancer. *RN, 60*(3), 41–44.

Griffith, C. J. (1995). Premenstrual syndrome: An update. *Journal of the American Academy of Physician Assistants, 8*(4), 31–2, 35–6.

Heaton, J. R., Morales, A., Adams, M. A., Johnson, B., & Rashidy, R.E. (1995). Recovery of erectile function by the oral administration of apomorphine. *Urology, 45*(3), 200–06.

Holm, K., Penckofer, S., & Chandler, P. J. (1995). Deciding on hormone replacement therapy. *American Journal of Nursing, 95*(8), 57–59.

Ivey, C. L. (1994). When your patient has ovarian cancer. *RN, 57*(11), 26–32.

Ivey, C. L., & Gordon, S. I. (1994). Breast reconstruction: New image, new hope. *RN, 57*(7), 48–54.

Kessenich, C. (1999). Myths & facts about menopause. *Nursing99, 29*(4), 67.

Kim, J. C., Lunati, F. P., Khan, S. A., & Waltzer, W. C. (1995). T-tube drainage of infected penile corporeal chambers. *Urology, 45*(3), 514–15.

Lepor, H. (1995). Long-term efficacy and safety of terazosin in patients with benign prostatic hyperplasia. *Urology, 45*(3), 406–13.

Lomano, J. M. (1994). A patient's guide to Taxol. *Oncology Nursing Forum, 21*(9), 1569–72.

MacDermott, B. L., Deglin, J. H. (1995). *Understanding basic pharmacology: Practical approaches for effective application.* Philadelphia: F. A. Davis.

Marieb, E. N. (1995). *Human anatomy and physiology* (3rd ed.). Redwood City, CA: Benjamin/Cummings Publishing.

Martini, F. H. (1995). *Fundamentals of anatomy & physiology* (3rd ed.). Englewood Cliffs, NJ: Prentice Hall.

Miller, K. (1999). Testicular torsion. *American Journal of Nursing, 99*(6), 33.

Mogus, M. (1997). Pelvic floor surgery? *RN, 60*(4), 36–41.

National Cancer Institute. (1994). *A mammogram could save your life* (NIH Publication No. 94-3418).

National Cancer Institute. (1993). *Take care of your breasts* (NIH Publication No. 93-3417).

National Cancer Institute. (1993). *What you need to know about ovarian cancer* (NIH Publication No. 94-1561).

National Cancer Institute. (1992). *What you need to know about cancer of the uterus* (NIH Publication No. 93-1562)

National Cancer Institute. (1991). *What you need to know about cancer of the cervix* (NIH Publication No. 91-2047).

North American Nursing Diagnosis Association. (1999). *NANDA nursing diagnoses: Definitions and classification 1999–2000.* Philadelphia: Author.

Otto, S. (1997). *Oncology nursing* (3rd ed.). St. Louis, MO: Mosby-Year Book.

Pickar, G. D. (1999). *Dosage calculations* (6th ed.). Albany, NY: Delmar Thomson Learning.

Reid, T. (1994). Treatment for infertility: Counting the cost. *Nursing Times, 90*(45), 27–8.

Rich, S. E. (1993). Tamoxifen and breast cancer—From palliation to prevention. *Cancer Nursing, 16*(5), 341–6.

Schnore, S., & Matsuda, K. (1997). Today's contraceptive choices. *RN, 60*(12), 30–37.

Shaw, K. (1995). Breast cancer and its treatment. *Journal of Practical Nursing, 45*(1), 21–9.

Shochey, C. (1994). Perimenopause and heavy menstrual flow: Standard treatments and alternative treatment modalities. *Nurse Practitioner: American Journal of Primary Health Care, 19*(9), 73–5.

Shurpin, K. (1997). Ovarian cancer. *American Journal of Nursing, 97*(4), 34–35.

Smeltzer, S. C., & Bare, B. G. (1996). Management of patients with disorders of the female reproductive system. In *Brunner and Suddarth's Medical-Surgical Nursing* (8th ed., pp. 1269–1301). Philadelphia: Lippincott.

Soper, D. E. (1994). Pelvic inflammatory disease. *Infectious Disease Clinics of North America, 8*(4), 821–40.

Speights, V. O., Jr., Brawn, P. N., Foster, D. M., Spiekerman, A. M., Kuhl, D., & Riggs, M. W. (1995). Evaluation of age-specific normal ranges for prostate-specific antigen. *Urology, 45*(3), 454–458.

Spratto, G., & Woods, A. (2000). *PDR for Nurses.* Albany, NY: Delmar Thomson Learning.

Taber, C. W. (1997). *Taber's cyclopedic medical dictionary* (18th ed.). Philadelphia: F. A. Davis.

Tamoxifen for breast cancer prevention. (1998, December 15). *Healthnews, 4*(15).

Twillie, D. A., Eisenberger, M. A., Carducci, M. A., Hseih, W. S., Kim, W. Y., & Simons, J. W. (1995). Interleukin-6: A candidate mediator of human prostate cancer morbidity. *Urology, 45*(3), 542–49.

Van Wynsberghe, D., Noback, C. R., & Carola, R. (1995). *Human anatomy & physiology* (3rd ed.). New York: McGraw-Hill.

vanLeeuwen, F., & Benraadt, J. (1994). Risk of endometrial cancer after tamoxifen treatment of breast cancer. *Lancet, 343*(8896), 448.

Wasaha, S., & Angelopoulos, F. (1996). What every woman should know about menopause. *American Journal of Nursing, 96*(1), 25–33.

Wolcott, J. (March, 1995). Locally refined therapy nipping prostate cancer. *Puget Sound Business Journal,* pp. 18–21.

Wolfe, S. (1997). The great mammogram debate, *RN, 60*(8), 41–44.

Zaccognini, M. (1999). Prostate cancer, *American Journal of Nursing, 99*(4), 34–35.

RESOURCES

American Association of Sex Educators, Counselors, and Therapists, P.O. Box 238, Mount Vernon, IA, 52314, fax 319-895-6203, AASECT@worldnet.att.net

American Cancer Society, Inc., 1599 Clifton Road, NE, Atlanta, GA, 30329, 404-320-3333, 800-ACS-2345, www.cancer.org

American College of Obstetricians and Gynecologists (ACOG), 409 12th Street SW, P.O. Box 96920, Washington, DC, 20090-6920, www.acog.org

American Society of Reproductive Medicine, 1209 Montgomery Highway, Birmingham, AL, 35216-2809

Association of Women's Health, Obstetrical, and Neonatal Nursing (AWHONN), 2000 L. Street NW, Suite 740, Washington, DC, 20036, www.awhonn.org

Cancer Information Service, National Cancer Institute, Building 31 Room 10 A 07, Bethesda, MD, 20892, (301) 496-5583, www.aoa.dhhs.gov

National Breast Cancer Hotline, 212 West Van Buren, Chicago, IL, 60016, 800-221-2141, www.y-me.org

National Osteoporosis Foundation (NOF), 1232 22nd St. NW, Washington, DC, 20037-1292, 202-223-2226, www.nof.org

North American Menopause Society (NAMS), Wolf H. Utain, M.D., 5900 Landerbrook Dr., Suite 195, Mayfield Heights, OH, 44124, 440-442-7550, e-mail: info@menopause.org, www.menopause.org

Older Women's League, 666 11th Street, N.W., Suite 700, Washington, DC, 20001, 202-783-6686

Recovery of Male Potency, Grace Hospital, 18700 Meyers Rd., Detroit, MI, 48235

RESOLVE, Inc., 5 Water Street, Arlington, MA, 02174-4814, 617-643-2424

CHAPTER 36
Nursing Care of the Client:
Sexually Transmitted Diseases

REFERENCES/SUGGESTED READINGS

Burton, A. A., Flynn, J. A., Neumann, T. M., Wilson, C., Quinn, T. A., & Hook, E. W. (1994, May–June). Routine serologic screening for syphilis in hospitalized patients: High prevalence of unsuspected infection in the elderly. *Sexually Transmitted Diseases, 21,* 133.

Centers for Disease Control and Prevention (CDC). (1999a, July). *Hepatitis B—Fact sheet* [On-line]. Available: www.cdc.gov/ncidod/diseases/hepatitis/b/fact.htm

Centers for Disease Control and Prevention (CDC). (1999b, July). *Hepatitis B vaccine—Fact sheet* [On-line]. Available: www.cdc.gov/ncidod/diseases/hepatitis/b/factvax.htm

Erickson, M. J. (1994, June). Chlamydial infections: Combating the silent threat. *American Journal of Nursing, 94,* 16B.

Hadley, J. (1999). *Culturally relevant behavioral intervention dramatically reduces STDs* [On-line]. Available: www.niaid.nih.gov/newsroom/std.htm

Jagger, J., & Perry, J. (1999). Power in numbers: Reducing your risk of blood borne exposures. *Nursing99, 29*(1), 51–52.

Lammon, C. B., Foote, A. W., Leli, P. G., Ingle, J., & Adams, M. H. (1995). *Clinical nursing skills.* Philadelphia: W. B. Saunders Company.

National Institute of Allergy and Infectious Diseases (NIAID) and National Institutes of Health (NIH). (1998a, June). *An introduction to sexually transmitted diseases* [On-line]. Available: www.niaid.nih.gov/factsheets/stdinfo.htm

National Institute of Allergy and Infectious Diseases (NIAID) and National Institutes of Health (NIH). (1998b, June). *Chlamydial infection* [On-line]. Available: www.niaid.nih.gov/factsheets/stdclam.htm

National Institute of Allergy and Infectious Diseases (NIAID) and National Institutes of Health (NIH). (1998c, June). *Gonorrhea* [On-line]. Available: www.niaid.nih.gov/factsheets/stdgon.htm

National Institute of Allergy and Infectious Diseases (NIAID) and National Institutes of Health (NIH). (1998d, June). *Vaginitis due to vaginal infections* [On-line]. Available: www.niaid.nih.gov/factsheets/stdvag.htm

National Institute of Allergy and Infectious Diseases (NIAID) and National Institutes of Health (NIH). (1998e, June). *Other important STDs* [On-line]. Available: www.niaid.nih.gov/factsheets/stdother.htm

National Institute of Allergy and Infectious Diseases (NIAID) and National Institutes of Health (NIH). (1998a, July). *Genital herpes* [On-line]. Available: www.niaid.nih.gov/factsheets/stdherp.htm

National Institute of Allergy and Infectious Diseases (NIAID) and National Institutes of Health (NIH). (1998b, July). *Human papillomavirus and genital warts* [On-line]. Available: www.niaid.nih.gov/factsheets/stdhpv.htm

National Institute of Allergy and Infectious Diseases (NIAID) and National Institutes of Health (NIH). (1998c, July). *Syphilis* [On-line]. Available: www.niaid.nih.gov/factsheets/stdsyph.htm

National Institute of Allergy and Infectious Diseases (NIAID) and National Institutes of Health (NIH). (1998, December). *Sexually transmitted diseases statistics* [On-line]. Available: www.niaid.nih.gov/factsheets/stdstats.htm

Sharts-Hopko, N. (1997). STDs in women: What you need to know. *American Journal of Nursing, 97*(4), 46–54.

RESOURCES

American College of Obstetricians and Gynecologists (ACOG), 409 Twelfth Street S.W., P.O. Box 96920, Washington, DC, 20090-6920, 202-863-2518, www.acog.org

American Public Health Association (APHA), 1015 Fifteenth Street N.W., Washington, DC, 20005, 202-789-5600, Fax: 202-789-5661, e-mail: comments@apha.org, www.apha.org/

American Social Health Association (ASHA), P.O. Box 13827, Research Triangle Park, NC, 27709-9940, 800-230-6089, Herpes Hotline: 919-361-8488, www.ashastd.org

Centers for Disease Control and Prevention (CDC), 1600 Clifton Road N.E., Atlanta, GA, 30333, 404-329-1388, www.cdc.gov

National Foundation for Infectious Diseases, 4733 Bethesda Avenue, Suite 750, Bethesda, MD, 20814

National Institute of Allergy and Infectious Diseases, National Institutes of Health, NIAID Office of Public Liaison, Building 31, Room 7A-50, 31 Center Drive MSC 2520, Bethesda, MD, 20892, www.niaid.nih.gov

Planned Parenthood Federation of America, Inc., 810 Seventh Avenue, New York, NY, 10019, 212-541-7800, www.plannedparenthood.org

U.S. Department of Health and Human Services (USDHHS), Public Health Service, 200 Independence Avenue S.W., Washington, DC 20201, 877-696-6775, www.os.dhhs.gov/

World Health Organization (WHO), Avenue Appia, CH 1211 Geneva 27, Switzerland, www.who.int/

CHAPTER 37
Nursing Care of the Client:
Endocrine System

REFERENCES/SUGGESTED READINGS

American Diabetes Association. (1996). Nutrition recommendations and principles for people with diabetes mellitus. Position Statement: American Diabetes Association. *Diabetes Care, 19*(1), 16–19.

American Diabetes Association. (1995). American Diabetes Association: Clinical practice recommendations 1995. *Diabetes Care, 18*(1).

American Diabetes Association. (1994). Nutrition recommendations and principles for people with diabetes mellitus. *Journal of the American Dietetic Association, 94*(5), 504–506.

American Diabetes Association. (1994). *Therapy for diabetes mellitus and related disorders* (2d ed.). Alexandria, VA.

Angelucci, P. A. (1995). Caring for patients with hypothyroidism. *Nursing, 25*(5), 60–61.

Baer, C. L., & Williams, B. R. (1996). *Clinical pharmacology and nursing* (3rd ed.). Springhouse, PA: Springhouse Corp.

Beare, P. G., & Myers, J. L. (Eds.). (1998). *Adult health nursing* (3rd ed.). St. Louis, MO: Mosby-Year Book, Inc.

Betz, J. L. (1995). Fast-acting human insulin analogs: A promising innovation in diabetes care. *The Diabetes Educator, 21*(3), 195–197.

Budinger, J. M., & Donnelly, S. S. (1994). Nursing care protocols for the kidney/islet cell transplant recipient. *ANNA Journal, 21*(2), 123–128.

Burton, M. (1997). Pheochromocytoma. *American Journal of Nursing, 97*(11), 57.

Carlisle, B.A. (1993, March). Treatment of diabetes in the elderly. *The Journal of Practical Nursing,* 23–31.

Centers for Disease Control and Prevention (CDC). (1999). The public health of diabetes in the United States [On-line]. Available: www.cdc.gov/diabetes/survl/surveil.htm

Centers for Disease Control and Prevention (CDC). (1998). Diabetes facts [On-line]. Available: www.cdc.gov/diabetes/pubs/facts98.htm

Chase, S. (1997). Oral hypoglycemics. *RN, 60*(12), 45–49.

Clayton, L., & Dilley, K. (1998). Cushing's syndrome. *American Journal of Nursing, 98*(7), 40–41.

Corsetti, A., & Buhl, B. (1994). Managing thyroid storm. *American Journal of Nursing, 94*(11), 39.

Depree, P. (1998). Lispro insulin. *Nursing98, 28*(11), 54–55.

Diabetes Control and Complications Trial Research Group. (1993). The effect of intensive treatment of diabetes on the development and progression of long-term complications in insulin-dependent diabetes mellitus. *The New England Journal of Medicine, 329*(14), 977–1036: Author.

5 tips for finger sticks. (1999). 5 tips for finger sticks. *Nursing99, 29*(5), 59.

Fleming, D. (1999). Challenging traditional insulin injection practices. *American Journal of Nursing, 99*(2), 72–74.

Freeland, B. (1998). Diabetic ketoacidosis. *American Journal of Nursing, 98*(8), 52.

Garrison, M. W. (1993). Identifying and treating common and uncommon infections in the patient with diabetes. *The Diabetes Educator, 19*(6), 522–529.

Halpin-Landry, J., & Goldsmith, S. (1999). Feet first: Diabetes care. *American Journal of Nursing, 99*(2), 26–33.

Heater, D. (1999a). If ADH goes out of balance: Diabetes insipidus. *RN, 62*(7), 42–46.

Heater, D. (1999b). If ADH goes out of balance: SIADH. *RN, 62*(7), 47–49.

Hernandez, D. (1998). Microvascular complications of diabetes. *American Journal of Nursing, 98*(6), 26–31.

Hutchinson, C., & Peppard, C. (1998). Hypoglycemia. *Nursing98, 28*(8), 68–69.

Ignatavicius, D. D., Workman, M. L., & Mishler, M.A. (1999). *Medical-surgical nursing across the health care continuum* (3rd ed.). Philadelphia: W. B. Saunders Co.

Jaffe, M. S. (1996). *Medical-surgical nursing care plans: Nursing diagnoses & interventions* (3d ed.). Stanford, CT: Appleton & Lange.

Kestel, F. (1994, July). Are you up to date on diabetes medications? *American Journal of Nursing,* 48–52.

Knight, J. (1998). Inserting an insulin catheter. *Nursing98, 28*(2), 58–60.

Lebovitz, H. A. (1994). *Therapy for diabetes mellitus and related disorders* (2d ed.). Alexandria, VA: American Diabetes Association.

LeMone, P. (1994). Responses of the older adult to the effects and management of diabetes mellitus. *MEDSURG Nursing, 3*(2), 122–127.

LeMone, P., & Burke, K. M. (1996). *Medical-surgical nursing: Critical thinking in client care.* New York: Addison-Wesley Nursing.

McCance, K. L., & Huether, S. E. (1998). *Pathophysiology: The biologic basis for disease in adults and children* (3d ed.). St. Louis, MO: Mosby-Year Book.

Monahan, F. D., & Neighbors, M. (1998). *Medical-surgical nursing: Foundations for clinical practice* (2d ed.). Philadelphia: W. B. Saunders Co.

Norris, J. (Senior Ed.). (1998). *Handbook of medical-surgical nursing* (2d ed.). Springhouse, PA: Springhouse Corp.

Oexmann, M. J. (1989). *Total available glucose—a diabetic food system.* New York: William Morrow.

Pagana, K. D., & Pagana, T. J. (1999). *Mosby's diagnostic and laboratory test reference* (4th ed.). St. Louis, MO: Mosby-Year Book.

Pickar, G. D. (1999). *Dosage calculations* (6th ed.). Albany, NY: Delmar Thomson Learning.

Reising, D. (1995, February). Acute hyperglycemia. *Nursing95,* (2), 33–40.

Reising, D. (1995, February). Acute hypoglycemia. *Nursing95,* (2), 41–48.

Robertson, C. (1998). When your patient is on an insulin pump. *RN, 61*(3), 30–33.

Siconolfi, L. A. (1994). The forgotten system: Endocrine dysfunction during multiple system organ dysfunction. *Critical Care Nursing Quarterly, 16*(4), 16–26.

Smeltzer, S. C., & Bare, B. G. (1996). *Brunner & Suddarth's textbook of medical-surgical nursing* (8th ed.). Philadelphia: Lippincott-Raven Publishers.

Spratto, G. R., & Woods, A. L. (2000). *PDR® nurses handbook.* Albany, NY: Delmar Thomson Learning.

Springhouse. (1999). *Illustrated guide to diagnostic tests* (2d ed.). Springhouse, PA: Springhouse Corp.

Strowig, S. M. (1995, June). Insulin therapy. *RN,* 30–37.

The Expert Committee on the Diagnosis and Classification of Diabetes Mellitus. (1997). Report of the expert committee on the diagnosis and classification of diabetes mellitus. *Diabetes Care, 20*(7), 1183–1197.

Thibodeau, G. A., & Patton, K. T. (1997). *The human body in health & disease* (2d ed.). St. Louis, MO: Mosby-Year Book.

Tomky, D. (1997). Diabetes: Taking a new look at an old adversary. *Nursing97, 27*(11), 41–45.

U.S. Department of Health and Human Services, National Center for Chronic Disease Control and Prevention, Division of Diabetes Translation (1992). *Diabetes in the United States: A strategy for prevention.* Washington, DC: U.S. Public Health Service.

Walpert, N. (1998). The highs and lows of autoimmune thyroid disease. *Nursing98, 28*(12), 58–60.

Weiss, R. (1994, September 13). Growth hormone provides no extra inches. *Washington (D. C.) Post,* Health Section, p. 7.

White, J. R. (1994, March). Update on oral hypoglycemics. *Journal of Practical Nursing,* 24–33.

Young, J. (1999). Myxedema coma. *Nursing99, 29*(5), 59.

RESOURCES

American Association of Diabetes Educators, 444 N. Michigan Avenue, Suite 1240, Chicago, IL, 60611, 800-832-6874, 312-644-2233

American Diabetes Association, ADA National Service Center, 1660 Duke Street, Alexandria, VA, 22314, 800-232-3472, 703-549-1500, www.diabetes.org

American Dietetic Association, 216 W. Jackson Boulevard, Chicago, IL, 60606-6995, 800-877-1600, 312-899-0040, www.eatright.org

Juvenile Diabetes Foundation International, 120 Wall Street, New York, NY, 10005-4001, 800-223-1138, 212-785-9500

National Diabetes Information Clearinghouse (NDIC), 1 Information Way, Bethesda, MD, 20842-3560, www.niddk.nih.gov

National Institutes of Health, 9000 Rockville Pike, Bethesda, MD, 20892, 301-496-4000, www.nih.gov/science/campus

CHAPTER 38
Nursing Care of the Client: Musculoskeletal System

REFERENCES/SUGGESTED READINGS

Altizer, L. (1995). Total hip arthroplasty. *Orthopaedic Nursing, 4,* 7–17.

Arthritis Foundation. (1998). Gout fact sheet [On-line]. Available: www.arthritis.org/resource/fs/gout.asp

Beare, P. G., & Myers, J. L. (1998). *Adult health nursing* (3rd ed.). St. Louis, MO: Mosby-Year Book.

Carpenito, L. J. (1999). *Nursing care plans and documentation* (3rd ed.). Philadelphia: J. B. Lippincott Company.

Darovic, G. (1997). Caring for patients with osteoporosis. *Nursing97, 27*(5), 50–51.

deWit, S. C. (1998). *Essentials of medical surgical nursing* (4th ed.). Philadelphia: W. B. Saunders Company.

Dowd, R. & Cavalieri, R. J. (1999). Help your patient live with osteoporosis. *American Journal of Nursing, 99*(4), 55–60.

Huston, C. J. (1994). Ruptured achilles tendon. *American Journal of Nursing, 12.*

Johnson, J., Anderson, C., Barrett, A., Duke, K., & Sharp, D. (1995). Roller traction: Mobilizing patients with acetabular fractures. *Orthopaedic Nursing, 1,* 21–24.

Leff, R. L., Kurent, J. E., & Dickoff, D. J. (1994). Polymyositis and dermatomyositis: Meeting the diagnostic challenge. *The Journal of Musculoskeletal Medicine, 4,* 57–65.

Monahan, F. D.,& Neighbors, M. (1998). *Medical-surgical nursing: Foundations for clinical practice* (2nd ed.). Philadelphia: W. B. Saunders Company.

Mourad, L. A., & Droste, M. M. (1993). *The nursing process in the care of adults with orthopaedic conditions* (3rd ed.). New York: Delmar Thomson Learning.

National Institute of Allergies and Infectious Diseases (NIAID). (1999). Lyme disease [On-line]. Available: www.niaid.nih.gov/publications/lyme

National Institute of Arthritis and Musculoskeletal and Skin Diseases (NIAMS). (1998, May). Genetics of osteoarthritis panel discussion [On-line]. Available: www.nih.gov.niams/reports/oabrief3.htm

National Institute of Arthritis and Musculoskeletal and Skin Diseases (NIAMS). (1998, October). Osteoporosis: progress and promise [On-line]. Available: www.nih.gov/niams/healthinfo/opbkgr/htm

National Institute of Arthritis and Musculoskeletal and Skin Diseases (NIAMS). (1999, January). Questions and answers about gout [On-line]. Available: www.nih.gov/niams/healthinfo/gout/htm

National Institute of Neurological Disorders and Stroke (NINDS). (1999, July). Carpal tunnel syndrome [On-line]. Available: www.ninds.nih.gov/patients/Disorder/CARPAL/carpal/HTM#moreinfo

National Osteoporosis Foundation (NOF). (1999a). Osteoporosis: Bone health [On-line]. Available: www.nof.org/osteoporosis/bonehealth.htm

National Osteoporosis Foundation (NOF). (1999b). Osteoporosis: Bone mass measurement [On-line]. Available: www.nof.org/osteoporosis/bonemass.htm

National Osteoporosis Foundation (NOF). (1999c). Osteoporosis: Fast facts [On-line]. Available: www.nof.org/osteoporosis/stats.htm

National Osteoporosis Foundation (NOF). (1999d). Osteoporosis: Men and osteoporosis [On-line]. Available: www.nof.org/osteoporosis/men_and_osteo.htm

Phipps, W. J., Sands, J. K., & Marek, J. F. (1999). *Medical-surgical nursing: Concepts and clinical practice* (6th ed.). St. Louis, MO: Mosby-Year Book.

Sipos, D. A. (1995). Carpal tunnel syndrome. *Orthopaedic Nursing, 1,* 17–20.

Smeltzer, S. C., & Bare, B. G. (1996). *Brunner and Suddarth's textbook of medical-surgical nursing* (8th ed.). Philadelphia: J. B. Lippincott Company.

Sparks, S. M., & Taylor, C. M. (1999). *Nursing diagnosis reference manual* (4th ed.). Springhouse, PA: Springhouse Corporation.

Taber, C. W. (1997). *Taber's cyclopedic medical dictionary* (18th ed.). Philadelphia: F. A. Davis Company.

Timby, B. K., Scherer, J. C., & Smith, N. E. (1999). *Introductory medical surgical nursing* (7th ed.). Philadelphia: J. B. Lippincott Company.

The TMJ Association. (1998). Changing the face of TMJ [On-line]. Available: www.tmj.org

Yarnold, B. (1999). Hip fracture. *American Journal of Nursing, 99*(2), 36–40.

RESOURCES

American Occupational Therapy Association, Inc., 4720 Montgomery Lane, P.O. Box 31220, Bethesda, MD, 20824-1220, 301-652-2682, Fax: 301-652-7711, http://www.aota.org/

American Physical Therapy Association, 1111 North Fairfax Street, Alexandria, VA, 22314, 703-684-2782, Fax: 703-684-7343, 800-999-2782, http://www.apta.org/

Arthritis Foundation, 1330 West Peachtree Street, Atlanta, GA, 30309, 800-283-7800, www.arthritis.org

National Amputation Foundation, 38-40 Church Street, Malverne, NY, 11565, 516-887-3600, Fax: 516-887-3667, http://www.va.gov/uso/naf.htm

National Easter Seal Foundation, Development Department, Easter Seal Society of Metropolitan Chicago, 14 E. Jackson Boulevard, Suite 900, Chicago, IL, 60604, 312-939-5115, www.eastersealchicago.org

National Institute of Arthritis and Musculoskeletal and Skin Diseases (NIAMS), NIAMS/National Institutes of Health, Bethesda, MD, 20892, 301-495-4484, www.nih.gov/niams

National Osteoporosis Foundation, 1232 22nd Street N.W., Washington, DC, 20037-1292, 202-223-2226, www.nof.org

Osteoporosis and Related Bone Diseases, National Resource Center, 1150 17th Street N.W. Suite 500, Washington, DC, 20036-4603, 800-624-2663, www.osteo.org

The TMJ Association, Ltd., P.O. Box 26770, Milwaukee, WI, 53226-0770, 414-259-3223, www.tmj.org

CHAPTER 39
Nursing Care of the Client: Immune System

REFERENCES/SUGGESTED READINGS

Aids Treatment Data Network. (1999, May). *Viral load tests* [On-line]. Available: www.aidsinfonyc.org/network/simple/viral.html

Arthritis Foundation. (1999a). *Arthritis types and prevalence* [On-line] Available: www.arthritis.org/resource/fs/arthritis%5Fprevalence.asp

Arthritis Foundation. (1999b). *Getting a grip on rheumatoid arthritis* [On-line]. Available: www.arthritis.org/resource/RAcampaign

Arthritis Foundation. (1999c). *Rheumatoid arthritis* [On-line]. Available: www.arthritis.org/offices/ae/about/rheumatoid.asp

Arthritis Foundation. (1999d). *Rheumatoid arthritis fact sheet* [On-line]. Available: www.arthritis.org/resource/fs/rheumatoid.asp

Arthur, V. (1994). Nursing care of patients with rheumatoid arthritis. *British Journal of Nursing, 3*(7), 325–327, 329–331.

Barbarito, C. (1999). Anaphylaxis. *American Journal of Nursing, 99*(1), 33.

Bertino, L. S., & Lu, L. C. (1993). The bite of the wolf: Systemic lupus erythematosus. *Rehabilitation Nursing, 16*(3), 173–178.

Burt, S. (1998). What you need to know about latex allergy. *Nursing98, 28*(10), 33–39.

Carpenito, L. J. (1997). *Nursing diagnosis: Application to clinical practice.* Philadelphia: J. B. Lippincott Company.

Centers for Disease Control and Prevention. (1996a). Update: Mortality attributable to HIV infection among persons aged 25–44 years—United States, 1994. *Morbidity and Mortality Weekly Report, 45*(6), 10–14.

Centers for Disease Control and Prevention. (1996b). Continued sexual risk behavior among HIV-seropositive, drug-using men—Atlanta; Washington, D.C.; and San Juan, Puerto Rico, 1993. *Morbidity and Mortality Weekly, 15*(7), 13–15.

Centers for Disease Control and Prevention. (1996c). AIDS associated with injecting drug use—United States, 1995. *Morbidity and Mortality Weekly Report, 45*(19), 37–42.

Centers for Disease Control and Prevention. (1995a). Questions and Answers: CDC DRAFT guidelines for HIV counseling and voluntary testing for pregnant women. *CDC HIV/AIDS prevention.* 1–5.

Centers for Disease Control and Prevention. (1995b). USPHS/IDSA Guidelines for the prevention of opportunistic infections in persons infected with human immunodeficiency virus: A summary. *Morbidity and Mortality Weekly Report, 44*(RR–8), 1–33.

Centers for Disease Control and Prevention. (1994). Guidelines for preventing the transmission of Mycobacterium tuberculosis in health-care facilities, 1994. *Morbidity and Mortality Weekly, 43*(RR–13), 1–132.

Finkelstein, D. M., Williams, P. L., Molenberghs, G., Feinberg, J., Powderly, W. G., Kahn, J., Dolin, R., & Cotton, D. (1996). Patterns of opportunistic infections in patients with HIV infection. *Journal of Acquired Immune Deficiency Syndromes and Human Retrovirology, 12,* 38–45.

Flaskerud, J. H., & Ungvarski, P. J. (1995). *HIV/AIDS: A guide to nursing care* (3d ed.). Philadelphia: W.B. Saunders Company.

Guyton, A. C., & Hall, J. E. (1996). *Textbook of medical physiology* (9th ed.). Philadelphia: W.B. Saunders Company.

Hardy, E. M., & Rittenberry, K. (1994). Myasthenia gravis: An overview. *Orthopaedic Nursing, 13*(6), 37–42.

Hausman, K. A. (1995). Interventions for clients with problems of the peripheral nervous system. In D. D. Ignatavicius, M. L. Workman, & M. A. Mishler (Eds.), *Medical-surgical nursing: A nursing process approach.* Philadelphia: W. B. Saunders Company.

Howard, J. (1997). *Myasthenia gravis: A summary* [On-line]. Available: www.myasthenia.org/information/summary.htm

Ignatavicius, D. D. (1999). Interventions for clients with connective tissue disease. In D. B. Ignatavicius, M.L. Workman, & M. A. Mishler (Eds.), *Medical-surgical nursing across the health-care continuum* (3d ed., pp. 405–445). Philadelphia: W. B. Saunders Company.

Johnson, B. (1999). Systemic lupus erythematosus. *American Journal of Nursing, 99*(1), 40–41.

Kaplan, L. D. (1990). The malignancies associated with AIDS. In M.A. Sande & P. A. Volberding (Eds.), *The medical management of AIDS* (2d ed., pp. 339–364). Philadelphia: W.B. Saunders Company.

Kirsten, V., & Whipple, B. (1998). Treating HIV disease: Hope on the horizon. *Nursing98, 28*(11), 34–39.

Kuper, B. C., & Failla, S. (1994). Shedding new light on lupus. *American Journal of Nursing, 94*(11), 26–32.

Lego, S. (1994). *Fear and AIDS/HIV: Empathy and communication.* Albany, NY: Delmar Publishers.

Lindberg, C.E. (1995). Perinatal transmission of HIV: How to counsel women. *Maternal Child Nursing, 20,* 207–212.

Lisanti, P., & Zwolski, K. (1997). Understanding the devastation of AIDS. *American Journal of Nursing, 97*(7), 27–34.

Lupus Foundation of America (LFA). (1995). *Causes, symptoms, testing, treatment* [On-line]. Available: www.lupus.org

Mahot, G. (1998). Rheumatoid arthritis. *American Journal of Nursing, 98*(12), 42–43.

Monahan, F. D. (1994). Nursing care of adults with immunodeficiency and hypersensitivity disorders. In F. D. Monohan, T. Drake, & M. Neighbors (Eds.), *Nursing care of adults* (pp. 313–351). Philadelphia: W.B. Saunders Company.

Mumu, R. D., Lyons, D. A., Borucki, M. J., & Pollard, R. B. (1994). *HIV manual for health care professionals.* Norwalk, CT: Appleton & Lange.

National Heart, Lung, and Blood Institute (NHLBI). (1999, July) *Use of autologous blood* [On-line]. Available: www.nhlbi.nih.gov/nhlbi/blood/transf/prof/transhc.htm

National Institute of Allergy and Infectious Diseases (NIAID). (1999a, July). *Asthma and allergy statistics* [On-line]. Available: www.niaid.gov/factsheets/allergystat.htm

National Institute of Allergy and Infectious Diseases (NIAID). (1999b, July). *Transplantation* [On-line]. Available: www.niaid.nih.gov/publications/womenshealth/transplant.htm

National Institute of Allergy and Infectious Diseases (NIAID) and National Institutes of Health (NIH). (1999, May). *HIV/AIDS statistics* [On-line]. Available: www.niaid.nih.gov/factsheets/hivstat.htm

National Institute of Allergy and Infectious Diseases (NIAID) and National Institutes of Health (NIH). (1999, March). *HIV infection and AIDS* [On-line]. Available: www.niaid.nih.gov/factsheets/hivinf.htm

National Institute of Allergy and Infectious Diseases (NIAID) and National Institutes of Health (NIH). (1997, May). *HIV wasting syndrome* [On-line]. Available: www.niaid.nih.gov/factsheets/hivwasting.htm

National Institute of Arthritis, Musculoskeletal, and Skin Diseases (NIAMS). (1999). *Systemic lupus erythematosus* [On-line]. Available: www.nih.gov/niams/healthinfo/slehandout

National Institute of Neurological Disorders and Stroke (NINDS). (1999a). *Myasthenia gravis* [On-line]. Available: www.ninds.nih.gov/patients/Disorders/myasthenia/myasthenia.htm

National Institute of Neurological Disorders and Stroke (NINDS). (1999b). *Neurological sequelae of lupus* [On-line]. Available: www.ninds.nih.gov/patients/Disorders/lupus/lupus.htm#moreinfo

Paar, D. P. (1994). Hepatitis. In R.D. Mumu, M. J. Borucki, D. A. Lyons. & R. B. Pollard (Eds.), *HIV manual for health care professionals* (pp. 77–86). Norwalk, CT: Appleton & Lange.

Pagana, K. D., & Pagana, T. J. (1999). *Mosby's diagnostic and laboratory test reference* (4th ed.). St. Louis, MO: Mosby-Year Book.

Price, A., & McCarley, P. B. (1994). Physical assessment for patients receiving therapeutic plasma exchange. *American Nephrological Nurses Association Journal, 21*(4), 149–201.

Stewart, K. (1998). Myasthenia gravis cholinergic crisis. *Nursing98, 28*(12), 33.

Thomson, J. M., McFarland, G. K., Hirsch, J. E., & Tucker, S. M. (Eds.) (1997). *Mosby's clinical nursing* (4th ed.). St. Louis, MO: Mosby-Year Book.

RESOURCES

AIDS Treatment Data Network: The Network, 611 Broadway, Suite 613, New York, NY, 10012, 800-734-7104, www.aidsinfonyc.org/network

The American Academy of Allergy, Asthma, and Immunology, 611 E. Wells Street, Milwaukee, WI, 53202, 414-272-6071, www.aaaai.org/

American Association of Blood Banks, 8101 Glenbrook Road, Bethesda, MD, 20814-2749, 301-907-6977, www.aabb.org

Arthritis Foundation, 1330 West Peachtree Street, Atlanta, GA, 30309, 800-283-7800, www.arthritis.org

Asthma and Allergy Foundation of America, 1233 Twentieth Street, N.W., Suite 402, Washington, DC, 20036, 800-7ASTHMA

Foundation for Latex Allergy Research and Education, Long Beach Memorial Hospital, 2501 Cherry Avenue, Suite 350, Long Beach, CA, 90806, 562-997-7888, www.flare.org

Latex Allergy News, 860-482-6869

Lupus Foundation of America, Inc., 1300 Piccard Drive, Suite 200, Rockville, MD, 20850-4303, 800-558-0121, 301-670-9292, www.lupus.org

Myasthenia Gravis Foundation, Inc., 123 West Madison, Suite 800, Chicago, IL, 60602-4503, 800-541-5454, www.myasthenia.org

CHAPTER 40
Nursing Care of the Client: Integumentary System

REFERENCES/SUGGESTED READINGS

Ashburn, M. A. (1995). Burn pain: The management of procedure-related pain. *Journal of Burn Care and Rehabilitation, 16*(3. Pt. 2): Supplement. 365–71.

Barczak, C., Barnett, R., Childs, E., & Bosley, L. (1997, July/August). Fourth national pressure ulcer prevalence survey. *Advances in Wound Care,* 10–14.

Beare, P., & Myers, J. L. (1998) *Principles and practice of adult health nursing* (3rd ed.). St. Louis, MO: Mosby-Year Book.

Bjorgen, S. (1998). Herpes zoster. *American Journal of Nursing, 98*(2), 46–47.

Bryant, R. A. (1999). *Acute and chronic wounds: Nursing management* (2nd ed.). St. Louis, MO: Mosby-Year Book.

Carpenito, L. J. (1997). *Nursing diagnosis: Application to clinical practice* (7th ed.). Philadelphia: J. B. Lippincott Company.

Carroll, P. (1995). Bed selection: Help patients rest easy. *RN, 58*(5), 44–50

Dennison, P. D., & Black, J. M. (1997). Nursing care of clients with peripheral vascular disorders. In J. M. Black & E. Matassarin-Jacobs (Eds.), *Luckmann and Sorensen's medical-surgical nursing: A psychophysiologic approach* (5th ed.). 1253–1313. Philadelphia: W. B. Saunders Company.

Deters, G. E. (1996). Management of patients with dermatologic problems. In S. C. Smeltzer & B. G. Bare (Eds.), *Brunner and Suddarth's textbook of medical-surgical nursing* (8th ed.). 1445–1500. Philadelphia: J. B. Lippincott Company.

Erwin-Toth, P., & Hocevar, B. (1995). Wound care: Selecting the right dressing. *American Journal of Nursing, 95*(2), 46–51.

Estes, M. E. Z. (1998). *Health assessment & physical examination*. Albany, NY: Delmar Publishers.

Fowler, A. (1994). Nursing management of a patient with burns. *British Journal of Nursing, 3*(21), 1105–1112.

Frantz, R. A., & Gardner, S. (1994). Clinical concerns: Management of dry skin. *Journal of Gerontological Nursing, 20*(9), 15–18, 45.

Fritsch, D. E., & Yurko, L. C. (1995). Management of persons with burns. In W. J. Phipps, V. L. Cassmeyer, J. K. Sands, & M. K. Lehman (Eds.), *Medical-surgical nursing: Concepts and clinical practice* (5th ed.). 2358–2397. St. Louis, MO: Mosby-Year Book.

Hill, M. (1998). Nursing management of adults with skin disorders. In P. G. Beare & J. L. Myers (Eds.), *Principles and practice of adult health nursing* (3rd ed.). 2089–2115. St. Louis, MO: Mosby-Year Book.

Jackson, L. (1995). Quick response to hypothermia and frostbite. *American Journal of Nursing, 95*(3), 52.

Kornfeld, H. S. (1995). Co-meditation: Guiding patients through the relaxation process. *RN, 58*(11), 57–59.

Kovach, T. (1995). The barrier defense: Skin hydration as infection control. *The Journal of Practical Nursing, 45*(1), 13–19.

Maklebust, J. (1995). Pressure ulcers: What works. *RN, 58*(9), 46–50.

Martini, F. (1992). *Fundamentals of anatomy and physiology* (2nd ed.). Englewood Cliffs, NJ: Prentice-Hall.

Mendez-Eastman, S. (1998). When wounds won't heal. *RN, 61*(1), 20–23.

Morton, O. (1993). Here comes the sun. *Nursing Times, 89*(29), 52–54.

Morykwas, M., & Argenta, L. (1995, May). An update on the use of negative pressure to promote healing of pressure sores and chronic wounds. *Proceedings of the 27th annual conference, Wound Ostomy and Continence Nurses,* Denver, CO.

National Decubitus Foundation. (1998). Cost savings through bedsore avoidance [On-line]. Available: www.decubitus.org/cost/cost.html

National Pressure Ulcer Advisory Panel (NPUAP). (1999). PUSH Tool [On-line]. Available: www.npuap.org/pushins.htm

Nicol, N. H. (1997). Nursing care of clients with integumentary disorders. In J. M. Black & E. Matassarin-Jacobs (Eds.), *Luckmann and Sorensen's medical-surgical nursing: A psychophysiologic approach* (5th ed.). 1955–1982. Philadelphia: W. B. Saunders Company.

Ogden, B. L. (1998). Nursing management of adults with burns. In P.G. Beare & J. L. Myers (Eds.), *Principles and practice of adult health nursing* (3rd ed.). 2117–2142. St. Louis, MO: Mosby-Year Book.

Sabatini, M. M. (1995). Skin cancer: The silent pandemic. *Dermatology Nursing, 7*(1), 45–50.

Schwartz, S., Shires, G., & Spencer, F. (1994). *Principles of surgery* (6th ed.). New York: McGraw-Hill.

Seeley, R. R., Stephens, T. D., & Tate, P. (1995) *Anatomy and physiology* (3rd ed.). St. Louis, MO: Mosby-Year Book.

Seymour, J. (1995). Skin care: Sun protection. *Nursing Times, 91*(25), 61, 63.

United States Department of Health and Human Services (USDHHS). (1992). *Pressure ulcers in adults: Prediction and prevention* (Publication Nos. 92-0047 and 92-0050). Rockville, MD: Public Health Service, Agency for Health Care Policy and Research.

Weaver, V. (1995). Management of persons with problems of the skin. In W. J. Phipps, V. L. Cassmeyer, J.K. Sands, & M. K. Lehman (Eds.), *Medical-surgical nursing: Concepts and clinical practice* (5th ed.). 2317–2357. St. Louis, MO: Mosby-Year Book.

RESOURCES

American Burn Association, 65 North Michigan Avenue, Suite 1530, Chicago, IL, 60611, 800-548-2876, ameriburn. org/home.htm

American Hair Loss Council, 401 North Michigan Avenue, Chicago, IL, 60611, 312-321-5128, 888-873-9714, www. ahlc.org/

Dermatology Foundation, 1560 Sherman Avenue, Suite 870, Evanston, IL, 60201-4802, 847-328-2256, www.dermfnd. org/

National Burn Victim Foundation, 246A Madisonville Road, P.O. Box 409, Basking Ridge, NJ, 07920, 908-953-9091, www.nbvf.org/

National Decubitus Foundation, 4255 South Buckley Road, Suite 228, Aurora, CO, 80013, www.decubitus.org

National Pressure Ulcer Advisory Panel (NPUAP), 11250 Roger Bacon Drive, Suite 8, Reston, VA, 20190-5202, 703-464-4849, www.iglou.com/npuap

National Psoriasis Foundation, 6600 SW 92nd, Suite 300, Portland, OR, 97223, 503-244-7404, www.psoriasis.org/

Skin Cancer Foundation, 245 Fifth Avenue, Suite 1403, New York, NY, 10016, 212-725-5176, www.skincancer.org

CHAPTER 41
Nursing Care of the Client: Nervous System

REFERENCES/SUGGESTED READINGS

American Academy of Neurology (AAN). (1997a). *Headache* [On-line], Available: www.aan.com/public/head/html

American Academy of Neurology (AAN). (1997b). *Tourette's syndrome* [On-line], Available: www.aan.com/public/head/html

Barinaga, M. (1995). Neurotrophic factors enter the clinic. *Science, 264,* 772–774.

Barinaga, M. (1995). Researchers broaden the attack on Parkinson's disease. *Science, 267,* 455–456.

Barr, M. L., & Kiernan, J. A. (1998). *The human nervous system: An anatomical viewpoint* (7th ed.). Philadelphia: J.B. Lippincott Company.

Beare, P. G., & Myers, J. L. (Eds.). (1998). *Principles and practice of adult health nursing* (3rd ed.). St. Louis, MO: Mosby-Year Book.

Buchanan, L. E., & Nawoczenski, D. A. (1987). *Spinal cord injury: Concepts and management approaches.* Baltimore: Williams and Wilkins.

Carpenito, L. J. (1997). *Handbook of nursing diagnosis* (7th ed.). Philadelphia: J. B. Lippincott Company.

Chipps, E. M., Clanin, N. J., & Campbell, V. G. (1992). *Neurologic disorders.* St. Louis, MO: Mosby-Year Book.

Cochran, I., Flynn, C. A., Goets, G., Potts-Nulty, S. E., Rece, J., & Sensenig, H. (1994). Stroke care: Piecing together the long-term picture. *Nursing94, 24*(6), 34–41.

Cox, H. C., Hinz, M. D., Lubno, M. A., Newfield, S. A., Ridenour, N.A., Slater, M. M., & Sridaromont, K. (1997). *Clinical applications of nursing diagnosis: Adult, child, women's, mental health, geriatric, and home health considerations.* (3rd ed.). Philadelphia: F.A. Davis.

Drucker, T. B., & Zeidman, S. M. (1994). Spinal cord injury: Role of steroid therapy. *Spine, 19,* 2281–2287.

Evans, M. J. (Ed.). (1995). (2nd ed.). *Neurological–neurosurgical nursing.* Springhouse, PA: Springhouse.

Fitzgerald, M. A. (1994). *Nursing health assessment: Concepts and activities.* Philadelphia: F.A. Davis.

Folstein, M., Folstein S., & McHugh, P. (1975). Mini-mental state: A practical method for grading the cognitive state of patients for the clinician. *Journal of Psychiatric Research, 12,* 189–198.

Frozena, C. (1997). Multiple Sclerosis. *American Journal of Nursing, 97*(11), 48–49.

Headache Classification Committee of the International Headache Society. (1988). Classification and diagnostic criteria for headache disorders, cranial neuralgias, and facial pain. *Cephalalgia, 8*(7), 9–96.

Hickey, J. V. (1997). *The clinical practice of neurological and neurosurgical nursing* (4th ed.). Philadelphia: J. B. Lippincott.

Huston, C. J., & Boelman, R. (1995). Autonomic dysreflexia. *American Journal of Nursing, 95*(6), 55.

Hyde, T. M., & Weinberger, D. R. (1995). Tourette's syndrome: A model neuropsychiatric disorder. *Journal of American Medical Association, 273,* 498–501.

Kalbach, L. R. (1991). Unilateral neglect: Mechanism and nursing care. *Journal of Neuroscience Nursing, 23,* 25–129.

Kurlan, R. (1998). *Current pharmacology of Tourette's Syndrome.* Bayside, NY: Tourette Syndrome Association. [On-line]. (Available) www.2mgh.harvard.edu/lsa/medsci/medicationsanddosages.html

Laskowski-Jones, L. (1993). Acute SCI: How to minimize. *American Journal of Nursing, 93*(12), 23–31.

Latham, L. (1994). When spinal cord injury complicates med/surg care. *RN, 57*(8), 26–30.

McCance, K. L., & Huether, S. E. (1998). *Pathophysiology: The biological basis for disease in adults and children* (3rd ed.). St. Louis, MO: Mosby-Year Book.

Meissner, J. E. (1994). Caring for clients with multiple sclerosis. *Nursing94, 24*(8), 60–61.

Mitiguy, J. (1991). The brain under attack. *HEADline, 2–8,* 10.

Mitsumoto, H., Ikeda, K., Klinlosz, B., Cedarbaum, J.M., Wong, V., & Lindasy, R. M. (1994). Arrest of motor neuron disease in wobbler mice cotreated with CNTF and BDNF. *Science, 265,* 1107–1110.

Monlus-Swift, C. (1998). Neurological disorders. In P.L. Swearingen (Ed.), *Manual of medical–surgical nursing care: Nursing interventions and collaborative management* (4th ed., pp. 181–319). St. Louis, MO: Mosby-Year Book.

National Spinal Cord Injury Statistical Center. (1998). *Spinal cord injury fact and figures.* Birmingham, AL: University of Alabama at Birmingham. (Supported by Grant No. HI33N50009-95A from National Institute on Disability and Rehabilitation Research, United States Department of Education.)

National Stroke Association Press Release. (March 13, 1995). *Stroke deaths increase for first time in 35 years.*

National Stroke Association. (1998a). *Stroke in America Campaign* [On-line], Available: www.stroke.org

National Stroke Association. (1998b). *Stroke prevention guidelines* [On-line], Available: www.stroke.org

New treatment for stroke victims. (1997, January). *The Journal Gazette.*

Raine, M. (1997, May 12). New technology eases the tremors caused by Parkinson's disease. *Corpus Christi Caller Times.* Corpus Christi, TX: Caller Times Publishing Co.

Reiman, E. M., Caselli, R. J., Yun, L. S., Chen, K., Bandy, D., Minoshima, S., Thibodeau, S. N., & Osborne, D. (1996). Preclinical evidence of Alzheimer's disease in person homozygous for the ε allele for apolipoprotein ε. *New England Journal of Medicine, 334,* 752–758.

Rudick, R. (1997). New approaches to multiple sclerosis. *Health News, 3*(17), 1–2. Waltham, MA: Massachusetts Medical Society.

Samuels, M. A. (Ed.). (1995). *Manual of neurological therapeutics* (5th ed.). Boston: Little Brown.

Selkoe, D. J. (1992). Aging brain, aging mind. *Scientific American, 267*(3), 134–142.

Smeltzer, S. C., & Bare, B. G. (Eds.). (1996). *Brunner and Suddarth's textbook of medical surgical nursing* (8th ed.). Philadelphia: J. B. Lippincott.

Taggart, H. M. (1998, March/April). Multiple sclerosis update. *Orthopaedic Nursing.*

Thelan, L. A., Davie, J. K., & Urden, L. D. (1998). *Critical care nursing: Diagnosis and management* (3rd ed.). St. Louis, MO: Mosby-Year Book.

RESOURCES

Alzheimer's Association, 919 North Michigan Avenue, Suite 1000, Chicago, IL, 60611, 1-800-272-3900, www.alz.org

Alzheimer's Disease Education and Referral Center, P.O. Box 8250, Silver Spring, MD, 20907-8250, 1-800-438-4380, www.alzheimer.org

American Academy of Neurology, 1080 Montreal Avenue, St. Paul, MN, 55116, 612-695-1940, www.aan.com

American Association of Spinal Cord Injury Nurses (AASCIN), 75-20 Astoria Boulevard, Jackson Heights, NY, 11370-1177, 718-803-3782

American Council for Headache Education, 1-800-255-ACHE (2243)

American Parkinson's Disease Association, Inc., 1250 Hylan Boulevard, Staten Island, NY, 10305, 718-981-8001, 1-800-223-2732, http://neurosurgery.mgh.harvard.edu/pd-suprt.htm#APDA

American Spinal Injury Association, 250 East Superior, Room 619, Chicago, IL, 60611, 312-908-6207

Epilepsy Foundation, 1000 Elmwood Avenue, Rochester, NY, 14620, 1-800-724-7930

Epilepsy Foundation of America, 4351 Garden City Drive, Suite 406, Landover, MD, 20785, 301-459-3700, 1-800-332-1000, www.efa.org

Guillain-Barré Foundation, International, P.O. Box 262, Wynnewood, PA, 19096, 610-667-0131, www.webmast.com/gbs

Huntington's Disease Society, 140 West 22 Street, 6th Floor, New York, NY, 10011-2420, 212-242-1968, 1-800-532-7667, http://neuro~www2msh.harvard.edu/hdsa/society.nclk

National Brain Injury Association, Inc., 105 North Alfred Street, Alexandria, VA, 22314, 703-236-6000

National Headache Foundation, 1-800-843-2256, www.headache.org

National Institute of Neurological Disorders and Stroke, Office of Scientific Health Reports, P.O. Box 5801, Bethesda, MD, 20824, 301-496-5751, 1-800-352-9424

National Multiple Sclerosis Society, 733 Third Avenue, New York, NY, 10017, 212-986-3240, 1-800-344-4867, www.nmss.org

National Parkinson's Foundation, 1501 N.W. Ninth Avenue, Miami, FL, 33136, 305-547-6666, 1-800-327-4545, www.parkinson.org

National Spinal Cord Injury Association, 545 Concord Avenue, Suite 29, Cambridge, MA, 02138, 617-441-8500, www.spinalcord.org

National Spinal Cord Injury Hotline, 1-800-526-3456

National Stroke Association, 96 Inverness Drive East, Suite 1, Englewood, CO, 80112-5112, 1-800-STROKES (787-6537), www.strokes.org

Parkinson's Disease Foundation, William Black Medical Res. Building, Columbia-Presbyterian Medical Center, 710 West 168th Street, New York, NY, 10032, 212-923-4700

Tourette Syndrome Association, 42-40 Bell Boulevard, Suite 205, Bayside, NY, 11361, 718-244-2999, www.2mgh.harvard.edu/tse/tsamain.nclk

CHAPTER 42
Nursing Care of the Client: Urinary System

REFERENCES/SUGGESTED READINGS

American Cancer Society (ACS). (1999a). Basic facts [On-line]. Available: www.cancer.org/statistics/basicfacts.html

American Cancer Society (ACS). (1999b). Selected cancers—bladder cancer [On-line]. Available: www.cancer.org/statistics/cff99/selectedcancers.html

American Society of Nephrology (ASN). (1999). Kidney disease facts & statistics [On-line]. Available: www.asn_online.com/facts/prevalence.html

Anderson, M. A., & Braun, J. V. (1995). *Caring for the elderly client.* Philadelphia: F. A. Davis Company.

Byers, J., & Goshorn, J. (1995). How to manage diuretic therapy. *American Journal of Nursing, 95*(2), 38.

Faller, N., & Lawrence, K. (1994). Obtaining a urine specimen from a conduit urostomy. *American Journal of Nursing, 94*(1), 37.

Goshorn, J. (1996). Kidney stones. *American Journal of Nursing, 96*(9), 40.

Kelly, M. (1996). Chronic renal failure. *American Journal of Nursing, 96*(1) 36.

Kelly, M. (1997). Acute renal failure. *American Journal of Nursing, 97*(3), 32–33.

King, B. (1994). Detecting acute renal failure. *RN, 57*(3), 34.

King, B. (1997). Preserving renal function. *RN, 60*(8), 34–39.

Lewis, S. M., & Collier, I. C. (1996). *Medical surgical nursing—assessment and management of clinical problems* (4th ed.). St. Louis, MO: Mosby-Year Book.

Loughrey, L. (1999). Taking a sensitive approach to urinary incontinence. *Nursing99, 29*(5), 60–61.

Marchiondo, K. (1998). A new look at urinary tract infection. *American Journal of Nursing, 98*(3), 34–38.

McKinney, B. (1996). When this rare cancer strikes. *RN, 59*(12), 36–40.

National Institute of Allergies and Infectious Diseases (NIAID). (1998, December). Biologic differences [On-line]. Available: www.niaid.nih.gov/publications/transplant/bio.htm

National Institute of Diabetes and Digestive and Kidney Diseases (NIDDK). (1998). Urinary incontinence in women [On-line]. Available: www.niddk.nih.gov/health/urolog/pubs/uiwomen/uiwomen.htm

National Institute of Diabetes and Digestive and Kidney Diseases (NIDDK). (1998a, February). Kidney stones in adults [On-line]. Available: www.niddk.nih.gov/health/kidney/pubs/stonadult/stonadult.htm

National Institute of Diabetes and Digestive and Kidney Diseases (NIDDK). (1998b, February). Polycystic kidney disease [On-line]. Available: www.niddk.nih.gov/health/kidney/pubs/polycyst/polycyst.htm

National Institute of Diabetes and Digestive and Kidney Diseases (NIDDK). (1999, January). Urinary tract infection in adults [On-line]. Available: www.niddk.nih.gov/health/kidney/pubs/utiadult/utiadult.htm

National Institute of Diabetes and Digestive and Kidney Diseases (NIDDK). (1999, May). Glomerular diseases [On-line]. Available: www.niddk.nih.gov/health/kidney/pubs/glomer/glomer.htm

National Institute on Aging (NIA). (1996). Urinary incontinence [On-line]. Available: www.nih.gov/nia/health/pub-pub/urinary.htm

National Kidney Foundation (NKF). (1997). About kidney disease [On-line]. Available: www.kidney.org/general/aboutdisease/index.cfm

National Kidney Foundation (NKF). (1998a, November). Ten facts about African-Americans and kidney disease [On-line]. Available: www.kidney.org/general/news/african-american.cfm

National Kidney Foundation (NKF). (1998b, November). The problem of kidney and urologic disease [On-line]. Available: www.kidney.org/general/news/problem.cfm

National Kidney Foundation (NKF). (1999, January). New study explains why cranberry juice may help UTI sufferers [On-line]. Available: www.kidney.org/general/news/cranberry.cfm

National Kidney Foundation (NKF). (1999, May). National Kidney Foundation releases nutrition guidelines for dialysis patients [On-line]. Available: www.kidney.org/general/news/nutguide.cfm

National Kidney Foundation (NKF). (1999a). End-stage renal disease in the United States [On-line]. Available: www.kidney.org/general/news/esrd.cfm

National Kidney Foundation (NKF). (1999b). Six warning signs of kidney and urinary tract disease [On-line]. Available: www.kidney.org/general/aboutdisease/warningsigns.cfm

Needham, J. (1993). *Gerontological nursing: A restorative approach*. Albany, NY: Delmar Publishers.

PDR Nurse's Handbook. (1999). Albany, NY: Delmar Publishers and Montvale, NJ: Medical Economics Company.

Resnick, B. (1993). Retraining the bladder after catheterization. *American Journal of Nursing, 93*(11), 46.

Restore your active lifestyle. (1995). Covington, GA: C. R. Bard.

Rice, J. (1998). *Medications and mathematics for the nurse* (8th ed.). Albany NY: Delmar Publishers.

Sasso, K. (1998). New options for stress incontinence. *RN, 61*(9), 36–39.

Scanlon, V. C., & Sanders, T. (1995). *Essentials of anatomy and physiology* (2nd ed.). Philadelphia: F.A. Davis Company.

Scherer, J. C., & Timby, B. K. (1995). *Introductory medical-surgical nursing* (6th ed.). Philadelphia: J.B. Lippincott Company.

Sosa-Guerrero, S., & Gomez, N. (1997). Dealing with end-stage renal disease. *American Journal of Nursing, 97*(10), 44–50.

Stockert, P. (1999). Getting UTI patients back on track. *RN, 62*(3), 49–52.

Thayer, D. (1994). How to assess and control urinary incontinence. *American Journal of Nursing, 94*(10), 42.

Townsend, C. (2000). *Nutrition and diet therapy* (7th ed.). Albany, NY: Delmar Publishers.

Walters, N. J., Estridge, B. H., & Reynolds, A. P. (1990). *Basic medical laboratory techniques* (2nd ed.). Albany, NY: Delmar Publishers.

Wood, J. M., & Bosley, C. L. (1995, March). Acute postrenal failure: Reversing the problem. *Nursing95, 48*(3).

RESOURCES

American Association of Kidney Patients, 100 South Ashley Drive, Suite 280, Tampa, FL, 33602, 800-749-2257, www.aakp.org

American Society of Nephrology, 1200 19th Street N.W. #300, Washington, D.C., 20036, 202-857-1190, www.asn-online.com

Bard Urological Division, C.R. Bard, Inc., Covington, GA, 800-526-2687

Bladder Health Control, c/o American Foundation for Urologic Disease, 1128 North Charles Street, Baltimore, MD, 21201, 410-468-1800, 800-242-2383, 877-OVERACT (877-683-7228), 410-468-1800, www.afud.org/oab

Interstitial Cystitis Association, 51 Monroe Street, Suite 1402, Rockville, MD, 20850, 301-610-5300, 800-HELP-ICA, www.ichelp.org

Medic Alert® Foundation, 2323 Colorado Avenue, Turlock, CA, 95382-2018, 209-668-3333, 800-IDALERT (800-432-5378), www.medicalert.org

National Association for Continence (NAFC), P.O. Box 8310, Spartanburg, SC, 29305-8310, 864-579-7900, 800-BLADDER (800-252-3337), www.nafc.org

National Kidney and Urologic Diseases Information Clearinghouse, 3 Information Way, Bethesda, MD, 20892-3580, 301-468-6345

National Kidney Foundation, 30 East 33rd Street, Suite 1100, New York, NY, 10016, 212-889-2210, 800-622-9010, www.kidney.org

Polycystic Kidney Research Foundation, 4901 Main Street, Suite 320, Kansas City, MO, 64112, 800-753-2873

The Simon Foundation for Continence, P.O. Box 835-F, Wilmette, IL, 60091, 847-864-3913 (Headquarters), 800-23-SIMON (Patient Information), www.simonfoundation.org

CHAPTER 43
Nursing Care of the Client: Sensory System

REFERENCES/SUGGESTED READINGS

Acute otitis media in adults. (1994). *Emergency Medicine, 26*(6), 44: Author.

A guide to assistive learning devices. (1993). *The Hearing Journal, 46*(2), 23: Author.

Dana, R. (1998, January 27). Dry eye syndrome. *Health News* 1, 3.

Kearney, K. (1997). Retinal detachment. *American Journal of Nursing, 97*(8), 50.

Maquen, E., Salz, J. J., Neoburn, A. B. (1994). Results of excimer laser photorefractive keratectomy for correction of myopia. *Ophthamology, 101*(9).

Roberts, A. (1994). Smell. *Nursing Times, 90*(6), 37–40.

Roberts, A. (1994). The senses: taste. *Nursing Times, 90*(15), 35–44.

Roberts, A. (1993). The ear and hearing, part 1. *Nursing Times, 89*(45), 10–16.

Roberts, A. (1993). The ear and hearing, part 2. *Nursing Times, 89*(49), 41–44.

Roberts, A. (1993). The ear and hearing, part 3. *Nursing Times, 90*(2), 12–18.

Silverstein, H., Wolfson, R. J., & Rosenberg, S. (1992). Diagnosis and management of hearing loss. *Clinical Symposia, 44*(3), 2–32.

Smeltzer, S. C., & Bare, B. G. (1996). *Brunner and Suddarth's Textbook of Medical-Surgical Nursing* (8th ed.). Philadelphia: J. B. Lippincott.

Sparks, S. M. & Taylor, C. M. (1998). *Nursing diagnosis reference manual* (4th ed.). Springhouse, PA: Springhouse Corporation.

Spencer, J. (1998, February 17). Coping with hearing loss. *Health News* 2, 1–2.

Tackling otitis media in adults. (1992). *Emergency Medicine, 24*(2), 67–8: Author.

Weiss, S. J. (1992). Measurement of the sensory qualities in tactile interaction. *Nursing Research, 41*(2), 82–6.

RESOURCES

Alexander Graham Bell Association for the Deaf, 3417 Volta Place NW, Washington, DC, 20007, 202-337-5220, www.agbell.org

American Academy of Ophthalmology, 655 Beach Street, San Francisco, CA, 94109, 415-561-8500, www.eyenet.org/

American Academy of Otolaryngology, Head and Neck Surgery, 1 Prince Street, Alexandria, VA, 22314, 703-836-4444, www.entnet.org

American Council of the Blind, 1155 15th Street NW, Suite 720, Washington, DC, 20005, 202-467-5081, 800-424-8666, http://acb.org/

American Foundation for the Blind, Inc., 11 Penn Plaza, Suite 300, New York, NY, 10011, 212-502-7600, http://www.afb.org, e-mail: afbinfo@afb.org

American Speech-Language-Hearing Association, 10801 Rockville Pike, Rockville, MD, 20852, 800-498-2071, 301-897-5700, http://www.asha.org

American Tinnitus Association, P.O. Box 5, Portland, OR, 97207, www.ata.org, 503-248-9985

Better Hearing Institute, 515 King St., Suite 420, Alexandria, VA, 22314, 800-327-9355

Better Vision Institute, Inc., 1655 North Fort Myer Drive, Suite 200, Arlington, VA, 22209, 703-243-1528, www.visionsite.org

Braille Institute, 741 N. Vermont Avenue, Los Angeles, CA, 90029-3594, 213-663-1111, 800-272-4553, www.healthy.net/pan/cso/cioi/BI.HTM, www.brailleinstitute.org

Guide Dogs for the Blind, P.O. Box 15200, San Rafael, CA, 94915, 415-499-4000, 800-295-4050, www.guidedogs.com

Guide Dog Users, Inc., 12 Riverside St., Apt. 1-2, Watertown, MA, 02172, 617-926-9198

Guiding Eyes for the Blind, 611 Granite Springs Road, Yorktown Heights, NY, 10598, 914-245-4024, www.guidingeyes.org

International Hearing Dog Inc., 5901 East 89th Avenue, Henderson, CO, 80640, 303-287-3277, www.ihdi.org

Leader Dogs for the Blind, 1039 South Rochester Road, Rochester, MI, 48307, 248-651-9011, www.leaderdog.org

Lion's International, 300 22nd St., Oak Brook, IL, 60523-8842, 630-571-5466, www.lionsclub.org

National Association for the Deaf, 814 Thayer Avenue, Silver Spring, MD, 20910, 301-587-1788 (TTY 301-587-1789), www.nad.org, e-mail: nadhg@juno.com

National Association for Visually Handicapped, 22 West 21st Street, New York, NY, 10010, 212-889-3141, www.navh.org/

National Board for Certification and Hearing Instruments, National Hearing Aid Helpline, 16880 Middlebelt Rd, Suite 4, Livonia, MI, 48154, 734-522-7200, 800-521-5247, www.hearingihs.org

National Society to Prevent Blindness, 500 East Remington Rd., Schaumburg, IL, 60173, 800-221-3004, www.preventblindness.org

Recording for the Blind, Inc., 20 Roszel Rd., Princeton, NJ, 08540, 609-452-0606, www.rfbd.org

Self Help for Hard of Hearing, 7910 Woodmont Avenue, Suite 1200, Bethesda, MD, 20814, 301-657-2248, www.shhh.org/

CHAPTER 44
Nursing Care of the Client: Responding to Emergencies

REFERENCES/SUGGESTED READINGS

American Heart Association. (1997). *Advanced cardiac life support*. Dallas, TX: Author.

Arbour, R. (1998). Aggressive management of intracranial dynamics. *Critical Care Nurse, 18,* 30–40.

Bowen, T., & Bellamy, R. (Eds.). (1998). *Emergency war surgery. United States Department of Defense*. Washington, DC: United States Government Printing Office.

Eliastam, M., Sternback, G., & Bresler, M. (1990). *Manual of emergency medicine*. Chicago: Year Book Medical Publishers.

Finley, D., & Kemp, E. (1993, February). The new CPR. *Texas EMS Magazine,* 8–16.

Miller-Keane, (1997). *Encyclopedia and dictionary of medicine, nursing, and allied health*. (6th ed.). Philadelphia: W.B. Saunders.

National Association of Emergency Medical Technicians. (1998). *PHTLS. Basic and advanced pre-hospital trauma life-support* (4th ed.). St. Louis, MO: Mosby Year Book.

Polaski, A., & Tatro, S. (1996). *Luckmann's core principles and practice of medical–surgical nursing*. Philadelphia: W. B. Saunders.

Sullivan, E., & Decker, P. (1997). *Effective leadership and management in nursing*. Menlo Park, CA: Addison Wesley.

Talbert, S., & Talbert, P. (1998). Flight nursing: Summary of strategies for managing severe traumatic brain injury during early posttraumatic phase. *Journal of Emergency Nursing, 24,* 254–257.

Upfal, M. (1993). *Chemical injury first aid pocket guide*. Schenectady, NY: Genium Publishing.

Weinmen, S. (1994). Trauma notebook: Straddle injury: A case study. *Journal of Emergency Nursing, 20,* 76–78.

RESOURCES

American Association of Critical Care Nurses (AACN), 101 Columbia, Aliso Viejo, CA, 92656, 949-362-2000, www.aacn.org/

American Red Cross, Attn: Public Inquiry Office, 11th Floor, 1621 North Kent Street, Arlington, VA, 22209, 703-248-4222, www.redcross.org

Emergency Nurses Association (ENA), 915 Lee Street, Des Plaines, IL, 60016, 800-243-8362, www.ena.org/

Salvation Army World Service Office, 615 Slaters Lane, Alexandria, VA 22313, 703-684-5528

CHAPTER 45
Nursing Care of the Client: Mental Illness

REFERENCES/SUGGESTED READINGS

Abraham, I. L., Neese, J. B., & Westerman, P. S. (1991). Depression: Nursing implications of a clinical and social problem. *Nursing Clinics of North America, 26*(3), 527–544.

Aguilera, D. C. (1997). *Crisis intervention theory and methodology* (8th ed.). St. Louis, MO: Mosby-Year Book.

American Psychiatric Association. (1994). *Diagnostic and statistical manual of mental disorders* (4th ed.). Washington, DC: Author.

Andresen, G. (1998). Assessing the older patient. *RN, 61*(3), 46–55.

Andrews, G. (1993). The benefits of psychotherapy. In N. Sartorius, G. Girolamo, G. A. Andrews, G. A. German, & L. Eisenberg (Eds.), *Treatment of mental disorders* (pp. 235–247). Washington, DC: American Psychiatric Press.

Badger, J. M. (1995). Reaching out to the suicidal patient. *American Journal of Nursing, 95*(3), 24–31.

Bailey, K. P. (1998). *Lippincott's need-to-know psychotropic drug facts*. Philadelphia: Lippincott.

Bolwig, T. (1993). Biological treatment other than drugs. In N. Sartorius, G. DeGeirdano, G. Andrews, G. A. German,

& L. Eisenberg (Eds.), *Treatment of mental disorders* (pp. 92–111). Washington, DC: American Psychiatric Press.

Burgess, A.W. (1990). *Nursing in the hospital and the community* (5th ed.). Norwalk, CT: Appleton & Lange.

Clark, C. C. (1997). Posttraumatic stress disorder: How to support healing. *American Journal of Nursing, 97*(8), 27–32.

Clark, M. J. (1999). Violence. In *Nursing in the community* (3rd ed.). Stamford, CT: Appleton & Lange.

Constantino, R. E., & Bricker, P. L. (1997). Social support, stress, and depression among battered women in the judicial setting. *Journal of the American Psychiatric Nurses Association, 3*(3), 81–88.

Deglin, J. H., & Vallerand, A. H. (1999). *Davis's drug guide for nurses* (6th ed.). Philadelphia: F. A. Davis.

DiVitto, S. (1998). Empowerment through self-regulation: Group approach for survivors of incest. *Journal of the American Psychiatric Nurses Association, 4*(3), 77–86.

Ellis, A. (1975). *A new guide to rational living.* Englewood Cliffs, NJ: Prentice-Hall.

Endler, N. S., & Persad, E. (1988). *Electroconvulsive therapy: The myths and the realities.* Toronto, Canada: Hans Huber Publishers.

Eskreis, T. R. (1998). Seven common legal pitfalls in nursing. *American Journal of Nursing, 98*(4), 34–41.

Eskreis-Nelson, T. R. (1997). Shedding some light on psychiatric care issues. *RN, 60*(2), 57–60.

Flowers, E. M. (1997). Recognition and psychopharmacologic treatment of geriatric depression. *Journal of the American Psychiatric Nurses Association, 3*(2), 32–39.

Frisch, N. C., & Frisch, L. E. (1998). *Psychiatric mental health nursing.* Albany, NY: Delmar Publishers.

Glod, C. A. (1997). Attention deficit hyperactivity disorder throughout the lifespan: Diagnosis, etiology, and treatment. *Journal of the American Psychiatric Nurses Association, 3*(3), 89–92.

Goldfried, R., Greenberg, L. S., & Marmar, C. (1990). Individual psychotherapy: Process and outcome. *Annual Review of Psychology, 41,* 659–688.

Goodwin, F. K., & Jamison, K. R. (1990). *Manic–Depressive illness.* New York: Oxford University Press.

Gorman, L. M., Sultan, D. F., & Raines, M. (1996). *Davis's manual of psychocial nursing for general patient care.* Philadelphia: F. A. Davis.

Hargreaves, W. A., & Shumway, M. (1989). Effectiveness of mental health services for the severely mental ill. In C. A. Taube & A. Hohmann (Eds.), *The future of mental health services research.* Washington, DC: U. S. Government Printing Office.

Hogarty, G. E., Anderson, C. M., Reiss D. J., Kornblith, S. J., Greenwald, D. P., Javna, C. D., & Madonia, M. J. (1986). Family psychoeducation, social skills training and maintenance chemotherapy. *Archives of General Psychiatry, 43,* 633–642.

Hyman, A., Schillinger, D., & Lo, B. (1995). Laws mandating reporting of domestic violence: Do they promote patient well-being? *JAMA, 273*(22), 1781–1787.

Isaacs, A. (1998). Depression & your patient. *American Journal of Nursing, 98*(7), 26–31.

Johnson, L., & Cheffer, N. D. (1996). Child sexual abuse: A case of intrafamilial abuse. *Journal of the American Psychiatric Nurses Association, 2*(4), 108–114.

Ladebauche, P. (1997). Childhood trauma: When to suspect abuse. *RN, 60*(9), 38–42.

Lynch, S. H. (1997). Elder abuse: What to look for, how to intervene. *American Journal of Nursing, 97*(1), 27–32.

McCloskey, J. C., & Bulechek, G. M. (1996). *Nursing interventions classification (NIC)* (2nd ed.). St. Louis, MO: Mosby.

McEnany, G. (1998). Sexual dysfunction in the pharmacologic treatment of depression: When "Don't Ask, Don't Tell" is an unsuitable approach to care. *Journal of the American Psychiatric Nurses Association, 4*(1), 24–29.

McGlashan, T. H. (1994). Psychosocial treatments of schizophrenia. In N. C. Andreasen (Ed.), *Schizophrenia, from mind to molecule* (pp. 189–215). Washington, DC: American Psychiatric Press.

Medical Education Group Learning Systems. (1995). *Domestic violence: A practical guide for physicians* [On-line]. Available: http://www.cme.edu/phydom/domes.html

Mohr, W. (1998). Updating what we know about depression in adolescents. *Journal of Psychosocial Nursing and Mental Health Services, 36*(9), 12–19.

Morris, R. (1998). Elder abuse: What the law requires. *RN, 61*(8), 52–53.

North, N. (1989). The effect of exercise on depression: A meta-analysis. *Dissertation Abstracts International, 49*(11-B), 5027–5028.

Peplau, H. E. (1962). Interpersonal techniques: The crux of psychiatric nursing. *American Journal of Nursing, 62*(6), 50–54.

Peplau, H. E. (1963). A working definition of anxiety. In S. Burd & M. Marshall (Eds.), *Some clinical approaches to psychiatric nursing.* New York: Macmillan.

Peplau, H. E. (1969). *Basic principles of patient counseling* (2nd ed.). Philadelphia: Smith, Kline, & French Laboratories.

Peplau, H. E. (1991). *Interpersonal relations in nursing.* New York: Springer.

Physician Desk Reference. (53rd ed.). (1999). Montvale, NY: Medical Economics.

Rogers, C. R. (1951). *Client centered therapy.* Boston: Houghton Mifflin.

Rogers, C. R., Gendlin, E. T., Kiesler, D. J., & Louax, C. (1967). *The therapeutic relationship and its impact.* Madison, WI: University of Wisconsin Press.

Romme, M. (1998). Listening to the voice hearers. *Journal of Psychosocial Nursing and Mental Health Services, 36*(9), 40–44.

Sexual assault glossary of terms [On-line]. (1996, December 27). Available: http://asucd.ucdavis.edu/organizations/other/rpep/terms.htm

Shea, C. A., Mahoney, M., & Lacey, J. M. (1997). Breaking through the barriers to domestic violence intervention. *American Journal of Nursing, 97*(6), 26–34.

Sullivan, G. H. (1998). Getting informed consent. *RN, 61*(4), 59–62.

Sundeen, S., Stuart, G. W., Rankin, E. A. D., & Cohen, S. A. (1998). *Nurse–Client interaction: Implementing the nursing process* (6th ed.). St. Louis, MO: Mosby.

Thobaben, M. (1989). State elder/adult abuse and protection laws. In R. Filinson & S. Ingman (Eds.), *Elder abuse practice and policy* (pp. 138–152). New York: Human Sciences.

Townsend, M. C. (2000). *Psychiatric mental health nursing: Concepts of care* (3rd ed.). Philadelphia: F. A. Davis.

Townsend, M. C. (1997). *Nursing diagnoses in psychiatric nursing: A pocket guide for care plan construction* (4th ed.). Philadelphia: F. A. Davis.

Travelbee, J. (1969). *Intervention in psychiatric nursing: Process in the one-to-one relationship.* Philadelphia: F. A. Davis.

Travelbee, J. (1971). *Interpersonal aspects of nursing* (2nd ed.). Philadelphia: F. A. Davis.

Truax, C. B., & Carkhuff, R. B. (1967). *Toward effective counseling and psychotherapy: Training and practice.* Chicago: Aldine Publishing.

United States Code Annotated, Title 42, The Public Health and Welfare, Chapter 67, Child Abuse Prevention and

Treatment and Adoption Reform; Subchapter 1, Child Abuse Prevention and Treatment; Definitions; Title II, Victims of Child Abuse Act of 1990; Subtitle D, Federal Victims' Protection and Rights; Section 226, Child Abuse Reporting. St. Paul, MN: West.

U. S. House of Representatives, Select Committee on Aging, (1981, April 3). *Elder Abuse (an examination of a hidden problem)* (Comm. Pub. No. 97–277). Washington, DC: U. S. Government Printing Office.

Ward-Collins, D. (1998). "Noncompliant": Isn't there a better way to say it? *American Journal of Nursing, 98*(5), 27–32.

Wilkinson, L. K. (1996). The martial arts: A mental health intervention? *Journal of the American Psychiatric Nurses Association, 2*(6), 202–206.

Women's Issues and Social Empowerment (W.I.S.E.). (1997, April 15). The dynamics of domestic violence [Online]. Available: http://www.infoxchange.net.au/wise/DVIM/DVDynamics.htm

Yamashita, M., & McNally-Forsyth, D. (1998). Family coping with mental illness: An aggregate from two studies, Canada and United States. *Journal of the American Psychiatric Nurses Association, 4*(1), 1–8.

RESOURCES

American Anorexia/Bulimia Association, 165 W 46th Street, S. 1108, New York, NY, 10036, 212-575-6200, www.aabainc.org

American Psychiatric Association, 1400 K Street N.W., Washington, DC, 20005, 202-682-6000, www.psych.org

American Psychiatric Nurses Association, 1200 19th Street N.W., Suite 300, Washington, DC, 20036-2422, 202-857-1133, www.apna.org

Anorexia/Bulimia Support, 3049 E. Genesee Street, Syracuse, NY, 13224, 315-445-1975

Anxiety Disorders Association of America, 11900 Parklawn Drive, Suite 100, Rockville, MD, 20852, 301-231-9350, www.adaa.org

Eating Disorders Awareness, 603 Stewart Street #803, Seattle, WA, 98101, 206-382-3587, members.aol.com/edapinc

NARSAD Research (National Alliance for Research on Schizophrenia and Depression), 60 Cutter Mill Road, Suite 404, Great Neck, NY, 11021, 516-829-0091, Fax: 516-487-6930, www.mhsource.com/narsad.html

National Alliance for the Mentally Ill (NAMI), 200 N. Glebe Road, Suite 1015, Arlington, VA, 22203-3754, 800-950-NAMI (6264), 703-524-7600, www.nami.org

National Association of Anorexia Nervosa and Associated Disorders, P.O. Box 7, Highland Park, IL, 60035, 847-831-3438, www.anad.org

National Center on Elder Abuse, American Public Welfare Association, 8101 1st Street N.E., Suite 500, Washington, DC, 20002, 202-682-2470, www.aoa.dhhs.gov/aoa/dir/143.html

National Depressive and Manic–Depressive Association, 730 North Franklin Street, Suite 501, Chicago, IL, 60610-3526, 800-826-3632, www.ndmda.org

National Institute of Mental Health, 6001 Executive Boulevard, Room 8184, MSC 9663, Bethesda, MD, 20892-9663, www.nimh.nih.gov

Parents Anonymous, The National Organization, 675 W. Foothill Blvd., Suite 200, Claremont, CA, 91711-3475, 909-621-6184, www.parentsanonymous-natl.org

Recovery, Inc.: The Association of Nervous and Former Mental Patients, 802 N. Dearborn Street, Chicago, IL, 60610, 312-337-5661, www.recovery-inc.com

Victims of Incest Can Emerge Survivors (VOICES), P.O. Box 148309, Chicago, IL, 60614, 800-786-4238, www.voices-action.org

CHAPTER 46
Nursing Care of the Client: Substance Abuse

REFERENCES/SUGGESTED READINGS

Alcoholics Anonymous. (1939). *Alcoholics Anonymous.* New York: Alcoholics Anonymous World Services.

Anderson, N. (1996). Decisions about substance abuse among adolescents in juvenile detention. *Image, 28*(1), 65–70.

Antai-Otong, D. (1995). Helping the alcoholic patient recover. *American Journal of Nursing, 95*(8), 22–29.

Crigger, N. (1998). Defying denial: Clues to detecting alcohol abuse. *American Journal of Nursing, 98*(8), 20–21.

Daley, D., Moss, H., & Campbell, F. (1993). *Dual disorders.* Center City, MN: Hazelden Foundation.

Jannke, S. (1994). When the mother-to-be drinks. *Childbirth Instructor.* New York: Cradle Publishing.

Johnson, V. (1973). *I'll quit tomorrow.* New York: Harper & Row.

Johnson, V. (1988). *Intervention: How to help someone who doesn't want help.* New York: New American Library.

Johnston, L., O'Malley, P., & Bachman, J. (1991). *Drug use among American high school seniors, college students and young adults 1975–1990.* Rockville, MD: National Institute on Drug Abuse, U.S. Department of Health and Human Services, Alcohol Drug Abuse, and Mental Health Administration.

Johnston, L., O'Malley, P., & Bachman, J. (1998). Drug use by American young people begins to turn downward [Online]. Available: www.isr.umich.edu/src/mtf/

Kasl, C. (1992). *Many roads, one journey: Moving beyond the twelve steps.* New York: Harper Collins.

Kendig, S. (1995). Women at risk for infection: The woman who is chemically dependent. *Journal of Obstetric, Gynecologic, and Neonatal Nursing, 24*(8), 776–781.

Kinney, J. (1991). *Clinical manual of substance abuse.* St. Louis, MO: Mosby-Year Book.

Kleber, H. (1994). Opioids detoxification. In M. Galanter & H. Kleber, *Textbook of substance abuse treatment.* Washington, DC: American Psychiatric Press.

Landau, E. (1995). *Hooked: Talking about addictions.* Brookfield, CT: The Millbrook Press.

Langone, J. (1995). *Tough choices.* Boston: Little, Brown and Company.

Lippman, H. (1992). Addicted nurses: Tolerated, tormented or treated. *RN, 55*(4), 36.

Marlatt, G. (1992). Substance abuse: Implications of a biopsychosocial model for prevention, treatment and relapse prevention. In J. Grabowski & G. Wanden Bos (Eds.), *Psychopharmacology: Basic mechanisms and applied interventions.* Washington, DC: American Psychological Association.

McFarland, R. (1993). *Drugs and your parents* (Rev. ed.). New York: Rosen Publishing Group.

National Institute on Alcohol Abuse and Alcoholism (NIAAA). (1999a). Age-specific number of deaths for cirrhosis with and without mention of alcohol, United States, 1970–95 [On-line]. Available: http\\:silk.nih.gov/silk/niaaa/database/cirmrt3a.txt

National Institute on Alcohol Abuse and Alcoholism (NIAAA). (1999b). Traffic crashes, traffic crash fatalities, and alcohol-related traffic crash fatalities, United States, 1977–96 [On-line]. Available: http\\:silk.nih.gov/silk/niaaa/database/crash01.txt

National Institute on Alcohol Abuse and Alcoholism (NIAAA). (1999c). Updated cost estimates for 1992 and inflation- and population-adjusted costs of alcohol and drug abuse for 1995 [in millions of current-year dollars] [On-line]. Available: http\\:silk.nih.gov/silk/niaaa/database/cost7.txt

National Institute on Drug Abuse (NIDA). (1997). Diagnosis and treatment of drug abuse in family practice [On-line]. Available: http://165.112.78.61/Diagnosis-Treatment/Diagnosis6.html

National Institute on Drug Abuse (NIDA). (1998a). Criteria for substance dependence diagnosis [On-line]. Available: www.nida.nih.gov/DSR.html

National Institute on Drug Abuse (NIDA). (1998b). Nicotine addiction [On-line]. Available: www.nida.nih.gov/researchreports/nicotine/nicotine.html

National Institute on Drug Abuse (NIDA). (1999a). Commonly abused drugs [On-line]. Available: www.nida.nih.gov/DrugsofAbuse.html

National Institute on Drug Abuse (NIDA). (1999b). Cigarettes and other nicotine products [On-line]. Available: www.nida.nih.gov/Infofax/tobacco.html

National Institute on Drug Abuse (NIDA). (1999c). Cocaine abuse and addiction [On-line]. Available: www.nida.nih.gov/ResearchReports/Cocaine/cocaine.html

National Institute on Drug Abuse (NIDA). (1999e). Ecstasy [On-line]. Available: www.nida.nih.gov/Infofax/ecstasy.html

National Institute on Drug Abuse (NIDA). (1999f). Heroin [On-line]. Available: www.nida.nih.gov/Infofax/heroin.html

National Institute on Drug Abuse (NIDA). (1999g). Heroin: Abuse and addiction [On-line]. Available: www.nida.nih.gov/ResearchReports/Heroin/heroin.html

National Institute on Drug Abuse (NIDA). (1999h). Inhalants [On-line]. Available: www.nida.nih.gov/Infofax/inhalants.html

National Institute on Drug Abuse (NIDA). (1999i). LSD [On-line]. Available: www.nida.nih.gov/Infofax/lsd.html

National Institute on Drug Abuse (NIDA). (1999j). Marijuana [On-line]. Available: www.nida.nih.gov/Infofax/marijuana.html

National Institute on Drug Abuse (NIDA). (1999k). Methamphetamine: Abuse and addiction [On-line]. Available: www.nida.nih.gov/ResearchReports/Methamph/methamph.html

National Institute on Drug Abuse (NIDA). (1999l). PCP (Phencyclidine) [On-line]. Available: www.nida.nih.gov/Infofax/pcp.html

National Institute on Drug Abuse (NIDA). (1999m). Steroids (Anabolic) [On-line]. Available: www.nida.nih.gov/Infofax/steroids.html

Navarra, T. (1995). Enabling behavior: The tender trap. *American Journal of Nursing, 95*(1), 50–52.

Phelps, G., & Field, P. (1992). Drug testing: Clinical and workplace issues. In M. Fleming & K. Barry. *Addictive disorders* (pp. 125–142). St. Louis, MO: Mosby-Year Book.

Santomier, J., & Hogan, P. (1991). Health implications of alcohol and other drug use. In M. Naegle (Ed.), *Substance abuse education in nursing* (Vol.1). New York: National League for Nursing.

Septien, A. (1993). *Everything you need to know about codependence.* New York: Rosen Publishing Group.

Waugfield, C. (1998). *Mental health concepts* (4th ed.). Albany, NY: Delmar Publishers.

Yates, J., & McDanier, J. (1994). Are you losing yourself in codependency? *American Journal of Nursing, 94*(4), 32–36.

Yoshuichi, E. (1992). Fetal alcohol syndrome. *Childbirth Instructor.* New York: Cradle Publishing.

RESOURCES

Al-Anon Al-Ateen Family Intergroup, 200 Park Avenue S., Room 814, New York, NY, 10003, 212-254-7236, 212-254-7230, 800-344-2666, 800-939-2770 (Spanish)

Alcoholics Anonymous (AA), P.O. Box 459, Grand Central Station, New York, NY, 10017, 212-870-3400, www.alcoholics-Anonymous.org

American Council for Drug Education, 164 W. 74th Street, New York, NY, 10023, 800-488-DRUG, 301-294-0600, www.acde.org

Cocaine Helpline, 800-662-HELP

Codependents Anonymous (CODA), P.O. Box 33577, Phoenix, AZ, 85607-3577, 602-277-7991, www.codependents.org

Drug Abuse Resistance Education (DARE), Local Police Department

Drug Enforcement Administration (DEA), Information Services Section (CPI), 700 Army-Navy Drive, Arlington, VA, 22202, 202-307-1000

Families Anonymous, (Families of Substance Abusers), Box 3475, Culver City, CA, 90231-3415, 800-736-9805

Mothers Against Drunk Driving (MADD), 511 E. John Carpenter Freeway, No. 700, Irving, TX, 75062, 214-744-6233, or, 3601 SW 29th, Topeka, KS, 66614, 800-443-6233, www.madd.org

Narcotics Anonymous (NA), World Service Office, P.O. Box 9999, Van Nuys, CA, 91409, 818-773-9999, www.na.org

National Clearinghouse for Alcohol and Drug Information, Box 2345, Rockville, MD, 20857, 301-468-2600, www.health.org

National Clearinghouse for Tobacco and Health, 170 Laurier Avenue West, Suite 1000, Ottawa, Ontario, Canada, K1P 5V5, 800-267-5234

National Cocaine Hotline, 1-800-COCAINE (262-2463)

National Council on Alcoholism, Inc., 12 West 21st Street, New York, NY, 10010, 212-206-6770

National Nurses Society on Addictions, 5700 Old Orchard Road, First Floor, Skokie, IL, 60077, 847-966-5010

National Self-Help Clearinghouse, 33 West 42nd Street, New York, NY, 10036, 212-840-1259

Office of Substance Abuse Prevention, 5600 Fishers Lane, Rockwall II, Rockville, MD, 20857, 301-443-0373

Students Against Driving Drunk (SADD) Inc., P.O. Box 800, Marlboro, MA, 01752, 508-481-3568, www.sadd.org/

Toughlove, P.O. Box 1069, Doylestown, PA, 18901, 215-348-7090

CHAPTER 47
Prenatal Care

REFERENCES/SUGGESTED READINGS

Callister, L., & Vega, R. (1998). Giving birth: Guatemalan women's voices. *JOGNN, 27*(3), 289–295.

Cefalo, R., & Moos, M. (1995). *Preconceptional health care: A practical guide* (2nd ed.). St. Louis, MO: Mosby-Year Book.

Dickason, E., Silverman, B., & Schult, M. (1994). *Maternal-infant nursing care* (3rd ed.). St. Louis, MO: Mosby-Year Book.

Dick-Read, G. (1933). *Natural childbirth.* London: Heinemann.

Dick-Read, G. (1944). *Childbirth without fear.* New York: Harper & Row.

Freda, M. (1998). Confronting the myths. *MCN, 23*(2), 107.

Gennaro, S., Kamwendo, L., Mbweza, E., & Kershbaumer, R. (1998). Childbearing in Malawi, Africa. *JOGNN, 27*(2), 191–196.

Guyer, B., et al. (1996). Annual summary of vital statistics— 1995. *Pediatrics, 98*(6), 1007–1019.

Howard, J., & Berbiglia, V. (1997). Caring for childbearing Korean women. *JOGNN, 26*(6), 665–671.

Hutchinson, M., & Baqi-Aziz, M. (1994, Nov.–Dec.). Nursing care of the childbearing Muslim family. *JOGNN, 23*(9), 767–771.

Jones, S. (1996, Nov.–Dec.). Genetics: Changing health care in the 21st century. *JOGNN, 25*(9), 777–783.

Ladewig, P., London, M., Olds, S. (1998). *Maternal-newborn nursing* (4th ed.). Menlo Park, CA: Addison-Wesley Longman, Inc.

Lamaze, F. (1965). *Painless childbirth.* New York: Dimon & Schuster.

Longobucco, D., & Freston, M. (1989, Nov.–Dec.). Relation of somatic symptoms to degree of paternal-role preparation of first-time expectant fathers. *JOGNN, 18,* 482.

Malnory, M. (1996). Developmental care of the pregnant couple. *JOGNN, 25*(6), 525–532.

Martinez, F., et al. (1994, Sept.). The effect of paternal smoking on the birthweight of newborns whose mothers did not smoke. The Health Medical Associates. *Am. J. Public Health, 84,* 1489–1491.

Nance, T. A. (1995). Intercultural communication: Finding common ground. *JOGNN, 24*(3), 249–255.

Nasso, J. (1997). Planning for pregnancy—A preconception health program. *MCN, 22*(3), 142–146.

Remich, M. (1997). Promoting a healthy pregnancy. In E. Q. Younkin & E. Q. Davis (Eds.), *Women's health: A primary care clinical guide* (2d ed.). Norwalk, CT: Appleton & Lange.

Rhodes, A. (1995). Liability for failure to offer prenatal AFP testing. *MCN, 20*(3), 169.

Robaire, B., & Hales, B. (1993, August). Paternal exposure to chemicals before conception. *BMJ, 307,* 341–342.

Rogers, J., & Davis, B. (1995). How risky are hot tubs and saunas for pregnant women? *MCN, 20*(3), 137–140.

Schneiderman, J. (1996). Postpartum nursing for Korean mothers. *MCN, 21*(3), 155–158.

Shapiro, P. (1995). *Basic maternal pediatric nursing.* Albany, NY: Delmar Publishers, Inc.

Spector, R. E. (1995). Cultural concepts of women's health and health-promoting behaviors. *JOGNN, 24*(3), 241–245.

Zwelling, E. (1996). Childbirth education in the 1990s and beyond. *JOGNN, 25*(5), 425–432.

RESOURCES

Association of Women's Health, Obstetric, and Neonatal Nurses (AWHONN), 2000 L Street N.W., Suite 740, Washington, DC, 20036, 800-673-8499 (U.S.), 800-245-0231 (Canada), www.awhonn.org/

March of Dimes, 1275 Mamaroneck Avenue, White Plains, NY, 10605, 888-MODIMES (663-4637), www.modimes.org/index.htm

CHAPTER 48
Complications of Pregnancy

REFERENCES/SUGGESTED READINGS

Acosta, P., & Wright, L. (1992). Nurses' role in preventing birth defects in offspring of women with phenylketonuria. *Journal of Obstetric, Gynecologic, and Neonatal Nursing, 21*(4), 270.

Anderson, B., & Shapiro, P. (1994). *Basic maternal newborn nursing* (6th ed.). Albany, NY: Delmar Publishers, Inc.

Bougere, M. (1998). Action stat: Abruptio placenta. *Nursing98, 28*(2), 47.

Dickason, E., Silverman, B., & Schult, M. (1998). *Maternal-infant nursing care* (3d ed.). St. Louis, MO: Mosby-Year Book.

Harvey, C. (1997). A look at electronic fetal monitoring update; the new terms. *Lifelines, 1*(6), 49–51.

Ladewig, P., London, M., & Olds, L. (1994). *Maternal-newborn nursing care: The nurse, the family, and the com-*

munity (4th ed.). Menlo Park, CA: Addison-Wesley Longman, Inc.

Mandeville, L. K., & Troiano, N. H. (1998). *High risk and critical care intrapartum nursing* (2nd ed.). Philadelphia: Lippincott.

Minnick-Smith, K., & Cook, F. (1997). Current treatment options for ectopic pregnancy. *American Journal of Maternal Child Nursing, 22*(1), 21–25.

NICHD (1997). Electronic fetal heart monitoring: Research guidelines for interpretation. The National Institute of Child Health and Human Development Research Planning Workshop. *Journal of Obstetric, Gynecologic, and Neonatal Nursing, 26*(6), 635–640.

Nursing98 Drug Handbook. (1998). Springhouse, PA: Springhouse Corporation.

Spratt, G., & Woods, A. (2000). *2000 PDR for nurses.* Albany, NY: Delmar.

Urbanski, T., Higgins, P., Murray, M., & Joffe, G. (1996). Caring for a woman with a hydatidiform mole and coexisting pregnancy. *American Journal of Maternal Child Nursing, 21*(2), 85–89.

RESOURCES

Association of Women's Health, Obstetric, and Neonatal Nurses (AWHONN), 2000 L Street NW, Suite 740, Washington, DC, 20036, 800-673-8499, www.awhonn.org

CHAPTER 49
The Birth Process

REFERENCES/SUGGESTED READINGS

Ahmed, S. (1994, December). *Culturally sensitive caregiving for Pakistani women.* Lecture presented at the Medical College of Virginia Hospitals, Richmond, VA.

Bergstrom, L., Seidel, J., Skellman-Hull, L., & Roberts, J. (1997). "I gotta push. Please let me push!": Social interactions during the change from first to second stage labor. *Birth, 24,* 173–180.

Blackburn, S., & Loper, D. (1992). *Maternal, fetal, and neonatal physiology.* Philadelphia: W. B. Saunders.

Bonica, J. J., & McDonald, J. (1990). The pain of childbirth. In J. J. Bonica (Ed.), *The management of pain* (2nd ed.) (pp. 1313–1334). Philadelphia: Lea & Febiger.

Burroughs, A. (1997). *Maternity nursing* (7th ed.). Philadelphia: W. B. Saunders.

Callister, L. (1995). Cultural meanings of childbirth. *Journal of Obstetric, Gynecologic, and Neonatal Nursing, 24*(4), 327–331.

Callister, L., & Vega, R. (1998). Giving birth: Guatemalan women's voices. *Journal of Obstetric, Gynecologic, and Neonatal Nursing, 27*(3), 289–295.

Cosner, K., & deJong, E. (1993). Physiologic second stage labor. *The American Journal of Maternal/Child Nursing, 18*(1), 38–43.

DeSeve, M. (1997). Keeping the faith: Jewish traditions in pregnancy & childbirth. *Lifelines, 1*(4), 46–49.

Dickason, L., Silverman, B., & Schult, M. (1997). *Maternal-infant nursing care* (3rd ed.). St. Louis, MO: Mosby-Year Book.

Fuller, B., Roberts, J., & McDay, S. (1993). Accoustical analysis of maternal sounds during the second stage of labor. *Applied Nursing Research, 6,* 7–13.

Gennaro, S., Kamwendo, L., Mbweza, E., & Kershbaumer, R. (1998). Childbearing in Malawi, Africa. *Journal of Obstetric, Gynecologic, and Neonatal Nursing, 27*(2), 191–196.

Gilbert, E., & Harmon, J. (1998). *Manual of high risk pregnancy and delivery* (2nd ed.). St. Louis, MO: Mosby-Year Book.

Gorrie, T., McKinney, E., & Murray S. (1998). *Foundations of maternal-newborn nursing* (2nd ed.). Philadelphia: W. B. Saunders.

Howard, J., & Berbiglia, V. (1997). Caring for childbearing Korean women. *Journal of Obstetric, Gynecologic, and Neonatal Nursing, 26*(6), 665–671.

Hutchinson, M., & Baqi-Aziz, M. (1994). Nursing care of the childbearing Muslim family. *Journal of Obstetric, Gynecologic, and Neonatal Nursing, 23*(9), 767–771.

Jordan, B. (1978). *Birth in four cultures.* St. Albans: Eden Press Women's Publications.

Ladewig, P., London, M., & Olds, S. (1998). *Maternal-newborn nursing care: The nurse, the family, and the community* (4th ed.). Menlo Park, CA: Addison-Wesley.

Lowdermilk, D., Perry, S., & Bobak, I. (1999). *Maternity nursing* (5th ed.). St. Louis, MO: Mosby-Year Book.

Lowe, N. (1996). The pain and discomfort of labor and birth. *Journal of Obstetric, Gynecologic, and Neonatal Nursing, 25*(1), 82–92.

Ludka, L., & Roberts, C. (1993). Eating and drinking in labor, a literature review. *Journal of Nurse Midwifery, 38*(4), 199.

Mattson, S. (1995). Culturally sensitive perinatal care for Southeast Asians. *Journal of Obstetric, Gynecologic, and Neonatal Nursing, 24*(4), 335–341.

McCartney, P. (1998a). The birth ball—Are you using it in your practice setting? *The American Journal of Maternal/Child Nursing, 23*(4), 218.

McCartney, P. (1998b). Caring for women with epidurals using the "laboring down" technique. *The American Journal of Maternal/Child Nursing, 23*(5), 274.

Menihan, C. A. (1996). Intrapartum fetal monitoring. In K. R. Simpson & P. A. Creehan (Eds.), AWHONN's *Perinatal Nursing*. Philadelphia: J. B. Lippincott.

O'Brian, W. F., & Cefalo, R. C. (1996). Labor and delivery. In S. G. Gabbe, J. R. Niehyl, & J. L. Simpson (Eds.). *Obstetrics: Normal and problem pregnancies* (3rd ed.). New York: Churchill Livingstone.

Perez, P., & Herrick, L. (1998). Doulas: Exploring their roles with parents, hospitals & nurses. *Lifelines, 2*(2), 54.

Petersen, L., & Besuner, P. (1997). Pushing techniques during labor: Issues and controversies. *Journal of Obstetric, Gynecologic, and Neonatal Nursing, 26*(6), 719–726.

Roberts, J., & Woolley, D. (1996). A second look at the second stage of labor. *Journal of Obstetric, Gynecologic, and Neonatal Nursing, 25*(5), 415–423.

Schmidt, J. (1997). Making the case for intrapartum amnioinfusion. *Lifelines, 1*(5), 47–51.

Schneiderman, J. (1998). Rituals of placenta disposal. *The American Journal of Maternal/Child Nursing, 23*(3), 142–143.

Scott-Ramos, I. (1995, January). *Culturally sensitive care giving for Latino women.* Lecture presented at the Medical College of Virginia Hospitals. Richmond, VA.

Sharts-Hopko, N. (1995). Birth in the Japanese context. *Journal of Obstetric, Gynecologic, and Neonatal Nursing, 24*(4), 343–351.

Shermer, R., & Raines, D. (1997). Positioning during the second stage of labor: Moving back to basics. *Journal of Obstetric, Gynecologic, and Neonatal Nursing, 26*(6), 727–734.

Simpson, K. (1997). Preterm birth in the United States: Current issues and future prospectives. *Journal of Perinatal Neonatal Nursing, 10*(4), 11.

Technical Working Group, World Health Organization. (1997). Care in normal birth: A practical guide. *Birth, 24*(2), 121.

Varney, H. (1997). *Varney's midwifery* (3rd ed.). Sudberry, MA: Jones & Bartlett.

Weber, S. (1996). Cultural aspects of pain in childbearing women. *Journal of Obstetric, Gynecologic, and Neonatal Nursing, 25*(1), 67–72.

RESOURCES

American College of Obstetricians and Gynecologists (ACOG), 409 12th Street S.W., P.O. Box 96920, Washington, DC, 20090-6920, 800-762-2264, www.acog.com

Association of Women's Health, Obstetric, and Neonatal Nurses (AWHONN), 2000 L Street N.W., Suite 740, Washington, DC, 20036, 800-673-8499, www.awhonn.org

Childbirth Graphics, P.O. Box 21207, Waco, TX, 76702, 800-229-3366

C/SEC, Inc. (Cesarean/Support Education and Concern), 22 Forest Road, Framingham, MA, 01701, 508-877-8266

Midwives Alliance of North America, c/o Concord Midwifery Service, 4805 Lawrence Ville Highway, Suite 116-279, Lilburn, GA, 30047, 888-923-6262, www.mana.org

National Association of Childbearing Centers, 3123 Gottschall Road, Perkiomenville, PA, 18074, 215-234-8068, www.BirthCenters.org

National Association of Parents and Professionals for Safe Alternatives in Childbirth (NAPSAC), Box 646, Route #4, Marble Hill, MO, 63764-9725, 573-238-2010

CHAPTER 50
Postpartum Care

REFERENCES/SUGGESTED READINGS

Albright, A. (1993). Postpartum depression: An overview. *Journal of Counseling Development, 71*(3), 316.

Ament, L. (1990). Maternal tasks of the puerperium reidentified. *Journal of Obstetric, Gynecologic, and Neonatal Nursing, 19*(4), 330.

American Academy of Pediatrics (AAP) & American College of Obstetricians and Gynecologists (ACOG). (1997). *Guidelines for perinatal care* (3rd ed.). Elk Grove Village, IL: American Academy of Pediatrics.

Bowes, W. (1996). Postpartum care. In S. Gabber, J. Niebyl, & J. Simpson (Eds.), *Obstetrics: Normal and problem pregnancies* (3rd ed.). New York: Churchill Livingstone.

Burroughs, A. (1997). *Maternity nursing* (7th ed.). Philadelphia: W. B. Saunders.

Callister, L., & Vega, R. (1998). Giving birth: Guatemalan women's voices. *Journal of Obstetric, Gynecologic, and Neonatal Nursing, 27*(3), 289–295.

Cunningham, F. G., MacDonald, P. C., Grant, N. F., Leveno, K. J., Gilstrap, L. C., & Hankins, G. D. V. (1997). *William's obstetrics* (20th ed.). Norwalk, CT: Appelton & Lang.

Ferguson, S., & Engelhard, C. (1996). Maternity length of stay and public policy: Issues and implications. *Journal of Pediatric Nursing, 11*(6), 392.

Ferketich, S. L., & Mercer, R. T. (1995). Paternal-infant attachment of experienced and inexperienced fathers during infancy. *Nursing Research, 44*(1), 31–37.

Gennaro, S., Kamwendo, L., Mbweza, E., & Kershbaumer, R. (1998). Childbearing in Malawi, Africa. *Journal of Obstetric, Gynecologic, and Neonatal Nursing, 27*(2), 191–196.

Gorrie, T., McKinney, E., & Murray, S. (1998). *Foundations of maternal-newborn nursing* (2nd ed.). Philadelphia: W. B. Saunders.

Green, S. E., & Adams, W. M. (1993). Chronic psychiatric illness and pregnancy: Nursing implications. *Journal of Perinatal, Neonatal Nursing, 7*(3), 7–18.

Ha, L. (1994, December). *Culturally sensitive caregiving for Vietnamese women.* Lecture presented at the Medical College of Virginia Hospitals, Richmond, VA.

Hamadeh, G., Dedmon, C., & Mozley, P. (1995). Postpartum fever. *American Family Physician, 52*(2), 531.

Havens, D., & Hannan, C. (1996). Legislation to mandate maternal and newborn length of stay. *Journal of Pediatric Health Care, 10*(3), 141.

Howard, J., & Berbiglia, V. (1997). Caring for childbearing Korean women. *Journal of Obstetric, Gynecologic, and Neonatal Nursing, 26*(6), 665–671.

Huml, S. C. (1995, April). Cracked nipples in the breastfeeding mother: Looking at an old problem in a new way. *Advance for Nurse Practitioners*.

Hutchinson, M., & Baqi-Aziz, M. (1994). Nursing care of the childbearing Muslim family. *Journal of Obstetric, Gynecologic, and Neonatal Nursing, 23*(9), 767–771.

Johnson & Johnson (1996). *Compendium of postpartum care*. Skillman, NJ: Johnson & Johnson Consumer Products.

Kaplan, H., Sadock, B., & Grebb, J. (1998). *Kaplan and Sadock's synopsis of psychiatry* (8th ed.). Baltimore: Williams & Wilkins.

Ladewig, P., London, M., & Olds, S. (1998). *Maternal-newborn nursing care* (4th ed.). Menlo Park, CA: Addison-Wesley.

Lowdermilk, D., Perry, S., & Bobak, I. (1999). *Maternity nursing* (5th ed.). St. Louis, MO: Mosby-Year Book.

Luegenbiehl, D., Brophy, G., Artigue, G., Phillips, K., & Flack, R. (1990). Standardized assessment of blood loss. *MCN, The American Journal of Maternal/Child Nursing, 15*(4), 241–244.

Martell, L. (1996). Is Rubin's "taking-in" and "taking-hold" a useful paradigm? *Health Care Women International, 17*(1), 1.

Mattson, S. (1995). Culturally sensitive perinatal care for Southeast Asians. *Journal of Obstetric, Gynecologic, and Neonatal Nursing, 24*(4), 335–341.

Rubin, R. (1961). Puerperal change. *Nursing Outlook, 9*(12), 743–755.

Ruchala, P., & Halstead, L. (1994). The postpartum experience of low-risk women: A time of adjustment and change. *Maternal Child Nursing Journal, 22*(3), 83.

Savoia, M. C. (1999). Bacterial, fungal, and parasitic disease during pregnancy. In G. N. Burrow & T. F. Ferris (Eds.), *Medical complications during pregnancy* (5th ed.). Philadelphia: W. B. Saunders.

Schneiderman, J. (1996). Postpartum nursing for Korean mothers. *The American Journal of Maternal/Child Nursing, 21*(3), 155–158.

Sharts-Hopko, N. (1995). Birth in the Japanese context. *Journal of Obstetric, Gynecologic, and Neonatal Nursing, 24*(4), 343–351.

Simpson, K., & Creehan, P. (1996). *AWHONN's Perinatal Nursing*. Philadelphia: Lippincott.

Smith-Hanrahan, C., & Deblois, D. (1995). Postpartum early discharge. *Clinical Nursing Research, 4*(1), 50.

Tiller, C. M. (1995). Father's parenting attitudes during a child's first year. *Journal of Obstetric, Gynecologic, and Neonatal Nursing, 24*(6), 508–514.

Visness, C., Kennedy, K., & Ramos, R. (1997). The duration and character of postpartum bleeding among breast-feeding women. *Obstetrics and Gynecology, 89*(2), 159.

Wilkerson, N. (1996). Appraisal of early discharge programs. *Journal of Perinatal Education, 5*(2), 1.

Wrasper, C. (1996). Discharge and timing and Rubin's concept of puerperal change. *Journal of Perinatal Education, 5*(2), 13.

Zlatnik, F. (1999). The normal and abnormal puerperium. In J. R. Scott, P. J. Di Saia, C. B. Hammond, & W. N. Spellacy (Eds.), *Danforths' obstetrics and gynecology* (8th ed.). Philadelphia: Lippincott.

RESOURCES

Association of Women's Health, Obstetric and Neonatal Nurses (AWHONN), 2000 L Street, N.W. Suite 740, Washington, DC, 20036, 800-673-8499, www.awhonn.org

Depression After Delivery (DAD) Support Network, P.O. Box 278, Belle Mead, NJ, 08502, 215-295-3994, 800-944-4773, www.behavenet.com/dadinc/

Health Science Consortium, 201 Silver Cedar Court, Chapel Hill, NC, 27514-1517, 919-942-8731

Hollister, Inc., 2000 Hollister Drive, Libertyville, IL, 60048, 800-323-4060, www.hollister.com

Johnson & Johnson Consumer Products, Inc., 199 Grandview Road, Skillman, NJ, 08558-9418, 908-874-1000

Postpartum Support International, 927 North Kellogg Avenue, Santa Barbara, CA, 93111, 800-967-7636

CHAPTER 51
Newborn Care

REFERENCES/SUGGESTED READINGS

Alexander, G. R., & Allen, M. C. (1996). Conceptualization, measurement, and use of gestational age: I. clinical and public health practice. *Journal of Perinatology, 16*(1), 53.

American Academy of Pediatrics (AAP). (1989). Report of the AAP task force on circumcision. *Pediatrics, 84*(4), 388–391.

American Academy of Pediatrics (AAP). Committee on Pediatrics and Committee on Genetics (1996). Newborn screening fact sheets. *Pediatrics, 98*(3), 473.

American Academy of Pediatrics (AAP). Work Group on Breastfeeding (1997). Breastfeeding and the use of human milk. *Pediatrics, 100*(6), 1035.

Ballard, J. L., Khoury, J. C., Wedig, K., Wang, L., Eilers-Walsman, B. L., & Lipp, R. (1991). New Ballard Score, expanded to include extremely premature infants. *Journal of Pediatrics, 19*(3), 417–423.

Baptist, E. C., & Amin, P. V. (1996). Perinatal testicular torsion and the hard testicle. *Journal of Perinatology, 16*(1), 67.

Behrman, R. E., Kliegman, R. M., & Aivin, A. M. (Eds.). (1996). *Nelson's textbook of pediatrics* (15th ed.). Philadelphia: W. B. Saunders.

Brazelton, T. B. (1984). *Neonatal behavioral assessment scale* (2nd ed.). London: Heineman.

Burroughs, A. (1997). *Maternity nursing* (7th ed.). Philadelphia: W.B. Saunders.

Callister, L., & Vega, R. (1998). Giving birth: Guatemalan women's voices. *Journal of Obstetric, Gynecologic, and Neonatal Nursing, 27*(3), 289–295.

Choudhry, U. (1997). Traditional practices of women from India: Pregnancy, childbirth, and newborn care. *Journal of Obstetric, Gynecologic, and Neonatal Nursing, 26*(5), 533–539.

Estes, M. E. Z. (1998). *Health assessment & physical examination*. Albany, NY: Delmar.

Fanaroff, A., & Martin, R. (1997). *Neonatal-perinatal medicine: Diseases of the fetus and infant* (6th ed.). St. Louis, MO: Mosby-Year Book.

Gennaro, S., Kamwendo, L., Mbweza, E., & Kershbaumer, R. (1998). Childbearing in Malawi, Africa. *Journal of Obstetric, Gynecologic, and Neonatal Nursing, 27*(2),191–196.

Gorrie, T., McKinney, E., & Murray, S. (1998). *Foundations of maternal-newborn nursing* (2nd ed.). Philadelphia: W. B. Saunders.

Howard, J., & Berbiglia, V. (1997). Caring for childbearing Korean women. *Journal of Obstetric, Gynecologic, and Neonatal Nursing, 26*(6), 665–671.

Hutchinson, M., & Baqi-Aziz, M. (1994). Nursing care of the childbearing Muslim family. *Journal of Obstetric, Gynecologic, and Neonatal Nursing, 23*(9), 767–771.

Krebs, T. (1998). Cord care: Is it necessary? *Mother Baby Journal, 3*, 5.

Ladewig, P., London, M., & Olds, S. (1998). *Maternal-newborn nursing care* (4th ed.). Menlo Park, CA: Addison-Wesley.

Letko, M. (1996). Understanding the Apgar score. *Journal of Obstetric, Gynecologic, and Neonatal Nursing, 25*(4), 299.

Lightfoot-Klein, H. G., & Shaw, E. (1990). Special needs of ritually circumcised women patients. *Journal of Obstetric, Gynecologic, and Neonatal Nursing, 20*(2), 102–106.

Lowdermilk, D., Perry, S., & Bobak, I. (1999). *Maternity nursing* (5th ed.). St. Louis, MO: Mosby-Year Book.

Lowe, N. K., & Reiss, R. (1996). Parturition and fetal adaptation. *Journal of Obstetric, Gynecologic, and Neonatal Nursing, 25*(4), 339–349.

Lund, C., Kuller, J., Lane, A., Lott, J., & Raines, D. (1999). Neonatal skin care: The scientific basis for practice. *Journal of Obstetric, Gynecologic, and Neonatal Nursing, 28*(3), 241–254.

Mattson, S. (1995). Culturally sensitive perinatal care for Southeast Asians. *Journal of Obstetric, Gynecologic, and Neonatal Nursing, 24*(4), 335–341.

Merenstein, G., Adams, K., & Weisman, L. (1998). Infections in the neonate. In G. Merenstein & S. Gardner (Eds.), *Handbook of neonatal intensive care* (4th ed.). St. Louis, MO: Mosby-Year Book.

Penny-MacGillivray, T. (1996). A newborn's first bath: When? *Journal of Obstetric, Gynecologic, and Neonatal Nursing, 25*(6), 481.

Schneiderman, J. (1996). Postpartum nursing for Korean mothers. *The American Journal of Maternal Child Nursing, 21*(3), 155–158.

Sharts-Hopko, N. (1995). Birth in the Japanese context. *Journal of Obstetric, Gynecologic, and Neonatal Nursing, 24*(4), 343–351.

Sherwen, L. N. (1995). Human immunodeficiency virus infection during the perinatal period. *Journal of Perinatology, 15*(1), 54.

Shorten, A. (1995). Female circumcision: Understanding special needs. *Holistic Nurse Practitioner, 9*(2), 66–73.

Tyrala, E. E. (1996). The infant of the diabetic mother. *Obstetric and Gynecologic Clinics of North America, 23*(1), 221.

Verma, R. P. (1995). Respiratory distress syndrome of the newborn infant. *Obstetric Gynecologic Survey, 50*(7), 542.

York, R., Bhuttarowas, P., & Brown, L. (1999). The development of nursing in Thailand. *The American Journal of Maternal Child Nursing, 24*(3), 145–150.

RESOURCES

Association of Women's Health, Obstetric and Neonatal Nurses AWHONN, 2000 L Street N.W., Suite 740, Washington, DC, 20036, 800-673-8499, www.awhonn.org

La Leche League International, 1400 Meacham Road, Schaumburg, IL, 60173-4048, 847-519-7730, http://lalecheleague.org

CHAPTER 52
Basics of Pediatric Care

REFERENCES/SUGGESTED READINGS

Abbott. K., Fowler-Kerry, S. (1995). The use of a topical refrigerant anesthetic to reduce injection pain in children. *Journal Pain Symptom Management, 10*(8), 584–590.

Ashwill, J. W., & Droske, S. C. (1997) *Nursing care of children: principles and practice.* Philadelphia: W. B. Saunders.

Ball, J., & Bindler, R. (1999). *Pediatric nursing* (2d ed.). Norwalk, CT: Appleton & Lange.

Behrman, R., Kliegman, R. M., & Jenson, H. B. (1999). *Nelson textbook of pediatrics* (16th ed.). Philadelphia: W. B. Saunders.

Brown. P. (1992). Saying goodbye. *Nursing Times, 89*(4), 26–29.

Eland, J. M., & Anderson, J. E. (1977). The experience of pain in children. In A. Jacox (Ed.), *Pain: A sourcebook for nurses and other health professionals.* Boston: Little, Brown.

Ellis, R. (1989). Once more into the void. *Contemporary Pediatrics, 6*(8), 164.

Faulkner, K. (1997). Talking about death with a dying child. *American Journal of Nursing, 97*(6), 64–69.

Gedaly-Duff, V., & Burns, C. (1992). Reducing children's pain-distress associated with injection using cold: A pilot study. *Journal of the American Academy of Nurse Practitioners, 4*(3), 95–99.

Kai, J. (1993). Parents' perceptions of taking babies' rectal temperature. *British Medical Journal, 307,* 660–662.

Marks, M. G. (1998). *Broadribb's introductory pediatric nursing* (5th ed.). Philadelphia: Lippincott.

Moldow, D., & Martinson, I. Home care for seriously ill children: A manual for parents. Children's Hospice International, 901 N. Washington Street, 7th Floor, Alexandria, VA 22314, (800) 24-CHILD.

Shelton, T., & Stepanek, J. (1994). Family-centered care for children needing specialized health and developmental services. Association for the Care of Children's Health. Bethesda, MD.

Visintainer, M., & Wolfer, J. (1975). Psychological preparation for surgical pediatric patient: The effect on children's and parents' stress response and adjustment. *Pediatrics, 56*(2), 187–202.

Wong, D. (1997). *Whaley & Wong's essentials of pediatric nursing.* St. Louis, MO: Mosby-Year Book.

Wong, D., Hockenberry-Eaton, M., Wilson, D., Winkelstein, M., Ahmann, E., & DiVito-Thomas, P. (1999). *Whaley & Wong's nursing care of infants and children* (6th ed.). St. Louis, MO: Mosby-Year Book.

Zuckerberg, A. L. (1994). Preoperative approach to child. *Pediatric Clinics of North America, 4*(1), 25.

RESOURCES

Association for the Care of Children's Health, 19 Mantua Road, Mount Royal, NJ, 08061, 609-224-1742, www.acch.org

Children's Hospice International, 2202 Mt. Vernon Avenue, Suite 3-c, Alexandria, VA, 22301, 1-800-24-CHILD, 703-684-0330, www.chionline.org

Compassionate Friends, P.O. Box 3696, Oak Brook, IL, 60522-3696, http://www.compassionatefriends.org/index.html

National Association of Pediatric Home and Community Care, 21 N. Quinsigamond Avenue, Shewsbury, MA, 01545, 508-856-1908, www.ummed.edu/dept/NAPHACC

National Father's Network, The Kindering Center, 16120 N.E. 8th Street, Bellevue, WA, 98008, www.fathersnetwork.org

Sibling Support Project, Children's Hospital and Medical Center, CL-09, P.O. Box 5371, Seattle, WA, 98105-0371, 206-368-4911, www.chmc.org/departmt/sibsupp

CHAPTER 53
Infants with Special Needs:
Birth to 12 Months

REFERENCES/SUGGESTED READINGS

The American SIDS Institute. (1999). *SIDS information* [Online]. Available: http://www.sids.org/rsearch/test/sld003.htm

Anderson, R. N., Kochanek, K. D., & Murphy, S. L. (1997). Report of final mortality statistics, 1995. *Monthly Vital*

Statistics Report, 4511 (Suppl. 2). Hyattsville, MD: National Center for Health Statistics.

Ashwill, J. W., & Droske, S. C. (1997). *Nursing care of children principles and practice.* Philadelphia: W. B. Saunders.

Balk, S. (1996). The environmental history: Asking the right questions. *Contemporary Pediatrics, 13*(2), 19–36.

Ball, J., & Bindler, R. (1999). *Pediatric nursing* (2nd ed.). Norwalk, CT: Appleton & Lange.

Barnett, E. D., Teele, D. W., Klein, J. O., Cabral, H. J., and Kharasch, S. J. (1997). Comparison of ceftriaxone and trimethoprim-sulfamethoxazole for acute otitis media. *Pediatrics, 99*(1), 23–28.

Beeber, S. (1996). Parental smoking and childhood asthma. *Journal of Pediatric Health Care, 10*(2), 58–62.

Behrman, R., Kliegman, R. M., & Arvin, A. M. (1996). *Nelson's textbook of pediatrics* (15th ed.). Philadelphia: W. B. Saunders.

Castiglia, P. (1998). Trisomy 21 syndrome: Is there anything new? *Journal of Pediatric Health Care, 12*(1), 35–37.

Comprehensive Sickle Cell Disease Program, Children's Medical Center of Dallas. (1995). *The infant and young child with sickle cell anemia.* Austin, TX: Texas Department of Health, Newborn Screening.

Cystic Fibrosis Foundation. (1998). *CPX study in adult patients moves to phase II* [On-line]. Available: http://www.cff.org/clinical03.htm

Duncan, B., Ey, J., Holberg, C. J., Wright, A. L., Martinez, F. D., and Taussig, L. M. (1993). Exclusive breast-feeding for at least 4 months protects against otitis media. *Pediatrics 91*(5), 867–872.

Eisenhauer, L. A., Nichols, L. W., Spencer, R. T., & Bergan, F. W. (1998). *Clinical Pharmacology and Nursing Management* (5th ed.). Philadelphia: Lippincott.

Fiel, S. B. (1995). Aerosol delivery of antibiotics to the lower airways of patients with cystic fibrosis. *Chest 107*(2), 61S–64S.

Green, S., & Rothrock, S. (1993). Single-dose intramuscular ceftriaxone for acute otitis media in children. *Pediatrics, 91*(1), 23–29.

Henley, S. N. (1996). *Sickle cell disease: A resource for the educator.* Austin, TX: Texas Department of Health, Newborn Screening Program.

Hoffman, J. I. (1990). Congenital heart disease: Incidence and inheritance, *Pediatric Clinics of North America, 37*(1), 31.

Kitchens, G. G. (1995). Relationship of environmental tobacco smoke to otitis media in young children. *Laryngoscope, 105*(5, Part 2), 1–13.

Knowles, M. R., Olivier, K. N., Hohneker, K. W., Robinson, J., Bennett, W. D., & Boucher, R. C. (1995). Pharmacologic treatment of abnormal ion transport in the airway epithelium in cystic fibrosis. *Chest, 107*(2), 71S–76S.

Lobo, M. L., Barnard, K. E., & Coombs, J. B. (1992). Failure to thrive: A parent–infant interaction perspective. *Journal of Pediatric Nursing, 7*(4), 251–261.

Marks, M. G. (1998). *Broadribb's introductory pediatric nursing* (5th ed.). Philadelphia: J. B. Lippincott.

Richard, M. (1991). Feeding the newborn with cleft lip and/or palate: The enlargement, stimulate, swallow, and rest (ESSR) method. *Journal of Pediatric Nursing, 6*(5), 317–321.

Richard, M. (1994). Common pediatric craniofacial reconstructions. *Nursing Clinics of North America, 29*(4), 791–799.

Saarinen, U. M., & Kajosaari, M. (1995). Breastfeeding as prophylaxis against atopic disease: Prospective follow-up study until 17 years old. *Lancet, 1995*(346), 1065–1069.

Sassen, M. L., Brand, R., & Grote, J. J. (1997). Risk factors for otitis media with effusion in children 0 to 2 years of age. *American Journal of Otolaryngology, 18*(5), 324–330.

Schuman, A. (1997). Disposable diapers? Definitely! *Contemporary Pediatrics, 14*(11), 131–139.

Shak, S. (1995). Aerosolized recombinant human Dnase I for the treatment of cystic fibrosis. *Chest, 107*(2), 65S–70S.

Shaw, G. M, Lamamer, E. J., Wassernman, C. R., O'Malley, C. D., & Tolarova, M. M. (1995). Risks of orofacial clefts in children born to women using multivitamins containing folic acid periconceptionally. *The Lancet, 346*(8972), 393.

Tully, S., Bar-Haim, Y., & Bradley, R. (1995). Abnormal tympanography after supine bottle feeding. *Journal of Pediatrics, 1995*(126), S105–S111.

Wahlgren, D., Hovell, M., Meltzer, S., Hofstetter, C., & Zakarian, J. (1997). Reduction of environmental tobacco smoke exposure in asthmatic children: A 2 year follow-up. *Chest, 111*(1), 81–88.

White, K. R., Munro, C. L., & Pickler, R. H. (1995). Therapeutic implications of recent advances in cystic fibrosis. *The American Journal of Maternal/Child Nursing, 20*(6), 58–64.

Winkelstein, M. (1995). Teaching pregnant adolescents to cope with environmental smoke. *Maternal Child Nursing, 20*, 38–42.

Wong, D. L. (1997). *Whaley & Wong's essentials of pediatric nursing* (5th ed.). St. Louis, MO: Mosby.

Wong, D. L., Hockenberry-Eaton, M., Winkelstein, M. L., Wilson, D., Ahmann, E., & DiVito-Thomas, P. A. (1999). *Whaley and Wong's nursing care of infants and children* (6th ed.). St. Louis, MO: Mosby.

Yetman, R., & Coody, D. (1997). Failure to thrive: A clinical guideline. *Journal of Pediatric Health Care, 11*(3), 134–137.

RESOURCES

American Cleft Palate–Craniofacial Association, 104 South Estes Drive, Suite 204, Chapel Hill, NC, 27514, 919-933-9044, www.cleft.com

American Lung Association, 1-800-LUNG USA (800-586-4872), www.lungusa.org

American Sickle-Cell Anemia Association, 10300 Carnegie Avenue, Cleveland, OH, 44106, 216-229-8600

Automotive Safety for Children Program, 575 West Drive, Room 004, Indianapolis, IN, 46202-5109, 317-274-2977 or 1-800-KID-N-CAR (in Indiana)

Cystic Fibrosis Foundation, 6931 Arlington Road, Bethesda, MD, 20814, 301-951-4422, 800-FIGHT CF, www.cff.org

Hydrocephalus Association, 870 Market Street, Suite 955, San Francisco, CA, 94102, 415-732-7040, www.neurosurgery. mgh.harvard.edu

La Leche League International, 1400 Meacham Road, Schaumburg, IL, 60173, 847-519-7730 (24-hour service), 800-LA-LECHE (for local number or catalog; 9 A.M.–3 P.M.)

National Association for Down Syndrome, 800-221-4602, www.nads.org

National Hydrocephalus Foundation, Route 1, River Road, Box 210, Joliet, IL, 60436, 815-467-6548

National Sudden Infant Death Syndrome Foundation, 1314 Bedford Avenue, Suite 210, Baltimore, MD, 21208, 800-638-7437

Spina Bifida Association of America, 4590 MacArthur Boulevard, NW, Suite 250, Washington, DC, 20007-4226, 202-944-3285 or 800-621-3141, www.sbaa.org

United Cerebral Palsy Association, Inc., 1600 L Street N.W., Suite 700, Washington, DC, 20036, 800-872-5827, www.ucpa.org, email: ucpnatl@ucpa.org

CHAPTER 54
Common Problems:
1–18 Years

REFERENCES/SUGGESTED READINGS

American Psychiatric Association. (1994). *Diagnostic and statistical manual of mental disorders* (4th ed.). Washington, DC: Author.

Ashwill, J. W., & Droske, S. C. (1997) *Nursing care of children principles and practice.* Philadelphia: W. B. Saunders.

Ball, J., & Bindler, R. (1999). *Pediatric nursing* (2nd ed.). Norwalk, CT: Appleton & Lange.

Behrman, R., Kliegman, R. M., & Arvin, A. M. (1996). *Nelson's textbook of pediatrics* (15th ed.). Philadelphia: W. B. Saunders.

Centers for Disease Control and Prevention (1994). General recommendations on immunization: Recommendations of the Advisory Committee on Immunization Practices (ACIP), *MMWR, 43*(RR-1), 1–38.

Centers for Disease Control and Prevention (1996). Update: vaccine side effects, adverse reactions, contraindications and precautions: Recommendations of the Advisory Committee on Immunization Practices (ACIP). *MMWR, 45*(RR-12), 1–35.

Center for Disease Control and Prevention (1997a). Rates of homicide, suicide, and firearm-related death among children—26 industrialized countries. *MMWR, 46*(5), 101–105.

Centers for Disease Control and Prevention (1997b). Status report on the childhood immunization initiative: National, state, and urban area vaccination coverage levels among children aged 19–35 months—United States, 1996. *MMWR, 46*(29), 657–664.

Eisenhauer, L., Nichols, L., Spencer, R., & Bergan, F. (1998). *Clinical pharmacology & nursing management* (5th ed.). Philadelphia: Lippincott.

Herrin, J. T., & Antoon, A. Y. (1996) Burn injuries. In R. Behrman, R. M. Kliegman, & A. M. Arvin (Eds.), *Nelson textbook of pediatrics* (15th ed., pp. 270–277). Philadelphia: W. B. Saunders.

Hurwitz, S. (1995). Acne treatment for the 90s. *Contemporary Pediatrics, 12*(8), 19–32.

Kelsch, R. C., & Sedman, N. J. (1993). Nephrotic syndrome. *Pediatrics in Review, 14*(1), 33.

Lund, C. C., & Browder, N. C. (1944). Estimation of burn size. *Surgery, Gynecology, and Obstetrics, 79,* 352–358.

Marks, M. G. (1998). *Broadribb's introductory pediatric nursing* (5th. ed.). Philadelphia, PA: J. B. Lippincott.

Ott, M. J., Horn, M., & McLaughlin, D. (1995). Pediatric TB in the 90s. *Maternal & Child Health Nursing, 20*(1), 16–20.

Thomas, E., & Buchwald, M. (1995). Child preferences for post-tonsillectomy diet. *International Journal of Pediatric Otorhinolaryngology, 31*(29), 33.

U.S. Department of Health and Human Services. (1990). *Healthy people 2000: National health promotion and disease prevention* (No. 91-502/2). Washington, DC: Author.

Wong, D. (1997). *Whaley & Wong's essentials of pediatric nursing.* St. Louis, MO: Mosby.

Wong, D., Hockenberry-Eaton, M., Winkelstein, M., Wilson, D., Ahmann, E., & DiVito-Thomas, P. (1999). *Whaley & Wong's nursing care of infants and children.* (6th. ed.). St. Louis, MO: Mosby.

RESOURCES

American Academy of Pediatrics (AAP), 141 Northwest Point Boulevard, Elk Grove Village, IL, 60007-1098, 800-433-9016; 847-228-5005, www.aap.org

American Anorexia / Bulimia Association, Inc., 165 West 46th Street, #1108, New York, NY, 10036, 212-575-6200

Autism Society of America (ASA), 7910 Woodmont Avenue, Suite 300, Bethesda, MD, 20814-3015, 301-657-0881, 800-3AUTISM x.150, www.autism-society.org.

Centers for Disease Control and Prevention, www.cdc.gov

Muscular Dystrophy Association of America, Inc., 3300 East Sunrise Drive, Tucson, AZ, 85718, 800-572-1717; FAX: 520-529-5300, www.mdausa.org/home.html

National Association of Anorexia Nervosa and Associated Disorders, Inc., P.O. Box 7, Highland Park, IL, 60035, 847-831-3438

National Association of Pediatric Nurses Associates and Practitioners (NAPNAP), 1101 Kings Highway, North, Suite 206, Cherry Hill, NJ, 08034-1912, 877-662-7627, www.napnap.org

National Hemophilia Foundation, 116 West 32nd Street, 11th Floor, New York, NY, 10001, 800-424-2634, www.hemophilia.org

The National Pediculosis Association, P.O. Box 610189, Newton, MA, 02161, 800-446-4NPA; 781-449-6487, www.headlice.org

National Scoliosis Foundation, Inc., 5 Cabot Place, Stoughton, MA, 02072

Scoliosis Association, Inc., P.O. Box 811705, Boca Raton, FL, 33481-1705, 800-800-0669

CHAPTER 55
Nursing Care of the Older Client

REFERENCES/SUGGESTED READINGS

American Association of Retired Persons. (1995). *A profile of older Americans.* Washington, DC: Department of Health and Human Services.

Andersen, C. (1999). *Antecedents, correlates, and impact of violent behaviors in the elderly VA client.* Unpublished thesis, University of Iowa, Iowa City, IA.

Andersen, C. F. (1999). *Nursing student to nursing leader: The critical path to leadership development.* Albany, NY: Delmar Publishers.

Bahr, Sr. R. T. (1994). An overview of gerontological nursing. In M. Hogstel (Ed.), *Nursing care of the older adult* (3rd ed., pp. 2–25). Albany: Delmar Publishers.

Campion, E. (1994). The oldest old. *New England Journal of Medicine, 330,* 1819–1820.

Dychtwald, K., & Flower, J. (1989). *Age wave: The challenges and opportunities of an aging america.* Los Angeles, CA: Jeremy T. Tarcher.

Fetters, C. (1994). *Standard of care on wandering.* Knoxville, IA: Department of Veterans Affairs Medical Center, Division of Nursing.

Gallo, G., Reichel, W., & Andersen, L. (1995). *Handbook of geriatric assessment* (2nd ed.). Gaithersburg, MD: Aspen Publishers.

Hogstel, M. (Ed.). (1994). *Nursing care of the older adult* (3rd ed.). Albany, NY: Delmar Publishers.

Hu, T.W. (1990). Impact of urinary incontinence on health-care costs. *Journal of American Geriatrics Society, 38*(3), 292–295.

Maas, M., Buckwalter, K., & Hardy, M. (1991). *Nursing diagnosis and new interventions for the elderly.* Redwood City, CA: Addison-Wesley.

McCloskey, J., & Bulechek, G. (1996). *Nursing interventions classifications (NIC)* (2nd ed.). St. Louis, MO: Mosby-Year Book.

Needham, J. F. (1995). *Gerontological nursing.* Albany, NY: Delmar Publishers.

Peskin, B. (1999). *Beyond the zone.* Houston, TX: Noble Publishing.

U.S. Senate Special Committee on Aging. (1990). *Aging America—Trends and projections.* Washington, DC: U.S. Department of Health and Human Services.

Yen, P. K. (1995). Maximizing calcium intake. *Geriatric Nursing, 16*(2), 92–93.

RESOURCES

Administration on Aging, U.S. Department of Health and Human Services, 330 Independence Avenue S.W., Washington, DC, 20201, 202-619-0724, www.aoa.dhhs.gov

American Association of Geriatric Psychiatry, 7910 Woodmont Avenue, Suite 1050, Bethesda, MD, 20814-3004, 301-654-7850, www.aagpgpa.org

American Association of Retired Persons (AARP), 601 East Street N.W., Washington, DC, 20049, 800-424-3410, www.aarp.org

American Nurses Association (ANA), Council on Gerontological Nursing Practice, 600 Maryland Avenue S.W., Suite 100W, Washington, DC, 20024, 800-274-4262, www.nursingworld.org

Department of Health and Human Services, Public Health Service, Agency for Health Care Policy and Research, Executive Office Center, 200 Independence Avenue, S.W., Washington, DC, 20201, 202-619-0257, 877-696-6775, www.dhhs.gov, www.ahcpr.gov

National Council on Aging, Inc., 409 3rd Street, S.W., Washington, DC, 20024, 800-424-9046, www.ncoa.org

CHAPTER 56
Rehabilitation, Home Health, Long-Term Care, and Hospice

REFERENCES/SUGGESTED READINGS

Abrams, W. B., Beers, M. H., & Berkow, R. (Eds.). (1995). *The Merck manual of geriatrics* (2nd ed.). Whitehouse Station, NJ: Merck Research Laboratories.

American Association of Retired Persons. (1995). *A profile of older Americans.* Washington, DC: U.S. Department of Health and Human Services.

American Health Care Association (AHCA). (1998). The looming crisis [On-line]. Available: www.ahca.org

Assisted Living Federation of America (ALFA). (1999). What is assisted living [On-line]. Available: www.alfa.org

Bailis, S. S. (1995). Accreditation: A necessary next step. *Provider, 21*(5), 55–56.

Barker, E. (1999). Life care planning. *RN, 62*(3), 58–61.

Benefield, L. (1996). Making the transition to home care nursing. *AJN, 96*(10), 47–49.

Boon, T. (1998). Don't forget the hospice option. *RN, 61*(2), 30–33.

Bral, E. (1998). Caring for adults with chronic cancer pain. *AJN, 98*(4), 26–32.

Buckwalter, K. C. (1995). Health care policy 101—what nurses and their clients need to know. *Journal of Gerontological Nursing, 21*(3), 5–6.

Diaz, D. (1995). Geriatric UPDATE 95. *Nursing95, 25*(3), 62–64.

Fisher, C. (1995). Coming home to assisted living. *Provider, 21*(10), 57–64.

Galarneau, L. (1993). An interdisciplinary approach to mobility and safety education for caregivers and stroke patients. *Rehabilitation Nursing, 18*(6), 395–398.

Glosner, G. W. (1995). How subacute care fills the gap. *Nursing95, 25*(3), 51.

Gresham, G. E., Duncan, P. W., Stason, W. B., et al. (1995, May). *Post stroke rehabilitation.* Clinical Practice Guide-line, No. 16, Rockville, MD: U.S. Department of Health and Human Services. Public Health Service Agency for Health Care Policy and Research. AHCPR Publication No. 95–0062.

Grove, N. (1997). Helping families select a nursing home. *RN, 60*(3), 37–40.

Habel, M. (Ed.). (1993). Rehabilitation nursing practice. *The specialty practice of rehabilitation nursing.* Skokie, IL: The Rehabilitation Nursing Foundation of the Association of Rehabilitation Nurses.

Health, Education, and Human Services Division. (1994). *Long-term care reform.* (GAO)/HEHS–94–227). Washington DC: U.S. General Accounting Office.

Hospice Education Institute (1999). Definition of palliative care [On-line]. Available: www.hospiceworld.org

Huey, F. L. (Ed.). (1995). Humpty dumpty: Good egg for rehab? *The Nursing Spectrum, 8*(25), 3.

Kazanowski, M. (1997). A commitment to palliative care: Could it impact assisted suicide? *Journal of Gerontologic Nursing, 23*(3), 36–42.

Lasky, W. F. (1995). Assisted living: A brand new world. *Nursing Homes, 44*(7), 40–41.

Meng, M. E. (1995). Starting an adult day care center. *Provider, 21*(12), 38–40.

Millea, K. (1995). Home health care UPDATE 95. *Nursing95, 25*(7), 57–59.

National Association for Home Care (NAHC). (1999). Hospice [On-line]. Available: www.nahc.org/HAA

National Hospice Organization (NHO). (1999). The basics of hospice [On-line]. Available: www.nho.org

National Institute on Aging (NIA). (1996). Planning for long-term care [On-line]. Available: www.nih.gov/nia/health/pubpub/longterm.htm

Puopolo, A. (1999). Gaining confidence to talk about end-of-life care. *Nursing99, 29*(7), 49–51.

Ufema, J. (1999). Reflections on death and dying. *Nursing99, 29*(6), 56–59.

Walsh, G. G. (1995). How subacute care fills the gap. *Nursing95, 25*(3), 51.

Wenckus, E. (1995). Working with an interdisciplinary team. *The Nursing Spectrum, 8*(6), 11–12.

RESOURCES

American Association of Homes and Services for the Aging, Suite 500, 901 E Street N.W., Washington, DC, 20004-2011, 202-783-2242, www.aahsa.org

American Association of Retired Persons (AARP), 601 E Street N.W., Washington, DC, 20049, 202-434-6190, 800-424-3410, www.aarp.org

American Health Care Association, 1201 L Street N.W., Washington, DC, 20005, 202-842-4444, www.ahca.org

American Hospital Association (AHA), Chicago Headquarters (CH), One North Franklin, Chicago, IL, 60606, 312-422-3000, www.aha.org

American Hospital Association, Washington Office (WO), 325 Seventh Street N.W., Washington, DC, 20004, 202-638-1100, 800-424-4301, www.aha.org

Assisted Living Federation of America, Suite 400, 10300 Eaton Place, Fairfax, VA, 22030, 703-691-8100, www.alfa.org

Association of Rehabilitation Nurses, 4700 W. Lake Avenue, Glenview, IL, 60025-1485, 800-229-7530, 847-375-4710, www.rehabnurse.org

Department of Health and Human Services, Public Health Service, National Institutes of Health, 200 Independence Avenue, S.W., Washington, DC, 20201, 202-619-0257, 877-696-6775, www.hhs.gov/

Foundation for Hospice & Home Care, 519 C Street N.E., Washington, DC, 20002, 302-547-6586

Health Care Financing Administration (HCFA), 7500 Security Boulevard, Baltimore, MD, 21244, 800-638-6833, www.hcfa.gov

Home Healthcare Nurses Association, 7794 Grow Drive, Pensacola, FL, 32514, 850-474-1066, 800-558-4462, www.hhna.org

Hospice Association of America (HAA), 228 Seventh Street S.E., Washington, DC, 20003, 202-546-4759, www.nahc.org/HAA

Hospice Education Institute, 190 Westbrook Road, Essex, CT, 06426-1510, 860-767-1620, 800-331-1620, www.hospiceworld.org

National Association for Home Care, 228 Seventh Street S.E., Washington, DC, 20003, 202-547-7424, www.nahc.org

National Citizens' Coalition for Nursing Home Reform, Suite 202, 1424 16th Street N.W., Washington, DC, 20036-2211, 202-332-2275, www.nccnhr.org

National Hospice Organization (NHO), 1901 North Moore Street, Suite 901, Arlington, VA, 22209, 703-243-5900, 800-658-8898, www.nho.org

National Rehabilitation Association, 633 S. Washington Street, Alexandria, VA, 22314, 703-836-0850, http://nationalrehab.org

National Rehabilitation Information Center (NARIC), 1010 Wayne Avenue, Suite 800, Silver Spring, MD, 20910-5633, 301-562-2400, 800-346-2742, www.naric.com

Nursing Home Information Service, National Council of Senior Citizens, 8403 Colesville Road, Suite 1200, Silver Spring, MD, 20910, 310-578-8938, www.ncscinc.org

CHAPTER 57
Leadership/Work Transition

REFERENCES/SUGGESTED READINGS

Bernzweig, E. P. (1995). *The nurse's liability for malpractice: A programmed course* (6th ed.). St. Louis, MO: Mosby-Year Book.

Bolles, R. N. (1997). *What color is your parachute? A practical manual for job-hunters & career-changers.* Berkeley, CA: Ten Speed Press.

Brent, N. J. (1997). *Nurses and the law: A guide to principles and application.* Philadelphia: Saunders.

Bureau of Labor Statistics. (1998). 1998–99 *Occupational outlook handbook.* Chicago, IL: Author.

Catalano, J. T. (1995). *Ethical and legal aspects of nursing* (2nd ed.). Springhouse, PA: Springhouse Corporation.

Catalano, J. T. (1996). *Contemporary professional nursing.* Philadelphia: Davis.

Guido, G. W. (1996). *Legal issues in nursing* (2nd ed.). Norwalk, CT: Appleton & Lange.

Haft, T. (1997). *Job notes: Resumes.* New York: Princeton Review Publishing, L.L.C.

Hansten, R. I., & Washburn, M. J. (1998). *Clinical delegation skills. A handbook for professional practice.* Gaithersburg, MD: Aspen Publishers.

Joint Commission on Accreditation of Healthcare Organizations. (1998). *Addressing staffing needs for patient care: Solutions for hospital leaders.* Oakbrook Terrace, IL: Author.

Marino, K. (1991). *Just resumes: 200 powerful and proven successful resumes to get that job.* New York: John Wiley & Sons.

Marquis, B. L., & Huston, C. J. (1996). *Leadership roles and management functions in nursing theory and application* (2nd ed.). Philadelphia: Lippincott-Raven.

Mattera, M. D. (Ed.). (1997). Ace the all-important job interview. *Nursing opportunities 1997.* Montvale, NJ: Medical Economics.

National Council of State Boards of Nursing. (1996). *Delegation: Concepts and decision-making process.* Chicago, IL

National Council of State Boards of Nursing, Inc. (1997a). *NCLEX candidate examination bulletin.* Chicago, IL: Author.

National Council of State Boards of Nursing, Inc. (1997b). *1996 profiles of member boards.* Chicago, IL: Author.

New York State Nurses Association. (1998a). LPNs and the practice of nursing. *Report the official newsletter of the New York State Nurses Association, 29*(9), 3.

New York State Nurses Association. (1998b). Responsibility for delegated and assigned care. *Report the official newsletter of the New York State Nurses Association, 29*(5), 3.

Office of the Professions. (1995). *Nursing handbook.* Albany, NY: New York State Education Department.

Parker, Y. (1996). *Damn good resume guide: A crash course in resume writing.* Berkeley, CA: Ten Speed Press.

Parkman, C. A. (1996). Delegation: Are you doing it right? *American Journal of Nursing, 96*(9), 43–47.

Trandel-Korenchuk, D. M. (1997). *Nurses and the law* (5th ed.). Gaithersburg, MD: Aspen Publishers.

Wilkinson, A. P. (1998, June). Nursing malpractice. *Nursing98, 28*(6), 34–38.

Appendix A: Recommended Childhood Immunization Schedule—United States, January–December 1999

Vaccines[1] are listed under routinely recommended ages. ⬜Bars *indicate range of recommended ages for immunization. Any dose not given at the recommended age should be given as a "catch-up" immunization at any subsequent visit when indicated and feasible.* ⬭Ovals *indicate vaccines to be given if previously recommended doses were missed or given earlier than the recommended minimum age.*

AGE ▶ VACCINE ▼	BIRTH	1 mo	2 mo	4 mo	6 mo	12 mo	15 mo	18 mo	4–6 yr	11–12 yr	14–16 yr
Hepatitis B[2]		Hep B									
			Hep B			Hep B				Hep B	
Diphtheria, Tetanus, Pertussis[3]			DTaP	DTaP	DTaP		DTaP[3]		DTaP	Td	
H. influenzae type b[4]			Hib	Hib	Hib	Hib					
Polio[5]			IPV	IPV	Polio[5]				Polio		
Rotavirus[6]			Rv[6]	Rv[6]	Rv[6]						
Measles, Mumps, Rubella[7]						MMR			MMR[7]	MMR[7]	
Varicella[8]						Var				Var[8]	

Approved by the Advisory Committee on Immunization Practices (ACIP), the American Academy of Pediatrics (AAP), and the American Academy of Family Physicians (AAFP).

[1]This schedule indicates the recommended ages for routine administration of currently licensed childhood vaccines. Combination vaccines may be used whenever any components of the combination are indicated and its other components are not contraindicated. Providers should consult the manufacturers' package inserts for detailed recommendations.

[2]*Infants born to HBsAg-negative mothers* should receive the 2nd dose of hepatitis B (Hep B) vaccine at least 1 month after the 1st dose. The 3rd dose should be administered at least 4 months after the 1st dose and at least 2 months after the 2nd dose, but not before 6 months of age for infants.

Infants born to HBsAg-positive mothers should receive hepatitis B vaccine and 0.5 mL hepatitis B immune globulin (HBIG) within 12 hours of birth at separate sites. The 2nd dose is recommended at 1 to 2 months of age and the 3rd dose at 6 months of age.

Infants born to mothers whose HBsAg status is unknown should receive hepatitis B vaccine within 12 hours of birth. Maternal blood should be drawn at the time of delivery to determine the mother's HBsAg status; if the HBsAg test is positive, the infant should receive HBIG as soon as possible (no later than 1 week of age).

All children and adolescents (through 18 years of age) who have not been immunized against hepatitis B may begin the series during any visit. Special efforts should be made to immunize children who were born in or whose parents were born in areas of the world with moderate or high endemicity of hepatitis B virus infection.

[3]DTaP (diphtheria and tetanus toxoids and acellular pertussis vaccine) is the preferred vaccine for all doses in the immunization series, including completion of the series in children who have received 1 or more doses of whole-cell DTP vaccine. Whole-cell DTP is an acceptable alternative to DTaP. The 4th dose (DTP or DTaP) may be administered as early as 12 months of age, provided 6 months have elapsed since the 3rd dose and if the child is unlikely to return at age 15 to 18 months. Td (tetanus and diphtheria toxoids) is recommended at 11 to 12 years of age if at least 5 years have elapsed since the last dose of DTP, DTaP, or DT. Subsequent routine Td boosters are recommended every 10 years.

[4]Three *Haemophilus influenzae* type b (Hib) conjugate vaccines are licensed for infant use. If PRP-OMP (PedvaxHIB® or ComVax® [Merck]) is administered at 2 and 4 months of age, a dose at 6 months is not required. Because clinical studies in infants have demon-

strated that using some combination products may induce a lower immune response to the Hib vaccine component, DTaP/Hib combination products should not be used for primary immunization in infants at 2, 4, or 6 months of age, unless FDA-approved for these ages.

[5]Two poliovirus vaccines currently are licensed in the United States: inactivated poliovirus (IPV) vaccine and oral poliovirus (OPV) vaccine. The ACIP, AAP, and AAFP now recommend that the first two doses of poliovirus vaccine should be IPV. The ACIP continues to recommend a sequential schedule of two doses of IPV administered at ages 2 and 4 months, followed by two doses of OPV at 12 to 18 months and 4 to 6 years. Use of IPV for all doses also is acceptable and is recommended for immunocompromised persons and their household contacts. OPV is no longer recommended for the first two doses of the schedule and is acceptable only for special circumstances such as: children of parents who do not accept the recommended number of injections, late initiation of immunization, which would require an unacceptable number of injections, and imminent travel to polio-endemic areas. OPV remains the vaccine of choice for mass immunization campaigns to control outbreaks due to wild poliovirus.

[6]Rotavirus (Rv) vaccine is shaded and italicized to indicate (1) health-care providers may require time and resources to incorporate this new vaccine into practice; and (2) the AAFP feels that the decision to use rotavirus vaccine should be made by the parent or guardian in consultation with their physician or other health care provider. The first dose of Rv vaccine should not be administered before 6 weeks of age, and the minimum interval between doses is 3 weeks. The Rv vaccine series should not be initiated at 7 months of age or older, and all doses should be completed by the first birthday.

[7]The 2nd dose of measles, mumps, rubella (MMR) vaccine is recommended routinely at 4 to 6 years of age but may be administered during any visit, provided at least 4 weeks have elapsed since receipt of the 1st dose and that both doses are administered beginning at or after 12 months of age. Those who have not previously received the second dose should complete the schedule by the 11- to 12-year-old visit.

[8]Varicella (Var) vaccine is recommended at any visit or after the 1st birthday for susceptible children; i.e., those who lack a reliable history of chickenpox (as judged by a health care provider) and who have not been immunized. Susceptible persons 13 years of age or older should receive 2 doses, given at least 4 weeks apart.

Courtesy of the Centers for Disease Control and Prevention

Appendix B: Abbreviations, Acronyms, and Symbols

ʒ	dram
℥	ounce
ℳ	minum
ā	before
AA	Alcoholics Anonymous
AAA	abdominal aortic aneurysm
AAFP	American Academy of Family Physicians
AaO₂	percentage saturation of hemoglobin with oxygen in arterial blood
AAOHN	American Association of Occupational Health Nurses
AAP	American Academy of Pediatrics
AARP	American Association of Retired Persons
ABC	airway, breathing, circulation
ABC	antigen-binding capacity
ABCD	asymmetry, border, color, diameter
ABG	arterial blood gases
ABVD	A combination of chemotherapy drugs: doxorubicin (Adriamycin), bleomycin sulfate (Blenoxane), vinblastine (Velban), dacarbazine (DTIC-Dome)
a.c.	before meals
ACE	angiotensin-converting enzyme
ACIP	Advisory Committee on Immunization Practices
ACKD	acquired cystic kidney disease
ACR	American College of Rheumatology
ACS	American Cancer Society
ACTH	adrenocorticotropic hormone
AD	Alzheimer's disease
AD	right ear
ad lib	freely, as desired
ADA	American Diabetes Association
ADA	American Dietetic Association
ADA	Americans with Disabilities Act
ADAMHA	Alcohol, Drug Abuse, and Mental Health Administration
ADC	AIDS dementia complex
ADD	attention deficit disorder
ADH	antidiuretic hormone
ADHD	attention deficit hyperactivity disorder
ADL	activities of daily living
ADN	associate degree nurse (nursing)
AEB	as evidenced by
AFB	acid-fast bacillus
AFP	alpha-fetoprotein
AGA	appropriate for gestational age
AGE	acute gastroenteritis
AGF	angiogenesis factor
AHA	American Hospital Association
AHCA	American Health Care Association
AHCPR	Agency Health Care Policy and Research
AHNA	American Holistic Nurses' Association
AI	adequate intake
AICD	automatic implantable cardioverter-defibrillator
AID	artificial insemination by donor
AIDS	acquired immunodeficiency syndrome
AIDS	autoimmune deficiency syndrome
AIH	artificial insemination by husband
AJN	*American Journal of Nursing*

AKA	above the knee amputation
ALFA	Assisted Living Federation of America
ALG	antilymphocytic globulin
ALL	acute lymphocytic leukemia
ALS	amyotrophic lateral sclerosis
ALT	alanine aminotransferase
AMA	against medical advice
AMA	American Medical Association
AML	acute myelocytic leukemia
ANA	American Nurses Association
ANA	antinuclear antibody
ANS	autonomic nervous system
AORN	Association of Operating Room Nurses
AP	anterior/posterior
AP	apical pulse
APA	American Psychiatric Association
APIC	Association for Practitioners in Infection Control and Epidemiology
APRN	advance practice registered nurse
APS	Adult Protective Services
APS	American Pain Society
APSGN	acute poststreptococcal glomerulonephritis
APTT	activated partial thromboplastin time
ARDS	adult respiratory distress syndrome
ARF	acute renal failure
AROM	active range of motion
AROM	artificial rupture of membranes
AS	left ear
ASA	acetylsalicylic acid
ASD	atrial septal defect
ASO	antireptolysin-O
ASPO	American Society for Psychoprophylaxis in Obstetrics
AST	aspartate aminotransferase
ATC	around the clock
ATG	antithymocytic globulin
ATN	acute tubular necrosis
ATP	adenosine triphosphatase
ATSDR	Agency for Toxic Substances and Disease Registry
AU	both ears
A-V	arteriovenous
AV	atrioventricular
AWHONN	Association of Women's Health, Obstetric, and Neonatal Nurses
AWS	alcohol withdrawal syndrome
BBA	Balanced Budget Act
BCG	bacilles *Calmette-Guérin*
BE	base excess
bid	twice a day
BKA	below the knee amputation
BMD	bone mineral density
BMI	body mass index
BMR	basal metabolic rate
BMT	bone marrow transplantation
B&O	belladonna and opium
BOW	bag of water
BP	blood pressure
BPD	biparietal diameter

BPD	bronchopulmonary dysplasia
BPH	benign prostatic hypertrophy
BPM	beats per minute
BRM	biologic response modifier
BSA	body surface area
BSE	breast self examination
BSI	body substance isolation
BSN	bachelor of science in nursing
BUBBLE	breasts, uterus, bladder, bowel, lochia, and episiotomy
BUN	blood urea nitrogen
BVI	bladder volume indicator
c	cup
c̄	with
Ca⁺	calcium ion
CABG	coronary artery bypass graft
CaCl₂	calcium chloride
CAD	coronary artery disease
CAHD	coronary artery heart disease
CAI	computer-assisted instruction
C & S	culture and sensitivity
cap	capsule
CAPD	continuous ambulatory peritoneal dialysis
CARF	Commission on Accreditation of Rehabilitation Facilities
CAT	computed axial tomography
CAT	computerized adaptive testing
CBC	complete blood count
CBD	common bile duct
CBE	charting by exception
cc	cubic centimeter
CCNS	cell-cycle nonspecific
CCRC	continuing care retirement community
CCS	cell-cycle specific
CCU	coronary care unit
CDC	Centers for Disease Control and Prevention
CEA	carcinoembryonic antigen
CEPN-LTC™	Certification Examination for Practical and Vocational Nurses in Long-Term Care
CEU	continuing education unit
CF	cystic fibrosis
CFTR	cystic fibrosis transmembrane regulator
C-H	crown–heel
CHAP	community health accreditation program
CHD	coronary heart disease
CHF	congestive heart failure
CHIP	Children's Health Insurance Program
CHO	carbohydrate (carbon, hydrogen, oxygen)
CHON	protein (carbon, hydrogen, oxygen, nitrogen)
CHOP	A combination of chemotherapy drugs: cyclophosphamide (Cytoxan), doxorubicin (Adriamycin), vincristine (Oncovin), prednisone (Deltasone)
CIN	cervical intraepithelial neoplasia
CIS	carcinoma *in situ*
CK or CPK	creatine kinase or creatine phosphokinase
Cl⁻	chloride ion
CLL	chronic lymphocytic leukemia
CLTC	certified in long-term care
cm	centimeter
CML	chronic myelocytic leukemia
CMS	circulation, movement, sensation
CMV	cytomegalovirus
CN	cranial nerve
CNA	certified nursing assistant
CNM	certified nurse midwife
CNO	community nursing organization
CNS	central nervous system

CNS	clinical nurse specialist
CO₂	carbon dioxide
CO₂⁻	carbon dioxide ion
COBRA	Comprehensive Omnibus Budget Reconciliation Act
COLD	chronic obstructive lung disease
COOH	carboxyl group
COPD	chronic obstructive pulmonary disease
COPP	A combination of chemotherapy drugs: cyclophosphamide (Cytoxan), vincristine (Oncovin), procarbazine (Matulanel), and prednisone (Deltasone)
CP	cerebral palsy
CPAP	continuous positive airway pressure
CPD	cephalopelvic disproportion
CPM	continuous passive motion
CPNP	Council of Practical Nursing Programs
CPR	cardiopulmonary resuscitation
CPR	computerized patient record
CPS	Child Protective Services
CPT	chest physiotherapy
C-R	crown–rump
CRF	chronic renal failure
CRNA	Certified Registered Nurse Anesthetist
CSF	cerebrospinal fluid
CSM	circulation, sensation, motion
CST	contraction stress test
CT	computed tomography
CVA	cerebrovascular accident
CVC	central venous catheter
CVP	A combination of chemotherapy drugs: cyclophosphamide (Cytoxan), vincristine (Oncovin), prednisone (Deltasone)
CVS	chorionic villi sampling
D₅W	dextrose 5% in water
DAI	diffuse axonal injury
D & C	dilatation and curettage
DAR	document, action, response
dc	discontinue
DDH	developmental dysplasia of the hip
DDS	doctor of dental surgery
DDST	Denver Developmental Screening Test
DEA	Drug Enforcement Agency
DES	diethylstilbestrol
DET	diethyltriptamine
DHHS	Department of Health and Human Services
DIC	disseminated intravascular coagulation
DICC	dynamic infusion cavernosometry and cavernosography
DJD	degenerative joint disease
DKA	diabetic ketoacidosis
dL	deciliter
DMARD	disease-modifying antirheumatic drug
DMD	doctor of dental medicine
DMD	Duchenne muscular dystrophy
DMT	dimethyltriptamine
DNA	deoxyribonucleic acid
DNR	do not resuscitate
DO	doctor of osteopathy
DOM	dimethyl-4-ethylamphetamine
DPAHC	durable power of attorney for health care
DPT	demerol, phenergan, thorazine
dr	dram, or ℨ
DRG	diagnosis-related group
DRI	dietary reference intake
DSM-IV	*Diagnostic and Statistical Manual of Mental Disorders,* 4th edition
DT	delirium tremens

DTaP	diphtheria, tetanus, acellular pertussis
DTP	diphtheria, tetanus, pertussis
DVT	deep vein thrombosis
EA	Emotions Anonymous
EABV	effective arterial blood volume
EAR	estimated average requirement
ECF	extended care facility
ECF	extracellular fluid
ECG (EKG)	electrocardiogram
ECT	electroconvulsive therapy
ED	emergency department
EDB	estimated date of birth
EDD	estimated date of delivery
EEG	electroencephalograph
EENT	eyes, ears, nose, and throat
EFM	electronic fetal monitoring
EGD	esophagogastroduodenoscopy
EKG	electrocardiogram
ELISA	enzyme-linked immunosorbent assay
elix	elixir
EMG	electromyogram
EMLA	eutectic (cream) mixture of local anesthetics
EMS	emergency medical services
EMT	emergency medical technician
EMT-P	emergency medical technician-paramedic
EPA	Environmental Protection Agency
EPO	exclusive provider organization
EPS	extrapyramidal symptom
ER	emergency room
ERCP	endoscopic retrograde cholangiopancreatogram
ERT	estrogen replacement therapy
ESR	erythrocyte sedimentation rate
ESRD	end-stage renal disease
esu	electrostatic unit
ESWL	extracorporeal shock wave lithotripsy
ET	endotracheal
ETT	endotracheal tube
EVAD	explantable venous access device
FAE	fetal alcohol effects
FAF	fibroblast activating factor
FAS	fetal alcohol syndrome
FAST	fetal acoustic stimulation test
FBD	fibrocystic breast disease
FBPP	fetal biophysical profile
FBS	fasting blood sugar
FDA	Food and Drug Administration
FHR	fetal heart rate
fl	fluid
FOBT	fecal occult blood test
4 Ps	passage, passenger, powers, pysche
FSBG	finger stick blood glucose
FSH	follicle-stimulating hormone
ft	foot
FTT	failure to thrive
g	gram
GAD	generalized anxiety disorder
GAS	general adaptation syndrome
GCS	Glasgow Coma Scale
GDM	gestational diabetes mellitus
GED	general education development
GER	gastroesophageal reflux
GFR	glomerular filtration rate
GGT	gammaglutamy transpeptidase
GH	growth hormone
GHb	glycosylated hemoglobin
GI	gastrointestinal
GIFT	gamete-intrafallopian transfer
GP/TPAL	gravida, para/term, preterm, abortions, living

GPA	Global Programme on AIDS
gr	grain
gtt	drop
GTT	glucose tolerance test
gtt/min	drops per minute
GU	genitourinary
h	hour(s)
H⁺	hydrogen ion
H$_2$CO$_3$	carbonic acid
H$_2$O	water
HAI	hemagglutination inhibition
H&H	hemoglobin and hematocrit
HAV	hepatitis A virus
HBIG	hepatitis B immune globulin
HBV	hepatitis B virus
HCFA	Health Care Financing Administration
hCG	human chorionic gonadotropin
HCl	hydrochloric acid
HCO$_3$⁻	bicarbonate ion
Hct	hematocrit
HCV	hepatitis C virus
HD	Hodgkin's Disease
HDL	high density lipoprotein
HDV	hepatitis D virus
Hep B	hepatitis B
Hgb F	fetal hemoglobin
Hgb	hemoglobin
HHNK	hyperosmolar hyperglycemic nonketotic syndrome
Hib	*haemophilus influenzae* type B
HICPAC	Hospital Infection Control Practices Advisory Committee
HIS	hospital information system
HIV	human immunodeficiency virus
HLA	human leukocyte antigen
HMO	health maintenance organization
hPL	human placental lactogen
HPV	human papillomavirus
HR	heart rate
HRSA	Health Resources and Services Administration
h.s.	hour of sleep
HSV	herpes simplex virus
HSV-2	herpes simplex virus type 2
IABP	intra-aortic balloon pump
IADL	instrumental activities of daily living
I&O	intake and output
IASP	International Association for the Study of Pain
IBD	inflammatory bowel disease
ICEA	International Childbirth Education Association
ICF	intermediate care facility
ICF	intracellular fluid
ICN	International Council of Nurses
ICU	intensive care unit
ID	identification
ID	intradermal
IDM	infant of a diabetic mother
IgG	immunoglobulin G
IgM	immunoglobulin M
IGT	impaired glucose tolerance
IHCT	interdisciplinary health care team
IHS	Indian Health Service
IM	intramuscular
in	inch
INR	International Normalized Ratio
IOL	intraocular lens
IOM	Institute of Medicine
IOP	intraocular pressure

IPV	inactivated polio vaccine
IQ	intelligence quotient
ISAM	infant of a substance abusing mother
ITP	idiopathic thrombocytopenic purpura
IUD	intrauterine device
IUGR	intrauterine growth retardation
IV	intravenous
IVAD	implantable vascular access device
IVF-ER	*in vitro* fertilization and embryo replacement
IVP	intravenous push, intravenous pyelogram
IVPB	intravenous piggyback
JA	juvenile arthritis
JCAHO	Joint Commission on Accreditation of Healthcare Organizations
JOGNN	*Journal of Obstetric, Gynecologic, and Neonatal Nursing*
K$^+$	potassium ion
kcal	kilocalorie
KCl	potassium chloride
kg	kilogram
KS	Kaposi's Sarcoma
KUB	kidneys/ureters/bladder
KVO	keep vein open
L	liter
L/S	lecithin/sphingomyelin
LAAM	levo-alpha-acetyl-methadol
LAD	left anterior descending
LAS	local adaptation syndrome
lb	pound
LDH	lactic dehydrogenase
LDL	low density lipoprotein
LDRP	labor, delivery, recovery, postpartum
LE	lupus erythematosus
LES	lower esophageal sphincter
LFT	liver function test
LGA	large for gestational age
LH	lactate hydrogenase
LH	luteinizing hormone
LHRH	luteinizing hormone releasing hormone
LLQ	left lower quadrant
LMA	left mentum anterior
LMP	last menstrual period
LMP	left mentum posterior
LMT	left mentum transverse
LOA	left occiput anterior
LOC	level of consciousness
LOP	left occiput posterior
LOT	left occiput transverse
LP/VN	licensed practical/vocational nurse
LPN	licensed practical nurse
LSA	left sacrum anterior
LSD	lysergic acid diethylamide
LSP	left sacrum posterior
LST	left sacrum transverse
LTB	laryngotracheobronchitis
LUQ	left upper quadrant
LVN	licensed vocational nurse
MAC	*myobacterium avium* complex
MADD	Mothers Against Drunk Driving
MAO	monoamine oxidase
MAOI	monoamine oxidase inhibitor
MAP	mean arterial pressure
MAR	medication administration record
mcg (or μg)	microgram
MCNS	minimal charge nephrotic syndrome
MD	doctor of medicine
MDI	metered-dose inhaler
MDMA	methylene dioxyamphetamine
MDR	multidrug-resistant

MDR-TB	multidrug-resistant tuberculosis
MDS	minimum data set
mEq	milliequivalent
mEq/L	milliequivalents per liter
mg	milligram
MG	myasthenia gravis
Mg^{++}	magnesium ion
MgCl	magnesium chloride
MgSO$_4$	magnesium sulfate
MI	myocardial infarction
min	minute
mL	milliliter
mm^3	cubic millimeter
mm Hg	millimeters of mercury
MMR	measles, mumps, rubella
MOM	Milk of Magnesia
MOPP	A combination of chemotherapy drugs: mechlorethamine or nitrogen mustard (Mustargen), vincristine (Oncovin), procarbazine hydrochloride (Matulane), prednisone (Deltasone)
mOsm/kg	milliosmoles/kilogram
MRI	magnetic resonance imaging
MRSA	methicillin-resistant *staphylococcus aureus*
MS	morphine sulfate
MS	multiple sclerosis
MSAFP	maternal serum alpha-fetoprotein
MSDS	material safety data sheet
MSH	melanocyte-stimulating hormone
MUGA	multi-gated acquisition
MVC	motor vehicle collision
N$_2$	nitrogen
NA	Narcotics Anonymous
Na$^+$	sodium ion
Na$_2$SO$_4$	sodium sulfate
NAACOG	Nurses Association of the American College of Obstetricians and Gynecologists
NaCl	sodium chloride
NaH$_2$PO$_4$	sodium dihydrogen phosphate
Na$_2$HPO$_4$	disodium phosphate
NAHC	National Association for Home Care
NaHCO$_3$	sodium bicarbonate
NaHPO$_4$	sodium monohydrogen phosphate
NANDA	North American Nursing Diagnosis Association
NaOH	sodium hydroxide
NAPNES	National Association of Practical Nurse Education and Service Inc.
NCHS	National Center for Health Statistics
NCLEX	National Council Licensure Examination
NCLEX-PN	National Council Licensure Examination—Practical Nurse
NCLEX-RN	National Council Licensure Examination—Registered Nurse
NCSBN	National Council of State Boards of Nursing
NF	*National Formulary*
NFLPN	National Federation of Licensed Practical Nurses, Inc.
NG	nasogastric
NGT	nasogastric tube
NH$_2$	amino group
NHL	non-Hodgkin's lymphoma
NHO	National Hospice Organization
NIA	National Institute on Aging
NIAID	National Institute of Allergies and Infectious Diseases
NIAMS	National Institute of Arthritis and Musculoskeletal and Skin Diseases
NIC	Nursing Interventions Classification

NIDA	National Institute on Drug Abuse
NIDDK	National Institute of Diabetes and Digestive and Kidney Diseases
NIH	National Institute of Health
NIS	nursing information system
NKF	National Kidney Foundation
NLEA	Nutrition, Labeling, and Education Act
NLN	National League for Nursing
NLNAC	National League for Nursing Accrediting Commission
NMDS	nursing minimum data set
NMS	neuroleptic malignant syndrome
NNRTI	nonnucleoside reverse transcriptase inhibitor
NOC	Nursing Outcomes Classification
NOF	National Osteoporisis Foundation
NP	nurse practitioner
NPO	*nil per os*, Latin for "nothing by mouth"
NPUAP	National Pressure Ulcer Advisory Panel
NREM	non-rapid eye movement
NRTI	nucleoside analog reverse transcriptase inhibitor
NS	normal saline
NSAID	nonsteroidal anti-inflammatory drug
NSF	National Sleep Foundation
NSR	normal sinus rhythm
NST	nonstress test
O$_2$	oxygen
OAM	Office of Alternative Medicine
O&P	ova and parasite
OBRA	Omnibus Budget Reconciliation Act
OCD	obsessive compulsive disorder
OD	right eye
OH	hydroxyl
OHL	oral hairy leukoplakia
OPV	oral polio vaccine
OR	operating room
ORIF	open reduction/internal fixation
OS	left eye
OSHA	Occupational Safety and Health Administration
OT	occupational therapist
OTC	over-the-counter
OU	both eyes
oz	ounce
p̄	after
P	pulse
PA	physician's assistant
PAC	premature atrial contractions
PaCO$_2$	partial pressure of carbon dioxide
PACU	postanesthesia care unit
PaO$_2$	partial pressure of oxygen
Pap	Papanicolaou test
PAT	paroxysmal atrial tachycardia
PBI	protein bound iodine
p.c.	after meals
PCA	patient-controlled analgesia
PCO$_2$ (PaCO$_2$)	partial pressure of carbon dioxide
PCP	phencyclidine
PCP	*pneumocystis carinii* pneumonia
PCP	primary care provider
PCR	polymerase chain reaction
PDA	patent ductus arteriosis
PDPH	postdural puncture headache
PEG	percutaneous endoscopic gastrostomy
PEM	protein energy malnutrition
PERRLA	pupils equal, round, reactive to light and accommodation
PFT	pulmonary function test
pH	potential hydrogen

PHS	Public Health Services
PI	peripheral intravenous
PICC	peripherally inserted central catheter
PID	pelvic inflammatory disease
PIE	problem, implementation, evaluation
PIH	pregnancy-induced hypertension
PKD	polycystic kidney disease
PKU	phenylketonuria
PLMD	periodic limb movement disorder
PMI	point of maximum intensity
PMN	polymorphonuclear leukocyte
PMR	progressive muscle relaxation
PMS	premenstrual syndrome
PNI	psychoneuroimmunology
PNS	peripheral nervous system
po	*per os*, Latin for "by mouth"
PO$_2$ (PaO$_2$)	partial pressure of oxygen
PO$_4^{--}$	phosphate ion
POMR	problem-oriented medical record
POR	problem-oriented record
PPBS	post prandial blood sugar
PPD	postpartum depression
PPD	purified protein derivative
PPG	post prandial glucose
PPO	preferred provider organization
PPS	prospective payment system
PRN	*pro re nata*, Latin for "as required"
PRO	peer review organization
PROM	passive range of motion
PROM	premature rupture of membranes
PSA	prostate specific antigen
PSDA	Patient Self-Determination Act
PSP	phenolsulfonphtalein
PSVT	paroxysmal supraventricular tachycardia
pt	pint
PT	physical therapist
PT	prothrombin time
PTCA	percutaneous transluminal coronary angioplasty
PTH	parathyroid hormone
PTSD	post-traumatic stress disorder
PTT	partial thromboplastin time
PTU	propylthiouracil
PUVA	psoralen ultraviolet
PVC	premature ventricular contraction
PVD	peripheral vascular disease
q	*quaque*, Latin for "every"
qd	every day
qh	every hour
qid	four times a day
qod	every other day
qs	quantity sufficient
q2h	every 2 hours
qt	quart
R	respiration
RA	rheumatoid arthritis
RAD	reactive airway disease
RAST	radio allergosorbent test
RBC	red blood count, red blood cell
RD	registered dietician
RDA	recommended dietary allowance
RDS	respiratory distress syndrome
REM	rapid eye movement
Resp	respirations
RF	rheumatoid factor
RhoGAM	RH immune globulin
RICE	rest, ice, compression, elevation
RIND	reversible ischemic neurological deficit
RLQ	right lower quadrant

RLS	restless leg syndrome	**TEFRA**	Tax Equity Fiscal Responsibility Act
RMA	right mentum anterior	**TENS**	transcutaneous electrical nerve stimulation
RMP	right mentum posterior	**THA**	total hip arthroplasty
RMT	right mentum transverse	**TIA**	transient ischemic attack
RN	registered nurse	**TIBC**	total iron binding capacity
RNA	ribonucleic acid	**t.i.d.**	three times a day
RNFA	registered nurse first assistant	**TIG**	tetanus immune globulin
ROA	right occiput anterior	**TIPS**	transjugular intrahepatic portosystemic shunt
ROM	range of motion	**TKA**	total knee arthroplasty
ROM	rupture of membranes	**TMJ**	temporomandibular joint
ROP	right occiput posterior	**TNM**	tumor, node, metastasis
ROS	review of systems	**t.o.**	telephone order
ROT	right occiput transverse	**TOF**	tetralogy of Fallot
RPCH	rural primary care hospital	**TPN**	total parenteral nutrition
RPh	registered pharmacist	**TPR**	temperature, pulse, respirations
RPR	rapid plasma reagin	**Tr or tinct**	tincture
RR	recovery room	**TRAM**	transplantation of the rectus abdominis muscle
RSA	right sacrum anterior		
RSP	right sacrum posterior	**TSE**	testicular self examination
RST	right sacrum transverse	**TSH**	thyroid-stimulating hormone
RSV	respiratory syncytial virus	**TSI**	thyroid-stimulating immunoglobulin
R/T	related to	**tsp**	teaspoon
RT	respiratory therapist	**TSS**	toxic shock syndrome
RTI	respiratory tract infection	**TTN**	transient tachypnea of the newborn
RUGS	resource utilization group system	**TULIP**	transurethral ultrasound-guided laser-induced prostatectomy
RUQ	right upper quadrant		
s̄	without	**TURP**	transurethral resection of the prostate
SA	sinoatrial	**U**	unit
SADD	Students Against Drunk Driving	**UA**	routine urinalysis
SaO₂	oxygen saturation	**UAP**	unlicensed assistive personnel
SBC	school-based clinic	**UC**	ulcerative colitis
SBP	systolic blood pressure	**UGI**	upper gasrointestinal tract
SC/SQ	subcutaneous	**UIS**	Universal Intellectual Standards
SCA	sickle-cell anemia	**UTI**	urinary tract infection
SCD	sequential compression device	**UL**	upper intake level
SCI	spinal cord injury	**UMLS**	Universal Medical Language System
SGA	small for gestational age	**U-100**	100 units insulin per cc
SGOT	serum glutamate oxaloacetate transaminase	**UPSIT**	University of Pennsylvania Smell Identification Test
SIADH	syndrome of inappropriate antidiuretic hormone		
		URQ	upper right quadrant
SIDS	sudden infant death syndrome	**USDHHS**	United States Department of Health and Human Services
SL	sublingual		
SLE	systemic lupus erythematosus	**USP**	*United States Pharmacopeia*
SMBG	self-monitor blood glucose	**USPHS**	United States Public Health Service
SNF	skilled nursing facility	**UTI**	urinary tract infection
SOAP	subjective data, objective data, assessment, plan	**UV**	ultraviolet
		VA	Veterans Administration, Veterans Affairs
SOAPIE	subjective data, objective data, assessment, plan, implementation, evaluation	**VAC**	vacuum assisted closure
		VAD	ventricular assist device, vascular access device
SOAPIER	subjective data, objective data, assessment, plan, implementation, evaluation, revision		
		var	varicella
SPF	sun protection factor	**VAS**	Visual Analog Scale
SROM	spontaneous rupture of membranes	**VBAC**	vaginal birth after cesarean
s̄s̄	one half	**VCD**	vacuum constriction device
SSRI	selective serotonin reuptake inhibitor	**VDRL**	venereal disease research laboratory
STAT	*statim,* Latin for "immediately"	**VF**	ventricular fibrillation
STD	sexually transmitted disease	**VLDL**	very low-density lipoprotein
supp	suppository	**VRE**	vancomycin-resistant enterococci
susp	suspension	**VS**	vital signs
SW	social worker	**VSD**	ventricular septal defect
T	temperature	**VT**	ventricular tachycardia
tab	tablet	**WBC**	white blood cell, white blood count
TAC	tetracaine, adrenaline, cocaine	**WHO**	World Health Organization
TB	tuberculosis	**WIC**	Women, Infants, and Children
Tbsp	tablespoon	**WNL**	within normal limits
TD	tardive dyskinesia	**WPM**	words per minute
Td	tetanus/diphtheria	**wt**	weight
TDD	telecommunication device for the deaf	**ZIFT**	zygote-intra-fallopian transfer
TEE	transesophageal echocardiography		

Appendix C: Recommended Dietary Allowances[a]

Category	Age (Yr) or Condition	Weight[b] (kg)	Weight[b] (lb)	Height[b] (cm)	Height[b] (in)	Kcal Per Day	Protein (g)	FAT-SOLUBLE VITAMINS Vitamin A (μg RE)[c]	Vitamin D (μg)[d]	Vitamin E (mg α-TE)[e]	Vitamin K (μc)
Infants	0.0–0.5	6	13	60	24	650	13	375	7.5	3	5
	0.5–1.0	9	20	71	28	850	14	375	10	4	10
Children	1–3	13	29	90	35	1,300	16	400	10	6	15
	4–6	20	44	112	44	1,800	24	500	10	7	20
	7–10	28	62	132	52	2,000	28	700	10	7	30
Men	11–14	45	99	157	62	2,500	45	1,000	10	10	45
	15–18	66	145	176	69	3,000	59	1,000	10	10	65
	19–24	72	160	177	70	2,900	58	1,000	10	10	70
	25–50	79	174	176	70	2,900	63	1,000	5	10	80
	Over 51	77	170	173	68	2,300	63	1,000	5	10	80
Women	11–14	46	101	157	62	2,200	46	800	10	8	45
	15–18	55	120	163	64	2,200	44	800	10	8	55
	19–24	58	128	164	65	2,200	46	800	10	8	60
	25–50	63	138	163	64	2,200	50	800	5	8	65
	Over 51	65	143	160	63	1,900	50	800	5	8	65
Pregnant						2,200	60	800	10	10	65
Lactating	1st 6 mo					2,700	65	1,300	10	12	65
	2nd 6 mo					2,700	62	1,200	10	11	65

WATER-SOLUBLE VITAMINS Vitamin C (mg)	Thiamin (mg)	Riboflavin (mg)	Niacin (mg NE)[f]	Vitamin B$_6$ (mg)	Folate (μg)	Vitamin B$_{12}$ (μg)	MINERALS Calcium (mg)	Phosphorus (mg)	Magnesium (mg)	Iron (mg)	Zinc (mg)	Iodine (μg)	Selenium (μg) 35
30	0.3	0.4	5	0.3	25	0.3	400	300	40	6	5	40	10
35	0.4	0.5	6	0.6	35	0.5	600	500	60	10	5	50	15
40	0.7	0.8	9	1.0	50	0.7	800	800	80	10	10	70	20
45	0.9	1.1	12	1.1	75	1.0	800	800	120	10	10	90	20
45	1.0	1.2	13	1.4	100	1.4	800	800	170	10	10	120	20
50	1.3	1.5	17	1.7	150	2.0	1,200	1,200	270	12	15	150	40
60	1.5	1.8	20	2.0	200	2.0	1,200	1,200	400	12	15	150	50
60	1.5	1.7	29	2.0	200	2.0	1,200	1,200	350	10	15	150	70
60	1.5	1.7	19	2.0	200	2.0	800	800	350	10	15	150	70
60	1.2	1.4	15	2.0	200	2.0	800	800	350	10	15	150	70
50	1.1	1.3	15	1.4	150	2.0	1,200	1,200	280	15	12	150	45
60	1.1	1.3	15	1.5	180	2.0	1,200	1,200	300	15	12	150	50
60	1.1	1.3	15	1.6	180	2.0	1,200	1,200	280	15	12	150	55
60	1.1	1.3	15	1.6	180	2.0	800	800	280	15	12	150	55
60	1.0	1.3	13	1.6	180	2.0	800	800	280	10	12	150	55
70	1.5	1.6	17	2.2	400	2.2	1,200	1,200	320	30	15	175	65
95	1.6	1.8	20	2.1	280	2.6	1,200	1,200	355	15	19	200	75
90	1.6	1.7	20	2.1	260	2.6	1,200	1,200	340	15	16	200	75

[a]The allowances, expressed as average daily intakes over time, are intended to provide for individual variations among most normal persons as they live in the United States under usual environmental stresses. Diets should be based on a variety of common foods to provide other nutrients for which human requirements have been less well defined.

[b]Weights and heights of reference adults are actual medians for the U.S. population of the designated age.

[c]Retinol equivalents: 1 RE = 1 μg retinol or 6 μg β-carotene.

[d]As cholecalciferol: 10 μg cholecalciferol = 400 U of vitamin D.

[e]Tocopherol equivalents: 1 mg d-α-tocopherol = 1-α-TE.

[f]Ne Niacin equivalent = 1 mg of niacin or 60 mg of dietary tryptophan.

From Recommended Dietary Allowances *(10th ed.), by Food and Nutrition Board, National Academy of Sciences—National Research Council, 1989, Washington, DC: The Council.*

Glossary

Abduction Lateral movement away from the body.

Ability Competence in an activity.

Abortion Termination of pregnancy before the age of fetal viability, usually 24 weeks.

Abruptio Placenta Premature separation, from the wall of the uterus, of normally implanted placenta.

Absorption Passage of a drug from the site of administration into the bloodstream; Process whereby the end products of digestion pass through the epithelial membranes in the small and large intestines and into the blood or lymph system.

Abuse Incident involving some type of violation to the client; Misuse, excessive, or improper use of a substance, the absence of which does not cause withdrawal symptoms.

Acceleration Short increase in fetal heart rate caused by fetal movement.

Accomodation Component of cognitive development that allows for readjustment of the cognitive structure (mindset) in order to take in new information.

Accountability Responsibility of actions and inactions performed by oneself or others.

Accreditation Process by which a voluntary, nongovernmental agency or organization appraises and grants accredited status to institutions and/or programs or services that meet predetermined structure, process, and outcome criteria.

Acculturation Process of learning norms, beliefs, and behavioral expectations of a group.

Acid Any substance that in a solution yields hydrogen ions bearing a positive charge.

Acidosis Condition characterized by an excessive number of hydrogen ions in a solution.

Acme Peak of a contraction.

Acquired Immunity Formation of antibodies (memory B cells) to protect against future invasions of an already experienced antigen.

Acquired Immunodeficiency Syndrome (AIDS) Progressively fatal disease that destroys the immune system and the body's ability to fight infection; caused by the human immunodeficiency virus (HIV).

Acrocyanosis Blue coloring of hands and feet.

Active Euthanasia Process of taking deliberate action that will hasten a client's death.

Active Listening Process of hearing spoken words and noting nonverbal behaviors.

Actively Suicidal Descriptor of an individual intent upon hurting or killing self and who is in imminent danger of doing so.

Activities of Daily Living Basic care activities that include mobility, bathing, hygiene, grooming, dressing, eating, and toileting.

Actual Nursing Diagnosis Nursing diagnosis that indicates that a problem exists; composed of the diagnostic label, related factors, and signs and symptoms.

Acupressure Technique of releasing blocked energy within an individual when specific points (tsubas) along the meridians are pressed or massaged by the practitioner's fingers, thumbs, and heel of the hands.

Acupuncture Technique of application of heat and needles to various points on the body to alter the energy flow.

Acute Pain Discomfort identified by sudden onset and relatively short duration, mild to severe intensity, and a steady decrease in intensity over several days or weeks.

Adaptation Ongoing process whereby individuals use various responses to adjust to stressors and change.

Adaptive Energy Inner forces that an individual uses to adapt to stress (phrase coined by Selye).

Adaptive Measure Measure for coping with stress that requires a minimal amount of energy.

Addiction Overwhelming preoccupation with obtaining and using a drug for its psychic effects; used interchangeably with dependence.

Adhesion Internal scar tissue from previous surgeries or disease processes.

Adjuvant Medication Drug used to enhance the analgesic efficacy of opioids, treat concurrent symptoms that exacerbate pain, and provide independent analgesia for specific types of pain.

Administrative Law Law developed by those persons who are appointed to governmental administrative agencies and who are entrusted with enforcing the statutory laws passed by the legislature.

Adolescence Developmental stage from the ages of 12 years to 20 years that begins with the appearance of the secondary sex characteristics (puberty).

Adult Day Care Provision of a variety of services in a protective setting for adults who are unable to stay alone, but who do not need 24-hour care.

Advance Directive Written instruction for health care that is recognized under state law and is related to the provision of such care when the individual is incapacitated.

Adventitious Breath Sound Abnormal sound, including sibilant wheezes (formerly wheezes), sonorous wheezes (formerly rhonchi), fine and course crackles (formerly rales), and pleural friction rubs.

Affect Outward expression of mood or emotions.

Affective Domain Area of learning that involves attitudes, beliefs, and emotions.

Afferent Nerve Pathway Ascending spinal cord pathway that transmits sensory impulses to the brain.

Afferent Pain Pathway Ascending spinal cord.

Afterpains Discomfort caused by the contracting uterus after the infant's birth.

Age of Viability Gestational age at which a fetus could live outside the uterus, generally considered to be 24 weeks.

Agent Entity capable of causing disease.

Agglutination Clumping together of red blood cells.

Agglutinin Specific kind of antibody whose interaction with antigens is manifested as agglutination.

Agglutinogen Any antigenic substance that causes agglutination by the production of agglutinin.

Agnosia Inability to recognize, either by sight or sound, familiar objects such as a hairbrush.

Agnostic Individual who believes that the existence of God cannot be proved or disproved.

Agranulocytosis Acute condition causing a severe reduction in the number of granulocytes (basophils, eosinophils, and neutrophils).

Airborne Precautions Measures taken in addition to Standard Precautions and for clients known to have or suspected of having illnesses spread by airborne droplet nuclei.

Airborne Transmission Transfer of an agent to a susceptible host through droplet nuclei or dust particles suspended in the air.

Aldrete Score Scoring system for objectively assessing the physical status of clients recovering from anesthesia; serves as a basis for dismissal from the postanesthesia care unit (PACU) and ambulatory surgery; also known as the post-anesthetic recovery score.

Algor Mortis Decrease in body temperature after death, resulting in lack of skin elasticity.

Alkalosis Condition characterized by an excessive loss of hydrogen ions from a solution.

Allergen Type of antigen commonly found in the environment.

Allergy Altered reaction of the tissues of some individuals to substances that in similar amounts are harmless to other people.

Alopecia Partial or complete baldness or loss of hair.

Alternative Therapy Therapy used instead of conventional or mainstream medical practices.

Ambulatory Surgery Surgical operation performed under general, regional, or local anesthesia and involving fewer than 24 hours of hospitalization.

Amenorrhea Absence of menstruation.

Amnesia Inability to remember things.

Amniocentesis Withdrawal of amniotic fluid to obtain a sample for specimen examination.

Amnion Inner fetal membrane originating in the blastocyst.

Amniotomy Artificial rupture of the membranes.

Amphiarthrosis Articulation of slightly movable joints such as the vertebrae.

Amputation Removal of all or part of an extremity.

Anabolism Constructive process of metabolism whereby new molecules are synthesized and new tissues are formed, as in growth and repair.

Analgesia Pain relief without producing anesthesia.

Analgesic Substance that relieves pain.

Analysis Breaking down the whole into parts that can be examined.

Analyte Substance that is measured.

Anaphylaxis Type I systemic reaction to allergens.

Anasarca Generalized edema.

Anesthesia Partial or complete absence of sensation.

Anesthesiologist Licensed physician educated and skilled in the delivery of anesthesia who also adds to the knowledge of anesthesia through research or other scholarly pursuits.

Anesthetist Qualified RN, dentist, or medical doctor who administers anesthetics under the direct supervision of an anesthesiologist or a surgeon.

Aneurysm Weakness in the wall of a blood vessel.

Anger Control Assistance Nursing intervention aimed at facilitating the expression of anger in an adaptive and nonviolent manner.

Angina Pectoris Chest pain caused by a narrowing of the coronary arteries.

Angiocatheter Intracatheter with a metal stylet.

Angioedema Allergic reaction consisting of edema of subcutaneous tissue, mucous membranes, or viscera.

Angiogenesis Formation of new blood vessels.

Angiography Visualization of the vascular structures through the use of fluoroscopy with a contrast medium.

Angioma Benign vascular tumor involving skin and subcutaneous tissue: most are congenital.

Anion Ion bearing a negative charge.

Annulus Valvular ring in the heart.

Anorexia Loss of appetite.

Anorexia Nervosa Psychiatric disorder of self-imposed starvation that results in a 15% or more loss of body weight.

Anosognosia Lack of awareness of own neurological deficits.

Anthropogenic State reflecting changes in the relationship between humans and their environment.

Anthropometric Measurements Measurements of the size, weight, and proportions of the body.

Antibiotic-Resistant Resistant to a previously effective antimicrobial agent.

Antibody Immunoglobulin produced by the body in response to bacteria, viruses, or other antigenic substances.

Anticipatory Grief Occurrence of grief work before an expected loss actually occurs.

Anticipatory Guidance Information, teaching, and guidance given to a client in anticipation of an expected event.

Antigen Any substance identified by the body as nonself.

Antineoplastic Agent that inhibits the growth and reproduction of malignant cells.

Antioxidant Substance that prevents or inhibits oxidation, a chemical process wherein a substance is joined to oxygen.

Antipyretic Drug used to reduce an abnormally high temperature.

Anxiety Subjective response that occurs when a person experiences a real or perceived threat to well-being; a diverse feeling of dread or apprehension.

Anxiolytic Antianxiety medication.

Aphasia Inability to communicate; often the result of a brain lesion.

Apheresis Removal of unwanted blood components.

Appendicitis Inflammation of the vermiform appendix.

Appropriate for Gestational Age Infant's weight falls between the 90th and 10th percentile for gestational age.

Areflexia Absence of reflexes.

Aromatherapy Therapeutic use of concentrated essences or essential oils that have been extracted from plants and flowers.

Arousal State of wakefullness and alertness.

Arterial Blood Gases Measurement of levels of oxygen, carbon dioxide, pH, partial pressure of oxygen (PO_2 or PaO_2), partial pressue of carbon dioxide (PCO_2 or $PaCO_2$), saturation of oxygen (SaO_2), and bicarbonate (HCO_3) in arterial blood.

Arteriography Radiographic study of the vascular system following the injection of a radiopaque dye through a catheter.

Arteriosclerosis Cardiovascular disease wherein plaque forms on the inside of artery walls, reducing the space for blood flow.

Arthroplasty Replacement of both articular surfaces within a joint capsule.

Ascites Abnormal accumulation of fluid in the peritoneal cavity.

Asepsis Absence of microorganisms.

Aseptic Technique Collection of principles used to control and/or prevent the transfer of pathogenic microorganisms from sources within (endogenous) and outside (exogenous) the client.

Aspiration Procedure performed to withdraw fluid that has abnormally collected or to obtain a specimen; also inhalation of regurgitated gastric contents into the pulmonary system.

Assault Threat to do something that may cause harm or be unpleasant to another person.

Assent Voluntary agreement to participate in a research project or to accept treatment.

Assessment First step in the nursing process; includes systematic collection, verification, organization, interpretation, and documentation of data.

Assessment Model Framework that provides a systematic method for organizing data.

Assignment Downward or lateral transfer of both responsibility and accountability for an activity.

Assimilation Component of cognitive development that involves taking in new experiences or information.

Assisted Living Combination of housing and services for persons who require assistance with activities of daily living.

Assisted Suicide Situation wherein another person provides a client with the means to end his own life.

Assumption Belief or attitude that one takes for granted in a situation that requires action or resolution.

Asthma Condition characterized by intermittent airway obstruction due to antigen–antibody reaction.

Astigmatism Asymmetric focus of light rays on the retina.

Ataxia Inability to coordinate voluntary muscle action.

Atelectasis Collapse of a lung or a portion of a lung.

Atheist Individual who does not believe in God or any other deity.

Atherosclerosis Cardiovascular disease of fatty deposits on the inner lining, the tunica intima, of vessel walls.

Atom Smallest unit of an element which still retains the properties of that element and which cannot be altered by any chemical change.

Atresia Absence or closure of a body orifice.

Attachment Long-term process that begins during pregnancy and intensifies during the postpartum period, which establishes an enduring bond between parent and child, and develops through reciprocal (parent to child and child to parent) behaviors.

Attitude Manner, feeling, or position toward a person or thing.

Attribute Characteristic that belongs to an individual.

Audible Wheeze Wheeze that can be heard without the aid of a stethoscope.

Auditory Hallucination Perception by an individual that someone is talking when no one in fact is there.

Auditory Learner Person who learns by processing information through hearing.

Augmentation of Labor Stimulation of uterine contractions after spontaneously beginning but having unsatisfactory progress of labor.

Aura Peculiar sensation preceding a seizure or migraine; may be a taste, smell, sight, sound, dizziness, or just a "funny feeling."

Auscultation Physical examination technique that involves listening to sounds in the body that are created by movement of air or fluid.

Autocratic Leadership style that is task oriented and based on the premise that the leader knows best.

Autoimmune Disorder Disease wherein the body identifies its own cells as foreign and activates mechanisms to destroy them.

Autologous From the same organism (person).

Automatic Implantable Cardioverter-defibrillator (AICD) Implantable device that senses a dysrythmia and automatically sends an electrical shock directly to the heart to defibrillate it.

Automatism Mechanical, repetitive motor behavior performed unconsciously.

Autonomic Nervous System That part of the peripheral nervous system consisting of the sympathetic and parasympathetic nervous systems and controlling unconscious activities.

Autonomy Self-direction; Ethical principle based on the individual's right to choose and the individual's ability to act on that choice.

Autopsy Examination of a body after death by a pathologist to determine cause of death.

Autosomal Pertaining to a condition transmitted by a non-sex chromosome.

Awareness Capacity to perceive sensory impressions through thoughts and actions.

Azotemia Nitrogenous wastes present in the blood.

Bacteremia Condition of bacteria in the blood.

Bactericide Bacteria-killing chemicals; found in tears.

Balanced Budget Act Federal law enacted in 1997 that replaced cost-based reimbursement for care in skilled nursing facilities with a prospective payment system based on client assessment within a resource utilization group system.

Ballottement Rebounding of the floating fetus when pushed upward though the vagina or abdomen.

Bands Immature neutrophils.

Barium Chalky-white contrast medium.

Barrier Precautions Use of personal protective equipment, such as masks, gowns, and gloves, to create a barrier between the person and the microorganisms and thus prevent transmission of the microorganism.

Basal Metabolism Energy needed to maintain essential physiological functions such as respiration, circulation, and muscle tone, when a person is at complete rest physically, digestively, and mentally.

Base Substance that when dissociated produces ions that will combine with hydrogen ions.

Baseline Level Lab value that serves as a reference point for future value levels.

Battery Unauthorized or unwanted touching of one person by another.

Behavioral Tolerance Compensatory adjustments of behavior made under the influence of a particular substance.

Beneficence Ethical principle based on the duty to promote good and prevent harm.

Benign Not progressive; favorable for recovery.

Bereavement Period of grief following the death of a loved one.

Bias Mental inclination or leaning.

Bioavailability Readiness to produce a drug effect.

Bioethics Application of general ethical principles to health care.

Biofeedback Measurement of physiological responses that yields information about the relationship between the mind and body and helps clients learn the way to manipulate these responses through mental activity.

Biologic Response Modifier Agent that destroys malignant cells by stimulating the body's immune system.

Biological Agent Living organism that invades a host, causing disease.

Biological Clock Internal mechanism capable of measuring time in a living organism.

Biopsy Excision of a small amount of tissue.

Blanching White color of the skin when pressure is applied.

Blastic Phase Intensified phase of leukemia that resembles an acute phase in which there is an increased production of white blood cells.

Bloody Show Expulsion of cervical secretions, blood-tinged mucus, and the mucus plug that blocked the cervix during pregnancy.

Body Image Individual's perception of physical self, including appearance, function, and ability.

Body Mass Index Measurement used to ascertain whether a person's weight is appropriate for height; calculated by dividing the weight in kilograms by the height in meters squared.

Body Mechanics Use of the body to move or lift objects.

Bodymind Inseparable connection and operation of thoughts, feelings, and physiological functions.

Bonding Rapid process of attachment, parent to infant, that takes place during the sensitive period, the first 30 to 60 minutes after birth.

Borborygmi High-pitched, loud, rushing sounds produced by the movement of gas in the liquid contents of the intestine.

Bradycardia Heart rate less than 60 beats per minute in an adult.

Bradykinesia Slowness of voluntary movement and speech.

Bradypnea Respiratory rate of 10 or fewer breaths per minute.

Braxton-Hicks Contractions Irregular, intermittent contractions felt by the pregnant woman towards the end of pregnancy.

Breakthrough Pain Sudden, acute, temporary pain that is usually precipitated by a treatment, a procedure, or unusual activity of the client.

Brief Dynamic Therapy Short-term psychotherapy that focuses on resolving core conflicts deriving from personality and living situations.

Bronchial Sound Loud, tubular, hollow-sounding breath sound normally heard over the sternum.

Bronchiectasis Lung disorder characterized by chronic dilation of the bronchi.

Bronchitis Inflammation of the bronchial tree accompanied by hypersecretion of mucus.

Bronchovesicular Sound Breath sound normally heard in the area of the scapula and near the sternum; medium in pitch and intensity, with inspiratory and expiratory phases of equal length.

Bruxism Grinding of teeth during sleep.

Buffer Substance that attempts to maintain pH range, or hydrogen ion concentration, in the presence of added acids or bases.

Bulimia Nervosa Psychiatric disorder characterized by episodic binge-eating followed by purging.

Burnout State of physical and emotional exhaustion that occurs when caregivers deplete their adaptive energy.

Butterfly Needle Wing-tipped needle.

Cachectic Being in a state of malnutrition and wasting.

Cachexia State of malnutrition and protein wasting.

Calculus Concentration of mineral salts in the body leading to the formation of stone.

Calorie Quantity of heat required to raise the temperature of 1 gram of water 1 degree Celsius.

Cancer Disease resulting from the uncontrolled growth of cells, which causes malignant cellular tumors.

Capitated Rate Preset fee based on membership rather than services provided; payment system used in managed care.

Caput Succedaneum Edema of the newborn's scalp which is present at birth, may cross suture lines, and is caused by head compression against the cervix.

Carcinogen Substance that initiates or promotes the development of cancer.

Carcinoma Cancer occurring in epithelial tissue.

Cardiac Output Volume of blood pumped per minute by the left ventricle.

Cardiac Tamponade Collection of fluid in the pericardial sac hindering the functioning of the heart.

Carrier Person who harbors an infectious agent but has no symptoms of disease.

Caseation Process whereby the center of the primary tubercle formed in the lungs as a result of tuberculosis becomes soft and cheese-like due to decreased perfusion.

Catabolism Destructive process of metabolism whereby tissues or substances are broken into their component parts.

Cataplexy Sudden loss of muscle control.

Cataract Condition in which the lens of the eye loses its transparency and becomes opaque.

Categorical Imperative Concept that states that one should act only if the action is based on a principle that is universal.

Catharsis Process of talking out one's feelings; "getting things off the chest" through verbalization.

Cation Ion bearing a positive charge.

Cavitation Process whereby a cavity is created in the lung tissue through the liquefaction and rupture of a primary tubercle.

Ceiling Effect Medication dosage beyond which no further analgesia occurs.

Cellular Immunity Type of acquired immunity involving T-cell lymphocytes.

Centering Process of bringing oneself to an inward focus of serenity; done before beginning an energetic touch therapy treatment.

Central Line Venous catheter inserted into the superior vena cava through the subclavian or internal or external jugular vein.

Central Nervous System System of the brain and spinal cord.

Cephalalgia Headache; also known as cephalgia.

Cephalhematoma Collection of blood between the periosteum and the skull of a newborn; appears several hours to a day after birth, does not cross suture lines, and is caused by the rupturing of the periosteal bridging veins due to friction and pressure during labor and delivery.

Cephalopelvic Disproportion Condition in which the fetal head will not fit through the mother's pelvis.

Certification Voluntary process that establishes and evaluates standards of care; mandatory for any health care services receiving federal funds.

Cerumen Ear wax.

Cervical Dilatation Enlargement of the cervical opening (os) from 0 to 10 cm (complete dilatation).

Cesarean Birth Birth of an infant through an incision in the abdomen and uterus.

Chadwick's Sign Purplish-blue color of the cervix and vagina noted about the eighth week of pregnancy.

Chain of Custody Documentation of the transfer of evidence (of a crime) from one worker to the next in a secure fashion.

Chain of Infection Phenomenon of the development of an infectious process.

Chalazion Cyst of the meibomian glands.

Chancre Clean, painless, syphilitic primary ulcer appearing 2 to 6 weeks after infection at the site of body contact.

Change Dynamic process whereby an individual's response to a stressor leads to an alteration in behavior.

Change Agent Person who intentionally creates and implements change.

Charting by Exception Documentation method that requires the nurse to document only deviations from preestablished norms.

Chemical Agent Substance that interacts with a host, causing disease.

Chemical Name Precise description of the drug's composition (chemical formula).

Chemical Restraint Medication used to control client behavior.

Chemoreceptor Receptor that monitors the levels of carbon dioxide, oxygen, and pH in the blood.

Chemotherapy Use of drugs to treat illness, especially cancer.

Cheyne-Stokes Respirations Breathing characterized by periods of apnea alternating with periods of dyspnea.

Child Abuse Any intentional act of physical, emotional, or sexual abuse or neglect committed by a person responsible for the care of a child.

Child Life Specialist Health care professional with extensive knowledge of psychology and early childhood development.

Chlamydia Sexually transmitted disease caused by the spherical bacterial organism *Chlamydia trachomatis*.

Chloasma Darkening of the skin of the forehead and around the eyes during pregnancy; also called "mask of pregnancy."

Cholecystitis Inflammation of the gallbladder.

Cholelithiasis Presence of gallstones or calculi in the gallbladder.

Cholesterol Sterol produced by the body and used in the synthesis of steroid hormones.

Chorea Condition characterized by abnormal, involuntary, purposeless movements of all musculature of the body.

Chorion Outer fetal membrane formed from the trophoblast.

Chronic Acute Pain Discomfort that occurs almost daily over a long period, has the potential for lasting months or years, and has a high probability of ending; also known as progressive pain.

Chronic Nonmalignant Pain Discomfort that occurs almost daily, has been present for a least 6 months, and ranges in intensity from mild to severe; also known as chronic benign pain.

Chronic Pain Discomfort generally identified as long term (lasting 6 months or longer) that is persistent, nearly constant, or recurrent, and that produces significant negative changes in a person's life.

Chronobiology Science of studying biorhythms.

Chvostek's Sign Abnormal spasm of the facial muscles in response to a light tapping of the facial nerve.

Chyme Acidic, semi-fluid paste found in the gastrointestinal tract.

Circadian Rhythm Biorhythm that cycles on a daily basis.

Circulating Nurse RN responsible and accountable for management of personnel, equipment, supplies, the environment, and communication throughout a surgical procedure.

Circumcision Surgical removal of the prepuce (foreskin) which covers the glans penis.

Circumoral Cyanosis Bluish discoloration surrounding the mouth.

Cirrhosis Chronic degenerative changes in the liver cells and thickening of surrounding tissue.

Civil Law Law that deals with relationships between individuals.

Claiming Process Process whereby a family identifies the infant's "likeness to" and the "differences from" family members, and the infant's unique qualities.

Clean Object Object on which there are microorganisms that are usually not pathogenic.

Cleansing Removal of soil or organic material from instruments and equipment used in providing client care.

Client Advocate Person who speaks up for or acts on behalf of the client.

Client Behavior Accident Mishap resulting from the client's behavior or actions.

Clinical Observing and caring for living clients.

Closed Reduction Repair of a fracture done without surgical intervention.

Coarse Crackle Moist, low-pitched crackling and gurgling lung sound of long duration.

Codependent Description for persons who live based on what others think of them.

Cognition Intellectual ability to think.

Cognitive Behavior Therapy Treatment approach aimed at helping a client identify stimuli that cause the client's anx-

iety, develop plans to respond to those stimuli in a non-anxious manner, and problem-solve when unanticipated anxiety-provoking situations arise.

Cognitive Domain Area of learning that involves intellectual understanding.

Cognitive Reframing Stress management technique whereby the individual changes a negative perception of a situation or event to a more positive, less threatening perception.

Coitus (Copulation) Sexual act that delivers sperm to the cervix by ejaculation of the erect penis.

Cold Stress Excessive heat loss.

Colic Condition of acute abdominal pain.

Colonization Multiplication of microorganisms on or within a host that does not result in cellular injury.

Colostomy Opening created anywhere along the large intestine.

Colostrum Antibody-rich yellow fluid secreted by the breasts during the last trimester of pregnancy and the first 2–3 days after birth; gradually changes to milk.

Combination Chemotherapy Administration of a combination of chemotherapy drugs over a set period of time.

Comedone Whitehead or blackhead.

Command Hallucination Perception by an individual of a voice or voices telling the individual to do something, usually to himself and/or someone else.

Communicable Agent Infectious agent transmitted to a client by direct or indirect contact, via vehicle, vector, or airborne route.

Communicable Disease Disease caused by a communicable agent.

Communication The sending and receiving of a message.

Comorbidity Simultaneous existence of more than one disease process within an individual.

Competency Specific skill or task needed for a particular position.

Complementary Therapy Therapy used in conjunction with conventional medical therapies.

Complete Protein Protein containing all nine essential amino acids.

Complicated Grief Grief associated with traumatic death such as death by homicide, violence, or accident; survivors suffer emotions of greater intensity than those associated with normal grief.

Compound Combination of atoms of two or more elements.

Comprehensive Assessment Type of assessment that provides baseline client data, including a complete health history and current needs assessment.

Compromised Host Person whose normal defense mechanisms are impaired and who is therefore susceptible to infection.

Computed Tomography Radiological scanning of the body with x-ray beams and radiation detectors to transmit data to a computer that transcribes the data into quantitative measurement and multidimensional images of the internal structures.

Concept Mental picture of abstract phenomena that serves to organize observations related to those phenomena.

Conditioning Teaching a person a behavior until it becomes an automatic response; method of conserving adaptive energy.

Conduction Loss of heat by direct contact with a cooler object.

Conductive Hearing Loss Condition characterized by the inability of sound waves to reach the inner ear.

Confabulation The making up of information to fill in memory gaps.

Confidential Private or secret.

Confidentiality Nondisclosure of the identity of or personal information about an individual.

Conflict Discord between two or more people that results from differences in ideas, values, or feelings.

Congruence Agreement between two things.

Conjunctivitis Inflammation of the conjunctiva.

Conscious Sedation Minimally depressed level of consciousness during which the client retains the ability to maintain a continuously patent airway and to respond appropriately to physical stimulation or verbal commands.

Consciousness State of awareness of self, others, and surrounding environment.

Constipation Condition characterized by hard, infrequent stools that are difficult or painful to pass.

Constitutional Law Law that defines and limits the power of government.

Contact Precautions Measures taken in addition to Standard Precautions for clients known to have or suspected of having illnesses easily spread by direct client contact or by contact with fomites.

Contact Transmission Physical transfer of an agent from an infected person to a host through direct contact with that person, indirect contact with an infected person through a fomite, or close contact with contaminated secretions.

Contraception Measure taken to prevent pregnancy.

Contract Law Enforcement of agreements among private individuals.

Contracture Permanent shortening of a muscle.

Contrast Medium Radiopaque substance that facilitates roentgen (x-ray) imaging of the body's internal structures.

Convalescent Stage Time period in which acute symptoms of an infection begin to disappear until the client returns to the previous state of health.

Convection Loss of heat by the movement of air.

Copulation (Coitus) Sexual act that delivers sperm to the cervix by ejaculation of the erect penis.

Cotyledon Subdivision on the maternal side of the placenta.

Couvade Development of physical symptoms by the expectant father such as fatigue, depression, headache, backache, and nausea.

Crackle Abnormal breath sound that resembles a popping sound, heard on inhalation and exhalation; not cleared by coughing.

Crenation Condition wherein cells decrease in size, shrivel and wrinkle, and are no longer functional when in a hypertonic solution.

Crepitus Grating or crackling sensation or sound.

Cretinism Congenital lack of thyroid hormones causing defective physical development and mental retardation.

Criminal Law Law concerning acts of offense against the welfare or safety of the public.

Crisis Acute state of disorganization that occurs when the individual's usual coping mechanisms are no longer effective. Stressor that forces an individual to respond and/or adapt in some way.

Crisis Intervention Specific technique used to assist clients in regaining equilibrium.

Critical Pathway Comprehensive, standard plan of care for a specific case situation.

Critical Period Time of the most rapid growth or development in a particular stage of the life cycle during which an individual is most vulnerable to stressors of any type.

Critical Thinking Mode of thinking—about any subject, content, or problem—whereby the thinker improves the quality of his or her thinking by skillfully taking charge of the structures inherent in thinking and imposing intellectual standards (or a level of degree of quality) upon them.

Cross-Tolerance Decreased sensitivity to other substances in the same category.

Crowning When the largest diameter of the fetal head is past the vulva.

Cryotherapy Use of cold applications to reduce swelling.

Cryptorchidism Failure of one or both testes to descend.

Cultural Assimilation Process whereby individuals from a minority group are absorbed by the dominant culture and take on the characteristics of the dominant culture.

Cultural Diversity Differences among people that result from racial, ethnic, and cultural variables.

Culture Dynamic and integrated structures of knowledge, beliefs, behaviors, ideas, attitudes, values, habits, customs, languages, symbols, rituals, ceremonies, and practices that are unique to a particular group of people. Growing of microorganisms to identify a pathogen.

Curative To heal or restore to health.

Curing Ridding one of disease.

Cutaneous Pain Discomfort caused by stimulation of the cutaneous nerve endings in the skin.

Cyanosis Bluish discoloration of the skin and mucous membranes observed in lips, nail beds, and earlobes.

Cycling Alteration in mood between depression and mania.

Cystitis Inflammation of the urinary bladder.

Cystocele Downward displacement of the bladder into the anterior vaginal wall.

Cytology Study of cells.

Cytomegalovirus One of the herpes type viruses: inhabits saliva, urine, blood, semen, and vaginal secretions.

Data Clustering Process of putting data together in order to identify areas of the client's problems and strengths.

Dawn Phenomenon Early morning glucose elevation produced by the release of growth hormone.

Death Rattle Breathing sound in the period preceding death caused by a collection of secretions in the larynx.

Debride To remove dead or damaged tissue or foreign material from a wound.

Decomposition Chemical reaction wherein the bonding between atoms in a molecule is broken and simpler products are formed.

Decrement Decreasing intensity of a contraction.

Defamation Use of words to harm or injure the personal or professional reputation of another person.

Defense Mechanism Unconscious operation that protects the mind from anxiety.

Defining Characteristics Collected data; also known as signs and symptoms, subjective and objective data, or clinical manifestations.

Deglutition Swallowing of food.

Dehiscence Complication of wound healing wherein the wound edges separate.

Dehydration Condition wherein more water is lost from the body than is being replaced.

Delegation Process of transferring to a competent individual the authority to perform a selected task.

Delirium Cognitive changes or acute confusion of rapid onset (less than 6 months).

Delusion False belief that misrepresents reality.

Dementia Organic brain pathology characterized by losses in intellectual functioning and a slow onset (longer than 6 months).

Democratic Leadership style in which all members have input in decision making.

Dental Caries Cavities.

Deontology Ethical theory that considers the intrinsic significance of an act as the criterion for determination of good.

Dependence Reliance on a substance to such a degree that abstinence causes functional impairment, physical withdrawal symptoms, and/or psychological craving for the substance. See also addiction.

Dependent Nursing Intervention Nursing action that requires an order from a physician or other health care professional.

Depersonalization Treating an individual as an object rather than as a person.

Depolarization Contraction of the heart.

Depression State wherein an individual experiences feelings of extreme sadness, hopelessness, and helplessness.

Detoxification Elimination of a substance from the body.

Development Behavioral changes in functional abilities and skills.

Developmental Tasks Certain goals that must be achieved during each developmental stage of the life cycle.

Dialysate Solution used in dialysis, designed to approximate the normal electrolyte structure of plasma and extracellular fluid.

Dialysis Mechanical means of removing nitrogenous waste from the blood by imitating the function of the nephrons; involves filtration and diffusion of wastes, drugs, and excess electrolytes and/or osmosis of water across a semipermeable membrane into a dialysate solution.

Diarthrosis Freely movable joint.

Didactic Systematic presentation of information.

Diet Therapy Treating a disease or disorder with a special diet.

Dietary Prescription/Order Order written by the physician for food, including liquids.

Differentiation Acquisition of characteristics or functions different from those of the original.

Diffusion Process whereby a substance moves from an area of higher concentration to an area of lower concentration.

Digestion Mechanical and chemical processes that convert nutrients into a physically absorbable state.

Diplopia Double vision.

Dirty Object Object on which there is a high number of microorganisms, some that are potentially pathogenic.

Discharge Planning Planning that involves critical anticipation and planning for the client's needs after discharge.

Discipline Branch of learning, field of study, or occupation requiring specialized knowledge.

Disciplined Trained by instruction and exercise.

Disenfranchised Grief "Grief that is not openly acknowledged, socially sanctioned, or publicly shared" (Doka, Rushton, & Thorstenson, 1994).

Disinfectant Chemical solution used to clean inanimate objects.

Disinfection Elimination of pathogens, with the exception of spores, from inanimate objects.

Dislocation Injury in which the articular surfaces of a joint are no longer in contact.

Disorientation State of mental confusion in which awareness of time, place, self, and/or situation is impaired.

Disseminated Intravascular Coagulation Abnormal stimulation of the clotting mechanism causing small clots throughout the vascular system and widespread bleeding internally, externally, or both.

Distraction Technique of focusing attention on stimuli other than pain.

Distress Subjective experience that occurs when stressors evoke an ineffective response.

Distribution Movement of drugs from the blood into various body fluids and tissues.

Diverticula Sac-like protrusion of the intestinal wall that results when the mucosa herniates through the bowel wall.

Diverticulitis Inflammation of one or more diverticula.

Diverticulosis Condition in which multiple diverticula are present in the colon.

Documentation Written evidence of: the interactions between and among health care professionals, clients and their families, and health care organizations; the administration of tests, procedures, treatments, and client education; and the result of or client's response to diagnostic tests and interventions.

Domestic Violence Aggression and violence involving family members.

Dominant Culture Group whose values prevail within a society.

Down Syndrome Congenital chromosomal abnormality; also called trisomy 21.

Droplet Precautions Measures taken in addition to Standard Precautions for clients known to have or suspected of having serious illnesses spread by large particle droplets.

Drug Allergy Hypersensitivity to a drug.

Drug Incompatibility Undesired chemical or physical reaction between a drug and a solution, between two drugs, or between a drug and the container or tubing.

Drug Interaction Effect one drug can have on another drug.

Drug Tolerance Reaction that occurs when the body becomes accustomed to a specific drug and requires larger doses of the drug to produce the desired therapeutic effects.

Ductus Arteriosus Fetal vessel connecting the pulmonary artery to the aorta.

Ductus Venosus Branch of the umbilical vein that enters the inferior vena cava.

Durable Power of Attorney for Health Care Legal document designating who may make health care decisions for a client when that client is no longer capable of decision making.

Duration Length of one contraction, from the beginning of the increment to the conclusion of the decrement.

Dysarthria Difficult and defective speech due to a dysfunction of the muscles used for speech.

Dysfunctional Grief Persistent pattern of intense grief that does not result in reconciliation of feelings.

Dysfunctional Labor Labor with problems of the contractions or of maternal bearing down.

Dysmenorrhea Painful menstruation.

Dyspareunia Painful intercourse.

Dysphagia Difficulty in swallowing.

Dysphasia Impairment of speech resulting from damage to the speech center in the brain.

Dysplasia Abnormal development.

Dyspnea Difficulty breathing as observed by labored or forced respirations through the use of accessory muscles in the chest and neck.

Dysrhythmia Irregularity in the rate, rhythm, or conduction of the electrical system of the heart.

Dystocia Long, difficult, or abnormal labor caused by any of the four major variables (4 Ps) that affect labor.

Dysuria Difficult or painful urination.

Early Deceleration Reduction in fetal heart rate that begins early in the contraction and virtually mirrors the uterine contraction.

Ecchymosis Large, irregular hemorrhagic area on the skin; also called a bruise.

Eclampsia Convulsion occurring in pregnancy induced hypertension.

Ectopic Pregnancy Pregnancy in which the fertilized ovum is implanted outside the uterine cavity.

Edema Detectable accumulation of increased interstitial fluid.

Effacement Thinning of the cervix.

Efferent Nerve Pathway Descending spinal cord pathway that transmits sensory impulses from the brain.

Effluent Liquid output from an ileostomy.

Electrocardiogram Graphic recording of the heart's electrical activity.

Electroconvulsive Therapy Procedure whereby clients are treated with pulses of electrical energy sufficient to cause brief convulsions or seizures.

Electroencephalogram Graphic recording of the brain's electrical activity.

Electrolyte Element or compound that, when dissolved in water or another solvent, dissociates (separates) into ions (electrically charged particles).

Element Basic substance of matter.

Emancipated Minor Child who has the legal competency of an adult because of circumstances involving marriage, divorce, parenting a child, living independently without parents, or enlistment in the armed services.

Embolus Mass, such as a blood clot or an air bubble, that circulates in the bloodstream.

Embryonic Stage Developmental stage that occurs during the first 2–8 weeks after fertilization of a human egg.

Emergency Medical or surgical condition requiring immediate or timely intervention to prevent permanent disability or death.

Emergency Medical Technician Health care professional trained to provide basic lifesaving measures prior to arrival at the hospital.

Emergency Nursing Care of clients who require emergency interventions.

Emotional Lability Loss of emotional control.

Empathy Capacity to understand another person's feelings or perception of a situation.

Emphysema Lung disease wherein air accumulates in the tissues of the lungs.

Empowerment Process of enabling others to do for themselves.

Empty Calories Calories that provide few nutrients.

Encephalitis Inflammation of the brain.

Encoding Laying down tracks in areas of the brain to enhance the ability to recall and utilize information.

Encopresis Passage of watery colonic contents around a hard fecal mass.

Endemic Occurring continuously in a particular population and having low mortality.

Endocrine Group of cells secreting substances directly into the blood or lymph circulation and affecting another part of the body.

Endometriosis Growth of endometrial tissue on structures outside of the uterus, within the pelvic cavity.

Endorphins Group of opiate-like substances produced naturally by the brain which raise the pain threshold, produce sedation and euphoria, and promote a sense of well-being.

Endoscopy Visualization of a body organ or cavity through a scope.

Energetic-Touch Therapy Technique of using the hands to direct or redirect the flow of the body's energy fields and thus enhance balance within those fields.

Engagement Condition of the widest diameter of the fetal presenting part (head) entering the inlet to the true pelvis.

Engorgement Distention and swelling of the breasts in the first few days following delivery.

Engrossment Parents' intense interest in and preoccupation with the newborn.

Enriched Descriptor for food in which nutrients that were removed during processing are added back in.

Enteral Instillation Administration of drugs through a gastrointestinal tube.

Enteral Nutrition Feeding method meaning both the ingestion of food orally and the delivery of nutrients through a gastrointestinal tube, but generally meaning the latter.

Entrainment Infant's ability to move in rhythm to the parent's voice.

Enzyme Globular protein produced in the body that catalyzes chemical reactions within the cells by promoting the oxidative reactions and synthesis of various chemicals.

Enzyme-Linked Immunosorbent Assay Basic screening test currently used to detect antibodies to HIV.

Epidemic Infecting many people at the same time and in the same geographic area.

Epidural Analgesia Analgesics administered via a catheter that terminates in the epidural space.

Episiotomy Incision in the perineum to facilitate passage of the baby.

Epistaxis Hemorrhage of the nares or nostrils; also known as nosebleed.

Epstein's Pearls Small, whitish-yellow epithelial cysts found on the hard palate.

Equipment Accident Accident resulting from the malfunction or improper use of medical equipment.

Erythema Redness of the skin that may be caused by inflammation of tissues or by sunburn.

Erythematous Characterized by redness of the skin.

Erythema Toxicum Neonatorum Pink rash with firm, yellow-white papules or pustules found on the chest, abdomen, back, and/or buttocks of a newborn.

Erythrocytapheresis Procedure that removes abnormal red blood cells and replaces them with healthy ones.

Erythropoiesis Production of red blood cells and their release by the red bone marrow.

Eschar Dry, dark, leathery scab composed of denatured protein.

Ethical Dilemma Situation wherein there is a conflict between two or more ethical principles.

Ethical Principle Widely accepted code, generally based on the humane aspects of society, that directs or governs actions.

Ethical Reasoning Process of thinking through what one ought to do in an orderly, systematic manner based on principles.

Ethics Branch of philosophy concerned with determining right from wrong on the basis of a body of knowledge.

Ethnicity Cultural group's perception of itself or a group identity.

Ethnocentrism Assumption of cultural superiority and an inability to accept other cultures' ways of organizing reality.

Etiology Related cause of or contributor to a problem.

Euglycemia Normal blood glucose level.

Euphoric Characterized by elation out of context to the situation.

Eupnea Easy respirations with a rate of breaths per minute that is age-appropriate.

Eustress Stress that results in positive outcomes.

Euthanasia Intentional action or lack of action that causes the merciful death of someone suffering from a terminal illness or incurable condition; derived from the Greek word *euthanatos,* which literally means "good or gentle death."

Evaluation Fifth step in the nursing process; involves determining whether client goals have been met, partially met, or not met.

Evaporation Loss of heat when water is changed to a vapor.

Evisceration Complication of wound healing characterized by a complete separation of wound edges accompanied by visceral protrusion.

Exacerbation Increase in the symptoms of a disease.

Exclusive Provider Organization Organization wherein care must be delivered by the plan in order for clients to receive reimbursement for health care services.

Excretion Elimination of drugs or waste products from the body.

Exophthalmos Marked protrusion of the eyeballs resulting from increased orbital fluid behind the eyeballs.

Expected Outcome Detailed, specific statement that describes the methods through which a goal will be achieved and that includes aspects such as direct nursing care, client teaching, and continuity of care.

Exposure Contact with an infected person or agent.

Expressed Contract Conditions and terms of a contract given in writing by the concerned parties.

External Respiration Exchange of gases between the atmosphere and the lungs.

External Version Manipulation of the fetus through the mother's abdomen to a presentation facilitating birth.

Extracellular Fluid Fluid outside of the cells; includes interstitial, intravascular, synovial, cerebrospinal, and serous fluids; aqueous and vitreous humor; and endolymph and perilymph.

Extravasation Escape of fluid into the surrounding tissue.

False Imprisonment Situation wherein a person is made to wrongfully believe that he cannot leave a place.

False Labor Contractions which do not cause the cervix to dilate.

Family-Centered Care Recognition that the family is the constant in a child's life while the service systems and support personnel within those systems change (Shelton & Stepanek, 1994).

Fasciculation Involuntary twitching of muscle fibers.

Fat-Soluble Vitamin Vitamin requiring the presence of fats for its absorption from the gastrointestinal tract into the lymphatic system and for cellular metabolism: vitamins A, D, E, and K.

Fee for Service System in which the health care recipient directly pays the provider for services as they are provided.

Feedback Response from the receiver of a message so that the sender can verify the message.

Felony Crime of a serious nature that is usually punishable by imprisonment in a state penitentiary or by death.

Ferguson's Reflex Spontaneous, involuntary urge to bear down during labor.

Fertilization Union of an ovum and a sperm.

Fetal Alcohol Syndrome Condition wherein fetal development is impaired by maternal consumption of alcohol.

Fetal Attitude Relationship of fetal body parts to one another, either flexion or extension.

Fetal Biophysical Profile Assessment of five variables: fetal breathing movement, fetal movements of body or limbs, fetal tone (flexion/extension of extremities), amniotic fluid volume, and reactive NST.

Fetal Lie Relationship of the cephalocaudal axis of the fetus to the cephalocaudal axis of the mother, either longitudinal or transverse.

Fetal Position Relationship of the identified landmark on the presenting part to the four quadrants of the mother's pelvis.

Fetal Presentation Determined by the fetal lie and the part of the fetus that enters the pelvis first.

Fetal Stage Intrauterine developmental period from 8 weeks to birth.

Fibrinolysis Process of breaking fibrin apart.

Fidelity Ethical concept based on faithfulness and keeping promises.

Fight-or-Flight Response State wherein the body becomes physiologically ready to defend itself by either fighting or running away from the danger.

Filtration Process of fluids and the substances dissolved in them being forced through the cell membrane by hydrostatic pressure.

Fine Crackle Dry, high-pitched crackling and popping lung sound of short duration.

First Assistant Associate of the surgeon, referring physician, or surgical resident who assists the surgeon to retract tissue, aids in the removal of blood and fluids at the operative site, and assists with hemostasis and wound closure.

Flashback Rushing of blood back into intravenous tubing when a negative pressure is created on the tubing. Reliving of an original trauma as if the individual were currently experiencing it.

Flora Microorganisms which occur or have adapted to live in a specific environment, such as intestinal, skin, vaginal, or oral flora.

Flow Rate Volume of fluid to infuse over a set period of time.

Fluoroscopy Immediate, serial images of the body's structure or function.

Focus Charting Documentation method using a column format to chart data, actions, and responses.

Focused Assessment Type of assessment that is limited in scope in order to focus on a particular need or health care problem or on potential health care risks.

Fomite Object contaminated with an infectious agent.

Fontanelle Membranous area where sutures meet on the fetal skull.

Foramen Ovale Flap opening in the atrial septum that allows only right to left movement of blood.

Foremilk Watery first milk from the breast, high in lactose, like skim milk, and effective in quenching thirst.

Forceps Metal instruments used on the fetal head to provide traction or to provide a method of rotating the fetal head to an occiput-anterior position.

Formal Contract Written contract that cannot be changed legally by an oral agreement.

Formal Teaching Teaching that takes place at a specific time, in a specific place, and on a specific topic.

Fortified Descriptor for food in which nutrients not naturally occurring in the food are added to it.

Fracture Break in the continuity of a bone.

Fraud Wrong that results from a deliberate deception intended to produce unlawful gain.

Free Radical Unstable molecule that alters genetic codes and triggers the development of cancer growth in cells.

Frequency Time from the beginning of one contraction to the beginning of the next contraction.

Friction Force of two surfaces moving against one another.

Fulguration Procedure to destroy tissue with long, high-frequency electric sparks.

Functional Area Specialized area of the brain.

Fundus Top of the uterus.

Funic Souffle Sound of blood pulsating through the umbilical cord; rate the same as the fetal heart beat.

Gastric Ulcer Erosion in the stomach.

Gastritis Inflammation of the stomach mucosa.

Gate Control Pain Theory Theory that proposes that the cognitive, sensory, emotional, and physiologic components of the body can act together to block an individual's perception of pain.

General Adaptation Syndrome Physiologic response that occurs when a person experiences a stressor.

General Anesthesia Method of producing unconsciousness; complete insensibility to pain; amnesia; motionlessness; and muscle relaxation.

Generic Name Name assigned by the U.S. Adopted Names Council to the manufacturer who first develops a drug.

Genuineness Sincerity.

Germicide Chemical that can be applied to both animate and inanimate objects for the purpose of eliminating pathogens.

Germinal Stage Developmental stage that begins with conception and lasts approximately 10 to 14 days.

Gerontological Nursing Specialty within nursing that addresses and advocates for the special care needs of older adults.

Gerontologist Specialist in gerontology in advanced practice nursing, geriatric psychiatry, medicine, and social services.

Gerontology Study of the effects of normal aging and age-related diseases on human beings.

Gingivitis Inflammation of the gums.

Glasgow Coma Scale Neurological screening test that measures a client's best verbal, motor, and eye response to stimuli.

Glucagon Hormone secreted by the alpha cells of the pancreas which stimulate release of glucose by the liver.

Gluconeogenesis Conversion of amino acids into glucose.

Glycogenesis Conversion of glucose into glycogen.

Glycogenolysis Conversion of glycogen into glucose.

Glycosuria Presence of excessive glucose in the urine.

Goal Objective that outlines the desired resolution of the nursing diagnosis over a longer period of time, usually weeks or months.

Goiter Enlargement of the thyroid gland.

Gonorrhea Sexually transmitted disease caused by the gram-negative bacterial organism *Neisseria gonorrhea*.

Good Samaritan Acts Laws that provide protection to health care providers by assuring them of immunity from civil liability when care is provided at the scene of an emergency and the caregiver does not intentionally or recklessly cause the client injury.

Goodell's Sign Softening of the cervix noted about the eighth week of pregnancy.

Gower's Sign Walking hands up legs to get from sitting to standing position (as in Duchenne muscular dystrophy).

Granulation Tissue Delicate connective tissue consisting of fibroblasts, collagen, and capillaries.

Graphesthesia Ability to identify letters, numbers, or shapes drawn on the skin.

Gravida Pregnancy, regardless of duration, including present pregnancy.

Grief Series of intense physical and psychological responses that occurs following a loss; a normal, natural, necessary, and adaptive response to a loss.

Grief Work Process whereby the bereaved experiences freedom from attachment to the deceased, becomes reoriented to the environment where the deceased is no longer present, and establishes new relationships.

Growth Quantitative (measurable) changes in the physical size of the body and its parts.

Gynecomastia Abnormal enlargement of one or both breasts in males.

Half-life Time it takes the body to eliminate half of the blood concentration level of the original dose of medication.

Halitosis Bad breath.

Hallucination Sensory perception that occurs in the absence of external stimuli and that is not based on reality.

Hallux Varus Placement of the great toe farther from the other toes.

Handwashing Rubbing together of all surfaces and crevices of the hands using a soap or chemical and water, followed by rinsing in a flowing stream of water.

Haustra Sac-like pouches of the colon.

Healing Process that activates the individual's recovery forces from within.

Healing Touch Energy-based therapeutic modality that alters the energy fields through the use of touch, thereby affecting physical, mental, emotional, and spiritual health.

Health According to the World Health Organization, the state of complete physical, mental, and social well-being, not merely the absence of disease or infirmity.

Health Care Delivery System Mechanism for providing services that meet the health-related needs of individuals.

Health Care Financing Agency Federal agency in charge of administering the Medicare program.

Health Care Surrogate Law Law enacted by some states that provides a legal means for decision making in the absence of advance directives.

Health Continuum Range of an individual's health, from highest health potential to death.

Health History Review of the client's functional health patterns prior to the current contact with a health care agency.

Health Maintenance Organization Prepaid health plan that provides primary health care services for a preset fee and focuses on cost-effective treatment methods.

Hearing Act or power of receiving sounds.

Heart Sound Sound heard by auscultating the heart.

Heberden's Nodes Enlargement and characteristic hypertrophic spurs in the terminal interphalangeal finger joints.

Hegar's Sign Softening of the uterine isthmus about the sixth week of pregnancy.

HELLP Syndrome Pregnancy-induced hypertension with liver damage characterized by hemolysis, elevated liver enzymes, and low platelet count.

Hemarthrosis Bleeding into the joints.

Hematemesis Vomiting of blood.

Hematocrit Percentage of red blood cells in a given volume of blood.

Hematopoiesis Process of blood cell production and development.

Hematuria Blood in the urine.

Hemiparesis Weakness of one side of the body.

Hemiplegia Paralysis of one side of the body.

Hemoconcentration Reduced volume of plasma water and the increased concentration of blood cells, plasma proteins, and protein-bound constituents.

Hemolysis Breakdown of red blood cells and the release of hemoglobin.

Hemorrhagic Exudate Discharge that has a large component of red blood cells.

Hemorrhoid Swollen vascular tissue in the rectal area.

Hemostasis Cessation of bleeding.

Hemothorax Condition wherein blood accumulates in the pleural space of the lungs.

Hepatitis Chronic or acute inflammation of the liver.

Hesitancy Difficulty initiating the urinary stream.

Hindmilk Follows foremilk, is higher in fat content, leading to weight gain, and is more satisfying.

Hirsutism Excessive body hair in a masculine distribution.

Histamine Substance released during allergic reactions.

History Study of the past, including events, situations, and individuals.

HIV-Wasting Syndrome Unexplained weight loss of more than 10% of body weight accompanied by weakness, chronic diarrhea, and fever in those infected with HIV.

Holistic Whole; includes physical, intellectual, sociocultural, psychological, and spiritual aspects as an integrated whole.

Homan's Sign Test to check for the presence of clots in the leg.

Homeostasis Balance or equilibrium among the physiologic, psychological, sociocultural, intellectual, and spiritual needs of the body.

Homologous From the same species.

Homonymous Hemianopia Loss of vision in half of the visual field on the same side of both eyes.

Hormone Substance that initiates or regulates activity of another organ, system, or gland in another part of the body.

Hospice Humane, compassionate care provided to clients who can no longer benefit from curative treatment, and have 6 months or less to live.

Host Simple or complex organism that can be affected by an agent.

Human Immunodeficiency Virus (HIV) Retrovirus that causes AIDS.

Human Leukocyte Antigen Antigen present in human blood.

Humoral Immunity Type of immunity dominated by antibodies.

Hydatidiform Mole Abnormality of the placenta wherein the chorionic villi become fluid filled, grape-like clusters; the trophoblastic tissue proliferates; and there is no viable fetus.

Hydramnios (Polyhydramnios) Excess amount of amniotic fluid.

Hydrocele Fluid around the testes in the scrotum.

Hydrostatic Pressure Pressure that a fluid exerts against a membrane; also called filtration force.

Hygiene Science of health.

Hyperbilirubinemia Excess of bilirubin in the blood.

Hyperemesis Gravidarum Excessive vomiting during pregnancy.

Hypergylcemia Condition wherein the blood glucose level becomes too high as a result of the absence of insulin.

Hyperopia Farsightedness.

Hypersensitivity Excessive reaction to a stimulus.

Hypersomnia Alteration in sleep pattern characterized by excessive sleep, especially in the daytime.

Hyperthermia Condition in which the core body temperature rises above 106°F.

Hypertonic Solution Solution that has a higher molecular concentration than the cell; also called a hyperosmolar solution.

Hypertrophy Increase in muscle mass.

Hyperuricemia Increased uric acid blood level.

Hyperventilation Breathing characterized by deep, rapid respirations.

Hypervigilant Condition of constantly scanning the environment for potentially dangerous situations.

Hypervolemia Increased circulating fluid volume.

Hypnosis Altered state of consciousness or awareness resembling sleep and during which a person is more receptive to suggestion.

Hypoglycemia Condition wherein the blood glucose level is exceedingly low.

Hypomania Mild form of mania without significant impairment.

Hypospadias Placement of the urinary meatus on the underside of the penis.

Hypothermia Condition in which the core body temperature drops below 95°F.

Hypotonia Lax muscle tone.

Hypotonic Solution Solution that has a lower molecular concentration than the cell; also called hypo-osmolar solution.

Hypoventilation Breathing characterized by shallow respirations.

Hypovolemia Abnormally low circulatory blood volume.

Hypoxemia Decreased oxygen level in the blood.

Iatrogenic Caused by treatment or diagnostic procedures.

Idiopathic Occuring without a known cause.

Idiosyncratic Reaction Highly unpredictable response that may be manifested by an overresponse, an underresponse, or an atypical response.

Ileal Conduit Implantation of the ureters into a piece of ileum, which is attached to the abdominal wall as a stoma so urine can be removed from the body.

Ileostomy Opening created in the small intestine at the ileum.

Illness Stage Time period when the client is manifesting specific signs and symptoms of an infectious agent.

Illusion Inaccurate perception or misinterpretation of sensory stimuli.

Imagery Relaxation technique of using the imagination to visualize a pleasant, soothing image.

Immune Response Body's reaction to substances identified as nonself.

Immunity Body's ability to protect itself from foreign agents or organisms.

Immunization Process of creating immunity or resistance to infection in an individual.

Immunotherapy Treatment to suppress or enhance immunological functioning.

Impaired Nurse Nurse who is habitually intemperate or is addicted to the use of alcohol or habit-forming drugs.

Implantable Port Device made of a radiopague silicone catheter and a plastic or stainless steel injection port with a self-sealing silicone-rubber septum.

Implantation Embedding of a fertilized egg into the uterine lining.

Implementation Fourth step in the nursing process; involves the execution of the nursing plan of care formulated during the planning phase.

Implied Contract Contract that recognizes a relationship between parties for services.

Impotence Inability of an adult male to have an erection firm enough, or to maintain it long enough, to complete sexual intercourse.

Incidence Frequency of disease occurrence.

Incident Report Risk-management tool used to describe and report any unusual event that occurs to a client, visitor, or staff member.

Incompetent Cervix Descriptor for when the cervix begins to dilate, usually during the second trimester.

Incomplete Protein Protein with one or more of the essential amino acids missing.

Increment Increasing intensity of a contraction.

Incubation Period Time interval between the entry of an infectious agent in the host and the onset of symptoms.

Independent Nursing Intervention Nursing action initiated by the nurse that does not require direction or an order from another health care professional.

Induction Dose Initial dose of chemotherapy.

Induction of Labor Stimulation of uterine contractions before contractions begin spontaneously for the purpose of birthing an infant.

Infancy Developmental stage from the end of the first month to the end of the first year of life.

Infection Invasion and multiplication of pathogenic microorganisms in body tissue that results in cellular injury.

Infectious Agent Microorganism that causes infection.

Infertility Inability or diminished ability to produce offspring.

Infiltration Seepage of foreign substances into the interstitial tissue, causing swelling and discomfort at the IV site.

Inflammation Nonspecific cellular response to tissue injury.

Informal Teaching Teaching that takes place any time, any place, and whenever a learning need is identified.

Informed Consent Legal form signed by a competent client and witnessed by another person that grants permission to the client's physician to perform the procedure described by the physician and that demonstrates the client's understanding of the benefits, risks, and possible complications of the procedure, as well as alternate treatment options.

Ingestion The taking of food into the digestive tract, generally through the mouth.

Initial Planning Development of a preliminary plan of care by the nurse who performs the admission assessment and gathers the comprehensive admission assessment data.

Insomnia Difficulty in falling asleep initially or in returning to sleep once awakened.

Inspection Physical examination technique that involves thorough visual observation.

Instrument of Healing Means by which healing can be achieved, performed, or enhanced.

Insulin Pancreatic hormone that aids in both the diffusion of glucose into the liver and muscle cells, and the synthesis of glycogen.

Intellectual Wellness Ability to function as an independent person capable of making sound decisions.

Intensity Strength of the contraction at the acme.

Interdependent Nursing Intervention Nursing action that is implemented in a collaborative manner with other health care professionals.

Internal Respiration Exchange of oxygen and carbon dioxide at the cellular level.

Interstitial Fluid Fluid in tissue spaces around each cell.

Interval Resting period between two contractions.

Intoxication Reversible effect on the central nervous system soon after the use of a substance.

Intracath Plastic tube for insertion into a vein.

Intracellular Fluid Fluid within the cells.

Intradermal Injection into the dermis.

Intramuscular Injection into the muscle.

Intraoperative Phase Time during the surgical experience that begins when the client is transferred to the operating room table and ends when the client is admitted to the postanesthesia care unit.

Intrapsychic Therapy Developmental approach based on an individual's unconscious processes.

Intrathecal Analgesia Administration of analgesics into the subarachnoid space.

Intravascular Fluid Fluid consisting of the plasma in the blood vessels and the lymph in the lymphatic system.

Intravenous Injection into a vein.

Intravenous Therapy Administration of fluids, electrolytes, nutrients, or medications by the venous route.

Intravesical Within the urinary bladder.

Intussusception Telescoping of one part of the intestine into another.

Invasive Accessing the body tissues, organs, or cavities through some type of instrumentation procedure.

Involution Return of the reproductive organs, especially the uterus, to their pre-pregnancy size and condition.

Ion Atom bearing an electrical charge.

Ischemia Oxygen deprivation, usually due to poor perfusion.

Ischemic Pain Discomfort resulting when the blood supply of an area is restricted or cut off completely.

Isolation Separate from other persons, especially those with infectious diseases.

Isotonic Solution Solution that has the same molecular concentration as does the cell; also called an isosmolar solution.

Isotopes Atoms of the same element that have different atomic weights (i.e., different numbers of neutrons in the nucleus).

IV Push (bolus) Method of administering a large dose of medication in a relatively short time, usually 1–30 minutes.

Jaundice Yellow discoloration of the skin, sclera, mucous membranes, and body fluids that occurs when the liver is unable to fully remove bilirubin from the blood.

Jet Lag Time required for the biological clock to adjust to a new time.

Job Description Written outline of job responsibilities.

Johnsonian Intervention Confrontational approach to a client with a substance problem that lessens the chance of denial and encourages treatment before the client "hits bottom."

Judgment Ability to evaluate alternatives to arrive at an appropriate course of action.

Justice Ethical principle based on the concept of fairness extended to each individual.

Justify To prove or show to be valid.

Kaposi's Sarcoma Vascular malignancy that can occur any place in the body, including internal organs.

Kardex Summary worksheet reference of basic client care information.

Keloid Abnormal growth of scar tissue that is elevated, rounded, and firm with irregular, clawlike margins.

Keratin Tough, fibrous protein produced by cells in the epidermis called keratinocytes.

Keratitis Inflammation of the cornea.

Kernicterus Severe neurologic damage resulting from a high level of bilirubin (jaundice).

Kernig's Sign Diagnostic test for inflammation in the nerve roots; the inability to extend the leg when the thigh is flexed against the abdomen.

Ketone Acidic byproduct of fat metabolism.

Ketonuria Presence of ketones in the urine.

Ketosis Condition wherein acids called ketones accumulate in the blood and urine, upsetting the acid–base balance.

Kilocalorie Equivalent to 1,000 calories.

Kinesthetic Learner Person who learns by processing information through touching, feeling, and doing.

Kyphosis Increased roundess of the thoracic spinal curve.

Laissez-faire Leadership style that is passive and nondirect.

Lanugo Fine hair covering the fetus's body.

Large for Gestational Age Infant's weight falls above the 90th percentile for gestational age.

Late Deceleration Reduction in fetal heart rate that begins after the uterus has begun contracting and increases to the baseline level after the uterine contraction has ceased.

Law That which is laid down or fixed.

Leadership Ability to direct or motivate others to achieve goals.

Learning Act or process of acquiring knowledge and/or skill in a particular subject.

Learning Disability Heterogenous group of disorders manifested by significant difficulties in the acquisition and use of listening, speaking, reading, writing, reasoning, or mathematical abilities.

Learning Plateau Peak in the effectiveness of teaching and depth of learning.

Learning Style Individual preference for receiving, processing, and assimilating information about a particular subject.

Lecithin Major component of surfactant.

Leopold's Maneuvers Series of specific palpations of the pregnant uterus to determine fetal position and presentation.

Let-Down Reflex Neurohormonal reflex that causes milk to be expressed from the alveoli into the lactiferous ducts.

Lethargy Decreased energy level.

Leukemia Cancer occurring in blood-forming tissues.

Leukocytosis Increased number of white blood cells.

Leukopenia Decreased number of white blood cells.

Liability Obligation one has incurred or might incur through any act or failure to act.

Libel Written words that harm or injure the personal or professional reputation of another person.

Libido Sexual energy.

Licensure Mandatory system of granting licenses according to specified standards.

Life Review Form of reminiscence wherein a client attempts either to come to terms with conflict or to gain meaning from life and die peacefully.

Ligation Application of a band or tie around a structure.

Lightening Descent of the fetus into the pelvis, causing the uterus to tip forward, relieving pressure on the diaphragm.

Linea Nigra Dark line on the abdomen from umbilicus to symphysis during pregnancy.

Lipid Organic compound that is insoluble in water but soluble in organic solvents such as ether and alcohol; also known as fats.

Lipodystrophy Atrophy or hypertrophy of subcutaneous fat.

Lipoma Benign tumor consisting of mature fat cells.

Lipoprotein Blood lipid bound to protein.

Liquefaction Necrosis Death and subsequent change of tissue to a liquid or semi-liquid state; often descriptive of a primary tubercle.

Listening Interpreting the sounds heard and attaching meaning to them.

Lithium Naturally occurring salt that is used as a mood-stabilizing medication in the treatment of bipolar disorder.

Litholapaxy Procedure involving crushing of a bladder stone and immediate washing out of the fragments through a catheter.

Lithotripsy Method of crushing a calculus any place in the urinary system with ultrasonic waves.

Liver Mortis Bluish-purple discoloration of the skin, usually at pressure points, that is a by-product of red blood cell destruction.

Living Will Legal document that allows a person to state preferences about the use of life-sustaining measures should she be unable to make her wishes known.

Local Adaptation Syndrome Physiologic response to a stressor (e.g., trauma, illness) affecting a specific part of the body.

Localized Infection Infection limited to a defined area or single organ.

Lochia Uterine/vaginal discharge after childbirth; initially bright red, then changing to a pink or pinkish brown, then to a yellowish white.

Locomotor Pertaining to movement or the ablility to move.

Logic Formal principles of a branch of knowledge (such as nursing).

Long-Term Care Facility Health care facility that provides services to individuals who are not acutely ill, have continuing health care needs, and cannot function independently at home.

Long-Term Goal Statement written in objective format and demonstrating an expectation to be achieved in resolution of the nursing diagnosis over a long period of time, usually weeks or months.

Lordosis Exaggeration of the curvature of the lumbar spine.

Loss Any situation, either actual, potential, or perceived, wherein a valued object or person is changed or is no longer accessible to the individual.

L/S Ratio Ratio of the surfactants lecithin and sphingomyelin; a 2:1 ratio indicates lung maturity in the fetus.

Lumbar Puncture Aspiration of cerebrospinal fluid from the subarachnoid space.

Lung Stretch Receptor Receptor that monitors the patterns of breathing and prevents overexpansion of the lungs.

Lymphokine Chemical substance released by sensitized lymphocytes (T cells) that assists in antigen destruction.

Lymphoma Tumor of the lymphatic system.

Macrosomia Excessive fetal growth characterized by a fetus weighing more than 4,000 g (8.8 lb.).

Magnetic Resonance Imaging Imaging technique that uses radiowaves and a strong magnetic field to make continuous cross-sectional images of the body.

Maintenance Therapy Small doses of chemotherapy given every 3 to 4 weeks to maintain remission.

Maladaptive Measure Measure used to avoid conflict or stress.

Malignant Becoming progressively worse and often resulting in death.

Malignant Hypertension Rapidly progressing form of hypertension with the diastolic pressure greater than 120 mm Hg.

Malpractice Negligent acts on the part of a professional; relates to the conduct of a person who is acting in a professional capacity.

Managed Care System of providing and monitoring care wherein access, cost, and quality are controlled before or during delivery of services.

Management Accomplishment of tasks through the effective use of people and resources.

Mania Extremely elevated mood with accompanying agitated behavior.

Maslow's Hierarchy of Needs Theory of behavioral motivation based on needs; includes physiologic, safety and security, love and belonging, self-esteem, and self-actualization needs.

Mastication Chewing food into fine particles and mixing the food with enzymes in saliva.

Mastitis Inflammation of the breast, generally during breast feeding.

Material Principle of Justice Rationale for determining those times when there can be unequal allocation of scarce resources.

Matter Anything that occupies space and possesses mass.

Maturation Process of becoming fully grown and developed; involves physiologic and behavioral aspects.

Maturational Loss Loss that occurs as a result of moving from one developmental stage to another.

Mechanism of Labor Series of movements of the fetus as it passes through the pelvis and birth canal.

Meconium Fecal material stored in the fetal intestines.

Meconium Ileus Impacted feces in the newborn, causing intestinal obstruction.

Median Survival Time Average length of life.

Medicaid Government title program (XIX) that pays for health services for the aged, poor, disabled, and low-income families with dependent children.

Medical Asepsis Practices that reduce the number, growth, and spread of microorganisms.

Medical Diagnosis Clinical judgment by the physician that identifies or determines a specific disease, condition, or pathological state.

Medical Model Traditional approach to health care wherein the focus is on treatment and cure of disease.

Medicare Amendment (Title XVIII) to the Social Security Act that helps finace the health care of persons over 65 years old and for permanently disabled younger persons who receive Social Security disability benefits.

Medigap Insurance Insurance plan for persons with Medicare that pays for health care costs not covered by Medicare.

Meditation Quieting of the mind by focusing the attention.

Melanin Pigment that gives skin its color.

Melena Stool containing partially broken down blood; usually black, sticky, and tar-like.

Menarche Onset of the first menstrual period.

Ménière's Disease State of hearing loss characterized by tinnitus and vertigo.

Meningitis Inflammation of the meninges.

Meningocele Saclike protrusion along the vertebral column filled with cerebrospinal fluid and meninges.

Menopause Cessation of menstruation.

Menorrhagia Excessively heavy menstrual flow.

Mental Disorder Clinically significant behavior or psychological syndrome or pattern that occurs in an individual and is associated with present distress or disability or with a significantly increased risk of suffering, death, pain, disability, or an important loss of freedom (APA, 1994).

Mental Illness Condition wherein an individual has a distorted view of self, is unable to maintain satisfying personal relationships, and is unable to adapt to the environment.

Mentation Ability to concentrate, remember, or think abstractly.

Metabolic Rate Rate of energy utilization in the body.

Metabolism Sum total of all the biological and chemical processes in the body.

Metacognition Process of examining the way we think.

Metastasis Spread of cancer cells to distant areas of the body by way of the lymph system or bloodstream.

Metritis Inflammation of the uterus including the endometrium and parametrium.

Metrorrhagia Vaginal bleeding between menstrual periods.

Microthrombi Very small clots.

Micturition Process of expelling urine from the urinary bladder; also called urination or voiding.

Middle Adulthood Developmental stage from the ages of 40 years to 65 years.

Milia Pearly white cysts on the face.

Minority Group Group of people that constitute less than a numerical majority of the population and who, because of their cultural, racial, ethnic, religious, or other characteristics, are often labeled and treated differently from others in the society.

Miscarriage Spontaneous abortion.

Misdemeanor Offense that is less serious than a felony and may be punished by a fine or by sentence to a local prison for less than 1 year.

Misuse Use of a legal substance for which it was not intended, or exceeding the recommended dosage of a drug.

Mitosis Cell division.

Mixed Agonist-Antagonist Compound that blocks opioid effects on one receptor type while producing opioid effects on a second receptor type.

Mixture Substances combined in no specific way.

Mnemonic Method to aid in association and recall; a memorable sentence created from the first letters of a list of items to be used to recall the items later.

Mode of Transmission Process that bridges the gap between the portal of exit of the infectious agent from the reservoir or source, and the portal of entry of the susceptible "new" host.

Modulation Central nervous system pathway that selectively inhibits pain transmission by sending signals back down to the dorsal horn of the spinal cord.

Molding Shaping of the fetal head to adapt to the mother's pelvis during labor.

Molecule Atoms of the same element that unite with each other.

Mongolian Spots Large patches of bluish skin on the buttocks of dark-skinned infants.

Mood Subjective report of the way an individual is feeling.

Moral Maturity Ability to decide for oneself what is "right."

Morbidity Illness.

Mortality Death.

Mortuary Funeral home.

Mourning Period of time during which grief is expressed and resolution and integration of the loss occur.

Mucous Fistula Stoma that secretes mucous.

Multigravida Condition of being pregnant two or more times.

Multipara Condition of having delivered twice or more after 24 weeks' gestation.

Myalgia Pain in muscles.

Myasthenia Gravis Autoimmune disease characterized by extreme muscle weakness and fatigue due to the body's inability to transmit nerve impulses to voluntary muscles.

***Mycobacterium Avium* Complex** Two closely related mycobacteria, *mycobacterium avium* and *mycobacterium intracellulare,* that are grouped together.

Myelomeningocele Saclike protrusion along the vertebral column that is filled with spinal fluid, meninges, nerve roots, and spinal cord.

Myocardial Infarction Necrosis (death) of the myocardium caused by an obstruction in a coronary artery.

Myocarditis Inflammation of the myocardium of the heart.

Myofascial Pain Syndrome Group of muscle disorders characterized by pain, muscle spasm, tenderness, stiffness, and limited motion.

Myopia Nearsightedness.

Myringotomy Surgical incision of the eardrum.

Myxedema Severe hypothyroidism in adults.

Narcolepsy Sleep alteration manifested as sudden uncontrollable urges to fall asleep during the daytime.

Narrative Charting Story format of documentation that describes the client's status, the interventions and treatments, and the client's response to treatments.

Necrosis Tissue death as the result of disease or injury.

Neglect Situation wherein a basic need of the client is not being provided.

Negligence General term referring to careless acts on the part of an individual who is not exercising reasonable or prudent judgement.

Neonatal Period First 28 days of life following birth.

Neonatal Transition First few hours after birth wherein the newborn makes changes to and stabilizes respiratory and circulatory functions.

Neonate Newborn from birth to 28 days of life.

Neoplasm Any abnormal growth of new tissue.

Nephrotoxic Quality of a substance that causes kidney tissue damage.

Nesting Surge of energy late in pregnancy when the pregnant woman organizes and cleans the house.

Neuralgia Paroxysmal pain that extends along the course of one or more nerves.

Neurogenic Shock Hypotensive situation resulting from the loss of sympathetic control of vital functions from the brain.

Neuropeptide Amino acid produced in the brain and other sites in the body that acts as a chemical communicator.

Neurotransmitter Chemical substance produced by the body that facilitates nerve-impulse transmission.

Neutral Thermal Environment Environment in which the newborn can maintain internal body temperature with minimal oxygen consumption and metabolism.

Nevi Pigmented areas in the skin; commonly known as birthmarks or moles.

Nevus Flammeus Large, reddish-purple birthmark usually found on the face or neck which does not blanch with pressure.

Nevus Vascularis Birthmark of enlarged superficial blood vessels, elevated and red in color.

Nociceptor Receptive neuron for painful sensations.

Nocturia Awakening at night to void.

Nocturnal Enuresis Incontinence that occurs during sleep.

Noninvasive Descriptor for procedure wherein the body is *not* entered with any type of instrument.

Nonmaleficence Ethical principle based on the obligation to cause no harm to others.

Nonshivering Thermogenesis Metabolism of brown fat; process unique to the newborn.

Nonverbal Communication Sending a message without words; sometimes called body language.

Nosocomial Originating in the hospital.

Nosocomial Infection Infection that is acquired in the hospital or other health care facility and was not present or incubating at the time of the client's admission.

Noxious Stimulus Underlying pathology that causes pain.

Nuchal Cord Condition of the umbilical cord being wrapped around the baby's neck.

Nuchal Rigidity Pain and rigidity in the neck.

Nullipara Condition of never having delivered an infant after 24 weeks' gestation.

Nursing An art and a science that assists individuals to learn to care for themselves whenever possible; also involves caring for others when they are unable to meet their own needs.

Nursing Audit Process of collecting and analyzing data to evaluate the effectiveness of nursing interventions.

Nursing Care Plan Written guide that organizes data about a client's care into a formal statement of the strategies that will be implemented to help the client achieve optimal health.

Nursing Diagnosis Second step in the nursing process; a clinical judgement about individual, family, or community (aggregate) responses to actual or potential health problems/life processes.

Nursing Intervention Action performed by a nurse that helps the client achieve the results specified by the goals and expected outcomes.

Nursing Intervention Classification Standardized language for nursing interventions.

Nursing Minimum Data Set Elements contained in clinical records and abstracted for studies on the effectiveness and costs of nursing care.

Nursing Outcomes Classification Standardized language for nursing outcomes.

Nursing Practice Act Statute that is enacted by the legislature of a state and that outlines the scope of nursing practice in that state.

Nursing Process Systematic method of providing care to clients, consisting of five steps: assessment, diagnosis, outcome identification and planning, implementation, and evaluation.

Nutrition All of the processes (ingestion, digestion, absorption, metabolism, and elimination) involved in consuming and utilizing food for energy, maintenance, and growth.

Nystagmus Constant, involuntary movement of the eye in various directions.

Obesity Weight that is 20% or more above the ideal body weight.

Objective Data Observable and measurable data that are obtained through standard assessment techniques performed during the physical examination and through laboratory and diagnostic tests.

Occult Blood Blood in the stool that can be detected only through a microscope or by chemical means.

Occult Blood Test (Guaiac) Test for microscopic blood done on stool.

Older Adulthood Developmental stage occurring from the age of 65 years until death.

Oligomenorrhea Decreased menstrual flow.

Oliguria Diminished production of urine.

Omnibus Budget Reconciliation Act Federal law first enacted in 1989 to provide for rights and clinical guidelines to ensure quality health services for older Americans.

Oncology Study of tumors.

Ongoing Assessment Type of assessment that includes systematic monitoring and observation related to specific problems.

Ongoing Planning Continuous updating of the client's plan of care.

Onset of Action Time it takes the body to respond to a drug after administration.

Oophoritis Inflammation of the ovary.

Open Reduction Surgical procedure that enables the surgeon to reduce (repair) a fracture under direct visualization.

Ophthalmia Neonatorum Inflammation of the newborn's eyes which results from passing through the birth canal when a gonorrheal or chlamydial infection is present.

Opinion Subjective belief.

Opioid Morphine-like compound that produces bodily effects such as pain relief, sedation, constipation, and respiratory depression.

Opisthotonos Complete arching of the body with only the head and feet on the bed.

Opportunistic Infection Infection in persons with a defective immune system that rarely causes harm in healthy individuals.

Oppression Condition wherein the rules, modes, and ideals of one group are imposed on another group.

Orchiectomy Removal of a testis.

Orientation Person's awareness of self in relation to person, place, time, and, in some cases, situation.

Orthopedics (Orthopaedics) Branch of medicine that deals with the prevention or correction of the disorders and diseases of the musculoskeletal system.

Orthopnea Difficulty breathing while lying down.

Orthostatic Hypotension Significant decrease in blood pressure that results when a person moves from a lying or sitting (supine) position to a standing position.

Osmolality Measurement of the total concentration of dissolved particles (solutes) per kilogram of water.

Osmolarity Concentration of solutes per liter of cellular fluid.

Osmosis Movement of a solvent, usually water, through a semipermeable membrane, from a region of higher concentration to a region of lower concentration.

Osmotic Pressure Pressure exerted against the cell membrane by the water inside a cell.

Osteoporosis Increase in the porosity of bone.

Otitis Externa Bacterial infection of the external ear canal.

Otitis Media Inflammation of the middle ear.

Otosclerosis Conductive hearing loss secondary to a pathologic change of the bones in the middle ear.

Overflow Incontinence Leaking of urine when the bladder becomes very full and distended.

Oxidation Chemical process of combining with oxygen.

Oxidized Joined with oxygen.

Pain Unpleasant sensory and emotional experience associated with actual or potential tissue damage or described in terms of such.

Pain Threshold Level of intensity at which pain becomes appreciable or perceptible.

Pain Tolerance Level of intensity or duration of pain that a person is willing to endure.

Palliative Relief of symptoms, such as pain, without altering the course of disease.

Palliative Care Care that relieves symptoms, such as pain, but does not alter the course of disease.

Pallor Abnormal paleness of the skin, seen especially in the face, conjunctiva, nail beds, and oral mucous membranes.

Palpation Physical examination technique that uses the sense of touch to assess texture, temperature, moisture, organ location and size, vibrations and pulsations, swelling, masses, and tenderness.

Palpitation Fluttering or pounding sensation in the chest.

Pancreatitis Acute or chronic inflammation of the pancreas.

Papanicolaou Test Smear method of examining stained exfoliative cells.

Para Condition of having delivered after 24 weeks' gestation, whether infant is born alive or dead or number of infants born.

Paracentesis Aspiration of fluid from the abdominal cavity.

Paradoxical Reaction Opposite effect of that which would normally be expected.

Paramedic Specialized health care professional trained to provide advanced life support to the client requiring emergency interventions.

Paraplegia Paralysis of lower extremities.

Parasomnia Condition characterized by profoundly disturbed sleep due to behavioral or physiologic events.

Parenteral Any route other than the oral-gastrointestinal tract.

Parenteral Nutrition Feeding method whereby nutrients bypass the small intestine and enter the blood directly.

Paresthesia Abnormal sensation such as burning, prickling, or tingling.

Paroxysmal Descriptor for a symptom that begins and ends abruptly.

Paroxysmal Nocturnal Dyspnea Condition of suddenly awakening, sweating, and having difficulty breathing.

Passive Euthanasia Process of cooperating with the client's dying process.

Patency Being freely opened.

Pathogen Microorganism that causes disease.

Pathogenicity Ability of a microorganism to produce disease.

Patient-Controlled Analgesia Device that allows the client to control the delivery of intravenous or subcutaneous pain medication in a safe, effective manner through a programmable pump.

Peak Plasma Level Highest blood concentration of a single dose of a drug until the elimination rate equals the rate of absorption.

Peer Assistance Program Rehabilitation program that provides an impaired nurse with referrals, professional and peer counseling support groups, and assistance and monitoring back into nursing.

Peptic Ulcer Erosion formed in the esophagus, stomach, or duodenum resulting from acid/pepsin imbalance.

Perception Ability to experience, recognize, organize, and interpret sensory stimuli.

Percussion Physical examination technique that uses short, tapping strokes on the surface of the skin to create vibrations of underlying organs.

Percutaneous Balloon Valvuloplasty Insertion of a balloon in a stenosed valve to expand the narrowed valvular space.

Perfectionism Overwhelming expectation of being able to get everything done.

Perfusion Blood flow through an organ or body part.

Pericardial Friction Rub Short, high-pitched squeak heard as two inflamed pericardial surfaces rub together.

Pericardiocentesis Removal of fluid from the pericardial sac.

Pericarditis Inflammation of the membrane sac surrounding the heart.

Perineal Care Cleansing of the external genitalia and perineum and the surrounding area.

Perioperative Period of time comprising the preoperative, intraoperative, and postoperative phases of surgery.

Peripheral Nervous System System of the cranial nerves, spinal nerves, and the autonomic nervous system.

Peripheral Resistance Pressure within a vessel that resists the flow of blood such as plaque buildup or vasoconstriction.

Peristalsis Coordinated, rhythmic, serial contraction of the smooth muscles of the gastrointestinal tract.

Peritonitis Inflammation of the peritoneum, the membranous covering of the abdomen.

Permeability Ability of a membrane to permit substances to pass through it.

Petechiae Pinpoint hemorrhagic spots on the skin.

Phantom Limb Pain Neuropathic pain that occurs after amputation with pain sensations referred to an area in the missing portion of the limb.

Pharmacokinetics Study of the absorption, distribution, metabolism, and excretion of drugs to determine the relationship between the dose of a drug and the drug's concentration in biological fluids.

Phimosis Condition wherein the opening in the foreskin is so small that it cannot be pulled back over the glans.

Phlebitis Inflammation in the wall of a vein without clot formation.

Phlebothrombosis Formation of a clot because of blood pooling in the vessel, trauma to the vessel's endothelial lining, or a coagulation problem with little or no inflammation in the vessel.

Phlebotomist Individual who performs venipuncture.

Phlebotomy Removal of blood from a vein.

Phospholipid Lipid composed of glycerol, fatty acids, and phosphorus; the structural component of cells.

Physical Agent Factor in the environment capable of causing disease in a host.

Physical Restraint Equipment that reduces the client's movement.

Physical Wellness Healthy body that functions at an optimal level.

Physically Aggressive Descriptor of an individual who threatens or actually harms someone.

Physiologic Anemia of Pregnancy Hemodilution caused by the increased maternal blood volume.

Phytochemical Physiologically active compound present in plants in very small amounts that gives plants flavor, odor, and color.

Pica Practice of eating substances not considered edible and which have no nutritive value such as laundry starch, dirt, clay, and freezer frost.

PIE Charting Documentation method using the problem, intervention, evaluation (PIE) format.

Piggyback Addition of an intravenous solution to infuse concurrently with another infusion.

Placenta Membranous vascular organ connecting the fetus to the mother, which produces hormones to sustain a pregnancy, supplies the fetus with oxygen and food, and transports waste products out of the fetal system.

Placenta Previa Condition in which the placenta forms over or very near the internal cervical os.

Planning Third step of the nursing process; includes both the formulation of guidelines that establish the proposed course of nursing action in the resolution of nursing diagnoses and the development of the client's plan of care.

Plateau Level at which a drug's blood concentration is maintained.

Pleural Effusion Collection of fluid within the pleural cavity.

Pleural Friction Rub Abnormal breath sound that is creaky and grating in nature and is heard on inspiration and expiration.

Pleurisy Condition arising from inflammation of the pleura, or sac, that encases the lung.

***Pneumocystis Carinii* Pneumonia** The most common opportunistic infection associated with advanced HIV.

Pneumonia Inflammation of the bronchioles and alveoli accompanied by consolidation, or solidification of exudate, in the lungs.

Pneumothorax Condition wherein air or gas accumulates in the pleural space of the lungs, causing the lungs to collapse.

Point-of-Care Charting Documentation system that allows health care providers to gain immediate access to client information at the bedside.

Poison Any substance that when taken into the body interferes with normal physiologic functioning; may be inhaled, injected, ingested, or absorbed by the body.

Policy Written description of employer's expectations for handling various situations.

Polydipsia Excessive thirst.

Polymenorrhea Menstrual periods that are abnormally frequent, generally less than every 21 days.

Polyp Abnormal growth of tissue.

Polyphagia Increased hunger.

Polypharmacy Problem of clients taking numerous prescription and over-the-counter medications for the same or various disease processes, with unknown consequences from the resulting combinations of chemical compounds and cumulative side-effects.

Polyuria Increased urination.

Port-a-Cath Port that has been implanted under the skin with a catheter inserted into the superior vena cava or right atrium through the subclavian or internal jugular vein.

Portal of Entry Route by which an infectious agent enters the host.

Portal of Exit Route by which an infectious agent leaves the reservoir.

Post Void Residual Urine that remains in the bladder after urination.

Post-mortem Care Care given immediately after death before the body is moved to the mortuary.

Postoperative Phase Time during the surgical experience that begins at the end of the surgical procedure and ends when the client is discharged from medical care by the surgeon, in addition to being discharged from the hospital or institution.

Postpartum Blues Mild transient condition of emotional lability and crying for no apparent reason, which affects up to 80% of women who have just given birth, and lasts about 2 weeks.

Postpartum Depression Condition similar to postpartum blues but which is more serious, intense, and persistent.

Postpartum Hemorrhage Blood loss of more than 500 mL after the third stage of labor or 1,000 mL following a cesarean birth.

Postpartum Psychosis Condition more severe than postpartum depression and characterized by delusions and thoughts of self harm or infant harm.

Postprandial After eating.

Postterm Delivery after 42 weeks' gestation.

Preadolescence Developmental stage from the ages of approximately 10 years to 12 years.

Precipitate Birth Birth occurring suddenly and unexpectedly without a CNM/physician present to assist.

Precipitate Labor Labor lasting less than 3 hours from the onset of contractions to the birth of the infant.

Preeclampsia Phase of pregnancy-induced hypertension prior to convulsions.

Preferred Provider Organization Type of managed care model wherein member choice is limited to providers within the system.

Prenatal Care Care of a woman during pregnancy, before labor.

Prenatal Period Developmental stage beginning with conception and ending with birth.

Preoperative Phase Time during the surgical experience that begins when the client decides to have surgery and ends when the client is transferred to the operating table.

Presbycusis Sensorineural hearing loss associated with aging.

Presbyopia Inablility of the lens of the eye to change curvature to focus near objects.

Preschool Period Developmental stage from the ages of 3 years to 6 years.

Prescriptive Authority Legal recognition of the ability to prescribe medications.

Presenting Part Part of the fetus in contact with the cervix.

Pressured Speech Rapid, intense style of speech.

Preterm Delivery after 24 weeks' gestation but before 38 weeks (full term).

Preterm Birth Birth that takes place before the end of the 37th week of gestation.

Preterm Labor Onset of regular contractions of the uterus that cause cervical changes between 20 and 37 weeks' gestation.

Prevention Hindering, obstructing, or thwarting a disease or illness.

Priapism Prolonged erection that does not occur in response to sexual stimulation.

Primary Care Care focused on promoting wellness and preventing illness.

Primary Care Provider Health care provider whom a client sees first for health care, typically a family practitioner (physician/nurse), internist, or pediatrician.

Primary Health Care Client's point of entry into the health care system; includes assessment, diagnosis, treatment, coordination of care, education, prevention services, and surveillance.

Primary Prevention All practices designed to keep health problems from developing.

Primary Source Major provider of information about a client.

Primary Tubercle Nodule that contains tubercle bacilli and forms within lung tissue.

Primigravida Condition of being pregnant for the first time.

Primipara Condition of having delivered once after 24 weeks' gestation.

Problem-Oriented Medical Record Documentation method focusing on the client's problem and using a structured, logical format to narrative charting, called SOAP (subjective data, objective data, assessment, plan).

Procedure Step-by-step instruction describing the process for performing various nursing tasks.

Process Series of steps or acts that leads to the accomplishment of a goal or purpose.

Procrastination Intentionally putting off or delaying something that should be done.

Prodromal Stage Time interval from the onset of nonspecific symptoms until specific symptoms of the infectious process begin to manifest.

Progressive Muscle Relaxation Stress management strategy in which muscles are alternately tensed and relaxed.

Projectile Vomiting Forceful ejection (up to 3 feet) of the contents of the stomach.

Prolapsed Cord Condition in which the umbilical cord lies below the presenting part of the fetus.

Prolapsed Uterus Downward displacement of the uterus into the vagina.

Prospective Payment Predetermined rate paid for each episode of hospitalization based on the client's age and principle diagnosis and the presence or absence of surgery or comorbidity.

Protocol Series of standing orders or procedures that should be followed under certain specific conditions.

Proxemics Study of the space between people and its effect on interpersonal behavior.

Pruritus Severe itching.

Pseudoaddiction Pattern of drug-seeking behavior in clients receiving inadequate pain management.

Pseudocyesis False pregnancy.

Pseudomenstruation Blood tinged mucus discharge from the vagina of a newborn caused by the withdrawal of maternal hormones.

Psychoanalysis Therapy focused on uncovering unconscious memories and processes.

Psychological Wellness Enjoyment of creativity, satisfaction of the basic need to love and be loved, understanding of emotions, and ability to maintain control over emotions.

Psychomotor Domain Area of learning that involves performance of motor skills.

Psychoneuroimmunology Study of the complex relationship among the cognitive, affective, and physical aspects of humans.

Psychoprophylaxis Mental and physical preparation for childbirth; synonymous with Lamaze.

Psychosis State wherein an individual has lost the ability to recognize reality.

Psychotherapy Treatment of mental and emotional disorders through psychological rather than physical methods.

Ptosis Drooping upper eyelid.

Puberty Emergence of secondary sex characteristics that signals the beginning of adolescence.

Public Law Law that deals with an individual's relationship to the state.

Pudendal Block Injection of a local anesthetic into the pudendal nerve to provide perineal, external genitalia, and lower vaginal anesthesia.

Puerperal (Postpartum) Infection Infection following childbirth occurring between the birth and 6 weeks postpartum.

Puerperium Term for the first 6 weeks after the birth of an infant.

Purpura Reddish-purple patches on the skin indicative of hemorrhage.

Purulent Exudate Discharge that occurs with severe inflammation accompanied by infection; also called pus.

Pulse Amplitude Measurement of the strength or force exerted by the ejected blood against the arterial wall with each contraction.

Pulse Deficit Condition in which the apical pulse rate is greater than the radial pulse rate.

Pulse Rate Indirect measurement of cardiac output obtained by counting the number of peripheral pulse waves over a pulse point.

Pulse Rhythm Regularity of the heart beat.

Pyelonephritis Bacterial infection of the renal pelvis, tubules, and interstitial tissue of one or both kidneys.

Pyorrhea Periodontal disease.

Pyuria Pus in the urine.

Quadriplegia Dysfunction or paralysis of both arms, both legs, and bowel and bladder.

Quickening Descriptor for when the mother first feels the fetus move, about 16 to 20 weeks' gestation.

Race Grouping of people based on biological similarities such as physical characteristics.

Radiation Loss of heat by transfer to cooler near objects, but not through direct contact.

Radiography Study of x-rays or gamma ray-exposed film through the action of ionizing radiation.

Radiotherapy Treatment of cancer with high-energy radiation.

Rapport Bond or connection between two people that is based on mutual trust.

Readiness for Learning Evidence of willingness to learn.

Reasoning Use of the elements of thought to solve a problem or settle a question.

Reconstructive To rebuild or reestablish.

Rectocele Anterior displacement of the rectum into the posterior vaginal wall.

Recurrent Acute Pain Discomfort marked by repetitive painful episodes that may recur over a prolonged period or throughout a client's lifetime.

Referred Pain Discomfort from the internal organs that is felt in another area of the body.

Reflective Introspective.

Reframing Technique of monitoring negative thoughts and replacing them with positive ones.

Regional Anesthesia Method of temporarily rendering a region of the body insensible to pain.

Rehabilitation Process designed to assist individuals to reach their optimal level of physical, mental, and psychosocial functioning.

Relapse Return to a previous behavior or condition.

Relaxation Technique Method used to decrease anxiety and muscle tension.

Religious Support System Group of ministers, priests, rabbis, nuns, or lay persons who are able to meet clients' spiritual needs in the health care setting.

REM Movement Disorder Condition wherein the paralysis normally occurring during REM sleep is absent or incomplete and the sleeper acts out the dream that is occurring.

Remission Decrease or absence of symptoms of a disease.

Renal Colic Severe pain in the kidney that radiates to the groin.

Repolarization Recovery phase of the cardiac muscle.

Reservoir Place where the agent can survive.

Resident Flora Microorganisms that are always present, usually without altering the client's health.

Residual Urine Urine remaining in the bladder after the individual has urinated.

Respect Acceptance of an individual as is and in a nonjudgmental manner.

Respiration Process of exchanging oxygen and carbon dioxide.

Respite Care Care and service that provides a break to caregivers and is utilized for a few hours a week, for an occasional weekend, or for longer periods of time.

Responsiveness Person's ability to perceive environmental stimuli and body reactions and then to respond with thought and action.

Rest State of relaxation and calmness, both mental and physical.

Restitution Rotation of the fetal head back to be in normal alignment with the shoulders after delivery of the fetal head.

Restless Leg Syndrome Condition characterized by uncomfortable sensations of tingling or crawling in the muscles, and twitching, burning, prickling, or deep aching in the foot, calf, or upper leg when at rest (lying or sitting).

Restraint Protective device used to limit the physical activity of a client or to immobilize a client or extremity.

Résumé Tool that summarizes employment qualifications.

Resuscitation Support measures implemented to restore consciousness and life.

Reticulocyte Immature red blood cell.

Retroperitoneal Behind the peritoneum outside the peritoneal cavity.

Retroplacental Behind the placenta.

Reverse Isolation Barrier protection designed to prevent infection in clients who are severely compromised and highly susceptible to infection; also known as protective isolation.

Reverse Tolerance Phenomenon whereby a smaller amount of substance will elicit the desired psychic effects.

Review of Systems Brief account of any recent signs or symptoms related to any body system.

Rheumatoid Arthritis Chronic, systemic auto-immune disease characterized by joint stiffness.

Rhinorrhea Watery nasal discharge.

Rigor Mortis Stiffening of the body that occurs 2 to 4 hours after death as a result of contraction of skeletal and smooth muscles.

Risk for Infection State wherein an individual is at increased risk for being invaded by pathogenic organisms.

Risk Nursing Diagnosis Nursing diagnosis indicating that a problem does not yet exist but that specific risk factors are present; composed of the diagnostic label followed by the phrase "Risk for" and a list of the specific risk factors.

Rooming-In Practice of staying with the client 24 hours a day to provide care and comfort.

Salpingitis Inflammation of the fallopian tube.

Salt Product formed when an acid and a base react with each other.

Sarcoma Cancer occurring in connective tissue.

Satiety Feeling of fulfillment.

School-Age Period Developmental stage from the ages of 6 years to 10 years.

Sclerotherapy Treatment which involves injecting a chemical into the vein, causing the vein to become sclerosed (hardened) so blood no longer flows through it.

Sclerotic Hardened tissue.

Scoliosis Lateral curvature of the spine.

Scrub Nurse RN, LP/VN, or surgical technologist who provides services under the direction of the circulating nurse and who is qualified by training or experience to prepare and maintain the integrity, safety, and efficiency of the sterile field throughout an operation.

Sebaceous cyst Sebaceous gland filled with sebum.

Sebum Oily substance secreted by the sebaceous glands of the skin.

Seclusion Confinement of a client to a single room.

Secondary Care Care focused on diagnosis and treatment after the client exhibits symptoms of illness.

Secondary Malignancy Second malignant condition that develops after successful treatment of an initial malignancy.

Secondary Prevention Early detection, diagnosis, screening, and intervention, generally before symptoms appear, to reduce the consequences of a health problem.

Secondary Source Data source other than the client; can include family members, other health care providers, or medical records.

Sedation Reduction of stress, excitement, or irritability via some degree of central nervous system depression.

Self-Awareness Consciously knowing how the self thinks, feels, believes, and behaves at any specific time.

Self-Care Deficit State wherein an individual is not able to perform one or more activities of daily living.

Self-Concept Individual's perception of self; includes self-esteem, body image, and ideal self.

Self-Efficacy Belief in one's ability to succeed in attempts to change behavior.

Semipermeable Membrane Membrane that allows passage of only certain substances.

Sensation Ability to receive and process stimuli received through the sensory organs.

Sensitivity Susceptibility of a pathogen to an antibiotic.

Sensorineural Hearing Loss Condition in which the inner ear or chochlear portion of cranial nerve VIII is abnormal or diseased.

Sensory Deficit Change in the perception of sensory stimuli; can affect any of the senses.

Sensory Deprivation State of reduced sensory input from the internal or external environment, manifested by alterations in sensory perception.

Sensory Overload State of excessive and sustained multi-sensory stimulation manifested by behavior change and perceptual distortion.

Sensory Perception Ability to receive sensory impressions and, through cortical association, relate the stimuli to past experiences and to form an impression of the nature of the stimulus.

Seroconversion Evidence of antibody formation in response to disease or vaccine.

Serosanguineous Exudate Discharge that is clear with some blood tinge; seen with surgical incisions.

Serous Exudate Discharge composed primarily of serum; is watery in appearance and has a low protein level.

Serum Lithium Level Laboratory test done to determine whether the client's lithium level is within a therapeutic range.

Shaman Folk healer-priest who uses natural and supernatural forces to help others.

Shamanism Practice of entering altered states of consciousness with the intent of helping others.

Shearing Force exerted against the skin by movement or repositioning.

Shock Condition of profound hemodynamic and metabolic disturbance characterized by inadequate tissue perfusion and inadequate circulation to the vital organs.

Short-Term Goal Objective that outlines the desired resolution of the nursing diagnosis over a short period of time, usually a few hours or days (less than a week).

Shroud Covering for the body after death.

Sibilant Wheeze Abnormal breath sound that is high pitched and musical in nature and is heard on inhalation and exhalation.

Sickled Condition in which red blood cells become crescent-shaped and elongated.

Single-Payer System Health care delivery model wherein the government is the only entity to reimburse.

Single Point of Entry Common feature of HMOs wherein the client is required to enter the health care system through a point designated by the plan.

Situational Loss Loss that occurs in response to external events that are usually beyond the individual's control.

Slander Words that are communicated verbally to a third party and that harm or injure the personal or professional reputation of another.

Sleep State of altered consciousness during which an individual experiences fluctuations in level of consciousness; minimal physical activity; and general slowing of the body's physiologic processes.

Sleep Apnea Syndrome wherein breathing periodically ceases during sleep for a period of 30–60 seconds; often associated with heavy snoring.

Sleep Cycle Sequence of sleep that begins with the four stages of no rapid eye movement (NREM) sleep in order, with a return to stage 3 and then stage 2, followed by passage into the first rapid eye movement (REM) stage.

Sleep Deprivation Prolonged inadequate quality and quantity of sleep.

Small for Gestational Age Infant's weight falls below the 10th percentile for gestational age.

Snellen Chart Chart containing various-sized letters with standardized numbers at the end of each line of letters.

Snoring Noisy breathing during sleep.

SOAP Charting Documentation method using subjective data, objective data, assessment, and plan.

Sociocultural Wellness Ability to appreciate the needs of others and to care about one's environment and the inhabitants of it.

Somatic Nervous System Nerves that connect the central nervous system to the skin and skeletal muscles and control conscious activities.

Somatic Pain Nonlocalized discomfort originating in tendons, ligaments, and nerves.

Somnambulism Sleepwalking.

Somogyi Phenomenon In response to hypoglycemia, the release of glucose-elevating hormones (epinephrine, cortisol, glucose) which produces a hyperglycemic state.

Sonorous Wheeze Abnormal breath sound that is low pitched and snoring in nature and is louder on expiration.

Source-Oriented Charting Narrative recording by each member (source) of the health care team on a separate record.

Specific Order Order written in a client's medical record or nursing care plan by a physician or nurse especially for that individual client; not used for any other client.

Spermatogenesis Production of sperm.

Spina Bifida Occulta Failure of the vertebral arch to close.

Spinal Shock Cessation of motor, sensory, autonomic, and reflex impulses below the level of injury; characterized by flaccid paralysis of all skeletal muscles, loss of spinal reflexes, loss of sensation, and absence of autonomic function below the level of injury.

Spiritual Wellness Inner strength and peace.

Spiritual Care Recognition of spiritual needs and the assistance given toward meeting spiritual needs.

Spiritual Needs Individual's desire to find meaning and purpose in life, pain, and death.

Spirituality Relationships with one's self, with others, and with a higher power or divine source.

Spore Bacteria in a resistant stage that can withstand unfavorable environments.

Sprain Injury to ligaments surrounding a joint caused by a sudden twist, wrench, or fall.

Stable Alert with vital signs within the client's normal range.

Staff Development Delivery of instruction to assist the nurse in achieving the goals of the employer.

Standard Level or degree of quality.

Standard Precautions Preventive practices to be used in the care of all clients in hospitals regardless of their diagnosis or presumed infection status.

Standards of Practice Guidelines established to direct nursing care.

Standing Order Standardized intervention written, approved, and signed by a physician that is kept on file within health care agencies to be used in predictable situations or in circumstances requiring immediate attention.

Startle Response Overreaction to minor sounds or noises.

Stasis Dermatitis Inflammation of the skin due to decreased circulation.

Station Relationship of the fetal presenting part to the ischial spines.

Status Asthmaticus Persistent, intractable asthma attack.

Status Epilepticus Acute, prolonged episode of seizure activity that lasts at least 30 minutes and may or may not involve loss of consciousness.

Statutory Law Law enacted by legislative bodies.

Steatorrhea Fatty stool.

Stent Tiny metal tube with holes in it that prevents a vessel from collapsing and keeps the atherosclerotic plaque pressed against the vessel wall; any material used to hold tissue in place or provide support.

Stereognosis Ability to recognize an object by feel.

Stereotyping Beliefs that all people within the same racial, ethnic, or cultural group act alike and share the same beliefs and attitudes.

Sterile Without microorganisms.

Sterile Conscience Individual's personal sense of honesty and integrity with regard to adherence to the principles of aseptic technique, including prompt admission and correction of any errors and omissions.

Sterile Field Area surrounding the client and the surgical site that is free from all microorganisms; created by draping of the work area and the client with sterile drapes.

Sterilization Total elimination of all microorganisms including spores.

Stock Supply Medications dispensed and labeled in large quantities for storage in the medication room or nursing unit.

Stoma Distal end of the gastrointestinal or urinary system brought to the outside of the body and sutured into place.

Stomatitis Inflammation of the oral mucosa.

Strabismus Inability of the eyes to focus in the same direction.

Strain Injury to a muscle or tendon due to overuse or overstretching.

Stress Nonspecific response to any demand made on the body (Selye, 1974).

Stress Incontinence Leakage of urine when a person does anything that strains the abdomen, such as coughing, laughing, jogging, dancing, sneezing, lifting, making a quick movement, or even walking.

Stress Test Measure of a client's cardiovascular response to exercise.

Stressor Any situation, event, or agent that produces stress.

Striae Gravidarum Reddish streaks frequently found on the abdomen, thighs, buttocks, and breasts; also called "stretch marks."

Stridor High-pitched, harsh sound heard on inspiration when the trachea or larynx is obstructed.

Stroke Volume Volume of blood pumped by the ventricle with each contraction.

Stye Pustular inflammation of an eyelash follicle or sebaceous gland on the eyelid margin.

Subacute Care Short-term, aggressive care for clients who are out of the acute stage of illness but who still require skilled nursing, monitoring, and ongoing treatment.

Subcutaneous Injection into the subcutaneous tissue.

Subinvolution Incomplete return of the uterus to its prepregnant size and consistency.

Subjective Data Data from the client's point of view, including feelings, perceptions, and concerns.

Subluxation Partial separation of an articular surface.

Substance A drug, legal or illegal, that may cause physical or mental impairment.

Suicidal Ideations Thoughts of hurting or killing oneself.

Suicide Purposefully taking one's own life.

Supine Hypotensive Syndrome Lowering of blood pressure in a pregnant woman when lying supine due to compression of the vena cava by the enlarged, heavy uterus.

Surfactant Phospholipids that are present in the lungs and lowers surface tension to prevent collapse of the airways.

Surgery Treatment of injury, disease, or deformity through invasive operative methods.

Surgical Asepsis Practices that eliminate all microorganisms and spores from an object or area.

Susceptible Host Person who lacks resistance to an agent and is thus vulnerable to disease.

Suture Thin, fibrous, membrane-covered space between skull bones.

Synarthrosis Immovable joint.

Syndactyly Fusion of two or more fingers or toes.

Synergism Result of two or more agents working together to achieve a greater effect than either could produce alone.

Synergy Two or more agents working together to achieve more than either could alone.

Synthesiasis Hearing colors and seeing sounds.

Synthesis Chemical reaction when two or more atoms, called reactants, bond and form a more complex molecular product. Putting data together in a new way.

Syphilis Sexually transmitted disease caused by the spirochete *Treponema pallidum*.

Systemic Infection Infection that affects the entire body with involvement of multiple organs.

Systemic Lupus Erythematosus Chronic, progressive, incurable autoimmune disease affecting multiple body organs.

Tachycardia Heart rate in excess of 100 beats per minute in an adult.

Tachypnea Respiratory rate greater than 24 beats per minute.

Talipes Equinovarus A congenital deformity in which the foot and ankle are twisted inward and cannot be moved to a midline position; also known as clubfoot.

Teaching Active process wherein one individual shares information with another as a means to facilitate learning and thereby promote behavioral changes.

Teaching Strategy Technique to promote learning.

Teaching–Learning Process Planned interaction that promotes a behavioral change that is not a result of maturation or coincidence.

Telangiectactic Nevi Birthmarks of dilated capillaries which blanch with pressure; also called stork-bites.

Telangiectasia Permanent dilation of groups of superficial capillaries and venules; commonly known as "spider veins."

Telemedicine Use of communications technology to transmit health information from one location to another.

Teleology Ethical theory that states that the value of a situation is determined by its consequences.

Tenesmus Spasmodic contradiction of the anal or bladder sphincter, causing pain and a persistent urge to empty the bowel or bladder.

Teratogen Agent such as radiation, drugs, viruses, and other microorganisms capable of causing abnormal fetal development.

Teratogenic Causing abnormal development of the embryo.

Teratogenic Substance Substance that can cross the placental barrier and impair normal growth and development.

Term Descriptor for a pregnancy between 38 and 42 weeks' gestation.

Tertiary Care Care focused on restoring the client to the state of health that existed before the development of an illness; if unattainable, then care directed to attaining the optimal level of health possible.

Tertiary Prevention Treatment of an illness or disease after symptoms have appeared so as to prevent further progression.

Tetany Sharp flexion of the wrist and ankle joints, involving muscle twitching or cramps.

Therapeutic Communication Communication that is purposeful and goal directed, creating a beneficial outcome for the client.

Therapeutic Massage Application of pressure and motion by the hands with the intent of improving the recipient's well-being.

Therapeutic Procedure Accident Accident that occurs during the delivery of medical or nursing interventions.

Therapeutic Touch Technique of assessing alterations in a person's energy fields and using the hands to direct energy to achieve a balanced state.

Thermogenesis Production of heat.

Thermoregulation Maintenance of body temperature.

Thoracentesis Aspiration of fluid from the pleural cavity.

Thrombectomy Surgical removal of a clot.

Thrombocytopenia Decrease in the number of platelets in the blood.

Thrombophlebitis Formation of a clot due to an inflammation in the wall of the vessel.

Thrombosis Formation of a clot in a vessel.

Thrombus Formed clot that remains at the site where it formed.

Time Management System to help meet goals through problem solving.

Tinnitus Ringing sound in the ear.

Tocolysis Process of stopping labor with medications.

Tocolytic Agent Medication that inhibits uterine contractions.

Toddler Period Developmental stage beginning at approximately 12 to 18 months of age, when a child begins to walk, and ending at approximately age 3 years.

Tolerance Decreased sensitivity to subsequent doses of the same substance; an increased dose of the substance is needed to produce the same desired effect.

Tophi Subcutaneous nodules of sodium urate crystals.

Tort Civil wrong committed by a person against another person or property.

Tort Law Enforcement of duties and rights among individuals and independent of contractual agreements.

Touch Means of perceiving or experiencing through tactile sensation.

Toxic Poisonous.

Toxic Effect Reaction that occurs when the body cannot metabolize a drug, causing the drug to accumulate in the blood.

Trade (Brand) Name Name assigned a drug by the pharmaceutical company. Always capitalized.

Transcutaneous Electrical Nerve Stimulation Process of applying a low-voltage electrical current to the skin through cutaneous electrodes.

Transducer Instrument that converts electrical energy to sound waves.

Transduction Noxious stimulus that triggers electrical activity in the endings of afferent nerve fibers (nociceptors).

Transesophageal Echocardiography Diagnostic ultrasonic imaging of the cardiac structures through the esophagus.

Transient Flora Microorganisms that attach to the skin for a brief period of time but do not continuously live on the skin.

Transmission Process whereby the pain impulse travels from the receiving nociceptors to the spinal cord.

Transmission-Based Precautions Practices designed for clients documented as, or suspected of, being infected with highly transmissible or epidemiologically important pathogens for which additional precautions beyond Standard Precautions are required to interrupt transmission in hospitals.

Trauma Wound or injury.

Triage Classification of clients to determine priority of need and proper place of treatment.

Trichomoniasis Sexually transmitted disease caused by a parasitic protozoan *Trichomonas vaginalis.*

Triglyceride Lipid compound consisting of three fatty acids and a glycerol molecule.

Trocar Sharply pointed surgical instrument contained in a cannula.

Trousseau's Sign Carpal spasm caused by inflating a blood pressure cuff above the client's systolic pressure and leaving it in place for 3 minutes.

Trust Ability to rely on an individual's character and ability.

Tumor Marker Substance found in the serum that indicates the possible presence of malignancy.

Turgor Normal resiliency of the skin.

Type and Cross-Match Laboratory test that identifies the client's blood type (e.g., A or B) and determines the compatibility of the blood between potential donor and recipient.

Ultrasound Use of high-frequency sound waves to visualize deep body structures; also called an echogram.

Umbilical Cord Structure which connects the fetus to the placenta.

Uncomplicated Grief Grief reaction that normally follows a significant loss.

Unilateral Neglect Failure to recognize or care for one side of the body.

Unit Dose Form System of packaging and labeling each dose of medication by the pharmacy, usually for a 24-hour period.

Urethrocele Downward displacement of the urethra into the vagina.

Urethrostomy Formation of a permanent fistula opening into the urethra.

Urge Incontinence Inability to suppress the sudden urge or need to urinate.

Urinary Incontinence Involuntary loss of urine from the bladder.

Urinary Retention Inability to void when there is an urge to void.

Urobilinogen Colorless derivative of bilirubin formed by the normal bacterial action of intestinal flora on bilirubin.

Urolithiasis Calculus or stone formed in the urinary tract.

Urticaria Allergic reaction causing raised pruritic, red, nontender wheals on the skin; also called hives.

Uterine Retraction Unique ability of the muscle fibers of the uterus to remain shortened to a small degree after each contraction.

Uterine Souffle Sound of blood pulsating through the uterus and placenta.

Utility Ethical principle that states that an act must result in the greatest degree of good for the greatest number of people involved in a given situation.

Vaccination Inoculation with a vaccine to produce immunity against specific diseases.

Value System Individual's collection of inner beliefs that guides the way the person acts and helps determine the choices the person makes.

Values Principles that influence the development of beliefs and attitudes.

Values Clarification Process of analyzing one's own values to better understand those things that are truly important.

Variable Deceleration Reduction in fetal heart rate that has no relationship to contractions of the uterus.

Variations Goals not met or interventions not performed according to the time frame; also called variances.

Varicosities Visibly prominent, dilated, and twisted veins.

Vasectomy Surgical resecton of the vas deferens.

Vasoconstriction Decrease in the diameter of a vessel.

Vasodilate Increase in the diameter of a vessel.

Vector-Borne Transmission Transfer of an agent to a susceptible host by animate means such as mosquitoes, fleas, ticks, lice, and other animals.

Vehicle Transmission Transfer of an agent to a susceptible host by contaminated inanimate objects such as food, milk, drugs, and blood.

Vein Ligation Tying off an involved section of a vein with suture.

Vein Stripping Introducing a wire into a vein to strip the walls of the vein.

Venereal Disease Disease usually acquired as a result of sexual contact; the preferred term currently in use is sexually transmitted disease.

Venipuncture Puncturing of a vein with a needle to aspirate blood.

Ventilation Movement of air into and out of the lungs.

Veracity Ethical principle based on truthfulness (neither lying nor deceiving others).

Verbal Communication Using words, either spoken or written, to send a message.

Verbally Aggressive Descriptor of an individual who says things in a loud and/or intimidating manner.

Vernix Caseosa White, creamy substance covering a fetus's body.

Vertigo Dizziness.

Vesicant Agent that may produce blisters and tissue necrosis.

Vesicular Breath Sound Soft, low breath sound heard over the majority of lung tissue.

Vesicular Sound Soft, breezy, low-pitched sound heard longer on inspiration than expiration that results from air moving through the smaller airways over the lung periphery, with the exception of the scapular area.

Villi Finger-like projections that line the small intestine.

Viral Load Test Test that measures copies of HIV RNA.

Virchow's Triad Three factors (pooling of blood, vessel trauma, and a coagulation problem) that lead to the formation of a clot.

Virulence Frequency with which a pathogen causes disease.

Visceral Pain Discomfort felt in the internal organs.

Visual Hallucination Perception by an individual that something is present when nothing in fact is.

Visual Learner Person who learns by processing information through seeing.

Vitiligo Depigmentation of the skin caused by destruction of melanocytes; appears as milk-white patches on the skin.

Void Process of urine elimination.

Volvulus Twisting of a bowel on itself.

Walking Rounds Reporting method used when members of the care team walk to each client's room and discuss care with each other and with the client.

Water Soluble Vitamin Vitamin that must be ingested daily in normal quantities because it is not stored in the body: vitamins C and B-complex.

Wellness State of optimal health wherein an individual moves toward integration of human functioning, maximizes human potential, takes responsibility for health, and has greater self-awareness and self-satisfaction.

Wellness Nursing Diagnosis Nursing diagnosis that indicates the client's expression of a desire to obtain a higher level of wellness in some area of function; composed of the diagnostic label preceded by the phrase "potential for enhanced."

Western Blot Test Confirmatory test used to detect HIV infection.

Wharton's Jelly Thick substance surrounding and protecting the vessels of the umbilical cord.

Whistleblowing Calling attention to unethical, illegal, or incompetent actions of others.

Windowing Cutting a hole in a plaster cast to relieve pressure on the skin or a bony area and to permit visualization of the underlying body part.

Witch's Milk A whitish fluid secreted by a newborn's nipples.

Withdrawal Symptoms produced when a substance on which an individual has dependence is no longer used by that individual.

Word Salad Nonsensical combination of words that is meaningless to others.

Wound Disruption in the integrity of body tissue.

Yin and Yang Opposing forces that, when in balance, yield health.

Young Adulthood Developmental stage from the ages of 21 years through approximately 40 years.

Zygote Fertilized ovum.

Index

Note: Page numbers in **bold** indicate boxed material; in *italics* indicate illustrations; page numbers followed by "t" indicate a table.